The 5-Minute Clinical Consult 2008 16th Edition features instant access to an interactive website at www.5mcc.com

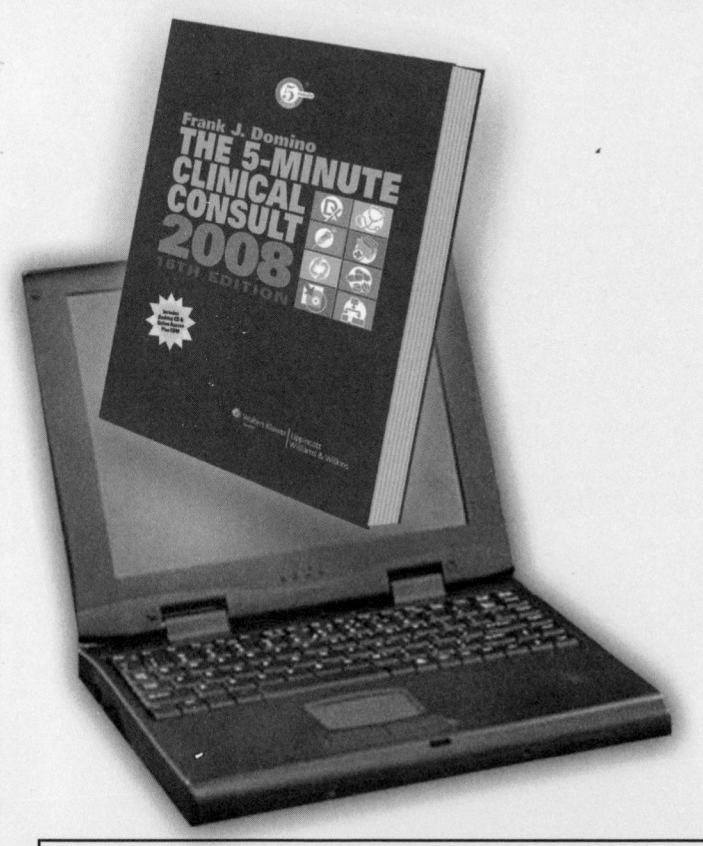

Online Text

Entire content of the book plus additional topics not covered in the book, online and fully searchable

Image Bank

Full color images from *Goodheart's Photoguide of Common Skin Disorders, Second Edition* searchable and downloadable

To gain access…obtain the CDROM from the inside front cover and install into your computer. This will automatically take you to a registration page to set up your username and password.

Once the username and password are set up you will no longer need the CDROM to gain access to the site and can utilize the CDROM for offline purposes.

Once you have completed your registration, go to **www.5mcc.com** and click on Gain Access to *The 5-Minute Clinical Consult 2008 Online Companion* where you will be prompted for your username and password.

Patient Handouts

178 English & 178 Spanish patient handouts from The American Academy of Family Physicians

Videos

Access to 15 videos of medical procedures including Exam Techniques, Joint Injections and more

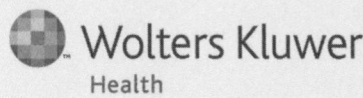 Wolters Kluwer | Lippincott Williams & Wilkins
Health

Your Partner in Education and Practice

THE 5-MINUTE CLINICAL CONSULT 2008

THE 5-MINUTE CLINICAL CONSULT 2008
16TH EDITION

Editor

Frank J. Domino, MD

Associate Professor
Clerkship Director
Department of Family Medicine and Community Health
University of Massachusetts Medical School
Worcester, Massachusetts

Wolters Kluwer | Lippincott Williams & Wilkins
Health
Philadelphia · Baltimore · New York · London
Buenos Aires · Hong Kong · Sydney · Tokyo

Acquisitions Editor: Ave McCracker
Managing Editor: Lauren Aquino
Project Manager: Rosanne Hallowell
Manufacturing Manager: Kathleen Brown
Marketing Manager: Kim Schonberger
Design Coordinator: Terry Mallon
Cover Designer: Becky Baxendell
Production Services: Aptara, Inc.
Printer: Quebecor World/Taunton

16th Edition

© 2008 by LIPPINCOTT WILLIAMS & WILKINS, a Wolters Kluwer business
530 Walnut Street
Philadelphia, PA 19106
LWW.com

Printed in the United States

ISBN: 0-7817-7608-2
ISBN 13: 978-0-7817-7608-0

10 9 8 7 6 5 4 3 2 1

PREFACE

Welcome to the 2008* edition of *The 5-Minute Clinical Consult*. I am again honored to be a part of this highly updated resource whose mission is to assist in your care of patients.

In this year's edition, you will find the time-honored features associated with this cornerstone reference. And thanks to your feedback, we have added a number of new components:

- Evidence-Based content of each chapter highlighted in the text
- Updated Health Maintenance section
- Inclusion of both Desktop and Online versions of the content, which include:
  - Additional topics not in the book
  - Video instruction on various physical diagnostic and treatment interventions.

Evidence-Based Health Care is the integration of the best medical information with the values of the patient *and your skill* as a clinician. Less harm comes to our patients if we respect the medical literature; we have improved our content and visibility of the best evidence, so you can focus on how to apply it.

The Health Maintenance recommendations included here have been updated through the end of 2006. This content is based on the U.S. Preventive Services Task Force, and has been organized by age into one-page recommendations. This summary will allow you to find the most current recommendations to improve health and prevent disease for each population of patients. Again, your feedback resulted in the inclusion of the Centers for Disease Control's immunization tables for quick reference.

* Why "2008 Edition" in the spring of 2007? To better meet your needs. To make this content fresh and current, we have moved the delivery of this book to the spring of each year. Included in your purchase is one year's subscription to electronic updates of its content. This will make your 5-Minute Clinical Consult the most useful, handy, and current resource you use.

Why a Desktop and Online version of this content? To respond to your needs for more content and access to your resources at the office, in the hospital, and at home. These new features include easy maneuverability between chapters and sections, extra content not in the book (including a large section on pediatric conditions), and, later this year, introduction of our unique Continuing Medical Education (CME) program. Additionally, you will be able to download updates to this content at no additional cost.

The CME software will collate your search topics, and periodically give you a listing of your searches. This represents the medical content *you* needed to know over the preceding months. Linked to this list will be an assortment of education resources you may use to address your educational needs. What could be better than very specific educational interventions tailored to your knowledge and informational needs?

To address your diagnostic challenges, the Signs and Symptoms section has been moved to the front of the book. Here, you can determine how to evaluate a patient complaint or finding by utilizing the evidence-based collection of assessment-based algorithms. On the Desktop and Web versions, these are hyperlinked to the appropriate chapters. I urge you to look through this section and recognize its utility in your approach to solving vexing patient questions.

So welcome to the 2008 edition of Lippincott Williams & Wilkins' 5-Minute Clinical Consult. Please never hesitate to drop me an e-mail at 5MinConsultFeedback@lww.com and share your thoughts, suggestions, and constructive criticism.

Frank J. Domino, MD
Associate Professor
University of Massachusetts Medical School
Worcester, Massachusetts

EVIDENCE-BASED MEDICINE

WHAT IS EVIDENCE-BASED MEDICINE AND WHY IS THIS NEW?

Think back on your early days of training: Were there interventions you performed that are no longer the standard of care? In my residency, we treated everyone who had a myocardial infarction with prophylactic lidocaine; this was based upon a logical series of assumptions. If you had an MI, you were prone to ventricular arrhythmias, and IV lidocaine could treat those life threatening rhythms. So why not give it prophylactically?

After years of this practice, researchers looked back on this "logical" but untested intervention and concluded that, despite its logic, the use of lidocaine resulted in worse outcomes than using it only if the patient developed those rhythms.

The underlying premise of Evidence-Based Medicine (EBM) is the evaluation of medical interventions, and the literature that supports those interventions, in a systematic fashion. EBM hopes to encourage treatments that are proven to be effective and safe. And when insufficient data exist, it hopes to inform you, the practitioner, on how you can safely proceed.

EBM uses as endpoints real patient outcomes, morbidity, mortality, and risk. It focuses less on intermediate outcomes (like bone density), and more on the patient's conditions (like hip fractures).

To incorporate Evidence-Based Medicine into practice, you must combine the best data with your clinical strengths and experience, as well as the patient's perspective. Implementing EBM *requires all three components*: The best medical evidence, the skill and experience of the provider, and the values of the patients. Should this patient be screened for prostate cancer? It depends on what is known about the utility of screening; what you know of its benefits and harms, and your ability to communicate that information; and that patient's ability to make an informed choice.

"All this in 15 minutes?" you ask. This is not an easy task. My goal is to provide you with the tools to assist in this process.

This book presents a number of evidence-based concepts as a first step to providing you with the absolute best information, coupled with some easy-to-interpret statistics to help you and the patient make decisions. While not every test or treatment has this level of detail, look for more of this content in future editions.

The language of medical statistics is useful to interpreting the concepts of Evidence-Based Medicine. Below is a list of these terms with examples to help take the confusion and mystery out of their use.

POPULATION INFORMATION

These terms are designed to help you and epidemiologists look at the "community" as a whole, and determine how commonly disease occurs.

Prevalence: *Proportion of people* in a population who have a disease at a certain point in time (often written as a percent)—e.g., in the US, "0.3% (3 in 1000) people over the age 50 have colon cancer."

Incidence: How many *new cases of a disease* occur in a population during a specified interval of time (#/10,000 patients/year)—e.g., "the estimated incidence of colon cancer in the US was 104,000 in 2005."

TESTING INFORMATION

We often hear the words *sensitivity* and *specificity* and cringe. They are, at a minimum, very confusing. These terms are characteristics of a test, but tell us little about the lab result we are holding in our hands. Rather, it is the *predicative value* that helps us interpret the test results we order, and what they mean to our patients.

ML is a 53 year old female whom you saw for a Health Maintenance visit; you ordered a *screening* mammogram and the report you hold demonstrates an irregular area of microcalcifications. She is waiting in your office to receive her test results; what can you tell her?

The data that follows comes from the

Sensitivity (Sn): Percent of People With Disease who test positive; for mammography, the Sensitivity is 71–96%.[*]

Specificity (Sp): Percent of People Without Disease who test negative; for mammography, the Specificity is 94–97%.

Does this help in your discussion with ML? No, because these tests refer to characteristics of people who are known to have disease (sensitivity) or those that are known not to have disease (specificity).

What you have is an abnormal test result in a woman who anxiously wants to know if she has cancer. To better explain this result to ML, you need to know the Positive Predictive Value.

Positive Predictive Value (PPV): Percent of *positive* test results that are truly positive; for this patient, the PPV for a woman between 50 and 59 years is about 22%.[†] So only 22% of abnormal screening mammograms in this age group truly identified cancer. The other 78% were false positives.

Negative Predictive Value (NPV): Percent of negative test results that are truly negative.

If we accept the best of this data, then 1 out of every 5 (20%) of abnormal mammograms correctly identify breast cancer. The other 4 out of 5 (80%) are false positives. The only way to determine which mammogram has identified cancer is to do further testing. When you tell ML that her mammogram is abnormal, you may both find some comfort knowing the chance that it is cancer is only 1 in 5.

The PPV and NPV are population dependent, while the Sensitivity and Specificity are characteristics of the test, and have little to do with the patient in front of you. Mammography PPV increases as our patients age.

---

* Agency for Health Research and Quality: http://www.ahrq.gov/clinic/3rduspstf/breastcancer/bcscrnsum1.htm.
† Per Skaane, MD, PhD, and Arnulf Skjennald, MD, PhD. Screen-Film Mammography versus Full-Field Digital Mammography with Soft-Copy Reading: Randomized Trial in a Population-based Screening Program—The Oslo II Study. *Radiology* 2004;232:197–204.

So when you receive an abnormal lab result, especially a screening test like mammography or PSA value, understand the limits of the test results based upon their PPV and NPV.

TREATMENT INFORMATION

In discerning the statistics of randomized, controlled trials of interventions, first consider an example. The Scandinavian Simvastatin Survival Study (4S)* found that using simvastatin in patients at high risk for heart disease for 5 years resulted in deaths in 8% of patients vs. 12% of those on placebo; this results in a Relative Risk of 0.70, a Relative Risk Reduction of 33%, and a Number Needed to Treat of 25. What does that mean?

There are two ways of considering the benefits of an intervention with respect to a given outcome. The Absolute Risk Reduction (ARR) is the difference in the percent of people with the condition before and after the intervention. Thus, if the incidence of MI was 12% for the placebo group and 8% for the simvastatin group, the ARR is 4% (12% − 8% = 4%).

The Relative Risk Reduction (RRR) reflects the improvement in the outcome as a percentage of the original rate. Thus, if the risk of MI were reduced by simvastatin from 12% to 8%, then the RRR would be 33% (4% ÷ 12% = 33%). Relative Risk Reduction is the usual way that results are reported and will often make small clinical improvements seem significant.

While RRR reflects *statistical* significance, ARR is usually a better measure of *clinical* significance. For instance, in one study, the treatment of mild hypertension has been shown to have a RRR of 40% over 5 years (40% fewer strokes in the treated group). However, the ARR was only 1.3%. Because mild hypertension does not regularly cause stroke, and is not strongly associated with strokes, preventing 40% of them yields only a small clinical benefit in that population.

It is important not to confuse Relative Risk Reduction with Relative Risk.

Absolute (or Attributable) Risk (AR): The percent of people in the placebo or the intervention group who reach a given endpoint; in this case, 8% of those on the medication died. Thus, the absolute risk of death on simvastatin was 8%.

Relative Risk (RR): The risk of disease of those treated or exposed to something (in this case, simvastatin) divided by those in the placebo group or who were untreated. It is interpreted as follows:

If RR < 1.0, it reduces risk—the smaller the number, the greater the risk reduction.

If RR > 1.0, it increases the risk—the greater the number, the greater the risk increase.

Despite their similarity of name, *Relative Risk is NOT the same as Relative Risk Reduction.*

Relative Risk Reduction (RRR): The relative decrease in risk of an endpoint compared to the percent of that endpoint in the placebo group.

If you are still confused, just remember the RRR is often an overestimation of the actual effect.

Number Needed to Treat (NNT): This is the number of people who need to be treated by an intervention to prevent one adverse outcome. This is a relative term. A "good" NNT can be a large number (>100) if risk of serious outcome is great. If the risk of

an outcome is not that dangerous, then lower (<25) NNTs are preferred.

The NNT should be compared to a similar statistic, the Number Needed to Harm (NNH). This is the number of people who have to be given treatment before one excess side effect or harm occurs. When the NNT is compared to the NNH, you and the patient can judge whether the benefit of the intervention is great enough to outweigh the risk of harm.

To help you interpret diagnostic and treatment recommendations within the *5-Minute Clinical Consult*, we have graded the best information within the text, and highlighted this content.

An "A" level designates the intervention as being of the highest quality. A "B" level implies that good, clinically trialed evidence exists, and a "C" level implies that this content is a common practice, but solid evidence does may not yet exist. The "C" level should be viewed as medical practice that has yet to be proven, but can also be the community standard of care.

For example, the American Cancer Society might recommend obtaining a serum PSA on all males over age 50. This test, while often performed, has yet to be proven as clearly beneficial to patients. A "C" level is not a negative grade, just an acknowledgment that definitive evidence to support this recommendation is lacking.

REFERENCES

Grading the quality of the research referenced for medical decision making is a new concept. This textbook will grade each reference to help you interpret how strong the medical evidence is that supports the chapter you are reading.

An "A Grade" means the reference is from the highest quality resource, like a Systematic Review. A systematic review is a summary of the medical literature on a given topic that uses strict, explicit methods to perform a thorough search of the literature and then provides a critical appraisal of individual studies, concluding in a recommendation. The most prestigious collection of systematic reviews is from the Cochrane Collaboration (www.cochrane.org).

A "B Grade" means the data referenced comes from high-quality randomized controlled trials that were performed to minimize bias in their outcome. Bias is anything that interferes with the truth; in the medical literature, it is often unintentional, but is much more common than we appreciate. In short, always assume some degree of bias exists in any research endeavor.

A "C Grade" implies that the reference used does not meet the A or B requirements; they are often treatments recommended by consensus groups (like the American Cancer Society) and are often the standards of care. But it is critical to factor into any decision based upon their recommendation that they often contain the bias of the author or the group that supports the reference. For example, the American Cancer Society's recommendation regarding screening for prostate cancer may not be as scientifically valid as the recommendation of the U.S. Preventive Services Task Force (www.ahrq.gov), the organization that determines which health maintenance interventions are reasonable and does so with the least bias.

BIAS

Bias is anything that interferes with the truth. There are many types of bias that should be considered by the publishers of medical

* Lancet. 1994 Nov 19;344(8934):1383–9.

information. Below are descriptions of a number of bias types that often affect our care without our being aware of their presence.

Publication Bias occurs when research is not published, such as when a study finds data that does *not* support an intervention. The motivation to publish information that "didn't work" is low, resulting in the researcher never writing or submitting the research. It is estimated that up to 40% of all medical research never gets published. So when you read of an intervention that "works," wonder what study was done that didn't.

Comparator Bias occurs when research compares an intervention to placebo, when placebo isn't the standard of care. Knowing a new antibiotic is more effective than placebo for treating acute sinusitis is not helpful if you typically use amoxicillin.

Why not release research comparing the new drug to the standard of care? Often, it has been done, and the new drug proved no better. If this study does not get published, you have an example of Publication Bias.

Selection Bias involves either using a tool that doesn't discriminate between populations selected, or just reporting a subset of study participants from a study. Either will result in the data being skewed because it can only be applied to a small subset of people. Selection bias is about including only certain subsets of participants in a study, or including everyone but just reporting on the subsets that received statistical benefit.

Attrition Bias and the Concepts of Intention to Treat. Attrition bias is when researchers do not fully acknowledge and address how a study deals with participants who do not adhere to the research protocol or drop out completely. Intention to Treat hopes to diminish Attrition Bias by statistically moving the non-adhering or dropped-out patients as unsuccessfully benefiting from the intervention. This hopefully limits Attrition Bias, but as there is no uniform method to Intention to Treat analysis, it can still hide manipulated data.

SUMMARY

I hope this brief introduction to Evidence-Based Medicine has been informative, clear, and helpful. If any of the information above seems unclear, or if you have a question, please drop me an email at 5MinConsultFeedback@lww.com.

Frank J. Domino, MD
Associate Professor
University of Massachusetts Medical School
Worcester, Massachusetts

ACKNOWLEDGMENTS

This year's *5-Minute Clinical Consult* brings you more content, new media (Desktop, Web), and a new editorial team. Leading our effort was our Point of Care editor, Ave Maria McCracken. Her "can do" attitude has been the energy that allowed 15 months of work to be completed in fewer than 8. Lauren Aquino was saddled with keeping me and our authors in line and my "In Box" full of work, all while responding to my daily e-mails of questions and new ideas. Our team's new minder, Mary Ann Geier, combined her wonderful insights and personality with her incredible organizational skills. I am deeply indebted to this team; without their dedication, you would not be holding this text. I am also indebted to the foresight and energy of Diane Harnish, Vice President and Publisher, Medicine, at Lippincott Williams & Wilkins, whose vision brings the best medical information to our hands, providing the tools that help us and our patients enjoy health.

The challenge of taking on a book that covers this broad a spectrum of medicine requires insights and skills far beyond my own. Bob Baldor, Alan Ehrlich, and Mark Quirk are an enormous support, always there to encourage, reassure, and impart wisdom.

Who does the hardest work when we are caring for our patients? Our families. Thanks to my wife, Sylvia, and my daughter, Molly. And welcome Milo (like the breakfast drink in Australia.)

Many in the academic and healthcare worlds are due thanks for support, insight, and friendship: Dan Lasser, Alan Chuman, Michele Pugnaire, Karen Rayla, Denise West, Phil Fournier, Erik Garcia, Jeff Stovall, Jim Comes, Len Levine, Jeremy Golding, J. Herb Stevenson, Lee Mancini, Jeanne Rousseau, Zainab Nawab, Melanie Mercurio, Cindy Lapan, Kim Koski, Carole Fahlin, Ryan Callery, and the faculty and students of the University of Massachusetts Medical School.

Medicine is a challenge that I have fortunately not had to meet alone. To my parents, Frank and Angela (Jean); my brother John and his family, Marylou, Cate, and Jane; Frank, Mary Anne, Diane, and David Christian; the Diana and Hymie Lipschitz family, and the Bob and Ruth Pabreza family—they are responsible for who I am and my survival and success in life.

I am blessed with the best of friends; without them, I would not be a physician. Thanks to Ron Jautz, Richard Onorato, John Horcher, Auguste Turnier, Bob Bacic, Antoinette and (Gary) Francis, Bob and Nancy Gallinaro, Drew and Jill Grimes, , Louay Toma, Laurie, Alan, Daniel, Jenny, and Matt Bugos, Teri and Andy Jennings, Mark Steenbergen, John and Kathleen Polanowicz, Phil Pettine, Steve Bennett, Vicki Triolo, and Amin Vidal.

CONTRIBUTING AUTHORS

George Abraham, MD, MPH
Clinical Associate Professor
Department of Medicine
University of Massachusetts Medical
    School;
Associate Program Director
Department of Internal Medicine
Saint Vincent Hospital
Worcester, Massachusetts

Muhanned Abu-Hijleh, MD, FCCP
Assistant Clinical Professor
Pulmonary and Critical Care Medicine
Brown Medical School;
Director
Interventional Pulmonary and Special
    Procedures Unit
Rhode Island Hospital
Providence, Rhode Island

**Abdulrazak Abyad, MD, PhD, MBA,
    MPH, AGSF**
Chairman
Middle-East Academy for Medicine of
    Aging Coordinator
Middle-East Primary Care Research
    Network;
President
Middle-East Association on Aging and
    Alzheimer's;
Director
Abyad Medical Center
Tripoli, Lebanon

Rodney D. Adam, MD
Professor
Department of Medicine and
    Microbiology/Immunology
University of Arizona College of
    Medicine;
Infectious Disease Physician
Department of Medicine
University Medical Center
Tucson, Arizona

Thomas Agresta, MD
Associate Professor
Department of Family Medicine
University of Connecticut
Farmington, Connecticut

Mohammad Alhabbal, MD
Resident
Department of Family Medicine
University of Massachusetts;
Resident
Department of Family Medicine
University of Massachusetts Memorial
    Medical Center
Worcester, Massachusetts

Ambareen Ali, MD
Physician
Family Practice and Obstetrics
Westside Health
Wilmington, Delaware

Richard W. Allinson, MD
Associate Professor
Department of Surgery
The Texas A & M System, Health
    Sciences Center
Temple. Texas;
Senior Staff Physician
Ophthalmology Section
Scott & White Clinic
Waco, Texas

Eric Alper, MD
Associate Professor
Department of Medicine
University of Massachusetts Medical
    School
Worcester, Massachusetts

**Maryellen Antonetti, MPH,
    PA-C, RN**
Assistant Professor
Clinical Director
Physician Assistant Program
Nova Southeastern University
Fort Lauderdale, Florida

Watson C. Arnold, MD
Director
Department of Pediatric Nephrology
Cook County Children's Medical
    Center
Fort Worth, Texas

Melissa Arthur, LCSW, MA
Assistant Professor
Department of Family Medicine
SUNY Upstate Medical University;
Director, Behavioral Science
Family Medicine Residency
St. Jospeh's Hospital
Syracuse, New York

Elizabeth L. Backer, MD
Clinical Associate Professor
Department of Family Medicine
University of Nebraska Medical Center;
Faculty
Department of Family Medicine
Nebraska Medical Center
Omaha, Mebraska

Colin R. Bamford, MD
Department of Neurology
University of Arizona College of Medicine
Tucson, Arizona

Benjamin Barankin, MD
Department of Medicine
Division of Dermatology
University of Alberta
Edmonton, Alberta, Canada

Brent J. Barber, MD
Assistant Professor
Department of Pediatrics
University of Arizona;
Department of Pediatrics
Arizona Health Sciences Center
Tucson, Arizona

Robert P. Baughman, MD
Professor of Medicine
Department of Internal Medicine
University of Cincinnati
Cincinnati, Ohio

Kay A. Bauman, MD, MPH
Medical Director
Department of Public Safety
Honolulu, Hawaii

Francesca L. Beaudoin, MS, MD
Resident
Department of Emergency Medicine
Brown Medical School
Rhode Island Hospital
Providence, Rhode Island

Paul Belliveau, PharmD, RPh
Associate Professor of Pharmacy Practice
Massachusetts College of Pharmacy and
    Health Sciences
Worcester, Massachusetts;
Clinical Pharmacist
Pharmacy
Concord Hospital
Concord, New Hampshire

Sheldon Benjamin, MD
Director of Psychiatric Education and
    Training
Director of Neuropsychiatry
Professor of Psychiatry and Neurology
University of Massachusetts Medical
    School
Worcester, Massachusetts

Katherine Berg, MD
Resident
Department of Internal Medicine
New England Medical Center
Boston, Massachusetts

George R. Bergus, MD
Professor
Department of Family Medicine
University of Iowa
Iowa City, Iowa

Garreth C. Biegun, MD
University of Massachusetts Medical
    School
Worcester, Massachusetts

Timothy L. Black, MD
Pediatric Surgeon
Department of Surgery
Cook Children's Medical Center
Fort Worth, Texas

Shawn H. Blanchard, MD
Assistant Professor
Department of Family Medicine
Oregon Health and Science University
Portland, Oregon

Alison H. Blatt, MD
Clinical Lecturer
Faculty of Medicine
Sydney University;
Provisional Fellow
Department of Urology
Concord Repatriation General Hospital
Sydney, Australia

Bruce Block, MD
Clinical Associate Professor
Department of Family Medicine
University of Pittsburgh School of
    Medicine;
Director
Primary Care Institute
UPMC-Shadyside Hospital
Pittsburgh, Pennsylvania

Jeremy S. Bordeaux, MD, MPH
Instructor
Department of Medicine
Division of Dermatology
University of Massachusetts Medical
    School;
Instructor
Department of Medicine
Division of Dermatology
Worcester, Massachusetts

Patricia Borman, MD
Director
Advanced Training for Geriatrics
Swedish Family Medicine
Seattle, Washington

Megan E. Bower, RN, MPH
School of Nursing
Boston College
Boston, Massachusetts

John C. Bradford, DO
Professor
Department of Emergency Medicine
Northeastern Ohio Universities College of
    Medicine
Rootstown, Ohio;
Interim Director
Department of Emergency Medicine
Akron General Medical Center
Akron, Ohio

Chad M. Braun, MD
Assistant Professor
Department of Family Medicine
University of Illinois-Chicago
Chicago, Illinois

Jacob R. Brodsky, MD
Resident Physician
Department of Otolaryngology and
    Communication Sciences
SUNY Upstate Medical University
Syracuse, New York

Stephen Bromley, MD
Research Affiliate
Smell and Taste Center
University of Pennsylvania
Philadelphia, Pennsylvania

James F. Broomfield, MD
Assistant Professor of Family Practice
University of Wyoming Family Practice
    Residency Program at Cheyenne
Cheyenne, Wyoming

Caroline K. Buckway, MD
Pediatric Endocrinologist
Department of Pediatrics
Providence Alaska Medical Center
Anchorage, Alaska

Kristin Burdick, MD
Resident
Family Medicine
Fletcher Allen Health Care
Burlington, Vermont

John R. Burk, MD
Private Practice
Pulmonology
Texas Pulmonary and Critical Care
    Consultants, PA
Sleep Consultants
Fort Worth, Texas

Delores Burroughs-Biron, MD
Associate Program Medical Director
Department of Family Medicine
University of Massachusetts Correctional
    Health Program
University of Massachusetts Medical
    School
Worcester, Massachusetts;
Medical Director
Health Services Unit
North Central Correctional Institution
Gardner, Massachusetts

Harold J. Bursztajn, MD
Associate Clinical Professor
BIDMC Psychiatry
Harvard Medical School;
Co-Founder, Program in Psychiatry and
    Law
BIDMC Psychiatry of Harvard Medical
    School
BIDMC
Boston, Massachusetts

David E. Burtner, MD
Vice Chairman and Professor
Department of Family and Community
    Medicine
Mercer University School of Medicine
Macon, Georgia

Brian D. Busconi, MD
Associate Professor
Department of Orthopaedic Surgery
University of Massachusetts Medical
    School;
Chief, Division of Sports Medicine
University of Massachusetts Memorial
    Medical Center
Worcester, Massachusetts

James N. Butera, MD
University Medicine Foundation, Inc.
Comprehensive Cancer Center
Rhode Island Hospital
Hematology/Oncology
Internal Medicine
Providence, Rhode Island

Nancy Byatt, MD, MBA
Psychiatry Resident
Office of Psychiatric Education and
    Training
University of Massachusetts Medical
    School
Worcester, Massachusetts

Jamie Byler, MD
Resident Physician
Department of Obstetrics and Gynecology
Akron General Medical Center
Akron, Ohio

Roger K. Cady, MD
Medical Director
Headache Care Center
Springfield, Missouri

Mitchell Cahan, MD
Assistant Professor of Surgery
Department of Surgery
University of Massachusetts School of
    Medicine;
Attending Surgeon
Department of Surgery
University of Massachusetts Memorial
    Medical Center
Worcester, Massachusetts

Lisa Capra, MD
Milford Regional Medical Center
Milford, Massachuchetts

Cynthia Gail Carmichael, MD
Department of Family Medicine
Contra Costa Health Service
Richmond, California

Laurie A. Carrier, MD
Resident
Department of Family
    Medicine/Psychiatry
University of Cincinnati;
Resident
Department of Family
    Medicine/Psychiatry
University Hospital
Cincinnati, Ohio

Katrina Carter, MD
Resident Physician
Department of Family Medicine
University of Nebraska Medical Center
Omaha, Nebraska

Roy R. Casiano, MD
Professor and Vice-Chair
Department of Otolaryngology;
Director
Division of General Otolaryngology
University of Miami School of Medicine
Miami, Florida

Daniel Casto, MD
Assistant Clinical Professor
Department of Family and Community
    Medicine
University of Arizona
Tucson, Arizona

Ximena M. Castro, MD
Resident
University of Massachusetts Medical
    School
University of Massachusetts Fitchburg
    Family Practice;
University of Fitchburg Family Practice
    Residency Program
Fitchburg, Massachusetts

Mary Cataletto, MD
Associte Professor of Clinical Pediatrics
Department of Pediatrics
SUNY Stony Brook
Stony Brook, New York;
Associate Professor of Pediatric
    Pulmonology
Department of Pediatrics
Winthrop University Hospital
Mineola, New York

Jeanne M. Cawse-Lucas, MD
University of Washington
Department of Family Medicine
University of Washington;
Resident
Department of Family Medicine
Swedish Medical Center
Seattle, Washington

Frank Celestino, MD
Associate Professor
Department of Family and Community
    Medicine
Wake Forest University School of
    Medicine
Winston-Salem, North Carolina

Jan Cerny, MD
Department of Medicine
Division of Hematology/Oncology
University of Massachusetts Medical
    School
Worcester, Massachusetts

Teresa V. Chan, MD
Resident Physician
Otolaryngology
Head and Neck Surgery
Boston Medical Center
Boston Massachusetts

Felix B. Chang, MD
Assistant Professor
Family Medicine and Community Health
University of Massachusetts Medical
    School
Worcester, Massachusetts;
Attending Physician
University of Massachusetts Fitchburg
    Family Practice
Residency Program
Fitchburg, Massachusetts

Phillip Chang, MD
Lecturer
Faculty of Medicine
University of New South Wales
Consultant, Otologist
ENT Department
St. Vincent's Hospital
Sydney, Australia

Daniel Chao, MD
University of Massachusetts Medical
    School
Worcester, Massachusetts

Jasmine Chao, MD
Adjunct Faculty Member
Department of Family Medicine
McGaw Medical Center of Northwestern
    University Family Practice Residency
Glenview, Illinois
Associate Member
Department of Family Medicine
Evanston Northwestern Healthcare
Evanston, Illinois

Jason Chao, MD, MS
Professor
Department of Family Medicine
Cast Western Reserve University;
Department of Family Medicine
University Hospitals of Cleveland
Cleveland, Ohio

J.C. Chave-Zimmerman, MD
Medical Director
St. Francis Family Practice Residency
Lincolnwood, Illinois

Eunice S. Chen, MD
Westlake Family Practice
Austin, Texas

Anthony W. Chow, MD, FRCPC, FACP
Professor of Medicine, Division of
    Infectious Diseases
Director/MD/PhD Program
Department of Medicine
University of British Columbia;
Consultant, Division of Infectious Diseases
Department of Medicine
Vancouver Hospital Health Sciences
    Center
Vancouver, British Columbia, Canada

Vasilios Chrisostomidis, DO
Assistant Professor
Department of Family Medicine
University of Massachusetts Medical
    School
Worcester, Massachusetts

Sara Cichowski, MD
Resident
Department of Family
    Medicine-Greenwood
Medical University of South Carolina
Charleston, South Carolina;
Faculty Physician
Department of Family Medicine
Self Regional Healthcare
Greenwood, South Carolina

Keri Clifford, MD
Division of Dermatology
University of Massachusetts
Worcester, Massachusetts

Richard D. Clover, MD
School of Public Health and Information
    Sciences
University of Louisville
Louisville, Kentucky

Irene C. Coletsos
University of Massachusetts Medical
    School
Worcester, Massachusetts

Dana Collaguazo, MD
Department of Emergency Medicine
The University of Iowa
Iowa City, Iowa

Jeremy Collins, MD
University of Massachusetts Medical
    School
Worcester, Massachusetts

Mary Ann Condon, NP, PhD
Binghamton University
Decker School of Nursing
Binghamton, NY

Donald S. Corenman, MD, DC
Steadman Hawkins Clinic
Vail, Colorado

Macario Corpuz, Jr., MD
Assistant Professor
Department of Family Medicine and
    Community Health
University of Massachusetts Medical
    School;
Medical Staff
Department of Family Medicine and
    Community Health
University of Massachusetts Memorial
    Hospital
Worcester, Massachusetts

Alan J. Cropp, MD, FCCP
Professor of Internal Medicine
Department of Pulmonary Medicine
Northeastern Ohio Universities College of
    Medicine
Rootstown, Ohio;
Assistant Director, Critical Care
Section Chief, Pulmonary Medicine
Department of Internal Medicine
St. Elizabeth Hospital
Youngstown, Ohio

Jason Cross, PharmD
Assistant Professor
Pharmacy Practice
Massachusetts College of Pharmacy and
    Health Sciences
Worcester, Massachusetts;
Clinical Pharmacist
Pharmacy
Baystate Medical Center
Springfield, Massachusetts

Hongyi Cui, MD, PhD
Senior Resident
Department of Surgery
University of Massachusetts
Worcester, Massachusetts

Paul T. Cullen, MD
Clinical Associate Professor
Department of Family Medicine
University of Pittsburgh
Pittsburgh, Pennsylvania;
Program Director
Washington Hospital Family Medicine
    Residency
Washington Hospital
Washington, Pennsylvania

Jennifer E. Cyrkler, MD
Resident
Department of Emergency Medicine
Highland General Hospital/Alameda
    County Medical Center
Oakland, California

Gregory R. Czarnecki, DO
Sports Medicine Fellow
Department of Family Medicine
University of Massachusetts Medical
    School;
Sports Medicine Fellow
Department of Sports Medicine
University of Massachusetts Memorial
    Medical Center
Worcester, Massachusetts

Sean J. Dacus, DO
Resident
University of Massachusetts Medical
    School
University of Massachusetts Fitchburg
    Family Practice;
University of Massachusetts Fitchburg
    Family Practice Residency Program
Fitchburg, Massachusetts

Mark R. Dambro, MD
Family Medicine
Fort Worth, Texas

Janice E. Daugherty, MD
Associate Professor of Medicine
Director of Predoctoral Education
The Brody School of Medicine at East
    Carolina University
Greenville, North Carolina

Konstantinos Deligiannidis, MD, MPH
Resident
Department of Family Medicine
University of Massachusetts Medical
    School
Worcester, Massachusetts

Bart M. Demaerschalk, MD, MSc
Assistant Professor
Department of Neurology
Mayo Clinic College of Medicine
Scottsdale, Arizona;
Director
Cerebrovascular Diseases Center
Mayo Clinic Hospital
Phoenix, Arizona

Mathew J. Devine, DO
Resident
Department of Family Medicine
University of Rochester;
Resident
Department of Family Medicine
Highland Hospital
Rochester, New York

Saritha Dhruvakumar, MD
Resident
Department of Medicine
University of Illinois
Chicago, Illinois

Nuhad D. Dinno, MD
Emeritus Clinical Professor
Department of Pediatrics
University of Washington Medical
    Center
Seattle, Washington

Robert Dobrzynski, MD
Clinical Instructor of Medicine
Department of Internal Medicine,
    Endocrinology
Brown University
Rhode Island Hospital
Providence, Rhode Island

Frank J. Domino, MD
Associate Professor
Clerkship Director
Department of Family Medicine and
    Community Health
University of Massachusetts Medical
    School
Worcester, Massachusetts

David J. Donahue, MD, FAAP
Medical Director
Department of Pediatric Neurosurgery
Cook Children's Hospital
Fort Worth, Texas

Justin Dorfman, DO
Sports Medicine Fellow
Department of Family Medicine
University of Massachusetts Medical
    School;
Sports Medicine Fellow
Department of Sports Medicine
University of Massachusetts Memorial
    Medical Center
Worcester, Massachusetts

Kaelen Dunican, RPh, PharmD
Assistant Professor
Pharmacy Practice
Massachusetts College of Pharmacy and
    Health
Worcester, Massachusetts

Stephen T. Earls, MD
Assistant Professor
Family Medicine and Community
    Health
University of Massachusetts Medical
    School
Worcester, Massachusetts;
Medical and Education Director
Barre Family Health Center
University of Massachusetts Memorial
    Healthcare
Barre, Massachusetts

Frank Ed, MD
Pediatric Ophthalmologist
University of Masschusetts Medical
    Center
Worcester, Massachusetts

Terence S. Edgar, MD
Chief
Department of Pediatric Neurology
Prevea Health
Green Bay, Wisconsin

Alan M. Ehrlich, MD
Assistant Clinical Professor
Department of Family Practice
University of Massachusetts Medical
    School
Worcester, Massachusetts

William G. Elder, Jr., PhD
Associate Professor
Department of Family and Community
    Medicine
University of Kentucky College of
    Medicine;
Chief of Behavioral Science
Department of Family and Community
    Medicine
University of Kentucky Chandler Medical
    Center
Lexington, Kentucky

Pamela I. Ellsworth, MD
Associate Professor of Urology
Department of Surgery/Urology
Brown University;
Urologist
Department of Surgery/Urology
Rhode Island Hospital/Hasbro Children's
    Hospital
Providence, Rhode Island

Teresa A. Everson, MD
Physician
Department of Family Medicine
Oregon Health and Science University;
Resident
Department of Family Medicine
Oregon Health and Science University
Portland, Oregon

Fady Faddoul, MD
Director
Advanced Education in General Dentistry
Case Western Reserve University School
    of Dentistry
Mayfield Village, Ohio

Kristyn Fagerberg, MD
West Lake Family Practice
Austin, Texas

Ramon Fakhouny, MD
Chief Resident
Department of Family Medicine
Grant Medical Center
Columbus, Ohio

Pang-Yen Fan, MD
Associate Professor of Clinical Medicine
University of Massachusetts Medical
    School
Worcester, Massachusetts

Andrew H. Fenton, MD
Associate Professor
Department of Surgery
Northeastern Ohio Universities College of
    Medicine
Rootstown, Ohio;
Medical Director
McDowell Cancer Center
Akron General Medical Center
Akron, Ohio

Warren J. Ferguson, MD
Associate Professor and Vice Chair
Family Medicine and Community Health
University of Massachusetts Medical
    School
Worcester, Massachusetts

Shawn M. Ferullo, MD
Sports Medicine Fellow
Department of Family Medicine
Boston University;
Sports Medicine Fellow
Department of Family Medicine
Boston Medical Center
Boston, Massachusetts

Scott A. Fields, MD
Professor and Vice Chair
Department of Family Medicine
Oregon Health and Science University
Portland, Oregon

Stenley Fineman, MD
Clinical Associate Professor
Department of Pediatrics
Emory University
Atlanta, Georgia

Jonathan M. Firnhaber, MD
Family Physician
Cholowinity Family Care
Cholowinity, North Carolina

Gene S. Fisch, PhD
Senior Research Statistician and
    Investigator
North Shore-Long Island Jewish
    Research Institute
New York, New York

Melissa A. Fischer, MD, MEd
Assistant Professor
Department of Internal Medicine
University of Massachusetts;
Assistant Professor
Department of Internal Medicine
University of Massachusetts Memorial
    Medical Center
Worcester, Massachusetts

Tim Fitzgibbons, MD
Fellow
Department of Cardiology
University of Massachusetts Medical
    School
Worcester, Massachusetts

Jonathan M. Flacker, MD
Director, Emma I. Darnell Geriatrics Center
Assistant Professor of Medicine
Division of Geriatric Medicine and
    Gerontology
Emory University School of Medicine
Atlanta, Georgia

Matthew J. Fleig, MD
Assistant Professor
Department of Family Medicine
University of Rochester
Highland Family Medicine
Rochester, New York

Joseph A. Florence, MD
Director of Rural Programs
Department of Family Medicine
James H. Quillen College of Medicine
East Tennessee State University
Johnson City, Tennessee

Jay Fong, MD
Assistant Professor
Pediatric Gastroenterology
University of Massachusetts Medical
    School;
Clinician
Pediatric Gastroenterology
University of Massachusetts Medical
    Center
Worcester, Massachusetts

Michael Ford, MD
Resident
Department of Surgery
University of Massachusetts Medical
    School
Worcester, Massachusetts

Grant C. Fowler, MD
Professor and Vice Chair
Department of Family and Community
    Medicine
University of Texas Medical School at
    Houston;
Assistant Chief
Department of Family Medicine
Memorial Hermann Hospital
Houston, Texas

Ryan Frankel, MD
Resident
Department of Urology
University of Massachusetts Medical
    Center
Worcester, Massachusetts

Drew A. Freilich, MD
Student
University of Massachusetts Medical
    School
Worcester, Massachusetts

Anatoli Freiman, MD
Dermatology Resident
McGill University
Montreal, Quebec, Canada

Nellie Freydin, PsyD
Primary Care Postdoctoral Fellow
Family Medicine and Community Health
University of Massachusetts Medical
    School
Worcester, Massachusetts

Brad Friedman, MD
Resident
Department of Pediatrics
University of Arizona Allied Health Center
Tucson, Arizona

Tyeese Gaines-Reed, DO, MA
Alumnus
Nova Southeastern University
College of Osteopathic Medicine
Fort Lauderdale, Florida

Eric P. Gall, MD
Professor and Chairman
Department of Medicine
Chicago Medical School
Rosalind Franklin University of Medicine
    and Science
North Chicago, Illinois

Fae Gwen B. Ganiron, BS, PharmD
Assistant Professor
Massachusetts College of Pharmacy
Worcester, Massachusetts;
Pharmacy MetroWest Medical Center
Framingham, Massachusetts

Leonard Ganz, MD
Director of Cardiac Electrophysiology
Pittsburgh Arrythmia Consultants
Pittsburgh, Pennsylvania

Erik Garcia, MD
Assistant Professor
Family and Community Medicine
University of Massachusetts;
Medical Director
Homeless Outreach and Advocacy Project
Community Healthlink
Worcester, Massachusetts

William G. Gardner, MD, MACP
Director of Internal Medicine
Family Medicine Residency Program
Southern Regional Area Health Education
    Center;
Infectious Diseases Staff
Department of Internal Medicine
Cape Fear Valley Medical Center
Fayetteville, North Carolina

Amit Garg, MD
Assistant Professor
Department of Medicine (Dermatology)
University of Massachusetts Medical
    School
Worcester, Massachusetts

William Garrison, MD
Professor of Pediatrics
Division of Developmental and Behavioral
    Pediatrics
University of Massachusetts Memorial
    Healthcare and University of
    Massachusetts Medical School
Worcester, Massachusetts

Elizabeth Gebhard, DO
Resident
University of Massachusetts Medical
    School
University of Massachusetts Fitchburg
    Family Practice;
University of Massachusetts Fitchburg
    Family Practice Residency Program
Fitchburg, Massachusetts

Mark Gerstberger, MD
Private Practice-Family Practice
Gerstberger Medical Clinic
Ulysses, Kansas

Dan Giang, MBA, PharmD
Adjunct Professor
Pharmacy Practice
Massachusetts College of Pharmacy and
    Health Sciences
Worcester, Massachusetts

Brent R. Gibson, MD, MPH
Teaching Fellow
Preventive Medicine and Biometrics
Uniformed Services University of the
    Health Sciences
Bethesda, Maryland

Jeff Ray Gibson, Jr., MD
Assistant Professor
Department of Anesthesiology
The Texas A & M University Health
    Sciences Center College of Medicine;
Senior Staff Anesthesiologist
Department of Anesthesiology
Scott & White Memorial Hospital
Temple, Texas

Keisha L. Gibson, MD
Fellow
Department of Pediatric Nephrology
University of North Carolina at Chapel Hill
Chapel Hill, North Carolina

Timothy Gibson, MD
Hospitalist
Hanshaw Pediatric Service
Worcester, Massachusetts

Javed M. Gilani, MD, FACP, FRCP
Clinical Assistant Professor
Internal Medicine
Jefferson Medical College
Philadelphia, Pennsylvania;
Attending Physician
Internal Medicine
Christiana Care Health System
Wilmington, Delaware

Noridelle Gilo, MD
Resident Physician
Department of Obstetrics and Gynecology
Akron General Medical Center
Akron, Ohio

Bruce G. Gilliland, MD
Professor of Medicine and Laboratory
    Medicine
Division of Rheumatology
University of Washington
Seattle, Washington

John R. Gimpel, DO, MEd
Clinical Assistant Professor
Department of Family Medicine
Georgetown University School of
    Medicine
Washington, D.C.;
Vice President for Clinical Skills Testing
National Board of Osteopathic Medical
    Examiners
Philadelphia, Pennsylvania

Paul R. Gittens, MD
Resident
Department of Urology
Thomas Jefferson University Hospital
Philadelphia, Pennsylvania

Jeremy Golding, MD
Assocaite Professor
Family Medicine Residency Program
Department of Family Medicine and
    Community Health
University of Massachusetts Memorial
    Medical Center;
Inpatient Services Director
Department of Family Medicine and
    Community Health
University of Massachusetts Memorial
    Hospital
Worcester, Massachusetts

Laura Goldman, MD
Assistant Professor
Department of Family Medicine
Boston University Medical School;
Department of Family Medicine
Boston Medical Center
Boston, Massachusetts

Keith T. Goldstein, MD
Medical Director of Critical Care
Department of Pulmonary and Critical
    Care Medicine
Hunterdon Medical Center
Flemington, New Jersey

Walter K. Goljan, MD
Private Practice
Worcester, Massachusetts

Leonard G. Gomella, MD
Professor and Chairman
Department of Urology
Jefferson Medical College
Philadelphia, Pennsylvania

Herbert P. Goodheart, MD
Assistant Clinical Professor
Department of Dermatology
Mount Sinai School of Medicine
New York, New York

Jeffrey L. Goodie, PhD
Assistant Professor of Family Medicine
Department of Family Medicine
Uniformed Services University of the
    Health Sciences;
Clinical Health Psychologist
Department of Psychology
National Navy Medical Center
Bethesda, Maryland

Geeta Gopalakrishnan, MD
Assistant Professor
Department of Medicine
Brown University
Providence, Rhode Island

Paul R. Gordon, MD, MPH
Associate Professor
Department of Family and Community
    Medicine
University of Arizona;
Department of Family Medicine
University Medical Center
Tucson, Arizona

R. Scott Gorman, MD
Community Internal Medicine
Mayo Clinic
Scottsdale, Arizona

Owen M. Gottfried, MD
Department of Neurosurgery
University of Utah Health Sciences Center
Salt Lake City, Utah

Theresa N. Grabo, PhD, APRN, BC, FNP
Graduate Program Director and Associate Professor
Decker School of Nursing
Binghamton University
Binghamton, New York;
Women's Healthcare Nurse Practioner
Valley Gyn Specialist
Luzern, Pennsylvania

Eric Grajkowski, DO
Family Medicine Resident
Department of Family Medicine
University of Nebraska Medical Center
Omaha, Nebraska

Heath A. Grames, PhD
Assistant Professor
Department of Family Medicine
University of Nebraska Medical Center
Omaha, Nebraska

Ellen Greenblatt, MD
Assistant Professor
Department of Obstetrics and Gynecology
University of Toronto
Clinical Director, Reproductive Biology and IVF Unit
Department of Obstetrics and Gynecology
Mount Sinai Hospital
Toronto, Ontario, Canada

Ronald A. Greenfield, MD
Professor of Medicine and Chief
Infectious Diseases Section
Department of Medicine
University of Oklahoma Health Sciences Center
Oklahoma City, Oklahoma

Samuel N. Grief, MD
Assistant Professor
Department of Family Medicine
University of Illinois at Chicago;
Assistant Professor Department of Family Medicine
University of Illinois Hospital
Chicago, Illinois

Pamela Lynn Grimaldi, DO
Assistant Professor
Department of Family Medicine and Community Health
University of Massachusetts Medical School;
Medical Staff
Department of Family Medicine
University of Massachusetts Memorial Hospital
Worcester, Massachusetts

Jill A. Grimes, MD
Clinical Instructor
University of Massachusetts Medical School
Worcester, Massachusetts;
University of Texas Health Services
Austin, Texas

Emily H. Groom, MD
Emergency Medicine Intern
Department of Emergency Medicine
University of Massachusetts
Worcester, Massachusetts

Rebecca Musher Gross, MD
Clinical Assistant Professor
Department of Family Medicine
Georgetown University Medical Center
Washington, D.C

John Guisto, MD
Associate Professor
Department of Emrgency Medicine
University of Arizona College of Medicine;
Medical Director
Department of Emergency Medicine
Arizona Health Sciences Center
Tucson, Arizona

Lisa S. Gussak, MD
Assistant Professor
Department of Family and Community Medicine
University of Massachusetts;
Attending Physician
Department of Family and Community Medicine
University of Massachusetts Memorial Hospital
Worcester, Massachusetts

Sarah Guzofski, MD
Resident
Department of Psychiatry
University of Massachusetts
Worcester, Massachusetts

Vladimir Hachinski, MD, DSc
Professor and Chair
Department of Clinical Neurological Sciences
The University of Western Ontario
London, Ontario, Canada

Diane M. Haleem, PhD, RN
Assistant Professor
Department of Nursing
East Stroudsburg University
East Stroudsburg, Pennsylvania

David E. Hall, MD
Clinical Associate Professor of Pediatrics
Emory University School of Medicine
Children's Healthcare of Atlanta at Scottish Rite
Atlanta, Georga

Wylie Hall, MD
Assistant Professor
Department of Neurology and Surgery
University of Massachusetts;
Director
Neurosciences Critical Care
University of Massachusetts Medical Center
Worcester, Massachusetts

Brian H. Halstater, MD
Assistant Clinical Professor
Program Director, Family Medicine Residency Program
Department of Community and Family Medicine
Duke University;
Attending Staff
Department of Community and Family Medicine
Duke University Hospital
Durham, North Carolina

Geoffrey R. Hamilton, MD
Clinical Assistant Professor
General Internal Medicine
Brown University
Providence, Rhode Island

John P. Haran, MD
University of Massachusetts Medical School
Worcester, Massachusetts

Adam J. Harner, MD
Resident
Department of Orthopaedics
University of Massachusetts Memorial Medical Center
Worcester, Massachusetts

Theodore R. Hartenstein, MD
Resident
Department of Medicine and Pediatrics
Baystate Medical Center
Springfield, Massachusetts

Syed Hasan, MD
University of Rochester Medical Center
Cardiology
Clinical Instructor
Strong Memorial Hospital
Rochester, New York

Brett Hassan, MD
Resident
University of Massachusetts School of
Medicine;
University of Massachusetts Memorial
Hospital
Worcester, Massachusetts

Fern R. Hauck, MD, MS
Associate Professor
Family Medicine and Public Health
Sciences
University of Virginia
Charlottesville, Virginia

Beverly N. Hay, MD
Assistant Professor of Pediatrics
Department of Pediatrics
University of Massachusetts Medical
School;
Chief, Division of Genetics
Department of Pediatrics
University of Massachusetts Memorial
Health Care
Worcester, Massachusetts

Julie A. Hayner, MD
University of Massachusetts
Worcester, Massachusetts

Rajneesh S. Hazarika, MD, MS
Resident
University of Massachusetts Medical
School
University of Massachusetts Fitchburg
Family Practice;
University of Massachusetts Fitchburg
Residency Program
Fitchburg, Massachusetts

Cathryn B. Heath, MD
Clinical Associate Professor
Department of Family Medicine
UMDNJ Robert Wood Johnson Medical
School
New Brunswick, New Jersey

Darell E. Heiselman, DO
Professor
Department of Internal Medicine
Northeastern Ohio Universities College of
Medicine
Rootstown, Ohio;
Critical Care Medicine
Department of Internal Medicine
Cuyahoga Falls General
Cuyahoga Falls, Ohio

Debra Heitman, MD
Assistant Professor
Division Chief, Undergraduate Education
Department of Emergency Medicine
University of Massachusetts Memorial
Medical Center
Worcester, Massachusetts

Thomas W. Hejkal, MD, PhD
Associate Professor
Department of Ophthalmology
University of Nebraska Medical Center
Omaha, Nebraska

David D. Henderson, MD
Assistant Professor
Department of Family Medicine
University of Connecticut School of
Medicine
Farmington, Connecticut;
Attending Physician
Department of Family Medicine
St. Francis Hospital
Hartford, Connecticut

Patrick C. Henderson, MD
Resident Physician
Department of Orthopaedic Surgery
University of Arizona
Tucson, Arizona

Scott T. Henderson, MD
Clinical Associate Professor
Department of Family Medicine
Carver College of Medicine, University of
Iowa;
Program Director
Mercy Family Medicine Residency
Mercy Medical Center-North Iowa
Mason City, Iowa

Pablo Hernandez, MD
Clinical Assistant Professor
Family Medicine and Community Health
University of Massachusetts Medical
School
Worcester, Massachusetts

Matthew P. Hill, MD
Clinical Fellow
Department of Internal Medicine
Harvard Medical School;
Resident
Department of Internal Medicine
Beth Israel Deaconess Medical Center
Boston, Massachusetts

Michael P. Hirsh, MD, FACS, FAAP
Professor
Department of Surgery and Pediatrics
University of Massachusetts Medical
School;
Chief
Divisions of Pediatric Surgery and
Trauma
Department of Surgery
University of Massachusetts Memorial
Health Center
Worcester, Massachusetts

Mary A. Hohenhaus, MD
Clinical Instructor
Department of Medicine
Brown University;
Internist
Department of Medicine
The Miriam Hospital
Providence, Rhode Island

David M. Holmes, MD
Clinical Assistant Professor
Department of Family Medicine
State University of New York at Buffalo;
Associate Vice Chair of Medical Student
Education
Department of Family Medicine
State University of New York at Buffalo
Buffalo, New York

Michael P. Hopkins, MD, MEd
Professor and Chair
Northeastern Ohio University College of
Medicine
Department of Obstetrics and
Gynecology
Rootstown, Ohio;
Director
Department of Obstetrics and
Gynecology
Aultman Health Foundation
Canton, Ohio

Mark C. Horattas, MD, FACS
Professor of Surgery
Department of Surgery
Northeastern Ohio Universities College of
Medicine
Rootstown, Ohio;
Professor of Surgery
Department of Surgery
Akron General Medical Center
Akron, Ohio

Felix Horng, MD, MBA
Assistant Clinical Professor
Department of Family Medicine
David Geffen School of Medicine at
    UCLA;
Assistant Clinical Professor
Department of Pediatrics and Family
    Medicine
Keck School of Medicine of USC
Los Angeles, California

Peter L. Hoth, MD
Sports Medicine Fellow
Department of Family Medicine
University of Massachusetts Medical
    School
Fitchburg, Massachusetts;
Sports Medicine Fellow
Family Medicine and Community Health
University of Massachusetts Memorial
    Hospital
Worcester, Massachusetts

Hans House, MD
Assistant Professor
Department of Emergency Medicine
University of Iowa;
Program Director
Department of Emergency Medicine
University of Iowa Hospitals and
    Clinics
Iowa City, Iowa

Jay U. Howington, MD
Assistant Professor of Surgery
Department of Surgery
Mercer University School of Medicine
Savannah, Georgia;
Stroke Director
Department of Neurosurgery
Memorial Health University Medical
    Center
Savannah, Georgia

Dennis E. Hughes, DO
Clinical Associate Professor
Department of Family and Community
    Medicine
University of Missouri School of Medicine
Columbia, Missouri;
Medical Director
Emergency Services
Coxhealth
Springfield, Missouri

Douglas Hunt, MD
University of Massachusetts Medical
    School
Worcester, Massachusetts

Ahntuan T. Huynh, DO
Resident Physician
Department of Obstetrics and Gynecology
Akron General Medical Center
Akron, Ohio

Robert Hyde, MD, MA, EMT-P
Resident
Department of Emergency Medicine
Mayo School of Graduate Medical
    Education
Rochester, Minnesota

Vivek Jain, MD
Department of Neurology
The Permanente Medical Group
Kaiser Permanente—Northern California
San Jose, California

Summer L. James, MD
Resident Physician
Department of Obstetrics and Gynecology
Akron General Medical Center
Akron, Ohio

Jamal Camilo Janania, MD
Resident
Family Medicine and Community Health
University of Massachusetts Medical
    School
Worcester, Massachusetts;
University of Massachusetts Fitchburg
    Family Practice Residency Program
Fitchburg, Massachusetts

Thomas Jaquith-Houston, MD
Resident
Family Medicine and Community Health
University of Massachusetts Medical
    School
Worcester, Massachusetts;
University of Massachusetts Fitchburg
    Family Practice Residency Program
Fitchburg, Massachusetts

Courtney Jarvis, PharmD
Assistant Professor of Pharmacy Practice
Massachusetts College of Pharmacy
Cllinical Assistant Professor of Family
    Medicine
University of Massachusetts Medical
    School
Worcester, Massachusetts;
Clinical Pharmacist
Department of Family Medicine and
    Community Health
University of Massachusetts Memorial
    Center
Worcester, Massachusetts

Carrie A. Jaworski, MD
Assistant Director
Resurrection Family Practice Residency
Resurrection Medical Center
Chicago, Illinois

Shannon B. Jenkins, MD
Assistant Professor
University Massachusetts Memorial
    Medical School

Eric L. Jenison, MD
Professor
Department of Obstetrics and Gynecology
Northeastern Ohio Universities College of
    Medicine
Rootstown, Ohio;
Chairman and Program Director
Department of Obstetrics and Gynecology
Akron General Medical Center
Akron, Ohio

Krista Johansen, MD
Resident
Department of Pathology
University of Massachusetts;
Resident
Department of Pathology
University of Massachusetts Memorial
    Healthcare
Worcester, Massachusetts

Ryan Johnson, MD
Resident
Department of Pediatrics
The University of Arizona
Tucson, Arizona

Marc Jeffrey Kahn, MD
Professor and Associate Dean
Department of Medicine
Tulane University School of Medicine
New Orleans, Louisiana

Daphne Karel, MD
Associate Professor
Department of Family Medicine
Greenwood Family Medicine Residency
    Program
Greenwood, South Carolina

Kristy Kedian, DO
Associate Professor
Family Medicine
University of Massachusetts Medical
    School;
Faculty
Department of Family Medicine
University of Massachusetts Memorial
    Hospital
Worcester, Massachusetts

Drew M. Keister, MD
Assistant Professor
Department of Family Medicine
University of Nebraska;
Associate Program Director
Family Medicine Residency
55th Medical Group
Offutt Air Force Base, Nebraska

Rick Kellerman, MD
Professor and Chair
Department of Family and Community
  Medicine
University of Kansas School of
  Medicine-Wichita
Wichita, Kansas

Bevin Kenney, MD
Intern
Department of Medicine
Brown University
Providence, Rhode Island

Robert M. Kershner, MD
President and CEO
Eye Laser Consulting
Boston, Massachusetts;
Clinical Professor of Ophthalmology
University of Utah Medical Center
Salt Lake City, Utah

Marc Jeffrey Khan, MD
Associate Dean for Student Affairs
Professor of Medicine
Section of Hematology and Medical
  Oncology
Tulane University Health Sciences Center
School of Medicine
New Orleans, Louisiana

Omar A. Khan, MD, MHS
Assistant Professor
Department of Family Medicine
University of Vermont
Burlington, Vermont;
Attending Physician
Department of Family Medicine
Christiana Care Health System
Wilmington, Delaware

George E. Kikano, MD
Chairman and Professor
Department of Family Medicine
Case Western Reserve University
University Hospitals of Cleveland
Cleveland, Ohio

Heather C. Killie, MD
Resident
Department of Orthopedic Surgery
University of Massachusetts Medical
  Center
Worcester, Massachusetts

Jane S. Kim, MD
Assistant Clinical Professor
Department of Medicine
University of Colorado
Denver, Colorado

Sam Kim, MD, MBBS, MedSc
Medical Student
Faculty of Medicine
University of New South Wales
Sydney, Australia

Mitchell S. King, MD
Associate Professor
Department of Family Medicine
Northwestern University Medical School
Northbrook, Illinois

Scott Kinkade, MD, MSPH
Assistant Professor
Department of Family and Community
  Medicine
University of Texas Southwestern Medical
  Center at Dallas Southwestern Medical
  School
Dallas, Texas

Cecilia M. Kipnis, MD
Intern
Department of Family Medicine
Naval Hospital Camp Pendleton
Camp Pendleton, California

Jeffrey T. Kirchner, DO
Clinical Associate Professor
Department of Family and Community
  Medicine
Temple University
Philadelphia, Pennsylvania;
Associate Director, Family Medicine
  Residency Program
Department of Family and Community
  Medicine
Lancaster General Hospital
Lancaster, Pennsylvania

Suzanne Klainer, MD
Resident
Department of Anesthesiology
Harvard University Medical School
Worcester, Massachusetts

Malgotzata Klonowska, MD
Chief Resident
Department of Neurology
University of Massachusetts Medical
  School
Worcester, Massachusetts

Aubrey L. Knight, MD
Professor
Department of Geriatric Medicine
The Virginia College of Osteopathic
  Medicine
Blacksburg, Virginia;
Vice President, Medical Affairs
The Hebrew Home of Greater Washington
Rockville, Maryland

Anjali Koka, MD
University of Massachusetts Medical
  School
Worcester, Massachusetts

Gargeyi Kommareddy, MD
Hospitalist, Auxillary Faculty Grant Family
  Practice Program
Grant Medical Center Medical Education
  Department
Grant Medical Center
Columbus, Ohio

Anya S. Koutras, MD
Assistant Professor
Department of Family Medicine
University of Vermont;
Family Medicine Attending
Department of Family Medicine
Fletcher Allen Health Care
University of Vermont
Burlington, Vermont

Peter Kozisek, MD
Family Medicine Residency of Idaho
Boise, Idaho

Jeffrey B. Kreher, MD
Primary Care Sports Medicine Fellow
Department of Family Medicine
Boston Medical Center
Boston University
Boston, Massachusetts

Nancy T. Kubiak, MD
Associate Professor
Internal Medicine
University of Louisville
Louisville, Kentucky

Dylan C. Kwait, MD
University of Massachusetts Medical
  School
Worcester, Massachusetts

Christ G. Kyriakedes, DO
Associate Professor of Clinical
  Emergency Medicine
Department of Emergency Medicine
Northeastern Ohio Universities College of
  Medicine
Rootstown, Ohio;
Residency Director
Department of Emergency Medicine
Akron General Medical Center
Akron, Ohio

Lars C. Larsen, MD
Professor
Department of Family Medicine
The Brody School of Medicine at East
  Carolina University
Greenville, North Carolina

Richard A. Larson, MD
Professor
Department of Medicine, Section of
  Hematology/Oncology
The University of Chicago
Chicago, Illinois

Margo Lauterbach, MD
Department of Psychiatry
University of Massachusetts Medical
  School
Worcester, Massachusetts

Jeanette Lavasta, MD
Resident
University of Massachusetts Medical
  School
University of Massachusetts Fitchburg
  Family Practice
Fitchburg, Massachusetts

Nicole R. Leboeuf, MD
University of Massachusetts Medical
  School
Worcester, Massachusetts

Cindy L. Lee, MD
Keck School of Medicine of USC
Los Angeles, California

Daniel J. Lee, MD
Chief, Otology and Neurotology
Assistant Professor
Department of Otolaryngology
University of Massachusetts Medical
  School
Worcester, Massachusetts

Daniel T. Lee, MD, MA
Associate Clinical Professor
Department of Family Medicine
David Geffen School of Medicine at UCLA
Los Angeles, California;
Staff Attending
Department of Family Practice
Santa Monica–UCLA Medical Center
Santa Monica, California

Monica Lee, MD
University of Massachusetts Medical
  School
Worcester, Massachusetts

Mark C. Leeson, MD, FACS
Professor
Department of Orthopedic Surgery
Northeastern Ohio Universities College of
  Medicine
Akron, Ohio

Matthew R. Leibowitz, MD
Assistant Clinical Professor
Division of Infectious Diseases
David Geffen School of Medicine at
  UCLA;
Attending Physician
Department of Medicine
UCLA Medical Center
Los Angeles, California

Karin S. Leschly, MD
Clinical Instructor
Department of Family Medicine
Boston Medical Center
Boston, Massachusetts

Richard P. Levy, MD
Adjunct Professor of Medicine
Department of Medicine
Dartmouth Medical School
Hanover, New Hampshire

James H. Lewis, MD
Professor of Medicine
Division of Gastroenterology
Georgetown University Medical Center
Washington, D.C.

Mian Li, MD, PhD
Assistant Professor
Department of Neurology
Georgetown University School of
  Medicine
Washington, D.C.

Peter Libby, MD
Mallinckrodt Professor of Medicine
Harvard Medical School
Chief, Cardiovascular Medicine
Department of Medicine
Brigham and Women's Hospital
Boston, Massachusetts

Leonard S. Lilly, MD
Associate Professor of Medicine
Harvard Medical School
Brigham and Women's Hospital
Boston, Massachusetts

Edward Liu, MD
Clinical Instructor of Medicine
Department of Internal Medicine
University of Medicine and Dentistry New
  Jersey
Robert Wood Johnson Medical School
New Brunswick, New Jersey;
Clinical Instructor
Department of Medicine
Division of Infectious Diseases
Jersey Shore University Medical Center
Neptune, New Jersey

Kimberly E. Liu, MD
Fellow, Reproductive Endocrinology and
  Infertility
Department of Obstetrics and Gynecology
University of Toronto
Toronto, Ontario, Canada

Nancy Liu, MD
Otolaryngology
Boca Raton, Florida

Philip P. Lobstein, MD
Private Practice
Cardiology
Fort Worth, Texas

Ana Vera Lopes, MD
Resident
University of Massachusetts Medical
  School
University of Massachusetts Fitchburg
  Family Practice Residency Program
Fitchburg, Massachusetts

Zhen Lu, MD
Chief Resident
Department of Family Medicine
University of Massachusetts Medical
  School
Worcester, Massachusetts

Rebecca S. Lundquist, MD
Assistant Professor
Department of Psychiatry
University of Massachusetts Medical
  School
Staff Psychiatrist
Department of Psychiatry
University of Massachusetts Medical
  Center
Worcester, Massachusetts

Christopher J. Lutrzykowski, MD
University of Massachusetts Fellow of
   Sports Medicine
Worcester, Massachusetts

Brock D. Lutz, MD
East Texas Infectious Disease
   Consultants
Tyler, Texas

Ann M. Lynch, PharmD, RPh
Assistant Professor of Pharmacy Practice
Massachusetts College of Pharmacy and
   Health Sciences
Worcester, Massachusetts

Paul Lyons, MD
Associate Professor
Associate Chair for Clinical Education
Department of Family and Community
   Medicine
Temple University School of Medicine
Philadelphia, Pennsylvania

Linda J. Machado, MD
Associate Professor
Department of Internal
   Medicine/Infectious Diseases
University of Oklahoma Health Sciences
   Center
Oklahoma City, Oklahoma

**D. W. MacPherson, MD, MSc (CTM),
   FRCPC**
Associate Professor
Department of Pathology and Molecular
   Medicine
McMaster University
Hamilton, Ontario, Canada

Jill D. Mahoney, MD
Family Practice Resident
Department of Family Medicine
University of Massachusetts Memorial
   Hospital
Worcester, Massachusetts

Jeffrey Mailhot, MD
Internal Medicine/Pediatrics Resident
Maine Medical Center
Portland, Maine

Barbara A. Majeroni, MD
Associate Professor of Clinical Family
   Medicine
Department of Family Medicine
State University of New York at Buffalo;
Attending Physician
Department of Family Medicine
Erie County Medical Center
Buffalo, New York

Samir Malkani, MD
Assistant Professor
Endocrinology
University of Massachusetts Medical
   School
Worcester, Massachusetts

Ronald L. Malm, DO
Assistant Professor
University of Wyoming;
Family Practice Residency Program
Cheyenne, Wyoming

Joshua M. V. Mammen, MD
Chief Resident
Department of Surgery
University of Cincinnati
Cincinnati, Ohio

Christopher S. Manasseh, MD
Associate Professor
Department of Family Medicine
Boston University School of Medicine;
Co-Director, Clinical Services
Department of Family Medicine
Boston University Medical Center
Boston, Massachusetts

Lee A. Mancini, MD, CSCS, CSN
Assistant Professor
Department of Family Practice
University of Massachusetts Medical
   School;
Family Practice Hospitalist, Sports
   Medicine Physician
Department of Family Practice
University of Massachusetts Medical
   Center
Worcester, Massachusetts

Atizazul Hassan Mansoor, MD
Resident
Department of Medicine
Boston University
Providence, Rhode Island

Geoffrey M. Margo, MD, PhD
Clinical Associate Professor
Department of Psychiatry
University of Pennsylvania Health System;
Director, Consultation/Liaison Psychiatry
Department of Psychiatry
Pennsylvania Hospital
Philadelphia, Pennsylvania

Katherine L. Margo, MD
Assistant Professor
Department of Family Medicine and
   Community Health
University of Pennsylvania School of
   Medicine;
Attending Physician
Department of Family Medicine and
   Community Health
Presbyterian Hospital
Philadelphia, Pennsylvania

Kathy Mariani, MD
Assistant Professor
Department of Family Medicine and
   Community Medicine
University of Massachusetts Medical
   School
Worcester, Massachusetts

Robert A. Marlow, MD, MA
Associate Professor of Clinical Family and
   Community Medicine
Department of Family and Community
   Medicine
University of Arizona
Tucson, Arizona;
Associate Director
Family Medicine Residency Program
Scottsdale Healthcare
Scottsdale, Arizona

Stephen A. Marin, MD, EdM
Instructor/Department of Family Medicine
   and Community Health
University of Massachusetts Medical
   School
Worcester, Massachusetts;
Staff Physician
Desmond Callan Community Health
   Center
Turners Falls, Massachusetts

Michael D. Mason, MD
Assistant Professor
University of Maine
Orono, Maine

Donnah Mathews, MD
Attending Physician
Rhode Island Hospital
Providence, Rhode Island

A. Raquel Matteo-Bibeau, MD
Infectious Disease Physician
Department of Medicine
St. Mary's Medical Center
Good Samaritan Medical Center
Columbia Hospital
West Palm Beach, Florida

Michele Matthews, PharmD
Assistant Professor of Pharmacy Practice
Massachusetts College of Pharmacy and
  Health Sciences;
Clinical Pharmacist
Department of Family Medicine
Hahnemann Family Health Center
Worcester, Massachusetts

Jennifer McCaul, MD
Assistant Professor
Department of Family Practice
St. Joseph's Hospital Family Practice
  Residency
Syracuse, New York

Timothy R. McCurry, MD
Clinical Assistant Professor
Department of Family Medicine
Stritch School of Medicine
Loyola University;
Program Director
Family Medicine Residency
Resurrection Medical Center
Chicago, Ilinois

K. Patricia McGann, MD
Palo Alto Medical Foundation
Associate Professor of Clinical Medicine
Stanford University School of Medicine
Los Altos, California

William T. McGee, MD, MHA
Assistant Professor of Medicine and
  Surgery
Tufts University School of Medicine
Boston, Massachusetts;
Intensivist
Critical Care Medicine
Baystate Medical Center
Springfield, Massachusetts

Brigid Barry McKenna, MD
Resident
Department of Internal Medicine and
  Pediatrics
University of Massachusetts Memorial
  Medical Center
Worcester, Massachusetts

Martha H. McLoughlin, MD
Resident
Department of Family Medicine
University of Massachusetts Memorial
  Medical Center
Worcester, Massachusetts

Erika McPhee, MD
University of Massachusetts Medical
  School
Worcester, Massachusetts

James T. McPhee, MD
University of Massachusetts Medical
  School
Worcester, Massachusetts

Bernadette Meade, MD
Geriatric Medicine and Internal Medicine
University of Massachusets Memorial
  Medical Center
Worcester, Massachusetts

Keith Medeiros, MD
Department of Internal Medicine
University of Massachusetts Medical
  School
Worcester, Massachusetts

Gary Mendese, MD
University of Massachusetts Memorial
  Medical Center
Worcester, Massachusetts

Frederico Milla, MD
Resident
Department of Surgery
University of Massachusetts Memorial
  Medical Center
Worcester, Massachusetts

Eric S. Miller, MD
Clinical Associate Professor
Department of Family Medicine
University of Pittsburgh School of
  Medicine;
Director
Family Practice Residency
Obstetrics and Gynecology Program
Pittsburgh, Pennsylvania

James P. Miller, MD
Medical Director
Department of Pediatric Surgery
Cook Children's Medical Center
Fort Worth, Texas

Katrina Miller, MD
Medical Director
Primary Care Physician Assistant Program
University of Southern California
Keck School of Medicine
Alhambra, California;
Visiting Assistant Professor
Department of Family Medicine
University of Southern California
Keck School of Medicine
Los Angeles, California

Nicholas Miller, MD
Resident
Department of Emergency Medicine
University of Connecticut
Hartford, Connecticut

Sandra Miller, MD
Clinical Assistant Professor
Department of Family and Community
  Medicine
University of Arizona;
Assistant Director
Family Medicine Residency
Banner Good Samaritan Medical Center
Phoenix, Arizona

Larry Millikan, MD
Professor and Chair Emeritus
Department of Dermatology
Tulane School of Medicine
New Orleans, Louisiana;
Professor and Chair Emeritus
Department of Dermatology
VA Biloxi
Biloxi, Mississippi

Jeffrey F. Minteer, MD
Associate Director
Family Practice Residency Program
The Washington Hospital
Washington, Pennsylvania

Reza Moattari, MD
Professor of Medicine
Head, Endocrinology Division
Northeastern Ohio Universities College of
  Medicine;
Chief
Endocrinology Section
Akron General Hospital
Akron, Ohio

Susan Louisa Montauk, MD
Professor
Department of Family Medicine
University of Cincinnati College of
  Medicine;
Medical Director
The Affinity Center
Cincinnati, Ohio

Phyllis Montellese, MD
Clinical Associate Professor
Department of Family Medicine
University of Pittsburgh;
Faculty
Department of Family Medicine Residency
  and Sports Medicine Fellowship
University of Pittsburgh Medical
  Center-Shadyside
Pittsburgh, Pennsylvania

T. Glendon Moody, MD
Clinical Lecturer
Department of Ophthalmology
University of Arizona College of
  Medicine-Tucson
Tempe, Arizona

Brian D. Moquin, MD
Gastrointestinal Fellow
University of Massachusetts Medical
    School;
Worcester, Massachusetts

Anna Morin, PharmD
Assistant Professor
Pharmacy Practice
Massachusetts College of Pharmacy and
    Health Sciences
Worcester, Massachusetts;
Clinical Pharmacist
Pharmacy
Westborough State Hospital
Westborough, Massachusetts

Frank Moskos, MD
Family Medicine Resident
Department of Family Medicine
Grant Medical Center
Columbus, Ohio

Herbert L. Muncie, Jr., MD
Professor
Department of Family Medicine
Louisiana State University;
Director, Predoctoral Education
Department of Family Medicine
Louisiana State University Health
    Sciences Center
New Orleans, Louisiana

Kerry J. Murphy, MD
Resident
Department of Medicine
Columbia University
New York, New York
Resident
Department of Medicine
New York Presbyterian Hospital
New York, New York

Mary E. Muscari, PhD, RN, CRNP, CS
Professor
Director of Forensic Health
University of Scranton
Scranton, Pennsylvania

Eleftherios Mylonakis, MD
Assistant Professor of Medicine
Harvard Medical School
Massachusetts General Hospital
Boston, Massachusetts

Smitha Nair, MD
Resident
University of Massachusetts Fitchburg
    Family Practice
University of Massachusetts Medical
    School;
University of Massachusetts Fitchburg
    Family Practice Residency Program
Fitchburg, Massachusetts

Leena Nathan, MD
Affiliate Residency Program of the David
    Geffen School of Medicine at UCLA
Resident Physician
Department of Family Medicine
Kaiser Permanente
Woodland Hills, California

Ramesh Nathan, MD
Assistant Clinical Professor
Department of Medicine
Division of Infectious Disease
David Geffen School of Medicine
University of California-Los Angeles
Los Angeles, California;
Staff Physician
Department of Medicine
Los Robles Hospital and Medical Center
Thousand Oaks, California

Zainab Nawab, MD
Family Medical Associates
Worcestor, Massachusetts

Donald A. F. Nelson, MD
Director of Medical Informatics
Family Practice Residency
Cedar Rapids Medical Education
    Foundation
Cedar Rapids, Iowa

Eric Nelson, MD
Resident
The Emory Clinic
Emory University School of Medicine
Atlanta, Georgia

Anne C. Nofziger, MD
Assistant Professor
Department of Family Medicine
University of Rochester School of
    Medicine
Rochester, New York

Nicole M. Nolan, PharmD
Assistant Professor
Department of Pharmacy Practice
Massachusetts College of Pharmacy and
    Health Sciences;
Clinical Pharmacist
VNA Care Network, Inc.
Worcester, Massachusetts

Laura L. Novak, MD
Department of Family Practice
Barberton Citizens Hospital
Barberton, Ohio

Cathryn B. Nowak, MD
Assistant Professor
Department of Pediatrics
University of Massachusetts Medical
    School
Worcester, Massachusetts;
Associate Physician in Chief
Department of Genetics
National Birth Defects Center
Waltham, Massachusetts

Kelly J. O'Callahan, MD
Instructor
Department of Medicine
University of Massachusetts Medical
    School;
Staff Physician
Department of Gastroenterology
University of Massachusetts Medical
    School
Worcester, Massachusetts

Jacqueline L. Olin, LS, PharmD, BCPS
Clinical Assistant Professor
Department of Pharmacy Practice and
    Administration
Ernest Mario School of Pharmacy at
    Rutgers University
Piscataway, New Jersey;
Clinical Coordinator
Department of Pharmacy
Hunterton Medical Center
Flemington, New Jersey

Douglas S. Parks, MD
Associate Professor
Family Practice Residency at Cheyenne
University of Wyoming;
Vice Chair
Department of Family Practice
United Medical Center
Cheyenne, Wyoming

Dhruv B. Pateder, MD
Chief Resident
Department of Orthopaedic Surgery
Johns Hopkins Hospital
Baltimore, Maryland

Matthew A. Pecci, MD
Assistant Clinical Professor
Department of Family Medicine
Boston Medical Center
Boston, Massachusetts

Liberto Pechet, MD
Professor Emeritus
Pathology and Medicine
University of Massachusetts Medical
  School;
Director, Hematology Labs
Hospital Laboratories
University of Massachusetts Medical
  Center
Worcester, Massachusetts

Ligia Peralta, MD
Associate Professor
Pediatrics
University of Maryland Medical Center
Chief of Adolescent and Adult Medicine
Director of Adolescent HIV Program
Baltimore, Maryland

Ruben Peralta, MD, FACS
Attending Surgeon
Department of Surgery
University of Massachusetts
Worcester, Massachusetts

Michael D. Perloff, MD, PhD
Resident
Department of Neurology
Boston Medical Center
Boston, Massachusetts

John R. Person, MD
Associate Clinical Professor
Department of Medicine/Section of
  Dermatology
University of Massachusetts Medical
  School;
Staff
Department of Medicine/Section of
  Dermatology
St. Vincent Hospital at Worcester Medical
  Center
Worcester, Massachusetts

Bobby Peters, MD, FAAEM
Assistant Professor
Department of Emergency Medicine
University of Iowa;
Assistant Clinical Professor
Department of Emergency Medicine
University of Iowa
Iowa City, Iowa

Brian D. Petroni, MD
University of Massachusetts Medical
  School
Worcester, Massachusetts

Nicole D. Pilevsky, MD
Private Practice
Obstetrics and Gynecology
Howard County General Hospital
Columbia, Maryland

Venu G. Pillarisetty, MD
Resident
Department of Surgery
University of Massachusetts;
Resident
University of Massachusetts Medical
  Center
Worcester, Massachusetts

Matthew J. Plante, MD
Assistant Clinical Instructor
Department of Orthopaedic Surgery
Brown Medical School;
Chief Resident
Department of Orthopaedic Surgery
Rhode Island Hospital
Providence, Rhode Island

Gregory A. Poland, MD
Professor
Department of Internal Medicine
Mayo Vaccine Research Group
The Mayo Clinic and Foundation
Rochester, Minnisota

David A. Pope, MD
Private Practice
Mayo Health System
Janesville, Minnesota

Stacy E. Potts, MD
Assistant Clinical Professor
Department of Family Medicine and
  Community Health
University of Massachusetts;
Family Physician
Department of Family Medicine and
  Community Health
University of Massachusetts Memorial
  Health Care
Worcester, Massachusetts

William A. Primack, MD
Clinical Professor of Medicine and
  Pediatrics
Department of Medicine
Division of Nephrology and Hypertension
University of North Carolina
Chapel Hill, North Carolina

Marlo W. Puleo II, MD
Hospitalist Auxillary Faculty Grant Family
  Practice Program
Grant Medical Center Medical Education
  Department
Grant Medical Center
Columbus, Ohio

Ronald E. Pust, MD
Professor and Director, Predoctoral
  Program
Department of Family and Community
  Medicine
University of Arizona College of Medicine
Tucson, Arizona

Jyoti Ramakrishna, MD
Assistant Professor
Department of Pediatrics, Division of
  Pediatric Gastroenterology
University of Massachusetts Medical
  School;
Acting Chief, Division of Pediatric
  Gastroenterology and Nutrition
Department of Pediatrics
University of Massachusetts Memorial
  Medical Center
Worcester, Massachusetts

Kiran V. Raman, MD
Resident
Department of Pediatrics
University of Rochester Medical Center;
Resident
Department of Pediatrics
Golisano Children's Hospital at Strong
Rochester, New York

J. Randall Richard, MD
Professor of Clinical Family Medicine
Northeastern Ohio Universities College of
  Medicine
Diector, Family Practice Residency
Barberton Citizens Hospital
Barberton, Ohio

Milisa Rizer, MD, MPH
Vice Chair for Clinical Affairs
Associate Professor of Clinical Family
  Medicine
Ohio State University Department of
  Family Medicine
Rardin Family Practice Center
Columbus, Ohio

Maya Roberts, BA
Medical Student
Yale University
New Haven, Connecticut

Duane C. Roe, MD
Professor
Department of Internal Medicine
Northeastern Ohio Universities College of
  Medicine
Rootstown, Ohio

Lewis C. Rose, MD
Coordinator of Procedural Training
Department of Family and Community
  Medicine
University of Texas Health Sciences
  Center at San Antonio
San Antonio, Texas

Montiel T. Rosenthal, MD
Assistant Clinical Professor
Director of Maternity Services
Department of Family Medicine
University of Cincinnati;
Medical Director-Prenatal Clinic
Department of Family Medicine
The Christ Hospital
Cincinnati, Ohio

Angie N. Ross, MD
Resident
Department of Internal Medicine
Emory University
Atlanta, Georgia

Bruce M. Rothschild, MD
Professor
Department of Medicine
Northeastern Universities College of
  Medicine
Rootstown, Ohio

Michael Rousse, MD, MPH
Corner Medical—Dartmouth Hitchcock
Lyndonville, Vermont

Marc G. Rucquoi, MD, FAAFP
Chocowinity Family Care
Chocowinity, North Carolina;
Attending Physician
Department of Family Medicine
Beaufort County Hospital
Washington, North Carolina

Christopher P. Ruisi, MD
Cardiology Fellow
Division of Cardiology
University of Massachusetts Medical
  Center
Worcester, Massachusetts

Laura J. Sacco, MD
Resident
Department of Obstetrics/Gynecology
Brown University;
Resident
Department of Obstetrics/Gynecology
Women and Infants Hospital
Providence, Rhode Island

Kia Saeian, MD
Associate Professor of Medicine
Department of Gastroenterology and
  Hepatology
Medical College of Wisconsin
Associate Professor fo Medicine
Department of Gastroenterology and
  Hepatology
Froedtert Memorial Lutheran Hospital
Milwaukee, Wisconsin

Richard F. Salmon, DO
Pediatric Hospitalist
Children's Healthcare of Atlanta
  at Scottish Rite
Atlanta, Georgia

Richard A. Samson, MD
Associate Professor
Department of Pediatrics
University of Arizona
Department of Pediatrics
Arizona Health Sciences Center
Tucson, Arizona

Arthur Sanders, MD
Professor
Department of Emergency Medicine
University of Arizona College of Medicine
Attending Physician
Department of Emergency Medicine
University Medical Center
Tucson, Arizona

John J. Santos, MD
Medical Student
University of Massachusetts Medical
  School
Worcester, Massachusetts

Benjamin L. Sapers, MD
Assistant Professor (Clinical)
Department of Medicine
Brown University;
Attending Physician
Department of General Internal Medicine
Rhode Island Hospital
Providence, Rhode Island

Wendy Satmary, MD, FACOG
Assistant Clinical Professor
Department of Obstetrics and Gynecology
University of California-Los Angeles
Los Angeles, California;
Physician
Department of Obstetrics and Gynecology
Kaiser Permanente
Woodland Hills, California

Jennifer L. Savitski, MD
Clinical Instructor
Department of Obstetrics and Gynecology
Northeastern Ohio University College of
  Medicine
Rootstown, Ohio;
Assistant Residency Program Director
Department of Obstetrics and Gynecology
Akron General Medical Center
Akron, Ohio

Karl M. Schmitt, MD
Assistant Director
Residency in Family Medicine
St. Elizabeth Hospital
Chairman
Department of Medicine
St. Elizabeth Medical Center
Edgewood, Kentucky

F. David Schneider, MD, MDPH
Associate Professor
Department of Family and Community
  Medicine
University of Texas Health Science
  Center of San Antonio
San Antonio, Texas

Michael T. Schnettler, MD
Resident
Department of Obstetrics and Gynecology
Aultman Hospital
Canton, Ohio

Jennifer L. Schott, MD
Instructor
Department of Pediatrics
University of Massachusetts Medical
  School;
Worcester, Massachusetts;
Pediatrician
Department of Pediatrics
Medical Associates Pediatrics
Leominster, Massachusetts

Lisa M. Schroeder, MD
Assistant Director
Barberton Family Practice Residency
  Program
Barberton, Ohio

Alexandra Schultes, MD
Associate Professor
Department of Family Practice
University of Massachusetts
Worcester, Massachusetts

Robert M. Schultz, MD
Medical Director
Prediatric Endocrine Associates, PC
Department of Endocrinology
Children's Hospital of Atlanta at Scottish
    Rite
Atlanta, Georgia

David P. Sealy, MD
Director, Sports Medicine
Clinical Professor and Director, Resident
    Education
Self Memorial Hospital Family Medicine
    Residency
Greenwood, South Carolina

W. Franklin Sease, Jr., MD
Steadman Hawkins Clinic of the Carolinas
Department of Orthopaedics
Greenville Hospital University Medical
    Center
Greenville, South Carolina

Sheila M. Seed, BS, Pharm, MPH, RPh
Assistant Professor
Department of Pharmacy Practice
Massachusetts College of Pharmacy and
    Health Sciences
Worcester, Massachusetts

Alexandra Sherman, BA
Medical Student
University of Massachusetts Medical
    School
Worcester, Massachusetts

Joseph Shrum, MD
Professor of Dermatology
Department of Dermatology
Tulane University Medical Center
New Orleans, Louisiana

Aamir Siddiqi, MD
Associate Director
St. Luke's Family Medicine Residency
Aurora Health Care;
Vice President Medical Staff
Aurora Sinai Medical Center
Milwaukee, Wisconsin

Hugh J. Silk, MD
Assistant Professor
Department of Family Medicine
University of Massachusetts Medical
    School;
Family Medicine Residency
Department of Family Medicine
Hahnemann Family Health Center
University of Massachusetts Memorial
    Medical Center
Worcester, Massachusetts

Gary J. Silko, MD, MS
Program Director
Family Medicine Residency
St. Vincent Health Center
Erie, Pennsylvania

Jason Silva, MD
Department of Orthopaedic Surgery
University of Massachusetts
Worcester, Massachusetts

Matthew Silva, PharmD, RPh, BCPS
Assistant Professor
Pharmacy Practice
Massachusetts College of Pharmacy and
    Health Sciences;
Consulting Pharmacist
Family Medicine
Family Health Center of Worcester
Worcester, Massachusetts

Manoj Singh, MD
Assistant Professor
Department of Family Medicine
University of Cincinnati
Attending Physician
Department of Family Medicine
The Christ Hospital
Cincinnati, Ohio

Taylor Sittler, MD
University of Massachusetts Medical
    School
Worcester, Massachusetts

W. Paul Slomiany, MD
Assistant Director
Family Practice Residency Program
Washington Hospital
Washington, Pennsylvania

Patrick Smallwood, MD
Assistant Professor of Psychiatry
Department of Psychiatry
University of Massachusetts Medical
    School;
Medical Director of Emergency/Mental
    Health and Consultation Liaison
    Psychiatry
Department of Psychiatry
University of Massachusetts Medical
    Center
Worcester, Massachusetts

Stanley G. Smith, MA, MB
Professor Emeritus
University of Western Ontario
Southwest Middlesex Health Centre
Mt. Brydges, Ontario, Canada

John C. Smulian, MD, MPH
Professor and Director
Division of Maternal Fetal Medicine
Department of Obstetrics, Gynecology,
    and Reproductive Sciences
UMDNJ Robert Wood Johnson Medical
    School
New Brunswick, New Jersey

Nancy Snapp, MD, MPH
Physician
International Community Health
Seattle, Washington

Veena Somani, MD
Resident
Family Medicine
Christiana Care Health System
Wilmington, Delaware

Weily Soong, MD
Alabama Allergy and Asthma Center
Birmington, Alabama

Jonathan M. Spector, MD
Assistant Professor
Department of Pediatrics
University of Massachusetts Medical
    Center;
Fellow in Neonatology
Department of Pediatrics
University of Massachusetts Medical
    Center
Worcester, Massachusetts

Nicholas J. Spirtos, DO
Associate Professor
Northeastern Ohio Universities College of
    Medicine;
Director
Northeastern Ohio Fertility Center
Northeastern Ohio Universities College of
    Medicine
Akron, Ohio

Joshua J. Spooner, PharmD, MS
Director
Clinical and Outcomes Services
Advanced Concepts Institute
University of the Sciences in Philadelphia
Philadelphia, Pennsylvania

Linda M. Spooner, PharmD, BCPS
Assistant Professor of Pharmacy Practice
Department of Pharmacy Practice
Massachusetts College of Pharmacy and
    Health Sciences-School of Pharmacy
Worcester, Massachusetts;
Clinical Pharmacy Specialist in Infectious
    Diseases
Department of Pharmacy
St. Vincent Hospital
Worcester, Massachusetts

Anirudh Sridharan, MD
Instructor
Department of General Internal Medicine
Johns Hopkins University School of
    Medicine Hospitalist
Department of Internal Medicine
Johns Hopkins Bayview Medical Center
Baltimore, Maryland

Mark Steenbergen, DO
Private Practice, Family Practice
Poughkeepsie, New York

Joseph R. Stenger, MD
Associate Professor
Department of Family Medicine and
    Community Health
University of Massachusetts Medical
    School
Worcester, Massachusetts;
Staff Physician
Department of Family Medicine
University of Massachusetts Memorial
    Health Care
Barre, Massachusetts

John Herbert Stevenson, MD
Assistant Professor
Department of Family Medicine
University of Massachusetts Medical
    School;
Director, Sports Medicine
Department of Family Medicine
University of Massachusetts Memorial
    Medical Center
Worcester, Massachusetts

Jeffrey Stovall,, MD
Assistant Professor
Department of Psychiatry and Family
    Medicine and Community Health
University of Massachusetts Medical
    School;
Director
Adult Outpatient Services
University of Massachusetts
Community Healthlink
Worcester, Massachusetts

Simone Stromer, MBBS
Associate Lecturer
Department of General Practice
University of Sydney
Sydney, Australia

David H. Stubbs, MD
The Iowa Clinic
Heart and Vascular Care
Iowa Methodist Medical Center
Des Moines, Iowa

Mark Su, MD
Clinical Instructor
Family Medicine
Tufts University School of Medicine
Boston, Massachusetts
Community Physician
Family Medicine
Anna Jaques Hospital
Newburyport, Massachusetts

Kim Subasick, MSN, RN
Professor
University of Scranton
Scranton, New York

Bhanu Sud, MD
Fellow Section of Infectious Diseases,
    Department of Medicine
University of Oklahoma Health Sciences
    Center
Oklahoma City, Oklahoma

Ryung Suh, MD, MPP, MBA, MPH
Professional Lecturer
Health Systems Administration
Georgetown University
Washington, D.C.;
Teaching Fellow and Resident
Department of Occupational and
    Environmental Medicine
Uniformed Services University of the
    Health Sciences
Bethesda, Maryland

Sandra Sulik, MD
Assistant Professor
Department of Family Medicine
St. Joseph's Family Practice Residency
    and Upstate Medical Center
Syracuse, New York

John F. Sullivan, MD
Resident
Department of Neuropsychiatry
University of Massachusetts Medical
    School;
Resident
Department of Neuropsychiatry
University of Massachusetts Memorial
    Medical Center
Worcester, Massachusetts

Karyn M. Sullivan, BSP, MPH, RPh
Assistant Professor of Pharmacy Practice
Massachusetts College of Pharmacy and
    Health Sciences
Worcester, Massachusetts;
Clinical Pharmacist
Department of Pharmacy
St. Vincent Hospital
Worcester, Massachusetts

Geoffrey R. Swain, MD, MPH
Associate Professor
Department of Family Medicine
University of Wisconsin School of
    Medicine and Public Health
Madison, Wisconsin;
Associate Medical Director
City of Milwaukee Health Department
Milwaukee, Wisconsin

E. James Swenson, MD
Assistant Professor, Primary Care Sports
    Medicine
Department of Orthopaedics
University of Rochester
Rochester, New York

Vassiliki Syriopoulou, MD
Professor of Pediatrics
First Department of Pediatrics
Athens University;
Chief of Infectious Disease
First Department of Pediatrics
Aghia Sophia Children's Hospital
Athens, Greece

Alfonso Tafur, MD
Resident
Internal Medicine
Mayo Clinic
Rochester, Minnesota

Sarah A. Tapyrik, MD
Department of Internal Medicine
Brown University;
Resident
Department of Internal Medicine
Rhode Island Hospital
Providence, Rhode Island

Poonam Thaker, MD
Family Medicine
Resurrection Family Practice
Chicago, Illinois

Margaret E. Thompson, MD
Associate Professor
Department of Family Practice
Michigan State University College of
    Human Medicine
East Lansing, Michigan

Rob Tiller, MD
Assistant Clinical Professor of Family
    Medicine
Family Practice Residency
Self Regional Healthcare
Montgomery Center for Family Medicine
University of South Carolina
Greenwood, South Carolina

William L. Toffler, MD
Professor
Department of Family Medicine
Oregon Health and Science University
Director of Predoctoral Education
Department of Family Medicine
Oregon Health and Science University
Portland, Oregon

Moshe S. Torem, MD, FAPA
Professor
Department of Psychiatry
Northeastern Ohio Universities College of
    Medicine
Medical Director
The Center for Mind-Body Medicine
Akron, Ohio

William A. Tosches, MD
Associate
Department of Neurology
University of Massachusetts Memorial
    Medical Center
Worcester, Massachusetts

Stephen E. Tosi, MD
Assistant Professor
Department of Surgery
University of Massachusetts Medical
    School;
Chief Medical Officer
University of Massachusetts Medical
    Center
Worcester, Massachusetts

Carol Lynn Touma, MD
Resident
Department of Internal Medicine
Brown University
Providence, Rhode Island

Tu-Mai Tran, MD, MSc
Faculty
Department of Family Medicine
Woodland Hills Kaiser Permanente Family
    Medicine Residency
Staff Physician
Department of Family Medicine
Kaiser Permanente
Woodland Hills, California

Nancy Tulathimutte, MD
House Staff
Department of Internal Medicine
University of Massachusetts Medical
    School
Worcester, Massachusetts

Michael Tutt, MD
Department of Internal Medicine
Fort Defiance Hospital
Fort Defiance, Arizona

Ana C. Tuya, MD
Assistant Professor
Division of Geriatrics
Brown University;
Attending Physician
Division of Geriatrics
Rhode Island Hospital
Providence, Rhode Island

Lawrence E. Udom, MD, MPH
Resident
Department of Family
    Medicine/Psychiatry
University of Cincinnati/Christ Hospital
Cincinnati, Ohio

Rohit Uppal, MD
Hospitalist
Department of Family Medicine
Grant Medical Center
Columbus, Ohio

Francisco G. Valencia, MD
Orthopaedic Surgeon
University of Orthopaedic Specialists
Tucson, Arizona

Michael M. Van Ness, MD
President
Gastroenterology Specialists, Inc.
Aultman Hospital
Canton, Ohio

Bruce T. Vanderhoff, MD
Clinical Associate Professor
Department of Family Medicine
Ohio State University;
Director of Medical Education
Grant Medical Center
Columbus, Ohio

Rimini Varghese, MD
House Officer
General Internal Medicine
Brown Medical School;
House Officer
General Internal Medicine
Rhode Island Hospital
Providence, Rhode Island

Rajiv R. Varma, MD
Associate Professor of Medicine
Department of Gastroenterology and
    Hepatology
Medical College of Wisconsin
Froedtert Memorial Lutheran Hospital
Milwaukee, Wisconsin

L. Cassandra Vawter, MD
Resident
Department of Psychiatry
University of Massachusetts Medical
    School
Worcester, Massachusetts

Brian P. Vickery, MD
Postdoctoral Fellow
Section of Allergy and Clinical
    Immunology
Yale University
New Haven, Connecticut

Richard Viken, MD
Professor
Department of Family Medicine
University of Texas Health Center at Tyler;
Chair
Department of Family Medicine
University of Texas Health Center at Tyler
Tyler, Texas

Kenton I. Voorhees, MD, FAAFP
Assistant Professor
Department of Family Medicine
University of Colorado
Littleton, Colorado;
Program Director
Swedish Family Medicine Residency
Swedish Medical Center
Englewood, Colorado

Kimberle Vore, MD
Clinical Assistant Professor of Family
    Medicine
Department of Family Medicine
University of Pittsburgh
Pittsburgh, Pennsylvania;
Clinical Instructor
Department of Family Medicine
The Washington Hospital
Washington, Pennsylvania

Anne Walsh, PA-C, MMSc
Clinical Instructor
Department of Family Medicine
Keck School of Medicine of USC
Los Angeles, California;
Physician Assistant
Department of
    Gastroenterology/Hepatology
Hertz and Associates in Gastroenterology
Los Alamitos, California

Amy Y. Wang, MD
Family Medicine
Chicago, Illinois

Sarita S. Warrier, MD
Resident Physician
Internal Medicine
Brown University
Providence, Rhode Island

Mitzi Wasik, PharmD, BCPS
Clinical Assistant Professor
College of Pharmacy
University of Illinois-Chicago;
Department of Family Medicine
University Medical Center
Chicago, Illinois

Donald E. Watenpaugh, PhD
Adjunct Professor
Department of Integrative Physiology
University of North Texas Health Science;
Director
Sleep Consultants, Inc.
Fort Worth, Texas

Aaron W. Way, DO
Resident
University of Massachusetts Medical
 School
University of Massachusetts Fitchburg
 Family Practice
Fitchburg, Massachusetts

Ramothea L. Webster, PhD
University of Massachusetts Medical
 School
Worcester, Massachusetts

Kurt J. Wegner, MD
Professor of Pediatrics
Neonatologist, Geneticist, and Pediatric
 Consultant
Northeastern Ohio Universities College of
 Medicine
Tod Children's Hospital
Youngstown, Ohio

Cheryl A. Wehler, MD
University of Massachusetts Medical
 School
University of Massachusetts Memorial
 Health Center
Worcester, Massachusetts

Martin E. Weinand, MD
Professor of Surgery
Division of Neurosurgery
University of Arizona College of Medicine
Tucson, Arizona

Barry D. Weiss, MD
Professor
Department of Family and Community
 Medicine
University of Arizona College of Medicine
Tucson, Arizona

Brett White, MD
Assistant Professor
Department of Family Medicine
University of Southern California;
Medical Director
Family Medicine
University of Southern California
Los Angeles, California

Christopher White, MD, JD
Clinical Instructor
Psychiatry and Family Medicine
University of Cincinnati;
Combined Resident
Psychiatry and Family Medicine
University of Cincinnati
Cincinnati, Ohio

Michelle Whitehurst-Cook, MD
Associate Professor
Department of Family Medicine
Virginia Commonwealth University
Richmond, Virginia

Alan L. Williams, MD
Adjunct Professor of Family Medicine
Department of Family Medicine
Uniformed Services University of the
 Health Sciences
Bethesda, Maryland

Pamela Williams, MD
Assistant Professor of Family Medicine
Department of Family Medicine
Uniformed Services University of the
 Health Sciences
Family Physician
University Family Health Center
Bethesda, Maryland

Christopher M. Wise, MD
W. Robert Irby Professor
Department of Internal
 Medicine-Rheumatology, Allergy and
 Immunology
Virginia Commonwealth University
VCH Health System
Richmond, Virginia

Fremont P. Wirth, MD
Assistant Clinical Professor of Surgery
Department of Surgery
Medical College of Georgia
Augusta, Georgia;
Staff
Department of Neurosurgery
St. Joseph's/Candler Health System
Savannah, Georgia

Jeffrey D. Wolfrey, MD
Clinical Professor
Department of Community and Family
 Medicine
University of Arizona College of Medicine
Tucson, Arizona;
Program Director
Family Medicine Residency
Banner Good Samaritan Medical Center
Phoenix, Arizona

Michael Wollin, MD
Clinical Associate Professor
University of Massachusetts Memorial
 Medical School
Worcester, Massachusetts

Frances Y. Wu, MD
Clinical Assistant Professor
Department of Family Medicine
UMDNJ-New Jersey Medical School
Newark, New Jersey
Assistant Director
Department of Family Medicine
Somerset Medical Center
Somerset, New Jersey

Jacqueline J. Wu, MD
General Surgery Resident
Department of Surgery
University of Massachusetts Medical
 School
Worcester, Massachusetts

James L. Young, MD
University of Massachusetts Medical
 School
Worcester, Massachusetts

Jane Y. Wu, MD
Staff Physician
Family Practice
Bridgewater Goddard Park Medical
 Associates
Brockton, Massachusetts

Kathleen Zeller, MD
Resident Physician
Department of Obstetrics and Gynecology
Akron General Medical Center
Akron, Ohio

Richard Kent Zimmerman, MD, MPH
Professor
Department of Family Medicine and
 Clinical Epidemiology
University of Pittsburgh
Pittsburgh, Pennsylvania

Gennine Zinner, RNCS, ANP
Adult Nurse Practitioner
Boston Health Care for the Homeless
Boston, Massachusetts

CONTENTS

Signs & Symptoms: An Algorithmic Approach

This section contains diagnostic flowcharts (or algorithms) to help the reader in the evaluation of a clinical problem. They are organized by the presenting clinical sign or symptom.

These diagnostic algorithms were designed to be used as an adjunct to the reader's clinical knowledge and impression. They are not an exhaustive review of the management of a problem, nor are they meant to be a complete list of diseases. They are meant to be a quick reference tool to aid the reader in the management of their patient.

Written by Robert A. Baldor, MD and Alan M. Ehrlich, MD, these algorithms address the most common problems in an ambulatory practice.

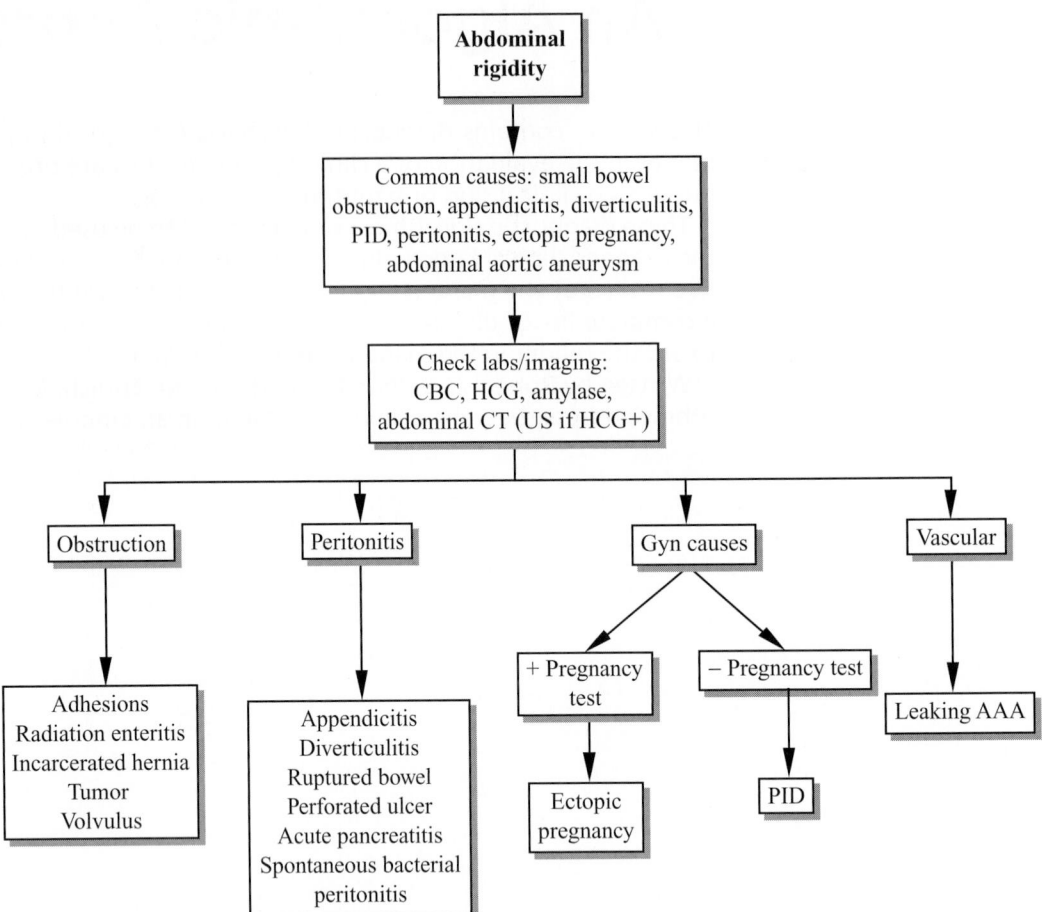

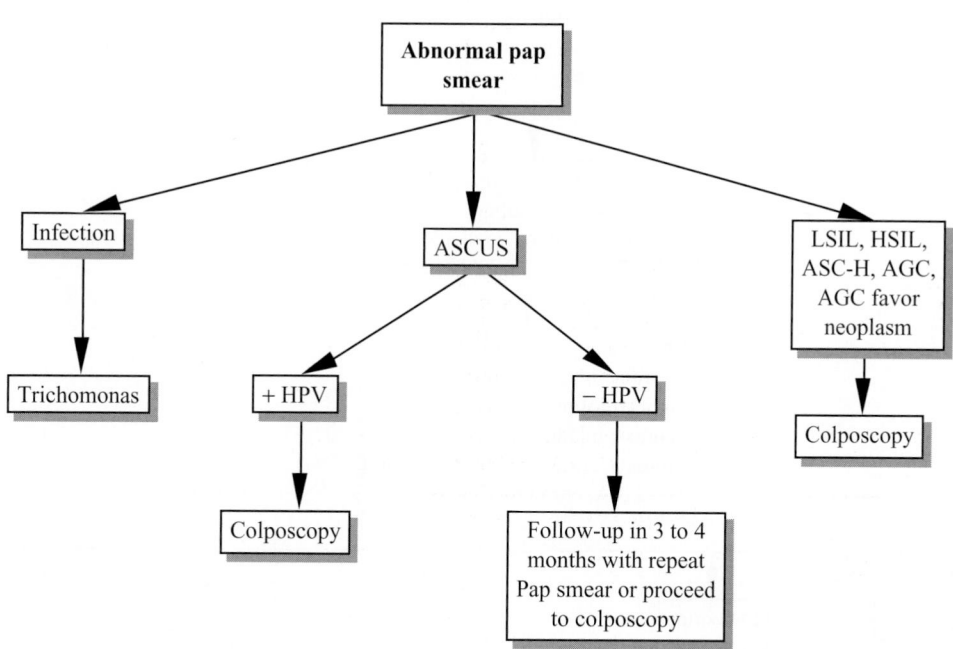

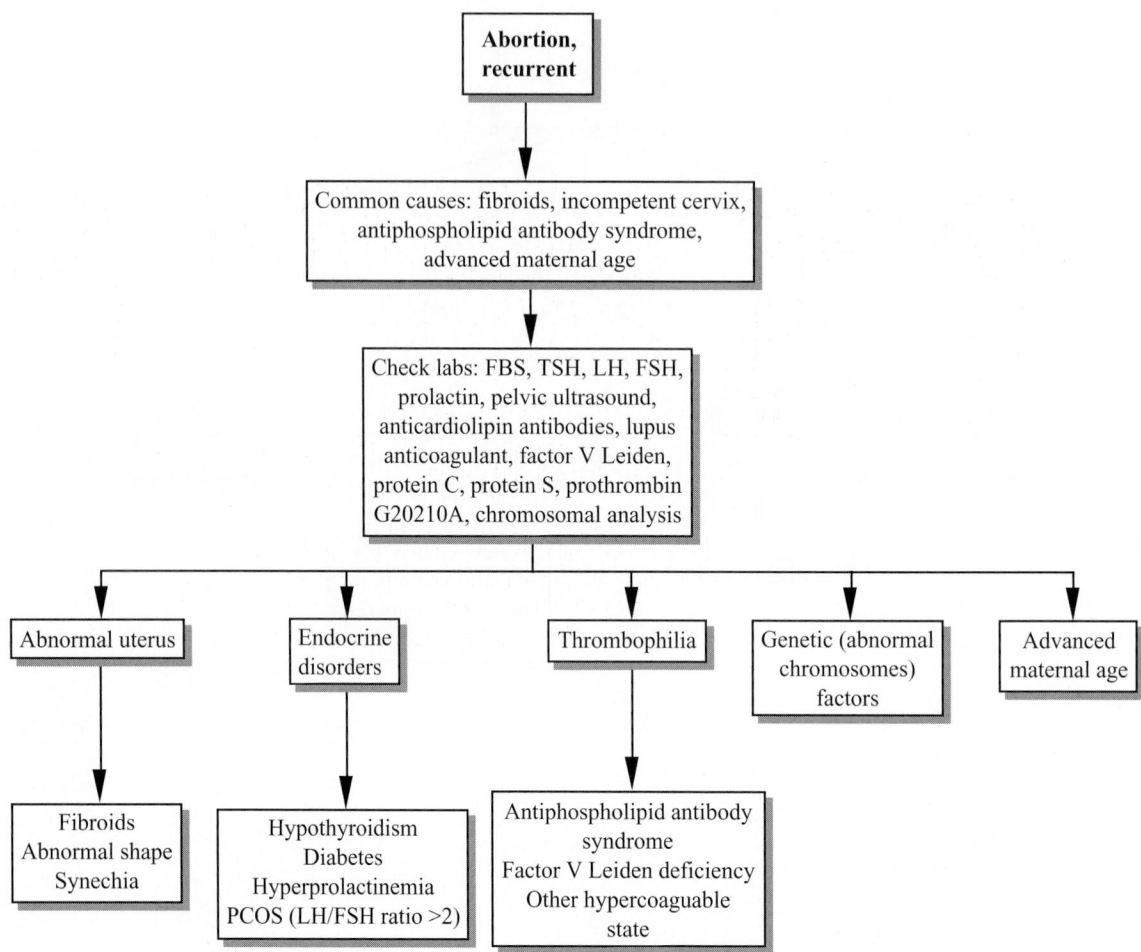

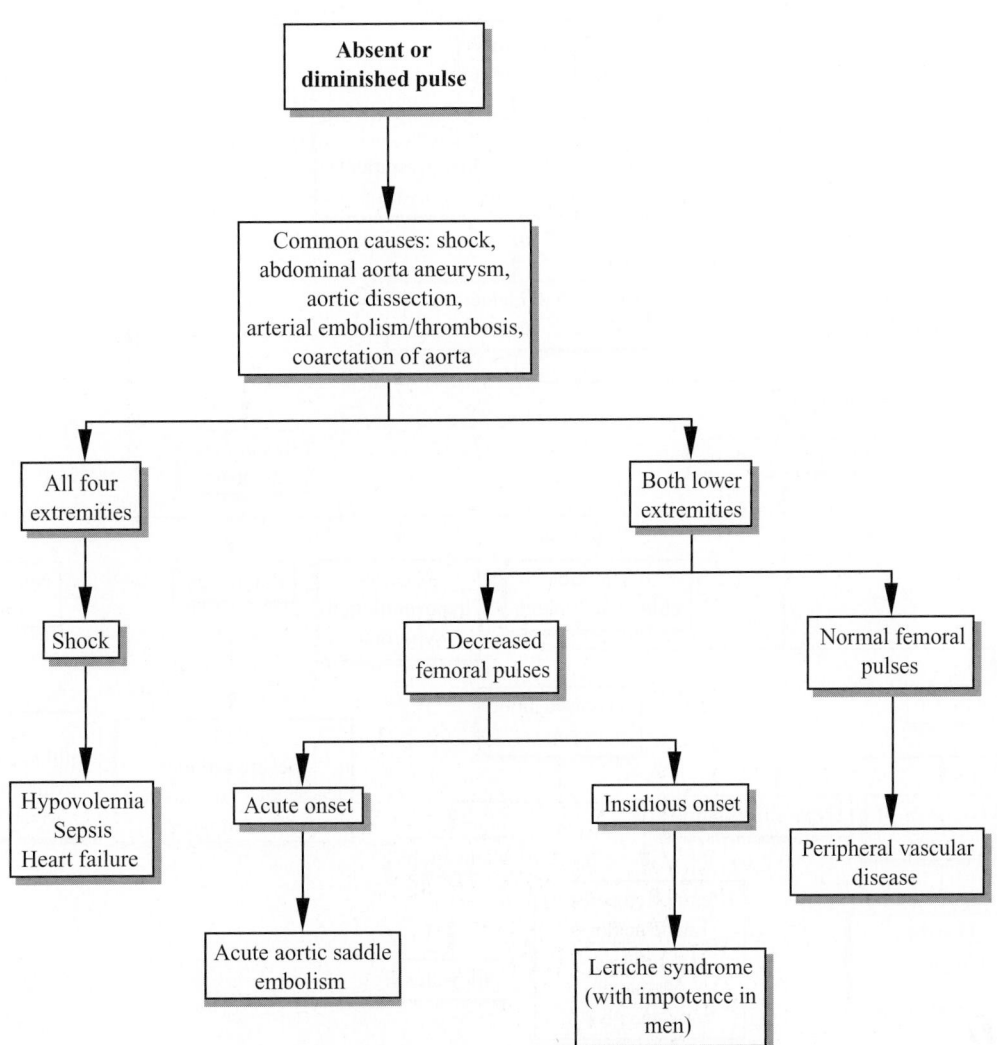

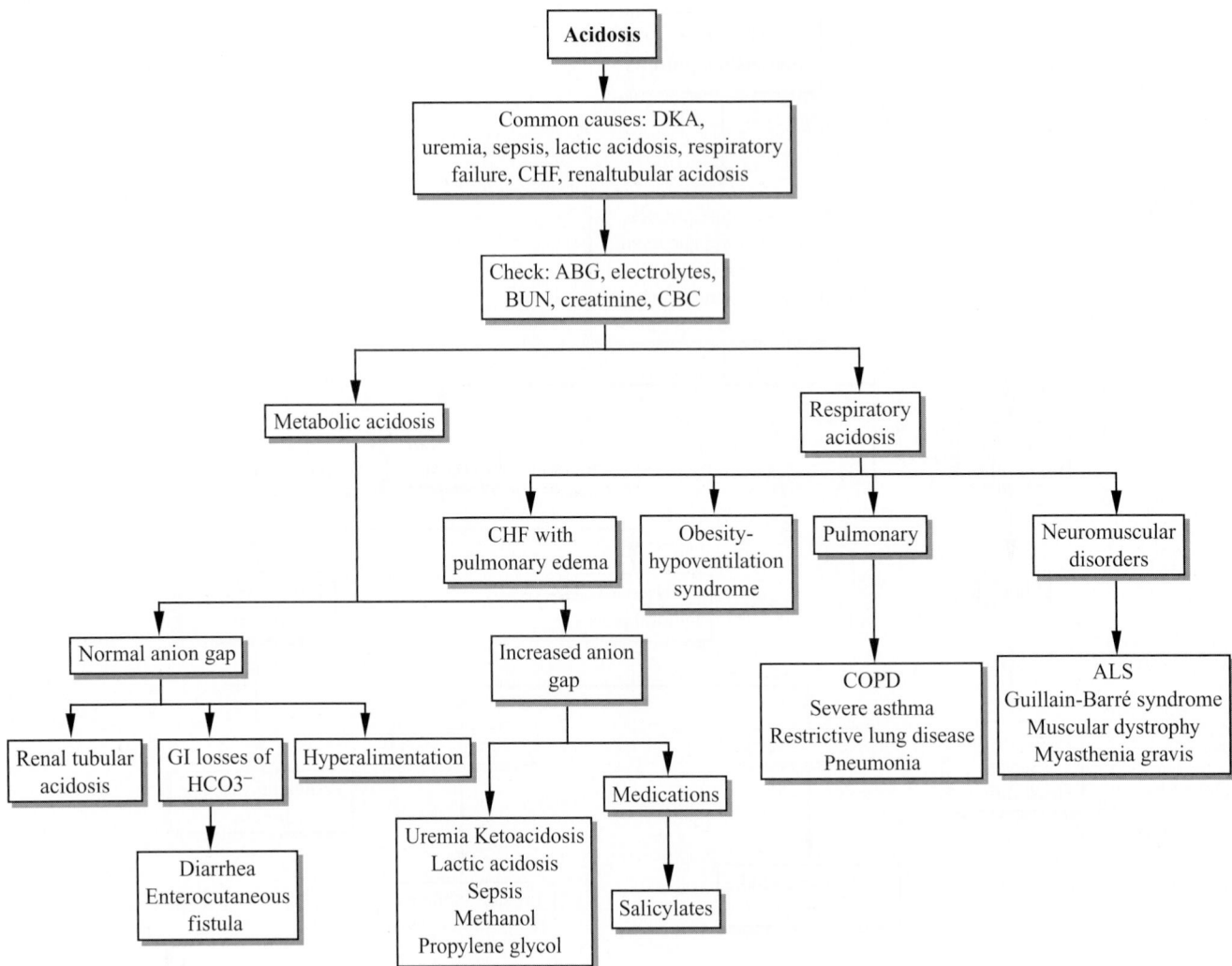

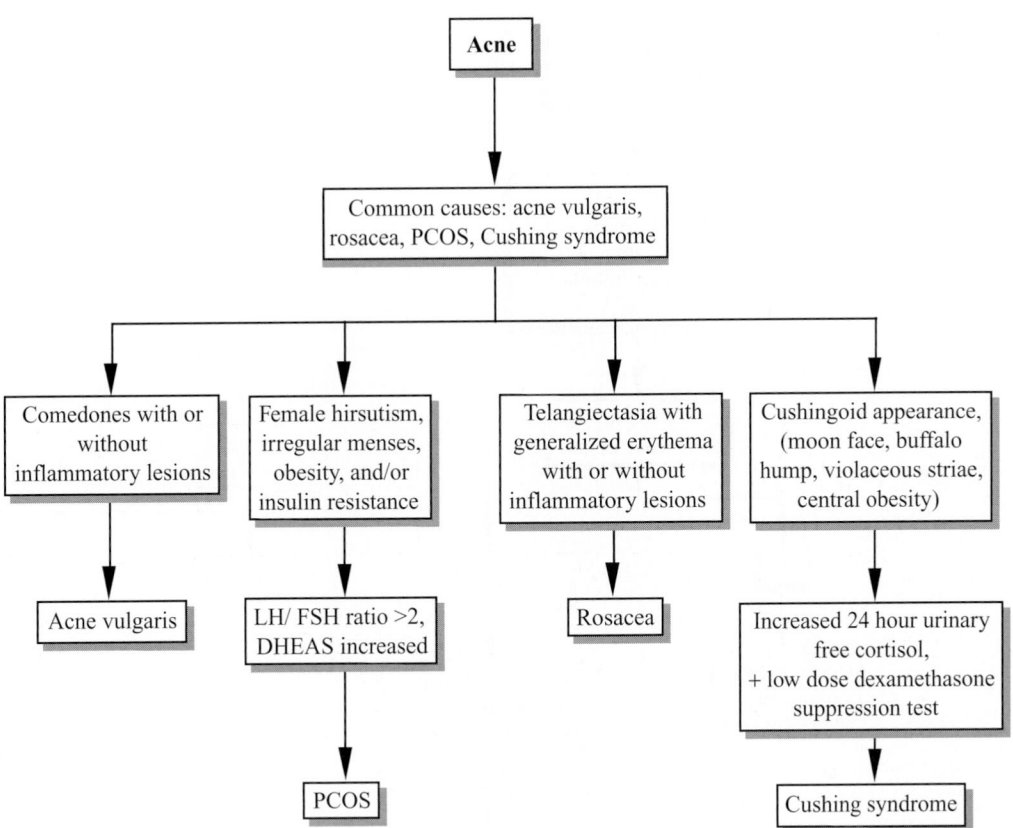

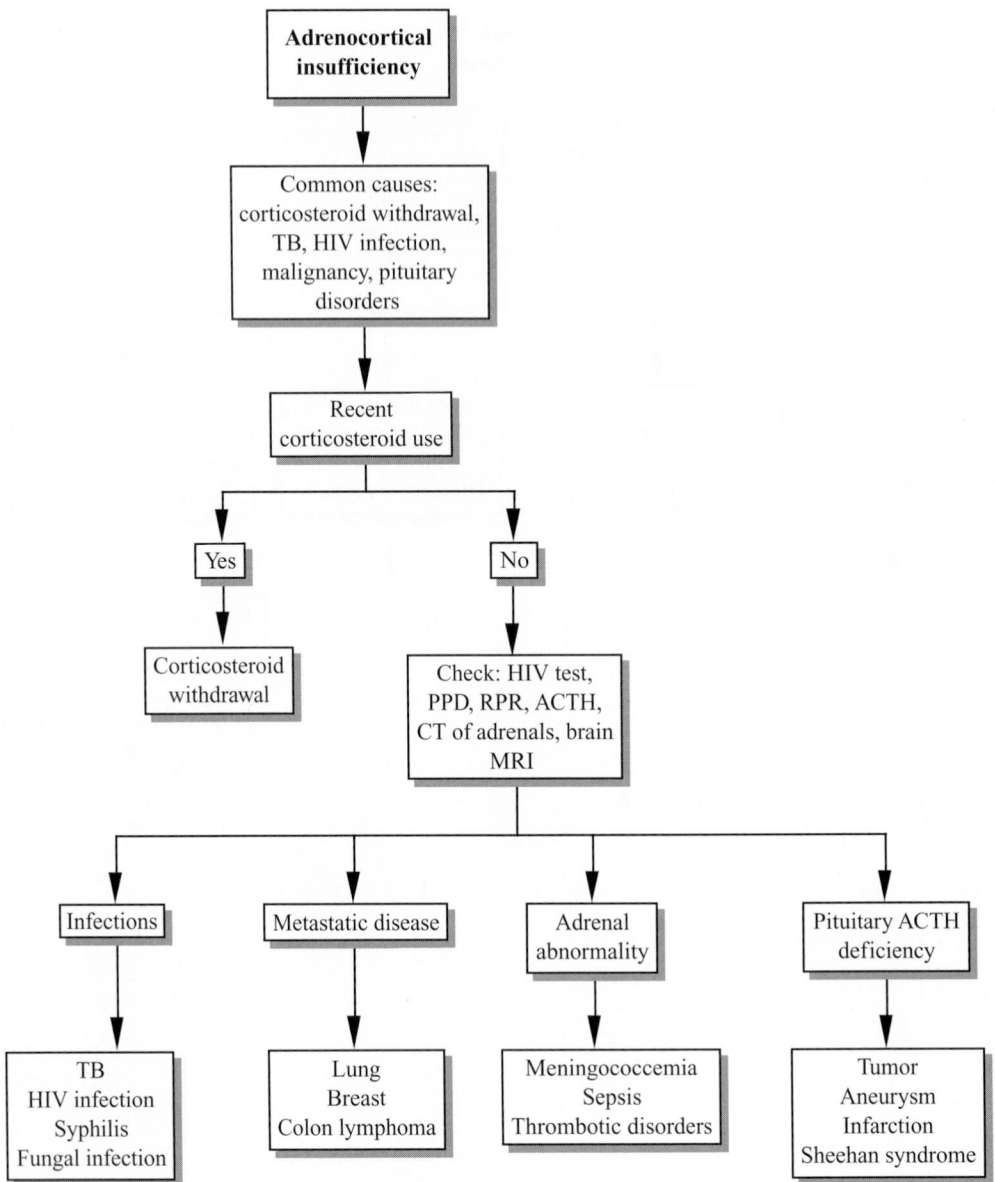

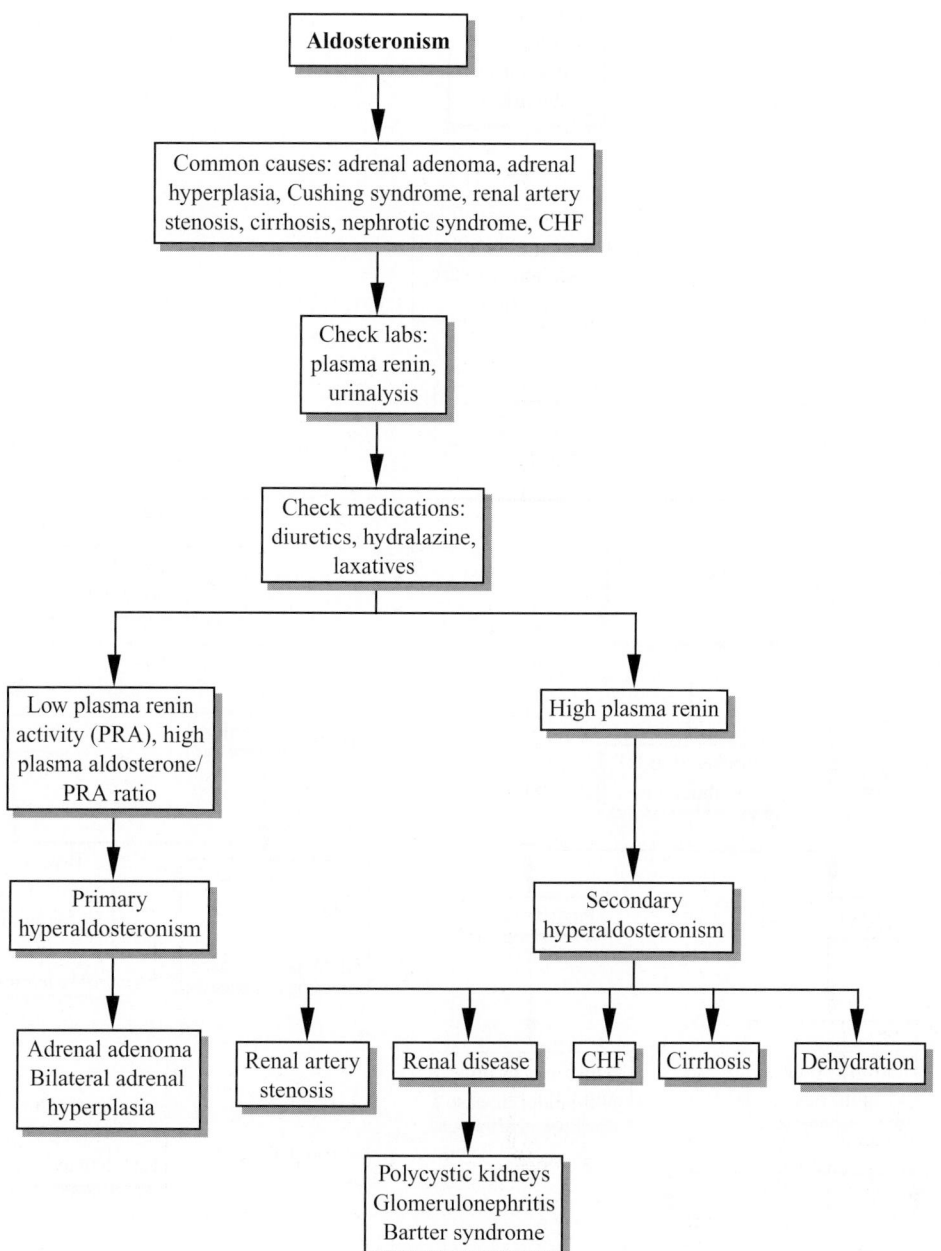

Aldosteronism

Common causes: adrenal adenoma, adrenal hyperplasia, Cushing syndrome, renal artery stenosis, cirrhosis, nephrotic syndrome, CHF

Check labs: plasma renin, urinalysis

Check medications: diuretics, hydralazine, laxatives

Low plasma renin activity (PRA), high plasma aldosterone/ PRA ratio

High plasma renin

Primary hyperaldosteronism

Secondary hyperaldosteronism

Adrenal adenoma Bilateral adrenal hyperplasia

Renal artery stenosis

Renal disease

CHF

Cirrhosis

Dehydration

Polycystic kidneys Glomerulonephritis Bartter syndrome

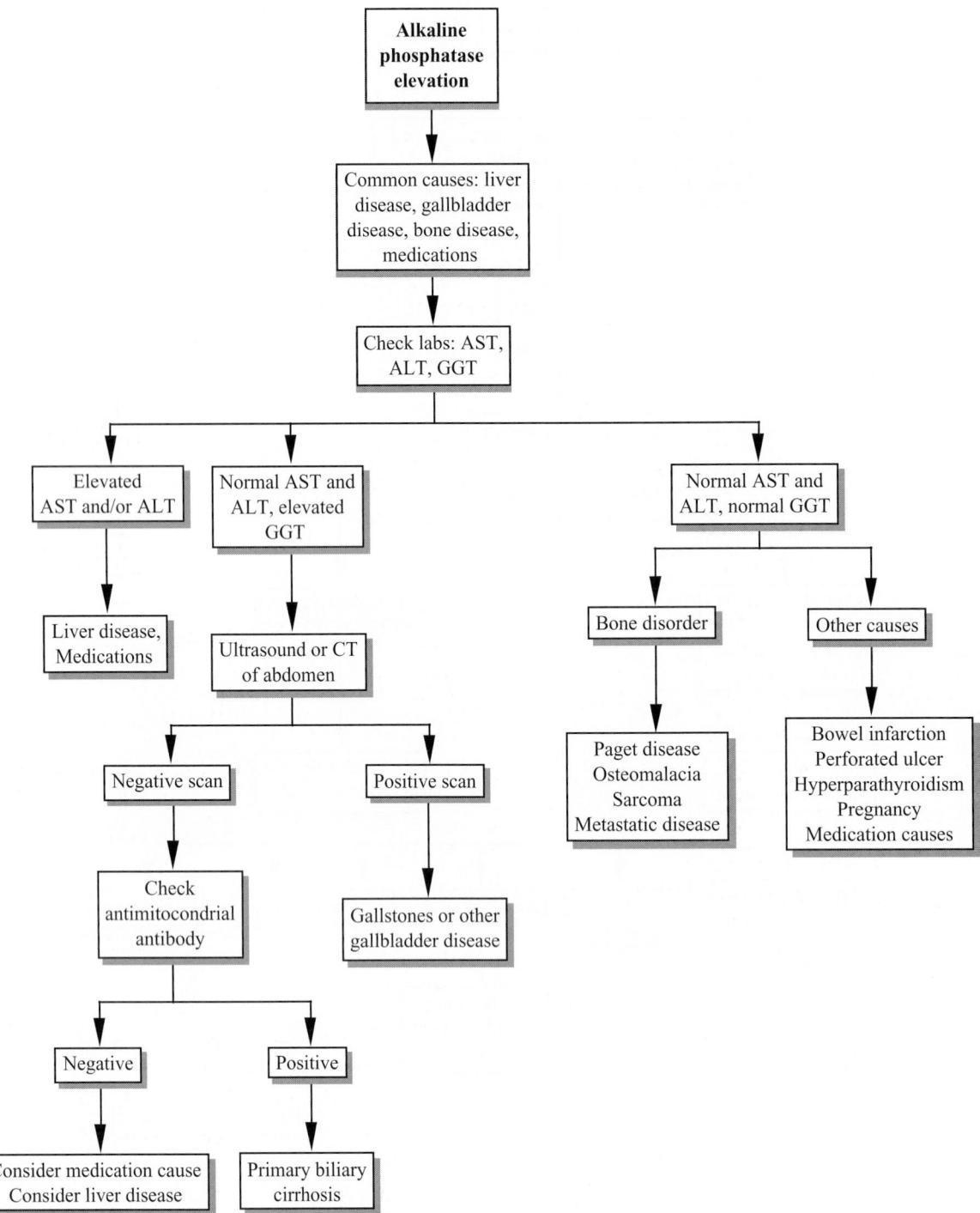

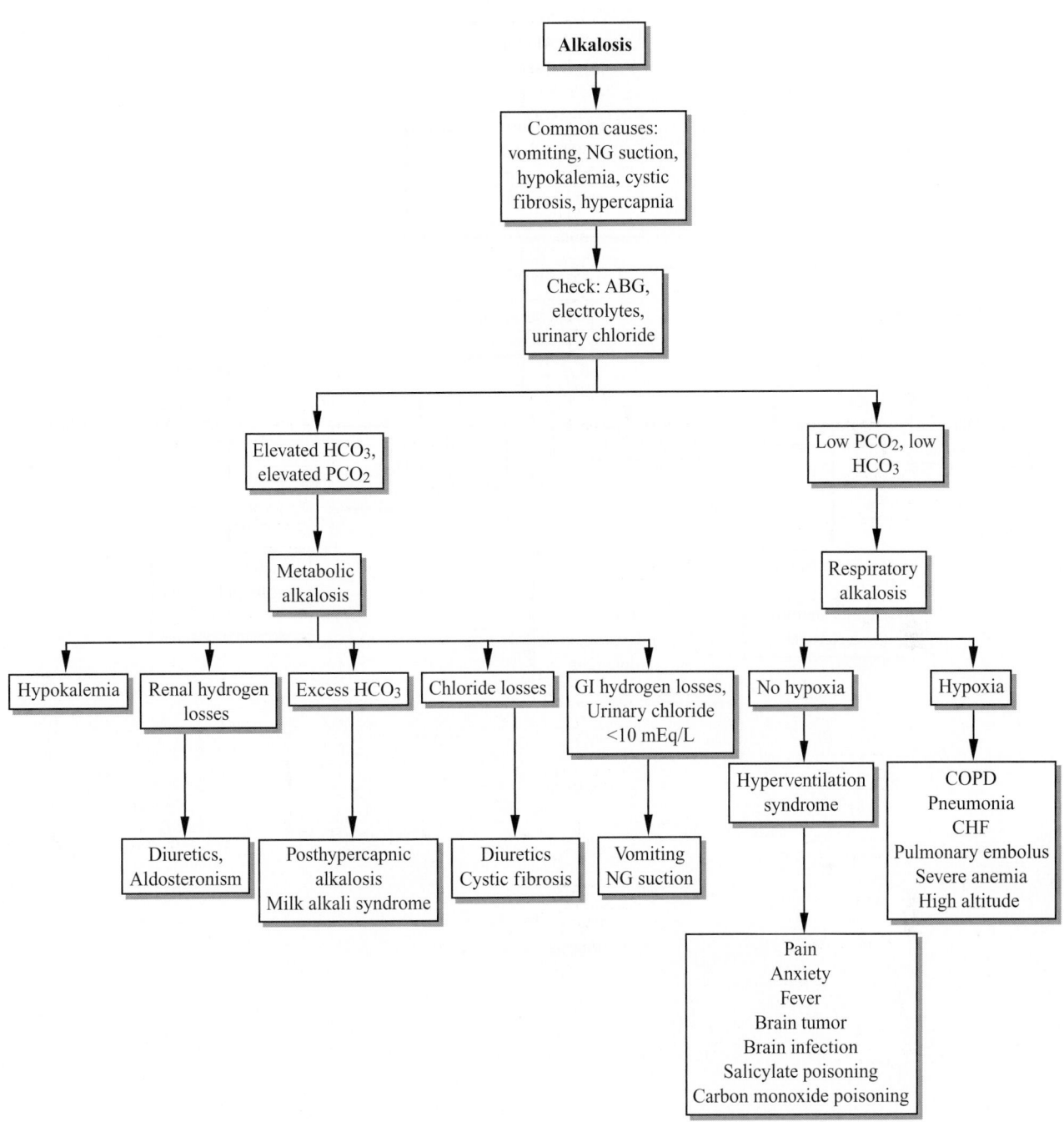

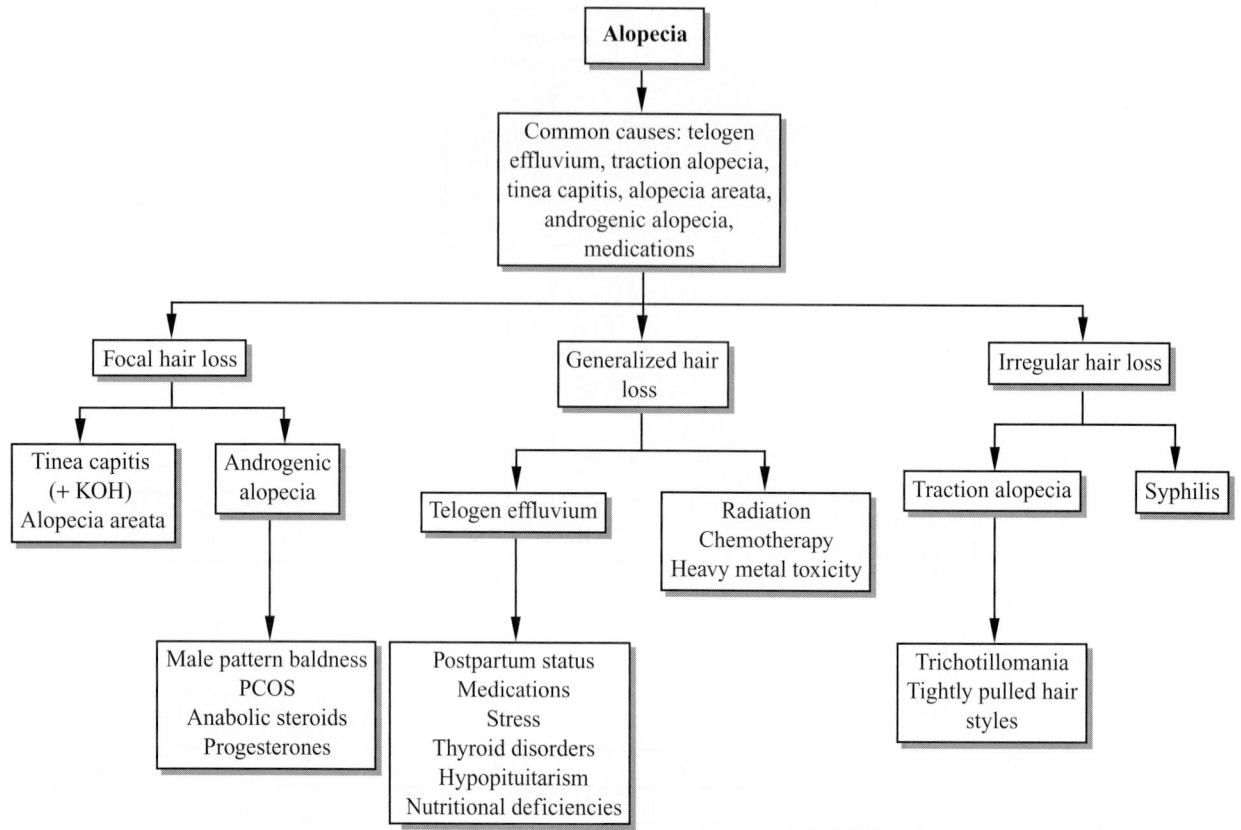

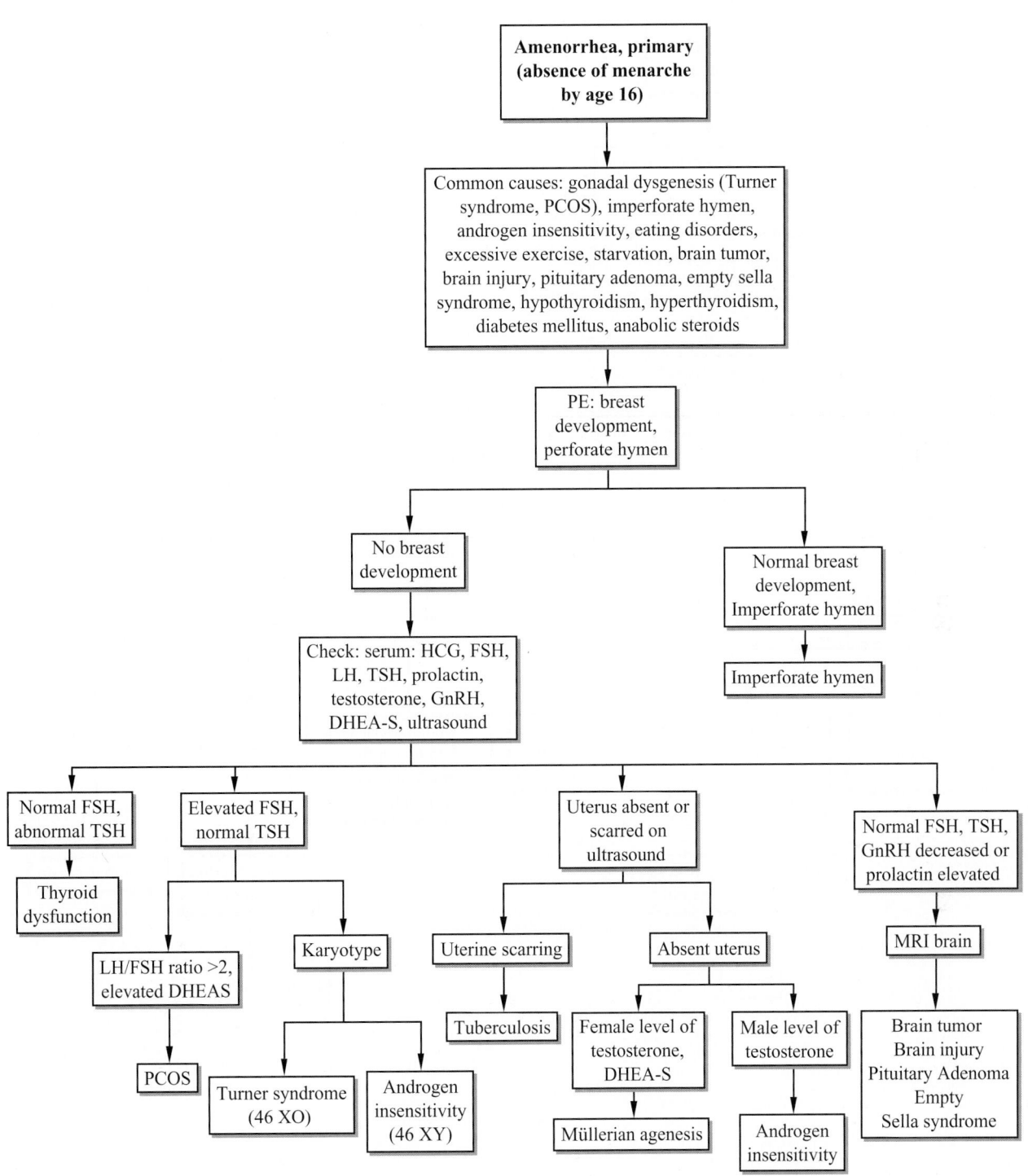

Amenorrhea, primary (absence of menarche by age 16)

Common causes: gonadal dysgenesis (Turner syndrome, PCOS), imperforate hymen, androgen insensitivity, eating disorders, excessive exercise, starvation, brain tumor, brain injury, pituitary adenoma, empty sella syndrome, hypothyroidism, hyperthyroidism, diabetes mellitus, anabolic steroids

PE: breast development, perforate hymen

No breast development

Normal breast development, Imperforate hymen

Imperforate hymen

Check: serum: HCG, FSH, LH, TSH, prolactin, testosterone, GnRH, DHEA-S, ultrasound

Normal FSH, abnormal TSH

Thyroid dysfunction

Elevated FSH, normal TSH

LH/FSH ratio >2, elevated DHEAS

PCOS

Karyotype

Turner syndrome (46 XO)

Androgen insensitivity (46 XY)

Uterus absent or scarred on ultrasound

Uterine scarring

Tuberculosis

Absent uterus

Female level of testosterone, DHEA-S

Müllerian agenesis

Male level of testosterone

Androgen insensitivity

Normal FSH, TSH, GnRH decreased or prolactin elevated

MRI brain

Brain tumor
Brain injury
Pituitary Adenoma
Empty
Sella syndrome

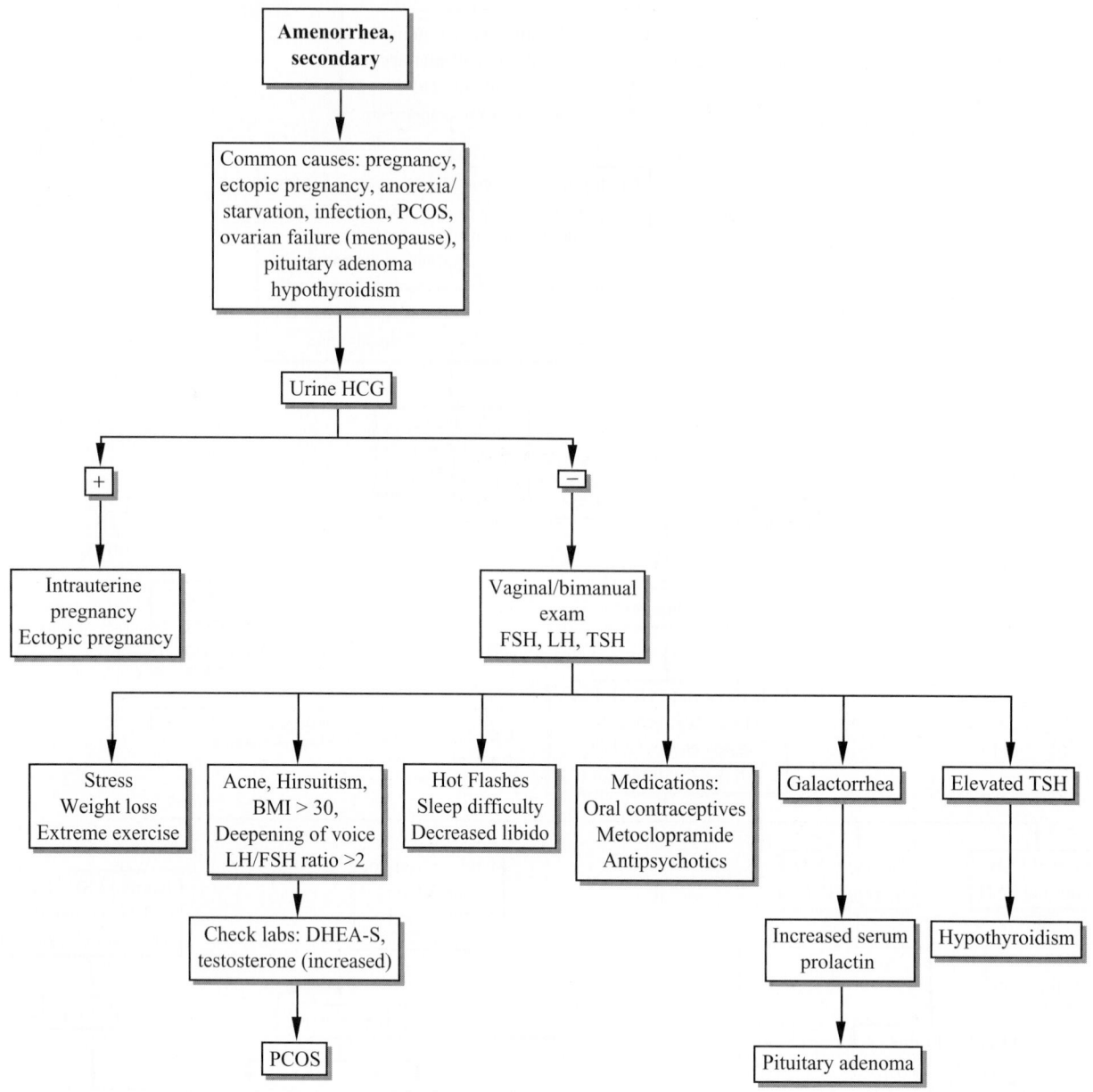

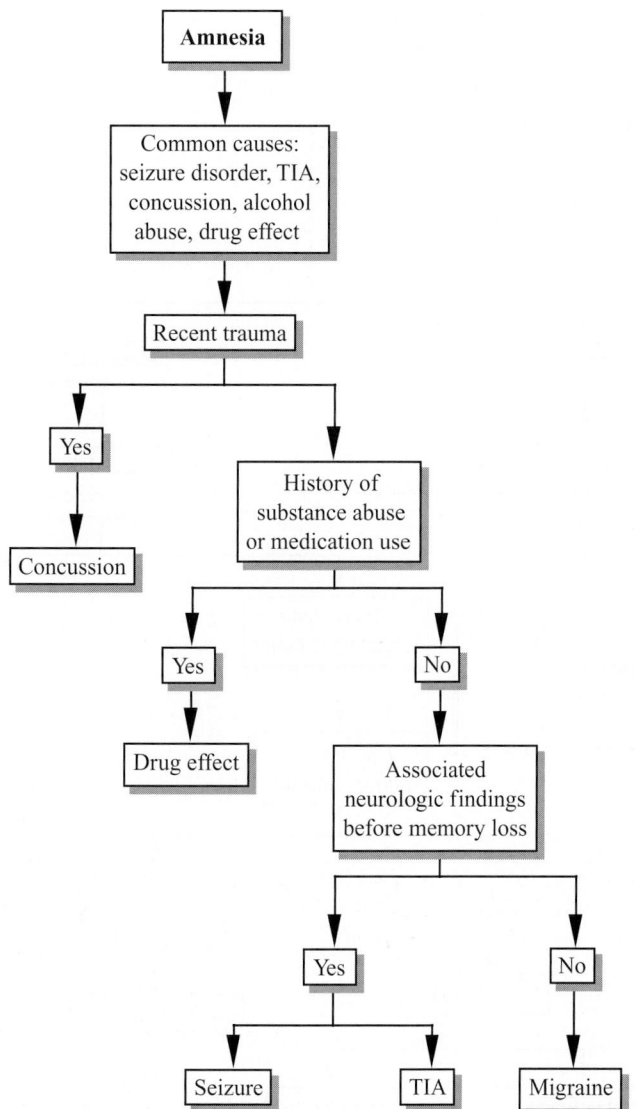

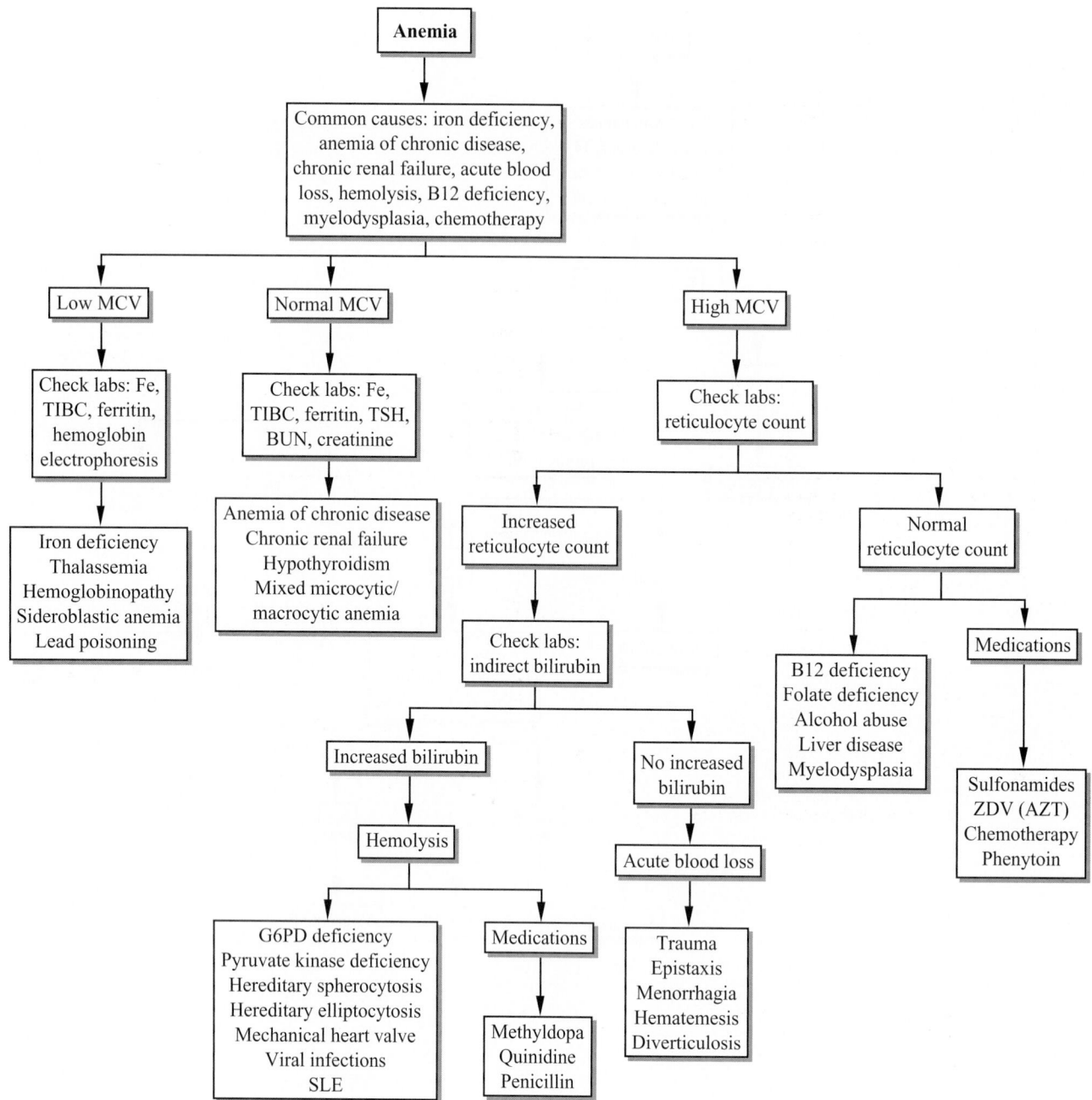

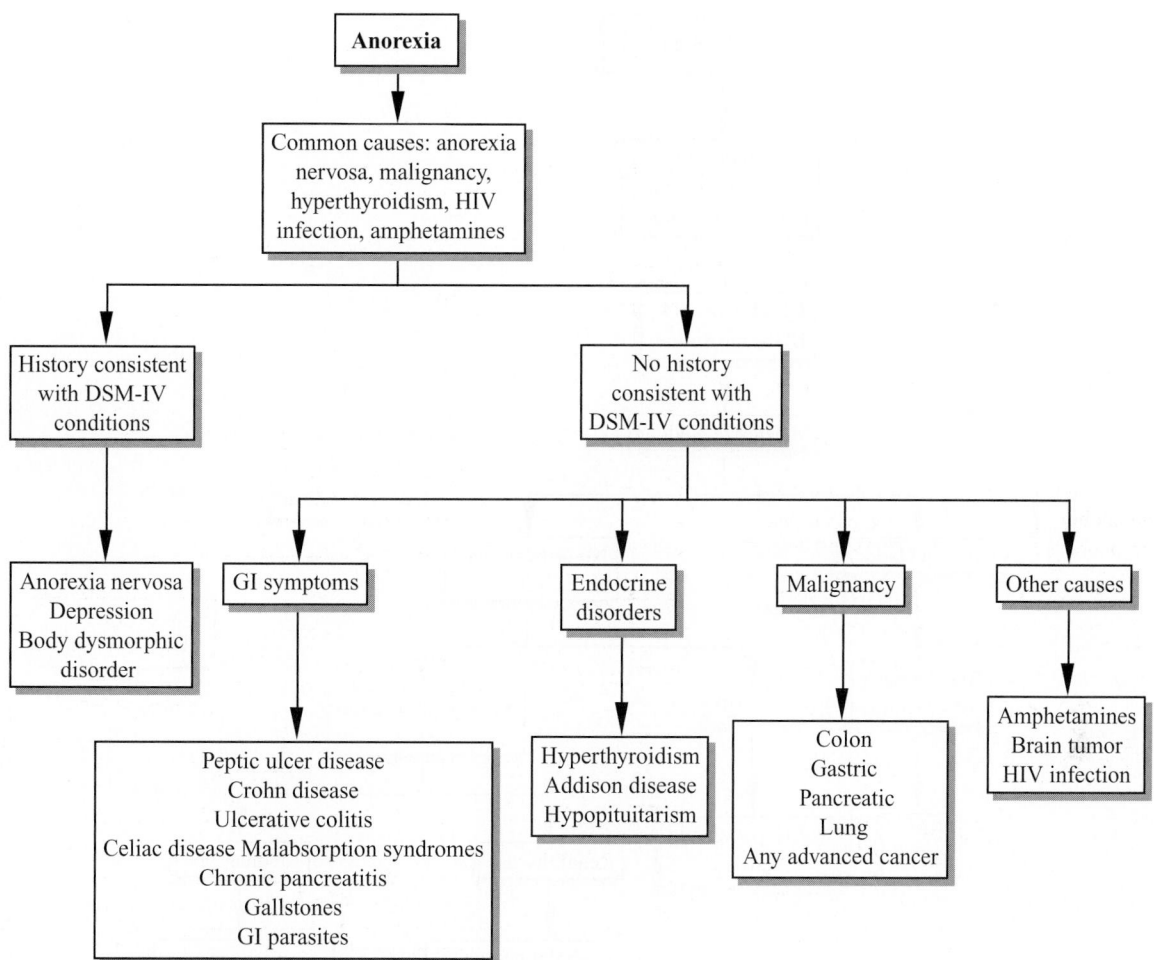

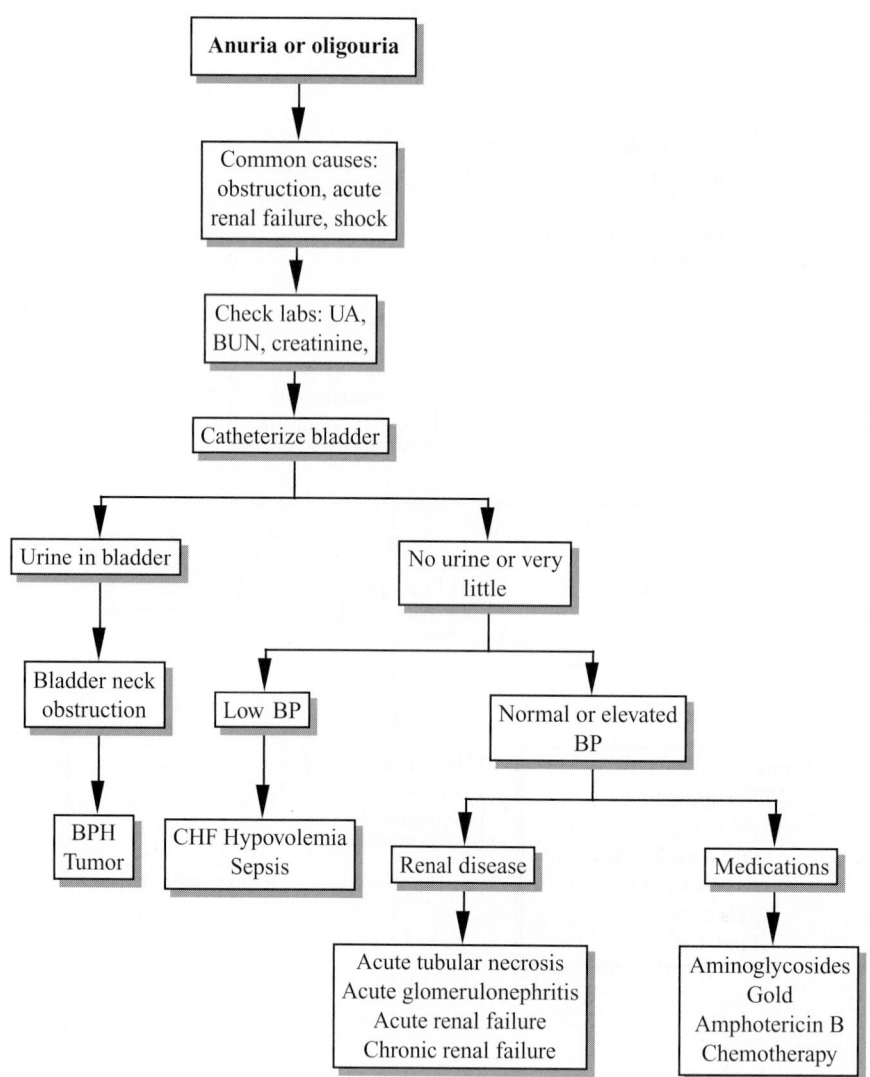

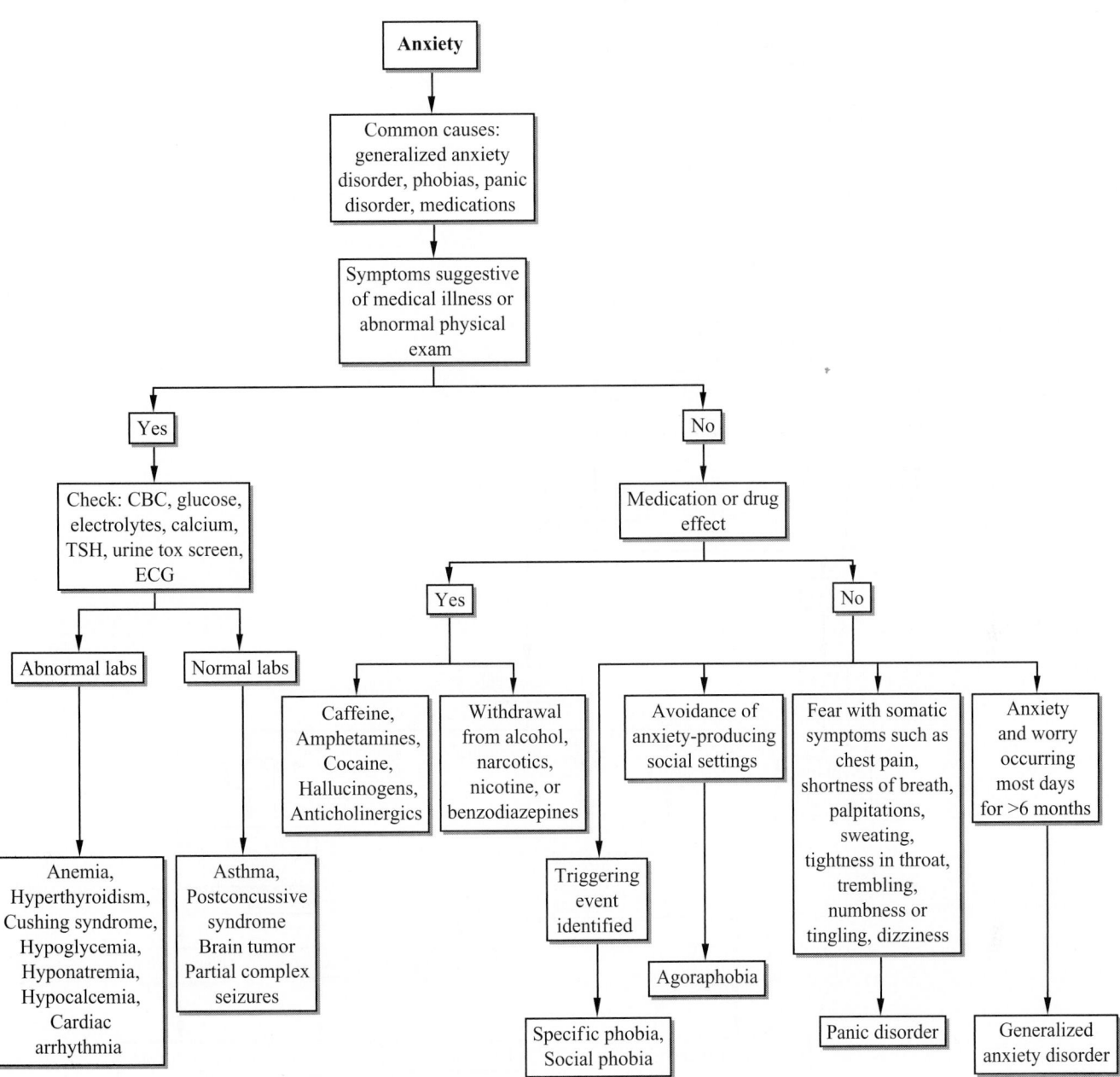

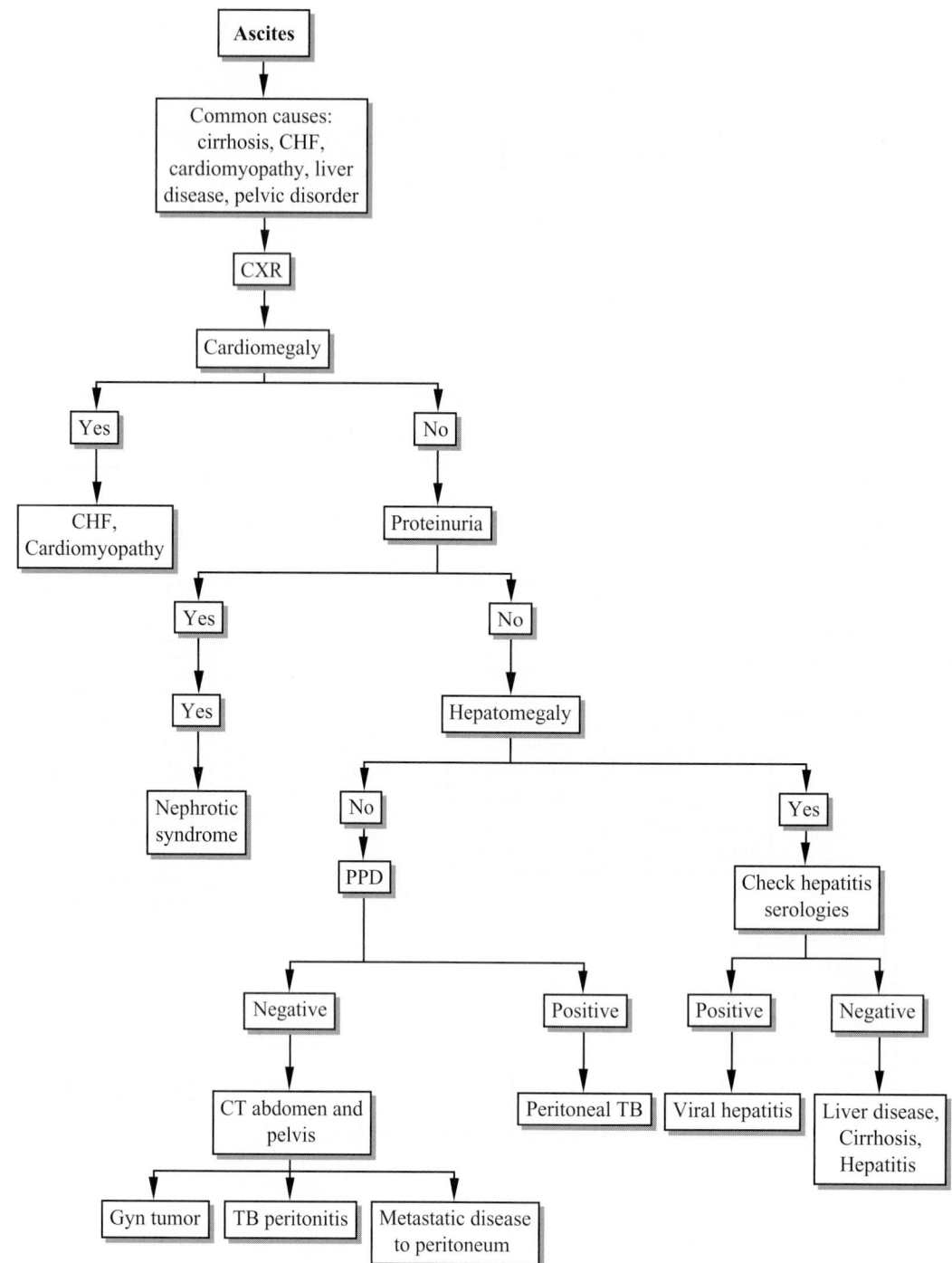

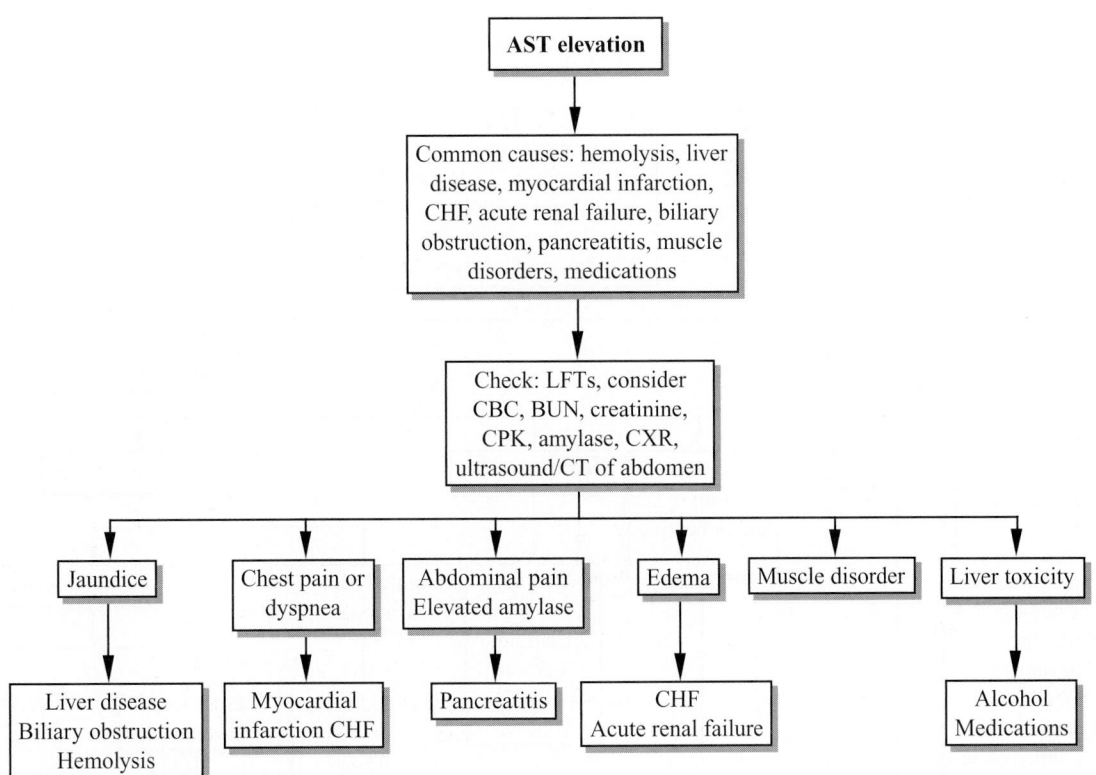

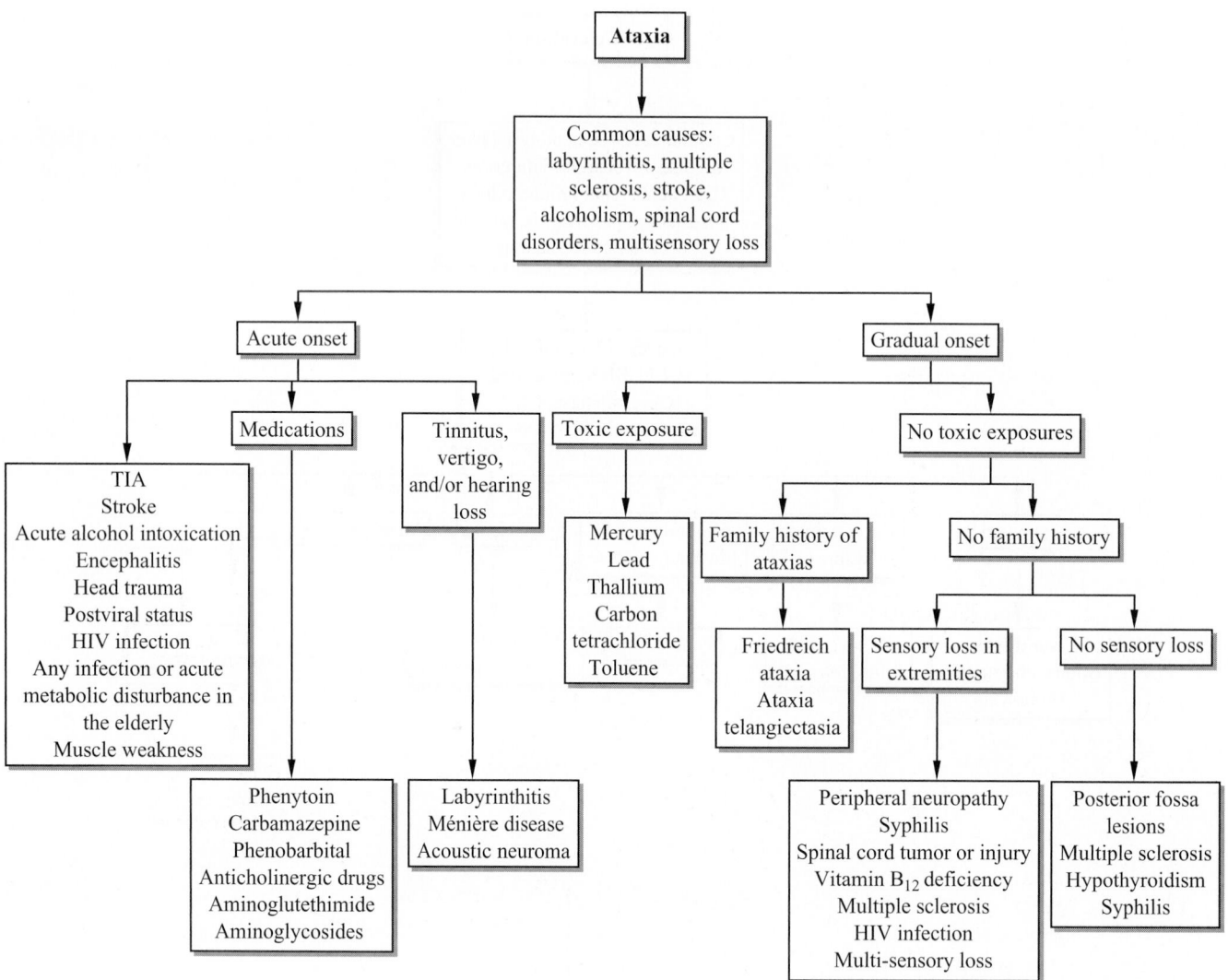

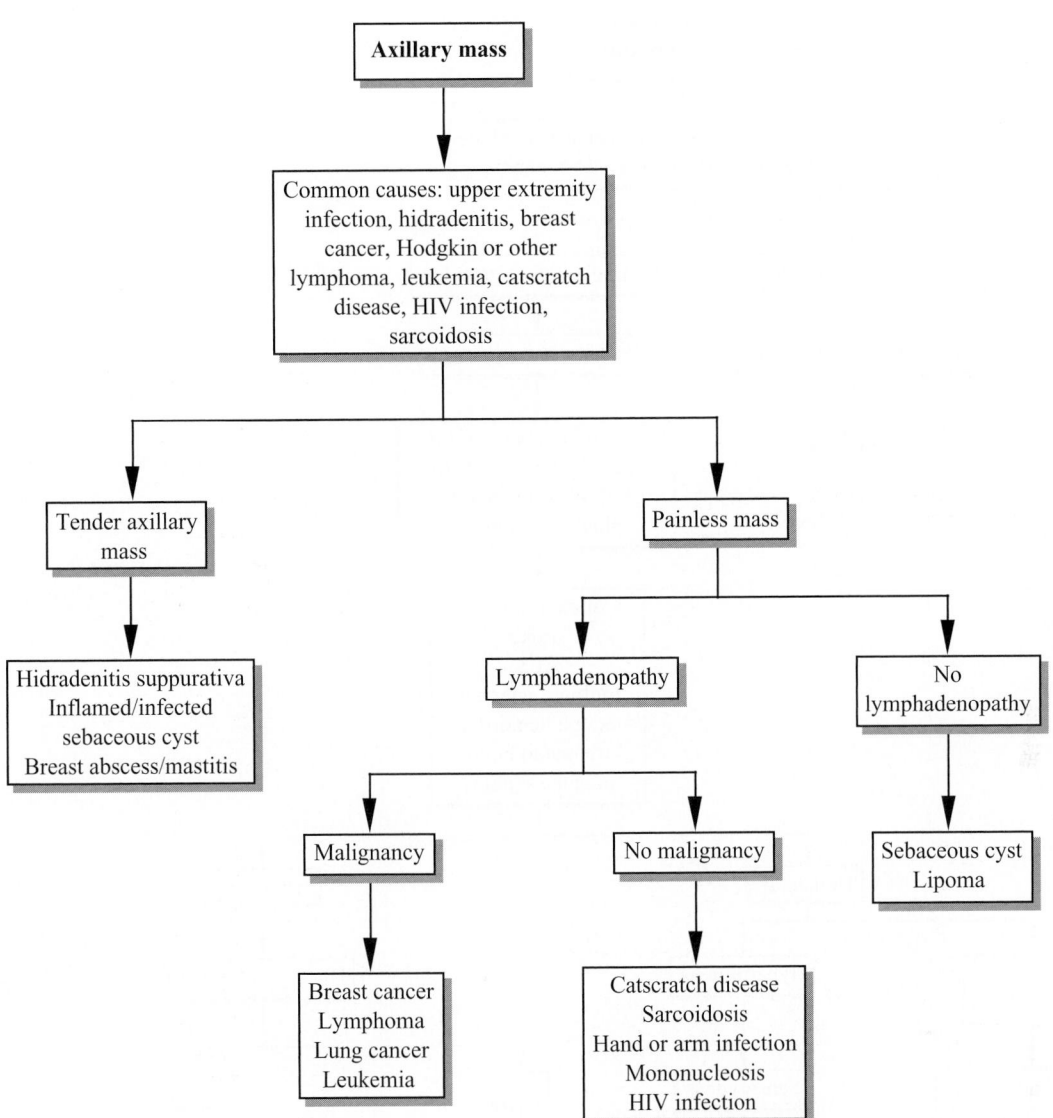

Axillary mass

Common causes: upper extremity infection, hidradenitis, breast cancer, Hodgkin or other lymphoma, leukemia, catscratch disease, HIV infection, sarcoidosis

Tender axillary mass

Painless mass

Hidradenitis suppurativa
Inflamed/infected sebaceous cyst
Breast abscess/mastitis

Lymphadenopathy

No lymphadenopathy

Malignancy

No malignancy

Sebaceous cyst
Lipoma

Breast cancer
Lymphoma
Lung cancer
Leukemia

Catscratch disease
Sarcoidosis
Hand or arm infection
Mononucleosis
HIV infection

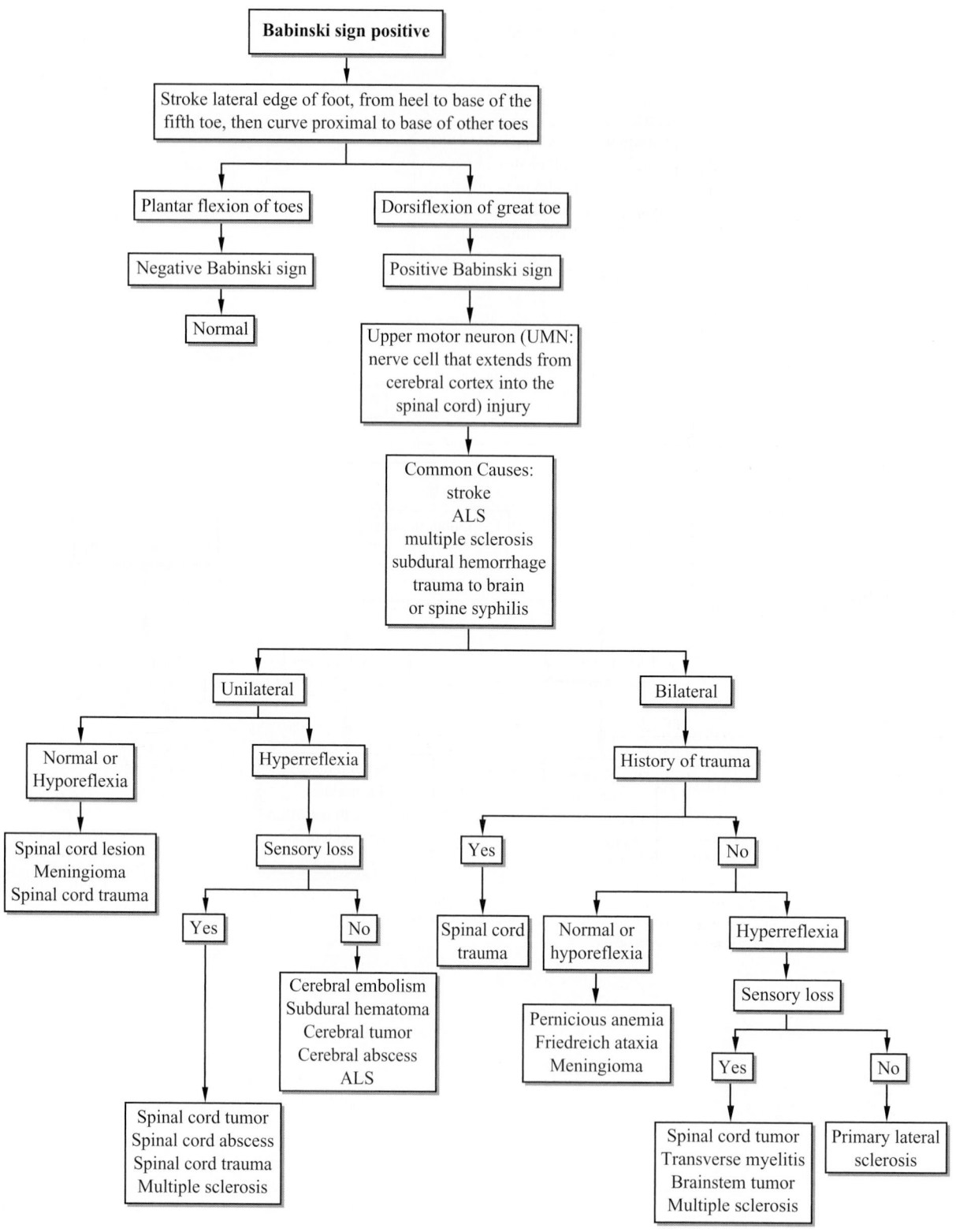

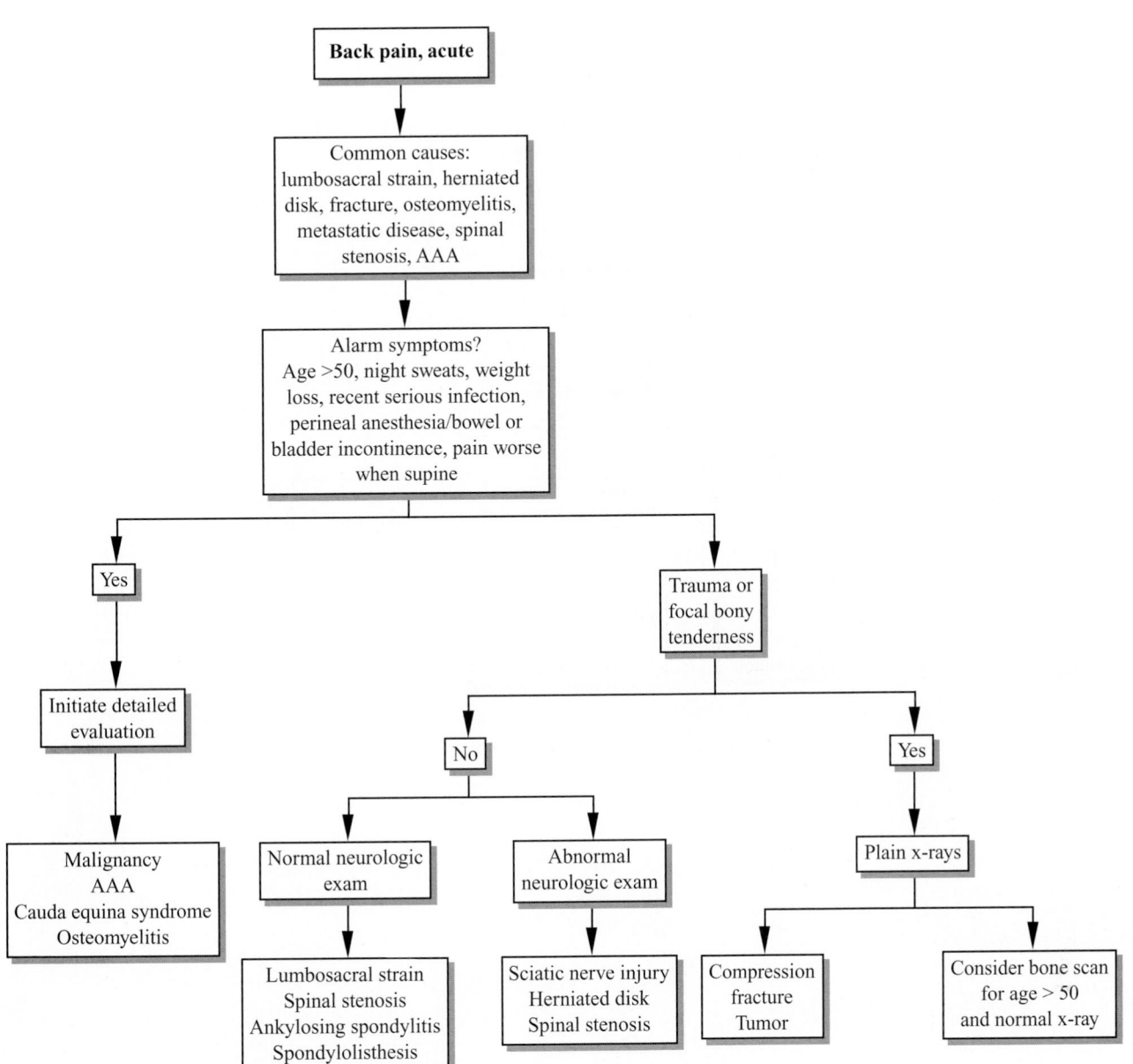

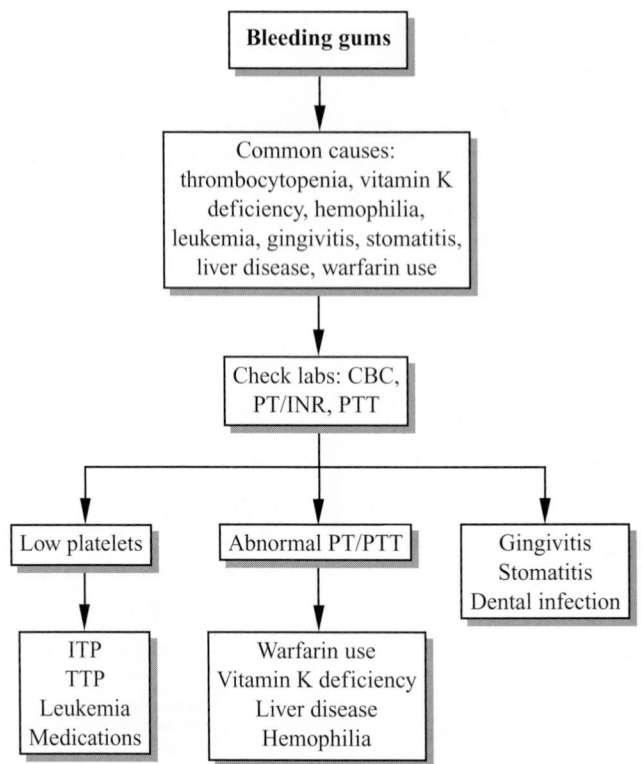

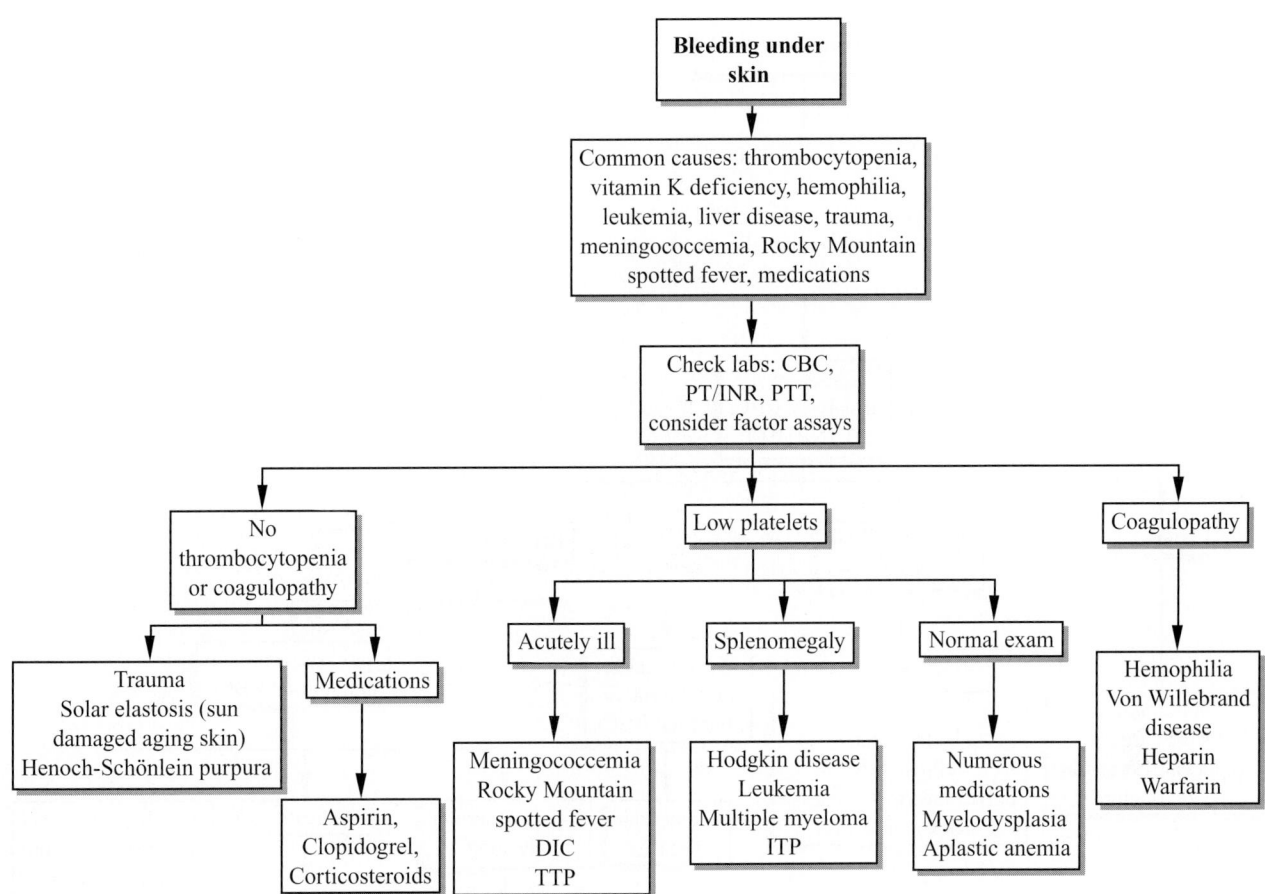

Bleeding under skin

↓

Common causes: thrombocytopenia, vitamin K deficiency, hemophilia, leukemia, liver disease, trauma, meningococcemia, Rocky Mountain spotted fever, medications

↓

Check labs: CBC, PT/INR, PTT, consider factor assays

No thrombocytopenia or coagulopathy

Trauma
Solar elastosis (sun damaged aging skin)
Henoch-Schönlein purpura

Medications

↓

Aspirin, Clopidogrel, Corticosteroids

Low platelets

Acutely ill

↓

Meningococcemia
Rocky Mountain spotted fever
DIC
TTP

Splenomegaly

↓

Hodgkin disease
Leukemia
Multiple myeloma
ITP

Normal exam

↓

Numerous medications
Myelodysplasia
Aplastic anemia

Coagulopathy

↓

Hemophilia
Von Willebrand disease
Heparin
Warfarin

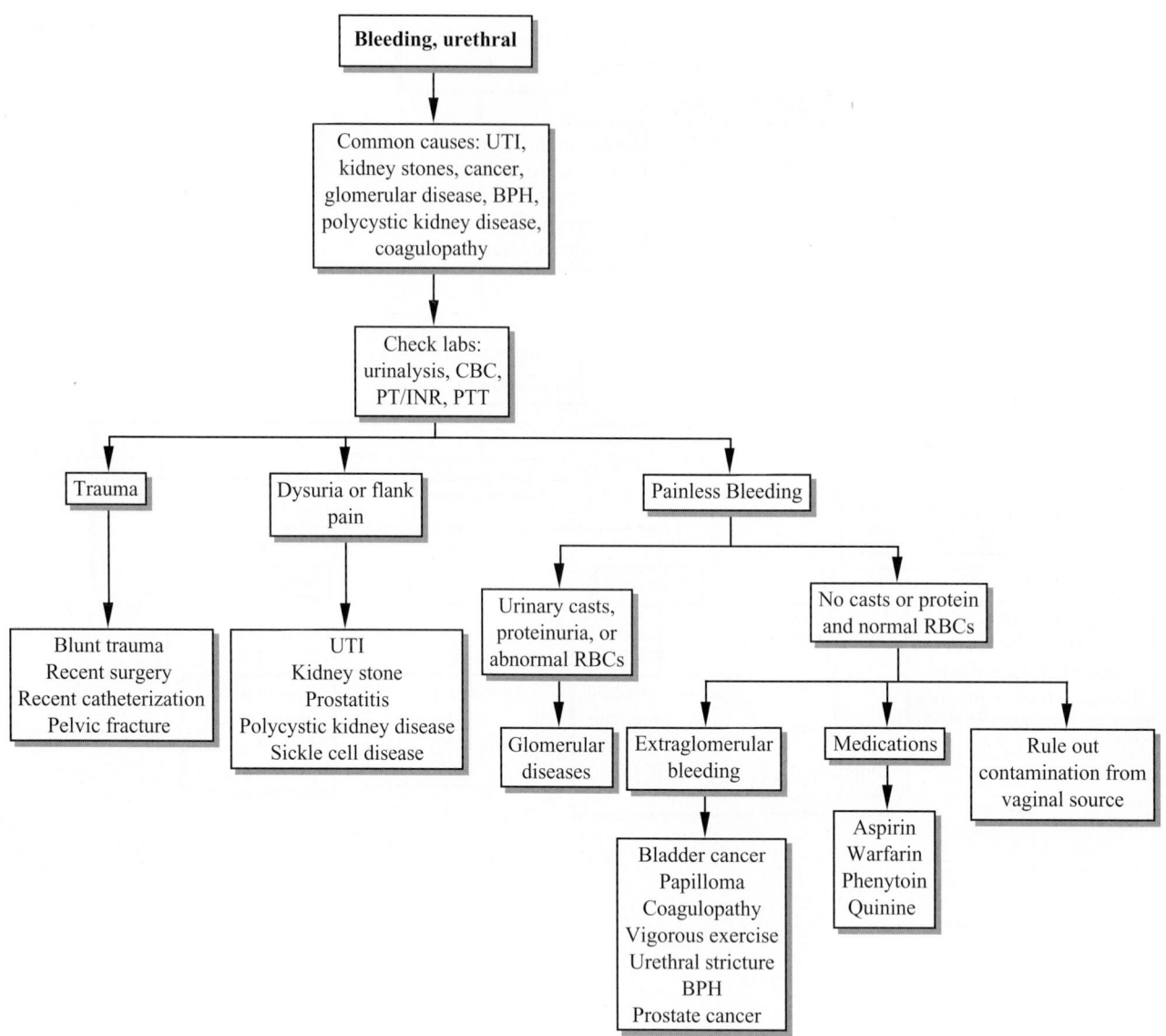

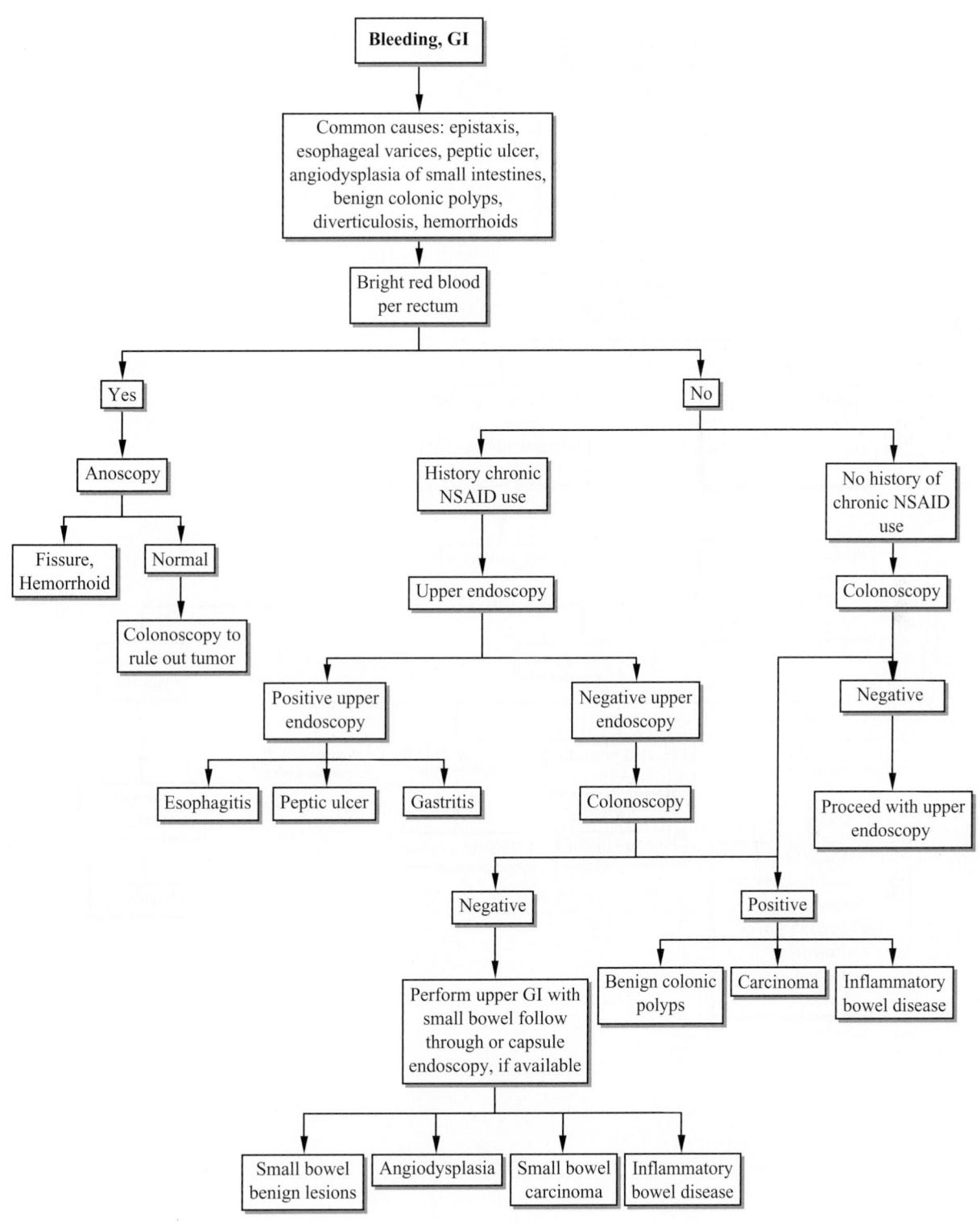

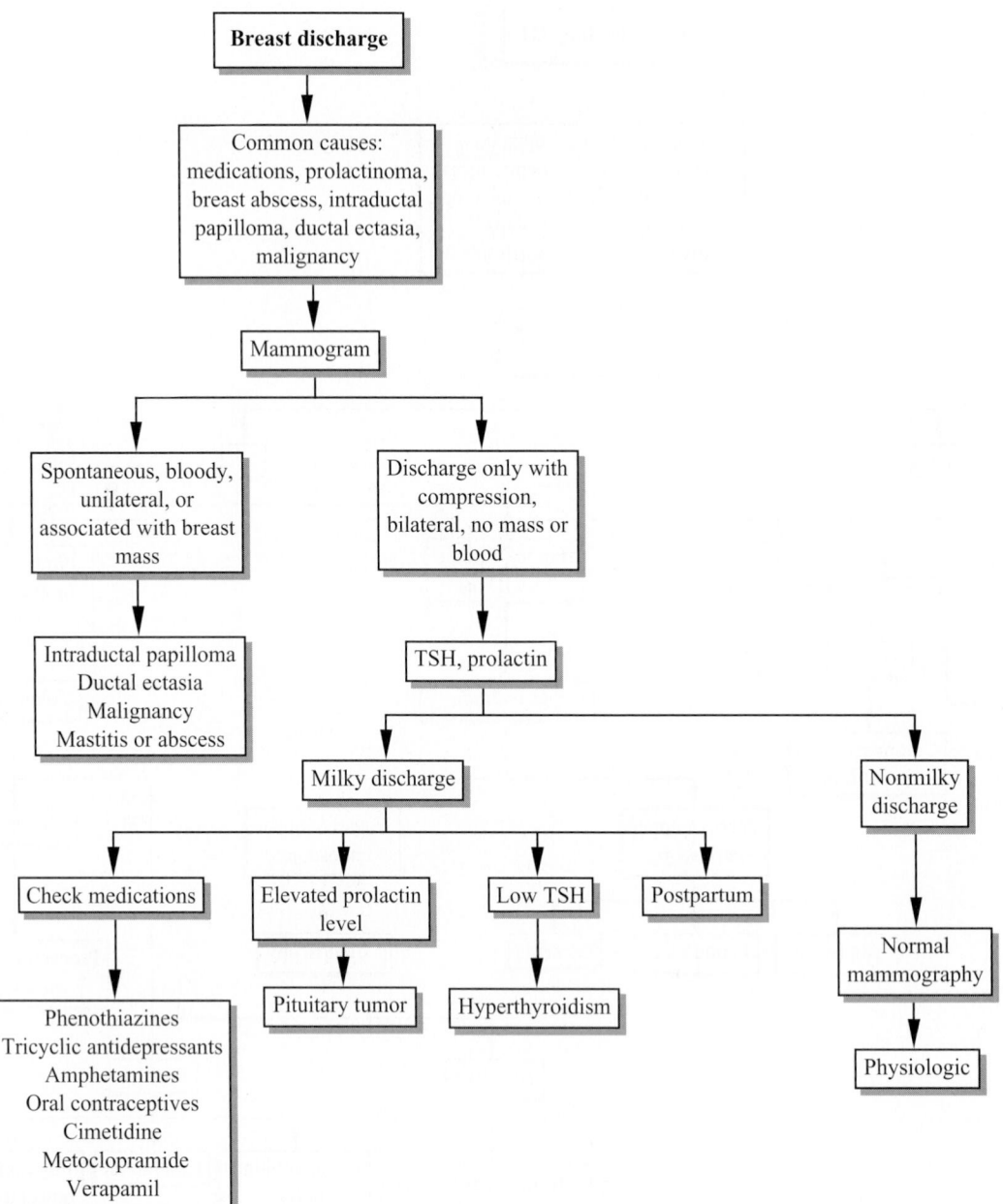

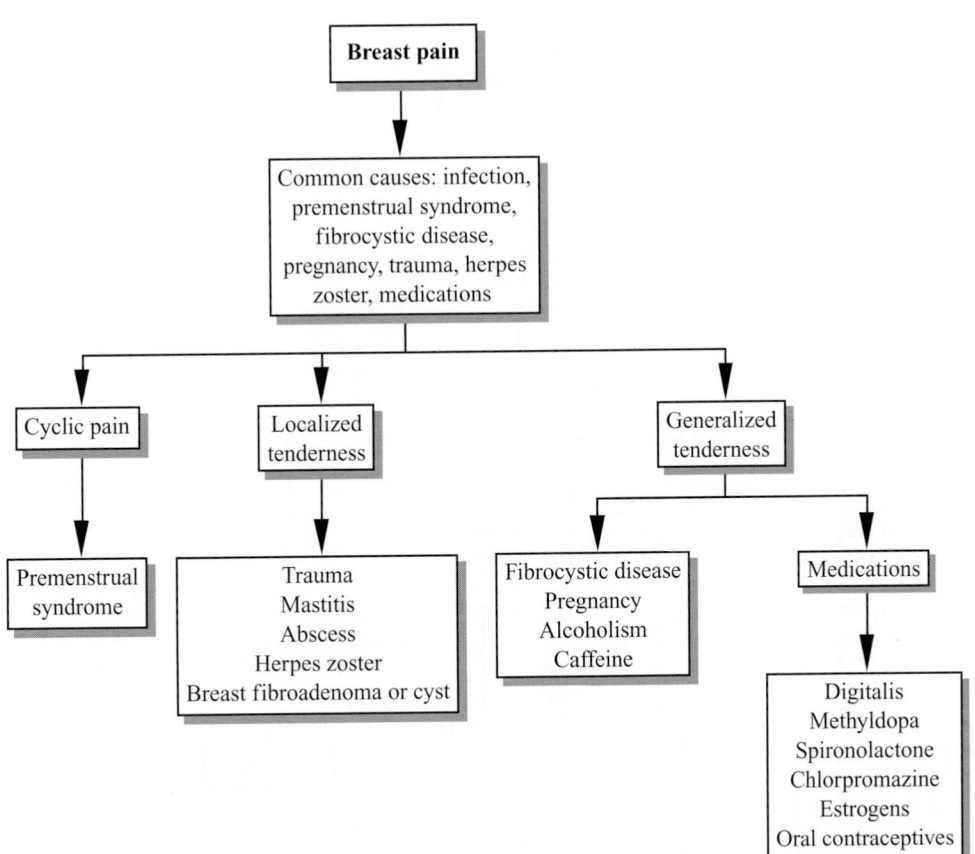

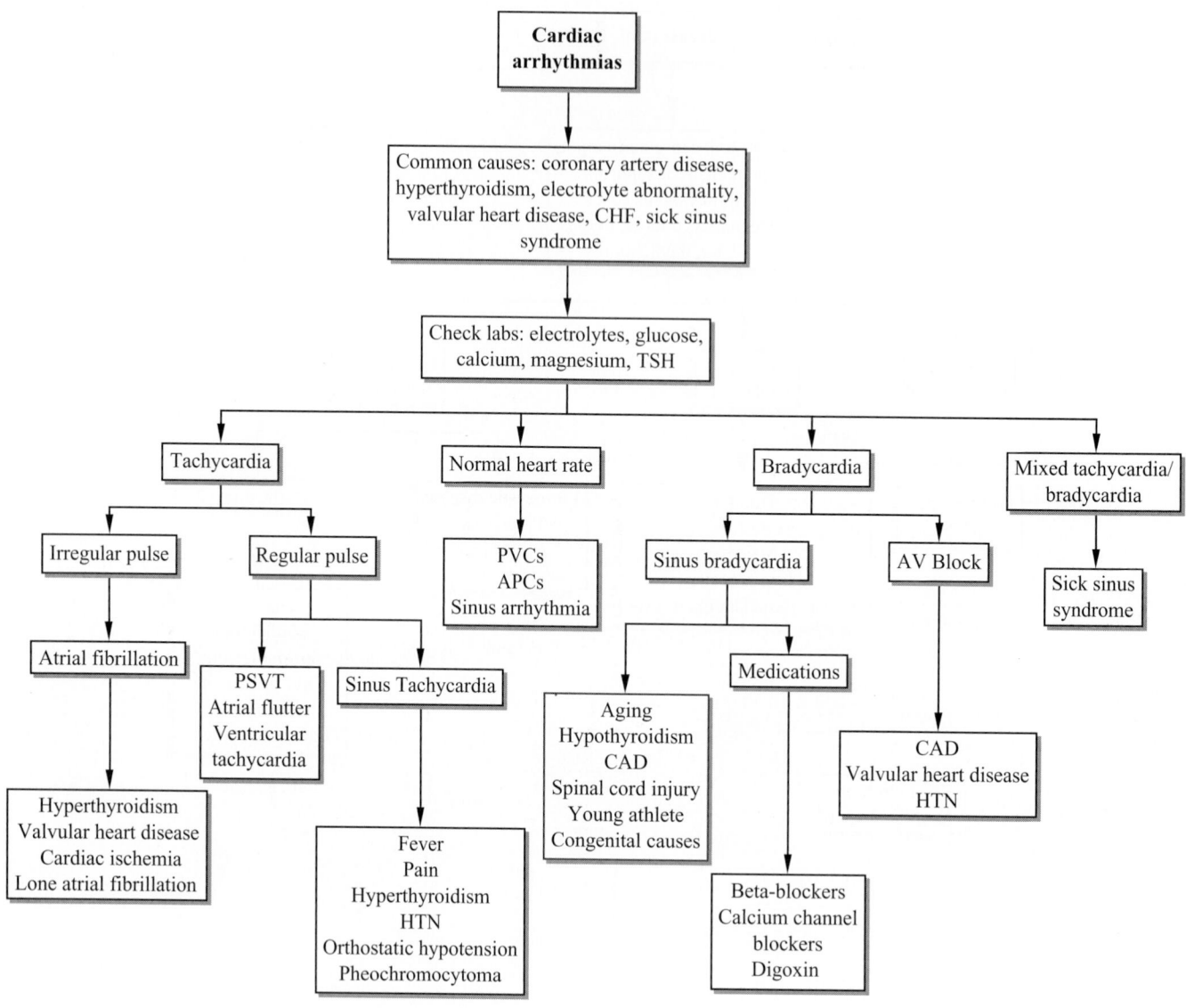

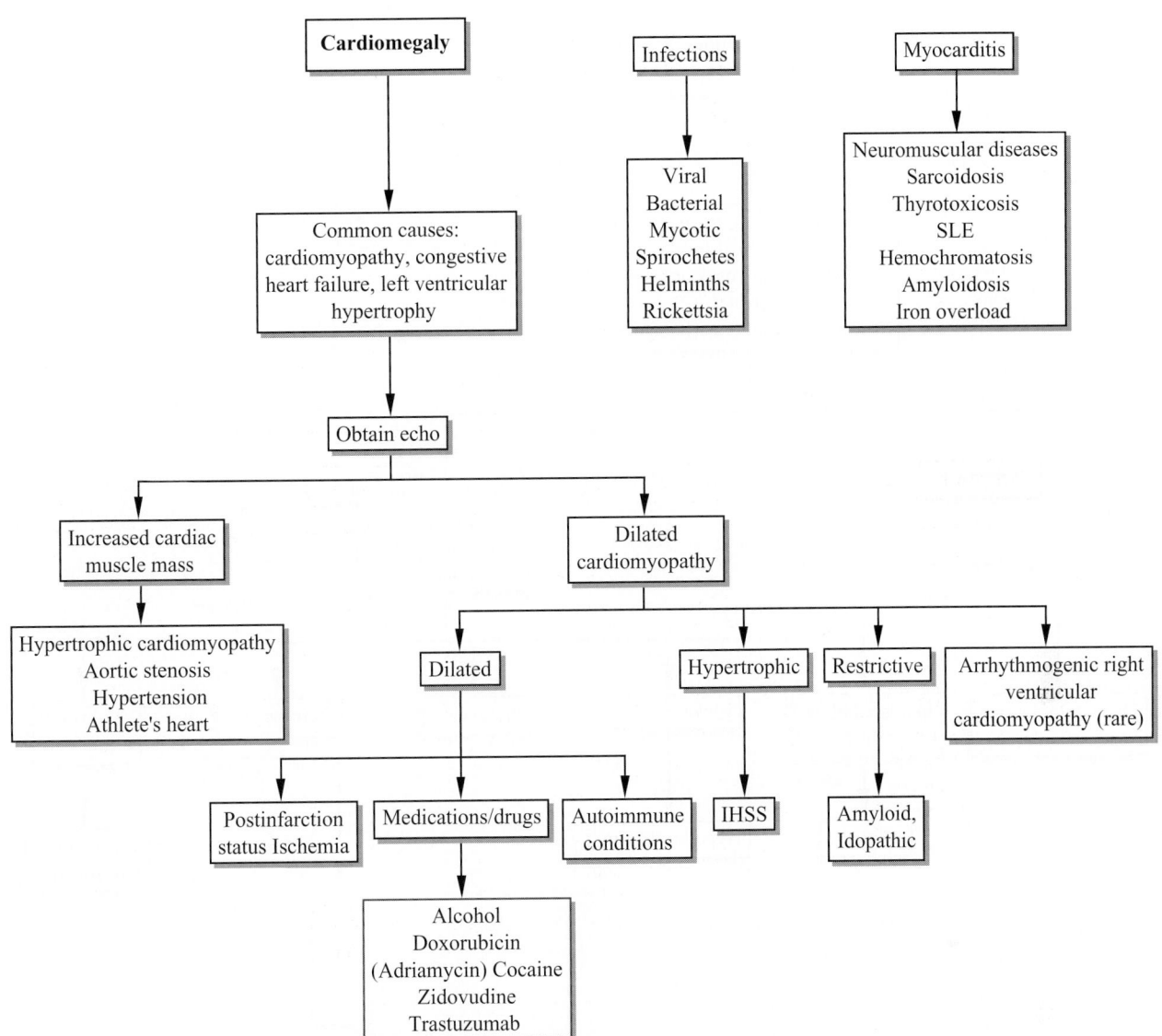

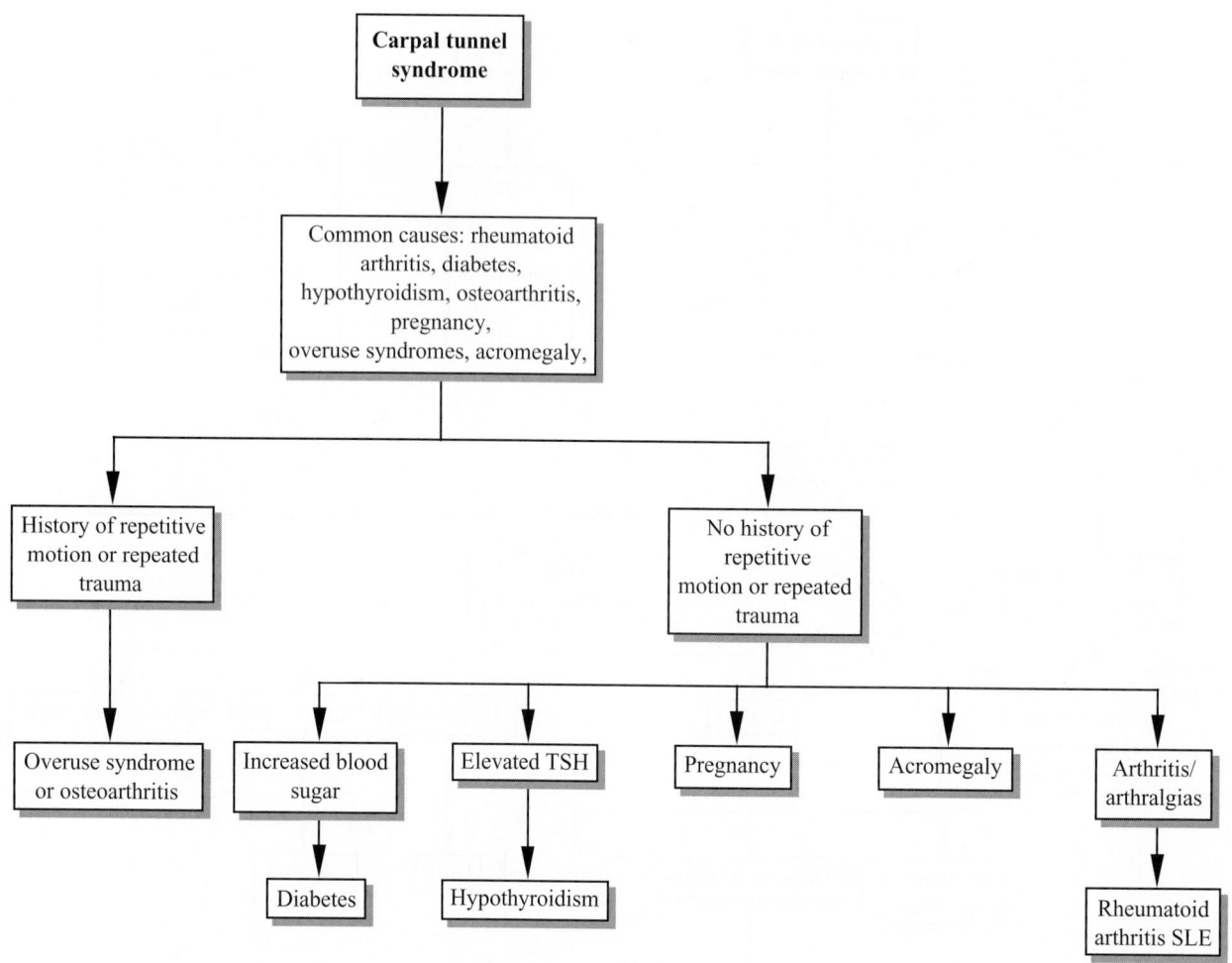

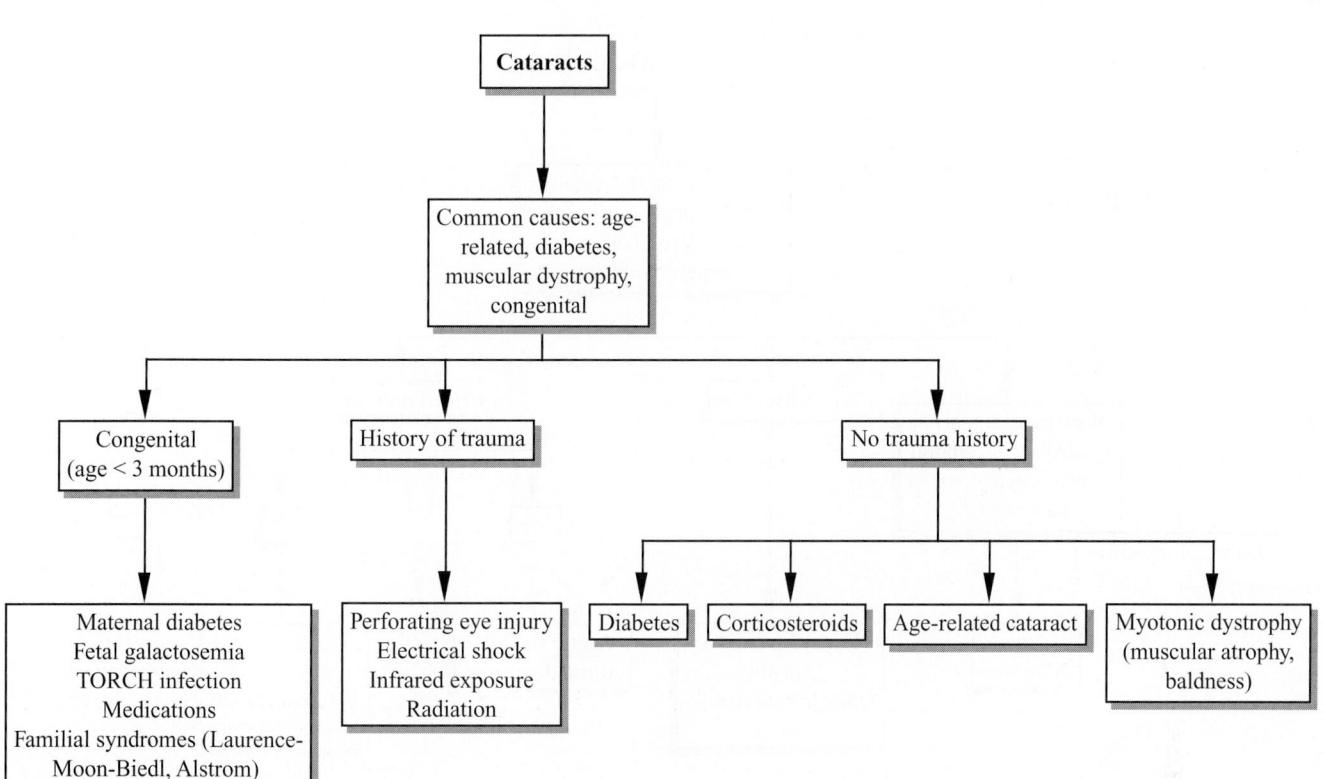

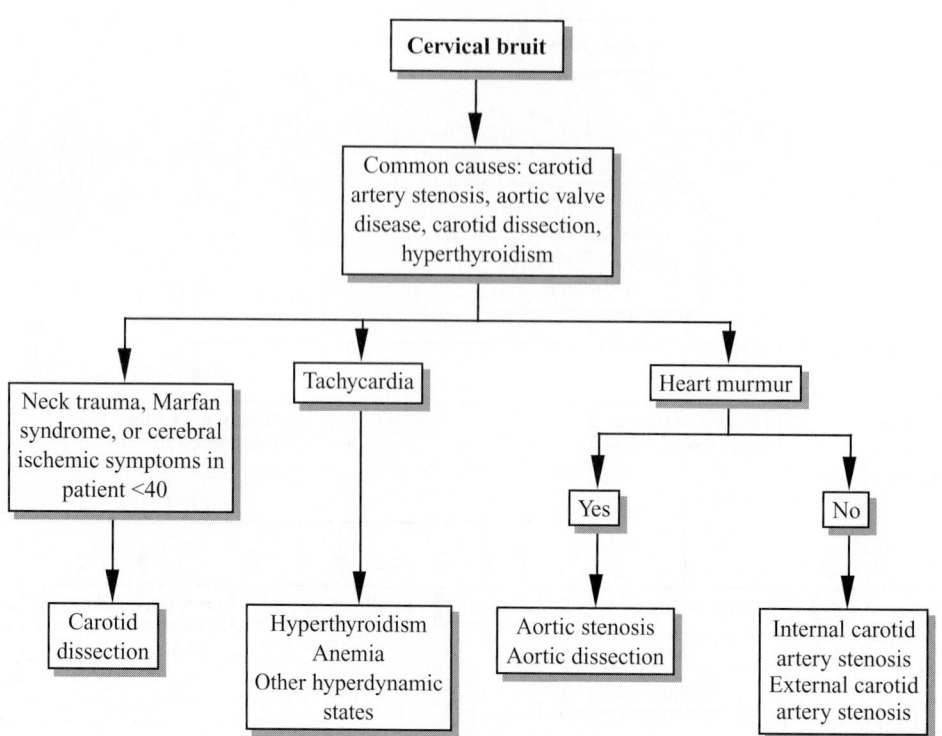

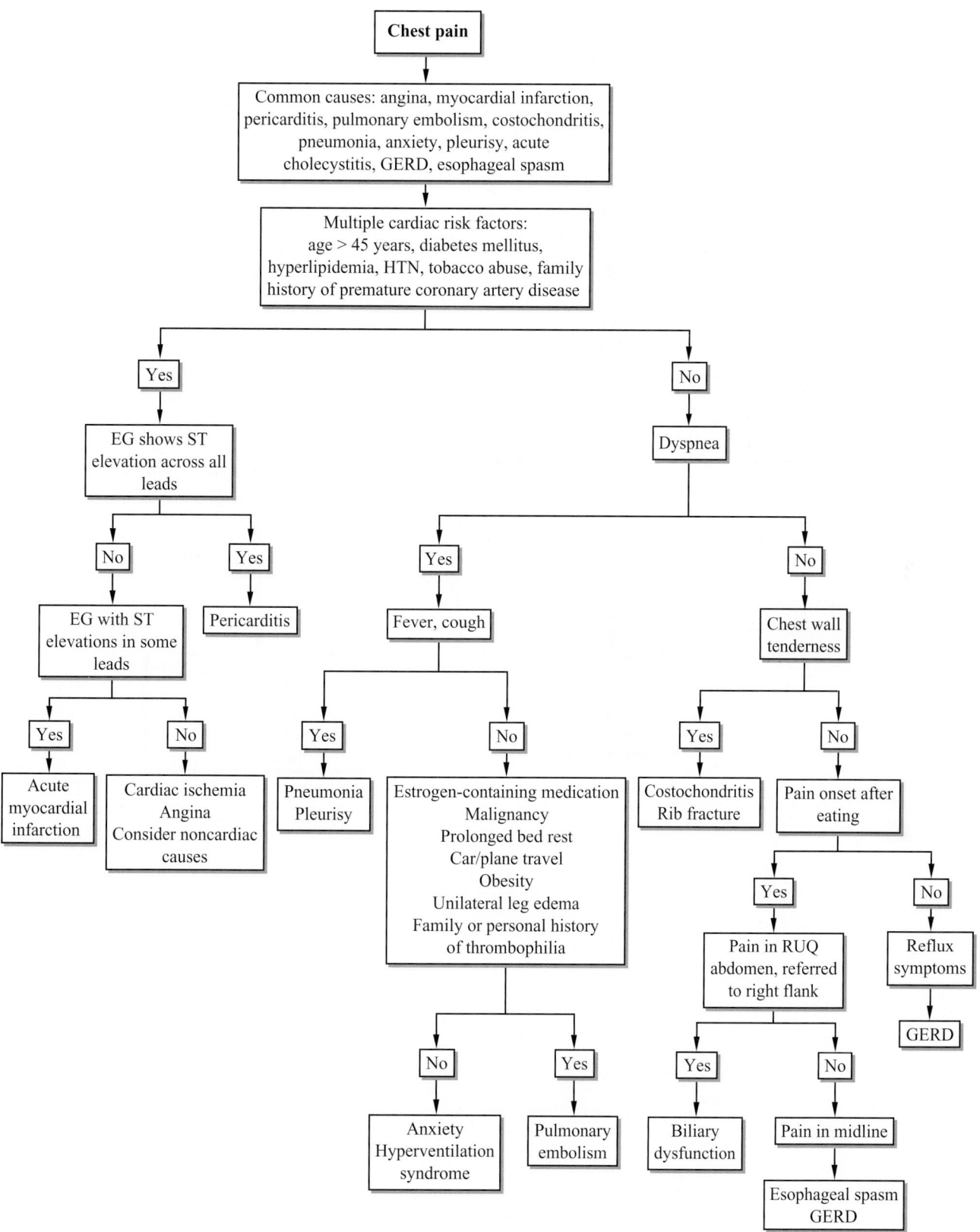

Chest pain

Common causes: angina, myocardial infarction, pericarditis, pulmonary embolism, costochondritis, pneumonia, anxiety, pleurisy, acute cholecystitis, GERD, esophageal spasm

Multiple cardiac risk factors: age > 45 years, diabetes mellitus, hyperlipidemia, HTN, tobacco abuse, family history of premature coronary artery disease

Yes

No

EG shows ST elevation across all leads

Dyspnea

No

Yes

Yes

No

EG with ST elevations in some leads

Pericarditis

Fever, cough

Chest wall tenderness

Yes

No

Yes

No

Yes

No

Acute myocardial infarction

Cardiac ischemia Angina Consider noncardiac causes

Pneumonia Pleurisy

Estrogen-containing medication Malignancy Prolonged bed rest Car/plane travel Obesity Unilateral leg edema Family or personal history of thrombophilia

Costochondritis Rib fracture

Pain onset after eating

Yes

No

Pain in RUQ abdomen, referred to right flank

Reflux symptoms

No

Yes

GERD

Anxiety Hyperventilation syndrome

Pulmonary embolism

Yes

No

Biliary dysfunction

Pain in midline

Esophageal spasm GERD

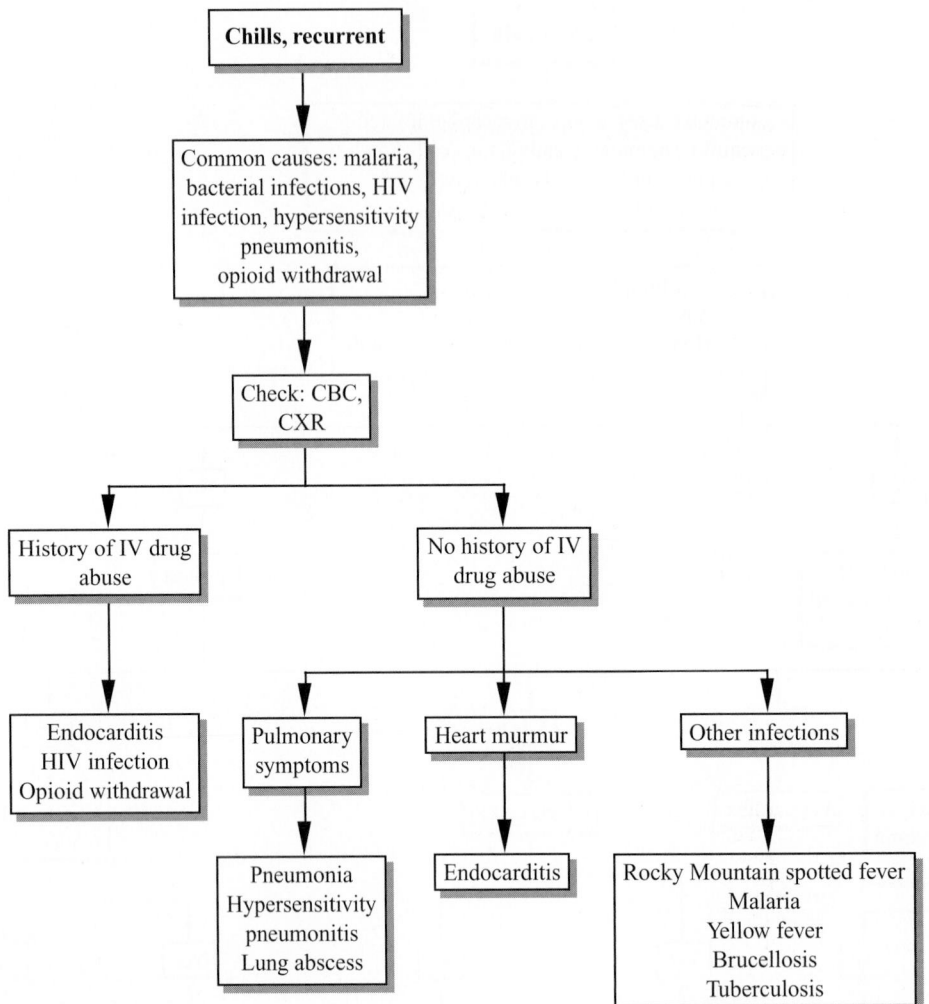

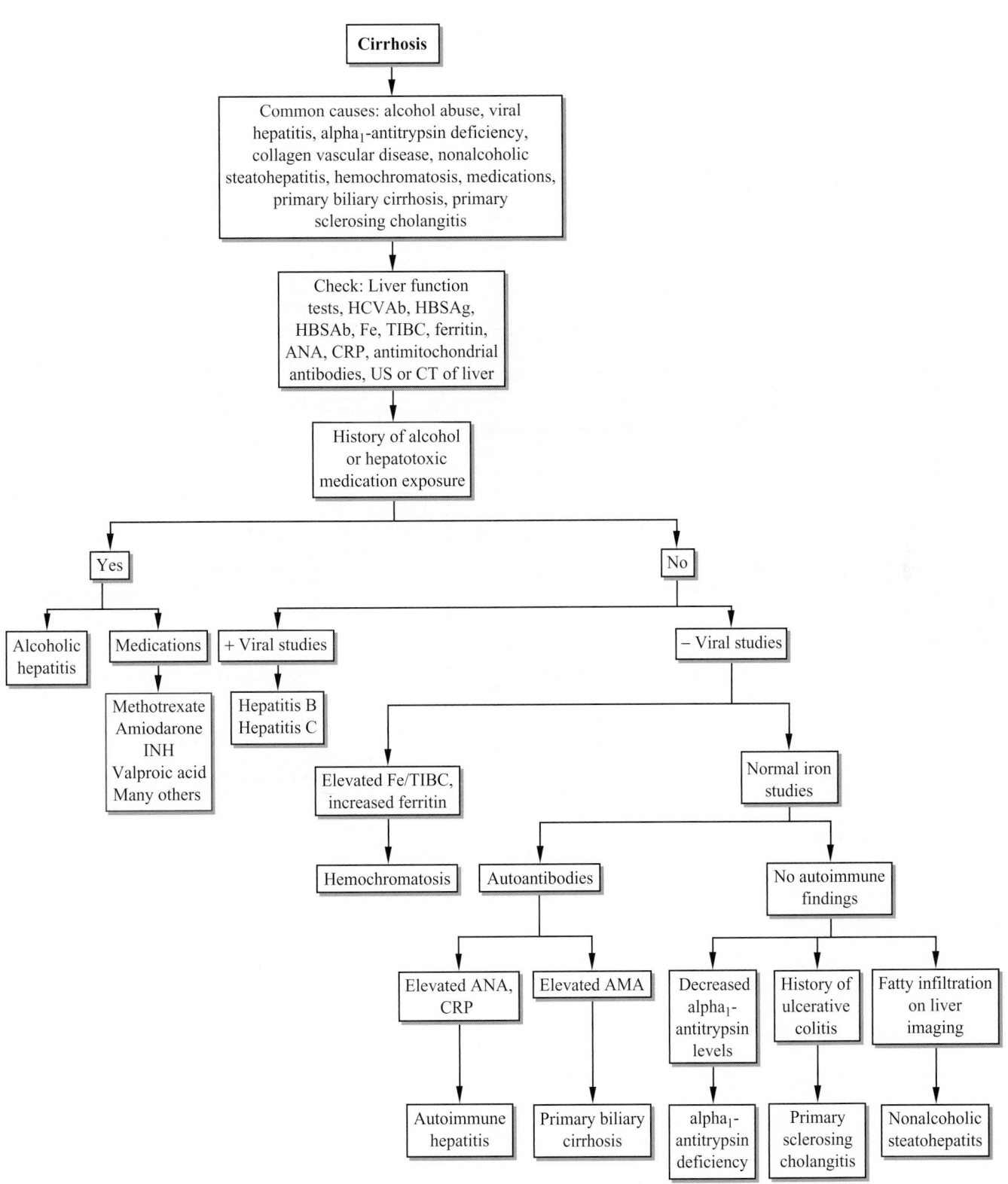

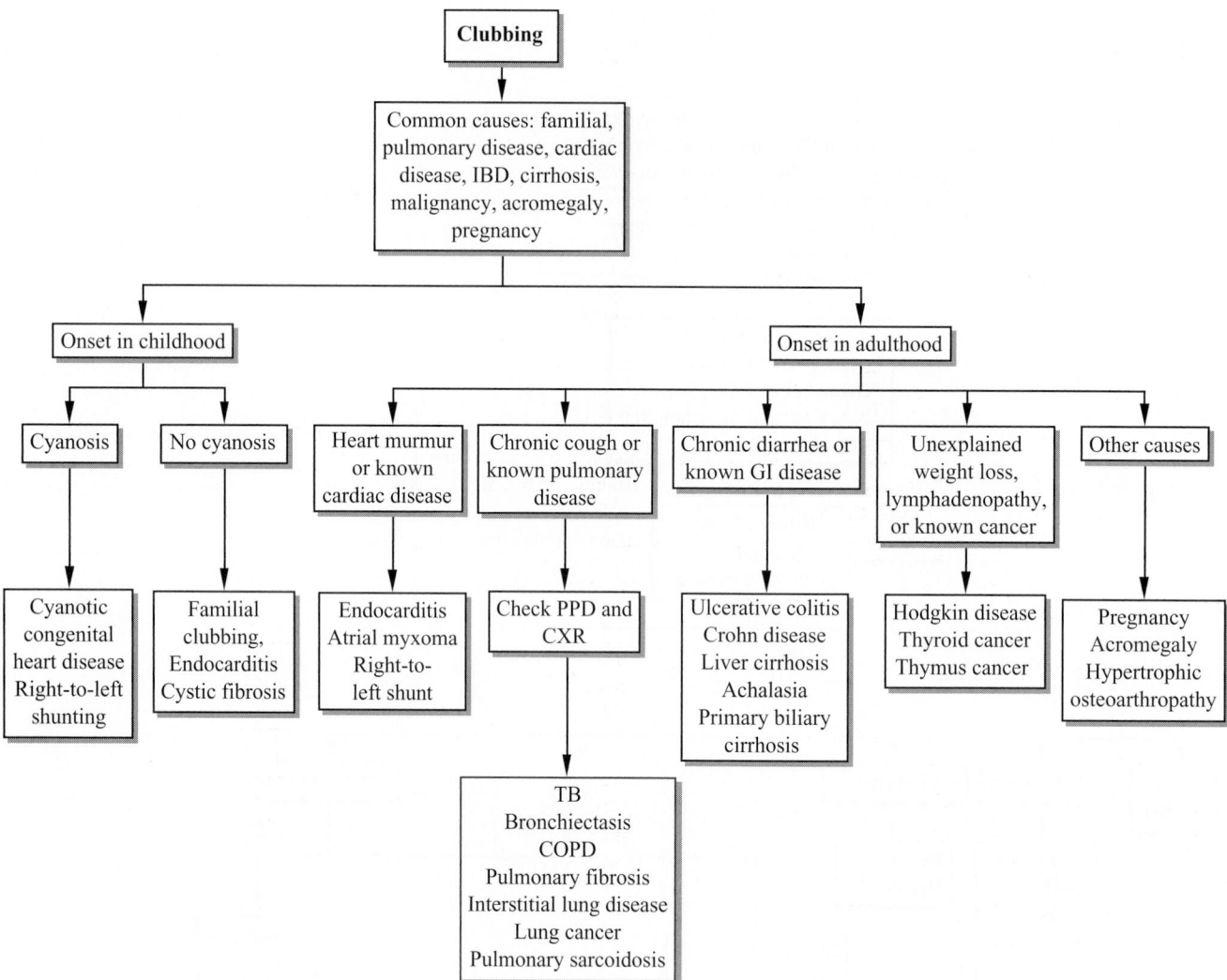

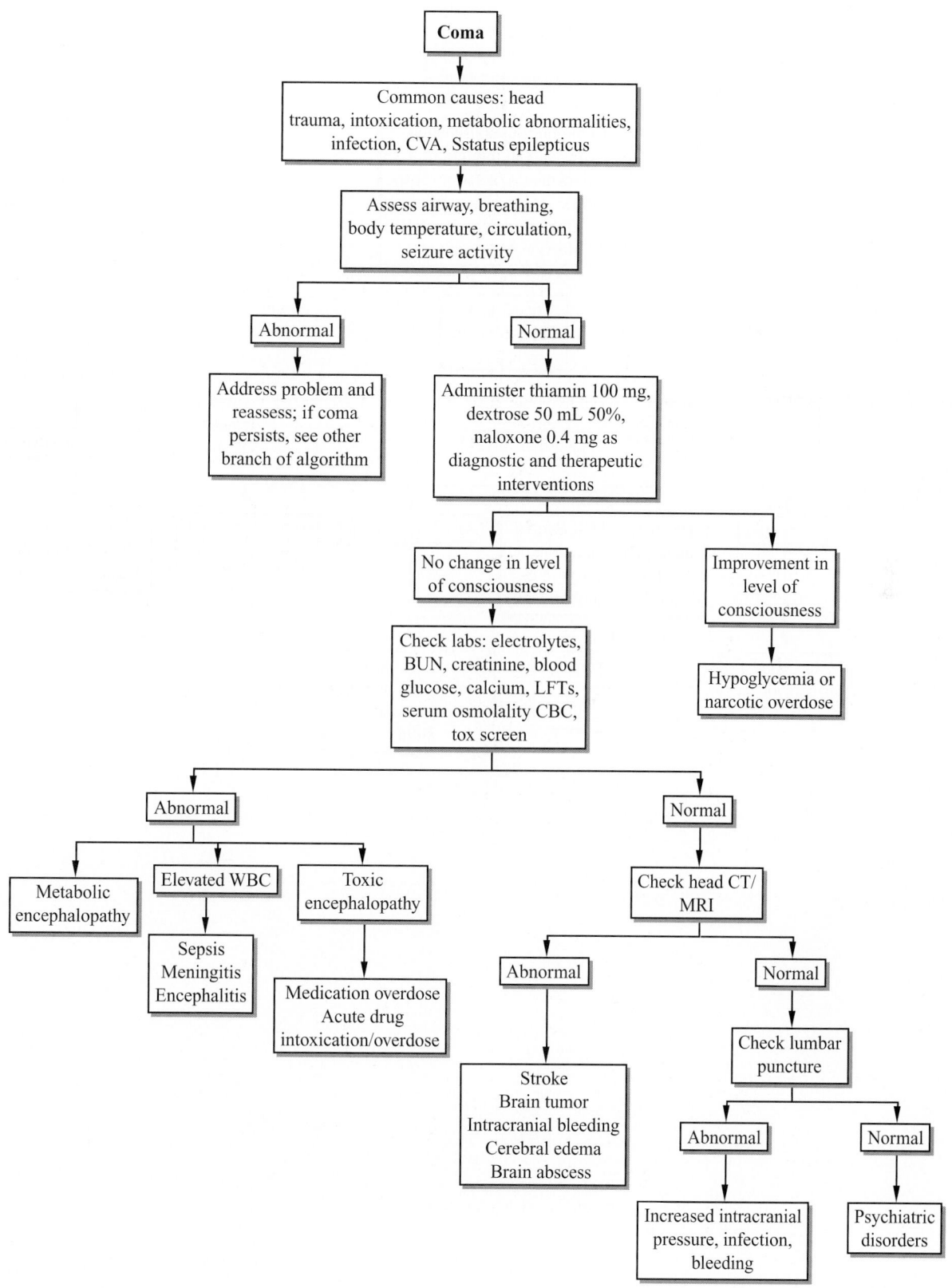

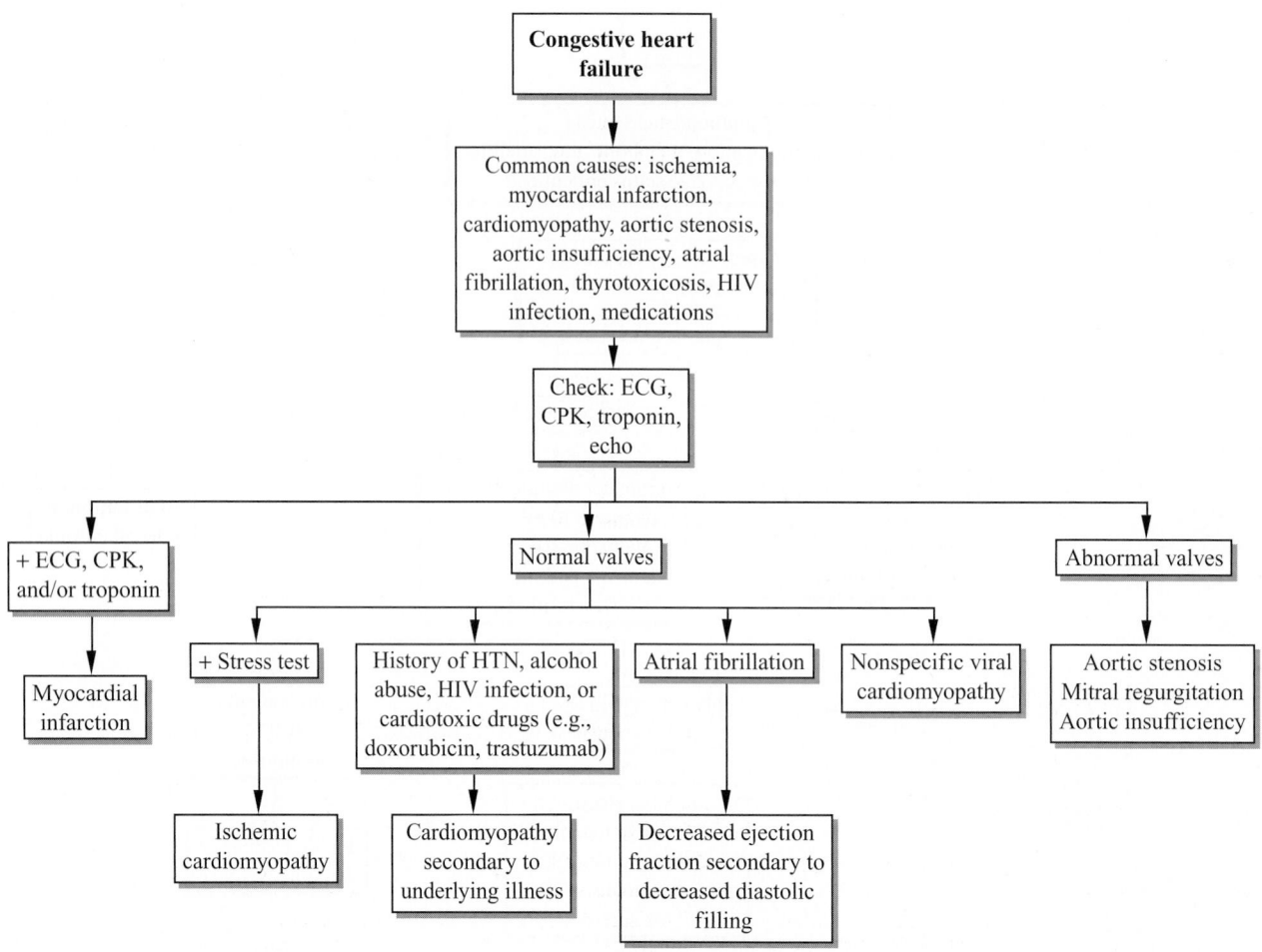

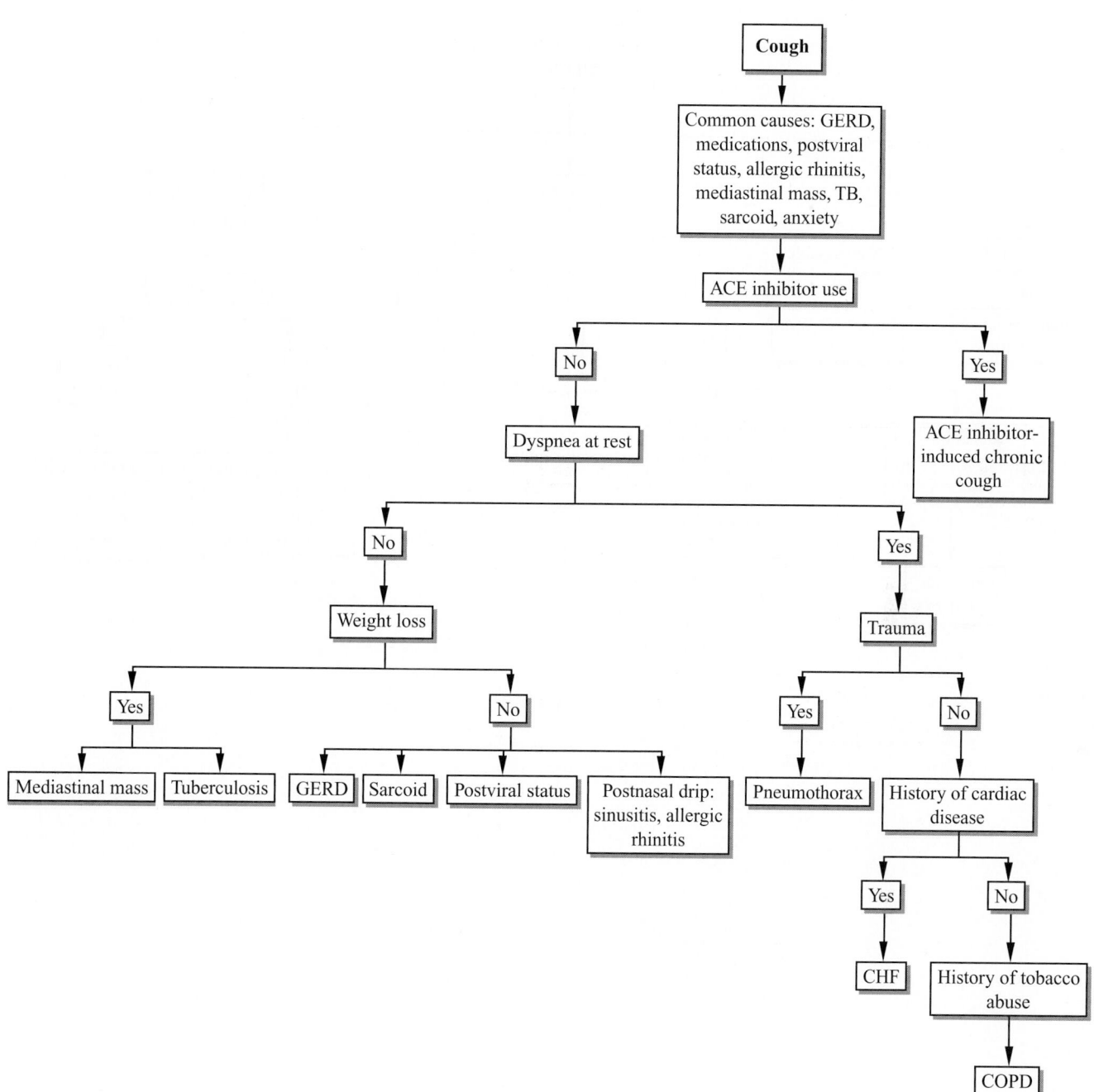

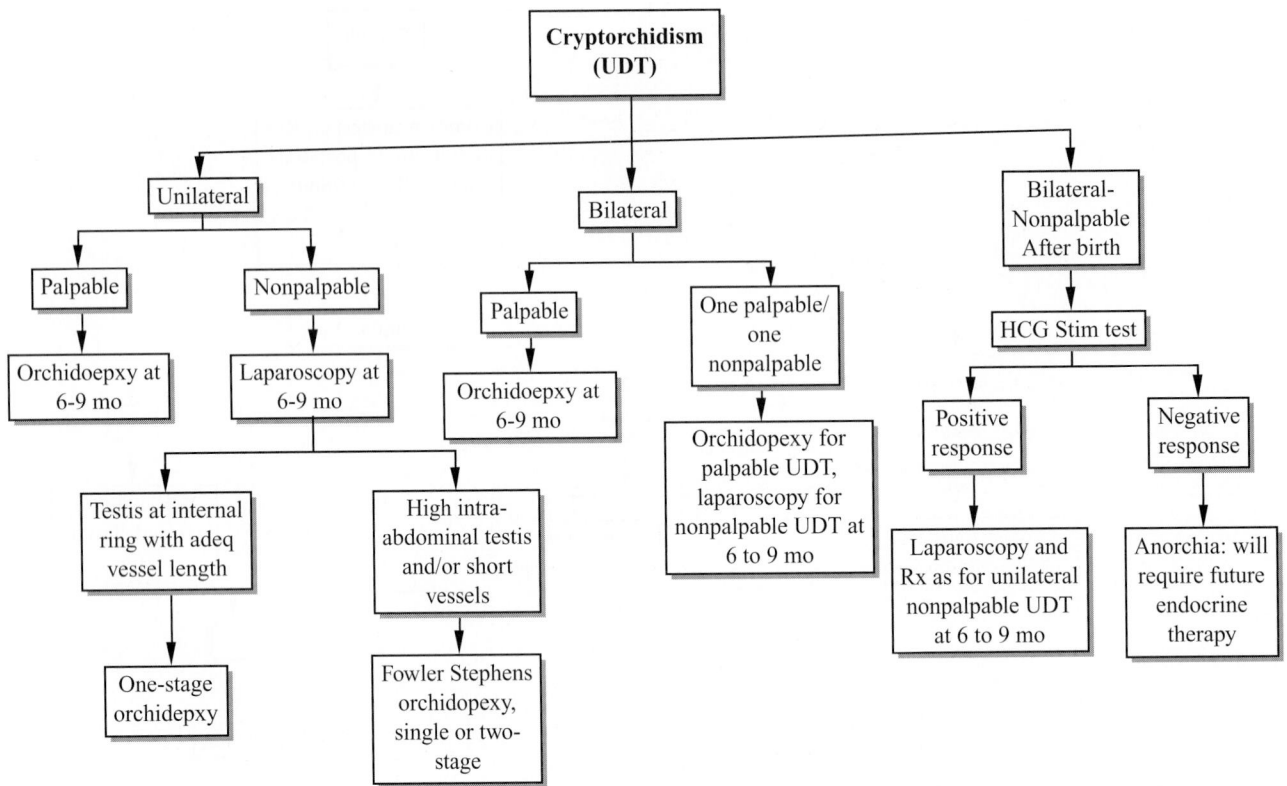

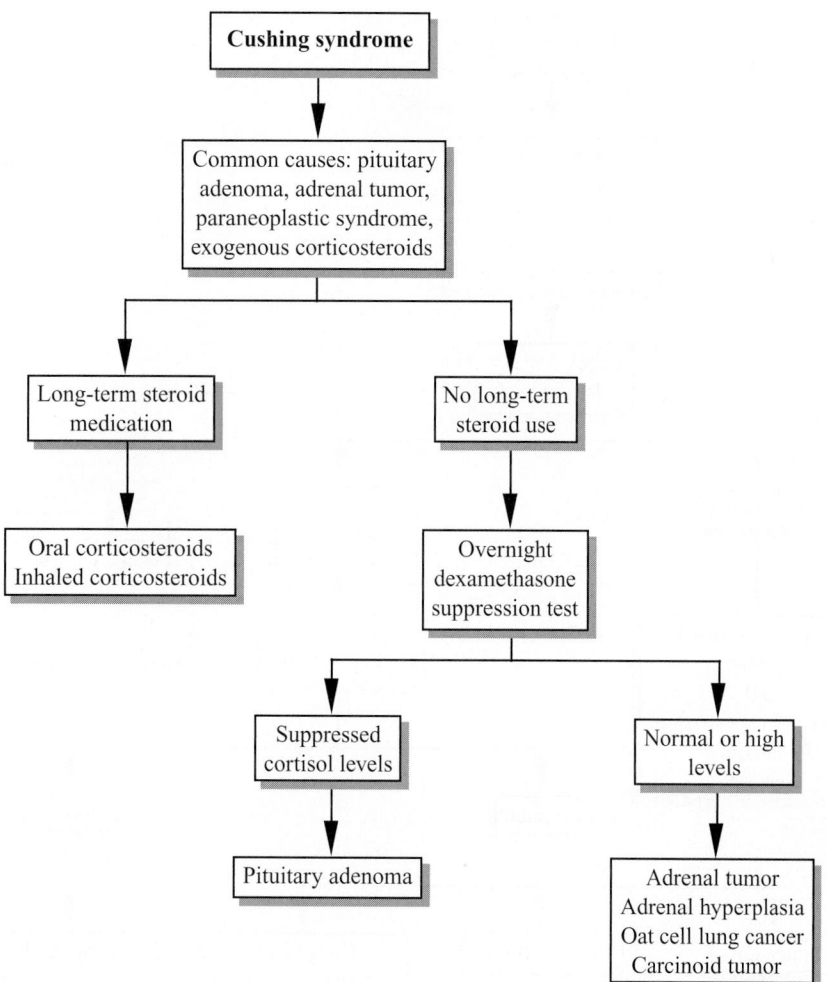

Cushing syndrome

↓

Common causes: pituitary adenoma, adrenal tumor, paraneoplastic syndrome, exogenous corticosteroids

Long-term steroid medication

No long-term steroid use

Oral corticosteroids
Inhaled corticosteroids

Overnight dexamethasone suppression test

Suppressed cortisol levels

Normal or high levels

Pituitary adenoma

Adrenal tumor
Adrenal hyperplasia
Oat cell lung cancer
Carcinoid tumor

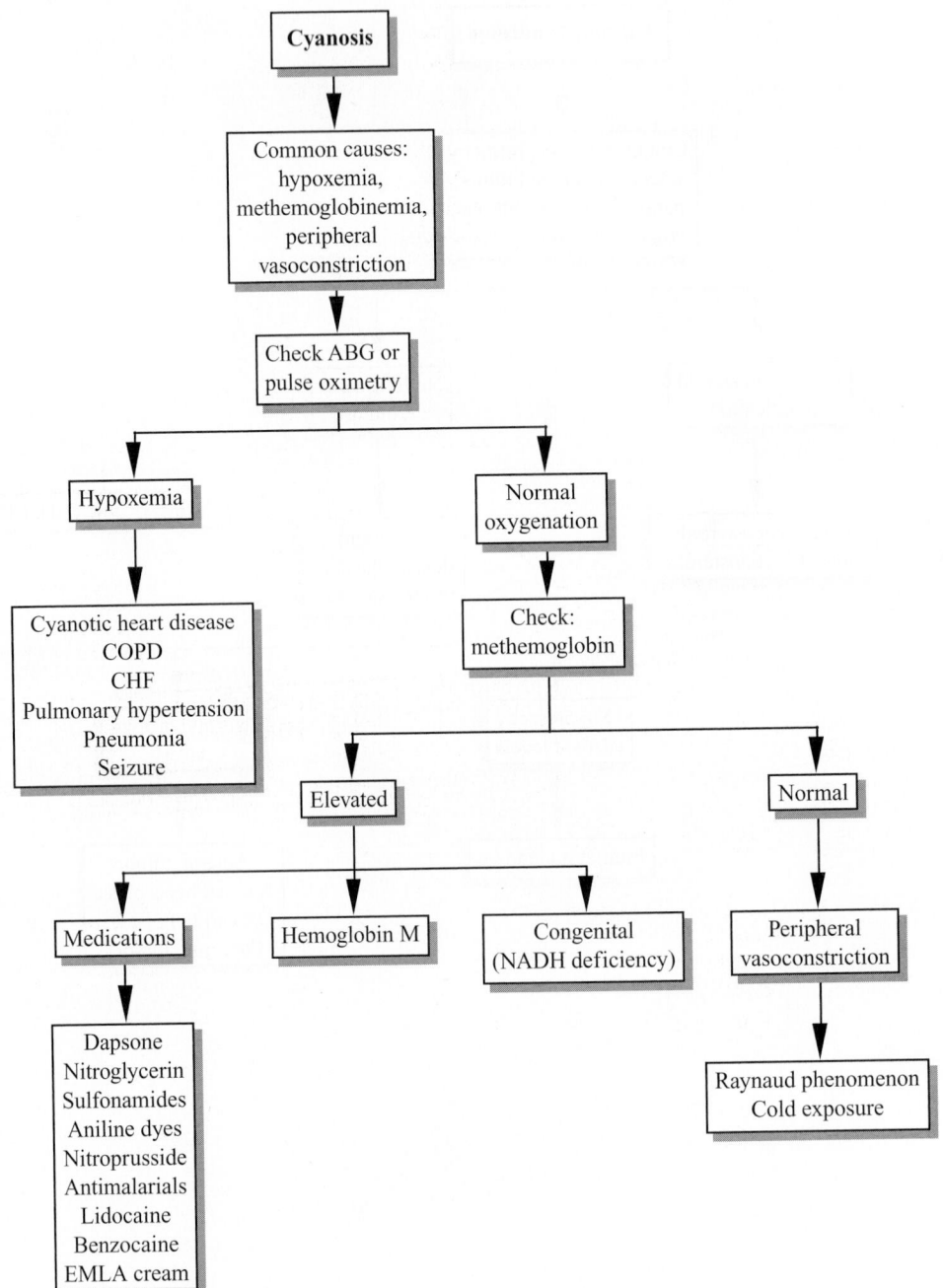

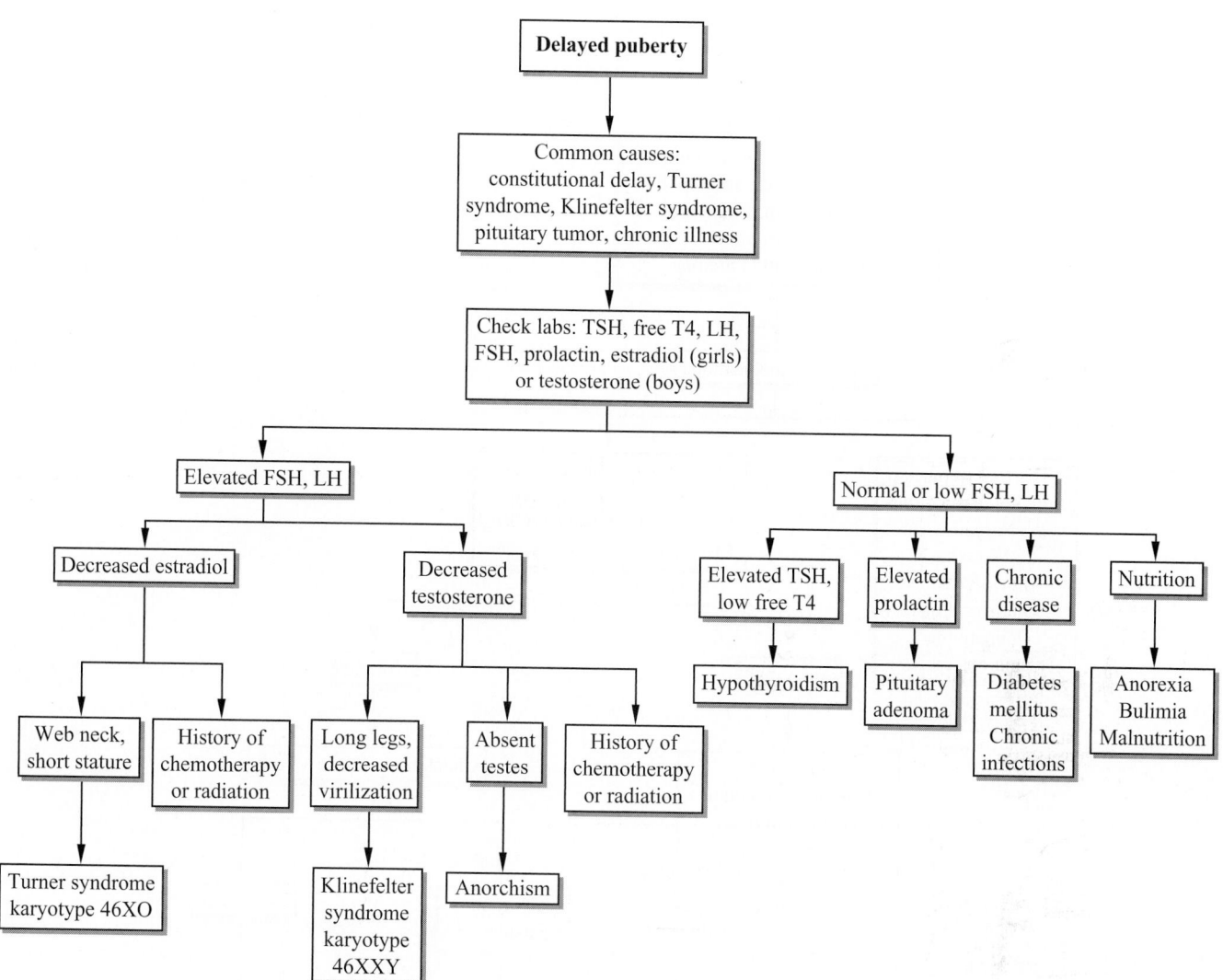

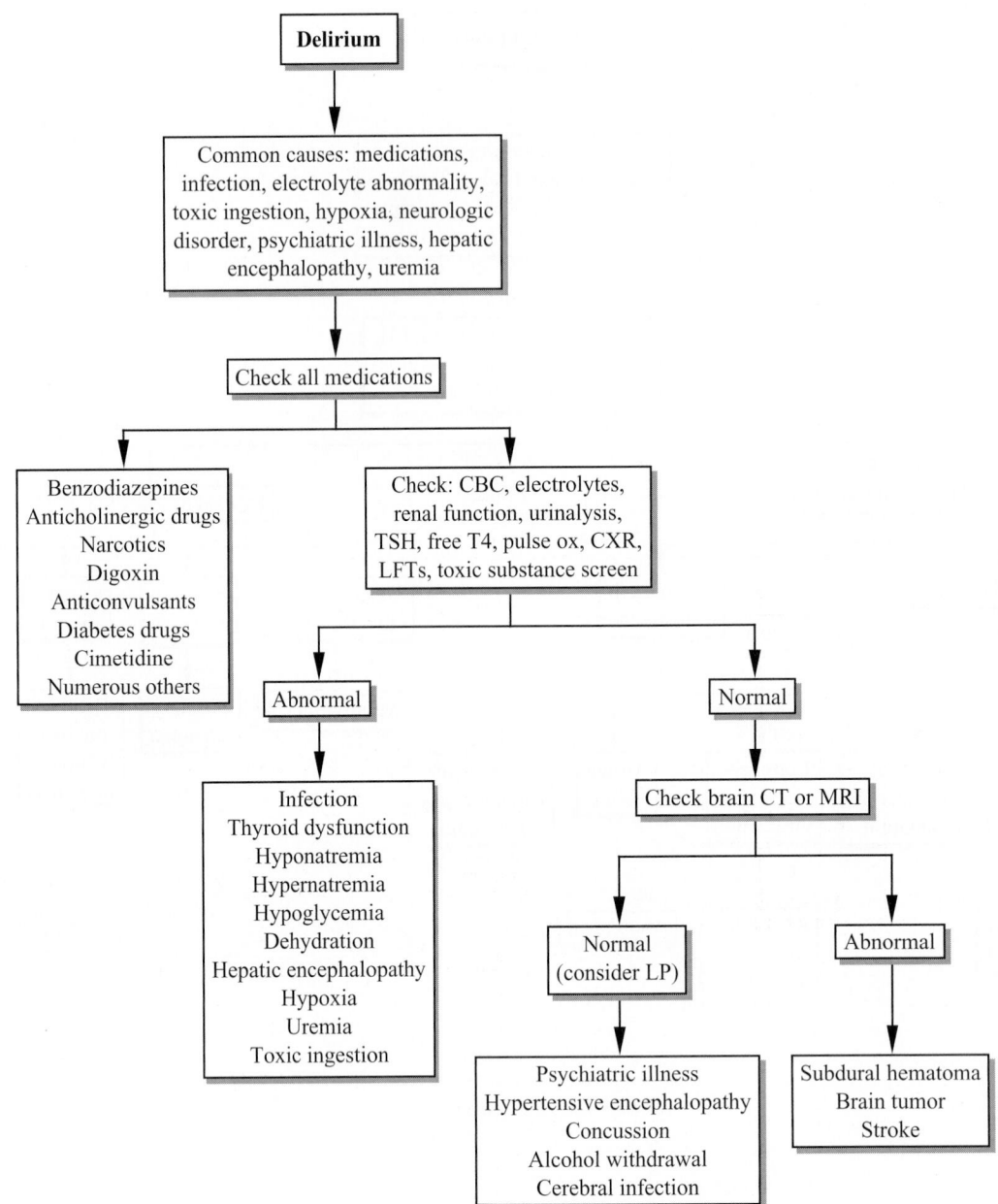

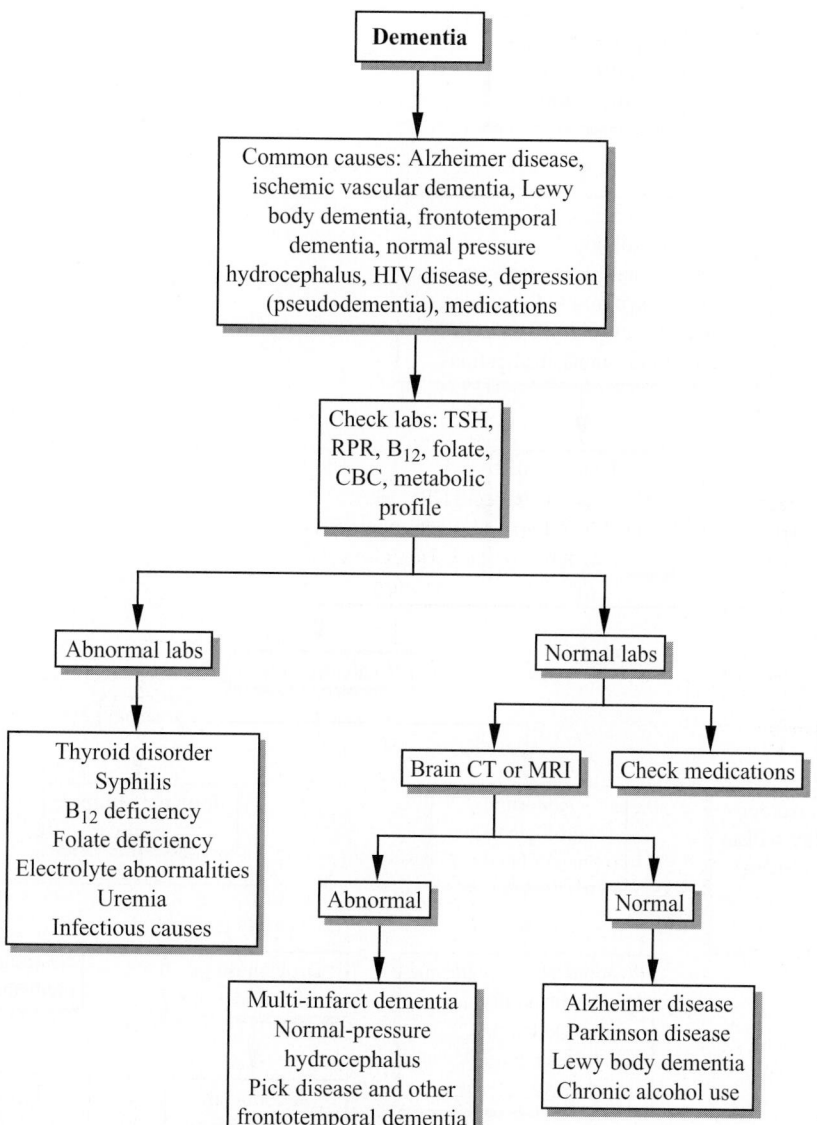

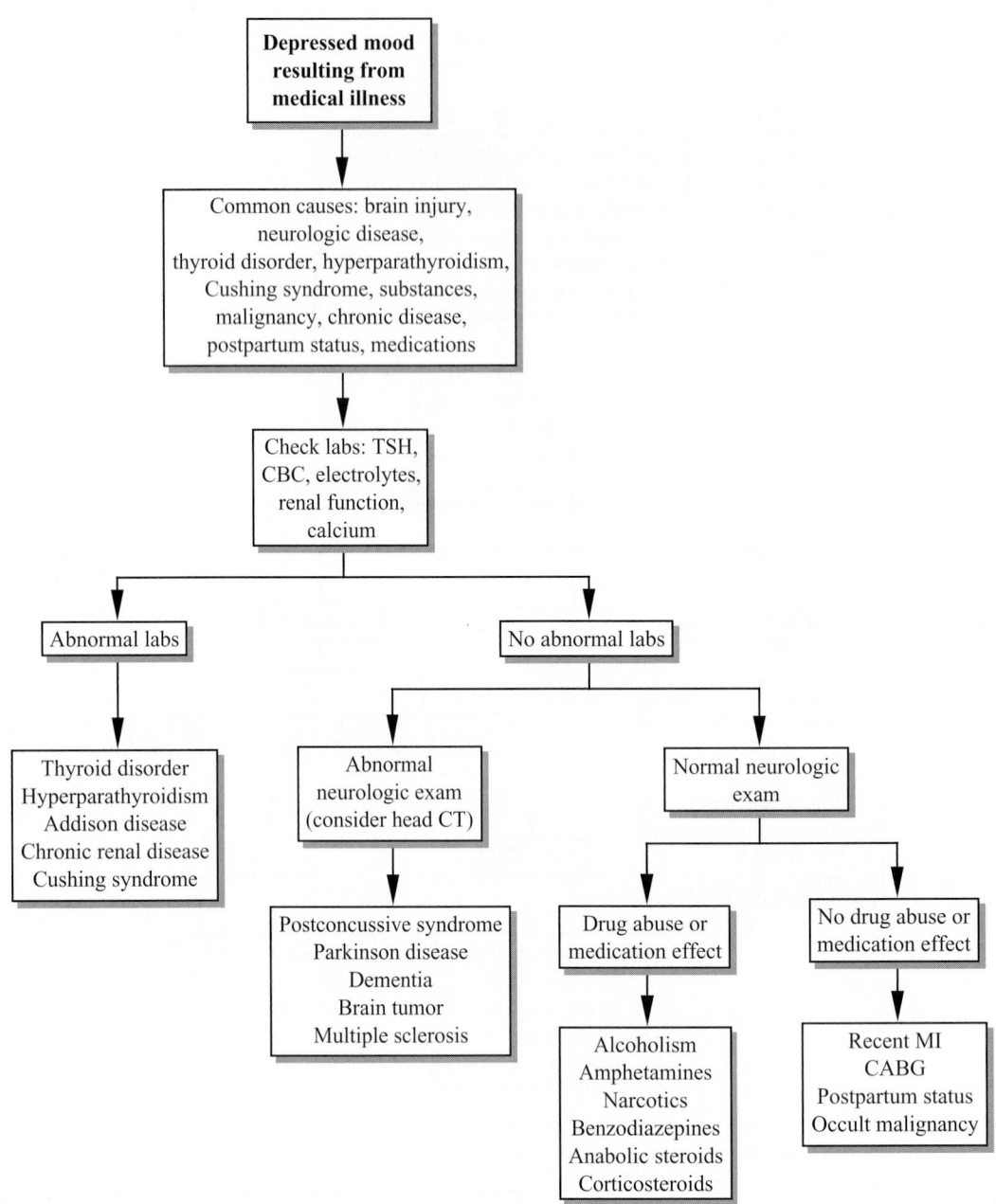

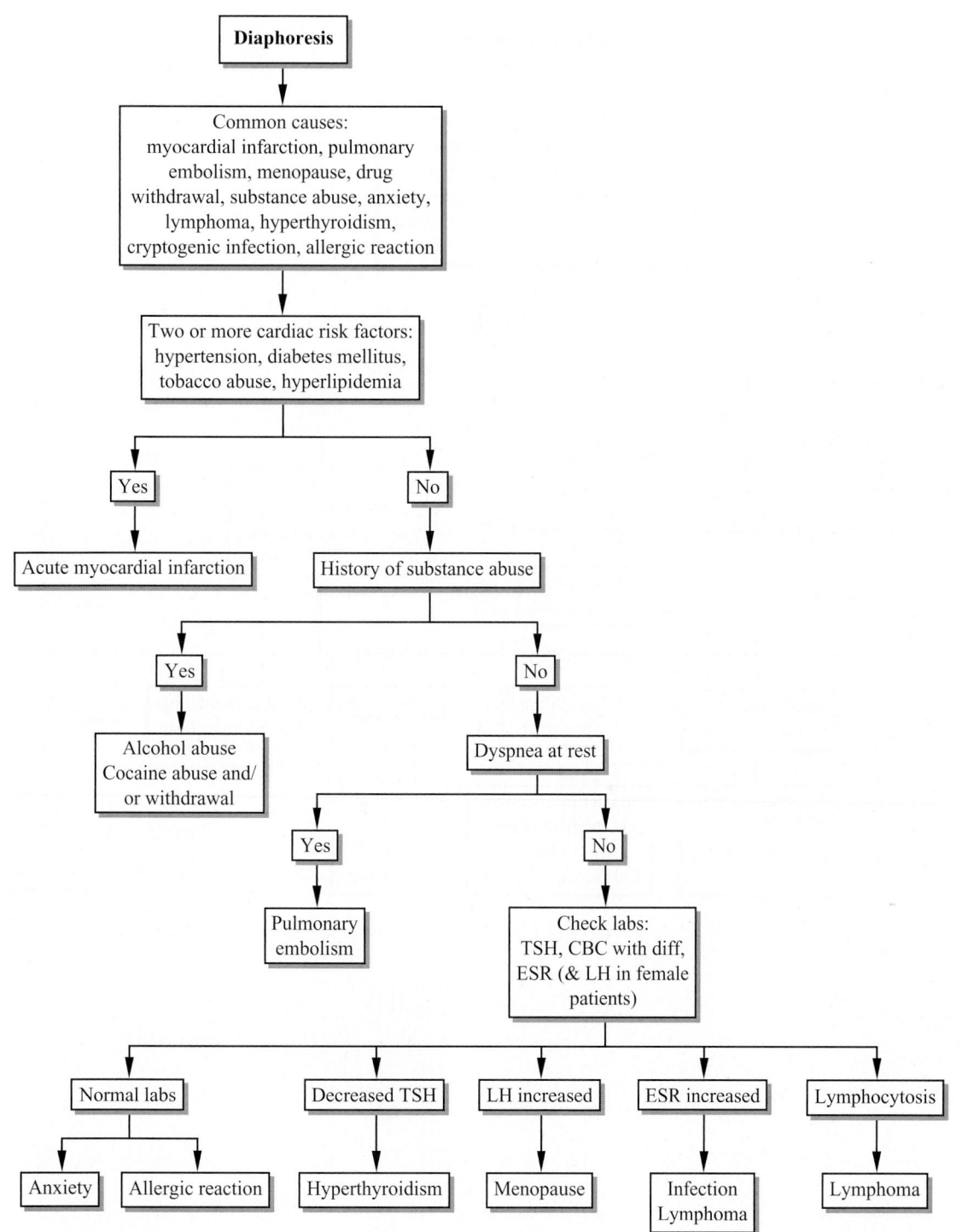

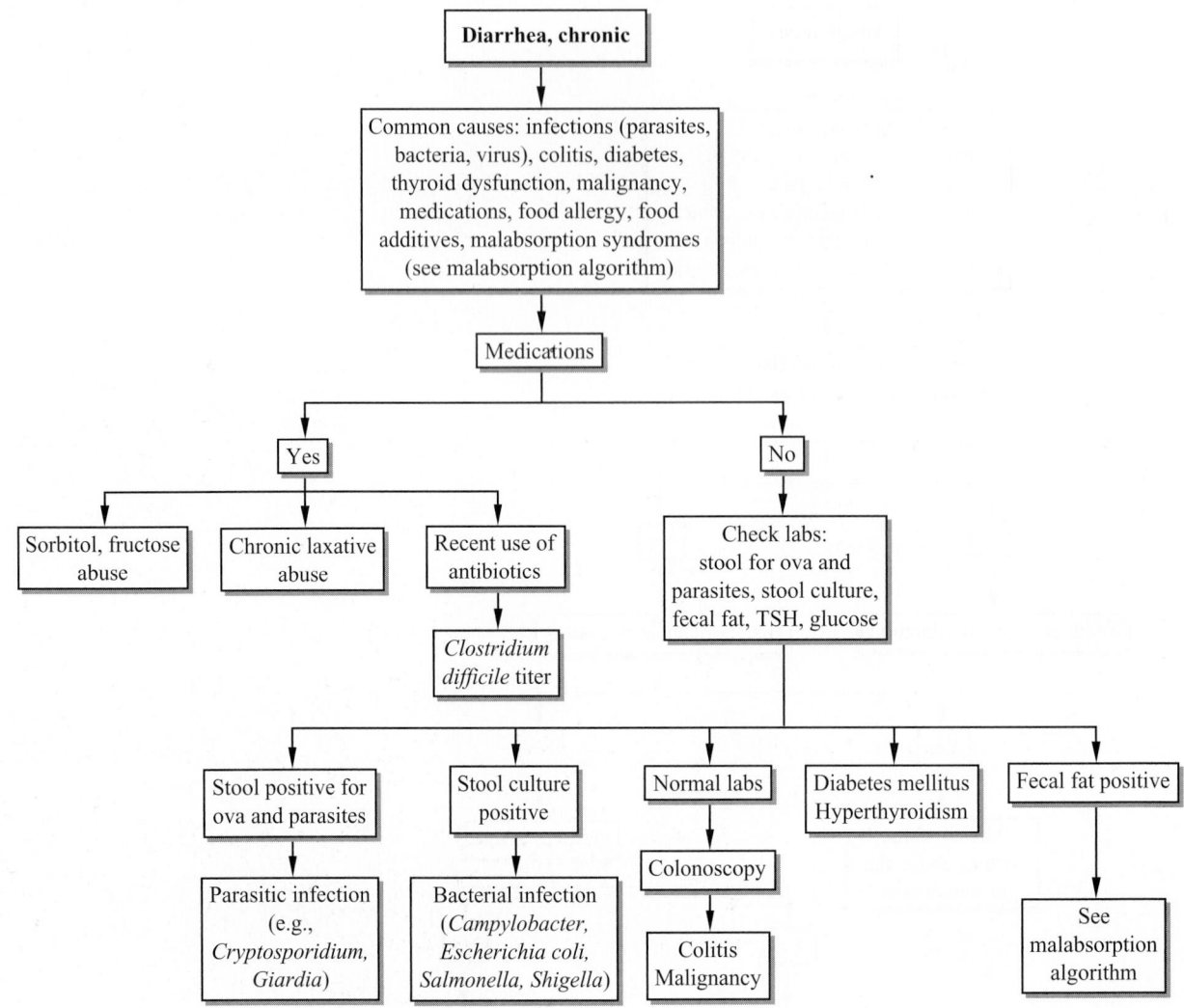

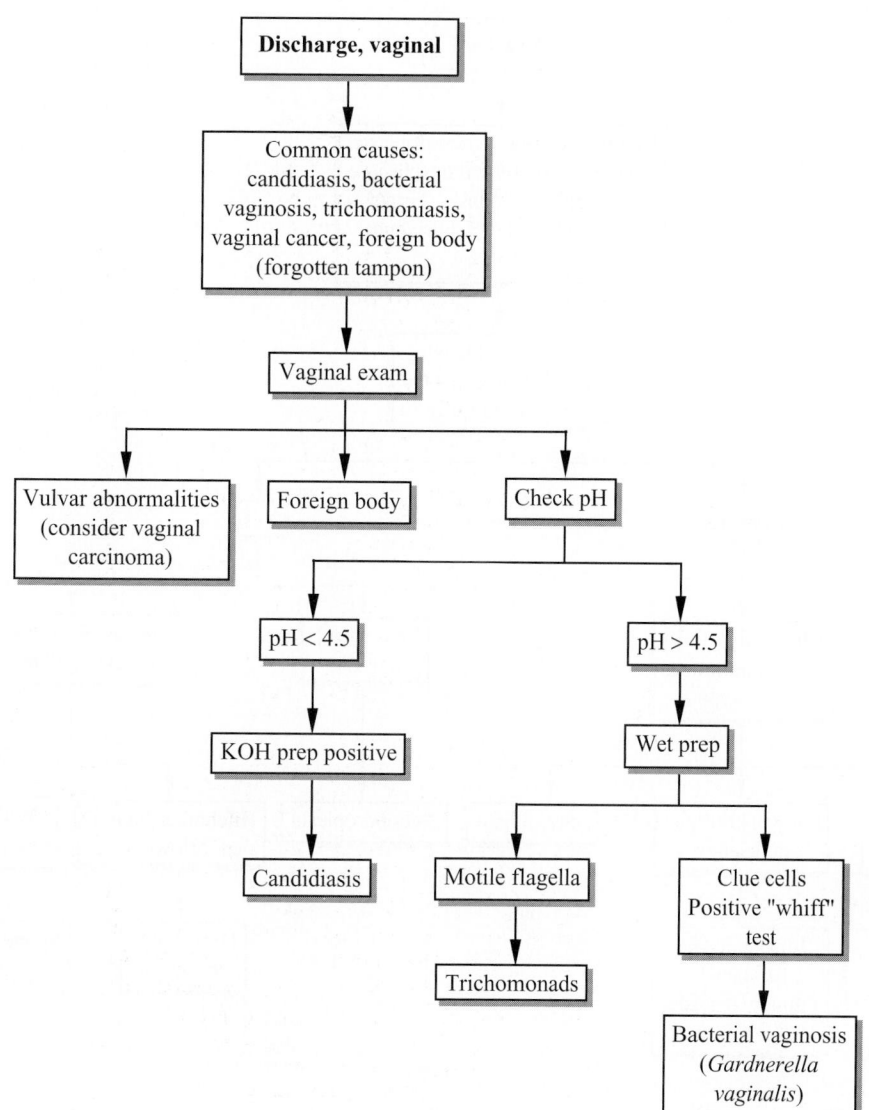

Discharge, vaginal

↓

Common causes:
candidiasis, bacterial
vaginosis, trichomoniasis,
vaginal cancer, foreign body
(forgotten tampon)

↓

Vaginal exam

Vulvar abnormalities
(consider vaginal
carcinoma)   Foreign body   Check pH

pH < 4.5   pH > 4.5

KOH prep positive   Wet prep

Candidiasis   Motile flagella   Clue cells
Positive "whiff"
test

Trichomonads   Bacterial vaginosis
(*Gardnerella
vaginalis*)

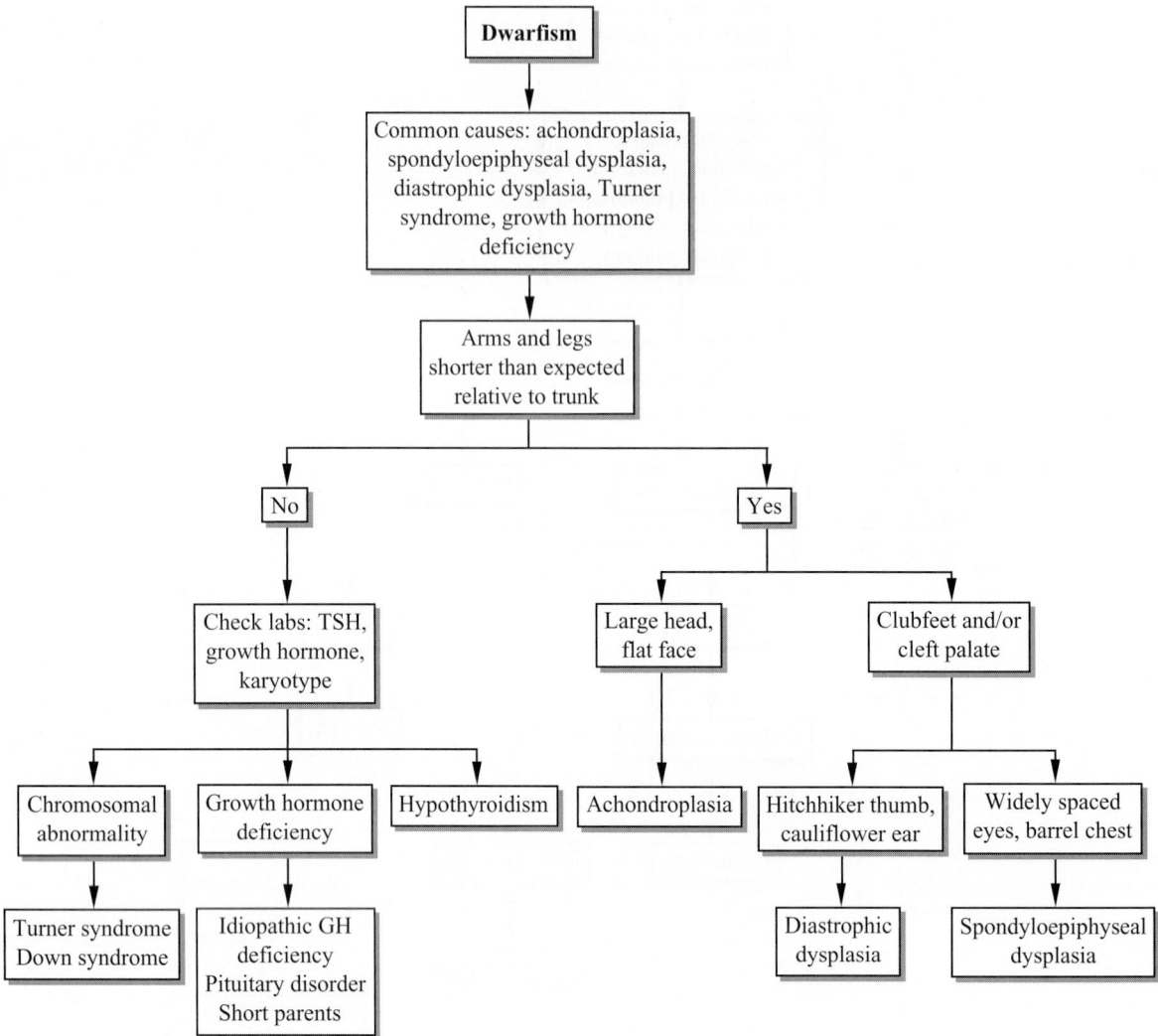

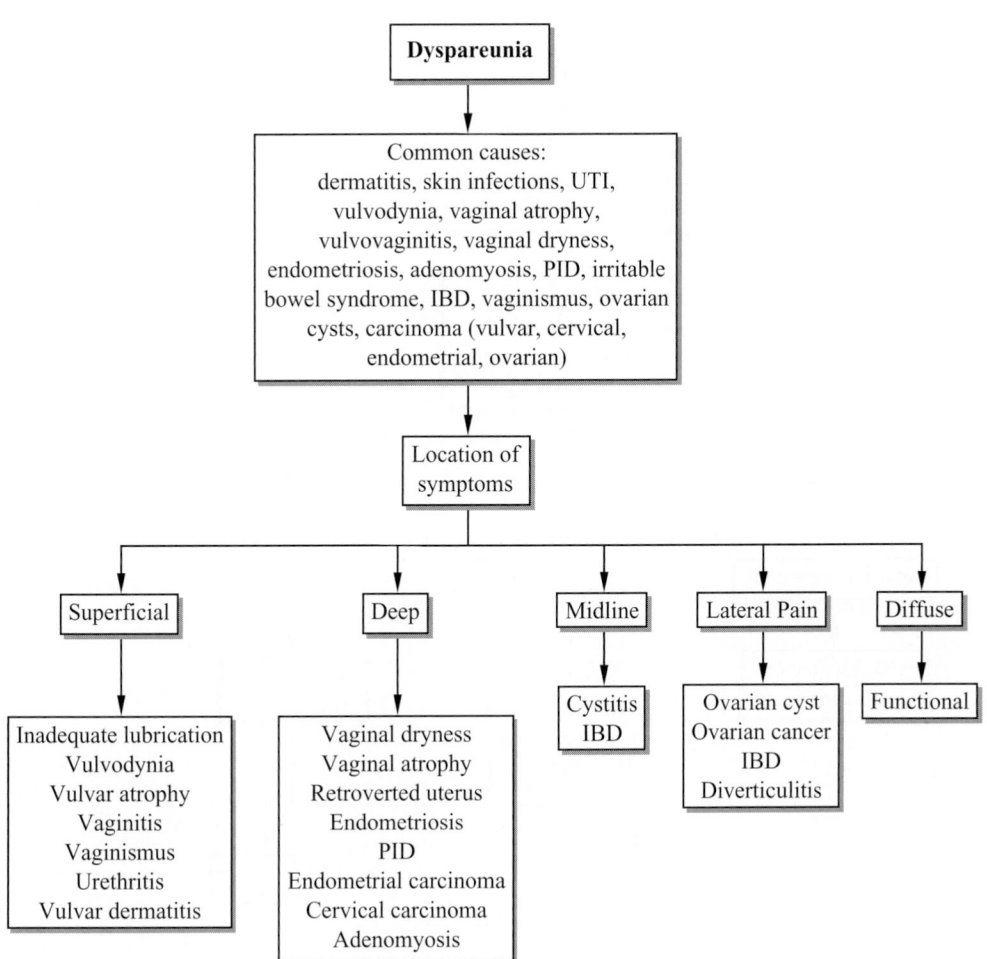

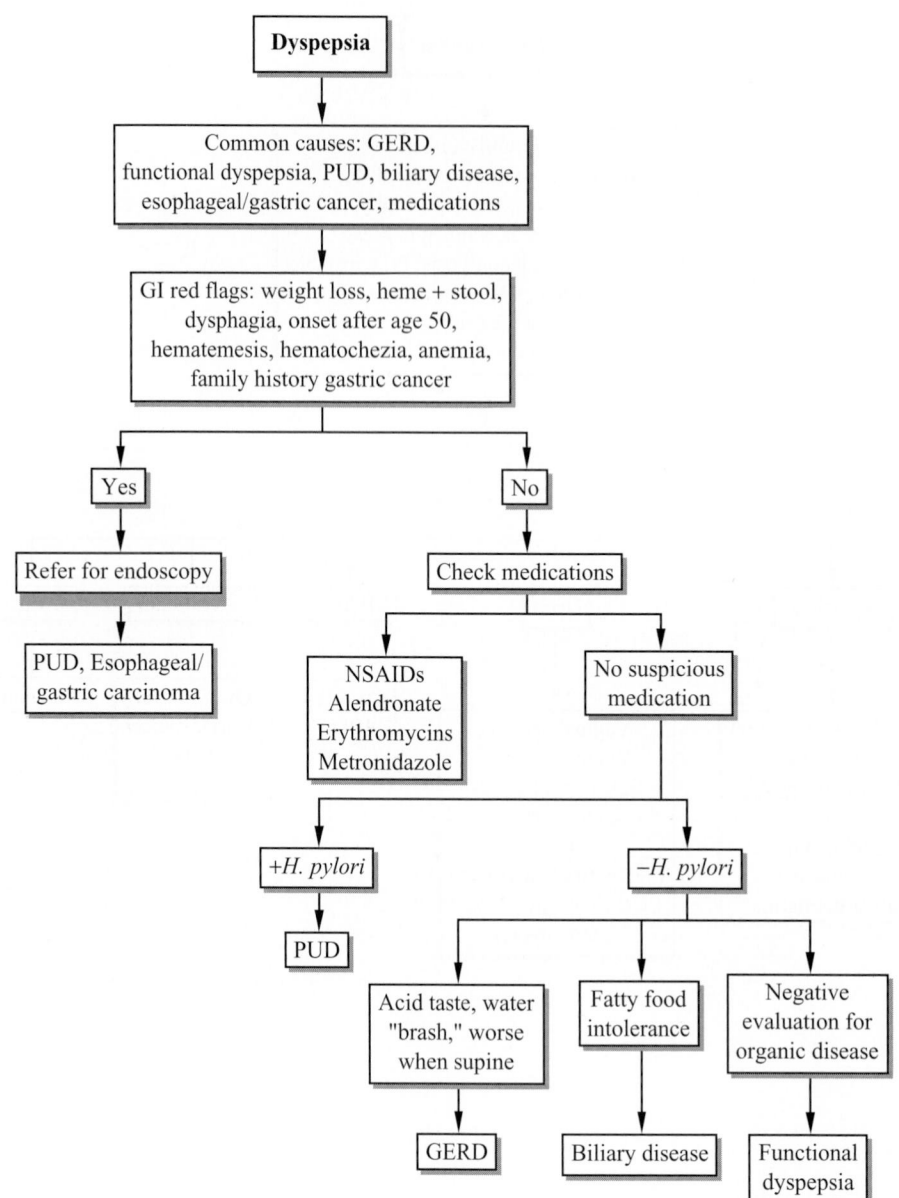

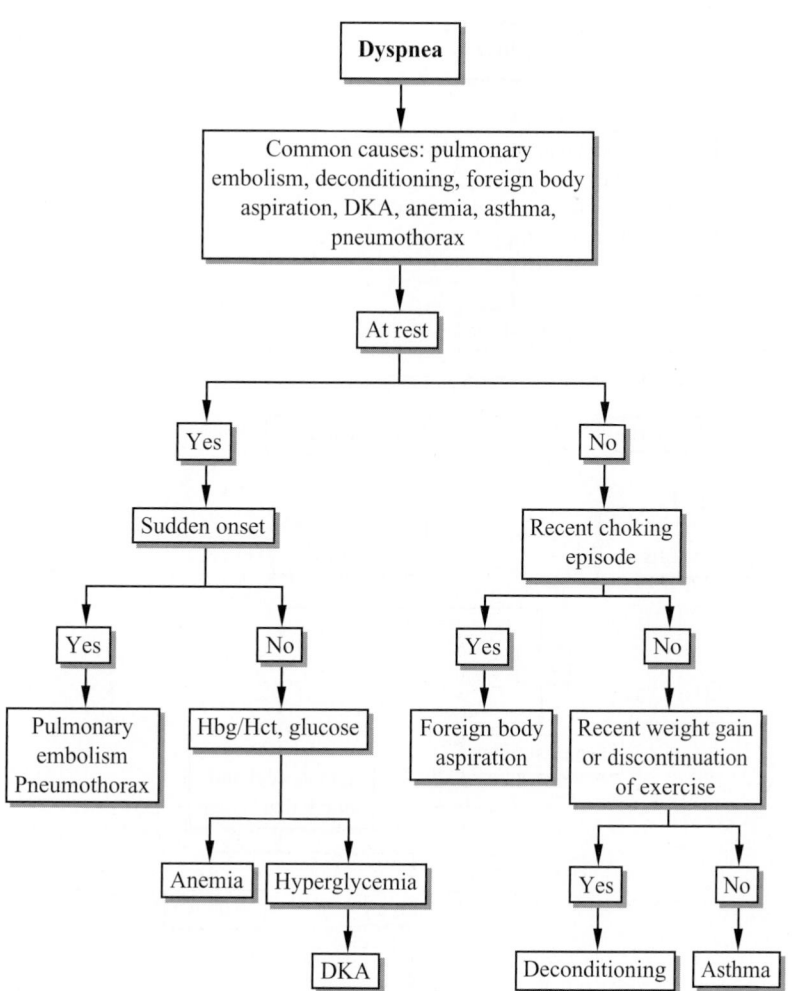

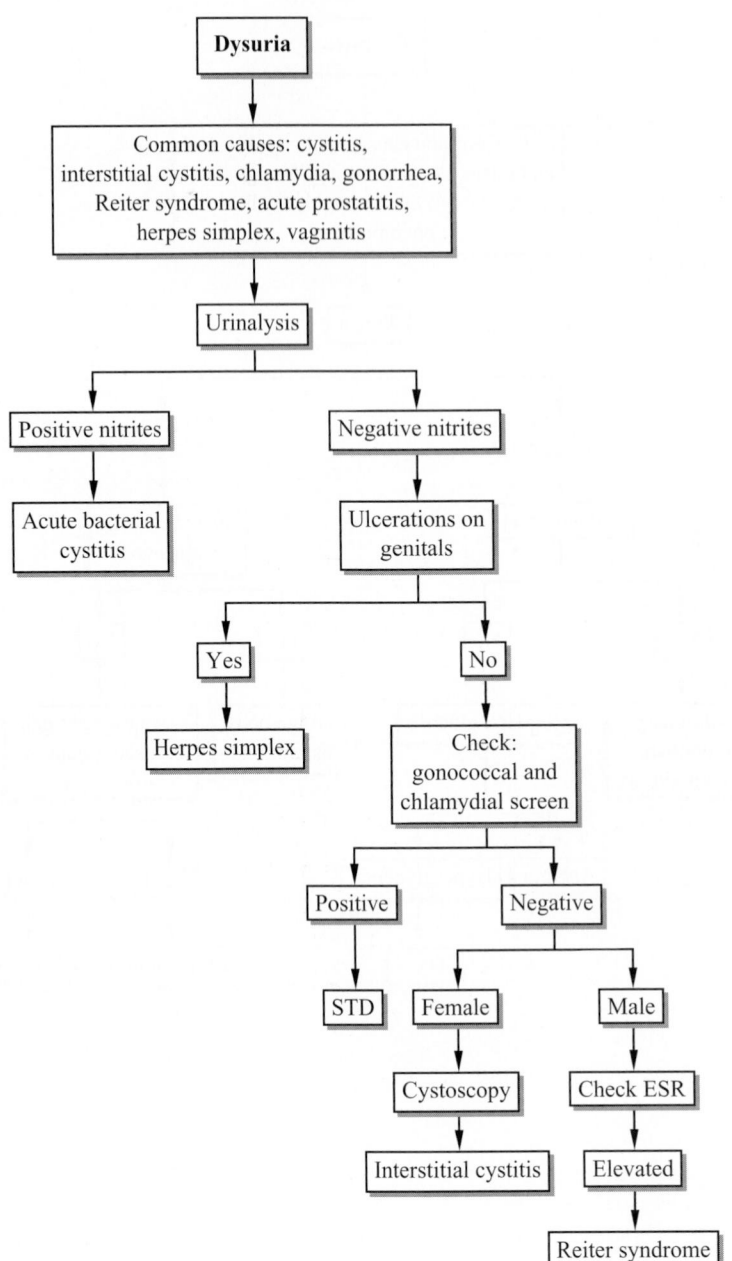

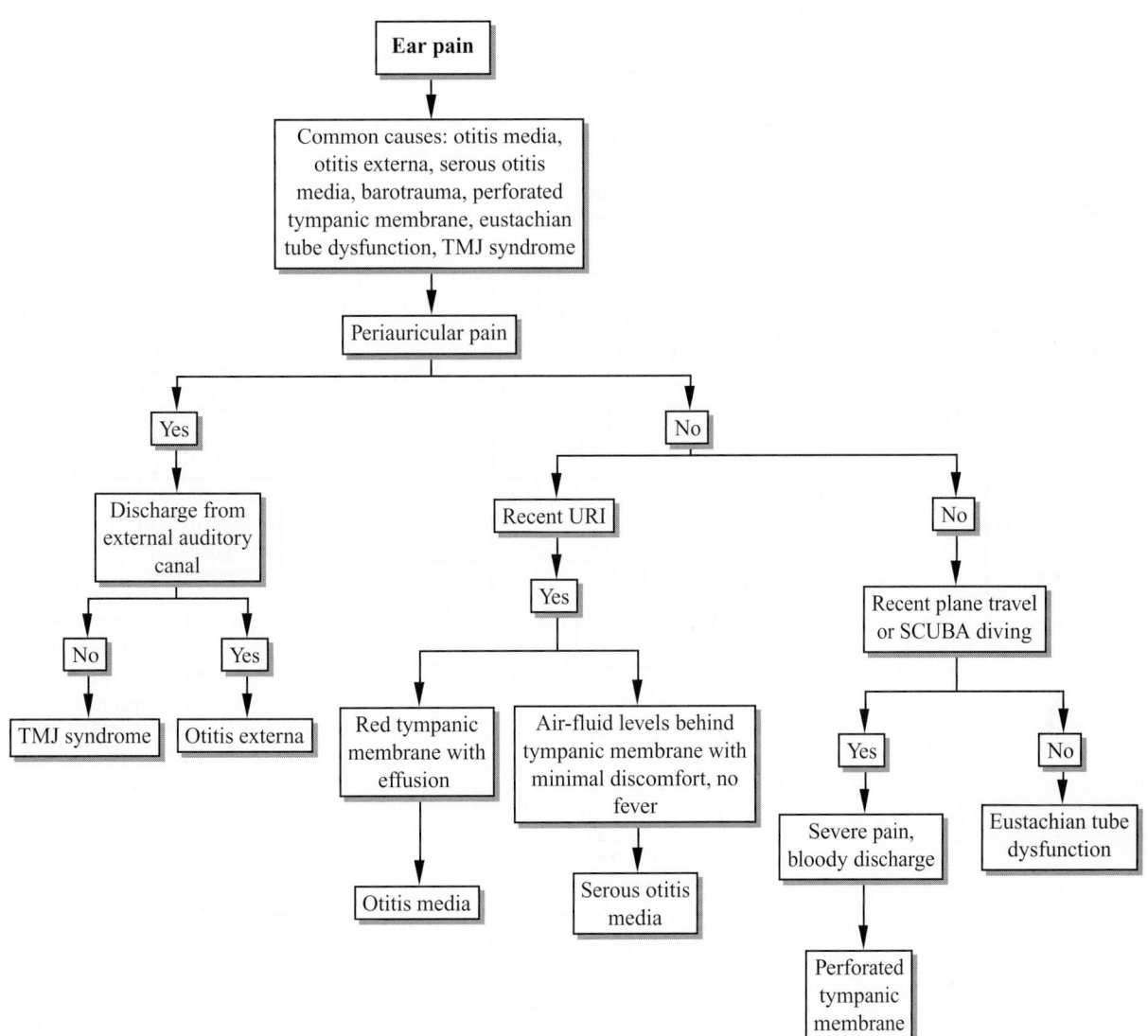

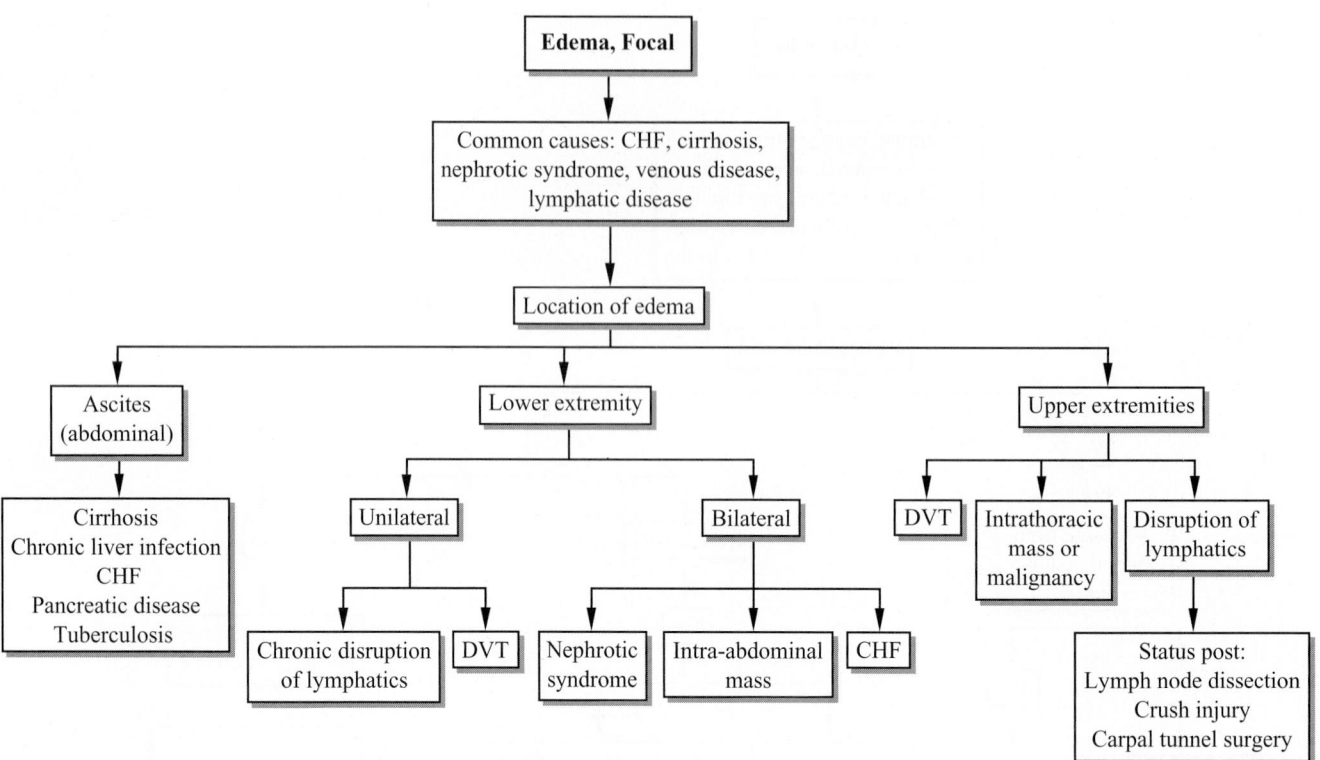

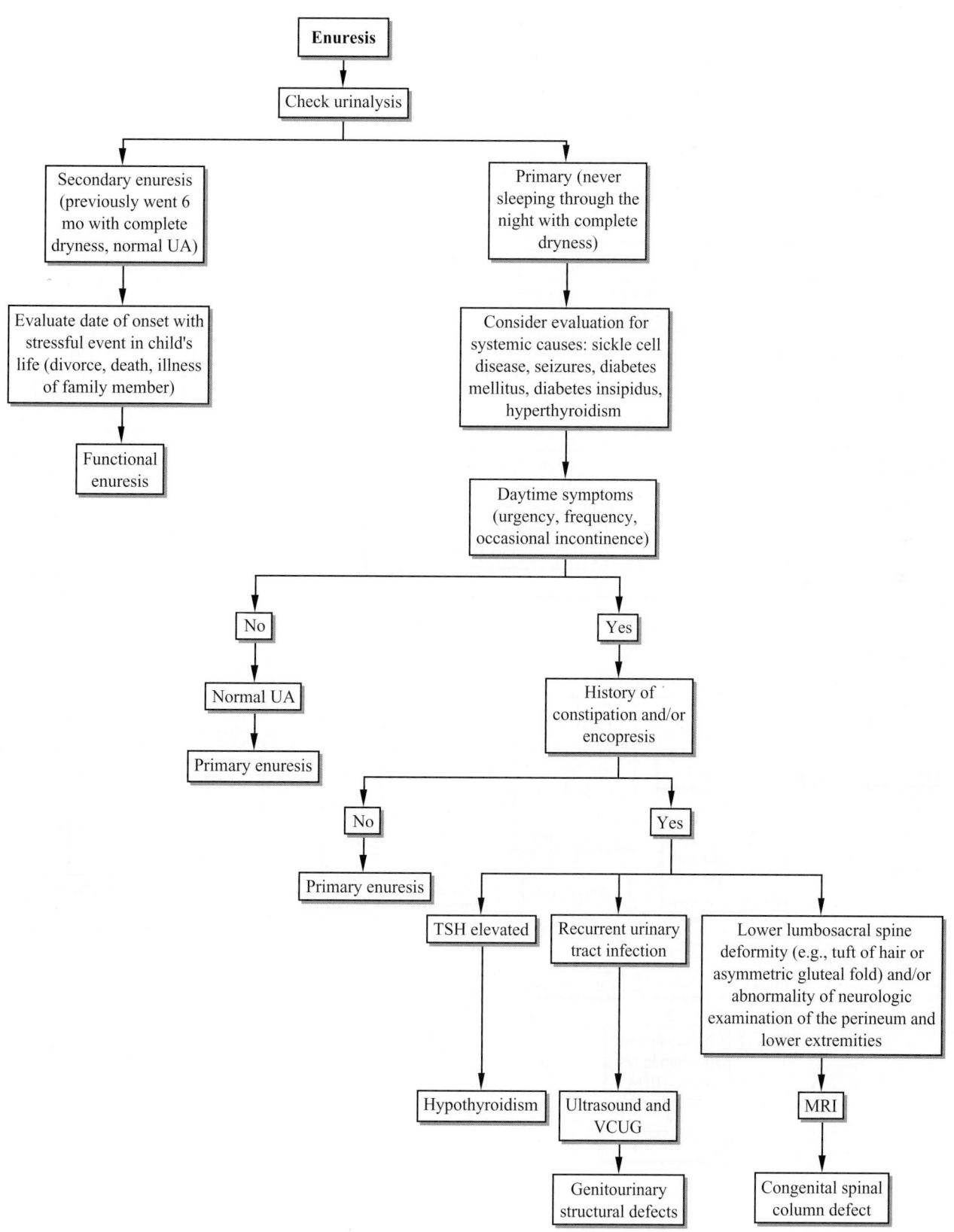

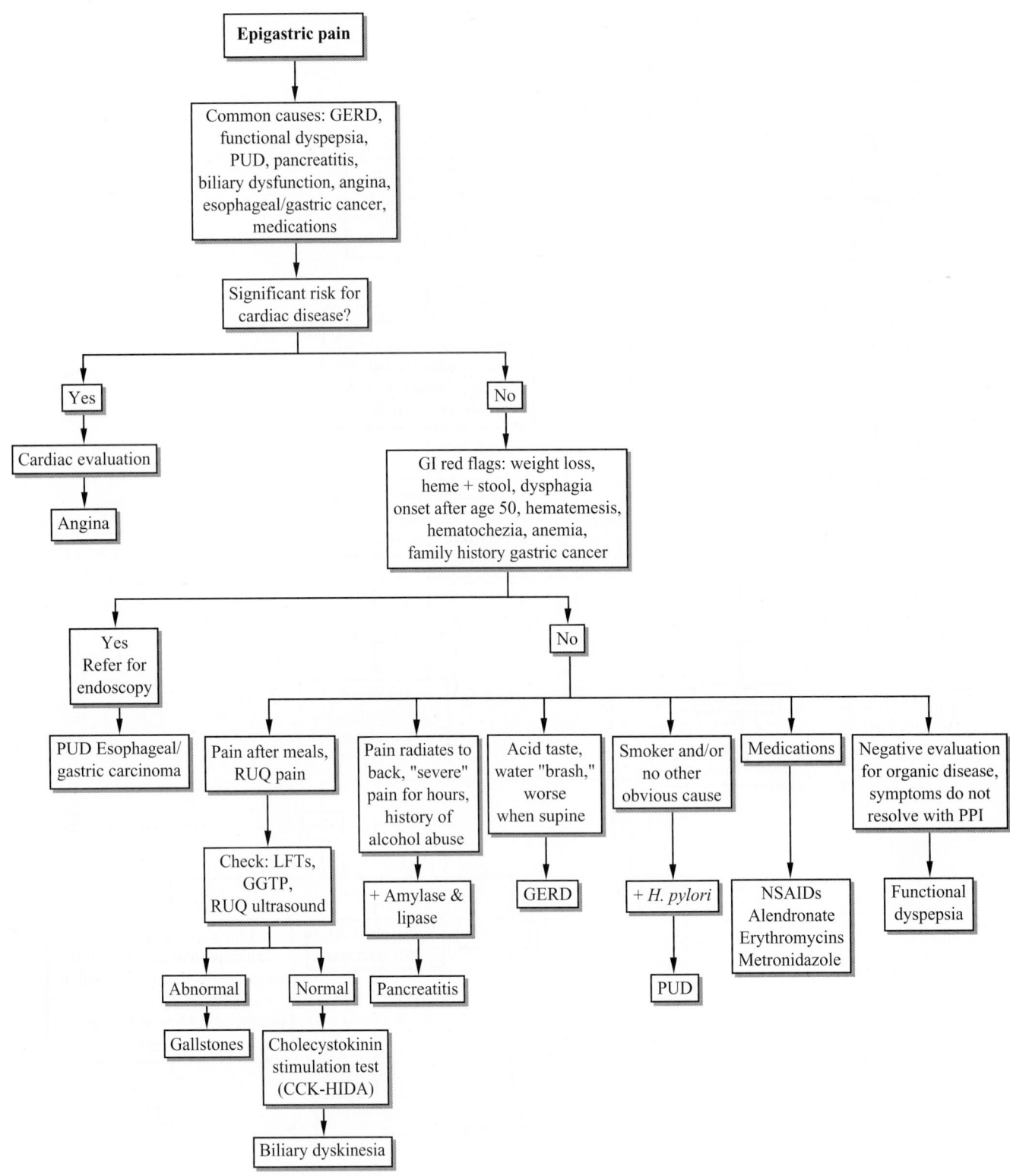

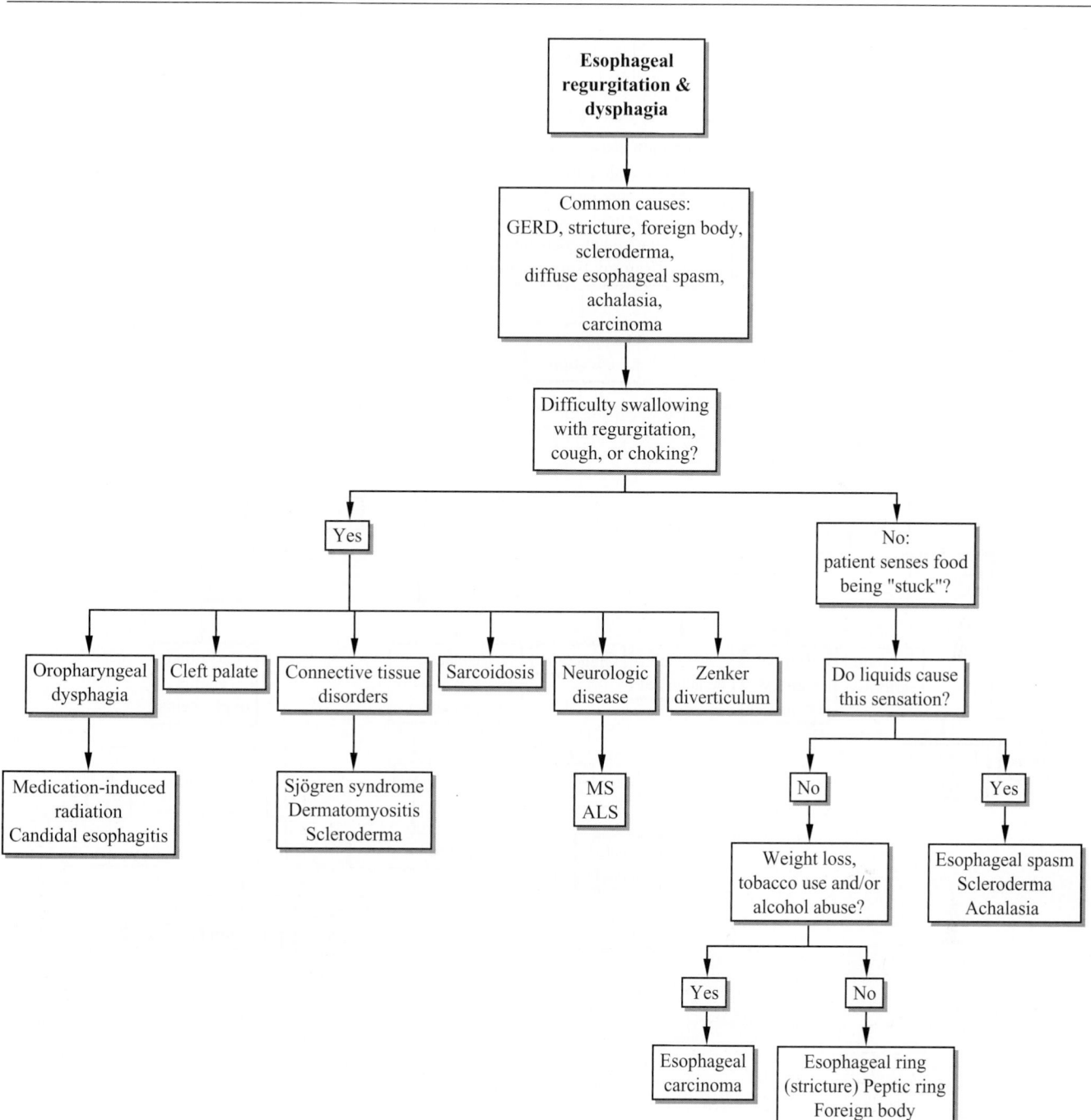

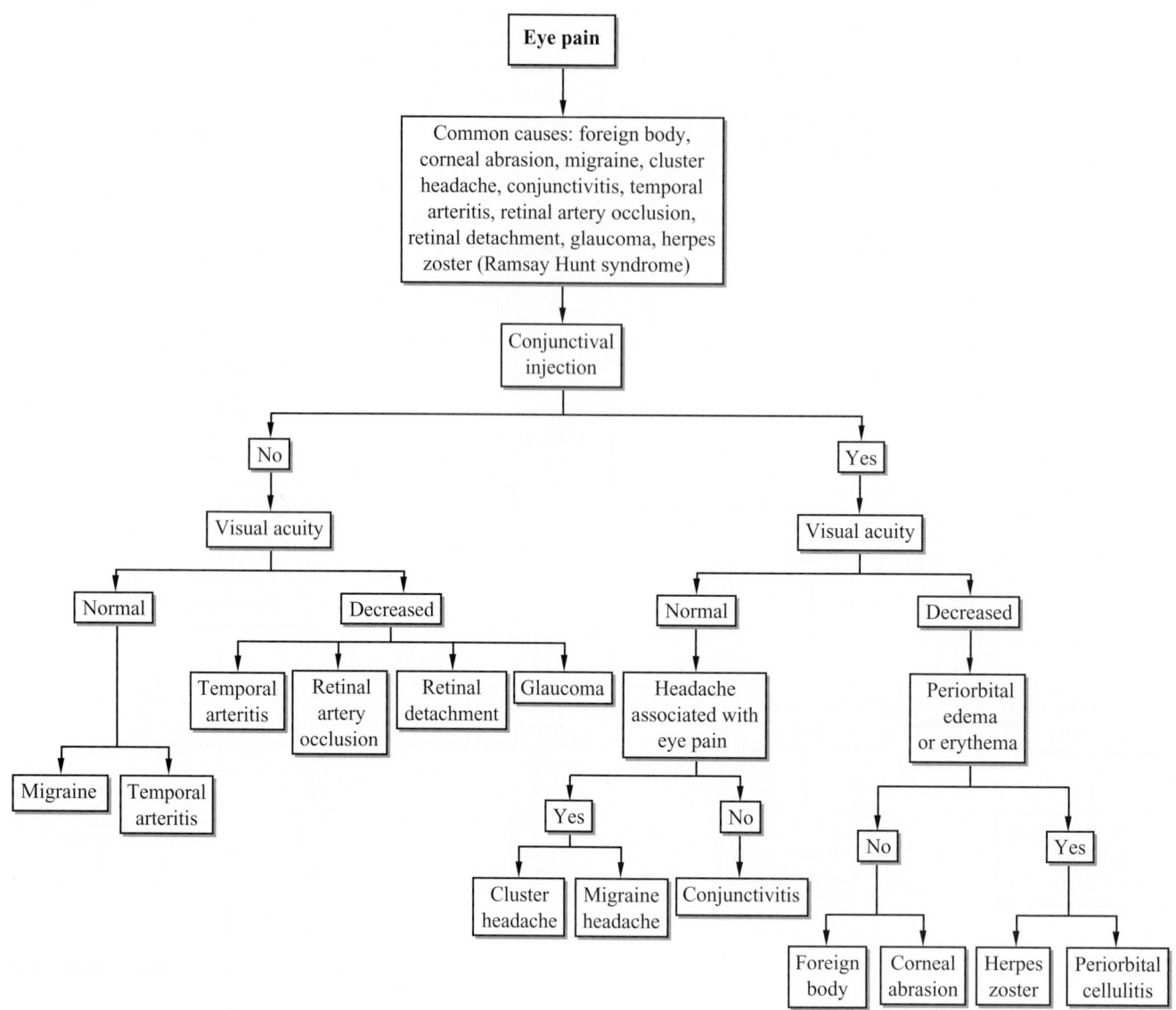

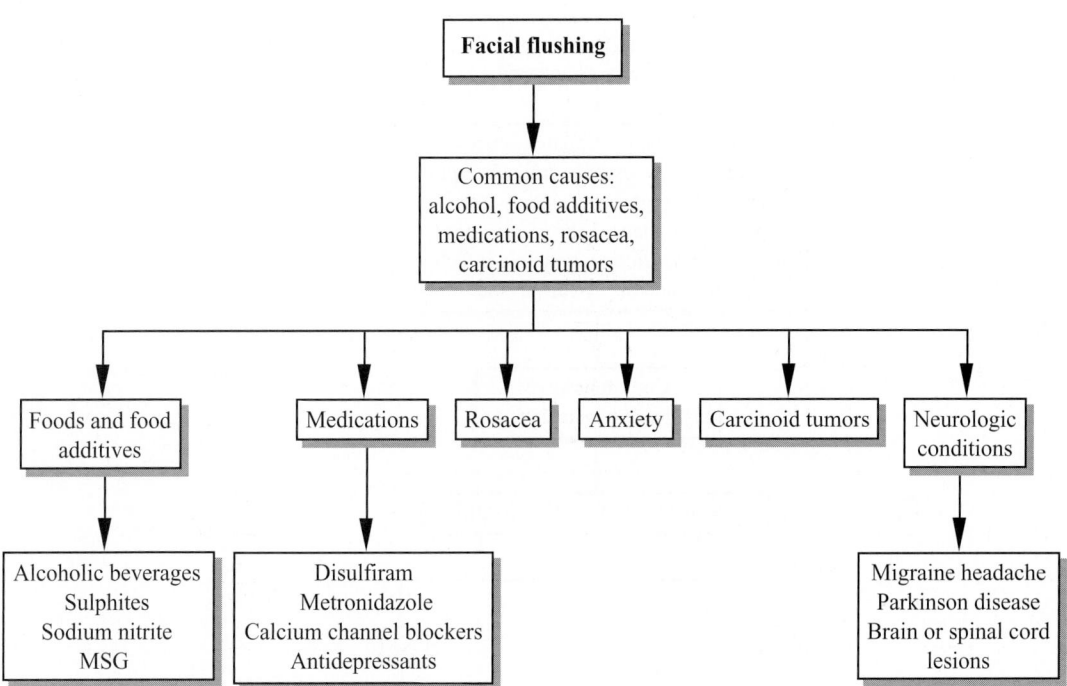

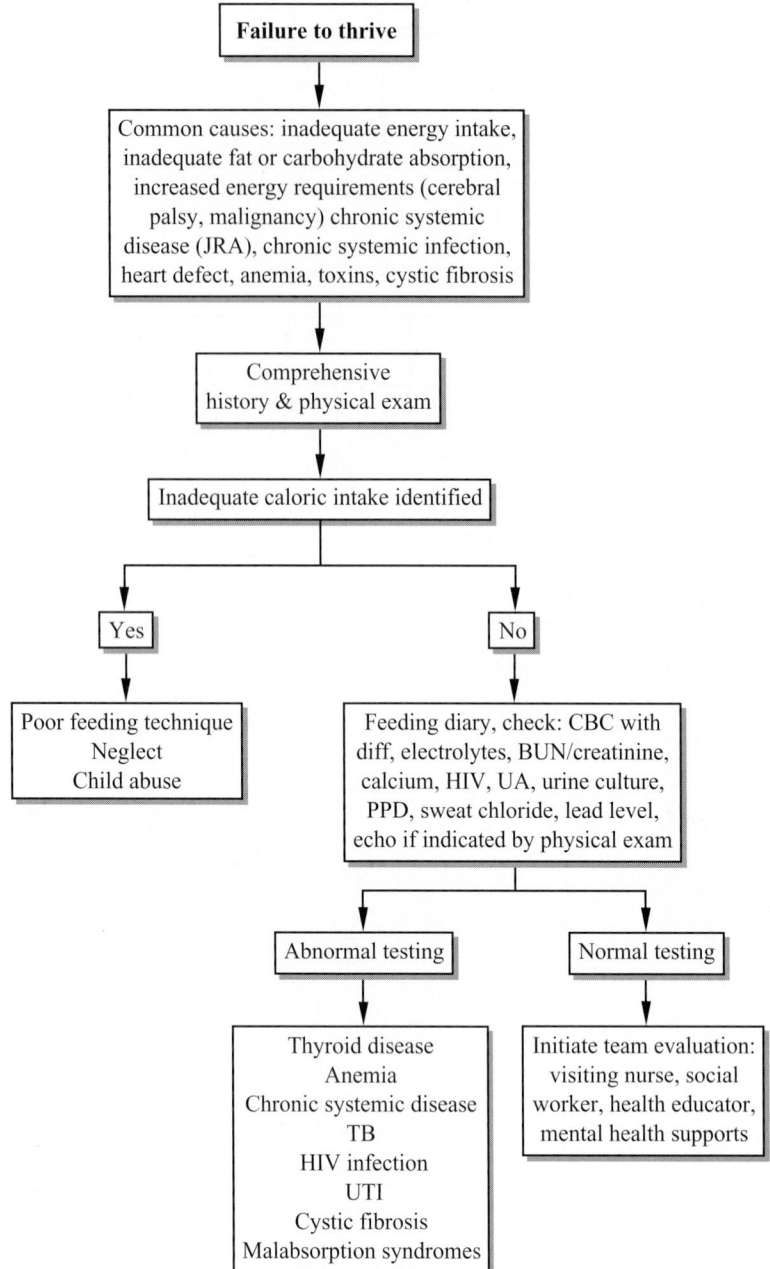

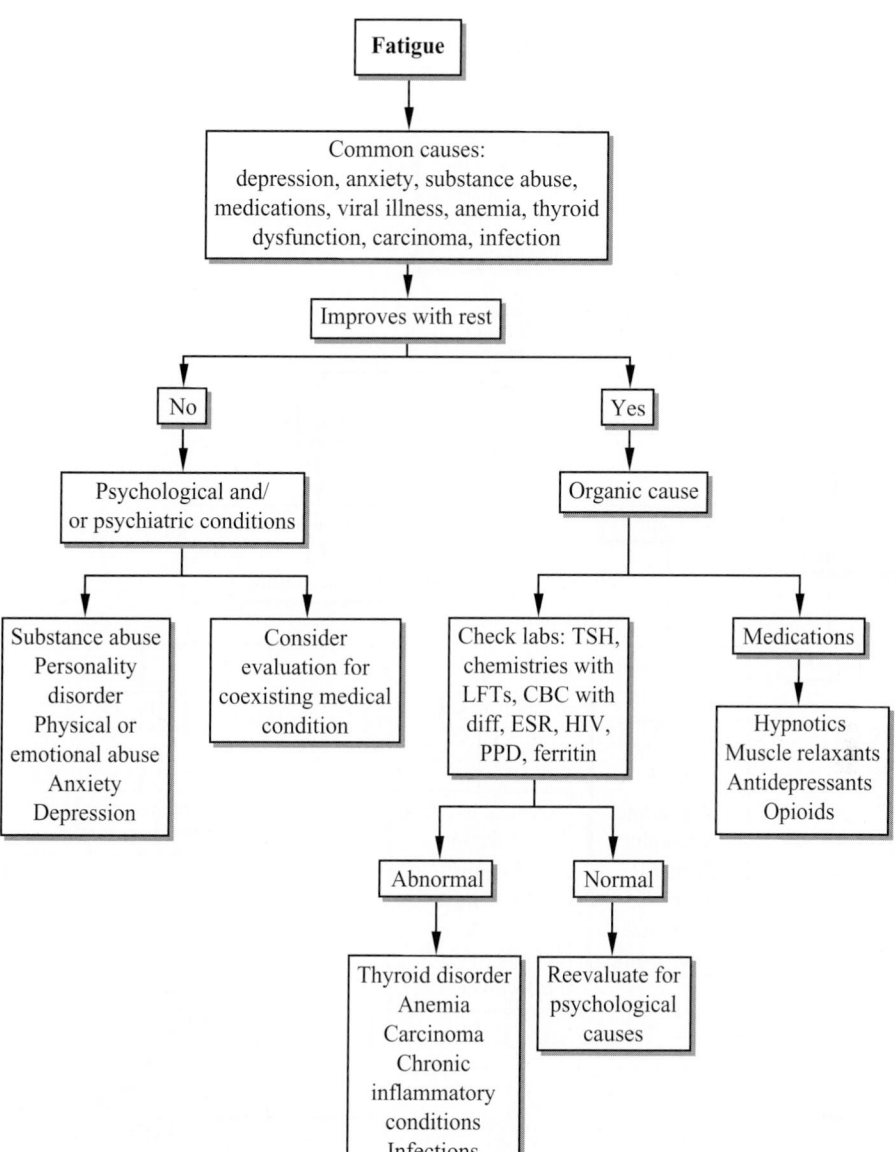

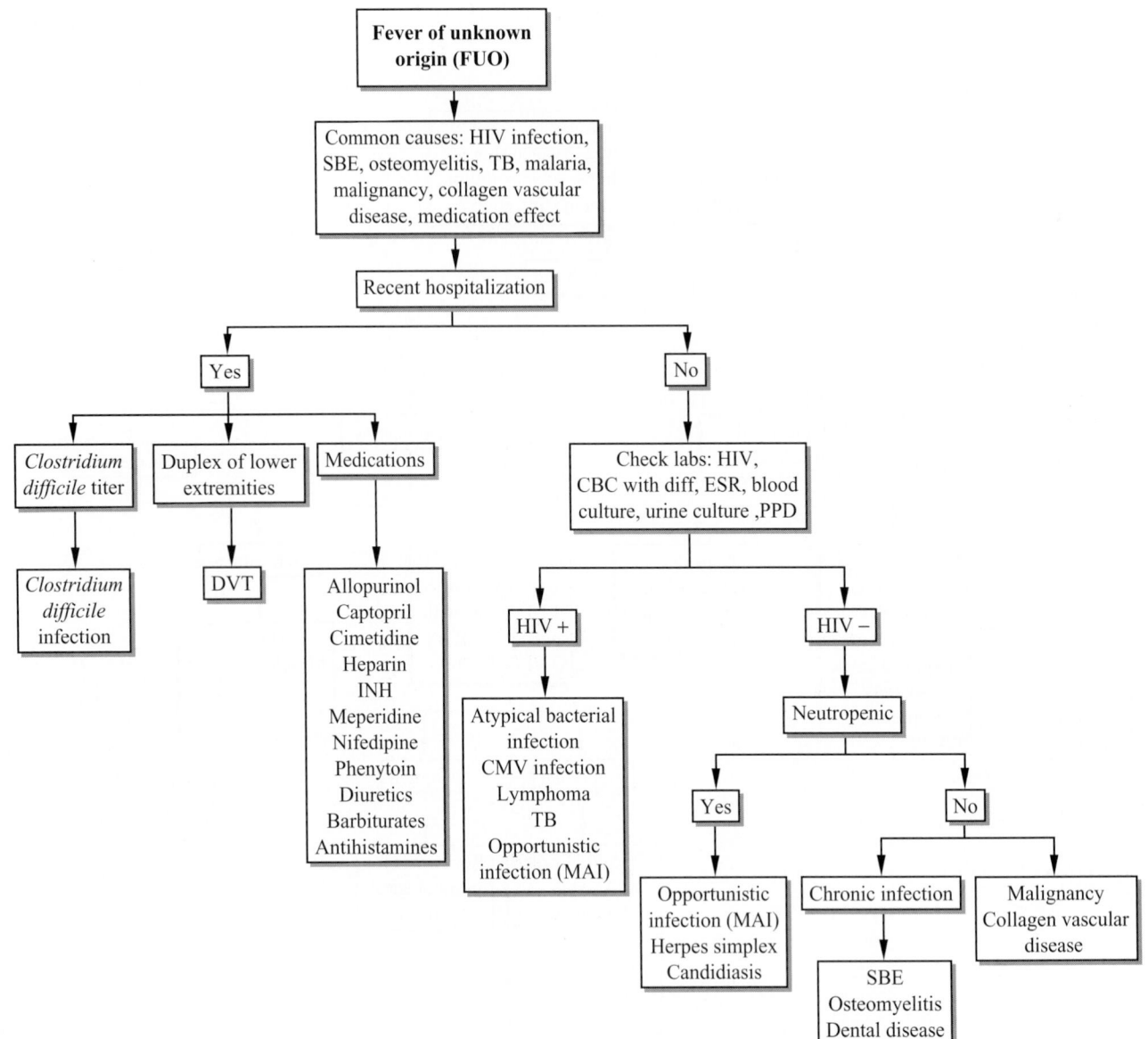

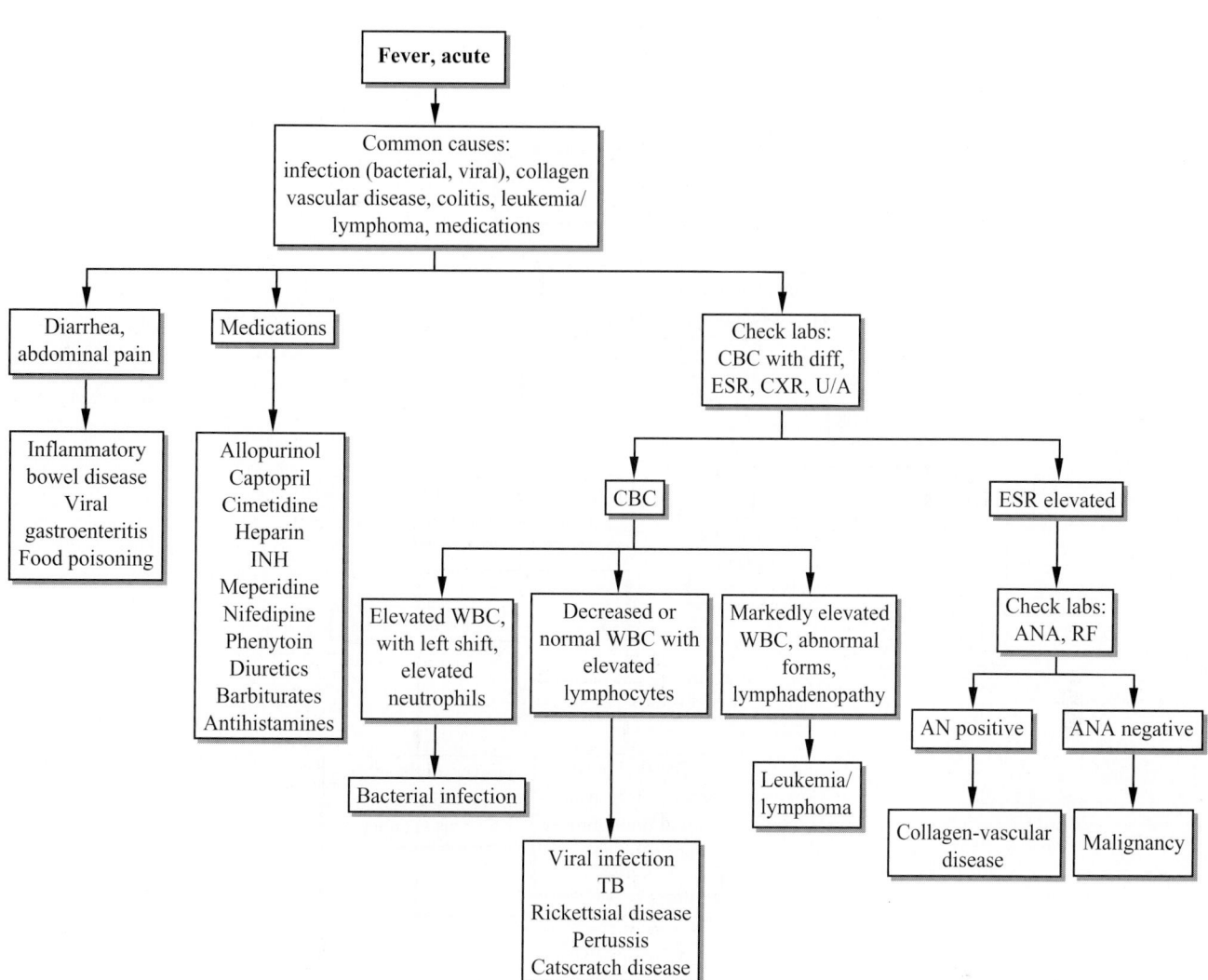

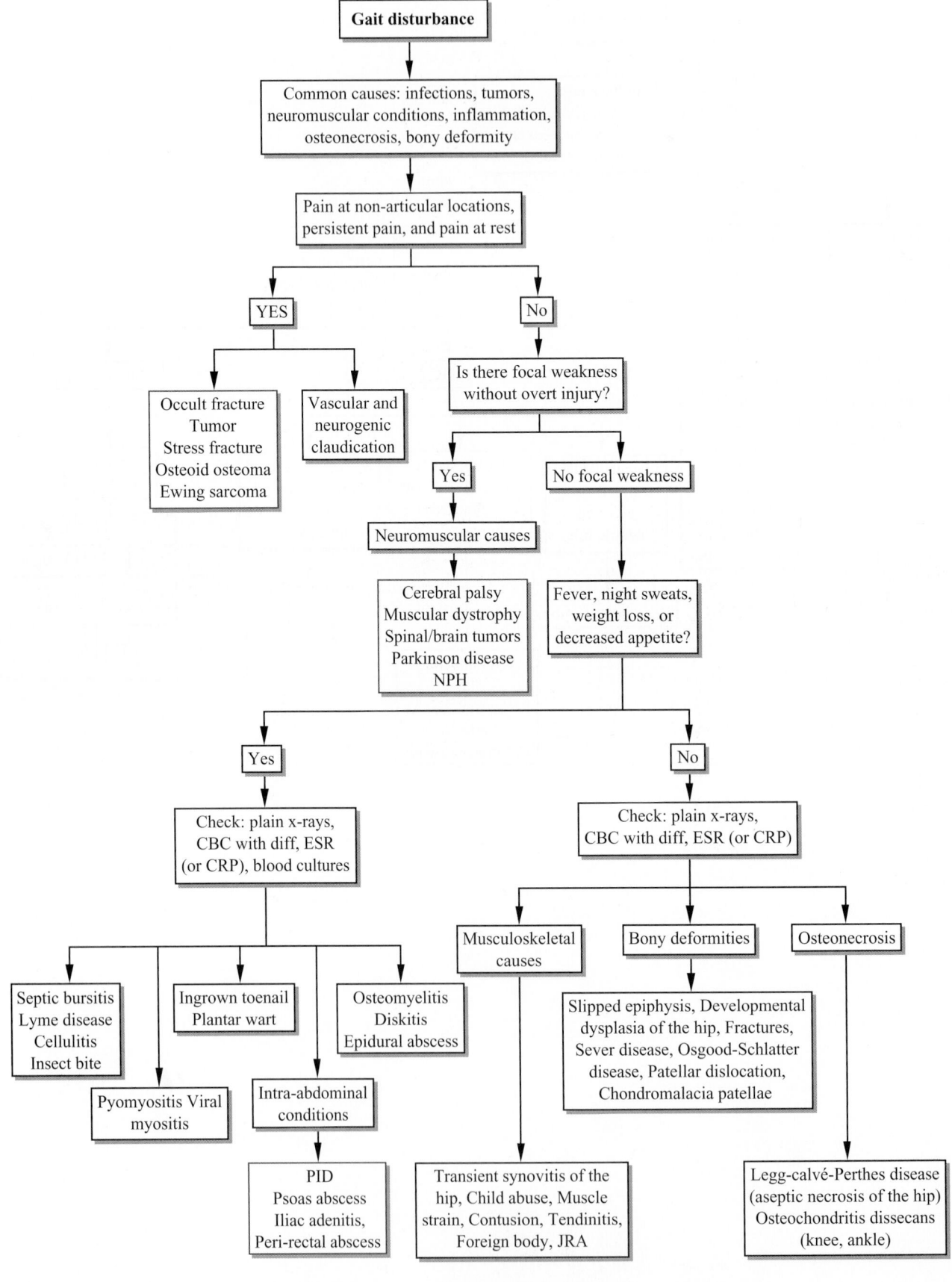

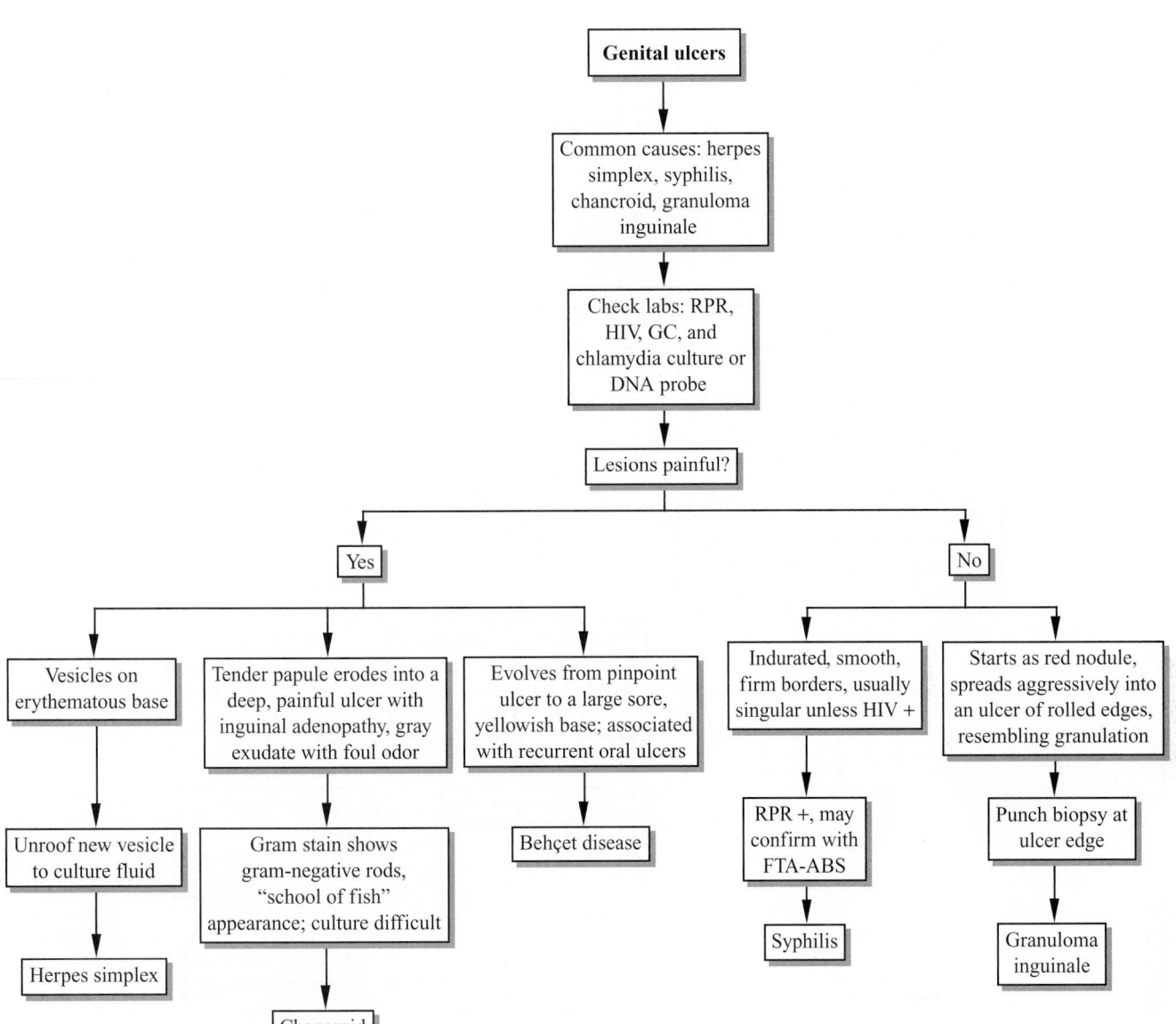

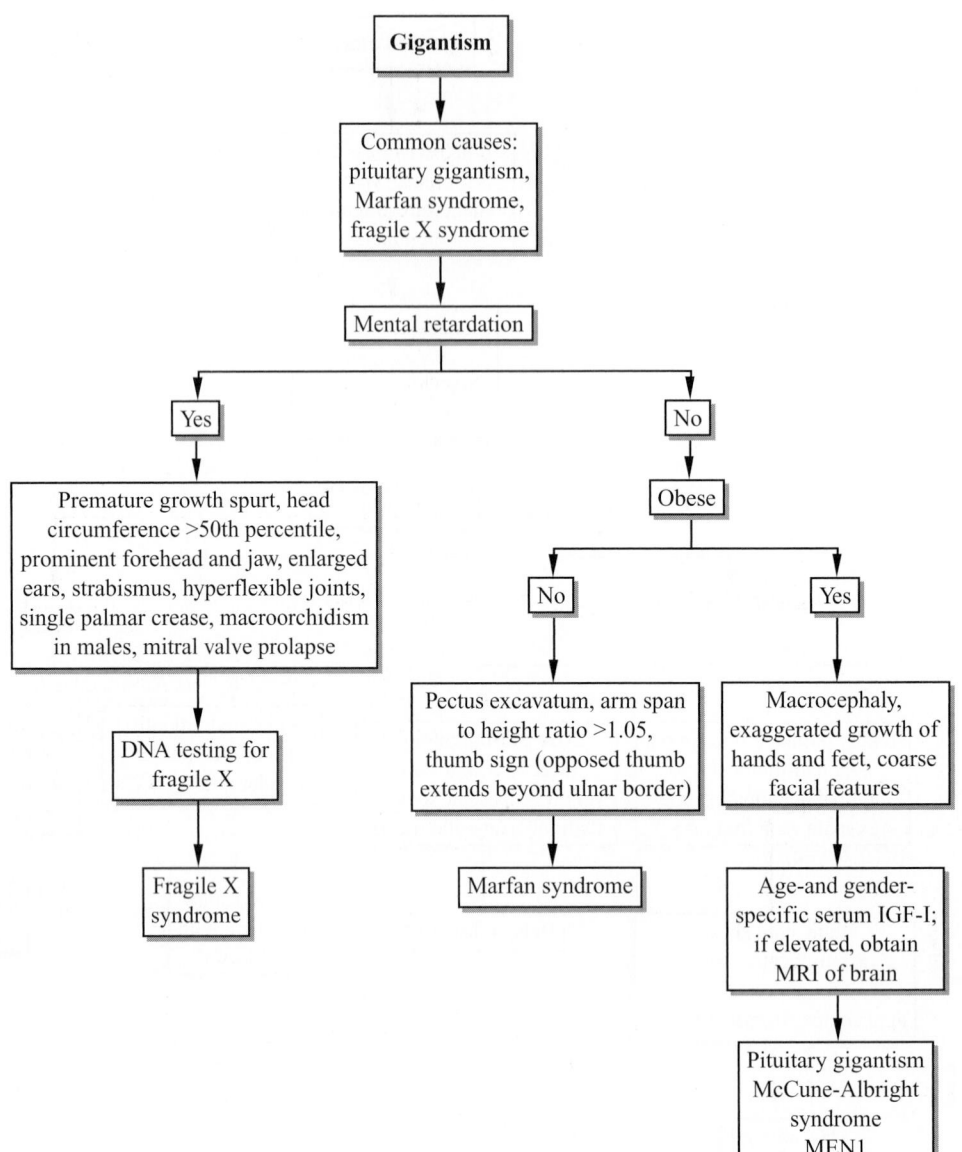

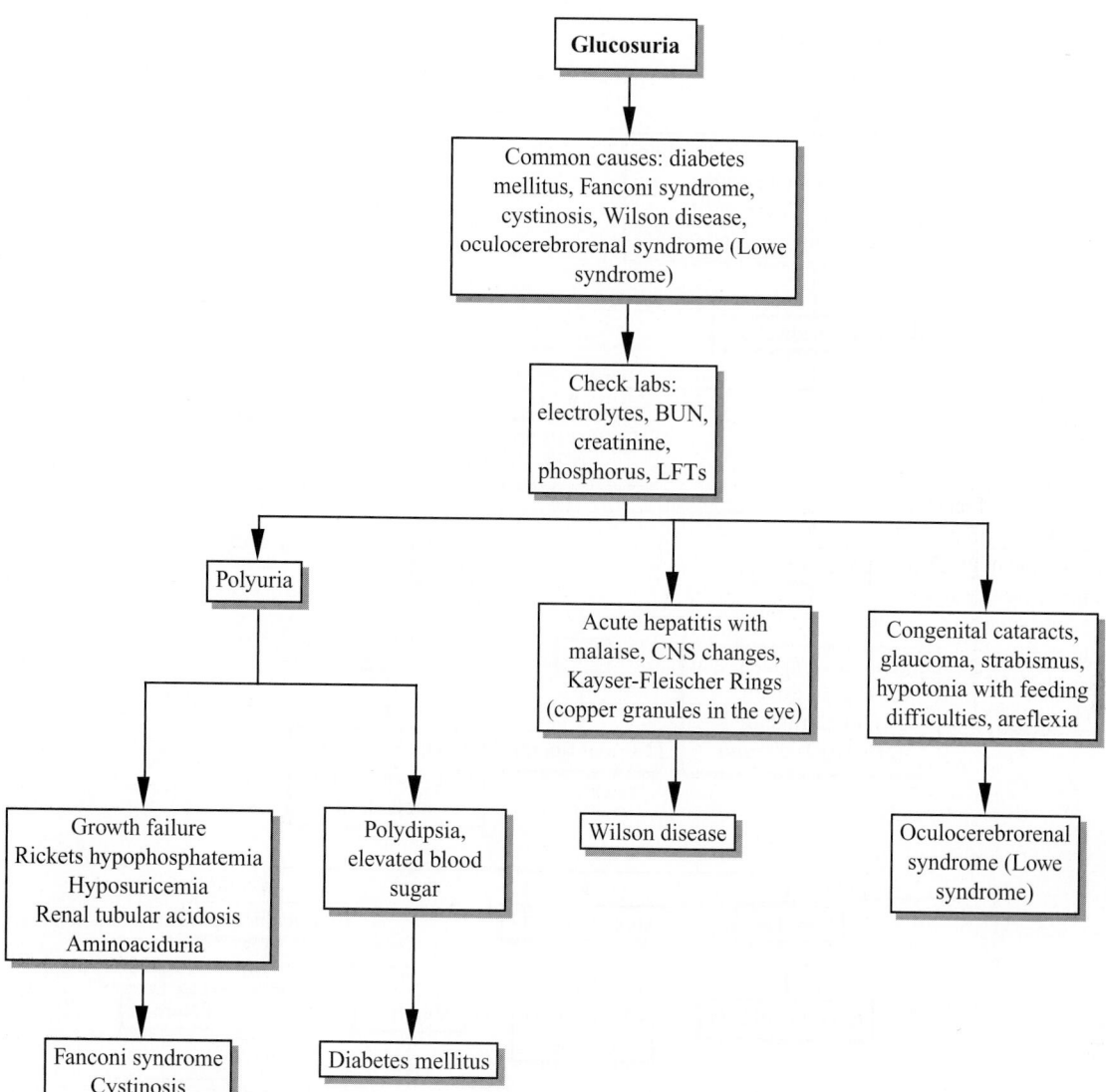

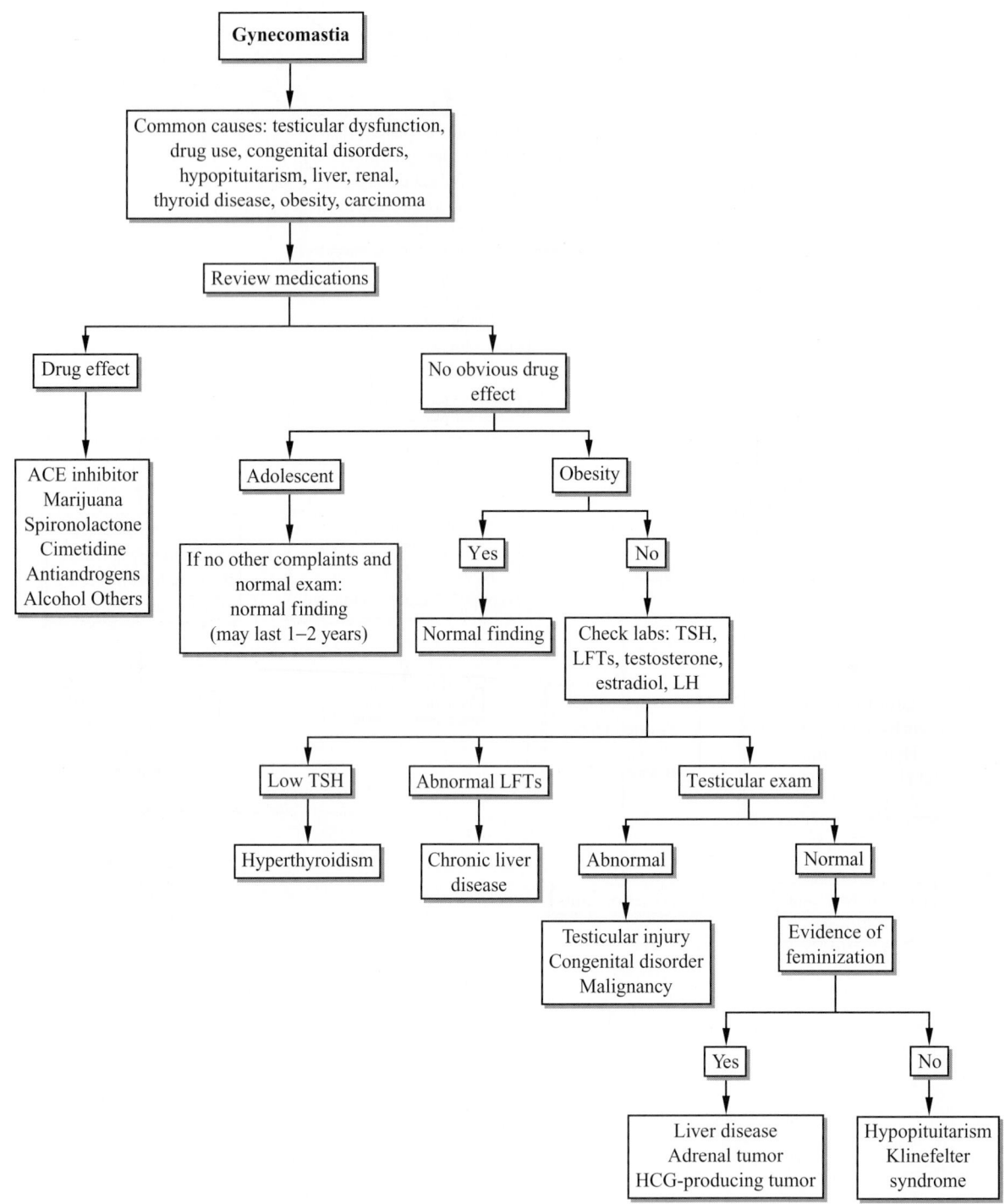

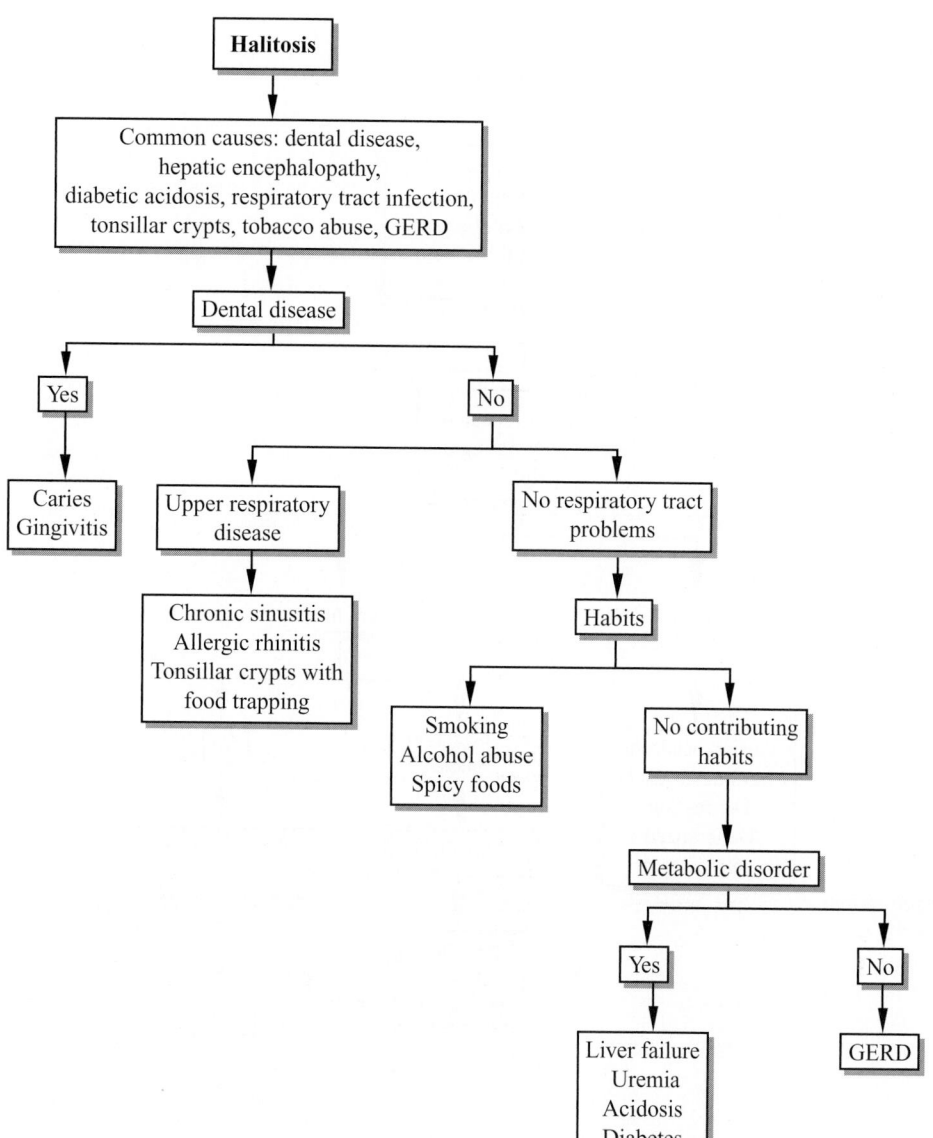

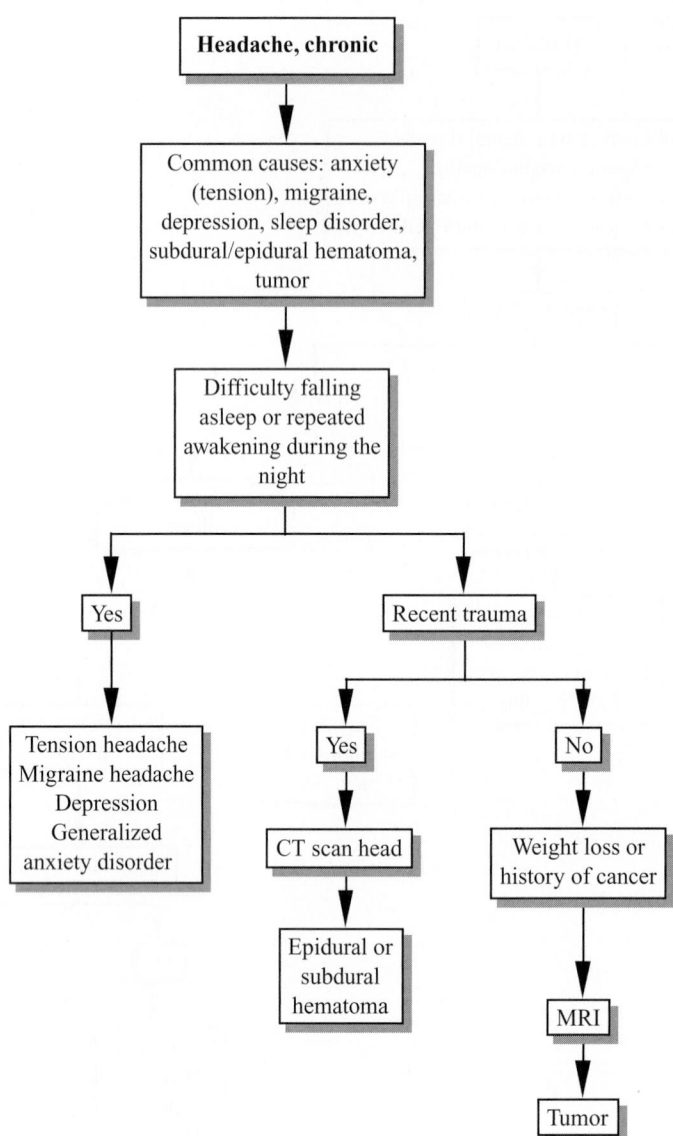

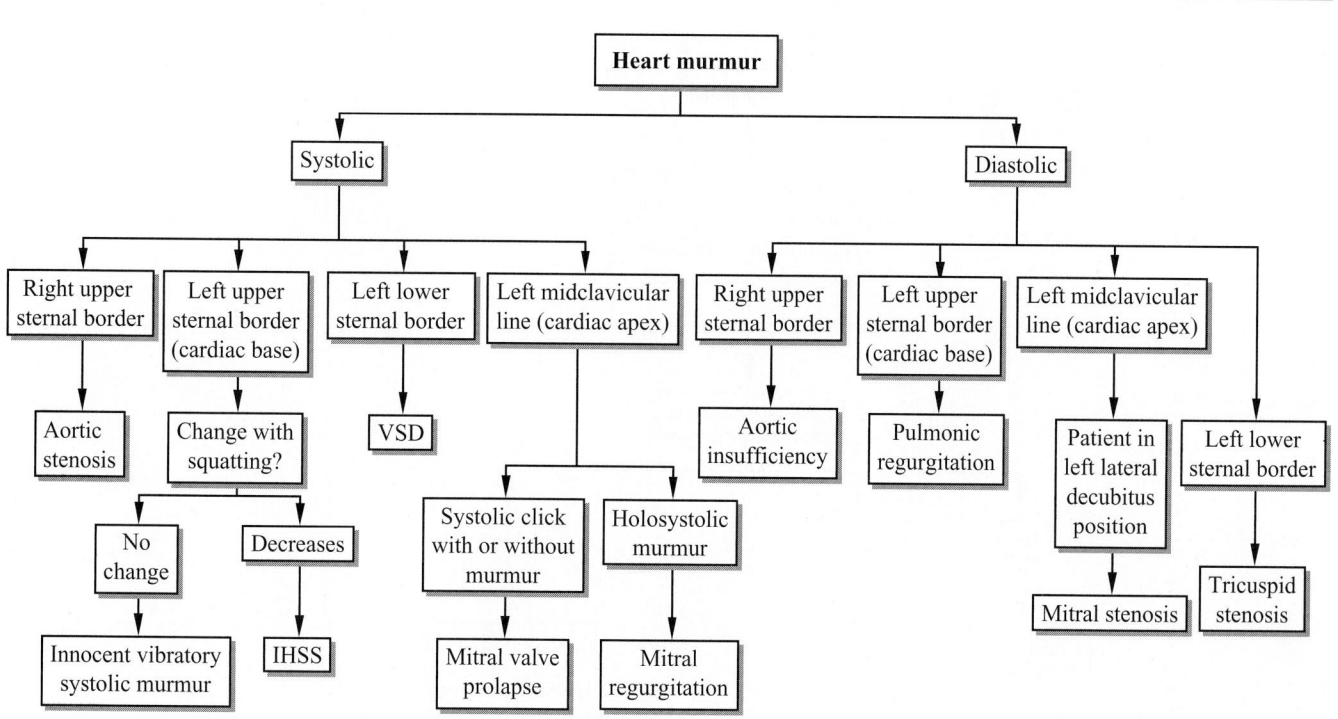

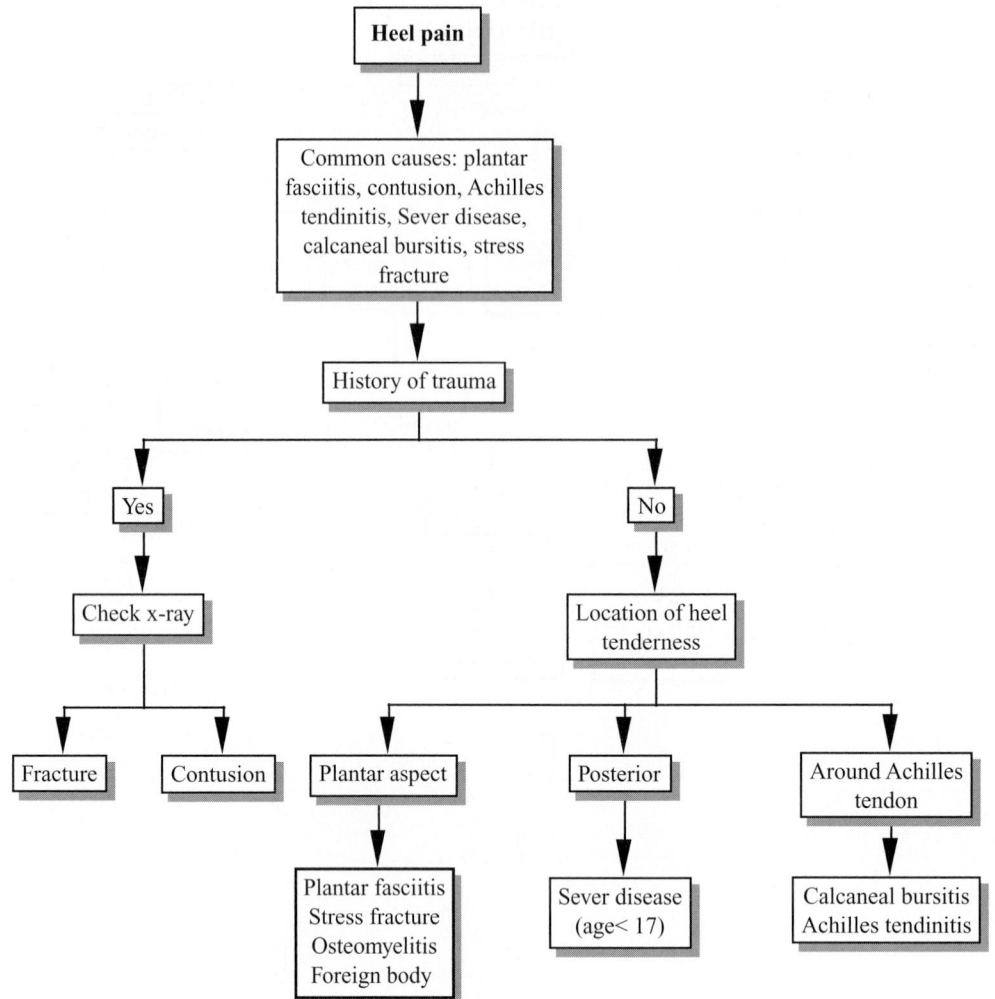

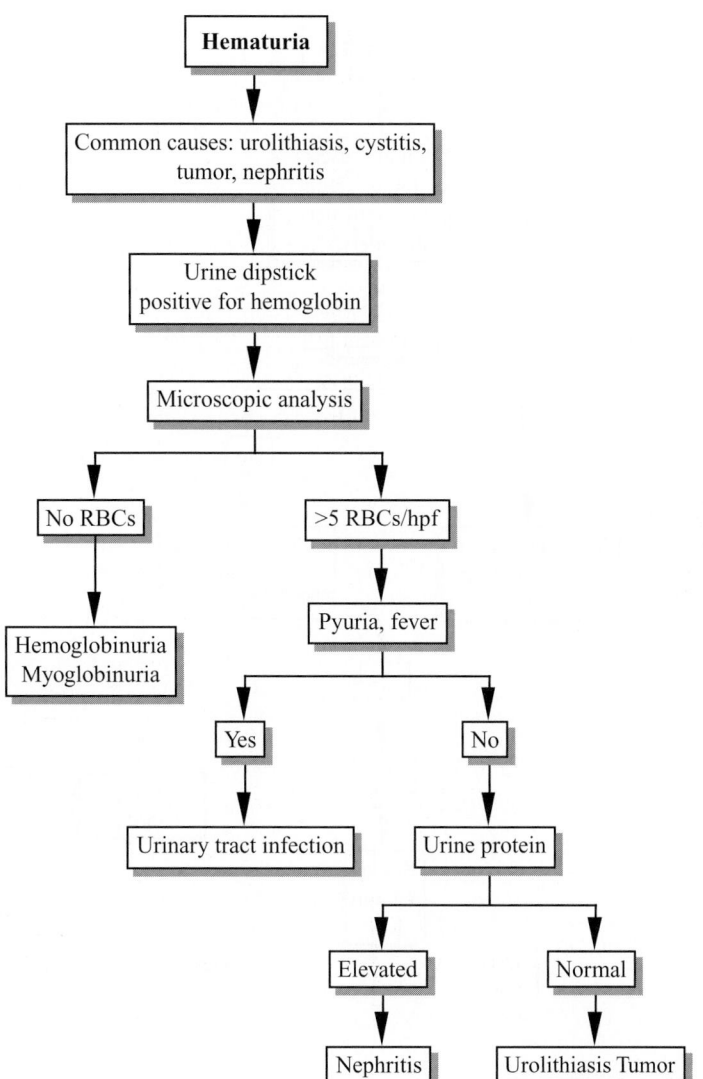

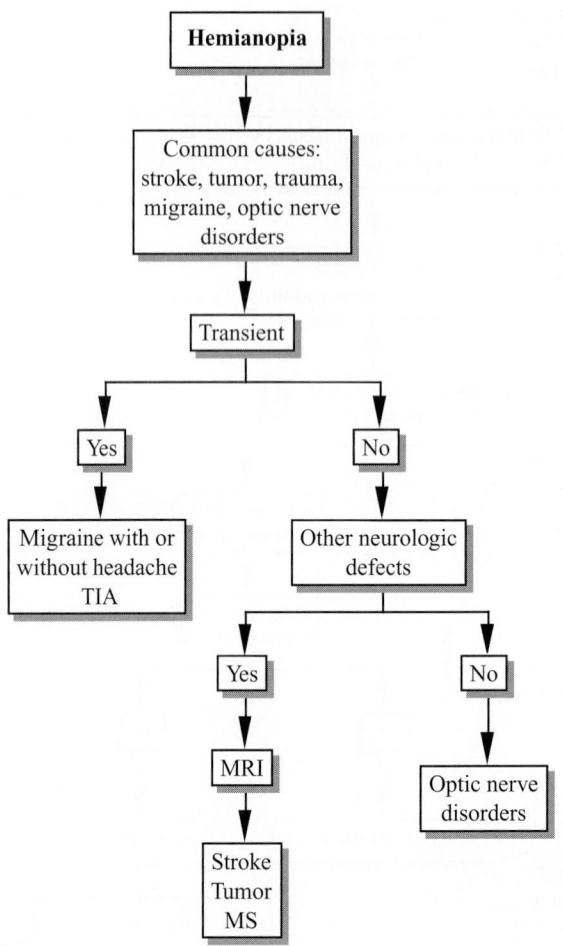

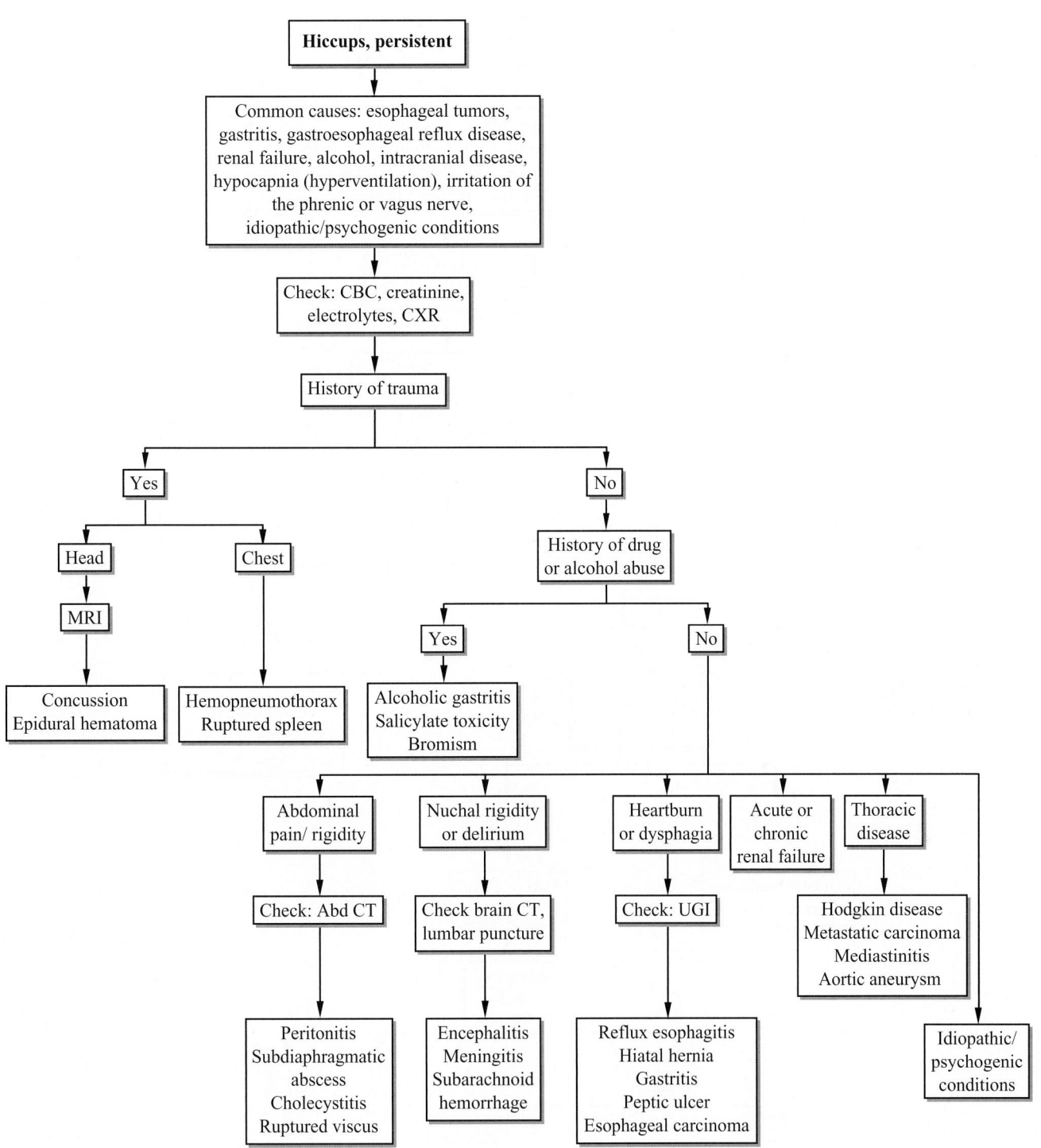

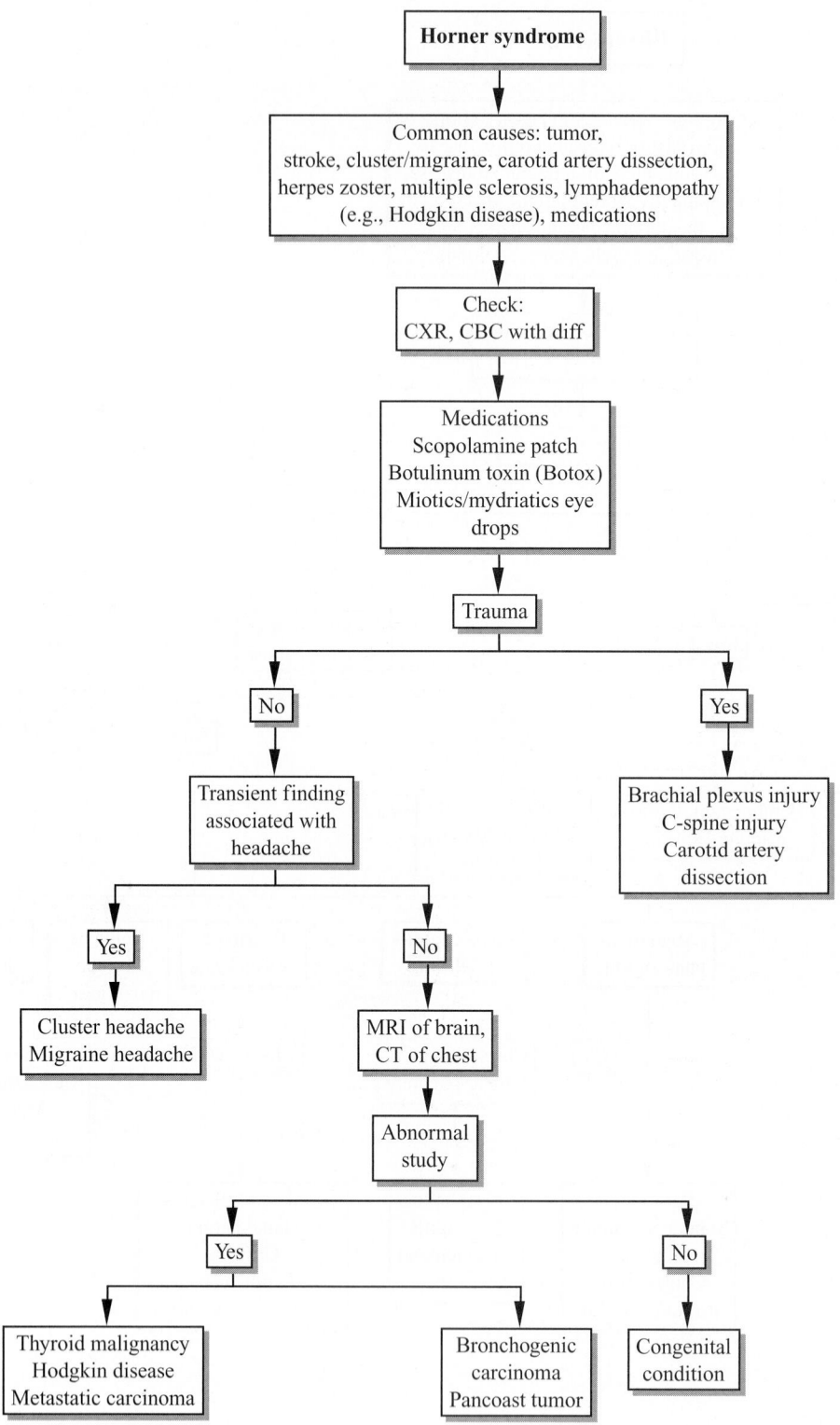

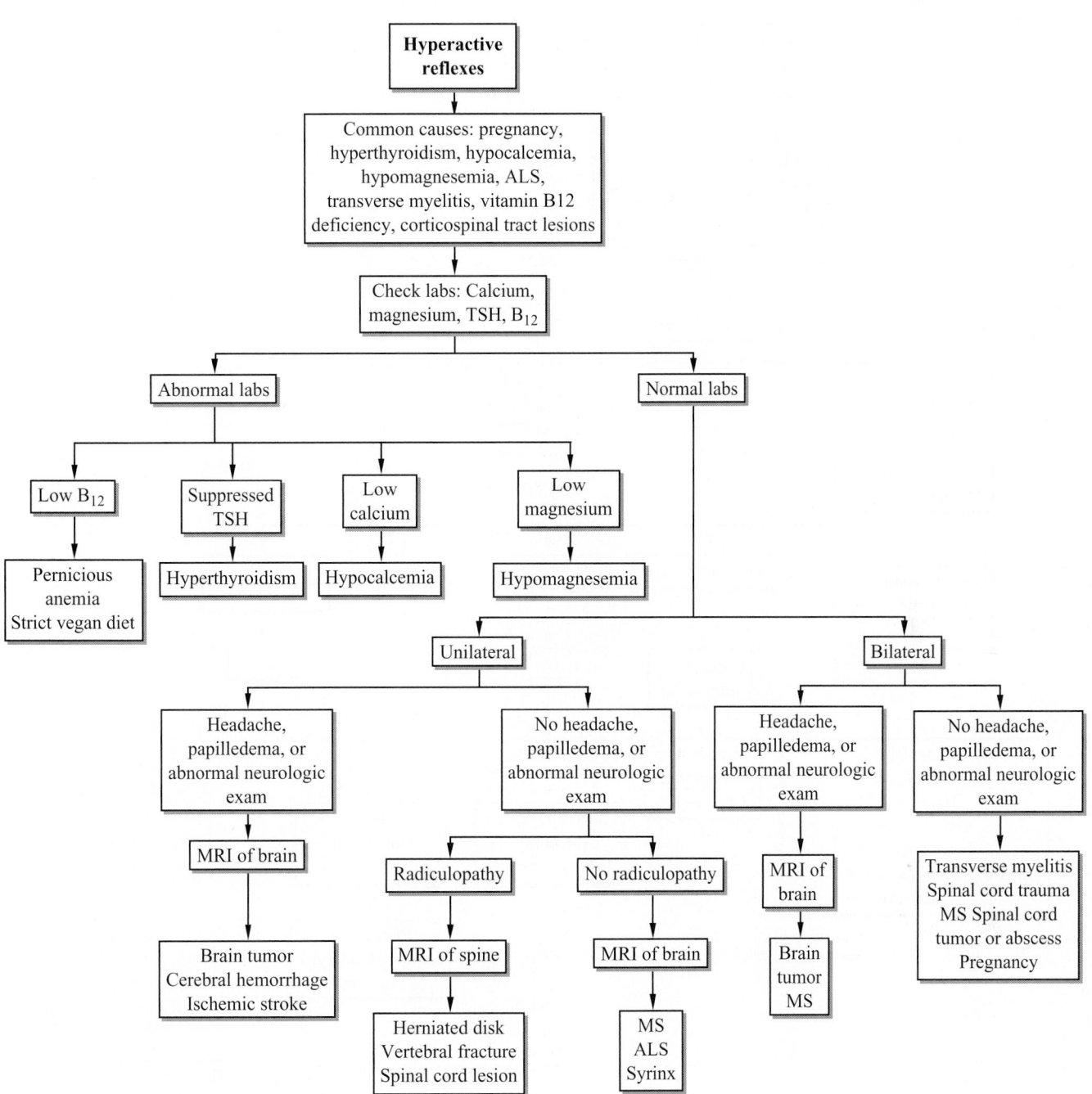

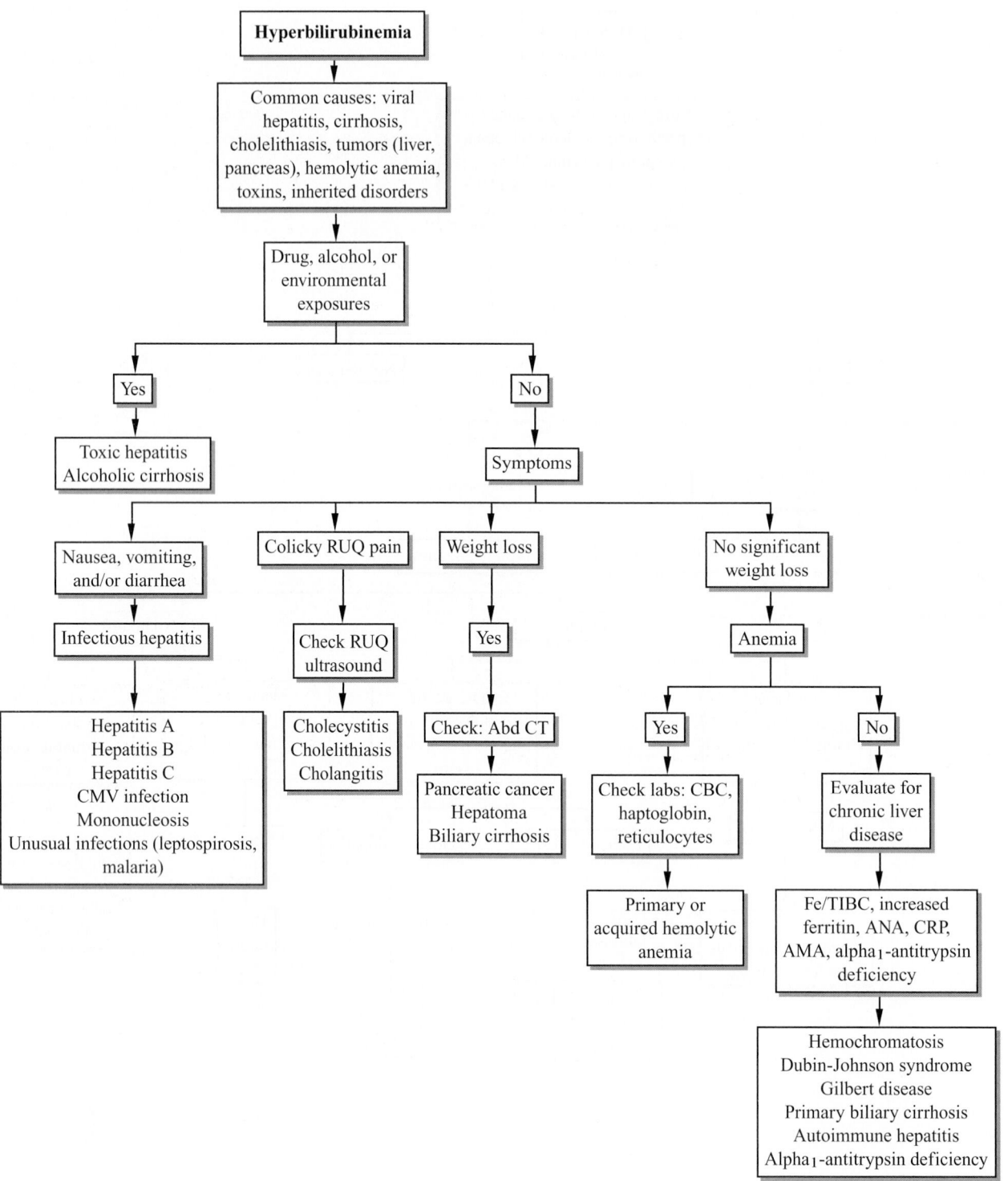

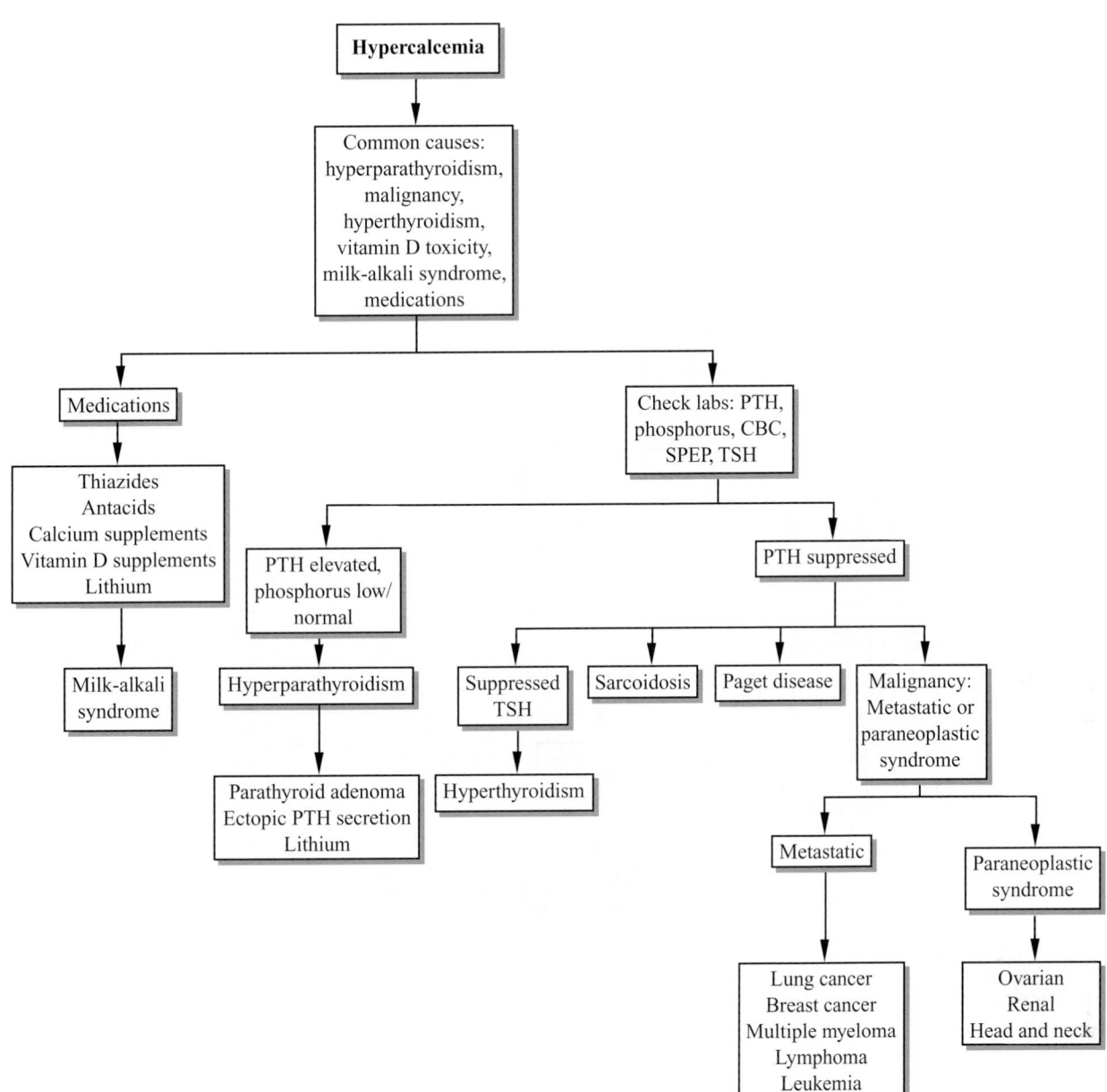

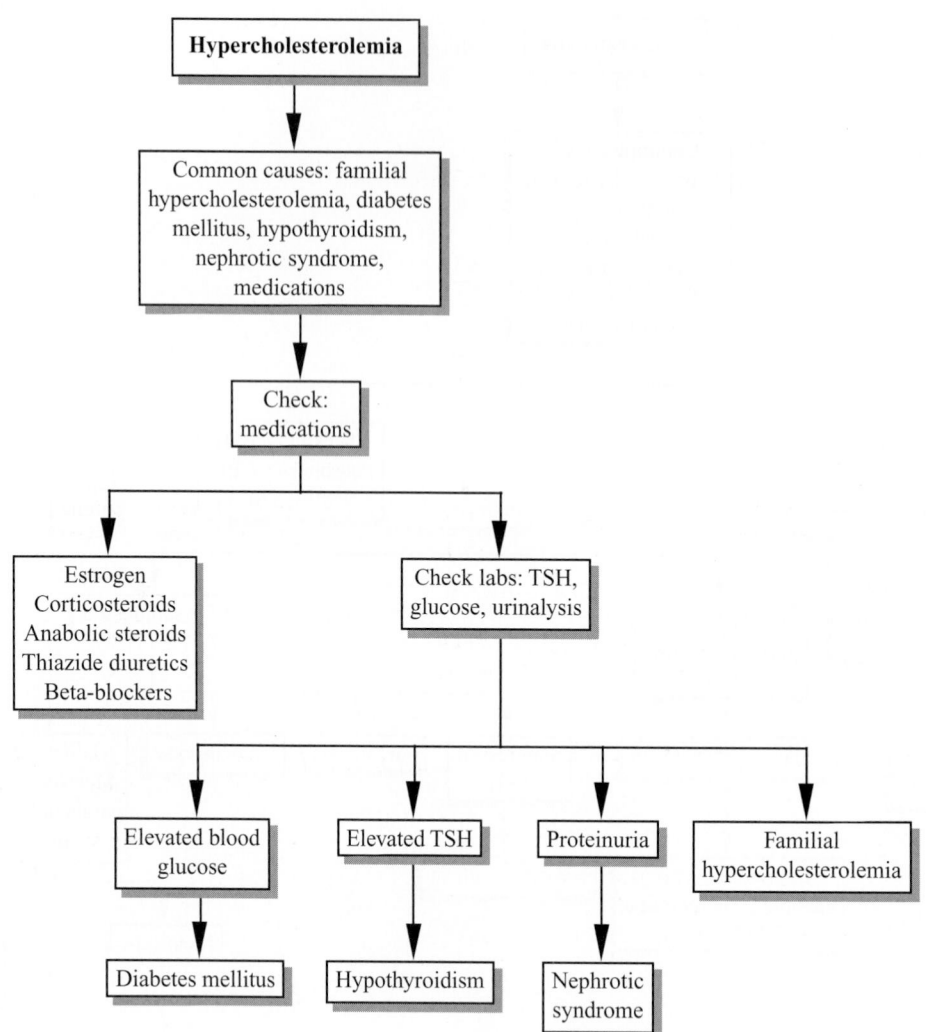

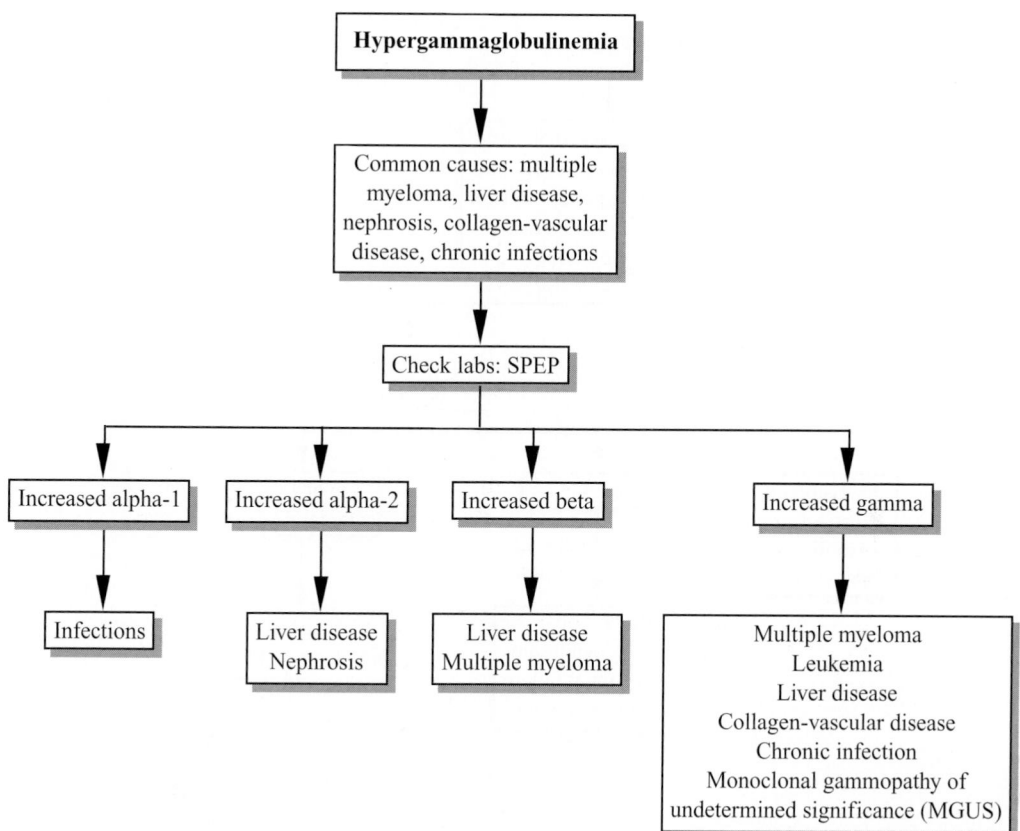

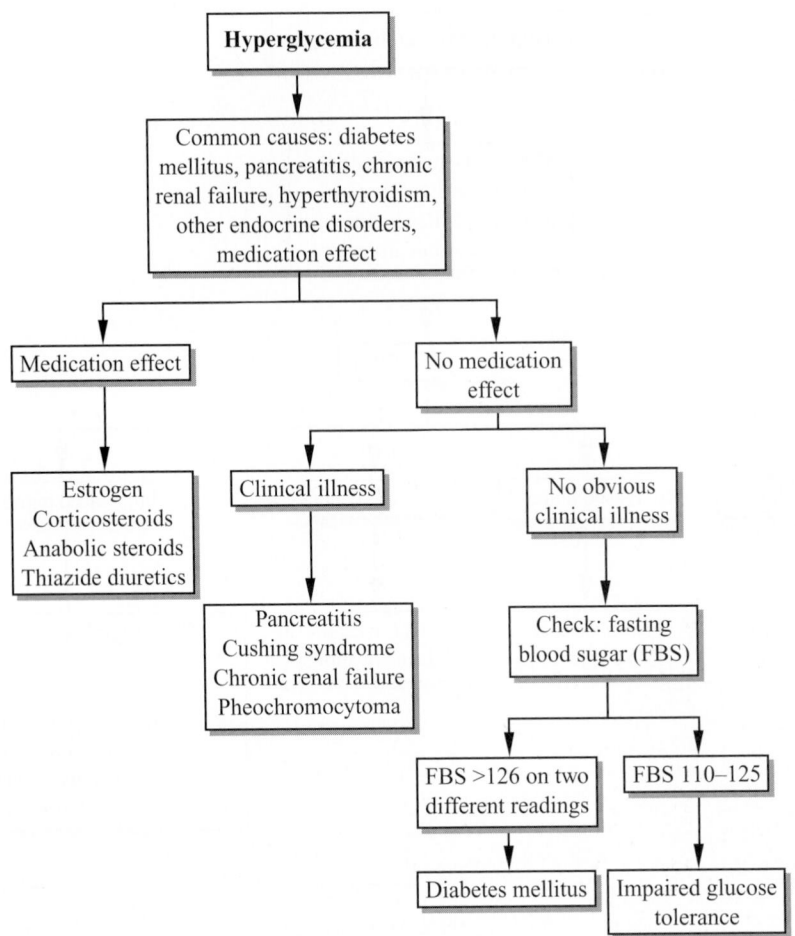

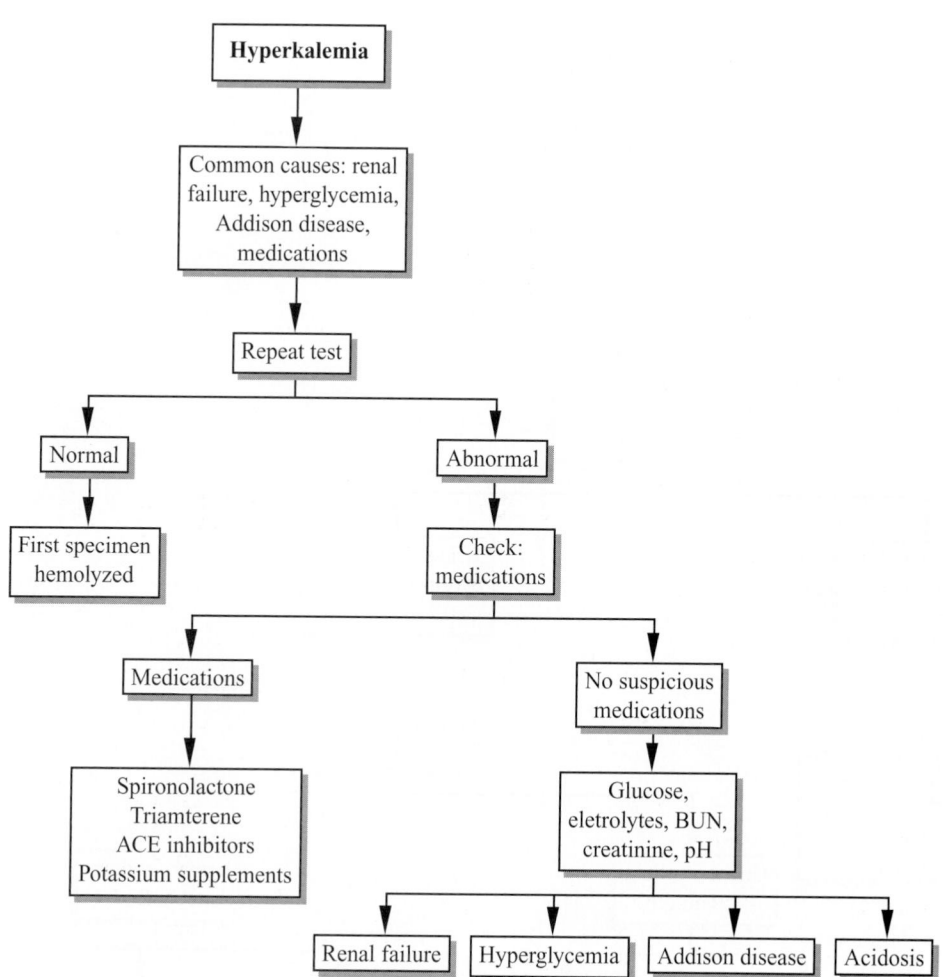

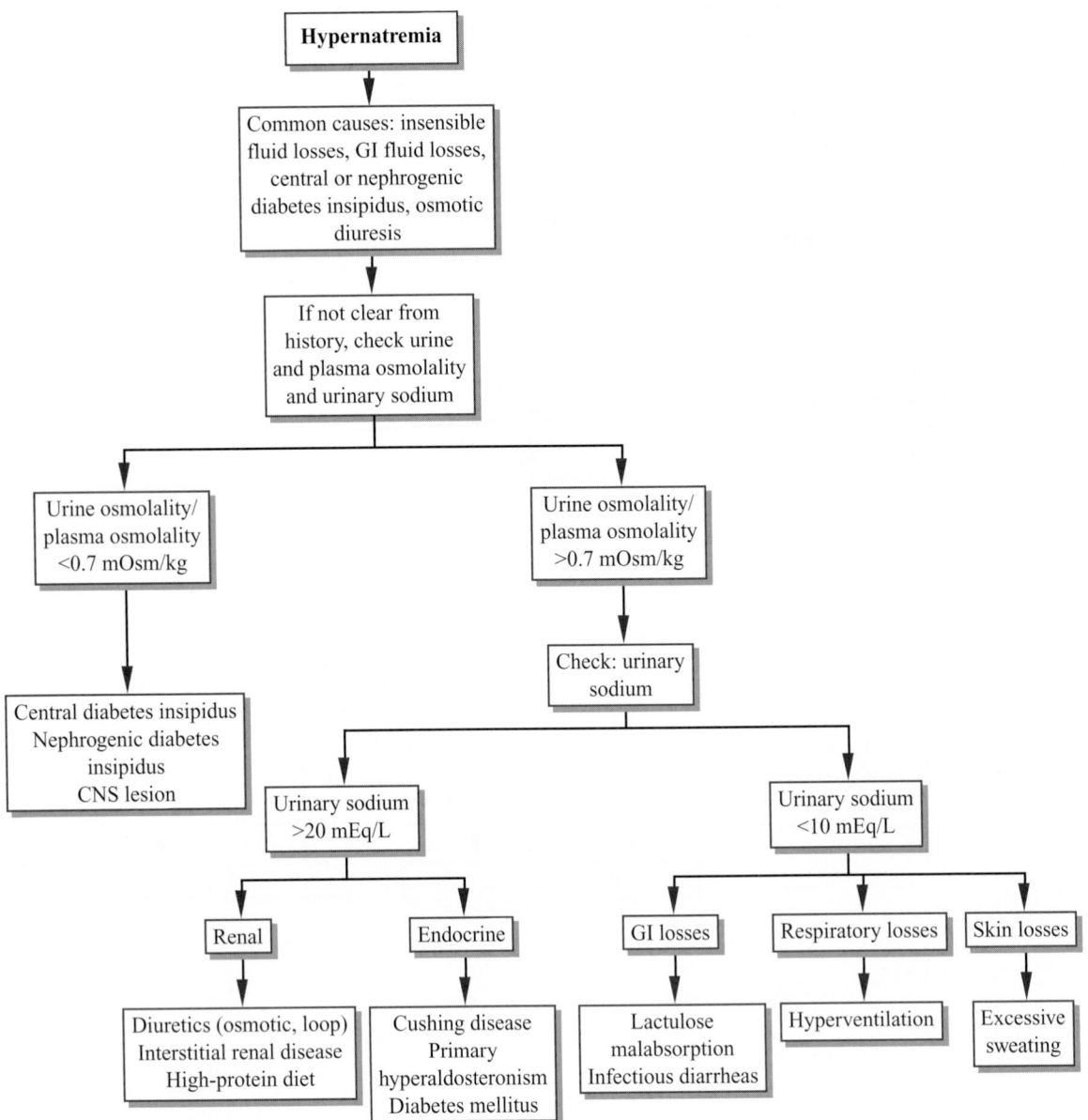

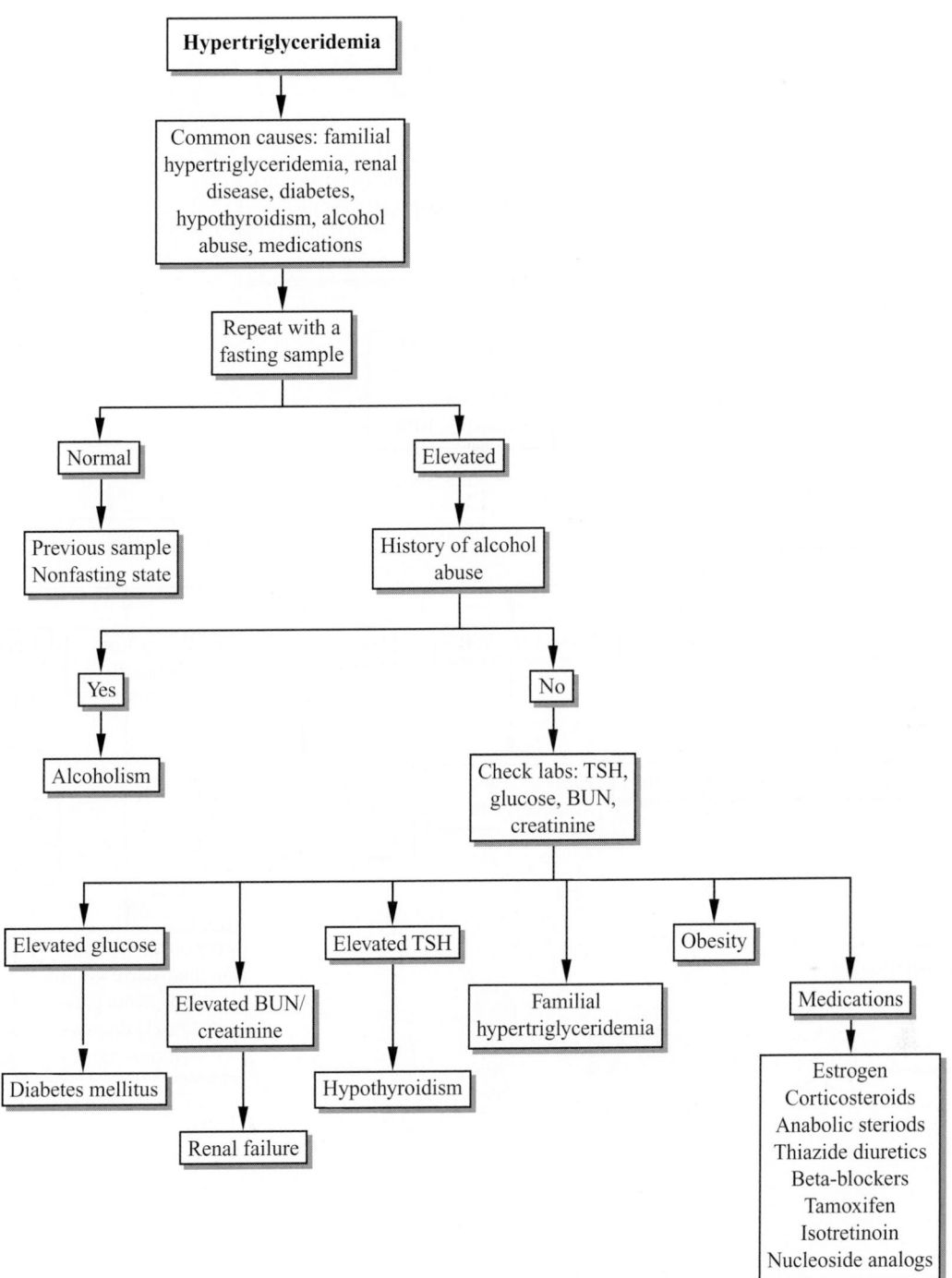

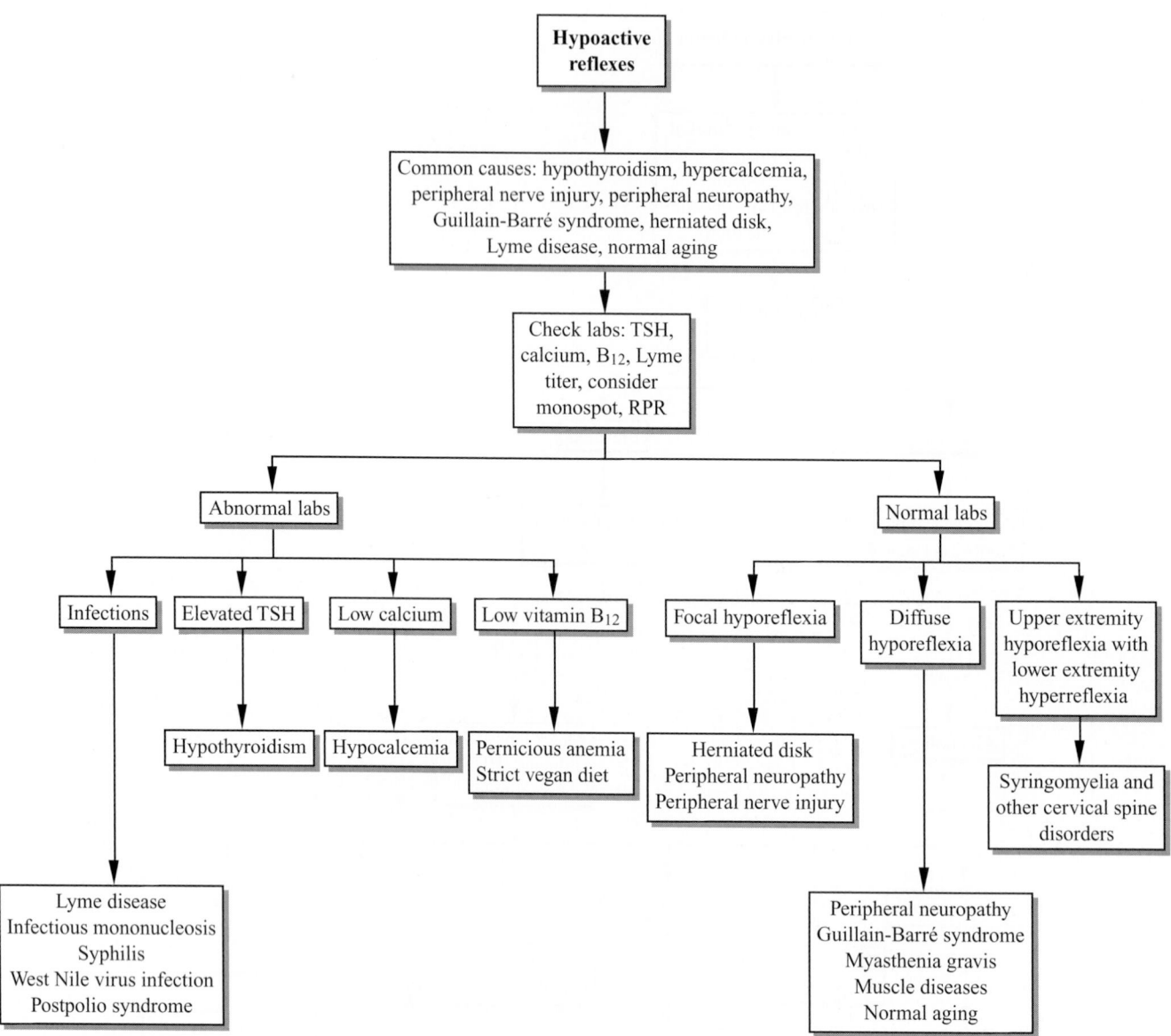

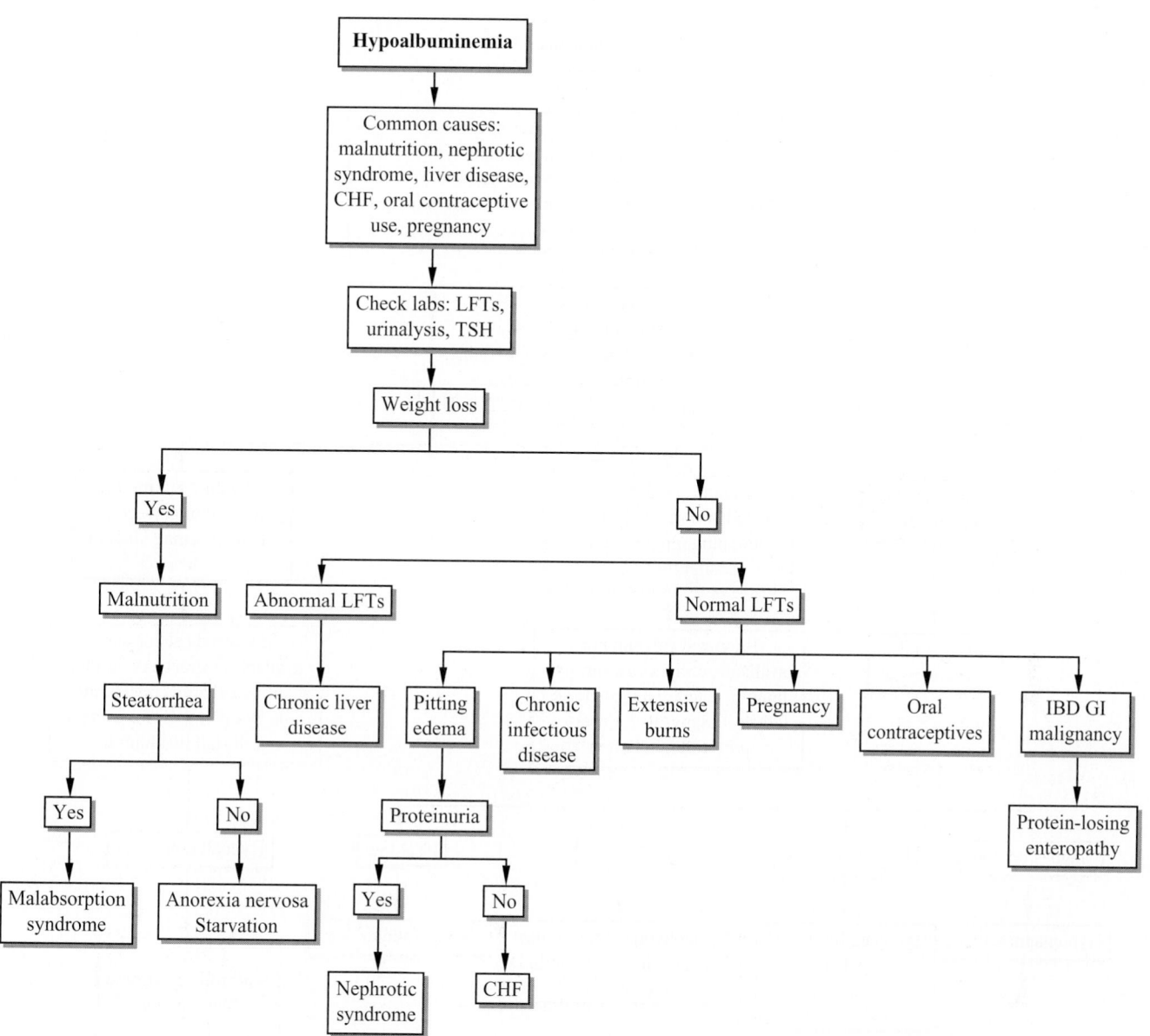

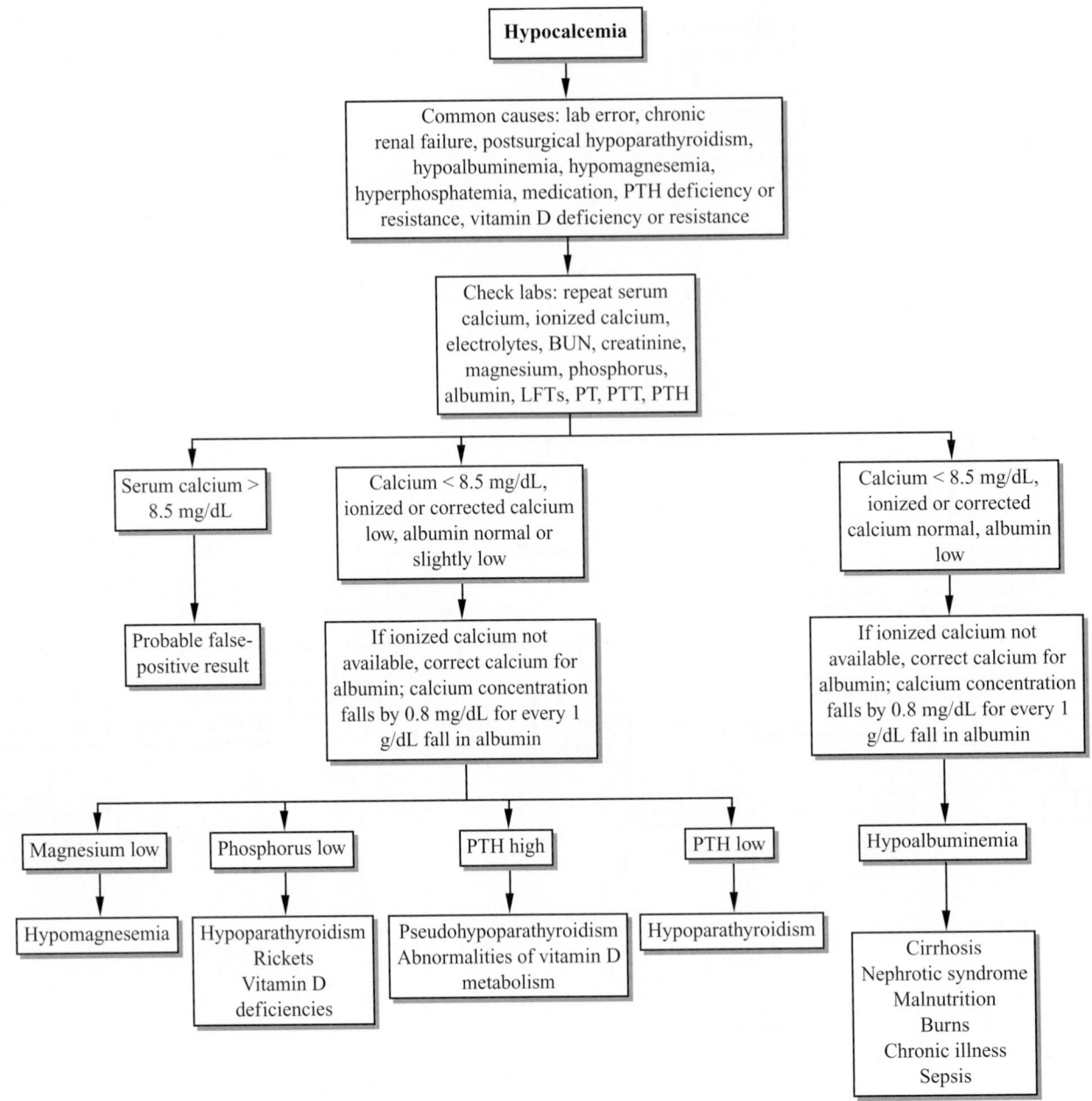

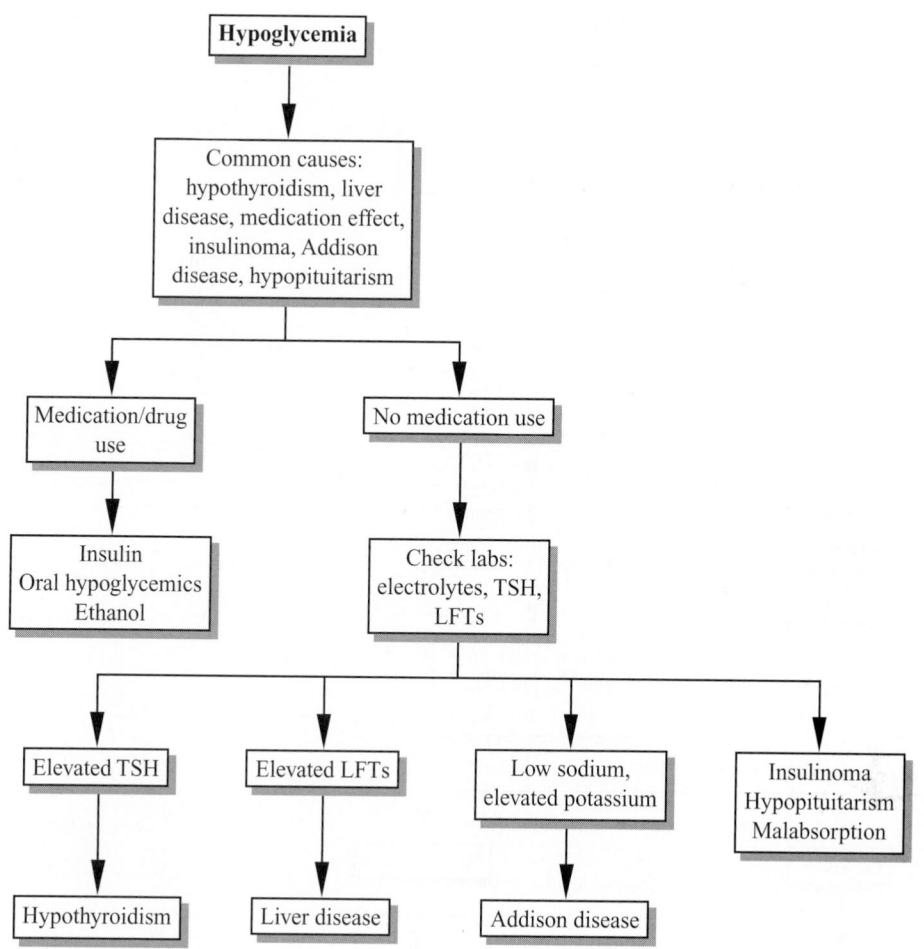

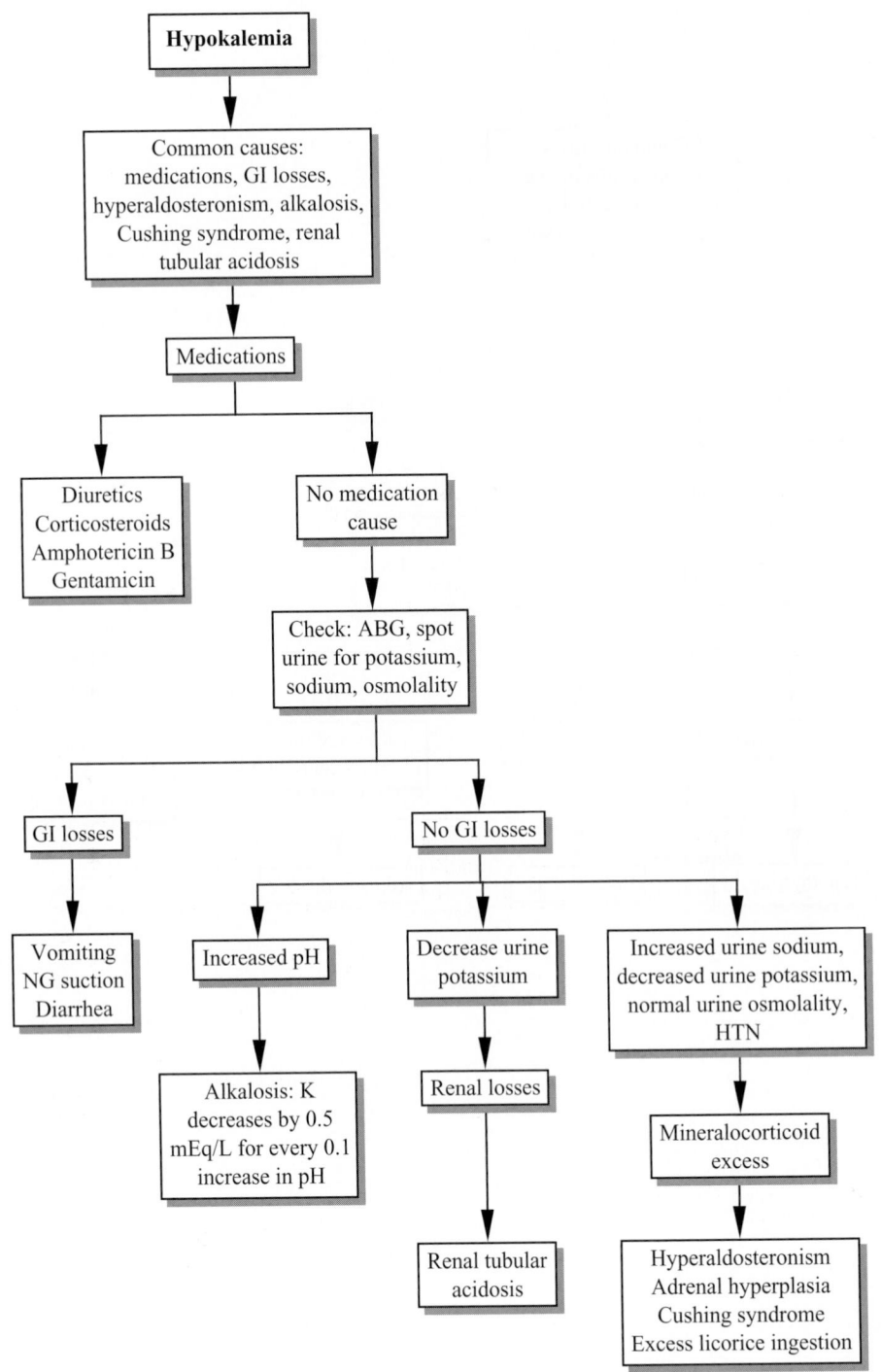

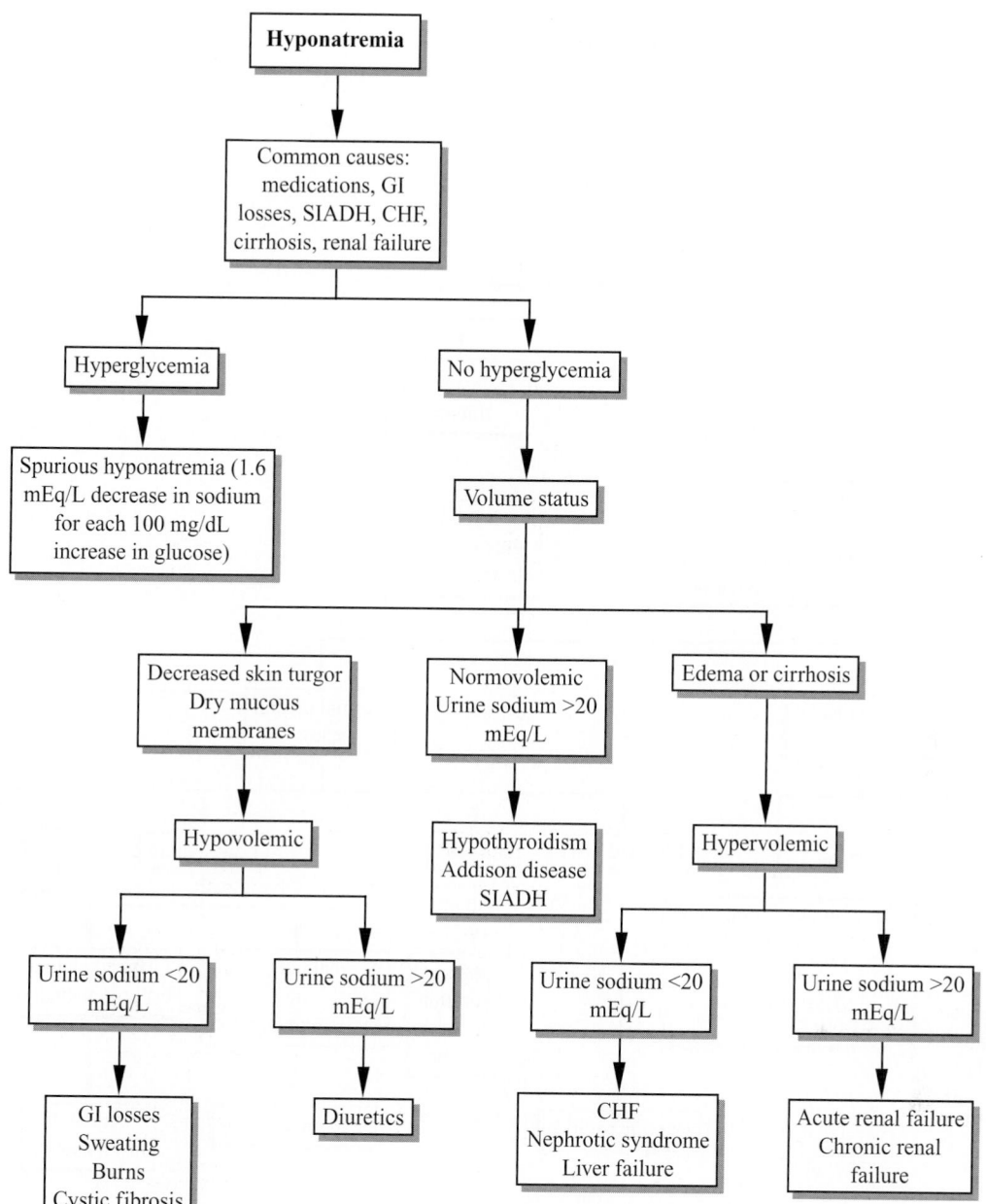

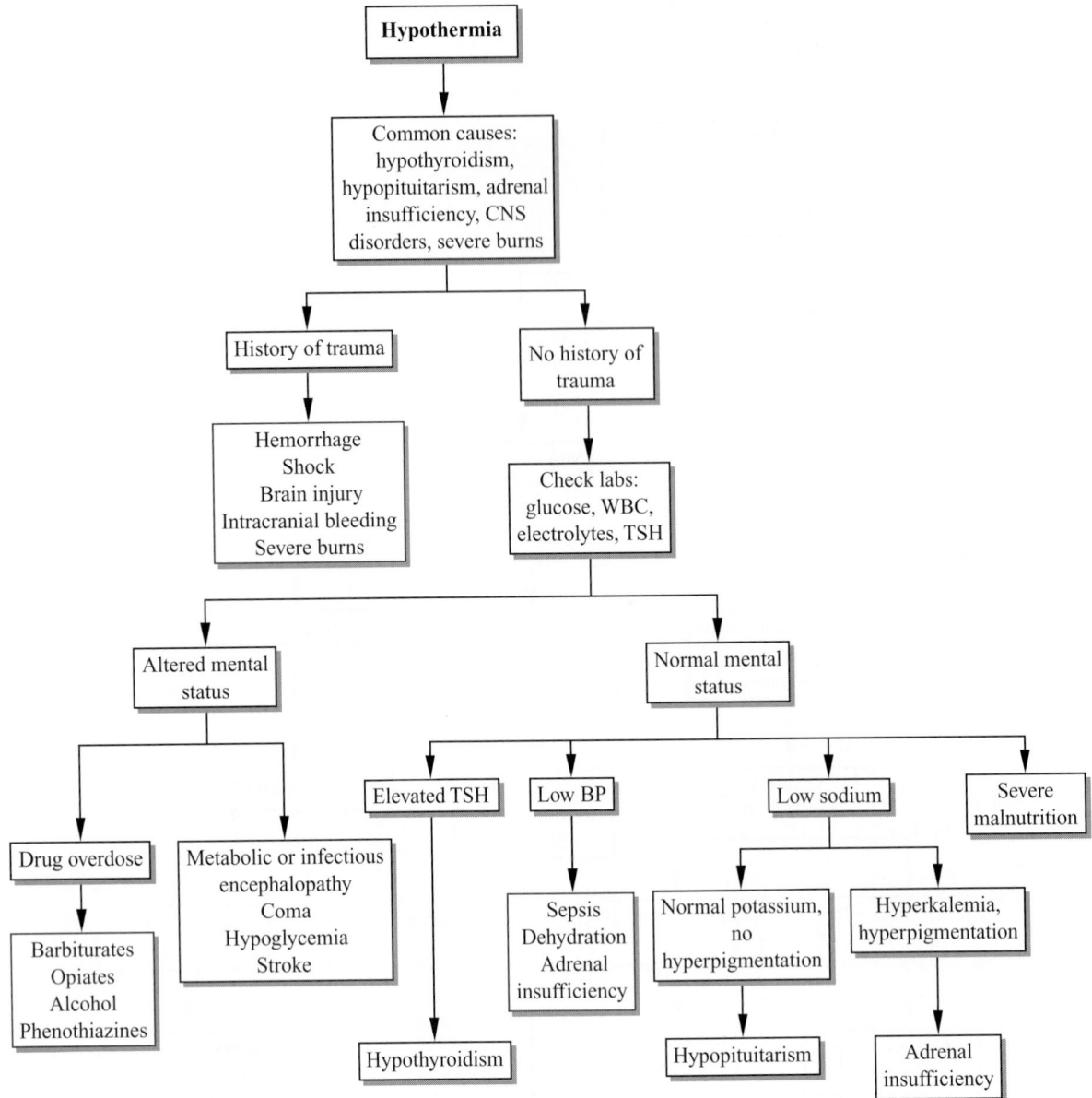

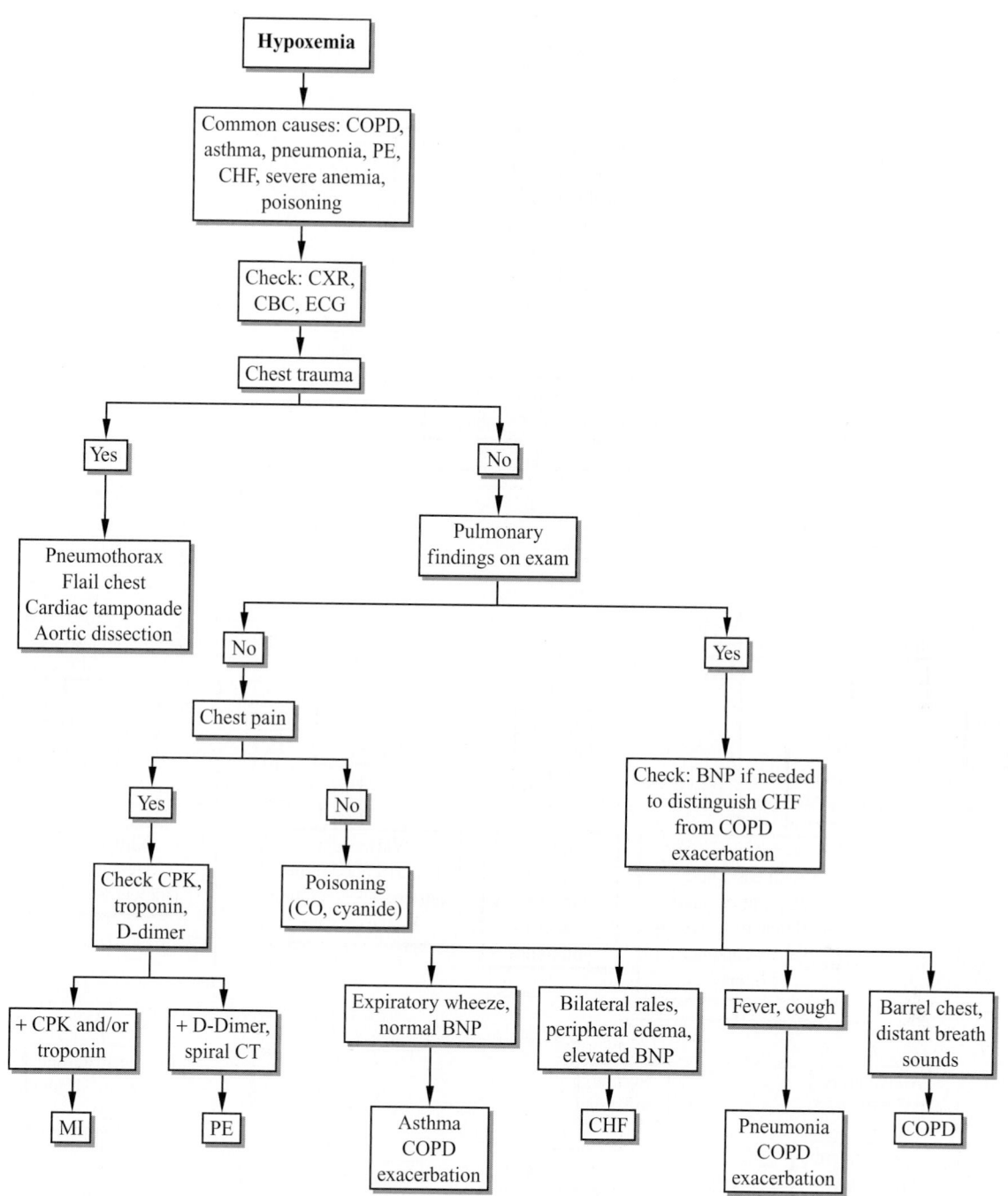

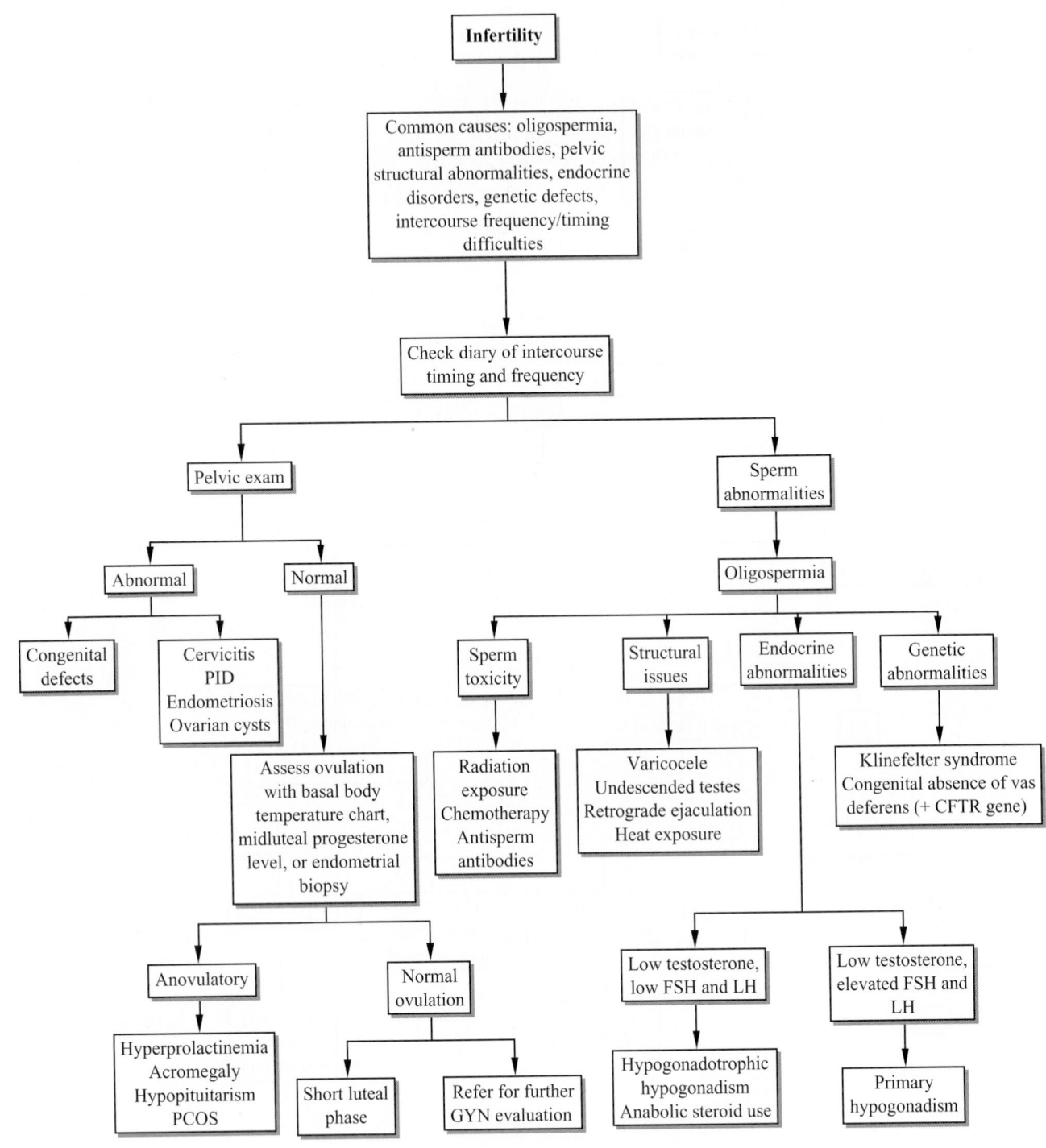

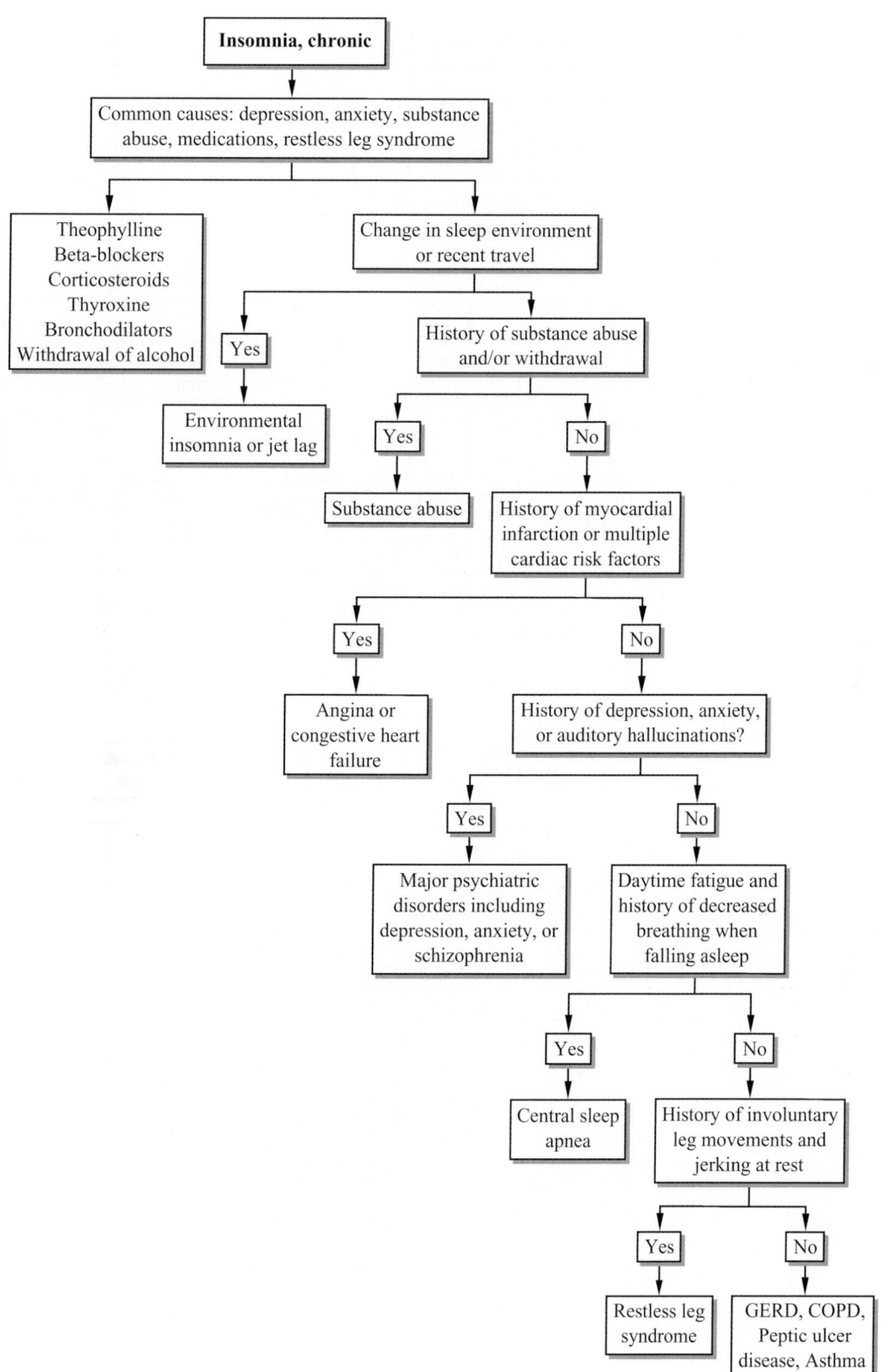

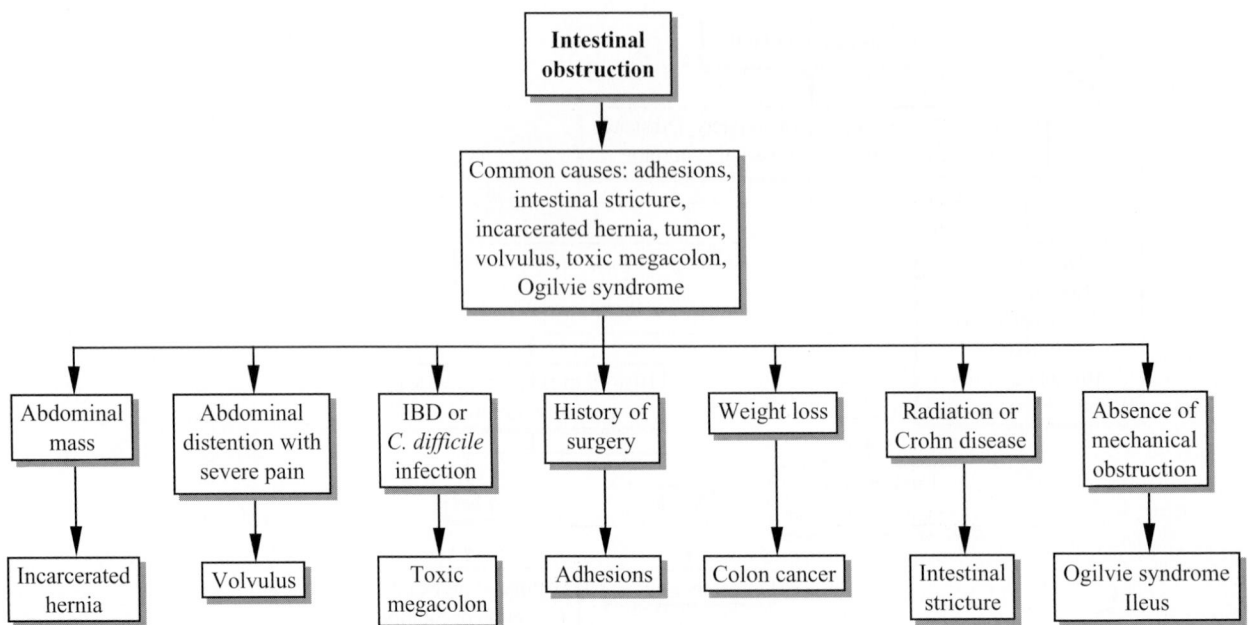

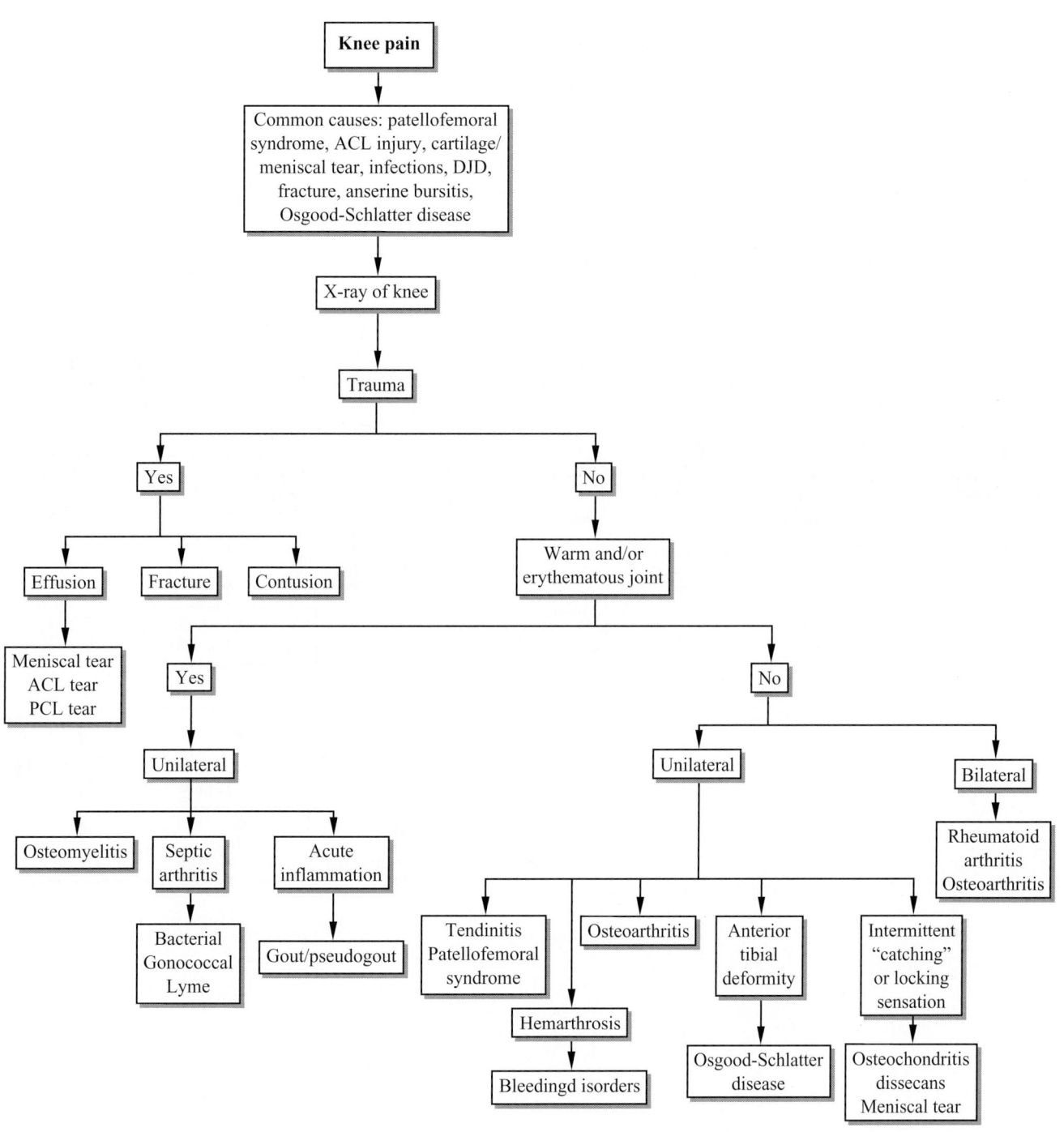

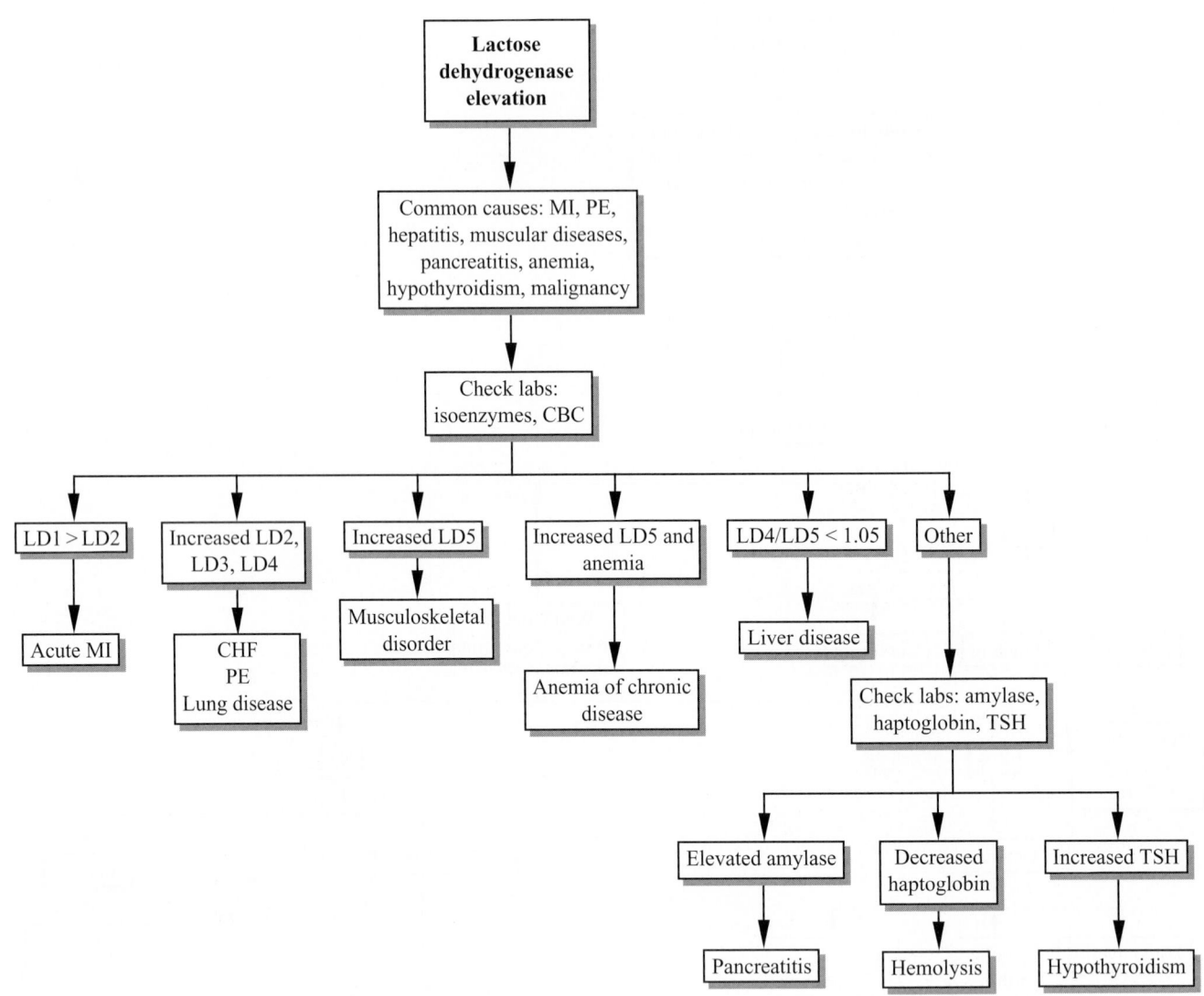

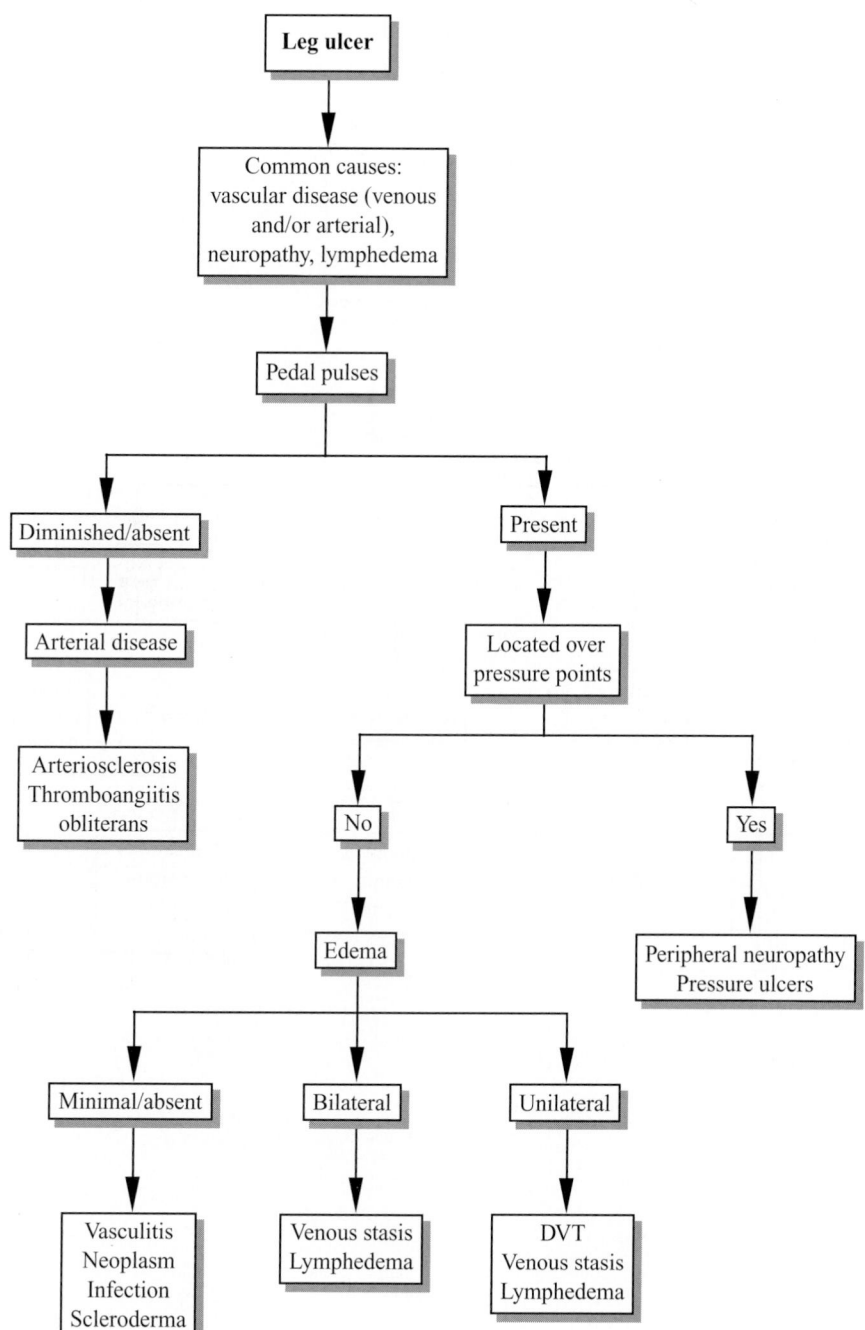

Leg ulcer

Common causes:
vascular disease (venous
and/or arterial),
neuropathy, lymphedema

Pedal pulses

Diminished/absent → Arterial disease → Arteriosclerosis
Thromboangiitis
obliterans

Present → Located over
pressure points

No → Edema

Yes → Peripheral neuropathy
Pressure ulcers

Minimal/absent → Vasculitis
Neoplasm
Infection
Scleroderma

Bilateral → Venous stasis
Lymphedema

Unilateral → DVT
Venous stasis
Lymphedema

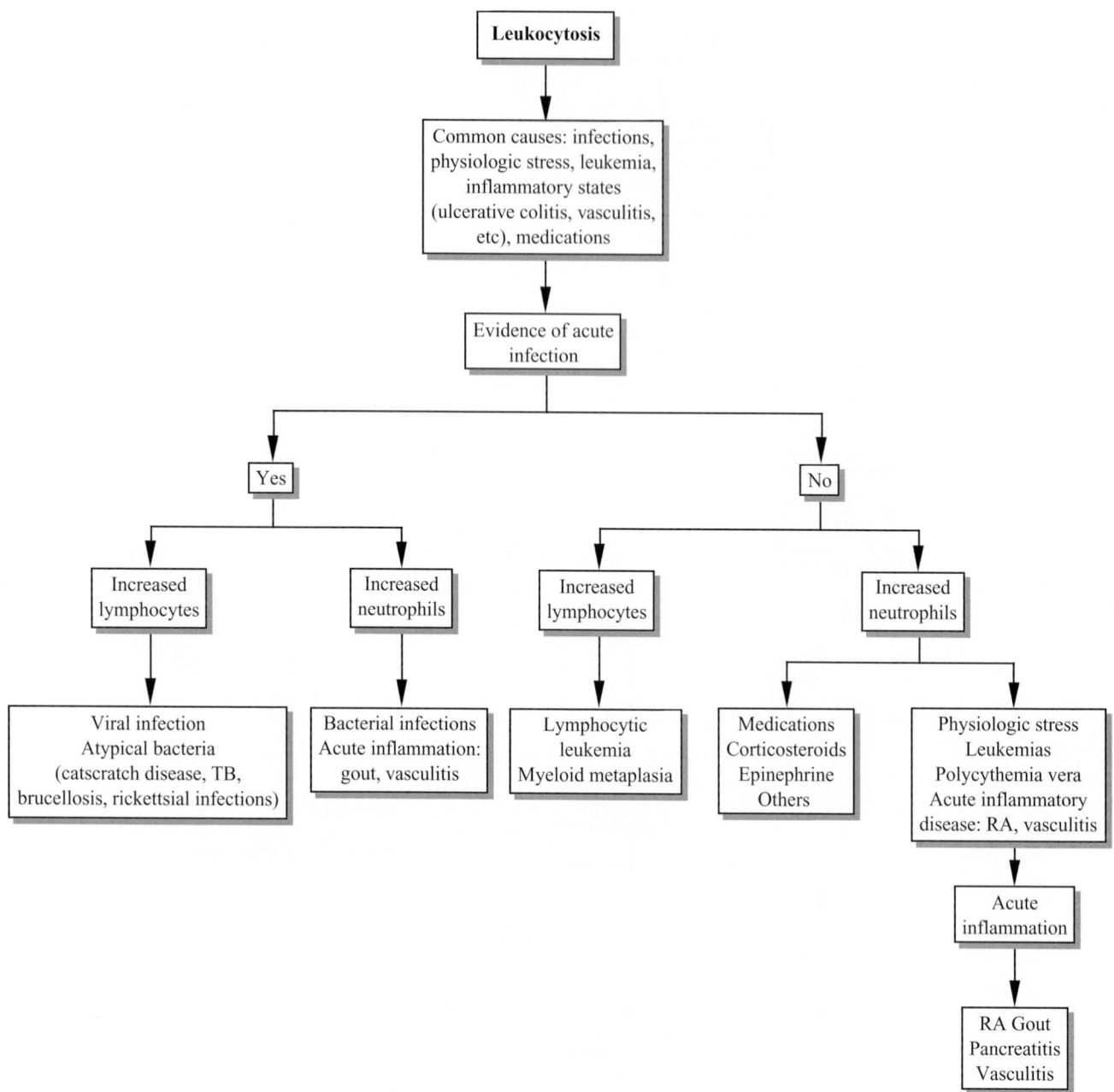

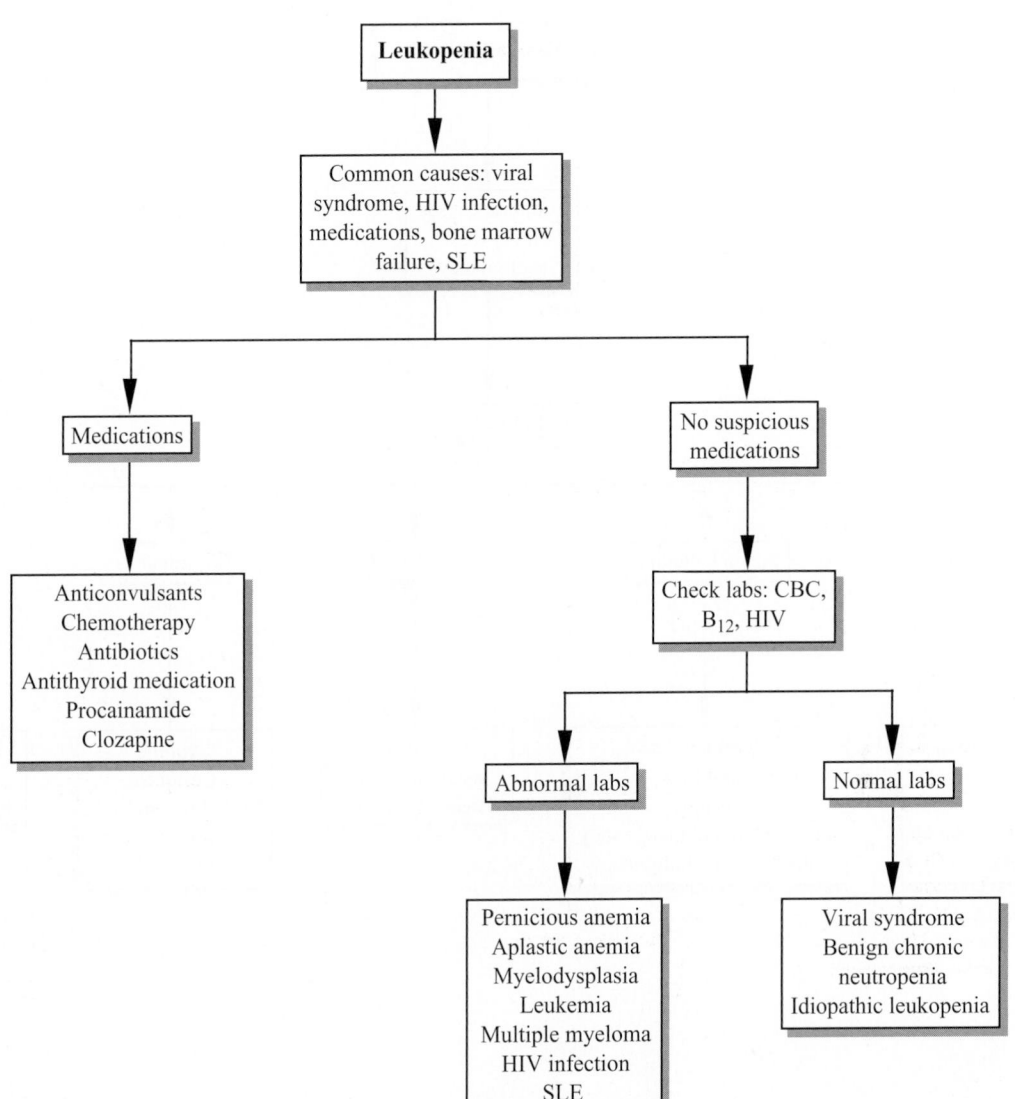

Lymphadenopathy

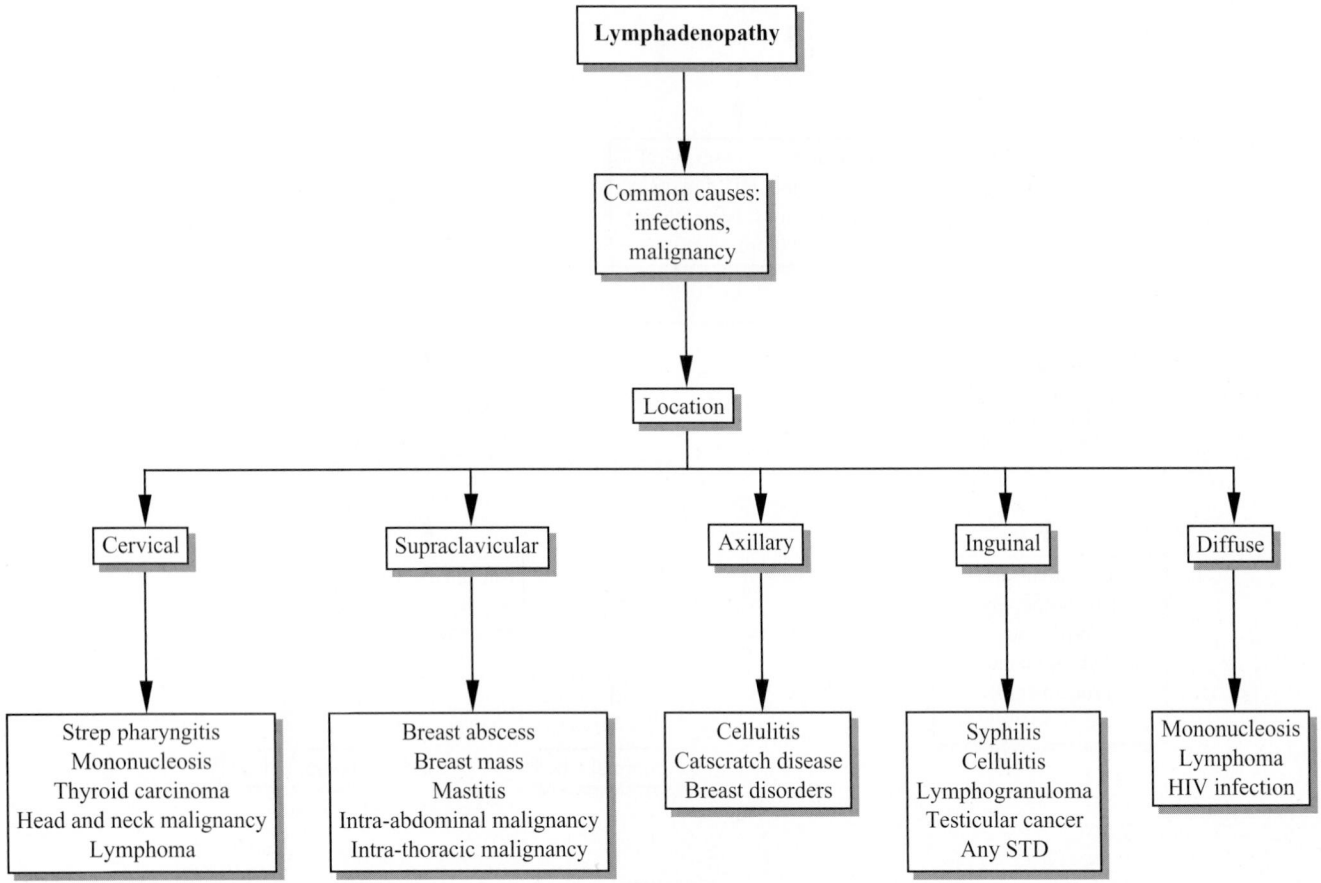

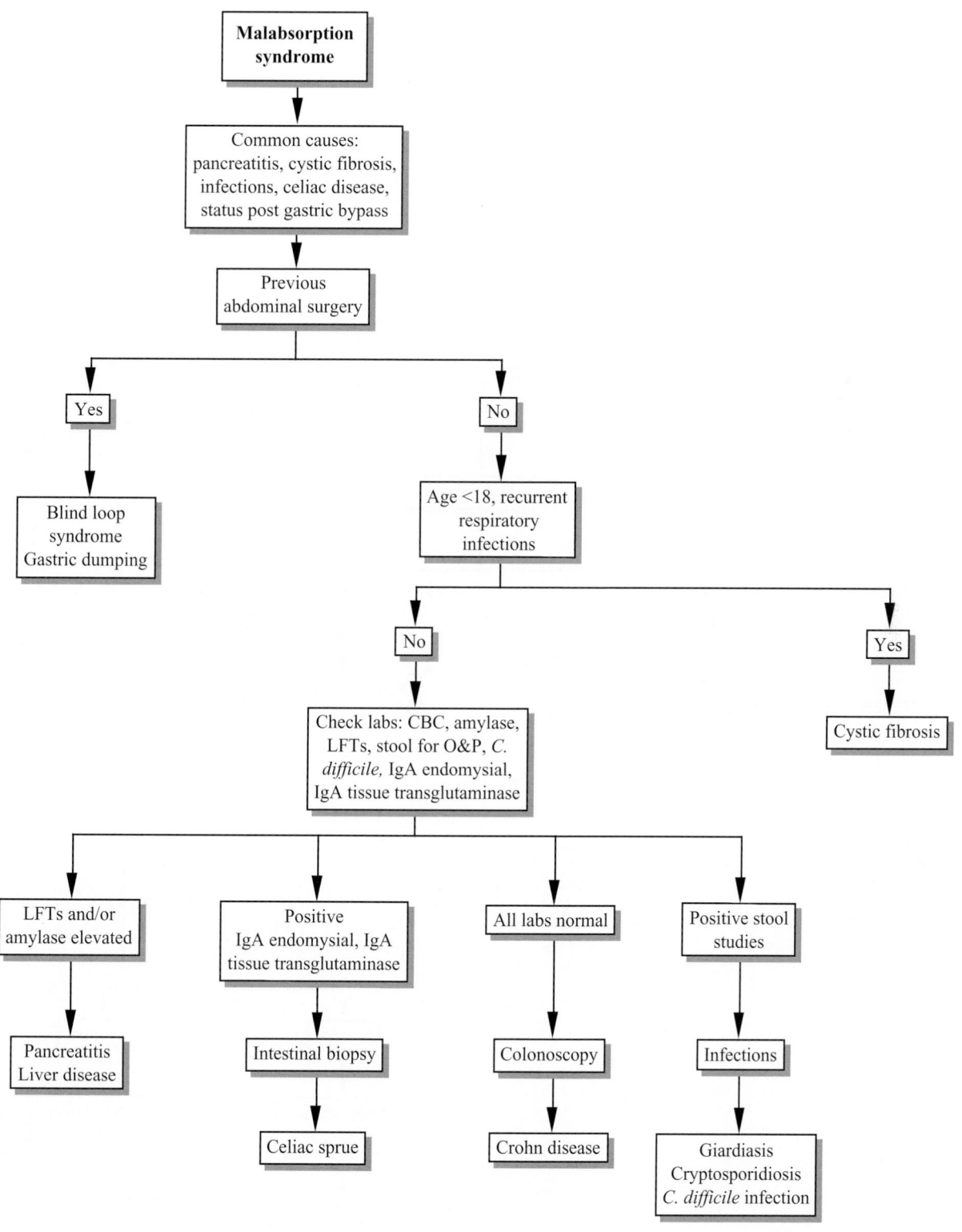

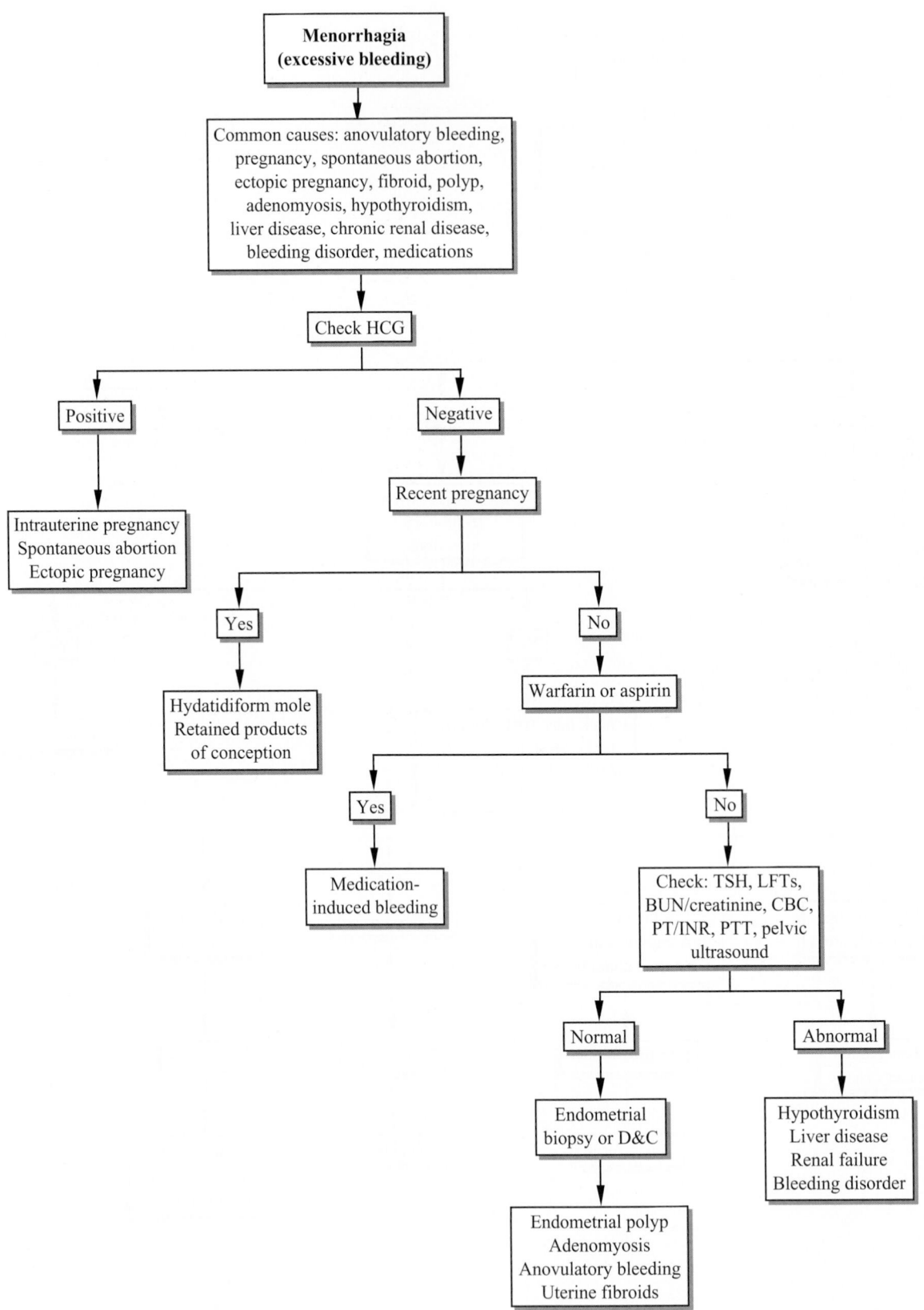

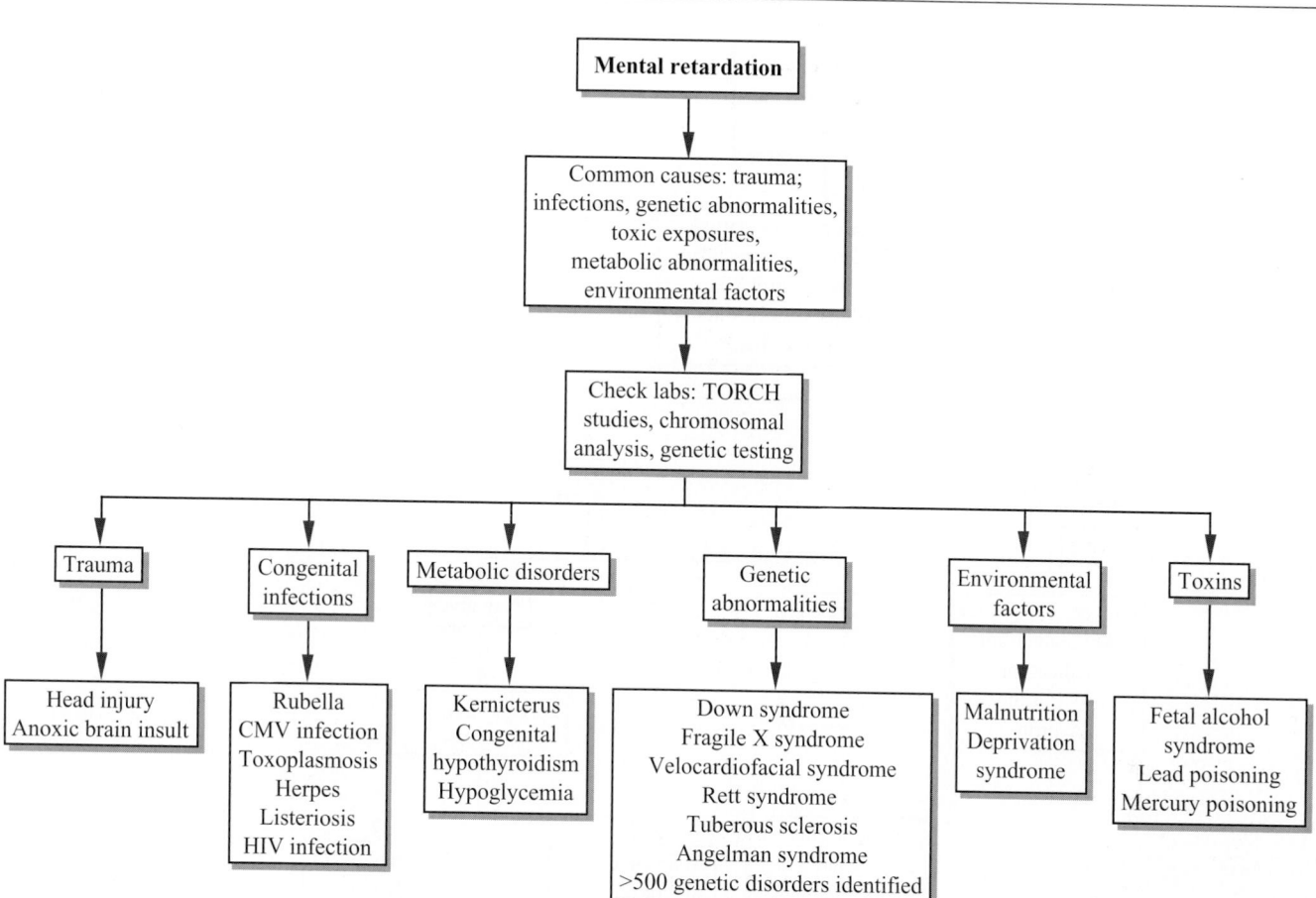

Mental retardation

↓

Common causes: trauma;
infections, genetic abnormalities,
toxic exposures,
metabolic abnormalities,
environmental factors

↓

Check labs: TORCH
studies, chromosomal
analysis, genetic testing

Trauma
Head injury
Anoxic brain insult

Congenital infections
Rubella
CMV infection
Toxoplasmosis
Herpes
Listeriosis
HIV infection

Metabolic disorders
Kernicterus
Congenital hypothyroidism
Hypoglycemia

Genetic abnormalities
Down syndrome
Fragile X syndrome
Velocardiofacial syndrome
Rett syndrome
Tuberous sclerosis
Angelman syndrome
>500 genetic disorders identified

Environmental factors
Malnutrition
Deprivation syndrome

Toxins
Fetal alcohol syndrome
Lead poisoning
Mercury poisoning

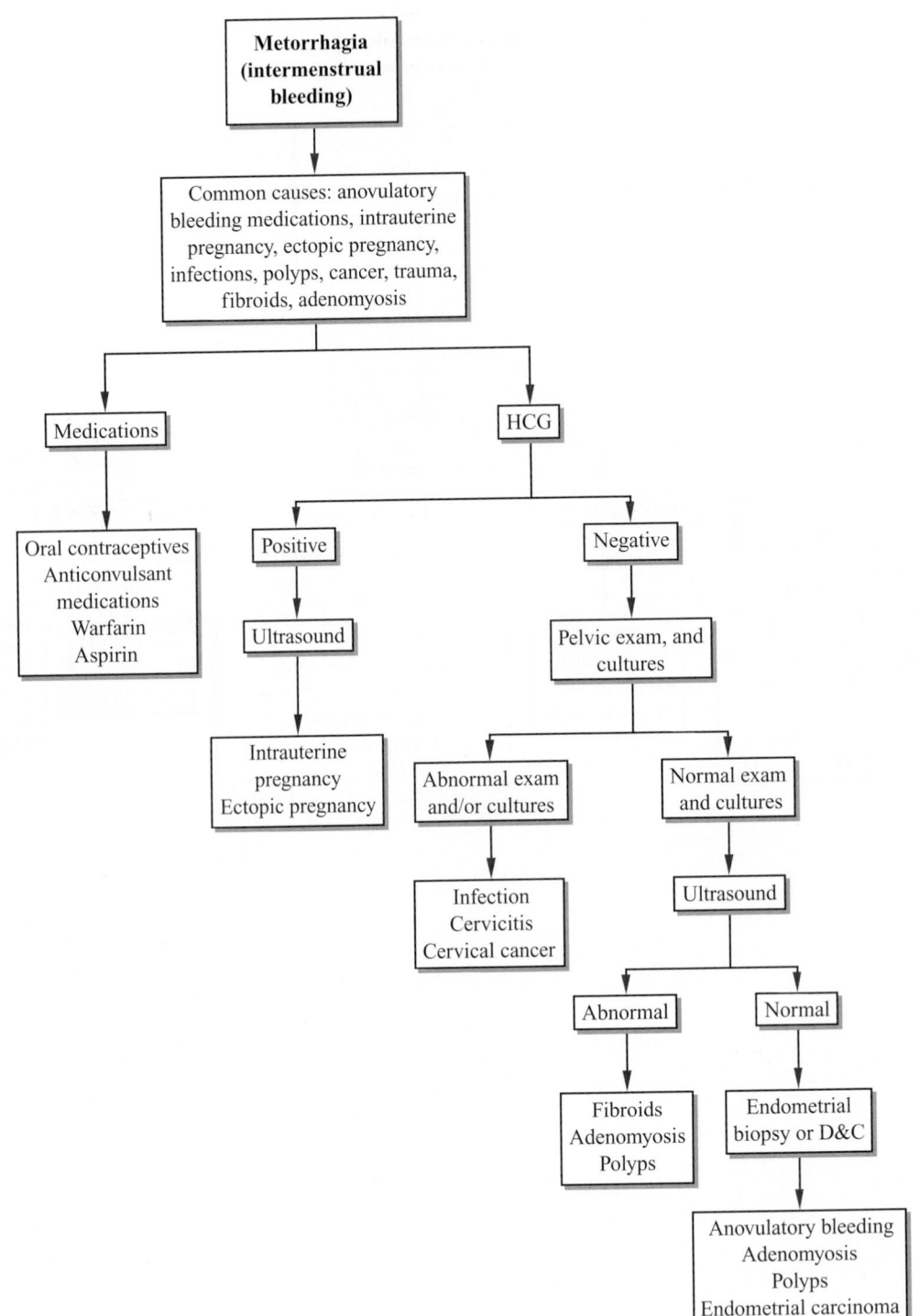

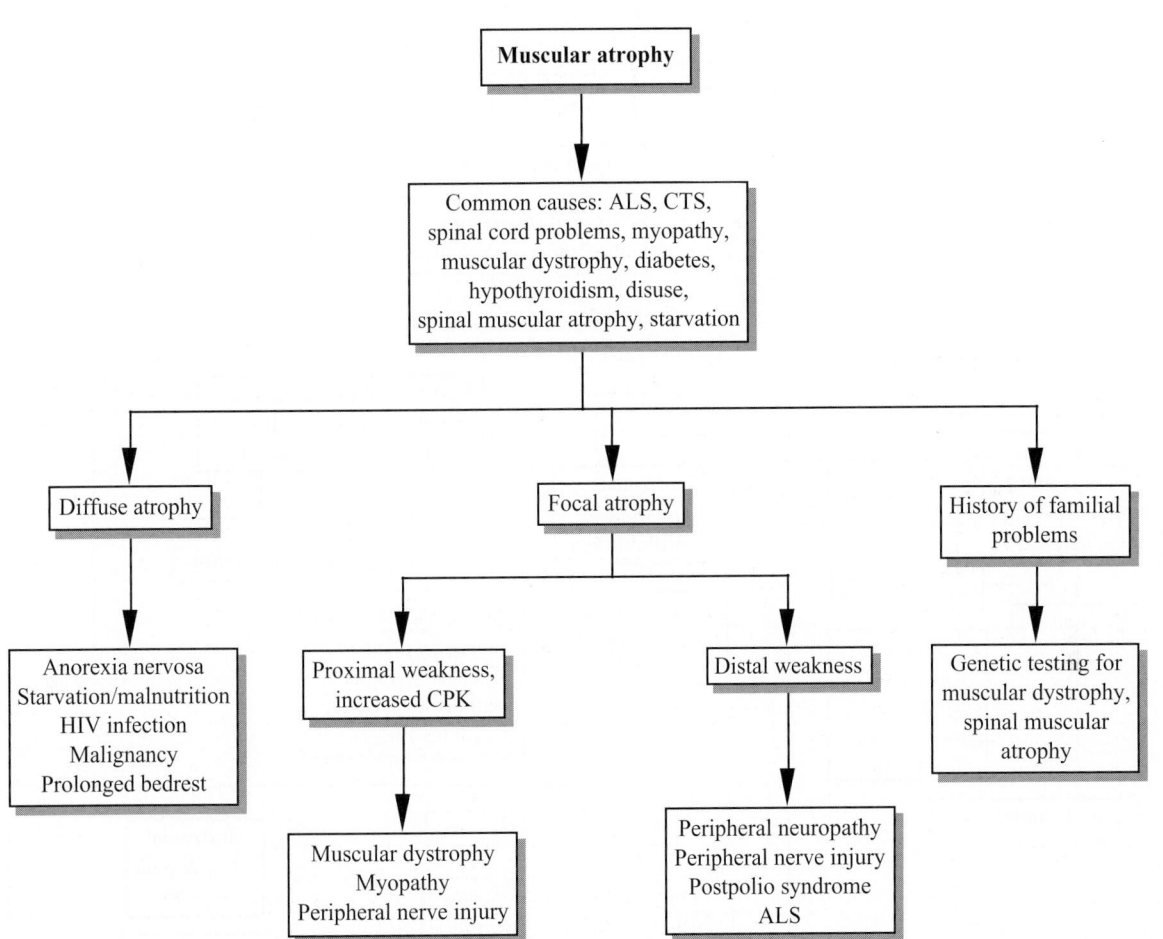

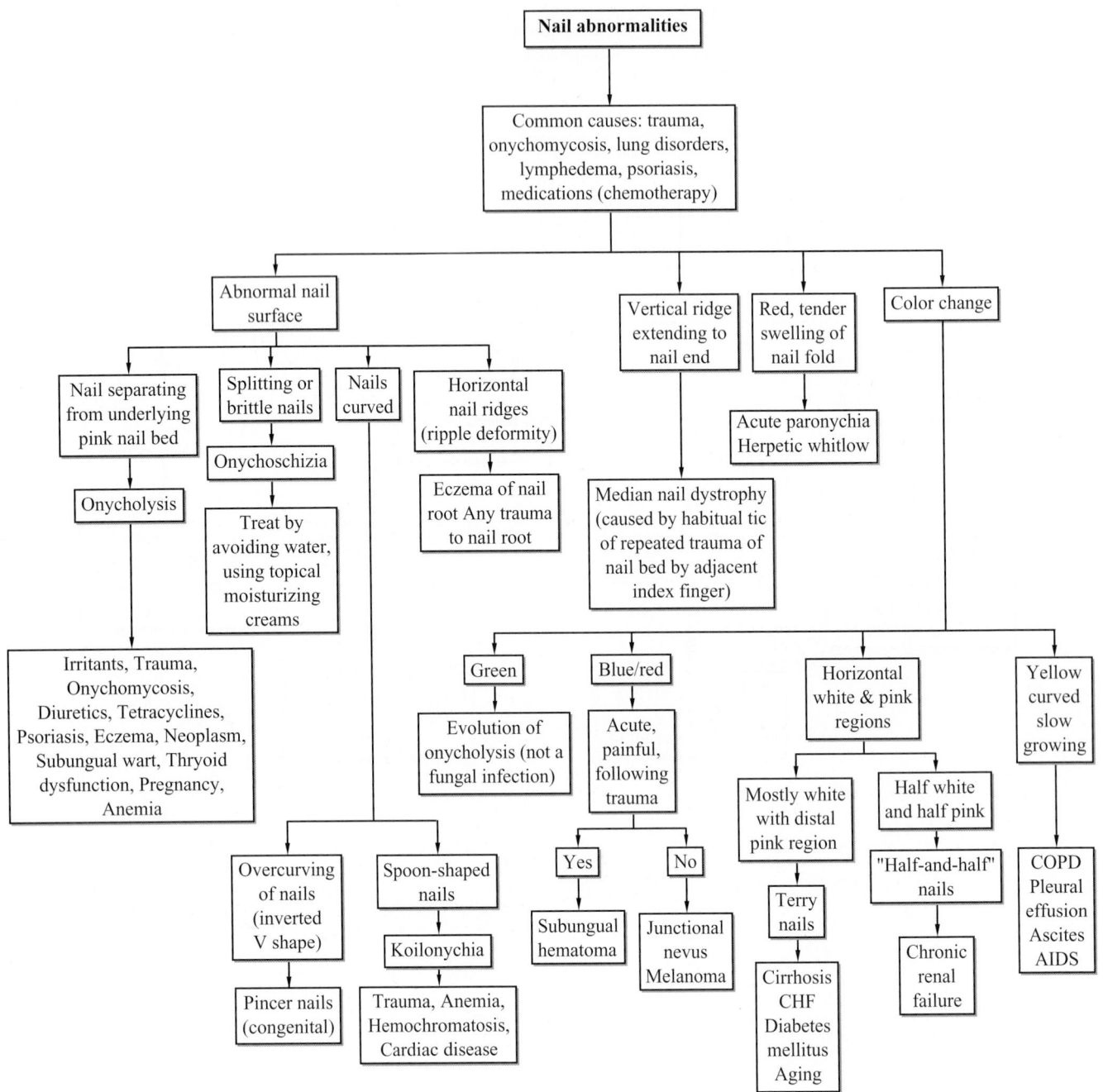

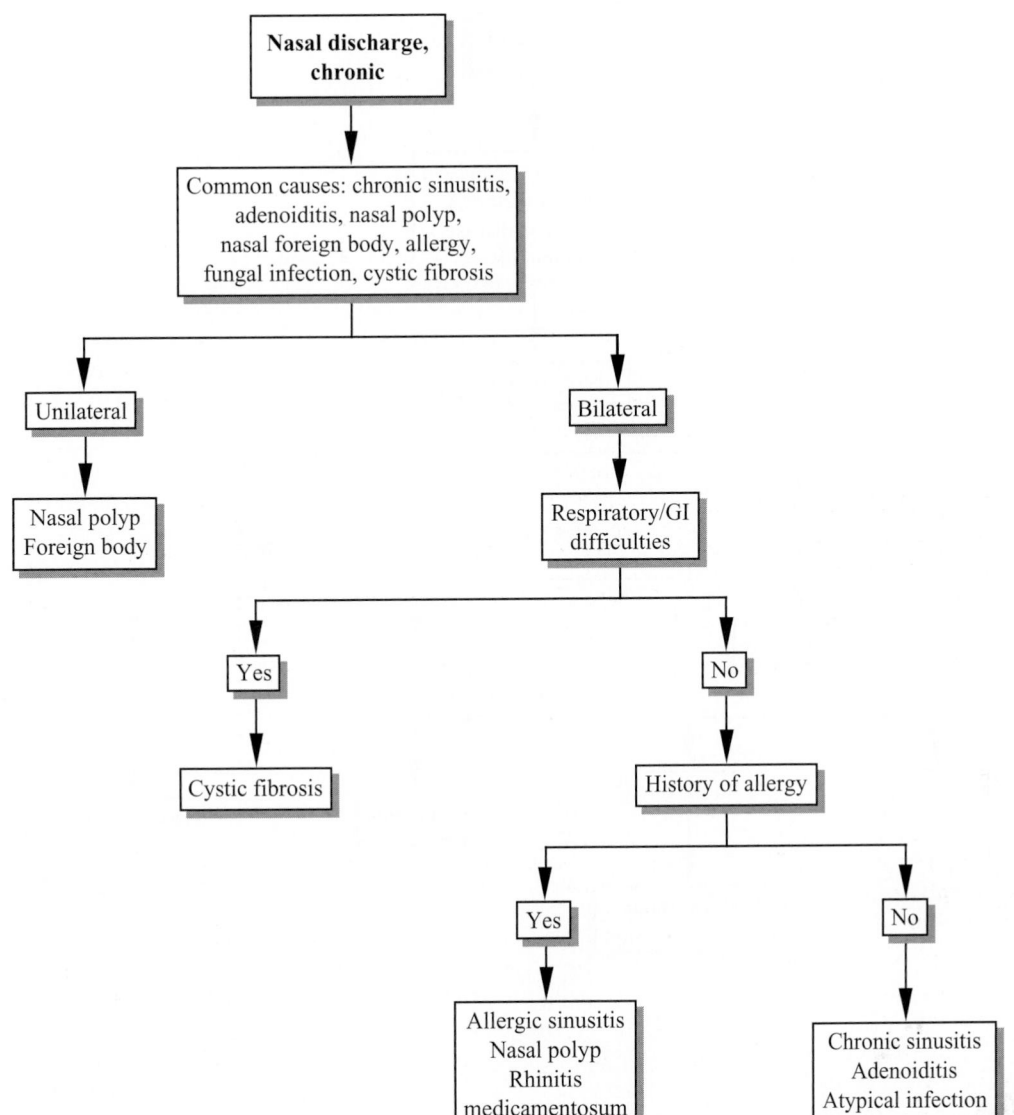

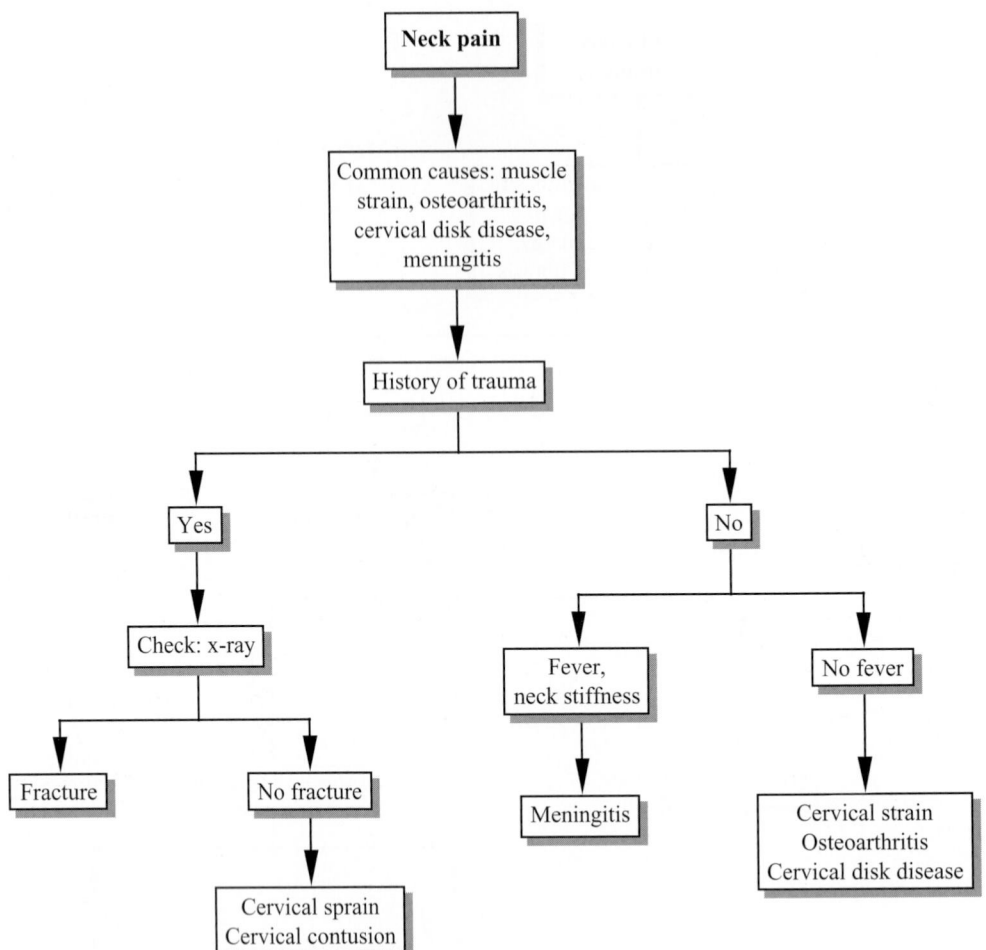

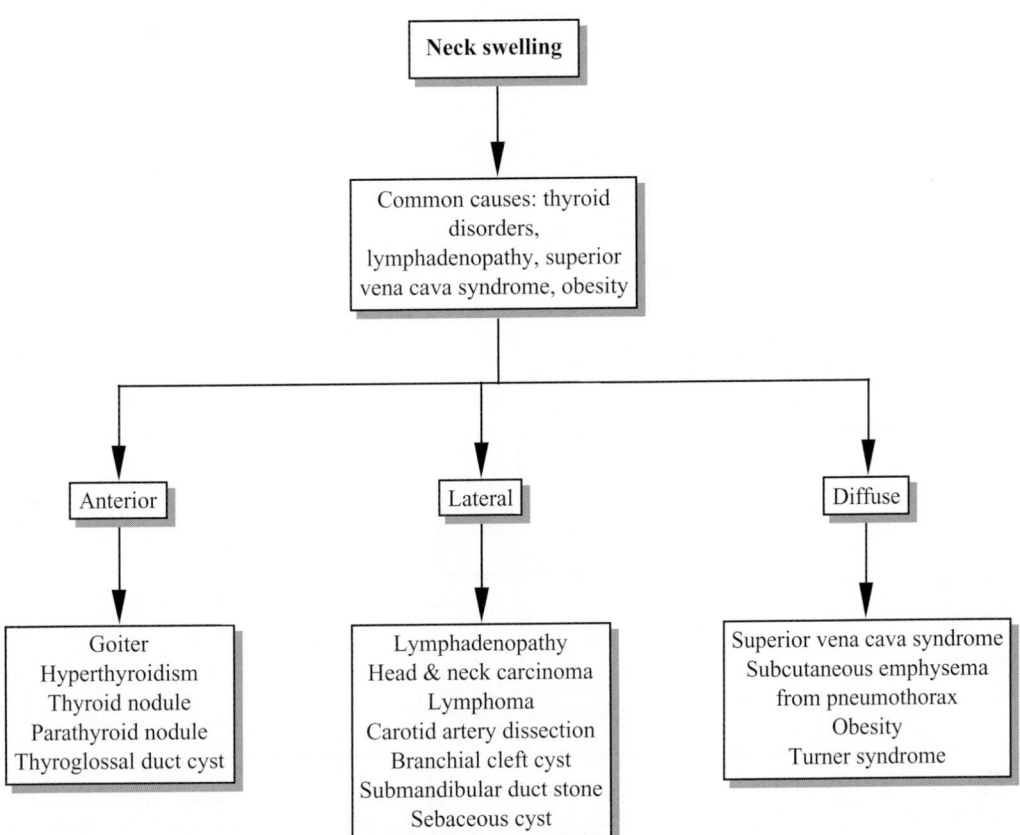

Neck swelling

Common causes: thyroid disorders, lymphadenopathy, superior vena cava syndrome, obesity

Anterior

Goiter
Hyperthyroidism
Thyroid nodule
Parathyroid nodule
Thyroglossal duct cyst

Lateral

Lymphadenopathy
Head & neck carcinoma
Lymphoma
Carotid artery dissection
Branchial cleft cyst
Submandibular duct stone
Sebaceous cyst

Diffuse

Superior vena cava syndrome
Subcutaneous emphysema
from pneumothorax
Obesity
Turner syndrome

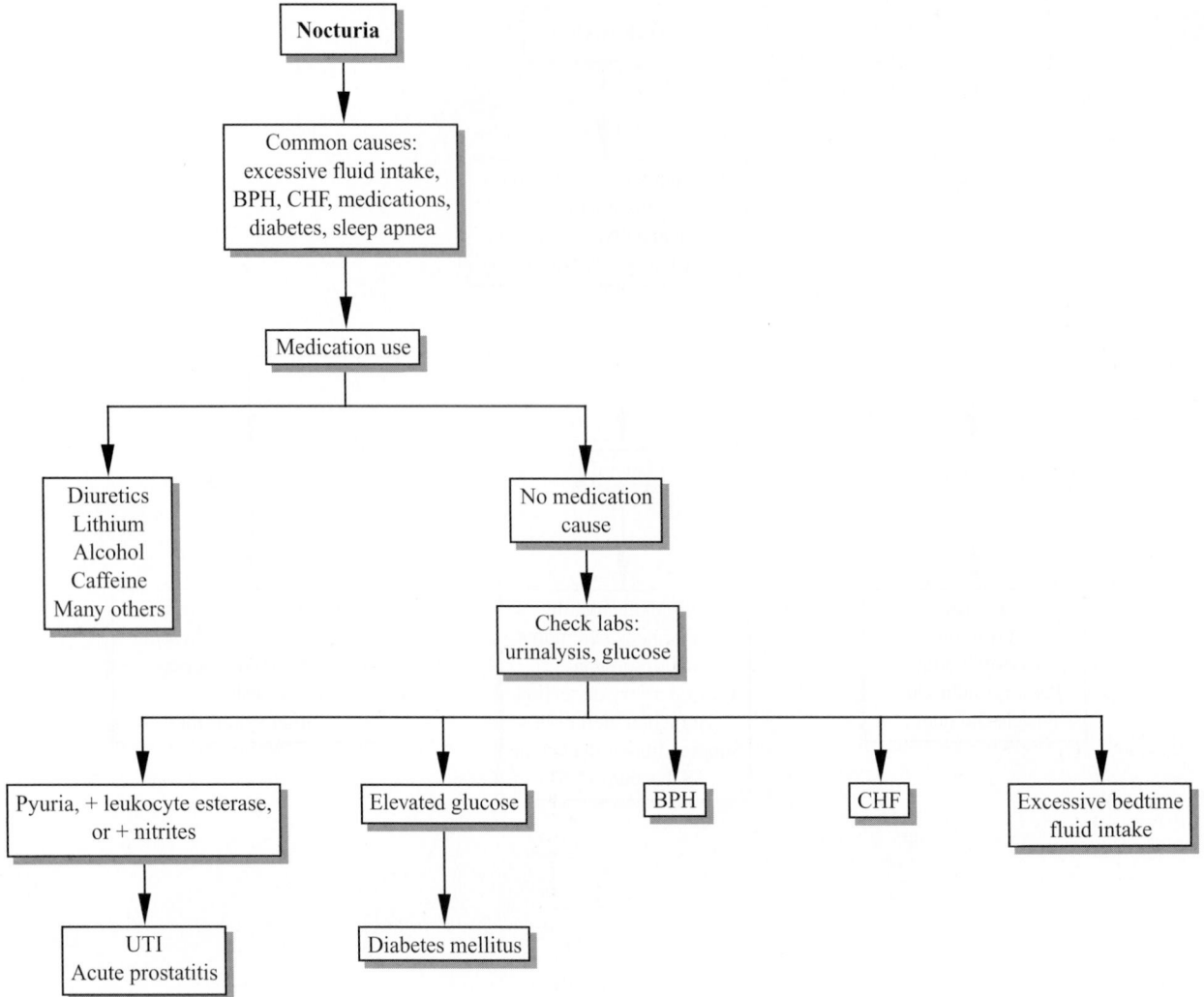

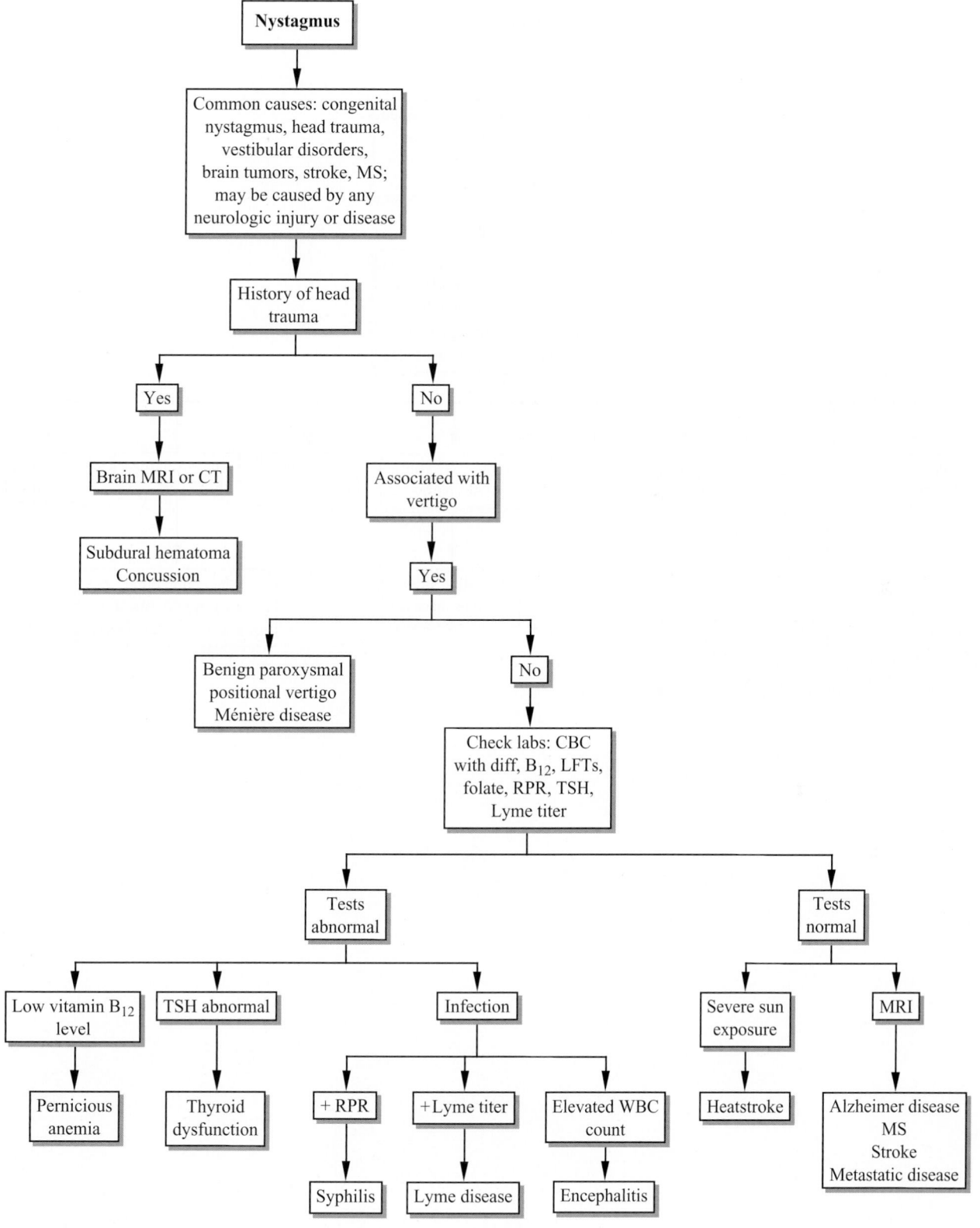

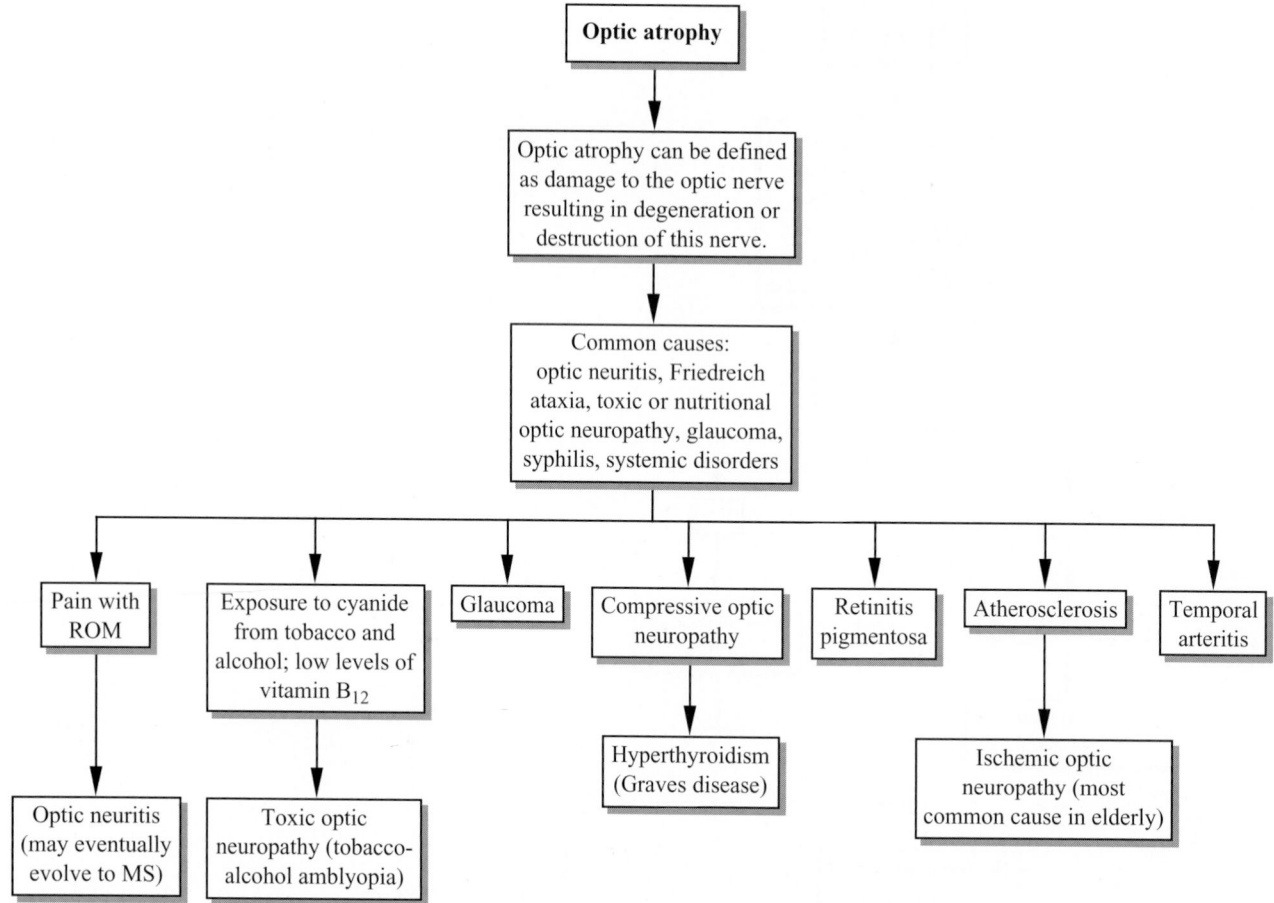

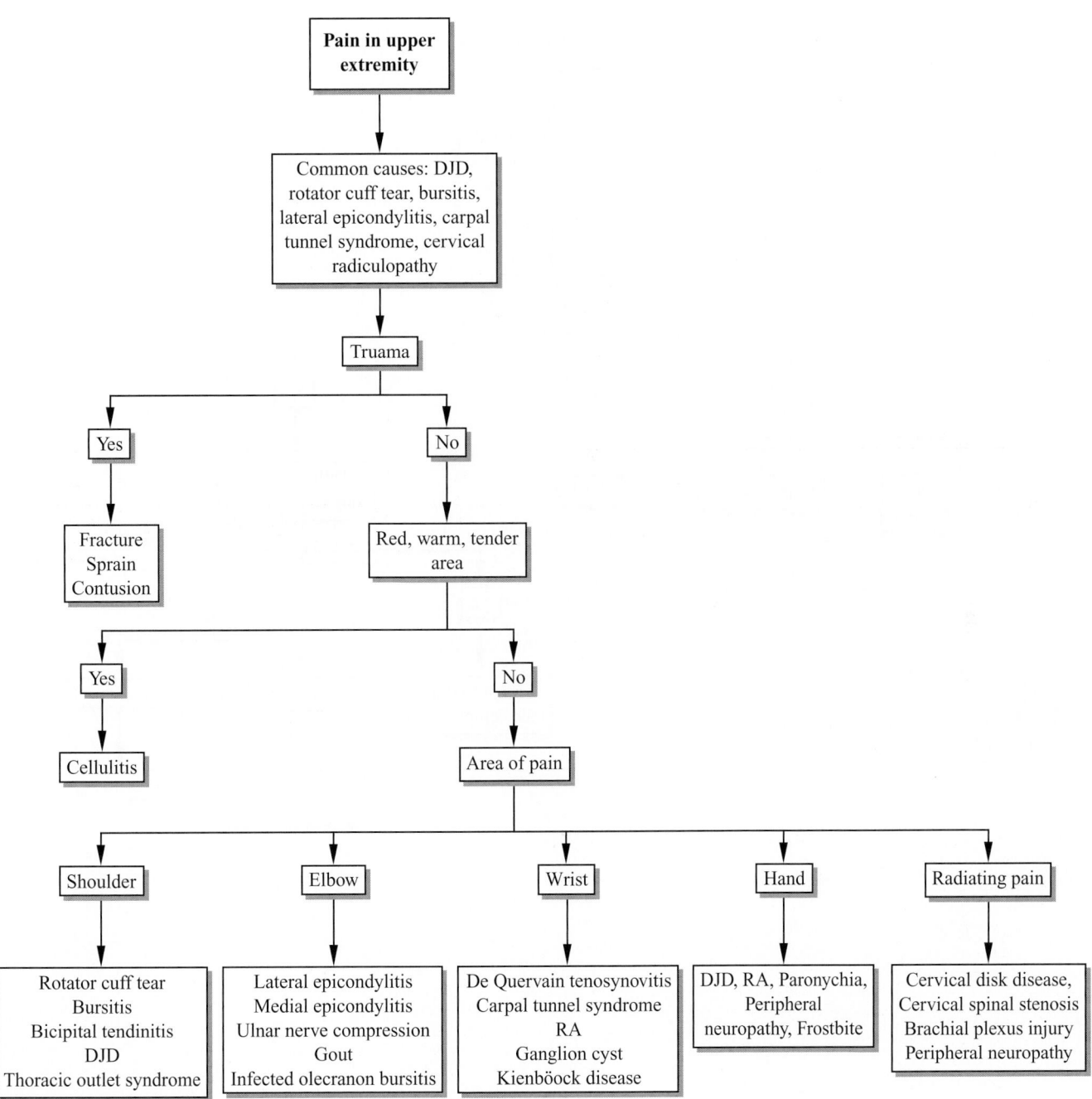

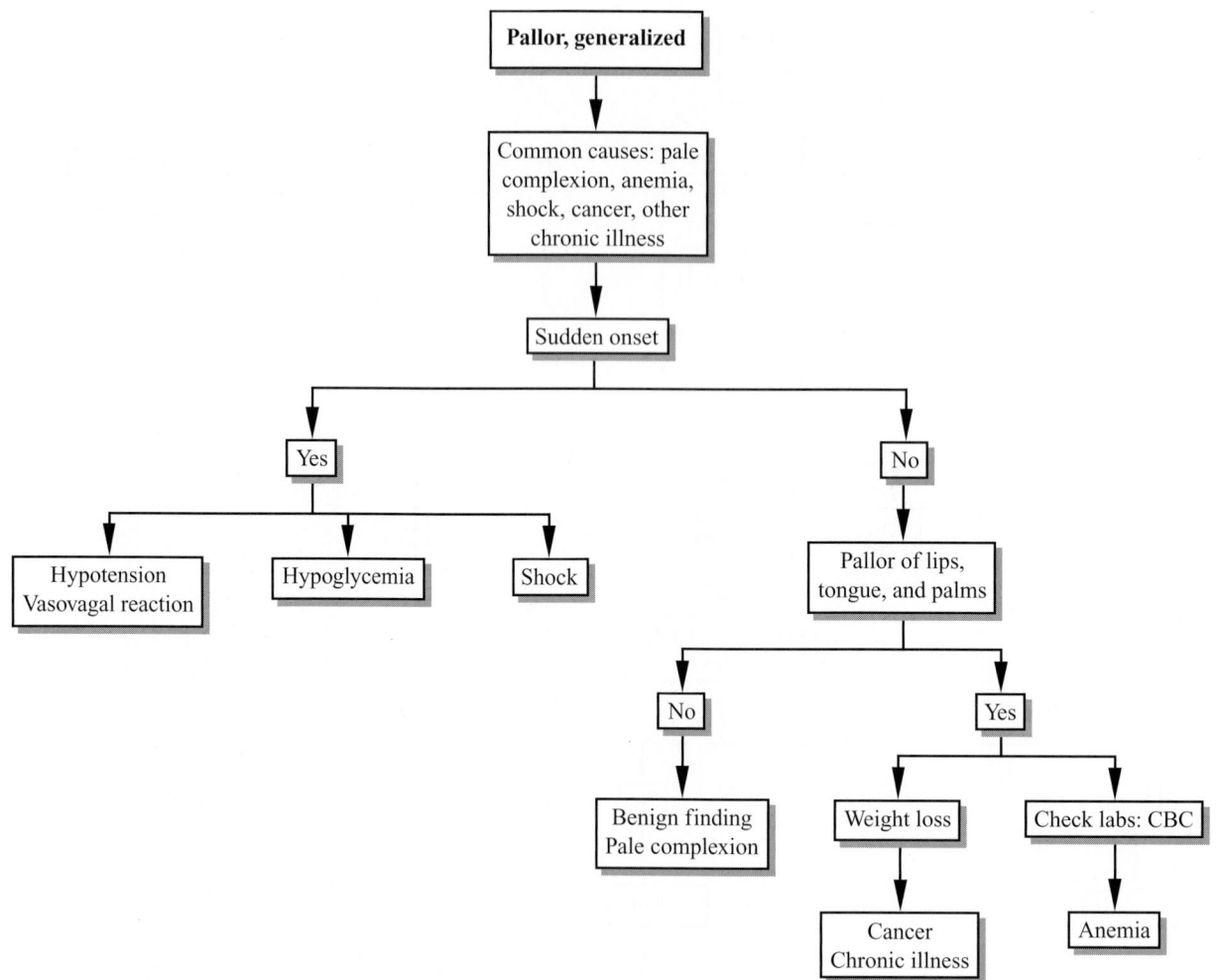

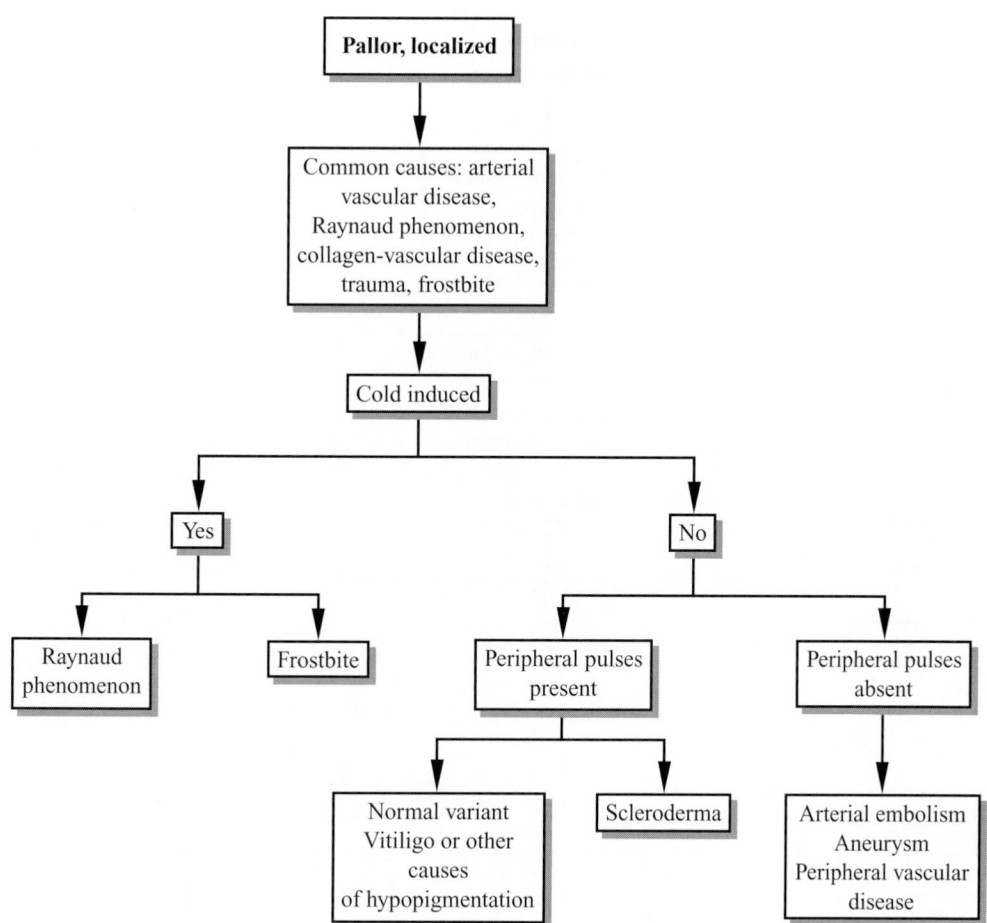

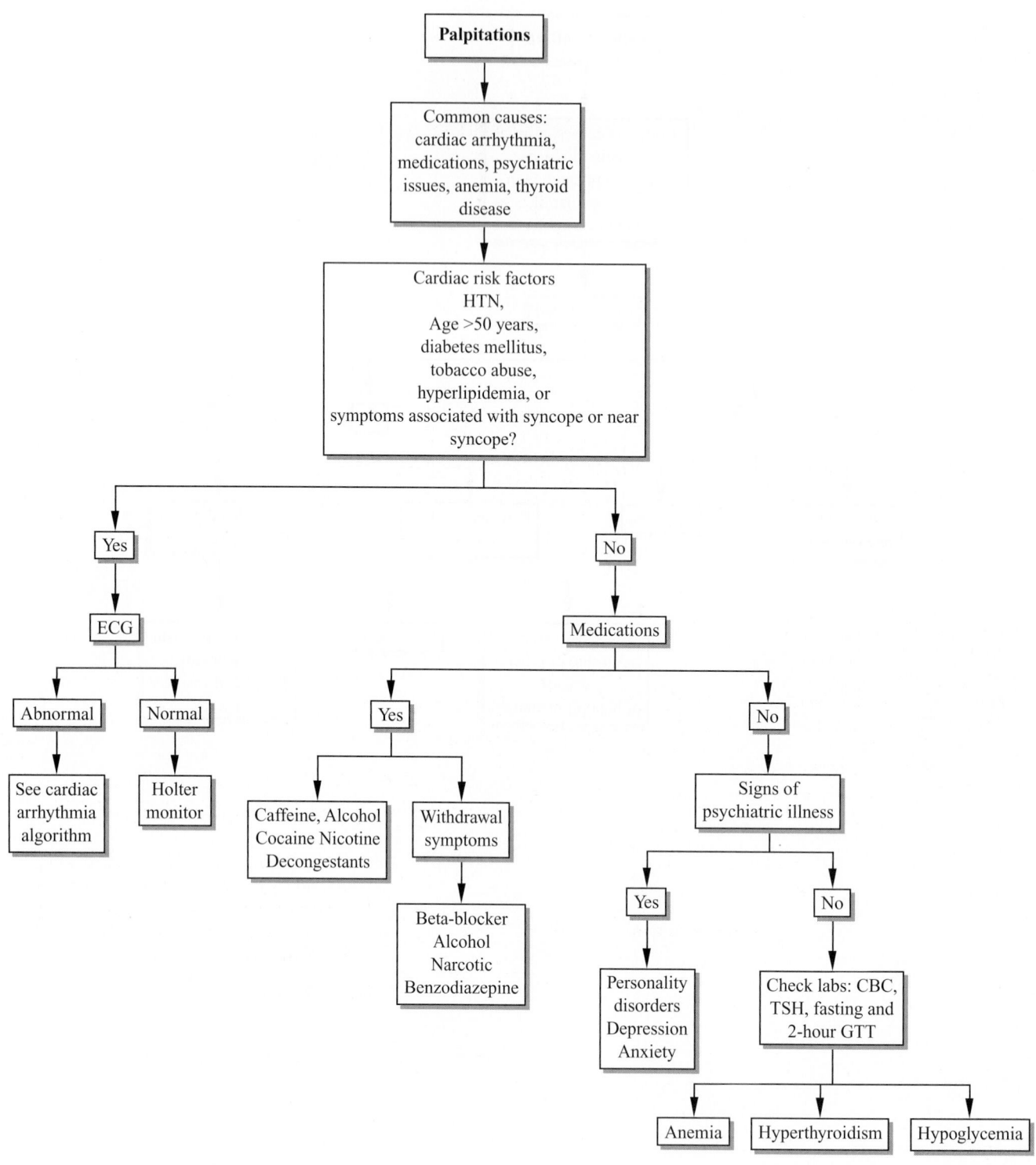

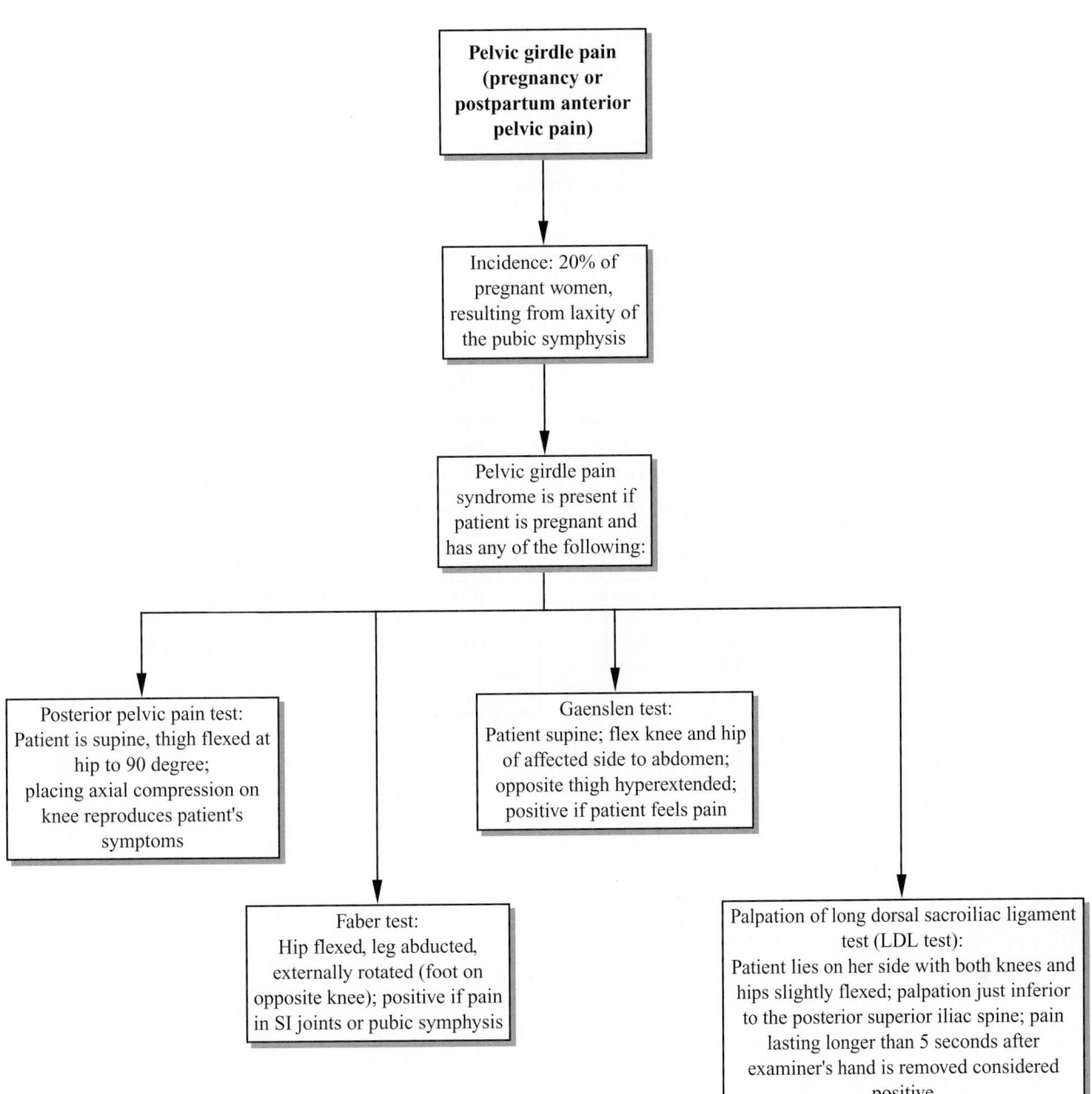

Pelvic girdle pain
(pregnancy or
postpartum anterior
pelvic pain)

↓

Incidence: 20% of
pregnant women,
resulting from laxity of
the pubic symphysis

↓

Pelvic girdle pain
syndrome is present if
patient is pregnant and
has any of the following:

Posterior pelvic pain test:
Patient is supine, thigh flexed at
hip to 90 degree;
placing axial compression on
knee reproduces patient's
symptoms

Faber test:
Hip flexed, leg abducted,
externally rotated (foot on
opposite knee); positive if pain
in SI joints or pubic symphysis

Gaenslen test:
Patient supine; flex knee and hip
of affected side to abdomen;
opposite thigh hyperextended;
positive if patient feels pain

Palpation of long dorsal sacroiliac ligament
test (LDL test):
Patient lies on her side with both knees and
hips slightly flexed; palpation just inferior
to the posterior superior iliac spine; pain
lasting longer than 5 seconds after
examiner's hand is removed considered
positive

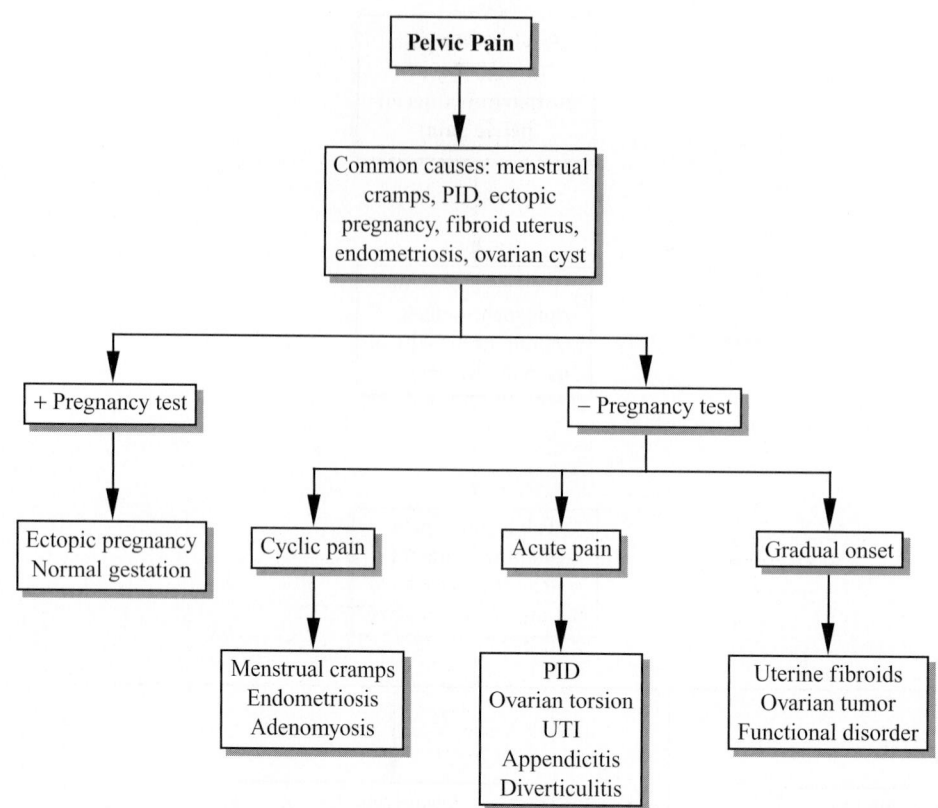

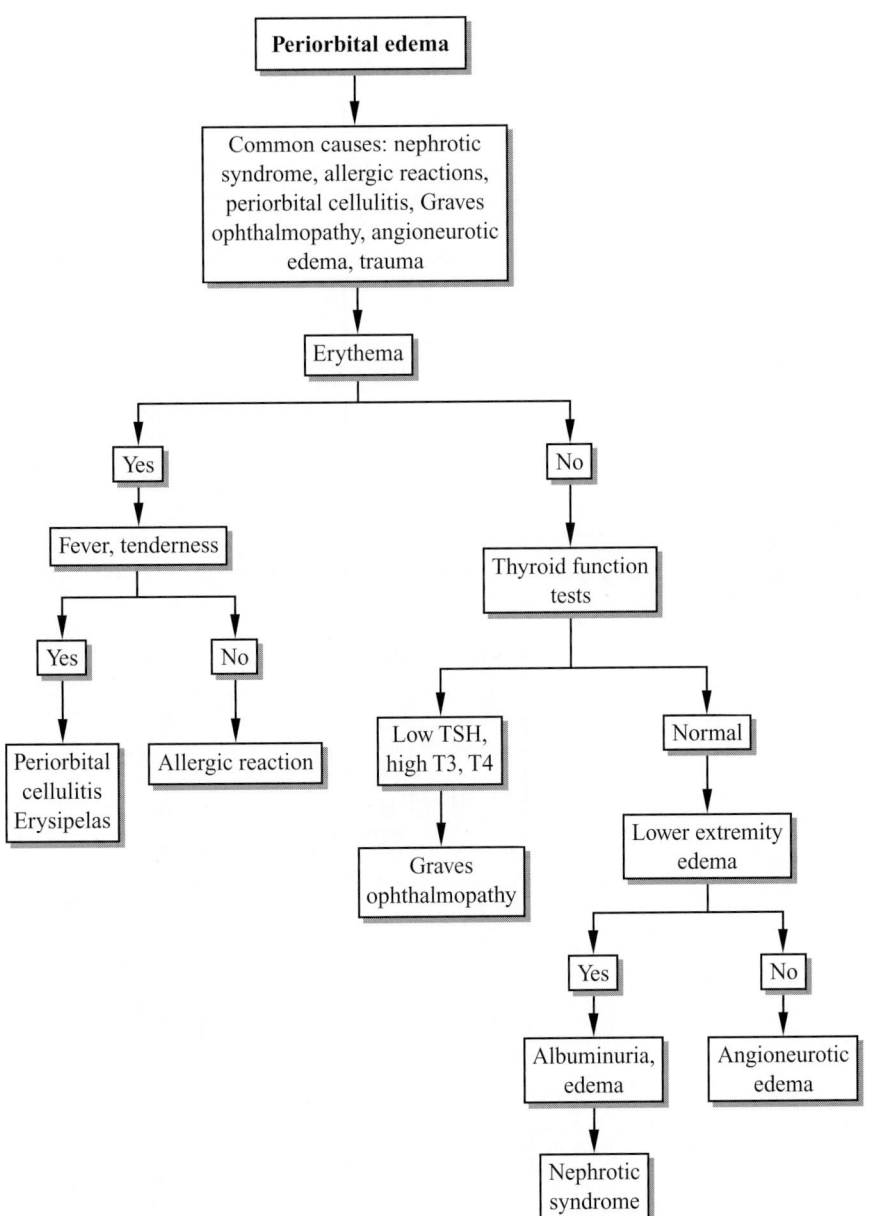

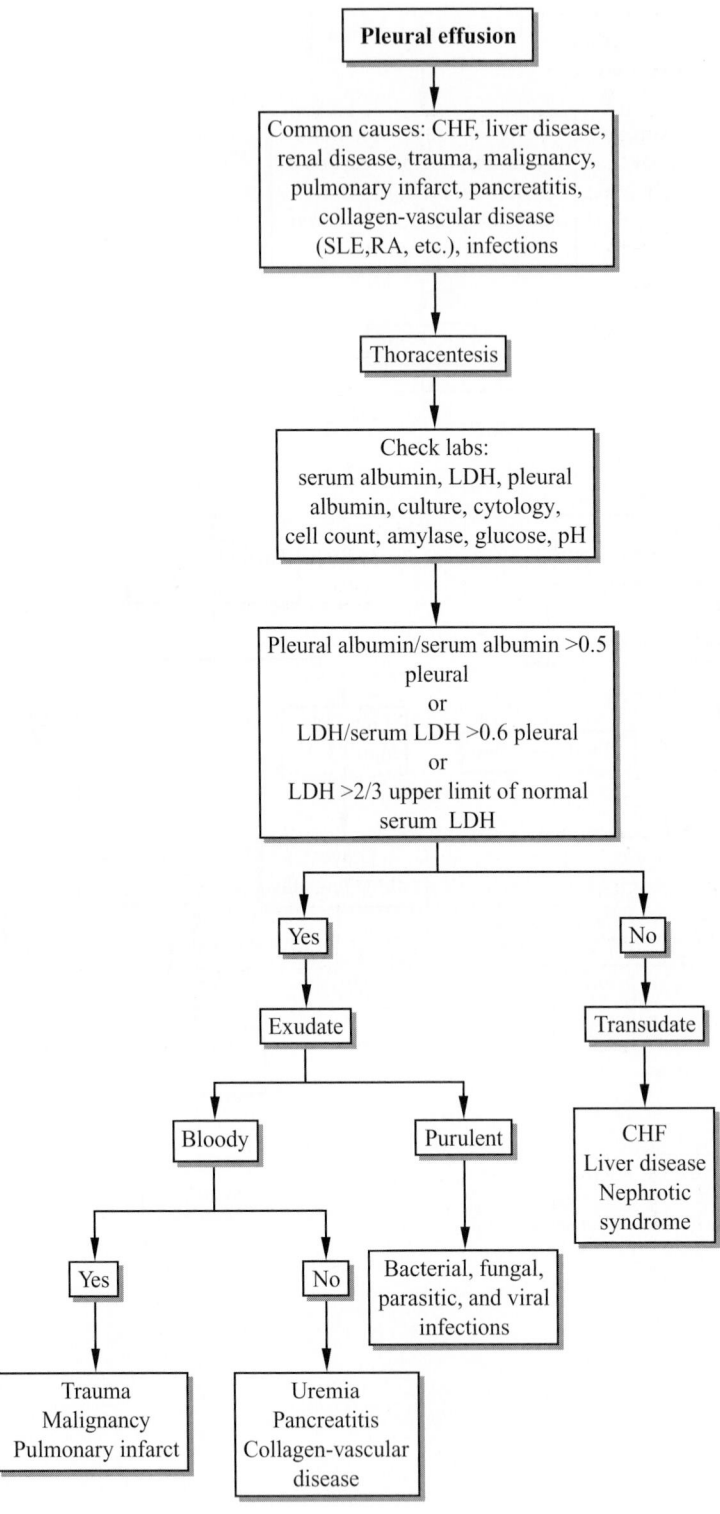

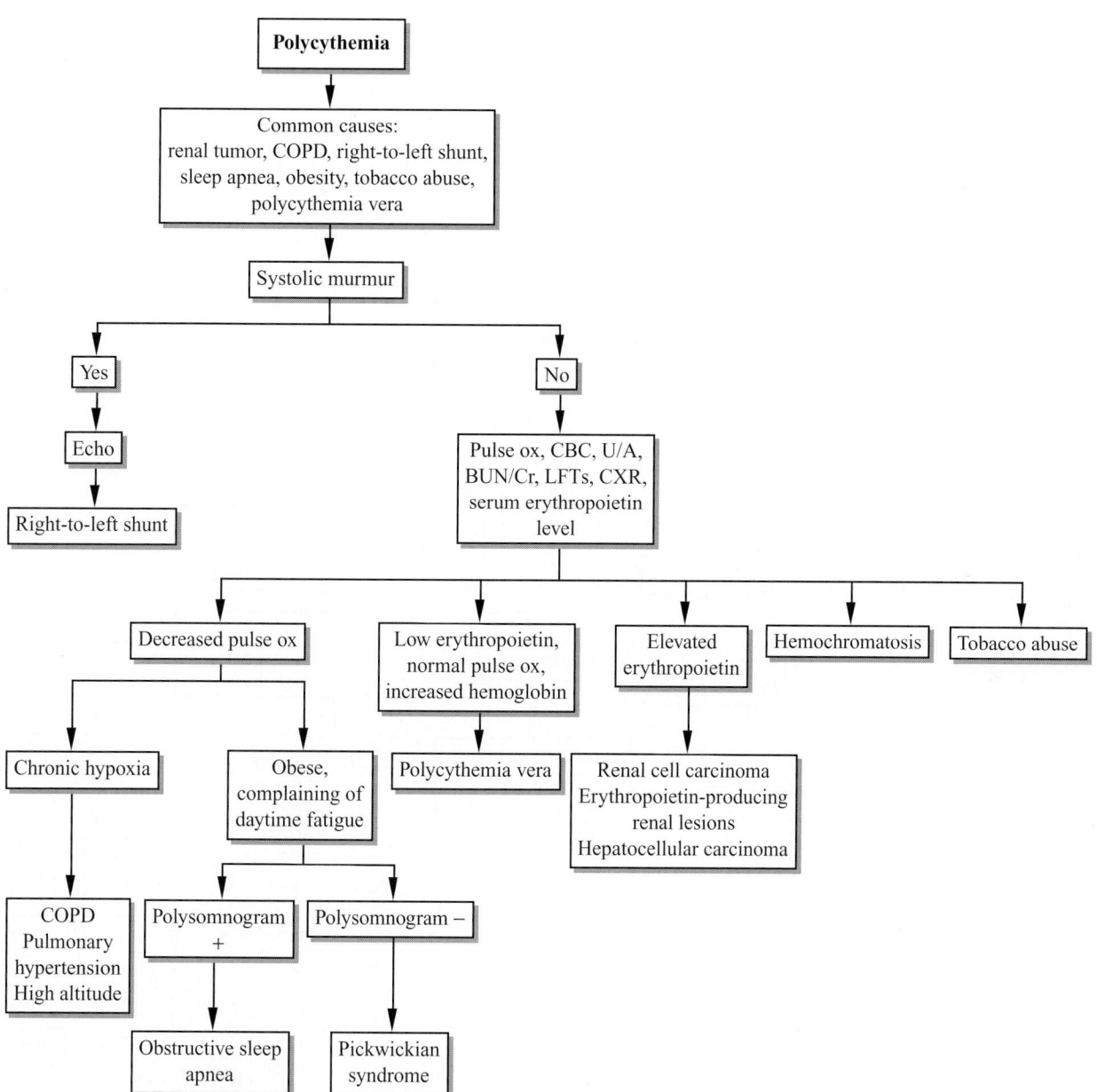

Polycythemia

Common causes:
renal tumor, COPD, right-to-left shunt,
sleep apnea, obesity, tobacco abuse,
polycythemia vera

Systolic murmur

Yes

Echo

Right-to-left shunt

No

Pulse ox, CBC, U/A,
BUN/Cr, LFTs, CXR,
serum erythropoietin
level

Decreased pulse ox

Low erythropoietin,
normal pulse ox,
increased hemoglobin

Elevated
erythropoietin

Hemochromatosis

Tobacco abuse

Chronic hypoxia

Obese,
complaining of
daytime fatigue

Polycythemia vera

Renal cell carcinoma
Erythropoietin-producing
renal lesions
Hepatocellular carcinoma

COPD
Pulmonary
hypertension
High altitude

Polysomnogram
+

Polysomnogram −

Obstructive sleep
apnea

Pickwickian
syndrome

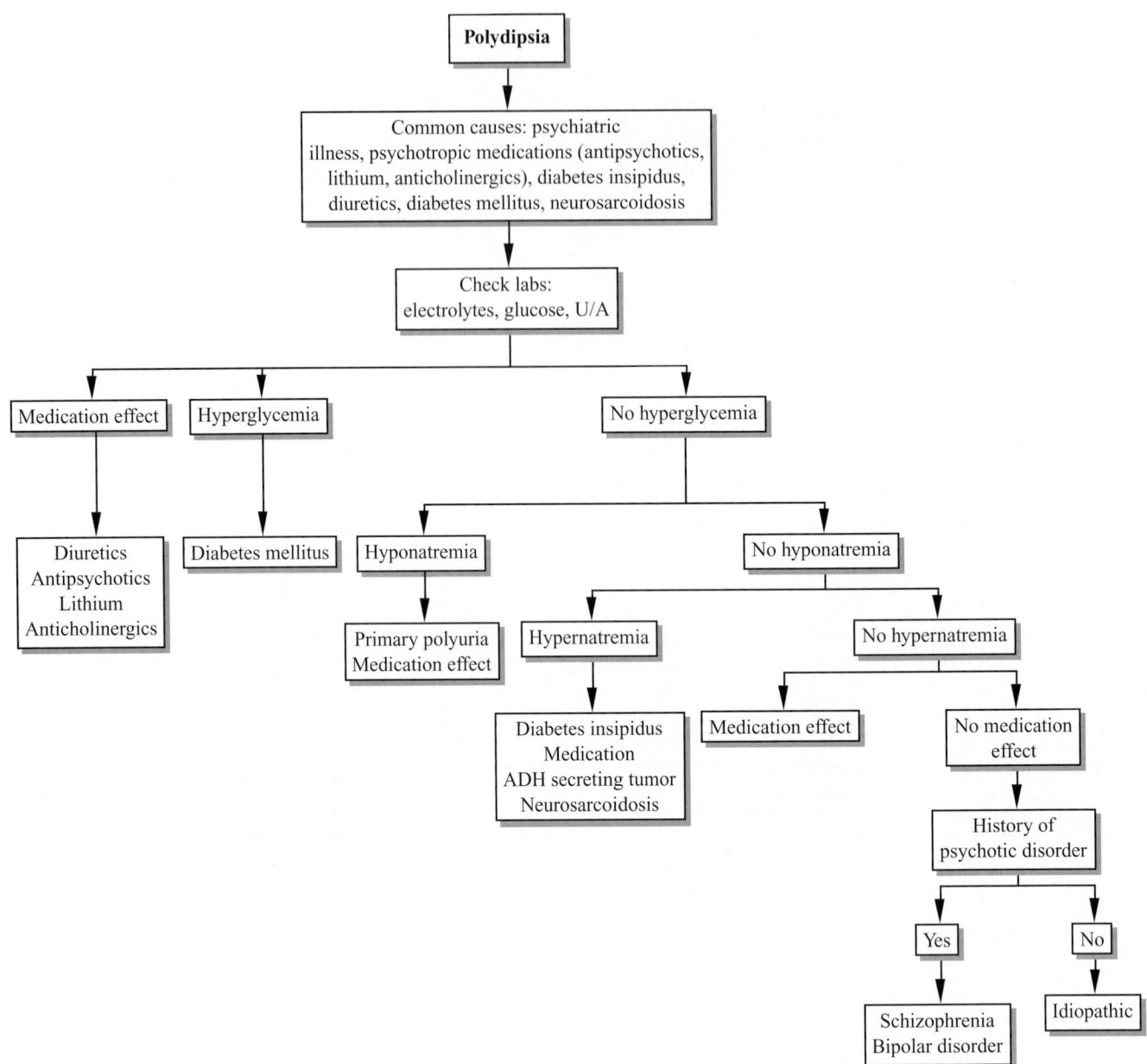

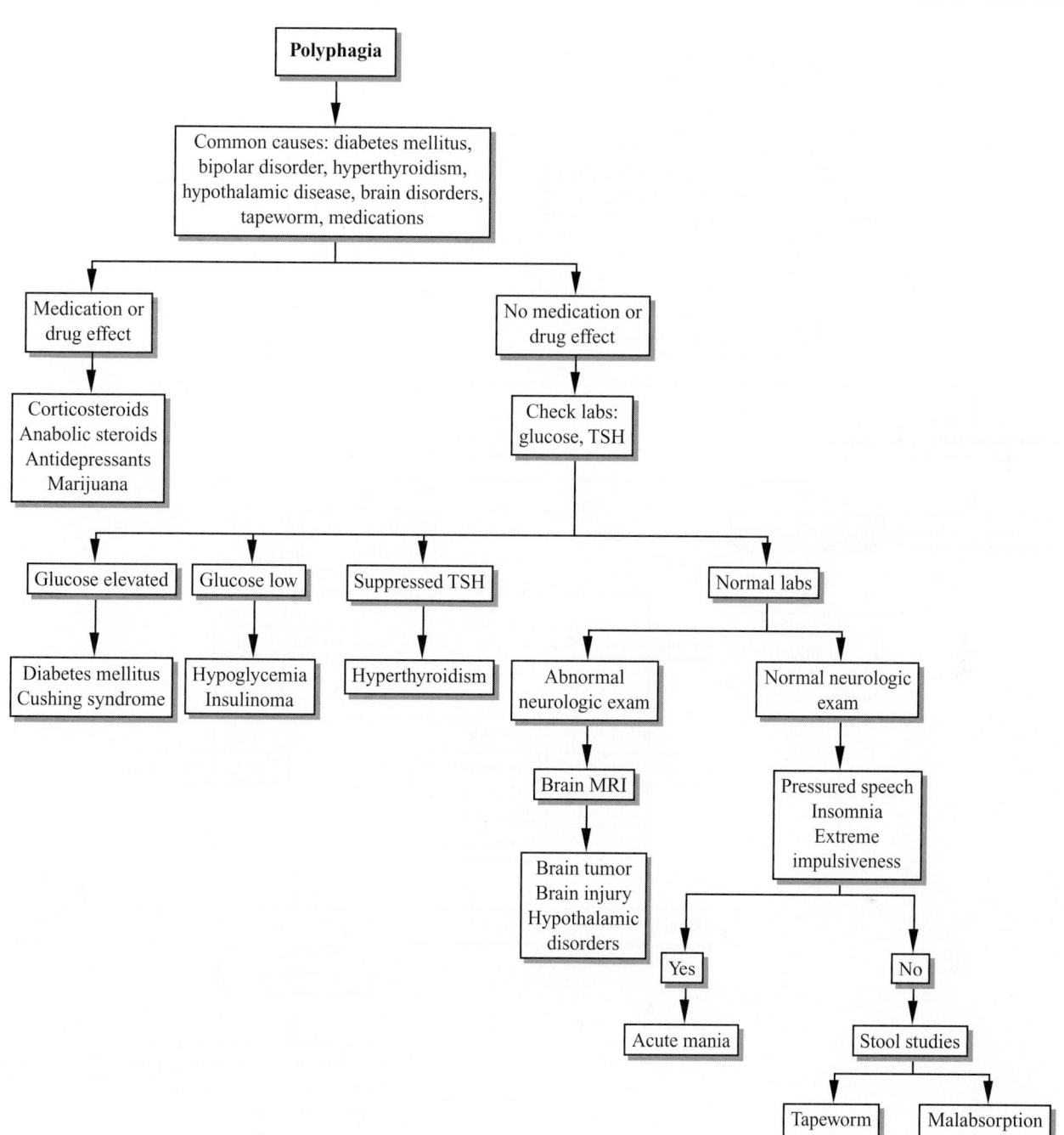

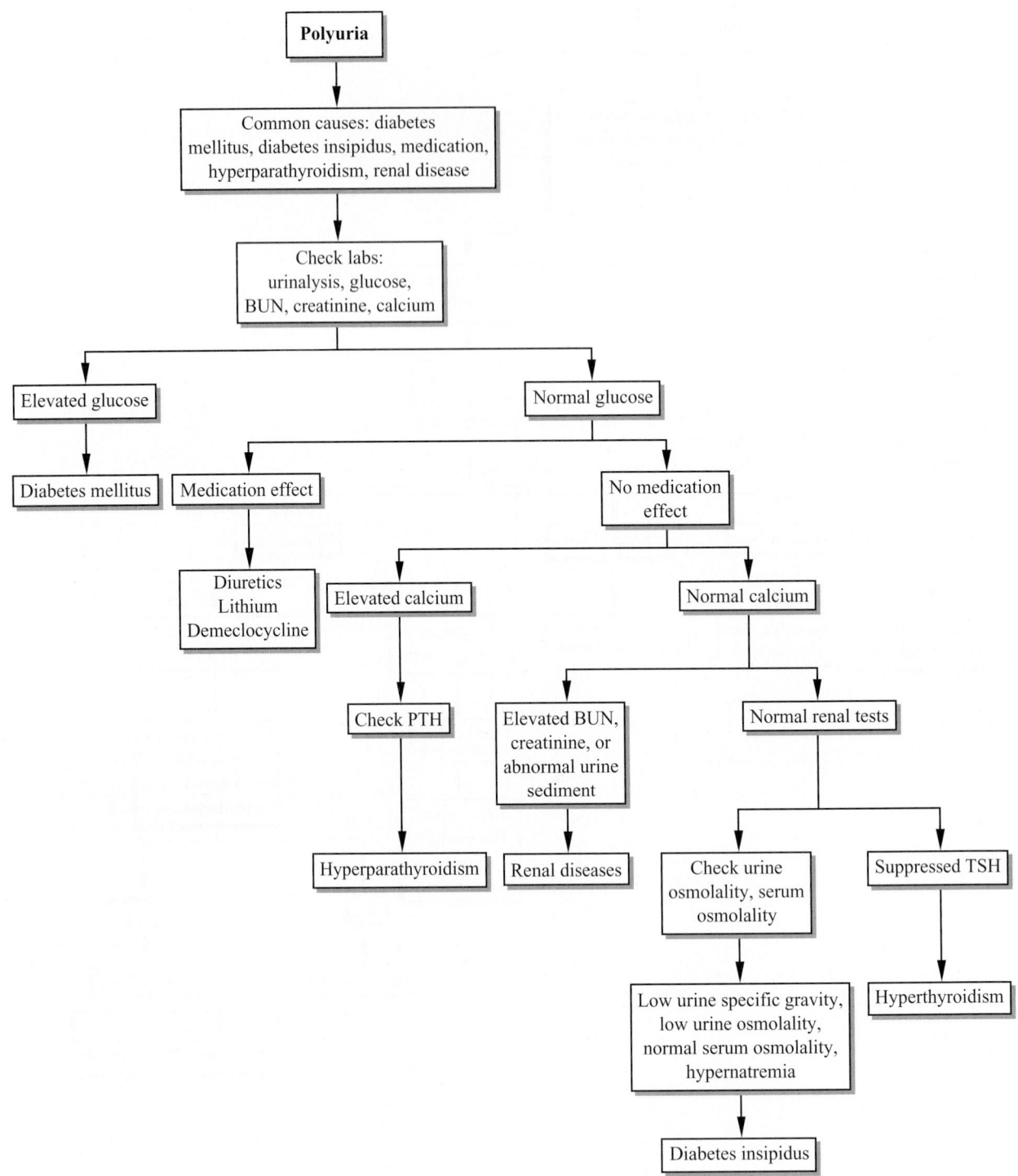

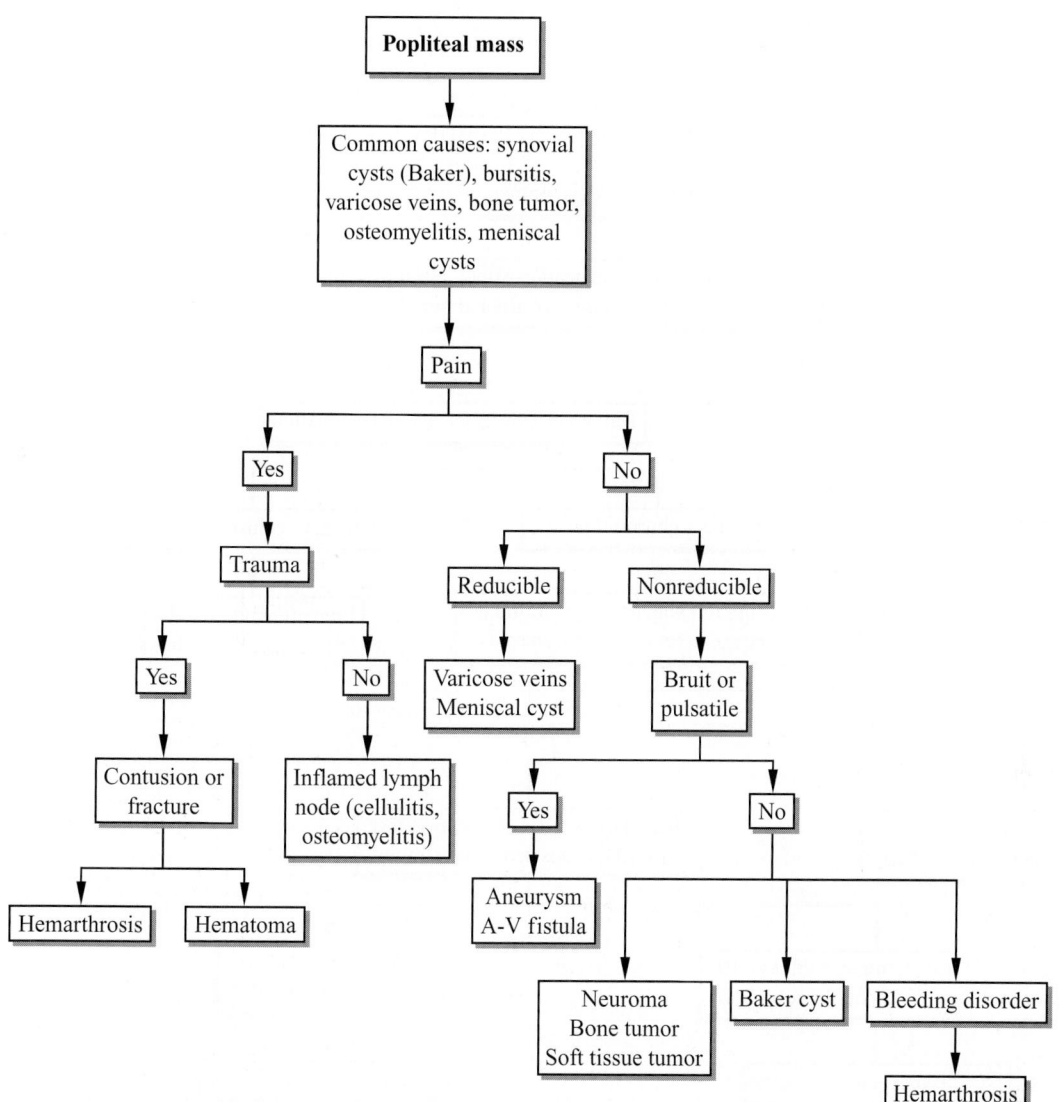

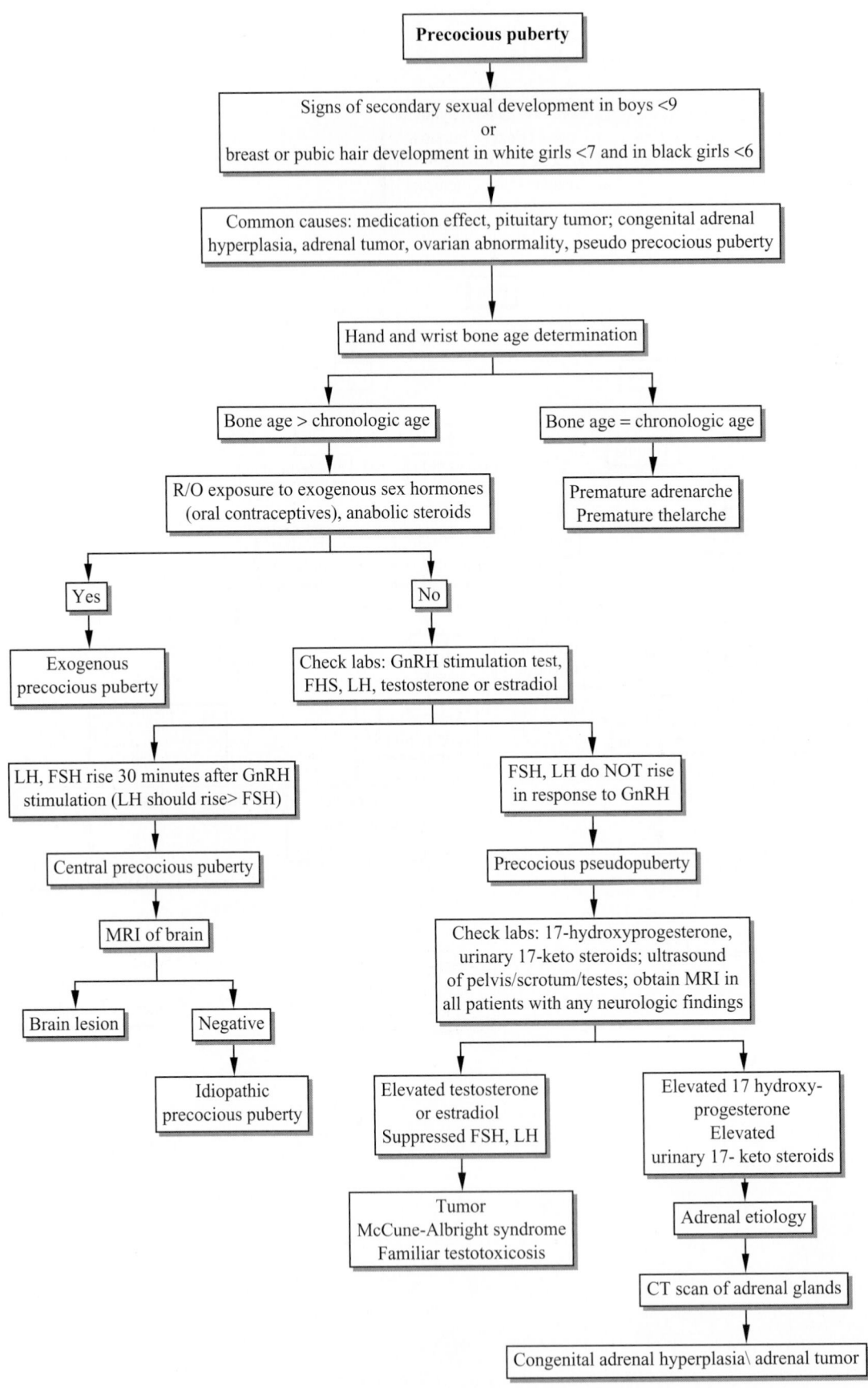

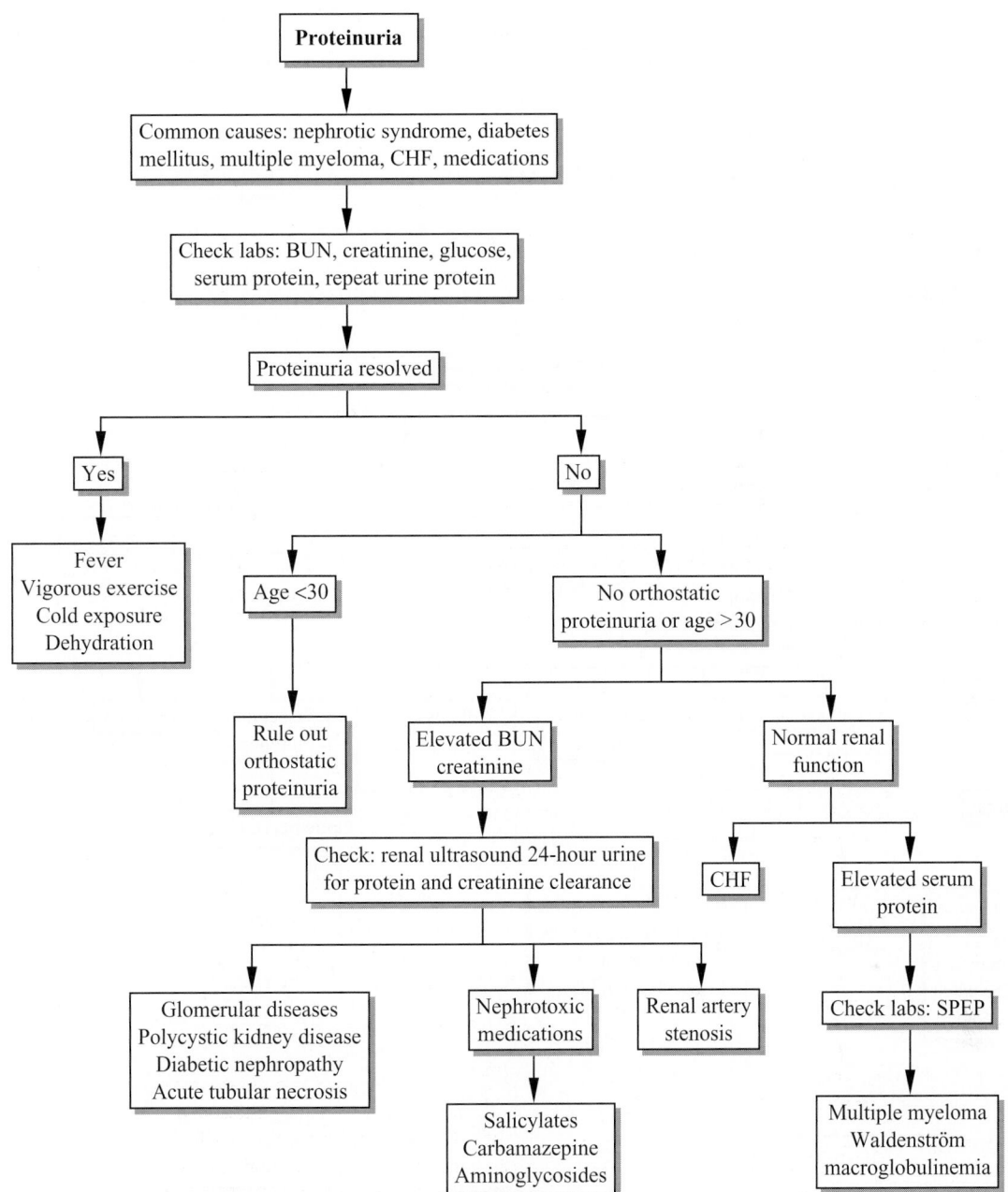

Proteinuria

↓

Common causes: nephrotic syndrome, diabetes mellitus, multiple myeloma, CHF, medications

↓

Check labs: BUN, creatinine, glucose, serum protein, repeat urine protein

↓

Proteinuria resolved

Yes

Fever
Vigorous exercise
Cold exposure
Dehydration

No

Age <30

↓

Rule out orthostatic proteinuria

No orthostatic proteinuria or age >30

Elevated BUN creatinine

↓

Check: renal ultrasound 24-hour urine for protein and creatinine clearance

Glomerular diseases
Polycystic kidney disease
Diabetic nephropathy
Acute tubular necrosis

Nephrotoxic medications

↓

Salicylates
Carbamazepine
Aminoglycosides

Renal artery stenosis

Normal renal function

CHF

Elevated serum protein

↓

Check labs: SPEP

↓

Multiple myeloma
Waldenström macroglobulinemia

Pupil Abnormalities

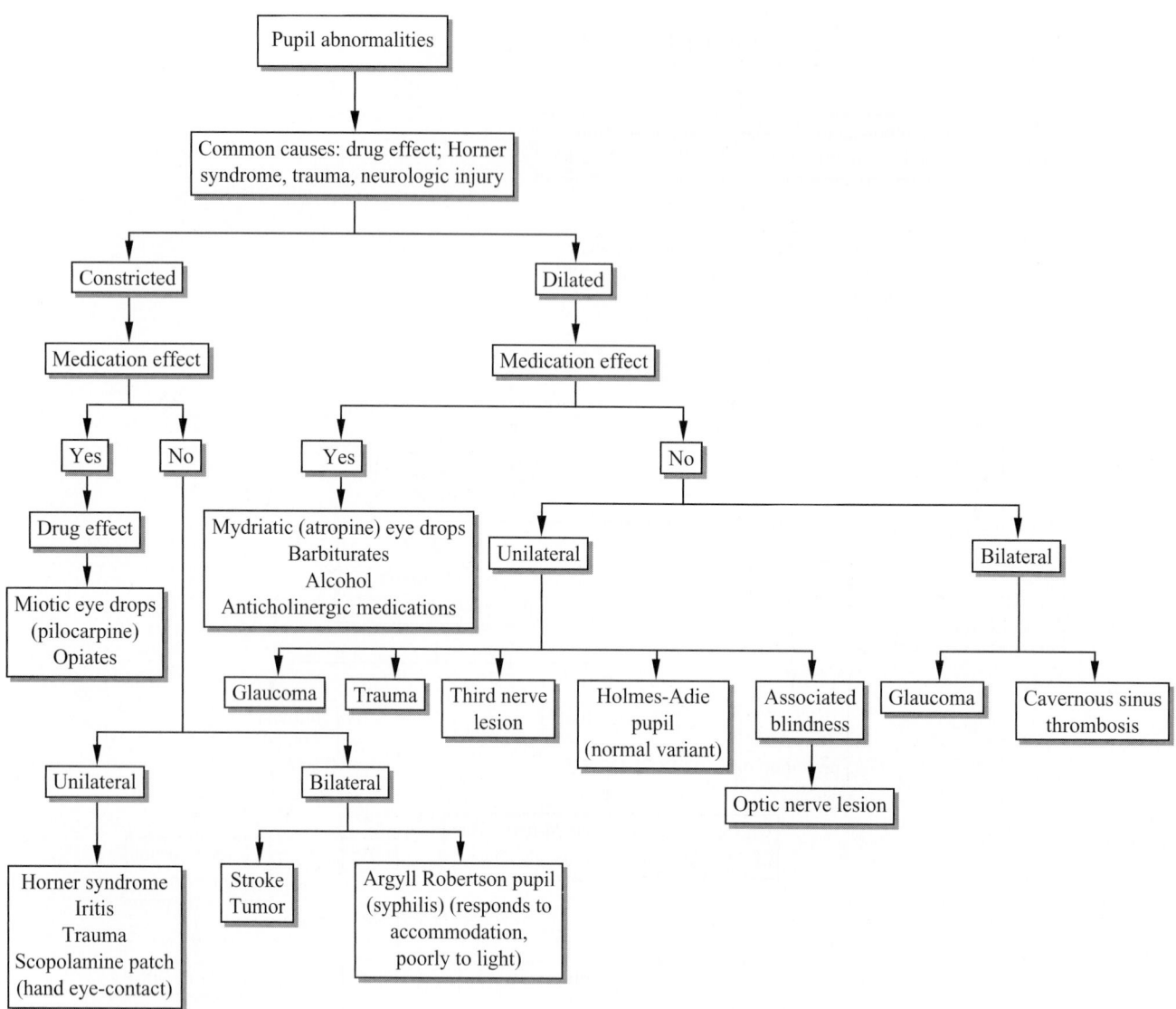

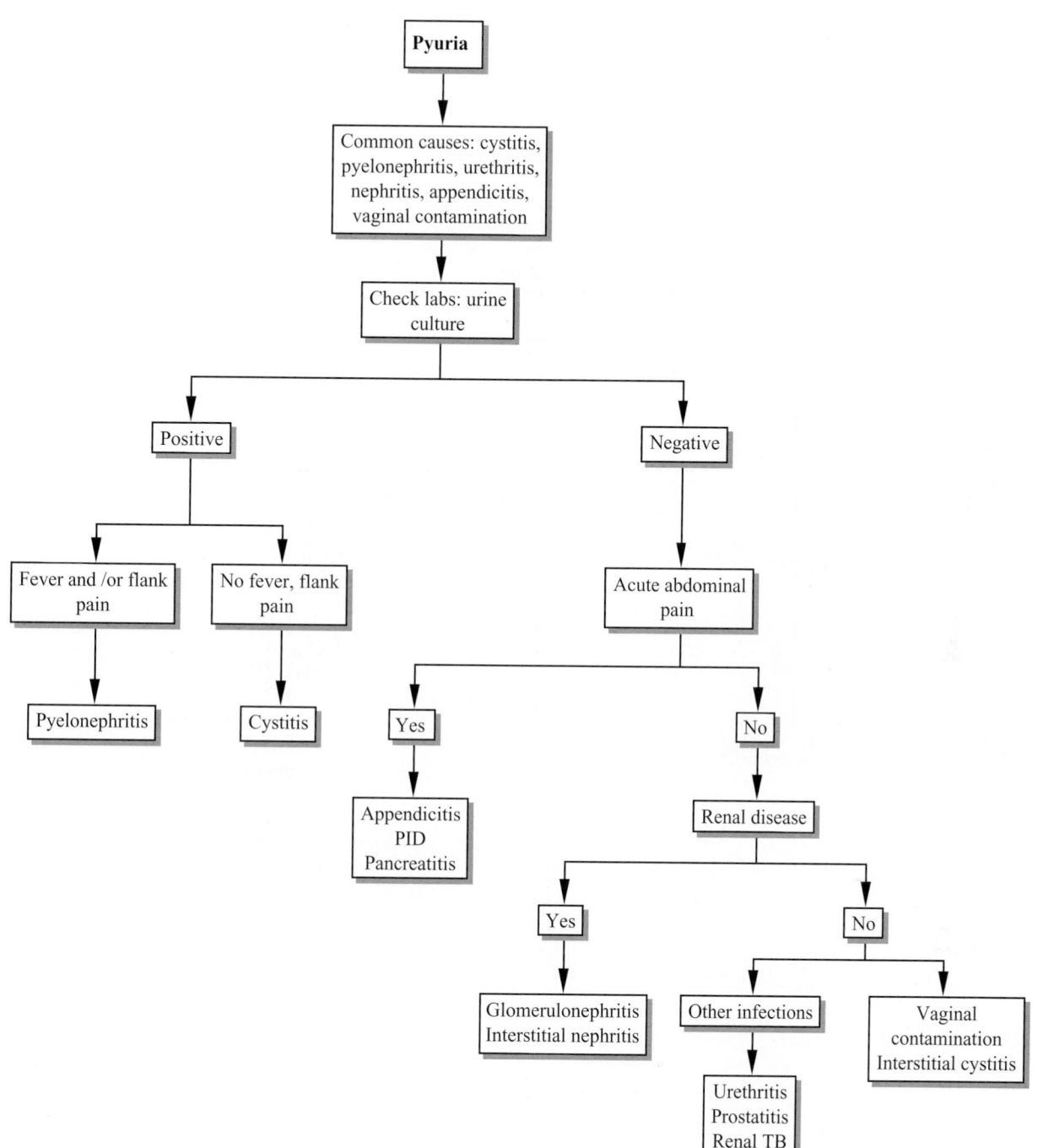

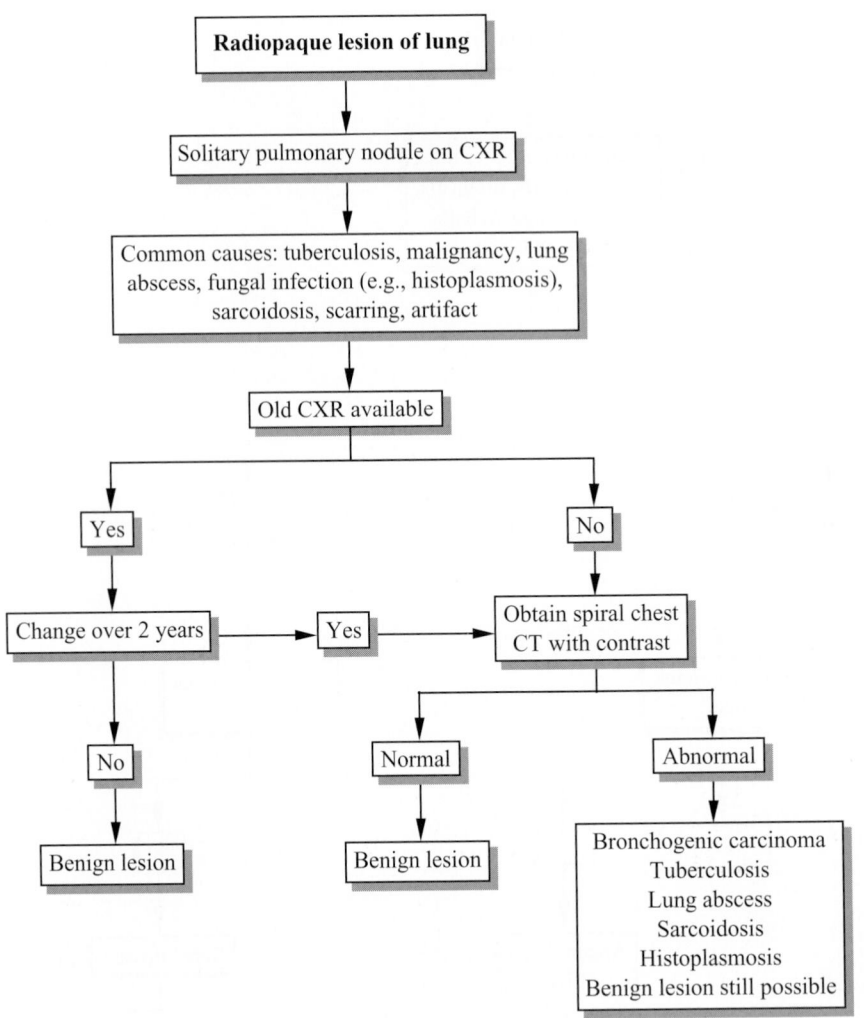

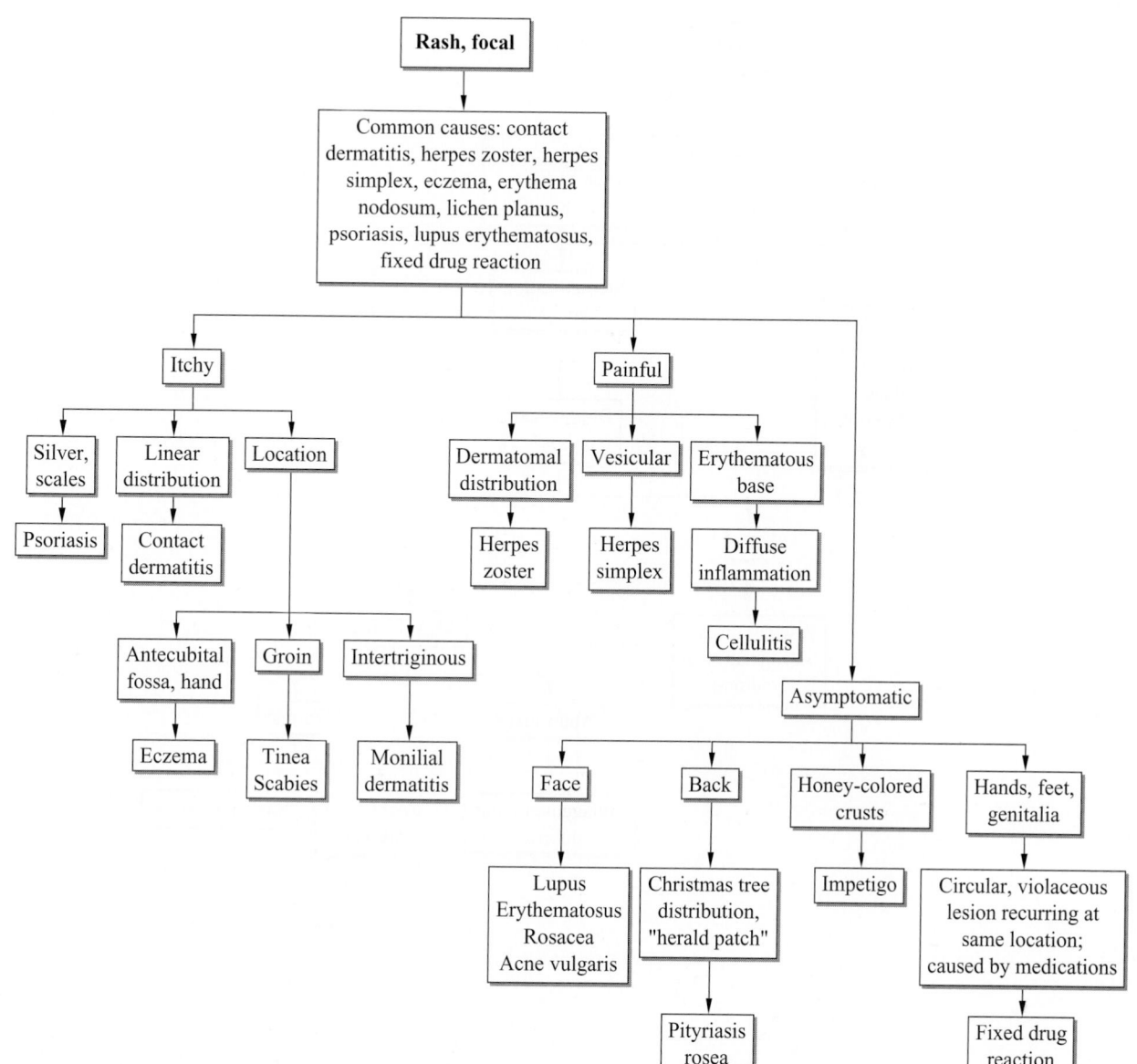

Rash, focal

Common causes: contact dermatitis, herpes zoster, herpes simplex, eczema, erythema nodosum, lichen planus, psoriasis, lupus erythematosus, fixed drug reaction

- **Itchy**
  - Silver, scales → Psoriasis
  - Linear distribution → Contact dermatitis
  - Location
    - Antecubital fossa, hand → Eczema
    - Groin → Tinea / Scabies
    - Intertriginous → Monilial dermatitis
- **Painful**
  - Dermatomal distribution → Herpes zoster
  - Vesicular → Herpes simplex
  - Erythematous base → Diffuse inflammation → Cellulitis
- **Asymptomatic**
  - Face → Lupus Erythematosus / Rosacea / Acne vulgaris
  - Back → Christmas tree distribution, "herald patch" → Pityriasis rosea
  - Honey-colored crusts → Impetigo
  - Hands, feet, genitalia → Circular, violaceous lesion recurring at same location; caused by medications → Fixed drug reaction

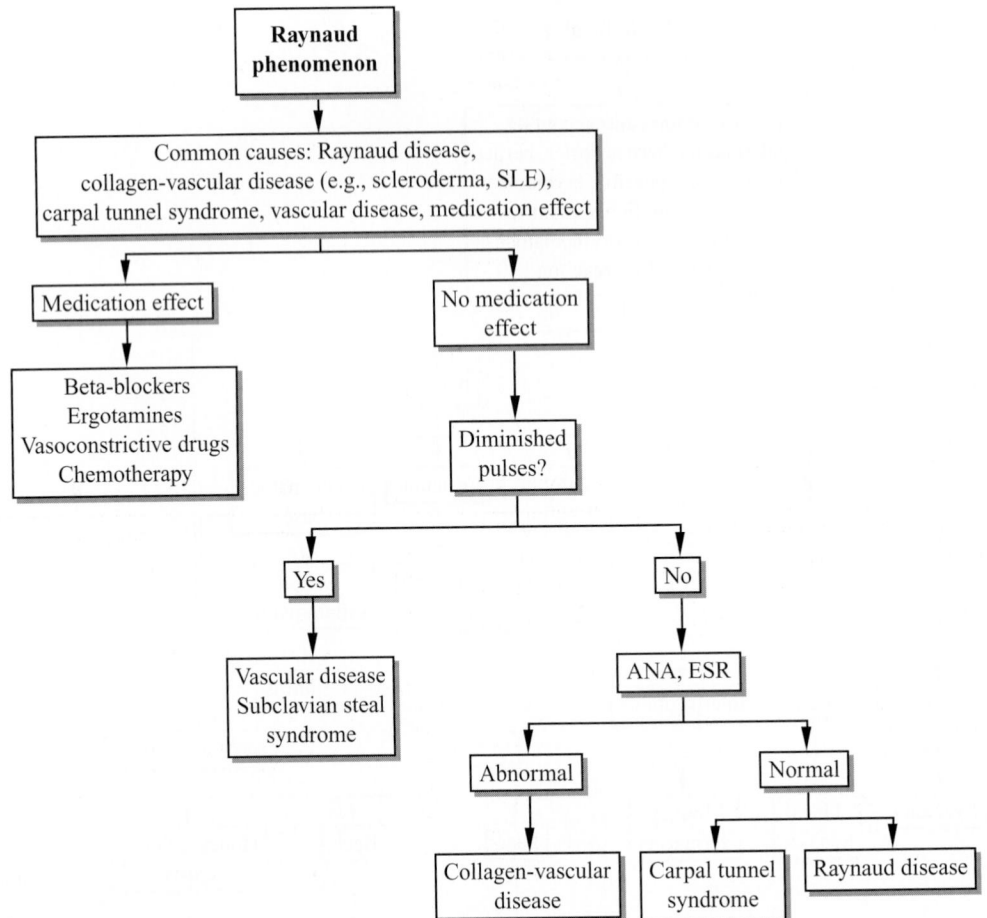

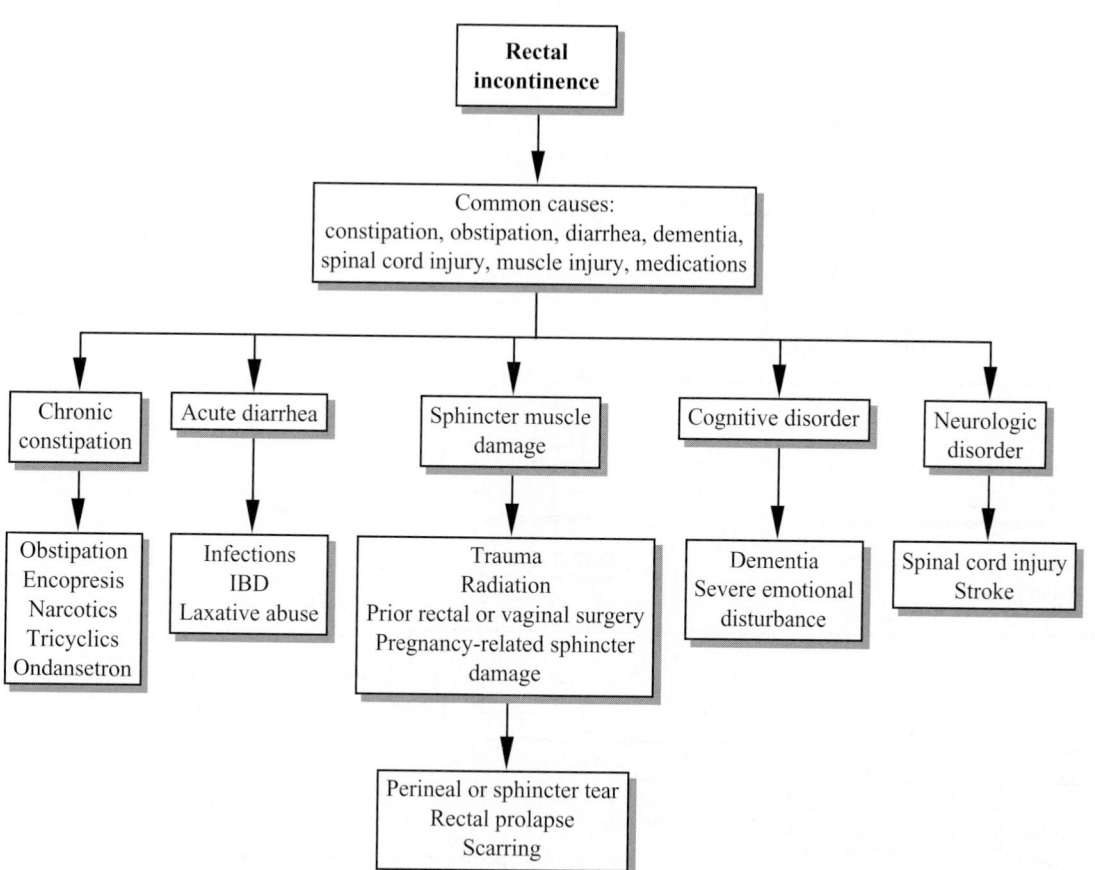

Rectal incontinence

↓

Common causes:
constipation, obstipation, diarrhea, dementia,
spinal cord injury, muscle injury, medications

Chronic constipation
↓
Obstipation
Encopresis
Narcotics
Tricyclics
Ondansetron

Acute diarrhea
↓
Infections
IBD
Laxative abuse

Sphincter muscle damage
↓
Trauma
Radiation
Prior rectal or vaginal surgery
Pregnancy-related sphincter damage
↓
Perineal or sphincter tear
Rectal prolapse
Scarring

Cognitive disorder
↓
Dementia
Severe emotional disturbance

Neurologic disorder
↓
Spinal cord injury
Stroke

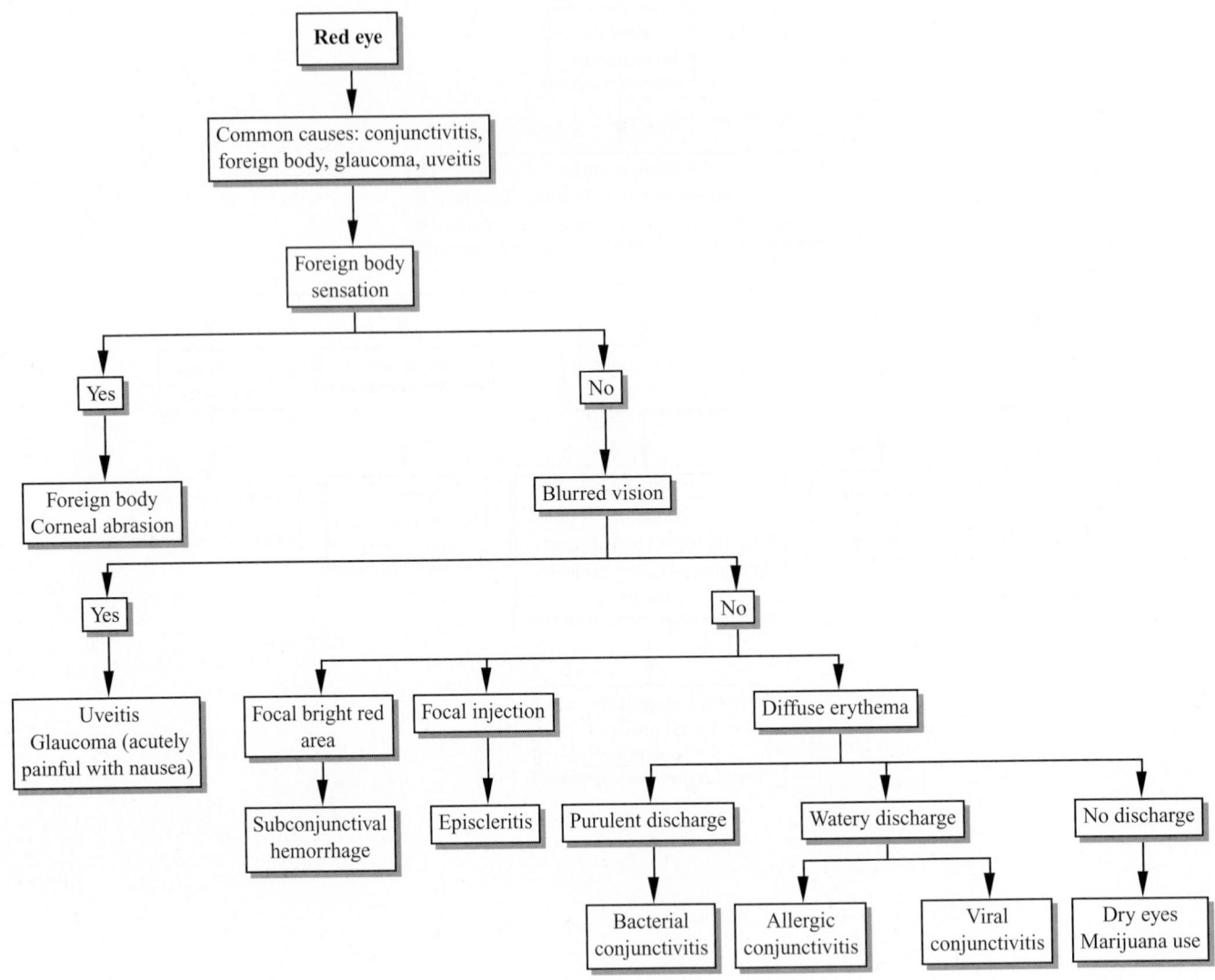

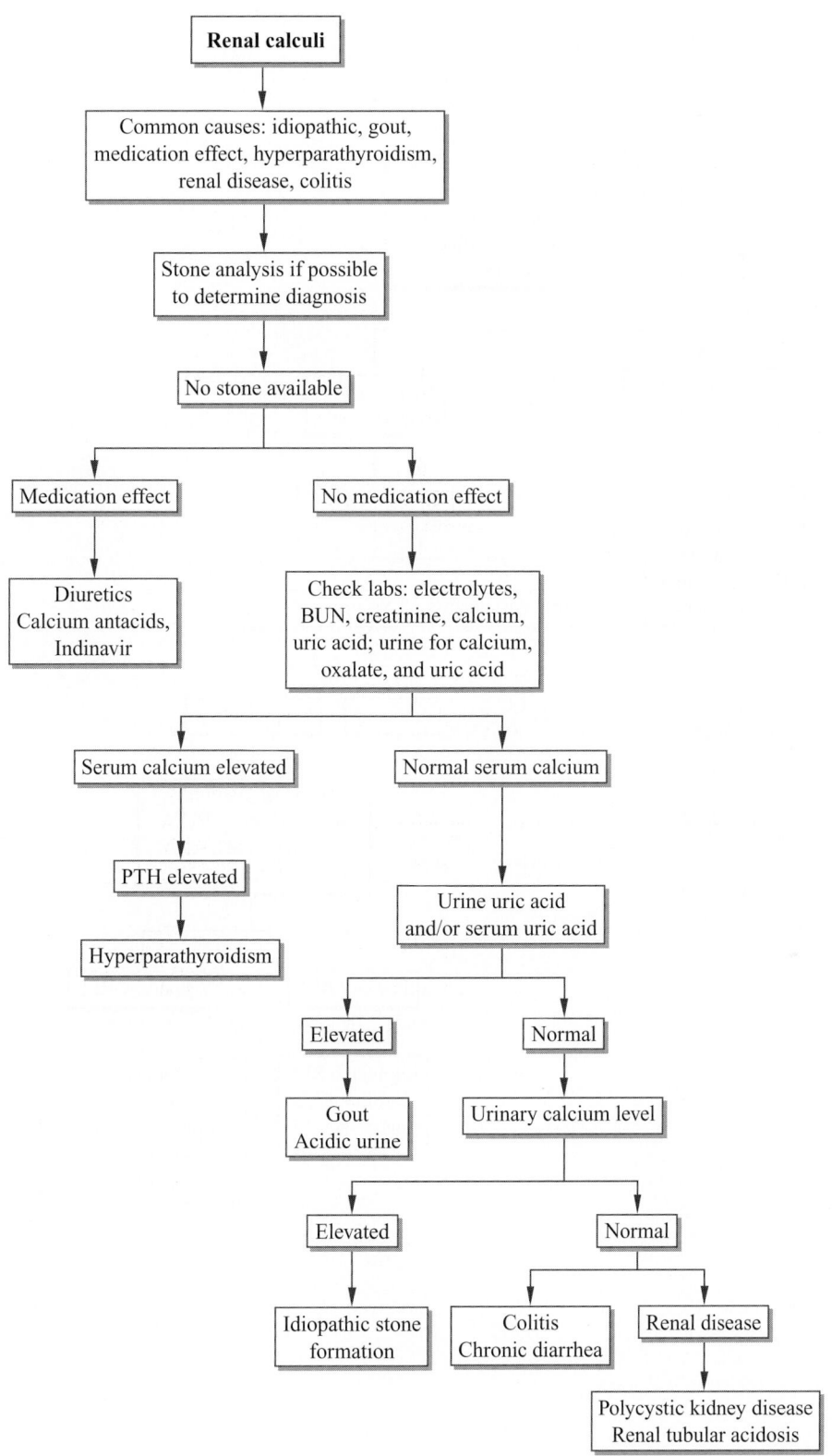

Renal calculi

↓

Common causes: idiopathic, gout,
medication effect, hyperparathyroidism,
renal disease, colitis

↓

Stone analysis if possible
to determine diagnosis

↓

No stone available

Medication effect | No medication effect

Diuretics
Calcium antacids,
Indinavir

Check labs: electrolytes,
BUN, creatinine, calcium,
uric acid; urine for calcium,
oxalate, and uric acid

Serum calcium elevated | Normal serum calcium

PTH elevated

↓

Hyperparathyroidism

Urine uric acid
and/or serum uric acid

Elevated | Normal

Gout
Acidic urine

Urinary calcium level

Elevated | Normal

Idiopathic stone
formation

Colitis
Chronic diarrhea | Renal disease

↓

Polycystic kidney disease
Renal tubular acidosis

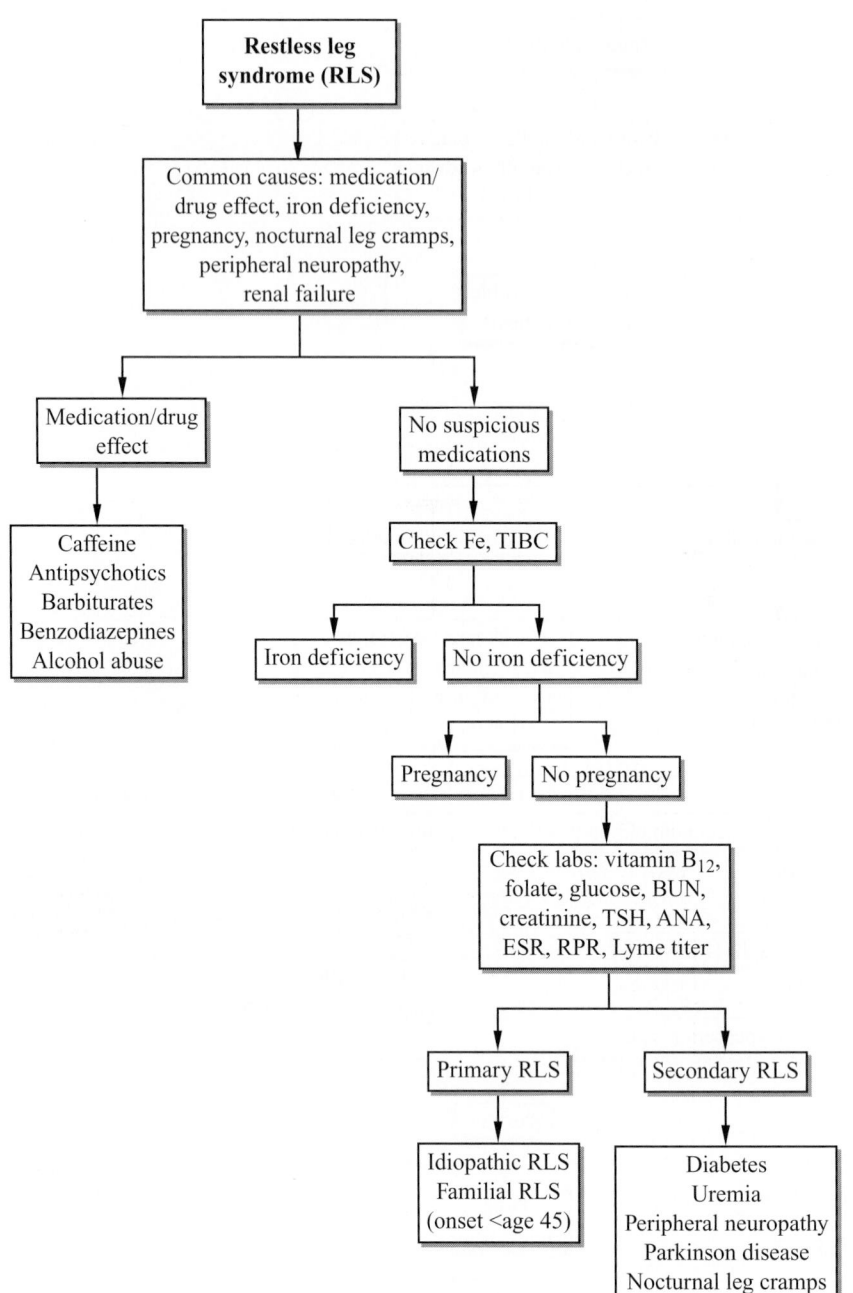

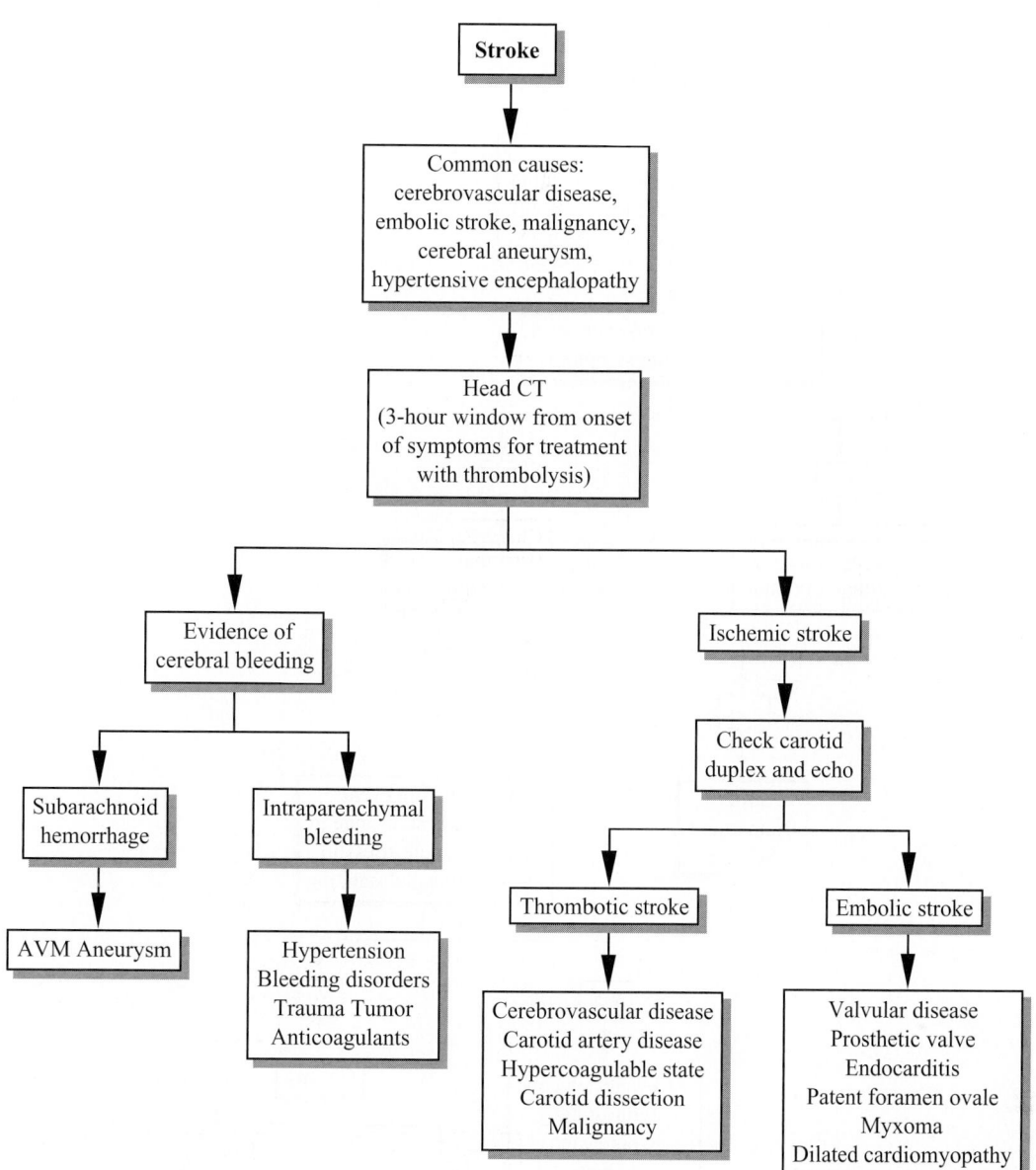

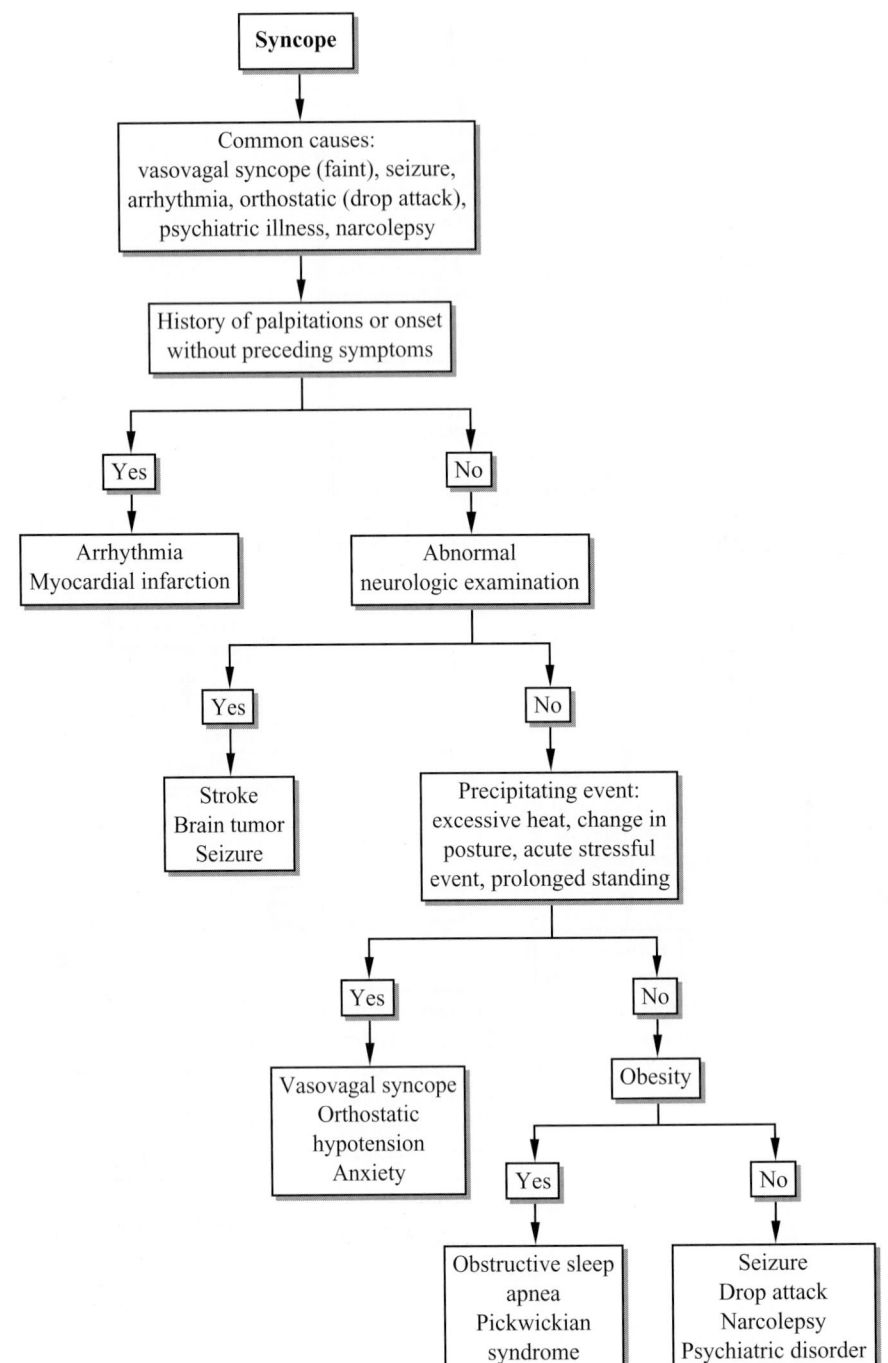

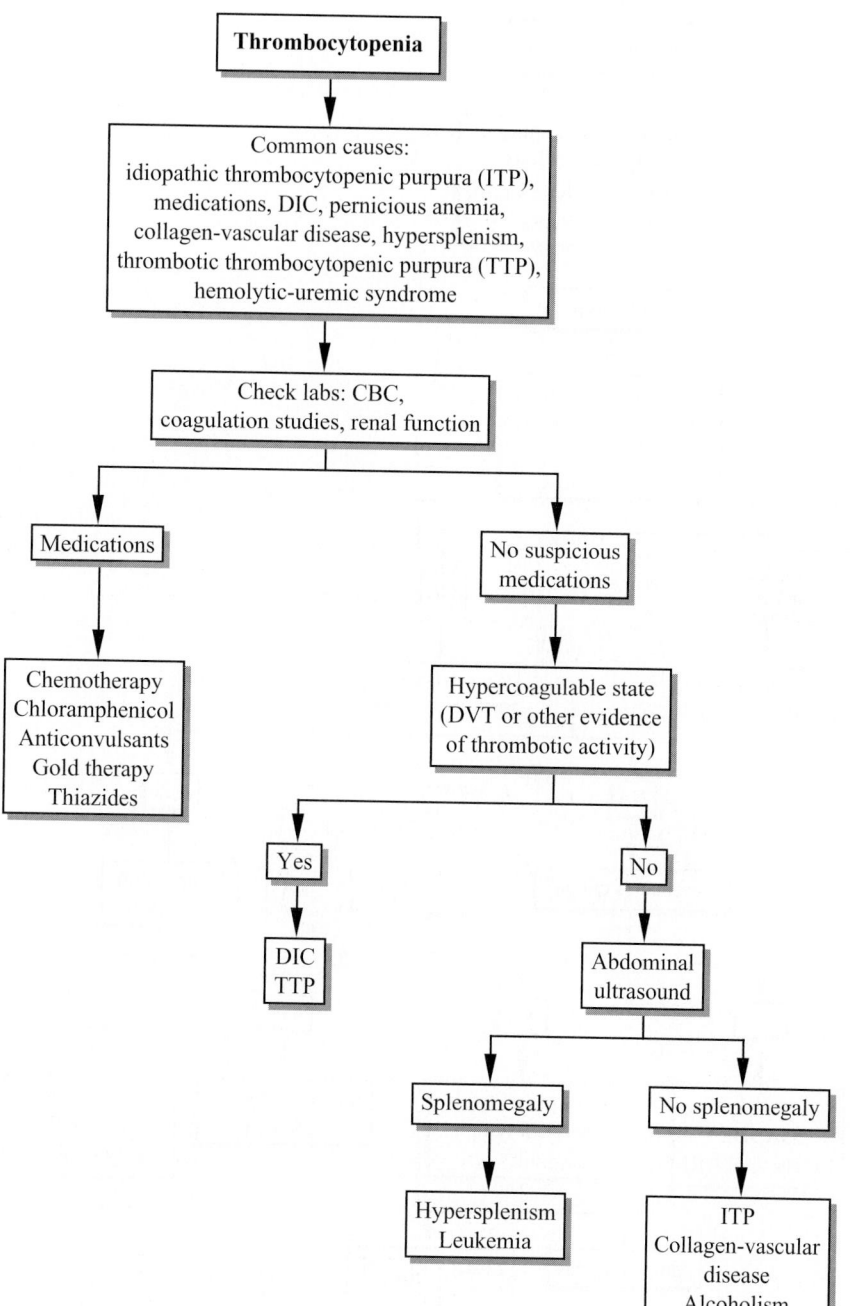

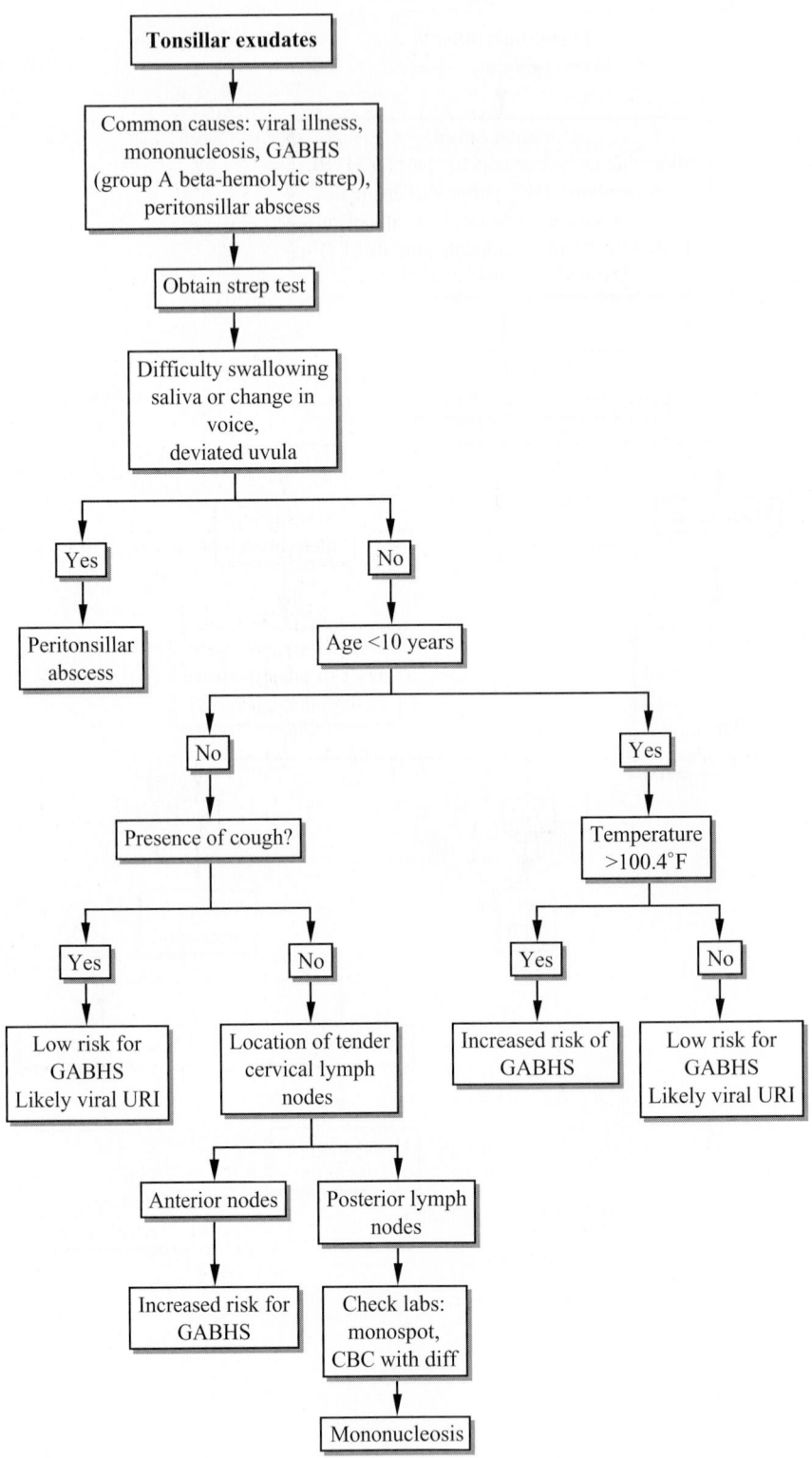

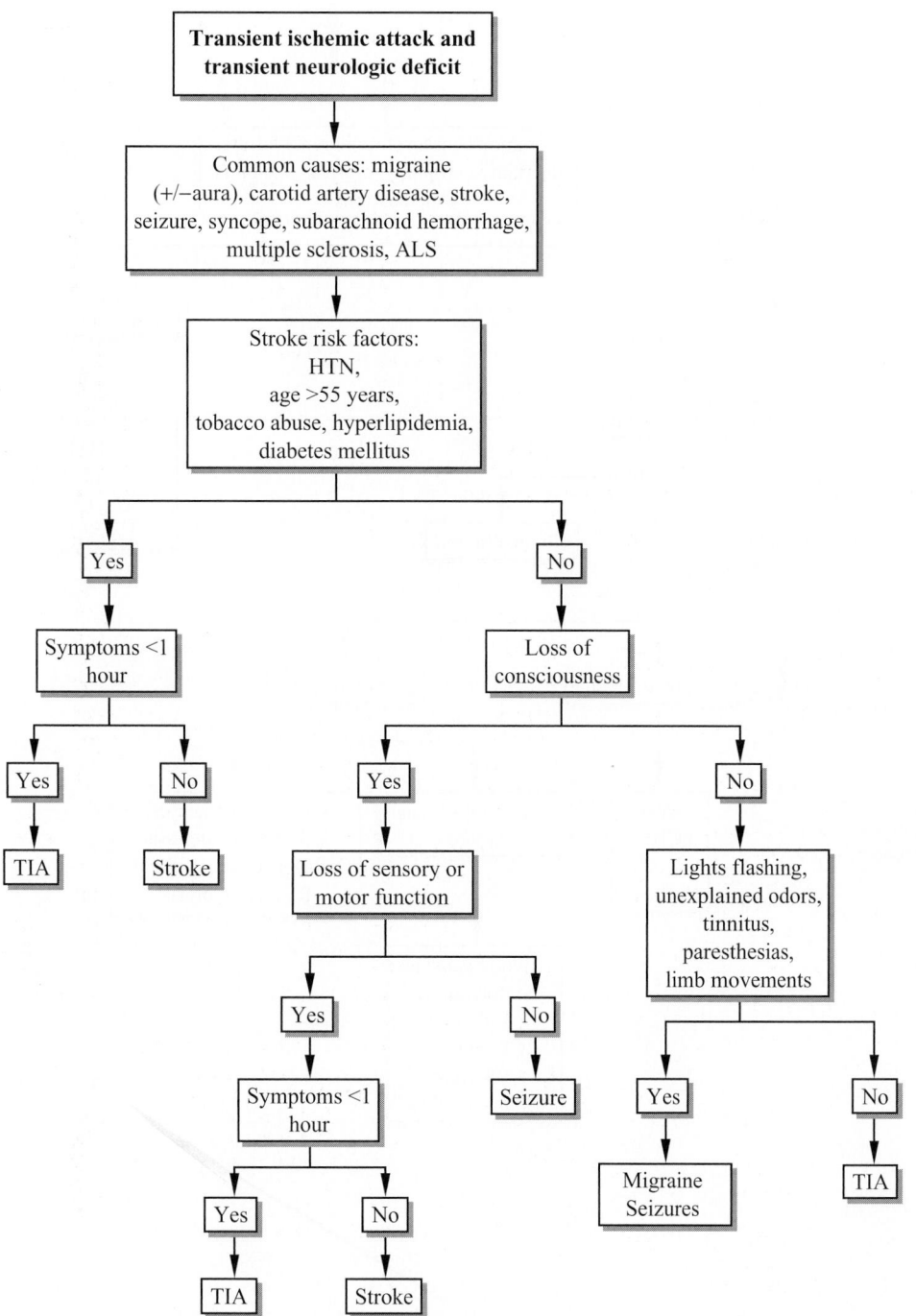

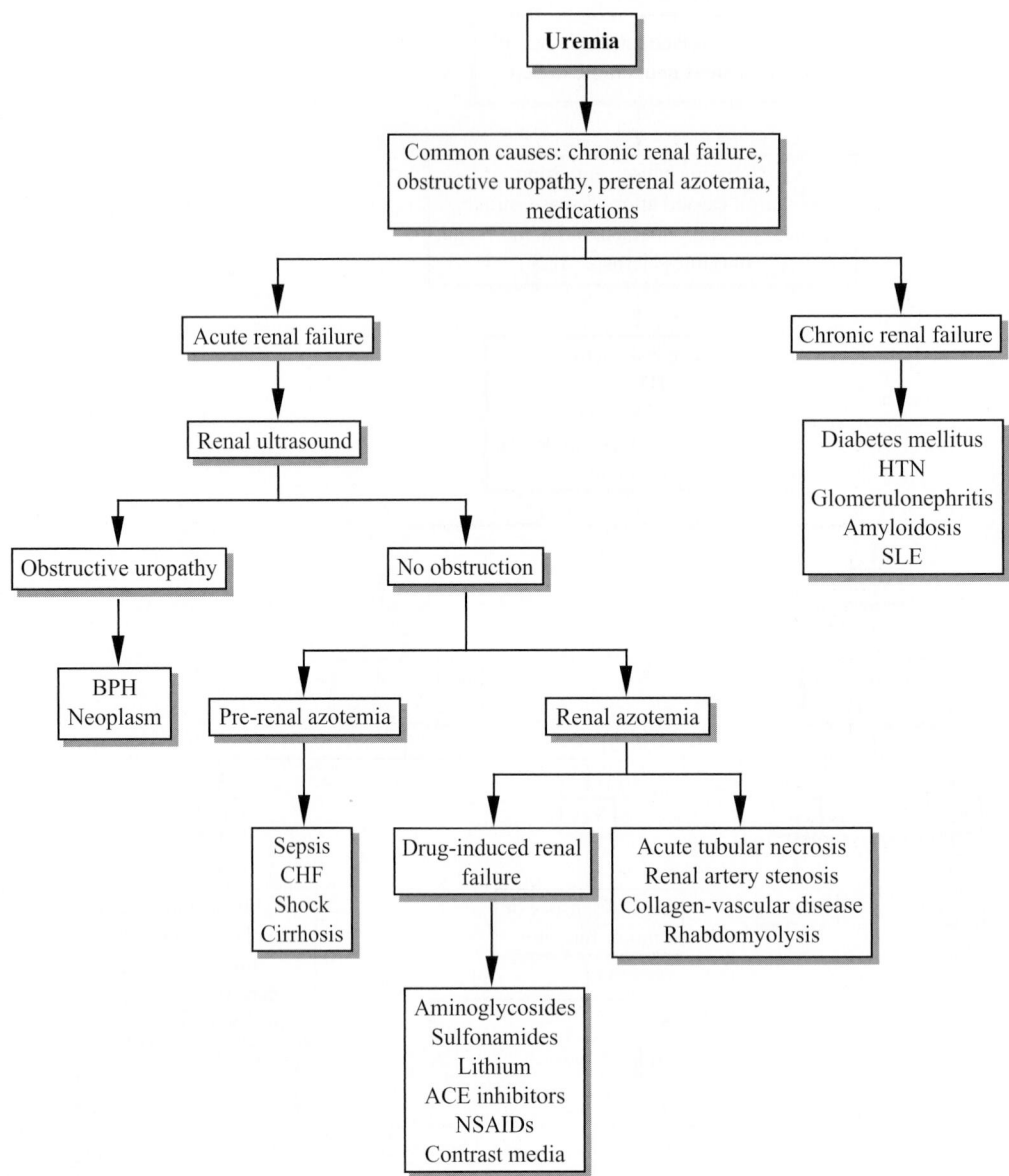

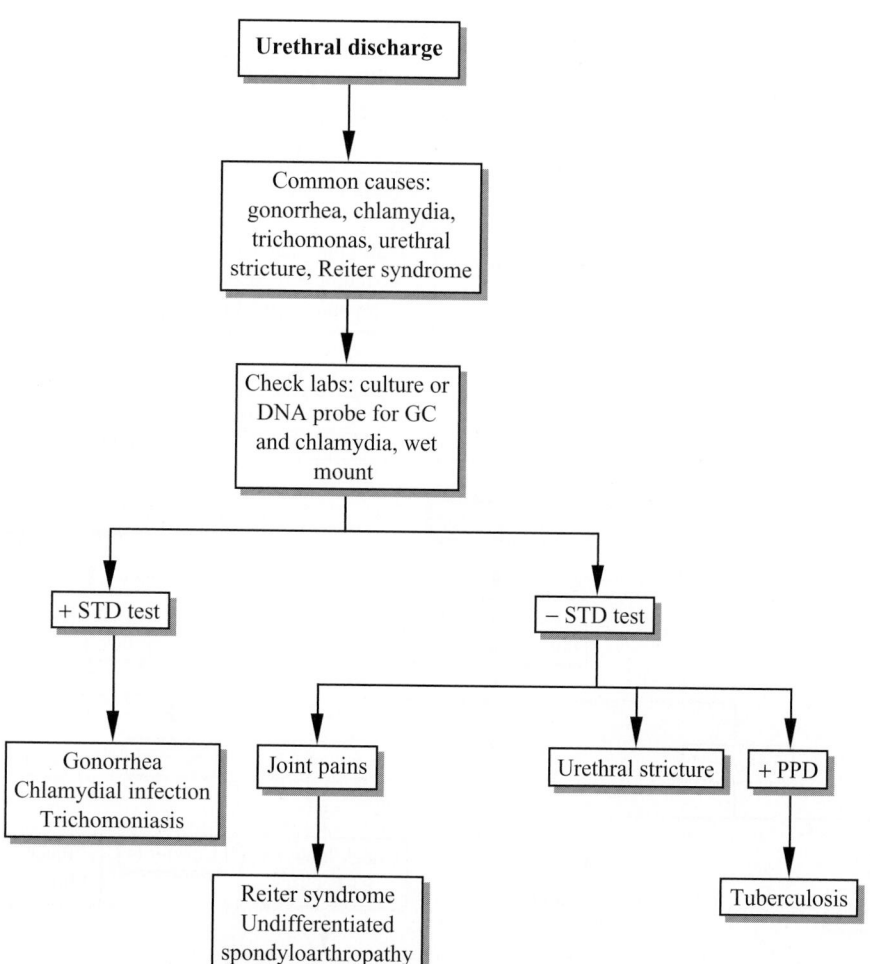

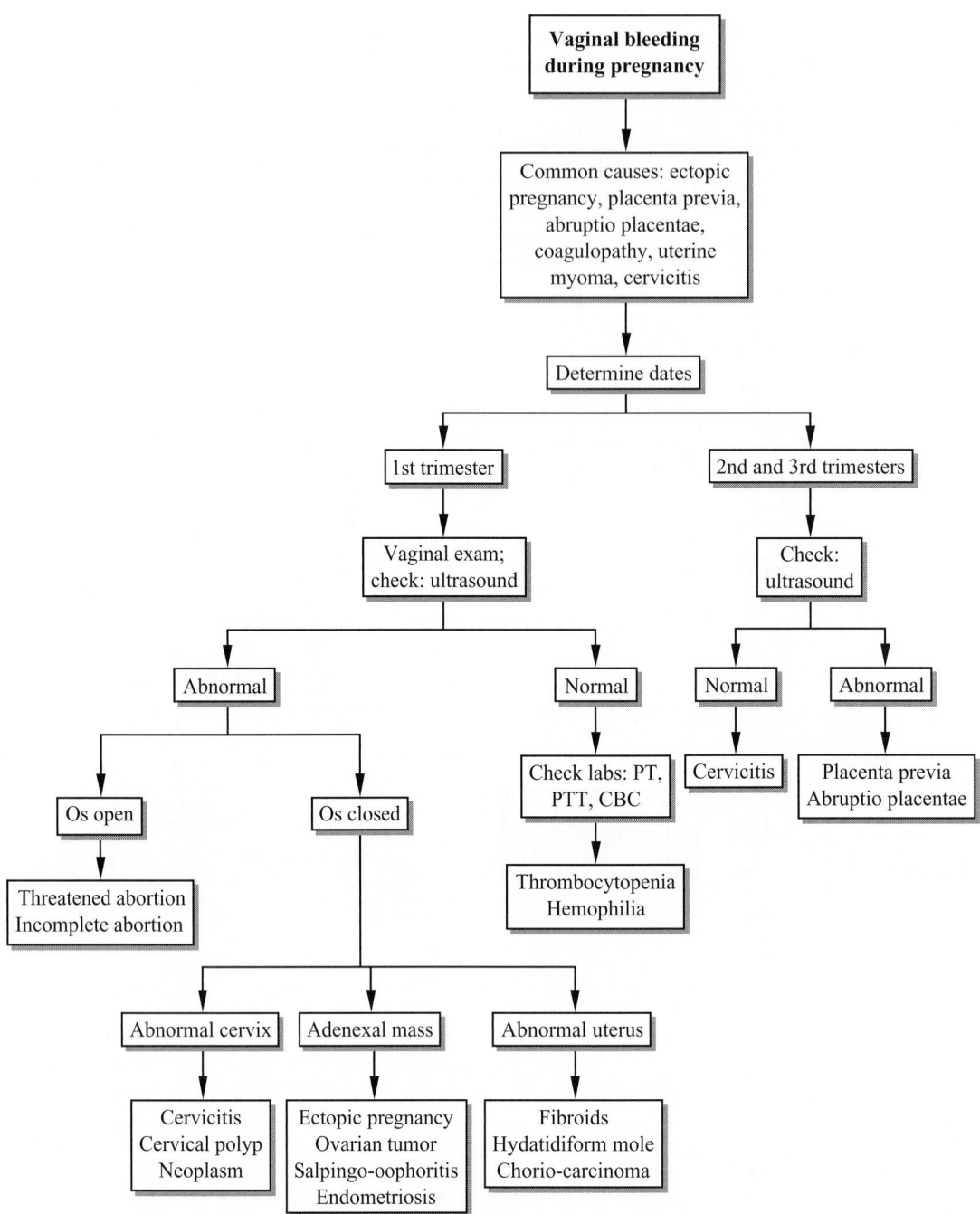

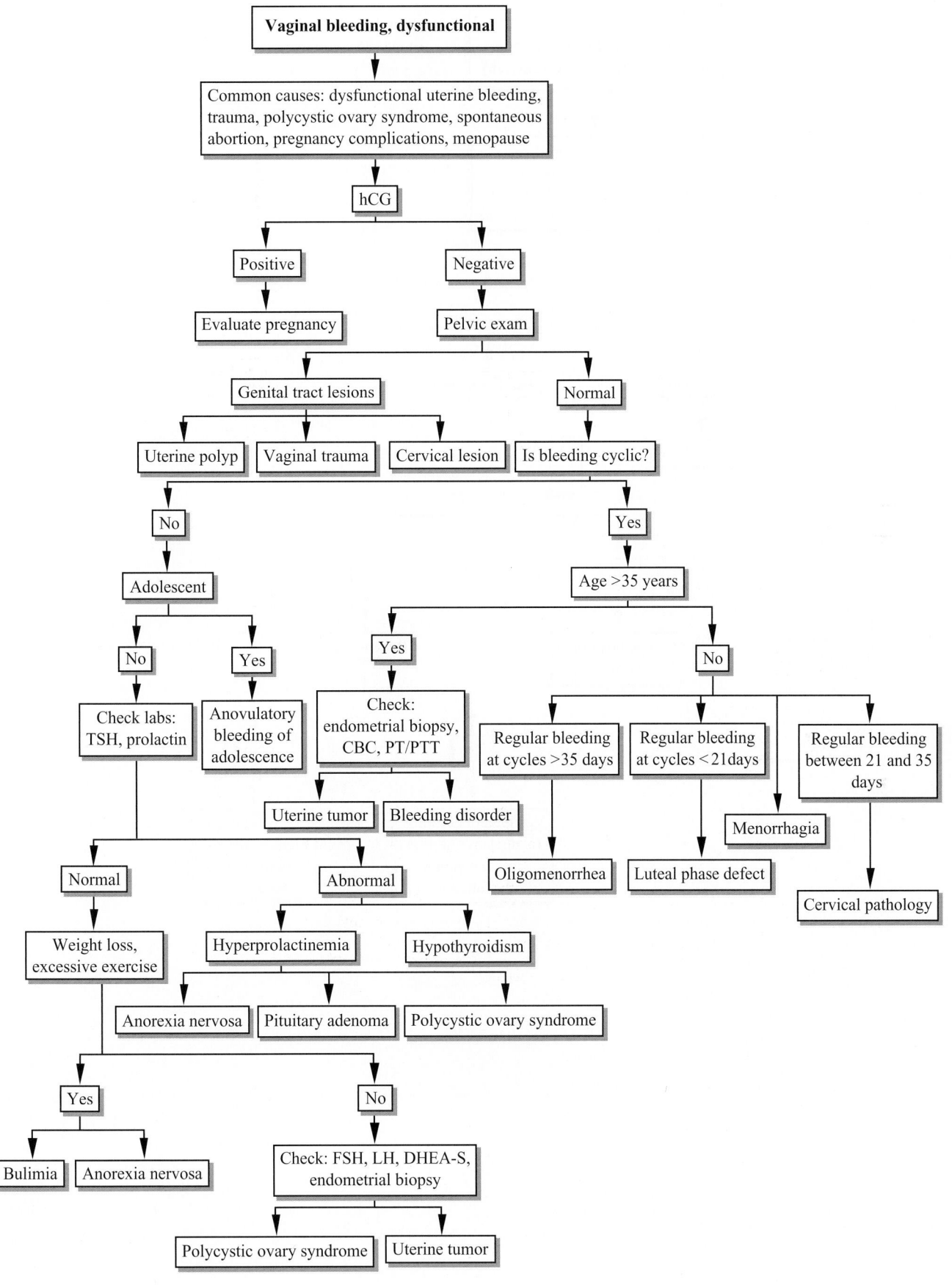

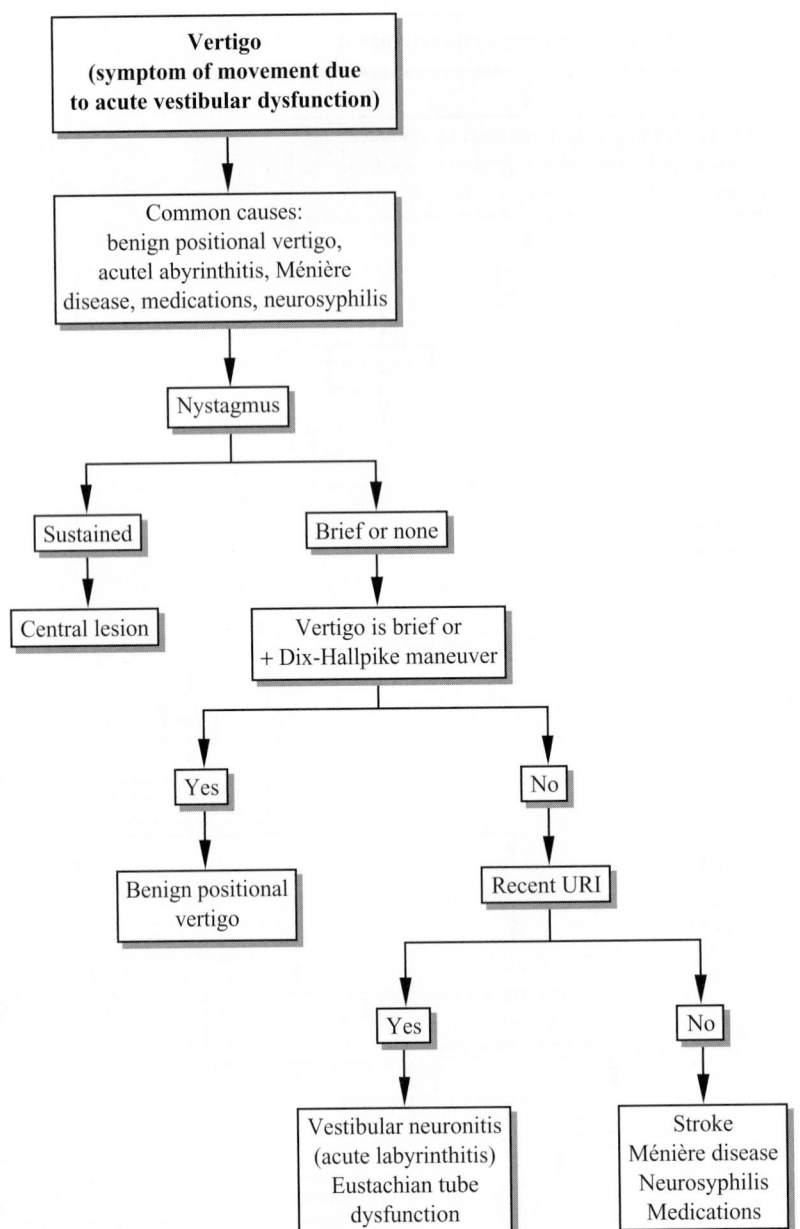

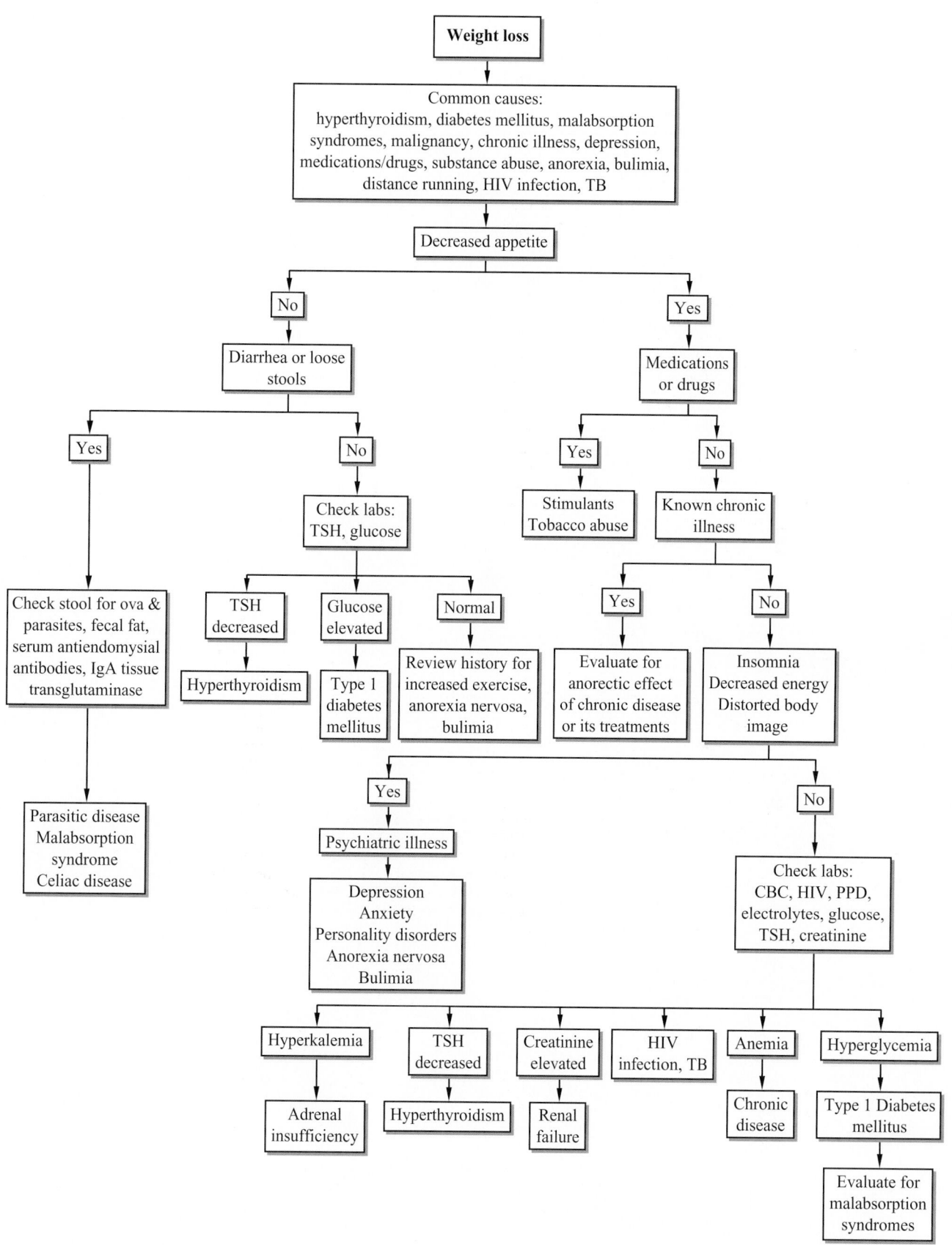

THE 5-MINUTE CLINICAL CONSULT 2008

ABNORMAL PAP/CERVICAL SMEAR

Jeremy Golding, MD

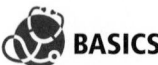 **BASICS**

DESCRIPTION
- The Papanicolaou (Pap) smear is a screening test for cervical cellular pathology. In many laboratories, automated cervical screening complements the Pap smear or supersedes it.
- Abnormal cervical smear results can range from benign cellular changes to suggestion of invasive cancer.
- System(s) Affected: Reproductive

ALERT
Cervical cancer arises from a sexually transmitted disease (STD) caused by human papilloma virus (HPV) (1)[A].

Geriatric Considerations
Less frequent, except in the unscreened population

Pediatric Considerations
Transient Pap smear abnormalities are very common in adolescents, but exceedingly rare before initiation of sexual activity.

Pregnancy Considerations
Squamous intraepithelial lesions can progress during pregnancy, but often regress postpartum.

GENERAL PREVENTION
- HPV Immunization of girls and women prior to sexual debut
- Delay 1st intercourse beyond early adolescence
- Monogamous relationship for both partners
- Smoking cessation
- Adequate antioxidant-rich food intake has been associated with decreased risk
- Obtain routine Pap smears; HPV changes occur ~3 years after initiation of sexual intercourse
- Use barrier methods of birth control if nonmonogamous relationship
- Discontinue Pap smears after age 65–70 in women with recent normal screening and not otherwise at high risk for cervical cancer

EPIDEMIOLOGY
Predominant age: Can occur at any age
- Incidence of CIN3 peaks between ages 25 and 29; invasive disease peaks 15 years later.

Incidence
- Low-grade squamous intraepithelial lesion ranges from 2–3% of all Pap smears
- High-grade squamous intraepithelial lesion and invasive cancer present on 1% of Pap smears
- Other reactive, reparative, and ASC-US (atypical squamous cells of undetermined significance) results are difficult to assess because of the lack of reporting mechanisms

RISK FACTORS
- Cigarette smoking
- Possible deficiency of antioxidants
- Early age of intercourse
- Multiple sexual partners
- Some correlation to low socioeconomic level
- Intercourse with a high-risk male partner
- Human papilloma virus (HPV) infection
- Immunosuppressed
- Human immunodeficiency virus (HIV) infection (associated with earlier and more rapidly progressive cervical disease)

ETIOLOGY
- HPV DNA is found in virtually all cervical carcinomas and precursor lesions worldwide (2)[C]:
  - HPV viral types 16, 18, 31, 35, 45, 51, 52, 56, and 58 are common high-risk or oncogenic virus types for cervical cancer.
  - HPV viral types 6, 11, 42, 43, and 44 are considered common low-risk types, and cause genital warts.
- HPV DNA of high-risk viral types is integrated into the human cervical cell DNA.

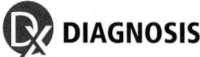 **DIAGNOSIS**

SIGNS AND SYMPTOMS
- Frequently no symptoms
- Occasionally external genital HPV lesions
- Occasionally vaginal discharge related to STD
- Rarely: Vaginal bleeding related to a malignant lesion

TESTS
Lab
- Bethesda System for reporting Pap/cervical smear results
  - Specimen adequacy
- Presence of endocervical cells
  - Negative for intraepithelial lesion or malignancy
  - Epithelial cell abnormalities
- ASC: Atypical squamous cells
- ASC-US: ASC of undetermined significance
- ASC-H: Atypical cells cannot exclude high-grade squamous intraepithelial lesion (SIL)
- LSIL: Low-grade SIL (Combines mild dysplasia and CIN1 with HPV)
- HSIL: High-grade SIL
- Squamous cell carcinoma
  - Glandular cells
- AGC: Atypical glandular cells
- AGCs of undetermined significance
- Atypical glandular cells, favor neoplasia
- Endocervical adenocarcinoma in situ

- Adenocarcinoma
- ThinPrep is a fluid-based collection and thin-layer preparation for cervical cancer screening.
- Sensitivity of a single Pap smear for HSIL ~70%; specificity of ~90%

Diagnostic Procedures/Surgery
- Colposcopy with visually directed biopsy generally recommended when any of the following are present
  - Initial Pap smear with LSIL or worse (adolescents may not require unless persistent)
  - ASC-US present on 2 Pap smears 4–6 months apart
  - ASC-US can be followed with (reflex) HPV hybrid capture 2 test
    - If positive for high-risk viral type: Colposcopy.
    - If negative for high-risk viral type: Repeat Pap smear in 1 year
  - ASC-H needs colposcopic evaluation
  - Any abnormal or suspicious lesion of the cervix or vagina that is visualized by the eye
  - Atypical glandular cells (mandate colposcopy and uterine sampling)
  - LSIL/CIN1 in an adolescent may be a self-limited HPV infection and can be followed with repeated Pap smear at 6 and 12 months
- HPV viral typing
  - Hybrid capture 2 test has 2 viral type probes: A low-risk probe and a high-risk probe.
  - High-risk probe can be used to identify patients with ASC-US who need colposcopy follow-up.
  - HPV typing may be used in combination with Pap smear for women ≥30. Women with negative cytology and negative for high-risk HPV may be followed every 3 years. Women with persistent positive high-risk HPV but negative cytology should undergo colposcopy.
- Loop electrosurgical excision procedure (LEEP)
- Cone biopsy
- Cervicography: Photographic evaluation of cervix

Pathological Findings
- Atypical squamous or columnar cells
- Coarse nuclear material
- Increased nuclear diameter
- Koilocytosis (HPV hallmark)

DIFFERENTIAL DIAGNOSIS
- Acute or chronic cervicitis
- HPV infection
- Cervical squamous intraepithelial neoplasia
- Cervical glandular neoplasia
- Invasive cervical malignancy
- Uterine malignancy (rare)

TREATMENT

GENERAL MEASURES
Office evaluation and observation
- Promote smoking cessation.
- Promote protected intercourse.

Diet
Promote increased intake of antioxidant-rich foods.

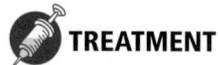 **MEDICATION (DRUGS)**

- Infective/reactive Pap smear
  - Metronidazole 250 mg t.i.d. PO for 7 days
- Condyloma acuminatum
  - Cryotherapy
  - Podophyllin topically every 1–2 weeks
  - Trichloroacetic acid, applied topically by a physician and covered for 5–6 days
- LSIL/CIN1: Observation with Pap smear repeated every 6 months may be appropriate for young women with LSIL, especially with confirmed CIN1.

SURGERY
- LSILs and HSILs and carcinoma in situ can be treated with outpatient surgery.
  - Cryotherapy, laser ablation, LEEP/large loop excision of transition zone, or LEEP or cold-knife conization
- If cervical malignancy, see "Cervical Malignancy" topic

 FOLLOW-UP

DISPOSITION
Outpatient

PROGNOSIS
- Generally excellent
- <1/2 of persistent infective, reactive, reparative, or ASC-US Pap/cervical smears will have more advanced lesions.
- Only a small percentage of LSILs will progress to more advanced lesion.
- Lesions discovered early are very amenable to treatment, with excellent results and few recurrences.

COMPLICATIONS
- Minor abnormalities on Pap/cervical smears can mask more advanced lesions.
- HSILs can progress to invasive cancer.

PATIENT MONITORING
High-risk HPV contact tracing

REFERENCES

1. Guide to Clinical Preventive Services: Report of the US Preventive Services Task Force 2003 update available at http://www.ahrq.gov/clinic/uspstf/uspscerv.htm
2. American Cancer Society guideline for the early detection of cervical neoplasia and cancer. *CA Cancer J Clin*. 2002;52(6):342–362.
3. Wright TC Jr, Cox JT, Massad LS, et al. ASCCP-Sponsored Consensus Conference. 2001 Consensus Guidelines for the management of women with cervical cytological abnormalities. *JAMA*. 2002;287:2120–2129. (Update expected Spring 2007; will be posted at http://www.asccp.org/consensus.shtml).
4. Solomon S, Davey D, Kurman R, et al. The 2001 Bethesda System: terminology for reporting results of cervical cytology. *JAMA*. 2002;287:2114–2119.
5. Bishop JW, Marshall CJ, Bentz JS. New technologies in gynecologic cytology. *J Reprod Med*. 2000;45: 701–719.
6. Canavan TP, Doshi NR. Cervical cancer. *Am Fam Phys*. 2000;61:1369–1376.
7. Apgar BS, Brotzman G. HPV testing in the evaluation of the minimally abnormal Papanicolaou smear. *Am Fam Phys*. 1999;59:2794–2801.

ADDITIONAL READING
ICSI: Management of abnormal pap smear: http://www.guideline.gov/summary/summary.aspx?doc id=8327

 MISCELLANEOUS

See also: Cervical malignancy; Condyloma acuminata; Failure to thrive; Trichomoniasis; Vulvovaginitis; Bacterial

CODES

ICD9-CM
- 795.00 Nonspecific abnormal Papanicolaou smear of cervix, unspecified
- 622.1 Dysplasia of cervix (uteri)

PATIENT TEACHING

Diet
Encourage increased intake of antioxidant-rich foods.

Activity
Promote protected intercourse.

Prevent
- Promote HPV immunization.
- Promote smoking cessation.
- Promote protected intercourse.
- Promote regular Pap smears according to recognized guidelines.
- Reschedule follow-up consultation for any abnormality.

 See Corresponding Diagnostic Algorithm

 See Patient Handout on CD

ABORTION, SPONTANEOUS

Paul Lyons, MD

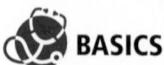 **BASICS**

DESCRIPTION

Abortion is the separation of products of conception from the uterus prior to the potential for fetal survival outside the uterus. Gestationally, the point at which potential fetal viability exists has been the subject of much legal and scientific debate, and definitions vary from state to state; however, a "potentially viable" fetus generally weighs at least 500 g and/or has a gestational age of >20 weeks.

- Spontaneous abortion
  - Expulsion of all (complete abortion) or part (incomplete abortion) of the products of conception from the uterus prior to the 20th completed week of gestation. The placenta, either in whole or in part, can be retained and leads to continuing vaginal bleeding (sometimes profuse). Abortion is considered "threatened" when vaginal bleeding occurs early in pregnancy, with or without uterine contractions, but without dilatation of the cervix, rupture of the membranes, or expulsion of products of conception. Cervical dilatation, rupture of membranes, or expulsion of products in the presence of vaginal bleeding portends "inevitable abortion." Differentiation between threatened and inevitable abortion is desirable because management differs.
- Missed abortion
  - Failed 1st-trimester pregnancy but without the usual signs and symptoms, such as bleeding or cramping
  - Term blighted ovum replaced by anembryonic gestation; ultrasound findings of "empty sac"
- Induced abortion
  - Evacuation of uterine contents or products of conception by either medical or surgical methodology
- Infected abortion
  - Infection involving the products of conception and the maternal reproductive organs
- Septic abortion
  - Dissemination of bacteria (and/or their toxins) into the maternal circulatory and organ system
- Habitual spontaneous abortion
  - 3 or more consecutive spontaneous abortions
  - Risk of another spontaneous abortion is ~25–30%, with 70% rate of successful pregnancy in subsequent pregnancy
- System(s) Affected: Endocrine/Metabolic; Reproductive
- Synonym(s): Miscarriage; Habitual abortion; Recurrent abortion

GENERAL PREVENTION

- Any vaginal bleeding in intrauterine pregnancy is abnormal and should be considered a "threatened" abortion. In reality, vaginal bleeding in early pregnancy is common (occurring in up to one-third of pregnancies), and often the bleeding source eludes diagnosis.
- All pregnant patients with first-trimester bleeding require evaluation for both threatened abortion and ectopic pregnancy
- In habitual abortion, the abortus should be sent for karyotyping. Explore other causes of habitual abortion with the couple to determine the best therapy.
- Special care and attention for the patient who has a subsequent pregnancy

EPIDEMIOLOGY

- Predominant age
  - Increases with advancing age, especially after 35 years of age
  - At age 40, the loss rate is twice that of age 20.
- Predominant sex: Female only

Prevalence

- ~10–15% of all clinically recognized pregnancies end in spontaneous abortion.
- Biochemical pregnancy manifests by the presence of β-human chorionic gonadotropin (HCG) in the blood 7–10 days after conception. When both clinical and biochemical pregnancies are considered, >50% of conceptions are spontaneously aborted.

RISK FACTORS

Most cases of spontaneous abortion occur in patients without identifiable risk factors.

- Chromosomal abnormalities
- Luteal phase defect
- Leiomyomas
- Incompetent cervix
- Infections
- Antifetal antibodies
- Autoimmune disease
  - Phospholipid syndrome
- Alloimmune disease (shared paternal antigens)
- Drugs, chemicals, noxious agents (alcohol, smoking, caffeine)
- X-irradiation
- Contraceptive intrauterine device

Genetics

~2/3 of 1st-trimester spontaneous abortions have significant chromosomal anomalies, with 1/2 of these being autosomal trisomies and the remainder being triploidy, tetraploidy, or 45X monosomies.

ETIOLOGY

See "Risk Factors".

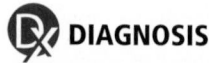 **DIAGNOSIS**

SIGNS AND SYMPTOMS

- Consider a diagnosis of spontaneous abortion in a woman of childbearing age presenting with abnormal vaginal bleeding.
- In a previously diagnosed intrauterine pregnancy
  - Vaginal bleeding
  - Uterine cramping
  - Cervical dilation
  - Ruptured membranes
  - Passage of nonviable products of conception

History

- In relation to the bleeding: Characteristics (amount, color, consistency, associated symptoms), onset (abrupt or gradual), duration, intensity/quantity, and exacerbating/precipitating factors
- In relation to prenatal course: Toxic or infectious exposures, family or personal history of genetic abnormalities, past history of ectopic pregnancy or spontaneous abortion

Physical Exam

- Fetal heart rate, uterine contractions
- Maternal heart rate, pulse, BP (including orthostatic changes), abdominal tenderness, pelvic examination for cervical dilation, blood, products of conception in os or vaginal vault, and uterine size and/or tenderness

TESTS
Lab

- Cultures: Gonorrhea and chlamydia
- CBC
- Rh type
- Urine HCG
- Serial serum β-HCG measurements can assess viability of the pregnancy. Normal gestations have an approximate 67% increase over 2-day interval. Abnormal gestations do not rise appropriately, plateau, or decrease in level before the 8th week of gestation.
- Serum progesterone level
  - >25 ng/mL: Consistent with normal intrauterine pregnancy; rarely seen in ectopic and/or nonviable pregnancy
  - <5 ng/mL: Indicator of nonviable intrauterine gestation or ectopic pregnancy

Imaging

- Ultrasound examination to evaluate fetal viability and to rule out ectopic pregnancy (1C)
  - Can be sensitive enough to confirm an intrauterine pregnancy in the 4th or 5th gestational week from last menstrual period
- Viable intrauterine pregnancy with fetal cardiac activity detected between 5 and 8 weeks from last menstrual period on transvaginal ultrasound
- Transvaginal ultrasound criteria for nonviable intrauterine gestation include 5-mm fetal pole without cardiac activity or 16-mm gestational sac without a fetal pole

Diagnostic Procedures/Surgery

Fetal heart tones can be auscultated with Doppler starting between 10 and 12 weeks' gestation from last menstrual period for a viable pregnancy.

Pathological Findings

Products of conception, Placental villi

DIFFERENTIAL DIAGNOSIS

- Ectopic pregnancy
  - A potentially life-threatening complication, difficult to distinguish from threatened abortion. Transvaginal ultrasonography can identify intrauterine gestational sacs at 32 days' gestation (at serum HCG levels of 1,500–2,000 IU/L). The absence of transvaginal ultrasound evidence of an intrauterine gestation with serum HCG >2,000 IU/L should be considered an ectopic pregnancy until proven otherwise.
- Cervical polyps, neoplasias, and/or inflammatory conditions can cause vaginal bleeding.
  - This bleeding is not usually associated with pain/cramping and is apparent on speculum exam.
- Hydatidiform mole pregnancy
  - Usually ends in abortion prior to the 20th week of pregnancy
  - Bloody discharge prior to abortion is common
  - An intrauterine grapelike-appearing mass on ultrasound is diagnostic ("snow storm" appearance)
  - Serum HCG is often high.
- Membranous dysmenorrhea
  - Characterized by bleeding, cramps, and passage of endometrial casts; can mimic spontaneous abortion
  - HCG is negative.
- HCG-secreting ovarian tumor

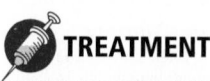 ## TREATMENT

GENERAL MEASURES

- Explore any 1st-trimester vaginal bleeding.
- Serial quantitative β-HCG determination and progesterone assay
- Transvaginal ultrasonography

Diet
No special diet

Activity
- If appropriate, bed rest
- Probably no effect on eventual outcome

IV Fluids
Hemodynamically unstable patients may require IV fluids and/or blood products to maintain BP.

 ## MEDICATION (DRUGS)

- Bleeding following uncomplicated dilatation and curettage (D&C) or spontaneous abortion usually controlled by the following
  - Carboprost (Hemabate): 250 μg IM
  - Oxytocin (Pitocin): 10 U IM or IV
  - Methylergonovine (Methergine): 0.2 mg IM
- Analgesics if needed
- RhoD immune globulin if mother is Rh negative
- Progesterone, if deficiency confirmed prior to pregnancy
- Precautions
  - Do not give methylergonovine IV
  - Refer to manufacturer's literature

Second Line
Rh-negative patients should be given Rh immune globulin following spontaneous abortion (1)[C]

SURGERY

- Inevitable or incomplete abortion: D&C (usually suction)
- When completeness of an abortion is uncertain, a D&C for retained products should be performed.
- Surgical management of incomplete abortion has been shown to improve outcomes compared to medical or expectant management (2)[A] (NNT = 3)

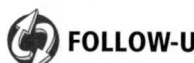 ## FOLLOW-UP

DISPOSITION
Outpatient or inpatient, depending on severity of symptoms (bleeding or pain)

Issues for Referral
Patients should be monitored for development of anxiety and/or depression for up to 1 year following spontaneous abortion. (1)[C]

PROGNOSIS

- If bleeding ceases, prognosis is excellent.
- Habitual abortion
  - Prognosis is dependent on etiology.
  - After 2 consecutive abortions, most couples want some investigation of the problem.
  - After 3 spontaneous abortions, evaluation is usually indicated.
  - Prognosis is still excellent, with up to 70% rate of success with subsequent pregnancy.

COMPLICATIONS

- Complications of D&C include uterine perforation, infection, and bleeding.
- Retained products of conception
- Depression and feelings of guilt (patient may need education and reassurance that she did not cause the miscarriage)

PATIENT MONITORING

- Identification of products of conception within material expelled from the uterus or D&C specimen
- If abortion is complete, observe the patient for further bleeding.
- Complete abortion usually indicated by decreased bleeding, closed cervix, intact or complete products of conception passed, and ultrasound findings of empty uterus and endometrial stripe. Follow HCG level weekly to zero to confirm complete evacuation of products of conception: May take 2 weeks. If levels plateau, suspect retained products of conception or ectopic pregnancy. Up to 6% of clinically diagnosed complete abortions are subsequently found to be ectopic pregnancies (3)[A].

REFERENCES

1. Greibel CP, Halvorsen J, Golemon TB, Day AA. Management of spontaneous abortion. *Am Fam Physician* 2005;72:1243–1250.
2. Sotiriadis A, Makrydimas G, Papatheodorou S, Ionnidis J. Expectant, medical or surgical management of first trimester miscarriage: a meta-analysis. *Obstetrics and Gynecology*. 2005;105:1104–1113.
3. Condous G, Khalid A, Bourne T. Do we need to follow up complete miscarriages with serum human chorionic gonadotropin levels? *Br J Obstet Gynaecol*. 2005;112(6):827–829.
4. Daily CA, Laurent SL, Nunley WC Jr. The prognostic value of serum progesterone and quantitative β-human chorionic gonadotropin in early human pregnancy. *Am J Obstet Gynecol*. 1994;171:380–384.
5. Ohno M, Maeda T, Matsunobu A. A cytogenic study of spontaneous abortion with direct analysis of chorionic villi. *Obstet Gynecol*. 1991;77:394–398.
6. Palmieri A, Moore G, et al. Ectopic pregnancy. In: Hacker and Moore, eds. *Essentials of Obstetrics and Gynecology*, 3rd ed. Philadelphia, PA: Saunders, 1998.
7. Rempen A. Diagnosis and viability of early pregnancy with vaginal sonography. *J Ultrasound Med*. 1990;9:711–716.
8. Simpson JL. Fetal wastage. In: Gabbe S, Niebyl J, et al., eds. *Obstetrics: Normal and Problem Pregnancies*, 3rd ed. New York, NY: Churchill Livingstone, 1996.

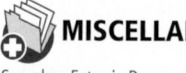 ## MISCELLANEOUS

See also: Ectopic Pregnancy

CODES

ICD9-CM
- 629.9 Unspecified disorder of female genital organs
- 632 Missed abortion
- 634.92 Spontaneous abortion without mention of complication, complete
- 634.91 Spontaneous abortion without mention of complication, incomplete
- 640.03 Threatened abortion, antepartum condition or complication

PATIENT TEACHING

Patient pamphlet (no. AP090) available from the American College of Obstetricians and Gynecologists 409 12th St., SW, Washington, DC 20090-6290; (800) 762-2264

 See Corresponding Diagnostic Algorithm

ABRUPTIO PLACENTAE

Cathryn B. Heath, MD

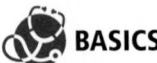 **BASICS**

DESCRIPTION

Premature separation of otherwise normally implanted placenta

- Grades
  - Grade 1: Minimal or no bleeding; detected as retroplacental clot after delivery of viable fetus. Mild uterine irritability (40% of cases)
  - Grade 2: Viable fetus with bleeding and tender, irritable uterus. Mild to moderate bleeding; fibrinogen level decreased (45% of cases)
  - Grade 3: Type A with dead fetus and no coagulopathy; type B with dead fetus and coagulopathy (A and B total 15% of all cases of abruptio placenta)
- Increased pelvic blood flow of pregnancy may enhance blood loss.
- Amniotic fluid embolism is rare but may present with disseminated intravascular coagulation and severe respiratory distress.
- If placenta is in anterior position, there is increased risk of fetal-maternal transfusion with trauma.
- System(s) Affected: Cardiovascular; Reproductive
- Synonym(s): Placental abruption; Premature separation of the placenta

GENERAL PREVENTION

Eliminate risk factors when possible.

EPIDEMIOLOGY

- Predominant age: Childbearing ages
- Predominant sex: Female only

Incidence

- 0.5–1.2% of all deliveries
- 15% if 1 prior episode
- 25% if 2 or more prior episodes
- 80% of cases occur prior to onset of delivery

RISK FACTORS

- Prior abruption (increases risk 10-fold)
- Blunt trauma
- Maternal smoking
- Severe small-for-gestational-age birth
- Hypertension: Pregnancy-induced and chronic
- Uterine anomalies
- Advanced maternal age
- Increased risk if hypertensive and parity >three
- Preterm rupture of membranes, especially if bleeding occurs during observation interval (1)[B]
- Vaginal bleeding before spontaneous rupture of membranes
- Factor V Leiden and other thrombophilic disorders
- Multiple gestation pregnancies (2)[B]

ETIOLOGY

- Cocaine use and abuse
- Trauma of variable amounts, especially blunt abdominal trauma in which external signs of trauma may be incongruent with fetal injury (motor vehicle collision or domestic violence)
- Sudden decompression of overdistended uterus, as in hydramnios or twin gestation

ASSOCIATED CONDITIONS

- Preeclampsia and other forms of hypertension in pregnancy
- Hypertension
- Postpartum hemorrhage
- Maternal and fetal organ damage from hypoperfusion

DIAGNOSIS

SIGNS AND SYMPTOMS

- Classic triad of vaginal bleeding, abdominal pain, and contractions
- 2nd- or 3rd-trimester vaginal bleeding of >1 pad or tampon per hour
- Back pain
- Abdominal pain
- Uterine tenderness, hypertonia, or high-frequency contractions
- Blood loss may be concealed
  - Clinical signs of shock may occur with little vaginal bleeding.
- Because blood volumes increase in pregnancy, volume lost may exceed 30% before signs of shock or hypovolemia occur.
  - Vital signs may be preserved even with significant loss.
- Fetal distress or demise
- Idiopathic preterm labor with or without fetal distress

TESTS

- Kleihauer-Betke for fetal-maternal transfusion
- Bedside clot test, with red-top tube of maternal blood with poor or nonclotting blood after 7–10 minutes indicating coagulopathy
- Apt test for fetal blood origin
  - Mix vaginal blood with small amount of tap water to cause hemolysis, centrifuge several minutes, mix pink hemoglobin–containing supernatant with 1 mL 1% sodium hydroxide (NaOH) for each 5 mL of supernatant; read color after 2 minutes, with fetal hemoglobin staying pink and adult turning yellow-brown
- Wright stain of vaginal blood
  - Observe for nucleated red blood cells (RBCs), usually of fetal origin
- Lecithin/sphingomyelin ratio if delay of delivery is an option and length of pregnancy is preterm

Lab

- Blood type, Rh, Coombs
- CBC with platelet count
- Prothrombin time
- Partial thromboplastin time
- Fibrinogen levels
- Cross-match at least 4 U packed RBCs
- Drugs that may alter lab results
  - Those that affect clotting parameters
  - RHoD immune globulin administered <12 weeks prior may affect antibody test
- Disorders that may alter lab results
  - Fibrinogen levels climb to 350–550 mg/dL (3.5–5.5 g/L) in 3rd trimester and must fall to 100–150 mg/dL (1.0–1.5 g/L) before partial thromboplastin time will rise.
  - Fibrin split or degradation products are elevated in pregnancy and are not very helpful in assessing disseminated intravascular coagulation.

Imaging

Although ultrasound may show sonolucent retroplacental clot, rounded placental margin, or thickened placenta, it is often not definitive, especially with posterior placement or mild abruption. However, ultrasound of the uterus, placenta and fetus may diagnose abruption placenta in 50% of cases. Large (>60 mL) are associated with a >50% fetal mortality.

Diagnostic Procedures/Surgery

External uterine monitoring often shows elevated baseline pressure and frequent low-amplitude contractions.

Pathological Findings

- Normocytic normochromic anemia with acute bleeding
- Elevated prothrombin time and partial thromboplastin time, fibrinogen levels below 100–150 mg/dL (1.0–1.5 g/L), platelets 20,000–50,000/μL if disseminated intravascular coagulation active
- Positive Kleihauer-Betke reaction if fetal-maternal transfusion has occurred
- Positive antibody if RhoD isosensitization has occurred

DIFFERENTIAL DIAGNOSIS

- Uterine rupture
- Placenta previa
- Vasa previa
- Marked bloody show
- Cervical and vaginal causes (e.g., chlamydia or gonorrhea with bloody, friable cervix)
- Masses
- Other painful conditions (e.g., appendicitis, pyelonephritis)
- Labor

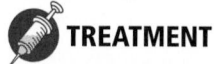 **TREATMENT**

GENERAL MEASURES
- History and physical exam with medical history, allergies, prior ultrasounds this gestation, and time of last meal
- In general, severe abruption best managed by delivery of fetus
- Grade 1: Usual labor protocol
- Grade 2: Rapid delivery, most often by cesarean delivery
- Grade 3: Vaginal delivery preferable if mother stable
- In trauma, monitor in the inpatient setting for at least 6 hours for evidence of fetal insult, abruption, fetal-maternal transfusion. If contractions or preterm labor occur, patient should be monitored for at least 24 hours. Risk factors for contractions with trauma include
  – Gestational age >35 weeks
  – Assaults
  – Pedestrian/vehicular collisions
  – Ejections from vehicle or lack of restraints (3)[B]
- Early aggressive restoration of maternal physiology to protect fetus and maternal organs from hypoperfusion/disseminated intravascular coagulation
- Stabilize vitals
- Maintain urine output >60 mL/h
- Bedrest with external fetal and labor monitoring, if fetus is viable
- Large-bore, 16- to 18-gauge IV crystalloid infusion
  – Central line placement only after coagulation status has been assessed
- Transfusions of whole blood and packed RBCs as necessary to maintain hematocrit >30%
- Fresh frozen plasma and platelet transfusions for coagulopathy, with cryoprecipitate and fibrinogen given if indicated
- Follow hemoglobin/hematocrit and coagulation status every 1–2 hours
- Place intrauterine pressure catheter, because fetal risk climbs with elevated pressure
- Role of amniotomy to prevent amniotic fluid embolism is debatable but will speed delivery
- Positioning on left side may enhance venous return and cardiac output
- Oxygen for all patients

Diet
NPO until status defined and possibility of cesarean delivery ruled out

Activity
Bed rest until status defined

SPECIAL THERAPY
IV Fluids
Saline or Ringer's lactate

 MEDICATION (DRUGS)

- May use oxytocin (Pitocin) augmentation to speed delivery
- Tocolytics such as terbutaline may be used in mild noncompromising preterm abruption.
- RhoD immune globulin IM for RhoD-negative mother if undelivered or indicated after delivery
- 300 μg RhoD immune globulin/15 mL fetal blood transfused, if Kleihauer-Betke test returns positive, administered IM
- Contraindications
  – Tocolytics should be withheld in preterm labor until abruption ruled out and fetal status defined
- Precautions
  – Suffusion of blood into myometrium with weakening may increase risk of uterine rupture with oxytocin (Pitocin) augmentation
  – Cryoprecipitate and fibrinogen may represent greater transfusion infection transmission risk

SURGERY
May need cesarean delivery after maternal stabilization if fetus is viable and the situation urgent

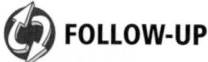 **FOLLOW-UP**

DISPOSITION
Hospitalize until stable

Discharge Criteria
If trauma without compromise after observation or small abruption and preterm, may observe outpatient, encouraging reduction of risk factors

PROGNOSIS
- 0.5–1% fetal mortality and 30–50% perinatal mortality
- With trauma and abruption, 1% maternal and 30–70% fetal mortality
- Labor typically more rapid, but hypotonus from blood suffusion may occur

COMPLICATIONS
- Infection transfusion risks: Hepatitis, cytomegalovirus, human immunodeficiency virus, and others
- Sensitization from blood product transfusion

PATIENT MONITORING
- If not delivered, monitor for intrauterine growth retardation
- See regularly and assess for preterm labor

REFERENCES
1. Ananth CV, Oyelese Y, et al. Preterm premature rupture of membranes, intrauterine infection, and oligohydramnios: risk factors for placental abruption. *Obst & Gynecol*. 2004;104(1): 71–77.
2. Salihu HM, Bekan B, et al. Perinatal mortality associated with abruptio placenta in singletons and multiples. *Am J Obstet Gynecol* 2005; 193(1):198–203.
3. Curet MJ, Schermer CR, et al. Predictors of outcome in trauma during pregnancy : identification of patients who can be monitored for less than 6 hours. *J Trauma*. 2000;49(1):18–24.

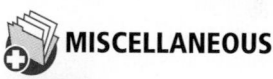 **MISCELLANEOUS**

CODES

ICD9-CM
641.20 Premature separation of placenta, unspecified

PATIENT TEACHING
- Call physician or proceed to hospital whenever patient experiences bleeding of >1 pad per hour or if severe uterine or back pain occurs
- Mayo Health: http://mayohealth.org

ACETAMINOPHEN POISONING

Lars C. Larsen, MD

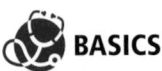 **BASICS**

DESCRIPTION

- A disorder characterized by hepatic necrosis following large ingestions of acetaminophen. Symptoms may vary from initial nausea, vomiting, diaphoresis, and malaise to jaundice, confusion, somnolence, coma, and death. The clinical hallmark is the onset of symptoms within 24 hours of ingestion of acetaminophen-only or -combination products.
- Acetaminophen poisoning is most often encountered following large single ingestions of acetaminophen-containing medications. Usual toxic doses are >7.5 g in adults and 150 mg/kg in children. However, poisoning also occurs after acute and chronic ingestions of lesser amounts in susceptible individuals, including those who regularly abuse alcohol, are chronically malnourished, or take medications that affect hepatic metabolism of acetaminophen.
- Therapeutic adult doses are 0.5–1 q4–6h; up to a maximum of 4 g/d. Therapeutic pediatric doses are 10–15 mg/kg q4–6h, not to exceed 5 doses in 24 hours.
- System(s) Affected: Cardiovascular; Gastrointestinal; Renal/Urologic
- Synonym(s): Paracetamol poisoning

Geriatric Considerations
Hepatic damage may be increased if taking hepatotoxic medications chronically.

Pediatric Considerations
Hepatic damage at toxic acetaminophen levels is decreased in children <6 years.

Pregnancy Considerations
- Increased incidence of spontaneous abortion, especially with overdose at early gestational age
- Incidence of spontaneous abortion or fetal death appears to be increased when N-acetylcysteine (NAC) treatment is delayed.

GENERAL PREVENTION
Parent/caregiver education essential:
- Education during well child exams regarding poisoning prevention
- Emergency telephone numbers

EPIDEMIOLOGY
- Predominant age: Children and adults at any age
- Predominant sex: No reported association

Incidence
- >131,700 ingestions of acetaminophen-containing medications reported by poison control centers in 2004
- 327 deaths in 2004, 3 in children <6 years

Prevalence
Approximately 31% of exposures are in children <6 years.

RISK FACTORS
- Age <6 years
- Concurrent oral poisoning with other substances
- Psychiatric illness
- History of previous toxic ingestions or suicide attempts
- Regular ingestion of large amounts of alcohol

ETIOLOGY
Accidental or intentional ingestion of acetaminophen or combination medications containing acetaminophen

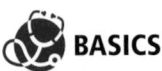 **DIAGNOSIS**

SIGNS AND SYMPTOMS
- Develop over the 1st 24 hours following large ingestions and may last as long as 8 days
- Severe symptoms indicate large ingestions or coingestants
- Fulminant hepatic failure occurs in <1% of adults and is very rare in children <6 years.
- Stage 1: 1st 24 hours
  - Nausea
  - Vomiting
  - Diaphoresis
- Stage 2: 24–48 hours
  - Right upper quadrant pain
  - Typically less nausea, vomiting, diaphoresis, and malaise than in stage 1
- Stage 3: 72–96 hours
  - Nausea, vomiting, malaise reappear
  - Severe poisonings may result in jaundice, confusion, somnolence, and coma
- Stage 4: 7–8 days
  - Resolution of clinical signs in survivors
- May develop gradually following long-term ingestion of near-therapeutic amounts of acetaminophen. Such patients may present in any stage 1–3, without a history of ingestion of the usual toxic doses.

TESTS
Lab
- Plasma acetaminophen levels should be drawn on all patients 4 hours or more after ingestion (levels prior to 4 hours not helpful).
- At least one additional acetaminophen level drawn 4–6 hours after the 1st level is recommended if the ingested acetaminophen is an extended-release product (e.g., Tylenol Extended Relief) or is not known to be an immediate-release product.
- If the second level is >1st level or is close to the "possible risk" level on the Rumack-Matthew nomogram, it may be prudent to obtain additional acetaminophen levels every 2 hours until the levels stabilize or decline.
- If coingestants include drugs that slow gastrointestinal motility, an acetaminophen level drawn 4–6 hours after the 2nd level may detect a late increase in serum acetaminophen concentration.
- Screens for suspected coingestants (aspirin, iron, and others) may be positive (especially when suicide is a possibility).
- With toxic ingestions, aspartate transaminase (AST; serum glutamic-oxaloacetic transaminase), alanine transaminase (serum glutamic-pyruvic transaminase), and bilirubin levels begin to rise in stage 2 and peak in stage 3. In severe poisonings, the prothrombin time will parallel these changes.
- AST levels >1,000 IU/L are consistent with the diagnosis, and levels of 20,000 IU/L are not uncommon.
- Laboratory abnormalities usually resolve by stage 4.
- Renal function abnormalities are common in patients with hepatotoxicity.
- Evidence of damage to the pancreas and heart may present following severe poisonings.
- Drugs that may alter lab results: None with clinically significant cross-reactivity with plasma acetaminophen assay
- Disorders that may alter lab results: Diseases or toxic substances that damage the liver, particularly alcohol

Imaging
No specific imaging required

Diagnostic Procedures/Surgery
None other than correlating plasma acetaminophen levels with the clinical presentation

Pathological Findings
Centrilobular hepatic necrosis

DIFFERENTIAL DIAGNOSIS
- Consider presence of coingestants, especially alcohol
- Other ingested toxins that produce severe acute hepatic injury, including the mushroom *Amanita phalloides* and products containing yellow phosphorus or carbon tetrachloride

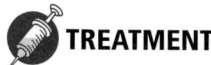 **TREATMENT**

INITIAL STABILIZATION

Contact a regional poison control center for management recommendations. In the United States, a local poison control center can be reached by calling (800) 222-1222.

GENERAL MEASURES

- Activated charcoal should be used (1,2)[C]; (3)[A], but preferably not within 1 hour of administration of the antidote NAC.

- The stomach of untreated patients may be emptied by gastric lavage if within 1 hour of ingestion.

- Ipecac is no longer recommended for routine use at home or in health care facilities (4)[C].

- NAC should be given (3)[A] when plasma acetaminophen concentrations measured 4 hours or more after ingestion are in the "possible risk" or higher levels on the Rumack-Matthew nomogram. This corresponds to acetaminophen levels >150 μg/mL (993 μmol/L), >75 μg/mL (497 μmol/L), and >40 μg/mL (265 μmol/L) at 4, 8, and 12 hours after ingestion, respectively.

- NAC therapy may be effective up to 36 hours or more after ingestion

Diet

No special diet except with severe hepatic damage

Activity

Restricted if significant hepatic damage has occurred

 MEDICATION (DRUGS)

First Line

- 2 classes of medicine
  - Activated charcoal
  - Acetylcysteine (NAC, Mucomyst)
- Emergency facility/hospital
  - Patients evaluated within 1 hour of ingestion may have their stomachs evacuated by gastric lavage.
  - Activated charcoal: 1 g/kg PO for initial dose; preferably not within 1 hour of NAC administration. Additional concurrent use during NAC therapy is controversial.
  - Acetylcysteine PO or IV
    ○ Oral loading dose of 140 mg/kg, followed by 70 mg/kg q4h for 17 additional doses. Whenever possible, NAC therapy should be initiated within 8 hours following the toxic ingestion.
    ○ IV loading dose of Acetadote 150 mg/kg over 15 minutes X 1 (some recommend the loading dose be given over 60 minutes to decrease incidence of anaphylactoid rxns). Maintenance doses: 50 mg/kg over 4 hours, followed by 100 mg/kg over 16 hours.
- Contraindications: Medication allergies
- Precautions
  - Oral NAC may cause significant nausea and vomiting due to its sulfur content; consider administration by nasogastric tube.
  - Nausea can be treated with metoclopramide (Reglan), 0.5–1 mg/kg IV, or ondansetron (Zofran), 0.15 mg/kg IV (for age >4 years, usually 4 mg/dose).
  - IV NAC (Acetadote) may cause anaphylactoid rxns including rash, bronchospasm, pruritis, angioedema, tachycardia, or hypotension.
- Reactions usually occur with loading dose. Slow or temporarily stop the infusion; may concurrently treat with antihistamines
- Significant possible interactions: Activated charcoal given within 1 hour of NAC may adsorb the NAC, thereby limiting its effectiveness.

Second Line

Oral racemethionine (methionine)

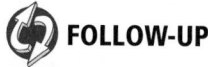 **FOLLOW-UP**

DISPOSITION

- All patients should be evaluated at a health care facility.
- Outpatient for nontoxic accidental ingestions

Admission Criteria

Toxic and intentional ingestions

Issues for Referral

Psychiatric follow-up after intentional ingestions

PROGNOSIS

- Complete recovery with early therapy
- $<1\%$ of adult patients develop hepatic failure.
- Hepatic failure is very rare in children <6 years.

COMPLICATIONS

Rare following recovery from acute poisoning

REFERENCES

1. Gaudreault P. Activated charcoal revisited. *Clin Ped Emerg Med.* 2005;6:76–80.
2. Heard K. Gastric Decontamination. *Med Clin N Am.* 2005;89:1067–1078.
3. Brok J, Buckley N, Glud C. Interventions for paracetamol (acetaminophen) overdoses. *The Cochrane Database of Systematic Reviews.* 2006; volume 1.
4. American Academy of Pediatrics Committee on Injury, Violence, and Poison Prevention. Poison treatment in the home. *Pediatrics.* 2003;112: 1182–1185.
5. Acetylcysteine (Acetadote) for acetaminophen overdosage. *The Medical Letter* 2005;47:70–71.
6. Watson WA, Litovitz TL, Rodgers GC Jr, et al. 2004 annual report of the American Association of Poison Control Centers Toxic Exposure Surveillance System. *Amer J Emerg Med.* 2005;23(pt 5)1: 589–666.

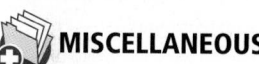 **MISCELLANEOUS**

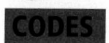

ICD9-CM

965.4 Poisoning by aromatic analgesics, NEC

PATIENT TEACHING

- Education of parents/caregivers during well child visits
- Anticipatory guidance for caregivers, family, and cohabitants of potentially suicidal patients
- Patient brochure (item no. 1515): *Child safety: keeping your home safe for your baby.* American Academy of Family Physicians (11400 Tomahawk Creek Parkway, Leawood, KS 66211-2672)
- Education of patients taking long-term acetaminophen therapy

ACNE ROSACEA

Larry Millikan, MD

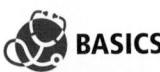 **BASICS**

DESCRIPTION

Chronic skin eruption with flushing and dilatation of small blood vessels in the face, especially nose and cheeks. Sometimes associated with ocular symptoms (ocular rosacea)

- System(s) Affected: Skin/Exocrine
- Synonym(s): Rosacea

ALERT

- Uncommon after age 60
- Unlikely in this age group
- Use of oral isotretinoin contraindicated

GENERAL PREVENTION

No preventive measure known

EPIDEMIOLOGY

- Predominant age: 30–50 years
- Predominant sex: Female > Male

Prevalence

Common

RISK FACTORS

Genetics

People of Northern European and Celtic background commonly afflicted

ETIOLOGY

- No proven cause
- Possibilities include
  - Thyroid and gonadal disturbance
  - Alcohol, coffee, tea, spiced food overindulgence (unproven)
  - Demodex follicular parasite (suspected)
  - Exposure to cold, heat, hot drinks
  - Emotional stress
  - Dysfunction of the gastrointestinal tract
  - Environmental trigger factors: Sun, wind, cold

ASSOCIATED CONDITIONS

- Seborrheic dermatitis of scalp and eyelids
- Keratitis with photophobia, lacrimation, visual disturbance
- Corneal lesions
- Blepharitis
- Uveitis

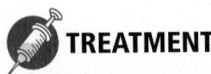 **DIAGNOSIS**

SIGNS AND SYMPTOMS

History

- Skin flush: Prominent at onset
- Redness: Lower half of nose, sometimes whole nose, forehead, cheeks, chin

Physical Exam

- Conjunctivae red: Sometimes
- Erythema, dusky: In advanced cases
- Blood vessels in involved area collapse under pressure
- Acne lesions form papules, pustules, and nodules
  - Comedones are rare.
- Telangiectasia
- Rhinophyma: Sometimes (more common in males)

TESTS

Diagnosis based on physical exam findings

Pathological-Findings

- Inflammation around hypertrophied sebaceous glands, producing papules, pustules, and cysts
- Absence of comedones and blocked ducts
- Vascular dilation and dermal lymphocytic infiltrate

DIFFERENTIAL DIAGNOSIS

- Drug eruptions (iodides and bromides)
- Granulomas of the skin
- Cutaneous lupus erythematosus
- Carcinoid syndrome
- Deep fungal infection
- Acne vulgaris
- Seborrheic dermatitis
- Steroid rosacea (abuse)

TREATMENT

GENERAL MEASURES

- Reassurance
- Treat psychological stress if present
- Avoid oil-based cosmetics
  - Others are acceptable and may help women tolerate the symptoms.
- Electrodesiccation or chemical sclerosis of permanently dilated blood vessels
- Possible evolving laser therapy

Diet

No restrictions

Activity

- No restrictions
- Support physical fitness

MEDICATION

First Line

- Low-dose oral tetracycline, 500–1,000 mg/d, or doxycycline, 50–150 mg/d, or minocycline, 75–200 mg/d; doxycycline, 20 mg PO b.i.d., 40 mg b.i.d. (oracea) if persistent
- Sulfur-containing local applications:
  – Alcohol-sulfur (Liquimat)
  – Sulfur (Fostril)
  – Resorcinol-sulfur (Rezamid)
  – Sulfacetamide-sulfur (Sulfacet-R, Nicosyn, Avar Gel, Avar Cleanser, Avar Green, Rosanil Cleanser, Plexion Cleanser, Ovace Wash, Clenia Emollient Cream, Clenia Foam Wash)
  – Urea-sulfacetamide-sulfur (Rosula)
- Azelaic acid (Finacea) topically
- Topical metronidazole (MetroGel) 0.75% gel:1% gel. Apply each morning and at bedtime after cleansing skin; also available as a cream and lotion, which may be better tolerated by some patients; or 1% cream formulation of metronidazole (Noritate), used once daily
- Topical erythromycin
- Topical clindamycin lotion preferred
- Possible utility of calcineurin inhibitors (tacrolimus, 0.1%; pimecrolimus, 0.1%)
- Topical steroids should not be used, as they may aggravate rosacea.
- Contraindications
  – Tetracycline: Not for use during pregnancy or in children <8 years
  – Isotretinoin: Teratogenic; not for use during pregnancy or in women of reproductive age who are not using reliable contraception
- Precautions: Tetracycline may cause photosensitivity; sunscreen recommended
- Significant possible interactions
  – Tetracycline: Avoid concurrent administration with antacids, dairy products, or iron
  – Broad-spectrum antibiotics: May reduce the effectiveness of oral contraceptives; barrier method recommended

Second Line

For severe cases, isotretinoin PO for 4 months

SURGERY

Surgical treatment of rhinophyma

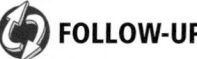 **FOLLOW-UP**

DISPOSITION

Outpatient treatment

PROGNOSIS

- Slowly progressive
- Subsides spontaneously (sometimes)

COMPLICATIONS

- Rhinophyma (dilated follicles and thickened bulbous skin on nose), especially in men
- Conjunctivitis
- Blepharitis
- Keratitis
- Visual deterioration

PATIENT MONITORING

- Occasional and as needed
- Close follow-up for women using isotretinoin

REFERENCES

1. Fitzpatrick TB, et al., eds. *Dermatology in General Medicine*, 5th ed. New York: McGraw-Hill, 1999.
2. Habif T. *Clinical Dermatology*, 4th ed. St. Louis MO: Mosby, 2004.
3. Powell FC. Clinical practice. Rosacea. *N Engl J Med*. 2005;352:793–803.

 MISCELLANEOUS

See also: Acne Vulgaris; Blepharitis; Dermatitis; Seborrheic; Lupus Erythematosus; Discoid; Uveitis

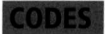 **CODES**

ICD9-CM

695.3 Rosacea

PATIENT TEACHING

American Academy of Dermatology (708) 330-0230

 See Corresponding Diagnostic Algorithm

 See Patient Handout on CD

ACNE VULGARIS

Katrina Miller, MD

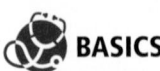 **BASICS**

DESCRIPTION
- Acne vulgaris is a disorder of the pilosebaceous units (PSU), caused by androgen-mediated hyperkeratinization and increased sebum production, resulting in plugging of the follicles and formation of comedones. When further inflammation occurs, lesions include papules, inflammatory pustules, nodules, and scarring.
- System(s) Affected: Skin/exocrine

Geriatric Considerations
Favre-Racouchot syndrome
Isotretinoin is a teratogenic; Pregnancy Class X

Pregnancy Considerations
- May result in a flare, or remission, of acne
- Erythromycin can be used in pregnancy; use topical agents when possible
- Avoid topical tretinoin, although no good evidence exists that its use is teratogenic.
- Contraindicated: Isotretinoin, tazarotene, tetracycline, doxycycline, minocycline

Pediatric Considerations
- Neonatal acne
- Infantile acne: Increased risk for severe teenage acne vulgaris.
- Rare in ages 1–7 years
  - Check for hyperandrogenemia of adrenal or ovarian origin
  - Do not use tetracyclines <8 years of age
- Adolescent acne
  - Often very significant to adolescent patient
  - Often an "entry ticket" for advice on lifestyle, contraception, physiology, etc.

EPIDEMIOLOGY
- Predominant age
  - Primarily early to late puberty, may persist into 3rd to 4th decades
  - Affected ages: All
- Predominant sex
  - Male > Female (adolescence)
  - Female > Male (adult)

Prevalence
- 17–50 million in the U.S. Varies geographically.
- Nearly 100% of adolescents affected. A smaller percentage will seek medical advice.
- 8% of 25–34 year olds, 3% of 35–44 year olds

RISK FACTORS
- Adolescence
- Increased endogenous androgenic effect
- Androgenic steroids (e.g., steroid abuse, some birth control pills)
- Possibly stress
- Oily cosmetics: Cleansing creams, moisturizers, and oil-based foundations; pomade
- Rubbing or occluding skin surface (e.g., sports equipment such as helmets and shoulder pads), telephone or hands against the skin
- Drugs
  - Androgens and androgenic stimulants
  - Anabolic steroids
  - Systemic corticosteroids
  - Long-acting progestins
  - Lithium, phenytoin, isoniazid, phenobarbital, ethionamide, azathioprine, disulfiram, cyclosporine, quinine, thiourea, and thiouracil
- Virilization disorders: PCOS
- Hot, humid climate

Genetics
- Familial association.
- If a family history exists, the acne may be more severe and occur earlier.

PATHOPHYSIOLOGY
- Androgens (testosterone and DHEA)
  - Stimulate sebum production and proliferation of keratinocytes in hair follicles
- Keratin plug obstructs follicle os, causing sebum accumulation and follicular distention
- *Propionibacterium acnes*, an anaerobe, colonizes and proliferates in the plugged follicle.
  - *P. acnes* promotes chemotactic factors and proinflammatory mediators, causing inflammation of follicle and dermis.

ETIOLOGY
Androgens, inflammation, and *P. acnes*

ASSOCIATED CONDITIONS
- Acne fulminans
- Pyoderma faciale
- Acne conglobata
- Hidradenitis suppurativa
- Pomade acne
- SAPHO syndrome: Synovitis, acne, pustulosis, hyperostosis, osteitis
- PAPA syndrome: Pyogenic sterile arthritis, pyoderma gangrenosum, cystic acne
- Dark-skinned patients: 50% keloidal scarring and 50% acne hyperpigmented macules (AHMs)

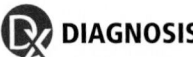 **DIAGNOSIS**

SIGNS AND SYMPTOMS
- Closed comedones (whiteheads)
- Open comedones (blackheads)
- Nodules or papules
- Pustules ("cysts")
- Scars: Ice pick, rolling, boxcar, atrophic macules, hypertrophic, depressed, sinus tracts
- Most common areas affected are: face, chest, back, and upper arms (areas of greatest concentration of sebaceous glands)
- Factors influencing symptomatology
  - Males later onset, greater severity
  - Females may worsen immediately prior to menses
- Grading system (American Academy of Dermatology, 1990)
  - Mild: Few papules/pustules; no nodules
  - Moderate: Some papules/pustules; few nodules
  - Severe: Numerous papules/pustules; many nodules
  - Very severe: Acne conglobata, acne fulminans, acne inversa

History
Duration, medications, cleansing products, stress, smoking, exposures, family history

Physical Exam
Type of lesions, number, location

TESTS
Lab
Testosterone, dehydroepiandrosterone sulfate (DHEA-S), luteinizing hormone (LH), and follicle-stimulating hormone (FSH) measure in rare cases when acne arises de novo in previously unaffected adult. High levels or LH:FSH ratio >2.5 suggests PCOS.

Pathological Findings
- Oiliness, thickening of the skin
- Hypertrophy of the sebaceous glands
- Perifolliculitis
- Scarring

DIFFERENTIAL DIAGNOSIS
- Folliculitis
- Acne (rosacea, cosmetica, steroid induced)
- Perioral dermatitis
- Chloracne
- Pseudofolliculitis barbae
- Drug eruption
- Verruca vulgaris and plana
- Keratosis pilaris
- Molluscum contagiosum

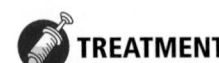 **TREATMENT**

GENERAL MEASURES
- Therapy goals
  - Lessen physical discomfort
  - Minimize scarring
  - Improve appearance
  - Avoid adverse psychologic impact
- Cleansing
  - Use mild soap, once or twice a day to control surface oiliness (frequent washing and abrasives can irritate the skin and increase sebum production and inflammation).
- *Comedonal acne (grade 1)*: Keratolytic agent preferred (1,3)[A]
- *Mild inflammatory acne (grade 2):* Topical antibiotic with benzoyl peroxide. Add keratinolytic agent if needed and tolerated (2,3)[A].
- *Moderate inflammatory acne (grade 3):* Systemic antibiotic added to regimen above for grade 2, or systemic antibiotic substituted for the topical treatment of benzoyl peroxide or topical antibiotic. Continue keratinolytic agent after completion of antibiotic for maintenance.
- *Severe inflammatory acne (grade 4):* As in Grade 3, or isotretinoin (1,3)[A]
- Apply topical agents to both lesions and surrounding area of affected skin.
- Topical retinoid plus antibiotic (topical or PO) is better than either alone (1,3)[A].
- Antibiotic therapy should be stopped after inflammatory lesions resolve.
- Oral antibiotics should generally be used for 6 months to prevent development of resistance. Topical antibiotic use should generally be limited to 3 months. Topical and oral antibiotics should not be used in combination.
- Recommended vehicle type
  - Cream: Dry or sensitive skin, better in cold, dry weather
  - Gel or solution: Oily skin, warmer, humid weather
  - Lotion: Hair bearing areas
- Avoid use of drying agents in combination with keratinolytic agents.
- Oilfree, noncomedogenic sun screens
  - Although UV light results in some improvement in untreated acne, it will react adversely with retinoids and tetracyclines.
- Stress management if acne flares with stress

Diet
- Good nutrition and hydration preferable
- Special diets do not diminish acne.

Activity
Cleansing after sweating

SPECIAL THERAPY
Phototherapy is effective for inflammatory lesions.

Complementary and Alternative Medicine
Zinc gluconate 30 mg/d may reduce inflammatory lesions (1)[B]

 ## MEDICATION (DRUGS)

- Keratinolytic agents (1)[A]
  - Side effects include dryness, erythema, scaling, and photosensitivity, which are dose related. Start with lower strength or frequency and increase as tolerated.
- Tretinoin (Retin-A, Retin A micro, Avita): Apply at bedtime; wash skin and let skin dry 30 minutes before topical application
  - Retin-A Micro and Avita are less irritating, less phototoxicity.
  - May cause an initial flare of lesions, which indicates a good initial response to treatment. May be eased by 14-day course of oral antibiotics
- Adapalene (Differin): Apply topically at night.

  - As effective and better tolerated than tretinoin (1,2)[A]

- Tazarotene (Tazorac): Apply at bedtime.
  - Highly effective
- Azelaic acid (Azelex): 20% topically, b.i.d.
  - Keratinolytic, antibacterial, and antiinflammatory
  - Reduces postinflammatory hyperpigmentation in dark-skinned individuals
  - Side effects: Erythema, dryness, scaling, hypopigmentation
- Salicylic acid: Less effective than tretinoin
- Alpha-hydroxy acids: Available OTC
- Antibiotics and anti-inflammatories (1)[A]
  - Daily to b.i.d. usage
- Topical benzoyl peroxide
  - Bactericidal through direct toxic effect
  - No P. acnes resistance noted
  - Benzoyl peroxide 2.5% as effective as stronger preparations
  - When used with tretinoin, apply benzoyl peroxide in morning and tretinoin at night
  - Side effects: Irritation; may bleach clothes
- Topical antibiotics (1)[A]
  - Erythromycin
  - Clindamycin
  - Metronidazole gel: Apply once daily
  - Azelaic acid (Azelex): 20% cream: Enhanced bactericidal effect and decreased risk of resistant P. acnes when used with zinc and benzoyl peroxide
  - Benzoyl peroxide-erythromycin (Benzamycin): Probably most effective topical antibiotic; especially effective with azelaic acid

  - Benzoyl peroxide-clindamycin (BenzaClin, DUAC, Clindoxyl): Better than either alone (2)[A]

  - Sodium sulfacetamide (Sulfacet-R, Novacet, Klaron): Useful in acne with seborrheic dermatitis or rosacea

- Systemic antibiotics (1)[A]

- Tetracycline: 500–2,000 mg/d, given b.i.d.–q.i.d.; begin at high dose, then taper in 4–6 months if good response; side effects include photosensitivity and esophagitis
  - Avoid use with antacids, iron
- Minocycline 50–200 mg/d, q.i.d.–b.i.d.; side effects include photosensitivity, urticaria, gray-blue skin color, vertigo, autoimmune hepatitis, pseudotumor cerebri, and lupus-like syndrome
- Doxycycline 50–200 mg/d, given b.i.d.–q.i.d.; side effects include photosensitivity
- Erythromycin: 500–1,000 mg/d; given b.i.d.–q.i.d.; decreasing effectiveness as a result of increasing P. acnes resistance
- Trimethoprim-sulfamethoxazole (Bactrim DS)

- Isotretinoin (Accutane) (1)[A]: 0.5–1.0 mg/kg/d b.i.d. PO; 60–90% cure rate; usually given for 12–20 weeks, 20% of patients relapse and require retreatment.
  - Side effects: Cheilitis, arthralgias, tendinitis, hyperlipidemia, pseudotumor cerebri, poor wound healing, highly teratogenic (severe central nervous system and cardiovascular anomalies and facial deformities)
  - Avoid tetracyclines or vitamin A preparations during isotretinoin therapy
  - Monitor for pregnancy, lipids and liver function tests at baseline, and every month.
  - Should be registered member of manufacturer's iPLEDGE program

- Acne hyperpigmented macules
  - Topical hydroquinones (1.5–10%)
  - Azelaic acid (20%) topically
  - Topical retinoids as above
- Other medications for women only

  - Oral contraceptives (1)[A]: More improvement with 35 mcg estradiol than lower dose.

  - Spironolactone (Aldactone); 25–200 mg/d; antiandrogen; reduces sebum production
  - Flutamide (Eulexin) 250–500 mg/d
  - Corticosteroids: Low dose, suppresses adrenal androgens. May be used in males with high-grade acne as well.

SURGERY
- Comedo extraction: Use a comedom extractor after incising the layer of epithelium over comedo
- Incision and drainage may be needed for abscesses
- Injection of large cystic lesions with 0.05–0.3 mL triamcinolone (Kenalog 2–5 mg/mL), use 30-gauge needle to inject and slightly distend cyst
- Acne scar treatment: Dermabrasion, chemical peels, laser resurfacing, grafting, subcutaneous incision, punch excision, punch elevation, tissue augmentation injections

FOLLOW-UP

Issues for Referral
Dermatology consultation recommended for the following: Refractory lesions despite appropriate therapy, consideration of isotretinoin therapy, management of acne scars

PROGNOSIS
Gradual improvement over time (usually within 8–12 weeks after beginning therapy)

COMPLICATIONS
- Acne conglobata: Severe confluent inflammatory acne with systemic symptoms
- Facial and psychological scarring
- Gram-negative folliculitis: Superinfection due to long-term oral antibiotic use, treatment with ampicillin, trimethoprim-sulfa, or isotretinoin

PATIENT MONITORING
- Monthly visits until adequate response
- Pretreatment and monthly lipids, liver function tests, and pregnancy tests when on isotretinoin
- Consider antibiotic resistance (60% overall) or gram-negative folliculitis if treatment fails

REFERENCES
1. Feldman S, Careccia RE, Barham KL, et al. Diagnosis and treatment of acne. *Am Fam Physician*. 2004;69(9):2123–2130.
2. Haider A, Shaw JC. Treatment of acne vulgaris. *JAMA*. 2004;292(6):726–735.
3. Webster G. Mechanism-based treatment of acne vulgaris: the value of combination therapy. *J Drugs and Dermatol*. 2005;4(3):281–288.

MISCELLANEOUS
See also: Acne rosacea

CODES
ICD9-CM
706.1 Other acne

PATIENT TEACHING
- Advise patient that no cure exists for acne; treatment only controls the lesions.
  - Most patients with acne believe it is curable, expect results quickly, and expect treatment to have a completion date.
- There may be a flare period (worsening of acne) during 1st 2 weeks of treatment.
- Any treatment measure takes a minimum of 4 weeks to show results.
- Topical agents can cause redness and drying of the skin.
- Picking at or popping lesions may increase inflammation and scarring.

 See Corresponding Diagnostic Algorithm

 See Patient Handout on CD

ACOUSTIC NEUROMA

Sam Kim, MD, MBBS, MedSc
Phillip Chang, MD

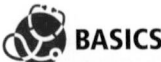 **BASICS**

DESCRIPTION

- Slow-growing benign Schwannoma, most often arising from the vestibular division of 8th cranial nerve
- Originates from Schwann cells of the nerve sheath
- Usually arise in the internal auditory canal near the cerebellopontine angle
- Most are unilateral; bilateral only seen in Neurofibromatos type II

EPIDEMIOLOGY

- 6–10% of all intracranial tumors
- 80–90% of cerebellopontine angle tumors
- 95% of cases are unilateral
- Present most commonly in the 5th–6th decade
- Female predominance
- Bilateral acoustic neuroma occurring in Neurofibromatosis II present before age of 30

Incidence

- 1/100,000 per year
- Asymptomatic lesions may be more common

Prevalence

3,000 diagnosed annually in the US

RISK FACTORS

Unknown

Genetics

- Unknown for unilateral acoustic neuroma
- Neurofibromatosis type II: Bilateral ANs
  - Autosomal domiant
  - Gene located on chromosome 22q1

PATHOPHYSIOLOGY

Exerts pressure on the surrounding structures

- Compression of acoustic and facial nerve when within internal acoustic canal
- Compression of brainstem, 4th ventricle and trigeminal nerve when at the cerebellar pontine angle

ETIOLOGY

Unknown

ASSOCIATED CONDITIONS

- Neurofibromatosis type II
- Pregnancy may accelerate the growth of the tumor

DIAGNOSIS

SIGNS AND SYMPTOMS

- Common
  - Sensorineural hearing loss (unilateral)
  - Tinnitus
  - Balance problems are common, but vertigo is less common.
- Less common
  - Weakness/loss of facial muscle functions
  - Headache with hydrocephalus and increased intracranial pressure
  - Trigeminal nerve involvement when tumor is large and compressing on CN V
  - Ataxia due to cerebellar or brainstem compression from very large tumor

History

- Hearing loss is often progressive
- Loss of speech discrimination

Physical Exam

- Examination with otoscope to exclude other causes of hearing loss (e.g., middle ear effusion, infection, wax, cholesteatoma or tympanic membrane rupture)
- Detailed neurological examination concentrating on the cranial nerves
- Weber and Rinne tests to confirm sensorineural hearing loss
- Evaluation of the contralateral ear in patients <30 years; suspect Neurofibromatosis type II

TESTS

- Pure-tone and speech audiometry (asymmetrical, high-frequency sensorineural hearing loss)
- Speech discrimination
- Stacked auditory brainstem response (ABR): 95% sensitivity and 88% specificity (1). Can detect tumors <1 cm
- Standard ABR: Can only detect tumors >1 cm.

Imaging

- MRI with gadolinium: Gold standard
  - 100% specificity
  - Detects tumors starting at 2 mm
  - Tumor has marked enhancement with Gadolinium
- Noncontrast T2-weighted fast spin-echo MRI:
  - 98% specificity
  - Cheaper than MRI with gadolinium
- CT
  - detect tumors as small as 1 cm
  - Up to 37% false negatives
  - Provides good information of surrounding bony structures of the tumor

Pathological Findings

- Well demarcated and encapsulated mass attached to neural structures without direct invasion
- Can be dense or cystic
- Microscopic: Densely packed spindle cells (Schwann cells) mixed in with myxoid and collagenous matrix
  - Zones of alternatively dense and sparse areas of Antoni A and B

DIFFERENTIAL DIAGNOSIS

- Cerebellopontine lesions
  - Meningioma
  - Glioma
  - Facial nerve Schwannoma
  - Epidermoid
  - Hemangioma
  - Arachnoid cyst
- Sensorineural hearing loss
  - Meniere's disease
  - Ototoxicity
  - Presbycusis
  - Cerebellar pathology

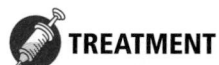 **TREATMENT**

SPECIAL THERAPY
Conservative management:

- Suitable for elderly patients contraindicated to surgery and radiotherapy
- Up to 57% of acoustic neuromas may show no growth (2)[A]
- Average growth rate is 1.9 mm per year (2)[A]
- Up to 20% of patients may eventually fail conservative management.

Radiotherapy
Stereotactic radiosurgery

- Gamma knife stereotactic radiosurgery
  – Performed on an outpatient basis
  – Alternative for those with smaller tumor (<3 cm) or contraindicated to microsurgery
  – Have shown to suppress tumor growth and provide good tumor control (3)[B]
  – Complications include trigeminal and/or facial nerve neuropathy from radiation damage.
- Fractionated stereotactic radiosurgery
  – Conformal radiation delivers a higher dose radiation within the tumor and less damage to surrounding healthy tissue.
  – Requires multiple treatment

 MEDICATION (DRUGS)

Chemotherapy has not yet been explored sufficiently.

SURGERY

- Recommended definitive treatment (A)
- Lowest rate of recurrence, with up to 97.5% complete tumor removal (4)[A]

- Intraoperative facial nerve monitoring is generally used.
- 3 standard approaches
  – Retromastoid/retrosigmoid: For any size
  – Middle cranial fossa: For small tumors with aim of preserving hearing
  – Translabirinthe: For larger tumors. Hearing not preserved. Completely exposes the distal internal auditory canal
- Surgical complications
  – Hearing loss
  – CSF leakage
  – Facial nerve injury
  – Headache
  – Meningitis

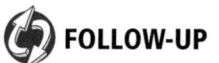 **FOLLOW-UP**

COMPLICATIONS
Due to pressure effect of a large tumor

- Cranial nerve compression
- Hydrocephalus
- Brainstem compression
- Cerebellar tonsil herniation

REFERENCES

1. Don M, et al. The stacked ABR: a sensitive and specific screening tool for detecting small acoustic tumors. *Audiol Neurootol.* 2005;274–290.
2. Smouha EE, et al. Conservative management of acoustic neuroma: A meta-analysis and proposed treatment algorithm. *Laryngoscope.* 2005; 450–454.
3. Lunsford LD, Niranjan A, Flickinger JC, et al. Radiosurgery of vestibular Schwannomas: Summary of experience in 829 cases. *J Neurosurg.* 2005;102 Suppl:195.
4. Kaylie DM, et al. A meta-analysis comparing outcomes of microsurgery and gamma knife radiosurgery. *Laryngoscope.* 2000;1850–1856.

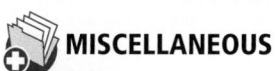 **MISCELLANEOUS**

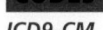 CODES

ICD9-CM
225.1 (M9560/0) Benign neoplasm of cranial nerves

PATIENT TEACHING

 See Corresponding Diagnostic Algorithm

ADDISON DISEASE

Rick Kellerman, MD
Mark Gerstberger, DO

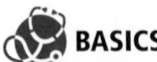 **BASICS**

DESCRIPTION

- Adrenal hypofunction from primary disease (partial or complete T-cell–mediated destruction of adrenal cells) of the adrenal gland with inadequate secretion of glucocorticoids and mineralocorticoids
- An autoimmune process is the most common cause (80% of the cases), followed by tuberculosis; AIDS is becoming a more frequent cause.
- Addison disease (primary adrenocortical insufficiency) is differentiated from secondary (pituitary failure) and tertiary (hypothalamic failure) causes of adrenocortical insufficiency (see Differential Diagnosis). Mineralocorticoid function usually remains intact in secondary and tertiary adrenocorticoid insufficiency
- Addisonian (adrenal) crisis: Acute complication of adrenal insufficiency (circulatory collapse, dehydration, hypotension, nausea, vomiting, hypoglycemia); usually precipitated by an acute physiologic stressor(s) such as surgery, illness, exacerbation of comorbid process, and/or acute withdrawal of long-term corticosteroid therapy
- System(s) Affected: Endocrine/metabolic
- Synonym(s): Adrenocortical insufficiency; Waterhouse-Frederickson syndrome (adrenal crisis); Corticoadrenal insufficiency; Primary adrenocortical insufficiency

Geriatric Considerations
Acute adrenal crisis is more likely in geriatric patients.

Pediatric Considerations
- Hydrocortisone and fludrocortisone doses are lower than adults
- More difficult to diagnose
- Occurs in siblings

GENERAL PREVENTION
- No preventive measures known for Addison disease.
- Prevention of complications
  - Anticipate adrenal crisis and treat before symptoms begin.
  - Elective surgical procedures require upward adjustment in steroid dose.

EPIDEMIOLOGY
- Predominant age: All ages; usually 3rd to fifth decade
- Predominant sex: Females > Males (slight)

Incidence
0.6:100,000

Prevalence
4:100,000

RISK FACTORS
- Family history of autoimmune adrenal insufficiency. ~40% of patients have a 1st- or 2nd-degree relative with associated disorders.
- Chronic steroid use, then experiencing severe infection, trauma, or surgical procedures

Genetics
Familial glucocorticoid insufficiency may have a recessive pattern; adrenomyeloneuropathy is X-linked. Frequent association with other autoimmune disorders. Increased risk with cytotoxic T lymphocyte antigen 4 (CTLA-4)

ETIOLOGY
- Autoimmune adrenal insufficiency (80% of cases in the U.S.)
- Tuberculosis (most common infectious cause worldwide)
- HIV (most common infectious cause in the U.S.)
- Waterhouse-Fredrickson syndrome (disseminated adrenal infection and subsequent infarction; meningococcemia most common; pseudomonas aeruginosa in children; CMV, cryptococcus, MAC in immunosuppressed, AIDS)
- Fungal disease (histoplasmosis, blastomycosis, coccidioidomycosis)
- Bilateral adrenal hemorrhage and infarction (anticoagulants; 50% are in the therapeutic range at the time of the hemorrhage)
- Antiphospholipid syndrome
- Metastatic (lung, breast, kidney, colon, melanoma), lymphoma, Kaposi sarcoma (tumor must destroy 90% of gland to produce hypofunction)
- Drugs (ketoconazole, etomidate)
- Shock
- Surgical adrenalectomy
- Radiation therapy
- Sarcoidosis
- Hemochromatosis
- Amyloidosis
- Adrenoleukodystrophy
- Adrenomyelodystrophy
- Polyglandular autoimmune endocrine syndromes
  - APS I (autoimmune polyglandular syndrome 1): Childhood onset (HLA-DR not associated), single gene mutation in APECED gene (APECED: Autoimmune polyendocrinopathy-candidiasis-ectodermal dystrophy)
  - APS II (autoimmune polyglandular syndrome II): Schmidt syndrome (50% of patients with Addison disease have Schmidt syndrome), adult onset (HLA-DR associated), adrenal failure with type I diabetes mellitus, and/or autoimmune thyroid disease (Hashimoto or Graves)
  - APECED (autoimmune polyendocrinopathy-candidiasis-ectodermal dystrophy): Autosomal recessive, any 2 of chronic mucocutaneous candidiasis, hypothyroidism or Addison disease
  - XPID (X-linked polyendocrinopathy, immune dysfunction, diarrhea): Rare; neonatal death
- Congenital (enzyme defects, hypoplasia, familial glucocorticoid insufficiency)
- Idiopathic

ASSOCIATED CONDITIONS
Diabetes mellitus, Grave disease, Hashimoto thyroiditis, Hypoparathyroidism, Hypercalcemia, Ovarian failure, Pernicious anemia, Myasthenia gravis, Vitiligo, Chronic moniliasis, Sarcoidosis, Sjögren syndrome, Chronic active hepatitis, Schmidt syndrome (multiple endocrine deficiency syndrome), Adrenoleukodystrophy

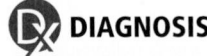 **DIAGNOSIS**

SIGNS AND SYMPTOMS
History
- Weakness, fatigue, tiredness
- Dizziness
- Anorexia, nausea, vomiting
- Abdominal pain
- Chronic diarrhea
- Depression (60–80% of patients)
- Decreased cold tolerance
- Salt craving

Physical Exam
- Weight loss
- Low BP, orthostatic hypotension
- Increased pigmentation (extensor surfaces, hand creases, dental-gingival margins, buccal and vaginal mucosa, lips, areola, pressure points, scars, "tanning," freckles)
- Vitiligo
- Hair loss in females

TESTS
- Basal plasma cortisol and ACTH (low cortisol and high ACTH indicative of Addison disease)
- Rapid ACTH stimulation test: Cosyntropin 0.25 mg IV, measure preinjection and baseline, 30-, and 60-minute postinjection cortisol levels. (Patients with Addison disease have low to normal values that do not rise.)
- Metapyrone test
- Insulin-induced hypoglycemia test
- CRH may help distinguish secondary from tertiary adrenal insufficiency.
- Autoantibody tests: 21-Hydroxylase (most common and specific), 17-hydroxylase, 17-alfa-hydroxylase (may not be associated), and adrenomedullin

Lab
- Low serum sodium
- Elevated serum potassium
- Elevated BUN, creatinine
- Elevated serum calcium
- Hypoglycemia when fasted
- Metabolic acidosis
- Low cortisol level (between 8 and 9 AM)
- Elevated ACTH level
- Moderate neutropenia
- Eosinophilia
- Relative lymphocytosis
- Anemia, normochromic, normocytic
- Adrenal-cortex autoantibody (ACA/21-hydroxylase)
- Low aldosterone levels
- TSH: Repeat when condition has stabilized
  - Thyroid hormone levels may normalize with the treatment of Addison disease.
- Drugs that may alter lab results: Digitalis.
- Disorders that may alter lab results: Diabetes mellitus

Imaging
- Abdominal CT scan
  - Small adrenal glands in autoimmune adrenalitis
  - Enlarged adrenal glands in infiltrative and hemorrhagic disorders
- Abdominal radiograph may show adrenal calcifications.
- CXR may show small heart size, and/or calcification of cartilage.

Diagnostic Procedures/Surgery
CT guided fine-needle biopsy of adrenal masses may be helpful.

Pathological Findings
- Atrophic adrenals in autoimmune adrenalitis
- Infiltrative and hemorrhagic disorders produce enlargement with destruction of the entire gland.

DIFFERENTIAL DIAGNOSIS
- Secondary adrenocortical insufficiency (pituitary failure)
  - Withdrawal of long-term corticosteroid use: Adrenal insufficiency from hypothalamic-pituitary axis depression from long-term corticosteroid use is much more common than Addison disease.
  - Sheehan syndrome (postpartum necrosis of pituitary)
  - Empty sella syndrome
  - Surgical excision of pituitary
  - Radiation to pituitary
  - Pituitary adenomas, carcinomas (rare), craniopharyngiomas
  - Infiltrative disorders of pituitary (sarcoidosis, hemochromatosis, amyloidosis, histiocytosis X)
  - Megestrol
- Tertiary adrenocortical insufficiency (hypothalamic failure)
  - Pituitary stalk transection
  - Trauma
  - Disruption of production of corticotropic releasing factor (CRF)
  - Hypothalamic tumors
- Myopathies
- Secretion of inappropriate antidiuretic hormone (SIADH)
- Heavy metal ingestion
- Severe nutritional deficiencies
- Sprue syndrome
- Hyperparathyroidism
- Neurofibromatosis
- Peutz-Jeghers syndrome
- Porphyria cutanea tarda
- Salt-losing nephritis
- Bronchogenic carcinoma
- Anorexia nervosa
- Other causes of hypoglycemia
- Depression

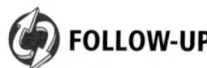 **TREATMENT**

INITIAL STABILIZATION
- Outpatient
- Inpatient during adrenal crisis

GENERAL MEASURES
- Treatment for adrenal insufficiency is with glucocorticoid and mineralocorticoid replacement.
  - The 5 S's of management of adrenal crisis: Salt, sugar, steroids, support, and search for a precipitating illness—usually infection, trauma, recent surgery, or not taking prescribed replacement therapy.
- Appropriate treatment for underlying cause

Diet
Diet to maintains water, sodium, and potassium balances.

Activity
As tolerated

 MEDICATION (DRUGS)

First Line
- Chronic adrenal insufficiency
  - Hydrocortisone 15–20 mg PO each morning on rising, and 10 mg at 4–5 PM each afternoon is the usual dosage (dosage may vary and is usually less in children's).
  - Fludrocortisone 0.05–0.2 mg PO once daily plus
  - Dehydroepiandrosterone 25–50 mg PO once daily (monitor lipid profile, breast or prostate cancer)
  - May require salt supplementation
- Acute adrenal insufficiency
  - Hydrocortisone 100 mg IV followed by 10 mg/h infusion
  - IV glucose, saline, and plasma expanders
  - Fludrocortisone 0.05 mg/d
- Acute illnesses (fever, stress, minor trauma):
  - Double the patient's usual steroid dose; taper the dose gradually over a week or more, and monitor VS and serum sodium.
- Supplement for surgical procedures: Administer 25–150 mg hydrocortisone or 5–30 mg methylprednisolone IV on the day of the procedure in addition to maintenance therapy. Taper gradually to the usual dose over 1–2 days.
- Precautions
  - Patients with hepatic disease may need a reduced dose of steroids.
  - Excessive corticosteroid doses or excessive duration of supplemental treatment of those who are acutely ill or undergoing surgery may increase the mortality rate.
  - Rifampin, phenytoin, and barbiturates may precipitate adrenal insufficiency in Addisonian patients by inducing steroid-metabolizing liver enzymes.
  - Patients on these drugs may require higher doses of corticosteroid due to increased steroid metabolism.
  - Refer to manufacturer's literature for other precautions
  - Significant possible interactions: Refer to manufacturer's literature

Second Line
Prednisone 5 mg in the morning and 2.5 mg at night plus fludrocortisone, and DHEA; dexamethasone 0.5 mg in the morning plus fludrocortisone plus DHEA

ALERT
Geriatric Considerations
Elderly should have a slightly reduced dose.

 FOLLOW-UP

PROGNOSIS
- Requires lifetime treatment
- Good outlook with appropriate treatment
- With adequate replacement therapy, life expectancy approximates normal.
- Without treatment, the disease is 100% lethal.

COMPLICATIONS
- Hyperpyrexia
- Psychotic reactions
- Complications from underlying disease
- Oversteroid or understeroid treatment
- Hyperkalemic paralysis (rare)
- Addisonian crisis

PATIENT MONITORING
- Verify adequacy of therapy: Normal BP, serum electrolytes normal, normal plasma renin, improvement of appetite and strength, increase in heart size to normal, and normal fasting blood glucose level
- Lifelong medical supervision for signs of adequate therapy and avoidance of overdose

REFERENCES
1. http://www.utdol.com/utd/content/topic.do?topicKey= adrenal/abstract.do?topicKey=adrenal/4314&refNum=12
2. King MS. Adrenal insufficiency: An uncommon cause of fatigue. *J Am Board Fam Pract*. 1999;12:386–390. (C)
3. Arlt W, Callies F, van Vlijmen JC, et al. Dehydroepiandrosterone replacement in women with adrenal insufficiency [see comments]. *N Engl J Med*. 1999;341:1013–1020. (A)

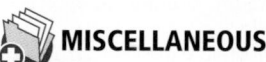 **MISCELLANEOUS**

CODES

ICD9-CM
255.4 Corticoadrenal insufficiency

PATIENT TEACHING
- For patient education materials, contact: National Adrenal Disease Foundation, 505 Northern Blvd., Suite 200, Great Neck, NY 11021, (516) 487-4992. (http://www.medhelp.org/nadf)
- Patient should wear or carry medical identification with information about the disease and the need for hydrocortisone or other replacement therapy.
- Instruct patient in self-administering of parenteral hydrocortisone for emergency situations (e.g., traveling in remote areas away from medical help)

See Corresponding Diagnostic Algorithm

ADENOVIRUS INFECTIONS

Ronald L. Malm, DO

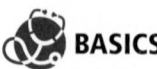BASICS

DESCRIPTION

Usually self-limited febrile illnesses characterized by inflammation of conjunctivae and the respiratory tract. Adenovirus infections occur in epidemic and endemic situations.

- Common types
  - Acute febrile respiratory illness, affecting primarily children
  - Acute respiratory disease, affecting adults
  - Viral pneumonia, affecting children and adults
  - Acute pharyngoconjunctival fever, affecting children, particularly after summer swimming
  - Acute follicular conjunctivitis, affecting all ages
  - Epidemic keratoconjunctivitis, affecting adults
  - Intestinal infections leading to enteritis, mesenteric adenitis, and intussusception
- Conjunctivitis, sometimes called *pink eye*
- System(s) Affected: Cardiovascular; Gastrointestinal; Hemic/Lymphatic/Immunologic; Musculoskeletal; Nervous; Pulmonary; Renal/Urologic

ALERT

Geriatric Considerations
Complications more likely

Pediatric Considerations
Viral pneumonia in infants may be fatal.

GENERAL PREVENTION

- Live types 4 and 7 adenovirus vaccine orally in enteric-coated capsules reduces incidence of acute respiratory disease.
- Frequent hand washing among office personnel and family members

EPIDEMIOLOGY

- Predominant age: All ages
- Predominant sex: Male = Female

Incidence

- Very common infection, estimated at 2–5% of all respiratory infections
- More common in infants and children

RISK FACTORS

- Large number of people gathered in a small area (e.g., military recruits, college students at the beginning of the school year, day care centers, community swimming pools, etc.)
- Immunocompromised at risk for severe disease

ETIOLOGY

- Adenovirus (DNA viruses 60–90 nm in size with 47 known serotypes; three types cause gastroenteritis); difficult to eliminate from skin and environmental surfaces
- Different serotypes have different epidemiologies.
- Most common known pathogens
  - Types 1, 2, 3, 5, and 7 cause respiratory illness.
  - Type 3 causes pharyngoconjunctival fever.
  - Types 4, 7, and 21 cause acute respiratory disease.
  - Several other types may cause epidemic keratoconjunctivitis.

ASSOCIATED CONDITIONS

- Hemorrhagic cystitis (can be caused by adenovirus)
- Viral enteritis
- Intussusception and mesenteric adenitis

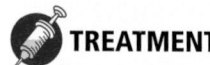DIAGNOSIS

SIGNS AND SYMPTOMS

History
Depends on type (see "Differential Diagnosis"). Common signs and symptoms with most respiratory forms

- Headache
- Malaise
- Sore throat
- Cough
- Fever (moderate to high)
- Vomiting
- Diarrhea

Physical Exam
- Mucosa exhibits patches of white exudates
- Cervical adenitis

TESTS
Cultures and serologic studies, if appropriate

Lab
- Viral cultures from respiratory, ocular, or fecal sources can establish diagnosis:
  - Pharyngeal isolate suggests recent infection.
- Antigen detection in stool for enteric serotypes is available.
- Serologic procedures such as complement fixation with a fourfold rise in serum antibody titer identify recent adenoviral infection.

Imaging
Radiographs: Bronchopneumonia in severe respiratory infections

Diagnostic Procedures/Surgery
Biopsy (lung or other) may be needed in severe or unusual cases

Pathological Findings
- Varies with each virus:
  - Severe pneumonia may be reflected by extensive intranuclear inclusions.
- Bronchiolitis obliterans may occur.

DIFFERENTIAL DIAGNOSIS
Early diagnosis depends on clinical evaluation. The following are the primary characteristics of the major adenovirus infections:

- Acute febrile respiratory illness
  - Nonspecific coldlike symptoms, similar to other viral respiratory illnesses (e.g., fever, pharyngitis, tracheitis, bronchitis, pneumonitis)
  - Mostly in children
  - Incubation period 2–5 days
  - May be pertussislike syndrome (rarely)
- Acute respiratory disease
  - Malaise, fever, chills, headache, pharyngitis, hoarseness, dry cough
  - Fever lasts 2–4 days
  - Illness subsides in 10–14 days
- Viral pneumonia
  - Sudden onset of high fever, rapid infection of upper and lower respiratory tracts, skin rash, diarrhea
  - Occurs in children aged a few days up to 3 years
  - Common; severe illness occurs in subset
- Acute pharyngoconjunctival fever
  - Spiking fever lasting several days, headache, pharyngitis, conjunctivitis, rhinitis, cervical adenitis
  - Conjunctivitis, usually unilateral
  - Subsides in 1 week
- Epidemic keratoconjunctivitis
  - Usually unilateral onset of ocular redness and edema, periorbital edema, periorbital swelling, local discomfort suggestive of foreign body
  - Lasts 3–4 weeks

TREATMENT

GENERAL MEASURES
- Treatment is supportive and symptomatic.
- Infections are usually benign and of short duration.

Diet
No special diet

Activity
Rest during febrile phases

SPECIAL THERAPY

Complementary and Alternative Medicine

Echinacea has not been shown to be better than placebo for treatment of viral upper respiratory infections. [A]

MEDICATION (DRUGS)

- Acetaminophen, 10–15 mg/kg/dose PO, for analgesia (avoid aspirin)
- Topical corticosteroids for conjunctivitis (after consulting an ophthalmologist)
- Cough suppressants and/or expectorants
- Antihistamine/decongestant combos may decrease cough. [B]

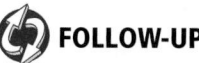 **FOLLOW-UP**

DISPOSITION
Admission Criteria
Severely ill infants or those with epidemic keratoconjunctivitis or infants with severe pneumonia

- Contact and droplet precautions during a hospitalization are indicated.

PROGNOSIS
- Self-limited, usually without sequelae
- Severe illness and death in very young and in immunocompromised hosts

COMPLICATIONS
Few if any recognizable long-term problems

PATIENT MONITORING
For severe infantile pneumonia and conjunctivitis, daily physical exam until well

REFERENCES

1. Barrett BP, Brown RL, Locken K, Maberry R, Bobula JA, D'Alessio D. Treatment of the common cold with unrefined echinacea. A randomized, double-blind, placebo-controlled trial. *Ann Intern Med.* 2002;137(12):939–946.
2. Pratter MR. Cough and the Common Cold, ACCP Evidence-Based Clinical Practice Guidelines *Chest.* 2006;129:72S–74S
3. Fahey T, Smucny J, Becker L, Glazier R. Antibiotics for acute bronchitis. *The Cochrane Database of Systematic Reviews* 2004, Issue 4. Art. No.: CD000245. DOI: 10.1002/14651858. CD000245.pub2.
4. Morris P, Leach A. Antibiotics for persistent nasal discharge (rhinosinusitis) in children. *The Cochrane Database of Systematic Reviews* 2002, Issue 4. Art. No.: CD001094. DOI: 10.1002/14651858. CD001094.
5. Spurling GKP, Del Mar CB, Dooley L, Foxlee R. Delayed antibiotics for symptoms and complications of respiratory infections. *The Cochrane Database of Systematic Reviews* 2004, Issue 4. Art. No.: CD004417. DOI: 10.1002/14651858.CD004417.pub2.

 MISCELLANEOUS

See also: Conjunctivitis; Intussusception; Pneumonia; Viral

CODES

ICD9-CM
- 079.0 Adenovirus
- 462 Acute pharyngitis
- 480.0 Pneumonia due to adenovirus

PATIENT TEACHING
- Avoid aspirin in children.
- Give instructions for nasal spray, cough preparations, frequent hand washing.

ALCOHOL USE DISORDERS

Geninne Zinner, RNCS, ANP

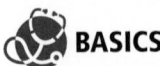 **BASICS**

DESCRIPTION

- Any pattern of alcohol use causing significant physical, mental, or social dysfunction; key features are tolerance, withdrawal, and persistent use despite problems.
- Alcohol abuse: Maladaptive pattern of alcohol use manifested by 1 (or more) of
  – Failure to fulfill obligations at work, school, or home
  – Recurrent use in hazardous situations
  – Recurrent alcohol-related legal problems
  – Continued use despite related social or interpersonal problems
- Alcohol dependence: Maladaptive pattern of use manifested by 3 (or more) of the following
  – Tolerance
  – Withdrawal
  – Using more than intended
  – Persistent desire or attempts to cut down/stop
  – Significant amount of time obtaining, using, or recovering from alcohol
  – Social, occupational, or recreational activities sacrificed for alcohol use
  – Continued use despite physical or psychological problems
- National Institute on Alcohol Abuse and Alcoholism (NIAAA) criteria for "at risk" drinking: Men >14 drinks a week, or >4 per occasion. Women: >7 drinks a week, or >3 per occasion.
- System(s) Affected: Nervous; Gastrointestinal
- Synonym(s): Alcoholism; Alcohol abuse; Alcohol dependence

ALERT

Geriatric Considerations
- Common in elderly; less likely to report problem. May exacerbate normal age-related cognitive deficits and disabilities.
- Multiple drug interactions
- Signs and symptoms may be different or attributed to chronic medical problem or dementia.
- Assessment tools may be inappropriate.

Pediatric Considerations
- Children of alcoholics at high risk
- In 2004, 28% of persons 12–20 years reported use in past month, 1 in 5 binge drink; binge drinkers are 7× more likely to report illicit drug use.
- Negative effect on maturation and development
- Early drinkers are 4 times more likely to develop a problem than those who begin >21.
- Depression, suicidal or disorderly behavior, family disruption, violence or destruction of property, poor school or work performance, sexual promiscuity, social immaturity, lack of interests, isolation, moodiness

Pregnancy Considerations
- Alcohol is teratogenic, especially during the 1st trimester; women should abstain during conception.
- 10–50% of children born to women who are heavy drinkers will have fetal alcohol syndrome.
- Women experience harmful effects at lower levels, and are less likely to report problems.

GENERAL PREVENTION
Counsel with family history and risk factors.

EPIDEMIOLOGY
- Predominant age: 18–25, but all ages affected
- Predominant sex: Male > Female (3:1)

Prevalence
- Lifetime prevalence: 13.6%
- 20% in primary care setting
- 48.2% of 21-year-olds in the US reported binge drinking in 2004.

RISK FACTORS
Family history, depression (40% with comorbid alcohol abuse), anxiety, other substance abuse, tobacco, male gender, low socioeconomic status, unemployment, peer/social approval, family dysfunction or trauma, PTSD, antisocial personality disorder, bipolar disorder, eating disorders, criminal involvement

Genetics
50–60% of risk is genetic.

PATHOPHYSIOLOGY
- Alcohol is a central nervous system depressant by facilitating γ-aminobutyric acid (GABA) inhibition and blocking N-methyl-D-aspartate receptors.
- Once tolerance has occurred, abrupt withdrawal results in hyperexcitability of these pathways.

ETIOLOGY
Multifactorial: Genetic, environment, psychosocial

ASSOCIATED CONDITIONS
- Cardiomyopathy
- Atrial fibrillation
- Hypertension
- PUD/gastritis
- Cirrhosis
- Fatty liver
- Cholelithiasis
- Hepatitis
- Diabetes mellitus
- Pancreatitis
- Malnutrition
- Upper GI malignancies
- Peripheral neuropathy
- Seizures
- Abuse
- Violence
- Trauma (falls, MVAs)

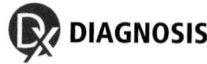 **DIAGNOSIS**

PRE HOSPITAL

Signs and Symptoms

- Behavioral
  - Anxiety, depression, insomnia;
  - Visual, auditory, tactile hallucinations 12–72 hours after last drink
  - Psychological and social dysfunction marital problems
  - Social isolation/withdrawal
  - Domestic violence
  - Alcohol-related legal problems
  - Repeated attempts to stop/reduce
  - Loss of interest in nondrinking activities
  - Employment problems (tardiness, absenteeism, decreased productivity, interpersonal problems, frequent job loss)
  - Blackouts
  - Complaints about alcohol-related behavior
  - Frequent trauma, MVAs, ED visits.
- Physical
  - Anorexia
  - Nausea, vomiting
  - Abdominal pain
  - Palpitations
  - Headache
  - Impotence
  - Menstrual irregularities
  - Infertility

Physical Exam

- General: Fever, agitation, diaphoresis
- HEENT: Plethoric, rhinophyma, poor oral hygiene, oropharyngeal malignancies
- Cardiovascular: Hypertension, dilated cardiomyopathy, tachycardia
- Respiratory: Aspiration pneumonia
- Gastrointestinal: Stigmata of chronic liver disease, peptic ulcer disease, pancreatitis, esophageal malignancies, varices
- Genitourinary: Testicular atrophy
- Musculoskeletal: Unhealed fractures, myopathy, osteopenia, bone marrow suppression
- Neurologic: Tremors, cognitive deficits (e.g., memory impairment), peripheral neuropathy, Wernicke-Korsakoff syndrome, grand mal seizures 2–48 hours after last drink, delirium tremens (DTs) begin 48–72 hours after last drink
- Endocrine/metabolic: Hyperlipidemias, cushingoid appearance, gynecomastia
- Dermatologic: Burns (e.g., cigarettes), bruises, poor hygiene, palmar erythema, spider telangiectasias, caput medusa, jaundice
- Physical exam may be completely normal
- Withdrawal symptoms begin 4–12 hours after alcohol is stopped/reduced; peak in intensity on day 2 of abstinence; and are mostly resolved by 4th or 5th day

TESTS

- CAGE Questionnaire: (Cut down, Annoyed, Guilty, and Eye opener): More than 2 "yes" answers is 74–89% sensitive, 79–95% specific for alcohol use disorder; less sensitive for early problem drinking, or heavy drinking (1)[A]
- Alcohol Use Disorders Identification Test: 10 items, if >4: 70–92% sensitive (1)[A]
- "Had 5 or more drinks on any 1 occasion in last 3 months" sensitive screen for problem drinking

Lab

- Blood alcohol concentration
  - >100 mg/dL in outpatient setting
  - >150 mg/dL without obvious signs of intoxication
  - >300 mg/dL at any time
- Levels suggestive if increased
  - AST/ALT ratio >2.0
  - γ-Glutamyl transferase (GGT)
  - Mean corpuscular volume
  - Prothrombin time
  - Uric acid
  - Triglycerides
  - Cholesterol (total)
- Often decreased
  - Calcium, magnesium, potassium, phosphorus
  - Blood urea nitrogen (BUN)
  - Hemoglobin, hematocrit
  - Platelet count
  - Serum protein, albumin

Imaging

- Radiograph: Multiple old rib fractures
- CT scan, MRI of brain: Cortical atrophy, lesions in thalamic nucleus and basal forebrain

Pathological Findings

- Liver: Inflammation or fatty infiltration (alcoholic hepatitis), periportal fibrosis (alcoholic cirrhosis occurs in only 10–20% of alcoholics)
- Gastric mucosa: Inflammation, ulceration
- Pancreas: Inflammation, liquefaction necrosis
- Heart: Dilated cardiomyopathy
- Immune system: Decreased granulocytes
- Endocrine organs: Elevated cortisol levels, testicular atrophy, decreased female hormones
- Brain: Cortical atrophy, enlarged ventricles

DIFFERENTIAL DIAGNOSIS

- Other substance use disorders
- Depression
- Dementia
- Cerebellar ataxia
- CVA
- Benign essential tremor
- Seizure disorder
- Hypoglycemia
- Diabetic ketoacidosis
- Viral hepatitis

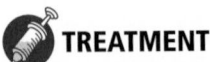

TREATMENT

PRE HOSPITAL
- Assess medical and psychiatric condition.
- Assess severity of withdrawal.

INITIAL STABILIZATION
- Airways, breathing, circulation
- Short-acting benzodiazepine for seizure
- Correct electrolyte imbalances, acidosis

GENERAL MEASURES
- Brief interventions by primary care physicians are highly effective for problem drinking (1)[A].
- Involve family, if feasible.
- Treat comorbid problems (sleep, anxiety, etc.); use caution if prescribing medications with cross-tolerance to alcohol (benzodiazepine).

Activity
Fall preventions or restrictions if delirious

Nursing
- Frequent vital signs during acute withdrawal
- Clinical Institute Withdrawal Assessment Scale for Alcohol (CIWA-Ar) very helpful (2,3)[A].

IV Fluids
Maintain fluids during withdrawal.

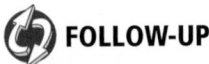

MEDICATION (DRUGS)

First Line
- Symptom-triggered regimens (benzodiazepine given only when CIWA-Ar score > 8) result in less total medication given and shorter duration of treatment than fixed-dose regimens (2,3)[A].
- In fixed-dose regimens, 1st dose of benzodiazepine should achieve sedation without respiratory compromise; drugs then are tapered daily as long as withdrawal symptoms are stable; CIWA-Ar is often used to guide dosing.
- Benzodiazepines reduce incidence of DTs and seizures (2,3)[A].
  - Chlordiazepoxide 50–100 mg PO/IM q6–8h, then taper (2–4)[A]
  - Diazepam 5–20 mg q6–8h (2–4)[A]
  - Lorazepam 1–4 mg q2–6h (2,3)[A]; in elderly, severe liver disease, or IV drip
  - Phenobarbital 60–120 mg q6–8h (4)[B] may be safer during pregnancy.
  - Carbamazepine 200 mg PO q.i.d., then taper over 5–7 days (efficacious for mild-moderate withdrawal, and is less sedating) (2)[A].
- Adjuncts to detoxification
  - β-Blockers for tachycardia or comorbid coronary artery disease (3)[B]
  - Clonidine 0.1–0.2 mg PO t.i.d. for autonomic hyperactivity (3,4)[C]
  - Antipsychotics for psychosis, agitation; haloperidol lowers seizure threshold (3)[C]
- Adjuncts to rehabilitation
  - Naltrexone 50–100 mg PO daily, or 380 mg IM once every 4 weeks: Opiate antagonist reduces craving and chance relapse (5)[A].
  - Acamprosate (Campral) 666 mg PO t.i.d. beginning after completion of withdrawal; reduces relapse of drinking (5)[A]
  - Topiramate (Topamax) 25–300 mg PO daily or divided b.i.d.; enhances abstinence (3)[B]
- Supplements to all
  - Thiamine 100 mg daily (1st dose IV prior to glucose to avoid Wernicke encephalopathy)
  - Folic acid 1 mg daily
  - Multivitamin daily
  - Magnesium sulfate 1 g IM/IV q4–6h (if history of DTs or seizure) (2)[C]
- Contraindications
  - Naltrexone: Pregnancy, hepatitis, hepatic failure. Monitor liver function tests.
- Precautions: Organic pain, organic brain syndromes
- Significant possible interactions: Alcohol, sedatives, hypnotics

Second Line
- Anticonvulsants gabapentin (Neurontin) and vigabatrin (Sabril) studied for detoxification (3)[B]
- Disulfiram 250–500 mg PO daily: Unproven efficacy; may provide psychologic deterrent
- Selective serotonin reuptake inhibitors (SSRIs) may be beneficial if comorbid depression exists.

FOLLOW-UP

DISPOSITION

Admission Criteria
Severe withdrawal symptoms (CIWA-Ar >14), prior DTs, withdrawal seizures, suicidal ideation or psychiatric symptoms, obstacles to follow-up, pregnancy, unstable living situation

Issues for Referral
Addiction specialist: 12-step or long-term program

PROGNOSIS
- Chronic relapsing disease; mortality rate > twice general population, death 10–15 years earlier
- Abstinence benefits survival, mental health, family, employment
- 12-step programs, cognitive-behavior and motivational therapies are effective during 1st year following treatment (1)[B].

COMPLICATIONS
- Cirrhosis
- GI malignancies
- Neuropathy
- Dementia
- Wernicke-Korsakoff syndrome
- CVA
- Ketoacidosis
- Infection
- Relapse
- Depression
- Suicide
- Trauma

PATIENT MONITORING
- Outpatient detoxification: Daily visits
- Early outpatient rehabilitation: Weekly visits
- Detoxification alone is not sufficient.

REFERENCES

1. Enoch MA, Goldman D. Problem drinking and alcoholism: Diagnosis and treatment. *Amer Fam Phys*. 2002;65:441–448.

2. Asplund CA, Aaronson JW, Aaronson HE. Three regimens for alcohol withdrawal and detoxification. *J Fam Pract*. 2004;53:545–554.

3. Bayard M, McIntyre J, Hill KR, et al. Alcohol withdrawal syndrome. *Amer Fam Phys*. 2004; 69(pt 6):1443–1450.

4. Kosten TR, O'Connor PG. Management of drug and alcohol withdrawal. *N Engl J Med*. 2003;348: 1786–1795.

5. Saitz R. Clinical practice. Unhealthy alcohol use. *N Engl J Med*. 2005;352–396.

6. Williams SH. Medications for treating alcohol dependence. *Amer Fam Phys*. 2005;72(pt 9): 1775–1780.

ADDITIONAL READING

• Substance Abuse and Mental Health Services Administration. (NSDUH series H-27, DHHS Publication No. SMA 05-4061). 2005. (http://oas.samhsa.gov/prevalence.htm)

• National Institute on Alcohol Abuse and Alcoholism: (NIH Publication No. 00-1583). 2000. (http://pubs. niaaa.nih.gov/publications/10report/intro.pdf)

• National Council on Alcoholism and Drug Dependence. NCADD Fact Sheet. Available online: ncadd.org/pubs/fsproblems.html

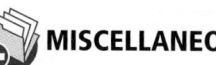 **MISCELLANEOUS**

See also: Substance use disorders

CODES

ICD9-CM

• 291.81 Alcohol withdrawal
• 303.00 Acute alcoholic intoxication, unspecified
• 303.90 Other and unspecified alcohol dependence, unspecified
• 305.00 Alcohol abuse, unspecified

PATIENT TEACHING

• American Council on Alcoholism: (800) 527-5344 or www.aca-usa.org (treatment facility locator, educational information)
• National Clearinghouse for Alcohol and Drug Information: (800) 729-6686 or www.health.org
• Center for Substance Abuse Treatment: (800) 662-HELP or www.csat.samhsa.gov (treatment facility locator)
• Alcoholics Anonymous: www.aa.org
• Rational Recovery: www.rational.org
• Secular Organizations for Sobriety: www.secularsobriety.org

 See Corresponding Diagnostic Algorithm

 See Patient Handout on CD

ALDOSTERONISM, PRIMARY

Mark C. Horattas, MD, FACS

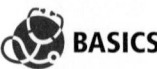 **BASICS**

DESCRIPTION
- The clinical syndrome of excess secretion of aldosterone is classically manifested by hypertension, hypokalemia, and depressed plasma renin activity (patients often present as normokalemic).
- Unilateral aldosterone-producing adenoma (APA): Cured with unilateral adrenalectomy
- Idiopathic hyperaldosteronism (IHA) due to bilateral adrenal hyperplasia: Not cured with surgery, medical management
- System(s) Affected: Endocrine/metabolic
- Synonym(s): Conn syndrome; Aldosteronoma; Hyperaldosteronism

ALERT
Pregnancy Considerations
Can be associated with toxemia during pregnancy or persistent hypertension following delivery. Treat hypertension with agents proven to be safe during pregnancy; avoid spironolactone and ACE inhibitors.

EPIDEMIOLOGY
Incidence
Involves 1% of the hypertensive population

Prevalence
- Usually diagnosed during 4th to 6th decades
- More common in women

RISK FACTORS
Genetics
Can be associated rarely with familial multiple endocrine neoplasia (MEN) syndromes.

ETIOLOGY
- Unilateral aldosterone-producing adenoma (APA)
- Idiopathic hyperaldosteronism (IHA)
- Other rare subtypes

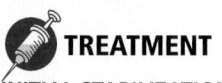 **DIAGNOSIS (2)[A]**

SIGNS AND SYMPTOMS
Physical Exam
- Usually asymptomatic
- Most patients are normokalemic.
- Marked hypokalemia may be associated with muscle weakness and cramping, intermittent paralysis, headaches, palpitations, polydipsia, polyuria, or nocturia.
- Mild to severe hypertension, one of the causes for secondary hypertension
- Funduscopy: Benign or grade 1–2
- Edema (rare)
- Hypokalemia (not required)
- Metabolic alkalosis
- Relative "hypernatremia"
- Impaired glucose tolerance

TESTS
- Screen for primary aldosteronism
  - Patients with hypertension and spontaneous hypokalemia
  - Patients with treatment-resistant hypertension
- Plasma aldosterone levels, plasma renin activity
- Special tests
  - Aldosterone suppression test with either a high salt diet or saline infusion
  - Spironolactone treatment trial

Lab
- Hypokalemia with inappropriate kaliuresis
- Insuppressible urine or plasma aldosterone levels
- Low ambulatory plasma renin activity
- High plasma aldosterone to renin ratio (>20 in ng/dL [>55 nmol/L] and ng/mL/h, respectively)
- Normal glucocorticoid excretion
- Drugs that may alter lab results: Diuretics, ACE inhibitors, spironolactone
- Disorders that may alter lab results: Malignant hypertension

Imaging
- Adrenal CT (preferred over MRI) with fine cuts
- Iodocholesterol (NP-59) scan with dexamethasone suppression
- Adrenal vein sampling (3)[A]

Diagnostic Procedures/Surgery (4)[A]
- Laparoscopic adrenalectomy if localized on CT scan
- Adrenal venous sampling for lateralization preoperatively if not localized by CT scan.

Pathological Findings
- Aldosteronoma usually a benign solitary adenoma.
- Idiopathic hyperaldosteronism (IHA) due to bilateral adrenal (zona glomerulosa) hyperplasia
- Aldosterone-producing adrenocortical carcinoma rarely

DIFFERENTIAL DIAGNOSIS
- Diuretic use
- Renovascular hypertension
- Pheochromocytoma
- Renin-secreting tumor
- Malignant hypertension
- Congenital adrenal hyperplasia
- Deoxycorticosterone-producing tumor
- Exogenous mineralocorticoid
- High-dose glucocorticoid therapy
- Apparent mineralocorticoid excess syndrome (congenital or acquired due to licorice ingestion)
- Liddle syndrome

TREATMENT

INITIAL STABILIZATION
- Appropriate health care
  - Unilateral APA: Unilateral adrenalectomy
  - Bilateral IHA: Chronic medical therapy
- Unilateral APA: Correct hypokalemia preoperatively with spironolactone
- Bilateral IHA: Low-sodium diet, regular isotonic exercise, maintenance of ideal body weight, tobacco avoidance, mineralocorticoid receptor antagonist, antihypertensive agent (e.g., calcium channel antagonist, ACE-inhibitor, low-dose thiazide diuretic)

Diet
Low sodium

MEDICATION (DRUGS)

- Potassium-sparing agent: Spironolactone (Aldactone) or amiloride (Midamor)
- Antihypertensive agent: Calcium channel antagonist, ACE inhibitor, angiotensin-II receptor antagonist, or low-dose thiazide diuretic
- Contraindications: Potassium-sparing agent and ACE inhibitors in renal failure, hyperkalemia, and pregnancy
- Precautions: Monitor serum potassium closely after any adjustment in potassium replacement or potassium-sparing agent.
- Significant possible interactions: Lithium and diuretics, NSAIDs with diuretics, and ACE inhibitors

SURGERY

The treatment of choice for patients with unilateral APA is adrenalectomy. Patients with bilateral IHA are treated medically.

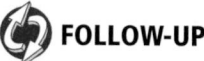 **FOLLOW-UP**

PROGNOSIS

- Surgical removal of an APA results in a cure of hypertension in ~30–60% of the cases.
- Hypertension does not resolve immediately postoperatively, but rather over 1–4 months.

COMPLICATIONS

Cardiac arrhythmia associated with severe hypokalemia

PATIENT MONITORING

- BP checks
- Serum potassium check
- 24-hour urine aldosterone following surgery

REFERENCES

1. Clark OH, Duh QY. *Textbook of Endocrine Surgery*. Philadelphia; WB Saunders, 2005.
2. Mulatero P, Stowasser M, Loh KC, et al. Increased diagnosis of primary aldosteronism, including surgically correctable forms, in centers from five continents. *J Clin Endocrinol Metab*. 2004;89:045 [PMID 15001583].
3. Young WF, Stanson AW, Thompson GB, et al. Role for adrenal venous sampling in primary aldosteronism. *Surgery*. 2004;136:1227 [PMID 15657580].
4. Mansmann G, Lau J, Balk E, et al. The clinically inapparent adrenal mass: update in diagnosis and management. *Endocr Rev*. 2004;25:309.

 MISCELLANEOUS

See also: Hypertension, essential, Hypokalemia

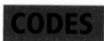 **CODES**

ICD9-CM
255 Primary aldosteronism

PATIENT TEACHING

 See Corresponding Diagnostic Algorithm

ALOPECIA

Aubrey L. Knight, MD

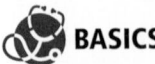 **BASICS**

DESCRIPTION

- Absence of the hair from skin areas where it normally is present. *Anagen* hairs are growing hairs. *Telogen* hairs are dead "resting" hairs.
- Telogen effluvium: Diffuse hair loss that (usually) results in temporarily decreased hair density but does not progress to complete baldness.
- Anagen effluvium: Diffuse shedding of hairs, including growing hairs, that may progress to complete baldness.
- Cicatricial alopecia: Also known as scarring alopecia; characterized by slick, smooth scalp without any evidence of follicular openings of hair.
- Androgenic alopecia: Hair loss occurring in either sex, caused by stimulation of the hair roots by male hormones, more common after age 50.
- Alopecia areata: Patchy, nonscarring hair loss.
- Traction alopecia: Patchy, initially nonscarring hair loss due to pulling on the hair.
- Tinea capitis: Patches of hair broken off close to the scalp ("Black dot"), with/without associated inflammation, caused by fungus infection.
- Trichotillomania: Intentional pulling out of otherwise healthy hair; is usually due to habit.

Pediatric Considerations
Tinea capitis is the only common form of alopecia.

Pregnancy Considerations
Postpartum hair loss is due to altered physiology during pregnancy.

EPIDEMIOLOGY

- Predominant age
  - Incidence of androgenic alopecia increases with age.
  - Tinea capitis and traction alopecia more common in children
- Predominant sex: Male > Female

Prevalence
- 50% of white men have noticeable male-pattern baldness by 50 years of age.
- 37% of postmenopausal females show some evidence of hair loss.

RISK FACTORS

- Positive family history of baldness
- Physical or psychologic stress
- Pregnancy
- Poor nutrition

Genetics
- In whites, androgenic alopecia follows a dominant trait with incomplete penetrance.
- Hereditary incidence notable in men and women with a strong family history of baldness

PATHOPHYSIOLOGY
See "Description"

ETIOLOGY

- Telogen effluvium
  - Postpartum
  - Drugs (oral contraceptives, anticoagulants, retinoids, β-blockers, chemotherapeutic agents, interferon)
  - Stress (physical illness, fever, or psychologic)
  - Hormonal (hypo- or hyperthyroidism, hypopituitarism)
  - Nutritional (malnutrition, iron deficiency, zinc deficiency)
  - Diffuse alopecia areata
- Anagen effluvium
  - Mycosis fungoides
  - X-ray treatment
  - Drugs (chemotherapeutic agents, allopurinol, levodopa, bromocriptine)
  - Poisoning (bismuth, arsenic, gold, boric acid, thallium)
- Cicatricial alopecia
  - Congenital and developmental defects
  - Infection (leprosy, syphilis, varicella zoster, cutaneous leishmaniasis)
  - Basal cell carcinoma
  - Epidermal nevi
  - Physical agents (acids and alkali, burns, freezing, radiodermatitis)
  - Cicatricial pemphigoid
  - Lichen planus
  - Discoid lupus erythematosus
  - Sarcoidosis
- Androgenic alopecia
  - Adrenal hyperplasia
  - Polycystic ovaries
  - Ovarian hyperplasia
  - Carcinoid
  - Pituitary hyperplasia
  - Drugs (testosterone, danazol, adrenocorticotropic hormone, anabolic steroids, progesterones)
- Alopecia areata
  - Unknown, but possibly autoimmune
- Traction alopecia
  - Trichotillomania (direct self-pulling of the hair)
  - Tight rollers or braids
- Tinea capitis
  - *Microsporum* sp.
  - *Trichophyton* sp.

ASSOCIATED CONDITIONS
Alopecia areata

- Down syndrome
- Vitiligo
- Diabetes

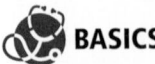 **DIAGNOSIS**

SIGNS AND SYMPTOMS

History
- Hair loss
- Pruritus (in tinea capitis)

Physical Exam
- Scaling of the scalp (in tinea capitis)
- Broken hairs (in tinea capitis and traction alopecia)
- Tapered hair at the borders of the patch of alopecia (in alopecia areata)
- Easily removable hairs at the periphery of the patch of alopecia (in alopecia areata)
- Inflammation (in tinea capitis)
- Hair-pull test: 3 cm above ear, pinch 20–40 hairs and exert slow, gentle traction while sliding fingersup hair shaft. Telogen(aka "club") hair bulbs are unpigmented and ovoid. Anagen hairs have elongated and possibly pigmented bulb with gelatinous root sheath.
- Light hair-pull test (positive if anagen hairs come loose easily; seen in alopecia areata)
- Hair pull test with >6 club hairs consistent with telogen effluvium

TESTS

Lab
Consider

- TSH
- CBC (may reflect an underlying immunologic disorder or anemia)
- Free testosterone and dehydroepiandrosterone sulfate in women with androgenic alopecia
- Serum ferritin
- VDRL or RPR for syphilis
- Lymphocyte T- and B-cell number (sometimes low in patients with alopecia areata)
- Drugs that may alter lab results:Thyroid drugs and iodine preparations (including topicals) will alter thyroid tests.

Diagnostic Procedures/Surgery
- Direct microscopic examination of the hair shaft
- Potassium hydroxide examination of the scale, if present (positive in tinea capitis)
- Fungal culture of the scale, if present
- Scalp biopsy (sometimes)
- Drugs that may alter lab results:Antifungal drugs may make potassium hydroxide examination falsely negative.

Pathological Findings
Scalp biopsy with routine microscopy and direct immunofluorescence will aid in the diagnosis of tinea capitis, diffuse alopecia areata, and the scarring alopecias due to lupus erythematosus, lichen planus, and sarcoidosis

DIFFERENTIAL DIAGNOSIS
Search for type of alopecia and then for possible reversible causes.

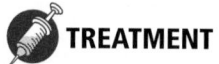 **TREATMENT**

INITIAL STABILIZATION
Outpatient treatment

GENERAL MEASURES
- Traction alopecia
  - Only with discontinuation of the hair pulling will the disorder resolve.
  - Psychologic or psychiatric intervention may be necessary.
  - Successful therapeutic approaches have included medications, behavior modification, and hypnosis.
- Tinea capitis
  - 6–8 weeks of oral therapy are often necessary. Topical medications are ineffective.
  - Careful hand washing and laundering of head wear and towels

Diet
No special diet

 MEDICATION (DRUGS)

- Androgenic alopecia: Topical minoxidil (Rogaine) 2%; finasteride (Propecia), 1 mg PO daily
- Alopecia areata: High-potency topical steroids, topical anthralin, intralesional steroids, psoralen with long-wave UV radiation, cyclosporine
- Tinea capitis: Griseofulvin (ultramicrosize) 250–375 mg/d PO in adults, 5.5–7.3 mg/kg/d in children. Alternatively, ketoconazole 200 mg/d PO. Treatment for 6–8 weeks.
- Contraindications
  - Griseofulvin: Pregnancy, porphyria, hepatocellular failure
  - Ketoconazole and cisapride (Propulsid) should not be used together.
  - Itraconazole and cisapride should not be used together.
- Precautions
  - Topical minoxidil
    o Burning and irritation of the eyes
    o Salt and water retention
    o Tachycardia
    o Angina (rare)
  - Topical steroids
    o Local burning and stinging
    o Pruritus
    o Skin atrophy
    o Telangiectasias
    o Hypothalamic-pituitary-adrenal (HPA) suppression if high-potency steroids used for prolonged duration
  - Griseofulvin
    o Photosensitivity reaction
    o Lupuslike syndrome
    o Oral thrush
    o Granulocytopenia
  - Ketoconazole
    o Anaphylaxis
    o Hepatotoxicity
    o Oligospermia
    o Neuropsychiatric disturbances
    o Gynecomastia
  - Itraconazole
    o Hepatotoxicity
    o Nausea, vomiting
  - Finasteride
    o Not indicated for use in women
    o Caution when there is liver disease

- Significant possible interactions
  - Griseofulvin and warfarin: Decreased activity of warfarin
  - Griseofulvin and barbiturates: Depressed activity of griseofulvin
  - Ketoconazole and warfarin: May enhance activity of warfarin
  - Ketoconazole and isoniazid, rifampin: Decreased activity of ketoconazole
  - Ketoconazole and phenytoin: May alter metabolism of either drug
  - Itraconazole and terfenadine: Prolonged QT and ventricular arrhythmias
  - Itraconazole and astemizole: Prolonged QT and ventricular arrhythmias
  - Itraconazole and cisapride: Contraindicated
  - Itraconazole and digoxin: May result in elevated levels of digoxin
  - H_2 blockers or antacids and ketoconazole: Decreased absorption of ketoconazole. If necessary, give H_2 blocker or antacids at least 2 hours after ketoconazole dose. Avoid using the proton pump inhibitor omeprazole for the same reason.

SURGERY
- Androgenic alopecia: Hair transplantation, scalp reduction, transposition flap, and soft-tissue expansion.
- Cicatricial alopecia: Only effective treatment is surgical (graft transplantation, flap transplantation, or excision of the scarred area).

 FOLLOW-UP

PROGNOSIS
- Telogen effluvium
  - Maximum shedding 3 months after the inciting event (medication, stress, nutritional deficiency) and recovery following correction of the cause
  - Rarely permanent baldness
  - Chronic effluvium uncommon
- Anagen effluvium
  - Shedding begins days to a few weeks after the inciting event, with recovery following correction of the cause.
  - Rarely permanent baldness
- Cicatricial alopecia
  - Hair follicles permanently damaged
- Androgenic alopecia
  - After 12 months of using topical minoxidil, 39% of subjects reported moderate to marked hair growth.
  - Prognosis depends on treatment response.
- Alopecia areata
  - Usually resolves within 3 years without treatment
  - Recurrence common
- Traction alopecia
  - Depends on behavior modification
- Tinea capitis
  - Usually complete recovery

PATIENT MONITORING
With ketoconazole, monitor liver enzymes

REFERENCES

1. Ross EK. Management of hair loss. *Dermatol Clin.* 2005;23(2):227–243.
2. University of Texas at Austin School of Nursing, Family Nurse Practitioner Program. Recommendations to diagnose and treat adult hair loss disorders or alopecia in primary care settings (non pregnant female and male adults). 2004 May. 21 pages. NGC:003722 at www.guidelines.gov
3. Fiedler VC, Alaiti S. Treatment of alopecia areata. *Dermatol Clin.* 1996;14:733–738.
4. Habif TP. *Hair Diseases: Clinical Dermatology*, 4th ed. 2004.
5. Jackson EA. Hair disorders. *Prim Care.* 2000;27:319–332.
6. Rietschel RL. A simplified approach to the diagnosis of alopecia. *Dermatol Clin.* 1996;14:691–695.
7. Sperling LC. Hair and systemic disease. *Dermatol Clin.* 2001;19:711–726.
8. Whiting DA. Chronic telogen effluvium. *Dermatol Clin.* 1996;14:723–731.

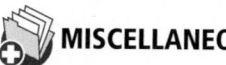 **MISCELLANEOUS**

See also: Lichen planus acrodermatitis enteropathica; Tinea capitis; Cutaneous T-cell lymphoma; Syphilis lichen planus; Cutaneous syphilis; Tinea capitis acrodermatitis enteropathica; Werner syndrome

CODES

ICD9-CM
- 704.00 Alopecia, unspecified
- 704.01 Alopecia areata
- 704.09 Diseases of hair and hair follicles, other
- 110.0 Dermatophytosis of scalp and beard

PATIENT TEACHING
National Alopecia Areata Foundation, 714 C St., San Rafael, CA 94901

 See Corresponding Diagnostic Algorithm

ALTITUDE ILLNESS
Robert Hyde, MD, MA, EMT-P

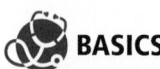 **BASICS**

DESCRIPTION
A spectrum of medical problems ranging from mild discomfort to fatal illness that may occur on ascent to higher altitude (elevations above 1,500 meters [4,921 feet]); is divided into 3 categories: High 1,500–3,500 m, very high 3,500–5,500 m, and extreme 5,500–8,850 m. (1) It can affect anyone, including the most experienced and fit individual. For most, is an unpleasant but self-limiting syndrome that will not require physician intervention.

- Acute mountain sickness (AMS): Symptoms associated with a physiologic response to a hypobaric, hypoxic environment. Onset occurs within 24 hours of arrival at altitude; often within 1–4 hours. Neurologic symptoms are predominant, and range from mild to moderate headache and malaise to severe impairment.
- High-altitude pulmonary edema (HAPE): Noncardiogenic pulmonary edema. Onset within 1–4 days at altitude. Rare below 8,000 feet (2,438 m).
- High-altitude cerebral edema (HACE): A potentially fatal neurologic syndrome; considered the end stage of AMS. Onset within 3–5 days at elevation as low as 2,750 m (9,022 feet), but may be more abrupt at higher altitudes. Death results from brain herniation.
- System(s) Affected: Nervous; Pulmonary
- Synonym(s): Mountain sickness

Geriatric Considerations
- Risk does not increase with age.
- Age alone should not preclude travel to high altitude; allow extra time to acclimate.
- Pre-existing medical problems made worse are referred to as altitude-exacerbated conditions.

Pediatric Considerations
- Altitude illness seems to have the same incidence in children as in adults, but diagnosis may be delayed in younger children.
- Any child who experiences behavioral symptoms after recent ascent should be presumed to be suffering from altitude illness.

Pregnancy Considerations
- The risk during pregnancy is unknown.
- No evidence that exposure to high altitude (1,500–3,500 m) poses a risk to a pregnancy
- It may be prudent to advise a low-altitude dwelling to any pregnant woman experiencing complications.

GENERAL PREVENTION
- General guidelines
  - Preacclimatization affords some protection against altitude illness.
  - Staged or graded ascent (rest day every 600–1,200 m) and a slow ascent rate (maximum 600 m/day) should allow adequate time for acclimatization.
  - Sleeping elevation: "Climb high and sleep low" is a prudent practice for anyone going above 3,500 m
  - Avoid heavy exertion for the 1st 1–3 days.

- Avoid respiratory depressants such as alcohol and soporifics.
- Pre-ascent physical conditioning is not preventive.
- Drug prophylaxis
  - Acetazolamide (if patient has a history of problems at altitude and/or plans to ascend >500 m/d). Dosage is usually 125–500 mg PO b.i.d. starting 2 days before ascent and continued for 3 days at maximum altitude. Patients with a drug allergy to sulfonamides should avoid acetazolamide.
  - Dexamethasone may significantly reduce the incidence and severity of acute mountain sickness. Dosage is 2–4 mg PO q6h, begun the day of ascent, continued for 3 days at the higher altitude, then tapered over 5 days. Adverse side effects are rare.
  - For HAPE only
    ○ Consider nifedipine 30 mg extended-release PO b.i.d. start prior to ascent and continue for 2 days at maximum altitude.
    ○ Consider beta-agonists (salmeterol, albuterol) 125 mcg inhaled b.i.d. starting 1 day before ascent and 2 days at maximum altitude.

EPIDEMIOLOGY
Most epidemiologic studies are limited to relatively homogenous populations of men.

Incidence
- AMS: 10–90% globally
- HAPE/HACE: 0.01–1% of sojourner ascents at typical mountain resorts, although incidence increases with rapid and higher ascents (2)

Prevalence
Unknown

RISK FACTORS
- Rapid rate of ascent
- Maximum altitude attained
- Increased duration at high altitude
- Failure to acclimatize at lower altitude
- Increased sleeping altitude
- Prior history of altitude illness
- Cardiac congenital abnormalities

PATHOPHYSIOLOGY
- Not completely understood
- Hypobaric hypoxia and hypoxemia are the pathogenetic precursors to altitude illness.
- Symptoms of AMS may be the result of cerebral swelling, either through vasodilatation induced by hypoxia or through cerebral edema.
- Other mechanisms include impaired cerebral autoregulation, release of vasogenic mediators, and alteration of the blood-brain barrier
- HAPE is a noncardiogenic pulmonary edema characterized by exaggerated pulmonary hypertension leading to vascular leakage through overperfusion, stress failure, or both.

ETIOLOGY
Individuals with a prior episode of HAPE have an increased risk of recurrence. (3)

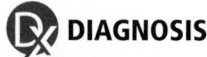 **DIAGNOSIS**

SIGNS AND SYMPTOMS
- AMS, mild to moderate symptoms
  - Headache, plus at least 1 of the following
    ○ Anorexia
    ○ Nausea or vomiting
    ○ Dizziness or lightheadedness
    ○ Insomnia
- AMS, severe symptoms
  - Increased headache
  - Irritability
  - Marked fatigue
  - Dyspnea with exertion
  - Nausea and vomiting
- HAPE (Lake Louise diagnostic criteria)
  - At least 2 of the following symptoms
    ○ Dyspnea at rest
    ○ Cough
    ○ Weakness
    ○ Decreased exercise performance
    ○ Chest tightness
    ○ Congestion
  - AND at least 2 of the following signs
    ○ Crackles or wheezing in at least 1 lung field
    ○ Central cyanosis
    ○ Tachycardia
    ○ Tachypnea
  - Note: Fatigue may be pulmonary edema
- HACE symptoms
  - Mental status changes (irrational behavior, lethargy, obtundation, coma)
  - Truncal ataxia
  - Papilledema, retinal hemorrhage, cranial nerve palsies
  - Focal neurologic deficits (rare)

TESTS
ECG may show sinus tachycardia, or right-sided heart strain.

Lab
- AMS: Laboratory studies are nonspecific and rarely required for diagnosis.
- HAPE: Severe hypoxemia demonstrated with oximetry or blood gas analysis.

Imaging
No radiographic feature is specific to HAPE.

DIFFERENTIAL DIAGNOSIS
Onset of symptoms >3 days at a given altitude, the absence of headache or the lack of rapid response to oxygen or descent suggest other diagnoses

- AMS/HACE
  - Subarachnoid hemorrhage; central nervous system (CNS) mass; cerebrovascular accident (CVA)
  - Migraine headache
  - Dehydration
  - Ingestion of toxins, drugs, or alcohol
  - Carbon monoxide exposure
  - CNS infection
  - Acute psychosis

- HAPE
  - Pneumonia
  - Cardiogenic pulmonary edema
  - Spontaneous pneumothorax
  - Pulmonary embolism
  - Asthma, bronchitis
  - Myocardial infarction
  - Hyperventilation syndrome

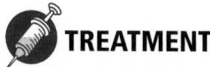 TREATMENT

INITIAL STABILIZATION
Outpatient treatment for mild cases

GENERAL MEASURES
- Therapy must be tailored to fit disease severity
- Early recognition is critical.
- Stop ascent, acclimatize at the same altitude and/or descend if symptoms do not improve over 24 hours. Definitive treatment is to descend to a lower altitude. Dramatic improvement accompanies even modest reductions in altitude.
- Oxygen helps relieve symptoms. Give continuously by cannula or mask initially, then titrate to SaO_2 >90%
- AMS
  - Acetazolamide is effective in reducing mild to moderate symptoms of AMS, but the optimum dosage is unknown. Consider 125–500 mg PO b.i.d. until symptoms resolve.
  - Dexamethasone may also be effective in treating moderate AMS. Consider 4 mg PO/IM/IV q6h.
  - Analgesics and antiemetics as needed for symptomatic relief
- HAPE
  - Oxygen therapy
  - Minimize exertion and keep patient warm
  - Immediate descent or evacuation to a lower altitude
  - Portable hyperbaric therapy (2–15 psi), such as the Gamow bag or Chamberlite, is an effective and practical alternative when descent is not possible.
  - Consider nifedipine 10 mg PO, then 20–30 mg extended release PO b.i.d.
- HACE
  - Immediate descent
  - Supplemental oxygen (highest flow available; maintain SaO_2 >90%)
  - Dexamethsone 8 mg IV/IM/PO initially, then 4 mg q6h
  - Hyperbaric therapy if unable to descend

Activity
Rest until symptoms clear

 MEDICATION (DRUGS)

First Line (4–6)[B]
- Oxygen: 2–15 L/min to maintain SaO_2 >90% until symptoms improve
- Acetazolamide:
  - Prevention of AMS: 125–500 mg PO b.i.d. starting 1 day before ascent and continued for 2 days at maximum altitude
  - Treatment of AMS: 125–500 mg PO b.i.d. until symptoms resolve
- Dexamethasone:
  - Prevention of AMS: 2 mg PO q6h or 4 mg PO q12h, starting 1 day before ascent and discontinued cautiously after 2 days at maximum altitude
  - Treatment of AMS: 4 mg PO/IV/IM q6h
  - Treatment of HACE: 8 mg PO/IV/IM initially, then 4 mg q6h
- Nifedipine (reduces pulmonary artery pressure):
  - Prevention of HAPE: 20–30 mg extended-release PO b.i.d. starting 1 day prior to ascent and continued for 2 days at maximum altitude
  - Treatment of HAPE: 10 mg, then 20–30 mg extended-release PO b.i.d.
- Salmeterol:
  - Prevention and possible treatment of HAPE: 125 mcg inhaled b.i.d. starting 1 day before ascent and continued for 2 days at maximum altitude
- NSAIDs:
  - Prevention and treatment of headache
  - Aspirin 325 mg PO q4h for total 3 doses
  - Ibuprofren 400–600 mg PO
  - Prevention of AMS: Dose unknown. Begin 1–5 days before ascent.
- Antiemetics:
  - Prochlorperazine 10 mg PO/IM q6–8h
  - Promethazine 25–50 mg PO/IM/PR q6h
- Contraindications: Refer to manufacturer's profile for each drug.
- Precautions: Refer to manufacturer's profile for each drug.
- Significant possible interactions: Refer to manufacturer's profile of each drug.

Second Line
Furosemide: Consider for treatment of AMS or HACE, 20–80 mg PO/IV q12h for total 2 doses. Currently out of favor; not recommended for prophylaxis; not established for use in HAPE

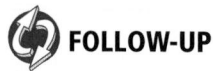 **FOLLOW-UP**

Admission Criteria
Severe cases

PROGNOSIS
Most cases of mild to moderate AMS are self-limiting and do not require physician intervention. Patients may resume ascent once symptoms subside. HAPE and HACE respond well to descent, evacuation, and/or pharmacologic treatment if identified early.

COMPLICATIONS
Patient may experience high-altitude retinal hemorrhage (HARH), which can cause visual changes, but is usually asymptomatic.

PATIENT MONITORING
- For mild cases, no follow-up needed.
- For more severe cases, follow until symptoms subside.

REFERENCES
1. Gallagher SA, Hackett PH. High-altitude Illness. *Emerg Med Clin N Am*. 2004;22:329–355.
2. Maloney JP, Broeckel U. Epidemiology, risk factors, and genetics of high-altitude-related pulmonary disease. *Clin Chest Med*. 2005;26:395–404.
3. Basnyat B, Murdoch DR. High-altitude Illness. *The Lancet*. 2003;361:1967–1973.
4. Hackett PH, Roach RC. High-Altitude Illness. *NEJM*. 2001;345(pt 2):107–114.
5. Barry PW, Pollard AJ. Altitude Illness. *BMJ*. 2003;326:915–919.
6. Dumont L, Mardirosoff C, Tramer MR. Efficacy and harm of pharmacological prevention of acute mountain sickness: quantitative systematic review. *BMJ*. 2000;321:267–272.
7. Rodway GW et al. High-altitude-related disorders, Part I: Pathophysiology, differential diagnosis and treatment. *Heart and Lung*. 2003;32(6):353–359.
8. Rodway GW, et al. High-altitude-related disorders, part II: Prevention, special populations and chronic medical conditions. *Heart and Lung*. 2003;33(1):3–12.

ADDITIONAL READING
For further information about hyperbaric therapies, oxygen systems, and protocols, visit http://www.ismmed.org and www.high-altitude-medicine.com.

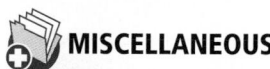 **MISCELLANEOUS**

CODES

ICD9-CM
993.2 Other and unspecified effects of high altitude

PATIENT TEACHING

 See Corresponding Diagnostic Algorithm

ALZHEIMER DISEASE

Jill A. Grimes, MD

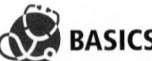 **BASICS**

DESCRIPTION

- Most common cause of dementia in the elderly.
- Degenerative neurologic disease characterized by progressive cognitive and behavioral impairment, usually occurring >65 years of age.
- Diagnosis of exclusion; cost in US >$110 billion/year.
- Usual course: Progressive and chronic
- System(s) Affected: Nervous
- Synonym(s): Presenile dementia; Senile dementia of the Alzheimer type

Geriatric Considerations
The US Preventive Services Task Force states evidence is lacking to recommend for or against routine screening for dementia in elderly patients without complaints of memory loss (5).

GENERAL PREVENTION

- Studies of NSAIDs, prednisone, estrogen, and vitamin E have not been shown to delay Alzheimer disease (1,2)[A].
- HRT is not recommended (6)[A].

- Intellectual challenge (puzzles) and regular physical exercise may offer preventive benefit.

EPIDEMIOLOGY

- Predominant age: >60
- Predominant sex: Female > Male (slightly)

Incidence
40% of those >85 are affected, which is 1,100/100,000 people.

RISK FACTORS

- Aging
- Low education level
- Down syndrome
- Positive family history
- Inheritance of the E4 allele of apolipoprotein E gene on chromosome 19 (E4 is a much less of a risk factor for African Americans and Hispanics)
- Smoking (2–4-fold increase)

Genetics
Positive family history in 50% of the cases, but 90% of AD cases are sporadic.

ETIOLOGY

- Unknown, but toxic β-amyloid deposits in neuritic plaques and arterial walls appear critical to pathogenesis.
- β-Amyloid precursor gene localized to chromosome 21

ASSOCIATED CONDITIONS

- Down syndrome
- Depression

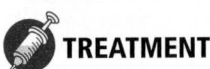 **DIAGNOSIS**

SIGNS AND SYMPTOMS

- No focal neurologic signs
- Short term memory loss
- Acalculia (e.g., cannot balance check book)
- Agnosia: Inability to recognize objects
- Apraxia: Inability to carry out movements
- Confabulation
- Delusions
- Impaired abstraction
- Decreased attention to hygiene
- Visuospatial distortion
- Late signs
  - Psychotic features
  - Mutism

History
Include family members in interview (helpful in assessment of behavioral changes, patients).

- Progressive memory loss
- Depression
- Apathy
- Anhedonia
- Intellectual decline
- Loss of interest; social withdrawal
- Occupational dysfunction
- Personality change
- Progressive cognitive impairment
- Restlessness
- Sleep disturbances
- Weight loss
- Incontinence

Physical Exam
- Complete neurologic exam to rule out other causes of dementia
- Folstein mini mental status exam

TESTS

- Lumbar puncture
- Neuropsychologic testing (if clinical picture is confusing or to help determine level of independence for skills such as balancing checkbooks, driving, or managing medicines)

Lab
- To help rule out other causes of dementia (3)[C].
- CBC
- Chemistry panel
- TSH
- Folate and B_{12} levels
- VDRL or RPR
- Sedimentation rate
- HIV antibody (selected cases)
- Family may have genetic testing for E4 allele of apolipoprotein E gene; not recommended.

Imaging
- Controversy exists concerning cerebral imaging (2,3)[C].
- An MRI or CT is needed to rule out other diagnoses, if cognitive decline is recent, there is history of stroke, or focal neurologic signs are present.
- CT/MRI: Moderate cortical atrophy, ventricular enlargement

- MRI: Hippocampal volumetry; positron emission tomography (PET) and single photon emission computed tomography (SPECT) not indicated.
- Medicare pays for PET to distinguish Alzheimer from frontotemporal dementia.

Pathological Findings
- Gross
  - Diffuse cerebral atrophy in hippocampus, amygdala, and some subcortical nuclei
- Micro
- Neuritic senile plaques
  - Neurofibrillary tangles
  - Pyramidal cell loss
  - Decreased cholinergic innervation (other neurotransmitters variably decreased)
  - Degeneration of locus ceruleus and basal forebrain nuclei of Meynert; amyloid angiopathy

DIFFERENTIAL DIAGNOSIS

- Vascular dementia; multi-infarct dementia
- Lewy body disease
- Dementia associated with Parkinson disease
- Normal pressure hydrocephalus
- Creutzfeldt-Jakob disease
- End-stage multiple sclerosis
- Brain-tumor: Primary or metastatic
- Subdural hematoma
- Progressive multifocal leukoencephalopathy
- Metabolic dementia (hypothyroidism)
- Drug reactions
- Alcoholism and other addictions
- Dementia pugilistica
- Depression
- Toxicity from liver and kidney failure
- Vitamin and other nutritional deficiencies
- Vasculitis
- Neurosyphilis

TREATMENT

GENERAL MEASURES

- Appropriate supportive care
- Outpatient, day care, assisted living, skilled nursing facility
- Optimize treatment of associated comorbidities
- Occupational therapy
- Music therapy
- Analyze environment for safety and security
- Assess needs of spouse/caregiver
- Advance directives planning

Diet
Nutritional supplements in later stages

Activity
- Exercise to reduce restlessness
- Continued cognitive challenge

Complementary and Alternative Medicine
- Randomized trials of *Ginkgo biloba* have produced conflicting results (1)[A].
- Coenzyme Q10, Huperzine not effective

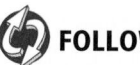 **MEDICATION (DRUGS)**

- Memory enhancement
  - Anticholinesterase inhibitors (1,2)[A]: Donepezil (Aricept) 5–10 mg/d, rivastigmine (Exelon) 3–6 mg b.i.d., or galantamine (Razadyne) 8–12 mg b.i.d.
  - Best in mild to moderate disease (Folstein MMSE scores 10–24); may show small benefit in more severe disease. Drugs may be effective in Lewy body dementia.
  - Only 30–40% of the patients will respond, either by modest improvement or slowed decline over 1–2 years. Unlike tacrine, no liver toxicity seen. Most common side effects are gastrointestinal.

First Line

- No specific drug therapy available for halting disease. Clinical studies are ongoing
- Use as few drugs as possible
- No drugs are helpful for wandering, restlessness, uncooperativeness, hoarding, and irritability. Use behavioral techniques and environmental modification (2)[C].
- For depression (occurs in 1/3 of patients), use selective serotonin reuptake inhibitors (SSRIs).
- Insomnia
  - Trazodone 25–100 mg at bedtime, zolpidem (Ambien) 5 mg at bedtime, zaleplon (Sonata) 5–10 mg at bedtime, ramelteon (Rozerem) 8 mg at bedtime.
  - Avoid diphenhydramine in elderly males, which can cause urinary retention.
- Moderate anxiety/restlessness
  - Consider low-dose, short-acting benzodiazepines, buspirone, or SSRIs, but efficacy unproven
- Severe aggressive agitation (especially if psychotic features present)
  - Risperidone (Risperdal) 0.25–1.0 mg b.i.d., olanzapine 2.5 mg/d b.i.d.; other newer atypical antipsychotic agents now preferred due to fewer side effects (2)[C].
  - Attempt periodic dose reductions or discontinuation, especially in a nursing home patient (see Omnibus Reconciliation Act [OBRA] 1987).
  - Anticholinesterase inhibitors also help behavioral symptoms (4,5)[A].
  - Carbamazepine (Tegretol) 100 mg b.i.d.–t.i.d., propranolol (Inderal) 10–40 mg b.i.d.–t.i.d., trazodone 200 mg/d, and valproic acid 250–1,500 mg/d (2)[C].
  - SSRIs are also being tried
  - Memantine (Namenda) (1)[A], 1st of new class of N-methyl-d-aspartate receptor antagonists; can be used as monotherapy or in combination with acetylcholinesterase inhibitors to enhance or preserve memory. Start 5 mg/d, titrating to target dose of 10 mg b.i.d. after 4 weeks. Shows efficacy in severe disease (MMSE 5–14).
- Contraindications
  - Avoid anticholinergic drugs, such as tricyclic antidepressants and antihistamines.
  - *Ginkgo biloba*: Avoid anticoagulants and aspirin

- Precautions
  - Benzodiazepines may produce paradoxical excitation or daytime drowsiness
  - Triazolam (Halcion) can produce confusion, memory loss, and psychotic behavior.
  - Atypical antipsychotic agents have been associated with hyperglycemia, ketoacidosis, increased stroke risk, and increased mortality in elders and dementia cases.
  - Anticholinesterase inhibitors provide only modest benefit for 1–2 years, after which decline continues at somewhat lesser rate than placebo. NNT is 7. No deterioration over 6–12 months is evidence of efficacy (1,2)[A].
  - Significant possible interactions
  - Antipsychotics: Lithium may induce extrapyramidal symptoms and disorientation.
  - Benzodiazepines may increase serum phenytoin concentration; cimetidine may increase the benzodiazepine concentration.
  - Donepezil (Aricept): Use with caution with anticholinergic medication or in patients with sick sinus syndrome or a history of peptic ulcers. Avoid paroxetine (Paxil), which causes increases donepezil levels.

Second Line

Studies reveal conflicting efficacy of selegiline 5 mg b.i.d., vitamin E, 1,000 b.i.d. or NSAIDS in slowing the progression of the disease (1,2)[A].

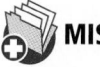 **FOLLOW-UP**

Issues for Referral

- Visiting nurse
- Social worker
- Physical therapist
- Occupational therapist
- Lawyer (living will, power of attorney)
- Support groups for patient and family
- Assess driving safety

PROGNOSIS

Poor: Average survival is 4–6 years

COMPLICATIONS

- Behavioral
  - Hostility, agitation, wandering, uncooperativeness
- Metabolic
  - Infection, dehydration, drug toxicity, malnutrition
- Other
  - Falls "Sundowning"
  - Depression (1/3 of patients)
  - Suicide: In early stages, if depressed

PATIENT MONITORING

- As often as necessary to treat poor nutrition, medical complications, provide support for family, assess need for placement
- Serial mental status testing potentially helpful, but bedside tests (MMSE) offer wide variability and lack of sensitivity
- Monitor caregiver burnout

REFERENCES

1. AHRQ report # 97. Pharmacological treatment of dementia. US Department of Health and Human Services, 2004.
2. Clark CM, Karlawish JH. Alzheimer disease: Current concepts and emerging diagnostic and therapeutic strategies. *Ann Intern Med*. 2003;138:400–410.
3. Knopman DS, Boeve BF, Petersen RC. Essentials of the proper diagnosis of MCI, dementia and major subtypes of dementia. *Mayo Clinic Proc*. 2003;78(10):290–308.
4. Sink KM, Holden KF, Yeffe K. Pharmacological treatment of neuropsychological symptoms of dementia. *JAMA*. 2005;293:596–608.
5. Trinh NH, Hoblyn J, Mohanty S, Yaffe K. Efficacy of cholinesterase inhibitors in the treatment of neuropsychiatric symptoms and functional impairment in Alzheimer disease: A meta-analysis. *JAMA*. 2003;289:210–216.
6. Hogervorst E, Yaffe K, Richards M, Huppert F. Hormone replacement therapy for cognitive function in postmenopausal women. Cochrane Database of Systematic Rev. 4, 2006.

 MISCELLANEOUS

See also: Alcohol use disorders; Hypothyroidism; Depression

CODES

ICD9-CM

- 290.0 Senile dementia, uncomplicated
- 290.10 Presenile dementia, uncomplicated
- 331.0 Alzheimer disease

PATIENT TEACHING

- Printed patient and family information available from: Alzheimer Association: 919 N. Michigan Ave., Suite 1000, Chicago, IL, http://www.alz.org/ (800) 272-3900
- Help family understand the progressive nature of the disease.
- Advance directives planning as early as possible; living will and health care POA

 See Corresponding Diagnostic Algorithm

See Patient Handout on CD

AMBLYOPIA

Robert M. Kershner, MD

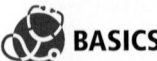 **BASICS**

DESCRIPTION

Amblyopia is the reduction in visual acuity in an eye due to not receiving adequate usage in early childhood; there is no structural or pathological abnormality of the eye, and it cannot be corrected by eye glasses or contact lens. Strabismus is the inability to align both eyes simultaneously under normal conditions.

- When seen in the geriatric population, the diagnosis has usually been made early in childhood.
- System(s) Affected: Nervous
- Synonym(s): Lazy eye

ALERT

Pediatric Considerations

More commonly seen in the pediatric age group early in life

GENERAL PREVENTION

None

EPIDEMIOLOGY

- Predominant age: May be present from birth or may be detected at any age
- Predominant sex: Male = Female

Prevalence

~2–2.5% in the general population

RISK-FACTORS

None identified

Genetics

Increased incidence in children with one parent with a history of amblyopia

PATHOPHYSIOLOGY

- Strabismic amblyopia is a loss of visual acuity in an individual due to suppression of the images in an eye, which turns out or in.
- Anisometropic amblyopia is present when 1 eye has a significantly different refractive error than the fellow eye, leading to visual blurring.
- Refractive amblyopia is due to uncorrected high refractive error, resulting in visual blurring in either or both eyes.
- Deprivation amblyopia (amblyopia ex anopsia) is due to relatively complete visual deprivation in one eye, which may be caused by a congenital abnormality such as a corneal scar or cataract.
- Deficiency amblyopia is also known as nutritional optic neuropathy or tobacco-alcohol amblyopia. Deficiencies of vitamins B_1 or B_{12}, or riboflavin, may be responsible.

ETIOLOGY

- See "Pathophysiology."

ASSOCIATED CONDITIONS

- Amblyopia is more common in families with a history of unequal refractive errors, high uncorrected refractive errors, and strabismus.

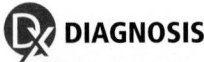 **DIAGNOSIS**

SIGNS AND SYMPTOMS

History

- Rubbing the eyes
- Sitting close to television or computer screen
- Problems in sports
- Preference for front-row seating
- Covering or closing an eye
- Squinting eye in bright light
- Eye turns "in" or "out"; wandering eye
- Poor vision in one eye without apparent explanation
- Poor vision that does not correct with glasses

Physical Exam

- Examination by an ophthalmologist to screen for unequal refractive error, outward or inward turning of the eye (strabismic amblyopia), and proper vision testing of the eye under monocular conditions.
- All children should have complete visual examinations prior to starting school, with each eye tested individually. Children from families with a known history of amblyopia or strabismus should have special exams by an ophthalmologist.

TESTS

Diagnostic Procedures/Surgery

A complete slit lamp and dilated funduscopic examination is necessary to exclude an organic cause for the decreased visual acuity.

DIFFERENTIAL DIAGNOSIS

The diagnosis of amblyopia can be confused with an organic lesion causing decreased visual acuity, and this must always be excluded before the diagnosis of amblyopia is considered.

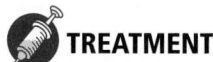 **TREATMENT**

INITIAL STABILIZATION
Outpatient treatment

GENERAL MEASURES
- Correction of the underlying disorder should be instituted at the earliest opportunity.
- Full refractive correction and/or patching of the stronger eye to encourage visual development of the amblyopic eye is warranted.
- Amblyopia never corrects itself spontaneously and will always require treatment. Children do not outgrow amblyopia.
- Deficiency amblyopia: Balanced diet, vitamins, and avoidance of alcohol and tobacco

Diet
No special diet

Activity
No restrictions

SURGERY
Surgical correction of an abnormal eye position may be required.

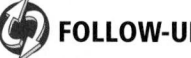 **FOLLOW-UP**

PROGNOSIS
A treatable condition in most cases if the diagnosis is made early
- Patching therapy, eyeglasses, and surgical correction of abnormal eye positions can result in near normalcy of vision when instituted early.
- Visual development occurs during 1st several years of life, and amblyopia therapy can be effective until ~age 12.

COMPLICATIONS
If there is failure to institute proper therapy early, permanent and profound visual loss can be expected.

PATIENT MONITORING
Once the diagnosis of amblyopia is made, the patient needs to be seen frequently at the discretion of the ophthalmologist until complete resolution of the problem occurs.

REFERENCES

1. American Academy of Ophthalmology. Binocular *Vision and Ocular Motility,* 1985–1986 (Ophthalmology Basic and Clinical Science Course, Section 6). San Francisco: American Academy of Ophthalmology, 1985.
2. Harley RD. *Pediatric Ophthalmology.* Philadelphia PA: Saunders,1983.

 MISCELLANEOUS

See also: Refractive Errors; Strabismus

CODES

ICD9
368.00 Amblyopia, unspecified

PATIENT TEACHING
Advise all parents to have children's eyes examined prior to their starting school.

AMEBIASIS

Rodney D. Adam, MD

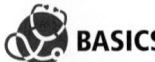 **BASICS**

DESCRIPTION

- Amebiasis is caused by the intestinal protozoan, *Entamoeba histolytica*. Infection results from ingestion of fecally contaminated food, such as garden vegetables, or by direct fecal-oral transmission. Most persons are asymptomatic or have minimal diarrheal symptoms; infection may be more severe in patients taking corticosteroids and other immunocompromised patients.
- In a few patients, invasive intestinal or extraintestinal (e.g., liver, and less commonly kidney, bladder, male or female genitalia, skin, lung, brain) infection results. Amebic abscess of the liver may develop during the acute attack or 1–3 months later; symptoms may be abrupt or insidious.
- *E. histolytica* has been divided into "pathogenic" and "nonpathogenic" strains. The pathogenic strains commonly cause invasive infection, while the noninvasive strains cause only asymptomatic intestinal infection. More recently, the nonpathogenic strains have been assigned to a separate species, *Entamoeba dispar*. Unfortunately, the species cannot be distinguished in a routine clinical laboratory.
- System(s) Affected: Gastrointestinal; Nervous; Renal/Urologic; Reproductive; Skin/Exocrine
- Synonym(s): Amebic colitis; Amebic dysentery

Geriatric Considerations
More severe in elderly

Pediatric Considerations
More severe in neonates

Pregnancy Considerations
- More severe in pregnancy
- Most agents are avoided in pregnancy (especially first trimester) because of concerns of teratogenicity, but invasive disease must still be treated
  - Paromomycin is sometimes recommended for noninvasive disease because it is not absorbed.
- Infectious disease consultation should be obtained.

GENERAL PREVENTION
- Avoid risk factors when possible.

EPIDEMIOLOGY
- Predominant age: All
- Predominant sex: Male > Female; probably because of greater occupational exposure

Prevalence
Probably <1% overall, but much higher in some risk groups, such as areas with large immigrant populations

RISK FACTORS
- Low socioeconomic status
- Institutional living
- Male homosexuality
- Invasive disease is more common in certain geographic locations, including some parts of Mexico, South Africa, and India.

ETIOLOGY
Infection with *E. histolytica* is transmitted through contaminated food or water or person-to-person contact.

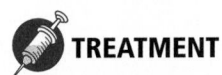 **DIAGNOSIS**

SIGNS AND SYMPTOMS
History
- Noninvasive infection (up to 99%) (characteristic of *E. dispar*)
  - Asymptomatic (90%)
  - Mild diarrhea
  - Abdominal discomfort
- Invasive intestinal infection
  - Abdominal pain and tenderness
  - Rectal pain
  - Diarrhea
  - Bloody stools
  - Fever (30%)
  - Systemic toxicity
- Extraintestinal infection
  - Fever
  - Systemic toxicity
  - Right upper quadrant abdominal pain and tenderness
  - Nausea and vomiting
  - Diarrhea (50%)
  - Hematuria, dysuria, urinary frequency and urgency

TESTS
Lab (1)[B], (2)[A]
- Stool for ova and parasites (unfortunately, the sensitivity of this exam is poor)
  - Diarrheal stool should be examined immediately for trophozoites in addition to fixed stool specimens (repeated as necessary).
  - In invasive intestinal infection, stools are bloody, but fecal leukocytes are usually absent.
- Serologic tests (especially indirect hemagglutination), positive in 85% of patients with colitis and most patients with extraintestinal disease
  - Serologic tests should be done in patients with idiopathic inflammatory bowel disease to rule out amebiasis.
- In bladder infections: Amoebae and/or cysts in urine
- Liver enzymes and alkaline phosphatase may be elevated in hepatic disease.
- Drugs that may alter lab results
  - Many drugs interfere with stool exams.

Imaging
CT scan or ultrasound for hepatic infection

Diagnostic Procedures/Surgery
- Rectosigmoidoscopy with biopsy
- Needle aspirate of hepatic lesions may be needed to rule out pyogenic infection or superinfection.

Pathological Findings
- Colon biopsy
  - Lysis of mucosal cells (flask ulcers)
  - Periodic acid–Schiff-stained trophozoites
  - Neutrophils at the periphery
- Liver biopsy
  - Necrosis surrounded by a rim of trophozoites
- Liver aspirate
  - Red-brown material (anchovy paste)

DIFFERENTIAL DIAGNOSIS
- Other infectious causes of colitis
  - Shigellosis
  - *Campylobacter* infection
  - Pseudomembranous colitis
  - Occasionally salmonellosis or *Yersinia* infection
- Noninfectious causes of colitis
  - Ulcerative colitis
  - Crohn colitis
  - Ischemic colitis
- Hepatic amebiasis must be distinguished from pyogenic liver abscess or superinfection of amebic abscess.

TREATMENT

INITIAL STABILIZATION
Outpatient treatment

GENERAL MEASURES
- Fluids and nutrition
- Electrolyte management

Diet
As tolerated

Activity
In accordance with illness of patient

MEDICATION (DRUGS) (1)[B]

First Line
- Noninvasive infection
  - Diiodohydroxyquin (also called iodoquinol): 650 mg t.i.d. PO for 20 days
- Invasive infection
  - Metronidazole (Flagyl): 750 mg t.i.d. PO for 5–10 days, followed by a 20-day course of diiodohydroxyquin to eliminate intestinal carriage
  - Tinidazole (Tindamax) 2 g daily for 3 days with food for intestinal infection and 2 g daily for 3–5 days for liver abscess
- Contraindications
  - Diiodohydroxyquin: Use cautiously in patients with thyroid diseases. Contraindicated in hepatic or renal dysfunction. May cause optic neuritis or peripheral neuropathy.
  - Known allergy to given medication
- Precautions
  - None of the agents have been proven safe during pregnancy, but pregnant women with invasive disease should still be treated.
- Significant possible interactions
  - Metronidazole and ethanol: Disulfiram reaction

Second Line
- Noninvasive infection
  - Diloxanide 500 mg PO t.i.d. for 10 days
  - Paromomycin 500 mg PO t.i.d. for 10 days
- Invasive infection
  - Dehydroemetine (as effective as metronidazole, but cardiotoxic): 1–1.5 mg/kg/d IM for 5 days
  - Chloroquine (less effective): 600 mg base/d PO for 2 days, then 200 mg/d PO for 2–3 weeks (pediatric dose: 10 mg/kg/d up to maximum of 300 mg/d)

SURGERY
With severe amebic colitis, surgery may be necessary for necrosis or perforation.

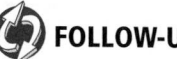 **FOLLOW-UP**

PROGNOSIS
- Untreated invasive amebiasis is frequently fatal.
- With treatment, improvement usually occurs within a few days.
- Some patients with amebic colitis have irritable bowel symptoms for weeks after successful treatment.
- Relapses possible

COMPLICATIONS
- Toxic megacolon with rupture
- Rupture of hepatic abscess, which may perforate into subphrenic space, right pleural cavity, or other nearby organs
- Bladder perforation, urethral strictures, vesicointestinal fistula

PATIENT MONITORING
- Patient signs and symptoms
- Stool for ova and parasite

REFERENCES
1. Haque R, Huston CD, Hughs M, Houpt E, Petri WA Jr. Amebiasis. *N Engl Journ Med*. 2003;348: 1565–1573.
2. Tanyuksel M, Petri WA Jr. Laboratory diagnosis of amebiasis. *Clin Microbiol Rev*. 2003;16:713–729.

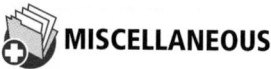 **MISCELLANEOUS**

See also: Diarrhea, Acute; Diarrhea, Chronic

CODES

ICD9-CM
- 006.0 Acute amebic dysentery without mention of abscess
- 006.3 Amebic liver abscess
- 006.4 Amebic lung abscess
- 006.5 Amebic brain abscess
- 006.6 Amebic skin ulceration
- 006.8 Amebic infection of other sites
- 006.9 Amebiasis, unspecified

PATIENT TEACHING
Avoid conditions of re-exposure

AMENORRHEA

Jeanne M. Cawse-Lucas, MD

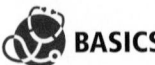 **BASICS**

DESCRIPTION
The absence of menses.

- Primary amenorrhea: No menses by age 14, with absence of secondary sexual characteristics, or no menses by age 16 with normal secondary characteristics
- Secondary amenorrhea: The cessation of menses for 3 cycles, or 6 months of amenorrhea
- System(s) Affected: Endocrine/metabolic; Reproductive

Pediatric Considerations
Primary amenorrhea by definition begins in this group.

Pregnancy Considerations
Pregnancy is the most common cause of secondary amenorrhea.

GENERAL PREVENTION
Maintenance of proper body mass index (BMI)

EPIDEMIOLOGY
Incidence
- Incidence of primary amenorrhea 0.3%
- Incidence of secondary amenorrhea 3.3%

Prevalence
Menarche to menopause

RISK FACTORS
- Overtraining (e.g., long-distance runner, ballet dancer) as part of the female athlete triad
- Eating disorders
- Psychosocial crisis

Genetics
No known genetic pattern

ETIOLOGY
- Primary amenorrhea
  - Imperforate hymen
  - Agenesis of the uterus and upper 2/3 of the vagina (Müllerian agenesis)
  - Turner syndrome
  - Constitutional delay
- Secondary amenorrhea
  - Physiological: Pregnancy, corpus luteal cyst, breast-feeding, menopause
  - Suppression of the hypothalamic-pituitary axis: Post-pill amenorrhea, stress, intercurrent illness, weight loss, and low BMI
  - Pituitary disease: Ablation of the pituitary gland, Sheehan syndrome, prolactinoma
  - Uncontrolled endocrinopathies: Diabetes, hypothyroidism, or hyperthyroidism
  - Polycystic ovarian syndrome (PCOS), (Stein-Leventhal syndrome)
  - Chemotherapy
  - Pelvic irradiation
  - Endometrial ablation (inducing Asherman syndrome)
  - Drug therapy: Systemic steroids, danazol, GRH-RH analogs, antipsychotics, OCPs
  - Premature ovarian failure
  - Female athlete triad (amenorrhea, osteoporosis, and disordered eating habits)

 DIAGNOSIS

SIGNS AND SYMPTOMS
History
The absence of periods

Physical Exam
- Galactorrhea
- Symptoms of hypothyroidism
- Symptoms of early pregnancy
- Signs of androgen excess
- Signs of estrogen deficiency
- Signs of congenital abnormalities such as imperforate hymen, absence of vagina or uterus

TESTS
- Progesterone challenge test: 10 mg of medroxyprogesterone acetate PO for 5 days: If withdrawal bleeding occurs, amenorrhea most likely due to chronic anovulation with estrogen (PCOS); if no bleeding, evaluate estrogen status with FSH
- FSH high: Ovarian failure
- FSH low or normal: Give cyclic estrogen and progesterone and, if menses start, diagnose chronic anovulation
- Estrogen absent (functional hypothalamic amenorrhea) or if menses doesn't start, diagnose Müllerian agenesis
- Prolactin high: Suspect prolactinoma, proceed with imaging the sella turcica

Lab
- If pregnancy test is negative
  - Serum prolactin
  - FSH
  - TSH
  - Blood sugar

ALERT
- Women <30 with ovarian failure should have karyotype analysis.
- Conditions that may alter lab results
  - Pregnancy
  - Menopause
  - Hyperprolactinemia
  - Ovarian suppression
  - Endocrinopathy

Imaging
- Ultrasound may show cysts undetectable during pelvic examination, presence or absence of uterus, and endometrial thickness.
- Radiologic evaluation of the sella turcica, if prolactinoma suspected (elevated serum prolactin) or functional hypothalamic amenorrhea suspected, because adenomas can occur even with normal prolactin levels

Diagnostic Procedures/Surgery
- Laparoscopy: Diagnosis of the streak ovaries of Turner syndrome or PCOS (not often done)
- Hysterosalpingogram: To rule out Asherman syndrome, if it is the appropriate clinical situation

Pathological Findings
Due to underlying disease

DIFFERENTIAL DIAGNOSIS
- Includes all causes listed in "Etiology"
- The most common cause of secondary amenorrhea is pregnancy.

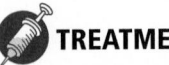 **TREATMENT**

INITIAL STABILIZATION
Outpatient

GENERAL MEASURES
- Definitive treatment depends on determining the cause of the amenorrhea.
- May not be necessary to treat all cases, especially if just temporary amenorrhea.

Diet
Correct overweight or underweight by dietary management

Activity
No restrictions

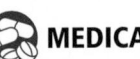 **MEDICATION (DRUGS)**

First Line
- Progesterone replacement: Medroxyprogesterone (Provera) 5 mg b.i.d. for 5 days, will result in a withdrawal bleed if the hypothalamopituitary-ovarian axis is intact and some endogenous estrogen production is present.
- Estrogen replacement: Conjugated estrogen, conjugated (Premarin) 0.625 mg for 25 days with progesterone added as above for the last 10 days will result in a withdrawal bleed, if the uterus and lower genital tract are normal.
- Use of hormonal therapies will not correct underlying problem. Other drugs might be required to treat specific conditions (e.g., bromocriptine for hyperprolactinemia).
- Use of hormonal replacement therapy is NOT recommended for long-term management of amenorrhea (1)[A]. It may be safe for short-term symptom management in young women (1)[C].
- Oral contraceptive pills or patches replace estrogen and prevent pregnancy and are probably the first-line drugs to use unless contraindicated. They also have a positive effect on bone mineral density in oligo/amenorrheic women (2)[B].
- Calcium supplementation 1,500 mg/d if cause is hypoestrogenism
- Because polycystic ovarian syndrome is related to insulin resistance, metformin (Glucophage) has been used (often starting at 500 mg b.i.d.) in an effort to correct metabolic abnormalities, improve ovulation (3)[A], and restore normal menstrual patterns (3)[B].

- Contraindications
  - Pregnancy
  - Thromboembolic disease
  - Previous myocardial infarct, cerebrovascular accident
  - Estrogen-dependent malignancy
  - Severe hepatic impairment or disease
- Precautions
  - Patients who are amenorrheic and wish to become pregnant should not be given hormone replacement therapy, but should receive treatment for infertility based on the specific cause.
  - Diabetes with insulin resistance
  - Seizure disorder
  - Migraine headache
  - Smoker >35
- Significant possible interactions
  - Barbiturates
  - Phenytoin
  - Rifampin
  - Corticosteroids
  - Theophyllines
  - Tricyclics
  - Oral anticoagulants (anticoagulant effect may be decreased)

SURGERY

- Hymenectomy, done as a day surgery, required for those whose primary amenorrhea is due to imperforate hymen
- Lysis adhesions in Asherman syndrome

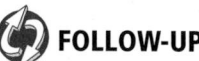 **FOLLOW-UP**

PROGNOSIS

- Reflects the underlying cause
- In secondary amenorrhea from hypothalamopituitary suppression, spontaneous resumption of menses with time (99% within 6 months) and correction of BMI

COMPLICATIONS

- Estrogen deficiency symptoms (e.g., hot flashes, vaginal dryness)
- Osteoporosis, in prolonged hypoestrogenic amenorrhea
- Increased risk of endometrial cancer in hyperestrogenism without progestin

PATIENT MONITORING

- Depends on the cause and treatment chosen
- If hormonal replacement is used, discontinuation after 6 months is advised to assess spontaneous resumption of menses.

REFERENCES

1. Farquhar CM, Marjoribanks J, et al. Long term hormonal therapy for perimenopausal and postmenopausal women. *The Cochrane Database of Systematic Reviews*, 2006.
2. Liu S, Lebrun C. Effect of oral contraceptive and hormone replacement therapy on bone mineral density in premenopausal and perimenopausal women: a systematic review. *British Journal of Sports Medicine*, 2006;40:11–24.
3. Andy C, Flake D. Do insulin-sensitizing drugs increase ovulation rates for women with PCOS? *The Journal of Family Practice*, 2005;54(2):156, 159–160.

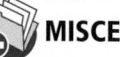 **MISCELLANEOUS**

See also: Diabetes mellitus, Type 1; Diabetes mellitus, Type 2; Hyperthyroidism; Hypothyroidism, adult; Osteoporosis; Polycystic ovary syndrome

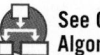 **CODES**

ICD9-CM

626.0 Absence of menstruation

PATIENT TEACHING

- Patient education consists of fully informing the patient of your findings, including the presence or absence of pregnancy, and of the underlying cause.
- Specific educational resources can be utilized as necessary (e.g., prenatal classes and menopause support groups).
- Specific information should be given about the expected duration of amenorrhea (temporary or permanent), effect on fertility, and the long-term sequelae of untreated amenorrhea (e.g., osteoporosis, vaginal dryness).
- Appropriate contraceptive advice should be given, as fertility returns before menses.
- Additional support may be needed if the amenorrhea is associated with a reduction in, or loss of, fertility.
- Society for Menstrual Cycle Research, 10559 N. 104th Place, Scottsdale, AZ 85258, (602) 451-9731.

See Corresponding Diagnostic Algorithm

AMYLOIDOSIS

Karin S. Leschly, MD

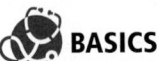 **BASICS**

DESCRIPTION

- A group of diseases characterized by increased deposition of amyloid fibrils in the tissues. Several different proteins may give rise to amyloid.
- These proteins are present due to their overproduction or decreased clearance. Their deposition may lead to compromise of vital organ function.
- Specific amyloid proteins aggregate mostly in specific organs.
- Primary or idiopathic (AL form): No associated disease
- Secondary, acquired, or reactive (AA form): Associated with chronic diseases, either infectious (tuberculosis, bronchiectasis, osteomyelitis, leprosy) or inflammatory (rheumatoid arthritis, granulomatous ileitis); Hodgkin disease; other tumors; and familial Mediterranean fever.
- Familial (hereditary) amyloidosis: Associated with distinctive types of neuropathy, nephropathy, and cardiopathy; may occur in almost every ethnic group
- Hemodialysis amyloidosis: Associated with renal hemodialysis
- Localized amyloidosis: Associated with Alzheimer disease
- System(s) affected: Cardiovascular; Endocrine/metabolic; Gastrointestinal; Musculoskeletal; Nervous; Pulmonary; Renal/urologic; Skin/exocrine

Geriatric Considerations
- In general, older individuals do less well.
- Age may precipitate familial amyloidosis, suggesting an age-related trigger.

EPIDEMIOLOGY

Incidence
- Primary amyloidosis: 1 per 100,000 person-years
- Secondary amyloidosis: Very rare
- Familial amyloidosis: 1 per million person-years

Prevalence
- Predominant age: 60–70
- Predominant sex: Male > Female (2:1)

RISK FACTORS
- Underlying plasma cell dyscrasia
- Underlying chronic inflammatory disease
- Familial Mediterranean fever
- Hemodialysis

Genetics
Only familial amyloidosis can be inherited. The genetics are variable but usually are autosomal dominant.

ETIOLOGY
- The cause of amyloid production and its deposition in tissues is unknown.
- In the different types of amyloidosis, etiologic mechanisms may vary. For example
  – Primary amyloidosis: The amyloid consists of immunoglobulin light chains, which are overproduced in plasma-cell disorders.
  – Secondary amyloidosis: The amyloid consists of amyloid fibrillary protein formed from serum amyloid protein, which is overproduced in chronic inflammatory conditions.
  – Familial (hereditary) amyloidosis: The amyloid consists of abnormal transthyretin protein or lysozyme protein produced in the liver.
  – Hemodialysis amyloidosis: The amyloid consists of β_2-microglobulin, which is normally cleared by the kidney, but not by hemodialysis.
  – Localized amyloidosis: Associated with hormonal proteins or aging, such as β-amyloid proteins in Alzheimer disease and other neurodegenerative diseases

ASSOCIATED CONDITIONS
Amyloid may bind Factor X, leading to bleeding problems.

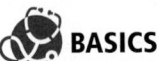 **DIAGNOSIS**

SIGNS AND SYMPTOMS
Manifestations are nonspecific, determined by the organ or system affected, and often are obscured by the underlying disease, which may be fatal before amyloidosis is suspected.

History
Fatigue, weight loss, gastroparesis, pseudo-obstruction, malabsorption, diarrhea, macroglossia

Physical Exam
- Nephrotic syndrome is the most striking manifestation: Early stages, slight proteinuria; late stages, anasarca, hypoproteinemia, and massive proteinuria
- Hepatic amyloid disease produces hepatomegaly, but rarely jaundice. Occasionally portal hypertension may occur, with esophageal varices and ascites.
- Cardiac involvement is common and may present as cardiomegaly, intractable heart failure, or any common arrhythmia.
- GI amyloid may cause esophageal motility abnormalities, gastric atony, small- and large-intestinal motility abnormalities, gastric atony, small- and large-intestinal motility abnormalities, malabsorption, bleeding, or pseudo-obstruction.
- Peripheral neuropathy, carpal tunnel syndrome
- Lung involvement may be characterized by focal pulmonary nodules, tracheobronchial lesions, or diffuse alveolar deposits. Patients may present with dyspnea, congestive heart failure, arrhythmia, angina pectoris, or sudden death
- Hilar adenopathy, mediastinal adenopathy
- Amyloid arthropathy may mimic rheumatoid arthritis: Symmetrical polyarthritis, rubbery periarticular soft-tissue swelling
- Skin lesions may be translucent or waxy; purpura (periorbital purpura) may result from amyloidosis of small cutaneous vessels, edema
- Dementia (may have role in Alzheimer disease)
- Macroglossia is common in primary and myeloma-related amyloidosis.

- A firm, symmetric, nontender goiter resembling Hashimoto or Riedel struma may result from amyloidosis of the thyroid gland.

TESTS
Specialized screening for mutant transthyretin

Lab
- Anemia may be present.
- Hypothyroidism may be present due to amyloidosis of the thyroid.
- Renal insufficiency is present in 50%.
- Proteinuria is present in ~80%.
- Primary amyloidosis
  – Elevated monoclonal protein level will be found in the serum and/or urine.
- Secondary amyloidosis
  – Tests to assess the underlying inflammatory disease will be useful.
- Familial amyloidosis
  – An abnormal transthyretin protein may be isolated.

Imaging
Echocardiography (if cardiac involvement is suspected)

Diagnostic Procedures/Surgery
- Amyloidosis is suspected on the basis of symptoms and signs, but can be diagnosed only by biopsy.
- Abdominal fat pad biopsy (up to 85% positive)
- Rectal biopsy (70% positive)
- Bone marrow biopsy (20% positive)
- Endomyocardial biopsy
- Renal biopsy

Pathological Findings
- Demonstration of amyloid deposits in tissues
- With Congo red staining, amyloid produces a green birefringence under polarized light.
- Electron microscopy is the definitive diagnostic tool.

DIFFERENTIAL DIAGNOSIS
- Peripheral neuropathy: Diabetes mellitus, alcoholism, vitamin deficiencies
- Carpal tunnel syndrome: Hypothyroidism, trauma, rheumatoid arthritis, late pregnancy
- Restrictive cardiomyopathy: Acute viral myocarditis, endomyocardial fibrosis, sarcoidosis, hemochromatosis
- Nephrotic syndrome: Glomerulonephritis, renal vein thrombosis
- Renal failure: Glomerulonephritis, obstructive uropathy, toxin- or drug-induced, acute tubular necrosis
- Symmetric polyarthritis: Rheumatoid arthritis, psoriatic arthritis, systemic lupus erythematosus
- Interstitial lung disease: Connective tissue diseases, infectious, sarcoidosis, drug-induced, pneumoconiosis
- Dementia: Alzheimer disease, multi-infarct dementia, Parkinson disease

TREATMENT

GENERAL MEASURES
- Therapy is 1st directed to underlying cause; such treatment may arrest amyloidosis.
- Management is generally symptomatic.
- Appropriate health care: Outpatient, except for serious complications (CHF, renal failure)
- Hemodialysis amyloidosis: Change to peritoneal dialysis (clears β_2-microglobulin).

Diet
- Low-protein, low-salt diet for renal failure patients
- Low-salt diet for CHF patients

Activity
- Fully active as tolerated
- Fatigue/shortness of breath may limit activity

MEDICATION (DRUGS)
- Primary amyloidosis
  - Treatment of the underlying plasma-cell disorder may or may not affect the outcome.
  - Melphalan and prednisone are among the drugs of choice for plasma-cell disorders.
  - Thalidomide also effective
  - The role of colchicine is considered less important; it may slow amyloid deposition.
- Secondary amyloidosis
  - Treatment of the underlying inflammatory process with disease-specific medications usually improves the outcome (i.e., isoniazid and rifampin for M. tuberculosis, methotrexate for rheumatoid arthritis).
  - Donepezil, galantamine, rivastigmine, and memantine have been approved for mild to moderate dementia caused by Alzheimer disease.
  - Colchicine, 0.6 mg b.i.d.–t.i.d. may prevent acute attacks in familial Mediterranean fever.
- Familial amyloidosis: None
- Hemodialysis amyloidosis: None
- Precautions
  - Melphalan: Bone marrow depression, including agranulocytosis, pancytopenia, thrombocytopenia, or aplastic anemia, may occur with prolonged administration. Monitor CBC periodically. Counsel patient to report symptoms/signs of infection (headache, sore throat, fever).
  - Thalidomide: Severe birth defects
  - Colchicine: Nausea, diarrhea, blood dyscrasia, rash, alopecia

SURGERY
- Splenectomy may ameliorate this condition by decreasing the amount of amyloid produced.
- Renal transplantation may improve the status of renal amyloidosis. However, amyloid will ultimately recur in a donor kidney.
- Liver transplantation or partial liver transplantation may cure familial (hereditary) amyloidosis.
- Other measures: Treatment of multiple myeloma with bone marrow transplantation is an option for some patients.
- A pacemaker may be indicated in those with amyloid-induced conduction defects.

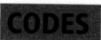 **FOLLOW-UP**

PROGNOSIS
- Primary amyloidosis
  - The prognosis depends on the underlying disease.
  - Once renal failure has developed, the prognosis is usually <1 year.
  - CHF has a 4-month prognosis.
  - Overall prognosis is poor; reported survival rates are 51% at 1 year and 16% at 5 years.
- Secondary amyloidosis
  - The prognosis is better, depending on ability to control the underlying process.
- Familial and hemodialysis amyloidosis
  - Highly variable
  - A liver transplant may be curative, but it is linked to the duration and severity of the pretransplant illness.
  - The deposition of amyloid in the heart may continue even after successful transplantation.

COMPLICATIONS
Despite intervention, worsening renal failure, heart failure, arthropathy, interstitial lung disease, and neuropathy are common.

PATIENT MONITORING
- Primary amyloidosis
  - Regular testing of monoclonal protein levels to assess response to therapy
  - Regular testing of renal function to assess response to therapy
- Secondary and hemodialysis amyloidosis
  - Follow-up to assess control of the underlying disease process
  - Regular testing of renal function to assess degree of impairment

REFERENCES

1. Cohen AS, Rubinow A, Anderson JJ, et al. Survival of patients with primary (AL) amyloidosis. Colchicine-treated cases from 1976–1983 compared with cases seen in previous years (1 961–1973). Am J Med. 1987;82:1182–1190.
2. Dember L, Sanchorawala V, Seldin DC, et al. Effect of dose-intensive melphalan and autologous blood stem-cell transplantation on AL amyloidosis-associated renal disease. Ann Intern Med. 2001;134:746–753.
3. Fiter J, Nolla JM, Valverde J, et al. Methotrexate treatment of amyloidosis secondary to rheumatoid arthritis. Clin Rev of Spain. 1995;195:390–392.
4. Falk RH, et al. The systemic amyloidosis. N Engl J Med. 1997;337:898–909.
5. Kyle RA, Greipp PR, O'Fallon WM. Primary systemic amyloidosis: multivariate analysis for prognostic factors in 168 cases. Blood. 1986;68:220–224.
6. Kyle RA, Gertz MA, Greipp PR, et al. Long-term survival (10 years or more) in 30 patients with primary amyloidosis. Blood. 1999;93:1062–1066.
7. Merlini G, Bellotti V. Molecular mechanisms of amyloidosis. N Engl J Med. 2003;349:583–596.
8. Skinner M. Amyloidosis. In: Kelley WN, Harris ED, et al, eds. The Textbook of Rheumatology. Philadelphia: WB Saunders; 1996:1409–1417.

 MISCELLANEOUS

See also: Multiple Myeloma

CODES

ICD9-CM
277.3 Amyloidosis

PATIENT TEACHING
- National Organization for Rare Disorders (NORD), Box 8923, New Fairfield, CT 06812.
- National Institute of Diabetes, Digestive and Kidney Disorders Information Clearinghouse, Bldg 31, Room 9A04, Bethesda, MD 20892.
- Amyloid Treatment and Research Program, Boston University School of Medicine. 715 Albany St., EB33, Boston, MA 02118
- Genetic information and counseling referrals:
- March of Dimes Birth Defects Foundation, 1275 Mamaroneck Ave., White Plains, NY 10605
- National Center for Education in Maternal and Child Health

See Corresponding Diagnostic Algorithm

AMYOTROPHIC LATERAL SCLEROSIS

Colin R. Bamford, MD

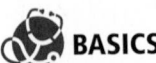 **BASICS**

DESCRIPTION

A degenerative disease (or group of diseases), that affects the upper and lower motor neurons

- Amyotrophic lateral sclerosis is the term applied to the sporadic and most common form of the disease. It includes a number of overlapping syndromes, such as pseudobulbar palsy, progressive bulbar palsy, progressive muscular atrophy, and primary lateral sclerosis.
- Familial ALS is an autosomal dominant or recessive disease, which is clinically similar to sporadic ALS but probably represents a distinct entity pathologically and biochemically.
- ALS-Parkinson-dementia complex of Guam is an ALS-like syndrome, often, but not always, associated with Parkinson syndrome and dementia, which is prevalent among the Chamorro Indians of Guam and very rare in the United States.
- System(s) Affected: Nervous
- Synonym(s): Motor neuron disease; Lou Gehrig disease; ALS

ALERT
Pediatric Considerations

- Infantile and juvenile spinal muscular atrophies are conditions that are distinct from amyotrophic lateral sclerosis both clinically and pathologically.
- Symptoms of ALS may inappropriately be attributed to age.

Pregnancy Considerations

- Uncommon among affected individuals
- Pregnancy would be unwise in any individual suffering from a disease with so poor a prognosis.
- If pregnancy did occur, the only foreseeable difficulties would be related to weakness.

EPIDEMIOLOGY
Incidence
0.4–2.0/100,000

Prevalence
- 5.0–8.0/100,000
- Predominant age: Uncommon before age 40
- Predominant sex: Male > Female

RISK-FACTORS
Age > 40

Genetics
Familial ALS

ETIOLOGY
- Sporadic ALS: Degeneration of the upper and lower motor neurons with their respective axons
  - Cause is unknown, but elevated levels of glutamate have been found in serum and cerebrospinal fluid (CSF)
  - High levels of glutamate are toxic; 90–95% of the cases of ALS are sporadic.

- Familial ALS: A genetically transmitted degenerative disease
  - Gene locus has been localized to the long arm of chromosome 21 and encodes the enzyme superoxide dismutase in 20% of familial ALS cases. 5–10% of the ALS cases are familial.
- ALS-Parkinson-dementia complex of Guam: Possible relationship to ingestion of the cycad nut or to some other environmental toxin

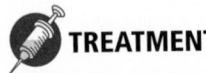 **DIAGNOSIS**

SIGNS AND SYMPTOMS
Physical-Exam
Variable combinations of

- Unexplained weight loss
- Focal wasting of muscle groups
- Limb weakness with variable symmetry and distribution
- Difficulty walking
- Difficulty swallowing
- Slurring of speech
- Inability to control affect
- Atrophy of muscle groups, initially in a myotomal distribution
- Fasciculations (other than calves)
- Hyperactive deep tendon reflexes (including jaw jerk)
- Spares cognitive, oculomotor, sensory, and autonomic functions

TESTS
Lab
- Elevated levels of glutamate in CSF and serum
- Anti-monosialoganglioside autoantibodies in low titer commonly found (of unclear significance)
- Possibly reduced levels of nerve growth factor
- There is no simple reliable laboratory test available that confirms the diagnosis of ALS.

Diagnostic Procedures/Surgery
- Electromyography: Denervation potentials (fibrillations, positive sharp waves) and often doublets are associated with prominent fasciculations, which suggest anterior horn cell dysfunction. Voluntary motor unit potentials have increased amplitude, long duration, and/or polyphasic pattern. The recruitment pattern is reduced for the force generated, and individual motor units have a high rate of discharge.
- Muscle biopsy: The biopsy will show groups of shrunken angulated muscle fibers (grouped atrophy) amid other groups of fibers with a uniform fiber type (fiber type grouping).

Pathological Findings
- Loss of Betz cells in the motor cortex
- Atrophic or absent anterior horn cells of spinal cord
- Atrophic or absent neurons within the motor nuclei of the medulla and pons

- Degeneration of the lateral columns of the spinal cord
- Atrophy of the ventral roots
- Grouped atrophy of muscle (motor units)

DIFFERENTIAL DIAGNOSIS
- Focal motor neuropathy
- Cervical spondylosis
- Lead intoxication
- Spinal muscular atrophy (adult form)
- Primary lateral sclerosis
- Familial spastic paraparesis
- Spinal multiple sclerosis
- Tropical spastic paraparesis

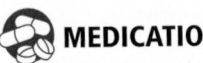 **TREATMENT**

GENERAL MEASURES
- Outpatient initially, may ultimately need nursing home placement and/or hospice
- Supportive care is necessary for complicating emergencies (aspiration, respiratory failure). Use of a respirator is a major ethical dilemma. Consideration should be given to those with selective respiratory dysfunction.
- Discussion of advance directive, focusing on patient's specific values about which interventions to be used, is critical to meeting the patients needs.
- Prosthetic devices (e.g., wheelchair)

Diet
Modify as tolerated; tube feedings may be necessary

Activity
As tolerated

SPECIAL THERAPY
Therapeutic trials of the efficacy of antioxidants (vitamins E and C and beta-carotene), nerve growth factor, gabapentin, myotrophin, and thyrotropin-releasing hormone have been undertaken. Reports are not encouraging.

MEDICATION

Riluzole produces a slight prolongation in life expectancy by decreasing the release of glutamate.

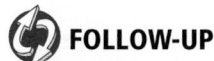 **FOLLOW-UP**

PROGNOSIS

- ALS usually results in death within 5 years.
- Patients who predominantly manifest progressive muscular atrophy have a better prognosis.
- There have been reports of spontaneous arrest of the disease.

COMPLICATIONS

- Aspiration pneumonia
- Decubitus ulcers
- Pulmonary embolism
- Nutritional deficiency

PATIENT MONITORING

- Initially every 3 months, frequency to be increased as needed for symptomatic therapy
- Patients with a presumed diagnosis of ALS should have imaging of the cervical spine and electrodiagnostic studies.

REFERENCES

1. Brown WF, Botton CF. *Clinical Electromyography*. 2nd ed. Boston, MA: Butterworth-Heinemann; 1993.
2. Rowland LD, ed. *Merritt's Textbook of Neurology*. 9th ed. Philadelphia, PA: Williams & Wilkins; 1995.

 MISCELLANEOUS

Also referred to as Mill's variant (unilateral involvement)

CODES

ICD9
- 335.29 Motor neuron disease, other
- 335.20 Amyotrophic lateral sclerosis

PATIENT TEACHING

Printed material for patients (and reference lists for physicians) available from:

- The Muscular Dystrophy Association: (520) 529-2000; (800) 572-1717; www.mdausa.org
- The ALS Association: (800) 782-4747; www.alsa.org
- Families of Spinal Muscular Atrophy: www.fsma.org

 See Corresponding Diagnostic Algorithm

ANAEROBIC AND NECROTIZING INFECTIONS

Ruben Peralta, MD, FACS
Hongyi Cui, MD, PhD

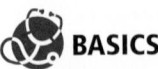 **BASICS**

DESCRIPTION
- Necrotizing infection of the skin and fascia are called necrotizing cellulitis and necrotizing fasciitis respectively.
- Anaerobic and necrotizing infections may be associated with gas in tissue.
- Necrotizing fasciitis is a rapidly spreading and potentially fatal soft-tissue infection located in the deep fascia, with secondary necrosis of the subcutaneous tissue. Organisms spread from the subcutaneous tissue along the deep fascial planes, presumably facilitated by bacterial enzymes and toxins.
- Type I necrotizing fasciitis is a mixed infection caused by the synergistic effect of both aerobic and anaerobic bacteria; Type II necrotizing fasciitis refers to a monomicrobial infection caused by *group A β-hemolytic streptococcus (GAS)*.
- Gas gangrene is a subset of necrotizing myositis usually caused by the *Clostridium* species with gas formation within the tissue.
- Necrotizing skin and soft-tissue infection is usually associated with extensive destruction of tissue, systemic toxicity, loss of limb, and even death.

ALERT
Geriatric Considerations
Increased risk with age >60

GENERAL PREVENTION
- Avoidance of trauma
- Good care of skin
- Control of diabetes
- Avoidance of tight orthopedic casts
- Follow routine surgical principles for skin closure

EPIDEMIOLOGY
- Predominant age: Any age
- Predominant sex: Male = Female

Incidence
Incidence of necrotizing faciitis 1,000–1,500 cases annually in the US

Prevalence
Rare

RISK FACTORS
- Tissue poor blood supply
- Old age
- Trauma
- Diabetes mellitus
- Malnutrition
- Immune suppression (e.g., HIV, malignancies, steroid use, etc.)
- Chickenpox
- Cigarette smoking
- Alcoholism
- Obesity
- Intravenous drug abuse
- Surgery

ETIOLOGY
Necrotizing fasciitis often begins as a cutaneous injury, which could be minor; a necrotizing process then begins below the dermis and spreads radially.

ASSOCIATED CONDITIONS
See "Risk Factors."

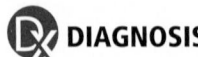 **DIAGNOSIS**

SIGNS AND SYMPTOMS
- Most important symptom is pain out of proportion to exam
- Malaise, anorexia

History
Most common predisposing conditions: Most cases arise from previous trauma or infection (surgical wound from open or laparoscopic procedure, ulcers, burns, IV drug injection site, abscess). May develop without apparent cause.

Physical Exam
The diagnosis of necrotizing fasciitis is clinical, based on physical exam
- Localized erythema and edema
- Skin discoloration with vesicle formation
- Foul odor
- Fever, often low grade early in the disease
- Tachycardia, hypotension
- Diaphoresis
- Rapidly spreading skin lesion

TESTS
Lab
- No test result is diagnostic, except frozen section biopsy of the fascia. Treatment should not be delayed while awaiting biopsy. Diagnosis is made clinically.
- Cultures and sensitivity tests for microorganisms reported to produce gas in human tissues
  - Gram-positive anaerobes
    - Cocci: *Peptostreptococcus* (anaerobic *Streptococcus*) (usually with group A streptococci [*Streptococcus pyogenes*, beta-hemolytic streptococci] or *Staphylococcus aureus*)
    - Bacilli: *Clostridium perfringens* and other clostridia
  - Gram-negative aerobes: Bacilli: *Escherichia coli, Klebsiella pneumoniae, Enterobacter* species, *Proteus* species (all usually in mixed infections)
  - Gram-negative anaerobes: Bacilli: *Bacteroides fragilis* (usually with other gram-negative bacilli)
- With severe gangrene, studies will reveal anemia and leukocytosis.
- Gram smears for many possible organisms
- Daily serum creatine kinase
- Elevated liver functions may result from release of bacterial toxins.
- Renal dysfunction may occur secondary to hypotension and myoglobinuria.
- Drugs that may alter lab results
  - Antibiotics before culture

Imaging
- Plain radiographs
  - Gas in tissues; foreign body if present
- CT
  - Soft-tissue swelling and presence of gas in tissues

Diagnostic Procedures/Surgery
Immediate surgical intervention, with longitudinal incisions of skin, superficial fascia, deep fascia, and muscles to look for and remove necrotic tissue and/or foreign bodies
- Multiple daily surgical interventions may be required.

Pathological Findings
Soft-tissue necrosis, with polymorphonuclear cells and vascular thrombosis

DIFFERENTIAL DIAGNOSIS
Other soft-tissue infection including abscess and post-surgical wound infection

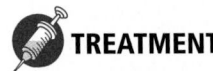 **TREATMENT**

GENERAL MEASURES
- Infectious disease consultation, if available
- IV fluids with electrolyte repletion, if indicated
- Daily complete blood count and electrolytes in acute phase
- Prophylaxis for tetanus
- Hyperbaric oxygen in selected cases

Diet
By mouth, as tolerated

Activity
Bed rest

SPECIAL THERAPY
Hyperbaric oxygen
- Unclear therapeutic value
- No delay of surgical intervention for hyperbaric oxygen therapy

MEDICATION (DRUGS)

- Initially broad-spectrum antibiotic regimen, then tailor to organisms identified by blood and wound cultures and organism sensitivities. (1)[B]
- Initial broad spectrum coverage should include penicillin, which will provide coverage of Streptococcus, and clindamycin, which works synergistically with penicillin when large bacterial load is present and also binds Group A Steptococcus toxin.
- Aminoglycosides will cover enteric Gram-negative organisms.
- Metronidazole is an alternative to clindamycin for treatment of anaerobic organisms.
- For vibrio species, tetracycline can be used.
- Retrospective studies suggest there may be a survival benefit with the use of Intravenous Immunoglobulin (IVIG) therapy. IVIG works by binding toxins and binds superantigens which suppresses pro-inflammatory mediators. (2)[B]
- Important: Do not delay treatment even if smear, cultures, and tests are negative.
- Unlike Clostridia perfingens and group A β-hemolytic streptococci, the Aeromonas species are uniformly resistant to penicillin-G but are reported highly sensitive to 3rd-generation cephalosporins.
- Precautions: Delay of operative treatment is an important determinant of increased morbidity and mortality.

SURGERY

- Necrotizing soft tissue infections are a surgical emergency. Patients should be taken to the operating room once the diagnosis is made.
- All necrotic tissue should be resected. Dissection should be carried along all involved fascial planes. Preservation of tissue should not take precedence over adequate debridement.
- If a limb is involved, amputation might be necessary because of extensive fascial and subcutaneous soft tissue necrosis and overwhelming systemic toxicity.
- Adequate surgical treatment can rarely be accomplished with a single operation. Debridement should continue until all necrotic tissue is removed. Multiple debridements is the norm.
- Negative pressure suction dressing (i.e., VAC dressing) may be utilized to improve wound care and assist with postoperative fluid management.
- Wound coverage and reconstruction can be undertaken once systemic sepsis has been controlled, all nonviable tissue has been removed and local bacterial control in the wound has been achieved.

 FOLLOW-UP

DISPOSITION

- Following surgical debridement, patients should be monitored and managed in an ICU setting if clinically indicated.
- Close contacts of patients and health care workers do not require chemoprophylaxis with antibiotics. (3)[B]

PROGNOSIS

- Mortality for necrotizing fasciitis decreased to 14% in 2002 from nearly 28% in 1994. (4)[B]
- Risk factors for mortality are associated with the following: Pre-existing and concurrent health conditions age >60 years, male, malnutrition, IV drug abuse, bacteremia, history of pulmonary or heart disease or carcinoma.

COMPLICATIONS

- Tissue and functional losses
- Amputation
- Fulminant course leading to death without treatment

PATIENT MONITORING

- As clinically indicated; may include following cultures, electrolytes, drug levels
- May require surgical critical care management in an ICU.
- Diligence required to recognize spreading gangrene

REFERENCES

1. Elliott D, Kufera JA, Myers RA. The microbiology of necrotizing soft tissue infections. *Am J Surg* 2000;361–366.
2. Norrby-Telund A, Low DE. Group A Streptococcal Toxic Syndrome and Necrotizing Fasciitis. *Current Treatment Options in Infectious Diseases* 2003;5,419–429.
3. Smith A. Invasive group A streptococcal disease: Should close contacts routinely receive antibiotic prophylaxis? *Lancet Inf Dis* 2005;5:494–500.
4. *MMWR*, 2005 51(53) 11 and *MMWR* 1994;43:401.

 MISCELLANEOUS

See also: Tetanus

CODES

ICD9-CM

- 785.4 Gangrene
- 040.0 Gas gangrene
- 136.9 Unspecified infectious and parasitic diseases
- 682.9 Cellulitis and abscess at unspecified site

ANAL FISSURE

Michael Rousse, MD, MPH

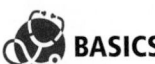 **BASICS**

DESCRIPTION
Anal fissure is a benign ano-rectal disease characterized by a knife-like tearing sensation upon defecation. An anal fissure is a tear in the lining of the anal canal distal to the dentate line, most commonly in the posterior midline.

GENERAL PREVENTION
Avoid local trauma or stretch of the anal canal. Soften stool by maintaining adequate hydration and fiber intake.

EPIDEMIOLOGY
- Very common ano-rectal condition. Often confused with hemorrhoids by lay person and primary care physicians.
- Predominant age: Early adult. Elderly are spared this affliction due to lower resting pressure in the anal canal.
- Predominant sex: Affects men and women equally but women more likely to get anterior midline tears (25% vs 8%). Any tear off of the midline, suspect a secondary cause.

Incidence
Exact incidence is unknown. Patients often treat with OTC and home remedies and do not seek the advice of a physician.

Prevalence
As many as 20% of patients, the majority of whom did not seek the advice of a physician, have symptoms referable to the ano-rectum.

Geriatric Considerations
Less common in the elderly because of lower resting anal sphincter tone

Pediatric Considerations
Not common in children, suspect abuse/trauma

RISK FACTORS
Constipation, passage of hard stool, high resting tone of internal anal sphincter, trauma, Crohn disease, HIV, syphilis, and TB

Pregnancy Considerations
Possible in pregnancy due to constipation and increased rectal pressure during and after pregnancy

Genetics
None known

PATHOPHYSIOLOGY
High resting pressure within the anal canal can lead to ischemia of the ano-dermal tissues; this increases the likelihood of splitting of the tissue with passage of stool. Thereafter, spasm of the internal anal sphincter results with or without passage of stool causing extreme, "knife-like," pain.

ETIOLOGY
Stretching and splitting of susceptible ano-dermal tissue

ASSOCIATED CONDITIONS
Crohn disease, TB, leukemia, and HIV

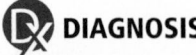 **DIAGNOSIS**

PRE HOSPITAL

ALERT
Knife-like pain with defecation, associated blood streaked bowel movement

SIGNS AND SYMPTOMS
Patients present with severe rectal pain, often with and following defecation, pain may be continuous. They may describe bright red blood on stool or streaking the paper when wiping. Occasional itch or perianal irritation.

History
Pain and bleeding with defecation

Physical Exam
Gentle spreading of the buttocks will reveal a tear in the ano-dermal tissue, typically posterior midline, occasionally anterior midline, rarely eccentric to midline. Minimal swelling or bleeding. Hypertrophic papillae/sentinel tag seen in chronic fissure.

Diagnostic Procedures/Surgery
None, avoid anoscopy or endoscopy
- Some cases may require exam under anesthesia.

Pathological Findings
Tear in ano-derm, hypertrophic papillae, and sentinel tag.

DIFFERENTIAL DIAGNOSIS
- Thrombosed external hemorrhoid—absence of swollen mass
- Peri-rectal abscess—fissure rather than a sinus
- Syphilis—Rare cause of recurrent fissures

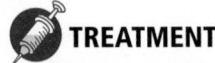 **TREATMENT**

GENERAL MEASURES
Stool softeners, analgesics, and anxiolytics

Diet
High fiber, extra fluids

Activity
No restrictions

Nursing
No restrictions

SPECIAL THERAPY
Sitz baths

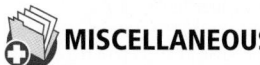
 MEDICATION (DRUGS)

Directed at reducing muscle spasm within the internal anal sphincter, softening stool to facilitate atraumatic passage, and pain relief. (1)[C]

First Line
- Stool softeners, fiber supplementation
- Analgesics
- Nitrates—topical nitroglycerin ointment 2% applied q.i.d.

Second Line
- Botulinum toxin—4 mL injected into the internal sphincter muscle
- Calcium channel blockers—oral or topical

SURGERY
- Reserved for failure of medical therapy, involves division of the internal sphincter muscle via various surgical approaches.
- Risk of fecal incontinence 45% in the short term, 6–8% in the long term. (2)[C]

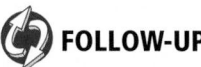 **FOLLOW-UP**

Issues for Referral
Medical therapy usually tried for 90 days, surgery is then considered

PROGNOSIS
Topical therapy is less likely to be successful for chronic fissures, ~40% failure rate. (2)[C]

COMPLICATIONS
Fecal incontinence and incontinence to flatus are primarily associated with surgery.

PATIENT MONITORING
- Once healed, most patients should have a colonoscopy to further work-up rectal bleeding.
- If <50, sigmoidoscopy may be sufficient.

REFERENCES
1. MacLeod J. *A Method of Proctology.* New York: Harper & Row,
2. Breen E, Bleday R. *Anal Fissure, Up To Date, 13.3.* Waltham, 2006.
3. Schwartz S. *Principles of Surgery,* 7th ed. New York, McGraw-Hill; 1999;1298–1299.

MISCELLANEOUS

PATIENT TEACHING
Avoid prolonged sitting during bowel movements; this creates extra pressure in the rectum. Drink plenty of liquids.

DIET
High fiber

ACTIVITY
No restrictions

ANAPHYLAXIS

Bobby Peters, MD, FAAEM

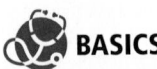 **BASICS**

DESCRIPTION
- An IgE mediated acute, systemic reaction following antigen exposure in a sensitized person
- A non-IgE mediated idiopathic anaphylactoid reaction also may occur. Anaphylactoid reactions are clinically indistinguishable from anaphylaxis and are treated in the same manner.
- System(s) Affected: Cardiovascular; Endocrine/Metabolic; Gastrointestinal; Hematologic/Lymphatic/Immunologic; Pulmonary; and Skin/Exocrine
- Synonym(s): Anaphylactoid reactions

GENERAL PREVENTION
- Avoid inducing drugs and foods.
- Carry a prefilled epinephrine syringe.
- Avoid areas where insect exposure likely. Avoid wearing insect attractants (e.g., perfumes, colored clothing); avoid bare feet outdoors.
- Carry or wear a medical alert ID about the anaphylaxis-causing substance or event.
- When radiologic contrast is unavoidable, use of low osmolar contrast agents (e.g., iothalamate) reduces the risk of contrast reactions to 3.1%.
  - Only 0.22% were considered severe.
  - Stop beta-blockers before administering contrast materials.
  - Pretreat with diphenhydramine (50 mg IV) and a steroid (e.g., methylprednisolone 60 mg IV q6h until procedure). Start methylprednisolone the day before the procedure is scheduled.
- Those with frequent (>6 per year) episodes of idiopathic anaphylaxis should be treated prophylactically with prednisone (40–60 mg/d in a single morning dose), hydroxyzine (25 mg t.i.d.), and albuterol (2 mg PO t.i.d.). The prednisone should be rapidly tapered to a every other day regimen.

ALERT
- Have a latex-free kit (gloves, etc) available for the treatment of latex-allergic patients. Some latex-allergic patients will react to tropical fruits, such as kiwi, bananas, avocados, and chestnuts.
- Avoid beta-blockers.

EPIDEMIOLOGY
- Predominant age: All ages
- Predominant sex: Male = Female

Incidence
- Up to 40,000 cases of idiopathic anaphylaxis occur per year with no identifiable cause.
- Drug-induced anaphylaxis in 1/2,700 hospitalized patients
- Anaphylaxis deaths: 0.3–0.7/100,000 per year

RISK FACTORS
- Previous anaphylaxis
- History of atopy or asthma

Genetics
Genetic predisposition for sensitization to antigens.

ETIOLOGY
- IgE-mediated mast cell degranulation
- Complement activation (C3a, C4a, C5a) by antigen–antibody complexes that contain complement-fixing antibodies.
- Other non-IgE–dependent anaphylaxis-like syndromes may be caused by modulators of arachidonic acid metabolism, sulfiting agents, exercise-induced anaphylaxis, and idiopathic recurrent anaphylaxis.
- Some important causes of anaphylaxis are:
  - Antimicrobials (e.g., penicillin)
  - Blood products (especially in IgA deficiency)
  - Iodinated contrast media
  - Ethylene oxide gas (dialysis tubing, other sterilized products)
  - Exercise
  - Foods (Common: Peanuts, nuts, fish, crustaceans, mollusks, cow milk, eggs, and soy)
  - Immunotherapy
  - Insect stings (e.g., honeybees, wasps, kissing bugs, and deer flies)
  - Latex rubber (gloves, catheters)
  - Macromolecules (e.g., chymopapain, insulin, dextran, glucocorticoid, and protamine)
  - Vaccines

ASSOCIATED CONDITIONS
- Asthma
- Atopy

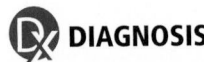 **DIAGNOSIS**

SIGNS AND SYMPTOMS
Physical Exam
- Pruritus, flushing, urticaria, angioedema
- Dyspnea, cough, rhonchi
- Rhinorrhea, bronchorrhea, wheezing
- Difficulty swallowing
- Nausea, vomiting, diarrhea, cramps, bloating
- Tachycardia, hypotension, shock, syncope
- Malaise, shivering
- Mydriasis

TESTS
Lab
- Hypoxemia, hypercarbia, acidosis
- Acidosis may cause apparent hyperkalemia by moving potassium extracellularly.
- Elevated serum tryptase, a mast cell enzyme for allergic and anaphylactic reactions. (11)[B]
- Drugs that may alter lab results: Epinephrine and albuterol may cause apparent hypokalemia by shifting K+ intracellularly.

DIFFERENTIAL DIAGNOSIS
- Anaphylactoid reactions
  - May occur after the 1st contact with substance, such as polymyxin, pentamidine, radiographic contrast media, and aspirin.
- Carcinoid syndrome
- Globus hystericus
  - May mimic pharyngeal edema

- Hereditary angioedema
  - C1q esterase deficiency with painless, pruritus-free angioedema without urticaria, flushing, or wheezing
- Pheochromocytoma
  - Paradoxically, because of beta-2 stimulation, some patients have hypotensive attacks accompanied by tachycardia.
  - Urticaria, angioedema, and wheezing are absent
- Pseudoanaphylactic reaction
  - After injection of procaine penicillin
  - Is a drug effect of procaine and not a penicillin allergy
- Scombroid poisoning
  - From ingestion of dark meat fish (e.g., tuna, mackerel, and mahi-mahi)
  - Histamine-like mediator: Symptoms include flushing, sweating, nausea, vomiting, diarrhea, headache, palpitations, dizziness, rash, swelling of face and tongue, respiratory distress, and vasodilatory shock.
- Serum sickness
  - Occurs several days after exposure
- Systemic mastocytosis
  - Benign or malignant overgrowth of mast cells
  - Urticaria pigmentosa seen in the benign form and the presence of reddish brown macular-papular cutaneous lesions, which urticate after trauma: Darier's sign.
- Vasovagal reactions
  - Bradycardia and hypotension without tachycardia, flushing, urticaria, angioedema, pruritus, and wheezing
- Pulmonary embolism, foreign body aspiration, and arrhythmia

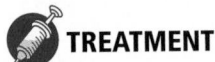 **TREATMENT**

GENERAL MEASURES
- Treatment depends on severity
- Maintain a patent airway
  - Endotracheal intubation and assisted ventilation may be necessary.
  - Possibly tracheostomy or needle cricothyrotomy in children <12 years
- Oxygen
- IV fluids (normal saline/lactated ringers)

Diet
Nothing until acute symptoms are controlled.

Activity
Bedrest until anaphylaxis clears and patient hemodynamically stable.

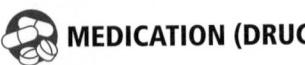 **MEDICATION (DRUGS)**

First Line
- Epinephrine
  - Less severe reaction: 0.3–0.5 mg (0.01 mg/kg in children) = (0.3–0.5 mL of a 1:1,000 solution, 0.01 mL/kg in children), SQ q20–30min as needed up to 3 doses

- – Life-threatening reactions: 0.5 mg (5 mL of a 1:10,000 solution) (for children: 0.05–0.1 mL/kg per dose) given IV slowly q5–10min as needed. If IV access is not possible, endotracheal or intraosseous may be effective.
- Diphenhydramine, an H_1 blocker: 25–50 mg intravenously (IM or PO:) q6h for 72 hours (children 1.25 mg/kg to 25 mg)
- Cimetidine, an H_2 blocker: 300 mg IV over 3–5 minutes (children 5–10 mg/kg per dose) and then 400 mg PO. b.i.d. is helpful and may be more effective than diphenhydramine.
- Corticosteroids: No immediate effect and unclear if they prevent recurrence.
  - – Hydrocortisone sodium succinate: 250–500 mg IV q4–6h (4–8 mg/kg for children) or
  - – Prednisone: 1 mg/kg in children, up to 60 mg
  - – Methylprednisolone: 60–125 mg IV in adults (1–2 mg/kg in children)
- Bronchodilator, if persistent bronchospasm
  - – Inhaled beta-2 agonists. Continuous nebulized albuterol of 10 mg per hour or 2.5 mg q15–20 min is safe, effective, and preferable to aminophylline as a first line.
- Laryngeal edema:
  - – Epinephrine: 5 mL 1:1,000 by nebulizer is more effective than racemic epinephrine and usually available.
- Persistent hypotension
  - – Dopamine: 200 mg in 500 mL of dextrose in water given by infusion pump; titrate to BP (3–20 mcg/ kg per minute)
  - – Glucagon: May be beneficial for resistant hypotension caused by concurrent beta-blockade therapy; 50 mcg/kg IV bolus over 1 minute, or alternatively, give as continuous infusion at 5–15 mcg/min
- Normal saline or Ringer's lactate: As necessary to maintain tissue perfusion
- Oral antihistamines and steroids for 72 hours

ALERT
Geriatric Considerations
Epinephrine may induce myocardial ischemia in those with cardiac disease, but is the drug of choice. Be alert for anticholinergic and CNS side effects after giving diphenhydramine or cimetidine.

Pediatric Considerations
Epinephrine could reduce the placental blood flow, but may save the life of the mother and fetus. It also increases risk of congenital malformation.

Second Line
- Several reports of tranexamic acid: 1,000 mg IV or sigma-aminocaproic acid for refractory anaphylaxis
- These drugs are not standard care; use only in patients who do not respond to other therapy.
- Aminophylline: 5–6 mg/kg IV in 100 cc D_5W over 20 minutes, then maintenance at 1 mg/kg/h drip
- Anti-IgE monoclonal antibody may have a role in long-term management of food-induced anaphylaxis. (12)[B]
- Venom immunotherapy has been effective in the prevention of sting anaphylaxis, but with a high side-effect risk. (13)[A]

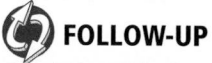 FOLLOW-UP

Admission Criteria
Moderate–severe anaphylaxis, admit for observation

Discharge Criteria
Outpatient: Patients with cutaneous angioedema, urticaria, and minimal bronchospasm may be released when symptoms and signs have cleared.

Issues for Referral
- Allergist referral, if anaphylaxis cause unclear
- Patients with anaphylaxis from insect stings benefit from desensitization immunotherapy.

PROGNOSIS
- Good prognosis if treated immediately; worse outcome with a delay of >30 minutes in administration of epinephrine
- Of those with idiopathic anaphylaxis, 60% are free of anaphylactic episodes at 2.5 years; most others were steroid-free

COMPLICATIONS
- Hypoxemia
- Cardiac arrest
- Death

REFERENCES
1. Anne S, et al. Risk of administering cephalosporin antibiotics to patients with histories of penicillin allergy. *Ann Allergy Asthma Immunol*.1995; 74:167.
2. The Diagnosis and Management of Anaphylaxis. Joint Task Force on Practice Parameters, American Academy of Allergy, Asthma and Immunology, American College of Allergy, Asthma and Immunology, and the Joint Council of Allergy. *Asthma and Immunology*. Allergy 1998;6.
3. Freeman TM. Allergy and Immunology. Anaphylaxis: Diagnosis and treatment. *Prim Care*. 1998;25:809.
4. Hoste S, Van Aken, Stevens E. Tranexamic acid in the treatment of anaphylactic shock. *Acta Anaesthesiologica Belgica*. 1991;42:113–116.
5. Patterson R, Hogan B, Yarnold PR, Harris KE. Idiopathic anaphylaxis: An attempt to estimate the incidence in the United States. *Arch Int ed*. 1995;155:869–871.
6. Sandler SG, Mallory, Malamut D, Eckrich R. IgA anaphylactic transfusion reactions. *Transfus Med Rev*. 1995;9:1–8.
7. Sloop GD, Friedberg C. Complications of blood transfusion: how to recognize and respond to noninfectious reactions. *Postgrad Med*. 1995;98: 159–162,166,169–172.
8. Tanus T, Mines D, Atkins PC, Levinson AL. Serum tryptase in idiopathic anaphylaxis: A case report and review of the literature. *Ann Emerg Med*. 1994;24:104–107.
9. Tintinalli JE, et al. *Emergency Medicine, A Comprehensive Study Guide*. 4th ed. New York, NY: McGraw-Hill; 1995.
10. Wittbrodt ET, Spinler A. Prevention of anaphylactoid reactions in high-risk patients receiving radiographic contrast media. *Ann Pharmacother*. 994;28:236–241.
11. Brown SG, Blackman KE, Heddle RJ. Can serum mast cell tryptase help diagnose anaphylaxis? *EMA*. 16;2:120–124.
12. Leung DY, Shanahan WR, Li XM, Sampson HA. New approaches for the treatment of anaphylaxis. *Novartis Foundation Symposium*. 257:248–260.
13. Brown SG, Wiese MD, Blackman KE, Heddle RJ. Ant venom immunotherapy: A double-blind, placebo-controlled, crossover trial. *Lancet*. 361;9362:1001–1006.

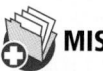 MISCELLANEOUS

Other Notes:
- Allergy to one species of legume (e.g., peanuts) or one type of seafood (e.g., shrimp) doesn't mean allergy to all products in that category. Skin testing is prudent.
- MMR vaccine can be safely administered to those with a history of egg allergy; most egg allergies are related to the albumin.
- Penicillin-allergic patients can generally tolerate second and third generation cephalosporins as well as monobactams (e.g., aztreonam). Generally, they will be allergic to carbapenems (e.g., imipenem) and 1st generation cephalosporins
- IgA-deficient patients should have washed red blood cells (RBCs) for transfusion.
- Those allergic to seafood are not allergic to iodine-based radiocontrast. Shellfish allergy is protein-related.

See also: Food Allergy; Insect Bites; Stings

 CODES

ICD9-CM
- 995.0 Other anaphylactic shock
- E947.8 Adverse effects in therapeutic use of other drugs and medicinal substances
- E947.9 Adverse effects in therapeutic use of unspecified drug or medicinal substance

PATIENT TEACHING
- Asthma & Allergy Foundation of America, 1717 Massachusetts Avenue, Suite 305, Washington, DC 20036; (800)7-Asthma or American Allergy Association, P.O. Box 7273, Menlo Park, CA 94026, (415) 322-1663.
- Medic-Alert type tags (Medic-Alert Foundation, Turlock, CA 95381-1009).
- Avoid beta-blockers, if possible.
- Instruct patient in the use of the bee sting kit.

ANEMIA, APLASTIC

Angie N. Ross, MD

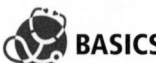 **BASICS**

DESCRIPTION
- Aplastic anemia is defined as pancytopenia and hypocellular bone marrow in the absence of abnormal cell infiltrate. The 2 forms of aplastic anemia include congenital and acquired.
- Congenital forms are seen mainly in the pediatric population and are associated with physical manifestations. The exception is an atypical presentation of Fanconi syndrome later in adult life, up to the 30s in males and up to 48 years in females.
- Acquired aplastic anemia has an insidious onset and is caused by exogenous insult triggering an autoimmune reaction. This form is usually responsive to immunosuppressive agents.
- System(s) affected: Hemic/lymphatic/immunologic
- Synonym(s): Hypoplastic anemia; Panmyelophthisis; Refractory anemia; Aleukia hemorrhagica; Toxic paralytic anemia

ALERT
- Prednisolone should not be used in treatment of patients with aplastic anemia (1)[C]
- Hematopoietic growth factors should not be used without close supervision in newly diagnosed patients (1)[C]

Geriatric Considerations
The elderly are more exposed to large numbers of drugs and, therefore, are more susceptible to secondary aplastic anemia.

Pediatric Considerations
- Congenital aplastic anemia requires a different treatment regimen (1)[B]
- Idiopathic aplastic anemia is more common in adolescents.
- Secondary aplastic anemia is seen in children exposed to ionizing radiation or treated with cytotoxic chemotherapeutic agents.

Pregnancy Considerations
Pregnancy may be rarely associated with aplastic anemia. Symptoms usual resolve after delivery. Supportive care is the mainstay and platelet count should be maintained above 20×10^9/L with platelet transfusion.

GENERAL PREVENTION
- Avoid possible toxic industrial agents.
- Use safety measures when working with radiation.

EPIDEMIOLOGY
- Predominant age
  - Congenital: Children and young adults
  - Acquired: Biphasic 10–25 and >60
- Predominant sex: Male = Female

Incidence
- 2 new cases per million in Europe and North America.
- The incidence is 3-fold in Thailand and China, when compared to the Western world

RISK FACTORS
- Viral illness/ Immunocompromised
- Toxin exposure
- Tumors of thymus (red cell aplasia)

Genetics
- A small number of patients with acquired and congenital forms have been found to have telomerase mutations. Mutations render carriers more susceptible to environmental insults to replicating stem cells. HLA-DR2 is twice as frequent than in the normal population.
- Autosomal recessive in congenital form

PATHOPHYSIOLOGY
- Injury to pluripotent stem cells causing markedly reduced hematopiesis and replacement of bone marrow by fat cells
- Current hypothesis supports stem cell destruction caused by activated autoimmune lymphocytes. Activation can arise from several causes mentioned below.
- Patients have high levels of interferon-γ gamma and fewer natural killer cells.
- Intact stromal function with normal to increased levels of cytokines and erythropoietin.

ETIOLOGY
- Idiopathic (~50% of the cases)
- Drugs (antibiotics, antirheumatics, anticonvulsants, chemotherapeutics, NSAIDs, sulfonamides.)
- Viral (HIV; EBV; postinfectious hepatitis-nonA, B, or C; parvovirus B_{19}, mostly in the immunocompromised; atypical mycobacterium)
- Toxic exposure (benzene, pesticides, arsenic)
- Radiation exposure
- Immune disorders(systemic lupus erythematous, eosinophilic fascitis, graft versus host disease)
- Pregnancy (rare)
- Congenital (Fanconi anemia, dyskeratosis congenita, Shwachman-Diamond syndrome, amegakaryocytic thrombocytopenia)

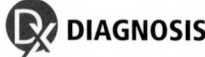 **DIAGNOSIS**

SIGNS AND SYMPTOMS
History
Recurrent infections

Physical Exam
- Mucosal hemorrhage, petechiae
- Pallor
- Fatigue, fever
- Hemorrhage, menorrhagia, occult stool blood, melena, epistaxis
- Dyspnea
- Palpitations
- Progressive weakness
- Retinal flame hemorrhages
- Systolic ejection murmur
- Weight loss
- Congenital
  - Short stature
  - Microcephaly
  - Radius and thumb anomalies
  - Renal anomalies
  - Skeletal anomalies
  - Hyperpigmentation (café au lait spots)
  - leukoplakia

TESTS
- Screening test to exclude other etiologies
- CBC and reticulocyte count
- Blood smear examination
  - Cytogenetic studies of peripheral lymphocytes if <35 to exclude fanconi anemia
  - Liver function test
  - Viral serology: Hepatitis A, B, C, EBV, CMV, HIV
  - Vitamin B_{12} and folate levels
  - Autoantibody screening ANA and anti-DNA
  - Flow cytometry or Ham test for PNH
  - Fetal hemoglobin in children
  - Red cell adenosine deaminase (pure red cell aplasia)
  - Cytogenetic analysis of bone marrow

Lab
- Pancytopenia
- Anemia
- Leukopenia
- Neutropenia
- Thrombocytopenia
- Decreased reticulocytes
- Increased serum iron secondary to transfusion
- Normal total iron binding capacity (TIBC)
- Borderline high mean corpuscular volume (MCV) >104
- CD 34$^+$ cells decreased in blood and marrow
- Hematuria
- Abnormal liver function tests (hepatitis)
- Increased fetal hemoglobin (Fanconi)
- Increased chromosomal breaks under specialized conditions (Fanconi)
- Molecular determination of abnormal gene (Fanconi)

Imaging
- CT of thymus region if thymoma-associated RBC aplasia suspected
- Radiographs of radius and thumbs (congenital anemia)
- Renal ultrasound (to rule out congenital anemia or malignant hematological disorder)
- Chest radiograph to exclude infection such as mycobacterial

Diagnostic Procedures/Surgery

Bone marrow aspirate and trephine biopsy

Pathological Findings

- Normochromic RBC
- Bone marrow
  - Decreased cellularity (<10%)
  - Decreased megakaryocytes
  - Decreased myelocytes
  - Decreased erythroid precursors
  - Prominent fat spaces
  - Prominent lymphocytes, macrophages and plasma cells

DIFFERENTIAL DIAGNOSIS

- Myelodysplastic disorders and acute myeloid leukemia; dysplastic cells of the granulocytic and megakaryocytic lineages, blast cells in the marrow
- Paroxysmal nocturnal hemoglobinuria, hemolytic anemia (dark urine), pancytopenia venous thrombosis (classically hepatic veins)
- Acute lymphoblastic leukemia-neutropenia more pronounced than pancytopenia, may have an increase in reticulin in the bone marrow
- Hairy cell leukemia; increased reticulin and infiltration of hairy cells
- Systemic lupus erythematosus
- Lymphomas; gene rearrangements
- Prolonged starvation or anorexia nervosa; bone marrow is gelatinous with loss of fat cells and increased ground substance
- Transient erythroblastopenia of childhood

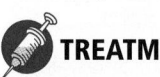 ## TREATMENT

INITIAL STABILIZATION

Inpatient. Referral to an institution that has experience in treating these patients is recommended.

GENERAL MEASURES

- Supportive measures: RBC and platelet transfusions. Use only CMV negative blood initially if patient is candidate for BMT.
- Oxygen therapy for severe anemia
- Good oral hygiene
- Control menorrhagia with norethisterone
- Avoid causative agents/isolation if necessary
- Human leukocyte antigen (HLA) testing on all patients and their immediate families
- Transfusion support (judiciously prescribed RBCs for severe anemia, consider leukocyte depleted units; platelets for severe thrombocytopenia; WBCs)
  - Transfuse when platelet count is $<10 \times 10^9$ or if $<20 \times 10^9$ with fever (1)[C]
- Immunosuppressive therapy (antithymocyte globulin [ATG] and cyclosporine) if no suitable donor

Diet

No special diet, but nutritious diet is important to improve resistance to infection.

Activity

Isolation procedures if neutropenic in addition to prophylactic antibiotic and antifungal

Nursing

If neutropenic, use antiseptic mouthwash such as chlorhexidine and give food low in bacterial content.

 ## MEDICATION (DRUGS)

- Antithymocyte globulin (ATG):
  - A horse serum containing polyclonal antibodies against human T cells. Skin test patients to determine any hypersensitivity.
  - Treatment for patients >40 and patient without a compatible donor. Consider in patients 30–40.
  - May be used as a single agent or in combination with cyclosporine. Increased efficacy with combination for children and patients with absolute neutropenia.
- Cyclosporine following initial ATG therapy for minimum of 6 months
  - Monitor through blood levels. Normal values for assays vary.
  - A 3–6 month trial may be necessary.
- Androgens
  - Clinical trials are inconclusive.
  - Useful for some patients lacking other options and less severe patients
- Oxymetholone: 1–2 mg/kg/d PO
  - A 2–3 month trial is usually necessary to assess the response.
- Prednisone for pure red cell anemia
- Note: Relapses may occur after the initial response to the immunosuppressive therapy if cyclosporine is discontinued too early.

SURGERY

- Bone marrow transplantation for patients with severe aplastic anemia and an HLA–identical donor, <30 years old. Consider in patients 30–40 in good general medical condition
  - Bone marrow stem cells and not mobilized peripheral stem cells should be used (B)
- Patients >40 have higher rates of graft versus host disease and graft rejection compared with children. Conditioning regimens are also poorly tolerated by older patients
- Unrelated donor transplants, if other therapy fails and/or <16 without HLA-matched sibling
- Thymectomy for thymoma

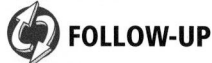 ## FOLLOW-UP

PROGNOSIS

- Bone marrow transplantation with HLA-matched sibling: Long-term survival 75–80%
- Immunosuppressive therapy using ATG and cyclosporin: Overall survival of 75%; 90% among responders at 5 years.

COMPLICATIONS

- Infection(fungal, sepsis)
- Graft versus host disease in bone marrow transplant recipients (acute 18% chronic 26%)
- Side effects of immunosuppressant medications
- Hemorrhage
- Transfusion hemosiderosis
- Transfusion hepatitis
- Heart failure
- Development of leukemia or myelodysplasia (15–19% risk at 6–10 years
- Refractory pancytopenia

PATIENT MONITORING

Close monitoring for all treatments is recommended. Drugs and other forms of treatment have numerous and severe side effects.

REFERENCES

1. Marsh Ball, et al. Guidelines for diagnosis and treatment of acquired aplastic anemia. *Br J Haematol*. 2003;123(5):782–801.
2. Young, Abkowitz, Luzzatto. New insights into the pathophysiology of acquired aplastic anemia. *Hematology*. 2000;18–38.
3. Young NS. Acquired aplastic anemia. *Ann Intern Med*. 2002;136(7):534–546.

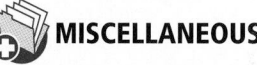 ## MISCELLANEOUS

See also: Leukemia, hairy cell; Myelodysplastic syndromes (MDS); Systemic lupus erythematosus (SLE)

CODES

ICD9-CM

284.9 Aplastic anemia, unspecified

PATIENT TEACHING

Printed patient information available from: Aplastic Anemia Foundation of America, P.O. Box 22689, Baltimore, MD 21203; (410) 955-2803.

 See Corresponding Diagnostic Algorithm

ANEMIA, AUTOIMMUNE HEMOLYTIC

Kerry J. Murphy, MD

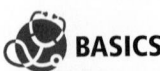 **BASICS**

DESCRIPTION
- Acquired anemia induced by binding of autoantibodies to RBC membrane antigens
- 3 main types defined by maximal binding temperature of the autoantibodies
  - Warm (37°C [98.6°F]) reacting IgG antibody
  - Cold (0–4°C [32–39.2°F]) reacting IgM antibody
  - Mixed type: Both warm IgG and cold C3 reacting antibodies
  - Drug induced: Mostly warm IgG reacting antibodies
  - System(s) Affected Hematopoietic/lymphatic/immunologic

GENERAL PREVENTION
None known

EPIDEMIOLOGY
- Predominant age: <50 years
- Predominant sex: Female > Male

Geriatric Considerations
Unusual in this age group; rule out neoplasia.

Pediatric Considerations
May occur in pediatric age group

Incidence
4/100,000 per year

RISK FACTORS
- Malignancy
- Autoimmune disorders
- Infection
- Medications
- Prior blood transfusion
- Prior hematopoietic cell transplant

Genetics
Unknown

PATHOPHYSIOLOGY
- Warm autoimmune hemolytic anemia (AIHA)
  - IgG attaches to RBCs, which are then ingested by macrophages of the spleen.
- Cold AIHA
  - IgM binds RBC surface temporarily, activates complement, deposits C3 on cell surface, and RBCs are ingested by macrophages of the liver.
  - Rarely, complete complement cascade activated with membrane attack complex insertion causing intravascular hemolysis.
- Mixed antibody AIHA: Both warm IgG and cold C3 involved.
- Drug induced
  - Hapten induced: Drug attaches to rbc membrane inducing IgG production.
  - Immune complex: Drug–IgM immune complex binds RBC membrane, activating complement.
  - Autoantibody: Drug induces production of anti-RBC IgG.

ETIOLOGY
- Warm antibody (48–70% cases)
  - Primary cause: Idiopathic
  - Secondary causes
    ○ Lymphoproliferative disorders (CLL, Hodgkin disease, NHL)
    ○ Autoimmune disorders
    ○ Viral infection (especially in children)
- Cold antibody
  - Cold agglutinin syndrome (CAS) (16–32%):
    ○ Acute: Infection (mycoplasma, mononucleosis, viral)
    ○ Chronic: Lymphoproliferative disorders (lymphoma)
  - Paroxysmal cold hemoglobinuria
    ○ Infection
- Mixed type
  - Idiopathic
  - Secondary to lymphoproliferative or autoimmune disorders
- Drug induced
  - Penicillin: Hapten induced
  - Quinine: Immune complex
  - α-Methyldopa: Autoantibody induced

ASSOCIATED CONDITIONS
- Evans syndrome
- Systemic lupus erythematosus
- Chronic lymphocytic leukemia
- Diffuse lymphomas

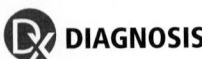 **DIAGNOSIS**

SIGNS AND SYMPTOMS

History
- Weakness/fatigue
- Exertional dyspnea
- Dizziness
- Palpitations
- Malaise
- Association with cold (CAS)

Physical Exam
- Pallor
- Jaundice
- Splenomegaly
- Hepatomegaly
- Tachycardia
- Flow murmur
- Blue gray discoloration of acral surfaces (CAS)

TESTS

Lab
- Direct Coombs' (DAT direct antiglobulin test)
  - Positive test indicates presence of antibodies or complement on RBC surface.
- CBC
  - Anemia (normocytic, normochromic); may be sudden and life threatening
  - Mild to moderate increase in mean corpuscular volume (MCV) depending on level of reticulocytosis
  - Increased mean cell hemoglobin concentration (MCHC)
  - Spherocytosis
  - Poikilocytosis
  - Anisocytosis
  - Rouleaux
  - Reticulocytosis
  - Nucleated RBC
  - Large polychromatophilic reticulocytes
- Hyperbilirubinemia (unconjugated)
- Decreased haptoglobin
- Elevated LDH
- Hemoglobinemia
- Serology
  - IgG antibody (warm, mixed, drug-induced, paroxysmal hemoglobinuria)
  - IgM antibody (cold)
- Urinalysis
  - Hemoglobinuria, hemosiderinuria

Pathological Findings
- Peripheral blood smear
  - Spherocytes, schistocytes
- Bone marrow biopsy
  - Bone marrow hyperplasia, increased marrow hemosiderin

DIFFERENTIAL DIAGNOSIS
- Other hemolytic anemias
- Autoimmune thrombocytopenic purpura (ITP)
- Evans syndrome
- Microangiopathic hemolytic disorders
- Aplastic anemia
- Megaloblastic anemia

TREATMENT

GENERAL MEASURES
- Warm antibody
  - Folic acid supplementation
  - Mild and moderate: See "Medications"
  - Severe
    - Plasmapheresis as a temporizing measure for refractory or life threatening anemia (1)[C]
    - Packed RBC transfusion for life-threatening anemia (difficult to cross-match; need special blood bank techniques; in emergency, use most compatible cross-match (2)[C]
- Cold antibody
  - Cold agglutinin syndrome
    - Avoid cold, maintain high temperatures indoors, wear additional clothing outdoors
    - Folic acid supplementation
    - Plasmapheresis as a temporizing measure for refractory or life-threatening anemia (1)[C]
    - Packed RBC transfusion for life-threatening anemia (2)[C]
- Paroxysmal cold hemoglobinuria
  - Supportive care
- Mixed
  - Steroids, splenectomy, and immunosuppressives as in warm AIHA
- Drug-induced
  - Stop the offending drug.
  - Plasmapheresis/exchange transfusion for severe life-threatening cases

Diet
No special diet

Activity
- Rest until asymptomatic.
- Avoid contact sports if splenomegaly is present.

MEDICATION (DRUGS)

First Line
- Warm antibody
  - Glucocorticoids: Prednisone 1 mg/kg/d PO in divided doses
    - 70–80% patients improve within 3 weeks
    - Taper gradually to 20 mg/d over 2 weeks
    - May require maintenance dose 10 mg every other day (1)[A]
  - Precautions: Significant side effects with long-term use
- Cold antibody
  - Malignancy induced: Chemotherapy
  - Rituximab for cold AIHA due to chronic lymphoproliferative disorders (1)[C]
- Mixed antibody
  - Prednisone as in warm AIHA

Second Line
- Warm antibody
  - Immunosuppressive drugs: Recommended for patients who fail splenectomy, relapse after splenectomy, cannot tolerate corticosteroids, and nonsurgical candidates
    - Cyclophosphamide 50 mg/kg/d for 4 days followed by GCSF for those with refractory anemia (2)[C]
    - Precautions: Monitor for marrow suppression
    - Azathioprine (Imuran) 1–2 mg/kg/d within 2 weeks of starting steroids if not responding (3)[C]
    - Cyclosporine 5–10 mg/kg/d in 2 divided doses
    - Rituximab (anti-CD20 monoclonal Ab) 375 mg/m^2 once weekly for 2–4 weeks for children and refractory cases
    - Mycophenolate mofetil 500–1000 mg/d in 2 divided doses; increase to 1–2 g daily (2)[C]
  - Other medical therapies for refractory cases
    - Danazol 600–800 mg/d PO
    - IVIG (1)[C]
- Mixed antibody
  - Immunosuppressives if refractory to steroids and splenectomy

SURGERY
- Warm antibody
  - Splenectomy is the preferred second-line treatment for warm AIHA for those who have failed steroids.
    - 50% initial response rate
    - Patients may require low-dose maintenance prednisone <15 mg daily
    - Post splenectomy: Vaccinate against encapsulated organisms such as pneumonococcus and meningococcus (2)[A]
- Cold antibody
  - Surgery not recommended
- Mixed antibody
  - Splenectomy

FOLLOW-UP

PROGNOSIS
- Good with appropriate treatment
- Determined by course of the primary disease If secondary to an underlying disorder

COMPLICATIONS
- Shock (severe anemia)
- Venous thromboembolism
- Thrombocytopenic purpura (Evans syndrome)
- Lymphoproliferative disorders in warm AIHA
- Post splenectomy sepsis syndrome

PATIENT MONITORING
- Monitor carefully if transfusion essential
- Use only warm IV fluids and blood products for cold AIHA
- Avoid hypothermic surgical procedures for cold AIHA

REFERENCES

1. Gehrs BC, Friedberg RC. Autoimmune hemolytic anemia. *Amer J Hematol*, 2002;69:258–271.
2. King KE, Ness PM. Treatment of autoimmune hemolytic anemia. *Sem in Hematology*, 2005; 42:131–136.
3. Pruss A, Salama A, Ahrens N, Hansen A, Kiesewetter H, Koscielny J, Dorner T. Immune hemolysis-serological and clinical aspects. *Clin Exp Med*, 2003;3:55–64.

MISCELLANEOUS

See also: Leukemia; Lymphoma, Non-Hodgkin, Systemic Lupus Erythematosus (SLE)

CODES

ICD9-CM
283.0 Autoimmune hemolytic anemias

PATIENT TEACHING

See Corresponding Diagnostic Algorithm

ANEMIA, IRON DEFICIENCY

Bruce Block, MD

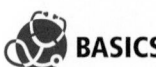 **BASICS**

DESCRIPTION
- Anemia due to decreased iron stores
- Poor iron utilization and poor iron re-utilization (e.g., anemia of chronic disease) are also due to iron deficiency, but iron stores are not depleted.
- Onset may be acute with rapid blood loss or chronic with poor diet or slow blood loss.
- Most common cause of anemia in the United States.
- System(s) Affected: Hemic/Lymphatic/Immunologic
- Synonym(s): Anemia of chronic blood loss; Hypochromic; Microcytic anemia; and Chlorosis

ALERT
Geriatric Considerations
60% of anemias in people >65 years
Pediatric Considerations
Frequent problem in infants whose major source of nutrition is cow's milk and juices.
Pregnancy Considerations
Common during pregnancy unless iron supplements are included in the diet.

GENERAL PREVENTION
- Good nutrition with adequate iron intake
- Correction of gynecologic or other problems causing excess blood loss

EPIDEMIOLOGY
- Predominant age: All ages, but especially toddlers and menstruating women.
- Predominant sex: Female > Male

Incidence
- Adults: 7–10%
- Infants and toddlers: 10–20%
- Pregnant patients: 15–45%

Prevalence
- Most likely in the poor and in underimmunized children

ETIOLOGY
- Blood loss (e.g., menses, GI bleed)
- Poor iron intake
- Poor iron absorption (e.g., postgastrectomy)
- Increased demand for iron (e.g., infancy, adolescence, and pregnancy)
- Hookworm infestation
- Gastric carcinoma

DIAGNOSIS

SIGNS AND SYMPTOMS
- Asymptomatic in most cases
- Cheilosis
- Dyspnea on exertion, fatigue, tachycardia, palpitation, or vasomotor disturbances
- Effects of underlying GI ulceration, neoplasm, uterine disorders, or bleeding varices
- Headache, inability to concentrate, irritability, listlessness
- Neuralgic pain, peripheral paresthesias
- Pica (dirt, paint, ice)
- Spoon-shaped, brittle nails
- Susceptibility to infection

TESTS
- Stool guaiac; if positive, GI endoscopy, stool for O & P, clotting studies
- Rule out thalassemia: Review prior CBCs for persisting mild anemia and marked micro-ovalocytosis, elevated hemoglobin A2 or hemoglobin F, family history, and especially high or high normal RBC count
- Rule out G6PD deficiency: Assay at least 6 weeks after last drop in hemoglobin
- Rule out poor re-utilization: Trial of iron (oral or parenteral), bone marrow aspiration, and iron stain
- Rule out gastric carcinoma, especially in the elderly

Lab
- Ferritin, repeat CBC with differential, peripheral smear
- Stainable iron in bone marrow aspiration is the gold standard
- Low serum ferritin is the best noninvasive test in adults, but it may miss some deficient patients, because ferritin is an acute phase reactant.
- Fe/total iron binding capacity (transferrin ratio) is no longer recommended, because it is less sensitive and less specific than ferritin.
- A peripheral smear usually shows hypochromia and microcytosis, but may be normal.
- Hemoglobin is usually lower than 12 g/dL, but patients with higher premorbid hemoglobin (such as smokers and patients with chronic hypoxemia) may be anemic at higher hemoglobin levels. Abnormal values for infants and toddlers, and for pregnant persons, are <10.5–11.0 g/dL.
- A low RBC count in chronic bleeding helps to distinguish it from thalassemia trait where the count is high or high-normal.

- Microcytosis with ovalocytosis and anemia unresponsive to iron suggest the thalassemia trait.
- A low MCV may be absent in mild anemia, or hidden by the population of larger cells (e.g., reticulocytes or macrocytes).
- An empiric trial of iron at 3 mg/kg/d may be the best way to diagnose decreased iron stores in infants and children, if reticulocytes are elevated in 7–10 days or hemoglobin is increased >1.0 g/dL after 4 weeks.
- Drugs that may alter lab results: Iron supplements or multivitamin–mineral preparations that contain iron
- Disorders that may alter lab results:
  - Ferritin elevated by acute liver disease, cirrhosis, Hodgkin disease, acute leukemia, solid tumors, fever, acute inflammation, renal dialysis
  - Hemoglobin may be elevated by smoking or chronic hypoxemia, thereby hiding anemia if standard anemia limits are used.

Imaging
GI endoscopy to discover occult bleeding sites

Pathological Findings
- Absent marrow iron stores
- Marrow: Hyperplastic, micronormoblastic

DIFFERENTIAL DIAGNOSIS
- Bone marrow aspiration
- Sigmoidoscopy
- Gastroscopy
- Colonoscopy
- Defective iron utilization (e.g., thalassemia trait, sideroblastosis, G6PD deficiency)
- Defective iron re-utilization (e.g., infection, inflammation, cancer, other chronic diseases)
- Hypoproliferation (e.g., decreased erythropoietin from hypothyroidism, renal failure, etc.)

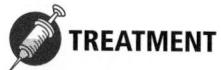 **TREATMENT**

INITIAL STABILIZATION
Outpatient

GENERAL MEASURES
- Search for the cause and correct it. There can be no excuse for not searching for a bleeding site.
- Avoid transfusions except in rare cases.

Diet
- Limit milk to 1 pint a day (adults).
- Emphasize protein-containing and iron-containing foods (meat, beans, and leafy green vegetables).
- Increase dietary fiber to decrease likelihood of constipation during iron replacement therapy.
- Do not consume milk, other dairy products, antacids, or tetracycline within 2 hours of the drug dosage.

Activity
Patients with hypoxemia, low cardiac output, or angina may require reduced activity prescriptions.

 MEDICATION (DRUGS)

FIRST LINE
- Ferrous sulfate 300 mg t.i.d. on an empty stomach 1 hour before meals is an ideal dose that provides 180 mg of elemental iron a day.
  - Dose can be reduced as needed for GI symptoms, which affect 15% of patients on standard iron therapy, or the dose can be taken with meals, which may reduce the delivery of iron by 50%.
  - People with a moderate anemia (hemoglobin = 10 g/dL) need only 1,500–2,000 mg of elemental iron replacement. Reducing the amount of iron per dose as much as necessary to abate symptoms will make parenteral iron therapy unnecessary in almost all cases.
  - Special iron formulations and compounds are very expensive and reduce symptoms only to the degree that they reduce the delivery of iron.
- Liquid iron preparations are useful for children with a recommended dose of 3 mg/kg/d given in a single dose. They can be also used in adults when low tolerance to iron pills requires a reduction of dosage.
- Vitamin C provides acidification to reduce the iron and thus increases absorption.
- Continued bleeding is often the cause for "failure to respond" to iron.
- Consider parenteral iron for patients with malabsorption, if higher doses and use of vitamin C fail.
- Contraindications
  - Antacids concomitantly
  - Tetracycline concomitantly
- Precautions
  - Iron preparations cause black bowel movements.
  - Iron overdose is highly toxic. Patients should be instructed to keep tablets and liquids out of the reach of small children.
- Significant possible interactions
  - Allopurinol
  - Antacids
  - Penicillamine
  - Tetracyclines
  - Vitamin E

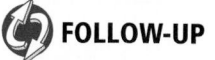 **FOLLOW-UP**

PROGNOSIS
Curable with iron therapy if the underlying cause can be discovered and cured

COMPLICATIONS
Neglecting to identify hidden bleeding points, particularly a bleeding malignancy

PATIENT MONITORING
Regularly after return to normal (in order to detect recurrences)

REFERENCES

1. Adams WG, et al. Anemia and elevated lead levels in underimmunized inner-city children. *Pediatrics*. 1998;101.
2. Farrell R, LaMont JT. Rational approach to iron-deficiency anaemia in premenopausal women. *Lancet*. 1998;352:1953–1954.
3. Fireman Z, Kopelman Y, Sternberg A. Endoscopic evaluation of iron deficiency anemia and follow-up in patients older than age 50. *J Clin Gastroenterol*. 1998;26:7–10.
4. Lee RG, Bithell TC, et al. *Wintrobe's Clinical Hematology*. 9th ed. Philadelphia, PA: Lea & Febiger; 1993.
5. Van den Broek, et al. Iron status in pregnant women: Which measurements are valid? *Br J Haematol*. 1998;103:817–824.
6. Waterbury L. Anemia. In: Barker LR, Burton JR, Zieve PD, eds. *Principles of Ambulatory Medicine*. 4th ed. Philadelphia, PA: Lippincott Williams & Wilkins; 1995:593–607.
7. Williams WJ, Beutler E, Erslev AJ, et al., eds. *Hematology*. 4th ed. New York, NY: McGraw-Hill; 1990.

 MISCELLANEOUS

CODES

ICD9-CM
280.9 Iron deficiency anemia, unspecified

PATIENT TEACHING

National Heart, Lung & Blood Institute, Communications & Public Information Branch, National Institutes of Health, Building 31, Room 41-21, 9000 Rockville Pike, Bethesda, MD 20892; (301) 251-1222.

 See Corresponding Diagnostic Algorithm

ANEMIA, PERNICIOUS

Abdulrazak Abyad, MD, PhD, MBA, MPH, AGSF

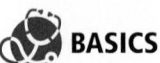 **BASICS**

DESCRIPTION

Pernicious anemia is a disorder due to vitamin B_{12} deficiency. It is invariably associated with atrophic gastritis and histamine-fast achlorhydria. Vitamin B_{12} cannot be absorbed in the terminal ileum without intrinsic factor (a secretion of the parietal cells of the gastric mucosa). Its usual course is slowly progressive.

- System(s) Affected: Gastrointestinal; Hematologic/Lymphatic/Immunologic; Nervous
- Synonym(s): Addison anemia; Megaloblastic anemia due to B_{12} deficiency

ALERT

Geriatric Considerations
More common in this age group and often in association with other autoimmune disorders, depression, and dementia

Pediatric Considerations
- Juvenile pernicious anemia occurs in older children and is the same in most respects as in adults.
- Congenital pernicious anemia is usually evident before 3 years of age.

Pregnancy Considerations
Untreated pernicious anemia in pregnancy may cause neural tube defects.

GENERAL PREVENTION
- Early detection of anemia
- Workup of anemia

EPIDEMIOLOGY
Predominant sex: Male = Female

Incidence
Unknown

Prevalence
Older adults (>60 years)

RISK FACTORS
- Vegetarian diet, without B_{12} supplementation
- Gastrectomy
- Blind loop syndrome
- Fish-tapeworm infestation
- Malabsorption syndromes
- Drugs: Oral calcium-chelating drugs, amino salicylic acid, and biguanides
- Chronic pancreatitis
- Alcoholism

Genetics
- HLA-DR2, HLA-DR4: Present in the rare form of pernicious anemia that is hereditary
- Endemic area: Northern Europe, including Scandinavia

ETIOLOGY
- Atrophic gastric mucosa
- Intrinsic factor deficiency
- Probable autoimmunity against gastric parietal cells
- Autoimmunity against intrinsic factor

ASSOCIATED CONDITIONS
- Autoimmune diseases including rheumatoid arthritis, IgA deficiency
- Graves disease
- Myxedema
- Iron deficiency
- Thyroiditis
- Vitiligo
- Idiopathic adrenocortical insufficiency
- Hypoparathyroidism
- Agammaglobulinemia
- Tropical sprue
- Celiac disease
- Crohn's disease
- Infiltrate disorders of the ileum and small intestine

DIAGNOSIS

SIGNS AND SYMPTOMS

History
- Anorexia, weight loss
- Depression
- Position sense: Decreased
- Prematurely gray-haired
- Tinnitus

Physical Exam
- Abnormal reflexes
- Ataxia
- Atrophic glossitis
- Babinski's sign: Positive
- Confusion
- Congestive heart failure
- Dementia
- Exertional dyspnea
- Extremity numbness
- Extremity paresthesias
- Hepatomegaly
- Hypoalgesia in "sock and glove" distribution
- Pallor
- Palpitations
- Poor finger coordination
- Purpura
- Romberg's sign: Positive
- Skin pigmentation increased
- Sore tongue
- Splenomegaly
- Tachycardia
- Vertigo
- Vibration sense: Decreased
- Vitiligo
- Weakness

TESTS
- Schilling test plus intrinsic factor: Normal vitamin B_{12} absorption
- Schilling test: Decreased vitamin B_{12} absorption
- Gastric analysis: Achlorhydria

Lab
- Achlorhydria
- Anisocytosis
- Haptoglobin decreased
- Howell-Jolly bodies
- Hypergastrinemia
- Hypersegmented neutrophils
- LDH increased
- Leukopenia
- Macrocytic anemia; MCV: 110–140
- Pentagastrin stimulation: Stomach pH >6
- Serum ferritin increased
- Serum vitamin B_{12} level <100 pg/mL (<74 pmol/L)
- Peripheral blood smear: Macro-ovalocytes
- Poikilocytes
- Thrombocytopenia
- Anti-intrinsic poikilocytosis factor antibody
- Anti-parietal cell antibody
- Direct hyperbilirubinemia
- Disorders that may alter lab results
  - Falsely elevated MCV
    - Cold agglutinins
    - Hyperglycemia
    - Marked hyperleukocytosis
  - Falsely normal serum vitamin B_{12} level
    - Myeloproliferative disorders
    - Liver disease
  - Falsely low serum B_{12} level
    - Multiple myeloma
    - Oral contraceptive intake
    - Pregnancy
    - Folate deficiency
    - Transcobalamin I deficiency
    - Recent isotope administration

Diagnostic Procedures/Surgery
- Bone marrow aspiration
- Detailed history and physical exam

Pathological Findings
- Bone marrow: Hypercellular, macrocytes, iron stores increased
- Nests of megaloblasts
- Giant metamyelocytes
- Macro-polymorpho-leukocytes
- Hypersegmented neutrophils
- Stomach: Atrophic gastritis, goblet cells increased
- Parietal cell atrophy
- Chief cell atrophy
- Gastric cytology: Cellular atypia
- Spinal cord: Myelin degeneration of the dorsal and lateral tracts
- Peripheral nerve degeneration
- Degenerative changes of the posterior root ganglia

DIFFERENTIAL DIAGNOSIS
- Folic acid deficiency
- Myelodysplasia
- Neurological disorders without B_{12} deficiency
- Liver dysfunction
- Hypothyroidism
- Hemolysis or bleeding
- Drug effects
- Alcoholism

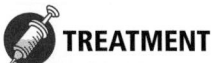 **TREATMENT**

GENERAL MEASURES
- Appropriate health care: Outpatient
- Treatment must be continued for life
- Identification and treatment of the underlying disorder

ALERT
Folic acid treatment without vitamin B_{12} in patients with pernicious anemia is contraindicated.

Diet
Emphasize meat, animal protein foods, and legumes unless contraindicated.

Activity
Unlimited

 MEDICATION (DRUGS)

- Parenteral Vitamin B_{12} (cyanocobalamin)
  - 1,000 mcg SQ for each dose
  - Administer daily for the 1st week
  - Administer weekly for 1 month
  - Monthly injections for remainder of life (patients may be taught to give self-injection)
- Precautions: Do not give folic acid supplements without vitamin B_{12}, may cause fulminant neurological deficit.

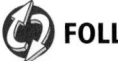 **FOLLOW-UP**

PROGNOSIS
- Anemia reversible with parenteral vitamin B_{12}
- Neurologic effects not reversible with parenteral vitamin B_{12}

COMPLICATIONS
- Hypokalemia may complicate the 1st week of treatment.
- Central nervous system symptoms may be permanent if patient is not treated in <6 months after the symptoms begin.
- Gastric polyps
- Stomach cancer
  - There is a 3-fold likelihood of developing gastric carcinoma.
  - Suggest endoscopy approximately every 5 years even if asymptomatic.

PATIENT MONITORING
- Monthly injections of vitamin B_{12}
- Endoscopy every 5 years to rule out gastric carcinoma

REFERENCES

1. Bennett JC, Plum F, eds. *Cecil Textbook of Medicine*. 20th ed. Philadelphia, PA: WB Saunders; 1996.
2. Chui CH, Lau FY, Wong R, et al. Vitamin B_{12} deficiency-need for a new guideline. *Nutrition*. 2001;17:917–920.
3. Wheby MS, ed. *The Medical Clinic of North America: Anemia. Vol. 76*. Philadelphia, PA: WB Saunders; 1992.
4. Williams WJ, Beutler E, Erslev AJ, et al., eds. *Hematology*. 4th ed. New York, NY: McGraw-Hill; 1990.

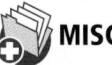 **MISCELLANEOUS**

See also: Tropical Sprue

CODES

ICD9-CM
- 281.0 Pernicious anemia
- 281.1 Other vitamin B_{12} deficiency anemia

PATIENT TEACHING

Griffith, HW: Instructions for Patients, WB Saunders, Philadelphia (instructions to photocopy for patient)

 See Corresponding Diagnostic Algorithm

ANEMIA, SICKLE CELL

Diane M. Haleem, PhD, RN

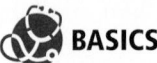 **BASICS**

DESCRIPTION

- A chronic hemoglobinopathy transmitted genetically; marked by moderately severe chronic hemolytic anemia, periodic acute episodes of painful "crises," and increased susceptibility to intercurrent infections, especially *Saccharomyces pneumoniae*.
- The heterozygous condition (Hb A/S) is called sickle cell trait and is usually asymptomatic with no anemia.
- System(s) Affected: Hematologic, Lymphatic/immunologic; Musculoskeletal
- Synonym(s): Sickle cell disease; Hb S disease

ALERT
Pediatric Considerations
- Sequestration crises and hand-foot syndrome seen only in infants/young children
- Functional asplenia in later childhood
- Adolescence/young adulthood
  - Frequency of complications and organ/tissue damage increase with age (except for strokes, which occur mostly in childhood).
  - Psychological complications: Body-image and sexual identity problems, interrupted schooling, career, restriction of activities, stigma of disease, low self-esteem
- Consider periodic transcranial Doppler ultrasound in all children ages 2–16

Pregnancy Considerations
- Usually complicated and hazardous, especially 3rd trimester and delivery
- Increased risk of crises, toxemia, infection, pulmonary infarction, phlebitis
- Fetal mortality 35–40%
- Partial exchange transfusion in 3rd trimester reduces maternal morbidity and fetal mortality.
- Chronic transfusions have been effective in diminishing episodes in pregnant women.

GENERAL PREVENTION
- Avoid conditions that precipitate sickling (hypoxia, dehydration, cold, infection, fever, acidosis, anesthesia).
- Granulocyte colony-stimulating factor is absolutely contraindicated.

EPIDEMIOLOGY
- Predominant age: All ages
- Predominant sex: Male = Female

Incidence
- ~1/500 African Americans and 1/1,000 Hispanics have sickle cell anemia.
- 10% African Americans have sickle trait.
- To a lesser extent, people from the Middle East, Mediterranean area, and aboriginal tribes in India

RISK FACTORS
- Vaso-occlusive crisis
  - Hypoxia
  - Dehydration, fever
  - Infection
  - Acidosis, cold
  - Anesthesia
  - Strenuous physical exercise
  - Smoking
- Aplastic crisis
  - Severe infections
  - Human parvovirus B_{19} infection
  - Folic acid deficiency
- Hyperhemolytic crisis
  - Acute bacterial infections
  - Exposure to oxidant drugs

Genetics
- Autosomal recessive, mostly in African Americans.
- Homozygous presence of a variant hemoglobin, Hb S, or sickle hemoglobin
- Heterozygous condition Hb A/S

ETIOLOGY
- At molecular level: Hb S is produced by substitution of valine for glutamic acid in the 6th amino acid position of the β-chains of the hemoglobin molecule. When deoxygenated, Hb S polymerizes and forms long rods that change RBC from biconcave to sickle shape.
- At cellular level: Sickle RBCs are inflexible; their odd shape and cell rigidity cause increased blood viscosity, stasis, mechanical obstruction of small arterioles and capillaries, and ischemia. Sickle RBCs are fragile, leading to hemolysis.
- At clinical level: Chronic anemia; "crises";
  - Vaso-occlusive crisis ("painful crisis"): Most common; pain results from tissue necrosis secondary to vascular occlusion and tissue hypoxia. Progressive organ failure and acute tissue damage result from repeated vaso-occlusive episodes.
  - Aplastic crisis: Suppression of RBC production by severe infection
  - Hyperhemolytic crisis: Accelerated hemolysis; increased RBC fragility/shortened lifespan
  - Sequestration crisis: Splenic sequestration of blood (only in infants/young children)
  - Susceptibility to infection: Impaired/absent splenic function; defect in the alternate pathway of complement activation

ASSOCIATED CONDITIONS
The psychosocial effects can result in low self-esteem, depression, and dependency.

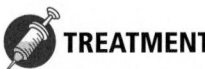 **DIAGNOSIS**

SIGNS AND SYMPTOMS
History
- Chronic hemolytic anemia
- Mild scleral icterus
- Increased infection risk, i.e., pneumococcal sepsis and *Salmonella* osteomyelitis
- Functional asplenia by ~5–6 years of age
- Delayed physical/sexual maturation

Physical Exam
- After 6 months of age, earliest symptoms are pallor and symmetric, painful swelling of the hands and feet (hand-foot syndrome).
- Often asymptomatic in early months of life
- Painful "crises" in bones, joints, abdomen, back, and viscera (90% of all hospital admissions)
- Acute chest syndrome S&S tachycardia, fever, bilateral infiltrates caused by decrease in hemoglobin and infarction of pulmonary vasculature (clinical picture consistent with pneumonia and/or infection)
- Many multisystem complications, especially in later childhood and adolescence

TESTS
Lab
- Hb electrophoresis
- Sickle cell anemia (FS pattern): 80–100% Hb S, variable amounts of Hb F and no Hb A. Sickle cell trait (FS pattern): 20–40% Hb S, 60–80% Hb A1, minimal Hb F.
- Screening tests: Sodium metabisulfite reduction test; "Sickledex" test
- Hemoglobin approximately 8 g/dL (1.24 mmol/L); RBC indices usually normal, but mean corpuscular volume (MCV) >75 m^3 (>75 fL)
- Reticulocytosis of 10–20%
- Leukocytosis; bands in absence of infection
- Thrombocytosis
- Peripheral smear: Sickled RBCs, nucleated RBCs, Howell-Jolly bodies
- Serum bilirubin mildly elevated (2–4 mg/dL [34–68 mol/L]); fecal/urinary urobilinogen high
- ESR low
- Serum LDH elevated
- Haptoglobin absent or very low
- Disorders that may alter lab results: Infection

Imaging
- Bone scan (to rule out osteomyelitis)
- CT/MRI (to rule out CVA)
- Chest radiograph: May show enlarged heart; diffuse alveolar infiltrates in acute chest syndrome
- Transcranial Doppler: Start at age 2; repeat yearly (1,2,3)[B]
- Echocardiography to detect pulmonary hypertension (2,3)[C]

Pathological Findings
- In moderate to severe cases, hyposplenism due to autosplenectomy is common.
- Hypoxia/infarction in multiple organs

DIFFERENTIAL DIAGNOSIS
- Anemia: Other hemoglobinopathies (e.g., Hb SC disease, Hb C disease, sickle cell-β thalassemia)
- Painful crises: Other causes of acute pain in bones, joints, and abdomen

TREATMENT

INITIAL STABILIZATION
General health maintenance: Assessment of growth/development, regular immunizations, vision/hearing screening, and dental care

GENERAL MEASURES
- Infections/fever: Treatment with antibiotics
- Minimize factors that enhance sickling
- Painful crises: Hydration (2X maintenance fluids); analgesics; oxygen if hypoxic
- Transfusion needed with aplastic crises, severe complications (i.e., CVA), before surgery
- Retinal evaluation starting at school age to detect proliferative sickle retinopathy
- Occupational therapy
- Cognitive and behavioral intervention: Include distraction, relaxation, and motivational therapy
- Support groups

- Special immunizations (1,3)[B]
  – Influenza vaccine yearly starting at age 2
  – Heptavalent conjugated pneumococcal vaccine at 2, 4, 6 months; booster at 15 months, 2 years, 5 years
  – 23-valent pneumococcal vaccine at 2 years; booster at age 5; always separate this by 8 weeks from heptavalent vaccine
  – Meningococcal vaccine after age 2

Diet
- Folic acid supplementation
- Avoid alcohol (leads to dehydration)

Activity
Bed rest with crises

Physical Therapy
To include heat, massage, and exercise

IV Fluids
2X maintenance fluids (NS preferred) for severe painful crises (2)[C]

 MEDICATION (DRUGS)

First Line
- Supplemental oxygen
- Painful crises (mild, outpatient)
  – Nonnarcotic analgesics (ibuprofen, tramadol) (1,2,3)[C]

- Painful crises (severe, hospitalized) (1,2,3)[B]
  – Parenteral narcotics (e.g., morphine on fixed schedule); (PCA pump may be useful.)
  – Corticosteroids (dexamethasone 0.3 mg/kg q12h for 4 doses in children) may be used for painful crisis or chest syndrome.

- Prevention of painful crisis
  – Hydroxyurea (increases hemoglobin F levels thus decreasing permanent formation of sickle cells.) in adult patients with ≥3 crisis/year. Start with 15 mg/kg/d single daily dose; titrate upward every 12 weeks if blood counts satisfactory. Increase in 5 mg/kg increments to maximum of 35 mg/kg/d. Reduces crisis and chest syndrome 50%; long-term safety unknown. Contraindicated in pregnancy (2–4)[A].
  – Inhaled nitric oxide, arginine butyrate (has anti-sticking properties; may enhance availability of nitric oxide) and combination of erythropoietin with hydroxyurea (2,4)[B].

- For infections prior to culture results (2,3)[C], prescribe an antibiotic that covers *S. pneumoniae*, *H. influenzae*, mycoplasma pneumoniae, and *Chlamydia pneumoniae*. If osteomyelitis, cover for *Staphylococcus aureus* and *Salmonella*.

- Prophylactic penicillin is indicated in all infants and children starting at 2 months (1,4)[A].
  – For 2–6 months of age: 62.5 mg b.i.d.
  – For 6 months–3 years: 125 mg b.i.d.
  – For 3–5 years: 250 mg b.i.d.
  – If no pneumococcal infections and no splenectomy stop at 6 years; if high risk remains, continue until puberty.
  – Alternative penicillin, benzathine IM 300,000 U/mo, ages 4 months–3 years, then 600,000 U/mo for 3–5 years
  – Rising pneumococcal resistance to penicillin may change future recommendations.

- Precautions: Avoid high-dose estrogen oral contraceptives; consider Depo-Provera.

Second Line
- Other NSAIDs
- Folic acid supplements (1,3)[C]
  – From 0–6 months: 0.1 mg/d
  – From 6–12 months: 0.25 mg/d
  – From 1–2 years: 0.5 mg/d
  – Beyond age 2: 1 mg/d

SURGERY
Bone marrow transplantation is curative, but the availability is limited.

 FOLLOW-UP

DISPOSITION
Admission Criteria
Severe pain, suspected infection or sepsis

PROGNOSIS
- Anemia is lifelong. In 2nd decade of life, patient usually experiences fewer crises, but complications are more frequent. Median age of death is 42 for men and 48 for women. Common causes are infections, thrombosis, pulmonary emboli, pulmonary hypertension, and renal failure.
- Children become anemic at infancy and begin to have sickle cell crisis at 1–2 years of age; some children die in their 1st year.

COMPLICATIONS
- Alloimmunization
- Bone infarct
- Aseptic necrosis of femoral head
- Cerebrovascular accidents (peak age 6–7)
  – In the 10% of patients who suffer these, transfusions q3–4 weeks will reduce the risk by 90%. Initiate based on abnormal transcranial Doppler. May require iron chelation therapy.
- Cardiac enlargement
- Pulmonary hypertension
- Cholelithiasis/abnormal liver function
- Chronic leg ulcers
- Poor wound healing
- Impotence
- Priapism
- Hematuria/hyposthenuria
- Renal concentrating and acidifying defects
- Retinopathy
- Acute chest syndrome (infection/infarction), leading to chronic pulmonary disease
- Infections (pneumonia, osteomyelitis, meningitis, pyelonephritis); sepsis
- Hemosiderosis (2° to multiple transfusions)
- Decreased intelligence, even without stroke
- Splenic infarction can occur by 10 years of age.
- Substance abuse related to chronic pain

PATIENT MONITORING
- Determined by number/severity of crises
- It is important to recognize and treat infections early. Parents and patients should be instructed that a temperature of ≥101°F (38.3°C) requires immediate medical attention.
- All febrile patients require cultures (blood/urine), chest radiograph, and CBC/reticulocytes.
- For patients who receive chronic transfusions, monitor for hepatitis and hemosiderosis.
- Begin periodic eye evaluations at age 5 to detect proliferative sickle retinopathy (1,3)[C].

REFERENCES

1. American Academy of Pediatrics, Section on Hematology/Oncology. Health supervision of children with sickle cell disease. *Pediatrics*. 2002;109:526–535.
2. Johnson CS, ed. Sickle cell disease. *Hematol Oncol Clin North Am*. 2005;19(5).
3. National Institutes of Health. The management of sickle cell disease, 4th ed. 2002. NH Publ# 02-2117.
4. Bonds DR. Three decades of innovation in the management of sickle cell disease. *Blood Rev*. 2005;19:99–110.
5. Stop Trial Investigators. Discontinuing prophylactic transfusions used to prevent stroke in sickle cell disease. *N Engl J Med*. 2005;353(26):2769–2778 .
6. Fischbach F. Nurse's Quick Reference to Common Laboratory and Diagnostic Tests, 3rd ed. Philadelphia: Lippincott, 2002.
7. Smeltzer SC, Bare BG, Hinkle JL, Cheever KH. Brunner & Suddarth's Textbook of Medical-Surgical Nursing, 11 ed. Philadelphia: Lippincott Williams & Wilkins, 2005.
8. Vichinsky EP. Pulmonary hypertension in sickle cell disease *N Engl J Med*. 2004;350(9):857–859.
9. Stuart MJ, Nagel RL. Sickle-cell disease. *Lancet*. 2004;364(9442):1343–1360.

CODES

ICD9-CM
282 Sickle cell disease, unspecified

PATIENT TEACHING
Prevention
- Guidelines for prompt management of fever, infections, pain, and specific complications should be reviewed at each visit.
- Stress importance of keeping well-hydrated.
- Teach early recognition of possible complications, especially priapism (persistent penile erection).
- Genetic counseling
- Avoidance of alcohol and smoking
- Stress importance of minimizing trauma, such as leg wounds; care using aseptic technique is imperative.

 See Corresponding Diagnostic Algorithm

ANEMIA, SIDEROBLASTIC

Anne C. Nofziger, MD

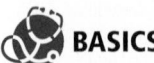 **BASICS**

DESCRIPTION
A heterogeneous group of disorders characterized by microcytic, hypochromic anemia, impaired heme biosynthesis causing ineffective erythropoiesis, and ringed sideroblasts in the bone marrow. Severity and course may range from severe progressive to indolent asymptomatic anemia; onset may be congenital or late in life.

GENERAL PREVENTION
Pyridoxine prophylaxis with INH therapy

EPIDEMIOLOGY
- As a group, sideroblastic anemias (SA) are uncommon, and specific incidence/prevalence information is difficult to find.
- Acquired forms more common than hereditary forms (1), usually occur in older adults; present in 25–30% of alcoholics with anemia (2)
- Several hundred X-linked cases described (3) Hereditary forms variably severe, usually manifest in childhood

RISK FACTORS
- Male gender (X-linked SA)
- Family history of hereditary SA
- Chronic alcohol abuse
- Gastric bypass surgery (1 case report) (4)

Genetics
- Usually X-linked
  - Defect in aminolevulinic acid synthase (ALAS-2 mutation), the first and rate-limiting enzyme in heme biosynthesis
  - With congenital ataxia: hABC7 gene mutations (mitochondrial transport protein)
- Rarely autosomal dominant or recessive; gene(s) unknown
- Mitochondrial cytopathy
  - Heterogeneous, involve deletions in mtDNA
  - Unpredictable maternal inheritance
- See "Etiology"

PATHOPHYSIOLOGY
- Impaired heme biosynthesis within mitochondria
- Ineffective erythropoiesis
- Increased GI absorption of iron (Fe overload)
- Enhanced apoptosis in bone marrow
- Possibly, reactive oxygen species play a role

ETIOLOGY
Acquired SA
- Reversible
- Drugs and toxins
  - Ethanol (SA is a later finding in multifactorial anemia related to alcoholism)
  - INH
  - Chloramphenicol
  - Cycloserine
  - Zinc toxicity (Cu deficiency)
- Nutritional deficiencies
  - Pyridoxine deficiency
  - Copper deficiency
    - Post-gastrectomy
    - Prolonged parenteral nutrition
    - Prolonged zinc supplementation
- Hypothermia
- Acquired idiopathic sideroblastic anemia (AISA)
  - Pure sideroblastic anemia (PSA)
    - Only the erythroid line affected
  - Refractory anemia with ringed sideroblasts (RARS)
    - Myelodysplasia, other cell lines also affected
  - Associated with hematologic malignancies, myeloproliferative disorders

Hereditary SA
- X-linked
- Autosomal dominant, recessive, maternal inheritance
- Mitochondrial cytopathy
  - Wolfram syndrome
  - Pearson syndrome

Congenital SA
Disproportionately male, sporadic, mild to severe, kindreds too small to analyze inheritance

ASSOCIATED CONDITIONS
- Alcoholism
- According to mutation, e.g., severe congenital ataxia (hABC7 mutation), pancreatic dysfunction (Pearson syndrome)
- Iron overload or "erythropoeitic hemochromatosis" (2) develops over time in all but reversible and x-linked/ataxia forms.
- Rarely, coexisting iron deficiency masks SA.

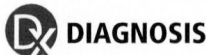 **DIAGNOSIS**

PRE HOSPITAL
Often an incidental finding

SIGNS AND SYMPTOMS
- Moderate to severe anemia
  - Fatigue
  - Dizziness
  - Diminished exercise tolerance
  - More symptomatic in older patients with comorbid conditions
- Specific to cause
  - Pyridoxine deficiency (peripheral neuropathy, dermatitis)
  - Alcoholism
- Manifestations of iron overload

History
- Toxin or drug exposures
- Family history of anemia, especially in men

Physical Exam
- No pathognomonic physical findings
- Mild-moderate hepatosplenomegaly at diagnosis in 1/3–1/2 of patients with AISA (2)

TESTS
Lab
- CBC
  - Low MCH
  - Low MCHC
  - Low MCV (may be normal or high, esp. in myelodysplasia)
  - High RDW
  - Hgb highly variable
  - Siderocytes in peripheral smear (occasional)
  - WBC normal; may be reduced if hypersplenism, myelodysplasia
  - Platelets normal; may be reduced if hypersplenism, myelodysplasia
  - Low reticulocyte count
- Iron studies
  - Ferritin increased
  - Transferrin saturation increased
  - Serum transferrin decreased
  - Reticuloendothelial iron increased

- Serum copper, ceruloplasmin, serum zinc if suspected as cause
- Liver enzyme derangements possible depending on cause (EtOH, cirrhosis, Fe overload)
- Molecular studies identify specific mutations causing hereditary SA syndromes
- Myelodysplasia: Morphologic and cytogenetic evaluation required for prognosis

Diagnostic Procedures/Surgery
- Bone marrow examination confirms diagnosis of SA
- Liver biopsy is best; test to assess degree of iron overload.
- See "Pathological Findings"

Pathological Findings
- Bone marrow examination is the key diagnostic modality (1)[C]
  - Normoblastic erythroid hyperplasia
  - Perls' Prussian blue iron stain: Ringed sideroblasts, >10% of erythroblasts with increased number of abnormally large granules ringing the nucleus
  - Electron microscopy: Iron-overloaded mitochondria within erythroblasts
  - Iron-laden macrophages
- Liver biopsy
  - Iron deposition as in hereditary hemachromatosis
  - Micronodular cirrhosis by 3rd or 4th decade

DIFFERENTIAL DIAGNOSIS
- Thalassemias
- Iron deficiency anemia
- Anemia of chronic disease
- Myelodysplastic syndromes
- Lead toxicity with anemia

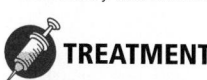 ## TREATMENT

GENERAL MEASURES
Treatment is largely supportive

- Pyridoxine supplementation improves symptoms in responsive cases (1)[B]
- Eliminate toxins, causative drugs
- Periodic transfusion: Maintain acceptable hemoglobin to alleviate symptoms and allow normal growth and development (children) (1)[B]
- Prevent end-organ damage from severe iron overload (1)[B]
  - Phlebotomy preferred modality if anemia is mild or moderate
  - Iron chelation in patients with more severe anemia, or requiring more transfusions

Diet
Address relevant nutritional deficiencies

Activity
As tolerated

SPECIAL THERAPY
Allogeneic stem cell transplantation has been successful in a few cases in younger patients with myelodysplastic syndromes.

IV Fluids
RBC transfusion when necessary

 ## MEDICATION (DRUGS)

First Line
- Trial of pyridoxine is indicated because it has few drawbacks and is very beneficial in responsive cases (1)[B]
  - Pyridoxine 50–100 mg PO daily
  - Maintenance: Minimum dose to maintain acceptable hgb.
  - Supplement folate to compensate for increased erythropoiesis if effective
  - Response likely if SA caused by alcohol abuse, pyridoxine antagonists, or some forms of hereditary x-linked SA.
- Chelation therapy for iron overload (1)[B]

- Deferoxamine 40 mg/kg/d in continuous 12–24-hour daily infusions
  - Limit ascorbate intake to 200 mg/d
  - Auditory/visual toxicity very rare
- Defirasirox is a new oral once-daily iron chelator
  - No long-term safety data
  - Main complications skin rash, GI upset
- Goal of therapy is to maintain serum ferritin <500 μg/L

Second Line
- Myelodysplasia: PSA and RARS
- Treatment considerations as above, though no expected response to pyridoxine
- Some respond to combination of erythropoeitin (EPO) and granulocyte colony-stimulating factor (G-CSF) (1)[C]
- Chemotherapeutic agents may have a role.

SURGERY
- Splenectomy is contraindicated due to frequent postoperative thromboembolic complications (2)[B].

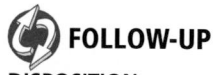 ## FOLLOW-UP

DISPOSITION
Admission Criteria
Generally managed in outpatient settings except for treatment of complications such as CHF, dysrhythmias.

Issues for Referral
- Hematology consultation is helpful for diagnosis and management, particularly if no reversible cause identified.
- Genetic counseling is important for patients with heritable cause of SA.

PROGNOSIS
- 75% of x-linked SA with ALAS-2 mutations are pyridoxine responsive (2)
- Prognosis better if iron overload prevented
- Aquired Idiopathic SA:
  - RARS: 1- and 5-year cumulative risk of acute leukemia are 20% and 38%, respectively (1)
  - When only the erythroid line is affected (PSA), course as in age-matched controls, transformation to leukemia not observed. (2)
  - If SA follows treatment for malignancy, leukemic transformation is common.

COMPLICATIONS
- Iron overload causing organ damage
  - Cardiac arrhythmia or CHF
  - Hepatic dysfunction
- Transfusion complications

PATIENT MONITORING
- Yearly ferritin and transferrin saturation to monitor for Fe overload
- Follow response to treatment: Reticulocytosis within 2 weeks, improved hgb within 1–2 months of response to pyridoxine, and correction of nutritional deficiency or withdrawal of reversible cause.

REFERENCES
1. Alcindor T, Bridges KR. Sideroblastic anaemias. Br J Haematol. 2002;116:733–743.
2. Bottomley SS. Sideroblastic anemias. In: Greer JP, Foerster J, Lukens J, et al., eds. Wintrobe's Clinical Hematology, 11th ed. Philadelphia: Lippincott, Williams and Wilkins; 2004.
3. http://ghr.nlm.nih.gov/ghr/ accessed February 2006
4. Almhanna K, Khan P, Schaldenbrand M, Momin F. Sideroblastic anemia after bariatric surgery. Am J Hematol. 2006;81(2):155–156.

ADDITIONAL READING
- See http://www.genetests.org for counseling information on specific heritable SA syndromes and availability of testing.
- http://ghr.nlm.nih.gov/ condition=xlinkedsideroblasticanemia

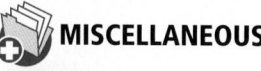 ## MISCELLANEOUS

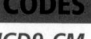 CODES

ICD9-CM
285.0 Sideroblastic anemia

 See Corresponding Diagnostic Algorithm

ANEURYSM OF THE ABDOMINAL AORTA

David H. Stubbs, MD

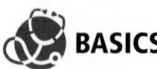 **BASICS**

DESCRIPTION

A permanent localized (i.e., focal) dilatation of the abdominal aorta having at least a 50% increase in diameter compared to the expected diameter of the artery. The clinical presentation of aneurysms relates to location, size, type, and comorbid factors affecting the patient. The majority of aneurysms are asymptomatic. Some present with rupture, others with embolism or thrombosis. The management and indications for surgical repair is dictated by the natural history of the aneurysm, the type, the consequences of repair, and the general status of the patient. There are two types, which are infrarenal (90%) and thoracoabdominal.

- System(s) Affected: Cardiovascular; Hemic/Lymphatic/Immunologic
- Synonym(s): Aortic aneurysms; AAA

ALERT
Geriatric Considerations
Familial aggregations exist, but pathogenesis relates to interaction of genetic, environmental, and biochemical factors.

- Marfan syndrome
- Ehlers-Danlos syndrome

Pediatric Considerations
Etiology more likely infectious or collagen disorders

GENERAL PREVENTION
Screening: 1-time ultrasound screening for AAA in male patients, ages 65–75 who have ever smoked >100 cigarettes

EPIDEMIOLOGY
- Predominant age: Elderly
- Predominant sex: Male > Female (4:1)

Incidence
- >15,000 deaths per year
- 10th leading cause of death in males >55
  - In men >60 years: 2–5%
  - In men >65 years: 6%
  - In men >75 years: 11%
- In women >65 years: 4%
- High risk groups
  - Coronary disease: 5–9%
  - Peripheral vascular disease: 10–15%
  - 1st degree relative with AAA: 25%
  - Males = 40% risk
  - Females = 15% risk
  - Obese patients >65 years
  - Presence of peripheral aneurysms

RISK FACTORS
- Hypertension
- Nicotine
- COPD
- Familial: Siblings of patients with AAA

ETIOLOGY
- Atherosclerosis
- Inflammatory (5–10%)
- Traumatic
- Genetic predisposition (Marfan, Ehlers-Danlos)

ASSOCIATED CONDITIONS
- Marfan syndrome
- Ehlers-Danlos syndrome

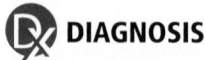 **DIAGNOSIS**

SIGNS AND SYMPTOMS
Physical Exam
Majority of patients with abdominal aortic aneurysm (AAA) are asymptomatic. Many are discovered during radiologic procedures performed for other reasons.

- Pulsatile epigastric mass
- Vague abdominal pain
  - May radiate to the back of flank
- Encroachment by aneurysm
  - Vertebral body erosion
  - Gastric outlet obstruction
  - Ureteral obstruction
- Lower extremity ischemia secondary to microembolization or macroembolization of mural thrombus
- The triad of shock, pulsatile mass, and abdominal pain should always suggest rupture of AAA
  - Shock may be absent if the rupture is contained.
  - Palpable pulsatile mass may be absent in up to 50% of the patients with rupture.
  - Pain may radiate to the back or into the groin.
  - Rupture associated with 90% mortality rate.
- Unusual presentations
  - Primary aortoenteric fistula: Erosion/rupture of AAA into duodenum
  - Aortocaval fistula: Erosion/rupture of AAA into vena cava or left renal vein
  - Inflammatory aneurysm: Encasement of aneurysm by thick inflammatory rind associated with chronic abdominal pain, weight loss, and elevated ESR
  - Surrounding viscera are densely adherent.

ALERT
Geriatric Considerations
More common in this age group and may present atypically

TESTS
Lab
Evaluation for concomitant CAD

- Selective evaluation for CAD is appropriate prior to elective AAA repair (i.e., cardiac clearance).
- Patients with mild, stable cardiac symptoms should have a noninvasive cardiac stress study.
- Coronary revascularization should be performed when the CAD would merit intervention on its own.

Imaging
Screening: 1–time ultrasound screening for AAA in male patients, ages 65–75, who have ever smoked >100 cigarettes

Diagnostic Procedures/Surgery
- Clinical examination
- Ultrasonography is the preferred initial diagnostic tool in suspected AAA, but is not reliable for a diagnosis of a rupture.
- CT scans are the preferred preoperative study. Avoid contrast if the patient has significant renal insufficiency. CT scans assist in the diagnosis of an inflammatory aneurysm.
- MRI: Similar to CT and avoids contrast. MR angiography may replace arteriograms.
- Aortography: Does not define outside dimensions of aneurysms.
- Indications for aortography
  - Associated renovascular hypertension
  - Symptoms of visceral angina
  - Significant iliofemoral occlusive disease
  - Peripheral aneurysms
  - Horseshoe or pelvic kidney
  - Prior colectomy

DIFFERENTIAL DIAGNOSIS
- Abdominal masses transmitting aortic pulse
- Other causes of abdominal pain (e.g., peptic ulcer disease)
- Other causes of back pain (e.g., arthritis, metastatic disease)

TREATMENT

INITIAL STABILIZATION
- The treatment of AAA is elective repair.
- The prevention of AAA is elective repair.

GENERAL MEASURES
- Control hypertension
- Treat atherosclerotic risk factors
- Stop smoking

SURGERY
- Repair when
  - Rupture occurs
  - Size >5.5 cm (or >6 cm in poor surgical risk patients)
  - Expansion >0.5 cm/6 months
  - Symptoms occur
- Poor surgical risk patients
  - Class III–IV angina; LVEF <30%; recent CHF or MI; severe valve disease
  - Serum creatinine >3 mg/dL
  - PaO_2 <50 mm Hg; FEV1<IL
  - Cirrhosis with ascites
  - Diffuse retroperitoneal fibrosis; hostile abdomen
  - Physiologic age > chronological age
- Endovascular aneurysm repair
  - There are currently 3 devices approved by the FDA for marketing. Late complications of these devices continue to occur.
  - Long-term CT surveillance is required.
  - Adequate iliac/femoral access
  - Infrarenal non-aneurysmal neck length of at least 1 cm at the proximal and distal ends of the aneurysm
  - Morphology suitable for endovascular repair
  - One of the following: A diameter >5 cm, a diameter of 4–5 cm, and an increase in size by 0.5 cm in the past 6 months.
  - Health status adequate to undergo the 2-hour plus implementation procedure

FOLLOW-UP

PROGNOSIS
- Aneurysms usually expand over time (Laplace's Law: T (wall tension) = Pressure × Radius. Wall tension is directly related to blood pressure and the radius of the artery.) When wall tension exceeds wall tensile strength, rupture occurs.
- **Surgical Outcomes:** Morbidity 32%; cardiac (MI) 11%; mortality 4.2%
- Risk of morbidity and mortality increase with age
- Operative mortality is inverse to surgeon volume, hospital volume, specialty (vascular vs general surgeon)
- Non-repair (natural history of AAA >5.5 cm); 57% mortality within 1.5 years
- Mean expansion is 0.4 cm per year
- Rupture risk is increased by:
  - Diastolic hypertension
  - Tobacco use
  - Diameter >6 cm
  - COPD
  - Familial history
- Ruptured aneurysms
  - 8% die before receiving definitive care and 50% of the remaining die during their treatment or hospitalization.

COMPLICATIONS
- Rupture
- Associated dissection
- Thrombosis
- Embolization distally

PATIENT MONITORING
- Hypertension control
- Lipid control
- Recurrent assessment of smoking status
- Perioperative complications
  - MI: 5%
  - Renal failure: 6%, chronic dialysis: 1%
  - Pulmonary failure: 5–8%
  - Microembolism (trash foot): 1–4%
  - Ischemic colitis: 0.5–1%
  - Wound infection: 2%
  - Graft infection: <0.5%
  - Stroke: 0.5–1%
  - Paraplegia: 0.2%
- Postsurgical monitoring
  - Anastomotic aneurysm
  - Graft infections
  - Aortoenteric fistula
  - Graft limb occlusion
  - Additional aneurysms: Thoracic, thoracoabdominal, femoral

REFERENCES
1. Irvin TT. Abdominal pain: A surgical audit of 1190 emergency admissions. *Br J Surg.* 1989;76:1121.
2. Johnston W, Rutherford RB, Tilson MD, et al. Suggested standards for reporting on arterial aneurysms. *J Vasc Surg.* 1991;13:452.
3. Lederle FA, Wilson SE, Johnson GR, et al. Aneurysm detection and management Veterans Affairs cooperative study group. Immediate repair compared with surveillance of small abdominal aortic aneurysms. *N Engl J Med.* 2002;346: 1437–1444.
4. Mason JJ, Owens DK, Harris RA, Cooke JP, Hlatky MA. The role of coronary angiography and coronary revascularization before non-cardiac vascular surgery. *JAMA.* 1995;273:1919.
5. Porter JM, ed. *The Year Book of Vascular Surgery.* New York, NY: Mosby-Year Book; 1997.
6. Rutherford B, ed. *Vascular Surgery.* 14th ed. Philadelphia: WB Saunders; 1995.
7. Szilagyi DE, Smith RF, DeRusso FJ, Elliott JP, Sherrin FW. Contribution of abdominal aortic aneurysmectomy to prolongation of life. *Ann Surg.* 1966;164:678.

MISCELLANEOUS

See also: Aortic Dissection; Ehlers-Danlos Syndrome; Giant Cell Arteritis; Marfan Syndrome; Polyarteritis Nodosa; Turner Syndrome

CODES

ICD9-CM
- 441.00 Dissection of aorta, unspecified site
- 441.4 Abdominal aneurysm without mention of rupture

PATIENT TEACHING

Diet
Low fat, low salt, and low caffeine

Activity
Regular aerobic exercise

 See Corresponding Diagnostic Algorithm

 See Patient Handout on CD

ANGINA

Philip P. Lobstein, MD

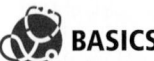 **BASICS**

DESCRIPTION

- Symptom complex resulting from mismatch of myocardial oxygen demand and supply:
  - Classic angina: A sense of choking or of pressure or heaviness deep to the precordium, usually brought on by exertion or anxiety and relieved by rest
  - Anginal equivalent: Exertional dyspnea or exertional fatigue, which results from myocardial ischemia and is relieved by rest or nitroglycerin
  - Variant angina: Also referred to as Prinzmetal angina; describes angina occurring at rest in atypical patterns such as after exercise or nocturnally. Prinzmetal angina is caused by coronary artery spasm, and is associated with ECG changes (usually ST elevation) during symptoms
  - Stable angina: Predictable chest discomfort that occurs in a consistent pattern at a certain level of exertion and is relieved with rest or nitroglycerin
  - Unstable angina: Pain that is new or is changed in character to become more frequent, more severe, or both. Unstable angina portends myocardial infarction in a certain percentage of patients.
- System(s) Affected: Cardiovascular
- Synonym(s): Heberden syndrome

ALERT

Geriatric Considerations
Patients may be very sensitive to the side effects of the medications.

Pediatric Considerations
Suspect familial dyslipidemias in children presenting with manifestations of coronary artery disease.

Pregnancy Considerations
Other diagnoses should be excluded, and the patient managed closely by an obstetrician or family physician and cardiologist: The metabolic demands of pregnancy will exacerbate symptoms and directly interfere with treatment.

GENERAL PREVENTION

- Discontinue tobacco, adherence to low fat/low cholesterol diet, regular aerobic exercise program
- Antilipidemics if indicated by current ATP guidelines
- Daily aspirin in those without contraindications

EPIDEMIOLOGY

- Predominant age: Most common in middle age and older men; postmenopausal women
- Predominant sex: Male > Female (before menopause)

Incidence
Presenting symptom of coronary artery
- Male: 38%
- Female: 61%

RISK FACTORS

- Family history of premature coronary artery disease (CAD)
- Hypercholesterolemia
- Hypertension
- Tobacco abuse
- Diabetes mellitus
- Male gender
- Advanced age
- Morbid obesity
- Hyperhomocysteinemia (possibly)

Genetics
Coronary artery disease has genetic implications.

ETIOLOGY

- Atherosclerosis of the coronary arteries
- Coronary artery spasm
- Aortic stenosis
- Hypertrophic cardiomyopathy
- Severe hypertension
- Aortic insufficiency
- Primary pulmonary hypertension

ASSOCIATED CONDITIONS

- Hypercholesterolemia
- Claudication, Peripheral vascular disease
- Arterial aneurysms
- Mitral regurgitation
- Papillary muscle dysfunction
- Ventricular aneurysm
- Abdominal aortic aneurysm
- Hypertrophic subaortic stenosis
- Primary hyperthyroidism
- Pernicious anemia and other high output states

DIAGNOSIS

SIGNS AND SYMPTOMS

- Precordial pressure or heaviness, radiating to the back, neck, or arms; brought on by exertion, emotional stress, meals, cold air, or smoking; and relieved by rest or nitrates
- Discomfort may radiate to the neck, lower jaw, teeth, shoulders, and inner aspects of the arms or back.
- Discomfort may be described with a clenched fist over the sternum (Levine sign).
- Dyspnea on exertion may present as the only symptom.
- A choking sensation on exertion is a classic symptom.
- Atypical symptoms are more likely in women, elderly, and diabetic patients.

History

- Quality of any previous anginal episodes and pattern over time
- Underlying history of heart disease or valvular disease
- Family history of MI, CAD, sudden death

Physical Exam
May see signs of dyslipidemia (xanthomas, xanthelasma, diminished peripheral pulses, carotid bruits).

TESTS

- ECG
  - May show evidence of ischemia or prior myocardial infarction; follow-up testing via angiography is warranted. Other findings are nonspecific and tracings are frequently normal.
  - Bundle branch block, Wolff-Parkinson-White syndrome, or intraventricular conduction delay may make the ECG unreliable.
- If normal ECG, exercise stress treadmill testing (ETT) based on probability is indicated.
  - ETT with imaging-via echocardiography or perfusion imaging with sestamibi.
  - In patients who cannot tolerate exercise, pharmacologic stress testing should be performed
  - Women have lower sensitivity and specificity with ETT than do men; exercise echocardiography is indicated
  - In Men
    - Low probability: ETT without imaging
    - Intermediate probability: ETT with imaging
    - High probability: ETT prior to angiography

Lab

- Total cholesterol: Frequently elevated
- HDL cholesterol: Frequently reduced
- LDL cholesterol: Frequently elevated
- CRP: Only useful (and offers no better predictive value than standard CHD risk factors) in those with Intermediate to high risk; should be measured at least twice over 2 weeks; is *not* predictive in low risk patients and in those on a β-blocker or statin.

Imaging

- Radionuclide scintigraphy
- Stress echocardiography
- Stress scintigraphy
- Coronary angiography

Diagnostic Procedures/Surgery

- Definitive evaluation requires coronary arteriography for confirmation and delineation of coronary disease, and direction of interventional therapy or surgery. Coronary artery stenting has proven very effective, with restenosis rates (in skilled hands) often <10%, eliminating need for surgery in many cases.
- Surgery in CAD not amenable to angioplasty, and stenting has proven to have a long-term benefit.

Pathological Findings
Atherosclerosis of the coronary arteries

DIFFERENTIAL DIAGNOSIS

- Esophagitis (GERD)
- Esophageal spasm
- Peptic ulcer disease
- Gastritis or nonulcer dyspepsia
- Cholecystitis
- Costochondritis
- Pericarditis
- Aortic dissection
- Pleurisy
- Pulmonary embolus
- Pulmonary hypertension
- Pneumothorax
- Radiculopathy
- Shoulder arthropathy
- Psychological: Anxiety and panic disorders

TREATMENT

PRE HOSPITAL

- EMS activation if chest discomfort unimproved or worsening 5 minutes after 1 nitroglycerin dose (1)[C]
  - EMS to initiate IV, O$_2$, and monitor
  - Aspirin administration if ACS suspected and not previously taken or contraindicated

GENERAL MEASURES

- The patient's symptoms should be brought under control medically. If symptoms are unstable, hospitalization is warranted.
- Treatment goal involves reducing myocardial oxygen demand or to increase oxygen supply.
- Noninvasive testing often is indicated as a means of stratifying the patient's risk for an event that might seriously compromise myocardial function.
- Quit smoking.
- Minimize emotional stress.
- Weight reduction in obese patients (2)[C]

Diet

Low-fat, low-cholesterol, low-salt diet

Activity

- As tolerated after consulting physician
- Exercise program after physician's approval; very effective if consistent

SPECIAL THERAPY

Complementary and Alternative Medicine

Relaxation/stress reduction therapy may help reduce anginal aggravations.

MEDICATION (DRUGS)

First Line

- Aspirin: 81–325 mg/d
- β-Blockers are effective in reducing heart rate and thereby decreasing oxygen consumption and reducing angina
  - Atenolol 25–100 mg/d, metoprolol 25–100 mg b.i.d., or bisoprolol 2.5–10/d
  - Adjust doses according to clinical response. Aim to maintain resting heart rate of 50–60 beats per minute.
  - Side effects are infrequent but include fatigue, exercise intolerance, erectile dysfunction, and exacerbation of peripheral vascular and obstructive pulmonary disease.
- Nitroglycerin 0.4 mg SL is the most effective therapy for acute anginal episodes
  - May repeat 2–3 times over a 10–15 minute period; if no relief, the patient should seek immediate medical attention.
- Long-acting nitrates (mononitrates or transdermal nitrates)
  - Should be used with a drug-free interval of 10–14 hours to prevent tolerance
  - Tachyphylaxis occurs rapidly.
  - Preload reduction and coronary vasodilatation
  - Side effects: Headaches and hypotension, tend to clear with continued usage.
  - A β-blocker or calcium channel blocker should be used in conjunction with the nitrates during the drug-free interval.
  - Caution patients not to use in conjunction with oral medicine for erectile dysfunction, such as sildenafil (Viagra).

- Long-acting calcium channel blockers: Verapamil 160–480 mg/d or diltiazem 90–360 mg/d, or nifedipine 30–120 mg/d, or amlodipine 5–20 mg/d. Drug of choice for variant angina. The various agents have their own individual side effects (i.e., verapamil, constipation; nifedipine, peripheral edema).
- HMG CoA reductase inhibitors (e.g., atorvastatin, pravastatin, lovastatin) for hypercholesterolemia: These drugs decrease incidence of symptomatic CAD and reduce both myocardial infarction and death from MI. LDL target levels below 100 mg/dL in diabetes mellitus and <130 mg/dL in low- to moderate-risk patients.
- ACE inhibitors (ramipril 10 mg) in patients with CAD or other vascular disease (3)[B], and particularly those with diabetes or left ventricular (LV) systolic dysfunction (3)[A] have been shown to reduce both cardiovascular death and MI.
- Heparin: Low-molecular-weight heparin should be initiated in patients hospitalized with unstable angina.
- Glycoprotein IIb/IIIa receptor antagonists (Integrilin): Indicated in certain patients hospitalized with unstable angina
- Combination therapy may be used (especially nitrates plus calcium antagonists with or without β-blockers).
- Contraindications:
  - Sildenafil (Viagra), vardenafil (Levitra), or tadalafil (Cialis) with nitrates should be avoided due to the risk of hypotension and possible death.
- Precautions: Avoid verapamil and diltiazem with compromised ventricular function (LV ejection fraction <40%) especially in conjunction with β-blockers.
- Significant possible interactions:
  - Combination therapies may impair LV function and precipitate heart failure.
  - β-Blockers and calcium channel blocker: May combine to produce symptomatic heart block, although either class of drug may act alone in producing this side effect
  - Niacin may worsen glucose intolerance.

Second Line

- Current ATP guidelines support the use of lipid-lowering drugs in patients with unfavorable lipid profiles and suspected or documented CAD with or without symptoms (4)[A].
- Consider adding clopidogrel (Plavix) to ASA for severe diffuse CAD. The use of Plavix is indicated after stent placement for at least 9 months to significantly reduce restenosis rates.

SURGERY

Coronary artery bypass graft surgery, angioplasty, stent placement, atherectomy in selected cases

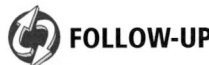

FOLLOW-UP

DISPOSITION

Admission Criteria

Unstable symptoms warrant hospitalization for evaluation.

PROGNOSIS

- Variable; depends on the extent of CAD as well as LV function
- Annual mortality is 3–4% overall

COMPLICATIONS

- Related to myocardial damage occurring during infarction
- Arrhythmia
- Cardiac arrest
- Congestive heart failure

PATIENT MONITORING

- Depends on the frequency and severity of the complaints
- Hospitalization is indicated in patients diagnosed with unstable angina

REFERENCES

1. Antman EM, Ane DT, Armstrong PW, et al. Guidelines for the management of patients with ST-elevation myocardial infarction—executive summary: a report of the American College of Cardiology/American Heart Association Task Force on Practice Guidelines. *Circulation.* 2004;110:588–636.
2. Gibbons RJ, Abrams J, Chatterjee K, et al. ACC/AHA 2002 guideline update for the management of patients with chronic stable angina—summary article: a report of the American College of Cardiology/American Heart Association Task Force on Practice Guidelines. *Circulation.* 2003;107:149–158.
3. Yusuf S, Sleight P, Pogue J, et al. Effects of an angiotensin-converting-enzyme inhibitor ramipril on cardiovascular events in high-risk patients. The HOPE Study Investigators. *N Engl J Med.* 2000;342:145–153.
4. Executive Summary of the Third Report of the National Cholesterol Education Program (NCEP) Expert Panel on Detection, Evaluation, and Treatment of High Blood Cholesterol in Adults (Adult Treatment Panel III). *JAMA.* 2001;285:2486–2497.

CODES

ICD9-CM

- 411.1 Intermediate coronary syndrome
- 413 Angina pectoris
- 413.1 Prinzmetal angina
- 413.9 Other and unspecified angina pectoris

PATIENT TEACHING

American Heart Association, 7320 Greenville Avenue, Dallas, TX 75231, (214) 373-6300.

 See Corresponding Diagnostic Algorithm

 See Patient Handout on CD

ANGIOEDEMA

Anatoli Freiman, MD

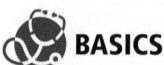 **BASICS**

DESCRIPTION

- Dermal (subcutaneous or submucosal) extravasation of fluid, leading to localized edema
- The release of inflammatory vasoactive mediators increases vascular permeability.
- The skin, gastrointestinal tract, and respiratory tract are most commonly involved. It is life threatening if the upper airway is affected. It usually resolves in hours to days.
- Can be idiopathic or induced by medications, allergens (e.g., food), or physical agents (e.g., vibration, cold)
- 2 rare but well-described categories of angioedema result from deficiency of C1 esterase inhibitor (C1 INH) of the compliment and kallikrein-kinin systems: Hereditary angioedema (HAE) and acquired angioedema (AAE).
  - HAE type I (80–85%): Due to hereditary deficiency of C1-INH; recurrent episodes of angioedema, involving both skin and mucous membranes or intestinal mucosa (25% mortality)
  - HAE type II (15–20%): Normal or elevated quantities of functionally impaired C1-INH
  - HAE type III: Rare, recently described estrogen-dependent form
  - AAE type I: Increased destruction of C1-INH, which occurs in patients with rheumatologic disorders and B-cell lymphoproliferative malignancies, such as leukemia, T-cell lymphoma, multiple myeloma, and essential cryoglobulinemia
  - AAE type I is also reported with carcinomas, infections, and vasculitides. Immune complexes continuously activate C1, leading to consumption of C1-INH and precipitating angioedema.
  - AAE type II: B cells secrete autoantibodies against C1-INH, leading to its inactivation
- Medication-induced angioedema
  - Immunologic hypersensitivity, as in penicillin reaction
  - Nonimmunologic, as in reactions to NSAIDs (e.g., aspirin)
  - Angiotensin converting enzyme (ACE) inhibitors decrease levels of angiotensin II and stimulate production of bradykinin, a potent vasodilator, thus leading to angioedema. This may occur immediately or months after starting the drug.
- System(s) Affected: Skin/Exocrine
- Synonym(s): Angioneurotic edema; Quincke edema

GENERAL PREVENTION

- If etiology known, avoidance
- Avoid ACE inhibitors in patients with a history of angioedema.

EPIDEMIOLOGY

- Predominant age
  - HAE: Infancy to second decade of life
  - AAE: Typically patients > 40 years old.
- Predominant sex: Male = Female (idiopathic)

Incidence

- 1 in 5,000
- Accompanies urticaria 40–50% of time

RISK FACTORS

- Medications and foods that can cause allergic reactions
- ACE inhibitors are contraindicated in patients with C1-INH deficiency

Genetics

HAE types I and II are inherited in autosomal dominant mode, whereas type III is X-linked. HAE occurs in 25% of the patients as a result of spontaneous mutations.

PATHOPHYSIOLOGY

Similar pathophysiology for urticaria and angioedema: Localized anaphylaxis causes vasodilatation and vascular permeability of superficial (urticaria) or subcutaneous/deeper dermal tissue (angioedema)

ETIOLOGY

- Idiopathic
- Medication-induced: ACE inhibitors, NSAIDs, antibiotics, or estrogen contraceptives
  - ACE inhibitors (ACEI) are ascribed to 10–25% of angioedema cases and mostly occur within the 1st 3–4 weeks of use. However, the 1st onset may be delayed years. Failure to react to re-challenge with drug does not rule out a cause–effect relationship between the ACEI and angioedema.
  - Losartan (Cozaar), valsartan (Diovan), and irbesartan (Avapro), which are all angiotensin receptor blockers (ARB), can also cause angioedema. It can occur within 24 hours to 16 months after initiating losartan therapy.
- Allergen-induced: Food allergens, such as fish, nuts, and preservatives
- Physically induced: Cold, pressure, vibration
- Hereditary or acquired C1-INH deficiency
- Thyroid autoimmunity has been reported to be associated with angioedema.

ASSOCIATED CONDITIONS

- Urticaria
- Anaphylaxis

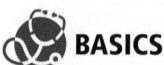 **DIAGNOSIS**

SIGNS AND SYMPTOMS

- Occurs alone or in association with urticaria in 50% of cases
- Angioedema usually does not cause itching in comparison to urticaria, but can cause burning.
- Relatively rapid onset of presentation; usually resolves spontaneously in <72 hours
- Skin
  - Localized swelling; may occur anywhere on body; usually face, extremities, or genitalia; often asymmetric
  - Frequently disfiguring and frightening to the patient
- Gastrointestinal
  - May present with intermittent unexplained abdominal pain
- Respiratory
  - May be associated with generalized anaphylactic reaction, potentially fatal if upper airway is compromised

History

- Acute onset of asymmetric localized swelling
- GI tract involvement may manifest as intermittent unexplained abdominal pain.
- In comparison to urticaria, angioedema is typically nonpruritic, but can cause burning.

Physical Exam

Subcutaneous swelling, usually of the face (eyelids, lips, ears, nose), and less often of the extremities or genitalia

TESTS

Lab

- If angioedema with urticaria and/or anaphylaxis, no testing is needed, but history should be directed to exposures: Foods, medications, exposures, etc.
- Without clear etiology and recurrence in angioedema and urticaria, CBC and ESR; macrocytosis implies a pernicious anemia; eosinophilia my imply atopy or rarely parasitic infection. Elevated ESR may imply systemic disorders.
- In recurrent angioedema without clear etiology and without urticaria, consider ordering C4. Low serum C4 is a very sensitive, but nonspecific, screening test for hereditary and acquired C1-INH deficiency. If C4 is normal, urticaria work-up is recommended.
- If C4 is low, C1-INH assay (immunoreactive) is performed for HAE type I and C1-INH assay (functional) for HAE type II.
- C1q is decreased in acquired C1-INH deficiency.
- If C4 and C1q are low (as in AAE), neoplastic and autoimmune work-up are warranted. Routine blood tests, a smear, protein electrophoresis, immunophenotyping of lymphocytes, and imaging studies are often undertaken to rule out hematological malignancies or cancer.
- May alter lab results
  - Antihistamines
  - H_2-blockers
  - Tricyclic antidepressants

Imaging
As part of neoplastic work-up if relevant

Diagnostic Procedures/Surgery
Skin biopsy (may be nonspecific)

Pathological Findings
Edema of deep dermis and subcutaneous tissue. Variable perivascular and interstitial infiltrate

DIFFERENTIAL DIAGNOSIS
- Urticaria
- Allergic contact dermatitis
- Connective tissue disease: Lupus, dermatomyositis
- Anaphylaxis
- Cellulitis, erysipelas
- Lymphedema
- Diffuse subcutaneous infiltrative process

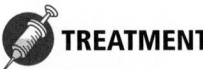 **TREATMENT**

PRE HOSPITAL
- Ensure airway patency 1st! Protect the airway if the mouth, tongue, and/or throat are involved.
- Perform CPR and transport to an emergency facility, if necessary.

INITIAL STABILIZATION
If anaphylaxis (circulatory collapse or airway compromise), consider epinephrine (1:1000) SC 0.3–0.5 q15min.

GENERAL MEASURES
- Symptomatic, supportive management
- Avoid known triggers.
- Cool, moist compresses to control itching or burning

 MEDICATION (DRUGS)

First Line
- 1st generation antihistamines for acute angioedema
  - Older children and adults: hydroxyzine (Vistaril 5 mg/5 cc, 25 tablets) 10–25 mg t.i.d. or diphenhydramine (Benadryl) 25–50 mg q6h
  - Children under 6 years of age: Diphenhydramine 12.5 mg (elixir) q6–8h (5 mg/kg/day)
- 2nd generation H_1 blockers are less sedating because they do not cross the blood–brain barrier.
  - Fexofenadine (Allegra) 60 mg b.i.d.
  - Loratadine (Claritin) 10 mg daily
  - Acrivastine (Semprex) 8 mg t.i.d.
  - Cetirizine (Zyrtec) 10 mg daily, which is more sedating than others in this class
- Anaphylaxis
  - Intubation if airway is threatened
  - Epinephrine 1:1,000, 0.2–0.3 mL IV or SQ
  - Specific HAE and AAE therapy
  - C1-INH concentrate
  - Attenuated androgens: Danazol or stanozolol are particularly effective for prevention of HAE because they increase the amount of active C1-INH. Give 200–600 mg daily for 1 month, then 5 days on, 5 days off. The side effects are headaches, weight gain, and hematuria.
  - Antifibrinolytic agents (plasmin inhibitors), such as tranexamic acid and aminocaproic acid, may also be used, but are not as effective as attenuated androgens in the management of HAE. On rare occasions they can cause thrombophlebitis, embolism, or myositis.
- Contraindications
  - Danazol not to be used in childhood, pregnancy, lactation, and prostate cancer
- Precautions
  - Drowsiness with 1st generation drugs
  - Second generation H_1 blockers should be used with caution in pregnancy and the elderly.

Second Line
Doxepin (Sinequan) may be effective for angioedema (10–25 mg at bedtime)

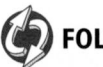 **FOLLOW-UP**

PROGNOSIS
Most patients with idiopathic angioedema do well. Chronic forms depend on underlying pathology.

COMPLICATIONS
- Anaphylaxis
- Respiratory compromise

PATIENT MONITORING
- Diagnostic work-up if symptoms are severe, persistent, or recurrent
- Protect airway if mouth, tongue, or throat is involved

REFERENCES
1. Bowen T, et al. Canadian 2003 international consensus algorithm for the diagnosis, therapy, and management of hereditary angioedema. *J Allergy Clin Immunol*. 2004;114(3):629–637.
2. Charlesworth EN. Differential diagnosis of angioedema. *Allergy Asthma Proc*. 2002; 23:337–339.
3. Frigas E, Nzeako UC. Angioedema. *Clin Rev Allerg Immunol*. 2002;23:217–231.
4. Heymann WR. Acquired angioedema. *J Am Acad Dermatol*. 1997;26:611–615.
5. Kim JS, Pongracic JA. Hereditary and aquired angioedema. *Allergy Asthma Proc*. 2004; 25:S47–S49.
6. Nzeako UC, Frigas E, Tremaine WJ. Hereditary angioedema: a broad review for clinicians. *Arch Intern Med*. 2001;161:2417–2429.

CODES

ICD9-CM
- 995.1 Angioneurotic edema
- 277.6 Other deficiencies of circulating enzymes

PATIENT TEACHING
- Educate HAE and AAE patients to inform health care providers of their disease.
- Avoid known trigger foods.
- HAE patients should avoid violent exercise and trauma.

 See Corresponding Diagnostic Algorithm

ANIMAL BITES

George R. Bergus, MD

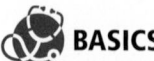 **BASICS**

DESCRIPTION
- Bite wounds to humans from dogs, cats, other animals including humans
- System(s) Affected: Endocrine/Metabolic; Hemic/Lymphatic/Immunologic; Nervous; Skin/Exocrine

ALERT
Geriatric Considerations
- Serious injury from any bite wound is more common >50 years old, those with wounds in the upper extremities, or those with puncture wounds.
- Increased risk of infection >50 years old

Pediatric Considerations
Young children are more likely to have severe bites.

GENERAL PREVENTION
- Instruct children and adults about animal hazards.
- Educate dog owners about responsible dog ownership.
- Strongly enforce animal control laws.

EPIDEMIOLOGY
Incidence
- Dog bites: 1,200/100,000
- Cat bites: 160/100,000
- Snake bites: 15/100,000 nonvenomous bites and 3/100,000 venomous bites per year
- Lifetime prevalence for animal bite: 50,000/100,000
- Dog bites are responsible for 1/3 million emergency room visits per year

Prevalence
- Predominant age: All ages, but children more likely to be affected
- Predominant sex: Male > Female

RISK FACTORS
- Dog bites are more common during warm weather.
- Male dogs are more likely to bite.
- Clenched-fist injuries are frequently associated with the use of alcohol.

ETIOLOGY
- Most bite wounds are from a domestic pet known to the victim.
- Large dogs are the most common source of bite wounds.
- Human bites are often the result of one person striking another in the mouth with a clenched fist.

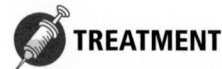 **DIAGNOSIS**

SIGNS AND SYMPTOMS
- Bite wounds can be tears, punctures, scratches, avulsions, or crush injuries.
- Dog bites (80–90% of bites)
  - In adults, hands are most commonly affected.
  - In children, the face is the most common site of injury, and involvement of the trunk is uncommon.
- Cat bites (10% of bites)
  - Predominantly involve the hands, followed by lower extremities, face, and trunk
  - Are more likely to become infected because of puncture nature of wounds

TESTS
Lab
- 85% of bite wounds will yield a positive culture, but culturing at time of injury is of little benefit
- Wound culture is essential in directing therapy.
  - Some pathogens are slow growing, so cultures should be kept for 7–10 days
  - Gram stain is sensitive but not specific for infecting organism
- Dog bites
  - *Pasteurella* species is present in 50% of bites.
  - Also found: *Streptococcus viridans*, *Staphylococcus aureus*, coagulase-negative Staphylococcus, *Bacteroides*, *Capnocytophaga canimorsus*, *Fusobacterium*
- Cat bites
  - *Pasteurella* species is present in 75% of bites.
  - The wound is often contaminated by other mixed bacteria, including several species of both aerobic and anaerobic organisms.
- Human bites
  - Streptococcus species, *Staphylococcus aureus*, *Eikenella corrodens*, and various anaerobic bacteria are very common.
- Other animal bites
  - Scant information on pathogens
- Drugs that may alter lab results
  - Previous antibiotic therapy

Imaging
- If bite wound is near a bone or joint, a plain radiograph is needed to check for bone injury and to use for comparison later if osteomyelitis is suspected.
- In human bite wounds from clenched-fist injuries, order plain-film radiographs to check for metacarpal or phalanx fracture.

Diagnostic Procedures/Surgery
- Consider rabies prophylaxis for bats, nondomestic dogs; rarely skunks, foxes and raccoon
- Surgical exploration may be needed to ascertain extent of injuries.
- Exploration should be performed on all serious hand wounds, especially clenched-fist injuries involving a joint.

DIFFERENTIAL DIAGNOSIS
Diagnosis is straightforward; what is of concern is judging the risk to the patient from the injury and resulting infection.

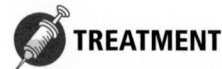 **TREATMENT**

GENERAL MEASURES
- Appropriate health care: Outpatient, unless patient has fulminant infection requiring systemic antibiotics, close observation, or surgery
- Elevation of the injured extremity to prevent swelling
- Contact the local health department and consult about the prevalence of rabies in the species of animal involved.

MEDICATION (DRUGS)

First Line

- Consider antirabies therapy.
- Use tetanus toxoid in those previously immunized, but >5 years since their last dose.
- Consider tetanus immune globulin (TIG) in patients without a full primary series of immunizations.
- Prophylactic therapy if wound seen in 1st 12 hours
  - Dog, cat, or animal: Amoxicillin-clavulanate 500–875 mg b.i.d. PO (pediatric: 20–40 mg/kg/d PO given t.i.d.)
  - Snake bite: If venomous, the patient needs rapid transport to a facility capable of definitive evaluation. If an envenomation has occurred, the patient will need to receive antivenin unless envenomation was only minimal. Be sure patient is stable for transport; consider measuring and or treating coagulation and renal status along with any anaphylactic reactions before transport.
  - Human bites: Amoxicillin-clavulanate (Augmentin) potassium, adult: 500 mg PO t.i.d. (pediatric: 20–40 mg/kg/d PO given t.i.d.)
- Established infection
  - After patient has developed a clinical infection, amoxicillin-clavulanate potassium (Augmentin) can be used pending culture reports
- Contraindications: Do not use penicillin-derived antibiotics in those with penicillin allergy.
- Precautions: Prescribe dosage of antibiotics by body weight and renal function.
- Significant possible interactions: Antibiotics may decrease efficacy of oral contraceptives

Second Line

- Alternative therapy for penicillin-allergic patients (for prophylaxis or empiric treatment)
  - ~10% cross-reactivity with cephalosporins in penicillin-allergic patients
  - Dog bite: Moxifloxacin 400 mg/day × 7 days in adults (pediatric: trimethoprim- sulfamethoxazole along with Clindamycin); avoid cephalexin due to resistant strains of *Pasteurella multocida*
  - Cat bite: As for dog bite
  - Human bite: Moxifloxacin 400 mg/day
- If hospitalized with established infection: Ampicillin-sulbactam (Unasyn) 1–2 g IV q6h or ticarcillin-clavulanate (Timentin) 3.1 g IV q4–6h

SURGERY

- Copious irrigation of the wound with normal saline via a catheter tip is needed to reduce risk of infection.
- Devitalized tissue needs debridement.
- Debridement of puncture wounds not advised.
- Consider surgical closure if the wound is clean after irrigation and bite is <12 hours old. Puncture wounds should be left open.
- Delayed primary closure in 3–5 days is an option for infected wounds.
- Splint hand if it is injured.
- Human bite wounds on the hands should not be primarily closed because of the high risk of infection. Large, gaping wounds should be reapproximated with widely spaced sutures or Steri-Strips.

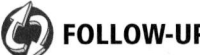 ## FOLLOW-UP

PROGNOSIS

Wounds should steadily improve and close over by 7–10 days.

COMPLICATIONS

- Septic arthritis
- Osteomyelitis
- Extensive soft tissue injuries with scarring
- Sepsis
- Hemorrhage
- Death
- Gas gangrene can take an exceedingly rapid course and should be treated very aggressively.

PATIENT MONITORING

- Patient should be re-checked in 24–48 hours if not infected at time of 1st encounter
- Daily follow-up is warranted with active infections.
- If antibiotics are used for an active infection, the duration of therapy should be 7–14 days, depending on the severity of the infection and the clinical response.

REFERENCES

1. Stevens DL, et al. Practice guidelines for the diagnosis and management of skin and soft-tissue infections. *Clin Infect Dis*. 2005;41(10):1373–1406.
2. Fleisher GR. The management of bite wounds. *N Engl J Med*. 1999;340:138–140.
3. Griego RD, et al. Dog, cat and human bites: A review. *J Am Acad Dermatol*. 1995;33:1019–1029.
4. Presutti RJ. Prevention and treatment of dog bites. *Am Fam Physician*. 2001;63(8):1567–1572, 1573–1574.
5. Sacks JJ, et al. Fatal dog attacks 1989–1994. *Pediatrics*. 1996;97:891–895.

 ## MISCELLANEOUS

Rabies

- Contact your local health department for information about the risk of rabies.
- Most human rabies are related to bat bites. See also: Bartonella Infections; Cellulitis; Rabies; Snake Envenomations; Crotalidae; Elapidae

CODES

ICD9-CM

- 879.8 Open wound(s) of unspecified site(s) without mention of complications
- 882.0 Open wound of hand except finger(s) alone without mention of complication
- 873.40 Open wound of face without mention of complications, unspecified site

PATIENT TEACHING

- Discussion with parents at well child checks should include education on how to avoid animal bites.
- KidsHealth at the AMA: www.ama-assn.org/insight/h focus/nemours/emer/whattodo/bites.htm
- AAFP: www.aafp.org/patientinfo/dogbite.html

 See Patient Handout on CD

ANKLE FRACTURES

Heather C. Killie, MD

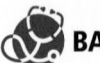 BASICS

DESCRIPTION
- Fractures involving the distal fibula (lateral malleolus) and/or distal tibia (medial malleolus and plafond)
- Includes a range of injuries to bones and ligaments of the ankle

GENERAL PREVENTION
- Proper shoe wear (i.e., flat, supportive shoes)
- Avoid running or walking on uneven or slick surfaces.

EPIDEMIOLOGY
- One of the most common fractures requiring orthopedic care
- Lateral malleolus more commonly involved (account for 2/3 of all ankle fractures)

Incidence
- Age-specific incidence increases in men >60 and women >50 years of age
- Highest incidence in elderly women (1)[B]

ALERT
Pediatric Considerations
- Pediatric will present with fractures involving the growth plates
- Most commonly a Salter-Harris I fracture of the distal fibula

RISK FACTORS
- Increased body mass index
- History of smoking
- No association between general health and risk for ankle fracture

PATHOPHYSIOLOGY
- The location and pattern of injury depend on foot position and the direction of force applied. Most commonly the foot is plantarflexed and inverted, and the force is external rotation.
- Axial load can cause a tibial plafond (a.k.a. *pilon*) fracture, which is an intra-articular fracture of the distal tibia where it articulates with the talus.

ETIOLOGY
Fall or twisting injury to the ankle

ASSOCIATED CONDITIONS
- Ankle sprains
- Syndesmosis injury
- Ankle or subtalar dislocation
- Fracture of the metatarsals, talus, calcaneus
- Osteochondral fracture (subchondral fracture of the distal tibia or talus)
- Neurovascular injury (very rare)

DIAGNOSIS

PRE HOSPITAL
- If ankle is obviously deformed, it should be reduced and provisionally splinted after adequate pain control is achieved.
- Place ice on ankle and elevate extremity

SIGNS AND SYMPTOMS
- Pain, swelling, and ecchymosis
- Pain or inability to bear weight
- Possible deformity

History
- Mechanism of injury
  – Fall or twisting injury
- Timing of injury
- Past history of ankle injuries
- Any other injuries sustained

Physical Exam
- Inspect the ankle and foot for swelling and ecchymosis.
- Inspect the skin for tenting or lacerations.
- Palpate dorsalis pedis and posterior tibial pulses
- Palpate medial and lateral malleoli, proximal leg, and foot
- Sensory and motor exam of ankle and foot
- Rule out compartment syndrome (very rare), especially of the deep posterior compartment of the leg.

TESTS
Lab
Routine lab studies are not needed unless the fracture is operative.

Imaging
- Ottawa Ankle Rules help the clinician determine when to get x-rays. (2)[A]

- X-rays when patient has pain at either malleoli and 1 or more of following:
  – Age >55
  – Inability to bear weight
  – Bony tenderness at posterior edge or tip of either malleoli
- 3 standard views: AP, Lateral, Mortise (15° internal rotation view)
- When foot pain present, get 3 views of foot

Diagnostic Procedures/Surgery
- Arthroscopy is an option in cases of persistent pain or suspicion of an OCD lesion.
- Open reduction, internal fixation in cases of instability (See "Treatment" section)

DIFFERENTIAL DIAGNOSIS
- Stress fracture
- Ankle sprain
- Osteochondral fracture
- Talus fracture
- 5th Metatarsal fracture
- Calcaneus fracture

TREATMENT

PRE HOSPITAL
- If ankle is obviously deformed, it should be reduced with adequate pain control and provisionally splinted per first-aid protocol.
- Ice and elevate the extremity.

INITIAL STABILIZATION
- As above if obvious deformity
- Place leg in a padded posterior splint to include toes to just below knee.
- If the fracture is open, remove any debris from the wound, place a moist dressing over the wound, and immediately contact an orthopedic surgeon.
- Obtain x-rays.

GENERAL MEASURES
Activity
- Non-weight bearing in all fractures
- EXCEPTION
  – Isolated avulsion fractures of the tip of the lateral malleolus may be weight bearing as tolerated.

Nursing
- Apply ice.
- Instruct patient to keep leg elevated
- Control pain.

SPECIAL THERAPY
Physical Therapy
Early range of motion is key to prevent stiffness.
- Encourage toe and knee motion as soon as possible.
- Start ankle ROM as soon as there is evidence of fracture healing (usually 6 weeks).

MEDICATION (DRUGS)

- In general, ankle fractures are painful, particularly in the 1st 5–7 days following an injury. As the swelling decreases, so does the pain.

First Line
- Acetaminophen
- Opiod analgesics (i.e., hydrocodone)
- Avoid NSAIDs acutely (may delay healing of fractures)

Second Line
Non-opiod analgesics (i.e., tramadol)

SURGERY
- Absolute surgical indications
  – Open fractures (fix within 6–8 hours)
- Relative surgical indications
  – Gross instability (i.e., dislocation on presentation, bi- or tri-malleolar ankle fractures)
  – Displacement after closed reduction attempt
  – Displaced, comminuted distal tibia fractures
- Surgical options
  – Open reduction internal fixation with plates and screws (most commonly)
  – External fixation for comminuted distal tibia fractures
- Timing of surgery
  – Within 6–8 hours if skin open
  – After swelling decreased in all other cases (preferably not >1 week)
- Length of recovery
  – In general, 6–8 weeks for healing
  – 6–8 weeks in a cast or splint (longer if fracture involves both medial and lateral malleoli)
  – 2–4 months for syndesmotic injury
  – Orthopedist may allow range of motion after 4 weeks and place in removable cast boot (fracture pattern and surgeon dependent)

 FOLLOW-UP

Most ankle fractures require close follow-up by an orthopedic surgeon (see "Referral" section)

DISPOSITION
- Patient should be transferred to the emergency department if
  – Open fractures
  – Dislocated ankle
  – Neurovascular injury
  – Possible compartment syndrome
- Otherwise, patient should be referred to an orthopedic surgeon

Admission Criteria
Admit to the hospital if
Open fracture
Neurovascular injury
Cannot maintain non-weight bearing status and requires physical therapy consultation
Concern of skin compromise
Concern of mechanism of injury (i.e., syncope, MI, head injury)

Discharge Criteria
When patient has completed the following
Able to ambulate with walker/crutches
Medical work-up (if needed) is completed
Appropriate orthopedic follow-up is arranged
Elderly patients may require a short stay in a rehabilitation facility.

Issues for Referral
- Most ankle fractures should be seen by an orthopedic surgeon within 5–7 days, earlier if a reduction is needed.
- Open fractures should be seen by an orthopedic surgeon immediately.

PROGNOSIS
- Good results can be achieved in most ankle fractures without surgery, provided the ankle mortise is maintained. (3)[B]

- Long term, some patients may develop ankle arthritis; timing is unpredictable.
- Effusion or pain can persist for up to 1 year.

COMPLICATIONS
- Non-operative
  – Displacement of the fracture
  – Malunion
  – Skin breakdown
  – DVT (rarely pulmonary embolism)
- Operative
  – Infection
  – Loss of fixation
  – Nonunion or malunion
  – Skin breakdown
  – DVT (rarely pulmonary embolism)

PATIENT MONITORING
- Serial x-rays should be performed weekly for 4 weeks if there is any question about stability.
- Otherwise, x-rays should be performed at 2 weeks, 4 weeks, and 8 weeks or until the fracture is healed.

REFERENCES

1. Court-Brown CM, McBirnie J, Wilson G. Adult ankle fractures—an increasing problem? *Acta Orthop Scand*. 1998;69(1):43–47.
2. Stiell IG, Greenberg GH, McKnight RD, et, al. Decision rules for the use of radiography in acute ankle injuries: Refinement and prospective validation. *JAMA*. Mar 1993;269:1127–1132.
3. Michelson JD. Ankle fractures resulting from rotational injuries. *J Am Acad Orthop Surg*. 2003;11:403–412.

ADDITIONAL READING

Bucholz RW, Heckman JD, eds. *Rockwood and Green's Fractures in Adults* 5th ed. Philadelphia: Lippincott Williams & Wilkins Publishers; 2001.

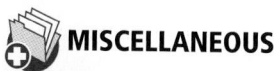 **MISCELLANEOUS**

 CODES

ICD9-CM
824.9 Fracture, ankle

PATIENT TEACHING

- It may take the bone 6–12 weeks for the fracture to heal.
- Ice and elevate the affected leg for 2–3 weeks following the injury to decrease swelling.
- Prevent splint/cast from getting wet.
- Do not scratch inside the splint/cast.
- Return to school/work only when you are not requiring narcotic pain medication.
- Use crutches/cane as instructed.
- Call your doctor if
  – Your swelling increases
  – Your toes become numb or painful
  – You have burning pain under the cast
  – You have increasing pain not helped by elevation and pain medication

ACTIVITY
- If fracture is stable, early weight bearing in a cast/protective boot is encouraged at 2–3 weeks.
- Most fractures should be non-weight bearing for 6–8 weeks or until there is evidence of healing.

PREVENT
- Avoid uneven surfaces for walking/running.
- Wear proper shoes.
- Avoid physical activity when fatigued.

ANKYLOSING SPONDYLITIS

Jane S. Kim, MD

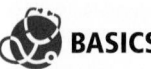 **BASICS**

DESCRIPTION
Ankylosing spondylitis (AS) is a chronic inflammatory seronegative arthritis affecting the axial skeleton with primary involvement of the sacroiliac joint.

- System(s) Affected: Musculoskeletal
- Synonym(s): Rheumatoid spondylitis; Marie-Strumpell disease

EPIDEMIOLOGY
- Predominant age: Onset usually in early 20s, rarely occurs after age >40 years of age
- Predominant sex: Male > Female (3:1)

Incidence
- In white males: 0.5–5 per 1,000
- Less common in women and African Americans

Prevalence
0.1–0.2% in United States

RISK FACTORS
- HLA-B27 (1% of HLA-B27-positive adults likely to have AS)
- Positive family history
  - 10% risk of developing AS for HLA-B27-positive child of spondylitic parent

Genetics
Familial clustering and higher than expected frequency of HLA-B27 tissue antigen

PATHOPHYSIOLOGY
Inflammation at the insertion of tendons causes new bone formation (enthesitis).

ETIOLOGY
Unknown

ASSOCIATED CONDITIONS
- Uveitis (25–30%)
- Iritis
- Psoriasis
- Aortic insufficiency (2%)

DIAGNOSIS

SIGNS AND SYMPTOMS
History
- Insidious onset
- Duration >3 months
- Morning stiffness
- Frequently awaken at night to "walk off" stiffness
- Improvement in stiffness with activity
- Increased symptoms with rest
- Hip, shoulder, or knee complaints
- Constitutional symptoms (fatigue, weight loss, low-grade fever)

Physical Exam
- Subgluteal or low back pain and/or stiffness
- Pleuritic chest pain often an early feature
- Diminished range of motion in the lumbar spine in all three planes of motion
- Loss of lumbar lordosis
- Thoracocervical kyphosis (rarely occurs before 10 years of symptoms)
- Aortic regurgitation murmur (1%)
- Acute anterior uveitis
- Osteoporosis
- Plantar fasciitis
- Peripheral arthritis (20–30%)

TESTS
- Synovial fluid: Mild leukocytosis, decreased viscosity
- EKG: Conduction defects
- Measurement of respiratory excursion of chest wall: <5 cm maximal respiratory excursion of chest wall measured at fourth intercostal space
- <2.5 cm is virtually diagnostic of ankylosing spondylitis
- Wright-Schober test for lumbar spine flexion is abnormal or <5 cm.
  - Mark the patient's back over the L5 spinous process and 10 cm above this point, then have the patient bend forward. The distance between the 2 marks should increase by 5 cm or more in normal persons.

Lab
- The HLA-B_{27} tissue antigen is present in 90% of White AS patients; there is a 5–8% incidence in the general population.
- ESR and CRP are elevated in the majority of the cases but correlate poorly with disease activity and prognosis. Mild elevation in serum IgA, creatine kinase, alkaline phosphatase, and complement may be seen.
- Absent rheumatoid factor
- Mild normochromic anemia (15%)

Imaging
- Sacroiliac joint early: Sclerosis on both sides of joint not extending >1 cm from articular surface = sacroiliitis
- Sacroiliac joint late
  - Ankylosis of sacroiliac joint
  - Osteopenia
- Spine
  - "Squaring" of vertebral bodies and ossification of annulus fibrosis giving appearance of "bamboo spine"
  - Ankylosis of facet joints
- Peripheral joint
  - Symmetric erosive changes in larger joints
  - Pericapsular ossification, sclerosis, loss of joint space
- Preferred position for imaging the SI joints with plain films is oblique projection. MRI of the SI joints may show increased signal from the bone and bone marrow suggesting osteitis and edema.

Diagnostic Procedures/Surgery
- Physical examination
- Radiographs: Sacroiliac joint films, lumbar spine series
- DEXA bone scan (high incidence of osteoporosis)
- MRI may show early enthesitis.

Pathological Findings
- Erosive changes coupled with new bone formation at the attachment of the tendons and ligaments to the bone resulting in ossification of periarticular soft tissues
- Synovial changes are indistinguishable from rheumatoid arthritis.
- Erosion of articular cartilage is less severe than in rheumatoid arthritis.

DIFFERENTIAL DIAGNOSIS
- Reactive arthritis
- Psoriatic arthritis
- Diffuse idiopathic skeletal hypertrophy (DISH)
- Spondylitis associated with inflammatory bowel disease
- Rheumatoid arthritis

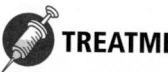 **TREATMENT**

GENERAL MEASURES

- Appropriate healthcare: Outpatient
- Posture training and range of motion exercises for spine are essential.
- Firm bed
- Sleep in supine position without a pillow
- Breathing exercises 2–3 × a day
- Smoking cessation

Activity

- Encourage active lifestyle. Swimming, tai chi, and walking are recommended.
- Avoid trauma/contact sports.
- Avoid prolonged standing.

SPECIAL THERAPY

Physical Therapy

Exercises to improve posture and flexibility

 MEDICATION (DRUGS)

First Line

- NSAIDs provide symptomatic relief, usually rapidly.
  – A dramatic response to NSAIDs can be diagnostic of AS.
- Selection is empiric, but traditionally indomethacin 50 mg t.i.d. or q.i.d. has been used.
- Intra-articular steroid injections may provide relief though systemic corticosteroids typically do not.
- Osteoporosis prophylaxis and treatment
- Injection of a long-acting corticosteroid into the sacroiliac joints may be beneficial in very symptomatic patients. Avoid systemic corticosteroids.
- Precautions
  – All patients on long-term NSAIDs should have their renal function monitored.
  – NSAIDs may aggravate peptic ulcer disease or cause gastritis.
  – NSAIDs should be used with caution in patients with a bleeding diathesis or patients requiring anticoagulants.
  – Refer to the manufacturer's profile of each drug for significant possible interactions.

Second Line

- Used when patients fail NSAIDs or become intolerant of them
- Sulfasalazine and methotrexate caused clinical improvement.
- Etanercept (anti-tumor necrosis factor alpha agent) showed rapid, significant, and sustained improvement and is now FDA-approved for AS. (2)[A]
- Infliximab can be efficacious and is also FDA-approved for AS. (4)[A]
  Thalidomide shows promise. (3)[C]
- Pamidronate may also help function and decrease
- disease activity. (3)[C]

SURGERY

- Total hip replacement should be considered to restore upright posture and to control pain in severe cases.
- Vertebral osteotomy can improve posture for those patients with severe cervical flexion.

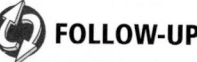 **FOLLOW-UP**

DISPOSITION

Issues for Referral

Rheumatologists will be experienced in diagnosing and treating AS.

PROGNOSIS

- Unpredictable course
- Prognosis good if mobility and upright posture maintained
- Usually progressive disability
- No difference in overall mortality

COMPLICATIONS

- Spine
  – Spinal fusion causing kyphosis
  – Cervical spine fracture (high mortality rate)
  – C1–C2 subluxation
  – Cauda equina syndrome (rare)
- Peripheral joint ankylosis
- Pulmonary
  – Restrictive lung disease
  – Upper lobe fibrosis (rare)
- Cardiac
  – Conduction defects
  – Aortic insufficiency
  – Aortitis
  – Pericarditis
- Uveitis and cataracts
- Renal
  – IgA nephropathy
  – Amyloidosis (rare)
- Cutaneous LCV (rare)
- Gastrointestinal: Illeal and colonic mucosal ulcerations, mostly asymptomatic

PATIENT MONITORING

Visits every 6–12 months to monitor posture and range of motion

REFERENCES

1. Bennett DL, Ohashi K, El-Khoury GY. Spondyloarthropathies: Ankylosing spondylitis and psoriatic arthritis. *Radiol Clin North Am*. 2004; 42(1):121–134.
2. Gorman JD, Sack KE, Davis JC Jr. Treatment of ankylosing spondylitis by inhibition of tumor necrosis factor alpha. *N Engl J Med*. 2002; 346:1349–1356.
3. Davis JC Jr, Huang F, Maksymowych W. New therapies for ankylosing spondylitis: Etanercept, thalidomide, and pamidronate. *Rheum Dis Clin North Am*. 2003;29:481–494.
4. De Keyser F, Baeten D, Van den Bosch F, Kruithof E, Mielants H, Veys EM. Infliximab in patients who have spondyloarpthropathy: Clinical efficacy, safety, and biological immunomodulation. *Rheum Dis Clin North Am*. 2003;29(3):463–479.
5. Kataria RK, Brent LH. Spondyloarthropathies. *Am Fam Phys*. 2004;69(12):2853–2860.

 MISCELLANEOUS

See also: Arthritis; Psoriatic; Arthritis; Rheumatoid (RA); Crohn Disease; Reiter Syndrome; Ulcerative Colitis

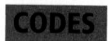 **CODES**

ICD9-CM

720.0 Ankylosing spondylitis

PATIENT TEACHING

- American Academy of Family Physicians Foundation: P.O. Box 8418, Kansas City, MO 64114, (800) 274-2237, ext. 4400 www.familydoctor.org.
- www.spondylitis.org

 See Corresponding Diagnostic Algorithm

ANORECTAL ABSCESS

Timothy L. Black, MD

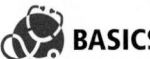 **BASICS**

DESCRIPTION

- Localized induration and fluctuance due to inflammation of the soft tissue near the rectum or anus
- 80% are perianal, the remainder are intrasphincteric or supra-levator (1)[C]
- System(s) Affected: Gastrointestinal; Skin/Exocrine

ALERT

Geriatric Considerations
A high pelvirectal abscess may cause no symptoms except lower abdominal pain and fever.

Pediatric Considerations
Common in first year of life

GENERAL PREVENTION

- Avoid constipation.
- Don't use enemas.
- Avoid rectal temperatures or medicines in immunocompromised patients.

EPIDEMIOLOGY

- Predominant age: All ages (most common in infants) (2)[C]
- Predominant sex: Male > Female (4:1)

Incidence
Common

RISK FACTORS

- Inciting trauma
  - Injections for internal hemorrhoids
  - Enema tip abrasions
  - Puncture wounds from eggshells or fish bones
  - Foreign objects
  - Prolapsed hemorrhoid
- Inflammatory bowel disease
- Chronic granulomatous disease
- Immunodeficiency disorders
- Hematologic malignancies (5–8% of these patients will have abscess at some time)
- Diabetes
- Chronic medical immunosuppression

ETIOLOGY

- Bacterial invasion of the anal glands found in the intersphincteric space, which may begin with an abrasion or tear in lining of anal canal, rectum, or perianal skin
- Organisms (usually mixed):
  - *Escherichia coli*
  - Proteus vulgaris
  - Streptococci
  - Staphylococci
  - Bacteroides
  - Pseudomonas aeruginosa

ASSOCIATED CONDITIONS

- Crohn's disease
- Other inflammatory disease (e.g., appendicitis, salpingitis, diverticulitis)
- Possibly perianal hidradenitis suppurativa, or HIV infection in patients with recurring perianal or ischiorectal abscesses

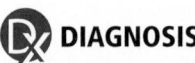 **DIAGNOSIS**

SIGNS AND SYMPTOMS

- Perirectal swelling for superficial abscesses
- Perirectal redness
- Perirectal tenderness
- Perirectal throbbing pain
- Fever and other toxic symptoms with deep abscesses
- If abscess is not accompanied by external swelling, digital rectal exam will reveal a swollen tender mass.
- Pain on defecation

Physical Exam
Digital rectal examination is mandatory

TESTS

Lab
Complete blood count: Leukocytosis

Imaging
- Barium enema (rarely needed)
- CT scan of pelvis and perineum indicated if horseshoe or ischiorectal abscess suspected (3)[C]

Diagnostic Procedures/Surgery
Only indicated if diagnosis in doubt
- Sigmoidoscopy: Rule out unusual causes
- Proctoscopy: Redness, induration of anus; tender mass

Pathological Findings
- Inflammation of anal mucosa
- Pus
- Inflammatory tissue

DIFFERENTIAL DIAGNOSIS

- Carcinoma
- Retrorectal tumors
- Crohn's disease
- Primary lesions of syphilis
- Tuberculous ulceration

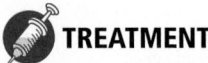 **TREATMENT**

GENERAL MEASURES
Appropriate health care

- Outpatient surgery with oral antibiotics (although in some cases, antibiotics may not be necessary) (4)[B]
- Inpatient surgery with IV antibiotics for supra-levator abscess or toxicity (3)[C]

Diet
Increase fiber and fluid intake.

Activity
Resume work and normal activity as soon as possible.

MEDICATION (DRUGS)

- Antibiotics
- Stool-softening laxatives
- Contraindications
  - Refer to manufacturer's literature
- Precautions
  - Refer to manufacturer's literature
- Significant possible interactions
  - Refer to manufacturer's literature

SURGERY

- Perianal abscess
  - Incise and drain abscess (4)[B]
  - Local anesthetic frequently appropriate
  - Pack wound with Iodoform gauze (24–48 hours).
- Ischiorectal abscess
  - Incise and drain abscess (4)[B]
  - General anesthetic usually required
  - Pack wound with Iodoform gauze or similar packing (removed gradually over several days).
  - Fistulectomy may be done at the same time in selected cases.
- Supralevator abscess
  - Incise and drain abscess into lower rectum or anal canal (3)[C]
  - General anesthesia required
- After surgery
  - Sitz baths q2–4h
  - Heating pad, heat lamp, or warm compress as needed for pain
  - Encourage moving legs as soon as possible
  - Prevent constipation.

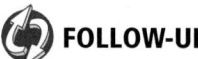 **FOLLOW-UP**

PROGNOSIS

- Slow healing depending on extent of disease and concurrent illnesses, complete healing by 6 months if no complications
- Healing in infants may be complete in 1–3 weeks.
- Drainage alone results in cure rate of 50% or more.

COMPLICATIONS

- Possible anorectal fistula (in 25% of patients) (2,3)[C]
- Possible rectovaginal fistula
- Fecal incontinence due to rupture through sphincter muscle
- Recurrence of abscess if underlying cause not corrected
- Necrotizing infection with rapid progression, sepsis, and death (3)[C]

PATIENT MONITORING

Routine postoperative care with attention to wound healing, which should progress from the inside out

REFERENCES

1. Fazio VW. Anorectal disorders. In: *Gastroenterology Clinics of North America*. Philadelphia: Saunders; 1987.
2. Ziegler M, Azizkhan R, Weber T, et al., eds. *Operative Pediatric Surgery*. New York: McGraw-Hill, 2003
3. Townsend C, Beauchamp RD, Evers BM, et al. eds. *Sabiston Textbook of Surgery*, 17 ed. Philadelphia: Elsevier Saunders, 2006
4. Whiteford MH, Kilkenny J, Hyman N, et al. Practice parameters for the treatment of perianal abscess and fistula-in-ano (revised). *Dis Colon Rectum* 2005;48:1337–1342.

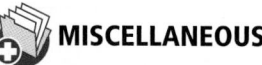 **MISCELLANEOUS**

See also: Anorectal Fistula

 CODES

ICD9-CM
566 Abscess of anal and rectal regions

PATIENT TEACHING

- Provide sitz bath instructions.
- Provide diet instructions.
- Provide dressing change instructions.
- Stress length of time to heal.
- Stress physical cleanliness.
- Watch for possible development of fistula-in-ano.
- Stress stool regularity.

ANORECTAL FISTULA

Timothy L. Black, MD

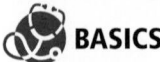 **BASICS**

DESCRIPTION

Inflammatory track with one opening in the anal canal and another in perianal skin. Fistulas occur spontaneously or secondary to perirectal abscess. Most fistulas originate in the anal crypts at the anorectal junction.

- Goodsall's rule
  - If external opening is anterior to an imaginary line drawn horizontally through anal canal, fistula usually runs directly into anal canal.
  - If external opening is posterior to line, fistula usually curves to posterior midline of anal canal.
  - For Goodsall's rule: Anterior fistulae, PPV is ~70%, for Posterior fistulae, PPV is ~40%.
  - In children, track is usually straight.
- Classification (1)[C]
  - Intersphincteric: Fistula is confined to the intersphincteric plane (most common).
  - Transsphincteric: Fistula connects intersphincteric plane with ischiorectal fossa by perforating the external sphincter.
  - Suprasphincteric: Fistula connects intersphincteric plane with ishiorectal fossa but loops over external sphincter.
  - Extrasphincteric: Fistula connects rectum to perineal skin but passes external to sphincter.
- System(s) Affected: Gastrointestinal; Skin/Exocrine
- Synonym(s): Fistula-in-ano; Anal fistula

ALERT

Geriatric Considerations
Constipation is a common complication.

Pediatric Considerations
- Most common in infants
- More frequent in males

GENERAL PREVENTION
Prevention or prompt treatment of anorectal abscess

EPIDEMIOLOGY
- Predominant age: All ages
- Predominant sex: Male = Female

Incidence
Common

RISK FACTORS
- Injection of internal hemorrhoids, puncture wound from eggshells or fish bones, foreign objects, enema tip injuries
- Ruptured anal hematoma
- Prolapsed internal hemorrhoid
- Acute appendicitis, salpingitis, diverticulitis
- Inflammatory bowel disease (chronic ulcerative colitis, Crohn disease)
- Previous perirectal abscess
- Radiation treatment to perineum/pelvis
- Trauma, either internal or external
- Carcinoma

ETIOLOGY
- Erosion of anal canal
- Extension from infection from a tear in lining of anal canal
- Infecting organism is commonly *Escherichia coli*

ASSOCIATED CONDITIONS
- Possibly associated with penetrating injury, intestinal tuberculosis, ulcerative colitis
- Hidradenitis suppurativa
- Crohn disease

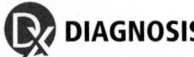 **DIAGNOSIS**

SIGNS AND SYMPTOMS
- Constant or intermittent drainage or discharge
- Firm tender perianal lump
- External anal sphincter pain during and after defecation
- Spasm of external anal sphincter during and after defecation
- Anal bleeding
- Discoloration of skin surrounding fistula
- Fistulous opening frequently granulose or scarred
- Possible fever
- Recurrent anorectal abscesses in identical locations

History
- History of perianal drainage
- History of perianal pain
- History of recurrent perianal abscesses

Physical Exam
- Perineal or perianal draining orifice
- Recurrent perianal abscesses in identical location
- Small palpable lesion sometimes identified on rectal exam at level of anal crypts

TESTS
Lab
- Complete blood count (usually not indicated)
- Prometheus first step serology for inflammatory bowel disease (if Crohn disease suspected)
- Consider RPR for recurrent fistulas in sexually active patients.

Imaging
- Lower gastrointestinal series if inflammatory bowel disease suspected
- Pelvic MRI or endorectal ultrasound may be useful in complex or recurrent fistulas

Diagnostic Procedures/Surgery
- Proctoscopy
- Sigmoidoscopy
- Probe inserted into tract to determine its course (be careful not to create an artificial opening)
- Injection of dilute methylene blue into abscess cavity may be helpful in demonstrating fistula (1)[C]

Pathological Findings
- Fistulous tract may be simple or multiple
- Fistulous tract has primary opening in anal crypt; secondary opening in anal skin, para-anal skin, perineal skin, or in rectal mucus membrane
- Anal sinus: Opens in anal crypt
- Termination of sinus is blind and located in para-anal or pararectal tissue.

DIFFERENTIAL DIAGNOSIS
- Pilonidal sinus
- Perianal abscess
- Urethroperineal fistulas
- Ischiorectal abscess
- Submucous or high muscular abscess
- Pelvirectal abscess (rare)
- Rule out: Crohn disease; carcinoma; retrorectal tumors

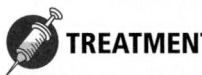 **TREATMENT**

GENERAL MEASURES
- Appropriate health care: Outpatient surgery
- Sitz baths 3–4 times per day until definitive surgery

Diet
Clear liquid diet until gastrointestinal function returns

Activity
Resume work and normal activity as soon as possible.

MEDICATION (DRUGS)

- Broad-spectrum antibiotic if active infection
  - Cephalexin (Keflex)
  - Cefadroxil (Duricef)
  - Ampicillin-sulbactam (Unasyn)
  - Amoxicillin-clavulanate (Augmentin)
- Stool-softening laxative
- Contraindications
  - Refer to manufacturer's literature
- Precautions
  - Refer to manufacturer's literature
- Significant possible interactions
  - Refer to manufacturer's literature

SURGERY

- Fistulotomy
  - Surgical incision of entire length of fistula (unroofing) (2)[A]
  - Mucosal tract should be cauterized or curetted
  - Sphincterotomy
- Fistulectomy
  - Complete excision of tract (rarely indicated, because of extensive tissue loss)
  - Sphincterotomy
- Consider Seton stitch placement (especially for suprasphincteric or transsphincteric fistulas). (2)[A]
- Endorectal advancement flap closure for complex fistulas. (2)[A]
- General anesthesia or regional anesthesia usually required (usually done as outpatient procedure in children)
- Consider use of fibrin glue in selected cases of anal fistulas (2)[A], (3)[C]
- Fistulas in Crohn Disease (2)[A]
  - Asymptomatic fistulas may not need treatment.
  - Simple fistulas treated with unroofing
  - Complex fistulas treated with advancement flap or long term setons
  - May require a stoma
- Postoperative: Sitz baths
- Avoid constipation.

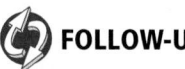 **FOLLOW-UP**

PROGNOSIS

- Surgical results usually excellent
- Postoperative healing
  - 4–5 weeks for perianal fistulas
  - 12–16 weeks for deeper fistulas
- Postoperative healing may occur within 2–3 weeks in children.
- Recurrence rates 2–9% in simple fistulas (2)[A]

COMPLICATIONS

- Constipation (urge to defecate may be suppressed due to pain)
- Rectovaginal fistula
- Partial incontinence of fecal material if sphincter is divided
- Delayed wound healing
- Low-grade carcinoma may develop in long-standing fistulas.
- Recurrent anorectal fistula if fistula is incompletely opened or excised
- Chronic intermittent infections
- Sepsis (rarely)

PATIENT MONITORING

Frequent follow-up examinations following surgery to ensure complete healing and assess continence

REFERENCES

1. Townsend C, Beauchamp RD, Evers BM, et al., eds. *Sabiston Textbook of Surgery*, 17th ed. Philadelphia: Elsevier Saunders; 2006.
2. Whiteford MH, Kilkenny J, Hyman N, et al. Practice parameters for the treatment of perianal abscess and fistula-in-ano (Revised). *Dis Colon Rectum*. 2005;48:1337–1342.
3. Hammond TM, Grahn MF, Lunniss PJ. Fibrin glue in the management of anal fistulae. *Colorectal Dis*. 2004;6:308–319.

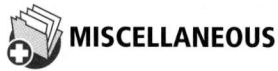 **MISCELLANEOUS**

See also: Anorectal Abscess; Crohn Disease

ANOREXIA NERVOSA (AN)

Mary Muscari, PhD, RN, CRNP, CS

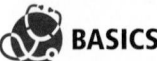 **BASICS**

DESCRIPTION
- Refusal to maintain normal body weight, with associated fear of weight gain, body image disturbance, and amenorrhea
- Restricting and binge-eating/purging subtypes
- System(s) Affected: Cardiovascular; Endocrine; Metabolic; Gastrointestinal; Nervous; Reproductive

GENERAL PREVENTION
Encourage rational attitude about nutrition and weight, minimize weight-related criticism and teasing, moderate overly high self-expectations, enhance self-esteem

EPIDEMIOLOGY
- Predominant age at onset: 13–18 years
- Predominant sex: Female > Male (20:1)
- Global distribution

Incidence
8–19 women, 2 men per 100,000 per year

Prevalence
<1% in women, <0.1% in men

RISK FACTORS
- Female gender
- Perceived body image distortions
- Perfectionism, obsessionality, rigidity
- Negative self-evaluation
- Academic and other achievement pressure
- Participation in sports or artistic activities that emphasize leanness or involve subjective scoring
  – Ballet, running, wrestling, figure skating, gymnastics, cheerleading, weight lifting
- Parental psychiatric disorder

Genetics
- Underlying genetic vulnerability likely, but not well understood
  – 1st-degree female relative with eating disorder increases risk 6- to 10-fold.

PATHOPHYSIOLOGY
Complex relationship between biologic, psychological, and social factors that results in an unrealistic perception of fatness. Subsequent malnutrition leads to disorder of multiple organs.

ETIOLOGY
- Serotonin neuronal systems are implicated.
- Multifactorial withpsychological, biological, genetic, environmental, and social factors

ASSOCIATED CONDITIONS
- Mood disorder
- Social phobia, obsessive-compulsive disorder
- Substance abuse disorder
- High rates of cluster C personality disorders

DIAGNOSIS

SIGNS AND SYMPTOMS
- Onset may be insidious or stress related
- Amenorrhea (primary or secondary)
- Report feeling fat even when emaciated
- Preoccupation with body size, weight control
- Elaborate food preparation and eating rituals
- Extensive exercise
- Weakness, fatigue, cognitive impairment
- Hypothermia, cold intolerance
- Constipation, bloating, early satiety
- Dry skin, scalp hair loss, peripheral edema
- Lanugo hair on extremities, face, and trunk
- Growth arrest, delayed puberty
- Hypotension, bradycardia, murmurs
- Decreased bone density, fractures

History
Ascertain fear of weight gain and/or distorted body image.

Physical Exam
- Often normal
- Vital signs: Bradycardia, orthostatic hypotension, body weight <85% expected
- Cardiac: Dysrhythmias, midsystolic click of mitral valve prolapse
- Skin/extremities: Dry, lanugo, hair loss, edema
- Neurologic and abdominal exams: To rule out other causes of weight loss and vomiting

TESTS
Lab
- No specific test for AN. Most findings are related directly to starvation, dehydration
  – All findings may be within normal limits.
- Low serum leuteinizing hormone, follicle-stimulating hormone; low T_4 with normal TSH
- Abnormal liver enzymes
- Altered blood urea nitrogen, creatinine clearance; electrolyte disturbances
- Hypoglycemia, hypercholesterolemia, hypercortisolemia, hypophosphatemia
- Low sedimentation rate
- Anemia, leukopenia, thrombocytopenia
- 12-lead ECG to assess for prolonged QT

Imaging
Dual-energy x-ray absorptiometry (DEXA) of bone only if underweight for >6 months to assess for diminished bone density

Diagnostic Procedures/Surgery
- DSM-IV-TR criteria
  – Refusal to maintain body weight at or above a minimally normal weight for age, height
  – Intense fear of gaining weight even though underweight
  – A disturbance in the way body weight/shape is experienced; undue influence of body on self-evaluation or denial of seriousness of low body weight
  – Specific types
    ○ Restricting: Not engaged in binge-eating or purging behaviors
    ○ Binge-eating/purging type: Regularly engages in binge-eating or purging behaviors (see Bulimia information related to these behaviors)
- Screening tools: SCOFF questionnaire, Eating disorder Screen for Primary Care (ESP), Eating Attitudes Test (EAT), Eating Disorder Inventory (EDI)

Pathological Findings
- Osteoporosis/osteopenia, pathologic fractures
- Sick euthyroid syndrome
- Cardiac impairment

DIFFERENTIAL DIAGNOSIS
- Hyperthyroidism,adrenal insufficiency
- Inflammatory bowel disease
- Immunodeficiency, chronic infections
- Malabsorption, diabetes
- CNS lesion
- Bulimia; body dysmorphic disorder
- Depressive disorders with loss of appetite
- Anxiety disorder, food phobia
- Conversion disorder, schizophrenic disorder

ALERT
AN may exist concurrently with chronic medical disorders, such as diabetes, cystic fibrosis.

TREATMENT

GENERAL MEASURES

- Initial treatment goal geared to weight restoration; most are managed as outpatients
- Outpatient treatment
  - Interdisciplinary team (primary care physician, mental health professional, nutritionist) (1,2)[B,C]
  - Average weekly weight gain goal: 0.5–1.0 kg (1)[C] with stepwise increase in calories
  - Cognitive behavioral and/or family-based therapy (2,3)[B]
  - Focus on health, not weight gain alone.
  - Build trust, treatment alliance ,
  - Involve patient in establishing diet and exercise goals.
  - Challenge fear of uncontrolled weight gain; help the patient to recognize feelings that lead to disordered eating.
  - In chronic cases, goal may be to achieve a safe weight rather than a healthy weight.
- Inpatient treatment
  - If possible, admit to specialized eating disorders unit (4)[C]
  - Monitor vital signs, cardiac function, watch for edema, rapid weight gain (fluid overload)
  - Initial bed rest with supervised meals may be necessary.
  - Stepwise increase in activity
  - Tube feeding or total parental nutrition used only as last resort
  - Supportive symptomatic care as needed

Diet

- Goal is stabilization at a healthy weight on a balanced diet with normal eating pattern
- Diminished ruminations about calories, weight; increased enjoyment

Activity

- Monitor activity.
- Stepwise increase as patient gains weight
- Focus on enjoyable activities rather than goal-oriented ones.

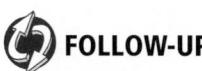 **MEDICATION (DRUGS)**

First Line

- No medications are available that effectively treat patients with AN, but antidepressants may benefit those with comorbid depression (5,6)[C].
- Selective serotonin-reuptake inhibitors such as fluoxetine (Prozac): 10–60 mg may
  - Help prevent relapse after weight gain
  - Treat comorbid depression or obsessive-compulsive disorder (1,4,6)[C]
  - Attend to black box warnings concerning antidepressants and conduct appropriate informed consent if antidepressants are prescribed

Second Line

- Management of osteopenia
  - Elemental calcium 1200–1500 mg/d plus MVI containing 800 IU of vitamin D (2,4)[C]
  - No indication for bisphosphonates in AN (2)[C]
  - Weak evidence for use of HRT (2)[C]
  - Psyllium (Metamucil) preparations (1 tbsp) to prevent constipation

 FOLLOW-UP

DISPOSITION

Admission Criteria

- Suggested physiologic values: Heart rate <40 bpm, BP <90/60, symptomatic hypoglycemia, potassium <3 mmol/L, temperature <97.0°F (36.1°C), dehydration, other cardiovascular abnormalities, weight <75% of the expected weight, rapid weight loss, lack of improvement while in outpatient therapy
- Suggested psychological indications: Poor motivation/insight, lack of cooperation with outpatient treatment, inability to eat, need for nasogastric feeding, suicidal plan or intent, severe coexisting psychiatric disease, problematic family environment

ALERT

Pediatric Considerations

- Children often present with nausea, abdominal pain, fullness, and inability to swallow.
- Additional indications for hospitalization: Heart rate <50 bpm, orthostatic BP, hypokalemia or hypophosphatemia, rapid weight loss even if weight not <75% below normal

Geriatric Considerations

Late-onset AN (>50) may be long-term disease, or triggered by death of loved one, marital discord, or divorce.

Discharge Criteria

Lower relapse rate when discharged at expected healthy weights

PROGNOSIS

- Prognosis: ~50% recover; 25% improved; 25% chronically ill
- Mortality: 5–7%

COMPLICATIONS

- Refeeding syndrome
- Cardiac arrhythmia; cardiac arrest
- Cardiomyopathy, congestive heart failure
- Delayed gastric emptying, necrotizing colitis
- Seizures, Wernicke encephalopathy, peripheral neuropathy, cognitive deficits
- Osteopenia, osteoporosis

Pregnancy Considerations

- Fertility may be affected.
- Increased risk for miscarriage, operative delivery, congenital malformations, and low-birth-weight infants; should be managed as high risk

PATIENT MONITORING

- Level of exercise activity
- Weigh weekly until stable, then monthly.
- Depression, self-esteem, suicidal ideation

REFERENCES

1. NICE. Eating disorders—core interventions in the treatment and management of anorexia nervosa, bulimia nervosa and related eating disorders. NICE Clinical Guideline no 9. London: NICE, 2004 (accessed 15 Feb 2006).
2. American Psychiatric Association. Practice Guideline for the Treatment of Patients with Eating Disorders, 3rd ed. 2006, June (accessed Dec 10, 2006).
3. Hay P, Bacaltchuk J, Claudino A, Ben-Tovim D, et al. Individual psychotherapy in the outpatient treatment of adults with anorexia. *Cochrane Database Syst Rev.* 2003;(4):CD003909.
4. Yager J, Anderson AE. Anorexia nervosa. *N Engl J Med.* 2005;353:1481–1488.
5. Berkman ND, Bulik CM, Brownley KA, et al. Management of eating disorders. Evidence report/technology assessment No. 135. (Prepared by the RTI International-University of North Carolina Evidence-Based Practice Center under Contract No. 290-02-0016.) AHRQ Publication No. 06-E010. Rockville, MD: Agency for Healthcare Research and Quality, April 2006.
6. Claudino A, Hay P, Lima M, et al. Antidepressants for anorexia nervosa. *Cochrane Database Sys Rev.* 2006;(1):CD04365.

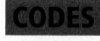 **MISCELLANEOUS**

See also: Amenorrhea; Osteoporosis; Bulimia

CODES

ICD9-CM
307 Anorexia nervosa

ICD10
F50.1 Anorexia nervosa

PATIENT TEACHING

Provide information on nutrition, metabolic balance, and natural history of the disorder.

Diet
Importance of continued adherence to prescribed diet

Activity
Importance of moderate activity for health, not thinness

Prevention
Focus on health lifestyle, not body image

ANTHRAX

Benjamin L. Sapers, MD

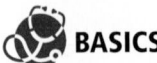 **BASICS**

DESCRIPTION

- Anthrax is a highly infectious disease of animals, especially ruminants (hooved animals such as cows, goats, sheep, etc.) that is caused by the bacteria *Bacillus anthracis*. Cutaneous (95% of US cases); inhalational, and gastrointestinal forms can be transmitted to man by contact with the animals or their products.
- Synonym(s) for skin anthrax: Charbon; Malignant pustule; Siberian ulcer; Malignant edema; Splenic fever; Milzbrand; Ragpicker disease
- Synonym(s) for chest anthrax: Woolsorter disease

GENERAL PREVENTION

- Anthrax vaccine protects against all forms of anthrax and is as safe as other vaccines, according to the Food and Drug Administration, the Centers for Disease Control and Prevention, and the National Academy of Sciences. A 2005 review by the Cochrane Infectious Disease Group concluded that the anthrax vaccine is effective in reducing the risk of contracting anthrax and has a low rate of adverse effects (1)[A].
- Vaccine is given in 6 doses (0, 2, and 4 weeks, and 6, 12, and 18 months) plus annual boosters.
  - If you get behind schedule, don't start the series over; begin where you left off (delays don't reduce the resulting protection).
  - Redness up to 1 inch (1 cm) wide occurs in 30% of men and 60% of women, and redness or other reactions >5 inches (4 cm) occur in ~1% of people (both male and female).
  - Anthrax vaccine often causes a nodule under the skin where the vaccine is injected; this can last from 2–3 months. These nodules eventually resolve.
  - The Advisory Committee on Immunization Practices recommends vaccination for the following groups
    - Persons who work directly with the organism in the laboratory
    - Persons who work with imported animal hides or furs in areas where standards are insufficient to prevent exposure to anthrax spores
    - Persons who handle potentially infected animal products in high-incidence areas
    - Military personnel deployed to areas with high risk for exposure to organisms (when used as a biologic warfare weapon)
    - Pregnant women should be vaccinated for anthrax only if absolutely necessary.
- Patients with a likely exposure history but no symptoms are candidates for postexposure prophylaxis with either ciprofloxacin 500 mg PO b.i.d. or doxycycline 100 mg PO b.i.d.

EPIDEMIOLOGY

- Cutaneous (skin): 95% of cases in the US; cases of cutaneous anthrax without occupational risk should raise concern for a terrorist attack. About 5–20% of untreated cases result in death.
- Gastrointestinal (GI): Very rare in the US (no documented case in the 20th century).
- Inhalational (chest) anthrax is very rare in US; must be considered a bioterrorist event in US until proven otherwise (the last US occupational case occurred in 1976). Death results in 99% of untreated cases, and in 45–80% of patients with severe symptoms who are treated in a state-of-the-art facility.
- Anthrax is most common in agricultural regions, where it occurs in animals. These regions include the Middle East, Asia, Southern and Eastern Europe, Africa, South and Central America, and the Caribbean.

RISK FACTORS

- Contact with infected animals or their products
- Bioterrorist event

PATHOPHYSIOLOGY

- *Bacillus anthracis* is a spore-forming, gram-positive bacterium found in the soil worldwide. The word *anthracis* is derived from a Greek word meaning "coal," which is used to describe the cutaneous form of the disease that leads to a characteristic black lesion.
- *B. anthracis* has 3 known virulence factors: An antiphagocytic capsule and 2 protein toxins (known as edema factor and lethal factor).
  - The capsule provides resistance to phagocytosis.
  - Lethal factor and edema factor are named for the effects they induce when injected into experimental animals.
  - A protein called protective antigen binds to the host cell's surface; when cleaved by a protease on the cell surface it creates a binding site to which the lethal factor and edema factor can bind; protective antigen is required for the action of the 2 protein toxins.
- *B. anthracis* spores introduced into the host are ingested at the exposed site by macrophages and then germinate into vegetative forms that produce the virulence factors.

ETIOLOGY

- Skin: Occurs when *B. anthracis* enters the skin through a cut or abrasion during the handling of animal products (such as meat, wool, or hides infected with *B. anthracis*)
- GI: Ingestion of bacillus-contaminated meat
- Chest: Inhalation of aerosolized *B. anthracis* spores

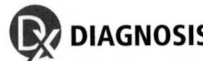 **DIAGNOSIS**

SIGNS AND SYMPTOMS

- Skin: Begins as a pruritic red-brown papule that enlarges with peripheral erythema, vesiculation, and induration, followed by black eschar formation within 7–10 days of the initial lesion. The papule, blister, and eschar are painless, and cutaneous symptoms may be accompanied by fever, malaise, and headache. A black eschar with massive edema is nearly pathognomonic for cutaneous anthrax.
- GI: Presents as 1 of 2 distinct syndromes—oropharyngeal and abdominal. Oropharyngeal syndrome presentation can include fever, edema, ulcer, severe sore throat, and lymphadenopathy resulting in marked unilateral or bilateral neck swelling. Abdominal syndrome may present with fever, malaise, hematemesis, anorexia, severe abdominal pain, and hematochezia or melena.
- Chest: Biphasic presentation, with initial phase featuring nonspecific influenzalike symptoms such as low-grade fever, chills, headache, nonproductive cough, diaphoresis, malaise, chest discomfort, nausea, vomiting, diarrhea, and abdominal pain. This initial phase is followed by the 2nd fulminant phase that includes abrupt onset of high fever, severe dyspnea, hypoxia, hypotension, and death.

History

- Skin: Crucial clinical clues are the rapid evolution of symptoms, lack of pain, occasional massive edema, and the near pathognomonic black eschar. Incubation period is usually immediate but may last up to 1 day.
- GI: Incubation period usually 1–7 days; 2–4 days after onset of symptoms, ascites develop as abdominal pain decreases. Shock and death occur within 2–5 days after onset of symptoms.
- Chest: Incubation period is usually <1 week, but may be as long as 2 months. 2nd portion of the biphasic presentation begins 1–5 days after onset of initial symptoms. There may be a 1–3 day period of improvement after the 1st phase and before the 2nd phase begins. Shock and death occur within 24–36 hours after onset of the 2nd phase.

Physical Exam

- Skin: Red-brown papule, vesicles, or black eschar
- GI: Acute abdomen with rebound tenderness may occur. Ascites present later in course
- Chest: Rhonchi may be present.

TESTS

Lab
Gram stain and culture. A presumptive diagnosis can be made if Gram-positive rods are present that are nonmotile, nonhemolytic, and encapsulated (usually seen with India ink). If antibiotics have been given for >24 hours, perform immunohistochemical staining and/or polymerase chain reaction.

Imaging
- Widened mediastinum on chest radiograph may be present in inhalational anthrax.
- Pleural effusions frequently present in chest anthrax; infiltrates are rare.
- GI: Mesenteric adenopathy on CT scan likely.

DIFFERENTIAL DIAGNOSIS
Skin
- Cellulitis
- Brown recluse spider bite
- Cat-scratch disease
- Rat bite fever
- Rickettsial spotted fever
- Carbuncle
- Cowpox
- Bullous erysipelas
- Tularemia vasculitides
- Ecthyma gangrenosum
- Orf (a transmissible viral disease of goats and sheep)

 TREATMENT

GENERAL MEASURES
Chest and GI anthrax is not known to spread from person to person, so communicability concerns are not an issue during management of the patient. For skin anthrax, avoid contact with the wound or wound drainage.

 MEDICATION (DRUGS)

First Line
- Skin: Ciprofloxacin 500 mg PO b.i.d. for 60 days or doxycycline 100 mg PO b.i.d. for 60 days. If systemic involvement, massive edema, or lesions on the head or neck, follow treatment recommendation per inhalational anthrax (2)[C].
- Chest and GI: IV ciprofloxacin 400 mg q12h or doxycycline 100 mg q12h AND 1 or 2 additional antimicrobials such as rifampin, vancomycin, penicillin, ampicillin, chloramphenicol, imipenem, clindamycin, and clarithromycin. May switch to PO when clinically appropriate. Must complete 60-day course (combined PO and IV) (2)[C].

Second Line
Patients being treated for anthrax may also benefit from vaccination as part of their regimen (3)[C].

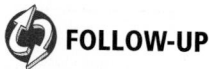 **FOLLOW-UP**

PROGNOSIS
- Skin: Death in 5–20% of untreated cases.
- GI: Mortality rates as high as 50% have been reported.
- Chest: Death in 99% of untreated cases.

PATIENT MONITORING
Must monitor patient for 60 days to ensure completion of the treatment course

REFERENCES
1. Jefferson T, Demicheli V, Deeks J, et al. Vaccines for preventing anthrax. [Systematic Review] Cochrane Infectious Diseases Group. *Cochrane Database of Systematic Rev.* 1, 2006.
2. Centers for Disease Control and Prevention. Update: Investigation of bioterrorism-related anthrax and interim guidelines for exposure management and antimicrobial therapy, October 2001. *MMWR Morb Mortal Wkly Rep.* 2001;50(42):909–919. Erratum in: *MMWR Morb Mortal Wkly Rep.* 2001;50(43):962.
3. Centers for Disease Control and Prevention. Use of anthrax vaccine in the United States, ACIP Recommendations. *MMWR Recommendations & Reports.* 2000;49(RR-15):1–20.

ADDITIONAL READING
- The anthrax vaccine immunization program. http://www.anthrax.mil
- Centers for Disease Control and Prevention, Emergency Preparedness and Response. http://www.bt.cdc.gov/agent/anthrax/
- Durning SJ, Roy MJ. Anthrax. In: Roy MJ, ed. Physician's Guide to Terrorist Attack. Totowa, NJ: Humana Press Inc.; 2003.

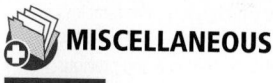 **MISCELLANEOUS**

CODES

ICD9-CM
- 022.0 Cutaneous Anthrax
- 022.1 Pulmonary Anthrax
- 022.2 Gastrointestinal Anthrax

ANTI-PHOSPHOLIPID ANTIBODY SYNDROME

Christopher S. Manasseh, MD

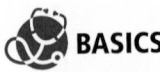 **BASICS**

DESCRIPTION

- An autoimmune thrombotic syndrome characterized by the presence of antiphospholipid antibodies in association with either recurrent venous or arterial thromboembolic events or repeated fetal loss
- Types
  - Primary
    - Occurs in patients without clinical evidence of another autoimmune disease
  - Secondary
    - Occurs in association with another disease such as systemic lupus erythematosus (SLE)
  - Catastrophic antiphospholipid syndrome
    - Differs from primary and secondary types in the caliber of vessels affected. Venous or arterial thrombosis of large vessels is less common, and patients present with acute thrombotic microangiopathy, kidney being the most commonly affected organ.
    - Disseminated intravascular coagulation which does not occur in primary or secondary forms is seen in up to 25% of patients with the catastrophic type.
- Synonym(s): Hughes syndrome

ALERT
Geriatric Considerations
Atherosclerosis and cancer are more frequent causes of thrombosis than is antiphospholipid antibody syndrome.

Pregnancy Considerations
- Increased frequency of recurrent fetal loss
- Increased risk of premature delivery due to pregnancy related hypertension and uteroplacental insufficiency

GENERAL PREVENTION
In pregnant women with h/o recurrent fetal loss, use low dose unfractionated heparin 5000 U SQ b.i.d.

- In all women with the syndrome and previous pregnancy loss, aspirin 325 mg/day may provide protection against future thrombosis.
- Modification of secondary risk factors for atherosclerosis include control of hypertension, diabetes, hyperlipidemia, and smoking cessation.

EPIDEMIOLOGY
1/2 of all patients with the syndrome have the primary form of the disease.

Incidence
- 15% of women with recurrent pregnancy loss have this syndrome
- 63% of patients have at least 1 valvular abnormality on echocardiogram

Prevalence
1–5% of otherwise young healthy adults have antiphospholipid antibodies
- 50–70% of patients with SLE who have the antiphospholipid antibodies may develop this syndrome

RISK FACTORS
- Smoking
- Oral contraceptive use
- Surgery
- Immobilization
- Pregnancy

PATHOPHYSIOLOGY
Any organ can be involved, and the extent of involvement depends on the
- Nature and size of vessel involved
- Acuteness or chronicity of the thrombotic process

ETIOLOGY
Antiphospholipid antibodies promote thrombosis by any of the following hypotheses
- Activation of endothelial cells
- Oxidant-mediated injury of the vascular endothelium
- Interference with the phospholipid binding proteins involved in the regulation of coagulation

ASSOCIATED CONDITIONS
- SLE
- Malignant hypertension
- Nephrotic syndrome

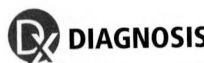 **DIAGNOSIS**

SIGNS AND SYMPTOMS
- Arthralgia
- Livedo reticularis

History
- Family history of rheumatic illness
- Personal history of thrombosis

Physical Exam
Look for deep vein thrombosis of the legs.
- Most common manifestation of the syndrome

TESTS
- ELISA test for anticardiolipin antibodies
- Clotting test for lupus anticoagulant

Lab
- Thrombocytopenia
- Leukopenia

Diagnostic Criteria
- The presence of at least ONE of the following clinical criteria
  - Vascular thrombosis
    - 1 or more clinical episodes of arterial, venous, or small vessel thrombosis, occurring within any tissue or organ
  - Complications of pregnancy
    - 1 or more unexplained deaths of morphologically normal fetuses at or after the 10th week of pregnancy OR
    - 1 or more premature births of morphologically normal neonates at or before the 34th week of pregnancy OR
    - 3 or more unexplained consecutive spontaneous abortions before the 10th week of pregnancy
- AND presence of at least ONE of the following laboratory criteria
  - Anticardiolipin antibodies
    - Anticardiolipin IgG or IgM antibodies present at moderate or high levels in the blood on 2 or more occasions at least 6 weeks apart
  - Lupus anticoagulant antibodies
    - Detected in the blood on 2 or more occasions at least 6 weeks apart

Pathological Findings
- Acute changes
  - Capillary congestion
  - Non-inflammatory fibrin thrombi
- Chronic changes
  - Ischemic hypoperfusion
  - Atrophy and fibrosis

DIFFERENTIAL DIAGNOSIS
- Other conditions that cause thrombotic microangiopathy, such as
  - Hemolytic-uremic syndrome
  - Thrombotic thrombocytopenic purpura
- Other thrombophilic conditions, such as
  - Deficiency of protein C, protein S
  - Deficiency of antithrombin III
  - Mutation of factor V Leiden
  - Prothrombin gene mutation
  - Homocysteinemia

MEDICATION (DRUGS)

First Line
Warfarin treatment of moderate intensity (to achieve an international normalized ratio (INR) of 2–2.9) significantly reduces the rate of recurrent thrombosis.
- Duration of treatment is lifelong.

Second Line
Corticosteroids and azathioprine for treatment of symptoms of lupus in patients with secondary form of the syndrome

SPECIAL THERAPY
In patients who develop new thromboses despite moderate intensity anticoagulant therapy and for patients with catastrophic antiphospholipid syndrome

- Plasmapheresis
- IV immune globulin

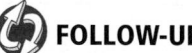 **FOLLOW-UP**

PROGNOSIS
- Pulmonary hypertension, neurologic involvement, myocardial ischemia, nephropathy, gangrene of extremities, and catastrophic APS are associated with a worse prognosis.
- Most patients experience recurrences months or years after the initial event.
- Mortality rate is ~50% in patients presenting with the catastrophic type, and death is due to multi-organ system failure.

COMPLICATIONS
Discontinuation of warfarin results in increased risk of thrombosis (even death), particularly in the 1st 6 months after stopping treatment.

PATIENT MONITORING
As warfarin therapy is lifelong, patients need to have regular monitoring to maintain INR in the therapeutic range (between 2 and 2.9).

REFERENCES

1. Lockshin M. Antiphospholipid antibody syndrome. In: Ruddy S, Harris ED, Sledge CB, ed. *Kelley's Textbook of Rheumatology*. Philadelphia: Saunders Company; 2001;1145–1152.
2. Erkan D, Yazici Y, Sobel R, Lockshin MD. Primary antiphospholipid syndrome. Functional outcome after 10 years. *J Rheumatol*. 2000;27:2817–2821.
3. Levine JS, Branch DW. The antiphospholipid syndrome. *N Eng J Med*. 2002;10:752–759.
4. Crowther MA, Ginsberg JS, et al. A comparison of two intensities of warfarin for the prevention of recurrent thrombosis in patients with antiphospholipid syndrome. *N Eng J Med*. 2003;12:1133–1138.

ADDITIONAL READING
The decade of autoimmunity: edited by Y. Shoenfeld, publication date 1999.

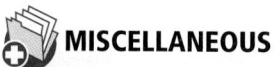 **MISCELLANEOUS**

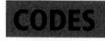 **CODES**

ICD9-CM
646.83/795.79

PATIENT TEACHING

Prevention
Avoid use of oral contraceptives.

 See Corresponding Diagnostic Algorithm

ANTITHROMBIN DEFICIENCY

Marc Jeffrey Kahn, MD

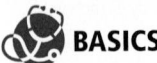 **BASICS**

DESCRIPTION

Antithrombin is a protease that inhibits thrombin by forming an irreversible complex. Antithrombin can also inhibit factors Xa, IXa, and XIa. This process is catalyzed by the presence of heparin. Patients deficient in antithrombin have an increased incidence of venous thrombosis including venous thrombosis. Arterial thrombosis is much less common in patients deficient in antithrombin.

- System(s) Affected: Cardiovascular; Nervous; Pulmonary; Reproductive; Hemic/Lymphatic/Immunologic
- Synonym(s): Antithrombin III deficiency

GENERAL PREVENTION

Patients with antithrombin deficiency without thrombosis do not require prophylactic treatment.

EPIDEMIOLOGY

- Predominant age: Mean age of 1st thrombosis is in the 2nd decade
- Predominant sex: Male = Female

Incidence
4% of patients with thrombophilia

Prevalence
0.16% of normal individuals

RISK FACTORS

- Oral contraceptives, pregnancy, and the use of hormone replacement therapy (HRT) increase the risk of venous thrombosis in patients with antithrombin deficiency.
- Patients with antithrombin deficiency and another prothrombotic state such as factor V Leiden or the prothrombin 20210 mutation have increased rates of thrombosis.

ALERT

Pregnancy Considerations
Increases thrombotic risk in patients with antithrombin deficiency

Genetics
- Autosomal dominant.
- Heterozygotes have an odds ratio of venous thrombosis of 10–20.

ETIOLOGY

Many mutations in the antithrombin gene have been identified.

- Type I deficiency is characterized by low levels of antigen. Type II deficiency is found when the antithrombin molecule is dysfunctional.
- Type II deficiencies are due to mutations in either the active center of antithrombin that binds the target enzyme or the heparin binding site.
- No patients homozygous for defects in the active center have been described, suggesting that this is a lethal condition. Patients heterozygous for mutations in the heparin binding site rarely have thrombotic episodes.

 DIAGNOSIS

SIGNS AND SYMPTOMS

- Deep or superficial venous thrombosis
- Recurrence rate of thrombosis is 12–17% per year.

TESTS

Lab
- Antithrombin levels in the presence of heparin
- Anti-thrombin–heparin cofactor assay
- Drugs that may alter lab results: Heparin and asparaginase can lower antithrombin levels.
- Disorders that may alter lab results
  – Liver disease, DIC, nephritic syndrome, and preeclampsia reduce antithrombin levels.
  – Acute thrombosis can lower antithrombin levels.

DIFFERENTIAL DIAGNOSIS

- Factor V Leiden
- Protein C deficiency
- Protein S deficiency
- Dysfibrinogenemia
- Dysplasminogenemia
- Homocysteinemia
- Prothrombin 20210 mutation
- Elevated factor VIII levels

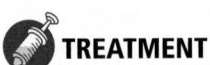 **TREATMENT**

INITIAL STABILIZATION
Outpatient

GENERAL MEASURES

- Routine anticoagulation for asymptomatic patients with antithrombin deficiency is not recommended. (1)[A]
- Patients with antithrombin deficiency and a 1st thrombosis should be anticoagulated initially with unfractionated heparin followed by oral anticoagulation with warfarin. (1)[A]

- The role of family screening for antithrombin deficiency is unclear, because most patients with this mutation do not have thrombosis. Screening may be considered for women considering using oral contraceptives or for pregnant women with a family history of factor protein S deficiency. (1)[C]

Diet
No restrictions

Activity
No restrictions

 MEDICATION

First Line

- Heparin initial bolus of 80 U/kg followed by infusion of 18 U/kg/h. Frequent monitoring of the PTT is important as nearly 1/2 of patients deficient in antithrombin require more than 40,000 U of heparin daily to adequately prolong the PTT. (1)[C] After the INR is 2–3, heparin can be stopped after 5 total days of therapy. (1)[A]
- Oral anticoagulant following the initial administration of heparin. Warfarin (Coumadin) 5 mg PO per day and adjusted to INR of 2–3. Patients should be maintained on warfarin for at least 6 months. (1)[A]
- Recurrent thrombosis requires indefinite anticoagulation. (1)[A]

- Contraindications
  – Active bleeding precludes anticoagulation; risk of bleeding is a relative contraindication to long-term anticoagulation.
- Precautions
  – Observe patient for signs of embolization, further thrombosis, or bleeding.
  – Avoid IM injections.
  – Periodically check stool and urine for occult blood and monitor CBCs including platelets.
  – Heparin-thrombocytopenia and/or paradoxical thrombosis with thrombocytopenia
- Significant possible interactions
  – Agents that intensify the response to oral anticoagulants: Alcohol, allopurinol, amiodarone, anabolic steroids, androgens, many antimicrobials, cimetidine, chloral hydrate, disulfiram, all NSAIDs, sulfinpyrazone, tamoxifen, thyroid hormone, vitamin E, ranitidine, salicylates, acetaminophen
  – Agents that diminish the response to oral anticoagulants: Aminoglutethimide, antacids, barbiturates, carbamazepine, cholestyramine, diuretics, griseofulvin, rifampin, and oral contraceptives

Second Line

- Argatroban 0.4–0.5 mcg/kg/min. Case reports describing the use of the direct thrombin inhibitor in patients with antithrombin deficiency have been published. (2)[C]
- Antithrombin III (ATnativ, Thrombate III) 50–100 IU/min IV titrated to antithrombin level desired. Precise role in therapy remains unclear. (1)[C]
- LMWH is difficult to manage in this population. (1)[C]

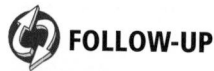 **FOLLOW-UP**

PROGNOSIS
The odds ratio of thrombosis in a patient with antithrombin deficiency is much higher than in patients with other thrombophilic conditions. The recurrence rate is similarly high. There is no difference in clinical severity between patients with type I defects and type II mutations.

COMPLICATIONS
Recurrent thrombosis (requires indefinite anticoagulation)

PATIENT MONITORING
Warfarin requires periodic (monthly after initial stabilization) monitoring of the INR.

REFERENCES

1. Vinazzer H. Hereditary and acquired antithrombin deficiency. *Semin Thromb Hemost*. 1999;25(3): 257–263.
2. Dager WE, Gosselin RC, Owings JT. Argatroban therapy for antithrombin deficiency and mesenteric thrombosis: Case report and review of the literature. *Pharmacotherapy*. 2004;24(5): 659–663.
3. Kottke-Marchant K, Duncan A. Antithrombin deficiency: Issues in laboratory diagnosis. *Arch Pathol Lab Med*. 2002;126(11):1326–1336.

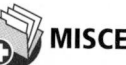 **MISCELLANEOUS**

See also: Thrombosis; Deep Vein (DVT); Protein C Deficiency; Protein S Deficiency; Prothrombin 20210 (Mutation); Factor V Leiden

CODES

ICD9-CM
286.9 Other and unspecified coagulation defects

PATIENT TEACHING
Patients should be educated about use of oral anticoagulant therapy if taking such. Avoid NSAIDs while on warfarin.

 See Corresponding Diagnostic Algorithm

ANXIETY

Mitzi Wasik, PharmD, BCPS

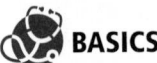 BASICS

DESCRIPTION (1)
A common acute or chronic, fearful emotion with associated physical symptoms. DSM-IV-R recognizes the following subtypes

- Acute situational anxiety: Response to recent stressful event, usually transient symptoms
- Generalized anxiety disorder (GAD): Persistent underlying anxiety or adjustment disorder with anxious mood and significant symptoms of motor tension, autonomic hyperactivity, and hypervigilance, lasting >6 months
- Panic disorder (PD): Recurrent unexpected attacks with at least one attack (or more) associated with persistent concern about additional attacks, worries about implications of the attack (losing control, having a heart attack), or a significant change in behavior related to the attack; often leads to agoraphobia
- Social phobia (Social Anxiety Disorder): Marked and persistent fear and avoidance of performance or social situations in which the person is exposed to unfamiliar people or scrutiny
- System(s) Affected: Nervous

GENERAL PREVENTION (2)
- Cognitive behavior therapy
- Management of stress, to extent possible
- Relaxation techniques
- Meditation

EPIDEMIOLOGY (3)
Predominant sex: Female > Male (2:1)

Incidence
- 15.7 million Americans suffer from anxiety disorders every year, 30 million will suffer at some point in their lives
- <30% of patients suffering from anxiety seek treatment.

Prevalence
- 12-month prevalence rate
  - Panic disorder:1.3–1.7%
  - Generalized anxiety disorder
    ○ All ages—12.1–12.7%
  - Social phobia: 1.7–3.7%
- Onset can occur anytime in life, from adolescent to adulthood
  - Women >age 45 are most frequently affected

RISK FACTORS
Social and financial problems, medical illness, family history, lack of social support

Genetics
Panic disorder: Increased concordance in monozygotic versus dizygotic twins

ETIOLOGY
- Panic disorder, social phobia, and obsessive compulsive disorder are associated with genetic factors.
- Mediated by abnormalities of neurotransmitter systems (serotonin, norepinephrine, and gamma-aminobutyric acid [GABA])

ASSOCIATED CONDITIONS
- Depression (commonly)
- Agoraphobia
- Alcohol or substance abuse
- Somatoform disorders

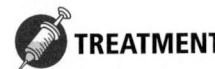 DIAGNOSIS (1,4)

SIGNS AND SYMPTOMS
History
Symptoms must occur for more days than not for 6 months

Physical Exam
- 3 (or more) criteria are required for diagnosis of GAD. Only one required in children
  - Restlessness or feeling keyed up or on edge
  - Easily fatigued
  - Difficulty concentrating or mind going blank
  - Irritability
  - Muscle tension
  - Sleep disturbances (difficulty falling or staying asleep)
  - Difficulty controlling worry
- Persistent worry must cause significant distress, impairment in social, occupational, or other areas of functioning
- Nonspecific signs and symptoms that may be present with different subtypes—unrealistic or excessive anxiety or worry, sense of impending doom, nervousness, instability, tachycardia, palpitations, systolic click murmur, hyperventilation, choking sensation, sighing respiration, nausea or abdominal distress, paresthesias, diaphoresis, dizziness or syncope, flushing, muscle tension, tremulousness, restlessness, headache, backaches, and muscle spasm

TESTS
EEG, ECG, etc.

Lab
Laboratory tests are often normal. See Differential Diagnosis for conditions to rule out.

Imaging
Usually none

Diagnostic Procedures/Surgery
Psychologic testing
- Anxiety Disorders Interview Schedule (ADIS), Hamilton's Anxiety Scale (HAM-A), Clinical Global Impression Scale (CGI), DSM-IV-R criteria

DIFFERENTIAL DIAGNOSIS
- Cardiovascular
  - Ischemic heart disease, valvular heart disease, cardiomyopathies, myocarditis, arrhythmias, mitral valve prolapse (most symptomatic cases are associated with panic disorder), congestive heart failure, or myocardial infarction
- Respiratory
  - Asthma, chronic obstructive pulmonary disease, pulmonary embolism, or pneumonia
- CNS
  - Stroke, seizures, dementia, migraine, Parkinson disease, neoplasms
- Metabolic and hormonal
  - Hyperthyroidism, pheochromocytoma, adrenal insufficiency, Cushing syndrome, hypokalemia, hypoglycemia, hyperparathyroidism
- Nutritional
  - Thiamine, pyridoxine, or folate deficiency, iron deficiency anemia

- Drug-induced anxiety
  - Alcohol, sympathomimetics (cocaine, amphetamines, caffeine)
- Withdrawal
  - Alcohol, sedative-hypnotics
- Other
  - Other psychiatric comorbidities

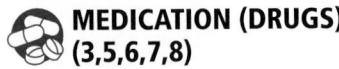 TREATMENT

GENERAL MEASURES
- Appropriate health care: Outpatient
- Based on careful workup and identification of etiology and subtype of anxiety disorders
- Identify coexistent substance abuse.
- Counseling or psychotherapy along with medications, biofeedback in selected cases
- Serial office visits

Diet
- Limit caffeine intake.
- Avoid alcohol (drug interactions).

Activity
Physical exercise

SPECIAL THERAPY
Complementary and Alternative Medicine
Kava was previously used but is no longer in favor due to liver toxicities.

MEDICATION (DRUGS) (3,5,6,7,8)

First Line
- Conditions

  - Acute situational anxiety: Short-term (up to 1 month) treatment with benzodiazepines (2)[B]

  - Generalized anxiety disorder

  - Escitalopram (Lexapro) 10 mg/day titrated by 10 mg every week to a max of 20 mg/day (10 mg/day max) (1)[A]
  - Paroxetine (Paxil) 10 mg daily titrated by 10 mg a week to a max 50 mg/day (20 mg/day most effective dose); (10 mg/day) (1)[A]
  - Venlafaxine (Effexor XR) 37.5–75 mg titrated to a max of 225 mg/day (1)[A]
  - Imipramine (Tofranil) 50 mg/day (max 200 mg/day, 100 mg in elderly) (1)[A]

  - Fluoxetine (Prozac) 10 mg daily up to max of 20–40 mg/day (2)[C]

  - Sertraline (Zoloft) 25 mg daily up to max of 200 mg/day (2)[B]
  - Buspirone (Buspar) 20–30 mg/day divided b.i.d. to t.i.d. (max 60 mg/day) (1)[A]
- Panic disorder and social phobia: SSRIs, TCAs (e.g., imipramine), buproprion, trazodone, and beta-blockers (2)[B]

Second Line
- Generalized anxiety disorder
  - Hydroxyzine 50–100 mg q6h (max 400 mg/day) (1) [A]
- BZDs (short-term use) (1)[A]
  - Alprazolam (Xanax) 0.25 mg b.i.d. to t.i.d. increase by 0.25 mg, if needed
  - Clonazepam (Klonopin) 0.5 mg t.i.d. to maximum of 1.5–4.5 mg per day
  - Diazepam (Valium) 2–5 mg b.i.d. increase by 2 mg if needed
  - Lorazepam (Ativan) 0.5 mg b.i.d. to t.i.d. increase by 0.5 mg if needed (response, if any, is slow, often 4–6 weeks)

- Panic disorder
  - BZDs may be used short term until TCA or SSRI takes effect (2–3 weeks)
  - BZDs may be helpful for initial control of symptoms until the SSRIs or TCAs are effective.

ALERT
Pediatric Considerations
- Reduced dosage of medications in adolescent
- Anxiety often comorbidly exists with ADHD

Geriatric Considerations
- Reduced dosage of medications
- Avoid TCAs and long-acting benzodiazepines.

Pregnancy Considerations
- BZDs: Contraindicated in 1st trimester of pregnancy, and with caution later in pregnancy and during lactation. May cause lethargy and weight loss in nursing infants; avoid breast-feeding if the mother is taking benzodiazepines chronically or in high doses.
- SSRIs: Taper and discontinue, if possible, in 1st trimester; may be used later in pregnancy (except paroxetine Class D).
- Precautions:
  - BZDs: Advanced age, renal insufficiency, suicidal tendency, open-angle glaucoma. Sudden discontinuation increases the risk of seizures, especially with alprazolam.
  - BZDs with short half-lives (e.g., alprazolam) increase the potential for dependency and protracted withdrawal symptoms; use with caution when patients with severe panic disorder are taking other CNS sedatives or with patients who have a history of substance abuse/dependence.
  - Buspirone: Hepatic and/or renal dysfunction
  - TCAs: Advanced age, glaucoma, benign prostate hypertrophy, hyperthyroidism, cardiovascular disease, liver disease, urinary retention, MAO inhibitor treatment
- Significant possible interactions
  - BZDs (CYP inhibitors/inducers): Cimetidine, ethanol, oral contraceptives, disulfiram, levodopa, rifampin
  - Buspirone: MAO inhibitors
  - TCAs: Amphetamines, barbiturates, guanethidine, clonidine, epinephrine, ethanol, norepinephrine, MAO inhibitors, propoxyphene, allow 14-day washout period before starting MAOIs after TCA d/c
  - SSRIs: MAO inhibitors (may cause fatal serotonin syndrome), may raise serum levels of other medications

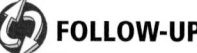 **FOLLOW-UP**

PROGNOSIS
With active treatment, excellent results can often be obtained.

COMPLICATIONS
- Impaired social/occupational functioning
- Drug dependence (benzodiazepines)
- Alcohol dependence

PATIENT MONITORING
- Watch for and treat associated psychiatric disorders.
- Monitor mental status on benzodiazepines and avoid drug dependence.
- Monitor blood pressure, heart rate, and anticholinergic side effects on TCAs.
- Monitor for suicidality with SSRIs, venlafaxine, and imipramine.

REFERENCES
1. American Psychiatric Association. *Diagnostic and Statistical Manual of Mental Disorders*, Fourth Edition, Text Revision. Washington, DC: American Psychiatric Association, 2000:429–484.
2. Rickels K, Moira R. Pharmacotherapy of generalized anxiety disorder. *J Clin Psychiatry*. 2002;63(suppl 14):9–16.
3. Lepine J. The epidemiology of anxiety disorders: Prevalence and societal costs. *J Clin Psychiatry*. 2002;63(suppl 14):4–8.
4. Kirkwood C, Melton S, Pharmacotherapy: A pathophysiologic approach. In: *Anxiety Disorders I: Generalized Anxiety, Panic, and Social Anxiety Disorders*. 6th ed. New York, NY; McGraw Hill: 2005.
5. Rickels K, Rynn M, Iyengar M, et al. Remission of generalized anxiety disorder: A review of the paroxetine clinical trials database. *J Clin Psychiatry*. 2006;67(1):41–47.
6. Goodman WK, Bose A, Wang Q. Treatment of generalized anxiety disorder with escitalopram: Pooled results from double-blind, placebo-controlled trials. *J Affect Disord*. 2005;87(2–3):161–167.
7. Mitte K, Noack P, Steil R, Hautzinger M. A meta-analytic review of the efficacy of drug treatment in generalized anxiety disorder. *J Clin Psychopharmacol*. 2005;25(2):141–150.
8. Briggs G. *Drugs In Pregnancy And Lactation: A Reference Guide to Fetal and Neonatal Risk*. 7th ed. Philadelphia, PA: Lippincott Williams & Wilkins; 2005.

ADDITIONAL READING
- Medline Plus, www.medlineplus.gov
- Mayo Clinic, www.mayoclinic.com

 MISCELLANEOUS

Abbreviations: DSM-IV-R, Diagnostic and Statistical Manual of Mental Disorders, 4th edition Text Revision; TCA, tricyclic antidepressant; SSRI, selective serotonin reuptake inhibitor; CYP, cytochrome P450 enzymes; BZD, benzodiazepine

CODES

ICD9-CM
300.00 Anxiety state, unspecified

PATIENT TEACHING
- American Academy of Family Physicians: 800-274-2237: www.familydoctor.org
- National Institute of Mental Health (NIMH): www.nimh.nih.gov/publicat/index.cfm
- Anxiety Disorders Association of America: www.adaa.org.

Prevention
Cognitive behavioral therapy
- Meditation
- Relaxation techniques
- Stress avoidance

 See Corresponding Diagnostic Algorithm

 See Patient Handout on CD

AORTIC DISSECTION

Jeremy Golding, MD

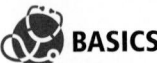 **BASICS**

DESCRIPTION
- Intimal tear in aorta resulting in hematoma formation. Accumulating blood in false lumen of arterial wall leads to propagation of this dissection.
- DeBakey classification: Based on origin site
  - Type I: Originates in ascending aorta, propagates at least as far as aortic arch
  - Type II: Involves only ascending aorta
  - Type III: Originates in descending aorta, may propagate proximately or distally
- Stanford classification: More widely used
  - Type A: Involves ascending aorta and aortic arch regardless of site of intimal tear
  - Type B: Involves descending aorta
- New classification, subdivisions of DeBakey or Stanford
  - 1. Classic
  - 2. Medial disruption with hematoma formation
  - 3. Discrete without hematoma
  - 4. Plaque rupture, ulceration
  - 5. Iatrogenic
- Synonym(s): Dissecting aneurysm

GENERAL PREVENTION
- Long-term control of hypertension
- Surveillance of aortic root and replacement when appropriate in patients with collagen disorders (e.g., Marfan, Ehlers-Danlos)

EPIDEMIOLOGY
- Predominant age: Depends on cause; commonly present in patients with Marfan syndrome in 3rd and 4th decades; otherwise most common between 6th and 8th decades
- Predominant sex: Male > Female (3:1)
- Mean age: Men 60 years, women 67 years

Incidence
2000 new cases diagnosed annually

Prevalence
US
- Diagnosed in 1 in 10,000 patients admitted to hospital
- Found in 1 in 350 patients at autopsy

RISK FACTORS
- Hypertension in 70% of patients
- Cystic medial necrosis
- Collagen abnormalities
  - Marfan syndrome
  - Ehlers-Danlos syndrome
- Inflammatory aortitis
- Takayasu arteritis
- Giant cell arteritis
- Congenital abnormalities
  - Bicuspid aortic valve
  - coarctation
- Pregnancy
- Chest trauma
- Cocaine use
- Cardiovascular surgery
- Elderly
- MDMA (ecstasy) use
- α_1-Antitrypsin deficiency
- Smoking

Genetics
Increased incidence among family members

ETIOLOGY
- Cystic medial necrosis
- Iatrogenic during arterial catheterization

ASSOCIATED CONDITIONS
- Ehlers-Danlos syndrome
- Marfan syndrome
- Aortic stenosis
- Coarctation of aorta
- Bicuspid valve
- Turner syndrome
- Osteogenesis imperfecta
- Syphilis
- Relapsing polychondritis
- During pregnancy: Possibly cystic medionecrosis of pregnancy; unclear whether pregnancy is originating factor or contributes to worsening of a pre-existing condition

DIAGNOSIS

SIGNS AND SYMPTOMS
- Abrupt onset of sharp or tearing pain
- Shearing anterior chest pain radiating to interscapular region
- Back pain
- Syncope
- Symptoms of CHF
- Stroke
- Limb ischemia
- Abdominal pain
- Acute myocardial infarction/angina
- Spinal cord syndromes/deficits
- Hypotension or hypertension
- Wide pulse pressure
- Murmur of aortic insufficiency
- Features of tamponade
- Dullness in left lung base (effusion)
- Pulse deficits or asymmetry
- Fever
- 96% of acute aortic dissections can be identified by abrupt onset of sharp thoracic or abdominal pain in the presence of mediastinal widening on chest radiograph and asymmetry of pulses

History
Typical patient is a hypertensive man in his 60s with abrupt onset of severe chest pain.

TESTS
- Electrocardiogram
  - Left ventricular hypertrophy
  - Nonspecific ST-T changes
  - Electrical alternans (in cardiac tamponade)
- Echocardiogram
  - Dilated aortic root
  - Increased aortic posterior or anterior wall thickness
  - Pericardial effusion
  - Oscillating intimal flap

Imaging
Chest radiograph, in stable patients
- Widening of superior mediastinum
- Left pleural effusion
- Haziness or enlargement of aortic knob
- Double density of descending aorta
- Irregular aortic contour: >5 mm separation of intimal calcification from outer aortic contour
- Rightward displacement of trachea
- Cardiomegaly

Diagnostic Procedures/Surgery
- (Sensitivity/specificity is indicated for each.)
- Chest CT (88/100%)
  - Demonstration of 2 lumens with hematoma formation
  - Detection of intimal flap
  - Differential flow between 2 lumens
  - Compression of true lumen by false lumen
- Spiral CT aortography; more sensitive and specific (99/99%)
- Aortogram (88/94%)
  - Demonstration of 2 lumens
  - Detection of intimal flap
  - Compression of true lumen
  - Ulcer-like projections of contrast
  - Altered flow patterns
- Transesophageal echocardiography (99/98%): Test of choice for unstable patients
- MRI: If available and patient hemodynamically stable, test of choice for delineation of vascular anatomy (>99/99%)
- Intravascular ultrasonography: May detect with negative transesophageal echocardiography

Pathological Findings
- ~60% of intimal tears occur in proximal ascending aorta. Remainder are between origin of left subclavian artery and ligamentum arteriosum, descending aorta (20%), aortic arch (10%), and abdominal aorta.
- Although medionecrosis is found in normal aging aortas, it is more extensive in patients who develop aortic dissection.
- Cystic medial necrosis is seen in patients with defects in elastin and connective tissue organization (e.g., Marfan, Ehlers-Danlos).
- Death usually is due to rupture and tamponade.

DIFFERENTIAL DIAGNOSIS
- Myocardial infarction
- Pulmonary embolism
- Pneumonia
- Pleurisy
- Pericarditis
- Pneumothorax
- Angina
- Acute pancreatitis
- Penetrating duodenal ulcer

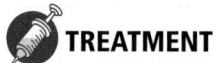 **TREATMENT**

GENERAL MEASURES

- Admit to ICU for assessment of hemodynamic stability, pain control, BP control
- Intubate; hemodynamically unstable patients
- Medical therapy
  - Treatment of choice for descending dissections without complications (Type III)
  - Based on decreasing BP and shearing forces of myocardial contractility (dp/dt) to decrease intimal tear and hematoma propagation
  - Survival is 60–80% at 4–5 years
- Arterial BP monitoring is critical.
- Careful observation for changes in mentation, neurologic signs, or evidence of organ dysfunction
- Foley catheter to follow urine output
- Swan-Ganz catheterization may be helpful in monitoring cardiac performance and filling pressures during use of vasoactive and cardiodepressive drugs.
- Pain control difficult despite use of narcotics.

Diet
NPO until surgical evaluation is complete and patient classified as medical therapy only

Activity
Bed rest

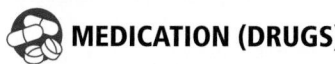 **MEDICATION (DRUGS)**

First Line
- Propranolol plus nitroprusside; dosing
  - Propranolol: 0.5–1 mg IV q5min until heart rate 60–70 bpm *and*
  - Nitroprusside: Titrated to reduce systolic BP to 100–110 mm Hg (13.3–14.6 kPa)
- Contraindications
  - Propranolol
    - Bronchial asthma
    - Diabetes mellitus
    - Raynaud disease
    - Sinus bradycardia
    - A-V heart block >1st degree
    - In presence of MAOIs
    - Cardiogenic shock
    - Acute CHF
    - Right ventricular failure from pulmonary hypertension
  - Nitroprusside
    - In treatment of compensatory hypertension, that is, arteriovenous shunt
    - In patients with inadequate cerebral circulation
    - For use during emergency surgery in moribund patients
- Precautions
  - Propranolol
    - Use cautiously in patients with angina pectoris, cardiac failure, impaired renal or hepatic function, thyrotoxicosis, pre-excitation syndromes, diabetes, or nonallergic bronchospasm.
    - Propranolol may produce bradycardia, heart block, or hypotension. Patients should not be suddenly withdrawn from β-blockers.
  - Nitroprusside
    - May not lower BP adequately; another agent may be required.

- In patients with renal or hepatic insufficiency, may cause cyanide toxicity through excessive production of serum thiocyanate. Confusion and hyper-reflexia are early signs of thiocyanate toxicity. Thiocyanate inhibits uptake and binding of iodine; caution with hypothyroidism. Check thiocyanate levels after 48 hours.
  - Administration via infusion pump.
  - Methemoglobinemia may be seen rarely.
- Significant possible interactions
  - Propranolol: Adenosine, albuterol, alfentanil, amiodarone, barbiturates, bromazepam, chlorothiazide, chlorpromazine, chlorpropamide, chlorprothixene, cimetidine, clonidine, dextroamphetamine, diazoxide, dihydroergotamine, diltiazem, disopyramide, tricyclic antidepressants, encainide, epinephrine, flecainide, fluvoxamine, furosemide, glipizide, halofenate, haloperidol, heparin, ibuprofen, indomethacin, insulin, isoniazid, isoproterenol, lidocaine, lidoflazine, methacholine, methyldopa, metoclopramide, naproxen, nifedipine, phenylpropanolamine, procainamide, quinidine, reserpine, rifampin, ritodrine, sulfonylureas, theophylline, thioridazine, tocainide, tubocurarine, verapamil, and warfarin
  - Nitroprusside: Clonidine and other antihypertensives may have hypotensive effects.

Second Line
- Labetalol: 10–20 mg IV bolus to a maximum of 300 mg total, then titrated to response with infusion
- Trimethaphan: Infusion rate 1–2 mg/min
- Reserpine: 0.5–2 mg IM q4–8h; onset of action 1–3 hours
- Methyldopa: 250–500 mg q6h; onset of action of 4–6 hours; duration 1–12 hours

SURGERY
- Treatment of choice for all ascending aortic dissections
- Surgical indications for Type III
  - Increasing size of hematoma
  - Impending rupture
  - Inability to control pain
  - Bleeding into pleural space
- Endovascular stents, fenestration, and stent grafting

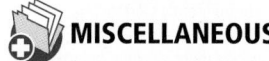 **FOLLOW-UP**

PROGNOSIS
- Mortality, untreated
  - 24 hours: 33%
  - 2 weeks: 60%
  - 3 months: 90%
- Hospital survival estimate, treated medically and surgically: 70%
- Mortality, ascending dissection treated early surgically: 29–38%
- 10-year survival, treated surgically (all): 40%
- Redissection risk
  - 5 years: 13%
  - 10 years: 23%

COMPLICATIONS
- Redissection
- Localized saccular aneurysm
- Cardiac tamponade
- Aortic valvular insufficiency
- Progressive aortic enlargement

PATIENT MONITORING
- Maintain systolic BP at 120 mm Hg (16 kPa) or below, as tolerated.
- Routine chest films and/or chest CT may be helpful for patient treated medically long term.
- Follow-up visit at 1 month, then at 3-month intervals. During follow-up, pay careful attention to signs and symptoms of aortic insufficiency, chest or back pain, and development of saccular aneurysms as displayed on chest films.

REFERENCES

1. Beckman JA, O'Gara PT. Diseases of the aorta. *Adv Intern Med*. 1999;44:267–291.
2. Erbel R, Alfonso F, Boileau C, et al. Diagnosis and management of aortic dissection. *Eur Heart J*. 2001;22:1642.
3. Hartnell GG. Imaging of aortic aneurysms and dissection: CT and MRI. *J Thorac Imaging*. 2001;16:35–46.
4. Lindsay JJ. Diagnosis and treatment of diseases of the aorta. *Curr Probl Cardiol*. 1997;22:485–542.
5. Manninen HI, Rasanen H. Intravascular ultrasound in interventional radiology. *Eur Radiol*. 2000;10:1754–1762.
6. Penco M, Paparoni S, Dagianti A, et al. Usefulness of transesophageal echocardiography in the assessment of aortic dissection. *Am J Cardiol*. 2000;86(4A):53G–56G.
7. Pretre R, von Segesser LK. Aortic dissection. *Lancet*. 1997;349:1461–1464.
8. Rogers FB, Osler TM, Shackford SR. Aortic dissection after trauma: Case report and review of literature. *J Trauma*. 1996;41:906–908.
9. Sommer T, Fehske W, Holzknecht N, et al. Aortic dissection: A comparative study of diagnosis with spiral CT, multiplanar transesophageal echocardiography, and MR imaging. *Radiology*. 1996;199:347–352.
10. Umana JP, Mitchell RS. Endovascular treatment of aortic dissections and thoracic aortic aneurysms. *Semin Vasc Surg*. 2000;13:290–298.
11. Vonkodolitsch Y, Schwartz AG, Nienaber CA. Clinical prediction of acute aortic dissection. *Arch Intern Med*. 2000;160:2977.

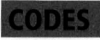 **MISCELLANEOUS**

See also: Ehlers-Danlos syndrome; Marfan syndrome

CODES

ICD9-CM
441 Dissection of aorta, unspecified site

PATIENT TEACHING

Depending on etiology, emphasis must be placed on risk factors and prevention of recurrence.

 See Corresponding Diagnostic Algorithm

AORTIC VALVULAR STENOSIS

Suzanne Klainer, MD

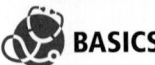 **BASICS**

DESCRIPTION
Acquired or congenital obstruction to left-ventricular outflow across aortic valve caused by decreased valve area. Is classified as mild, moderate, or severe based on measured area.

GENERAL PREVENTION
Prevention of Rheumatic Heart Disease for acquired postinflammatory aortic stenosis.

EPIDEMIOLOGY
- Predominant age (1)
  - <30 years: Congenital
  - 30–70 years: Congenital or rheumatic
  - >70 years: Degenerative calcification of aortic valve
- Predominant sex: Male > Female, 2:1

Prevalence (2)
- 1.3% of 65–74 years
- 2.4% of 75–84 years
- 4% of >84 years
- Bicuspid aortic valve: 0.8% of population (3)

Geriatric Considerations
Increased incidence of degenerative calcific aortic stenosis

RISK FACTORS
- Unicommissural valve
- Bicuspid valve
- Prior rheumatic fever
- Advanced age
- Hypercholesterolemia
- Metabolic disease (SLE, Fabry)

PATHOPHYSIOLOGY
Resistance to outflow at the aortic orifice causes increased afterload. The left ventricle responds to this pressure overload with thickening of myocardial wall, resulting in left ventricular (LV) dysfunction and CHF as well as increased myocardial oxygen demand.

ETIOLOGY
- Congenital
  - Unicuspid valve
  - Bicuspid valve: Not inherently stenotic, but becomes so as a result of wear-and-tear thickening and calcification; calcified bicuspid valve is most common cause of isolated aortic stenosis in adults.
  - Tricuspid valve with fusion of commissures
  - Hypoplastic annulus
- Acquired
  - Rheumatic fever (or, rarely, other inflammatory disease)
  - Degenerative calcific aortic stenosis in elderly

ASSOCIATED CONDITIONS
- Coronary artery disease (present in 50% of patients)
- Aortic regurgitation (particularly in calcified bicuspid valves and rheumatic disease)
- Mitral valve disease (primarily in rheumatic heart disease)
- LV dysfunction and CHF
- A-fibrillation associated with CHF

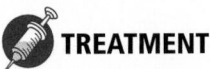 **DIAGNOSIS**

SIGNS AND SYMPTOMS
- Angina pectoris: Most frequent symptom
- Near syncope
- Syncope: Often exertional
- Exertional dyspnea
- Orthopnea
- Paroxysmal nocturnal dyspnea
- Palpitations
- Fatigue
- Neurologic events (transient ischemic attack or cerebrovascular accident) owing to embolization
- Systolic crescendo-decrescendo murmur: Usually best heard at 2nd right sternal border (may have associated thrill); may radiate into carotid arteries
- Ejection (early systolic) click
- Prolonged ejection time
- Delayed, small carotid upstroke
- Delayed/decreased intensity of A2
- Paradoxical splitting of S2
- LV heave
- High-pitched diastolic blow: May be present at left sternal border (associated aortic regurgitation)

History
Above symptoms in elderly patient or one with history congenital heart defect or rheumatic fever

Physical Exam
- Cardiac
  - Systolic crescendo-decrescendo murmur RSB, radiating to carotids
  - Delayed carotid upstroke
  - Left ventricular heave
  - Increased intensity of A2

TESTS
ECG
- Conduction defects
- Left-atrial enlargement
- Ventricular arrhythmias
- LV hypertrophy
- ST segment depression

Lab
Elevated BNP

Imaging
- Chest radiograph
  - May be normal in compensated, isolated valvular aortic stenosis
  - Cardiac hypertrophy early, later cardiomegaly
  - Poststenotic dilatation of ascending aorta
  - Calcification of aortic valve cusps (may require fluoroscopy to visualize)
- Echocardiography
  - Aortic valve morphology, thickening, calcifications
  - Decreased aortic valve excursion
  - Planimetry of aortic valve area
  - LV hypertrophy
  - LV ejection fraction
  - Chamber dimensions
  - Presence or absence of wall-motion abnormalities suggesting coronary artery disease
- Doppler echocardiography
  - Transvalvular gradient
  - Valve area
  - Diastolic function
  - Associated aortic regurgitation

Diagnostic Procedures/Surgery
Cardiac catheterization: Recommended for patients undergoing AV replacement at risk for CAD and for assessment of severity when AVR is planned or noninvasive studies are inconclusive (A)
- Identifies transvalvular gradient, valve area, LV ejection fraction, concomitant CAD

Pathological Findings
- LV hypertrophy
- Myocardial interstitial fibrosis
- Aortic valvular calcification in older patients
- 50% incidence of concomitant CAD

DIFFERENTIAL DIAGNOSIS
- Mitral regurgitation
  - Either primary or secondary to underlying coronary artery disease or dilated cardiomyopathy
  - Usually an apical, high-frequency, pansystolic murmur, often radiating to axilla
- Hypertrophic obstructive cardiomyopathy
  - Also systolic crescendo-decrescendo murmur, but best heard at left sternal border and may radiate into axilla
  - However, characteristically intensified by changing from squatting to standing and/or by Valsalva maneuver, lessened by changing from standing to squatting
- Aortic supravalvular stenosis
- Discrete subaortic stenosis

TREATMENT

INITIAL STABILIZATION
Outpatient care except for surgical intervention or comorbid condition requiring hospital care

GENERAL MEASURES
- Asymptomatic patient with noncritical aortic stenosis: Because aortic stenosis is progressive, follow closely with appropriate evaluation.
- All patients should receive endocarditis prophylaxis prior to dental work or invasive procedures regardless of age, cause, or severity of stenosis. (4)[C]
- Patients with stenosis of rheumatic cause should receive (in addition to endocarditis prophylaxis prior to dental work or invasive procedures) rheumatic fever prophylaxis, especially if <35 years or in close contact with young children.
- Screen for and treat comorbid diseases.
  - Commonly HTN, CAD, CHF, and A-fib.

ALERT
Pregnancy Considerations
- Severe critical aortic stenosis responds poorly to hemodynamic changes in pregnancy, labor, and delivery.
- Pregnancy should be avoided with critical aortic stenosis; may need Cesarean section for delivery of baby.

Diet
Only restriction is low-sodium diet in presence of CHF

Activity
In known or suspected severe aortic stenosis, vigorous physical activity contraindicated

MEDICATION (DRUGS)

- ACE I is beneficial for treatment of LV dysfunction and associated heart failure, but can cause hypotension in patients with baseline low blood pressure (5) [B].
- Statins: Anecdotal evidence suggest that statins slow progression of AS, however, recent RCT failed to support this claim (6).
- Prophylactic antibiotics for
  - Bacterial endocarditis
  - Rheumatic fever, where indicated
  - See "General Measures"

ALERT
Use antihypertensives cautiously, because they potentially can cause hypotension in AS.

SURGERY
- Aortic valve replacement indicated in

  - Patients with symptomatic severe AS, patients with severe AS undergoing CABG, or patients with severe AS undergoing aortic or other valve surgery (4)[A].
  - Moderate AS undergoing cardiac surgery (4)[B]

  - Asymptomatic patients with critical AS (aortic valve area <0.6.0 cm^2), LV dysfunction, abnormal response to exercise, ventricular tachycardia, or increasing cardiomegaly ($\geq$15 mm) (4)[C]
- Surgical valve replacement consists of removal of stenotic, native valve and placement of prosthetic mechanical or tissue valve.
- Balloon angioplasty of stenotic aortic valves

  - May benefit pediatric patient with congenital disease (4)[A]
  - In elderly as a bridge to AV replacement, for palliation in patients with serious comorbid conditions, and in patients who require urgent noncardiac surgery (4)[B]

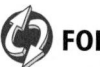 **FOLLOW-UP**

DISPOSITION
Admission Criteria
See criteria for comorbid conditions.

Discharge Criteria
See criteria for comorbid diseases.

PROGNOSIS
- Mortality following onset of symptoms (7)
  - 26% at 1 year
  - 57% at 3 years
- Risk of sudden death is 0.4% per year (4)

COMPLICATIONS
- Progressive stenosis
- Sudden death
- Congestive heart failure
- Angina
- Syncope
- Hemolytic anemia
- Bleeding disorder (acquired vWF d/o) (8)
- Infective endocarditis

PATIENT MONITORING
- Symptomatic patients should be examined frequently.
- ECG every 2–5 years to assess progression in the asymptomatic patient with mild/moderate disease, respectively (4)[C]
- Advise patient to immediately report any symptoms referable to AS.

REFERENCES
1. Subramanian E. Surgical pathology of pure aortic stenosis. A study 374 cases. *Mayo Clin Proc.* 1984;59:683.
2. Stewart et al. Clinical factors associated with calcific aortic valve disease. *J Am Coll Cardiol.* 1997;29:630.
3. Otto CM, Burwash, Legget, et al. Prospective study of asymptomatic valvular aortic stenosis. Clinical, echocardiographic and exercise predictors of outcome. *Circulation.* 1997;95:2262.
4. Bono et al. ACC/AHA task force report. *J Am Coll Cardiol* 1998;32:1486.
5. Chockalingam et al. SCOPE-AS. *Am Heart J.* 2004;147(4):E19.
6. Crowell et al. SALTIRE. *N Engl J Med.* 2005;352:2389–2397.
7. Chizner et al. The natural history of aortic stenosis in adults. *Am Heart J* 1980;99(4):419–424.
8. Vincentelli, et al. Acquired von Willebrand in aortic stenosis. *N Engl J Med.* 2003;349:343.
9. Nistri, et al. Frequency of bicuspid aortic valves in young male conscripts by echocardiogram. *Am J Cardiol.* 2005;96:718.

 MISCELLANEOUS

LV is relatively noncompliant in aortic stenosis, thus

- Atrial contraction is important component of diastolic filling.
- Loss of atrial contraction with onset of atrial fibrillation can cause acute clinical and hemodynamic deterioration.

 CODES

ICD9-CM
424.90 Endocarditis, valve unspecified, unspecified cause

PATIENT TEACHING
- Educate patient about symptoms; instruct to report symptoms promptly should they occur.
- Inform patient when prophylactic antibiotics are needed for medical or dental procedures.

 See Corresponding Diagnostic Algorithm

APPENDICITIS, ACUTE

Andrew H. Fenton, MD

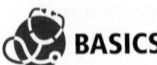 **BASICS**

DESCRIPTION
Acute inflammation of the vermiform appendix
- 1st described by Fitz in 1886
- McBurney described point of maximal tenderness

EPIDEMIOLOGY
- Predominant age
  – Ages 10–30: Male > Female (3:2)
  – Over age 30: Male = Female
  – Rare in infancy
- Predominant sex: Slight male predominance

Incidence
Lifetime incidence 1 in every 15 persons (7%)

Prevalence
- 10/100,000
- Most common acute surgical condition of abdomen

ALERT
Pregnancy Considerations
- Most common extrauterine surgical emergency
- 1 in 2,000 pregnancies
- Difficult diagnosis
- Appendix displaced superolaterally by gravid uterus
- Fetal mortality rate: 2–8.5%

RISK FACTORS
- Adolescent males
- Familial tendency
- Intra-abdominal tumors

Genetics
Unknown

PATHOPHYSIOLOGY ETIOLOGY
Obstruction of appendiceal lumen
- Fecaliths (most common)
- Lymphoid tissue hypertrophy
- Inspissated barium
- Vegetable, fruit seeds and other foreign bodies
- Intestinal worms (ascarids)
- Strictures

DIAGNOSIS

SIGNS AND SYMPTOMS
- Abdominal pain (100%): Periumbilical, then right lower quadrant; lessened with flexion of thigh
- Muscle guarding
- Anorexia (almost 100%)
- Nausea (90%)
- Vomiting (75%); mild
- Obstipation
- Diarrhea; mild
- Sequence of symptom appearance (95%): Anorexia, then abdominal pain, then vomiting
- Slight temperature elevation (1°C)
- Slight tachycardia
- Patient frequently lies motionless with right thigh drawn up
- Maximal tenderness at McBurney point
- Direct and referred right-lower-quadrant tenderness
- Voluntary and involuntary guarding
- Cutaneous hyperesthesia at T10–12
- Rovsing sign: Right-lower-quadrant pain with palpatory pressure in left lower quadrant
- Psoas sign: Pain with right thigh extension
- Obturator sign: Pain with internal rotation of flexed right thigh
- Retrocecal appendix: Flank tenderness in right lower quadrant
- Pelvic appendix: Local and suprapubic pain on rectal exam

ALERT
Pediatric Considerations
- Decreased diagnostic accuracy
- Higher fever, more vomiting

Geriatric Considerations
Decreased diagnostic accuracy

History
Cornerstone of diagnosis, with clinical findings

Physical Exam
- Diagnostic laparoscopy: Consider in young adult females
- Rectal and pelvic examinations
- May need intensive in-hospital observation to allow serial examination

TESTS
Lab
- Moderate leukocytosis: 10,000–18,000/mm³ in 75%
- Moderate polymorphonuclear predominance
- hCG to rule out ectopic pregnancy
- Urinalysis
  – Elevated specific gravity
  – Hematuria (sometimes)
  – Pyuria (sometimes)
  – Albuminuria (sometimes)
- Drugs that may alter lab results
  – Antibiotics
  – Steroids

Imaging
- Used in differential diagnosis and to detect complications
- CT scan: Diagnostic test of choice; also for abscess (1)[B]

Diagnostic Procedures/Surgery
Diagnostic laparoscopy, especially in fertile women (1)[A]

Pathological Findings
- Acute appendix inflammation
- Local vascular congestion
- Obstruction
- Gangrene
- Perforation with abscess (15–30%)

DIFFERENTIAL DIAGNOSIS
- Any cause of acute abdomen
- 75% of erroneous diagnoses accounted for by
  – Acute mesenteric lymphadenitis
  – No organic pathologic condition
  – Acute pelvic inflammatory disease
  – Ovarian cyst torsion
  – Ruptured graafian follicle
  – Acute gastroenteritis
- Also consider
  – Urologic causes
  – Testicular torsion
  – Inflammatory bowel disease
  – Colonic disorders
  – Other gynecologic diseases

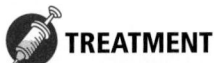 **TREATMENT**

GENERAL MEASURES
- For nonsurgical patients, antibiotic coverage (e.g., quinolone and metronidazole)
- Recurrence rate too high in other patients to recommend antibiotics as a primary therapy

Diet
NPO

Nursing
Pre-op preparation

SPECIAL THERAPY
IV Fluids
- Fluid resuscitation with LR
- Correct fluid and electrolyte deficits.

 MEDICATION (DRUGS)

First Line
- Uncomplicated acute appendicitis: 1 preoperative dose of broad-spectrum antibiotic (2)[A]
  - Cefoxitin (Mefoxin)
  - Cefotetan (Cefotan)

- Gangrenous or perforating appendicitis
  - Broadened antibiotic coverage for aerobic and anaerobic enteric pathogens
  - Adjust dosage and choice of antibiotic based on intraoperative cultures.
  - Continue antibiotics for 7 days postoperatively or until patient becomes afebrile with normal white count.
  - Pathogens usually sensitive to ampicillin, gentamicin, and clindamycin
- Contraindications: Documented allergy to specific antibiotic
- Precautions: Adjust antibiotic dosages for elderly and patients with renal failure.
- Significant possible interactions: Refer to manufacturer's literature for each drug.

Second Line
- Metronidazole (Flagyl): Anaerobic coverage only
- Ampicillin-sulbactam (Unasyn)
- Ticarcillin-clavulanate (Timentin)
- Piperacillin-tazobactam (Zosyn)

SURGERY
Inpatient surgery is appropriate measure

- Immediate appendectomy; laparoscopic favored unless perforation (3)[A]

- Drainage of abscess, if present

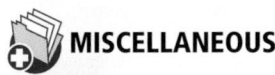 **FOLLOW-UP**

DISPOSITION
Admission Criteria
Complicated appendicitis

Discharge Criteria
Tolerating PO; return of bowel function; afebrile; normal WBC

Issues for Referral
Follow-up with surgeon 1–2 weeks

PROGNOSIS
- Generally uncomplicated course in young adults with nonruptured appendicitis
- Factors increasing morbidity and mortality
  - Extremes of age
  - Appendiceal rupture
- Morbidity rates
  - Nonperforated appendicitis: 3%
  - Perforated appendicitis: 47%
- Mortality rates
  - Unruptured appendicitis: 0.1%
  - Ruptured appendicitis: 3%
  - Patients >60 years of age: 50% of deaths from appendicitis
  - Elderly patient with ruptured appendix: 15%

ALERT
Pediatric Considerations
- Rupture earlier
- Rupture rate: 15–50%

Geriatric Considerations
Rupture rate: 67–90%

COMPLICATIONS
- Wound infection

- Intra-abdominal abscess; lower rate with antibiotic prohylaxis [2A]

- Fecal fistula
- Intestinal obstruction
- Incisional hernia
- Liver abscess (rare)
- Paralytic ileus

PATIENT MONITORING
Routine visits at 2 and 6 weeks after surgery

REFERENCES
1. Mun S, Ernst RD, Chen K, et al. Rapid CT diagnosis of acute appendicitis with IV contrast material. *Emerg Radiol.* 2005;17:1–4 [e-pub ahead of print]
2. Andersen BR, Kallehaue FL, Andersen HK. Antibiotics versus placebo for prevention of postoperative infection after appendectomy. The Cochrane Database of Systematic Reviews 2006 issue 1. *John Wiley & Sons, Ltd.*
3. Sauerland S, Lefering R, Neugebauer EAM. Laparoscopic versus open surgery for suspected appendicitis. The Cochrane Database of Systematic Reviews 2006 issue 1. *John Wiley & Sons, Ltd*

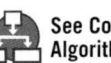 **MISCELLANEOUS**

CODES

ICD9-CM
- 540.0 Acute appendicitis with generalized peritonitis
- 540.9 Acute appendicitis without mention of peritonitis

PATIENT TEACHING
Contact physician for postoperative development of
- Anorexia
- Nausea
- Vomiting
- Abdominal pain
- Fever
- Chills

Diet
Regular

Activity
Restrict activity for 4–6 weeks after surgery.

See Corresponding Diagnostic Algorithm

ARTERIAL EMBOLUS AND THROMBOSIS

Jeremy Golding, MD

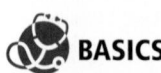 **BASICS**

DESCRIPTION
- Acute loss of perfusion distal to occlusion of major artery owing to
  - Embolus that migrates to point of occlusion or
  - Clot intrinsic to point of occlusion (thrombosis)
- Both are true emergencies.
- Following obstruction of artery, soft coagulum forms both proximally and distally in areas of stagnant flow.
- As clot extends, collateral pathways become involved, and process becomes self-propagating.
- Ultimately, venous circulation can become involved.
- Extent of vascular compromise is critical and determines "golden" period of 4–6 hours. After this time, the profound ischemia leads to irreversible cellular death.
- Distribution of emboli
  - Femoral artery: 30%
  - Iliac artery: 15%
  - Aortic bifurcation: 10%
  - Popliteal artery: 10%
  - Brachial: 10%
  - Mesenteric arteries: 5%
  - Renal: 5%
  - Cerebral (estimated): 15–20%
- System(s) Affected: Cardiovascular; Hematologic/lymphatic/immunologic

GENERAL PREVENTION
- Anticoagulation in atrial arrhythmia
- Reduction of atherosclerosis risk factors

EPIDEMIOLOGY
- 50–100/100,000 hospital admissions
- A leading cause of limb loss in elderly
- Predominant age: Elderly
- Predominant sex: Male > Female
- Rare in children and during pregnancy

RISK FACTORS
Drug abuse

Genetics
Can be associated with inheritable hypercoagulable and premature atherosclerotic syndromes

ETIOLOGY
- Emboli
- Cardiac
  - Atrial flutter/fibrillation
  - Valve disease
  - Myocardial infarction
  - Cardiomyopathy
  - Cardiac tumors
  - Endocarditis
- Aneurysms: Cardiac, aortic, peripheral
- Thrombosis
  - Atherosclerotic occlusive disease
  - Aortic and peripheral aneurysms, especially popliteal
  - Hypercoagulable states
  - Venous gangrene
  - Drug abuse
  - Heparin allergy (heparin-induced thrombocytopenia)
  - Vascular bypass

- Trauma
  - Blunt
  - Penetrating
  - Vascular and cardiac interventional procedures
- Venous thrombosis with patent foramen ovale (paradoxical embolus)

ASSOCIATED CONDITIONS
- Acute mesenteric ischemia
- Renal infarction
- Carotid/cerebrovascular accident
- Multiple emboli
- Digital microembolization

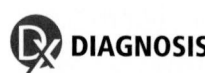 **DIAGNOSIS**

SIGNS AND SYMPTOMS
- To estimate occlusion location
  - Symptoms typically start 1 joint below occlusion.
  - Palpable pulses absent below occlusion and accentuated above.
- The 5 *P*s: If any one is present, frequent re-evaluations indicated. Proximal occlusions lead to more rapid progression of findings. Occlusion at aortic bifurcation can produce bilateral findings.
  - Pain: Diffuse in distal area. If persists, crescendo in nature. Predominates as 1st symptom in embolism. Not alleviated by change of position.
  - Pulselessness: Mandatory for diagnosis of embolism or thrombosis. Pedal pulses subject to observer error. Always compare to opposite limb.
  - Pallor: Skin color pale early, cyanotic later. Check extremity temperature left to right and top to bottom. Look for signs of chronic ischemia: skin atrophy, loss of hair, thick nails.
  - Paresthesia: Numbness early with thrombosis. Light touch 1st to be lost. Not reliable in diabetics. Loss of pain and pressure indicate advanced ischemia.
  - Paralysis: Motor defect occurs after sensory and indicates profound ischemia.

TESTS
- EKG
- Special tests
- Noninvasive/indirect
  - Doppler: Presence or absence of flow
  - Ankle/arm index (AAI; aka ankle/brachial index [ABI]) = dorsal pedal/posterior tibial pressure divided by brachial pressure;
  - AAI >0.30 favorable (normal >1)

Lab
For preoperative evaluation, elucidation of cause, or documentation of ischemia severity
- Myocardial/muscle isoenzymes
- Coagulation parameters
- Blood pH/bicarbonate
- Urine myoglobin
- Electrolytes

Imaging
Noninvasive/direct: Duplex imaging if time permits

Diagnostic Procedures/Surgery
Arteriography
- Rarely indicated preoperatively in threatened limb
- May help differentiate thrombosis from embolus in nonthreatened limb
- Useful with occluded grafts

DIFFERENTIAL DIAGNOSIS
- Emboli vs. thrombosis
- Emboli
  - Myocardial diseases: Myocardial infarction, arrhythmias (e.g., atrial fibrillation), aneurysms
  - Pain as 1st symptom
- Thrombosis
  - Absence of heart disease: Infarction, arrhythmias
  - Chronic vascular history
  - Bilateral changes of chronic ischemia
  - Numbness rather than pain as 1st symptom
  - Vascular procedures: Bypass/interventional
- Other conditions
  - Acute aortic dissection (chest or back pain)
  - Acute deep vein thrombosis (massive swelling and warm skin)
  - Low flow states

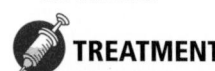 **TREATMENT**

GENERAL MEASURES
- Time is of the essence.
  - Unless contraindicated, systemic heparinization to decrease clot propagation and prophylaxis against further emboli
  - Resuscitation and stabilization of patient to extent permitted by time
  - Triage, based on detailed exam, history, and Doppler examination, determines appropriate therapy.
- Early subcritical stenosis criteria
  - Mild ischemic pain
  - Normal neurologic exam
  - Capillary refill present
  - Arterial signals present by Doppler in distal extremity
  - Ankle/arm index >0.30
  - Treatment
    ○ Heparin (see "Medications")
    ○ Arteriography
  - Embolism
    ○ Surgical removal if acceptable operative risk, for example, balloon embolectomy
    ○ Anticoagulation versus intra-arterial thrombolytics if prohibitive risk
  - Thrombosis
    ○ Trial of thrombolytics and correction of arterial defect if good risk
    ○ Anticoagulation if poor risk or thrombolytics contraindicated

- Critical stenosis criteria
  - Ischemic pain
  - Mild neurologic deficit
  - Weakness of dorsiflexion
  - Minimal sensory loss: Light touch and/or vibratory
  - No pulsatile flow by Doppler
  - Venous flow present
  - Treatment
    ○ Time to intervention is critical
    ○ Heparin (see "Medications")
    ○ Arteriography
    ○ Individualize thrombolysis and/or operative procedure (depending on extent of thrombosis and amenability for surgical removal)
    ○ Thrombolysis to optimize alternatives
    ○ Adjunctive operative therapy
    ○ Intraoperative lytic therapy: Bypass, patch angioplasty
- Late (nonsalvageable) criteria
  - Profound sensory loss
  - Muscle paralysis
  - Absent capillary refill
  - Skin marbling
  - Muscle rigor
  - No arterial or venous signals by Doppler
  - Treatment
    ○ Arteriography usually not warranted
    ○ Attempts at reperfusion contraindicated
    ○ Anticoagulation
    ○ Definitive amputation, if possible

 ## MEDICATION (DRUGS)

First Line
- Heparin
  - 80–100 U/kg IV loading dose (~5,000–10,000 U)
  - Continuous infusion sufficient to double PTT, generally 18 U/kg/h
- Contraindications
  - Heparin:
    ○ Allergy
    ○ Bleeding diathesis
    ○ Trauma (e.g., head injury)
    ○ Hematuria/hemoptysis
    ○ Acute aortic dissection
  - tPA/Urokinase
    ○ Nonsalvageable ischemia
    ○ Recent MI
    ○ Aneurysm
    ○ Aortic dissection
    ○ Trauma
    ○ Uncontrolled hypertension
    ○ Recent operative procedure

Second Line
Multiple thrombolytics in development

SURGERY
Angioplasty, Thromboembolectomy

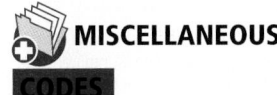 ## FOLLOW-UP

PROGNOSIS
- 90% good outcome with prompt treatment
- Delayed/untreated associated with high mortality and limb loss
- 20–30% hospital mortality associated with causative factors

COMPLICATIONS
- Acidosis
- Myoglobinuria and acute renal failure
- Hyperkalemia
- Recurrent occlusion
- Failure to remove clot/obstruction
- Compartment syndromes/reperfusion syndrome, delayed or acute: Predisposing factors include
  - Combined arterial injury
  - Profound and prolonged ischemia
  - Hypotension
- Clinical findings of compartment syndrome
  - Severe pain
  - Pain with passive muscle movement
  - Hypesthesias of nerves in compartment
  - Paralysis of nerves, especially peroneal foot drop
  - Tender, tense edema
  - Compartment pressure >30–45 mm Hg
- Consequences of unrecognized compartment syndrome
  - Acute
    ○ Amputation
    ○ Sepsis
    ○ Myoglobin renal failure
    ○ Shock
    ○ Multiple organ failure
  - Delayed
    ○ Ischemic contracture
    ○ Infection
    ○ Causalgia
    ○ Gangrene
- Treatment of compartment syndrome is fasciotomy.

PATIENT MONITORING
Postoperative monitoring

- Anticoagulation
- Establish brisk diuresis.
- Continued resuscitation and diagnosis, including echocardiography and other studies (see "Causes" and "Risk Factors")
- Monitor perfusion stability.
- Treat/eliminate causative factors.

REFERENCES

1. Antithrombotic therapy in peripheral arterial occlusive disease: the Seventh ACCP Conference on Antithrombotic and Thrombolytic Therapy. Chest.2004 Sep;126(3 Suppl):609S–26S. Available at www.ngc.gov.
2. *Townsend. Sabiston Textbook of Surgery*, 17th ed. Boston: Saunders, 2004.
3. Brewster DC, Chin AK, Fogarty TJ. Arterial thrombosis. In: Rutherford RB, ed. *Vascular Surgery*, 3rd ed. Philadelphia: WB Saunders; 1989.
4. Miller DC, Roon AJ, eds. *Diagnosis and Management of Peripheral Vascular Diseases*. Menlo Park, CA: Addison-Wesley; 1982.
5. Rutherford RB, Flannigan DP, Gupta SK, et al. Suggested standards of reports dealing with lower extremity ischemia. *J Vasc Surg*. 1986;64:80–94.

 ## MISCELLANEOUS

CODES

ICD9-CM
- 444.0 Arterial embolism and thrombosis of abdominal aorta
- 444.21 Arterial embolism and thrombosis of arteries of upper extremity
- 444.22 Arterial embolism and thrombosis of arteries of lower extremity
- 444.81 Arterial embolism and thrombosis of iliac artery
- 444.9 Arterial embolism and thrombosis of unspecified artery

PATIENT TEACHING

Prevention
- Quit smoking
- Antithrombotic or anticoagulant therapy

 See Corresponding Diagnostic Algorithm

See Patient Handout on CD

ARTERIAL GAS EMBOLISM

Jacqueline J. Wu, MD
Ruben Peralta, MD, FACS

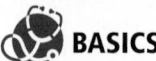 **BASICS**

DESCRIPTION

- Arterial gas embolisms are caused by the entry of gas into the pulmonary veins or directly into the arteries of the systemic circulation.
  - Gas may enter arteries as a result of overexpansion of lungs by decompression barotraumas.
  - May result from paradoxical embolus
- Emboli can travel to any artery, but the most serious consequences occur when they affect the cerebral or coronary circulation.
- Synonym(s): Gas embolism; Air embolism

ALERT

Any diver who has an onset of new symptom(s) or sign(s) after recently completing a Self-Contained Underwater Breathing Apparatus. SCUBA dive of any type, to any depth, for any period of time: Serious consideration must be given that such a patient sustained a dive-related injury.

GENERAL PREVENTION

- Strict adherence to diver safety protocols, especially including the buddy system
- No diving after any dive injury or with any medical condition until evaluated and approved by a physician knowledgeable about diving medicine

EPIDEMIOLOGY

- Predominant age: Young adult
- Predominant sex: Male > Female

Prevalence

Estimated (based on injury/mortality reports collected by Divers Alert Network) to occur in approximately 4 per 100,000 sport divers per year

RISK FACTORS

- Surgery: Recent craniotomy with patient in upright position, cardiothoracic (with cardiopulmonary bypass), hip replacement, Caesarian section
- SCUBA: Arterial gas embolism is the most serious and rapidly fatal of all SCUBA diving injuries and is second only to drowning as the leading cause of death associated with sport diving. Arterial gas embolism occurs on ascent; from alveolar rupture; time to the manifestation of symptoms is nearly always <10 minutes.
- History of patent foramen ovale has been associated with a >4-fold increase in decompression illness events and 2-fold more ischemic brain lesions than in divers without this condition.

ETIOLOGY

- Cerebral air embolism
  - Air bubbles occlude the brain vasculature
  - ICP increases
  - Unequal distribution of blood in the brain causes hyperemia and ischemia
  - Small bubbles irritate vascular wall causing breakdown of blood-brain barrier; small size allows rapid absorption and may cause only brief interruption of cerebral blood flow.
  - Larger air bubbles take longer to absorb (up to several hours) and can cause primary ischemic injury with diffuse brain edema and increased ICP.
- Coronary air embolism: Caused by obstruction of coronary arteries by an air bubble
  - Temporary ischemia of myocardium
  - Labile BP
  - Dysrhythmias
  - Cardiac failure and/or arrest
- Obstruction is possible in any artery.
  - Small emboli in the vessels of skeletal muscles and viscera are well-tolerated.
  - Arterial gas embolisms to coronary and cerebral arteries are especially serious or fatal because of the vulnerability of heart and brain to short periods of ischemia.

ASSOCIATED CONDITIONS

- Pulmonary barotrauma leading to arterial gas embolism can also cause pneumomediastinum, subcutaneous emphysema, pneumopericardium, pneumothorax, and pneumoperitoneum.
- Always consider the possibility of decompression sickness in addition to arterial gas embolism in any SCUBA diver who has recently completed a dive.

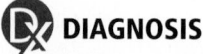 **DIAGNOSIS**

SIGNS AND SYMPTOMS

- Cerebral air embolism
  - Dizziness
  - Chest pain
  - Cardiac arrythmia
  - Paresthesias
  - Minor motor weakness
  - Convulsions
  - Paralysis
  - Nausea
  - Visual disturbances
  - Gas bubbles in vessels of retina
  - Headache
  - Asymmetric pupils
  - Hemianopia
  - Bradypnea
  - Cheyne-Stokes breathing
  - Aphasia
  - Mental status changes ranging from subtle to total lack of consciousness
- Coronary arterial embolism
  - Cardiac arrythmias
  - Cardiac arrest

ALERT

Anesthesia and/or analgesics alter the symptomatology and may complicate evaluation of the patient's clinical status. Delayed recovery from general anesthesia may be a clue to cerebral arterial embolism.

TESTS

Lab

- Hematocrit: Increased, indicating volume depletion and extravascular shift of fluid into injured tissues
- Serum creatine kinase: Correlation between creatine kinase activity and outcome suggests that elevated serum level of this enzyme may be a marker for size and severity of arterial gas embolism.
- Urinalysis: Increased specific gravity indicates volume depletion.

Imaging

- Chest radiograph to rule out pneumothorax
- ECG
- CT scan: Changes often very subtle
- MRI: Can sometimes show increased volume of water in injured tissue (not very reliable)

DIFFERENTIAL DIAGNOSIS

Decompression sickness

TREATMENT

PRE HOSPITAL
- General
  - Life-saving measures (e.g., CPR) must take precedence to sustain life.
  - Endotracheal intubation for somnolent or comatose patient
  - Highest possible concentration of oxygen: Eliminates gas in the bubbles by establishing diffusion gradient that favors egress of gas from bubbles
  - Place patient in flat, supine position (head down position may aggravate cerebral edema that develops).
- Hyperbaric oxygen
  - 1st-line treatment of choice for arterial gas embolism: Immediate transport to a suitable hyperbaric chamber for recompression as soon as possible; do not delay because of nonessential procedures
  - 100% oxygen at pressure above that of the atmosphere at sea level
  - Decreases bubble size
  - Prevents cerebral edema
  - For assistance and advice in locating the nearest treatment chamber in your area (worldwide), call Divers Alert Network (DAN) at any hour (919) 684-4326.
- IV fluids
  - To counteract hemoconcentration seen in gas embolism
  - Colloids preferred over crystalloid (latter may promote cerebral edema)
  - Goal is normovolemia

INITIAL STABILIZATION
- See "Treatment" and "General Measures."
- Hospital-based hyperbaric chamber capable of performing a U.S. Navy Table 6A recompression (165 feet of seawater)

GENERAL MEASURES
- CPR
- Keep patient recumbent while maintaining patent airway.
- Maintain hydration with IV fluids.
- Frequent neurologic checks in the acute pretreatment and treatment phases

Diet
Nothing to be consumed until after treatment

Activity
None until after treatment

SPECIAL THERAPY
IV Fluids
- Colloids preferred over crystalloid
- Achieve normovolemia

MEDICATION (DRUGS)

First Line
Oxygen
- As high a concentration as possible
- Transfer to facility with hyperbaric chamber as soon as possible

Second Line
- Heparin
  - Prevents platelet clumping
  - Studies of its use are inconsistent.
- Barbituates (if indicated)
  - For suppression of seizures
  - Reduce ICP
  - Decrease cerebral oxygen consumption
- Lidocaine
  - Decreases ICP
  - Improves recovery of somatosensory evoked potential following cerebral air embolism
  - Preserves cerebral blood flow

FOLLOW-UP

PROGNOSIS
Complete to partial resolution with adequate treatment

COMPLICATIONS
- Long-term serious neurologic impairments
- Death

PATIENT MONITORING
Complete neurologic assessment at 1, 3, 6, and 12 months

REFERENCES
1. Muth CM, Shank ES. Gas embolism. *N Engl J Med*. 2000; 342:476–482.
2. Vann RD, Dovenbarger JA. Reports on decompression illness. Diving fatalities and project dive exploration, the Divers Alert Network Annual Review of Recreational Scuba Driving Injuries and Fatalities. *2002 Data Durham: Divers Alert Network*. 2004:1–152.
3. Van Hulst RA, Klein J, Lachmann B. Gas embolism: Pathophysiology and treatment. *Clin Physiol Funct Imaging*. 2003;23:237–246.
4. Davis J. *Medical Examination of Sport Scuba Divers*, 2nd ed. San Antonio, TX: Medical Seminars; 1986.

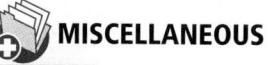

MISCELLANEOUS

CODES

ICD9-CM
958.0 Air embolism

PATIENT TEACHING

Divers Alert Network (DAN)
- Diving emergency hotline for medical emergencies only: 919-684-8111 or 919-684-4DAN (collect); 24 hours, 365 days a year
- Medical information line for nonemergency questions: 919-684-2948 M–F (9–5 EST)
- DAN America information line: 800-446-2671 or 919-684-2948 M–F (9–5 EST); website www.diversalertnetwork.org
- On-Site Neurologic Exam by Ed Thalmann; website www.diversalertnetwork.org/medical/neuroexam.asp

ARTERIOSCLEROTIC HEART DISEASE

Felix B. Chang, MD
Alfonso Tafur, MD

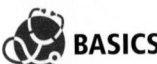 **BASICS**

DESCRIPTION

- Arteriosclerosis is a group of diseases characterized by thickening and loss of elasticity of arterial walls that progressively block coronary arteries and their branches. Arteriosclerosis is the most common form of coronary arteriosclerosis. Process is chronic, occurring over many years, and is the most common cause of cardiovascular disability and death. Other forms of arteriosclerosis include arteriolosclerosis and calcific stenosis, both of which are uncommon in coronary vasculature.
- Subclinical cardiovascular disease (CVD) is defined as a plaque occurrence in carotid arteries with ≥25% stenosis, ankle-brachial blood pressure index (ABI) <0.9 and, coronary calcification based on Agatston calcium score ≥200
- Synonym(s): Coronary artery disease; Coronary heart disease; Coronary arteriosclerosis

GENERAL PREVENTION

See "Treatment: General Measures"

EPIDEMIOLOGY

- Leading cause of death in the US and Europe
- Predominant sex: Male > Female
- Predominant age for peak clinical manifestations
  - Men: 50–60
  - Women: 60–70
- Rare in pregnancy

Incidence

Greatest incidence in geriatric population

Prevalence

Common

RISK FACTORS

- Primary risk factors
  - Diabetes mellitus (considered AHD equivalent)
  - Male age >45 or female >55
  - Family history of premature coronary heart disease (1st degree relative: Male <55 years, female <65 years)
  - BP >140/90 or hypertension on medication
  - Active cigarette abuse
  - HDL cholesterol <40 mg/dL (HDL >60 mg/dL is a negative factor)
- Secondary risk factors
  - Elevated LDL cholesterol
  - Obesity

ETIOLOGY

- Inflammation including autoimmunity
- Atherosclerosis
- Narrowing of coronary arteries
- Embolism compromising coronary arteries at orifices
- Subintimal atheromas in large and medium vessels

ASSOCIATED CONDITIONS

- Obesity
- Hypertension
- Diabetes
- Hypercholesterolemia

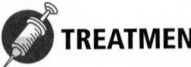 **DIAGNOSIS**

SIGNS AND SYMPTOMS

- Variable: May remain clinically asymptomatic even in advanced disease states, for example, silent ischemia
- Clinical manifestations
  - Substernal chest pain
  - Exertional dyspnea
  - Orthopnea
  - Paroxysmal nocturnal dyspnea
  - Cardiac arrhythmias
  - Systolic murmur
  - Cardiomegaly
  - Pedal edema

Physical Exam

- Brachial artery pressures for ABI: When the 2 brachial artery pressures differ by 10 mm Hg or more, the highest brachial artery pressure is used as the denominator. For each lower extremity, the highest pressure (dorsalis pedis or posterior tibial) is used an numerator.
- 5 ABI categories: <0.90 (definite peripheral arterial disease [PAD]); 0.90–0.99 (borderline ABI); 1,00–1,09 (low-normal ABI); 1.10–1.29 (normal ABI); and >1.30 (high ABI)

TESTS

- ECG: Variable; may be normal or may see ST-segment elevation/depression and/or T-wave inversion
- Exercise stress test: Positive

Lab

- Elevated triglycerides
- Elevated total cholesterol
- Elevated LDLs
- Decreased HDLs
- Elevated cholesterol/HDL ratio
- American Heart Association statement currently supports C reactive protein is no more predictive of AHD than traditional risk factors.

Imaging

- Angiography: Narrowed coronary arteries
- Echocardiography: Wall-motion abnormalities
- Pharmacologic stress tests (dobutamine, dipyridamole, adenosine): Positive
- Stress thallium test: Positive
- Noninvasive CAD detection with multislice CT or MRI

Pathological Findings

- Gross: Narrowed coronary arteries
- Micro: Cholesterol plaques on intima of coronary vessels
- Fibrotic subendothelial connective tissue of intima with plaque

TREATMENT

GENERAL MEASURES

- Outpatient for management of risk factors
- Inpatient care for acute ischemic syndromes
- CHC or CHD risk equivalents (10 years risk >20%) has a LDL c goal <100 mg/dL
- Prevention of further disease progression
  - Smoking cessation
  - Treatment of hypercholesterolemia (diet, drugs)
  - Increase HDL (diet, exercise)
  - Control of BP (<140/90; if DM or renal disease, <130/80) (4)[C]
  - Diabetes mellitus treated early and adequately
  - Exercise 30–40 minutes 5 times/week (4)[C]
  - Prophylactic aspirin
  - Stress reduction
  - Diet changes
  - Weight loss (BMI <25) (4)[C]
- Treatment of complications: Covered elsewhere under individual topics (e.g., angina pectoris, myocardial infarction, heart failure, stroke, and peripheral arterial occlusion)
- Preventive measures can begin early (e.g., proper nutrition, exercise, weight control, smoking deterrent programs).

Diet

- Low fat: 20–30 g of fat per day
- Weight-loss diet, if obesity a problem
- Increase soluble fiber.

Activity

Exercise may be helpful in preventing clinical coronary disease and useful for therapeutic measures; 30–40 minutes 3 times/week.

MEDICATION (DRUGS)

First Line

- Aspirin/ASA: 160–325 mg/d (clopidogrel if ASA is contraindicated; some data reflect both beneficial if history of acute coronary syndrome)
- ACE Inhibitors in all with increased risk factors, DM, or know CAD
- Cholesterol-lowering agents
  – HMG-CoA reductase inhibitors (dose varies with product): atorvastatin (10–80 mg PO once daily), fluvastatin (20–80 mg/d), lovastatin (10–80 mg/d), pravastatin (10–80 mg/d), simvastatin (20–40 mg once daily), rosuvastatin (5–40 mg once daily)
- Statins also have anti-inflammatory and immunomodulatory effects by reducing monocyte adhesion to EC and endothelial secretion of cytokines and MHC call II expression.
- ω-3 Acid ethyl esters2-4 g EPA+DHA daily
- To increase HDL cholesterol
  – Niacin: 2–6 g/d in divided doses (efficacious, but restricted by side effects)
- Gemfibrozil : 600 mg 2 b.i.d.
- Fenofibrate: 67–200 mg/d
- Probucol: 500 mg 2 b.i.d.
- Colesevelam: 3.75–4.375 g/d
- Ezetimibe: 10 mg/d
- Contraindications: Refer to manufacturer's literature.
- Precautions: Slow-release form of niacin may be linked to hepatotoxicity. Refer to manufacturer's literature.
- Significant possible interactions: Refer to manufacturer's literature.

Second Line

Ticlopidine, Dipyridamole, Clopidogrel—antiplatelet activity

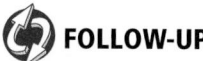 **FOLLOW-UP**

When starting HMG-CoA reductase inhibitors monitor LFT initially, follow-up ~12 weeks after starting therapy, then annually or more frequently if it is indicated.

PROGNOSIS

Guardedly favorable. Many risk factors can be modified.

COMPLICATIONS

- Myocardial infarction
- Ventricular fibrillation
- CHF
- Angina pectoris
- Sudden cardiac death

PATIENT MONITORING

- Monitor cholesterol and triglyceride levels.
- Encourage participation in other preventive programs (weight loss, smoking cessation).

REFERENCES

1. Dewey M, Teige R, Schanapauff D, et al. Noninvasive detection of coronary artery stenoses with multislice computed tomography or magnetic resonance imaging. *Ann Intern Med.* 2006;145:407–415.
2. Zouridakis E, Avanzas P, Arroyo-Espliquero R, et al. Markers of inflammation and rapid coronary artery disease progression in patient with stable angina pectoris. *Circulation.* 2004;28:110(13):1747–1753.
3. Doria A, Sherer Y, Meroni P, et al. Inflammation and accelerated atherosclerosis: Basic mechanisms. *Rheum Dis Clin N Am.* 2005;31:355–362.
4. Smith SC, et al. AHA/ACC guidelines for preventing heart attack and death in patients with atherosclerotic cardiovascular disease: 2001 update—A statement for healthcare professionals from the American Heart Association and the American College of Cardiology. *J Am Coll Cardiol.* 2001;38:1581–1583.

ADDITIONAL READING

Knoflach M, Maryl B, Mayerl C. et al. Atherosclerosis is a paradigmatic disease or the elderly: Role of the immune system. *Immunol Allergy Clin N Am.* 2003;23:117–132.

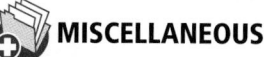 **MISCELLANEOUS**

See also: Angina; Atherosclerosis; Myocardial Infarction

 CODES

ICD9-CM

414.00 Coronary atherosclerosis of unspecified type of vessel, native or graft

PATIENT TEACHING

For patient education materials favorably reviewed on this topic, contact: American Heart Association, 7320 Greenville Avenue, Dallas, TX 75231, (214) 373–6300.

Prevention

- Quit Smoking, exercise, decrease caloric and fat intake, weight and hypertension control
- Life style changes are indicated when lifestyle-related factors (obesity, physical inactivity, increased triglycerides, decreased HDL, or metabolic syndrome are present) regardless of LDL.

See Patient Handout on CD

ARTHRITIS, INFECTIOUS, BACTERIAL

Bruce M. Rothschild, MD

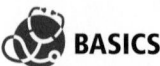 **BASICS**

DESCRIPTION
- Invasion of joints by live micro-organisms or their fragments. One of the few curable causes of arthritis. May allow early recognition of systemic infection/disease.
- System(s) Affected: Musculoskeletal
- Synonym(s): Suppurative arthritis; Septic arthritis

GENERAL PREVENTION
Condoms and discretion for STD protection

EPIDEMIOLOGY
- Predominant age (1, 2, 3)[A]
  - Neisserial: Especially 15–40 years of age; can occur at any age
  - Non-Neisserial
    ○ Years <2: 27% Staphylococcus, 20% Streptococcus, 33% Haemophilus, and 13% other Gram-negative rods, 7% miscellaneous
    ○ Years 2–14: 34% Staphylococcus, 29% Streptococcus, 13% Haemophilus, and 13% other Gram-negative rods, 11% miscellaneous
    ○ Adult: 34% Staphylococcus, 38% Streptococcus, 2% Haemophilus, and 26% other Gram-negative rods
- Predominant sex
  - Neisserial: Female > Male (4:1)
  - Non-Neisserial: Male > Female (2:1)
  - Subacute bacterial endocarditis-related: Male = Female

Prevalence
- Neisserial
  - Responsible for 50% of infectious arthritis
  - 0.6% of the 3% of women with gonorrhea
  - 0.1% of the 0.7% of men with gonorrhea
  - Arthritis occurs in 7% of individuals with *Neisseria meningitidis*
- Non-Neisserial: Half as frequent as Neisserial

RISK FACTORS
- Young patient with venereal exposure
- Concurrent extra-articular infection
- Prior arthritis in infected joint
- Trauma
- Joint puncture or surgery
- Prosthetic joint (4)[A]
- Prior antibiotic, corticosteroid, or immunosuppressive therapy
- Serious chronic illness (e.g., diabetes, liver disease, malignancy, primary immunodeficiency)
- Defective phagocytic mechanisms (e.g., chronic granulomatous disease)
- IV drug abuse
- Unusual travel/habitat history
- Sickle cell anemia
- C8 deficiency
- Systemic infection; infection elsewhere
- Immunodeficiency; immunosuppression
- Rheumatoid arthritis

ETIOLOGY
- Hematogenous invasion (80–90%)
- Contiguous spread (10–15%)
- Direct penetration of microorganisms secondary to trauma or joint injection

DIAGNOSIS

SIGNS AND SYMPTOMS
- Predominantly monoarticular (90%). (Haemophilus may be pauciarticular and Mycoplasma often a migratory polyarthritis.)
- Limited or loss of joint use/motion
- Joint effusion, tenderness
- Joint warmth: Present in <50%
- Joint redness: Present in <50%
- Tenosynovitis
- Sudden flare of 1 or 2 joints in patient with underlying joint disease
- Fever: In 90% during course of infection
- Chills
- Malaise
- Cutaneous lesions
- Peripheral neuropathy
- Back pain: Subacute bacterial endocarditis (5)[A]
- Hypertrophic osteoarthropathy: Rare, secondary to endocarditis
- Dermato-arthritis
  - Usually pustular skin lesions in gonorrhea
  - Usually petechial rash in meningococcemia
- Bacteremic phase: Migratory polyarthritis, Tenosynovitis, high fever, chills, pustules
- Localized phase:
  - Usually monoarticular
  - Low-grade fever (80%)

TESTS
Lab

Synovial fluid (6)[A]

- Synovial fluid is usually cloudy with >50,000 WBC/HPF. (Caveat: Cell count must be performed within 1 hour of obtaining specimen to be valid.)
- Synovial-fluid white count can be recognized as elevated (in presence of trauma) if RBC/WBC ratio is significantly less than 700.
- Polymorphonuclear leukocytes usually predominate in synovial fluid.
- Synovial-fluid glucose is often more than 40 mg/dL (2.22 mmol/L) less than simultaneously obtained serum glucose value (in fasting patient).
- Decreased levels of complement
- Crystals (e.g., urate or calcium pyrophosphate) do not exclude infectious arthritis.
- Joint fluid: For Gram stain (positive in 50%); culture (positive in 50–70%)
- Serum cidal level assessment of antibiotic is suggested (10-fold margin suggested)

Serum Testing

- Westergren erythrocyte sedimentation rate: Often elevated, but normal in 20%
- Rheumatoid factor: Positive in 50%, if endocarditis present and in viral arthritis
- Elevated peripheral white blood cell count in 50–90% of the patients
- Cryoglobulins
- Immune complexes
- Febrile agglutinins (to include Brucella and rickettsial-related titers)
- Antistreptolysin O titer usually normal, exclusive of streptococcal infections

- Depressed serum levels of complement
- Microscopic hematuria in subacute bacterial endocarditis (5)[A]
- Blood, orifice, urine cultures
- "Bedside culture" is recommended to enhance isolation of fastidious organisms.
- All cultures should be preserved and observed for 3 days to 2 weeks (3, 6–8)[A].
- Neisserial infection generally requires use of special agars (e.g., chocolate or Thayer Martin)
- Drugs that may alter lab results: Antibiotics
- Countercurrent immunoelectrophoresis or complement fixation for specific bacterial antigens
- Polymerase chain reaction for specific bacterial DNA (8,9)[A]

Imaging
- X-ray (8)[A]
  - Soft-tissue swelling
  - Juxta-articular osteoporosis
  - Radiolucent area (gas) in a joint space from gas-forming organisms (Caveat: May be normal as a "vacuum phenomenon.")
  - Effacement of obturator fat pad (with hip involvement)
  - X-ray changes usually a late phenomenon
  - Rarefaction of subchondral bone may occur
  - Joint-space loss (secondary to cartilage destruction) may occur in 4–10 days.
  - Erosions
  - Joint destruction with ankylosis may occur.
- Other imaging techniques
  - Technetium joint scans: Reveal distribution of inflammation; sensitive, not specific
  - Gallium or Ceretec WBC scan, Indium scans: Reveal inflammation as well as infection
  - CT: To identify sequestration
  - MRI: Effusion, perhaps early cartilage damage, osteomyelitis

Diagnostic Procedures/Surgery
- Arthrocentesis with Gram stain and culture: Positive in 50–70% (7)[A]
  - Must always be done when possibility of infectious arthritis considered
  - Arthrocentesis should probably be performed within 12 hours of suspicion.
- Arthrocentesis approach must avoid contaminated tissue (e.g., overlying cellulitis).

Pathological Findings
Synovial biopsy will reveal polymorphonuclear leukocytes and possibly the causative organism, if synovial fluid and blood cultures are negative.

DIFFERENTIAL DIAGNOSIS
- Gout
- Pseudogout (calcium pyrophosphate deposition disease)
- Spondyloarthropathy (Reiter syndrome, psoriatic arthritis, ankylosing spondylitis, arthritis of inflammatory bowel disease)
- Juvenile rheumatoid arthritis
- Type IIa hyperlipoproteinemia
- Foreign-body synovitis

- Rheumatoid arthritis
- Rheumatic fever
- AIDS
- Cellulitis
- Palindromic rheumatism
- Neuropathic arthropathy
- Lyme arthritis
- Sarcoidosis
- Granulomatous arthritis

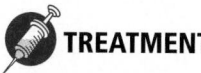 **TREATMENT**

GENERAL MEASURES
- Hospitalization for parenteral therapy
- Outpatient treatment rarely possible for extremely compliant patient with known organism
- Repeat arthrocentesis to drain joint as fluid re-accumulates.
- Avoid anti-inflammatory therapy to allow assessment of therapeutic response to antibiotic.
- If joint prosthesis is present in an infection, removal of the prosthesis must be considered.
- Continue treatment for 1–2 weeks after total resolution of all signs of inflammation, 3–4 weeks for Gram-negative organisms, and 6–8 weeks, if joint was previously diseased.
- Intra-articular antibiotics not required and may actually aggravate the arthritis

Diet
No special diet

Activity
Limit activity or splint joint initially. Alternative approach: Continuous passive motion

 MEDICATION (DRUGS)

First Line
- Neisserial (3,8)[A]
  - Ceftriaxone 1 g IM or IV every day for 14 days (but at least 7 days after symptoms resolve)
  - Spectinomycin 2 g IM q12h × 10 days
- Non-Neisserial (3,8)[A]
  - Gram-positive cocci in chains or clumps: Nafcillin 150 mg/kg per day q4–6h IV/IM
  - Gram-positive diplococci: Penicillin G 1.4 million units q6h
  - Gram-negative bacilli: Neonates, penicillin and gentamicin; ages 6 months–4 years, cefuroxime; adult, penicillin or cephalosporin plus gentamicin, all at full dose. Add clindamycin, at full dose, in presence of retroperitoneal or pelvic abscess.
  - Gram-negative pleomorphic organisms: Clindamycin at full dose (clindamycin has Gram-negative activity only against anaerobes)
  - No bacteria seen on smear: Penicillin or cephalosporin plus gentamicin

- Contraindications: Tetracycline not for use in pregnancy or children <8 years

- Precautions
  - Observe for allergic reactions/serum sickness
  - Tetracycline may cause photosensitivity; sunscreen recommended
- Significant possible interactions
  - Tetracycline: Avoid concurrent administration with antacids, dairy products, or iron
  - Broad-spectrum antibiotics: May reduce effectiveness of oral contraceptives; barrier method recommended

Second Line
- Non-Neisserial
  - In children age 6 months–4 years: Ampicillin; chloramphenicol may be required to cover resistant Haemophilus
  - Infectious disease consult strongly advised to supplement rheumatologist input for Haemophilus infections
- Neisserial and Non-Neisserial:
  - Quinonlones (e.g., ciprofloxacin)

SURGERY
Arthrotomy indicated only if fluid accumulated is loculated and/or not amenable to needle drainage

 FOLLOW-UP

PROGNOSIS
- Early treatment should allow cure.
- Delayed recognition/treatment complicated by morbidity and mortality

COMPLICATIONS
- Death (9–33% in elderly)
- Limited joint range of motion
- Flail or fused or dislocated joint
- Carpal tunnel syndrome
- Septic necrosis
- Sinus formation
- Ankylosis
- Osteomyelitis
- Postinfectious synovitis
- Shortening of limb (in children)

PATIENT MONITORING
- Recurrent arthrocentesis as fluid re-accumulates to verify sterilization of joint and reversion of inflammatory signs to normal
- If no improvement within 48 hours, reevaluate.
- Complete blood count, liver and kidney function, and urinalysis twice a week while on antibiotics (with creatinine when gentamicin used)
- Gentamicin levels
- Essential to follow up 1 week and 1 month after stopping antibiotics to detect any relapse

REFERENCES
1. Dubost JJ, Soubrier M, De Champs C, et al. No changes in distribution of organisms responsible for septic arthritis over a 20 year period. *Ann Rheum Dis*. 2002;61:257–260.
2. Garcia-De La Torre I. Advances in the management of septic arthritis. *Rheum Dis Clin N Am*. 2003;29:61–75.
3. Gonzalez-Juanatey C. Rheumatic manifestations of infective endocarditis in non-addicts: A 12-year study. *Medicine*. 2001;80:9–19.
4. Gershwin ME, Robbins DL. *Musculoskeletal Diseases of Children*. New York, NY: Grune & Stratton; 1983.
5. Gupta MN, Sturrock RD, Field M. Prospective comparative study of patients with culture proven and high suspicion of adult onset septic arthritis. *Ann Rheum Dis*. 2003;62:327–331.
6. Khachatourians AG, Patzakis MJ, Roidis N, Holtom PD. Laboratory monitoring in pediatric acute osteomyelitis and septic arthritis. *Clin Orthop*. 2003;(409):186–194.
7. Ross JJ, Hu LT. Bacterial and Lyme arthritis. *Curr Infect Dis Rep*. 2004;5:380–387.
8. Tarkin IS, Dunman PM, Garvin KL. Improving the treatment of musculoskeletal infections with molecular diagnostics. *Clin Orthop Rel Res*. 2005;437:83–88.
9. Wilkinson NZ, Kingsley GH, Jones HW, et al. The detection of DNA from a range of bacterial species in the joints of patients with a variety of arthritides using a nested, broad-range polymerase chain reaction. *Rheumatol*. 1999;38:260–266.
10. Zimmerli W, Trampuz A, Ochsner PE. Prosthetic joint infections. *N Engl J Med*. 2004;351:1645–1654.

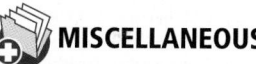 **MISCELLANEOUS**

See also: Reiter Syndrome

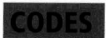 **CODES**

ICD9-CM
711.00 Pyogenic arthritis, site unspecified

PATIENT TEACHING
Rothschild BM. Diagnosing and treating infectious arthritis. *Geriatric Consultant*. 1986;5:14–15.

 See Patient Handout on CD

ARTHRITIS, INFECTIOUS, GRANULOMATOUS

Bruce M. Rothschild, MD

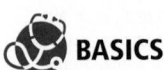 **BASICS**

DESCRIPTION
- Invasion of joints by live microorganisms or their fragments. One of the few curable causes of arthritis. May allow early recognition of systemic infection/disease.
- System(s) Affected: Musculoskeletal
- Synonym(s): Fungal arthritis

GENERAL PREVENTION
Prophylaxis in presence of predisposing joint condition

EPIDEMIOLOGY
- Occurs in 1–3% of patients with tuberculosis infections
- Predominant age: Diffuse
- Predominant sex
  - Male > Female (Brucella and mycobacterial)
  - Female > male (fungal)

Prevalence
- 1 in 3,000,000
- Infrequent in pediatric population

RISK FACTORS
- Concurrent acquired immunodeficiency disease
- Concurrent extra-articular infection
- Prior arthritis in infected joint
- Trauma
- Rheumatoid arthritis
- Joint puncture or surgery
- Prosthetic joint
- Prior antibiotic, corticosteroid, or immunosuppressive therapy
- Serious chronic illness (e.g., diabetes, liver disease, malignancy, primary immunodeficiency)
- Defective phagocytic mechanisms (e.g., chronic granulomatous disease)
- Intravenous drug abuse
- Exposure history (e.g., unpasteurized milk)
- Farmers, butchers, veterinarians
- Travel/habitat history
- Gardening, especially for sporotrichosis

ETIOLOGY
- Hematogenous invasion by microorganisms (80–90%)
- Contiguous spread (10–15%)
- Direct penetration of microorganisms secondary to trauma

ASSOCIATED CONDITIONS
- Systemic infection
- Infection elsewhere
- Immunodeficiency (e.g., from medications)
- Immunosuppression

ALERT
Geriatric Considerations
- Grave in elderly
- Tuberculosis much more likely to occur

DIAGNOSIS

SIGNS AND SYMPTOMS
- Predominantly monoarticular (90%). Fungal may present as a migratory polyarthritis. (1,2)
- Joint tenderness
- Limited joint use/motion; especially in children
- Joint effusion
- Joint warmth; present in less than 50%
- Joint redness; present in less than 50%
- Loss of joint motion
- Tenosynovitis
- Sudden flare of single joint in patient with underlying joint disease
- Fever; in 50% at some time during course of infection
- Chills
- Malaise
- Cutaneous lesions
- Peripheral neuropathy
- Back pain; especially in tuberculosis and brucellosis
- Hypertrophic osteoarthropathy
- Fretfulness; especially in children
- Doughy swelling, with minimal tenderness
- Dactylitis
- Diaphoresis
- Headache
- Hepatosplenomegaly
- Lymphadenopathy
- Erythema nodosum
- Iritis (with mycobacterial arthritis)

TESTS
Lab
- Arthrocentesis (3, 4)[A], (5), (6)[A]
  - Bacterial: For Gram stain, silver, and acid-fast stain and culture, cell count and differential, glucose
  - Mycobacterial: Acid fast (positive in 20%), culture (positive in 80%)
  - Must be done in all patients when possibility of infectious arthritis considered
  - Synovial fluid usually cloudy with >20,000 WBC/HPF, but may have fewer white blood cells present or over 100,000 (Caveat: Cell count must be performed within 1 hour of obtaining specimen to be valid.)
  - Synovial-fluid white count can be recognized as elevated (in presence of trauma) if the RBC/WBC ratio is significantly less than 700.
  - Polymorphonuclear leukocytes usually predominate in synovial fluid (although granulomatous and viral arthritis may have a mononuclear cell predominance).
  - Synovial-fluid glucose often more than 40 mg/dL (2.22 mmol/L) less than in simultaneously obtained serum glucose value (in fasting patient). However, arthrocentesis should not be delayed simply to obtain fasting synovial fluid glucose level.
  - Synovial-fluid eosinophilia may occasionally be seen in the healing phase of infection, but parasitic (e.g., guinea-worm) infection must also be considered.
  - Approach must avoid contaminated tissue (e.g., overlying cellulitis).
  - Drug-sensitivity testing recommended

- The presence of crystals in the synovial fluid (e.g., urate or calcium pyrophosphate) does not exclude infectious arthritis.
  - Depressed synovial fluid levels of complement
- Synovial membrane: Biopsy and culture
- Blood, urine, sputum cultures
  - Fungal blood cultures
  - Polymerase chain reaction for specific microorganisms
  - All cultures should be held for 2 weeks; acid-fast cultures for 6 weeks
- Gastric lavage for acid fast: Increases yield 7%
- Serum testing
  - Polymerase chain reaction DNA analysis for tuberculosis
  - Westergren erythrocyte sedimentation: Often elevated, but normal in 20%
  - Rheumatoid factor positive in 50% if endocarditis present
  - Elevated peripheral white blood cell count
  - Cryoglobulins
  - Immune complexes
  - Febrile agglutinins (to include Brucella- and rickettsial-related titers)
  - Antistreptolysin-O titer usually normal
  - Decreased serum complement levels
- Other
  - Disorders that may alter lab results: Diabetes
  - Drugs that may alter lab results: Insulin, antibiotics

Imaging
- X-ray (1,2),(4)[A],(5),(6–8)[A]
  - X-ray changes usually a late phenomenon
  - Soft-tissue swelling
  - Osteoporosis
  - Effacement of the obturator fat pad (with hip involvement) or psoas shadow
  - Rarefaction of subchondral bone
  - Joint-space loss
  - Erosions
  - Joint destruction with ankylosis
  - Subchondral erosion with preservation of joint space strongly suggests granulomatous infection.
- Technetium joint scans: Reveal distribution of inflammation, not just infection
- Gallium scan, Ceretec or indium WBC scans: Reveal inflammation as well as infection
- Computerized tomography: To identify sequestration
- Magnetic resonance imaging: Perhaps early cartilage damage, osteomyelitis (1),(4)[A]

Pathological Findings
Synovial biopsy may reveal granulomas and possibly the causative organism.

DIFFERENTIAL DIAGNOSIS
- Gout
- Pseudogout (calcium pyrophosphate deposition disease)
- Spondyloarthropathy (Reiter syndrome, psoriatic arthritis, ankylosing spondylitis, arthritis of inflammatory bowel disease)
- Juvenile rheumatoid arthritis
- Type IIa hyperlipoproteinemia
- Foreign body synovitis
- Rheumatoid arthritis
- Rheumatic fever

- AIDS
- Cellulitis
- Palindromic rheumatism
- Neuropathic arthropathy
- Lyme arthritis
- Sarcoidosis
- Pyogenic arthritis

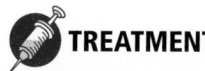 TREATMENT

GENERAL MEASURES

- Appropriate care
  - Fungal: Initial hospitalization for parenteral therapy
  - Mycobacterial: Outpatient, once diagnosed
  - Brucella: Outpatient, once diagnosed
- Repeat arthrocentesis to drain joint as fluid reaccumulates.
- Avoid adding anti-inflammatory therapy to avoid compromising the assessment of the therapeutic response to the antibiotic.
- Infection associated with prosthetic joints may be difficult to eradicate without removal.
- For Brucella or fungal infections, continue treatment for 1–2 weeks after total resolution of all signs of inflammation, and 6–8 weeks if joint was previously diseased (e.g., arthritis).
- Antigranulomatous therapy requires a long program (see Tuberculosis).
- Intra-articular antibiotics are not indicated.
- Infectious-disease consultation may be helpful.

Diet
As tolerated

Activity
Limit/splint joint initially, while pursuing full passive range of motion Alternative approach: Continuous passive motion.

MEDICATION (DRUGS)

- Medications based on sensitivity of organisms
- Mycobacterial infection (4)[A], (5,7)[A], (8)
  - Use combination of isoniazid, rifampin, and pyrazinamide/ethambutol.
  - Isoniazid 5 mg/kg, up to 300 mg PO every day
  - Rifampin 10 mg/kg, up to 600 mg PO every day
  - Pyrazinamide 15–30 mg/kg up to 2 g per day. After 2 months, replace with ethambutol 15 mg/kg
  - Continue therapy for 9–24 months.
  - Request infectious-disease consultation.
- Brucella (6)[A]
  - Tetracycline plus streptomycin or trimethoprim-sulfamethoxazole or rifampin (for dosage, see manufacturer's literature)
- Fungal infection (5)
  - Choice of medication depends on organism
  - Amphotericin B
  - Ketoconazole
  - Flucytosine (5-fluorocytosine)
- Contraindications
  - Tetracycline not for use in pregnancy or children <8 years

- Precautions
  - Observe for allergic reactions/serum sickness
  - Tetracycline may cause photosensitivity; sunscreen recommended
- Significant possible interactions
  - Tetracycline: Avoid concurrent administration with antacids, dairy products, or iron
  - Ketoconazole: Multiple drug interactions
- Alternative drugs: See Tuberculosis.

SURGERY
Arthrotomy indicated only if fluid accumulated is loculated and/or not amenable to needle drainage

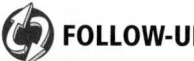 FOLLOW-UP

PROGNOSIS
- Early initiation of treatment should allow cure.
- Delayed recognition/treatment complicated by increased morbidity and mortality

COMPLICATIONS
- Limited joint range of motion
- Flail or fused joint
- Carpal-tunnel syndrome
- Septic necrosis
- Sinus formation
- Ankylosis
- Joint dislocation
- Osteomyelitis
- Shortening of limb (in children)

PATIENT MONITORING
- Verify sterilization of joint and reversion of inflammatory signs to normal
- Treatment of mycobacterial arthritis requires monthly complete blood count, assessment of liver and kidney function, and urinalysis.
- Essential to follow up frequently after stopping antibiotics to detect relapse.
- As dictated by therapy protocols (e.g., amphotericin B)

REFERENCES

1. Resnick D. *Diagnosis of Bone and Joint Disorders*. Philadelphia, PA: WB Saunders Co.; 2002:2375–2612.
2. Rothschild BM, Martin L. *Skeletal Impact of Disease Pathology*. Albuquerque, NM: New Mexico Museum of Natural History; 2006.
3. Fukushima M, Kakinuma K, Hayashi H, et al. Detection and identification of mycobacterial species isolated by DNA microarray. *J Clin Microbiol*. 2003;41:2605–2615.
4. Hus C-Y, Shih TT-F. Tuberculous infection of the wrists: MRI features. *Am J Roentgenol*. 2004;183:623–628.
5. Kelly WW, Harris ED Jr, Ruddy S, Sledge CB. *Textbook of Rheumatology*. Philadelphia, PA: WB Saunders Co.; 1997.
6. Yilmaz E, Parlak M, Akalin H, et al. Brucella spondylitis: Review of 25 cases. *J Clin Rheumatol*. 2004;10:300–307.
7. Papagelopoulos PJ, Papadopoulos EC, Mavrogenis AF, et al. Tuberculous sacroiliitis. A case report and review of the literature. *Eur Spine J*. 2005;14:683–688.
8. Sawlani V, Chandra T, Mishra RN, Aggarwal A, Jain UK, Gujral RB. MRI features of tuberculosis of peripheral joints. *Clin Radiol*. 2003;58:755–762.
9. Gershwin ME, Robbins DL. *Musculoskeletal Diseases of Children*. New York, NY: Grune & Stratton; 1983.
10. Rothschild BM, Rothschild C. Recognition of hypertrophic osteoarthropathy in skeletal remains. *J Rheum*. 1998;25:2221–2228.

MISCELLANEOUS

- Other notes: Infectious arthritis may be caused by many other organisms including bacterial (particularly neisseria), rickettsial, parasitic, fungal, and viral agents. Much of the information contained in this profile applies to these other organisms as well as to granulomatous infections.
- See also: Brucellosis

CODES

ICD9-CM
- 023.9 Brucellosis, unspecified
- 031.8 Other specified mycobacterial diseases
- 115.99 Histoplasmosis, unspecified other

PATIENT TEACHING
- Rothschild BM. Diagnosing and treating infectious arthritis. *Geriatric Consultant*. 1986;5:14–15.
- Arthritis Foundation, 1314 Spring Street, NW Atlanta, GA 30309 (404) 872–7100.

 See Patient Handout on CD

ARTHRITIS, JUVENILE RHEUMATOID

Jason Silva, MD

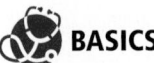 **BASICS**

DESCRIPTION

- Most common form of chronic arthritis in children and a major cause of musculoskeletal disability.
- General characteristics
  - Age of onset <16 years
  - Signs of arthritis
    ○ Joint swelling, decreased range of motion, pain
  - >6 weeks of symptoms
- 3 subtypes exist, determined by clinical characteristics seen in 1st 6 months of illness
  - Systemic: Occurs in 10–20% of affected children; usually characterized by febrile onset and evanescent rash with multiple physical and laboratory abnormalities
  - Polyarticular: Occurs in 30–40% of affected children; multiple (>4) joint involvement and minimal systemic features; large and small joints affected
  - Pauciarticular: Occurs in 40–50% of affected children; involvement of ≤4 joints, usually larger joints, especially of lower extremities; risk for chronic uveitis in young girls and axial skeletal involvement in older boys
- System(s) Affected: Hematologic/lymphatic/immunologic; Musculoskeletal
- Synonym(s): Juvenile chronic arthritis; Juvenile arthritis; Juvenile idiopathic arthritis; Still disease

GENERAL PREVENTION
No known preventive measures

EPIDEMIOLOGY
- Predominant age: 1–4 years and 9–14 years
- Predominant sex
  - Poly/Pauciarticular: Female > Male
  - Systemic: Female = Male

Incidence
1/10,000 children

Prevalence
~1/1,000 children

RISK FACTORS
- HLA-B27 in pauciarticular juvenile rheumatoid arthritis increases risk of spondyloarthropathy
- Rheumatoid factor positivity increases risk for severe arthritis in polyarticular JRA
- ANA positivity increases risk for uveitis in pauciarticular and polyarticular JRA

Genetics
- HLA-B27 histocompatibility antigen associated with risk of evolving spondyloarthropathy in older boys with pauciarticular JRA
- Weaker HLA associations exist for other subtypes (HLA-DR5, HLA-DR8, HLA-DR4)
  - DR 4: Polyarticular
  - DR 5, 8: Pauciarticular

ETIOLOGY
Multifactorial, including
- Abnormal immune response
- Genetic predisposition
- Environmental triggers, possibly infectious
- Immunoglobulin or complement deficiency

ASSOCIATED CONDITIONS
- Other autoimmune disorders
- Increased prevalence of autoimmune thyroiditis, subclinical hypothyroidism, and celiac disease (1)[B]

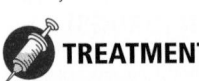 **DIAGNOSIS**

SIGNS AND SYMPTOMS
- Systemic
  - Arthralgias/arthritis
  - Fever: Spiking and remitting, may be >39°C
  - Rash: Salmon, macular, nonpruritic rash over trunk and extremities
  - Chest pain, pericardial friction rub
  - Dyspnea
  - Fatigue
  - Hepatosplenomegaly
  - Lymphadenopathy
  - Myalgias
  - Weight loss
- Polyarticular
  - Arthralgia/arthritis
  - Growth retardation
  - Hand weakness/difficulty writing
  - Malaise
  - Morning stiffness
  - Rheumatoid nodules
  - Synovial thickening
  - Weight loss
- Pauciarticular
  - Abnormal gait
  - Eye pain, redness
  - Joint swelling
  - Leg-length abnormality
  - Morning stiffness
  - Photophobia
  - Flexion contractures

Pregnancy Considerations
Unpredictable effect on disease activity

Physical Exam
Atlantoaxial instability/subluxation

TESTS

Lab
- Leukocyte count normal or markedly elevated (systemic), lymphopenia
- Hemoglobin normal or low (especially systemic)
- Platelet count normal or elevated
- Joint-fluid aspiration and analysis helpful in excluding infection
- ANA positive (>1:80): 40% (polyarticular or pauciarticular): increased risk of uveitis in female patients
- Rheumatoid factor positive: 10–15% (usually polyarticular): Poor prognosis
- TSH
- HLA-B27 positive: 70% in pauciarticular boys
- ESR
  - Systemic: Always elevated
  - Polyarticular: Usually elevated
  - Pauciarticular: May be within normal range
- Drugs that may alter lab results
  - Anti-inflammatories may alter CBC and ESR.
  - Anticonvulsants, antiarrhythmics may increase ANA
- Disorders that may alter lab results: Hemoglobinopathies may alter ESR.

Imaging
- Radiograph of affected joint(s)
- Early radiographic changes
  - Soft-tissue swelling
  - Periosteal reaction
  - Juxta-articular demineralization
- Later changes include
  - Joint-space loss
  - Articular surface erosions
  - Subchondral cyst formation
  - Sclerosis
  - Joint fusion
- Echocardiography (pericarditis)
- Radionuclide scans (infection, malignancy)
- CT, MRI helpful in identifying early erosions

Diagnostic Procedures/Surgery
- Synovial biopsy occasionally indicated
- Arthrocentesis

Pathological Findings
Synovium shows hyperplasia of synovial cells, hyperemia, and infiltration of small lymphocytes and mononuclear cells.

DIFFERENTIAL DIAGNOSIS
- Other rheumatic diseases, especially SLE and dermatomyositis
- Atypical bacterial or viral infections
  - Septic arthritis, osteomyelitis
- Hemoglobinopathies
- Malignancy: Leukemia
- Vasculitis
- Rheumatic fever
- Lyme disease
- Postinfectious arthritis
- Musculoskeletal
  - Legg-Calve-Perthes, toxic synovitis
- Pain syndromes

TREATMENT

GENERAL MEASURES
- Treatment goal: Control active disease and extra-articular manifestations to maintain musculoskeletal function as normal as possible.
- Outpatient care except for initial diagnostic workup of systemic juvenile rheumatoid arthritis disease and complications for all subtypes
- Patients require regular (every 4 months in young patients with pauciarticular disease) ophthalmic exams to uncover asymptomatic eye disease, at least for 1st 3 years.
- Moist heat, sleeping bag, or electric blanket to relieve morning stiffness
- Splints for contractures

Diet
Regular diet with special attention to adequate calcium, iron, protein, and caloric intake

Activity
- Full activity as tolerated
- Regular school; may need modified physical education program

SPECIAL THERAPY

Physical Therapy
- Include daily home exercise program, required for joints with limited motion.
- Orthotics for support

MEDICATION (DRUGS)

First Line

- NSAIDs adequate in ~50% of patients, symptoms often improve within days, full efficacy 2–3 months
- Average of 2 or 3 trials needed to determine most effective drug for an individual patient; change NSAID if no clinical response within 3 weeks of initiating treatment
- Drugs for children include
  – Ibuprofen (Motrin, Advil, Nuprin): 30–40 mg/kg/d, divided q.i.d.
  – Naproxen (Naprosyn, Aleve): 10–20 mg/kg/d divided b.i.d.
  – Tolmetin sodium: 15–30 mg/kg/d; t.i.d. or q.i.d.
- Contraindications to NSAIDs: Known allergies
- Precautions: May worsen a bleeding diathesis; use caution with all NSAIDs in renal insufficiency and hypovolemic states
- Significant possible interactions: NSAIDs may lower serum levels of digitalis and anticonvulsants and blunt the effect of loop diuretics. NSAIDs may increase serum methotrexate levels.

Second Line

- 30–40% of patients will require addition of disease-modifying antirheumatic drugs, including methotrexate, sulfasalazine, antimalarials, leflunomide
- Methotrexate: Standard dose 8–12.5 mg/m^2/wk
- Plateau of efficacy reached with parenteral administration of 15 mg/m^2/wk; further increase in dosage is not associated with any additional therapeutic benefit (2)[B]
- Other agents
  – Corticosteroids for serious cardiac involvement or unresponsive uveitis
  – Intra-articular corticosteroids
  – Etanercept (Enbrel)
  – Immune globulin intravenously
  – Cyclosporine (Neoral)
- Alternative drugs
  – Other NSAIDs
  – Salicylates: Avoid salicylate therapy during serious viral illness or varicella exposure secondary to risk of Reye syndrome
  – Analgesics for pain control

SURGERY

- Total hip and/or knee replacement may be needed for severe disease.
- Soft tissue release, if splinting, traction unsuccessful
- Limb length or angular deformity corrections
- Synovectomy is rarely performed.

Pediatric Considerations

Behavioral and compliance problems frequent in toddlers and teenagers

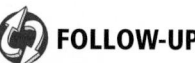 **FOLLOW-UP**

DISPOSITION

Admission Criteria

- Patient loses ambulatory ability
- Signs/symptoms of pericarditis

PROGNOSIS

- 50–60% ultimately remit, but functional ability depends on adequacy of long-term therapy (disease control, maintaining muscle and joint function).
- Poorest prognosis in patients who have polyarticular juvenile arthritis with positive rheumatoid factor, or patients with systemic JRA

COMPLICATIONS

- Blindness
- Band keratopathy
- Glaucoma
- Short stature
- Debilitating joint disease
- DIC, hemolytic anemia
- Patient on NSAIDs
  – Peptic ulcer
  – Gastrointestinal hemorrhage
  – CNS reactions
  – Renal disease
  – Leukopenia
- Patient on disease-modifying antirheumatic drug
  – Bone-marrow suppression
  – Hepatitis
  – Renal disease
  – Dermatitis
  – Mouth ulcers
  – Retinal toxicity (antimalarials); rare
- Osteoporosis
- Macrophage activation syndrome
  – Decreased blood cell precursors secondary to histiocyte degradation of marrow

PATIENT MONITORING

Determined by medication

- NSAIDs: Periodic CBC, urinalysis
- Aspirin and/or other salicylates: Transaminase and salicylate levels, weekly for 1st month, then every 3–4 months
- Methotrexate: Monthly LFTs, CBC
- Antimalarials: Ophthalmologic monitoring

REFERENCES

1. Stagi S, et al. Thyroid function, autoimmune thyroiditis and coeliac disease in juvenile idiopathic arthritis. *Rheumatology (Oxford)*. 2005;44(4): 517–520.
2. Ruperto N, et al. A randomized trial of parenteral methotrexate comparing an intermediate dose with a higher dose in children with juvenile idiopathic arthritis who failed to respond to standard doses of methotrexate. *Arthritis Rheum*. 2004;50(7): 2191–201.
3. Hashkes PJ, Laxer RM. Medical treatment of juvenile idiopathic arthritis. *JAMA*. 2005;294(13): 1671–1684 .

 MISCELLANEOUS

CODES

ICD9-CM

- 714.30 Polyarticular juvenile rheumatoid arthritis, chronic or unspecified
- 714.31 Polyarticular juvenile rheumatoid arthritis, acute
- 714.32 Pauciarticular onset juvenile rheumatoid arthritis
- 714.33 Monoarticular onset juvenile rheumatoid arthritis

PATIENT TEACHING

- Ongoing education of patients and families needed with special attention to
  – Psychosocial needs
  – Behavioral strategies for dealing with pain and noncompliance
  – Use of health care resources
- Printed and audiovisual information available from local Arthritis Foundation

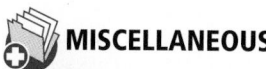 **See Patient Handout on CD**

ARTHRITIS, OSTEO

Bruce C. Gilliland, MD

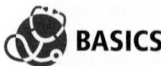 **BASICS**

DESCRIPTION
Most common form of joint disease. Involves progressive loss of articular cartilage and reactive changes at joint margins and in subchondral bone

- Primary
  - Idiopathic
  - Divided into subsets depending on clinical features
- Secondary
  - Childhood anatomic abnormalities (e.g., congenital hip dysplasia, slipped femoral epiphyses)
  - Inheritable metabolic disorders (e.g., alkaptonuria, Wilson disease, hemochromatosis)
  - Neuropathic arthropathy (Charcot joints)
  - Hemophilic arthropathy
  - Acromegalic arthropathy
  - Paget disease
  - Hyperparathyroidism
  - Noninfectious inflammatory arthritis (e.g., rheumatoid arthritis, spondyloarthropathies)
  - Gout, calcium pyrophosphate deposition disease (pseudogout)
  - Septic or tuberculous arthritis
  - Post-traumatic
- System(s) Affected: Musculoskeletal
- Synonym(s): Osteoarthrosis; Degenerative joint disease

EPIDEMIOLOGY
- Predominant age
  - Symptomatic disease: >40
  - Leading cause of disability in those >65
  - Radiographic evidence (estimates): 33% to almost 90% in those >65
- Predominant sex: Male = Female

Prevalence
- ~ 60 million patients
- Increases with age
- Almost universal >65 (by x-ray study but not clinically)

RISK FACTORS
- Age >50
- Obesity (weight-bearing joints)
- Prolonged occupational or sports stress
- Injury to a joint from trauma
- Injury to a joint from pre-existing inflammatory arthritis or infectious arthritis

Genetics
Genetic transmission unknown, but a woman with distal interphalangeal joint osteoarthritis is more likely to have a mother or sister with similar joint involvement

ETIOLOGY
Biomechanical, biochemical, inflammatory, and immunologic factors all implicated in pathogenesis

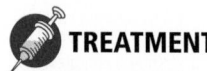 **DIAGNOSIS**

SIGNS AND SYMPTOMS
- Slowly developing joint pain
- Pain that follows use of a joint
- Stiffness of <15 minutes duration (especially morning and after sitting)
- Joint bony enlargement (e.g., Heberden nodes of distal interphalangeal joints)
- Decreased range of motion
- Tenderness usually absent; may be associated with synovitis and occur along joint margin
- Crepitation as late sign
- Local pain and stiffness with osteoarthritis of spine, with radicular pain (if there is compression of nerve roots)

TESTS
Lab
- Usually not helpful in diagnosis (sedimentation rate not increased)
- May be useful in monitoring treatment with NSAIDs (renal insufficiency and GI bleeding)
- Disorders that may alter lab results: In secondary osteoarthritis, underlying disorder may have abnormal lab results, for example, hemochromatosis (abnormal iron studies).

Imaging
- X-ray films usually normal early
- Later often show
  - Narrowed joint space
  - Osteophyte formation
  - Subchondral bony sclerosis
  - Cyst formation
- Erosions may occur on surface of distal and proximal interphalangeal joints when osteoarthritis is associated with inflammation (erosive osteoarthritis).

Diagnostic Procedures/Surgery
- Joint aspiration
  - May be helpful in distinguishing between osteoarthritis and chronic inflammatory arthritides
  - Osteoarthritis: Cell count usually <500 cells/mm^3, predominantly mononuclear
  - Inflammatory: Cell count usually >2,000 cells/mm^3, predominantly neutrophils

Pathological Findings
- Synovial fluid may have slight leukocytosis, predominantly mononuclear.
- Calcium pyrophosphate dihydrate and/or apatite crystals may occasionally be seen in effusions; require polarized light microscopy or special techniques to see.
- Subchondral bone trabecular microfractures
- Degradation response produced by release of proteolytic enzymes, collagenolytic enzymes, prostaglandins, and immune responses

DIFFERENTIAL DIAGNOSIS
- Distinguish from other types of arthritis by
  - Absent systemic findings
  - Minimal articular inflammation
  - Distribution of involved joints (e.g., distal and proximal interphalangeal joints, not wrist and metacarpophalangeal joints)
- In spine, distinguish from
  - Osteoporosis
  - Metastatic disease
  - Multiple myeloma
  - Other bone disease

TREATMENT
GENERAL MEASURES
- Outpatient
- Reassure patient of absence of generalized systemic disease, but recognize potential disability.
- Weight reduction if obese
- General fitness program
- Heat (e.g., local, tub baths)
- Physical therapy to maintain or regain joint motion and muscle strength. Quadriceps-strengthening exercises can relieve knee pain and disability.
- Protect joints from overuse (e.g., cane, crutches, walker, neck collar, elastic knee support)

Diet
No special diet

Activity
As active as tolerated

MEDICATION (DRUGS)

First Line

For management of pain and inflammation

- Acetaminophen 1,000 mg q.i.d. most effective for OA of knee; useful for other sites as 1st line for relief of pain
- If not effective, add nonacetylated salicylates (e.g., salsalate, choline-magnesium salicylate) or low-dose ibuprofen ≤1,600 mg/day.
- Other NSAIDs have similar efficacy; prolonged use associated with renal insufficiency, hypertension, leg edema, and GI bleeding. Because pain in osteoarthritis varies from day to day, brief courses of an NSAID are preferable.
- Cyclooxygenase-2 specific inhibitors are somewhat less likely to cause GI ulcers, but work as well as NSAID's in reducing arthritis inflammation and pain. They are much more expensive than conventional NSAID's and should be reserved for patients who are at higher risk for stomach ulcers and bleeding.
- Opioid analgesics (e.g., codeine, oxycodone, propoxyphene) should be restricted for treatment of acute episodes of pain.

Contraindications

- NSAIDs contraindicated in patients with
  - Renal disease
  - Congestive heart failure
  - Hypertension
  - Active peptic ulcer disease
  - Previous hypersensitivity to an NSAID or aspirin (asthma, nasal polyps, urticaria/angioedema, hypotension)
- Combinations of NSAIDs are contraindicated due to risk of adverse reactions without concomitant improved efficacy.
- Oral or parenteral adrenal corticosteroids are contraindicated.

Precautions

- In patients with history of peptic ulcer disease or risk factors for upper GI bleeding, acetaminophen is recommended.
- If NSAID is necessary because of inadequate response to acetaminophen, it should be given with misoprostol or with proton pump inhibitor.
- Risk factors for upper GI bleeding: Previous history of bleeding or peptic ulcer, ≥65 years of age, and concomitant use of oral corticosteroids or anticoagulants. In these patients, risk of stomach ulcers can be reduced by such drugs as misoprostol (Cytotec) and the proton pump inhibitors. Be cautious in patients at high risk of coronary artery disease or stroke, given possible increased risk with COX2 inhibitors.

Significant possible interactions

- NSAIDs reduce effectiveness of ACE inhibitors and diuretics; may induce renal insufficiency.
- Aspirin and NSAIDs (except COX2 inhibitors) may increase effects of anticoagulants.
- Increased hypoglycemic effects of oral hypoglycemics with aspirin
- Avoid concomitant use of aspirin with NSAIDs.
- Salicylates reduce effectiveness of spironolactone (Aldactone) and uricosurics.
- Corticosteroids and some antacids increase salicylate excretion, whereas ascorbic acid and ammonium chloride reduce salicylate excretion and may cause toxicity.

Second Line

- Judiciously use intra-articular injections of corticosteroids for selected acute flare-ups of joints (no more than 3 per year up to a maximum of 12 injections per joint). If used excessively, can accelerate joint deterioration
- Series of injections of hyaluronic acid preparation into painful knee may provide relief of pain and improve function.
- Local application of capsaicin cream for pain relief; most effective in small joints of hand; may cause local burning

ALERT

Pregnancy Considerations

- Acetylsalicylic acid (ASA) and NSAIDs: Some risk to fetus during 1st and 3rd trimester of pregnancy
- Compatible with breast feeding

SURGERY

May be indicated in advanced disease (e.g., osteotomy, débridement, removal of loose bodies, joint replacement, fusion)

FOLLOW-UP

PROGNOSIS

- Tends to be progressive
- Early in course, pain relieved by rest; later, pain may occur at rest and at night.
- Joint effusions may occur, especially in knees.
- Joint enlargement occurs later in course owing to bony enlargement.
- Osteophyte (spur) formation, especially at joint margins, as disease progresses
- Advanced stage with full-thickness loss of cartilage down to bone

COMPLICATIONS

- Decompensated CHF, GI bleeding, decreased renal function on NSAIDs or ASA
- Hypoglycemic reactions (rare) in diabetic patients taking oral hypoglycemic agents
- Infection or accelerated cartilage loss with intra-articular corticosteroids

PATIENT MONITORING

- Follow range of motion and functional status at regular intervals.
- Watch for GI blood loss and follow cardiac, renal, and mental status in older patients on NSAIDs or ASA.
- Periodic CBC, renal function tests, stool for occult blood

REFERENCES

1. Brandt KD. Management of osteoarthritis. In: Ruddy S, Harris ED, Sledge CB, eds. *Kelley's Textbook of Rheumatology*. 5th ed. Philadelphia: WB Saunders; 2001:1419–1432.
2. Golden BD, Abramson SB. Selective cyclooxygenase-2 inhibitors. *Rheumatic Dis Clin N Am*. 1999;25:359–378.
3. Hochberg MC, Altman RD, Brandt KD. Guidelines for the medical management of osteoarthritis. Part I. Osteoarthritis of the hip. *Arthritis Rheum*. 1995;38:1535–1540.
4. Hochberg MC, Altman RD, Brandt KD. Guidelines for the medical management of osteoarthritis. Part II. Osteoarthritis of the knee. *Arthritis Rheum*. 1995;38:1541–1546.
5. Mankin HJ, Brandt KD. Pathogenesis of osteoarthritis. In: Ruddy S, Harris ED, Sledge CB, eds. *Kelley's Textbook of Rheumatology*. 5th ed. Philadelphia: WB Saunders; 2001:1391–1407.
6. Solomon L. Clinical features of osteoarthritis. In: Ruddy S, Harris ED, Sledge CB, eds. *Kelley's Textbook of Rheumatology*. 5th ed. Philadelphia: WB Saunders; 2001:1409–1417.

MISCELLANEOUS

CODES

ICD9-CM

715.90 Osteoarthrosis, unspecified whether generalized or localized, site unspecified

PATIENT TEACHING

- For a listing of sources for patient education materials favorably reviewed on this topic, physicians may contact: American Academy of Family Physicians Foundation, P.O. Box 8418, Kansas City, MO 64114, (800) 274-2237, ext. 4400. Also see www.familydoctor.org.
- Arthritis Foundation, P.O. Box 7669, Atlanta, GA 30357-0669; (800) 283-7800

See Corresponding Diagnostic Algorithm

ARTHRITIS, PSORIATIC

Michael Tutt, MD
Jeremy Golding, MD

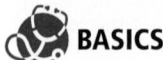 **BASICS**

DESCRIPTION

Arthritis associated with psoriasis. Serologic tests for rheumatoid factor usually are negative. Patients exhibit sausage-shaped digits and characteristic radiologic changes. Psoriatic arthropathy occurs in ~5% of individuals with psoriasis, especially those with psoriatic nail disease. Several forms have been described, although separation into these forms is not distinct. Different authors call them by different descriptive terms.

- Forms of psoriatic arthropathy
  - Psoriatic nail disease and distal interphalangeal involvement (classic psoriatic arthritis). Characteristics
    - Nail pitting
    - Transverse depressions
    - Subungual hyperkeratosis
    - Distal interphalangeal arthritis
- Arthritis mutilans: Destructive, resorptive arthropathy; produces so-called opera-glass hand
- Symmetric polyarthropathy resembling rheumatoid arthritis (RA): May be indistinguishable from RA, and may be coincidental RA in a patient who has psoriasis
- Asymmetric oligoarthropathy (more common type): Little relationship between joint and skin activity; joints involved may be both large and small
- Psoriatic spondylitis: Asymmetrical spondylitis and sacroiliitis
- System(s) Affected: Musculoskeletal; Skin/exocrine, Visual
- Synonym(s): Psoriasis, arthropathic

EPIDEMIOLOGY

- Typical onset age 30–35
- Not commonly seen in pediatric population
- Predominant sex: Female > Male (slightly)

Prevalence

- Prevalence 1–2 individuals per 1000 population.
- 5–20% of individuals with psoriasis will develop joint disease.

RISK FACTORS

- Psoriasis
- Positive family history

Genetics

- HLA-B27 usually present in patients with spondylitis-type psoriatic arthropathy
- Psoriasis itself is associated with HLA-B13, HLA-Bw17, HLA-Cw6, HLA-Bw38, HLA-DR4, and HLA-DR7.

ETIOLOGY

- Unknown
- Probably genetically related
- Pathogenesis: In contrast to ameliorating affect of AIDS (HIV infection) on RA, AIDS is associated with more aggressive joint disease in psoriatic arthritis. Theoretically, then, CD4 cells, which seem to "drive" RA, are not involved in pathogenesis of psoriatic arthritis.

ASSOCIATED CONDITIONS

Psoriasis

DIAGNOSIS

SIGNS AND SYMPTOMS

- Joint swelling, tenderness, warmth, restricted movement
- Dactylitis
- Distribution of arthritis depends on form of psoriatic arthritis
- Nail changes
  - Pitting
  - Transverse ridging
  - Onycholysis
  - Keratosis
  - Yellowing
  - Destruction of entire nail
- Fever
- Malaise
- Psoriasis: Variable severity
- Arthritic symptoms are worse in geriatric population.
- Some individuals develop uveitis.

TESTS

Lab

- Serum rheumatoid factor: Negative
- Elevated ESR
- Elevated uric acid
- Anemia
- HLA B27 (if spondylitis)

Imaging

- Radiographs
  - Gross destructive changes of isolated small joints
  - Peripheral arthritis mutilans
  - Erosions, ankylosis
  - Extensive bone resorption to cause opera-glass hand
  - Fluffy periostitis
  - Atypical spondylitis with syndesmophyte formation
  - Acro-osteolysis, "pencil-in-cup" appearance
  - Asymmetric sacroiliitis
  - Absence of osteoporosis
- MRI is sensitive in detecting sacroiliitis, joint synovitis, erosions, and enthesitis.

Pathological Findings

Synovitis (resembling RA)

DIFFERENTIAL DIAGNOSIS

- Psoriasis
- Seropositive inflammatory polyarthritis
- RA
- Osteoarthritis
- Gout
- Reiter syndrome
- Ankylosing spondylitis

TREATMENT

GENERAL MEASURES

Outpatient

- Immobilizing splints
- Isometric exercises and swimming later
- Paraffin baths or other heat therapy
- Protection of affected joints
- Regular, moderate exposure to sun
- Psoriatic skin care

Diet

No special diet

Activity

Encourage exercise (particularly swimming) to maintain strength and flexibility.

MEDICATION (DRUGS)

First Line

- Several options available, depending on involvement of skin and joints
  - NSAIDs in usual doses; no evidence for superiority of any one NSAID. NSAIDs are usually 1st-line treatment.
  - Local corticosteroid injection
  - Low-dose systemic steroids, if necessary
  - Topical therapy including steroids for skin
  - PUVA therapy may be helpful for skin lesions
- Disease-modifying agents may be useful if disease remains active despite of NSAIDs, and should be introduced early if aggressive, deforming, or erosive disease is present:
  - Methotrexate, for severe or extensive disease may be effective
  - Leflunomide
  - Gold salts
  - Antimalarials (controversial)
  - Sulfasalazine
  - Immunosuppressives in resistant cases
  - Cyclosporine (Neoral) in resistant cases
  - Combination of methotrexate and cyclosporine or sulfasalazine under guidance of rheumatologist
- Contraindications
  - NSAIDs may flare psoriasis.
  - Methotrexate is contraindicated in HIV-positive patients.
- Precautions
  - Phenylbutazone may cause bone-marrow depression.
  - NSAIDs and aspirin may cause gastritis and renal failure.
  - Refer to manufacturer's literature.
- Significant possible interactions: NSAIDs may impair methotrexate excretion and cause methotrexate toxicity. Refer to manufacturer's literature.

Second Line

Etretinate 0.5–1.0 mg/kg/d in 2 divided doses

ALERT

Pregnancy Considerations

Avoid medications (e.g., methotrexate, gold, antimalarials, sulfasalazine, cyclosporine, etretinate) during pregnancy.

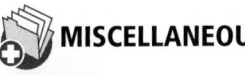 ## FOLLOW-UP

PROGNOSIS

- Course: acute, intermittent
- More favorable than for RA (except for 20% of patients who develop arthritis mutilans)
- Treatment of skin lesions can sometime improve arthritic symptoms.
- Joint surgery is at least as successful as for RA; infectious complications are more common.

COMPLICATIONS

- Chronicity
- Severe deforming arthritis (arthritis mutilans)
- Spondylitic form of arthritis with sacroiliitis and spinal involvement
- Corticosteroids may destabilize psoriatic lesions.
- Antimalarials can provoke exfoliative dermatitis.

PATIENT MONITORING

Frequent follow-up for medication adjustment and encouragement

REFERENCES

1. Gladman D. Psoriatic arthritis. Up To Date 2006.
2. Kelley WN, Harris ED, Ruddy S, et al. *Textbook of Rheumatology*, 5th ed. Philadelphia: WB Saunders, 1997.
3. Kippel JH, Dippe PA, eds. *Rheumatology*. St. Louis: Mosby, 1994.
4. Koopman WJ, ed. *Arthritis and Allied Disorders*, 13th ed. Philadelphia: Lea & Febiger, 1997.
5. Salvariniet et al. Psoriatic arthritis. *Curr Opin Rheumatol*. 1998;10:299–305.

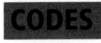 ## MISCELLANEOUS

CODES

ICD9-CM

696.0 Psoriatic arthropathy

PATIENT TEACHING

- Stress noncontagious nature of condition.
- For a listing of sources for patient education materials favorably reviewed on this topic, physicians may contact: American Academy of Family Physicians Foundation, P.O. Box 8418, Kansas City, MO 64114, (800) 274-2237, ext. 4400. Also see www.familydoctor.org.
- Arthritis Foundation, 1314 Spring Street N.W., Atlanta, GA 30309, (404) 872-7100 or http://www.arthritis.org/conditions/diseasecenter/psoriaticˉarthritis.asp

ARTHRITIS, RHEUMATOID (RA)

Konstantinos Deligiannidis, MD, MPH
Joseph R. Stenger, MD

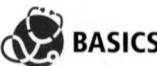 **BASICS**

DESCRIPTION

Chronic systemic inflammatory disease (typically joint-involving) of unknown cause. Articular inflammation may be remitting, but if continued, usually results in joint damage and disability. Characteristic extra-articular manifestations include rheumatoid nodules, arteritis, neuropathy, scleritis, pericarditis, and splenomegaly.

- System(s) Affected: Musculoskeletal; Hematologic/lymphatic/immunologic; Cardiovascular; Nervous; Pulmonary; Renal

Geriatric Considerations

- Increased contribution/interaction of age-related comorbidities; pericarditis, septic arthritis, Sjögren syndrome more common
- Less tolerance to drugs; increased incidence of hydroxychloroquine-associated maculopathy, D-penicillamine rash, and sulfasalazine-induced nausea/vomiting

Pregnancy Considerations

- Use effective contraception with DMARDs. Modify regimen with pregnancy or breast-feeding.
- Labor/delivery pose no serious problems, unless severe mechanical joint disease.
- >75% improve during pregnancy, but relapse in 6 months. Occasionally, 1st episodes occur during pregnancy.
- Fetal abnormalities not increased

EPIDEMIOLOGY

- Predominant age: 3rd–6th decades
- Predominant sex
  - Female > Male (2:1; overall incidence and prevalence of articular manifestations)
  - Male > Female (systemic disease)

Prevalence

- US population: 0.3–1.5%
- Native Americans: 3.5–5.3%

RISK FACTORS

- HLA-DR4
- Family history
- Native American ethnicity
- Age 20–50 years

Genetics

- Seropositive RA aggregates in families
- Increased relative risk of 4–5 times for HLA-DR4 positive person; African Americans tend not to exhibit this tendency.

ETIOLOGY

Antibody-complement complex results in intra-articular inflammation.

ASSOCIATED CONDITIONS

- Sjögren syndrome
- Felty syndrome
- Increased incidence of infections, lymphomas, renal and cardiovascular disease
- Renal disorders from therapy.
- Amyloidosis from chronic inflammation

DIAGNOSIS

SIGNS AND SYMPTOMS

- American College of Rheumatology diagnostic criteria (5 of the 7 must be present; 1st 4 must be continuous >6 weeks)
  - Morning stiffness >1 hour's duration
  - Arthritis of 3 or more joint groups with soft-tissue swelling or fluid
  - Swelling involving 1 or more of the following joint groups: wrists, proximal interphalangeal, metacarpophalangeal
  - Symmetrical joint swelling
  - Subcutaneous nodules
  - Positive rheumatoid-factor test
  - Radiographic changes consistent with RA
- General
  - Joints: Wrists, knees, elbows, shoulders, ankles, and subtalar joints (most often involved) with swelling, heat, deformity, pain on passive motion, morning stiffness. 70% show radiologic signs of joint damage within 3 years of onset.
  - Systemic: Fatigue, depression, malaise, anorexia, rheumatoid nodules, ocular disease, lymphadenopathy, splenomegaly, entrapment neuropathies, osteoporosis.
  - Patients experience symptoms an average of 36 weeks before diagnosis.

TESTS

Lab

- Hematocrit: Mild anemia (of chronic disease)
- ESR: Usually elevated
- C-reactive protein: Direct measure of impact of IL-6 on liver cells
- Rheumatoid factor: >1:80 in 70–80% of patients with RA
  - RF tests are assays for IgM Ab.
  - Poor screening tool with positive predictive value of only 20% in asymptomatic persons. In patients with rheumatologic symptoms, positive predictive value is 80%.
  - Not useful for monitoring course of illness
- Antinuclear antibody: Present in 20–30%
- Electrolytes, creatinine, liver function, urinalysis to assess organ comorbid states
- Synovial fluid
  - Yellowish-white, turbid, poor viscosity
  - Mucin clot poor owing to degradation of hyaluronic acid by lysosomal enzymes
  - WBC increased (3,500–50,000)
  - Protein: ~4.2 g/dL (42 g/L)
  - Serum-synovial glucose difference ≥30 mg/dL (≥1.67 mmol/L)
- Drugs that may alter lab results: Prior treatment with immunosuppressives may "normalize" results.
- Disorders that may yield false-positive RF results: Sjögren syndrome, mixed cryoglobulinemia, parasitic infections (e.g., malaria), liver disease, endocarditis, acute viral infections (e.g., mononucleosis, influenza, rubella)

Imaging

- Radiograph films are useful in following disease progression.
- Bone scan is appropriate if aseptic necrosis suspected.
- CT/MRI are useful in specific situations such as cervical-spine symptoms.

DIFFERENTIAL DIAGNOSIS

- Sjögren syndrome
- Sarcoidosis
- Systemic lupus erythematosus
- Psoriatic arthritis
- Vasculitis
- Gout/pseudogout
- Seronegative polyarthritis
- Polymyositis
- Erosive osteoarthritis
- Reiter syndrome
- Behçet syndrome
- Lyme disease
- Scleroderma
- Chronic infection
- Occult malignancy

TREATMENT

GENERAL MEASURES

- Key elements include ongoing evaluation of
  - Disease activity and extent of synovitis
  - Structural damage
  - Psychosocial functional status
- Intervene before joint damage occurs.
- Emphasize
  - Exercise and mobility
  - Reduction of joint stress
  - General health care

Activity

Encourage full activity, but patient should avoid heavy work or exercise during active phases.

MEDICATION (DRUGS)

First Line

- No one disease-modifying antirheumatic drug (DMARD) is consistently better than another, but methotrexate, hydroxychloroquine, sulfasalazine, and leflunomide preferred over gold, D-penicillamine, azathioprine, and cyclosporine, based on relative risks/benefits.
- Combinations of DMARDs may be more effective than individual drugs.
- Start DMARDs within 2 months if patient has ongoing joint pain/morning stiffness, active synovitis, or persistent increase in ESR and/or C-reactive protein despite appropriate-dose NSAIDs.
- Early disease or acute/chronic inflammations
  – Aspirin or other NSAID; try various classes.
  – Prednisone/prednisolone: 5–15 mg/d for severe disease or to minimize disease activity while waiting for DMARDs to act, when temporary decrease in activity is anticipated, or to control active disease when NSAIDs/DMARDs have failed. Generally to be used only for short periods, or intermittently. Low-dose prednisolone is more effective than NSAIDs (1)[A].
- Persistent disease activity (chronic synovitis, morning stiffness, increased ESR and/or C-reactive protein, extra-articular disease): Add DMARDs to above-mentioned anti-inflammatories; hydroxychloroquine or sulfasalazine often are 1st choice. When second-line agent's therapeutic level is reached, decrease prednisone slowly.
  – Minocycline: Effective with active mild/moderate disease (2)[A], and twice as effective as hydroxychloroquine in patients also treated with low-dose prednisone. Serious problems are rare.
  – Intra-articular steroids: Rarely used.
  – Antimalarials: Hydroxychloroquine (Plaquenil) 400 mg qhs for 2–3 months, then 200 mg at bedtime; 6-month trial usual (3)[A].
  – Auranofin (Ridaura): 6–10 mg/d PO; re-evaluate in 6 months or 1 g total
  – Injectable gold (Aurolate): Weekly for 22 weeks, then every 2–4 weeks
  – Sulfasalazine: 500 mg/d, increase to 2 g/d over 1 month; max: 2–3 g/d; 6-month trial (4)[A].
  – Penicillamine (D-penicillamine): 250 mg/d, increase slowly to 750–1,000 mg/d; 9-month trial with 8–12 weeks at maximum dosage. However, has dose-related side-effects (5)[A].
  – Azathioprine: Because of toxicity, reserve for persons not responsive to other DMARDs.
  – Methotrexate (Rheumatrex): 5–15 mg per week PO; 3–6-month trial. For steroid-dependent disease or after other measures fail. The DMARD with most predictable benefit. Has many significant side effects (6)[A] but the addition of folate to methotrexate reduces liver toxicity and allows reduction of methotrexate without lessening effectiveness, although it requires 10–20% increase in dosage.
  – Protein A immunoadsorption (Prosorba): For moderate to severe RA in patients failing other DMARDs; removes antibodies responsible for RA activity. Majority respond in 9–21 weeks; costly.

– Hyaluronate (Hyalgan, Hyalgan G-F20): Hyaluronic acid substitute. For pain relief; variable responses. Currently limited to knee disease. Exact role in RA unclear; expected therapy duration 6–12 months.
– Infliximab (Remicade), adalimumab (Humira), and etanercept (Enbrel): Tumor necrosis factor inhibitors. Administered intravenously bimonthly (infliximab), biweekly (adalimumab), or twice weekly subcutaneously (etanercept). Optimal dosage and duration of treatment unclear. Short- and long-term toxicity low. Adalimumab is more beneficial with persistent disease activity, whereas infliximab and etanercept also can be used in early disease. Adalimumab with methotrexate is effective, but unclear with other DMARDs (7–9)[B]. Costly. Check PPD prior to treatment.
– Leflunomide (Arava): Modifies T-cell function to decrease autoimmune activity. Benefits similar to sulfasalazine and methotrexate, but overall difference in side effects are not statistically significant from sulfasalazine, but are slightly increased compared to methotrexate (10)[A]. Dose: 20 mg/d. For patients not responding to traditional agents or for whom use of traditional agents has been limited by side effects.
– Interleukin-1 receptor antagonist (Anakinra): Dose 100 mg/d SQ. Adverse reactions include rash, pruritus, neutropenia, and severe infections. TNF inhibitors may be more effective. Costly.
- Contraindications: Avoid leflunomide in pregnancy.
- Precautions
  – Consider proton pump inhibitors for patients on chronic NSAID therapy; give folic acid (1–2/d) for patients on methotrexate.
  – Avoid NSAID combinations.

Second Line

- Combinations that may be useful for resistant disease
  – Methotrexate and cyclosporine
  – Gold salts and prednisone
  – Methotrexate and hydroxychloroquine

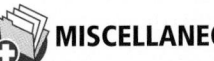 **FOLLOW-UP**

PROGNOSIS

- Progressive decline in function.
- Complete remission defined as absence of
  – Symptoms of active inflammatory joint pain
  – Morning stiffness
  – Fatigue
  – Synovitis on physical exam
  – Progression of damage shown on radiograph films
  – Elevation of ESR
- Poor prognostic findings
  – Moderate to severe disease: Persistent swelling of proximal interphalangeal joints, flexor tenosynovitis of hands, high ESR, RF, or C-reactive protein, large number of swollen joints, extra-articular disease, bone erosions or cartilage loss, subcutaneous nodules, and early decline in function
  – Inheritance of shared epitope: RA homozygous for shared epitope on DR1 or DR4 HLA class 11 β-chains have poor prognosis. However, impractical to assay routinely for these sequences
  – Early or advanced age at disease onset
- 50% cannot function in primary job within 10 years of onset.

COMPLICATIONS

- Erosive arthritis and joint destruction
- Skin vasculitis
- Pericarditis
- Intracardiac rheumatoid nodules causing valvular, conduction abnormalities
- Pleural, subpleural disease; interstitial fibrosis
- Mononeuritis multiplex, median nerve entrapment
- Sjögren syndrome, scleral rheumatoid nodules
- Felty syndrome

REFERENCES

1. Gotzsche PC and Johansen HK. Short-term low-dose corticosteroids vs placebo and nonsteroidal anti-inflammatory drugs in rheumatoid arthritis. *The Cochrane Database of Systematic Reviews* 1, 2006.
2. Tilley BC. et al. Minocycline in rheumatoid arthritis. A 48-week, double-blind, placebo-controlled trial. *Ann Intern Med* 1995;122:81–89.
3. Suarez-Almazor ME, Belseck E, et al. Antimalarials for treating rheumatoid arthritis. [Systematic Review] Cochrane Musculoskeletal Group Cochrane Database of Systematic Reviews. 1, 2006.
4. Suarez-Almazor ME, Belseck E, et al. Sulfasalazine for treating rheumatoid arthritis. *The Cochrane Database of Systematic Reviews* 1, 2006.
5. Suarez-Almazor ME, Belseck E, Spooner CH. Penicillamine for treating rheumatoid arthritis. *The Cochrane Database of Systematic Reviews* 1, 2006.
6. Suarez-Almazor ME, Belseck E, et al. Methotrexate for treating rheumatoid arthritis. *The Cochrane Database of Systematic Reviews* 1, 2006.
7. Blumenauer BBTB, Burls A, et al. Infliximab for the treatment of rheumatoid arthritis. *The Cochrane Database of Systematic Reviews* 1, 2006.
8. Blumenauer B, Judd M, et al. Etanercept for the treatment of rheumatoid arthritis. *The Cochrane Database of Systematic Reviews* 1, 2006.
9. Navarro-Sarabia F, Ariza-Ariza R, et al. Adalimumab for treating rheumatoid arthritis. *The Cochrane Database of Systematic Reviews* 1, 2006.
10. Osiri M, Robinson VA, et al. Leflunomide for treating rheumatoid arthritis. *The Cochrane Database of Systematic Reviews* 1, 2006.

 MISCELLANEOUS

Functional ability classification

- Class I: None
- Class II: Moderate
- Class III: Marked restriction, inability to perform most of usual activities
- Class IV: Incapacitation

CODES

ICD9-CM

- 714.0 Rheumatoid arthritis
- 714.1 Felty syndrome

PATIENT TEACHING

See Corresponding Diagnostic Algorithm

ARTIFICIAL INSEMINATION

Jennifer E. Cyrkler, MD
Megan E. Bower, RN, MPH

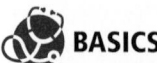

BASICS

DESCRIPTION

- Artificial insemination is the placement of washed sperm into the female reproductive tract.
- Placement can be intracervical, intrauterine, intraperitoneal, or intrafollicular.
- Most common is intrauterine insemination (IUI).
- Sperm are washed to reduce antigenicity.
- Insemination can be with partner's sperm or therapeutic insemination with donor sperm (TID).
- Fecundity is inversely related to maternal age.
- Contraindications to artificial insemination
  - Infection (acute cervicitis, endometritis, acute prostatitis, epididymitis, salpingo-oophoritis)
  - Anovulation
  - Pregnancy
  - Unexplained uterine bleeding
- System(s) affected: Endocrine/metabolic; Reproductive
- Synonym(s): Therapeutic insemination; Intrauterine insemination

EPIDEMIOLOGY

Predominant age: Reproductive-age women (18–45)

Incidence

Varies, depending on etiology of infertility

RISK FACTORS

- Male factor: 35%
- Cervical factor: 10%
- Testicular trauma from vasectomy, prostatitis, or a genetic predisposition can predispose to serum antibody production.
- Cervical trauma from cryotherapy, loop electrosurgical excision procedure, conization, or laser therapy can cause poor sperm–cervical mucous interaction.

ETIOLOGY

Indications for intrauterine insemination

- Absence of a male partner
- Male factor infertility: Oligospermia, asthenospermia, hypospadias, retrograde ejaculation, coital dysfunction
- Female factor indications include: Cervical mucous abnormalities
- Male factor with sexually transmissible virus with a seronegative partner
- Unexplained infertility

ASSOCIATED CONDITIONS

Causes of infertility

DIAGNOSIS

SIGNS AND SYMPTOMS

Inability to conceive

History

- Coital frequency
- Use of contraception
- Prior pregnancies from either partner
- Prior pelvic infections
- Gynecologic history
- Medication history

TESTS

Lab

- Semen analysis
- Sperm antibody testing
- Special tests
  - Zona-free hamster sperm-penetration assay
  - Bovine cervical mucus sperm-penetration test
- Drugs that may alter lab results
  - Clomiphene citrate (Clomid) can cause poor cervical mucus secondary to its antiestrogenic effects at the level of the cervix.
- Disorders that may alter lab results
  - Abnormal pH of vagina or cervical mucus
  - Bacterial infection semen/mucus

Imaging

Hysterosalpingogram

Diagnostic Procedures/Surgery

Postcoital test (out of use, recent literature has discredited its effectiveness) (1,2)

Pathological Findings

- Chronic cervicitis
- Chronic prostatitis

DIFFERENTIAL DIAGNOSIS

- Primary female factor?
- Primary male factor?

TREATMENT

INITIAL STABILIZATION

Outpatient

GENERAL MEASURES

- Intrauterine insemination should be closely timed with ovulation. Ovulation prediction kits detect the luteinizing hormone (LH) surge that precedes ovulation by 12–36 hours. Intrauterine insemination is performed the day of and/or the day after the LH surge.
- The volume of inseminate that can be transferred into the uterus is 0.25–0.5 mL. Small amounts are used to avoid cramping and flushing the oocyte out of the tube. The volume is also limited by space within the uterus.
- Intrauterine insemination is an office procedure. 1st, the position of the uterus is determined. A speculum is placed in the vagina and the cervix is visualized. The sample of washed sperm is placed into the uppermost portion of the uterine cavity using an insemination catheter with a disposable tuberculin syringe. Avoid touching the uterine fundus with the catheter tip. Occasionally a tenaculum is needed on the anterior lip of the cervix, to straighten the endocervical canal. Cervical dilatation or paracervical block is rarely required. The sample is injected slowly over 30–60 seconds.

SPECIAL THERAPY

Complementary and Alternative Medicine

Recent studies have supported the use of acupuncture as adjuvant therapy to IVF (3,4).

MEDICATION (DRUGS)

First Line

- Clomiphene (Clomid), FSH r human menopausal gonadotropins
  - Menotropins may be used for controlled ovarian hyperstimulation, and ovulation may be initiated by the administration of human chorionic gonadotropin (HCG), a LH-like molecule.
- A recombinant LH product, choriogonadotropin-α (Ovidrel), may be used subcutaneously for final follicular maturation and ovulation.
  - Intrauterine insemination is performed 24–36 hours after HCG administration.
- Clomiphene predisposes to poor cervical mucus, which can adversely alter sperm/mucus interaction. Clomiphene may induce luteal-phase defects.
- Dosages
  - Clomiphene: 50 mg/d for 5–7 days to induce ovulation
  - FSH (Bravelle, Follistim, Gonal-F); 150 IU/d IM for 5 days to induce ovulation
  - Menotropins (Pergonal, Repronex, Gonal-F, Follistim), utilized for superovulation induction: Dosage and length of administration depends on patient response
- Contraindications
  - Uncontrolled thyroid and adrenal dysfunction
  - Intracranial lesion
  - High follicle-stimulating hormone (FSH) level, indicating primary ovarian failure
  - Abnormal bleeding of undetermined etiology
  - Ovarian cysts of unknown origin
  - Hypersensitivity
  - Pregnancy
- Precautions
  - Multiple births: Clomiphene 8%, menotropins 25%
  - Severe ovarian hyperstimulation (ascites, pleural effusion, dehydration, electrolyte imbalance, pain)
  - Ovarian torsion

Second Line

Estrogen in follicular phase of cycle to improve mucus (conjugated equine estrogen 1.25–2.5 mg/d cycle days 5–12 or Estraderm patches 0.1–0.2 mg/d cycle days 5–12)

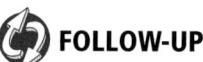

FOLLOW-UP

PROGNOSIS

- Virtually all resulting pregnancies occur within the 1st 6 treatment cycles. A 6-month treatment interval usually represents an adequate therapeutic trial.
- There is a significant but small effect of IUI therapy alone in treating unexplained infertility (5A). IUI has been shown to be effective when cervical factor is present (5, 6)[A].
- There is a documented increase in efficacy with combination of intrauterine insemination and controlled ovarian hyperstimulation (5, 6)[B].
- The highest success rates are seen with idiopathic or cervical factor problems.
- The poorest outcome is with male factor.
- Monthly fecundities of 14% have occurred with therapeutic inseminations utilizing fresh semen.

COMPLICATIONS

- Uterine cramping
- Mild vasomotor symptoms
- Infection
- Theoretical but unproven risk is development of antisperm antibodies in response to increase exposure of the immune system to sperm antigens

PATIENT MONITORING

- Patients on Clomiphene require an ultrasound or a bimanual exam on a monthly basis.
- Patients on menotropins require at least serum estradiol measurements and pelvic sonography to monitor ovarian response.

REFERENCES

1. Oei SG, Helmerhorst FM, Bloemenkamp KWM, et al. Effectiveness of the postcoital test: a randomized controlled trial. *Br Med J.* 1998;317:502.
2. Helmerhorst FM, Van Vliet HA, Gornas T, et al. Intra-uterine insemination versus timed intercourse for cervical hostility in subfertile couples. 2005 Oct 19;(4): CD002809.
3. Dieterle S, Ying G, Hatzmann W, Neuer A. Effect of acupuncture on the outcome of in vitro fertilization and intracytoplasmic sperm injection: A randomized, prospective, controlled clinical study. Fertility Sterility. 2006.
4. Westergaard LG, Mao Q, et al.Acupuncture on the day of embryo transfer significantly improves the reproductive outcome in infertile women: A prospective, randomized trial. *Fertility Sterility.* 2006.
5. Practice Committee of the American Society for Reproductive Medicine. Effectiveness and treatment for unexplained infertility. *Fertility Sterility.* 2004;82(Suppl 1):S160–163.
6. Cohlen BJ. Should we continue performing intrauterine inseminations in the year 2004? *Gynecol Obstet Invest.* 2005;59(1):3–13. Epub 2004 Aug 27. Review.

ADDITIONAL READING

Johnson K, Posner SF, Biermann J, et al. Recommendations to improve preconception health and health care—United States. A report of the CDC/ATSDR Preconception Care Work Group and the Select Panel on Preconception Care. *MMWR Rec.* 2006;55(RR–6):1-23.

MISCELLANEOUS

For donor insemination, only frozen semen is used and only after a 6-month period of "quarantine" to minimize danger of transmission of HIV and other sexually transmitted diseases.

CODES

ICD9-CM

- 606.9 Male infertility, unspecified
- 628.3 Female infertility of uterine origin
- 628.4 Female infertility of cervical or vaginal origin

PATIENT TEACHING

No vaginal lubricants or douching

Prevention

If taking Clomiphene, signs and symptoms of ovarian hyperstimulation syndrome (OHSS) include swelling of the hands or legs, abdominal pain and swelling, shortness of breath, weight gain, and nausea or vomiting. Seek medical attention.

ASBESTOSIS

Ruben Peralta, MD, FACS
Sarah Guzofski, MD

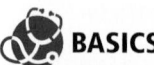 **BASICS**

DESCRIPTION

- Slowly progressive lung disease caused by inhalation of dust from the fibrous silicate asbestos
- Asbestos is used in insulation and other building products, cement, and textiles.
- Nodular interstitial fibrotic lung disease caused by cascade of inflammatory responses to inhaled asbestos fibers. Pleural fibrosis, pleural plaques and interstitial fibrosis develop. Lung cancer risk is increased.
- Synonym(s): Asbestos pneumoconiosis

GENERAL PREVENTION

- Asbestos has been federally regulated by the Occupational Health and Safety Administration since 1972. Primary responsibility of employers to provide safe work environment.
- Exposure control: Substitution of safer material or adoption of control technologies
- During high-exposure periods such as building repair, use fit-tested personal respirators for workers.
- World Health Organization (WHO) recommendations for regular health screening of exposed workers
  - Chest radiograph film at baseline
  - For workers with <10 years since 1st exposure: Chest radiograph every 3–5 years
  - >10 years: Chest radiograph every 1–2 years
  - >20 years: Chest radiograph annually
  - All workers: Annual respiratory symptom questionnaire, physical examination, and spirometry (alternatively can be done on chest radiograph schedule)
- Reporting of new cases to health authorities

EPIDEMIOLOGY

- In the US, an estimated 1.3 million people who work in maintenance and construction are at risk for exposure (1)[B].
- Predominant age: <Middle age (40–75 years)
- Predominant sex: Male > Female, owing to exposure pattern

RISK FACTORS

- Professional exposures most common in construction; those who mine, mill, or remove asbestos; ship builders; textile workers; railroad workers
- Office workers, teachers, and students in buildings with asbestos in place have exposure orders of magnitude below those of construction workers.
- Cigarette smoking markedly increases risk of radiographic changes and eventual lung cancer risk, thought to be due to decreased clearance of asbestos fibers.

Genetics
No known genetic pattern

ETIOLOGY

- Asbestos fibers are inhaled. Macrophages engulf the fibers and release inflammatory mediators. Inflammatory mediators cause fibroblast proliferation, leading to fibrosis and remodeling of interstitial lung tissue, including intra-alveolar fibrosis and loss of alveolar capillary units (1)[B].
- Disease continues to slowly progress over the course of years, even if exposure is not ongoing.
- The degree of fibrosis depends on amount of asbestos exposure.
- Symptoms may be related to impaired gas exchange and/or a pattern of restrictive lung disease.

DIAGNOSIS

- Credible history of exposure (ask about intensity and duration of exposure).
- Delay from exposure to detection (typically becomes clinically apparent 10–15 years after exposure).
- Typical radiographic findings
- Restrictive pattern of lung disease
- Impaired diffusion capacity
- Lung biopsy or bronchoalveolar lavage (BAL) can reveal asbestos fibers or asbestos bodies. May help diagnostically in cases with history of minimal exposure or with atypical clinical or radiographic features. Transbronchial biopsy is less reliable than BAL or open lung biopsy in establishing diagnosis (1)[B].

SIGNS AND SYMPTOMS

- Insidious onset
- Progressive dyspnea is the most common symptom.
- Dry cough
- Progressive exercise intolerance
- Pleuritic chest pain
- Inspiratory crackles (may be best heard laterally)
- Wheeze with forced exhalation
- Digital clubbing and cyanosis in advanced disease
- Right-sided heart failure

TESTS
Pulmonary function test
- Not diagnostically specific
- Useful for following level of impairment
- Restrictive, mixed, or obstructive pattern
- Reduction in diffusing capacity to carbon monoxide (2)[B]

Lab
No pathognomonic lab findings

Imaging

- Chest radiograph (sensitivity 90%, specificity 93%) (1)[B]
  - Most common findings are bilateral pleural thickening and circumscribed calcified pleural plaques.
  - Pleural plaques usually posterior-lateral, may also involve diaphragm (3)[B]
  - As disease progresses, irregular, linear opacities most often in middle or lower lung fields
  - Less common: Rounded atelectasis (Blesovsky syndrome) when fibrosis of visceral pleura extends into parenchyma (4)[B]
  - Classification scheme available through International Labour Office
- High-resolution CT may increase sensitivity to near 100%; improves detection of interstitial fibrosis.

Pathological Findings

Pleural plaques are found in parietal pleura; made up of collagen bundles with rare inflammatory cells. Pleural thickening involves the visceral pleura (3)[B].

DIFFERENTIAL DIAGNOSIS
Other pneumoconioses
- Idiopathic pulmonary fibrosis
- Hypersensitivity pneumonitis
- Sarcoidosis
- Other pneumoconiosis, including mixed exposures

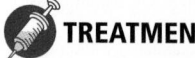 **TREATMENT**

GENERAL MEASURES
- No effective treatment to reverse course
- Approach directed at elimination of progression, amelioration of symptoms, reduction of risk of associated disorders
- Withdrawal from exposure (3)[B]. Workers with no symptoms and only chest radiographic changes may make an informed choice to continue employment using maximum environmental and personal protection.
- Pneumococcal and influenza vaccines
- Chest physiotherapy
- Home oxygen
- Smoking cessation: Cigarette smokers have more radiographic signs of disease and have a significantly increased risk for lung cancer.

Diet
High calorie, high protein with advanced disease

Activity
Graded exercise

MEDICATION (DRUGS)

First Line
- No specific pharmacologic treatment
- Oxygen
- Bronchodilators for pulmonary toilet

Second Line
- Antibiotics for respiratory infections
- Diuretics if cor pulmonale develops

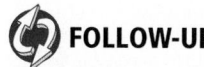 ## FOLLOW-UP

PROGNOSIS
- Severity depends on duration and intensity of exposure.
- Lung disease irreversible
- Increased risk for lung cancer (synergistic increase with cigarette smoking) and mesothelioma (2)[B]

COMPLICATIONS
- Mesothelioma
  - Related to dose, time elapsed from exposure (usually 25–40 years after exposure).
  - Risk is higher with exposure to amphibole fibers rather than chrysotile fibers.
  - Insidious but progressive. Median survival for mesothelioma is 8–18 months (5)[B]
  - Pleural effusion in 80–95% (4)[B]
- Lung cancer risk is associated with asbestos exposure whether asbestosis is present or not; synergistically increased risk in asbestos workers who smoke.
- Gastrointestinal cancer risk may be increased

PATIENT MONITORING
- Chest radiograph
- Occasional pulmonary function tests
- Prompt treatment of infections

REFERENCES

1. American Thoracic Society. Diagnosis and initial management of nonmalignant diseases related to asbestos. *Am J Respir Crit Care Med* 2004;170:691–715.
2. Glazer CS, Newman LS. Occupational interstitial lung disease. *Clin Chest Med* 2004;25.
3. Huggins JT, Sahn SA. Causes and management of pleural fibrosis. *Respirology* 2004;9:441.
4. Cugell DW, Kamp DW. Asbestos and the pleura. *Chest*, 2004;125:1103–1117.
5. Martino D, Pass HI. Integration of multi-modality approaches in the management of malignant pleural mesothelioma. *Clin Lung Cancer* 2004;5:290–298.
6. www.atsdr.cdc.gov/medical_community/ working_with_patients/_downloads/ overviewclin_32205_hi.pdf (accessed 5/25/2006) (C)

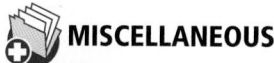 ## MISCELLANEOUS

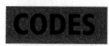 **CODES**

ICD9-CM
501 Asbestosis

PATIENT TEACHING

Printed patient information available from National Cancer Institute: http:// ww.cancer.gov/cancertopics/ factsheet/Risk/asbestos

ASCITES

Anne Walsh, PA-C, MMSc

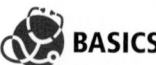 **BASICS**

DESCRIPTION
Accumulation of fluid >25 mL in abdominal cavity. May occur in any condition that causes generalized edema.

GENERAL PREVENTION
Varies with etiology

EPIDEMIOLOGY
- Determined by etiology
- Children: Nephrotic syndrome and malignancy most common
- Adults: Cirrhosis, heart failure, nephrotic syndrome, peritonitis most common

RISK FACTORS
Those associated with possible causes

ETIOLOGY
- Peritoneal infection and inflammation
  - Tuberculosis
  - Fungal disease
  - Bacterial infection (foreign body, fistula)
  - Perforated viscus
  - Granulomatous peritonitis (e.g. sarcoidosis)
  - Parasitic infection
- Metabolic diseases
  - Cirrhosis
  - Prehepatic and posthepatic portal hypertension
  - Myxedema
  - Nephrogenous
  - Dialysis-related
  - Protein malnutrition (hypoalbuminemia <2 g/dL)
- Cardiac congestion
  - Congestive heart failure
  - Constrictive pericarditis
  - Tricuspid stenosis or insufficiency
- Traumatic
  - Pancreatic or biliary fistula
  - Lymphatic tear (chylous ascites)
  - Hemoperitoneum (trauma, ectopic pregnancy, tumor)
- Malignancy
  - Peritoneal seeding: Ovarian, colon, pancreas, others
  - Primary peritoneal carcinoma
  - Leukemia, lymphoma

ASSOCIATED CONDITIONS
Listed in "Etiology"

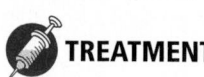 **DIAGNOSIS**

SIGNS AND SYMPTOMS
- Abdominal pain
- Abdominal distention
- Shortness of breath
- Anorexia
- Nausea
- Early satiety
- Heartburn
- Flank pain/bulging
- Weight gain
- Dyspnea/orthopnea
- Abdominal fluid wave
- Shifting dullness or "puddle sign" (dull over dependent abdomen)
- Penile/scrotal edema
- Umbilical/inguinal herniae
- Pleural effusion
- Pedal edema
- Rales
- Tachycardia
- Flatulence
- Palmar erythema, spider angiomata in cirrhosis

History
(As pertinent to underlying cause)

Physical Exam
Include abdominal, pelvic, rectal, cardiac, lungs, lymph nodes, skin, mental status. Positive findings listed above.

TESTS
Lab
Ascitic fluid should be sampled in all new-onset or new-to-treat cases.

- Obtain in all
  - Culture via blood culture bottles
  - Total cell count
  - Polymorphonuclear leukocytes: >250 mm^3 suggests infection requiring antibiotics
  - Albumin in both serum and ascites: Calculate SAAG (serum to-ascites albumin gradient)
    - <1.1 g indicates exudate, i.e., inflammatory, biliary/pancreatic, carcinomatosis
    - >1.1 g indicates transudate/portal hypertension
  - Protein: >2 g (some sources cite 2.5 g) indicates exudate
- Of use in specific circumstances
  - Amylase, triglycerides, glucose
  - Lactate dehydrogenase
  - Acid-fast or fungal cultures/smears
  - Cytology only if exudate

Blood tests
- BUN/creatinine
- Electrolytes
  - Sodium levels in single sample
    - <10 mEq/L (<10 mmol/L) diuretic response unlikely
    - >10–70 mEq/L (>10–70 mmol/L) diuretic response likely
    - >70 mEq/L (>70 mmol/L) diuretics unnecessary
- Other labs as indicated by underlying condition (liver enzymes, tumor markers, etc.)
- Drugs/disorders that may alter lab results
  - Refer to laboratory test reference

Imaging
- Abdominal ultrasound highly sensitive
- CT scan to rule out intra-abdominal pathology
- MRI best for evaluation of liver disease

Diagnostic Procedures/Surgery
- Diagnostic paracentesis
- Diagnostic laparoscopy

Pathological Findings
- Peritoneal biopsy may reveal tuberculosis or malignancy; of no value in other types of fluid
- Culture may reveal organism(s) responsible for inflammatory disease (e.g., TB)
- Cytology may reveal malignant cells from metastatic disease
  - Typically adenocarcinoma (ovary, breast, GI tract)
  - Rarely primary peritoneal carcinoma

DIFFERENTIAL DIAGNOSIS
- Obesity
- Bowel obstruction (air and liquid in distended intestine)
- Pregnancy in reproductive-age female
- Fluid type, transudate: Likely causes include
  - Congestive heart failure
  - Constrictive pericarditis
  - Cirrhosis
  - Nephrotic syndrome
  - Protein malnutrition/hypoalbuminemia
- Fluid type, exudate: Likely causes include
  - Neoplasm
  - Tuberculosis
  - Pancreatitis
  - Myxedema
  - Biliary pathology
  - Budd-Chiari syndrome

TREATMENT

GENERAL MEASURES
- Care may be outpatient or inpatient, depending on physical condition
- For all patients
  - Sodium restriction required:
  - 2 g daily until renal excretion improves, usually required 3–6 months. Consultation with dietician helpful to increase patient compliance
  - Water restriction only necessary if serum sodium <130 mEq/L
  - Persistent elevation of creatinine >2.5 mg/dL should lead to decreasing diuretic doses and therapeutic paracentesis.
  - Daily record of weight to monitor gains and losses
- For ascites with edema
  - Salt restriction and diuretics usually effective
  - Maximum weight loss of 5 pounds per day
  - Weekly electrolytes on serum during rapid weight loss
- For ascites without edema
  - Dietary restrictions and diuretics as above
  - Maximum weight loss of 2 pounds per day
  - Refractory ascites
- Confirm patient compliance with adequate sodium restriction (most common cause)

- Diuretic-intractable ascites: (worse despite max doses spironolactone [300 mg/day] and furosemide [160–200 mg/day] and Na restriction OR progressive rise in creatinine to 2)
  - Start paracentesis 5–10 L per session
    ○ Complication: Hemodynamic collapse and renal failure
    ○ Replace albumin IV for all removals >5 L at rate of 8 g albumin for each liter removed
  - Continue diuretics at 1/2 previous dose

Diet
Consultation with dietician helpful
- Sodium restriction, 2 g/day monitor
- Adequate nutrition
- Protein restriction not likely beneficial but often recommended; avoid high-protein diet (can precipitate hepatic encephalopathy if cirrhosis)
- Fluid restriction (1–1.5 L/day) only if dilutional hyponatremia (Na <125 mmol/L).

Activity
Bed rest only if heart failure and/or prominent leg edema

Comp-Alt-Medicine
Caution patients to avoid herbs and other supplements unless approved by physician (risk drug interactions, hepatotoxicity, coagulopathy)

 ## MEDICATION (DRUGS)

First Line
- Diuretics needed in nearly all patients
  - Spironolactone 100–300 mg/day PO in single dose best for cirrhotic ascites; typical initial dose is 100–200 mg given in AM
  - Furosemide 20–120 mg/day PO best for all other etiologies; typical initial dose is 40 mg given in AM
  - May use spironolactone and furosemide together
  - Dose should be sufficient to obtain net sodium loss in urine
  - Discontinue NSAIDs except 81 mg dose of aspirin. Follow body weight daily. If there is a <2-pound loss in the next 4 days, increase either spironolactone by 100 mg or furosemide by 40 mg. If the 2-pound weight loss continues in the next 4 days, continue with the same dose. Emphasize sodium restriction.
  - Spot sodium in mEq/L × estimated urine output (1 L if no information) should equal estimated dietary sodium. Increase diuretics daily until this goal attained. Measure serum electrolytes before each dose change.
- Contraindications: Consult manufacturer
- Precautions
  - In hospital, or when rapid diuresis, observe creatinine weekly. NSAIDs may worsen or initiate oliguria or azotemia. Potassium supplements usually required when diuresis exceeds 1 pound per day.
  - Spironolactone or amiloride may increase potassium; monitoring necessary after 1st week of therapy and at least monthly thereafter.
  - Observe patients closely for signs of volume depletion, encephalopathy, and renal insufficiency.
- Significant possible interactions: Avoid concomitant potassium supplements if spironolactone used alone

Second Line
- Only rarely do alternative diuretics lead to success if combinations of spironolactone and furosemide fail or result in increased BUN/creatinine
  - Most commonly used in cases of GI intolerance or allergic reactions
  - Alternatives to spironolactone: Amiloride up to 10 mg/day; triamterene up to 200 mg/day in divided doses
  - Alternatives to furosemide: Torsemide up to 100 mg per day; ethacrynic acid 50 mg IV (may be effective when oral drugs cannot be used)

SURGERY
- TIPS (transjugular intrahepatic portosystemic shunt; radiological procedure); effective for intractable ascites
  - At time of placement, measured portal pressure should drop ≥20 mm Hg or to <12 mm Hg, and ascites should be readily controlled with diuretics. Conduct yearly ultrasonographic study to confirm functional shunt.
  - Dilation/replacement may be required after 2+ years. Encephalopathy is a possible complication of TIPS.
- Surgical portacaval shunt: An 8–10 mm mesenteric caval shunt often is effective.
  - Significant operative mortality, morbidity, encephalopathy; most experts prefer TIPS instead.
- When recurrent pleural effusion present in patient with chronic ascites, fusing of pleural surfaces is sometimes used. Alternative is TIPS.
- Liver transplant referral should be considered in all patients with decompensated liver disease, regardless of whether ascites is present/controlled.

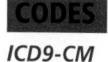 ## FOLLOW-UP

PROGNOSIS
- Varies depending on underlying cause
- Rarely life-threatening in itself but may be a symptom of life-threatening disease (e.g., cancer, end-stage liver disease)
  - Conservative therapy usually successful if cause is reversible or treatable (e.g., infection)

COMPLICATIONS
- Overly aggressive diuresis may lead to hypokalemia, worsening encephalopathy, intravascular volume depletion, azotemia, renal failure, and death.
- Hepatorenal syndrome: Urine volume <500 mL/day, decreasing urine sodium, rising blood urea, and creatinine >1.5 mg/dL
  - Stop all diuretics. IV fluid challenge of 1.5 L plasma expander after 1 day if no improvement.
  - Vasopressors (e.g., terlipressin IV every q4–6h) may resolve renal failure in 50% of patients.
- Spontaneous bacterial peritonitis: Ascitic fluid cell count >250 polymorphonuclear leukocytes, fever, clinical deterioration. Treat with 3rd generation cephalosporin or comparable antibiotic; combined antibiotic treatment plus IV albumin results in improved survival in some patients.
- Hydrothorax: Always on right side; cell and lab properties same as ascites. Do not place chest tube. Treat ascites vigorously; if hydrothorax does not disappear, consider TIPS.
- Other complications may be associated with specific etiologies of ascites.

PATIENT MONITORING
- Daily body weight
- Weekly electrolytes when appreciable diuresis present (>1 pound weight loss/day) and 1 week post change in dose/type of diuretic
- Mental status to assess for encephalopathy
- Monitor underlying disease as indicated (comprehensive panel, CBC, etc.).

REFERENCES

1. Russo MW, Jacques PF, Mauro M, Odell P, Brown RS Jr. Predictors of mortality and stenosis after transjugular intrahepatic portosystemic shunt. *Liver Transpl*. 2002;8:271–277.
2. Runyon BA. Management of adult patients with ascites due to cirrhosis. *Hepatology*. 2004; 39:841–856.
3. Gines P, Uriz J, Calahorra B, Garcia-Tsao G, et al. Transjugular intrahepatic portosystemic shunting versus paracentesis plus albumin for refractory ascites in cirrhosis. *Gastroenterology*. 2002; 123:139–147.
4. Nietsch H. Management of portal hypertension. *J Clin Gastroenterol*. 2005:39:232–236.
5. Saadeh S, Davis GL. Management of ascites in patients with end-stage liver disease. *Rev Gastroenterol Disord*. 2004;4:175–185.
6. Talwalker J, Kamath P. Influence of recent advances in medical management on clinical outcomes of cirrhosis. *Mayo Clin Proc*. 2005;80:1501–1508.

 ## MISCELLANEOUS

See also: Cirrhosis of the Liver; Congestive Heart Failure; Nephrotic Syndrome

CODES

ICD9-CM
789.5 Ascites

PATIENT TEACHING

See Corresponding Diagnostic Algorithm

ASPERGILLOSIS

Rodney D. Adam, MD

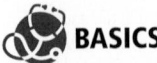 **BASICS**

DESCRIPTION
Disease caused by a ubiquitous mold; primarily involves lungs. Frequently lethal in neutropenic and bone marrow transplant (BMT) patients. Syndromes include:

- Allergic aspergillosis
  - Extrinsic allergic alveolitis: Hypersensitivity pneumonitis in individuals repeatedly exposed to fungus
  - Allergic bronchopulmonary aspergillosis: (1,2)[C]
  - Pulmonary infiltrates, mucous plugging; secondary to allergic reaction to fungus (3)[C]
- Aspergillomas: "Fungus ball" saprophytic colonization within pre-existing pulmonary cavities
- Invasive aspergillosis: Most common and severe in BMT and neutropenic patients. Also occurs with increased frequency in other immunocompromised persons, such as those with AIDS, solid-organ transplant, or high-dose corticosteroids; commonly fatal (3,4)[C]
- System(s) Affected: Cardiovascular; Gastrointestinal; Musculoskeletal; Nervous, Pulmonary
- Synonym(s): Hypersensitivity pneumonitis; Fungus ball

GENERAL PREVENTION
- Allergic: Avoid exposure.
- Aspergillomas: Treatment of underlying diseases (e.g., chronic obstructive pulmonary disease [COPD])

EPIDEMIOLOGY
- Predominant age: Depends on subtype:
  - Allergic: Tends to occur in patients <35 years
  - Aspergillomas: Older patients with chronic lung disease
  - Invasive: All ages
- Predominant sex: Male = Female

Prevalence
Rare

RISK FACTORS
- Allergic
  - Exposure
  - Asthma
- Aspergillomas
  - COPD
  - Bronchiectasis
  - Tuberculosis (TB)
  - Malignancy
- Invasive
  - Neutropenia
  - Corticosteroid therapy
  - Graft Versus Host disease in recipients of bone marrow transplant
  - AIDS

Genetics
No known genetic pattern

ETIOLOGY
Aspergillus species in decreasing order of frequency
- *Aspergillus fumigatus*
- *Aspergillus flavus*
- *Aspergillus niger*

ASSOCIATED CONDITIONS
- Allergic: Asthma
- Aspergillomas
  - COPD
  - TB
  - Pulmonary mycoses
  - Silicosis
  - Sarcoidosis
  - Nontuberculous mycobacteria
  - Ankylosing spondylitis
  - Malignancy
- Invasive: Neutropenia

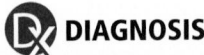 **DIAGNOSIS**

SIGNS AND SYMPTOMS
- Allergic
  - Cough
  - Wheezing
  - Constitutional symptoms
  - Plug expectoration
- Aspergillomas
  - Hemoptysis
  - Manifestations of underlying disease
- Invasive
  - Fever
  - Cough
  - Rales
  - Rhonchi
  - Toxicity
  - CNS signs
  - GI bleeding

TESTS
- Allergic bronchopulmonary aspergillosis
- Invasive: None

Lab
- Allergic bronchopulmonary aspergillosis
  - Eosinophilia
  - Immediate skin reactivity to *Aspergillus* antigen
  - Precipitating-serum antibodies (precipitins) against *Aspergillus* antigens
  - Elevated serum IgE concentrations
  - Elevated serum IgE and IgG antibodies specific to *Aspergillus fumigatus*
- Invasive
  - Sputum culture
  - Cultures of bronchoalveolar lavage or bronchial washings
  - Biopsy is definitive.
  - Blood cultures almost never positive

Imaging
Chest radiographs
- Fleeting infiltrates (allergic bronchopulmonary aspergillosis)
- Round intracavity mass (aspergillomas)
- Nodular or patchy infiltrates progressing to diffuse consolidation and cavitation (invasive)
- Nodular, cavitary, or pleural-based wedge-shaped lesions

Diagnostic Procedures/Surgery
- Bronchoscopy, bronchial washings, bronchoalveolar lavage, or transthoracic needle aspiration may be helpful in isolating organism in invasive disease.
- Open lung biopsy is diagnostic but often not possible in severely ill, ventilated patients.

Pathological Findings
- Necrotizing pneumonia
- Hemorrhagic infarcts
- Blood vessel invasion
- Branching septate hyphae if organism seen microscopically

DIFFERENTIAL DIAGNOSIS
- Allergic: Other causes of asthma and hypersensitivity pneumonitis
- Aspergillomas
  - Neoplasm
  - TB
- Invasive
  - Bacterial pneumonia
  - Pulmonary hemorrhage
  - Drug toxicity
  - Malignancy
  - Mucor (sinuses)

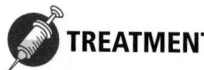 TREATMENT

GENERAL MEASURES
- Allergic
  - Usually outpatient
  - Extrinsic allergic alveolitis: Drug therapy, exposure avoidance
  - Allergic bronchopulmonary aspergillosis: Corticosteroids
- Aspergillomas
  - Usually outpatient
  - Individualized therapy ranging from no therapy to surgical resection of cavities in cases of severe hemoptysis
  - Systemic antifungal therapy seldom useful
- Invasive
  - Inpatient
  - High-dose intravenous antifungal therapy (prognosis tends to be poor)
  - Treatment of underlying disease
  - Adjunctive cytokine therapy to reverse neutropenia

Diet
No special diet

Activity
As tolerated

 MEDICATION (DRUGS)

First Line
- Allergic
  - Extrinsic allergic alveolitis: Bronchodilators, cromolyn, steroids
  - Allergic bronchopulmonary aspergillosis: Steroids are the mainstay of therapy. Antifungal agents (itraconazole or voriconazole) are being used increasingly as adjunctive agents.
- Aspergillomas: None
- Invasive: High-dose lipid formulation of amphotericin B (5 mg/kg/day and frequently higher). The lipid formulations of amphotericin B (Abelcet, Ambisome) are preferred over standard amphotericin because of reduced nephrotoxicity in view of high doses required, and perhaps better efficacy.
- Caspofungin: Echinocandin approved for patients with aspergillosis unresponsive to other therapy or who have unacceptable toxicity to other agents. Micafungin and anidulafungin are other echinocandins that have been approved for treatment of candidiasis and are expected to have efficacy for treatment of aspergillosis.
- Voriconazole: Superior to conventional amphotericin in a large study; well absorbed orally
- Contraindications: Refer to manufacturer's literature.
- Precautions
  - Amphotericin B (including the lipid formulations) can cause significant renal insufficiency and electrolyte abnormalities. Saline infusion at time of amphotericin B administration may decrease nephrotoxicity.
  - Itraconazole: Normal, low gastric pH necessary for absorption
- Significant possible interactions
  - Amphotericin B: Other nephrotoxic drugs (e.g., aminoglycosides, cyclosporine) accelerate development of renal insufficiency.
  - Amphotericin B: Diuretics accelerate electrolyte depletion.
  - Voriconazole: Hepatically metabolized drugs, serum levels may be altered
  - Itraconazole: Hepatically metabolized drugs, serum levels altered

Second Line
- Itraconazole occasionally useful as alternative agent
- Note: Because of frequent failure of single-drug therapy, combination therapy is frequently proposed.

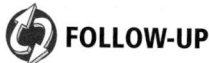 **FOLLOW-UP**

PROGNOSIS
- Allergic
  - With treatment: Good
  - Untreated: Can progress to severe fibrosis, COPD
- Aspergillomas: Prognosis more related to underlying disease
- Invasive: Poor

COMPLICATIONS
- Allergic
  - Bronchiectasis
  - Pulmonary fibrosis
  - Obstructive lung disease
- Aspergillomas: Hemoptyses
- Invasive
  - Metastatic infection of CNS, GI tract, and other organs
  - Death

PATIENT MONITORING
- Allergic
  - Extrinsic allergic alveolitis: Spirometry
  - Allergic bronchopulmonary aspergillosis: Chest radiograph, IgE levels
- Aspergillomas: Chest radiograph, symptoms
- Invasive: Chest radiograph, CBC

REFERENCES
1. Greenberger PA. Allergic bronchopulmonary aspergillosis. *J Allergy Clin Immunol*. 110:685–692.
2. Zander DS. Allergic bronchopulmonary aspergillosis: An overview. *Arch Pathol Lab Med*. 129:924–928,l.
3. Soubani AO, Chandrasekar PH. The clinical spectrum of pulmonary aspergillosis. *Chest*. 2002;121:1988–1999.
4. Lin S, Schranz J, Teutsch S. Aspergillosis case-fatality rate: Systematic review of the literature. *Clin Infect Dis*. 2001;32:358–366.
5. Herbrecht R, Denning DW, Patterson TF, et al. Invasive Fungal Infections Group of the European Organisation for Research and Treatment of Cancer and the Global Aspergillus Study Group. Voriconazole versus amphotericin B for primary therapy of invasive aspergillosis. *N Engl J Med*. 2002;347:408–415.

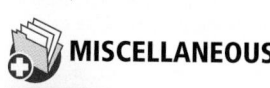 **MISCELLANEOUS**

CODES

ICD9-CM
117.3 Aspergillosis

PATIENT TEACHING
Directed to specifics of individual circumstances

ASTHMA

Mary Cataletto, MD

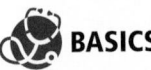 **BASICS**

DESCRIPTION

- Disorder of tracheobronchial tree characterized by mild to severe obstruction to airflow that is at least partially reversible. Symptoms vary, generally episodic or paroxysmal, but may be persistent. Clinical hallmark is wheezing, but cough or chest tightness may be predominant symptom.
- Acute symptoms characterized by narrowing of large and small airways owing to spasm of bronchial smooth muscle, edema, and inflammation of bronchial mucosa, and production of mucus.
- Classification
  - Mild intermittent:
    Day symptoms: $</= 2$ days/week; Night symptoms: $</= 2$ nights/month
  - Mild Persistent:
    Day symptoms: >2 days/week, <1/day; Night symptoms: >2 nights/month
  - Moderate Persistent:
    Day symptoms: Daily
    Night symptoms: >1 night/week
  - Severe Persistent:
    Day symptoms: continuous
    Night symptoms: >1 night/week
- Occurs in setting in which asthma is likely, and other, rarer conditions have been excluded
- System(s) affected: Pulmonary
- Synonym(s): Bronchial asthma; Reactive airway disease

Pregnancy Considerations
- ~50% of asthma patients have no changes, 25% seem to improve, and 25% develop worse symptoms.
- Stress prevention.
- Avoid medications with contraindications.

GENERAL PREVENTION
- Patient and/or family partnership with health care provider
  - Patient understanding of medication, inhalers, nebulizers, peak flow meters, triggers
  - Monitor symptoms: Peak flow monitoring may also be helpful.
  - An asthma action plan may be helpful
- Investigate and control triggering factors (pollutants, exercise, house-dust mites, roaches, molds, animal dander)
- Evaluate and treat comorbidities (GERD, atopy, sinus disease)
- Annual influenza immunization
- Avoid cigarette exposure.
- Avoid aspirin, NSAIDs, β-blockers, sulfites, if sensitive.
- Regular follow-up

EPIDEMIOLOGY
- Leading cause of missed school days: 7.5 million per year
- Predominant age
  - 50% of cases: Children <10 years
  - Young adult (16–40 years), but may occur at any age. Unusual for initial episode to occur in geriatric population
- Predominant sex
  - Children <10: Male > Female
  - Puberty: Male = Female
  - Adult onset: Female > Male

Incidence
- 10 million new cases each year; however, confusion exists owing to lack of uniform definition
- 50% of new cases of asthma occur in children <10 years.

Prevalence
7–19% of children

RISK FACTORS
- Positive family history of asthma or atopy
- Viral lower-respiratory infection during infancy
- Environmental tobacco smoke
- Inner-city dwelling

Genetics
- Search for an asthma gene under way
- Familial association of reactive airway disease, atopic dermatitis, and allergic rhinitis

ASSOCIATED CONDITIONS
- Reflux esophagitis
- Sinusitis
- Atopy

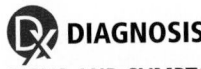 **DIAGNOSIS**

SIGNS AND SYMPTOMS
- Variation in pattern of symptoms: Paroxysmal, versus constant,
- Abnormal pulmonary function tests may occur without symptoms
  - Wheezing
  - Cough
  - Chest tightness
  - Chest pain
  - Exercise-induced wheezing or cough
  - Prolonged expiration
  - Nocturnal attacks
  - Pulsus paradoxus
  - Tachycardia
  - Hypoxia
  - Accessory respiratory muscle use
  - Flattened diaphragms
  - Growth usually normal

History
- Pattern
- Triggers
- Exposures (pets, tobacco smoke)
- Comorbidities
- Severity
- Medications
- Family history of asthma and allergy

Physical Exam
Focus on general appearance; upper, middle, and lower airway; and skin

TESTS
- Pulmonary function tests with methacholine challenge: Reversible airway obstruction (increased airway resistance, decreased airflow rates). If pulmonary function tests are within normal limits and no bronchodilator response is seen, airway challenge with cold air, methacholine, or exercise may be helpful in establishing diagnosis.
- Allergy testing

Lab
- CBC: Peripheral eosinophilia in atopic patients
- Immunoglobulins
  - Screen for immunodeficiency (IgA, IgG subclasses) for patients with recurrent infections or severe allergies.
  - IgE is elevated in atopic patients and markedly elevated in allergic bronchopulmonary aspergillosis.
- Sweat test in chronic childhood asthmatics to rule out cystic fibrosis
- Arterial blood gases may be helpful in status asthmaticus.
- Antihistamines may alter allergy skin testing.

Imaging
Chest radiograph: Valuable at time of initial diagnosis to rule out other serious intrathoracic pathology, but should not be routine with each exacerbation
- Right middle lobe atelectasis may occur
- Hyperinflation
- Air leak syndromes: Pneumothorax, pneumomediastinum may occur

Diagnostic Procedures/Surgery
- Spirometry: Decreased FEV_1
- Bronchoscopy: Rarely indicated

Pathological Findings
- Smooth-muscle hyperplasia
- Mucosal edema
- Thickened basement membrane
- Inflammatory response
- Hyperinflated lungs
- Mucus plugging

DIFFERENTIAL DIAGNOSIS
- Foreign-body aspiration: Always consider, especially with unilateral wheeze.
- Cystic fibrosis
- Viral respiratory infections (croup, bronchiolitis)
- Epiglottitis
- Bronchopulmonary aspergillosis
- Tuberculosis
- Hyperventilation syndrome
- Habit cough
- Congestive heart failure
- Chronic obstructive pulmonary disease
- Hypersensitivity pneumonitis
- Vascular anomalies
- Mediastinal mass
- Tracheobronchomalacia
- Vocal cord dysfunction

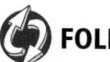 **TREATMENT**

INITIAL STABILIZATION

- Relieve bronchospasm: Administer short acting β_2 agonist
- Administer supplemental oxygen for severe exacerbation
- IV fluids if necessary
- Oral corticosteroids if exacerbation
  - Adult: 60–80 mg/d prednisone
  - Pediatric: 1–2 mg/kg/d prednisone (1)

Diet
Avoid foods with preservatives, known allergic triggers and those with sulfites

Activity
- Early diagnosis and appropriate treatment facilitate unrestricted activity.
- Be aware of known triggers
  - Allergic factors
    - Airborne pollens
    - Molds
    - House dust (mites)
    - Cockroaches
    - Animal dander
    - Feather pillows
  - Other factors
    - Tobacco smoke and other pollutants
    - Infections, especially viral
    - Aspirin
    - Exercise
    - Cold air
    - Sinusitis
    - Gastroesophageal reflux
    - Sleep (peak expiratory flow rate lowest at 4 am)
- Current research focuses on inflammatory response (including abnormal release of chemical mediators, eosinophil chemotactic factor, neutrophil chemotactic factor, and leukotrienes).

Nursing
Care should be culturally sensitive

SPECIAL THERAPY
IV Fluids
May be necessary if patient is tachypneic, unable to tolerate oral feeds, or is dehydrated.

 MEDICATION (DRUGS)

First Line
- Asthmatics should have an action plan for exacerbations. Patients with mild intermittent asthma do not require daily treatment and should keep a short-acting β_2 agent available for symptomatic relief. Patients with persistent asthma require daily medication. The drug regimen of choice for patients with persistent asthma includes an inhaled corticosteroid. The preferred regimens are as follows for persistent asthma:
- Mild persistent asthma: Low-dose inhaled corticosteroid
- Moderate persistent asthma: Low-dose inhaled corticosteroid plus a long-acting β-agonist. Medium-dose inhaled corticosteroids also can be used.
- Severe persistent asthma: High-dose inhaled corticosteroids plus a long-acting β-agonist.
- Alternatives exist in each category.

 FOLLOW-UP

DISPOSITION
Admission Criteria
- Respiratory distress
- Complications including pneumonia, pneumothorax, significant atelectasis
- Need for supportive care (e.g., dehydration)
- Poor control of symptoms or poor response to treatment

Discharge Criteria
- Support systems in place
- Patient and family education
- Control of exacerbation
- Stable clinical status

Issues for Referral
- For patients <5 years
  - Required for step 3 and 4 care and may be considered for step 2 care. Referral also should be considered when specialized testing or treatment is required, when the diagnosis is in question, and when further education is requested or required.
- For patients ≥5 years
  - Required for step 4 care; should be considered for step 3 care when specialized testing or treatment is required, when the diagnosis is in question, or when additional educational intervention is needed.

PROGNOSIS
- Excellent, with attention to general health and use of medications to control symptoms
- Mortality risk increases with
  - >3 emergency room visits per year
  - Nocturnal symptoms
  - History of ICU admission
  - Mechanical ventilation
  - >2 hospitalizations per year
  - Systemic steroid dependence
  - History of syncope with asthma
  - History of noncompliance
- Mortality rates are increasing.
- If response to treatment is poor, review diagnosis and compliance prior to adding more potent therapy.

COMPLICATIONS
- Respiratory failure
- Atelectasis: Most common in right middle lobe
- Flaccid paralysis after exacerbation (self-limited and rare)
- Death
- Air-leak syndromes (e.g., pneumothorax)
- Syndrome of inappropriate secretion of antidiuretic hormone (SIADH)
- Altered theophylline metabolism
- Steroid myopathy
- Inhaled steroid safety has been established.

PATIENT MONITORING
- Peak expiratory flow rate at home
- Office spirometry with periodic full pulmonary function tests done in PFT lab
- For ED patients consider
  - Oximetry
  - Arterial blood gases
  - Electrolytes: Frequent albuterol lowers potassium.
  - Exhaled nitric oxide
  - PEFR or FEV_1 measurements

- Written and periodically revised action plan is helpful.
- Periodically drug and device training should be reviewed.

REFERENCES

1. Expert Panel Report. Guidelines for the diagnosis and management of asthma. NHLBI, 2002. NIH Publication 97-4051A.
2. Williams SG, Schmidt DK, et al. Key clinical activities for quality asthma care. Recommendations of the National Asthma Education and Prevention Program, *MMWR*. 2003;March 28.

ADDITIONAL READING
http://www.nhlbi.nih.gov.guidelines/asthma/index/htm

 MISCELLANEOUS

See also: Bronchiolitis; Bronchitis, acute; Chronic obstructive pulmonary disease and emphysema; Congestive heart failure; Cystic fibrosis; Epiglottitis; Hypersensitivity pneumonitis; Immunodeficiency diseases; Laryngotracheobronchitis; Tuberculosis

CODES

ICD9-CM
- 493.00 Extrinsic asthma, unspecified
- 493.10 Intrinsic asthma, unspecified
- 493.90 Asthma, unspecified

PATIENT TEACHING
- American Lung Association, 1740 Broadway, New York, NY 10019, (212) 315-8700
- Asthma and Allergy Foundation of America, Suite 305, Washington, DC 20036, (800) 7-ASTHMA, (800) 727-8462

 See Corresponding Diagnostic Algorithm

See Patient Handout on CD

ATELECTASIS

Taylor Sittler, MD
Deborah Heitmann, MD

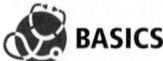 BASICS

DESCRIPTION
- Atelectasis (lung collapse) is a portion of lung that is nonaerated, but otherwise normal.
- May be an asymptomatic finding on chest radiograph
- Pulmonary blood flow to the area of atelectasis is usually reduced, which limits shunting and arterial hypoxemia.
- Diagnosis and therapy are directed at the etiology.
- Synonym(s): Lung collapse

GENERAL PREVENTION
- Avoid 100% inspired oxygen, which can be rapidly absorbed and cause atelectasis
- Foreign body/aspiration precautions
- Postoperative mobilization and/or rotation several times per hour
- Chest physiotherapy and incentive spirometry as preventive maneuvers in high-risk patients. Shown to be effective and cost-effective preceding pulmonary lobectomy (1)[C] and following myocardial revascularization (2)[C].

EPIDEMIOLOGY
- Predominant age: All ages
- Predominant sex: Male = Female

Incidence/Prevalence
Incidence/prevalence poorly documented: Very common postoperatively, particularly following thoracic/upper abdominal surgery, general anesthesia, and in intensive care with high-inspired oxygen concentrations

RISK FACTORS
- Atelectasis following anesthesia is increased in smokers, obese individuals, and individuals with short, wide thoraces.
- Increased risk in the elderly and in neonates
- Asthma—right middle lobe most common

ALERT
High oxygen content of inspired air increases risk

Genetics
Depends on basic condition (e.g., cystic fibrosis, chronic obstructive pulmonary disease, asthma, congenital heart disease, and congestive heart failure)

ETIOLOGY
- Obstructive (most common)
  - *Resorptive*: Due to airway obstruction from luminal blockage (mucus, tumor, foreign body), airway wall abnormality (edema, tumor, bronchomalacia, deformation), or extrinsic airway compression (cardiac, vascular, tumor, adenopathy)

- Non-obstructive
  - *Surfactant Impairment*: Due to pulmonary edema, infection, primary surfactant deficiency
  - *Compression*: Lobar emphysema, tumor, abscess, cardiomegaly. Right middle lobe atelectasis from chronic inflammation and bronchial compression by lymph nodes
  - *Relaxation*: Loss of contact between parietal and visceral pleura due to fluid or air in the pleural space (pneumothorax, effusion, empyema, hemothorax, chylothorax)
  - *Chest wall restriction*: Due to skeletal deformity and/or muscular weakness (scoliosis, neuromuscular disease, phrenic nerve paralysis, anesthesia)
  - *Parenchymal scarring*: Granulomatous disease, necrotizing pneumonia, asbestosis (more common in elderly), toxic inhalation, drug-induced fibrosis (e.g., amiodarone)

Geriatric Considerations
Increased risk. Primary and secondary lung tumors are sometimes associated.

Pediatric Considerations
- Increased risk. Congenital airway obstruction due to mediastinal cysts, tumor, or vascular rings
- Foreign body aspiration

ASSOCIATED CONDITIONS
- Cystic fibrosis
- Asthma
- Adult respiratory distress syndrome (ARDS)
- Neonatal respiratory distress syndrome
- Pulmonary edema
- Pulmonary embolism
- Neuromuscular disorders
- General anesthesia
- Mechanical ventilation

DIAGNOSIS

SIGNS AND SYMPTOMS
History
- Small atelectasis
  - Commonly asymptomatic
  - Produces no change in the overall clinical presentation
- Large atelectasis
  - Tachypnea
  - Cough
  - Pain

Physical Exam
- Hypoxia
- Dullness to percussion
- Absent breath sounds if airway is occluded
- Bronchial breathing if airway is patent
- Diminished chest expansion
- Tracheal or precordial impulse displacement
- Wheezing may be heard with focal obstruction.

TESTS
Lab
Sputum culture if infection is suspected

Imaging
- Chest CT or MRI may be indicated to visualize airway and mediastinal structures and to distinguish cause of atelectasis
- Chest radiograph (posterior-anterior and lateral)
  - May demonstrate linear, round, or wedge-shaped densities.
  - Right middle lobe and lingular atelectasis will obscure the ipsilateral heart border.
  - Lower lobe atelectasis will obscure the diaphragm.
  - Raised diaphragm, flattened chest wall, movement of mediastinal structures and diaphragm toward the atelectatic region
  - Unaffected lung may show compensatory hyperinflation.
- Obstructive findings
  - Air bronchograms usually absent
  - Wedge-shaped densities
- Nonobstructive findings
  - Evidence of airway compression, pleural fluid, or air should be sought.
  - Diffuse microatelectasis in surfactant deficiency may progress to a patchy or diffuse reticular granular pattern, then to a pulmonary edema-like pattern, and finally to bilateral opacification in severe cases.
  - *Round atelectasis*: Pleural-based round density on chest radiograph with a comet tail of vessel and airway; usually indicates asbestosis.

Diagnostic Procedures/Surgery
- Bronchoscopy to assess airway patency in unexplained or refractory cases
- Echocardiography to assess cardiac status in cardiomegaly
- Barium swallow to assess mediastinal vascular compression

Pathological Findings
- Needle biopsy is rarely needed for diagnosis.
- Pathology varies with the cause.
- Obstructive atelectasis—nonaerated lung without inflammation or infiltration

DIFFERENTIAL DIAGNOSIS
- Atelectasis is not a specific diagnosis, but rather a result of disease or distorted anatomy. The differential is, therefore, found under Etiology.
- The radiographic differential includes pneumonia, fluid accumulation, lung hypoplasia, tumor, and interstitial lung disease.

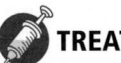 **TREATMENT**

GENERAL MEASURES

- Suction and vigorous coughing to remove obstruction, then physical therapy, and bronchoscopy to remove obstruction if previous measures fail
  - Bronchoscopy as therapy is controversial other than for obstruction removal.
- Ensure adequate oxygenation (arterial O_2 saturation >90%) and humidification.
- Incentive spirometry
- Initiate intubation and mechanical ventilation with positive end-expiratory pressure (PEEP) in severe respiratory distress or hypoxemia.
  - Lower tidal volume (6 mL/kg) and lower end-inspiratory values (<30 mm Hg) associated with reduced mortality (3)[B]
  - PEEP 15–20 mL may be necessary to maintain arterial O_2 saturation in surfactant-impaired states (3)[B]
- CPAP 5–15 cm H_2O in recurrent atelectasis or with neuromuscular weakness
- Ensure patient is lying on the unaffected side to promote drainage.
- Maximize patient mobility and encourage frequent coughing and deep breathing every hour. See also "Physical Therapy" section.

Diet
No special diet

Activity
Encourage activity and mobilization as tolerated.

SPECIAL THERAPY
Physical Therapy
Chest physiotherapy with percussion and postural drainage. Deep breathing every hour.
- Consider adding treatments using new airway clearance techniques such as PEEP mask.

 MEDICATION (DRUGS)

- Bronchodilator therapy (β-agonist aerosol); efficacy controversial
- Empiric, broad-spectrum antibiotics for infection if atelectasis occurs outside the hospital setting see "C ommunity-acquired Pneumonia"
- Analgesia for pain control to permit deep inspiration and coughing
- Other therapies directed at basic cause: Antibiotics, foreign-body removal, tumor therapy, cardiac medication, and steroids in asthma

SURGERY
Only for respectable disease (e.g., tumor)

 FOLLOW-UP

PROGNOSIS
- Resolution with medical therapy
- Surgical therapy needed only for resectable causes or if chronic infection and bronchiectasis supervene

COMPLICATIONS
- Atelectasis is rarely life threatening and usually resolves spontaneously.
- Acute atelectasis
  - Hypoxemia and respiratory failure
  - Postobstructive drowning of the lung
  - Sepsis
- Chronic atelectasis
  - Acute pneumonia
  - Bronchiectasis
  - Pleural effusion and empyema

PATIENT MONITORING
- Varies with cause and patient status
- In simple atelectasis associated with asthma or infection, monthly visits are adequate.

REFERENCES
1. Varela G, Ballesteros E, et al. Cost-effectiveness analysis of prophylactic respiratory physiotherapy in pulmonary lobectomy. *Eur J Cardiothorac Surg* 2006;29(2):216–20. Epub 2006 Jan 11.
2. Leguisamo CP, Kalil RAK, Furlani AP. Effectiveness of a preoperative physiotherapeutic approach in myocardial revascularization. *Brazil J Cardiovasc Surg* 2005;20(2):134–141.
3. McCunn M, Sutcliffe AJ, et al. Guidelines for management of mechanical ventilation in critically injured patients. *TraumaCare* 2004;14(4):147–151.

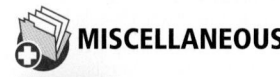 **MISCELLANEOUS**

CODES

ICD9-CM
518 Pulmonary collapse

PATIENT TEACHING
- Encourage activity as appropriate.
- Instruct in basic cause and its therapy.

ATHEROSCLEROSIS

Manoj Singh, MD

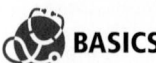

BASICS

DESCRIPTION
The common form of arteriosclerosis in which deposits of yellowish plaques (atheromas) containing cholesterol, lipoid material, and lipophages are formed within the intima and inner media of large and medium-sized arteries

ALERT
Geriatric Considerations
- Atherosclerosis happens to all who live long enough.
- Effects and complications can be minimized and/or delayed by avoiding all risk factors possible.

Pediatric Considerations
Fatty streaks and deposits in the intima of the aortas of all children begin as early as 3 years of age.

GENERAL PREVENTION
Treat or control modifiable risk factors.

EPIDEMIOLOGY
- Incidence/prevalence in the United States
  - Common, but declining steadily
  - The effects on the brain, heart, kidneys, extremities, and other vital organs form the leading cause of morbidity and mortality in the United States and most Western countries.
  - Complications of atherosclerosis account for half of all deaths, and one third of the deaths in persons 35–65 years of age.
- Predominant age: 35 and older
- Predominant sex: Male > Female

RISK FACTORS
- Modifiable
  - Hypertension
  - Tobacco smoking
  - Diabetes mellitus (considered equivalence of CHD)
  - Obesity
  - Physical inactivity
  - Decreased high-density lipoprotein (HDL) cholesterol
  - Increased low-density lipoprotein (LDL) cholesterol
  - Comorbidities that may increase risk
    - Hypothyroidism
    - Elevated homocysteine levels
    - High testosterone levels in women
    - Low testosterone levels in men
- Nonmodifiable
  - Male gender
  - Increasing age
  - Family history of *premature* atherosclerosis

Genetics
There is a probable genetic link; many risk factors for atherosclerosis (lipid metabolism, hypertension, and diabetes) are clearly inheritable.

ETIOLOGY
- Biochemical, physiologic, environmental factors that lead to thickening and occlusion of the lumen of arteries
- Aging (some degree of atherosclerosis is universal)
- One or more of the risk factors listed under "Risk Factors"

ASSOCIATED CONDITIONS
- Essential hypertension
- Coronary arteriosclerosis
- Congestive heart failure
- Cerebrovascular accident
- Atrial arrhythmias
- Ventricular arrhythmias
- Renal failure, chronic
- Aortic dissection
- Thrombosis and embolism, arterial
- Atherosclerotic occlusive disease

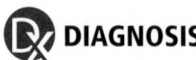

DIAGNOSIS

SIGNS AND SYMPTOMS
- Characteristically silent until atheromas produce
  - Stenosis
  - Thrombosis
  - Aneurysm
  - Embolus
- For lists of possible symptoms see the following topics
  - Essential hypertension
  - Coronary arteriosclerosis
  - Congestive heart failure
  - Cerebrovascular accident
  - Atrial arrhythmias
  - Ventricular arrhythmias
  - Renal failure, chronic
  - Dissecting aneurysm
  - Thrombosis and embolism, arterial

TESTS
Lab
- Associated with elevated serum cholesterol
- Elevated LDL and low HDL

Imaging
Extensively calcified atherosclerotic plaques may be identified in major blood vessels on radiography.

Diagnostic Procedures/Surgery
- Associated with hypercholesterolemia; elevated LDL and low HDL
- Arterial Doppler studies (carotid, renal)
- Angiography
- Ankle-brachial index (ABI)

Pathological Findings
- Early changes (simple), potentially reversible
  - Accumulation of lipid-laden cells in the intimal layer of the artery (usually monocytes/macrophages from circulating blood)
  - Lipid streaks in aorta and coronary arteries
- Late changes (complicated) usually reversible
  - Atheromatous plaques with necrosis, fibrosis, calcification
  - Weakening of elastic lamellae
  - Neovascularization
  - Arterial obstruction
  - Thrombosis
- Oxidized low-density lipoprotein induces vascular smooth muscle cell apoptosis and cell death.
- Alteration of endothelial function involving mostly nitrous oxide pathways promotes platelet adhesion and aggregation, local clotting, and vascular growth and alters vascular tone.
- Decrease in elastin with aging along with collagen degeneration and increased intima-media thickness of arterial wall

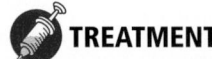

TREATMENT

INITIAL STABILIZATION
- Outpatient until complications occur
- Emphasis on prevention

GENERAL MEASURES
For details, see the following topics
- Essential hypertension
- Congestive heart failure
- Cerebrovascular accident
- Renal failure, chronic
- Dissecting aneurysm
- Thrombosis and embolism, arterial
- Diabetes
- Hyperlipidemia
- Hypothyroidism

Diet
American Heart Association Dietary recommendations are controversial, and have not been proven effective at lowering atherosclerotic risk
- Initial diet, step 1
  - Total fat <30% of total calories; saturated fat <10%
  - Carbohydrates 50–60% of total calories
  - Protein 10–20% of total calories
  - Cholesterol <300 mg a day
  - Total calories—amount required to achieve and maintain desirable weight
  - Sodium 1,650–2,400 mg
  - Alcohol <30 g
- Initial diet, step 2
  - Total fat <30% of total calories; saturated fat <7%
  - Carbohydrates 50–60% of total calories
  - Protein 10–20% of total calories
  - Cholesterol <200 mg per day
  - Total calories—amount required to achieve and maintain desirable weight
  - Sodium 1,650–2,400 mg
  - Alcohol <30 g
  - Antioxidants (vitamins A, E, C)

Activity
Encourage physical fitness as this will may progression (5)[B]

Complementary and Alternative Medicine
- Omega-3 fatty acids 1000 mg/d may be effective in lowering risk, but data are conflicting. (6)[C]
- Good evidence exists showing the following do NOT lower atherosclerotic risk:
- Vitamin E [I]
- lowering homocysteine levels (8)[I]
- Chelation therapy (9)[I]
- Anticoagulation (10)[D]
- Garlic (11)[I]
- No evidence that testosterone treatment is beneficial for aortic atherosclerosis (12)[D]

MEDICATION (DRUGS)

For details, see the following topics
- Essential hypertension
- Coronary arteriosclerosis
- Congestive heart failure
- Stroke
- Atrial arrhythmias
- Ventricular arrhythmias
- Renal failure, chronic
- Dissecting aneurysm
- Thrombosis and embolism, arterial
- Angina
- Myocardial infarction
- Arteriosclerotic heart disease
- Atherosclerotic occlusive disease
- Hypothyroidism
- Hyperlipidemia

SURGERY
- Angioplasty
- Stent
- Carotid endarterectomy
- Rotational atherectomy (13)[C]

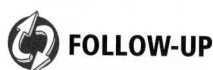 ## FOLLOW-UP

PROGNOSIS
Avoiding risk factors has greatly decreased mortality rates in the past decade.

COMPLICATIONS
- Coronary artery disease
- Renal failure
- Cerebrovascular accidents
- Dissecting or ruptured aneurysms
- Congestive heart failure
- Arterial thrombosis
- Gangrene
- Cardiac arrhythmias
- Sudden death

REFERENCES

1. Fauci AS, ed. *Harrison's Principles of Internal Medicine*. 14th ed. New York, NY: McGraw-Hill; 1998.
2. Guidelines for cardiopulmonary resuscitation and emergency cardiac care. *JAMA*. 1992;268:28.
3. Hunninghake D, ed. Lipid disorders. *Med Clin North Am*. 1994;78.
4. Hurst JW, et al. *The Heart*. 8th ed. New York, NY: McGraw-Hill; 1994.
5. Nordstrom CK, et al. Leisure time physical activity and early atherosclerosis: The Los Angeles Atherosclerosis Study. *Am J Med*. 115:19–25.
6. Omega-3 fatty acids for intermittent claudication. *The Cochrane Database of Systematic Reviews*. 2006, Issue 1.
7. Vitamin E for intermittent claudication. *The Cochrane Database of Systematic Reviews*. 2006, Issue 1.
8. Homocysteine lowering interventions for peripheral arterial disease and bypass grafts. *The Cochrane Database of Systematic Reviews*. 2006, Issue 1.
9. Chelation therapy for atherosclerotic cardiovascular disease. *The Cochrane Database of Systematic Reviews*. 2006, Issue 1.
10. Anticoagulants for intermittent claudication. *The Cochrane Database of Systematic Reviews*. 2006, Issue 1.
11. Garlic for peripheral vascular disease. *The Cochrane Database of Systematic Reviews*. 2006, Issue 1.
12. Steroid sex hormones for lower limb atherosclerosis. *The Cochrane Database of Systematic Reviews*. 2006, Issue 1.
13. PTRA for coronary artery disease. *The Cochrane Database of Systematic Reviews*. 2006, Issue 1.

 ## MISCELLANEOUS

- See also: Aortic Dissection; Arterial Embolus and Thrombosis; Atherosclerotic Occlusive Disease; Congestive Heart Failure; Hypertension, Essential; Renal Failure, Chronic; Stroke (Brain Attack)

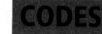 **CODES**

ICD9-CM
414.00 Coronary atherosclerosis of unspecified type of vessel, native, or graft

PATIENT TEACHING

- Crucial parts of preventing and treating atherosclerosis involve nutrition, fitness, and smoking cessation and treating modifiable risk factors.
- Extensive educational materials are available from many agencies (e.g., American Heart Association, U.S. Government Printing Office, National Cholesterol Education Program). Use these to help teach patients how to avoid or eliminate risk factors.

 See Corresponding Diagnostic Algorithm

ATRIAL FIBRILLATION

Leonard Ganz, MD
Leonard S. Lilly, MD

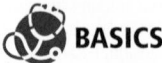 **BASICS**

DESCRIPTION
- Chronic or paroxysmal arrhythmia is characterized by chaotic atrial electrical activity.
- Clinical pattern
  - Paroxysmal AF (PAF)—episodes are self-terminating.
  - Persistent—sinus rhythm can be restored through pharmacologic or direct current (DC) cardioversion
  - Permanent sinus rhythm cannot be restored for meaningful period of time
- Electrophysiologic mechanism is most likely multiple re-entrant wavelets within the atria.
- In some patients, triggering premature atrial beats and/or bursts of tachycardia emanate from the pulmonary venous ostia or other sites.
- Because the atrioventricular node is bombarded with nearly continuous atrial electrical impulses, the ventricular response is irregular and usually rapid (may exceed 160 beats per minute).
- Symptoms vary from none to mild (palpitations, lightheadedness, fatigue, poor exercise capacity) to severe (angina, dyspnea, syncope). Symptoms are frequently more serious in patients with structural heart disease.
- In some patients with Wolff-Parkinson-White syndrome, atrial fibrillation may be extremely rapid and degenerate into ventricular fibrillation.

ALERT
Geriatric Considerations
Both the incidence of atrial fibrillation and the stroke risk of atrial fibrillation increase with age.

Pediatric Considerations
Uncommon in children with normal hearts; seen in congenital heart disease and in surgical repair.

Pregnancy Considerations
- Atrial fibrillation is unusual during pregnancy in the absence of structural heart disease.
- The use of digoxin is safe; beta-blockers, procainamide, and quinidine are probably safe. Limited information regarding calcium blockers
- The risk of fetal hemorrhage makes anticoagulation problematic; moreover, warfarin causes fetal anomalies. SC heparin is best choice if long-term anticoagulation is necessary.
- Direct current cardioversion does not harm fetus.

GENERAL PREVENTION
- Ethanol may trigger atrial fibrillation in some.
- In cardiomyopathy/heart failure, hemodynamic decompensation may trigger atrial fibrillation.

EPIDEMIOLOGY
- Incidence/prevalence increases with age.
- Predominant sex: Male > Female

Prevalence
- Estimated at 1 per 1,000 adults per year; estimated at 2–4% of adult population
- Approximately 2–4% of septuagenarians, 5–10% of octogenarians

RISK FACTORS
- Hypertension
- Diabetes mellitus
- Left ventricular hypertrophy
- Coronary artery disease

- Congestive heart failure
- Rheumatic heart disease
- Hyperthyroidism
- Post-surgical state (cardiothoracic surgery)

Genetics
There is no specific genetic pattern.

ETIOLOGY
- Hypertensive heart disease
- Valvular/rheumatic heart disease
- Coronary artery disease
- Acute myocardial infarction
- Pulmonary embolus
- Cardiomyopathy
- Congestive heart failure
- Infiltrative heart disease
- Pericarditis
- Ingestion (e.g., ethanol in "holiday heart")
- Hyperthyroidism
- Postoperative (e.g., cardiothoracic surgery)
- Sick sinus (tachy-brady) syndrome
- Idiopathic (including "lone" atrial fibrillation)

ASSOCIATED CONDITIONS
- Wolff-Parkinson-White syndrome
- Sick sinus syndrome
- Atrial flutter
  - A related arrhythmia with regular atrial electrical activity, typical rate 250–350, manifested as sawtooth "flutter" waves on ECG. 2:1 or 4:1 conduction through the atrioventricular node to the ventricle is usual, so the pulse is frequently regular.
  - Patients may have atrial fibrillation and flutter.
  - Management for both arrhythmias is similar; atrial flutter is more difficult to control pharmacologically and more easily electrically cardioverted than is atrial fibrillation.
  - Although atrial flutter alone may pose a lower a risk of thromboembolism than atrial fibrillation, guidelines for anticoagulation of atrial flutter and atrial fibrillation are the same.
  - Radiofrequency catheter ablation to cure atrial flutter is widely applied.

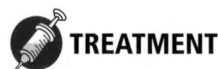 **DIAGNOSIS**

SIGNS AND SYMPTOMS
- Irregular pulse
- Tachycardia
- Heart failure
- Hypotension
- Palpitations
- Lightheadedness
- Poor exercise capacity
- Fatigue
- Dyspnea
- Angina
- Near syncope/syncope
- Stroke
- Arterial embolization

History
- Palpitations, dyspnea, lightheadedness, etc.
- Cardiac risk factors common

Physical Exam
Irregularly irregular pulse, frequently tachycardia

TESTS
- ECG is diagnostic; low amplitude fibrillatory waves without discrete P waves; irregularly irregular pattern of QRS complexes
- The Holter monitor and event monitor are helpful in diagnosing paroxysmal atrial fibrillation.

Lab
- TSH to screen for hyperthyroidism
- INR/PT in patients treated with warfarin

Imaging
- Chest x-ray for cardiopulmonary disease
- Echocardiogram for structural heart disease
- Spiral chest CT scan (or other tests such as D-dimer, ventilation-perfusion scan, or pulmonary angiography) if pulmonary embolus suspected
- Transesophageal echocardiography to detect left atrial appendage thrombus if cardioversion

Diagnostic Procedures/Surgery
- Evaluation for ischemia not generally indicated unless sign/symptoms are present
- Evaluation for pulmonary embolus not indicated unless signs/symptoms are present

Pathological Findings
- Atrial dilatation
- Atrial injury (chronic or acute)
- Atrial thrombus, especially in atrial appendage
- Sclerosis/fibrosis of sinoatrial node
- Coronary artery disease, valvular/rheumatic disease, cardiomyopathy, pulmonary embolus

DIFFERENTIAL DIAGNOSIS
- Multifocal atrial tachycardia
- Sinus tachycardia with frequent atrial premature beats
- Atrial flutter (see "Associated Conditions")

TREATMENT

INITIAL STABILIZATION
- Inpatient if
  - Significant symptoms
  - Extremely rapid ventricular rate
  - Initiating antiarrhythmic therapy
  - Atrial fibrillation triggered by acute process (acute myocardial infarction, congestive heart failure, pulmonary embolus)
  - High risk for stroke (rheumatic heart disease, prior transient ischemic attack/stroke)
- Outpatient management for low-risk patients

GENERAL MEASURES
- Avoid potential triggers.
  - Avoid ethanol, caffeine, and nicotine.
  - Manage underlying structural heart disease.
- Prevent complications.
  - Anticoagulation to reduce the risk of embolic complications
  - Antibiotic prophylaxis if atrial fibrillation is due to valvular heart disease
- Therapy strategies
  - Ventricular rate control with atrioventricular nodal blocking agents

- Restore and maintain sinus rhythm with antiarrhythmic drugs.
- Nonpharmacologic therapies

Diet
As appropriate for underlying heart disease

Activity
- As tolerated
- When treated, minimal impairment in patients

ALERT
- Clinical risk factors for stroke
  - Age >65
  - Diabetes
  - Hypertension
  - History of stroke or transient ischemic attack
  - History of congestive heart failure
- Echocardiographic risk factors for stroke
  - Left atrial enlargement
  - Mitral regurgitation
  - Left ventricular dysfunction

Nursing
Monitor vital signs, symptoms

 ## MEDICATION (DRUGS)

- Anticoagulation
  - Unless contraindicated, patients with atrial fibrillation with any risk factors for stroke should receive warfarin to maintain an international normalized ratio of 2.0–3.0.
  - Patients in whom warfarin is contraindicated should receive aspirin 325 mg/day—appropriate in low-risk patients (e.g., age <65 years with no risk factors for stroke)
  - Paroxysmal atrial fibrillation treatment same as for chronic atrial fibrillation
- Routine use of antiarrhythmic drugs to maintain sinus rhythm has not proved beneficial. Antiarrhythmic drugs may be used when a specific indication for sinus rhythm maintenance exists.
- Control of ventricular rate:
  - Beta-blockers (propranolol, metoprolol, atenolol, nadolol)
  - Non-dihydropyridine calcium channel blockers (diltiazem and verapamil)
  - Cardiac glycosides (digoxin), which might be less effective than other agents in controlling ventricular response
- Conversion to/maintenance of sinus rhythm
  - DC cardioversion
  - Antiarrhythmic therapy for chemical cardioversion and maintenance of sinus rhythm following cardioversion carries a risk of pro-arrhythmia.
  - Ibutilide, an intravenous type III agent, for chemical cardioversion of atrial fibrillation and flutter of short duration (<90 days)
  - If duration of atrial fibrillation is >24–48 hours or unknown, treat with warfarin for ≥3 weeks before and 4 weeks after cardioversion. Or, once anticoagulation is established, perform transesophageal echocardiography. If no atrial thrombus, may cardiovert. Anticoagulation should be continued for ≥4 weeks thereafter.
  - Long-term, and perhaps indefinite, anticoagulation should be considered.

- Chronic oral antiarrhythmic therapy to suppress atrial fibrillation recurrences
  - Type IA (procainamide, disopyramide, quinidine)
  - Type IC (flecainide, propafenone) in patients with structurally normal hearts or mild hypertensive heart disease
  - Type III (sotalol, amiodarone, dofetilide)
- Acute therapy for hemodynamically compromised patients
  - Heparin for anticoagulation
  - IV beta or calcium channel blocker for control of ventricular rate
  - Pharmacologic and/or direct current cardioversion

Contraindications
- Active bleeding precludes anticoagulation; the risk of bleeding is a relative contraindication to long-term anticoagulation.
- Warfarin is contraindicated in patients with a history of warfarin skin necrosis.
- Type IC drugs are contraindicated in patients with coronary artery disease and cardiomyopathy.
- Type IA drugs (sotalol, ibutilide, and dofetilide) should not be used in patients with torsade de pointes history.

Precautions
- With type IA drugs, the risk of torsade de pointes increases with the extent of QT interval prolongation (i.e., the QTc).
  - Avoid other drugs that prolong QT interval, such as phenothiazines, tricyclic antidepressants, terfenadine, astemizole, and erythromycin.
  - Avoid hypokalemia and hypomagnesemia.
  - Torsade de pointes due to drug-induced long QT syndrome is said to be "pause dependent" as the risk increases with bradycardia, heart block, and sinus pauses.
- With type IC drugs, stress testing to exclude exercise-induced arrhythmia or QRS widening.
- With amiodarone, careful surveillance for hepatic, thyroid, pulmonary, skin, and ophthalmologic adverse effects is necessary.
- In many patients, adequate medical therapy of atrial fibrillation will cause bradycardia necessitating a permanent pacemaker.

Significant possible interactions
- Quinidine increases digoxin levels.
- Amiodarone increases digoxin levels and enhances effects of warfarin.

SURGERY
- Radiofrequency catheter ablation procedures to prevent atrial fibrillation recurrence in patients with both paroxysmal and persistent AF. Reserve catheter ablation for highly symptomatic patients who have failed drug therapy.
- Cardiac surgery (e.g., the "maze procedure") may be considered in severely symptomatic, medically refractory patients.
- Permanent dual chamber pacing may reduce the incidence of new onset atrial fibrillation and reduces the frequency of episodes of PAF in patients with sick sinus syndrome.
- Radiofrequency catheter ablation of atrioventricular node with pacemaker implantation in symptomatic medically refractory patients
- Consider implantable defibrillators to cardiovert atrial fibrillation in selected patients.

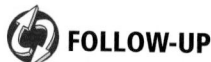 ## FOLLOW-UP

PROGNOSIS
- The stroke risk is low with anticoagulation.
- Atrial fibrillation increases the risk of morbidity and mortality, but prognosis is a function of underlying heart disease.

COMPLICATIONS
- Embolic stroke
- Peripheral arterial embolization
- Complications of pharmacologic therapy (bradyarrhythmias and torsade de pointes)
- Bleeding with anticoagulation

PATIENT MONITORING
- ECG/Holter to monitor rhythm
- Maintain INR at 2.0–3.0
- ECG to monitor QTc interval if on antiarrhythmic therapy
- Careful follow-up of antiarrhythmic drug

REFERENCES
1. ACC/AHA/ESC. Guidelines on the management of patients with atrial fibrillation. *J Am Coll Cardiol*. 2001;38:1231–1265.
2. Falk RH. Atrial fibrillation. *N Engl J Med*. 2001;344:1067–1078.
3. Prystowsky EN, Benson DW, Fuster V, et al. Management of patients with atrial fibrillation. *Circulation*. 1996;93:1262–1277.
4. Riley RD, Pritchell ELC. Pharmacologic management of atrial fibrillation. *J Cardiovasc Electrophysiol*. 1997;8:818–829.

 ## MISCELLANEOUS

- Other notes: The risk of stroke is extremely low in young patients without structural heart disease, so called "lone atrial fibrillation."
- See also: Atrial Flutter

CODES

ICD9-CM
- 427.31 Atrial fibrillation
- 427.32 Atrial flutter

 See Corresponding Diagnostic Algorithm

ATRIAL FLUTTER

Drew M. Keister, MD

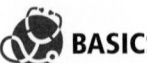 **BASICS**

DESCRIPTION
- Atrial flutter (A. Flutter) is a cardiac arrhythmia resulting in a narrow-QRS tachycardia with an atrial rate of 250–350 beats per minute.
  - "Saw-toothed" P-waves are classic.
    - Usually most prominent in lead V1
  - Ventricular rate is dependent upon AV node conduction (see Pathophysiology).
- System(s) Affected: Cardiac

EPIDEMIOLOGY
- Predominant age: Most patients >55 years old
- Predominant sex: 2.5:1 Male predominance

Incidence
88 per 100,000 person-years

Prevalence
Range: 0.2% in young adults −0.9% in 65+

RISK FACTORS
- Heart disease (e.g. left ventricular (LV) dysfunction, LV hypertrophy, valvular heart disease (especially rheumatic), coronary artery disease (CAD), acute MI, atrial fibrillation (A Fib), pericarditis, history of congenital heart disease, recent cardiac surgery, atrial scarring)
- Pulmonary disease (e.g. COPD, pulmonary embolism, pneumonia)
- Hypertension (HTN)
- Hyperthyroidism
- Obesity

PATHOPHYSIOLOGY
Most commonly caused by a rapid re-entrant circuit around the tricuspid valve (specifically, the cavotricuspid isthmus)
- AV node conduction is variable
  - 2:1 most common; rate usually 150 bpm
  - 3:1 possible; rate approx 100 bpm
  - 1:1 rare; ventricular rate 200+ bpm
  - Irregular conduction can cause irregularly irregular pulse, mimicking A Fib

ETIOLOGY
- Most cases associated with a predisposing factor (see "Risk Factors")
- Lone A. Flutter; no predisposing factor
  - 1.7% of patients with atrial flutter
- Digitalis toxicity; rare cause

ASSOCIATED CONDITIONS
- See "Risk Factors"
- Occurs in ~ 30% of patients with A Fib

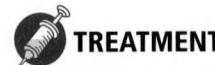 **DIAGNOSIS**

SIGNS AND SYMPTOMS
History
- Common
  - Palpitations
  - Shortness of breath
  - Fatigue
  - Light-headedness
- Less common
  - Chest pain
  - Near-syncope
  - Insidious onset with fatigue or worsening of a chronic cardiac/pulmonary disease
- Rare
  - Syncope
  - Symptoms/signs of acute embolic stroke

Physical Exam
- Common: Often fairly normal exam
  - Tachycardia
    - May be regular or irregularly irregular
  - Mild dyspnea
  - Evidence of a predisposing factor
- Less common
  - Moderate dyspnea
  - Congestive heart failure
    - More common in elderly or with prior history
- Rarely, hemodynamic compromise occurs
  - Hypotension
  - Severe dyspnea or respiratory failure
  - Hypoxia with cyanosis or pallor
  - Decreased level of consciousness

TESTS
Lab
- A serum TSH is indicated to exclude hyperthyroidism.
- When clinically indicated
  - CBC if at risk for anemia
  - Metabolic panel if renal disease, HTN
  - Digoxin level
  - PTT/PT/INR if considering anticoagulation

Imaging
- Chest x-ray to exclude lung disease or CHF
- Echocardiogram to assess LV function

Diagnostic Procedures/Surgery
- 12-lead ECG
  - Narrow-complex tachycardia with classic saw-toothed P-waves in V1 or inferior leads
  - Assess for signs of ischemia/infarction
- When clinically indicated
  - Holter monitor: If symptoms are concerning, but rhythm not present at time of evaluation
  - Electrophysiologic studies should be considered in patients with recurrent atrial flutter to map the source of the arrhythmia for possible ablation.

DIFFERENTIAL DIAGNOSIS
- A Fib
- Paroxysmal supraventricular tachycardia
- Sinus tachycardia
- Junctional tachycardia
- Multifocal atrial tachycardia
- Wolff-Parkinson-White Syndrome

TREATMENT

PRE HOSPITAL
- Support ABCs
- Consider immediate cardioversion for hemodynamically unstable patients, if available.
- Initiate O_2, IV; monitor throughout transport.
- Consider calcium channel blocker or beta-blocker for rate control, if available.

INITIAL STABILIZATION
First priority is to determine stability of patient
- Hemodynamically stable
  - Continue ABC support.
  - Consider calcium channel blocker or beta-blocker for rate control. (1)[C]
- Hemodynamically unstable (see "Physical Exam—hemodynamic compromise"):
  - DC cardioversion is best treatment. (1)[C]
  - Begin with dose of 50 joules and increase as needed. (1)[C]
  - Atrial overdrive pacing is also effective. (1)[C]

GENERAL MEASURES
- Identify and treat underlying causes first.
- A. flutter often self-resolves within days.
  - Watchful waiting may be appropriate in hemodynamically stable patients, particularly with a reversible predisposing cause and normal left atrial size.
- Restoration of normal sinus rhythm is generally the goal of therapy. (1)[C]
  - Self-limited A. flutter related to an underlying cause rarely requires chronic therapy. (1)[C]
  - >50% of patients with chronic or recurrent A. flutter experience recurrence within 1 year of successful cardioversion. (2)

Diet
NPO unless heart rate controlled, hemodynamically stable and no plan to ablate

Activity
Bed rest until heart rate controlled and patient hemodynamically stable

Nursing
Strict I/Os to assess for fluid retention/CHF

SPECIAL THERAPY
IV Fluids
- If hemodynamic unstable, use fluid boluses to maintain blood pressure
- Caution in LV dysfunction: avoid CHF
- If NPO, use appropriate maintenance fluid

MEDICATION (DRUGS)

EMBOLIC STROKE PREVENTION

- Use anticoagulation (coumadin or heparin) for stroke prevention before cardioversion and when A. flutter persists >48 hours, except in patients <65 with lone A. flutter. (3)[C]

First Line
Rate Control Agents

- Rate control agents useful in the initial management, but generally not efficacious in controlling chronic or recurrent arrhythmia. (1)[C]
- Calcium-channel blockers
  - Diltiazem (Cardizem)
    - Initial dose: 0.25 mg/kg IV × 1, may give 0.35 mg/kg IV × 1 after 15 min if needed
    - Maintenance: 5–15 mg/h IV up to 24 h
    - Rate control usually achieved in 30 min (1)
  - Verapamil (Isoptin, Calan, Verelan)
    - Initial dose: 2.5–5 mg IV over 2 minutes, may repeat 5–10 mg dose after 15–30 minutes to max dose of 20 mg
    - Pediatric dose
      <1 yr: 0.1–0.2 mg/kg IV over 2 min, may repeat × 1 in 30 min;
      1–15 years: 0.1–0.3 mg/kg (max 5 mg) IV over 2 min; repeat (max 10 mg) in 30 min
    - As efficacious as diltiazem; increased hypotension (1)
  - Contraindications: Hypotension, documented sensitivity, 2nd or 3rd degree AV block, severe CHF, sick sinus syndrome
  - Precautions: Use caution with CHF, LV dysfunction, liver or kidney disease
  - Interactions: May increase digoxin levels; with amiodarone or beta-blockers may severely decrease cardiac output
  - Adverse reactions: Hypotension, CHF, peripheral edema, AV block
- Beta-blockers
  - Rate control usually achieved in 30 min (1)
  - Metoprolol (Lopressor)
    - Initial: 5 mg IV, repeat q5min; Max: 15 mg
    - Maintenance: 5–15 mg IV q3–6h
  - Esmolol (Breviblock)
    - Initial dose: 500 mcg/kg IV over 1 min, repeat q4min to total of 3 doses if needed
    - Maintenance: 50 mcg/kg/min, increased by 50 mcg/kg/min q4min prn—max of 200 mcg/kg/min
    - Half-life approx 8 min; good choice for patients at risk for complications
  - Contraindications: Hypotension, documented sensitivity, 2nd or 3rd degree AV block, severe CHF, sick sinus syndrome
  - Precautions: Use caution with CHF, LV dysfunction, kidney disease, asthma
  - Interactions: Bradycardia with digoxin; with amiodarone or beta-blockers may severely decrease cardiac output
  - Adverse reactions: Hypotension, CHF, peripheral edema, AV block

- Digoxin (Lanoxin)
  - Initial dose: 0.75 mg–1.25 mg PO or 0.5–1 mg IV divided 50% initially, then 25% × 2q6–12h
  - Maintenance: 0.125–0.5 mg PO per day or 0.1–0.4 mg IV per day
  - Therapeutic level: 0.8–2 ng/mL
  - Contraindications: Documented sensitivity, sick sinus syndrome, IHSS
  - Precautions: Use caution with electrolyte abnormalities (especially hypokalemia, hypercalcemia), impaired renal function, thyroid disease, acute MI, AV block
  - Interactions: Unpredictable effects with many anti-arrhythmics; additive bradycardia with calcium-channel blockers, beta-blockers
  - Adverse reactions: AV block, bradycardia, mental disturbances, nausea
  - Rate control usually achieved in 4 hours (1)

Second Line
Anti-Arrhythmics

- Pure Class III Anti-arrhythmics
  - Ibutilide (Corvert)
    - Initial dose: <60 kg: 0.01 mg/kg over 10 minutes; 60 kg: 1 mg over 10 minutes; may repeat in 10 minutes prn
  - Dofetilide (Tykosyn)
    - Dosing: Dependent on QTc interval and creatinine clearance, see package insert
    - Oral medication
  - Contraindications: Documented sensitivity, QTc > 440 ms, use of a class I or III anti-arrhythmic within 4 hours, structural heart disease, sinus node disease
  - Precautions: Correct hypokalemia and hypomagnesium prior to use; use caution in AV block, CHF, QT prolongation, renal/hepatic disease, elderly patients
  - Interactions: Many anti-arrhythmics have unpredictable effects with digoxin; additive bradycardia with calcium-channel blockers, beta-blockers
  - Adverse reactions: Polymorphic VT/torsades de pointes (1.5–3%), AV block, QT prolongation, CHF, renal failure, allergy, hypotension, hypertension, headache (4%)
  - Efficacy = 38–76% (1)
- Class 1a and 1c anti-arrhythmics, sotalol, beta-blockers, calcium channel blockers, and amiodarone have limited utility in converting A. flutter to sinus rhythm. (1)

SURGERY

Catheter ablation is the treatment of choice for patients with recurrent or chronic A. flutter. (1)[A]

- 80% remain in sinus rhythm at 21 months compared to 36% with anti-arrhythmics. (1)
- To prevent rehospitalization with ablation compared to anti-arrhythmics, NNT is 2.2. (1)
- Catheter ablation results in improved symptoms and improved quality of life. (1)

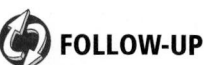

FOLLOW-UP

DISPOSITION

Admission Criteria

- Most patients with first diagnosis of persistent A. flutter require admission for cardiac monitoring.
- All patients who cannot be rate controlled in the outpatient setting should be admitted.
- Patients with hemodynamic compromise may require ICU admission.

Discharge Criteria

Hemodynamically stable patients with normal heart rates may be discharged in A. flutter, but most patients admitted until sinus rhythm restored

Issues for Referral

Cardiology consult suggested for refractory cases and for patients with multiple comorbidities

PROGNOSIS

Incidence of embolization with A. flutter is similar to A. fib, 1.7–7%. (1)

COMPLICATIONS

- Acute stroke/other embolic events
- Congestive heart failure
- Acute cardiopulmonary failure

PATIENT MONITORING

Patients with chronic atrial flutter require monitoring of anticoagulation and LV function.

REFERENCES

1. Blonstrom-Lundqvist C, Schienman MM, et al. ACC/AHA/ESC guidelines for the management of patients with supraventricular arrhythmias-executive summary. *J Am Coll Cardiol*. 2003;42(8):1493–1531.
2. Crijns HJ, Van Gelder IC, Tieleman RG, et al. Long-term outcome of electrical cardioversion in patients with chronic atrial flutter. *Heart*. 1997;77(1):56–61.
3. Scholten MF, Thornton AS, Mekel JM, et al. Anticoagulation in atrial fibrillation and flutter. *Europace*. 2005;7(5):492–499.

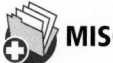 MISCELLANEOUS

See also: Atrial Fibrillation

 CODES

ICD9-CM
427.32 Atrial Flutter

PATIENT TEACHING

Activity

Patients with chronic or recurrent A. flutter may perform activity as tolerated if rate-controlled.

See Corresponding Diagnostic Algorithm

ATRIAL SEPTAL DEFECT (ASD)

Ryan Johnson, MD
Brent J. Barber, MD

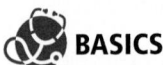 **BASICS**

DESCRIPTION
- A defect or opening in the atrial septum allowing flow of blood between the two chambers
- Shunting
  - Typically left to right; occurs in late ventricular systole and early diastole
  - Degree depends on size of the defect and relative compliance of the two ventricles
  - Can be minimal right-to-left shunting in early ventricular systole, especially during inspiration
- Symptoms typically occur due to right ventricular and pulmonary vascular volume overload, sometimes with resultant pulmonary hypertension
- Types
  - Ostium secundum occurs in the region of the fossa ovalis (most common).
  - Sinus venosus occurs in the superior-posterior septum, usually associated with partial anomalous pulmonary venous return.
  - Ostium primum occurs in the inferior portion of the septum (often associated with cleft mitral valve).
- System(s) Affected: Cardiovascular, Pulmonary

ALERT
Geriatric Considerations
Defects may still be closed surgically.

Pediatric Considerations
Most frequently appears in this age group

Pregnancy Considerations
Evaluate prior to pregnancy, because condition may worsen.

GENERAL PREVENTION
Evaluate prior to pregnancy

EPIDEMIOLOGY
- Predominant age: Newborn, but may be diagnosed at any age
- Predominant sex: Female > Male (2:1)

Incidence
Accounts for 10% of congenital heart defects

RISK FACTORS
- Congenital heart disease
- Family history

Genetics
Congenital, associated with multiple syndromes, rarely familial

ETIOLOGY
Unknown

ASSOCIATED CONDITIONS
- Mitral stenosis
- Mitral regurgitation
- Anomalous pulmonary venous return
- Multiple congenital syndromes

 DIAGNOSIS

SIGNS AND SYMPTOMS
- Easy fatigability, dyspnea on exertion, heart failure (late)
- Signs vary according to extent of shunting
  - Prominent precordial bulge
  - Right ventricular lift
  - Palpable pulmonary artery pulse
  - Fixed, widely split S2
  - Pulmonic flow murmur
  - Low-pitched diastolic murmur at left lower sternal border
  - Cyanosis and clubbing (with severe pulmonary hypertension: Eisenmenger syndrome)
  - Stroke due to paradoxical emboli

ALERT
Pediatric Considerations
Childhood symptoms
- Usually minimal
- Can include failure to thrive and frequent pulmonary infections

TESTS
Lab
- ECG findings
  - Ostium secundum: Rightward axis, right ventricular hypertrophy, rSR' pattern in V1
  - Sinus venosus: Leftward axis, inverted P wave in lead III
  - Ostium primum: Leftward axis
    Note: All may be associated with PR prolongation.

Imaging
- X-ray: Varying degrees of cardiac enlargement, increased pulmonary vascular workings
- Cardiac magnetic resonance imaging
- Cardiac catheterization (indicated in select patients) demonstrates right ventricle enlargement and location of the shunt.
- Echocardiography

Diagnostic Procedures/Surgery
- Cardiac magnetic resonance imaging
- Cardiac angiography
- Echo and Doppler
- Transesophageal echo in adults

Pathological Findings
- Gross defect in atrial septum
- Dilated right atrium, right ventricle
- Enlarged pulmonary artery

DIFFERENTIAL DIAGNOSIS
Other congenital heart disease, right bundle branch block (for widely split S2)

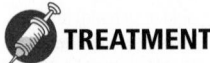 **TREATMENT**

GENERAL MEASURES
- Appropriate health care: Referral/evaluation by a cardiologist
- Majority of small ASDs will close spontaneously, however, close follow-up is warranted. (1,2) [B]

Activity
As tolerated

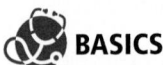 **MEDICATION (DRUGS)**

- Antibiotic prophylaxis (not for secundum atrial septal defect)
- Anticoagulation if paradoxical emboli

SURGERY
- Closure via percutaneous transcatheter device or surgery(particularly when the pulmonary systemic flow ratio is $\geq 1.5:1$, or evidence of right heart enlargement)
- Percutaneous transcatheter device closure of secundum atrial septal defects and patent foramen ovale is now considered a standard and low-risk procedure that has widely replaced the surgical approach. (3)[A]
- Closure is usually delayed until preschool age (2–4 years), except for large defects to be repaired earlier.
- Closure in adult patients with stroke reduces the risk of further neurologic events. (4)[B] However, device closure of a patent foramen ovale in the adult population remains controversial.
- New evidence suggests symptomatic migraine relief following patent foramen ovale closure. (5)[B]

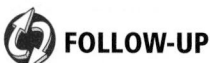 **FOLLOW-UP**

PROGNOSIS
- Course: chronic
- 50% mortality by age 50 years in untreated patients with large defects
- Favorable in surgically treated symptomatic patients

COMPLICATIONS
- Congestive heart failure
- Cyanosis
- Late-onset arrhythmias 10–20 years after surgery (5%)
- Stroke
- Pulmonary hypertension
- Eisenmenger syndrome
- Infective endocarditis

PATIENT MONITORING
- Until defect has closed
- Routine echocardiography follow-up

REFERENCES

1. Helgason H, Jonsdottir G. Spontaneous closure of atrial septal defects. *Pediatr Cardiol*. 1999;20:195–199.
2. McMahon CJ, Feltes TF, Fraley JK, et al. Natural history of growth of secundum atrial septal defects and implications for transcatheter closure. *Heart*. 2002;87:256–259.
3. Holzer R, Hijazi ZM. Interventional approach to congenital heart disease. *Curr Opin Cardiol*. 2004;19:84–90.
4. Onorato E, Melzi G, Casilli F, et al. Patent foramen ovale with paradoxical embolism: Mid-term results of transcatheter closure in 256 patients. *J Interv Cardiol*. 2003;16:43–50.
5. Morandi E, Anzola GP, Angeli S, et al. Transcatheter closure of patent foramen ovale: A new migraine treatment? *J Interv Cardiol*. 2003;16:39–42.
6. Friedman WF, Perloff JK Congenital heart disease in infancy and childhood. In: Braunwald E, ed. *Heart Disease*. 4th ed. Philadelphia: WB Saunders; 1992.
7. Hillis DL, Lange RA, Winniford MD, Page RL. *Manual of Clinical Problems in Cardiology*. New York: Little, Brown; 1995.

 MISCELLANEOUS

See also: Aortic Valvular Stenosis; Coarctation of the Aorta; Complete Atrioventricular (AV) Canal; Patent Ductus Arteriosus; Pulmonic Valvular Stenosis; Tetralogy of Fallot; Ventricular Septal Defect (VSD)

CODES

ICD9-CM
429.71 Acquired cardiac septal defect

PATIENT TEACHING

For patient education materials on this topic, contact: American Heart Association, 7320 Greenville Avenue, Dallas, TX 75231, (214) 373-6300.

ATTENTION DEFICIT/HYPERACTIVITY DISORDER

Laura L. Novak, MD

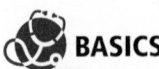 **BASICS**

DESCRIPTION
- Behavior problem characterized by a short attention span, distractibility, low frustration tolerance, impulsivity, and hyperactivity. Attention deficit disorder (ADD) is ADHD without the impulsivity and hyperactivity.
- Can result in poor school performance, difficulty in peer relationships, and parent/child conflict
- System(s) Affected: Nervous
- Synonym(s): Attention deficit disorder; Hyperactivity

GENERAL PREVENTION
- Children are at risk for abuse, depression, and social isolation.
- Parents need regular support and advice.
- Establish contact with teacher each school year.

EPIDEMIOLOGY
- Predominant age
  - Onset <7 years old
  - Lasts into adolescence and adulthood
  - 50% meet diagnostic criteria by age 4 years.
- Predominant sex: Male > Female (5:1); ADD without hyperactivity may be more common in girls

Incidence
5% of school-aged children

RISK FACTORS
- Family history
- Comorbid conditions (associated with, but not caused by)
  - Learning disabilities
  - Mood disorders
  - Oppositional defiant disorder
  - Conduct disorder

Genetics
Familial pattern

ETIOLOGY
Multifactorial

ASSOCIATED CONDITIONS
See "Risk Factors"

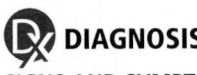 **DIAGNOSIS**

SIGNS AND SYMPTOMS
- The AAP guidelines recommend using the *DSM-IV* criteria to establish the diagnosis of ADHD.
- *DSM-IV*: 6 or more inattention criteria and/or 6 or more hyperactivity/impulsivity criteria. Symptoms must begin by age 7 years, be present for >6 months, and be noticed in 2 settings (e.g., home and school).
- Inattention
  - Careless mistakes in tasks
  - Difficulty sustaining attention
  - Doesn't seem to listen
  - Doesn't follow through or finish tasks
  - Difficulty organizing tasks
  - Avoids tasks that require sustained mental effort
  - Loses things
  - Easily distracted
  - Forgetful

- Hyperactivity/Impulsivity
  - Fidgets
  - Difficulty remaining seated
  - Runs or climbs excessively
  - Difficulty playing quietly
  - Acts as if "driven by a motor"
  - Talks excessively
  - Blurts out answers before question is complete
  - Has difficulty awaiting turn
  - Interrupts others

History
- Birth and development history
  - Good psychosocial evaluation of home environment
- School performance history

TESTS
- Behavioral testing
  - Behavior rating scales (Connors, others) should be completed by parents and teachers. They are repeated after therapy is started to gauge differences (*DSM-IV* criteria can be used).
  - Testing for learning disability (e.g., dyslexia) through the school

Lab
Rarely needed, can check lead level

Diagnostic Procedures/Surgery
- Diagnosis is by *DSM-IV* criteria.
- Electroencephalogram not needed unless symptoms are highly suggestive of seizure disorder (e.g., absence seizures)

Pathological Findings
Motor tics can be present (e.g., cough, noises, twitching).

DIFFERENTIAL DIAGNOSIS
- Refer to *DSM-IV* (see References).
- Activity level appropriate for age
- Dysfunctional family situation
- Learning disability (e.g., dyslexia)
- Hearing/vision disorder
- Oppositional/defiant disorder (see *DSM-IV*)
- Conduct disorder (see *DSM-IV*)
- Lead poisoning
- Medication reaction (decongestant, antihistamine, theophylline, phenobarbital)
- Tourette syndrome—motor tics and coprolalia
- Pervasive developmental delay (autism)
- Asberger syndrome—high functioning autism
- Absence seizures (attention deficit only)

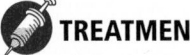 **TREATMENT**

GENERAL MEASURES
- Parent/school/patient education
- Work closely with teacher.
- Avoid unproved therapies.

Diet
No dietary changes have been proven to help attention deficit/hyperactivity disorder.

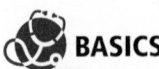 **MEDICATION (DRUGS)**

First Line
The American Academy of Pediatrics has recommended in their guideline (1)[C] that stimulant medications should be the first line in treatment of ADHD. It also recommends that a second type of stimulant be tried if the first treatment fails. As of this writing, the FDA is considering applying a "black box" warning to stimulants based on some reported cases of sudden death seen in patients using stimulant medications.
- Stimulant
  - Methylphenidate (Ritalin, Concerta, Metadate CD, Ritalin LA, others): Ritalin 5–20 mg in the morning, at noon, and at 4 pm; maximum dose 60 mg/d (short-acting); Concerta 18, 36, 54 mg in the morning; Metadate CD 40 mg in the morning; Ritalin LA 20, 30, 40 mg in the morning (long-acting)
- Precautions
  - If not responding, check compliance and consider another diagnosis. (1)[C]
  - Some children experience withdrawal (tearfulness, agitation) after a missed dose.
  - Methylphenidate has become a drug of abuse and should be monitored carefully: 20 mg nongeneric has highest street value
  - Drug holidays should only be given if family/peer relationships are not harmed.
- Significant possible interactions
  - Stimulants may increase levels of anticonvulsants, selective serotonin reuptake inhibitors, tricyclics, and warfarin.

ALERT

Pregnancy Considerations
Medications used in ADHD are category C—caution in pregnancy

Second Line
- Amphetamine (stimulant)
- Adderall carries a "black box" warning for potential drug abuse
  - Adderall: 2.5–20 mg q4–6h
  - Adderall XR: 5–30 mg every morning; ≥ 6 years
- Nonstimulant
  - Atomoxetine carries a "black box" warning regarding potential exacerbation of suicidality (similar to selective serotonin reuptake inhibitors). Because of this, the manufacturer recommends weekly visits for 4 weeks, then every other week visits for four sessions, then every 12 week visits. Atomoxetine has also been associated with hepatic injury in a small number of cases, and the manufacturer recommends checking liver enzymes if symptoms (jaundice, fatigue, malaise) develop.
  - Atomoxetine (Strattera); selective norepinephrine reuptake inhibitor; 0.5–2 mg/kg/d every morning (10 mg, 18 mg, 25 mg, 40 mg, 60 mg). Maximum dose 1.4 mg/kg/d or 100 mg/d, whichever is less.
  - Slower onset of efficacy; gastrointestinal side effects and sedation. Not addictive
  - Atomoxetine interacts with paroxetine (Paxil), fluoxetine (Prozac), and quinidine

- Other nonstimulant drugs (e.g., clonidine, tricyclic antidepressants, selective serotonin reuptake inhibitors): Due to the mixed efficacy and high side effects of these drugs, they are not recommended for use without a consultant.

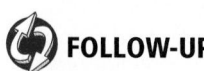

FOLLOW-UP

PROGNOSIS

- May last through school years and into adulthood
- May become easier to control with increasing age
- Encourage career choices that allow autonomy and mobility
- With treatment, there is no increased incidence of delinquency unless other comorbid features exist (e.g., conduct disorder).
- Encourage parents to subtract 2 years from their child's chronological age when allowing privileges (e.g., treat a 16-year-old like a 14-year-old, delay driving until age 18).

COMPLICATIONS

- Untreated attention deficit/hyperactivity disorder can lead to failing school, parental abuse, social isolation, and poor self-esteem.
- If appetite poor, offer food morning and evening
- Some children experience withdrawal (tearfulness, agitation) after a missed medication dose.

PATIENT MONITORING

- Parent/teacher rating scales initially, in 2 weeks, and regularly
- Office visits to monitor side effects and efficacy: End point is improved grades, improved rating scales, acceptable family interactions, and improved peer interactions.
  - Monitor growth and blood pressure.

REFERENCES

1. American Academy of Pediatrics (AAP) Clinical Practice Guidelines—treatment of schoolafed children with ADHD. *Pediatrics.* 2001;108(4):1033–1044.
2. American Psychiatric Association. *Diagnostic and Statistical Manual of Mental Disorders.* 4th ed. Revised. Washington, DC: American Psychiatric Association; 2000.
3. Rappley, MD. Attention Deficit-Hyperactivity Disorder. *N Engl J Med.* 2005;352(2):165–173.
4. Brown RT, Amler RW, Freeman WS, et al. Treatment of Attention Deficit/Hyperactivity Disorder: Overview of the evidence. *Pediatrics.* 2005;115(6):e749–e757.

ADDITIONAL READING

Barkley RA. *ADHD: A Handbook for Diagnosis and Treatment.* 2nd ed. New York: Guilford Press; 1998.

 MISCELLANEOUS

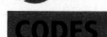

ICD9-CM

- 314.00 Attention deficit disorder without mention of hyperactivity
- 314.01 Attention deficit disorder with hyperactivity

PATIENT TEACHING

- Key points for parents
  - 50% of attention deficit/hyperactivity disorder children have one parent with attention deficit/hyperactivity disorder; modify education sessions with parents accordingly.
  - Behavior therapy such as token systems may be helpful. (1)[A]
  - Reinforce good behavior (with rewards and attention).
  - Make eye contact with each request.
  - Give one task at a time.
  - Stop behavior before it escalates.
  - Find things child is good at and emphasize these.
  - Some families benefit from "anger training," "social training," and family therapy.
  - Refer to advocacy and support groups.
  - Coordinate homework with teachers using daily assignment notebook.
- Support groups
  - Children and Adults with Attention Deficit Disorder (CHADD):chadd.org; 800-233-4050
  - Attention Deficit Disorder Warehouse: addwarehouse.com; 800-233-9273
  - Learning Disabilities Association (LDA): LDAlearning.com
  - National Information Center for Children & Youth with Disabilities: www.nichcy.org

AUTISM

Brigid Barry McKenna, MD

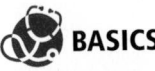 BASICS

DESCRIPTION
- Autism is a pervasive developmental disorder of early childhood, characterized by
  - Severe impairment in effective social skills
  - Absent or impaired communication skills
  - Repetitive and/or stereotyped activities and interests, especially inanimate objects
- System(s) Affected: Nervous
- Synonym(s): Early infantile autism; Childhood autism; Kanner autism; Pervasive developmental disorder

ALERT
Pediatric Considerations
Onset seen only in children <3 years.

Pregnancy Considerations
May be increased risk of autism with complications of pregnancy, labor, and delivery

EPIDEMIOLOGY
- Predominant age: Onset prior to age 3 years, but generally abnormal development is apparent well before
- Predominant sex: Male > Female (4:1)

Incidence
Estimated 1/500 children (1)

RISK FACTORS
- Certain medical conditions, including fragile X syndrome, tuberous sclerosis, congenital rubella syndrome, and untreated phenylketonuria (PKU)
- Sibling with autism

Genetics
- High concordance in monozygotic twins
- Increased recurrence risk (3–7%) in subsequent siblings (2)

ETIOLOGY
- No single cause has been identified. It is generally believed that autism is caused by abnormalities in brain structure or function. Research continues to investigate the links between heredity, genetics, and medical problems.
- No documented scientific evidence exists that proves vaccines (specifically thimerosal preservative) cause autism.

ASSOCIATED CONDITIONS
- Mental retardation (common)
- Attention deficit/hyperactivity disorder (common)
- PKU, tuberous sclerosis, and fragile X syndrome (Rare)
- Anxiety
- Depression
- Obsessional behavior
- Seizures (common)

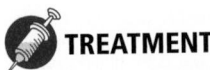 DIAGNOSIS

SIGNS AND SYMPTOMS
- Impairment in social interaction
  - Poor eye contact (1)
  - Does not seem to know how to play with toys (1)
  - Does not smile (1)
  - Loss of social skills (1)
- Communication impairment
  - Does not babble, point, or make meaningful gestures by 1 year of age (1)
  - Does not speak one word by 16 months (1)
  - Does not combine 2 words by 2 years (1)
  - Does not respond to name (1)
- Repetitive and stereotyped patterns of behavior
  - Excessively lines up toys or other objects (1)
  - Unusually attached to one particular toy or object (1)
  - Odd movements (toe walking) (1)

History
- Pregnancy, neonatal, and developmental history
- Seizure disorder
- Family history of autism or any genetic disorders

Physical Exam
Macrocephaly in 25% (2)

TESTS
- Screening tests
  - Checklist for Autism in Toddlers (CHAT) is used to screen for autism at 18 months of age
  - Modified Checklist for Autism in Toddlers (M-CHAT) to screen for autism at 24 months
  - The Screening Tool for Autism in Two-Year-Olds (STAT)
  - Autism Screening Questionnaire has been used with children age 4 years and older.
- Diagnostic testing
  - Evaluation by multidisciplinary team that includes a psychiatrist, a neurologist, a psychologist, a speech therapist, and other autism specialists
  - Childhood Autism Rating Scale (CARS)
  - Autism Diagnosis Interview Revised (ADI-R)
  - Autism Diagnostic Observation Schedule (ADOS-G)
  - Intellectual level needs to be established and monitored, as it is one of the best measures of prognosis.

Lab
- Lead screening
- PKU screening
- Chromosomal analysis (fragile X, others)

Imaging
MRI could be useful in ruling out associated conditions.

Diagnostic Procedures/Surgery
EEG, as autistic children have a markedly higher incidence of epilepsy, which increases with age

DIFFERENTIAL DIAGNOSIS
- Other mental and central nervous system disorders
  - Schizophrenia
  - Elective mutism
  - Language disorder
  - Mental retardation
  - Stereotyped movement disorder
- Other pervasive developmental disorders
  - Rett disorder
  - Childhood disintegrative disorder
  - Asperger disorder

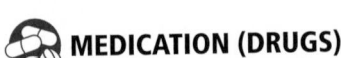 TREATMENT

GENERAL MEASURES
- Comprehensive structured educational programming of a sustained and intensive design, most commonly applied behavioral analysis therapy (ABA)
- There is currently no cure for autism. Early diagnosis and initiation of multidisciplinary intervention will help enhance functioning in later life.
- Early Intervention for ages 3 and under
- School-based special education
- Find alternative methods of communication
  - Sign language
  - Picture exchange communication system (PECS)
- Consider consults
  - Ophthalmology
  - Otolaryngology
  - Metabolic testing
  - Genetic screening for Fragile X
  - Wood's lamp exam (for tuberous sclerosis)
- Parent support groups and respite programs

Diet
Gluten- and casein-free diets show some reduction in autistic traits; however, large scale, good quality RCTs are needed. (3)

Activity
As tolerated by the child

SPECIAL THERAPY
Complementary and Alternative Medicine
Vitamin B_6-Magnesium has shown some improvement in speech and language; however, due to the small number of studies and small sample size, no recommendations exist for its use. (4)

MEDICATION (DRUGS)

- Stimulant medications such as methylphenidate are efficacious in treating concomitant symptoms of attention deficit disorder, such as impulsiveness, hyperactivity, and inattention; however, the magnitude of response is less than in typically developing children, and adverse effects are more frequent. (5)[A]
- Fluvoxamine, an SSRI, has shown some help in reducing ritualistic behavior and improving mood and language skills. (6)[B]
- Risperidone (Risperdal) has been shown to be effective for short-term treatment of tantrums, aggression, and self-injurious behavior. Improvements in stereotyped behavior and hyperactivity have also been noted. Given the risk of serious side effects, it should be reserved for moderate to severe behavioral problems. (7)[A]

- Precautions
  - Risperidone may be associated with hyperglycemia and ketoacidosis. Risperidone may cause neuroleptic malignant syndrome and extrapyramidal reactions. (7)

FOLLOW-UP

PROGNOSIS
- Those who begin treatment at a young age have significantly better outcomes.
- Prognosis is closely related to initial intellectual abilities, with only 20% functioning above the mentally retarded level.
- Communicative language development before 5 years of age is also associated with a better outcome.
- The general expected course is for a life-long need for supervised structured care.

COMPLICATIONS
- Increasing incidents of seizure disorders in up to 1 in 4 children with autism (1)
- Increased risk for physical and sexual abuse in autistic children

PATIENT MONITORING
- Constant by caregivers
- As indicated by physician, prescribed medical management
- Intellectual and language testing every 2 years in childhood

REFERENCES

1. Strock M. Autism spectrum disorders (pervasive developmental disorders). NIH Publication No. NIH-04-5511. Bethesda, MD: National Institute of Mental Health, National Institutes of Health, U.S. Department of Health and Human Services; [updated 2004 April; cited 2006 Mar 2]. Available from: http://www.nimh.nih.gov/publicat/autism.cfm
2. Committee on Children with Disabilities. The Pediatrician's role in the diagnosis and management of autistic spectrum disorder in children. *Pediatrics*. 2001;107:1221–1226.
3. Milward C, Ferriter M, Calver S, et al. Gluten- and casein-free diets for autistic spectrum disorder. *Cochrane Database of Systematic Reviews*. 1,2006.
4. Nye C, Brice A. Combined vitamin B_6-magnesium treatment in autism spectrum disorder. *Cochrane Database of Systemic Reviews*. 1,2006.
5. Research Units on Pediatric Psychopharmacology Autism Network. Randomized, controlled, crossover trial of methylphenidate in pervasive developmental disorders with hyperactivity. *Arch Gen Psychiatry*. 2005;62:1266–1272.
6. McDougle CJ, Naylor ST, Cohen DJ, et al. A double-blind, placebo-controlled study of fluvoxamine in adults with autistic disorder. *Arch Gen Psychiatry*. 1996;53:1001–1008.
7. Research Units on Pediatric Psychopharmacology Autism Network. Risperidone in children with autism and serious behavioral problems. *N Eng J Med*. 2002;347:314–321.

 MISCELLANEOUS

See also: Anxiety; Attention Deficit/Hyperactivity Disorder; Depression; Fragile X Syndrome; Mental Retardation; Schizophrenia; Seizure Disorders

CODES

ICD9-CM
299.0 Infantile autism

PATIENT TEACHING

- Autism Society of America, 7910 Woodmont Ave., Bethesda, MD 20814-3007; 800-autism; www.autism-society.org.
- The Center for Disease Control and Prevention, Autism Information Center. www.cdc.gov/ncbddd/dd/ddautism.htm

AVIAN FLU

Sheila M. Seed, BS, Pharm, MPH, RPH
Walter K. Goljan, MD

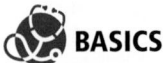 **BASICS**

DESCRIPTION
Avian influenza A subtype H5N1 is highly pathogenic and aggressive form of influenza. Presents with influenza-like symptoms, with lower respiratory tract symptoms (limited upper respiratory tract symptoms). Has a high mortality rate in elderly and very young.

GENERAL PREVENTION
- Consider with any patient with influenza-like symptoms who has had close contact with H5N1 or ill poultry.
- Chemoprophylaxis with antivirals should be considered if H5N1 circulating in community.

EPIDEMIOLOGY
Predominate age: All age groups

Prevalence
Rare

RISK FACTORS
- Direct contact with H5N1 virus.
- Contact with infected poultry
- Close contact with infected person

ETIOLOGY
- Infected poultry (domesticated ducks, turkeys, chickens)
- Low incidence of human-to-human transmission in household clusters and health care workers

ASSOCIATED CONDITIONS
Severe respiratory distress (common in severe cases)

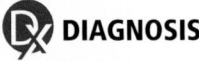 **DIAGNOSIS**

PRE HOSPITAL
- Respiratory infection (incubation period 7 days).
- Standard precautions during transport.

SIGNS AND SYMPTOMS
- Primary phase (1–5)[A]
  - Influenza-like symptoms with lower respiratory tract symptoms.
  - Temp >100.4°F (38°C)
  - Cough
  - Sore throat
  - Shortness of breath
  - Diarrhea (watery without blood)
  - Pleuritic pain
  - Bleeding of nose and gums
  - Conjunctivitis (rare)
- Secondary acute phase
  - Severe respiratory distress
  - Pneumonia not responsive to antibiotics
  - Multiorgan dysfunction

History
- Known close contact with suspected or confirmed case.
- Close contact with infected poultry
- Travel within 10 days in high-risk area

Physical Exam
- Lab abnormalities (1,3,5)[A]
  - Leukopenia (mainly lymphopenia)
  - Thrombocytopenia (mild to moderate)
  - Elevated aminotransferases (slight-moderate)
  - Disseminated intravascular coagulation
  - Decreased leukocyte, platelet, and lymphocyte counts (associated with increase risk of death)
- Chest radiograph (1,3,5)[A]
- Consolidation-bilateral and multifocal
  - After 7 days-patchy lobar and interstitial infiltrates.
  - Pleural effusions with cavitation (less common)
- Respiratory (1,3,5)[A]
  - Respiratory distress
  - Tachypnea
  - Inspiratory crackles

TESTS
Lab
- CBC with differential
- Liver profile
- Chemical profile
- Blood culture

Imaging
Chest radiograph

Diagnostic Procedures/Surgery
- Lab confirmation of H5N1 virus is done case-by-case and requires one of the following (1,4)[A]
  - Positive influenza A/H5 (Asian lineage) virus-real time reverse transcription polymerase chain reaction (LRN labs)
  - Positive immunofluorescence test for antigen with use of monoclonal antibody against H5.
  - Positive viral culture
  - 4-fold rise in H5-specific antibody titer in paired serum samples.

DIFFERENTIAL DIAGNOSIS
- Acute respiratory syndrome
- Influenza
- Pneumonia
- SARS

 TREATMENT

PRE HOSPITAL
Standard and droplet precautions

INITIAL STABILIZATION
- Ventilatory support within 48 hours (1,3)[B]
- Broad-spectrum antibiotics, antivirals agents, with or without corticosteroids until lab confirmation of H5N1 virus (5)[A]

GENERAL MEASURES
Nursing
- Use standard and droplet precautions.
- N-95 masks

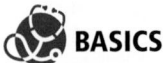 **MEDICATION (DRUGS)**

All patients should receive neuraminidase inhibitors as soon as possible pending results of diagnostic lab tests.

ALERT
The use of amantadine (Symmetrel) and rimantadine (Flumadine) are not considered beneficial unless access to newer agents are unavailable. No vaccine is commercially available.

First Line
- Treatment of mild-moderate cases (1,5)[C]: Oseltamivir (Tamiflu) 75 mg PO b.i.d. for 5 days
- Treatment of severe cases (1,5)[C]: Oseltamivir(Tamiflu) 150 mg b.i.d. for 7–10 days
- Postexposure prophylaxis (1,5)[C]: Oseltamivir (Tamiflu) 75 mg PO once a day for 7–10 days
- Adverse effects: Generally well tolerated; nausea, vomiting, diarrhea, abdominal pain, headache, insomnia, bronchitis, vertigo.
- Drug interactions: Not metabolized by CYP450; drug interactions with drugs metabolized by this system are unlikely. Does not affect metabolism of acetaminophen.

Pediatric Considerations
- Pediatric treatment is weight-based. Safety and efficacy not established for children <1 year of age (1,5)[C]
  - Oseltamivir 30 mg PO b.i.d. for 5 days ≤15 kg.
  - Oseltamivir 45 mg PO b.i.d. for 5 days >15–23 kg
  - Oseltamivir 60 mg PO b.i.d. for 5 days >23–40 kg
  - Oseltamivir 75 mg PO b.i.d. for 5 days >40 kg
- Postexposure prophylaxis (1,5) [C]
  - Dosing is weight-based as above but administered once daily for 7–10 days.

Geriatric Considerations
- Renal impairment (1,5)[C]
  - Creatinine clearance 10–30 mL/min
    - Treatment: Oseltamivir 75 mg PO daily.
    - Postexposure prophylaxis: Oseltamivir 75 mg PO every other day or 30 mg PO daily
- Hepatic impairment (1,5)[C]
  - No dosage adjustment needed.

Pregnancy Considerations
- Oseltamivir is Category C
- Use with caution only if potential benefits outweigh possible risk.
- Unknown if distributed in breast-milk

Second Line

- Zanamivir (Relenza) is considered second-line agent. Not recommended for patients with underlying respiratory disease (asthma, COPD) (5)[C]
- Treatment (ages 13–≥65 years)
  – Zanamivir 10 mg (2 inhalations) b.i.d. for 5 days.
- Postexposure prophylaxis (ages 13–≥65)
  – Zanamivir 10 mg (2 inhalations) once daily for 7–10 days.
- Adverse effects
  – Hypersensitivity reactions: Bronchospasms and allergic-like reactions have occurred.
  – Diarrhea, nausea, vomiting, headache, dizziness, sinusitis, cough, throat infections
  – Some adverse effects due to lactose in powder of inhaler
- Drug interactions: Not metabolized by CYP450; drug interactions with drugs metabolized by this system are unlikely.

Pediatric Considerations

- Zanamivir is not licensed for use in children <7 years of age for treatment and <5 years for prophylaxis (5)[C].
- Treatment (7–13 years of age): Zanamivir 10 mg (2 inhalations) b.i.d. for 5 days.
- Prophylaxis (5–13 years of age): Zanamivir 10 mg (2 inhalations) once daily 7–10 days.

Geriatric Considerations

No dosage adjustment for renal or hepatic impairment (5)[C]

Pregnancy Considerations

- Zanamivir is Category C
- Use with caution only if potential benefits outweigh possible risk.
- Unknown if distributed in breast-milk
- Other medications (1,5)[C]
  – Broad-spectrum antibiotics: Follow hospital protocols for community-acquired pneumonia.
  – Corticosteroids: No clear evidence of benefits
  – Interferon-α: No basis for use

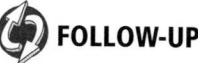 FOLLOW-UP

DISPOSITION

Admission Criteria

If known H5N1 activity in community, or if patient has traveled to country with H5N1 activity, admission should be considered if patient presents with

- Severe acute respiratory illness
- Serious unexplained illness (encephalopathy or diarrhea)

Discharge Criteria

If discharged early, family requires education of proper personal hygiene and infection-control measures. Postexposure prophylaxis given to family members.

PROGNOSIS

Mortality rate is high (some reports >50%). Median time to death was 9 days (range 6–17 days) with or without treatment.

COMPLICATIONS

- Multiorgan failure, acute (1–4)[C]
- Renal dysfunction
- Cardiac compromise
- Cardiac dilatation, supraventricular tachyarrhythmias
- Ventilator-associated pneumonia
- Pulmonary hemorrhage
- Pneumothorax
- Pancytopenia
- Reye syndrome
- Sepsis syndrome without documented bacteremia.

PATIENT MONITORING

Clinical deterioration is rapid.

REFERENCES

1. Beigel JH, Farrar J, et al. Avian influenza A (H5N1) infections in humans. *N Engl J Med.* 2005;350: 1374–1385.
2. World Health Organization. WHO international guidelines on clinical management of humans infected by influenza A (H5N1). February 20, 2004. Accessed Sep 19, 2006 at http://who.int/csr/disease/avian_influenza/guidelines/Guidelines_Clinical%20Management_H5N1_rev.pdf.
3. Chotpitayasunondh T, Ungchusak K, Hanshaoworakul W, et al. Human disease from influenza A (H5N1), Thailand, 2004. *Emerg Infect Dis.* 2005;11:201–209.
4. Hien TT, Liem NT, Dung NT, et al. Avian influenza A (H5N1) in 10 patients in Vietnam. *N Engl J Med.* 2004;350:1179–1188.
5. World Health Organization. WHO Rapid advice guidelines on pharmacological management of humans infected with avian influenza A (H5N1) virus. May 2006. Accessed Sep 19, 2006 at http://who.int/csr/disease/avian_influenza/guidelines/pharmamanagement/en.

ADDITIONAL READING

Centers for Disease Control and Prevention CDC: Question & Answers about Avian Influenza http://www.cdc.gov/flu/avian/gen-info/qa.htm.

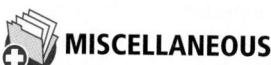 MISCELLANEOUS

Report any cases to public health officials surveillance is necessary to monitor for possible pandemic.

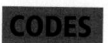 **CODES**

ICD9-CM

487.1-Influenza

BABESIOSIS

Eleftherios Mylonakis, MD
Vassiliki Syriopoulou, MD

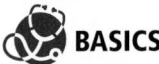 **BASICS**

DESCRIPTION
- Babesiosis is a tick-borne hemolytic disease that is caused by intra-erythrocytic protozoan parasites of the genus *Babesia*.
- Rarely reported outside the United States. Sporadic cases have been reported from a number of countries, including France, Italy, the former Yugoslavia, the United Kingdom, Ireland, the former Soviet Union, and Mexico. In the United States, infections have been reported in many states, but the most endemic areas are the islands off the coast of Massachusetts (including Nantucket and Martha's Vineyard), New York (including Long Island, Shelter Island, and Fire Island), and in Connecticut. In these areas, asymptomatic human infection seems to be common. (1–4, 6–9)
- Incubation period of babesiosis varies from 5–33 days. Most patients do not recall recent tick exposure. After an infected blood transfusion, the incubation period can be up to 9 weeks.
- System(s) Affected: Cardiovascular Gastrointestinal; Hemic/Lymphatic/Immunologic; Musculoskeletal; Nervous; Pulmonary; Renal/Urologic

ALERT
Geriatric Considerations
Morbidity and mortality is higher in patients >65.

GENERAL PREVENTION
- Avoid endemic regions during the peak transmission months of May to September (especially relevant for asplenic or immunocompromised persons, in whom babesiosis can be a devastating illness).
- Using insect repellant is advised during outdoor activities, especially in wooded or grassy areas
  – Products with 10–35% N-diethyl-*meta*-toluamide (DEET) will provide adequate protection under most conditions.
- Early removal of ticks is important; the tick must remain attached for at least 24 hours before the transmission of *Babesia microti* occurs. Daily self-examination is recommended for persons who engage in outdoor activities in endemic areas.
- Pets must be examined for ticks because they may carry ticks into the home.

EPIDEMIOLOGY
Predominant age: All ages; most patients present in their 40s or 50s.

Incidence
- Between 1968 and 1993, >450 *Babesia* infections were confirmed in the United States by blood smears or serologic testing. Prevalence is difficult to estimate because of lack of surveillance, and because infections are often asymptomatic (1,2).
- In a recent 1-year seroconversion study of patients in New York State who were at high risk for tick-borne diseases, antibodies to *Babesia microti* were seen in 7 of 671 participants (1%). (3)

Prevalence
High-level parasitemia is more common in asplenic patients. Such patients have been treated successfully with exchange transfusion in addition to drugs.

RISK FACTORS
- Exposure to endemic areas
- Transfusion-associated babesiosis and transplacental/perinatal transmission have been reported.

ETIOLOGY
- *Babesia microti* (in the United States) and *Babesia divergens* and *Babesia bovis* (in Europe) cause most infections in humans. Recently, one case of *Babesia divergens* was reported in the United States.
- A previously unknown species of *Babesia* (WA-1) was isolated from an immunocompetent man in Washington State who had clinical babesiosis. Researchers also described another probable new babesial species (MO1) associated with the first reported case of babesiosis acquired in the state of Missouri. MO1 is probably distinct from *B. divergens*, but the two share morphologic, antigenic, and genetic characteristics.
- Ixodid (or hard-bodied) ticks, in particular, *Ixodes dammini* (*Ixodes scapularis*) and *Ixodes ricinus*, are the vectors of the parasite.

ASSOCIATED CONDITIONS
- Coinfection with *Borrelia burgdorferi* and *Babesia microti* is relatively common in endemic areas.
- Coinfection with *Ehrlichia* species may also be seen. Three species of *Ehrlichia* have been described that infect humans, *Ehrlichia chaffeensis*, *Ehrlichia phagocytophila*, and *Ehrlichia ewingii*. Typically, patients have a nonspecific febrile illness. Rash is uncommon with human granulocytic ehrlichiosis but common with human monocytic ehrlichiosis. Laboratory findings often include leukopenia, thrombocytopenia, and increases in serum hepatic enzyme activities. (4)

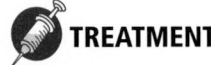 **DIAGNOSIS**

SIGNS AND SYMPTOMS (3)
- Asymptomatic
- High fever (up to 40°C [104°F])
- Chills
- Diaphoresis
- Gastrointestinal (anorexia, nausea, abdominal pain, vomiting, diarrhea)
- Generalized weakness
- Fatigue
- Myalgia
- Respiratory (cough, shortness of breath)
- Headache
- Hepatomegaly and splenomegaly or evidence of shock
- Rash (uncommon)
- Central nervous system involvement includes headache, photophobia, neck and back stiffness, altered sensorium, and emotional lability
- Jaundice and dark urine may develop later in course of illness

TESTS
Lab
- Mild to severe hemolytic anemia (common nonspecific finding)
- Normal to slightly depressed leukocyte count (common nonspecific finding)
- Typical morphologic picture on the blood smear
- A Wright- or Giemsa-stained peripheral blood smear is most commonly used to demonstrate the presence of intraerythrocytic parasites.
- Rarely, tetrads of merozoites are visible.
- Serologic evaluation with the indirect immunofluorescent antibody test with use of *Babesia microti* antigen is available in a few laboratories. The cut-off titer for determination of a positive result varies with the particular laboratory protocol used, but in most laboratories, titers of more than 1:64 are considered consistent with *Babesia microti* infection. Tenfold to 20-fold higher titers can be observed in the acute setting, with a gradual decline over weeks to months. The correlation between the level of the titer and the severity of symptoms is poor.
- Detection of *Babesia microti* by polymerase chain reaction (PCR) is more sensitive and equally specific for the diagnosis of acute cases, in comparison with direct smear examination and hamster inoculation. PCR-based methods may also be indicated for monitoring of the infection.

Diagnostic Procedures/Surgery
Based on typical morphologic picture on the blood smear in conjunction with epidemiologic information

DIFFERENTIAL DIAGNOSIS
- Bacterial sepsis
- Hepatitis
- Lyme disease
- Ehrlichiosis
- Leishmaniasis
- Malaria

TREATMENT

GENERAL MEASURES
- Appropriate health care: Outpatient or inpatient, depending on symptoms
- Supportive care

MEDICATION (DRUGS)

First Line

- Atovaquone (Mepron): Suspension 750 mg b.i.d. plus azithromycin (Zithromax) 500–1,000 mg/d (5)[B]

- Combination of quinine (Quinamm): 650 mg of salt orally t.i.d. and clindamycin (Cleocin) 600 mg orally t.i.d., or 1.2 g parenterally b.i.d. for 7–10 days is the most commonly used treatment. (Pediatric: Dosage is 20–40 mg/kg/d for quinine and 25 mg/kg/d for Clindamycin.)

- In areas endemic for Lyme disease and ehrlichiosis, it may be advisable to add doxycycline (Vibramycin) 100 mg b.i.d. PO in the management of patients with babesiosis until serologic testing is completed.

- Exchange transfusion, together with antibabesial chemotherapy, may be necessary in critically ill patients. This treatment is usually reserved for patients who are extremely ill (blood parasitemia >10%, massive hemolysis and asplenia).

- Precautions: Clindamycin can lead to *Clostridium difficile* associated diarrhea.

Second Line

Several other drugs have been evaluated, including tetracycline, primaquine, sulfadiazine (Microsulfon), and pyrimethamine (Fansidar). Results have varied. Pentamidine (Pentam) has proved to be moderately effective in diminishing symptoms and decreasing parasitemia.

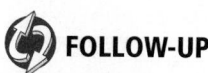 **FOLLOW-UP**

PROGNOSIS

- When left untreated, silent babesial infection may persist for months or even years.
- 139 hospitalized cases in New York State between 1982 and 1993 (3)
  - 9 patients (6.5%) died.
  - 1/4 of the patients were admitted to the ICU.
  - 1/4 of the patients required hospitalization for more than 14 days.
- Alkaline phosphatase levels greater than 125 U/L, white blood cell counts greater than 5×10^9/L, history of cardiac abnormality, history of splenectomy, presence of heart murmur, and parasitemia values of 4% or higher were associated with disease severity.

COMPLICATIONS

- Congestive heart failure
- Disseminated intravascular coagulation
- Acute respiratory distress syndrome (can occur even a few days after the onset of effective antimicrobial treatment)
- Renal failure and myocardial infarction also have been associated with severe babesiosis.

PATIENT MONITORING

Monitor for complications (congestive heart failure, etc.) and follow parasitemia as needed.

REFERENCES

1. Quick RE, Herwaldt BL, Thomford JW, et al. Babesiosis in Washington State: A new species of *Babesia*? *Ann Intern Med*. 1993;119:284–290.
2. Persing DH, Herwaldt BL, Glaser C, et al. Infection with a *Babesia*-like organism in northern California. *N Engl J Med*. 1995;332:298–303.
3. White DJ, Talarico J, Chang HG, et al. Human babesiosis in New York State: A review of 139 hospitalized cases and analysis of prognostic factors. *Arch Intern Med*. 1998;158:2149–2154.
4. Mylonakis E. When to suspect and how to monitor babesiosis. *Amer Fam Physician*. 2001;63:1969–1974.
5. Krause PJ, Lepore T, Sikand VK, et al. Atovaquone and azithromycin for the treatment of babesiosis. *N Engl J Med*. 2000 Nov 16;343(20):1454–8.
6. Beattie JF, Michelson ML, Holman PJ. Acute babesiosis caused by *Babesia divergens* in a resident of Kentucky. *N Engl J Med*. 2002;29;347(9):697–698.
7. Gelfand JA. Babesia species. In: Mandell GL, Douglas RG, Bennett JE, Dolin R, eds. *Mandell, Douglas, and Bennett's Principles and Practice of Infectious Diseases*. 6th ed. New York, NY: Churchill Livingstone, 2005:3209–3215.
8. Gutman JD, Kotton CN, Kratz A. Case records of the Massachusetts General Hospital. Weekly clinicopathological exercises. Case 29-2003. A 60-year-old man with fever, rigors, and sweats. *N Engl J Med*. 2003;349(12):1168–1175.
9. Pruthi RK, Marshall WF, Wiltsie JC, Persing DH. Human babesiosis. *Mayo Clin Proc*. 1995;70:853–862.

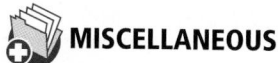 **MISCELLANEOUS**

See also: Lyme Disease

CODES

ICD9-CM
088.82 Babesiosis

PATIENT TEACHING

AAFP patient handout:
www.aafp.org/afp/20010515/1976ph.html

BAKER CYST

Gregory R. Czarnecki, DO
John Herbert Stevenson, MD

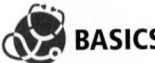 **BASICS**

DESCRIPTION
- Aka popliteal cyst; a fluid-filled synovial-lined sac (cyst) arising in the popliteal fossa
- Can be unilateral or bilateral
- Found in both children and adults

EPIDEMIOLOGY
Bimodal distribution: Children 4–7 and adults increasing with age

Prevalence
- Varies by study
- 2.4% in asymptomatic children in 1 prospective study (1)[B]
- 5% in adults by MRI in 1 prospective study; up to 58% in others, limited by sample population and largely retrospective data (2)[B]

RISK FACTORS
- Knee osteoarthritis
- Rheumatoid arthritis
- Meniscal degeneration/tear
- Advancing age

ETIOLOGY
- Extension or herniation of synovial membrane of the knee joint capsule or connection of normal bursa with the joint capsule. This may be the result of increased intraarticular pressure and is commonly seen in association with knee effusions. Direct trauma to the bursa may be the primary cause in children.
- A valvelike mechanism has been described with this connection of bursa and joint allowing primary one-way passage of fluid from the joint to the bursal connection.
- Associated intraarticular pathological findings are rare in children but common in adults—up to 50%. (3)[B]
- Bursa under the medial head of the gastrocnemius or semimembranosus bursa most commonly involved

ASSOCIATED CONDITIONS
- Osteoarthritis
- Rheumatoid arthritis
- Meniscal tear, notably posterior horn of medial meniscus

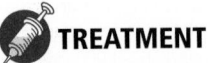 **DIAGNOSIS**

History
- (Often) painless mass arising in the popliteal fossa
- May complain of restricted range of motion or tightness with knee flexion
- Ruptured cyst typically painful with associated swelling causing pseudothrombophlebitis
- Large cysts may cause entrapment neuropathy of the tibial nerve.
- Vascular compression may produce claudication.

Physical Exam
- Examine in full extension and 90° flexion. Mass increases with extension and may disappear on flexion (Foucher sign).
- Most commonly found in medial popliteal fossa
- Mass may be fluctuant or tender
- Transillumination to distinguish cystic vs. solid

TESTS
Imaging
- Ultrasound readily confirms presence and size.
- MRI allows further characterization of association with joint capsule.
- May also detect on arthrography or CT scan
- Radiographs may show soft tissue density posteriorly.

Diagnostic Procedures/Surgery
Arthrography may demonstrate communication with joint capsule.

DIFFERENTIAL DIAGNOSIS
- Aneurysm
- Deep venous thrombosis
- Infection/abscess
- Lipoma
- Fibroma
- Fibrosarcoma
- Hematoma
- Vascular tumor
- Xanthoma
- Any condition causing synovitis

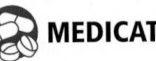 **TREATMENT**

GENERAL MEASURES
- No treatment if aysmptomatic
- Compressive wrap or sleeve may be used for comfort
- Treat underlying cause if present, (e.g., intraarticular derangement)

Activity
No restrictions

SPECIAL THERAPY
- Aspiration for symptom relief, recurrance common
- Injection with corticosteroid directly into cyst following aspiration, or intraarticular if communicating cyst. If joint communication is present, intraarticular corticosteroid injection may assist regression of cyst. (3)[B]

Physical Therapy
Physical therapy is helpful in improving knee range of motion and strength. It is also helpful if co-existing knee arthritis or stable meniscal tear.

MEDICATION (DRUGS)

Analgesics, NSAIDS for symptomatic relief.

SURGERY
Excision via arthroscopy or open procedure often requires treatment of intraarticular pathology (when present) to prevent recurrence of cyst. (3)[B]

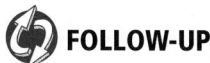 **FOLLOW-UP**

Routine monitoring providing diagnosis is clear. Size of cyst may vary depending on degree of knee effusion and joint communication.

Issues for Referral
Consider whether definitive treatment desired. Despite surgical removal, some cysts recur; treatment of underlying intraarticular pathology, if present, is imperative.

PROGNOSIS
- Variable
- Many cysts remain asymptomatic, and some will regress or resolve with treatment of associated cause without direct treatment of the cyst; in others, size may remain stable or expand; recurrence is common.
- In children, most resolve without treatment.

COMPLICATIONS
- Compartment syndrome in ruptured cyst
- Pain with cyst expansion/dissection or rupture
- Frequent recurrence

PATIENT MONITORING
See above

REFERENCES
1. Seil R, Rupp S, et al. Prevalence of popliteal cysts in children: A sonographic study and review of the literature. *Arch Ortho Traum Su*. 1999;119:73–75.
2. Rupp S, Seil R, et al. Popliteal cysts in adults: prevalence, associated intraarticular lesions, and results after arthroscopic treatment. *Am Sport Med*. 2002;30(1):112–115.
3. Handy JR. Popliteal cysts in adults: A review. *Semin Arthritis Rheu*. 2001;31(2):108–118.
4. Canale. *Campbell's Operative Orthopaedics*, 10th ed., Mosby, Inc. 2003;894–903.

 MISCELLANEOUS

CODES

ICD9-CM
- 727.5 (Rupture of synovium)
- 727.51 (Baker cyst)

PATIENT TEACHING
Popliteal cyst is a benign entity that is often associated with other knee pathology. Though most are asymptomatic, they can be quite painful if rupture occurs or cause compressive symptoms if enlarging.

Activity
No restrictions

 See Corresponding Diagnostic Algorithm

 See Patient Handout on CD

B

BALANITIS

James P. Miller, MD
Timothy L. Black, MD

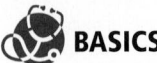 **BASICS**

DESCRIPTION
- Balanitis: Inflammation of glans penis
- Posthitis: Inflammation of the foreskin
- System(s) Affected: Reproductive; Skin/Exocrine

ALERT
Geriatric Considerations
Condom catheters can predispose to balanitis.

Pediatric Considerations
Oral antibiotics predispose male infants to *Candida balanitis*.

GENERAL PREVENTION
- Proper hygiene and avoidance of allergens
- Circumcision

EPIDEMIOLOGY
- Predominant age: Adult
- Predominant sex: Male only

RISK FACTORS
- Presence of foreskin
- Morbid obesity
- Poor hygiene
- Diabetes
- Nursing home environment

ETIOLOGY
- Allergic reaction (condom latex, contraceptive jelly)
- Infections (*Candida albicans, Borrelia vincentii*, streptococci, trichomonas)
- Fixed drug eruption (sulfa, tetracycline, barbital)
- Plasma cell infiltration (*Zoon balanitis*)
- Autodigestion by activated Pancreatic transplant exocrine enzymes

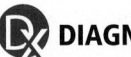 **DIAGNOSIS**

SIGNS AND SYMPTOMS
History
- Pain
- Drainage
- Dysuria

Physical Exam
- Erythema
- Edema
- Discharge
- Ulceration
- Plaque

TESTS
Lab
- Microbiology culture
- Wet mount
- Serology for syphilis
- Serum glucose

Diagnostic Procedures/Surgery
Biopsy, if persistent

Pathological Findings
Plasma cells infiltration with *Zoon balanitis*

DIFFERENTIAL DIAGNOSIS
- Leukoplakia
- Lichen planus
- Psoriasis
- Reiter syndrome
- Lichen sclerosus et atrophicus
- Erythroplasia of Queyrat
- Balanitis xerotica obliterans (BXO)

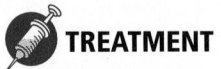 **TREATMENT**

GENERAL MEASURES
- Appropriate health care: Outpatient
- Warm compresses or sitz baths
- Local hygiene

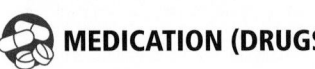 **MEDICATION (DRUGS)**

- Fungal
  - Clotrimazole (Lotrimin) 1% b.i.d.
  - Nystatin (Mycostatin) b.i.d.–q.i.d.
  - Fluconazole 150 mg single dose (1)[B]
- Bacterial
  - Bacitracin q.i.d.
  - Neomycin-polymyxin B-bacitracin (Neosporin) q.i.d.
  - If cellulitis, cephalosporin or sulfa drug PO or parenteral
  - Dermatitis
  - Topical steroids q.i.d.
  - *Zoon balanitis*
  - Topical steroids q.i.d.
- BXO
  - 0.05% Betamethasone b.i.d. (2)[B]
  - 0.1% Tacrolimus b.i.d. (3)[C]
- Contraindications: Refer to manufacturer's profile for each drug.
- Precautions: Refer to manufacturer's profile for each drug.
- Significant possible interactions: Refer to manufacturer's profile for each drug.

SURGERY
Consider circumcision as preventive measure

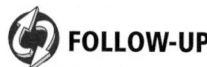 FOLLOW-UP

DISPOSITION

Admission Criteria
- Uncontrolled diabetes
- Sepsis

Discharge Criteria
Resolution of problem

Issues for Referral
Recurrent infections or development of meatal stenosis

PROGNOSIS
Should resolve with appropriate treatment

COMPLICATIONS
- Meatal stenosis
- Premalignant changes from chronic irritations
- Urinary tract infections

PATIENT MONITORING
- Every 1–2 weeks until etiology has been established
- Persistent balanitis may require biopsy to rule out malignancy or BXO

REFERENCES

1. Stary A, Soeltz-Szoets J, Kiegler C, et al. Comparison of the efficacy and safety of oral fluconazole and topical clotrimazole in patients with candida balanitis. *Genitourin Med.* 1996;72:98–102.
2. Kiss A, Csontai A, Pirot L, et al. The response of Balanitis xerotica obliterans to local steroid application compared to placebo in children. *J Urol.* 2001;165:219–220.
3. Pandher BS, Rustin HMA, Kaisary AV. Treatment of Balanitis Xerotica Obliterans with topical tacrolimus. *J Urol.* 2003;170:923.

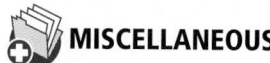 MISCELLANEOUS

See also: Reiter Syndrome

CODES

ICD9-CM
- 607.1 Balanitis
- 112.2 Candidiasis of other urogenital sites
- 099.8 Other specified venereal diseases

PATIENT TEACHING
- Need for appropriate hygiene
- Avoidance of known allergens

Diet
Weight reduction, if obese

Prevention
Proper hygiene

BAROTITIS MEDIA

Tyeese Gaines-Reid, DO, MA

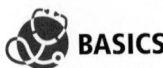 **BASICS**

DESCRIPTION
- Inflammation of the middle ear space (tympanic cavity, eustachian tube, and mastoid air cells) secondary to changes in negative pressure between the external canal and middle ear
- Caused by the inability of the eustachian tube to adequately equilibrate the middle ear air pressure with the moment-to-moment changes in environmental atmospheric pressures while descending or ascending in air (flight) or in water (diving)
  - Causes the retraction or protraction of the tympanic membrane, with subsequent inflammation and/or rupture
  - May cause asymmetric pressure stimulation of the inner ear and vestibular end organ
  - Negative pressure can also cause serous fluid or blood to pool in the middle ear.
- System(s) Affected: Nervous; ENT
- Synonym(s): Dysbarism; Aerotitis; Otitic barotrauma; Middle ear barotrauma

ALERT
Valsalva maneuver can spread nasopharyngeal infection into the middle ear.

Pediatric Considerations
Children have difficulty dilating the eustachian tube even at small pressure changes and therefore are at higher risk (especially with upper-respiratory infection).

Pregnancy Considerations
The nasal congestion often associated with pregnancy increases risk of barotitis media.

GENERAL PREVENTION
- Avoid altitude changes when any risk factors are present for eustachian tube dysfunction.
- Use methods of autoinflation during pressure changes.

EPIDEMIOLOGY
- Predominant age: All ages
- Predominant sex: Male = Female

Incidence
- The most common medical disorder experienced by SCUBA divers
- Also highly prevalent among aircraft flight personnel (especially high-performance jet aircraft), passengers, and sky divers

RISK FACTORS
- Participating in high-risk activities without adequate eustachian tube autoinflation (Valsalva maneuver, swallowing, yawning)
- Any causes of eustachian tube and external ear canal dysfunction
  - SCUBA diving
  - Airplane flight (especially high performance)
  - Sky diving
  - High-altitude mountain traveling
  - High-altitude elevator rides
  - Hyperbaric oxygen chamber therapy
  - High-impact sports
- Infants and young children (especially with upper-respiratory infection)
- Upper respiratory infections
- Nasal congestion or allergic rhinitis
- Pregnancy
- Anatomic obstruction in the nasopharynx

ETIOLOGY
- Rapid descent or ascent with eustachian tube obstruction
  - Upper-respiratory infections: Sinusitis, rhinitis, tonsillitis, adenoiditis, otitis media
  - Overzealous forceful Valsalva maneuver (in ascent with vestibular stimulation)
  - Allergic rhinitis
  - Nonallergic rhinitis with eosinophilia
  - Obstructing nasal polyps
  - Deviated nasal septum
  - Congenital abnormalities of inner/middle ear (cleft palate)
  - Nasopharyngeal tumors
- Rapid descent or ascent with external ear canal occlusion
  - Otitis externa (swimmer's ear)
  - Impacted cerumen
  - Ear plugs
- Trauma to external and middle ear
  - Boxing, soccer, water skiing, accidents, etc.
  - Overzealous use of cotton swab in cleaning ear canals
- Otalgia and hearing loss occurs as a result of stretching and malformation of the tympanic membrane.

ASSOCIATED CONDITIONS
- Aerosinusitis
- Aerodontalgia
- Face mask squeeze
- Epistaxis
- Alternobaric vertigo
- Unequal caloric stimulation vertigo
- Anxiety (leading to panic attack)
- Temporomandibular joint syndrome
- Inner ear cochlear damage and/or perilymph fistula

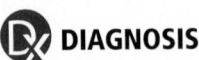 **DIAGNOSIS**

SIGNS AND SYMPTOMS
- Abrupt onset
- Otalgia (ear pain)
- Feeling of fullness or pressure in ear
- Conductive hearing loss
- Dizziness
- Tinnitus, pulsating or constant
- Vertigo
- Nausea and vomiting
- Transient facial paralysis
- With tympanic membrane rupture, leakage of air or fluid from the ear during sneezing or Valsalva
- Crying in children (which is a means of autoinflation)

TESTS
Tympanometry

Imaging
Only to rule out suspected nasopharyngeal tumor or sinusitis

Diagnostic Procedures/Surgery
- Otoscopic exam
- Audiogram: Conductive (middle ear) vs. mixed (inner ear) hearing loss
- Surgical exploration to rule out inner ear involvement if suspected

Pathological Findings
- Tympanic membrane retraction or protraction with hemotympanum or rupture
- Edema of mucosal lining and capillary engorgement with transudation of middle ear effusion
- Inner ear involvement with rupture of the round or oval windows and leakage of perilymph into the middle ear and perilymphatic fistula development

DIFFERENTIAL DIAGNOSIS
- Inner ear barotrauma
- Serous otitis media
- Acute and chronic otitis media
- External otitis
- Myringitis bullosa
- Temporomandibular joint syndrome

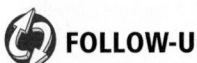 **TREATMENT**

GENERAL MEASURES

- Prevention/avoidance is best
  - Avoid flying or diving while risk factors exist, if possible
- Autoinflate the eustachian tube during pressure changes
  - Valsalva method (1)[B]
    - Patient occludes nose with thumb and index finger pressure on nasal alae, then carefully exhales with mouth closed until ears "pop." This will equalize pressures, relieve pain, and restore hearing. This usually must be repeated several times during descent or ascent.
  - Infants: Breastfeeding, or sucking on pacifier or bottle
  - ≥4 years: Chewing gum
  - ≥8 years: Blowing up a balloon
  - Adults: Chewing gum, sucking hard candy, or yawning
- Nasal balloon (1)[B]
- If the suggested maneuvers are unsuccessful, return to baseline altitude if possible; autoinflate then resume ascent/descent
- If associated bacterial upper respiratory infection, treat with appropriate antibiotics
- If inner ear exposed, bed rest with head of bed elevated to help drainage

Diet
Avoid food allergens that cause rhinitis.

Activity
- No flying or diving until complete resolution of all signs and symptoms and Valsalva maneuver can be performed
- In severe cases, bed rest

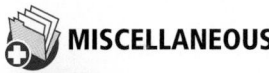 **MEDICATION (DRUGS)**

First Line
- Antihistamines
  - Pseudoephedrine. Start 30–60 minutes prior to exposure
    - Studies showed oral pseudoephedrine decreased otalgia in adults but not in children (2)[C].
  - Oxymetazoline nasal spray (Afrin, Afrin 12-Hour)
    - Beware of rebound congestion after 3–5 days of use
    - No statistical significance that it prevents symptoms (2)[C]
  - Phenylephrine nasal spray (Neo-Synephrine)
  - Antihistamines for allergic component (no data demonstrate benefit except to relieve allergy symptoms)
    - Diphenhydramine (Benadryl)
    - Loratadine (Claritin)
    - Fexofenadine (Allegra)
- Precautions
  - All medications must be used on the ground to rule out idiosyncratic reactions that could incapacitate in an airplane or underwater environment.
  - Elderly are more susceptible to drug side effects, especially with diphenhydramine
  - Caution with hypertension
- Analgesics for pain control
- Tinnitus can be treated with high-dose steroids if given within 3 weeks of onset (3)[C].

SURGERY
If necessary, myringotomy or tympanoplasty

 FOLLOW-UP

DISPOSITION

Admission Criteria
Patients with complicating emergencies (e.g., incapacitating pain requiring myringotomy, large tympanic perforation requiring tympanoplasty)

Issues for Referral
Refer to otolaryngology if
- Inner ear is exposed
- Perilymphatic fistula
- Sensorineural hearing loss

PROGNOSIS
- Untreated, simple barotitis media resolves on its own unless secondary to diving.
- Ear block: Hours–days, with complete resolution and return to flight or diving within days–weeks
- Tympanic rupture: Recovery within weeks–months

COMPLICATIONS
- Permanent hearing loss
- Ruptured tympanic membranes
- Serous otitis media
- Chronic tinnitus, vertigo
- Bruising of or bleeding into tympanic membrane
- Fluid exudate in middle ear
- Perilymphatic fistula
- Sensorineural hearing loss

PATIENT MONITORING
- Otoscopic until symptoms clear
- In severe cases, audiograms

REFERENCES
1. Stangerup SE, Klokker M, Yesterhauge S. Point prevalence of barotitis and its prevention and treatment with nasal balloon inflation: A prospective, controlled study. *Otol Neurol.* 2004;25(2):89–94.
2. Mirza S, Richardson H. Otic barotrauma from air travel. *J Laryngol Otol.* 2005;119(5):366–370.
3. Duplessis C, Hoffer M. Tinnitus in an active duty navy diver: A review of inner ear barotrauma, tinnitus, and its treatment. *Undersea Hyperbaric Med.* 2006;33(4):223–230.

ADDITIONAL READING
Internet references
- Emedicine, www.emedicine.com
- MedlinePlus Medical Encyclopedia www.medlineplus.gov
- Up to Date, www.uptodate.com

 MISCELLANEOUS

CODES

ICD9-CM
- 993.0 Barotrauma, otitic
- 993.1 Barotrauma, sinus

PATIENT TEACHING
- Teach Valsalva maneuver.
- Educate on how to create allergy-free environment.
- American Academy of Pediatrics Travel Safety Tips www.aap.org
- Divers Alert Network of Duke University Medical Center, information line, (919) 684-2948

See Patient Handout on CD

BARRETT ESOPHAGUS

Laura Goldman, MD

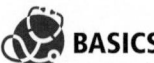 **BASICS**

DESCRIPTION
- Replacement of normal squamous epithelium of the distal esophagus with abnormal columnar epithelium as a consequence of gastric acid reflux
- Precursor of adenocarcinoma of the esophagus
- Divided into long (≥3 cm) and short segments (<3 cm)

GENERAL PREVENTION
- Case-controlled studies have shown that aspirin, and NSAIDs may prevent esophageal cancer, but no randomized trials to date (1)[B]
- No evidence that gastric acid-suppression reduces cancer risk (medical or surgical) (1)[A]
- Epidemiological evidence that weight loss, cessation of smoking, and eating fruits and vegetables can decrease cancer risk (2)[C]

EPIDEMIOLOGY
- Most common in white men >55
- Uncommon in Blacks and Asians, Hispanics similar to Caucasians
- Can affect children, but rarely occurs before the age of 5

Prevalence
- Estimates vary widely in studies
  - Most patients with Barrett esophagus are not diagnosed (3)[B]
  - In patients without gastroesophageal reflux disease (GERD) symptoms 0–25%
  - In patients with chronic GERD symptoms, 10%

RISK FACTORS
- Chronic GERD symptoms
- Male
- White
- Most frequent in 55–65 years of age

PATHOPHYSIOLOGY
- Reflux of gastric contents injures mature cells and triggers metaplastic transformation from squamous cells to more resistant columnar cells called specialized intestinal metaplasia
- Columnar cells have higher malignant potential than squamous cells
- Annual incidence of esophageal cancer in patients with Barrett's is 0.5% per year
- A few studies have demonstrated no difference in overall survival in patients with Barrett esophagus compared to the general population. One observational study showed only 4 of 409 patients affected died of esophageal cancer in 10 years. (3)[B]
- Cancers evolve through a sequence of DNA changes that can be recognized by the pathologist as dysplasia, categorized as low grade or high grade depending on severity of changes.
- Develops to full extent over a relatively short period of time, <1 year

ETIOLOGY
Caused by chronic reflux of gastric contents

ASSOCIATED CONDITIONS
- Esophageal cancer is the most rapidly increasing cancer in the United States, with 0.4% annual increase
- Specialized intestinal metaplasia may also be found in the esophagogastric junction, with lower incidence of cancer, but differentiating between this and Barrett's may be difficult.

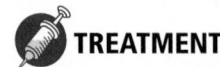 **DIAGNOSIS**

SIGNS AND SYMPTOMS
- Barrett esophagus causes no symptoms
- Most patients seen for GERD symptoms

History
- Heartburn, regurgitation, and dysphagia are the most common symptoms of GERD.
- Less common include chest pain, odynophagia, chronic cough, water brash, globus sensation, laryngitis, and asthma
- Weight loss, anorexia, dysphagia, odynophagia, or bleeding may indicate complications of GERD or cancer

Physical Exam
Normal

TESTS
Upper endoscopy with random multiple biopsies is the only test recommended for diagnosis.

Lab
H. pylori testing not indicated; it does not infect the esophagus, and it does not increase the risk of Barrett's or esophageal cancer

Imaging
None

Diagnostic Procedures/Surgery
- Specialized intestinal metaplasia (reddish, velvety appearance) can be seen at endoscopy
- Multiple biopsies are taken of this area.
- Multiple experimental techniques to identify dysplasia have not been shown in studies to increase accuracy of diagnosis (dysplasia is not visible). (1)[A]

Pathological Findings
- Histologic examination must reveal specialized intestinal metaplasia (also called specialized columnar epithelium) to diagnose Barrett esophagus
- Biopsies may or may not demonstrate low-grade or high-grade dysplasia

DIFFERENTIAL DIAGNOSIS
- Erosive esophagitis may make biopsies inadequate, and repeat study after treatment may be necessary.
- Pathology may show 2 types of columnar epithelium that DO NOT have malignant potential: Cardiac epithelium and gastric-fundic type.
- Intraobserver agreement among experienced pathologists for low-grade dysplasia is 50%, while for high-grade dysplasia it is 85%; second expert pathologist opinion is recommended (4)[A]

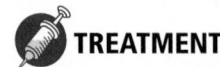 **TREATMENT**

GENERAL MEASURES
- The goal of treatment is to control GERD symptoms and detect and treat dysplasia and cancer.
- The efficacy of treatments in reducing the number of deaths from cancer has not been established. (1)[A]

Diet
- Avoid foods that can cause reflux.
- Avoid other acidic foods if known to trigger symptons: Colas, red wine, orange juice
- Weight loss if obese

Activity
- Avoid supine position after eating; avoid tight fitting clothes.
- Smoking cessation

SPECIAL THERAPY
- Treatment of high-grade dysplasia is controversial.
- Esophagectomy is usually recommended. (4)[B] There are multiple endoscopic procedures now available, but none has been shown to decrease long-term risk of cancer. (5)[A] They may be considered in patients who are poor operative candidates (4,5)
  - Photodynamic therapy (PDT) is available in some academic centers; efficacy is not established; cancer has been shown to recur after treatment and strictures occur in 40%. (1,5)
  - Other endoscopic ablative procedures (thermal, photochemical, radiofrequency); again efficacy unknown and cancers have been reported post-treatment. (5)
  - Endoscopic mucosal resection: Involves excision of mucosa down to submucosa; its efficacy is unknown; can be paired with PDT; remains experimental (1)[A]
  - Intensive surveillance with endoscopy every 3–6 months and treatment of cancer if it arises; little data to support safety and efficacy (5)[A]

MEDICATION (DRUGS)

- Goal of therapy is the control of the symptoms of GERD (5)[A] and the maintenance of healed mucosa
- Therapy usually does not result in reversal of Barrett esophagus. (4)[A]

First Line

- Once a day proton-pump inhibitor (PPI) therapy for long-segment disease (5)[B]
- H_2-receptor antagonist may be sufficient for short-segment disease (5)[B]

Second Line

- If once a day PPI does not control symptoms, b.i.d. dosing is recommended. (4)[A]
- If H_2-receptor antagonist does not control symptoms, step-up to PPI. (4)[A]

SURGERY

- Fundoplication is an option to control GERD symptoms, but it has not been shown to reverse Barrett esophagus or decrease risk of cancer (5)[A]
- Esophagectomy is the only treatment of high-grade dysplasia that guarantees cancer-free survival (5)
- Mortality rate from esophagectomy is 8–23%, and 30–50% develop serious post-op complications

ALERT
Geriatric Considerations
If the patient is a poor operative candidate for PDT or other endoscopic ablative procedure, surveillance or no treatment may be preferable; treatment must be individualized.

 FOLLOW-UP

- Surveillance is controversial; aim is to detect high-grade dysplasia or early carcinoma
- Only evidence to support improved survival in patients undergoing surveillance is from non-randomized, retrospective studies (1,3)
- Vast majority (96% in one study) of patients with adenocarcinoma of esophagus are NOT known to have Barrett esophagus before diagnosis of cancer (6)[B]

ALERT
Geriatric Considerations
Surveillance should only be done if there is reasonable life expectancy and ability to tolerate treatment of esophageal cancer (4)

DISPOSITION

- American College of Gastroenterology Guidelines for surveillance in Barrett esophagus (4)[C]
  – If no dysplasia on 2 consecutive endoscopies with biopsies, 3-yr interval is appropriate
  – If low-grade dysplasia, and repeat endoscopy again shows low-grade, yearly endoscopy until no dysplasia
  – If high-grade, repeat Esophagogastroduodenoscopy (EGD) w/biopsies to rule out cancer, expert pathologist confirmation; intervention or EGD every 3 months

Issues for Referral

- Patients should be treated with a PPI prior to endoscopy
- Diagnosis of high-grade dysplasia should be confirmed by a second expert pathologist. (4)[A]
- Patients considering esophagectomy should be referred to a high-volume institution; mortality and morbidity rates have been shown to be inversely related to volume. (4)[A]

PROGNOSIS

- Annual incidence of esophageal cancer in patients with Barrett esophagus is 0.5% per year.
- Low-grade dysplasia may be transient: 7% progress to cancer in 3–7 yrs
- High-grade progresses to cancer in 22% (3–7 yrs) (4)[B]

COMPLICATIONS

Same as GERD: Stricture, bleeding, ulceration

REFERENCES

1. Sampliner RE. Managing Barrett esophagus esophagus: What is new in 2005? *Dis Esophagus.* 2005;18:17–20.
2. Wang et al. AGA medical position statement: Role of gastroenterologist in the management of EsoCa *Gastroenterology.* 2005;128.
3. Sharma P, Sidorenko EI. Are Screening and surveillance for Barrett esophagus really worthwhile? *Gut.* 2005;54:27–32.
4. Sampliner RE and the Practice Parameters Committee of the American College of Gastroenterology. Updated guidelines for the diagnosis, surveillance, and therapy of Barrett Esophagus. *Am J of Gastroenterology.* 2002;97:1888–1895.
5. Spechler SJ. Barrett Esophagus. *N Eng J Med.* 2002;346:836–842.
6. Corley DA, Levin TR, et al. Surveillance and survival in Barrett's adenocarcinomas: A population based study. *Gastroenterology.* 2002;122:3:633–40.

 MISCELLANEOUS

ADDITIONAL READING

UpToDate Online 13.3 has an excellent evidence-based review.

CODES

ICD9-CM
530.85 Barrett Esophagus

PATIENT TEACHING

- Increases risk of esophageal cancer, 0.5% per year
- However, the vast majority of people with Barrett esophagus die of another condition
- Much research is ongoing, and treatment recommendations may change.

Diet

- Avoid foods that make symptoms worse; especially acidic foods like orange or tomato juice, carbonated beverages
- Avoid lying down after eating
- Place blocks under head of bed to elerate
- Quit smoking

Prevention

- There is no evidence to suggest that treating GERD symptoms will reverse Barrett esophagus or prevent cancer.
- The use of aspirin or NSAIDs MAY prevent cancer, but this has not been proven.

See Patient Handout on CD

BARTONELLA INFECTIONS

Mary H. Hohenhaus, MD

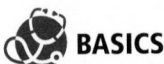 **BASICS**

DESCRIPTION
- Fastidious intracellular Gram-negative bacilli
  - At least 20 distinct species, 8 known to cause disease in humans
  - *Bartonella henselae* and *B. quintana* most common in North America
- Infections manifest in 2 broad categories
  - Localized skin lesions and prominent regional lymphadenitis (cat scratch disease [CSD])
  - Bacteremia with localized vascular lesions in various organs and potential for persistent disseminated infection
- System(s) Affected: Cardiovascular; Gastrointestinal; Hemic/Lymphatic/Immunologic; Musculoskeletal; Nervous; Pulmonary; Skin/exocrine
- Synonym(s): Bartonellosis

GENERAL PREVENTION
Vector avoidance

EPIDEMIOLOGY
- CSD: Predominantly children
- Others: Predominantly adults

Incidence
- Carrión disease: 12.7/100 person-years in endemic areas
- CSD: Estimated 9.3/100,000 in US (~25,000 cases annually)
- Endocarditis: Estimated 3–4% of cases, up to 1/3 of "culture negative" cases
- Others: Unknown

Prevalence
- Seroprevalence studies of *B. henselae* suggests many childhood infections are asymptomatic.
- Studies of *B. quintana* in homeless populations suggest seroprevalence of 10%.

RISK FACTORS
- Vector exposure with cutaneous inoculation
  - *B. bacilliformis*: Lutzomyia sandflies, limited to Andean South America
  - *B. quintana*: Human body louse, typically in alcoholic, homeless men
  - *B. henselae*: Domestic cat (especially scratch/bite from kitten)
  - Others: Unknown
- Cell-mediated immune dysfunction (particularly in bacillary angiomatosis/bacillary peliosis)
  - HIV infection, especially with CD4+ lymphocyte count <100/mcL
  - Chronic steroid, immunosuppressant, or alcohol use

PATHOPHYSIOLOGY
- Erythrocyte and endothelial cell invasion
- Stimulation of angiogenesis

ETIOLOGY
- *B. bacilliformis*: Carrión disease
- *B. quintana*: Trench fever, bacillary angiomatosis (subcutaneous and osseous lesions), bacillary peliosis, endocarditis
- *B. henselae*: CSD, acute and persistent bacteremia, bacillary angiomatosis (hepatosplenic lesions), bacillary peliosis, endocarditis (preexisting valvular disease), neurologic manifestations
- *B. clarridgeiae, B. elizabethae, B. grahamii, B. vinsonii, B. washoensis*: Case reports of CSD, bacteremia, endocarditis, myocarditis, others

DIAGNOSIS

- Diagnosis of typical CSD traditionally requires at least 3 of the following
  - Animal contact (usually cat) resulting in a scratch, abrasion, or ocular lesion
  - Positive serologic test
  - Characteristic lymph node pathology
  - No evidence of other cause
- Diagnosis of other syndromes requires high clinical suspicion and identification of compatible syndrome; if test results are not helpful, response to appropriate antibiotics may be suggestive.

SIGNS AND SYMPTOMS
- Carrión disease (aka Bartonellosis; usually has 2 distinctive stages: An acute, life-threatening illness associated with high fever, hemolytic anemia, and a chronic, benign cutaneous eruption consisting of raised, reddish-purple nodules.
  - Oroya fever (acute bacteremia): In severe cases, abrupt onset 3 weeks after inoculation. Profound anemia, many complications, may be fatal.
  - Asymptomatic persistent bacteremia: <15% of untreated Oroya fever survivors
  - Verruga peruana: Crops of nodular angiomatous skin lesions months after Oroya fever; mucosal and internal lesions also; involute in months to years
- Typical CSD (up to 90% of cases)
  - Days after inoculation 2–3-mm nontender papules develop at the trauma site; progress to reddened then crusted vesicles
  - Tender regional adenopathy 1–8 weeks postinoculation; fever, malaise, headache
  - Usually involves nodes of upper extremities, neck, head
  - Suppuration of nodes common, but only 10% require drainage
  - Resolution in 2–4 months for majority
- Atypical CSD
  - Parinaud oculoglandular syndrome: Unilateral granulomatous conjunctivitis and preauricular lymphadenitis
  - Neuroretinitis: Abrupt, painless unilateral vision loss; macular star exudate, papilledema; self-limited, with return of visual acuity
  - Encephalopathy: Rapid progression from headache to lethargy, coma, and seizure; sequelae rare

- Other manifestations self-limited, sequelae rare: Granulomatous hepatitis/splenitis, osteolysis, atypical pneumonitis, fever of unknown origin, mononucleosis-type syndrome, others
- Bacteremia (short-term mortality uncommon)
  - *B. quintana* (urban trench fever, Wolhynia fever, shin-bone fever, quintan fever): Incubation days–weeks; sudden onset of fever, headache, leg pain; self-limited illness may be brief (4–5 days), prolonged (2–6 weeks), most commonly paroxysmal (3–5 episodes of 5 days' duration). Insidious course in HIV.
  - *B. henselae*: If HIV-infected, insidious onset of fatigue, malaise, aches, weight loss, recurring fevers, headache; localizing findings uncommon. If HIV-uninfected, abrupt onset of fever (may persist or relapse), myalgias, arthralgias, headache; localizing findings unusual; may persist without symptoms.
- Endocarditis: Fever, dyspnea, murmur, embolic phenomena; aortic valve involvement most common
- Bacillary angiomatosis: Mostly immunocompromised hosts (e.g., HIV-infected); involves skin (crops of subcutaneous or dermal nodules and/or skin-colored to purple papules; may ulcerate with serous or bloody drainage and crusting), regional lymph nodes, internal organs
- Bacillary peliosis: Involves liver and spleen in immunosuppressed persons; can involve lymph nodes; nonspecific clinical manifestations
- Neurologic syndromes in HIV: Cognitive dysfunction, behavioral disturbances; may be mistaken for dementia, psychiatric disease

TESTS
Lab
- Skin testing reagents: Not recommended
- Giemsa-stained blood smear may show *B. bacilliformis* adherent to erythrocytes
- Non-*bacilliformis* species
  - Indirect fluorescent antibody and enzyme immunoassay tests are available
    - Interpretation complicated by variable correlation between titers and disease stage, lack of uniformity among serologic tests, and cross-reactivity among *Bartonella* species and other bacteria.

ALERT
Advise lab if *Bartonella* infection is suspected so that blood, tissue, and cerebrospinal fluid cultures are prepared with appropriate media under optimal conditions; prolonged incubation required.

- Polymerase chain reaction (PCR) and immunohistochemical labeling primarily research tools, although PCR of valve tissue can aid diagnosis of endocarditis
- Drugs that may alter lab results: Antibiotics (cultures falsely negative)

Imaging
Ultrasonography, CT, or ECG as indicated

Diagnostic Procedures/Surgery
- Biopsies for histology/culture of nodules, lymph nodes, or internal organs
- Lumbar puncture if CNS involvement

B

Pathological Findings

- Verruga peruana: Neovascular proliferation; bacteria uncommonly are identified.
- CSD: Granulomas, stellate necrosis, mixed inflammatory infiltrates; bacilli in tissue may be demonstrable by silver impregnation stains (e.g., Warthin-Starry).
- Endocarditis: Warthin-Starry–stained bacilli may be seen in vegetations.
- Bacillary angiomatosis
  - Lobular proliferations of small blood vessels are seen, containing cuboidal endothelial cells interspersed with inflammatory cells, mostly neutrophils.
  - Warthin-Starry stain or electron microscopy may show clusters of bacilli
- Bacillary peliosis: Blood-filled cystic structures. Warthin-Starry stain may show surrounding clumps of bacilli.

DIFFERENTIAL DIAGNOSIS

- Typical CSD: Sporotrichosis, histoplasmosis, plague, tularemia, brucellosis, mycobacteria, staphylococci, streptococci, other agents associated with injection drug use; lymphoma; metastatic malignancy
- Atypical CSD: Other agents causing similar syndromes
- Non-*bacilliformis* bacteremia syndromes
  - Immunocompromised: *Cryptococcus neoformans*, *Histoplasma capsulatum*, *Coccidioides immitis*, *Mycobacterium avium*-complex
  - Arthropod exposure: Rickettsial infections, tularemia, plague, babesiosis, borreliosis
  - Cat/dog scratch/bite: *Pasteurella*
  - Influenza, infectious mononucleosis, hepatitis
- Endocarditis: Other slow-growing bacteria (*Haemophilus, Actinobacillus, Cardiobacterium, Eikenella, Kingella, Coxiella*)
- Bacillary angiomatosis/bacillary peliosis: Kaposi sarcoma; pyogenic granuloma, hemangioma
- Neurologic syndrome in HIV: Tertiary syphilis, cryptococcal meningitis, toxoplasmosis, progressive multifocal leukoencephalopathy, alcohol or drug abuse

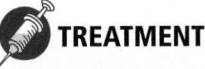 TREATMENT

INITIAL STABILIZATION

- Outpatient for uncomplicated infection
- Initial hospitalization may be necessary for IV antibiotics or complications.

GENERAL MEASURES

- CSD: Supportive therapy (e.g., aspiration suppurative nodes)
- Systemic syndromes (including CSD-associated neuroretinitis and encephalopathy): Antibiotics

Activity

Fully active if uncomplicated

 MEDICATION (DRUGS)

First Line

- Oroya fever: Chloramphenicol 500 mg (pediatric dose 50–75 mg/dg/d) PO/IV q.i.d. + β-lactam for 14 days (not available in US) (1) [B]; ciprofloxacin 500 mg (250 mg for children 7–12 years) PO b.i.d. for 10 days
- Verruga peruana: Rifampin 10/mg/kg/d (not to exceed 600 mg/d in children) for 10 days (1) [B]
- Typical CSD: No clear benefit, although oral azithromycin may speed resolution of extensive lymphadenopathy: Adults and children >45.5 kg: 500 mg on day 1; 250 mg daily on days 2–5; children ≤45.5 kg: 10 mg/kg on day 1; 5 mg/kg daily on days 2–5 (1) [A]
- Retinitis: Doxycycline 100 mg PO b.i.d. + rifampin 300 mg PO b.i.d. for 4–6 weeks (1) [B]
- Trench fever or chronic *B. quintana* bacteremia: Doxycycline 200 mg PO daily for 4 weeks + gentamicin 3 mg/kg IV daily for 2 weeks (1) [A]
- Bacillary angiomatosis: Erythromycin 500 mg (pediatric dose 40 mg/kg/d to maximum daily dose of 2 g/d) PO q.i.d. or doxycycline 100 mg PO b.i.d. for 3 months; consider longer course if immunocompromised (1) [B]
- Bacillary peliosis: Erythromycin 500 mg (pediatric dose 40 mg/kg/d to maximum daily dose of 2 g/d) PO q.i.d. or doxycycline 100 mg PO b.i.d. for 4 months; consider longer course if immunocompromised (1) [B]
- Endocarditis (culture positive): Gentamicin 3 mg/kg IV daily for 2 weeks + doxycycline 100 mg PO b.i.d. for 6 weeks (1) [B]
- Endocarditis (culture negative): Gentamicin 3 mg/kg IV daily for 2 weeks + ceftriaxone 2 g IV/IM daily for 6 weeks +/– doxycycline 100 mg PO/IV b.i.d. for 6 weeks (1) [B]

SURGERY

Valve replacement if indicated in endocarditis

 FOLLOW-UP

PROGNOSIS

- CSD: Spontaneous resolution usually in 2–4 months without specific therapy
- Other syndromes: With proper treatment, full resolution; if relapse, consider long-term suppressive antibiotics after retreatment

COMPLICATIONS

Relapse, especially in HIV infection

PATIENT MONITORING

Close follow-up after completion of antibiotics to monitor for relapse

REFERENCES

1. Rolain JM, Brouqui P, Koehler JE, et al. Recommendations for treatment of human infections caused by *Bartonella* species. *Antimicrob Agents Chemother* 2004;48(6):1921–1933.

ADDITIONAL READING

- Agan BK, Dolan MJ. Laboratory diagnosis of *Bartonella* infections. Clin Lab Med. 2002;22:937–962.
- Dehio C. Molecular and cellular basis of *Bartonella* pathogenesis. Ann Rev Microbiol. 2004;58:365–390.
- Slater LN, Welch DF. *Bartonella*, including cat-scratch disease. In: Mandell, Bennett, Dolin, eds. *Principles and Practice of Infectious Diseases*, 6th ed. Philadelphia: Churchill Livingstone, 2005.

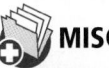 MISCELLANEOUS

CODES

ICD9-CM

- 078.3 Cat-scratch disease
- 083.1 Trench fever
- 083.8 Other diagnoses, including bacillary angiomatosis/bacillary peliosis
- 088.0 Bartonellosis

PATIENT TEACHING

 See Corresponding Diagnostic Algorithm

 See Patient Handout on CD

BASAL CELL CARCINOMA

Melissa A. Fischer, MD, MEd

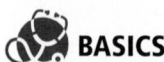 **BASICS**

DESCRIPTION
- Basal Cell Carcinoma (BCC) is a common malignant tumor of the skin originating from the basal cells of the epidermis and its appendages
- Rarely metastasizes, but capable of local tissue destruction

ALERT
Geriatric Considerations
Greater frequency in geriatric patients (age 55–75 have 100× incidence of age <20)

Pediatric Considerations
Rare in children, but childhood sun exposure important in adult disease

GENERAL PREVENTION
- Sunscreens (though likely more effective for squamous cell carcinoma) (1)[B]
- Hats, long-sleeve shirts
- Avoid tanning and sunburn, especially during childhood

EPIDEMIOLOGY
- Incidence/prevalence in United States: ~900,000 cases/year
- Predominant age: Generally >40, but incidence is increasing in younger populations
- Predominant sex: Males > Female (although incidence is increasing in females)

Incidence
- Lifetime risk of caucasion North American: 30%

RISK FACTORS
- Chronic sun exposure (UV radiation)
- Light complexion
- Tendency to sunburn
- Male sex, although increasing risk in women due to lifestyle changes such as tanning beds/salons
- Family history of skin cancer, basal cell nevus syndrome (rare autosomal dominant)
- 3–4 decades after chronic arsenic exposure, 2 decades after therapeutic radiation, chronic immunosuppression

PATHOPHYSIOLOGY
- UV-induced inflammation and Cyclooxygenase activation in skin
- Patched, Drosophila, Homolog of tumor suppressor gene mutations (familial and sporadic)
- Cytochrome P-450 CYP2D6 and glutathione S-transferase detoxifying enzyme gene mutations (especially in truncal BCC)

ASSOCIATED CONDITIONS
- Xeroderma pigmentosum
- Nevoid BCC syndrome

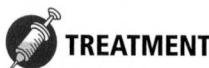 **DIAGNOSIS**

SIGNS AND SYMPTOMS
- 70% facial, 15% truncal
- Nodular: Most common (60%), presents as pinkish, pearly papule often with telangiectatic vessel and ulceration, usually on face
- Superficial: (30%) light red, scaly papule or plaque with atrophic center, ringed by translucent micropapules, usually on trunk; more common in men
- Morpheaform: (5–10%) firm, smooth, flesh-colored papule with ill-defined borders
- As the nodules enlarge, central ulceration and crusting can occur

History
Exposure to risk factors, family history

TESTS
Diagnostic Procedures/Surgery
Biopsy and pathologic examination mandatory to confirm diagnosis

Pathological Findings
- Nidus of basal cells extending into dermis
- Characteristic cells resemble normal basal cells with large basophilic, oval nuclei.
- Rare mitoses
- Tumor cells arranged in palisades at periphery

DIFFERENTIAL DIAGNOSIS
- Sebaceous hyperplasia
- Epidermal inclusion cyst
- Intradermal nevi (pigmented and nonpigmented)
- Molluscum contagiosum
- Squamous cell carcinoma
- Nummular dermatitis
- Psoriasis
- Melanoma (pigmented lesions)

TREATMENT

PRE HOSPITAL
Outpatient unless extensive lesion

GENERAL MEASURES
Activity
No restrictions except to avoid overexposure to sun

MEDICATION (DRUGS)

Topical antibiotics after excision for 24–48 hours (optional)

SURGERY
- Generally first choice, specific treatment selection varies with extent and location of lesion, tumor border distinctiveness (2)[A]

- High-risk areas
  - Inner canthus, Nasolabial sulcus, Philtrum, Preauricular area, Retroauricular sulcus, Lip, Temple
- Curettage and electrodesiccation
  - Nodular lesion <1 cm, in low-risk area, if not deeply invasive
  - Requires specialized training and experience in surgical technique
- Excision
  - Useful for lesions in high-risk areas, not as dependent on lesion size
  - Poor choice if multiple lesions
  - Requires appropriate training
- Cryosurgery
  - Reserved for small lesions in low-risk area
  - Requires specialized training and equipment
  - May want pre- and post-treatment biopsies
- Mohs surgery
  - The preferred microsurgically controlled surgical treatment for lesions in high-risk area, for recurrent lesion, if there is an aggressive growth pattern
  - Requires referral to appropriately trained dermatologic surgeon

RADIATION
- Useful for large lesions, very elderly (life expectancy <15 years) or patients who could not tolerate minor surgical procedures
- Also may be used when preservation of local tissue important, such as near lips and eyelids

MEDICAL
5-Fluorouracil (3)[C]
- inhibits thymidylate synthetase interrupting DNA synthesis
- for superficial lesions in low-risk areas
- primary treatment only
- 5% applied b.i.d. for 3–10 weeks
  Other non-surgical treatments under investigation: Imiquimod, photodynamic therapy, interferon

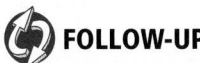 **FOLLOW-UP**

PROGNOSIS
- Proper treatment yields 90–95% cure
- Most recurrences happen within 5 years
- Development of new BCCs: Patients (36%) will develop a new lesion within 5 years

COMPLICATIONS
- Local recurrence and spread
- Usually recurrences will appear within 5 years.
- Metastasis (rare, <0.1%), but metastatic disease usually fatal within 8 mos

PATIENT MONITORING
- Every month for 3 months, then twice yearly for 5 years; yearly thereafter
- Increased risk of other skin cancers (4)[C]

REFERENCES

1. Green A, Williams G, Neale R, et al. Daily sunscreen application and betacarotene supplementation in prevention of baseal-cell and squamous-cell carcinomas of the skin: A randomized controlled trial. *Lancet.* 1999;354: 723.
2. Bath FJ, Bong J, Perkins W, Williams HC. Interventions for basal cell carcinoma of the skin. *Cochrane Database Syst Rev.* 2003;CD003412.
3. Goette DK. Topical chemotherapy with 5-Fluorouracil. A review. *J Am Acad Dermatol.* 1981;4:633.
4. Friedma GD, Tekawa IS. Association of basal cell skin cancers with other cancers (United States). *Cancers Cause Control.* 2000;11:891.

 MISCELLANEOUS

Related terms: Basal cell epithelioma; Rodent ulcer

CODES

ICD9-CM
- 173.3 Other malignant neoplasm of skin of other and unspecified parts of face
- 173.4 Other malignant neoplasm of scalp and skin of neck
- 173.5 Other malignant neoplasm of skin of trunk, except scrotum
- 173.6 Other malignant neoplasm of skin of upper limb, including shoulder
- 173.7 Other malignant neoplasm of skin of lower limb, including hip
- 173.9 Other malignant neoplasm of skin, site unspecified

PATIENT TEACHING
- Teach patient appropriate sun avoidance techniques, sunscreens, etc.
- Skin self-exam

 See Patient Handout on CD

BEHÇET SYNDROME

Bruce M. Rothschild, MD

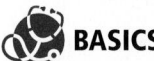 **BASICS**

DESCRIPTION

- Rare multisystem, chronic disease characterized by oral and genital mucocutaneous ulcerations, skin rashes, arthritis, thrombophlebitis, uveitis, colitis, and neurologic symptoms (1–6)[A]
- Endemic in Japan and Northeastern Mediterranean region
- Synonym(s): Ucocutaneous ocular syndrome; Franceschetti-Valero syndrome

ALERT

Geriatric Considerations
Rare

Pediatric Considerations
Rare

Pregnancy Considerations (7)[B]
- Thalidomide contraindicated in pregnancy
- Possible increase in thrombosis and fetal demise

GENERAL PREVENTION
Avoid English walnuts

EPIDEMIOLOGY
- Predominant age: 3rd to 4th decades
- Predominant sex: Male > Female frequently twice as often, whereas as some studies suggest equal frequency

Prevalence (6,8)[A]
- 1/100,000 prevalence in the United States
- In other countries, per 100,000
  - Japan: 10
  - Iran: 16–100
  - Germany: 2
  - Saudi Arabia: 20

RISK FACTORS
See "Etiology"

Genetics
- One report in a mother and newborn (9)
- Very rarely familial

ETIOLOGY (2–6)[A], (9)[A]
Unknown:
- Classified as vasculopathy or autoimmune
- HLA-B5 alloantigen relationship
- Possible environmental toxin: Heavy metals, pesticides
- Possibly English walnuts or Ginkgo nuts
- Fibrinolysis abnormality
- 1 report associated with HIV infection (10)

ASSOCIATED CONDITIONS
- Amyloid
- Sweet syndrome

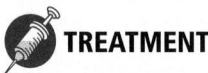 **DIAGNOSIS**

SIGNS AND SYMPTOMS (2–6)[A], (8)[A]
- Aphthous stomatitis
- Genital ulcers: Painful in the male, usually painless in the female
- Dermal: Papulovesicular, erythema nodosum, pathergy, erythema multiforme, vasculitis, pyoderma
- Ocular: Liritis, iridocyclitis, chorioretinitis, hypopyon, hemorrhage, papilledema, optic atrophy (8)[A]
- Morning stiffness: In 1/3 of patients
- Polyarthritis: Self-limited and predominantly affecting lower extremities
- Thrombophlebitis: Peripheral, pulmonary, cerebral, Budd Chiari syndrome (11)[A]
- Neurologic: Cranial nerve palsy, hemiplegia, intracranial hypertension, meningomyelitis and recurrent meningitis, confusional state (12)[A], (13)[A]
- GI: Aphthous ulcers, colitis, melena
- Pulmonary infiltrates—possibly related to thrombosis
- Myopathy/myositis: Rare
- Peripheral gangrene: Rare
- Epididymitis
- Glomerulonephritis: Rare

TESTS (2–6)[A], (8)[A]
- Erythrocyte sedimentation rate elevation, but can be normal
- Immune complexes detected by Raji cell and C1q solid phase assays, but not clinically useful
- Cryoglobulin
- Hypergammaglobulinemia
- Circulating anticoagulation (rare)
- Depression of plasma antithrombin III levels with active disease
- Increased fibrinolytic activity during attacks
- Antineutrophil cytoplasmic antigen antibodies, perinuclear variety
- Demyelinating antibodies in neuro-Behçet syndrome
- Anticardiolipin antibodies (rare), lupus anticoagulants
- Antiendothelial antibodies
- Pathergy

Diagnostic Procedures/Surgery
- Careful history and physical and frequent reevaluation
- Synovial fluid: Inflammatory effusion
- Arteriography: For aneurysms or thrombosis

Pathological Findings
- May be no recognizable changes
- Mononuclear perivascular infiltration
- Mononuclear infiltrate in synovium
- Endothelial cell swelling
- Partial obliteration of vascular lumen
- Neutrophilic dermatitis (Sweet syndrome) (rarely)

DIFFERENTIAL DIAGNOSIS
- Reiter syndrome and other forms of spondyloarthropathy
- Inflammatory bowel disease (Crohn disease and ulcerative colitis)
- Syphilis
- Erythema nodosum
- Aphthous stomatitis
- Herpes simplex
- Stevens-Johnson syndrome
- Vasculitis
- Multisystem disease
- Thrombophlebitis related to coagulation factor deficiency
- Mollaret meningitis

TREATMENT

INITIAL STABILIZATION
- Usually outpatient
- Inpatient usually required for neurologic complications

GENERAL MEASURES
According to body system involved

Diet
No special diet

Activity
As tolerated

💊 MEDICATION (DRUGS)

First Line (2–6)[A], (14–15)[A], (16)[B]

- Colchicine: 0.6 mg b.i.d.
- Topical ocular steroids
- Prednisone: 1 mg/kg for severe involvement, especially central nervous system
- Azathioprine: 2–3 mg/kg/d PO
- Methotrexate: Use lowest possible dose; perhaps 7.5 mg per week
- Cyclosporine: 1–4 mg/kg, but monitor liver function, creatinine, magnesium, and lipids every 2 weeks for 3 months, then every month (17)[A]
- Resistant cases may require
  – Tacrolimus (FK 506) 0.09–0.15 mg/kg/d
  – Thalidomide 300 mg/d
  – Interferon alpha (15)[A]
  – Anticoagulants for patients with anticardiolipin antibodies: Warfarin (Coumadin) to establish PT international normalized ratio 3.0 to 3.5.
- Contraindications
  – Thalidomide contraindicated during pregnancy
  – Refer to manufacturer's literature
- Precautions
  – Refer to manufacturer's literature
  – Absorption of drugs such as amitriptyline, diazepam, carbamazepine, phenytoin, and acetaminophen may be reduced in Behçet syndrome. (14)[A]
- Significant possible interactions: Refer to manufacturer's literature.

Second Line

- Levamisole: 100–150 mg 2 days per week
- Chlorambucil: But concern with respect to toxicity, especially its malignant potential
- Cyclophosphamide: 50–100 mg per day in morning.
- The patient should drink 8–10 glasses of water per day and report any blood in the urine.
- Tumor necrosis factor inhibitors (18)[A]
- Stem cell transplantation (19)[B]
- Anti-CD52 antibody (16)[B]

⚡ FOLLOW-UP

PROGNOSIS

- Normal life expectancy, except with neurologic involvement
- Possible vision impairment

COMPLICATIONS (2–6), 8[A]

- Death
- Blindness
- Paralysis
- Embolism/thrombosis—pulmonary, vena cava, peripheral
- Aneurysms
- Amyloidosis
- Thrombotic events, especially when anticardiolipin antibodies present

PATIENT MONITORING

Dependent on severity of system involvement and medication monitoring

REFERENCES

1. International diagnostic study group for Behçet's disease. Evaluation of ("classification") criteria in Behçet's disease—Towards internationally agreed criteria. *Br J Rheumatol*. 1992;31:299–308.
2. Kaklamani VG, et al. Behçet's disease. *Semin Arthritis Rheu*. 1998;27:197–217.
3. Lockwood CM, Hale G, Waldman H, Jayne DR. Remission induction in Behçet's disease following lymphocyte depletion by the anti-CD52 antibody CAMPATH 1-H. *Rheumatology (Oxford)*. 2003;42:1539–1544.
4. Pacor ML, et al. Cyclosporin in Behçet's disease. *J Rheumatol*. 1994;13:224–227.
5. Shimizu T, et al. Behçet disease. *Semin Arthritis Rheu*. 1979;8:223–260.
6. Zouboulis CC, Vaiopoulos G, Marcomichelakis N, et al. Onset signs, clinical course, prognosis, treatment and outcome of adult patients with Adamantiades-Behçet's disease in Greece. *Clin Exp Rheumatol*. 2003;21(suppl 30):19–26.
7. Sushan JJ, Sela EY, Ozcan C. Behçet's disease and pregnancy. *Acta Obstet Gynecol Scand* 2005;84:939–944 [B].
8. Yoshida A, Kawashima H, Motoyama Y, et al. Comparison of patients with Behçet's disease in the 1980's and 1990's. *Ophthalmology* 2004;111:810–815 [A].
9. Fam A. Neonatal Behçet syndrome in an infant of a mother with the disease. *Ann Rheumatic Dis*. 1981;40:509–512.
10. Stein C. *J Rheumatol*. 1991;18:1427–1428.
11. Huong DL, et al. Arterial lesions in Behçet's disease. *J Rheumatol*. 1995;22:2103–2113.
12. Akman-Demir G, et al. Seven-year follow-up of neurologic involvement in Behçet syndrome. *Arch Neurol*. 1996;53:691–768.
13. Gerber S, et al. Long-term MR follow-up of cerebral lesions in neuro-Behçet's disease. *Neuroradiology*. 1996;38:761–768.
14. Chaleby K. Decreased drug absorption in a patient with Behçet's syndrome. *Clin Chem*. 1987;33:1679–1681.
15. Hamuryudan V, et al. Systemic interferon alpha-2b treatment in Behçet syndrome. *J Rheumatol*. 1994;21:1098–1100.
16. Mauer B, Hensel M, Max R, et al. Autologous haematopoietic stem cell transplantation for Behçet's disease with pulmonary involvement: Analysis after 5 years of followup. *Ann Rheumatic Dis*. 2006;65:127–129 [B].
17. Sakane T, Takeno M, Suzuki N, Inaba G. Behçet's disease. *N Engl J Med*. 1999;341:1284–1291.
18. Hassard PV, Binder SW, Nelson V, Vasiliauskas EA. Anti-tumor necrosis factor monoclonal antibody therapy for gastrointestinal Behçet's disease: a case report. *Gastroenterology*. 2001;120:995–999.
19. Melikoglu M, Fresko I, Mat C, et al. Short-term trial of etanercept in Behçet's disease: A double blind, placebo controlled study. *J Rheumatol* 2005;32:98–105 [B].
20. O'Duffy JD. Behçet's disease. *Curr Opin Rheumatol*. 1994;6:39–43.

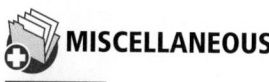 MISCELLANEOUS

CODES

ICD9-CM
136.1 Behçet syndrome

PATIENT TEACHING

American Behçet Association, 421 21st Avenue SW, Rochester, MN 55902; (507) 281-3059.

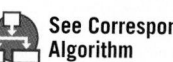 **See Corresponding Diagnostic Algorithm**

BELL PALSY

Dylan C. Kwait, MD

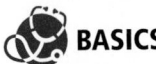 **BASICS**

DESCRIPTION
- Peripheral lower motor neuron facial palsy, usually unilateral, which arises secondary to inflammation and subsequent swelling and compression of the 7th (facial) cranial nerve and the associated vasa nervorum.
- Synonym(s): Idiopathic facial paralysis

EPIDEMIOLOGY
- Accounts for 60–75% of all cases of unilateral facial paralysis (1)[A]
- Predominant age
  - Median age of onset is 40 years, but affects all ages (2)[A].
- Predominant sex: Male = Female (2)[A]

Incidence
- Incidence in the US is 20–30 cases per 100,000 people per year (2)[A].
- Incidence is lowest in children ≤10 years of age; highest in people ≥70 years of age (2)[A].
- Incidence is higher among pregnant women (1)[A].
- Occurs with equal frequency on the left and right sides of the face (2)[A].

Prevalence
Affects 40,000 Americans every year (3)[A].

RISK FACTORS
- Pregnancy
- Diabetes mellitus
- Age >30
- Exposure to cold temperatures
- Upper respiratory infection (e.g., coryza, influenza)

Genetics
A genetic predisposition may be associated with Bell palsy, but it is unclear which factors are inherited.

ETIOLOGY
- Results from damage to the 7th (facial) cranial nerve
- Inflammation of the 7th nerve causes swelling and subsequent compression of both the nerve and the associated vasa nervorum
- May arise secondary to reactivation of latent herpes virus (herpes simplex virus type 1 and herpes zoster virus) in cranial nerve ganglia (1)[A].
- May arise secondary to ischemia from arteriosclerosis associated with diabetes mellitus (2)[A].

ASSOCIATED CONDITIONS
- Lyme disease
- Diabetes mellitus
- Hypertension
- Herpes simplex virus
- Herpes zoster virus
- Ramsay Hunt syndrome
- Sjögren syndrome
- Sarcoidosis
- Eclampsia
- Amyloidosis

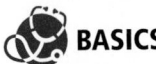 **DIAGNOSIS**

SIGNS AND SYMPTOMS
- Weakness on affected side of face, often sudden in onset
- Pain in or behind the ear in 50% of cases (may precede the palsy in 25% of cases) (2)[A]
- Subjective numbness on the ipsilateral side of the face
- Alteration of taste on the ipsilateral anterior 2/3 of the tongue (chorda tympani branch of the facial nerve)
- Hyperacusis (nerve to the stapedius muscle)
- Decreased tear production

History
It is vital to elicit
- Time course of the illness (e.g., rapid vs. slow onset)
- Any predisposing factors (e.g., recent viral infection, trauma, new medications, hypertension, diabetes mellitus)
- Presence of hyperacusis or history of recurrent Bell palsy (both associated with poor prognosis)
- Any associated rash (suggestive of herpes zoster, Lyme disease, or sarcoid)

Physical Exam
- Neurologic examination to determine if the weakness is due to a problem in either the central or peripheral nervous systems
  - Flaccid paralysis of muscles on the affected side, including the forehead
    ○ Impaired ability to raise the ipsilateral eyebrow
    ○ Impaired closure of the ipsilateral eye
    ○ Bell phenomenon: Upward diversion of the eye with attempted closure of the lid
    ○ Impaired ability to smile, grin or purse the lips
  - Patients may complain of numbness, but on sensory testing, no deficit is present.
  - Examine for involvement of other cranial nerves.
- HEENT
  - Carefully examine head, neck, and oropharynx to exclude masses.
  - Perform pneumatic otoscopic examination.
- Skin
  - Examine for erythema migrans (Lyme disease) and vesicular rash (herpes zoster virus).

TESTS
- Electromyography
  - Nerve conduction on affected and nonaffected sides can be compared to determine extent of nerve injury.
- Electroneurography
  - Evoked potentials of affected and nonaffected sides can be compared.
- CSF analysis
  - Not routinely indicated
  - CSF protein is elevated in 1/3 of cases.
  - CSF cells show mild elevation in 10% of cases with a mononuclear cell predominance.

Lab
- Lyme titer and IgM, IgG, and IgA for *B. burgdorferi*
- Salivary PCR for herpes simplex virus type 1 or herpes zoster virus (these tests are largely reserved for research purposes) (1)[A]
- IgM, IgG, and IgA titers for varicella zoster virus, cytomegalovirus, rubella, hepatitis A, hepatitis B, and hepatitis C
- ESR
- Blood glucose level
- CBC
- RPR test
- HIV test

Imaging
- Facial radiographs
  - Rule out fractures
- CT
  - Rule out fractures
  - Rule out stroke
- Brain MRI
  - Not routinely indicated
  - Rule out central pontine, temporal bone, and parotid neoplasms (2)[A]

Diagnostic Procedures/Surgery
Invasive diagnostic procedures are not indicated, because biopsy could further damage the 7th nerve (4)[A].

Pathological Findings
- Dilatation of the vasa nervorum
- Edema of the facial nerve with infiltration of mononuclear cells and possible atrophy

DIFFERENTIAL DIAGNOSIS
- Infectious
  - Lyme disease
  - Herpes zoster (Ramsay-Hunt syndrome)
  - Acute or chronic otitis media
  - Malignant otitis externa
  - Osteomyelitis of the skull base
  - Infectious mononucleosis
  - Leprosy
- Trauma injury
  - Temporal bone fracture
  - Mandibular bone fracture

- Neoplastic (should be considered in cases where onset of palsy is slow and progressive and accompanied by additional cranial nerve deficits and/or headache) (1)[A]
  - Tumors of the parotid gland
  - Cholesteatoma
  - Skull-base tumor
  - Carcinomatous meningitis
  - Leukemic meningitis
- Cerebrovascular
  - Brainstem stroke involving antero-inferior cerebellar artery
  - Aneurysm involving carotid, vertebral or basilar arteries
- Other
  - Multiple sclerosis
  - Myasthenia gravis (should be considered in cases of recurrent or bilateral facial palsy) (2)[A]
  - Guillain-Barré syndrome (may also present with bilateral facial palsy) (2)[A]
  - Sjögren syndrome
  - Sarcoidosis
  - Amyloidosis
  - Melkersson-Rosenthal syndrome
  - Polyneuritis

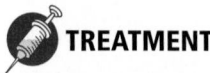

TREATMENT

GENERAL MEASURES
- Artificial tears should be used to lubricate the cornea.
- The ipsilateral eye should be patched and taped shut at night to avoid drying and infection.

Diet
No restrictions

Activity
No restrictions

MEDICATION (DRUGS)

No evidence suggests that pharmacologic intervention (with anti-inflammatory and/or antiviral agents) or decompression surgery is any more beneficial than watchful waiting in terms of treatment or prevention of long-term effects. (4)[A]

ALERT

Pregnancy Considerations
Steroids should be used cautiously in pregnancy; consult with an obstetrician.

First Line
- Corticosteroids
  - Prednisone (5)[B]: Total from 410 mg over 10 days to 760 mg PO over 16 days, tapering dose (adults only)
  - Treatment should begin immediately after onset, and should not be instituted if symptoms have been present for >7 days.
  - May reduce edema around the 7th cranial nerve; small benefit in adult patients, but use remains controversial.

- Antivirals
  - Acyclovir (5)[B]: 400 mg PO 5 times per day for 10 days (adults only)
  - Should be instituted within 72 hours, but may be started up to 7 days after onset of symptoms.
  - Combination acyclovir and prednisone therapy may improve recovery rates when compared with prednisone alone. (5)[B]
- Contraindications
  - Documented hypersensitivity
  - Pre-existing infections including tuberculosis and systemic mycosis
- Precautions: Use with discretion in pregnancy, peptic ulcer disease, and diabetes.
- Significant possible interactions: Measles-mumps-rubella, oral polio virus vaccine, and other live vaccines

SURGERY
- Surgical treatment of Bell palsy remains controversial and is reserved for intractable cases (1)[A].
- The 7th cranial nerve is surgically decompressed at the entrance to the meatal foramen where the labyrinthine segment and geniculate ganglion reside. (2)[A]
- Decompression surgery should not be performed >14 days after the onset of paralysis because severe degeneration of the facial nerve is likely irreversible after 2–3 weeks. (2)[A]

FOLLOW-UP

DISPOSITION
Issues for Referral
Patients may need to be referred to an ear, nose, and throat specialist or a neurologist.

PROGNOSIS
- Most achieve complete spontaneous recovery within 2 weeks (3)[A].
- 85% of untreated patients will experience the 1st signs of recovery within 3 weeks of onset. (5)[C].
- Over 80% recover within 3 months (3)[A].
- 16% are left with a partial palsy, motor synkinesis, and autonomic synkinesis (1)[A].
- 5% experience severe sequelae, and a small number of patients experience permanent facial weakness and dysfunction (1)[A].
- Poor prognostic factors include
  - Age >60 years
  - Complete facial weakness
  - Hypertension
  - Ramsay-Hunt syndrome
  - Absence of recovery at 3 weeks

COMPLICATIONS
- Corneal abrasion or ulceration
- Steroid-induced psychological disturbances; avascular necrosis of the hips, knees, and/or shoulders
- Steroid use can unmask subclinical infection (e.g., tuberculosis).

PATIENT MONITORING
- Patients should start treatment immediately and be followed for 12 months.
- Patients who do not recover complete facial nerve function should be referred to an ophthalmologist for tarsorrhaphy.

REFERENCES
1. Holland NJ, Weiner GM. Recent developments in Bell's palsy. Br Med J. 2004;329:553–557.
2. Gilden DH. Bell's palsy. N Engl J Med. 2004;351:1323–1331.
3. Holten K. How should we manage Bell's palsy? J Fam Pract. 2004;53(10):797–798.
4. Atkin PA. Diagnosis and the management of Bell's palsy. Practitioner. 2003;247(1642):36.
5. Peitersen E. The natural history of Bell's palsy. Am J Otol. 1982;4(2):107–111.

ADDITIONAL READING
Piercy J. Bell's palsy. Br Med J. 2005;330:1374.

MISCELLANEOUS

See also: Herpes simplex virus; Herpes zoster virus; Ramsay-Hunt syndrome; Sjögren syndrome; Sarcoidosis; Amyloidosis; Lyme disease; Diabetes mellitus; Melkersson-Rosenthal syndrome

CODES

ICD9-CM
351.0 Bell's palsy

PATIENT TEACHING

 See Patient Handout on CD

BIPOLAR DISORDER

Susan Louisa Montauk, MD

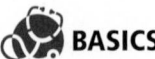 **BASICS**

DESCRIPTION
- A psychiatric disorder characterized by at least one episode of mania and often involving dramatic "mood swings"; episodes of mania and/or hypomania, and major depression that cause marked impairment and/or hospitalization.
- The symptoms must not be due to a substance (e.g., drug), treatment (e.g., ECT or light therapy), a general medical condition (e.g., hyperthyroidism), or medication

ALERT
Geriatric Considerations
New onset in seniors demands a workup for organic or chemically induced pathology

Pediatric Considerations
- Signs and symptoms must be placed into a developmental context
- There is a large overlap with symptoms of Attention Deficit Hyperactivity Disorder (ADHD) and Oppositional Defiant Disorder
- Children and adolescents experience more rapid cycling and mixed states than adults
- Depression often presents as irritable mood

Pregnancy Considerations
No medications currently used for bipolar I disorder are category A or B

EPIDEMIOLOGY
Incidence
No overall incidence data have been reported.

Prevalence
1.0–1.6% (1)

RISK FACTORS
Genetics (2,3)
- Monozygotic twin concordance 40–70%
- Heritability estimate 0.93
- Several chromosomes implicated
- likely many gene set variations

PATHOPHYSIOLOGY
- Neurotransmitters known to be involved
- Serotonin
- Norepinephrine
- Dopamine
- Brain structures most involved
- MRI findings suggest that abnormalities in prefrontal cortical areas, striatum, and amygdala predate illness onset

ETIOLOGY
- Genetic predisposition (major)
- Life stressors

ASSOCIATED CONDITIONS
Substance abuse (60%) (4), ADHD, Anxiety disorders (e.g., Anorexia nervosa, Bulimia nervosa, Generalized anxiety disorder, Obsessive compulsive disorder, Panic disorder, Post-traumatic stress disorder, Social phobia)

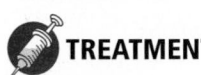 **DIAGNOSIS**

DSM-IV-R CRITERIA
- Bipolar I disorder requires at least one manic or mixed episode (simultaneous mania and depression). There may be episodes of hypomania or major depression as well.
- Mania
  - Distinct period of abnormally and persistently elevated, expansive, or irritable mood, lasting at least 1 week (or any duration if hospitalization is necessary)
  - During the period of mood disturbance, 3 or more of the DIGFAST 1 symptoms must persist (4 if the mood is only irritable) and must be present to a significant degree
- Depression
  - 5 or more of the 9 symptoms (see Sns and Sxs) must have been present during the same 2-week period and represent change from previous functioning; at least 1 of the symptoms is either (1) or (2).
  - Bipolar II (More common in primary care) requires a major depression and at least one hypomanic episode.

SIGNS AND SYMPTOMS
- **Mania** (DIGFAST)
  - **D**istractibility (attention too easily drawn to unimportant or irrelevant external stimuli)
  - **I**nsomnia, decreased need for sleep (e.g., feels rested after only 3 hours of sleep)
  - **G**randiosity or inflated self-esteem
  - **F**light of ideas or subjective experience that thoughts are racing
  - **A**gitation or increase in goal-directed activity (socially, at work or school, or sexually)
  - **S**peech pressured/more talkative than usual
  - **T**aking risks: Excessive involvement in pleasurable activities that have a high potential for painful consequences (e.g., financial or sexual)
- **Hypomania**
  - A distinct period of persistently elevated, expansive, or irritable mood, lasting throughout at least 4 days, that is different from usual non-depressed mood but is not severe enough to cause marked impairment in social or occupational functioning
- **Depression** (DSM)
- Depressed mood most of the day
  - Markedly diminished interest or pleasure activities most of the day
  - Significant weight loss when not dieting or weight gain
  - Insomnia or hypersomnia
- Psychomotor agitation or retardation
- Feel worthless
- Excessive/inappropriate guilt
- Diminished concentration; indecisiveness
- Recurring thoughts of death; suicidal ideation/plan

- **Signs and Symptoms More Likely in Bipolar than in Unipolar Depression (5,6)**
- Agitation
- Atypical depression symptoms (subjectively restless, leaden paralysis, hypersomnia)
- Feelings of worthlessness
- Hyperphagia
- Hypersomnia
- Melancholia
- Psychomotor retardation
- Suicidal ideation/planning
- Minimal tearfulness

History
- Collateral information makes diagnostics more complete and is often the best source for a clear history.
- HOPI (major points)
  - Mood-Mood Disorder Questionnaire and an interview
  - Sleep: Longest awake without stimulants and without sleepiness?
  - Coexistent conditions? Psychosis?
  - Suicide/violence risk

Physical Exam
Base focused exam on history and review of systems

TESTS
- Mood Disorder Questionnaire
  - Sensitivity for mania/hypomania 0.73, specificity 0.90 (7)
- Child Behavior Checklist
  - For Juvenile Bipolar Disorder
- "Dementia" workup if new onset in seniors

Lab
- No labs help rule in bipolar disorder
- Consider drug/alcohol screen if may help assist in future psychoeducation
- Many mood stabilizer medications must have regular blood draw monitoring

DIFFERENTIAL DIAGNOSIS
Other disorders with mania
- Brain tumors
- Drug intoxications
- Organic mood disorders
- Schizoaffective disorder

TREATMENT

PRE HOSPITAL
- Medication
- Psychotherapy
- Psychoeducation
- Cognitive Behavioral Therapy
- Social Rhythm Therapy

INITIAL STABILIZATION
Safe environment plus appropriate medication. Useful comparative studies not done

GENERAL MEASURES
Although experts agree that adopting a "healthy lifestyle" is key to better outcomes, there are few clinical trials to access specific diet or exercise effects

MEDICATION (DRUGS)

First Line
Maintenance therapy for Bipolar Disorder often consists of 3–4 of the following psychoactive medications. (8)

Antiseizure Medications
NOTE: Taper any antiseizure med discontinued for reasons other than major side effects.

- Carbamazepine (Carbatrol, Equetro, Tegretol, generic):
  – FDA approval: Equetroonly for acute mania and mixed episodes
  – Selected warnings: Do not use with TCA or MAOI/Caution with renal or cardiac disease. (Aplastic anemia/agranulocytosis/Preg Cat D)
  – Monitoring: Baseline and q3–6 months
- Divalproex sodium (Depakote, generic)
  – FDA approval: None
  – Selected warnings: Do not use with hepatic or urea cycle disorders. Pancreatitis, polycystic ovary syndrome Preg Cat D. *Dose-related* hepatic failure and low platelets
  – Monitoring: Baseline and q6 months
- Lamotrigine (Lamictal)
  – FDA approval: Only for maintenance therapy
  – Selected warnings: Titrate slowly (rash). Caution with renal, hepatic, or cardiac impairment. Blood dyscrasias, acute multiorgan failure, deadly hypersensitivity. Chronic ophthal. Preg Cat C.
  – Monitoring: Baseline
- Oxcarbazepine (Trileptal)
  – FDA approval: None
  – Selected warnings: Caution if hypersensitivity to carbamazepine. Severe rash, hyponatremia/Preg Cat C adjust for CrCl.
  – Monitoring: Baseline
- Topiramate (Topamax)
  – FDA approval: None
  – Adult dose: 25 mg/d; increase by 25–50 mg q3–14 days prn/as tolerated. Adjust for CrCl.
  – Selected warnings: Possible acidosis in predisposed states. Renal stones, low serum bicarb, acute myopia, oligohidrosis. Preg Cat C.
  – Monitoring: Baseline and as needed (prn)

Atypical Antipsychotics
NOTE: All of these drugs have the following possible major side effects: Orthostatic hypotension, Poor ability to reduce core body temperature, Negatively effect glucose regulation, Negatively affect lipid metabolism, Tardive dyskenesia, Increased mortality in elderly with dementia-related psychosis, Seizures, Neuroleptic malignant syndrome, Weight gain. All except aripiprazole may increase prolactin Preg Cat C.
NOTE: All of these drugs need the following

- Monitoring: Blood work and weight at baseline then 4, 8, and 12 weeks; then q3 months
- Aripiprazole (Abilify):
  – FDA approval: Acute mania, mixed episodes, and maintenance
  – Selected warnings: CVAs in seniors with dementia
- Olanzapine (Zyprexa)
  – FDA approval: Acute mania, mixed episodes, and maintenance therapy (Zydis ODT contains phenylalanine)
  – Selected warnings: CVAs in seniors with dementia

- Quetiapine (Seroquel)
  – FDA approval: Acute mania
  – Selected warnings: Cataracts, hypothyroidism
  – Monitoring: Eye exam at baseline, then prn
- Risperidone (Risperdal)
  – FDA approval: Acute mania and mixed episodes
  – Selected warnings: M tabs contain phenylalanine
- Ziprasidone (Geodon)
  – FDA approval: Acute mania and mixed episodes

Lithium
Lithium (Lithobid, Eskalith, generic)

- FDA approval: Adult acute mania and maintenance therapy
- Selected warnings: Use with caution in patients with significant renal or cardiovascular disease, in severely debilitated or dehydrated patients, and sodium-depleted patients (diuretics, Angiotensin Converting Enzyme Inhibitors (ACEIs). Toxicity can lead to diabetes insipidus, seizures, encephalopathic syndrome, arrhythmias, hypothyroidism. Preg Cat D.
- Monitoring: At baseline, with dose change, then in 5 days, then q2–3 months × 3, then q6–12 months

Second Line
- Antidepressants (not until mood stabilizers are on board) for some patients
- Benzodiazepines

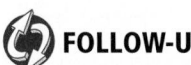 FOLLOW-UP

Admission and Discharge Criteria
Both primarily determined by safety

Issues for Referral
- Experience and comfort level of physician
- Stability of patient

PROGNOSIS
- Most untreated persons will experience manic and/or depression episodes across their lifespan
- Treatment reduces frequency and severity

COMPLICATIONS
In general, the most extreme "complication" is violence toward self or others

PATIENT MONITORING
- Careful medication monitoring
- Regularly scheduled visits to help support medication adherence and healthy lifestyle

REFERENCES

1. Kessler RC, et al. Lifetime and 12-month prevalence of DSM-III–R psychiatric disorders in the United States: Results from the National Comorbidity Study. *Arch Gen Psychiatry.* 1994;51:8–19.
2. Kieseppa T, et al. High concordance of bipolar I disorder in a nationwide sample of twins. *Am J Psychiatry.* 2004;161(10):1814–21.
3. Craddock N, Jones I. Molecular genetics of BD. *Br J Psychiatry.* 2001;41(suppl):128–133.
4. Rush J. Toward an Understanding of BD and Its Origin. *J of Clinical Psychiatry* 2003;64(suppl 6): 4–8.
5. Keck PE. Evaluating Treatment decisions in Bipolar Depression. CME. Medsacpe. www.medscape.com
6. Mitchell PB, Wilhelm K, Parker G, et al. The clinical features of bipolar depression: A comparison with matched major depressive disorder patients. *J Clin Psychiatry.* 2001;62:212–216.
7. Hirshfeld RM. Validation of the Mood Disorder Questionnaire *Bipolar Depression Bulletin.* July 2004.
8. Post RM. Practical approaches to polypharmacy in the long-term management of bipolar disorder. *Drug Benefit Trends.* 2004;16:329–342.
9. Ketter TA, Ed. Advances in Treatment of Bipolar Disorder. Review of Psychiatry, Vol 24 Amer Psychiatric Publishing
10. Working Group on BD. Practice guidelines for the treatment of patients with BD. *Am J Psychiatry* 2002;159(Suppl 4):1–50.
11. Vieta E, Goikolea JM. Atypical antispyhotics: Newer options for mania and maintenance therapy. *BD* 2005;7(Suppl 4):21–33.

ADDITIONAL READING
- Hirschfeld RM, Vomik LA. Rscognition and diagnosis of bipolar disorder. *J Clin Psychiatry.* 2004;65(Suppl 15):5–9.
- Vieta E, Pacchiarotti I, Scott J, et al. Evidence-based research on the efficacy of psychologic interventions in bipolar disorders: a critical review. *Curr Psychiatry Rep.* 2005;7(6):449–455.

 MISCELLANEOUS

CODES

ICD9-CM
(Partial List of the 29 related codes)
- 296.00 Bipolar I disorder, single manic episode, unspecified
- 296.40 Bipolar I disorder, most recent episode (or current) manic, unspecified
- 296.50 Bipolar I disorder, most recent episode (or current) depressed, unspecified

PATIENT TEACHING

Prevention
Healthy lifestyle choices and careful adherence to treatment can decrease mania and/or depression episodes.

 See Corresponding Diagnostic Algorithm

 See Patient Handout on CD

BLADDER CANCER

Margaret E. Thompson, MD

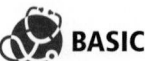 **BASICS**

DESCRIPTION

Primary malignant neoplasms arising in the urinary bladder

- Most common type is transitional cell carcinoma (90%)
- Other types include adenocarcinoma, small cell carcinoma, and squamous cell carcinoma.
- Rhabdomyosarcoma of the bladder may occur in children

GENERAL PREVENTION

Smoking cessation

EPIDEMIOLOGY

Incidence increases with age (median age at diagnosis = 73 years)

- More common in men than in women (4:1)
- More common in Whites than Asians or African Americans

Incidence

- 36.0 per 100,000 men per year (1)
- 9.1 per 100,000 women per year

Prevalence

As of January 1, 2002, 367,550 men and 131,649 women in the United States (1)

RISK FACTORS

- Smoking is the single greatest risk factor
- Other risk factors
  - Occupational carcinogens in dye, rubber, paint, plastics, metal, and automotive exhaust
  - Schistosomiasis in Mediterranean (squamous cell cancer)
  - History of pelvic irradiation
  - Chronic lower urinary tract infection
  - Chronic indwelling urinary catheter
  - Cyclophosphamide exposure
  - High-fat diet
  - Chronic low fluid intake
  - Slight increase in risk with prostate cancer

Genetics

Hereditary transmission unlikely, though transitional cell carcinoma pathophysiology is related to oncogenes; in particular, p56

PATHOPHYSIOLOGY

- 70–80% is superficial (in lamina propria or mucosa):
  - Usually highly differentiated with long survival
- Initial event seems to be activation of an oncogene on chromosome 9
- 20% of tumors are invasive (deeper than lamina propria) at presentation:
  - Tend to be high grade with worse prognosis

ETIOLOGY

- See "Risk Factors"
- Activation of oncogene on chromosome 9

ASSOCIATED CONDITIONS

Cigarette smoking

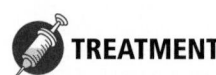 **DIAGNOSIS**

PRE HOSPITAL

Diagnosis depends on biopsy results obtained by cystoscopy, which is often performed in ambulatory site or as outpatient surgery

SIGNS AND SYMPTOMS

- Hematuria—gross or microscopic, usually painless
- May have urinary frequency, urgency, nocturia
- Abdominal or pelvic pain in advanced disease

History

- Hematuria (gross or microscopic) (85–90%)
- Urinary symptoms—frequency, urgency
- Exposures (see "Risk Factors")

Physical Exam

- Normal in early cases
- Pelvic or abdominal mass in advanced disease
- Wasting in systemic disease

TESTS

Urinalysis is the initial test in patients presenting with gross hematuria or urinary symptoms

Lab

- Macroscopic hematuria (55% sensitivity, PPV 0.22 for urologic cancer) (2)[A]
- Urine cytology 54% sensitivity over all, (lower in less-advanced tumors), 94% specific (3)[A]
- Other urine markers
  - NMP22: 67% sensitive, 78% specific (3)[A]
  - BTA stat: 70% sensitive, 75% specific (3)[A]
- Bottom line: None of the urine markers is sensitive enough to rule out bladder cancer on its own. Cytology is the most specific. (3)[A]

Imaging

Done for staging and evaluating extent of disease, but not for diagnosis itself

- IV push to look at upper tracts if there is suspicion of disease there
- For invasive disease, metastatic workup should include chest x-ray, liver function tests, alkaline phosphatase
- Bone scan should be performed if the patient has bone pain or if alkaline phosphatase is elevated (4)[B]
- Urologic CT scan (abdomen, pelvis, with and without contrast) or MRI 40–98% accurate, with MRI slightly more accurate (4)[B]: Recommended if metastasis is suspected

Diagnostic Procedures/Surgery

- Cystoscopy is the gold standard for diagnosis, but one study showed that 33% of patients had residual tumor after transurethral resection of superficial tumor (4)[B]
- Transurethral resection of the bladder tumor (TURBT) with bladder washings
  - Sensitivity of cytology on bladder washings for carcinoma in situ is nearly 100%

ALERT

Any patient who smokes and presents with microscopic or gross hematuria, or irritative voiding symptoms such as urgency and frequency, should be evaluated by cystoscopy for the presence of a bladder neoplasm.

Pathological Findings

- Characterized as superficial or invasive
- 70–80% present as superficial lesion
- Superficial lesions
  - Carcinoma-in-situ (CIS, Tis): Flat lesion, high grade
  - Ta—Non-invasive papillary carcinoma (Ta)
  - T1—Extends into submucosa, lamina propria
- Invasive cancer
  - T2—Invasion into muscle
    - pT2a—invasion into superficial muscle
    - pT2b—invasion into deep muscle
  - T3—Invasion into perivesical fat
    - pT3a—microscopic
    - pT3b—macroscopic
  - T4—invasion into adjacent organs
    - aT4a—invades prostate, uterus, or vagina
    - aT4b—invades abdominal or pelvic wall
  - N1–N3—invades lymph nodes
  - M—metastasis to bone or soft tissue

DIFFERENTIAL DIAGNOSIS

Includes differential diagnosis for hematuria

- Other urinary tract neoplasms
- UTI
- Prostatism
- Bladder instability
- Interstitial cystitis
- Urolithiasis
- Interstitial nephritis
- Papillary urothelial hyperplasia

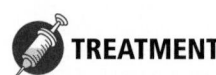 **TREATMENT**

INITIAL STABILIZATION

Generally, hematuria from bladder cancer is not significant enough to cause hemodynamic compromise.

GENERAL MEASURES

Radiotherapy

- In the United States, used for patients with muscle-invasive cancer who are not surgical candidates
- Treatment of choice for muscle-invasive cancer in some European and Canadian centers:
  - 65–70 Gy over 6–7 weeks is standard
- Chemotherapy with cis-platin combined with radiotherapy may preserve bladder function

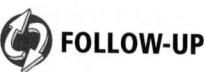 **MEDICATION (DRUGS)**

- Intravesical Bacillus Calmette-Guerin (BCG) after TURBT in high grade lesions has been shown to decrease recurrence in Ta or T1 tumors (5)[A]
  - Common regimen is weekly for 6 weeks, then monthly for 6–12 months

- Intravesical mitomycin C also used

First Line
Chemotherapy is the first-line treatment for metastatic bladder cancer

- Methotrexate-vinblastine-doxorubicin-cisplatin (MVAC) is preferred regimen

SURGERY
- Diffuse carcinoma in situ is treated with intravesical therapy (see Medication)
- Superficial cancer
  - TURBT sometimes followed by intravesical therapy
- Invasive cancer
  - Radical cystectomy for invasive disease that is confined to the bladder more effective than radical radiotherapy. (6)[A] Urine is diverted via an ileal loop with ostomy or neobladder constructed with intestine.
  - Neoadjuvant chemotherapy with cisplatin-methotrexate-vinblastine prior to surgery used by some centers

 FOLLOW-UP

- Superficial cancers
  - Urine cytology alone has not been shown to be sufficient for follow up
  - Cystoscopy every 3 months for 18–24 months, every 6 months for the next 2 years, then annually (7)[C]
- Follow-up for invasive cancers is dependent on the approach to treatment
- Patients treated with BCG require life-long follow-up

Admission Criteria
Need for surgery or intensive therapy

Issues for Referral
Patients with microscopic or gross hematuria should be referred to a urologist for cystoscopy

PROGNOSIS
- Superficial bladder cancer
  - BCG treatment prevents recurrence vs TURBT alone, difference 30%, NNT 3.3 (7)[A]
  - BCG prevents progression vs TURBT alone, difference 8% (7)[A]

- Invasive cancer
  - T2 disease—radical cystectomy results in 60–75% 5-year survival
  - T3 or T4 disease—radical cystectomy results in 20–40% 5-year survival
  - Neoadjuvant chemotherapy with cystectomy has led to varying degrees of increased survival.
  - Radiation with chemotherapy has led to varying degrees of increased survival.
- Metastatic cancer
  - MVAC resulted in mean survival of 12.5 months (8)[C]

COMPLICATIONS
- Superficial bladder cancer
  - Local symptoms
    ○ Dysuria, frequency, nocturia, pain, passing debris in urine
    ○ Bacterial cystitis
    ○ Perforation
  - General symptoms
    ○ Flu-like symptoms
    ○ Systemic infection
- Invasive cancer
  - Symptoms related to definitive treatment, including incontinence, bleeding
  - Patients with neobladder at risk for azotemia and metabolic acidosis

PATIENT MONITORING
See "Follow-Up"

REFERENCES

1. National Cancer Institute. SEER Cancer fact sheet, Ries LAG, Eisner MP, Kosary CL, et al., eds. *SEER Cancer Statistics Review*, 1975–2002, National Cancer Institute. Bethesda, MD. Available at: http://seer.cancer.gov/csr/1975˙2002. Accessed February 10, 2006.
2. Buntinx F, Wauters H. The diagnostic value of macroscopic haematuria in diagnosing urological cancers: A meta-analysis. *Fam Pract*. 1997;14: 63–68.
3. Glas AS, Roos D, Deutekom M, et al. Tumor markers in the diagnosis of primary bladder cancer. A systematic review. *J Urol*. 2003;169:1975–1982.
4. Kirkali Z, Chan T, Manoharan, M, et al. Bladder cancer: epidemiology, staging, and grading, and diagnosis. *Urology*. 2005;66(Suppl 6A):4–34.
5. Shelley MD, Court JB, Kynaston H, et al. Intravesical Bacillus Calmette-Guerin in Ta and T1 bladder cancer (Cochrane Review). In: *The Cochrane Library, Issue 4, 2005*. Chichester, UK: John Wiley and Sons, Ltd.
6. Shelley MD, Barber J, Wilt T, Mason MD. Surgery versus radiotherapy for muscle invasive bladder cancer (Cochrane Review). In: *The Cochrane Library, Issue 4, 2005*. Chichester, UK: John Wiley and Sons, Ltd.
7. Smith JA, Labasky RF, Montie JE, Rowland RG, Cockett, ATK, Fracchia JA. Report on the management of non-muscle invasive bladder cancer. American Urologic Association monograph. Baltimore, MD: American Urology Association, Inc. 1999.
8. Loehrer PJ, Einhorn LH, Elson PJ, et al. A randomized comparison of cisplatin alone or in combination with methotrexate, vinblastine, and doxorubicin in patients with metastatic urothelial carcinoma: A cooperative group study. *J Clin Oncol* 1992;10:1066.
9. U.S. Preventive Services Task Force. Screening for bladder cancer in adults: Recommendation statement. Rockville, MD: Agency for Healthcare Research and Quality; 2004.

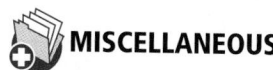 **MISCELLANEOUS**

See also: Hematuria

CODES

ICD9-CM
188.0 to 188.9

PATIENT TEACHING
Hematuria should be reported to physician immediately

Prevention
Smoking cessation

See Corresponding Diagnostic Algorithm

BLADDER INJURY

Mitchell Cahan, MD
Michael Ford, MD

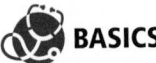 **BASICS**

DESCRIPTION
- Injury to the bladder is the result of trauma, either blunt or penetrating.
- Rupture is associated with a full bladder and blunt injury.
- Very rarely, an operative complication or nontraumatic etiology is the cause.
- Classification
  - Intraperitoneal rupture
  - Extraperitoneal (retroperitoneal) rupture
- Associated ureter/urethral injury

GENERAL PREVENTION
Seat belts

Incidence
~0.5% of trauma patients (1)
- Blunt injuries are associated with pelvic fracture in over 95% of cases.

RISK FACTORS
- High-energy mechanism (fall, MVA)
- Pelvic fracture
- Penetrating wound
- Prior bladder/pelvic surgery
- Pelvic radiotherapy

PATHOPHYSIOLOGY
Rupture can lead to urinoma or peritonitis

ETIOLOGY
- High-energy trauma
- Rupture due to increased pressure in nondistensible (full) bladder
- Laceration due to bone fragment or penetrating object (knife, bullet)

ASSOCIATED CONDITIONS
- Pelvic fracture
- Ureteropelvic disjunction
- Urethral injury; almost exclusively in males
- Peritonitis is unusual in bladder injury.

DIAGNOSIS

PRE HOSPITAL
Isolated bladder injury is rare. Typically patient has other serious injuries.

SIGNS AND SYMPTOMS
- Pelvic/suprapubic pain
- Blood at meatus
- Urinary retention

History
- High-energy deceleration injury (fall, MVA)
- Penetrating trauma
  - Recent abdominal/pelvic surgery

Physical Exam
- Suprapubic tenderness to palpation
- Blood at meatus
- Scrotal/urethral hematoma
  - Free-floating prostate
  - High-riding prostate

TESTS
Lab
Blood on urinalysis
- Serum creatinine and K + are elevated and Na + is decreased in intraperitoneal ruptures.
- Serum labs are unchanged in extraperitoneal ruptures (3).

Imaging
- Cystography is the gold standard for diagnosis.
- High-resolution CT scans also are acceptable.

ALERT
Retrograde urethrography must be performed before placing a Foley catheter when urethral injury is suspected.

Diagnostic Procedures/Surgery
- Intraperitoneal ruptures and penetrating injuries require urgent operative management.
- Extraperitoneal ruptures may be treated with Foley catheter drainage alone.
  - Consider suprapubic tube if drainage is needed for >10 days.

Pathological Findings
- Perivesicular hematoma
- Perforation at dome of bladder (in trigone, near urachus)
- Jagged tear in bladder

DIFFERENTIAL DIAGNOSIS
- Isolated urethral injury
- Isolated pelvic fracture
- Isolated ureteral injury
- Other visceral rupture

TREATMENT

PRE HOSPITAL
- Cervical spine precautions
- Stabilize hemodynamics.
- Stabilize pelvis.

INITIAL STABILIZATION
Stabilize pelvis.

GENERAL MEASURES
- Foley catheter placement
- Pain control
- Antibiotics
- Antispasmodics (Ditropan)
- Imaging diagnosis

Diet
No restrictions

Activity
No restrictions

Nursing
Foley to gravity

Physical Therapy
May be necessary for associated pelvic fractures

IV Fluids
Ringer's lactated solution or normal saline for initial resuscitation

MEDICATION (DRUGS)

- Analgesics
- Antibiotics
- Antispasmodics

First Line
- Narcotic pain control (i.e., morphine, hydromorphone); titrate to effect
- Broad-spectrum antibiotics, such as ciprofloxacin 500 mg b.i.d.
- Ditropan 5–10 mg t.i.d. p.r.n. for spasm

ALERT
There is concern about fluoroquinolones causing damage to cartilage in children.

Second Line
- Broad-spectrum antibiotics
- Antispasmodics (i.e., flavoxate)

SURGERY
- Urgent surgery is indicated for intraperitoneal bladder rupture.
- Extraperitoneal rupture usually is manageable conservatively.

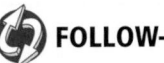 **FOLLOW-UP**

Admission Criteria
Admit all patients with bladder rupture for surgery or observation.

Discharge Criteria
- Stable for transfer to rehab or can perform ADLs
- Extraperitoneal ruptures controlled with indwelling Foley catheter if rupture not healed
- No evidence of infection
- Pain controlled

Issues for Referral
- All bladder ruptures should be evaluated by a urologist or surgeon immediately.
- Patient should be seen in follow-up by a urologist.

PROGNOSIS
Full return to normal function

COMPLICATIONS
- Infection
- Peritonitis
- Stricture is a rare complication
- Death

REFERENCES
1. Inaba K, McKenney M, Munera F, et al. Cystogram follow-up in the management of traumatic bladder disruption. *J Trauma.* 2006;60(1):23–28.
2. Lunetta P, Penttila A, Sajantila A. Fatal isolated ruptures of bladder following minor blunt trauma. *Ugeskr Laeger.* 2005;167(49):4654–4659.

 MISCELLANEOUS

CODES

ICD9-CM
- 569.9 Unspecified disorder of bladder
- 569.6 Ruptured bladder, nontraumatic

PATIENT TEACHING
- Return to regular lifestyle is expected.
- No special instructions are needed.

Diet
Regular

Activity
No restrictions

BLASTOMYCOSIS

William G. Gardner, MD, MACP

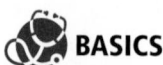 **BASICS**

DESCRIPTION

- An uncommon, systemic infection caused by the dimorphic fungus Blastomyces dermatitidis
- System(s) Affected: Pulmonary; Skin/subcutaneous; Bone/joint; Genitourinary; Central nervous system (CNS)
- Synonym(s): North American blastomycosis

ALERT

Geriatric Considerations
Prognosis is worse in elderly patients with significant underlying pulmonary or renal disease.

Pediatric Considerations
Uncommon in children

Pregnancy Considerations
- Amphotericin B is drug of choice
- Azoles should not be used during pregnancy.

GENERAL PREVENTION
- Unknown
- Condoms for sexual encounters

EPIDEMIOLOGY
- Incompletely understood
- Predominant age: Adults, but 10–20% of cases in children in endemic areas
- Predominant sex: Male > Female

Incidence
Ranges from 0.3–1.5 cases per 100,000 population per year

Prevalence
Higher prevalence in endemic areas

- Midwestern, Southcentral US, Great Lakes region of US and Canada
- Large outbreak occurred in Wisconsin
- Sporadic cases around the world

RISK FACTORS
- Occupational or recreational exposure to soil containing spores of Blastomyces dermatitidis
- Residence in endemic areas
- HIV/AIDS or other immunocompromised states (corticosteroids, blood malignancies)

Genetics
No genetic predisposition known

ETIOLOGY
- Infection acquired by respiratory route
- Inhalation of spores of Blastomyces dermatitidis into lungs with lymphohematogenous dissemination to other organ systems
- Primary inoculation of skin may occur rarely.
- Female infection results from sexual contact.
- Reactivation of latent infection or reinfection may occur in immunocompromised patients

ASSOCIATED CONDITIONS
- Most infected persons have no predisposing conditions
- Occasionally occurs in HIV-infected or immunocompromised persons

DIAGNOSIS

SIGNS AND SYMPTOMS
- Acute pulmonary infection
  - Onset may be abrupt or insidious
  - Incubation period 30–45 days
  - Presents as a non-specific flu-like illness
  - Fever, chills, myalgias, arthralgias
  - Cough nonproductive
  - Often self-limiting
  - Severe disease and respiratory failure occurs in <10% of cases
- Chronic pulmonary infection
  - Chronic pneumonia, indolent onset
  - Weight loss, fever, night sweats
  - Productive cough, purulent sputum
  - Hemoptysis uncommon
  - May mimic tuberculosis, other fungal pneumonias, and cancer
- Cutaneous blastomycosis
  - Most common extrapulmonary type: <80%
  - May occur with or without pulmonary disease
  - 2 types of lesions
    ○ Verrucous lesions begin as small papulopustular lesions, become crusted, and have sharp borders, central clearing, scar formation, depigmentation, and microabscesses at periphery.
    ○ Ulcerative lesions (initially pustules) form shallow ulcers with raised edges and granulating base.
  - May be mistaken for pyoderma gangrenosum, squamous cell carcinoma, and other chronic infectious lesions (e.g., Sporotrichosis, atypical mycobacteria)
  - SC nodules may suppurate forming chronic ulcers.
  - Regional adenopathy (uncommon)
- Skeletal blastomycosis
  - 10–50% of extrapulmonary cases
  - Long bones, vertebrae, ribs, cranium most commonly involved
  - Well-circumscribed osteolytic lesions
  - May present with contiguous soft tissue abscesses and/or sinus tracts
  - Paraspinous abscess in vertebral disease
  - Acute or chronic arthritis may result from joint involvement, usually large joints.
- Genitourinary blastomycosis
  - Occurs in 10–30% of cases
  - Involves prostate, epididymis, and testes
  - Enlarged, tender prostate
  - May cause outflow obstruction
  - Involvement of female genitalia uncommon but can be acquired through sexual contact
- Other
  - CNS involvement with acute or chronic meningitis, epidural or cerebral abscesses: More common in AIDS
  - Liver, spleen, pericardium, thyroid, gastrointestinal tract, and adrenal gland involved

TESTS
- Special staining of tissue with Gomori methenamine silver stain
- Periodic acid-Schiff's stain colors cell wall pink or red
- Mucicarmine stain helps differentiate from encapsulated Cryptococcus

Lab
- Culture of Blastomyces dermatitidis from tissue or body secretions on Sabouraud's media
  - Slow growing
  - Identify by highly specific DNA probes
- Yeast forms (5–15 μm in diameter, with refractile cell wall, broad-based budding, and no capsule) in tissue or secretions by wet mount
- In pulmonary disease, potassium hydroxide prep of sputum reveals organism in >50%
- Serologic tests have variable sensitivity and low specificity and are not helpful in the diagnosis.
- Skin testing with Blastomycin is not useful.
- Disorders that alter lab results: Lidocaine inhibits growth in bronchoscopic cultures.

Imaging
- CT scan of head for CNS lesions
- CT scan or MRI of spine for vertebral lesions
- Bone scan for skeletal lesions
- Chest x-ray
  - Acute pulmonary disease
    ○ Alveolar or interstitial infiltrates
  - Chronic pulmonary disease
    ○ Upper lobe fibronodular infiltrates in 50%
    ○ Mass lesions in 30%
    ○ Pulmonary nodules ± without cavitation
    ○ Pleural effusion in <10%
    ○ Mediastinal adenopathy in <20%

Diagnostic Procedures/Surgery
- Aspiration of abscess for wet mount and culture
- Needle or surgical biopsy of involved tissue for histology and culture

Pathological Findings
- Early response with polymorphonuclear leukocytes followed by granuloma formation with lymphocytes and macrophages
- Granulomas do not show caseation necrosis.
- Yeast is often found attached to or inside monocytes, macrophages, and giant cells.

DIFFERENTIAL DIAGNOSIS
- Pulmonary
  - Acute bacterial pneumonia
  - Tuberculosis
  - Other fungal diseases
  - Bacterial lung abscess
  - Empyema
  - Bronchogenic carcinoma
- Cutaneous
  - Pyoderma gangrenosum
  - Bacterial pyoderma
  - Cutaneous mycobacterial infection
  - Other cutaneous fungal infections (sporotrichosis, histoplasmosis, or ocryptococcosis)
  - Squamous cell carcinoma
- Bone
  - Bacterial osteomyelitis
  - Tuberculosis
  - Neoplastic disease
- Genitourinary
  - Bacterial prostatitis
  - Prostate cancer
  - Other fungal infections
  - Tuberculosis

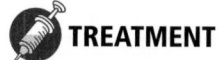 **TREATMENT**

INITIAL STABILIZATION
- Acute non-life-threatening pulmonary infection may be treated with itraconazole as an outpatient.
- Severe life-threatening infection, CNS disease, or disease in immunocompromised host should be treated initially with intravenous amphotericin B in the hospital.

GENERAL MEASURES
- Systemic antifungal therapy is indicated for all cases of extrapulmonary blastomycosis.
- Systemic antifungal therapy is indicated for all but very mild or asymptomatic pulmonary cases, in which a trial of observation may be appropriate.

Activity
No restrictions after patient is released from hospital

Nursing
Routine care

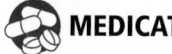 **MEDICATION (DRUGS)**

First Line
- Milder forms
  - Itraconazole (Sporanox): 200 mg PO b.i.d. for at least 6 months. Take with food; antacids or hydrogen blockers result in lower serum levels. Little drug is excreted in urine; thus genitourinary disease is more resistant to therapy.
  - Pediatrics: Non-life-threatening disease treat with itraconazole 5–7 mg/kg/d. Life-threatening or CNS disease treat with amphotericin B.
- Severe forms
  - Amphotericin B (Fungizone): 0.5–0.8 mg/kg IV over 4–6 hours daily for a cumulative dose of 1.5–2.5 g (1st dose of amphotericin B is given as a test dose of 1 mg in 200 mL 5% dextrose in sterile water IV over 2–4 hours). If tolerated, give maintenance dose of 0.5–0.8 mg/kg/d. Rigors can be prevented by preinfusion dose of meperidine 50 mg. To reduce infusion-related fever, preinfusion acetaminophen and diphenhydramine.
- Contraindications
  - Life-threatening intolerance to amphotericin such as anaphylaxis
  - CNS disease: Amphotericin B (total dose 2 g); alternative fluconazole 800 mg/d because of good CNS penetration
- Precautions
  - Monitor for hypotension during the infusion.
  - Monitor renal function, serum sodium, potassium, and magnesium, complete blood count twice weekly
  - Replace potassium and magnesium prn.
  - When serum creatinine rises to 1.6 mg/dL (141 μmol/L) or greater, dosage interval should be changed to 48 hours.
  - Watch for phlebitis at infusion site.
  - Consider peripherally inserted central catheter for infusion.
- Significant possible interactions
  - Avoid use of potentially nephrotoxic drugs such as aminoglycosides, which may potentiate nephrotoxicity of amphotericin B.
  - Itraconazole: Concurrent use of rifampin, phenytoin, or carbamazepine may increase hepatic metabolism, resulting in lower-serum drug levels and treatment failure.

Second Line
- Efficacy of alternative regimens not well established by controlled studies
  - Fluconazole 400 mg daily for 6 months for non-life-threatening blastomycosis
  - Ketoconazole (Nizoral): 400–800 mg PO daily for 6 months
- Lipid preparations of amphotericin B have not been adequately evaluated in human blastomycosis; they provide an alternative for patients unable to tolerate amphotericin B.

SURGERY
- Surgical débridement of bone lesions if there are areas of devitalized bone
- Surgical drainage of contiguous abscesses, cutaneous abscesses, or pleural empyema

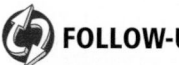 **FOLLOW-UP**

DISPOSITION
Specialty referral
- Immunocompromised or HIV patients
- Severe pulmonary disease
- Deep abscesses
- Children

Admission Criteria
- Severe pulmonary disease
- Immunocompromised or AIDS patient with severe disease

Discharge Criteria
Clinically stable and responding to therapy

Issues for Referral
Follow-up with infectious diseases physician and primary care physician.

PROGNOSIS
- Cure in >90% with appropriate therapy
- Relapse in <10% of cases
- Immunocompromised and AIDS patients have a poorer prognosis

COMPLICATIONS
- Adverse reactions with amphotericin B are frequent and significant.
- Treatment-induced nephrotoxicity, electrolyte imbalance, and anemia

PATIENT MONITORING
- Monitor closely during early therapy.
- Monitor serum electrolytes, creatinine, and CBC twice weekly during amphotericin B therapy.
- Post-therapy follow-up every 3 months for 2 years, then twice yearly

REFERENCES
1. Chapman SW, et al. Practice guidelines for the management of patients with blastomycosis. *Clin Infect Dis*. 2000;30:679–683.
2. Pappas PG. Blastomycosis. *Sem Resp Crit Care M*. 2004;25:113–120.
3. Patel RG, et al. Clinical presentation, radiographic findings, and diagnostic methods of pulmonary blastomycosis: A review of 100 consecutive cases. *South Med J*. 1999;92:289–295.
4. Crampton TL, et al. Epidemiology and clinical spectrum of blastomycosis diagnosed at Manitoba hospitals. *Clin Infect Dis*. 2002;34:1310–1316.

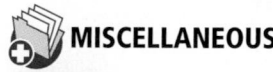 **MISCELLANEOUS**

CODES

ICD9-CM
116.0 Blastomycosis

PATIENT TEACHING
Counsel patient and family on potential adverse effects associated with antifungal therapy, duration of therapy, and potential for relapse or chronic infection.

Diet
Normal diet

Activity
Restrictions based on location and severity of disease

Prevention
No special measures

BLEPHARITIS

Joshua J. Spooner, PharmD, MS
A. Raquel Matteo-Bibeau, MD

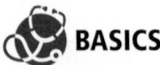

BASICS

DESCRIPTION
- An inflammatory reaction of the eyelid margin
  - Usually occurs as seborrheic or as staphylococcal blepharitis.
  - Multiple types may coexist.
- System(s) Affected: Skin/Exocrine
- Synonym(s): Granulated eyelids

EPIDEMIOLOGY
- Predominant age: Adult
- Predominant sex: Male = Female

Incidence
One of the most common ocular disorders

RISK FACTORS
- Seborrheic dermatitis
- Contact dermatitis
- Herpes simplex dermatitis
- Varicella-zoster dermatitis
- Acne rosacea
- Diabetes mellitus
- Immunocompromised state (e.g., AIDS, chemotherapy)
- Isotretinoin use
- Dry eye syndromes

ETIOLOGY
- Seborrheic
  - Accelerated shedding of skin cells with associated sebaceous gland dysfunction
  - *Malassezia furfur* (formerly Pityrosporum ovale) yeasts often colonize
- Staphylococcal
  - Superinfection of Zeis glands of lid margin and meibomian glands posterior to lashes with *Staphylococcus aureus*
  - Usually part of mixed blepharitis
- Meibomian gland dysfunction
  - Obstruction and inflammation of the meibomian glands
    ○ Associated with acne rosacea, acne vulgaris, and oral retinoid therapy
- Other types of blepharitis
  - Ulcerative blepharitis
    ○ More severe blepharitis with small marginal ulceration and destruction of the hair follicles
  - Contact dermatitis/blepharitis
    ○ Develops from type IV hypersensitivity; common causes include ocular medications, topical anesthetics, antivirals, and cosmetics
    ○ May occur with secondary *Staphylococcus* infection
  - Eczematoid blepharitis
    ○ Caused by hypersensitivity reaction to exotoxins and antigens from local flora
    ○ Strong association with eczema, asthma
    ○ Staphylococcal infection common
  - Angular blepharitis
    ○ Often caused by *Staphylococcus* or *Moraxella* infection

ASSOCIATED CONDITIONS
See "Risk Factors"

DIAGNOSIS

SIGNS AND SYMPTOMS
- Frequently reported in all types of blepharitis
  - Burning
  - Itching
  - Eyelid erythema
  - Conjunctival injection (red eyes)
  - Lacrimation, tearing
  - Tear deficiency
  - Foreign body sensation
  - Photophobia (light sensitivity)
  - Impaired vision
- Staphylococcal
  - Recurrent stye (external or internal hordeolum)
  - Missing, broken, or, misdirected eyelashes (trichiasis)
  - Eyelid deposits: Matted, hard scales; collarettes (ringlike formation around the lash shaft)
  - Ulcerations at base of eyelashes (rare)
  - Eyelid scarring may occur
- Seborrheic blepharitis
  - Eyelid deposits: Dry flakes, oily or greasy secretions on lid margins and/or lashes
  - Associated dandruff of scalp, eyebrows
- Meibomian gland dysfunction
  - Eyelash misdirection may occur with longstanding disease
  - Eyelid deposits: Fatty deposits; may be foamy
  - Eyelid margin thickening
  - Plugged meibomian gland orifices
  - Chalazion (sometimes multiple)
  - Eyelid scarring with long-term disease
- Mixed blepharitis
  - Signs and symptoms of more than 1 type of blepharitis may be present

History
- Duration of symptoms (1)[C]
- Unilateral or bilateral presentation (1)[C]
- Note any exacerbating conditions (e.g., smoke, allergens, wind, contact lenses, etc.) (1)[C]
- Symptoms related to systemic diseases (1)[C]
- Current and recent medication use (1)[C]
- Recent exposure to infected individuals (1)[C]

Physical Exam
- Test of visual acuity (1)[C]
- External examination (skin and eyelids) (1)[C]

TESTS
Lab
Special tests
- Cultures in atypical blepharitis
- Biopsy in atypical cases for carcinoma

Imaging
Slit-lamp biomicroscopy (1)[C]
- Examine tear film, eyelid margins, eyelashes, tarsal and bulbar conjunctiva, and cornea:
  - Reveals loss of lashes (madarosis), whitening of the lashes (poliosis), trichiasis, crusting, eyelid margin ulcers, and lid irregularities

DIFFERENTIAL DIAGNOSIS
- Masquerade syndrome:
  - Persistent inflammation and thickening of eyelid margin may indicate squamous cell, basal cell, or sebaceous cell carcinoma masquerading as blepharitis.
    ○ These carcinomas may also mimic styes or chalazia.
  - Sebaceous carcinoma of the eyelid has a 22% fatality rate. Up to 1/2 of these potentially fatal sebaceous cell carcinomas may resemble benign inflammatory diseases, particularly chalazia and chronic blepharoconjunctivitis.
  - Consider this in all cases of recurrent, persistent, or atypical chalazion; chronic unilateral unresponsive blepharoconjunctivitis; diffuse or nodular tumors of the eyelid; orbital mass developing after removal of an eyelid or caruncular tumor; and any tumor developing in a person with a history of ocular radiotherapy (2)[C].

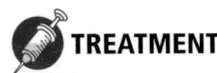

TREATMENT

Best evidence treatment
- American Academy of Ophthalmology Cornea/External Disease Panel, Preferred Practice patterns Committee. Preferred Practice Pattern: Blepharitis. San Francisco: AAO. 2003.

GENERAL MEASURES
- Appropriate health care: Outpatient
- Promote proper eyelid hygiene (1)[C]
  - Apply warm compresses for several minutes once daily to soften adherent encrustations
  - The eyelid margins are then gently scrubbed with eyelid cleanser or diluted baby shampoo twice a day, to remove adherent material and clean the meibomian gland orifices (3)[C]
- Brief, gentle massage of the eyelids can help express meibomian secretions in patients with meibomian gland dysfunction (1)[C]
- Discontinue soft contact lenses use during an acute case of blepharitis.
  - Chronic recurrent blepharitis requires referral to ophthalmologist for evaluation as to whether patient should continue in lenses.

MEDICATION (DRUGS)

First Line

- Topical treatment to lid, if *Staphylococcus* likely: Follow eye hygiene with application of bacitracin 500 u/g or (second choice) erythromycin 0.5% ophthalmic ointment:
  – Apply with a cotton-tipped applicator
  – The frequency and duration of treatment guided by the severity (1)[C].
- Topical corticosteroids (short-term) may be useful for eyelid or ocular surface inflammation.
  – The minimum effective dose should be used; long-term use avoided if possible (1,4)[C]
- For patients with meibomian gland dysfunction inadequately controlled with eyelid hygiene, consider: Doxycycline 100 mg/d or tetracycline 1000 mg/d in divided doses, tapered after clinical improvement (2–4 weeks) to doxycycline 50 mg/d or tetracycline 250–500 mg/d (1)[C].
- As aqueous tear deficiency is common in blepharitis, use twice-daily artificial tears in addition to eyelid hygiene and medications.
- Contraindications: Allergy to medication; tetracyclines are not for use in pregnancy, nursing women, or in children <8 years.
- Precautions: Tetracyclines may cause photosensitivity; sunscreen recommended. Corticosteroids may increase intraocular pressure and risk of cataract.
- Significant possible interactions: Tetracyclines; avoid concurrent administration with antacids, dairy products, or iron. May potentiate the effect of warfarin. Broad-spectrum antibiotics may reduce the effectiveness of oral contraceptives; barrier method recommended.

Second Line

- Topical fluoroquinolones (gatifloxacin 0.3%, levofloxacin 0.5%, or moxifloxacin 0.5%) may be helpful for persistent or recurrent staphylococcal blepharitis or for those patients who prefer a solution.
- Seborrheic blepharitis may respond to antifungal agents, such as a short course of itraconazole (5)[C].

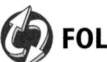 **FOLLOW-UP**

PROGNOSIS

- Symptoms can frequently be improved but are rarely eliminated.
- Long-term eyelid hygiene required for control.

COMPLICATIONS

- Stye and chalazion
- Scarring of eyelid margin
- Corneal infection

PATIENT MONITORING

- Patients should schedule a return visit if their condition worsens despite treatment.
- Return visit intervals for patients with severe disease vary.
- If corticosteroid prescribed, re-evaluate within a few weeks to measure intraocular pressure and determine response to therapy.

REFERENCES

1. *American Academy of Ophthalmology Cornea/External Disease Panel, Preferred Practice patterns Committee*. Preferred Practice Pattern: Blepharitis. San Francisco: AAO. 2003.
2. Tsai T, O'Brien JM. Masquerade syndromes: Malignancies mimicking inflammation in the eye. *Int Ophthalmol Clin* 2002;41:115–131.
3. McCulley JP, Shine WE. Changing concepts in the diagnosis and management of blepharitis. *Cornea* 2000;19:650–658.
4. Abelson MB, Cohane K, Fink K. Blepharitis: Hiding in plain sight. *Rev Ophthalmol* May 15. 2004.
5. Ninoyima J, et al. A case of seborrheic blepharitis: Treatment with itraconazole. *Nippon Ishinkin Gakkai Zasshi* 2002;43:189–191.

ADDITIONAL READING

- Lemp MA. Contact lenses and associated anterior segment disorders: Dry eye, blepharitis, and allergy. Ophthalmol Clin North Am 2003;16:463–469.
- McCulley JP, Shine WE. Eyelid disorders: The meibomian gland, blepharitis, and contact lenses. Eye & Contact *Lens* 2003;29(1S):S93–95.
- Rao NA, Hidayat AA, McLean IW, Zimmerman IE. Sebaceous carcinomas of the ocular adnexa: A clinicopathologic study of 104 cases, with five year follow-up data. Hum Pathol 1982;13:113–122.
- Frucht-Pery J, Sagi E, Hemo I, Ever-Hadani O. Efficacy of doxycycline and tetracycline in ocular rosacea. Am J Ophthalmol 1993;116:88–92.

 MISCELLANEOUS

See also: Conjunctivitis; Dry eye syndrome (keratoconjunctivitis sicca)

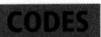 **CODES**

ICD9-CM

373.00 Blepharitis, unspecified

PATIENT TEACHING

- Blepharitis "Fact Sheet" from American Academy of Ophthalmology
- Advise patient that blepharitis is a chronic condition, prone to recurrence if eyelid hygiene is not maintained after antibiotic treatment is discontinued.

 See Corresponding Diagnostic Algorithm

 See Patient Handout on CD

BODY DYSMORPHIC DISORDER

Jennifer L. Schott, MD

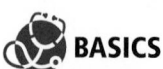 **BASICS**

DESCRIPTION
According to the DSM-IV-TR, body dysmorphic disorder is a preoccupation with an imagined defect in appearance that causes clinically significant distress or impairment in social, occupational, or other important areas of function that is not accounted for by another mental disorder. If there is a minor physical anomaly, the concern is excessive. (1)

EPIDEMIOLOGY
- May be equally common in men and women
- Different cultural beliefs may influence or amplify preoccupations.
- Usually begins during adolescence with an average age of onset of 17 years (1)
  - Adolescents usually present similar to adults
  - Can present in childhood, often with refusing to attend school or planning suicide (2)
- Onset can be gradual or abrupt
- Often a delay in diagnosis until 10–15 years after the onset (1)

Prevalence
- 0.7% in the general community
- 5–40% in individuals with Anxiety or Depressive Disorders (3)
- 6–15% in cosmetic surgery patients and in dermatologic clinics (1)

RISK FACTORS
- Genetic predisposition
- Shyness, perfectionism, or anxious temperament
- Childhood adversity
  - Teasing or bullying
  - Poor peer relationships
  - Social isolation
  - Lack of support of family
  - Sexual abuse
- History of dermatological or other physical stigmata
- Being more aesthetically sensitive than average
- Low self esteem (3)

PATHOPHYSIOLOGY
- Not known
- A cognitive behavioral model has been described in which an external representation of the person's appearance creates a distorted mental image that through selective attention increases the awareness of the image and its specific features. The preoccupation of the distorted image is maintained by different safety and submissive behaviors to decrease the scrutiny by others but actually tends to increase the individual's doubts and reinforces the behavior.
- Possible lesions in the frontostriatal connections, which cause abnormal verbal and nonverbal encoding strategies leading to executive memory deficits (3)

ETIOLOGY
Not known but likely multifactorial involving genetic, biological, and environmental factors

ASSOCIATED CONDITIONS
- Depression
- Social phobia
- Bipolar disorder
- Eating disorders
- Obsessive-compulsive disorder
- Suicide
- Delusional disorder, somatic type (1)

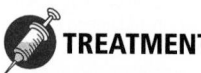 **DIAGNOSIS**

SIGNS AND SYMPTOMS
- Preoccupation that 1 or more of their features are unattractive, ugly, or deformed
- Can involve any part of the body but usually involves the skin, hair, or facial features (1)
  - Women are more likely to be preoccupied with their weight, hips, legs, and breasts
  - Men are more likely to be preoccupied with their height, body hair, body build, and genitals (4,5)
- Nature of the preoccupation can change with time
- Have little insight
- Tend to display delusions of reference
- Large amounts of time are consumed by behaviors to examine the perceived defect repeatedly, disguise it, or improve it
  - Mirror gazing
  - Excessive grooming
  - Camouflaging the "defect"
  - Skin picking
  - Reassurance seeking
  - Dieting
  - Pursuing dermatological treatment or cosmetic surgery
- Tend to avoid social interactions
- Trouble staying in school, maintaining a job, or maintaining significant relationships
  - Tend to be unhappy with results of dermatologic and cosmetic procedures (1)

History
- Determine and validate the patient's concern
- Determine the severity of the disorder
- Quantify the amount of time spent worrying about the "distorted" appearance
- Determine what is done to hide or eliminate the problem
- Determine the degree to which the defect affects their school, job, or social life
- Rule out other psychiatric disorders (6)

Physical Exam
- Important to do a mental status examination
  - Look for
    - Depression
    - Suicidal ideation
    - Anxiety
  - Rule out organic factors by reviewing
    - Orientation
    - Memory
    - Ability to concentrate
- Rule out actual physical pathology

DIFFERENTIAL DIAGNOSIS
- Normal concerns about appearance
- Eating disorders
- Gender identity disorder
- Major depressive episode
- Narcissistic personality disorder
- Avoidant personality disorder
- Social phobia
- Schizophrenia
- Obsessive-compulsive disorder
- Trichotillomania
- Hypochondriasis
- Delusional disorder, somatic type
- Koro: A culture-related syndrome seen in Southeast Asia
  - Involves a preoccupation that the genitals (penis, labia, nipples, or breast) is shrinking and is disappearing into the abdomen (1)

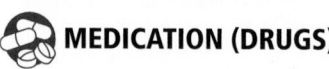 **TREATMENT**

SPECIAL THERAPY
- Refer to a psychiatrist for diagnosis and therapy

- Cognitive behavior therapy has been shown to be very effective (7)[B]
  - Behavioral experiments
  - Graded exposure tasks
  - Imagery rescripting
  - Cognitive restructuring
  - Reverse role playing
  - Relaxation

- Support groups (7)[C]
- Psychotherapy may be effective (7)[C]
- Therapy with and for family members, spouses, or significant others

MEDICATION (DRUGS)

First Line
Selective Serotonin-reuptake inhibitors (SSRI) (7)[B]
- Not an approved use by the FDA
- Patients with and without a delusional disorder did equally well with an SSRI
- Maximum tolerated dose should be taken for at least 12–16 weeks
- Dosages may need to be higher than typically recommended for an eating disorder (3,6,7)

Second Line
Adding a low dose antipsychotic drug to an SSRI if there is failure to respond to 2 or more SSRIs (2)[C]

SURGERY
Cosmetic surgery and dermatologic procedures may have potential benefits or no benefit
- Difficult patients for dermatologists and plastic surgeons due to tendency to insist on repeated procedures, are often unhappy with the results, and require repeated reassurance (3)

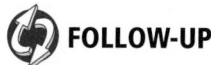 **FOLLOW-UP**

PROGNOSIS
Continuous course with periods of waxing and waning in the intensity of symptoms
- The longer the duration and the more severe the symptoms, the less the chance of partial or full remission (8)

COMPLICATIONS
- Repeated surgical or dermatological procedures
- Suicide
- Comorbid conditions
- Poor social relations
- Poor self esteem
- Inability or limited ability to function in society

PATIENT MONITORING
- Close monitoring by psychiatrist
- Regular counseling

REFERENCES
1. American Psychiatric Association: *Diagnostic and Statistical Manual of Mental Disorders, Fourth Addition, Text Revision*. Washington, DC: American Psychiatric Association, 2000;507–510.
2. Albertini RS, Philips KA. Thirty-Three cases of body dysmorphic disorder in children and adolescents. *J Am Acad Child Psy*. 1999;38:453–459.
3. Veale D. Body dysmorphic disorder. *Postgrad Med J*. 2004;80:67–71.
4. Perugi G, Akiskal H, Giannotti D, Frare F, Di Vaio S, Cassano G. Gender-related differences in body dysmorphic disorder. *J Ner Ment Dis*. 1997; 185:578–582.
5. Philips KA, Diaz SF. Gender differences in body dysmorphic disorder. *J Ner Ment Dis*. 1997; 185:570–577.
6. Slaughter JR, Sun SM. In pursuit of perfection: A primary care physician's guide to body dysmorphic disorder. *Am Fam Physician*. 1999;60:1738–1742.
7. Ipser JC, Stein DJ. Pharmacotherapy and psychotherapy for body dysmorphic disorder. *The Cochrane Library*. 2005;4.
8. Philips KA, Pagano ME, Menard W, Fay C, Stout RL. Predictors of remission from body dysmorphic disorder: A prospective study. *J Ner Ment Dis*. 2005;193:564–567.

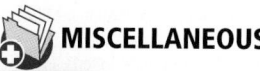 **MISCELLANEOUS**

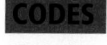

ICD9-CM
F45.2

PATIENT TEACHING
Important to maintain an ongoing relationship with one's psychiatrist and/or counselor

BONE TUMOR, PRIMARY MALIGNANT

Mark R. Dambro, MD

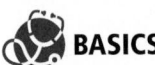

BASICS

DESCRIPTION
- Primary malignant bone tumors are rare. 4 types make up the majority
  - Malignant fibrous histiocytoma (malignant fibrous histiocytoma): A pleomorphic sarcoma of storiform pattern without differentiation.
  - Osteosarcoma: Similar to malignant fibrous histiocytoma with differentiation to osteoid production
  - Chondrosarcoma: Cellular cartilaginous lesion with abundant binucleate cells, myxoid areas, and pushing borders
  - Ewing sarcoma: Small, blue-round cell neoplasm
- System(s) Affected: Musculoskeletal

ALERT
Pregnancy Considerations
- Increased growth of musculoskeletal malignancies during pregnancy
- Soft-tissue desmoid tumors have estrogen and progesterone receptors.

GENERAL PREVENTION
None identified

EPIDEMIOLOGY
- Predominant age
  - Malignant fibrous histiocytoma: Teens and elderly
  - Osteogenic sarcoma: Teens and early 20s
  - Chondrosarcoma: Very young and very old
  - Ewing sarcoma: Children, teens, and early 20s
- Predominant sex: Male = Female

Incidence
- Rare
- 5,000 bone and soft-tissue sarcomas diagnosed per year in the US
- A practicing orthopedic surgeon may see 1 primary malignant tumor of bone in every 5 years of practice.
- Ewing sarcoma is less common in African Americans.

RISK FACTORS
- Multiple enchondromatosis (Ollier disease): Chondrosarcoma
- Multiple hereditary exostosis: Chondrosarcoma
- Previous irradiation, risk factor for malignant fibrous histiocytoma
- Previous history of bilateral retinoblastoma: Osteosarcoma

Genetics
- Ewing sarcoma has 11/22 chromosomal translocation and EW5-FLI-1 fusion protein.
- Osteosarcoma shows loss of retinoblastoma and p53 suppressor genes and amplification of the genes C-myc, mdm-2, SAS, and cyclin-dependent kinase.

ETIOLOGY
- Generally unknown
- Malignant fibrous histiocytoma often follows irradiation or arises in old bone infarct.
- Osteosarcoma has association with loss of suppressor retinoblastoma and p53 genes.
- Chondrosarcoma may arise in pre-existing enchondroma or exostosis.

ASSOCIATED CONDITIONS
- A higher incidence of chondrosarcoma is seen in patients with multiple hereditary exostosis, multiple enchondromatosis (Ollier disease), and patients with enchondromatosis and hemangiomatosis (Maffucci syndrome).
- Patients with enchondromatosis more often die of gastrointestinal (GI) malignancies than of metastatic chondrosarcoma.

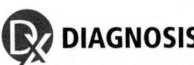

DIAGNOSIS

SIGNS AND SYMPTOMS
- Pain with weight bearing, at rest, and at night
- Swelling
- Tenderness
- Fracture with minor trauma
- Minor injury may bring attention to lesion

TESTS
- A rectal exam should be done to exclude prostate nodules
- Open biopsy or needle biopsy. Needle biopsies may not provide enough tissue for frozen section, touch prep, permanent section, snap freezing, electron microscopy, cytogenetic and molecular studies, DNA indices, immunoperoxidase staining, and immunophenotyping (lymphoma).
- Biopsy of associated soft-tissue mass may lessen the risk of pathologic fracture.
- Biopsy tract should be excised in continuity with the tumor at the time of resection.

Lab
- 50% of osteosarcomas have an elevated alkaline phosphatase.
- Ewing sarcoma may be associated with an elevated ESR and lactate dehydrogenase.
- Prostatic-specific antigen to exclude prostatic carcinoma
- Calcium, phosphate, alkaline phosphatase
- Thyroid function tests to exclude thyroid carcinoma
- Elevated ESR and WBCs in osteomyelitis
- Serum protein electrophoresis and urine electrophoresis to exclude myeloma

Imaging
- Plain films provide the most important information regarding the nature of the lesion and guide further testing.
- Bone scan is done prior to biopsy, to look for other lesions.
- CT scan for cortical destruction and internal calcification or ossification. Abdominal CT, MRI, or renal ultrasound to exclude hypernephroma
- MRI scan determines the extent of marrow involvement and associated soft-tissue mass.
- Chest radiograph and chest CT for metastatic disease
- Mammogram to exclude breast carcinoma

Diagnostic Procedures/Surgery
Bone biopsy

Pathological Findings
- Histology and special studies in combination with radiographic findings confirm the diagnosis.
- Ewing sarcoma expresses MIC-2 protein (CD99).
- Electron microscopy
  - Glycogen granules in Ewing sarcoma
  - Neurosecretory granules in neuroectodermal tumors
  - Birbeck bodies in histiocytosis-X
- Osteosarcoma may express Her-2/neu, indicating, if present, a more aggressive tumor, but one that may respond more favorably to trastuzumab (Herceptin).

DIFFERENTIAL DIAGNOSIS
- Solitary metastatic lesion or myeloma, especially in patients >40 years
- Lymphoma at any age
- Benign bone tumors and benign bone tumors that look aggressive (aneurysmal bone cyst, giant cell tumor, eosinophilic granuloma)
- Infection (osteomyelitis)
- Metabolic bone disease (osteopenia, Paget, hyperparathyroidism)
- Synovial diseases (pigmented villonodular synovitis, synovial chondromatosis, degenerative or inflammatory synovitis)
- Myositis ossificans and repair reaction to trauma
- Avascular necrosis

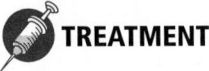

TREATMENT

Inpatient surgery

GENERAL MEASURES
Diet
No special diet

Activity
Varies with stage of disease and treatment

MEDICATION (DRUGS)

First Line

- These drugs are administered according to specific protocols. Other protocols may be appropriate.
- Malignant fibrous histiocytoma and osteosarcoma
  - Doxorubicin (Adriamycin)
  - Intra-arterial and intravenous cisplatin
  - High-dose methotrexate with leucovorin rescue
  - Ifosfamide (with mesna to protect against hemorrhagic cystitis)
  - Cyclophosphamide (Cytoxan)
  - Dactinomycin (actinomycin-D)
  - Bleomycin
- Liposome-encapsulated muramyl tripeptide phosphatidylethanolamine immune-modulating agent for osteosarcoma (under trial in Cancer Center Support Group and Pediatric Oncology Group studies)
- Ewing sarcoma
  - Cyclophosphamide
  - Vincristine
  - Actinomycin D
  - Doxorubicin (Adriamycin)
  - Ifosfamide
  - Etoposide
- Contraindications: Refer to manufacturer's literature.
- Precautions
  - Left ventricular dysfunction with Adriamycin. Cumulative dose >450 mg/m^2 increases risk. Follow with serial echocardiograms and/or nuclear multiple-gated acquisition ventriculogram scans when cumulative dose >250 mg/m^2.
  - With high-dose methotrexate, hydration, alkalinization of the urine, and close monitoring of plasma levels are needed.
- Significant possible interactions
  - Myelosuppression
  - Renal tubular dysfunction with ifosfamide
  - Renal and hepatic dysfunction and GI mucositis with methotrexate
  - Nephrotoxicity and ototoxicity with cisplatin

Second Line

Ondansetron (Zofran), dronabinol (Marinol), metoclopramide (Reglan), and others for nausea control.

SURGERY

- Resection with adequate margin is required to minimize risk of local persistence.
- For malignant fibrous histiocytoma and osteosarcoma, preresection neoadjuvant chemotherapy treats micrometastatic disease immediately, allows time for ordering replacement prosthesis and bone graft, allows for an in vivo assessment of the chemotherapy responsiveness of the tumor, and may facilitate limb salvage by allowing a "safer" close margin.
- Chondrosarcoma in the extremities should be treated exclusively by surgery unless it is of the mesenchymal or dedifferentiated high-grade variety.

- Ewing sarcoma was traditionally treated with chemotherapy, and surgery was limited to those lesions that were extremely large, associated with pathologic fracture, or involved an expendable bone. Most Ewing sarcoma lesions were irradiated. However, despite irradiation, local recurrence is common in up to 25% with pelvic lesions. Therefore, surgery with limb salvage is increasingly accepted. A dramatic decrease in size in Ewing sarcoma occurs after initial chemotherapy, and a decision can then be made after restaging as to whether to irradiate or to resect the primary lesion.
- The treatment goal is to minimize local recurrence while preserving function. Limb salvage is employed whenever a safe margin can be obtained.

 FOLLOW-UP

PROGNOSIS

- With amputation alone, 80% of patients with osteosarcoma had pulmonary metastatic disease by 2 years. With chemotherapy, the 5-year disease free survival rate is 50–85%.
- Favorable prognostic factors for malignant fibrous histiocytoma and osteosarcoma include responsiveness to chemotherapy, distal portions of the extremities, small size, age >10 years.
- Most chondrosarcomas are of lower grade and have a low risk of metastatic spread and low incidence of local recurrence after adequate surgery.
- Malignant fibrous histiocytoma, osteosarcoma, and Ewing sarcoma have an overall 50% survival with combined treatment modalities.

COMPLICATIONS

- Limb salvage with any primary malignant bone tumor is fraught with potential complications.
- Micrometastatic disease may have occurred at the time of presentation and can appear at any time during the course of treatment or follow-up.
- Local recurrence risk for osteosarcoma with limb salvage is <10%.
- Leg-length discrepancy, infection, wound dehiscence, skin coverage problems, arterial and nerve injury, nonunion of bone grafts, and mechanical loosening of prosthetic implants can occur.
- Thoracotomy and continued chemotherapy are often recommended for metastatic disease to the lung.
- Ewing sarcoma, metastatic to the lung, is quite diffuse and is less amenable to thoracotomy.

PATIENT MONITORING

- Patients who require adjuvant chemotherapy are treated with maintenance chemotherapy after resection of the tumor.
- Blood counts for myelosuppression
- Serial echocardiograms when Adriamycin is being used; G-CSF often used to minimize neutropenia
- Chest radiographs obtained every 2 months for the 1st year, every 3 months for the 2nd year, and every 4 months in the 3rd year
- CT scans of the lungs are initially repeated every 6 months during 1st 2 years.
- Ewing sarcoma may recur >5 years after diagnosis.

REFERENCES

1. Enneking WF. *Musculoskeletal Tumor Surgery, Vols. 1 and 2.* New York: Churchill Livingstone, 1983.
2. Mendelsohn J. Jeremiah Metzger Lecture. Targeted cancer therapy. *Trans Amer Clin Climatol Assoc.* 2000;111:95–110.
3. Schajowicz F, McGuire MH. Diagnostic difficulties in skeletal pathology. *Clin Orthop Rel Res.* 1991;240:281–310.
4. Longhi A, Pasini E, Bertoni F, et al. Twenty-year follow-up of osteosarcoma of the extremity treated with adjuvant chemotherapy. *J Chemother.* 2004;16(6):582–588.
5. Velez-Yanguas MC, Warrier RP. The evolution of chemotherapeutic agents for the treatment of pediatric musculoskeletal malignancies. *Orthop Clin North Amer.* 1996;27:545–549.
6. Womer RB. The cellular biology of bone tumors. *Clin Orthop Rel Res.* 1991;262:1221.

 MISCELLANEOUS

- Osteosarcoma variants such as parosteal, periosteal, and intraosseous osteosarcoma are lower-grade lesions with a more favorable prognosis; they often do not require chemotherapy. Other variants, postirradiation, and post-Paget osteosarcoma metastasize early.
- Chordoma: Rare malignant bone tumor that develops from the remnants of the primitive notochord. May be located in the sacrum or near the base of the skull. Usual course: Slowly progressive; recurrent; cure possible.

CODES

ICD9-CM

Malignant neoplasm of bone and articular cartilage, site unspecified

PATIENT TEACHING

Refer to local branch of American Cancer Society for information and support groups.

See Corresponding Diagnostic Algorithm

BORDERLINE PERSONALITY DISORDER

Heath A. Grames, PhD

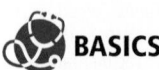 **BASICS**

DESCRIPTION

Beginning no later than adolescence or early adulthood, a consistent and pervasive pattern of an unstable affect and sense of self, impulsivity, and volatile interpersonal relationships. (1)[C]

- Common behaviors and variations (1)[C]
  - Self mutilation (pinching, scratching, cutting)
  - Suicide (ideation, history of attempts, plans)
  - Splitting (idealizing then devaluing people and relationships)
  - Presentation of helplessness or victimization
  - Emotional pain (may look for physical diagnoses)
  - May be high utilizer of medical services

ALERT

Geriatric Considerations
Illness (acute and chronic) may exacerbate borderline personality disorder behaviors and may lead to intense feelings of fear and helplessness. Manifestations may decrease with age. (1)[C]

Pediatric Considerations
Diagnosis is rarely made for children (1)[C]. Must 1st rule out Axis I disorders and behavior related to a general medical condition or to the developmental cycle of the child. For diagnosis, baseline behaviors must be representative of borderline personality disorder.

Pregnancy Considerations
Physical and social changes may induce stress or increase fears, causing increased borderline behaviors.

GENERAL PREVENTION
Tends to be a multi-generational problem. Children, caregivers, and significant others should have time and activities away from the borderline individual, which may help protect them from the disorder.

EPIDEMIOLOGY
- Predominant age: Onset no later than adolescence or early adulthood (may go undiagnosed for years) (1)[C]
- Predominant sex: Female > Male (1)[C]

Prevalence
- General population = ~2% (1)[C]
- Estimated lifetime prevalence = 10–13% (1)[C]
- Estimates of 20–30% (all personality disorders) prevalence in primary care outpatient settings (2)[C]

RISK FACTORS
Physical illness and external social factors may exacerbate borderline personality behaviors.

Genetics
1st-degree relatives are at greater risk for also having this disorder (3)[C] (undetermined whether risk is due to genetics or psychosocial factors).

ETIOLOGY
Undetermined, but generally accepted, that is due to a combination of the following (2)[C]
- Hereditary tempermental traits
- Environment (i.e., history of neglect and abuse, ongoing conflict in home)
- Developmental traits

ASSOCIATED CONDITIONS
- Mood disorders, common (1)[C]
- Anxiety disorders, common (1)[C]
- Substance-related disorders, common (1)[C]
- Eating disorders, common (1)[C]
- PTSD, common (1)[C]
- Co-occurring personality disorders, frequent (1)[C]

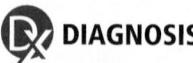 **DIAGNOSIS**

PRE HOSPITAL
- Assess suicide ideation and self-harm behavior
- Assess for psychosis

SIGNS AND SYMPTOMS
See "Description"

History
- Clinic visits for problems that do not have biological findings
- Problems with medical staff members
- Idealizing or unexplained anger at physician
- History of unrealistic expectations of physician (e.g., "I know you can take care of me." "You're the best, unlike my last provider.")

Physical Exam
Scarring from self-mutilating (look on arms and legs where hidden by clothing, but can occur on other parts of the body)

TESTS

Diagnostic Procedures/Surgery
Patient must meet at least 5 of the following (1)[C]
- Attempt to avoid abandonment
- Volatile interpersonal relationships
- Identity disturbance
- Impulsive behavior
  - In at least 2 areas
  - Impulsive behavior is self-damaging
- Suicidal or self-mutilating behavior
- Mood instability
- Feeling empty
- Unable or difficult to control anger
- Paranoid or dissociative when under stress

DIFFERENTIAL DIAGNOSIS
- Mood disorders (1)[C]
  - Look at baseline behaviors when considering borderline vs. mood disorder
- Psychotic disorder (1)[C]
  - With borderline, only occurs under intense stress and is not characteristic of disorder
- Other personality disorder (1)[C]
  - Consider patients thoughts, feelings, and behavior to differentiate borderline from other personality disorders
  - High co-occurrence of borderline and other personality disorders

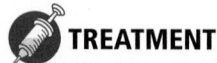 **TREATMENT**

PRE HOSPITAL
- Appropriate psychiatric care must be available.
- Patient may need to be on suicide watch
- Inpatient hospitalization is ineffective in changing Axis II disorder behaviors.
- Inpatient hospital services for conditions related to Axis II disorder should be limited and of short duration to decrease dependence (increased dependence may decrease likelihood of behavior change)
- Hospitalization should be considered for the following
  - Adjust medications
  - Implement psychotherapy for crisis intervention
  - Stabilize patient (psychosocial stressors)

INITIAL STABILIZATION
If psychotic, consider antipsychotic medications (2)[C]

GENERAL MEASURES
- Focus on patient management rather than "fixing" behaviors.
- Schedule follow-up to relieve patient stress. (4)[C]
- Meet with and rely on treatment team to avoid splitting of team by patient and to provide opportunity for team to discuss issues with patient
- As necessary, refer patient to mental health therapist

Nursing
Nurses can be helpful in managing patient and calling the patient as needed (contact with the patient helps relieve patient stress)

SPECIAL THERAPY
Consider referring patient for specialty mental health services, such as Dialectic Behavioral Therapy (DBT)

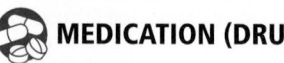 **MEDICATION (DRUGS)**

- There are no medications that treat borderline personality disorder
- Treat symptoms and Axis I disorders (2)[C]

First Line
- Depression/anxiety (4)[C]
  - SSRI, Selective Serotonin-reuptake Inhibitors
- Impulsive, aggressive, or history of bi-polar disorder (2)[C]
  - Mood stabilizer
- Psychosis, paranoid or hostile behavior, debilitating anxiety (2)[C]
  - Atypical antipsychotic

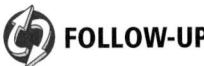 **FOLLOW-UP**

- Schedule routine follow-up with patient (relieves patient anxiety about medical care relationship with physician) (4)[C]
- Focus should be on medical conditions and co-morbid Axis I disorders (4)[C]

Admission Criteria
Refer to inpatient or outpatient psychiatry services if harm to self or others is expressed

- Call police or admit for inpatient services immediately if patient is psychotic and/or presents risk of harm to self or others

Discharge Criteria
- Patient should not present risk of harm to self or others
- Patient should have safety plan
- Routine follow-up should be scheduled with psychiatrist, mental health therapist, or primary care provider

Issues for Referral
- If hospitalized, probably for suicide risk, mood or anxiety disorders, or substance-related disorders
- Urgency for scheduled follow-up depends on community resources (i.e., do outpatient day programs for suicidal patients exist? What substance abuse programs are available?)
  – With increased risk for self harm or self-defeating behaviors and low community resources, the patient can/will use increased need for frequent visits
- Treatment of Axis II disorder should include psychotherapy and/or psychiatry.

PROGNOSIS
- Borderline behaviors may decrease with age (1)[C]
- Treatment is complex and takes time
- Medical focus is on patient management and caring for medical and Axis I disorders (5)[C]

PATIENT MONITORING
Monitor for suicidal or other self-harm behaviors

REFERENCES

1. American Psychiatric Association. *Diagnostic and Statistical Manual of Mental Disorders*, 4th ed.. Washington, DC: American Psychiatric Association; 1994.
2. Ward RK. Assessment and management of personality disorders. *American Family Physician*. 2004;70:1505–1512.
3. Koenigsberg HW, Woo-Ming AM, Siever LJ. Pharmacological treatments of personality disorders. In: Nathan PE, Gorman JM, eds. *A guide to treatments that work*, 2nd ed. New York, NY: Oxford University Press; 2002:625–641.
4. Feder A, Robbins SW, Ostermeyer B. Personality disorders. In: Feldman MD, Christensen JF, eds. *Behavioral medicine in primary care: A practical guide*, 2nd ed. New York, NY: McGraw-Hill; 2003:231–252.
5. Makela EH, Moeller KE, Fullen JE, Gunel E. Medication utilization patterns and methods of suicidality in borderline personality disorder. *The Ann Pharmacother*. 2006;40:49–52.

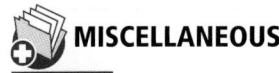 **MISCELLANEOUS**

CODES

ICD9-CM
- 301.8 (Other Personality Disorders)
- 301.83 (Borderline Personality Disorder)

PATIENT TEACHING
Activity
- Exercise to decrease stress
- Find time to relax: Remove self from daily problems (teaches self-management)

BOTULISM

John C. Bradford, DO

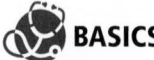 **BASICS**

DESCRIPTION
- An intoxication-producing paralytic disease caused by neurotoxins of *Clostridium botulinum,* the most toxic substances known to science
- The toxin prevents acetylcholine release at presynaptic membranes, blocking neuromuscular transmission in cholinergic nerve fibers.
- 5 forms exist
  - Food-borne botulism
  - Infantile botulism
  - Wound botulism
  - Hidden or intestinal botulism
  - Inadvertant botulism
  - Inhalation (potential sixth form through deliberate release of toxin)
- System(s) Affected: Endocrine/Metabolic; Gastrointestinal (GI); Nervous
- Synonym(s): Sausage poisoning; Kerner disease

ALERT
Pediatric Considerations
Avoid honey in the 1st year of life.

GENERAL PREVENTION
- Avoid giving honey to infants.
- Do not eat or taste food from bulging cans, or if food smells "off."

EPIDEMIOLOGY
- Predominant age
  - Food-borne: All ages
  - Infantile: 2–4 months (rare after 6 months)
  - Wound: Usually younger adult
  - Inadvertent: >1 year
- Predominant sex
  - Food-borne and infantile: Male = Female
  - Wound: Male > Female
  - Inadvertent: Female > Male

Incidence
- Average of 110 cases per year (25% food-borne, 72% infant)
- Wound botulism incidence increasing due to IV heroin use and cocaine abuse
- Hidden or intestinal: More common in disorders of the GI tract, such as prior surgery, Crohn disease, or recent antibiotic use
- Inhalation: Only a single incident involving 3 laboratory workers has been described.

RISK FACTORS
- Food-borne: Ingestion of home-canned or prepared foods
- Infantile: From ingestion of honey; breastfeeding (controversial)
- Wound: IV drug use (e.g., black tar heroin) or "skin popping." Sinusitis secondary to cocaine use also reported.

ETIOLOGY
- Ingestion of *C. botulinum* neurotoxins (A, B, and E most common)
- Food-borne, usually from home-canned vegetables, prepared foods, or foods incubated in anaerobic conditions
- Infantile from ingestion of spores in environment or occasionally in honey
- Wound due to contamination with toxin-producing *C. botulinum*
- Hidden or intestinal (source yet identified)
- Inadvertent—IM injections of botulinum toxin

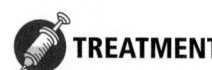 **DIAGNOSIS**

SIGNS AND SYMPTOMS
- Food-borne
  - Onset 2–36 hours after ingestion, as long as 14 days
  - Nonspecific findings early (nausea, vomiting, malaise, dizziness, and abdominal distension)
  - Dry mouth
  - Constipation, urinary retention
  - Symmetric descending weakness or paralysis of motor and autonomic nerves, usually beginning with the cranial nerves
  - Cranial nerve paralysis (ptosis; extraocular muscle paresis; fixed, dilated pupils; dysphagia)
  - Postural hypotension
  - Muscle weakness, respiratory paralysis (no sensory deficits)
  - Afebrile
  - Progression over several days
- Infantile
  - Constipation (early sign)
  - Loss of head control
  - Loss of suck
  - Loss of facial expression and verbalization
  - Symmetric descending weakness and cranial nerve paresis similar to food-borne form
  - Diminished or absent deep tendon reflexes
  - Autonomic dysfunction
  - Afebrile
  - Usual progression over 2–5 days; can be short as a few hours
- Wound
  - Onset 4–14 days postinjury
  - Findings similar to food-borne botulism, but GI symptoms less common
  - May be febrile
- Hidden
  - Possible adult variant of infant botulism
  - Findings similar to infant botulism
  - Inadvertent
  - Moderate to marked clinical weakness following IM therapeutic injections
  - Autonomic nervous system deficits also reported
  - Inhalation
  - Likely as irritant upper airway prodrome followed by variable degrees of paralysis

TESTS
- Stool contains organism and toxin
- Serum toxin present in food-borne form

Lab
- Routine tests—check for hypokalemia
- CSF testing—normal helps differentiate from Guillain-Barré syndrome
- Toxin detected in gastric contents, blood, feces, and suspected food and containers
- Confirmation available at Centers for Disease Control and prevention (CDC) and some state laboratories
- Pulmonary function testing
- Disorders that may alter lab results
  - Underlying myoneural disease

Diagnostic Procedures/Surgery
Electrophysiology testing can provide presumptive evidence of botulism in patients with the clinical picture and in whom bioassay studies are negative. The most consistent finding is a smaller amplitude evoked muscle action potential on repetitive nerve stimulation with incremental response.

Pathological Findings
Nonspecific

DIFFERENTIAL DIAGNOSIS
- Guillain-Barré syndrome
- Encephalitis
- Tick paralysis
- Myasthenia gravis
- Eaton Lambert myasthenic syndrome
- Basilar artery stroke
- Congenital neuropathy or myopathy
- Sepsis
- Hypokalemic periodic paralysis
- Polio
- Other poisonings (organophosphate, shellfish, *Amanita* mushrooms, atropine, and aminoglycosides)
- Miller Fisher variant of Guillian-Barré syndrome
- Diphtheritic neuropathy

TREATMENT

Advanced medical and nursing supportive care with special attention to respiratory status; aggressive airway management for those at risk for respiratory failure

GENERAL MEASURES
- Meticulous airway management
- Monitor pulmonary function
- Physical therapy with range of motion exercise and assisted ambulation as tolerated
- Prevention of decubiti

Diet
Nasogastric feedings, if needed

Activity
Bed rest initially

MEDICATION (DRUGS)

First Line
- Antitoxin therapy with trivalent A-B-E antitoxin—Call CDC Assistance, (770) 488-7100 for help in locating and acquiring the antitoxin. A single vial IV provides adequate serum levels.
- Most benefit from antitoxin in cases with rapidly progressive paralysis.
- Early administration important
- Horse serum derived: Up to 20% reaction incidence. Consider skin testing or pretreatment with steroids or antihistamines.
- Infantile
  - Treatment with Human Botulism Immune Globulin recommended by some authors
  - Available only through the California State Health Department (510) 540-2646
- Wound
  - Antitoxin therapy with trivalent A-B-E antitoxin, one vial IV and one vial IM, repeat in 2–4 hours if persistent symptoms
  - Antibiotics unproven by clinical trial but widely used and recommended
    - Penicillin G (3 million units IV q4h in adults)
    - Metronidazole (500 mg IV q8h) for penicillin-allergic patients
  - Vaccine—pentavalent vaccine available
    - Efficiency in terrorist attack is unknown
    - Newer vaccines being developed
- Contradictions: Previous reaction to horse serum–containing medications represents a relative contraindication to trivalent antitoxin. Human Botulism Immune Globulin has a greatly decreased risk of hypersensitivity reactions.

SURGERY
Wound excision débridement

 ## FOLLOW-UP

PROGNOSIS
- Delay in administering toxin is the most important factor that affects clinical course and outcome
- Mortality: 10–40%
- Mortality for patients >60 years twice that of younger patients
- Full recovery may take months.

COMPLICATIONS
- Aspiration pneumonia
- Nosocomial infection
- Hypoxic tissue damage
- Death

PATIENT MONITORING
Cardiorespiratory monitoring during illness

REFERENCES
1. Horowitz BZ. Botulinum toxin. *Crit Care Clin*. 2005;21:825–839.
2. Cherington M. Botulinum: Update and review. *Semin Neurol*. 2004;24(2):155–163.
3. Arnon SS. Botulinum toxin as a biological weapon. *JAMA*. 2001;285(8):1059–1070.
4. Coffield JA. Botulinum neurotoxin: The neuromuscular junction revisited. *Crit Rev Neurobiol*. 2003;15(3–4):175–196.

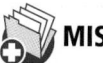 ## MISCELLANEOUS

- Other notes
  - Organism present in stools of 1–2% of healthy individuals
  - Release of toxins in the gut may worsen symptoms of infantile botulism by bacterial lysis.
- See also: Food Poisoning; Bacterial

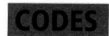 ### CODES

ICD9-CM
005.1 Botulism

PATIENT TEACHING
- When preserving food at home, kill *Clostridiumbotulinum* spores by pressure cooking at 250°F (120°C) for 30 minutes.
- Toxin can be destroyed by boiling for 10 minutes or cooking at 175°F (80°C) for 30 minutes
- Avoid honey in 1st year of life

BRAIN ABSCESS

Peter Kozisek, MD

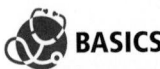 **BASICS**

DESCRIPTION
- Single or multiple abscesses within the brain, usually occurring secondary to a focus of infection outside the central nervous system
- May mimic brain tumor, but evolves more rapidly (days to a few weeks)
- Starts as a cerebritis, becomes necrotic, and subsequently becomes encapsulated
- Synonym(s): Cerebral abscess

ALERT
Geriatric Considerations
Age does not affect outcome as much as the abscess size and state of neurological dysfunction at presentation.

Pediatric Considerations
- About 1/3 of the cases in pediatric age group
- Rarely found in infants <1 year of age
- Cyanotic congenital heart disease frequently associated

GENERAL PREVENTION
- Adequate treatment of otitis media, mastoiditis, dental abscess, other predisposing factors
- Prophylactic antibiotics after compound skull fracture or penetrating head wound

EPIDEMIOLOGY
- Incidence/prevalence in the US: Infrequent
- Predominant age: Median age 30–40 years
- Predominant sex: Male > Female (2:1)

RISK FACTORS
- AIDS
- Immunocompromised
- IV drug abuse

Genetics
No known genetic pattern

ETIOLOGY
- Direct extension from otitis, mastoiditis, sinusitis, or dental infection
- Cranial osteomyelitis
- Penetrating skull trauma
- Prior craniotomy
- Bacteremia from lung abscess, pneumonia
- Bacterial endocarditis
- Fungal infection of the nasopharynx
- *Toxoplasma gondii* (in AIDS patients)
- Cyanotic congenital heart disease
- IV drug use
- No source found in 20%
- Most common infective organisms: Streptococci, staphylococci, enteric Gram-negative bacilli and anaerobes (usually same as source of infection), *Nocardia*

ASSOCIATED CONDITIONS
- AIDS
- Congenital heart disease

 DIAGNOSIS

SIGNS AND SYMPTOMS
History
- Recent onset of headache becoming severe
- Nausea and vomiting
- Mental changes progressing to stupor and coma
- Afebrile or low-grade fever
- Neck stiffness
- Seizures
- Papilledema
- Focal neurological signs depending on location

Physical Exam
- Lumbar puncture often contraindicated
- Search for primary source of infection (chest radiograph, skull film for fracture, or sinus films)

TESTS
- WBC may be normal or mildly elevated
- Culture of abscess contents, predominant organisms include Toxoplasma (AIDS), Staphylococcus (trauma), aerobic or anaerobic bacteria, fungi (rare)
- Blood studies: Mild polymorphonuclear leukocytosis; elevated sedimentation rate
- Special test: Surgical burr hole with aspiration to make a specific bacteriologic diagnosis

ALERT
Clinical Considerations
Drugs that may alter lab results: Prior administration of antibiotics

Imaging
- CT or MRI are the diagnostic methods of choice. The findings are dependent on stages of the abscess.
- Radionuclide [117]In-labeled leukocytes may distinguish abscess from neoplasm

Pathological Findings
- Suppuration, liquefaction, and encapsulation, depending on stage of evolution
- Fibrosis

DIFFERENTIAL DIAGNOSIS
- Brain tumors
- Cysticercosis
- Stroke
- Resolving intracranial hemorrhage
- Subdural empyema
- Extradural abscess
- Encephalitis

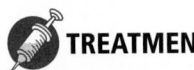 **TREATMENT**

PRE HOSPITAL
Inpatient for close observation, diagnostic evaluation, and specialty consultation (neurology, neurosurgery, or infectious disease)

GENERAL MEASURES
- Palliative and supportive
- Medical therapy
  - For surgically inaccessible, multiple abscesses
  - For abscesses in early cerebritis stage
  - Small (<2.5 cm) abscess
  - Therapy directed toward most likely organism

Diet
IV fluids if nausea and vomiting present

Activity
Bed rest until infection controlled and abscess evacuated or resolving, then up as tolerated

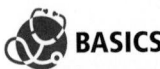 **MEDICATION (DRUGS)**

- Antibiotics according to organism if known
- If organism unknown, begin with penicillin G and metronidazole, or chloramphenicol (Chloromycetin), if metronidazole cannot be used
- Add oxacillin or nafcillin if trauma or IV drug user (use vancomycin in penicillin-sensitive patients)
- If Gram-negative organism suspected (otic, GI, GU organ), add 3rd-generation cephalosporin
- Abscess associated with HIV infection assumed to be due to *Toxoplasma gondii*
  - Daily doses of sulfadiazine and pyrimethamine
  - Therapy will be lifelong in AIDS patients.
- Anticonvulsants
  - Phenytoin until abscess resolved or perhaps longer
  - Obtain anticonvulsant levels
- Following a surgical procedure, use corticosteroids to reduce edema, such as Dexamethasone. Taper rapidly. Use is usually limited to 1 week. Continue antibiotics for 6–8 weeks.
- Contraindications: Sensitivity or allergy to any prescribed medications
- Precautions
  - Sulfadiazine poorly water-soluble. Patients must maintain adequate hydration or risk developing crystalluria.
  - Decrease dosage of penicillin in patients with renal dysfunction
  - Monitor serum levels of anticonvulsants.
  - A dose of pyrimethamine is required for the treatment of toxoplasmosis, which may approach toxic levels. The patient should be observed for folic acid deficiency and treated with folinic acid (leucovorin), 5–15 mg (PO, IM, IV) if necessary.
- Significant possible interactions: Refer to the manufacturer's literature.

SURGERY
Surgical therapy
- Mandatory when neurologic deficits are severe or progressive
- Used when the abscess is in the posterior fossa
- Abscess drainage via a needle under stereotactic CT guidance through a burr hole under local anesthesia is the most rapid and effective surgical method of treatment and may be repeated if needed.
- Craniotomy: If abscess is large or multilocular
- Abscess resulting from trauma

B

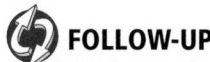 **FOLLOW-UP**

PROGNOSIS
Survival: >80% with early diagnosis and treatment

COMPLICATIONS
• Permanent neurological deficits
• Surgical complications
• Recurrent abscess
• Seizures

PATIENT MONITORING
• Postsurgical monitoring as needed
• Serial CT or MRI: To confirm progressive resolution, early detection, and management of complications

REFERENCES

1. Graham DI, Lantos PL, eds. *Greenfield's Neuropathology.* 9th ed. London: Arnold; 2002.
2. Osenbach RK, Loftus CM. Diagnosis and management of brain abscess. *Neurosurg Clin North Am.* 1992;3:403–420.
3. Rakel RE, ed. *Conn's Current Therapy.* Philadelphia, PA: Elsevier Saunders; 2005.
4. Ropper A, Victor M, eds. *Adams and Victor's Principles of Neurology.* 8th ed. New York, NY: McGraw-Hill; 2005.
5. Rowland LD, ed. *Merritt's Textbook of Neurology.* 10th ed. Baltimore, MD: Williams & Wilkins; 2000.

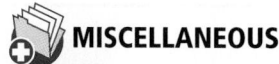 **MISCELLANEOUS**

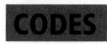 **CODES**

ICD9-CM
324.0 Intracranial abscess

PATIENT TEACHING
For patient education materials favorably reviewed on this topic, contact the Brain Research Foundation, 208 S. LaSalle Street, Suite 1426, Chicago, IL 60604; (312) 782-4311.

 See Corresponding Diagnostic Algorithm

BRAIN INJURY, TRAUMATIC

John Herbert Stevenson, MD

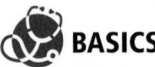 **BASICS**

DESCRIPTION
- Frequently related to rapid deceleration, as occurs ins motor vehicle accidents or diving accidents; may also be due to blunt trauma.
- Traumatic brain injury (TBI) is a dynamic process with initial bleeding followed by secondary injury due to cerebral edema, continued intracranial bleeding, etc.
- Predicting outcome initially is difficult, and patients may improve for years.
- System(s) Affected: Cardiovascular; Endocrine/Metabolic; Nervous
- Synonym(s): Head injury

ALERT
Geriatric Considerations
- Poorer prognosis with increasing age
- Subdural hematomas are common after fall or blow; symptoms may be subtle.

Pediatric Considerations
Outcome for children is more positive, except in severe TBI.

GENERAL PREVENTION
- Safety education
- Seat belts, bicycle and motorcycle helmets
- Protective headgear for contact sports

EPIDEMIOLOGY
- Predominant age: 15–24 years
- Predominant sex: Male > Female

Incidence
- 200/100,000
- 500,000 hospitalizations and 75,000 deaths per year

RISK FACTORS
Alcohol, prior head injury, contact sports; "heading" soccer balls may cause long-term cognitive loss.

ETIOLOGY
- Motor vehicle accident (50%)
- Falls
- Assault
- Child abuse
  - Consider if dropped or fell <4 feet (e.g., off bed, couch) and significant injury present
  - Subdural more likely to be abuse
  - Any retinal hemorrhage (retinal hemorrhage is not caused by seizures or simple head trauma)

ASSOCIATED CONDITIONS
Alcohol and drug abuse

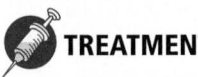 **DIAGNOSIS**

SIGNS AND SYMPTOMS
Variable and dependent on degree of injury

History
- Loss of consciousness (LOC)
- External signs of head injury
- Headache
- Vomiting
- Amnesia
- Epidural hemorrhage from blunt trauma is generally acute, 30% with a "lucid interval" (initial loss of consciousness [LOC] followed by recovery of consciousness, then LOC secondary to the intracranial bleed)
- Subdural hemorrhage usually has a slower onset and may present weeks after the initial injury, especially in the elderly.

Physical Exam
- Focal signs and symptoms
- Evidence of increased intracranial pressure (ICP) (elevated BP, decreased pulse rate, or slow or irregular breathing [Cushing triad])—only 30% have all 3
- Decorticate or decerebrate positioning (both bad prognostic signs)
- Seizures
- Signs of basilar skull fracture: Raccoon eyes, battle sign, hemotympanum, CSF rhinorrhea or otorrhea (see "Tests")
- Unilateral dilated pupil in an alert patient is not consistent with impending herniation, because such patients are always unconscious.

TESTS
- Neuropsychometric testing when able
- CSF rhinorrhea
  - Contains glucose, whereas nasal mucus does not
  - Check also for the double-halo sign: Put a drop of nasal discharge on filter paper. If it contains CSF and blood, 2 rings appear, a central ring followed by a paler ring.

Lab
- Evaluate for coagulopathy.
- Drug and alcohol screening

Imaging
- CT, noncontrast, is study of choice to review bone windows, tissue windows, and subdural space
  - NEXUS II study has demonstrated 8 clinical criteria that, if all absent, indicate a low likelihood of significant TBI
    - Evidence of significant skull fracture (depressed, basilar, or diastatic)
    - Altered level of alertness
    - Neurologic deficit
    - Persistent vomiting
    - Presence of scalp hematoma
    - Abnormal behavior
    - Coagulopathy
    - Age >65
- Skull radiographs are not helpful in most cases, but can be done to document child abuse.

Diagnostic Procedures/Surgery
- Placement of ICP monitor when indicated
- Serial neurologic exams

Pathological Findings
- Epidural, subdural, or intraparenchymal hemorrhage
- Coup or contra-coup injury
- Evolving, diffuse axonal injury is a principal cause of neurologic sequelae with mild head trauma.

DIFFERENTIAL DIAGNOSIS
Other causes of coma (e.g., drug overdose, infection, metabolic, vascular causes)

TREATMENT

INITIAL STABILIZATION
- ABCs take priority over head injury.
- C-spine immobilization should be considered in all head trauma.

GENERAL MEASURES
- Acute management depends on severity of injury. Most patients need no interventions.
- Immediate goal: Determine who needs further therapy, imaging studies (CT), and hospitalization to prevent further injury.
- For the severely injured patient
  - Avoid hypotension or hypoxia. Head injury causes increased ICP secondary to edema, and perfusion pressure must be maintained.
  - Use normal saline for resuscitation fluid.
  - Hyperventilation is controversial, but current literature suggests a short duration of hyperventilation, not below $Paco_2$ 30 mm Hg may be beneficial. Prophylactic hyperventilation for those without signs or symptoms of increased intracranial pressure is contraindicated and may cause additional injury secondary to vasoconstriction.
  - Hypothermia: Although no difference is seen in mortality, may have marginal benefit especially in patients with elevated ICP refractory to other methods.
  - Seizure prophylaxis does not change outcomes (such as death rates) but may prevent seizures. Consider phenytoin for 1 week postinjury.
  - Manage breakthrough seizures with lorazepam.

Diet
As tolerated

Activity
See "Activity" under topic "Postconcussive Syndrome" for sports activity management.

MEDICATION (DRUGS)

First Line
- Pain: Morphine 12 mg IV p.r.n.
- Increased ICP
  - 0.252 g/kg (0.251 g/kg in children) given over 30–60 minutes in patients with adequate renal function; should not be used unless there is evidence of increased ICP; prophylactic use is associated with worse outcomes.
  - 20–40 mg IV to promote diuresis
  - Neither furosemide or mannitol should be given to a hypotensive patient.
  - Hypertonic saline 2 mL/kg IV decreases ICP without adverse hemodynamic status and may have beneficial effects on immune system and excitatory neurotransmitters.
- Sedation
  - Preferred due to short duration of action allowing serial neurologic exams
- Seizures
  - 15 mg/kg IV (1 mg/kg/min IV, not to exceed 50 mg/min). Stop infusion if QT interval increases by >50% () 15 mg/kg IV, not to exceed 150 mg/min, if need rapid infusion due to active seizures
  - () 12 mg (0.1 mg/kg in children) IV. Preferred over diazepam.
  - 15 mg/kg IV at 25–50 mg/min. May give IM.
- Contraindications: Allergy

Second Line
- Diuretics and IV β-blockers (e.g., esmolol or labetalol) can be used to maintain mean arterial pressure between 130–70 mm Hg, which may be helpful. However, nitrates may increase ICP.
- Antibiotics (e.g., cefazolin) should be given if penetrating trauma is present. Prophylactic antibiotics are not useful in basilar skull fractures.

SURGERY
Depends on neurosurgical consult

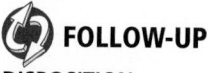 **FOLLOW-UP**

DISPOSITION
Discharge Criteria
- Abnormal CT
- Abnormal Glasgow coma scale
- Clinical evidence of basilar skull fracture
- Persistent neurological deficits (e.g., confusion, somnolence)
- Patient with no competent adult at home for observation
- Possibly admit: LOC, amnesia, etc.

Discharge Criteria
Normal hemocrit with return to normal mental status and responsible adult to observe patient at home (see "Patient Monitoring")

Issues for Referral
Consult neurosurgery for
- All penetrating head trauma
- All abnormal head CTs

PROGNOSIS
- Gradual improvement for many
- 30–50% of severe head injuries may be fatal.
- Prolonged coma may be followed by satisfactory outcome.
- Rehabilitation indicated following a significant acute injury. Set realistic goals.

COMPLICATIONS
- Delayed hematomas
- Chronic subdural hematoma, which may follow even "mild" head injury, especially in the elderly. Often presents with headache and decreased mentation.
- Delayed hydrocephalus
- Emotional disturbances and psychiatric disorders resulting from head injury may be refractory to treatment.
- Seizure disorders—in 50% of penetrating head injuries, in 20% of severe closed head injuries, and in <5% of head injuries overall. Hematomas significantly increase risk of epilepsy.
- Second-impact syndrome occurs when the central nervous system loses autoregulation. An individual with a minor head injury is returned to a contact sport and, following even minor trauma (e.g., whiplash), the patient will lose consciousness and herniate within 12 minutes, with a 50% mortality. A similar syndrome of "malignant edema" can occur in children with even a single injury.

PATIENT MONITORING
- Any patient discharged should have "head injury instructions" to watch for symptoms indicating the need for further intervention (e.g., changing mental status, worsening headache, focal findings). Give to a competent surrogate who will observe the patient. A patient who deteriorates is not likely to remember or act on any instructions.
- Schedule regular follow-up.
- The *postconcussion syndrome* can follow mild head injury without LOC and includes headaches, dizziness, fatigue, and subtle cognitive or affective changes.
- Proper counseling, symptomatic management, and gradual return to normal activities is essential to prevent a posttraumatic neurosis that can become refractory to treatment.

 MISCELLANEOUS

- Other notes: The Glasgow coma scale is not a linear scale; a score of 14 (normal being 15) represents a moderately severe injury category.
- See also: Brain injury—post acute care issues; Postconcussive syndrome; Seizure disorders

CODES

ICD9-CM
- 800.00 Fracture of vault of skull, closed without mention of intracranial injury, unspecified state of consciousness
- 850.9 Concussion, unspecified
- 851.xx Cerebral laceration or contusion
- 852.00 Subarachnoid hemorrhage following injury without mention of open intracranial wound, unspecified state of consciousness
- 854.00 Intracranial injury of other and unspecified nature, without mention of intracranial wound, unspecified state of consciousness

PATIENT TEACHING

 See Corresponding Diagnostic Algorithm

 See Patient Handout on CD

BRAIN INJURY—POST ACUTE CARE ISSUES

Bart M. Demaerschalk, MD, MSc

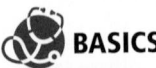 **BASICS**

DESCRIPTION
Traumatic brain injury (TBI) is broadly defined as brain injury due to externally inflicted trauma and may result in significant impairment of an individual's physical, cognitive, and psychosocial functioning.

- System(s) Affected: Nervous; Pulmonary; Skin/Exocrine; Endocrine/Metabolic; Renal/Urologic; Gastrointestinal (GI); Musculoskeletal

GENERAL PREVENTION
Improved safety standards and programs designed to minimize injury from vehicular-related events (motor vehicle, motorcycle, bicycle, pedestrian), falls, violence, sports, and recreation provide the best prevention against TBI. (1,2)[C]

EPIDEMIOLOGY
- Predominant age: Highest incidence persons 15–24 years of age and those >75 years, with additional smaller peak in children <5 years.
- Predominant sex: Male > Female (2:1)

Incidence
An estimated 1.2 million–1.7 million Americans sustain TBI per year. Incidence of TBI is 100/100,000 in the US, 230,000 hospitalizations, 50,000 deaths per year, and an estimated 80–90,000 sustain long-term disabilities.

Prevalence
Prevalence estimates range from 2.5 million–6.5 million individuals living with consequences of TBI.

RISK FACTORS
See "Brain Injury, Traumatic"

ETIOLOGY
Motor vehicle, bicycle, or pedestrian-vehicle incidents (50%), falls, acts of violence and assault, and sports and recreation–related injuries are the leading causes of TBI.

ASSOCIATED CONDITIONS
- Psychosis
- Suicide attempts
- Substance abuse
- ADD

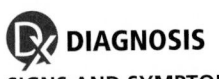 **DIAGNOSIS**

SIGNS AND SYMPTOMS
- Consequences of TBI often influence human functions along a continuum from altered physiological functions, through neurological, psychological, cognitive, and behavioral impairments, to medical problems and disabilities that affect the individual, family, and community.
- Nonneurological complications include pulmonary, metabolic and endocrinological, nutritional, gastrointestinal, musculoskeletal, genitourinary, dermatologic, and chronic pain.
- Most neurological complications are apparent within the 1st days or months following injury. Long-term sequelae include seizures, headache, visual defects, and movement and sleep disorders.
- Cognitive consequences include memory impairment, difficulties in attention and concentration, language deficits, visual perception problems, and poor executive skills, problem solving, reasoning, insight, judgment, planning, information processing, and organization.

- Behavioral problems include decreased ability to initiate responses, verbal and physical aggression, agitation, learning difficulties, shallow self-awareness, altered sexual functioning, impulsivity, and social disinhibition.
- Psychological consequences include mood disorders, personality changes, altered emotional control, depression, and anxiety.
- Social consequences include risk of suicide, divorce, unemployment, economic strain, and alcohol/substance abuse.

Pediatric Considerations
- Interactions of physical, cognitive, and behavioral sequelae interfere with new learning. The effect of early TBI may not become apparent until later in the child's development.

TESTS
- Evoked potentials (auditory, visual, and somatosensory)
- Behavioral assessment, neuropsychological testing, and vocational assessment
- Cognitive test for orientation and arousal; use Western Neuro Sensory Stimulation Profile or Galvest. Orient. Amnesia Test
- EEG

Lab
- CBC, electrolytes, blood urea nitrogen creatinine, calcium, albumin, vitamin B_{12}, folate, thyroid stimulating harmone, alkaline phosphatase, aspartate aminotransferase (AST), alanine amino-transferase (ALT), morning cortisol level, urine culture
- Culture, ova, and parasites for diarrhea
- Skin culture
- Culture tracheal site
- Endocrine workup as indicated

Imaging
- Bone scan: Heterotopic ossification
- CT: Hydrocephalus, atrophy, hematoma
- Video pharyngeal fluoroscopic swallowing study
- MRI to evaluate diffuse axonal injury

Diagnostic Procedures/Surgery
- Altered arousal—visual, auditory, and somatosensory evoked potentials
- Neurogenic bladder-check post-void residuals 3–4 times. If >50 cc or 20% of voided volume, urodynamics
- Ultrasound of bladder and kidney: Urolithiasis and hydronephrosis
- Endoscopy: Cause of dysphagia
- Contractures and spasticity: Examination under anesthesia
- Respiratory and neurologic: Sleep/oxygen saturation study, bronchoscopy for stricture

Pathological Findings
- Hydrocephalus with periventricular edema
- Joint contractures results in collagen cross linking: Decreased range of motion
- Heterotopic ossification: Disorganized osteoid calcification in soft tissue

DIFFERENTIAL DIAGNOSIS
Differential Diagnosis of Pain after TBI: (5)
The diagnosis of pain following TBI can be difficult in light of the limitations imposed by cognitive,

language, and behavioral deficits. The differential diagnosis includes
- Dysautonomia: Characterized by episodes of tachypnea, hypertension, painful posturing/contractions, and diaphoresis
- Neuropathic pain: Described as burning, shock-like, or pins and needles; Allodynia/hyperpathia. The 3 most common forms are complex regional pain syndrome, central pain syndrome, and peripheral neuropathy.
- Spasticity or spastic dystonia
- Headache: Posttraumatic headache
- Myofascial pain syndrome
- Neurogenic Heterotopic Ossification: Bone formation in soft tissue
- Deep Venous Thrombosis
- Constipation and urinary retention
- Trauma: Fractures, musculoskeletal injuries
- Shoulder: Subluxation, acromioclavicular separation, rotator cuff tendonitis/tear

Differential Diagnosis of Alteration in Functional Capacity/Level after TBI:
Chronic infection (UTI, aspiration pneumonia, GI), depression, hypothyroidism or hydrocephalus, intracerebral hemorrhage, epilepsy/seizures, fractures, tracheal stricture, pain, alcohol or drugs, polypharmacy and/or central nervous system depressant/psychoactive drugs

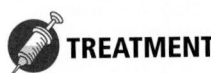 **TREATMENT**

GENERAL MEASURES
- Diminished level of arousal: Identify best modality for communication, assess functional skills (proper seating, hand function), behavioral or neuropsychologist. Social work (to assist with family education and long-term planning) and nursing
- Reduce sedatives
- Neurogenic bladder—treat UTI
  - If post-void residual <50 cc, then trial of regular voiding routine q2h
  - If still incontinent, add oxybutynin
  - If still incontinent, try condom catheter during the day; incontinent pads at night.
  - If high post-void residuals or high pressure bladder or dyssynergic bladder on urodynamics: Intermittent catheter q4–6h
- Neurogenic bowel: Regular bowel routine
- Contractures and spasticity: Stretching
  - If no progress after 4 weeks, consider serial casting or custom made orthotic
  - Contractures >45°: Consider tendon release
- Heterotopic ossification: Stretch soft tissue to decrease maturation of osteoid, consider orthotics/splinting, bone scan at baseline
- Skin: q2h turning, avoid sitting such as in bed at 45°, observe for erythema around tube sites and rule out latex allergy
- Respiratory: Night humidification if has a tracheotomy, may require suctioning
- Endocrine: Monitor fluid balance
- Dental: Assessment and x-rays
- Rehabilitative practices: Rehabilitative programs should be interdisciplinary, comprehensive, and include cognitive and behavioral assessment and intervention. (1) [C]

- Non-pharmacological therapeutic interventions
  - Cognitive exercises (including computer-assisted strategies), compensatory devices (memory books, paging systems), psychotherapy, behavior modification, vocational rehabilitation, school setting rehabilitation, nutritional support, music and art therapy, and therapeutic recreation (4)[C]

Diet
- Consult with dietitian
- Ensure adequate hydration; 2–2.5 L of water/day. More if outside or in hot weather.
- Bolus feeds preferred if fed by gastrostomy
- Upright and quiet for 1/2 hour following feeds, as aspiration can occur even with a g-tube

Activity
As tolerated: Outings in wheelchair can be beneficial; skin very sensitive to sun/wind

 ## MEDICATION (DRUGS)

- Psychostimulants may affect speed of cognitive processing, mood, and behavior, but effects on attention, distractibility, and memory are less clear. Methylphenidate 20–40 mg/d in 2 divided doses; Dextroamphetamine. (9)[B]

- Agitation
  - Treat epilepsy or depression
  - Minimize the use of antipsychotics and benzodiazepines, as they worsen cognition.

  - If necessary, use antipsychotics of the atypical class (Clozapine, Olanzepine, Quetiapine, Risperidone, Ziprasidone). (8)[B]

- Abulia and lack of initiative: Amantadine (Symmetrel), bromocriptine, methylphenidate, levodopa (8)[C]

- Epilepsy: American Academy of Physical Medicine and Rehabilitation does not recommend antiepileptic drugs for preventing late (>7 days post TBI) posttraumatic seizures. [B] If epilepsy occurs, avoid phenytoin and phenobarbital—too sedating. (6)

- Spasticity caution: Be aware of potential negative consequences of all agents. Dantrolene sodium 25–200 mg/day divided t.i.d.; Baclofen; intrathecal Baclofen; Diazepam, Clonidine, Tizanidine, and Gabapentin; Botulinum toxin injections for focal spasticity. (7)[B]

- Neurogenic bladder: Oxybutynin 2.5 mg t.i.d.–10 mg q.i.d. if bladder pressures low and/or post-void residuals low [B]

- Bowel routine: Stool softener such as docusate sodium (daily) combined with laxative (night before suppository), high fiber and suppository (every other day) to induce bowel movement [C]

- Heterotopic ossification: Indomethacin 25–50 mg t.i.d. If severe, progressive, or history of GI ulceration, then etidronate (Didronel) 20 mg/kg for 6 months or alendronate 20 mg once a day. [C]

- Neurobehavioral problems: Weak evidence that psychostimulants are effective in the treatment of inattention, apathy, and slowness; high-dose beta-blockers in the treatment of agitation and aggression; and anti-convulsants and anti-depressants in the treatment of agitation and aggression with an affective disorder. (3,4)[B]

- Contraindications: Refer to manufacturers' literature

- Precautions: Medications may have significant adverse effects in persons with TBI and can impede rehabilitation progress.
- Significant possible interactions: Refer to manufacturers' literature.

SURGERY
Tendons releases; fundoplasty or gastrostomy; tracheostomy; ventriculoperitoneal or ventriculoatrial shunt

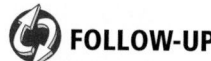 ## FOLLOW-UP

PROGNOSIS
- Most rapid return of function is during 1st 2 years, but some improve slowly for 5–10 years
- Highly variable (80% of individuals with severe injuries become independent in dressing and self-care at 1 year)
- Negative prognostic factors
  - Age >40
  - Abnormal pupillary responses
  - Prolonged coma (i.e., GCS <9, seven days after injury)
  - Abnormal evoked potentials
  - Extraocular eye movement abnormalities

COMPLICATIONS
- Major affective disorder (depression, psychosis) in up to 50% of patients
- Family and caregiver burn out
- Substance abuse
- Social isolation
- May be at higher risk of dementia
- Latex allergy to g-tube, catheters
- Dental caries
- Osteoporosis
- Falls
- Aspiration pneumonia
- Pressure ulcers
- Dysphagia, esophagitis
- Bladder incontinence
- Contractures/spasticity

PATIENT MONITORING
- Patients make slow steady gains. Ongoing outcome assessments determine progress (or not) in abilities and medication efficacy.
- Review medical status monthly

REFERENCES
1. NIH Consensus Development Panel on Rehabilitation of Persons with Traumatic Brain Injury. Rehabilitation of persons with traumatic brain injury. *JAMA*. 1999;282(10):974–983.
2. Lovasik D, Kerr M, Alexander S. Traumatic brain injury research: A review of clinical studies. *Crit Care Nurs Q*. 2001;23(4):24–41.
3. Shoumitro D, Crownshaw T. The role of pharmacotherapy in the management of behaviour disorders in traumatic brain injury patients. *Brain Injury*. 2004;18(1):1–31.
4. Glenn MB. A differential diagnostic approach to the pharmacological treatment of cognitive, behavioral, and affective disorders after traumatic brain injury. *J Head Trauma Rehab*. 2002;17(4):273–283.
5. Ivanhoe CB, Hartman ET. Clinical caveats on medical assessment and treatment of pain after TBI. *J Head Trauma Rehab*. 2004;19(1):29–39.

6. Bushnik T, Englander J, Duong T. Medical and social issues related to posttraumatic seizures in persons with traumatic brain injury. *J Head Trauma Rehab*. 2004;19(4):296–304.
7. Zafonte R, Elovic EP, Lombard L. Acute care management of post-TBI spasticity. *J Head Trauma Rehab*. 2004;19(2):89–100.
8. Elovic EP, Lansang R, Li Y, Ricker JH. The use of atypical antipsychotics in traumatic brain injury. *J Head Trauma Rehab*. 2003;18(2):177–195.
9. Whyte J, Vaccaro M, Grieb-Neff P, Hart T. Psychostimulant use in the rehabilitation of individuals with traumatic brain injury. *J Head Trauma Rehab*. 2002;17(4):284–299.

 ## MISCELLANEOUS

- Rehabilitation program guidelines
  - Individualized goals: Behavioral approach emphasizing reinforcement of task behavior
  - Flexible: Alter to meet changing needs
  - Functional (based on activities of daily living): Self care activities involve range of motion exercises
  - Consider patient's attention span and best time of day when planning
  - Allow for as patient control and choice when able (e.g., choice of clothes, music, etc.)
  - Consistency and familiarity
  - Quality of life issues vital (e.g., comfort measures, sensory stimulation, address spiritual and/or cultural needs, and positioning)
  - For agitated behavior, consider consult with behavioral psychologist to design program integrating medications and behavior therapy techniques. Minimize use of punishment and reinforce correct behavior.
- See also: Brain Injury, Traumatic; Constipation; Dysphagia; Fecal Impaction; Gastroesophageal Reflux Disease; Hemorrhoids; Osteoporosis; Pressure Ulcer; Seizure Disorders; Sleep Apnea, Obstructive; Stomatitis; Stroke (Brain Attack); Stroke Rehabilitation

CODES

ICD9-CM
- 530.10 Esophagitis, unspecified
- 750.6 Congenital hiatus hernia
- 787.1 Heartburn
- 733.00 Osteoporosis, unspecified
- 707.0 Decubitus ulcer
- 345.3 Epilepsy, grand mal status

PATIENT TEACHING
- For information and family support groups: http://www.tbinet.org/or http://www.biausa.org/
- Families need support, advocacy, education, information (verbally and written [e.g., audio tape meetings]), opportunities to have input regarding priorities and treatment plans, and the opportunity to discuss limits of treatment for patient (advance directive)

 See Corresponding Diagnostic Algorithm

BRANCHIAL CLEFT FISTULA

Timothy L. Black, MD

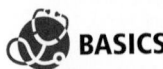 **BASICS**

DESCRIPTION
- A congenital, abnormal tract connecting the skin of the neck with an internal structure, resulting from failure of closure of a branchial cleft
- May involve branchial clefts I–IV, which develop in the 4th gestational week
- System(s) Affected: Skin/Exocrine

ALERT
Pediatric Considerations
Almost all occur in the pediatric age group.

EPIDEMIOLOGY
- Predominant age: By definition, all are present at birth, although they may remain unnoticed for some time. (Branchial cleft cysts may not present until later childhood.) (1)[C]
- Predominant sex: Unknown

Incidence
Unknown

Prevalence
Unknown

RISK FACTORS
Positive family history

Genetics
10% have family history.

ETIOLOGY
- The 1st branchial cleft contributes to the tympanic cavity and eustachian tube. Related fistulae are very rare and tend to be infra- or retroauricular. (Preauricular cysts and sinuses are not thought to be of branchial cleft origin.)
- The 2nd branchial cleft forms the hyoid bone and tonsillar fossa. Related fistulae (most common variant) course between the internal and external carotid arteries. Internal opening usually at level of tonsillar fossa. External opening along anterior border of sternocleidomastoid muscle. (1)[C]
- 3rd and 4th branchial clefts form parathyroid glands, thymus, and portions of thyroid (parafollicular cells). Fistulae are rare; those from 3rd cleft course posterior to carotid artery; both should have external ostia on lower anterior neck. Sinus tracts (also called *pyriform sinuses*) originate in the pyriform sinus and course adjacent to the thyroid cartilage. (2)[C]

ASSOCIATED CONDITIONS
Microtia and aural atresia occur with failure of development of 1st branchial cleft. (3)[C]

 DIAGNOSIS

SIGNS AND SYMPTOMS
- Presence of tiny external opening usually on lower neck along anterior border of sternocleidomastoid muscle
- Spontaneous mucoid drainage
- External openings may also be marked by a skin tag or cartilage.
- Infection may rarely be the presenting sign, with erythema, swelling, pain, or fever.
- 10% are bilateral. (3)[C]

History
History of drainage from cervical area

Physical Exam
Small orifices located in the mid neck, most commonly along the anterior border of the sterno-cleidomastoid muscle (less commonly in the lower neck or post-auricular)

TESTS
Lab
Culture if signs of infection.

Diagnostic Procedures/Surgery
- Sinogram or fistulogram may be done, but is of little value.
- CT of neck with IV contrast occasionally beneficial in 3rd and 4th branchial cleft fistulas/sinus (2)[C]
- Pharyngoscopy may occasionally be useful

Pathological Findings
- Lined by stratified squamous epithelium, may contain hair follicles, sweat glands, sebaceous glands, or cartilage (3)[C]
- Some are lined by ciliated columnar epithelium

DIFFERENTIAL DIAGNOSIS
- External sinuses
- Cystic hygroma
- Dermoid cysts
- Lymphadenopathy

TREATMENT

- Surgical excision
- Outpatient status usually appropriate

SURGERY
- Small transverse incision at external ostium with careful dissection of fistula (1)[C]
- Stepladder incisions may be needed (3)[C]
- End of fistula ligated flush with pharyngeal mucosa. 1st branchial cleft lesions may require larger incision (1)[C]
- Methylene blue injection into fistula may be useful
- Drains are not used.
- Antibiotics only for infection

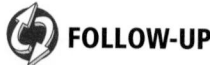

FOLLOW-UP

PROGNOSIS
Good

COMPLICATIONS
- Facial nerve injury
- Infection
- Carotid artery injury
- Possible recurrence if any epithelium remains
- Neoplastic degeneration of branchial remnants (~250 reported cases) if not resected

PATIENT MONITORING
- Follow at weekly intervals, if infected, until resolution, then excision
- Postoperative visit at 2 weeks

REFERENCES

1. Roback SA, Telander RL. Thyroglossal duct cysts and Branchial cleft anomalies. *Sem Ped Surg.* 1994;3:142–146.
2. Liberman M, Kay S, Emil S, et al. Ten years of experience with third and fourth branchial remnants. *J Ped Surg.* 2002;37:685–690.
3. Ashcraft KW, Murphy JP, Sharp RJ, eds. *Pediatric Surgery.* 3rd ed. Philadelphia, PA: WB Saunders; 2000.

MISCELLANEOUS

Branchial cleft remnants, sinuses, and cysts are also the result of failure of branchial cleft to complete its normal development.

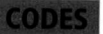 **CODES**

ICD9-CM
744.41 Branchial cleft sinus or fistula

PATIENT TEACHING

 See Corresponding Diagnostic Algorithm

B

BREAST ABSCESS

Anya S. Koutras, MD
Kristen Burdick, MD

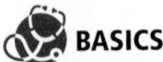 **BASICS**

DESCRIPTION
- Collection of pus, usually localized.
- Can be associated with lactation or fistulous tracts secondary to squamous epithelial neoplasm or duct occlusion
- System(s) Affected: Skin/Exocrine
- Synonym(s): Mammary abscess; Peripheral breast abscess; Subareolar abscess; Puerperal abscess

ALERT
Pregnancy Considerations
Most commonly associated with postpartum lactation

GENERAL PREVENTION
- Prevention of mastitis
- Early treatment of mastitis with milk expression and cold compresses
- Early treatment with antibiotics

EPIDEMIOLOGY
- Predominant age
  - Puerperal abscess: Premenopausal
  - Subareolar abscess: Postmenopausal
- Predominant sex: Female

Incidence
- 0.1–0.5% of breast-feeding women
- Puerperal abscess rare after 1st 6 weeks of lactation

RISK FACTORS
- Puerperal mastitis: 5–11% go on to abscess (most often due to inadequate therapy). Risk factors for mastitis are those that result in milk stasis (infrequent feeds, missing feeds)
- Poor latch, damaged nipple, illness in mother or baby, rapid weaning, breast pressure, blocked nipple pore or duct, maternal stress or fatigue, maternal malnutrition
- General factors: Diabetes, rheumatoid arthritis,
- Steroids, silicone/paraffin implants, lumpectomy with radiation, heavy cigarette smoking,
- Nipple retraction

ETIOLOGY
- Delayed treatment of mastitis
- Puerperal abscesses: Blocked lactiferous duct
- Subareolar abscess: Squamous epithelial neoplasm with keratin plugs or ductal extension with associated inflammation
- Peripheral abscess: Stasis of the duct

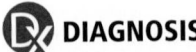 **DIAGNOSIS**

SIGNS AND SYMPTOMS
- Tender breast lump, fluctuant, usually unilateral
- Erythema
- Draining pus
- Local edema
- Systemic malaise (though usually less malaise than with mastitis)
- Fever
- Nipple and skin retraction
- Proximal lymphadenopathy

TESTS
Lab
- Leukocytosis
- Elevated sedimentation rate
- Culture and sensitivity of drainage to identify pathogen, usually Staphylococci or Streptococci. *E. coli* is 3rd most common. Nonlactational abscess associated with anaerobic bacteria.

Imaging
- Ultrasound
- Mammogram

Diagnostic Procedures/Surgery
- Aspiration for culture
- Fine-needle aspiration not accurate to exclude carcinoma

Pathological Findings
- Squamous metaplasia of the ducts
- Intraductal hyperplasia
- Epithelial overgrowth
- Fat necrosis
- Duct ectasia

DIFFERENTIAL DIAGNOSIS
- Carcinoma (inflammatory or primary squamous cell))
- Tuberculosis (may be associated with HIV infection)
- Actinomycosis
- Typhoid
- Sarcoid
- Granulomatous disease
- Syphilis
- Foreign body reactions (e.g., to silicone and paraffin)
- Mammary duct ectasia
- Hydatid cyst
- Sebaceous cyst

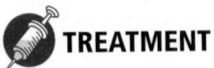 **TREATMENT**

PRE HOSPITAL
Outpatient, unless systemically immunocompromised or septic

GENERAL MEASURES
- Cold compresses for pain control
- Important to continue to breast-feed or express milk

Diet
- No restrictions
- Lecithin supplementation

Activity
No restrictions

MEDICATION (DRUGS)

- Must combine antibiotics with drainage for cure
- Culture mid-stream sample of milk for mastitis, abscess fluid for breast abscess.
- NSAIDs
- Start with dicloxacillin 500 mg q.i.d. for 10–14 days
- If no response in 24–48 hours, switch to:
- Cephalexin 500 mg q.i.d. for 10–14 days
  – Or amoxicillin-clavulanate (Augmentin) 250 mg t.i.d.
- Clindamycin 300 mg t.i.d. if anaerobes suspected
- Contraindications: Allergy to the antibiotic
- Precautions: Refer to manufacturer's profile for each drug
- Significant possible interactions: Refer to manufacturer's profile for each drug

SURGERY

- Aspiration under ultrasound guidance (1,2)[B], (3)[C]
- If aspiration and antibiotics fail, incision and drainage with removal of loculations
- Biopsy of all nonpuerperal abscesses to rule out carcinoma
- Open all fistulous tracts, especially in nonlactating abscesses

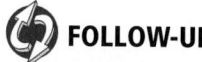 **FOLLOW-UP**

PROGNOSIS

- Good. Complete healing expected in 8–10 days
- Subareolar abscess frequently reoccur, even after I + D and antibiotics; may require surgical removal of ducts.

COMPLICATIONS

Fistula

PATIENT MONITORING

Ensure resolution to exclude carcinoma.

REFERENCES

1. Dener C, Inan A. Breast abscesses in lactating women. *World J Surgery*. 2003;27:130.
2. Schwarz, RJ, Shrestha R. Needle aspiration of breast abscesses. *Am J Surgery*. 2001;182:117.
3. Christensen AF, Al-Suliman N, et al. Ultrasound-guided drainage of breast abscesses: Results in 151 patients. *Br J Radiol*. 2005 Mar; 78(927):186–188.

ADDITIONAL READING

- Cibele B, Schwartz K, Foxman B. Lactation mastitis. JAMA. 2003;289:1609–1612.
- Ng C, Jahanfar S, Teng CL. Antibiotics for mastitis in breastfeeding women (Protocol). Cochrane Database of Systematic Reviews, 2005;(3): CD005458.

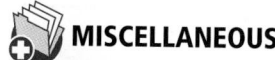 **MISCELLANEOUS**

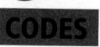 **CODES**

ICD9-CM

- 611.0 Inflammatory disease of breast
- 675.1 Puerperal, postpartum

PATIENT TEACHING

- Care of wound
- Breast-feeding precautions

 See Corresponding Diagnostic Algorithm

BREAST CANCER

Alexandra Sherman, BA

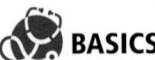 **BASICS**

DESCRIPTION
- Malignant neoplasm in the breast
- Classified as carcinoma in situ (CIS) or invasive; <70% of all breast cancers possess a component of invasion.
- Age-specific incidence of breast cancer increases sharply until menopause and continues to increase at a slower rate in the geriatric population.

ALERT
Geriatric Considerations
Higher percentage of estrogen receptor–positive tumors (80%) in the geriatric population; correlates with improved disease free survival.

Pregnancy Considerations
- Breast cancer occurs infrequently during pregnancy (2.8%).
- Delay in diagnosis is common, and most series report poorer survival related to advanced stage at diagnosis.

GENERAL PREVENTION
- Mammography to screen for disease
  - The U.S. Preventive Services Task Force recommends a mammography with or without clinical breast examination every 1–2 years for women >40.
  - The American Cancer Society recommends mammography and a clinical breast examination every year after age 40 and a clinical breast examination every 3 years for ages 20–39.
  - The ACOG and AMA recommend mammogram every 1–2 years and an annual clinical breast examination starting at age 40 and then annual mammograms at age 50.
  - Albeit controversial, mammography may reduce mortality by 30% in women 50–69; the reduction in mortality is less impressive for women <50 or >70 years.
- Tamoxifen reduces invasive and noninvasive breast cancers by 50% in high-risk women but has significant risk of thromboembolic events and uterine cancer.
  - Recently reported results from the STAR trial showed that raloxifene (Evista) was as effective as tamoxifen in preventing invasive breast cancer in postmenopausal women but was associated with less risk for DVT (NNT = 455), pulmonary emboli, and uterine cancer (NNT=370).

EPIDEMIOLOGY
- Breast cancer is the most common malignancy in women in North America.
- Predominant age: 30–80 with peak age 45–65; 77% of cases occur in women >50
- Predominant sex: Female > Male (1% occurs in males)

Incidence
The American Cancer Society estimates that 212,930 new cases will be diagnosed in 2005, with 40,870 deaths (including 460 men).

Prevalence
One in 7 women will develop breast cancer within her lifetime.

RISK FACTORS
- Increased risk occurs in 1st-degree relatives (relative risk 1.7– 2.5), with bilateral disease in premenopausal relatives (relative risk = 10.5), or bilateral disease in postmenopausal relatives (relative risk = 5.0).
- Hormonal risk factors include early menarche, late menopause, nulliparity, 1st full-term pregnancy after age 30, postmenopausal HRT.
- Women with a history of breast cancer or previous breast biopsies revealing atypical changes are at increased risk (5–10 times) for subsequent cancer.
- Exogenous estrogen use, especially in conjunction with progestins, increases risk.
  - Premenopausal oral contraceptives have not been shown to increase risk.
- Radiation exposure has been associated with an increased risk of breast cancer.

Genetics
- 10–20% of the patients have a significant family history of breast cancer.
- Women who inherit a mutated BRCA1, a tumor suppressor gene, have a 60–80% lifetime risk of breast cancer and a 33% risk of ovarian cancer. BRCA2 is associated with increased risk of breast cancer in men and women.
  - Family history suggestive of breast cancer susceptibility genes include multiple 1st-degree and 2nd-degree relatives with early breast cancer diagnosis and the presence of ovarian cancer.
  - 1 in 400 U.S. women carry a germ-line mutation for BRCA1.
- Her-2,neu is an oncogene whose overexpression plays a role in 25–30% of breast cancers; Her-2,neu confers a poor prognosis and has treatment implications.

ASSOCIATED CONDITIONS
Organ disease at metastatic sites

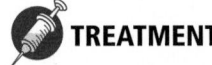 **DIAGNOSIS**

SIGNS AND SYMPTOMS
- Palpable mass (55%)
- Abnormal mammogram without a palpable mass (35%)
- Color, size (enlargement or shrinkage), or shape changes
- Lymphedema (peau d'orange)
- Dimpling
- Nipple retraction, tenderness, or pain
- Axillary mass
- Bone pain (rare)
- Discharge (bloody discharge is more ominous)

History
Any personal or family history of breast cancer, previous breast biopsy, or recent changes in breasts

TESTS
Bone scan, CT, or ultrasound of abdomen if widespread or recurrent disease is suspected

Lab
Initial lab tests include CBC, liver function tests, chest radiograph, bilateral mammography ± ultrasound, estrogen and progesterone receptor determination, FISH for her-2,neu status and S-phase determination. Consider MRI.

Imaging
- Mammography (sensitivity = 50–80% depending on analog versus digital, age, menstrual status, and breast density; positive predictive value = 5–20%)
  - Most common abnormalities: Irregular mass, spiculated density, microcalcifications (35%), or architectural distortion.
- Ultrasound may confirm whether a suspicious lump is solid or cystic and help define its size and extent.

Diagnostic Procedures/Surgery
- Nonpalpable lesions: Core biopsy or open excisional biopsy
- Palpable abnormality: Fine-needle aspiration or core-needle biopsy.

Pathological Findings
- Noninvasive cancers: Intraductal (DCIS) or intralobular (LCIS) (carcinoma in situ)
  - Intraductal cancers: Micropapillary, cribriform, solid, or comedo. The comedo growth pattern is considered more aggressive.
- Invasive cancers
  - Ductal NOS (70%), lobular (5%), Paget disease (2%), inflammatory and miscellaneous (metaplastic, neuroendocrine, or squamous cell carcinomas [1%])
  - Patients with invasive intraductal histologies with medullary (6%), colloid/mucinous (3%), tubular, papillary, and adenoid cystic (2%) subtypes have improved survival.

DIFFERENTIAL DIAGNOSIS
- Benign breast disorders, such as abscesses, hematomas, fibroadenomas, fibrocystic change, ductal or lobular hyperplasia, or sclerosing adenosis
- Malignant breast diseases, including sarcomas, lymphomas, or metastatic disease to breast

TREATMENT

Patients treated by a team consisting of a medical oncologist, a surgeon, and a radiation oncologist

GENERAL MEASURES
- Early breast cancer treatment (stage I/II)
  - Lumpectomy (wide excision with breast conservation), sentinel node biopsy, hormonal therapy, and radiotherapy is the treatment of choice.
  - Combination chemotherapy is also indicated, because most patients have subclinical metastases.
- Treatment of locally advanced breast cancer (stage III)
  - Usually multidisciplinary treatment consisting of mastectomy, axillary dissection, radiation, and chemotherapy ± tamoxifen
- Treatment of advanced or recurrent disease (stage IV)
  - Surgical resection if possible, plus chemotherapy, radiation, hormonal therapy.

Activity
As tolerated.

SPECIAL THERAPY
Radiotherapy

- Postlumpectomy radiation is the mainstay of adjuvant local therapy and has been shown to decrease local recurrence compared to lumpectomy and hormonal therapy alone (1)[A].

- The indications for postmastectomy radiation therapy to the chest wall include patients with ≥4 positive lymph nodes, the presence of extracapsular extension, and tumor stage of T3 or more.

 MEDICATION (DRUGS)

- Combination chemotherapy (most common regimens: CMF, AC or AC + Taxol) reduces the risk of recurrence and improves overall survival in women with tumors >1cm and positive nodes.

  – Chemotherapy, notably AC + Taxol improves overall survival by 16.7% in ER⁻ women compared to 4% in ER⁺ women (2)[B].

- Adjuvant tamoxifen (Nolvadex) (20 mg/d) reduces the risk of recurrence and death for women of all ages by 5–11%, especially in postmenopausal, ER/PR⁺ women.

- An aromatase-inhibitor, anastrazole (Arimidex) (1 mg/d) may be more effective (NNT = 40 recurrent disease) and better tolerated (NNT = 166 endometrial cancer, NNT = 125 DVT) in ER/PR⁺, postmenopausal women with localized disease than tamoxifen, although it does increase risk of musculoskeletal problems (NNH = 30 fracture) compared to tamoxifen (3)[A].

- Trastuzumab (Herceptin) (4 mg/kg loading dose, 2 mg/kg maintenance infusion) improves mortality by 1/3 when combined with chemotherapy for early stage HER-2,neu + breast cancer (4)[A].

- Contraindications: Strict hematologic, renal, hepatic, and cardiac guidelines must be followed for the administration of cytotoxic chemotherapy. Arimidex should not be given to pregnant women.

- Adverse events: See manufacturer' literature. Herceptin associated with CHF.

- Precautions: Monitor for infections and infusion reactions in chemotherapy patients. See "Complications" section for discussion of tamoxifen.

- Significant possible interactions: Drug interactions are common and depend on combinations used. Refer to manufacturer's literature.

First Line
All drugs mentioned above may be used as first-line treatments.

SURGERY

Breast-conserving surgery is appropriate for most breast cancers, because no difference in long-term survival is noted when comparing mastectomy to breast conservation (5)[A]. Axillary node dissection is indicated with all invasive tumors and large noninvasive ones. Identification and biopsy of sentinel nodes may be preferred over axillary dissection because of its lower morbidity rate, but is only appropriate for patients with early-stage breast cancer with clinically negative axillary nodes.

 FOLLOW-UP

PROGNOSIS
- 5-year survival
  – Stage 0 (noninvasive): 100%
  – Stage I (2 cm, no spread): 98%
  – Stage II (>2 cm, or spread to axillary lymph nodes): 76–88%
  – Stage III (>5 cm or fixed nodes, metastatic disease to the skin, inflammatory changes, chest wall extension, or supraclavicular lymph nodes): 49–56%
  – Stage IV (distant metastatic disease): 16%
- The status of the axillary lymph nodes is the most important indicator for disease relapse.
  – If any axillary nodes are positive, 60–70% risk of relapse within 5 years.
  – If all axillary nodes are negative, 70–80% chance of a long-term cure

COMPLICATIONS
- Postoperative: Lymphedema (<5% in modified radical mastectomy), seroma, wound infection, and limited shoulder motion
- Chemotherapy: Nausea, vomiting, alopecia, leukopenia, bladder irritation, stomatitis, fatigue, and menstrual abnormalities
- Tamoxifen: Hot flushes, menstrual irregularities including menopause, vaginal discharge, hypercalcemia, skin rashes, endometrial carcinoma, DVTs, CVAs and interactions with warfarin, erythromycin, cyclosporin, nifedipine, and diltiazem.
- Irradiation: Skin reaction, fatigue, fibrosis (1%), brachial plexopathy (1%), rib fracture (1%), arm edema, pulmonary fibrosis (1%), and rarely 2nd breast malignancy

PATIENT MONITORING
- Up to 60% of patients with invasive disease will relapse within 5 years despite initial therapy.
  – Diagnosis of relapse does not impact survival.
- Surveillance for recurrent disease should include physical examination every 4–6 months for 5 years, then yearly. Mammography and routine chemistries should be done annually. Women on tamoxifen should have annual pelvic exams.
- The workup of a suspected recurrence should include CBC, liver function tests, chest radiograph, bone scan, a CT of the affected area, mammogram, and/or a biopsy.

REFERENCES

1. Fisher B, Anderson S, Bryant J, et al. Twenty-year follow-up of a randomized trial comparing total mastectomy, lumpectomy, and lumpectomy plus irradiation for the treatment of invasive breast cancer. *NEJM* 2002;347:1233–1241.
2. Berry D, Cirrincione C, Henderson C, et al. Estrogen receptor status and outcomes of modern chemotherapy for patients with node positive breast cancer. *JAMA* 2006;295:1658–1667.
3. Howell A, Cuzick J, Baum M, et al. Results of the ATAC (Arimidex, Tamoxifen, Alone or in Combination) trial after completion of 5 years' adjuvant treatment for breast cancer. *Lancet* 2005;365(9453):60–62.
4. Romond E, Perez E, Bryant J, et al. Trastuzumab plus adjuvant chemotherapy for operable her-2 positive breast cancer. *NEJM* 2005;353:1673–1684.
5. Veronesi U, Cascinelli N, Mariani L, et al. Twenty-year follow-up of a randomized study comparing breast-conserving surgery with radical mastectomy for early breast cancer. *NEJM* 2002;347:1227–1232.

 **MISCELLANEOUS**

CODES

ICD9-CM
- 174.9 Malignant neoplasm of female breast, unspecified
- 175.9 Malignant neoplasm of male breast, other and unspecified sites

PATIENT TEACHING

Patients should be reminded of the importance of regular mammography +/− BSE in the early detection of breast cancer.

 See Corresponding Diagnostic Algorithm

 See Patient Handout on CD

BREAST-FEEDING

Kathy Mariani, MD

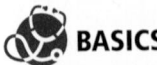 **BASICS**

DESCRIPTION

Breast-feeding is the natural process of feeding an infant human milk. Nursing an infant directly at the breast is usually done, but in many circumstances the milk may be expressed by hand or a pump to be fed to the infant at another time.

- Maternal benefits include
  - Easier postpartum weight loss
  - Decreased postpartum bleeding due to oxytocin release
  - Increased bonding
  - Convenience of feeding
  - Delayed postpartum fertility
  - Increased sense of well being (endorphin response)
  - More rapid and complete reversion of mother's pelvis and uterus to prepuerperal state
  - Decreased risk of breast cancer
  - Possible decreased risk of osteoporosis
  - Economical
- Infant benefits include
  - Maternal antibody protection
  - Decreased incidence of otitis media
  - Decreased upper respiratory infection and sepsis
  - Fewer respiratory and gastrointestinal infections
  - Decreased incidence of obesity
    - Ideal food—easily digestible, nutrients well absorbed, less constipation
  - Increased attachment between mother and baby
  - Decreased incidence of allergies in childhood
- Contraindications
  - HIV infection
  - Active tuberculosis
  - Hepatitis is not a contraindication.
  - Substances of abuse will pass into human milk; see reference on drugs in lactation
- Physiology
  - Stimulation of areola causes secretion of oxytocin.
  - Oxytocin is responsible for let-down reflex when milk is ejected from cells into milk ducts.
  - Sucking stimulates secretion of prolactin, which triggers milk production. Thus milk is made in response to nursing and increases supply.

- Technique
  - Initiate immediately after birth
  - Get in comfortable position, usually sitting or reclining with baby's head in crook of mother's arm (side-lying position often useful following cesarean-section delivery)
  - Bring baby to mother to decrease stress on back.
  - Baby's belly and mother's belly should face each other or touch (belly to belly).
  - Initiate the rooting reflex by tickling baby's lips with nipple or finger. As baby's mouth opens wide, mother guides her nipple to back of her baby's mouth while pulling the baby closer. This will ensure that the baby's gums are sucking on the areola, not the nipple.
  - Feed every 2–4 hours, 20 minutes per side
- System(s) Affected: Endocrine/Metabolic; Skin/Exocrine

EPIDEMIOLOGY

- Predominant age: 16–45 years
- Predominant sex: Female only

Incidence

According to Healthy People 2010, in 2002, 70% of new mothers initiated breast-feeding, and 29% were doing at least some breast-feeding at 6 months of age. The national goal is 75–50%, respectively

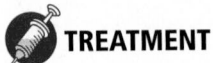 **TREATMENT**

INITIAL STABILIZATION
Outpatient

GENERAL MEASURES
See "Patient Teaching."

Diet

- Adequate calorie and protein intake while nursing.
- Drinking cow's milk is not necessary.
- Drink plenty of fluids (8–12 oz. glasses/day).
- Continue prenatal vitamins.
- Fluoride supplement unnecessary
- New National Academy of Science guidelines recommend that children get at least 200 IU/d of vitamin D beginning in the newborn period to prevent rickets. For exclusively breast-fed babies, this will require taking a vitamin supplement such as PolyViSol or Vi-Daylin vitamin drops, 1/2 cc/d.

Activity
No restrictions

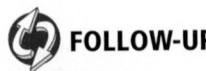 **FOLLOW-UP**

PROGNOSIS
Healthy baby

COMPLICATIONS

- Plugged ducts (mother is well except for) sore lump in 1 or both breasts without fever
  - Use moist hot packs on lump prior to and during nursing; more frequent nursing on affected side; ensure good technique
- Mastitis
  - Sore lump in 1 or both breasts plus fever and/or redness on skin overlying lump
  - Use moist hot packs on lump prior to and during nursing; more frequent nursing on affected side; antibiotics covering for *Staphylococcus aureus* (the most common organism) for at least 7 days
  - Patients can be quite ill with mastitis.
  - Other possible sources of fever should be ruled out—endometritis, pyelonephritis in particular. Mother should get increased rest, use acetaminophen (Tylenol) as necessary. Fever should resolve within 48 hours or consider changing antibiotics. Lump should also resolve. If it continues, an abscess may be present, requiring surgical drainage.
- Milk supply inadequate
  - Check weight gain
  - Review signs of adequate supply; review technique, frequency, and duration of nursing.
  - Check to see if mother has been supplementing, thereby decreasing her own milk production.
- Sore nipples
  - Check technique
  - Baby should be taken off the breast by breaking the suction with a finger in the mouth.
  - Air-dry nipples after each nursing; no breast creams and do not wash nipples with soap and water; check for signs of thrush in baby and mother
- Engorgement
  - Usually develops after milk 1st comes in (day 3 or 4)
  - Signs are warm, hard, sore breasts.
  - To resolve, offer baby more frequent nursing; may have to hand express a little milk to soften areola enough to let baby latch on; nurse long enough to empty breasts; generally resolves within a day or 2.
- Flat or inverted nipples
  - When stimulated, inverted nipples will retract inward, flat nipples remain flat; should check for this on initial prenatal physical
  - Nipple shells, a doughnut-shaped insert, can be worn inside the bra during the last month of pregnancy to gently force the nipple through the center opening of the shell.
  - Babies can nurse successfully even if the shell does not correct the problem before birth. A lactation consultant or La Leche League member may be a good resource in this situation. Another source: *J Human Lactation*. 1993;9:27–29.

PATIENT MONITORING
See mother and baby within a few days of hospital discharge if she is a 1st-time breast-feeder.

REFERENCES

1. Berlin CM, Briggs GG. Drugs and chemicals in human milk. *Semin Fetal Neonatal Med*. 2005; 10(2):149–159.

2. Meek J, ed. *New Mother's Guide to Breastfeeding*. American Academy of Pediatrics. 2002

3. Moreland J, Coombs J. Promoting and supporting breast-feeding. *Amer Fam Physician*. 2000; 61:2093–2100, 2103–2104.

4. Sinusas K, Gagliardi A. Initial management of breast-feeding. *Amer Fam Physician*. 2001; 15;64:981–988.

PATIENT TEACHING

- Antepartum
  - Regular promotion of advantages of breast-feeding
  - Discuss woman's postpartum plans (i.e., if going to work). Emphasize possibility of nursing part-time after returning to work or nursing until weaning the week before returning to work.
  - Emphasize importance of only breast-feeding for 1st 3 weeks of life to allow adequate buildup of sufficient milk supply. Substitution of a bottle feed can occur after this time and still allow for continued nursing.
  - Counsel women on technique.
- Natural history
  - Colostrum present in breast at birth but may not be seen
  - Milk will not come in before 3rd day postpartum.
  - Frequent nursing (at least 9 times or more per 24 hours) will lead to milk coming in sooner and in greater quantities.
  - Allow baby to determine duration of each nursing; baby will lose weight the 1st few days and may not get back to birth weight until day 10.

- Postpartum
  - Immediate breast-feeding after the birth
  - Rooming-in to encourage on-demand feeding
  - Observation of a nursing session by experienced physician, nurse, or lactation consultant
  - Avoid formula or water supplementation.
  - Review expectations, techniques. Be very encouraging.
  - See in office within a few days of discharge, especially if 1st-time nursing
- Signs of adequate nursing
  - Breasts become hard before and soft after feeding.
  - 6 or more wet diapers in 24 hours.
  - Baby satisfied; appropriate weight gain (average 1 oz/d in 1st few months)
  - Growth spurts—anticipate these around 10 days, 6 weeks, 3 months, and 4–6 months. Baby will nurse more often at these times for several days. This will increase milk production to allow for further adequate growth.
  - Supplemental baby vitamins are unnecessary unless the baby has very limited exposure to sun (then needs vitamin D).
- Weaning
  - Breast milk alone is adequate food for 1st 6 months
  - Solids may be introduced at 4–6 months
  - For mothers going to work, start switching the baby to bottle feeding during the hours mother will be gone about a week ahead of time. Do this by dropping a breast-feed every few days and substituting pumped breast milk or formula, preferably given by another caregiver.
  - To increase the likelihood that baby will take a bottle occasionally, introduce it at 3–4 weeks and give once or twice a week.

- Family planning
  - Frequent nursing increases the duration of postpartum amenorrhea; however, breast-feeding is not a completely reliable form of contraception.
  - Options include barrier methods, implants, Depo-Provera, oral contraception, intrauterine devices, and the lactational amenorrhea method.
  - There is some disagreement on estrogen's effect on milk supply, so some providers use progesterone-only birth control pills in the early postpartum period.

BREECH BIRTH

Kimberle Vore, MD

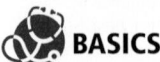 **BASICS**

DESCRIPTION
- At the time of delivery, the fetal buttocks are the presenting part in the maternal pelvis
  - Frank breech presentation: The fetal hips are flexed and the knees are extended with the feet near the shoulders; accounts for 60–65% of breech presentations at term.
  - Incomplete breech presentation: 1 or both of the fetal hips are incompletely flexed, resulting in some part of the fetal lower extremity as the presenting part. Thus the terms single footling, double footling, knee presentation. Accounts for 25–35% of breech presentations.
  - Complete breech: Similar to frank breech except that knees are flexed rather than extended. Accounts for 5% of breech presentations.
- System(s) Affected: Reproductive

Pregnancy Considerations
A problem of pregnancy

GENERAL PREVENTION
- External cephalic version
  - Conversion of breech to vertex can be attempted after 36 weeks of gestation and if successful allows for vaginal vertex delivery. Success rates 48–78%, with reversion rates back to breech of 2%.
  - External cephalic version associated with risk (1–2%) of umbilical cord entanglement, abruptio placenta, preterm labor, premature rupture of membranes, fetal brachycardia, fetal-maternal hemorrhage, and severe maternal discomfort
  - Prior to procedure, tocolytics are usually administered and RhoGAM is given to Rh-negative mothers.
  - External cephalic version should only be attempted with continuous fetal heart monitoring in the delivery suite, where immediate cesarean delivery can be done
  - External cephalic version requires 2 operators, 1 to monitor fetal cardiac activity via ultrasound and holding fetal position, while the 2nd person lifts the buttocks out of the pelvis by abdominal manipulation and then guides the fetal head into the pelvis.
  - Contraindications to external cephalic version include multiple pregnancy, nonreassuring fetal monitoring, placenta previa, premature rupture of membranes, abruption, previous uterine surgery, uterine malformation, oligohydramnios, maternal cardiac disease, or major fetal anomalies.
  - Successful external cephalic version factors include multiparity, relaxed abdominal wall, adequate amniotic fluid, nonfrank breech, floating presenting part, posterior placenta, and average maternal body weight.
  - Failure of external cephalic version associated with maternal obesity, nulliparity, anteriorly located placenta, large fetus, decreased amniotic fluid, frank breech that is engaged in pelvis
- Prevention of fetal anomalies by tight glucose control in diabetics
- Antenatal folate therapy to decrease risk of neural tube detects

EPIDEMIOLOGY
Predominant sex: Female only (affects only women in terms of pregnancy, but affects both sexes of fetuses)

Prevalence
- 3–4% of singleton-term deliveries and up to 15–30% of low-birth-weight infants (<2,500 g)
- Breech presentation is common in early pregnancy. At 25–26 weeks, ~20–30% of singleton fetuses are in breech position, but this decreases near term.

RISK FACTORS
- Fetal anomalies including anencephaly, hydrocephalus, trisomy 21 and 21, fetal alcohol syndrome, Potter syndrome, myotomic dystrophy
- Uterine anomalies including bicornate uterus
- Uterine relaxation associated with great parity
- Uterine overdistension as in polyhydramnios or multiple gestation
- Placenta previa
- Placental implantation in cornual-fundal region
- Low-birth-weight or premature infant
- Macrosomia
- Pelvic contractions or irregularly shaped pelvis—such as android or platypelloid pelvis
- Pelvic tumors
- Nulliparity
- Previous history of breech birth

Genetics
Fetal anomalies including anencephaly, hydrocephalus, and trisomy 21 and 18 have higher incidences of breech birth.

ETIOLOGY
Probably a combination of 1 or more of the risk factors listed above

ASSOCIATED CONDITIONS
- See "Risk Factors"
- Congenital hip dislocation is more common in 1st-born (breech) females.

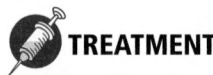 **DIAGNOSIS**

SIGNS AND SYMPTOMS
- Anus palpable on digital vaginal exam
- Leopold maneuver reveals ballottable head in fundal region
- Mother reports kicking in lower abdomen
- Presenting part not palpable in pelvis near term

TESTS
Imaging
- Ultrasound—confirms presenting part
- Radiograph—flat plate of abdomen and pelvimetry to determine extent of head flexion and pelvic measurements (rarely done)

Diagnostic Procedures/Surgery
- Near-term women should be examined to determine presenting part.
- If breech is suspected, an ultrasound should be done to confirm presenting part.
- When breech presentation is confirmed, the option for external version or elective cesarean section should be discussed with the patient.

Pathological Findings
- Congenital malformation among term breech infants: Overall incidence 6–9%
- There is a higher incidence of congenital hip dislocation in infants with breech presentation at term.

DIFFERENTIAL DIAGNOSIS
- In labor, diagnosis is made by vaginal exam and confirmed by ultrasound. Can be confused with face presentation on digital vaginal exam
- In breech presentation, greater trochanter and anus form a straight line. In face presentation, mouth and malar bones form a triangle.

💉 **TREATMENT**

Inpatient for labor and delivery

GENERAL MEASURES
- Continuous electronic fetal monitoring during labor
- Breech presentation may be converted by external version (see "General Prevention"), but this is not always successful and has risks.
- Currently, the American College of Obstetricians and Gynecologists (ACOG) recommends external version at term and planned cesarean delivery for persistent breech presentation. This recommendation is based on a large randomized clinical trial showing decreased perinatal and neonatal morbidity and mortality in planned breech cesarean delivery (1) [NNT 30] vs planned breech vaginal delivery. There was no difference in maternal morbidity or mortality. (1)[B]

Diet
NPO until delivery accomplished

Activity
Bed rest during labor

SURGERY
- Breech delivery is accomplished either vaginally or by cesarean section
- Most physicians and patients opt for elective cesarean delivery for breech presentation near term, which is usually planned for the 39th week of pregnancy.
- When a patient presents in labor with the fetus in breech position, a decision about a trial of labor or immediate cesarean section must be made. Preferably this decision is made prior to onset of labor.
- Obtain ultrasound to document fetal presentation, check for fetal abnormalities, and estimate fetal weight in deciding candidacy for vaginal delivery.
- The selection for vaginal breech delivery could include
  - Breech presentation in advanced labor
  - Delivery of a 2nd twin in nonvertex presentation
  - Fetus too immature to survive
  - Fetus with congenital defects incompatible with life

- Cesarean section procedure
  - Prepare for cesarean section by starting IV fluids and obtaining blood type and screen, in all patients, in case needed for emergency.
  - A low transverse cesarean section may need to be extended vertically if there is difficulty with head entrapment (this extension produces a weak scar).
  - General anesthesia with isoflurane can rapidly relax the uterus and allow delivery of an entrapped after-coming head.
  - Delivery is usually accomplished with spinal anesthesia.
  - Cord blood gases should be obtained following delivery.
- Vaginal delivery procedures
  - Currently not recommended, but may be an option in limited circumstances (see above)
  - The candidate for vaginal delivery needs to be attended by a birth attendant skilled in breech delivery, a scrubbed assistant, an anesthesiologist capable of rapid induction of general anesthesia, and an individual skilled in neonatal resuscitation.
  - Epidural is preferred anesthesia
  - Leave membranes intact as long as possible, to prevent possible cord prolapse
  - The patient should not push until fully dilated, due to risk of partial delivery through a cervix that is not fully dilated, which can lead to head entrapment.
  - Consider cutting a large episiotomy to allow sufficient room for delivery.
  - Use abdominal guidance of fetal head to keep it flexed as it descends into the pelvis.
  - The infant should not be touched before the umbilicus crosses the maternal perineum. Traction prior to this point constitutes a complete breech extraction and is associated with higher risk of perinatal morbidity and mortality.
  - With the fetal back anterior, maintain downward traction while grasping the fetal hips until the scapula becomes visible.
  - Check for nuchal arm.
  - As one axilla becomes visible, rotate the infant until the shoulders are oriented anteriorly and posteriorly, allowing their delivery.
  - The fetal head is delivered in a face-down position with either piper forceps or manual flexion of the head.
  - Cord blood gases should be obtained following delivery.

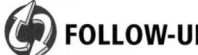 **FOLLOW-UP**

PROGNOSIS

- Perinatal morbidity and mortality are much higher in breech births. A large proportion of the deaths are related to congenital abnormalities.
- Successful external cephalic version at term significantly lowers cesarean rate. (2)[A]
- For infants 750–1500 g or <32 weeks gestational age, there is a much higher rate of cerebral hemorrhage and perinatal death associated with vaginal compared to cesarean delivery.

COMPLICATIONS

- Trauma to the head, soft tissue, brachial plexus, and spinal cord—not always prevented by cesarean
- Asphyxia secondary to cord compression or prolapse
- Congenital hip dislocation

PATIENT MONITORING

- Continuous fetal heart rate monitoring should be done during labor and delivery.
- 6-weeks postpartum care as for other deliveries

REFERENCES

1. Term Breech Trial. *Lancet*. 2000;356(9239):1375
2. External Cephalic Version. ACOG practice bulletin. Num. 13, February. 2000.
3. Committee on Obstetric Practice. ACOG committee opinion. Mode of term singleton breech delivery. Number 265, December 2001. American College of Obstetricians and Gynecologists. *Int J Gynaecol Obstet*. 2002;77:65–66.
4. Scorza W. Intrapartum management of breech presentation. *Clin Perinatol*. 1996;23:31–49.

 MISCELLANEOUS

- Other notes: Maneuvers of cesarean breech delivery are similar to vaginal breech extraction and can be associated with severe trauma to the infant.
- See also: Placenta Previa; Premature Labor

CODES

ICD9-CM

- 652.20 Breech presentation without mention of version, unspecified
- 763.0 Breech delivery and extraction
- 763.4 Cesarean delivery

PATIENT TEACHING

- Educate patient about increased risk of fetal distress and fetal trauma in both cesarean and vaginal breech delivery compared to vaginal vertex delivery.
- Vaginal breech delivery is associated with increased risk of prolapsed cord and/or cord compression; fetal hypoxia; nuchal arm, with attendant risk of trauma including humerus fracture, clavicle fracture, and nerve palsies; and entrapment of fetal head.
- External version may allow for vaginal vertex delivery with decreased risk of infant and maternal morbidity (see "General Prevention").
- When planned elective cesarean breech delivery is the chosen mode of delivery, the patient should be instructed to go to the hospital at the 1st signs of labor, if she goes into labor prior to scheduled cesarean section, which is usually scheduled at 39–40 weeks gestation.
- Risks of cesarean delivery including infection, bleeding, and possible damage to maternal bladder or bowel. Slightly increased risk of maternal morbidity and mortality compared to vaginal vertex delivery.

BRONCHIECTASIS

Dylan C. Kwait, MD

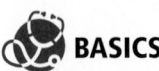 **BASICS**

DESCRIPTION

Irreversible dilatation of 1 or more airways accompanied by recurrent bronchial infection/inflammation and chronic mucopurulent sputum production; generally classified into cystic fibrosis (CF) and non-cystic fibrosis (non-CF) bronchiectasis.

ALERT

Geriatric Considerations

Elderly are more likely to need hospitalization for treatment.

Pediatric Considerations

Associated with childhood respiratory infections, CF, and other congenital conditions.

GENERAL PREVENTION

- Immunize against
  - Pertussis, measles, *Haemophilus influenza* type B (in childhood)
  - Viral illnesses (influenza)
  - Pneumococcal pneumonia
- Genetic counseling in cases in which a congenital condition may increase the likelihood of developing bronchiectasis
- Adequate treatment of all pneumonias

EPIDEMIOLOGY

- Still a significant cause of respiratory morbidity
- Predominant age: Most commonly presents in 6th decade of life (1)[A]
- Predominant sex: Female > Male (1)[A]

Incidence

Incidence has decreased in the US secondary to widespread childhood vaccination against pertussis (2)[A] and the effective treatment of childhood respiratory infections with antibiotics (1)[A].

Prevalence

- Prevalence in the adult US population estimated to be at least 110,000 (1)[A].
- Prevalence is 5 to 10 times higher in those >55 years of age (3)[B]

RISK FACTORS

- Severe respiratory infection in childhood (measles, adenovirus, influenza, pertussis, or bronchiolitis)
- Predisposing congenital condition
- Systemic diseases (e.g., rheumatoid arthritis and connective tissue disorders)
- Chronic rhinosinusitis
- Recurrent pneumonia
- Aspirated foreign body
- Immunodeficiency

PATHOPHYSIOLOGY

"Vicious cycle hypothesis": Transmural infection, generally by bacterial organisms, causes inflammation and obstruction of airways. Damaged airways and dysfunctional cilia foster bacterial colonization, which leads to further inflammation and obstruction (2)[A].

ETIOLOGY

- CF bronchiectasis
- Non-CF bronchiectasis
  - Most cases are idiopathic (4)[B].
  - The etiologic agent most commonly associated with non-CF bronchiectasis is childhood respiratory infection (2)[A].
  - May be associated with many conditions.

ASSOCIATED CONDITIONS

- Mucociliary clearance defects
  - Primary ciliary dyskinesia
  - Young syndrome (secondary ciliary dyskinesia)
  - Kartagener syndrome
- Other congenital conditions
  - α_1-Antitrypsin deficiency
  - Marfan syndrome
  - Cartilage deficiency (Williams-Campbell syndrome)
- Chronic obstructive pulmonary disease
- Postinfectious conditions
  - Bacteria (*H. influenzae* and *Pseudomonas aeruginosa*)
  - Mycobacterial infections (TB and MAC)
  - Whooping cough
  - Aspergillus species
  - Viral (HIV, adenovirus, measles, influenza virus)
- Immunodeficient conditions
  - Primary
    - Hypogammaglobulinemia
  - Secondary
    - Allergic bronchopulmonary aspergillosis
    - Post-transplantation
- Sequelae of toxic inhalation or aspiration (e.g., chlorine, luminal foreign body)
- Rheumatic/chronic inflammatory conditions:
  - Rheumatoid arthritis
  - Sjögren syndrome
  - Systemic lupus erythematosus
  - Inflammatory bowel disease
- Miscellaneous
  - Yellow nail syndrome

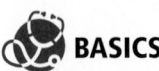 **DIAGNOSIS**

SIGNS AND SYMPTOMS

Symptoms are commonly present for many years and include

- Chronic cough (90%) (1)[A]
- Sputum: copious and purulent (90%) (1)[A]
- Rhinosinusitis (60–70%) (1)[A]
- Fatigue, may be a dominant symptom (70%) (1)[A]
- Dyspnea (75%) (2)[A]
- Chest pain, may be pleuritic (20–30%)(1)[A]
- Hemoptysis (20–30%) (1)[A]
- Wheezing (20%)(1)[A]

History

It is vital to elicit

- Time course of illness
- Any predisposing factors (either congenital, infectious, and/or exposure-related)
- Immunization history

Physical Exam

- Bi-basal crackles (60%) (1)[A]
- Wheezing (34%) (2)[A]
- Rhonchi (44%) (2)[A]
- Digital clubbing (3%) (2)[A]

TESTS

- Spirometry
  - Limited use in diagnosis
  - Characterized by moderate airflow obstruction and hyperresponsive airways (1)[A]
  - FEV1<80% predicted and FEV1/FVC <0.7 (3)[B]
- Special tests
  - Ciliary biopsy by electron microscopy

Lab

- Sputum culture
  - *H. influenzae*, nontypeable form (42%) (1)[A]
  - *P. aeruginosa* (18%) (1)[A]
  - Cultures may also be positive for *Streptococcus pneumoniae*, *Moraxella catarrhalis*, MAC, and *Aspergillus* (1)[A]
  - 30–40% of all isolates will show no growth (1)[A]
- Special tests
  - Sweat test for CF
  - PPD test for TB
  - Skin test for *Aspergillus*
  - HIV test
  - Serum immunoglobulins to test for humoral immunodeficiency

Imaging

- CT scan

  - Noncontrast high-resolution CT (HRCT) is the most important tool used to diagnose bronchiectasis (2)[A].
  - Bronchi are dilated and do not taper; varicose constrictions and ballooned cysts may also be appreciated (2)[A].

- Chest radiograph

  - Nonspecific findings; sensitivity and specificity are too low to confirm the diagnosis (3)[B]
  - Increased lung markings (1)[A]
  - May be normal

Diagnostic Procedures/Surgery

Interventional bronchoscopy

- Used to obtain culture and evacuate sputum

Pathological Findings

- Dilatation of airways (2)[A]
- Thickened bronchial walls with necrosis of bronchial mucosa (2)[A]
- Peribronchial scarring (2)[A]

DIFFERENTIAL DIAGNOSIS

- Chronic obstructive pulmonary disease
- Asthma
- CF
- Chronic bronchitis
- Pulmonary tuberculosis
- Allergic bronchopulmonary aspergillosis

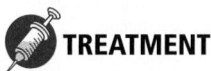 TREATMENT

Treatment of non-CF bronchiectasis involves determining the cause of exacerbations, promoting good bronchopulmonary hygiene through daily airway clearance, and surgical resection of damaged lung when necessary.

INITIAL STABILIZATION

Hemoptysis, although rare, may occur and can be life threatening. Appropriate measures must be taken to minimize blood loss.

GENERAL MEASURES

- Dry powder mannitol improves tracheobronchial clearance (1)[A]
- Maintain hydration (nebulized saline may be used) (2)[A]
- Noninvasive positive-pressure ventilation (2)[A]

Diet

No dietary restrictions

Activity

Regular exercise is recommended.

Physical Therapy

Sputum clearance techniques

- Physiotherapy (percussion and postural drainage)
- Pulmonary rehabilitation (improves exercise tolerance, but does not benefit from Inspiratory muscle training) (1)[A]

 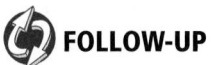 MEDICATION (DRUGS)

First Line

- Antibiotics

  - May be used in acute exacerbations

  - Chronic therapy decreases sputum volume and purulence, but does not diminish the frequency of exacerbations (5)[A].
  - Patients may require twice the usual dose and should receive long courses of treatment (7–14 days) (3)[B].

  - Selection is complicated by the wide range of pathogens involved and the existence of resistant organisms (culture should be used to direct therapy).

  - Augmentin (3)[B]: 500 mg PO q8–12h for 7–10 days (pediatric: Base dosing protocol on amoxicillin content)
  - Trimethoprim–sulfamethoxazole (3)[B]: 160 mg TMP/800 mg SMZ PO q12h for 10–14 days (pediatric: ≥2 months, 8 mg/kg TMP and 40 mg/kg SMZ PO per 24 hours, administered in 2 divided doses q12h for 10 days)
  - Doxycycline and cefaclor given orally are also effective (3)[B].
  - Nebulized aminoglycosides (tobramycin): 300 mg by aerosol b.i.d. (6)[B]
  - Macrolides appear to have immunomodulatory benefits (1)[A].

  - Antibiotics should be administered IV in cases of severe infection.

- Bronchodilators

  - Chronic use of β-2 agonists (e.g., albuterol) effectively reverses airflow obstruction (1)[A].

- Inhaled corticosteroids

  - Decrease sputum and tend to improve lung function (3)[B]

  - Fluticasone: 110–220 mcg inhaled b.i.d.
- Contraindications: Documented hypersensitivity
- Precautions: Cross-allergy and organ impairment
- Significant possible interactions: Broad-spectrum antibiotics may reduce efficacy of oral contraceptives

Second Line

Other broad-spectrum antimicrobials including antipseudomonals.

SURGERY

Surgery should be considered in cases in which disease is localized and symptoms remain intolerable despite medical therapy. Surgery effectively improves symptoms in 80% of these cases (1)[A].

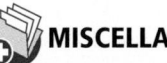 FOLLOW-UP

PROGNOSIS

- Mortality rate is 13% (death due directly to bronchiectasis) (1)[A].
- *Pseudomonas* infection is associated with poorer prognosis (1)[A].

COMPLICATIONS

- Hemoptysis
- Recurrent pulmonary infections
- Pulmonary hypertension
- Cor pulmonale
- Lung abscess

PATIENT MONITORING

- Serial spirometry, performed every 2–5 years, should be used to monitor the course of the disease (1)[A].
- Routine microbiological sputum analysis (1)[A].
- Annual influenza and pneumococcal immunizations (3)[B].

REFERENCES

1. King P, Holdsworth S, Freezer N, Holmes P. Bronchiectasis. *Intern Med J.* 2006;36(11):729.
2. Barker AF. Bronchiectasis. *N Engl J Med.* 2002;346:1383–1393.
3. Bradley J, Lavery K, Rendall J, Elborn JS. Managing bronchiectasis. *Practitioner.* 2006;250(1681):194.
4. Pasteur MC, Helliwell SM, Houghton SJ, et al. An investigation into the causative factors in patients with bronchiectasis. *Am J Respir Crit Care Med.* 2000;162:1277–1284.
5. Evans DJ, Bara AI, Greenstone M. Prolonged antibiotics for purulent bronchiectasis. *Cochrane Database of Sys Rev.* 2006;(4):CD00284.
6. Lobue PA. Inhaled tobramycin: Not just for cystic fibrosis anymore? *Chest.* 2005;127:1098.

 MISCELLANEOUS

See also: Cystic fibrosis; Chronic obstructive pulmonary disease; Asthma; Pulmonary tuberculosis; Aspergillosis; Kartagener syndrome

CODES

ICD9-CM

- 494.0 Bronchiectasis without acute exacerbation
- 494.1 Bronchiectasis with acute exacerbation

PATIENT TEACHING

Printed patient information available from www.lungusa.org or the American Lung Association, 1740 Broadway, New York, NY 10019; (212) 315-8700.

See Corresponding Diagnostic Algorithm

BRONCHIOLITIS

Dennis E. Hughes, DO

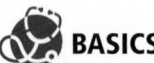 **BASICS**

DESCRIPTION
- Inflammation and obstruction of small airways and reactive airways. May be seasonal (winter and spring) and often occurs in epidemics
- Usual course: Insidious; acute; progressive

ALERT
Pediatric Considerations
Most common in infants

GENERAL PREVENTION
- Hand washing
- Contact isolation of infected babies
- Persons with colds should keep contacts with infants to a minimum
- Palivizumab (Synagis), a monoclonal product, administered monthly, October–May, 15 mg/kg IM; used for respiratory syncytial virus prevention in high-risk patients
  - 28–32 week gestation and <6 months old; once begun, continue through end of season regardless of age attained
  - <28 weeks gestation and <12 months old
  - Moderately severe bronchopulmonary dysplasia and up to 2 years old
  - Hemodynamically significant congenital heart disease (until age 6 months)
- Respiratory syncytial virus immune globulin, a human blood product, can also be used in at-risk patients. Monthly infusions of 750 mg/kg, October–May (1).

EPIDEMIOLOGY
- Leading cause of hospitalizations in infants and children.
- Predominant age: Newborn to 2 years (peak age <6 months). Neonates are not protected despite transfer of maternal antibody.
- Predominant sex: Male > Female

Incidence
21% in North America; 3% of children hospitalized with bronchiolitis. Increasing since 1980 (1).

RISK FACTORS
- Smoking
- Low birth weight
- Immunodeficiency
- Formula feeding (not breastfed)
- Contact with infected person
- Children in day care environment
- Heart-lung transplantation patient
- Adults: Exposure to toxic fumes, connective tissue disease

ETIOLOGY
- Respiratory syncytial virus (70%)
- Parainfluenza
- Adenovirus
- Rhinovirus
- Influenza virus
- Chlamydia
- Eye, nose, mouth inoculation
- Necrosis and lysis of epithelial cells and subsequent release of inflammatory mediators. This results in edema, mucus secretion, combined with necrotic debris, and loss of cilia, resulting in luminal obstruction.

ASSOCIATED CONDITIONS
- Common cold
- Conjunctivitis
- Pharyngitis
- Otitis media
- Diarrhea

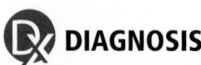 **DIAGNOSIS**

SIGNS AND SYMPTOMS
- Anorexia
- Cough
- Cyanosis
- Apnea
- Fever
- Grunting
- Irritability
- Noisy breathing (due to rhinorrhea)
- Vomiting

Physical Exam
- Tachypnea
- Rhinorrhea
- Wheezing
- Retractions

TESTS
- Arterial O_2 saturation by pulse oximetry (<92% significant)
- Respiratory viral antigens (not usually necessary during RSV season because the disease is managed symptomatically)
- Urine culture is advised as there is a clinically relevant rate of UTI (1).
Sepsis work up not usually necessary if clinical picture is consistent with bronchiolitis

Imaging
Chest radiograph
- Patchy infiltrates
  - Focal atelectasis—right upper lobe common
  - Air trapping
  - Flattened diaphragm
  - Increased anteroposterior diameter
  - Peribronchial cuffing

Pathological Findings
- Abundant mucous exudate
- Mucosal: Hyperemia, edema
- Submucosal lymphocytic infiltrate, monocytic infiltrate, plasmacytic infiltrate
- Small airway debris, fibrin, inflammatory exudate, fibrosis
- Peribronchiolar mononuclear infiltrate

DIFFERENTIAL DIAGNOSIS
- Asthma
- Vascular ring
- Foreign body
- Heart failure
- Bacterial pneumonia
- Gastroesophageal reflux
- Aspiration
- Cystic fibrosis
- Pertussis
- Croup

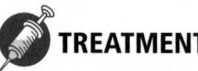 **TREATMENT**

- Most patients can be treated at home.
- Inpatient treatment is indicated for a patient with increased respiratory distress, cyanosis, and dehydration or inability to feed.

GENERAL MEASURES
- Most critical phase is the 1st 48–72 hours after onset. Treatment is usually symptomatic.
- Fluid at maintenance (after correcting for any dehydration); add for respiratory fluid loss.
- Mechanical ventilation in respiratory failure
- Isolation: Contact; hand washing most important
- Cardio-respiratory monitoring

Diet
- Frequent small feedings of clear liquids
- If hospitalized, a patient may require intravenous fluids.

Activity
- Avoid exposure to crowds, viral illness for 2 months
- Avoid smoke

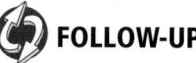

MEDICATION (DRUGS)

First Line
- Oxygen
- Nebulized Albuterol (0.15 mg/kg) may be effective for acute symptoms; a trial of therapy is reasonable. No benefit noted in several high quality studies (1, 2)[B].
- Epinephrine aerosols (0.5 mL of 2.25% solution in 3 mL NS) also may be tried. Caution, because a "rebound phenomena" may occur (child is sent home and worsens: monitor for 2 hours). Benefit remains unproven (3)[B].
- Ribavirin
  - Controversial (cost, unclear efficacy)
  - Inhaled antiviral agent active against respiratory syncytial virus
  - May be indicated in patients with underlying cardiopulmonary disease, young age (<6 weeks), immunosuppressed (AIDS, organ transplant patients), or premature infants
  - Nebulize via small-particle aerosol generator
  - Pregnant women should not be exposed (1).
- Corticosteroids
  - Oral dexamethasone (1mg/kg loading dose, then 0.6 mg/kg b.i.d. for 5 days) reduced subsequent hospitalization (4)[B].
  - Nebulized dexamethasone (2–4 mg in 3 mL NS) may have anecdotal benefit; studies show mixed results (1).

Second Line
- Antibiotics only if secondary bacterial infection present (rare)
- Heliox therapy(70% helium–30% oxygen) maybe of benefit in moderate to severe bronchiolitis (5)[C].

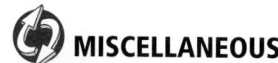

FOLLOW-UP

DISPOSITION
Admission Criteria
- Respiratory rate >70/min with respiratory distress or apnea
- Ill or toxic appearance
- Underlying heart or respiratory condition
- Dehydrated or unable to feed
- Uncertain home care

PROGNOSIS
- In most cases, recovery is complete within 7–14 days.
- Mortality statistics differ, but probably <1%
- High-risk infants (bronchopulmonary dysplasia, congenital heart disease) may have a prolonged course.

COMPLICATIONS
- Bacterial superinfection
- Bronchiolitis obliterans
- Apnea
- Respiratory failure
- Death
- Increased incidence of reactive airway disease

PATIENT MONITORING
- If the patient is receiving home care, follow daily by telephone for 2–4 days; the patient may need frequent office visits.
- For a hospitalized patient, monitor as needed depending on the severity of the infection. Bronchiolitis can be associated with apnea. Hospitalization is usually only required if oxygen is a requirement.

REFERENCES

1. King VJ, et al. Pharmacologic treatment of bronchiolitis in infants and children: A systematic review. *Arch Pediatr Adolesc Med* 2004;158(2): 127–137.
2. Patel H, et al. A randomized, controlled trial of the effectiveness of nebulized therapy with epinephrine compared with albuterol and saline in infants hospitalized for acute viral bronchiolitis. *J Ped* 2002;141(6):818–824.
3. Mull cc, et al. A randomized trial of nebulized epinephrine vs albuterol in the emergency department of bronchiolitis. *Arch Pediatr Adolesc Med* 2004;158(2):113–118.
4. Schuh S, et al. Efficacy of oral dexamethasone in outpatients with acute bronchiolitis. *J Ped* 2002;140(1):27–32.
5. Martinon-Torres F, et al. Heliox therapy in infants with acute bronchiolitis. *Pediatrics* 2002;109(1):68–73.

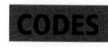

MISCELLANEOUS

CODES

ICD9-CM
466.1 Acute bronchiolitis

PATIENT TEACHING
- American Academy of Pediatrics Website: www.aap.org
- American Academy of Family Physicians Website: www.familydoctor.org

BRONCHIOLITIS OBLITERANS AND ORGANIZING PNEUMONIA

David A. Pope, MD

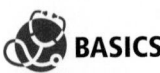 **BASICS**

DESCRIPTION
- A primary or secondary process of the lungs characterized by granulation-like tissue involving the distal airways and alveoli
- A specific reaction of lung tissue to a variety of injuries
- It may occur as patchy infiltrates, or it may be nodular or secondary to another lung disease.
- The process may also appear to be a migrating one.
- It may have a gradual or sudden onset.
- Lungs show a pattern of multiple patchy pneumonia, which are seen on the chest radiograph as patchy alveolar or ground glass opacifications with or without interstitial infiltrates; there may be air bronchograms as well.
- Most cases will respond to corticosteroids, which may have to be given for a year or more
- Synonym(s): Intraluminal fibrosis of distal airways; Idiopathic bronchiolitis obliterans and organizing pneumonitis; Cryptogenic organizing pneumonia; Obliterative bronchiolitis

Geriatric Considerations
More common than originally thought and may be sudden and very severe

Pediatric Considerations
Rare, but has been reported after viral pneumonia (adenovirus influenza):
- Characteristics include delayed recovery, persistent cough, crackles, or wheezing after pneumonia
- Laboratory findings generally not helpful
- Imaging shows: Ventilation-perfusion ratio matched defects; high-resolution CT, bronchiectasis, bronchogram, pruned tree appearance
- Diagnosis confirmed by biopsy
- Treatment includes steroids: 1 mg/kg q24h for 1 month, followed by weaning over several months

GENERAL PREVENTION
Except for prevention of relapse, none known

EPIDEMIOLOGY
- Incidence/prevalence in United States: Unknown
- Predominant age: Reported cases range age 0–70, mean age: 50s

Incidence
Unknown

Prevalence
Unknown

RISK FACTORS
- AIDS
- Immunocompromised patients, including transplant patients
- More likely in smokers

ETIOLOGY
Idiopathic. A complex response to a variety of injuries, such as toxic inhalation; post mycoplasma, viral and bacterial infection; aspiration; immunologic factors; drugs

ASSOCIATED CONDITIONS
- Drug-induced pneumonitis
  - Paraquat poisoning
  - Amiodarone toxicity
  - Acebutolol toxicity
  - Amphotericin B
  - Bleomycin
  - Caramazepine
  - Cephalosporins
  - Gold
  - Minocycline
  - Nitrofurantoin
  - Phenyltoin
  - Sulphamethoxypyridazine
  - Sulphasalazine
  - Ticloppidine
  - Freebase cocaine pulmonary toxicity
  - Overdose of L-tryptophan
- Infections
  - Chronic infectious pneumonia
  - Malaria
  - Chlamydia
  - Legionella
  - Mycoplasma
  - Pneumocystis
  - Cryptococcus
- Immunocompromise: Bone marrow, lung, renal, transplantation
- Connective tissue diseases
  - Rheumatic lung
  - Sjögren syndrome
  - Polymyositis
  - Scleroderma
  - Essential mixed cryoglobulinemia
- Miscellaneous
  - Cystic fibrosis
  - Bronchopulmonary dysplasia
  - Renal failure
  - CHF
  - Adult respiratory distress syndrome
  - Chronic eosinophilic pneumonia
  - Hypersensitivity pneumonitis
  - Histiocytosis X
  - Sarcoidosis
  - Pneumoconioses
  - Radiation pneumonitis

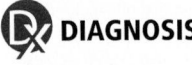 **DIAGNOSIS**

Think of the possibility

SIGNS AND SYMPTOMS
- Most patients present with a flu-like illness that lasts 4–10 weeks or longer. Most have been treated with antibiotics without success.
- Fever
- Dry cough
- Weight loss
- Dyspnea may be severe
- Bilateral crackles
- Fatigue

TESTS
- Leukocytosis with a normal differential
- Elevated erythrocyte sedimentation rate:
- Negative cultures
- Negative serology for mycoplasma, *Coxiella*, *Legionella*, psittacosis, and fungus
- Negative viral studies
  - Pulmonary function shows a restrictive/obstructive pattern.
  - Flow-volume loop shows terminal airway obstruction.
  - Chest radiograph may show patchy alveolar opacities, often in the middle or upper lung area, a ground glass pattern that may have air bronchograms
  - The involved area may seem to migrate.
  - Ventilation-perfusion ratio scan: Matched patchy defects

Imaging
- Chest radiograph: Often appears more normal than the physical examination
- CT scans more accurately define the distribution and extent of the patchy alveolar opacities with areas of hyperlucency.
- Diagnosis is difficult by CT only

Diagnostic Procedures/Surgery
- Open lung biopsy
- Transbronchial biopsy
- It may be wise to use a trial of steroids as a diagnostic trial, although not all would agree.
- If a diagnostic trial is successful, be prepared to treat the patient for at least 1 year.

Pathological Findings
- Intraluminal fibrosis of distal airspaces is the major pathologic feature.
- Fibroblasts and plugs of inflammatory cells and loose connective tissue fill these distal airways.
- Inflammatory cells are mainly lymphocytes and plasma cells.
- Interstitial fibrosis is present.
- Plugs of edematous granulation tissue in the terminal and respiratory bronchioles and alveolar ducts do not cause permanent damage.

DIFFERENTIAL DIAGNOSIS
- Usual interstitial pneumonitis
- Noninfectious diseases
- Tuberculosis
- Sarcoidosis
- Histoplasmosis
- Berylliosis
- Goodpasture syndrome
- Neoplasm
- Polyarteritis nodosa
- Systemic lupus erythematosus
- Wegener granulomatosis
- Sjögren syndrome
- Chronic eosinophilic pneumonia
- Cryptogenic bronchiolitis

TREATMENT

Inpatient may be required

GENERAL MEASURES
• Monitor blood gases or pulse oximetry.
• Oxygen as necessary

Diet
No special diet

Activity
As tolerated

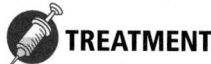 **MEDICATION (DRUGS)**

First Line
Prednisone
• For 1–3 months, 60 mg/d
• Then taper over a few weeks to 20 mg (this dose may later be given as alternate-day therapy). Increase length of taper for patients on long-term therapy to avoid precipitating Addisonian crisis.
• Treatment may be needed for 1 year or more.
• Contraindications: Refer to the manufacturer's literature.
• Precautions: Be aware of the patient's Mantoux status and history of peptic ulcer disease. Long-term steroid treatment is associated with significant adverse effects including Cushing syndrome, fluid retention, osteoporosis, hyperkalemia, and poor wound healing.
• Significant possible interactions: Refer to the manufacturer's literature.

Second Line
• Steroids other than prednisone may be used.
• 1 paper reported the use of erythromycin 600 mg a day for 3–4 months after initial control with prednisone.
• Prescribe antimicrobials, if the original infection is persistent. The proper choice depends on the pathogen.

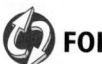 **FOLLOW-UP**

PROGNOSIS
Complete recovery, but individual case management is mandatory

COMPLICATIONS
• Bronchiectasis
• Death, but with proper treatment, recovery is usually complete without permanent sequelae

PATIENT MONITORING
• Frequent visits, weekly at 1st
• Prednisone must be continued because of the chance of relapse
• Monitor the lung disease and the side effects of prednisone therapy (Mantoux, monthly CBC, funduscopic exam every 3–6 months, serial dual energy x-ray absorptiometry (DEXA) scans for osteoporosis)

REFERENCES

1. Cordier JF, Loire R, Brune J. Idiopathic bronchiolitis obliterans organizing pneumonia. *Chest*. 1989; 96:999–1004.
2. Epler GR, Colby TV, et al. Bronchiolitis obliterans organizing pneumonia. *N Engl J Med*. 1985; 312:152–158.
3. Hardy KA, Schidlow D, Zaeri N. Obliterative bronchiolitis in children. *Chest*. 1988;93:460–466.
4. Lynch DA. Imaging of small airways diseases. *Clin Chest Med*. 1993;14:623–634.
5. Mueller NL, Staples CA, Miller RR. Bronchiolitis obliterans organizing pneumonia: CT features in 14 patients. *AJR*. 1990;154:983–987.
6. St John RC, Dorinsky PM. Cryptogenic bronchiolitis. *Clin Chest Med*. 1993;14:667–675.
7. http://www.epler.com/boop1.html
8. http://www.emedicine.com/radio/byname/ bronchiolitis-obliterans-organizing-pneumonia.html

 MISCELLANEOUS

• Other notes: This disease behaves differently than bronchiolitis obliterans. Bronchiolitis obliterans and organizing pneumonia is a restrictive problem; bronchiolitis obliterans is an obstructive problem. Bronchiolitis obliterans causes permanent lung damage; bronchiolitis obliterans and organizing pneumonia is completely reversible.
• See also: Sjögren Syndrome

CODES

ICD9-CM
491.8 Other chronic bronchitis

PATIENT TEACHING

Emphasize the need to continue prednisone because of the chance of a relapse.

BRONCHITIS, ACUTE

Alan J. Cropp, MD, FCCP

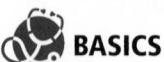 **BASICS**

DESCRIPTION
- Inflammation of trachea, bronchi, and bronchioles resulting from a respiratory tract infection or chemical irritant (1,2)
- Cough is the predominant symptom (3,4)
- Generally self-limited with complete healing and full return of function
- Most infections viral if no underlying cardiopulmonary disease is present
- Synonym(s): Tracheobronchitis

ALERT
Geriatric Considerations
Can be a serious illness in this age group, particularly if part of influenza or with underlying chronic obstructive pulmonary disease (COPD)

Pediatric Considerations
- In this age group, usually occurs in association with other conditions of upper and lower respiratory tract (trachea usually involved)
- Some children seem to be more susceptible than others (if repeated attacks, child should be evaluated for anomalies of the respiratory tract including immune deficiencies or for chronic asthma)
- If acute bronchitis is caused by respiratory syncytial virus, it may be fatal.

GENERAL PREVENTION
- Avoid smoking
- Control underlying risk factors (asthma, sinusitis, and reflux)
- Avoid exposure especially daycare
- Vaccinations, specifically pneumovax, influenza

EPIDEMIOLOGY
- Predominant age: All ages
- Predominant sex: Male = Female

Incidence
~5% of adults per year

Prevalence
Results in 10–12 million office visits per year

RISK FACTORS
- Chronic bronchopulmonary diseases
- Chronic sinusitis
- Bronchopulmonary allergy
- Hypertrophied tonsils and adenoids in children
- Immunosuppression
- Air pollutants
- Elderly
- Infants
- Smoking
- 2nd-hand smoke
- Alcoholism
- Gastroesophageal reflux disease (GERD)
- Tracheostomy
- Environmental changes
- Immunoglobulin deficiency
- HIV

Genetics
No known genetic pattern

PATHOPHYSIOLOGY
Acute bronchitis causes an injury to the epithelial surfaces resulting in an increase in mucous production (2)

ETIOLOGY
- Adenovirus
- Influenza A and B
- Parainfluenza
- *Chlamydia pneumoniae* (TWAR agent)
- *Bordetella pertussis*
- Respiratory syncytial virus
- Coxsackievirus
- Herpes simplex
- *Haemophilus influenzae*
- Possibly fungi
- *Mycoplasma*
- Secondary bacterial infection as part of an acute upper respiratory infection
- *Streptococcus pneumoniae*
- *Moraxella catarrhalis*
- *Mycobacterium tuberculosis*
- Rhinovirus
- Coronavirus (types 1–3)
- Chemical irritants

ASSOCIATED CONDITIONS
- Asthma
- Epiglottitis; rare but can be rapidly fatal
- Coryza
- Pharyngitis
- Croup
- Influenza
- Smoking
- Pneumonia
- Emphysema
- Sinusitis
- Bronchial obstruction
- GERD

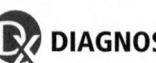 **DIAGNOSIS**

PRE HOSPITAL
Usually treated as outpatient unless comorbidity exists

SIGNS AND SYMPTOMS
- Cough
- Fever
- Fatigue
- Aching (i.e., myalgia)
- Hemoptysis
- Chest burning
- Dyspnea (sometimes)

History
- Preceding respiratory tract infection, such as a common cold with coryza, malaise, chills, slight fever, sore throat, back and muscle pain
- Cough, initially dry and unproductive, then productive; later, mucopurulent sputum, which may indicate secondary infection

Physical Exam
- Rales, rhonchi, wheezing
- No evidence of pulmonary consolidation
- Pharynx injected
- Fever
- Tachypnea

TESTS
- Arterial blood gases: Hypoxemia (rarely)
- Leukocytosis
- Sputum culture/gram stain
- Viral titers
- Mycoplasma titers
- Pulmonary function tests (seldom needed during acute stages): Increased residual volume, decreased maximal expiratory rate (2)

Imaging
Chest radiograph
- Lungs normal if uncomplicated
- Helps rule out other diseases (pneumonia) or complications

Diagnostic Procedures/Surgery
Rarely indicated

DIFFERENTIAL DIAGNOSIS
- Asthma
- Allergy
- Eosinphilic Pneumonitis
- Influenza
- Bronchopneumonia
- Bronchiectasis
- Acute sinusitis
- Aspiration
- Cystic fibrosis
- Reactive airways dysfunction syndrome
- Bacterial tracheitis
- Retained foreign body
- Inhalation injury
- Heart failure
- Bronchogenic carcinoma
- GERD

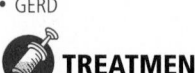 **TREATMENT**

PRE HOSPITAL
Aerosolized bronchodilator may be helpful if patient has bronchospasm

INITIAL STABILIZATION
- Outpatient unless elderly or complicated by severe underlying disease
- May require supplemental oxygen in selected cases

GENERAL MEASURES
- Rest
- Steam inhalations
- Vaporizers
- Antibiotics if complicated by comorbidity (e.g., COPD, severe asthma, etc.) (overused in United States)
- Adequate hydration
- Stop smoking
- Treat associated illnesses (e.g., GERD)
- Antitussives

Diet
Increased fluids (3–4 L/d) while febrile

Activity
Rest until fever subsides.

Nursing
Ensure patient comfort and moniter for signs of deterioration, especially if underlying lung disease exists.

SPECIAL THERAPY
IV Fluids
May be helpful if patient is dehydrated.

Complementary and Alternative Medicine
Throat lozenges for pharyngitis

 ## MEDICATION (DRUGS)

First Line
- Meta-analysis has demonstrated the lack of efficacy of antibiotics in uncomplicated acute bronchitis. (5)[A]
- Amantadine or rimantadine therapy if influenza A suspected; most effective if started within 24–48 hours of development of symptoms (also consider tamiflu or relenza)
- Decongestants if accompanied by sinus condition (1)[B]
- Antipyretic analgesic such as aspirin or ibuprofen
- Antibiotics (Amoxicillin 500 mg q8h or TMP/SMX DS b.i.d) for more severe symptoms (high fever persists, concomitant COPD, purulent discharge)
- Amoxicillin: 500 mg q8h or trimethoprim-sulfamethoxazole DS q12h for routine infection
- Doxycycline: 100 mg/d for 10 days if *Moraxella*, *Chlamydia*, or *Mycoplasma* suspected
- Clarithromycin (Biaxin): 500 mg q12h or azithromycin (Zithromax) Z-pack for PCN or sulfa allergy or mycoplasma infection
- Quinolone for more serious infection or other antibiotic failure or in elderly or multiple comorbidities
- Cough suppressant for troublesome cough (not with COPD); guaifenesin with codeine or dextromethorphan (4)[A]
- Inhaled beta agonist (e.g., albuterol) or in combination with steroids (2)[B]
- Consider steroids for bronchospasm
- Watch for theophylline toxicity with macrolides and quinolones. Macrolides also interfere with oral contraceptives.
- Significant possible interactions: Refer to the manufacturer's literature.

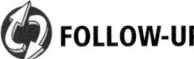 ## FOLLOW-UP

DISPOSITION
Usually a self-limited disease not requiring follow-up

Admission Criteria
Severe exacerbation of underlying disease

Discharge Criteria
Improvement in symptoms

Issues for Referral
Complications such as pneumonia

PROGNOSIS
- Usual: Complete healing with good return of function
- Can be serious in the elderly or debilitated
- Cough may persist for several weeks after an initial improvement (2)
- Postbronchitic reactive airways disease (rare)
- Bronchiolitis obliterans and organizing pneumonia (rare)

COMPLICATIONS
- Bronchopneumonia
- Acute respiratory failure
- Bronchiectasis
- Chronic cough
- Hemoptysis
- Superinfection

PATIENT MONITORING
- Oximetry until no longer hypoxemic
- Recheck for chronicity

REFERENCES

1. Flaherty K, Saint S, Fenfrick AM, Martinez F. The spectrum of acute bronchitis. *Postgrad Med*. 2001;109:39–47.
2. Knutson D, Braun C. Diagnosis and management of acute bronchitis. *Am Fam Physician*. 2002; 65:2039–2044.
3. Snow V, Mottur-Pilson C, Gonzales R. Principles of appropriate antibiotic use for treatment of acute bronchitis in adults. *Ann Intern Med*. 2001; 134:518–20.
4. Gonzales R, Bartlett J, Besser R, et al. Principles of appropriate antibiotic use for treatment of uncomplicated acute bronchitis: Background. *Ann Intern Med*. 2001;134:521–529.
5. MacKay DN: Treatment of acute bronchitis in adults without underlying lung disease. *J Gen Intern Med*. 1996;11(9):557–562.

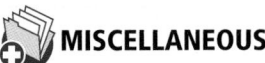 ## MISCELLANEOUS

See also: Asthma; Chronic Obstructive Pulmonary Disease; and Emphysema

 CODES

ICD9-CM
466.0 Acute bronchitis

PATIENT TEACHING
- For patient education materials favorably reviewed on this topic, contact American Lung Association, 1740 Broadway, New York, NY 10019, (212) 315-8700. www.lungusa.org
- American Academy of Family Physicians: www.familydoctor.org

 See Corresponding Diagnostic Algorithm

 See Patient Handout on CD

BRUCELLOSIS

Nancy Snapp, MD, MPH

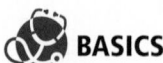 **BASICS**

DESCRIPTION
- Systemic bacterial infection caused by *Brucella* species in infected animal products, or vaccine
- Incubation period usually 5–60 days, but highly variable and may be several months
- Characterized by intermittent or irregular fevers, with symptoms ranging from subclinical disease to infection of almost any organ system
- Bone and joint involvement common
- May be chronic or recurrent
- System(s) Affected: Cardiovascular; Endocrine/Metabolic; Gastrointestinal; Musculoskeletal; Nervous; Pulmonary; Renal/Urologic; Skin/Exocrine
- Synonym(s): Undulant fever; Malta fever

Pediatric Considerations
May be mild, subclinical

Pregnancy Considerations
High rates of miscarriage or abortion (can occur in subclinical cases). Early antibiotic treatment is preventive.

GENERAL PREVENTION
- Avoid infected dairy products.
- For occupational exposure, use caution, animal vaccination, protective goggles, protective gloves. There is a possibility of future human vaccine.
- Postexposure prophylaxis same as treatment in large-scale exposure such as bioterrorism
- Susceptible to heat, disinfectant, but can survive in dust, soil, or water for weeks

EPIDEMIOLOGY
- Predominant age: All ages, but especially ages 20–60 years (occupational exposure), sometimes children (milk-related outbreaks)
- Predominant sex:
  – Male > Female (occupational exposure)
  – Female ≥ Male (milk exposure)

Incidence
~100 per year (0.34/100,000), but probably underreported (1,2)

Prevalence
- Common in developing countries; consider in immigrants
- Highest rates in Hispanic population, along US–Mexico border
- Considered a potential biological terror agent in aerosolized form
- Reportable in all states except Nevada

RISK FACTORS
- In the US, from occupational exposure to infected animals (especially cattle, sheep) veterinarians, meat processors, farm workers who may experience accidental exposure to vaccine.
- Consumer exposure to unpasteurized milk products, cheese, especially in Hispanics along US–Mexico border
- Exposure while traveling in countries where endemic (Mediterranean, Middle East, North and East Africa, Central Asia, India, Mexico, and Central and South America)

- Worse in chronically ill, immunosuppressed, and malnourished
- Iron deficiency increases susceptibility

Genetics
- Some evidence for intrauterine transmission
- Some complications may have genetic predisposition (2)

ETIOLOGY
- *Brucella* ingestion from tissue or milk
- Worst disease: *B. melitensis*, *B. suis*; also *B. canis*, *B. abortus*. Enters through mucous membrane or broken skin; occasionally inhaled.
- Facultative intracellular parasite
- Person-to-person transmission rare; sexual, vertical, and possibly breast milk; case report of neonatal brucellosis from a blood transfusion
- Potential air-borne biologic weapon

 **DIAGNOSIS**

SIGNS AND SYMPTOMS
- Fever (may be undulant, increased in afternoon and evening, maximum 101–104°F daily); weakness; headache; sweating; chills; generalized aching; arthralgia (90%) (2)[A]
- Also common: Weight loss, depression, irritability, hepatosplenomegaly (20–30%)
- Hepatic dysfunction (abnormal liver function test): 30–60%
- Gastrointestinal symptoms (unusual)
- Lymphadenopathy, especially cervical, inguinal (12–21%)
- Orchitis, epididymitis (normal urinalysis) (2–40%)
- Nephritis, prostatitis (rare)
- Cystitis
- Pulmonary—cough or other pulmonary symptoms; radiograph may be normal (15–25%)
- Cutaneous—many transient, nonspecific rashes have been described; also, purpura from thrombopenia (5%)
- Visual disturbances, eye pain
- Chronic fatigue syndrome and various neuropsychiatric symptoms described. Relationship is unclear.
- Also localized suppurative infections (see "Complications")
- Malodorous perspiration (2)

History
Exposure

TESTS
Echocardiogram, depending on location

Lab
- Isolation of organism from blood, discharge, bone, or other tissue (3)[C]
  – Fastidious and slow growing
  – Watch for 3–4 weeks, with periodic subcultures
  – Automated systems shorten time, but not all recognize brucellosis.
  – Polymerase chain reaction (PCR) accurate, including nonblood samples, but not available in most clinical labs (3)[C]
  – Skin tests not standardized, not recommended for diagnosis

- Acute illness: Blood culture positive 70%, bone marrow 90%
- May have thrombocytopenia, disseminated intravascular coagulation; granulopenia, lymphopenia, lymphocytosis. 30–60% with abnormal liver function test. Up to 70% may have normal labs.
- Serology: Use at least 2 tests to confirm (4)[C]
  – *Brucella* standard tube agglutination paired sera, >1:160 or 4× rise (cheapest)
  – Easy, accurate, and rapid dipstick for IgM now exists for developing countries
- More effective enzyme-linked immunosorbent assay (ELISA), indirect fluorescent antibody test, Coombs tests, immunocapture-agglutination (Brucellacapt). With ELISA, IgM, IgG, or IgA may be present at low levels >1 year even if treated
- IgM increased initially for several weeks, declines by 3 months
- IgG begins to rise in 2 weeks, may stay up (low levels) >1 year if treated or not treated (though IgM increase may be lower or gone by 6 months if treated, can also persist >1 year at low levels). IgG titer rises again with reinfection or reactivation. IgG and IgA titer >1:160 at 1 year implies ongoing disease. (4)[C]
- New research: Gene cloning and amplification for discriminatory markers detection and strain differences; PCR-ELISA
- Drugs that may alter lab results
  – None
- Disorders that may alter lab results
  – Serologic cross-reaction with *F. tularensis*, *Yersinia enterocolitica*, *V. cholerae*, or vaccinated patients
  – Has been misdiagnosed in culture as *Moraxella phenylpyruvica*

Imaging
- Bone scan, CT, depending on location
- Chest radiograph—pleural effusion, lung cavitation
- Joint radiographs frequently normal, requiring scan or MRI

Diagnostic Procedures/Surgery
Biopsy, aspiration, depending on location

Pathological Findings
- Facultative intracellular Gram-negative coccobacillus; can survive inside phagocytic cells, circulate to regional lymph nodes, and into circulation
- Variable tissue reaction depending on site, organisms. Causes local microabscesses; noncaseating granulomas; (1) possibly some immune reaction in arthritis, including elevated C3, C4; antinuclear antibody, and rheumatoid factor.

DIFFERENTIAL DIAGNOSIS
- Many nonspecific systemic febrile illnesses; a great mimic
- Tularemia
- Psittacosis
- Rickettsial disease
- Tuberculosis
- Visceral leishmaniasis
- Other disease of infected organs
- HIV infection

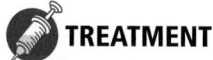 TREATMENT

- Outpatient in mild cases, hospitalization in severe illness
- Cardiac care unit for patients with complicating cardiac disease

GENERAL MEASURES

- Supportive care
- In milk-related or occupational outbreak, look for other cases.

Diet

- No special diet
- May need to provide supplemental foods, such as milk shakes, to counter weight loss

Activity

Bed rest during febrile periods and restricted activity in acute cases

Nursing

Patient comfort, education

IV Fluids

If cardiac complications

 MEDICATION (DRUGS)

First Line

- Optimal therapy includes 2 drugs, at least 1 with good intracellular penetration. In some cases, 3 drugs may give a better long-term cure.
- Longer courses (months) may improve relapse rate in complicated disease.
- Rifampin 600–900 mg and doxycycline 200 mg given together every day for at least 6 weeks (possibly for several months with severe complications); 5–10% relapse rate, not related to drug resistance—use same drugs for relapse. Usual cause is localized sequestration of organisms or noncompliance with medication (5)[C].
- Steroids in Herxheimer reaction, severe illness, and pancytopenia
- Contraindications
  – Avoid doxycycline in children and pregnant women (affects bone).
- Precautions:
  – May get Herxheimer reaction when therapy initiated
- Significant possible interactions:
  – Rifampin is a potent inducer for the hepatic P450 enzyme system, and may increase metabolism of many drugs metabolized by the liver.
  – Doxycycline: Antacids, anticoagulants, barbiturates, carbamazepine, hydantoins, cimetidine, digoxin, insulin, iron salts, lithium, methoxyflurane, oral contraceptives, penicillins, sodium bicarbonate

Second Line

- In recent studies, ciprofloxacin 1 g daily and rifampin 600 mg/d for 30 days as effective as rifampin/doxycycline for 4–5 weeks (2,6)[A]
- Doxycycline PO b.i.d. and streptomycin by injection—very effective (streptomycin currently not available in the US except by special request from Centers for Disease Control and Prevention); slightly more effective than doxycycline/rifampin, especially with spondylitis, but more toxic and less convenient (5)
- In children and pregnant women, rifampin 15 mg/kg for 4–5 weeks plus cotrimoxazole for 6 weeks or gentamicin for 7 days or netilmicin 5–6 mg/kg IM. Significant cotrimoxazole resistance in some countries (1,6)[C]
- Ofloxacin plus rifampin effective in recent study
- Sensitivities frequently don't reflect in vivo action (2)[C]

SURGERY

Specific complications may require surgical drainage or valve replacement (endocarditis).

 FOLLOW-UP

PROGNOSIS

- Untreated case fatality <2%
- Most cases resolve with treatment in 2–3 weeks in acute uncomplicated cases, but at least 6 weeks treatment recommended

COMPLICATIONS

- Relapse rate overall: 5–10% (6)[C]
- Complications present 10–15% (4)[C]
- Localized suppurative infections—osteo-articular (20–85%). Includes arthritis (possibly also immune effect), bursitis, tenosynovitis, osteomyelitis, sacroiliitis, vertebral or paraspinous abscess
- Endocarditis—rare, but main cause of death in brucellosis
- Thrombophlebitis
- Neuro-brucellosis—most are meningeal. Also peripheral neuritis (usually single; bilateral is possible), encephalitis, myelitis, radiculopathy. Possibly neuropsychiatric symptoms
- Intrinsic ocular lesions—uveitis, retinal thrombophlebitis, nummular keratitis
- Pneumonitis with pleural effusion
- Hepatitis
- Cholecystitis
- Chronic infection. Persistent (>1 year) signs of infection, elevated titers, occasional bacteria in blood or tissue. Chronic fatigue syndrome with everything negative is controversial.

PATIENT MONITORING

- Check serology at 6 months and 1 year for chronic disease (difficult to evaluate if continuing exposure).
- Investigate any evidence of complication or recurrence.
- PCR recently shown to be sensitive and specific for monitoring treatment relapse

REFERENCES

1. Sauret J, Vilissova N. Human brucellosis. *J Amer Board Fam Pract.* 2002;15:401–406.
2. Pappas, Georgios, et al. Brucellosis. *N Eng J Med.* 2005;352(22);2325–2336.
3. Al Dahouk S, Tomaso H, et al. Laboratory-based diagnosis of brucellosis—a review of the literature. Part I: Techniques for direct detection and identification of *Brucella* spp. *Clin Lab.* 2003; 49:487–505.
4. Al Dahouk S, Tomaso H, et al. Laboratory-based diagnosis of brucellosis—a review of the literature. Part II: Serological tests for brucellosis. *Clin Lab.* 2003;49:577–589.
5. Montejo JM, et al. Open randomized therapeutic trial of six antimicrobial regimens in brucellosis. *Clin Infect Dis.* 1993;16:671–676.
6. Pappas, Georgios, et al. New approaches to the antibiotic treatment of brucellosis. *Intl J Antimicrob Ag.* 2005;26(2);101–105.

 MISCELLANEOUS

See also: Abortion, Spontaneous; Chronic Fatigue Syndrome; Thrombosis, Deep Vein (DVT)

CODES

ICD9-CM

023.9 Brucellosis, unspecified

PATIENT TEACHING

Food Safety and Inspection Service, Office of Public Awareness, Department of Agriculture, Room 1165-S, Washington, DC 20205, (202) 447-9351.

See Corresponding Diagnostic Algorithm

BULIMIA NERVOSA

Jeffrey L. Goodie, PhD
Pamela Williams, MD

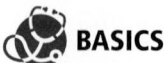 **BASICS**

DESCRIPTION
- A pattern of uncontrolled eating during discrete periods followed by compensatory behaviors.
- System(s) Affected: Oropharyngeal, Endocrine/Metabolic, Gastrointestinal, Dermatologic, Cardiovascular, Nervous

GENERAL PREVENTION
- Encourage realistic weight management strategies and attitudes
- Moderate overly high self-expectations
- Decrease anxiety/depressive symptoms
- Improve stress management

EPIDEMIOLOGY
- Predominant age: Adolescents and young adults; mean age of onset: 18–19
- Predominant sex: Female > Male (10:1 to 20:1)

Incidence
28.8 women, 0.8 men per 100,000 per year

Prevalence
- 1–2% in women 16–35 years old
- 0.1% in young men

RISK FACTORS
- Female gender
- History of obesity and dieting
- Body dissatisfaction
- Critical comments by family or others about weight, body shape, or eating
- Severe life stressor; achievement pressure; competition stressors
- Low self-esteem
- Perceived pressure to be thin
- Perfectionistic or obsessional thinking
- History of anorexia nervosa
- Environment that stresses thinness or physical fitness (e.g., armed forces, ballet, cheerleaders, gymnastics, or models)
- Family history of substance abuse, affective disorders, eating disorder, or obesity
- Type I diabetes
- Poor impulse control, alcohol misuse
- Sexual abuse is not causally related to bulimia.

ETIOLOGY
Combination of biological, genetic psychological, environmental, and social factors. Unique contribution of any specific factor remains unclear.

ASSOCIATED CONDITIONS
- Major depression and dysthymia
- Anxiety disorders
- Substance abuse/dependence
- Bipolar disorder
- Obsessive-compulsive disorder
- Schizophrenic disorder
- Borderline personality disorder

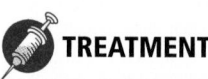 **DIAGNOSIS**

DSM IV TR CRITERIA
- Recurrent episodes of binge eating (2 times per week for 3 months)
  – Eating in a discrete period of time more than most people would eat during that time
  – Perceived lack of control during binge
- Recurrent inappropriate compensatory behavior (2 times per week for 3 months)
- Purging and nonpurging subtypes
  – Purging: Often by self-induced vomiting, laxatives, diuretics
  – Nonpurging: Binges followed by sharply restricted diet and/or vigorous exercise
- Body shape and weight significantly affect self-evaluation.

SIGNS AND SYMPTOMS
- Unhappiness and/or preoccupation with weight and diet attempts
- Pattern of restricting diet, binge eating, and purging behaviors
  – Binge is context specific; amount can vary
    ○ Average binge between 1,000–2,000 kcals[2]
  – Vomiting (often with little effort)
  – Vigorous aerobic exercise
  – Distress/shame related to loss of control
- Requesting weight loss help
- Menstrual disturbance
- Fatigue and lethargy
- Abdominal pain, bloating, constipation, diarrhea, irritable bowel syndrome, rectal prolapse
- Enamel erosion, parotid swelling, sore throat
- Onset may be stress related
- Mildly underweight to overweight
- Frequent fluctuations in weight
- Diet pill, diuretic, laxative, ipecac, and thyroid medication use/abuse
- Omission/underdosing insulin in diabetes patients
- Depressed mood and self-depreciation following the binges
- Relief and increased ability to concentrate following the purges

History
Corroborate with parent/relative

Physical Exam
- Often normal
- Eroded tooth enamel
- Asymptomatic, non-inflammatory salivary gland (parotid) enlargement
- Calluses, abrasions, bruising on hand, thumb
- Peripheral edema

TESTS
Lab
- All results may be within normal limits and are not necessary for diagnosis.
- Hypokalemia, hypochloremia
- Hypomagnesemia, hyponatraemia, hypocalcaemia, hypophosphataemia
- Alkalosis
- Leukopenia
- Elevated blood urea nitrogen
- Elevated basal serum prolactin
- Mild elevation in serum amylase

Imaging
Not indicated

Diagnostic Procedures/Surgery
Psychological self-report screening
- Eating Attitudes Test
- Eating Disorder Inventory
- Eating Disorder Screen for Primary Care
- Bulimia Test—Revised
- Bulimia Investigatory Test Edinburgh
- SCOFF (sick, control, one, fat, food) questionnaire

Pathological Findings
- Esophagitis
- Pseudo-Bartter syndrome
- Acute pancreatitis
- Cardiomyopathy and muscle weakness due to ipecac abuse

DIFFERENTIAL DIAGNOSIS
- Anorexia, binge eating/purging type
- Major depressive disorder
- Psychogenic vomiting
- Hypothalamic brain tumor
- Epileptic equivalent seizures
- Kleine-Levin syndrome
- Body dysmorphic disorder
- Borderline personality disorder

TREATMENT

GENERAL MEASURES
- Most patients can be treated as outpatients.
- Outpatient
  – Build trust, increase motivation for change
  – Assess psychological and nutritional status
  – Consider evidence-based self-help program
  – Cognitive behavioral therapy (1–3)[A]
    ○ Involve patient in establishing target goals
    ○ Use self-monitoring techniques of food intake, frequency of binges/purges, related antecedents, consequences, and thoughts
    ○ Self-monitoring weight once per week along with emotional and thought reactions
    ○ Educate about ineffectiveness of purging for weight control and adverse outcomes
    ○ Establish prescribed eating plan to develop regular eating habits; realistic weight goal
    ○ Gradually introduce feared foods into diet
    ○ Problem solve how to cope with triggers
    ○ Address calories, weight, and purging ruminations
    ○ Challenge fear of loss of control
    ○ Establish relapse prevention plan
  – Gradual laxative withdrawal
  – Interpersonal therapy (1,3)[C]
  – Family therapy for adolescents
  – Nutritional education, relaxation techniques
  – After vomiting, avoid brushing teeth and consider using non-acidic mouthwash (1)
  – Limiting acidic foods, beverages to meal time

- Inpatient
  - If possible, admit to eating disorders unit
  - Supervised meals and bathroom privileges
  - Monitor weight and physical activity
  - Monitor electrolytes
  - See outpatient recommendations
  - Gradually shift control to patients as they demonstrate responsibility

Diet
- Balanced diet, normal eating pattern
- Reintroduce feared foods

Activity
- Monitor excess activity
- Encourage enjoyable activities

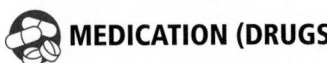 **MEDICATION (DRUGS)**

First Line
- Selective serotonin reuptake inhibitors (SSRIs), particularly fluoxetine (Prozac) at 60 mg, are effective in reducing symptoms with relatively few side effects. Higher doses than standard doses for depression are often needed. (1)[B]

- Tricyclic antidepressants (amitriptyline, desipramine, and imipramine) and monoamine oxidase inhibitors: Phenelzine (Nardil) 60–90 mg/d have been shown to decrease binging and vomiting. (1,2)[C] Patients with atypical depression may respond to monoamine oxidase inhibitors and not SSRIs.
- Augment with buspirone (BuSpar) if desired. To prevent relapse, maintain antidepressant medication at full therapeutic dose for at least 1 year.
- Note: Misrepresentation and non-adherence may be more likely in this population.
- Contraindications: Hypersensitivity
- Precautions
  - Serious toxicity following overdose is common.
  - Patients may vomit medications.
- Significant possible interactions
  - Monoamine Oxidase Inhibitor should not be combined with SSRI or tricyclic medication
  - Lithium and tricyclic medication can be lethal when administered to hypokalemic patients.

Second Line
- Ondansetron (Zofran) 4–8 mg t.i.d. between meals can help prevent vomiting.
- Psyllium (Metamucil) preparations 1 tbs qhs with glass of water, can prevent constipation during laxative withdrawal.

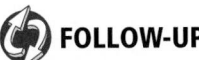 **FOLLOW-UP**

DISPOSITION
Admission Criteria
Hospitalize if severe malnutrition, dehydration, electrolyte disturbances, cardiac dysrhythmia, uncontrolled binging and purging, psychiatric emergency, or failed outpatient treatment.

PROGNOSIS
- Following effective treatment
  - 50% asymptomatic after 2–10 years, 30% remissions, relapses, or subclinical behaviors; 20% no significant change
- Untreated
  - Likely to remain chronic/relapsing problem
- Greater weight fluctuations, other impulsive behaviors, and personality disorder diagnoses may predict poor prognosis.

COMPLICATIONS
- Suicide
- Drug and alcohol abuse
- Infarction and perforation of the stomach
  - Gastric dilatation
  - Mallory-Weiss tears
  - Spontaneous pneumomediastinum
- Potassium depletion; cardiac arrhythmia; cardiac arrest
- Maternal and fetal problems if pregnant
  - Binging/purging behaviors may change with pregnancy

PATIENT MONITORING
- Binge-purge activity, including antecedents and consequences
- Level of exercise activity
- Self-esteem, comfort with body and self
- Ruminations and depression
- Repeat any abnormal lab values weekly or monthly until stable

REFERENCES
1. NICE. Eating disorders—core interventions in the treatment of anorexia nervosa, bulimia nervosa, and related eating disorders. NICE Clinical Guideline no 9. London: NICE, 2004: Available at: http://www.nice.org.uk. Accessed January 20, 2006.
2. Bacaltchuk J, Hay P, Trefiglio R. Antidepressants versus psychological treatments and their combination for bulimia nervosa. *Cochrane Database Sys Rev.* 2001(4):CD003385.
3. Hay PJ, Bacaltchuk J. Psychotherapy for bulimia nervosa and binging. *Cochrane Database Syst Rev.* 2003(1):CD000562.
4. Fairburn CG, Harrison PJ. Eating disorders. *Lancet.* 2003;361:407–416.
5. Mehler, PS. Bulimia nervosa. *N Engl J Med.* 2003;349:875–881.

ADDITIONAL READING
McCabe RE, McFarlane TL, Olmstead MP. *Overcoming bulimia: your comprehensive, step-by-step guide to recovery.* 2003; Oakland, CA: New Harbinger.

 MISCELLANEOUS

See also: Anorexia nervosa; Hyperkalemia; Laxative abuse; Salivary gland tumors

CODES

ICD9-CM
307.51 Bulimia Nervosa

ICD10
F50.2 Bulimia Nervosa

PATIENT TEACHING
Review outpatient treatment recommendations

 See Corresponding Diagnostic Algorithm

 See Patient Handout on CD

BURNS

Timothy L. Black, MD
James P. Miller, MD

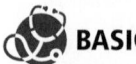

BASICS

DESCRIPTION
- Tissue injuries caused by application of heat, chemicals, electricity, or irradiation to the tissue
- Extent of injury (depth of burn) is result of intensity of heat (or other exposure) and duration of exposure
  - Partial thickness: 1st degree involves superficial layers of epidermis. 2nd degree involves varying degrees of epidermis (with blister formation) and part of the dermis.
  - Full thickness: 3rd degree involves destruction of all skin elements with coagulation of subdermal plexus
- System(s) Affected: Endocrine/Metabolic; Skin/Exocrine

Geriatric Considerations
- Prognosis poorer for severe burns
- Patients >60 years of age account for 11% of burns. (1)[C]

Pediatric Considerations
Consider child abuse or neglect when dealing with hot water burns in children
- Observe distribution of burns.
- Pay attention to straight lines, especially if bilateral.

GENERAL PREVENTION
Skin grafts or newly epithelialized skin is highly sensitive to sun exposure and thermal extremes.

EPIDEMIOLOGY
- Predominant age: All ages
  - Average age is 30 years
  - 13% are infants, and 11% are >60 years of age
- Predominant sex: Males account for 70%

Incidence
Per year in US
- Total population: 1.2–2 million burns, 700,000 emergency room visits, 45,000–50,000 hospitalizations, 3,900 deaths due to burn-related complications (1,2)[C]
- In children: 250,000 burns, 15,000 hospitalizations, 1,100 deaths
- Estimated total cost of $2 billion annually for burn care in the United States (1)[C]
- 75% of burn related deaths are the result of house fires (1)[C]

RISK FACTORS
- Water heaters set too high
- Workplace exposure to chemicals, electricity, or irradiation
- Young children and elderly adults with thin skin are more susceptible to injury.
- Carelessness with burning cigarettes
- Inadequate or faulty electrical wiring
- Lack of smoke detectors

ETIOLOGY
- Open flame and hot liquid are most common (heat usually ≥15–45°C)
- Caustic chemicals or acids (may show little signs or symptoms for the first few days)
- Electricity (may have significant injury with very little damage to overlying skin)
- Excess sun exposure

ASSOCIATED CONDITIONS
Smoke inhalation syndrome
- Occurs within 72 hours of burn
- Should be suspected in all burns occurring in an enclosed space
- Intubation, ventilation with positive end-expiratory pressure assistance

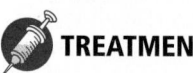

DIAGNOSIS

SIGNS AND SYMPTOMS
- 1st degree
  - Erythema of involved tissue
  - Skin blanches with pressure
  - Skin may be tender
- 2nd degree
  - Skin is red and blistered
  - Skin is very tender
- 3rd degree
  - Burned skin is tough and leathery
  - Skin is not tender

History
- History of source of burn
- In children, check for consistency between the history and the burn's physical characteristics

Physical Exam
- Careful documentation of extent of burn and the estimated depth of burn
- Check for any signs suggestive of potential airway involvement: Singed nasal hair, facial burns, carbonaceous sputum, progressive hoarseness, or tachypnea

TESTS
- Children: Glucose (hypoglycemia may occur in children because of limited glycogen storage)
- Smoke inhalation: Arterial blood gas, carboxyhemoglobin
- Electrical burns: ECG, urine myoglobin, creatine kinase isoenzymes

Lab
- Hematocrit
- Type and cross
- Electrolytes, including blood urea nitrogen and creatinine
- Urinalysis
- Disorders that may alter lab results: Preexisting cardiac disease

Imaging
- Chest radiograph
- Xenon scan may be useful in suspected smoke inhalation.
- Other radiographs if other trauma involved

Diagnostic Procedures/Surgery
Bronchoscopy may be necessary in smoke inhalation to evaluate lower respiratory tract.

Pathological Findings
- 1st degree
  - Devitalization of superficial layers of epidermis
  - Congestion of intradermal vessels
- 2nd degree
  - Coagulation necrosis of varying depths of epidermis
  - Clefting of epidermis (blister)
  - Coagulation of subdermal plexus
  - Skin appendages intact
- 3rd degree
  - Necrosis of all skin elements
  - Coagulation of subdermal plexus

DIFFERENTIAL DIAGNOSIS
- Toxic epidermal necrolysis
- Scalded skin syndrome

TREATMENT

- Hospitalization for all serious burns
  - 2nd-degree burns >10% body surface area, any 3rd-degree burn
  - Burns of hands, feet, face, or perineum
  - Electrical/lightning burns
  - Inhalation injury
  - Chemical burns
  - Circumferential burn
- Transfer to burn center for (1,2,3)[C]
  - 2nd- and 3rd-degree burns >10% body surface area in patients <10 years and >50 years of age
  - 2nd-degree burns >20% body surface area and full thickness burns >5% BSA in any age range
  - Burns of hands, feet, face, or perineum
  - Electrical/lightning burns
  - Inhalation injury
  - Chemical burns
  - Circumferential burn
  - Chemical burns with threat of functional impairment

PRE HOSPITAL (1)[C]
- Remove patient from source of the burn
- Extinguish and remove all burning clothing
- Remove all rings, watches, and jewelry
- Room-temperature water may be poured onto burn but only in the 1st 15 minutes following burn exposure
- Wrap patient to prevent hypothermia
- All patients should receive 100% O_2 by face mask

GENERAL MEASURES

- Based on depth of burns and accurate estimate of total body surface area involved (rule of nines)
- Rule of nines (1)[C]
  - Each upper extremity: Adult and child 9%
  - Each lower extremity: Adult 18%; child 14%
  - Anterior trunk: Adult and child 18%
  - Posterior trunk: Adult and child 18%
  - Head and neck: Adult 10%; child 18%
- Quick estimate (for smaller burns): The surface area of the patient's hand is ~1% of the body surface area.
- Tetanus prophylaxis (if not current)
- Remove all rings, watches, and other items from injured extremities to avoid tourniquet effect.
- Remove clothing and cover all burned areas with dry sheets.
- Flush area of chemical burn (for ~2 hours)
- 100% oxygen administration for all major burns; consider early intubation
- Do not apply ice to burn site.
- Nasogastric tube (high risk of paralytic ileus)
- Foley catheter
- Pain relief
  - IV meperidine (Demerol), morphine, or methadone for severe pain
  - Oral analgesics, such as acetaminophen (Tylenol) with codeine, acetaminophen with oxycodone (Percocet), or acetaminophen with hydrocodone (Lortab) for moderate pain
- ECG monitoring in 1st 24 hours following electrical burn
- Whirlpool hydrotherapy followed by silver sulfadiazine (Silvadene) occlusive dressings in severe burns
- Once- or twice-a-day cleansing with dressing changes
- Epilock or Elasto-Gel may be used as dressing in selected patients (especially useful for outpatient treatment of minor burns)
- Burn fluid resuscitation (1,2,3)[C]
  - Calculate fluid resuscitation from time of burn, not from time treatment begins
  - 2–4 mL Ringer's lactate × body weight (kg) × % body surface area burn (1/2 given in 1st 8 hours, 1/4 in 2nd 8 hours, and 1/4 in 3rd 8 hours). In children, this is given in addition to maintenance fluids and is adjusted according to urine output and vital signs.
  - Colloid solutions are not recommended during the 1st 12–24 hours of resuscitation (1,2)[C], (4)[A]
- Other: Use of biological membranes or skin substitutes may be indicated for burn coverage.

Diet

- High-protein, high-calorie diet when bowel function resumes
- Nasogastric tube feedings may be required in early postburn period
- Total parenteral nutrition if NPO expected for >5 days

Activity

Early mobilization is the goal.

MEDICATION (DRUGS)

First Line

- Morphine small frequent IV doses (0.1 mg/kg/dose in children; 2.5–20 mg q2–6h in adults)
- Silver sulfadiazine (Silvadene) topically to burn site (can cause leukopenia)
- Electrical burn with myoglobinuria will require alkalinization of urine and mannitol
- No indication for prophylactic antibiotics.
- Consider H_2 blockers (cimetidine, ranitidine, famotidine, or nizatidine) for stress ulcer prophylaxis in severely burned patients.
- Contraindications
  - Specific drug allergies
- Precautions
  - Be alert for respiratory depression with narcotics.
- Significant possible interactions
  - Refer to manufacturer's profile for each drug.

Second Line

- Mafenide (Sulfamylon)—full-thickness burn (caution: Metabolic acidosis)
- Silver nitrate 0.5% (messy, leaches electrolytes from burn, and causes water toxicity)
- Povidone–iodine (Betadine) may result in iodine absorption from burn, "tan eschar." Makes débridement more difficult.
- Travase—enzymatic débridement

SURGERY

- Escharotomy may be necessary in constricting circumferential burns of extremities or chest.
- Tangential excision with split-thickness skin grafts

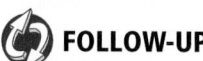 FOLLOW-UP

PROGNOSIS

- 1st-degree burn: Complete resolution
- 2nd-degree burn: Epithelialization in 10–14 days (deep 2nd-degree burns will probably require skin graft)
- 3rd-degree burn: No potential for re-epithelialization, skin graft required
- Length of hospital stay and need for ICU care depend on extent of burn, smoke inhalation, and age
- A 50% survival rate can be expected with a 62% burn in ages 0–14 years, 63% burn in ages 15–40 years, 38% burn in age 40–65 years, 25% burn in patients >65 years (1,2,3)[C]
- 90% of survivors can be expected to return to an occupation as remunerative as their preburn employment.

COMPLICATIONS

- Gastroduodenal ulceration (Curling ulcer)
- Marjolin ulcer—squamous cell carcinoma developing in old burn site
- Burn wound sepsis—usually gram-negative organisms
- Pneumonia
- Decreased mobility with possibility of future flexion contractures
- Hypertrophic scarring common with burns

PATIENT MONITORING

According to extent of burn and treatment

REFERENCES

1. Teague H, Sweneki SA, Tang A. The burned patient: Assessment, diagnosis, and management in the ED. *Trauma Reports*. 2005;6:1–12.
2. Townsend C, Beauchamp RD, Evers BM, et al. eds. *Sabiston Textbook of Surgery* 17 ed. Philadelphia, PA: Elsevier Saunders, 2006.
3. Gillespie RW, Dimik AR, Hallberg PW. *Advanced Burn Life Support Course Provider's Manual*. Lincoln, NE: Nebraska Burn Institute; 1990.
4. Roberts I, Alderson P, Bunn F, et al. Colloids versus crystalloids for fluid resuscitation in critically ill patients (Review). *Cochrane Database Sys Rev.* 2006; Vol 1.

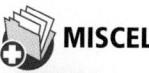 MISCELLANEOUS

CODES

ICD9-CM

- 940.9 Unspecified burn of eye and adnexa
- 941.00 Unspecified degree burn of face and head, unspecified site
- 942.00 Unspecified degree burn of trunk, unspecified site
- 948.0 Burn, any degree <10% of body surface area (fifth digit can indicate body surface area involved in third degree burn)
- 949.0 Unspecified burn, unspecified degree
- 949.1 Unspecified burn, erythema [first degree]
- 949.2 Unspecified burn, blisters, epidermal loss [second degree]
- 949.3 Unspecified burn, full thickness skin loss [third degree NOS]

PATIENT TEACHING

- Use of sunscreen
- Access to electrical cords/outlets
- Isolate household chemicals
- Use low temperature setting for water heater
- Household smoke detectors with special emphasis on maintenance
- Family/household evacuation plan
- Proper storage and use of flammable substances

 See Corresponding Diagnostic Algorithm

 See Patient Handout on CD

BURSITIS

John Herbert Stevenson, MD
Christopher Lutryzkowski, MD
Peter L. Hoth, MD

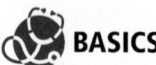 **BASICS**

DESCRIPTION

- A bursa is a sac that is formed or found in areas subject to friction, such as locations where tendons pass over bony landmarks. Most common sites are subdeltoid, olecranon, prepatellar, trochanteric, radiohumeral. They essentially lubricate the region with synovial fluid.
- Large bursae usually communicate with joints and are responsible for retaining the synovial fluid in place.
- Bursae are fluid-filled sacs that serve as a cushion between tendons and bones.
- Bywaters, an English rheumatologist, found at least 78 bursae symmetrically placed on each side of the body.
- System(s) Affected: Musculoskeletal

ALERT

Pediatric Considerations
Bursitis less common in the pediatric population.

GENERAL PREVENTION

- Appropriate warm-up and cool-down maneuvers, avoidance of overuse, or inadequate rest between workouts
- Range-of-motion exercises
- Maintain high level of fitness and general good health.

EPIDEMIOLOGY

Predominant age
- 15–50 years (most common in skeletally mature)
- Traumatic bursitis more likely in patients <35 years of age

Incidence
- Common
- Trochanteric pain: 1.8 per 1000 per year (6)[B]

RISK FACTORS

Individuals who engage in repetitive and vigorous training or others who suddenly increase their level of activity (e.g., "weekend warriors")

ETIOLOGY

- Bursitis may be acute or chronic.
- Many types of bursitis, including infectious, traumatic, inflammatory, and gouty
- Less often rheumatoid disease or tuberculosis as well as gout and pseudogout

ASSOCIATED CONDITIONS

- Tendinitis
- Sprains, strains
- Associated stress fractures

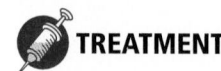 **DIAGNOSIS**

SIGNS AND SYMPTOMS

- Pain/tenderness
- Decreased range of motion of affected region (rare except at shoulder)
- Erythema if infection present
- Swelling
- Crepitus sometimes found

TESTS

ECG (if shoulder pain mimics cardiac pain)

Lab
- The following may help in differentiating soft-tissue disease from rheumatic and connective tissue disease
  - CBC
  - ESR
  - Serum protein electrophoresis
  - Rheumatoid factor
  - Serum uric acid
  - Phosphorus
  - Alkaline phosphatase
  - Blood testing for syphilis
  - Joint fluid analysis and culture (when indicated)
- Drugs that may alter lab results
  - ESR rate may be increased with coexistent use of methyldopa, methysergide, penicillamine, theophylline, vitamin A.
  - ESR may be decreased with coexistent use of quinine, salicylates, and drugs that cause a high glucose level.

Imaging
- MRI may prove beneficial if diagnosis is unclear
- Calcific deposits may be seen on plain radiograph.
- Ultrasound (1)[B]

Diagnostic Procedures/Surgery
- Aspiration of swollen bursa and evaluation of synovial fluid
- The clinician must differentiate infected from inflammatory bursitis. Fluid analysis and culture help make the diagnosis. If the Gram stain and culture yield an infective cause, treat with appropriate antibiotics. If the etiology is inflammatory, give local care.

Pathological Findings
- Acute with early inflammation: Bursa is distended with watery or mucoid fluid.
- Infection: Purulent fluid
- Chronic
  - Bursal wall is thickened, and inner surface is shaggy and trabeculated.
  - The space is filled with granular, brown, inspissated blood admixed with gritty, calcific precipitations.
  - Upper extremity tendonitis and bursitis are usually the result of repetitive microtrauma, probably resulting in disruption of fibers leading to pain, spasm, and disability.

DIFFERENTIAL DIAGNOSIS

- Septic arthritis
- Gout, pseudogout
- Rheumatic disorders
- Osteoarthritis
- Tendinitis, strains, and sprains
- Lyme arthritis

TREATMENT

Outpatient; refer only difficult cases.

INITIAL STABILIZATION
GENERAL MEASURES

- Conservative therapy consists of rest, ice, and local care; elevation, gentle compression (often referred to as RICE therapy [rest-ice-compression-elevation]).
- Compression with Ace wrap or neoprene sleeve
- Bursa aspiration
- Corticosteroid injection if infectious etiology ruled out
- Treatment of any underlying infection

Diet
Consider changes if bursitis is directly related to obesity/crystalline deposition.

Activity
Rest and elevation of affected extremity

MEDICATION (DRUGS)

First Line
- NSAIDs or aspirin (2,4,5)[C], (9)[C]
- Antibiotic therapy if infection present; cover for staph and strep species (most common) (8)[B]
- Contraindications: Refer to manufacturer's profile of each drug.
- Precautions: Refer to manufacturer's profile of each drug.
- Significant possible interactions: Refer to manufacturer's profile of each drug.

Second Line
- Injectable corticosteroids once infectious etiology ruled out (2,4,5)[C], 3[B], (9)[B]
- Systemic steroids provide limited short-term benefit (7)[B].

SURGERY
Surgical excision in severe cases unresponsive to conservative treatments (8)[B]

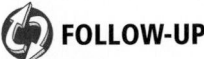 FOLLOW-UP

PROGNOSIS
- Most bouts of bursitis heal without sequelae.
- Repetitive acute bouts may lead to chronic bursitis, necessitating repeated joint/bursal aspirations or eventually surgical excision of involved bursa.

COMPLICATIONS
- Septic bursitis may extend to the nearby joint.
- Acute bursitis may progress to chronic.
- Severe long-range limitation of motion

PATIENT MONITORING
- Discontinue NSAIDs as soon as possible to avoid side effects
- Some patients may require repeated injections (usually no more than 3) of a corticosteroid and lidocaine (2,4,5)[C].

REFERENCES

1. Finlay K, Friedman L. Ultrasonography of the lower extremity. *Orthop Clin North Am.* 2006;37(3): 245–75,v.
2. Talia, Alfred H., Cardone, Dennis. Diagnostic and Therapeutic injection of the shoulder region. *Am Fam Phys.* 2003;67(6): 1271–1278.
3. Buchbinder R, et. al. Corticosteroid injection for shoulder pain. *Cochrane Database Sys Rev.* Jan. 1, 2003.
4. Cardone D, Tallia AH. Diagnostic and therapeutic injection of the elbow. *Am Fam Phys.* 2002;66(11):2097–3100.
5. Cardone D, Tallia AH. Diagnostic and therapeutic injection of the hip and knee. *Am Fam Phys.* 2003;67(10):2147–2153.
6. Lieviense A, et al. Prognosis of trochanteric pain in primary care. *Br J Gen Pract.* xxx;55(512): 199–204.
7. Buchbinder R, et. al. Short course prednisolone for adhesive capsulitis (frozen shoulder or stiff painful shoulder): A randomized, double blind, placebo controlled trial. *Ann Rheum Dis.* 2004;63(11): 1460–1469.
8. Small LN. Suppurative tenosynovitis and septic bursitis. *Infect Dis Clin North Am.* 2005;19(4): 991–1005, xi.
9. McFarland EG. Miscellaneous conditions about the elbow in athletes. *Clin Sports Med.* 2004;23(4): 743–763, xi–xii.

MISCELLANEOUS
See also: Tendinitis

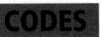 CODES

ICD9-CM
727.3 Other bursitis

ICD10

PATIENT TEACHING

 See Corresponding Diagnostic Algorithm

 See Patient Handout on CD

CANDIDIASIS

Brock D. Lutz, MD
Ronald A. Greenfield, MD

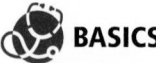 BASICS

DESCRIPTION

Candida albicans and related species cause a variety of infections

- Cutaneous syndromes include erosio interdigitalis blastomycetica, folliculitis, balanitis, intertrigo, paronychia, onychomycosis, diaper rash, perianal candidiasis, and the syndromes of chronic mucocutaneous candidiasis.
- Mucous membrane infections include oral candidiasis (thrush), esophagitis, and vaginitis.
- The most serious manifestations of candidiasis are candidemia and hematogenously disseminated invasive candidiasis.

The remainder of this chapter discusses candidemia and hematogenously disseminated candidiasis.

GENERAL PREVENTION

- Polyenes, azoles, and echinocandins reduce the incidence of candidiasis in patients undergoing induction therapy for acute leukemia or bone marrow or stem cell transplantation. (4)[A]
- Fluconazole prophylaxis in high-risk ICU patients reduces the incidence of invasive candidiasis. (6)[A]

EPIDEMIOLOGY

- Predominant age: All ages are susceptible to hematogenously disseminated candidiasis; premature neonates are at particularly high risk.
- Predominant sex: Male = Female (hematogenously disseminated candidiasis)

Incidence

≥20/100,000 persons per year

RISK FACTORS

- Neutropenia
- Corticosteroid treatment
- HIV infection
- Diabetes mellitus
- Mucocutaneous colonization/infection
- Broad-spectrum antibacterial chemotherapy
- Indwelling intravascular access devices
- Cardiothoracic or abdominal surgery
- Parenteral nutrition
- Prolonged hospital stay
- ICU stay
- Burns
- Premature birth

PATHOPHYSIOLOGY

An acute suppurative infection in which polymorphonuclear host defense is the critical element.

ETIOLOGY

- *Candida albicans* is the most frequent pathogen. Other important human pathogens include *C. tropicalis, C. krusei, C. stellatoidea, C. pseudotropicalis, C. guilliermondi, C. parapsilosis, C. lusitaniae, C. rugosa, C. lambica,* and *C. glabrata.*

- *Candida* species colonize human mucocutaneous surfaces; most infections are endogenously acquired from this reservoir.
- Human-to-human transmission of *Candida* occurs in some settings.

ASSOCIATED CONDITIONS

See "Risk Factors."

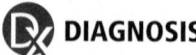 DIAGNOSIS

SIGNS AND SYMPTOMS

- Fever
- Malaise
- Tachycardia
- Hypotension
- Altered mental status
- Hepatosplenomegaly
- Maculopapular or nodular skin rash

ALERT

Pediatric Considerations

For an infant with thrush, be sure to also check for candidal diaper dermatitis. Also, there is often a concomitant infection.

TESTS

- The diagnosis is established by isolating the causative organism from blood cultures or other normally sterile body sites, or by demonstration of organisms in histopathologic specimens of normally sterile tissues.
- Isolation of *Candida* from multiple sites should raise the diagnostic suspicion of hematogenously disseminated invasive candidiasis.
- *Candida* species isolated from a normally sterile site should be identified to the species level. (4)[A]
- Because fluconazole-resistant *C. albicans* and particularly non-albicans species are reported with increasing frequency, fluconazole susceptibility testing should be performed before treatment with fluconazole. (4)[B]

Imaging

- Generally not specifically useful in diagnosis of hematogenously invasive disseminated candidiasis.
- In the syndrome of hepatosplenic candidiasis (chronic systemic candidiasis) imaging of the liver and spleen by liver scan, ultrasound, CT, or MRI may suggest this syndrome as the cause of persistent fever and liver dysfunction in patients who have recently recovered from neutropenia.

Diagnostic Procedures/Surgery

- If blood cultures remain consistently negative, aspiration or excisional biopsy of sites of focal infection may be useful in diagnosis.
- Aspiration and biopsy of skin lesions occasionally seen with hematogenously disseminated candidiasis are also useful.

Pathological Findings

Characteristic histopathology of lesions of Candida invasion of visceral organs is microabscess formation.

DIFFERENTIAL DIAGNOSIS

Includes a variety of cryptic bacterial infections and, in the neutropenic host, multiple opportunistic infections.

TREATMENT

Inpatient for hematogenously disseminated invasive candidiasis

GENERAL MEASURES

- Fluid and electrolyte therapy are often required.
- Hemodynamic and respiratory support may be required in seriously ill patients.
- The removal of potentially infected intravascular access devices is imperative.

Diet

No special diet

Activity

As tolerated

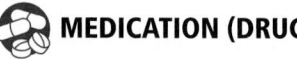 MEDICATION (DRUGS)

First Line

- Caspofungin

  - An initial therapy of choice for any patient with candidemia (4)[A].

  - Administer 70 mg IV dose on day 1 followed by 50 mg IV daily for 2 weeks after last positive sterile site culture if no evident metastatic infection
  - Modify dose for severe hepatic insufficiency.
  - *C. parapsilosis* has reduced sensitivity to echinocandins.

- Fluconazole

  - An initial therapy of choice for some patients (4)[A]

  - Because it is fungistatic rather than fungicidal, it should not be used for treatment of patients with severe neutropenia or severe immunosuppression.
  - It should only be used after confirmation of *in vitro* susceptibility in patients with azole therapy in prior 3 months
  - Should be used empirically only in institutions with a very low prevalence of resistance
  - Useful for switch therapy after demonstration of *in vitro* susceptibility after initial therapy with amphotericin or an echinocandin.
  - For 1st week, administer daily 400–800 mg intravenously, followed by additional IV or oral therapy at the same dose for ≥2 weeks after the last positive blood culture or last evidence of infection. Higher doses of fluconazole may be required if non-*albicans* species are known or suspected, because they carry a higher likelihood of drug resistance.
  - *C. krusei* and many *C. glabrata* are resistant to fluconazole.

- Liposomal amphotericin B
  - An initial therapy of choice for any patient with candidemia (4)[A]
  - Usual dosage is 3 mg/kg IV daily.
  - Substantially more expensive than conventional amphotericin B deoxycholate, but also substantially less toxic
    - *C. lusitaniae* may be resistant.
  - Consider higher doses for *C. krusei* or *C. glabrata* (5–10 mg/kg/day).

Second Line
- Although caspofungin is the only echinocandin approved by the FDA for this indication, preliminary data suggest that micafungin and anidulafungin have similar efficacy and safety for treatment of hematogenously disseminated invasive candidiasis. (B)
- Other azole antifungals depending on activity and safety (itraconazole and voriconazole). (B)
- Contraindications
  - The safety of amphotericin B therapy in pregnant patients has not been established.
  - Echinocandins are pregnancy category C.
- Precautions
  - Liposomal amphotericin B
    - The toxicity is less common than with conventional amphotericin B, but may still be formidable. Acute reactions (fever, rigors, and hypotension) may occur during the initiation of therapy. Ameliorate or eliminate by premedication with acetaminophen or ibuprofen. Use meperidine if needed to abort rigors.
    - Azotemia may occur; there may be an indication for reducing dose in some patients (to reduce toxicity). Maintenance of optimal fluid status and prevention of dehydration help minimize the risk of azotemia. "Sodium loading" with 77 mEq (77 mmol) sodium daily (= 1 L half-normal saline) may decrease renal toxicity.
    - Significant hypokalemia and renal tubular acidosis may develop. Significant hypomagnesemia may worsen hypokalemia.
    - Anemia commonly develops in patients on protracted therapy, but is almost always reversible.
    - Headache and phlebitis are common.
    - Leukopenia, thrombocytopenia, and liver function abnormalities are rarely encountered.

- Itraconazole, voriconazole, and caspofungin and other echinocandins do not enter the urinary stream in sufficient concentrations to treat UTIs.
- Significant possible drug-drug interactions
  - Caspofungin and other echinocandins
    - Potentially important interactions with carbamazepine, phenytoin, cyclosporine, tacrolimus, sirolimus, non-nucleoside reverse transcriptase inhibitors, and rifampin
  - Liposomal amphotericin B
    - Concomitant therapy with cyclosporine or other nephrotoxic agents, such as aminoglycosides or vancomycin, may increase the risk of amphotericin-induced nephrotoxicity.
  - Fluconazole and other azoles
    - Potentially important drug-drug interactions may occur in patients receiving oral hypoglycemics, coumarin-type anticoagulants, phenytoin, cyclosporine, rifampin, theophylline, or terfenadine or astemizole.
    - These drug-drug interactions are more likely with itraconazole and voriconazole than with fluconazole.

 FOLLOW-UP

Patients should receive followup visit approximately 6 weeks after end of therapy and be screened for metastatic infection complications by history and physical exam

PROGNOSIS
Overall mortality for patients with hematogenously disseminated candidiasis is 40–75%, with mortality attributable to candidemia being 15–37%.

COMPLICATIONS
- Systemic inflammatory response syndrome
- Pyelonephritis
- Endophthalmitis
- Endocarditis, myocarditis, pericarditis
- Arthritis, chondritis, osteomyelitis
- Pneumonitis
- Central nervous system infection

PATIENT MONITORING
- Evaluate CBC, serum electrolytes, and serum creatinine at least twice weekly in patients on liposomal amphotericin B therapy.
- If blood cultures are positive, they should be repeated until negative.

REFERENCES
1. Benjamin DK Jr., Stoll BJ, Fanaroff AA, et al. Neonatal candidiasis among extremely low birth weight infants: Risk factors, mortality rates, and neurodevelopmental outcomes at 18 to 22 months. *Pediatrics*. 2006;117:84–92.
2. Golan Y, Wolf MP, Pauker SG, Wong JB, Hadley S. Empirical anti-Candida therapy among selected patients in the intensive care unit: a cost-effectiveness analysis. *Ann Intern Med*. 2005;143:857–869.
3. Ostrosky-Zeichner L, Pappas PG. Invasive candidiasis in the intensive care unit. *Crit Care Med*. 2006;34:857–863.
4. Spellberg BJ, Filler SG, Edwards JE Jr. Current treatment strategies for disseminated candidiasis. *Clin Infect Dis*. 2006;42:244–251.
5. Uzon D, Anaissie EJ. Predictors of outcome in cancer patients with candidemia. *Am Oncol*. 2000;11:1517–1521.
6. Varadakas KZ, Samonis G, Michalopoulos A, et al. Antifungal prophylaxis with azole in high-risk, surgical intensive care unit patients: A meta-analysis of randomized, placebo-controlled trials. *Crit Care Med*. 2006;34:1216–1224.

 MISCELLANEOUS

- Other candidal infections
  - Intraperitoneal infection in patients with major abdominal surgery
  - Biliary tract candidiasis
  - Isolated lower UTI
- See also: Candidiasis; Mucocutaneous; Vulvovaginitis; Candidal

CODES

ICD9-CM
- 112.5 Candidiasis, disseminated
- 112.9 Candidiasis of unspecified site

PATIENT TEACHING
Advise patients of the nature of the infection and the toxicities associated with therapy.

 See Corresponding Diagnostic Algorithm

 See Patient Handout on CD

CANDIDIASIS, MUCOCUTANEOUS

Susan Louisa Montauk, MD

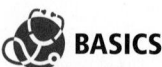

BASICS

DESCRIPTION
A mucocutaneous disorder caused by infection with various species of Candida. Areas include
- *Candida* vulvovaginitis: Vaginal mucosa and/or cutaneous aspects of the vulva
- *Candidal* Balanitis: Glans penis
- *Candidal* Paronychia: Nail bed of a digit
- Oropharyngeal candidiasis: Oral cavity (thrush) and/or pharynx
- *Candida* esophagitis: Esophagus (commonly associated with immunosuppression)
- Gastrointestinal candidiasis: Gastritis, sometimes with ulcers, usually associated with thrush; may affect the small and large bowel
- Angular cheilitis: Fissures at mouth corners
- System(s) Affected: Gastrointestinal; Skin/Exocrine; Genitourinary
- Synonym(s): Monilia; Thrush; Yeast

ALERT
Vaginal antifungal creams and suppositories can weaken condoms and diaphragms.

Pregnancy Considerations
- No known fetal complications of maternal *Candida*
- Miconazole is usually the drug of choice.

GENERAL PREVENTION
- Antibiotics may potentiate candidiasis.
- *Candida* overgrowth is more likely with pH changes from douching, chemicals (such as spermicides), or other vaginitides.
- Moist environments are conducive to overgrowth of *Candida*. Cotton underwear may help deter some *Candida* infections.

EPIDEMIOLOGY
- Common in the United States, very common in with immunodeficiency and/or uncontrolled diabetes
- Predominant age
  - Infants and seniors for thrush and cutaneous infections (infant diaper rash)
  - Women of childbearing age predominate for vaginitis. It is uncommon to see prepubertal or postmenopausal yeast vaginitis because of atrophic changes in the vaginal wall.
- Predominant sex: Female > Male (because of vaginitis)

Incidence
Not well studied, but some estimate 50/100,000

Prevalence
Candida colonizes more than 1/2 of U.S. population

RISK FACTORS
- Immunosuppression (includes chronic medications such as corticosteroids and immune modulators for transplants or rheumatologic dz
- Antibacterial therapy
- Douches, chemical irritants, and other vaginitides can predispose to yeast vaginitis
- Dentures
- Birth control pills
- Hyperglycemia

Genetics
- *Chronic mucocutaneous candidiasis* is a heterogeneous, genetic syndrome that usually presents in childhood, but it's mode of inheritance has not been clarified.

- Family analysis has identified an isolated form of mucocutaneous candidiasis, as well as its chromosomal region, which affects nails only.

ETIOLOGY
C. albicans and, less frequently, *C. tropicalis*

ASSOCIATED CONDITIONS
- HIV and other leukopenias
- Diabetes mellitus
- Cancer and other immunosuppressive disorders
- Disorders that call for steroids (oral or intranasal) (1) and other immunosuppressive chemotherapy

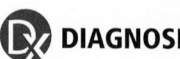

DIAGNOSIS

NOTE: Candida is normally present, in very small amounts, in the oral cavity, gastrointestinal tract, and female genital tract.

SIGNS AND SYMPTOMS
- In children
  - Oral: White, raised, painless, distinct patches within the mouth
  - Perineal: Erythematous maculopapular rash with white "satellite" pustules
  - Angular cheilitis—painful fissures in mouth corners
- In adults: Vulvovaginal lesions; thin to thick whitish "cottage cheese-like" discharge; erythematous patches in the vagina or on the perineum; symptoms range from none to intense pruritus with "burning" irritation
- In immunocompromised hosts
  - Oral lesions: White, raised, painless, distinct patches; erythematous, slightly raised patches; thick, dark-brownish coating; deep fissures
  - Esophagitis: Dysphagia, odynophagia, retrosternal pain; usually associated with thrush
  - Gastrointestinal symptoms: Ulcerations, pain
  - Balanitis: Erythema, linear erosions, scaling
  - Angular cheilitis (see "In children")

TESTS
Lab
- Potassium hydroxide 10% microscopic slide preparation (KOH prep): Breaks down epithelial cell walls; allows yeast forms to be visualized
  - Best if heated
  - Lack of slide identification does not rule out
  - A scant number of fungal forms without symptoms does not imply pathogenesis
- Culture: Blood or Sabouraud agar is present; a positive test may be the result of normal flora.
- Drugs that may alter lab results
  - Douches and spermicides
  - Inadequately dosed antifungal medications
- Disorders that may alter lab results: Other vaginitides (may obscure vaginal slide findings)

Imaging
Barium swallow—esophageal candidiasis may reveal a "cobblestone" appearance, fistulas or esophageal dilatation (from denervation)

Diagnostic Procedures/Surgery
- KOH prep—a sample of the discharge or "coating" of the infected area or ulcer is needed.

- Esophagitis may require an endoscopic biopsy.
- HIV seropositivity plus thrush with dysphagia relieved by antifungal treatment is acceptable criteria for the diagnosis of *Capital* esophagitis.

Pathological Findings
Slide preparation: Mycelia (hyphae) or pseudomycelia (pseudohyphae) yeast forms; *Candida* does not induce a heightened polymorphonuclear leukocyte response

DIFFERENTIAL DIAGNOSIS
- Baby formula can mimic thrush.
- Hairy leukoplakia—does not rub off to erythematous base; usually on lateral tongue.
- Bacterial vaginitis
- Angular Cheilitis from vitamin B or iron deficit, other microbes, or edentulous "over" closure
- Symptoms of *Trichomonas vaginalis* that are similar to those of *Candida* vaginalis include
  - Initial symptoms appearing postmenstrually
  - Marked vulvar irritation
  - Labial erythema
  - External dysuria
  - Vaginal tenderness
- Iron deficiency and staph infections can mimic angular cheilitis

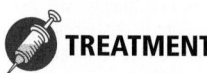

TREATMENT

GENERAL MEASURES
Screen both well infants and patients with severe immunodeficiency at routine visits.

Diet
A few authorities say rectal colonization may be decreased with active-culture yogurt or other live lactobacillus; evidence is not yet strong.

Complementary and Alternative Medicine
Probiotics—certain gut bacteria, in particular species of Lactobacillus and Bifidobacterium, may exert beneficial effects in the oral cavity by inhibiting cariogenic streptococci and *Candida sp.* (2)

MEDICATION (DRUGS) (3,4,5) [A,B]

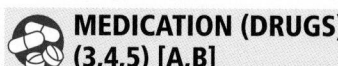

First Line
Vaginal (choose one):
- **Miconazole** (Monistat) 2% cream: One applicator or one 100–200 mg suppository, intravaginally q.h.s. × 7 days
- **Clotrimazole** (Gyne-Lotrimin, Mycelex): Intravaginal tablets (100 mg q.h.s. × 6–7 days, 200 mg q.h.s. × 3 days; 500 mg daily × 1), or 1% cream (one applicator q.h.s. × 6–7 days)
- **Nystatin** (Mycostatin, Nilstat): 100,000 U/g cream (one applicator) or 100,000 U tablets (one tablet) intravaginally 1 × day × 7–14 days
- **Fluconazole** (Diflucan): 150 mg tablet × 1

Oropharangeal
- **Clotrimazole** (Mycelex): 10 mg troche, suck on over 20 minutes 5 × day × 7–14 days*
- **Nystatin pastilles**: 1–2 q.i.d. × 7–14 days*

*Two days after disappearance of thrush

C

Esophagitis
Fluconazole:100 mg/d × 14–21 days, load w/200 mg)
Itraconazole (Sporanox)

- Solution: 1–200 mg daily × 7–14 days
- Capsules: 200 mg/d (take with food) × 2–3 weeks

Gastrointestinal
Therapy not well defined

- Contraindications
  - Vaginal antifungal creams and suppositories can decrease protective aspects of condoms and diaphragms.
  - Any drug is contraindicated if it causes a severe allergic response or severe adverse reaction.
  - Ketoconazole, itraconazole, or nystatin (if swallowed): Severe hepatotoxicity
  - Amphotericin B: Renal failure
- Precautions
  - Miconazole: Usually pregnancy drug of choice
  - Fluconazole: Renal excreted; rare hepatotoxicity; resistance has often been noted
  - Itraconazole: Doubling the dosage results in ~3-fold increase in itraconazole plasma concentrations.
- Possible interactions (rarely seen with creams, lotions, or suppositories)
  - Fluconazole
    - Rifampin: Decreased fluconazole concentrations
    - Tolbutamide: Decreased tolbutamide concentrations
    - Warfarin, phenytoin, cyclosporine: Altered metabolism; check levels
- Itraconazole: This potent cytochrome P450 3A4 isoenzyme system (CYP3A4) inhibitor may increase plasma concentrations of the many drugs metabolized by that pathway and cause serious cardiovascular events. Carefully assess all co-administered medications.

Second Line
Oropharyngeal

- **Nystatin oral suspension** (100,000 U/mL): Children: 5–10 mL q.i.d. × 10 days directly to oral lesions); Adults: Swish "for as long as reasonable" and swallow 5–10 mL q.i.d. × 14 days); prophylaxis = above dosages 2–5 × day.
- **Fluconazole**: 100 mg/d × 7–14 days (load immunocompromised patient with 200 mg)
- **Itraconazole** (Sporanox) Suspension: 200 mg (20 mL) daily swish and swallow × 7–14 days* Capsules: 200 mg/d (take with food) × 2–4 wks*
- **Amphotericin B** (Fungizone) oral suspension (100 mg/mL): 1 mL q.i.d., swish "for as long as reasonable" and swallow; use between meals
- **Ketoconazole**: 200–400 mg PO daily for 14–21 days

Esophagitis: Amphotericin B (variable dosing)
Vaginal:

- Terconazole (Terazol), particularly for recurrent cases that may involve imidazole resistance: 0.4% cream (one applicator intravaginally q.h.s. × 7 days); 0.8% cream/80 mg suppositories (1 applicator or 1 suppository intravaginally q.h.s. × 3 days)
- Itraconazole 200 mg capsule 1 b.i.d. × 1 day
- Any of the antifungal creams or suppositories can be tried every month for a few days near menses to help curb recurrent infections.

*Two days after disappearance of thrush

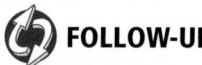 **FOLLOW-UP**

DISPOSITION
Issues for Referral

- Patients without obvious reasons for recurrent superficial candidal infections (e.g., HIV, diabetes) may have chronic mucocutaneous candidiasis.
- GI candidiasis

PROGNOSIS
For immunocompetent individuals, a benign course and excellent prognosis are the norm. In immunosuppressed persons, *Candida* may become an "AIDS-defining illness" by the Centers for Disease Control and Prevention criteria and chronicity may cause much morbidity.

COMPLICATIONS

- Major complications rarely develop in immunocompetent persons.
- In immunosuppressed persons, complications depend on the severity of the immune status. Moderate immunosuppression (e.g., CD4 200–500 cells/mm^3) may be associated with chronic candidiasis. In severe immunosuppression (e.g., CD4 <100 cells/mm^3), thrush may lead to esophagitis, then a full-systemic infection involving every organ system, particularly renal.

PATIENT MONITORING
Immunocompromised persons may benefit from regular symptom evaluation plus "routine" KOH preps during vaginal and oral exams.

REFERENCES

1. Kyrmizakis DE, et al. Acute candidiasis of the oro- and hypopharynx as the result of topical intranasal steroids administration. *Rhinology*. 2000;38(2):87–89.
2. Strus M. et al. The in vitro activity of vaginal Lactobacillus with probiotic properties against Candida. *Infect Dis Obstet Gynecol*. 2005;13(2):69–75.
3. Rex JH, et al. Practice guidelines for the treatment of candidiasis. Infectious Diseases Society of America. *Clin Infect Dis*. 2000;30(4):662–678. Epub 2000 Apr 20.
4. Eggimann P, Garbino J, Pittet D. Management of Candida species infections in critically ill patients. *Lancet Infect Dis*. 2003;3(12):772–785. Review.
5. Pappas PG, et al. Guidelines for treatment of candidiasis. *Clin Infect Dis*. 2004;38:161–189.
6. Friedlander SF, Rueda M, Chen BK, Caceres-Rios, HW. Fungal, protozoal, and helminthic infections. In: Schachner LA, Hansen RC, eds. *Pediatric Dermatology*. Edinburgh: Mosby; 2003:1093.

ADDITIONAL READING

- Betts RF, et al. *A Practical Approach to Infectious Diseases*. Boston, MA: Little, Brown & Co; 2002.
- Kauffman CL, Barnhill RL, eds. Fungal infections. In: *Textbook of Dermatopathology*, New York, NY: McGraw-Hill; 2004.

 MISCELLANEOUS

- Other notes
  - Transmission from person to person is rare.
  - Occasionally *Candida* vaginitis may be sexually transmitted.
  - Rarely, oral *Candida* leukoplakia may be precancerous.
  - Skin testing is positive in 70–85% of individuals randomly checked in studies.
- See also: Candidiasis; HIV Infection; AIDS; Vulvovaginitis; Candidal

CODES

ICD9-CM

- 112.0 Candidiasis of mouth
- 112.1 Candidiasis of vulva and vagina
- 112.9 Candidiasis of unspecified site

PATIENT TEACHING

- Advise patients at risk for recurrence about antibacterial therapy overgrowth 1[B]

- Inform appropriate patients of over-the-counter vaginitis medications and their use or contraindication during pregnancy.

Diet
Daily ingestion of live lactobacillus may decrease candida colonization by increasing healthy flora in the GI tract.

 See Corresponding Diagnostic Algorithm

CARBON MONOXIDE POISONING

Felix B. Chang, MD

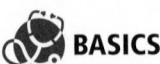 **BASICS**

DESCRIPTION
- Carbon Monoxide (CO) is the leading cause of poisoning death in the us CO is an odorless, tasteless, colorless, gas, produced by combustion of carbon-containing compounds.
- CO inhalation leads to displacement of oxygen from binding sites on hemoglobin.
- CO has about 250 times the affinity for hemoglobin that oxygen has.
- Detrimental effects are related to tissue hypoxia from decreased oxygen content and a shift of the oxyhemoglobin dissociation curve to the left.
- CO binds to cytochrome oxidase, impairing mitochondrial function and to cytochrome oxidase, affecting muscle function.
- CO binding to myoglobin affects muscle activity.
- System(s) Affected: Cardiovascular; Musculoskeletal; Nervous

ALERT
Tissue hypoxia includes the fetus. CO poisoning may cause significant fetal abnormalities, depending on the developmental stage. However, adult hemoglobin holds to oxygen less tightly than does fetal hemoglobin. Therefore, a pregnant mother potentially may be unaffected while the fetus is affected.

EPIDEMIOLOGY
- 40,000 emergency department visits annually
- 5,000 to 6,000 deaths annually in the US
- Inadvertent CO poisoning likely causes 500 deaths annually.
- Unintended poisoning is most common during winter month in cold climates.
- 10,000 individuals miss 1 or more days of work due to CO poisoning.

RISK FACTORS
- Cigarette smoking
- Smoke inhalation
- Being in a closed space with a faulty furnace or stove or running engine
- Employment in coal mine, as an auto mechanic, paint stripper, or in the solvent industry
- Improper vented fuel-burning devices
  - Kerosene heaters, charcoal grills, camping stoves, gasoline-power generators, wood stoves
  - Open air exposure to motorboat exhaust
  - Underground utility electrical cable fires

PATHOPHYSIOLOGY
- CO is rapidly absorbed in lungs.
- CO binds to hemoglobin to form carboxyhemoglobin (COHb), resulting in impaired oxygen carrying capacity, utilization, and delivery.
  - Leftward shift of the oxyhemoglobin dissociation curve occurs.
  - CO interferes with peripheral oxygen utilization by inactivating cytochrome oxidase.
- Delayed neurologic sequelae, probably involves lipid peroxidation by toxic oxygen species generated by xanthine oxidase.

- The half-life of CO while the patient is breathing room air is ~300 minutes, while breathing high-flow oxygen via a nonrebreathing face mask is ~90 minutes, and with 100 % hyperbaric oxygen is ~30 minutes.

ETIOLOGY
- CO inhalation
- Inhaled or ingested methylene chloride (from paint remover) (dichloromethane) is metabolized to CO by the liver, causing CO toxicity in the absence of ambient CO.

ASSOCIATED CONDITIONS
CO and cyanide poisoning can occur simultaneously following smoke inhalation (synergistic effect).

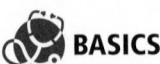 **DIAGNOSIS**

- Acute CO poisoning is suggestive by history, physical examination, and an elevated COHb
- Chronic CO intoxication is difficult to diagnose.
- Pulse oximetry cannot screen for CO exposure, because it does not differentiate carboxyhemoglobin from oxyhemoglobin.

PRE HOSPITAL
Patients often present in clusters, with similar symptoms and a common environment.

SIGNS AND SYMPTOMS
- Headaches
- Tinnitus
- Nausea
- Dizziness
- Weakness
- Confusion
- Fatigue
- Flushing
- Vomiting
- Central nervous system depression
- Syncope
- Angina
- Tachycardia
- Tachypnea
- Cardiac dysrhythmias
- Nystagmus
- Ataxia
- Seizures
- Coma
- Diarrhea
- Cardiopulmonary arrest

Physical Exam
- A careful neurologic examination is crucial.
- In absence of trauma or burns, look for altered mental status.
- "Cherry red" appearance of the lips and skin
- Impaired judgment, respiratory depression, arrhythmias, hypotension
- Cyanosis
- Visual field defects, blindness, papilledema

TESTS
Lab
- Measurement of COHb.
- Check CO level via co-oximetry of arterial or venous blood.
- Check acid-base status on blood gas.
- EKG in all patients
- Cardiac enzymes in
  - ≥ 65 years
  - Patient with cardiac risk factors
  - Younger patients with chest pain or symptoms suggestive of ischemia

Imaging
Head CT scan is helpful to rule out other causes of neurologic decompensation.

Pathological Findings
Hemorrhagic infarction of the globus pallidus and deep white matter have been reported (rare).

DIFFERENTIAL DIAGNOSIS
- Cyanide toxicity
- Acute viral syndrome
- Other causes of mental status changes: Metabolic, drugs, infectious, trauma

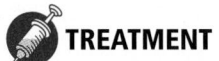 ## TREATMENT

INITIAL STABILIZATION
- ED for mild poisoning
- Inpatient treatment for moderate or severe poisoning

GENERAL MEASURES
- Removal from offending source
- Rapid reduction in tissue hypoxia with 100% oxygen to reduce the half-time of elimination of CO to 40 minutes
- Supportive care as necessary
- Intubation and mechanical ventilation may be necessary for severe intoxication.
- Volume resuscitation

Activity
Rest until carboxyhemoglobin reduced and symptoms abate

SPECIAL THERAPY
- 100% oxygen by tight-fitting nonrebreathing mask
- Hyperbaric oxygen for severe poisoning
- For mild poisoning (carboxyhemoglobin levels <30%); no signs or symptoms of cardiovascular or neurologic dysfunction
  - Treatment: Admission if carboxyhemoglobin >25%
  - Symptomatic medication for headache
  - 100% oxygen by nonrebreathing mask until carboxyhemoglobin <5%
  - Patients with underlying heart disease should be admitted regardless of level of carboxyhemoglobin.
- For moderate poisoning (carboxyhemoglobin 30–40%); no signs or symptoms of cardiovascular or neurologic dysfunction
  - Treatment: Admission
  - Cardiovascular status should be followed closely, even in the absence of clear cardiac effects.
  - Determination of acid–base status: Corrected by oxygen
  - 100% oxygen by nonrebreathing mask until carboxyhemoglobin <5%
- For severe poisoning (carboxyhemoglobin >40%); cardiovascular or neurologic functional impairment at any carboxyhemoglobin level
  - Treatment: Admission
  - Cardiovascular function monitoring
  - Acid–base status monitoring
  - 100% oxygen by nonrebreathing mask until carboxyhemoglobin <5%
  - Hyperbaric oxygen immediately if available; if unavailable, treat as in moderate poisoning
  - If no improvement occurs in cardiovascular or neurologic function within 4 hours, transport the patient to the nearest facility with hyperbaric oxygen, regardless of distance.

 ## MEDICATION (DRUGS)

First Line
- Institution of 100% oxygen by high-flow mask or endotracheal tube
- 100% normobaric oxygen for all suspected victims of CO poisoning, regardless of pulse oximetry or arterial Po$_2$ (1)[B].

 ## FOLLOW-UP

DISPOSITION
Admission Criteria
Patients whose symptoms do not resolve, who demonstrate ECG or laboratory evidence of severe poisoning, or who have other medical or social cause of concern should be hospitalized.

Discharge Criteria
Patient with mild symptoms from accidental poisoning can be managed in the ED and safely discharged.

PROGNOSIS
Most survivors recover completely, with only a minority developing chronic neuropsychiatric impairment.

COMPLICATIONS
- Myocardial infarction
- Pulmonary edema (CHF)
- Pneumonia (aspiration)
- Anoxic encephalopathy
- Long-term neuropsychiatric complications
  - Intellectual deterioration
  - Memory impairment
- Dysrhythmia
- Shock
- Rhabdomyolysis, personality changes
  - Irritability
  - Aggressiveness
  - Violence
  - Moodiness

ALERT
Geriatric Considerations
- Higher incidence of cardiovascular and neurologic disease, increasing complications.
- Atherosclerosis with chronic exposure

PATIENT MONITORING
- Measurement of carboxyhemoglobin levels
- Arterial blood gases
- Psychiatric evaluation and follow-up for intentional exposure

REFERENCES

1. Hampson NB, Scott KL, Zmaeff JL. Carboxyhemoglobin measurement by hospitals: Implications for the diagnosis of carbon monoxide poisoning. *J Emerg Med.* 2006;31:13.
2. Kao LW, Nanagas KA. Carbon monoxide poisoning. *Emerg Med Clin North Am.* 2004;22:985.
3. Satran D, Henry CR, Adkinson C, et al. Cardiovascular manifestations of moderate to severe carbon monoxide poisoning. *J Am Coll Cardiol.* 2005;45:1513.

ADDITIONAL READING
- Internet resources available at: www.cpsc.gov.
- Insufficient evidence to establish usefulness of hyperbaric oxygen for carbon monoxide poisoning. Cochrane Library 2005;1:CD002041.
- Juurlink D, Buckley N, Stanbrook M, et al. Hyperbaric oxygen for carbon monoxide poisoning. Cochrane Database Syst Rev 2005;CD002041.

 ## MISCELLANEOUS

CODES

ICD9-CM
986 Toxic effect of carbon monoxide

PATIENT TEACHING
Professional installation and maintenance of combustion devices1-800-638-2772; Consumer Products Safety Commission hotline

Activity
Rest until symptoms abate

Prevention
- CO detectors
- Public education
- Appropriate ventilation of areas with devices
- Determination of the mechanism of exposure is critical in cases of accidental poisoning in order to limit the risk

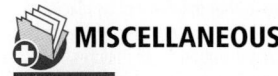 **See Corresponding Diagnostic Algorithm**

CARDIAC ARREST

Bobby Peters, MD, FAAEM

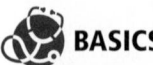

BASICS

DESCRIPTION
- Absence of effective mechanical cardiac activity
- This section is not a substitute for an American Heart Association–approved Advanced Cardiac Life Support (ACLS) course and is intended only as a quick reference.
- Synonym(s): Code Blue

ALERT
Geriatric Considerations
Poor risk for survival and long-term outcome

Pediatric Considerations
Bradycardia is the most common initial form of cardiac arrest. Most frequently, it is a response to underlying pulmonary disease and hypoxia. Adequate oxygenation and ventilation are especially important.

Pregnancy Considerations
- Displace the uterus either manually or by placing a rolled towel or pad under the right hip. If the patient cannot be resuscitated within 5–15 minutes, consider emergency C-section to relieve uterine obstruction and increase blood return to the heart. This may also be done to save the fetus if at a viable age.
- Consider amniotic fluid embolism or eclampsia-related seizures as precipitating factors.

GENERAL PREVENTION
Treat underlying disease

EPIDEMIOLOGY
- Predominant age: Increases with age
- Predominant sex: Male > Female

Prevalence
In the United States: 200:100,000 (per year)

RISK FACTORS
- Male gender
- Increasing age
- Hypercholesterolemia
- Hypertension
- Cigarette smoking
- Family history of atherosclerosis
- Diabetes

ETIOLOGY
- Asystole (confirm in two leads; 11% actually fine ventricular fibrillation [VF])
- VF
- Pulseless ventricular tachycardia (VT)
- Pulseless electrical activity (PEA, previously known as electrical mechanical dissociation [EMD])

ASSOCIATED CONDITIONS
- Coronary artery disease (cardiac arrest may be first presenting symptom)
- Valvular heart disease
- Hypertension

DIAGNOSIS

SIGNS AND SYMPTOMS
- Loss of consciousness secondary to central nervous system hypoperfusion
- Absence of pulses in large arteries
- Apnea or agonal breathing
- Cyanosis or pallor

History
Find out how patient coded
- Witness or unwitnessed?
- Seizure activity?
- History or risk factors?

Physical Exam
- Check pupils: Dilated may indicate drug overdose
- Check pulse, hydration status, diaphoretic? (i.e., reasons for tachycardia)
- Check lungs (i.e., did person have respiratory decline before cardiac decline?)

TESTS
ECG

Lab
- Arterial blood gases
- Electrolytes
- CBC
- Drug levels (check toxicology screen, Tylenol level, also digoxin level or antiepileptic levels of history of specific medication use, etc.)
- Prothrombin time (international normalized ratio), partial thromboplastin time, type, and cross, if indicated
- Lab results may be altered by
  – Digoxin toxicity: May cause hyperkalemia
  – Hypo- or hyperventilation: Changes oxygen partial pressure and carbon dioxide partial pressure
  – Acidosis: Increases serum potassium

Imaging
Chest radiograph for endotracheal tube (ET) placement, pneumothorax; consider echocardiogram for pericardial effusion

Diagnostic Procedures/Surgery
- If PEA secondary to tamponade, may need paracardiocentesis
- If coding, probably needs airway intubation
- May need central line for IV access
- May need chest tube for pneumothorax

Pathological Findings
Based on underlying cause

DIFFERENTIAL DIAGNOSIS
- Adverse reaction to drugs: Barbiturates, narcotics, calcium channel blockers, beta-blockers, and tricyclic antidepressants
- Shock: Septic or blood-loss induced
- Hypothermia
- Pulmonary embolism
- Cardiac tamponade
- Pneumothorax
- Acidosis
- Electrolyte abnormality
- Carbon monoxide poisoning

TREATMENT

INITIAL STABILIZATION
- Prehospital emergency medical service personnel, ED, "cardiac arrest team," intensive care setting
- If response time is >5 minutes, improved outcome noted in patients when CPR started before defibrillation in Vfib. (1)[A]

GENERAL MEASURES
- Perform defibrillation 1st
  – Adults: 200, 300, or 360 J
  – Children: Use largest paddles that will fit on child, even adult size if good contact can be achieved.
  – Defibrillate at 2 J/kg once. Increase to 4 J/kg twice.
- Administer 100% oxygen by bag-valve-mask or ET (preferred)
- Start 2 IV lines as close to the heart as possible (central line okay, but do not waste time). Large-bore peripheral lines can deliver fluid more quickly than a central line, especially important in PEA secondary to hypovolemia.
- Perform CPR, including closed-chest compression. Intermittent abdominal compression and active compression/decompression show no survival advantage.
- Keep patient, especially a child, warm if possible.
- Monitor pulse after 3 initial defibrillations. Check monitor between each defibrillation and after any intervention.
- Use an end-tidal CO_2 monitor to assess gas exchange, if available. Esophageal intubation will produce a very low end-tidal CO_2 and requires proper reintubation.

MEDICATION (DRUGS)

First Line
- Lidocaine, atropine, naloxone, and epinephrine may all be given by ET. Follow with 10 mL of normal saline or sterile water, followed by bagging.
- Epinephrine: 1 mL = 1 mg (1:1,000); 1 mL = 0.1 mg (1:10,000)
- Adults: VT and pulseless VT. Use in order listed below
  - Defibrillate (nonsynchronized setting) 3 times at 200, 300, and 360 J.
    - Check monitor rhythm.
    - Follow each drug administration with repeated defibrillation at 360 J.
    - Check monitor and pulses after each subsequent intervention.
- Epinephrine: 1 mg IV every 3–5 minutes or a vasopressin 40 U IV single dose, 1 time only; may choose to resume epinephrine if no response after a single dose of vasopressin (high-dose epinephrine is permissible, but discouraged and may actually worsen outcomes).
- Amiodarone: 300 mg IV push may be used prior to lidocaine
- Lidocaine: 1.5 mg/kg IV, repeat in 5 minutes to total dose of 3 mg/kg
- Magnesium sulfate: 1–2 mg IV in suspected torsades de pointes or refractory VF/VT
- Procainamide: 30 mg per minute IV in refractory VF/VT (maximum dose: 17 mg/kg) is permissible. However, because the time to a useful level by infusion is so long, it is discouraged and is unlikely to be of any benefit. No improvement in survival to discharge.
- Bicarbonate: 1 mEq/kg IV only in known preexisting bicarbonate-responsive acidosis or to alkalinize the urine in known tricyclic overdose

Adults: Asystole
- CPR
- Confirm in 2 leads.
- Consider possible causes, including hypoxia, hyperkalemia, hypokalemia, preexisting acidosis, drug overdose, and hypothermia.
- Consider defibrillation, as for VT/VF, since VF may be mistaken for asystole.
- Consider immediate transcutaneous pacing.
- Epinephrine: 1 mg IV push repeated q3–5min; may use intermediate-dose or high-dose epinephrine (2–5 mg IV or 0.1 mg/kg IV) q3–5min
- Atropine: 1 mg IV push q3–5min to total dose of 0.04 mg/kg; shorter atropine dosing intervals acceptable (q1–2min)
- Consider termination of efforts if no reversible underlying cause is found.

For Pulseless Electrical Activity
- Includes EMD, idioventricular rhythms, ventricular escape rhythms, bradycardic-asystolic rhythms, and postdefibrillation idioventricular rhythms
- Assess blood flow by Doppler ultrasound if available.
- Consider possible reversible causes: Cardiogenic shock (weak pump), cardiac tamponade, tension pneumothorax, severe hypovolemia, pulmonary embolism (consider thrombolytics), hypothermia, hypoxia, acidosis, hyperkalemia, or overdose of drugs such as beta-blockers, calcium channel blockers, tricyclics, and digoxin (pnemonic 5H and 5Ts).
- Epinephrine: 1 mg IV push and repeat q3–5min; may use intermediate-dose or high-dose epinephrine (2–5 mg IV or 0.1 mg/kg IV, respectively) q3–5min, but this shows no proven improvement in survival
- Atropine: 1 mg IV q3–5min to total dose of 0.04 mg/kg if absolute bradycardia (<60 beats per minute) or relative bradycardia; may decrease interval to 1–2min if desired

Children (drugs listed in alphabetical order):
- Amiodarone for pulseless VF/VT, 5 mg/kg IV or intraosseous (IO) rapid bolus; for perfusing tachyarrhythmias, loading dose of 5 mg/kg IV or IO over 20–60 minutes, maximum dose 15 mg/kg/d
- Atropine: 0.01–0.02 mg/kg per dose; minimum dose is 0.1 mg, maximum single dose is 0.5 mg in child, 1.0 mg in adolescent
- Epinephrine
  - For bradycardia: 0.01 mg/kg IV/IO or 0.1 mg/kg ET (1:1,000)
  - For asystolic or pulseless arrest: 1st dose is 0.01 to 0.03 mg/kg IV/IO. Doses as high as 0.2 mg/kg may be effective.
  - Infusion: 0.1 μg/kg per minute. Titrate to desired effect (0.1–1.0 μg/kg per minute).
- Lidocaine:
  - Bolus: 1 mg/kg per dose (maximum 3 mg/kg)
  - Infusion: 20–50 μg/kg per minute
- Sodium bicarbonate: 1 mEq/kg per dose or 0.3 × kg × base deficit; infuse slowly and only if ventilation is adequate
- Contraindications and precautions
  - There are contraindications during an arrest.
  - Calcium may be used if known (preexisting) hyperkalemia precipitated arrhythmia; calcium is contraindicated in hyperkalemia secondary to digoxin.
  - Magnesium is relatively contraindicated in renal failure, but given the consequences of not terminating rhythm; this is only a relative contraindication in this setting.

Second Line
Asystole: Aminophylline 250 mg IV bolus has been effective in uncontrolled trials, but should be used only when conventional therapy has failed.

SURGERY
If indicated
- Pericardiocentesis to treat cardiac tamponade
- Needle decompression (second intercostal space midclavicular line), then chest tube insertion to treat tension pneumothorax

 FOLLOW-UP

PROGNOSIS
- Outcome is related to underlying disease, age, duration of arrest, and other factors.
- Outcome is poor if
  - >4 minutes to CPR or >8 minutes to ACLS
  - Arrest occurs in field
  - Resuscitation effort >30 minutes
- About 14% survive in-hospital arrest, fewer after field arrest

COMPLICATIONS
- Significant neurologic, hepatic, renal, or cardiac ischemic injury
- Rib fractures or pneumothorax from CPR

PATIENT MONITORING
Intensive care setting on continuous monitor to look for precipitating cause, including serial ECGs and enzymes to rule out myocardial infarction

REFERENCES

1. Wik L, Hansen TB, Fylling F, et al. Delaying defibrillation to give basic cardiopulmonary resuscitation to patients with out-of-hospital ventricular fibrillation: A randomized trial. *JAMA.* 2003;289(11):1389–1395.
2. Graber MA. Emergency medicine. In: Graber MA, Lanternier ML, Graber M, eds. *The Family Practice Handbook.* St. Louis, MO: Mosby-Yearbook; 1997.
3. The American Heart Association in collaboration with the International Liaison Committee on Resuscitation. Guidelines 2000 for cardiopulmonary resuscitation and emergency cardiovascular care. *Circulation.* 2000;102(suppl 8):I95–I104.

 MISCELLANEOUS

Make sure patient is not listed as Do Not Resuscitate.

CODES

ICD9-CM
427.5 Cardiac arrest

PATIENT TEACHING

See Corresponding Diagnostic Algorithm

CARDIAC TAMPONADE

Keith Medeiros, MD

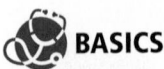 **BASICS**

DESCRIPTION

- Rapid or slow compression of cardiac chambers by pressure on the heart secondary to an increase in pericardial fluid.
- Tamponade can be acute or subacute depending on the etiology.
- As fluid accumulates, pressure primarily affects the compliant cardiac wall and transmits the pressure transmurally, resulting in increased ventricular pressure. This decreases ventricular filling and reduces cardiac output by reducing stroke volume.
- The compensatory mechanisms for tamponade are increased peripheral resistance, central venous pressure, and heart rate.
- In some patients, pulsus paradoxus (10 mm Hg drop in systolic blood pressure between inspiration and expiration) and equalization of pressures may not occur, the absence of which does not rule out tamponade.
- In patients with elevated left ventricular (LV) diastolic pressures (as with chronic hypertension), resistance to LV filling is constant. Throughout the cardiac cycle, equalization of pressures in these patients may only be noted in the right heart chambers, with LV pressures being higher than right ventricular (RV) pressures.
- Variants include low pressure and regional tamponade.
- System(s) Affected: Cardiovascular

RISK FACTORS

Cardiac tamponade should be suspected in the hemodynamically unstable patient

- With known pericarditis
- Following blunt or penetrating chest trauma
- Following open heart surgery or cardiac catheterization
- With known or suspected intrathoracic neoplasm
- With suspected dissecting aortic aneurysm
- With renal failure on dialysis

PATHOPHYSIOLOGY

Fluid accumulation in the pericardial space leading to compression of cardiac chambers as the heart has to compete with increased pericardial contents for the fixed intrapericardial space. Cardiac filling is reduced, limiting cardiac output and eventually causing hypotension and shock. This can occur rapidly in cases of acute tamponade, usually resulting from trauma or surgery, or over weeks to months with slowly developing effusions that allow the pericardial compliance to increase gradually (1)[A].

ETIOLOGY

- Uremia
- Neoplasm: Breast, lung, lymphoma, leukemia
- Occurs in <1% of fibrinolytic-treated acute MI and is associated with increased 30-day mortality (2)[A].
- Postoperative
- HIV
- Other viruses: Coxsackie group B, influenza, ECHO, herpes
- Bacterial infection: *Staphylococcus aureus*, *Mycobacterium tuberculosis*, *Streptococcus pneumoniae* (rare)
- Fungal infection: *Histoplasmosis capsulatum*
- Lupus and rheumatologic disease
- Trauma
- Placement of central venous catheter, pacer wires
- Hypothyroidism
- Drug effects

ASSOCIATED CONDITIONS

- Myocardial infarction
- Aortic aneurysm

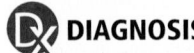 **DIAGNOSIS**

SIGNS AND SYMPTOMS

- Acute
  - Patients may complain of chest pain or dyspnea
  - Markedly elevated JVP
  - Signs of cardiogenic shock: Cyanosis, cool extremities, and oliguria
- Subacute
  - Most common complaints are intolerance to minimal activity and dyspnea. Agitation, central nervous system depression, coma, and cardiac arrest may develop later.

History

History of renal failure, surgery, neoplasm, or trauma

Physical Exam

- Beck triad: Distant heart sounds, hypotension, distended neck veins
- Narrow pulse pressure
- Pulsus paradoxus: >10 mm Hg drop in systolic blood pressure between inspiration and expiration
- Neck veins may be distended and reveal a rapid systolic (X) descent and attenuated or absent diastolic (Y) descent
- Tachycardia: A compensatory mechanism to maintain output
- Right upper quadrant tenderness due to hepatic engorgement
- Increased area of cardiac dullness outside the apical point of maximum impulse

TESTS

ECG

- May show sinus tachycardia, low-voltage QRS complexes, diffuse ST segment elevation, and PR segment depression of pericarditis
- Electrical alternans (QRS and/or R wave variation from beat to beat) seen in 10–20% of cases of tamponade; 50–60% of these are neoplastic in origin

Lab

- CBC
- Sedimentation rate
- Cardiac enzymes to rule out acute myocardial infarction
- Antinuclear antibodies
- Rheumatoid factor
- BUN/creatinine
- Pericardial fluid for culture of bacteria, fungus, mycobacteria, Gram stain, hematocrit, cell count, cytology, glucose, protein, rheumatoid factors, complement levels

Imaging

- Chest radiograph: May show enlargement of cardiac shadow (if >200 mL fluid present)
- Echocardiogram:
  - Diagnostic of cardiac compression
  - RA collapse is a sensitive sign of increased intrapericardial pressure but, diastolic RV collapse is more specific for tamponade (3,4)[A].
  - Doppler: May show respiratory variation in transvalvular flow velocities, LV ejection, and LV isovolumetric times (3,4)[A].

Diagnostic Procedures/Surgery

Right heart catheterization:

- Equalization (within 2–3 mm) of right atrial, pulmonary artery diastolic, pulmonary capillary wedge, left atrial, and left ventricular diastolic pressures
- The intracardiac diastolic pressure will approximate the intrapericardial pressure.
- The dip and plateau pattern of constriction or restriction pericardial disease is absent.
- Loss of Y descent on atrial waveform

Pathological Findings

Pericardial blood usually does not clot, but occasionally will.

DIFFERENTIAL DIAGNOSIS

- Tension pneumothorax
- Acute RV failure
- COPD
- Constrictive pericarditis
- Acute acceleration of chronic bronchitis
- Acute pulmonary embolus
- Fat embolus
- Excessive or rapid administration of fluids
- Abdominal distention from ascites or ileus
- Increased intrathoracic pressure from pneumothorax, hemothorax, airway obstruction, or mechanical ventilation
- Administration of vasopressors

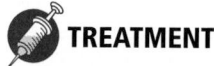 **TREATMENT**

INITIAL STABILIZATION
Inpatient

GENERAL MEASURES
- Maintain hemodynamic stability until definitive correction of the pericardial tamponade
- All patients should have BP, heart rate, and at a minimum, central venous pressure measurement every 15 minutes. Strong consideration should be given to placement of a Swan-Ganz catheter if time allows.
- Fluids may be of temporary benefit, but rising filling pressures may further compromise coronary perfusion

Diet
As tolerated

Activity
Bed rest

 MEDICATION (DRUGS)

Inotropic support with or without vasodilators is controversial partly due to maximal endogenous inotropic stimulation present during acute tamponade (1)[A].

SURGERY
Pericardiocentesis:
- Indications
  - Rapid deterioration of hemodynamic function
  - A delay in operation for traumatic effusion
  - Diagnosis
- If rapid reaccumulation is anticipated (as in malignancy), it may be helpful to insert a long-term drainage catheter. Also consider instillation of sclerosing agents.
- Surgery should be performed under the most optimal circumstances available, as the patient's condition allows.
- Blind pericardiocentesis should be performed only in life-threatening emergencies.
- Ideally, echocardiography can be brought to the bedside to assist in needle placement and progress of fluid removal.
- Invasive monitoring is also helpful to follow decrease in pericardial pressures.
- Fluoroscopy may also be used.
- ECG guidance using the "V" lead to avoid contact with the epicardium may be useful.
- 20% of patients with tamponade will have a negative tap because the pericardial sac contains coagulated material. Hemorrhagic pericardial effusions usually do not clot.

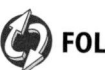 **FOLLOW-UP**

Follow-up echocardiography should be used to evaluate for recurrence of effusions (3,4)[A].

PROGNOSIS
Good results are expected with the appropriate treatment.

COMPLICATIONS
- Cardiac perforation and/or laceration at time of pericardiocentesis
- Pneumothorax at time of pericardiocentesis
- Constriction of pericardium

PATIENT MONITORING
Close monitoring until stable with telemetry to monitor for cardiac arrhythmia

REFERENCES

1. Spodck DH, Acute cardiac tamponade. *N Engl J Med* 2003 Aug 14;349(7):684–690.
2. Patel MR et al. Cardiac tamponade in the fibrinolytic era: Analysis of >100,000 patients with ST-segment elevation myocardial infarction. *Am Heart J* 2006 Feb;151(2):316–322.
3. Cheitlin MD, et al. ACC/AHA/ASE 2003 guideline update for the clinical application of echocardiography: Summary article: a report of the American College of Cardiology/American Heart Association Task Force on Practice Guidelines for the Clinical Application of Echocardiography, *Circulation*. 2003;108:1146.
4. Cheitlin MD, et al, *ACC/AHA Guidelines for the Clinical Application of Echocardiography. Circulation* 1997;95:1686–1744.

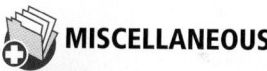 **MISCELLANEOUS**

CODES

ICD9-CM
423.9 Unspecified disease of pericardium

PATIENT TEACHING

 See Corresponding Diagnostic Algorithm

C

CARDIOMYOPATHY, END-STAGE

Tim Fitzgibbons, MD
Theo E. Meyer, MD, DPhil

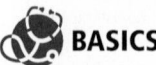 **BASICS**

DESCRIPTION

In 1995, the WHO defined cardiomyopathy as a "disease of the myocardium associated with cardiac dysfunction." They proposed a classification system based on pathophysiology. Each class may be caused by many disorders, and some disorders may overlap classes.

- Classification of cardiomyopathy
  - Dilated (*systolic*)
    - Characterized by dilation and reduced systolic function of one or both ventricles
  - Hypertrophic (*diastolic*)
    - Left and or right ventricular hypertrophy with normal to reduced end diastolic volumes
    - May include asymmetric septal hypertrophy
    - Cause of SCD in young athletes
  - Restrictive (*diastolic*)
    - Restrictive filling and reduced diastolic volume of either or both ventricles
    - Systolic function may be near normal
    - Etiology: Idiopathic, amyloidosis, etc.
  - Arrhythmogenic right ventricular (RV) dysplasia
    - Fibrofatty replacement of the RV
    - May present with arrhythmia or SCD in the young
  - Unclassified
    - Cases that do not fit easily into 1 group (i.e., non compacted myocardium)
  - Specific: Includes patients with cardiomyopathy in association with a known systemic disorder, for example
    - Ischemic
    - Valvular
    - Hypertensive
    - Inflammatory
    - Metabolic
    - Peripartum
- "End-stage" cardiomyopathy patients have "Stage D" heart failure, or severe symptoms at rest refractory to standard medical therapy.
- System(s) Affected: Cardiovascular; Renal

ALERT

Pediatric Considerations
Etiology: Idiopathic, viral, congenital heart disease, and familial.

Pregnancy Considerations
May occur in women postpartum

GENERAL PREVENTION
Reduce salt and water intake; home blood pressure measurement and a daily weight

EPIDEMIOLOGY
Predominant age: Ischemic cardiomyopathy is the most common etiology; predominantly patients >50 years. Consider uncommon causes in young.

Incidence
- 60,000 patients <65 die each year from end-stage heart disease.
- From 35,000–70,000 of the population might benefit from cardiac transplant or chronic support.

Prevalence
Most rapidly growing form of heart disease

RISK FACTORS
- Hypertension
- Hyperlipidemia
- Obesity
- Diabetes mellitus
- Smoking
- Physical inactivity
- Excessive alcohol intake
- Dietary sodium

Genetics
Hypertrophic, dilated cardiomyopathy, and arrhythmogenic RV dysplasia may present as familial syndromes with autosomal dominant inheritance.

ETIOLOGY
- Ischemic heart disease: Most common etiology; up to 66% of patients
- Hypertension
- Familial cardiomyopathies
- Congenital heart disease
- Peripartum/postpartum
- Toxic/metabolic causes
  - Alcoholism
  - Radiation
  - Beriberi
  - Kwashiorkor
  - Cobalt
  - Selenium deficiency
  - Hemosiderosis
  - Thyrotoxicosis
- Infectious causes
  - Viral (e.g., HIV, coxsackievirus)
  - Diphtheria
  - Toxoplasmosis
  - Trichinosis
  - Trypanosomiasis
  - Acute rheumatic fever
- Inherited disorders of metabolism
  - Glycogen storage disease
  - Pompe disease
  - Hurler syndrome
  - Hunter syndrome
  - Fabry disease
- Inherited neuromuscular disorders
  - Duchenne muscular dystrophy
  - Friedreich ataxia
- Drugs
  - Chemotherapy: Anthracyclines, cyclophosphamide, Herceptin
- Inflammatory causes
  - Giant cell myocarditis
  - Loeffler eosinophilia
  - Sarcoidosis
- Idiopathic
- Other causes
  - Tachycardia-mediated cardiomyopathy
  - Amyloidosis
  - Valvular heart disease
  - Endomyocardial fibrosis

DIAGNOSIS

SIGNS AND SYMPTOMS
- Dyspnea at rest or with exertion
- Paroxysmal nocturnal dyspnea
- Orthopnea
- Postprandial dyspnea
- Fatigue
- Syncope
- Tachypnea

Physical Exam
- Low pulse pressure
- Cool extremities
- Jugular venous distention
- Bibasilar rales
- Tachycardia
- S3 gallop
- Hepatosplenomegaly
- Ascites
- Edema

TESTS
- ECG: LV hypertrophy, interventricular conduction delay, atrial fibrillation, evidence of prior Q-wave infarction.
- Cardiopulmonary exercise testing: Maximal oxygen consumption <10 mL/kg/mm correlates with 50% 1-year mortality, and >18 mL/kg/mm correlates with >90% 1-year survival. Used in stable outpatients to estimate prognosis and prior to cardiac transplant referral.

Lab
- Hyponatremia
- Prerenal azotemia
- Anemia
- Elevated BNP or pro-BNP
- Mild hyperbilirubinemia
- Elevated liver function tests
- Elevated uric acid

Imaging
- Chest radiograph
  - Cardiomegaly
  - Increased vascular markings to the upper lobes
  - Pleural effusions may or may not be present
- ECG
  - In dilated cardiomyopathy 4-chamber enlargement and global hypokinesis are present.
  - In hypertrophic cardiomyopathy, severe left ventricular (LV) hypertrophy is present.
  - Segmental abnormalities in contraction of the LV are indicative of previous localized myocardial infarction.
- Cardiac MRI
  - May be useful to characterize particular nonischemic cardiomyopathies

Diagnostic Procedures/Surgery
Cardiac catheterization:

- Helpful to rule out ischemic heart disease
- PA catheters may be reasonable in patients with refractory HF to help guide management (3)[C].

DIFFERENTIAL DIAGNOSIS
- Severe pulmonary disease
- Primary pulmonary hypertension
- Recurrent pulmonary embolism
- Hypothyroidism
- Some advanced forms of malignancy

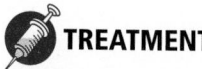 TREATMENT

GENERAL MEASURES
- Reduction of filling pressures
- Treatment of electrolyte disturbances

Diet
Low fat, low salt, fluid restriction

 MEDICATION (DRUGS)

First Line
- Systolic failure syndromes
  - ACE inhibitors
    - Lisinopril 5–40 mg/d or captopril 6.25–50 mg t.i.d. (3)[A]
  - Loop diuretics
    - May need to be given IV initially, and then orally as patient stabilizes
    - Furosemide 40–120 mg/d or t.i.d.(3)[A]
  - β-Blockers:
    - Use with caution in acutely decompensated or low cardiac output states
    - Metoprolol succinate 12.5–200 mg/d, carvedilol 3.125–25 mg b.i.d., or bisoprolol 1.25–10 mg/d (3)[A]
  - Aldosterone antagonists
    - Patients with NYHA III-IV CHF, EF<35%, on standard therapy
    - Spironolactone 12.5–25 mg/d (3)[A]
  - Digoxin 0.125–0.250 mg/d for symptomatic patients on standard therapy (3)[A]
  - BiDil (hydralazine/nitrates)
    - BiDil 1 tablet t.i.d is recommended in addition to standard treatment in African American patients with Class III–IV symptoms (3)[A]
- Diastolic failure
  - Few evidence-based therapies for diastolic heart failure. Empiric management goals include
    - Management of hypertension
    - Reduction of congestive states (i.e., diuretics)
    - Prevention of progression of LVH (i.e., RAAS blockade)
    - Maintenance of sinus rhythm

- Contraindications
  - β-Blockers: Low cardiac output, 1st- or 2nd-degree heart block
  - Aldosterone antagonists: Oliguria, anuria, renal dysfunction
  - Loop diuretics: Hypokalemia, hypomagnesemia
  - ACE inhibitors: Pregnancy, angioedema
- Precautions
  - In patients with CKD, digoxin dosage should be 0.125 mg/d, and drug levels followed carefully.
  - Closely monitor electrolytes
  - ACE inhibitors: Initiate with care if blood pressure is low. Begin with low-dose captopril, such as 6.25 mg t.i.d.
  - β-Blockers: Avoid in patients with evidence of poor tissue perfusion; they may further depress systolic function.
  - Milrinone, amrinone: Contraindicated for long-term use due to increased mortality

Second Line
- Nesiritide .01 mcg/kg/min IV for 48 hours in HF patients with dyspnea at rest (3)[C]
- Angiotensin receptor blockers as an alternative to, or in addition to ACE inhibitors

SPECIAL THERAPY
- Prophylactic ICD should be considered for patients with an LVEF <30% (3)[A].
- Biventricular pacing should be considered for patients with QRS interval >120 ms, LVEF <35%, and Class III CHF despite medical therapy(3)[A].

- Patients with severe, refractory HF with no reasonable expectation of improvement should not be considered for an ICD (3)[C].

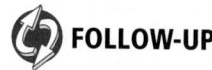 FOLLOW-UP

DISPOSITION
Issues for Referral
- Consider referral to a heart failure center.
- Management by a heart failure team improves outcomes and facilitates early transplant referral.

PROGNOSIS
20–40% of patients in New York functional class IV die within 1 year. With a transplant, a 1-year survival is as high as 94%.

COMPLICATIONS
Worsening congestive heart failure, syncope, arrhythmias, or sudden death

REFERENCES
1. Richardson P. Report of the 1995 WHO on the definition and classification of cardiomyopathies. *Circulation.* 1996;93:841–842.
2. Noria A, Stevenson LW. Medical management of advanced heart failure. *JAMA.* 2002;287:628–640.
3. Hunt SA, et al. ACC/AHA 2005 guideline update for the diagnosis and management of chronic heart failure in adults. *J Am Coll Cardiol.* 2005;46:1116–1143.

 MISCELLANEOUS

See also: Alcohol use disorders; Amyloidosis; Diabetes mellitus, type 1; Diabetes mellitus, type 2; Hypertension; Hypothyroidism, adult; Idiopathic hypertrophic subaortic stenosis; Malnutrition, protein-calorie; Rheumatic fever; Sarcoidosis

CODES

ICD9-CM
- 425.4 Other primary cardiomyopathies
- 425.5 Alcoholic cardiomyopathy

PATIENT TEACHING
See Corresponding Diagnostic Algorithm

CAROTID SINUS SYNDROME

Jeremy Golding, MD

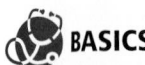 **BASICS**

DESCRIPTION

- In carotid sinus syndrome, stimulation of one or both of the hypersensitive carotid sinuses at the bifurcation of the common carotid arteries produces brief episodes of faintness or loss of consciousness. 4 types are described
  - Cardioinhibitory: Vagally mediated, causing bradycardia, sinus arrest, or atrioventricular block for >3 seconds
  - Vasodepressor: A sudden drop of peripheral vascular resistance leads to a >50 mm Hg decrease in systolic blood pressure (BP) without change in heart rate or to a >30 mm Hg symptomatic drop in systolic BP.
  - Mixed: Combined cardioinhibitory and vasodepressor changes
  - Cerebral: Extremely rare; carotid sinus hypersensitivity occurs without bradycardia or hypotension.
- System(s) Affected: Cardiovascular; Nervous
- Synonym(s): Hypersensitive carotid sinus syndrome; Carotid sinus syncope; Carotid sinus hypersensitivity

ALERT

Geriatric Considerations

- More likely to occur in elderly
- Associated with atheromata secondary to coronary artery disease. Should be considered in elderly patients with frequent falls.

GENERAL PREVENTION

- Avoidance of pressure on the neck
- Support hose may be helpful for some patients with vasodepressor type.

EPIDEMIOLOGY

- Predominant age: Elderly
- Predominant sex: Male > Female

Incidence

64 of 132 consecutive patients (48.5%) >65 evaluated for dizziness, falls, or syncope were found to have carotid sinus–type sensitivity.

RISK FACTORS

- Diffuse atherosclerosis
- Wearing tight collars
- Shaving over region of carotid sinus
- Emotional upheaval
- Head movement

ETIOLOGY

- Unknown etiology
- Stimulation of the hypersensitive baroreceptors in the carotid sinus affects vagus and sympathetic nerve outflow.
- Carotid body tumors
- Inflammatory and malignant lymph nodes in the neck
- Metastatic cancer
- Coronary artery disease

ASSOCIATED CONDITIONS

- Sick sinus syndrome
- Atrioventricular block
- Coronary artery disease

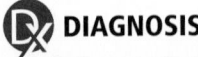 **DIAGNOSIS**

SIGNS AND SYMPTOMS

Paroxysmal

- Dizziness
- Syncope
- Falls
- Blurred vision
- Vertigo
- Tinnitus
- Bradycardia
- Hypotension
- Pallor
- Sweating
- Tachypnea
- No postictal symptoms

TESTS

Special tests

- With the patient in the supine position and while the ECG is monitored, manual pressure ("massage") of the carotid sinus causes asystole of >3 seconds (cardioinhibitory) and/or a drop in systolic BP as described in Description. Diagnostic yield may be increased by combining with tilt-table testing.

Diagnostic Procedures/Surgery

- Unilateral carotid sinus pressure ("massage") (check for potential contraindications before performing massage, including carotid bruits, known carotid hypersensitivity, and demonstrated carotid artery disease). Direct steady pressure is applied over the carotid sinus for 10 seconds.
- Orthostatic vital signs (exclude orthostatic hypotension)
- Electrophysiologic studies
- ECG
- Carotid duplex scan

DIFFERENTIAL DIAGNOSIS

- Vasovagal syncope
- Postural hypotension
- Primary autonomic insufficiency
- Hypovolemia
- Arrhythmias
- Sick sinus syndrome
- Syncope secondary to reduced cardiac output (e.g., aortic stenosis)
- Cerebrovascular insufficiency
- Emotional disturbances
- Other causes of syncope

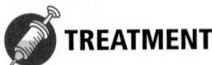 **TREATMENT**

Outpatient. No treatment is required for asymptomatic individuals.

GENERAL MEASURES

Cardiac pacing (dual chamber) is the treatment of choice for recurrent episodes.

Diet

No special diet

Activity

No restrictions

MEDICATION (DRUGS)

First Line
- Anticholinergics: Atropine (acutely) for the cardioinhibitory type
- Sympathomimetics: Ephedrine
- Theophylline
- In one study, selective serotonin reuptake inhibitors were successful in controlling symptoms.
- Contraindications: Refer to manufacturer's instructions.
- Precautions: Concomitant usage of digitalis, β-blockers, clonidine, and -methyldopa may accentuate response to carotid sinus massage.
- Significant possible interactions: Refer to manufacturer's instructions.

Second Line
Fludrocortisone has been used in clinical trials for patients with vasodepressor carotid sinus syndrome.

SURGERY
- Carotid sinus denervation by surgery or radiation therapy for selected patients
- Implantation of a permanent pacemaker helps prevent recurrent symptoms in patients with cardioinhibitory component.
- Surgery for selected patients with atheromata

 FOLLOW-UP

DISPOSITION
Admission Criteria
Syncope of uncertain etiology

PROGNOSIS
May be serious if syncope is associated with atheromatous narrowing of sinus artery or basilar artery

COMPLICATIONS
- Prolonged confusion
- Frequent falls, leading to injuries and fractures

PATIENT MONITORING
Follow as an outpatient.

REFERENCES

1. ACC/AHA/NASPE 2002 Guideline update for implantation of cardiac pacemakers and antiarrhythmia devices: Summary article. A report of the American College of Cardiology/American Heart Association task force on practice guidelines (ACC/AHA/NASPE committee to update the 1998 pacemaker guidelines). *Circulation*. 2002;106:2145.
2. Braunwald E, ed. *Heart Disease: A Textbook of Cardiovascular Medicine*, 6th ed. Philadelphia: WB Saunders, 2001.
3. Isselbacher KJ, et al., eds. *Harrison's Principles of Internal Medicine*, 14th ed. New York: McGraw-Hill, 1998.
4. McIntoch SJ, Lawson J, Kenny RA. Clinical characteristics of vasopressor, cardioinhibitory, and mixed carotid sinus syndrome in the elderly. *Am J Med*. 1993;95:203–208.

 MISCELLANEOUS

- See also: Atherosclerosis
- It is clinically important to distinguish carotid sinus syndrome from sick sinus syndrome.

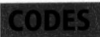 **CODES**

ICD9-CM
337.0 Idiopathic peripheral autonomic neuropathy

C

CARPAL TUNNEL SYNDROME

Jay U. Howington, MD
Fremont P. Wirth, MD

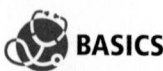 **BASICS**

DESCRIPTION
- The most common cause of peripheral nerve compression
- The median nerve is compressed as it traverses the carpal tunnel in the wrist and hand. The tunnel is composed of the carpal bones dorsally and the transverse carpal ligament ventrally. It contains flexor tendons and the median nerve.
- Symptoms tend to affect the dominant hand, but more than half of patients experience bilateral symptoms.
- System(s) Affected: Musculoskeletal; Nervous

Pregnancy Considerations
May occur during pregnancy

GENERAL PREVENTION
Take a break once an hour when doing repetitive work involving hands.

EPIDEMIOLOGY
- Predominant age: 40–60
- Predominant sex: Female > Male (3:1 to 10:1) (1)

Prevalence
Most common entrapment neuropathy. Most recent estimates of prevalence indicate that the disorder occurs in 346/100,000 population.

RISK FACTORS
- No clear evidence that repetitive flexion and extension of the wrist may influence the development of carpal tunnel syndrome.
- Occupation as a seamstress or computer operator may exacerbate carpal tunnel syndrome. There is, however, no universal agreement that carpal tunnel syndrome is job related.

Genetics
Unknown; however a familial type has been reported.

ETIOLOGY
- Disorders affecting the musculoskeletal system in the region of the wrist, including
  - Trauma or Colles fracture
  - Degenerative joint disease
  - Rheumatoid arthritis
  - Ganglion cyst
  - Scleroderma
- Hypothyroidism and diabetes are frequently associated with this condition, which also occurs with increased frequency during pregnancy.
- Other miscellaneous causes include acromegaly, lupus erythematosus, leukemia, pyogenic infections, sarcoidosis, primary amyloidosis, and Paget disease.
- Hyperparathyroidism, hypocalcemia

ASSOCIATED CONDITIONS
- Diabetes
- Obesity
- Pregnancy

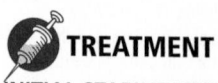 **DIAGNOSIS**

SIGNS AND SYMPTOMS
- Symptoms characteristically are relieved by shaking or rubbing the hands.
- During waking hours symptoms occur when driving the car, reading the newspaper, and occasionally when using the hands for repetitive maneuvers.
- The altered sensation is characteristically confined to the thumb and the index and middle finger, but many patients do not distinguish this localization and feel the entire hand is affected
  - Tingling or prickling sensations in the fingers
  - Burning pain in the fingers particularly at night (acroparesthesias)
  - Arm pain
  - Finger sensory loss
  - Positive Tinel sign
  - Positive Phalen sign
  - Wasting of the thenar and hypothenar muscles is a late sign.
  - Weakness of the hand, however, for such tasks as opening jars is often noted by the patient early in the disorder.

TESTS
- Special tests
  - Electromyography
    - Will be abnormal in >85% of cases
    - Prolonged distal latency of the median motor nerves may be seen.
    - The most sensitive indicator is the median sensory distal latency, which is prolonged. Further, the sensory nerve action potential may be reduced or unobtainable.
    - Not required as a diagnostic test where clinical symptoms are well defined or to predict surgical outcome (2)[A].
  - Stimulation of the ulnar nerve should be done as well to exclude generalized polyneuropathy.

Lab
- No one laboratory test is diagnostic.
- Normal thyroid function studies and normal glucose metabolism studies may be helpful in excluding these conditions, which may be associated with carpal tunnel syndrome.

Imaging
- Special radiographic views of the carpal tunnel may be obtained. These are of limited usefulness unless heterotopic calcification can be identified.
- Magnetic resonance neurography may be used to confirm compression of the median nerve in the carpal tunnel and to assess the success of surgical decompression.

Diagnostic Procedures/Surgery
- Tinel sign—tapping of the wrist proximal to the carpal tunnel may produce electric sensation perceived by the patient, a sign of nerve compression (50% sensitivity and 77% specificity (2)[A].
- Phalen sign—holding the wrist flexed for 60 seconds—may precipitate the paresthesias experienced by the patient (68% sensitivity and 73% specificity) (2)[A].
- A blood pressure tourniquet to cut off circulation to the arm may precipitate symptoms promptly.

DIFFERENTIAL DIAGNOSIS
- Cervical spondylosis
- Generalized peripheral neuropathy
- Brachial plexus lesion
- Pronator syndrome
- Anterior Interosseous syndrome

TREATMENT

INITIAL STABILIZATION
- Outpatient
- Outpatient surgery

GENERAL MEASURES
- Splinting of the wrist in extension while sleeping may provide significant relief of symptoms. Prolonged use of splinting if possible may allow some symptoms to resolve.
- Injection of the carpal tunnel with hydrocortisone (Medrol 40 mg/mL); 1 mL + 1% lidocaine (1 mL) may provide significant temporary relief. This is particularly useful during pregnancy.
- The combination of splinting and steroid injections provide long-term relief in only 10% of cases and is not better than either treatment in isolation (3)[A].

Diet
No special diet

Activity
As tolerated

MEDICATION (DRUGS)

First Line

Nonsteroidal anti-inflammatory agents such as ibuprofen 400 mg b.i.d. or t.i.d. or naproxen sodium 500 mg b.i.d. will provide significant relief of symptoms in many patients.

- Contraindications: Gastrointestinal intolerance
- Precautions: Gastrointestinal side effects of nonsteroidal anti-inflammatory drugs may preclude their use in selected patients.
- Significant possible interactions: Refer to manufacturer's literature.

Second Line

Other nonsteroidal anti-inflammatory drugs

SURGERY

- Surgical decompression of the carpal tunnel by dividing the transverse carpal ligament completely provides almost total relief of symptoms in >95% of patients.
- Surgical decompression is usually done as an outpatient procedure under local anesthesia.
- Healing of the incision generally takes 2 weeks; an additional 2 weeks of recuperation may be required before the hand can be fully used for tasks requiring strength.
- Recent randomized, controlled studies indicate that surgery is more effective than splinting at 18 months. (4)[A]

 FOLLOW-UP

PROGNOSIS

Untreated, the condition can be expected to lead to numbness and weakness in the hand with atrophy of hand muscles and permanent loss of function of the extremity.

COMPLICATIONS

- Postop infection (rare)
- Injury to recurrent branch of the nerve

PATIENT MONITORING

- Patients treated with wrist splints or other palliative measures such as cortisone injections will require follow-up in the ensuing 4–12 weeks to assess the success of treatment modalities.
- Patients treated surgically rarely experience recurrence of the disorder. Routine follow-up once healing of the incision has occurred is not necessary.

REFERENCES

1. Nordstrom DL, DeStefano F, Vierkant RA, et al. Incidence of diagnosed carpal tunnel syndrome in a general population. *Epidemiology.* 1998;9: 342–345.
2. Jordan R, Carter T, Cummins C. A systematic review of the utility of electrodiagnostic testing in carpal tunnel syndrome. *Br J General Practice.* 2002;52: 670–673.
3. Graham RG, Hudson DA, et al. A prospective study to assess the outcome of steroid injections and wrist splinting for the treatment of carpal tunnel syndrome. *Plas Reconst Surg.* 2004;113:550–556.
4. Gerritsen AA, de Vet HC, Scholten RJ, et al. Splinting vs surgery in the treatment of carpal tunnel syndrome: A randomized controlled trial. *JAMA.* 2002;288:1245–1251.
5. Cudlip SA, Howe FA, Clifton A, et al. Magnetic resonance neurography studies of the median nerve before and after carpal tunnel decompression. *J Neurosurg.* 2002;96:1046–1051.

 MISCELLANEOUS

See also: Arthritis; Rheumatoid (RA); Hypoparathyroidism; Scleroderma; Systemic Lupus Erythematosus (SLE)

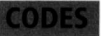 **CODES**

ICD9-CM

354.0 Carpal tunnel syndrome

PATIENT TEACHING

Carpal Tunnel Syndrome Foundation. For patient education materials favorably reviewed on this topic, contact: American Academy of Family Physicians Foundation, P.O. Box 8418, Kansas City, MO 64114, (800) 274-2237, Ext. 4400.

 See Corresponding Diagnostic Algorithm

 See Patient Handout on CD

C

CATARACT

T. Glendon Moody, MD

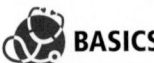

BASICS

DESCRIPTION
- Any opacity of the lens, either localized or generalized
- Single largest cause of blindness in the world, blinding an estimated 17 million people
- Types include
  - Age-related ("senile"): 90%
  - Congenital 1/250 newborns: 10–38% of childhood blindness
  - Toxic/nutritional
  - Systemic disease associated, such as myotonic dystrophy, atopic dermatitis
  - Metabolic diabetes (accelerated sorbitol pathway), hypocalcemia, Wilson disease
  - "Complicated"—secondary to associated eye disease, such as uveitis (juvenile rheumatoid arthritis, sarcoid). Also secondary to occult tumor (melanoma, retinoblastoma)
  - Trauma heat (infrared), electrical shock, radiation, concussion, perforating eye injuries, or intraocular foreign body
- System(s) Affected: Nervous

Geriatric Considerations
92% of people >75 years have cataracts.

Pediatric Considerations
See information on congenital cataracts.

Pregnancy Considerations
See information on congenital cataracts (e.g., rubella syndrome).

GENERAL PREVENTION
- Use of ultraviolet protecting glasses in sunny climates may slow progression of cataract, but this is not proven by controlled studies to date.
- Antioxidants (vitamins C, E, others) theoretically beneficial, but not proven

EPIDEMIOLOGY
- Predominant age: Depends on type of cataract
- Predominant sex: Male = Female

Prevalence
- 5% of age 52–62
- 46% of age 75–85 have significant vision loss (20/30 or worse).
- 92% of age 75–85 have some cataract changes

RISK FACTORS
- Aging
- Patient with one of the predisposing diseases

Genetics
- Age-related cataract has no clear pattern.
- Congenital sometimes associated (e.g., heredofamilial systemic disorders [Laurence-Moon-Biedl syndrome], chromosomal disorders [Down syndrome])

ETIOLOGY
- Age-related cataract
  - Continual addition of layers of lens fibers throughout life creates hard, dehydrated lens nucleus that impairs vision (nuclear cataract).
  - Aging alters biochemical and osmotic balance required for lens clarity; outer lens layers hydrate and become opaque, affecting vision.
- Congenital
  - Usually obscure
  - Drugs (corticosteroids in first trimester, sulfonamides)
  - Metabolic diabetes in mother, galactosemia in fetus
  - Intrauterine infection during first trimester (e.g., rubella, herpes, mumps)
  - Maternal malnutrition
- Other cataract types
  - Have in common that a biochemical/osmotic imbalance disrupts lens clarity
  - Local changes in lens protein distribution lead to light scattering manifesting as lens opacity.

ASSOCIATED CONDITIONS
- Diabetes
- Ocular diseases

DIAGNOSIS

SIGNS AND SYMPTOMS
- Age-related cataract
  - Blurred vision, distortion, or "ghosting" of images
  - Problems with visual acuity in bright light or night driving (glare)
  - Falls or accidents
  - Injuries (e.g., hip fracture)
  - Signs on eye examination: A lens opacity consistent with the symptoms
- Congenital: Lens opacity present at birth or within 3 months after birth
- Often asymptomatic or parents notice child's visual inattention or strabismus (lazy eye):
  - Leukocoria (white pupil reflex), strabismus, nystagmus, associated syndrome signs (as in Down or rubella syndromes)
  - Visual acuity tests abnormal for one or both eyes
  - Note: Must always rule out ocular tumor. Early diagnosis and treatment of retinoblastoma may be lifesaving.
- Other types of cataract
  - May present with decreased visual acuity complaint
  - Appropriate history or signs to help in diagnosis

TESTS
- Visual quality assessment: Glare testing, contrast sensitivity are sometimes indicated. (Hyperglycemic state as in poor diabetic control creates osmotic change within lens and may alter measurement of visual acuity and refractive state.)
- Retinal/macular function assessment: Potential acuity meter testing, fluorescein retinal angiography sometimes required

Diagnostic Procedures/Surgery
See special tests noted above.

Pathological Findings
Consistent with lens changes found in the type of cataract

C

DIFFERENTIAL DIAGNOSIS

An opaque-appearing eye may be due to surface opacities of the cornea (scarring), lens opacities, tumor, retinal detachment, or gliotic retinal scar. Biomicroscopic examination (slit lamp) or careful ophthalmoscopic exam should provide diagnosis. A visual acuity worse than 20/30, not easily correctable by glasses and explainable by the degree of cataract noted on examination makes the diagnosis

- In the elderly, visual impairment often due to multiple factors, such as cataract and macular degeneration, both contributing to visual loss
- Age-related cataract significant if symptoms and ophthalmic exam support cataract as major cause of vision impairment
- Congenital lens opacity in absence of other ocular pathology such as tumor, nerve glioma, or retinopathy of prematurity may be consistent with the visual loss. It may cause severe amblyopia.
- Note: No cataract produces an afferent pupillary reaction defect (Marcus Gunn pupil). Abnormal pupillary reactions mandate further evaluation for other pathology.

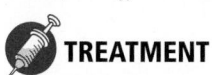

TREATMENT

Outpatient or inpatient surgery

MEDICATION (DRUGS)

There is no medication at present to prevent or slow the progression of cataracts.

SURGERY

- Age-related cataract
  - Surgical removal of the cataract: Indicated if visual impairment–producing symptoms distressing to the patient or interfering with lifestyle or occupation, or posing risk of fall or injury
  - Because significant cataract may develop gradually, the patient may not be aware of how it has changed his or her lifestyle. Physician may note a significant cataract, and patient reports "no problems." Thus, the evaluation requires physician/patient exchange of information.

  - Surgical technique: Cataracts are not removed by laser. Most surgical techniques include implantation of a plastic intraocular lens immediately following cataract extraction.
  - Anesthesia: Usually local, with anesthesiologist monitoring vital signs
  - Presurgical evaluation: By the primary care physician includes physical exam, lab work (e.g., CBC, electrolytes, ECG). Patients on anticoagulants may need to temporarily discontinue 1 week before surgery if possible. Not always necessary, so need to discuss with ophthalmologist.
  - Postoperative care: Usually protective eye shield as directed, topical antibiotic and steroid ophthalmic medications. Avoid lifting or bending over for a few weeks.
- Congenital cataract
  - Treatment is surgical removal of cataract. Newborn may need surgery within days to reduce risk of severe amblyopia. Use of implant lenses is controversial.
  - Postoperative care: Long-term patching program for good eye to combat amblyopia; refractive correction of operative eye, with multiple repeat examinations; very difficult challenge for physician and parents

FOLLOW-UP

PROGNOSIS

- Ocular prognosis good after cataract removal if no prior ocular disease
- In congenital cataracts, prognosis is often poor because of the high risk of amblyopia.

COMPLICATIONS

Blindness

PATIENT MONITORING

- As cataract progresses, the ophthalmologist may change spectacle correction to maintain vision. When this is no longer practical or successful, surgery is recommended.
- Following surgery, spectacle correction may be required to maximize visual acuity for the patient's need. It is usually measured several weeks after surgery.

REFERENCES

1. Tasman W, ed. *Duane's Ophthalmology*. Philadelphia, PA: JB Lippincott; 2002.

 MISCELLANEOUS

Other notes: If patient has cataract and symptoms do not seem to support recommended surgery, a second opinion by another ophthalmologist may be indicated.

CODES

ICD9-CM
- 366.19 Other and combined forms of senile cataract
- 743.30 Congenital cataract, unspecified

PATIENT TEACHING

See "Surgery."

 See Corresponding Diagnostic Algorithm

CELIAC DISEASE

Jeremy Golding, MD

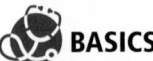 **BASICS**

DESCRIPTION
- Classically, a chronic diarrheal disease characterized by intestinal malabsorption of virtually all nutrients and precipitated by eating gluten-containing foods. Multiple forms exist. Nondiarrheal form may actually be most common (intestinal villous atrophy produces vitamin and mineral malabsorption).
- System(s) Affected: Gastrointestinal
- Synonym(s): Sprue; Gluten enteropathy; Celiac sprue

ALERT
Pediatric Considerations
Failure to thrive and delayed growth with short stature may be early manifestations. A few children may outgrow intolerance to wheat after prolonged glutenfree diets, but should be cautioned to watch for signs of recurrence in middle age.

Pregnancy Considerations
Celiac disease may be an underappreciated cause of male and female infertility. Consider celiac disease in pregnant women with severe anemia.

GENERAL PREVENTION
Avoid all gluten-containing products (wheat, barley, rye, and possibly oat products).

EPIDEMIOLOGY
- Disease primarily of individuals of Northern European ancestry.
- Predominant sex: Female > Male (3:2)

Prevalence
- 1 in 120–300 persons in North America

RISK FACTORS
- 1st-degree relatives 10% incidence
- 71% in monozygotic twins

Genetics
HLA-DQ2 and/or DQ8 closely associated (testing may be indicated if indeterminate small bowel pathology)

ETIOLOGY
Sensitivity to gluten, specifically gliadin fraction

ASSOCIATED CONDITIONS
- May have secondary lactase deficiency
- Extraintestinal manifestation may include marked decrease in bone density
- Dermatitis herpetiformis common
- Autoimmune thyroiditis
- Diabetes, type 1 (prevalence of celiac disease in type 1 diabetes is 3–8%)
- Elevated AST and ALT

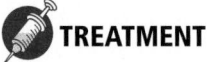 **DIAGNOSIS**

SIGNS AND SYMPTOMS
- Diarrhea
- Steatorrhea
- Muscle cramps
- Iron deficiency anemia
- Nervousness
- Weight loss
- Failure to thrive (slowing velocity of weight gain)
- Weakness
- Lassitude
- Fatigue
- Large appetite
- Abdominal distention
- Explosive flatulence
- Abdominal pain, nausea, vomiting rare
- Recurrent aphthous stomatitis

Lab
- Elevated liver function tests
- Positive IgA antiendomysial antibodies and IgA tissue transglutaminase (sensitivity 90–98%, specificity 98%) when on normal (non–glutenfree) diet.
- IgA-deficient patients have false-negative IgA ti-endomysial and IgA ti-transglutaminase antibodies.
- 72-hour fecal fat showing >7% fat malabsorption
- D-Xylose test showing malabsorption of this sugar
- Decreased calcium
- Increased prothrombin time
- Decreased neutral fats
- Decreased cholesterol
- Decreased vitamin A
- Decreased vitamin B_{12} (rare)
- Decreased vitamin D
- Decreased vitamin C
- Decreased folic acid
- Decreased iron (common)
- Decreased total protein
- Anemia (common)
- Evaluate for osteoporosis

Imaging
Upper GI series showing flocculation of barium, edema, and flattening of mucosal folds.

Diagnostic Procedures/Surgery
Endoscopy with diagnostic biopsy of the duodenal mucosa with repeat endoscopy and normal biopsy on a gluten-free diet is necessary before a firm diagnosis can be made. In general, diagnosis should not be made based on serology alone.

Pathological Findings
Small bowel biopsy: Flattened villi, hyperplasia and lengthening of crypts, infiltration of plasma cells and lymphocytes in lamina propria.

DIFFERENTIAL DIAGNOSIS
Rule out
- Short bowel syndrome
- Pancreatic insufficiency
- Crohn disease
- Whipple disease
- Hypogammaglobulinemia
- Tropical sprue
- Lymphoma
- AIDS
- Acute enteritis
- Giardiasis
- Eosinophilic gastroenteritis
- Pancreatic disease

TREATMENT

- Outpatient
- Immunization with pneumococcal vaccine is appropriate, because hyposplenism is common in patients with celiac disease.

GENERAL MEASURES
- Removal of gluten from the diet. Rice, corn, and soybean flour are safe, palatable substitutes.
- Levels of IgA antigliadin normalize with gluten abstinence.

Diet
Removal of gluten: Wheat, rye, barley, and those with gluten additives. This is a difficult diet, and should be coordinated with a skilled dietician.

Activity
No restrictions

MEDICATION (DRUGS)

First Line
- Usually none: Diet is treatment
- Prednisone, 40–60 mg/d PO in cases of refractory sprue
- In refractory disease, consider
  - Steroids
  - Azathioprine
  - Cyclosporine
  - Possible future role of infliximab (Remicade)
- Contraindications
  - History of tuberculosis, fungus, or herpes infections
- Precautions
  - Use with caution in congestive heart failure, diabetes, peptic ulcer, and myasthenia gravis.
- Significant possible interactions
  - Diuretics taken concomitantly may lead to potassium depletion.

Second Line
Patients may require supplemental calcium, calcium carbonate, 500 mg PO b.i.d., and vitamin D (ergocalciferol) 10–100 g/d; in severe malabsorption, up to 2.5 mg/d may be required.

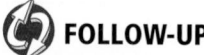 **FOLLOW-UP**

PROGNOSIS
- Good with correct diagnosis and adherence to gluten-free diet
- Patient should feel better in 7 days.
- All symptoms usually disappear in 4–6 weeks.
- It is unknown whether strict dietary adherence decreases cancer risk.

COMPLICATIONS
- Malignancy: <10% of patients (50% of whom have small bowel lymphoma)
- Refractory sprue
  - May respond to prednisone 40–60 mg/d PO
  - Refractory sprue unresponsive to corticosteroid therapy raises the specter of adult-onset autoimmune enteropathy or cryptic T-cell lymphoma. In this circumstance, screening for antienterocyte autoantibodies and careful scrutiny of the small intestine, including retroperitoneal lymph node biopsy with full-thickness small bowel biopsy, may be needed.
- Chronic ulcerative jejunoileitis
  - Associated with multiple ulcers, intestinal bleeding, strictures, perforation, obstruction, and peritonitis
  - 7% mortality
- Osteoporosis secondary to decreased vitamin D and calcium absorption
- Dehydration
- Electrolyte depletion
- Refractory cases may need total parenteral nutrition
- Death (rare)

PATIENT MONITORING
Repeat endoscopy after 6–8 weeks on a gluten-free diet (in selected cases).

REFERENCES

1. AGA Guideline. Celiac sprue. *Gastroenterology.* 2001;120:1522.
2. Carroccio A, Soresi M, Di Prima L, et al. Screening for celiac disease in patients with chronic liver disease. *Gastroenterology.* 2003;125:1289.
3. Kaukinen K, Halme L, et al. Celiac disease in patients with severe liver disease: Gluten-free diet may reverse hepatic failure. *Gastroenterology.* 2002;122:881–888.
4. McClave S. Celiac and tropical sprue. In: Chobanian SJ, Van Ness MM, eds. *A Manual of Clinical Problems in Gastroenterology*, 2nd ed. Boston: Little-Brown, 1993.
5. Ryan BM, Kelleher D. Refractory celiac sprue. *Gastroenterology.* 2000;119:243–251.

 MISCELLANEOUS

The most common cause of refractory diarrhea is noncompliance with a glutenfree diet.

CODES

ICD9-CM
579.0 Celiac disease

PATIENT TEACHING
- Clinical dietitian
- Copy of gluten-free diet materials
- Possible lay self-help group
- American Celiac Society, 45 Gifford Avenue, Jersey City, NJ 07304, (201) 432-1207
- Gluten Intolerance Group (206) 325-6980

 See Corresponding Diagnostic Algorithm

See Patient Handout on CD

CELLULITIS

Abdulrazak Abyad, MD, PhD, MBA, MPH, AGSF

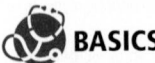 **BASICS**

DESCRIPTION

An acute spreading infection of the dermis and subcutaneous tissue. Several entities are recognized

- Cellulitis of the extremities: An expanding, red, swollen, tender, or painful plaque with an indefinite border that may cover a wide area
- Recurrent cellulitis of the leg after saphenous venectomy: Patients have an acute onset of swelling and erythema of the legs arising months to years after coronary artery bypass (i.e., surgery using lower extremity veins for bypass grafts).
- Dissecting cellulitis of the scalp: Recurrent painful, fluctuant dermal and subcutaneous nodules
- Facial cellulitis in adults: Rare; patients usually develop pharyngitis, followed by high fever, rapidly progressive anterior neck swelling, tenderness, and erythema associated with dysphagia.
- Facial cellulitis in children: Potentially serious; swelling and erythema of the cheek develop rapidly, usually unilaterally.
- Perianal cellulitis: Bright perianal erythema extending from the anal verge approximately 2–3 cm onto the surrounding perianal skin
- Pseudomonas cellulitis: May be a localized phenomenon or it may occur during *Pseudomonas* septicemia
- System(s) Affected: Skin/Exocrine

ALERT
Geriatric Considerations
In cellulitis of lower extremities, older patients are more prone to develop thrombophlebitis.

GENERAL PREVENTION
- Treat tinea pedis with antifungal agent (e.g., clotrimazole) to prevent recurrent cellulitis of the legs in patients who have had coronary bypass.
- Avoid trauma.
- Avoid swimming with skin abrasion.
- Avoid human or animal bites.
- Wear support stockings to lessen peripheral edema.
- Maintain good skin hygiene.
- Achieve and maintain glycemic control.
- For recurrent cellulitis: Prophylactic penicillin G (250–500 mg PO b.i.d.)
- *H. influenzae* cellulitis: Rifampin prophylaxis for entire family of index case or in day care classroom in which one or two children exposed. Dosage: 20 mg/kg/d (maximum: 600 mg/d) for 4 days

EPIDEMIOLOGY
- Predominant age
  - Perianal cellulitis: Principally in children
  - Facial cellulitis: In adults, usually older than 50 years. In children, between 6 months and 3 years
- Predominant sex: Male = Female (perianal cellulitis more common in boys)

Incidence
Unknown

Prevalence
Unknown

RISK FACTORS
General

- Previous trauma (e.g., laceration, puncture, human or animal bite)
- Underlying skin lesion (e.g., furuncle, ulcer)
- Surgical wound
- After coronary artery bypass in patients whose saphenous veins have been removed
- Lower extremity lymphedema secondary to radical pelvic surgery, radiation therapy, and/or neoplastic involvement of pelvic lymph nodes
- Mastectomy
- Diabetes mellitus
- IV drug use
- Immunocompromised host
- Burns
- Environmental and occupational factors

ETIOLOGY
By site

- Cellulitis of the extremities: group A *streptococcus*, *Staphylococcus aureus*
- Recurrent cellulitis of the leg: non-group A *β*-hemolytic *Streptococci* (groups C, G, and B)
- Dissecting cellulitis of the scalp: *S. aureus*
- Facial cellulitis in adults: *Haemophilus influenzae* type B
- Facial cellulitis in children: *H. influenzae* type B, patients >3 years with portal of entry: Staphylococcal and streptococcal
- Synergetic necrotizing cellulitis: Mixed aerobic-anaerobic flora
- Intravenous drug use: *S. aureus*, streptococci, Enterobacteriaceae, *Pseudomonas*, fungi
- Synergetic necrotizing cellulitis: Mixed aerobic-anaerobic flora
- Specific diseases
  - Diabetes mellitus: *S. aureus*, streptococci, Enterobacteriaceae, anaerobes
  - Human bites: *Eikenella corrodens*
  - Animal bites (e.g., cat, dog): Staphylococci, *Pasteurella multocida*
- Patient groups
  - Neonates: group B *streptococcus*
  - Immunocompromised:
    ○ Bacteria (e.g., *Serratia, Proteus*, and other Enterobacteriaceae)
    ○ Fungi (e.g., *Cryptococcus neoformans*)
    ○ Atypical mycobacterium
  - Children with nephrotic syndrome: *Escherichia coli*
  - Environmental and occupational exposures:
    ○ *Erysipelothrix rhusiopathiae*
    ○ *Vibrio* sp.
    ○ *Aeromonas hydrophila*
- Rare causes
  - Anaerobic
  - *Clostridium perfringens* (in gas-forming cellulitis)
  - Tuberculosis
  - Syphilitic gumma
  - Fungal causes: Mucormycosis, aspergillosis

ASSOCIATED CONDITIONS
- Facial cellulitis in children
  - Upper respiratory tract infection
  - Unilateral or bilateral otitis media in 68% of patients
  - Meningitis in 8% of patients
- Perianal cellulitis
  - Pharyngitis may precede infection.
- Frontal sinus in adult
  - Subacute bacterial endocarditis
  - Scarlet fever
  - Vaccinia
  - Herpes simplex
  - Herpes zoster

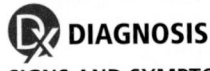 **DIAGNOSIS**

SIGNS AND SYMPTOMS
- General
  - Local tenderness
  - Pain
  - Erythema
  - Malaise
  - Fever, chills
  - Involved area is red, hot, and swollen.
  - Borders of the area are not elevated and not demarcated.
  - Regional lymphadenopathy is common.
- Recurrent cellulitis
  - Same as general cellulitis
  - Edema
  - High fever, chills, and toxicity
- Dissecting cellulitis of the scalp
  - Purulent drainage from burrowing interconnecting abscesses
- Facial cellulitis in adults
  - Malaise
  - Anorexia
  - Vomiting
  - Itching
  - Burning
  - Dysplasia
  - Anterior neck swelling
- Facial cellulitis in children
  - Irritability
  - Upper respiratory tract infection symptoms
- Perianal cellulitis
  - Intense perianal erythema
  - Pain on defecation
  - Blood-streaked stools
- Perianal pruritus

TESTS
Lab
- Aspirates from the point of maximum inflammation: Yield a 45% positive culture rate compared with a 5% rate from leading edge culture
- Blood cultures: Potential pathogens isolated in 25% of patients
- Mild leukocytosis with a left shift
- Mildly elevated erythrocyte sedimentation rate

- Complete blood chemistry
- Serial serologic testing with antistreptolysin O, antideoxyribonuclease B, and antihyaluronidase tests may be successful in diagnosing cellulitis caused by group A, C, or G hemolytic streptococci.
- Sinus drainage and culture of aspirate
- Drugs that may alter lab results: Previous antibiotic therapy may alter lab results.

Imaging
Gas-forming cellulitis

- Plain radiographs show gas bubbles in the soft tissue.
- CT shows gas and myonecrosis.

Diagnostic Procedures/Surgery
- Skin biopsy
- Lumbar puncture should be considered for all children with *H. influenzae* type B cellulitis.

Pathological Findings
Biopsy of skin shows marked infiltration of the dermis with eosinophils and inflammatory changes.

DIFFERENTIAL DIAGNOSIS
- Perianal cellulitis
  - Candida intertrigo
  - Psoriasis
  - Pinworm infection
  - Inflammatory bowel disease
  - Behavioral problem
  - Child abuse
- Others
  - Acute gout
  - Fasciitis or myositis
  - Mycotic aneurysm
  - Ruptured Baker cyst
  - Thrombophlebitis
  - Osteomyelitis
  - Herpetic whitlow
  - Cutaneous diphtheria
  - Pseudogout
  - Chronic venous stasis dermatitis

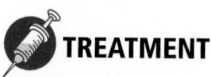 TREATMENT

GENERAL MEASURES
- Immobilization and elevation of the involved limb to reduce swelling may be needed in *H. influenzae* type B.
- Sterile saline dressings to decrease local pain
- Moist heat to localize the infection
- Cool aluminum acetate (Burow solution) compresses for pain relief

Diet
Regular diet

Activity
Ambulatory in mild infection; bed rest in severe infection

 MEDICATION (DRUGS)

First Line
Treat 10–30 days, guided by culture results whenever possible.

- Mild early suspected streptococcal etiology: Aqueous penicillin G, 600,000 units, then IM procaine penicillin at 600,000 units q8h–q12h
- Staphylococcal infection or no confirmed etiology: Penicillinase-resistant penicillin (e.g., oxacillin 0.5–1.0 g PO q6h)
- Severe infection: Penicillinase-resistant penicillin (e.g., nafcillin 1.0–1.5 g IV q4h)
- Gram-negative bacillus as possible etiology: Aminoglycoside (gentamicin) plus a semisynthetic penicillin
- Rapidly progressive cellulitis after an injury in fresh water: Penicillinase-resistant penicillin plus gentamicin or chloramphenicol
- Human bites: Amoxicillin-clavulanate (Augmentin)
- Animal bites (cellulitis at the saphenous site): Penicillin or nafcillin, at high dosage, IV for 7 days before switching to PO therapy
- Facial cellulitis in adults and children: (*H. influenza* B) Cefotaxime IV
- Gas-forming cellulitis: Aqueous penicillin G 10–20 million units/d IV
- Diabetes mellitus: Cefoxitin or, if toxic, clindamycin and gentamicin
- IV drug abuse: Vancomycin and gentamicin
- Compromised hosts: Clindamycin and gentamicin
- Burn patients: Vancomycin and gentamicin
- Contraindications: Allergies to the antibiotic
- Precautions: Renal failure, other organ failure
- Significant possible interactions: Refer to manufacturer's literature.

Second Line
- Mild infection
  - Penicillin allergy: erythromycin, 500 mg PO q6h
- Severe infection
  - Vancomycin 1.0–1.5 g/d IV
  - Human bite and animal bites: IV cefoxitin
- Gas-forming cellulitis
  - Metronidazole 500 mg IV q6h
  - Clindamycin 600 mg IV q8h
- Fluoroquinolones (adults)

SURGERY
- Débridement for gas and purulent matter collections
- Intubation or tracheotomy may be needed for cellulitis of the head or neck.
- Hand infections: Wide filleting incision in necrotizing cellulitis

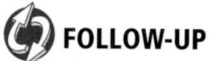 FOLLOW-UP

PROGNOSIS
With adequate antibiotic treatment, outlook is good.

COMPLICATIONS
- Bacteremia
- Local abscesses
- Superinfection with gram-negative organisms
- Lymphangitis, especially in recurrent cellulitis
- Thrombophlebitis or venous thrombosis of lower extremities in older patients
- Dissecting cellulitis of the scalp: Scarring, alopecia
- Facial cellulitis in children: Meningitis in 8% of patients
- Gas-forming cellulitis: Gangrene, amputation, 25% mortality

PATIENT MONITORING
- Take a blood culture at the end of treatment to ensure cure effected.
- Repeat needle aspirate culture.
- Repeat blood count if patient was toxic.
- Repeat lumbar puncture in case of meningitis.
- Consider prophylaxis of deep vein thrombosis.

REFERENCES
1. Habif T. *Clinical Dermatology*. 4th ed. St. Louis, MO: Mosby; 2004.
2. Mandell GL, ed. *Principles and Practice of Infectious Diseases*. 5th ed. New York, NY: Churchill Livingstone; 2000.

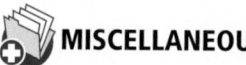 **MISCELLANEOUS**

See also: Animal Bites; Cellulitis; Periorbital and Orbital; Erysipelas; Thrombophlebitis; Superficial;

CODES

ICD9-CM
682.9 Cellulitis and abscess at unspecified site

PATIENT TEACHING
- Good skin hygiene
- Avoid skin traumas.
- Report early skin changes to physician.

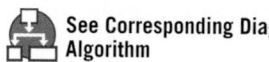 **See Corresponding Diagnostic Algorithm**

CELLULITIS, PERIORBITAL AND ORBITAL

Abdulrazak Abyad, MD, PhD, MBA, MPH, AGSF

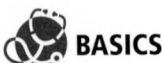 **BASICS**

DESCRIPTION

An acute spreading infection of the dermis and subcutaneous tissue. Several entities have been recognized. Cellulitis around the eyes is a potentially dangerous periorbital and orbital infection.

- System(s) Affected: Nervous; Skin/Exocrine

ALERT

Newborns may acquire orbital cellulitis resulting from intrauterine infection.

GENERAL PREVENTION

- Avoid dermatologic trauma.
- Avoid swimming in fresh water or salt water with skin abrasion.
- In *Haenophilus influenzae* cellulitis: Rifampin prophylaxis for the entire family of a confirmed case. Rifampin prophylaxis in day-care classroom in which 1–2 children exposed. Dosage: 20 mg/kg/24 hours (maximum of 600 mg a day) for 4 days.

EPIDEMIOLOGY

Predominant sex: Male = Female

Incidence

Unknown

Prevalence

Unknown

RISK FACTORS

- Trauma
- Chronic sinusitis (i.e., anaerobic pathogen)
- Acute sinusitis (i.e., aerobic pathogen)
- Retained orbital foreign bodies
- Puncture wound
- Surgical procedure: Exploration for orbital tumor, retinal detachment procedure, strabismus operation
- Acute dacryocystitis
- Dental or intracranial infection
- Bacteremia

Genetics

No known genetic pattern

ETIOLOGY

- Cellulitis around the eye in adults
  - *Staphylococcus aureus* most common
  - *Streptococcus pyogenes*
  - *Streptococcus pneumoniae*
  - Mixed infection
- Cellulitis around the eye in children <5 years old
  - *H. influenzae* most common

ASSOCIATED CONDITIONS

Sinusitis and ethmoiditis observed in children (in 84% of patients)

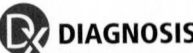 **DIAGNOSIS**

SIGNS AND SYMPTOMS

- Lid edema
- Rhinorrhea
- Orbital pain, tenderness
- Headache
- Conjunctival hyperemia
- Chemosis
- Ptosis
- Limited ocular motion
- Increased intraocular pressure
- Sensation of disorder in cornea
- Congestion of retinal veins
- Chorioretinal stria
- Gangrene and sloughing of lids

TESTS

Serial serologic testing with antistreptolysin O, antideoxyribonuclease B, and antihyaluronidase tests may be successful in diagnosing cellulitis caused by groups A, C, or G hemolytic streptococci.

Lab

- Aspiration of fluid from the orbit is contraindicated.
- Blood culture more likely to be positive in children <5 years old.
- Culture of discharge from nasal mucosa, nasopharynx, and conjunctiva
- Drugs that may alter lab results: Previous antibiotic therapy

Imaging

- B-scan ultrasound
- Plain orbital and sinus films
- CT is the most accurate modality and provides the most information.
- MRI is the imaging modality of choice in diagnosing suspected cases of cavernous sinus thrombosis.

Diagnostic Procedures/Surgery

- Skin biopsy
- Lumbar puncture should be considered for all children with *H. influenzae* type B cellulitis.

DIFFERENTIAL DIAGNOSIS

- Retro-orbital cellulitis
- Abscess

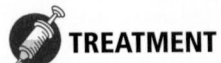 **TREATMENT**

INITIAL STABILIZATION

Outpatient for mild cases, inpatient for severe infections

GENERAL MEASURES

Diet

Regular diet

Activity

- Ambulatory in mild infection
- Bed rest in severe infection

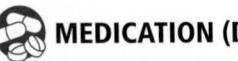 **MEDICATION (DRUGS)**

First Line

- In adults, nafcillin or oxacillin 1.5 g q4h
- In children, ampicillin 200 mg/kg/d in divided doses IV plus nafcillin or oxacillin (100 mg/kg/d)
- Sinus decongestion: Nasal sprays, oral decongestants, and oral antihistamines
- Contraindications
  - Allergies to the antibiotic
  - Previous history of allergy to the drug
- Precautions: Renal failure, other organ failure
- Significant possible interactions: Refer to manufacturer's literature.

Second Line
- In adults, cefotaxime, clindamycin, chloramphenicol, or vancomycin
- In children, if strain of *H. influenzae* resistant to ampicillin: 3rd-generation cephalosporin, cefotaxime, or chloramphenicol
- In immunocompromised patients: Piperacillin and gentamicin
- Fluoroquinolones (adults)
- Linezolid (Zyvox) in complicated or resistant cases, often requiring infectious disease consultation

SURGERY
- Surgical débridement and/or drainage is needed if abscess develops or if clinical situation deteriorates despite adequate therapy in 24–48 hours or if visual acuity decreases.
- In orbital mucormycosis, surgical débridement of devitalized tissue is extremely important.

 FOLLOW-UP

PROGNOSIS
With adequate antibiotic treatment, outlook is good.

COMPLICATIONS
- Osteomyelitis
- Strabismus
- Afferent pupillary defect
- Chronic draining sinus
- Scarred upper eyelid
- Profound visual loss
- Blindness
- Ophthalmoplegia
- Cavernous sinus thrombosis
- Meningitis
- Intracranial abscess
- Acute infarction of retina and choroid

PATIENT MONITORING
Repeat imaging in patients with orbital cellulitis

REFERENCES
1. Habif T. *Clinical Dermatology*. 4th ed. St. Louis, MO: Mosby; 2004.
2. Mandell GL, ed. *Principles and Practice of Infectious Diseases*. 5th ed. New York, NY: Churchill Livingstone; 2000.
3. Morgan SJ. Purulent orbital cellulitis. *Eye*. 2002;16:215.

 MISCELLANEOUS

See also: Animal Bites; Cellulitis; Erysipelas Thrombophlebitis; Superficial

CODES

ICD9-CM
376.01 Orbital cellulites

C

PATIENT TEACHING
- Maintain good skin hygiene.
- Avoid skin trauma.
- Report early skin changes to health care professional.

CEREBRAL PALSY

Terence S. Edgar, MD

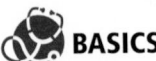 **BASICS**

DESCRIPTION
A persistent disorder of posture and movement, caused by nonprogressive defects or lesions of the immature brain. Includes several forms
- Hemiplegic Cerebral Palsy (CP)
- Diplegic CP
- Quadriplegic CP
- Monoplegic CP
- Dyskinetic CP
- Mixed types

GENERAL PREVENTION
Optimal antenatal and perinatal care.

EPIDEMIOLOGY
Incidence
150–250/100,000 live births

Prevalence
300–400/100,000 of the population

RISK FACTORS
- Prenatal
  - Maternal infection, illness, and chemical or alcohol dependency
  - Prenatal anoxia due to placental dysfunction or maternal cardiorespiratory disease
  - Multiple births
  - Polyhydramnios
  - Bleeding in the 3rd trimester
- Perinatal
  - Chorioamnionitis
  - Low-birth-weight infants
  - Hypoxic ischemic encephalopathy
  - Stroke
    ○ Grade IV intraventricular hemorrhage (IVH)
  - Hyperbilirubinemia
- Postnatal
  - Traumatic brain injury
  - Meningitis and encephalitis
  - Stroke
  - Asphyxia

ETIOLOGY
- In most cases, the exact cause is unknown, but is most likely multifactorial.
- Hemiplegic CP
  - 70–90% are congenital and 10–30 acquired (e.g., vascular, congenital, traumatic).
  - Most commonly the vascular territory of the middle cerebral artery (L > R).
  - Other structural brain abnormalities: Hemibrain atrophy, posthemorrhagic porencephaly
- Diplegic CP
  - In premature infant
    ○ Periventricular leukomalacia (PVL)
    ○ Grade IV IVH
  - Term infant: Multifactorial
- Quadriplegic CP
  - Frequently multifactorial
  - Structural brain abnormalities
  - Cerebral hypoperfusion and watershed infarcts
- Dyskinetic CP
  - Hypoxic brain injury
  - Kernicterus

ASSOCIATED CONDITIONS
- Seizures
- Learning difficulties
- Scoliosis
- Speech difficulties
- Feeding difficulties
- Constipation
- Incontinence
- Mental retardation
- Visual impairments
  - Strabismus
  - Homonymous hemianopia
  - Optic atrophy

ALERT
Optimization of prenatal and perinatal care will potentially reduce the incidence of CP.

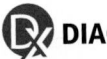 **DIAGNOSIS**

SIGNS AND SYMPTOMS
History
- Ask the following questions
  - Any complications during pregnancy or delivery?
  - Did the child have low tone as an infant?
  - Is there evidence for delayed gross motor development?
  - Early hand preference
- Review prenatal and perinatal history for risk factors.
- The presence of unexplained regression excludes the diagnosis of CP.
  - Consider neurodegenerative disease.

Physical Exam
- Persistence of primitive reflexes
- Poor trunk and head control with impaired fine motor control
- Hemiplegic CP
  - Unilateral spasticity: Arm > leg
  - Relative weakness on 1 side
  - Observe for homonymous hemianopia and strabismus
  - Possible unilateral sensory deficits
- Diplegic CP
  - Spasticity: Legs > arms
  - Scissoring gait
    ○ Flexed hips and knees
    ○ Toe walker
  - Seizures and learning difficulties less common
- Quadriplegic CP
  - Significant fluctuation of tone
  - Stimulant-induced spasms and strong extensor drive
  - Weak trunk and poor head control
  - Speech and swallow difficulties
  - Involvement of all 4 extremities
  - (If arms more involved than legs, categorized as a double hemiplegic)
- Dyskinetic CP
  - Poor trunk and head control
  - Frequently hypotonic, spasticity less pronounced
  - Oromotor dysfunction
  - Arms usually more involved than legs

TESTS
Lab
- A 2004 American Academy of Neurology practice parameter suggests further studies if
  - The clinical history or findings on neuroimaging do not determine a specific structural abnormality.
  - Additional or atypical features are present in the history or clinical examination.
  - A brain malformation is detected in a child with CP.
- Other tests
  - Diagnostic testing for coagulation disorders if a cerebral infarction is seen
  - Routine EEG is not recommended unless seizures are clinically suspected.

Imaging
- Early neonatal period
  - Cranial ultrasound: Helpful in the medically unstable infant
  - Head CT: Identifies congenital malformations, intracranial hemorrhage, and PVL
- MRI is recommended in the older infant and child.
- Normal MRI does not preclude the diagnosis of CP, but rules out an underlying metabolic or genetic etiology.

Pathological Findings
PVL: Focal areas of coagulative necrosis involving the periventricular white matter adjacent to the lateral ventricles

DIFFERENTIAL DIAGNOSIS
- Rett syndrome
- Inherited metabolic disorders
- Benign congenital hypotonia
- Hydrocephalus
- Familial spastic paraparesis
- Tethered cord syndrome
- HIV
- Congenital cytomegalovirus infection
- Mitochondrial myopathy
- Neuronal migration disorder

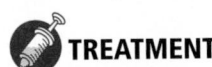 **TREATMENT**

GENERAL MEASURES
Goals
- Prevent contractures
- Minimize spasticity
- Facilitate the patient's ability to ambulate, perform activities of daily living, and participate in meaningful social interactions

SPECIAL THERAPY
- Physical therapy
  - Is used to enhance motor skills, improve muscle strength, and prevent contractures
- Occupational therapy
  - Enhances skills required for daily living
- Speech therapy
  - Assists communication in children with speech impairments
- Special education
  - Assists children with special learning needs

MEDICATION (DRUGS)

First Line
- Baclofen
  - Gamma-aminobutyric acid agonist, facilitates central nervous system (CNS) inhibition
  - Adults: Initial dose is 5 mg t.i.d. and increase over a period of 10 days to a maintenance dose of 20 mg t.i.d. Not to exceed 80 mg/d divided q.i.d.
  - Pediatric dose: Not established
  - Intrathecal baclofen: Very effective in patients with severe spasticity and stimulus-induced spasms
- Diazepam
  - Is a GABA agonist, facilitating CNS inhibition
  - Adult dose: 5–10 mg PO q4–6h
  - Pediatric dose (<12 yrs): 0.12–0.5 mg/kg/24 hrs PO, divided q6–8h
- Botulinum toxin type A and B
  - Causes reversible presynaptic blockade of the neuromuscular junction and reduces tone
  - Effective treatment of focal spasticity

Second Line
- Dantrolene
- Tizanidine
- Gabapentin
- Anticholinergic agents (Trihexphenidyl)
- Dopamine agonists

SURGERY
- Orthopedic intervention for tendon-lengthening procedures and scoliosis management
- Dorsal root rhizotomy
  - Consider in diplegic CP with good trunk strength, and no associated dyskinesia

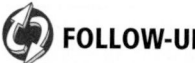 **FOLLOW-UP**

PROGNOSIS
Patients with severe forms of CP have a reduced life span. However, many patients experience a typical life expectancy.

REFERENCES

1. Ashwal S, Russman BS, Blasco PA, et al. Practice parameter: Diagnostic assessment of the child with cerebral palsy: Report of the Quality Standards Subcommittee of the American Academy of Neurology and the Practice Committee of the Child Neurology Society. *Neurology.* 2004;62(6): 851–863.
2. Dodd KJ, Taylor NF, Graham HK. A randomized clinical trial of strength training in young people with cerebral palsy. *Dev Med Child Neurol.* 2003;45:652–657.
3. Ubhi R, Bhakta BB, Ives HL, et al. Randomized double blind placebo controlled trial of the effect of botulinum toxin on walking in cerebral palsy. *Arch Dis Child.* 2000;83:481–487.
4. Van Schaeybroeck P, Nuttin B, Lagae L, et al. Intrathecal baclofen for intractable cerebral spasticity: A prospective placebo-controlled, double-blind study. *Neurosurgery.* 2000; 46:603–609.
5. Shevell M, Ashwal S, Donley D, et al. Practice parameter: Evaluation of the child with global developmental delay. Report of the Quality Standards Subcommittee of the American Academy of Neurology and the Practice Committee of the Child Neurology Society. *Neurology.* 2003; 60:367–380.
6. Russman BC. Early diagnosis and interventional therapy in cerebral palsy. *Neurology.* 2001; 57–1526.

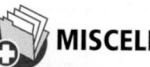 **MISCELLANEOUS**

CODES

ICD9-CM
- 343.0 Infantile cerebral palsy; diplegic
- 343.1 Infantile cerebral palsy; hemiplegic
- 343.2 Infantile cerebral palsy; quadriplegic
- 343.3 Infantile cerebral palsy; monoplegic
- 343.8 Other specified infantile cerebral palsy
- 343.9 Infantile cerebral palsy, unspecified

PATIENT TEACHING

 See Corresponding Diagnostic Algorithm

C

CERVICAL DYSPLASIA

Martha H. McLoughlin, MD

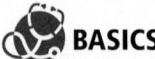 **BASICS**

DESCRIPTION

Preinvasive neoplastic epithelial changes in the transformation zone of the uterine cervix often associated with human papilloma virus (HPV) infections

- Mild dysplasia (cervical intraepithelial neoplasia [CIN] I or squamous intraepithelial lesion [SIL] low grade): Cellular changes are limited to the lower 1/3 of the squamous epithelium.
- Moderate dysplasia (CIN II or SIL high grade): Cellular changes are limited to the lower 2/3 of the squamous epithelium.
- Severe dysplasia (CIN III or SIL high grade or carcinoma in situ): Cellular changes involve the full thickness of the squamous epithelium.
- System(s) Affected: Reproductive

Geriatric Considerations
Less frequent

Pediatric Considerations
Very rare

Pregnancy Considerations
Dysplasia may progress during pregnancy

- It is important to determine the severity and to exclude the presence of invasive carcinoma.
- Definitive treatment is not required.
- Dysplasia by itself is not an indication for cesarean section.

GENERAL PREVENTION

- Annual Pap smears
- Ability to obtain skilled colposcopy service as needed
- Patient education (individually or by community services) to emphasize the need for protected intercourse and annual Pap smears
- Education of medical care providers to make patient referrals for the screening service, unless they provide it themselves
- Smoking cessation
- An HPV vaccine has been developed, but is not yet available for clinical use

EPIDEMIOLOGY

- Predominent age: The median age for carcinoma in situ is 28 years. Earlier lesions can be expected at younger ages.
- Predominent sex: Affects females only; usually a problem for women in the reproductive age group.

Incidence
Difficult to assess because of wide variability in false-negative Pap smear reporting and uneven distribution of qualified colposcopy practitioners

Prevalence
3,600 in 100,000 women aged 27–28 years

RISK FACTORS

- Multiparity and pregnancy before age 20 years
- Multiple sexual partners
- Early age at 1st sexual intercourse
- Condyloma acuminatum infection elsewhere in the body
- Cigarette smoking
- Prostitution
- Lower socioeconomic status
- Folate/beta carotene deficiency
- Oral contraceptive use

ETIOLOGY
There is strong linkage with infections by HPV types 16, 18, 31, 33, and 35. Other types of the same virus have also been implicated.

ASSOCIATED CONDITIONS

- Condyloma acuminatum
- Carcinoma of the cervix
- HIV

DIAGNOSIS

SIGNS AND SYMPTOMS

- Frequently none
- Occasionally associated with condyloma acuminata in the vulva, vagina, or anus
- Occasionally there are coexisting sexually transmitted diseases in the lower reproductive tract (e.g., chlamydia and/or gonorrhea).

TESTS

Lab

- Pap smear: Results may be affected by surgical lubricants (e.g., K-Y Jelly).
- HPV testing
- Viral DNA hybridization (ViraPap) and others
- PAPNET system to review negative Pap smears
- Cytyc 2000 ThinPrep Pap test (replacement of current Pap preparations)

Diagnostic Procedures/Surgery

- Pap smear with speculum examination
- Colposcopy and directed cervical biopsies
- Cone biopsy (by cold knife, laser, or loop excision)
- Endocervical curettage (not performed during pregnancy)
- Loop electrosurgical excision procedure (LEEP)
- Cervicography
- Use of HPV DNA typing to select certain cases with borderline abnormalities (e.g., atypical squamous cells of undetermined significance), for closer follow-up and colposcopy

Pathological Findings

- Clumping of the nuclear chromatin material
- Reversal of the nuclear/cytoplasmic ratio
- Koilocytosis
- Hyperchromasia

DIFFERENTIAL DIAGNOSIS

- Invasive carcinoma of the cervix
- Condyloma acuminatum

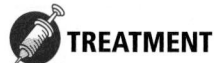

TREATMENT

GENERAL MEASURES
- Outpatient
- Office evaluation and observation

Diet
No restriction

Activity
Four weeks of pelvic rest after cone biopsy

MEDICATION (DRUGS)

Treatment is primarily surgical.

First Line
- Supplemental therapy to surgery: Fluorouracil (Efudex) once or twice daily as 5% vaginal cream
- Contraindication: Hypersensitivity to 5-fluorouracil
  - If hand is used in application, wash hands immediately afterward.
  - Avoid contact with eyes, nose, and mouth.

SURGERY
Outpatient: Cryotherapy, laser ablative or excisional cone, cold knife cone, LEEP of transformation zone

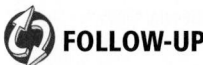

FOLLOW-UP

PROGNOSIS
- Generally excellent. 73–90% of patients with cervical dysplasia are cured with a single treatment (cryotherapy, laser, LEEP).
- May persist as a result of incomplete excision
- There may be recurrence due to the inability to eradicate HPV in the patient's body or prevent new infections.
- Immunocompromised patients, especially those with HIV, have a recurrence rate of >50%.

COMPLICATIONS
- Some severe dysplasia will progress to invasive carcinoma of the cervix.
- Possible complications following cone biopsy of the cervix
  - Hemorrhage
  - Infection
  - Cervical stenosis
  - Cervical incompetence
  - Infertility
  - Incomplete excision of dysplastic tissue
  - Recurrence

PATIENT MONITORING
Repeat Pap smears every 4 months during the 1st year after cone excision for severe dysplasia; every 6 months thereafter. For lesser lesions, repeat Pap smear yearly. Probe endocervical canal to ensure patency.

REFERENCES

1. American College of Obstetricians and Gynecologists www.acog.org
2. Block BB, Branham RA. Efforts to improve the follow-up of abnormal Papanicolaou test results. *J Am Board Fam Pract*. 1998;11:1.
3. Bosch FX, Manos MM, Munoz N, et al. Prevalence of human papilloma virus in cervical cancer–worldwide perspective. *J Natl Cancer Inst*. 1995;87:796.
4. Cox JT. Management of cervical intraepithelial neoplasia. *Lancet*. 1999;353:857.
5. Disaia PJ, Creasman WT. *Clinical Gynecologic Oncology*. 4th ed. St. Louis, MO: CV Mosby Co; 1993.
6. Herbst AL, Mishell DR, Stenchever MA, Droegemueller W. *Comprehensive Gynecology*. 2nd ed. St. Louis, MO: CV Mosby Co; 1992.
7. Korn AP. Management of abnormal cervical/vaginal Pap smears. *Medscape Women's Health*. 1996; 1(3)1.
8. Koss LG. Reducing the error rate in Papanicolaou smears. *Physician Assist*. 1994;18:48–52.
9. Koutsky LA, Ault KA, Wheeler CM, et al. A controlled trial of a human papillomavirus type 16 vaccine. *N Engl J Med*. 2002;347:1645.
10. Kurman RJ, ed. *Blaustein's Pathology of the Female Genital Tract*. 3rd ed. New York, NY: Springer-Verlag; 1987.
11. Maiman M, Fruchter RG, Serur E, et al. Human immunodeficiency virus infection and cervical neoplasia. *Gynecol Oncol*. 1990;38:377.
12. Manos M, Kinney W, Hurley L, Sherman M, Shich-Ngai J, Kurman R. Identifying women with cervical neoplasia, using human papilloma virus DNA testing for equivocal Papanicolaou results. *JAMA*. 1999;281:1605–1610.
13. Novak ER, Woodruff JD. *Novak's Gynecologic and Obstetric Pathology with Clinical and Endocrine Relations*. 8th ed. Philadelphia, PA: WB Saunders; 1979.
14. Richart R, Jones HW III, Reid R. Classification and interpretation of Pap smears. *ACOG Update*. 1993;10:1–10.
15. Sherman ME, Mango LJ, Kelly D, et al. PAPNET analysis of reportedly negative smears preceding the diagnosis of high-grade intraepithelial lesion or carcinoma. *Modern Pathol*. 1994;7:578–581.
16. Trevathan E, Layde P, Webster LA, et al. Cigarette smoking and dysplasia and carcinoma in situ of the uterine cervix. *JAMA*. 1983;250:499.
17. Update: National Breast and Cervical Cancer Early Detection Program: July 1991–September 1995. *MMWR*. 1996;45:484–487.
18. Ursin G, Peters RK, Henderson BE, et al. Oral contraceptive use and adenocarcinoma of the cervix. *Lancet*. 1994;344:1390.
19. Wright TC, Richart RM, Ferencz A. *Electrosurgery for HPV-related Diseases of the Lower Genital Tract*. New York, NY: Arthur Vision, Inc & Biovision, Inc; 1992.

MISCELLANEOUS

See also: Abnormal Pap Smear; Cervical Malignancy; Condyloma Acuminate; SIL is in Reference to Pap Smear Only

CODES

ICD9-CM
622.1 Dysplasia of cervix (uteri)

C

PATIENT TEACHING
See "Follow-Up"

See Corresponding Diagnostic Algorithm

See Patient Handout on CD

CERVICAL HYPEREXTENSION INJURIES

Vasilios Chrisostomidis, DO

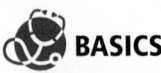

BASICS

DESCRIPTION
- Results from upward or backward injury to frontal head, jaw, and face. May involve the following
  - Soft-tissue injury around cervical spine: Whiplash or acute cervical musculoligamentous strain or sprain
  - Vertebral structures: Fractures, dislocations, ligamentous tears, and disc disruption/subluxation
  - Spinal cord: Acute central cord syndrome (CCS) secondary to cord compression or vascular insult
  - Vascular: Vertebral artery or carotid artery dissection
- System(s) Affected: Musculoskeletal; Nervous; Vascular

GENERAL PREVENTION
- Wear seat belts.
- Use proper equipment when participating in sports activities.

EPIDEMIOLOGY
- Predominant age: Trauma and sports injuries most common in young adults, average age 29.4 years; CCS most common among older people, average age 53 years
- Predominant sex: Male > Female

Incidence
About 25% of spinal injuries caused by hyperextension

RISK FACTORS
Present in 65% of cases of CCS
- Spinal stenosis
  - Congenital
  - Acquired: Prior trauma, spondylosis
- Spinal rigidity
  - Klippel-Feil syndrome
  - Ankylosing spondylitis

Genetics
Related to predisposing factors like ankylosing spondylitis associated with HLA-B27

ETIOLOGY
Trauma
- Mostly motor vehicular accidents
- Sports injuries
- Falls
- Assaults

DIAGNOSIS

SIGNS AND SYMPTOMS
- Neck pain, stiffness, and tenderness
- Headaches
- Paresthesia
- Numbness
- Shoulder pain, spasms, and tenderness; range of motion limitation; radicular signs
- Classically, with forehead, face, or jaw abrasion, laceration, or contusion
- CCS
  - Typically distal upper extremity weakness or paralysis worse than proximal upper extremity, worse than lower extremity
  - Variable sensory changes below level of lesion and sphincter dysfunction (including urinary retention)
  - Horner syndrome if C8–T11 involved
  - Lhermitte sign (7% of cases): Defined as electrical sensation in the spine or limbs after neck flexion

TESTS

Imaging
- Plain cervical spine films remain primary initial diagnostic modality
- Follow NEXUS or Canadian Cervical Spine Rules.
  - Static: Cervical spine series with minimum of 2 views; lateral view reveals posttrauma abnormalities in 70–83% of cases, addition of anteroposterior and open-mouth views increases sensitivity; may show prevertebral soft-tissue swelling without other radiologic signs in CCS, craniocervical soft-tissue swelling in C2 fractures or bony abnormalities.
  - Dynamic: Flexion/extension, only if asymptomatic neck and no neurologic deficits or mental impairment, evaluates ligamentous integrity in acute setting, also evaluates spine stability and union by amount of movement in fractures during or after treatment.
- CT scan or tomograms: Better delineation of fractures, spinal canal status. Becoming more common as availability increases.
- CT myelogram: Alternative to MRI; delineates neural impingement
- MRI: Diagnostic procedure of choice in CCS with direct visualization of traumatic cord lesions (edema or hematomyelia), soft tissue compressing cord, and stenosis of canal. It also detects a high percentage of occult discs and ligamentous or soft-tissue abnormalities, but modality is poor with fractures.

ALERT

Geriatric Considerations
- Degenerative disease of cervical spine may be confused with acute traumatic change on imaging.
- Osteoporosis increases risk of fracture.

Pediatric Considerations
Consider spinal cord injury without radiographic abnormality, which has a high incidence at <9 years. MRI may help detect the injury.

Diagnostic Procedures/Surgery
Discussed in other sections of topic; care must be taken to avoid overlooking subtle hyperextension injuries.

Pathological Findings
- Acute cervical strain/sprain based on animal, cadaver, and postmortem studies
- Muscle tears of the sternocleidomastoid or partial avulsion of the longus colli muscle
- Stretching or rupture of anterior longitudinal ligament
- Injuries to intervertebral discs and facet joint capsules
- Rarely, retropharyngeal hematoma
- Vertebral fractures: See "General Measures."
- CCS: Secondary to cord compression or vascular insult
- Traditionally reported as central gray matter injury with hemorrhage
- Central hemorrhage is seen with more severe injuries.
- It is currently thought that there is predominantly white matter injury with involvement of the lateral column, particularly the corticospinal tracts.
- Pathological hallmark is diffuse axonal disruption.

DIFFERENTIAL DIAGNOSIS
- Herniated discs
- Arthritis
- Radiculopathy
- Myelopathy
- For CCS
  - Bell cruciate palsy
  - Bilateral brachial plexus injuries
  - Carotid artery dissection
  - Vertebral artery dissection

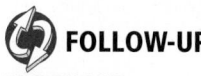 **TREATMENT**

INITIAL STABILIZATION
- Outpatient or inpatient as required by injury
- ATLS protocol with backboard and collar

GENERAL MEASURES
- Whiplash; depending on severity
  - Soft or rigid collar (6)[C]
  - Medicines: Analgesics, muscle relaxants and anti-inflammatory agents
  - After resolution of spasms, repeat flexion/extension lateral cervical spine views to confirm stability.
- CCS
  - See "Medications."
  - If no instability, bed rest with soft collar for 4–6 weeks followed by mobilization with collar for another 4–6 weeks
- Fractures: Stability determined by usual radiologic criteria; surgical decompression and stabilization are indicated in
  - Patients with incomplete spinal cord injuries and spinal canal compromise resulting from bone, disc, subluxation, or hematoma
  - Those whose condition deteriorates or does not improve on conservative therapy
- Hangman fracture: Traumatic spondylolisthesis of the axis with bilateral fractures through the C2 pedicles, often with anterior subluxation of C2 over C3
  - Usually stable, managed with sternal-occipital-mental orthosis
  - Unstable if C2 subluxation over C3; >50% of vertebral body of C3 in anteroposterior diameter
  - Unstable if excessive angulation of C2 over C3
  - Treated with halo vest immobilization for 8–14 weeks until repeated flexion/extension films taken
  - If stable, use rigid collar for additional 8–12 weeks.
- Odontoid fracture: Treated according to type
  - I: Through apex, may be unstable and require surgical fusion
  - II: Most common type, at base of dens, usually unstable; nonunion rates of about 30% with immobilization alone, especially with increased dens displacement >6 mm in patients >7 years
  - III: Through C2 body, usually stable; immobilized in halo for 8–14 weeks, rigid collar for 8–14 weeks, then mobilization
- C3–C7 hyperextension fractures
  - If stable, rigid collar for 8–14 weeks, then mobilization
  - If unstable, halo brace: Make serial lateral cervical spine films from supine to upright; if still unstable, surgical stabilization is required.
  - Postoperatively, follow-up with radiographs until trabeculation across fracture site or interbody fusion is achieved.
  - Dissection-vertebral artery versus carotid artery requires a cerebral angiogram or MRA and anticoagulation to prevent further ischemic embolic events.

Diet
No special diet

Activity
- Activity restriction with increases after patient improvement
- Rest and immobilization until pain is controlled; followed by gradual mobilization and rehabilitation exercises if needed

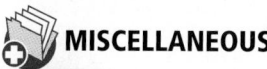 MEDICATION (DRUGS)

First Line
CCS

- Methylprednisolone IV 30 mg/kg over 1 hour, followed by IV 5.4 mg/kg/h for 23 hours (continue for 47 hours if started >8 hours after injury). It improves neurologic outcome, as well as motor and sensory function at 6 weeks, 6 months, and 1 year after incomplete spinal cord injury (4)[B].

SURGERY
- CCS
  - In acute cases, surgery is associated with deterioration and increased complications and therefore contraindicated.
  - Surgery may be indicated in patients whose health improves, but then begins to deteriorate.
  - Otherwise, surgical decompression and stabilization are performed only when neurologic function has reached a plateau or maximum recovery without surgical intervention.
- Fractures: See "General Measures."

FOLLOW-UP

PROGNOSIS
- Most important prognostic factor is the initial neurologic status (4)[C].
- Whiplash: Most patients recover well; mild symptoms resolve within 6 months
  - On average, more severe injuries without disc involvement resolve in 21 months.
  - 30 months for injuries with degenerative changes
  - At 2 years, 42% complete recovery, 15% mild discomfort, 43% significant discomfort affecting work
- CCS
  - Most patients recover motor strength within 2 weeks.
  - Younger patients have better prognosis.
  - Leg, bowel, and bladder functions return first.
  - Return of arm strength follows, then that of hand.
  - Upper extremities recover less well, and fine finger movements usually are not regained completely.
  - With cord contusion but no hematomyelia, 50% recover enough strength and sensation to ambulate independently, although usually with spasticity.
- Fracture-dislocation
  - Hangman fracture: 93–100% fusion rate after 8–14 weeks external immobilization
  - Odontoid fracture: Type III, 90% fusion with immobilization

COMPLICATIONS
- Persistent symptoms
- Nonunion of fractures
- Persistent instability requiring additional procedure
- Reactions and infection related to orthosis

PATIENT MONITORING
- Patients under observation should be checked with radiographs every 3–4 weeks for about 3 months, at which point bone healing is usually adequate.
- Halo is then replaced with rigid collar for next 3 months, or rigid collar is replaced with soft collar for comfort of patient.

REFERENCES

1. Eichler ME, Vollmer DG. Cervical spine trauma. In: Youmans JR, ed. *Neurological Surgery*, 4th ed. Philadelphia: WB Saunders. 1996;1939–1946.
2. Greenberg MS. *Handbook of Neurosurgery*, 4th ed. Lakeland, FL: Greenberg Graphics, 1997.
3. McDowell GS, Cammisa FP, Eismont FJ. Hyperextension injuries of the cervical spine. In: Levine AM, Eismont FJ, Garfin SR, et al., eds. *Spine Trauma*. Philadelphia: WB Saunders, 1998:367–386.
4. McKinley W, et al. Outcomes of surgical management versus late or no surgical intervention after acute spinal cord injury. *Arch Phys Med Rehabil*. 2004;85:1818–1825.
5. Platzer P, et al. Delayed of missed diagnosis of cervical spine injuries. *J Trauma*. 2006;61:150–155.
6. Rechtine, G. Nonoperative management and treatment of spine injuries. *Spine*. 2006;31:22–27.
7. Sonntag VKH, Francis PM. Controversies in spinal cord syndromes. In: Garfin SR, Northup BE, eds. *Surgery for Spinal Cord Injuries*. New York: Raven Press; 1993:15–31.
8. Travis RL. Hyperextension and hyperflexion injuries of the cervical spine. In: Youmans JR, ed. *Neurological Surgery*, 4th ed. Philadelphia: WB Saunders, 1996:2037–2042.
9. Wong WB, Parjabi MM, White AA. Mechanisms of injury in the cervical spine. In: Clark CR, ed. *The Cervical Spine*, 3rd ed. Philadelphia: Lippincott-Raven; 1998:79.

MISCELLANEOUS

CODES

ICD9-CM
- 952.00 Cervical spinal cord injury without evidence of spinal bone injury, C1-C4 level with unspecified spinal cord injury
- 847.00 Neck-Anterior longitudinal ligament, atlanto-axial joints, whiplash injury.
- 805.00 Fracture of vertebral column without mention of spinal cord injury.

PATIENT TEACHING

For patient instruction on prevention: THINK FIRST Foundation, 26 South La Grange Road, Suite 103. La Grange, IL 60525
1-800-844-6556. www.thinkfirst.org.

See Patient Handout on CD

CERVICAL MALIGNANCY

Martha H. McLoughlin, MD

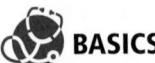 **BASICS**

DESCRIPTION
- Invasive cancer of the uterine cervix
- Commonly involves the vagina, parametria, and pelvic side walls
- In advanced cases, the cancer may invade the bladder, rectum, or other pelvic sites.
- System(s) Affected: Reproductive
- Synonym(s): Cancer of the uterine cervix; Cervical cancer; Cervical carcinoma

ALERT
Geriatric Considerations
Because >1/2 the invasive cancer cases are seen in the >65 age group, efforts should be concentrated on expanding the availability of Pap smear screening to the geriatric population.

GENERAL PREVENTION
- Smoking cessation
- Avoidance of sexually transmitted diseases (STDs)
- Regular Pap smears and pelvic exams; appropriate intervals (according to American College of Obstetricians and Gynecologists and American Cancer Society):
  – All women who are or who have been sexually active or who have reached age 18 should undergo an annual Pap test and pelvic examination.
  – After a woman has had 3 or more consecutive satisfactory annual examinations with normal findings, the Pap smear may be performed less frequently at the discretion of her physician.
  – Women who have had a history of cervical cancer, or women at an increased risk of developing cancer should continue to be screened annually.

EPIDEMIOLOGY
Affects only women

Incidence
The peak incidence of cervical cancer occurs in women aged 45–49 years. Only 10% of cases occur in women aged ≥75.

Prevalence
In the US, there are an estimated 10,370 new cases of invasive cervical cancer diagnosed annually, with 3,710 deaths due to the disease.

RISK FACTORS
- Multiple sexual partners
- Male partner with multiple sexual partners
- Male partner who has had a partner with cervical carcinoma
- Early age at 1st sexual intercourse
- Current or previous HPV infections, Human Papilloma virus (e.g., condyloma acuminatum, cervical intraepithelial neoplasia)
- History of STDs
- Smoking
- Immunosuppression from drugs or HIV infection
- Diethylstilbestrol offspring
- Unprotected sex
- High parity

Genetics
Not an inherited disease

ETIOLOGY
Unknown; strong association with genital infection by the oncogenic strains of HPV 16 and 18

ASSOCIATED CONDITIONS
Condyloma acuminatum, Preinvasive/invasive lesions of the vulva and vagina

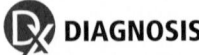 **DIAGNOSIS**

SIGNS AND SYMPTOMS
- Abnormal vaginal bleeding
- Postcoital vaginal bleeding
- Pelvic, leg, and/or back
- Dyspareunia
- Hematuria
- Rectal bleeding
- Foul vaginal discharge
- Cervical ulcer, crater, or fungating mass
- Extension of the cervical mass into upper vagina and/or parametria, with induration, nodularity, and fixation to surrounding tissue
- Can often be asymptomatic

Physical Exam
Most women have a visible cervical lesion on exam

TESTS
Lab
- For initial diagnosis: Pap smear and cervical biopsies
- Pap smears are not obscured by vaginal lubricants, but can be compromised by vaginitis or excessive vaginal bleeding.
- CBC
- Blood urea nitrogen, creatinine

Imaging
- CT scans of the abdomen and pelvis, if needed, for detection of lymph node metastasis and for evaluation of planned radiation therapy
- Lymphangiography, if needed, for detection of pelvic and para-aortic lymph node metastasis
- Chest radiograph
- Excretory pyelogram

Diagnostic Procedures/Surgery
- Colposcopy, if indicated
- Endocervical curettage
- Cervical conization, if indicated; can resolve the question of early invasion and, if present, can determine the depth of invasion and presence of lymphatic and vascular involvement
- Liver function tests
- Cystoscopy
- Sigmoidoscopy
- Selection of surgical therapy in younger women with early stages of cancer provides ovarian conservation.

Pathological Findings
- Invasive squamous cell carcinoma is the major cell type (80%)
- Invasive adenocarcinoma is becoming increasingly evident, especially in women <35.
- Other cell types are also present in the minority (e.g., adenosquamous, neuroendocrine, small cell)

DIFFERENTIAL DIAGNOSIS
- Marked cervicitis and erosion
- Cervical polyp
- Cervical condyloma
- Metastasis from endometrial carcinoma or gestational trophoblastic disease
- Cervical pregnancy
- Nabotian cysts
- Glandular hyperplasia

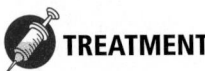 **TREATMENT**

INITIAL STABILIZATION
According to the depth of invasion and clinical staging

GENERAL MEASURES
- Improve the patient's nutritional state, correct any anemia, and treat any vaginal and/or pelvic infections.
- Chemotherapy has been used extensively as adjuvant therapy for metastatic disease and more recently as neoadjuvant therapy.

Pregnancy Considerations
- Generally, the choice of treatment depends on the length of gestation, the patient's wish to continue pregnancy to attainment of fetal lung maturity, and the treating physician's comfort level in delaying definitive therapy and the severity of the abnormal Pap smear.
- If treatment is delayed, the patient must receive close follow-up care with its frequency dependent on the severity of the disease.
- Selection of the mode of therapy is based on clinical staging, as noted previously.

Diet
As appropriate

Activity
As tolerated

MEDICATION (DRUGS)

First Line

- Cisplatin, hydroxyurea, and fluorouracil have been used as adjuvant sensitizer to radiation therapy.
- Cisplatin/carboplatin, etoposide (VP-16), ifosfamide, and bleomycin have been used as adjuvant therapy for recurrent, metastatic disease.
- Contraindications, precautions, and possible interactions: Refer to the manufacturer's profile for each drug.

Second Line

Prescribe Ondansetron (Zofran), dronabinol (Marinol), metoclopramide (Reglan), Prednisone, and others for nausea control.

SURGERY

- Stage IA1 (lesions with <3-mm invasion from basement membrane): Cervical conization with total hysterectomy later when patient's family is completed; otherwise, total hysterectomy by either the abdominal or vaginal route
- Stage IA2 (lesions with >3-mm but <5-mm invasion from the basement membrane) and stages IB1, IB2, IIA: Patient has the option of radical hysterectomy, bilateral pelvic lymphadenectomy, and para-aortic node sampling or primary radiation with brachytherapy and teletherapy
- Stage IVA (lesions limited to central metastasis to the bladder and/or rectum): Pelvic exenteration may be feasible.
- Radiotherapy
  - For stage IA2 or higher
    - Brachytherapy with intracavitary radium or cesium or interstitial cesium needles to treat the central tumor sites
    - Teletherapy with external megavoltage radiation to treat tumor metastasis in the pelvic walls
  - For localized persistent or recurrent disease, radiation therapy or pelvic exenteration as appropriate

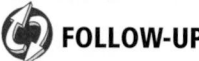 **FOLLOW-UP**

PROGNOSIS

After commonly accepted surgical and radiation treatments, 5-year survival

Stage	5-yr Survival (%)
1	80
2	65
3	30
4	15

COMPLICATIONS

- Hemorrhage
- Pelvic infection
- Bladder dysfunction
- Genitourinary fistula
- Ureteral obstruction with renal failure
- Bowel obstruction
- Lymphocyst
- Pulmonary embolism
- Loss of ovarian function from radiotherapy, or indication for bilateral oophorectomy

PATIENT MONITORING

- With completion of definitive therapy, each patient is evaluated with physical/pelvic examinations and Pap smears at the following intervals:
  - Every 3 months for 1–2 years
  - Every 6 months until the 5th year
  - Yearly thereafter
- The 3 most common signs of cancer recurrence are unexplained weight loss, leg edema, and pelvic or thigh pain.

REFERENCES

1. Jemal A, Murray T, Ward E, et al. Cancer statistics 2005. *CA Cancer J Clin.* 2005;55:10.
2. McMeekin DS, McGonigle KH, Vasilev SA. Cervical cancer prevention: Towards cost effective screening. *Medscape Women's Heal.* 1997;2.
3. Nanda K, McCrory D, Myers E, Bastian L, Hasselblad V, Hickey J. Accuracy of the Papanicolaou test in screening for and follow-up of cervical cytological abnormalities: A systematic review. *Ann Intern Med.* 2000;132:810–819.
4. National Cancer Institute. *Cancer Statistics Review 1973–1987.* Bethesda, MD: National Cancer Institute; 1990. Publication no. (NIH) 90–2789.
5. Parke SL, Tong T, Bolden S, Wingo PA. Cancer statistics, 1997. *CA Cancer J Clin.* 1997;47:527.
6. Vizcaino AP, Moren V, Bosch FX, et al. International trends in the incidence of cervical cancer. *Int J Cancer.* 1998;75:536.

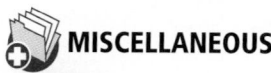 **MISCELLANEOUS**

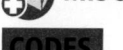 **CODES**

ICD9-CM

180.0 Malignant neoplasm of body of cervix uteri, endocervix

PATIENT TEACHING

Refer patient to the American Cancer Society for more information: 1599 Clifton Rd., Atlanta, GA 30329; (404) 320-3333. Web site: www.cancer.org.

 See Corresponding Diagnostic Algorithm

 See Patient Handout on CD

CERVICAL POLYPS

Nicole D. Pilevsky, MD

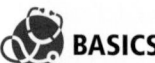 **BASICS**

DESCRIPTION
Pedunculated masses, usually single, that vary in size from a few millimeters to 3 cm, protrude from the cervix, and may bleed
- System(s) Affected: Reproductive

Geriatric Considerations
Rare

Pediatric Considerations
Rare

Pregnancy Considerations
Delay removal of polyps until postpartum unless bleeding or cervical dilation found.

GENERAL PREVENTION
None known

EPIDEMIOLOGY
- Predominant age: 40–60 years
- Predominant sex: Female only

Incidence
Common

RISK FACTORS
None

PATHOPHYSIOLOGY
Hyperplastsic proliferation of cervical or endometrial cells

ETIOLOGY
- Unknown for most cases
- Secondary reaction to cervical inflammatory or hormonal stimulation

ASSOCIATED CONDITIONS
None commonly

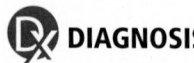 **DIAGNOSIS**

SIGNS AND SYMPTOMS
- Painless
- Intermenstrual bleeding
- May cause postcoital or postmenopausal bleeding
- Leukorrhea

History
Abnormal vaginal bleeding or discharge

Physical Exam
Polyp evident on speculum exam

TESTS
Lab
Send polyp for pathologic analysis

Diagnostic Procedures/Surgery
Perform Papanicolaou smear before treatment

Pathological Findings
- Benign hyperplastic endocervical epithelium, often with a large number of blood vessels involved
- Extremely rare incidence of dysplasia or malignancy
- Case reports of lymphoma and sarcoma botryoides [C]

DIFFERENTIAL DIAGNOSIS
- Prolapsed submucous myoma or endometrial polyp
- Other causes of intermenstrual bleeding
- Decidualized endometrium

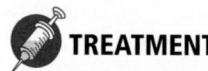 **TREATMENT**

INITIAL STABILIZATION
Outpatient management usually, but larger polyps may require removal in an operating room.

GENERAL MEASURES
Diet
General diet

Activity
Following removal, avoid sexual intercourse, tampons, and douching for 2 weeks.

MEDICATION (DRUGS)

None

SURGERY
Simple surgical excision in office with traction or electrocautery; control bleeding with silver nitrate, Monsel's solution, or cautery; larger polyps may require ligature

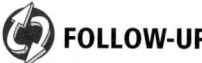 **FOLLOW-UP**

DISPOSITION
Admission Criteria
Uncontrolled hemorrhage

Issues for Referral
Refer to a gynecologist for removal

PROGNOSIS
Recurrence not likely with complete excision

COMPLICATIONS
Bleeding and mild pain with removal

PATIENT MONITORING
Recheck at routine appointments or as needed.

REFERENCES

1. Rittenbach J, Cao JD, Weiss LM, et al. Primary diffuse large B-cell lymphoma of the uterus presenting solely as an endometrial polyp. *Int J Gynecol Pathol*. 2005;24(4):347–351.
2. Miyamoto T, Shiozawa T, Nakamura T, et al. Sarcoma botyoides of the uterine cervix in a 46-year-old woman: Case report and literature review. *Int J Gynecol Pathol*. 2004;23(1):78–82.

 MISCELLANEOUS

CODES

ICD9-CM
622.7 Mucous polyp of cervix
ICD10
N84.1 Mucous polyp of cervix

PATIENT TEACHING
See Corresponding Diagnostic Algorithm

CERVICAL SPINE INJURY

Ruben Peralta, MD, FACS
Sarah Guzofski, MD

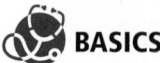 **BASICS**

DESCRIPTION

Patients with spinal cord injuries present a significant diagnostic challenge. A high index of suspicion is required to detect injury as well as other medical and surgical conditions that may be masked by the spinal cord injury.

The ultimate functional outcome for the patient with cervical spine trauma is dependent on the degree and level of spinal cord injury. Early identification of unstable injuries and prevention of injury must be a priority.

Cervical spine injuries may involve bony structures and/or the spinal cord itself.

Cervical Spine Bony Injuries

Anatomically, the cervical spine is classified by anatomic location or by mechanism of injury and can be divided into 2 regions:

- Axial (C1–C2)
  – C1 ring fracture (Jefferson fracture)
  – C2 (Hangman's)
- Sub-axial (C3–C7)
  – Cervical body fractures: Include lateral mass fracture and facet joint dislocation

  By mechanism of injury: Flexion, flexion-rotation, extension, or compression

Spinal Cord Injury

- The American Spinal Injury Association Scoring System (which motor and sensory deficits) is recommended for use in all suspected spinal cord injuries.
- Spinal cord injuries can be divided into complete and incomplete
  – Complete: Neurologic deficit in all sensory and motor modalities
  – Incomplete
    ○ Central cord syndrome: Most common incomplete injury; motor deficits greater in upper than lower extremities, due to watershed injury affecting long fiber tracts; may be because of hyperextension causing edema or ischemia
    ○ Anterior cord syndrome: Posterior columns spared; affects spinothalamic, corticospinal, anterior and lateral columns; loss of pain, temperature, motor with preserved vibration, and position sense below the lesion
    ○ Posterior cord syndrome: Sensory deficits more pronounced than motor; due to contusion of posterior columns
    ○ Brown sequard syndrome: Ipsilateral motor loss and vibration sensation deficits with contralateral loss of pain and temperature sensation; hemisection of cord most often due to penetrating trauma

EPIDEMIOLOGY

- Predominant age: Most common 16–25
- Predominant sex: Male > Female

Incidence

250,000 people in US living with spinal cord injury

Prevalence

- Cervical spine injuries account for 12,000 deaths in the US each year. 1/2 of these result from motor vehicle accidents.
- 11,000 people hospitalized for spinal cord injury annually.
- 1990 study indicates 6% of hospitalizations for injury are due to vertebral injury, whereas only 1% were due to spinal cord injury
- Although spinal cord injuries are relatively rare, they have a significant economic and social impact (e.g., need for intensive initial hospital care, long-term rehabilitation, and, at times, life-long care).

RISK FACTORS

- Motor vehicle collisions
- Diving accidents
- Falls
- Substance abuse

ETIOLOGY

- Trauma
- In people <65, motor vehicle collisions most common cause; >65, falls

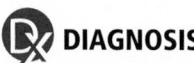 **DIAGNOSIS**

SIGNS AND SYMPTOMS

- In a trauma setting, a high index of suspicion for spinal cord injury should be maintained until such injuries can be excluded by clinical examination and imaging studies.
- As per Adult Trauma Life Support (ATLS) protocol, a complete neurologic exam, including rectal examination, must be performed as part of the initial evaluation.
- Pain, stiffness, and/or tenderness in an alert patient

TESTS

Imaging

- CT scan is the most reliable screening tool for cervical spine trauma; however, it provides little information about nerve or ligamatous injury.
- MRI is used for the evaluation of spinal cord and ligamentous injury.
- Lateral cervical spine plain radiography has become less prominent as an evaluation tool in the acute trauma setting (even though it remains part of the ATLS protocol).

DIFFERENTIAL DIAGNOSIS

- Osteoarthritis
- Cervical spondylosis

 TREATMENT

PRE HOSPITAL

- Immediate immobilization of cervical spine for every victim of trauma with neck pain or tenderness, high-impact mechanism of injury, and patient with altered level of consciousness
- High cervical spine injuries can require early intubation due to loss of phrenic nerve function (C3–C5)

INITIAL STABILIZATION

- Begin with ATLS protocol
- Arterial oxygen should be measured immediately. Adequate oxygenation in cord injury helps prevent further damage and aids recovery.
- In all documented spinal cord injuries, a thorough clinical and radiographic evaluation must be undertaken to rule out any other concomitant injuries.
- Supportive care (e.g., airway management, ventilation support for high cervical spinal injury, blood pressure support)

GENERAL MEASURES

- Spinal shock: Transient loss of all neurologic function occurring below the level of the spinal cord injury; distinct from neurogenic shock, which is characterized by hypotension and bradycardia from loss of sympathetic function secondary to spinal cord injury
- Usually traumatic brain injuries alone do not cause hypotension, but can cause hypertension, except in extremes of life with head laceration with undermined time of injury
- In patients with hypotension, consider other injuries that could cause hypotension (e.g., blood loss, pericardial tamponade, tension pneumothorax, cardiac contusion)
- Prophylaxis of deep venous thrombosis (DVT) and stress gastritis
- Skin care for prevention of pressure ulcers

Activity

- C spine immobilization
- Bed rest until thoracic and lumbar spine injuries have been ruled out

Physical Therapy

Physical therapy should be initiated as soon as injuries have been ruled out.

MEDICATION (DRUGS)

First Line
- Steroid treatment
  - For incomplete cord injury
  - Based on time elapsed from injury. recommendation is for steroid treatment if within 8 hours of injury.
  - Methylprednisolone: Bolus: 30 mg/kg, 5.4 mg/kg/h for the next 23 hours if <3 hours; if >3 hours but <8 hours, treat for total of 48 hours (1)[B]

- Contraindications
  - Sepsis or other serious infection

SURGERY
Indications for emergency surgery

- Controversial, but in general emergent decompressive surgery with spinal stabilization is indicated for incomplete injury with persistent or progressive spinal cord compression as demonstrated by clinical findings and radiologic studies. Controversy exists regarding the indications for early decompressive surgery for complete lesions. (2)[C]

 FOLLOW-UP

PROGNOSIS
In cases of significant spinal cord injuries, the prognosis is guarded. Development of newer orthopedic devices can stabilize the spine and allow early mobilization, but do not help to reverse neurologic damage if sustained.

COMPLICATIONS
- Complications associated with high level spinal cord injury include bradycardia and acute respiratory failure from diaphragmatic paralysis.
- DVT
- Spasticity
- Constipation
- Bladder dysfunction
- Pressure ulcers
- Osteoporosis
- Depression
- Autonomic dysreflexia

PATIENT MONITORING
Critical care facilities must be available initially; physical and occupational therapy units with special skills in spinal cord injuries will be required later.

REFERENCES

1. Bracken MB, et al. A randomized control trial of methylprednisolone or naloxone in the treatment of acute spinal cord injury. Results of the second acute spinal cord injury study. *N Engl J Med*. 1990; 322:1405–1411.
2. Fehlings M, Perrin R. The role and timing of early decompression for cervical spinal cord injury: Update with a review of recent clinical evidence. *Injury*. 2005;36:S13–S26.
3. Bracken MB, et al. Efficacy of methylprednisolone in acute spinal cord injury. *JAMA*. 1984;251:45–52.
4. Diaz JJ, Aulino JM, Collier B, et al. The early work-up for isolated ligamentous injury of the cervical spine: Does computed tomography have a role? *J Trauma*. 2005;59:897–903.
5. Hurlbert RJ. The role of steroids in acute spinal cord injury: An evidence-based analysis. *Spine*. 2001; 26:S39–S46.
6. Spencer MT, Bazarian JJ. Are Corticosteroids effective in Traumatic Spinal Cord Injury? *Ann Emerg Med*. 2003;41:409–413.

 MISCELLANEOUS

Spinal cord injury without any radiographic abnormality common in children, mostly due to ligamentous laxity

CODES

ICD9-CM
- 952.00 Cervical spinal cord injury without evidence of spinal bone injury, C1-C4 level with unspecified spinal cord injury
- 806.00
- 805.00

PATIENT TEACHING

Activity
Patients should be taught technique for self-catheterization.

See Corresponding Diagnostic Algorithm

C

CERVICAL SPONDYLOSIS

Erika McPhee, MD
Ruben Peralta, MD, FACS

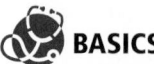 BASICS

DESCRIPTION

- Cervical spondylosis (degeneration & possible fusion of vertebrae) is a degenerative process of the cervical spine occurring as a natural consequence of aging.
- Degeneration of the discs with loss of disc height alters the biomechanics of the vertebral body and facet joints resulting in facet joint arthritis and osteophyte formation.
- Subsequent pathologic changes manifest in several ways including axial neck pain, radiculopathy, and myelopathy. Patients may have any combination of these manifestations.

GENERAL PREVENTION

The midcervical spine is the area usually involved in spondylosis. This portion will develop a flexion deformity, causing extension of the upper spine as the body tries to keep the head erect.

EPIDEMIOLOGY

- Predominant age: Above age 40, the incidence increases with each passing decade
- Predominant sex: Male > Female (3:2)

Incidence

Population >40 years: 30 to 40%

Prevalence

66% of adults experience neck pain in their lifetime and 5% are highly disabled by it.

RISK FACTORS

- Incidence higher in those who carry loads on their head compared to those who do not.
- Role of trauma in the etiology is controversial.

Genetics

A congenital decrease in the anterior-posterior (AP) diameter of the spinal canal may be a predisposition for cervical myelopathy.

ETIOLOGY

- Axial neck pain: May be multifactorial. Sources of pain include the intervertebral disc, facet joints, vertebral bodies, spinal ligaments, and paraspinal musculature.
- Cervical spondylotic radiculopathy: Pain, weakness, or sensory deficit resulting from compression of nerve roots secondary to soft tissue/disc and/or bony impingement.
- Cervical spondylotic myelopathy: Long-tract signs resulting from a decrease in the space available for the spinal cord

ASSOCIATED CONDITIONS

Lumbar spine degeneration

DIAGNOSIS

SIGNS AND SYMPTOMS

- Axial neck pain: pain or soreness usually in the paramedian neck muscles posteriorly, with radiation toward the occiput or into the shoulder and periscapular regions. Headaches are common.
- Cervical spondylotic radiculopathy: symptoms in a specific dermatomal distribution in the upper extremity. Symptoms are typically sharp pain, tingling, or burning sensation. There may be a sensory or motor deficit in the involved nerve root. Symptoms may be intensified by neck movement.
  - Common cervical radiculopathy patterns
    - C2: Posterior occiptital headaches, temporal pain.
    - C3: Occipital headache, retro-orbital or retro-auricular pain.
    - C4: Base of neck, trapezial pain
    - C5: Lateral arm pain, deltoid weakness, decreased biceps reflex
    - C6: Pain in radial forearm, thumb and index fingers, weakness of biceps and wrist extension, decreased brachioradialis reflex
    - C7: Pain in middle finger, weakness of triceps and wrist flexion, decreased triceps reflex
    - C8: Pain in ring and little fingers, weakness of finger flexors
    - T1: Pain in ulnar forearm, weakness of hand intrinsics
- Cervical spondylotic myelopathy: Lower-extremity gait disturbances, loss of upper extremity fine motor control, and bowel/bladder dysfunction (late finding).
- Loss of neck extension (common)
- Lateral flexion of the cervical spine is limited in the erect position, but greatly increased when lying down. (Functional disorders are not improved by lying down.)

ALERT

Pregnancy Considerations

Symptoms may be worse in pregnancy.

History

- In cervical spondylotic myelopathy, commonly a history of a progressive stepwise deterioration of neurological status.
- Patient may report difficulty with grasping, holding, worsening handwriting.
- Increasing difficulty with balance and gait.

Physical Exam

- Axial neck pain: Localized areas of muscular tenderness may be present.
- Cervical spondylotic radiculopathy
  - Shoulder abduction sign: Pain relieved when holding arm on the affected side over the head with the wrist resting on top of the head
  - Spurling maneuver: Aggravation of symptoms with extension or lateral rotation of the head to the affected side.

- Cervical spondylotic myelopathy
  - Brisk reflexes, clonus, presence of pathologic reflexes
    - Positive Babinski: Up-going toes with scratching of plantar foot
    - Hoffman's sign: Flicking of the volar surface of the flexed middle finger distal phalanx causes pathologic flexion of the thumb and index finger
    - Finger escape sign: Inability to maintain the ulnar digits extended and adducted
    - Inverted radial reflex: Brachioradialis reflex is diminished but causes spastic contraction of the finger flexors

TESTS

Imaging

- Radiographs of the cervical spine, anteroposterior, lateral open-mouth odontoid, and both oblique views should be obtained. Osteophytes and/or joint space narrowing will be evident.
- Computed tomography (CT) with or without myelography vs. magnetic resonance imaging (MRI) scans
  - Valuable when surgery is contemplated or the diagnosis is in doubt
  - Not indicated in the great majority of cases as a careful history and physical examination coupled with routine cervical spine radiographs will make the diagnosis
  - The decision as to which is better, CT or MRI, is controversial. MRI depicts cord changes, enlargement, compression, or atrophy well, whereas CT, especially in conjunction with myelography, shows bony changes, especially in foramina involvement. MRI has the obvious advantage of not requiring a myelogram and is the study of choice for diagnosis of cervical radiculopathy or myelopathy.
  - Postoperatively, MRI is excellent in evaluating patients who have failed to obtain relief from surgery or have developed new symptoms. If this does not demonstrate a cause, then a CT scan with contrast may be obtained.

Diagnostic Procedures/Surgery

- Nerve root injections may be helpful in the case of cervical spondylotic radiculopathy
- Indications for surgery for radiculopathy include severe or progressive weakness/numbness, and failure of conservative measures
- Surgical intervention has been shown to improve functional outcomes by stopping the progression of neurologic deficits and should be considered for myelopathy unless case is mild or in those who pose a prohibitive surgical risk.

DIFFERENTIAL DIAGNOSIS

- Cervical disk disease (the two often coexist)
- Pancoast tumor of lung
- Rheumatoid arthritis
- Neurologic disorders such as multiple sclerosis

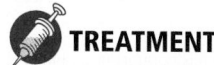 TREATMENT

GENERAL MEASURES

- Initial treatment is conservative and should include soft cervical collar, analgesics, and muscle relaxants, as well as restriction of activity.
  - Ultrasonic treatments especially combined with gentle muscle stimulation (US-MS) for 15 to 20 minutes daily or 2 times a day may be helpful.
  - Physical therapy
- Chronic
  - No treatment is necessary except the prescription of non-narcotic analgesics for symptoms.
  - Any type of activity or work that causes strain of the neck should be avoided.

Diet

No special diet

Activity

Any activity that does not cause symptoms should be encouraged, as the disease is chronic. Needless restrictions may lead to unnecessary decline in function.

 MEDICATION (DRUGS)

First Line

- Acetaminophen (Tylenol) 1000 mg q.i.d.:
  - Safest regimen. Studies have shown it to be at least as effective as nonsteroidal anti-inflammatory drugs (NSAIDs).
- NSAIDs
  - Aspirin 1 g q.i.d. is effective in many cases.
  - If aspirin fails, any of the other NSAIDs may used; all have about the same success rate.
- Cortisone
  - Should not be used in long-term management
  - Occasional injections to trigger zones with 40 mg methylprednisolone (Depo-Medrol) may be given, but should be saved for severe exacerbations.
- Lidocaine 1%
  - Trigger point injection into "hot areas," especially the scapular area
  - Often as effective in relieving symptoms alone as when combined with methylprednisolone
- For select cases amitriptyline can be used for chronic pain.

SURGERY

- Indications: Severe pain unresponsive to conservative measures, significant or progression of neurologic deficits, long tract signs, vertebral artery syndrome
- Most common surgery is anterior interbody fusion with excision of disk and any accessible osteophytes
- The decision to use an anterior versus posterior surgical approach will depend on the patient's individual nature and location of pathology

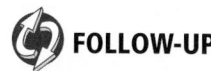 FOLLOW-UP

PROGNOSIS

- Fortunately, the prognosis is for a benign course in the overwhelming majority of cases, though for most of their lives, patients will be plagued by pain that exacerbates often with no known cause.
- In the case of myelopathy, the goal of operative intervention is to halt the progression of the pathology. Patients will not necessarily regain any lost function.
- Poor prognostic indicators include positive Babinski and bowel/bladder symptoms.

COMPLICATIONS

Loss of motion, especially extension, may require adjustments to certain occupations to prevent uncommonly significant muscle loss, instability of gait, or bladder or bowel function loss

PATIENT MONITORING

Patients should be seen in 3 to 4 weeks for an evaluation of their neurologic status; if unchanged, follow-up at intervals of 3 to 6 months, depending on the severity of their symptoms.

REFERENCES

1. Emery SE, Bohlman HH, Bolesta MJ, Jones PK: Anterior cervical decompression and Arthrodesis for the treatment of cervical spondylotic myelopathy: Two to seventeen-year follow-up. *J Bone Joint Surg Am* 1998;80:941–951.
2. Rao R. Neck pain, cervical radiculopathy, and cervical myelopathy. Pathophysiology, natural history, and clinical evaluation. *J Bone Joint Surg Am*. 2002;84:1872–1881.
3. Riew KD, Rhee JM. Cervical degenerative disk disorders. In: Koval KJ, editor. *Orthopaedic knowledge update*. 7th edition. Rosemont (IL): AAOS;2002;609–619.
4. Roh JS, Teng AT, Yoo JU, Davis J, Furey C, Bohlman HH. Degenerative disorders of the lumbar and cervical spine. *Orthop Clin N Am*. 2005;36:255–262.

 MISCELLANEOUS

CODES

ICD9-CM

- 722.4 Degeneration of cervical intervertebral disc
- 721.0 Cervical spondylosis without myelopathy
- 721.1 Cervical spondylosis with myelopathy

PATIENT TEACHING

- Instruct (or have a therapist instruct) the patient in the proper use of orthopedic appliances.
  - Cervical collars should produce a slight flexion of the neck, as should traction.
  - Avoid extension in all situations.
- Instruct the patient to report any weakness, numbness, paresthesias,, or bladder or bowel incontinence immediately.

 See Corresponding Diagnostic Algorithm

CERVICITIS

Barbara A. Majeroni, MD

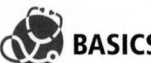 **BASICS**

DESCRIPTION
- Inflammation or infection of the uterine cervix
- System(s) Affected: Reproductive
- Synonym(s): Mucopurulent cervicitis

Geriatric Considerations
- Chronic cervicitis in postmenopausal women may be related to lack of estrogen.
- The possibility of infectious cervicitis should not be overlooked in geriatric patients, as many remain sexually active.

Pediatric Considerations
Infectious cervicitis in children should lead to an investigation for possible sexual abuse.

Pregnancy Considerations
Screen all pregnant women for infectious cervicitis, because of the risk of transmission to the fetus.

GENERAL PREVENTION
Often related to sexually transmitted disease (STD)
- Abstinence only method for complete prevention
- "Safe sex practices," such as using of condoms, can decrease the risk.
- Screening of sexually active women <25 has been advocated.

EPIDEMIOLOGY
- Predominant age: Infectious cervicitis is most common in women age 15–19, but may be seen at any age.
- Predominant sex: Affects only females

Incidence
- Gonorrhea: 166/100,000; 2.3% of sexually active women <30
- Chlamydia: 290/100,000; 5–35% of women
- Trichomoniasis: 1200/100,000; 5–25% of women

RISK FACTORS
- Multiple sexual partners
- Unprotected sex
- History of STD
- Postpartum period
- Smoking

ETIOLOGY
- Infectious cervicitis may be caused by *Chlamydia trachomatis*, *Neisseria gonorrhoeae*, herpes simplex, Mycoplasma genitalum, Ureaplasmas, Herpes simplex, or *Trichomonas vaginalis*.
- Chronic cervicitis is characterized by inflammation of the cervix without an identified pathogen.

ASSOCIATED CONDITIONS
Patients with infectious cervicitis should be screened for other STDs: Syphilis, trichomoniasis, HIV, and Hepatitis.

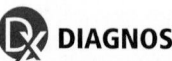 **DIAGNOSIS**

SIGNS AND SYMPTOMS
- Mucopurulent (yellow) discharge from the cervix
- Cervical erosion or erythema
- Easily induced endocervical mucosal bleeding (friability)
- Tenderness of cervix
- Postcoital bleeding
- Frequently asymptomatic

History
- Vaginal discharge in setting of risk factors
- Pelvic pain
- Itching
- Post-coital bleeding

TESTS
Lab
- Endocervical gram stain: >10 white blood cells per high power field suggests cervicitis
- Cervical cultures for *C. trachomatis*, *N. gonorrhoeae*
- Nucleic acid amplification tests: More sensitive and may also be used on urine as well as endocervical specimens. (1)[A] (sensitivity 94%, specificity 99% fo N. gonorrhea; sensitivity 83%, specificity 99% for Chlamydia trachomatis
- Vaginal wet mount for *Trichomonas vaginalis*
- If ulcerations are present, culture for herpes simplex virus.

- Venereal Disease Research Laboratory or rapid plasma reagin to rule out concurrent syphilis
- Consider testing for concurrent HIV and Hepatitis B and C.
- Lab results may be altered by a recent antibiotic treatment.

Diagnostic Procedures/Surgery
Colposcopy is indicated in chronic inflammation, with a biopsy of suspicious areas.

Pathological Findings
Inflammatory changes on a Pap smear: Infectious cervicitis may cause abnormal Pap smear and may be associated with cervical cancer.

DIFFERENTIAL DIAGNOSIS
- Vaginal infections with *Candida albicans* or *Trichomonas vaginalis* extending into the cervix
- Bacterial vaginosis
- Carcinoma of the cervix

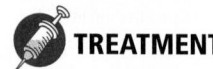 **TREATMENT**

GENERAL MEASURES
Chronic cervicitis with negative cultures and biopsies may be treated with cryosurgery

Diet
No special diet

Activity
Full activity

MEDICATION (DRUGS)

First Line

- If infectious cervicitis suspected, treat without awaiting culture results: Ceftriaxone (Rocephin) 125 mg single dose IM followed by either doxycycline (Vibramycin) 100 mg PO b.i.d. for 7 days or azithromycin (Zithromax) 1 g single dose (2,3)[A]
  - Option of Rocephin and azithromycin removes patient compliance factor, because they are 1-time doses
- For trichomoniasis: Metronidazole (Flagyl) 2 g single dose
- For herpes: Acyclovir (Zovirax) 200 mg PO 5 times daily (or 400 mg t.i.d.) for 7 days
- Chronic cervicitis associated with postmenopausal vaginal atrophic changes may respond to topical estrogen creams.
- Contraindications
  - Doxycycline should not be used in pregnant or nursing mothers.
- Precautions
  - Doxycycline should not be taken with milk, antacids, or iron-containing preparations.
- Significant possible interactions
  - Doxycycline may reduce effectiveness of warfarin (Coumadin) and oral contraceptives.

Second Line

- Any of the following may be substituted for ceftriaxone for *N gonorrhoea:* (quinolones should not be used for gonorrhea in patients who have traveled to Hawaii, California, or Southeast Asia because of high levels of resistance) Ouinolones are contraindicated in pregnancy. (4)[A]
  - Cefixime 400 mg PO single dose
  - Ofloxacin (Floxin) 400 mg PO single dose
  - Ciprofloxacin (Cipro) 500 mg PO single dose
  - Levofloxacin (Levaquin) 250 mg PO single dose
  - Amoxicillin 3 g PO given 30 minutes after probenacid 1 g PO.
- Doxycycline or azithromycin for Chlamydia may be substituted with
  - Erythromycin base or stearate 500 mg PO q.i.d.
  - Erythromycin ethylsuccinate 800 mg PO q.i.d.

 FOLLOW-UP

Often follow-up cultures are recommended to document adequate infection eradication. Follow-up nucleic acid amplification tests should not be done <3 weeks after treatment because of false positives due to dead organisms.

DISPOSITION
Admission Criteria
Only considered if refractory pelvic inflammatory disease (PID)

PROGNOSIS
- Infectious cervicitis usually responds to systemic antibiotics.
- Chronic cervicitis may be resistant to treatment and should be monitored closely for cervical dysplasia.

COMPLICATIONS
- Cervicitis due to *C. trachomatis* or *N. gonorrhoeae* is associated with an 8–10% risk of developing subsequent PID.
- Moderate to severe inflammation is associated with increased risk of Human Pappiloma Virus infection and cervical carcinoma.

PATIENT MONITORING
- Repeat cultures after treatment for chlamydia or gonorrhea are indicated in pregnant or high-risk patients.
- Annual Pap smears in sexually active patients to screen for chronic cervicitis

REFERENCES
1. Cook RL, Hutchison SL, Østergaard L, Braithwaite RS, Ness RB. Systematic review: Noninvasive testing for chlamydia trachomatis and neisseria gonorrheae. *Ann Int Med*. 2005;142:914–925.
2. Centers for Disease Control and Prevention. Sexually transmitted diseases: Treatment guidelines 2002. *MMWR Recomm Rep*. 2002;5:32–42.
3. Lau C-Y, Qureshi AK. Azithromycin versus doxycycline for genital chlamydial infections: A meta-analysis of randomized clinical trials. *Sex Trans Dis*. 2002;29:497–502.
4. Brocklehurst P. Antibiotics for gonorrhea in pregnancy. *The Cochrane Database of Systematic Reviews*. 2006;1. Accessed February 20, 2006.

ADDITIONAL READING
Simpson T, Oh MK. Urethritis and cervicitis in adolescents. *Adolescent Med Clin* 2004;15:153–271.

 MISCELLANEOUS

- Other notes
  - The presence of *Trichomonas* does not rule out other concurrent infection.
  - Positive results for *N gonorrhoeae* of Chlamydia may need to be reported to local or state health department.
  - Adolescents remain a high-risk group for STDs.
- See also: Cervical Dysplasia; Cervicitis; Ectropion and True Erosion; Chlamydial Sexually Transmitted Diseases; Gonococcal Infections; Trichomoniasis

CODES

ICD9-CM
- 618.9 Cervicitis
- 098.15 Acute gonococcal cervicitis
- 079.88 Chlamydia infection
- 099.53 Other venereal diseases due to *Chlamydia trachomatis*, lower genitourinary sites

PATIENT TEACHING

- Advise patient to use condoms consistently and include discussion of abstinence.
- If infectious etiology, advise patient to inform her partners so they can seek treatment.

Prevention
Patients with more than one sexual partner should be advised to use condoms at every encounter.

 See Corresponding Diagnostic Algorithm

See Patient Handout on CD

CERVICITIS, ECTROPION AND TRUE EROSION

Martha H. McLoughlin, MD

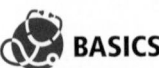

BASICS

DESCRIPTION
- Cervicitis: Inflammatory changes of the cervix due to infections, generally in other parts of the reproductive tract
- Ectropion: Eversion of the cervical columnar cells; often seen during pregnancy
- True erosion: Loss of overlying vaginal epithelium due to trauma (e.g., forceful insertion of vaginal speculum in patient with atrophic mucosa)
- System(s) Affected: Reproductive

Geriatric Considerations
Menopause

Pregnancy Considerations
- Ectropion
- Azithromycin should be used with caution.
- Doxycycline should not be used during pregnancy.

GENERAL PREVENTION
- Sexually transmitted infection (gonorrhea, chlamydia, trichomoniasis): Treat sexual partners; advise use of condom during coitus.
- Estrogen deficiency: Estrogen replacement therapy

EPIDEMIOLOGY
- Predominant age: Sexually active women
- Predominant sex: Female only

Incidence
- Cervicitis: Increasingly common in sexually active women
- Ectropion: Often with oral contraceptive use; very common in pregnant women
- True erosion: Occasionally seen in postmenopausal women

RISK FACTORS
- Cervicitis
  - Sexual contact with infected partner(s), recurrence due to inadequate therapy
  - Other reproductive tract infections: Vaginitis, pelvic inflammatory disease
  - Foreign objects: Pessary, diaphragm, cervical cap, etc.
- Ectropion: Pregnancy
- True erosion: Estrogen deficiency, trauma

ETIOLOGY
- Cervicitis: *Chlamydia trachomatis*, *Trichomonas vaginalis*, Herpes Simplex Virus (HSV)
- Non-sexually transmitted cervicitis can be caused by beta hemolytic streptococcus or *E. Coli*
- Ectropion
  - Hormonal changes with oral contraceptive use (especially with progesterone) or pregnancy
  - Resulting from cervical laceration during childbirth
- True erosion: Injury to atrophic epithelium due to estrogen deficiency in menopause

ASSOCIATED CONDITIONS
- Gonorrhea/Chlamydia
- Bacterial vaginosis

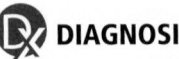

DIAGNOSIS

SIGNS AND SYMPTOMS
- Cervicitis: Purulent vaginal discharge, vulvar pruritus, metrorrhagia, dyspareunia, post-coital bleeding, dysuria, spotting
- Ectropion: Cervix turns red owing to color of the columnar epithelium
- True erosion: Vaginal bleeding, sharply defined ulcers of cervix

Physical Exam
- Cervical motion tenderness may be appreciated on bimanual pelvic exam
- Cervix may appear erythematous, enlarged/edematous; purulent discharge may be seen with cervicitis
- With cervicitis, signs of sexually transmitted disease (STD) may be seen (ulceration with HSV; punctate hemorrhages with Trichomonas; purulent discharge and friabilty with gonorrhea and chlamydia)

TESTS
Lab
- Saline and potassium hydroxide preparation of cervical and vaginal smears
- Culture of cervical discharge
- Papanicolaou smear of the cervix
- Chlamydia DNA probe
- Gonorrhea DNA probe

Imaging
None

Diagnostic Procedures/Surgery
Colposcopy

Pathological Findings
- Cervicitis: Acute and chronic inflammatory changes, presence of infective organisms
- Ectropion: None/squamous metaplasia
- True erosion: Sharply defined ulcer borders, loss of epithelium

DIFFERENTIAL DIAGNOSIS
- Cervical dysplasia
- Carcinoma of the cervix

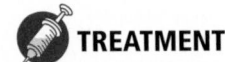

TREATMENT

INITIAL STABILIZATION
Outpatient

MEDICATION (DRUGS)

First Line

- Trichomoniasis: Metronidazole 500 mg b.i.d. for 7 days *or* 2 g once or 1 g b.i.d. for 2 doses
- Chlamydial infection: For nonpregnant women, doxycycline 100 mg b.i.d. PO for 7 days; for pregnant women, erythromycin base 500 mg q.i.d. PO for 7 days, or erythromycin ethylsuccinate 800 mg q.i.d. for 7 days
- Ectropion: None, unless patient is extremely symptomatic with copius discharge. Then acid-buffered vaginal jelly can be used to decrease discharge. Cautery can be used, but is generally considered overly invasive.
- True erosion: Estrogen, conjugated vaginal cream daily for 2 weeks, followed by estrogen replacement therapy
- Contraindications
  - Metronidazole: Use during 1st trimester of pregnancy
  - Doxycycline: Pregnancy or lactation
  - Estrogen: See extended list of contraindications to estrogen use in standard texts.
- Precautions
  - Metronidazole: Possible fetal harm if used during 1st trimester of pregnancy, disulfiram reaction with ethanol ingestion
  - Doxycycline: Possible fetal harm if used during pregnancy; staining of the infant's teeth if used during breast-feeding; allergy; photosensitization
  - Erythromycin: Nausea or vomiting
  - Estrogens: History of estrogen-dependent neoplasms; history of thromboembolic diseases: See extended list of contraindications to estrogen therapy in standard texts.
- Significant possible interactions
  - Metronidazole: Ethanol
  - Doxycycline: Dairy products, iron preparations, warfarin, and oral contraceptives (advise use of alternative contraceptive method)
  - Erythromycin: Astemizole, may increase latter's levels with subsequent electrocardiographic changes.
  - Erythromycin: Theophylline (elevated theophylline level)
  - Estrogen: N/A

Second Line

- Metronidazole: Sulfanilamide-aminacrine-allantoin cream (AVC cream)
- Doxycycline: Erythromycin or azithromycin
- Erythromycin: Clindamycin
- Estrogen: Lubricant, same as is used for vaginal speculum examination
- Azithromycin: 1 g for only 1 dose (pregnancy category B)
- Ofloxacin: 300 mg b.i.d. for 7 days
- Amoxicillin-clavulanate (Augmentin): 250 mg PO q8h for 7 days

SURGERY

Chronic cervicitis that does not respond to medical treatment may be treated with electrocautery or loop excision. Adverse effects of cautery can include cervical stenosis, which can affect fertility.

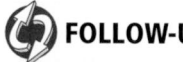 FOLLOW-UP

PROGNOSIS

- Cervicitis: Excellent healing after infection is eradicated
- Ectropion: Spontaneous regression postpartum, cessation of use of oral contraceptives
- True erosion: Spontaneous healing

PATIENT MONITORING

- Trichomoniasis: Repeat vaginal smear until infection is cleared.
- Chlamydial infection: Repeat culture after antibiotic therapy complete.
- Estrogen deficiency: Re-examine in 1 month to confirm healing.

REFERENCES

1. Disaia PJ, Creasman WT. *Clinical Gynecologic Oncology*. 3rd ed. St. Louis, MO: Mosby; 1989.
2. Herbst AL, Mishell DR, Stenchever MA, et al. *Comprehensive Gynecology*. 2nd ed. St. Louis, MO: Mosby; 1992.
3. Kurman RJ, ed. *Blaustein's Pathology of the Female Genital Tract*. 3rd ed. New York, NY: Springer-Verlag; 1987.
4. Novak ER, Woodruff JD. *Novak's Gynecologic and Obstetric Pathology with Clinical and Endocrine Relations*. 8th ed. Philadelphia, PA: WB Saunders; 1979.
5. Lebhere TB. In: Hacker NF, Moore JG, eds. *Essentials Obstetrics and Gynecology*. 2nd ed. Philadelphia, PA: WB Saunders; 1992.
6. Iglesias E, Alderman E, Fox A. Use of wet smear to screen for sexually transmitted disease. *Infect Med*. 2000;17:175–185.

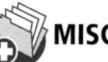 MISCELLANEOUS

Lubricants (e.g., KY Jelly) do not alter Pap smear results, so not of concern when performing vaginal exam

CODES

ICD9-CM
616.0 Cervicitis and endocervicitis

PATIENT TEACHING

Provide printed material about STDs and about estrogen deficiency and estrogen replacement therapy.

C

CHANCROID

Jeffery T. Kirchner, DO

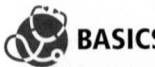 **BASICS**

DESCRIPTION

A sexually transmitted disease characterized by painful genital ulcerations and inflammatory inguinal adenopathy. Although uncommon in the US, is found worldwide. Chancroid is endemic in developing countries and a co-factor for HIV transmission.

- System(s) Affected: Reproductive; Skin/Exocrine
- Synonym(s): Soft chancre; Ulcus

Pregnancy Considerations

Mother-infant transmission has not been reported.

EPIDEMIOLOGY

- Predominant age: Teenagers and adults
- Predominant sex: Male predilection

Prevalence

<100 cases reported to the Centers for Disease Control and Prevention (CDC) in 2000–2002. Actual numbers are considered higher owing to underreporting.

RISK FACTORS

- Multiple sexual partners
- Uncircumcised men
- Prostitutes are often carriers.

ETIOLOGY

Haemophilus ducreyi (gram-negative bacterium)

ASSOCIATED CONDITIONS

- Syphilis: Concurrent in 10% of patients (according to new CDC data)
- Herpes simplex virus or HIV infection

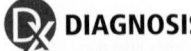 **DIAGNOSIS**

SIGNS AND SYMPTOMS (1,2)

- Tender genital papule that progresses to a pustular stage and ruptures after 2–3 days to form an ulcer
- Irregularly edged painful ulcer(s)
- Ulcers may be 1 mm–5 cm
- Ulcers may occur on the shaft of the penis, glans, and meatus in men.
- Ulcers in women most commonly occur in labia majora, but are also seen in labia minora, perineum, thigh, and cervix.
- Painful inguinal adenopathy with abscess (bubo) formation in 50% of patients
- Atypical presentations include folliculitis and foreskin abscess.

TESTS

Lab

- Serologic testing for antibody to *H. ducrey* with enzyme-linked immunosorbent assay. Gram stain; culture of organism on Mueller-Hinton agar with incorporated vancomycin. Polymerase chain reaction where modality available
- Drugs that may alter lab results
  – Previous antibiotic therapy
- Disorders that may alter lab results
  – None expected

Diagnostic Procedures/Surgery (1)

- Gram stain and culture of ulcer exudate
- Aspiration of inguinal bubo (lymph node)
- Polymerase chain reaction testing of ulcer exudate for *Haemophilus ducrey* DNA
- Dark-field examinations of exudate to rule out *Treponema pallidum* infection
- Culture or polymerase chain reaction testing for herpes simplex virus (HSV)

Pathological Findings

"School of fish" pattern on Gram stain

DIFFERENTIAL DIAGNOSIS

- Syphilis (classically a painless ulceration)
- HSV-1 and -2
- Lymphogranuloma venereum
- Granuloma inguinale

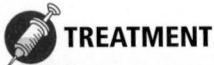 **TREATMENT**

INITIAL STABILIZATION

Outpatient treatment

GENERAL MEASURES

- Saline or Burrow solution to soak ulcers
- Aspiration of buboes if >5 cm; approached through adjacent uninvolved skin

ALERT

HIV disease may affect treatment response.

Activity

Refrain from sexual intercourse until genital lesions are fully resolved.

MEDICATION (DRUGS)

First Line

- Azithromycin: 1 g PO single dose (more expensive than other treatments) (1,3)[A]

- Ceftriaxone: 250 mg IM single dose

- Ciprofloxacin: 500 mg PO b.i.d. for 3 days (1,3)[A]

- Erythromycin base: 500 mg q.i.d. for 7 days (1,3)[A]

- Contraindications
  – Allergy to the medication
  – Ciprofloxacin during pregnancy and lactation, and patients <18 years

- Precautions: Refer to manufacturer's profile of each drug.

- Significant possible interactions: Refer to manufacturer's profile of each drug.

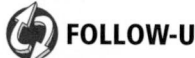 ## FOLLOW-UP

PROGNOSIS

- Full clinical resolution with appropriate treatment
- 5% relapse after treatment
- Primary infection is not believed to provide immunity.

COMPLICATIONS

- Phimosis
- Balanoposthitis
- Rupture of buboes with fistula formation and scarring

PATIENT MONITORING

- Avoidance of sexual activity until ulcers resolved
- Patient should be observed during follow-up until all clinical signs of infection resolved.
- Should see symptomatic improvement within 3 days and objective improvement by day 7
- Baseline syphilis serology and at 3 months
- HIV testing at baseline and at 3 months post treatment

REFERENCES

1. Lewis DA. Chancroid: Clinical manifestations, diagnosis, and management. *Sex Transm Inf*. 2003;79:68–71.
2. Montero JA. Chancroid: An update. *Infect Med*. 2002;191:174–178.
3. Centers for Disease Control and Prevention. Sexually transmitted diseases treatment guidelines—2002. *Morbidity and Mortality Weekly Report*. 2002;51:1–80.

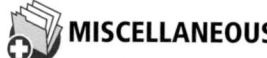 ## MISCELLANEOUS

- See also: Syphilis
- Other notes: Chancroid has been shown to be an established risk factor for acquisition of HIV infection.

 CODES

ICD9-CM
099.0 Chancroid

PATIENT TEACHING

- Sexual counseling
- Use of condoms
- Local wound care
- Treatment of all sexual partners with same regimen as index case
- HIV testing

C

CHARCOT JOINT

Jason A. Silva, MD

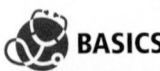 **BASICS**

DESCRIPTION

- A progressive destructive arthritis secondary to peripheral neuropathy and loss of pain sensation. The affected joints are subjected to repeated stress that is unrecognized by the patient, therefore causing continuous damage to the underlying bone and cartilage.
- Most often seen in tarsal and tarsometatarsal joints, less in metatarsophalangeal and talotibial joints. May also be seen in knee, hip, spine. Upper extremity joints rarely is involved.
- Diabetes mellitus is the most common cause in the U.S.
- 3 stages are identified
  - Fragmentation/destruction
  - Coalescence
  - Consolidation/resolution
- Patients suspected to have a Charcot neuropathy should be referred to an orthopaedic foot and ankle surgeon or podiatrist for follow-up and treatment.
- System(s) Affected: Musculoskeletal; Endocrine; Neurologic
- Synonym(s): Neuropathic joint disease; Neuropathic arthropathy

GENERAL PREVENTION

- Excellent control of blood sugar
- Diabetic foot care

EPIDEMIOLOGY

- Primarily seen in 5th and 6th decades
- Male = Female
- Bilateral involvement in ~20% of cases

Incidence

0.5–2.5% in patients with diabetes mellitus

Prevalence

0.1% in all patients, up to 13% in high-risk diabetes foot clinics

RISK FACTORS

- >15-year history of diabetes
- Poor blood sugar control
- Poor foot hygiene; poor-fitting shoes, socks

Genetics

Family history of diabetes mellitus

PATHOPHYSIOLOGY

Exact cause unknown, 2 major theories

- Autonomic neuropathy
  - Autonomic neuropathy leads to local increase in blood flow, which leads to osteopenia secondary to increased osteoclastic activity
- Neurotraumatic
  - Repetitive microtrauma unsensed by the patient leads to osseous destruction and progressive damage to ligaments, articular surfaces, and may lead to fractures and subluxation.

ETIOLOGY

Many causes of peripheral neuropathy

- Diabetes mellitus
- Syphilis/tabes dorsalis
- Syringomyelia, upper extremity disease
- Meningomyelocele
- Frequent intra-articular steroid injections
- Alcoholism
- Pernicious anemia
- Charcot-Marie-Tooth disease
- Leprosy (Hansen disease)
- Renal dialysis
- Chronic insensitivity to pain
- Amyloidosis

ASSOCIATED CONDITIONS

Other sequelae of diabetes

- Retinopathy, nephropathy

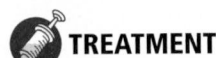 **DIAGNOSIS**

SIGNS AND SYMPTOMS

- Findings frequently confused with cellulitis
- Symptoms usually unilateral
- Significant swelling
- Local increased warmth: 3–7°C higher than unaffected extremity
- Skin erythema
- Effusion in joint
- Loss of distal sensation
- Skin intact
- Decreased pain, proprioception in affected limb
- Laxity/instability of joint

History

- Long-standing diabetes
- May recall predisposing trauma, such as ankle twist/sprain, object dropped on foot

Physical Exam

- Localized warmth, swelling, erythema
- Elevating the foot should resolve swelling
- Neurologic exam
  - Findings normally symmetric, sensory, and distal
  - Decreased or absent reflexes
  - Loss of pain, proprioception, and vibratory sensation
- Foot deformities
  - Corns/calluses
  - Collapse of arch
  - Collapse of tarsal bones causing rocker bottom foot
  - Protruding osteophytes
- Peripheral circulation often normal

TESTS

Lab

- Blood sugar, hemoglobin A1c
- WBC may be elevated in osteomyelitis.
- ESR: Elevated in osteomyelitis
- Basic metabolic panel: BUN, creatinine to rule out renal disease
- B_{12}/folate, hematocrit, MCV
- RPR, FTA-ABS to rule out syphilis
- Elevated alkaline phosphatase, calcium, PTH, and low phospate to rule out metabolic bone disease

Imaging

- Radiographs
  - Early changes
    - Slight fracture with joint subluxation
    - Joint effusion
    - Joint space narrowing
    - Sclerosis of subchondral bone
    - Bone fragmentation
  - Late changes
    - Marked articular destruction
    - Fractures
    - Hypertrophic changes
    - Bone resorption
    - Subluxation
    - Intra-articular loose bodies
    - Osteolysis
    - Large osteophytes
- May be difficult to differentiate radiograph findings from those of osteomyelitis
- MRI: Assists in ruling out osteomyelitis
- Bone scan: Assists in ruling out osteomyelitis
  - Indium[111] more specific than technetium[99]

Diagnostic Procedures/Surgery

Arthrocentesis

- Fluid for culture and sensitivity if osteomyelitis suspected
- Presence of WBC, CPPD crystals

DIFFERENTIAL DIAGNOSIS

- Cellulitis
- Osteomyelitis
- Osteonecrosis
- Advanced osteoarthritis
- Calcium pyrophosphate dihydrate crystal deposition disease (CPDD)

TREATMENT

PRE HOSPITAL

- Early recognition of diabetic foot pathology
- Non-weightbearing on affected extremity

INITIAL STABILIZATION

- Immobilization of joint is initial treatment
  - Casting:
    - Provides full immobilization
    - Casts must be checked weekly for correct fit, especially if underlying ulceration of skin
    - Casts should be changed every 1–2 weeks
    - Time in cast determined by clinical and radiographic measures
    - Total-contact cast better disperses pressure
  - Brace/orthotic
    - Alternative to casting
    - Removable
    - Patients may be noncompliant, and may not be able to sense a poor fitting brace
- Immobilization needed for minimum of 6 months; possibly 1 year or longer
- Also necessary to reduce stress on affected joint by limiting pressure
  - Non-weightbearing preferred, partial weightbearing at minimum

GENERAL MEASURES

- Goal of treatment is to restore joint stability and limit progression of disease.
- After casting, various braces are used to protect affected extremity
  - Ankle-foot orthotic (AFO), rocker-bottom shoes, Charcot restraint orthotic walker, custom prescription footwear
- Strict blood sugar control to limit progression of peripheral neuropathy

Diet
Diabetic diet recommended

Activity
Non- or partial weightbearing initially

SPECIAL THERAPY
Protective treatment with bracing, orthotics

Radiotherapy
Radiotherapy does not appear to benefit healing of acute Charcot feet in diabetes (2)[B].

 MEDICATION (DRUGS)

- Because pathophysiology is thought to involve increased osteoclastic activity, bisphosphonates have been used to halt progression of disease
  - Pamidronate, alendronate shown to give clinical improvement (1)[A]

First Line
- Bisphosphonates
- Diabetic medications

SURGERY
- Surgical treatment is reserved for severe cases and/or failure of conservative treatment.
- Surgery is indicated when a risk of skin ulceration, unstable fracture, or dislocation is present, or failure of medical therapy.
- Procedures performed vary depending on joints involved and surgeon experience
  - Exostosectomy of bony projections
  - Open reduction internal fixation (ORIF)
  - Osteotomy
  - Arthrodesis with or without tendon lengthening
  - Amputation
- Any surgical treatment should be delayed until after early fragmentation and inflammatory stages.
- Patients treated surgically often have long healing times.

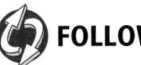 **FOLLOW-UP**

Regular follow-up with podiatrist, diabetician to maintain strict foot care

DISPOSITION
Admission Criteria
Foot ulceration, suspicion of associated osteomyelitis, fractures

PROGNOSIS
- Patients often are immobilized for several months.
- Total healing may take years to achieve.
- Patients must be vigilant about preventing further injury, receiving regular footcare, examining feet daily, noting swelling and/or temperature of joints.
- Maintain strict diabetic control.

COMPLICATIONS
- Unidentified fractures can lead to debilitating joint deformities and skin ulcerations, increasing risk of infection.
- Collapse and inversion of arch into clubfoot or rocker bottom foot
- Amputation

PATIENT MONITORING
- Regular monitoring of blood sugar, HB A1C
- Regular care with podiatrist

ALERT
Geriatric Considerations
Because most cases occur in patients >50, diabetic patients in this age group should be counseled about the symptoms and signs of neuropathic joint disease. The benefits of good blood sugar control should be discussed.

REFERENCES

1. Anderson JJ, et al. Bisphosphonates for the treatment of Charcot neuroarthropathy. *J Foot Ankle Surg*. 2004;43(5):285–289.
2. Chantelau E, Schnabel T. "Palliative radiotherapy for acute osteoarthropathy of diabetic feet: A preliminary study. *Pract Diabetes Int*. 1997;14(6): 154–156.
3. *Wheeless' Textbook of Orthopaedics*. Charcot Changes in the Diabetic Foot and Ankle
4. Canale ST, et al. *Campbell's Operative Orthopaedics*, 10th ed. Chicago: Mosby, 2002.
5. Jude EB, Boulton AJ. Medical treatment of Charcot's arthropathy. *J Am Podiatric Med Assoc*. 2002;92(7):381–383.

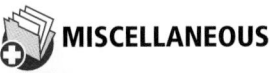 **MISCELLANEOUS**

CODES

ICD9-CM
- 713.5 Arthropathy associated with neurological disorders
  - Charcot's arthropathy associated with diseases classifiable elsewhere
  - Neuropathic arthritis associated with diseases classifiable elsewhere
- Neuropathic joint disease [Charcot's joints]
  - 094.0—NOS
  - 250.6—Diabetic
  - 336.0—Syringomyelic
  - 094.0—Tabetic [Syphilitic]

PATIENT TEACHING
- Importance of strict blood sugar control
- Multidisciplinary team approach

Diet
Diabetic diet is prudent.

Activity
Non-weightbearing when signs of Charcot joint are present

Prevention
- Well-fitting footwear with adequate support
- Frequent examination of feet for signs of pressure sores or ulcerations
- Good foot hygiene

C

CHICKENPOX (VARICELLA ZOSTER)

Kay A. Bauman, MD, MPH

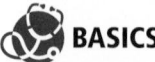

BASICS

DESCRIPTION
A common, highly contagious generalized exanthem characterized by the development of crops of pruritic vesicles on the skin and mucous membranes

- Virus is spread by respiratory (airborne) droplets, direct contact with varicella vesicles, or rarely zoster lesions
- Virus establishes latency in the dorsal root ganglia; reactivation results in herpes zoster or "shingles"
- Outbreaks tend to occur late winter to early spring in temperate climates.
- The usual incubation period is 14–16 days (range, 10–21). Patients are infectious from ~48 hours before appearance of the rash until the final lesions have crusted. Most people acquire chickenpox during childhood and develop lifelong immunity. (1)
- System(s) Affected: Nervous, Skin/Exocrine
- Synonym(s): Varicella

ALERT
Geriatric Considerations
- Infection more severe than in children
- Latent varicella infection may reactivate and cause the exanthem known as shingles or zoster.
- Most common cause of death: Primary viral pneumonia

Pediatric Considerations
- Neonates born to mothers who develop chickenpox 5 days before or 2 days after delivery are at risk for serious disease. Must give varicella-zoster immune globulin
- Varicella bullosa seen mainly in children <2 years. Lesions appear as bullae instead of vesicles. The clinical course does not change.
- Most common cause of death: Septic complications and encephalitis
- Avoid aspirin/acetylsalicylic acid in children because of link to Reye disease

Pregnancy Considerations
- Risk of transplacental infection after maternal infection is 25%.
- Congenital malformations are seen in 2% (1) of patients when the fetus is infected during the 1st or 2nd trimesters; characterized by limb atrophy and scarring of the skin of the extremities and occasional CNS and eye manifestations
- Morbidity is increased in women infected during pregnancy (e.g., pneumonia).

GENERAL PREVENTION
- Exposed, susceptible people should be considered at risk and potentially infectious for 21 days.
- Isolation of hospitalized patients
- Passive immunization with IM varicella-zoster immune globulin given within 96 hours (preferably within 72 hours) of exposure to ensure efficacy. (1) Recommended for people exposed to chickenpox or shingles within 96 hours who are immunocompromised, ≥15 years old without prior history of chickenpox, newborns of mothers with onset of chickenpox <5 days before delivery or <2 days after delivery. Exposure criteria: Continued household contact, prolonged face-to-face contact (same room), or indoor playmate >1 hour

- Active immunization after exposure: Shown to prevent or reduce significantly the severity of varicella if given within 72 hours postexposure.
- Active immunization: Varicella virus vaccine (Varivax): Live attenuated vaccine approved by the Federal Drug Administration in 1995 for pediatrics immunization and recommended by the Advisory Committee on Immunization Practices for immunization of healthy patients ≥12 months who have not had chickenpox
  - 12 months–12 years old: Single dose 0.5 mL SC. Seroconversion rates: 95% (1)
  - ≥13 years: 2 0.5-mL SC doses 4–8 weeks apart, seroconversion rates 78–82% after 1 dose, 99% after 2 doses (1)
  - May be considered for a subset of HIV-positive children in Centers for Disease Control and Prevention class I with CD4 >25% (1)
- Vaccine recipients should avoid contact with immunocompromised people and pregnant women who have never had chickenpox and their newborns, for up to 6 weeks after vaccination.

EPIDEMIOLOGY
- Predominant age: Peak incidence pre-schoolers to 9 years, but may occur at any age
- Predominant sex: Male = Female

Incidence
- Decreasing in incidence since vaccine available: Reported US varicella cases 1991: 147,076; reported for 2003: 20,948 (2,3)
- Prior to vaccine availability, approximately 100 deaths in the US/year were reported; for 2003 and the 1st 1/2 of 2004, only 8 deaths were reported (4).

RISK FACTORS
- No prior history of varicella infection
- Immunosuppressed patients (especially children with leukemia/lymphoma in remission or receiving high-dose corticosteroids)

Genetics
No known genetic pattern

ETIOLOGY
Varicella-zoster virus is a member of the alpha Herpesviridae subfamily; a double-stranded DNA virus; reservoir: Humans

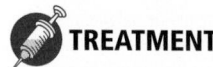

DIAGNOSIS

SIGNS AND SYMPTOMS
- Prodromal symptoms: Fever, malaise, anorexia, and mild headache
- Characteristic rash: Crops of "teardrop" vesicles on erythematous bases
- Lesions erupt in successive crops.
- Progress from macule to papule to vesicle, then begin to crust
- Pruritic rash present in various stages of development.
- Lesions may be present on mucous membranes, both oral and vaginal.
- Malaise, muscle aches, arthralgias, and headache more common in adults (5)
- Subclinical in ~4% of cases (5)

TESTS
Generally used for complicated cases and epidemiologic studies

- Visualization of the virus by electron microscopy, tissue culture (costly), and various methods of acute and convalescent sera collection: Latex agglutination (most available), enzyme immunoassay, indirect immunofluorescence antibody, fluorescent antibody to membrane assay, or polymerase chain reaction assay, which can detect wild from vaccine viral strains (1)

Lab
- Leukocyte count may be normal, low, or mildly increased.
- Marked leukocytosis suggests secondary infection.
- Multinucleated giant cells visible on Tzanck smear from scrapings of vesicles
- Isolated virus from human tissue culture

Pathological Findings
- Skin lesions identical histologically to those of herpes simplex virus
- In fatal cases, intranuclear inclusions can be found in the endothelium of blood vessels and most organs.

DIFFERENTIAL DIAGNOSIS
- Herpes simplex virus infection
- Herpes zoster
- Impetigo
- Coxsackievirus infection
- Scabies
- Dermatitis herpetiformis
- Drug rash
- Rickettsialpox infection

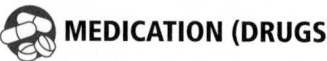

TREATMENT

Outpatient except for complicating emergencies

GENERAL MEASURES
- Supportive/symptomatic treatment
- Good hygiene to avoid secondary infection

Diet
No special diet

Activity
As tolerated. Children may return to school when lesions have scabbed over, temperature is normal, and sense of well-being has returned.

MEDICATION (DRUGS)

First Line
- Antipyretics for fever; avoid aspirin in children
- Local and/or systemic antipruritic agents for itching
- In immunocompromised patients: Varicella-zoster immune globulin available for passive immunization. Varicella-zoster immune globulin must be given within 96 hours after exposure to be beneficial. After 4th day postexposure, wait for rash to develop, then give acyclovir 500 mg/m²/d q8h for 7 days.
- Acyclovir: Decreases duration of fever and shortens time of viral shedding. Recommended for adolescents, adults, and high-risk patients. Most beneficial if initiated early in the disease (≤24h).
  - 2–16-year-old patients: 20 mg/kg/dose (max. 800 mg/dose), q.i.d. for 5 days

– Adults: 800 mg, 5× daily.
• Contraindications
  – Hypersensitivity to the drug
• Precautions
  – Possible renal insufficiency with acyclovir
• Significant possible interactions
  – Concurrent administration of probenecid increases half-life; increased effects with zidovudine (e.g., drowsiness, lethargy)

Second Line
• Famciclovir: 500 mg t.i.d. for 7–10 days
• Valacyclovir: 1 g t.i.d. for 7–10 days

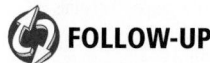 FOLLOW-UP

PROGNOSIS
• In the healthy child, chickenpox is rarely serious and recovery is complete.
• Confers lifelong immunity
• 2nd attack rare, but subclinical infection can occur; happens occasionally after vaccination in children
• Infection latent and may recur years later as herpes zoster in adults (and sometimes in children)
• Fatalities rarely occur from complications.

COMPLICATIONS
• Although only 2% of cases are reported after 2nd decade, 35% of deaths occur in the age group. (5)
• Secondary bacterial infection: Cellulitis, abscess, erysipelas, sepsis, septic arthritis/osteomyelitis, or staphylococcal pyomyositis
• Pneumonia: 20–30% of adults with chickenpox have lung involvement, 1/400 are hospitalized (5)
• Encephalitis (the most common central nervous system complication); meningitis
• Reye syndrome
• Purpura
• Thrombocytopenia
• Glomerulonephritis
• Arthritis
• Hepatitis

PATIENT MONITORING
Usually none needed in mild cases. If complications occur, intensive supportive care may be required.

REFERENCES
1. American Academy of Pediatrics. *Report of the Committee on Infectious Diseases (Red Book)*. Elk Grove Village, IL: American Academy of Pediatrics; 2003.
2. Centers for Disease Control and Prevention. Summary of Notifiable Diseases, United States, 1991. *Morbidity and Mortality Weekly Report*. 1992;40(No. 53).
3. Centers for Disease Control and Prevention. Summary of Notifiable Diseases, United States, 2003. *Morbidity and Mortality Weekly Report*. 2005;52(No. 54).
4. Centers for Disease Control and Prevention. Varicella-Related Deaths—United States, January 2003–June 2004. *Morbidity and Mortality Weekly Report*. 2005;54:272–274.
5. Goldman L, Bennett JC, ed. *Cecil Textbook of Medicine*, 21st Edition, Philadelphia, PA: WB Saunders 2000.

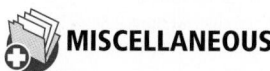 MISCELLANEOUS

See also: Herpes Zoster; Immunizations

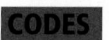 CODES

ICD9-CM
052.9 Varicella without mention of complication

C

CHILD ABUSE

Emily H. Groom, MD

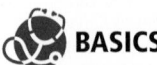 **BASICS**

DESCRIPTION
- May encompass emotional abuse, psychological abuse, physical abuse, sexual abuse, neglect, or any combination thereof
- System(s) Affected: Gastrointestinal (GI) Endocrine/Metabolic; Musculoskeletal, Nervous; Renal; Reproductive; Skin/Exocrine
- Synonym(s): Battered child syndrome; Suspected non-accidental trauma; Child maltreatment

ALERT
Pregnancy Considerations
Emergency contraception reduces rate of pregnancy after rape or sexual abuse if given in timely fashion.

- Levonorgestrel 1.5 mg (2 split doses 12 hours apart or a single dose) and low- and mid-doses (25–50 mg) of mifepristone offer high efficacy (1)[A]

GENERAL PREVENTION
- Early detection of abuse and intervention whenever possible
- Education of children and caregivers to recognize abuse

EPIDEMIOLOGY
- All ages affected
- Predominant sex: Male = Female

Prevalence
- An estimated 906,000 children in the US were victims of child abuse or neglect in 2003. (2)
- Rate of victimization 12.4 per 1,000 children in the US in 2003 (2)

RISK FACTORS
- May be many
- Poverty, parental substance abuse, lower educational status, parental history of abuse, mentally ill parent, poor social support network, or domestic violence

ETIOLOGY
Not well defined

ASSOCIATED CONDITIONS
- Failure to thrive
- Developmental deficits
- Poor school performance
- Poor social skills

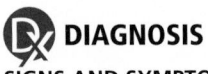 **DIAGNOSIS**

SIGNS AND SYMPTOMS
- Absence of physical findings does not indicate that the child's history is incorrect.
- Nonspecific symptoms of abuse
  - Behavior changes
  - Anxiety and/or depression
  - Sleep disturbances, night terrors
  - School problems
  - Self-destructive behaviors
- Physical abuse
  - Skin markings (e.g., lacerations, burns, ecchymoses, linear/shaped contusions, bites)
  - Immersion injuries with clearly distinguished outlines (e.g., from boiling water)

- Oral trauma (e.g., torn frenulum, loose teeth)
- Ear trauma (e.g., signs of ear pulling)
- Eye trauma (e.g., hyphema, hemorrhage)
- Abdominal blunt trauma
- Fractures
- Head trauma
- Sexual abuse
  - Abuse often consists of contact not likely to produce detectable injuries (e.g., fondling)
  - Unexplained penile, vaginal, hymenal, perianal, or anal injuries/bleeding/discharge
  - Pregnancy or sexually transmitted diseases (STDs)
  - Sperm is a definitive finding of child abuse
- Neglect
  - Child may be undersized or unkempt
  - Rashes
  - Fearful or too trusting
  - Clinging to or avoiding caregiver
  - Flat or balding occiput
  - Abnormal development or growth parameters

History
- Use non-judgmental, open-ended questions
- Red flags: Injuries don't match the history, the story changes, the history given by caregiver does not match the child's history, mechanism of injury inconsistent with child's developmental stage, or there is a considerable delay in seeking treatment for injuries
- There is insufficient evidence to support routine screening of caregivers for the physical abuse/neglect of children (3)

Physical Exam
- General assessment for signs of physical abuse, neglect, self-injurious behaviors (4)[C]
- Thorough physical exam is indicated, including
  - Skin
  - Head, eyes, ears, nose, and mouth
  - Chest/abdomen
  - Genital/perianal
  - Extremities with focus on inner arms and legs (note bruises) as well as skeletal trauma
  - Growth data
- Consider examination under sedation with careful monitoring (4)[C]
- Maintain high index of suspicion for occult head, chest, and abdominal trauma
- Suspected sexual abuse: Examine the mouth, breasts, genitals, perineal region, buttocks, and anus for bruises, scars, bite marks, burns, or discharge. (4)[C]
- Note and interpret abnormailities. (4)[C]
- Consider photographs and diagrams. (4)[C]
- Consultation with an expert physician may be advisable. (4)[C]

TESTS
Lab
- Lab testing should be directed by history and physical exam
  - Urinalysis (e.g., abdominal/flank/back/genital trauma)
  - Complete blood chemistry and coagulation studies including prothrombin time, partial thromboplastin time, bleeding time, and platelet count (e.g., rule out bleeding disorder, abdominal trauma)

- Electrolytes, creatinine, blood urea nitrogen, glucose
- Liver and pancreatic function tests (e.g., abdominal trauma)
- In cases of suspected neglect
  - Stool exam, calorie count, purified protein derivative and anergy panel, sweat test, lead and zinc levels
- In cases of suspected sexual abuse
  - STD testing: Gonorrhea, Chlamydia, Trichomonas (4)[C]
  - Testing for other STDs, HIV, herpes, hepatitis B/C, and syphilis may be considered. (4)[C]
  - Serum pregnancy test (4)[C]
- Disorders that may alter lab results
  - See "Differential Diagnosis"

Imaging
- Imaging should be directed by history and physical exam
- Radiographic series
  - Anterioposterior (AP)/lateral skull, lateral cervical spine, AP/lateral/oblique ribs, AP pelvis, Lateral thoracic— Lumbar spine, AP upper and lower extremities, oblique hands, AP feet (5)[C]
- CT abdomen
- CT head w/o contrast
- Consider bone scan
- Consider MRI as adjunct to head CT (5)[C]

Diagnostic Procedures/Surgery
- As clinically indicated
- Lumbar puncture for suspected subarachnoid hemorrhage (may require prior head CT to determine risk of herniation)
- Sexual abuse
  - Consider photocolposcopy
  - <72 hours from time of abuse: Collect samples for the forensic laboratory (contact authorities for appropriate protocol) (4)[C]
  - >72 hours from time of abuse (without acute injury): Maintain child's safety and evaluate at earliest convenient time (4)[C]

Pathological Findings
- Spiral fractures in nonambulatory patients
- Chip or bucket-handle fractures
- Epiphysial or metaphysial rib fractures in infants
- Rupture of liver/spleen in abdominal blunt trauma
- Retinal hemorrhages in shaken baby syndrome
- See "Signs and Symptoms"

DIFFERENTIAL DIAGNOSIS
- Physical trauma (including but not limited to)
  - Accidental injury
  - Bleeding disorders (e.g., classic hemophilia)
  - Metabolic diseases
  - Congenital conditions
  - Toxic ingestion
  - Conditions with skin manifestations (e.g., mongolian spots, Henoch-Schönlein purpura, meningococcemia, erythema multiforme, hypersensitivity, car seat burns, staphylococcal scalded skin syndrome, chickenpox, impetigo)
  - Cultural practices (e.g., cupping, coining)

- Neglect (including but not limited to)
  - Endocrinopathies (e.g., diabetes mellitus)
  - Constitutional
  - GI (e.g., clefts, malabsorption, irritable bowel disease)
  - Central nervous system (CNS) abnormalities/seizure disorder
  - Sudden Infant Death Syndrome (SIDS)
- Skeletal trauma (including but not limited to)
  - Obstetrical trauma
  - Nutritional: Metabolic defects (e.g., scurvy, rickets)
  - Infection (e.g., congenital syphilis, osteomyelitis)
  - Osteogenesis imperfecta
  - Neoplasm

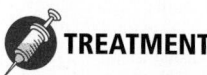 TREATMENT

INITIAL STABILIZATION
- Acute episodes, especially of sexual abuse, are often best managed in an ED equipped for collecting forensic specimens and maintaining chain of evidence.
- Follow current BLS and PALS/ATLS guidelines for resuscitation.
- Mandatory reporting to child protective authorities
- Consultation with local child abuse specialist is advisable.

GENERAL MEASURES
- Always explain what the physical exam will involve and why certain procedures are necessary.
- Examine child in a comfortable setting
- Allow child to choose who will be in the room
- Use appropriate positions to examine the anal and genital areas of young children (4)[C]
- Test for STDs before treatment (4)[C]

Diet
As clinically indicated

Activity
As clinically indicated

 MEDICATION (DRUGS)

First Line
Antibiotics as indicated for treatment of documented STDs or infection.

Second Line
Post-coital contraceptive drugs: Refer to "Alert" on "Pregnancy Considerations"

SURGERY
As clinically indicated

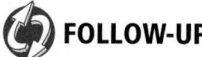 FOLLOW-UP

DISPOSITION
Admission Criteria
- Moderate to severe injuries
- Unstable
- Acute psychological trauma
- If safety of child outside the hospital cannot be guaranteed

Discharge Criteria
Child should be sent to another relative or into foster care if the suspected abuser lives with the child

Issues for Referral
- Counseling for individual and family
- After initial evaluation, consider referral to sexual assault center.

PROGNOSIS
Without intervention, child abuse is often a chronic and escalating phenomenon.

COMPLICATIONS
- Long-term physical and psychological damage
- Death

PATIENT MONITORING
- Refer to the state protective services
- Observe as clinically indicated
- Monitor injury healing over time
- Follow-up assessment for STDs that may not present acutely (e.g., HPV, herpes) (4)[C]

REFERENCES
1. Cheng L, Gülmezoglu AM, Van Oel CJ, Piaggio G, Ezcurra E, Van Look PFA. Interventions for emergency contraception. *The Cochrane Database of Systematic Reviews* 2004, Issue 3.
2. Department of Health and Human Services, Administration on Children, Youth, and Families (ACF). *Child maltreatment 2003 [online].* Washington, DC: Government Printing Office; 2005.
3. U.S. Preventive Services Task Force. Screening for family and intimate partner violence: Recommendation statement. *Ann Fam Med.* 2004;2(2):156–160.
4. Nancy Kellogg and the Committee on Child Abuse and Neglect. The evaluation of sexual abuse in children. *Pediatrics.* 2005;116:506–512.
5. Sirotnak AP, Grigsby T, Krugman RD. Physical abuse of children. *Pediatr Rev.* 2004;25(8):264–277.
6. Maguire S, Mann MK, Sibert, Kemp A. Are there patterns of bruising in childhood which are diagnostic or suggestive of abuse? A systematic review. *Arch Dis Child.* 2005;90:182–186.

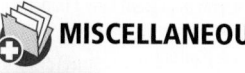 MISCELLANEOUS

CODES

ICD9-CM
- 995.50 Child abuse, unspecified
- 995.51 Child emotional/psychological abuse
- 995.52 Child Neglect (nutritional)
- 995.53 Child sexual abuse
- 995.54 Child physical abuse
- 995.55 Shaken Infant Syndrome
- 995.59 Other child abuse and neglect

PATIENT TEACHING

 See Corresponding Diagnostic Algorithm

 See Patient Handout on CD

C

CHLAMYDIA PNEUMONIAE

John R. Gimpel, DO, MEd

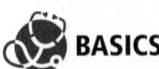 **BASICS**

DESCRIPTION

- *Chlamydia pneumoniae*, an obligate intracellular bacteria, has been established as an important cause of adult respiratory disease including pneumonia, bronchitis, sinusitis, and pharyngitis, and is capable of causing persistent latent infection. Humans are the only known reservoir.
- System(s) Affected: Respiratory
- Synonym(s) TWAR agent; 1 cause of "atypical pneumonia"

GENERAL PREVENTION

- As transmission is via contact with respiratory secretions, advise hand washing and avoid exposure to infected persons.
- Flu and pneumococcal vaccines for high-risk groups

EPIDEMIOLOGY

- Incubation period is ~30 days.
- Predominant age: More common in elderly; less common in children 2 months to 5 years of age
- Serologic evidence of acute and chronic infection found in ~1/3 of patients with acute cardio obstructive pulmonary disease (COPD) exacerbation, often together with other concurrent bacterial infection

Incidence

- Accounts for 6–10% of community-acquired pneumonia in adults requiring hospitalization, (1)[C], and 3–6% of bronchitis cases. Numbers do not necessarily apply to all areas. Incidence of subclinical infection is much greater.
- Most cases occur sporadically, though intrafamilial spread also occurs.

Prevalence

Estimated incidence 100–200 cases of community acquired pneumonia/100,000/year

- No particular seasonal variation
- Country-wide epidemics have been documented in Scandinavian countries.
- Outbreaks have occurred among groups of military recruits, university students, and nursing home residents.

Pediatric Considerations

Uncommon in children 2 months to 5 years of age

PATHOPHYSIOLOGY

Infection with *C. pneumoniae* and resultant host responses may lead to mucus production in the nasal passages, sinuses, bronchial tree, and alveoli, along with nasopharyngeal and airway inflammation and bronchospasm.

ASSOCIATED CONDITIONS

- COPD, including Asthma
- HIV infection
- Cystic fibrosis
- Diabetes mellitus

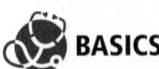 **DIAGNOSIS**

PRE HOSPITAL

Generally diagnosis and treatment is empiric in nature, and diagnostic workup only required in patients who are extremely ill, those with significant comorbidities or those who are otherwise immunocompromised

Geriatric Considerations

- Usually more severe disease in older adults, and more common in the elderly who also have concomitant disease
- Elderly patients less likely to exhibit respiratory symptoms with pneumonia, and may present with altered mental status or history of falls.

SIGNS AND SYMPTOMS

- 70–90% of infections are mild or subclinical.
- Severe illness uncommon but possible

History

- Onset often gradual with delayed presentation
- Sore throat and hoarseness may precede cough by a week or more, giving biphasic appearance to illness, and are very common (uncommon in Legionella, less common in Mycoplasma, Strep pneumoniae, and *Haemophilus influenzae*)
- Cough (often prominent with scant sputum)
- Fever (usually early in illness, usually low grade), chills common
- Rhinitis
- Headache
- Malaise
- Myalgias
- Sinus congestion
- Nausea
- Altered mental status

Physical Exam

- General appearance usually nontoxic, unless extremely ill
- Fever (positive likelihood ratio 2.2 for pneumonia)
- Tachypnea (positive likelihood ratio 2.0 for pneumonia) (2)[A]
- Tachycardia (positive likelihood ratio 1.6 for pneumonia) (2)[A]
- Diminished breath sounds (positive likelihood ratio 2.3 for pneumonia) (2)[A]
- Crackles or wheezing (positive likelihood ratio 2.0 for pneumonia) (2)[A]
- Bronchial breath sounds (positive likelihood ratio 3.3 for pneumonia) (2)[A]
- Percussion dullness and egophony less sensitive but more specific for pneumonia (positive likelihood ration 3.0 and 4.1, respectively, for pneumonia) (2)[A]
- Pharyngeal erythema (without exudates)
- Retropharyngeal lymphoid granulation

TESTS

Generally not required or cost-effective, unless patient is extremely ill and requires hospitalization

Lab

- Leukocyte count usually normal or low, may be mildly elevated, although nonspecific
- Blood cultures recommended if toxic and requiring hospitalization
- Liver function tests and electrolytes usually normal
- Sputum (no longer recommended as required) is often negative by gram stain and routine culture
- Most easily cultured in HL or HEp2 cells (culture is 10–80% sensitive and >95% specific) (3)[A]
- Testing with microimmunoflourescence (MIF) is recommended by the Centers for Disease Control and Prevention as enzyme immunoassay testing is less specific; however, MIF testing for *C. pneumoniae* may also lack specificity and sensitivity. (3)[A]
- Every effort should be made to obtain paired sera. The convalescent sera should be obtained 3 weeks after disease onset.
- 4-fold antibody rise diagnostic of acute infection (10–100% sensitivity) (3)[A]
- Presence of IgM antibody (≥1:16) or of high IgG antibody titers (≥1:512) by MIF suggests a recent or acute infection
- Early treatment with tetracycline may blunt IgG antibody response
- Complement fixation (CF) for chlamydia widely available, but cannot distinguish *C. pneumonia* from *Chlamydophila psittaci*
- Polymerase chain reaction (PCR) from pharyngeal swab or broncheoalveolar lavage specimen (30–95% sensitivity, >95% specificity) (3)[A]

Imaging

- Patients with suspected community-acquired pneumonia should be evaluated with a chest x-ray (3)[A]
- Chest x-ray may be abnormal even in clinically mild disease
- Variable radiographic abnormalities include unilateral and bilateral infiltrates and pleural effusions. Single, subsegmental funnel-shaped or circumscribed infiltrate is common.

Diagnostic Procedures/Surgery

While serology is 95% specific, definitive diagnosis requires a positive culture or PCR testing. (3)[A]

DIFFERENTIAL DIAGNOSIS

- Other causes of atypical pneumonia, including *Mycoplasma pneumoniae* and *Legionella pneumophila*
- Other bacterial causes of pneumonia, including *Streptococcus pneumoniae*. H. Influenzae, *Moraxella catarrhalis*, and *Staph aureus*
- Respiratory viruses, including adenovirus, influenza A, influenza B, parainfluenza virus, and respiratory syncytial virus
- Endemic fungal pathogens, such as blastomycosis, coccidiodomycosis, and histoplasmosis
- Bioterrorism agents: Anthrax, plague, and tularemia
- Conditions that mimic community-acquired pneumonia: ARDS, atelectasis, idiopathic pulmonary fibrosis, neoplasm, pulmonary embolus, sarcoidosis, CHF

TREATMENT

PRE HOSPITAL

Usually outpatient care for most; those with severe pneumonia or coexisting illness may require hospitalization:

- Pneumonia Severity Index or other validated prediction rule can assist in predicting those patients with community-acquired pneumonia with higher morbidity and those requiring hospitalization (4)[A]
  - Elderly, male sex, and nursing home residents have higher mortality
  - Patients with altered mental status, respiratory rate >30 bpm, systolic BP <90 mm Hg, temperature <35°C(95°F) or >40°C (104°F), all are associated with increased mortality
  - Lab abnormalities associated with increased morbidity and mortality: Arterial pH <7.35, blood urea nitrogen >64 mg/dL, sodium <130 mEq/L, glucose >250 mg/dL, hematocrit <30%, oxygen saturation <90% or partial pressure of arterial oxygen <60 mm Hg pleural effusions also signify a higher mortality rate

GENERAL MEASURES

Infection in debilitated or hospitalized patients can be severe

Diet

No special diet; increased fluids generally recommended

Activity

Usually reduced activity and increased rest during acute illness

Complementary and Alternative Therapies

- Herbal, Chinese, and homeopathic remedies widely utilized to loosen secretions and help with bronchodilation in the treatment of respiratory illnesses
- Manipulative treatment in small studies shown to reduce duration of IV antibiotic treatment and days in the hospital for hospitalized elderly patients with pneumonia (5)[C]

MEDICATION (DRUGS)

- Broad-spectrum antibiotics may reduce the effectiveness of oral contraceptives; barrier method recommended

- Beta-lactam antibiotics and sulfasoxazole not effective for *C. pneumoniae*; however, an advantage in clinical efficacy or mortality by empiric coverage of atypical pathogens in patients with community acquired pneumonia has not been shown (6)[A]

First Line

- Azithromycin 500 mg on day 1, then 250 mg on days 2–5 or
- Clarithromycin 500 mg q12h for 10–14 days or
- Doxycycline 100 mg q12h for at least 14 days
  - Tetracycline not for use during pregnancy or in children <8 years
  - Tetracycline may cause photosensitivity; sunscreen recommended
  - Tetracyclines may increase the anticoagulant effect of warfarin.

ALERT

Pregnancy Considerations

Tetracyclines and flouroquinolones contraindicated

Second Line (3,7)[A]

- Alternative drugs: Erythromycin base 250–500 mg q.i.d. for 14–21 days
- Levofloxacin 250–500 mg/d (PO or IV) or other respiratory flouroquinolones have good bioavailability and the convenience of once daily dosing, but are recommended for use only when patients have failed treatment with a 1st line drug, or have had recent antibiotics, significant comorbidities, or allergies to alternatives

FOLLOW-UP

- Weekly patient monitoring until well
- Follow-up chest x-ray for resolution
  - Reinfection is possible
  - There have been reports of individuals who are persistently culture-positive despite antibiotic treatment.

Discharge Criteria

Reversal of the above-noted criteria, with the patient tolerating oral medications, otherwise stable medically, and stable for discharge per the clinical judgment of the physician

PROGNOSIS

- Pneumonia is especially life-threatening in older adults and patients with other illnesses that affect the lungs (e.g., asthma, COPD) or the immune system (e.g., diabetes), with an overall 0.5–29% mortality rate.
- Estimated mortality rate from *C. pneumoniae* is 9%, but this may be an overestimate due to the number of subclinical cases.
- Death usually from secondary infection or underlying comorbidity

COMPLICATIONS

- Reactive airway disease
- Erythema nodosum
- Otitis media
- Endocarditis
- Pericarditis or Myocarditis
- Meningoencephalitis
- Associated with atherosclerotic disease: TP C. pneumoniae has been cultured from atherosclerotic plaque in patients with coronary artery disease, but treatment has not been shown to effect mortality.

REFERENCES

1. File TM Jr, et al. Clinical characteristics of Chlamydia pneumoniae infection as the sole cause of community-acquired pneumonia. *Clin Infect Dis.* 1999;29:426–428.
2. McGee S. *Evidence-Based Physical Diagnosis.* Philadelphia, PA: WB Saunders; 2001.
3. Lutfiyya MN, Henley E, Chang LF, Reyburn SW, Diagnosis and treatment of community-acquired pneumonia. *AFP.* 2006;73:3:442–450.
4. Fine MJ, Auble TE, Yearly DM, et al. A prediction rule to identify low-risk patients with community-acquired pneumonia. *NEJM.* 1997;336:243–250.
5. Noll DR, Shores JH, Gamber RG, Herron KM, Swift J. Benefits of osteopathic manipulative treatment for hospitalized elderly patients with pneumonia. *JAOA.* 2000;100(12):776–782.
6. Shefet D, Robenshtok PM, Leibovici L. Empiric antibiotic coverage of atypical pathogens for community acquired pneumonia in hospitalized adults. 2006. *The Cochrane Database of Systematic Reviews* 2006 Issue 1. Available at: www.cochrane.org/reviews/en/ab004418.html. Accessed February 3, 2006.
7. Thibodeau KP, Viera AJ. Atypical pathogens and challenges in community-acquired pneumonia. *AFP.* 2004;69:7:1701–1706.
8. Miyashita N, Fukano H, Okimoto N, et al. Clinical presentation of community-acquired Chlamydia pneumonia in adults. *Chest.* 2002;121: 1176–1181.

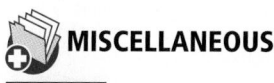

MISCELLANEOUS

CODES

ICD9-CM

078.88 Other specified diseases due to chlamydiae

PATIENT TEACHING

American Family Physician (www.familydoctor.org).

See Patient Handout on CD

C

CHLAMYDIAL SEXUALLY TRANSMITTED DISEASES

Geoffrey R. Swain, MD, MPH

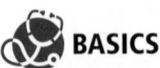 **BASICS**

DESCRIPTION

- An obligate intracellular membrane-bound prokaryotic organism, *Chlamydia trachomatis* causes an estimated 3 million new sexually transmitted infections in the United States each year.
- In 1994, chlamydial sexually transmitted diseases (STDs) in the US cost an estimated $2 billion per year, mainly due to costly complications such as pelvic inflammatory disease (PID), infertility, and ectopic pregnancy.
- Currently, many more women than men are screened, resulting in a larger male reservoir.
- System(s) Affected: Reproductive

Clinical Considerations
Studies indicate that 75–90% of women and 50–90% of men with chlamydial STDs are asymptomatic; persons with asymptomatic infection can remain infectious for years.

Pregnancy Considerations
Perinatal acquisition may result in neonatal pneumonia and/or conjunctivitis. Tetracycline and ofloxacin are contraindicated during pregnancy; consider erythromycin or azithromycin.

GENERAL PREVENTION
- Populations with prevalence >5% should be screened at least annually. (1)[C] These include those with the following characteristics
  - New or >1 sex partner in past 6 months
  - Attending an adolescent or family planning clinic or an STD or abortion clinic
  - Attending a jail or other detention center clinic
  - Rectal pain, discharge, or tenesmus
  - Testicular pain
- All sexually active woman <25 years old should be screened. (1)[A]
- Consider screening all sexually active men <25 years old (studies are pending). (2,3)[A]

EPIDEMIOLOGY
- Predominant age: 15–25 years
- Inversely proportional to age (after onset of sexual activity)
- Predominant sex: Male = Female

Prevalence
- Of the general medical population: 3–5%
- Of teens and young adults: 5–15%
- Of patients at STD clinics: 10–20%

RISK FACTORS
Risk correlates
- With number of sexual partners
- Inversely with age

Genetics
Unknown

ETIOLOGY
C. trachomatis serotypes D–K

ASSOCIATED CONDITIONS
- PID
- Epididymitis
- Cervicitis
- Urethritis

- Diseases caused by other chlamydial species:
  - Psittacosis: *Chlamydia psittaci*
  - Pneumonia: *Chlamydia pneumoniae*; *C. trachomatis* (infants)
  - Lymphogranuloma venereum: *C. trachomatis* serotypes L1–L3
  - Trachoma: *C. trachomatis* serotypes A–C

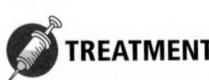 **DIAGNOSIS**

SIGNS AND SYMPTOMS
A substantial majority of cases are asymptomatic. Of those with symptoms, the most common are

- In males
  - Urethritis
  - Epididymitis
  - Proctitis
  - Reiter syndrome
- In females
  - Cervicitis, typically mucopurulent
  - Urethral syndrome
  - Bartholinitis
  - Endometritis
  - Salpingitis/PID
  - Fitz-Hugh-Curtis perihepatitis syndrome
- In infants
  - Conjunctivitis
  - Pneumonitis
  - Carriage: Pharynx/gastrointestinal tract
- Symptoms most strongly associated with chlamydia include urethral or cervical discharge and pelvic or testicular pain. Persons with such symptoms, or with rectal pain, discharge, or tenesmus, should be tested for chlamydia.
- Although chlamydia (and gonorrhea) can cause mucopurulent cervicitis (MPC), these organisms cannot be isolated from most cases of MPC, and most women who have these organisms do not have MPC. Therefore, neither women with MPC nor their partners should be treated empirically for chlamydia in the absence of other evidence supporting such treatment.

History
- Complete sexual history, including
  - Number of sex partners past 30 days
  - Use of barrier protection
  - Exchange of money or drugs for sex
  - Oral or anal receptive intercourse
- Symptom history, with onset date for each symptom

Physical Exam
- Men and women
  - External genitalia (rash? lesions?)
  - Urethra (discharge?)
  - Inguinal lymph nodes
  - Pharynx and perianal area, if history indicates
- In addition, for women
  - Cervix (discharge? motion tenderness?)
  - Uterus, ovaries, adnexa

TESTS
Lab
- Chlamydial cell culture
  - Sensitivity 50–70%
  - Specificity 100%
  - Takes up to 7 days
- Antigen detection and enzyme immunoassay Sensitivity 50–90%

- Direct fluorescent antibody detection
  - Sensitivity ~75% in an experienced lab technician's hands
  - Specificity >99%
- Amplified molecular testing (e.g., polymerase chain reaction, ligase chain reaction, specific dynamic action, human chorionic somatotropin, thyroid microsomal antigen)
  - Sensitivity ~95%
  - Specificity ~99%
  - Rapid turnaround times
  - Urine or swab specimens are relatively expensive.
  - Lab tests may remain positive for as long as 3 weeks after successful treatment.
  - Many tests are not approved for rectal or pharyngeal chlamydia.

Diagnostic Procedures/Surgery
Specimens should contain cell scrapings rather than inflammatory discharge, because the organism lives only inside the epithelial cells.

DIFFERENTIAL DIAGNOSIS
- *Neisseria gonorrhea*
  - Urethritis
  - Proctitis
  - Epididymitis
  - Cervicitis
  - PID
  - Bartholin abscess
  - Perihepatitis
- *Mycoplasma*, or *Ureaplasma urealyticum*
  - Urethritis, epididymitis
  - Reiter disease
  - PID
- *C. trachomatis* (serotypes L1–L3)
  - Lymphogranuloma venereum
  - Proctitis

TREATMENT

INITIAL STABILIZATION
Outpatient treatment, unless patient is moderately or severely ill with PID or other complications

GENERAL MEASURES
- All patients with known or suspected chlamydia should be tested for gonorrhea, infectious hepatitis, syphilis, and HIV (the latter requires individual counseling and consent). (1)[C]
- Some experts recommend that all patients treated for chlamydia should be treated empirically for gonorrhea simultaneously, unless they are known to be negative for gonorrhea by sensitive lab testing.
- All partners of patients treated for chlamydia should be tested if possible but treated empirically regardless, rather than waiting for test results.
- Some experts recommend treating partners of men being treated for nonspecific urethritis; others recommend testing partners and waiting for test results.
- Neither women with MPC nor their partners should be treated empirically for chlamydia in the absence of other evidence supporting such treatment. (1)[C]

Activity
Abstinence from sexual contact until diagnosis and treatment complete for patient and all partners

MEDICATION (DRUGS)

First Line
- For urethritis, cervicitis, and sexual partners of infected persons
  - Doxycycline: 100 mg PO b.i.d. for 7 days
  - Azithromycin: 1 g PO in a single dose
  - In pregnant women: Erythromycin base 250 mg PO q.i.d. for 14 days
- For other chlamydial syndromes
  - Epididymitis: Tetracycline, doxycycline (as listed above), or erythromycin for 10–14 days
  - PID: Doxycycline for 10–14 days to cover the chlamydial component (gonorrhea and anaerobic organisms must be treated as well; see Centers for Disease Control and Prevention recommendations: Ceftriaxone 250 mg once IM, cefoxitin, other 3rd-generation cephalosporin, or a quinolone). Erythromycin for 10–14 days may be needed in pregnant or tetracycline-intolerant females to treat chlamydial component.
- Tetracyclines (e.g., doxycycline) and quinolones (e.g., ofloxacin, levofloxacin) are contraindicated in children and pregnant women.
- Tetracyclines may cause photosensitivity; sunscreen is recommended.
- Avoid concurrent administration of tetracyclines with antacids, dairy products, or iron.
- Broad-spectrum antibiotics may reduce the effectiveness of oral contraceptives; barrier method is recommended.
- Practitioners may elect to give azithromycin and ceftriaxone together to the patient in the office to reduce patient noncompliance.

Second Line
- Erythromycin base: 500 mg PO q.i.d. for 7 days
- Erythromycin ethylsuccinate: 800 mg PO q.i.d. for 7 days
- Ofloxacin: 300 mg PO b.i.d. for 7 days
- Levofloxacin: 500 mg PO daily for 7 days

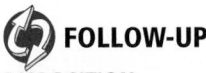 **FOLLOW-UP**

DISPOSITION
Admission Criteria
- High fever or dehydration
- Failure to improve with outpatient antibiotics

PROGNOSIS
Prognosis is good with early and compliant therapy; however, because of the asymptomatic nature of the early disease and the population affected, symptomatic PID still accounts annually for 2.5 million outpatient visits and more than 250,000 hospitalizations.

COMPLICATIONS
- Both sexes: Enhancement of transmission of and susceptibility to HIV
- Males
  - Transient oligospermia
  - Postepididymitis urethral stricture (rare)
- Females
  - Tubal infertility
  - Tubal (ectopic) pregnancy
  - Chronic pelvic pain

PATIENT MONITORING
- It is not routine to test the patient to see if a cure has been obtained, although it is reasonable to retest persons treated with erythromycin 1–2 months after treatment.
- Sexual partners need to be evaluated and treated empirically, if necessary, to prevent passing the disease back and forth between partners. Partnerships with local public health departments should be fostered to assist with partner tracing.
- Lack of resolution or recurrence of symptoms must be immediately reported to the physician.
- Severe cases of urethritis/cervicitis as well as the chlamydial syndromes should be seen in follow-up after the completion of therapy.
- Up to 25% of asymptomatic patients screened for chlamydia may not return for treatment post–chlamydia culture results. Strategies must be developed to ensure treatment can be instituted.

REFERENCES
1. Centers for Disease Control and Prevention. Sexually transmitted disease treatment guidelines 2002. *Mortality and Mordality Weekly Report*. 2002;51:32–36.
2. Turner CF, Rogers SM, Miller HG, et al. Untreated gonococcal and chlamydial infection in a probability sample of adults. *JAMA*. 2002;287:726–733.
3. Leighton K, St. Louis M, Farshy F, et al. Risk behaviors, medical care, and chlamydial infection among young men in the United States. *Am J Pub Health* 2002;92:1140–1143.
4. Heath C, Heath J. Chlamydia trachomatis infection update. *Am Fam Physician*. 1995;52:1455–1461.
5. Stamm WE. Chlamydia trachomatis: The persistent pathogen. *Sex Transm Dis*. 2001;28:684–689.
6. Stamm WE, Holmes KK. Chlamydia trachomatis Infections in the adult. In: Holmes KK, Mardh PA, Sparling PF, et al., eds. *Sexually Transmitted Diseases*. 2nd ed. New York, NY: McGraw-Hill; 1990:181–193.
7. Swain GR, McDonald RA, Pfister JR, Gradus MS, Sedmak GV, Singh A. Decision analysis: Point-of-care chlamydia testing vs. laboratory-based methods. *Clin Med Res*. 2004;2:29–35.
8. U.S. Preventive Services Task Force. Screening for chlamydial infection: Recommendations and rationale. *Am J Prev Med*. 2001;20(suppl 3):90–94.

 MISCELLANEOUS

See also: Cervicitis; Epididymitis; Gonococcal Infections; HIV infection and AIDS; Pelvic Inflammatory Disease; Syphilis; Urethritis

CODES

ICD9-CM
- 615.9 Unspecified inflammatory disease of uterus, except cervix
- 616.0 Cervicitis and endocervicitis
- 616.10 Vaginitis and vulvovaginitis, unspecified

PATIENT TEACHING
- Suggest risk reduction counseling and encourage abstinence outside of marriage.
- Encourage safe sex practices, such as barrier protection.
- Inform about serious sequelae of chlamydial disease, such as tubal infertility or chronic pelvic pain.
- Stress the need to finish entire course of antibiotics.
- For a listing of sources for patient education materials favorably reviewed on this topic, contact the American Academy of Family Physicians Foundation, P.O. Box 8418, Kansas City, MO 64114; (800) 274-2237, ext. 4400; Web site: www.familydoctor.org.

 See Corresponding Diagnostic Algorithm

C

CHOLANGITIS (ACUTE)

Mark Horattas, MD

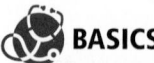 **BASICS**

DESCRIPTION
- Bacterial infection of the bile duct system that is associated with obstructive biliary duct pathology
- System(s) Affected: Gastrointestinal

GENERAL PREVENTION
Cholangiography when indicated at time of cholecystectomy with endoscopic, radiographic, or surgical clearance of retained CBD stones

EPIDEMIOLOGY
- Predominant age: 55–70 years; rare in children, more common in adults
- Predominant sex: Female > Male

RISK FACTORS
- Cholelithiasis
- Endoscopic or surgical manipulation
- Foreign bodies such as parasites, biliary stents

ETIOLOGY
- Biliary tract obstruction from
  - Stones
  - Tumor (pancreatic, CBD, ampulla, metastatic)
  - Benign strictures (postsurgical, primary sclerosing cholangitis)
  - Parasites (*Ascaris*)
  - Pancreatitis
  - Blood clots
- Reflux of small bowel bacteria
  - Choledochoenterostomy
  - Sump syndrome
- Other causes
  - Cholecystitis
  - Bacteremia
  - Surgical, radiographic, or endoscopic manipulation
  - Biliary stent

ASSOCIATED CONDITIONS
- Choledocholithiasis
- Malignant tumors
- Benign strictures
- Biliary-enteric anastomosis
- Invasive procedures
- Foreign bodies
- Parasites
- Secondary sclerosing cholangitis

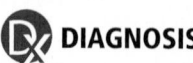 **DIAGNOSIS**

SIGNS AND SYMPTOMS
Patient may have only 1 or 2 of the following symptoms, and the abdominal exam may be unrevealing:
- Right upper quadrant pain, not severe
- Jaundice
- Chills and fever
  - Previous 3 items referred to as Charcot's triad
- Shock
- Central nervous system depression

TESTS
Lab
- Increased white blood cells with left shift
- Hyperbilirubinemia in 90% of cases
- Alkaline phosphatase increased in 90% of cases
- Positive blood culture in 50% of cases (Gram-negative aerobes and some anaerobes)

Imaging
Ultrasound will diagnose gallstones and CBD size but will demonstrate CBD calculi in <15% of cases

Diagnostic Procedures/Surgery
- Need to delineate underlying biliary tract abnormality
- Cholangiography is definitive test
- Percutaneous transhepatic cholangiography or endoscopic retrograde cholangiopancreatography

Pathological Findings
In acute toxic disease, pus under pressure in the CBD

DIFFERENTIAL DIAGNOSIS
- Acute cholecystitis: Pain and tenderness are invariably present. (May be very difficult to distinguish between cholangitis and acute cholecystitis.)
- Pyogenic liver abscess
- Hepatitis
- Acute pancreatitis
- Perforated duodenal ulcer
- Pelvic inflammatory disease with peritonitis
- Kidney stones
- Pancreatitis

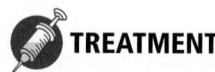 **TREATMENT**

INITIAL STABILIZATION
Inpatient treatment

GENERAL MEASURES
Control sepsis, then evaluate with cholangiography and treat underlying biliary tract pathology. Urgent bile duct decompression may be necessary.

Diet
NPO until acute phase is terminated

Activity
As tolerated

MEDICATION (DRUGS)

First Line

Antibiotic regimen should cover Gram-negative aerobes, enterococci, and anaerobes.

- Ampicillin: 1 g q6h IV (substitute ciprofloxacin or levofloxacin in penicillin allergic patient) *plus*
- Aminoglycoside (e.g., tobramycin 1–1.7 mg/kg q8h IV; amikacin is an alternative but is expensive) plus
  – Metronidazole: 500 mg q8h IV
- For contraindications and possible drug interactions, refer to the manufacturer's profile for each drug.
- Renal toxicity may occur with aminoglycoside therapy; check peak and trough levels.

Second Line

- Piperacillin-tazobactam (Zosyn) *or*
- Ampicillin-sulbactam (Unasyn) *or*
- Ticarcillin-clavulanate (Timentin)

SURGERY

- Patients who do not respond to antibiotics and supportive care require emergency decompression of the biliary duct system. This may be accomplished by surgery, endoscopy, or transhepatic cholangiography.
- In case of obstruction secondary to stones, endoscopic papillotomy and stone extraction will drain the duct, may be definitive treatment of the underlying cause, and are shown to reduce mortality.

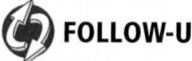 **FOLLOW-UP**

PROGNOSIS

- Acute cholangitis: Good
- Acute toxic cholangitis: Mortality is high

COMPLICATIONS

- Hepatic abscess
- Sepsis
- Hepatic dysfunction

PATIENT MONITORING

Requires careful monitoring of hemodynamic parameters

REFERENCES

1. Boeg JH, Way LW. Acute cholangitis. *Ann Surg.* 1980;191:264.
2. Nahrwold DL. Cholangitis. In: Sabiston DC, ed. *Textbook of Surgery.* 15th ed. Philadelphia, PA: WB Saunders 1996.
3. Pitt HA, Longmire WP Jr. Suppurative cholangitis. In: Hardy JM, ed. *Critical Surgical Illness.* 2nd ed. Philadelphia, PA: WB Saunders 1980.

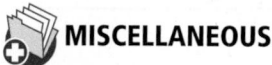 **MISCELLANEOUS**

See also: Cholelithiasis

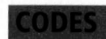 **CODES**

ICD9-CM

576.1 Cholangitis

PATIENT TEACHING

For patient education materials favorably reviewed on this topic, contact National Digestive Diseases Information Clearinghouse, Box NDDIC, Bethesda, MD 20892, (301) 468-6344.

 See Corresponding Diagnostic Algorithm

C

CHOLECYSTITIS

Thomas Agresta, MD

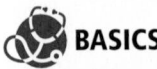 **BASICS**

DESCRIPTION
- Inflammation of the gallbladder occurring acutely or chronically, often secondary to previously asymptomatic gallstones
- System(s) Affected: Gastrointestinal

GENERAL PREVENTION
- Ursodeoxycholic acid (Ursodiol) 10 mg/kg/d following bariatric surgery or very low-calorie diets
- Daily cholecystokinin (100 kcal) during total parenteral alimentation (TPN) for >1 month
- Physical activity 30 minutes 5 days/week

EPIDEMIOLOGY
- Predominant age: 5th and 6th decades
- Predominant sex: Female > Male (2:1)

Incidence
Symptomatic gallstones 47–183/10,000 person years

Prevalence
- Increased in Native Americans and Whites
- Less prevalent in African Americans
- Increases with age and body mass index (BMI)
- Prevalence by ultrasound surveys
  - By age 30, 30% of Native Americans
  - By age 60, 80% of Native Americans
  - By age 60, 30% of Whites
  - By age 60, 20% of African Americans

RISK FACTORS
- Current gallstones (see Cholelithiasis)
- Cardiac surgery
- Trauma
- Obesity: BMI >30 Relative Risk (RR) = 3.7
- 1st-degree relative with gallstones RR = 2.2
- Estrogen use (NNH per year 323–500) (1)[A]
- Rapid weight loss >1.5 kg per week
- Prolonged parenteral alimentation
- Pregnancy

ETIOLOGY
- Gallstones: 90–95% of cases
  - Obstruction of the cystic duct, leads to acute cholecystitis
  - May obstruct the common bile duct (CBD), causing jaundice
  - May obstruct the pancreatic duct, causing pancreatitis
- Gallbladder sludge is a viscous material, insoluble in bile, that layers on sonogram
  - Occasionally produces cholecystitis
  - Occurs in most pregnant women, patients on TPN, and patients with rapid weight loss
- Acalculous cholecystitis (5% cases)
  - Associated with severe stressors, including cardiac surgery and multiple trauma
  - May be associated with ischemic damage to the gallbladder wall
- Bacteria present in 20–30% cases
  - Usually enteric (*E. Coli*, *Klebsiella*, *Enterobacter*, *Enterococcus*, *Pseudomonas*)
  - Usually do not initiate the inflammation but are important in the complications of empyema and ascending cholangitis
  - In emphysematous cholecystitis, *Clostridia* likely responsible
- CBD neoplasms and strictures: Usually associated with cholangitis and pancreatitis

ASSOCIATED CONDITIONS
- Pancreatitis
- Hemolytic anemias such as sickle cell disease and spherocytosis
- Cirrhosis, hypersplenism

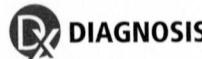 **DIAGNOSIS**

Geriatric Considerations
Sometimes difficult to diagnose in the elderly, as pain may seem less severe and may not be able to generate fever or leukocytosis

SIGNS AND SYMPTOMS
- Asymptomatic: Only 5–10% of people with gallstones become symptomatic each year
- Acute cholecystitis
  - Abdominal pain: Sudden onset, intense, in epigastrium or right upper quadrant, radiates to shoulder or back. Pathognomonic feature is "biliary colic," a pain rising over 2–3 minutes to an intense plateau that is maintained for >20 minutes.
  - Nausea and vomiting
  - Recurrent attacks 1–6 hours after meals, lasting >12 hours until patient recovers—usually <3 days
  - Elevated temperature: Mild to moderate
  - Local tenderness, rarely diffuse
  - Murphy's sign: Inspiratory arrest elicited when palpating right upper quadrant while patient inhales deeply Positive LR 2.8
  - Palpable gall bladder in 5% of cases
- CBD stone
  - Jaundice in 50% of cases
  - Biliary colic in 60% of cases
  - Fever and chills in 30% of cases
  - Pruritus in 10% of cases
  - Loose bowel movements, light color
  - Hepatomegaly in >80% of cases
  - Palpable gall bladder in 10% of cases
  - Tenderness (infrequent)
- Gallstone ileus (rare)
  - Gallstone >3 cm that fistulizes into bowel and obstructs at ileocecal area
  - Antecedent pain, often over weeks, with nonbiliary colic
  - Abdominal distention, mild tenderness
  - Air in biliary passages on plain radiograph
  - Intestinal obstruction at level of terminal ileum
- Pancreatitis
  - Pain over upper abdomen
  - Nausea and vomiting
- Empyema
  - Insidious weight loss, mild wasting
  - Gradual onset of occult infection signs, fever, and anorexia
  - Mass usually present
  - Tenderness usually absent
- Chronic cholecystitis
  - Associated with gallstones, often asymptomatic; 20% become symptomatic over 15–20 years
  - Mild dyspepsia following fatty meals

TESTS
Lab
- Acute cholecystitis
  - Leukocytosis: 12,000–15,000 white blood cells/mm^3
  - Liver tests usually abnormal: Alanine aminotransferase (ALT), aspartate aminotransferase (AST) slightly elevated; alkaline phosphatase, gamma-glutamyl transferase (GGT) elevated with CBD obstruction
- CBD stone
  - High bilirubin in 50% of cases; in 100% >10 days
  - Elevated alkaline phosphatase and GGT in 85% of cases
  - Positive blood culture in 15% of cases
  - Barely abnormal ALT, AST
  - Leukocytosis if infection
  - Serum amylase may be elevated; if >1,000 U, concomitant pancreatitis should be considered
- Drugs that may alter lab results
  - Steroids
  - Immunosuppressive drugs: May mask leukocytosis and early signs of inflammation
- Conditions that may alter lab results
  - Advanced age, malnutrition
  - Lymphoma, other immunocompromised states

Imaging
- Ultrasonography: 1st test of choice
  - Best technique to diagnose gallstones: High sensitivity = 95%; high specificity = 98%
  - Less sensitive (60%) and specific (77%) to diagnose acute cholecystitis. Findings include thick gallbladder wall (>3 mm), gallbladder distention, sludge in lumen, and pericholecystic fluid.
  - Endoscopic ultrasound is superior to endoscopic retrograde cholangiopancreatography (ERCP) in detecting CBD stones.
- Hepatobiliary technetium Tc 99 m iminodiacetic acid scan
  - Highly sensitive (97%) for diagnosis of acute cholecystitis
  - HIDA derivatives are taken up by hepatocytes, excreted in bile, and concentrated in gallbladder.
  - Failure to see gallbladder in 1 hour is highly suspicious for acute cholecystitis.
  - Usually abnormal in acalculous cholecystitis
  - Perform during acute pain
- Plain radiographs (upright):
  - 20% of gallstones are radiopaque.
  - Emphysematous cholecystitis: Air in the gallbladder wall or in lumen
- CT scan
  - No advantage over ultrasonography in gallstone/acute cholecystitis diagnosis
  - Better than ultrasonography in detecting enlargement of pancreas. Helpful in the diagnosis of abscess formation
  - Better than ultrasonography for dilated CBD
- ERCP: Useful to see status of biliary and pancreatic ducts, can also remove ampula stones
- Percutaneous transhepatic cholangiography: Gives more detail about intrahepatic biliary system
- MRI: Almost as sensitive as ERCP in detecting CBD stones

Diagnostic Procedures/Surgery

Laparotomy if unable to make diagnosis by less invasive means

DIFFERENTIAL DIAGNOSIS

- Acute pancreatitis
- Peptic ulcer
- Diverticulitis
- Pyelonephritis
- Pneumonitis
- Hepatic abscess
- Hepatic tumor
- Irritable bowel disease
- Nonulcer dyspepsia

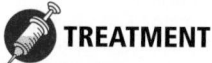 **TREATMENT**

PRE HOSPITAL
Outpatient treatment for mild symptoms

INITIAL STABILIZATION
Ascending cholangitis is a surgical emergency. Laparotomy or drainage by ERCP or transhepatic cholangiography is required.

GENERAL MEASURES
Start IV fluids and nasogastric suction

Diet
- NPO during acute cholecystitis
- Avoid fatty meals to reduce attacks.

Activity
As tolerated by the patient

SPECIAL THERAPY
- Dissolution therapy: Use only if laparoscopic cholecystectomy can not be performed
  - Ursodeoxycholic acid (Actigall) 10 mg/kg is the drug of choice.
  - To be effective, there must be a functioning gallbladder on oral cholecystography, few small stones without calcium
  - Alternative drug is chenodeoxycholic acid (Chenodiol) 12–15 mg/kg/d.
- Lithotripsy: Possible in chronic cholecystitis

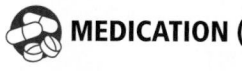 **MEDICATION (DRUGS)**

First Line
- For mild attack
  - Diclofenac: 75 mg IV or IM may be abortive.

  - Ampicillin: 4–6 g/d or cefazolin (Ancef) 2–4 g per day (2)[A]

- For severe attack: Gentamicin 3–5 mg/kg/d and clindamycin 1.8–2.7 g per day. No significant improvement in outcome proven. [C] Penicillin may be added if needed.
- Gallstone formation with rapid weight loss after bariatric surgery or severe diets is prevented by ursodiol (ursodeoxycholic acid) 10 mg/kg/d.
- Gallstone formation in prolonged parenteral alimentation is prevented by daily feeding of 100 kcal or daily injection of cholecystokinin.
- Contraindications: Hypersensitivity reactions
- Precautions
  - Aminoglycosides: Nephrotoxicity, ototoxicity
  - Adjust dosage for renal failure.
- Significant possible interactions: Refer to the manufacturer's profile of each drug.

Second Line
For acute cholecystitis: 3rd-generation cephalosporins

SURGERY
- Laproscopic cholecystectomy performed early (<72 hours) is the preferred treatment for symptomatic cholecystitis (3)[A]
  - Laparotomy is an acceptable alternative.
  - Delay only if surgery is contraindicated
  - Mortality rate: 0.1% in patients <50 years, 0.8% in those >50 years
- If there is jaundice, evaluate the CBD by intraoperative cholangiogram or ERCP.
- Laparoscopic cholecystostomy
  - As an alternative to surgical drainage
  - If the patient is a poor risk, the gallbladder or biliary passages can be drained by radiologic or endoscopic techniques.
- Other indications for emergency surgery
  - Toxic patient
  - Perforation or abscess

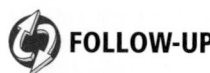 **FOLLOW-UP**

DISPOSITION
Admission Criteria
Biliary colic lasting >6 hours and/or showing toxicity, jaundice, or fevers and chills.

PROGNOSIS
- Generally good for gallbladder disease. Deaths are mainly a result of comorbidities, especially coronary artery disease
- Untreated symptomatic gallstones usually have recurrent symptoms in 3–6 months.
- After cholecystectomy, stones may recur in the bile ducts.

COMPLICATIONS
Occur in ~5% cases of acute cholecystitis and include
- Perforation with peritonitis
- Pancreatitis
- Abscess formation
- Fistula formation (intestine, colon, cutaneous)
- Gangrene of gallbladder
- Empyema
- Cholangitis
- Hepatitis
- Gallstone ileus

PATIENT MONITORING
Post cholecystectomy: Follow through postoperative period for complications.

ALERT
Geriatric Considerations
- Complications more likely
- Cholecystectomy mortality rate higher

REFERENCES
1. Cirillo D, Wallace R, Rodabough R, et al. Effect of Estrogen Therapy on Gallbladder Disease. *JAMA*. 2005;293:330–339.
2. Paul M, Silbiger I, Grozinsky S, Soares-Weiser K, Leibovici L. Beta lactam antibiotic monotherapy versus beta lactam-aminoglycoside antibiotic combination therapy for sepsis. *The Cochrane Database of Systematic Reviews* 2006, Issue 1.
3. Papi C, Catarci M, D'Ambrosio L, et al. Timing of Cholecystectomy for Acute Calculous Cholecystitis: A Meta-Analysis. *Am J Gastroenterology* 2004;99:147–155.
4. Bellow C, Berger D, Crass R. Management of Gallstones. *Am Fam Physician* 2005;72:637–642.
5. Trowbridge RL, Rutkowski NK, Shojania KG. Does this patient have acute cholecystitis? *JAMA*. 2003;289:80–86.
6. Bingener J, Schwesinger W, Chopra S, Richards M, Sirinek K. Does the correlation of acute cholecystitis on ultrasound and at surgery reflect a mirror image? *Am J Surgery*. 2004;188:703–707.

 MISCELLANEOUS

See also: Cholangitis (Acute); Choledocholithiasis; Cholelithiasis

CODES
ICD9-CM
- 574.00 Calculus of gallbladder with acute cholecystitis, without mention of obstruction
- 574.01 Calculus of gallbladder with acute cholecystitis, with obstruction
- 575.10 Cholecystitis, unspecified

PATIENT TEACHING

 See Corresponding Diagnostic Algorithm

C

CHOLEDOCHOLITHIASIS

Taylor Sittler, MD
Debra Heitmann, MD

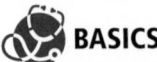

BASICS

DESCRIPTION
- Stones in common bile duct (CBD)
- 3 types: Cholesterol stones (majority), calcium bilirubinate or pigment stones, and mixed stones
- Pigment stones may form de novo in the CBD
- System(s) Affected: Gastrointestinal
- Synonym(s): CBD stones; CBD calculi

GENERAL PREVENTION
- Operative exploration at time of cholecystectomy to identify and remove CBD stones
- T-tube cholangiogram after operative bile duct exploration

EPIDEMIOLOGY
Incidence
- 10–15% of patients with gallstones have choledocholithiasis discovered at time of cholecystectomy
- Increases with age (30–50% of patients >60 years old with gallstones have CBD stones)

Prevalence
Predominant sex: Female > Male

RISK FACTORS
- Cholelithiasis (almost 50% of CBD stones migrate from the gallbladder [GB])
- Pancreatitis (30%)
- Obesity
- Chronic hemolysis
- Prior cholecystectomy

ALERT
Pregnancy Considerations
Cholestasis of pregnancy may lead to choledocholithiasis

Genetics
- MDR3 defects may predispose to bile sludge formation, cholelithiasis, cholestasis of pregnancy, and subsequent choledocholithiasis (3,4)[C].
- Increased prevalence in Hispanic population

ETIOLOGY
- Cholelithiasis: Majority of stones
- Chronic hemolytic states
- Formation of de novo pigment stones
  - Dilated, sclerosed, or strictured ducts (e.g., from recurrent cholangitis)
  - Hepatobiliary parasitism (*Ascaris lumbricoides* or *Clonorchis sinensis*)

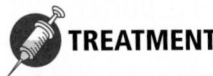

DIAGNOSIS

SIGNS AND SYMPTOMS
May be asymptomatic (30–50%)

History
- Right upper quadrant pain (60%)
  - Moderate/intense spasmodic pain, often intermittent, transient, recurrent
  - Pain not relieved by antacids
- Secondary effects of obstruction
  - Hepatomegaly (80%)
  - Clay-colored stool (50%)
  - Tea-colored urine (50%)
  - Jaundice (50%)
  - Nausea / vomiting (15%)
  - Pruritus
  - Pancreatitis (epigastric pain radiating to back, etc.)
- Infection that may progress to cholangitis and septic shock
  - Fever, chills (30%)
  - Hypotension, flushing
- History of CBD strictures, recurrent or sclerosing cholangitis, sphincter of Oddi dysfunction, cystic dilation
- Weight loss

Physical Exam
- Right upper quadrant tenderness on palpation
- Jaundice
- Anorexia
- Palpable GB (less common)

TESTS
Lab
- Leukocytosis
- Increased alkaline phosphatase
- Hypercholesterolemia (when associated with chronic cholestasis)
- Increased liver transaminases
- Direct hyperbilirubinemia (with total serum bilirubin >3 mg/dL)

Imaging
Imaging is the most effective way to confirm suspected choledocholithiasis
- Transabdominal ultrasound
  - Fastest modality
  - Can confirm but not exclude stones (sensitivity 15–50%, specificity 75%)
  - Can detect dilation of CBD
- Magnetic resonance cholangiopancreatography (MRCP) (sensitivity 92%, specificity 97%)
  - Most accurate noninvasive test, no contrast required (5)[A]
  - Preferred by patients over endoscopic cholangiopancreatography (ERCP), no associated morbidity, and may be less costly than diagnostic ERCP (6)[A]
- Abdominal CT
  - Less sensitive than MRCP but much faster
  - Good at detecting CBD dilation, complications, and delineating surrounding structures (e.g., pancreas)
- Cholescintigraphy (HIDA/DISIDA scan): CBD radionuclide imaging. Isotope derivatives taken up by hepatocytes and excreted into biliary tree
  - May be combined with CCK to observe GB function and estimate GB "ejection fraction"

Diagnostic Procedures/Surgery
- Cholangiography is the gold standard for determining presence of CBD stones.
  - ERCP (sensitivity 90–95%, specificity 95%): Most common diagnostic modality. Allows for papillotomy/stone extraction at time of diagnosis
  - Percutaneous transhepatic cholangiography (PTC): Puncture of hepatic duct by needle, injection of radiopaque dye, and subsequent radiograph imaging of abdomen. Used in place of ERCP in patients with extensive bile duct stone disease or in whom ERCP would be difficult
  - Intraoperative cholangiography: Contrast inserted via opening in cystic duct during cholecystectomy
- Endoscopic ultrasound
  - More likely to detect stones than transabdominal route (sensitivity 85–93%, specificity 97%)
- Intraoperative intraluminal ultrasonography
  - Can be performed during laparoscopic or open procedures
  - May be indicated in patients with contrast dye allergy
- Postoperative studies
  - ERCP and PTC are common postoperatively
  - T-tube cholangiography
  - Choledochoscopy (very sensitive)

Pathological Findings
- Dilated bile ducts
- Bile plugging
- Small bile duct proliferation
- Cholesterol gallstones

DIFFERENTIAL DIAGNOSIS
- Biliary stricture
- Narrowed biliary–enteric anastomosis
- Cholangitis (acute or primary sclerosing)
- Cholangiocarcinoma
- Sphincter of Oddi dysfunction
- Biliary parasites
- Papillary stenosis
- Blood clots

TREATMENT

GENERAL MEASURES
Diet
NPO

Activity
As tolerated

SPECIAL THERAPY
Lithotripsy: Shock-wave lithotripsy to break up stones, leaving smaller fragments in the CBD that can be passed into the intestine or removed by procedure. High complication rate.
- Typically used as an adjunct to surgery or ERCP to fragment large stones (>2 cm)

MEDICATION (DRUGS)

- Stress Ulcer Prophylaxis
  - Sucralfate
  - H₂ antagonists
  - Proton pump Inhibitors
- Antibiotics are indicated if infection of the biliary tract is suspected (see also "Cholangitis")

First Line
- Broad coverage antibiotics. Prescribed for prophylaxis (substitute fluoroquinolones for penicillin allergic patients):
  - Piperacillin-tazobactam (Zosyn) 3.375 g IV q6h
  - Ampicillin-sulbactam (Unasyn) 1.5–3.0 g (1–2 g ampicillin + 0.5–1 g sulbactam) IV/IM q 6–8h; not to exceed 8 g/d ampicillin or 4 g/d sulbactam
  - Ticarcillin-clavulanate (Timentin) 3.1 g IV q4h
  - Mezlocillin 3–4 g IV/IM q4–6h
- Fluoroquinolones have good biliary penetration
  - Levofloxacin 250–500 mg IV or PO once daily
  - Ciprofloxacin 200 mg IV/PO b.i.d.
- Duration of therapy depends on rapidity of response, subsequent surgery, and presence of bacteremia
- Addition of metronidazole for anaerobic coverage in sepsis/infection, elderly patients, and patients with previous biliary manipulation (not necessary with newer broad-spectrum penicillins)
  - Metronidazole 500 mg IV q8h

Second Line
Less common due to bacterial resistance
- Ampicillin 1 g IV q6h *plus*
- Tobramycin 1–1.7 mg/kg IV q8h; amikacin is an alternative but expensive

MEDICAL TREATMENTS

- Endoscopic CBD stone removal: Often performed following endoscopic cholangiography or following stone identification by other modalities.
  - Relatively low complication rate
- PTC with extraction: Common when CBD stones are identified via PTC. An external catheter is placed for stone removal at a later date. (success rate 75–85%)

SURGICAL TREATMENTS
- Surgical CBD stone removal: High success rate (75–95%) and few complications
  - Laparoscopic: Often performed at the time of cholecystectomy. May be preferable to pre-/postoperative ERCP once laparoscopy has been initiated. (7([A], (8)[B]
  - Open choledochotomy: Rarely used. Only for complex cases where laparoscopic and endoscopic techniques fail
- Surgical drainage via external catheter or by papillotomy through ampulla of Vater
  - Indications for drainage include sphincter of Oddi sclerosis or dysfunction, multiple or primary CBD stones, or previous stone

ALERT
Geriatric Considerations
If the patient is elderly, surgery may prevent or delay the need for a cholecystectomy. Higher mortality is associated with open choledochotomy in the elderly.

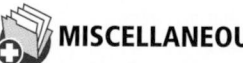 FOLLOW-UP

PROGNOSIS
- With surgical treatment, prognosis is good
- Untreated, 55% of patients experience complications

ALERT
Geriatric Considerations
The prognosis is guarded in the elderly, particularly in an emergent setting. Elderly patients are twice as likely to develop complications (40–60%), and have increased mortality following CBD surgery.

COMPLICATIONS
- Cholangitis: Most frequent (60%)
- Retained CBD stones (2–10%)
- Pancreatitis
- Biliary enteric fistula
- Hemobilia
- Liver dysfunction

PATIENT MONITORING
- Routine postoperative care
- Liver function tests and bilirubin levels.

REFERENCES
1. Jacquemin E. Role of multidrug resistance 3 deficiency in pediatric and adult liver disease: One gene for three diseases. *Semin Liver Dis* 2001;21(4):551–562. (C)
2. Lammert F, Wang DQ, et.al. Spontaneous cholecysto- and hepatolithiasis in Mdr2-/- mice: a model for low phospholipid-associated cholelithiasis. *Hepatology* 2004;39(1):117–128. (C)
3. Romagnuolo J, Bardou M, et al. Magnetic resonance cholangiopancreatography: A meta-analysis of test performance in suspected biliary disease. *Ann Intern Med* 2003;139(7):547–557. (A)
4. Kaltenthaler E, Vergel YB, et al. A systematic review and economic evaluation of magnetic resonance cholangiopancreatography compared with diagnostic endoscopic retrograde cholangiopancreatography. *Health Technol Assess* 2004;8(10):iii, 1–89. (A)
5. Tranter SE, Thompson MH. Comparison of endoscopic sphincterotomy and laparoscopic exploration of the common bile duct. *Br J Surg* 2002;89(12):1495–504. (A)
6. Nathanson LK, O'Rourke NA, et al. Postoperative ERCP versus laparoscopic choledochotomy for clearance of selected bile duct calculi: A randomized trial. *Ann Surg* 2005;242(2):188–192. (B)
7. Clinical manifestations of gallstone disease. In: *Sleisenger and Fordtran's Gastrointestinal and Liver Disease*. Philadelphia: WB Saunders, 2004.
8. Calculous biliary disease. In: Sabiston DC, ed. *Textbook of Surgery*. Philadelphia: WB Saunders, 2002.

ADDITIONAL READING
eMedicine: choledocholithiasis

MISCELLANEOUS

See also: Gallbladder Adenocarcinoma; Cholangitis (acute); Cholecystitis; Cholelithiasis; Jaundice

CODES

ICD9-CM
- 574.30 Calculus of bile duct with acute cholecystitis, without mention of obstruction
- 574.50 Calculus of bile duct without mention of cholecystitis, without mention of obstruction

PATIENT TEACHING
- Contact National Digestive Diseases Information Clearinghouse, Box NDDIC, Bethesda, MD 20892; (301) 468-6344.
- Medline Encyclopedia: http://www.nlm.nih.gov/medlineplus/ency/article/000274.htm

See Corresponding Diagnostic Algorithm

CHOLELITHIASIS

Hongyi Cui, MD, PhD
Ruben Peralta, MD, FACS

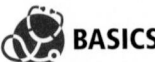 **BASICS**

DESCRIPTION
- Cholesterol, pigment, or mixed stones formed and contained in the gallbladder
- Synonym(s): Gallstones

Pediatric Considerations
- Uncommon <10 years of age
- Associated with blood dyscrasia
- Most gallstones in pediatric population are pigment stones.

GENERAL PREVENTION
- Ursodiol (Actigall) taken during rapid weight loss prevents stone formation.
- Low-fat diet is advisable but not proven to prevent gallstone formation.

EPIDEMIOLOGY
Incidence
- Increased in Native Americans and Hispanics
- Increases with age by 1–3% per year; peak at 6th decade
- 2% of the US population develops gallstones annually.

Prevalence
- Population: 8–10% of US
- Predominant sex: Female > Male (2:1)

RISK FACTORS
- Short gut syndrome
- Terminal ileal resection
- Vagotomy
- Inflammatory bowel disease
- Multiparity
- Long-term total parenteral nutrition
- Cirrhosis (for pigment stones)
- Hemolytic disorders
  - Hereditary spherocytosis
  - Sickle cell anemia
- Obesity
- Hyperlipidemia
- Rapid weight loss
- Diabetes (for complications)
- Age (peak in 60s)
- Caucasian, Hispanic, or Native American descent
- Female gender
- Early use of birth control pills; estrogen replacement therapy at high doses

Genetics
Animal studies indicate that gallstone formation is a dominant trait determined by at least 2 genes; susceptible strains fail to down-regulate cholesterol synthesis during cholesterol feeding.

ETIOLOGY
- Production of bile supersaturated with cholesterol
- Decrease in bile content of either phospholipids or bile acids
- Biliary stasis or impaired gallbladder motility
- Hemolytic diseases
- Biliary infection

ASSOCIATED CONDITIONS
90% of people with gallbladder carcinoma have gallstones.

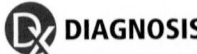 **DIAGNOSIS**

SIGNS AND SYMPTOMS
- Mostly asymptomatic (80%)
  - 5–10% become symptomatic each year
  - Over their lifetime, <1/2 of the patients with gallstones develop symptoms.
- Episodic right upper quadrant or epigastric pain radiating to the back (biliary colic), usually postprandially
- Nausea
- Vomiting
- Fatty food intolerance (not proven)
- Indigestion or bloating sensation

Physical Exam
Physical exam is usually normal

TESTS
Lab
No lab study is specific for cholelithiasis.

Imaging
- Hepatobiliary radionuclide scan
- Ultrasound (best technique to diagnose gallstones and differentiate from cholecystitis)
- Oral cholecystogram
- CT scan (no advantage over ultrasound)
- 10–30% of gallstones are radiopaque. Calcium or pigment-containing gallstones are more likely to be visible on plain x-ray. A "porcelain gallbladder" is a calcified gallbladder, visible by x-ray; associated with gallbladder cancer (25%).

Pathological Findings
- Pure cholesterol stones have a white or slightly yellow color.
- Pigment stones may be black or brown. Black stones contain calcium bilirubinate, most often secondary to cirrhosis or hemolysis and almost always form in the gallbladder. Brown stones are associated with biliary tract infection, caused by bile stasis, and as such may form either in the bile ducts or gallbladder.

DIFFERENTIAL DIAGNOSIS
- Peptic ulcer
- Hepatitis
- Pancreatitis
- Coronary artery disease
- Appendicitis
- Pneumonia
- Gallbladder cancer
- Renal stones
- Stricture
- Gallbladder polyps
- Biliary sludge
- Acalculous cholecystitis
- Biliary dyskinesia
- Choledocholithiasis
- Choledochocyst

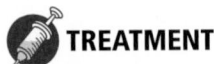 **TREATMENT**

Geriatric Considerations
Age alone should not alter the therapy plan.

INITIAL STABILIZATION
Inpatient for surgical procedures

GENERAL MEASURES
- Treat only symptomatic gallstones
- Advise patient of presence of stones
- Observe asymptomatic stones
- Oral dissolution: Rarely used
- During pregnancy, attempt conservative therapy, but perform surgery if indicated.
- Prophylactic cholecystectomy for bariatric surgery, pediatric gallstones, congenital hemolytic anemia, gallstone >2.5 cm in diameter, calcified (porcelain) gallbladder, poor access to medical care

Diet
A low-fat diet may be helpful.

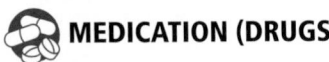 **MEDICATION (DRUGS)**

First Line
- Analgesics for pain relief
- Oral dissolution therapy is an option for nonsurgical care for cholelithiasis. These treatments are rarely used today.

Second Line
NSAIDs may have a role in pain relief, given that prostaglandins are important in the development of pain.

SURGERY
- Surgical intervention should be considered for patients who have symptomatic cholelithiasis or complications such as cholecystitis. (1)[B]
- Laparoscopic cholecystectomy is currently the standard of care for most cases (2)[B]
  - Surgery-related complications include common bile duct injury (0.5%), right hepatic duct/artery injury, cystic duct leak, or biloma formation.
  - Conversion to open procedure based on the judgment of the operating surgeon
  - Intraoperative cholangiogram (IOC) may help delineate bile duct anatomy when dissection proves difficult. Selective or routine use of IOC is a topic of debate but may be associated with earlier recognition and decreased incidence of bile duct injury. (3)[B]
- Open cholecystotomy
- Direct contact dissolution
  - For only a small subset of patients
  - High recurrence rate
- Extracorporeal shock wave lithotripsy
  - Role of this modality is unclear; currently under study
- Percutaneous cholecystostomy in high-risk patients

FOLLOW-UP

PROGNOSIS

- <1/2 of patients with gallstones become symptomatic.
- Cholecystectomy: Mortality 0.5% elective, 3–5% emergency; morbidity <10% elective, 30–40% emergency
- ~10–15% of the patients will have associated choledocholithiasis.
- After cholecystectomy, stones may recur in the bile duct.

COMPLICATIONS

- Acute cholecystitis (90–95% secondary to gallstones)
- Gallstone pancreatitis
- Acute cholangitis
- Common bile duct stones with obstructive jaundice
- Gallstone ileus
- Liver abscess
- Biliary-enteric fistula
- Peritonitis
- Gallbladder cancer
- Mirizzi syndrome (bile duct obstruction caused by gallstones lodged in Hartmann's pouch of gallbladder)

PATIENT MONITORING

- Medical attention if asymptomatic stones become symptomatic
- Patients on oral dissolution agents should be followed up with liver enzyme, serum cholesterol, and imaging studies.

REFERENCES

1. Bellows CF, Berger DH, Crass RA. Management of gallstones. *Am Fam Physician*. 2005;72:637–642.
2. Shamiyeh A, Wayland W. Current status of laparoscopic therapy of cholelithiasis and common bile duct stones. *Dig Dis*. 2005;23:119–126.
3. Connor S, Garden OJ. Bile duct injury in the era of laparoscopic cholecystectomy. *Br J Surg*. 2006; 93:158–168.

 MISCELLANEOUS

- Other notes: Laparoscopic cholecystectomy has become the most frequently used procedure. (Lithotripsy may be considered in rare circumstances.)
- See also: Cholangitis (Acute); Cholecystitis; Choledocholithiasis; Jaundice

CODES

ICD9-CM

- 574.00 Calculus of gallbladder with acute cholecystitis, without mention of obstruction
- 574.10 Calculus of gallbladder with other cholecystitis, without mention of obstruction
- 574.20 Calculus of gallbladder without mention of cholecystitis, without mention of obstruction
- 575.0 Acute cholecystitis
- 575.10 Cholecystitis, unspecified
- 574.01 Calculus of gallbladder with acute cholecystitis, with obstruction

PATIENT TEACHING

 See Corresponding Diagnostic Algorithm

See Patient Handout on CD

CHOLERA

Abdulrazak Abyad, MD, PhD, MBA, MPH, AGSF

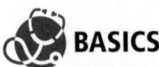 **BASICS**

DESCRIPTION

An acute infectious disease caused by *Vibrio cholerae* (El Tor type is responsible for current epidemic; the other type, classic, is found only in Bangladesh). Characteristics include severe diarrhea with extreme fluid and electrolyte depletion, and vomiting, muscle cramps, and prostration. (New serotype now in Bangladesh, India [0139]. Important because of lack of efficacy of standard vaccine.)

- Usual course: Acute, chronic, and relapsing
- Clinical course is 3–5 days, and in the early stages a severely affected patient can lose 1 L/h.
- Endemic areas: India, Southeast Asia, Africa, Middle East, Southern Europe, Oceania, South and Central America
- System(s) Affected: Gastrointestinal
- Synonym(s): Asiatic cholera; Epidemic cholera; Rice-water diarrhea; Cholera gravis

Pediatric Considerations

- Breast-feeding protects against cholera.
- Vaccine not recommended for children <6 months

GENERAL PREVENTION

- Water purification
- Careful food selection (e.g., no unpeeled raw fruits or vegetables, no raw or undercooked seafood)
- Enteric precautions
- Tetracycline for social contacts of an index case
- Natural infection confers long-lasting immunity.
- Prophylactic vaccine
  - 50% effective for 3–6 months
  - Not recommended unless required by destination country, and if so, a single dose is sufficient
  - Concomitant administration with yellow fever vaccine may result in reduced vaccine response to yellow fever.
  - Invariably associated with local side effects
  - Systemic side effects of fever and malaise
  - A new vaccine shows promise, but remains in the testing stage.

EPIDEMIOLOGY

- Predominant age: All ages
- Predominant sex: Male = Female

Prevalence

About 0.01 cases/100,000. The few cases in the United States have been found in returning travelers or are associated with food brought into this country illegally.

RISK FACTORS

- Traveling or living in epidemic/endemic areas
- Exposure to contaminated food or water
- Person-to-person transmission (rare)
- In endemic areas, children <5 years
- Attack more severe in patients with blood group O compared with AB
- People with low gastric acid secretion
- Gastrectomy
- Patients on acid-suppressing medications

ETIOLOGY

- Enterotoxin elaborated by Gram-negative bacteria
- *Cholerae* (O-group 1)
- Human host
- Contaminated food
- Contaminated water
- Contaminated shellfish

ASSOCIATED CONDITIONS

Increased risk of disease with gastric achlorhydria

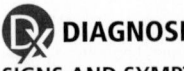 **DIAGNOSIS**

SIGNS AND SYMPTOMS

- Abdominal discomfort
- Anorexia
- Anuria
- Apathy
- Cholera gravis
- Cyanosis
- Decreased skin turgor
- Dehydration
- Diarrhea, painless
- Distant heart sounds
- Diuresis, sudden
- Dysrhythmias
- Fever
- Hypotension
- Hypothermia
- Hypovolemic shock
- Increased or decreased bowel sounds
- Lethargy
- Listlessness
- Malaise
- Oliguria
- Rice-water diarrhea
- Seizures
- Sunken eyes
- Tachycardia
- Thirst
- Vomiting
- Washerwoman's fingers
- Weak peripheral pulses
- Weakness

TESTS
Lab
- Stool culture: On selective media (thiosulfate citrate bile salts sucrose [TCBS])
- Typed antisera specific agglutination
- Dark-field microscopy: Characteristic vibrio motility in stool
- Increased vibriocidal antibodies in nonimmunized patient
- Laboratory abnormalities of severe dehydration
  - Acidemia
  - Acidosis
  - Hypokalemia
  - Hyponatremia
  - Hypochloremia
  - Hypoglycemia
  - Increased specific gravity
  - Polycythemia
  - Mild neutrophilic leukocytosis

Imaging
- Abdominal film: Ileus
- Chest radiograph: Microcardia

Diagnostic Procedures/Surgery
Physical examination and medical history that includes recent travel

Pathological Findings
- Electron microscopy: Organism adheres to mucosa
- Intact mucosa
- Increased cellularity of lamina propria
- Increased cellularity of mucosa
- Vascular congestion
- Lymphoid hyperplasia of Peyer patches
- Lymphoid hyperplasia of mesenteric lymph nodes
- Lymphoid hyperplasia of spleen
- Cerebral edema
- Acute tubular necrosis
- Vacuolar hypokalemic nephropathy
- Pulmonary edema
- Hyaline membranes
- Bronchopneumonia
- Focal myocardial damage
- Lipid-depleted adrenals
- Tubularization of zona fasciculata

DIFFERENTIAL DIAGNOSIS
Other causes of severe diarrhea and dehydration (e.g., infection with *Shigella*, *Escherichia coli*, venous viruses)

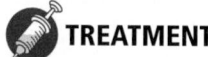 TREATMENT

INITIAL STABILIZATION
Outpatient for mild cases, inpatient for moderate to severe cases

GENERAL MEASURES
- Determination of the amount of fluid loss (may compare patient's previous with current weight)
- Rehydration therapy: Oral for mild to moderate cases. Patients with severe dehydration may require IV fluid replacement.

Diet
Small, frequent meals when vomiting stops and appetite returns

Activity
Bed rest until symptoms resolve and strength returns

 MEDICATION (DRUGS)

First Line
- Oral rehydration therapy

For mild disease

- Oral rehydration solution (ORS) commercial brands available (Pedialyte, Rehydralyte, Resol, Rice-Lyte) *or*
- Oral rehydration solution formula from World Health Organization, per liter
  - Sodium chloride 3.5 g
  - Potassium chloride 1.5 g
  - Glucose 20 g
  - Trisodium citrate 2.9 g
- Parenteral rehydration

Rehydration for severely dehydrated patients

- IV rehydration (Ringer lactate) is followed by oral or nasogastric administration of glucose or sucrose-electrolyte solution.
- Antibiotics
  - For older children and adults: Doxycycline (Vibramycin): 300 mg once or 100 mg b.i.d. for 3 days or tetracycline 50 mg/kg/d for 3 days
  - For young children: trimethoprim-sulfamethoxazole (SMX-TMP, Bactrim, Septra) 8 mg/kg trimethoprim plus 40 mg/kg sulfamethoxazole per day, divided q12h. This dosage is equivalent to 1 mL/kg of trimethoprim-sulfamethoxazole suspension.
  - In pregnant patients: Furazolidone 100 mg q.i.d. for 7–10 days
- Contraindications
  - Tetracycline: Not for use in pregnant patients or children <8 years old.
  - Furazolidone and alcohol in combination may cause disulfiram-like reaction.
- Precautions
  - Tetracycline: May cause photosensitivity; sunscreen recommended.
- Significant possible interactions
  - Tetracycline: Avoid concurrent administration with antacids, dairy products, or iron.

Second Line
In young children: Furazolidone (Furoxone) 5–10 mg/kg/d divided q6h for 3 days

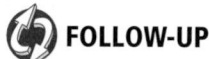 FOLLOW-UP

PROGNOSIS
- Prompt PO or IV treatment can save lives.
- Appropriate disposal of human waste
- Antibiotic treatment reduces duration and infectivity of disease.
- Mortality <1% with appropriate supportive care
- Mortality higher with untreated hypovolemic shock

COMPLICATIONS
- Hypovolemic shock
- Chronic biliary infection
- Up to 50% mortality with untreated shock
- Intermittent stool shedding

PATIENT MONITORING
Observe patient until symptoms are resolved.

REFERENCES
1. Mandell GL, ed. *Principles and Practice of Infectious Diseases*. 4th ed. New York, NY: Churchill Livingstone; 1995.
2. Warren KS, Mahmoud AA, eds. *Tropical and Geographical Medicine*. New York, NY: McGraw-Hill; 1990.
3. Dhiman BR, Greenough CB III, eds. *Cholera*. New York, NY: Plenum Publishing; 1992.
4. Shears P. Recent developments in cholera. *Curr Opin Infect Dis*. 2001;14:553–558.

 MISCELLANEOUS

- US Centers for Disease Control and Prevention do not expect a major outbreak of cholera in the United States, but has issued a "Cholera Preparedness Plan" outlining steps for proper surveillance, treatment, laboratory diagnosis, investigation of outbreaks, and public education.
- See also: Diarrhea, Acute; Oral Rehydration

 CODES

ICD9-CM
001.9 Cholera, unspecified

PATIENT TEACHING
- Centers for Disease Control and Prevention. Traveler's Information Hotline: (404) 332-4559 (available 24 hours via a touch-tone telephone).
- International Association for Medical Assistance to Travelers, 417 Center St., Lewiston, NY 14092; (716) 754-4883

C

CHRONIC COUGH

Jacqueline L. Olin, MS, PharmD, BCPS

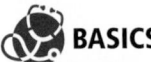 **BASICS**

DESCRIPTION

- Chronic cough persists >8 weeks in adults.
- Subacute cough describes cough lasting 3–8 weeks.
- In children, chronic cough is defined as >4 weeks in duration.
- Patients present because of fear of the causative illness (e.g., cancer), as well as annoyance, self-consciousness, and hoarseness. Patients with stress urinary incontinence may find cough particularly troubling.
- Chronic obstructive pulmonary disease and smoking-related cough are most common causes at the PCP level.
- System(s) Affected: Gastrointestinal; Pulmonary

EPIDEMIOLOGY

- Predominant age: All age groups
- Predominant sex: Male = Female

Incidence

Recurrent cough has been reported at 3–40% by various population estimates.

RISK FACTORS

Although various conditions may contribute to chronic cough, the main causes include

- Smoking
- Pulmonary diseases

Genetics

No genetic basis exists as a cause.

PATHOPHYSIOLOGY

Varies with findings and disorders implicated

ETIOLOGY

- Often multiple etiologies, but most are related to bronchial irritation. Most frequent etiologies (account for >90% of cases) in nonsmokers include
  - Upper airway cough syndrome (UACS) (postnasal drip syndrome)
  - Asthma
  - Gastroesophageal reflux disease
  - Nonasthmatic eosinophilic bronchitis (NAEB)
- Other causes
  - Angiotensin-converting enzyme (ACE) inhibitor therapy
  - Aspiration
  - Bronchiectasis
  - Cystic fibrosis
  - Chronic interstitial lung disease
  - Lung neoplasm or laryngeal cancer
  - Pertussis
  - Psychogenic (habit cough)
  - Restrictive lung disease
  - TB, atypical mycobacterium, and other chronic lung infections

ASSOCIATED CONDITIONS

Patients with UACS, asthma, and GERD may present with chronic cough as the only symptom, and not the usual symptoms associated with the diagnoses

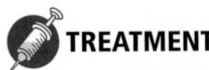 **DIAGNOSIS**

SIGNS AND SYMPTOMS

- Variable and related to the underlying cause
- Usually nonproductive cough with no other signs or symptoms
- Possible signs and symptoms of UACS, sinusitis, GERD, congestive heart failure, connective tissue disorders
- Absence of additional signs/symptoms of a particular condition not necessarily helpful (75% of GERD patients have no other signs or symptoms)

ALERT
Pediatric Considerations
Habitual cough is more likely in school-age children.

History
The age of the patient, presence of associated signs/symptoms, medical history, medication (ACE inhibitor), environmental exposures, potential for aspiration, and smoking history may make some causes more likely.

Physical Exam
The character of cough is rarely helpful in diagnosis.

TESTS
Extensive testing only if indicated by the history and physical. Simple testing (chest radiograph, sinus studies) followed by empiric therapy directed at likely underlying etiology.

Pediatric Considerations
Children with chronic cough should undergo, as a minimum, spirometry and chest radiograph (if age appropriate).

Lab
- Sweat chloride testing
- Sputum for eosinophils and cytology

Imaging
- Chest radiograph
- Chest CT if needed
- Upper GI series

Diagnostic Procedures/Surgery
If diagnosis suspected and inadequate response to initial measures, procedures can be considered:

- Pulmonary function testing
- Purified protein derivative skin testing
- 24-hour esophageal pH monitor
- Bronchoscopy if necessary
- Endoscopic or videofluoroscopic swallow evaluation
- Sinus imaging
- ECG
- Barium esophagram

Pathological Findings
Specific to underlying cause

TREATMENT

- Best evidence treatment:
  - In patients with chronic cough, considerations for potential etiology should include asthma (2)[B] or UACS (2)[C].
  - In patients with chronic cough who complain of heartburn and regurgitation, GERD should be considered as a potential etiology (2)[C].
  - When indicated, ACE inhibitor therapy should be switched in patients in whom intolerable cough occurs (2)[A].
  - 90% of patients will have resolution of cough after smoking cessation (2)[A]
  - With chronic cough, empiric treatment should be directed at the most common causes (UACS, asthma, GERD, NAEB) (2)[C].
  - Oral antihistamine/decongestant therapy with a first-generation antihistamine should be initial empiric treatment (2)[C].
  - In patients with cough associated with the common cold, nonsedating antihistamines were not found to be effective in reducing cough (2)[C].
  - In stable patients with chronic bronchitis, therapy with ipratropium bromide may reduce chronic cough (1)[C].
  - Central cough suppressants (codeine, dextromethorphan) are recommend for short-term symptomatic relief of coughing in patients with chronic bronchitis (1)[C]. These agents have limited efficacy in cough due to upper respiratory infections (1)[C].
  - For cough associated with lung cancer, the use of narcotic cough suppressants is recommended (1)[C].

ALERT
Pediatric Considerations

- The American Academy of Pediatrics does not recommend central cough suppressants for treating any kind of cough (2)[B].

- In children <14 years old, when pediatric recommendations are not available, adult recommendations should be used with caution (2)[C].

GENERAL MEASURES
- Directed at most likely etiology
- Eliminate smoking and ACE inhibitors
- Often empiric treatment of postnasal drip and gastroesophageal reflux disease
- Attempt maximal therapy for single most likely cause for several weeks, then search for coexistent etiologies.

Diet
Patients with GERD may benefit by avoiding ethanol, caffeine, nicotine, citrus, tomatoes, chocolate, and fatty foods.

Activity
Patients with GERD may benefit from elevation of head of bed and elimination of meals at bedtime.

SPECIAL THERAPY
Physical Therapy
Chest physiotherapy is recommended to increase mucus clearance in patients with cystic fibrosis. Its long-term benefits are unknown.

MEDICATION (DRUGS)

Treatments (antacids, bronchodilators, proton pump inhibitors, antibiotics) should be directed at the specific cause of the cough.

First Line
- In adults, oral antihistamine/decongestant therapy with a 1st-generation antihistamine should be initial empiric treatment. Multiple formulations are available over the counter. Example:
  - Dexbrompheniramine 6 mg/pseudoephedrine 120 mg q12h: Age >12 years
- Central cough suppressants for short-term symptomatic relief of nonproductive cough
  - Dextromethorphan (Delsym) 30 mg b.i.d.: Age >6 years
  - Narcotics: Codeine 15–30 mg q6h, hydrocodone (Vicodin) 5 mg q6h

ALERT
Pediatric Considerations
Cough suppressants and other over-the-counter cough medicines are not recommended in young children.

Second Line
For patients with cystic fibrosis
- Amiloride may increase cough clearance

SURGERY
- Fundoplication may be effective for cough secondary to refractory GERD.
- Cough secondary to chronic sinusitis

 FOLLOW-UP

DISPOSITION
This condition is generally handled on an outpatient basis.

Issues for Referral
Refer based on specific diagnosis for cough

PROGNOSIS
- >80% of patients can be effectively diagnosed and treated using a systematic approach.
- Cough from any cause may take weeks to months until resolution, and resolution depends greatly on efficacy of treatment directed at underlying etiology.

COMPLICATIONS
- Cardiovascular: Arrhythmias, syncope
- Stress urinary incontinence
- Abdominal and intercostal muscle strain
- Gastrointestinal: Emesis, hemorrhage, herniation
- Neurological: Dizziness, headache, seizures
- Respiratory: Pneumothorax, laryngeal or tracheobronchial trauma
- Skin: Petechiae, purpura, disruption of surgical wounds
- Medication side effects

PATIENT MONITORING
- Frequent follow-up is necessary to assess the effectiveness of the treatment and the addition of other medications as needed.
- Consider stepwise withdrawal of medications after resolution of the cough.

REFERENCES

1. Bolser DC. Cough suppressant and pharmacologic protussive therapy: American College of Chest Physicians (ACCP) evidence-based clinical practice guidelines. *Chest* 2006;129(Suppl): 238S–249S.
2. Irwin RS. Baumann MH. Bolser DC, et al. and American College of Chest Physicians (ACCP). Diagnosis and management of cough executive summary: ACCP evidence-based clinical practice guidelines. *Chest* 2006;129:1S–23S.
3. Morice AH, Kastelik JA. Cough. 1: Chronic cough in adults. *Thorax* 2003;58:901–907.

 MISCELLANEOUS

See also: Asthma; Bronchiectasis; Congestive heart failure; Eosinophilic pneumonias; Gastroesophageal reflux disease; Laryngeal cancer; Lung, primary malignancies; Pertussis; Pulmonary edema; Rhinitis, allergic; Sinusitis; Tuberculosis

CODES

ICD9-CM
- 786.2 Cough
- 306.1 Physiological malfunction arising from mental factors, respiratory
- 491.0 Simple chronic bronchitis

PATIENT TEACHING
- Reassure patient that most cases do not have life-threatening causes and that the condition can usually be managed effectively.
- Counsel that several weeks to a month may be needed for significant reduction or total elimination of cough.
- Prepare the patient for the possibility of multiple diagnostic tests and therapeutic regimens, because the treatment is very often empiric.

Diet
Patients with GERD may benefit by avoiding foods likely to cause symptoms.

Prevention
90% of patients will have resolution of cough after smoking cessation

C

CHRONIC FATIGUE SYNDROME

Sarah Guzofski, MD
Ruben Peralta, MD

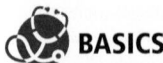 **BASICS**

DESCRIPTION
Chronic fatigue syndrome is characterized primarily by profound mental and physical exhaustion, in association with multiple systemic and neuropsychiatric symptoms that last at least 6 months. The disorder must have a new or definite onset (not lifelong), not be relieved by rest, and result in a >50% reduction in previous activities (occupational, educational, social, and personal).

EPIDEMIOLOGY
- Predominant age: 20–50
- Predominant sex: Female > Male
- All socioeconomic groups

- Initially reported to be most common in Caucasian population, but these were clinic-based studies; community-based studies have found at least as high risk among Latino, African American, and Native American populations, suggesting earlier findings related to health care access. (1)[B]

Incidence
10/100,000

RISK FACTORS
Possibly higher risk if history of childhood physical or sexual abuse

ETIOLOGY
- Unknown
- Multiple immunologic and infectious processes have been investigated. Currently thought to be multifactorial with interaction between genetic predisposition, an initiating stressor, and perpetuating factors (such as resultant disruption in work and social relationships).

- Virus (either as a physiologic stressor or environmental trigger) could be precipitant. Many patients with chronic fatigue recall significant stressors (e.g., major medical procedure, loss of a loved one, loss of employment) in months before symptoms began. (2,3)[B]
- Neuroendocrine abnormalities have been found, including diminished cortisol response to increased corticotropin concentrations and upregulation of the serotonin system, but the implications are not clear. (3)[B]

ASSOCIATED CONDITIONS
Common comorbidities include (1): Fibromyalgia, Irritable bowel syndrome, Temporomandibular joint disorder, Anxiety disorders, including panic, Major depression

DIAGNOSIS

SIGNS AND SYMPTOMS
Centers for Disease Control and Prevention Diagnostic Criteria: At least 6 months of fatigue sufficient to "substantially reduce" patient's level of activity—4 or more of the following (4)[C]
- Poor memory/concentration
- Sore throat
- Tender lymph nodes
- Myalgias
- Arthralgias
- Recent-onset headache
- Unrefreshing sleep
- Excessive tiredness with exercise

May also be associated with (3)[B]
- Low-grade fever
- Dizziness
- Nausea
- Anorexia
- Night sweats
- Irritability
- Symptoms should have clear onset

TESTS
Lab
- Initial lab studies
  - Chemistry panel
  - CBC
  - Urinalysis
  - Thyrotropin
  - Erythrocyte sedimentation rate (ESR)

- Additional studies, if clinically suspected (5)[B]
  - Anti-nuclear antibodies (if + ESR)
  - Creatine kinase
  - Rheumatoid factor (if + ESR)
  - Purified protein derivative
  - Serum cortisol
  - HIV
  - Lyme serology

DIFFERENTIAL DIAGNOSIS
- Malignancies
- Autoimmune disease
- Localized infection (occult abscess)
- Chronic or subacute bacterial disease (endocarditis)
- Lyme disease
- Fungal disease (histoplasmosis, coccidioidomycosis)
- Parasitic disease (amebiasis, giardiasis, helminth infestation)
- HIV-related disease
- Psychiatric disorders
  - Drug dependency or abuse, including prescription drugs
  - Depression
  - Hypochondriasis
  - Anxiety disorders
  - Somatization disorder
- Chronic inflammatory disease (sarcoidosis, Wegener granulomatosis)
- Known chronic viral disease (HIV)
- Neuromuscular disease (multiple sclerosis, myasthenia gravis)
- Endocrine disorder (hypothyroidism, Addison, Cushing, diabetes mellitus)
- Iatrogenic (e.g., medication side effects)
- Toxic agent exposure
- Other known or defined systemic disease (chronic pulmonary, cardiac, hepatic, renal, or hematologic disease)
- Physiologic (inadequate or disrupted sleep, menopause)

 TREATMENT

GENERAL MEASURES

- 2 treatments have been shown effective (2,3,6)[B]
  - Cognitive behavioral therapy: Exercise program plus re-structuring of counterproductive cognitions. Challenge fatigue-related cognition. Plan social and occupational rehabilitation
  - Graded exercise protocols: Based on a physiologic approach to reconditioning. Does not address cognitive understanding of symptoms
- Both involve a carefully planned balance between activity and rest.
- Patients learn that activity will not worsen their illness.
- Improve functional capacity and diminish sense of fatigue.
- The duration of illness does not predict treatment outcome, so this approach can be applied to patients with chronic symptoms.

Activity
- Gradual increase in physical exercise
- Avoid extended periods of rest.

 MEDICATION (DRUGS)

Medications are generally not considered helpful. Studies have been conducted with antidepressants, immunoglobulins, and hydrocortisone, and none have shown clear benefit. (2,6)[B]

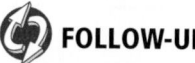 FOLLOW-UP

DISPOSITION

Issues for Referral
- Psychiatrist to assess for comorbid disorders
- Occupational health physician may be able to help in planning program of recovery

PROGNOSIS
- Indolent; condition comes and goes
- Generally, improvement is slow with a course of months to years.

COMPLICATIONS
- Depression
- Unemployment. Although studies document improvement with treatment, <1/3 of patients in trials return to work. (7,8)[B]

PATIENT MONITORING
Although no consensus exists, periodic re-evaluation is appropriate for support, relief of symptoms, and assessment for possible other causes of debility.

REFERENCES

1. Afari N, Buchwald D. Chronic fatigue syndrome: A review. *Am J Psychiat.* 2003;160:221–236.
2. Rimes KA, Chalder T. Treatments for chronic fatigue. *Occup Med-Oxford.* 2005;55:32–39.
3. Prins JB, van der Meer JWM, Bkeijenberg G. Chronic fatigue syndrome. *Lancet.* 2006;367: 346–355.
4. Fukuda K, Straus S, Hickie I, et al. The chronic fatigue syndrome: A comprehensive approach to its definition and study. *Ann Intern Med.* 1994;84: 118–121.
5. Viner R, Christie D. Fatigue and somatic symptoms. *BJM.* 2005;330:1012–1015.
6. Margo KL, Margo GM. Two therapies lift mood in chronic fatigue syndrome. *Current Psychiatry.* 2006;5:91–100.
7. Cairns R, Hotopf M. A systematic review describing the prognosis of chronic fatigue syndrome. *Occup Med-Oxford.* 2005;55:20–31.
8. Ross SD, Estok RP, Frame D, et al. Disability and the chronic fatigue syndrome. *Arch Intern Med.* 2004;164:1098–1107.

 MISCELLANEOUS

Chronic fatigue syndrome, its etiology, diagnosis, and management are all controversial topics.

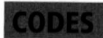 CODES

ICD9-CM
780.71 Chronic Fatigue syndrome

PATIENT TEACHING
- Chronic Fatigue and Immune Dysfunction Syndrome Association of America
- http://www.cfids.org/

Activity
Gradual increase in exercise, scheduled rest and avoidance of prolonged rest

 See Patient Handout on CD

C

CHRONIC OBSTRUCTIVE PULMONARY DISEASE AND EMPHYSEMA

Alan J. Cropp, MD, FCCP

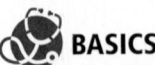 **BASICS**

DESCRIPTION

- Chronic obstructive pulmonary disease (COPD) encompasses: Several diffuse pulmonary diseases including chronic bronchitis, asthma, cystic fibrosis, bronchiectasis, and emphysema. The term usually describes a mixture of chronic bronchitis and emphysema; characterized by airflow limitation that is not fully reversible.
- Chronic bronchitis is defined clinically by increased mucus production and recurrent cough present on most days for at least 3 months during at least 2 consecutive years.
- Emphysema is the destruction of interalveolar septa; it occurs in the distal or terminal airways and involves both airways and lung parenchyma.

GENERAL PREVENTION

Avoidance of smoking is the most important preventive measure. Passive smoke also has been shown to be harmful. Early detection may be useful in preserving remaining lung function.

EPIDEMIOLOGY

- Predominant age: >40
- Predominant sex: Male > Female

Geriatric Considerations

Relative risk is 1.2–2.3 times greater than in a younger person. Disease is unusual in anyone <25 unless antiprotease deficiency is present. Incidence increases as age nears 60.

Pediatric Considerations

Repeated childhood respiratory illnesses increases risk of COPD.

Incidence

~10–20% of adults; >100,000 deaths/year in the US

Prevalence

- 14 million people have chronic bronchitis; 2 million people have emphysema.
- 4th leading cause of death in US

RISK FACTORS

- Passive smoking, especially adults whose parents smoked
- Severe viral pneumonia early in life
- Aging
- Ethyl alcohol consumption
- Airway hyperactivity

Genetics

- Chronic bronchitis is not a genetic disorder.
- Antiprotease deficiency (due to alpha-1 antitrypsin deficiency), is an inherited, rare disorder due to 2 autosomal codominant alleles.

PATHOPHYSIOLOGY

Impaired gas (CO_2 and O_2 exchange 1)

- Destruction of lung parchyma in emphysema
- Airway obstruction by mucus in chronic bronchitis

ETIOLOGY

- Cigarette smoking
- Air pollution
- Antiprotease deficiency (alpha-1 antitrypsin)
- Occupational exposure (firefighters, jobs around a great deal of dust)
- Infection possibly (viral)
- Occupational pollutants (cadmium, silica)

ASSOCIATED CONDITIONS

Lung cancer, Coronary artery disease, Peptic ulcer disease, Chronic sinusitis, Malnutrition, Laryngeal carcinoma, Acute bronchitis

DIAGNOSIS

SIGNS AND SYMPTOMS

- Chronic bronchitis
  - Cough
  - Sputum production
  - Frequent infections
  - Intermittent dyspnea
  - Hemoptysis
  - Morning headache
  - Pedal edema
- Emphysema
  - Minimal cough
  - Scant sputum
  - Dyspnea
  - Often significant weight loss
  - Occasional infections

History

Patient's habits with regard to tobacco and alcohol use should be verified and discussed to assist in immediate diagnosis. Also should discuss causes of exacerbation (i.e., recent infection). (1)

Physical Exam

- Chronic bronchitis
  - Cyanosis
  - Wheezing
  - Weight gain
  - Diminished breath sounds
  - Distant heart sounds
- Emphysema
  - Barrel chest
  - Minimal wheezing
  - Use of accessory muscles of respiration
  - Pursed lip breathing
  - Cyanosis slight or absent
  - Breath sounds diminished

TESTS

Lab

- Chronic bronchitis
  - Hypercapnia
  - Polycythemia
  - Hypoxia can be moderate to severe
- Emphysema
  - Normal serum hemoglobin or polycythemia
  - Normal $PaCO_2$; unless forced expiratory volume in 1 secord (FEV1) <1 L, in which case it can be elevated
  - Mild hypoxia, especially at night
- Drugs that may alter lab results: Sedatives, including alcohol
- Disorders that may alter lab results: Obesity, concurrent restrictive lung dysfunction, primary pulmonary hypertension, acute infections, anemia, pulmonary embolism, sleep apnea, congestive heart failure (CHF)

Imaging

- Chronic bronchitis chest x-ray: Increased bronchovascular markings and cardiomegaly.
- Emphysema CXR: Small heart, hyperinflation, flat diaphragms and possibly bullous changes
- CAT may show bullous changes.

Diagnostic Procedures/Surgery

- Pulmonary function testing
  - Not indicated during acute exacerbation (1)
  - Decreased (FEV1) with concomitant reduction in FEV1/forced vital capacity (FVC) ratio
  - Poor or absent reversibility to bronchodilators
  - Normal or reduced FVC
  - Normal or increased total lung capacity
  - Increased residual volume
  - Diffusing capacity is normal or reduced
- Nocturnal oximetry

Pathological Findings

- Chronic bronchitis
  - Bronchial mucous gland enlargement
  - Increased number of secretory cells in surface epithelium
  - Thickened small airways from edema and inflammation
  - Smooth muscle hyperplasia
  - Mucus plugging
  - Bacterial colonization of airways
- Emphysema
  - Entire lung affected
  - Bronchi usually clear of secretions
  - Anthracotic pigment
  - Alveoli enlarged with loss of septa
  - Cartilage atrophy
  - Bullae

DIFFERENTIAL DIAGNOSIS

Acute bronchitis, Asthma, Bronchiectasis, Bronchogenic carcinoma, Acute viral infection, Normal aging of lungs, Occupational asthma, Chronic pulmonary embolism, Sleep apnea, Primary alveolar hypoventilation, Chronic sinusitis, Reactive airways dysfunction syndrome, CHF

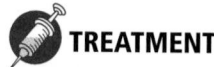 ## TREATMENT

INITIAL STABILIZATION
- Outpatient treatment is usually adequate; hospitalization may be required for exacerbation, infection, or procedures (lung biopsy).
- Acute respiratory failure may require an ICU and mechanical ventilation.

GENERAL MEASURES
- Smoking cessation
- Aggressive treatment of infections
- Treat any reversible bronchospasm
- Reduce secretions through good pulmonary hygiene.
- Cor pulmonale may necessitate use of home oxygen.
- Institute pulmonary rehabilitation.
- Give appropriate vaccinations.
- Maintain adequate hydration.

Diet
A high-protein diet is suggested. Decreased carbohydrates may benefit those with hypercarbia.

Activity
- As tolerated
- Full activity should be encouraged.

Nursing
Teach proper inhaler use

SPECIAL THERAPY
Adequate hydration, supplemental oxygen, antibiotics when indicated, mucolytic agents, pulmonary rehabilitation, and pulmonary hygiene

Physical Therapy
Pulmonary rehabilitation may be of benefit.

 ## MEDICATION (DRUGS)

First Line

- Sympathomimetics (2)[A]: Metaproterenol (Alupent), albuterol (Proventil, Ventolin), pirbuterol (Maxair), 1–2 puffs from the metered dose inhaler q4–6h. Frequency may be increased to q3h. Use of spacer device (AeroChamber, Inspirease) may be beneficial (up to 4 puffs recommended by some). Long-acting sympathomimetics, such as salmeterol (Serevent, 1 inhalation b.i.d.) or formoterol (Foradil, 1 inhalation q12h), may be considered.
- Anticholinergics (2)[A]
  - Ipratropium (Atrovent): 2 puffs (36 μg) q.i.d. may take additional inhalations not to exceed 12 in 24 hrs
  - Tiotropium (Spiriva): 1 inhalation daily
- Corticosteroids (3)[B]: Prednisone (Deltasone) given orally 7.5–15 mg/d. Consider pulse dosing (40 mg/day) with taper depending on length of therapy. Most useful in bronchitis with some reversibility; inhaled corticosteroids may be beneficial with less side effects.
- Theophylline (2)[B]: (Theo-Dur, Unidur, Uniphyl): 400 mg/d; increase by 100–200 mg in 1–2 weeks, if necessary.

- Mucolytic agents may improve secretions.
- Purified human alpha-1 antitrypsin for patients with this deficiency: 60 mg/kg weekly to maintain level exceeding 80 mg/dL
- Contraindications
  - Theophylline: Hypersensitivity
  - Sympathomimetics: Cardiac arrhythmias, hypersensitivity

- Anticholinergics: Hypersensitivity to atropine or its derivatives
- Corticosteroids: Systemic fungal infections; hypersensitivity
- Precautions
  - Theophylline: Reduce dosage in patients with impaired renal or liver function, >55; CHF. Therapeutic drug level is 10–20 μg/mL (55.5–111 μmol).
  - Rifampin may decrease theophylline levels by increasing theophylline metabolism. Monitor serum theophylline level.
  - Sympathomimetics: Excessive use may be dangerous. May need to reduce dosage in patients with cardiovascular disease, hypertension, hyperthyroidism, diabetes, or convulsive disorders.
  - Anticholinergics: Narrow angle glaucoma, prostatic hypertrophy, bladder-neck obstruction
  - Corticosteroids may mask infection or predispose to infection, especially fungal; subcapsular cataracts; glaucoma; adrenocortical insufficiency; psychic derangements; gastrointestinal bleeding; diabetes mellitus, reactivation of tuberculosis
- Significant possible interactions
  - Theophylline: Lithium carbonate; propranolol; erythromycin; cimetidine; ranitidine; rifampin; ciprofloxacin
  - Addition of cimetidine, ciprofloxacin, or erythromycin will decrease theophylline clearance and cause theophylline levels to rise. Careful monitoring of serum theophylline levels is warranted. Note: Cimetidine is now an OTC drug.
  - Sympathomimetics, monoamine oxidase inhibitors, or tricyclic antidepressants
  - Anticholinergics: Refer to the manufacturer's instructions.
  - Corticosteroids: NSAIDs (indomethacin, aspirin), synthetic thyroid hormone

Second Line
- Sympathomimetics may be given as aerosolized solution (albuterol, metaproterenol [Metaprel], levalbuterol, isoetharine) when mixed with saline; PO (Alupent, Proventil, Brethine, Ventolin) or subcutaneously (terbutaline)
- Anticholinergics: Atropine sulfate, glycopyrrolate. Ipratropium (Atrovent) now available in aerosolized solution and may be mixed with albuterol.
- Corticosteroids may be given IV (hydrocortisone, methylprednisolone) or inhaled (beclomethasone, flunisolide, triamcinolone acetonide).
- Home oxygen

SURGERY
- Lung reduction surgery (selected cases)
- Lung transplantation (selected cases)

 ## FOLLOW-UP

DISPOSITION
Admission Criteria
Acute decompensation due to exacerbation from infection or need for mechanical ventilation.

Discharge Criteria
- Patient should have adequate gas exchange.
- Hypoxia can be treated with home O_2.

Issues for Referral
Severe exacerbation or frequent hospitalizations

PROGNOSIS
- Patient's age and postbronchodilator FEV1 are the most important predictors of prognosis. Young age and FEV1 >50% predicted to have a good prognosis. Older patients do worse.
- Supplemental oxygen, when indicated, shown to increase survival.
- Smoking cessation important for improved prognosis
- Malnutrition, cor pulmonale, hypercapnia, and pulse >100 indicate a poor prognosis.

COMPLICATIONS
- Infection is common.
- Cor pulmonale, secondary polycythemia, bullous lung disease, acute or chronic respiratory failure, pulmonary hypertension, malnutrition, pneumothorax, poor sleep quality, arrhythmias, acute respiratory failure

PATIENT MONITORING
- Severe or unstable patients should be seen monthly. When stable, see biannually.
- Check theophylline level with dose adjustment, then check every 6–12 months.
- With home oxygen, check arterial blood gases yearly or with change in condition. Monitor oxygen saturation (pulse oximetry) more frequently.
- Some patients only desaturate at night and thereby only need nocturnal oxygen.
- Avoid travel at high altitude.
- Discuss advance directive and proxy.

REFERENCES
1. Snow V, Lasher S, Mottur-Pilson C. Evidence base for management of acute exacerbations of chronic obstructive pulmonary disease. *Ann Intern Med*. 2001;134:595–599.
2. Iqbal A, Schloss S, George D, Isonaka S. Worldwide guidelines for chronic obstructive pulmonary disease: A comparison of diagnosis and treatment recommendations. *Respirology*. 2002;7:233–239.
3. Pauwels RA. Global strategy for the diagnosis, management, and prevention of chronic obstructive pulmonary disease. *Am J Respir Crit Care Med*. 2001;163:1256–1276

 ## MISCELLANEOUS

CODES

ICD9-CM
- 496 Chronic airway obstruction, NEC
- 492.8 Other emphysema

PATIENT TEACHING
Printed material available from National Jewish Hospital in Denver, CO. Local branch of American Lung Association also has informational material.

 See Corresponding Diagnostic Algorithm

See Patient Handout on CD

CIRRHOSIS OF THE LIVER

Anne Walsh, PA-C, MMSc

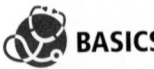 **BASICS**

DESCRIPTION

Cirrhosis is a chronic disease in which liver cell injury causes inflammation, necrosis, and stellate cell activation. Fibrosis replaces normal liver tissue and destroys the liver's vascular and lobular architecture, progressively diminishing blood flow and decreasing its normal function. The end result is liver failure and/or cancer.

Geriatric Considerations
Jaundice and encephalopathy more common

Pediatric Considerations
Inborn errors of metabolism may cause congenital liver injury; some treatable with diet and surgery

GENERAL PREVENTION
Counsel patients to prevent risk factors for chronic liver disease (e.g., alcohol abuse); majority of chronic liver disease is preventable

EPIDEMIOLOGY
- Predominant age: Peak incidence ages 40–50
- Predominant sex: Male > Female; but more females get cirrhosis from alcohol abuse.
- 15th leading cause of death ages 45–54 and 12th leading cause of death in all US adults.

Genetics
Hemochromatosis, Wilson disease, and alpha-1-antitrypsin deficiency in adults

ETIOLOGY
Toxins, viruses, bile stasis, autoimmune disease, or metabolic disorders

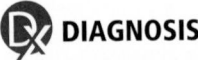 **DIAGNOSIS**

SIGNS AND SYMPTOMS
Typically asymptomatic until end-stage disease
- Signs
  - Skin changes
    - Spider angiomata, xanthoma
    - Hyperpigmentation
    - Jaundice, scleral icterus
    - Ecchymoses
    - Excoriation
    - Palmar erythema
    - Caput medusa
  - Organomegaly
    - Hepatomegaly if fatty liver, alcohol, or viral
    - Splenomegaly, if portal hypertension
    - Cirrhotic liver is typically small and hard
  - Central obesity/body mass index >30
  - Gynecomastia
  - Dupuytren's contractures
  - Asterixis

- Symptoms
  - Fatigue, malaise, weakness
  - Anorexia
  - Weight loss (gain if ascites/edema)
  - Right upper abdominal tenderness
  - Absent/irregular menses
  - Diminished libido, erectile dysfunction
  - Tea-colored urine
  - Clay-colored stools
  - Leg edema
  - Abdominal swelling/bloating
  - Easy bruising
  - Abnormal bleeding
  - Hematemesis, hematochezia, or melena
  - Pruritis
  - Night blindness

History
Risk factors for any cause of liver disease must be determined. (e.g., family history of alcoholic abuse, primary liver cancer, autoimmune disease).

Physical Exam
See positive findings under "Diagnosis, Signs."

TESTS
- Liver biopsy: Definitive diagnostic test. If International Normalized Ratio (INR) <1.5 and is no ascites. Otherwise, transjugular biopsy.
- Liver-spleen scan: Used to diagnose portal hypertension in presumed cirrhosis if patient cannot be safely biopsied.
- Endoscopy (EGD) for all patients with portal hypertension to screen for esophageal varices/portal hypertensive gastropathy paracentesis: Diagnostic or therapeutic

Lab
- Changes of hepatocyte injury
  - Alanine aminotransferase and aspartate aminotransferase levels commonly mildly elevated; typically aspartate aminotransferase > aldnine aminotransferase. NOTE: Liver enzymes normalize as cirrhosis progresses.
- Changes of cholestasis
  - Alkaline phosphatase levels elevated
  - 5'-nucleotidase liver-specific
  - Gammaglutamyl transpeptidase elevated
  - Total bilirubin levels elevated. NOTE: Direct bilirubin indicates bile stasis; indirect bilirubin indicates Gilbert disease.
  - Cholesterol/triglycerides typically elevated when insulin resistance/fatty liver is present
- Changes of impaired synthetic liver function
  - Low albumin and cholesterol
  - Prolonged INR; prothrombin time (PT), partial thromboplastin time
- Changes suggesting portal hypertension with enlarged spleen
  - Decreased platelet count
  - Low-normal range is significant and may indicate advanced fibrosis
- Changes of progressive cirrhosis
  - Elevated ammonia level; decreased blood urea nitrogen, sodium, and potassium

- Specific tests to determine etiology
  - Viral hepatitis panel
    - Hepatitis B surface antigen, core antibody, surface antibody (to determine need for vaccine); hepatitis B quantitative DNA (viral load) if sAg positive
    - Hepatitis C antibody, hepatitis C quantitative RNA (viral load) if positive
    - Hepatitis A antibody (determine need for vaccine)
  - Serum ethanol in patients suspected of ongoing alcohol abuse
- Elevated gamma-glutamyl transpeptidase
  - Antimitochondrial antibody to screen for primary biliary cirrhosis
  - Antismooth muscle and antinuclear antibodies to screen for chronic active (autoimmune) hepatitis
  - Iron saturation >50% and markedly increased ferritin levels to screen for hemochromatosis
  - Ceruloplasmin to screen for Wilson disease;
  - Alpha fetoprotein to screen for hepatocellular carcinoma (HCC).

Imaging
- Abdominal ultrasound to assess liver size, contour. Determines presence of hepatic steatosis, gallstones, bile duct dilatation, splenomegaly, ascites, or mass; liver biopsy.
- Doppler ultrasound of hepatic/portal veins.
- Abdominal CT with contrast to differentiate abnormalities seen on ultrasound (e.g., scars related to cirrhosis vs. primary neoplasm, metastatic disease, focal fatty sparing).
- MRI to clarify patency of blood vessels and collaterals; best test for HCC if alpha-fetoprotein high and/or liver mass seen on ultrasound
- If status of extrahepatic bile ducts uncertain by CT/MRI, or if bile duct biopsy required, endoscopic retrograde cholangiopancreatography may be indicated

Diagnostic Procedures/Surgery
History, examination, labs, and imaging provide diagnosis in >50% of cases. Liver biopsy is performed in 80% of cases.

Pathological Findings
- Fibrosis and regenerative nodules are general features of cirrhosis.
- Alcoholic liver disease: Steatosis, polymorphonuclear leukocyte (PMN) infiltrate, ballooning degeneration of hepatocytes, Mallory bodies, giant mitochondria
- Nonalcoholic steatohepatitis: Nearly identical to alcoholic liver disease, thus confirmed by history.
- Biliary cirrhosis: PMN infiltrate in wall of bile ducts, inflammation increased in portal spaces, progressive loss of bile ducts in portal spaces
- Hemochromatosis: Intrahepatic iron stores increased (iron stain or weighted biopsy tissue)
- Alpha-1-antitrypsin deficiency: Positive periodic acid-Schiff bodies in hepatocytes
- Hepatitis B and C: Periportal lymphocytic inflammation

DIFFERENTIAL DIAGNOSIS
- Diffuse hepatic parenchymal disease
- Other causes of portal hypertension
- Metastatic or multifocal cancer in the liver
- Vascular congestion (e.g., cardiac cirrhosis)
- Reversible (e.g., acute alcoholic hepatitis)

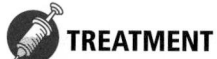 **TREATMENT**

PRE HOSPITAL
Outpatient care except for major gastrointestinal (GI) bleeding, hepatic encephalopathy, sepsis/infection, rapidly progressing hepatic decompensation, renal failure

GENERAL MEASURES
- Treat the underlying cause if possible.
- Patients MUST abstain from alcohol, drugs, and nutritional supplements with no benefit.
- Immunize for pneumococcal disease, hepatitis A and B if seronegative, influenza.
- Hemochromatosis: Phlebotomy until iron stores depleted per decreased ferritin
- Non-alcoholic fatty liver disease: Weight reduction, exercise, control of lipid and diabetes

Diet
Maintain nutritious diet:1–1.5 g protein/kg of body weight, high fiber, daily multivitamin (without iron) and <2 g/d sodium (essential if ascites/edema). Branched-chain amino acid supplementation improves quality of life and survival in patients with decompensated cirrhosis. [B]

Activity
Regular conditioning may help fatigue.

Complementary and Alternative Medicine
- Milk thistle (silymarin) taken according to manufacturer's recommendations may improve symptoms and without adverse effects. NOTE: Some preparations contain substances that interfere with INR and transaminases.
- Milk thistle has no effect on overall mortality (6).

 MEDICATION (DRUGS)

As indicated to treating the underlying cause
- Hepatitis C: Combination therapy with pegylated-interferon alpha 2a/2b subcutaneously once weekly plus ribavirin 200 mg 2–3 pills PO b.i.d. for 6–12+ months (eradicates virus permanently in 50% of patients; sustained viral response seen in 80–90% of genotype 2 or 3 patients).
- Hepatitis B: Lamivudine 100 mg PO daily, adefovir 10 mg PO daily, or entecavir 0.5–1 mg PO daily until resistance develops (usually several years); alternatively peg-interferon for 48 weeks.
- Biliary cirrhosis: Ursodeoxycholic acid 10 mg/kg PO daily, indefinitely [A]
- Wilson disease: Penicillamine 1–3 g/d as tolerated or tetrathiomolybdate, 100–400 mg/d. After 1 year, zinc acetate alone 250 mg b.i.d. used for maintenance.
- Autoimmune (chronic active) hepatitis: Prednisone 5–20 mg/d with or without azathioprine (Imuran) 0.5–1 mg/kg for at least 2 years. Use smallest dose steroids necessary to maintain stable transaminases.

PREVENTING/TREATING COMPLICATIONS
- Esophageal varices: Propranolol 40–160 mg or nadolol 10 mg daily, to lower portal pressure by 20 mm Hg or pulse rate by 25%. [A] Ascites/edema: Low-sodium (<2 g/day) and spironolactone 100–400 mg PO daily with furosemide 40–160 mg PO daily. Torsemide may substitute for furosemide.
- Encephalopathy: Lactulose 15 mL b.i.d., titrate to cause 2–3 loose bowel movements daily.
- Renal insufficiency: Stop diuretics, nephrotoxic drugs; normalize electrolyte; hospitalize for plasma expansion or dialysis
- Prophylactic antibiotics recommended for invasive procedures, GI bleeding [A]
- Patients with esophageal varices requiring banding or portal hypertensive gastropathy should be maintained on a proton pump inhibitor. [C]
- Recombinant factor VIIa rapidly corrects bleeding associated with hepatic coagulopathy

SURGERY
- Varices: Endoscopic ligation; 4–6 treatments typical (will also need beta blocker). Consider a transjugular intrahepatic shunt (TIPS).
- Ascites: Paracentesis every 2 weeks or more
- Transplantation: Either cadaveric (orthotopic) liver or living donor partial transplant
- Hepatocellular carcinoma. Cure if small with partial resection of liver

PROGNOSIS
- At diagnosis of cirrhosis, expect 5–20 years of asymptomatic disease
  – 5% per year develop HCC
- Life expectancy is shortened
  – 50% of compensated cirrhotics develop ascites over 10 years
  – 50% 5-year survival if ascites develops
  – Acute variceal bleed carries 30% mortality
- At onset of complications, expect death within 5 years without transplant
  – With transplant, 85% survive 1 year; death occurs at ~5% per year
- Fewer than 25% of eligible patients are transplanted, due to donor organ shortage.

COMPLICATIONS
- Ascites
  – Umbilical/ventral hernia
  – Dyspnea
- Edema
- Muscle wasting
- Depression
- Encephalopathy
- Coagulopathy
  – GI bleed: Esophageal varices, gastropathy, colopathy
- Hepatocellular carcinoma
- Susceptibility to infections
- Spontaneous bacterial peritonitis
- Heptorenal syndrome
- Fulminant hepatic failure

PATIENT MONITORING
- Patients should be referred for gastroenterologist/hepatologist consult.
- Once stable, monitor liver enzymes, platelets, and PT every 6–12 months.
- Patients >55 years, with hepatitis B or C, decreased prothrombin level (by elevated INR), or low platelets are highest risk for HCC. Check alpha-fetoprotein every 6–12 months, and yearly ultrasound for screening
- Endoscopy at diagnosis and every 2 years [C]
- Influenza vaccine, Pneumovax, and Hepatitis A and B immunizations (if seronegative)

REFERENCES
1. Talwalker J, Kamath P. Influence of recent advances in medical management on clinical outcomes of cirrhosis. Mayo Clin Proc. 2005;80:1501–1508.
2. Muto Y, Sato S, Watanabe A, et al. Effects of oral branched-chain amino acid granules on event-free survival in patients with liver cirrhosis. Clin Gastroenterol Hepatol. 2005;3:705–713.
3. Saadeh S, Davis GL. Management of ascites in patients with end-stage liver disease. Rev Gastroenterolo Disord. 2004;4:175–185.
4. Nietsch H. Management of portal hypertension. J Clin Gastroenterol. 2005;39:232–236.
5. Rambaldi A, Jacobs BP, Iaquinto G, Gluud C. Milk thistle for alcoholic and/or hepatitis B or C virus liver diseases. The Cochrane Database of Systematic Reviews. 2006;1.
6. Rambaldi A, Jacobs BP, Iaquinto G, et al. Milk thistle for alcoholic and/or hepatitis B or C virus liver diseases. Cochrane Hepato-Biliary Group Cochrane Database of Systematic Reviews. 4, 2006.

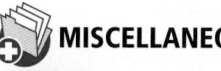 **MISCELLANEOUS**

CODES

ICD9-CM
- 571.2 Alcoholic cirrhosis of liver
- 571.5 Cirrhosis of liver without mention of alcohol

PATIENT TEACHING
- Educate caregivers on possible complications
- Educate/support patient in maintaining general good health
- Avoid crowds and sick contacts.
- No drugs/herbs/vitamins etc. without review
- Hepatitis B/C should be taught transmission precautions (e.g., sharps, no sharing of razors/toothbrushes, safer sex practices)
- Refer to community support groups (e.g., Hepatitis C, Alcoholics Anonymous).

 See Corresponding Diagnostic Algorithm

 See Patient Handout on CD

CLAUDICATION

Ruben Peralta, MD, FACS
James T. McPhee, MD

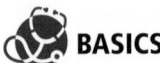 BASICS

DESCRIPTION
- Claudication is exercise-induced cramping muscle pain in the lower extremities.
- Claudication is the most common symptom of patients with aorto-iliac disease.
- <10% of patients with known lower extremity atherosclerosis develop claudication.

ALERT
Geriatric Considerations
Condition more commonly seen in the elderly

GENERAL PREVENTION
- Patients should initiate walking program as soon as possible.
- Smoking cessation

EPIDEMIOLOGY
- Claudication is more common in men >55 years of age and in women >60 years of age.
- Male > Female; <2:1 ratio.

Incidence
Bimodal peak in incidence (Framingham study): .07% in men 35–44 years and 1.4% in men >65 years; diabetic patients 4–6 times that of nondiabetic patients.

Prevalence
~1.7–2.2% among older patients

RISK FACTORS
- Cigarette smoking and hypertension are most closely linked with worsening claudication symptoms.
- The primary risk factors include
  - Cigarette smoking: ~90% of all patients with claudication smoke cigarettes.
  - Diabetes mellitus
  - Hypertension
  - Hypercholesterolemia
  - Family history
  - Obesity
  - Preexisting heart disease

Genetics
Genetic loci have not yet been determined.

ETIOLOGY
- Sites affected depend on vasculature involved
- Aortoiliac disease: Pain may extend from buttocks to thigh.
- Femoropopliteal disease: Pain may extend from calves to feet.
- Superficial femoral artery occlusion accounts for most cases of claudication involving lower-extremity claudication symptoms.
- Subclavian, axillary, and brachial artery blockages may lead to claudication symptoms in upper extremity.
- Other causes of arterial occlusion to consider, which may cause similar pain syndromes: Emboli, popliteal entrapment, adventitious cystic disease of the popliteal arteries, and thromboangiitis obliterans (Buerger disease)

ASSOCIATED CONDITIONS
- Other manifestations of arteriosclerotic vascular disease
  - Myocardial infarction(s)
  - Carotid artery occlusive disease
  - Renovascular occlusive disease
  - Hypertension
- Of all patients with peripheral artery disease (PAD), 25–68% have concurrent CAD and 34–50% have a concomitant cerebrovascular diagnosis (1)[B].

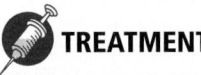 DIAGNOSIS

SIGNS AND SYMPTOMS
- Cold feet are an early warning symptom.
- Sudden or gradual onset
- Patients will limit their walking based on their symptoms.
- Symptom continuum ranges from calf muscle fatigue to severe cramps and pain.
- Rubor evident in dependent limbs
- Leg color may be normal when horizontal, but may darken to a dusky crimson when in lowered position.
- Lower extremities are hairless.
- Poorly palpable or absent lower extremity pulses
- Paresthesias or numbness are later symptoms.
- Patients with diabetes less likely to report pain.
- Nonhealing ulcer is associated with poor circulation.
- Can lead to marked limitation of daily activities (1)[B].

History
History of relevant risk factors
- Cigarette smoking
- Hypertension
- Preexisting heart disease
- Diabetes mellitus
- Obesity
- Hypercholesterolemia
- Restricted walking distance due to pain (relieved by rest)
- The Rose questionnaire asks whether calf pain while walking is relieved by 10 minutes of rest or whether pain is exacerbated by an increased pace or walking uphill, or is relieved by tapering or stopping the activity. Other items include persistent pain if walking continues and absence of calf pain while sedentary. If physicians' diagnosis of claudication is the standard criterion, the Rose questionnaire has a specificity of ~99% and a sensitivity of 66%.
- The Edinburgh is a modified Rose questionnaire that takes into account that some patients might continue to walk through calf pain. This questionnaire has a sensitivity of ~91% for the detection of patients with claudication.

Physical Exam
- Signs of peripheral vascular disease: Abnormal skin coloration (pallor, rubor), cool feet, atrophy of nails, delayed capillary refill, loss of hair
- Diminished or absent femoral, popliteal, dorsalis pedis or posterior tibial pulses (2)[B].

TESTS
Lab
No pathognomonic lab findings

Imaging
- Duplex ultrasound: Reliable in suprainguinal and thigh region, unacceptable in knee region.
- Digital subtraction angiography remains the gold standard.
- Contrast enhanced magnetic resonance angiography (MRA): Good alternative to angiography in suprainguinal and thigh region. MRA superior to duplex in the knee region. May overestimate degree of stenoses (3)[B].

Diagnostic Procedures/Surgery
- The ankle-brachial index (ABI) is the systolic blood pressure at the ankle divided by that of the higher of 2 systolic pressures taken in the bilateral brachial arteries. Normal indices are minimally ≥1. ABI <0.9 correlates with at ≥50% stenosis of at least 1 vessel (4)[B].
  - An ABI between 0.4 and 0.9 suggests stenosis, and correlates with clinical claudication.
  - ABI <0.5 suggests multisegmental arterial stenoses.
  - An ABI of <0.3 correlates with probable tissue death and/or rest pain.
- Given that calcified vasculature impairs compressibility, and ankle-brachial indexes cannot be measured conventionally in these patients, photoplethysmography is another diagnostic option to evaluate blood pressure in the toes.
- 2 useful claudication screening tools are the Rose and Edinburgh questionnaires.

DIFFERENTIAL DIAGNOSIS
- Neither pseudoclaudication nor osteoarthritis affects ABI.
- Pseudoclaudication is attributed to spinal cord impingement or spinal stenosis. Sitting or squatting helps relieve symptoms of pseudoclaudication.
- Osteoarthritis: Weight bearing worsens the pain.

TREATMENT

GENERAL MEASURES
- Elimination of risk factors whenever possible
- Smoking cessation is critical to success and is the single most important intervention.
- Optimization of diet with low-fat and low-cholesterol regimen.
- Exercise is essential to management, significantly improving maximal walking time, distance to claudication and calf blood flow (5)[B].

Diet
Low-fat, low-cholesterol diet

Activity
Six-month exercise program with 30-minute sessions 3 times a week improves exercise performance, glycemic control, and lipid profiles (1)[B].

MEDICATION (DRUGS)

First Line

- Antiplatelet treatment, most often using aspirin, should be considered for all patients to address their overall risk. It has no proven benefit for decreasing lower-extremity claudication; may be beneficial for other conditions due to atherosclerotic disease (e.g., coronary and cerebral).
- Statins reduce incidence of new intermittent claudication, and increase painfree walking time (5)[B].
- Pentoxifylline (Trental) reduces blood viscosity and improves erythrocyte flexibility, dose 400–800 mg b.i.d.– t.i.d. Administer for at least 6–8 weeks to determine whether therapy is effective.
- Cilostazol (Pletal) improves maximal and pain-free walking distance. 50–100 mg b.i.d.
- Contraindications: Cilostazol is contraindicated in patients with symptoms of congestive heart failure; Pentoxifylline is contraindicated in patients with recent cerebral or retinal hemorrhage.
- Precautions: Headache occurs in >30% of patients taking cilostazol.
- Significant possible interactions: Cilostazol is metabolized through the cytochrome P-450 isoenzymes. Use caution during coadministration of other inhibitors of CYP3A4 (grapefruit juice, ketoconazole, itraconazole, erythromycin and diltiazem), and during coadministration of inhibitors of CYP2C19 (omeprazole); Pentoxifylline may cause theophylline levels to rise; concurrent use of β-blockers in patients with coexisting cardiovascular disease does not appear to worsen claudication symptoms in affected patients.

Second Line

- Ticlopidine (Ticlid)
- Vasodilators
- Calcium channel blockers
- Anticoagulants are of no benefit in claudication.
- Role of PGE1 and PGI2 analogues and stimulants (AS-103, iloprost, beraprost, defibrotide) continues to be investigated.

SURGERY

- Most patients do not require surgical management.
- Angioplasty and stenting are gaining favorability as a 1st-line treatment modality that does not preclude secondary successful surgical bypass.
- Arterial bypass surgery is considered gold standard by most vascular surgeons (6)[B].

 FOLLOW-UP

- Peripheral noninvasive vascular studies every 6 months
- If findings suggest condition of patient is worsening, this would be indication for surgery.

PROGNOSIS

- Patients should experience gradual improvement with the use of medical therapy and walking program and diminution or complete elimination of risk factors. Some patients may require revascularization. Disease progression may include rest pain, tissue loss, and gangrene.
- Chronic intermittent ischemia may cause lasting defects in muscle function, producing weakness that could be an early sign of PAD.

COMPLICATIONS

- Tissue/limb loss predominantly affects patients with diabetes as disease progresses.
- Complications of reperfusion
  – Compartment syndrome
- Venous thrombosis is induced by low-flow state, which may flush to right side of heart to pulmonary circulation.

REFERENCES

1. Hiatt, WR. The U.S. experience with cilostazol in treating intermittent claudication. *Atherosclerosis Supplements* 2006;6:21–31.
2. Kahn NA, et al. Does the clinical examination predict lower extremity peripheral arterial disease? *JAMA* 2006;295:536–546.
3. Gjonnaess E, et al. Gadolinium-enhanced magnetic resonance angiography, colour duplex and digital subtraction angiography of the lower limb arteries from the aorta to the tibio-peroneal trunk in patients with intermittent claudication. *Eur J Vasc Endovasc Surg* 2006;31: 53–58.
4. Feringa HHH, et al. The long-term prognostic value of the resting and postexercise ankle brachial index. *Arch Intern Med* 2006;166:529–535.
5. Hankey, GJ. Medical treatment of peripheral arterial disease. *JAMA* 2006;295:547–553.
6. Black JH, et al. Contemporary results of angioplasty-based infrainguinal percutaneous interventions. *J Vasc Surg* 2005;42:932–939.

 MISCELLANEOUS

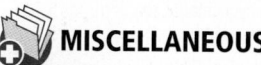 **CODES**

ICD9-CM
443.9 Peripheral vascular disease, unspecified

PATIENT TEACHING

Patient teaching Prevention
Encourage an exercise program, smoking cessation, healthy dietary choices, management of blood glucose levels in diabetic patients, and hypertension control.

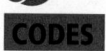 **See Corresponding Diagnostic Algorithm**

C

CLOSTRIDIUM DIFFICILE INFECTION

Dan K. Giang MBA, PharmD
Brian D. Moquin, MD

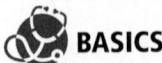 **BASICS**

DESCRIPTION

- *Clostridium difficile* is a Gram-positive, spore-forming anaerobic bacillus.
- Infection caused by *C. difficile* is usually linked to broad-spectrum antibiotic use.
- Severity of infection can range from diarrhea to colitis to perforation to death.
- System(s) Affected: Gastrointestinal
- Synonyms(s): *Clostridium difficile*–associated disease or diarrhea (CDAD); Antibiotic-associated diarrhea, *C. diff*

GENERAL PREVENTION

- Implementation of a comprehensive infection control program has resulted in a decrease in the incidence of *C. difficile* infection (1).
- Disinfection with hypochlorite solution
- Hand washing with soap and water
- Use of disposable rectal thermometers
- Reduction of unnecessary broad-spectrum antibiotic use
- If possible, isolation of infected patients
- Education of hospital personnel
- Use of contact precautions

EPIDEMIOLOGY

Incidence

- Most cases of *C. difficile* infection occur in hospitals or long-term care facilities at a rate of 25–60 per 100,000 occupied bed-days (2).
- For outpatient setting, the rate is ~7.7 cases per 100,000 person-years (2).

Prevalence

- *C. difficile* causes ~25% of all cases of antibiotic-associated diarrhea (2).
- *C. difficile* causes pseudomembranous colitis in >95% of patients (3).

RISK FACTORS

- Exposure to all antimicrobial agents (except aminoglycosides) is associated with *C. difficile* infection.
- Patients in health care settings have a higher risk of developing *C. difficile* infection.
- Age >65 years
- Duration of stay in the hospital
- Nasogastric intubation
- Severe primary illness
- Controversial: Use of antiulcer medications
- Chemotherapy

ALERT

Geriatric Considerations

C. difficile is the most common cause of acute diarrheal illness in long-term care facilities. These patients are older and receive more antibiotics and antacids than the general public; thus, it is difficult to determine which factors contribute most to this increased risk.

Pediatric Considerations

Neonates have a higher rate of *C. difficile* colonization (25–80%), yet neonates are much less likely to be symptomatic than adults, possibly due to immature toxin receptors.

Genetics

No known genetic factors

PATHOPHYSIOLOGY

- *C. difficile* can thrive in the colon and cause infection if disruption of the normal flora and ingestion of *C. difficile* occur.
- Ingestion of *C. difficile*–resistant spores can also cause infection.
  - *C. difficile* spores can survive for months.
- Host factors such as the presence of antibodies to *C. difficile* toxins can reduce the severity and prevent recurrences of infection.
- *C. difficile* produces toxins that are essential for disease to occur.
  - Toxins A (enterotoxin) and B (cytotoxin) attract neutrophils and monocytes and degrade colonic epithelial cells, causing colitis, pseudomembrane colitis, and watery diarrhea.
  - Binary toxin produces a virulent form of disease (different from toxin A or B); this may have resulted in increased rates of colectomies and mortality.
  - Binary toxin has been identified in ~6% of clinical *C. difficile* isolates obtained in the US and Europe.

ETIOLOGY

- Altered colonic mucosa
- *C. difficile* spore ingestion
- Active toxin release

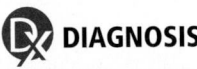 **DIAGNOSIS**

SIGNS AND SYMPTOMS

- Mild disease
  - Mild lower abdominal cramping pain
- Moderate disease
  - Fever
  - Nausea and vomiting
- Severe disease
  - Peritonitis
  - Ileus
  - Hypovolemia

History

- Recent antibiotic use
- Diarrhea which is watery, foul-smelling
- Fever (typically <10%)
- Recent hospitalizations or nursing facility

Physical Exam

- Mild abdominal tenderness to peritonitis depending on severity
- Hypovolemia

TESTS

Lab

- ELISA for toxins
  - Available within 2–6 hours
  - Sensitivity 63–99%
  - Specificity 75–100%
  - Some labs only test for toxin A, others test for A and B
- Tissue culture cytotoxicity assay
  - Takes 24–48 hours for results; labor intensive
  - Sensitivity 67–100%
  - Specificity 85–100%
- Microbiology culture
  - Nontoxin producing strains also detected
  - Mostly used to evaluate epidemiology studies
- PCR-based testing is currently research-based.

Imaging

- Plain films may show thumbprinting, colonic distension.
- CT radiography may show mucosal wall thickening, thickened colonic wall, pericolonic inflammation.

Diagnostic Procedures/Surgery

- Endoscopy can be used to evaluate for pseudomembranes and exclude other conditions.
- Flexible sigmoidoscopy may miss 15–20% of pseudomembranes that may be present more proximal in the colon.
- Colonoscopy evaluates the entire colon
  - Used when diagnosis is in doubt or severity demands rapid diagnosis

Pathological Findings

Pseudomembranes consist of inflammatory and cellular debris that forms visible exudates that can obscure the underlying mucosa. These exudates have a yellow to grayish color

DIFFERENTIAL DIAGNOSIS

- Food poisoning
- Enteric infections
- Antibiotic-associated diarrhea

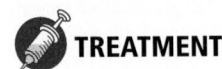 **TREATMENT**

INITIAL STABILIZATION

- Current nonessential antibiotic therapy should be discontinued if possible (1–4)[A].
- Institute supportive therapy with fluids and electrolytes if needed (1, 2)[A].

GENERAL MEASURES

Avoid antimotility agents and opiates (1–4)[A].

Diet

No restrictions; as tolerated.

Activity

Bed rest during acute phase.

Nursing

See "General Prevention."

SPECIAL THERAPY

IV Fluids

- Infuse to keep patient euvolemic.
- Once over acute phase, patient can be weaned off IV fluids.

Complementary and Alternative Therapies

Use of probiotics in conjunction with antibiotic therapy can decrease risk of antibiotic-associated diarrhea and *C. difficile* disease (5, 6)[A].

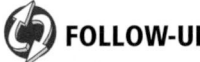 **MEDICATION (DRUGS)**

If clinically indicated (moderate to severe diarrhea, fever, significant leukocytosis, abdominal pain, etc.), consider antimicrobial against *C. difficile* (1–4)[A].

First Line

Metronidazole (1–4)[A]

- Drug of choice due to low cost and prevention of the emergence of vancomycin-resistant organisms.
- 250 mg PO q.i.d. or 500 mg PO t.i.d. for 10–14 days.
- If patient is unable to take oral medications, then IV metronidazole or intraluminal vancomycin can be used.

Second Line

- Vancomycin (1, 2, 4)[A]
  - 125 mg PO q.i.d. for 10–14 days.
  - Indicated for patients who cannot tolerate or failed metronidazole therapy, and for those who are pregnant.
- Alternative drugs
  - Bacitracin (1, 2, 4)[A]
    - 20,000 to 25,000 U PO q.i.d. for 7–10 days.
    - Reserved for unusual situations in which metronidazole and vancomycin cannot be used.
    - Use caution in patients with renal deficiency or renal failure.

SURGERY

If *C. difficile* infection progresses to toxic megacolon, peritonitis, or sepsis after initiation of treatment, other therapeutic options should be explored, including a surgical consult (3,4)[A].

FOLLOW-UP

DISPOSITION

Many patients can be treated as outpatients.

Admission Criteria

- Hypovolemia
- Comorbid conditions
- Inability to keep up with enteric losses
- Hematochezia
- Electrolyte disturbances

Discharge Criteria

- Improved diarrhea severity and frequency
- Tolerating both medications and PO
- Afebrile

PROGNOSIS

- Majority of patients will improve with conservative management and antibiotics.
- 1–3% of patients will develop severe colitis requiring emergency colectomy.
- Binary toxin strain has recently appeared, which results in fulminate disease outbreaks (7).

PATIENT MONITORING

- Relapses of colitis will occur in 15–30%.
- Relapses typically occur 2–10 days after discontinuation of antibiotics.
- Repeat treatment with 14-day course of antibiotics will result in 40% cure rate.
- The management of a 1st relapse following therapy for *C. difficile* diarrhea and colitis does not differ substantially from treatment of the initial episode.
- Administration of vancomycin or metronidazole every other day or every 3rd day would allow the spores to germinate on the off days and then be killed when the antibiotics are taken again.
- One report described 22 patients with multiple relapses of *C. difficile* colitis who were treated with the following oral vancomycin regimen
  - Week 1: 125 mg q.i.d.
  - Week 2: 125 mg b.i.d.
  - Week 3: 125 mg/d
  - Week 4: 125 mg every other day
  - Weeks 5 and 6: 125 mg every 3 days
  - All patients responded symptomatically; no relapses occurred during a mean follow-up period of 6 months.
- If continued infection; consider pulse therapy with vancomycin

REFERENCES

1. Aslam S, Hamill RJ, et al. Treatment of *Clostridium difficile*-associated disease: Old therapies and new strategies. *Lancet Infect Dis*. 2005;5:549–557.
2. Mylonakis E, Ryan ET, et al. *Clostridium difficile*-associated diarrhea. *Arch Intern Med*. 2001;161:525–533.
3. Sunenshine RH, McDonald LC. *Clostridium difficile*-associated disease: New challenges from an established pathogen. *Cleve Clin J Med*. 2006;73:187–197.
4. McFarland LV. Alternative treatments for *Clostridium difficile* disease: What really works? *J Med Micro*. 2005;54:101–111.
5. McFarland LV. Meta-analysis of probiotics for the prevention of antibiotic associated diarrhea and the treatment of *C. difficile* disease. *Am J Gastroenterol*. 2006;101(4):812–822.
6. Bricker E, Garg R, et al. Antibiotic treatment for *Clostridium difficile*-associated diarrhea in adults. *Cochrane Database Sys Rev*. 2005;1:CD004610. DOI: 10.1002/14651858.CD004610.pub2.
7. McDonald L. An epidemic, toxin gene-variant strain of *Clostridium difficile*. *N Engl J Med*. 2005;353(23):2433–2441.

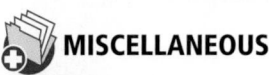 **MISCELLANEOUS**

CODES

ICD9-CM
008.45 Clostridium difficile

PATIENT TEACHING

Patients should be kept informed of the progress of disease and taught to practice good hygiene (i.e., hand washing).

Prevention

Use of probiotics (*Lactobacillus* and *Bifidobacterium*)

COARCTATION OF THE AORTA

Timothy McCurry, MD
Poonam Thaker, MD

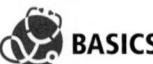

BASICS

DESCRIPTION
A constriction (discrete or of varying lengths) of the aorta usually located just distal to the left subclavian artery at the junction of the ligamentum arteriosum. Primarly effects are cardiovascular.

Pregnancy Considerations
- Condition is commonly seen in infants.
- There is a greater risk of complications if correction is delayed beyond early childhood. Often the diagnosis itself is delayed.

Pregnancy Considerations
Uncorrected coarctation or restenosis carries high risk of aortic rupture or dissection and cerebral hemorrhage (aneurysm of circle of Willis rupture), but smaller risk of preeclampsia than with other forms of hypertension.

EPIDEMIOLOGY
Predominant age: Frequently seen in infants.
Predominant sex: Male > Female 1.7:1

Incidence
64/100,000 in patients <1 year of age

RISK FACTORS
Genetics
No mendelian inheritance, but is commonly seen in association with Turner syndrome. Family history of left ventricular outflow tract obstruction is a risk factor.

ETIOLOGY
- Turner syndrome
- Congenital left heart abnormalities
- Takayasu arteritis

ASSOCIATED CONDITIONS
- Bicuspid aortic valve 85%
- Patent ductus arteriosus 65%
- Ventricular septal defect 30–35%
- Aortic stenosis and insufficiency
- Subvalvular aortic stenosis
- Mitral valve abnormalities (common)
- Transposition of great vessels or double outlet right ventricle
- Aneurysm of circle of Willis
- Neurofibromatosis I
- Acquired intercostal aneurysms

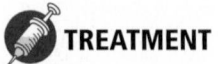

DIAGNOSIS

SIGNS AND SYMPTOMS
- Headaches
- Leg fatigue and pain on exertion
- Prominent neck pulsations
- Epistaxis
- Hypertension
- Pulse disparity: Radial-femoral pulse delay and increased amplitude in brachial versus femoral pulse
- Funduscopy: Corkscrew tortuosity of retinal arterioles
- Delayed, weak, or absent pulse
- Prominent left ventricular impulse
- Murmur (aortic stenosis or insufficiency, ventricular septal defect, rarely mitral valve)
- S4 systolic ejection click
- Bruit (coarctation, collaterals, patent ductus arteriosus)
- Cyanosis, rarely
- In infancy, may also have heart failure, failure to thrive, irritability, tachypnea, and dyspnea
- Extensive collaterals develop from branches of the subclavian, internal mammary, superior intercostal, and axillary arteries.

Physical Exam
Blood pressures: All 4 extremities show upper limb systemic hypertension and differential of <10 mm Hg.

TESTS
Imaging
- Doppler examination of pulses reveals disparity.
- Chest x-ray may show rib notching, "3" sign, rarely cardiomegaly
- Electrocardiogram may show left ventricular hypertrophy.
- Echocardiography for coarctation and coexisting cardiac anomalies
- Transesophageal echocardiography
- MRI

Diagnostic Procedures/Surgery
Cardiac catheterization and angiography: Poststenotic dilation

Pathological Findings
- Segmental tubular hypoplasia
- Discrete obstruction with medial thickening
- Distal aneurysm

DIFFERENTIAL DIAGNOSIS
- Takayasu arteritis
- Neurofibromatosis
- Pseudocoarctation (with or without hypertension, peripheral vascular disease)

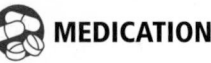

TREATMENT

GENERAL MEASURES
Usually requires surgery on an inpatient basis
Diet
No special diet required

Activity
Exercise may exacerbate hypertension, but normal activity is nonetheless recommended after correction.

MEDICATION (DRUGS)

- Alprostadil (prostaglandin E1), for patency of ductus arteriosus
- Antibiotic prophylaxis (for dental and/or invasive procedures) on a lifelong basis even after correction
- Antihypertensives if needed
- Preload and afterload reduction if heart failure develops
- Contraindications: Refer to manufacturer's profile of each drug.
- Precautions
  – Lowering BP in upper extremity may cause hypoperfusion of lower extremities.
  – Lowering BP is not advised in pregnancy unless mandated by emergency.

SURGERY
- Inpatient surgery is required.
- Surgical correction or balloon angioplasty can be done in infancy if urgently needed. Best results when performed in patients aged 1–2 years.
- Surgery should be done in childhood and adulthood as soon as coarctation is diagnosed to prevent later complications.
- 3 common surgical procedures for correction of coarctation include
  – End-to-end anastomosis
  – Patch aortoplasty (insertion of Dacron patch)
  – Subclavian flap procedure
- Balloon angioplasty of coarctation offers good results for primary treatment and for postoperative restenosis.
- Stent placement
- May prevent unnecessary dilation of coarctation during angioplasty
- May further prevent late recoarctation than angioplasty alone

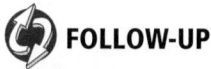 **FOLLOW-UP**

PROGNOSIS
- Depends on age of repair and presence of other cardiac abnormalities
- Residual or restenosis (6–33%)
- Subsequent cardiac surgery (11%)
- Hypertension (25%)
- Survival after surgery: 10 years (91%), 20 years (84%), 30 years (72%)
- Uncorrected, 80% mortality before age 50 years

COMPLICATIONS
Most common with late or no correction
- Heart failure
- Aneurysm of circle of Willis, rupture possible
- Hypertension
- Rupture or dissection of aortic aneurysm
- Endarteritis or endocarditis (need antibiotic prophylaxis)
- Aortic valve disease (stenosis or insufficiency)
- Postcoarctectomy syndrome: Recurrence, hypertension, atherosclerotic heart disease, aneurysm at site of coarctectomy, progressive aortic stenosis and/or regurgitation
- Fistula formation between aorta and airways leading to hemoptysis

PATIENT MONITORING
Frequent postoperative follow-up for evidence of restenosis (check for hypertension and pulse disparities) and late complications

REFERENCES
1. Fuster V, ed. *Hurst's: The Heart*. 10th ed. New York, NY: McGraw-Hill; 2001.
2. Chizer MA. *Classic Teachings in Cardiology*. Cedar Grove, NJ: Laennec Publishing; 1996.
3. Braunwald E, et al. *Heart Disease*. 6th ed. Philadelphia, PA: WB Saunders; 2001.
4. Rosenthal E. Stent Implantation of aortic coarctation: The treatment of choice in adults? *J Am Cardiol*. 2001;38:1524–1527.
5. Ledesma M, et al. Results of stenting for ortic coarcatation. *Am J Cardiol*. 2001;88:460–462.
6. Manganas C, et al. Reoperation and coarctation of the aorta: The need for lifelong surveillance. *Ann Thorac Surg*. 2001;7:1222–1224.
7. Heikkinen LO, et al. Aortopulmonary fistula after coarctation repair. *Ann Thorac Surg*. 2002; 73:1634–1636.

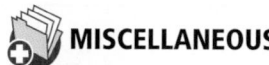 **MISCELLANEOUS**

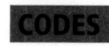 **CODES**

ICD9-CM
- 747.10 Coarctation of the aorta
- 747.11 Interruption of aortic arch

PATIENT TEACHING
- Discuss postcoarctation syndrome with patient.
- Patients should be encouraged to lead normal lives and pursue usual activities after coarctation correction.
- For favorably reviewed patient education materials on this topic, contact: American Heart Association, 7320 Greenville Avenue, Dallas, TX 75231; (214) 373-6300.

 See Corresponding Diagnostic Algorithm

 See Patient Handout on CD

C

COCCIDIOIDOMYCOSIS

Sandra Miller, MD

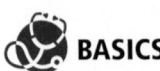 **BASICS**

DESCRIPTION
A pulmonary fungal infection endemic to the southwestern desert of the US. Can rarely progress to involve extrapulmonary sites (<1%), including bone, CNS, and skin, endocrine/metabolic, musculoskeletal, nervous, pulmonary, skin, and exocrine systems. Sometimes called "the great imitator." Incubation period is 1–4 weeks after initial exposure. Known locally as "cocci" or "Valley Fever."

Pregnancy Considerations
Increased risk for dissemination, especially if contracted late in gestation

GENERAL PREVENTION
- Not contagious between host and contacts
- Cultures in lab are highly contagious through inhalation; lab personnel must be cautious when handling specimens.
- High-risk populations (see "Risk Factors") should consider avoiding potentially high-risk activities, such as construction, archaeologic digs, and others involving soil.

EPIDEMIOLOGY
It affects patients of all ages, and there is no gender predilection.

Incidence
In the US: 100,000 cases per year (0.5% extrapulmonary)

RISK FACTORS
- Members of certain groups are more prone to dissemination: Immunocompromised people, pregnant women, African Americans, Filipinos.
- CNS involvement is more common in young white men.
- Immunosuppression: Chemotherapy and/or immunosuppressive drugs for cancer or transplant patients. Previously infected patients can experience relapse years later through the mechanism of cell-mediated immune deficiency.
- Diabetes mellitus
- AIDS
- Long-term steroid use
- Aging

Genetics
Nothing is known about its genetic makeup.

ETIOLOGY
Coccidioides immitis is a soil-dwelling fungus especially well adapted to arid conditions. Liberated spores are inhaled when soil is disturbed in any sort of digging, construction sites, archaeologic sites, dust storms, and in cave exploration.

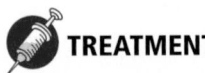 **DIAGNOSIS**

SIGNS AND SYMPTOMS
Primary pulmonary
- Anorexia
- Arthralgias
- Chest pain, pleurisy
- Chills
- Cough, dry or productive
- Cyanosis
- Dyspnea
- Erythema nodosum
- Fatigue
- Fever
- Headache
- Malaise
- Night sweats
- Pleural friction rub
- Rash
- Sore throat
- Tachycardia
- Toxic erythema
- Weight loss

NOTE: Over 1/2 of cases are subclinical. Disseminated cases may involve CNS symptoms, bone pain, fungal skin lesions, etc.

History
Travel history is essential when working up or providing therapy for any pulmonary infection not responding to normal measures.

TESTS
Lab
- Serology: Immunodiffusion measures precipitin antibodies (IgM) that rise within 2 weeks and fall after 2 months; complement fixation antibodies (IgG) rise at 1–3 months; patients with mild symptoms may never be detected serologically. Initially, negative serology may represent a falsely negative "window" between falling IgM and rising IgG levels.
- May have elevated erythrocyte sedimentation rate and peripheral eosinophilia
- Culture of sputum, wound and joint aspirate; fungus unlikely to grow in urine, blood, or pleural fluid.
- No disorders have been demonstrated to alter lab results.

Imaging
Chest radiograph findings include normal, infiltrate(s), nodule(s), cavity, adenopathy mediastinal or hilar, pleural effusion

Diagnostic Procedures/Surgery
- Biopsy of affected tissue (lung nodule, skin lesion)
- If unable to establish diagnosis from serology and/or biopsy: Bronchoscopy, fine-needle biopsy, open lung biopsy, pleural biopsy, bone/skin/node biopsy, CSF stain, serology, or culture

Pathological Findings
Fungal elements, spherules

DIFFERENTIAL DIAGNOSIS
Pulmonary
- Pneumonia of all etiologies
- Lung carcinoma
- Sarcoidosis
- Histoplasmosis, infection by other fungi
- Lung abscess
- Tuberculosis
- Lymphoma
- All other causes of cough, fever, or fatigue
- Old cocci granulomas can be mistaken for tumors.

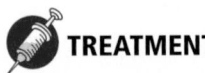 **TREATMENT**

INITIAL STABILIZATION
- Outpatient except in severe cases
- Persistent or severe cases should receive antifungal treatment and should generally be referred to a pulmonary or infectious disease specialist. Although there are no controlled studies and each case is considered individually, expert consensus guidelines include (1)[C]:
- Symptoms lasting >8 weeks
- IgG ≥1:16
- Bilateral pneumonia
- Extensive unilateral pneumonia
- Weight loss >10%
- Extreme fatigue/work disability
- All high-risk patients should be considered for treatment even with mild disease (1)[C]

GENERAL MEASURES
- Cool mist humidifier for dry cough or sore throat, antitussives
- Rest
- Supportive therapy

Diet
No special diet

Activity
As tolerated

MEDICATION (DRUGS)

- In mild cases, treat for symptomatic relief of cough with antitussives; treat pleuritic pain with nonsteroidal antiinflammatory drugs.
- For persistent, progressive, or disseminated disease, the following drugs are indicated. No significant random controlled trials exist; most studies involve small numbers of patients with advanced disease and significant relapse rates. Most treating physicians should seek expert consultation, as drug choice and therapy duration (generally 3–6 months for nondisseminated disease) remain controversial. Consensus guidelines suggest (1)[C]
  – Ketoconazole: 400 mg/d
  – Fluconazole: 400 mg/d. Fluconazole is also the treatment of choice for coccidioidomeningitis with a usual dose of 800 mg/d
  – Itraconazole: 200 mg b.i.d.
  – Severe and rapidly progressive disease, including late pregnancy, may require amphotericin B
- Contraindications: Avoid steroid therapy.
- Precautions: Amphotericin is highly nephrotoxic.
- Significant possible interactions
  – Ketoconazole-H_2 blockers decrease absorption of ketoconazole (ketoconazole requires an acidic pH for absorption).
  – Azole antifungals: Prolongation of QT segment and ventricular arrhythmias

 ## FOLLOW-UP

If serology provides negative result but index of suspicion remains high, repeat every 2 weeks. With positive serologic result, follow titers every 2 weeks until titers are dropping and the patient has clinical improvement or resolution. Observe and repeat abnormal chest radiographs until findings are resolved or scarring process is complete.

PROGNOSIS
- Most cases are self-limited and resolve within a few months. Progressive and disseminated disease can be difficult to eradicate.
- Prognosis poor if weak cell-mediated immunity response or high IgG
- Relapse of extrapulmonary or disseminated disease is common

COMPLICATIONS
- Severe cases are fatal, especially if associated with meningitis. Coccidioidomycosis can cause destruction of pulmonary tissue due to scarring, cavities, and other factors.
- Hemoptysis

REFERENCES

1. Galgiana JN, Ampel NM. Practice guidelines for the treatment of coccidioidomycosis, *Clin Infect Dis*. 2000;30(4):658–661.
2. Galgiani JN. Primary coccidioidal infection. UpToDate Clinical Reference. Available at: http://www.uptodate.com. Accessed June 21, 2005.
3. Hedges E, Miller S. Coccidioidomycosis: Office diagnosis and treatment. *Am Fam Physician*. 1990;5:1499–1506.

 ## MISCELLANEOUS

 CODES

ICD9-CM
114.9 Coccidioidomycosis, unspecified

PATIENT TEACHING

For favorably reviewed patient education materials on this topic, contact: American Lung Association, 1740 Broadway, New York, NY 10019; (212) 315-8700

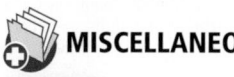 **See Corresponding Diagnostic Algorithm**

See Patient Handout on CD

C

COLIC, INFANTILE

Daniel T. Lee, MD, MA

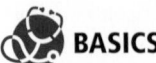 **BASICS**

DESCRIPTION
Colic is defined as excessive crying in an otherwise healthy baby. A commonly used criteria is the Wessel criteria or the "rule of 3": crying lasts for >3 hours a day, >3 days a week, and persists >3 weeks. Many clinicians have dropped the criterion of persistence for >3 weeks, as few parents or clinicians will wait that long before evaluation or intervention. Some clinicians feel colic represents the extreme end of the spectrum of normal crying, while most feel colic is a distinct clinical entity.

- System(s) Affected: Gastrointestinal; Nervous

Pediatric Considerations
This is a problem during infancy.

GENERAL PREVENTION
Colic is normally not preventable.

EPIDEMIOLOGY
- Predominant age: 2 weeks–4 months of age
- Predominant sex: Male = Female

Prevalence
Probably between 10% and 25% of infants, though wider ranges of 3–43% have been quoted

RISK FACTORS
Physiologic predisposition in infant, but no definitive risk factors have been established

Genetics
None known

ETIOLOGY
The cause is unknown. Factors that may play a role include
- Swallowing air during the process of crying, feeding, or sucking
- Overfeeding or feeding too quickly. Underfeeding also has been proposed.
- Inadequate burping after feeding
- Family tension
- Parental anxiety, depression, and/or fatigue
- Parent-infant interaction mismatch
- Allergies to cow's milk or breast milk protein
- Esophageal reflux
- Baby's inability to console itself when dealing with stimuli
- Increased gut hormone, motilin, causing hyperperistalsis
- Tobacco smoke exposure
- Fruit juice intolerance

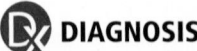 **DIAGNOSIS**

SIGNS AND SYMPTOMS
- Protracted, paroxysmal, intense crying
- High-pitched screams
- Inconsolability
- Flushed face with occasional circumoral pallor
- Fist clenching
- Back arching
- Drawing up of legs to abdomen with periodic extension of legs
- Abdomen distended and tense
- Arms stiff, tight, and extended (elbows may also be flexed)
- May have excessive flatus
- Symptoms may occur more often in late afternoon and evening

History
The colicky episodes may have a clear beginning and end. The crying is generally spontaneous without preceding events triggering the episodes. The crying is typically different from normal crying. Colicky crying may be louder, more turbulent, variable in pitch, and appear more like screaming. The infant acts normally when not colicky.

Physical Exam
Exam is normal

TESTS
Lab
No lab tests

Imaging
No imaging tests

Diagnostic Procedures/Surgery
A thorough history and physical examination should be performed to rule out other causes. Otherwise, no diagnostic procedures or surgery is indicated.

Pathological Findings
None

DIFFERENTIAL DIAGNOSIS
Any organic cause for excessive or qualitatively different crying in infants (e.g., meningitis, sepsis, strangulated hernia, occult fracture, digit or penile hair tourniquet, foreign bodies, corneal abrasion, constipation, otitis media, intussusception, gastroesophageal reflux, lactose intolerance, UTI, anal fissure, child abuse)

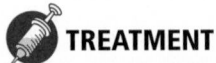 **TREATMENT**

INITIAL STABILIZATION
Outpatient management

GENERAL MEASURES
- Soothe by holding and rocking the baby (1)[C]
- Use pacifier (1)[C]
- Use of gentle rhythmic motion (e.g., strollers, infant swings, car rides) (1)[C]
- Place near "white noise" (e.g., vacuum cleaner, clothes dryer, white noise machine) (1)[C]
- Crib vibrators or car ride simulators have not been shown helpful (1,2)[B]
- Increased carrying or use of infant carrier did not improve colic (1,2)[B]
- Employ the 5 "S's" (Need to be done concurrently)
  1) Swaddling—tight wrapping with blanket
  2) Side/Stomach—laying baby on side or stomach
  3) Shushing—loud white noise
  4) Swinging—rhythmic, jiggly motion
  5) Sucking—sucking on anything (e.g., nipple, finger, pacifier) (1)[C]

Diet
- If formula feeding, consider a 1-week trial of switching to hypoallergenic formulas, such as whey hydrolysate (e.g., Good Start) or casein hydrolysate (e.g., Alimentum, Nutramigen, Pregestamil). (2,3)[B]
- Switching to soy formula may also be beneficial. (2,3)[B]
- Herbal teas containing mixtures of chamomile, vervain, licorice, fennel, and balm mint used up to t.i.d. may be beneficial. (1–3)[B]
- Supplementing with sucrose solution may be helpful. (2,3)[B]
- Use of lactase enzymes in formula, breast milk, or given directly to the infant has no therapeutic benefit. (2)[B]
- Adding fiber to the formula has not been shown helpful. (2,4)[B]

Nursing
- If breast feeding, continue to do so. Switching to formula probably will not help. (1)[C]
- Possible therapeutic benefit from eliminating milk products, eggs, wheat, and nuts from the diet of breastfeeding mothers. (1,2)[B]

SPECIAL THERAPY
Physical Therapy
Infant massage has not been shown to be helpful. (1)[B]

Complementary and Alternative Medicine
- Use of music may help. (4,5)[C]
- Chiropractic treatment has shown no benefit over placebo. (1)[C]

MEDICATION (DRUGS)

First Line
None

Second Line
- Dicyclomine (Bentyl) has been proven beneficial, but the potential serious adverse effects such as apnea, seizures, and syncope have precluded its use. Further, the manufacturer has made the medication contraindicated for infants <6 months. (1–3)[B]
- Simethicone has not been shown beneficial. (1–3)[B]

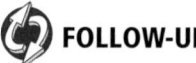 **FOLLOW-UP**

PROGNOSIS
- Usually subsides by 3–6 months of age
- Despite apparent abdominal pain, colicky infants eat well and gain weight normally.
- Colic has no bearing on the baby's intelligence or future development.

COMPLICATIONS
Colic is self-limiting and does not result in lasting effects to maternal mental health. (6)[C]

PATIENT MONITORING
Frequent outpatient visits as needed for parental reassurance, education, and to ensure the health of the infant and parents

REFERENCES
1. Roberts DM, Ostapchuk M, O'Brien JG. Infantile colic. *Am Fam Physician*. 2004;70:735–740, 741–742.
2. Garrison MM, Christakis DA. A systematic review of treatments for infant colic. *Pediatrics*. 2000; 106:184–190.
3. Wade S, Kilgour T. Extracts from "clinical evidence": infantile colic. *BMJ*. 2001;323:437–440.
4. Clemons RM. Issues in newborn care. *Primary Care*. 2000;27:251–267.
5. McCollough M, Sharieff G. Common complaints in the first 30 days of life. *Emerg Med Clin North Am*. 2002;20:27–48.
6. Clifford TJ. Sequelae of infant colic: Evidence of transient infant distress and absence of lasting effects on maternal mental health. *Arch Pediatr Adolesc Med*. 2002;156:1183–188.

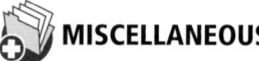 **MISCELLANEOUS**

Two books to consider recommending to parents include
- Karp, H. *The Happiest Baby on the Block: The new way to calm crying and help your newborn baby sleep longer*. New York, NY: Random House, Inc.; 2002.
- Lester B, Grace CO. *Why Is My Baby Crying? The Parent's Survival Guide for Coping with Crying Problems and Colic*. New York, NY: Harper Collins Pub. Inc.; 2005.

 CODES

ICD9-CM
789.0 Abdominal pain

PATIENT TEACHING
- Explain spectrum of crying behavior. Reassure parents that colic is not the result of bad parenting.
- The American Academy of Pediatrics 141 Northwest Point Boulevard Elk Grove Village, IL 60007-1098; (847)434-4000, (847)434-8000 (Fax)

Activity
- Avoid overfeeding or underfeeding
- Instruct better feeding techniques, use improved bottles (low air, curved), sufficient burping after feeding
- Explain that employing various specific colic-management techniques may not provide benefits beyond routine advice, support, and reassurance. (1)[B]
- Prevent caregiver burnout by advising parents get proper rest breaks, sleep, and help in caring for infant.

See Patient Handout on CD

COLORECTAL MALIGNANCY (CRC)

Marc G. Rucquoi, MD, FAAFP

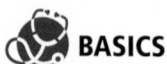 **BASICS**

DESCRIPTION

A malignant neoplasm arising from the luminal surface of the colon, rectum, or anus. The 4th most common type of malignancy in the US and the 2nd most common cause of cancer-related deaths.

- Adenocarcinoma: 95% of colorectal cancers are carcinomas, and ~95% of these are adenocarcinomas unequally distributed, with 38% in proximal colon and 62% in distal colon or rectum. Precursor adenomas include tubular, tubulovillous, and villous adenomas (with varying degrees of dysplasia)
- Carcinoid: Uncommon, rising from enterochromaffin cells; usually located in appendix or rectum; not likely to metastasize unless >2 cm in diameter
- Squamous cell carcinoma: Uncommon form; located in the anal canal; also called epidermoid or cloacogenic carcinoma
- Melanoma: Rare; usually presents as pigmented lesion adjacent to dentate line

Geriatric Considerations
Coexistence of other medical illness may complicate postoperative course.

Pediatric Considerations
Adenocarcinoma of colon rarely occurs in children; prognosis is poor in pediatric patients.

EPIDEMIOLOGY
Predominant age: 90% of adenocarcinoma occurs in people >50 years of age, with peak incidence in the 7th decade. No gender predilection has been found.

Incidence
In the US: ~155,000 new cases/year

Summary of Prevention Evidence:
- The US Preventive Services Task Force (USPSTF) found good evidence that periodic fecal occult blood testing (FOBT) starting at age 50 years reduces mortality from colorectal cancer. And fair evidence suggests that sigmoidoscopy alone or in combination with FOBT reduces mortality.

- Colonoscopy with removal of adenomatous polyps may reduce the risk of CRC. (3)[A]
- Fiber supplementation and diets low in fat and high in fiber, fruits, and vegetables do not reduce the rate of adenoma recurrence over a 3–4-year period. (1)[B]
- Epidemiologic, experimental (animal), and clinical investigations suggest diets high in total fat, protein, calories, alcohol, and meat (both red and white) and low in calcium and folate are associated with an increased incidence of CRC. (3)[A]

RISK FACTORS
- Adenocarcinoma
  - 2/3 of patients are >50 years old.
  - Pancolonic ulcerative colitis: 2% per year after 10 years active disease
  - Familial polyposis: 100%
  - Hereditary nonpolyposis colorectal cancer (HNPCC) (family history)
  - Benign adenomas: Tubular 3%; villous 9–12%
  - Coexisting (synchronous) colon cancer (5%)
  - Previous (metachronous) colon cancer: 2–5%
- Carcinoid
  - Multiple endocrine adenopathy (MEA), rare
  - Other organs with carcinoid (small bowel, bronchial)
- Squamous cell carcinoma
  - Bowen disease
  - Paget disease
  - Average risk (>50 years):
    ○ Flexible sigmoidoscopy every 5 years
    ○ Colonoscopy every 10 years
    ○ Barium enema every 5 years
  - High risk (history of polyps, personal history of colorectal cancer, family history of colorectal cancer, history of inflammatory bowel disease, familial adenomatous polyposis, hereditary nonpolyposis colon cancer):
    ○ Colonoscopy
  - Schedules vary depending on underlying risk.

Genetics
- Hereditary colon and rectal cancer accounts for ~15–20% of cases of colorectal cancer.
- Ras oncogene mutations are seen in 40–50% of adenocarcinoma; alterations of suppressor genes also seen in 75%, especially involving chromosomes 17 and 18.

ETIOLOGY
- Undetermined; both genetic and environmental factors may contribute.
- Cultural: High levels of dietary animal fat, low dietary fiber

ASSOCIATED CONDITIONS
Colonic carcinoid: Multiple endocrine neoplasia types I and II

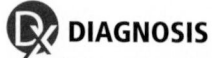 **DIAGNOSIS**

SIGNS AND SYMPTOMS
- Vary with location
- Early lesions are frequently asymptomatic
- Right-sided adenocarcinoma
  - Anemia
  - Pain and/or mass in right lower quadrant
  - Occult blood in stool
  - Change in appearance of stool (infrequent)
- Left-sided adenocarcinoma
  - Change in bowel habits (constipation or diarrhea)
  - Reduced caliber of stool
  - Red blood mixed in stool
- Rectal adenocarcinoma
  - Bright red rectal bleeding
  - Tenesmus
  - Mass on digital exam
- Carcinoid
  - Often incidental finding
  - Appendicitis-like if located in appendix
  - Rectal bleeding
  - Cramping abdominal pain
  - Carcinoid syndrome occurs with metastases to liver; includes facial flushing, abdominal cramps, diarrhea
- Squamous cell carcinoma
  - Painful defecation
  - Rectal bleeding
  - Mass or ulcer in anal canal
  - Nonhealing anal fissure

TESTS
Lab
Carcinoembryonic antigen levels are usually elevated with bulky tumor or metastases, useful finding in postoperative assessment

- Any positive result to FOBT must be evaluated by colonoscopy
- Iron deficiency anemia
- Urinary 5-hydroxyindoleacic acid; elevated in carcinoid
- Elevated plasma carcinoembryonic antigen (may also relate to renal failure)
- Drugs that may alter lab results
  - Medications containing aspirin and other nonsteroidal anti-inflammatory drugs: False-positive FOBT test may result
  - Smoking: Increased carcinoembryonic antigen
- Disorders that may alter lab results
  - Peptic ulcer disease, ulcerative colitis, hemorrhoids, benign polyps: Positive FOBT result

Imaging for Patients with CRC
- CT: Used for staging CRC. ~50% of colon cancer patients will be diagnosed with hepatic metastases, either at the time of initial presentation or as a result of disease recurrence.
- Transrectal ultrasound: Used in defining extent of involvement by rectal lesions

Diagnostic Procedures/Surgery
- Anoscopy: Useful for anal canal visualization, biopsies
- Colonoscopy with biopsy: Used for primary diagnosis, screening of high-risk patients, and post-resection surveillance

Pathological Findings
- Adenocarcinoma
  - May appear as ulcerated, polypoid, or fungating mass. May extend to local structures or metastasize by blood, lymphatics; staging of tumor reflects level of penetration
  - Tumor-node-metastasis staging
    - Stage I invades to muscularis propria.
    - Stage II invades serosa or adjacent organs.
    - Stage III involves regional nodes.
    - Stage IV shows distant metastases.
- Carcinoid
  - Tends to be multicentric
  - Metastasizes by blood, lymphatics
- Squamous cell carcinoma
  - Most are ulcerative but size may vary greatly.
  - Metastasize to inguinal lymphatics

DIFFERENTIAL DIAGNOSIS
- Strictures (ischemic, Crohn, diverticulosis)
- Other neoplasms (prostatic carcinoma, lipoma, leiomyoma, sarcoma, among others)
- Infectious/inflammatory lesions (ameboma, tuberculoma, hemorrhoids)
- Extrinsic masses (abscesses, cysts/pseudocysts, phlegmons)

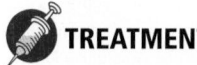

TREATMENT
GENERAL MEASURES
Diet
Usually normal; avoidance of gas-producing foods (cabbage, beans, onions, alcoholic beverages) may be helpful in patient with ostomies

Activity
Usually normal; may be slightly modified for patient with stoma

MEDICATION (DRUGS)

- Steroids or somatostatin may palliate symptoms of carcinoid syndrome.
- Stage III colon adenocarcinoma: Fluorouracil plus folinic acid (leucovorin) plus oxaliplatin or CPT-11
- Stage II and III rectal: 5-fluorouracil + radiation
- Contraindications: Peptic ulcer disease (steroids)

SURGERY
- Colonic polyps should be removed and examined microscopically. If benign, surveillance colonoscopy should be performed after 3 years, and if normal, every 5 years.
- Surgical procedures: Radical resection of tumor with wide margins; includes segments of normal colon, mesentery, and lymph nodes
- Right hemicolectomy for proximal tumors
- Left hemicolectomy for descending colon cancers
- Sigmoid colectomy for sigmoid cancers
- Abdominoperineal resection with colostomy for cancers of distal rectum (within 5–7 cm of dentate line)
- Preoperative or postoperative radiotherapy and chemotherapy: May improve outcome when used for rectal carcinoma
- For carcinoma of anus: Combined chemotherapy (5-fluorouracil and mitomycin C) and radiotherapy. Convert to abdominoperineal resection for residual or recurrent tumor or consider salvage chemotherapy (5-fluorouracil + cisplatin).

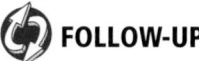 FOLLOW-UP

PROGNOSIS
- Adenocarcinoma: The overall 5-year survival is 50% and varies with age and race. As expected, mortality decreases with advanced stage
  - Stage 1 (Duke A)
  - Stage II A & B (Duke B)
  - Stage III A-C (Duke C)
  - Stage IV (Duke D)
- Carcinoid
  - Overall 5-year survival is 65%
  - Relates to tumor stage as in adenocarcinoma
- Squamous cell carcinoma
  - Overall 5-year survival rate is 79%

COMPLICATIONS
- After resections
  - Mortality: 5–10%
  - Wound infection: 5–15%
  - Anastomotic stricture/leak/abscess: 2–5%
  - Pneumonia: 5–10%
  - Urinary tract infection: 5–20%
- During chemotherapy or radiation therapy
  - Stomatitis
  - Proctitis/diarrhea
  - Temporary alopecia

PATIENT MONITORING
- Adenocarcinoma after remainder of colon is cleared of all lesions:
  - Colonoscopy: Repeat in 1 year, then every 3 years.
  - Carcinoembryonic antigen test, liver chemistries, fecal occult blood test: Every 3 months for 2 years; then every 4 months for year 3; then every 6 months for year 4; then annually
- Carcinoid
  - 5-Hydroxyindole acetic every 6 months for 2 years, then annually
- Squamous cell carcinoma
  - Clinical evaluation every 4 months for 1 year, then annually
  - Biopsy is mandatory for suspicious areas in anus and groin.

Screening Guidelines
- Screening begins in asymptomatic adults at 50 years of age.
- Screening begins in patients with a 1st-degree affected relative 10 years prior to affected relative's diagnosis, or 40 years of age, whichever is earlier.
- Digital rectal exam with single stool card is not recognized by USPSTF as a screening modality for CRC.
- USPSTF-recommended screening options (Testing intervals recommended by the American Cancer Society for asymtomatic individuals)
  - Home stool cards ×3 (annually)
  - Sigmoidoscopy (every 5 years)
  - Dual contrast barium enema (every 5 years)
  - Colonoscopy (every 10 years)
- "Virtual Colonoscopy: No USPSTF recommendations for this modality

REFERENCES
1. Benson AB, et al. NCCN Practice guidelines for colorectal cancer. *Oncology.* 2000;14:203–212.
2. U.S. National Institutes of Health, National Cancer Institute, Colon and Rectal Cancer resources page. Available at: http://www.cancer.gov/cancertopics/types/colon-and-rectal. Accessed May 30, 2006.
3. U.S. Preventive Services Task Force, Screening for colorectal cancer. Available at: http://www.ahrq.gov/clinic/uspstf/uspscolo.htm. Accessed May 30, 2006.

C

 MISCELLANEOUS

CODES

ICD9-CM
- 153.9 Malignant neoplasm of the colon, unspecified
- v12.72 Personal history of colonic polyps
- v76.51 Screening for malignancy of colon

PATIENT TEACHING
- National Cancer Institute, Department of Health And Human Services, Public Inquiries Section, Office of Cancer Communications, Building 31, Room 101-18, 9000 Rockville Pike, Bethesda, MD 20892; (301) 496-5583. (http://www.cancer.gov/cancertopics/pdq/treatment/colon/patient)
- American Cancer Society, (800) ACS-2345, www.cancer.org

 See Corresponding Diagnostic Algorithm

 See Patient Handout on CD

COMMON COLD

Lisa M. Schroeder, MD

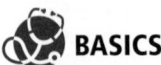 **BASICS**

DESCRIPTION
Inflammation of nasal passages resulting from infection with various respiratory viruses; called an upper respiratory infection.
Usually not serious; most cases are self-treated.
- System(s) Affected: ENT; Pulmonary

GENERAL PREVENTION
Frequent hand washing and avoiding touching one's face may help prevent colds.

EPIDEMIOLOGY
- Predominant age: Children > Adults
- Predominant sex: Male = Female

Incidence
- Preschool children: 6–10 colds per year; kindergarten 12 per year; school children: 7 per year; adolescents/adults: 2–4 per year
- National Ambulatory Survey: 31 episodes per 100 persons per year (counting only colds that lead to medical attention or at least 1 day of restricted activity)

RISK FACTORS
- Exposure to infected people
- Touching one's nose or conjunctiva with contaminated fingers
- Allergic disorders
- Smoking

Genetics
Native Americans and Innu are at higher risk than other ethnic groups and have more frequent complications such as otitis media.

ETIOLOGY
- Usually due to 1 of 200 virus strains from 6 virus families; many strains present within the same geographic region or patient family
  - Rhinovirus, with >200 serotypes
  - Influenzavirus types A, B, C
  - Parainfluenza viruses
  - Respiratory syncytial viruses
  - Coronaviruses
  - Adenoviruses
  - Certain enteric cytopathogenic human orphan viruses
- In 40% of cases, no pathogen can be identified.

ASSOCIATED CONDITIONS
- Pharyngitis
- Sinusitis
- Bronchitis
- Bronchiolitis
- Pneumonia
- Croup
- Asthma

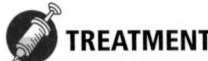 **DIAGNOSIS**

SIGNS AND SYMPTOMS
- Nasal stuffiness and/or obstruction (80–100%)
- Sneezing (50–70%)
- Scratchy throat (50%)
- Cough (40%)
- Hoarseness (30%)
- Malaise (20–25%)
- Headache (25%)
- Fever exceeding 100°F/37.7°C (0–1%)

TESTS
Lab
In some health care centers, rapid antigen tests for various respiratory viruses are available for those patients who require hospitalization or for the purposes of research.

Imaging
Not indicated unless concern is present about superinfection of the sinuses, supraglottic region, trachea, or lungs.

Diagnostic Procedures/Surgery
In rare cases, clinicians may want to culture virus from nasal washing or identify it by enzyme-linked immunosorbent assay or radioimmunoassay.

Pathological Findings
- Rhinovirus infects the ciliated epithelium lining the nose. Edema and hyperemia of nasal mucous membranes result.
- Exudation of serous and mucinous fluid containing immunoglobulins
- Histology: Edema of subepithelial connective tissue and a scanty cellular infiltrate containing neutrophils, plasma cells, lymphocytes, and eosinophils
- Rhinovirus causes a "nondestructive" inflammation of the mucous membranes, in contrast to influenza and parainfluenza, which denude epithelium to the basement membrane.

DIFFERENTIAL DIAGNOSIS
- Allergic rhinitis
- Mumps
- Rubeola
- Cytomegalovirus
- Epstein-Barr virus
- *Mycoplasma pneumoniae*
- Influenza virus: Systemic symptoms, including myalgias, malaise, severe headache, and ocular symptoms, overshadow respiratory complaints.

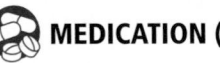 **TREATMENT**

INITIAL STABILIZATION
Generally self-care on an outpatient basis

GENERAL MEASURES
- Rest, fluids, and palliation of symptoms
- Reassure patient and family that usual course is 6–10 days.
- Home cool mist humidifier, or heated humidified air
- Discontinue use of tobacco and alcohol.
- In infants, clear nasal passages with a bulb syringe, position the mattress at 45°, and use saline nasal drops.

Diet
Encourage consumption of fluids.

Activity
Normal activities as tolerated, but with extra rest during the 1st few days

MEDICATION (DRUGS)

First Line
No cure or practical preventive measure documented. Medications targeting a particular symptom reduce the likelihood of adverse systemic effects.
- Topical decongestants (sympathomimetics) reduce edema and swelling of the nasal mucosa, promote drainage, and reduce nasal airflow resistance. Preferred over oral type because of minimal systemic effects. Sprays preferred over drops in patients >6 years old.
- Oxymetazoline
  - Adults and children aged 6–12: 0.05% solution, 2–3 sprays in each nostril b.i.d.
  - Children aged 2–6 years: 0.025% solution, 2–3 drops in each nostril b.i.d.
  - Rebound congestion (rhinitis medicamentosa) unlikely if used <5 days
- Topical anticholinergics control rhinorrhea, but do not relieve nasal congestion or sneezing
  - Ipratropium: Adults and children >11 years old: 0.06% solution, 2 sprays to each nostril t.i.d. for 4 days
- Oral decongestant (sympathomimetic) advantages over topical decongestants: Longer duration of action, lack of local irritation, and no risk of rhinitis medicamentosa
- Pseudoephedrine
  - Adults: 60 mg q4–6h (120 mg sustained release q12h)
    - ○ Superior to placebo in short term use (1,2)[A]
  - Children aged 6–12 years: 30 mg q4–6h
  - Children aged 2–5 years: 15 mg q4–6h
    - ○ Insufficient data to recommend in children (2)
- Antihistamines: Safe and mildly effective in alleviating sneezing and rhinorrhea. Their benefit may come from anticholinergic effects, which dry nasal and pharyngeal secretions and promote rest through sedative effects.

- Chlorpheniramine
  - Adults: 4 mg q4–6h (or 8 mg t.i.d., 12 mg b.i.d.)
  - Children aged 6–12 years: 2 mg q4–6h
  - Children aged 2–6 years: 1 mg q4–6h
- Cough suppressants: Cough due to irritation of tracheobronchial receptors by postnasal drip and may therefore benefit from decongestants. If cough is nonproductive or if it interferes with sleep or normal activities, a cough suppressant is indicated. Codeine and dextromethorphan exhibit comparable, but minimal efficacy. Adverse effects: Drowsiness and gastrointestinal upset.
- Codeine
  - Adults: 10–20 mg q4–6h
  - Children aged 6–12: 5–10 mg q4–6h
  - Children aged 2–6: 2.5–5 mg q4–6h
- Dextromethorphan
  - Adults: 10–30 mg q4–6h
  - Children aged 6–12: 15 mg q4–6h
  - Children aged 2–6: 2.5–7.5 mg q4–6h
- Expectorants: Although commonly employed, efficacy has not been proven
- Guaifenesin
  - Adults: 100–400 mg q4h
  - Children aged 6–12 years: 100–200 mg q4h
  - Children aged 2–5 years: 50–100 mg q4h
- Contraindications
  - Patients receiving monoamine oxidase inhibitors or selegiline should not take oral decongestants.
- Precautions
  - Oral decongestants
    - Affect all vascular beds and may increase blood pressure. They are cardiac stimulants and may result in arrhythmias. They may increase glucose levels in patients with glucose intolerance or diabetes mellitus.
    - Other adverse effects include headache, nervousness, sleeplessness, and dizziness.
    - Should be used with caution in patients also taking guanethidine
- Antihistamines
  - Nasal blockage and sinus congestion may worsen.
- Cough suppressants
  - Misuse and dependence can occur with codeine, but dextromethorphan abuse by adolescents has also been reported.
- Expectorants
  - Liquid preparations may contain high concentrations of alcohol.
  - Nausea, vomiting, or abdominal pain are common adverse effects.

Second Line
- Many mouthwashes, gargles, and lozenges are promoted to relieve the pain of sore throat. The demulcent effects of hard candy, gargling with warm saline, and products with anesthetics (benzocaine or phenol) may provide pain relief.
- Aromatic oils (menthol, camphor, eucalyptus), when applied topically or taken in a lozenge, produce a sensation of increased airflow in the absence of a significant change in airflow resistance.
- Antibacterials are of no value. (3)[A]
- Antivirals
  - Zinc chloride prevents viral replication in vitro, but the efficacy of lozenges remains unproved.

Complementary and Alternative Medicine
- Vitamin C (ascorbic acid)
  - No preventive effects and only a modest (average, 23%) reduction in severity and duration of symptoms. (4)[A]
  - Precipitation of urate, oxalate, or cystine stones has been seen: Urine glucose monitoring may be inaccurate in people taking large doses of vitamin C.
  - High-dose vitamin C prophylaxis proven beneficial in those exposed to heavy exertion and cold stress. Zinc and high dose vitamin C prophylaxis and treatment should not be recommended for the general population. Conflicting evidence exists for the use of echinacea (7,8,9)

Geriatric Considerations
Medications commonly produce adverse effects in older people.

Pregnancy Considerations
- Decongestants: No clear association has been determined between use of this drug group and congenital defects.
- Antihistamines: No clear association has been confirmed between use of this drug group and congenital defects.
- Codeine: Indiscriminate use during pregnancy may pose a risk to the fetus.

Pediatric Considerations
- Medications are likely to produce adverse effects or toxicity in young children
- Incidence of colds is highest in this age group.

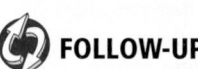 **FOLLOW-UP**

Patients should contact the PCP's office if they develop fever associated with systemic symptoms, difficulty breathing, dyspnea, or purulent draining.

COMPLICATIONS
- Lower respiratory tract infection
- Bronchial hyperreactivity
- May lead to decompensation in patients with asthma and chronic lung disease
- Otitis media (2% of colds)
- Acute sinusitis (0.5% of colds)
- Pneumonia
- Rhinitis medicamentosa

PATIENT MONITORING
Complete recovery should be expected within 3–10 days.

REFERENCES
1. Eccles R, Jawad MS, Jawad SS, et al. Efficacy and safety of single and multiple doses of pseudoephedrine in the treatment of nasal congestion associated with common cold. *AM J Rhinol*. 2005;19(1):25–31.
2. Taverner D, Latte J, Draper M. Nasal decongestants for the common cold. *The Cochrane Database of Systematic Reviews*. 2004, Issue 3. Art No CD001953.
3. Arroll B, Kenealy T. Antibiotics for the common cold and acute purulent rhinitis. *The Cochrane Database of Systematic Reviews* 2002, Issue 4.
4. Hemila H, Chalker E, D'Souza RRD, et al. Vitamin C for preventing the common cold. *The Cochrane Database of Systemic Reviews* 2004, Issue 4.
5. Turner RB, Bauer R, Woelkaret K, et al. An evaluation of Echinacea angustifolia in experimental rhinovirus infections. *N Engl J Med*. 2005;353(4):341–348.
6. Melchart D, Linde K, Fischer P, et al. Echinacea for preventing and treating the common cold. *The Cochrane Database of Systematic Reviews* 1999, Issue1.
7. Marshall I. Zinc for the common cold. Cochrane Acute Respiratory Infections Group Cochrane Database of Systematic Reviews 4, 2006.
8. Douglas RM, Hemila H, Chalker E, D'Souza RRD, Treacy B. Vitamin C for preventing and treating the common cold. Cochrane Acute Respiratory Infections Group Cochrane Database of Systematic Reviews 4, 2006.
9. Linde K, Barrett B, Wolkart K, Bauer R, Melchart D. Echinacea for preventing and treating the common cold. Cochrane Acute Respiratory Infections Group Cochrane Database of Systematic Reviews 4, 2006.

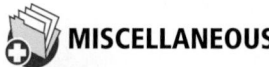 **MISCELLANEOUS**

CODES

ICD9-CM
- 460 Acute nasopharyngitis (common cold)
- 465.9 Acute URI NOS

PATIENT TEACHING
- Reassure patient and family that colds are ubiquitous and a normal part of human existence.
- Spread is primarily through hand-to-hand transmission of virus-contaminated nasal secretions; people with colds touch their nose and eyes and then other people.
- Small-particle aerosols released in talking, coughing, and sneezing do not travel far and contain only a low concentration of rhinovirus.
- Rhinovirus survives for hours on hands and on hard surfaces, but it does not survive long on porous surfaces such as facial tissue.
- Individual susceptibility to colds depends in large part on preexisting antibody levels.
- Serum immunity lasts for years, but most people gain little protection against future colds due, in part, to the large number of viral serotypes and the antigenic drift that occurs over time in some viral types (rhinovirus, influenza).
- Educate patient and family about the expected course of the disease and symptomatic measures.
- Advise patients and family to contact your office if they develop dyspnea, productive cough, a temperature exceeding 102°F (38.9°C), or shaking and chills.
- Patient information at www.niaid.nih.gov/factsheets/cold.htm

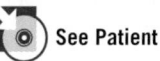 **See Patient Handout on CD**

COMPLEMENTARY AND ALTERNATIVE MEDICINE (CAM)

William G. Elder Jr., PhD
Andrew Bentley

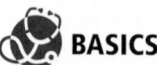 **BASICS**

DESCRIPTION

- CAM is a group of diverse medical and health care systems, practices, and products that are not presently considered to be part of conventional medicine.
- CAM use is increasing. Out of pocket expenditures for CAM exceed those for conventional outpatient medical care. Patient values and preferences influence their treatment choices.
- New rigorously designed research findings are available on positive and negative effects of CAM treatments.
- Health care providers must be prepared to advise patients regarding CAM based on evidence for efficacy and safety.

EPIDEMIOLOGY

- Monthly prevalence for visits to CAM providers is 6.5%, vs. 11.5% to a PCP
- All ages use CAM
- 25% of patients with cancer use 7 or more therapies

CAM Treatments
10 most common CAM therapies (2002)
- Prayer/self, 43%
- Prayer/others, 24.4%
- Natural products 18.9%
- Deep breathing, 11.6%
- Prayer group, 9.6%
- Meditation, 7.6%
- Chiropractic, 7.5%
- Yoga, 5.1%
- Massage, 5%
- Diets, 3.5%

Predictors of CAM Use
- Gender ratio: Female predominance 2.5:1
- College graduation and residence in western states
- 10% of patients use CAM to address a medical condition with the exception that 37% of patients with "distant" cancers seek cure (rr = 11).
- Most common uses are to control pain and to increase wellness (e.g., boost the immune system)
- Trends associated with increasing use include cultural diversity and pluralism in health care, insurance/legislative changes that recognize CAM approaches, and increasingly informed and activist patients.

Common Patient Beliefs Regarding CAM
- CAM is safe and will not hurt.
- It must work if they can advertise it.
- My doctor will judge me for using—only 33% of patients tell their doctor about CAM use.
- CAM use may be consistent with world view, including religious beliefs
- Patients often prefer the warmth, interest, and extra time they receive from CAM providers. It may help them to feel more in control.
- Many CAM approaches are significantly less expensive and invasive than traditional approaches.

PATIENT-CENTERED APPROACH TO CAM USE
- Use evidence for
  - Efficacy
  - Safety
- To place therapy on continuum of approach
  - Recommend
  - Accept
  - Discourage

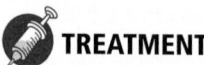 **TREATMENT**

Evidence Supports Both Safety and Efficacy
Clinical therapies
- Manipulation and mobilization for acute low-back pain posterior neck pain
- Mind-body techniques for migraines, chronic pain, and insomnia
- Riboflavin for migraine prophylaxis
- Black cohash for hot flashes in menopause
- Glucosamine and chondroitin sulfate for osteoarthritis and knee pain

Evidence Supports Safety, but Evidence Regarding Efficacy is Inconclusive
Clinical examples
- Acupuncture for chronic pain
- Homeopathy for seasonal rhinitis
- Dietary fat reduction for certain types of cancer
- Mind-body techniques for metastatic cancer

Evidence Supports Efficacy, but Evidence Regarding Safety is Inconclusive
Clinical examples
- St. John's Wort for depression
- Saw palmetto for benign prostatic hyperplasia (benefit is of statistical significance, but provides little clinical difference)
- Ginko biloba for cognitive function in dementia

Evidence Indicates Serious Risk
Clinical examples
- Dangerous delay or replacement of curative conventional treatments; injections of unapproved substances; use of toxic herbs or substances; known herb-drug interactions

Inefficacy
Acupuncture for chemotherapy-induced nausea and dental pain

COMPLICATIONS
Potentially Toxic Herbs with Mechanisms of Toxicity
- Bitter orange: Sympathomimetic; increases heart rate, BP
- California poppy: May cause respiratory depression; contains opioids
- Cascara sagrada: Depletes serum potassium
- Chaparral: Hepatotoxic
- Ephedra: Sympathomimetic; increases heart rate, BP
- Ginkgo: Extravasation, increased bleeding time
- Guarana: Tachycardia, hypertension; contains caffeine
- Kava: Decreases utilization of niacin; possibly hepatotoxic
- Licorice: Long-term use depletes serum potassium
- Lilly of the valley: Cardiac glycosides
- Poke root: Strong gastric irritant, may cause sedation
- Senna: Depletes serum potassium
- Snakeroot (*Aristolochia species*): Nephrotoxic
- Wormwood: Elevates serotonin level, may raise BP
- Yohimbe: Elevates BP

Important Herbal-Medication Interactions
- Angelica: Additive effect with CA channel blockers
- Cascara sagrada: Shortens transit time of intestinally absorbed drugs
- Chamomile: Antagonistic interaction with benzodiazepines
- Dong Quai: Additive effect with CA channel blockers
- Echinacea: May counteract with immunosuppressants
- Garlic: Modest anticoagulant effect; decreases levels of saquinavir
- Ginkgo: Dangerous synergistic effect with anticoagulants
- Ginseng: Potentiates dopaminergic drugs; counteracts with phenothiazines
- Kava: Additive effect with sedatives
- Kelp: May interfere with thyroxine and liothyronine
- Licorice: Increases potential for digoxin toxicity
- Lobelia: Potentially counteracts beta 2 adrenergic bronchodilators
- Meadowsweet: Increases action of anticoagulants; contains salicylates
- Motherwort: Can potentiate digoxin; contains cardiac glycosides
- Milk thistle: Might accelerate clearance of liver-metabolized drugs
- Pumpkin seed: Elevates levels of androgenic drugs
- Red clover: Antagonistic interaction with estrogens
- Saw palmetto: May potentiate or antagonize androgenic drugs
- Soy isoflavones: Antagonistic interaction with estrogens
- St. John's Wort: Induces CYP450 pathways, inactivating many drugs
- Tobacco: May counteract beta-blockers
- Uva Ursi: Interferes with action of other diuretics
- Valerian: Potential for interference with valproic acid derivatives
- Willow bark: Additive effect with anticoagulants; contains salicylates

DEFINITIONS AND ADDITIONAL TERMS

- Complementary medicine: Treatments used together with conventional medicine
- Alternative medicine: Unrelated group of non-orthodox therapeutic practices, often with explanatory systems that do not follow conventional biomedical explanations
- The National Institutes of Health have categorized CAM modalities into 5 domains
  - Biologically Based Therapies: Diets, herbals, and vitamins
  - Manipulative and Body-Based Methods: Massage, chiropractic, and osteopathy
  - Mind-Body Medicine: Yoga, spirituality/prayer, and relaxation
  - Alternative Medical Systems: Homeopathy, naturopathy, and ayurveda
  - Energy Therapies: Reiki, magnets, and qi gong

REFERENCES

1. Barnes P, Powell-Griner E, McFann K, Nahin R. CDC Advance Data Report #343. *Complementary and Alternative Medicine Use Among Adults: United States,* 2002. May 27, 2004.
2. Blumenthal M, Goldberg A, Brinckman J. *Herbal Medicine: Expanded Commission E Monographs. Newton, MA: Integrative Medicine Communications;* 2000.
3. Duke JA. *Handbook of Phytochemical Constituents of GRAS Herbs and Other Economic Plants.* Boca Raton, FL: CRC Press; 1992.
4. Elder WG. Complementary and Alternative Medicine. Evidence-based Review. *Presented at: 37th Annual Family Practice Review Course;* February 2006; Lexington, KY.
5. Green LA, Yawn BP, Lanier D, Dovey SM. The ecology of medical care revisited, *N Engl J Med.* 2001;344(26):2021–2025.
6. Kennedy J. Herb and supplement use in the US adult population. *Clin Ther,* 2005;27(11): 1847–1858.
7. Rakel D, Faas N. *Complementary Medicine in Clinical Practice.* Boston, MA: Jones and Bartlett, 2005.
8. Sherman KJ, Cherkin DC, Deyo RA, et al. Diagnosis and treatment of chronic back pain by acupuncturists, chiropractors, and massage therapists. *Clin J Pain,* 2006;22(3);227–234.
9. Weiger WA, Smith M, Boon H, Richardson MA, Kaptchuk TJ, Eisenerg DM. Advising patients who seek complementary and alternative medical therapies for cancer. *Ann Intern Med.* 2002;137(11): 889–2003.

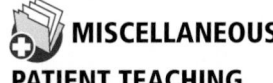

MISCELLANEOUS

PATIENT TEACHING

- The National Center for Complementary and Alternative Medicine: Public Information Clearinghouse (http://nccam.nih.gov/health/clearinghouse)
  - Description: NCCAM Public Information Clearinghouse, designed to be the public's point of contact for obtaining scientifically based information on CAM.
- National Library of Medicine: Alternative Medicine (http://www.nlm.nih.gov/nccam/camonpubmed.html)
  - Description: This version of PubMed, the National Library of Medicine's interface to the MEDLINE database, automatically limits to the complementary medicine journal subset.
- Dr. Weil.com (http://www.drweil.com)
  - Description: This popular guru of integrative medicine offers many aspects of information on balanced living, wellness, and herbal medicine.
- Kentucky Integrative Care Project (http://www.mc.uky.edu/cam/resources gov sites.htm)
  - Description: Site of University of Kentucky's CAM education effort, Web-based bibliography of links for the public and health care providers

 See Patient Handout on CD

C

COMPLEX REGIONAL PAIN SYNDROME (CRPS)

Dennis E. Hughes, DO

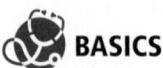 **BASICS**

DESCRIPTION

Pain syndrome after injury to bone and soft tissue. Pathogenesis is obscure. Evidence suggests that these syndromes involve areas of the brain and nervous system.

- Type I: No nerve injury (reflex sympathetic dystrophy [RSD])
- Type II: Associated with a demonstrable nerve injury (causalgia)
- System(s) Affected: Nervous
- Synonym(s): Traumatic erythromelalgia; Weir Mitchell causalgia; Causalgia; Reflex sympathetic dystrophy; Posttraumatic neuralgia; Sympathetically maintained pain

EPIDEMIOLOGY

- Predominant age: Mean age 36–46 (1)
- Predominant sex: Female predilection (60–81%) (1)

Incidence
Unknown

Prevalence
Unknown

RISK FACTORS
Minor or severe trauma

- Surgery
- Lacerations
- Burns
- Frostbite
- Casting
- Penetrating injury

Genetics
No known genetic pattern

ETIOLOGY
Other than known nerve injury (type II or causalgia), no known definitive pathogenesis

ASSOCIATED CONDITIONS
- Serious injury to bone and soft tissue
- Herpes zoster
- Postherpetic neuralgia results from partial or complete damage to afferent nerve pathways.
- Pain occurs in dermatomes as a sequela of herpes zoster.

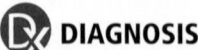 **DIAGNOSIS**

SIGNS AND SYMPTOMS
Type I and Type II

- Hypersensitivity to light touch
- Thermal hypersensitivity
- Osteoporosis
- Hair loss
- Mottled skin
- Muscle spasms
- Nail brittleness
- Burning pain
- Paroxysms of pain
- Partial motor paralysis
- Worse with emotional stress
- Hyperhydrosis

History
Inciting injury ranging from a minor sprain to severe trauma

Physical Exam
Patient adopts a protective posture to guard the affected extremity; many use a glove or stocking to protect from thermal or mechanical stimulation

TESTS
Imaging
- Electromyography and nerve conduction velocity studies to evaluate peripheral nerve function
- 3-phase bone scan to delineate presence of demineralization or occult osteomyelitis (1)
- Plain radiographs may show patchy osteoporosis within 2 weeks of onset of CRPS. (1)

Diagnostic Procedures/Surgery
- May use drop of acetone on skin of involved limbs to evaluate thermal hypersensitivity
- Thermography to measure skin temperatures between the affected and contralateral extremity (1,2)

Pathological Findings
- Partial or complete damage to afferent nerve pathways and probably reorganized central pain pathways
- Nerves most commonly involved are median and sciatic.
- Atrophy in affected muscles
- Incomplete nerve plexus lesion

DIFFERENTIAL DIAGNOSIS
- Infection
- Hypertrophic scar
- Bone fragments
- Neuroma
- CNS tumor or syrinx

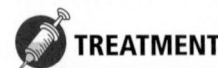 **TREATMENT**

INITIAL STABILIZATION
- Outpatient, except for operative procedures or IV sympathetic nerve blockade
- Avoid mobilization after injury.
- Avoid nerve damage during surgical procedures.

GENERAL MEASURES
- Available information about treatment is based on small studies or treatment reports; therefore, therapy remains largely empiric.
- Treatment response can be predicted by diagnosis (type I vs. type II)
- Type I
  – Physical therapy
  – Transcutaneous nerve stimulation
  – Biofeedback
  – Psychotherapy
- Type II
  – Sympathetic blocks
  – Sympathectomy
- Anesthetic blockade (chemical or surgical) of sympathetic nerve function: Transient relief suggests that chemical or surgical sympathectomy will be helpful. (1)[C]
- IV regional sympathetic block with guanethidine or reserpine by pain specialist or anesthetist
- Transcutaneous electric nerve stimulation (controversial)
- Inject myofacial painful trigger points.

Diet
No special diet

Activity
Maintain as high a level of physical and intellectual activity as possible.

SPECIAL THERAPY
Physical Therapy
- Physical therapy essential during all phases of treatment. Various modalities, including heat, cold massage, and contrast baths have proven benefical. (1,2)
- Work hardening and occupational rehabilitation many times can help the patient become functional.

Complementary and Alternative Medicine
- Briskly rub the affected part several times per day.
- Try acupuncture.
- Hypnosis can be suggested.
- Relaxation training (alternate muscle relaxing and contracting)
- Biofeedback
- Discourage maladaptive behaviors.
- After 2 months duration of the illness, psychological evaluation is generally indicated to indentify and treat any comorbid conditions. (1)

MEDICATION (DRUGS)

First Line

No single drug or combination of drugs has produced consistent results; early therapy is beneficial.

- α-Adrenergic blockers
  - Phenoxybenzamine: 40–120 mg/d, PO in divided doses. The initial dose should not exceed 10 mg.
- Miscellaneous
  - Prednisone: 30 mg/d PO for 2–3 weeks, then tapered over 2–4 weeks. (3)[B]
- Tricyclic antidepressants (response to each may be variable; therefore, several should be considered (2,3)[C]
  - Amitriptyline (Elavil): 25–100 mg/d at bedtime
  - Nortriptyline (Pamelor): 25–100 mg/d
- Anticonvulsants (serum drug level monitoring may be needed, except for clonazepam; individualize doses)
  - Carbamazepine (Tegretol): 200–1,000 mg/d PO
  - Phenytoin (Dilantin): 100–300 mg/d PO
  - Clonazepam (Klonopin): 1–10 mg/d PO
  - Valproic acid (Depakene): 750–2,250 mg/d PO, maximum of 60 mg/kg
  - Gabapentin: 100 mg/d at bedtime up to 600–1,200 mg t.i.d. (2,3)[B]
- Skeletal muscle relaxant
  - Baclofen: 10–40 mg/d PO; may act synergistically with carbamazepine and phenytoin (2)
- Contraindications
  - Refer to manufacturer's literature.
- Precautions
  - Refer to manufacturer's literature.
- Significant possible interactions
  - Many exist with this group of drugs. Refer to manufacturer's literature.

Geriatric Considerations

Pain perception is frequently more prominent in older patients. Start with smaller than usual doses of drugs.

Pregnancy Considerations

Many useful drugs are contraindicated in pregnant patients.

Second Line

Narcotics: Only after all nonopioid therapies are exhausted. It may be necessary to use to allow patient to engage in physical therapy. (3)[C]

SURGERY

Sympathectomy sometimes necessary

 ## FOLLOW-UP

DISPOSITION

Issues for Referral

Refer the patient to a specialty pain clinic in difficult cases.

PROGNOSIS

- Splinting of an injured extremity for sufficient time
- Adequate analgesics during recovery from injuries
- Course: Variable, chronic, and remitting
- Outlook only satisfactory: May need several attempts at different treatment modalities. No 1 form of therapy is superior to others. Failure to respond to one form does not suggest lack of success with another.
- Those patients receiving workers' compensation for an injury or secondary gain from family or friends are in a separate category and may never get well.

COMPLICATIONS

- Drug mishaps
- Joint contractures
- Contralateral spread of symptoms

PATIENT MONITORING

- Watch carefully for adverse reactions to medications.
- Several different forms of therapy may need to be tried.

REFERENCES

1. Ghai B, Dureja G. Complex regional pain syndrome: a review. *J Postgrad Med*. 2004;50:300–307.
2. Rho RH, Brewer RP, Lamer TJ, et al. Complex regional pain syndrome. *Mayo Clin Proc*. 2002;77:174–180.
3. Harden RN. Pharmacotherapy of complex regional pain syndrome. *Am J Phys Med Rehab* 2005; 84:s17–s28.
4. Atkins RM. Complex regional pain syndrome. *J Bone Joint Surg Br*. 2003;85:1100–1106.

 ## MISCELLANEOUS

See also: Arterial Embolus and Thrombosis; Herpes Zoster

CODES

ICD9-CM

- 337.21 Reflex sympathetic dystrophy of the upper limb
- 337.22 Reflex sympathetic dystrophy of the lower limb
- 354.4 Causalgia of upper limb
- 355.71 Causalgia of lower limb

PATIENT TEACHING

- Stress staying active physically.
- Instruct carefully about any prescribed medications.
- Internet: Reflex Sympathetic Dystrophy Syndrome Association www.rsds.org; (203) 877-3790 or American RSD Hope Group www.rsdhope.org; (207) 583-4589

See Patient Handout on CD

C

CONCUSSION

John Herbert Stevenson, MD
Christopher Lutryzkowski, MD
Peter L. Hoth, MD

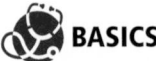 **BASICS**

DESCRIPTION
- A complex pathophysiological process affecting the brain, induced by traumatic biomechanical forces.
- Concussion severity can only be determined in retrospect.
- System(s) Affected: Cardiovascular; Endocrine/metabolic; Nervous; Psychiatric
- Synonym(s): Mild traumatic brain injury (TBI).

ALERT
Pediatric Considerations
Children (age 5–18) should not be allowed to return to training or play that same day and not until completely symptom free (1)[C].

GENERAL PREVENTION
- Safety education
- Rule enforcement in sports (e.g., penalties for spearing or head-to-head contact
- Consideration of rule changes in sports to decrease dangerous plays
- Current protective headgear for contact sports decreases facial injuries but has not been shown to decrease the overall concussion risk.

EPIDEMIOLOGY
- Predominant age: 12–24 years
- Predominant sex: Male > Female
- Usually seen with accidents versus sports-related

Incidence
- 0.14–3.66 injuries per 100 player season at the high school level
- 0.5–3.0 injuries per 1,000 athlete exposures at the collegiate level (2)[C]
- Average annual incidence 503:100,000.
- ~1.5 million cases of TBI in US annually, 85% of which are considered mild TBI
- ~10% of TBIs are related to sports or cycling injuries
- Among the 5–14 age group, 26.4% of mild TBI is related to sports or cycling (3)[B].

RISK FACTORS
Contact sports, history of recent concussion, substance use.

PATHOPHYSIOLOGY
Concussion represents a functional brain injury rather than a structural brain injury. The neurobiologic cascade has been shown to include excitatory amino acid release, ionic flux, hyperglycolysis, and reduced cerebral blood flow (4)[B].

ETIOLOGY
- Falls
- Sports-related
- Motor vehicle accidents

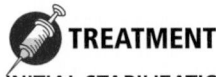 **DIAGNOSIS**

SIGNS AND SYMPTOMS
Variable and dependent on degree of injury
History
- Cognitive symptoms
  - Confusion
  - Posttraumatic amnesia (PTA)
  - Retrograde amnesia (RGA)
  - Loss of consciousness (LOC)
  - Disorientation
  - Feeling "in a fog," "zoned out"
  - Inability to focus
  - Delayed verbal and motor responses
  - Slurred/incoherent speech
  - Excessive drowsiness
- Somatic
  - Headache
  - Fatigue
  - Disequilibrium, dizziness
  - Visual disturbances
  - Phonophobia
- Affective
  - Emotional lability
  - Irritability

Physical Exam
- ABCs if seen acutely
- External evidence of major trauma
- Focal neurologic signs and symptoms
- Musculoskeletal: Evaluate for possible C-spine injury and stability
- Detailed neurologic exam including
  - State of alertness
  - Orientation
  - 3 or 5 word recall at 5 minutes
  - Concentration/attention (serial 3's or 7's)
  - Cerebellar function (Romberg)

TESTS
- The Sideline Assessment of Concussion (SAC) scale has been validated to drop from baseline after a concussion and return to baseline once symptoms clear (5)[B].
- Serial cognitive evaluations should be done by an experienced health care provider using the neurologic exam listed above or by using other assessment tools such as the SCAT Card (Sport Concussion Assessment Tool) (1)[C].
- Computerized neurocognitive testing to date lacks sufficient evidence on validity and cost effectiveness to warrant global usage (6)[B].
- Current gold standard is evaluation and treatment by a trained physician. Until improved outcomes, validity, and cost-effectiveness of computerized testing are established, use should be limited to experimental situations or possibly in management of complex concussions (1)[C].

Lab
Generally not necessary.

Imaging
- Structural neuroimaging is usually normal in the setting of concussion.
- Consider MRI or CT with prolonged LOC, focal neurologic deficit, or overall worsening symptoms in setting of complex concussion.
- Role of functional MRI is largely experimental and unvalidated at this time (1)[C].

Diagnostic Procedures/Surgery
Serial neurologic exams at least every 10–15 minutes until symptoms are clearing and patient is stabilizing or patient has been transported to hospital for further evaluation.

DIFFERENTIAL DIAGNOSIS
- Simple concussion: Symptoms from this injury typically resolve completely within 7–10 days.
- Complex concussion: This injury may exhibit persistent symptoms, encompasses prolonged LOC, and may show extended cognitive impairment after the initial injury.

TREATMENT

INITIAL STABILIZATION
- ABCs take priority over head injury and concussion.
- C-spine immobilization should be considered in all head trauma.

GENERAL MEASURES
- Acute management depends on severity of injury. Most patients need only physical and cognitive rest, serial clinical evaluations, to include neurologic checks, and a plan for follow-up evaluation (2)[C].
- Prolonged LOC, abnormal neurologic exam, or deteriorating symptoms necessitate urgent or emergent referral to the hospital for further evaluation (2)[C].

Diet
As tolerated.

Activity
- Complete rest until symptom free.
- Cognitive rest (including video games)
- May then begin gradual reintroduction of activity as long as symptom free (1)[C]
  - Light aerobic exercise
  - Sport specific exercise
  - Noncontact training drills
  - Full contact training
  - Game play
- If postconcussive symptoms occur (exertional headache, visual disturbance, or disequilibrium), decrease level of activity and try asymptomatic progress again in 24 hours.
- Return To Play Guidelines (Colorado) (8)

Symptoms	Grade	1st Concussion
Sx <15 min, no PTA	1	RTP when Sx free x 20 min
PTA <30 min, No LOC	2	RTP when Sx free x 1 mo
Any LOC	3	Transport to hospital

Sx, Symptoms; PTA, Post Trauma Amnesia; RTP, Return to Play; LOC, Loss of Consciousness

C

 MEDICATION (DRUGS)

- Simple concussion: Ibuprofen or acetaminophen may be use as adjunct pain management for headache (1)[C].
- Complex concussion: Prolonged symptomology with complex concussion such as sleep disturbance or anxiety may benefit from appropriate pharmacologic treatment for symptom relief (1)[C].

SURGERY
Generally not indicated, unless signs of more severe TBI present, with increased intracranial pressure or large bleed.

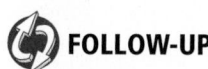 **FOLLOW-UP**

DISPOSITION
Admission Criteria
- Progressive neurologic symptoms including: Deterioration of mental status, seizures, and focal neurologic signs.
- No competent adult at home.

Discharge Criteria
- Improving mental status at or near baseline
- Competent adult at home for patient observation (see "Patient Monitoring")

Issues for Referral
- Simple concussions can be managed by most primary care physicians using the standard guidelines for return-to-play; generally, referral to a specialist is not needed (1)[C].
- Patients with a complex concussion should be referred to a sports medicine physician or neurologist for management and clearance prior to returning to sports activities (1)[C].

COMPLICATIONS
- Delayed hematomas, including subdural hematomas, can present minutes to hours after initial injury, necessitating serial neurologic checks and close observation.
- Postconcussion syndrome occurs when symptoms of concussion, such as headache, fatigue, memory changes, or emotional lability, are persistent and last >1–3 months (7)[B].
- Recurrent concussions can lead to 2nd-impact syndrome, or can occur with less and less impact force. Symptoms can persist longer than a 1st concussion, and progression to chronic cognitive and psychiatric symptoms is possible.
- 2nd-impact syndrome describes an additional insult or injury to a brain after a concussion and before the brain has had adequate time to completely recover. A rare, but life-threatening cerebral edema after a repeated head injury can occur. The etiology is thought to be due to loss of regulation of either cerebral circulation or glucose metabolism in the concussed brain.

PATIENT MONITORING
- Written instructions regarding postconcussion management should be given to a competent adult describing signs to watch for and when to bring the patient back for further evaluation.
- Have a follow-up plan prior to discharge to home, ideally to be seen within a few days.
- Instruct patients and families regarding postconcussive symptoms including the cognitive, somatic, and affective symptoms listed earlier.
- Ensure adequate rest and symptomfree return to both school and sports-related activities.

REFERENCES
1. McCrory P, Johnston K, Meeuwisse W, et al. Summary and agreement statement of the 2nd International Conference on Concussion in Sport, Prague 2004. *Br J Sports Med*. 2005;39:196–204.
2. Concussion (Mild Traumatic Brain Injury) and the Team Physician: A Consensus Statement. *Med Sci Sports Exerc*. 2006;38(2):395–399.
3. Bazarian JJ, McClung J, Shah MN, et al. Mild traumatic brain injury in the United States, 1998–2000. *Brain Injury*. 2005;19:85–91.
4. Giza CC, Hovda DA. The neurometabolic cascade of concussion. *J Athl Train*. 2001;36:228–235.
5. McCrea M, Kelly JP, Randolph C, et al. Standardized assessment of concussion (SAC): On-site mental status evaluation of the athlete. *J Head Trauma Rehab*. 1998;13(2):27–35.
6. Randolph C, McCrea M, Barr W. Is neuropsychological testing useful in the management of sport-related concussion? *J Athletic Train*. 2005;40(3):136–151.
7. Ryan LM, Warden DL, Post concussion syndrome. *Intern Rev Psychiatry*. 2003;15:310–316.
8. Colorado Medical Society School and Sports Medicine Committee. Guidelines for the management of concussion in sports. *Colo Med*. 1990;87:4.

 MISCELLANEOUS

See also: Traumatic brain injury; Brain injury—post acute care issues; Postconcussive syndrome; Seizure disorders

CODES

ICD9-CM
- 850.9 Concussion, unspecified
- 854.00 Intracranial injury of other and unspecified nature, without mention of intracranial wound, unspecified state of consciousness
- 310.2 Post-concussion syndrome

PATIENT TEACHING

Prevention
Useful website: www.thinkfirst.ca

 See Patient Handout on CD

CONDYLOMATA ACUMINATA

Carrie A. Jaworski, MD
Syed Hasan, MD

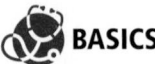 **BASICS**

DESCRIPTION

Condylomata acuminata are soft, skin-colored, fleshy warts that are caused by human Papillomavirus (HPV). More than 100 known types of HPV exist; types 6, 11, 16, 18, 31, 33, and 35 have been associated with condylomata acuminata. The disease is highly contagious; the warts may appear singly or in groups, small or large. They may appear in the vagina, on the cervix, around the external genitalia and rectum, and in the urethra and anus. Reports have been made of conjunctival, nasal, oral and laryngeal warts, and occasionally, of those affecting the throat. Incubation period may be from 1–6 months.

- System(s) Affected: Skin/Exocrine; Reproductive

Pregnancy Considerations
Consider sexual abuse if seen in children; although they can be infected by other means (e.g., transfer from wart on another child's hand).

Pregnancy Considerations
- Warts often grow larger during pregnancy and regress spontaneously after delivery. Use cryotherapy.
- Virus does not cross the placenta. Treatment during pregnancy is somewhat controversial. C-section is not absolutely indicated.
- Few documented cases of HPV transmission to infant at time of delivery have resulted in laryngeal papillomas, a rare and life-threatening condition.

GENERAL PREVENTION
- Use of condoms by male sexual partners of people who have been treated for HPV infection
- Use of condoms by infected men (preventive effects not adequately evaluated; 40% of infected men have scrotal warts)
- Abstinence by women until treatment completed
- Circumcision may prevent recurrence in some men.
- HPV vaccine: Phase II trial in progress, results appear encouraging.

EPIDEMIOLOGY
- Most common viral sexually transmitted disease (STD) in the US
- ~1% of the sexually active people in the United States carry the virus.
- 26% transmission after single encounter
- Predominant age: 15–30 years of age
- Predominant sex: Male = Female

Incidence
- ~750,000 new cases per year: Rates are increasing.
- Venereal warts are increasing in an ever-younger population. A recent study of 487 college women showed an infection rate of 48%.
- Increased size and number in immunocompromised patients

Prevalence
- Peak prevalence in ages 17–33
- Minimum of 10–20% of sexually active women may be infected with HPV. Studies in men suggest a similar prevalence.
- Pregnancy and immunosuppression favor recurrence and increasing growth of lesions.

RISK FACTORS
- Young adult
- Sexually active
- Not using condoms
- Possibly subclinical infection
- Young age of commencing sexual activity
- Cigarette smoking: Tobacco smoke has been shown to reduce cellular protection by decreasing cervical keratinocyte production.
- Poor hygiene
- Pregnancy
- White race
- History of genital warts

ETIOLOGY
Human Papillomaviruses, which are circular double-stranded DNA molecules. There are >70 HPV subtypes. Types 6 and 11 cause common venereal warts. Cervical dysplasia and carcinoma in situ are likely caused by types 16, 18, 31, 33, and 35.

ASSOCIATED CONDITIONS
- 90% of cervical cancer contains evidence of HPV infection.
- Gonorrhea
- Syphilis
- AIDS
- Chlamydia
- Other STD

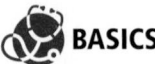 **DIAGNOSIS**

SIGNS AND SYMPTOMS
- Tumors may be soft, sessile
- Surface may be smooth or rough
- Multiple fingerlike projections
- Perianal condylomata acuminata usually rough and cauliflower-like
- Penile lesions often smooth and papular
- Penile lesions often occur in groups of 3 or 4.
- Male sites include frenulum, corona, glans, prepuce, meatus, shaft, and scrotum.
- Female sites include labia, clitoris, periurethral area, perineum, vagina, and cervix (flat lesions).
- Pruritus
- Irritation characterized by burning and redness
- Bleeding (result of trauma)
- Perianal area (both sexes)
- Subclinical HPV infection
- May be detected by test

History
Details regarding sexual history, contraception use, and other lifestyle issues must be explored.

Physical Exam
Acetowhitening: Subclinical lesions can be visualized by wrapping the penis with gauze soaked with 5% acetic acid for 5 minutes. Using a 10× hand lens or colposcope, warts appear as tiny white papules. A shiny white appearance of the skin represents foci of epithelial hyperplasia (subclinical infection). Not highly specific, low positive predictive value.

TESTS
Lab
- Serologic tests for syphilis negative
- Pap smear

Diagnostic Procedures/Surgery
Biopsy with highly specialized identification techniques rarely useful. HPV DNA detected through polymerase chain reaction

- Colposcopy
- Antroscopy
- Anoscopy
- Urethroscopy may be required to visualize intraurethral lesions.

Pathological Findings
- Possible cervical dysplasia
- Benign
- Well-organized basal layer
- Underlying infiltration of lymphocytes
- Plasma cells
- Hyperplastic epithelial changes
- Basement membrane intact
- Sometimes difficult to differentiate from squamous cell carcinoma

DIFFERENTIAL DIAGNOSIS
- Condylomata lata (flat warts of syphilis)
- Lichen planus
- Normal sebaceous glands
- Seborrheic keratosis
- Molluscum contagiosum
- Keratomas
- Scabies
- Crohn disease
- Skin tags
- Melanocytic nevi
- Vulvar intraepithelial neoplasia
- Buschke-Lowenstein tumor

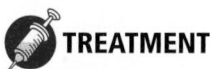 TREATMENT

PRE HOSPITAL
Disease is always seen on outpatient basis.

GENERAL MEASURES
- May resolve spontaneously
- Treatment determined by location, size of warts
- Small warts may be treated with topical applications of pharmacotherapeutic agents.
- Cryotherapy
- Change therapy if no improvement after 3 treatments, no complete clearance after 6 treatments, or therapy's duration or dosage exceeds manufacturer's recommendations.
- Appropriate screening and counseling of partners

Diet
No special diet

Activity
No restrictions, except for sexual contact

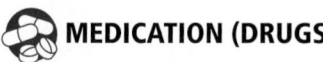 MEDICATION (DRUGS)

First Line
- Imiquimod (Aldara): 5% cream applied overnight 3 times weekly until warts resolve for up to 16 weeks
- Cryotherapy: Liquid nitrogen is applied to warts in 5–10-second bursts. Usually requires 2–3 weekly sessions
- Podophyllin in tincture of benzoin. Apply directly to warts. Leave on for 1–4 hours, then wash off. Repeat treatment every 7 days until gone (in-office procedure) or
- Podofilox (Condylox): Apply to external warts (affected area) q12h (allowing to dry) for 3 consecutive days. May repeat after 4 days (home application).
- Trichloroacetic acid: 25–85%. Apply only to warts. Use powder/talc to remove unreacted acid. Repeat in office at weekly intervals.
- Topical cidofovir gel: Undergoing phase III trials; applied once daily for 5 days every other week for maximum of 6 cycles
- Intralesion interferon has been shown to be effective in refractory cases and should be reserved for such cases.
- Contraindications
  – Podophyllin: Do not use in pregnant patients or on oral, cervical, urethral, or perianal warts. Can use on limited number of vaginal warts with careful drying after application.
  – Cryotherapy: Cryoglobulinemia

- Precautions
  – Podophyllin: To minimize local and systemic reactions, wash treated areas 1–4 hours after application and use ointments to protect surrounding skin from contact with podophyllin.
  – Cryotherapy: None
  – Electrocautery: Do not use in patients with pacemaker.

Second Line
- External (penile and perianal)
  – Podophyllin
  – Podofilox (Condylox) self-treatment
  – Intralesional interferon
  – Small study of topical use of Calmette-Guérin bacillus for penile lesions
- Urethral meatus
  – Podophyllin
  – Topical fluorouracil
- Anal
  – Trichloroacetic acid: Apply weekly.
  – Topical fluorouracil
- Oral
  – Trichloroacetic acid is ideal for isolated lesions in pregnant women.
  – Oral cimetidine: 30–40 mg/kg divided t.i.d. for 3 months in children with genital and perigenital condyloma. It is used as a primary and adjunctive therapy.

SURGERY
- Larger warts require laser treatment or electrocoagulation.
- Surgical excision for large warts
- Intraurethral, external (penile and perianal), anal and oral lesions can be treated with fulgurating CO_2 laser. Oral or external penile/perianal lesions can also be treated with electrocautery or surgery.

 FOLLOW-UP

PROGNOSIS
- Warts will clear with treatment or resolve spontaneously.
- Recurrences are frequent and may necessitate repeated treatment.
- Some studies identified 3 independent risk factors for condylomatous relapse: Positive HIV status, male gender, and Langerhans' Cell level: Cell level per mm of anal tissue (15 vs. 30)
- Without treatment, may remain stable, worsen, or resolve completely
- Asymptomatic infection persists indefinitely.

COMPLICATIONS
- Cervical dysplasia
- Malignant change: Progression to cancer rarely, if ever, occurs.
- Male urethral obstruction
- The prevalence of high-grade dysplasia and cancer in anal canal is higher in HIV-positive than in HIV-negative patients, probably because of HPV activity.

PATIENT MONITORING
- Patients must be seen every 2 weeks until lesions resolve and have annual Pap test for foreseeable future.
- Persistent warts require biopsy.
- Sexual partners require monitoring.
- Treatment does not decrease transmissible infectivity.

REFERENCES
1. Beutner KR, Wiley DJ, Douglas JM, et al. Genital warts and their treatment. *Clin Infect Dis.* 1999;28(suppl 1):537–556.
2. Bohle A, Buttner H, Jocham D, et al. Primary treatment of condylomata acuminata with viable bacillus Calmette-Guerin. *J Urol.* 2001;165: 834–836.
3. Edwards L. Imiquimod in clinical practice. *Aust J Dermatol.* 1998;39(suppl 1):S14–S16.
4. Fitzpatrick TB, et al. *Color atlas and synopsis of clinical dermatology.* New York, NY: McGraw-Hill; 1992.
5. Franco I. Oral cimetidine for the management of genital and perigenital warts in children. *J Urol.* 2000;164(suppl 3 pt 2):1074–1075.
6. Sobhani I, Vuagnat A, Walker F, et al. Prevalence of high-grade dysplasia and cancer in the anal canal in human papillomavirus-infected individuals. *Gastroenterology.* 2001;120:857–866.

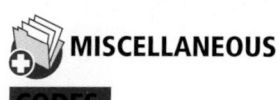 MISCELLANEOUS

CODES

ICD9-CM
078.11 Condyloma acuminata

PATIENT TEACHING
- Explain preventive measures and chronic nature of the infection.
- Numerous pamphlets on HPV, STD prevention, condom use
- Emphasize the need for women to get regular Pap smears.

See Patient Handout on CD

C

CONGENITAL MEGACOLON

Timothy L. Black, MD

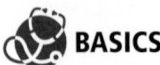 **BASICS**

DESCRIPTION
Congenital disease of the colon, characterized by functional obstruction, accumulation of feces, and massive dilatation of colon.

- System(s) Affected: Gastrointestinal; Nervous
- Synonym(s): Aganglionic megacolon; Hirschsprung disease; Zuelzer-Wilson disease (total colonic aganglionosis)

Pediatric Considerations
Occasionally infants have only mild or intermittent constipation with intervening bouts of diarrhea. These cases may not be diagnosed until later in infancy or childhood.

EPIDEMIOLOGY
- Predominant age: Infancy
- Predominant sex
  – Males > Females for short segment (8:2)
  – Males > Females for long segment (5:4)

Incidence
1 in 2,000–5,000 births in the US (white 91%, black 8%, Asian 0.5%)

RISK FACTORS
- Family history of Hirschsprung disease
- Offspring risk if parent has short segment, 2%; if parent has long segment, up to 50%
- Sibling risk if male affected: Female has 0.6% risk (short segment)
- Sibling risk if female affected: Male has 18% risk (long segment)

Genetics
- Familial 50 times base rate
- Sometimes associated with Down syndrome
- Dominant mutations in the RET gene is found in 50% of familial patients with Hirschsprung disease and in 15–35% of patients with sporadic Hirschsprung disease (10q11.2 locus). Other gene mutations have also been implicated.

ETIOLOGY
- Congenital absence of Auerbach and Meissner autonomic plexuses in bowel wall (usually limited to the colon)
- Aganglionosis results in the lack of propagation of propulsive waves of muscle contraction and absence of relaxation of the internal anal spincter.

ASSOCIATED CONDITIONS
- Associated anomalies are found in 11–30% of patients (especially neurologic, and cardiovascular, urologic, and gastrointestinal) (1,2)[C]
- Chagas disease (secondary aganglionic megacolon may be a late complication of Chagas)
- Megacolon, acquired, functional, usually begins in 3rd or 4th year of life
- Down syndrome (3% of patients with Hirschsprung 4 times the expected incidence of Down syndrome in the normal population)
- Cardiovascular defects (6%)
- Urogenital anomalies (11%)
- Dandy-Walker syndrome
- Cataract, coloboma, microphthalmia, etc.
- Cleft palate
- Congenital small or large bowel atresia
- Waardenburg syndrome
- Ondine syndrome
- Sipple syndrome (medullary throid carcinoma, hyperparathyroidism, Cushing disease, Hirschsprung disease),
- MEN-IIB syndrome
- Prematurity in 7% (1)[C]

DIAGNOSIS

SIGNS AND SYMPTOMS
- Early infancy
  – Onset early in infancy, newborn fails to pass meconium in 24–48 hours after birth
  – Obstipation
  – May have diarrhea
  – Marked abdominal distention
  – Colonic peristalsis visible
  – Vomiting
  – Palpable fecal mass
  – Growth retardation (possible)
- Older infants
  – Failure to thrive
  – Anorexia
  – Severe constipation
  – Lack of physiologic urge to defecate
  – Empty rectum on digital examination
  – Palpable colon
  – Visible peristalsis
  – Hypoalbuminemia

History
- Constipation
- Poor feeding habits
- Vomiting

Physical Exam
- Abdominal distension
- Palpable fecal mass on abdominal exam
- Empty rectum
- Explosive diarrhea on rectal exam possible

TESTS

Lab
- Electrolytes, albumin, CBC, urinalysis, thyroid function
- Proctoscopy: Ampulla empty of feces
- Biopsy: Absence of ganglia in wall of narrowed rectum
- Anorectal manometry

Imaging
Radiograph-barium enema (unprepped) shows

- Large ovoid fecal mass mottled by small, irregular gas shadows
- Dilatation of sigmoid colon above narrowed distal sigmoid or rectum
- Narrowed portion rippled or segmented
- Typical transition zone between narrowed distal colon and dilated proximal bowel
- Fluid levels within proximal bowel loops
- Diaphragm may be elevated

Diagnostic Procedures/Surgery
- Suction aspiration biopsy of bowel wall (2 cm above dentate line)
  – Can be done without anesthesia at bedside
- Full-thickness biopsy may be required if suction biopsy equivocal
- Barium enema
- Proctosigmoidoscopy (not often of value without biopsy)
- Laparoscopy: Normal proximal colon dilatation
- Anorectal manometry: Internal sphincter relaxation failure

Pathological Findings
- Congenital absence of Auerbach and Meissner autonomic plexuses in myenteric plexus of colon wall
- Obstruction may begin at anus and may extend proximally to involve varying portions of the colon and small bowel (rarely may involve entire small bowel).
- Enormous dilatation and hypertrophy of all layers proximal to involved colon
- Aganglionosis of involved bowel
- Submucosal hypertrophied nerve bundles

DIFFERENTIAL DIAGNOSIS
- Megacolon, secondary (to Chagas disease)
- Megacolon, acquired, functional
- Functional constipation
- Hypoganglionosis
- Meconium plug syndrome
- Small left colon syndrome
- Meconium ileus

TREATMENT

INITIAL STABILIZATION
- Early workup (ambulatory or hospital)
- Inpatient for surgery

GENERAL MEASURES
- Treatment may be symptomatic or definitive.
- May need emergency correction of fluid and electrolyte imbalance
- Removal of fecal accumulation: Retention enemas of 3–4 ounces (90–120 mL) of mineral oil followed by repeated colonic irrigations with isotonic saline solution. Avoid use of other solutions (e.g., water, soapsuds, enemas).
- May require manual disimpaction for short segment Hirschsprung disease.

Diet
- Diet will not control the obstipation of Hirschsprung.
- Postoperative diet: Standard for age when bowel function returns

 MEDICATION (DRUGS)

First Line
- None recommended for treatment
- Preliminary to surgery: Bowel prep

Second Line
Metronidazole (Flagyl) for bowel preparation

SURGERY
- Inpatient surgery
  - Proximal colostomy and resection of aganglionic bowel is gold standard (and necessary when there is significant proximal dilation)
  - Definitive pull-through procedure (Duhamel, Soave, or Swenson) when dilation has resolved (usually 2–4 months) (3)[C]
  - Single-stage procedure may be possible in infants
  - Transanal endorectal pull-through in infants if proximal bowel not too dilated (4)[C]
- This is usually done without a protective colostomy.
  - Laparoscopic technique may be used alone or combined with transanal endorectal pull-through.
- Confirmation of normal ganglion cells mandatory at colostomy site and proximal resection site prior to anastomosis
- Total colon Hirschsprung disease may require other procedures, including Martin's modification of Duhamel's pull-through (5)[C]
  - Cecal patches have also been used.

 FOLLOW-UP

PROGNOSIS
- Favorable
  - Decreasing mortality over past 25 years, now estimated at ≤3% (2)[C]
- Requires long-term follow-up
- Requires aggressive management of any suspected Hirschsprung enterocolitis with
  - Rectal irrigation
  - IV antibiotics
  - Nasogastric decompression

COMPLICATIONS
- Toxic enterocolitis, possibly fatal
  - Enterocolitis may occur before or after definitive pull-through
  - Enterocolitis may be rapidly progressive
- Bleeding and/or perforation

PATIENT MONITORING
Closely until recuperated fully from surgical intervention

REFERENCES
1. Ryan ET, Ecker JL, Christakis NA, et al. Hirschsprung's disease: Associated abnormalities and demography. *J Pediatr Surg.* 1992;27:76–81.
2. Suita S, Taguchi T, Ieiri S, et al. Hirschsprung's disease in Japan: Analysis of 3852 patients based on a nationwide survey in 30 years. *J Ped Surg.* 2005;40:197–202.
3. Salch W, Rasheed K, Mahaidly MA, et al. Management of Hirschsprung's disease: A comparison of Soave's and Duhamel's pull-through methods. *Pediatr Surg Int.* 2004;20:590–593.
4. Elhalaby EA, Hashish A, Elbarbary MM, et al. Transanal one-stage endorectal pull-through for Hirschsprung's Disease: A multicenter study. *J Ped Surg.* 2004;39:345–351.
5. Wildhaber BE, Teitelbaum DH, Coran AG. Total colonic Hirschsprung's disease: A 28-year experience. *J Ped Surg.* 2005;40:203–207.

 MISCELLANEOUS

ALERT
- Other notes: Diagnosis must be made as early as possible to prevent toxic enterocolitis
- See also: Constipation

CODES

ICD9-CM
751.3 Hirschsprung disease and other congenital functional disorders of colon

PATIENT TEACHING
- After surgery, instruct parents to detect and report dehydration, decreased urinary output, sunken eyes, poor skin turgor, vomiting, or fever.
- Encourage bonding with parents by having parents participate in their child's care as much as possible including participation in colostomy care.
- Request enterostomal therapist to teach family appropriate colostomy care.

 See Patient Handout on CD

C

CONGESTIVE HEART FAILURE

Dennis E. Hughes, DO

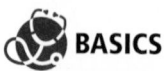 **BASICS**

DESCRIPTION

Affecting both the cardiovascular and pulmonary systems, congestive heart failure is the principal complication of heart disease. It is a pathophysiologic state produced by an abnormality in cardiac pump function, either transient or prolonged. The heart is unable to transport blood in a sufficient flow to meet metabolic needs.

- 2 physiologic components explain most of the clinical findings of congestive heart failure
  - An inotropic abnormality, often due to myocardial infarction, resulting in diminished systolic emptying (systolic dysfunction). Ejection fraction <45%.
  - A compliance abnormality, normally due to hypertensive cardiomyopathy, in which the ability of the ventricles to accept blood is impaired (diastolic dysfunction). Ejection fraction >45% (1).

ALERT
Geriatric Considerations
- Medications may need dosage adjustment.
- Age-related cardiomyopathy

Pediatric Considerations
Usually associated with forms of congenital heart disease

Pregnancy Considerations
If condition develops during pregnancy, it will require special care.

GENERAL PREVENTION
Treat underlying disorders when possible.

EPIDEMIOLOGY
Incidence
- Affects 4.8 million in US; 500,000 new cases annually.
- Primarily a disease of the elderly; 75% of hospital admission for HF in persons >65.
- Incidence and prevalence not decreased in 2 decades (2).

RISK FACTORS
- Iatrogenic reduction of intensity of therapy
- Inappropriate sodium and/or fluid excess
- Patient noncompliance with therapy
- Intercurrent arrhythmia (e.g., atrial fibrillation)
- Administration of drug with negative inotropic effects
- Excessive physical, emotional, or environmental stress
- Thyrotoxicosis, pregnancy, or any condition associated with increased metabolic demand
- Recent pregnancy (postpartum cardiomyopathy)

ETIOLOGY
- Coronary artery disease
- Myocardial infarction
- Cardiomyopathy
  - Alcoholism
  - Viral
  - Long-standing hypertension
  - Drugs (e.g., chemotherapeutic agents)
  - Muscular dystrophy
  - Amyloidosis
  - Postpartum state

- Valvular abnormalities
  - Aortic stenosis or regurgitation
  - Rheumatic heart disease (mitral and aortic valvular disease)
- Renal artery stenosis, usually bilateral, may cause recurrent "flash" pulmonary edema
- Volume overload
- Cardiac depressants; negative inotropes (e.g., β-blockers, IV amiodarone)
- Arrhythmias (atrial fibrillation)
- High output states
  - Hyperthyroidism
  - Beriberi-related heart disease
  - Anemia
- HIV

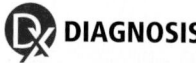 **DIAGNOSIS**

SIGNS AND SYMPTOMS
- Dyspnea on exertion—cardinal sign of left heart failure
- Deteriorating exercise capacity
- Easy fatigue
- Difficulty breathing
- Weakness
- Nocturia
- Nocturnal nonproductive cough
- Orthopnea
- Paroxysmal nocturnal dyspnea
- Wheezing, especially nocturnal in absence of history of asthma or infection (cardiac asthma)
- Anorexia
- Fullness or dull pain in right upper quadrant
- Anxiety
- Cool extremities owing to peripheral vasoconstriction
- Edema
- Cerebral dysfunction
- Abdominal bloating (ascites)
- Cyanosis
- Hypotension
- Anasarca
- Frothy and/or pink sputum
- Cardiac cachexia
- Cheyne-Stokes respirations

Physical Exam
- Positive hepatojugular reflux
- Rales
- Hepatomegaly
- S3 gallop
- Ascites
- Peripheral edema

TESTS
Lab
- β-type natriuretic peptide may be helpful in
  - Titrating treatment because its value changes rapidly
  - ED setting to help differentiate the cause of dyspnea

- β-type natriuretic peptide is a useful marker of ventricular dysfunction. It is a cardiac neurohormone secreted from the ventricles in an increasing amount in response to abnormal pressure overload and increasing volume. β-type natriuretic peptide has been shown to better predict the presence or absence of CHF than any set of clinical or lab measures of the cause of dyspnea. A level of <100 pg/mL essentially rules out heart failure (NPV ~99%) as a cause of dyspnea. Patients with BNP values >500 pg/mL have a high probability (PPV ~70%) of heart failure as a cause of clinical dyspnea (3).
- BNP values may be increased in older patients, renal failure, women, pulmonary disease, systemic hypertension, and hypothyroidism among others (3).
- Lab findings in early and mild to moderately severe congestive heart failure
  - Respiratory alkalosis
  - Mild azotemia
  - Decreased erythrocyte sedimentation rate
  - Proteinuria (usually <1 g/24 h that clears with treatment)
- Lab findings
  - Increased creatinine
  - Hyperbilirubinemia in severe cases
  - Dilutional hyponatremia

Imaging
- Echocardiographic studies are most useful to determine ejection fraction and valvular abnormalities.
- Nuclear imaging to evaluate left and right ventricular size and systolic function
- Radiograph
  - Increased heart size
  - Interstitial edema
  - Kerley B lines
  - Subpleural effusions
  - Alveolar edema
  - Butterfly pattern of pulmonary edema

Diagnostic Procedures/Surgery
- Complete pulmonary function tests.
- Cardiac catheterization, both right and left, for full diagnosis and prognosis
- Heart valve surgery may be needed if defective heart valve is responsible; mitral valve repair especially helpful if mitral regurgitation is aggravating condition.
- Cardiac transplantation to be considered in patients <55 and without other disqualifying medical problems who are developing CHF unresponsive to other therapeutic maneuvers, and who are considered to have a life expectancy of <1 year.
- Biventricular pacing

Pathological Findings
- Early and acute
  - Firm lungs with microscopic revealing engorged capillaries with thickening of the alveolar septa with extravasation of red cells and edema fluid
  - Liver is engorged, firm, and fluid-filled. Microscopic analysis reveals dilated central hepatic veins and sinusoids.
- Late and chronic
  - Hemosiderin deposits in lungs.
  - "Nutmeg" liver with centrilobular necrosis
  - Occasionally, hemorrhagic nonbacterial enterocolitis with hemorrhagic necrosis secondary to mesenteric vasoconstriction

DIFFERENTIAL DIAGNOSIS
- Simple dependent edema
- Exertional asthma
- Severe diffuse coronary artery disease
- Occult chronic obstructive pulmonary disease
- Nephrotic syndrome
- Cirrhosis
- Venous occlusive disease with subsequent peripheral edema

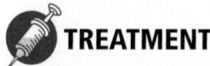 TREATMENT

INITIAL STABILIZATION
Inpatient care needed in severe cases

GENERAL MEASURES
- Treat heart failure immediately.
- Search for underlying correctable conditions.
- Eliminate contributing factors when possible.
- Supply supplemental oxygen.
- Antiembolism stockings
- Restrict fluids and sodium. Educating patient about this is imperative for long-term control. Maintaining weight daily guides overall therapy.
- Identify and control underlying correctable conditions (e.g., acute myocardial infarction, valvular disease, hyperthyroidism, but most commonly inadvertent salt and/or fluid overload).

Diet
- Restrict sodium (initially 4 g/d).
- Reduce weight if needed.
- Follow low-fat diet to retard CAD.
- Restrict fluids as needed.

Activity
Cardiac rehabilitation to increase functional capacity as well as long-term prognosis and quality of life (1).

 MEDICATION (DRUGS)

First Line
For acute symptoms, use of nitroglycerine (0.4 mg sublingual) is effective in quickly vasodilating and reducing preload and afterload. Followed by use of a short-acting ACE inhibitor and a loop diuretic can profoundly improve the clinical picture.
- ACE inhibitors
  - Used to decrease afterload: Shown to increase survival Improve general symptomatology and overall exercise capacity (4)[B].
  - Angiotensin receptor blockers
  - Less side effects than ACE inhibitors
  - Equivalency to ACE inhibitors not established.
  - Valsartan only ARB to have FDA approval for HF treatment (2,4).
- β-Blockers used in systolic HF
- Carvedilol: 3.125 mg b.i.d. to a maintenance of 25 mg b.i.d.
- Metoprolol extended release: 12.5 mg/d to a maximum of 200 mg/d (2).
- Digoxin reduces symptoms, but has not shown any effect on mortality
  - Effects similar in all age groups.
  - In patients with preserved renal function (creatine clearance >50 cc/min), the recommended dose is 0.125 mg/d (2).
- Diuretics helpful to manage volume overload
  - Furosemide (Lasix): 20–80 mg IV/IM/PO.
  - Metolazone (Zaroxolyn): 5–0 mg PO per day.
  - Spironolactone (only diuretic to reduce mortality when added to standard therapy): 12.5–25 mg PO per day. Maximum 50 mg PO per day. (2)[A].
- Vasodilators
  - IV nitroglycerin may be of short-term benefit to decrease preload, afterload, and systemic resistance.
  - The combination of hydralazine (75 mg/d) and isosorbide dinitrate (40 mg q.i.d.) is effective in persons unable to take ACE inhibitors or an ARB (2).
- Contraindications: Refer to manufacturer's literature.

Second Line
- Dobutamine can be used on an intermittent outpatient basis with intermittent infusions. However, despite possibly improving quality of life, it reduces short-term survival.
- Natrecor is approved for short term use in decompensated heart failure. It is a recombinant form of human brain nature tic peptide. It is given in a bolus followed by a continuos infusion for 24–48 hours (5).

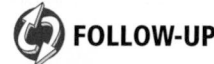 FOLLOW-UP

PROGNOSIS
- Result of initial treatment is usually good, whatever the cause.
- Long-term prognosis variable. Mortality rates range from 10% with mild symptoms to 50% with advanced, progressive symptoms.

COMPLICATIONS
- Electrolyte disturbance
- Atrial and ventricular arrhythmias
- Mesenteric insufficiency
- Protein enteropathy
- Digitalis intoxication

PATIENT MONITORING
- Variable depending on clinical circumstances. Initially every 2–3 weeks after patient stabilized.
- Home visits by trained home health nurses have shown decreased hospitalizations.

REFERENCES
1. Clark AL. Origin of symptoms in chronic heart failure. *BMJ Heart.* 2006;92(10):12–16.
2. Rich MW. Drug therapy of heart failure in the elderly. *Am J Geriatr Cardiol.* 2003;12(4):235–242.
3. Bettencourt PM. Clinical usefulness of B-type natriuretic peptide measurements: Present and future perspectives. *BMJ Heart.* 2005;91(11):1489–1494.
4. Eisenberg MJ, Gioria LC. Angiotensen II receptor blockers in congestive heart failure. *Cardiol Rev.* 2006;14(1):26–34.
5. Shatsky M. Nesiritide (Natrecor) for acute decompensated heart failure. *Am Fam Phy.* 2006;73(4):687–688.
6. Tang WH, et al. Aldosterone receptor antagonists in the medical management of chronic heart failure. *Mayo Clin Proc.* 2005;80(2):1623–1630.

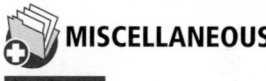 MISCELLANEOUS

CODES

ICD9-CM
428.0 Congestive heart failure, unspecified

PATIENT TEACHING
- Printed patient information available from:
- American Heart Association, 7320 Greenville Avenue, Dallas, TX 75231, (214)373-6300
- American College of Cardiology, 911 Old Georgetown Road, Bethesda, MD 20814, (301) 897-5400

 See Corresponding Diagnostic Algorithm

 See Patient Handout on CD

CONJUNCTIVITIS, ACUTE

Frances Y. Wu, MD

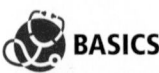**BASICS**

DESCRIPTION
- Inflammation of the bulbar and/or palpebral conjunctiva <4 weeks duration
- System(s) Affected: Nervous; Skin/Exocrine
- Synonym(s): Pink eye

Geriatric Considerations
More likely to have autoimmune, systemic, or irritative conditions

Pediatric Considerations
- Neonatal conjunctivitis may be gonococcal, chlamydial, irritative, or related to dacryocystitis. Gonococcal ophthalmia neonatorum requires emergency admission and consultation.
- Daycare regulations often require any child with presumed conjunctivitis be treated with an antibiotic prior to readmission, despite the lack of evidence to support their need.

GENERAL PREVENTION
Wash hands frequently.

EPIDEMIOLOGY
- Predominant age: Pediatric: Viral Adult: Viral, bacterial, allergic
- Predominant sex: Male = Female

Incidence
In the US: Variable, but accounts for 1–2% of all ambulatory office visits

RISK FACTORS
- History of contact with infected persons; bacterial or viral conjunctivitis
- Sexually transmitted disease (STD) contact: Gonococcal, chlamydial, syphilis, or herpes
- Use of contact lenses: Pseudomonal
- Epidemic bacterial (streptococcal) conjunctivitis reported in school settings

ETIOLOGY
- Viral
  - Adenovirus (common cold)
  - Coxsackie
  - Enterovirus (acute hemorrhagic conjunctivitis)
  - Herpes simplex, primary and recurrent
  - Herpes zoster or varicella
  - Molluscum contagiosum
  - Measles, mumps, or influenza
- Bacterial
  - *Staphylococcus aureus*
  - *Staphylococcus epidermidis*
  - *Streptococcus pneumoniae*
  - *Haemophilus influenzae* (especially in children)
  - Pseudomonas species (in contact lens users; frequently progresses to corneal ulcers)
  - *Neisseria gonorrhoeae*
  - *Neisseria meningitidis*
  - *Chlamydia trachomatis* causes a chronic conjunctivitis: Gradual onset >4 weeks
- Allergic
  - Hay fever, seasonal allergies
  - Vernal conjunctivitis/atopy
- Nonspecific
  - Irritative: Topical medications, wind, or dry eye, ultraviolet light exposure, smoke
  - Autoimmune: Sjögren, pemphigoid, Wegeners granulomatosis
  - Rare: Rickettsial, fungal, parasitic, tuberculosis, syphilis, Kawasaki disease, Grave disease, gout, carcinoid, sarcoid, psoriasis, Stevens-Johnson, Reiter syndrome

ASSOCIATED CONDITIONS
- Viral infection (e.g., common cold)
- STDs

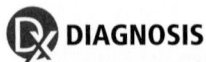**DIAGNOSIS**

SIGNS AND SYMPTOMS
- General: Common to all conjunctivitis
  - Red eye, conjunctival injection
  - Foreign body sensation
  - Eyelid sticking or crusting, discharge
  - Normal visual acuity and papillary reactivity (otherwise see: "Differential Diagnosis")
- Viral
  - Watery mucous discharge
  - Inferior palpebral conjunctival follicles
  - Palpable preauricular lymphadenopathy
  - Severe viral: Herpes simplex or zoster
    ○ Burning sensation, rarely itching
    ○ Unilateral, with concurrent herpetic skin vesicles on eyelid or in distribution of ophthalmic branch of trigeminal nerve if herpes zoster
    ○ Palpable preauricular node
- Bacterial, nongonococcal: May be epidemic
  - Mild pruritus, mild discharge
  - Conjunctival chemosis/edema
  - No preauricular adenopathy
  - If contact lens user, must rule out pseudomonal keratitis
- Bacterial, gonococcal hyperacute infection
  - Rapid onset 12–24 hours
  - Severe purulent discharge
  - Chemosis/conjunctival edema
  - May have rapid growth of superior corneal ulceration
  - Eyelid swelling
  - Preauricular adenopathy
  - History or signs of other STDs (chlamydia, HIV, etc.)
- Allergic
  - Itching most dominant symptom
  - Watery discharge
  - History of seasonal or dander allergies
  - Chemosis/conjunctival edema
  - Eyelids edematous and red
  - No preauricular adenopathy
- Nonspecific irritative
  - Dry eyes with intermittent redness and mucus
  - Irritation after a chemical exposure or drug reaction
  - Foreign body: May still have redness and discharge 24 hours after removal

History
- Any change in visual acuity implies complications, not just conjunctivitis.
- Viral: Personal or contact with upper respiratory infection
  - May start with one eye, then progress to both
  - If herpetic, may have history of recurrences or burning sensation with vesicles
- Bacterial: Difficult to distinguish from viral, unless contact lens user
- Allergic: Itching is predominant symptom in eye and nose
  - Seasonal or dander allergies
  - Family history of atopy or asthma
- Irritative: Feels dry, exposure to wind, chemicals, or drug
- Foreign body: Redness may persist 24 hours after removal

Physical Exam
- Must note visual acuity
- Skin: Look for herpetic vesicles, nits, or styes
- Limbal flush at corneal margin if uveitis
- Discharge but no injection if blepharitis

TESTS
Lab
- Usually not needed initially for the most common causes of conjunctivitis
- Culture swab if thought to be bacterial or if contact lens user

Imaging
- Diagnostic procedures/surgery
- Fluorescein staining to detect foreign bodies, corneal ulcers, or punctate keratitis and look for dendritic lesions of herpes simplex or zoster

DIFFERENTIAL DIAGNOSIS
- Uveitis (iritis, iridocyclitis, choroiditis): Limbal flush (red band at corneal margin, less on other areas of conjunctiva), hazy anterior chamber, and decreased visual acuity
- Penetrating ocular trauma: Ophthalmologic emergency; hospitalize
- Acute glaucoma (ophthalmologic emergency): Headache, corneal clouding, decreased visual acuity
- Corneal ulcer(s) or foreign body: Abnormal fluorescein exam
- Dacryocystitis: Tenderness and swelling over tear sac (near nasal bridge)
- Scleritis and episcleritis: Red injected vessels are radially oriented, sectoral (pie wedge) inflammation, sometimes with nodularity of sclera
- Ophthalmia neonatorum: Neonates in 1st 2 days of life (gonococcal; 5–12 days of life): Chlamydial, consider herpes simplex virus (HSV) if maternal cultures were positive for herpes simplex. Consider specialty consultation. All of these require systemic therapy.

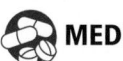

TREATMENT

GENERAL MEASURES
- Appropriate health care: Outpatient
- Cool compresses and eyelid cleansing with wet cloth up to q.i.d.
- Discontinue use of contact lenses for duration of inflammation
- Patching of eye not beneficial
- Try to avoid irritants such as smoke, dry wind, and prolonged sun exposure.

MEDICATION (DRUGS)

First Line
- Viral (nonherpetic)
  - Artificial tears for symptomatic relief
  - Vasoconstrictor/antihistamine (e.g., Naphazoline/Pheniramine) q.i.d. for severe itching
  - Consider inexpensive, topical antibiotic ointments for social reasons (e.g., return to daycare required) (1)[C]
  - Erythromycin ophthalmic 0.5% ointment b.i.d. for 5 days or
  - 10% sodium sulfacetamide ophthalmic drops 2 drops q4h for 5 days.
  - Tobramycin ophthalmic 0.3% drops, 2 drops q6h for 5 days
- Viral (herpetic): Should be supervised by opthalmologist
  - Triflumidine: 1% drops 1 q2h (1)[C].
  - Acyclovir oral: 400 mg 5 times a day for HSV (use 800 mg for Zoster) × 7 days.
- Bacterial (nongonococca INNT 5 to reduce symptoms by 1–2 days. Usually self-limited 5–7 days, so treatment is optional except for chlamydial (by history) (2)[B], (3)[A]
  - Bacitracin ophthalmic: 1/2 inch b.i.d.–q.i.d. for 5 days or
  - Erythromycin ophthalmic ointment: 1/2 inch b.i.d.–q.i.d. for 5 days or
  - Sodium sulfacetamide (10% solution:) 2 drops q4h (while awake) for 5 days
  - Tobramycin ophthalmic 0.3% drops: 2 drops q6h for 5 days
  - Chlamydial in neonates requires oral erythromycin ethyl succinage 30 mg/kg daily q6h PO × 14 d, max 3 g/d
- Bacterial (gonorrheal)
  - Consider emergent ophthalmologic consultation and hospitalization for IV ceftriaxone.
  - If no corneal lesions, ceftriaxone 1 g IM as single dose and topical bacitracin ophthalmic ointment 1/2 inch q.i.d.
  - Avoid aminoglycoside drops and neomycin ointments, as they can cause a reactive keratoconjunctivitis after a few days of use.
- Allergic and atopic
  - Artificial tears, 4–8 times per day
  - Vasoconstrictor/antihistamine q.i.d.
  - Ketotifen 1 drop b.i.d.
  - Olopatadine (Patanol) b.i.d.–t.i.d.
  - Azelastin 1 drop b.i.d. (4)[C]
  - Cromolyn (Opticrom) 4%, q.i.d. (4)[C]

- Oral non-sedating antihistamines (Zyrtec (cetirizine) 10 mg/d, Allegra (fexofenadine) 60 mg b.i.d., etc. have shown similar efficacy to topical agents and treat nasal and urticarial symptoms as well
- Oral antihistamine (e.g., diphenhydramine 25 mg t.i.d.) in severe cases
- Contraindications: Avoid use of topical steroids unless in ophthalmologic setting and able to monitor intraocular pressure
- Precautions
  - Do not allow dropper to touch eye or skin to avoid contamination. Discard old eye cosmetics after an infection.
  - Vasoconstrictor/antihistamine: Rebound vasodilation after prolonged use
  - Avoid topical steroids in nonophthalmologic setting, as patients must be monitored for development of steroid-related cataracts and glaucoma. If superior shield ulcer of vernal conjunctivitis is present, refer to ophthalmology for steroids.

Second Line
- Viral and allergic: Numerous OTC and prescription topical vasoconstrictors and antihistamines
- Bacterial
  - Polymyxin-gramicidin

FOLLOW-UP

DISPOSITION
Admission Criteria
Penetrating ocular trauma; emergency consultation

Issues for Referral
Decreased visual acuity, herpetic keratitis, or contact lens-related bacterial conjunctivitis: Recommend specialty consultation.

PROGNOSIS
- Viral: 5–10 days for pharyngitis with conjunctivitis
- Several weeks for epidemic keratoconjunctivitis
- Herpes simplex: 2–3 weeks
- Bacterial: Self-limited treated, 4 days, untreated 5–7 days

COMPLICATIONS
- Corneal scars with herpes simplex
- Neonatal herpes simplex could include encephalitis.
- Lid scars or entropion with Varicella zoster
- Bacterial superinfection
- Chronic marginal blepharitis
- Conjunctival scar if membrane develops
- Corneal ulcers or perforation, very rapid with gonococcal
- Hypopyon: Pus in anterior chamber
- Chlamydial neonatal ophthalmia: Could have concomitant pneumonia

PATIENT MONITORING
- Referral if worse in 24 hours
- Bacterial: Expect improvement in 24 hours and resolution in 2–5 days.

REFERENCES
1. Greenberg MF, Pollard ZF. The red eye in childhood. *Pediatr Clin North Am.* 2003;50:105–124.
2. David SP. Should we prescribe antibiotics for acute conjunctivitis? *Am Fam Physician.* 2002;66: 1649–1650.
3. Sheikh A, Hurwitz B Topical antibiotics for acute bacterial conjunctivitis: A systematic review. *Br J Gen Pract.* 2001;467;473–477.
4. Bielory L, et al. Efficacy and tolerability of newer antibistamines in the treatment of allergic conjunctivitis. *Drugs.* 2005;65(2):215–228.
5. Martin M, Turco JH, Zegans ME, et al. An outbreak of conjunctivitis due to atypical Streptococcus pneumoniae. *N Engl J Med.* 2003;348:1112–1121.
6. Rietveld, RP, et al. Predicting bacterial cause in infectious conjunctivitis: Cohort study on informativeness of combinations of signs and symptoms, *BMJ.* 2004;329;206–210.

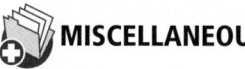

MISCELLANEOUS

See also: Rhinitis; Allergic

CODES

ICD9-CM
- 077.99 Unspecified diseases of conjunctiva due to viruses
- 372.50 Conjunctival degeneration, unspecified
- 372.14 Other chronic allergic conjunctivitis

PATIENT TEACHING

Prevention
Demonstrate eye dropper techniques: While eye is closed, and head tipped back, drop several drops in a lake at nasal margin; then patient can open eyes to allow liquid to enter. Never touch tip of applicator to skin or eye.

 See Corresponding Diagnostic Algorithm

 See Patient Handout on CD

CONSTIPATION

Abdulazrak Abyad, MD, PhD, MBA, MPH, AGSF

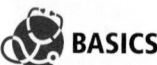

BASICS

DESCRIPTION
A combination of changes in the frequency, size, consistency, and ease of stool passage, which leads to an overall decrease in the volume of bowel movements. Highly subjective interpretation, with each person having an individual threshold to define the term. Affects gastrointestinal (GI) system. Obstipation is often used to mean intractable constipation.

Geriatric Considerations
* People who have enjoyed regular bowel movements throughout their lives, seldom suffer constipation owing to age alone.
* People with a lifelong tendency to constipation often encounter increasing difficulty with advancing age.
* Increased incidence of colorectal neoplasms with age may be associated with constipation.

Pediatric Considerations
Consider Hirschsprung disease.

Pregnancy Considerations
Women with a tendency to constipation may find the condition more troublesome in the 3rd trimester and require dietary adjustment and supplements.

GENERAL PREVENTION
Because for some patients a tendency to constipation is habitual, instruction in proper diet, bowel training, and use of bulk-forming supplements must be reinforced.

EPIDEMIOLOGY
Predominant age: May affect all ages, but more pronounced in children and older people. Affects most people at some point in course of life.
Predominant sex: Female > Male

RISK FACTORS
* Extremes of life (very young and very old)
* Neurosis
* Polypharmacy
* Sedentary lifestyle or condition
* Improper diet and inadequate or improper fluid intake

Genetics
Unknown, but condition may be familial

ETIOLOGY
* Electrolyte abnormalities
  – Hypercalcemia
  – Hypokalemia
* Hormonal abnormalities
  – Hypothyroidism
  – Diabetes
* Congenital impediments (e.g., aganglionic megacolon [Hirschsprung disease] or excessively elongate, redundant, capacious bowel [dolichocolon])
* Congenital or acquired neuromuscular bowel impairment (pseudo-obstruction)
* Concomitant illness, injury, or debility
* Mechanical bowel impediment (obstruction or ileus, resulting from any cause)
* Inadequate fluid intake

* Side-effect of drugs (e.g., anticholinergic agents, opiates)
* Chronic abuse of laxatives or cathartics
* Psychiatric, cultural, emotional, environmental factors
* Painful fecal evacuation resulting from anal disease (e.g., fissures)

ASSOCIATED CONDITIONS
Debility, either general as in the aged, or that imposed by specific underlying illness

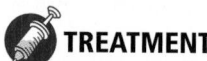

DIAGNOSIS

SIGNS AND SYMPTOMS
* Lower frequency of defecation than the patient perceives as normal (normal is 3–5 times per week)
* Harder stool than normal
* Smaller stools than normal (average <35 g/d is abnormal)
* Impaction of hard stool
* Inspissated stool
* Lack of consistent urgency to evacuate bowels
* Difficulty expelling feces from the rectum
* Painful evacuation of feces
* Lingering sense of incomplete emptying of the bowel
* Abdominal fullness or a feeling of malaise secondary to inadequate bowel evacuation
* Tenesmus

TESTS
Lab
Only necessary when other disorders are being considered
* Complete blood chemistry to detect anemia that may indicate colorectal neoplasm
* Thyroid functions
* Electrolytes, glucose, and calcium

Imaging
* Plain frontal spine film of the abdomen may help to discern the extent and nature of the problem.
* Barium enema or barium swallow with small-bowel follow-through looking for anatomic defects (mass lesions, ileus)
* Cineradiography of passage of barium, instilled in, then expelled from, the rectosigmoid segment (defecography), may help define evacuation disorders in some cases.

Diagnostic Procedures/Surgery
* Endoscopic evaluation
  – Flexible sigmoidoscopy
  – Colonoscopy
* In selected cases of long-standing constipation, timed measure of passage of ingested stool markers may help discern differing impediments.
* Anorectal motility in patients with suspected Hirschsprung disease or anorectal motility disorders
* Digital rectal exam is needed to rule out a rectal mass; check for blood in the stool and define stool consistency
* Sigmoidoscopy or colonoscopy is seldom required, unless to define an abnormality discovered by barium enema or when evidence of iron deficiency anemia or blood in the stool is present.

Pathological Findings
* None in common, functional constipation
* Paucity or absence of intramural enteric ganglia in certain cases of congenital or acquired megacolon
* Neuromuscular abnormalities in certain cases of pseudo-obstruction

DIFFERENTIAL DIAGNOSIS
* Congenital
  – Hirschsprung disease/syndrome
  – Hypoganglionosis
  – Congenital dilation of the colon
  – Small left colon syndrome
* Meconium ileus
* Normal evacuation with overanxious patient or parent
* Illnesses predisposing to constipation
  – Dehydration
  – Hypothyroidism
  – Hypokalemia
  – Hypercalcemia
* Other causes of abdominal pain

TREATMENT

INITIAL STABILIZATION
Outpatient in most cases, except when investigation discloses an underlying lesion or obstruction that requires hospitalization

GENERAL MEASURES
* Attempt to eliminate medications that may cause or worsen constipation.
* Increase fluid intake.
* Modify diet.
* Enemas if other methods fail

Diet
* If no anatomic abnormalities have been found, increase fiber to ~15 g/d (bran, fruit, green vegetables, and whole grain cereals and breads).
* Encourage liberal intake of fluids.

Activity
Encourage exercise and physical activity.

MEDICATION (DRUGS)

First Line

- Hydrophilic colloids (bulk-forming agents, thus not really drugs)
  - Psyllium (Konsyl, Metamucil, Perdiem Fiber): 1 rounded tsp in liquid PO daily up to t.i.d.
  - Methylcellulose (Citrucel): 1 rounded tsp in 8 oz cold water PO daily up to t.i.d.
  - Polycarbophil (Mitrolan, FiberCon): 1 g PO q.i.d.
- Osmotic laxatives: Appropriate for short-term use. The usual dosage is 15–30 mL daily to b.i.d.
  - Milk of magnesia
  - Magnesium citrate
  - Phosphate of soda
  - Lactulose (Chronulac)
  - Sorbitol
  - Alumina-magnesium (Maalox, Mylanta)
  - Polyethylene glycol (MiraLax) (0.8 mg/kg/d): Max is 17 g
- Stool softeners:
  - Docusate sodium (Colace): 100 mg b.i.d.
- Contraindications
  - Any impediment to bowel transit, such as an obstructing lesion or ileus. Osmotic laxatives may result in overdistension or bowel perforation.
  - Any acute intra-abdominal inflammatory condition
  - Renal failure/disease and heart failure are relative contraindications.
- Precautions: Advise patient against chronic use of irritant and osmotic laxatives.
- Significant possible interactions
  - Laxatives that contain magnesium
    ○ Bind tetracyclines and prevent their absorption
    ○ Reduce effectiveness of digitalis and phenothiazines
    ○ Sodium polystyrene sulfonate (Kayexalate) binds and prevents neutralization of bicarbonate, leading to systemic alkalosis, which may be severe.

Second Line

- Lubricants (e.g., mineral oil) are unpalatable to many patients, subject to leakage, and impose the risk of aspiration.
- Emollient suppositories are useful and may be helpful in alleviating or palliating anorectal pain.
- Irritant cathartics (stimulants)
  - Ricinoleic acid or castor oil (Neoloid): 30–60 mL/d
  - Bisacodyl (Dulcolax, Modane): 2–3 tablets PO or 1 suppository b.i.d.
- Motor and secretory properties
  - Anthraquinones: Senna (Ex-Lax in various formulations, Senokot): 1–2 capsules or 15–30 mL at bedtime
- Enemas (avoid soap suds, which may lead to colitis)
  - Sodium phosphate (Fleet enema)
- Suppositories
  - Osmotic: Sodium phosphate
  - Lubricant: Glycerin
  - Stimulatory: Bisacodyl
- Prokinetic agents

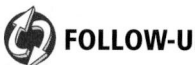 **FOLLOW-UP**

PROGNOSIS

Constipation that is only occasional, brief, and responsive to simple measures is harmless. That which is habitual can be a lifelong nuisance.

COMPLICATIONS

- Volvulus
- Cancer risk
- Acquired megacolon: In severe, long-standing cases
- Cathartic colon: Repeated laxative abuse
- Fluid and electrolyte depletion: Laxative abuse
- Rectal ulceration (stercoral ulcer) related to recurrent fecal impaction
- Anal fissures

PATIENT MONITORING

What seems to be simple, functional constipation, if it persists, should be further investigated for a possible organic cause.

REFERENCES

1. Abyad A, Mourad F. Constipation: Common-sense care of the older patient. *Geriatrics*. 1996;51: 28–36.
2. Devroede G. Constipation. In: Sleisenger MH, Fordtran JS, eds. *Gastrointestinal Disease*. 4th ed. Philadelphia, PA: WB Saunders; 1989.
3. Goroll AH, et al. Approach to the patient with constipation. In: Goroll AH, Mulley AG, eds. *Primary Care Medicine*. Philadelphia, PA: JB Lippincott; 1987.
4. Haubrich WS. Constipation. In: Berk JE, et al. eds. *Bockus Gastroenterology*. 4th ed. Philadelphia, PA: WB Saunders; 1985.
5. Lennard-Jones JE. Clinical management of constipation. *Pharmacology*. 1993;47(suppl 1): 216–223.
6. Nunez M, Robinson B. Management of constipation in the older patient. *J Florida Med Assoc*. 1991;78:829–831.
7. Rogers AI. Constipation. In: Berk JE, Haubrich WS, eds. *Gastrointestinal Symptoms: Clinical Interpretation*. Philadelphia, PA: BC Decker; 1991.
8. Wald A. Approach to the patient with constipation. In: Yamada T, ed. *Textbook of Gastroenterology*, vol 1. Philadelphia, PA: JB Lippincott; 1991.

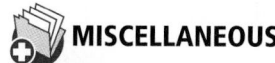 **MISCELLANEOUS**

CODES

ICD9-CM

- 564.00 Constipation, unspecified
- 564.7 Megacolon, other than Hirschsprung
- 564.89 Other functional disorders of intestine
- 751.3 Hirschsprung disease and other congenital functional disorders of colon

PATIENT TEACHING

- Define constipation and normal variations.
- Occasional mild constipation is normal.
- Instruction in consistent bowel training; that is, allowing adequate time for bowel evacuation in a quiet, unhurried environment; instruction in facilitating posture on commode, for example, thighs flexed toward abdomen
- Parent sometimes needs more treatment/advice than the constipated child

 See Corresponding Diagnostic Algorithm

 See Patient Handout on CD

C

CONTRACEPTION

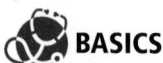

Leena Nathan, MD
Tu-Mai Tran, MD, MSc

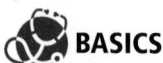 **BASICS**

DESCRIPTION
Methods to prevent pregnancy; mechanisms include preventing implantation, ovulation, or entry of sperm into uterus. Natural family planning's objective is to limit coitus around the time of ovulation. The most effective method is permanent sterilization. Although sterilization may be reversed, it is uncommon.

ALERT
Geriatric Considerations
Healthy nonsmokers may use oral contraceptives until 50. Use another contraceptive method during this period.

Pediatric Considerations
Use of estrogen prior to pubertal growth spurt may reduce ultimate height owing to epiphysial closure.

Pregnancy Considerations
- Pregnancy may occur with any method
  - After permanent sterilization: Indicates failure of procedure; consider ectopic pregnancy.
  - With an intrauterine device, remove device if string is visible. If string not seen, leave in position; slight increase in risk of spontaneous abortion.
  - With oral contraceptive: Stop pill. Only very slight chance of virilization of female fetus.
- Progestin-only is the preferred OCP for 1st 6 weeks of breast-feeding, because combined estrogen-progestin can suppress milk production.
- Lactation delays resumption of ovulation postpartum due to prolactin-induced inhibition of GNRH release, but should not be used exclusively for contraception.

EPIDEMIOLOGY
Incidence
- ~98% of women of reproductive age have used some form of contraception, but 1/3 of pregnancies are unplanned or unwanted.
- Oral contraceptives are leading method (31% of women), followed by tubal sterilization.
- Factors in choice of contraceptive method include efficacy, convenience, adverse effects, and affordability.
- Contraception efficacy:
- Pregnancy rate (%) during 1st year of use

	Typical Use	Perfect Use
No method	85	85
Cervical Cap	40	26
Condom		
Male	15	2
Female	21	5
Diaphragm with spermicide	16	6
Sponge	40	20
Rhythm (calendar)	13	5
Symptothermal	13–20	2
Withdrawal	27	4
Depot-Provera	3	<1
IUD, Copper T or Mirena	<1	<1
Patch	8	<1
OCPs	8	<1
Ring	8	<1
Female Sterilization	<1	<1
Vasectomy	<1	<1

- Emergency contraception
  - Pills: Pregnancy rate decreases by 75–89%
  - Depending on regimen (lower rate for levonorgestrel alone versus estrogen-progestin pills)
  - IUD: Pregnancy rate decreased by 99%

Prevalence
- Predominant age
  - Female: 11–52 years
  - Male: Any age after reaching puberty
- Predominant sex: Female.

RISK FACTORS
For pregnancy
- Any ovulating woman who engages in intercourse with a fertile male
- Young adolescents
- Lower socioeconomic population or those with limited knowledge and access to reproductive services

 DIAGNOSIS

TESTS
Lab
- Female
  - Cervical cytology
  - Cultures for *Neisseria gonorrhoeae* and *Chlamydia*
  - Blood pressure monitoring
  - Blood lipids, blood sugar
  - Pregnancy test (if hormonal contraception is not initiated at time of menses)
- Male
  - None, except routine preoperative studies made before vasectomy
  - Semen analysis after vasectomy; aspermia will require up to 15 ejaculations.

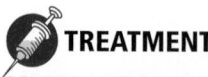 **TREATMENT**

GENERAL MEASURES
- Nondrug methods
- Latex condom
- Diaphragm: Needs fitting.
- Intrauterine device: Contraindications include pregnancy, history of PID, undiagnosed genital bleeding, uterine anomalies, large fibroids.
- Periodic abstinence
  - Calendar method: Track length of last 6 cycles; fertility period is calculated by subtracting 18 from the number of days of shortest cycle and 11 from number of days in longest cycle. Example, if shortest cycle is 28 days and longest cycle is 31 days, fertile period is from day 10 to 20.
  - Symptothermal method: Calculate the 1st day of abstinence by subtracting 21 from the length of the shortest menstrual cycle in the previous 6 months, or the 1st day cervical mucus is detected, whichever comes first. End calculated as 3 days after body temperature rises 1°C.
  - Withdrawal method: Male partner withdraws from vagina before ejaculation. Failure occurs if withdrawal is not timed accurately or if the pre-ejaculatory fluid contains sperm.

 MEDICATION (DRUGS)

- Spermicides
  - All contain nonoxynol-9
- Sponge
  - 2-inch circular disk that contains nonoxynol-9. Moisten with water before insertion in vagina; effective for 24 hours.
- Oral contraceptives
  - Side effects minimized with pills having <50 μg estrogen. Oral contraceptives with 35 μg of ethinyl estradiol provide the same blood hormone levels as 50 μg of mestranol.
  - Triphasics contain less total progestogen and are less likely to adversely affect lipid profile.
  - The progesterone (derivatives of testosterone) varies. Newer progestogens are less androgenic and have less affect on lipoproteins. Possible increased risk of stroke with desogestrel.
  - Continuous pill (i.e., seasonal with 84 active days and 7 inactive) used for endometriosis and premenstrual dysphoric disorder.
  - If adverse effects occur, pill may be changed by trial and error.
- Weekly hormonal patch (Ortho-Evra)
  - Patch must be changed weekly; contains 20 mcg ethinyl estradiol and 150 mcg norelgestromin. Patch may cause irritation. Not a reliable in women >90 kg.
- Vaginal contraceptive ring (NuvaRing)
  - Flexible polymer ring containing 15 mcg ethinyl estradiol and 120 mcg etonogestrel; inserted into vagina for 3 weeks per cycle.
- Medroxyprogesterone (Depo-Provera)
  - 150 mg IM every 3 months
  - Contraceptive levels of hormone persist for up to 4 months (2–4 week margin of safety)

- Intrauterine device
- (Copper T): Insert during menses (ensures patient is not pregnant); interferes with sperm transport and ova fertilization; effective for 10 years.
- Levonorgestrel intrauterine system (Mirena)
  - T-shaped intrauterine device that releases 20 mcg of levonorgestrel per day.
  - Effective for up to 5 years.
  - Expect menstrual irregularities initially and then possibly amenorrhea.
- Emergency contraception: Start within 72 hours for maximum effectiveness
  - Estradiol/levonorgestrel (Preven, Ovral, Ogestrel): 50 mg/0.25 mg. 2 tablets q12h (4 tablets total). Note: Antinausea medication (e.g., Phenergan) given 1–2 hours before the doses
  - Levonorgestrel (Plan B): 0.75 mg. 1 tablet q12h (2 tablets total). Less nausea and slightly more effective.
  - Copper-bearing intrauterine device. Insert 5 days after intercourse; over 99% effective in preventing pregnancy and continues to provide contraception for up to 10 years.
- Contraindications
  - Hormonal contraceptives (WHO Medical Eligibility Criteria for Contraceptive Use)
    - History of CAD or multiple risk factors (age >55, smoking, HBP, DM)
    - History of DVT/PE
    - History of CVA
    - History of migraines at age >35 or migraine at any age with aura
    - Current or past breast cancer
    - Active liver disease or hepatic tumor
    - Pregnancy
    - Unexplained, abnormal uterine bleeding without further investigation
  - Relative contraindication: Smokers >35
- Significant possible interactions due to increased metabolism of hormones (add barrier method)
  - Certain anticonvulsants such as phenytoin (Dilantin)
  - Rifampin

SURGERY
- Permanent sterilization
  - Tubal sterilization in the female
  - Hysteroscopic sterilization via polyester fibers (Essure): Polyester fibers with a coiled spring are introduced into each fallopian tube by transcervical route. Requires another contraceptive be used for 3 months after procedure.
  - Vasectomy in the male

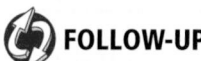 FOLLOW-UP

COMPLICATIONS
- Hormonal contraceptives, serious
  - Thromboembolism.
  - Hypertension
  - Myocardial infarction
- Oral contraceptives, minor
  - Nausea and vomiting: Take after eating.
  - Breakthrough bleeding: Usually self-limiting after 3 months; if persists, change pill
  - Amenorrhea: Pregnancy must be ruled out
  - Cyclic weight gain: Use smallest dose of estrogen available.
  - Breast tenderness: Rare with low-dose pill
  - Depression: Rare with low-dose pill
  - Chloasma: Stop pill or cover with makeup
  - Acne or hirsutism: Change to a less androgenic progesterone
  - Cholestatic jaundice: Stop pill; do not restart
  - Weight gain throughout cycle: Use triphasic pill to minimize dose of progesterone or use newer progesterone
- Injectable contraceptive (Depo-Provera)
  - Irregular bleeding no treatment needed
  - Amenorrhea: Common after 1 year of use
  - Possible increased bone resorption and decreased bone mineral density (BMD). FDA recommends BMD for use >2 years and to consider periodic estrogen
- Sponge and diaphragm
  - Associated with toxic shock syndrome.
- Intrauterine device
  - PID or salpingitis: Remove device and start antibiotic therapy
  - Heavy bleeding and cramps: Remove device
  - Although overall risk is low, possible ectopic pregnancy may occurs.

PATIENT MONITORING
- Pelvic exam, Pap smear, and HPV testing annually or every 3 years for patients with negative pap/HPV on past 3 Paps
- Check for intrauterine device 1 month after insertion.
- Oral contraceptive users: 3 months after starting for hypertension, then annually

REFERENCES

1. CDC National Center for Health Statistics. Use of Contraception and Use of Family Planning Services: United States:1992–2002. Hyattsville, MD, 2004.
2. Hatcher RA, Zietman M, Cwiak C, et al. *A Pocket Guide to Managing Contraception*, 8th Ed. Tiger, GA: Bridging the Gap Foundation, 2005.
3. Berek JS, et al. *Novak's Gynecology*, 12th ed. Baltimore: Williams & Wilkins; 1996.
4. Ellertson C, Trussell J, Stewart F, et al. Emergency contraception. *Semin Reprod Med*. 2001;19:323–330.
5. Nordenberg T. Protecting against unintended pregnancy: a guide to contraceptive choices. *FDA Consum*. 2000;34.
6. Speroff L, et al. *Clinical Gynecologic Endocrinology and Infertility*, 5th ed. Baltimore: Williams & Wilkins, 1994.
7. *Contraceptive Technology*, 18th edition, 2004.

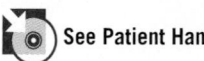 MISCELLANEOUS

- Other benefits of oral contraception
  - Clearly established benefits: Reductions in ovarian cancers, endometrial cancers, ectopic pregnancies, and PID; less dysmenorrhea and anemia; reduced functional ovarian cysts, and a regular menstrual cycle; improvement in acne
  - Relationship to breast cancer unclear, possible slight increase risk, especially in women with strong family history, >40 years old, smokers, and Asian race
- Barrier contraceptives: Lowers risk of sexually transmitted diseases (STDs).

PATIENT TEACHING
- Condoms: Water-based lubricants reduce the risk of breakage. Withdraw penis before becomes flaccid.
- IUD: Check string periodically.
- Diaphragm
  - Refit after childbirth or if weight changes by more than 10%.
  - Before inserting, 1 tablespoon of water-soluble spermicidal jelly or cream should be placed in the dome.
  - Leave in at least 6 hours after coitus.
  - If coitus is repeated before 6 hours, insert another teaspoon of spermicidal jelly into the vagina without removing the diaphragm.
- Female condom
  - New condom required for each sex act
- Oral contraception
  - Pill should be taken same time each day.
  - If a pill is missed, take 2 the following day, but use a barrier method until next period.
- Printed materials available from ACOG (1-800-673-8444)
- Emergency contraception (EC) prevents pregnancy via several proposed mechanisms including inhibition of sperm motility, alterations in tubal transport, unfavorable uterine receptivity, and/or fertilization inhibition. EC does not affect an established pregnancy. (Telephone information available at 1-888-NOT-2-LATE.)

See Patient Handout on CD

COR PULMONALE

Angie N. Ross, MD

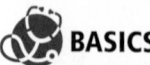 **BASICS**

DESCRIPTION

- Right ventricular enlargement, dysfunction, and failure caused by pulmonary hypertension (increased right ventricular afterload) secondary to diseases of the lung, thorax, and resistant pulmonary vasculature
- Acute cor pulmonale: Acute dilatation or overload of the right ventricle secondary to massive pulmonary embolism
- Chronic cor pulmonale: Hypertrophy and dilatation of the right ventricle resulting from diseases of the pulmonary parenchyma and/or pulmonary vasculature (most commonly chronic obstructive pulmonary disease [COPD])
- System(s) Affected: Cardiovascular; Pulmonary; Renal; Urologic

ALERT
Geriatric Considerations
Metabolism of sedatives and narcotics is slowed, thus the respiratory drive of these patients may be affected for prolonged periods.

Pregnancy Considerations
Increased demand for placental perfusion may be severe.

GENERAL PREVENTION
- Discontinue tobacco use.
- Limit exposure to inhalational irritants and allergens.

EPIDEMIOLOGY
Usually patients are >45 years; male predilection

Incidence
Difficult to assess incidence/prevalence due to risk of performing right heart catheterization on patients at risk.

RISK FACTORS
- Tobacco use
- Living at high altitudes
- Industrial exposures

PATHOPHYSIOLOGY
Chronic cor pulmonale

- The pathophysiology is secondary to pulmonary hypertension. In chronic respiratory disease, pulmonary hypertension results from increased pulmonary vascular resistance (PVR).
- The PVR increases as a result of alveolar hypoxia. Acute hypoxia causes vasoconstriction in small precapillary arteries, whereas chronic hypoxia causes pulmonary vascular remodeling. The increased PVR causes increased work for the right ventricle and subsequent right ventricular hypertrophy (RVH) and dilation. Pulmonary hypertension may worsen with exercise, sleep, and acute COPD exacerbations.

ETIOLOGY
- Air flow limitation
  - COPD (80–90%)
    - Emphysema
    - Chronic bronchitis
  - Cystic fibrosis
- Restrictive lung disease
  - Kyphoscoliosis
  - Idiopathic pulmonary fibrosis
  - Connective tissue disorders
- Central respiratory insufficiency
  - Obesity-hypoventilation syndrome
  - Sleep apnea
- Neuromuscular disease
  - ALS
  - Myasthenia gravis
  - Guillain-Barré syndrome
- Pulmonary circulation
  - Pulmonary thromboembolism
  - Primary pulmonary hypertension
  - Sickle cell disease

ASSOCIATED CONDITIONS
Left heart failure

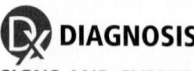 **DIAGNOSIS**

SIGNS AND SYMPTOMS
- Acute cor pulmonale is usually due to thromboembolic disease
  - Severe dyspnea
  - Pallor
  - Diaphoresis
  - Jugular venous distention with inspiration (Kussmaul sign)
  - Systolic murmur loudest at left sternal border (tricuspid regurgitation)
  - Distended, tender, pulsatile liver
  - S3 gallop
  - Hypoxemia
- Chronic cor pulmonale
  - Peripheral edema is most common sign of right heart failure (RHF) but nonspecific. May be caused by hypercapnic acidosis and hypoxemia triggering renal compensation vs. true RHF.
  - Dyspnea, fatigue, lethargy, exertional syncope, reflecting poor cardiac output
  - Exertional angina, either from compression of left main coronary artery or subendocardial ventricular ischemia
  - Hoarseness secondary to compression of the left recurrent laryngeal nerve by enlarged pulmonary vessels (Ortner syndrome)
  - Productive or nonproductive cough

Physical Exam
- Right-sided murmurs
  - Increased intensity of pulmonic component of 2nd heart sound
  - Pansystolic-tricuspid regurgitation
  - Early diastolic-pulmonary regurgitation
- RVH
  - Heave, 4th heart sound, prominent A and V waves

TESTS
Lab
- Acute cor pulmonale: Ventilation/perfusion mismatch with hypoxia and hypercapnia
- Chronic cor pulmonale: Pulmonary function testing shows airflow obstruction with reduced Po_2 and possibly elevated hematocrit levels.
  - Arterial blood gas may show hypercapnic acidosis and hypoxemia.
  - BNP and cardiac troponins may be elevated

Imaging
- Chest radiograph
  - Heart size may be normal in mild to moderate disease.
  - There may be counterclockwise cardiac rotation and loss of aortic knob prominence with severe disease.
  - In the posteroanterior view, the left heart border is mostly composed of the right ventricle.
- Doppler echocardiography with saline contrast to estimate tricuspid regurgitation is the most reliable noninvasive estimation of pulmonary artery pressure (PAP). Limitation in COPD patients. 80% accuracy in patients with mild disease, and 75% accuracy in patients with COPD.
- MRI can be used more specifically to characterize right ventricular size, mass morphology, and function.
- ECG often shows normal results, but findings can include signs of right ventricular strain or hypertrophy
  - RVH is indicated by clockwise rotation of electrical axis, right axis deviation, and P pulmonale (increased P wave amplitude in II, III, and aVF).

Diagnostic Procedures/Surgery
- Right heart catheterization is the gold standard for quantitation of ventricular and pulmonary pressures and exclusion of congenital heart disease as etiology of RHF. This procedure is reserved for the following individuals
  - ECHO fails to measure tricuspid regurgitation to r/o pulmonary HTN
  - Precise measures of PVR for vasodilator therapy is needed.
  - Left heart catheterization also is required.
- Lung biopsy also helpful in discriminating among granulomatous and collagen-vascular diseases

DIFFERENTIAL DIAGNOSIS
- Primary disease of the left side of the heart
- Congenital heart disease with left-to-right shunting
- Primary pulmonary HTN
- Pulmonary thromboembolic disease
- All of the above would show a PAP >40 mm Hg vs. COPD, in which PAP is 20–35 mm Hg at rest.

TREATMENT

INITIAL STABILIZATION
- Acute cor pulmonale: ICU setting
- Chronic cor pulmonale: Outpatient therapy

GENERAL MEASURES
- Vigorous antibiotic treatment of acute respiratory tract infections
- Avoidance of airway irritants (e.g., tobacco smoke), sedatives, and tranquilizers
- Treatment of underlying pulmonary disease, including
  - Chronic obstructive pulmonary disease
    ○ Bronchodilators to relieve obstruction
    ○ Supplemental oxygen to correct hypoxia and acidemia
    ○ Vasodilators, diuretics, and phlebotomy (when hematocrit levels reach 55–60%) are possibly useful.
  - Ventilatory abnormalities (e.g., sleep apnea)
    ○ Continuous positive airway pressure or biphasic positive airway pressure
    ○ Progestins
    ○ Tracheostomy
  - Acute or chronic thromboembolic disease
    ○ Appropriate anticoagulation and hemodynamic support

Diet
Moderate reduction of salt intake

Activity
As tolerated

MEDICATION (DRUGS)

First Line
- Oxygen
  - Long-term therapy to maintain arterial oxygen >60 mm Hg (>8.0 kPa), if possible, to reduce pulmonary vascular resistance and improve myocardial dynamics.
  - Renal vascular vasoconstriction also may be relieved.
  - Excess oxygen depresses respiratory drive in patients with carbon dioxide retention.
- Diuretics
  - Can improve function of both ventricles if RV volume is elevated.
  - Combinations of loop diuretics and spironolactone are efficacious.
  - Furosemide (20–80 mg PO/IV)
    ○ Monitor for excess volume depletion with regular BUN and creatinine measurements. Avoid metabolic alkalosis as this can suppress ventilation.
  - Theophylline
    ○ Bronchodilator, increases right ventricular ejection fraction by increasing myocardial contractility. Diaphragm endurance also is enhanced; decreases pulmonary and systemic vascular resistance to some degree.

- β-Adrenergic agonists
  - During acute, short-term administration, terbutaline is beneficial, probably by increasing right ventricular ejection fraction and lowering pulmonary vascular resistance.
- Bronchodilators
  - Ipratropium (500 mcg nebulized), metaproterenol (0.2–0.3 mL 5% solution in 2.5 mL normal saline [NS] nebulized), and albuterol (2.5–5 mg nebulized) used q6h and more often if necessary to maintain airway patency and arterial oxygen saturation
- Vasodilators
  - Hydralazine (25 mg PO t.i.d. up to 100 mg t.i.d.), nifedipine (30–60 mg PO q.i.d. up to 120 mg q.i.d.), diltiazem, and prazosin.
  - Reserved for patients with persistent disease (oxygen and bronchodilator failure).
  - No evidence of efficacy beyond 3–6 month use.
  - Success with these agents can be accurately assessed only with invasive monitoring.
- Preliminary data with oral sildenafil show it is an effective and selective pulmonary vasodilator that increases cardiac output without increasing wedge pressure in patients with pulmonary hypertension.
- In patients with pulmonary arterial HTN and WHO class III or IV symptom severity, bosentan (Tracleer) administered at 125 mg PO b.i.d. has been shown to improve exertional tolerance and walking distance.
  - Bosentan also has been shown to improve cardiac function and reduce PVR, PAP, and mean right atrial pressure.
  - Bosentan is an endothelin-1 receptor antagonist.
  - Liver function tests must be monitored while patients are on this medication because it has been associated with liver toxicity. If ALA or ALT levels exceed 3 times the upper limit of normal on therapy, it must be discontinued.
  - The use of bosentan is absolutely contraindicated in pregnant patients because of the high likelihood of inducing teratogenic effects.
- Contraindications: Avoid sedatives and respiratory depressants.

Second Line
- Digoxin is no longer recommended; it increases right heart contractility, but also induces pulmonary vasoconstriction, which may exacerbate RHF. Because of hypoxia and diuretic use, dangerous arrhythmias may develop.
- Other therapies being tested include inhalational nitric oxide, IV epoprostenol, and endothelin receptor blockers.

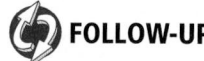 ## FOLLOW-UP

Admission Criteria
Acute cor pulmonale: ICU setting for therapy

PROGNOSIS
- Prevalence of RVH has dramatically decreased with the application of long-term oxygen therapy.
- The PAP level is a good indicator of prognosis. In patients with COPD and mild disease (PAP 20–35 mm Hg), 5-year survival is 50%.
- Prognosis is poor in patients with severe pulmonary HTN.

PATIENT MONITORING
Regular arterial blood gas monitoring for patients with advanced disease

REFERENCES

1. Weitzenblum E. Chronic cor pulmonale. *Heart.* 2003;89:225-230(A).
2. Piazza, Goldhaber. The acutely decompensated right ventricle. *Chest.* 2005;128:1836–1852(B).
3. Hoves, Deane. The effects of oxygen and dopamine on renal and aortic blood flow in COPD with hypoxia and hypercapnia. *Am J Respir Crit Care Med.* 1995;1(2pt1):378–383(B).
4. Clozel. The effects of bosentan on cellular processes involved in pulmonary arterial hypertension: do they explain the lung benefit?. *Ann Med.* 2003;35(8):605–613(B).
5. Wikins, Paul, Strange. Sildenafil vs. Endothelin Receptor Antagonist for Pulmonary Hypertension (SERADH). *Am J Respir Crit Care Med.* 20051;171(11):1292–1297(A).

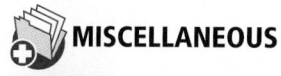 ## MISCELLANEOUS

CODES

ICD9-CM
- 415.0 Acute cor pulmonale
- 416.9 Chronic pulmonary heart disease, unspecified

PATIENT TEACHING
- Teach patient to
  - Recognize signs of COPD exacerbation
  - Recognize sudden unilateral swelling of lower extremity in patient with hypercoagulability
  - Recognize signs of edema
  - Report any signs of infections to physician.
  - Avoid use of nonprescription medications, especially sedatives
- Stress the need for adequate rest.
- Referral to social service agency for home care help (oxygen, suctioning, etc.)

Diet
Diet restriction

C

CORNEAL ABRASION

Felix Horng, MD, MBA
Brian Halstater, MD

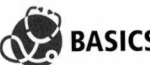 **BASICS**

DESCRIPTION

Corneal abrasion result from scratching, denuding, abrading, or cutting of the outermost layer of the eye

- Minor abrasions tend to heal quickly
- Deeper injuries may take 24–72 hours to heal.
- Corneal scarring is a potential complication, requiring corneal transplant for impaired vision.

GENERAL PREVENTION

- Use eye protection while working with dust, sand or debris, or playing contact sports. [C]
- Avoid extended contact lens use. [C]
- Artificial tears for those with inability to blink [C]
- Environmental interventions (i.e., clip children's fingernails, remove low-lying tree branches) [C]

EPIDEMIOLOGY

Incidence

Most common ophthalmologic visit to ER

RISK FACTORS

- Younger, active individuals
- Extended contact lens use
- Inability to blink (e.g., Bell Palsy, general anesthesia)

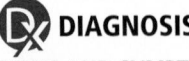 **DIAGNOSIS**

SIGNS AND SYMPTOMS

- Acute eye pain
- Photophobia
- Foreign body sensation
- Tearing
- Blepharospasm
- Other less common
  - Blurred vision
  - Headache

History

Possible history includes

- Recent ocular trauma
- Extended contact lens use
- Blowing dust, sand, or debris

Physical Exam

- Use topical anesthetic, such as proparacaine 0.5%, for easier examination, especially if blepharospasm is present.
- Fluorescein staining
  - Fluorescein uptake revealed in areas of damage via Wood lamp or Cobalt blue slit lamp
- Conjunctival injection often present
- Visual acuity usually normal
  - Acuity may be abnormal if abrasion lies in the central visual axis or if abrasion is large

TESTS

Lab

Bacterial cultures if corneal ulcer suspected

DIFFERENTIAL DIAGNOSIS

- Corneal ulcer (e.g., herpetic)
  - Dendritic corneal ulcer, hallmark sign
  - May have vesicular skin rash on initial presentation
  - Stromal keratitis in severe presentations
  - Refer immediately to ophthalmology.
- Bilateral or true idiopathic lesions may suggest basement membrane dystrophy.

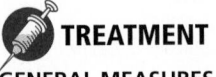 **TREATMENT**

GENERAL MEASURES

- Consider topical NSAIDS, which are moderately useful for reducing pain. (1,2)[A]

- Apply topical antibiotics, usually for 5–7 days (1)[C]
  - Ointment preferred over drops as it is considered more lubricating and protective
  - Consider antipseudomonal coverage for contact lens wearers (1)[C]
- Avoid use of topical anesthetics after initial examination, as it may cause corneal toxicity and retard healing. (1)[C]

- Eye patching is no longer recommended. (1,3,4,5)[A]
  - No healing improvement with metaanalysis of 5 randomized control trials.
- Mydriatics are no longer recommended for ciliary spasm. (1,6)[B]

- Oral analgesics are generally not necessary. [C]

MEDICATION (DRUGS)

- Topical NSAIDS
- Topical antibiotics
  - Consider antipseudomonal coverage for contact lens wearers. (1)[C]

First Line
- Topical NSAIDS
  - Diclofenac 0.1% 1 drop q.i.d.
  - Ketorolac 0.5% 1 drop q.i.d.
- Topical antibiotics
  - Gentamycin 0.3% ointment or solution. 1/2 inch ribbon t.i.d. or 1–2 drops q4h
  - Erythromycin 0.5% ointment 1/2 ribbon b.i.d.–q.i.d.

Second Line
Topical antibiotics
- Ciprofloxacin 0.3% solution 1–2 gtts q.i.d.
- Ofloxacin 0.3% 1–2 gtts q1–6h

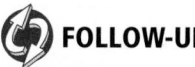 **FOLLOW-UP**

DISPOSITION
Issues for Referral
Referral to ophthalmologist is indicated for
- Retained foreign bodies
- Suspected corneal ulcerations/deep eye injuries
- Recurrent corneal erosions
- Persistent symptoms after 72 hours
- Non-improving or worsening symptoms

PROGNOSIS
Very good: Minor lesions usually heal within 24–72 hours

COMPLICATIONS
Complications are rare, however
- Recurrent corneal erosions may occur at original injury site.
- Scarring may occur, especially with deeper injuries, possibly requiring corneal transplant for impaired vision.

PATIENT MONITORING
Re-evaluate in 24 hours. (1)[C]
- If lesion is not healed, re-evaluate within 72 hours. (1)[C]

REFERENCES

1. Wilson SA, Last A. Management of corneal abrasions. *Am Fam Physician*. 2004; 70(1):123–128.
2. Weaver CS, Terrell KM. Evidence-based emergency medicine. Update: do ophthalmic non-steroidal anti-inflammatory drugs reduce the pain associated with simple corneal abrasion without delaying healing? *Ann Emerg Med*. 2003;41:134–140.
3. Michael JG, Hug D, Dowd MD. Management of corneal abrasion in children: A randomized clinical trial. *Ann Emerg Med*. 2002;40:67–72.
4. Le Sage N, Verreault R, Rochette L. Efficacy of eye patching for traumatic corneal abrasions: A controlled clinical trial. *Ann Emerg Med*. 2001; 38:129–134.
5. Flynn CA, D'Amico F, Smith G. Should we patch corneal abrasions? A meta-analysis. *J Fam Practice*. 1998;47:264–270.
6. Carley F, Carley S. Towards evidence based emergency medicine: best BETs from the Manchester Royal Infirmary. Mydriatics in corneal abrasion. *Emerg Med*. 2001;18:273.

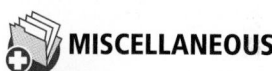 **MISCELLANEOUS**

CODES

ICD9-CM
918.1

PATIENT TEACHING

 See Corresponding Diagnostic Algorithm

 See Patient Handout on CD

C

CORNEAL ULCERATION

Alan M. Ehrlich, MD

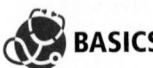 ## BASICS

DESCRIPTION
- Corneal ulcers usually represent an infection of the cornea by bacteria, virus, or fungi as a result of breakdown in the protective epithelial barrier. If left untreated, corneal ulcers can result in blindness.
- Ulcerations may be central or marginal.
- System(s) Affected: Nervous

ALERT
Geriatric Considerations
Ring ulceration more common

GENERAL PREVENTION
Avoid corneal abrasion or injury and improper contact lens handling.

EPIDEMIOLOGY
- Predominant age: None
- Predominant sex: Male = Female

Prevalence
Common in the US

RISK FACTORS
- Any abrasive injury
- Contact lenses (especially soft lenses)
- Chronic topical steroid use
- Abuse of topical anesthetics
- Autoimmune disorders
- Vitamin A deficiency
- Chronic corneal exposure (exophthalmos or Bell palsy)
- Recent eye surgery, including LASIK

ETIOLOGY
- Corneal ulcers are predisposed by the presence of an entry to the external eye through dry eye, burns, abrasion, contact lenses, inappropriate use of topical anesthetics, antibiotics, or antiviral drops, immunosuppressant drugs, diabetes, immunodeficiency.
- Causative agents
  - Gram-positive organisms (staphylococci, streptococci, and bacilli)
  - Anaerobes (cocci, bacilli)
  - Gram-negative organisms (diplococcus, rods, and anaerobes)
  - Pseudomonas
  - Viruses such as herpes
  - Fungal organisms (Candida, Aspergillus, Fusarium) in agricultural workers or associated with ocular corticosteroid use
    - Peripheral ulcerative keratitis usually caused by autoimmune disorders such as RA, SLE, scleroderma, etc.
    - Vitamin A deficiency may cause corneal necrosis or keratomalacia

ASSOCIATED CONDITIONS
- Chronic ulcerations may be associated with neurotrophic keratitis owing to lack of 5th nerve innervation of the cornea. Individuals with thyroid disease, diabetes, or immunosuppressive conditions are particularly at risk.
- Any cause of fat malabsorption may be associated with Vitamin A deficiency

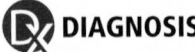 ## DIAGNOSIS

SIGNS AND SYMPTOMS
- Eyelid and conjunctiva become inflamed.
- Mucopurulent discharge
- The corneal epithelium will be absent, with underlying ulceration and infiltration of the corneal stroma with leukocytes.
- Foreign body sensation
- Blurred vision
- Light sensitivity
- Pain

History
- Red painful eye
- Contact lens user, dry eyes, or history of trauma from foreign body or chemical burn
- Connective tissue disorders

Physical Exam
- Impaired visual acuity in affected eye
- Conjunctival inflammation
- White patch on cornea
- Location of ulcer (central versus peripheral)

TESTS
Lab
- Culture the ulcer.
- Culture contact lens if applicable.
- Drugs that may alter lab results: Pretreatment with topical antibiotics or corticosteroids may delay diagnosis.

Diagnostic Procedures/Surgery
- Scrapings of the corneal ulcer for culture and sensitivities ideally should be done before beginning local antibiotics. The sample should be plated onto the culture media directly.
- Fluorescein staining to detect foreign bodies, corneal ulcers, or punctate keratitis, and to look for dendritic lesions of herpes simplex or zoster.

Pathological Findings
Scrapings for Gram and Giemsa stain may demonstrate bacteria, yeast, or intranuclear inclusions that may aid in the diagnosis.

DIFFERENTIAL DIAGNOSIS
- Foreign bodies
- Corneal abrasions
- Keratitis
- Herpes simplex or zoster

TREATMENT

GENERAL MEASURES
- Appropriate health care
  - Outpatient or inpatient for severe ulcer or noncompliant patient
  - All cases of corneal ulceration should be promptly referred to an ophthalmologist.
- Aggressive topical antibiotic treatment directed toward the causative agent should be instituted immediately while culture studies are pending.
- Supplemental topical cycloplegia reduces the inflammation and aids in patient comfort.
- Bandaging the eye should be avoided, and topical steroids should never be used. Daily evaluation is necessary and prompt consultation with an ophthalmologist or corneal specialist is advised.

Activity
Reduced, until vision returns to normal and healing is complete

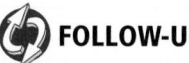 **MEDICATION (DRUGS)**

First Line

- Consultation with an ophthalmologist is indicated to help determine initial therapy.
- Topical quinolones (e.g., ciprofloxacin [Ciloxan] 0.3%, gatifloxacin (Zymar), levofloxacin (Quixin), moxifloxacin (Vigamox).
- Topical gentamicin and tobramycin are effective against Pseudomonas, Enterobacter, Klebsiella, and aerobic gram-negative organisms, cephalosporins (e.g., cefazolin 50 mg/mL) may also be used
- Fungal keratitis must be treated with parenteral amphotericin B for Candida and Aspergillus; clotrimazole, miconazole, econazole, and ketoconazole also may be required.
- Herpetic keratitis should initially be treated with trifluridine or acyclovir topically [C]
- Contraindications: Refer to manufacturer's profile of each drug.
- Precautions: Refer to manufacturer's profile of each drug.
- Significant possible interactions: Refer to manufacturer's profile of each drug.

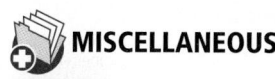 **FOLLOW-UP**

DISPOSITION

Issues for Referral

Evaluation by an ophthalmologist to scrape the ulcer for culture and guide antibiotic selection is appropriate.

PROGNOSIS

- Corneal ulcerations should improve daily and heal with appropriate therapy.
- If healing does not occur or the ulcer extends, then consideration should be given to an alternative diagnosis and treatment.

COMPLICATIONS

Scarring of the cornea and loss of vision

PATIENT MONITORING

The patient should be monitored at least daily until healed.

REFERENCES

1. Wirbelauer C. Management of the red eye for the primary care physician. *Am J Med*. 2006;119(4):302–6 [C].
2. Karp CL, Forster RK. The Corneal Ulcer In: *Cornea*, 2nd ed. Philadelphia: Elsevier Mosby 2005: 353–357 [C].
3. Biswell R. Cornea. In: *General Ophthalmology*, 15th ed. Stamford CT: Appleton and Lange, 1999:120–131 [C].
4. Squirrell DM, et al. Peripheral ulcerative keratitis "corneal melt" and rheumatoid arthritis: a case series. *Rheumatology*. 1999;117(10):1423–1427 [C].

MISCELLANEOUS

CODES

ICD9-CM
370.00 Corneal ulcer, unspecified

PATIENT TEACHING

Prevention
Prevention of abrasions and proper handling of contact lenses can prevent recurrence of corneal ulcers.

C

COSTOCHONDRITIS

Scott A. Fields, MD

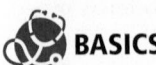 **BASICS**

DESCRIPTION

Anterior chest wall pain associated with pain and tenderness of the costochondral and costosternal regions. The musculoskeletal system is affected. It is also called costosternal syndrome, parasternal chondrodynia, anterior chest wall syndrome, Tietze disease and syndrome, and chondrocostal junction syndrome.

Pediatric Considerations
Pay special attention to psychogenic chest pain with children who perceive family discord.

Pregnancy Considerations
Unknown

GENERAL PREVENTION
Avoid any activity that increases pain.

EPIDEMIOLOGY
- Predominant age: 20–40 years
- Predominant sex: Female

Incidence
About 10% of chest pain complaints; 15–20% of teenagers with chest pain may have costochondritis

RISK FACTORS
- Unusual physical activity or overuse
- Recent upper respiratory infection (URI)

Genetics
Unknown

ETIOLOGY
- Not fully understood
- Trauma
- Overuse

ASSOCIATED CONDITIONS
URI

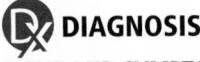 **DIAGNOSIS**

SIGNS AND SYMPTOMS
- Insidious onset
- Pain usually sharp, sometimes pleuritic
- Pain involves multiple locations, the 2nd–5th costal cartilage most often involved.
- Pain worsens with movement and breathing.
- Heat often relieves pain.
- Chest tightness is often associated with the pain.
- Pain sometimes radiates into arm.
- Nonsuppurative edema and tenderness at rib articulations
- Redness and warmth at sites of tenderness

History
A complete and thorough history is mandatory for the diagnosis.

Physical Exam
A complete physical examination is mandatory for the diagnosis.

Geriatric Considerations
Often presents with multiple problems capable of causing chest pain, making a thorough history and physical exam imperative

TESTS
Lab
The diagnosis of costochondritis is primarily based on a complete and thorough history and physical examination. Laboratory exams should be used only if concern exists regarding other elements of the differential diagnosis. ESR is inconsistently elevated.

Imaging
No imaging is indicated for the diagnosis of costochondritis; chest radiograph normal

Diagnostic Procedures/Surgery
None indicated for the diagnosis of costochondritis

Pathological Findings
Costochondral joint inflammation

DIFFERENTIAL DIAGNOSIS
- Cardiac
  - Coronary artery disease
  - Aortic aneurysm
  - Mitral valve prolapse
  - Pericarditis
  - Myocarditis
- Gastrointestinal
  - Gastroesophageal reflux
  - Peptic esophagitis
  - Esophageal spasm
  - Gastritis
- Musculoskeletal
  - Fibromyalgia
  - Slipping rib syndrome involves the lower ribs
  - Costovertebral arthritis
  - Painful xiphoid syndrome
  - Rib trauma with swelling
  - Thoracic disc compression
  - Ankylosing spondylitis
  - Epidemic myalgia
  - Precordial catch syndrome
- Psychogenic
  - Anxiety disorder
  - Panic attacks
  - Hyperventilation
- Respiratory
  - Asthma
  - Pneumonia
  - Chronic cough
  - Pneumothorax
- Other
  - Herpes zoster
  - Spinal tumor
  - Metastatic cancer
  - Substance abuse (cocaine)

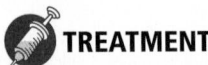 **TREATMENT**

GENERAL MEASURES
Patient reassurance, rest and heat

Diet
Normal

Activity
As possible

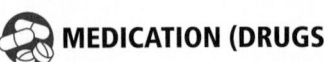 **MEDICATION (DRUGS)**

First Line
NSAIDs (aspirin, ibuprofen, naproxen, or diclofenac). Other analgesics may be used as needed. (1–3)[C]
- Contraindications
  - History of anaphylaxis to aspirin
  - Peptic ulcer disease
  - Renal insufficiency
- Precautions
  - Peptic ulcers may occur with chronic use of NSAIDs
  - Acute interstitial nephritis
  - Drug accumulation with renal insufficiency
  - Liver function abnormalities in up to 15% of patients
- Significant possible interactions: NSAIDs
  - Albumin-bound drugs: Displacement of either drug
  - Warfarin: Increased prothrombin time (PT). Monitor PT closely and adjust warfarin dosage as needed. Monitor lithium levels and adjust lithium dosage as needed. The patient may need to increase lithium dosage when therapy with NSAIDs has been discontinued.
  - Lithium: Increased lithium plasma level
  - Furosemide: Decreased natriuretic effect and increased risk of acute renal failure secondary to decreased renal blood flow
  - Propranolol: Decreased antihypertensive effect

Second Line
Acetaminophen (1–3)[C]

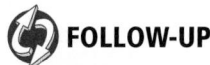 **FOLLOW-UP**

DISPOSITION

Admission Criteria
Only indicated if differential diagnosis is unclear and cardiac or other more serious etiology of chest pain is being considered (4)[C]

Discharge Criteria
When diagnosis is established

PROGNOSIS
- Self-limited illness, although sometimes chronic
- Often recurs

COMPLICATIONS
Incomplete attention to differential diagnosis or inappropriate interventions in a desire to ensure that a more life-threatening diagnosis is not missed

PATIENT MONITORING
Follow-up in 1 week

REFERENCES

1. Gregory PL, Biswas AC, Batt ME. Musculoskeletal problems of the chest wall in athletes. *Sports Med*. 2002;32:235–250.
2. Jensen S. Musculoskeletal causes of chest pain. *Aust Fam Physician*. 2001;30:834–839.
3. Mukamel M, Kornreich L, Horev G, et al. Tietze's syndrome in children. *J Pediatr*. 1997;131: 774–775.
4. Disla E, Rhim HR, Reddy A, et al. Costochondritis. A prospective analysis in an emergency department setting. *Arch Intern Med*. 1994;154:2466–2469.
5. An exploratory report of chest pain in primary care. A report from ASPN. *J Am Board Fam Pract*. 1990;3:143–150.
6. Klinkman MS, Stevens D, Gorenflo DW. Episodes of care for chest pain: A preliminary report. From MIRNET. Michigan Research Network. *J Fam Pract*. 1994;38:345–352.

 MISCELLANEOUS

CODES

ICD9-CM
733.6 Tietze disease

PATIENT TEACHING
Educate the patient in regard to the self-limited nature of the illness. Instruct patient on proper physical activity regimens to avoid overuse syndromes. Also stress the importance of avoiding sudden, significant changes in activity.

 See Corresponding Diagnostic Algorithm

 See Patient Handout on CD

C

CROHN DISEASE

Ruben Peralta, MD, FACS
Venu G. Pillarisetty, MD

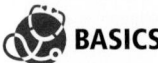 **BASICS**

DESCRIPTION
- Idiopathic inflammatory disease of the alimentary tract that may present anywhere in the GI tract, but is most commonly found in the terminal ileum (60%), but may be limited to the colon in 15–20%, proximal small bowel 10%
  - Transmural disease
  - May involve multiple regions of the intestine with normal sections in between (skip lesions)

EPIDEMIOLOGY
Incidence
- Annual incidence of 3–7 cases per 100,000
- Race: In US more common in whites than African Americans or Asians
- Predominant age:15–25 years, 2nd smaller peak in ages 55–65 years
- Predominant sex: Female > Male

Prevalence
20–100 per 100,000

RISK FACTORS
Cigarette smoking (2 times higher risk in smokers)

Genetics
15% of patients have 1st-degree relatives with inflammatory bowel disease. Family members develop the disease with similar patterns and similar age of onset.

PATHOPHYSIOLOGY
- Segmental disease with patchy distribution and variable severity
- Strictures commonly present and occasionally prevent passage of the endoscope

ETIOLOGY
- Idiopathic, immune-mediated
- No infectious etiology has been identified.
- Aggravated by bacterial infection
- Aggravated by inflammatory cascade
- Aggravated by smoking cessation

ASSOCIATED CONDITIONS
- Viral gastroenteritis can be a more severe illness in these patients.
- Arthritis of 2 types: Similar to rheumatoid and spondylitis
- Variety of skin lesions, erythema nodosum, nonspecific rashes, pyoderma gangrenosum
- Uveal tract disease rare but related
- Sclerosing cholangitis in ~10%
- Pigment gallstones are increased with ileal disease
- Increased risk of both colorectal cancer and small bowel cancer

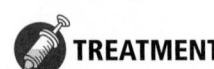 **DIAGNOSIS**

SIGNS AND SYMPTOMS
- Depends on the areas of intestinal involvement
- All forms of Crohn
  - Diarrhea occurs in most patients
  - Abdominal pain in 2/3
  - Weight loss, malaise
  - Abdominal tenderness
  - Low-grade fever
  - Abdominal mass (occasionally)
  - Fistula: Perirectal, bladder, skin, vagina
  - Extraluminal disease (10%): Skin, iritis, arthritis, sclerosing cholangitis
- Small-bowel disease only (15–30%)
  - Diarrhea prominent, including nocturnal
  - Vague abdominal pain frequent
  - Intestinal obstruction (1/3): Cramping abdominal pain precedes for months.
  - Bleeding in 20%, rarely massive
  - Perianal disease, including fistulae
  - Internal fistulae
- Colon disease only (25–30%)
  - Diarrhea prominent, including nocturnal
  - Hematochezia
  - Abdominal pain in 50%, relieved by stooling
  - Perianal disease in 40%, fistulae
  - Weight loss prominent
  - Megacolon in 10%
  - Intestinal obstruction occasional
- Colon and small-bowel disease (40–60%)
  - Intestinal obstruction much more common than in other types

TESTS
- Colonoscopy is most helpful.
- Constellation of barium-identified distribution of lesions, endoscopic findings, and biopsies usually establish the diagnosis.

Lab
- Anemia common
- Albumin level decreased in severe cases
- Serum electrolytes imbalance
- Steatorrhea
- Sedimentation rate, C-reactive protein
- Vitamin levels to evaluate specific nutrient deficiency (Vitamin B_{12}, fat-soluble vitamins)
- pANCA (perinuclear antineutrophil cytoplasmic antibody) titer
  - Elevated in ulcerative colitis (85%) and Crohn disease (15%)
- Antiglycan antibody titer
  - Elevated in Crohn disease (75%) and ulcerative colitis (5%)

Imaging
- Barium radiographs: enema and small bowel
  - Loss of smooth mucosa, undermined ulcers
  - Narrowed lumen in most involved segments of small bowel (string sign)
  - Fistulae from involved segment to other bowel loops, bladder, or vagina or external site
  - Skip areas, multiple lesions common
  - Failure to reflux into ileum on barium enema
  - Ulcers undermining mucosa
  - Narrowed lumen
  - Fistula to other parts of intestine

- CT scans
  - Thickening of bowel wall, strictures, and dilatation
  - Defines abscess cavities and fistulae
  - Identifies extensive perirectal disease

Diagnostic Procedures/Surgery
- Ileoscopy and enteroscopy
- Biopsy of mucosa, helpful but not diagnostic
  - Helps rule out other causes

Pathological Findings
- All layers of intestinal wall, with inflammation in at least focal areas in >95% of cases
- Skip areas (a normal segment between 2 involved segments)
- Granuloma in up to 50% of resected specimen
- Fat hypertrophy following mesenteric vessels in 50% of cases of small-bowel disease

DIFFERENTIAL DIAGNOSIS
- Appendicitis
- Ulcerative colitis
- Indeterminate colitis
- Pelvic inflammatory disease
- Endometriosis
- Irritable bowel syndrome
- Ischemic colitis (older age group)
- Enteric pathogens: Amebiasis, tuberculosis, *Yersinia*, *Campylobacter*, gonorrhea, *Clostridium difficile* toxin, *Shigella*, *Salmonella*, lymphogranuloma venereum (LGV), and non-LGV chlamydia, fungi (e.g., actinomycosis)
- Malignancy: Lymphoma, adenocarcinoma
- Radiation enteritis
- Caustic enemas (e.g., hydrogen peroxide)
- Small-bowel disease
  - Drugs (e.g., NSAIDs)
  - Eosinophilic gastroenteritis

TREATMENT

GENERAL MEASURES
- Attention to maintaining weight and nutrition
- Physical rest and relief of emotional stress
- Monitor severe cases for fat malabsorption.
- Perirectal disease: Sitz baths, soap and water after stooling, surgical drainage of perirectal abscesses, surgical treatment of recurrent fistulae if medical management fails

Diet
- If fat malabsorption, diminish fat in diet
- If strictures or recurrent obstruction, avoid highly fibrous substances
- If diarrhea prominent, increase dietary fiber (sometimes recommended), decrease fat
- Enteral nutrition preferred over parenteral

Activity
Full activity as tolerated

MEDICATION (DRUGS)

First Line

- Because the etiology is unknown, directed treatment at underlying cause is not possible. Medical treatment consists of symptomatic measures and supportive care (e.g., antispasmodic and anti-diarrheals).
- Naive patient, relapse, major symptoms
  – Prednisone: 20–60 mg/d PO
    ○ Most appropriate for small bowel Crohn
  – Sulfasalazine and mesalamine
    ○ Start at same time as prednisone.
- If tenesmus or bleeding prominent
  – Mesalamine enema or hydrocortisone enema maintenance therapy
  – Mesalamine, methotrexate, or azathioprine
    ○ Prolong remission and delay surgery
- Predominantly perirectal disease with fistulae
  – Metronidazole (Flagyl) 250 mg t.i.d. for maximum of 8 weeks
- Patients who relapse with prednisone tapering or fail to respond
  – Add azathioprine 2–2.5mg/kg/d or mercaptopurine (6-MP) If good response, taper steroid.
  – If inadequate response, maintain patient on immunosuppressant and start a course of anti-TNF-α monoclonal antibody
- Patients with symptomatic fistula failing to heal with conservative therapy
  – Infliximab permits healing in 50%.
- Patients with joint, eye, and skin extraintestinal manifestations
  – Unresponsive to mesalamine, occasionally responsive to prednisone
  – Usually responsive to infliximab
- For all well-controlled patients
  – Loperamide (Imodium) 2 mg to control diarrhea to avoid interference with daily life
  – Watch for thrombocytopenia and pancytopenia.

Second Line

- Budesonide can be administered topically or orally; synthetic glucocorticoid with reduced bioavailability
  – Alternate to prednisone in patients requiring long-term steroid
  – Partially avoids steroid complications
- Methotrexate 25 mg IM weekly as an alternative to 6-MP or azathioprine
- Cyclosporine has assisted in closing fistulae when other measures fail.
- Etanercept (tumor necrosis factor inhibitor), is being increasingly used.
- Natalizumab, an integrin-blocking agent, may have benefit; appropriate use not yet defined.

SURGERY

- Palliative, not curative
- Indications
  – Failure of medical management
  – Total or recurrent intestinal obstruction
  – Perforation
  – Symptomatic fistulae other than rectal
  – Inability to thrive, growth retardation
  – Abscess
  – Toxic megacolon or extensive disease
  – Failure of ostomy to function after ≥1 year
  – Cancer or suspected cancer

FOLLOW-UP

PROGNOSIS

- Chronic condition with variable but nearly certain progression
- Average patient has surgery every 7 years
  – Short-bowel syndrome common after more than 4 surgeries
- Recurrence common
- Most are able to maintain normal life

COMPLICATIONS

- Recurrence usually in gut segment most proximal to anastomoses
- Fistulae (15%): Perirectal, cutaneous, enterovaginal, and enterovesicular
- Extraluminal disease (10%)
  – Skin, uveal tract, joint, and biliary tract
- Extensive colon disease associated with increased risk of adenocarcinoma
- Colon perforation
- Toxic megacolon
- Gallstones occur in >25%.
- Osteoporosis commonly occurs; more frequent and severe when chronic use of steroids.

PATIENT MONITORING

- Regular assessment (every 3–6 months if patient is stable) of symptoms, particularly status of weight, pain, diarrhea, hemoglobin, and sedimentation rate
- To assess the relative response to therapy, Crohn's Disease Activity Index (CDAI) is an objective measure for recording disease activity that can be used to assess response to therapy.
- Endoscopy and further images if changes in symptoms and signs
- Check liver tests yearly.
- Check vitamin B_{12} level in those with ileal disease or ileal resection.
- Check folate level in all on 5-aminosalicylate; use supplements in all.

REFERENCES

1. Jess T, Gamborg M, Matzen P, et al. Increased risk of intestinal cancer in Crohn's disease: A meta-analysis of population-based cohort studies. *Am J Gastroenterol*. 2005;100:2724–2729.
2. Korzenik JR, Podolsky DK. Evolving knowledge and therapy of inflammatory bowel disease. *Nat Rev Drug Discovery*. 2006;5(3):197–209.
3. Yantiss RK, Odze RD. Histopathology. 2006;48:116–132.

MISCELLANEOUS

CODES

ICD9-CM

- 555.0 Regional enteritis of small intestine
- 555.1 Regional enteritis of large intestine
- 555.9 Regional enteritis of unspecified site

PATIENT TEACHING

- An important part of management
- Crohn and Colitis Foundation of America, Inc., 11th floor, Park Ave. South, NY 10016, Phone (800) 343-3637. Joining local chapters recommended

See Corresponding Diagnostic Algorithm

See Patient Handout on CD

CRYPTOCOCCOSIS

Cynthia Gail Carmichael, MD

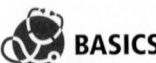 **BASICS**

DESCRIPTION
- Infection caused by *Cryptococcus neoformans*, which is a fungus that rarely causes disease in hosts with normal immune function
- Cryptococcal meningitis is 1 of the more common AIDS-defining infections in HIV-seropositive persons.
- Multisystemic involvement possible
- System(s) Affected: Nervous; Pulmonary; Skin/Exocrine; Endocrine/Metabolic
- Synonym(s): Torulosis

GENERAL PREVENTION
- Life-long antifungal medication generally required for suppression
  - Without suppression, relapse is common (50% in AIDS patients within 1 year).
  - Suppress with fluconazole 200 mg PO daily.
  - Alternative suppression: Itraconazole 200 mg PO daily
  - May consider discontinuing suppressive fluconazole when patients respond to antiretroviral therapy with CD4 count >100–200 cells/mm^3 for >6 months.
  - Restart suppressive fluconazole if CD4 cell count decreases to <100–200.
- Primary prophylaxis with fluconazole (100–200 mg/d or 3 times a week) or 400 mg per week in selected patients with CD4 count <50–100 cells/mm^3 decreases the incidence
  - Consider cost, possible drug resistance, and drug interactions. Most HIV specialists do not routinely recommend primary prophylaxis.

EPIDEMIOLOGY
- Predominant age: Generally adults
- Predominant sex: More common in males (reflects HIV prevalence)

Incidence
- Decreasing in recent years
- 5–8% of opportunistic infections in AIDS patients

RISK FACTORS
- Immunosuppression (CD counts <50–100)
  - Results in reactivation of latent infection (usually foci in lungs)
- Exposure to bird roosts

ETIOLOGY
- Cryptococcus fungus is ubiquitous.
- Person-to-person transmission is rare.

ASSOCIATED CONDITIONS
- HIV infection
- AIDS

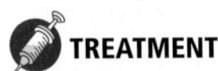 **DIAGNOSIS**

SIGNS AND SYMPTOMS
- Cryptococcal meningitis
  - Insidious onset with subtle findings
  - Frontal or temporal headache (80–95%)
  - Fever (60–80%)
  - Impaired mentation/lethargy/memory loss
  - Seizures or focal neurologic signs (less common)
  - Meningismus/photophobia in 1/3–1/4 of patients may be absent (80%).
  - Death within 1st few weeks of diagnosis is often related to increased intracranial pressure.
- Pulmonary cryptococcus
  - May be asymptomatic
  - Cough
  - Shortness of breath
  - Fever
  - Hemoptysis
  - Frequently disseminates in immunosuppressed patients
- Disseminated cryptococcus
  - Painless skin nodules (5–10%)
  - Erythematous papules, vesicles, macules, or ulcers
  - Heart, bone, kidney, adrenals, eyes, prostate, and lymph nodes may harbor infection with symptoms referable to affected organ.

TESTS
Lab
- Serum cryptococcal antigen
  - If positive, search for dissemination and perform lumbar puncture
- Cerebrospinal fluid (CSF) cryptococcal antigen
  - Positive in 95% of culture-proven cases
- India ink preparation of CSF
  - 50% positive in non-AIDS patients
  - 80% (bronchoalveolar lavage) positive in AIDS patients
- Culture of CSF, sputum, blood, and urine

Imaging
- Cryptococcal meningitis
  - CT of brain is negative unless focal cryptococcomas present
- Pulmonary cryptococcosis
  - Chest radiograph may show infiltrates, nodules, mass lesions (with rare cavitation), miliary spread, hilar adenopathy (10%), or pleural effusions (<5%).

Diagnostic Procedures/Surgery
- Lumbar puncture in cryptococcal meningitis
- Imperative to check opening pressure initially); significantly increased intracranial pressure associated with poor prognosis; may require repeat lumboperitoneal (LP) or surgical shunt/drain to decrease intracranial pressure
  - In non-AIDS patients: Elevated opening pressure, elevated CSF protein, decreased glucose, and lymphocytic pleocytosis
  - In AIDS patients: Abnormal CSF findings in 40% of patients; high opening pressure (>200 mm H$_2$O) in 70% of patients
- Biopsies of skin lesions may be diagnostic.

Pathological Findings
- Inflammation
- Granuloma formation (may caseate and cavitate)
- Basilar meningitis with mucoid exudate

DIFFERENTIAL DIAGNOSIS
- CNS disease
  - Toxoplasmosis
  - Lymphoma
  - AIDS dementia complex
  - Progressive multifocal leukoencephalopathy
  - Herpes encephalitis
  - Other fungal disease
- Pulmonary disease
  - Tuberculosis
  - *Pneumocystis carinii*
  - Histoplasmosis
  - Coccidioidomycosis
  - Kaposi sarcoma
  - Lymphoma
- Disseminated disease
  - Tuberculosis
  - Histoplasmosis
  - Lymphoma
  - Coccidioidomycosis

TREATMENT

GENERAL MEASURES
Diet
As tolerated

Activity
As tolerated

MEDICATION (DRUGS)

First Line
- Amphotericin B (0.7 mg/kg/d IV) or liposomal Amphotericin B (see "Second Line Medications") plus flucytosine (100 mg/kg/d) until patient is clinically improving (2–3 weeks); followed by fluconazole
- Fluconazole (Diflucan) 400 mg/d (PO or IV) until 8 weeks of primary therapy have been completed
- Precautions
  – With Amphotericin B, permanent renal impairment, hypokalemia, or hypomagnesemia may occur.
  – Fever, chills, and headache during infusion possible: Pretreat with diphenhydramine, acetaminophen to decrease fever and chill.
  – Add heparin 500 U and hydrocortisone 50 mg to IV amphotericin B to decrease phlebitis.

Second Line
- Liposomal amphotericin (Ambisome) 4 mg/kg/d IV for 14 days followed by fluconazole
- Combination fluconazole 400–800 mg/d PO for less severe disease.
- Fluconazole 400–800 mg PO or IV daily plus flucytosine 25 mg/kg PO q.i.d. for 4–6 weeks. Due to toxicity, use only when patient is intolerant or unresponsive to 1st line treatment.
- For patients with elevated intracranial pressure, aggressive serial lumbar punctures or surgical shunts or drains is indicated.

ALERT
Pregnancy Considerations
Avoid fluconazole during the 1st trimester of pregnancy due to potential teratogenic effects. Consider Amphotericin instead.

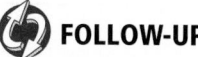 **FOLLOW-UP**

PROGNOSIS
- Fatal without treatment
- No statistics available on survival

COMPLICATIONS
- Cryptococcal infections are fatal unless treated.
- Increased intracranial pressure

PATIENT MONITORING
- Patients with cryptococcal meningitis require lifelong suppression with fluconazole after treatment unless CD4 cell count increases to >100–200. (See "General Prevention").
- Monitor clinical status and repeat lumbar puncture indicated.
- Foci in the prostate may be difficult to eliminate

REFERENCES

1. Aberg JA, Powderly WG. Cryptococcosis. In: Cohen PT, Sande MA, Volberding PA, eds. AIDS Knowledge Base.
2. Centers for Disease Control and Prevention. Guidelines for Preventing Opportunistic Infections Among HIV-Infected Persons—2002 Recommendations of the U.S. Public Health Service and the Infectious Disease Society of America. MMWR 2002;51(No. rr-8)
3. Centers for Disease Control and Prevention. Treating opportunistic infections among HIV-infected adults and adolescents: Recommendations from CDC, the National Institutes of Health, and the HIV Medicine Association/Infectious Disease Society of America. MMWR 2004;53(No. RR15)
4. Chetchotisakd P, Sungkanuparph S, Thinkhamrop B, et al. A multicentre, randomized, double-blind, placebo-controlled trial of primary cryptococcal meningitis prophylaxis in HIV-infected patients with severe immune deficiency. HIV Med. 2004;5: 140–143.
5. Graybill JR, Sobel J, Saag M, et al. Diagnosis and management of increased intracranial pressure in patients with AIDS and cryptococcal meningitis. Clin Inf Dis 2000;30:47–54.
6. Van der Horst CM, Saag MS, Cloud GA, et al. Treatment of cryptococcal meningitis associated with the acquired immunodeficiency syndrome. N Engl J Med. 1997;337:15–21.

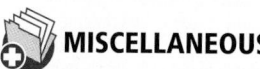 **MISCELLANEOUS**

See also: HIV Infection; AIDS

 CODES

ICD9-CM
117.5 Cryptococcosis

C

CRYPTORCHIDISM

Pamela I. Ellsworth, MD

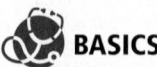 **BASICS**

DESCRIPTION

- Incomplete or improper descent of 1 or both testicles. Normally, descent is in the 7th–8th month of gestation. The cryptorchid testis (UDT) may be palpable or nonpalpable.
- Types of cryptorchidism
  - Abdominal: Located inside the internal ring
  - Canalicular: Located between the internal and external ring
  - Ectopic: Located outside the normal path of testicular descent from abdominal cavity to scrotum; may be ectopic to perineum, femoral canal, superficial inguinal pouch (most common), suprapubic area and opposite hemiscrotum
  - Retractile: Fully descended testis that moves freely between the scrotum and the groin
  - Iatrogenic: Previously descended testis becomes undescended secondary to scar tissue after inguinal surgery, such as an inguinal hernia repair or hydrocelectomy
- System(s) Affected: Reproductive
- Synonym(s): Undescended testes

Pediatric Considerations

- This problem is usually detectable at birth or soon thereafter.
- If surgery is to be the treatment, it should be performed during the 1st 6–9 months of life. (1)
- Puberty: If unilateral cryptorchidism is discovered at or after puberty, the usual treatment is orchiectomy.

EPIDEMIOLOGY

- Predominant age: Premature newborns
- Predominant sex: Male only

Prevalence

In the US, cryptorchidism occurs in 3% of full-term and 33% of premature newborn males. Spontaneous testicular descent occurs by age 1–3 months in 50–70% of full-term males with cryptorchidism. Descent at 6–9 months of age is rare.

RISK FACTORS

- Family history of cryptorchidism: Boys with UDTs: 4% of their fathers and 6.2–9.8% of their brothers have UDTs. (C)
- The following may be associated with an increased risk of cryptorchidism
  - 1st-born child
  - Cesarean section delivery
  - Toxemia of pregnancy
  - Hypospadias
  - Congenital subluxation of hip
  - Low birth weight
  - Pre-term birth
  - Advanced maternal age
  - Maternal obesity
  - Consumption of cola-containing drinks during pregnancy

Genetics

Occurrence of undescended testes in siblings as well as fathers suggests a genetic etiology.

ETIOLOGY

- Not fully known
- May involve alterations in mechanical factors (gubernaculum, length of vas deferens and testicular vessels, groin anatomy, epididymis, cremasteric muscles, and abdominal pressure), hormonal factors (gonadotropin, testosterone, dihydrotestosterone, and Müllerian inhibiting substance), and neural factors (ilioinguinal nerve and genitofemoral nerve)

ASSOCIATED CONDITIONS

- Inguinal hernia
- Hemiscrotum
- Hydrocele
- Abnormalities of vas deferens and epididymis
- Klinefelter syndrome
- Hypogonadotropic hypogonadism
- Germinal cell aplasia
- Müllerian inhibiting factor deficiency
- 5-Alpha-reductase deficiency
- True hermaphrodite
- Prune belly syndrome
- Meningomyelocele
- Hypospadias
- Wilms tumor
- Kallmann syndrome
- Prader-Willi syndrome
- Cystic fibrosis

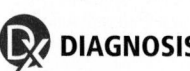 **DIAGNOSIS**

SIGNS AND SYMPTOMS

One or both testicles in a site other than the scrotum; may be an isolated defect or associated with other congenital anomalies

TESTS

Lab

- In boys ≤3 months with bilateral non-palpable UDTs, luteinizing hormone, follicle stimulating hormone, and testosterone helpful to determine whether testes present
- >3 months of age, human chorionic gonadotropin (HCG) stimulation test to determine presence/absence of testicular tissue (HCG 2000 IU daily for 3 days, and check testosterone pre- and post-stimulation)

Imaging

- Ultrasonography has a sensitivity of 76%, a specificity of 100%, and an accuracy of 84% in the dx on nonpalpable UDT, whereas MRI has a sensitivity of 86%, a specificity of 79%, and an accuracy of 85% (2)[C]
- CT scan findings in children are inconsistent.

Diagnostic Procedures/Surgery

- Physical exam
- Performed with warm hands, with child in sitting, standing, and squatting positions
- A Valsalva maneuver and applied pressure to lower abdomen may help identify the testes, especially a gliding testis.
- Failure to palpate a testis after repeated exams suggests an intra-abdominal or atrophic testis.
- An enlarged contralateral testis in the presence of a nonpalpable testis suggests testicular atrophy/absence.
- Laparoscopy is useful in a child with impalpable cryptorchidism to accurately confirm testicular absence or presence and to determine the feasibility of performing a standard orchiopexy (3)[C]

Pathological Findings

- Higher incidence of carcinoma in undescended testis and alterations in spermatogenesis
- Histologic changes occur by 1.5 years of age and include smaller seminiferous tubules, fewer spermatogonia, and more peritubular tissue

DIFFERENTIAL DIAGNOSIS

- Retractile testis (hypermobile testis): A normally descended testis that ascends into the inguinal canal because of an active cremasteric reflex (more common in males 4–6 years old)
- Atrophic testis: May occur as a result of neonatal torsion

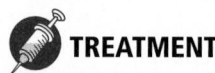 **TREATMENT**

GENERAL MEASURES

- Appropriate health care: Outpatient until surgery performed
- Rule out retractile testis
- Administration of chorionic gonadotropin may cause testicular descent in some boys. Reports of efficacy are inconsistent.

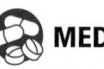 **MEDICATION (DRUGS)**

- The International Health Foundation recommends biweekly HCG injections for 5 weeks: 250 (IU) for infants, 500 IU for children ≤6 years of age, and 1,000 IU for ≥6 years of age.
- Success rates for descent into the scrotum range from 0–55%. (4)[B] The more distal the testis, the more likely the descent.
- Contraindications: HCG therapy contraindicated in patients with a clinically apparent inguinal hernia, those with a history of previous ipsilateral groin surgery, or in ectopic testicles. Also refer to manufacturer's literature.
- Precautions: May induce precocious puberty; discontinue drug, effects should reverse in 4 weeks; premature epiphyseal closure
- Significant possible interactions: Refer to manufacturer's literature.

SURGERY

- Reasons to consider: Avoids torsion, averts trauma, decreases but does not eliminate risk of malignancy, and prevents further alterations in spermatogenesis
- Orchiopexy should be performed by age 1. Alterations in germ cell count in the cryptorchid testis have been identified by age 2.

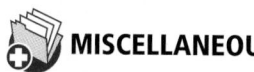

FOLLOW-UP

PROGNOSIS

- Disorder usually corrected with medical or surgical therapy; however, possible life-long consequences
- If testicle is absent or orchiectomy required, may consider placement of testicular prosthesis

COMPLICATIONS

Progressive failure of spermatogenesis, if left untreated. Even with orchiopexy, the fertility rate is still reduced, especially with bilateral undescended testicles. Spermatogenesis is related to the duration of cryptorchidism and the location of the testis. Formerly bilaterally cryptorchid men have a greater decrease in fertility compared to unilateral cryptorchid male and to the general male population. Abnormalities have also been identified in the contralateral descended testis, although less severe.

ALERT

Clinical

- 4–7 times higher risk of developing testicular cancer in male with hx UDT (5)[C]
- Hernia development (25%)

PATIENT MONITORING

- Patients should be followed after surgery to evaluate testicular growth.
- Testicular tumors occur mainly during or after puberty and thus, these children should be taught self-examination when they are older.

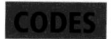

REFERENCES

1. Lee P. Fertility after cryptorchidism: epidemiology and other outcome studies. *Urology* 2005;66:427–31.
2. Kanemoto K, Hayashi Y, Kojima Y, Maruyama T, Ito M, Kohri K. Accuracy of ultrasonography and magnetic resonance imaging in the diagnosis of non-palpable testis. *Int J Urol.* 2005;12:668–672.
3. Patil KK, Green JSA, Duffy PG. Laparoscopy for impalpable tesits. *BJU.* 2005;95:704–708.
4. Henna MR, Del Nero RGM, Sampaio CZS, et al. Hormonal cryptorchidism therapy: Systematic review with metanalysis of randomized trials. *Pediatr Surg Int.* 2004;20(5):357–359.
5. Cortes D. Cryptorchidism: Aspects of pathogenesis, histology and treatement. *Scan J Nephrol.* 1998; 9:54.

MISCELLANEOUS

See also: Hydrocele; Meningomyelocele; Wilms Tumor

CODES

ICD9-CM

752.51 Undescended testis

C

PATIENT TEACHING

Discuss with parents about causes, available treatments, and possible effects on patient's reproductive potential; also increased risk for testicular cancer and need for self-examination

CUBITAL TUNNEL SYNDROME

Lee A. Mancini, MD, CSCS, CSN

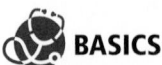 **BASICS**

DESCRIPTION
Compression of the ulnar nerve on the medial aspect of the elbow where it enters the cubital tunnel.

GENERAL PREVENTION
- Sleep with elbows straight and avoid sleeping with arms overhead.
- Keep proper posture when working at a desk.
- Avoid long periods of time with elbows bent or pressure on elbows.

EPIDEMIOLOGY
- Predominant sex: Male (3–8× more common)
- Elbow is most common site of compression of ulnar nerve
- 2nd most common nerve compression of upper extremity (1)

RISK FACTORS
- Patients with end-stage renal disease on hemodialysis
- Pre-existing polyneuropathy
- Athletes in throwing sports, racquet sports, weight-lifting, and skiing
- Patients who sleep with their elbows bent, their arms overhead, or both

PATHOPHYSIOLOGY
- Cubital tunnel is a fibroosseus canal formed by medial condyle, ulnar collateral ligament, and flexor carpi ulnaris muscles
- Elbow flexion increases distance from medial epicondyle to olecranon 5 mm for every 45°
- Elbow flexion places stress on medial collateral ligament and overlying retinaculum.
- Shape of cubital tunnel changes from a circle to an oval with a 2.5-mm loss of height with elbow flexion
- Loss of height of cubital tunnel with elbow flexion decreases tunnel volume by 55%, which doubles intraneural pressure on the ulnar nerve from 7–14 mm Hg.
- Maximal pressure on the ulnar nerve in cubital tunnel is created by shoulder abduction, elbow flexion, and wrist extension.

ETIOLOGY
- Caused by constricting fascial bands, subluxation of ulnar nerve over medial epicondyle, cubitus valgus, bony spurs, hypertrophied synovium, tumors, ganglia, or direct compression of ulnar nerve as it crosses cubital tunnel
- Elbow flexion decreases volume of cubital tunnel, causing compression of ulnar nerve
- Compression of ulnar nerve causes pain at medial aspect of elbow, and symptoms at forearm and hand

ASSOCIATED CONDITIONS
- Ulnar nerve subluxation
- Osteoarthritis of elbow joint

DIAGNOSIS

SIGNS AND SYMPTOMS
- Paresthesias along lateral forearm, wrist, and 4th and 5th digits
- Paresthesias may be intermittent at 1st and then become more constant
- Nocturnal elbow pain
- Medial elbow pain
- McGowan Grade I: No wasting or weakness of intrinsic muscles, feeling of clumsiness in affected hand, mild paresthesias in ulnar nerve distribution
- McGowan Grade II: Intermediate lesions with weak interossei and muscle wasting
- McGowan Grade III: Severe lesions with paralysis of interossei and a marked weakness of the hand
- Chronic symptoms: Loss of grip strength and loss of fine motor skills in hand

History
- History of trauma over the area
- Repetitive elbow flexion and extension activities (such as in hammering)
- Overhead throwing athlete with repetitive elbow motion

Physical Exam
- Inspect carrying angle of both elbows
- Palpate medial epicondyle and cubital tunnel for areas of tenderness or ulnar nerve subluxation
- Check elbow range of motion
- Positive Hoffman-Tinel test (tapping over ulnar nerve) (2)
- Pain on palpating over ulnar nerve
- Atrophy of intrinsic muscles
- Loss of sensation at ulnar side of 5th digit
- May be wasting of hypothenar muscles and flexion contracture of 4th and 5th digits (ulnar claw)
- Wartenburg sign is clawing or abduction of the 5th digit with extension
- Assess ability to cross 2nd and 3rd digits
- Evaluate grip and pinch strength for weakness
- Check vibration and light touch sensation

TESTS
- Hoffman-Tinel test performed by tapping over the ulnar nerve at the cubital tunnel. A positive Tinel test may be present in 24% of the asymptomatic population.
- Elbow flexion test is the most diagnostic test for cubital tunnel syndrome. The patient flexes the elbow >90°, supinates the forearm, and extends the wrist. Results are positive if pain is recreated or if paresthesias occurs within 60 seconds. Shoulder abduction can also be added to enhance diagnostic ability.

Imaging
X-rays may reveal osteophytes impinging on the area. Include anterior posterior (AP) lateral, and cubital tunnel views. (2)
- Cubital tunnel view: Elbow is maximally flexed and x-ray beam is shot as an AP view of the distal humerus
- CXR if patient has history of smoking and ulnar nerve symptoms (to exclude Pancoast tumor in apical lung)
- MRI shows inflammation and irritation of ulner nerve
- High-resolution ultrasound

Diagnostic Procedures/Surgery
- Corticosteroid injection into ulnar groove
- Electromyogram (EMG) is not essential when diagnosis is obvious on clinical exam. EMG should be used to determine the efficacy of conservative treatment or when the diagnosis is unclear.
- EMG is considered positive if motor conduction delay across the elbow <50 m/s or difference between motor velocity across elbow and below the elbow >10 m/s
- Nerve conduction studies

Pathological Findings
Inflammation and swelling of ulnar nerve

DIFFERENTIAL DIAGNOSIS
- Cervical disc lesion
- Thoracic outlet syndrome
- Carpal tunnel syndrome
- Medial epicondylitis
- Thoracic outlet syndrome
- Pancoast's syndrome
- Metabolic disorders creating peripheral neuropathies
- Multiple sclerosis and other myelopathies

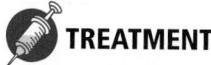 **TREATMENT**

INITIAL STABILIZATION
- Rest
- Avoidance of aggravating activities

GENERAL MEASURES
- Conservative treatment is initial approach if no motor weakness
- Patient instructed to avoid periods of prolonged elbow flexion
- Patient instructed to avoid long periods of pressure and compression on the ulnar nerve at the elbow
- Patients to change how they get out of bed
- Ice/heat for symptom relief
- Splint or brace while sleeping to keep affected elbow in extension and take pressure off cubital tunnel
- Work place modifications (e.g., correct posture, avoid long periods of time with elbows bent)

Activity
- Avoid any activities that bring about symptoms.
- Otherwise activity as tolerated

SPECIAL THERAPY
- Corticosteroid injection into ulnar groove
- Use 1 mL lidocaine and 20–40 mg methylprednisolone injected into ulnar groove, parallel to ulnar nerve (2)

Physical Therapy
Hand therapy and custom splint prescription

Complementary and Alternative Therapies
Vitamin B_6 (100 mg daily)

 MEDICATION (DRUGS)

First Line
NSAIDs or other analgesic

Second Line
Corticosteroid (injection)

SURGERY
- Goal of surgery is to create more space for ulnar nerve (3)
- Simple cubital tunnel decompression (3,4)[C]
- Ulnar nerve transposition: Moves the ulnar nerve in front of the medial epicondyle so it does not catch or stretch when the elbow is bent. The nerve is moved just beneath the skin or muscle. (3,4)[C]
- Medial epicondylectomy: Surgically removes the medial epicondyle, allows ulnar nerve to glide back and forth (3,4)[C]

 FOLLOW-UP

Issues for Referral
Failure of conservative treatment, loss of grip strength, flexion contracture of 4th and 5th digits, positive EMG for motor conduction delay

PROGNOSIS
- Both conservative and surgical methods result in 85–90% good-to-excellent results
- For McGowan Grade III: Anterior intramuscular transposition has best outcome (4)[C]

COMPLICATIONS
Anterior transposition may have recurrent subluxation of the ulnar nerve.

REFERENCES
1. Fernandez E, Pallini R, Lauretti L, Scogna A, La Marca F. Neurosurgery of the peripheral nervous system: Cubital tunnel syndrome. *Surg Neurol*. 1998;50:83–85.
2. Chumbley EM, O'Connor FG, Nirschl RP. Evaluation of overuse elbow injuries. *Am Fam Physician*. 2000;61:691–702.
3. Mowlavi A, Andrews K, Lille S, Verhulst S, Zook EG, Milner S. The management of cubital tunnel syndrome: A meta-analysis of clinical studies. *Plast Reconst Surg*. 2000;106:327–334.
4. Bartels RHMA, Menovsky T, Van Overbeeke JJ, Verhagen WIM. Surgical management of ulnar nerve compression at the elbow: An analysis of the literature. *J Neurosurg*. 1998;89:722–727.

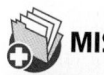 **MISCELLANEOUS**

CODES

ICD9-CM
354.2 Ulnar nerve neuropathy

PATIENT TEACHING
- In severe cases, the nerve damage may be permanent, and the patient may not recover.
- The longer the nerve has been irritated, the more difficult it is to recover fully.

Prevention
See "General Prevention"

CUSHING SYNDROME AND CUSHING DISEASE

Alan M. Ehrlich, MD

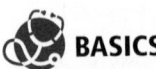 **BASICS**

DESCRIPTION
- Clinical abnormalities associated with chronic exposure to excessive amounts of cortisol (the major adrenocorticoid)
- Cushing disease occurs when Cushing syndrome is due to a pituitary adenoma. This is the most common cause of primary Cushing syndrome.
- System(s) Affected: Endocrine/metabolic; Musculoskeletal; Skin/exocrine; Cardiovascular

ALERT
Pediatric Considerations
- Rare in infancy and childhood
- Most cases in children <8 years are a result of malignant adrenal tumors.

Pregnancy Considerations
Pregnancy may exacerbate disease.

GENERAL PREVENTION
Avoid excessive corticosteroid treatment when possible.

EPIDEMIOLOGY
- Predominant age: All ages
- Predominant sex: Females > Males

Incidence
Uncommon: 0.7–2.4 per million per year

Prevalence
In difficult to control diabetic patients with obesity and hypertension, prevalence has been reported at 2–5% (1)[B].

RISK FACTORS
- Prolonged use of corticosteroids
- Pituitary tumor
- Adrenal mass
- Neuroendocrine tumor (e.g., bronchial carcinoid)

Genetics
- Multiple endocrine neoplasia type I
- Carney complex (an inherited multiple neoplasia syndrome)
- McCune-Albright syndrome (mutation of GNAS1 gene)

PATHOPHYSIOLOGY
Pituitary tumor causing excess adrenocorticotropic hormone (ACTH) (corticotropin)

ETIOLOGY
- Exogenous glucocorticoids and/or ACTH
- Endogenous ACTH-dependent hypercortisolism
  – ACTH-secreting pituitary tumor: 70%
  – Ectopic ACTH production (e.g., small cell carcinoma of lung, bronchial carcinoid): 15%
- Endogenous ACTH-independent hypercortisolism: 15%
  – Adrenal adenoma
  – Adrenal carcinoma
  – Macronodular or micronodular hyperplasia

ASSOCIATED CONDITIONS
Tumors of the pituitary
- Multiple endocrine neoplasia type I
- Carney complex

DIAGNOSIS

SIGNS AND SYMPTOMS
History
- Weight gain: 95%
- Decreased libido: 90%
- Menstrual irregularity: 80%
- Hirsutism: 75%
- Depression/emotional lability: 70%
- Easy bruising: 65%
- Proximal muscle weakness: 60%

Physical Exam
- Obesity: 95%
- Facial plethora: 90%
- Moon face (facial adiposity): 90%
- Thin skin: 85%
- Hypertension: 75%
- Skeletal growth retardation in children: 70–80%
- Diabetes or glucose intolerance: 60%
- Purple striae on the skin
- Increased adipose tissue in neck and trunk
- Acne

TESTS
Lab
- Elevated late-night salivary cortisol sensitivity: 90–95%; specificity 90–95%
- 24-hour urinary free cortisol level: sensitivity 41–70%, with specificity approaching 100%
- Plasma cortisol (morning and evening)
- Plasma ACTH concentration
- Dynamic endocrine testing (e.g., dexamethasone suppression test): Sensitivity 95%, specificity 70%
- CBC, electrolytes, and serum glucose
- Urinalysis
- Possible findings include
  – Glycosuria
  – Neutrophilia
  – Lymphopenia
  – Hyperglycemia
  – Hyperlipidemia
  – Hypokalemia

Imaging
- Chest radiograph
- Lumbar spine radiograph
  – Osteoporosis is common
- Pituitary MRI scan if pituitary tumor suspected
- Abdominal CT scan if adrenal disease suspected
- Chest CT scan if ectopic ACTH secretion is suspected and inferior petrosal sinus sampling rules out pituitary source (2)[C]
- Octreotide scintigraphy to look for occult ACTH secreting tumor

Diagnostic Procedures/Surgery
- Diagnostic procedure depends on circumstances and judgment
- Inferior petrosal sinus sampling with CRH stimulation if ACTH-dependent tumor suspected (2)[C]

Pathological Findings
- Hyalinization of basophilic cells (anterior pituitary)
  – Crooke cell changes
- Muscular atrophy
- Nephrosclerosis
- Corticotroph pituitary tumor
- Ectopic ACTH-secreting tumor
- Adrenal adenoma or carcinoma
- Micronodular or macronodular hyperplasia

DIFFERENTIAL DIAGNOSIS
- Obesity
- Diabetes mellitus
- Hypertension
- Hypercortisolism secondary to alcoholism (pseudo-Cushing)

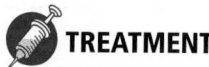 ## TREATMENT

GENERAL MEASURES
- Depends on cause
- Surgery is the treatment of choice.
- Persistent disease may require radiation, drug therapy, or surgery.
- Medical treatment with adrenocortical inhibitors
  - Has not been very successful
  - Use only when other methods fail and in consultation with an experienced clinician.

Diet
- Potassium supplements
- High protein

Activity
Determined by patient's symptoms and form of treatment used

Radiotherapy
As indicated

 ## MEDICATION (DRUGS)

Consultation with an endocrinologist is helpful in determining treatment.

First Line
- Adjunctive management considerations
  - Inhibit cortisol production: Ketoconazole 400–600 mg b.i.d. (dosages higher than conventionally recommended)
  - Glucocorticoid replacement following pituitary surgery: Discontinue in 3–12 months in most cases.
  - Bisphosphonates for prevention of osteoporosis (3)[C]

Second Line
- Mitotane
- Aminoglutethimide
- Metyrapone

SURGERY
- Primary hypersecretion of ACTH
  - Trans-sphenoidal microsurgery
  - Bilateral adrenalectomy as an adjunct for patients not cured
- Adrenocortical tumors
  - Surgical removal when possible
  - Poor prognosis for adrenocortical carcinoma
- Ectopic ACTH production
  - Removal of neoplastic tissue
  - Metastatic spread makes surgical cure unlikely/impossible
  - Bilateral adrenalectomy

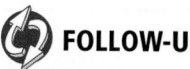 ## FOLLOW-UP

PROGNOSIS
- Generally chronic course with cyclic exacerbations and rare remissions
- Guardedly favorable prognosis with surgery
- 20% long-term recurrence rate after surgery
  - Poor with malignancy

COMPLICATIONS
- Osteoporosis
- Increased susceptibility to infections
- Metastases of malignant tumors
- Increased cardiovascular risk even after treatment
- Lifelong glucocorticoid dependence following treatment with bilateral adrenalectomy
- Nelson syndrome (pituitary rumor) after treatment with bilateral adrenalectomy

PATIENT MONITORING
- Individualize depending on therapy.
- Check regularly for signs of adrenal hypofunction.

REFERENCES

1. Newell-Price J, et al, Cushing's syndrome. *Lancet*. 2006;367:1605–1617[B].
2. Findling JF, Raff H. Cushing's syndrome: Important issues in diagnosis and management. *J Clin Endocrinol Metabol*. 2006;10:3746–3753 [C].
3. DiSomma C, et al. Effectiveness of chronic treatment with alendronate in the osteoporosis of Cushing's disease. *Clin Endocrinol*. 1998;48(5):655–662[C].
4. Isidori AM, et al. The ectopic adrenocorticotropin syndrome: Clinical features, diagnosis, management and long term follow up. *J Clin Endocrinol Metabol*. 2006;91(2):371–377. [C].

 ## MISCELLANEOUS

CODES

ICD9-CM
255.0 Cushing syndrome

PATIENT TEACHING
- Comprehensive teaching to help patient cope with lifelong treatment (if needed)
  - Drug therapy
  - Diet
  - Activity
  - Early treatment of infections
  - Need to monitor weight daily
  - Emotional lability prevention
- Refer to National Adrenal Disease Foundation: NADF; 505 Northern Blvd., Great Neck, NY 11021; (516)407-4992; e-mail: nadf@aol.com.

 See Corresponding Diagnostic Algorithm

CUTANEOUS DRUG REACTIONS

Jeremy Golding, MD

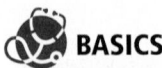 **BASICS**

DESCRIPTION

- Cutaneous or mucocutaneous eruptions are the most common adverse reactions to oral or parenteral drug therapy.
- Reactions may be immunologically mediated, either IgE dependent, immune complex dependent, cytotoxic, or delayed-type hypersensitivity (type 4 hypersensitivity). Most immunologic drug reactions are type 4.
- Nonimmunologic reactions are common. The majority of reactions occur within 1 week of initiation of drug therapy but may occur up to 4 weeks after initiation of therapy. Mechanisms include drug accumulation, idiosyncratic reactions (e.g., amoxicillin in infectious mononucleosis), direct release of mast-cell mediators, Jarisch-Herxheimer phenomenon, overdosage, and phototoxic dermatitis.
- Morphologically, morbilliform (maculopapular) and urticarial eruptions are the most common, but multiple morphologic types of reactions may occur.
- System(s) Affected: Hemic/lymphatic/immunologic; Skin/exocrine
- Synonym(s): Drug eruptions; Dermatitis medicamentosa

ALERT

Geriatric Considerations
- Possibly more likely in this age group, due to greater number of medications
- Severe systemic reactions less well tolerated

Pediatric Considerations
May occur in this age group

GENERAL PREVENTION
- Future avoidance of specific drugs and any analogs
- Be aware of any potential cross reactions (e.g., 8–10% incidence of reactions of cephalosporins in patients sensitized to penicillins and the crossover for the anticonvulsive drugs hydantoin, barbiturates, and carbamazepine [Tegretol]).
- Always question patients about prior drug reactions, specific type of reaction, and use of OTC medicines.

EPIDEMIOLOGY
- Predominant age: All ages affected
- Predominant sex: Female > Male (specific ratio unknown)

Incidence
- In the US: 2–5% of inpatients develop drug eruptions.
- Severe and life-threatening reactions may affect 1 in 1000 inpatients.
- Likelihood of developing a cutaneous reactions greater in patients with HIV.

Prevalence
Approximately 125 million Americans regularly use prescription drugs as outpatients; the overall prevalence in this group is unknown.

ETIOLOGY
- Acneform: Oral contraceptive pills (OCPs), corticosteroids, iodinated compounds, hydantoins, and lithium
- Erythema multiforme: Sulfonamides, penicillins, barbiturates, hydantoins, NSAIDs, tetracycline, Cefaclor, and Terbinafine
- Erythema nodosum: OCPs, sulfonamides, and penicillins
- Fixed drug eruptions: OCPs, barbiturates, salicylates, tetracycline, sulfonamides, and sulfonylureas
- Lichenoid: Gold, antimalarials, and tetracycline
- Photosensitivity: Phenothiazines, griseofulvin, sulfonamides, and tetracycline
- Vasculitis: Thiazides, gold, sulfonamides, NSAIDs, and tetracycline
- Bullous: NSAIDs, thiazides, barbiturates, and captopril
- Skin necrosis: Warfarin

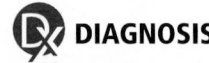 **DIAGNOSIS**

SIGNS AND SYMPTOMS
- Maculopapular (morbilliform) eruptions (exanthems)
  - Most frequent cutaneous reaction
  - May be indistinguishable from viral exanthem
  - Erythematous macules and papules
  - Often confluent and symmetric
  - Pruritus common
  - Mucous membranes, palms, and soles
  - Onset typically 7–21 (~10) days after initiation of drug
- Urticaria
  - Pruritic red wheals distributed anywhere on the body, including mucous membranes
  - Individual lesions fade within 24 hours, but new urticaria may develop.
  - May be mediated by anaphylactic or accelerated IgE reactions, serum sickness, or nonimmunologic histamine reactions
  - Deep dermal and subcutaneous swelling constitute angioedema and, when mucous membranes are involved, may be life-threatening
- Acneform eruptions
  - Pustular lesions, but unlike true acne (no comedones)
- Eczematous reactions
  - Pruritic scalelike erythematous lesions typically on flexor surfaces of arms or legs
- Erythema multiforme
  - Target lesions
  - Bullous lesions
  - Mucous membrane involvement (Stevens-Johnson syndrome)
- Exfoliative erythroderma
  - Generalized erythema and scaling
  - Potentially life threatening
- Fixed drug eruptions
  - Single or multiple, round, sharply defined, dark red plaques
  - Appear shortly after drug exposure and reappear in the same location after drug ingestion; lesions can occur anywhere: Glans penis common in men (especially with tetracycline).
  - Onset usually 2 hours after ingestion of drug
  - Some patients have a refractory period during which the drug fails to activate lesions.
- Lichen planuslike eruptions
  - Violaceous papules on extensor wrist surfaces
  - Reticular pattern, buccal mucosa
- Lupus erythematosuslike reactions
  - Malar erythema
- Photosensitivity reaction
  - Phototoxic reactions within 24 hours of light exposure
  - Photoallergic reactions; less common
- Vasculitis
  - Petechiae or purpura concentrated on lower legs
- Vesiculobullous eruptions
  - Small, isolated bullae, erythema multiforme, toxic epidermal necrolysis (potentially fatal)

- Acute generalized exanthematous pustulosis (AGEP)
  - Generalized scarlatiniform erythema with many small, sterile, nonfollicular pustules
  - Clinical presentation is similar to pustular psoriasis, but AGEP has more marked hyperleukocytosis with neutrophilia and eosinophilia.
  - Often caused by drugs (antibiotics) in 1st days of administration.

History

- Detailed drug-use history, including all OTC medicines, duration of therapy, medications used within the past 4 weeks

Physical Exam

- Accurate observation and morphologic description of all conditions facilitates differential diagnosis.
- **Describe location and morphology of all lesions. Examine mucus membranes.**
- Nikolsky sign (epidermis sloughs with lateral pressure; indicates serious eruption that may constitute a medical emergency)

TESTS

Lab

- Routine laboratory tests generally are nonspecific and usually not helpful.
- Eosinophilia: Possible in certain allergic reactions but generally of little value clinically
- Special tests
  - Skin testing (useful in IgE-mediated reactions)
  - IgG and IgM: Hemagglutination assays can detect drug-specific antibodies, but not routinely useful
- Cultures may be useful to exclude infectious causes.
- Drugs that may alter lab results: Procainamide, hydralazine (positive antinuclear antibodies)

Diagnostic Procedures/Surgery

- Withdrawal of suspected offending agent and observation for resolution of rash
- Selective special testing for suspected IgE-mediated reactions
- Punch biopsy sometimes helpful for fixed drug eruptions, which show certain characteristic histologic features (e.g., lichen planus-like or erythema multiforme)

Pathological Findings

Pathologic findings depend on type of reaction; they may be nonspecific.

DIFFERENTIAL DIAGNOSIS

- Viral exanthem: Because maculopapular eruptions are the most common form of drug reaction, these are often difficult to distinguish from viral exanthems. Presence of fever, lymphocytosis, and other systemic findings may help differentiate.
- Drug eruptions manifest as many types of dermatosis (as previously listed); consider a primary dermatosis in the differential diagnosis. Resolution of the eruption upon withdrawal of a drug will help to clarify diagnosis. The histopathology of skin biopsy also can be helpful in persistent cases.
- Skin reactions in young children may be due to the dye in liquid antibiotics.

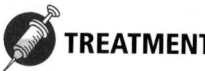 **TREATMENT**

GENERAL MEASURES

- Appropriate health care
  - Urticaria, angioedema, or bullous lesions, and generalized erythroderma are all potentially more serious than other types of reactions; therefore, possible offending medications should be discontinued immediately, and these patients should be seen as soon as possible for evaluation.
  - Consider inpatient treatment for anaphylactic reactions, Stevens-Johnson syndrome, extensive bullous reactions, or toxic epidermal necrolysis (TEN).
- Discontinue the suspected offending agent. In patients with multiple medications, the decision to discontinue each medication should be based on the likelihood of each individual medication causing the reaction (e.g., 7% for penicillins, sulfonamides) and the risk/benefit ratio of continuing each medication.
- Rechallenge with specific medications thought to have caused urticaria, angioedema, anaphylaxis, erythema multiforme, or other bullous lesions is potentially dangerous
- Medications may be continued if necessary through morbilliform eruptions unless the eruption is severe or unless accompanied by blistering, sloughing, or mucus membrane involvement.

Activity

- No specific restrictions in general
- For acute eczematous or urticarial reactions with intense pruritus, tepid bathing and avoidance of perspiration may be helpful.
- For TEN, admit to burn unit

 MEDICATION (DRUGS)

- Specific therapy depends on the type of drug eruption. Most require no specific therapy.
- Symptomatic therapy is helpful for pruritus, xeroses, urticaria, and angioedema.
- For pruritus (possibly also improve some eruptions): Antihistamines (e.g., diphenhydramine [Benadryl] 25–50 mg q6h, hydroxyzine [Atarax] 10–25 mg q6–8h)
- Anaphylaxis or widespread urticaria: Epinephrine 1:1,000, 0.01 mL/kg (0.3 mL maximum) SC
- For anaphylaxis, severe urticaria, erythema multiforme: Corticosteroids parenterally as indicated by patient's condition; or on tapering PO schedule (10–14 days).
- Therapy of TEN is controversial; the majority do not favor use of systemic corticosteroids; IV IgG therapy can be life-saving.
- Topical lubricants, emollients for eczematous reactions
- Topical corticosteroids (Groups I–III) for limited eczematous-type eruptions or for lichenoid eruptions
- Systemic corticosteroids (for urticaria, angioedema, and anaphylaxis): Prednisone 40–60 mg/d for 5–10 days. It is also useful in severe diffuse eczematous reactions.
- Contraindications: Refer to manufacturer's information
- Precautions: Refer to manufacturer's information
- Significant possible interactions: Refer to manufacturer's information

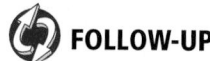 **FOLLOW-UP**

PROGNOSIS

- Eruptions generally fade within days after removing offending agent.
- Urticaria, angioedema, and bullous reactions are potentially more serious, even life threatening.

COMPLICATIONS

- Anaphylaxis
- Laryngeal edema
- Possible associated bone marrow suppression
- Hepatitis and hematologic changes (dapsone, hydantoin)
- Possible cross-reaction to chemically similar agents with future exposure

PATIENT MONITORING

- For urticarial, bullous, or erythema multiformelike lesions, close patient follow-up is indicated to ensure no progression occurs.
- Patients with systemic anaphylaxis or widespread bullous lesions, including TEN, should be admitted to hospital until condition improves.
- Maintain at least telephone follow-up until the eruption has completely cleared.
- Label the patient's chart with the suspected agent and the specific type of reaction.

REFERENCES

1. Blume, et al. Drug eruptions. *e-Medicine* Sept 2006.
2. Bigby M. Rates of cutaneous reactions to drugs. *Arch Dermatol.* 2001;137(6):765–770.
3. Daoud MS, et al. Recognizing cutaneous drug eruptions. *Post Grad Med.* 1998;104(1):101–115.
4. Habif T. *Clinical Dermatology*, 4th ed. St. Louis: CV Mosby, 2004.
5. Heller HM. Adverse cutaneous drug reactions in patients with human immunodeficiency virus-1 infection. *Clin Dermatol.* 2000;18(4):485–489.
6. Lazarou J, et al. Incidence of adverse drug reactions in hospitalized patients. *JAMA.* 1998;279: 1200–1205.
7. Roujeau JC. Treatment of severe drug eruptions. *J Dermatol.* 1999;26(11):718–722.
8. Yates AB, deShazo RD. Allergic and nonallergic drug reactions. *South Med J.* 2003;96(11): 1080–1087.

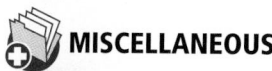 **MISCELLANEOUS**

CODES

ICD9-CM

693.0 Dermatitis due to drugs or medicines taken internally

PATIENT TEACHING

Printed patient information: American Academy of Dermatology, 930 N. Meacham Rd., P.O. Box 4014, Schaumberg, IL 60168-4014; (708) 330–0230

C

CUTANEOUS SQUAMOUS CELL CARCINOMA

Herbert P. Goodheart, MD

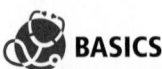 **BASICS**

DESCRIPTION

- Squamous cell carcinoma (SCC) is a malignant epithelial tumor arising from keratinocytes of the epidermis.
- Cutaneous (nonmucous membrane) SCC is the 2nd most common form of skin cancer.
- Lesions most frequently occur on sun-exposed sites of elderly, fair-skinned individuals: The head, neck, ears, forearms and hands.
- The majority of SCCs arise in solar keratoses *(actinic keratoses)*. Such SCCs that develop from solar keratoses are slow growing, minimally invasive, unaggressive, and the prognosis is usually excellent because distant metastases are extremely rare.
- An SCC may appear de novo without a preceding solar keratosis
- SCCs may also develop from causes other than sun exposure. For example, a SCC may arise in an old burn scar, or from sites previously exposed to ionizing radiation. A SCC may also emerge from pre-existing human papilloma virus infection *(verrucous carcinoma)*.
- When metastases from SCC do occur, they are more likely to result from lesions that appear on the ears or on the vermillion border of the lips or from tumors larger than 2 cm in diameter (1).
- Metastases are even more apt to arise from lesions on
  - Mucous membranes
  - Sites that received ionizing radiation
  - The skin of organ transplant recipients
  - Chronic inflammatory lesions (e.g., discoid lupus erythematosus)
  - Long-standing scars or cutaneous ulcers (e.g., venous stasis ulcers) or other nonhealing wounds.
- System(s) affected: Skin/exocrine
- Synonym(s): Squamous cell carcinoma of the skin; Epidermoid carcinoma; Prickle cell carcinoma

GENERAL PREVENTION

- Sun-avoidance measures
  - Sunscreens, hats, etc.
  - Sunglasses with UV protection
  - Tinted windshields and side windows in cars
  - Sun-protective garments
- Avoidance of contact with known carcinogenic compounds

EPIDEMIOLOGY

- Predominant age: Elderly population
- Predominant sex: Males > Females

Incidence

- The incidence is highest in Australia and in the Sun Belt of the US
- SCCs are rare in dark-skinned individuals

RISK FACTORS

- Older age
- Male sex: Although incidence is increasing in females due to lifestyle changes (e.g., suntan parlors, shorter dresses, etc.)
- Chronic sun exposure: SCC is noted more frequently in those with a greater degree of outdoor activity (e.g., farmers, sailors, gardeners).
- Family history of skin cancer
- Irish-Scottish-British descent
- Fair complexion, fair hair
- Light blue or green eyes
- Poor tanning ability with tendency to burn
- Organ transplant recipients
- Long-term phototherapy recipients of PUVA (an oral psoralen with ultraviolet A light)

ETIOLOGY

- Exact mechanisms not established
- Epidemiologic and experimental evidence suggests the following as causative agents
  - Sunlight (solar radiation)
  - Radiation exposure
  - Tanning parlors, PUVA phototherapy exposure
  - Inorganic arsenic exposure
  - Exposure to coal tar and other oil and tar derivatives
  - Immunosuppression by medications or disease such as HIV

ASSOCIATED CONDITIONS

- Solar keratosis (some investigators consider a solar keratosis to be an early squamous cell carcinoma)
- Keratoacanthoma
- Cutaneous horn
- Actinic cheilitis (solar keratoses of the mucous membranes of the lips)
- Leukoplakia of lip
- Xeroderma pigmentosum
- Immunosuppression
- Vitiligo
- Albinism
- Chronic skin ulcers
- Chronic thermal burns

DIAGNOSIS

SIGNS AND SYMPTOMS

- Lesions occur chiefly on in chronically **sun-exposed areas**
  - The face, especially on the nose, temples, forehead, backs of the forearms, and hands.
  - Bald areas of the scalp and top of ears in men
  - The sun-exposed "V" of the neck, as well as the posterior neck below the occipital hairline.
  - In elderly females, lesions tend to occur on the legs and other sun-exposed locations.
  - In African Americans: Equal frequency in sun-exposed and unexposed areas.
- Clinical appearance
  - Generally slow-growing, firm papules, nodules, or plaques
  - Lesions may have a smooth, verrucous, or papillomatous surface.
  - Varying degrees of ulceration, erosion, crust, or scale
  - Color is often red to brown, tan or pearly. May be indistinguishable from basal cell carcinoma.

SIGNS AND SYMPTOMS

Most SCCs are asymptomatic, although bleeding, pain, and tenderness may be noted.

PROGNOSIS

- The ability to produce scale *(keratinization)* indicates a tendency to be more differentiated and less likely to metastasize.
- Softer, nonkeratinizing lesions are not as well differentiated and are more likely to spread.

History

Often a family history of skin cancer

TESTS

Diagnostic Procedures/Surgery

- Surgical biopsy to ensure diagnosis
  - Shave biopsy
  - Excisional biopsy

Pathological Findings

- In the *in situ* type of SCC (*Bowen disease*), only the full thickness of the epidermis is involved. Atypical keratinocytes (squamous cells) show a loss of polarity and an increased mitotic rate. The basement membrane remains intact.
- An invasive squamous cell carcinoma penetrates through the basement membrane into the dermis. It has various levels of anaplasia, and may manifest relatively few to multiple mitoses and display varying degrees of differentiation, such as keratinization.
- SCCs proliferate first by local invasion. Metastases, when they do occur, spread via local lymph ducts to local lymph nodes.

DIFFERENTIAL DIAGNOSIS

- Solar keratosis *(actinic keratosis)*. An early SCC lesion that is often clinically difficult to distinguish from a precursor solar keratosis.
- Verruca vulgaris. A wart may also resemble a SCC.
- Seborrheic keratosis. An extremely common benign skin growth that becomes apparent >40 years of age.
  - They have virtually no malignant potential.
  - The typical seborrheic keratosis lesion has a warty, "stuck-on" appearance that ranges from tan to dark brown to black.
- Keratoacanthoma. This lesion also may be clinically impossible to differentiate from a SCC.
  - Occurs in the elderly >65 years.
  - It is fast growing.
  - Usually has a typical central crater
  - If ignored, lesions may regress spontaneously.
  - Resembles an SCC histologically, and is considered by some dermatologists and dermatopathologists to be a low-grade variant of an SCC. (Some investigators feel that it should be treated as an SCC.)
- Basal cell carcinoma may be indistinguishable from an SCC, particularly if the lesion is ulcerated.
- Melanoma
  - An amelanotic melanoma (lacking typical pigmentation)
  - An ulcerated melanoma may also be impossible to distinguish from a SCC.
- Clinical variants
  - Bowen disease *(squamous cell carcinoma in situ)* is a solitary lesion that resembles a scaly psoriatic or eczematous plaque.
    - This lesion often arises in non–sunexposed sites such as the trunk or extremities. Atypical cells fill the epidermis. When an SCC in situ occurs on the penis, it is known as **erythroplasia of Queyrat.** Untreated, these lesions may become invasive.
    - **Bowen disease** and frank squamous cell carcinoma are 2 of the few skin cancers that should be considered as a diagnosis in blacks. These non–sun-related skin cancers tend to arise on the extremities de novo, or in an old scar or in a lesion of discoid lupus erythematosus.
  - Cutaneous horn
    - **SCC with an overlying cutaneous horn.** A cutaneous horn represents a fingernail platelike keratinization produced by the SCC. Bowen disease may also produce a cutaneous horn on its surface.
  - Keratoacanthoma
    - Craterlike nodular lesions that resemble SCCs.

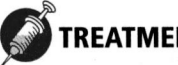 TREATMENT

SURGERY

- Electrocautery (electrodesiccation) and curettage
  - For small lesions (generally smaller than 1 cm) on flat surfaces (e.g., forehead, cheek) and SCC in situ (Bowen disease)
- Cryosurgery with LN$_2$ in selected lesions
- Total excision, which is the preferred method of therapy for SCC, permitting histologic diagnosis of the tumor margins
- Micrographic (Mohs') surgery may be indicated for
  - Excessively large or invasive carcinomas
  - Recurrent lesions
  - Lesions with a poorly delineated clinical border
  - SCC within an orifice (e.g., ear canals or nostrils).
  - Locations where preservation of normal tissue is extremely important (e.g., tip of the nose, eyelids, ala nasi, ears, lips, and glans penis)
  - Bone or cartilage invasion
  - A lesion in an area of late radiation change

SPECIAL THERAPY
Radiotherapy
- Suitable for larger, advanced lesions.
- Also used for those patients who are physically debilitated or are unable to, or refuse to undergo, excisional surgery

ALERT
Clinical
- An SCC arising on a mucous membrane, one arising from a chronic ulcer, or one arising in an immunocompromised patient should be regarded as potentially metastatic.
- A subungual SCC can easily be mistaken for a verruca.
- High-risk SCCs may require imaging studies
- Lymph node biopsy is indicated for suspected nodal involvement.

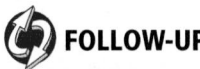 MEDICATION (DRUGS)

Imiquimod 5% cream for Bowen disease *(squamous cell carcinoma in situ)* (2)[A]

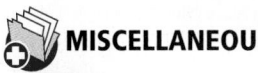 FOLLOW-UP

PROGNOSIS
- 90–95% cure rate with appropriate treatment
- Lesions ≥2 cm more prone to recur
- Head and neck lesions have better prognosis (3).

COMPLICATIONS
- Untreated, SCC becomes indurated, with a tendency to ooze, ulcerate, or bleed.
- Local recurrence
- Metastatic disease

PATIENT MONITORING
After therapy, periodic skin exam every month for 3 months, 6 months after treatment, and then yearly.

REFERENCES

1. Schmults CD. High-risk cutaneous squamous cell carcinoma: Identification and management.
2. Patel GK, Goodwin R. Imiquimod 5% cream monotherapy for cutaneous *squamous cell carcinoma in situ (*Bowen's disease): A randomized, double-blind, placebo-controlled trial. *J Am Acad Dermatol.* 2006;54(1):25–32.
3. Adv Dermatol 2005;21:133–152 Clayman GL, Lee JJ, Holsinger FC, et al. Mortality risk from squamous cell skin cancer. *J Clin Oncol.* 2005;23(4):759–765.

MISCELLANEOUS

CODES
ICD9-CM
- 173.3 Other malignant neoplasm of skin of other and unspecified parts of face
- 173.4 Other malignant neoplasm of scalp and skin of neck
- 173.5 Other malignant neoplasm of skin of trunk, except scrotum
- 173.6 Other malignant neoplasm of skin of upper limb, including shoulder
- 173.7 Other malignant neoplasm of skin of lower limb, including hip
- 173.9 Other malignant neoplasm of skin, site unspecified

PATIENT TEACHING

- Skin self-exam
- Sun avoidance techniques, sunscreens, etc.
- Follow-up visits to dermatologist
- Materials available from American Cancer Society

Prevention
Appropriate sun avoidance measures such as sunscreen and protective clothing

 See Patient Handout on CD

CUTANEOUS T-CELL LYMPHOMA

Keri Clifford, MD
Amit Garg, MD

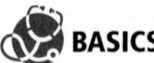 **BASICS**

DESCRIPTION
- Cutaneous T-cell lymphomas are a heterogeneous group of relatively uncommon extranodal non-Hodgkin lymphomas
- This section focuses on mycosis fungoides, the most common type of cutaneous lymphoma. For other subtypes, please consult the reference section.

EPIDEMIOLOGY
- Median age at diagnosis is 55–60, however it can occur in children and young adults
- Male : Female = 1.6–2:1

Incidence
0.36 cases per 100,000

RISK FACTORS
No compelling evidence that mycosis fungoides is caused by viral infection or chemical exposure

Genetics
- Clonal T-cell receptor gene rearrangements are detected in most cases.
- No recurrent, mycosis fungoides-specific chromosomal translocations have been identified.
- Loss at 10q and abnormalities in p15, p16, and p53 are common.

PATHOPHYSIOLOGY
- Malignancy of CD4$^+$ helper T cells
- Malignant cells have a high affinity to the epidermis.
- Malignant T cells are also activated T cells (CD45RO$^+$) and produce cytokines, such as IL-4 and IL-5, which can lead to eosinophilia and atopylike symptoms.

ETIOLOGY
Unknown

DIAGNOSIS

SIGNS AND SYMPTOMS
- Rash
- Skin tumors or ulcers
- Pruritus

Physical Exam
- Pink scaly patches and plaques, typically in sun-protected areas such as the buttocks, thighs, and breasts
- Cutaneous tumors and ulcerations
- Exfoliative erythroderma (>80% of total body surface area is red and scaly)
- Palmoplantar keratoderma (thickened scaly skin on palms and soles)
- Lymphadenopathy can be present in later stages.
- Hepatosplenomegaly can be present at late stages.

TESTS
Lab
- CBC with differential and platelets
- PCR of peripheral blood to detect clonal rearrangement of the T-cell receptor
- Flow cytometry
- Sézary cell count
  - A CD4:CD8 ratio of >10, a circulating clonal T-cell population, and a Sézary cell count of >1000/mm^3, and loss of T-cell antigens are all consistent with leukemic involvement

Imaging
CT of the chest, abdomen, and pelvis or PET/CT for advanced disease (IIb and later)

Diagnostic Procedures/Surgery
- Skin biopsy: Diagnostic procedure of choice
- Lymph node biopsy if there is clinical adenopathy or advanced disease
- Bone marrow biopsy for advanced disease

Pathological Findings
Skin biopsy
- Superficial bandlike infiltrate
- Epidermotropism of lymphocytes, Pautrier microabscesses
- Atypical lymphocytes with cerebriform nuclei (Sézary cells)
- Dermal infiltrates of atypical cells in tumors
- Cells are usually CD3$^+$, CD4$^+$, CD45RO$^+$, CD8$^-$
- Loss of T cell antigens such as CD2, CD3, CD5, and CD7 is often seen.

DIFFERENTIAL DIAGNOSIS
- Patches and plaques (T1–2)
  - Parapsoriasis
  - Atopic dermatitis
  - Nummular eczema
  - Psoriasis
  - Contact dermatitis
- Tumor
  - Cutaneous B-cell lymphoma
  - Cutaneous metastases
- Staging is done based on physical examination and pathology.
  - T1: Patches or plaques involving <10% of total body surface area
  - T2: Patches or plaques involving >10% of total body surface area
  - T3: Cutaneous tumors
  - T4: Erythroderma
  - N0: Lymph nodes clinically uninvolved
  - N1: Lymph nodes clinically enlarged but not histologically involved
  - N2: Lymph nodes clinically normal but histologically involved
  - N3: Lymph nodes clinically enlarged and histologically involved
  - M0: No visceral disease
  - M1: Visceral disease
- Stage groups
  - IA: T1N0M0
  - IB: T2N0M0
  - IIA: T1–2N1M0
  - IIB: T3N0–1M0
  - III: T4N0–1M0
  - IVA: T1–4N2–3M0
  - IVB: T1–4N0–3M1
- Sézary syndrome (leukemic phase of cutaneous T cell lymphoma) is defined by
  - Erythroderma
  - Lymphadenopathy
  - Peripheral blood involvement

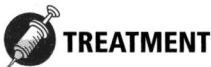 **TREATMENT**

GENERAL MEASURES
- Most patients are managed on an outpatient basis.
- Treatment should be individualized for each patient, based on their extent of disease and side effects of possible therapies.

Activity
No limitations

SPECIAL THERAPY
Radiotherapy
Localized or total skin electron-beam therapy can be used in most stages of disease, either as monotherapy or in combination with other agents.

 MEDICATION (DRUGS)

First Line
- Therapy must be individualized. No universally accepted standard approach exists to treatment of this disease. The stage of disease dictates the aggressiveness of therapy.
- T1 and T2 disease
  - Topical potent corticosteroids
  - Topical mechlorethamine (nitrogen mustard)
  - Topical Bis-chlor nitrosourea
  - Topical bexarotene
  - Phototherapy: Psoralen and ultraviolet A light (PUVA) or narrow band UVB
  - Oral retinoids (bexarotene)
  - Oral methotrexate
- T3 disease
  - Oral retinoids (bexarotene)
  - Interferon α-2b
  - Denileukin diftitox
  - Chemotherapy
- T4 disease and Sézary syndrome
  - Oral retinoids
  - Denileukin diftitox
  - Phototherapy
  - Extracorporeal photopheresis
  - Chemotherapy
  - Bone marrow transplantation

 FOLLOW-UP

DISPOSITION
Issues for Referral
- Dermatology referral for management of early disease
- Hematology-oncology is involved for later stage disease.
- Radiation oncology for XRT

PROGNOSIS
- Mycosis fungoides is a chronic disease; cure is very uncommon and not the usual goal of treatment.
- 10-year disease-specific survival rates
  - T1: 97–98%
  - T2: 83%
  - T3: 42%
  - T4: Similar to T2
  - 20% for patients with lymph node involvement

COMPLICATIONS
Immunosuppression from the disease and treatments can lead to infections and secondary malignancies.

PATIENT MONITORING
Must be individualized

REFERENCES

1. Willemze R, Jaffe ES, Burg G, et al. WHO-EORTC classification for cutaneous lymphomas. *Blood*. 2005;105:3768–3785.
2. Girardi M, Heald PW, Wilson LD. The pathogenesis of mycosis fungoides. *N Engl J Med*. 2004;350:1978–1988.

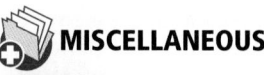 **MISCELLANEOUS**

CODES

ICD9-CM
202.80 Other malignant lymphomas, unspecified site, extranodal and solid organ sites

PATIENT TEACHING
- Patient information can be found at:
- American Academy of Dermatology website www.aad.org
- Cutaneous Lymphoma Foundation website www.clfoundation.org

CYSTIC FIBROSIS

Ann M. Lynch, PharmD, RPh

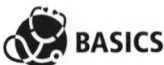 **BASICS**

DESCRIPTION
- Cystic fibrosis (CF) is an autosomal-recessive genetic condition that most prominently affects the lungs and pancreas.
- The intestinal track, liver, reproductive organs, and skin can all be involved.
- Initially a pediatric disease, CF has become an adult medical condition as improvements in medical care have led to a dramatic increase in long-term survival.

GENERAL PREVENTION
Genetic analysis of siblings of known CF patients is recommended.

EPIDEMIOLOGY
CF is the most common lethal inherited disease in the Caucasian population, and is found in every ethnic and racial group.

Incidence
Number of infants born with CF in relation to the total number of live-births in the US
- 1 in 3,200 Caucasians
- 1 in 9,500 Hispanics
- 1 in 15,000 African-Americans
- 1 in 31,000 Asian-Americans

Prevalence
- >22,700 patients with CF living in the US per the 2004 CF Foundation Patient Registry.
- ~900 new diagnoses are made annually

RISK FACTORS
The risk is based on genetic inheritance factors.

Genetics
The CFTR gene (cystic fibrosis transmembrane conductance regulator)
- Located on the long arm of chromosome 7
- CFTR protein acts as a chloride channel for ion and water transport.
- Over 1,000 mutations exist that can cause phenotypic CF.
- Most common mutation is loss of the phenylalanine residue at 508th position (ΔF508).
- ΔF508 accounts for ~2/3 of affected alleles in the CF population in the US.

PATHOPHYSIOLOGY
- Abnormal CFTR function leads to abnormally viscous secretions that alter organ function.
- The lungs
  - Histologically, the lungs are normal at birth
  - A combination of obstruction, infection, and inflammation begins to negatively impact upon lung growth, structure, and function
    - Highly viscous secretions lead to decreased mucociliary clearance.
    - Endobronchial infection begins early in life.
    - Infection is accompanied by an intense neutrophilic response in and around the bronchi and bronchioles.
    - Degradation of supporting airway tissues causes bronchiectasis, then respiratory insufficiency and eventual failure.

ASSOCIATED CONDITIONS
- Extrapulmonary manifestations
- The gastrointestinal tract
  - Pancreatic exocrine insufficiency
    - Malabsorption of fat and protein and insufficient absorption of fat-soluble vitamins (A, D, E, and K)
    - 85–90% of patients
  - Hepatobiliary disease
    - Focal biliary cirrhosis (5% of patients)
    - Cholelithiasis
  - Meconium ileus at birth
    - 10–15% of patients
  - Distal intestinal obstruction syndrome (DIOS)
    - Also known as *meconium ileus equivalent*
    - Intestinal blockage that typically occurs in older children and adults
- Endocrine
  - CF-related diabetes (CFRD)
  - Increasing incidence with advancing age
- Reproductive organs
  - Congenital absence of the vas deferens
    - Obstructive azoospermia in 98% of males

ALERT
Pregnancy Considerations
- Females have slight decrease in fertility.
- Pulmonary disease is worse during pregnancy.

DX **DIAGNOSIS**

PRE HOSPITAL
- Prenatal testing for CF genetics is offered routinely to mothers in the US.
  - Most useful in those with strong family history
- Prenatal ultrasound: Hyperechoic bowel pattern suggestive of CF
  - Fetal intestinal obstruction

SIGNS AND SYMPTOMS
- General (any age)
  - Family history
  - Chronic/recurrent respiratory symptoms
  - Persistent infiltrates on chest radiographs
  - Hypochloremic metabolic acidosis
- Neonatal
  - Meconium ileus
  - Prolonged jaundice
- Infancy
  - Failure to thrive
  - Chronic diarrhea
  - Anasarca/hypoproteinemia
  - Pseudotumor cerebri (vitamin A deficiency)
  - Hemolytic anemia (vitamin E deficiency)
- Childhood
  - Recurrent sinusitis
  - Steatorrhea
  - Rectal prolapse
  - DIOS
- Adolescence and adulthood
  - Allergic bronchopulmonary aspergillosis (ABPA)
  - Chronic sinusitis
  - Bronchiectasis
  - Hemoptysis
  - Pancreatitis
  - Portal hypertension
  - Azoospermia

History
The diagnosis of CF should be suspected in any child with failure to thrive, steatorrhea, and recurrent respiratory problems.

Physical Exam
- Respiratory
  - Rhonchi and/or crackles
  - Hyperresonance on percussion
  - Nasal polyps
- Gastrointestinal
  - Hepatosplenomegaly when cirrhosis present
- Other
  - Digital clubbing
  - Growth retardation
  - Delayed puberty

Lab
- Newborn screening programs for CF is included in 34 states as of October 2006
  - Immunoreactive trypsinogen (IRT) elevated in blood spots of most infants with CF
- Sweat test (gold standard)
  - Sweat chloride
    - >60 mmol/L is positive for CF
    - <40 mmol/L is normal
- CFTR mutation analysis
  - Limited panel testing
    - Identifies >90% of mutations
    - Finite chance of false negative (especially patients of non-European decent)
  - Full sequence testing
    - Costly and time consuming

TESTS
- Sputum culture (common CF organisms)
  - *Staphylococcus aureus*
  - Nontypeable *Haemophilus influenzae*
  - *Pseudomonas aeruginosa*
    - Nonmucoid and mucoid
  - *Burkholderia cepacia*
    - At least 10 genomovars identified
    - Associated with worsening pulmonary disease
  - Atypical mycobacteria
  - *Aspergillus fumigatus*
    - May lead to allergic bronchopulmonary aspergillosis (ABPA)
- Pulmonary function tests (PFTs)
  - FEV1 assesses for obstructive lung disease
- 72-hour fecal fat
  - Assessment for fat malabsorption
- Stool elastase
  - Assessment of pancreatic exocrine function

Imaging
- Chest radiography
  - Hyperinflation early in disease
  - Bronchial thickening and plugging
  - Nodular densities, patchy atelectasis, and confluent infiltrates
  - Bronchiectasis
- Chest CT (not routine)
  - Defines disease more extensively
  - Useful when unusual findings noted on CXR

Diagnostic Procedures/Surgery
Flexible bronchoscopy
- Bronchoalveolar lavage (BAL)
  - Occasionally used for identification of lower airway bacterial pathogens

DIFFERENTIAL DIAGNOSIS
- Pulmonary
  - Difficult-to-manage asthma
  - Chronic bronchitis
  - Recurrent pneumonia
  - Chronic/recurrent sinusitis
- Gastrointestinal
  - Celiac disease
  - Protein-losing enteropathy
  - Pancreatitis of unknown etiology
  - Shwachman-Diamond syndrome

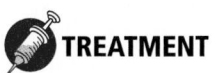 TREATMENT

PRE HOSPITAL
Oral antibiotics and increased chest physiotherapy often are utilized with increased pulmonary symptoms (cough and increased sputum production).

INITIAL STABILIZATION
Nasal-canula oxygen is beneficial when the patient is hypoxic (SaO$_2$ <90%).

GENERAL MEASURES
- Yearly Influenza vaccination is encouraged for all CF patients and family members.
- Infection control
  - Use contact precautions for any patient known to harbor MRSA, *B. cepacia*, or multidrug resistant *P. aeruginosa*.
- Avoidance of smoke

Diet
- Restrictions are highly discouraged in CF.
- High-calorie, high-fat diet with added salt

Activity
Routine exercise is critical in prevention

Nursing
- Familiarity with nursing staff improves overall care and comfort of patients with chronic diseases.
- Nursing assignments should involve only one CF patient per nurse for isolation purposes.

SPECIAL THERAPY
- Airway clearance techniques (1)
- Chest physiotherapy with postural drainage
  - VEST (airway clearance system)
  - Flutter valve or acapella

Physical Therapy
In-hospital physical therapy may be helpful because time spent with reduced mobility in the hospital adds to joint stiffness and pain.

IV Fluids
Avoid over-zealous IV fluids with worsening lung disease.

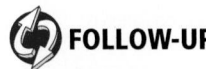 MEDICATION

- *Pulmonary*
- Antibiotics
  - Oral
    - *S. aureus*: Bactrim or cephalexin
    - *P. aeruginosa*: Fluoroquinolones
    - Azithromycin (chronic use/anti-inflammatory properties) (2)
    - Inhaled
    - TOBI (tobramycin 300 mg/dose via nebulizer)
    - Colistin (more commonly used in Europe)
  - IV
    - *S. aureus*: Zosyn or nafcillin
    - MRSA: Vancomycin or linezolid
    - *P. aeruginosa*: β-Lactam (Zosyn or ceftazidime) plus aminoglycoside (tobramycin) (3)
    - *B. cepacia*: 3 or more drugs based on synergy studies
- Inhalation therapy
  - β-Agonist in conjunction with chest physiotherapy (4)
  - Recombinant human DNAse (mucolytic) (5)
  - Hypertonic saline
    - May cause bronchoconstriction
- Anti-inflammatory agents
  - Oral steroids
    - Useful in setting of ABPA
  - Ibuprofen
- *Gastrointestinal*
- Pancreatic enzymes
  - Use in pancreatic insufficient patients
  - Name brand should not be substituted
- Vitamin supplementation
  - Fat-soluble vitamins (A,D,E, and K)
- Liver disease (cholestasis)
  - Ursodeoxycholic acid
- *Endocrine*
- CF-related diabetes
  - SQ insulin
  - Dietary restrictions should be avoided

SURGERY
- Lung transplantation
  - Reserved for patients with severe pulmonary impairment and limited life expectancy (FEV1 <30% predicted)
  - 5-year posttransplant survival: 50%
  - Outcomes improved at established transplant centers
- Liver transplantation
  - Reserved for cases of progressive liver failure and/or portal hypertension leading to gastrointestinal bleeding

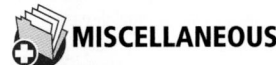 FOLLOW-UP

DISPOSITION
Admission Criteria
- Pulmonary exacerbation (most common reason for admission)
  - Increased cough, sputum production, and decreased pulmonary function
  - Change in lung examination (rales, retractions, tachypnea)
  - New abnormalities on chest film
  - Decreased appetite and weight loss
  - Decreased energy level
  - Fever, leukocytosis
- Bowel obstruction (DIOS)
- Pancreatitis (in pancreatic sufficient patients)

Discharge Criteria
- Pulmonary exacerbations often last 2 weeks
- Home IV antibiotics for select patients
Issues for Referral
Upon discharge for a pulmonary exacerbation, follow-up with their CF provider within 2–4 weeks
PROGNOSIS
- Most recent median survival is ~37 years, as of 2005 CF Foundation Patient Registry.
- Progression of lung disease usually determines length of survival.
PATIENT MONITORING
- It is recommended by the CF Foundation that all patients be followed in an accredited CF Center.
- Routine clinic visits every 3 months

REFERENCES
1. Main E, Prasad A, Schans C. Conventional chest physiotherapy compared to other airway clearance techniques for cystic fibrosis. *Cochrane Database Sys Rev.* 2005(1):CD002011.
2. Saiman L, Marshall BC, Mayer-Hamblett N, et al. Azithromycin in patients with cystic fibrosis chronically infected with *Pseudomonas aeruginosa*: a randomized controlled trial. *JAMA.* 2003;290(13):1749–1756.
3. Noone PG, Knowles MR. *Standard therapy of CF lung disease.* Philadelphia: Lippincott-Raven, 1999.
4. Halfhide C, Evans HJ, Couriel J. Inhaled bronchodilators for cystic fibrosis. *Cochrane Database Sys Rev.* 2005(4):CD003428.
5. Jones AP, Wallis CE. Recombinant human deoxyribonuclease for cystic fibrosis. [Update of Cochrane Database Sys Rev. 2000;(2):CD001127; PMID: 10796748]. Cochrane Database Sys Rev. 2003(3):CD001127.

 MISCELLANEOUS

CODES
ICD9-CM
- 277.00 CF w/o meconium ileus
- 277.01 CF w/ meconium ileus
- 277.02 CF w/ pulmonary manifestations
- 277.03 CF w/ gastrointestinal manifestations

PATIENT TEACHING
- Home treatment is critical to better outcomes.
- Individualize routine home therapy is important to meet patient's medical needs and potential for success.

See Corresponding Diagnostic Algorithm

CYTOMEGALOVIRUS INCLUSION DISEASE

Douglas Hunt, MD

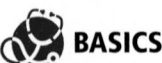 **BASICS**

DESCRIPTION

- β-Herpesvirus
- Primary infection usually inapparent and may remain latent throughout a person's life, rarely reactivating without immunocompromise
- Severe disease can result from primary infection of newborns and reactivation in setting of immunocompromise or organ transplantation
- Name derives from the infected cells, which are large and bear intranuclear inclusions described as "owl's eye" inclusions.
- Not highly contagious.
  - Spread via close personal contact with persons shedding virus from saliva, urine, blood, breast milk, or semen
  - Also acquired via infected transplant organs
- Infection may be in almost any organ
- Categories of CMV infections include the following
  - Congenital: Vary greatly from mild cytomegaloviremia in a normal infant to the cause of abortion, stillbirth, postnatal death from hemorrhage, anemia, or liver or CNS damage.
  - Acute infection in a normal host: Symptomatic infection commonly presents with acute mononucleosis syndrome (1)
  - Infection in bone marrow and solid organ transplant patients
    ○ Bone marrow transplant: Usually interstitial pneumonia
    ○ Liver transplant: Hepatitis
    ○ Kidney transplant: CMV syndrome
  - Infection in patients with AIDS: Most commonly retinitis, 2nd most commonly colitis, followed by esophagitis and neurologic disease (2)
  - Infections in other immunocompromised patients: Pulmonary, gastrointestinal, or renal disease
- System(s) affected: Ophthalmic; Pulmonary; Gastrointestinal; Neurologic; Renal; Skin/exocrine
- Synonym(s): Giant cell inclusion disease; CID CMV; Salivary gland virus disease

ALERT

Pregnancy Considerations
- CMV infection during pregnancy can be hazardous to the fetus.
- May lead to stillbirth, brain damage, birth defects, or to severe neonatal illness

Pediatric Considerations
May occur congenitally or postnatally

GENERAL PREVENTION

- Handwashing and basic hygiene (3)[A]
- Avoid immunosuppression (when possible)
- Highly active anti retroviral therapy (HAART) is the best method to prevent infection in high-risk HIV patients (4)[A]
- Chronic maintenance therapy for life in HIV patients with CMV end-organ disease unless successfully treated with ART (1)[A]. Options include
  - Parenteral or oral ganciclovir (1)[A]
  - Parenteral foscarnet (1)[A]
  - Combined parenteral ganciclovir and foscarnet (1)[A]
  - Parenteral cidofovir (1)[A]
  - Ganciclovir administration via intraocular implant or repetitive intravitreous injection of fomivirsen (1)[A]
- CMV antibody+, HIV+ children who are severely immunosuppressed require oral ganciclovir 30 mg/kg t.i.d. (3)[C]
- Antiviral suppression of CMV reactivation in CMV+transplant recipients or recipients of CMV+ organs
  - Solid organ transplant: Prophylactic or preemptive treatment with oral ganciclovir, valganciclovir (5)[A]
  - Bone marrow transplant: IV ganciclovir
- Immunization with live-attenuated CMV vaccine decreases severity of disease in renal transplant patients (6)[A]
- CMV immunoglobulins decrease rate of severe disease after liver transplant (7)[A] and decrease incidence of disease after renal transplant (8)[A]

EPIDEMIOLOGY

Incidence
- Common, but frequently asymptomatic
- <2–3 cases of end-organ disease per 100 person-years in HIV patients
- CMV infection is even more prevalent in populations at higher risk for HIV infection (IV drug users 75%, homosexual males 90%).
- Predominant age: All ages, peaks at <3 months; 16–40 years, and 40–75 years
- Predominant sex: Males > Females

Prevalence
- Occurs worldwide
- 40–100% of the general US population is seropositive from prior exposure during childhood or early adulthood (4):
- 20% of children in the US are seropositive before reaching puberty (4)
- Most common perinatally transmitted infection: 0.2–2.2% of births in US (9)

RISK FACTORS

- HIV infection, with specific risks including
  - CD4 count <50 cells/μL (2)[B]
  - Absence of treatment with or failure to respond to ART (2)[B]
  - Previous opportunistic infections (2)[B]
  - HIV viral load >100,000 (2)[B]
- Organ transplantation
- Blood transfusion
- Immunocompromise
- Living in closed population
- Corticosteroid therapy
- Day care environment—infant or geriatric (3)[B]
- For congenital infection—maternal infection during pregnancy
- Low socioeconomic status (9)[C]

ETIOLOGY

- Primary infection
- Reinfection with different CMV strains
- Reactivation of latent virus in patients who are immunosuppressed

ASSOCIATED CONDITIONS

- AIDS
- Corticosteroid therapy
- Leukemia
- Lymphoma

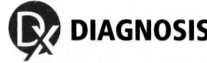 **DIAGNOSIS**

SIGNS AND SYMPTOMS

- Congenital
  - Asymptomatic cytomegaloviremia
  - Symptomatic: Small for gestational age, purpura/petechiae, jaundice, hepatosplenomegaly, chorioretinitis, microcephaly, intracranial calcifications, hearing impairment
  - 90% have late complications: Sensorineural hearing loss (most common), mental retardation, chorioretinitis, optic atrophy, seizures, learning disabilities (9)
- Acquired: Acute infection in a normal host
  - Usually asymptomatic
  - Mononucleosis syndrome: Fever, malaise, sore throat, headache, antibiotic rash (1)
  - Less common: Exudative pharyngitis, splenomegaly, cervical adenopathy, rash (1)
- Infections in AIDS patients
  - Retinitis: Usually unilateral, floaters, scotomata, peripheral field defects. Diagnosis made when characteristic retinal changes noted by ophthalmologist on funduscopic exam (2)
  - Colitis: Fever, weight loss, anorexia, abdominal pain, diarrhea, malaise. Hemorrhage and perforation rare but serious (2)
  - Esophagitis: Fever, odynophagia, nausea, abdominal discomfort (2)
  - Pneumonitis: Shortness of breath, dyspnea on exertion, nonproductive cough, hypoxemia (2)
  - Neurologic disease: Dementia, lethargy, confusion, fever, focal neurological signs (2)
- Infections in transplant recipients
  - Persistent fever (most common) (3)
  - Bone marrow transplant: Interstitial pneumonia (5)
  - Liver transplant: Hepatitis (5)
  - Kidney transplant: CMV syndrome (fever, leucopenia, atypical lymphocytes, hepatomegaly, myalgia, arthralgia) (5)

TESTS

Lab

- Acute infection in a normal host
  - Elevated liver transaminases in 92%, though transaminases rarely increase to >5 times normal ranges (1)
  - Anemia (1)
  - Thrombocytopenia (1)
  - Positive cold agglutinins (1)
  - Lymphocytosis with >10% atypical (1)
  - Negative heterophil antibody test (rules out EBV mononucleosis) (1)
  - Positive CMV IgM antibodies; may not peak until 4–7 weeks after acute infection (1)
  - CMV IgG should increase 4-fold during acute infection (1)
- Congenital/infant
  - <12 months: Positive CMV antibody indicates maternal infection, but not necessarily child infection (3)
  - >12 months: Positive CMV antibody assay or culture indicates previous infection, but not necessarily active disease (3)
  - Recovery of virus from tissue in symptomatic patient (GI or pulmonary tissue) indicates infection, though 1–6 weeks are required for distinctive cytopathic events to occur (3)
  - Quantitative DNA PCR evidences disease and can be used to monitor therapy (3)
  - Direct hyperbilirubinemia >3 mg/dL (3)
  - Thrombocytopenia (<75,000/mL) (9)
  - Elevated liver transaminases (9)
- Immunocompromised
  - Viremia: PCR, antigen assays (pp65 lower-matrix protein in leukocytes), blood culture, although viremia can be present without CMV disease (2)[A]
  - Serum CMV antibodies not useful; can be falsely negative due to immunosuppression (2)[C]
  - Neurologic disease: CMV detected in CSF or brain tissue clinches diagnosis. Enhanced by PCR analysis (2)[A]

Imaging

- Head CT or MRI: Periventricular enhancement (CMV neuro disease)
- Chest radiograph: Interstitial infiltrates (CMV pneumonitis)

Diagnostic Procedures/Surgery

- Bronchoscopy: Identification of CMV inclusion bodies in lung tissue in context of pulmonary infiltrates (pneumonitis)
- Endoscopic of gastrointestinal tract: Mucosal ulcerations and colonoscopic, rectal, or esophageal biopsy (colitis, esophagitis) (2)[B]

Pathological Findings

Giant cells with basophilic inclusion bodies (owl's eye)

DIFFERENTIAL DIAGNOSIS

- Congenital: Toxoplasmosis, rubella, herpes, syphilis
- Acquired in immunocompetent: EBV mononucleosis, viral hepatitis
- Acquired immunocompromised: Other viral, bacterial, fungal opportunistic infections

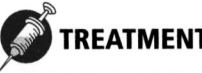

TREATMENT

GENERAL MEASURES

Diet

Normal

Activity

Bed rest

MEDICATION (DRUGS)

First Line

- Congenital disease: Ganciclovir 12 mg/kg intravenously q12h for 6 weeks (9)[B]
- Pediatric disseminated disease: IV ganciclovir (1)[A]

- CMV mononucleosis/asymptomatic viremia: No treatment (2)[D]
- Retinitis: Effective treatments include the following and should be chosen in consultation with a specialist
  - Oral valganciclovir (for peripheral lesions) (2)[A]
  - Intravenous ganciclovir followed by oral valganciclovir (2)[A]
  - Intravenous foscarnet (2)[A]
  - Intravenous cidofovir (2)[A]
  - Ganciclovir intraocular implant with oral or intravenous valganciclovir (2)[A]
  - Treat until CD4 >100 for 3–6 months (2)[A]
- Colitis or esophagitis: IV ganciclovir or foscarnet for 21–28 days or until symptom resolution (2)[B]
- Neurologic disease: Prompt treatment with ganciclovir and foscarnet (2)[B]
- CMV disease in transplant patients: IV ganciclovir for 2–4 weeks (5)[B]

Second Line

- Adult CMV retinitis: Fomivirsen (9)[A]
- Pediatric disseminated disease: Foscarnet 60 mg/kg q8h for 14–21 days (9)[A], Combination ganciclovir and foscarnet (9)[B]
- CMV disease in transplant patients: Valganciclovir (5)[C]
- CMV in bone marrow transplant patients
  - Prophylaxis: Valacyclovir (5)[B]
  - Preemptive: Foscarnet (5)[B]

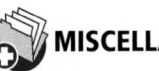

FOLLOW-UP

PROGNOSIS

Severe disease with primary infection in newborns and reactivation in immunocompromised

COMPLICATIONS

- Congenital: Hearing loss, mental retardation, optic atrophy, seizures, learning disabilities
- Colitis: Hemorrhage and perforation

PATIENT MONITORING

- CMV urine culture at birth for all HIV-infected or -exposed (3)[C] and annual testing for CMV seronegative/HIV+ children (3)[C]
- Patients with CD4 counts <50 should have ophthalmologic screening every 3–6 months (3)[C]

REFERENCES

1. Taylor GH. Cytomegalovirus. *Am Fam Phys* 2003;67(3):519–524.
2. Benson CA, Kaplan JE, Masur H, et al. Treating opportunistic infections among HIV-infected adults and adolescents: Recommendations from the CDC, the National Institutes of Health, and the HIV Medicine Association/Infectious Diseases Society of America. *Morbid Mortal Weekly Rep* 2004;53 (RR15):1–112.
3. Cohen J, Powderly WG. *Infectious diseases*, 2nd ed. New York: Elsevier, 2004.
4. Salzberger B, Hartmann P, Hanses F, et al. Incidence and prognosis of CMV disease in HIV-infected patients before and after introduction of combination antiretroviral therapy. *Infection* 2005;33(5):345–349.
5. Razonable RR, Emery VC. IHMF management recommendations: management of CMV infection and disease in transplant patients. *Herpes* 2004;11(3):77–86.
6. Patel R, Paya CV. Infections in solid-organ transplant recipients. *Clin Microbiol Rev* 1997;10:86–124.
7. Arbo MD, Snydman DR, Wong JB, et al. Cytomegalovirus immune globulin after liver transplantation: A cost-effectiveness analysis. *Clin Transplant* 2000;14(1):19–27.
8. Snydman DR, Werner BG, Heinze-Lacey B, et al. Use of cytomegalovirus immune globulin to prevent cytomegalovirus disease in renal-transplant recipients. *N Engl J Med* 1987;317:1049–1054.
9. Mofenson LM, Oleske J, Serchuck L, et al. Treating opportunistic infections among HIV-exposed and infected children: Recommendations from the CDC, the National Institutes of Health, and the HIV Medicine Association/Infectious Diseases Society of America. *Morbid Mortal Weekly Rep* 2004;53(RR14):1–63.

MISCELLANEOUS

CODES

ICD9-CM

078.5 Cytomegaloviral disease

PATIENT TEACHING

See Corresponding Diagnostic Algorithm

DE QUERVAIN TENOSYNOVITIS

Justin Dorfman, DO
John Herbert Stevenson, MD

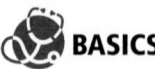

BASICS

DESCRIPTION
De Quervain tenosynovitis is a stenosis of the 1st dorsal compartment of the wrist including the extensor pollicis brevis (EPB) and abductor pollicis longus (APL). It is an inflammation or thickening of the tendon sheath that surrounds EPB and the APL, which leads to pain with certain movements of the thumb.

GENERAL PREVENTION
Avoidance of repetitive actions of the thumb associated with forceful grasping or repetitive wrist ulna/radial deviation (e.g., hammering)

EPIDEMIOLOGY
- Predominant age: 30–50
- Predominant sex: Female (6–10× more likely than men)

RISK FACTORS
- Women age 30–50
- Pregnancy
- Individuals participating in golf, fly fishing, and racquet sports
- Repetitive motions with the hand/thumb requiring forceful grasping or wrist ulna/radial deviation; often seen in carpenters

PATHOPHYSIOLOGY
Repetitive actions of the wrist and the thumb results in microtrauma and thickening of the surrounding tendon (EPB, APL). This thickening causes inflammation and pain with movements of the thumb and wrist and may elicit pain over the radial styloid as they rub over the prominence.

ETIOLOGY
- Repetitive movements of the wrist and thumb and activities that require forceful grasping
- Trauma
- Systemic diseases (e.g., rheumatoid arthritis)

DIAGNOSIS

SIGNS AND SYMPTOMS
- Pain and swelling over the radial styloid, which may be exacerbated when patients move their thumb or make a fist
- Crepitus with movement of the thumb may be felt or heard.
- Occasionally slight swelling at the base of the thumb and wrist is noted.
- Decreased range of motion of the thumb

History
- Patients may complain of gradual worsening pain along their thumb and radial aspect of their wrist with certain movements including ulnar deviation of the wrist.
- Usually insidious in onset
- There is usually no associated trauma.

Physical Exam
- Swelling and tenderness may be appreciated over the distal radius.
- Pain over the 1st extensor compartment on resisted thumb abduction or extension
- There may be associated crepitus with movement of the thumb.

TESTS
Finkelstein's test is pathognomonic for De Quervain tenosynovitis. This test involves patients flexing their thumb in their palm, while the examiner ulnar deviates the wrist. The test is positive if patients' symptoms are reproduced.

Lab
No labs are indicated.

Imaging
This disease is primarily a clinical diagnosis, but if the diagnosis is questionable, then x-rays of the wrist may be indicated to rule out other pathology. MRI is the test of choice to rule out co-existing soft tissue injury or wrist joint pathology.

Pathological Findings
Inflamed and thickened retinacular sheath of the tendon

DIFFERENTIAL DIAGNOSIS
- Fracture of the scaphoid
- Dorsal wrist ganglion
- Osteoarthritis of the first carpometacarpal joint
- Flexor carpi radialis tendonitis
- Infectious tenosynovitis
- Tendonitis of the wrist extensors
- Intersection syndrome
- Trigger thumb

TREATMENT

INITIAL STABILIZATION
- Splinting of the thumb (thumb spica splint or dorsal hood splint)
- Rest
- Ice (15–20 minutes 5–6× a day)
- Anti-inflammatory medications

GENERAL MEASURES
- Rest and immobilization may be helpful early in the disease process. This is achieved with the use of a thumb spica splint.
- NSAIDS may help along with the splint to decrease the inflammation.
- If full relief is not being achieved, a corticosteroid injection of the tendon sheath along with hand therapy has been shown to have high cure rates. Additional injections may be required for refractory cases.
- Anatomical variants may complicate treatment, including 2 tendon sheaths in the 1st compartment or the EPB tendon may travel in a separate compartment.
- Surgery is only indicated for severely persistent cases.

Diet
As tolerated

Activity
Avoidance of repetitive activities and motions that aggravate the pain

SPECIAL THERAPY
Physical Therapy
- Hand therapy along with iontophoresis/phonophoresis may help improve outcomes for moderate cases.
- Patients may incorporate thumb-stretching exercises into their rehabilitation.

Complementary and Alternative Therapies
Corticosteroid injection of the tendon sheath has shown significant cure rates. An 83% success rate after single injection has been reported. (1)[B] Additional injections are sometimes required.

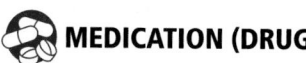 **MEDICATION (DRUGS)**

First Line
Immobilization and NSAIDS

Second Line
Corticosteroid injection

SURGERY
Only indicated for patients who have failed conservative treatment. Surgical release has shown cure rates of up to 91%. (2)[B]

 FOLLOW-UP

Additional corticosteroid injection may be performed at 4–6 weeks if symptoms are not significantly reduced.

DISPOSITION
Issues for Referral
Referral to a hand surgeon is indicated if there is no improvement after conservative treatments.

PROGNOSIS
Prognosis is extremely good with conservative treatments. 95% success rates have been shown with conservative therapy over 1 year, although up to 1/3 of patients will have recurrence. (3)[A] Surgery has shown success in 91% of patients who did not improve with conservative therapy.

COMPLICATIONS
- Most complications are secondary to the treatment modalities. This includes gastrointestinal, renal, and hepatic injury secondary to NSAIDs.
- Nerve damage may occur during surgery.
- Hypopigmentation, fat atrophy, bleeding, and infection are potential adverse events from corticosteroid injections.
- If not treated correctly, loss of flexibility of the thumb due to fibrosis may occur.

REFERENCES
1. Richie CA, Briner WW. Corticosteroid Injection for Treatment of De Quervain's Tenosynovitis: A Pooled Quantitative Literature Evaluation. *Journal of the American Board of Family Practice*. 2003;16: 102–106.
2. Ta KT, Eidelman D,Thomson JG. Patient satisfaction and outcomes of surgery for de Quervain's tenosynovitis. *J Hand Surg-Am*. 1999;24(5): 1071–1077.
3. Jirarattanaphochai K, Saengnipanthkul S, et al. Treatment of De Quervain Disease with triamcinolone injection with or without nimesulide: A randomized double-blind, placebo-controlled trial. *J Bone Joint Surg*. 2004; 86(12):2700–2706.
4. Rossi R, Cellocco P, et al. De Quervain Disease in volleyball players. *Am J Sport Med*. 2005;33: 424–427.
5. Rettig AC. Athletic injuries of the wrist and hand. Part II overuse injuries of the wrist and traumatic injuries of the hand. *Am J Sport Med*. 2004;32: 262–273.
6. Tallia AF, Cardone DA. Diagnostic and therapeutic injection of the wrist and hand region. *Am Fam Physician*. 2003;67:745–750.
7. Mellion MB, Walsh WM, Madden C, et al. *Team Physician's Handbook*, 3rd Ed. Philadelphia, PA: Hanley & Belfus, Inc. 2002;438.

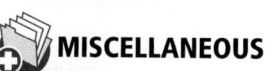 **MISCELLANEOUS**

CODES

ICD9-CM
727.04

PATIENT TEACHING
Modification of activities eliciting pain

DECOMPRESSION SICKNESS

Darell E. Heiselman, DO

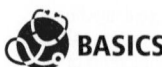 **BASICS**

DESCRIPTION

- Metastatic dissolution of gas bubbles (usually nitrogen) into tissues caused by a relatively rapid decrease in the environmental pressure
- 5 types based on symptomatology
  - Limb bends
    ○ Development of minute gas bubbles in tissues owing to rapid decompression, causing a poorly localized pain-only syndrome
    ○ May herald more serious disease (shoulder most common).
  - Cerebral bends
    ○ Strokelike picture owing to paradoxic arterial gas embolism (via atrioventricular or intracardiac shunt), de novo arterial gas formation, and/or cerebral edema.
  - Spinal cord bends
    ○ Transverse paresis caused by retrograde venous thrombosis with patchy necrosis and edema of the spinal cord.
    ○ Predilection for high lumbar nerve roots owing to lack of collateral circulation
  - Inner ear bends
    ○ Development of bubble formation and hemorrhage in labyrinthine fluid spaces and vasculature
  - Lung bends (chokes)
    ○ Excessive venous bubbles develop and release vasoactive substances, causing pulmonary irritation and bronchoconstriction.
    ○ Primary symptoms are substernal chest pain (worse with inspiration), dyspnea, and cough.
- Decompression sickness (DCS)
  - Type I (mild)
    ○ Mild pain (70–85%): Increases with time; shoulder most common
    ○ Rash
    ○ Pruritus
  - Type II (serious)
    ○ Pulmonary (2%): Nonproductive cough, chest discomfort on inspiration, severerespiratory distress.
    ○ Nervous system: Spinal cord is the most common: Paresthesia, paresis, paralysis, loss of bladder or bowel control
- Synonym(s): Bends; Paretic bends; Caisson disease

ALERT

Pregnancy Considerations

- Pregnant patient with decompression sickness a priority, because fetus also may be affected
- No contraindication to recompression

GENERAL PREVENTION

- Follow decompression tables (Navy, National Association for Underwater Instructors [NAUI], Professional Association for Diving Instructors [PADI]) for diving to depth (>33 feet).
- Use dive computers that calculate nitrogen content of various tissues.
- Allow adequate time between diving and flying to altitude (24 hours).

EPIDEMIOLOGY

- Predominant age: 20–29 years
- Predominant sex: 95% Males, although no evidence suggests increased susceptibility based on sex.

Incidence

13.4 per 100,000 dives

Prevalence

Uncommon: <1% even in high-density diving areas and areas of caisson work

RISK FACTORS

- Prolonged dive at depth >33 feet
- Obesity
- Multiple repetitive scuba dives
- Cold-water diving
- Poor physical conditioning
- Vigorous physical activity
- Dehydration
- Local injury
- Patent foramen ovale (for neurologic symptoms)
  - Routine screening not recommended

ETIOLOGY

- Rapid ascent from scuba diving (depth >33 feet)
- Rapid ascent/decompression in an airplane
- Tunnel work suggests caisson disease.
- Inadequate pressurization/denitrogenation when flying
- Flying to high altitude too soon after scuba diving

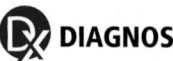 **DIAGNOSIS**

PRE HOSPITAL

- Variable clinical manifestations
- Most important diagnostic clue is recent decompression.
- 71% of nervous system decompression sickness presents as skin or limb bends.
- Limb bends with musculoskeletal complaints frequently diagnosed as malingering owing to vague nature
- Only way to exclude the diagnosis in patient at risk is a negative test of pressure

SIGNS AND SYMPTOMS

- 95% present in 3–4 hours, but may be delayed for 24 hours or more.
- Burning blebs (skin bends), lymphedema
- Painful pruritic red rash (cutis marmorata)
- Vague, poorly localized pain
- Headache, visual field deficits
- Ataxia, nystagmus
- Delirium
- Coma
- Convulsions
- Confusion
- Patchy numbness
- Respiratory chokes in 2%
- Coughing paroxysms (Behnke sign)
- Arrhythmia
- Bradycardia or tachycardia
- Hypotension
- Tachypnea, hemoptysis
- Subcutaneous emphysema along tendon sheaths (rare)
- Rapidly ascending paraplegia
- Negative or positive scotomata
- Sharply defined area of pallor on tongue (Liebermeister sign)
- Air in retinal vessels

TESTS

Electroencephalogram

- Irregular slowing with cerebral bends

Lab

- Arterial blood gases
  - May show decreased P_{O_2}, decreased P_{CO_2}, and metabolic acidosis
- CBC
  - Increased hematocrit in severe cases owing to dehydration
  - Thrombocytopenia.
- Coagulation tests
  - May see increased fibrin split products
  - May see increased prothrombin time

Imaging

- Chest radiograph
  - Pneumothorax
  - Mediastinal emphysema
  - Right-sided heart enlargement
- Plain radiograph or ultrasound
  - Gas bubbles in joints, tendons, bursae, muscles
- CT scan
  - For all patients with history of trauma or neurologic signs

Diagnostic Procedures/Surgery

Test of pressure

- Trial of recompression to 2.8 atmosphere absolute (ata)/100% oxygen for 10 minutes

Pathological Findings

- Skin lesions
  - Painful, pruritic, blotchy red rash on torso
  - Burning blebs on skin
  - Lymphedema
- Joints
  - Erythema and edema on periarticular surfaces

DIFFERENTIAL DIAGNOSIS

- Arterial gas embolism
- Traumatic injury to extremity
- Cerebrovascular accident
- Musculoskeletal strains
- Urticaria
- Malingering

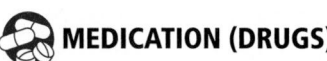 **TREATMENT**

PRE HOSPITAL
- Referral through Divers' Alert Network (DAN; 919-684-8111) to nearest hyperbaric facility for recompression test
- Treatment is based on the procedures 1st established in the armed services (e.g., U.S. Navy Table 6).

GENERAL MEASURES
- 100% oxygen via tight nonrebreathing mask
- Rapid referral to hyperbaric chamber facility
- Position recumbent, not Trendelenburg

Diet
Normal

Activity
Bed rest when neurologic involvement present

SPECIAL THERAPY
- Hyperbaric decompression
- Transport via ground, low-altitude airplane, or aircraft pressurized to sea level.

IV Fluids
Fluid resuscitation
- Avoid D_5W or hypotonic IV solutions with cord injury.
- No experimental or clinical studies support use of volume expanders (dextran, albumin); they are not without risk.

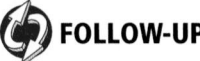 **MEDICATION (DRUGS)**

First Line
- Diazepam: 5–15 mg IV (IM absorption unpredictable) for inner ear decompression sickness
  – Relieves vertigo, nausea, and vomiting
- Steroids
  – Advocated by some for the assumed vasogenic edema seen in decompression sickness
  – Controversial and not proven in controlled clinical trials
  – If prescribed, do not use for >4 days for neurologic symptoms.
- Contraindications: Hypersensitivity to benzodiazepines and acute narrow-angle glaucoma
- Precautions
  – Monitor respiratory status, BP, and heart rate.
  – Reduce dose in elderly and patients with hepatic dysfunction.
- Significant possible interactions: Benzodiazepines potentiate the effects of other central nervous system depressants.

Second Line
Adjunctive therapy
- Digitalization for CHF/tachycardia
- Aminophylline *not* useful for chokes
- Roles of steroids and heparin not determined

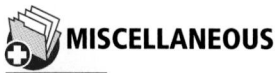 **FOLLOW-UP**

Discharge Criteria
Patients may be sent home when cutaneous symptoms only are present, if the appropriate response to therapy is observed in the emergency department.

PROGNOSIS
- Excellent for early symptomatic presentation, referral, and treatment
- Related to duration and severity of symptoms prior to treatment
- Although recompression therapy is best administered early as possible, some patients may still benefit even 6–9 days after the incident; referral is critical, even if symptoms resolve.
- 25% of patients relapse.

COMPLICATIONS
- Oxygen toxicity with seizures (infrequent and unpredictable)
- Neurologic sequelae for nonresponders
- Long-term risk of aseptic necrosis

PATIENT MONITORING
Symptomatic assessment for relapse/progression

REFERENCES
1. Bove A, Davis JC. *Diving Medicine*, 2nd ed. Philadelphia: WB Saunders, 1990.
2. Catron PW, Flynn ET. Adjuvant drug therapy for decompression sickness: A review. *Undersea Biomed Res*. 1982;9:161–173.

MISCELLANEOUS

CODES

ICD9-CM
993.3 Caisson disease

PATIENT TEACHING
Scuba divers should be certified by an appropriate diving agency: NAUI, PADI, SSI, or YMCA.

Prevention
Sport divers who have not been diving for >6 months should review diving principles/skills via a refresher course.

D

DEEP VEIN THROMBOPHLEBITIS (DVT)

Rob Tiller, MD

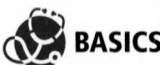 **BASICS**

DESCRIPTION

Development of single or multiple blood clots within the deep veins of the extremities or pelvis, usually accompanied by inflammation of the vessel wall. The major clinical consequence is embolization, usually to the lung, which is frequently life threatening.

- System(s) Affected: Cardiovascular
- Synonym(s): Deep vein thrombosis

GENERAL PREVENTION

- Avoid prolonged immobility.
- Low-estrogen birth control pills when possible
- Surgical patients need active prophylaxis: Low-dose SC heparin with dosage adjusted to slightly prolong the activated partial thromboplastin time (aPTT), low-dose warfarin, low-molecular-weight heparin (LMWH), and intermittent mechanical compression of the legs reduce the risks of DVT.

EPIDEMIOLOGY

- Predominant age: Mean age of 60 years (increasing age is an independent risk factor)
- Predominant sex: Male > Female (1.2:1)

ALERT
Geriatric Considerations
More common because predisposing conditions are more common

Incidence
Common (~250,000 hospitalizations and 50,000 deaths from complications of venous thromboembolic disease)

RISK FACTORS

- Clinical risk factors
  - Increasing age
  - Trauma, especially long bone fractures or crush injuries
  - Surgery (most commonly orthopedic, gastrointestinal, and genitourinary)
  - Prolonged immobility
  - Pregnancy, especially the puerperium
  - Indwelling central venous catheters
  - Travel (>4 hours)
  - Hormone replacement therapy
  - Tamoxifen therapy
  - Selective estrogen receptor modulator therapy (raloxifene [Evista])
  - High altitude (>14,000 feet)
- Pathologic risk factors
  - Prior DVT or pulmonary embolism
  - Inherited hypercoagulable states (thrombophilic states)
    - Factor V Leiden mutation resulting in resistance to activated protein C
    - Prothrombin mutation (G20210A)
    - Hyperhomocysteinemia
    - Protein C deficiency
    - Protein S deficiency
    - Antithrombin III deficiency
    - Homocysteinuria (rare)
  - Other hypercoagulable states
    - Antiphospholipid syndrome (lupus anticoagulant, anticardiolipin antibodies)
    - Elevated factor VIII, IX, XI
    - Elevated fibrinogen
    - Elevated von Willebrand factor
  - Malignancy
  - Obesity
  - Nephrotic syndrome
  - Polycythemia vera
  - Homocystinuria (rare)
  - *Campylobacter jejuni* bacteremia (very rare)
  - Myeloproliferative disorders
  - Vitamin deficiencies (B_6, B_{12}, folate)
  - Heparin-induced thrombocytopenia
  - Acute myocardial infarction
  - Neurologic disease with paralysis (acute spinal cord injury, cerebrovascular accident)

Pediatric Considerations
In this age group, patients with DVT in absence of preceding trauma should be worked up for inherited coagulopathy.

Genetics
Inherited thrombophilic states increase risk for venous thromboembolic disease.

ETIOLOGY

- Venous stasis
- Injury to vessel wall
- Abnormalities of coagulation

ASSOCIATED CONDITIONS

Malignant neoplasm (1/5 of all venous thromboembolic disease), Mild to moderate hyperhomocysteinemia, Inherited thrombophilias, Antiphospholipid antibody syndrome, Budd-Chiari syndrome (hepatic vein thrombosis), Renal vein thrombosis

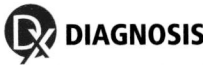 **DIAGNOSIS**

SIGNS AND SYMPTOMS
- Many cases are completely asymptomatic, diagnosed after embolization.
- Physical exam is only 30% accurate for DVT
- Limb pain (common)
- Limb swelling (common)
- Leg pain on dorsiflexion of the foot (Homan sign; unreliable test for DVT, only ~50% sensitivity)
- Palpable tender cord in affected limb (uncommon)
- Warmth of skin over area of thrombosis (uncommon)
- Redness of skin over area or thrombosis (uncommon)
- Fever (uncommon, except in septic thrombophlebitis)
- Nontender swelling of collateral superficial veins (uncommon)
- Massive edema with cyanosis and ischemia; a medical emergency (phlegmasia cerulea dolens, rare)
- Pain on percussion of the medial tibia (Lisker sign)
- Pain on compression of calf against tibia in the anteroposterior plane (Bancroft or Moses sign)

TESTS
Lab
- D-dimer (sensitive but not specific; has a high negative predictive value)
- Baseline labs: CBC, platelet count, aPTT, prothrombin time (PT)/International Normalized Ratio (INR)
- Labs for idiopathic (no known inciting event) DVT
  - 1st tier of testing: Factor V Leiden, G20210A prothrombin, serum homocysteine, factor VIII level, and lupus anticoagulant
  - 2nd tier of testing: Protein C and S antigen levels, antithrombin activity, and anticardiolipin antibodies
- Drugs that may alter lab results: Heparin, estrogens may lower antithrombin III levels. Coumadin affects protein C and protein S function, so it may interfere with functional assays of these proteins.
- Disorders that may alter lab results: Thrombosis itself lowers antithrombin III levels, so any workup for antithrombin III deficiency must be performed after patient has completed therapy. Syphilis and systemic lupus erythematosus are associated with increased antiphospholipid antibodies.

Imaging
- Compression ultrasonography: Noninvasive, highly sensitive, and specific for popliteal and femoral thrombi. Disadvantages include poor ability to detect calf vein thrombi, does not identify clots in pelvic veins or vena cava, is operator dependent, does not distinguish acute from chronic thrombi, and is difficult to distinguish extrinsic vein compression from intravenous clot.
- Contrast venography: The gold standard test but should not be the initial screening tool. Disadvantages include discomfort, technical difficulty, and small risk of morbidity.
- Impedance plethysmography (IPG): Probably as accurate as duplex ultrasound, less operator dependency, but poor at detecting calf vein thrombi; not widely available
- Magnetic resonance venography: As accurate as contrast venography. May be useful for patients with contraindications to IV contrast material
- ^{125}I-fibrinogen scan: Detects only active clot formation; very good at detecting ongoing calf thrombi. Major disadvantage: Takes 4 hours for results. It has generally been supplanted by contrast ultrasonography and IPG.

Pathological Findings
- Clot consisting predominantly of red blood cells, with some platelets and fibrin attached to vessel wall at 1 end with proximal end floating free in the lumen. Varying degrees of inflammation of the vessel wall are present.
- DVT may be the sentinel event for an underlying malignancy or thrombophilia.

DIFFERENTIAL DIAGNOSIS
- Cellulitis
- Ruptured synovial cyst (Baker cyst)
- Lymphedema
- Extrinsic compression of vein by tumor or enlarged lymph nodes
- Pulled, strained, or torn muscle
- Compartment syndrome
- Localized allergic reaction
- Filariasis (in developing countries)

D

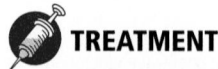

TREATMENT

INITIAL STABILIZATION
Patients with complicated DVT should usually be admitted; others can be managed as outpatients.

GENERAL MEASURES
For hospitalized patients: IV anticoagulation; close observation for embolic events

Diet
Patients taking warfarin must be aware that foods high in vitamin K can affect prothrombin time.

Activity
Gradual resumption of normal activity, with avoidance of prolonged immobility

MEDICATION (DRUGS)

DVT may be complicated if any of these is present: Evidence of pulmonary embolism, recent surgery, peptic ulcer disease, malignant hypertension, increased risk of falling, extensive proximal DVT, heparin allergy or history of heparin-induced thrombocytopenia, known bleeding disorder, active bleeding, comorbid illness with high risk of bleeding, renal insufficiency, pregnancy, known protein C or S deficiency, noncompliance, poor follow-up, inadequate home support, inaccessibility to outpatient monitoring, morbid obesity, age <18 years, age >75 years, and severe leg pain and swelling

First Line
- Uncomplicated DVT
  - LMWH (can be administered in an outpatient setting: Enoxaparin (Lovenox) 1 mg/kg/dose b.i.d. SC; dalteparin (Fragmin). No lab monitoring is required.
- Complicated DVT
  - Heparin 80 U/kg IV bolus followed by continuous infusion starting at 18 U/kg/h. Adjust dosage to aPTT of 2–3 × control; or
  - Enoxaparin (Lovenox) either 1 mg/kg/dose b.i.d. SC or 1.5 mg/kg daily SC. No lab monitoring is required.
- Maintenance therapy
  - Warfarin (Coumadin) may be started on the 1st day; once therapeutic anticoagulation is reached, 5 mg daily and adjusting based on PT with a target PT of 1.5–2 × control. Continue heparin until target PT level is achieved (INR 2–3). For patients with contraindications to warfarin, LMWH or heparin can be continued SC for the duration of treatment.
  - Dalteparin (Fragmin) is approved for DVT prophylaxis.
- Contraindications
  - Severe active bleeding, neurosurgical procedure within 30 days, pregnancy (warfarin only), previous adverse reaction to the drug (other than bleeding, which is a known side effect)
  - Relative contraindications: Recent hemorrhage, recent surgical procedure other than neurosurgery, history of significant peptic ulcer disease, or recent nonembolic stroke

- Precautions
  - Observe patient for signs of embolization, further thrombosis, or bleeding.
  - Avoid IM injections. Periodically check stool and urine for occult blood; monitor CBC including platelets.
  - Heparin—thrombocytopenia and/or paradoxical thrombosis with thrombocytopenia
  - Warfarin—necrotic skin lesions (typically breasts, thighs, and buttocks)
  - LMWH—adjust dosage in renal insufficiency
- Significant possible interactions
  - Agents that intensify the response to oral anticoagulants: Alcohol, allopurinol, amiodarone, anabolic steroids, androgens, many antimicrobials, cimetidine, chloral hydrate, disulfiram, all NSAIDs, sulfinpyrazone, tamoxifen, thyroid hormone, vitamin E, ranitidine, salicylates, acetaminophen
  - Agents that diminish the response to anticoagulants: Aminoglutethimide, antacids, barbiturates, carbamazepine, cholestyramine, diuretics, griseofulvin, rifampin, and oral contraceptives

Second Line
- Thrombolytic agents (urokinase, streptokinase, alteplase [tissue plasminogen activator]): Effective in dissolving clots and are currently investigational for treatment of DVT. In current clinical practice they should be reserved for massive thromboembolic disease. The same contraindications apply as for anticoagulants.
- If warfarin is contraindicated, heparin can be given in the ambulatory setting by intermittent SC self-injection.

Pregnancy Considerations
- Warfarin (Coumadin) is a teratogen and is therefore contraindicated in pregnancy. Treat pregnant women with DVT with full-dose heparin initially, followed by SC heparin starting at 15,000 units b.i.d. with target aPTT of 1.5 to 2× control.
- Warfarin is safe with breast-feeding
- Septic thrombophlebitis, usually associated with childbirth, requires antibiotic therapy as well as anticoagulation.

SURGERY
When anticoagulants and thrombolytics are contraindicated, filtering devices ("umbrellas") can be inserted into the vena cava to "trap" emboli before they reach the lungs. Very large clots can be surgically removed in certain circumstances.

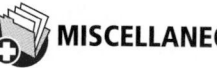 FOLLOW-UP

PROGNOSIS

- 20% of untreated proximal (e.g., above the calf) DVTs progress to pulmonary emboli, and 10–20% of those are fatal. With aggressive anticoagulant therapy, mortality is decreased 5–10-fold.
- DVT confined to the infrapopliteal veins has a small risk of embolization, but these can propagate into the proximal system. Follow with serial IPG or duplex ultrasound. Some recommend full anticoagulation therapy for all patients with calf vein DVT because of a 25% 1-year risk of developing chronic venous insufficiency.
- Skin necrosis is a possibility in patients with protein C deficiency who also take warfarin.

COMPLICATIONS

- Pulmonary embolism (fatal in 10–20%)
- Arterial embolism (paradoxical embolization) with AV shunting
- Chronic venous insufficiency
- Postphlebitic syndrome (pain and swelling in affected limb without new clot formation)
- Treatment-induced hemorrhage
- Soft tissue ischemia associated with massive clot and high venous pressures—phlegmasia cerulea dolens (rare but is a surgical emergency)

PATIENT MONITORING

- Heparin: Activated partial thromboplastin time (PTT) monitored several times a day until dose stabilizes. Discontinue heparin if platelets <75,000
- Warfarin: PTT/INR daily until target achieved, then weekly for several weeks, then (if stable) monthly
- Duration of treatment with warfarin after venous thrombotic event
  - 3 months of warfarin: Event provoked by surgery, trauma, or immobilization
  - 6 months of warfarin
    - 1st unprovoked event
    - Event provoked by pregnancy, peripartum, or oral contraceptive pills/hormone replacement therapy
    - Proximal vein thrombosis
    - Pulmonary embolism provoked by surgery, trauma, or immobilization
    - Age >45 years with DVT
    - Heterozygous for factor V Leiden with event
    - Heterozygous for G20210A prothrombin mutation with event
  - 6–18 months of warfarin: Active cancer, continued immobilization, venous insufficiency, protein C/S deficiency, or elevated factor VIII
  - Indefinite treatment with warfarin
    - Recurrent DVT, PE, or other thrombotic event
    - Life-threatening event (large pulmonary embolism, limb-threatening DVT)
    - Cerebral or visceral vein thrombosis
    - Antithrombin deficiency with event
    - Homozygous for factor V Leiden with event
    - Combined clotting disorders (e.g., factor V Leiden plus elevated homocysteine) with event
    - Antiphospholipid antibodies with event
- Monitoring with LMWH: No monitoring is required; however, in selected patients (e.g., those with severe renal insufficiency, morbid obesity), an anti-factor Xa activity level may help guide titration of therapy. This assay is limited by controversy over its correlation to therapeutic efficacy and ability to predict hemorrhage in high-risk patients.
- Investigate significant bleeding (e.g., hematuria or gastrointestinal hemorrhage), because anticoagulant therapy may unmask a pre-existing lesion (e.g., cancer, peptic ulcer disease, or arteriovenous malformation).

REFERENCES

1. Brown DF. Treatment options for deep venous thrombosis. *Emerg Med Clin North Amer.* 2001;19:913–923.
2. Collet JP, Montalescot G, Fine E, et al. Enoxaparin in unstable angina patients who would have been excluded from randomized pivotal trials. *J Amer Coll Cardiol.* 2003;41:8–14.
3. Heit JA: Risk factors for venous thromboembolism. *Clin Chest Med.* 2003;24:1–12.
4. Hull RD: Peripheral venous disease. In: Goldman L, Bennett JC, eds. *Cecil Textbook of Medicine.* Philadelphia, PA: WB Saunders; 2000.

MISCELLANEOUS

See also: Antithrombin Deficiency; Factor V Leiden; Protein C Deficiency; Protein S Deficiency; Prothrombin 20210 (Mutation); Pulmonary Embolism

CODES

ICD9-CM

- 289.81 Primary hypercoagulable state
- 289.82 Secondary hypercoagulable state
- 415.19 Pulmonary embolism and infarction, other
- 451.19 Phlebitis and thrombophlebitis of deep vessels of lower extremities, other
- 453.8 Embolism and thrombosis of other specified veins

PATIENT TEACHING

- Advise women taking estrogen of risks and common symptoms of thromboembolic disease, especially with concominant tobacco use.
- Advise women with an inherited or acquired thrombophilia or history of thrombosis to avoid oral contraceptives and hormone replacement therapy. Women with personal or family history of thrombosis should be offered screening for inherited or acquired thrombophilias (clotting disorders).

 See Corresponding Diagnostic Algorithm

 See Patient Handout on CD

DEHYDRATION

Keisha L. Gibson, MD
William A. Primack, MD

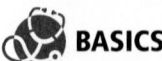 **BASICS**

DESCRIPTION
A state of negative fluid balance

GENERAL PREVENTION
Patient/parent education on the early signs of dehydration

EPIDEMIOLOGY
Cause of 10% of all pediatric hospitalizations in the US

RISK FACTORS
- Age <5
- The elderly
- Neurologic compromise

PATHOPHYSIOLOGY
Negative fluid balance occurs when ongoing fluid losses exceed fluid intake. Fluid losses can be insensible (sweat, respiration), obligate (urine, stool), or abnormal (diarrhea, vomiting, osmotic diuresis in diabetic ketoacidosis). Negative fluid balance can ultimately lead to severe intravascular volume depletion and ultimately end organ damage from inadequate perfusion.

ETIOLOGY
- Most commonly diarrheal illnesses.
- Other excessive losses including vomiting,
- sweating, frequent urination
- Decreased intake

ASSOCIATED CONDITIONS
- Hyponatremia
- Hypernatremia
- Hyperkalemia
- Hyperglycemia
- Shock
- Renal failure

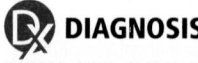 **DIAGNOSIS**

SIGNS AND SYMPTOMS
Calculate % Dehydration = (pre-illness weight − illness weight)/pre-illness weight × 100 or see table

Degree of Dehydration	Clinical Signs
MILD Children (5–10%) Adults (3–5%)	Normal pulse, normal BP, normal respirations, tacky or slightly dry buccal mucosa, normal anterior fontanelle, normal eyes, normal skin turgor, mildly reduced urine output, increased thirst
MODERATE Children (10–15%) Adults (5–10%)	Rapid pulse, normal to low BP, deep/increased respirations, dry buccal mucosa, sunken anterior fontanelle, reduced skin turgor, cool skin, markedly reduced urine output, listlessness or irritability
SEVERE Children (>15%) Adults (>10%)	Rapid/weak pulse, low BP (shock), deep or tachypneic respirations, parched buccal mucosa, markedly sunken anterior fontanelle, skin tenting, cool, mottled, acrocyanotc skin, anuria, grunting, lehthargy, coma

History
- Intake (include description and amount)
- Diarrhea (frequency, consistency, mucous, blood)
- Vomiting (bilious/non-bilious)
- Fever
- Urination pattern
- Sick contacts
- Mental status
- Medication history (e.g., diuretics, laxatives)

Physical Exam
- Vitals: Pulse, BP, temperature
- Weight loss: <5%, 10%, or >15%
- Mucous membranes (tacky, dry, or parched)
- Eyes (normal tears, decreased tears, sunken)
- Capillary refill (normal, delayed >3 seconds)

TESTS
Lab
- Generally not necessary for mild dehydration but consider electrolytes, blood urea nitrogen, creatinine
- Urinalysis (specific gravity, hematuria, glucosuria)

DIFFERENTIAL DIAGNOSIS
- Gastroenteritis
- Intestinal obstruction
- Diabetes/DKA
- Diabetes insipidus
- Sepsis
- Anorexia
- Malabsorption
- Metabolic disorder
- Decreased intake due to inadequate thirst response

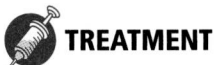 **TREATMENT**

PRE HOSPITAL
See chapter on "Oral Rehydration"

INITIAL STABILIZATION
- 1st stabilize airway, breathing, and circulation
- If mild dehydration, may try oral rehydration therapy: See chapter on "Oral Rehydration"
- If excessive vomiting or severe dehydration with shock, start IV access and fluids as described by the following.

SPECIAL THERAPY
IV Fluids
- Stage I: For moderate to severe dehydration in children: Isotonic saline or lactate ringer solution bolus of 10–20 ccs/kg. May repeat up to 60 cc/kg; if still hemodynamically unstable, consider colloid replacement (blood, albumin, fresh frozen plasma) and address other causes for shock. In adults, use isotonic saline or lactate ringer 20 cc/kg/h until normal state of consciousness returns or vital signs stabilize. Also consider colloid replacement if continued fluids required beyond 3 L.
- Stage II: Replace fluid deficit along with maintenance over 48 hours. Fluid deficit = Pre-illness weight–illness weight.

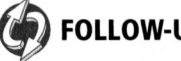 **FOLLOW-UP**

Admission Criteria
- Electrolyte abnormalities, including hyponatremia or hypernatremia
- Intractable vomiting limiting ability to maintain adequate oral hydration.

COMPLICATIONS
- Shock
- Seizures
- Cardiovascular arrest

REFERENCES
1. Steiner MJ, DeWalt DA, Byerley JS. Is this child dehydrated? *JAMA.* 2004;291:2746.
2. American Academy of Pediatrics, Provisional Committee on Quality Improvement, Subcommittee on Acute Gastroenteritis. Practice parameter: The management of acute gastroenteritis in young children. *Pediatrics.* 1996;97:424.
3. Allison SP, Lobo DN. Fluids and electrolytes in the elderly. *Curr Opin Clin Nutr Metab Care.* 2004;7(1):27–33.
4. Behrman H, Kliegman R, Jenson H. *Nelson Textbook of Pediatrics.* 17th ed. 2004;246–251.
5. Liebelt E. Clinical and laboratory evaluation and management of children with vomiting, diarrhea, and dehydration. *Curr Opin Pediatr.* 1998; 10(5):461–469.

 MISCELLANEOUS

PATIENT TEACHING
- Patients should be advised to seek care from nearest emergency facility or call 911 if they or their child feels faint or dizzy when rising from a sitting or lying position, becomes lethargic and/or confused, or complains of a rapid heart rate.
- Patients should be advised to call their physician if an illness is combined with the inability to keep down any fluids, vomiting has been going on >24 hours in an adult or >12 hours in a child, diarrhea has lasted >2 days in an adult or child, your infant or child is much less active than usual or is irritable, of if you or your child have excessive urination, especially if there is a history or family history of diabetes or you are taking diuretics.

D

DELIRIUM

Jonathan M. Flacker, MD

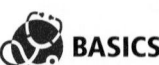 **BASICS**

DESCRIPTION
- A neurologic complication of illness and/or medication(s) especially common in older patients
- A medical emergency requiring immediate evaluation to decrease morbidity and mortality
- System(s) Affected: Nervous
- Synonym(s): Acute confusional state; Altered mental status; Organic brain syndrome; Acute mental status change

GENERAL PREVENTION
Follow treatment approach

EPIDEMIOLOGY
- Predominant age: Older persons
- Predominant sex: Male = Female

Incidence
- 25–60%
- >50% in high-risk older patients

Prevalence
10–40% in hospitalized older patients

RISK FACTORS
Predisposing risk factors
- Advanced age
- Prior cognitive impairment
- Functional impairment
- High blood urea nitrogen (BUN): Creatinine ratio
- Dehydration
- Malnutrition
- Hearing or vision impairment
- Frailty

Precipitating risk factors
- Severe illness in any organ system(s)
- Need for a urinary catheter
- >3 medications
- Pain
- Any adverse iatrogenic event
- Medications, especially long-acting sedative hypnotics (e.g., diazepam and flurazepam), narcotics (especially meperidine), and anticholinergics (especially diphenhydramine)

PATHOPHYSIOLOGY
- Neuropathophysiology is not clearly defined
- Multicomponent approach addressing contributing factors can reduce incidence and complications

ETIOLOGY
Usually multifactorial
- Often interaction between predisposing and precipitating risk factors
- With more predisposing factors (i.e., the frailer the patients), fewer precipitating factors needed to produce delirium
- If few predisposing factors (e.g., very robust patients) more precipitating factors needed to manifest delirium

ASSOCIATED CONDITIONS
Multiple, but most common are
- New medicine or medicine changes
- Infections (especially lung and urine, but meningitis needs consideration as welll)
- Toxic-metabolic (especially low sodium, elevated calcium, renal failure and hepatic failure)
- Heart attack
- Stroke
- Alcohol or drug withdrawal

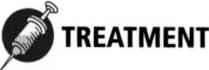 **DIAGNOSIS**

PRE HOSPITAL
The Confusion Assessment Method (CAM) may be applied either pre-hospital or in hospital, and has been adapted for the ICU setting (CAM-ICU)

ALERT
Clinical
- Key diagnostic features comprise the CAM. (1)
  - Acute change in mental status that fluctuates
  - Abnormal attention and **either** disorganized thinking **or** altered level of consciousness
- Any of the following nondiagnostic symptoms may be present
  - Short- and long-term memory problems
  - Sleep-wake cycle disturbances
  - Hallucinations and/or delusions
  - Emotional lability
  - Tremors and asterixis
- Subtypes based on level of consciousness
  - Hyperactive delirium (15%): Patients are loud, rambunctious, and disruptive.
  - Hypoactive delirium (20%): Quietly confused; may sit and not eat, drink, or move
  - Mixed delirium (50%): Features of both hyperactive and hypoactive delirium
  - Normal consciousness delirium (15%): Still display disorganized thinking, along with acute onset, inattention, and fluctuation.

History
- Time course of mental status changes
- Recent medication changes
- Symptoms of infection
- New neurologic signs

Physical Exam
- Good cardiorespiratory exam essential
- Focal neurologic signs usually absent
- Mini-mental state exam helpful as structured interview and to follow course over time

TESTS
ECG as necessary

Lab
- CBC
- Electrolytes, BUN, and creatinine
- Urinalysis, urine culture
- If needed
  - Arterial blood gases
  - Drug screen
  - Liver function tests

Imaging
- Chest radiograph
- Non–contrast-enhanced head (CT) scan if
  - Unclear diagnosis
  - Recent fall
  - Receiving anticoagulants
  - New focal neurologic signs
  - To rule out increased intracranial pressure before lumbar puncture

Diagnostic Procedures/Surgery
Lumbar puncture
- Rarely necessary
- Perform if clinical suspicion of a CNS bleed or infection is high.

DIFFERENTIAL DIAGNOSIS
- Depression (slow onset, disturbance of mood, normal level of consciousness, and fluctuates over weeks to months)
- Dementia (insidious onset, memory problems, normal level of consciousness, and fluctuates over days to weeks)
- Psychosis (rarely sudden onset in older adults)

TREATMENT

PRE HOSPITAL
- Stabilize vitals if needed.
- Ensure immediate evaluation.

INITIAL STABILIZATION
As needed

GENERAL MEASURES
- Postoperative patients should be monitored and treated for the following
  - Myocardial infarction/ischemia
  - Pulmonary complications/pneumonia
  - Pulmonary embolism
  - Urinary or stool retention (attempt catheter removal by postoperative day 2)
- Anesthesia route (general epidural) does not affect the risk of delirium

- Multifactorial treatment: Identify contributing factors and provide pre-emptive care to avoid iatrogenic problems (2–4)[A] with special attention to

  - CNS oxygen delivery (attempt to attain the following)
    - Sao_2 >90% with goal of SaO_2 >95%
    - Systolic blood pressure <2/3 of baseline or >90 mm Hg
    - Hematocrit >30%
- Fluid/electrolyte balance
  - Sodium, potassium, and glucose normal (glucose <300 mg/dL in diabetics)
  - Treat fluid overload or dehydration
- Treat pain
  - Schedule acetaminophen (1 g q.i.d.) if daily pain
  - Morphine or oxycodone for breakthrough pain if acetaminophen ineffective

ALERT
Avoid meperidine (Demerol)

- Eliminate unnecessary medications
  - Investigate new symptoms as potential medication side effects
- Regulate bowel/bladder function
  - Bowel movement at least every 48 hours
  - Screen for urinary retention or incontinence, especially after catheter removal
- Prevent major hospital-acquired problems
  - 6-inch-thick foam mattress overlay or a pressure-reducing mattress
  - Avoid urinary catheter
  - Incentive spirometry, if bed bound
  - SC heparin 5,000 U b.i.d., if bed fast
- Environmental stimulation
  - Glasses and hearing aids
  - Clock and calendar
  - Soft lighting
  - Radio, tapes, and television, if desired
- Sleep
  - Quiet environment
  - Soft music
  - Therapeutic massage
- Restraints do not reduce risk of falls/injury
  - Use only in the most difficult-to-manage patients, as briefly as possible

Diet
- Dentures used properly
- Proper positioning for meals
- Assistance with meals when necessary
- Nutritional supplements (1–3 cans daily) if intake is poor
- Temporary nasogastric tube if unable to eat and bowels working

Activity
- As tolerated
- Early physical therapy consultation to prevent deconditioning

Nursing
- Institute skin care program for patients with established incontinence
- Turning regimen if at risk of pressure ulcers

SPECIAL THERAPY
Physical Therapy
Early mobilization critical

- Out of bed on hospital day 2 (or postoperative day 1) if no contraindications
- Out of bed several hours daily if able
- Daily therapy if not ambulating independently
- Daily therapy if not functionally independent

IV Fluids
As needed for dehydration

 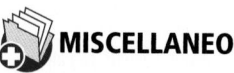

MEDICATION (DRUGS)

- Nonpharmacologic approaches are preferred for initial treatment
- Medications often treat only the symptoms and do not address the underlying cause

First Line
- Neuroleptics
  - Haloperidol (Haldol): Initially, 0.25–0.5 mg PO/IM/IV unless urgent sedation needed
  - Quetiapine (Seroquel): 25 mg/d to b.i.d.
- Short-acting benzodiazepines, if neuroleptics do not work or should be avoided:
  - Lorazepam (Ativan): Initially, 0.25–0.5 mg PO/IM/IV q6–8h, may need to adjust to effect (caution in patients with impaired liver function).
- Risperidone (Risperdal): 0.25–0.5 mg/d PO
- Contraindications: Avoid neuroleptics in patients with parkinsonism or Parkinson disease.
- Precautions: Neuroleptics may cause extrapyramidal effects, and benzodiazepines may lead to sedation. Both increase the risk of falls.

Second Line
Olanzapine (Zyprexa): 2.5–5.0 mg/d PO

 FOLLOW-UP

DISPOSITION
Admission Criteria
New delirium is a medical emergency and requires admission except in the setting of palliative home care

Discharge Criteria
- Resolution of precipitating factor(s)
- Safe discharge site if still delirious

Issues for Referral
- If delirium at discharge, will usually be followed in post-acute facility
- If no delirium at discharge, follow-up with primary care physician in 1–2 weeks

PROGNOSIS
Usually improves with treatment of underlying condition, but may become chronic.

COMPLICATIONS
- Falls
- Pressure ulcers
- Malnutrition
- Functional decline
- Versedation
- Polypharmacy

PATIENT MONITORING
- Evaluate and assess mental status daily.
- Depends on specific conditions present.

REFERENCES

1. Inouye SK, van Dyck CH, Alessi CA, et al. Clarifying confusion: The confusion assessment method. *Ann Intern Med*. 1990;113:941–948.
2. Inouye SK, Bogardus ST, Baker DI, et al. The hospital elder life program: A model of care to prevent cognitive and functional decline in older hospitalized patients. *J Am Geriatr Soc*. 2000; 48:1697–1706.
3. Marcantonio ER, Flacker JM, Wright RJ, et al. Reducing delirium after hip fracture: A randomized trial. *J Am Geriatr Soc*. 2001;49:516–522.
4. Naughton B, Saltzman S, Ramadan F, et al. A multifactorial intervention to reduce prevalence of delirium and shorten hospital stay. *J Am Geriatr Soc* 2005;53:18–23.
5. Pandharipande P, Jackson J, Ely E. Delirium: Acute cognitive dysfunction in the critically il. *Curr Opin Crit Care* 2005;11:360–368.

 MISCELLANEOUS

See also: Alcohol use disorders; Dementia; Depression; Restlessness

CODES
ICD9-CM
- 290.3 Senile dementia with delirium
- 290.11 Presenile dementia with delirium
- 291.0 Alcohol withdrawal delirium
- 291.1 Alcohol amnestic syndrome
- 292.0 Drug withdrawal syndrome
- 292.81 Drug-induced delirium
- 293.0 Acute delirium
- 293.1 Subacute delirium
- 293.89 Other specified transient organic mental disorders
- 780.09 Alterations of consciousness, other

PATIENT TEACHING

Diet
None, but must ensure nutrition

Activity
None, but must ensure activity

See Corresponding Diagnostic Algorithm

DEMENTIA

Aubrey L. Knight, MD

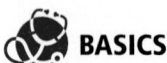 BASICS

DESCRIPTION
- A pathologic process defined as a persistent impairment of a prior level of intellectual functioning
- Alzheimer dementia (AD)
  - Characterized by relentless deterioration of higher cortical functioning
  - Variable rate of deterioration
- Vascular dementia (VaD)
  - Formerly multi-infarct dementia
  - Caused by clinical or subclinical cerebral infarcts secondary to atherosclerosis
  - Stepwise deterioration with periods of clinical plateaus
- Dementia with Lewy bodies (DLB)
  - Early-onset dementia with associated psychosis, depression
- Frontotemporal dementia (FTD)
  - Insidious change in personality with cognitive dysfunction
  - Onset usually >65 years of age

Geriatric Considerations
Begin drugs with small doses and increase slowly.

GENERAL PREVENTION
Ischemic-vascular dementia: General stroke prevention (lipid, diabetes, BP control)

EPIDEMIOLOGY
- Predominant age: Increasing incidence with increasing age
- Predominant sex: Male = Female

Incidence
- Between ages 60–64 years: 0.5%
- Between ages 80–90 years: 3.2%
- 1,480/100,000

Prevalence
In the US, 1.2 million people have severe dementia and another 2.5 million have moderate illness.

RISK FACTORS
- Increasing age
- Prevalence of atherosclerotic disease (VaD)
- History of head trauma
- History of CNS infection
- Midlife depression (VaD)

Genetics
- At least 15% of patients with AD will report a positive family history
- Persons with Trisomy 21 (Down syndrome) who survive into their 20s and 30s will inevitably develop a progressive dementia

ETIOLOGY
- AD
  - Genetic predisposition in >15%
- VaD
  - Cerebral atherosclerosis or emboli with clinical or subclinical infarcts (1)[B]
- Secondary dementias: Causes include hypothyroidism, vitamin B deficiency, normal pressure hydrocephalus, AIDS, syphilis, and various medications.

DIAGNOSIS

DSM-IV Codes
- 290.10—AD, early onset, uncomplicated
- 290.11—AD, early onset with delirium
- 290.12—AD, early onset with delusions
- 290.13—AD, early onset with depression
- 290.00—AD, late onset, uncomplicated
- 290.30—AD, late onset with delirium
- 290.20—AD, late onset with delusions
- 290.21—AD, late onset with depressed mood
- 290.40—VaD, uncomplicated
- 290.41—VaD with delirium
- 290.42—VaD with delusions
- 290.43—VaD with depressed mood
- 290.10—FTD
- 294.8—Dementia NOS
- 294.9—Cognitive disorder NOS

SIGNS AND SYMPTOMS
- Impaired short-term and long-term memory
- Impaired abstract thinking
- Impaired judgment
- Aphasia
- Apraxia
- Agnosia
- Anomia
- Personality change, emotional outbursts, wandering, restlessness, hyperactivity, especially with FTD
- Sleep disturbances
- Mood disturbances
- Urinary incontinence (usually late in AD or normal pressure hydrocephalus)
- Fecal incontinence (late)
- Rigidity
- Tremor (especially with DLB)
- Hallucinations (especially with DLB)
- Delusions
- Overt paranoid behavior
- Weight loss
- Seizures

TESTS
- Mental status testing
- Neuropsychologic testing
- Electroencephalogram for patients with altered consciousness or associated seizures

Lab
Done primarily to rule out potentially reversible causes
- Thyroid function tests
- Syphilis serology
- Serum B_{12} and folate levels
- CBC and screening metabolic profile
- Drugs that may alter lab results: Thyroid hormone replacement and iodine preparations may affect thyroid function tests.
- Disorders that may alter lab results: False positive syphilis serology with acute infections, leprosy, subacute bacterial endocarditis, and autoimmune disorders

Imaging
- Head CT if history suggestive of a mass, or focal neurologic signs or in patient with dementia of brief duration 2[A]
- MRI (2)[A]
  - More sensitive than CT for detection of soft-tissue lesions (small infarcts, mass lesions, atrophy of the brainstem, and other subcortical structures).
  - May also clarify ambiguous CT findings.
- Isotope cisternography if suspicious of normal pressure hydrocephalus
- Positive emission tomography shows cortical hypometabolism (2)[C]

Pathological Findings
- AD
  - Diffuse cerebral atrophy in association areas, hippocampus, amygdala
  - Granulovesicular degeneration
  - Neurofibrillary tangles
  - Senile neuritic plaques
  - Microvascular amyloid
- VaD
  - Old infarcts, lacunes
  - Manifestations of atherosclerotic disease

DIFFERENTIAL DIAGNOSIS
- Delirium
- Normal aging
- Mild cognitive impairment
- Depression
- Schizophrenia
- Chronic alcoholism
- Postsurgical and/or postanesthesia state
- Normal pressure hydrocepahalus

TREATMENT

GENERAL MEASURES
- Daily schedules and written directions
- Support and education of caregivers
- Emphasis on nutrition, personal hygiene, personal safety (accident-proofing the home), and supervision
- Discussions with the family concerning advance directives
- Socialization (adult day care)
- Sensory stimulation (prominent displays of clocks and calendars)
- Improvement in sleep hygiene
- Pharmacotherapy should be reserved for specific behavioral symptoms after non-pharmacologic therapy has failed.

Diet
No special diet

Activity
Fully active with direction and supervision

MEDICATION (DRUGS)

- Appropriately treat secondary causes, such as hypothyroidism or vitamin B_{12} deficiency.
- With other causes, drugs are used to treat behavioral symptoms after nonpharmacologic therapy has failed.
- Minimize medication use
- Aggressive behaviors: Antipsychotics such as risperidone (Risperdal) 0.5–1.0 mg, olanzapine (Zyprexa) 2.5 mg, or quetiapine (Seroquel) 25 mg PO at bedtime are reasonable choices in a non-emergency situation (3)[B]. Other options include carbamazepine (Tegretol) 100 mg b.i.d.–t.i.d. or Valproic acid 250–1,500 mg/d in divided dose (3)[C].
- Depression: Use serotonin reuptake inhibitors: Sertraline (Zoloft), fluoxetine (Prozac), paroxetine (Paxil), citalopram (Celexa), or escitalopram (Lexapro) all orally. Start with 1/2 the usual starting dose.
- Sleep disturbance: Intermittent use of temazepam (Restoril) 7.5–15 mg, zolpidem (Ambien) 5 mg, trazodone (Desyrel) 25–50 mg, or mirtazapine (Remeron) 7.5 mg at bedtime is occasionally warranted

- Cognitive dysfunction: Donepezil (Aricept) 5–10 mg daily, rivastigmine (Exelon) 1.5–6 mg b.i.d., galantamine (Reminyl) 4–12 mg (4)[B], memantine (Namenda) 5–20 mg/d PO (5)[C]
- Contraindications
  – Avoid anticholinergic drugs including tricyclic antidepressants and antihistamines
- Precautions
  – Hypnotics should not be used on a regular basis.
  – Antipsychotics
    ○ Risperidone may be associated with hyperglycemia and ketoacidosis.
  – Cholinesterase inhibitors (Aricept, Exelon, Reminyl)
    ○ Use with caution if the patient is at risk for gastrointestinal ulcers.
    ○ Use with caution if the patient suffers with sick sinus syndrome or other supraventricular cardiac conduction conditions.
  – Selective serotonin reuptake inhibitors (SSRIs)
    ○ Weight loss
    ○ Might decrease seizure threshold
- Significant possible interactions
  – Antipsychotics
    ○ Lithium may induce extrapyramidal symptoms and disorientation.
  – Benzodiazepines
    ○ Increased serum phenytoin concentration
    ○ Cimetidine may increase the benzodiazepine concentration.
  – SSRIs
    ○ Do not use in combination with monoamine oxidase inhibitors
    ○ May increase warfarin effect
    ○ Monitor lithium levels closely in those patients on lithium when a SSRI is added.

FOLLOW-UP

DISPOSITION
- Outpatient except when complications warrant hospitalization
- Nursing home or assisted living if disease progresses to the point that long-term care becomes necessary

PROGNOSIS
- AD: A progressive disease with variable rates of progression, but inevitably leading to profound cognitive impairment.
- VaD: Less likely to be progressive, but cognitive improvement is unlikely.
- Secondary dementias: Treatment of the underlying condition may lead to improvement

PATIENT MONITORING
- Periodic mental status testing to assess progression and predict prognosis
- Periodic monitoring of nutritional status
- Periodic monitoring of the caregiver status to assess for caregiver stress
- Periodic assessment of the environment for safety

REFERENCES

1. Newman AB, Fitzpatrick AL, Lopez O, et al. Dementia and Alzheimer's disease incidence in relationship to cardiovascular disease in the cardiovascular health study cohort. *JAGS*. 2005;52:1101–1107.
2. Geldmacher DS. Differential diagnosis of dementia syndromes. *Clin Geriat Med*. 2004;20(1):27–43
3. Kawas CH. Early Alzheimer's disease. *N Engl J Med*. 2003;349(11)1056–1063.
4. Trinh NH, Hoblyn J, Mohanty S, Jaffe K. Efficacy of cholinesterase inhibitirs in the treatment of neuropsychiatric symptoms and functional impairment in Alzheimer's disease. *JAMA*. 2003;289:210–216.
5. Cummings JL. Alzheimer's disease. *N Engl J Med*. 2004;351(1):56–67.
6. Tariot PN, Farlow MR, Grossberg GT, et al. Memantine treatment in patients with moderate to severe Alzheimer's disease already receiving donepezil: A randomized controlled trial. *JAMA*. 2004;291(3):317–324.

MISCELLANEOUS

See also: Alcohol use disorders; Alzheimer disease; Down syndrome; Huntington disease; Hypothyroidism, Adult; Parkinson disease; Stroke (brain attack); Syphilis

CODES

ICD9-CM
- 290.0 Senile dementia, uncomplicated
- 290.10 Presenile dementia, uncomplicated
- 290.40 Arteriosclerotic dementia, uncomplicated
- 331.0 Alzheimer disease

PATIENT TEACHING
- Mace N, Rabins Peter. *The 36-Hour Day*. 3rd ed. New York, NY: Warner Books Inc; 2001.
- Printed material available from the Alzheimer Association, 225 N. Michigan Ave. Floor 17 Chicago, IL 60601-7633; (800) 621-0379, www.alz.org.

 See Corresponding Diagnostic Algorithm

DEPENDENT PERSONALITY DISORDER

Heath A. Grames, PhD

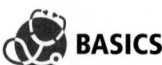 **BASICS**

DESCRIPTION
Beginning no later than adolescence or early adulthood, a consistent and pervasive pattern of dependency on others to make even the most trivial decisions for them, feelings of incompetence, and an excessive need for others to take care of them. (1)[C]

- Common behaviors and variations (1)[C]
  - Can be very clingy to caregivers
  - May isolate contact they have with other people to interactions with caregivers
  - May be very agreeable or submissive with others (even when they don't agree) out of fear of losing support/approval from others
  - May experience large amounts of distress when faced with decisions
  - May experience fear when alone
  - Lack of independence/fear of independence

Geriatric Considerations
Illness (acute and chronic) may exacerbate dependent personality disorder behaviors and may lead to intense feelings of fear and helplessness. (2)[C]

Pediatric Considerations
Diagnosis is rarely made for children/adolescence (may not be appropriate due to dependency needs of children/adolescence). Must 1st rule out Axis I disorders and behavior related to a general medical condition or to the developmental cycle of the child. For diagnosis, baseline behaviors must be representative of dependent personality disorder. (1)[C]

Pregnancy Considerations
Physical and social changes may induce stress or increase fears, which may result in increased dependent behaviors. Distinguish this disorder from increased dependency due to pregnancy (i.e., when there is no/poor support system).

GENERAL PREVENTION
Children with chronic illness or handicap may be more susceptible to dependent personality disorder. (1)[C] When possible, foster appropriate independence in the face of disability.

EPIDEMIOLOGY
- Predominant age: Onset no later than adolescence or early adulthood (may go undiagnosed for years) (1)[C]
- Predominant sex: Female > Male (1)[C]

Prevalence
Estimates of 20–30% of all personality disorders prevalence in primary care outpatient settings (3)[C]

- Dependent personality disorder is among most common in mental health clinics (1)[C]

RISK FACTORS
- Chronic or severe illness or disability in children (1)[C]
- Childhood/adolescent separation anxiety (1)[C]
- Parenting style that does not encourage age-appropriate independence

ETIOLOGY
Undetermined, but generally accepted, that it is due a combination of the following (3)[C]

- Hereditary temperamental traits
- Environment (e.g., not allowed independence (age appropriate)
- Developmental traits

ASSOCIATED CONDITIONS
- Mood disorders, increased risk (1)[C]
- Anxiety disorders, increased risk (1)[C]
- Adjustment disorders, increased risk (1)[C]
- Co-occurring personality disorders, frequent (1)[C]

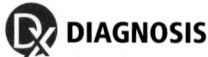 **DIAGNOSIS**

PRE HOSPITAL
Due to high co-occurrence with other Axis II disorders, assess suicide ideation and self-harm behavior

SIGNS AND SYMPTOMS
See "Disorder, Description"

History
- Difficulty making decisions (even trivial decisions) without great deal of reassurance and coaxing (1)[C]
- Seek physician to make decisions for him/her
- Dramatic/urgent demands for medical attention (even when symptoms are not painful or life-threatening)
- May actively attempt to prolong illness or seek unnecessary medical procedures (2)[C]
- Perception that he/she needs to be taken care of
- Clingy/demanding
- Once physician is in role of caregiver, may become submissive, agreeable (fear of losing relationship)

Diagnostic Procedures/Surgery
- Patient must meet at least 5 of the following (1)[C]
- Indecisive—needs support/reassurance from others to make decisions
- Defers personal responsibility (decision making, life choices) to others
- Does not voice disagreement with others without difficulty, out of fear of losing relationship
  - Not including realistic fears of abuse/retribution
- Difficulty starting/doing projects independently
- Seeks nurturance/support from others, even at great personal costs
- Experiences discomfort with solitude—fears having to care for self

DIFFERENTIAL DIAGNOSIS
- Mood disorders (1)[C]
  - Consider baseline behaviors when considering dependent vs. mood disorder
- Anxiety disorders (1)[C]
  - With dependent, baseline behaviors will suggest personality disorder (chronic, does not only occur at moments of stress or with Axis I disorders)
- Adjustment disorder (1)[C]
  - Differentiate in that dependence from stressor is not chronic and is related to stressor
- Other personality disorder (1)[C]
  - Consider patients thoughts, feelings, and behavior to differentiate dependent from other personality disorders
  - High co-occurrence of dependent and other personality disorders, especially borderline, histrionic, and avoidant
    - Chronic substance abuse (2)[C]

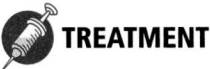 **TREATMENT**

PRE HOSPITAL
- Inpatient hospitalization is ineffective in changing Axis II disorder behaviors
- Inpatient hospital services for conditions related to Axis II disorder should be limited and of short duration to decrease dependence (decreasing likelihood of behavior change)
- Hospitalization should be considered for the following
  - Adjust medications
  - Implement psychotherapy for crisis intervention
  - Stabilize patient (psychosocial stressors)
- If suicidal, may need to be on suicide watch and receive appropriate psychiatric care

GENERAL MEASURES
- Focus on patient management rather than fixing or curing behaviors. (3)[C]
- Schedule follow-up to relieve patient stress.
- Meet with and rely on treatment team to avoid burnout and to provide opportunity for team to discuss issues with patient
- As necessary, refer patient to mental health therapist.

Nursing
Nurses can be helpful in managing the patient and calling the patient as needed (contact with the patient help relieve patient stress).

SPECIAL THERAPY
Consider referring patient for specialty mental health services.

 MEDICATION (DRUGS)

- There are no medications that treat dependent personality disorder
- Treat symptoms and Axis I disorders (3)[C]

First Line
Depression/anxiety (3)[C]
- Serotonin reuptake inhibitor
  - Benzodiazepine (short-term) if needed for anxiety symptom relief

 FOLLOW-UP

- Schedule routine follow-up with patient (relieves patient anxiety about medical care relationship with physician)
- Focus should be on medical conditions and co-morbid Axis I disorders

Admission Criteria
Refer to inpatient or outpatient psychiatry services if harm to self or others is expressed

Issues for Referral
Treatment for Axis II disorder should include psychotherapy and/or psychiatry.

PROGNOSIS
Medical focus is on patient management and caring for medical and Axis I disorders (2)[C]

REFERENCES
1. American Psychiatric Association. *Diagnostic and Statistical Manual of Mental Disorders*, 4th ed. Washington, DC: American Psychiatric Association; 1994.
2. Feder A, Robbins SW, Ostermeyer B. Personality disorders. In: Feldman, Christensen, JF, eds. *Behavioral medicine in primary care: A practical guide*, 2nd ed. New York, NY: McGraw-Hill; 2003;231–252.
3. Ward RK. Assessment and management of personality disorders. *Am Fam Physician*, 2004;70:1505–1512.

 MISCELLANEOUS

CODES

ICD9-CM
301.6 (Dependent Personality Disorder)

D

DEPRESSION
Nellie Freydin, PsyD

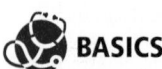 **BASICS**

DESCRIPTION
- Primary mood disorder characterized by a depressed mood and/or a decrease in interest in things that used to give pleasure (anhedonia) during the same 2-week period and represents a change from previous functioning.
- 4th most common reason to visit the family physician
- Physicians must have a high index of suspicion.
- Dysthymic disorder may be differentiated from major depression as a chronically depressed mood occurring for more days than not over a 2-year period.
- Bipolar disorder, a different clinical entity, may 1st present as an episode of depression.
- Also known as unipolar affective disorder.
- System(s) Affected: Nervous

ALERT
Geriatric Considerations
- Depression is not a normal part of aging
- More common in elderly, and difficult to precisely diagnose due to medical comorbidities (highest rates of depression are associated with stroke, coronary artery disease, cancer, Parkinson disease, and Alzheimer disease)
- Depression frequently coexists with dementia or delirium, with disorientation, memory loss, and distractibility most prominent

Pediatric Considerations
Depression occurs in children and can present with the following symptoms: Somatic complaints, irritability (versus depressed mood), and social withdrawal.

Pregnancy Considerations
- Use caution in prescribing psychoactive medications and paroxetine.
- SSRIs have been used successfully, although they are category C.
- Untreated depression can put both mother and fetus at risk.

EPIDEMIOLOGY
Prevalence
~5–20% will experience a significant depression at some time.

RISK FACTORS
- Gender
  - Twice as common in females
  - History of depression, dysthymia, or postpartum depression increases risk
- Age
  - 1st onset usually in late 20s (earlier in women than men)
- Strong family history (depression, suicide, alcoholism, other substance abuse)
- Presence of chronic disease
- Migraine headaches
- Chronic pain (especially back pain)
- Recent myocardial infarction
- Stroke
- Peptic ulcer disease
- Insomnia
- Domestic abuse or violence
- Adolescence
- Behavioral disorders, especially hyperactivity

- Substance abuse and dependence
- Menopause
- Losses and stressors

Genetics
Possible defect on chromosome II, X, or 12q

PATHOPHYSIOLOGY
- Changes in receptor–neurotransmitter relationship in the limbic system
  - Serotonin and norepinephrine are the primary neurotransmitters involved; dopamine, acetylcholine, and γ-aminobutyric acids have also been involved
- Increased pump uptake of the neurotransmitters. As action potential is passed on, the neurotransmitter is (a) reabsorbed into the neuron where it is either destroyed by an enzyme or actively removed by a reuptake pump and stored until needed or (b) destroyed by monoamine oxidase (MAO) in the mitochondria.
- Lack of neurotransmitters causes symptoms (e.g., decreased norepinephrine causes dullness and lethargy, while decreased serotonin causes irritability, hostility, and suicide ideation)

ETIOLOGY
- Impaired synthesis of the neurotransmitters
- Increased metabolism of neurotransmitters
- Environmental factors and learned behavior may affect neurotransmitters and/or have an independent influence on depression

ASSOCIATED CONDITIONS
- Manic depression (bipolar)
- Schizophrenia
- Schizo-affective disorders
- Psycho-physiological disorders
- Physical disorders
- Cyclothymic and grief reactions
- Alcoholism

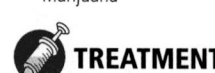 **DIAGNOSIS**

SIGNS AND SYMPTOMS
- Depressed mood most of the day, nearly every day
- Anhedonia
- Depression is probable when at least 4 of the following exist in addition to depressed mood or anhedonia
  - Appetite: Significant weight gain or loss when not dieting (change of >5% of body weight in 1 month)
  - Sleep disturbance: Insomnia or hypersomnia nearly every day
  - Fatigue: Out of proportion to the amount of energy expended
  - Psychomotor retardation or agitation: Restlessness, irritability, or withdrawal
  - Poor self-image: Worthlessness, excessive or inappropriate guilt
  - Concentration: Diminished thinking or concentration, poor memory, indecisiveness
  - Suicidal ideation: Recurrent thoughts of death; sometimes as patients begin to recover they gain enough energy to think about and sometimes attempt suicide

History
Common mnemonic for screening SIGECAPS
- S-sleep disturbance (falling asleep or recurrent wakening)
- I-interest loss; anhedonia
- G-guilt; inordinate feelings or responsibility
- E-energy; loss of energy
- C-concentration; loss of ability to focus
- A-appetite changes; over eating *or* loss of appetite
- P-psychomotor changes; decrease (flat affect) and agitation (manic episodes)
- S-suicidal/homicidal thoughts

TESTS
- Depression is primarily a clinical diagnosis by eliciting family, social, and psychosocial factors.
- Validated standard rating scales can assist
  - Zung Self-rating Depression Scale
  - BDI-2: Beck Depression Inventory
  - CES-D Scale: Criteria for Epidemiologic Studies—Depression Scale
  - CDI: Children's Depression Inventory
  - Yesavage Geriatric Depression Scale
- ECG
  - Diagnosis of arrhythmia
- EEG
  - Only if organic brain disease is suspected

Lab
- Used to rule out other diagnoses; e.g., TSH.
- All psychoactive drugs may alter lab results

Imaging
CT or MRI of brain, if organic brain syndrome (OBS) included in differential

DIFFERENTIAL DIAGNOSIS
- Organic brain diseases
- Endocrine diseases, such as hypothyroid and hyperthyroid diseases
- Diabetes mellitus
- Liver failure
- Renal failure
- Malignancy
- Chronic fatigue syndrome
- Lupus
- Vitamin deficiency
  - Pernicious anemia
  - Pellagra
- Medication side effects
  - Many drugs cause or worsen depression
- Medication overdose
- Medication abuse
- Withdrawal from medication
- Substance abuse and dependence
- Withdrawal from abused substance
  - Alcohol, anxiolytics, amphetamine, cocaine
  - Marijuana

TREATMENT

GENERAL MEASURES
- Psychotherapeutic interventions act synergistically with pharmacologic therapy.
- Psychotherapy and/or daily aerobic exercise can be as effective as oral antidepressants for mild to moderate depression.
- Electroconvulsive therapy (ECT) can be very effective in refractory cases.

Diet
As tolerated

Activity
No restrictions

SPECIAL THERAPY
Complementary and Alternative Medicine
- Hypericum perforatum (St. John's Wort)
  - Use in mild depression; evidence is inconsistent (5)[A]
- SAM-e (S-adenosyl methionine)
  - 400–1600 mg/d; may cause insomnia, lack of appetite, constipation, dry mouth, diaphoresis, dizziness, and anxiety (4)[A]
- Acupuncture: Insufficient evidence that it is useful in management of depression (6)[B]

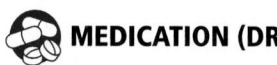 **MEDICATION (DRUGS)**

ALERT
Geriatric Considerations
- Decrease beginning dose by 1/2 and treat for a longer period than younger adults (4)[A]
- Higher risk of side effects or drug interactions due to decreased renal and hepatic function (4)[A]

Pediatric Considerations
- Decrease beginning dose by 1/2
- Recent evidence links SSRIs (especially Paroxetine) with suicide in adolescents (4)[A]
- Tricyclics not useful in children before puberty and are of moderate benefit at most for adolescents; safety also unclear (3)[A]

First Line
- All are equally efficacious for depression. Selection is based on side effects profile.
  - SSRIs: May cause insomnia, anxiety, headache, sexual dysfunction; overdose less likely to be fatal
    - Fluoxetine (Prozac): 20 mg–80 mg/d every am
    - Sertraline (Zoloft): 50–200 mg/d every am
    - Paroxetine (Paxil): 10–40 mg/d every am
    - Paroxetine CR: 12.5–37.5 mg/d every am
    - Citalopram (Celexa): 20–40 mg every am
    - Escitalopram (Lexapro): 10–20 mg every am
  - Others
    - Venlafaxine (Effexor): 75–150 mg/d (divided doses); increases serotonin and norepinephrine; can cause insomnia, anxiety, and anorexia
    - Bupropion (Wellbutrin): 100–300 mg/d (divided doses) (catecholamine reuptake inhibitor); increased seizure risk
    - Duloxetine (Cymbalta):40–60 mg/d
- Contraindications: Refer to manufacturer's profile of each drug
- Precautions
  - Avoid paroxetine in pregnancy (4)[A]
  - Polycyclic antidepressants can be fatal with overdose, may produce arrhythmias and lower seizure threshold
  - Venlafaxine
    - 2 weeks washout before instituting therapy
  - Selective serotonin reuptake inhibitors (SSRIs)
    - Fluoxetine, sertraline, or paroxetine are best given in the morning
    - Abrupt discontinuation may result in withdrawal symptoms

- Significant possible interactions: Monoamine oxidase inhibitors (MAOIs)

Second Line
- Clomipramine (Anafranil): 25–200 mg/d
  - Used to treat obsessive–compulsive disorder
- Fluvoxamine (Luvox): 50–300 mg/d divided
  - Indicated for obsessive-compulsive disorder
- MAOIs
  - Significant drug and food interactions limit use, but can be useful in refractory cases
- Polycyclic (TCAs) antidepressants with sedating properties (also have anticholinergic properties, potential for fatal overdose)
  - Amoxapine (Asendin): 50–400 mg/d (divided doses). Maximum hs dose 300 mg
  - Amitriptyline (Elavil, Endep): 150–300 mg/d at bedtime
  - Maprotiline (Ludiomil): 75–225 mg/d (useful with associated anxiety)
  - Mirtazapine (Remeron): 15–45 mg/d at bedtime
  - Nortriptyline (Pamelor, Aventyl): 75–150 mg/d at bedtime (a metabolite of amitriptyline)
  - Doxepin (Adapin, Sinequan): 75–300 mg/d at bedtime
  - Trimipramine (Surmontil): 75–300 mg/d at bedtime (divided doses)
  - Trazodone (Desyrel): 150–300 mg/d at bedtime (divided doses) Maximum hs dose 600 mg
- Polycyclic antidepressants with activating properties (also have anticholinergic properties, insomnia, anxiety, potentially fatal overdose)
  - Imipramine (Tofranil): 150–300 mg/d
  - Desipramine (Norpramin, Pertofrane): 100–300 mg/d
  - Protriptyline (Vivactil): 15–60 mg/d (divided doses)

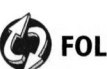 **FOLLOW-UP**

DISPOSITION
Admission Criteria
Inpatient care is indicated for seriously depressed, psychotic, or suicidal patients.

PROGNOSIS
- 70% significant improvement.
- Anticipate recurrences

COMPLICATIONS
- Suicide
- Failure to improve

PATIENT MONITORING
- See within 2 weeks after starting medication.
- During follow-up, evaluate the side effects, dosage, and effectiveness of the medication.
- Follow every 2 weeks until improvement.
- Follow every 3 months thereafter.
- Explain treatment must continue for at least 6 months–2 years; longer with family history of depression and the very young.
- The relationship (therapeutic alliance) between the patient and health care professional is important in success of treatment

REFERENCES
1. Abkevich V, et al. Predisposition locus for major depression at chromosome 12q22-1223.2. *Am J Hum Genet* 2003;73(6):1271–1281.
2. American Psychiatric Association. Diagnostic and statistical manual of mental disorders DSM-IV-TR (4th ed., text revision). Washington, DC: American Psychiatric Publishing, 2000.
3. Hazell P, O'Connell D, Heathcote D, Henry D. Tricyclic drugs for depression in children and adolescents. Cochrane Database of Systematic Reviews 2002; Issue 2. Art. No.: CD002317. DOI: 10.1002/14651858.CD002317.
4. Institute for Clinical Systems Improvement. Major depression in adults in primary care. Bloomington, MN: Institute for Clinical Systems Improvement, 2006.
5. Linde K, Mulrow CD, Berner M, Egger M. St. John's Wort for depression. Cochrane Database of Systematic Reviews 2005, Issue 2, Art. No.: CD000448. DOI: 10.1002/14651858. CD000448.pub2.
6. Smith CA, Hay PPJ. Acupuncture for depression. Cochrane Database of Systematic Reviews 2004, Issue 3. Art. No.: CD004046. DOI: 10.1002/14651858.CD004046.pub2.
7. Wilson K, Mottram P, Sivanranthan A, Nightingale A. Antidepressants versus placebo for the depressed elderly. Cochrane Database of Systematic Reviews 2001, Issue 1. Art. No.: CD000561. DOI: 10.1002/14651858.CD000561.

 MISCELLANEOUS

CODES

ICD9-CM
- 311 Depressive disorder, not elsewhere classified
- 296.20 Major depressive disorder, single episode, unspecified
- 296.30 Major depressive disorder, recurrent episode, unspecified

PATIENT TEACHING
- Educate about mental health: Depression is a medical illness, not a character defect.
- Educate about efficacy of treatment: Effective for nearly all patients.
- Educate about medications and side effects
- Consider referral to mental health professional and support groups, such as the National Depression Manic Depression Association (DMDA): (800) 82-MDMDA
- Stress need for long-term treatment and follow-up, which includes lifestyle changes
- Recommended reading for patients
  - Addis ME, Martell CR. Overcoming Depression One Step at a Time: The New Behavioral Activation Approach to Getting your Life Back. Oakland, CA: New Harbinger Publications, 2004
  - *Depression*. Mayo Clinic. http://www.mayoclinic.com/health/depression/DS00175

Activity
Aim for 30 minutes of moderate–intensity exercise, 3–5 days per week for healthy adults (4)[A]

Prevention
Patient and family should be alert to early signs and symptoms of recurrence and seek treatment early if depression returns.

 See Corresponding Diagnostic Algorithm

 See Patient Handout on CD

DERMATITIS, ATOPIC

Dennis E. Hughes, DO

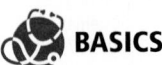 BASICS

DESCRIPTION
- Chronic pruritic eczematous condition affecting characteristic sites
- System(s) Affected: Skin/Exocrine
- Synonym(s): Eczema; Disseminated neurodermatitis; Atopic eczema; Atopic neurodermatitis; Constitutional dermatitis; Besnier prurigo

GENERAL PREVENTION
Smallpox vaccine should be avoided in patients with atopy, because of risk of eczema herpeticum.

EPIDEMIOLOGY
Incidence
Mainly childhood disease; affects 10% of all children, usually appearing in the 1st year of life and gradually subsiding over subsequent years.

Prevalence
Common; increased since 1970

RISK FACTORS
- Skin infections
- Emotional stress
- Irritating clothes and chemicals
- Excessively hot or cold climate
- Food allergy in children (controversial)
- Exposure to tobacco smoke
- Family history of atopy
  - Asthma
  - Allergic rhinitis

Genetics
Genetic predisposition
- Family history positive in 2/3 of cases

ETIOLOGY
- Unknown
- Genetically determined, nonallergic disease

ASSOCIATED CONDITIONS
- Asthma
- Allergic rhinitis
- Hyper-IgE syndrome (Job syndrome)
  - Atopic dermatitis
  - Elevated IgE
  - Recurrent pyodermas
  - Decreased chemotaxis of mononuclear cells

DIAGNOSIS

SIGNS AND SYMPTOMS
- Pruritus is the most common symptom
- Distribution of lesions
  - Infants: Trunk, face, and extensor surfaces
  - Children: Antecubital and popliteal fossae
  - Adults: Face, neck, upper chest, and genital areas
- Morphology of lesions
  - Infants: Erythema and papules; may develop oozing, crusting vesicles
  - Children and adults: Lichenification and scaling are typical with chronic eczema.
- Associated features
  - Facial erythema, mild to moderate
  - Perioral pallor
  - Infraorbital fold (Dennie sign/Morgan line)
  - Dry skin
  - Increased palmar linear markings
  - Pityriasis alba (hypopigmented asymptomatic areas on face and shoulders)
  - Keratosis pilaris

History
- Family history of atopic dermatitis may be more useful than morphology in making the diagnosis
- In adults with limited distribution of lesions, a history of childhood eczema is a clue to diagnosis

Physical Exam
Involves the flexor skin creases

TESTS
Diagnosis based on clinical findings

Lab
Serum IgE levels frequently are elevated but are rarely needed and do not assist in diagnosis or treatment

Diagnostic Procedures/Surgery
Skin biopsy shows nonspecific eczematous changes (biopsy is rarely required because diagnosis is made on clinical grounds)

Pathological Findings
- Epidermis thickened and hyperkeratotic
- Perivascular inflammation of dermis

DIFFERENTIAL DIAGNOSIS
- Photosensitivity rashes
- Contact dermatitis (especially if only the face is involved)
- Scabies
- Seborrheic dermatitis (especially in infants)
- Psoriasis or lichen simplex chronicus if only localized disease is present in adults
- Rare conditions of infancy
  - Histiocytosis X
  - Wiskott-Aldrich syndrome
  - Ataxia-telangiectasia syndrome
- Ichthyosis vulgaris

TREATMENT

INITIAL STABILIZATION
Generally outpatient, using topical corticosteroids

GENERAL MEASURES
- Decrease stress if possible
- Avoid agents that may cause irritation (e.g., wool, perfumes)
- Minimize sweating
- Lukewarm (not hot) baths
- Minimize use of soap (superfatted soaps best)
- Frequent systemic lubrication with thick emollient creams (e.g., Eucerin) over moist skin
- Sun exposure may be helpful
- Humidify the house
- Avoid excessive contact with water
- Avoid lotions that contain alcohol
- If very resistant to treatment, search for a coexisting contact dermatitis

Diet
- The role of food allergies and exacerbations of atopic dermatitis is controversial
- Most common suspicious foods are eggs, milk, wheat, and peanuts
- Consider elimination diets (e.g., for 3–4 weeks) and food challenges
- Consider delaying introduction of the common suspicious foods until an infant is 6 months old

Activity
No restrictions

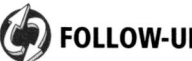 MEDICATION (DRUGS)

Pediatric Considerations
Chronic potent fluorinated corticosteroid use may cause striae, hypopigmentation, or atrophy, especially in children.

First Line
Frequent systemic lubrication with thick emollient creams (e. g., Eucerin) over moist skin

- Infants and children: 0.5–1% topical hydrocortisone creams or ointments
- Hypopigmentation can happen even with short-term use.
- Adults: Higher potency (over 1%) topical corticosteroids in areas other than face and skin folds
- Short-course higher-potency corticosteroids for flares, then return to the lowest potency (creams preferred) that will control dermatitis. (1)[C]

Second Line
- Topical immunomodulators (tacrolimus or pimecrolimus) for episodic use for children >2 years. Black box warning from the FDA regarding potential cancer risk. (2,3)
- Antihistamines for pruritus (e.g., hydroxyzine, 10–25 mg at bedtime and as needed)
- Plastic occlusion in combination with topical medication to promote absorption
- For severe atopic dermatitis, consider systemic steroids for 1–2 weeks (e.g., prednisone 2 mg/kg/d PO (maximum 80 mg/d) initially, tapered over 7–14 days.
- Topical tricyclic doxepin as a 5% cream may decrease pruritus
- Evening primrose oil (includes high content of fatty acids)
  – May decrease prostaglandin synthesis
  – May promote conversion of linoleic acid to omega-6 fatty acid
- Modified Goeckerman regimen (tar and UV light)
- Immune modifiers (methotrexate, azathioprine, cyclosporine)
- Probiotics may reduce the severity of the condition, reducing medication use. (4)[C]

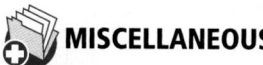 FOLLOW-UP

PROGNOSIS
Chronic disease
- Declines with increasing age
- 90% of patients have spontaneous resolution by puberty.
- Localized eczema (e.g., chronic hand or foot dermatitis, eyelid dermatitis, or lichen simplex chronicus) may continue in some adults.

COMPLICATIONS
- Cataracts are more common in patients with atopic dermatitis.
- Skin infections (usually *Staphylococcus aureus*); sometimes subclinical
- Eczema herpeticum
  – Generalized vesiculopustular eruption caused by infection with herpes simplex or vaccinia virus
  – Causes acute illness requiring hospitalization
- Atrophy and/or striae if fluorinated corticosteroids are used on face or skin folds
- Systemic absorption may occur if large areas of skin are treated, particularly if high-potency medications and occlusion are combined.

PATIENT MONITORING
Individualize depending on severity of disease

REFERENCES

1. Williams HC. Atopic dermatitis. *NEJM*. 2005;352: 2314–2324.
2. Eichenfield LF, Hanifin JM, Luger TA, et al. Consensus conference on pediatric atopic dermatitis. *J Am Acad Dermatol*. 2003;49: 1088–1095.
3. Trammell D, Shakil A, Wilder L. What is the role of tacrolimus and pimecrolimus in atopic dermatitis? *J Fam Prac*. 2005;54:714–716.
4. Weston S, et al. Effects of probiotics on atopic dermatitis: A randomized controlled trial. *Arch Disease Child*. 2005;90:892–897.
5. Tofte SJ, Hanifin JM. Current management and therapy of atopic dermatitis. *J Am Acad Dermatol*. 2001;44[Suppl]:S13–S16.

D

 MISCELLANEOUS

 CODES

ICD9-CM
691.8 Other atopic dermatitis and related conditions

PATIENT TEACHING
- Goal is control, not cure (although many patients will outgrow their disease)
- See www.niams.nih.gov/hi/topics/dermatitis

See Corresponding Diagnostic Algorithm

See Patient Handout on CD

DERMATITIS, CONTACT

Julie A. Hayner, MD

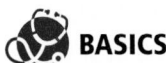 **BASICS**

DESCRIPTION
- The cutaneous reaction to an external substance.
- Primary irritant dermatitis (80%) is due to direct injury of the skin. It affects individuals exposed to specific irritants and generally produces discomfort immediately after exposure.
- Allergic contact dermatitis (ACD) (20%) affects only individuals previously sensitized to the contactant. It represents a delayed hypersensitivity reaction, requiring several hours for the cascade of cellular immunity to be completed to manifest itself.
- System(s) Affected: Skin/Exocrine
- Synonym(s): Dermatitis venenata

GENERAL PREVENTION
- Avoid causative agents.
- Use of protective gloves (with cotton lining) may be helpful.

EPIDEMIOLOGY
Incidence
Occupational contact dermatitis: 20.5/100,000 workers (1)[B].

Prevalence
- Contact dermatitis represents >90% of all occupational skin disorders.
- Predominant sex: Male = Female
  - Variations due to differences in exposure to offending agents as well as normal cutaneous variations between male and female (eccrine and sebaceous gland function and hair distribution)

ALERT
Geriatric Considerations
Increased incidence of irritant dermatitis secondary to skin dryness

Pediatric Considerations
Increased incidence of positive patch testing due to better delayed hypersensitivity reactions; usual cautions with medications

RISK FACTORS
- Occupation
- Hobbies
- Travel
- Cosmetics
- Jewelry

Genetics
Increased frequency of ACD in families with allergies

PATHOPHYSIOLOGY
Hypersensitivity reaction to a substance generating cellular immunity response

ETIOLOGY
- Plants
  - Rhus-urushiol (poison ivy, oak, sumac)
  - Primary contact: Plant (roots/stems/leaves)
  - Secondary contact: Clothes/fingernails (not blister fluid)
- Chemicals
  - Nickel: Jewelry, zippers, hooks, and watches
  - Potassium dichromate: Tanning agent in leather
  - Paraphenylenediamine: Hair dyes, fur dyes, and industrial chemicals
  - Turpentine: Cleaning agents, polishes, and waxes
  - Soaps and detergents

- Topical medicines
  - Neomycin: Topical antibiotics
  - Thimerosal (Merthiolate): Preservative in topical medications
  - Anesthetics: Benzocaine
  - Parabens: Preservative in topical medications
  - Formalin: Cosmetics, shampoos, and nail enamel

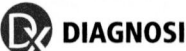 **DIAGNOSIS**

SIGNS AND SYMPTOMS
- Acute
  - Papules, vesicles, bullae with surrounding erythema
  - Crusting and oozing
  - Pruritus
- Chronic
  - Erythematous base
  - Thickening with lichenification
  - Scaling
  - Fissuring
- Distribution
  - Where epidermis is thinner (eyelids, genitalia)
  - Areas of contact with offending agent (e.g., nail polish)
  - Palms and soles more resistant
  - Deeper skin-folds spared
  - Linear arrays of lesions
  - Lesions with sharp borders and sharp angles are pathognomonic.

History
Exposure to irritating substance

Physical Exam
Well-demarcated area with a papulovesicular rash

TESTS
Diagnostic Procedures/Surgery
Patch tests for allergic contact dermatitis (systemic corticosteroids or recent, aggressive use of topical steroids may alter results) (2)[B]

Pathological Findings
- Intercellular edema
- Bullae

DIFFERENTIAL DIAGNOSIS
- Based on clinical impression
  - Appearance, periodicity, and localization
- Groups of vesicles
  - Herpes simplex
- Diffuse bullous or vesicular lesions
  - Bullous pemphigoid
- Photodistribution
  - Phototoxic/allergic reaction to systemic allergen
- Eyelids
  - Seborrheic dermatitis
- Scaly eczematous lesions
  - Atopic dermatitis
  - Nummular eczema
  - Lichen simplex chronicus
  - Stasis dermatitis
  - Xerosis

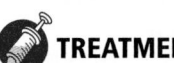 **TREATMENT**

GENERAL MEASURES
- Removal of offending agent
  - Avoidance
    - Work modification
    - Protective clothing
    - Barrier creams
- Topical soaks with cool tap water, Burow's solution (1:40 dilution), or saline (1 tsp/pint water), or silver nitrate solution
- Lukewarm water baths
- Aveeno (oatmeal) baths
- Chronic
  - Emollients (white petrolatum, Eucerin)

Diet
No special diet

Activity
Stay active, but avoid overheating

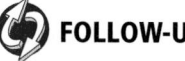 **MEDICATION (DRUGS)**

First Line
- Topical medications
  - Shake lotion of zinc oxide, talc, menthol 0.25%, phenol 0.5% (Gold Bond, others)
  - Corticosteroids for allergic contact dermatitis (3)[A], but not for irritant dermatitis (4)[B]
    - High-potency steroids: Fluocinonide (Lidex) 0.05% ointment t.i.d.–q.i.d.
    - Caution regarding face/skin folds: Use lower-potency steroids and avoid prolonged usage. Switch to lower-potency topical steroid once the acute phase is resolved.
- Calamine lotion
- Topical antibiotics for secondary infection (bacitracin, gentamicin, erythromycin)
- Systemic
  - Antihistamine
    - Hydroxyzine: 25–50 mg PO q.i.d.
    - Diphenhydramine: 25–50 mg PO q.i.d.
  - Corticosteroids
    - Prednisone: Taper starting at 60–80 mg/d PO, tapered over 10–14 days
  - Antibiotics for secondary infection
    - Erythromycin: 250 mg PO q.i.d.
    - Dicloxacillin: 250 mg PO q.i.d. for 7–10 days
    - Amoxicillin-clavulanate (Augmentin): 500 mg PO b.i.d. for 7–10 days
  - Precautions
    - Antihistamines may cause drowsiness
    - Prolonged use of potent topical steroids may cause local skin effects (atrophy, stria, telangiectasia)

Second Line
Other topical or systemic antibiotics, depending on organisms and sensitivity

ALERT
Pregnancy Considerations
Usual cautions with medications

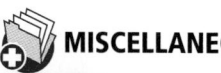 **FOLLOW-UP**

DISPOSITION
Admission Criteria
Rarely will need hospital admission

Issues for Referral
May need referral to a dermatologist if refractory to conventional treatment

PROGNOSIS
- Self-limited
- Benign

COMPLICATIONS
- Generalized eruption secondary to autosensitization
- Secondary bacterial infection

PATIENT MONITORING
- As necessary for recurrence
- Patch testing for etiology after resolved

REFERENCES

1. Incidence and prevalence rates for occupational contact dermatitis in an Australian suburban area. *Contact Dermatitis*. 2005;52:254–259.
2. Saripalli YV, Achen F, Belsito DV. The detection of clinically relevant contact allergens using standard screening tray of 23 allergens. *J Am Acad Dermatol*. 2003;49:65–69.
3. Hachem JP, De Paepe K, Vanpee E, et al. Efficacy of topical corticosteroids in nickel-induced contact allergy. *Clin Exp Dermatol*. 2002;27:47–50.
4. Levin C, Zhai H, Bashir S, et al. Efficacy of corticosteroids in acute experimental irritant contact dermatitis. *Skin Res Technol*. 2001;7:214–218.

 MISCELLANEOUS

CODES

ICD9-CM
- 692.0 Contact dermatitis and other eczema due to detergents
- 692.9 Contact dermatitis and other eczema due to unspecified cause

PATIENT TEACHING
- Avoidance of irritating substance
- Cleaning of secondary sources (nails, clothes)
- Fallacy of blister fluid spreading disease

See Corresponding Diagnostic Algorithm

D

DERMATITIS, DIAPER

Dennis E. Hughes, DO

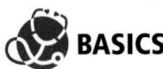

BASICS

DESCRIPTION
- Diaper dermatitis is a rash occurring under the covered area of a diaper. The rash may be an irritant contact dermatitis, candidiasis, atopic dermatitis, or seborrheic dermatitis.
- System(s) Affected: Skin/Exocrine
- Synonym(s): Diaper rash

Geriatric Considerations
Incontinence

GENERAL PREVENTION
See: "General Measures"

EPIDEMIOLOGY
- Predominant age: Infants; highest incidence 9–12 months
- Predominant sex: Male = Female

Incidence
Common in the US

Pediatric Considerations
Problem most common in this age group

RISK FACTORS
- Infrequent diaper changes
- Waterproof diapers
- Improper laundering
- Family history of dermatitis
- Hot, humid weather
- Recent treatment with oral antibiotics
- Diarrhea

ETIOLOGY
Irritation to skin from prolonged contact with urine or feces (1)

ASSOCIATED CONDITIONS
Contact (allergic or irritant) dermatitis, Seborrheic dermatitis, Psoriasis, Candidiasis, Atopic dermatitis

DIAGNOSIS

SIGNS AND SYMPTOMS
- Irritant contact diaper dermatitis
  - Prominent rash on buttocks and pubic skin
  - Creases of skin are relatively spared
  - Rash is dusky red and shiny
  - Skin seems chapped
  - Weeping, crusting, and excoriations are not prominent.
- Candidiasis diaper rash
  - Initial involvement of creases with rapid extension
  - Color: Bright red
  - Accompanying edema
  - Isolated satellite papules and pustules at margins of inflammatory plaques
  - Excoriations are prominent.
  - Positive potassium hydroxide (KOH) preparation
  - Positive cultures
- Atopic diaper dermatitis
  - Distribution spares creases
  - Genitalia frequently involved
  - Itch-scratch cycle with excoriations are prominent.
  - Child scratches vigorously at night
  - Weeping, crusting, excoriations sometimes present; secondary bacterial infection can occur
- Seborrheic diaper dermatitis
  - Dusky-red patches and plaques deep within skin creases
  - Nonintertriginous skin is relatively spared
  - Weeping, crusting, excoriations: Not prominent
  - Other sites of seborrheic dermatitis are frequently present: Retroauricular, axillary folds, scalp

TESTS
- KOH preparation
- Culture pustules, if present

Lab
Culture will reveal *Candida*, if present

Diagnostic Procedures/Surgery
- Culture lesions
- KOH preparation

Pathological Findings
Varying inflammation is the most prominent finding

DIFFERENTIAL DIAGNOSIS
- Contact dermatitis
- Seborrheic dermatitis
- Candidiasis
- Atopic dermatitis
- Scabies
- Acrodermatitis enteropathica
- Letterer-Siwe disease
- Congenital syphilis
- Child abuse
- Streptococcal infection
- Kawasaki disease
- Biotin deficiency
- Psoriasis

TREATMENT

GENERAL MEASURES
- Appropriate health care: Outpatient
- Expose the buttocks to air as much as possible. (1)
- Don't use waterproof pants during treatment (day or night); they keep skin wet and subject to rash or infection.
- Change diapers frequently, even at night if the rash is extensive (2)
- Super-absorbable diapers beneficial (1,2)
- Discontinue using baby lotion, powder, ointment, or baby oil (except zinc oxide).
- Zinc oxide ointment or other barrier cream to the rash at the earliest sign, and b.i.d. or t.i.d (like Desitin or Balmex). Thereafter apply to clean, thoroughly dry skin (1)
- Use mild soap and pat dry.

Activity
Protect from overheating.

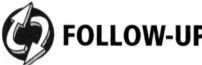 **MEDICATION (DRUGS)**

First Line

- If candidiasis suspected or diaper rash persistent, use an antifungal such as miconazole nitrate 2% cream, miconazole powder, econazole (Spectazole), clotrimazole (Lotrimin), or ketoconazole (Nizoral) cream, at each diaper change. (1)
- If inflammation is prominent, consider very-low-potency steroid cream, such as hydrocortisone 0.5–1% t.i.d. along with an antifungal cream and/or a combination product such as clioquinol-hydrocortisone (Vioform–hydrocortisone) cream. (1)
- If a secondary bacterial infection is suspected, use an anti-Staphylococcal oral antibiotic or mupirocin (Bactroban) ointment topically.
- Precautions: Avoid high- or moderate-potency steroids often found in combination steroid-antifungal mixtures. (1)

Second Line

Sucralfate paste for resistant cases

 FOLLOW-UP

PROGNOSIS

Quick, complete clearing with appropriate treatment

COMPLICATIONS

- Secondary bacterial infection
- Secondary yeast infection

PATIENT MONITORING

Recheck weekly until clear, then at times of recurrence

REFERENCES

1. Scheinfeld N. Diaper dermatitis: A review and brief survey of eruptions of the diaper area. *Am J Clin Derm*. 2005;6:273–281.
2. Jannniger CK Thomas IT. Diaper dermatitis: An approach to prevention employing effective diaper care. *Cutis*. 1993;52:153–155.
3. Kazaks EL, Lane AT. Diaper dermatitis. *Pediatr Clin North Amer*. 2000;47(4):909–919.

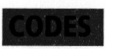 **MISCELLANEOUS**

- 2 or more types of diaper dermatitis can exist concomitantly. If so, treat each accordingly.
- See also: Candidiasis; Dermatitis, atopic; Dermatitis, contact' Psoriasis

CODES

ICD9-CM

691.0 Diaper or napkin rash

D

DERMATITIS, EXFOLIATIVE (ED)

Herbert P. Goodheart, MD

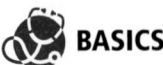 BASICS

DESCRIPTION
- ED, or *erythroderma*, is a generalized (often >90% of body) scaling eruption of the skin.
- ED may arise idiopathically or secondary to an underlying cutaneous or systemic disease or as a reaction to medications.
- Cutaneous involvement consists of redness and/or scaling of the skin.
- When fulminant, this reaction is potentially life threatening.
- ED is a rare disorder that may appear suddenly or gradually, occasionally accompanied by fever, chills, and lymphadenopathy.
- System(s) Affected: Skin/Exocrine
- Synonym(s): Erythroderma; Exfoliative erythroderm; Red man syndrome (*homme rouge*); Pityriasis rubra

EPIDEMIOLOGY
- Predominant age: 75% of patients are >40 years
- Predominant sex: Male > Female (2–4:1)

Incidence
In the US: Rare; estimated 1% of hospitalizations for skin disease

RISK FACTORS
- Underlying diseases as noted below
- Male sex
- Age >40 years

PATHOPHYSIOLOGY
This varies and depends on the underlying cause
- A marked loss of exfoliated epidermis occurs (uncontrolled desquamation) due to an increased mitotic rate
- This may contribute to hypoalbuminemia, edema, heat loss, and hypothermia

ETIOLOGY
- The most common associated conditions or diseases that have been reported to present with or develop into ED include
  - In adults, psoriasis, most frequently
  - In children, ED is most often secondary to severe atopic dermatitis
  - Drug reactions
  - ED is idiopathic in up to 20–30% of cases
- Less commonly, ED has been noted as a finding in the following skin disorders
  - Allergic contact dermatitis
  - Stasis dermatitis with secondary autoeczematization
  - Pityriasis rubra pilaris (a rare disorder of keratinization)
  - Graft-versus-host disease
  - Seborrheic dermatitis (Leiner's disease) in infants
  - Ichthyosiform dermatoses
  - Pemphigus foliaceus
  - Papulosquamous dermatitis of AIDS
  - Fungal disease with id reaction
- Other rare reported associations include
  - Reiter syndrome
  - Systemic lupus erythematosus
  - Hailey-Hailey disease
  - Norwegian scabies
  - Sarcoidosis
  - Lichen planus
  - Systemic lupus erythematosus
  - Dermatomyositis
- Medications: May occur as a reaction to the following drugs: Allopurinol, antimalarials, aspirin, barbiturates, captopril, codeine, cefoxitin, cimetidine, dapsone, gold salts, hydantoins, isoniazid, lithium, NSAIDS, omeprazole, para-aminosalicylic acid, penicillins, phenybutazone, phenothiazines, St. John's Wort, sulfonamides, sulfonylureas, thalidomide, and vancomycin
- May occur as a complication or presenting symptom of the following malignancies
  - Mycosis fungoides (cutaneous T-cell lymphoma)
  - Sézary syndrome (leukemic variant of mycosis fungoides)
  - Hodgkin disease
  - Non-Hodgkin lymphoma and leukemia

DIFFERENTIAL DIAGNOSIS
- Extensive acute eczematous dermatoses, such as contact dermatitis and drug eruptions
- Toxic epidermal necrolysis
- Staphylococcal scalded skin syndrome
- Erythema multiforme major

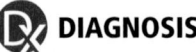 DIAGNOSIS
- Diagnosis of ED is made on a clinical basis. Determination of the underlying cause is often elusive
- Infrequently, clinical findings, such as the characteristic lichenification of atopic dermatitis or nail pitting that suggests psoriasis, may be found

SIGNS AND SYMPTOMS
- There is marked generalized erythema followed by scaling
- Pruritus may be severe
- Edema and increased warmth of the skin
- Pedal or pretibial edema
- Lymphadenopathy, usually a reactive type (*dermatopathic lymphadenopathy*) is often present
- Nail dystrophy in 40%
- Fever in 40–50%
- Chills
- Malaise/weakness
- Eosinophilia (30%)
- Hepatomegaly (20%)
- Splenomegaly when underlying lymphoma/leukemia present
- Alopecia
- Hypoproteinemia
- Dehydration
- High-output cardiac failure
- Tachycardia (40%)
- In time, lichenification may occur
- Postinflammatory dyspigmentation (hyper or hypopigmented areas of the skin)

History
Eliciting a history of drug ingestion or a pre-existing dermatosis or disease may be valuable.

TESTS
Lab
None diagnostic. May have elevated WBC count with eosinophilia, anemia, elevated erythrocyte sedimentation rate, decreased albumin, and electrolyte abnormalities

Imaging
Chest radiograph and other imaging procedures as indicated to investigate any underlying disease process

Diagnostic Procedures/Surgery
- Laboratory testing can provide serologic evidence of Sézary syndrome or leukemia
- Patch testing during a period of remission may uncover a contact allergen
- Skin biopsy (lymph node or bone marrow), as indicated to investigate an underlying disease process
- Further tests are performed if suggested by the review of systems and physical examination

Pathological Findings
- May have characteristics of an underlying cutaneous disease; however, findings are most often nonspecific and consist of
  - Hyperkeratosis, parakeratosis, and acanthosis in the epidermis; and edema, vasodilation, and perivascular infiltrates with lymphocytes, histiocytes, and eosinophils in the dermis
- Repeated or multiple biopsies are sometimes helpful

TREATMENT

- Cool tap water dressings
- Application of intermediate-strength topical steroids (e.g., triamcinolone cream 0.025–0.1%) beneath wet dressings
- Cool colloid baths with oatmeal (e.g., Aveeno)
- Local bland, moisturizing ointments/lotions
- Systemic antibiotics if signs of secondary infection are observed
- Antihistamines act primarily as sedatives

ALERT
Systemic steroids may be helpful in some cases, but should be avoided in suspected cases of psoriasis.

GENERAL MEASURES
- Outpatient care except in those cases with complications of secondary infection, dehydration, or heart failure
- Withdrawal of any implicated medications or treatment of any identified underlying infection/disease
- Protection from development of hypothermia
- Because ED may evolve rapidly, the patient frequently requires hospitalization, where measures such as fluid replacement, temperature control, and expert topical skin care are available

Diet
- Increased fluid intake
- Ensure adequate nutrition with emphasis on sufficient protein intake

Nursing
- Bed rest, cool compresses, lubrication with emollients, antipruritic therapy with oral antihistamines, and low- to intermediate-strength topical steroids are applied

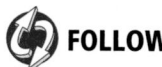 MEDICATION (DRUGS)

First Line
- Mid-potency topical steroids
- In addition, treatment specific to any underlying infection or disease should be provided
- Systemic steroids: Initial dosage equivalent to prednisone 40 mg/d with increases in dosage by 20 mg/d if there is no response after 3–4 days. Subsequently, dosage should be tapered as symptoms are controlled.
- Contraindications: Psoriasis as the underlying cause of the exfoliative dermatitis, whereas oral retinoids are an excellent choice for this disease.

Second Line
- When psoriasis is the underlying cause, cyclosporine, methotrexate, etretinate, phototherapy, photopheresis, photochemotherapy, as well as monoclonal antibodies such as infliximab and alemtuzumab may be effective
- Photochemotherapy may also be useful therapy for treating ED associated with mycosis fungoides
- Isotretinoin has been used when pityriasis rubra pilaris is the underlying cause
- Antimetabolites/cytotoxic drugs
- Bexarotene

 FOLLOW-UP

DISPOSITION
Admission Criteria
- Impending or actual heart failure
- Inability to control ED on an outpatient basis

PROGNOSIS
- The prognosis of ED depends largely on underlying etiology
- In patients with an identified underlying cause, the course and prognosis will generally parallel the primary disease
- ED due to a drug eruption usually clears when the drug is stopped
- Acute, severe episodes, particularly in elderly persons or in persons with preexisting heart disease, have more guarded prognosis
- In patients with idiopathic ED, the prognosis is poor and recurrences are not uncommon

COMPLICATIONS
- Secondary infection
- Sepsis
- Hypothermia
- Dehydration/electrolyte disturbances
- High-output heart failure

REFERENCES
1. Rongioletti F, Borenstein M, Kirsner R, Kerdel F. Erythrodermic, recalcitrant psoriasis: Clinical resolution with infliximab. *J Dermatolog Treat* 2003;14:222–225.
2. Heald P. The treatment of cutaneous T-cell lymphoma with a novel retinoid. *Clin Lymphoma*. 2000;1S45–1S49.
3. Alonso-Llamazares J, Dietrich SM, Gibson LE. Bullous pemphigoid presenting as exfoliative erythroderma. *J Am Acad Dermatol*. 1998;39: 827–830.
4. Pruszowski A, Bodemer C, Fraitag S, et al. Neonatal and infantile erythrodermas: A retrospective study of 51 patients. *Arch Dermatol*. 2000;136:875–880.

MISCELLANEOUS

CODES

ICD9-CM
695.89 Other specified erythematous conditions, other

D

DERMATITIS, HEPETIFORMIS

Amit Garg, MD

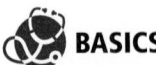

BASICS

DESCRIPTION
- Dermatitis herpetiformis (DH) is a chronic intensely pruritic papulovesicular eruption primarily involving extensor skin surfaces and the scalp. DH is distinguished from other bullous diseases by characteristic histologic and immunologic findings, as well as associated gluten-sensitive enteropathy (1).
- System(s) Affected: Skin
- Synonym(s): Duhring disease

EPIDEMIOLOGY
Incidence
- Occurs most frequently in those of Northern European descent. Rare in personas of Asian or African American descent.
- Mean age of onset is in the 4th decade.
- Predominant sex: Male > Female (1.4:1)

Prevalence
11 per 100,000 in US population. As high as 10 per 100,000 internationally.

RISK FACTORS
- Gluten-sensitive enteropathy
- Family history of dermatitis herpetiformis

Genetics
High incidence of human leukocyte antigen A1, B8, DR3, DQ2

PATHOPHYSIOLOGY
IgA antibodies against epidermal transgluaminase-3 result in recruitment of neutrophils and complement in the dermal papillae

ETIOLOGY
Unknown

ASSOCIATED CONDITIONS
- Gluten-sensitive enteropathy
- Gastric atrophy
- Gastric hypochlorhydria
- Pernicious anemia
- Gastrointestinal lymphoma
- Non-Hodgkin lymphoma
- Hyperthyroidism
- Hypothyroidism
- Thyroid nodules
- Thyroid cancer
- Glomerulopathy
- Autoimmune disorders including systemic lupus erythematosus, dermatomyositis, Sjögren's disease, rheumatoid arthritis, Raynaud phenomenon, diabetes mellitus, myasthenia gravis, Addison disease, vitiligo

History
Waxing and waning, intensely pruritic rash with tiny vesicles. Eruption may worsen with gluten intake. GI symptoms may be absent or may not be reported until prompted.

SIGNS AND SYMPTOMS
- Symmetric, grouped, intensely pruritic, erythematous papules with vesicles
- Elbows, extensor forearms, and scalp are the most common site of involvement. Buttocks, knees, upper back, and posterior neck also frequently are affected.
- Oral lesions are rare. Palms and soles are spared
- Vesicles are often excoriated to erosions at the time of exam.
- Those with associated enteropathy are most often asymptomatic. <10% complain of bloating or diarrhea and have malabsorption with steatorrhea.

TESTS
Lab
- Antibodies to tissue transglutaminase, which shares significant homology to epidermal translutaminase-3.
- IgA endomysial antibodies are most specific for gluten sensitivity and may be found in patients with DH (2).
- CBC, LFTs, glucose-6-phosphate dehydrogenase (G6PD) levels in anticipation of dapsone therapy

Diagnostic Procedures/Surgery
Skin biopsy

Pathological Findings
- H&E staining reveals subepidermal blisters with neutrophilic microabscesses in the dermal papillae
- Direct immunofluorescence on skin, the most reliable diagnostic criterion, reveals a granular pattern of IgA deposition in the papillary dermis (3)

DIFFERENTIAL DIAGNOSIS
- Scabies
- Bullous pemphigoid
- Linear IgA disease
- Transient acantholytic dermatosis
- Papular urticaria
- Erythema multiforme
- Eczema
- Excoriations

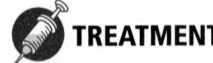

TREATMENT

GENERAL MEASURES
- Control of disease achieved with dietary regulations, medications, or both.
- Outpatient care with a dermatologist.
- Consultation with gastroenterologist and dietician.
- No large, randomized controlled trials evaluate medication or dietary regulations in the treatment of dermatitis herpetiformis

Diet
- Improvement in cutaneous disease and normalization of small bowel mucosa result from strict compliance with a gluten free diet in most patients (4,5)[C]
- Gluten is present in barley, rye, and wheat.
- Rice and oats are well tolerated.

MEDICATION (DRUGS)

First Line

- Dapsone is the only medication FDA approved for use in this disease. Adult doses range from 25–400 mg/d with improvement in symptoms within 24–48 hours. Use minimum effective dose. Average maintenance dose is 1 mg/kg/d. Minor outbreaks on face and scalp are common even with treatment.
- Contraindications: See manufacturer's profile for each drug.
- Precautions
  - Common side effects include nausea, vomiting, headache, dizziness, weakness. A drop in Hgb of 1–2 g is characteristic with dapsone 100 mg/d. G6PD deficiency increases severity of hemolytic stress. Dose-related methemoglobinemia occurs, typically with doses >100 mg/d. Other adverse events include toxic hepatitis, cholestatic jaundice, hypoalbuminemia, sensory and motor neuropathy, psychosis, infectious mononucleosis syndrome with fever and lymphadenopathy, agranulocytosis, aplastic anemia, leukopenia, exfoliative dermatitis, erythema multiforme, erythema nodosum, and urticaria
  - Dapsone is secreted in breast milk and will produce hemolytic anemia in infants.
- Significant possible interactions: See manufacturer's profile for each drug.

ALERT

Pediatric Considerations

- <2 years: Dosing not established.
- >2 years: 0.5–1.0 mg/kg/d PO

Pregnancy Considerations

- Dapsone is Category C. Safety during pregnancy is not established
- Adherence to a strict glutenfree diet 6–12 months before conception should be considered with the hope of eliminating need for dapsone during pregnancy.

Second Line

- Sulfapyridine
- Colchicine, prednisone, tetracycline plus nicotinamide, cyclosporine, prednisone, and topical steroids are third-line medications.

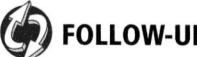 **FOLLOW-UP**

PROGNOSIS

- Lifelong disease. Remission in 10–20%
- Skin disease responds quickly to dapsone.
- Strict adherence to a glutenfree diet improves clinical symptoms and decreases dapsone requirement. Glutenfree diet is the only sustainable method of eliminating cutaneous and gastrointestinal disease. Dapsone does not alter GI mucosal pathology.
- Occasional new lesions (2–3 per week) are to be expected and are not an indication for altering daily dosage.
- Risk of lymphoma may be decreased in those who maintain a glutenfree diet.

PATIENT MONITORING

- Baseline CBC and liver function studies should be obtained.
- G6PD should be quantified prior to initiating dapsone in Asians, African Americans, and those of southern Mediterranean descent.
- CBC should be checked weekly for 1st month, monthly for the next 5 months, and semiannually thereafter.
- Chemistry profile should be checked every 6 months.
- Patient should be made aware of potential hemolytic anemia and the signs associated with methemoglobinemia.

REFERENCES

1. Smith EP, Jone JJ. Dermatitis herpetiformis and linear IgA bullous dermatosis. *Dermatol Clin.* 1993;3:511–526.
2. Buetner EH, Chorzelski TP, Kumar V, et al. Sensitivity and specificity of IgA class antiendomysial antibodies for dermatitis herpetiformis and findings relevant to their pathogenic significance. *J Am Acad Dermatol.* 1986;15:467–473.
3. Zone JJ, Meyer LJ, Petersen MJ. Deposition of granular IgA relative to clinical lesions in dermatitis herpetiformis. *Arch Dermatol.* 1996;132:912–918.
4. Garioch JJ, Lewis HM, Sargent SA, et al. 25 years' experience of a gluten free diet in the treatment of dermatitis herpetiformis. *Br J Dermatol.* 1994;131:541–545.
5. Reunala T, Blomqvist K, Tarpila S, et al. Gluten free diet in dermatitis herpetiformis. Clinical response of skin lesions in 81 patients. *Br J Dermatol.* 1977;97:472–480.

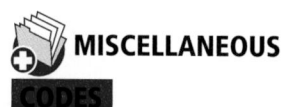 **MISCELLANEOUS**

CODES

ICD9-CM
694.0 Dermatitis herpetiformis

PATIENT TEACHING

- American Academy of Dermatology, 930 N. Meacham Rd., P.O. Box 4014, Schaumburg, IL 60168-4014; (708) 330-0230
- Gluten Intolerance Group of North America, 31214 – 124 Ave SE, Auburn WA 98092. Phone 206.246.6652, Fax 206.246.6531. http://www.gluten.net/diet

 See Corresponding Diagnostic Algorithm

 See Patient Handout on CD

D

DERMATITIS, SEBORRHEIC

Dennis E. Hughes, DO

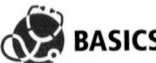 **BASICS**

DESCRIPTION
Chronic, superficial, inflammatory condition affecting hairy regions of the body, especially scalp, eyebrows, and face.

EPIDEMIOLOGY
- Predominant age: Infancy, adolescence, and adulthood (1)
- Predominant sex: Males > Female

Incidence
Common

Prevalence
Common

RISK FACTORS
- Parkinson disease
- AIDS (disease severity correlated with progression of immune deficiency)
- Emotional stress

Genetics
Positive family history common

PATHOPHYSIOLOGY
Chronic inflammatory disease with different characteristics for different age groups; scale is typically present; can occur from infancy through old age.

ETIOLOGY
- Skin surface yeasts (*Pityrosporum ovale*) may be a contributing factor (1,2)
- Genetic and environmental factors
  - Flares are common with stress or illness.
- Parallels increased sebaceous gland activity in infancy and adolescence or as a result of some acnegenic drugs

ASSOCIATED CONDITIONS
- Parkinson disease
- AIDS

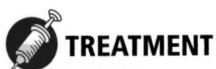 **DIAGNOSIS**

SIGNS AND SYMPTOMS
- Infants
  - Cradle cap: Greasy scaling of scalp, sometimes with associated mild erythema (1)
  - Diaper and/or axillary rash
  - Age at onset typically ~1 month
  - Usually resolves by 8–12 months
- Adults
  - Red, greasy, scaling rash in most locations, consisting of patches and plaques with indistinct margins
  - Red, smooth, glazed appearance in skin folds
  - Minimal pruritus
  - Chronic waxing and waning course
  - Bilateral and symmetric
  - Most commonly located in hairy skin areas with numerous sebaceous glands: Scalp and scalp margins, eyebrows and eyelid margins, nasolabial folds, ears and retroauricular folds, presternal area, and mid-upper back

Physical Exam
Greasy scaley skin of scalp with cervical adenopathy (posterior)

TESTS
Diagnostic Procedures/Surgery
Consider biopsy if
- Usual therapies fail
- Petechiae are noted
- Histiocytosis X suspected
- Fungal cultures in refractory cases or when pustules and alopecia present (1)

Pathological Findings
Nonspecific changes of eczematous dermatitis

DIFFERENTIAL DIAGNOSIS
- Atopic dermatitis
  - Distinction may be difficult in infants
- Psoriasis
  - Usually the knees, elbows, and nails will be involved.
  - Scalp psoriasis will be more sharply demarcated than seborrhea, with crusted, infiltrated plaques rather than mild scaling and erythema.
- Candida
- Tinea cruris or capitis
  - Suspect these when usual medications fail or if there is hair loss.
- Eczema of auricle or otitis externa
- Rosacea
- Discoid lupus erythematosus
- Histiocytosis X
  - May appear as seborrheic-type eruption
- Dandruff
  - Scalp only, noninflammatory

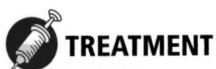 **TREATMENT**

INITIAL STABILIZATION
Outpatient care

GENERAL MEASURES
- Increase frequency of shampooing
- Sunlight in moderate doses may be helpful.
- Cradle cap
  - Frequent shampooing with a mild, nonmedicated shampoo
  - Remove thick scale by applying warm olive or mineral oil and then wash off several hours later with a mild soap and a soft-bristle toothbrush or terry cloth washcloth (3)
- Adults
  - Wash all affected areas with antiseborrheic shampoos. Start with OTC brands (Tegrin, Selsun Blue) and increase to more potent preparations (containing coal tar, sulfur, selenium, or salicylic acid), if no improvement is noted. (3)
  - For dense scalp scaling, 10% Liquor Carbonic Detergens in Nivea Oil may be used at bedtime, covering the head with a shower cap. This should be done nightly for 1–3 weeks.

Diet
No special diet

Activity
Full activity

MEDICATION (DRUGS)

First Line
- Cradle cap
  - The patient may use a coal tar shampoo or ketoconazole (Nizoral) shampoo, if the nonmedicated shampoo is ineffective (3)
- Adults
  - Ketoconazole (Nizoral) cream may be used to clear scales in other areas, followed by an application of steroids to reduce inflammation. Begin with 1% hydrocortisone and advance to more potent (fluorinated) steroid preparations as needed. Avoid continuous use of the more potent steroids to reduce the risk of skin atrophy, hypopigmentation, or systemic absorption (especially in infants and children).
  - 1% ciclopirox shampoo twice weekly (2)[B]
  - Once controlled, washing with zinc soaps or selenium lotion with periodic use of low potentcy steroid cream will help maintain remission (3)
  - Benyoyl peroide washes are helpful in controlling seborrhea of the trunk (3)
- Precautions: Fluorinated corticosteroids and higher concentrations of hydrocortisone (e.g., 2.5%) may cause atrophy or striae if used on the face or on skin folds.

Second Line
- Severe seborrhea nonresponsive to topical therapy in adults
- Isotretinoin: 0.1–0.3 mg/kg/d
- Use with caution

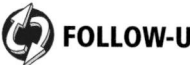 **FOLLOW-UP**

PROGNOSIS
- In infants, seborrheic dermatitis usually remits after 6–8 months.
- In adults, seborrheic dermatitis is usually chronic and unpredictable, with exacerbations and remissions. Disease is usually easily controlled with shampoos and topical steroids.

COMPLICATIONS
- Skin atrophy or striae possible from fluorinated corticosteroids, especially if used on the face
- Glaucoma can result from use of fluorinated steroids around the eyes.
- Photosensitivity occasionally caused by tars
- Herpes keratitis is a rare complication of herpes simplex
  - Instruct patient to stop eyelid steroids if herpes simplex develops

PATIENT MONITORING
Every 2–12 weeks as necessary, depending on disease severity and degree of patient sophistication

REFERENCES

1. Williams JV, et al. Prevalence of scalp scaling in prepubertal children. *Pediatrics*. 2005;115:1–6.
2. Shuster S, et al. Treatment and prophylaxis of seborrheic dermatitis of the scalp with antipityrospral 1% ciclopirox shampoo. *Arch Derm*. 2005;141:47–52.
3. Johnson BA, Nunley JR. Treatment of seborrheic dermatitis. *Am Fam Physician*. 2000; 61:2703–2710, 2713–2714.

 MISCELLANEOUS

See also: Dermatitis, atopic; Tinea capitis; Tinea cruris

CODES

ICD9-CM
690.10 Seborrheic dermatitis, unspecified

PATIENT TEACHING
- Goal of treatment is control, rather than cure, of disease
- Seborrheic dermatitis does not cause hair loss

D

DERMATITIS, STASIS

Joseph A. Florence, MD

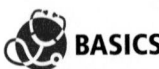 **BASICS**

DESCRIPTION
Chronic, erythema, scaling, and noninflammatory edema of the lower extremities accompanied by cycle of scratching, excoriations, weeping, crusting, and inflammation in patients with chronic venous insufficiency, due to impaired circulation and other factors (nutritional edema)
- Clinical skin manifestation of chronic venous insufficiency usually appearing late in the disease (1)
- System(s) Affected: Skin/Exocrine
- Synonym(s): Gravitational eczema; Varicose eczema; Venous dermatitis

GENERAL PREVENTION
- Use compression stockings to avoid recurrence of edema.
- Topical lubricants b.i.d. to prevent fissuring and itching

EPIDEMIOLOGY
- Predominant age: Adult, geriatric
- Predominant sex: Female > Male

Incidence
In the US: Common in patients >50 years of age (6–7% of patients >50 years old)

Geriatric Considerations
Common in this age group
- It is estimated to affect 15–20 million patients >50 years in the US

RISK FACTORS
- Atopy
- Superimposition of itch-scratch cycle
- Trauma
- Previous deep vein thrombosis (DVT)
- Previous pregnancy
- Prolonged medical illness
- Obesity
- Secondary infection
- Low-protein diet
- Old age
- Deposition of fibrin around capillaries
- Microvascular abnormalities
- Ischemia
- Genetic propensity
- Edema
- Wearing of tight garments that constrict the thigh
- Vein stripping
- Vein harvesting in patients requiring coronary artery bypass grafting
- Previous cellulitis

Genetics
Familial link probable

ETIOLOGY
- Incompetence of perforating veins causing blood to backflow to the superficial venous system leading to venous hypertension and cutaneous inflammation
- Continuous presence of edema in ankles, usually present because of venous valve incompetency (varicose veins)
- Weakness of venous walls in lower extremities
- Trauma to edematous, eczematized skin
- Itch may be caused by inflammatory mediators (from mast cells, monocytes, macrophages, or neutrophils) liberated in the microcirculation and endothelium (1)[A]

ASSOCIATED CONDITIONS
- Varicose veins
- Other eczematous disease

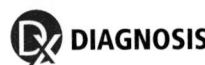 **DIAGNOSIS**

History
- Erythema, scaling, and edema of the lower extremities
- Puritis
- Excoriations
- Weeping, crusting, and inflammation of the skin
- Noninflammatory edema precedes the skin eruption and ulceration
- Edema initially develops around the ankle
- Itching, pain, and burning may precede skin signs, which are aggravate during evening hours (2)[A]
- Insidious onset
- Usually bilateral
- Patients may describe their legs as aching or heavy.

Physical Exam
- Evaluation of the lower extremities reveals
  - Scaly, eczematous patches
  - Violaceous (sometimes brown), erythematous-colored lesions due to deoxygenation of venous blood (postinflammatory hyperpigmentation and hemosiderin deposition within the cutaneous tissue)
- Distribution: Medial aspect of ankle with frequent extension onto the foot and lower leg
- Brawny induration
- Stasis ulcers (frequently accompany stasis dermatitis) secondary to cuts, bruises, and excoriations to the weakened skin around the ankle
- Mild puritis, pain (if ulcer present)
- Varicosities are often associated with ulcers
- Clinical inspection reveals erythematous color with increased pigmentation, swelling, and warmth.
- Skin changes are more common in the lower 3rd of the extremity and medially

TESTS
Lab
Culture stasis ulcers if bacterial infection is suspected

Imaging
Consider Venous Doppler studies if DVT is suspected.

Diagnostic Procedures/Surgery
Rule out arterial insufficiency.

Pathological Findings
Chronic inflammation, characterized histologically by proliferation of small blood vessels in the papillary dermis

DIFFERENTIAL DIAGNOSIS
- Other eczematous diseases, such as
  - Atopic dermatitis
  - Uremic dermatitis
  - Contact dermatitis (due to topical agents used to self-treat)
  - Neurodermatitis
  - Arterial insufficiency
  - Sickle cell disease causing skin ulceration
  - Cellulitis
- Tinea dermatophyte infection
- Pretibial myxedema
- Nummular eczema
- Lichen simplex chronicus
- Xerosis
- Asteatotic eczema

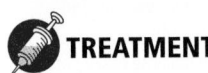 **TREATMENT**

GENERAL MEASURES
- Primary role of treatment is to reverse effects of venous hypertension
- Appropriate health care
  - Outpatient
  - Inpatient for vein stripping, sclerotherapy, or skin grafts
  - Venous ulcer treatment includes autolytic, biologic, chemical, mechanical, and surgical
    ○ Autolytic: Hydrogels, alginates, hydrocolloids, foams, and films
    ○ Biologic: Topical application of granulocyte macrophage colony-stimulating factor promotes healing of ulcers
    ○ Chemical: Enzyme débriding agents
    ○ Mechanical: Wet to dry dressings, hydrotherapy, and irrigation
    ○ Surgical modifying cause of venous hypertension, treat ulcer by graft
- Reduce edema
  - Leg elevation: Heels higher than knees, knees higher than hips
  - Compression therapy: Elastic bandage wraps: Ace bandages or Unna paste boot (zinc gelatin) if lesions are dry or compression stockings (Jobst or nonfitted type)
  - Pneumatic compression devices
  - Diuretic therapy
- Treat infection
  - Débride the ulcer base of necrotic tissue
  - Improvement of lipodermatosclerosis

Diet
- No special diet
- Lose weight, if overweight

Activity
- Avoid standing still
- Stay active and exercise regularly
- Elevate foot of bed unless contraindicated

MEDICATION (DRUGS)

First Line

- Use of antibiotics topically or systemically is controversial, as stasis ulcer may not be infected. Antibiotics are indicated if bacterial infection is present or may be used empirically if bacterial infection is suspected.
- If secondary infection, treat with oral antibiotics for Staphylococcus or Streptococcus organisms (e.g., dicloxacillin 250 mg q.i.d., cephalexin 250 mg q.i.d. or 500 mg b.i.d., or levofloxacin 250 mg q.i.d.)
- *Staphylococcus aureus* or β-hemolytic Streptococcus: Treat with oral antibiotics.
- Gram-negative colonization: Treat with topical antimicrobial agents (e.g., benzoyl peroxide, acetic acid, silver nitrate, or Hibiclens) or broad-spectrum topical antibiotics (e.g., neomycin or bacitracin-polymyxin B [Polysporin])
- 5% Aluminum acetate (Burow's solution) wet dressings and cooling pastes
- Topical triamcinolone 0.1% (Kenalog, Aristocort) cream/ointment t.i.d. or topical betamethasone
- Betamethasone valerate (Valisone) 0.1% cream/ointment/solution t.i.d. (3)[A]
- Topical antipruritic: Pramoxine, camphor, menthol, and doxepin
- Systemic steroids for severe cases
- Calcium dobesilate has been shown to be an effective adjuvant therapy (4)[A]
- Precautions
  – Refer to the manufacturer's literature.

Second Line

- Consider antibiotics on basis of culture results of exudate from ulcer craters
- Lubricants when dermatitis is quiescent
- Chronic stasis dermatitis can be treated with topical emollients (e.g., white petroleum, lanolin, Eucerin).
- Antipruritic medications (e.g., diphenhydramine, cetirizine hydrochloride, desloratadine)

SURGERY

Sclerotherapy and surgery may be required.

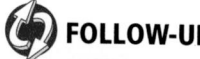 ## FOLLOW-UP

PROGNOSIS

- Chronic course with intermittent exacerbations and remissions
- The healing process for ulceration is often prolonged and may take months

COMPLICATIONS

- Sensations of itching, pain, and burning have negative impact on the quality of life (2)[A]
- Secondary bacterial infection
- DVT
- Bleeding at dermatitis sites
- Squamous cell carcinoma in edges of long-standing stasis ulcers
- Scarring, which in turn leads to further compromise to blood flow and increased likelihood of minor trauma

PATIENT MONITORING

If Unna bootis used: Cut off and reapply boot once a week (restricts edema and prevents scratching).

REFERENCES

1. Antignani PL. Classification of chronic venous insufficiency: A review. *Angiology*. 2001;52(Suppl): S17–S26.
2. Duque MI, Yosipovitch G, et al. Itch, pain, and burning sensation are common symptoms in mild to moderate chronic venous insufficiency with an impact on quality of life. *J Am Acad Dermatol*. 2005;53(3):504–508.
3. Weiss SCA. Randomized controlled clinical trial assessing the effect of betamethasone valerate 0.12% foam on the short term treatment of stasis dermatitis. *J Drugs Dermatol*. 2005;4(3):339–345.
4. Kaur C, Sarkar R, et al. An open trial of calcium dobesilate in patients with venous ulcers and stasis dermatitis. *Int J Dermatol*. 2003;42:147–152.

ADDITIONAL READING

- Theodosat A. Skin diseases of the lower extremities in the elderly. *Dermatol Clin*. 2004;22(1):13–21.
- Valencia IC, Falabella A, Kirsner RS, Eaglstein WH. Chronic venous insufficiency and venous leg ulceration. *J Amer Acad Dermatol*. 2001;44(3): 401–421.

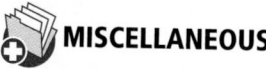 ## MISCELLANEOUS

See also: Varicose veins

CODES

ICD9-CM

- 454.1 Varicose veins of lower extremities with inflammation
- 459.81 Venous (peripheral) insufficiency, unspecified

PATIENT TEACHING

- Stress staying active to keep circulation and leg muscles in good condition. Walking is ideal.
- Keep legs elevated while sitting or lying.
- Don't wear girdles, garters, or pantyhose with tight elastic tops.
- Don't scratch.
- Elevate foot of bed with 2- to 4-inch blocks.

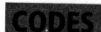

D

DIABETES INSIPIDUS

Keith Medeiros, MD

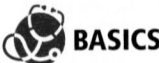 **BASICS**

DESCRIPTION
- Defective regulation of water balance secondary to decreased pituitary secretion of (central DI), or failure of response to (nephrogenic DI), vasopressin
- System(s) Affected: Endocrine/Metabolic

GENERAL PREVENTION
- Avoid marked increase in water loss.
- Take fluids as dictated by thirst with no water restriction.

EPIDEMIOLOGY
Incidence
18.3% following transsphenoidal microsurgery (1)

Prevalence
- Vasopressin deficiency may occur at any age, including infancy and childhood.
- Nephrogenic diabetes insipidus (DI) is usually manifest in infancy.
- Nephrogenic DI is encountered in males with rare exception, reflecting its X-linked recessive mode of inheritance.

RISK FACTORS
- Intracranial neoplasm
- Following surgery
- Patients using lithium

Genetics
- Central DI
  - Familial cases of vasopressin deficiency have been reported (commonly autosomal dominant; >20 mutations have been identified), but the disease is usually isolated, and often secondary to other disorders.
- Nephrogenic DI
  - Most common is an X-linked defect in the V2 receptor that binds ADH.
  - Autosomal dominant or recessive defects in the aquaporin-2 gene that encodes an ADH responsive water channel.

PATHOPHYSIOLOGY
- Central DI
  - Inadequate secretion of vasopressin may be due to loss of or malfunction of the neurosecretory neurons that make up the neurohypophysis (posterior pituitary) and the pituitary stalk.
- Nephrogenic DI
  - Insensitivity to vasopressin
  - A disorder of renal tubular function resulting in inability to respond to vasopressin in absorption of water

ETIOLOGY
- Central DI
  - Inadequate secretion of vasopressin due to pathologic condition, which may be idiopathic or familial
    - Trauma
    - Neurosurgery
    - Tumors (craniopharyngioma, lymphoma, metastasis)
    - Idiopathic
    - Infections (meningitis, encephalitis)
    - Granulomas (sarcoid, histiocytosis)
    - Vascular disorders

- Nephrogenic DI (insensitivity to vasopressin):
  - Genetic defect in resorption of water in renal tubule (collecting ducts)
  - Drugs (2)[A]
    - Lithium, demeclocycline, dexamethasone, dopamine, ifosfamide, ofloxacin, amphotericin B, orlistat
  - Hypercalcemia
  - Hypokalemia

ASSOCIATED CONDITIONS
- Potassium depletion
- Chronic hypercalcemia
- Tumors
- Infection
  - Encephalitis
  - Tuberculosis
  - Syphilis
- Xanthomatosis
- Pyelonephritis
- Renal amyloidosis
- Sjögren syndrome
- Sickle cell anemia
- Wolfram syndrome (DIDMOAD: DI, diabetes mellitus, optic atrophy, and deafness)

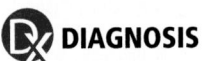 **DIAGNOSIS**

SIGNS AND SYMPTOMS
- Thirst/polydipsia (with a particular preference for cold or iced drinks)
- Polyuria
- Nocturia
- Dehydration
- Headache
- Visual disturbance

History
- Rate of onset of polydipsia is more rapid in central DI versus nephrogenic
- Family history of polyuria

TESTS
- Water restriction test to evaluate the ability to concentrate urine
  - Water is withheld and urine and plasma osmolality are measured at hourly intervals.
  - A rise in urine osmolality indicates an intact ADH response.
  - A rise in plasma osmolality or stable urine osmolality indicates poor ADH response.
  - Perform the test during the day, not overnight to avoid serious volume depletion or hypernatremia.
  - If the results support the diagnosis, desmopressin should be administered to test renal concentrating ability.
- Urine/plasma osmolal ratio and plasma vasopressin concentrations
  - Results may be difficult to interpret: Low ratios may be found in patients with primary polydipsia

Lab
- Urine electrolyte levels
  - Hypernatremia (usually <150 mEq/L because of increased thirst)
- Urine osmolality
  - Inability to concentrate urine (measure by osmolality, rather than specific gravity)
  - Hypokalemia and hypercalcemia alter ability to concentrate urine
- Urinary glucose
  - Rule out diabetes mellitus
- Plasma vasopressin or urinary vasopressin following osmotic stimulus, such as fluid restriction or administration of hypertonic saline
- Drugs that may alter lab results: Lithium, demeclocycline, and methoxyflurane may produce vasopressin insensitivity.
- Disorders that may alter lab results: Hypokalemia and hypercalcemia alter ability to concentrate urine

Imaging
If the diagnosis of DI is made, appropriate studies for cause, including imaging of the brain must be performed.

Diagnostic Procedures/Surgery
Fluid deprivation to concentrate urine

Pathological Findings
Degeneration and death of neurosecretory neurons in the neurohypophysis

DIFFERENTIAL DIAGNOSIS
- Diabetes mellitus and other causes of polydipsia and polyuria
- Increased solute load for excretion as occurs with high salt intake
- Psychogenic polydipsia (ultimately impairs vasopressin secretion)

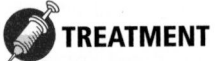 **TREATMENT**

GENERAL MEASURES
- Control fluid balance and prevent dehydration
- Check weight daily.
- Provide good skin and mouth care.
- Nephrogenic DI
  - Correct hypercalcemia and hypokalemia and discontinue causative medications (3)[A].

Diet
- Normal, with free access to fluids
- Young infants with nephrogenic DI may benefit from low-solute formula.
- A low-sodium, low-protein diet may reduce urine output in nephrogenic DI

Activity
Not restricted

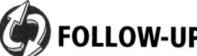 **MEDICATION (DRUGS)**

First Line
- Central (vasopressin deficient) DI
  - Desmopressin (DDAVP) (a derivative of vasopressin)
    - Intranasally 1– 2 times a day in dosage necessary to control polyuria or polydipsia (usually 5–20 μg)
    - Orally starting at 100 μg 2–4 times a day on an empty stomach titrated to 200–600 μg 2–4 times a day (4)[B]
- Nephrogenic DI
  - Hydrochlorothiazide 25 mg once or b.i.d.
  - Amiloride can be added to HCTZ for an additive effect.
- Contraindications: Use desmopressin with caution in the immediate postoperative period for intracranial lesions because of possible cerebral edema.
- Precautions: An overdose of desmopressin may produce water intoxication and hyponatremia in patients with excessive water intake.

Second Line
- Central DI
  - Chlorpropamide (Diabinese): 125–250 mg once or b.i.d. enhances renal response to ADH.
  - Clofibrate (Atromid-S): 500 mg q6h may increase ADH release.
  - Hydrochlorothiazide: 25 mg once or b.i.d.
- Precautions: Chlorpropamide is an oral hypoglycemic agent that can cause hypoglycemia in elevated doses.

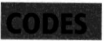 **FOLLOW-UP**

- Initial diagnosis and management may require hospitalization.
- Continuing care is provided on an outpatient basis with self-medication.

PROGNOSIS
- Most reversible cases of nephrogenic DI are caused by medications, and patient symptoms improve with removal of the offending agent (2)[A]
  - Lithium may cause irreversible DI (2)[A]
- Generally good prognosis depending on underlying disorder

COMPLICATIONS
- Dilatation of the urinary tract has been observed (probably secondary to large volume of urine).
- Complications of the primary disease (tumor histiocytosis, etc.) should be anticipated.
- In congenital nephrogenic DI, an associated retardation of mental development may occur in some patients (cause undetermined).
- Without treatment, dehydration can lead to confusion, stupor, and coma.
- Subnormal growth rate

PATIENT MONITORING
- Regular follow-up at 2–3-week intervals initially and 3–4 months later
- Adjust treatment on the basis of urine and electrolyte concentrations and the patient's symptoms.

REFERENCES
1. Nemergut EC, Zuo Z, Jane JA Jr, Laws ER Jr. Predictors of diabetes insipidus after transsphenoidal surgery: a review of 881 patients. *J Neurosurg* 2005 Sep;103(3):448–454.
2. Garofeanu CG, Weir M, Rosas-Arellano MP, et al. Causes of reversible nephrogenic diabetes insipidus: a systematic review. *Am J Kidney Dis* 2005 Apr;45(4):626–637. Review.
3. Makaryus AN, McFarlane SI. Diabetes insipidus: diagnosis and treatment of a complex disease. *Cleve Clin J Med* 2006 Jan;73(1):65–71.
4. Fukuda I, Hizuka N, Takano K. Oral DDAVP is a good alternative therapy for patients with central diabetes insipidus: experience of five-year treatment. *Endocr J* 2003 Aug;50(4):437–443.

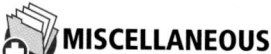 **MISCELLANEOUS**

See also: Sjögren syndrome

CODES

ICD9-CM
253.5 Diabetes insipidus

PATIENT TEACHING
- Administration and dosage of intranasal desmopressin
- Importance of having access to fluids as thirst dictates
- Wear a medical identification neck tag or bracelet

 See Corresponding Diagnostic Algorithm

 See Patient Handout on CD

D

DIABETES MELLITUS, TYPE 2

Ramothea L. Webster, PhD

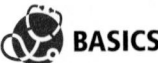 **BASICS**

DESCRIPTION
- Nonketotic hyperglycemia, insulin resistance, and relative impairment in insulin secretion; accounts for 80% of diabetic cases
- System(s) Affected: Endocrine/metabolic; Nervous; Renal/urologic; Cardiovascular

Geriatric Considerations
Common in the elderly and is a significant contributing factor to blindness, renal failure, and lower limb amputations.

Pediatric Considerations
Incidence in children is increasing dramatically, possibly related to increases in childhood obesity.

Pregnancy Considerations
- Intensive management by an endocrinologist in conjunction with a perinatologist may be helpful in decreasing the risk of maternal complications and fetal wasting.
- C-section or vaginal delivery after a C-section are not contraindicated.

GENERAL PREVENTION
- Avoidance of weight gain and obesity
- Maintain regular physical activity

EPIDEMIOLOGY
Incidence
300/100,000; Males: 230/100,000, Females: 340/100,000

Prevalence
- 5,000/100,000; within race: 7.2% whites, 9% Hispanics, 11.2% blacks, and 35% Pima Indians
- Typically occurs after age 40, however, if diagnosed before age 40, average reduction in life-years is 12 years (M) and 19 years (F).
- Lifetime risk of developing diabetes for individuals born in 2000 is 33% (Males) and 39% (Females).

RISK FACTORS
- Family history: 1st-degree relative
- Gestational diabetes (GDM)
- Obesity: Induces resistance to insulin-mediated peripheral glucose uptake
- Ethnicity: African American, Latino, Native American, Asian American, and Pacific Islander
- BP >140/90 mm Hg
- HDL <35 mg/dL (0.9 mmol/L) and/or triglycerides >250 mg/dL (2.82 mmol/L)
- Impaired fasting glucose (IFG) or impaired glucose tolerance (IGT)
- Polycystic ovary syndrome (PCOS)
- Acanthosis nigricans (AN)
- Vascular disease

Genetics
- Strong polygenic familial susceptibility
- Concordance is nearly complete in identical twins.
- Hispanic, Polynesian, Native American, or African American ancestry

PATHOPHYSIOLOGY
Progressive defects in insulin secretion and peripheral insulin action ("insulin resistance")

ETIOLOGY
- Genetic factors
- Obesity
- Drug or chemical Induced (e.g., medications used for psychosis, HIV, or transplant recipients)

ASSOCIATED CONDITIONS
- Hypertension (HTN)
- Hyperlipidemia (HLD)
- Impotence
- Infertility
- Syndrome X/ metabolic syndrome
- Renal insufficiency/failure
- Cardiovascular disease
- Retinopathy
- Stroke
- Pancreatic cancer

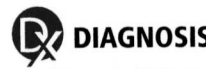 **DIAGNOSIS**

SIGNS AND SYMPTOMS
- Related to hyperglycemia and complications, including nephropathy, neuropathy, and retinopathy
- Polyuria, polydipsia, polyphagia, weight loss, weakness, fatigue, and frequent infections

TESTS
- Glucose tolerance test usually not necessary, except when diagnosing gestational diabetes
- Hemoglobin A1c not recommended for diagnosis, but helpful in management

Lab
- Criteria for diagnosis
  - Symptoms of diabetes (polyuria, polydipsia, weight loss) plus casual (random) plasma glucose ≥200 mg/dL (11.1 mmol/L) or
  - Fasting plasma glucose (FPG) ≥126 mg/dL (7.0 mmol/L) on two occasions or
  - 2-hour plasma glucose ≥200 mg/dL (11.1 mmol/L) during oral glucose tolerance test (OGTT) with 75 g glucose load (1)[A]
- Drugs that may alter lab results: Newer, atypical antipsychotics (Zyprexa, Clozaril, etc.), pentamidine, nicotinic acid, glucocorticoids, thyroid hormone, diazoxide, β-adrenergic agonists, thiazides, Dilantin, α-interferon, some fluoroquinolones, and some 2nd-generation (atypical) antipsychotics

DIFFERENTIAL DIAGNOSIS
- Type 1 diabetes mellitus
- Gestational diabetes mellitus
- Other specific types of diabetes mellitus
  - Genetic defects of β-cell function
  - Genetic defects in insulin action
  - Diseases of exocrine pancreas
  - Endocrinopathies
  - Drug or chemical induced
  - Infections
  - Immune mediated
  - Genetic syndromes sometimes associated with diabetes
  - Hemochromatosis

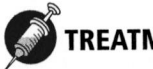 **TREATMENT**

GENERAL MEASURES
- Home monitoring of blood glucose
- Hemoglobin A1c every 3–6 months
- Regular examination for complications
- Foot examination every visit to check for neuropathy, arterial insufficiency, and foot ulcers
- Nephropathy: Urine analysis to check microalbumin yearly
- Retinopathy: Yearly eye exams
- NCEP Adult Treatment Panel III recommends an LDL-cholesterol goal of below 100 mg/dL by using a lipid-lowering agent, if necessary.
- Strict control of hypertension (goal blood pressure below 130/80 mm Hg) reduces the risk of complications and death related to diabetes.
- Low-dose aspirin is recommended for all adults with diabetes, unless there is a contraindication.
- ACE (ARB if ACE intolerant) use as a first-line HTN drug (1)[A]; if contraindicated consider a CCB.

Diet
American Diabetes Association (ADA) diet
- Mild caloric restriction to achieve mild to moderate weight loss (5–10 kg).
- Food choices are similar to Dietary Guidelines for Americans and the Food Guide Pyramid
  - Calories from protein: 10–20%
  - <10% of calories each from saturated and polyunsaturated fat
  - Remainder of calories from monounsaturated fat and carbohydrates, depending on individual patient factors
  - Sugar is not specifically prohibited

Activity
Regular aerobic exercise can improve glucose tolerance and decrease medication requirements. At least 30 minutes per day of "moderate exercise" is appropriate (e.g., brisk walking).

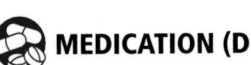 **MEDICATION (DRUGS)**

First Line
- General
- Sulfonylureas was used as initial treatment, but data support metformin as the preferred first medication for type II DM patients due to its effects on weight loss and insulin resistance
- If 1 drug does not produce adequate control, add another drug from a different class
- If 2 agents are not adequate, insulin might be the next best addition or another oral agent
- If HbA1c >8%, then start patient with 2 oral agents simultaneously because each agent has the potential to decrease the HbA1c by 1.5–2% points, with a goal of <7% according to the ACE and <6.5% according to the AACE
- The following classes of agents may be used alone or in combination.
  - Biguanides
    ○ Metformin (Glucophage): 500–850 mg b.i.d.–t.i.d. or long-acting per day
    ○ Avoid situations that increase risk for lactic acidosis: renal insufficiency, radiocontrast agents, surgery, or acute illnesses such as liver disease, cardiogenic shock, pancreatitis, or hypoxia

- Caution with congestive heart failure, alcohol abuse, elderly patients, or with tetracycline
  - Sulfonylureas
    - Glimepiride (Amaryl): 1–8 mg/d
    - Glipizide (Glucotrol): 2.5–mg/d in 1–2 doses; 1st dose, 20 mg q a.m.
    - Glipizide extended-release: 5–20 mg/d
    - Glyburide (DiaBeta, Micronase): 1.25–20 mg/d in 1 or 2 doses; 1st dose 10 mg every a.m.
    - Note: Sulfonylureas may be taken w/meals, except glipizide: 30 minutes before meals.
    - Caution with renal, liver, or thyroid disease, sulfa allergy, Cr CL <50, pregnancy near term
  - Thiazolidinediones
    - Pioglitazone (Actos): 15–45 mg/d
    - Rosiglitazone (Avandia): 2–4 mg b.i.d.
    - Monitor serum transaminase every 2 months for the 1st year, contraindicated for liver disease patients
  - α-Glucosidase inhibitors
    - Acarbose (Precose): 25–100 mg t.i.d.
    - Miglitol (Glyset): 25–100 mg t.i.d.
    - Taken at beginning of meals to decrease postprandial glucose peaks
    - Poor patient compliance due to GI symptoms; last drug of choice
    - Avoid use in renal insufficiency, inflammatory bowel disease, colonic ulceration, or partial bowel obstruction.
  - Insulin: rapid (Aspart, Lispro, Glulisine), short (Regular Insulin), intermediate (NPH), and long/peakless (Glargine)
    - Can be given up to t.i.d
    - May be used in combo with oral agents, or with an insulin of a different half-life.
    - Most often required in late stages of type II DM when oral agents fail to control glucose levels (1,2)[A].
  - Pramlintide (Symlin): 60–120 mcg qAC (3)[C]
    - Synthetic analog of human neuroendocrine hormone amylin
    - Produced in the pancreas to assist in postprandial glucose control.
    - Works by modulating gastric emptying, preventing increase in serum glucagon, and increasing the feeling of satiety.
    - Preprandial, short-acting, or rapid-acting insulins should be reduced by 50% at initiation of drug.
    - Drug interactions: Anticholinergic drugs or agents that slow intestinal absorption of nutrients
    - Contraindicated in patients with gastroparesis
  - Exenatide (Byetta): 5–10 mcg b.i.d. 60 minutes before morning and evening meal (3)[C]
  - Stimulates the production of insulin in response to high blood glucose after meals, and slows the rate of gastric emptying
  - Synthetic version of exendin, a substance found in gila monster saliva
  - Sulfonylureas should be empirically decreased to reduce the chance of hypoglycemia
  - Advised to take other oral medications 1 hour before injecting Exenatide
- Combination agents
  - Fixed-dose combinations of metformin with glipizide, glyburide, or rosiglitazone
  - Premixed doses of insulin: Standard (NPH/Regular insulin) or analog (intermediate/rapid analog).
- Contraindications to oral agents: Type I (insulin dependent) diabetes mellitus, ketotic patients, pregnancy, history of specific drug allergy; use caution in liver or renal disease, acute infection or stress
- Precautions: Warn patients of signs of hypo- and hyperglycemia
- Significant possible interactions
  - Drugs that may potentiate sulfonylureas Salicylates, clofibrate, warfarin (Coumadin), chloramphenicol, ethanol, and angiotensin-converting inhibitors
  - Thiazides can cause impaired glucose tolerance.
  - Gatifloxacin can cause either severe hypoglycemia or hyperglycemia.
  - Thiazolidinedione pioglitazone may decrease effectiveness of oral contraceptives.
  - Drug binders, such as cholestyramine resin, should be taken at least 2 hours apart from α-glucosidase inhibitors.

Second Line
- Meglitinides
  - Repaglinide (Prandin): 0.5–4 mg before meals t.i.d.; may be useful in patients with sulfa allergy or renal impairment.
  - Nateglinide (Starlix): 60–120 mg before meals t.i.d. (1, 2)[A]
- Older, 1st-generation sulfonylureas
  - Chlorpropamide (Diabinese): 100–500 mg/d
  - Tolazamide (Tolinase): 100–1000 mg/d in 1–2 doses
  - Tolbutamide (Orinase): 500–3000 mg/d in 2–3 doses

 ## FOLLOW-UP

PROGNOSIS
- Maintenance of normal blood sugar levels may delay or prevent complications of diabetes
- In susceptible individuals, complications begin to appear 10–15 years after onset, but can be present at time of diagnosis since disease may go undetected for years

COMPLICATIONS
- Appear to be due to effects of DM on macro- and microvascular arterial cell walls (1)[A]
- Peripheral neuropathy
- Proliferative retinopathy
- Nephropathy and chronic renal failure
- Atherosclerotic cardiovascular and peripheral vascular disease
- Hyperosmolar coma
- Gangrene of extremities
- Blindness
- Glaucoma
- Cataracts
- Skin ulceration
- Charcot joints

PATIENT MONITORING
- Frequency of follow-up depends on compliance and degree of metabolic control; every 2–4 months is typical
- Home blood glucose monitoring *may* help slow progression of microvascular disease in highly motivated patients
- Hemoglobin A1c twice a year for glycemic controlled patients, and quarterly for uncontrolled or change in therapy patients
- Each patient should have a complete yearly physical exam (1)[A].

REFERENCES
1. Standards of Medical Care in Diabetes – 2006. *Diabetes Care* 2006;29(Supp 1):S4–42.
2. DeWitt DE, Hirsch IB. Outpatient insulin therapy in type 1 and type 2 diabetes mellitus: scientific review. *JAMA* 2003;289(17):2254–2264.
3. New Drugs: Symlin and Byetta. *Pharmacist's Letter/Prescriber's Letter* 2005;21(6):210–603.
4. Diagnosis and classification of diabetes mellitus. *Diabetes Care* 2006;29(Supp 1):S43–48.

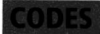 ## MISCELLANEOUS

- Hyperglycemia that is not sufficient to meet diagnostic criteria for DM is called either impaired fasting glucose (IFG) or impaired glucose tolerance (IGT); both are states that increase patient's risk for DM or CVD.
- See also: Diabetes Mellitus, Type 1; Diabetic Ketoacidosis (DKA); Hypertension, Essential

CODES

ICD9-CM
- 250.00 Diabetes mellitus without mention of complication, type 2 or unspecified type, not stated as uncontrolled
- 250.02 Diabetes mellitus without mention of complication, type 2 or unspecified type, uncontrolled

PATIENT TEACHING
- Support groups/classes certified by the ADA
- Patient education materials are available from the American Diabetes Association, 430 North Michigan Ave., Chicago, IL 60611

 See Corresponding Diagnostic Algorithm

 See Patient Handout on CD

DIABETES MELLITUS, TYPE 1

Robert M. Schultz, MD

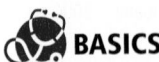 **BASICS**

DESCRIPTION

Chronic disease caused by pancreatic insufficiency (deficiency) of insulin production

- Results in hyperglycemia and end-organ complications (e.g., accelerated atherosclerosis, neuropathy, nephropathy, and retinopathy)
- Features include the following
  - Patients insulinopenic and require insulin
  - Ketosis
  - Usually rapid onset
  - Nutritional status: Normal or thin physique
  - Disease lability
  - Response to oral drugs uncommon
  - Seasonal: January–April are peak onset periods (children <6 years have greater degree of seasonal risk)
- System(s) Affected: Endocrine/Metabolic

Pregnancy Considerations
- Consultation with a perinatalogist may be helpful in the management of the pregnancy.
- During embryogenesis, hyperglycemia increases the incidence of congenital malformations. Tight control of blood sugar before conception is important.
- A safe pregnancy is possible with vaginal delivery of a term baby. Close monitoring of blood sugar during labor is important.

EPIDEMIOLOGY
- Mean age of onset 8–12 years, peaking in adolescence
- Onset is ~1.5 years earlier in girls than boys.
- Rapid decline in incidence after adolescence

Incidence
- 15/100,000 per year
- Racial predilection for whites
- African Americans have lowest overall incidence

Pediatric Considerations
- More prevalent in children
- Over the past 10 years, a larger percentage of very young children (<5 years) present with diabetes.

RISK FACTORS
- Certain human leukocyte antigen (HLA) types
- Presence of a specific 64,000 mw protein that may be responsible for antibody formation
- Family history
- Dietary factors: Breast-feeding may provide a degree of protection against the disease, whereas diets high in dairy products are associated with an increased risk of the disease.
  - Insulin-dependent or non–insulin-dependent diabetes in any 1st-degree relatives
  - Slightly greater risk of a child if the father has type 1 diabetes

Genetics
- Mode of genetic expression not clear
- Genes located on major histocompatibility complex on chromosome 6
- HLA DR3 and DR4 are individually associated with an increased risk; if a person is carrying both susceptibility genes, the relative risk is increased.
- HLA B_8 and B_{15} associated with increased risk

PATHOPHYSIOLOGY
- Alteration in immunologic integrity, placing the beta cell at special risk for inflammatory damage
- The mechanism of damage is autoimmune.

ETIOLOGY
- Inherited defect
- Environmental factors
  - Viruses (such as mumps, Coxsackie, cytomegalovirus, and hepatitis viruses)
  - Diet high in nitrosamines
  - Environmental toxins
  - Emotional and physical stress

ASSOCIATED CONDITIONS
- Autoimmune diseases, such as hypothyroidism and Addison Disease
  - Screening regularly for hypothyroidism is particularly important in females.
- Diabetes mellitus can also be seen as part of multiple endocrine adenomatosis.

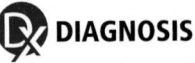 **DIAGNOSIS**

SIGNS AND SYMPTOMS
- Polyuria and polydipsia
- Polyphagia is classic, but not common
- Anorexia is commonly observed.
- Weight loss 10–30%
  - Often almost devoid of body fat at diagnosis
- Increased fatigue
- Decreased energy levels and lethargy
- Muscle cramps
- Irritability and emotional lability
- Vision changes, such as blurriness
- Altered school and work performance
- Headaches
- Anxiety attacks
- Abdominal discomfort and pain
- Nausea, diarrhea, or constipation

TESTS

Lab
- World Health Organization: Fasting glucose >126 mg/dL or random of >200 mg/dL
- Oral glucose tolerance test
  - If diagnosis is questionable
- IV glucose test
  - Early detection of subclinical diabetes
- Consider HLA-typing
- Blood glucose
- Electrolytes
- Venous pH
- Urinalysis
  - Evaluate glucose and ketones
- CBC (WBC may be elevated)
- Hemoglobin A1c level
- C-peptide insulin level
- Islet-cell antibodies
- T4 and thyroid antibodies
- Glutamic acid dearboxylase (GAD) antibodies
- Drugs that may alter lab results (particularly in patients prone to diabetes): The following may cause hyperglycemia
  - Hormones
  - Glucagon, glucocorticoids, growth hormone, epinephrine, estrogen and progesterone (oral contraceptives), thyroid preparations

- Medications: Thiazide diuretics, furosemide, acetazolamide, diazoxide, beta-blockers, alpha-agonists, calcium channel blockers, phenytoin, phenobarbital sodium, nicotinic acid, cyclophosphamide, L-asparaginase,
- Epinephrine-like drugs (decongestants and diet pills), fish oils

Pathological Findings
Inflammatory changes, lymphocytic infiltration around the Islets of Langerhans or islet cell loss

DIFFERENTIAL DIAGNOSIS
- Benign renal glycosuria
- Glucose intolerance
- Type 2 non–insulin-dependent diabetes mellitus
  - Children might have MODY (maturity-onset diabetes of the young)
  - Incidence rising
- Infantile-onset diabetes mellitus
- Secondary diabetes
  - Pancreatic disease (pancreatitis, cystic fibrosis)
  - Hormonal disorders (pheochromocytoma, multiple endocrine adenomatosis)
  - Inborn errors of metabolism (glycogen storage disease, type I)
  - Genetic disorders with insulin resistance (acanthosis nigricans)
  - Hereditary neuromuscular disease
  - Progeroid syndromes
  - Obesity (Prader-Willi syndrome)
  - Cytogenetic syndromes (trisomy 21, Klinefelter, and Turner syndromes)
  - Drug- or chemical-induced glucose intolerance
  - Acute poisonings (salicylate poisoning can cause hyperglycemia and glycosuria, and may mimic diabetic ketoacidosis)

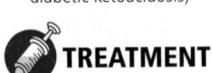 **TREATMENT**

INITIAL STABILIZATION
- Initial care: Inpatient stabilization vs. outpatient management
- Majority of care done by family. Encourage child to do as much self-care as possible.
- Diabetic ketoacidosis
  - IV fluids and IV insulin until stable
  - Restore electrolyte and acid-base balance
  - Correct hyperglycemia
  - Prevent hypoglycemia and hypokalemia
  - Risk of cerebral edema

GENERAL MEASURES
- Overall "control" of carbohydrate metabolism for the very young child
  - Normoglycemia (adjusted for age): "Tight" control with striving for blood glucose levels in range of 80–150 mg/dL (4.4–8.3 mmol/L) all the time, might be dangerous (risk of repeated hypoglycemia).
  - Hemoglobin A1c level close to normal (nondiabetic) range
- Overall good health
  - Asymptomatic
  - Normal appearance
  - Try to keep lipid profile normal
- Normal growth and development
  - Reach optimal height for genetic potential
  - Appropriate and timely pubertal maturation
  - Coping psychosocial development: Normal school or work attendance and performance; normal goals and career plans.

- Prevent acute complications
  - Hypoglycemic insulin reactions
  - Ketoacidosis
- Delay or prevent chronic complications

Diet
- Appropriate American Diabetic Association exchange diet
- Carbohydrate counting: Necessary when on lantus/humalog or novologinsulin regimen with multiple daily injections. Allows patient flexibility of eating and ability to eat almost anything

Activity
- All normal activities, including full participation in sports activities
- Regular aerobic exercise is preferable.

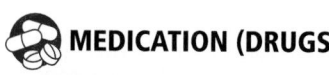 ## MEDICATION (DRUGS)

First Line
- Newest insulin regimen using insulin glargine (Lantus): Humalog or NovoLog at breakfast, lunch, and supper and before snacks
  - Dosage based on a determined insulin/carbohydrate ratio and correction factor for elevated blood sugar, plus Lantus insulin (a 24-hour nearly "peakless" insulin, providing basal insulin throughout the day)
  - This insulin regimen is physiologic and gives the profiles similar to the insulin pump. It offers the advantage of allowing patients to eat "whenever" and "whatever" they desire.
  - Insulin pump (external) therapy: Insulin pump therapy with Medtronic Minimed, Animas, or Cozmo Pumps: Used much more commonly in diabetic patients these days (adults and children); basal insulin is given continuously (rates preset), and bolus doses are given before meals and snacks. Based on insulin/carbohydrate ratios; ALL insulin is Humalog or NovoLog.
- Insulin
  - Source: DNA-recombinant human insulin is the main source of insulin in recent years
  - Types: Lantus (insulin glargine), Humalog, Novolog, NPH, Regular, Premixtures of 70/30 and 75/25 (these mixtures are not commonly used in children)
- Standard insulin regimens (Given SC by syringe; or pen devices such as Humalog pen, Novolog Flexpen, and Opticlix pen (for Lantus)
  - 2 doses: NPH/Lente and Regular/Humalog/NovoLog in a 2:1 ratio given before breakfast and before supper
  - Morning dose usually 1/2–2/3 of total daily dose (other than for newly onset diabetics, this 2-dose regimen will not achieve optimal glycemic control)
  - 3 doses: NPH/Lente and Regular/Humalog/NovoLog at supper; and a bedtime dose of NPH/Lente
  - This may prevent nighttime hypoglycemia and the dawn (Somogyi) phenomenon.
  - 4 doses: Humalog or NovoLog insulin at breakfast, lunch, and supper, and NPH/Lente at bedtime
- Precautions: Avoid hypoglycemia, the dawn phenomenon, and Somogyi syndrome (rebound hyperglycemia).
- Significant possible interactions: Beta-blockers may mask symptoms of hypoglycemia and delay return to normoglycemia.

Second Line
- Oral hypoglycemics not indicated in type 1 diabetes (unless an obese patient, who may have MODY; or a combination of type 1 and type 2)
  - Metformin (Glucophage)
- Immunosuppressants
  - Cyclosporine: Reduces rate of autoimmune beta cell destruction, must be started in initial weeks after initial diagnosis (studies: At 1 year, 20% of cyclosporine-treated patients on no insulin, compared to 12–15% of placebo controls; after 1 year, progressive decline in beta cell function and loss of remission). Side effects include renal disease, hypertension, and lymphoma.
  - Other interventional drugs being studied Azathioprine, steroids, and nicotinamide

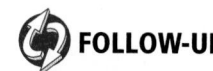 ## FOLLOW-UP

PROGNOSIS
- Initial remission or "honeymoon" phase with decreased insulin needs and easier control, usually 3–6 months and rarely beyond a year
- Progression to "total diabetes" when endogenous insulin is insignificant; usually is gradual, but stress or illness initiate it suddenly
- Current prognosis
  - Increasing longevity and "quality of life" with careful blood glucose monitoring and improvement in insulin delivery regimens
  - At this time, reduced life expectancy, but has improved over the past 20 years

COMPLICATIONS
- Microvascular disease (retinopathy, nephropathy, neuropathy)
- Hyperlipidemia
- Macrovascular disease (coronary and cerebral artery disease)
- Foot problems
- Hypoglycemia
- Diabetic ketoacidosis
- Excessive weight gain
- Psychologic problems of chronic disease

PATIENT MONITORING
- Initially, frequent outpatient follow-up visits until stable; every 2–3 months thereafter
  - Monitor height, weight, and sexual maturation
- Daily home blood glucose monitoring with home blood glucose meter: One Touch Ultra and Ultrasmart; Accuchek Advantage, Compact, and Aviva; Precision X-tra or QID; Freestyle; Ascensia Contour; BD Logic. Several of the insulin pumps have meters that attach to the pump and transmit readings directly to pump.
  - Blood tests should be done 4–6 times daily for optimal monitoring with adjustment of insulin.
- Quarterly measurement of hemoglobin A1c
- Yearly serum lipids and thyrotropin
- Dietary management
  - Adjust for increased caloric needs for age, level of physical activity, pubertal growth spurt, and changes in weight

REFERENCES
1. Travis L, et al. *Diabetes Mellitus in Children and Adolescents*. Philadelphia, PA: WB Saunders, 1987.
2. Pediatric Clinics of North America. *Pediatric and Adolescent Endocrinology. Vol. 34*. Philadelphia, PA: W.B. Saunders; 1987.
3. Lebovitz HE, ed. *Therapy for Diabetes Mellitus and Related Disorders*. Washington, DC: American Diabetes Association; 1991.
4. Clark CM, et al. Prevention and treatment of the complications of diabetes mellitus. *N Engl J Med*. 1995;332:1210–1217.

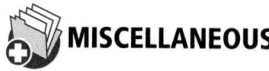 ## MISCELLANEOUS

See also: Diabetes mellitus, type 2; Diabetic ketoacidosis (DKA)

CODES

ICD9-CM
- 250.00 Diabetes mellitus without mention of complication, type 2 or unspecified type, not stated as uncontrolled
- 250.01 Diabetes mellitus without mention of complication, type 1, not stated as uncontrolled
- 250.03 Type I Diabetes, poorly controlled

PATIENT TEACHING
- Complete initial education and ongoing education for patient and family
  - The team approach is ideal, if available.
- For a listing of sources, physicians may contact: American Academy of Family Physicians Foundation, P.O. Box 8418, Kansas City, MO 64114; (800) 274-2237, Ext. 4400.

 See Corresponding Diagnostic Algorithm

 See Patient Handout on CD

D

DIABETIC KETOACIDOSIS (DKA)

Francesca L. Beaudoin, MS, MD

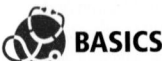 BASICS

DESCRIPTION
- A true medical emergency secondary to severe insulin deficiency and characterized by hyperglycemia, ketosis, and metabolic acidosis
- System(s) Affected: Endocrine/Metabolic

GENERAL PREVENTION
- Close monitoring of glucose during stressful situations
- Careful insulin control
- Educational program for sick-day management instructions

EPIDEMIOLOGY
- Predominant age: 0–19 years of age
- Predominant sex: Male = Female

Incidence
In US: 46 episodes/10,000 diabetic patients; 2 per 100 patient years of type 1 diabetes mellitus

RISK FACTORS
- Type 1 > Type 2 diabetes
- Younger patients at higher risk

PATHOPHYSIOLOGY
A relative or absolute deficiency of insulin, exacerbated by an increase in counter-regulatory hormones (catecholamines, cortisol, glucagon, growth hormone) leading to a hyperglycemic crisis.

ETIOLOGY
- Insufficient insulin/medication noncompliance
- Infection: 30–40%
- 1st presentation of DM: 10–20%
- Myocardial infarction: 5–7%
- No cause identified: 10–30%
- Cerebrovascular accident
- Medications (corticosteroids, thiazides)
- Drugs (cocaine)
- Trauma
- Surgery
- Emotional stress

ASSOCIATED CONDITIONS
Complications of chronic diabetes such as nephropathy, neuropathy, and retinopathy

DIAGNOSIS

SIGNS AND SYMPTOMS
- Polyuria, nocturia
- Polydipsia
- Generalized weakness
- Malaise, lethargy
- Nausea, vomiting
- Abdominal pain
- Decreased perspiration
- Coma
- Confusion
- Fever
- Anorexia or increased appetite

Physical Exam
- Hypotension
- Tachycardia
- Hypothermia or fever
- Tachypnea, Kussmaul respirations
- Decreased reflexes
- Abdominal tenderness
- Decreased bowel sounds
- Fruity odor to breath (acetone smell)
- Dry mucus membranes, poor skin tugor
  - Attempt to find precipitating cause (i.e., source of infection).

TESTS
- ECG (may show myocardial infarct or electrolyte abnormalities)
  - Usually shows sinus tachycardia
- Urine and blood cultures
- Consider lumbar puncture (LP) if suspected meningitis
- CBC, electrolytes, blood urea nitrogen (BUN), Cr, Mg, Phos
- Serum β-HB or ketones
- Arterial blood gases

Lab
- Hyperglycemia (usually 250–800 mg/dL [13.88–44.4 mmol/L] range)
- Serum ketosis: Check beta-hydroxybutyrate instead of ketones to evaluate ketosis (1)[B]
  - With concomitant lactic acidosis, acetoacetate production may be inhibited in presence of high levels of beta hydroxybutyrate. Nitroprusside reaction, which measures only acetoacetate, may not be strongly positive.
- Urine ketosis (may initially be falsely negative, urinalysis may only identify acetoacetate, and not beta hydroxybutyrate).
- Glycosuria
- Hyponatremia
  - Very low serum sodium (<110 mmol/L) suggests an artifact due to severe hyperglycemia and/or hypertriglyceridemia.
- Hyperamylasemia
- Hypertriglyceridemia/Hypercholesterolemia
- Increased creatinine and BUN
  - Markedly increased serum ketones may cross-react and cause a falsely high serum creatinine.
- $HCO_3 \leq 15$ mEq/L
- Decreased calculated total body K^+
  - Severe acidosis gives an artificially high K^+ level.
- Metabolic acidosis on arterial blood gasses
- Increased serum osmolality
- Increased anion gap
- Elevated base deficit

Imaging
Chest radiograph to rule out pulmonary infection

Diagnostic Procedures/Surgery
Only if surgical problem is the underlying precipitant (e.g., appendicitis).

DIFFERENTIAL DIAGNOSIS
- Hyperosmolar non-ketotic coma
- Alcoholic ketoacidosis
- Starvation ketosis
- Toxic ingestions (e.g., salicylates)
- Lactic acidosis
- Acute hypoglycemic coma
- Uremia/Chronic renal failure

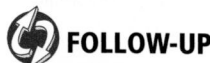 TREATMENT

PRE HOSPITAL
- Oxygen and airway management, as needed
- Establish IV access
- Start isotonic crystalloid solution (0.9% saline)
- Fingerstick glucose testing
- Empiric naloxone if altered mental status

GENERAL MEASURES
- All but mild cases require inpatient management; severe DKA requires an ICU setting.
- Goals
  - Fluid resuscitation
  - Insulin therapy
  - Correction of electrolytes
- Laboratory testing during management
  - Serum glucose q1–2h until stable
  - Electrolytes, phosphorous, and venous pH q2–6h prn

ALERT
Pediatric Considerations
Occasionally children/adolescents exhibit marked mental deterioration, including development of coma q4–6h after therapy has begun; mortality is high. Think of cerebral edema 2° to rapid IV hydration.
- Diagnose by CT scan
- Treat with IV bolus of mannitol 1 g/kg in 20% solution.
- If no response, hyperventilation to a pCO$_2$ of 28 mm Hg

Geriatric Considerations
Must be careful with impaired renal function or CHF when correcting fluid and electrolyte abnormalities

Pregnancy Considerations
Pregnancy itself is diabetogenic. It also results in a compensated respiratory alkalosis (HCO$_3$ 19–20) with theoretically reduced buffering capacity. Therefore, pregnant patients are more susceptible to DKA.
- Euglycemic DKA
- Increased risk of pre-eclampsia and fetal death
- β-tocolytics, corticosteroids can trigger DKA
- Perinatal mortality is between 9% and 35%

Diet
- NPO initially
- Advance to pre-ketotic diet when nausea and vomiting are controlled.

Activity
Bed rest

SPECIAL THERAPY
IV Fluids
- 10–20 mL/kg over the 1st hour, then ~500 mL/h (~7 mL/kg/h) × 4 hours or until dehydration improves, then 250 mL/h (3.5 mL/kg/h) until tolerating PO.
- Switch to 5% dextrose in 0.45% saline at maintenance rate when serum glucose <250 mg/dL. Maintain blood glucose between 150–250 mg/dL.
  - Too rapid correction of fluid balance may precipitate cerebral edema. (2)[C]

Pediatric Considerations
- 100 mL/kg for 1st 10 kg, 50 mL/kg for 2nd 10 kg, and 20 mL/kg thereafter.
- Fluid deficit: Multiply patient's body weight by percentage dehydration; replace maintenance and deficit evenly over 48 hours

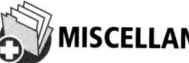 MEDICATION (DRUGS)

- Insulin: IV infusion of regular insulin at 0.1 U/kg/h May use IM or SC route, but IV recommended for moderate to severe DKA. (1,2)[B]
- Potassium: Falsely elevated 2° acidosis, start replacement when K$^+$ ≤5.0 and urine output is adequate. Start 30–40 mEq/L IV fluids. Increase rate (up to 60 mEq/L) if K$^+$ ≤ 3.5. (1,2)[A]
  - Hold insulin if K$^+$ ≤ 2.5, give IV potassium 1 mEq/kg over 1 hour.
  - For each 0.1 unit of pH, serum K$^+$ will change by ~0.6 mEq in opposite direction
- Phosphorus: Routine replacement may lead to hypocalcemia; if low, give 1/3 of K$^+$ replacement as KPhos. [B]
- Sodium bicarbonate: No demonstrable benefit from bicarbonate with a pH >7.0. (1,2)[B] Rehydration usually leads to resolution of acidosis.
- Magnesium: If Mg ≤1.8 mg/dL and symptomatic, consider replacement.
- Precautions
  - If the patient is on an insulin pump, it should be stopped.
  - Double insulin if no response in serum glucose over 1st 2 hours
  - Continue IV insulin until acidosis resolves, then taper and switch to SQ regular insulin when patient is eating.
  - If using bicarbonate, add 50 mg NaHCO$_3$ to 1 L 0.45% saline and give over 2 hours
  - If blood glucose does not fall by ~75 mg q2h, increase insulin rate

 FOLLOW-UP

DISPOSITION
Admission Criteria
ADA admission guidelines: Blood glucose >250 mg/dL; pH < 7.3; HCO$_3$ ≤15 mEq/L; ketones in urine. ICU setting for severe DKA (3)

Discharge Criteria
Reversal of acidosis; tolerating PO intake; resumption of home medication regimen; identification and treatment of any underlying precipitant (e.g., infection).

PROGNOSIS
- 16% of all diabetes related fatalities
- Mortality 1–2%
- In children <10 years old, DKA causes 70% of diabetes-related fatalities

COMPLICATIONS
- Cerebral edema
- Pulmonary edema
- Vascular thrombosis
- Hypokalemia
- Cardica dysrhythmia
- Myocardial infarction
- Acute gastric dilatation
- Late hypoglycemia
- Erosive gastritis
- Infection, mucormycosis
- Respiratory distress
- Hypophosphatemia

PATIENT MONITORING
- Monitor mental status, vital signs, urine output q30–60 min until improved, then q2–4h every 24 hours
- Blood sugar q1h until <300 mg/dL (16.65 mmol/L), then q2–6h
- Potassium, bicarbonate, sodium, anion gap q2h
- Phosphate, calcium, magnesium; q4–6h

REFERENCES
1. Kitabchi AE et al. Hyperglycemic crises in diabetes. *Diabetes Care.* 2004;27(S1):S94–S102.
2. Agus MS, Wolfsdorf JI. Diabetic ketoacidosis in children. *Pediatr Clin North Am.* 2005;52(4):1147–1163.
3. American Diabetes Association. Hospital admission guidelines for diabetes. *Diabetes Care.* 2004;27(S1):S103.
4. Carroll MA, Yeomans ER. Diabetic ketoacidosis in pregnancy. *Cri Care Med.* 2005; 33(10 Suppl):S347–S353.
5. Trachtenbarg DE. Diabetic ketoacidosis. *Am Fam Physician.* 2005;71(9):1705–1714.

MISCELLANEOUS

See also: Diabetes mellitus, type 1

CODES

ICD9-CM
- 250.1 Diabetes with ketoacidosis, unspecified
- 250.12 Diabetes with ketoacidosis, type 2
- 250.13 Diabetes with ketoacidosis, type 1

PATIENT TEACHING
Prevention
- Careful control of the blood glucose level (usually HgbA1c ≤7%).
- Monitor glucose carefully during periods of stress, infection, and trauma.

See Corresponding Diagnostic Algorithm

DIABETIC POLYNEUROPATHY

Kim A. Subasic, MD

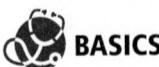 BASICS

DESCRIPTION
- Several distinct patterns described.
- Symmetric polyneuropathy
  - Distal sensory or sensorimotor
  - Proximal lower-extremity polyneuropathy
  - Autonomic neuropathies
- Focal and multifocal neuropathy
  - Cranial neuropathy
  - Focal limb neuropathy
  - Diabetic amyotrophy
  - Truncal
  - Chronic inflammatory demyelinating polyneuropathy (CIDP)

GENERAL PREVENTION
Maintenance of blood glucose at near normal levels

EPIDEMIOLOGY
Diabetes is the most common cause for polyneuropathy in general clinical practice.

Prevalence
- Prevalence increases with diabetes duration.
- Generalized polyneuropathy
  - 10% at diabetes diagnosis
  - 50% at 25 years
  - Cross-sectional prevalence 15% by symptoms; 50% by nerve conduction
- Autonomic neuropathy
  - 16.7% in a U.K. study

RISK FACTORS
- Poor glycemic control
- Duration of diabetes
- Older age
- Presence of retinopathy
- Hyperlipidemia
- Hypertension
- Obesity

PATHOPHYSIOLOGY
>1 pathogenetic factor may operate
- Vasculopathy causing nerve ischemia
  - Likely in mononeuropathies
- Metabolic derangement due to hyperglycemia
  - Aldose reductase converts excess glucose to sorbitol, which causes nerve damage.
  - Sorbitol flux through sorbitol dehydrogenase leads to increased nicotinamide adenine dinucleotide/nicotinamide adenine dinucleotide ratio.
  - Nonenzymatic glycation of neural proteins and lipids form damaging products.
  - Oxidative stress occurs from excessive production of reactive oxygen species.
  - Advanced glycation end products (AGEs) and advanced lipoxidation end products (ALEs) play a role in vascular abnormalities.
  - Protein kinase C activation leads to vascular endothelial defects.

DIAGNOSIS

PRE HOSPITAL
History
- Symmetric distal sensory or sensorimotor polyneuropathy
  - Most common form
  - Distressing numbness, tingling, pain of legs/feet, usually worse at night
  - Sometimes silent and unnoticed by patient
  - Ataxia due to proprioceptive loss
  - Neuropathic foot ulcers due to analgesia and repetitive injury
  - Neuropathic degeneration of foot joints
  - Hands involved late
  - Distal muscle involvement usually mild
- Symmetric proximal polyneuropathy
  - Slow proximal leg weakness, wasting
  - Iliopsoas, quadriceps, and hamstrings
  - Rarely, muscles of shoulder girdle involved
  - Pain and sensory changes less prominent
- Focal cranial or limb mononeuropathy
  - May involve 3rd, 4th, 6th, or 7th cranial nerve :
    ○ 3rd cranial nerve palsy leads to ophthalmoplegia and pain; ptosis, diplopia
    ○ 6th cranial nerve palsy leads to diplopia on lateral gaze
    ○ Femoral, sciatic, or peroneal neuropathy Motor weakness or pain in nerve distribution
    ○ Any major peripheral nerve can be involved
- Truncal neuropathies
  - Painful radiculopathy over dermatomes
- Diabetic amyotrophy (this term is used for a lumbar radiculoplexopathy)
  - Unilateral hip, thigh pain
  - Pelvic girdle, thigh weakness, atrophy
  - Recovery over months
- Chronic inflammatory demyelination polyneuropathy (CIPD)
  - Progressive, severe motor loss
- Diabetic autonomic neuropathy (DAN)
  - Gastrointestinal dysfunction Nocturnal watery diarrhea, sometimes alternating with constipation; gastroparesis with postprandial fullness nausea and vomiting
  - Cardiovascular Autonomic Neuropathy (CAN) Postural dizziness; increased risk for coronary event; exercise intolerance
  - Urogenital Urinary hesitancy, overflow incontinence; erectile dysfunction; vaginal dryness; sexual dysfunction
  - Sudomotor: Anhidrosis or hyperhydrosis; gustatory sweating of head and upper body

Physical Exam
- Symmetric distal polyneuropathy
  - "Stocking-and-glove" distal sensory loss
  - Large-fiber neuropathy: Light touch and vibration loss
  - Small-fiber involvement: Temperature and pinprick
  - Absent ankle reflexes
  - Wasting, weakness of small muscles in foot, changes to arch of foot or toes
  - Sometimes, with small fiber involvement, lack of objective sensory deficit despite pain

- Symmetric proximal polyneuropathy
  - Proximal leg, arm wasting and weakness
  - Loss, patellar reflexes
- Focal cranial or limb mononeuropathy
  - 3rd cranial nerve palsy. Painful ophthalmoplegia and ptosis; preserved pupillary reflexes (in contrast to compressive palsies)
  - 6th cranial nerve Lateral gaze palsy
  - Femoral neuropathy Weakness of lower leg extension; hip flexion; quadriceps wasting; absent patellar reflex; sensory loss anterior thigh
  - Sciatic neuropathy Pain or sensory loss in back of thigh and leg; weakness of hamstrings; lower leg muscles
  - Peroneal neuropathy foot drop
- Truncal neuropathies
  - Pain or sensory loss
- Lumbar radiculoplexopathy (amyotrophy)
  - Weakness and wasting pelvic girdle and thigh
  - Sensory loss in L2–L3
  - Absent patellar reflex
- Autonomic neuropathy
  - Cardiovascular Resting tachycardia; orthostatic hypotension
  - Gastroparesis Postprandial distension; gastric splash

TESTS
Usually none required, except where features are atypical or another etiology is likely.

Lab
- Fasting plasma glucose to diagnose diabetes
- Hemoglobin A1c to assess glycemic control
- Postprandial glucose
- Serum B_{12} levels
- Thyroid function
- Creatinine and BUN
- Syphilis testing
- In mononeuropathy/mononeuritis, multiplex tests for vasculitis, paraproteinemia, and sarcoid

Imaging
In radiculopathy or mononeuropathy, imaging studies to exclude compressive lesions

Diagnostic Procedures/Surgery
- Nerve conduction testing
  - Sensory involvement with or without motor involvement is seen.
  - Useful to confirm mononeuropathy
  - Useful to distinguish chronic inflammatory demyelinating polyneuropathy from rapidly progressive diabetic neuropathy
  - In small unmyelinated fiber painful neuropathy, test may be normal.
- Electromyogram
  - Picture of acute and chronic denervation of affected muscles seen

Pathological Findings
- In peripheral nerve, wallerian degeneration, focal axonal swellings containing neurofilaments, axonal atrophy, and demyelination are seen.
- Thick neural capillary basement membrane
- It is unclear whether changes are a result of ischemic injury or metabolic damage.
- Asymmetric neuropathy and mononeuropathy often are associated with obliterative microvascular lesions and perivascular inflammation.

DIFFERENTIAL DIAGNOSIS
- The following also cause symmetrical polyneuropathy
- Uremic polyneuropathy
- Drug induced
  - Antineoplastic drugs: Cisplatin, Vincristine
  - Isoniazid
  - Amiodarone
- Toxic
  - Chronic arsenic poisoning
  - n-hexane, methyl-n-butyl ketone
- Nutritional deficiency
  - Usually associated with alcoholism
- Paraneoplastic polyneuropathy
- Hypothyroidism

 ## TREATMENT
GENERAL MEASURES
- Maintain blood glucose close to normal.
- Provide appropriate footwear to prevent pressure damage to insensate feet.

Diet
Appropriate to maintain glycemic control

Activity
- Limit weightbearing on neuropathic ulcer.
- Administer stress test prior to starting exercise program.

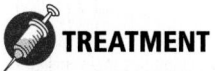 ## MEDICATION (DRUGS)

For sensory symptoms, some antidepressants and anticonvulsant medications help; the addition of analgesics may be required for better pain relief.

First Line
- Management of painful and sensory neuropathy
  - Tricyclic antidepressants (1,5) [A]
    - Analgesia may be related to effects on sodium channels
    - Amitriptyline is most commonly used
    - Dose 25–150 mg at bedtime (4)
    - Anticholinergic side effects may occur
    - Nortriptyline (75–150 mg) and desipramine (75–200 mg) have less troublesome side effects.
  - Anticonvulsants (Gabapentin) (1,3) [A]
    - Least side effects and favorable trial data cause it to be the most used drug.
    - Acts on subunits of voltage-gated calcium channels (same site as pregabalin).
    - Dose titration is from 300–1,200 mg t.i.d.
    - Reduce dose in renal insufficiency.
    - Adverse effects are dizziness and fatigue.
- Management of autonomic neuropathy
  - Orthostatic hypotension
    - Fludrocortisone: Increased risk of heart failure
    - Midodrine
  - Gastroparesis
    - Metoclopramide or domperidone
  - Adverse effects to CNS
    - Erythromycin
  - Diabetic diarrhea
    - Loperamide
    - Clonidine: To treat severe diarrhea
    - Octreotide
    - Antibiotics for bacterial overgrowth

- Erectile dysfunction
  - Phosphodiesterase-5 inhibitors
  - Prostaglandin E1 injection
  - Mechanical devices
- Hyperhidrosis
  - Propantheline

Second Line
- Antidepressants
  - Duloxetine [A]
    - Selective serotonin and norepinephrine uptake inhibitor
    - Usual dose is 60–120 mg once daily (1)
    - Adverse effects are nausea and dizziness
  - Selective serotonin reuptake inhibitors [B]
    - Not as effective as tricyclic antidepressants
- Anticonvulsants
  - Pregabalin (1,2,4,5) [A]
    - Binds Ca^{++} channel associated protein, inhibits neurotransmitter release
    - Usual dose 150–600 mg
    - Adverse effects are dizziness and edema
  - Carbamazepine [B]
    - Alleviates pain by blocking sodium channels
    - Dose 400–1200 (1000–1600) mg daily
  - Lamotrigine/Topiramate [B]
    - 200–600 mg (1)
    - Adverse effects: Skin rash, necrolysis
- Topical therapies
  - Capsicin [B]
    - Depletes C fibers in skin of substance-P
    - 0.075% cream applied t.i.d.
  - Lignocaine patches [B]
    - Causes sodium channel blockade
    - 5% (700 mg) patches applied daily to feet
- Opiate analgesia
  - Tramadol
    - Nonnarcotic medication, binds opiate receptors, fewer opiate side effects
    - Usual dose 200–400 mg (1)
  - Oxycodone
    - Controversial due to dependence potential
- Topical nitrates [B]
  - In small studies, spray or patch show benefit
- α-Lipoic acid [B]
  - 2 small trials have shown benefit
  - 600 mg (1)
  - IV route to initiate therapy
- Protein kinase C inhibitors
  - Ruboxistaurin
    - Slows progression of disease process
    - Anticipated availability 2007 (2)[A]
- Evening primrose oil
  - Active ingredient is α-linoleic acid
- Benfotiamine (2)[C]
  - Allithiamine
  - Pilot studies have shown significant benefit

Geriatric Considerations
Anticholinergic effects of tricyclics may cause urinary retention, arrhythmias.

SPECIAL THERAPY
- Acupuncture [C]
- Transcutaneous electrical nerve stimulation
- Percutaneous nerve stimulation
- Electrical spinal cord stimulation

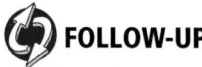 ## FOLLOW-UP
PROGNOSIS
- Generalized symmetric polyneuropathies
  - Usually slow chronic progression
  - Insensitive but painless foot as pain lessens
- Acute mononeuropathy and focal neuropathies: Recovery over months–years

COMPLICATIONS
- Neurotropic ulceration
  - Painless ulcers on weightbearing area
  - Callus formation precursor to ulceration
- Neuropathic arthropathy
  - Results in complete disorganization of joint structure in foot, "Charcot joint"

REFERENCES
1. Duby JJ, Campbell RK, Setter SM, et al. Diabetic neuropathy: an intensive review. Am J Health-System Pharmacists. 2004;61:160–173.
2. Wu S, Armstrong DG. Pharmacological management of diabetic neuropathy: an evaluation. Podiatr Manag. 2005;159–160,162,164–165.
3. Poncelet AN. Diabetic polyneuropathy: risk factors, patterns of presentation, diagnosis and treatment. Geriatrics. 2003;58(6):16–25,30.
4. Bolton AJ, Vinik AI, Arezzo JC, et al. Diabetic neuropathies: a statement by the American Diabetes Association. Diabetes Care. 2005;28(4):956–962.
5. Stillman M. Cleve Clin J Med. 2006;73(8):726–739.

ADDITIONAL READING
Ropper AH, Brown RH. Adam and Victor's Principles of Neurology, 8th ed. New York: McGraw-Hill Medical Publishing, 2005.

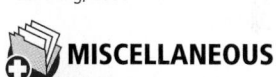 ## MISCELLANEOUS
CODES
ICD9-CM
Polyneuropathy in diabetes (manifestation)

PATIENT TEACHING

 See Corresponding Diagnostic Algorithm

 See Patient Handout on CD

DIARRHEA, ACUTE

Laura J. Sacco, MD

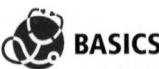 **BASICS**

DESCRIPTION
- Abrupt-onset diarrhea in a healthy individual is most often related to an infectious process.
- A variety of symptoms often are observed, including frequent passage of loose or watery stools, fever, chills, anorexia, vomiting, and malaise.
- Acute viral diarrhea (50–70%)
  - Most common form; usually occurs for 1–3 days; self-limited
  - Causes changes in small intestinal cell morphology, such as villous shortening and an increase in the number of crypt cells
- Bacterial diarrhea (15–20%)
  - May be suspected if history of similar and simultaneous illness is present in individuals who have shared contaminated food with the patient
  - Diarrhea developing within 12 hours of the meal is most likely due to ingestion of a preformed toxin
- Protozoal infections (10–15%)
  - Cause prolonged, watery diarrhea that often afflicts travelers returning from endemic areas with contaminated water supply
- Traveler's diarrhea
  - Typically begins 3–7 days after arrival in a foreign location and is generally quite acute
- System(s) Affected: Endocrine/metabolic, Gastrointestinal

GENERAL PREVENTION
- Frequent oversights during foreign travel include brushing teeth with contaminated water, ingesting ice cubes, or eating cold salads or meats.
- Avoid uncooked or undercooked seafood or meat, buffet meals left out for several hours, or food served by street vendors.

EPIDEMIOLOGY
Predominant age: All ages

RISK FACTORS
- Individual from an industrialized country visiting a developing country
- Immunocompromised host
- Antibiotic use
- Day care attendance

ETIOLOGY
- Bacterial
  - *E. coli*
  - *Salmonella*
  - *Shigella*
  - *Campylobacter jejuni*
  - *Vibrio parahaemolyticus*
  - *Vibrio cholerae*
  - *Yersinia enterocolitica*
  - *C. difficile*
- Viral
  - Rotavirus
  - Norwalk virus
- Parasitic
  - *Giardia lamblia*
  - *Cryptosporidium*
  - *Entamoeba histolytica*

Pediatric Considerations
- Rotavirus is a common cause of viral diarrhea in the winter months and is accompanied by vomiting.
- Other etiologies include overfeeding, medications, cystic fibrosis, and malabsorption.

Geriatric Considerations
Watery diarrhea with chronic constipation may be caused by fecal impaction or obstructing neoplasm.

ASSOCIATED CONDITIONS
- Diabetes mellitus
- Ileal resection
- Gastrectomy
- Hyperthyroidism

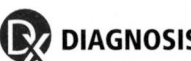 **DIAGNOSIS**

SIGNS AND SYMPTOMS
- Loose liquid stools ± blood or mucus
- Fever
- Abdominal pain and distension
- Headache
- Anorexia
- Malaise
- Vomiting
- Myalgia
- With Giardia: Cramping, pale-greasy stools, fatigue, weight loss, chronicity

History
- Assess stool characteristics: Frequency and quantity, presence of mucous or blood, consistency (1)[A]
- Travel history, day care attendance, ingestion of raw or undercooked meat, raw seafood, unpasteurized milk, sick contacts (1)[A]

Physical Exam
- Determine hydration status; look for decreased skin turgor, dry mucous membranes, hypotension, or decreased urination. In children: Absence of tears, depressed fontanelles, dry diapers.
- Abdominal exam to rule out surgical causes of diarrhea such as appendicitis or pelvic abscess

TESTS
Lab
- Consider testing if diarrhea is prolonged
- CBC
  - Increased WBC with a left shift may indicate an infectious process.
  - A decreased hemoglobin/hematocrit may indicate anemia from blood loss.
- Serum electrolytes
  - Increased sodium from dehydration
  - Decreased potassium from diarrhea
- Blood urea nitrogen, creatinine: Elevated in dehydration
- pH: Hyperchloremic acidosis

- Stool sample
  - Occult blood present in inflammatory bowel disease, bowel ischemia, bacterial infections
  - Fecal leukocytes present in diarrhea caused by *Salmonella, Campylobacter, Yersinia*
  - For community-acquired or traveler's diarrhea >1 day or accompanied by fever or bloody stools: Culture or test for *Salmonella, Shigella, Campylobacter, E. coli* O157:H7. If antibiotics or chemotherapy in recent weeks, *C. difficile* toxin A and B (1)[B]
  - For nosocomial diarrhea (onset ≥3 days in hospital): Test for *C. difficile* toxins A and B. Also consider bacterial cultures listed above in patients with bloody stools or infants (1)[B]
  - For diarrhea >7 days: Stool ova and parasites plus bacterial cultures if immunocompromised (1)[B]
  - *Giardia* ELISA: >90% sensitive in at-risk population, consider prior to O&P

Imaging
Abdominal radiographs (flat plate and upright) indicated with abdominal pain or evidence of obstruction to rule out toxic megacolon and bowel ischemia

Diagnostic Procedures/Surgery
Sigmoidoscopy indicated with bloody diarrhea or suspected pseudomembranous or ulcerative colitis

Pathological Findings
- Viral diarrhea: Changes in small intestine cell morphology that include villous shortening, increased number of crypt cells, and increased cellularity of the lamina propria
- Bacterial diarrhea: Bacterial invasion of colonic wall leads to mucosal hyperemia, edema, and leukocytic infiltration

DIFFERENTIAL DIAGNOSIS
- Inflammatory bowel disease
- Drugs (cholinergic agents, magnesium-containing antacids)
- Pseudomembranous colitis secondary to antibiotic use
- Diverticulitis
- Spastic (irritable) colon
- Fecal impaction
- Malabsorption
- Zollinger-Ellison syndrome
- Ischemic bowel
- Gastrinoma

TREATMENT

INITIAL STABILIZATION

Outpatient health care except for complicating emergencies (dehydration)

GENERAL MEASURES

- Replacement of lost fluid and electrolytes (1)[A]
  - Clear liquids at room temperature, such as tea, broth, carbonated beverages (without caffeine), and rehydration fluids (e.g., Gatorade) to replace lost fluid
  - Packets of rehydration salts (1 packet to be diluted in 1 quart of water); drink until thirst is quenched (helps replace electrolytes); treatment of choice for pediatric patients
  - IV fluids if patient cannot tolerate oral rehydration

ALERT

Pregnancy Considerations

Dehydration may lead to preterm labor.

Diet

- Early refeeding is encouraged
- During periods of active diarrhea, avoid coffee, alcohol, dairy products, most fruits, vegetables, red meats, and heavily seasoned foods.
- Begin by eating clear soup with rice, salted crackers, dry toast or bread, and sherbet.
- As stooling rate decreases, slowly add to diet baked potato and chicken soup with noodles.
- As stool begins to retain shape, add to diet baked fish, poultry, applesauce, and bananas.

Activity

As tolerated

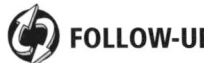 MEDICATION (DRUGS)

First Line

- Loperamide: 4 mg followed by 2 mg capsule after each unformed stool or bismuth subsalicylate, 30 mL every 1/2 hour until 8 doses, may be helpful in mild diarrhea
- In children with acute infectious diarrhea treatment with *Lactobacillus* is safe and effective for reducing the duration and frequency of diarrhea (2)[A].
- In patients being treated with antibiotics, administration of a probiotic such as *Lactobacillus* is effective for preventing diarrhea (3)[A].
- If diarrhea persists, and a bacterial or parasitic organism is identified, antibiotic therapy should be started
  - *Giardia*: Metronidazole 250 mg t.i.d. for 5 days
  - *E. histolytica*: Metronidazole 750 mg t.i.d. for 10 days
  - *Shigella*: Trimethoprim-sulfamethoxazole 160 mg and 800 mg, respectively, b.i.d. for 5 days, or ciprofloxacin (Cipro) 500 mg b.i.d. for 3 days
  - *Campylobacter*: Erythromycin 500 mg q.i.d. for 5 days or ciprofloxacin (Cipro) 500 mg b.i.d. day for 3 days
  - *C. difficile*: Discontinue antibiotics if possible. Consider metronidazole 500 mg t.i.d. for 10–14 days if diarrhea persists or worsens.
  - Traveler's diarrhea: Ciprofloxacin (Cipro) 750 mg 1 dose or, if severe, 500 mg divided PO b.i.d. for 3 days (4)[A] *or* TMP/SMX (Bactrim) DS 1 tab b.i.d. for 3 days
- Contraindications
  - Antibiotics are contraindicated in *Salmonella* infections unless caused by *S. typhosa* or the patient is severely ill (5)[A].
  - Avoid alcoholic beverages with metronidazole due to the possibility of a disulfiram reaction.
  - Antibiotics are not indicated in food-borne toxigenic diarrhea.
- Precautions
  - Antiperistaltic agents (e.g., loperamide) should be used with caution in patients suspected of having infectious diarrhea (especially if *E. coli* 0157:H7 suspected) or antibiotic-associated colitis.
  - Doxycycline, sulfamethoxazole-trimethoprim, and ciprofloxacin may cause photosensitivity; use sunscreen.
- Significant possible interactions
  - Salicylate absorption from bismuth subsalicylate can cause toxicity in patients already taking aspirin-containing compounds and may alter anticoagulation control in patients taking Coumadin.
  - Ciprofloxacin and erythromycin increase theophylline levels.

Second Line

- Doxycycline: 100 mg b.i.d. for 3 days
- Diphenoxylate-atropine in nonpregnant adults
- Tinidazole or secnidazole for *E. histolytica*
- *Oral* Vancomycin for *C. difficile* infections

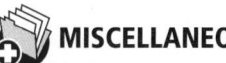 FOLLOW-UP

PROGNOSIS

This common problem is rarely life-threatening if adequate hydration is maintained.

COMPLICATIONS

- Dehydration
- Sepsis
- Shock
- Anemia

PATIENT MONITORING

If diarrhea continues for 3–5 days with or without blood or mucus, consult a physician.

REFERENCES

1. Guerrant RL, Van Gilder T. Practice guidelines for the management of infectious diarrhea. *Clin Infect Dis 2001 Feb* 1;32(3):331–351.
2. Lactobacillus is safe and effective for treating children with acute infectious diarrhea. *ACP Journal Club* 2002;137(3):96.
3. Probiotics are effective in preventing antibiotic-associated diarrhea. *ACP Journal Club* 2002;137(3):95.
4. Single-dose ciprofloxacin stemmed traveler's diarrhea. *ACP Journal Club* 1995;122:43.
5. Antibiotics have no effect on diarrhea and increase bacteriologic relapse in *Salmonella* intestinal infection. *ACP Journal Club* 1999;130:15.
6. Diskin, A. Gastroenteritis. http://www.emedicine.com/emerg/topic213.htm.

 MISCELLANEOUS

See also: Botulism; Cholera; Food poisoning; Bacterial

CODES

ICD9-CM

- 005.9 Food poisoning, unspecified
- 558.2 Toxic gastroenteritis and colitis
- 558.9 Other and unspecified noninfectious gastroenteritis and colitis
- 787.91 Diarrhea

PATIENT TEACHING

See guidelines in "Prevention" section

 See Corresponding Diagnostic Algorithm

See Patient Handout on CD

D

DIARRHEA, CHRONIC

Jeremy Golding, MD

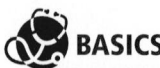 BASICS

DESCRIPTION
- A decrease in fecal consistency for >4 weeks (American Gastroenterological Association)
- Causes include inflammatory diarrhea, osmotic diarrhea (malabsorption), secretory diarrhea (endogenous and exogenous), and intestinal dysmotility.
- System(s) Affected: Gastrointestinal

Geriatric Considerations
Patients with life-long diarrhea may suffer increasing difficulty with advanced age.

GENERAL PREVENTION
Refrain from dietary or pharmacologic agents that may precipitate a diarrhea event.

EPIDEMIOLOGY
Incidence
Reliable data on incidence is lacking, but ∼5% of the population is affected in the US

Prevalence
- Predominant age: Determined by certain illnesses
- Predominant sex: Female > Male

RISK FACTORS
- Inflammatory
  - AIDS
  - Infections
  - Radiation
  - Family history
- Osmotic
  - Infectious
  - Abdominal surgery including cholecystectomy, resection (gastric and small bowel), vagotomy
  - Chronic alcohol abuse
  - Sorbitol, fructose, gluten
- Secretory: Distal ileal surgery
- Altered intestinal motility
  - Diabetes
  - Fecal impaction
  - Neurological diseases
- Factitious: Laxative use

Genetics
- Celiac sprue and inflammatory bowel disease may be familial
- Lactose intolerance: Increased incidence in certain geographic regions

ETIOLOGY
- Functional diarrhea
- Inflammatory diarrhea
  - Inflammatory bowel disease (ulcerative colitis and Crohn disease)
  - Radiation enterocolitis
  - Eosinophilic gastroenteritis
  - Hypersensitivity (e.g., food allergy)
  - AIDS: Mucosal and submucosal inflammation with possible impairment in absorption and excessive secretion

- Infectious diarrhea
  - Parasites (e.g., *Giardia lamblia, Isospora*)
  - Helminths (e.g., *Strongyloides*)
  - Bacterial (e.g., *Mycobacterium avium intracellulare, Clostridium difficile*)
- Osmotic diarrhea
  - Pancreatic insufficiency (e.g., alcohol-induced, cystic fibrosis)
  - Bacterial overgrowth
  - Celiac disease
  - Thyrotoxicosis
  - Lactase deficiency
  - Whipple disease
  - Abetalipoproteinemia
  - Postsurgical (short gut, PUD surgery)
  - Drugs: Osmotically active agents (e.g., antacids, Milk of Magnesia), antibiotics, NSAIDs, prostaglandins, colchicine, metformin, digoxin, selective serotonin reuptake inhibitors, and antineoplastic agents
  - Herbal products: St. John's Wort, *Echinacea*, feverfew, garlic, saw palmetto, ginseng, cranberry extract, pokeroot tea, aloe vera
- Secretory diarrhea
  - Carcinoid syndrome
  - Zollinger-Ellison syndrome
  - Vasoactive intestinal peptide-secreting pancreatic adenomas
  - Medullary carcinoma of thyroid
  - Villous adenoma of rectum
  - Microscopic colitis
  - Choleraic diarrhea: Excessive secretion of electrolytes
  - Diabetic
  - Laxatives (phenolphthalein, cascara, senna, aloe)
  - Toxins (arsenic, mushrooms, insecticides, alcohol)
- Altered intestinal motility (most common in clinical practice)
- Irritable bowel syndrome (most common in young females)
- Fecal impaction
- Neurologic diseases
- Diabetes: Increased transit and possible bacterial overgrowth
- In children: Diarrhea secondary to dietary products (e.g., fructose and apple juice)

ASSOCIATED CONDITIONS
Immune-complex mediated extra-intestinal complications of inflammatory bowel disease:
- Arthritis
- Uveitis
- Pyoderma gangrenosum
- Nephritis

℞ DIAGNOSIS

SIGNS AND SYMPTOMS
Frequent loose stools, fever, abdominal pain, weight loss, tenesmus, flatus, bulky stools plus
- Inflammatory: Blood (must rule out colonic neoplasm), anemia, abdominal pain
- Osmotic: Steatorrhea, azotorrhea, weight loss, improves with fasting
- Altered intestinal motility: Alternating diarrhea and constipation, passage of mucus and incomplete evacuation, bloating, anxiety, depression (not nocturnal)
- Factitious: Peripheral edema, weakness, nausea, nocturnal, hypokalemia
- Malabsorption: Pale, greasy, voluminous, foul-smelling stools (lactose intolerance, celiac, chronic pancreatitis, bacterial overgrowth)

History
- Onset, pattern (intermittent vs continuous), duration, travel, exposures, weight loss
- Rome criteria for IBS

Physical Exam
Thorough physical exam helpful

TESTS
Special tests
- Inflammatory: Colonic biopsies
- Fecal fat stool collections
- Breath test for labeled CO_2 to assess fat, carbohydrate, and bile salt malabsorption
- Blood and urine hormone levels in endocrine diseases
- Malabsorption: Small bowel biopsies

Lab
- CBC with differential, electrolytes, total protein, albumin, TSH, anti-endomysial antibody (AEA), and transglutimase antibody (TGA) if sprue suspected
- Stool ova and parasites
- Stool fat, osmolality, pH, leukocytes, and occult blood
- Stool for *C. difficile* toxin
- Screen for laxative abuse (e.g., phenolphthalein)
- When tumor syndrome seems likely based on presentation or finding on radiography: Gastrin, calcitonin, vasoactive intestinal polypeptide, somatostatin, urine excretion of 5-hydroxy acetic acid, metanephrine, and histamine.

Imaging
- Barium enema
- CT to rule out pancreatic cancer or chronic pancreatitis if abnormal pancreatic enzymes or evidence of malabsorption.

Diagnostic Procedures/Surgery
- Colonoscopy/sigmoidoscopy for inflammatory lesions; if occult blood in stool ± iron deficiency
- If barium enema is negative and diarrhea persists, biopsies are indicated.
- EGD with small bowel biopsies if malabsorption disorder is suspected

Pathological Findings

- When present, the findings are those of the associated or underlying disease.
- None seen in functional disorder
- Melanosis coli suggests cathartic abuse

DIFFERENTIAL DIAGNOSIS

- Functional disorder
- Inflammatory bowel disease: Look for systemic illness or extraintestinal manifestations (arthritis, pyoderma gangrenosum, erythema nodosum, uveitis, or vasculitis)
- Factitious: Psychiatric disease, or past history of
- Irritable bowel syndrome: Alternating diarrhea and constipation, psychiatric overtones
- Tropical sprue
- Tuberculosis enteritis
- Chronic radiation enterocolitis
- Colonic neoplasm
- Diverticular disease

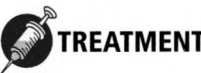 TREATMENT

- Best evidence suggests that opioids and opioid agonist should be considered as first-line symptomatic relief of diarrhea (1)[C]
- Octreotide (Sandostatin): Used in carcinoid and other peptide-secreting tumors, dumping syndrome. and chemotherapy-induced diarrhea (2)[C]
- Cholestyramine (Questran) for bile salt malabsorption and certain postsurgical patients (3)[C]
- Bismuth is of unproven efficacy (4)[C].
- Psyllium may alter stool consistency, but does not decrease volume (5)[C].

GENERAL MEASURES

- Unless the patient is hypotensive or an electrolyte abnormality or deconditioning is present, outpatient therapy is adequate.
- Fluids with electrolyte supplementation

Diet

- Abstain from gluten products, sorbitol, lactose-containing products, and food allergens.
- In irritable bowel syndrome, may need to add dietary fiber (bulking agents); (e.g., 20–30 g/d supplemental fiber).

Complementary and Alternative Medicine

Some herbal remedies commonly cause chronic diarrhea: St. John's Wort, *Echinacea*, feverfew, garlic, saw palmetto, ginseng, cranberry extract, pokeroot tea, aloe vera

 MEDICATION (DRUGS)

First Line

- Opiates
  - Diphenoxylate-atropine (Lomotil): 5–20 mg/d or loperamide (Imodium) 4–16 mg/d, doses calculated and timed according to patient's individual needs
    - Contraindicated in infectious diarrheas, because of possible organism enhancement of tissue
    - Avoid in ulcerative colitis toxic megacolon
- Octreotide (Sandostatin: 200–300 SC mcg/d in 2–4 divided doses
  - Can be switched to IM depot form (Sandostatin LAR) 20 mg intragluteally q4 weeks. Revaluate after 2 months
- Cholestyramine (Questran) 4–8 grams t.i.d.
  - May interfere with absorption of fat soluble vitamins and other medications
- Lactase (Lactaid, Lactrase) for lactose intolerance Chew/swallow 3 original strength tablets or 1 Fast-Acting Tablet with 1st bite of food containing dairy products
- Steroids and sulfasalazine derivatives in inflammatory bowel disease

SURGERY

For villous adenomas, hormone producing tumors, and refractory ulcerative colitis

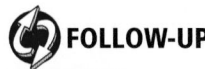 FOLLOW-UP

PROGNOSIS

Variable, from a short (factitious and altered intestinal motility) and treatable course, to a chronic illness (e.g., Crohn disease, ulcerative colitis)

COMPLICATIONS

- Fluid and electrolyte abnormalities
- Malnutrition
- Anemia

REFERENCES

1. Schiller LR. Review article: anti-diarrheal pharmacology and therapeutics. *Aliment Pharmacol Ther*. 1995;9:87.
2. Eherer AJ, Santa Ana, CA, Porter J, Fordtran JS. Effect of psyllium, calcium polycarbophil, and wheat bran on secretory diarrhea induced by phenolphthalein. *Gastroenterology*. 1993;104:1007.
3. Schiller LR, Hogan RB, Morawski SG, et al. Studies of the prevalence and significance of bile acid malabsorption in a group of patients with idiopathic chronic diarrhea. *Gastroenterology*. 1987;92:151.
4. Yeoh EK, Horowitz M, Russo A, et al. Gastrointestinal function in chronic radiation enteritis-effects of loperamide-N-oxide. *Gut*. 1993;34:476.
5. DuPont HL. Bismuth subsalicylate in the treatment and prevention of diarrheal disease. *Drug Intell Clin Pharm*. 1987;21:687.

 MISCELLANEOUS

See also: Crohn disease; Cryptococcosis; Diarrhea, acute; Irritable bowel syndrome; Ulcerative colitis; Uveitis

CODES

ICD9-CM

- 558.2 Toxic gastroenteritis and colitis
- 558.9 Other and unspecified noninfectious gastroenteritis and colitis
- 787.91 Diarrhea

PATIENT TEACHING

- Explain in simple terms of bowel physiology
- Reassure that normal frequency varies widely
- Restrict colon stimulants

Diet

Dietary consult when appropriate

 See Corresponding Diagnostic Algorithm

 See Patient Handout on CD

D

DIFFUSE INTERSTITIAL LUNG DISEASE

Jacqueline L. Olin, MS, PharmD, BCPS
Keith T. Goldstein, MD

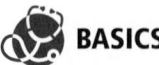 **BASICS**

DESCRIPTION
Interstitial lung diseases (ILDs) represent a diverse group of chronic progressive lung diseases associated with alveolar inflammation and/or potentially irreversible pulmonary fibrosis. More than 200 individual diseases may present with similar characteristics, which has made ILD difficult to classify. A classification scheme proposed by the American Thoracic Society and European Respiratory Society includes these subtypes:

- Known causes (environmental, occupational, or drug-associated disease)
- Systemic disorders (including sarcoidosis, Wegener granulomatosis, collagen vascular disease, etc.)
- Rare lung diseases (including pulmonary histiocytosis, lymphangioleiomyomatosis, etc.)
- Idiopathic interstitial pneumonias (IIPs)
- Based on clinical, radiologic, and histologic features, IIPs are further subclassified into the following diagnoses
  - Idiopathic pulmonary fibrosis (IPF), which is characterized by progressive dyspnea, cough, restrictive lung disease, and a specific histopathological pattern
  - IIPs other than IPF (including nonspecific interstitial pneumonia [NSIP], respiratory bronchiolitis-associated ILD [RBILD], acute interstitial pneumonia [AIP], etc.)

GENERAL PREVENTION
Avoiding environmental or occupational exposure to organic or inorganic dusts, and smoking cessation may reduce incidence or improve clinical course in patients with established ILD.

EPIDEMIOLOGY
Due to lack of consistency in disease presentation and definition, epidemiologic data are not well-defined. Incidence and prevalence statistics are from a population-based registry in New Mexico (4).

Incidence
Annual incidence
- 31.5 per 100,000 – Males
- 26.1 per 100,000 – Females

Prevalence
- Although IPF usually occurs after the age of 50, an earlier onset may occur with some other subtypes.
- Annual prevalence
  - 80.9/100,000 – Males
  - 67.2/100,000 – Females

RISK FACTORS
- Environmental or occupational exposure to inorganic or organic dusts
- 66–75% with smoking history
- Due to diversity of diseases, age is not a reliable predictor of pathology.

Genetics
Some studies suggest that some subtypes of ILD may be associated with specific predisposing genes and environmental exposures; however the role of genetic factors is unknown at this time; ~10% of IPF cases are inherited.

PATHOPHYSIOLOGY
Alveolar inflammation may progress into irreversible fibrosis. Varying degrees of ventilatory dysfunction occur among the ILD subtypes. ILD associated with collagen vascular disease and systemic connective disorders can manifest involvement of skin, joints, muscular, and ocular systems.

ETIOLOGY
Some types of ILD are associated with specific exposures

- Medications (including amiodarone, antibiotics [especially nitrofurantoin], chemotherapy agents, gold, illicit drugs)
- Inorganic dusts (including silicates, asbestos, talc, mica, coal dust, graphite)
- Organic dusts (including moldy hay, inhalation of fungi, bacteria, animal proteins)
- Metals (including tin, aluminum, cobalt, iron, barium)
- Gases, fumes, vapors, aerosols

ASSOCIATED CONDITIONS
Many systemic disorders and primary diseases are associated with ILD. A partial list includes

- Collagen vascular disease
- Sarcoidosis
- Amyloidosis
- Pulmonary-renal (including Goodpasture syndrome)
- Vasculitides (including Churg-Strauss syndrome, Wegener granulomatosis)

DIAGNOSIS

SIGNS AND SYMPTOMS
- Progressive exertional dyspnea
- Nonproductive cough
- Abnormal chest radiograph (compare with previous)
- May also present with
  - Hemoptysis (idiopathic alveolar hemosiderosis)
  - Fatigue
  - Weight loss

History
Obtaining a history of illness duration (acute vs. chronic), potential environmental or occupational exposures, travel, and medical conditions (including systemic diseases) is important in assessing cause of the ILD

Physical Exam
Findings are usually nonspecific. Some common features include
- Rales; may have "Velcro" quality
- Inspiratory "squeaks"
- Clubbing of the digits
- Cyanosis in advanced disease

TESTS
Lab
- Arterial blood gas
- If systemic disorder suspected consider obtaining antinuclear antibodies, rheumatoid factor, erythrocyte sedimentation rate, antineutrophil cytoplasmic antibodies
- If indicated, hypersensitivity pneumonitis panel, plasma angiotensin converting enzyme concentration (sarcoidosis)

Imaging
- Chest radiography
- High-resolution computed tomography (HRCT) of the chest
  - Most useful tool for distinguishing between ILD subclasses

Diagnostic Procedures/Surgery
- Pulmonary function testing (spirometry, lung volumes, carbon monoxide diffusing capacity)
  - Commonly demonstrates a restrictive defect (decreased vital capacity and total lung capacity)
  - Very low baseline carbon monoxide diffusing capacity may predict mortality
- Bronchoscopy
  - Bronchoalveolar lavage (BAL) cellular analysis studies may be useful in distinguishing some subtypes (including sarcoidosis, cancer) but overall usefulness is limited
  - Fiberoptic transbronchial lung biopsy may help diagnose sarcoidosis and, on occasion, sufficiently supportive of other ILD diagnoses
- Thoracoscopic surgery for lung biopsy has the greatest diagnostic specificity for ILDs but is infrequently used.

Pathological Findings
- The diagnostic classifications of IIPs are based on histopathologic patterns seen on lung biopsy.
- Characteristic changes on HRCT may help to distinguish between subtypes. Honeycombing, and ground-glass opacities may be seen.

DIFFERENTIAL DIAGNOSIS
- Acute pulmonary edema
- Diffuse hemorrhage
- Atypical pneumonia

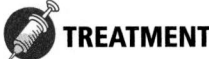 **TREATMENT**

- Evidence does not support routine use of any specific therapy for ILD in general and especially IPF. There is no evidence that any pharmacological therapies improve survival or quality of life (4).
- Corticosteroids have a role in some ILD subtypes for which pulmonologist referral is recommended.
- Current evidence does not clearly support routine use of noncorticosteroid anti-inflammatory agents including cyclosporine, azathioprine, colchicines, cyclophosphamide, cytokines, methotrexate, or interferon (3).

GENERAL MEASURES

- Avoiding or minimizing offending environmental or occupational exposures
- Cessation of culprit medications
- Smoking cessation

 MEDICATION (DRUGS)

First Line

- Corticosteroids have been the mainstay of treatment regimens for ILD; however, response rates have been variable across and within subtypes. The optimal dose and duration of therapy is unknown.
- Common starting dose of prednisone 0.5–1 mg/kg once daily for 4–12 weeks, with potential up-titration to 0.5 mg/kg based on patient response.

Second Line

- Azathioprine or cyclosporine have been used for IPF alone or in combination with steroids with limited success rates.
  - Azathioprine was studied at 2–3 mg/kg/d (not to exceed 200 mg/d; adjusted to the nearest 25-mg dose increment) in combination with prednisone and ultimately as a steroid-sparing agent.
  - Cyclophosphamide is commonly used in treatment of Wegener granulomatosis. It is given 1.5–2 mg/kg PO per day for 6 months–2 years.
- Methotrexate has been used in treatment of mild Wegener granulomatosis in combination with corticosteroids. A studied dosing regimen consisted of an initial methotrexate dose of 0.3 mg/kg (maximum dose of 15 mg) once weekly, with 2.5 mg titration each week (maximum dose of 25 mg/wk.)
- The addition of acetylcysteine (1800 mg/d for 12 months) to therapy with azathioprine and prednisone in IPF was studied in a double-blind, placebo-controlled trial. Improvements in vital capacity and carbon monoxide diffusing capacity were noted in the acetylcysteine-treated patients.

SURGERY

Single- or double-lung transplantation may be a treatment of last resort in some patients. However some ILDs associated with systemic disease may recur in the recipient lung.

 FOLLOW-UP

DISPOSITION

- All patients need pulmonary referral.
- Follow-up testing should include pulmonary function tests, cardiopulmonary stress test, pulse oximetry, and chest radiograph.

PROGNOSIS

Overall prognosis is varied between subtypes. IPF confers the worst prognosis (50–80% mortality in 5 years). Some entities, including hypersensitivity pneumonitis, nonspecific interstitial pneumonia, and cryptogenic organizing pneumonia, have a good prognosis.

COMPLICATIONS

- Progressive respiratory failure
- Cor pulmonale
- Pneumothorax

REFERENCES

1. American Thoracic Society. European Respiratory Society International multidisciplinary consensus classification of idiopathic interstitial pneumonias. *Am J Respir Crit Care Med* 2002;165:277–304.
2. Collard HR, King TE Jr. Demystifying idiopathic interstitial pneumonia. *Arch Intern Med* 2003;163:17–29.
3. Davies HR, Richeldi L, Walters EH. Immunomodulatory agents for idiopathic pulmonary fibrosis. *Cochrane Database of Systematic Reviews* 2006;(3).
4. King TE Jr. Clinical advances in the diagnosis and therapy of the interstitial lung diseases. *Am J Respir Crit Care Med* 2002;172:268–279.
5. Martinez FJ and Keane MP. Update in diffuse parenchymal lung diseases 2005. *Am J Respir Crit Care Med* 2006;173:1066–1071.

ADDITIONAL READING

1. Dermedts M, Behr J, Buhl R, et al. High-dose acetylcysteine in idiopathic pulmonary fibrosis. *N Engl J Med* 2005;353:2229–2242.

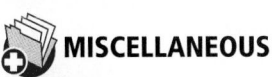 **MISCELLANEOUS**

CODES

ICD9-CM

495 Extrinsic allergic alveolitis
496 Chronic airway obstruction

DIGITALIS TOXICITY

Mario W. Puleo II, MD
Bruce T. Vanderhoff, MD

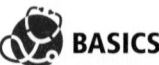 **BASICS**

DESCRIPTION
- May result from digitalis overdosage, hypokalemia, advanced degenerative heart disease with conduction disturbances, or a combination of factors
- Toxicity may develop even when serum levels are within normal range.
- Usual course: Acute; occasionally chronic
- System(s) Affected: Cardiovascular; Gastrointestinal; Nervous

GENERAL PREVENTION
- Store digitalis safely
- Monitor for toxicity
- Fluid plus electrolyte therapy according to need as determined by periodic studies, particularly of potassium level
- If there is a documented recent exposure, consider gastric decontamination by lavage and administer activated charcoal.
- A poison control center or toxicologist might best manage symptomatic overdose patients.
- Educate regarding potential for drug interactions
- Onset of vague symptoms should raise suspicion of toxicity.
- Be aware of conditions that predispose a patient to toxicity, such as heart failure and dehydration.

EPIDEMIOLOGY
- Predominant age: Middle age to elderly (40–75 years)
- Predominant sex: Male = Female

Incidence
In US, it occurs in 5–23% of patients sometime during their therapy.

RISK FACTORS
- Anoxia
- Catecholamines
- Decompensating heart failure
- Diuretics
- Hypercalcemia
- Myocardial infarction
- Recent cardiac surgery
- Renal failure
- Suicide attempt
- Acute and chronic renal failure

Genetics
No known genetic pattern

ETIOLOGY
- Alkalosis
- Amiodarone
- Broad spectrum antibiotics
- Cor pulmonale
- Diltiazem
- Hemodialysis
- Hypernatremia
- Hypokalemia
- Hypomagnesemia
- Hypothyroidism
- Macrolides
- Myocarditis
- Overdosage
- Poisoning with plants containing cardiac glycosides (e.g., oleander, foxglove)
- Procaine
- Quinidine
- Reserpine
- Spironolactone
- Steroids

ASSOCIATED CONDITIONS
- Chronic heart failure
- Acute pulmonary edema

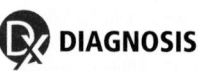 **DIAGNOSIS**

SIGNS AND SYMPTOMS
- Abdominal pain
- Anorexia
- Bilateral central scotomata
- Bizarre mental symptoms in elderly patients
- Blurred vision
- Bradycardia
- Confusion
- Delirium
- Depression
- Diarrhea
- Disorientation
- Drowsiness
- Fatigue
- Hallucinations
- Halos around lights
- Headache
- Hypotension
- Impaired color vision
- Irregular pulse
- Lethargy
- Loss of visual acuity
- Mydriasis
- Nausea
- Neuralgia
- Nightmares
- Personality changes
- Photophobia
- Restlessness
- Vertigo
- Vomiting
- Weakness

TESTS
EKG (Note that no arrhythmia is unique to digitalis toxicity; thus, any sudden change in cardiac rhythm suggests possible toxicity)
- Accelerated junctional rhythms
- Atrial flutter
- Atrial premature contractions
- Atrial tachycardia with atrioventricular block
- Bidirectional tachycardia
- Bundle branch block
- Junctional premature beats
- Sinus bradycardia
- Sinus bradycardia with junctional tachycardia
- Ventricular fibrillation
- Ventricular premature contractions
- Wenckebach's block with junctional premature beats
- P-R changes
- Q-T changes

Lab
- Eosinophilia
- Increased digitalis level, especially if ≥4 ng/mL (≥5.1 nmol/L)
  - Digoxin levels may not correlate with amount taken in acute ingestion
- Potassium
  - Hyperkalemia with acute ingestion
  - Hypokalemia with chronic ingestion of excess or chronic renal failure
- Drugs that may alter lab results: Any digitalis drug
- Disorders that may alter lab results: Many cardiac abnormalities

DIFFERENTIAL DIAGNOSIS
- Heart block
- Renal disease
- Other causes of life-threatening arrhythmia

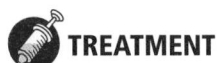 TREATMENT

INITIAL STABILIZATION
Inpatient—coronary care unit

GENERAL MEASURES
- Maintain airways
- Continuous cardiac monitoring
- Discontinue digitalis
- Check serum electrolytes
  - Maintain potassium in high-normal range: Treat hyperkalemia (K >5.5) with NaHCO$_3$ (1 mEq/kg) glucose (0.5 g/kg), and insulin 0.1 U/kg; do not use calcium, as it may worsen ventricular arrhythmias.
- Correct calcium and magnesium abnormalities.
- Avoid quinidine, which may increase serum digoxin levels by displacing digoxin from its binding sites and by decreasing renal and nonrenal excretion.
- Avoid beta-adrenergic blocking drugs and isoproterenol.
- Procainamide may be used.
- If the patient is hemodynamically stable with primarily enhanced vagal activity (1st-degree or 2nd-degree atrioventricular block) and if the peak digitalis effect has been reached, no acute therapy is required.
- Must monitor for 24 hours after ingestion

Diet
Low salt, low fat

Activity
Bed rest with monitoring

 MEDICATION (DRUGS)

First Line
- Fluid plus electrolyte therapy
- Correct acidosis
- Digoxin Immune Fab (Digibind)
  - Indicated for treatment of severe, life-threatening arrhythmias due to digoxin or digitoxin overdosage
  - Obtain a digoxin level before administration; be aware that the digoxin level may be falsely high if measured <6 hours after ingestion.
  - Do not draw another digoxin level for 4 days after digoxin antibody (Digibind) administration, because the drug's half-life is up to 20 hours in patients with normal renal function.
  - For adults and children ingesting an unknown amount of digoxin, administer 10 vials of digoxin Immune Fab in 50 mL of normal saline IV over 30 minutes; however, if there is a life-threatening arrhythmia, give as bolus. Observe response and administer an additional 10 vials if clinically indicated. Watch for volume overload in children.
  - For toxicity during chronic therapy: Adults, 15 vials digoxin Immune Fab in 50 mL normal saline IV over 30 minutes; children, <20 kg, 1 vial should suffice.
- For ventricular arrhythmias use
  - Lidocaine: 50–100 mg IV (for ventricular arrhythmias), repeated in 3–5 minutes if needed, up to a total of 300 mg. Give no more than 300 mg in 1 hour. 1 protocol calls for an initial bolus of lidocaine followed by 20–50 mcg/kg/min infusion for maintenance.
  - Phenytoin: 100 mg q3–5min up to 1,000 mg
  - Magnesium
  - Digoxin Immune Fab (Digibind)
  - Activated charcoal
    - Safe, efficacious, can lower serum digoxin level by 30–40%
    - May require multiple dosing for maximal efficacy, a "gastrointestinal dialysis"
    - Consider especially in acute or overdose settings
- Treat bradycardia and heart block with atropine 0.5–2 mg IV. There is a controversy as to whether pacing should be done, as it is associated with a high complication rate in digoxin intoxicated patients and should be used for those in whom Fab is ineffective.
- Contraindications: Refer to the manufacturer's literature.
- Precautions: Refer to the manufacturer's literature.
- Significant possible interactions: Refer to the manufacturer's literature.

Second Line
Consider atropine, cholestyramine

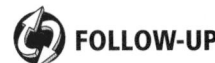 FOLLOW-UP

PROGNOSIS
Recovery likely if patient survives 24 hours

COMPLICATIONS
- Death
- Conduction defects
- Life-threatening rhythm disturbances

PATIENT MONITORING
- Close EKG monitoring, potassium and digitalis levels throughout total treatment
- Monitor kidney function

REFERENCES
1. Beller GA, et al. Digitalis intoxication: a prospective clinical study with serum level correlations. *N Engl J Med.* 1971;284:989.
2. Borron SW, et al. Advances in the management of digoxin toxicity in the older patient. *Drugs and Aging.* 1997;10:18–33.
3. Burroughs Wellcome Co. Digibind product information. *Research Triangle Park, NC;* 1991.
4. Dec GW. Digoxin remains useful in the management of chronic heart failure. *Med Clin North Am.* 2003;87(2):317–337.
5. Dyer S. Plant exposures: Wilderness medicine. *Med Clin North Am.* 2004;22(2); vii, 299–313.
6. Gaudreault P. Activated charcoal revisited. *CPEM.* 2005;6:76–80.
7. Shlipak MG. Renal function, digoxin therapy, and heart failure outcomes; evidence from the digoxin intervention group trial. *J Am Soc Nephrol.* 2004;15(8):2195–2203.
8. Carter BL, et al. Monitoring digoxin therapy in two long-term facilities. *J Am Geriatr Soc.* 1981;29:263.
9. Cauffield JS, et al. The serum digoxin concentration. 10 questions to ask. *Am Fam Phys.* 1997;56:495–503.
10. Duhme DW, et al. Reduction of digoxin toxicity associated with measurement of serum levels. *Ann Int Med.* 1974;80:516.
11. Marcus FI. Diagnosing digitalis intoxication. *Hospital Med.* 1990;7:75.
12. Olson K, et al. *Poisoning and Drug Overdose.* Norwalk, CT: Appleton & Lange, 1994.

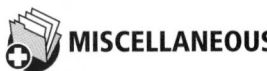 MISCELLANEOUS

See also: Ventricular tachycardia (VT)

CODES

ICD9-CM
972.1 Poisoning by cardiotonic glycosides and drugs of similar action

 See Corresponding Diagnostic Algorithm

D

DIPHTHERIA

Richard Kent Zimmerman, MD, MPH
Gregory A. Poland, MD

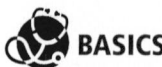 **BASICS**

DESCRIPTION

- Acute respiratory tract infection caused by *Corynebacterium diphtheriae*, usually producing a membranous pharyngitis
- Incubation period 2–5 days. Infection usually occurs during fall and winter in temperate regions. In the tropics, seasonal trends are less distinct.
- Transmission by respiratory route from infected person or carrier. Humans are the only reservoir.
- Several forms occur
  - Membranous pharyngotonsillar diphtheria: The membrane is gray, adheres to the pharynx, and is surrounded by erythema. The underlying mucosa bleeds when the membrane is removed.
  - Nasal diphtheria: Unilateral discharge
  - Obstructive laryngotracheitis: Complication when membrane descends into larynx or bronchial tree. When it breaks up in young children, total obstruction of the airway may occur.
  - Cutaneous diphtheria: Punched-out ulcer covered by gray membrane (particularly in tropics and among homeless). Peaks August–October in southern US.
- System(s) Affected: Cardiovascular; Nervous; Pulmonary; Skin/Exocrine

GENERAL PREVENTION

Prevention is by immunization

- Children age 6 weeks up to 7 years of age should receive doses at 2, 4, 6, and 15–18 months and 4–6 years of age with 0.5 mL of DTaP vaccine IM. If the pertussis component is contraindicated, then pediatric diphtheria tetans (DT) should be used. A booster dose of adult should be given at age 11–12 years.
- Unimmunized persons ≥7 years should receive 2 doses of adult Td 4–8 weeks apart with a 3rd dose 6–12 months later. 0.5 mL of Td should be given. 1 of these doses may be Tdap.
- Subsequently, booster doses with Tdap should be given every 10 years to all individuals without a contraindication. An alternative strategy after the booster at age 11–12 years is a single adult booster at 50 years of age, in addition to following the recommendations for Td boosters in the event of an injury or wound.
- Immunized individuals may develop diphtheria, but their course is milder; immunization protects against the toxin, not infection or microbial carriage in the nose, pharynx, or skin.
- Disinfect all articles in contact with patient
- Close contacts should be cultured and given antibiotic prophylaxis regardless of immunization status. Previously immunized contacts should receive a booster of diphtheria toxoid unless vaccinated within the past 5 years. Unimmunized contacts should begin the series: Erythromycin prophylaxis for 7 days.

EPIDEMIOLOGY

- Predominant age: Children <15 years of age and poorly immunized adults
- Predominant sex: Male = Female

Incidence

In the US: For noncutaneous form, 1.6 in 100 million. Diphtheria is a rare condition in the US today. Fairly recent outbreaks have occurred in the new independent states of the former Soviet Union.

RISK FACTORS

- Crowded living conditions
- Inadequate immunization. In the US, 22–62% of people ages 18–39 years and 41–84% of people >60 years of age lack protective levels of antibody.
- Lower socioeconomic status
- Native Americans
- Alcoholism
- Travelers: Outbreaks have occurred in the Ukraine and Russia.

ETIOLOGY

Corynebacterium diphtheriae

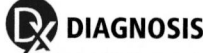 **DIAGNOSIS**

SIGNS AND SYMPTOMS

- Membranous pharyngotonsillar diphtheria
  - Initially, white to yellow membrane, which is easily removed
  - Adherent, whitish-gray, leathery membrane on tonsils or pharynx
  - Removing membrane causes bleeding of mucosa
  - Injected pharynx
  - Membrane may become black due to hemorrhage
  - Sore throat
  - Cervical adenopathy with swelling
  - Malaise and prostration
  - Enlarged, tender cervical and submandibular lymph nodes
  - May progress to edematous, swollen neck (bull neck)
  - Paralysis of soft palate
  - Low-grade fever of 37.8–38.8°C (100–100.9°F)
  - Thrombocytopenia and purpura
- Nasal diphtheria
  - Serosanguineous or seropurulent discharge and excoriations
  - Often discharge is unilateral
  - Often chronic, mild course
- Obstructive laryngotracheitis
  - Hoarseness
  - Croupy cough
  - Progresses to dyspnea and stridor
  - Labored breathing
  - Thick speech
- Cutaneous diphtheria
  - On skin, conjunctiva, vulva, vagina, and penis
  - Primary cutaneous diphtheria: Starts as tender pustule on lower extremity and becomes deep, round, punched-out ulcer covered by grayish membrane
  - Secondary infection of preexisting wound Purulent exudate, partial membrane

TESTS

Lab

- Gram-positive rods in the pathognomonic Chinese character configuration
- Moderate leukocytosis
- Thrombocytopenia
- Transient albuminuria
- In experienced hands, methylene-blue stains can assist in a presumptive diagnosis.
- Culture from nose and throat beneath membrane and have plated on special media; inform lab that diphtheria is suspected
- Should test for toxigenicity of strain
- Serial ECGs and cardiac enzymes to detect myocarditis
- Delayed peripheral nerve conduction velocities
- Culture on Loeffler or tellurite medium is positive in 8–12 hours if not previously treated with an antibiotic. Laboratory must be alerted to use 1 of the special media.
- Drugs that may alter lab results
  - If an antibiotic was used, then 5 days or more may be required for the culture to grow on Loeffler medium.

Diagnostic Procedures/Surgery

- Culture throat or lesions
- Smear of exudate for gram stain

Pathological Findings

- Pleomorphic Gram-positive rods
- Necrotic epithelium
- Hyaline degeneration

DIFFERENTIAL DIAGNOSIS

- Bacterial pharyngitis including group A Streptococcus
- Viral pharyngitis
- Mononucleosis
- ral syphilis
- Candidiasis
- Vincent angina
- Acute epiglottitis

TREATMENT

GENERAL MEASURES

- Appropriate health care
  - Inpatient, initially hospitalized in unit that can monitor cardiac and respiratory status (must act on presumptive diagnosis because therapy cannot wait for culture confirmation)
  - Isolation until cultures on 2 consecutive days are negative. The 1st culture must be taken at least 24 hours after the cessation of antibiotic therapy.
- Have intubation or tracheostomy readily available. For laryngeal disease, laryngoscopy is desirable. Intubation or tracheostomy should be considered early for laryngeal disease.
- Avoid hypnotics and sedatives while monitoring respiratory status.
- Physical therapy in convalescence for range-of-motion exercises to prevent contractions

Diet
Liquid to soft as tolerated

Activity
Rest (for at least 3 weeks, until risk of developing myocarditis has passed)

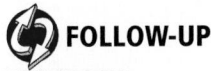 MEDICATION (DRUGS)

First Line
- Both antitoxins and antibiotics are needed for noncutaneous diphtheria.
- Diphtheria antitoxin, equine: Use 20,000–40,000 units of antitoxin for laryngeal or pharyngeal disease of <48 hours' duration; 40,000–60,000 units for nasopharyngeal lesions; 80,000–120,000 units for extensive disease ≥3 days or swelling of the neck (bull neck). Administer antitoxin by IV infusion over 60 minutes and/or by IM injection. Some experts recommend treating cutaneous disease with 20,000–40,000 units of antitoxin, while others doubt its value when there are no signs of systemic disease. Antitoxin is obtained from the US Centers for Disease Control and Prevention.
- Erythromycin parenterally or PO, 40–50 mg/kg/d; maximum of 2 g/d for 14 days
- Precautions
  - Equine antitoxin: 7% of patients are sensitive to equine antitoxin and need desensitization. Always test for hypersensitivity to antitoxin prior to its administration.
  - 1st, a drop of 1:100 dilution of antitoxin is placed on a scratch on the forearm. If negative, an intradermal skin test is done with 1:1,000 dilution (0.02 mL). A positive reaction is the development of urticaria within 20 minutes of injection.
  - If no reaction to 1st intradermal, then repeat test with a 1:100 dilution
  - If the person has a negative history for animal allergy, has not previously received animal serum and had a negative scratch test, then 1:100 dilution may be used initially.

Second Line
- Penicillin G IM, 100,000–150,000 U/kg/d q.i.d. up to 600,000 U/d
- DL-carnitine 100 mg/kg/d b.i.d. PO in children for 4 days in myocarditis (experimental)

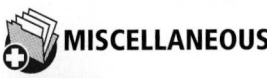 FOLLOW-UP

PROGNOSIS
- <5% mortality rate
- Prognosis guarded until recovery
- In convalescing patients, 5–10% persistence in nasopharynx

COMPLICATIONS
- Myocarditis (10–25%) may occur early
- Cranial and peripheral neuropathy (2–6 weeks after onset)
- ECG abnormalities in 2/3 of patients, including bundle branch block, tachycardia, atrial or ventricular fibrillation, and extrasystoles
- Right-sided heart failure
- Local paralysis of soft palate and posterior pharynx demonstrated by regurgitation of fluids through the nares
- Peripheral and cranial neuropathy affecting primarily motor nerve functions. Motor dysfunction starts proximally and extends distally. It usually resolves slowly.
- Syndrome like Guillain-Barré

PATIENT MONITORING
- ECG, cardiac enzymes, and respiratory status. Serial ECG 2–3 times per week for 4–6 weeks to detect myocarditis
- Elimination of the organism should be documented by 3 negative cultures at least 24 hours apart. The 1st culture should be at least 24 hours after the completion of antimicrobial therapy.
- During convalescence, patients should be immunized against diphtheria, because infection does not necessarily confer immunity.

REFERENCES
1. Atkinson W, Hamborsky J, Wolfe S, eds. *Epidemiology and Prevention of Vaccine-Preventable Diseases (Pink Book)*. 9th ed. Washington, DC: Public Health Foundation; 2006.
2. Red Book Report of the Committee on Infectious Diseases, 2007. Elk Grove Village, IL: American Academy of Pediatrics; 2007.

MISCELLANEOUS

CODES

ICD9-CM
- 032.0 Faucial diphtheria
- 032.1 Nasopharyngeal diphtheria
- 032.2 Anterior nasal diphtheria
- 032.3 Laryngeal diphtheria
- 032.81 Conjunctival diphtheria
- 032.82 Diphtheritic myocarditis
- 032.83 Diphtheritic peritonitis
- 032.84 Diphtheritic cystitis
- 032.85 Cutaneous diphtheria
- 032.89 Other specified diphtheria, other
- 032.9 Diphtheria, unspecified

PATIENT TEACHING
Explain aspects of illness and complications.

D

DISSEMINATED INTRAVASCULAR COAGULATION (DIC)

Jan Cerny, MD

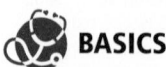 **BASICS**

DESCRIPTION

- Massive systemic intravascular activation of coagulation, leading to widespread deposition of fibrin in the circulation. Contributes to multiple organ failure by compromising the blood supply. Ongoing consumption of platelets and coagulation proteins may induce bleeding.
- Occurring in complications of obstetrics (e.g., abruptio placentae, fetus retention), infection (especially Gram-negative), malignancy (metastatic tumor or leukemia), trauma, and other severe illnesses.
- System(s) Affected: Hematologic/Lymphatic/Immunologic
- Synonym(s): Consumptive coagulopathy; DIC

GENERAL PREVENTION
No preventive measures known

EPIDEMIOLOGY
Incidence
Unknown

Prevalence
- Predominant age: None
- Predominant sex: Male = Female

RISK FACTORS
- Pregnancy
- Prostatic surgery
- Head injury
- Inflammatory states

ETIOLOGY
- Coagulation disorder due to widespread activation of clotting mechanism.
- Systemic formation of fibrin is the result of the simultaneous coexistence of
  - Increased thrombin generation
  - Suppression of the physiologic anticoagulant pathways
  - Impaired fibrinolysis
  - Activation of the inflammatory pathway
- Causes can be classified as acute or chronic, systemic or localized
  - Obstetric complications
  - Severe infection
  - Neoplasms (acute promyelocytic leukemia)
  - Intravascular hemolysis
  - Vascular disorders; thrombosis
  - Snake bite
  - Massive tissue injury
  - Trauma
  - Hypoxia
  - Liver disease
  - Infant and adult respiratory distress syndrome
  - Purpura fulminans
  - Thermal injury

ASSOCIATED CONDITIONS
Thromboembolic phenomena is associated with venous thrombosis, thrombotic vegetations on the aortic heart valve, arterial emboli, neonatal purpura fulminans (homozygous protein C or protein S deficiency).

ALERT
Pediatric Considerations
Neonatal purpura fulminans is associated with disseminated intravascular coagulation and protein C or protein S deficiency (homozygous).

 DIAGNOSIS

SIGNS AND SYMPTOMS
- Bleeding from at least 3 unrelated sites is suggestive of DIC.
- Epistaxis
- Gingival bleeding
- Mucosal bleeding
- Hemoptysis
- Hematemesis
- Metrorrhagia
- Retinal hemorrhages
- Fever
- Confusion
- Disorientation
- Stupor
- Cough
- Dyspnea
- Localized rales
- Tachypnea
- Pleural friction rub
- Blood in stool
- Hematuria
- Oliguria
- Anuria
- Skin petechiae
- Thrombosis
- Skin petechiae
- Purpura
- Ecchymosis
- Skin hemorrhagic necrosis
- Peripheral cyanosis

History
- Symptoms related to the underlying disease process.
- History of blood loss or hypovolemia.
- Symptoms of large-vessel thrombosis, such as deep venous thrombosis, and of microvascular thrombosis (e.g., renal failure).

Physical Exam
- Acute DIC: Findings of underlying disease process; petechiae on the soft palate and legs from thrombocytopenia and ecchymosis at the venipuncture sites and traumatized areas
- Chronic DIC: Signs of venous thromboembolism may be present.

TESTS
Lab
- Thrombocytopenia
  - Increased partial thromboplastin time
  - Increased prothrombin time
  - Increased thrombin time
  - Decreased fibrinogen (serial levels)
  - Increased fibrin degradation product
  - Decreased antithrombin III
  - Positive D-Dimer assay
  - Increased bleeding time
  - Schistocytes in peripheral blood
  - Microangiopathic hemolytic anemia
- Leukocytosis
  - Increased lactate dehydrogenase
  - Increased blood urea nitrogen
  - Decreased factor V
  - Decreased or increased factor VIII (can help differentiate DIC vs. liver failure)
  - Decreased factor X
  - Decreased factor XIII
  - Hemoglobinemia
  - Hematuria
  - Guaiac-positive stools
  - Decreased protein C

Imaging
Chest radiograph: Bilateral perihilar soft density

DIFFERENTIAL DIAGNOSIS
- Fulminant liver failure or massive hepatic necrosis
- Vitamin K deficiency
- Thrombotic thrombocytopenic purpura
- Hemolytic-uremic syndrome
- Heparin-induced thrombocytopenia
- Primary fibrinolysis
- HELLP syndrome in pregnancy (hemolysis, elevated liver function, and low platelets)

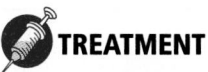

TREATMENT

GENERAL MEASURES
- Appropriate health care: Inpatient
- Treat underlying condition (e.g., evacuation of uterus in abruptio placenta): Broad-spectrum antibiotics for Gram-negative sepsis
- Replacement of blood loss
  - Fresh frozen plasma
  - Platelet concentrates
  - Cryoprecipitate or fibrinogen concentrates
- Anticoagulants remain very controversial
- Restoration of anticoagulant pathways
  - Antithrombin III in selected cases, but also controversial
  - Recombinant human activated protein C (benefit only in patients at high risk of death from sepsis).
  - Activated factor VII use remains controversial

Diet
No special diet

Activity
As tolerated

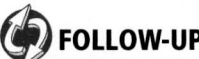

MEDICATION (DRUGS)

First Line
- Treat underlying disorder.
- For selected cases use recombinant human activated protein C.
- Broad-spectrum antibiotics for sepsis
- Significant possible interactions: Refer to the manufacturer's literature.

FOLLOW-UP

PROGNOSIS
Related to severity of cause

COMPLICATIONS
- Acute renal failure
- Shock
- Cardiac tamponade
- Hemothorax
- Intracerebral hematoma
- Gangrene and loss of digits

PATIENT MONITORING
- Monitor closely until much improved.
- Serial coagulation tests and fibrinogen levels.

REFERENCES

1. Isselbacher KJ, et al, eds. Harrison's Principles of Internal Medicine, 13th ed. New York: McGraw-Hill, 1994.
2. Stites DP, Stobo JD, Wells JV, eds. Basic and Clinical Immunology, 8th ed. New York: Appleton & Lange, 1994.
3. Franchini M, Lippi G, Manzato F. Recent acquisitions in the pathophysiology, diagnosis and treatment of disseminated intravascular coagulation. *Thromb J*. 2006;4:4.
4. Vincent JL, Bernard GR, Beale R, et al. Drotrecogin alfa (activated) treatment in severe sepsis from the global open-label trial ENHANCE: further evidence for survival and safety and implications for early treatment. *Crit Care Med*. 2005;33(10):2266–2277.

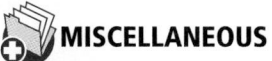

MISCELLANEOUS

CODES

ICD9-CM
286.6 Defibrination syndrome

PATIENT TEACHING

Recommend the following to patients: Moore S, ed. Griffith's Instructions for Patients, 6th ed. Philadelphia: WB Saunders, 1999.

See Corresponding Diagnostic Algorithm

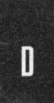

D

DISSOCIATIVE DISORDERS

Moshe S. Torem, MD, FAPA

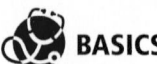 **BASICS**

DESCRIPTION

A sudden change in state of consciousness, identity, motor behavior, thoughts, feelings, and perception of external reality to such an extent that these functions do not operate congruently. Many pathologic symptoms can be found, but the patient experiences dysphoria, suffering, and maladaptive functioning.

- Disorders include: Dissociative amnesia, Dissociative fugue, Dissociative identity disorder, Depersonalization disorder, Dissociative disorder not otherwise specified. Authors may include somnambulism (sleep-walking disorder), conversion reactions, pseudo-epilepsy, and (in some cultures) a variety of possession syndromes.
- System(s) Affected: Nervous
- Synonym(s): Hysterical neurosis, dissociative type; Ganser syndrome

ALERT

Geriatric Considerations
Decrease in dissociative disorders; medication side effects more likely

Pediatric Considerations
Suspect abuse or neglect

GENERAL PREVENTION
- Child abuse prevention via parent education and community agency intervention
- Crisis intervention following individual trauma or disasters for prevention of chronic morbidity/disability

EPIDEMIOLOGY
- Predominant age: Adolescents and young to middle-age adults; rare as a new illness in elderly. If untreated, may linger from childhood into adult and old age
- Predominant sex: Female > Male (2:1)

Prevalence
- Transient symptoms of depersonalization or derealization in the general population are common with a lifetime prevalence rate of 26–74% with 31–66% occurring at the time of a traumatic event. 8–10% of the general population, are psychiatrically ill. As many as 70% of young adults report short periods of dissociative experiences that are self-limiting and resolve spontaneously.

RISK FACTORS
- Exposure to neglect, abuse, and trauma in childhood
- Tendency to cope with life stresses by excessively using an escape mechanism of daydreaming and/or dissociation
- Physical, emotional, verbal, or sexual abuse in childhood
- Sudden and severe trauma or threat to one's psychologic or physical integrity
- Sudden and unexpected exposure to watching others being killed or severely injured (as in an industrial or car accident)
- A preponderance of coping with trauma and internal or interpersonal conflicts by the use of dissociation
- Psychologic/social support to cope with the trauma/abuse was unavailable.

ETIOLOGY
Uncertain

ASSOCIATED CONDITIONS
See "Risk Factors"

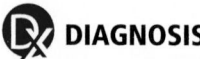 **DIAGNOSIS**

SIGNS AND SYMPTOMS
- All disorders share symptoms that
  - Cause significant distress or impairment in social, occupational, or other important areas of functioning
  - Are not due to the direct physiologic effects of a substance (e.g., drug of abuse, a medication) or a general medical condition (e.g., temporal lobe epilepsy)
- Dissociative amnesia
  - 1 or more episodes of inability to recall important personal information that is too extensive to be explained by ordinary forgetfulness
  - Not occurring during another psychiatric illness and not due to effects of chemical substance (drug abuse or medication)
  - Not due to a neurologic or other medical condition (e.g., head trauma)
- Dissociative fugue
  - Sudden unexpected travel away from home or one's customary place of work with an inability to recall one's past
  - Confusion about personal identity or assumption of a new identity (partial or complete)
  - Above symptoms do not occur exclusively during course of dissociative identity disorder.
  - Symptoms cause significant distress or impairment in social, occupational, or other important areas of functioning with activities of daily living.
- Dissociative identity disorder
  - Presence of 2 or more distinct identities or personality states (each with its own relatively enduring pattern of perceiving, relating to, and thinking about environment and self)
  - At least 2 of these identities or personality states recurrently take control of the person's behavior.
  - Inability to recall important personal information (too extensive to be explained by ordinary forgetfulness)
  - Reports of time distortion, lapses, and discontinuities
  - Experiencing voices from inside one's head
  - Chronic headaches
  - History of severe emotional or physical abuse as a child
  - Referring to self as "he/she," "we," "us"
  - Eating disorders
  - Flashbacks
  - Feelings of derealization
  - Feelings of depersonalization
  - Amnesia about important childhood events
  - Personal objects and belongings that cannot be accounted for
  - Disowning unrecalled behaviors
  - Different handwriting styles
  - Different signatures and names found in personal diary
  - Sudden mood changes
  - Sudden behavioral changes (e.g., from adult to young child)
  - Episodes of déjà vu
  - Feeling controlled by "another person" from within
  - Self-inflicted violence such as wrist cutting

- Depersonalization disorder
  - Persistent or recurrent experiences of feeling detached from, and as if one is an outside observer of, one's mental processes or body (e.g., feeling like one is in a dream)
  - During the depersonalization experience, reality testing remains intact.
  - The depersonalization experience does not occur exclusively during the course of another mental disorder, such as schizophrenia, panic disorder, acute stress disorder, or another dissociative disorder.
- Dissociative disorder, not otherwise specified Predominant feature is a dissociative symptom (e.g., a disruption in the usually integrated functions of consciousness, memory, identity, or perception of the environment) that does not meet the criteria for any specific dissociative disorder.
  - Clinical presentations similar to dissociative identity disorder that fail to meet the full criteria for this disorder. Examples include (a) there are not 2 or more distinct personality states or (b) amnesia for important personal information does not occur.
  - Derealization unaccompanied by depersonalization in adults
  - States of dissociation that occur in individuals who have been subjected to periods of prolonged and intense coercive persuasion (e.g., brainwashing, thought reform, or indoctrination while captive)
  - Dissociative trance disorder: Single or episodic disturbances in the state of consciousness, identity, or memory that are indigenous to particular locations and cultures. Dissociative trance involves narrowing of awareness of immediate surroundings or stereotyped behaviors or movements that are experienced as being beyond one's control.
  - Possession trance: Involves replacement of the customary sense of personality identity, attributed to the influence of a spirit or power and associated with stereotyped "involuntary" movements or amnesia
  - Loss of consciousness, stupor, or coma not attributed to a general medical condition
  - Ganser syndrome: The giving of approximate answers to questions (e.g., "2 + 2 = 5") when not associated with dissociative amnesia or dissociative fugue

TESTS
- EEG to rule out epilepsy and sleep disorders
- Polysomnogram to rule out sleep apnea

Lab
- Toxicology screening may be helpful.
- Drugs that may alter lab results: Lithium carbonate may produce hypothyroidism.
- Disorders that may alter lab results
  - Patients (especially those with dissociative identity disorder) may present with medical oddities such as fast healing of broken bones, x-rays resembling brain atrophy, brain infarcts, lupus, or abnormal pulmonary function tests.
  - A variety of symptoms (e.g., blurred vision, nausea and vomiting, rapid heart beat, palpitation, extreme bradycardia, urinary frequency and urgency, and extreme changes in levels of blood glucose) may lead to erroneous diagnosis.

Imaging
CT scan and MRI of the head to rule out multiple infarct dementia, brain tumors, and some forms of encephalopathy

Diagnostic Procedures/Surgery
- Neuropsychologic testing to rule out learning disabilities and cognitive deficits due to early dementia or borderline mental retardation
- Psychologic testing to identify specific disorders, personality structure, and dynamics
- Dissociation scales help assess the tendency to dissociate in daily living activities.
- Amobarbital (Amytal) interviews (narcoanalysis) and special interviews under hypnosis are useful in selected cases.
- Clinician reviews patient's diary for handwriting and signature changes

DIFFERENTIAL DIAGNOSIS
- Other mental/CNS disorder: Schizophrenia, depression, anxiety disorder, mania, obsessive/compulsive disorder, identity disorder, phobic disorders, and eating disorders
- Other: Extreme sensory deprivation, epilepsy; early phases of dementia, encephalitis, head trauma, migraine, cerebral vascular disease, brain tumors
- Endocrinopathy: Hypoglycemia, hypothyroidism, and hyperthyroidism
- Miscellaneous: Huntington disease, carbon monoxide poisoning, mescaline intoxication, botulism, and hyperventilation
- Obstructive sleep apnea, nocturnal myoclonus

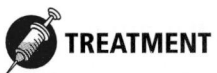

TREATMENT
INITIAL STABILIZATION
- Outpatient, individual psychotherapy
- At times of crisis: Intensive hospital-based treatment (as a protection for patients with suicidal or homicidal impulses, and/or self-inflicted violence)
- Use inpatient care to verify diagnosis with special tests and begin treatment program that continues on outpatient basis.
- NOTE: Treatment emphasis should be on progress in the adaptive functions with daily living activities, symptom alleviation, ego strengthening, and preventing regressions.

GENERAL MEASURES
- Individual psychotherapy plus behavior modification, narcoanalysis and narcosynthesis, and hypnoanalysis and hypnotherapy
- Adjuncts: Support groups, group therapy, expressive art therapy, occupational and recreational therapy
- Bibliotherapy and graphotherapy are useful.

Activity
Based on patient's condition

MEDICATION (DRUGS)

First Line
- No medications are specifically curative. The following have been helpful
  - Antidepressants: Depression
  - Benzodiazepines: Anxiety and insomnia
  - Propranolol 80–400 mg/d: Flashbacks and other dissociative symptoms
  - Neuroleptics (in low doses): Self-abusive behavior. Haloperidol 2–5 mg/d; perphenazine 4–16 mg/d or risperidone 1–4 mg/d
  - Severe agitation, droperidol 1–5 mg IM (effective in producing calm sleep/stopping agitation)
  - Mood swings, in dissociative disorders, do not respond to the use of lithium carbonate, carbamazepine, or valproic acid unless the patient has comorbid bipolar disorder.
- Precautions
  - Short-acting benzodiazepines abuse potential
  - Overdose/suicide potential with tricyclic antidepressants (TCAs)
  - Very low doses of neuroleptics can be used without producing tardive dyskinesia (try to avoid higher doses)
  - Risperidone may be associated with hyperglycemia and ketoacidosis.
- Significant possible interactions
  - Avoid monoamine oxidase inhibitors with TCAs or selective serotonin reuptake inhibitors.

Second Line
- Anxiety symptoms
  - Buspirone (Buspar) 30–80 mg/d for anxiety
- Obsessive compulsive symptoms
  - Clomipramine (Anafranil) 75–200 mg/d
  - Fluvoxamine (Luvox) 100–300 mg/d
  - Fluoxetine (Prozac) 20–80 mg/d
  - Paroxetine (Paxil) 20–60 mg/d
  - Sertraline (Zoloft) 50–200 mg/d
- Alternative neuroleptics have recently been found useful for the control of self-inflicted violence
  - Risperidone (Risperdal) 0.5–4 mg/d
  - Olanzapine (Zyprexa) 2.5–10 mg/d
  - Quetiapine (Seroquel) 25–200 mg/d
  - Aripiprazole (Abilify) 5–15 mg/d
  - Ziprasidone (Geodon) 40–100 mg/d

FOLLOW-UP

PROGNOSIS
- Ranges from spontaneous improvement, in cases of dissociative amnesia, dissociative fugue, and depersonalization disorder, to acute and chronic morbidity in others
- Without treatment, a dissociative identity disorder patient may have a healthy functioning facade, with episodes of depression, confusion, mood swings, etc. With age, the intensity/frequency of dissociative experiences may decrease and crystallize around 1–2 major personality states.
- Effective treatment produces partial or full recovery for many patients.

COMPLICATIONS
Self-inflicted violence, suicide attempts, substance abuse, and chemical dependency

PATIENT MONITORING
- Outpatients: Psychotherapy (1–4 hours per week) to avoid hospitalization
- Inpatients: More intensive treatment (e.g., daily psychotherapy)

REFERENCES

1. American Psychiatric Association. *Diagnostic and Statistical Manual of Mental Disorders*. 4th ed. Washington, DC: American Psychiatric Association. 1994:477–491.
2. Chefetz RA. Reassociating psychoanalysis and dissociation: A review of *Dissociation of Trauma: Theory, Phenomenology, and Technique*. *Contemp Psychoanal*. 2004;40(1):123–133.
3. Chu JA, et al. Memories of childhood abuse; dissociation, amnesia, and corroboration. *Amer J Psychiatry*. 1999;156:749–755.
4. Dell PF. Dissociative phenomenology of dissociative identity disorder. *J Nerv Ment Dis*. 2002;190(1):1–15.
5. Fine CG, Berkowitz AS. The wreathing protocol: The imbrication of hypnosis and EMDR in the treatment of dissociative identity disorder and other dissociative responses. *Amer J Clin Hypn*. 2001;43(3–4):275–290.
6. Kluft RP, Fine CG. *Clinical Perspectives on Multiple Personality Disorder*. Washington, DC: American Psychiatric Press; 1993.
7. Lipsanen T, et al. Visual distortions and dissociation. *J Nerv Ment Dis*. 1999;187: 109–112.
8. Maldonado JR, Butler LD, Spiegal D. Treatment for dissociative disorders. In: Natham P, Gorman JM, eds. *A Guide to Treatments That Work*. 2nd ed. London, England: Oxford University; 2002; 463–496.
9. Markowitsch HJ. Psychogenic amnesia. *Neuroimage*. 2003;20[Suppl 1]:S132–S138.
10. Meares R. The contribution of Hughlings Jackson to an understanding of dissociation. *Amer J Psychiatr*. 1999;156(12):1850–1855.
11. Merckelbach H, Muris P. The causal link between self-reported trauma and dissociation: A critical review. *Behav Res Ther*. 2001;39(3):245–254.
12. Michelson LK, Ray WJ, eds. *Handbook of Dissociation*. New York: Plenum; 1996.
13. Moskowitz A. Dissociation and violence: A review of the literature. *Trauma Violence Abuse*. 2004;5(1):21–46.
14. Nijenhuis ER. Somatoform dissociation: Major symptoms of dissociative disorders. *J Trauma Dissoc*. 2000;1(4):7–29.

15. Putnam FW. *Diagnosis and Treatment of Multiple Personality Disorder*. New York, NY: Guilford; 1989.
16. Spiegel D. Trauma, dissociation, and memory. *Ann NY Acad Sci*. 1997;821:225–237.
17. Spitzer C, Spelsberg B, Grabe HJ, Mundt B, Freyberger HJ. Dissociative experiences and psychopathology in conversion disorders. *J Psychosom Res*. 1999;46:291–294.
18. Steinberg M. *Handbook for the Assessment of Dissociation: A Clinical Guide*. Washington, DC: American Psychiatric Press; 1995.
19. Steinberg M. Hughlings Jackson and dissociation. *Amer J Psychiatry*. 2001;158(1):145–146.
20. Steinberg M. Updating diagnostic criteria for dissociative disorders: Learning from scientific advances. 2001;2(1):59–63.
21. Torem MS. Medications in the treatment of dissociative identity disorder. In: Spira JL, ed. *Treating Dissociative Identity Disorder*. San Francisco, CA: Jossey-Bass; 1996:99–132.

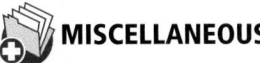 **MISCELLANEOUS**

ICD9-CM

- 300.15 Dissociative disorder or reaction, unspecified
- 301.50 Histrionic personality disorder, unspecified

PATIENT TEACHING

- Self-hypnosis, relaxation exercises, and guided imagery
- Encourage patients to read about their condition and be inspired by others who have been diagnosed, treated, and recovered
  – Sizemore C. *A Mind of My Own*. New York, NY: W. Morrow; 1989.

 See Patient Handout on CD

D

DIVERTICULAR DISEASE

Brett Hassan, MD

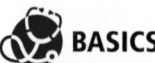 **BASICS**

DESCRIPTION

- Diverticulosis of colon and its varied clinical consequences
  - Diverticula develop in countries where people eat a low-fiber diet and are much more prevalent in western societies.
- Diverticula of colon: Sac-like protrusion of the abdominal wall at the sites of blood vessel penetration (1)
  - In western societies, 90% are found in the sigmoid colon, while right-sided colonic involvement is more common in Asian populations (1)
  - Diverticula increase in numbers with age, but risk of complication other than bleeding does not (2)
- Diverticular hemorrhage: Occurs in 3–5% of patients with diverticular disease (1)
  - Accounts for >40% of lower gastrointestinal (GI) bleeds (1)
- Diverticulitis: The most usual clinical complication of diverticular disease, affects 10–25% of patients, an abscess or peridiverticular inflammation initiated by the rupture of a mucosal microscopic abscess into the mesentery; this can progress into complicated diverticulitis
- Complicated diverticulitis includes associated abscess, perforation, fistula, or stricture (2)
- Uncomplicated can be prevented from becoming complicated by early diagnosis and treatment (2)
  - Develops in about 5% of subjects with diverticulosis each year
- System(s) Affected: Gastrointestinal

GENERAL PREVENTION

High-fiber diet, psyllium, agar, methylcellulose

EPIDEMIOLOGY

Incidence
- 2,200–3,000/100,000 (diverticulitis)
- Diverticula in up to 20% in general population, but increases progressively with age reaching up to 2/3 of people by the 8th decade (1)
- Yearly mortality rate: 2.5/100,000 per year (3)

Prevalence
- Predominant age: < 10% of people < 40 years old, 2/3 of people in their 80s have diverticuli (1)
- Predominant sex: Male = Female

ALERT

Pediatric Considerations
Very rare

Geriatric Considerations
- More common
- May sometimes be difficult to diagnose

RISK FACTORS
- Age >40
- Low-fiber diet
- Sedentary lifestyle (3)
- Previous diverticulitis
- Number of diverticula in the colon

Genetics
No known genetic pattern

ETIOLOGY
Causes are speculative/not clearly proven

- Increased colonic wall resistance due to connective tissue changes (1)
- Disordered colonic motility causing increased luminal pressures (1)
- Low-fiber diet: Increases segmentation and causes higher intraluminal pressure
- Defects in colonic wall strength
- Bleeding is caused by medial thinning of the vasa recta and weakening of the artery resulting in rupture. Causes of these changes are not known (1)

ASSOCIATED CONDITIONS
Often occurs in conjunction with spastic colon

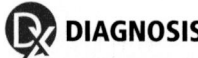 **DIAGNOSIS**

SIGNS AND SYMPTOMS

- Diverticulosis: 2 types: Asymptomatic and symptomatic
  - 80–85% of patients remain asymptomatic. Of the 15–20% with symptoms, 1–2% will need hospitalization, and 0.5% will need surgery (3)
  - Pain: Dull, colicky, mostly in left lower quadrant, can be worse after eating, some relief following bowel movement or passage of flatus
  - Diarrhea or constipation
  - Abdomen may be distended and tympanitic
  - Absent signs of peritoneal inflammation
  - Melena, hematochezia if diverticula bleed
- Diverticulitis: Uncomplicated and complicated
  - Pain: Acute onset, mostly localized in left lower quadrant; prominently associated with tenderness in same region.
  - Fever with chills as severity increases
  - Anorexia, nausea, or vomiting
  - Constipation or diarrhea
  - Rebound tenderness, involuntary guarding, or boardlike rigidity
  - Palpable mass that is tender, firm, or fixed
  - Abdomen distended and tympanitic
  - Bowel sounds depressed or could be exaggerated if obstruction ensues
  - Dysuria, frequency if bladder involved
  - Pneumaturia, fecaluria if colovesical fistula develops
  - Rectal exam may reveal tenderness, induration, or mass in the cul-de-sac
  - Enterocutaneous, enterovaginal, and perirectal fistulae may be the initial manifestation

TESTS
Lab
- WBC normal in diverticulosis, elevated with immature polymorphs in diverticulitis
- Hemoglobin low, if bleeding is a symptom
- Sedimentation rate elevated in diverticulitis
- Urine analysis may be abnormal with microscopic pyuria, hematuria, pneumaturia, or fecaluria possibly suggesting fistula formation (2)
- Urine culture: Persistent infection in colovesical fistula
- Blood culture: Positive in diverticulitis with generalized peritonitis
- Drugs that may alter lab results
  - Steroids
  - Other immunosuppressive drugs
- Disorders that may alter lab results
  - Severe malnutrition

Imaging
- Plain film abdomen supine and upright; useful in peritonitis and perforation
- Barium enema: Should be avoided in diverticulitis due to risk of extravasation into the peritoneum (2); has been used for diagnosis of diverticulosis
- Water-soluble contrast enema can be used and can show diverticulosis, mucosal thickening or spasm (2)
- Diverticula may be seen on endoscopy, but less sensitive than Barium enema, and endoscopy should be avoided in diverticulitis due to risk of perforation (2)
- Patients with suspected diverticulitis should have a CT scan with IV and oral contrast to rule out complicated disease. (2)[C] CT could also show fat streaking or diverticula (2)
- CT scan can show degree of acute perforation and assist in surgical planning (4)
- Angiography: Diagnostic as well as therapeutic in diverticular bleeding
- Fistulograms
- Other imaging studies
  - 99 mTc labeled RBC scan for bleeding (rarely used) and/or angiography (2)
  - Gallium or indium labeled leukocytes to localize abscess (rarely used)

Diagnostic Procedures/Surgery
- Colonoscopy and flexible sigmoidoscopy: Helpful in diagnosis of diverticulosis and extremely valuable in differential diagnosis to prove or rule out cancer; do not perform in acute diverticulitis due to risk of perforation
  - Ulcerative or ischemic colitis can uniformly be diagnosed by these modalities.
- Cystoscopy: In colovesical fistula

Pathological Findings
- Surgical and autopsy studies show colonic muscular hypertrophy (4)
- Electron microscopy shows increased elastin content in the taenia coli (4)
- Multiple diverticula: Spastic colon diverticulosis, simple massed diverticulosis, right-sided diverticulosis
- Solitary diverticulum: Giant sigmoid diverticulum
- Diverticulitis: Inflammation, necrosis, and perforation
- Diverticulitis: Earliest stage, rupture of a mucosal abscess into mesentery; does not start with obstruction of the neck as does appendicitis

DIFFERENTIAL DIAGNOSIS
- Irritable bowel syndrome
- Lactose intolerance
- Carcinoma of distal colon
- Complicated ulcer disease
- Ulcerative colitis, Crohn disease
- Gall bladder disease
- Incarcerated hernia
- Angiodysplasia (for rectal bleed)
- Ischemic or infectious colitis
- Acute appendicitis
- Ectopic gestation when pregnancy is suspected
- Other gynecologic and urologic disorders (5)

ALERT
Pediatric Considerations
- Rule out ectopic pregnancy.
- Careful selection of antibiotic use in pregnant women due to teratogenic effects of certain medications.

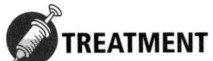

TREATMENT
GENERAL MEASURES
- Appropriate health care
  - Diverticulosis: Outpatient with fiber supplements to soften stools
  - Outpatient diverticulitis: Pain, tenderness, leukocytosis, but no toxicity or peritoneal signs; treat with antibiotics
  - ~1–2% of subjects require hospitalization (3) for toxicity, septicemia, peritonitis, or failure of the symptoms to be resolved in a few days; ~50% of these patients will require surgery.
  - Toxic patients require hospitalization and IV antibiotics at least until there is a positive response.
- General measures
  - IV fluids, analgesics, nasogastric suction
  - 0.5% of patients may require surgery (3)

Diet
- NPO during acute diverticulitis; progress to fluids, then to high fiber as normal bowel function returns
- Patients with known diverticulosis should eat a high-fiber diet to prevent symptomatic disease. (5)[C]
- High-fiber diet has yet to show role in treatment, but role in prevention is well established (6)

Activity
Fully active in diverticulosis, restricted activity in diverticulitis

MEDICATION (DRUGS)

First Line

- Diverticulosis
  - Pain syndromes may be treated with antispasmodics or short-acting narcotics high-fiber diet
  - Constipation and diarrhea: Manage as indicated for irritable bowel disease
- Diverticulitis
  - Oral antibiotics for outpatient treatment of mild disease: Cover for anaerobes and Gram-negative rods with metronidazole (Flagyl) and Augmentin, a quinolone, or Bactrim (5)[C]
  - More severe cases in hospitals use IV antibiotics: Flagyl or clindamycin along with an aminoglycoside, monobactam, or 3rd-generation cephalosporin (5)[C]
  - Diverticular bleeding
  - Vasopressin 0.2–0.3 units/min through selective intra-arterial catheter; used when bleeding demonstrated at angiography
- Contraindications
  - Hypersensitivity reaction
- Precautions
  - Avoid morphine and other opiates that may increase intraluminal pressure, except for Demerol.
  - Watch for renal toxicity and ototoxicity with aminoglycosides.
- Significant possible interactions: Refer to the manufacturer's profile of each drug.

Second Line

Tobramycin and metronidazole, 3rd-generation cephalosporins

SURGERY

- Indication for emergent surgery: Generalized peritonitis, uncontrolled sepsis, visceral perforation, colonic obstruction or acute deterioration (2)
- Surgery other than for emergent reasons is controversial.
- Elective surgery after acute diverticulitis: After a 1st bout of diverticulitis, there is a 33% chance in a 2nd bout. After a 2nd bout, there is a 66% chance of a 3rd bout (7), so patients should be referred for surgical consultation after the 2nd time (5)
- Large abscesses are usually drained radiologically and, when resolved, the most involved segment of the colon resected (2)

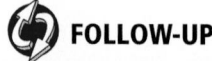 ## FOLLOW-UP

PROGNOSIS

- The prognosis is good with early detection and treatment of the complications.
- Risk of diverticulitis recurrence increases with each bout. (2)
- Of those with diverticular bleeding, re-bleeding occurs in up to 6% of patients (1)

COMPLICATIONS

- Hemorrhage
- Perforation
- Peritonitis
- Bowel obstruction
- Abscess: Paracolic, subhepatic, subphrenic
- Fistula: Colovesical, colovaginal, colocutaneous

PATIENT MONITORING

- Some physicians would not do any invasive studies; others have recommended a repeat barium enema every 3 years if the symptoms are infrequent or absent, or following corrective surgery.
- Patients with symptomatic diverticular disease should have a colonoscopy to exclude underlying malignancy. (5)[C]

REFERENCES

1. Stollman N, Raskin B. Seminar: Diverticular Disease of the Colon. *The Lancet*. 2004;363:631–639.
2. Boulos, PB. Complicated diverticulosis. *Best Pract Res Cl Ga*. 2002;16(4):649–662.
3. Colecchia A, et al. Diverticular disease of the colon: New perspectives in symptom development and treatment. *World J Gastroentero*. 2003;9(7):1385–1389.
4. Lohrmann, C. et al. CT in acute perforated sigmoid diverticulitis. *Eur J Radiol*. 2005;56:78–83.
5. Salzman H, Lillie D. Diverticular disease: Diagnosis and treatment. *Am Fam Physician*. 2005;72(7):1229–1235.
6. Murray CDR, Emmanuel, AV. Medical Management of Diverticular Disease. *Best Pract Res Cl Ga*. 2002;16(4):611–620.
7. Janes S, Meagher A. Frizelle FA. Elective surgery after acute diverticulitis. *Brit J Surg*. 2005;92:133–142.

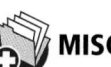 **MISCELLANEOUS**

See also: Irritable bowel syndrome

CODES

ICD9-CM

- 562.10 Diverticulosis of colon (without mention of hemorrhage)
- 562.11 Diverticulitis of colon (without mention of hemorrhage)

PATIENT TEACHING

- Additional material may be obtained from National Digestive Diseases Information Clearinghouse, Box NDDIC, Bethesda, MD 20892; (301) 468-6344.
- Emphasize the importance of a high-fiber diet and recognizing the symptoms of complications at the early stage.

 See Corresponding Diagnostic Algorithm

 See Patient Handout on CD

DOWN SYNDROME

Cathryn B. Nowak, MD
Beverly N. Hay, MD

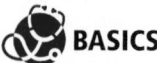 **BASICS**

DESCRIPTION

- A congenital condition associated with mental retardation and an increased risk of multisystem medical problems. One of the most common causes of mental retardation. It is caused by excess chromosome 21 material (Trisomy 21). The syndrome occurs in all races with equal frequency.
- System(s) Affected: Neurologic (100%); Cardiac (40–50%); Gastrointestinal (8–12%)

Synonym(s): Trisomy 21; Down syndrome

ALERT

Pediatric Considerations
- Balanced approach is critical when giving initial diagnosis because it impacts bonding and parental expectations.
  - Have infant with family and refer to baby by name.
  - Mention positive aspects along with differences.
  - Congratulate family on birth.
- Congenital heart disease is major cause of morbidity/mortality. Murmur may not be present. Delay in recognition may lead to irreversible pulmonary hypertension.
- Early treatment of subclinical thyroid disease may improve growth and development (1)[B].

Geriatric Considerations
- Life expectancy is increasing
- Age-related health issues occur at earlier age than in general population. Communication difficulties interfere with prompt recognition of
  - Alzheimer disease and other psychiatric illness
  - Thyroid/autoimmune disorders
  - Cataracts/hearing loss

Pregnancy Considerations
- Most DS males are infertile
  - Few case reports of successful paternity
- Females are subfertile but can conceive
  - 36% of reported offspring have DS
- Ascertain if pregnancy achieved voluntarily
- Assess mental and physical fitness to carry pregnancy/care for child

GENERAL PREVENTION
- No prevention of DS occurring at conception
- Preimplantation diagnosis with IVF or prenatal diagnosis and termination are current options

EPIDEMIOLOGY
- Predominant age: Most identified at birth
- Predominant sex: Male = Female

Incidence
In the US 1 in 800 births

Prevalence
350,000 persons in the US

RISK FACTORS
Increases with mother's age
- 1 in 1,445, age 20 y
- 1 in 270, age 35 y
- 1 in 100, age 37 y
- 1 in 25, age 45 y

Genetics
- As in "Description." See also "Etiology."
- Inheritance
  - Chance to have another child with DS is
    - 1% (or age-risk, whichever is greater) after 1 child with nondisjunction trisomy 21
    - 10–15% for mothers and 3–5% for fathers who carry a balanced translocation. *Except* if the parental translocation is 21:21(45,t [21:21]), the recurrence is 100%.
  - Unclear after child with mosaic DS, but ~1%

ETIOLOGY
- Chromosomal: Trisomy 21: An extra chromosome 21 is found in all cells in 95% of patients due to nondisjunction (failure of normal chromosome sorting) usually in maternal meiosis.
- Translocation DS: Extra chromosome 21q material is translocated to another chromosome (usually 13, 14, or 21) in 3% of patients. For translocation trisomy 21, 2/3 are new, 1/3 have a parental carrier.
  - Translocation DS more likely if mother <30 years of age
- Mosaic trisomy 21: 2 or more cell populations found (usually normal and trisomy 21) in 2% of patients. Manifestations often milder.

ASSOCIATED CONDITIONS
- Cardiac
  - Congenital heart defects: (40–50%)
    - Mostly endocardial cushion or VSD
- Gastrointestinal/growth
  - Structural defects: (12%)
    - Duodenal or anal atresia/stenosis, Hirschsprung disease, annular pancreas
  - Gastroesophageal reflux
  - Constipation
  - Altered growth pattern
- Pulmonary
  - Tracheal stenosis/tracheoesophageal fistula
  - Pulmonary hypertension
  - Obstructive apnea
- Genitourinary
  - Cryptorchidism
  - Hypospadias
  - Renal anomaly
- Hematologic/neoplastic
  - Macrocytosis (66%)
  - Transient leukemoid reaction: (10%)
    - Self-resolves generally but can be preleukemic in 20–30%
  - Leukemia: (0.5–1%)
  - Decreased risk of most solid tumors; risk of germ cell tumors is increased
- Endocrine
  - Acquired hypothyroidism (20–40%)
    - Congenital hypothyroidism also increased
  - Diabetes
  - Hypogonadism
- Skeletal
  - Atlantoaxial instability (15%); 2% symptomatic
  - Ligamentous laxity
  - Scoliosis (some cases have adulthood onset)
  - Hip (8%)
    - Dysplasia/dislocation, slipped capital femoral epiphyses, avascular necrosis

- Immune/rheumatologic
  - Abnormal immune function
    - Increased rate of and mortality from infection, especially respiratory
  - Increased risk autoimmune disorders
    - Thyroid, celiac disease, lupus
- Neurologic
  - Mental retardation
    - Range from near normal to severe with average being moderate retardation
  - Seizures
    - Infantile spasms (5–10%)
    - Increased risk child/adult onset seizures
  - Alzheimer disease: 100% have neuropathologic changes, though not all develop symptoms
- Psychiatric
  - Emotional/conduct disorders (25–33%)
  - Depression: Up to 10% of adults
- Sensory
  - Hearing loss: (60%)
    - Mostly conductive due to high frequency of asymptomatic middle ear effusion
  - Visual impairment (60–70%)
    - Mostly strabismus, nystagmus, cataracts
- Dermatologic: Worsens with increasing age.
  - Palmoplantar hyperkeratosis (>75%), atopic or seborrheic dermatitis (50%), onychomycosis (50%) syringomas (30%), furunculosis/folliculitis (15%)

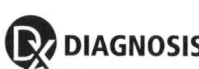 **DIAGNOSIS**

SIGNS AND SYMPTOMS

History
- Maternal age and prenatal diagnostic studies
- Additional directed questions are crucial for timely recognition and treatment of associated conditions.

Physical Exam
- DS specific growth curves should be used
- Infants and children
  - Brachycephaly (100%)
  - Hypotonia (80%)
  - Small ears, often low set and simplified
  - Upslanting palpebral fissure (90%)
  - Epicanthic folds (90%)
  - Depressed nasal bridge
  - Short neck, often with increased nuchal folds
  - Abnormal dermatoglyphics, including transverse palmar crease, single flexion crease on 5th finger
  - Increase space between toes 1–2; 5th finger clinodactyly; brachydactyly
- Adults
  - Features may become less obvious

TESTS

Lab
- A chromosome test is definitive and should always be done at the time of clinical suspicion. Parental chromosome study only indicated if translocation DS found in child.
- Other studies as indicated for surveillance or for clinical suspicion of associated conditions.

Imaging

- ECG at the time of diagnosis. A ventricular septal defect (VSD)/endocardial cushion defect may not be apparent at birth.
- Radiographs of neck currently recommended for all children, once between ages 3–5 years.
  - Repeat for minor trauma, neck pain, long-tract symptoms, or breathing problems.

Diagnostic Procedures/Surgery

Repair of congenital anomalies is appropriate.

DIFFERENTIAL DIAGNOSIS

- Other chromosomal anomalies
- Zellweger peroxisomal disorder: Similar facial features and severe hypotonia
- Upslanted palpebral fissures, epicanthic folds, 5th-finger clinodactyly and transverse palmar crease may each be a benign familial feature. Unilateral transverse palmar crease seen in 4% of general population and bilateral in 1%.

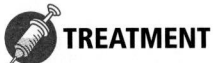

TREATMENT

GENERAL MEASURES

- Appropriate health care
- Genetic evaluation and counseling
- Most important is to educate parents and to address their fears.

Diet

- No special diet. Programs suggesting megavitamin therapy have not been proven.
- Caloric needs are lower in adolescents/adults.

Activity

- Fully active unless heart disease
- A supervised environment is needed for the majority of older children and adults.

SPECIAL THERAPY

- Infant stimulation programs
- Special needs educational supports
  - Inclusion programs generally work well

Physical Therapy

Physical/occupational/speech therapy

Complementary and Alternative Medicine

- Use of piracetam is controversial.
- Vitamin E, selenium, and zinc may be beneficial (3)[C]

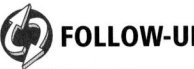

FOLLOW-UP

DISPOSITION

Discharge Criteria

If the social situation dictates adoption, there are families specifically seeking to adopt DS children.

Issues for Referral

Development of associated conditions may require subspecialty referral.

PROGNOSIS

- Associated congenital anomalies are the immediate concern during the newborn period, and severity may affect prognosis.
- Enriched/nurturing environment is critical.
- Life expectancy for current adults is shortened but is expected to equal general population over the next generation.
- Adults can often work in protected situations; a few are largely independent.
- Earlier onset of age-related health issues
  - Clinical Alzheimer disease in at least 1/3 of patients after age 35 years.

PATIENT MONITORING

- Surveillance recommendations (2)[C] (4)[C] (repeat additionally for clinical suspicion).
- Echocardiogram for all newborns regardless of murmur. Repeat periodically adolescent/adult.
- Thyroid: Initial newborn screen
  - Repeat at 6 months, 12 months, and then annually
- C-spine flexion/extension films once at 3–5 years of age and as indicated by clinical issues
- Hematologic
  - CBC as newborn, then repeat as adolescent
- Celiac: Initial screen at 2 years
  - Consider rescreening periodically.
- Vision: Assess for strabismus, cataracts, and nystagmus at birth and on each routine visit.
  - Refer to ophthalmologist by 6 months and every 2 years in early childhood, annually in later childhood into adulthood
- Hearing: Neonatal screen with ABR or OAE, then audiogram every 6 months until age 3 years, then annual hearing assessment

REFERENCES

1. van Trotsenburg ASP, et al. The effect of thyroxine treatment started in the neonatal period on development and growth of two-year-old Down syndrome children. *J Clin Endocrinol Metab* 2005;90:3304–3311.
2. Cohen WI. Current dilemmas in Down syndrome clinical care. *Am J Med Genet* 2006;142C: 141–148.
3. Roizen NJ. Complementary and alternative therapies for Down syndrome. *MRDD Res Rev* 2005;11:149–155.
4. Smith DS. Health care management of adults with Down syndrome. *Am Fam Physician* 2001;64: 1031–1038.

D

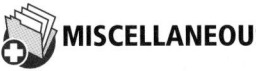 MISCELLANEOUS

- Mongolism is a term no longer used.
- Other notes: Families report that physicians are too pessimistic when giving the diagnosis.

CODES

ICD9-CM

758.0 Down syndrome

PATIENT TEACHING

- National Down Syndrome Congress (800) 232-NDSC www.ndsccenter.org
- National Down Syndrome Society (800) 221-4602 www.ndss.org

 See Corresponding Diagnostic Algorithm

DUMPING SYNDROME

Hongyi Cui, MD, PhD
Ruben Peralta, MD, FACS

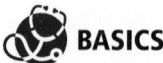 **BASICS**

DESCRIPTION
- Gastrointestinal symptoms resulting from rapid gastric emptying. Usually occurs following gastric surgery (gastrectomy, vagotomy, pyloroplasty).
- Synonym(s): Early postgastrectomy syndrome

GENERAL PREVENTION
- Eating frequent, small, dry meals that contain no refined carbohydrates.
- Restrict fluids to between meals.

EPIDEMIOLOGY
- Predominant age: Middle age to elderly
- Predominant sex: Male = female

Incidence
In the US
- 0.9% of proximal gastric vagotomy without any drainage procedure; 10–22% truncal vagotomy and drainage
- After partial gastrectomy, 14–20% of patients develop symptoms of dumping.

RISK FACTORS
Surgical drainage procedures, particularly gastrectomy; antiulcer surgery; antireflux surgery in pediatric patients.

ETIOLOGY
Multifactorial, including
- Alterations in the storage function of the stomach and/or the pyloric emptying mechanism, leading to rapid delivery of hyperosmolar material into the intestine. This results in fluid shifts from the intravascular compartment into the bowel lumen, leading to rapid small-bowel distention and an increase in the frequency of bowel contractions.
- Supraphysiologic release of various GI peptides/vasoactive mediators, leading to paradoxical vasodilation in a relatively volume-contracted state.
- Reactive hypoglycemia secondary to hyperinsulinemia caused by high concentration of carbohydrates in the proximal small intestine and rapid absorption of glucose.

ASSOCIATED CONDITIONS
- Peptic ulcer disease
- Reactive hypoglycemia
- Gastrectomy/vagotomy/pyloroplasty
- After Nissen fundoplication for reflux disease in pediatric population

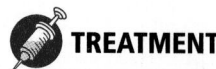 **DIAGNOSIS**

SIGNS AND SYMPTOMS
- Abdominal discomfort, crampy pain
- Diarrhea (postprandial)
- Borborygmi
- Bloating or epigastric fullness
- Nausea
- Palpitations
- Diaphoresis
- Weight loss
- Faintness, fatigue, and headache
- Flushing
- Light-headedness and desire to lie down
- Confusion and syncope

TESTS
Lab
- Postprandial hypoglycemia
- Anemia
- Hypoalbuminemia
- Drugs that may alter lab results: Insulin
- Disorders that may alter lab results: Diabetes mellitus

Imaging
- Upper gastrointestinal series: Barium rapidly emptying from stomach
- Nuclear medicine gastric emptying study
- Endoscopy (exclude mechanical obstruction)

Diagnostic Procedures/Surgery
- Dumping syndrome is diagnosed based on typical symptoms in patients who have undergone gastric surgery.
- Signs and symptoms can be elicited with the glucose challenge test.
- Hydrogen breath test after oral ingestion of glucose is also a sensitive test in patients with dumping syndrome.

DIFFERENTIAL DIAGNOSIS
- Mechanical obstruction
- Gastroenteric fistula
- Celiac sprue
- Crohn disease
- Pancreatic exocrine insufficiency
- Neuroendocrine tumors (e.g., carcinoid)
- Irritable bowel syndrome
- Lactose intolerance

TREATMENT

GENERAL MEASURES
Most patients can be managed conservatively with dietary modification and medical treatment. Surgery is only the last resort.

Diet
- Low-carbohydrate diet
- Milk or milk products also should be avoided
- Frequent small meals with minimal liquid
- Drink fluids between meals only
- High-protein diet
- Add dietary fiber
- Adequate caloric intake

Activity
- No restrictions
- Lying down after eating or when symptoms occur

MEDICATION (DRUGS)

First Line

- Octreotide (Sandostatin) 200–500 μg subcutaneous, given in divided doses q8h. Can be very expensive (1)[B].

- Late dumping symptoms can be ameliorated by the α-glucosidase inhibitor acarbose (100–200 mg, PO t.i.d.), which lowers blood glucose by delaying GI absorption of carbohydrates.
- Pectin/guar gum

Second Line

Anticholinergics: Results generally are disappointing.

SURGERY

- Surgery only if dietary and medical management unsuccessful and symptoms debilitating; the results are variable and unpredictable.
- Options of surgery include Roux-en-Y conversion, pyloric reconstruction, reversed intestinal segment, and conversion of Billroth II to Billroth I anastomosis.
- Patients with refractory dumping symptoms after loop gastrojejunostomy may benefit from simple takedown of the anastomosis; conversion to Roux-en-Y gastrojejunostomy is a reasonable option for patients with disabling dumping after distal gastrectomy. Other procedures have been attempted with limited success.

 ## FOLLOW-UP

PROGNOSIS

Favorable

COMPLICATIONS

- Hypoglycemia
- Malnutrition
- Electrolyte disturbances including hypokalemia

PATIENT MONITORING

Follow to be sure of adequate nutrition.

REFERENCES

1. Ukleja A. Dumping syndrome: pathophysiology and treatment. *Nutr Clin Pract* 2005;20:517–525.
2. Penning C, Vecht J, Masclee AA. Efficacy of depot long-acting release octreotide therapy in severe dumping syndrome. *Aliment Pharmacol Ther* 2005;22:963–969.
3. Bouras EP, Scolapio JS. Gastric motility disorders: Management that optimizes nutritional status. 2004;38:549–557.

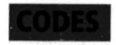 ## MISCELLANEOUS

See also: Diarrhea, chronic; Hypoglycemia, nondiabetic; Peptic ulcer disease

CODES

ICD9-CM
564.2 Postgastric surgery syndromes

PATIENT TEACHING

National Digestive Diseases Information Clearinghouse, Box NDDIC, Bethesda, MD 20892, (301) 468-6344

D

DUPUYTREN CONTRACTURE

Jeffrey F. Minteer, MD

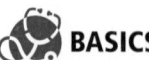 ## BASICS

DESCRIPTION
- Contracture of the palmar fascia due to fibrous proliferation, resulting in flexion deformities and loss of function
- Similar change may rarely occur in plantar fascia; it usually appears simultaneously.
- System(s) Affected: Musculoskeletal

GENERAL PREVENTION
None known. Avoid risk factors when possible.

EPIDEMIOLOGY
- Predominant age: Age 50 (males); 60 (females)
- Predominant sex: Male > Female (ranges from 2:1–10:1)

Prevalence
- Unknown in US
- Norway: 9% males and 3% females

Geriatric Considerations
Occurs primarily in this age group

RISK FACTORS
- Smoking (mean 16 pack-years, odds ratio 2.8)
- Increasing age
- Male/Caucasian
- Workers exposed to vibration
- Diabetes mellitus (1/3 affected, increases with time, usually mild; middle and ring finger involved)
- Epilepsy
- Chronic illness (e.g., pulmonary tuberculosis, liver disease)
- Hypercholesterolemia
- Liver disease
- HIV infection

Genetics
- Autosomal dominant with variable penetrance
- 68% of male relatives of affected patients develop disease at some time

ETIOLOGY
- Unknown
- Possibly a T-cell mediated autoimmune disorder

ASSOCIATED CONDITIONS
- Alcoholism
- Epilepsy
- Diabetes mellitus
- Chronic lung disease
- Occupational hand trauma (vibration white finger)
- Shoulder-hand syndrome
- Status postmyocardial infarction
- Hypercholesterolemia

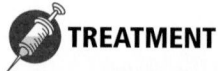 ## DIAGNOSIS

SIGNS AND SYMPTOMS
- Typical
  - Caucasian male aged 50–60 years
  - Bilateral, with 1 hand more involved
  - Family history
  - Unilateral or bilateral (50%)
  - Right hand more frequent
  - Ring finger more frequent
  - Ulnar digits more affected than radial digits
  - Mild pain early
  - Later, painless plaques or nodules in palmar fascia
  - Extends into a cord-like band in the palmar fascia
  - Skin adheres to fascia and becomes puckered
  - Nodules can be palpated under the skin
  - Digital fascia becomes involved as disease progresses
  - Web space contractures
  - Dupuytren diathesis can involve plantar (Ledderhose—10%) and penile (Peyronie—2%) fascia
  - Knuckle pads
- Atypical
  - No age, gender differences
  - No family history
  - May have systemic disease (see "Risk Factors")
  - May have a history of trauma
  - More common unilateral
  - No ectopic manifestations (Ledderhose or Peyronie)
  - Nonprogressive

TESTS

Imaging
MRI can assess cellularity of lesions that correlate with higher recurrence after surgery

Pathological Findings
- Myofibroblasts
- 1st stage (proliferative): Increased myofibroblasts
- 2nd stage (residual): Dense fibroblast network
- 3rd stage (involutional): Myofibroblasts disappear

DIFFERENTIAL DIAGNOSIS
- Early for callosity
- Tendon abnormalities
- Camptodactyly: Early teens; tight fascial bands on ulnar side of small finger
- Diabetic cheiroarthropathy
- Volkmann ischemic contracture

TREATMENT

INITIAL STABILIZATION
- Outpatient monitoring and physical therapy
- Inpatient if surgery indicated

GENERAL MEASURES
- Steroid injection for acute tender nodule
- Physiotherapy alone is ineffective
- Isolated involvement of palmar fascia can be followed
- Metacarpophalangeal (MP) joint involvement can be followed if flexion contracture is <30°
- Clostridial collagenase injections in phase 2 trial look promising

Diet
No special diet

Activity
No restrictions

SPECIAL THERAPY
Physical Therapy
Postsurgery: Start 3–5 days after surgery (passive and active exercises, posterior dynamic extension splints)

MEDICATION (DRUGS)

First Line
- Steroid injection for an acute tender nodule, painful knuckle pad
- Clostridial collagenase injections may also be effective. (Phase II trail)

Second Line
- Topical high-potency steroids: Case report of improvement with clobetasol 0.1% b.i.d. and at bedtime for 2–4 weeks
- Prophylactic external beam radiation

SURGERY
- Selective fascial ray release
- Indications
  - Any involvement of the proximal interphalangeal (PIP) joints
  - Metacarpophalangeal (MCP) joints are contracted at least 30°.
  - Positive Hueston tabletop test: When the palm is placed on a flat surface, the digits cannot be simultaneously placed fully on the same surface as the palm because of flexion contractures.
- May require skin grafts for wound closure with severe cutaneous shrinkage
- 80% have full range of movement if operated on early
- Continuous elongation technique is useful to prepare a severely contracted PIP joint for surgery. The digit can frequently be completely extended; however, it will relapse if surgery is not performed.
- Amputation of little finger, if severe and deforming
- MCP joints respond better than PIP joints, especially if contracted >45°

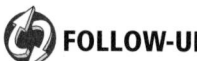 **FOLLOW-UP**

PROGNOSIS
- Typical
  - Unpredictable, but usually slowly progressive
  - Patients likely to have aggressive disease if 1 or more of the following are present: Age <40 years at onset, knuckle pads, positive family history, bilateral disease involving radial side of hand
  - Reports of clinical regression with continuous passive skeletal traction in extension and under a skin graft
  - Recurrence rate after surgery is 10–34%
  - Prognosis better for MP joint vs. PIP joint after surgery
- Atypical
  - Nonprogressive
  - Surgery rarely needed
  - Recurrence unlikely if surgery performed

COMPLICATIONS
- Postsurgery development of reflex sympathetic dystrophy
- Postoperative recurrence or extension in 46–80%
- Postoperative hand edema and skin necrosis
- Digital infarction

PATIENT MONITORING
Follow patient in early stages of disease

REFERENCES
1. Attali P, Ink O, Pelletier G, et al. Dupuytren's contracture, alcohol consumption and chronic liver disease. *Arch Intern Med*. 1987;147:1065–1067.
2. Hill N, Hurst L. Dupuytren's contracture. *Hand Clin*. 1989;5:349–357.
3. Hueston JT. Repression of Dupuytren's contracture. *J Hand Surg*. 1992;17:453–457.
4. Hunt TR III. What is the appropriate treatment for Dupuytren contracture? *Cleve Clin J Med*. 2003; 70:96–97.
5. McFarlane RM. The current status of Dupuytren's disease. *J Hand Surg*. 1995;8:181–184.
6. Rayan G. Clinical presentation of Dupuytren's disease. *Hand Clin*. 1999;15:87–96.
7. Way LW. *Current Surgical Diagnosis and Treatment*. 8th ed. Los Altos, CA: Lange; 1989.

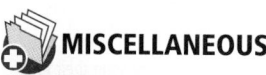 **MISCELLANEOUS**

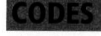

ICD9-CM
728.6 Contracture of palmar fascia

PATIENT TEACHING
- Regular follow-up by physician every 6 months–1 year
- Avoid risk factors, especially with a strong family history

D

DYSFUNCTIONAL UTERINE BLEEDING

Jeanne M. Cawse-Lucas, MD

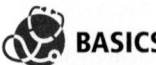 **BASICS**

DESCRIPTION

Abnormal uterine bleeding, usually associated with anovulatory cycles, in the absence of other detectable organic lesions. This unit deals with women of reproductive age.

- 3 major categories
  - Estrogen breakthrough bleeding
  - Estrogen withdrawal bleeding
  - Progestin breakthrough bleeding
- System(s) Affected: Endocrine/Metabolic, Reproductive

EPIDEMIOLOGY

- Predominant age: 12–45 years
- Predominant sex
  - Female only
- Early postpubertal females and those in their later reproductive years are most often affected.

Prevalence

Widespread, with no specific geographic variation

RISK FACTORS

See "Etiology".

Genetics

Unclear; tendency to have familial characteristics

PATHOPHYSIOLOGY

- Anovulation: 90% of DUB is anovulatory. Production of estrogen unaccompanied by cyclic surges of luteinizing hormone (LH) or secretion of progesterone from the corpus luteum.
- Midcycle spotting: Decreased estrogen at midcycle following ovulation
- Frequent menses: Short follicular phase owing to inappropriate feedback at pituitary/hypothalamic level
- Deficiency of luteal phase: Insufficient corpus luteum prematurely decreases progesterone; associated with premenstrual spotting or polymenorrhea
- Prolonged corpus luteum activity: Persistent progesterone production results in prolonged cycles or protracted episodes of bleeding
- Other: Uterine lesions, leiomyomata, polyps, carcinoma, vaginal infection, foreign body, ectopic pregnancy, hydatid mole, endocrine dysfunction (especially thyroid), blood dyscrasias

ETIOLOGY

- Carcinomas of the vagina, cervix, uterus, and ovaries always must be considered.
- Multiple organic pathologies can present as abnormal vaginal bleeding
  - Thrombocytopenia
  - Hypothyroidism
  - Hyperthyroidism
  - Liver disease
  - Hypertension
  - Diabetes mellitus
  - Adrenal disorders
- Pregnancy
- Trauma to the cervix, vulva, or vagina
- Other causes of DUB include
  - Structural disorders, such as functional ovarian cysts, cervicitis, endometritis, salpingitis, leiomyomas, polyps
  - Polycystic ovary disease
  - Vaginal infection
  - Ectopic pregnancy
  - Hydatidiform mole
  - Blood dyscrasias
  - Iatrogenic (anticoagulants, SSRIs, antipsychotics, steroids, hormonal medications)
  - Excessive weight gain
  - Increased exercise performance
  - Stress

ASSOCIATED CONDITIONS

See "Etiology".

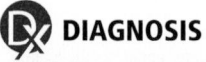 **DIAGNOSIS**

SIGNS AND SYMPTOMS

- Uterine bleeding
  - Unrelated to menses
  - In excess of normal menstrual flow
  - Occurring in an irregular pattern
  - Rarely painful
- Absence of
  - Other systemic symptoms
  - Unusual bleeding from other areas
  - Urinary or gastrointestinal irregularities
  - Evidence of thyroid disease
  - Galactorrhea
  - Pregnancy (especially ectopic)
  - Evidence for reproductive tract malignancy

History

- Careful history of bleeding, with graphic display of cycles, is often helpful.
- Medication history, especially aspirin or anticoagulants and hormonal preparations

Physical Exam

Pelvic examination

TESTS

- Determination of ovulatory status
  - Menstrual cycle charting
  - Basal body temperature monitoring
  - Measurement of the serum progesterone concentration in the midluteal phase 18–24 days after the onset of menses: Normal midluteal phase progesterone levels: 6–25 ng/mL. A single level >6 ng/mL usually indicates a normal luteal phase. LH pulses render a single low value unreliable.
- Pap smear
- Endometrial biopsy in selected patients
  - All patients older than 35 years of age
  - Obese patients
  - Patients with diabetes mellitus
  - Patients with hypertension
  - Patients with suspected polycystic ovary syndrome

Lab

- Human chorionic gonadotropin (rule out pregnancy and/or hydatiform mole)
- TSH (1B)
- PT/PTT
- CBC
- Prolactin

Imaging

- Transvaginal ultrasound to measure endometrial thickness and to look for leiomyomata and masses
  - May be considered in addition to endometrial biopsy, has high sensitivity for endometrial carcinoma (1)[A]
  - Consider if there is suspicion of pregnancy, anatomic abnormalities, or polycystic ovarian syndrome.

Diagnostic Procedures/Surgery
- Endometrial biopsy
  - Perform in all women >35 years of age with menorrhagia to rule out endometrial cancer or a premalignant lesion.
  - Also consider in women aged 18–35 with abnormal uterine bleeding with risk factors for endometrial cancer, including obesity, diabetes, chronic anovulation, history of breast cancer, tamoxifen use, and family history of endometrial, ovarian, breast, or colon cancer.
  - Perform at or beyond day 18; secretory endometrium confirms ovulation occurred in that cycle.
  - Will not diagnose leiomyosarcoma or leiomyoma because these lesions are deep to the endometrial lining
- Saline-infusion sonohysterography with endometrial biopsy
  - Highly sensitive for identification of endometrial abnormalities (1)[B]
- Dilatation and curettage in those who have higher risk for endometrial hyperplasia and carcinoma (consider more strongly over endometrial biopsy if the suspected diagnosis is endometritis, atypical hyperplasia, or carcinoma)
  - Heavy, uncontrolled bleeding
  - Histologic examination is necessary, but biopsy is contraindicated.
  - Medical curettage fails.

Pathological Findings
Vary depending on the disease process present. Pathological review of endometrial sampling specimens is mandatory in all patients.

ALERT
Geriatric Considerations
Pursue uterine bleeding in a postmenopausal female as if there were carcinoma or other significant pathology present.

Pregnancy Considerations
May be confused with ectopic pregnancy, hydatidiform mole

DIFFERENTIAL DIAGNOSIS
See "Etiology".

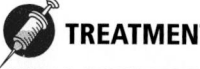 TREATMENT

INITIAL STABILIZATION
Almost always outpatient; hospitalization for hemodynamic instability due to heavy bleeding

GENERAL MEASURES
Diet
Normal; correct anemia with supplemental iron.

Activity
As tolerated

 MEDICATION (DRUGS)

First Line
- Acute, emergent, non-ovulatory
  - Conjugated equine estrogens (25 mg/IV) q4h for a maximum of 6 doses, then OCP or progestin for cycle regulation
- Acute, non-emergent, non-ovulatory
  - 35 mcg estrogen plus progesterone pill 2–4 times daily for 5–7 days until cessation of bleeding, then taper to 1 pill daily for 3–6 months
- Nonacute, non-ovulatory
  - Oral contraceptives: 20–35 mcg estrogen plus progesterone (mono- or triphasic)
  - Progestin: Medroxyprogesterone acetate (Provera) 10 mg/d for 5–10 days per month for cycle regulation is less effective than IUD or NSAIDS (see below). Daily progesterone for 21 days per cycle results in significant less blood loss (2)[A].
  - NSAIDS (e.g., naproxen sodium (Naprosen 500 mg b.i.d.), mefenamic acid (Ponstel, 500 mg t.i.d.), ibuprofen (Advil, Motrin, 600–1200 mg/d): Decreases amount of blood loss compared to placebo. (3)[A]
  - Progesterone-releasing intrauterine devices (Mirena) are more effective and have greater satisfaction than cyclical progesterone but have more side effects. (2)[A], (4)[A], (5)[A]
  - Gonadotropin-releasing hormone (GnRH) agonists: Create a hypogonadotropic state; provide only short-term benefits (6–9 months), are expensive, and have multiple side effects.
- Contraindications
  - Therapy should not be instituted until a reasonable attempt at diagnosis has been made and other causes of uterine bleeding have been considered.
  - "Blind" hormonal therapy is ill-advised and potentially dangerous.
  - Advise women >35 years of age who smoke of OCP risk
- Precautions
  - Absence of withdrawal bleeding requires workup.
  - Exclude endometrial hyperplasia and carcinoma before administering estrogen to perimenopausal or otherwise at-risk women.

Second Line
- Danazol (Danocrine 200–400 mg/dL) is more effective than NSAIDS but is expensive and has more side effects (3)[A].
- Antifibrinolytics like tranexamic acid (Cyclokapron, 1g q.i.d. days 1–5 of cycle) are very effective and without increased side effects but very expensive (6)[A].

SURGERY
- Hysterectomy if endometrial cancer or if medical therapy fails
- Endometrial ablation is less expensive than hysterectomy with high satisfaction rates but often requires repeat treatment (7)[A]

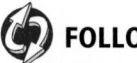 FOLLOW-UP

PROGNOSIS
- Varies with pathophysiologic process
- In young women, most anovulatory cycles can be treated confidently and successfully with physiologically sound therapeutic regimens, without surgical intervention.

COMPLICATIONS
- Anemia
- Adenocarcinoma of the uterus if prolonged unopposed estrogen stimulation in women with intact uterus

PATIENT MONITORING
- All women treated for AUB with estrogens should maintain a menstrual calendar to document the pattern of bleeding abnormalities and their relation to therapy.

REFERENCES
1. Albers J, Hill S, Wesley R. Abnormal uterine bleeding. *American Family Physician*. 2004; 69:8.
2. Lethaby A, Irvine G, Cameron I. Cyclical progestogens for heavy menstrual bleeding. *The Cochrane Database of Systematic Reviews*. 2004.
3. Lethaby A, Augood C, Duckitt K. Nonsteroidal anti-inflammatory drugs for heavy menstrual bleeding. *Cochrane Database of Systematic Reviews*. 2004.
4. Lethaby A, Cook I, Rees M. Progesterone or progesterone-releasing intrauterine systems for heavy menstrual bleeding. *Cochrane Database of Systemic Reviews*. 2005.
5. Marjoribanks J, Lethaby A, Farquhar C. Surgery versus medical therapy for heavy menstrual bleeding. *Cochrane Database of Systematic Reviews*. 2004.
6. Lethaby A, Farquhar C, Cooke I. Antifibrinolytics for heavy menstrual bleeding. *Cochrane Database of Systematic Reviews*. 2004.
7. Lethaby A, Sheppard S, Cooke I, Farquhar C. Endometrial resection and ablation versus hysterectomy for heavy menstrual bleeding. *Cochrane Database of Systematic Reviews*. 2004.

 MISCELLANEOUS

See also: Dysmenorrhea, Ectopic pregnancy, Menorrhagia

 CODES

ICD9-CM
- 626.8 Disorders of menstruation and other abnormal bleeding from female genital tract, other

PATIENT TEACHING
- Thorough yet easily comprehended explanation of diagnostic approach and plan of treatment is important. Many questions regarding fertility, cancer, and infectious disease
- Discuss ways for patient to avoid prolonged stress or emotional turmoil.
- American College of Obstetricians and Gynecologists (ACOG), 409 12th St. SW, Washington, DC 20024-2188, (800)762-ACOG

See Corresponding Diagnostic Algorithm

D

DYSHIDROSIS

Tyeese Gairies-Reed, DO, MA

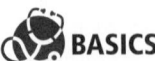BASICS

DESCRIPTION
- Dyshidrotic eczema
  - Recurrent, nonerythematous, vesicular eruption primarily of the palms, soles, and interdigital areas
  - The term *pompholyx* (Greek, "bubble") is generally reserved for cases of deep-seated pruritic vesicles.
  - It is generally associated with, but not caused by, hyperhidrosis (excessive sweating).
- Lamellar dyshidrosis
  - A fine, spreading exfoliation of the superficial epidermis in the same distribution as described above.
  - Hyperhidrosis may or may not be associated.
- System(s) Affected: Skin/Exocrine; Immunologic
- Synonym(s): Pompholyx; Cheiropompholyx; Keratolysis exfoliativa; Dyshidrotic eczema; Vesicular palmoplantar eczema; Hand eczema; Desquamation of interdigital spaces; Palmar pompholyx reaction

GENERAL PREVENTION
- Control emotional stress
- Avoid sweating
- Avoid irritants
- Treatment for psychological factors, if appropriate

EPIDEMIOLOGY
- Predominant age: Usually <40 years
- Predominant sex: Male = Female
- Comprises 5–20% of hand eczema cases
- More common in warmer weather

Prevalence
20 cases per 100,000

RISK FACTORS
- Other skin conditions
  - Atopic dermatitis
  - Contact dermatitis
  - Dermatophytosis
  - Bacterial infections
- Sensitivity to
  - Foods
  - Drugs such as aspirin or other salicylates
  - Nickel

Genetics
- 50% of patients with dyshidrotic eczema have a familial or personal history of atopy
- Twin studies showed simultaneous breakouts

PATHOPHYSIOLOGY
Exact mechanism unknown

ETIOLOGY
- Exact cause not known
- Commonly associated with
  - Hot weather
  - Nickel sensitivity
  - Irritating compounds and solutions
  - Atopy
  - Stress
  - Dermatophyte infection
  - Hyperhidrosis
  - Not considered a cause of dyshidrosis
  - Patients experience relief from dyshidrosis after botulism toxin, which is also treatment for hyperhidrosis.
  - Excessive sweating may worsen pruritus and burning.

DIAGNOSIS

SIGNS AND SYMPTOMS
- Dyshidrotic eczema
  - Small fluid-filled vesicles of the palms and soles
  - Most common along the edges of the fingers, toes, palms, and soles
  - Scaling, fissures, and lichenification may follow vesicle formation.
  - Burning and itching
  - Bilateral and frequently symmetric lesions
  - Vesicles may sometimes coalesce to form larger vesicles or bullae.
  - Vesicles may rupture, leading to a fine scaling similar to tinea.
- Lamellar dyshidrosis:
  - Small white macules that spread peripherally
  - Central area begins to scale
  - Desquamation of the horny layer of the skin that continues to spread

History
- Emotional stress
- Atopy, familial or personal
- Exposure to allergens or irritants
- Costume jewelry
- IV immunoglobulin therapy

TESTS
Lab
Skin culture in suspected secondary infection

Diagnostic Procedures/Surgery
- Diagnosis is usually based on clinical exam.
- Skin biopsy
- Patch test (allergic)
- KOH wet mount (dermatophyte)

Pathological Findings
- Dyshidrotic eczema
  - Fine 1–2-mm spongiotic vesicles intraepidermally
  - Sweat ducts are not involved.
- Lamellar dyshidrosis
  - Exfoliation of the horny layer of the epidermis

DIFFERENTIAL DIAGNOSIS
- Tinea manuum or pedis
- Id reaction
- Contact dermatitis (allergic or irritant)
- Atopic dermatitis
- Drug reaction
- Dermatophytid
- Dyshidrosiform pemphigoid
- Pustular psoriasis
- Seborrheic dermatitis
- Acrodermatitis continua
- Pustular bacterid

TREATMENT

INITIAL STABILIZATION
Outpatient care

GENERAL MEASURES
- Avoidance of possible causative factors (see "Risk Factors" and "Etiology").
- Avoid, when possible, stress or excessive sweating.
- Avoid excess detergents and water.
- Moisturizers for symptomatic relief
- Hand care (1)[C]
  - Avoid soaking hands in water
  - Avoid potential irritants
    - Polishes, solvents, cleansers, fragranced chemicals, fruits and vegetables, shampoo, unknown chemicals
  - Pat hands dry
  - Avoid overcleaning or scrubbing
  - Use lukewarm, not hot, water
  - Wear protective gloves
- Foot care
  - Wear shoes with leather rather than rubber soles (e.g., sneakers).
  - Wear socks made of cotton instead of synthetic materials.
  - Remove shoes and socks whenever possible, to allow sweat evaporation and to apply lubricants.

Diet
No restrictions

Activity
Decrease activity until bullae heal

SPECIAL THERAPY
Complementary and Alternative Medicine
- Burrow solution compress (aluminum acetate)
- Application of coal tar preparations (for lamellar dyshidrosis)

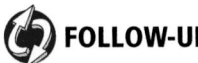

MEDICATION (DRUGS)

- Lamellar dyshidrosis
  - IM corticosteroids
  - Keratolytics are sometimes helpful.

First Line

- Mild cases (1)[C]
  - Topical steroids (medium-/high-potency)
    o Ointments more effective than creams
- Moderate to severe cases (2,3)[A]
  - Psoralens and ultraviolet therapy (UVA-1)
- Recurrent cases (1)[C]
  - Systemic steroids at onset of itching prodrome
  - Single morning dose of 60 mg for 3–4 days every 2–4 months

Second Line

- Botulinum toxin A (4)[A]
- Oral alitretinoin (5)[B]

- Immunosuppressants

  - Tacrolimus shown effective in combination with mometasone (6)[A]

- Antihistamines (1)[C]
- Antibiotics (1)[C]
  - For secondary bacterial infections
- Nickel chelators if needed

FOLLOW-UP

DISPOSITION
Issues for Referral

- Psychologist (stress modification)
- Allergist (allergen testing)

PROGNOSIS

- Condition is benign.
- Usually heals without scarring
- Lesions will often resolve spontaneously, but heal faster with appropriate treatment.
- Recurrence is common.

COMPLICATIONS

- Secondary bacterial infections
- Dystrophic nail changes

PATIENT MONITORING

- Dyshidrotic Eczema Area and Severity Index can be used to monitor progress
  - Number of vessels per square inch
  - Erythema
  - Desquamation
  - Severity of itching
  - Areas affected
- Monitor blood pressure in patients receiving systemic corticosteroids.

REFERENCES

1. Petering H, Breuer C, Herbst R. Comparison of localized high-dose UVA1 irradiation versus topical cream psoralen-UVA for treatment of chronic vesicular dyshidrotic eczema. *J Am Acad Dermatol.* 2004;50:68–72.
2. Polderman MC, Govaert JC, le Cessie S. A double-blind placebo-controlled trial of UVA-1 in the treatment of dyshidrotic eczema. *Clin Exper Dermatol.* 2003;28:584–587.
3. Wollina U, Karamfilov T. Adjuvant botulinum toxin A in dyshidrotic hand eczema: a controlled prospective pilot study with left-right comparison. *J Eur Acad Dermatol Venereol.* 2002;16:40–42.
4. Schnopp C, Remling R, Mrenschlager M. Topical tacrolimus (FK506) and mometasone furoate in treatment of dyshidrosis palmar eczema: A randomized, observer-blinded trial. *J Am Acad Dermatol.* 2002;46:73–77.
5. Ruzicka T, Larsen FG, Galewicz D. Oral alitretinoin (9-cis-retinoic acid) therapy for chronic hand dermatitis in patients refractory to standard therapy. *Arch Dermatol.* 2004;140:1453–1459.
6. Warshaw EM. Therapeutic options for chronic hand dermatitis. *Dermatol Ther.* 2004;17:240–250.

ADDITIONAL READING

Internet references

- Emedicine at www.emedicine.com
- MedlinePlus Medical Encyclopedia at http://www.medlineplus.gov

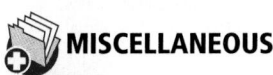

MISCELLANEOUS

CODES

ICD9-CM
705.81 Dyshidrosis

PATIENT TEACHING

- Instructions on self-care, complications, and avoidance
- Explain the association between stress and dyshidrosis, and suggest counseling if appropriate.

D

DYSMENORRHEA

Janice E. Daugherty, MD

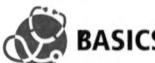 **BASICS**

DESCRIPTION
- Pelvic pain occurring at or around the time of menses; a leading cause of absenteeism for women <30 years
- Primary dysmenorrhea—without pathologic physical findings
- Secondary dysmenorrhea—often more severe than primary, having a secondary pathologic (structural) cause
- System(s) Affected: Reproductive
- Synonym(s): Menstrual cramps

GENERAL PREVENTION
- Primary: Choose a diet low in animal fats, dairy products, and eggs. Increase vegetables, raw seeds, and nuts to increase production of beneficial prostaglandins.
- Secondary: Reduce risk of sexually transmitted diseases (STDs)

EPIDEMIOLOGY
- Predominant age
  - Primary: Teens to early 20s
  - Secondary: 20s–30s
- Predominant sex: Female only

Prevalence
- >50% of adult females have menstrual pain.
- 10% are incapacitated for 1–3 days each cycle.

RISK FACTORS
- Primary
  - Nulliparity
  - Obesity
  - Cigarette smoking
  - Positive family history
- Secondary
  - Pelvic infection
  - STDs
  - Endometriosis

Genetics
Not well studied

PATHOPHYSIOLOGY
See "Etiology".

ETIOLOGY
- Primary: Elevated production (2–7 times normal) of prostaglandins and other mediators in the uterus that produce uterine ischemia through
  - Platelet aggregation
  - Vasoconstriction
  - Dysrhythmic contractions with pressures higher than the systemic BP
- Secondary
  - Congenital abnormalities of uterine or vaginal anatomy
  - Cervical stenosis
  - Pelvic infection
  - Adenomyosis
  - Endometriosis
  - Pelvic tumors, especially leiomyomata
  - Uterine polyps
  - Intrauterine device (IUD)

ALERT
Pediatric Considerations
Onset with 1st menses raises probability of genital tract anatomic abnormality, such as transverse vaginal septum, and uterine anomalies.

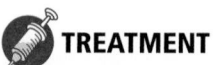 **DIAGNOSIS**

SIGNS AND SYMPTOMS
- Mild: Pelvic discomfort or cramping or heaviness on 1st day of bleeding, with no associated symptoms
- Moderate: Discomfort occurring on 1st 2–3 days of menses and accompanied by mild malaise, diarrhea, and headache
- Severe: Intense, cramplike pain lasting 2–7 days; often with nausea, diarrhea, back pain, thigh pain, and headache

TESTS
Lab
- Urine hCG to rule out ectopic pregnancy
- Cervical cultures to rule out infection
- WBC if suspect severe pelvic inflammatory disease (PID) or ectopic pregnancy
- Drugs that may alter lab results
  - Antibiotics

Imaging
- Primary: Consider ultrasound to rule out secondary abnormalities if history is not characteristic
- Secondary: Ultrasound or laparoscopy to define anatomy

Diagnostic Procedures/Surgery
- Primary
  - History is characteristic
  - Physical examination should be normal.
  - Response to NSAIDs helps confirm diagnosis.
- Secondary
  - History of onset at least 18–24 months after menarche
  - Physical examination may reveal anatomic abnormalities or tenderness.
  - Laparoscopy (rarely needed)

Pathological Findings
- Primary
  - None
- Secondary
  - Uterine enlargement
  - Leiomyomata
  - Ligamentous thickening
  - Fixation of pelvic structures
  - Endometritis
  - Salpingitis

DIFFERENTIAL DIAGNOSIS
- Primary
  - History is characteristic.
- Secondary
  - Pelvic or genital infection
  - Complication of pregnancy
  - Missed or incomplete abortion
  - Ectopic pregnancy
  - Uterine or ovarian neoplasm
  - Endometriosis
  - Urinary tract infection
  - Complication of uterine device

ALERT
Pediatric Considerations
Consider ectopic pregnancy in differential diagnosis of pelvic pain with vaginal bleeding.

TREATMENT

INITIAL STABILIZATION
- Primary: Outpatient care
- Secondary: Usually outpatient care

GENERAL MEASURES
- General physical conditioning, exercise to raise endorphins
- Transcutaneous electrical nerve stimulator
- Secondary dysmenorrhea: Treatment of infections; suppression of endometrium if endometriosis is suspected
- Acupuncture may be effective.

Diet
- Dietary supplementation with vitamin B_1 (thiamine) 100 mg PO daily has been found effective when used for at least 90 days.
- Dietary supplementation with fish oil capsule daily has been found effective when used for 2 months.
- Low-fat vegetarian diet significantly decreases pain.

Activity
Normal

MEDICATION (DRUGS)

First Line
- Ibuprofen 400–600 mg q4–6h, *or*
- Naproxen sodium 550 mg q12h, *or*
- Other NSAIDs
- Oral contraceptives in monthly or 3-monthly cycles
- Contraindications
  - Platelet disorders
  - Gastric ulceration or gastritis
  - Thromboembolic disorders
  - Vascular disease
  - Contraindications to oral contraceptives
- Precautions
  - Gastrointestinal irritation
  - Lactation
  - Coagulation disorders
  - Impaired renal function
  - CHF
  - Liver dysfunction
- Significant possible interactions
  - Coumarin-type anticoagulants
  - Aspirin with other NSAIDs
  - Methotrexate
  - Furosemide
  - Lithium

Second Line
- Mefenamic acid 500 mg at once, then 250 mg q6h may be tried if other NSAIDs are ineffective, as it blocks production of prostaglandins as well as already-formed prostaglandins.
- Tramadol (Ultram) for severe symptoms
- Progestin-containing IUD in suitable candidates

SURGERY
Adenomyosis may require hysterectomy.

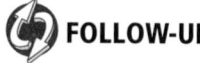 ## FOLLOW-UP

PROGNOSIS
- Primary: Improves with age and parity
- Secondary: Likely to require therapy based on underlying cause

COMPLICATIONS
- Primary: Anxiety and/or depression
- Secondary: Infertility from underlying pathology

REFERENCES

1. Chavez ML, DeKorte CJ. Valdecoxib: A review. *Clin Ther*. 2003;25:817–851.
2. Coco AS. Primary dysmenorrhea. *Am Fam Physician*. 1999;60:489–496.
3. Harel Z, Biro FM, Kottenhahn RK, et al. Supplementation with omega-3 polyunsaturated fatty acids in the management of dysmenorrhea in adolescents. *Am J Ob Gyn*. 1996;174: 1335–1338.
4. Lethaby A, Augood C, Duckitt K. Nonsteroidal anti-inflammatory drugs for heavy menstrual bleeding (Cochrane Review). In: *The Cochrane Library*. Issue 4. Chichester, U.K. John Wiley & Sons Ltd; 2003.
5. Marjoribanks J, Proctor ML, Farquhar C. Nonsteroidal anti-inflammatory drugs for primary dysmenorrhoea (Cochrane Review). In *The Cochrane Library*. Issue 4. Chichester, U.K. John Wiley & Sons; 2003.
6. Milson I, Hedner N, Mannheimer C. A comparative study of the effect of high-intensity transcutaneous nerve stimulation and oral naproxen on intrauterine pressure and menstrual pain in patients with primary dysmenorrhea. *Am J Obstet Gynecol*. 1994;170(1 pt 1):123–129.
7. Morgan PJ, Kung R, Tarshis J. Nitroglycerin as a uterine relaxant: A systematic review. *J Obstet Gynaecol Can*. 2002;24:403–409.
8. Nigam S, Benedetto C, Zonca M, et al. Increased concentrations of eicosanoids and platelet-activating factor in menstrual blood from women with primary dysmenorrhea. *Eicosanoids*. 1991;4:137–141.
9. Proctor ML, Roberts H, Farquhar CM. Combined oral contraceptive pill (OCP) as treatment for primary dysmenorrhoea (Cochrane Review). In: *The Cochrane Library*. Issue 4. Chichester, U.K.: John Wiley & Sons; 2003.
10. Proctor ML, Smith CA, Farquhar CM, Stones RW. Transcutaneous electrical nerve stimulation and acupuncture for primary dysmenorrhoea (Cochrane Review). In: *The Cochrane Library*. Issue 4. Chichester, U.K. John Wiley & Sons; 2003.
11. Stones RW, Mountfield J. Interventions for treating chronic pelvic pain in women (Cochrane Review). In: *The Cochrane Library*. Issue 4. Chichester, U.K.: John Wiley & Sons; 2003.
12. Transdermal nitroglycerin in the management of pain associated with primary dysmenorrhea: A multinational study. *J Int Med Res*. 1997;25: 41–44.
13. Smith RP. Cyclic pelvic pain and dysmenorrhea. *Obstet Gynecol Clin North Am*. 1993;20: 753–764.
14. White AR. A review of controlled trials of acupuncture for women's reproductive health care. *J Fam Plan Reprod Health Care*. 2003;29:233–236.
15. Ziaei S, Faghihzadeh S, Sohrabvand F, et al. A randomised placebo-controlled trial to determine the effect of vitamin E in treatment of primary dysmenorrhoea. *BJOG*. 2001;108:1181–1183.

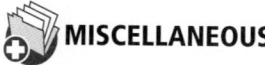 ## MISCELLANEOUS

See also: Endometriosis

CODES

ICD9-CM
625.3 Dysmenorrhea

PATIENT TEACHING

- Reassure patient that primary dysmenorrhea is treatable with use of NSAIDs prior to menses and/or oral contraceptives, and that it will usually abate with age and parity.
- Vitamin E 500 IU daily 2 days prior to menses and 3 days after onset, magnesium, and fish oil supplements have all shown to be slightly better than placebo in small studies and may be considered for primary dysmenorrhea.

 See Patient Handout on CD

DYSPAREUNIA

Eunice S. Chen, MD

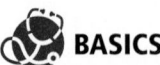 **BASICS**

DESCRIPTION
- Persistent or recurrent pain with attempted or complete vaginal entry and/or intercourse. Dyspareunia may be the result of organic, emotional, or psychogenic causes.
- Primary: Present throughout one's sexual history
- Secondary: Arising from some specific event or condition (e.g., menopause, infection, medications)
- Superficial: Pain at or near the introitus or vulvar vestibule associated with penetration
- Deep: Pain after penetration located at the cervix or lower abdominal area
- Complete: Present under all circumstances
- Situational: Occurring selectively with specific situations
- System(s) Affected: Reproductive; Psychological

GENERAL PREVENTION
- Avoidance of alcohol and tobacco products
- With vulvar vestibulitis: Proper vulvar hygiene including avoidance of soaps, perfumes, or pantiliners (1)[A].

EPIDEMIOLOGY
- Predominant age: All ages
- Predominant sex: Female > Male

Prevalence
- Most sexually active women will experience dyspareunia at some time in their lives.
- ~15% (4–40%) of adult women will have dyspareunia on a few occasions during a year.
- ~1–2% of women will have painful intercourse on a more-than-occasional basis.
- Male prevalence is ~1%.

ALERT
Geriatric Considerations
The incidence increases dramatically in the postmenopausal woman, due to vaginal atrophy.

RISK FACTORS
- Diabetes
- Estrogen deficiency
- Alcohol/marijuana use
- Menopause
- Medroxyprogesterone use
- Stress
- Fatigue or overwork
- Lactation
- Vaginal surgery
- Radiation treatment
- Medication side effects (antihistamines, tamoxifen, bromocriptine, low-estrogen oral contraceptives, depo-medroxyprogesterone, desipramine)

PATHOPHYSIOLOGY
See "Etiology."

ETIOLOGY
- Disorders of vaginal outlet
  - Hymenal ring abnormalities
  - Postmenopausal atrophy
  - Decreased lubrication
  - Episiotomy scars
  - Vulvar vestibulitis/vulvodynia
  - Infections
  - Trauma
  - Adhesions
  - Clitoral irritation
  - Vulvar papillomatosis
- Disorders of vagina
  - Infections
  - Vaginismus
  - Masses or tumors
  - Decreased lubrication
  - Pelvic relaxation resulting in rectocele, uterine prolapse, or cystocele
  - Inflammatory or allergic response to foreign substance
  - Abnormality due to surgery or radiation
  - Congenital malformations
- Disorders of pelvic structures
  - Pelvic inflammatory disease
  - Endometriosis
  - Malignant or benign tumors of uterus
  - Ovarian pathology
  - Pelvic adhesions
  - Prior pelvic fracture
  - Levator ani myalgia
  - Pelvic venous congestion
- Disorders of the gastrointestinal (GI) tract
  - Inflammatory bowel disease
  - Crohn disease
  - Diverticular disease
  - Constipation
  - Hemorrhoids
  - Fistulas
- Disorders of the urinary tract
  - Interstitial cystitis
  - Ureteral or vesical lesions
- Male
  - Genital muscle spasm
  - Infection and irritation of penile skin
  - Cancer of penis
  - Phimosis
  - Penile anatomy disorders
  - Prostate infections and enlargement
  - Infection of seminal vesicles
  - Testicular disease
  - Torsion of spermatic cord
  - Musculoskeletal disorders of pelvis and lower back
  - Urethritis
- Psychologic disorders
  - Fear
  - Depression
  - Anxiety
  - Phobic reactions
  - Conversion reactions
  - Hostility toward partner
  - Psychologic trauma

ASSOCIATED CONDITIONS
- Vaginismus
- Vulvar vestibulitis

Pregnancy Considerations
- Pregnancy is a potent influence on sexuality dyspareunia is common.
- Episiotomies are not protective (2)[A].
  - Mediolateral episiotomies increase risk compared with no episiotomy (3)[B].

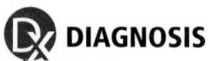 **DIAGNOSIS**

SIGNS AND SYMPTOMS
- Pelvic pain
- Pain with penetration
- Anorgasmia
- Burning
- Vaginal discharge
- Vaginal tears
- Vaginal dryness
- Urinary incontinence
- Depression

History
A comprehensive medical and psychosexual history including inquiry of (4)[A]
- Detailed review of systems
- Sexual abuse history
- Depression
- Substance abuse
- Pelvic trauma
- Arousal disorders
- Psychosocial history
- Recurrent yeast infections

Physical Exam
An external genital exam with pelvic exam

TESTS
Lab
- Gonorrhea culture
- Wet mount
- Chlamydia culture
- Herpes culture
- Urinalysis
- Urine culture
- Pap smear to assess estrogen status
- Fasting blood glucose
- TSH
- Total and free testosterone

Imaging
- Voiding cystourethrogram if urinary tract involved
- GI contrast studies if GI symptoms

Diagnostic Procedures/Surgery
- Colposcopy if vaginal/vulvar lesions
- Laparoscopy if complex deep penetration pain
- Cystoscopy if urinary tract involvement
- Sigmoidoscopy if GI involvement

DIFFERENTIAL DIAGNOSIS
- Vaginismus
- Vulvo-vaginal candidiasis
- Cervicitis
- Vaginal atrophy
- Lichen simplex chronicus
- Lichen sclerosis
- Genital herpes simplex

TREATMENT

GENERAL MEASURES

- Organic causes can be identified during the initial evaluation and specific treatment initiated.
- Once organic causes are ruled out, initiate individual and/or couple behavioral therapy.
- Behavioral therapy
  - Designed to systemically desensitize to intercourse through a series of interventions over a period of weeks
- Individual therapy: Help patient with intrapersonal issues and assess role of partner
- Couple therapy
  - Indicated to help resolve interpersonal problems
  - May involve short-term structured intervention or sexual counseling.

Diet

High-fiber diet if constipation is the cause.

Activity

Routine; sitz baths may relieve painful inflammation.

Physical Therapy

- Pelvic floor physiotherapy
- EMG biofeedback

MEDICATION (DRUGS)

Depending on the etiology, antibiotics, antifungals, or antivirals for infection; estrogen for vaginal atrophy; analgesics and topical anesthetics for pain; and lubricants for dryness

First Line

Vulvar vestibulitis/vulvodynia may respond to tricyclic antidepressants, venlafaxine, or anticonvulsants such as gabapentin.

Second Line

Botulinum toxin type A for pelvic floor spasm (5)[B]

SURGERY

- Reserved for the most refractive cases.
- Vestibulectomy, vestibuloplasty, or perineoplasty (6)[C]

 ## FOLLOW-UP

PROGNOSIS

- Depends on etiology
- Complications
- Marital discourse
- Depression

REFERENCES

1. Farage M, Galask R. Vulvar vestibulitis syndrome: a review. *Eur J Obstet Gynecol Reprod Biol.* 2005;123(1):9–16.
2. Carroli G, Belizan J. Episiotomy for vaginal birth. *The Cochrane Library,* Issue 4. Chichester, U.K.: John Wiley and Sons, Ltd., 2005.
3. Satore A, De Seta F, Maso G, et al. The effects of mediolateral episiotomy on pelvic floor function after vaginal delivery. *Obstet Gynecol.* 2004;103:669–673.
4. Basson R. Summary of the recommendations on sexual dysfunctions in women. *J Sexual Med.* 2004;1(1).
5. Abbott JA, et al. Botulinum toxin type A for chronic pain and pelvic floor spasm in women: a randomized controlled trial. *Obstet Gynecol.* 2006;108(4):915–923.
6. Goldstein A, et al. Surgical treatment of vulvar vestibulitis syndrome: outcome assessment derived from a postoperative questionnaire. *J Sexual Med.* 2006;3(5): 923.

ADDITIONAL READING

Hay-Smith EJC. Therapeutic ultrasound for postpartum perineal pain and dyspareunia. The Cochrane Library, Issue 4. Chichester, U.K.: John Wiley and Sons, Ltd., 2005.

Heim LJ. Evaluation and differential diagnosis of dyspareunia. *Am Fam Phys.* 2001;63:1535–1544.

 ## MISCELLANEOUS

See also: Balanitis; Endometriosis; Pelvic inflammatory disease (PID); Sexual dysfunction in women; Vaginismus; Vulvovaginitis, candidal; Vulvovaginitis; Estrogen deficient

CODES

ICD9-CM

- 302.76 Psychosexual dysfunction with functional dyspareunia
- 625.0 Dyspareunia
- 608.89 Other specified disorders of male genital organs, other

PATIENT TEACHING

- www.dyspareunia.org
- Kegel exercise information (Our Bodies, Ourselves for the New Century: A Book by and for Women. New York: Simon & Schuster, Boston Women's Health Collective.
- Provide couples with information about sexual arousal techniques. Our Bodies, Ourselves for the New Century: A Book by and for Women. New York: Simon & Schuster, Boston Women's Health Collective, 1998.

See Corresponding Diagnostic Algorithm

DYSPEPSIA, FUNCTIONAL

K. Patricia McGann, MD, MSPH

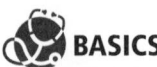 **BASICS**

DESCRIPTION

- An ill-defined condition characterized by the presence of chronic intermittent symptoms for at least 3 months of epigastric pain, postprandial fullness, early satiety, or epigastric burning without mucosal lesions or other structural abnormalities of the gastrointestinal (GI) tract
- Analogous to irritable bowel syndrome (IBS) of the upper GI tract
- System(s) Affected: Gastrointestinal
- Synonym(s): Nonulcer dyspepsia; Moynihan dyspepsia; Pseudo-ulcer dyspepsia; Phantom ulcer; Nonorganic dyspepsia; Nervous dyspepsia

GENERAL PREVENTION

Avoid foods and habits known to exacerbate symptoms (see "Treatment")

EPIDEMIOLOGY

Incidence
- Common in US, affecting 15–20% of patients referred to gastroenterologists
- Accounts for 60% of patients with dyspepsia

Prevalence
- Predominant age: Adults, but can be seen in children
- Predominant sex: Females > Males

RISK FACTORS
- Other functional disorders
- Anxiety
- Depression

Genetics
Possible link to G-protein beta-3 subunit 825 CC genotype

ETIOLOGY
- Often unknown; may be of several different etiologies
- Evanescent ulcers (20–30% go on to develop ulcers)
- Gastric motility disorder (delayed or accelerated)
- Visceral hypersensitivity
- Impaired gastric accommodation
- Controversial relationship to *Helicobacter pylori*
- Adverse drug effects
- Carbohydrate malabsorption
- Food intolerance
- Psychosocial factors

ASSOCIATED CONDITIONS
Other functional bowel disorders

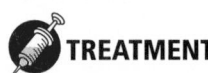 **DIAGNOSIS**

SIGNS AND SYMPTOMS
- Belching
- Aerophagia, gaseousness, abdominal distension
- Borborygmus
- Epigastric pain, gnawing or burning; eating may improve or worsen symptoms
- Substernal pain, gnawing or burning
- Early satiety
- Anorexia, nausea, or vomiting
- Change in bowel habits
- Abdominal tenderness
- No anatomic abnormalities

ALERT

Pediatric Considerations
Look for family system dysfunction.

Pregnancy Considerations
Pregnancy may exacerbate condition.

Geriatric Considerations
Cancer risk is higher.

History
Careful history

Physical Exam
Careful physical exam

TESTS
Rarely needed; diagnosis is clinical
- Esophageal manometry
- 24-hour intraesophageal pH monitoring

Lab
- CBC
- Chemistry panel
- Stool for occult blood
- Certain drugs may alter results.

Imaging
- Recommended in patients
  - >55 years at onset of symptoms
  - With symptoms and signs suggesting more serious disease
  - Who need added reassurance
  - Who are younger and do not respond rapidly to empiric treatment
- Usual
  - Endoscopy
  - Upper GI series
- Sometimes
  - Barium enema
  - Gallbladder studies (e.g., ultrasound or oral cholecystogram)
  - Nuclear medicine gastric emptying study (in selected cases)

Diagnostic Procedures/Surgery
Normal studies of esophagus, stomach, and duodenum (particularly in patients >45 years)

Pathological Findings
None (by definition)

DIFFERENTIAL DIAGNOSIS
- Gastroesophageal reflux
- Cholecystitis
- Peptic ulcer disease
- Gastric cancer
- Esophageal spasm
- Malabsorption syndromes
- Pancreatic disease
- IBS
- Aerophagia
- Ischemia heart disease
- Diabetes mellitus
- Thyroid disease
- Connective tissue disorders
- Conversion disorder

TREATMENT

GENERAL MEASURES
- Appropriate health care: Outpatient
- Supportive measures
  - Reassurance
  - Do not investigate excessively.
  - Dietary changes (see Diet)
  - Elevate head of bed (where applicable).
  - Maintain ideal body weight.
  - Explore psychological issues.

Diet
- Avoid foods known to exacerbate symptoms.
- Frequent small meals
- Avoid regular and decaffeinated coffee.
- Avoid tea, cocoa, and chocolate.
- Avoid heavy alcohol use.
- Avoid cigarette smoking.
- Avoid aspirin-containing compounds and NSAIDs.

Activity
Stress reduction
- Relaxation techniques
- Physical exercise
- Reflux precautions where applicable

MEDICATION (DRUGS)

First Line

- 40% of the patients improve with placebo.
- Acid reduction drugs
  - H_2 antagonists
  - Antacids
  - Proton pump inhibitors (PPIs), rarely needed
- *H. pylori* eradication not proven beneficial.
- Contraindications
  - Avoid magnesium-containing antacids in patients with significant renal dysfunction.
- Precautions
  - Adjust H_2 antagonist and PPI dosages in patients with renal disease.
  - Calcium-containing antacids may precipitate the formation of kidney stones.
- Significant possible interactions
  - H_2 blockers interact with drugs metabolized by and affecting the liver.
  - Antacids compete with digoxin, iron salts, tetracycline, fluoroquinolones, and other drugs for absorption from the stomach.

Second Line

- Gastric motility drugs
  - Metoclopramide (Reglan); although side effects are significant
  - Erythromycin
- Amitriptyline: 50 mg at bedtime
- Selective serotonin-reuptake inhibitors
- Itopride (dopamine D_2-antagonist)
  - Placebo-controlled trial showed symptom improvement
  - Mechanism unknown, requires more studies

SPECIAL THERAPY

Complementary and Alternative Medicine

- Cognitive behavioral therapy
- Hypnotherapy
- Psychotherapy

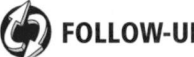 **FOLLOW-UP**

PROGNOSIS

Long-term or chronic symptoms with symptom-free periods

COMPLICATIONS

Undiagnosed serious pathology

PATIENT MONITORING

- Usual duration of medication is 4 weeks, then 2 weeks intermittently for exacerbations. If chronic medication use is needed, use imaging to rule out serious pathology.
- Continue observation to provide support and reassurance.
- Minimize diagnostic studies unless disabling symptoms persist or new problems arise.

REFERENCES

1. Choung RS, Talley NJ. Novel mechanisms in functional dyspepsia. *W J Gastroenterol*. 2006;12(5): 673–677.
2. Dickerson LM, King DE. Evaluation and management of nonulcer dyspepsia. *Am Fam Phys*. 2004;70(1):107–114.
3. Drossman DA, et al., eds. Rome III: The Functional Gastrointestinal Disorders, 3rd ed. McLean, VA: Degnon Assoc., 2006. Accessed online Jan 2, 2007,at: http://www.romecriteria.org/RomeCritieraLaunch.pdf.
4. Fisher RS, Parkman HP. Management of nonulcer dyspepsia. *N Engl J Med*. 1998;339(19): 1376–1381.
5. Holtmann G, Talley NJ, et al. A placebo-controlled trial of itopride in functional dyspepsia. *N Engl J Med*. 2006;354(8):832–840.
6. Meurer LN. Treatment of peptic ulcer disease and nonulcer dyspepsia. *JFP*. 2001;50(7):614–619.
7. Moayyedi P, Delaney BC, et al. The efficacy of proton pump inhibitors in nonulcer dyspepsia: a systematic review and economic analysis. *Gastroenterol*. 2004;127:1329–1337.

 MISCELLANEOUS

See also: Dyspepsia, gastritis; Irritable bowel syndrome

CODES

ICD9-CM

536.8 Dyspepsia and other specified disorders of function of stomach

PATIENT TEACHING

Diet

See "Diet" section under "Treatment"

Activity

See "Activity" section under "Treatment"

Prevention

Continued health habits listed under treatment (i.e., avoid activities known to exacerbate problems, maintain healthy lifestyle, continue stress reduction techniques)

 See Corresponding Diagnostic Algorithm

D

DYSPHAGIA

Ana C. Tuya, MD

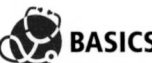 **BASICS**

DESCRIPTION
- The sensation of difficulty swallowing
- A disorder of transferring the food bolus from oropharynx to esophagus or of impairment in transport of the bolus through the esophagus
- Commonly divided into oropharyngeal and esophageal types
- System(s) Affected: Gastrointestinal; Nervous

GENERAL PREVENTION
- Observe feeding of infants closely for aspirations; have suction available.
- Advise for correction of poorly fitting dentures in the elderly patient.
- Avoid drinking alcohol with meals.
- Give consideration to positioning during meals, texture of foods being eaten.

EPIDEMIOLOGY
- Predominant age: All ages; increasing prevalence with age
- Predominant sex: Male = Female

Incidence
In US: 7% incidence lifetime

Prevalence
- 7–10% of people >50
- 30–40% of nursing home residents
- 25% of hospitalized patients

RISK FACTORS
- Children: Hereditary and/or congenital malformations
- Adults: Age >50 years, esophageal cancer more likely
- Smoking
- Long history of gastroesophageal reflux disease (GERD)
- Medications (quinine, potassium chloride, vitamin C, tetracycline, NSAIDs, and others)
- Neurological events or diseases (CVA, neuromuscular disease, Parkinson disease)

ETIOLOGY
- In children
  - Malformations: Congenital (esophageal atresia, choanal atresia)
  - Malformations: Acquired (corrosive or herpetic esophagitis)
  - Neuromuscular/neurologic: Delayed maturation, cerebral palsy, muscular dystrophy
  - GERD
- In adults: Esophageal
  - Structural: Tumors (cancer or benign), strictures (peptic, chemical, trauma, radiation), rings and webs, extrinsic compression, vascular anomaly (goiter), foreign body
  - GERD
  - Neuromuscular: Achalasia, diffuse esophageal spasm, scleroderma, myasthenia gravis, nutcracker esophagus
- In adults: Oropharyngeal
- Cerebrovascular accident (CVA)
- Parkinson disease
- Degenerative diseases (multiple sclerosis, amyotrophic lateral sclerosis, Huntington disease)
- Zenker diverticulum

- Myasthenia gravis
- Cervical spondylosis
- Obstructive lesions (tumors, inflammatory masses)

ALERT
Pediatric Considerations
Congenital malformations

Geriatric Considerations
- Poor dentition and/or dentures
- Drug induced

ASSOCIATED CONDITIONS
- Esophageal carcinoma
- GERD
- Dysphagia lusoria
- Achalasia
- Symptomatic diffuse esophageal spasm
- Scleroderma
- Myasthenia gravis
- CVA

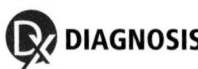 **DIAGNOSIS**

ALERT
Rapidly progressive symptoms and/or profound weight loss indicative of malignant process; requires immediate attention.

SIGNS AND SYMPTOMS
- Oropharyngeal type
  - Choking with swallowing
  - Coughing with swallowing
  - Nasal speech
  - Aspiration pneumonia
  - Weight loss
  - Dysarthria
  - Localize to cervical region
  - Nasopharyngeal regurgitation
- Esophageal type
  - Pressure sensation in mid-chest (localizing below suprasternal notch highly likely to be esophageal disorder); narrow the diagnostic possibilities by asking if this occurs for solids, liquids, or both.
  - Aspiration pneumonia
  - Weight loss
  - Symptoms of GERD

History
- Is the dysphagia for solids, liquids, or both?
- Where does the food bolus feel stuck?
- Are there symptoms of oropharyngeal dysfunction?
- Is the dysphagia intermittent or progressive?
- Is there a history of chronic heartburn?
- Are there associated symptoms like weight loss or chest pain?
- What medications are being taken?
- Is there odynophagia?

Physical Exam
- Neck and oral cavity for lesions, masses, goiter
- Signs of collagen vascular disease
- Detailed neurologic exam, especially cranial nerves (CVA, neuromuscular disease, Parkinson)

TESTS
- In infants/children
  - Observe sucking/eating
  - Attempt to pass nasogastric tube to assess esophageal patency

- Radiography of neck and chest
- Contrast radiography
- Endoscopy
- In adults
  - Barium swallow
  - Endoscopy
  - Barium cine/video esophagogram
  - Ambulatory, 24-hour pH testing
  - Esophageal manometry
  - Videofluoroscopy

Lab
As per differential diagnosis (thyroid panel, infectious causes)

Imaging
- Barium swallow
- CT scan of chest

Diagnostic Procedures/Surgery
- Endoscopy with biopsy
- Esophageal manometry
- Esophageal pH monitoring

Pathological Findings
- Squamous cell or adenocarcinoma
- Barrett metaplasia
- Fibrous tissue of a ring, web, or stricture
- Acute or chronic inflammatory changes
- Oropharyngeal lesions

DIFFERENTIAL DIAGNOSIS
- Cardiac chest pain
- Globus hystericus

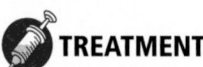 **TREATMENT**

INITIAL STABILIZATION
- Outpatient for conditions where patient is able to maintain nutrition and where there is little risk of complication
- Hospitalization may be required for either infants or adults where dysphagia is associated with total or near total obstruction of esophageal lumen.
- Endoscopy and/or esophageal dilatation may be needed for stenoses and strictures (often recur).
- Surgery may be needed in either benign or malignant processes.

GENERAL MEASURES
- Exclude cardiac disease.
- Ensure airway and pulmonary function.
- Assess nutritional status.
- Speech therapy evaluation is helpful.

Diet
Depends on etiology and severity.

Activity
No restriction

Nursing
Monitor for aspiration

SPECIAL THERAPY
Physical Therapy
Speech therapy for swallowing assessment, dietary and positioning recommendations, and muscle strengthening exercise

IV Fluids
For dehydrated, hypovolemic patients

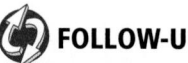 **MEDICATION (DRUGS)**

- For spasms
  - Calcium channel blockers (nifedipine [Procardia]10–30 mg t.i.d.) poor efficacy rates
- For esophagitis
  - Antacids
  - H₂-blockers (cimetidine [Tagamet], ranitidine [Zantac], nizatidine [Axid], famotidine [Pepcid])
  - Proton pump inhibitors (omeprazole [Prilosec], lansoprazole [Prevacid]), rabeprazole (AcipHex), esomeprazole (Nexium), pantoprazole (Protonix)
  - Prokinetic agents: Metoclopramide (Reglan)
- Contraindications
  - Anticholinergics: Obstructive uropathy, glaucoma, myasthenia gravis, achalasia, dementia/delirium, advanced age
  - Nitrates: Early myocardial infarction, severe anemia, increased intracranial pressure, hypotension
- Precautions: May need to use liquid forms of medications
- Significant possible interactions: Refer to the manufacturer's profile of each drug.

SURGERY

- Esophageal dilatation (pneumatic or bougie)
- Esophageal stent; laser for cancer palliation
- Treatment for underlying problem (e.g., thyroid goiter, esophageal atresia)
- Photodynamic therapy (cancer)
- Surgery for Zenker diverticulum, refractory strictures, or myotomy for achalasia

 FOLLOW-UP

DISPOSITION

Admission Criteria
- Complete or partial esophageal obstruction with malnutrition or hypovolemia/dehydration
- Comorbid conditions complicating etiology of dysphagia

Discharge Criteria
- Correction of dysphagia
- Tolerating adequate diet
- Control of pain syndrome

Issues for Referral
- Need for endoscopy, refractory: Gastroenterology
- Failure of dilation or medications: Surgery

PROGNOSIS
Course and prognosis varies with specific diagnosis (cancer, poor; esophageal peptic stricture, good)

COMPLICATIONS
- Aspiration/aspiration pneumonia
- Esophageal "asthma"
- Malnutrition
- Death

PATIENT MONITORING
Related to specific etiology of the dysphagia

REFERENCES

1. Lind CD. Dysphagia: evaluation and treatment. *Gastroenterol Clin North Am.* 2003;32(2): 553–575.
2. Saud BM, Szyjkowski RD. A diagnostic approach to dysphagia. *Clin Fam Pract.* 2004;6(3):525–546.[C]
3. Hammond CA, Goldstein LB. Cough and aspiration of food and liquids due to oral-pharyngeal dysphasia: ACCP evidence-based clinical practice guidelines. *Chest.* 2006;129;154–168. [C]

ADDITIONAL READING

Spechler SJ. Esophageal disorders. In: ACP Medicine Gastroenterology I, WebMD Inc.,2003; www.acponline.com

MISCELLANEOUS

See also: Esophageal tumors; Gastroesophageal reflux disease

CODES

ICD9-CM
- 787.2 Dysphagia
- 438.82 Dysphagia, late effects CVA
- 530.3 Esophageal stricture/stenosis
- 530.0 Achalasia

D

PATIENT TEACHING

Diet
- Counsel the patient on avoiding irritating drugs.
- Counsel the patient on the importance of chewing food well.
- Speech therapy texture recommendations

Activity
- Sit upright for meals, stay upright after
- Strengthening exercises for post CVA

Prevention
- In infants/children: Discuss underlying problem and therapy for recurrent aspiration.
- Positioning and texture in older adults, dentures, supervision to prevent aspiration

ECLAMPSIA (TOXEMIA OF PREGNANCY)

Konstantinos Deligiannidis, MD, MPH
Stacy E. Potts, MD

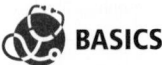 **BASICS**

DESCRIPTION

Seizure activity or coma in an obstetric patient with pre-eclampsia, without underlying neurologic disease. Most postpartum cases occur within 48 hours of delivery, but can occur up to 4 weeks postpartum.

- A complication of pregnancy
- System(s) Affected: Hematologic/Lymphatic/ Immunologic; Nervous; Reproductive
- Synonym(s): Pregnancy-associated seizures; Toxemic seizures

ALERT
Pediatric Considerations
Adequate neonatal care/facilities are essential.

GENERAL PREVENTION
- Adequate prenatal care
- Good control of pre-existing hypertension
- Recognition and treatment of pre-eclampsia
- Aspirin has been suggested to lower fetal death; recent evidence in a large randomized, controlled trial showed no benefit.
- Calcium supplementation has been shown to reduce the risk of pre-eclampsia by 30% (9 randomized, controlled trials).
- Some evidence suggests vitamin C (1,000 mg/d) plus E (400 U/d) reduces risk for pre-eclampsia.

EPIDEMIOLOGY
Predominant age: Most cases occur in younger women because of the higher incidence of pre-eclampsia in younger (nulliparous) women. However, older (>40 years) pre-eclamptic patients have 4 times the incidence of seizures compared with patients in their 20s.

Incidence
- Incidence of pregnancy-induced hypertension affects approximately 6% of pregnancies, with pre-eclampsia complicating 2–4%. Of pre-eclamptic patients, eclampsia develops in 1 in 2,000 deliveries in developed countries. In developing countries, estimates range from 1 in 100 to 1 in 1,700.
- Younger patients have highest incidence.

RISK FACTORS
- Nulliparity: 5:1
- Age >40 years: 3:1
- African American: 1.5:1
- Family history of pregnancy-induced hypertension: 5:1
- Chronic hypertension: 10:1
- Chronic renal disease: 20:1
- Antiphospholipid syndrome: 10:1
- Diabetes: 2:1
- Women who are carrying twins: 4:1
- High BMI: 3:1

Genetics
There does seem to be some genetic predisposition. The single-gene model best explains the frequency of about 25%, but multifactorial inheritance also is possible.

PATHOPHYSIOLOGY
- Presumably, the placenta and fetal membranes play a role in the development of pre-eclampsia because of the prompt resolution of the disease following delivery.

- A common pathway thought to be associated with the development of pre-eclampsia is uteroplacental ischemia:
  – Uteroplacental ischemia is postulated to predispose to the production and release of biochemical mediators that enter the maternal circulation, causing widespread endothelial dysfunction and generalized arteriolar constriction and vasospasm.
- Systemic derangements in eclampsia include the following:
  – Cardiovascular: Generalized vasospasm, increased peripheral vascular resistance, increased left ventricular stroke work index, decreased central venous pressure, decreased pulmonary wedge pressure
  – Hematologic: Decreased plasma volume, increased blood viscosity, hemoconcentration, coagulopathy
  – Renal: Decreased glomerular filtration rate, decreased renal plasma flow, decreased uric acid clearance
  – Hepatic: Periportal necrosis, hepatocellular damage, subcapsular hematoma
  – Central nervous system: Cerebral edema, cerebral hemorrhage

ETIOLOGY
- Exact cause of seizures remains unclear.
- Trophoblastic tissue seems to be required and somehow results in widespread vasospasm.
- Severe cerebral vasoconstriction and hemorrhages occur owing to failure of the constriction to limit perfusion pressure in the capillaries, with consequent rupture and vasogenic cerebral edema and ring hemorrhages.
- Now considered to be primarily an endothelial disorder

ASSOCIATED CONDITIONS
None

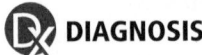 **DIAGNOSIS**

SIGNS AND SYMPTOMS
- Tonic-clonic seizure activity (focal or generalized)
- Headache, visual disturbance, and epigastric or right upper quadrant pain often precedes seizure.
- Seizures may occur once or repeatedly.
- Postictal coma, cyanosis (variable)
- Temperatures >39°C, consistent with central nervous system hemorrhage
- Disseminated intravascular coagulation (DIC), thrombocytopenia, liver dysfunction, renal failure associated
- Normal blood pressure, even in response to treatment, does not rule out potential for seizures. Up to 30% may not have edema, 20% may not have proteinuria.
- Hemoconcentration: Predisposition to pulmonary and/or cerebral edema with fluid therapy. Actually an excess of extracellular fluid is inappropriately distributed to the extracellular spaces.

TESTS
Fetal monitoring depends on other clinical factors. Consider nonstress testing weekly to twice weekly when diagnosis is established and if clinical condition/laboratory testing indicates progressive disease.

Lab
- Complete blood count/platelets
- 24-hour urine for protein/creatinine clearance
- Creatinine
- Serum transaminase
- Serum albumin
- Lactate dehydrogenase, uric acid
- Coagulation profiles: Abnormalities suggest severe disease.
- Serum markers such as human chorionic gonadotropin, leptin, and inhibin A have not proved to be useful as screening tests.
- Drugs that may alter lab results: Concurrent treatment with phenytoin, barbiturates (not with magnesium)

Imaging
- Ultrasound is used to monitor growth, cord blood flow, and Bishop score. Perform as indicated based on clinical stability and laboratory findings.
- CT or MRI can evaluate for mass lesions, infarct, and hemorrhages, but are rarely used when usual clinical picture is present. Should be considered if focal findings persist or uncharacteristic signs/symptoms are present

Diagnostic Procedures/Surgery
- No additional procedures are generally applicable.
- Electroencephalogram is rarely useful.
- Cerebral spinal fluid studies are of no value unless other causes (e.g., meningitis) are seriously considered in differential diagnosis.

Pathological Findings
Cerebral edema, hyperemia, focal anemia, thrombosis, and hemorrhage; cerebral lesions account for 40% of eclamptic deaths.

DIFFERENTIAL DIAGNOSIS
- Epilepsy
- Cerebral tumors
- Meningitis/encephalitis
- Ruptured cerebral aneurysm
- Until other causes are proven, however, all pregnant women with convulsions should be considered to have eclampsia.

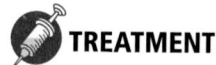 **TREATMENT**

INITIAL STABILIZATION
Inpatient management

GENERAL MEASURES
- Control of convulsions, correction of hypoxia and acidosis, lowering of blood pressure, steps to effect delivery as soon as convulsions are controlled
- See "Medication (Drugs)."
- Indications for delivery
  - Gestational age >38 weeks
  - Platelet count <100,000
  - Progressive deterioration in liver/renal function
  - Suspected abruption
  - Persistent severe neurologic symptoms
  - Severe growth retardation
  - Nonreassuring fetal testing results
  - Oligohydramnios
- Women with severe disease who are between 32 and 37 weeks gestation and have worsening clinical/fetal status merit delivery, preferably after an attempt to demonstrate/promote fetal lung maturity.

Diet
NPO until stable, then usual seizure precautions.

Activity
Bed rest

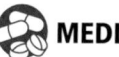 **MEDICATION (DRUGS)**

First Line
Recent randomized trials: Magnesium sulfate is superior to phenytoin in treatment and prevention of eclampsia and probably more effective and safer than diazepam. Compared to diazepam, magnesium sulfate has a significant reduction in risks of maternal death, recurrence of seizures, and in Apgar scores of <7 at 1 minute, and <7 at 5 minutes (1)[A]. Compared to phenytoin, magnesium sulfate has a significant reduction in recurrence of seizures (2)[A].

- Magnesium sulfate
  - 2–4 g IV, repeated every 15 minutes to a maximum of 6 g to achieve resolution of an ongoing convulsion
  - Magnesium then is continued at 1–3 g/h, with the amount given based on the neurologic examination and patellar reflex.
  - Levels of 6–8 mEq/mL are considered therapeutic, but clinical status is most important and must ensure that (a) patellar reflex is present, (b) respirations are not depressed, (c) urine output is ≥25 mL/h.
  - May be given safely, even in presence of renal insufficiency
- Fluid therapy
  - Ringer lactated solution with 5% dextrose at 60–120 mL/h, with careful attention to fluid-volume status
  - Invasive monitoring may be needed.
  - Earlier transfusion may be considered because of attenuated intravascular volume and hemoconcentration.
- Hypertension, if present and severe (e.g., >160/110 mm Hg) also should be treated
  - Hydralazine—5 mg IV, then 5–10 mg boluses as needed every 20 minutes, or
  - Labetalol—10–20 mg IV, then double dose at 10-minute intervals up to 80 mg; maximum total cumulative dose of 220–230 mg (e.g., 20-40-80-80 or 10-20-40-80)
- Contraindications
  - Previous sensitivity/intolerance to a specific drug
  - Avoid diuretics, which may decrease the already lowered intravascular volume.
  - Hyperosmotic agents are dangerous owing to capillary leakage.
- Precautions
  - Careful monitoring of neurologic status, urine output, respirations, and fetal status
- Significant possible interactions
  - Combinations of medications may cause respiratory depression.
- Calcium carbonate (1 g administered slowly IV) may reverse magnesium-induced respiratory depression.

Second Line
- Diazepam 2 mg/min until resolution or 20 mg given, or lorazepam 1–2 mg/min up to total of 10 mg, or phenytoin 18–20 mg/kg at a rate of 20–40 mg/min, or phenobarbital 100 mg/min to a total of 20 mg/kg given
- Nifedipine may be added to magnesium sulfate, but is not yet standard therapy.

SURGERY
If fetal distress is evident or maternal condition is at high risk of deterioration in spite of medical therapy, cesarean section may be indicated. Patient is still at some risk for postpartum eclampsia, however.

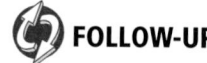 **FOLLOW-UP**

PROGNOSIS
- 25% of eclamptic women will have hypertension in subsequent pregnancies, but only 5% of these will be severe and only 2% will be eclamptic again.
- Eclamptic, multiparous women may be at higher risk for subsequent essential hypertension.
- Multiparous women with eclampsia have higher mortality in subsequent pregnancies than do primiparous women.
- Racial factors are unclear because the higher incidence of essential hypertension in blacks may predispose them to higher rates of hypertension postpartum, rather than a history of eclampsia.

COMPLICATIONS
- 56% have transient deficits including cortical blindness.
- Most women do not have long-term sequelae from eclampsia.
- Death from toxemia or its complications
- Death of fetus

PATIENT MONITORING
Blood pressure, neurologic examination, condition of fetus

REFERENCES
1. Duley L, Henderson-Smart D. Magnesium sulfate versus diazepam for eclampsia. *Cochrane Database of Systematic Reviews* 2006;1.
2. Duley L, Henderson-Smart D. Magnesium sulfate versus phenytoin for eclampsia. *Cochrane Database of Systematic Reviews* 2006;1.

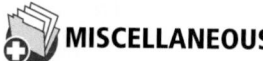 **MISCELLANEOUS**

See also: Pre-eclampsia

CODES

ICD9-CM
- 642.40 Mild or unspecified pre-eclampsia, unspecified
- 642.50 Severe pre-eclampsia, unspecified
- 642.60 Eclampsia, unspecified
- 642.90 Unspecified hypertension complicating pregnancy, childbirth, or the puerperium, unspecified
- 780.39 Other convulsions

PATIENT TEACHING
- Explain to the patient and partner/family what has happened and the need for the prompt actions necessary to ensure the safety of the mother and infant.
- Additional materials from American College of Obstetricians and Gynecologists, 409 12th St. SW, Washington, DC 20024-2188, (800) 762-ACOG

ECTOPIC PREGNANCY

Martha H. McLoughlin, MD

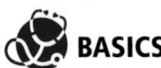 **BASICS**

DESCRIPTION

Extrauterine pregnancy: Any pregnancy existing outside the confines of the uterine cavity

- Tubal pregnancy: Pregnancy existing within the different portions of the fallopian tubes, (e.g., ampullary, isthmic, fimbrial, interstitial)
- Ovarian pregnancy: Pregnancy existing within the confines of an ovary
- Abdominal pregnancy: Pregnancy existing in the abdominal (peritoneal) cavity, most commonly within the cul-de-sac. Occasionally it may implant on the intestines, pelvic side walls, omentum, or even on the surfaces of the liver or spleen.
- Cervical pregnancy: Pregnancy is implanted in the substance of the cervix below the level of the internal os.
- Intraligamentary pregnancy: After a tubal pregnancy ruptures, the surviving embryo secondarily implants within the confines of the anterior and posterior leaves of the broad ligament.
- System(s) Affected: Reproductive
- Synonym(s): Extrauterine pregnancy; Tubal pregnancy; Ovarian pregnancy; Abdominal pregnancy; Cervical pregnancy; Intraligamentary pregnancy

GENERAL PREVENTION

- Reliable contraception
- Repeat tubal pregnancies occur in ~12%. For a patient who becomes pregnant again, use ultrasound to verify intrauterine pregnancy.
- Screening and treatment of sexually transmitted diseases (gonorrhea, chlamydia) that can cause pelvic inflammatory disease (PID) and scarring

EPIDEMIOLOGY

- Predominant age: >40% occur in women between ages 20–29.
- Predominant sex: Female only

Incidence

- 108,800 cases in 1992 in the US
- 16.8 per 1,000 pregnancies (live birth, legally induced abortions, and ectopic pregnancies)

RISK FACTORS

- Previous tubal surgery
- Previous ectopic pregnancy
- Previous PID
- Pelvic adhesions
- Previous uterine surgery
- Use of an intrauterine device (IUD)
- History of endometritis
- Recipients of assisted reproductive technologies (e.g., in vitro fertilization, embryo transfer)
- Diethylstilbestrol exposure in utero

PATHOPHYSIOLOGY

- Most ectopic pregnancies (>95%) are located in the fallopian tube
  - The most common site is the ampullary portion of the tube, where 70% occur.
  - The next most common sites are the isthmic segment of the tube (12%), the fimbria (11%), and the cornual and interstitial region of the tube (2%).

- Nontubal sites of ectopic pregnancy are a rare occurrence, with abdominal pregnancies accounting for 1.3% of ectopic pregnancies and ovarian and cervical sites accounting for 0.2% each.

ETIOLOGY

- Tubal pregnancy
  - Previous tubal pregnancy
  - PID
  - Endometriosis
  - Previous tubal surgery
  - Salpingitis isthmica nodosa
  - Pelvic adhesions
  - Pelvic tumors
- Ovarian pregnancy
  - Implantation of the fertilized ovum on the ovarian surface
  - Tubal abortion with secondary implantation of the embryo on the tubal surface
- Abdominal pregnancy
  - Tubal abortion with secondary implantation
  - Uteroperitoneal fistula following rupture of cesarean section or myomectomy scars
  - External transmigration theory
  - Menstrual regurgitation of a fertilized ovum theory
- Cervical pregnancy
  - Endometrium unreceptive to implantation due to infection
  - Uterine myomas
  - Atrophic endometrium
  - Septate uterus
  - Presence of IUD
  - Scarring of the endometrium
  - Oral contraceptive use
- Intraligamentary pregnancy: Rupture of a tubal pregnancy and secondary implantation between the anterior and posterior leaves of the broad ligament

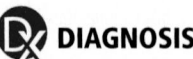 **DIAGNOSIS**

SIGNS AND SYMPTOMS

- Tubal pregnancy
  - Pelvic pain
  - Amenorrhea followed by irregular vaginal bleeding
  - Abdominal tenderness
  - Adnexal tenderness or mass
  - Tenesmus
  - Shoulder pain
  - Syncope
  - Passage of decidual cast
- Ovarian pregnancy
  - Pain and cramps
  - Pelvic mass
  - Vaginal bleeding after a period of amenorrhea
  - Clinical shock after rupture
- Abdominal pregnancy
  - History suggestive of tubal abortion or rupture
  - Pregnancy complicated by unusual gastrointestinal symptoms
  - Fetal movements very marked or painful
  - Easy palpation of the fetal parts or movements
  - Pregnancy described by a multiparous woman as "different"
  - False labor near term
  - High-lying fetus in abnormal presentation, often transverse
  - Displacement of a firm, long cervix
  - Palpation of the fetal parts through the vaginal fornix

- Cervical pregnancy
  - A soft and disproportionately enlarged cervix equal to or greater than the uterine corpus (hourglass effect)
  - Extrusion of dark tissue through the external os
  - Continuous vaginal bleeding after amenorrhea
- Intraligamentary pregnancy
  - History suggestive of tubal abortion or rupture
  - Unilateral pelvic mass associated with pain

TESTS
Lab
- Urine pregnancy test
- Human chorionic gonadotropin (HCG): Serial quantitative serum beta should demonstrate a 66% increase q48h; if <66% increase, consider ectopic pregnancy until proven otherwise.
- Serial blood counts to quantify blood loss
- Serum progesterone level

Imaging
- Vaginal and abdominal ultrasonography
- CT scan
- MRI
- Endovaginal color Doppler flow imaging

Diagnostic Procedures/Surgery
- Culdocentesis
- Endometrial biopsy and/or dilatation and curettage
- Laparoscopy
- Laparotomy

Pathological Findings
- Tubal pregnancy: Presence of chorionic villi within the tubal wall
- Ovarian pregnancy (Spiegelberg criteria)
  - The pregnancy must occupy the position of the ovary.
  - The pregnancy must be connected to the uterus by the utero-ovarian ligament.
  - The ipsilateral oviduct must be normal.
  - The pregnancy sac must show the presence of ovarian tissue.
- Abdominal pregnancy—primary form
  - Both ovaries and oviducts must be normal.
  - There is no uteroperitoneal fistula.
  - Attachment of the conceptus is exclusively to the peritoneal surface.
- Abdominal pregnancy–secondary form: Fetal or placental tissue is found within the abdominal cavity beyond the ovaries or oviducts.
- Cervical pregnancy
  - Chorionic villi are implanted within the substance of the uterine cervix below the level of the internal os.
  - The uterine cavity above the internal os is free of the products of conception.
- Intraligamentary pregnancy: The products of conception are within the confines of the broad ligament.

DIFFERENTIAL DIAGNOSIS
- Uterine (missed) abortion
- Appendicitis
- Salpingitis
- Ruptured corpus luteum cyst
- Cornual myoma or abscess
- Ovarian tumor
- Endometrioma
- Cervical cancer
- Cervical phase of uterine abortion
- Placenta previa

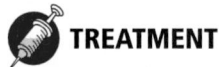 **TREATMENT**

INITIAL STABILIZATION
- Outpatient for most evaluation and treatment
- Outpatient surgery for unruptured tubal pregnancy
- Inpatient surgery for unstable hemodynamic conditions after resuscitation

GENERAL MEASURES
Diet
Variable

Activity
Variable

 MEDICATION (DRUGS)

First Line
- Methotrexate is a folic acid antagonist that inhibits DNA synthesis and cell reproduction. It is used as primary treatment for unruptured tubal pregnancy and for persistent disease after salpingostomy.
- With methotrexate, best results are obtainable when unruptured tubal pregnancy is <3 cm diameter or HCG <5,000 mIU/mL, and before ultrasound evidence of fetal heart beats. With properly selected patients, the success rate is ~90%.
- Methotrexate as supplementary treatment for retained placenta after delivery of the fetus in abdominal pregnancy
- Dosage: Either single- or multi-dose treatment. Single dose is typically used for tubal pregnancies, while multi-dose is used for interstitial or cervical pregnancy
  - Single: IM methotrexate: 50 mg/m^2 of body surface area; may repeat once if unsatisfactory response
  - Multi-dose: Methotrexate 1 mg/kg IM/IV every other day, with leucovorin 0.1 mg/kg IM in between. Administer maximum of 4 doses of methotrexate. Course may be repeated 7 days after last dose if necessary.
- Contraindication
  - Pregnant women with psoriasis
  - Hemodynamic instability
  - Poorly compliant patients
- Precautions
  - Methotrexate has toxic effects on the hematologic, renal, gastrointestinal, pulmonary, and neurologic systems.
- Significant possible interactions
  - Refer to the manufacturer's profile of each drug.

Second Line
Dactinomycin (variable dosing)

SURGERY
- Indications for surgery include ruptured tubal pregnancy, contraindications to medical treatment, or failed medical treatment.
- The surgical treatment of choice is laparoscopic surgery. Randomized trials have shown that laparoscopic surgery results in less blood loss, less anesthesia, shorter hospital stays, and is cheaper than laparotomy.
- When possible, salpingostomy is preferable to salpingectomy, as fertility is preserved. Salpinectomy should be used if there is uncontrolled bleeding, recurrent ectopic pregnancy at the same site, or a very large ectopic pregnancy is present.
- Careful curettage, packing of the cervix and uterine cavity, bilateral internal iliac artery ligations, or even hysterectomy may be necessary as treatment for cervical pregnancy.

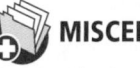 **FOLLOW-UP**

PROGNOSIS
With early diagnosis and treatment, rupture is unlikely to occur.

COMPLICATIONS
- Hemorrhage and hypovolemic shock
- Infection
- Loss of reproductive organs after complicated surgery
- Infertility
- Urinary and/or intestinal fistulas after complicated surgery
- Need for blood transfusions with associated hazards
- Disseminated intravascular coagulation

PATIENT MONITORING
- Serial serum quantitative β-HCG until level drops to near zero
- Follow-up pelvic ultrasonogram for persistent or recurrent masses
- Follow-up imaging studies for retained placenta in abdominal pregnancy (e.g., ultrasonography, CT scan, MRI)

REFERENCES

1. American College of Obstetricians and Gynecologists practice bulletin. Medical management of tubal pregnancy. Clinical management guidelines for obstetrician-gynecologists. *Int J Gynaecol Obstet.* 1999;65:97–103.
2. Durfee RB, Pernoll ML. Early pregnancy risks. In: Pernoll M, Benson RC, eds. *Current Obstetric and Gynecologic Diagnosis and Treatment.* 7th ed. Norwalk, CT: Appleton and Lange; 1991.
3. Emerson DS, Cartier MS, Altieri LA, et al. Diagnostic efficacy of endovaginal color Doppler flow imaging in an ectopic pregnancy screening. *Radiology.* 1992;183:413–420.
4. Hajenius PJ, Mol BW, Bossuyt PM, et al. Interventions for tubal ectopic pregnancy. *Cochrane Database Syst Rev.* 2000;CD000324.
5. Herbst AL, Mishell DR, Stenchever MA, Droegemueller W. *Comprehensive Gynecology.* 2nd ed. St. Louis, MO: The CV Mosby Co; 1992.
6. Kadar N, Bohrer M, Kemmann E, Shelden R. The discriminatory HCG zone for endovaginal sonography, a prospective randomized study. *Fertil Steril.* 1994;61:1016–1020.
7. Kurman RJ, ed: *Blaustein's Pathology of the Female Genital Tract.* 3rd ed. New York, NY: Springer-Verlag; 1987.
8. Pellerito JS, Taylor KJ, Quedens-Case C, et al. Ectopic pregnancy: Evaluation with endovaginal color flow imaging. *Radiology.* 1992;183:407–411.
9. Stovall TG, Ling FW. Gonadotrophin in screening for ectopic pregnancy. *Hum Reprod.* 1992;7:723–725.
10. Stovall TG, Ling FW. Single dose methotrexate, an expanded clinical trial. *Am J Obstet Gynecol.* 1993;168:1759–1765.
11. Tay J, Moore J, Walker J. Ectopic pregnancy: regular review. *BMJ.* 2000;320:916–919.
12. Tulandi, T. Current protocol for ectopic pregnancy. *Contemp Obstet Gynecol.* 1999;44:42.
13. Yao M, Tualndi T. Current status of surgical and non-surgical treatment of ectpoic pregnancy. *Fertil Steril.* 1997;67:421.

 MISCELLANEOUS

See also: Abortion, spontaneous

CODES

ICD9-CM
633.90 Unspecified ectopic pregnancy without intrauterine pregnancy

PATIENT TEACHING

American College of Obstetricians and Gynecologists (ACOG), 409 12th St. SW, Washington, DC 20024-2188: (800) 762-ACOG, www.acog.org

See Corresponding Diagnostic Algorithm

E

EJACULATORY DISORDERS

Bruce Block, MD

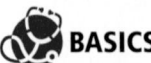

BASICS

DESCRIPTION

- Premature ejaculation: Inability to constantly control the ejaculatory reflex is a common sexual disorder affecting all age groups
  - Definition criteria vary (e.g., inability to maintain an erection of sufficient duration to satisfy a partner, or ejaculation that occurs before individual wants it to)
  - Natural biologic response is to ejaculate within 2 minutes after vaginal penetration
  - Ejaculatory control is an acquired behavior that increases with experience.
- Retarded ejaculation: A condition in which erection is normal or prolonged but ejaculation does not occur
- Retrograde ejaculation: The valve at the base of the bladder fails to close during ejaculation, and the ejaculate is forced backward into the bladder. Erection and sexual pleasure are usually not diminished.
- System(s) Affected: Nervous; Reproductive
- Synonym(s): Premature ejaculation; Retarded ejaculation; Retrograde ejaculation; Inhibited orgasm in males

GENERAL PREVENTION

Better sexuality education may reduce problems.

EPIDEMIOLOGY

- Premature ejaculation is common (particularly in the adolescent)
- Predominant age: All age groups
- Predominant sex: Male only

Prevalence

20%

RISK FACTORS

See "Etiology."

Genetics

No known genetic pattern

PATHOPHYSIOLOGY

See "Etiology."

ETIOLOGY

- Never any ejaculate
  - Congenital structural disorder (müllerian duct cyst, wolffian abnormality)
  - Acquired (radical prostatectomy, postinfectious, posttraumatic, T10–12 neuropathy)
- Retrograde ejaculation
  - Transurethral resection of the prostate (25%)
  - Surgery on the neck of the bladder
  - Extensive pelvic surgery
  - Retroperitoneal lymph node dissection for testicular cancer (also may produce failure of emission)
  - Neurologic disorders (e.g., multiple sclerosis)
  - Drugs (e.g., amoxapine, desipramine, imipramine)
- Retarded ejaculation
  - Rarely may be caused by an underlying painful disorder (e.g., prostatitis, seminal vesiculitis)
  - May be psychogenic as part of erectile dysfunction
  - Sympathectomy (e.g., spinal cord injury, diabetes mellitus)
  - Some drugs may impair ejaculation (e.g., certain monoamine oxidase inhibitors, selective serotonin reuptake inhibitors [SSRIs], α-blockers, antipsychotics, tricyclic antidepressants)
- Premature ejaculation
  - Sexual inexperience
  - High level of sexual arousal
  - Fear of sexually transmitted disease
  - Anxiety
  - Guilty feelings about sex
  - Interpersonal maladaptation (e.g., marital problems, unresponsiveness of mate)
  - Lack of privacy

ALERT

Geriatric Considerations

Age alone does not cause ejaculation problems.

ASSOCIATED CONDITIONS

- Neurologic disorders (e.g., multiple sclerosis)
- Prostatitis
- Psychologic disorders
- Interpersonal disorders

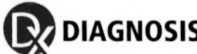

DIAGNOSIS

SIGNS AND SYMPTOMS

- Ejaculation occurring before individual wishes
- Ejaculation does not occur following normal stimulation (including masturbation)

History

- Detailed sexual history
- Many men do not distinguish initially between erection and ejaculation.
- Some men have unrealistic expectations of ejaculatory response and frequency.
- Include the sexual partner in the interview, especially if the patient expresses a belief that he is not meeting the partner's needs.

Physical Exam

Look for multiple sclerosis, spinal cord injury, and emotional disorders (as above).

TESTS

Look for diabetes.

Lab

- Laboratory test results are usually normal
- Postejaculate urinalysis will confirm retrograde ejaculation when infertility is a concern.

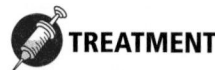

TREATMENT

INITIAL STABILIZATION
Outpatient care

GENERAL MEASURES
- Identification of any medical cause (even if not reversible) helps patient accept condition
- Improve partner communication.
- Reduce performance pressure through reassurance.
- Use sensate focus therapy.
- Techniques to learn ejaculatory control (e.g., coronal squeeze technique or start-and-stop technique)
- Use of a variety of resources may be necessary (e.g., psychiatrists, psychologists, sex therapists, vascular surgeons, urologists, endocrinologists, neurologists).
- If drugs are a possible cause, consider discontinuing or changing the dosage.
- Retrograde ejaculation may be helped if intercourse occurs when bladder is full.

Diet
No special diet, except for patients with diabetes

Activity
No restrictions

MEDICATION (DRUGS)

- Premature ejaculation may respond to topical anesthetic gel applied under a condom for 30 minutes prior to intercourse.
- Clomipramine or sertraline have been shown to delay ejaculation for 4–6 minutes after treatment for 4 weeks.
- A majority of men can discontinue the drug treatment after 7 months and maintain a normal ejaculatory delay.
- Intermittent use has been effective in some men when used 3–4 hours prior to intercourse. An initial 3 week continuous treatment may increase success with subsequent intermittent use.
- Switching antidepressants to bupropion, nefazodone, mirtazapine, or possibly trazodone often eliminates drug-induced ejaculatory disturbance.
- Retarded orgasm and ejaculation in patients who must continue SSRI drugs may respond to sildenafil.

FOLLOW-UP

PROGNOSIS
Often improves with therapy and counseling

COMPLICATIONS
Psychologic impact on some males—signs of severe inadequacy, self-doubt, additional anxiety, and guilt

PATIENT MONITORING
As needed depending on type of therapy

REFERENCES

1. Antidepressants and sexual dysfunction: A patient-centered approach. *J Clin Psychiatry (Monograph Series)*. 1999;17.
2. Hendry WF. Disorders of ejaculation: Congenital, acquired and functional. *Br J Urol*. 1998;82: 331–341.
3. Kamischke A, Nieschlag E. Update in medical treatment of ejaculatory disorders. *Int J Androl*. 2002;25:333–344.
4. Montague, DK, Jarow, J, Broderick, GA, et al. AUA guideline on the pharmacologic management of premature ejaculation. *J Urol*. 2004;172:290.
5. Segraves RT. Effects of psychotropic drugs on human erection and ejaculation. *Arch Gen Psychiatry*. 1989;46:275–284.
6. Stine CC, Collins M. Male sexual dysfunction. *Prim Care*. 1989;16:1031.
7. Vale J. Ejaculatory dysfunction. *BJU Int*. 1999; 83:557–563.
8. Walsh PC, Gittes RF, Perlmutter AD, eds. *Campbell's Urology*. 6th ed. Philadelphia, PA: WB Saunders; 1992.
9. Yaffe M, Fenwick E. *Sexual Happiness: A Practical Approach*. New York, NY: H Holt & Co; 1988.

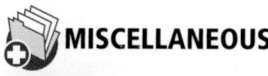

MISCELLANEOUS

CODES

ICD9-CM
- 302.75 Psychosexual dysfunction with premature ejaculation
- 306.59 Physiological malfunction arising from mental factors, genitourinary, other
- 608.89 Other specified disorders of male genital organs, other

PATIENT TEACHING
See "General Measures."

ENCEPHALITIS, VIRAL

Mary Cataletto, MD

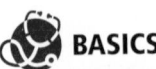 **BASICS**

DESCRIPTION

- Acute brain inflammation caused by viral invasion or by a viral-mediated inflammatory response in the brain following an acute, systemic infection
- May be accompanied by meningeal, spinal cord, or peripheral nerve involvement
- Most cases are rare complications of common systemic viral infections
- Post-viral encephalitis usually occurs via immune-mediated mechanisms and has onset 2–12 days after the primary viral infection.
- System(s) Affected: Nervous
- Synonym(s): Meningoencephalitis

GENERAL PREVENTION

- Use of appropriate insect repellants, protective clothing, and avoidance and removal of ticks
- Human vaccines are available for Yellow fever and Japanese encephalitis virus
- West Nile Virus (WNV): Vaccine available for horses

EPIDEMIOLOGY

- Predominant age: Age extremes at highest risk, especially for herpes simplex encephalitis
  - WNV encephalitis found to have age-related susceptibility with advanced age.
- Predominant sex: Male = Female

Incidence

- Uncommon in US: 117 cases reported to Centers for Disease Control and Prevention (CDC) in 2000; estimated 20,000 cases per year overall, most of which are mild
- Herpes simplex virus encephalitis (most common) estimated incidence is 1 in 250,000 per year

Prevalence

- Seasonal variation
- Arthropod-borne diseases (e.g., arboviruses) are predominantly spring and summer
- Enteroviruses peak in late summer, early fall (most common cause of viral meningitis in the US and responsible for up to 20% of viral encephalitis)
- Mumps and varicella prevalent in spring
- Most others (e.g., herpes simplex virus) are not seasonal.

RISK FACTORS

- Many agents produce more severe disease in newborns and the elderly
- Travel to endemic areas; contact with animals
- Exposure to vectors (e.g., culicine mosquitoes)
- Poor hygiene (principal mode of transmission of enteroviruses is fecal-oral, although respiratory transmission is important for some enteroviruses)
- HIV infection
- Immunosuppression

ALERT

Geriatric Considerations

May be at risk for severe disease

Pediatric Considerations

- Enteroviruses are a major cause of encephalitis in children (e.g., Coxsackieviruses A2, 4–7, 9, 10, 16 and B1–5; echoviruses 1–9, 11–25,27,30 & 33 and enterovirus 71
- Newborns are at higher risk for severe herpes simplex virus and enteroviral CNS disease.

- Pediatric cases of WNV CNS infection are uncommon.
- Children are more commonly symptomatic from arboviral infection than are adults.

Pregnancy Considerations

- Risk of herpes simplex virus infection in an infant delivered vaginally to a mother with a primary genital infection is ~40%; drops to 3–5% in reactivation genital lesions
- Enteroviruses may be transmitted transplacentally to fetus; cause of neonatal disease if mother infected just prior to delivery
- Intrauterine transmission of WNV is suspect. The CDC is collecting data.

ETIOLOGY

- Epidemic
  - Arboviruses (e.g., St. Louis encephalitis, Japanese encephalitis, eastern equine encephalitis, western equine encephalitis, Venezuelan equine encephalitis, West Nile fever) most important cause of severe encephalitis worldwide
  - Enteroviruses (most commonly Coxsackie B viruses, but also includes poliovirus, echovirus)
  - Nipah virus
  - Mumps
  - Varicella-zoster
  - Influenza
  - Human T-lymphotropic virus type III (HTLV-III)
- Endemic
  - Herpes simplex virus types 1 and 2
  - Epstein-Barr virus
  - Varicella-zoster virus
  - Adenovirus
  - Rabies
  - Dengue
  - Benign lymphocytic choriomeningitis V
  - Infectious mononucleosis
  - California encephalitis virus
  - St. Louis encephalitis virus
  - Russian spring-summer encephalitis
  - Murray Valley encephalitis
  - Lacrosse encephalitis
  - Powassan encephalitis

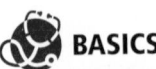 **DIAGNOSIS**

SIGNS AND SYMPTOMS

- Nonspecific symptoms (e.g., malaise, skin rash, fever, myalgia) may precede neurologic symptoms.
- Mental status changes/confusion
- Meningeal involvement is signified by stiff neck and headache.
- Photophobia, lethargy progressing to coma, seizures, and focal neurologic deficits may be observed.
- Progression is variable; may be rapid or follow a more indolent course
- Temporal lobe involvement by herpes simplex leads to temporal lobe seizures, aphasia, and anosmia.
- Presence of postural or kinetic tremors, myoclonus, and weakness is not common in most encephalitis. Presence of these symptoms should raise concern about the possibility of WNV, St. Louis encephalitis, and Japanese encephalitis.

TESTS

- Electroencephalographic findings are usually abnormal, with slowing or epileptiform activity present. Temporal lobe abnormalities, particularly periodic lateralized epileptic form discharges, should suggest a diagnosis of herpes simplex virus encephalitis.
- Most viral encephalitis cases have specific diagnosis made by measurement of acute and convalescent (2–3 weeks) serum antibody concentrations for the specific pathogen. A 4-fold change in titer is suggestive of the diagnosis.
- Cerebrospinal fluid (CSF) antibody index can be used to ascertain specific CNS production of antibody against the infecting agent: Serum and CSF IgG antibody and serum and CSF albumin concentrations are determined. Infection may be suggested by a higher specific antibody: Albumin ratio in CSF than in serum.
- Antigen detection in CSF by polymerase chain reaction has been useful in cases of herpes simplex virus and enteroviral disease, but is available only in some centers.
- Enteroviruses may be recovered from CSF viral culture in ~60% of cases, but most other viral agents are present in quantities too low to be detected by these techniques.
- CSF WNV IgM antibodies are diagnositic of WNV CNS infection. Negative results during the 1st 72 hours do not eliminate the diagnosis. Most patients (>90%) with WNV CNS infection will be positive by day 8. IgM antibody response may persist postinfection.

Lab

- Standard laboratory studies (e.g., CBC, serum chemistries) are usually normal or nonspecifically abnormal.
- CSF examination is essential
  - WBC count is usually increased (10–2,000 cells/mm^3) but may be normal, especially in immunocompromised host; neutrophils predominate early, then a shift to mononuclear cells is seen
  - RBC count usually normal (more likely elevated in herpes simplex infections)
  - Protein may be normal or mildly elevated.
  - Glucose may be normal or mildly decreased.
  - Enzyme-linked immunosorbent assay detection of IgM is helpful retrospectively to determine the causative agent.
  - Polymerase chain reaction to amplify viral DNA is the diagnostic choice for herpes simplex virus (particularly in neonatal cases), cytomegalovirus, human herpesvirus 6, and enterovirus infections. Availability is limited.
- Drugs that may alter lab results: Steroid therapy may mask CSF inflammatory findings.
- Disorders that may alter lab results: Immunocompromised patients may have normal CSF findings.

Imaging

- Imaging studies (e.g., CT scan, MRI, brain scan) may be normal early; later, nonspecific abnormalities are seen (Exception: Herpes simplex encephalitis)
- Temporal lobe pathology suggests the diagnosis of herpes simplex virus
- MRI more sensitive than CT in viral encephalidities May increase yield by T2 weighted imaging and FLAIR sequences.
- Single-proton emmission CT, may be considered in cases where MRI is normal, EEG is nondiagnostic, and HSE is still strongly suspected.

Diagnostic Procedures/Surgery

Brain biopsy, coupled with immunohistochemistry, may be useful in certain cases, particularly to identify treatable causes.

Pathological Findings

- Varies according to etiology
- Usually have prominent perivascular inflammation
- Swelling and degenerative changes of neural elements
- Negri bodies may be seen in brain, conjunctiva, and skin from the base of the neck in rabies patients

DIFFERENTIAL DIAGNOSIS

- Bacterial infection
- Rickettsial infection
- Spirochetal infection
- Other infectious agents
  – Naegleria, Acanthamoeba
- Intracranial hemorrhage
- Intracranial tumor
- Trauma
- Thromboembolism
- Systemic lupus erythematosus
- Toxic ingestion
- Hypoglycemia

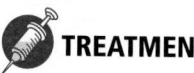 TREATMENT

GENERAL MEASURES

- Appropriate health care: Inpatient with symptomatic and supportive therapy as needed
- Maintenance of adequate respiratory and circulatory support
- Control cerebral edema if necessary (hyperventilation, osmotic diuresis).
- Anticonvulsant as needed
- Monitor for syndrome of inappropriate antidiuretic hormone secretion.
- Prevent bed sores.

Diet

- As indicated by clinical condition
- May need fluid restriction for syndrome of inappropriate antidiuretic hormone secretion or cerebral edema

Activity

As indicated by clinical condition

 MEDICATION (DRUGS)

First Line

Specific antiviral therapy is not available for many of the etiologic agents described. However consideration should be given to the following antiviral agents when the causative organism is identified (when available, consultation with an infectious disease specialist is recommended):

- Acyclovir for herpes simplex encephalitis (NB resistance may be seen in immunocompromised hosts)
- Pleconaril (Picovir) for enteroviral encephalitis
- Amantadine or Rimantidine for Influenza A:
  – Oseltamivir for Influenza B
- Foscarnet (Foscavir) is an effective option in patients with acyclovir resistant herpes simplex virus.
- Vidarabine (adenine arabinoside) for acyclovir-resistant herpes simplex virus; has been used in combination with acyclovir

 FOLLOW-UP

PROGNOSIS

- Generally difficult to predict; somewhat based on infecting agent (e.g., herpes simplex virus-2, severe; varicella, mild) and age
- WNV encephalitis (based on 2002 and 2003 epidemics) overall mortality 12–15% but up to 35% in patients >65 years old.
- With disseminated neonatal herpes simplex virus, early antiviral therapy reduces mortality rate to 60% (85% without therapy), but subsequent neurologic impairment is ~40%.
- With CNS neonatal herpes simplex virus disease only, mortality is ~15% (50% without therapy). Unfortunately, antiviral therapy has had no impact on the morbidity of survivors; 65% have neurologic impairment.

COMPLICATIONS

- Varies with etiologic agent
- Herpes simplex virus encephalitis has the highest morbidity and mortality of the the common viral encephalitides (untreated mortality, 70%; <5% of survivors have normal neurologic function).

PATIENT MONITORING

Intracranial pressure monitoring may be needed for severe cases.

REFERENCES

1. Feigin R, Cherry I, *Textbook of pediatric infectious diseases*, 5th ed., Saunders; 2004.
2. Griffin DE, Johnson RT. Encephalitis, myelitis, and neuritis. In: Mandell GL, et al, eds. *Principles and Practice of Infectious Diseases*. 4th ed. New York, NY: Churchill Livingstone; 1995.
3. Hinson VK, Tyou WR. Update on viral encephalitis. *Curr Opin Neurol*. 2001;14:369–374.
4. Read SJ. Laboratory diagnosis of common viral infections of the central nervous system by using a single multiplex PCR screening assay. *J Clin Microbiol*. 1999;37:1352–1355.
5. Redington J, Tyler KL. Viral infections of the nervous system. *Arch Neurol*. 2002;59:712.
6. Romero JR, Newland JG. Viral meningitis and encephalitis: Traditional and emerging viral agents. *Sem Ped Inf Dis*. 2003;14:72–82.
7. Tyler, KL. West Nile Infection in the United States. *Arch Neurol* 2004;61:1190–1195.
8. Whitley RJ. Viral encephalitis. *New Engl J Med*. 1990;323:242.
9. Whitley RJ. Viral encephalitis. *Pediatr Rev*. 1999; 20:192–198.

ADDITIONAL READING

Interim guidelines for the evaluation of infants born to mothers infected with West Nile Virus during pregnancy, *MMWR*. 2004;53:154–157

 MISCELLANEOUS

See also: HIV infection and AIDS; Meningitis; viral

CODES

ICD9-CM

- 047.9 Unspecified viral meningitis
- 049.9 Unspecified non-arthropod-borne viral diseases of central nervous system

PATIENT TEACHING

Prevention

- DEET (N, N diethyl meta toluamide)-containing mosquito repellents
- Avoidance of outdoor activities during periods of peak mosquito activity (near dawn and dusk)
- Use of protective clothing
- Removal of potential mosquito breeding sites (e.g., stagnant water)
- The above recommendations are especially important to help prevent WNV infection during pregnancy.
- Vaccines when available

 See Corresponding Diagnostic Algorithm

E

ENCOPRESIS

Jay Fong, MD
William Garrison, MD

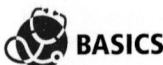

BASICS

DESCRIPTION
- The regular and uncontrolled passage of fecal material into clothes or other inappropriate places by a child >4 years.
- System(s) Affected: Gastrointestinal
- Synonym(s): Soiling

GENERAL PREVENTION
- Optimal feeding practices
- Normal bowel function and recommendations for bowel training
- Early detection of problems
- Avoid Karo syrup.
- Prompt treatment of perianal dermatitis to avoid painful defecation
- Look for signs of relapse, which include large-caliber stools, decrease in frequency of defecation, and soiling
- Avoid over-reliance on diapers and pull-ups after 3rd year of life

EPIDEMIOLOGY
- Predominant age: 70% have onset <5 years of age
- Predominant sex: Males > Females (1.5:1)

Prevalence
1.3% of all children >4 years of age

RISK FACTORS
- Boys are more often affected.
- Difficulty with bowel training, including pressure related to early daycare placement
- Unresolved fecal retention and impaction
- Recurrent discomfort or pain associated with bowel movements

Genetics
None known

PATHOPHYSIOLOGY
- In most cases, encopresis develops as a consequence of chronic constipation with resulting overflow incontinence, which typically is termed *retentive encopresis*.
- Chronic constipation due to irregular and incomplete evacuation results in progressive rectal distension and stretching of both the internal and external anal sphincters.
- As the child habituates to chronic rectal distension, he may no longer sense the normal urge to defecate. Eventually, soft or liquid stool begins to leak around the retained fecal mass, resulting in fecal soiling.
- Many children voluntarily withhold stool in response to physical urge to defecate.

ETIOLOGY
- Psychologic
  - Difficulty with toilet training, including unusual anxiety or broad pattern of conflict with parent around sleeping, eating, clothing.
  - Resistance to using toilet facilities, such as school bathrooms or outdoor toilets during camping trips
  - Association with sexual abuse in boys
- Anatomic
  - Anal fissure
  - Painful defecation of any kind
  - Muscle hypotonia
  - Slow intestinal motility
  - Aganglionic megacolon or Hirschsprung disease
  - Spinal cord defects
  - Anal stenosis
  - Anterior displacement of the anus: Determined by anogenital index, which is the distance from the posterior aspect of the vagina or scrotum to the anus divided by the full distance to the tip of the coccyx, should be >0.34 females and >0.45 males
  - Postsurgical stricture of anus or rectum
  - Pelvic mass
  - Neurofibromatosis
- Dietary or metabolic
  - Lack of fiber
  - Excessive protein or milk intake
  - Inadequate water intake
  - Hypothyroidism
  - Cystic fibrosis

ASSOCIATED CONDITIONS
- Perianal dermatitis
- Urinary tract infections (UTI)
- Sexual abuse in boys

DIAGNOSIS

SIGNS AND SYMPTOMS
- Constipation (retentive encopresis) usually accompanies encopresis
- Unrecognized constipation and/or stool retention often precedes the symptom presented to the care provider.
- Large amount of fecal material on abdominal, pelvic, or rectal exam
- Pasty stool found on underclothes
- Fecal or foul odor surrounds the child
- Often intermittent periumbilical pain
- Occasional passage of a voluminous stool
- History of painful bowel movements
- Some children seem shy and withdrawn.
- Some children may act out or display aggressive behavior.
- Some have had recurrent UTIs.
- Overlap with attention-deficit disorders is common in children >5 years.
- Abrupt onset after age 5 years more likely to be associated with psychosocial trauma

Physical Exam
- Detailed history and complete physical exam
- Neurologic examination of lower extremities
- Genital area
- Digital rectal
- Abdominal radiograph

TESTS
Lab
- Urinalysis and urine culture may be indicated.
- Thyroid function studies

Imaging
Abdominal plain films are occasionally necessary if an impaction is suspected but not detected by abdominal or rectal examination.

Diagnostic Procedures/Surgery
History of constipation <1 month of age is almost always present with aganglionic megacolon, and that history would warrant a barium enema and/or rectal biopsy.

DIFFERENTIAL DIAGNOSIS
- Not difficult when brought to provider's attention
- Suspect when examination detects soiling of underclothes
- Must look for underlying treatable causes of constipation

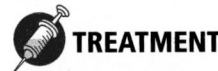

TREATMENT

INITIAL STABILIZATION
Hospital admission and abdominal films may be necessary to ensure complete removal of impaction. The most common factors leading to a need for additional clean-outs is lack of a daily maintenance plan that includes stool softening medication, and no plan for outpatient follow-up within 1 week's time.

GENERAL MEASURES
- Anticipatory guidance relative to toilet training beginning at 18 months, with special attention to when children should reduce reliance on diapers or pull-ups during the daytime hours.
- The impaction must be eliminated before starting maintenance treatment.
- Avoid redevelopment of an impaction.
- Avoid frequent and repeated digital examinations, enemas, and suppositories, especially in infants.
- Biofeedback training has been used in conjunction with standard treatment, but is limited by noncompliance and age of the child
- Once stools seem regular in frequency, child to sit on toilet b.i.d. at the same time each day for 10–15 minutes, and 10–15 minutes after meals, including during daycare or school time.
- *Adequate fluid intake*

Diet
- Avoid excessive milk, bananas, apples, and gelatin.
- Increased fiber

Activity
Unrestricted

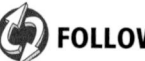 **MEDICATION (DRUGS)**

- Remove stool impaction (before starting maintenance treatment program)
- Give 1 oz (28.4 g) of mineral oil the 1st day
- On the next day, give 1–3 enemas until clear; this may need to be repeated on 1–2 subsequent days
  - Give an oil retention enema.
  - Follow the oil retention enema with hypophosphate enemas (e.g., sodium phosphate [Fleet] 1 oz [28.4 g] per 20 lb [9.1 kg]) of body weight *or*
  - Normal saline enemas: 2 tsp table salt per quart (946 mL) of warm water and give 2 oz (60 mL) per year of age to a maximum of 16 oz (480 mL)
  - A bisacodyl (Dulcolax) suppository may be inserted to assist the evacuation.
- Alternative: Give an oral solution of polyethylene glycol (Colyte, NuLYTELY) at 20 mL/kg/h for 4 hours on 2 consecutive days or PEG 3350 at 1.5 g/kg/d on 2 consecutive days.
- Maintenance treatment
  - ≥6 months to keep stool soft and mobile
  - Can give PEG 3350 maintenance therapy at 0.75 g/kg/d
  - Give mineral oil (may mix with orange juice to make palatable; *avoid in infants to avoid aspiration and lipoid pneumonia*
  - Fiber or other hydrophilic agents may be used to soften the stool (e.g., lactulose, methylcellulose, psyllium, polycarbophil, malt soup extract).
  - Multivitamins must be given between doses of mineral oil to ensure absorption of fat-soluble vitamins (A, D, E, K).
- Contraindications: Refer to the manufacturer's profile for each drug.
- Precautions
  - Avoid bedtime doses of mineral oil, to decrease risk of aspiration
  - Alert caregiver(s) of the possibility of anal leakage of mineral oil, which may affect compliance, especially during initial days of treatment.
- Significant possible interactions: Refer to the manufacturer's profile for each drug.

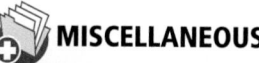 **FOLLOW-UP**

PROGNOSIS

- Usually responds well, although relapses may occur if daily maintenance schedule is not followed.
- Children with psychosocial or emotional problems that preceded the encopresis are more recalcitrant to treatment. The most common are oppositional, attention-deficit, and anxious children.
- Outcomes will be affected by not addressing common parental fears regarding use and duration of stool softening medications. Noncompliance after a few days or weeks is not uncommon.

COMPLICATIONS

- Excessive enemas or suppositories may cause colitis.
- Perianal dermatitis
- Anal fissure

PATIENT MONITORING

- Continue the maintenance treatment program for at least 6 months; possibly for as long as 1–2 years.
- Visits every 4–10 weeks for support and to ensure compliance; more often with oppositional or anxious children.
- Telephone availability to prevent problems and adjust doses
- Redevelopment of impaction must be removed.
- Chief target behaviors in a behavior plan for such children are (a) compliance with medication, (b) compliance with "sits", and (c) self-initiation of bathroom visits.
- Children who do not progress with a behavior plan should be referred for more in-depth mental health evaluation and counseling.

REFERENCES

1. Hatch TF. Encopresis and constipation in children. *Pediatr Clin North Amer*. 1988;35:257–278.
2. Kuhn BR, Marcus BA, Pitner SL. Treatment guidelines for primary nonretentive encopresis and stool toileting refusal. *Am Fam Physician*. 1999;59:2172–2178.
3. Clinical Practice Guideline, Evaluation and Treatment of Constipation in Infants and Children: Recommendations of the North American Society for Pediatric Gastroenterology, Hepatology and Nutrition. *J Pediatr Gastroenterol Nutrit*. 2006;43:e1e13.

 MISCELLANEOUS

CODES

ICD9-CM
787.6 Incontinence of feces

DSM-IV
- 787.6 Encopresis with constipation and overflow incontinence
- 307.7 Encopresis without constipation and overflow incontinence

PATIENT TEACHING

- Education and demystifying of the process
- Careful and full explanation of the treatment plan
- Allay the guilt and avoid punishment for soiling
- In children >4 years, explain to parents how over-reliance on diapers and pull-ups, while convenient, can prolong the problem.
- Always attempt to use positive reinforcement first for successful toilet sits and medication compliance.
- If a positive approach is unsuccessful, suggest removing daily privileges (e.g., TV, video games, etc.) for noncompliance with behavioral plan (i.e., taking medication, agreeing to sit, alerting parents to soiled underwear, etc.)

See Corresponding Diagnostic Algorithm

E

ENDOCARDITIS, INFECTIVE

Nancy Tulathimutte, MD

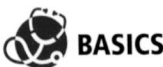 **BASICS**

DESCRIPTION

- Disease resulting from infection primarily of the valvular endocardium and occasionally the mural endocardium
- System(s) Affected: Cardiovascular; Endocrine/Metabolic; Hematologic/Lymphatic/Immunologic; Pulmonary; Renal/Urologic; Skin/Exocrine
- Synonym(s): Bacterial endocarditis; Subacute bacterial endocarditis; Acute bacterial endocarditis

GENERAL PREVENTION

- Treat dental caries while patient is treated for endocarditis/maintain good oral hygiene
- Antibiotic prophylaxis to patients undergoing procedures that may cause transient bacteremia
- For dental/oral/upper respiratory tract procedures (may be used in patients with prosthetic valves). (1)[C]
  - Amoxicillin: 3 g PO (penicillin allergic, clindamycin 600 mg PO) 1 hour prior procedure
  - Alternative: Ampicillin 2 g IV/IM (penicillin-allergic patients: Clindamycin 600 mg IV) 30 minutes before procedure
- For gastrointestinal (GI)/genitourinary (GU) procedures (1)[C]
  - Ampicillin or amoxicillin 2 g IV (or IM) 30 minutes before procedure and 1g IV/PO 6h post-procedure plus gentamicin 1.5 mg/kg IV (or IM) (not to exceed 120 mg) 30 minutes before procedure
  - If penicillin-allergic: Vancomycin 1 g IV infused over 2 hours plus gentamicin 1.5 mg/kg IV (or IM) (not to exceed 120 mg); complete infusion 30 minutes before procedure

EPIDEMIOLOGY

- Predominant age: All ages
- Predominant sex: Male > Female (slightly)

Incidence

In the US: 1.7 to 4.2/100,000; 0.32–1.3/1,000 hospital admissions

RISK FACTORS

- High risk (1)[C]
  - Prosthetic cardiac valves, including bioprosthetic and homograft valves
  - Previous bacterial endocarditis
  - Most congenital cardiac malformations
  - Surgically constructed systemic pulmonary shunts or conduits
- Moderate risk (1)[C]
  - Rheumatic and other acquired valvular dysfunction, even after valvular surgery
  - Mitral valve prolapse with regurgitation
  - Hypertrophic cardiomyopathy
  - Indwelling intravascular devices
- Procedures requiring prophylaxis
  - Oral/Upper respiratory tract: Gingival irritation, including cleaning, tonsillectomy and/or adenoidectomy, rigid bronchoscopy

- GI/GU: Sclerotherapy of esophageal varices, esophageal dilatation, gallbladder surgery, cystoscopy, urethral dilatation, urethral catheterization in the presence of infection, urinary tract surgery, prostatic surgery, vaginal hysterectomy, vaginal delivery in the presence of infection
- Skin: Incision and drainage of infected tissue

ETIOLOGY

- Acute endocarditis
  - Gram-positive: *Staphylococcus aureus*, streptococcus groups A, B, C, G, *Streptococcus pneumoniae, Staphylococcus lugdunensis, Enterococcus* spp (*E. faecalis, E. faecium, E. durans*)
  - Gram-negative: Haemophilus influenzae or parainfluenzae, Neisseria gonorrhoeae
- Subacute endocarditis
  - Gram-positive: Alpha-hemolytic streptococci (Viridans Group Strep), *Streptococcus bovis, Enterococcus* spp, *S. aureus*
  - *HACEK* organisms: *Haemophilus aphrophilus* or *paraphrophilus, Actinobacillus actinomycetemcomitans, Cardiobacterium hominis, Eikenella corrodens, Kingella kingae*
- Endocarditis in intravenous drug-abusers (often involves the tricuspid valve)
  - Gram-positive: *S. aureus, Enterococcus* spp
  - Gram-negative: *Pseudomonas aeruginosa, Burkholderia cepacia*, other bacilli
  - *Candida* spp
- Early prosthetic valve endocarditis (<60 days after valve implantation)
  - Gram-positive: *S. aureus, Staphylococcus epidermidis*
  - Gram-negative bacilli
  - Fungi: *Candida* spp, *Aspergillus* spp
- Late prosthetic valve endocarditis (>60 days after valve implantation)
  - Gram-positive: Alpha-hemolytic streptococci, *Enterococcus* spp, *S. epidermidis*
  - Fungi: *Candida* spp, *Aspergillus* spp
- Culture-negative endocarditis
- Abiotrophia (formerly B_6 deficient streptococci):
  - *Bartonella quintana* (homeless people)
  - *Bartonella henselae* (cat owners)
  - Fastidious organism: *Brucella* spp, fungi, *Coxiella burnetii* (Q fever), *Chlamydia trachomatis, Chlamydia psittaci*, HACEK organisms

DIAGNOSIS

SIGNS AND SYMPTOMS

Modified Duke Criteria for Diagnosis of Infective Endocarditis (2)[B] (Definite: 2 major criteria, or 1 major and 3 minor criteria, or 5 minor criteria; Possible: 1 major and 1 minor criteria, or 3 minor criteria)

- Major clinical criteria
  - Positive blood culture: (a) Typical microorganism for infective endocarditis from 2 separate blood cultures, or (b) persistently positive blood culture. Defined as recovery of a microorganism consistent with infective endocarditis from: Blood cultures drawn >12 hours apart, or all of 3 or a majority of 4 or more separate blood cultures, with 1st and last drawn at least 1 hour apart

- Single positive blood culture for *C. burnetii* or anti-phase-1 IgG antibody titer >1:800
- Positive echocardiogram (transoesophageal echocardiogram recommended with prosthetic valves and "possible IE," or with complicated IE; (a) Oscillating mass on valve or supporting structures, or in the path of regurgitant jets, or on implanted material or (b) periannular abscess, or (c) new partial dehiscence of prosthetic valve
- New valvular regurgitation (change in pre-existing murmur not sufficient)

- Minor criteria
  - Predisposing heart condition or IV drug use
  - Fever ≥38.0°C (100.4°F)
  - Vascular phenomena: Major arterial emboli, septic pulmonary infarcts, mycotic aneurysm, intracranial hemorrhage, conjunctival hemorrhage, Janeway lesions
  - Immunologic phenomena: Glomerulonephritis, Osler nodes, Roth spots, rheumatoid factor
  - Microbiologic evidence: Positive blood culture, but not of major criterion (excluding single positive cultures for coagulase-negative staphylococci and organisms that do not cause endocarditis) or serologic evidence of infection with organism consistent with infective endocarditis

TESTS

Lab

- Positive blood cultures drawn >2 hours apart
- Leukocytosis in acute endocarditis
- Anemia in subacute endocarditis
- Elevated erythrocyte sedimentation rate
- Decreased C3, C4, CH50 in subacute endocarditis
- Hematuria, microscopic or macroscopic
- Rheumatoid factor in subacute endocarditis
- Consider serologies for Chlamydia, Q fever, and Bartonella in "culture-negative" endocarditis

Imaging

- Trans-thoracic or transesophageal echocardiography
- CT scan may be useful in locating abscesses

Pathological Findings

- Vegetations are composed of platelets, fibrin, and colonies of micro-organisms. Destruction of valvular endocardium, perforation of valve leaflets, rupture of chordae tendineae, abscesses of myocardium, rupture of sinus of Valsalva, pericarditis may occur.
- Emboli, infarction, abscesses, and/or infarction may be found in any organ.
- Immune-complex glomerulonephritis possible

DIFFERENTIAL DIAGNOSIS

- Connective tissue diseases
- Fever of unknown origin
- Intra-abdominal infections
- Rheumatic fever
- Salmonellosis
- Tuberculosis
- Atrial myxoma

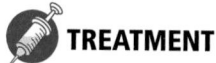

TREATMENT

GENERAL MEASURES
- Outpatient home IV antibiotic therapy in selected stable and reliable patients
- Treat CHF if it occurs

Activity
- Bed rest is indicated initially.
- Ambulation when clinically improved

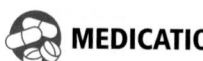

MEDICATION (DRUGS)

First Line
- Penicillin-susceptible streptococci: Penicillin G 12–18 million U/d IV either continuously or in 4–6 equally divided doses for 4 weeks (preferred in patients >65 or patients with renal or cranial nerve VIII impairment) OR ceftriaxone 2 g/d IV/IM in 1 dose for 4 weeks (3)[A]
  - Pediatric dose: Penicillin 200,000 U/kg/d IV in 4–6 equally divided doses or ceftriaxone 100 mg/kg/d IV/IM in 1 dose (4)[A]
- Penicillin-resistant Streptococci and Enterococci: Penicillin 18–30 million U/d IV either continuously or in 6 equally divided doses OR Ampicillin 12g/d IV in 6 equally divided doses for 4–6 weeks, both plus Gentamicin 3mg/kg/d IV/IM in 3 equally divided doses. If Gentamicin-resistant, use Penicillin plus Streptomycin 15 mg/kg/d IV/IM in 2 equally divided doses (3)[A]
- Staphylococcus on native valve
  - Oxacillin-sensitive: Oxacillin or nafcillin 2 g IV q4h for 6 weeks +/− gentamicin 3 mg/kg/d IV/IM in 2–3 equally divided doses for the 1st 3–5 days 3[A].
  - Oxacillin-resistant: Vancomycin 30 mg/kg/d IV in 2 equally divided doses for 6 weeks (3)[B]
- Staphylococcus of prosthetic valve
  - Oxacillin-sensitive: Oxacillin or Nafcillin 12g/d IV in 6 equally divided doses plus Rifampin 900 mg/d IV/PO in 3 equally divided doses, both for 6 wks, plus gentamicin 3 mg/kg/d IV/IM in 2–3 equally divided doses for the 1st 2 weeks (3)[B]
  - Oxacillin-resistant: Vancomycin 15 mg/kg (usual dose 1 g) IV infused over 1h q12h, plus rifampin 300 mg IV/PO q8h, both for 6 weeks, plus gentamicin 3 mg/kg/d IV/IM in 2–3 equally divided doses for the 1st 2 weeks (3)[B]
- HACEK organisms: Ceftriaxone 2 g IM or IV q24h for 4 weeks (3)[B] OR Ampicillin-Sulbactam 12 g/d IV in 4 equally divided doses for 4 weeks (3)[B] OR Ciprofloxacin 1 g/d PO or 800 mg/d IV in 2 equally divided doses for 4 weeks (3)[C]

- Precautions
  - In patients with renal impairment, dosage adjustment should be made for penicillin G, gentamicin, cefazolin, and vancomycin
  - Rapid infusion of vancomycin <1 hour may cause "red-man syndrome"; due to histamine release, not an allergic reaction; will disappear when rate of infusion is reduced
- Significant possible interactions
  - Vancomycin plus gentamicin increases renal toxicity.
  - Rifampin increases the requirement for coumadin and oral hypoglycemic agents.

Second Line
For patients allergic to penicillin
- Penicillin-susceptible streptococcioI

- Penicillin G 12–18 million U/d continuously or in 6 divided doses OR ceftriaxone 2 g IV, both plus gentamicin 3 mg/kg in 2–3 divided doses per day for 2 weeks (3)[B] (not to be used in patients with immediate type hypersensitivity to penicillin), or vancomycin 15 mg/kg (not to exceed 2g/d) IV over 1 hour q12h for 4 weeks (6 weeks for prosthetic valve endocarditis)
- Enterococci: Desensitization to penicillin should be considered. Vancomycin 15 mg/kg (usual dose 1 g) IV infused over 1 hour q12h, plus gentamicin or streptomycin for 4–6 weeks (6 weeks for prosthetic valve endocarditis). (3)[B]
- Staphylococcus of native valve: Cefazolin 2 g IV q8h (not to be used in patients with immediate-type hypersensitivity to penicillin) with option of gentamicin 3 mg/kg/d in 2–3 equally divided doses for the 1st 3–5 days (3)[B], or vancomycin 15 mg/kg (usual dose 1 g) IV infused over 1 hour q12h, for 6 weeks (3)[B]

SURGERY
Surgical therapy should be considered in the following scenarios

- CHF due to valve incompetence (3)[B]
- Embolic event in 1st 2 weeks of antibiotic therapy (3)[B]
- Persistent bacteremia after 1 week of antibiotic therapy, or infection caused by resistant organisms, e.g., fungus, Pseudomonas aeruginosa, S. marcescens (3)[B]
- Valve dehiscence, perforation, rupture or fistula, or large perivalvular abscess. (3)[B] Anterior mitral valve leaflet vegetation >10 mm in size, persistent vegetation after systemic embolization (3)[B], or increase in vegetation size despite antibiotic therapy (3)[C]

FOLLOW-UP

PROGNOSIS
- Staphylococcal endocarditis: Fever and positive blood cultures may persist up to 10 days after appropriate treatment started
- Streptococcal endocarditis: Clinical response within 48 hours of antibiotic treatment and blood cultures negative soon after start of antibiotics

COMPLICATIONS
- Arterial emboli and infarcts (e.g., myocardial infarction, mesenteric, splenic, cerebral infarct)
- Infectious emboli (e.g., abscesses of heart, lung, brain, meninges, bone, pericardium)
- Inflammatory/immune disorders (e.g., arthritis, myositis, glomerulonephritis)
- Miscellanous complications (e.g., CHF, ruptured valve cusp, sinus of Valsalva aneurysm, cardiac arrhythmia, intra- and extracranial mycotic aneurysms)

PATIENT MONITORING
- Check gentamicin peak (~3 μg/mL) and trough (<1 μg/mL) levels if used for >5 days, and in patients with renal dysfunction.
- Check vancomycin trough (<10 μg/mL) levels in patients with renal dysfunction.

- Perform twice weekly blood urine nitrogen (BUN) and serum creatinine while the patient is receiving gentamicin.
- Consider audiometry baseline and follow-up during long-term aminoglycoside therapy.

REFERENCES

1. Ramsdale D, Turner-Stokes, L. Prophylaxis and treatment of infective endocarditis in adults. *Clinical Medicine*, 2004;4(6):545–550.
2. Li J, et al. Proposed modifications to the Duke criteria for the diagnosis of infective endocarditis. *Clin Infect Dis*. 2000;30:633–638.
3. Baddour L, et al. Infective endocarditis: Diagnosis, antimicrobial therapy, and management of complications. *Circulation*. 2005;111:e394–e434.
4. Watanakunakorn C, Burkert T. Infective endocarditis at a large community teaching hospital, 1980–1990. A review of 210 episodes. *Medicine* 1993;72:90–102.

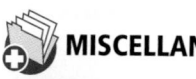

MISCELLANEOUS

CODES

ICD9-CM
- 421.0 Acute and subacute bacterial endocarditis
- 421.9 Acute endocarditis, unspecified
- 996.61 Infection and inflammatory reaction due to cardiac device, implant, and graft

PATIENT TEACHING

Prevention
- Importance of dental hygiene
- Appropriate antibiotic prophylaxis
- Give patient American Heart Association (AHA) wallet card listing antibiotic regimens for prophylaxis. Obtain AHA wallet card, 78-1005 (CP), from local chapters of the AHA.

See Corresponding Diagnostic Algorithm

ENDOMETRIAL CANCER AND UTERINE SARCOMA

Michael P. Hopkins, MD, MEd
Kathleen Zeller, MD
Eric L. Jenison, MD

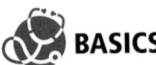

BASICS

DESCRIPTION
- Endometrial cancer: Malignancy of the endometrial lining of the uterus. Tumor grade: Low, moderate, high. Cell types: Adenocarcinoma, adenosquamous (malignant squamous elements), clear cell, and papillary serous.
- Sarcomas
  - Mixed Müllerian sarcoma (carcinosarcoma): Heterologous sarcoma elements not native to the Müllerian system (e.g., cartilage or bone); homologous sarcoma elements native to the Müllerian system.
  - Endometrial stromal sarcoma develops from the stromal component of the endometrium.
  - Leiomyosarcoma develops in the myometrium or in a myoma (fibroid).
- System(s) Affected: Reproductive
- Synonym(s): Uterine cancer; Endometrial cancer; Corpus cancer

Pregnancy Considerations
This malignancy is not associated with pregnancy.

GENERAL PREVENTION
- In young women who are obese or anovulatory, the risk of endometrial cancer can be reduced by cyclic progesterone to prevent unopposed estrogen, taking birth-control pills, or permanently losing weight.
- Estrogen replacement therapy should always include progestational agents unless the woman has undergone a hysterectomy.

EPIDEMIOLOGY
- Predominant age
  - Endometrial cancer: The majority are postmenopausal. It can also occur in younger women in their 20s and 30s with polycystic ovarian syndrome, chronic anovulation, or severe obesity.
  - Sarcomas: Majority of patients are aged 40–69 years.
- Predominant sex: Female only

Incidence
Most common gynecologic malignancy: 40,000 new cases per year, 7,000 deaths per year

Prevalence
500,000 women in the US

RISK FACTORS
- Early menarche
- Late menopause
- Nulliparity
- Personal or family history of colon or reproductive system cancer
- Metabolic syndrome
- Obesity
- Diabetes mellitus
- Hypertension
- Polycystic ovarian syndrome
- Endometrial hyperplasia
- Unopposed estrogens
- Tamoxifen
- Age
- Prior pelvic irradiation (sarcoma)

Genetics
- Endometrial: Lynch Syndrome (hereditary nonpolyposis colorectal cancer)
- Sarcoma: African American

ETIOLOGY
- Endometrial: Unopposed estrogen due to
  - Polycystic ovarian disease
  - Obesity
  - Chronic anovulation
  - Estrogen replacement therapy (estrogen replacement without concomitant progesterone increases the risk. When progesterone is added, the risk does not decrease to 0 but does decrease to that of the general population.)
  - Tamoxifen: Increases risk similar to that of unopposed estrogen.
- Sarcomas: Etiology unknown

ASSOCIATED CONDITIONS
- Obese patients with endometrial cancer should be screened annually because of increased risk of breast and colon cancer.
- Patients who have breast or colon cancer are at increased risk for endometrial cancer.
- Granulosa cell tumors of the ovary produce estrogen so that these patients will have an increased risk of endometrial cancer.

DIAGNOSIS

SIGNS AND SYMPTOMS
- Endometrial cancer
  - Postmenopausal bleeding is the most frequent sign. Any spotting or abnormal discharge mandates evaluation.
  - Pap smear is rarely positive
  - Occasionally, a patient will pass tissue that will confirm a diagnosis.
- Sarcoma
  - Mixed Müllerian sarcoma: Bleeding and prolapsing tissue, pain
  - Leiomyosarcoma: Increasing size of presumed uterine myomas, pain
  - Dilation and curettage is rarely diagnostic.

History
- Heavy or irregular bleeding
- Post-menopausal bleeding or discharge

TESTS
Any that may be indicated preoperatively

Lab
- Liver and renal function tests
- Levels of cancer antigen 125 may be elevated when intra-abdominal disease is present.
- Disorders that may alter lab results
  - A biopsy of a pregnant uterus can produce tissue that looks hyperplastic or premalignant.

Imaging
- Chest x-ray: Most common site of metastases is the lungs. (Rarely this malignancy will go to the bone or the liver.)
- CT scan, bone scan, liver spleen scan: Not part of the routine evaluation, but may be needed if suspected metastasis.
- Mammogram (endometrial cancer is associated with breast cancer)
- Consider colonoscopy (endometrial cancer is associated with colon cancer)
- MRI has been reported to show the depth of myometrial penetration accurately (not always cost effective).
- Vaginal ultrasound usually shows increased endometrial thickening, which can lead to diagnosis.

Diagnostic Procedures/Surgery
- Office endometrial biopsy (90% accurate). If this is negative, a dilation and curettage is necessary. Endometrial stromal sarcoma and leiomyosarcoma are rarely diagnosed preoperatively.
- Fractional dilation and curettage is 99% accurate except in cases of sarcoma.

Pathological Findings
- Stage I (confined to corpus)
  - A. Confined to endometrium
  - B. <50% myometrial invasion
  - C. >50% myometrial invasion
- Stage II
  - A. Endocervical superficial involvement
  - B. Cervical stromal invasion
- Stage III
  - A. Uterine serosal/adnexal involvement/positive result on peritoneal cytologic washings
  - B. Vaginal metastases
  - C. Involved pelvic/para-aortic lymph nodes
- Stage IV
  - A. Extension to involve the mucosa of the bladder or rectum
  - B. Distant metastatic disease or inguinal node involvement
- Stages are also subgrouped according to histologic grade
  - G1: Well differentiated
  - G2: Moderately differentiated
  - G3: Poorly differentiated

DIFFERENTIAL DIAGNOSIS
- Atypical complex hyperplasia (a premalignant lesion of the endometrium)
- Bleeding resulting from cervical cancer
- Ovarian cancer invading the uterus
- Adenocarcinoma of the cervix
- Endometriosis
- Adenomyosis

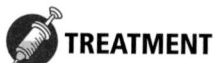 TREATMENT

INITIAL STABILIZATION
According to comorbidities.

GENERAL MEASURES
- Main treatment for uterine cancer is surgery.
- Radiation is used to prevent tumor recurrence at the vaginal cuff.

Diet
As tolerated and according to comorbidities.

Activity
Patients are usually ambulatory and able to resume full activity by 6 weeks postsurgery.

SPECIAL THERAPY
Radiotherapy

- Nonoperative candidates: Radiation therapy alone. (1)[A]
- Low risk: No adjuvant radiation therapy (1)[A]
- Intermediate risk: Consider adjuvant vaginal brachytherapy. Reduces local recurrences but has no effect on overall survival (1)[A]

- High risk: Chemotherapy and radiation therapy in some cases

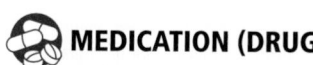 MEDICATION (DRUGS)

First Line
- Endometrial

  – Chemotherapy for high risk or metastatic disease—the 2 regimens include (2–4)[A]
    ○ Doxorubicin + Cisplatin
    ○ Paclitaxel + Carboplatin

  – Hormonal therapy

    ○ Medroxyprogesterone acetate: For recurrence or metastases (2,4)[A]

    ○ Tamoxifen or aromatase inhibitors
    ○ Megestrol (Megace) 160 mg daily for 3 months for women with premalignant lesions, atypical complex hyperplasia, or well differentiated endometrial cancer desiring continued fertility. Follow with dilation and curettage to determine cancer resolution.
- Sarcoma
  – Chemotherapy

    ○ Doxorubicin combinations (5)[A]

  – Hormonal
    ○ Tamoxifen or aromatase inhibitors
    ○ Progesterones

Second Line
Ondansetron (Zofran), dronabinol (Marinol), metoclopramide (Reglan), and others to control nausea from chemotherapy

SURGERY
Surgical staging followed by chemotherapy, radiation therapy, if indicated
- Cytologic washings
- Extrafascial hysterectomy and bilateral salpingoophorectomy
- Pelvic and para-aortic lymph node dissection
- Omental sampling as indicated
- Optimal tumor debulking

ALERT
Geriatric Considerations
Older (especially obese) patients may be at high risk for surgery. Alternative radiation therapy can be considered.

 FOLLOW-UP

DISPOSITION
Issues for Referral
Patients should be referred to gynecologic oncologist, radiation oncologist, and medical oncologist as indicated.

PROGNOSIS
5-year survival rate for uterine malignancy

Grade	Survival (%)
Ia G1	98
Ib G2	85
Ic G3	60
IIa/b	60
III	40
IV	15

COMPLICATIONS
- Surgical: Excessive bleeding, wound infection, lymphedema, deep vein thrombosis (DVT), and damage to the urinary or intestinal systems
- Radiation: Diarrhea, ileus, bowel obstruction or fistula, radiation cystitis, proctitis, vaginal stenosis, DVT
- Chemotherapy: Per the drug given

PATIENT MONITORING
- Pap smear every 4 months for 2 years, then every 6 months for 3 years
- Chest x-ray annually

REFERENCES

1. Einhorn N, Trope C, Ridderheim M, Boman K, Sorbe B, Cavallin-Stahl E. A systematic overview of radiation therapy effects in uterine cancer (corpus uteri). *Acta Oncol.* 2003;42(5–6):557–561.
2. Polyzos NP, Pavlidis N, Paraskevaidis E, Ioannidis JP. Randomized evidence on chemotherapy and hormonal therapy regimens for advanced endometrial cancer: An overview of survival data. *Eur J Cancer.* 2006;42:319–326.
3. Humber C, Tierney J, Symonds P, et al. Chemotherapy for advanced, recurrent or metastatic endometrial carcinoma. *Cochrane Database Syst Rev.* 2005;(4):CD003915.
4. Martin-Hirsch PL, Jarvis G, Kitchener H, Lilford R. Progestagens for endometrial cancer. *Cochrane Database Syst Rev.* 2000;(2):CD001040.
5. Bramwell VH, Anderson D, Charette ML; Sarcoma Disease Site Group. Doxorubicin-based chemotherapy for the palliative treatment of adult patients with locally advanced or metastatic soft tissue sarcoma. *Cochrane Database Syst Rev.* 2003;(3):CD003293

 MISCELLANEOUS

See also: Cervical malignancy

CODES

ICD9-CM
- 180.0 Malignant neoplasm of body of cervix uteri, endocervix
- 182.0 Malignant neoplasm of corpus uteri, except isthmus
- 182.1 Malignant neoplasm of body of uterus, isthmus
- 182.8 Malignant neoplasm of other specified sites of body of uterus

PATIENT TEACHING
- The American Cancer Society in the local community
- American Cancer Society, www.cancer.org
- American College of Obstetricians & Gynecologists (ACOG), 409 12th St., SW, Washington, DC 20024-2188; (800) 762-ACOG

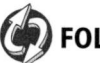 See Patient Handout on CD

E

ENDOMETRIOSIS

Nicholas J. Spirtos DO

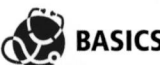 **BASICS**

DESCRIPTION
- Heterotopic islands of uterine mucosa (endometrium) found in many locations
- Pelvic sites: Peritoneal surfaces (bladder, cul-de-sac, pelvic side walls, broad ligaments, uterosacral ligaments, fallopian tubes, and uterus), lymph nodes, ovaries, and bowel
- Distant sites: Vagina, cervix, abdominal wall, arm, leg, pleura, lung, diaphragm, kidneys, spleen, gallbladder, nasal mucous membranes, spinal canal, stomach, and breast
- System(s) Affected: Reproductive
- Synonym(s): Endometriosis externa

GENERAL PREVENTION
- Pregnancy seems to have a temporary ameliorating effect on the course of the disease.
- Endometriosis is generally a recurring disorder that may persist even into early menopause.

EPIDEMIOLOGY
- Predominant age: Women of reproductive age and possibly in menopausal women, with signs and symptoms aggravated by hormone replacement therapy
- Predominant sex: Female only

Prevalence
May be as high as 25% in women of reproductive age

RISK FACTORS
- Hereditary/genetic predisposition
- Delayed childbearing
- Luteinized unruptured follicle syndrome (granulosa/theca cells undergo luteinization, but actual follicular rupture fails to occur, thereby predisposing to limited progesterone secretion into peritoneal cavity, thus allowing refluxed endometrial cells to implant and proliferate)

ETIOLOGY
- Retrograde menstruation (Sampson's theory)
- Lymphatic/vascular metastases (Halban's theory)
- Direct implantation
- Coelomic metaplasia (coelomic epithelium undergoes metaplasia, forming functioning endometrium)

ASSOCIATED CONDITIONS
- Pelvic endometriosis is rarely associated with endometrioid carcinoma of the ovary.
- Hematuria with bladder involvement
- Rectal bleeding with bowel involvement
- Hemoptysis with lung involvement

DIAGNOSIS

SIGNS AND SYMPTOMS
- Infertility (30–40% of patients with endometriosis)
- Dyspareunia
- Dysmenorrhea
- Dyschezia
- Chronic pelvic pain
- Premenstrual spotting
- Spontaneous abortion (theoretic)
- Luteinized unruptured follicle syndrome

TESTS
Cancer antigen 125 (CA-125) test

Lab
No special value, but CA-125 levels may be elevated

Imaging
- Vaginal/abdominal ultrasound (identify only endometriomas of ovaries)
- MRI for pelvic masses (endometriomas)
- Hysterosalpingography for tubal occlusion proximally or distally and periadnexal adhesions

Diagnostic Procedures/Surgery
Laparoscopy

Pathological Findings
Biopsy of endometriotic lesions usually demonstrates both endometrial glands and stroma

DIFFERENTIAL DIAGNOSIS
Differential diagnosis of pelvic pain includes all causes of acute abdomen, including
- Complications of intrauterine and extrauterine pregnancy
- Urinary tract infection
- Irritable bowel syndrome
- Ulcerative colitis
- Crohn disease
- Pelvic adhesions
- Acute salpingitis
- Ruptured ovarian cyst
- Intussusception
- Malignancies
- Other conditions

TREATMENT

INITIAL STABILIZATION
Diagnose and treat early to prevent sequelae such as infertility and pelvic pain

GENERAL MEASURES
Diet
No special diet

Activity
Activity may be limited, depending on severity of pelvic pain.

MEDICATION (DRUGS)

First Line
- Gonadotropin-releasing hormone (GnRH) agonists such as
  - Nafarelin (Synarel) intranasal 400 μg/d divided as 2 inhalations per day, 1 in each nostril. If patient continues with menses after 2 months of treatment, dose may be increased to 800 μg.
  - Leuprolide acetate (Lupron, Lupron Depot) 0.5–1.0 mg/d or 3.75–7.5 mg/month, respectively
  - Goserelin (Zoladex) implant 3.6 mg SC every 4 weeks for 6 months
- Maintenance
  - 6–9 months of therapy followed by active attempts at pregnancy or maintenance therapy with oral contraceptive agents
  - Calcium supplementation 1,000–1,500 mg/d is recommended when using GnRH analog therapy to prevent calcium loss as women become severely hypoestrogenic
- Contraindications
  - Any contraindication to the drug itself or of hypoestrogenemia
- Precautions
  - Calcium loss secondary to hypoestrogenemia
  - Hot flashes secondary to hypoestrogenemia
  - Paresthesias of face and upper extremities
  - Contraception measures should be used by sexually active women because ovulation may not be suppressed even if menses cease.
- Significant possible interactions
  - Refer to the manufacturer's literature

Second Line
- Danazol (Danocrine) 400–800 mg/d for 6–9 months
- Medroxyprogesterone (Provera) 30 mg/d for 6–9 months
- Megestrol (Megace) 40 mg/d for 6–9 months
- "Continuous" oral contraceptives (e.g., ethinyl estradiol-norgestrel [Lo/Ovral, Ovral]) until childbearing is desired if no medical contraindications

SURGERY
- At the time of laparoscopy, attempt laser vaporization or fulguration of implants, drainage/resection of ovarian endometriomas, and lysis of pelvic adhesions.
- Consider uterosacral ligament laser vaporization/fulguration for presacral neurectomy for severe pelvic pain or dysmenorrhea. Microsurgery or in vitro fertilization or gamete intrafallopian tube transfer may be necessary when laparoscopic surgery followed by superovulation induction with human menopausal gonadotropins, pure follicle-stimulating hormone, and artificial intrauterine insemination have failed to achieve pregnancy.

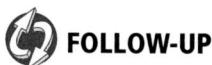 **FOLLOW-UP**

Pregnancy Considerations
Refer to board-certified reproductive endocrinologist or gynecologist with expertise in infertility

Geriatric Considerations
Endometriosis may persist even during early menopause and may be exacerbated with estrogen replacement therapy.

PROGNOSIS
- Pregnancy should occur, but depends on the severity of the disease
- Signs and symptoms generally regress with the onset of menopause but can usually be controlled during the reproductive years.

COMPLICATIONS
- Infertility/subfertility
  - Endometriosis of the intramural portion of the fallopian tube may cause isthmic proximal tubal obstruction and infertility.
  - Infertility may be related not only to anatomic disruption of pelvic structures but to liberation of peritoneal macrophages, which may predispose to gamete phagocytosis
  - Immune disorders, such as production of antiendometrial antibodies, can also be associated with reproductive dysfunction.
- Sterility
- Chronic pelvic pain
- Total abdominal hysterectomy and bilateral salpingo-oophorectomy
- Intussusception

PATIENT MONITORING
- Monitor serum estradiol levels until <10 pg/mL (37 pmol/L) when using GnRH analogs
- Monitor patient's pain response with history and physical exams every 8–12 weeks
- Monitor size of ovarian endometriomas with ultrasound every 8–12 weeks
- May need additional surgery depending on patient's fertility and/or pelvic pain

REFERENCES
1. Berger DL, Mohammadkhani MS. Weekly clinicopathological exercises: Case 13-2000: A 26-year-old women with bouts of abdominal pain, vomiting, and diarrhea. *N Engl J Med*. 2000; 342:1272–1278.
2. Speroff L, Glass RH, Kase NG: Endometriosis and infertility. In: Brown CL, ed. *Clinical Gynecologic Endocrinology and Infertility*. 5th ed. Baltimore, MD: Williams & Wilkins; 1994.

 MISCELLANEOUS

See also: Appendicitis; acute; Ectopic pregnancy
- Other notes
  - Educate female patients of reproductive age as to the signs and symptoms of pelvic endometriosis, especially teenagers complaining of dysmenorrhea and/or dyspareunia.

CODES

ICD9-CM
- 617.0 Endometriosis of uterus
- 617.3 Endometriosis of pelvic peritoneum

PATIENT TEACHING
- Prevention of disease is difficult but may be maintained in quiescent state with oral contraceptive agents
- Printed materials available from The American Fertility Society, 2140 11th Ave South, Suite 200, Birmingham, AL 35205-2800; (205) 933–8494

 See Corresponding Diagnostic Algorithm

See Patient Handout on CD

E

ENURESIS

Paul R. Gittens, MD
Leonard G. Gomella, MD

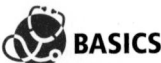 **BASICS**

DESCRIPTION
- Nocturnal enuresis (NE): The involuntary passage of urine while asleep after the anticipated age of bladder control (age 5).
- Classified: Primary NE and secondary NE
  - Primary NE (1% of adult population; 87.4% of all cases): Child/adult who has never been continent at night for at least 6 months
  - Secondary NE (11.6% of cases): Return of loss of urine after a period of 6 months or more of urinary control
- Also categorized as
  - Monosymptomatic NE: Bed wetting with normal daytime urination (80–85% of NE)
  - Polysymptomatic NE: Bed wetting with other symptoms (frequency, urgency)
- Adult-onset NE with absent daytime incontinence is a serious symptom; it usually signifies significant urethral obstruction and a high incidence of bladder diverticulum, hydronephrosis, and vesicoureteral is reflux. Complete urologic evaluation and therapy are warranted. Urodynamic studies needed to assess for lower urinary tract dysfunction (anatomic or neurologic).
  - Usually associated with diurnal symptoms, voiding dysfunction, and UI
- System(s) Affected: Nervous; Renal/Urologic
  - DSM-IV describes NE as a child >5 years with repeated voiding of urine in the bed or clothes at least twice a week for at least 3 consecutive months.
- Synonym(s): Bed wetting; Sleep enuresis; Nocturnal incontinence; Primary nocturnal enuresis

GENERAL PREVENTION
No measures known

EPIDEMIOLOGY
- American children achieve toilet training readiness skills by ~22–30 months
- Girls get bladder control sooner than boys
- ~5% of school age children bed wet every night of the week
- Predominant sex: Male > Female (2:1)

Prevalence
- 15% of children wet the bed at 5 years of age
- Ages 7 and 10 years
  - 9% and 7% in boys
  - 6% and 3% in girls
- Spontaneous resolution: 15% per year
- >18 prevalence is 0.5–2%

Pediatric Considerations
Relatively common problem

Geriatric Considerations
Infrequent; often associated with diurnal enuresis (incontinence)

RISK FACTORS
- Family history
- Stressors (emotional, environmental) common in secondary enuresis (e.g., divorce, death, etc.)
- Constipation and encopresis
- Organic disease
  - 1% of monsymptomatic NE (e.g., UTI, posterior urethral valves, ectopic ureter, constipation, diabetes, spinal cord pathology, sleep apnea)
- Psychological disorders
  - Comorbid disorders are highest with secondary NE
  - Conduct disorder, hyperkinetic syndrome, internalizing disorders
  - Association with attention deficient hyperactivity disorder
  - Abuse; victims may present with NE
  - NE can precipitate a child or elderly/dependent to become abused.
- Altered mental status or impaired mobility

Genetics
- Nocturnal bladder control is more heritable in boys than in girls
- Most commonly, NE is an autosomal dominant inheritance pattern with high penetrance (90%)
  - 1/3 of all cases are sporadic.
  - 4 loci associated with NE identified
  - Higher rates in monozygotic vs. dizygotic twins
  - 75% of children with enuresis have a 1st-degree relative with the condition
  - If both parents had NE, risk in child is 77%; 44% if 1 parent affected
  - 15% of children with no parental history

ETIOLOGY
- Both functional and organic causes; many theories, none absolutely confirmed
- Some suggests NE is caused by a mismatch in nocturnal urine production and small functional bladder capacity.
- Increased bladder instability
- Deficiency of arginine vasopressin (AVP); due to decreased inherent nocturnal AVP or decreased AVP stimulation secondary to an empty bladder (bladder distention stimulates AVP)
- No evidence of sleep disorders/alterated sleep pattern. NE occurs in all stages of sleep.
- Maturational delay of central nervous system
- Organic urologic causes in 1–4% of enuresis in children: UTI, occult spina bifida, ectopic ureter, lazy bladder syndrome, irritable bladder with wide bladder neck
- Organic non-urologic causes: Epilepsy, diabetes mellitus, food allergies, obstructive sleep apnea

Pregnancy Considerations
Voiding changes common, may resolve after birth

ASSOCIATED CONDITIONS
See "Risk Factors."

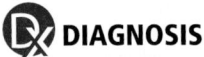 **DIAGNOSIS**

SIGNS AND SYMPTOMS
- Bed wetting
- Lower urinary tract symptoms
- Posturing to hold urine
- Children may be withdrawn and shy; some show aggressive behaviors; both may be secondary to enuresis and not primary behaviors.
- Stress factors (intrafamilial discord, significant life events, psychosocial or emotional problems)

History
- Distinguish primary or secondary NE
- Lower urinary tract symptoms
- Constipation and encopresis
- Intake daily with voiding and elimination
- General medical history, allergies, and medication
- Psychosocial history
- Family history of enuresis

Physical Exam
- Genital urinary exam
  - Males: Meatal stenosis, hypospadias, epispadias, phimosis
  - Females: Vulvitis, vaginitis, labial adhesions, ureterocele at introitus. Wide vaginal orifice with scar or healed laceration, may be evidence of abuse.
- Anatomic anomalies may predispose to UTI
- Dimpling or tufts of hair on sacrum
- Neurological exam
- Rectal exam: Tone and constipation

TESTS
- Urodynamic testing may be beneficial in adults and polysymptomatic NE; more urodynamic study findings than in children (28–70%)
- Detrusor instability and/or reduced bladder capacity most common findings
- Uroflow and residual urine indicated when day symptoms are present or are not able to be excluded and adult onset NE

Lab
- Urinalysis sufficient in monosymptomatic
- Urinalysis and culture: UTI, pyuria, hematuria, proteinuria, glycosuria, and poor concentrating ability (low specific gravity) may suggest organic etiology, especially in adults.
- Blood urea nitrogen and creatinine: Renal insufficiency
- Urine cytology if bladder carcinoma suspected
- Drugs that may alter lab results: Diuretics may cause low urinary-specific gravity.

Imaging

- Urinary tract imaging is usually not necessary; findings are similar in normal population
- If abnormal clinical findings or adult onset
- IV pyelogram, renal ultrasound, voiding cystourethrogram, or retrograde pyelogram as indicated; may detect anomalies
- Spine radiographs for spina bifida occulta

DIFFERENTIAL DIAGNOSIS

- Primary NE
  - Delayed physiologic urinary control
  - UTI (both)
  - Spina bifida occulta
  - Obstructive sleep apnea (both)
  - Idiopathic detrusor instability
  - Previously unrecognized myelopathy or neuropathy (e.g., multiple sclerosis, tethered cord, epilepsy)
  - Anatomic urinary tract abnormally (e.g., ectopic ureter)
- Secondary NE
  - Bladder outlet obstruction
  - Neurological disease, neurogenic bladder (e.g., spinal cord injury)

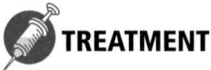 TREATMENT

Pediatric Considerations

Self-concept and self-esteem are adversely affected by enuresis in children; therefore, early successful treatment is advocated. Very rare

GENERAL MEASURES

- Pharmacotherapy, psychotherapy, and behavioral modifications
- Counseling care provider and child regarding enuresis, its occurrence, and prognosis
- Address correctable cause (e.g., UTI, constipation, encopresis, diabetes mellitus)
- Psychotherapy requires participation of child together with the entire family
- Behavioral modifications
  - Self-monitoring and record keeping are primary techniques to improve enuresis.
  - Motivation and responsibility training: Child responsible for cleaning bed linen
  - Calendar with "star" rewards for dry nights and some reward system
  - Efficacy of 25%, with 5% relapse rate
  - Penalties for wetting counterproductive
- Bladder training: Exercises to increase bladder capacity (biofeedback); variable results
- Enuresis alarms: 70% success; 30% relapse. They appear more effective than drugs by the end of treatment.
- Alternative treatments: Acupuncture (traditional and laser), hypnosis

Diet

- Restricting liquids after 6 p.m. may help.
- Avoid caffeinated beverages (diuretic effect).
- Low calcium and sodium dietary content in late afternoon and nighttime meals
- Avoid foods that appear to cause urinary problems (e.g., spicy foods, certain fruits).

Activity

No restrictions

 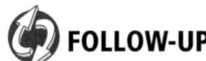 MEDICATION (DRUGS)

First Line

- Imipramine (Tofranil): Tricyclic antidepressant, anticholinergic effects; increases bladder capacity, antispasmodic properties
- Imipramine used primarily in adults; use in children reserved for resistant cases
- Dose: Adults, 25–75 mg and children >6 years, 10–25 mg PO at bedtime; increase by 10–25 mg at 1–2 week intervals, treat for 2–3 months, then taper; 25–30% success when used >3 months
- Desmopressin (DDAVP): Synthetic analog of vasopressin, decreases nocturnal urine output. Intranasally 20–40 ug
  - Child >6 years old, 20 μg intranasally at bedtime
  - Oral DDAVP: 0.2 mg, titrate to 0.6 mg
  - 10–60% success; safe even when used for >12 months; high relapse rate after discontinuation without a structured withdrawal program
- Oxybutynin (Ditropan, Ditropan XL, Oxytrol patch): anticholinergic—smooth muscle relaxant, antispasmodic; may increase functional bladder capacity and aids in timed voiding
  - Ditropan: Adults and children >5 years, 5 mg PO t.i.d.–q.i.d.; children 1–5 years old, 0.02 mg/kg/dose b.i.d.– q.i.d. (syrup 5 mg/5 mL)
  - Ditropan XL: Adults, 5 mg/d PO; increase to 30 mg/d PO (5, 10-mg tabs)
  - Oxytrol patch: 1 patch every 3–4 days (3.9 mg/patch) (w/drug holidays)
  - Ditropan 5–10 mg nighttime dose: 30–50% success, 50% relapse after stopped
- Tolterodine (Detrol, Detrol LA): Anticholinergic, fewer side effects than Ditropan.
  - Detrol: 1–2 mg PO b.i.d.
  - Detrol LA: 2–4 mg/d
- Precautions
  - Oxybutynin: Glaucoma, myasthenia gravis, gastrointestinal or genitourinary obstruction, ulcerative colitis, megacolon. Use a decreased dose in the elderly.
  - Tolterodine: Urinary retention, gastric retention, or uncontrolled narrow-angle glaucoma; significant drug interactions with CYP2D6, CYP3A3/4 substrates
  - DDAVP: Avoid in patient at risk for electrolyte changes or fluid retention (CHF, renal insufficiency)
  - Imipramine: Do not use with monoamine oxidase inhibitor, hypotension and arrhythmias; low toxic therapeutic ratio
- Refer to the manufacturer's profile for each drug.

Second Line

- Combination therapy with DDVAP and oxbutynin has shown to have better results than individual use.
- Prostaglandin inhibitors (indomethacin) studied; may increase in bladder capacity

SURGERY

Only in surgically correctable cause (e.g., tethered cord, ectopic ureter, benign prostatitic hypertrophy, obstructive sleep apnea)

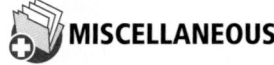 FOLLOW-UP

PROGNOSIS

In children, NE usually self-limiting; 1% will persist as adult; evaluate for organic causes

COMPLICATIONS

UTI, perineal excoriation, psychological problems (especially in children)

PATIENT MONITORING

Follow until enuresis resolved; monitor therapy

REFERENCES

1. Berberich HJ, Neubauer H. Urological dysfunction after sexual abuse and violence. *Urologe A.* 2004;43:273–237.
2. Can G, et al. Child abuse as a result of enuresis. *Pediatr Int.* 2004;46:64–66.
3. Diehr S, Bercaw D. How effective is desmopressin for primary nocturnal enuresis? *Fam Pract.* 2003;52:568–569.
4. Djurhuus JC, Rittig S. Nocturnal enuresis. *Curr Opin Urol.* 2002;12:317–320.
5. Hjalmas K et al. Nocturnal enuresis: An international evidence based mananagement strategy. *Journal of Urol.* 2004;171:2545–2561.
6. Glazener CM, Evans JH, Peto RE. Alarm interventions for nocturnal enuresis in children. *Cochrane Database Syst Rev.* 2003: CD002911.
7. Lee T, Comparison of effects of treatment of primary nocturnal enuresis with oxybutynin plus desmopressin, desmopressin alone, migraine alone: A randomized controlled clinical trial. *J Urol.* 2005;174:1084–1087.
8. Mammen AA, Ferrer FA: Nocturnal enuresis: Medical management. *Urol Clin N AM.* 2004;31:491–498.
9. NieldL. S, Kamat D. Enuresis: How to evaluate and treat. *Clin Pediatrics.* 2004;43:409–415.
10. Rawashdeh YF et al. Demographics of enuresis patients attending a referral centre. *Scand J Urol Nephrol*
11. Sakamoto K, Blaivas JG. Adult onset nocturnal enuresis. *Urology.* 2001;165(6 pt 1):1914–1917.

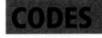 MISCELLANEOUS

See also: Urinary incontinence

CODES

ICD9-CM

- 307.6 Enuresis
- 788.30 Urinary incontinence, unspecified

PATIENT TEACHING

- Explain to parents that most cases of childhood enuresis resolve spontaneously.
- Limit fluids near bedtime

 See Corresponding Diagnostic Algorithm

E

EOSINOPHILIC PNEUMONIAS

George E. Kikano, MD

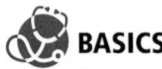 **BASICS**

DESCRIPTION
- Eosinophilic pneumonias are characterized by eosinophilic lung infiltrates with or without peripheral blood eosinophilia.
- They are classified as acute or chronic and can be either idiopathic or secondary to other causes.
- Included are
  - Löffler syndrome (simple pulmonary eosinophilia)
  - Allergic bronchopulmonary aspergillosis
  - Drug-induced pulmonary eosinophilia
  - Tropical pulmonary eosinophilia
  - Chronic or prolonged pulmonary eosinophilia
  - Hypereosinophilic syndrome
  - Churg-Strauss syndrome (polyarteritis nodosa) or allergic angiitis
- System(s) Affected: Pulmonary
- Synonym(s): Löffler syndrome; Pulmonary infiltrates with eosinophilia syndrome (PIE)

GENERAL PREVENTION
Avoid exposure to offending agent

EPIDEMIOLOGY
Incidence
In the US: Rare

Prevalence
- Predominant age: Any age
- Predominant sex: Male = Female (male in 4th decade; female in 6th decade)

RISK FACTORS
- Patients with chronic disorders (e.g., asthma, cystic fibrosis)
- Living or traveling in certain geographical areas (e.g., India, Ceylon, Burma, Malaysia, Indonesia, tropical Africa, South America, South Pacific)
- Cigarette smoking has recently been suggested.

Genetics
No known genetic pattern

ETIOLOGY
- Idiopathic (though hypersensitivity suspected) in 1/3 of cases
- Drugs/toxins (penicillin, nitrofurantoin, isoniazid, chlorpropamide, sulfonamides, antituberculous therapy [para-aminosalicylic acid (PAS)], gold, aspirin, hydralazine)
- Tropical
  - Parasites
  - *Toxocara* larvae
  - Filariae
  - Nematodes (*Strongyloides, Ascaris, Ancylostoma*)
- *Aspergillus fumigatus* (asthmatic pulmonary eosinophilia)
- Systemic vasculitis

ASSOCIATED CONDITIONS
- Asthma
- Hypersensitivity pneumonitis
- Wegener granulomatosis

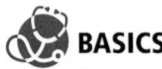 **DIAGNOSIS**

SIGNS AND SYMPTOMS
- Dyspnea
- Fever in acute cases
- Cough with sputum
- Chills
- Hypoxia
- Wheezing in some patients
- Anorexia
- Decreased localized breath sounds
- Tachycardia
- Malaise
- Symptoms may be mild or life-threatening

History
With particular emphasis on drug intake, recent travel to tropical areas

Physical Exam
With particular emphasis on systemic symptoms

TESTS
- Bronchoscopy with broncho alveolar lavage
- Lung biopsy when diagnosis uncertain or clinical course is severe (rare)
- Pulmonary function studies

Lab
- Leukocytosis
- Eosinophilia in peripheral blood and lungs
- *A. fumigatus* found in sputum
- Positive filarial complement fixation
- Elevated IgE levels
- Increased WBC
- Elevated erythrocyte sedimentation rate
- Stool examination for parasites

Imaging
High-resolution CT, chest x-ray: Migratory infiltrates, small pleural effusion; transient infiltrates; interstitial opacities

Diagnostic Procedures/Surgery
Bronchoscopy with broncho-alveolar lavage

Pathological Findings
Lung
- Alveolar eosinophilic filling
- Septal eosinophilic infiltration

DIFFERENTIAL DIAGNOSIS
- Tuberculosis
- Sarcoidosis
- Hodgkin lymphoma
- Other lymphoproliferative disorders
- Eosinophilic granuloma of the lung
- Desquamative interstitial pneumonitis
- Hypereosinophilic syndrome
- Wegener granulomatosis
- Interstitial lung disease

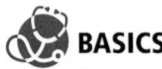 **TREATMENT**

GENERAL MEASURES
- Appropriate health care
  - Outpatient for milder cases
  - More severe cases may require inpatient care.
- Evaluate for secondary causes
- Mild cases may require no specific therapy.
- Coughing and deep breathing exercises to clear secretions
- Discontinuing offending drug
- Treatment of underlying parasite infestation

Diet
High calorie, high protein, soft diet

Activity
As tolerated

MEDICATION (DRUGS)

First Line
- Corticosteroid therapy
  - In chronic pulmonary eosinophilia, 20–40 mg prednisone daily
  - In Churg-Strauss syndrome, may require large doses (e.g., 40–60 mg of prednisone daily)
  - Withdrawal should be possible after recovery; in chronic conditions, treatment should continue for 6–12 months
- Treat asthma, if present
- Piperazine for *Ascaris* infestation
- Diethylcarbamazine (available only from the manufacturer) 6–8 mg/kg PO for 10–14 days for tropical pulmonary eosinophilia
- Appropriate vermifuges for helminthic infections
- Contraindications
  - Refer to the manufacturer's literature
- Precautions
  - Refer to the manufacturer's literature.
- Significant possible interactions
  - Refer to the manufacturer's literature.

Second Line
- In Churg-Strauss syndrome and cases resistant to corticosteroid therapy, adding azathioprine or cyclophosphamide may be helpful.
- Some patients may require oxygen therapy.

 FOLLOW-UP

PROGNOSIS
- Excellent in the milder forms
- Corticosteroid therapy is dramatically effective in more severe cases.

ALERT
Geriatric Considerations
More morbidity, probably due to decreased lung capacity and likelihood of concomitant diseases

COMPLICATIONS
- Some patients may show evidence of dysfunction in the small airways.
- Delay in treatment of tropical pulmonary eosinophilia may result in irreversible pulmonary fibrosis.

PATIENT MONITORING
Physical examinations and chest x-rays until resolved

REFERENCES
1. Murray JF, Nadel JA, eds. *Textbook of Respiratory Medicine*. 3rd ed. Philadelphia, PA: W.B. Saunders; 2000.

 MISCELLANEOUS

See also: Aspergillosis; HIV-associated; Roundworms; Tissue; Tuberculosis; Wegener granulomatosis

CODES

ICD9-CM
518.3 Pulmonary eosinophilia

PATIENT TEACHING

Provide information about activity, diet, and symptoms of recurrence and advise patient to avoid exposure of offending agent, if possible.

E

EPICONDYLITIS

Shawn M. Ferullo, MD

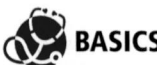 **BASICS**

DESCRIPTION
- Tendon injury characterized by pain and tenderness at the tendinous origins of the wrist flexors/extensors on the epicondyles of the humerus.
- May be acute (traumatic) or chronic (overuse)
- 2 types
  - Medial epicondylitis or "Golfer's Elbow"
    - Involvement of the wrist flexors and pronators on the medial epicondyle
  - Lateral epicondylitis or "Tennis Elbow"
    - Involvement of the wrist extensors and supinators on the lateral epicondyle
- May be caused by many different athletic or occupational activities
- Common in carpenters, plumbers, gardeners
- Usually occurs unilaterally on the epicondyles of the dominant arm
- Lateral > Medial

GENERAL PREVENTION
- Limit overuse of the wrist flexors, extensors, pronators, and supinators.
- Use proper techniques when working.
- Use lighter tools.

EPIDEMIOLOGY
- Predominant age: >40
- Predominant sex: Male = Female

Incidence
- Very common site of overuse injury
- Lateral > Medial

RISK FACTORS
- Repetitive wrist motions
  - Flexion/pronation → medial
  - Extension/supination → lateral

PATHOPHYSIOLOGY
- Acute (tendonitis)
  - Inflammatory response to injury
- Chronic (tendonosis)
  - Overuse injury
  - Tendon degeneration, fibroblast proliferation, microvascular proliferation, lack of inflammatory response

ETIOLOGY
- Repetitive wrist motions
- Tool/racquet gripping
- Shaking hands
- Sudden maximal muscle contraction
- Direct blow

DIAGNOSIS

SIGNS AND SYMPTOMS
- Localized pain just proximal to the affected epicondyle
- Increased pain with wrist flexion/pronation (medial)
- Increased pain with wrist extension/supination (lateral)
- Pain with gripping
- Sensation of mild forearm weakness

History
- Occupational activities
- Sport participation
- Direct trauma
- Duration of symptoms
- Treatments or medication use

Physical Exam
- Medial epicondylitis
  - Tenderness at origin of wrist flexor tendons
  - Increased pain with resisted wrist flexion and pronation
  - Normal elbow range of motion
  - Increased pain with gripping
- Lateral epicondylitis
  - Tenderness at origin of wrist extensors
  - Increased pain with resisted wrist extension/supination
  - Normal elbow range of motion
  - Increased pain with gripping

TESTS
Imaging
- None required
- Anterior–posterior/lateral radiograph if decreased range of motion or trauma
- MRI for recalcitrant cases

Diagnostic Procedures/Surgery
Local injection of anesthetic to document resolution of symptoms

DIFFERENTIAL DIAGNOSIS
- Osteoarthritis
- Fractures of the epicondyles
- Posterior Interosseous nerve entrapment (lateral)
- Ulnar neuropathy (medial)
- Synovitis

TREATMENT

GENERAL MEASURES
- May take weeks to months to resolve
- Majority of patients will improve with conservative treatment
- Relative rest with reduction of aggravating activities
- Changing technique of activities
- Ice to area for 10 minutes b.i.d.
- Elbow straps during activity. (1)[B]

Activity
Relative rest

SPECIAL THERAPY
Physical Therapy
- Begin once acute pain resolved
- Focus on eccentric strength training
- Grip exercises
- Ultrasound (2)[B]
- Corticosteroid iontophoresis

Complementary and Alternative Therapies
- Accupuncture
- Botulinum toxin injections (3)[B]

MEDICATION (DRUGS)

First Line
NSAIDs: Good for short term relief. There are no data to support long-term usefulness. (4)[B]

Second Line
Corticosteroid injections (5)[B]

- Help relieve pain in acute setting, no effect in long-term outcome

SURGERY
- May be indicated in refractory cases
- Involves débridement and release of the involved tendons
- Can be performed open or arthroscopically (1)[B]

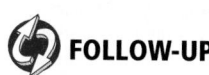 **FOLLOW-UP**

DISPOSITION
Issues for Referral
Failure of conservative therapy

PROGNOSIS
Good; majority resolve with conservative care

REFERENCES

1. Dunkow PD, Jatti M, Muddu BN. A comparison of open and percutaneous techniques in the surgical treatment of tennis elbow. *J Bone Joint Surg[Br]*. 2004;86-B:701.
2. Smidt N et al., Corticosteroid injections, physiotherapy or a wait-and-see policy for lateral epicondylitis: A randomized controlled trial. *Lancet*. 2002;359:657–662.
3. Wong SM et al., Treatment of lateral epicondylitis with botulinum toxin: A randomized, double blind, placebo-controlled trial. *Ann Intern Med*. 2005; 143(11):793–797.
4. Green S et al., Non-steroidal anti-inflammatory drugs for treating lateral elbow pain in adults. *Cochrane Database Syst Rev*. 2001;(4):CD002267.
5. Assendelft WJ et al.,Tennis elbow (lateral epicondylitis). *Clinical Evidence*. 2002; 8:1290–1300.
6. Wilson JJ, Best TM. Common overuse tendon problems a review and recommendations for treatment. *Am Fam Physician*. 2005; 72(5):811–818.

 MISCELLANEOUS

CODES

ICD9-CM
- 726.31 Medial Epicondylitis
- 726.32 Lateral Epicondylitis

PATIENT TEACHING

 See Corresponding Diagnostic Algorithm

 See Patient Handout on CD

E

EPIDIDYMITIS

Peter T. Nieh, MD

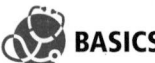 **BASICS**

DESCRIPTION
Inflammation of the epididymis resulting in scrotal pain, swelling and induration of the posterior-lying epididymis, and eventual scrotal wall edema, involvement of the adjacent testicle, and hydrocele formation (1)[C]
- System(s) Affected: Reproductive
- Synonym(s): Epididymo-orchitis

GENERAL PREVENTION
- Vasectomy or vasoligation during transurethral surgery
- Antibiotic prophylaxis for urethral manipulation
- Early treatment of prostatitis
- Avoid vigorous rectal examination with acute prostatitis

EPIDEMIOLOGY
- Predominant age: Usually younger, sexually active men or older men with urinary infection, but may also rarely occur in prepuberal boys
- Predominant sex: Male only

Incidence
Common

Prevalence
Common

RISK FACTORS
- Urinary tract infection (UTI), particularly prostatitis
- Indwelling urethral catheter
- Urethral instrumentation or transurethral surgery
- Urethral stricture
- Transrectal prostate biopsy (2)[C]
- Prostate brachytherapy (seeds) for prostate cancer
- Anal intercourse
- HIV-immunosuppressed patient
- Severe Behçet disease

PATHOPHYSIOLOGY
Epididymitis most often is owing to the retrograde extension of organisms from the prostate or urethra via thevas deferens and is rarely the result of hematogenous spread. The causative organism is identified in 80% of patients and varies according to the age of the patient.

ETIOLOGY
- <35 years
  – Usually chlamydia or *Neisseria gonorrhoeae*
  – Look for serous urethral discharge (chlamydia) or purulent discharge (gonorrhea).
- >35 years
  – Coliform bacteria usually, but sometimes *Staphylococcus aureus* or *S. epidermidis*
  – Often associated with distal urinary tract obstruction
  – Tuberculosis, if sterile pyuria and nodularity of vas deferens
  – Sterile urine reflux after transurethral prostatectomy
  – Granulomatous reaction following bacillus Calmette-Guérin intravesical therapy for superficial bladder cancer
- Prepubertal boys
  – Usually coliform bacteria
  – Evaluate for underlying congenital abnormalities, such as vesicoureteral reflux, ectopic ureter, or anorectal malformation (rectourethral fistula).
- At any age: Amiodarone, an antiarrhythmic agent, may cause noninfectious epididymitis that resolves with decreasing the drug dosage.
- Syphilis, brucellosis, blastomycosis, coccidioidomycosis, and cryptococcosis are rare causes of epididymitis.
- Nonbacterial epididymitis and epididymo-orchitis are not rare. Their cause is not clear, but may be secondary to retrograde extravasation.

ASSOCIATED CONDITIONS
- Prostatitis
- Urethritis

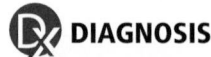 **DIAGNOSIS**

Pediatric Considerations
- In prepubertal patients, may be postinfectious inflammatory condition treated with analgesics and usually no antibiotics (3)[C]
- Bacteremia from *Haemophilus influenzae* infection may produce acute epididymitis.
- In adolescent males, must rule out acute testicular torsion

Geriatric Considerations
Diabetic patients with sensory neuropathy may have little pain despite severe infection/abscess.

SIGNS AND SYMPTOMS
- Scrotal pain, sometimes extending to the groin region, may begin relatively acutely over several hours.
- Urethral discharge or symptoms of UTI, such as frequency of urination, dysuria, cloudy urine, or hematuria
- Initially, only the posterior-lying epididymis, usually the lower-most tail section, is very tender and indurated.
- Elevation of the testes/epididymis improves the discomfort.
- Entire hemiscrotum becomes swollen, the testis becomes indistinguishable from the epididymis, the scrotal wall becomes thick and indurated, and reactive hydrocele may occur.
- Fever and chills occur with severe infection and abscess formation.

TESTS
Lab
- Pyuria on urinalysis
- Leukocytosis
- Gram stain urethral discharge

Imaging
- Ultrasound of scrotum
- Radionuclide scan

Diagnostic Procedures/Surgery
Scrotal exploration or aspiration of epididymis (rarely performed)

Pathological Findings
- Gross abscesses and microabscesses
- Organisms reach the epididymis through the lumen of the vas deferens.
- Interstitial congestion
- Fibrous scarring

DIFFERENTIAL DIAGNOSIS
- Epididymal congestion following vasectomy
- Testicular torsion
- Torsion of appendix testis
- Mumps orchitis
- Testicular tumor
- Testicular trauma
- Epididymal cyst
- Spermatocele
- Hydrocele
- Varicocele
- Epididymal adenomatoid tumor
- Epididymal rhabdomyosarcoma

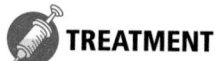 **TREATMENT**

INITIAL STABILIZATION
- Outpatient care, usually
- Inpatient, if septic or if surgery is scheduled

GENERAL MEASURES
- Scrotal elevation
- Ice pack
- Spermatic cord block with local anesthesia in severe cases

Diet
No restrictions, but force fluids

Activity
Bed rest for minimum of 1–2 days

Nursing
No special considerations

 MEDICATION (DRUG)

First Line
- <35 years, for chlamydia: Doxycycline 100 mg PO b.i.d. for 10 days and ceftriaxone 250 mg IM. Be sure to treat the sexual partner.
- If penicillin allergic or participates in insertive anal intercourse: Ciprofloxacin (Cipro) 500 mg PO b.i.d. or ofloxacin (Floxin) 200 mg PO b.i.d. for 10 days
- Older men with bacteriuria
  - Ciprofloxacin (Cipro) 500 mg PO b.i.d. or Ciprofloxacin (Cipro XL) 1,000 mg daily for 10–14 days
  - Levofloxacin (Levaquin) 250 mg PO b.i.d. for 10–14 days
  - Trimethoprim-sulfamethoxazole (Bactrim, Septra) double strength PO b.i.d. for 10–14 days
  - Amoxicillin/clavulanate (Augmentin) 500/125–875/125 mg PO b.i.d. for 10 days
- Analgesia
  - NSAIDs (e.g., naproxen or ibuprofen) for mild to moderate pain
  - Acetaminophen-codeine or acetaminophen-oxycodone for moderate to severe pain
- Septic or toxic patient
  - 3rd-generation cephalosporin (ceftriaxone 1–2 g IV/IM q24h; cefoperazone 1–2 g IV/IM q12h; ceftazidime 1 g IV/IM q8–12h (adjust for renal function)
  - Aminoglycoside (gentamicin 1 mg/kg IV/IM q8h, adjusted for renal function) after a loading dose of 2 mg/kg
  - Ampicillin/sulbactam (Unasyn) 1.5–3 g IV/IM q6h (adjust for renal function)
  - Ticarcillin/clavulanate (Timentin) 3.1 g IV q4–6h (adjust for renal function)
  - Piperacillin/tazobactam (Zosyn) 3.375 g IV q6h (adjust for renal function)
- Contraindications: None
- Precautions: Refer to the manufacturer's profile of each drug.
- Significant possible interactions: Refer to the manufacturer's profile of each drug.

Second Line
- Trimethoprim-sulfamethoxazole (Bactrim, Septra) double strength PO bid for 10–14 days; increasing bacterial resistance may limit effectiveness
- Other aminoglycosides or 3rd-generation cephalosporin depending on specific pathogen
- Add rifampin (rifampicin) or vancomycin as required.

SURGERY
- Aspiration of hydrocele to assist examination of scrotal contents and relieve discomfort
- Vasostomy to drain infected material
- Scrotal exploration, if uncertain whether condition is epididymitis or testicular torsion
- Drainage of abscesses, epididymectomy, or epididymo-orchiectomy in severe cases that do not respond to antibiotics

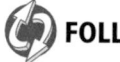 **FOLLOW-UP**

DISPOSITION
Admission Criteria
- Intractable pain
- Sepsis
- Purulent drainage

Discharge Criteria
- Comfortable with analgesics
- Afebrile or low-grade fever

Issues for Referral
If concerned about a urethral stricture, referral in 1–2 weeks with urologist to consider cystoscopy

PROGNOSIS
- Pain improves within 1–3 days, but induration may take several weeks/months to completely resolve
- If bilateral involvement, sterility may result.

COMPLICATIONS
- Recurrent epididymitis
- Infertility
- Fournier gangrene (necrotizing synergistic infection)

PATIENT MONITORING
Office visits until all signs of infection have cleared

REFERENCES
1. Berger RE. Acute epididymitis. *Semin Urol*. 1991;9:28.
2. Donzella JG, et al. Epididymitis after transrectal ultrasound-guided needle biopsy of prostate gland. *Urology*. 2004;63:306–308.
3. Somekh E, Gorenstein A, Serour F. Acute epididymitis in boys: Evidence of a post-infectious etiology. *J Urol*. 2004;171:391–394.

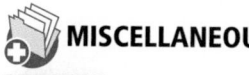 **MISCELLANEOUS**

CODES

ICD9-CM
604.90 Orchitis and epididymitis, unspecified

PATIENT TEACHING
- Stress completing course of antibiotics, even when asymptomatic.
- Early recognition and treatment of UTI or prostatitis

 See Patient Handout on CD

EPIGLOTTITIS

Vassiliki Syriopoulou, MD

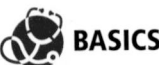 **BASICS**

DESCRIPTION

An illness with acute onset characterized by inflammation and edema of the supraglottic structures, epiglottis, vallecula, arytenoepiglottic folds, and arytenoids. (1,2)

- System(s) Affected: Pulmonary
- Synonym(s): Supraglottitis

GENERAL PREVENTION

- *Haemophilus influenzae* vaccine is effective although not 100% protective. (1–7)
- Rifampin prophylaxis (20 mg/kg/d for 4 days, maximum daily dose 600 mg) for all household and day care contacts. Family and close contacts may be asymptomatic carriers of *H. influenzae*.

EPIDEMIOLOGY

Predominant age

- In the prevaccine era, the most commonly affected group were children 2–4 years old.
- With increasing use of *H. influenzae* type b (Hib) vaccine, the predominant age is shifting to older children (median age, 7 years) and adults. (1,3,5,8)
- Predominant sex: Male > Female (1.8:1)

Incidence

- Has decreased dramatically since the introduction of the Hib vaccine (1,2,4)
- In adults: 1–3 in 100,000

Pediatric Considerations

Rare since introduction of Hib vaccine

Geriatric Considerations

Rare

PATHOPHYSIOLOGY

- In epiglottitis, usually a local invasion of the epiglottis occurs followed by bacteremia
- The epiglottis, aryepiglottic folds, false vocal cords, and supraglottic structures become inflamed and edematous, leading to narrowed airway and respiratory compromise.
- Inspiratory airway occlusion often occurs prior to total occlusion from supraglottic edema.

ETIOLOGY

- Bacterial
  – Hib
  – *Streptococcus pyogenes*
  – *Streptococcus pneumoniae*
  – *Staphylococcus aureus*
- Fungal
- Viral
- Traumatic: Caustic ingestion
- Allergic reactions

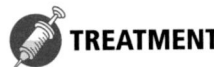 **DIAGNOSIS**

SIGNS AND SYMPTOMS

- Sudden onset and fulminant course
- Fever
- Sore throat
- Dysphagia, drooling
- Cervical adenopathy
- Airway obstruction resulting in respiratory distress
- "Tripod" position (sitting propped up on hands with head forward and tongue out)
- Muffled voice/cry (vs. hoarseness in croup)
- Minimal cough (vs. barking cough in croup)
- Toxic appearance/shock (occasionally, owing to associated septicemia)
- Stridor softer and less prominent than in croup
- Usually no history of prodromal upper respiratory infection (vs. positive history in croup)
- In adults, presentation is more indolent (sore throat is the predominate symptom).

TESTS

Lab

- Blood culture (positive in >75–90% of children with Hib acute epiglottitis). See under "Diagnostic Procedures/Surgery"—should not visualize/swab epiglottis except in controlled environment (e.g., operating room). Blood tests are also contraindicated until airway secured.
- Epiglottic swab culture (positive in 70%)
- CBC: Leukocytosis with left shift
- Hib antigen test in blood/urine useful in children with previous antibiotic treatment
- Hypoxia, usually not present until airway obstructed

Imaging

- Neck radiographs are contraindicated if epiglottitis is suspected because of danger of sudden complete airway obstruction, although lateral neck films are often obtained (ensure adequate staff in case complete airway obstruction occurs).
- Chest radiographs after intubation to check position of endotracheal tube and to rule out pneumonia, which may occur as a complication in ≤25% of cases

Diagnostic Procedures/Surgery

- Visualization of epiglottis with tongue depressor is contraindicated because of danger of sudden complete airway obstruction.
- Controlled visualization of epiglottis at intubation in OR is diagnostic (cherry red, edematous epiglottis)
- Lumbar puncture is indicated if there is clinical suspicion of meningitis
- In an adult, indirect laryngoscopy is generally safe

DIFFERENTIAL DIAGNOSIS

- Viral croup (laryngotracheobronchitis)
- Acute angioneurotic edema (no fever)
- Aspirated foreign body
- Bacterial tracheitis (pseudomembranous croup)
- Retropharyngeal or peritonsillar abscess
- Diphtheria in an unimmunized patient (often an adult)
- Sepsis from other cause

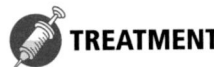 **TREATMENT**

INITIAL STABILIZATION

Acute epiglottitis is a medical emergency. During acute illness, hospitalize patient in ICU. (1,2)[C]

GENERAL MEASURES

- Each institution should have an emergency protocol involving a team of emergency room physicians, pediatricians, anesthesiologists, surgeons, pediatric intensivists, and pediatric ICU nurses (principles are similar for pediatric and adult patients).
- Call anesthesiologist to bedside
- Have equipment for intubation and needle cricothyrotomy or percutaneous tracheostomy at bedside
- Notify OR
- Notify pediatric surgeon or ear, nose, and throat specialist for standby in OR in case tracheostomy becomes necessary.
- Keep patient quiet, calm, sitting up (in parent's arms)
- Avoid venipuncture, blood gases, oxygen masks, IV lines, injections, monitors, and radiographs.
- Judicious use of sedation that does not depress respirations may be appropriate.
- Racemic epinephrine is without benefit
- Avoid examining the pharynx.
- Transport patient and parent together to OR in a wheelchair
- Intubate all patients, preferably in OR under controlled circumstances by experienced anesthesiologist with surgeon or ear, nose, and throat specialist on standby for emergency tracheostomy
- Tracheostomy not indicated unless intubation unsuccessful (1,2,5)[C]
- Tape airway securely in place, and use a bite block if indicated
- Splint elbows and restrain arms to avoid self-extubation
- Use humidity in a tent and avoid T piece (traction increases risk of accidental extubation)
- Continuous positive airway pressure, mechanical ventilation, and sedation usually unnecessary
- Pay attention to supervision and pulmonary toilet/suctioning to minimize risk of endotracheal tube plugs

Diet

IV fluid initially, then nasogastric feedings while intubated

MEDICATION (DRUGS)

First Line
- Begin empiric antibiotic promptly after blood and epiglottic cultures are obtained. Use antibiotics guided by cultures thereafter. Duration of antimicrobial: 7 days. (1,2)[C]
- Cefotaxime (Claforan) 100–200 mg/kg/d q8h IV (1,2)[C]
- Ceftriaxone (Rocephin) 50–100 mg/kg/d q12h IV (1,2)[C]
- Ampicillin-sulbactam (Unasyn) 150 mg/kg/d q6h IV (1,2)[C]
- Amoxicillin-clavulanate 100 mg/kg/d q8h IV
- Contraindications
  – Refer to the manufacturer's profile.
- Precautions
  – Refer to the manufacturer's profile.
- Significant possible interactions
  – Refer to the manufacturer's profile.

Second Line
- Ampicillin 100 mg/kg/d divided q6h IV and chloramphenicol 100 mg/kg/d divided q6h. Follow levels. May stop chloramphenicol only if Hib is sensitive to ampicillin. (1,2)[C]
- Steroids and racemic epinephrine are of no benefit. (3)[C]
- Antipyretics if necessary

SURGERY
Emergency tracheotomy may be necessary (2,5)[C]

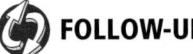 **FOLLOW-UP**

PROGNOSIS
- Most patients can be extubated after 24–48 hours.
- Morbidity and mortality are low with appropriate intervention.

COMPLICATIONS
- Pneumonia, meningitis, cervical adenitis, septic arthritis, pericarditis, and cellulitis (rare)
- Epiglottic abscess
- Septic shock (in ~1%)
- Pneumothorax, pneumomediastinum (very rare)
- Death from asphyxia

PATIENT MONITORING
- Rule out secondary foci of infection
- Observe swallowing ability and presence of an air leak around endotracheal/nasotracheal tube
- Follow-up laryngoscopy prior to extubation (advocated by some)
- Observe in ICU for 24 hours following extubation

REFERENCES

1. Burns JE, Hendley JO. In: Mandell GL, Bennett JE, Dolin R, eds. *Mandell, Douglas, and Bennett's Principles and Practice of Infectious Diseases*. 6th ed. New York, NY: Churchill Livingstone, 2005: 784–786.
2. Chery JD. Epiglottitis (supraglottitis). In: Feigin RD, et al, eds. *Textbook of Pediatric Infectious Diseases*. 5th ed. Philadelphia, PA: WB Saunders; 2004: 241–251.
3. Frantz TD, Rasgon BM, Quesenberry CP Jr. Acute epiglottitis in adults. Analysis of 129 cases *JAMA*. 1994;272:1358–1360.
4. Gonzalez Valdepena H, et al. Epiglottitis and Haemophilus influenzae immunization: The Pittsburgh experience—a five-year review. *Pediatrics*. 1995;96:424–427.
5. Mayo-Smith MF, et al. Acute epiglottitis. An 18-year experience in Rhode Island *Chest*. 1995;108:1640–1647.
6. McEwan J, et al. Pediatric acute epiglottitis: Not a disappearing entity. *J Pediatr Otorhinolaryngol*. 2003;67:317–321.
7. Shah RK, Roberson DW, Jones DT. Epiglottitis in the hemophilus type B vaccine era: Changing trends. *Laryngoscope*. 2004;114:557–560.
8. Berger G, et al. The rising incidence of adult acute epiglottitis and epiglottic abscess. *Am J Otolaryngol*. 2003;24:374–383.

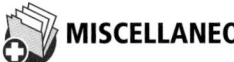 **MISCELLANEOUS**

See also: Immunizations

CODES

ICD9-CM
- 464.30 Acute epiglottitis without mention of obstruction
- 464.31 Acute epiglottitis with obstruction

PATIENT TEACHING
Reassurance about treatment and outcome

E

EPISTAXIS

Phyllis Montellese, MD

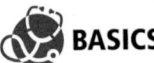 **BASICS**

DESCRIPTION
- Hemorrhage from the nose involving either the anterior or posterior mucosal surfaces
- Synonym(s): Nosebleed

GENERAL PREVENTION
- Liberal application of petroleum jelly (Vaseline) to nostril to prevent drying and picking
- Humidification at night
- Cut fingernails

EPIDEMIOLOGY
Incidence
- In the US: Common
- Bimodal with peaks in children up to 15 and in adults >50

Prevalence
10% of the population; by some reports as many as 60% in certain age groups

RISK FACTORS
Genetics
Possible male predominance noted by some

ETIOLOGY
- Idiopathic
- Local inflammation/irritation
  - Infection
  - Irritant inhalation
  - Topical steroid use
  - Septal deviation (more air movement on one side)
  - Low humidity
- Trauma
  - Epistaxis digitorum (nose picking)
  - Foreign bodies
  - Septal perforation
  - Sinus fracture

ASSOCIATED CONDITIONS
- Vascular malformation/telangiectasia
- Neoplasm
- Systemic
  - Coagulopathy primary or iatrogenic
  - Thrombocytopenia
  - Elevated international normalized ratio
  - Cirrhosis
  - There is no proven association with hypertension (1)[B]

 DIAGNOSIS

SIGNS AND SYMPTOMS
- Blood loss through 1 or both nostrils in the majority of cases due to anterior nasalseptal bleeding.
- Insidious blood loss from posterior nasal blood loss can present with hematemesis, hemoptysis, anemia, melena and even cardiovascular compromise.

TESTS
Lab
- CBC, platelet count, protime
- Cross-match when appropriate
- Toxicology screen when nasal use of illicit drugs is suspected

Imaging
MRI to evaluate for neoplasm when indicated

Diagnostic Procedures/Surgery
Nasal endoscopy

DIFFERENTIAL DIAGNOSIS
- Diagnosis usually apparent; the differential for the etiology is key
- Posterior bleeding needs to be included in the differential for any chronic blood loss.

TREATMENT

GENERAL MEASURES
- Resuscitation as indicated
- Examiner to wear protective gear, including gown, gloves, and goggles
- Patient to be seated, head forward, to avoid blood going down the posterior pharynx
- Patient applies direct pressure by pinching the lower part of the nose for 10–15 minutes without a break. This will stop the active bleeding in the majority of patients.
- An ice pack placed over the dorsum of the nose may help with hemostasis.
- Inspect the nasal septum for the bleeding site.
- The affected nare should be sprayed with lidocaine and phenylephrine
- If an anterior septal site is visualized, this may be treated with gentle and specific silver nitrate cautery for ~10 seconds.
- Diffuse oozing is suggestive of a systemic etiology.

Packing–Anterior
- Layering of Vaseline ribbon gauze
  - For gauze packing, be certain both ends of the ribbon gauze protrude from the nostril.
  - The packing is layered from the floor upward.
  - Secure packing with gauze across the outside of the nostril
- Nasal tampon may be used after lubricating the tip with KY Jelly or antibiotic cream or ointment
- Remember to initially angle the tampon up but then horizontally along the direction of the nasal cavity.
- Additional saline may be needed to expand the tampon if the bleeding has slowed.

Packing–Posterior
- Frequently requires an ear, nose, and throat consultation
- In the emergent setting, this may be attempted utilizing a foley catheter or a specific posterior packing balloon.
- With both methods, the tubing is introduced through the nose similar to the passage of a nasogastric tube. Once it reaches the posterior oral pharynx, the balloon is inflated and the tubing is pulled back outward to tamponade the posterior bleeding source. If using a Foley catheter (10–14 French), the balloon can be inflated with 10 mL of saline. Traction is maintained with an umbilical cord clamp with adequate padding between the clip and the nose to avoid injury.

Packing Duration
Twenty-four-hour minimum; some authors recommend 3–5 days. The latter recommendation carries the risk of mucosal injury and toxic shock syndrome (TSS). The former has the risk of re-bleed, which usually occurs between 24–48 hours.

Pediatric Considerations
More likely anterior bleed

Geriatric Considerations
More likely posterior bleed

Activity
Dependent on the severity of the bleed and necessity to pack

MEDICATION (DRUGS)

First Line

- Acute: Vasocontrictors, primarily phenylephrine, and oxymetazoline
  - Anesthetic: Lidocaine spray
- Chronic
  - Antibiotic cream bid as effective as cautery in multiple small clinical trials in prevention of recurrence
  - Iron if indicated
- Contraindication
  - Previous adverse drug reaction
- Precaution
  - Monitor BP in patients with hypertension for adverse reaction to vasoconstrictors

Second Line

- Acute: Vasoconstrictors (e.g., cocaine, epinephrine [risk of medical error].
- Anesthetic: Cocaine, tetracaine
- Chronic: Vaseline or bacitracin, as it is not clear that the antibiotic or the vehicle helps in prevention, as there was no control group in studies reviewed (3,4)[B]

SURGERY

- Especially with posterior bleeding, endoscopic laser or electro-cauterization
- Angiography with arteriolar embolization

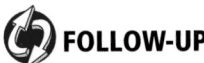 **FOLLOW-UP**

PROGNOSIS
Good results with proper treatment

COMPLICATIONS
- Septal perforation
- Alar ischemia
- Pressure-induced tissue necrosis of the nasal mucosa

PATIENT MONITORING
- When significant blood loss, hemodynamic monitoring
- If packing to remain >36–48 hours, need to watch for signs/symptoms of infection including TSS

REFERENCES

1. Fuchs FD, et al. Absence of association between hypertension and epistaxis: A population-based study. *Blood Pressure*. 2003;12(3):145–148.
2. Leong SCL, Roe RJ, Karkanevatos A. No frills management of epistaxis. *Emerg Med J*. 2005; 22:470–472.
3. Kubba H, et al. A prospective, single-blind, randomized controlled trial of antiseptic cream for recurrent epistaxis in childhood. *Clin Otolaryngol*. 2001;26:465–468.
4. Murthy P, et al. A randomized clinical trial of antiseptic nasal carrier cream and silver nitrate cautery in the treatment of recurrent anterior epistaxis. *Clin Otolaryngol*. 1999;24:228–231.
5. Kucik CJ, Clenney T. Management of epistaxis. *American Family Physician*. 2005:7(2).

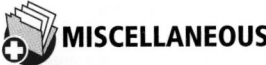 **MISCELLANEOUS**

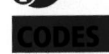 CODES

ICD9-CM
784.7 Epistaxis

PATIENT TEACHING

- Demonstrate proper pinching pressure techniques.
- Avoidance of trauma or irritants is key. Management of systemic illness and proper use of medication

 See Corresponding Diagnostic Algorithm

E

EPSTEIN-BARR VIRUS (EBV) INFECTIONS

Dennis E. Hughes, DO

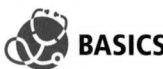 **BASICS**

DESCRIPTION

- EBV is tropic for B lymphocytes, which are infected in the oropharynx through salivary exchange; infected B cells then circulate in the blood and are distributed to the bone marrow and lymphoreticular system.
- EBV can also be found in infected epithelial cells of the buccal mucosa, salivary glands, tongue, and endocervix; this suggests that chronic epithelial replication brings about continuous reinfection of B lymphoid cells.
- Immune T cell responses to latently infected B cells account for the clinical findings.
- All seropositive persons actively shed the virus in the saliva.
- System(s) Affected: Hemic/Lymphatic/Immunologic

EPIDEMIOLOGY

Incidence

Worldwide, infects >90% of people. (1)

Prevalence

- Military and college student groups have the most active infection rate.
- Predominant age
  - Older children, adolescents, and young adults
  - By young adult life, 60–90% of persons are antibody positive (to EBV); antibodies persist for lifetime of the person. (1)
- Predominant sex: Male = Female

RISK FACTORS

- Age
- Sociohygienic level
- Geographic location
- Close, intimate contact

ETIOLOGY

EBV, a member of the herpesvirus (DNA virus) group

ASSOCIATED CONDITIONS

- Infectious mononucleosis: The symptomatic primary EBV infection seen in otherwise healthy older children, adolescents, and young adults
  - Clinical features variable in severity and duration: In children, generally mild; in adults, more severe and protracted
  - Incubation period is 30–50 days
- X-linked lymphoproliferative syndrome (Duncan disease)
- Lymphoproliferative syndromes due to EBV infections in transplant patients
- Lymphomas (B cell lymphoblastic, T cell)
- Lymphocytic interstitial pneumonitis
- Hairy leukoplakia of the tongue and CNS lymphomas in AIDS patients
- Burkitt lymphoma
- Nasopharyngeal carcinoma
- Parotid carcinoma
- Hodgkin lymphoma

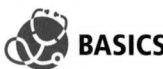 **DIAGNOSIS**

SIGNS AND SYMPTOMS

- May begin abruptly or insidiously
- In adults, temperature may rise to 103°F (39.4°C) and gradually fall over a variable period of 7–10 days; in severe cases temperature elevations of 104–105°F (40.0–40.6°C) may persist for 2 weeks
- Children usually have a low-grade fever or may be afebrile.
- Diffuse hyperemia and hyperplasia of oropharyngeal lymphoid tissue
- Gelatinous, grayish-white exudative tonsillitis persists for 7–10 days in 50%
- Petechiae develop at border of hard and soft palates in 60%
- Tender lymphadenopathy (cervical nodes are most commonly enlarged)
- Axillary, epitrochlear, popliteal, inguinal, mediastinal and mesenteric nodes may also be affected.
- Lymph node enlargement subsides over days or weeks
- Splenomegaly in 50%
- Abnormal hepatic enzymes in 80% of patients for several weeks after onset; hepatomegaly in 15–20%
- Pneumonitis
- Chest pain (myocarditis and pericarditis)
- Hilar adenopathy may be observed in infectious mononucleosis cases having extensive lymphoid hyperplasia
- Neurologic (rare)
  - Aseptic meningitis
  - Bell palsy
  - Meningoencephalitis
  - Guillain-Barré syndrome
  - Transverse myelitis
  - Cerebellar ataxia
  - Acute psychosis
- Hematologic (rare)
  - Thrombocytopenia, slight to moderate, early in illness
  - Hemolytic anemia with marked neutropenia during early weeks
  - Aplastic anemia
  - Agammaglobulinemia
- Skin manifestations: 3–16%
  - Erythematous macular or maculopapular rash
  - Petechial and purpuric exanthems have been reported
  - Rash location: Trunk and upper arms; occasionally the face and forearms involved
  - Urticarial lesions on the abdomen, arms, legs

ALERT

Pediatric Considerations

- Infection during infancy and childhood usually subclinical and inapparent
- Clinical infectious mononucleosis more common in older children and young adults

Geriatric Considerations

Heterophile-positive infectious mononucleosis has been reported in an elderly patient 5 weeks after a blood transfusion.

Pregnancy Considerations

Testing for EBV important to rule out cytomegalovirus or HIV infectins, as the latter are associated with significant pregnancy complications. (2)

Physical Exam

Fever, lymphadenopathy, pharyngitis in >50% with palatal petchiae and heptospleenomegally ~10% (1)

TESTS

Lab

- Lymphocytes and atypical lymphocytes
  - Increased numbers of lymphocytes and atypical lymphocytes (may be up to 70% of leukocytes) in peripheral blood
  - In 1st week after onset, WBC count is normal or moderately decreased. By the 2nd week, lymphocytosis develops with >10% atypical lymphocytes
  - During early illness, atypical lymphocytes are B cells transformed by the EBV; later, atypical cells are primarily T cells having an immunoregulatory function.
- Antibodies
  - Heterophil antibodies in 80–90% of adults
  - Responsible heterophile antibody is an IgM response, which appears during the 1st or 2nd week of illness and persists for 3–6 months.
  - In general, agglutinin titer is higher in infectious mononucleosis than in other disorders; an unabsorbed heterophile titer >1:128 and 1:40 or higher after absorption is significant.
- Specific antibodies to EBV-associated antigens
  - Develop regularly in infectious mononucleosis
  - Viral capsid-specific IgM and IgG are present early in illness; viral capsid-IgM responses disappear after several months, whereas viral capsid-IgG antibodies persist for life.
- Disorders that may alter lab results: Atypical lymphocytes are not specific for Epstein-Barr infections and may be present in other clinical conditions including rubella, infectious hepatitis, allergic rhinitis, asthma, and primary atypical pneumonia. In infectious mononucleosis, increased numbers of atypical forms are present in peripheral blood; in other disorders, quantitative percentage is usually less

Imaging

Ultrasound, splenomegaly

Diagnostic Procedures/Surgery

See "Lab."

Pathological Findings

- Widespread focal and perivascular aggregates of mononuclear cells are found throughout the body.
- Mononuclear infiltrations involve lymph nodes, tonsils, spleen, lungs, liver, heart, kidneys, adrenal glands, skin, and CNS.
- Bone marrow hyperplasia develops regularly, and small granulomas may be present; these are non-specific and have no prognostic significance.
- A polyclonal B cell proliferative response is characteristic of infectious mononucleosis. Relatively few circulating lymphocytes are infected by EBV and represent <0.1% of circulating mononuclear cells in the acute illness.

DIFFERENTIAL DIAGNOSIS
- Streptococcal pharyngitis and tonsillitis
- Diphtheria
- Blood dyscrasias
- Rubella
- Measles
- Viral hepatitis
- Cytomegalovirus
- Toxoplasmosis

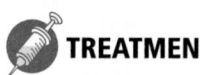 **TREATMENT**

INITIAL STABILIZATION
Outpatient, usually

GENERAL MEASURES
- The treatment is chiefly supportive.
- During acute stage, rest in bed

Diet
- Maintain adequate fluid intake.
- Low-fat, high-carbohydrate diet
- Avoid alcohol for 6–8 months.

Activity
- Decided on an individual basis during convalescence
- Excess exertion, heavy lifting, and participation in contact sports are prohibited during acute illness and also in the presence of splenomegaly.

ALERT
Rupture of the spleen may be fatal if not recognized and requires blood transfusions, treatment for shock, and splenectomy.

 MEDICATION (DRUGS)

First Line
- Antimicrobial agents (usually a penicillin) if throat culture is positive for Group A, beta-hemolytic streptococci (2)
- Warm saline gargles for the pain of pharyngeal involvement and enlarged lymph nodes
- Corticosteroids:
  – Consider in severe pharyngotonsillitis with oropharyngeal edema and airway encroachment. Dexamethasone (0.3 mg/kg/d) may be used for 1–3 days. (2,4)[C]
  – Also for patients with marked toxicity or major complications (e.g., hemolytic anemia, thrombocytopenic purpura, neurologic sequelae, myocarditis, and pericarditis. (1)
- Precautions: Refer to the manufacturer's literature.
- Significant possible interactions: Refer to the manufacturer's literature.

SURGERY
With profound thrombocytopenia, refractory to corticosteroid therapy, splenectomy may be necessary.

 FOLLOW-UP

PROGNOSIS
- Infectious mononucleosis: Usually mild or moderate severity
- Acute symptoms 2–3 weeks with full recovery in 4–8 weeks

COMPLICATIONS
- Airway obstruction
- Hematologic or neurologic complications
- Toxemia
- Splenic rupture (rare); greatest risk is during 2nd–3rd week
- Hypersensitivity rash
  – Develops 7–10 days after initiation of ampicillin (or its analogues and other penicillins) treatment; generalized erythematous maculopapular eruption occurs mainly over trunk and extremities, including palms and soles. Rash persists for a week; desquamation may continue for several days

PATIENT MONITORING
- Avoid contact sports, heavy lifting, and excess exertion until spleen and liver have returned to normal size.
- Eliminate alcohol or exposure to other hepatotoxic drugs until liver function studies return to normal.
- Monitor patients closely during the 1st 2–3 weeks after the onset of symptoms. Thereafter, follow patients until their symptoms subside.
- Rarely, laboratory results resolve more slowly and symptoms (malaise, fatigue, intermittent sore throat, lymphadenopathy) may persist for several months

REFERENCES
1. Cohen J. Epstein-Barr virus infection. *New Engl J Med* 2000;343:481–492.
2. Halstead ME, Bernhardt DT. Common infections in the young athlete. *Pediatr Ann* 2002;31:42–48.
3. Roy M, et al. Dexamethasone for the treatment of sore throat in children with suspected infectious mononucleosis. *Arch Pediatr Adolesc Med*. 2004;158:250–254.
4. Thompson SK, et al. Infectious mononucleosis and corticosteroids: Management practices and outcomes. *Arch Oto-Head and Neck Surg*. 2005; 131:900–904.

 MISCELLANEOUS

CODES

ICD9-CM
075 Infectious mononucleosis

PATIENT TEACHING
Reassurance and support

E

ERECTILE DYSFUNCTION

Bruce Block, MD

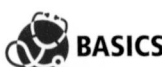

BASICS

DESCRIPTION
- Dissatisfaction with size, rigidity, or duration of erection
- Male sexual dysfunction encompasses an even larger group of complaints and disorders of arousal, desire, orgasm, sensation, and relationship.
- Transient periods of impotence occur in ~1/2 of adult males and are not considered dysfunctional.
- System(s) Affected: Cardiovascular; Nervous; Renal/Urologic; Reproductive
- Synonym(s): Impotence

GENERAL PREVENTION
Because erectile dysfunction is multifactorial, referral to a sex therapist or couples therapist may help to speed recovery and prevent future problems.

EPIDEMIOLOGY
Incidence
In US, involves ~10% of men, but is underreported by patients

Prevalence
- Predominant age
  - Patients with psychologic, gender, and primary organic problems often present themselves for help between adolescence and the 3rd decade.
  - Patients with relationship problems, but concerned mainly about physical problems, tend to seek care in the 6th decade.
  - Most patients with physical problems are in the 7th and 8th decade, but rarely seek help.
- Predominant sex: Male only

RISK FACTORS
- Prior pelvic surgery
- Medication use
- Trauma
- Diabetes

Genetics
Rarely related to chromosomal disorders

ETIOLOGY
- Endocrine
- Neurologic
- Vascular
- Medication(s)
- Psychological
- Structural

ALERT
Geriatric Considerations
Aging alone is not a cause.

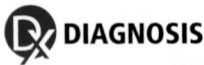

DIAGNOSIS

SIGNS AND SYMPTOMS
- Reduction of erectile size and rigidity
- Inability to maintain erection
- Inability to achieve erection
- Reduced body hair
- Thyromegaly
- Gynecomastia
- Testicular atrophy or absence
- Deformed penis
- Peripheral vascular disease
- Neuropathy

TESTS
- Nocturnal penile tumescence testing
- Consider the following only in rare circumstances, when indicated
  - 24-hour urine zinc
  - Dorsal nerve somatosensory–evoked potentials
  - Sacral evoked response
  - Penile-brachial BP
  - Aortogram
  - Selective pudendal angiogram
  - Dynamic cavernosography
  - Penile BP

Lab
- CBC
- Basic metabolic panel (glucose, K+, Na+, blood urea nitrogen, creatinine)
- Albumin
- Thyroid-stimulating hormone
- Prolactin
- Free testosterone (morning sample)

Imaging
Doppler, angiogram, cavernosogram

Diagnostic Procedures/Surgery
Response to papaverine or alprostadil injection

Pathological Findings
Most men >55 will have some test abnormality, medication or risk factor, but it is not necessarily the cause of the erectile dysfunction.

DIFFERENTIAL DIAGNOSIS
- Endocrine
  - Low or high thyroxine
  - Low testosterone
  - High prolactin
  - Diabetes
  - High estrogen effect
  - Renal failure
  - Zinc deficiency
- Neurological
  - Central
  - Spinal
  - Peripheral
- Vascular
  - Arterial insufficiency
  - Cavernosal insufficiency
  - Venous insufficiency
- Medication
  - Beta-blockers, thiazides
- Psychological
  - Depression
  - Schizophrenia
  - Relationship disorders
  - Personality disorders
  - Anxiety
- Structural
  - Microphallus
  - Chordee and Peyronie disease
  - Cavernosal scarring
  - Phimosis
  - Hypospadias
  - Postsurgical sequelae

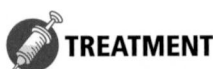

TREATMENT

INITIAL STABILIZATION
Appropriate health care: Because erectile dysfunction is multifactorial, outpatient evaluation by a generalist

GENERAL MEASURES
- Early use of penile implants is now discouraged, because of success with vacuum erectile devices, sensate focus therapy, injection therapy, and oral therapy.
- Improve partner communication
- Reduce performance pressure
- Use sensate focus therapy
- Try vacuum erectile device or oral therapy (can be used in conjunction with intracavernous injections).
- Use of psychiatrists, psychologists, sex therapists, vascular surgeons, urologists, endocrinologists, neurologists, or plastic surgeons is often necessary for refractory cases.

Diet
Control diabetes, if present

Activity
No restrictions

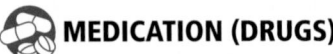

MEDICATION (DRUGS)

First Line
- Erection induction: Phosphodiesterase type 5 (PDE-5) inhibitors
  - Sildenafil (Viagra): 25 mg, 50 mg, or 100 mg tablets. Usual dose, 50 mg 1/2 hour prior to sexual activity. Duration up to 4 hours. On empty stomach.
  - Vardenafil (Levitra): 2.5 mg, 5 mg, 10 mg, or 20 mg tablets. Usual dose, 10 mg 1/2 hour prior to sexual activity. Duration up to 4 hours. On empty stomach.
  - Tadalafil (Cialis): 5 mg, 10 mg, or 20 mg tablets. Usual dose, 10 mg 1 hour prior to sexual activity. Duration up to 36 hours. Without regard to food intake.

Second Line
- Erection induction: Prostaglandins
  - Intracavernous injection (1/2-inch, 30-gauge needle), starting with 0.1 mL
- Alprostadil/Papaverine/Phenotolamine (Trimix) (1mL solution containing alprostadil 5.8 μg/mL plus papaverine 17.64 mg/mL plus phentolamine 0.58 mg/mL).

Compounded Intracavernousal Solution

Drug	Amt	Conc/mL
PGE-1 (500 mcg/mL)	50 mcg	6.6 mcg
Papaverine (300mg/10mL)	150 mg	20 mg
Phentolamine	5 mg	0.67 mg
Bacteriostatic NaCl QS	7.5 mL	
Compounds	7.5 mL; usual dose	0.1–0.5 mL

- Alprostadil (Caverject): 10–20 μg/mL; inject into the dorsolateral aspect of proximal 3rd of penis. Do not exceed 60 mg dose. Do not use >3 times a week or more than once in 24 hours. Patient to notify physician if erection lasts >6 hours for immediate attention.
  or
- Alprostadil (Muse) urethral suppository: 125 mg, 250 mg, 500 mg, and 1,000 mg pellets. Maximum of 2 uses in 24 hours.
- Miscellaneous
  – Testosterone cypionate: 200 mg IM every 2 weeks when hypogonadism is present. Testosterone patch or gel is also available.
  – Bromocriptine: 2.5 mg 2 b.i.d. a day up to 40 mg/d when hyperprolactinemia is present
- Cabergoline: Usual starting dose of 0.25 mg biweekly to a maximum dose of 1 mg biweekly. Some studies have shown efficacy even with once-a-week dosing when hyperprolactinemia is present
- Contraindications
  – Avoid injections in patients with bleeding disorders, sickle cell disease or trait, and penile deformities.
  – Avoid use in patients with known allergies to constituents.
  – Nitroglycerin (or other nitrates) and phosphodiesterase inhibitors: Potential for severe, potentially fatal, hypotension
- Precautions
  – Testosterone: Urinary retention, acne, sodium retention, and gynecomastia
  – Bromocriptine and cabergoline: Self-limited nausea, vomiting
  – Injection therapy: Priapism, fibrosis, hypotension, and nausea
  – Urethral suppositories: Penile pain and irritation, as well as testicular pain; no reports yet of priapism
  – Sildenafil: Hypotension (caution for patients on nitrates)
  – PDE-5 inhibitors: Use caution with congential prolonged QT syndrome, class Ia or II antiarrhythmics, nitroglycerin, alpha-blockers (e.g., terazosin, tamsulosin), retinal disease, unstable cardiac disease, liver and renal failure
- Significant possible interactions
  – PDE-5 inhibitor concentration is affected by CYP3A4 inhibitors (e.g., erythromycin, indinavir, ketoconazole, ritonavir, amiodarone, cimetidine, clarithromycin, delavirdine, diltiazem, fluoxetine, fluvoxamine, grapefruit juice, itraconazole, nefazodone, nevirapine, ritonavir, saquinavir, and verapamil). Serum concentrations and/or toxicity may be increased. When used with these drugs, reduce the dose of a PDE-5 inhibitor (1/2 of the usual initial dose every 3 days).
  – PDE-5 inhibitor concentration may be reduced by rifampin and phenytoin.

Complementary and Alternative Medicine
Positive evidence exists for the use of yohimbine to improve erectile function. However, its use has fallen out of favor with the development of phosphodiesterase type 5 inhibitors. (9)

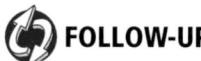 **FOLLOW-UP**

PROGNOSIS
- Given that the majority of patients have unspecified causes of their erectile disorders, vacuum erection device, injection, or suppository therapy with alprostadil, oral sildenafil, and a penile implant have improved the outlook greatly.
- Expect 20% failure rate of vacuum erection device, high drop-out rate from injection therapy, and a 10–30% non-use rate for penile implants.
- Spontaneous cure rate is ~15%
- Studies indicate a response rate of 40–60% for urethral alprostadil compared to 85–90% for the injection.
- Sildenafil and other PDE-5 inhibitors are effective in 70% of men at maximum dose, but are less effective in patients with diabetes and those who have had a prostatectomy for cancer.

COMPLICATIONS
Specific to therapy

PATIENT MONITORING
Meet with the patient and, if possible, his partner, as required by the cause, therapy, and response.

REFERENCES
1. Evans C. The use of penile prostheses in the treatment of impotence. *Brit J of Urology.* 1998;81:591–598.
2. Gholami SS, et al. Peyronie's disease: A review. *J Urol.* 2003;169:1234–1241.
3. Gingell JC. New developments in self-injection therapy for erectile dysfunction. *Brit J of Urology.* 1998;81:599–603.
4. Lue TF. Erectile dysfunction. *New Engl J Med.* 2000;342:1802–1813.
5. Montague D. *Disorders of Male Sexual Dysfunction.* Boca Raton, FL: Year Book Medical Publishers; 1988.
6. Schover LR, et al. The use of treatments for erectile dysfunction among survivors of prostate carcinoma. *Cancer.* 2002;95:2397–2407.
7. Segraves RT, Schoenberg HW. *Diagnosis and Treatment of Erectile Disturbances.* New York, NY: Plenum, 1985.
8. Wagner G, Green R. *Impotence.* New York, NY: Plenum; 1981.
9. Ernst E, Pittler MH. Yohimbine for erectile dysfunction: A systematic review and meta-analysis of randomized clinical trials. *J Urol* 1998;159(2): 433–436.

E

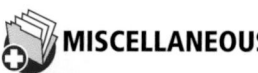 **MISCELLANEOUS**

CODES

ICD9-CM
- 302.70 Psychosexual dysfunction, unspecified
- 302.71 Psychosexual dysfunction with inhibited sexual desire
- 302.72 Psychosexual dysfunction with inhibited sexual excitement
- 302.9 Unspecified psychosexual disorder
- V41.7 Problems with sexual function
- 607.84 Impotence of organic origin

PATIENT TEACHING
Recommend *The New Male Sexuality* by Bernie Zilbergeld, PhD, Bantam Books, 1992, as well as problem-specific handouts.

 See Patient Handout on CD

ERYSIPELAS

Felix B. Chang, MD
Ana Vera Lopes, MD

BASICS

DESCRIPTION
- Acute, well demarcated superficial bacterial skin infection with lymphatic involvement caused by group A streptococci. Usually acute, but a chronic recurrent form also exists.
- System(s) Affected: Skin/Exocrine
- Synonym(s): Saint Anthony's fire; Ignis sacer

GENERAL PREVENTION
- Maintenance antibiotics for chronic recurrent cases.
- Consider suppressive prophylactic antibiotics therapy in patients with ≥2 episodes in a 12-month period
- Men who shave within 5 days of facial erysipelas are more likely to have a recurrence.
- In recurrent cases, search for other possible source of streptococcal infection (e.g., tonsils, sinuses, teeth, toenails)

EPIDEMIOLOGY
- Predominant age: Infants and adults >40 years. Greatest in elderly (>75 years)
- Predominant sex: Male = Female

Incidence
Unknown

Prevalence
Unknown

RISK FACTORS
- Skin barrier disruption (surgical incisions, insect bites, eczematous lesions, local trauma, abrasions, fungal infections, toe web intertrigo)
- Fissured skin (especially at the nose and ears)
- Leg ulcers/stasis dermatitis
- Venous or lymphatic compromise (radiotherapy, saphenectomy, lymphadenectomy)
- Chronic diseases (diabetes, malnutrition, nephrotic syndrome)
- Immunocompromised or debilitated individual
- Alcohol abuse
- Morbid obesity
- Recent streptococcal pharyngitis
- No portal of entry can be found in most cases

ETIOLOGY
- Group A β-hemolytic streptococci primarily; occasionally other streptococcus groups C or G.
- Rarely, group B streptococci or *Staphylococcus aureus* may be involved.

ALERT
Pediatric Considerations
Group B streptococcus may be a cause in neonates/infants.

DIAGNOSIS

PRE HOSPITAL
Systemic prodromal symptoms that may include chills, malaise, moderate to high-grade fever, headache, vomiting, anorexia, usually in the 1st 48 hours.

SIGNS AND SYMPTOMS
- Acute onset of erythematous patch
- Sharply demarcated, raised border, deeply erythematous, shiny plaque that spreads circumferentially over hours–days
- Center of lesion clears as periphery spreads.
- Lesion is characteristically hot, indurated (peau d'orange), marked swelling
- Headache and vomiting may be prominent.
- Arthralgias
- Pruritus
- Skin discomfort
- Vesicles and bullae may form but are not uniformly present
- Facial redness
- Desquamation may occur.
- Lower extremity most commonly involved (70–80%)
- Face involvement is less common (5–20%), especially nose and ears.
- Chronic form may recur hours to years after initial episode.
- Chronic form usually recurs at site of the previous infection.
- Fever is usually the differentiating factor among similar skin manifestations.
- Patients on systemic steroids may be more difficult to diagnose because signs and symptoms of the infection may be masked by anti-inflammatory action of the steroids.
- Systemic toxicity resolves rapidly with treatment; skin lesions desquamate on days 5–10 but usually heal without scarring.

ALERT
Pediatric Considerations
- Abdominal involvement more common in infants
- Face, scalp, and leg common in older children
- Umbilical stump

Geriatric Considerations
- Fever may not be as prominent.
- More prone to complications
- High-output cardiac failure may occur in debilitated patients with underlying cardiac disease.
- Face and lower extremity most common areas

Physical Exam
- Vital signs: Moderate to high-grade fever with resultant tachycardia. Hypotension may occur.
- Integument: Hot, tender, erythematous superficial plaque with sharply demarcated borders at palpation. Typically presents in a butterfly pattern in facial involvement. Pustules characteristically absent.
- Lymphatics: Regional lymphadenopathy rare, lymphangitic streaking, peau d'orange

TESTS
Lab
- Classic erysipelas can be diagnosed and treated without laboratory workup. Reserve diagnostic for severely ill, toxic patients or those who are immunosuppressed.
- Leukocytosis (usually >15,000 cells/mm^3)
- Streptococci may be cultured from exudate or noninvolved sites.
- Antistreptolysin, streptozyme, anti-DNase may be helpful
- Blood culture (<5% positive)
- High antihyaluronidase, anti-DNAse, ASO titers

Pathological Findings
- Edema
- Vasodilation and enlarged lymphatics
- Infiltration of polymorphonuclear leukocytes, lymphocytes, and other inflammatory cells
- Endothelial cell swelling
- Rare bacterial invasion of local blood vessels
- Gram-positive cocci

DIFFERENTIAL DIAGNOSIS
- Erysipeloid (little toxicity)
- Cellulitis (less clearly margins)
- Erythema annulare centrifugum
- Contact dermatitis (no fever)
- Giant urticaria
- Angioneurotic edema (no fever)
- Scarlet fever (usually more widespread without edema)
- Lupus (of the face; less fever, positive antinuclear antibodies)
- Polychondritis (of the ear)
- Dermatophytes
- Tuberculoid leprosy
- Inflammatory breast cancer
- Necrotizing fasciitis
- Herpes zoster

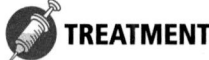

TREATMENT

Infectious Diseases Society of America guidelines on the diagnosis and management of skin and soft tissue infections recommends penicillin, either orally or parenterally, depending on clinical severity as the treatment of choice for erysipelas.

INITIAL STABILIZATION
Outpatient care

GENERAL MEASURES
- Symptomatic treatment of aches and fever
- Adequate fluid intake
- Local treatment with cold compresses

Diet
No special diet

Activity
Bed rest, with activity based on severity of illness

IV Fluids
IV therapy if systemic toxicity unable to tolerate PO

MEDICATION (DRUGS)

First Line
- Adults: Penicillin V (Pen-Vee K) for 10–14 days (improvement in 24–48 hours). 250–500 mg PO q6h or penicillin G procaine 0.6–1.2 million U IM b.i.d. or 10 days for severe or complicated cases (2)[A]
  - Pediatric dose: Penicillin VK <12 years: 25–50 mg/kg/d PO div. q6–8h or; >12 years adults dose or penicillin G procaine <30 Kg: 300,000 U/d IM, >30 kg: adult dose
- Nafcillin or oxacillin 2.0 g q4h IV or penicillin G parenterally is recommended for severe or complicated cases (1 million–2 million units q4–6h).
- In chronic recurrent infections, some authors recommend lower-dose daily maintenance/prophylactic treatment after the acute infection resolves.
- Contraindications: Refer to the manufacturer's profile of each drug.
- Significant possible interactions: Refer to the manufacturer's profile of each drug.

Second Line
- Macrolides in penicillin allergic patients:
  - Erythromycin
    - Children: 30–40 mg/kg/d q6h;
    - Adults: 250–500 mg/dose q6h
  - Azithromycin 500 mg on day one, then 250 mg/d or Clarithromycin 500 mg b.i.d.
- Cephalosporins: 1st-generation cephalosporins for suspected staphylococcal infections (2)[A]
  - Cephalexin Adults:250–500 mg PO q6h; pediatric dose: 25–50 mg/kg/d PO divided q6h
  - Cefazolin 1–2 g IV q8h (adults)
  - Contraindications: Allergy
  - Pregnancy category B
- Consider penicillinase-resistant penicillin, such as dicloxacillin 500 mg q6h in facial involvement owing to possible staphylococcal infection or 1st-generation cephalosporin. A-III
- Recurrent erysipelas in adults:
  - Pen V 250 mg PO b.i.d.
  - Erythromycin 500 mg/d PO
  - Azithromycin 500 mg/d PO or
  - Clarithromycin 500 mg/d PO

DISPOSITION
Admission Criteria
- Patient with systemic toxicity
- Patient with high risk factors (lymphedema, postsplenectomy, diabetes, etc.)

Discharge Criteria
No evidence of systemic toxicity, with improvement or erythema and swelling

Issues for Referral
Recurrent infection, treatment failure

PROGNOSIS
- Adequate treatment results in full recovery.
- Chronic edema/scarring may result from chronic recurrent cases.
- Rarely, elephantiasis may result from chronic recurrent cases.
- Bulla formation suggest longer disease course
- Untreated cases sometimes resolve spontaneously.

COMPLICATIONS
- Bacteremia
- Scarlet fever
- Pneumonia
- Abscess
- Embolism
- Gangrene
- Meningitis
- Sepsis
- Toxic shock syndrome
- Tendonitis
- Septic arthritis
- Death

PATIENT MONITORING
Patients should be treated until all symptoms and skin manifestations have resolved.

REFERENCES

1. Bonnetblanc JM, Bedane C. Erysipelas: recognition and management. *Am J Clin Dermatol.* 2003;4(3):157–163.
2. Stevens DL, Bisno AL, Chambers HR, et al. Practice guidelines for the diagnosis and management of skin and soft tissue infections. *Clin Infect Dis.* 2005;41:1973.
3. Morris A. Cellulitis and erysipelas. *Clin Evid.* 2002;1483.

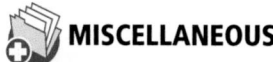

MISCELLANEOUS

CODES

ICD9-CM
035 Erysipelas

ICD10
A46 erysipelas

PATIENT TEACHING
Stress importance of completing medication regimen prescribed

Activity
Bed rest with elevation of extremity during acute infection, then activity as tolerated

Prevention
Appropriate management of underlying medical condition that might predispose to the condition: tinea pedis, stasis dermatitis, etc.

 See Corresponding Diagnostic Algorithm

E

ERYTHEMA MULTIFORME

Lewis C. Rose, MD

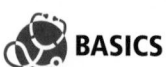 **BASICS**

DESCRIPTION

- An acute self-limited hypersensitivity reaction involving the skin and sometimes the mucus membranes
  - Erythema multiforme minor (also called the *erythema multiforme Hebra*) is a mild form that appears as a pleomorphic rash and includes target lesions, but not large vesicles or petechia, affecting the skin with or without involving 1 mucus membrane site
- Erythema multiforme major is a more severe form, involving >1 mucus membrane site.
- Although many authors consider erythema multiforme to be the same as Stevens-Johnson syndrome, there appears to be a growing consensus that the 2 are unrelated.
- System(s) Affected: Skin/Exocrine
- Synonym(s): Erythema exudativum multiforme

GENERAL PREVENTION

- Known or suspected etiologic agents should be avoided.
- Acyclovir may help prevent herpes-related erythema multiforme.
- Tamoxifen has been shown to prevent premenstrual-related disease.

EPIDEMIOLOGY

Incidence

The incidence in the US is not known. In Germany, the incidence of erythema multiforme major, Stevens Johnson syndrome, and toxic epidermal necrolysis combined appears to be 0.189/100,000 persons per year.

Prevalence

- Predominant age: Peak incidence in 20s and 30s; rare <age 3 and >age 50
- Predominant sex: Male > Female (3:2)

ALERT

Pediatric Considerations

More severe forms of the disease tend to occur in younger males; it is rare in children <3 years of age.

Geriatric Considerations

Rarely seen in people >50

RISK FACTORS

- Previous history of erythema multiforme
- Male sex

Genetics

Possibly associated with HLA-B15

ETIOLOGY

- Most cases appear to be due to a preceding infection. Drugs seem to be an infrequent cause
- Viral infections, particularly herpes simplex; also Epstein-Barr, Coxsackie, echovirus, varicella, mumps, and poliovirus
- Bacterial infections, including brucellosis, diphtheria, borreliosis
- Mycoplasma appears to more often precede Stevens-Johnson syndrome.
- Protozoan infections
- Fungal infection, including *Trichophyton rubrum*
- Collagen vascular diseases
- Malignancy
- Pregnancy
- Premenstrual hormone changes
- Consumption of beer
- Reiter syndrome
- Sarcoidosis
- Vaccines: Tetanus/diphtheria, bacillus Calmette-Guérin, oral polio vaccine
- Medications: The accepted list includes sulfonamides, penicillins, anticonvulsants, and salicylates, but many of these were actually associated with Stevens Johnson syndrome when it was considered to be a type of erythema nodosum major.
- Radiotherapy

ASSOCIATED CONDITIONS

Any of the infections or diseases listed under "Etiology"

ALERT

Pregnancy Considerations

Reported as a possible etiologic condition

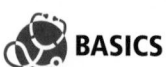 **DIAGNOSIS**

SIGNS AND SYMPTOMS

- Typical pleomorphic eruption is a mixture of macules of various sizes and target lesions. These consist of a central inflamed and superficially necrotic area, surrounded by a halo of less inflamed skin, enclosed within an outer erythematous rim
  - Purpuric lesions are uncommon, and vesicles may be related to antecedent herpes 1 infections.
  - Rash occurs on the palms, soles, dorsum of the hands, and extensor surface of the extremities and the face; often recurrent, following a viral infection
- Involvement of mucus membranes is quite common, which caused confusion with Stevens-Johnson syndrome. In erythema multiforme, mucus membrane involvement consists of target lesions of the lips or herpetic lesions without extensive necrosis.

- Pruritus is usually absent.
- The skin may feel normal, or there may be a mild burning sensation.
- Corneal ulceration is a serious complication.

ALERT

Clinical Considerations

Because it is an immunologic reaction, drug-related erythema multiforme will not occur until 7–14 days after exposure to the offending agent, unless the patient has had the medication previously.

TESTS

Diagnostic Procedures/Surgery

Skin biopsy

Pathological Findings

A predominantly inflammatory pattern characterized by a lichenoid infiltrate, which is of high density and rich in T-lymphocytes, and epidermal necrosis that mainly affects the basal layer

DIFFERENTIAL DIAGNOSIS

- Stevens-Johnson syndrome
- Urticaria
- Necrotizing vasculitis
- Drug eruptions
- Contact dermatitis
- Pityriasis rosea
- Secondary syphilis
- Ringworm
- Pemphigus vulgaris
- Pemphigoid
- Dermatitis herpetiformis
- Herpes gestationis
- Septicemia
- Serum sickness
- Viral exanthems
- Rocky Mountain spotted fever
- Collagen vascular diseases
- Mucocutaneous lymph node syndrome
- Meningococcemia
- Lichen planus
- Behçet syndrome
- Recurrent aphthous ulcers
- Herpetic gingivostomatitis
- Granuloma annulare

 **TREATMENT**

INITIAL STABILIZATION
Care at home, unless mouth herpes precludes oral intake

GENERAL MEASURES
- Treatment of any underlying or causative disease
- Withdrawal of any causative drugs
- For mild cases, symptomatic treatment is sufficient. For more severe cases, be meticulous regarding wound care and the use of Burow's solution or Domeboro solution dressings.
- Oral lesions can be treated with mouthwashes with warm saline or a solution of diphenhydramine, lidocaine (Xylocaine), and Kaopectate to provide symptomatic relief and oral hygiene and to facilitate oral intake.

Diet
As tolerated with increased fluid intake

Activity
As tolerated

 **MEDICATION (DRUGS)**

First Line
- Steroid use is controversial. Patients who have recurrent herpes-induced erythema mulitforme may benefit from acyclovir, by reducing the number of herpetic episodes. Other causative infections should be treated appropriately.
- Contraindications: Some underlying infections or health problems, such as diabetes, may contraindicate the use of steroids.
- Precautions: Refer to the manufacturer's profile of each drug.
- Significant possible interactions: Refer to the manufacturer's profile of each drug.

Second Line
None have been shown to be useful.

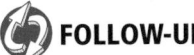 **FOLLOW-UP**

PROGNOSIS
- Rash evolves over 1–2 weeks and subsequently resolves within 2–3 weeks, generally without scarring or sequelae.
- Following resolution, there may be some post-inflammatory hyperpigmentation.
- Risk of recurrence may be as high as 37%.

COMPLICATIONS
Corneal ulceration is a serious complication of Stevens-Johnson syndrome. It is not clear whether this can occur in true erythema multiforme. Although there may be complications of the underlying disease, there are no other complications of erythema multiforme.

PATIENT MONITORING
- The disease is self-limiting.
- Complications are rare with no mortality.

REFERENCES
1. Assier H, et al. Erythema multiforme with mucous membrane involvement and Stevens-Johnson syndrome are clinically different disorders with distinct causes. *Arch Dermatol*. 1995;131: 539–543.
2. Cote B, et al. Clinicopathological correlation in erythema multiforme and Stevens-Johnson syndrome. *Arch Dermatol*. 1995;131: 1268–1272.
3. Kakourou T, et al. Corticosteroid treatment of erythema multiforme major (Stevens-Johnson syndrome) in children. *Eur J Pediatr*. 1997;156: 90–93.
4. Paquet P, Pierard GE. Erythema multiforme and toxic epidermal necrolysis: A comparative study. *Am J Dermatopath*. 1997;19:127–132.
5. Rahman SA, et al. Erythema multiforme associated with superficial fungal disease. *Cutis* 1995;55:329–351.
6. Revuz JE, Roujeau JC. Advances in toxic epidermal necrolysis. *Seminars in Cutaneous Medicine & Surgery*. 1966;15:258–266.
7. Rzany B, et al. Epidemiology of erythema exudativum multiforme majus, Stevens-Johnson syndrome, and toxic epidermal necrolysis in Germany (1991–1992): Structure and results of a population-based registry. *J Clin Epidemiol*. 1996;49:769–773.
8. *Saunders Electronic Atlas of Dermatology*. Philadelphia, PA: WB Saunders; 1996.
9. Tay YK, et al. Mycoplasma pneumonia infection is associated with Stevens-Johnson syndrome, not erythema multiforme (von Hebra). *J Am Acad Dermatol*. 1996;35:757–760.
10. Vaness MJ, Dwyer PK. Erythema multiforme-like reaction associated with radiotherapy. *Australian Radiology*. 1996;40:334–347.
11. Weston WL, et al. Target lesions on the lips: Childhood herpes simplex associated with erythema multiforme mimics Stevens-Johnson syndrome. *J Am Acad Dermatol*. 1997;37: 848–850.

 MISCELLANEOUS

See also: Dermatitis; Herpetiformis; Herpes gestationis; Urticaria

CODES

ICD9-CM
695.1 Erythema multiforme

PATIENT TEACHING
- Patients should be reassured that the disease is self-limited, but that recurrences are possible.
- Encourage avoidance of any identified etiologic agent.

E

ERYTHEMA NODOSUM

Gargeyi Kommareddy, MD

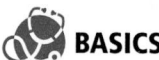 **BASICS**

DESCRIPTION
- Clinical pattern of multiple, bilateral, cutaneous, inflammatory, nonulcerating, and nonscarring eruptions that undergo characteristic color changes ending in temporary bruiselike areas
- Occurs most commonly on the extensor surface of the shins, less common on thighs and forearms
- Often idiopathic, but may be seen as a response to a variety of clinical entities
- Usually subsides in 3–6 weeks without scarring or atrophy
- Synonym(s): Dermatitis contusiformis

ALERT
Pediatric Considerations
Incidence equal, male and female

Pregnancy Considerations
May have repeat outbreaks during pregnancy

EPIDEMIOLOGY
- Predominant age: 20–30 years
- Predominant sex: Female > Male (3:1)

Incidence
Unknown

Prevalence
Unknown

RISK FACTORS
Listed under "Etiology"

ETIOLOGY
- Idiopathic: 37–60%
- Bacterial: Streptococcal infections (most common cause in children), tuberculosis, leprosy, *Yersiniaenterocolitica*, tularemia, *Campylobacter*, salmonella, *Shigella*, gonorrhea
- Sarcoid
- Drugs: Sulfonamides, oral contraceptives, bromides
- Pregnancy
- Deep fungal: Dermatophytes, coccidioidomycosis, histoplasmosis, blastomycosis
- Viral/chlamydial: Infectious mononucleosis, lymphogranuloma venereum, paravaccinia
- Enteropathies: Ulcerative colitis, Crohn disease, Behçet disease (6), Celiac disease (7)
- Malignancies: Lymphoma/leukemia, sarcoma, post radiation therapy

ASSOCIATED CONDITIONS
See "Etiology"

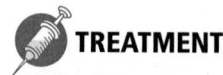 **DIAGNOSIS**

SIGNS AND SYMPTOMS
- Initially raised, warm, tender, brightly erythematous nodules on anterior shins. Lesions become bluish and fluctuant, gradually fading to yellowish resembling a bruise.
- Can also occur on any area with subcutaneous fat
- Diameter 1–15 cm
- Fever, malaise, chills
- Hilar adenopathy
- Episcleral lesions
- Eruptions often preceded by symptoms of upper respiratory infection
- Headache
- Arthralgias (rare)

TESTS
Lab
- Elevated erythrocyte sedimentation rate
- CBC: Mild leukocytosis
- Throat culture, antistreptolysin O titers (throat culture usually not positive because infection typically resolves before lesions appear)
- Stool culture and leukocytes, if indicated
- Skin testing for mycobacteria, if indicated
- Drugs that may alter lab results: Antecedent antibiotics may affect cultures.

Imaging
Chest radiograph for hilar adenopathy or infiltrates related to sarcoidosis or tuberculosis

Diagnostic Procedures/Surgery
Deep skin excisional biopsy including subcutaneous fat; usually not necessary.

Pathological Findings
- Septal panniculitis
- Neutrophilic infiltrate in septa of fat tissue, early in course
- Fibrosis, periseptal granulation tissue, lymphocytes, and multinucleated giant cells predominate late in course
- Lower dermis/subcutis involvement and septal fibrosis may occur.

DIFFERENTIAL DIAGNOSIS
- Superficial thrombophlebitis
- Cellulitis
- Septic emboli
- Erythema induratum (cold, ulcerating nodules on calves)
- Nodular vasculitis (warm, ulcerating nodules)
- Weber-Christian disease (violaceous, scarring nodules)
- Lupus panniculitis
- Cutaneous polyarteritis nodosa
- Sarcoidosis granulomata
- Cutaneous T cell lymphoma
- Erythema nodosum leprosum

TREATMENT

INITIAL STABILIZATION
Outpatient

GENERAL MEASURES
- Wet dressings (hot soaks and topical medications are not useful)
- Discontinue potentially causative drugs
- Treat underlying disease

Diet
No restrictions

Activity
- Bed rest, keep legs elevated
- Elastic wraps or support stockings may be helpful if patients want to be up and around.

MEDICATION (DRUGS)

First Line
- Medication usually more effective after initial onset versus with chronic disease
- Condition often self-limited
- NSAIDs
  - Indomethacin: 75–150 mg/d, divided 3 times a day
  - Naproxen (Naprosyn): 500–1000 mg/d, divided b.i.d.
  - Aspirin: 325 mg 8–12 times per day; use enteric coated to decrease GI upset. Titrate to blood levels.
- Contraindications
  - Active or recent peptic ulcer disease
  - History of hypersensitivity to NSAIDs
- Precautions
  - GI upset/bleeding
  - Fluid retention
  - Dose reduction in elderly, especially those with renal disease, diabetes, or heart failure
  - May mask fever
  - NSAIDs may elevate liver function tests
- Significant possible interactions
  - May blunt antihypertensive effects of diuretics and beta-blockers
  - NSAIDs can elevate plasma lithium levels.
  - Caution advised with naproxen or any highly protein-bound drug, because it may compete for albumin binding and elevate levels
  - NSAIDs can cause significant elevation and prolongation of methotrexate levels.

Second Line
- Potassium iodide 400–900 mg/d, divided 2–3 times a day for 3–4 weeks (for persistent lesions)
- Corticosteroids only in very severe, refractory cases
- Other NSAIDs
- Recent reports of improvement with colchicine 0.6–1.2 mg b.i.d.
- Vitamin B_{12} replacement trial (8)

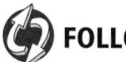 **FOLLOW-UP**

PROGNOSIS
- Individual lesions resolve over 3–6 weeks.
- Total time course of 6–12 weeks, but may vary with etiologic disease, if present
- Joint aches and pains may persist for years.
- Lesions do not scar.
- 1 or more recurrences in 12–14% of cases
  - Occur over variable periods, averaging several years
  - Seen most often with sarcoid, streptococcal infection, pregnancy, and oral contraceptives

COMPLICATIONS
- Vary according to underlying disease
- None expected from lesions of erythema nodosum

PATIENT MONITORING
Monthly follow-up or as dictated by underlying disorder

REFERENCES
1. Fitzpatrick TB, et al. eds. *Dermatology in General Medicine*. 5th ed. New York, NY: McGraw-Hill; 1999.
2. Habif T. *Clinical Dermatology*. 4th ed. St. Louis, MO: CV Mosby; 2004.
3. Hannuksela M. Erythema nodosum. *Clin Dermatol*. 1986;4:88–95.
4. Gonzalez-Gay MA, et al. Erythema nodosum: A clinical approach. *Clin Exp Rheumatol*. 2001; 19:365–368.
5. Requena L, Requena C. Erythema nodosum. *Dermatol Online J*. 2002;8:4.
6. Erythema nodosum: Underlying conditions. *Clin Rheumatilogy* 2000;19:212.
7. Erythema nodosum in asoociation with celiac disease. *Pediatr Dermatol*. 2004;21(3):227–230.
8. Successful treatment of chronic erythema nodosum with vitamin B_{12}. *J Am Board of Family Practice*. 2005;18:6.

 MISCELLANEOUS

Other notes
- Lofgren syndrome (erythema nodosum and hilar adenopathy) is seen with multiple etiologies and does not exclusively indicate sarcoid.
- The clinical variant of erythema nodosum migrans (subacute nodular migratory panniculitis) is often unilateral with nodules fewer in number, smaller in size, and longer lasting that extend radially by division into smaller nodules.
- In patients with a history of Hodgkin lymphoma, erythema nodosum is a warning of impending recurrence.

 CODES

ICD9-CM
695.2 Erythema nodosum

PATIENT TEACHING
- Lesions will resolve over a few months.
- No scarring is anticipated.
- Joint aches and pains may persist.
- <20% recur.

 See Corresponding Diagnostic Algorithm

E

ERYTHROBLASTOSIS FETALIS

Donald A. F. Nelson, MD

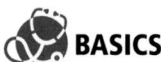 **BASICS**

DESCRIPTION
- Hemolytic anemia of the fetus or newborn caused by transplacental transmission of maternal antibody
- When severe, the anemia may result in extramedullary hematopoiesis, secondary organ dysfunction, heart failure, hydrops, and death.
- The name *erythroblastosis* refers to the presence of immature erythrocytes in the peripheral blood from accelerated hematopoiesis.
- System(s) Affected: Cardiovascular; Hemic/Lymphatic/Immunologic; Nervous
- Synonym(s): Erythroblastosis neonatorum; Hemolytic disease of the newborn; Congenital anemia of the newborn; Immune hydrops fetalis; Icterus gravis neonatorum

ALERT
Pediatric Considerations
Affects fetus and neonate exclusively

GENERAL PREVENTION
- Rho(D) immune globulin (RhIG, RhoGAM, Gamulin Rh) given prophylactically to unsensitized, Rh-negative pregnant women at risk. Usually at 28–32 weeks' gestation and at birth if infant is Rh positive (see: "Rh Incompatibility").
- Artificial insemination with sperm from antigen-negative donor for isoimmunized woman whose partner is antigen positive

EPIDEMIOLOGY
- Predominant age: Fetus and newborn
- Predominant sex: Male = Female

Pregnancy Considerations
- ~9% of pregnancies have an Rh-negative mother with an Rh-positive fetus.
- With Rho(D) immune globulin prophylaxis, risk of sensitization is reduced to <1% of susceptible pregnancies. (2)

RISK FACTORS
- Prior transfusion with incompatible blood
- Any Rh-positive pregnancy in Rh-negative woman
- Without prophylactic immunotherapy (Rh immune globulin), risk of Rh sensitization is up to 16% during or after term pregnancy, ~3% for spontaneous abortion, and 5–6% for surgical abortion.
- Sensitization by exposure to fetal blood may also occur with ectopic pregnancy, amniocentesis, chorionic villus sampling, placental trauma or manipulation, and placental abruption.
- Prophylaxis with Rh immune globulin greatly reduces but does not eliminate the risk.

Genetics
May occur when the fetus inherits a paternal blood group antigen lacking in the mother. The Rh D antigen is most frequently implicated (for more on inheritance of Rh antigens, see "Rh Incompatibility").

ETIOLOGY
- Maternal isoimmunization to Rh antigen by transfusion of Rh-positive blood
- Maternal isoimmunization from exposure to fetal Rh antigens in prior pregnancy or current pregnancy
- Maternal isoimmunization to other blood group antigens (e.g., Kell Duffy, Kidd M, Diego S) is unusual but may cause serious disease. (3)

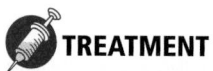 **DIAGNOSIS**

SIGNS AND SYMPTOMS
Physical Exam
- Pallor
- Respiratory distress
- Hepatomegaly
- Splenomegaly
- Ascites
- Hypotension/shock
- Edema/anasarca/hydrops
- Jaundice of newborn
- Purpura/bleeding problems
- Fetal death in utero

TESTS
- Elevated amniotic fluid bilirubin (δ OD 450)
- Paternal blood typing may exclude pregnancy from being at risk.

Lab
- Positive indirect Coombs test (antibody screen) during pregnancy
- Positive direct Coombs test in fetus or newborn
- Anemia in fetus or newborn
- Reticulocytosis
- Nucleated RBCs on differential count
- Hyperbilirubinemia (indirect bilirubin)
- Thrombocytopenia
- Drugs that may alter lab results
  - Prior administration of Rho(D) immune globulin may lead to weakly (false) positive indirect Coombs test in mother and direct Coombs test in infant.

Imaging
- Ultrasonography may demonstrate hepatomegaly, abdominal enlargement, ascites, or signs of hydrops.
- Doppler flow studies of fetus are experimental in assessing degree of anemia
- Fetus may be severely affected without hydrops; ultrasound is poor at predicting need for intervention

Diagnostic Procedures/Surgery
- Amniocentesis
- Umbilical cord blood sampling

Pathological Findings
- Erythroid hyperplasia of bone marrow
- Extramedullary hematopoiesis
- Hepatomegaly
- Splenomegaly
- Cardiac enlargement
- Pulmonary hemorrhages
- Enlargement, edema of placenta

DIFFERENTIAL DIAGNOSIS
- Fetal blood loss anemia
- Twin-to-twin transfusion
- Arteriovenous or cardiac malformations
- Hereditary hemolytic anemias
- Drug-induced hemolytic anemia
- Nonimmune fetal hydrops
- Hemolysis from intrauterine infection (syphilis, toxoplasmosis, cytomegalovirus, others)

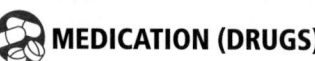 **TREATMENT**

INITIAL STABILIZATION
- Affected pregnancies are usually managed at the tertiary care level by perinatologists because of the specialized, somewhat hazardous, treatment measures involved.
- Delivery should occur in an institution capable of performing exchange transfusion, even if only mild involvement of the infant is expected.
- Infants with moderate or severe disease require neonatal intensive care.

GENERAL MEASURES
- See "Patient Monitoring"
- Depending on severity of involvement, treatment of infant may include
  - Phototherapy
  - Transfusion after delivery
  - Exchange transfusion
  - Diuretics and digoxin for hydrops
  - Early delivery
  - Intrauterine transfusion: Intravascular approach via the umbilical vein is becoming preferred over the intraperitoneal approach and appears to be more effective.

MEDICATION (DRUGS)
- Diuretics or inotropic agents may be used in addition to transfusion to manage heart failure in the newborn.
- Immune globulin infusion and erythropoietin have been used experimentally in combination with intrauterine transfusion to reduce the number of transfusions needed. (1,4)[C]
- Promethazine, corticosteroids, and plasmapheresis have been tried as alternatives to invasive treatments but have not been effective.

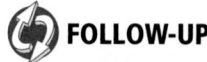

FOLLOW-UP

PROGNOSIS

- 50% of affected infants have mild disease and require no treatment (or treatment of anemia and jaundice only after delivery), and can be delivered at or near term.
- 30% have moderate disease with anemia and hepatomegaly. They require close follow-up of the pregnancy for signs of deterioration, which may require early delivery after 32–34 weeks or intrauterine transfusion prior to that age. After delivery, exchange transfusion is likely to treat anemia and hyperbilirubinemia.
- 20% have fetal hydrops, require intrauterine transfusion, and delivery as early as 32–34 weeks.
- Disease severity tends to worsen in successive affected pregnancies.
- Hydrops is associated with poorer prognosis.
- Without treatment, overall perinatal mortality is ~50%.
- With appropriate monitoring and treatment, most infants do well, even those requiring intrauterine transfusion, and perinatal mortality has been reduced to 2–3%. (2)
- Fortunately, universal screening for Rh sensitization and widespread use of Rh immune globulin in 3rd trimester and/or birth have made disease relatively rare.

COMPLICATIONS

- Fetal distress requiring emergent delivery
- Fetal death in utero
- Disseminated intravascular coagulation (DIC)
- Pregnancy loss from umbilical blood sampling
- Pregnancy loss from intrauterine transfusion
- Asphyxia
- Neonatal hemolytic anemia, mild to severe
- Neonatal anemia from hematopoietic suppression after intrauterine transfusion
- Pulmonary edema
- CHF
- Shock
- Neonatal jaundice, mild to severe
- Kernicterus

PATIENT MONITORING

- Maternal antibody titer measured by 20 weeks and every 4 weeks during pregnancy. A titer of 1:16 or greater, particularly if rising, indicates need for further testing. (3)[C]
- Periodic amniocentesis for photometric determination of amniotic fluid bilirubin levels in pregnancies with elevated antibody titers. Results estimate the extent of fetal hemolysis and the need for cord blood sampling. (3)[C]
- Percutaneous umbilical blood sampling (PUBS, cordocentesis) for fetal blood type, hematocrit, reticulocyte count, presence of erythroblasts (3)[C]
- Fetal heart rate testing/ultrasonography to assess fetal status [C]
- Amniocentesis for fetal lung maturity at the point of pregnancy where early delivery is a management option, especially after 34 weeks (3)[C]

REFERENCES

1. Alcock GS, Liley, H. Immunoglobulin infusion for isoimmune haemolytic jaundice in neonates. Cochrane Database of Systematic Reviews. 1, 2006.
2. Bowman J. Thirty-five years of Rh prophylaxis. *Transfusion* 2003;43:1661–1666.
3. Management of isoimmunization in pregnancy. ACOG Educational Bulletin 227. Aug 1996.
4. Ovali F, Samanci N, Dagoglu T. Management of late anemia in Rhesus hemolytic disease: Use of recombinant human erythropoietin (a pilot study). *Pediatric research*. 1996 May;39(5):831–834.

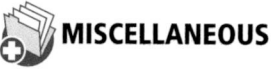

MISCELLANEOUS

See also: Rh incompatibility

CODES

ICD9-CM

- 773.0 Rh hemolytic disease in fetus or newborn
- 773.1 ABO hemolytic disease in fetus or newborn
- 773.2 Other hemolytic disease in fetus or newborn
- 773.3 Isoimmune hydrops fetalis
- 773.4 Kernicterus due to isoimmunization
- 773.5 Isoimmune late anemia

E

ESOPHAGEAL VARICES

Kelly J. O'Callahan, MD

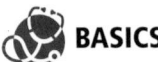 **BASICS**

DESCRIPTION

- Dilated collateral veins in the lamina propria of the distal esophagus connecting the portal and systemic circulations
- Result from chronic hypertension in the portal circulation due to increased resistance to blood flow
- Increased pressure and turbulent flow within these vessels as well as their superficial location in the distal esophagus make them prone to rupture with significant morbidity and mortality

GENERAL PREVENTION

Endoscope esophagus annually in patients with cirrhosis

- Consider use of non-selective beta-blockers or obliteration of varices with esophageal banding for those intolerant of medication to prevent bleeding

EPIDEMIOLOGY

- Esophageal varices occur in ~50% of patients with cirrhosis.
- 50% of patients with esophageal varices bleed during their lifetime.
- Bleeding from esophageal varices is associated with a 15–25% mortality.
- Predominant sex: Male > Female

RISK FACTORS

- Cirrhosis of the liver
- Inherited thrombotic conditions such as anti-thrombin III, substance S or R deficiencies
- Prolonged use of estrogen-progesterone

Genetics

No known pattern

ETIOLOGY

- Cirrhosis accounts for >90% of cases. Alcohol and hepatitis C are the most common etiologies.
- Hemochromatosis, hepatitis B, nonalcoholic fatty liver disease, biliary cirrhosis, and autoimmune cirrhosis account for remainder. Extrahepatic portal vein thrombosis from umbilical vein infection, trauma, chronic pancreatitis, thrombotic conditions, and polycythemia.
- Malignant invasion of liver sinusoids or portal vein; seen in lymphoma, leukemia, hepatocellular carcinoma, and pancreatic carcinoma.
- Metabolic diseases altering liver sinusoids— amyloid, Gaucher disease, fatty liver
- Budd-Chiari syndrome
- Veno-occlusive disease

ASSOCIATED CONDITIONS

- Portal hypertensive gastropathy
- Gastric varices, may occur after eradication
- Hemorrhoids

DIAGNOSIS

SIGNS AND SYMPTOMS

- GI bleeding
  - 75% of time, painless hematemesis and/or melena
  - Occult bleeding with anemia 25%
- Signs of cirrhosis

History

- Generally a history of cirrhosis or liver disease
- Painless hematemesis or melena

Physical Exam

- Possible hypotension/tachycardia
- Small, hard liver
- Splenomegaly
- Ascites
- Visible abdominal periumbilical collateral circulation (Caput medusae)
- Spider angiomata on upper chest/back
- Palmar erythema

TESTS

Lab

- Anemia related to blood loss
- Possibly abnormal liver function tests, thrombocytopenia, prolonged prothrombin time or low albumin-reflecting cirrhosis

Imaging

- Barium swallow
  - Demonstrates advanced varices, but is insensitive to small ones
  - Precludes possible urgent endoscopy
- Doppler sonography: Demonstrates patency, diameter, and flow in portal vein, and splenic vein, and large collaterals intra-abdominally
- MRI
  - Demonstrates large vascular channels intra-abdominally, and in the mediastinum
  - Can demonstrate patency of the intrahepatic portal vein and splenic vein
- Venous phase celiac arteriography: Demonstrates portal vein and its collaterals, also can diagnose hepatic vein occlusion

Diagnostic Procedures/Surgery

- Esophagoscopy as part of esophagogastroduodenoscopy
  - Can identify and treat varices that appear as protruding submucosal veins in the distal 3rd of the esophagus
  - Can identify actively bleeding varices as well as those with stigmata of recent hemorrhage
  - Can treat actively bleeding vessels with sclerotherapy or esophageal band ligation or can obliterate vessels to prevent rebleeding. Can also identify associated conditions, including gastric varices and portal hypertensive gastropathy.
- Endoscopic ultrasound is particularly sensitive to gastric varices.
- Portal pressure measurement
  - Radiologist introduces a catheter retrograde into the hepatic vein in a wedged position to occlude flow
  - The catheter is withdrawn to a free position and pressure again measured. The difference between wedged and free is the portal pressure. If <12 mm Hg, bleeding is less likely. Progressive increases above 12 correlate with the likelihood of hemorrhage.
  - This is sometimes used to monitor successful treatment with beta adrenergic blocking agent though it is not widely available.
- Transjugular intrahepatic portasystemic shunt (TIPS)
- Surgical portocaval shunts

Pathological Findings

- Extensive collateral circulation in the mediastinum and in the abdomen in addition to large vessels in the submucosa of the esophagus
- When bleeding occurs, these large veins explode into the submucosa of esophagus and rupture into the lumen.

DIFFERENTIAL DIAGNOSIS

- Upper GI bleeding
  - Pulmonary bleeding; hemoptysis
  - Peptic ulcer disease
  - Gastric or esophageal malignancy
  - Artenovenous malformation (AVM)
  - Nosebleed
- Lower GI bleeding
  - Hemorrhoids
  - Colonic neoplasia
  - Diverticulosis
  - AVMs

TREATMENT

Inpatient for acute bleeding

GENERAL MEASURES
- Treat comorbidities, generally related to cirrhosis
- Hospital management of bleeding varices
  - Appropriate resuscitation and maintenance of blood volume
  - Treat coagulopathy, if necessary.

  - IV somatostatin to lower portal venous pressure usually used as adjuvant to endoscopic management. Begin with IV bolus of 50 mg followed by drip of 50 mg/h. (1)[A]
  - Urgent upper endoscopy for diagnosis and treatment. Variceal band ligation or sclerotherapy for bleeding varices or those nonbleeding, which are medium to large in size to decrease risk of bleeding. Variceal band ligation are preferred due to better bleeding cessation with fewer complications. (2)[A]

  - Repeat ligation or sclerosant injection if bleeding recurs.
  - If endoscopic treatment fails to stop bleeding or cannot be accomplished, may need to use Senstaken Blakemore or Minnesota tube to stabilize patient for a transjugular intrahepatic portosystemic shunt
- Management of nonbleeding varices
  - If ligation started, usually in medium to large varices (grade 2–4), repeat banding at 1–3 week intervals. 4–6 treatments are usually required to obliterate varices.

  - For those not treated endoscopically, begin non-selective beta-blockers such as propranolol or nadolol. Increase dose for goal of heart rate reduction of 25% of baseline (SBP >90, HR >50). For those who do not tolerate the side effects of this regimen, proceed with endoscopic variceal band ligation as primary prophylaxis. (3)[A]
  - If bleeding recurs, or portal pressure measurement shows portal pressure still >12 mm Hg, isosorbide mononitrate may be added, though endoscopic band ligation preferred if possible. (4)[B]
  - Refractory bleeding may require use of TIPS, or portocaval shunt (5)[B]
  - Refer for liver transplantation where appropriate.

Diet
Will be dictated by other comorbidities

Activity
No restrictions

 MEDICATION (DRUGS)

- For varices
  - Propranolol: 40 mg b.i.d. increase until heart rate decreased by 25% from baseline
  - Nadolol 80 mg daily, increase as above
  - Isosorbide mononitrate further reduces portal pressure and can be used in conjunction with beta-blocking agents. Begin at 20 mg b.i.d.
  - During banding or sclerotherapy: Proton pump inhibitor, such as lansoprazole 30 mg/d until varices obliterated
- During bleeding, consider antibiotic prophylaxis for spontaneous peritonitis and other infections with ciprofloxacin for 7–10 days.
- Contraindications: Severe asthma with beta-blockers
- Precautions: Symptomatic hypotension

First Line
Beta-blockers, proton pump inhibitors, antibiotics

Second Line
Isosorbide mononitrate

SURGERY
- Portacaval shunt
- Esophageal transection
- Liver transplantation

 FOLLOW-UP

DISPOSITION
Admission Criteria
Clinically significant GI bleeding

Discharge Criteria
Cessation of bleeding, stability of other comorbidities

Issues for Referral
Primarily those associated with liver transplantation

PROGNOSIS
- Depends heavily on ability to treat or reverse underlying condition
- In those with cirrhosis, 1 year survival for those who are alive 2 weeks after variceal bleed is ~50%.

COMPLICATIONS
- Bleeding
- Gastric or other uncommon varices may occur following successful eradication of esophageal varices.
- Esophageal varices can recur after obliteration.

PATIENT MONITORING
- Edoscopic variceal ligation, repeated every 1–4 weeks until varices eradicated
- Repeat esophagogastro duedenoscopy annually to watch for recurrence.
- If transjugular intrahepatic portasystemic shunt or other portacaval shunt, repeat endoscopy only if clinically bleeding
- If transjugular intrahepatic portasystemic shunt present, follow-up as recommended by radiologist; usually Doppler sonogram each 6 months

REFERENCES

1. Zhou Y, et al. Comparison of the efficacy of octreotide, vasopressin, and omeprazole in the control of acute bleeding in patients with portal hypertensive gastropathy: A controlled study. *J Gastroenterol Hepatol*. 2002;17:973–979.
2. Laine L, et al. Endoscopic ligation compared with sclerotherapy for the treatment of bleeding esophageal varices. *Ann Intern Med*. 1993; 119:1–7.
3. Boyer TD. Primary prophyaxis for variceal bleeding: Are we there yet? *Gastroenterology*. 2005;128: 1120–112.
4. Merkel C, et al. Randomised trial of nadolol alone or with isosorbide mononitrate for primary prophylaxis of variceal bleeding in cirrhosis. *Lanc*. 1996;348:1677.
5. Sanyal AJ, et al. Transjugular intrahepatic portosystemic shunts for patients with active variceal hemorrhage unresponsive to sclerotherapy. *Gastroenterology*. 1996;111:138.

 MISCELLANEOUS

See also: Cirrhosis of the liver; Hemorrhoids; Portal hypertension

CODES

ICD9-CM
- 456.0 Esophageal varices with bleeding
- 456.1 Esophageal varices without mention of bleeding

PATIENT TEACHING
- Appropriate to cirrhosis
- National Digestive Information Clearinghouse, 2 Information Way, Bethesda, MD 20892 or American Liver Foundation, 1425 Pompton Way, Cedar Grove, NJ 07009

See Corresponding Diagnostic Algorithm

E

ESSENTIAL TREMOR SYNDROME

Cynthia Brown, MD

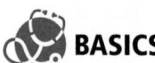 ## BASICS

DESCRIPTION

- A postural tremor that is slow, rhythmic, and primarily affecting the hands, head, and voice, with a frequency of 4–12 Hz.
- It may be familial, sporadic, or associated with other movement disorders.
- It can begin at any age, but the incidence and prevalence increases with age.
- The tremor can be exacerbated by emotional or physical stresses, fatigue, and caffeine.

EPIDEMIOLOGY

Can occur at any age but onset peaks during teenage years and 50s

Incidence

0.4–5% of the general population

RISK FACTORS

Genetics

Can be familial, autosomal dominant in ~50% of cases

ETIOLOGY

Genetic association

PATHOPHYSIOLOGY

Unknown

ASSOCIATED CONDITIONS

Can be present in 10% of patients with Parkinson disease

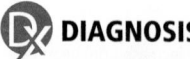 ## DIAGNOSIS

SIGNS AND SYMPTOMS

Postural tremor that worsens with movement

History

- The tremor can worsen with age.
- Tremor often decreases after ingestion of alcohol.

Physical Exam

- Tremor can affect upper limbs (~95% of patients).
- Less commonly, the tremor affects head (~34%), lower limbs (~30%), voice (~12%), tongue (~7%), face (~5%), and trunk (~5%).

TESTS

Rule out Wilson disease and thyroid dysfunction

Lab

- Check ceruloplasmin and serum copper to rule out Wilson disease.
- Check thyroid stimulating hormone.

Imaging

Brain MRI usually is not necessary or indicated unless Wilson disease is found, or examination implies central lesion.

Diagnostic Procedures/Surgery

Electromyogram usually is not necessary.

Pathological Findings

Posture-related tremor

DIFFERENTIAL DIAGNOSIS

- Wilson disease
- Hyperthyroidism
- Psychogenic tremor
- Medication effect

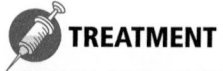 ## TREATMENT

GENERAL MEASURES

Diet

Avoid caffeine

Activity

Adequate rest is important.

MEDICATION (DRUGS)

First Line
- Propanolol 60–240 mg/d in divided doses is effective in ~50% of patients, or primidone 25 mg initially titrated upward as needed p.r.n. to maximum of 250 mg t.i.d.
- Sotalol and atenolol are alternatives.

Second Line
- Topiramate up to 400 mg/d
- Gabapentin up to 400 mg t.i.d.
- Clonazepam and alprazolam should be used with caution due to abuse potential.
- Clozapine is recommended only for refractory cases of limb tremor due to potential of agranulocytosis.

SURGERY
- Deep brain stimulation may be used to treat medically refractory limb tremor and has fewer adverse effects than thalamotomy.
- Unilateral thalamotomy may be used to treat limb tremor that is refractory to medical management.
- Bilateral thalamotomy is not recommended.

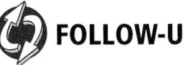 **FOLLOW-UP**

DISPOSITION
Issues for Referral
Referral to a neurologist can help differentiate those with dystonia, neuropathic tremor, Parkinson disease, or drug-induced tremor.

PROGNOSIS
Tremor tends to worsen with age, increasing in amplitude.

REFERENCES
1. Zesiewicz TA, et al. Practice parameter: therapies for essential tremor: Report of the Quality Standards Subcommittee of the American Academy of Neurology. 2005;28;64(12):2008–2020.

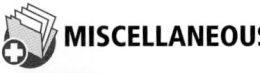 **MISCELLANEOUS**

CODES

ICD9-CM
- 333.1 Essential and other specified forms of tremor
- 781.0 Abnormal involuntary movements

PATIENT TEACHING
- Avoid caffeine
- Somewhat relieved by rest

 See Corresponding Diagnostic Algorithm

E

EUSTACHIAN TUBE DYSFUNCTION

David J. Lee, MD

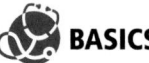 **BASICS**

DESCRIPTION
- Eustachian tube is either too open or too closed, associated with abnormal pressure at either end.
- Eustachian tube dysfunction (ETD) is classically, a *blockage* of the eustachian tube.
- Acute ETD may occur in the setting of pressure changes (e.g., plane travel) or acute upper airway inflammation (e.g., URI, sinusitis).
- Chronic ETD may lead to negative middle ear pressure, retracted tympanic membrane, serous effusions, otitis media, adhesive otitis media, or cholesteatoma.
- Patulous ET (PET), a distinct entity, is failure of the eustachian tube to close.
  - Often manifested as autophony
  - See other references dedicated to PET
- System(s) Affected: Auditory
- Synonym(s): Auditory tube dysfunction; Eustachian tube disorder; Blocked eustachian tube; Patulous eustachian tube

ALERT
- Sudden single-sided deafness can masquerade as ETD.
- A simple 512-Hz tuning fork test lateralizes to the opposite ear in sudden sensorineural hearing loss and to the affected ear in ETD with conductive hearing loss.
- Any sudden sensorineural hearing loss is a medical emergency and should be referred to an otolaryngologist immediately.
- Treatment with high-dose steroids should begin ASAP, ideally within 10 days of onset.

GENERAL PREVENTION
- Control sources of upper airway inflammation most commonly allergies, GERD, upper respiratory infections
- Avoid autoinsufflation of middle ear (blow against pinched nostril and closed mouth).
- Avoid exposure to pressure changes (plane flight, scuba diving) in the setting of URI.
- Avoid exposure to environmental irritants:
  - Smoking and 2nd-hand smoke

Pediatric Considerations
- ETD is common in this age group.
- Associated with URI or adenoid hypertrophy
- Referral to an otolaryngologist if hearing loss or recurrent or chronic middle ear infections.

EPIDEMIOLOGY
- Most common in children <5 (1)
- Associated with low SES (1)
- Slightly more common in males (1)
- Race: Native American, Inuit, Australian Aborigines (1)
- Similar incidence among African Americans and Caucasians (1)

Incidence
70–90% before age 2, decreases with age (1)

Geriatric Considerations
- No studies thus far have looked at the incidence or prevalence in this population.
- Compliance in ET changes with aging (3).

RISK FACTORS
- Adult and pediatric
  - Tobacco and pollutant exposure
  - Gastroesophageal reflux disease
  - Allergy
  - Chronic sinusitis
  - Sleep apnea with CPAP use
  - Adenoid hypertrophy or nasopharyngeal mass
  - Neuromuscular disease
  - Family history
  - Altered immunity
  - Early onset or history of ETD as a child
  - Native American, Inuit, Australian Aborigine
- Pediatric
  - 2nd-hand smoke
  - Prematurity and low birth weight
  - Young age
  - Craniofacial abnormalities (e.g. cleft palate, Down syndrome)
  - Day care, exposure to many other children
  - Crowded living conditions
  - Low socioeconomic status
  - Use of pacifier
  - Prone sleeping position
  - Short period of breastfeeding
  - Prolonged bottle use

Pregnancy Considerations
- Eustachian tube dysfunction may be exacerbated by rhinitis of pregnancy.
- Previous otologic history and concurrent smoking are predisposing factors.
- Symptoms typically resolve postpartum.

Genetics
- Twin studies show genetic component (1).
- Specific genetic cause still undefined.

PATHOPHYSIOLOGY
- Eustachian tube functions
  - Ventilation/regulation of middle ear pressure
  - Protection from nasopharyngeal secretions
  - Drainage of middle ear fluid
  - Palate, nasal cavities, nasopharynx at the tube's proximal end, and middle-ear and mastoid gas cell system at its distal end
  - Eustachian tube is closed at rest, opens with yawning, swallowing, sneezing.
- Cycle of dysfunction
  - Structural or functional obstruction of the ET compromises 3 functions of this system:
  - Negative pressure develops in middle ear.
  - Serous exudate is drawn from middle ear mucosa by negative pressure or refluxed into the middle ear if the ET opens momentarily.
  - Infection of static fluid causes edema and release of inflammatory mediators, which exacerbates cycle of inflammation/obstruction.

ETIOLOGY
- In children, horizontally oriented tube predisposes to difficulties with ventilation and drainage (1).
- Shorter tube predisposes to reflux (1).
- Adenoid hypertrophy can block the torus tubaris (proximal opening of the ET) (1).
- In adults, paradoxical closing with swallowing has been noted in a majority of cases (1).

ASSOCIATED CONDITIONS
- Hearing loss
- Tympanic membrane retraction
- Middle ear effusion
- Cholesteatoma
- Allergic rhinitis
- Chronic sinusitis
- Upper respiratory infection
- Adenoid hypertrophy
- Obesity
- Cleft palate
- Down syndrome
- Nasopharyngeal carcinoma or other tumor

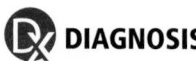 **DIAGNOSIS**

SIGNS AND SYMPTOMS
- Fullness, pressure, clogged feeling in the ear
- Otalgia or ear discomfort
- Hearing loss
- Tinnitus
- Dizziness

ALERT
Unilateral symptoms and/or recent onset of symptoms in the absence of identifiable cause for ETD warrants workup for nasopharyngeal process such as benign or malignant tumor (1)[A].

History
- Recent onset versus chronic life-long problem
- History of previous ear infections
- Previous ear surgeries including tubes
- Subjective hearing loss
- Sidedness, unilateral or bilateral
- Associated dizziness versus vertigo:
  - Duration, timing, exacerbating, and alleviating factors
- Constant versus waxing waning symptoms
- Smoking history
- Antecedent URI
- Difficulty breathing through nose
- Allergic symptoms
- Trauma
- Throat pain
- Voice change
- Weight loss

Physical Exam
- Pneumatic otoscopy: Retracted tympanic membrane, decreased movement, effusion
- Tuning fork tests: 512-Hz fork lateralizes to affected ear in setting of conductive hearing loss
- Toynbee maneuver: View changes of the drum while patient autoinsufflates against closed lips and pinched nostrils.
- Nasopharyngoscopy: Adenoid hypertrophy or nasopharyngeal mass
- Anterior rhinoscopy: Nasal obstruction, turbinate hypertrophy
- TMJ nontender

TESTS

Lab
None in clinical practice

Imaging
- Radiologic studies are not routinely performed if clinical signs/symptoms suggest ETD without middle ear/mastoid sequelae.
- CT scan may show middle ear/mastoid opacification or other sequelae of chronic ETD.

Diagnostic Procedures/Surgery
- Audiogram may show conductive hearing loss.
- Tympanometry: Type B or C tympanograms indicate fluid or retraction, respectively. Negative middle ear peak pressures seen even with normal (Type A) tympanograms.

Pathological Findings
- Blockage of the ET orifice by mucopurulent nasal discharge or edema
- Compression of the orifice by adenoid tissue
- Hypertrophy of the peritubal tonsil
- Paradoxical tube closure when swallowing
- Atrophy of the orifice
- In over 1/3 of patients, endoscopic findings were normal (5).

DIFFERENTIAL DIAGNOSIS
- Sudden single-sided deafness (a medical emergency)
- Tympanic membrane perforation
- Barotrauma
- TMJ disorder
- Ménière disease
- Superior semicircular canal dehiscence
- Skull base tumor

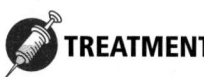 **TREATMENT**

GENERAL MEASURES
Reduce cycle of inflammation with decongestants, antihistamines, topical steroids, antireflux medications, and antibiotics when indicated.

Diet
- Generally no restrictions. Avoid foods that would exacerbate reflux symptoms.
- In newborns, breastfeeding has been associated with a lower incidence of ETD (1)[A].

Activity
Avoid scuba diving, plane flights with URI (1)[C]

Complementary and Alternative Therapies
Zinc nasal spray (Zicam) may help reduce length of URI but may cause anosmia.

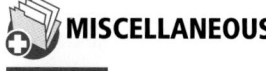 **MEDICATION (DRUGS)**

First Line
- Medication is tailored to individual patient's symptoms.
- Decongestants (1)[C]
  – Phenylephrine (Neo-synephrine)
- Nasal steroids (1)[B]
  – Beclomethasone (Beconase, Vancenase)
  – Budesonide (Rhinocort)
  – Flunisolide (Nasarel, Nasolide)
  – Fluticasone (Flonase), others
- 2nd-generation H$_1$ antihistamines (1)[B]
  – Loratadine (Claritin)
  – Desloratadine (Clarinex)
  – Fexofenadine (Allegra)
  – Cetirizine (Zyrtec)
- Other nasal sprays:
  – Oxymetazoline (Afrin)
  – No proven efficacy; avoid in children (1)[B]
  – Astelin (Azelastiline) (antihistamine)
- Antireflux, proton pump inhibitors (1)[B]
  – Omeprazole (Prilosec)
  – Pantoprazole (Protonix)
- Antibiotics, not routinely used unless associated with acute pain and fever
  – Amoxicillin, 1st line (1)[A]
  – Treatment for 10 days is most effective (1)[B].
  – Consider topical antibiotic drops with topical steroid in setting of discharge alone (1)[A].
  – Neomycin-polymyxin-hydrocortisone suspension (Cortisporin)
  – Ciprofloxacin hydrocortisone suspension (Cipro HC), others
- Pain control, anti-inflammatory:
  – Acetaminophen, NSAIDs

Second Line
- 1st-generation antihistamines
  – Diphenhydramine (Benadryl), others
- Antireflux, H$_2$ blockers
  – Ranitidine (Zantac), others

SURGERY
- Myringotomy and pressure equalization tube placement to ventilate middle ear, relieve pressure, and prevent sequelae of chronically retracted drum (1)[A]
- Adenoidectomy if tissue is present
  – In children, first set of tubes alone, then adenoidectomy if problems recurs (1)[A]
- Direct nasopharyngoscopy and biopsy if mass
- Mastoidectomy for associated sequelae (e.g., chronic otomastoiditis, cholesteatoma):
  – Culture-directed IV antibiotics is 90% effective in treating chronic suppurative otitis media (CSOM) and mastoiditis (1)[B].

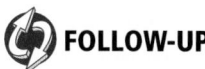 **FOLLOW-UP**

- Monitor pressure equalization tubes every 3 months in children and every 6 months in adults.
- Monitor tympanic membrane retraction pocket for progression every 6–12 months to allow for early intervention for erosion or cholesteatoma.

DISPOSITION
Typically, outpatient management

Issues for Referral
Refer to otolaryngologist if conservative first-line medications have provided no relief of symptoms.

PROGNOSIS
- Chronic disorder; current treatments provide symptomatic relief; usually require prolonged use

COMPLICATIONS
- Morbidity related to hearing compromise
- Mortality rare. Related to sequelae of untreated middle ear disease

REFERENCES
1. Bluestone CD. Studies in otitis media: Children's Hospital of Pittsburgh-University of Pittsburgh progress report–2004. *Laryngoscope.* 2004;114(11 Pt 3 Suppl 105):1–26. Review.
2. Takasaki K, Sando I, Balaban CD, et al. Histopathological changes of the eustachian tube cartilage and the tensor veli palatini muscle with aging. *Laryngoscope* 1999;109:1679–1683.
3. Kaneko A, Hosoda Y, Doi T, et al. Tubal compliance—changes with age and in tubal malfunction. *Auris Nasus Larynx* 2001;28:121–124.
4. Grimmer JF. Poe DS. Update on eustachian tube dysfunction and the patulous eustachian tube. *Curr Opin Otolaryngol Head Neck Surg.* 2005;13(5):277–282.
5. Takahashi H, Honjo I and Fujita A. Endoscopic findings at the pharyngeal orifice of the eustachian tube in otitis media with effusion. *Eur Arch Oto-Rhino-Laryngol.* 1996;253 (1-2).
6. Butler CC, Van Der Voort JH. Oral or topical nasal steroids for hearing loss associated with otitis media with effusion in children. *Cochrane Database Syst Rev.* 2002;(4):CD001935. Review.

ADDITIONAL READING
- Bluestone CD, Hebda PA, Alper CM et al. Recent advances in otitis media: Eustachian tube, middle ear and mastoid anatomy, physiology, pathophysiology and pathogenesis. Ann Otol Rhinol Laryngol Suppl. 2005;194: 16–30.
- National Institute on Deafness and Other Communication Disorders (NIDCD): http://www.nidcd.nih.gov/health/hearing/
- Sudden Deafness: www.suddendeafness.org

 MISCELLANEOUS

CODES

ICD9-CM
- 381.7 Patulous Eustachian tube
- 381.81 Eustachian tube dysfunction
- 381.9 Eustachian tube disorder, NOS

See Patient Handout on CD

E

FACTITIOUS DISORDER/MÜNCHHAUSEN SYNDROME

Irere C. Coletsos, MD
Harold J. Bursztasn, MD

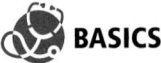 BASICS

DESCRIPTION
- Factitious disorders are challenging to diagnose and, once suspected, it is difficult to deliver compassionate care.
- These patients are aware they are not ill, but will try to mimic illnesses because of an unresolved need to be taken care of (1).
- Patients may make themselves ill to produce symptoms. Thus, the symptoms may be real.
- If questioned, patients will deny the illness was self-inflicted, although they are aware that this is the case (2).
- Their goal is to maintain a sick role (vs. malingering, in which the goal may be more concrete, such as avoiding work). They are aware that they are not physically ill and/or they have caused their own illnesses (vs. somatoform disorders, including conversion disorder, in which patients feel the symptoms they are reporting and believe they are physically ill. They are not consciously responsible for the illnesses' etiology).
- Types of factitious disorders include
  – Factitious disorder with predominantly physical signs and symptoms
    ○ Often occurs after a major stress
    ○ Typically simulates *1* physical disease (3). Münchhausen syndrome (an extreme form) is named after an 18th-century German nobleman who served in the Russian military and told tall tales of his adventures upon return. These patients spend a majority of their lives seeking medical care from different providers and hospitals (changing when treatment is refused) and are willing to undergo painful procedures and surgeries to maintain their sick role.
  – Factitious disorder with predominantly psychological signs and symptoms
    ○ Patients with this disorder mimic the behavior of people with mental illnesses, claiming they are hearing voices or having visual hallucinations; give wrong answers to simple questions to mimic psychosis; act confused or bizarre. This is also known as Ganser syndrome, for the 20th-century German psychiatrist Sigbert Joseph Maria Ganser, who described this behavior in some prisoners. This is a rare disorder, and care must be taken to differentiate it from physical causes of psychotic-like symptoms, such as stroke, head injury, or chronic alcoholism.
  – Factitious disorder with combined psychological and physical signs and symptoms
    ○ Patients claim to have both symptoms—neither the physical nor the psychological predominate.

EPIDEMIOLOGY
Incidence
Unknown

Prevalence
- Factitious disorder with predominantly physical signs and symptoms: ~1–5% of people presenting with medical illness, according to some studies, but hard to estimate due to the secretive nature of the disorder.
- Factitious disorder with predominantly psychological signs and symptoms or the combined disorder: Thought to be much more rare.

RISK FACTORS
- Abuse/deprivation in childhood.
- Childhood traumas, including hospitalizations or the experience of growing up with ill or emotionally unavailable caretakers.

Genetics
None known at this time.

ETIOLOGY
The theoretical psychological basis of factitious disorder is thought to be an unresolved sense of deprivation from childhood that, in a time of stress in adulthood, leads a patient to falsely claim (or even self-inflict) medical illness in order to get medical care. In Münchhausen, this behavior is chronic.

ASSOCIATED CONDITIONS
- History of many medical procedures
- Substance abuse
- Suicide attempts
- Psychiatric comorbidities, including adjustment disorder, borderline personality disorder, depression, somatoform disorder

DIAGNOSIS

SIGNS AND SYMPTOMS
A patient will relate a history of disease symptoms, often with "classic" textbook details, but has no signs of disease on examination. Or, if signs are noted, there may be evidence they were self-inflicted or are not medically caused (2)[C].

History
Careful elicitation of the patient's developmental history may reveal the patient's earlier abuse or deprivations (1)[B], (4)[C].

Physical Exam
- Normal, or evidence of self-inflicted wounds, such as scars
- Abscesses
- Rashes
- Old wound with fresh bleeding (4)[C]
- Tenderness on palpation (and no tenderness noted by patient when the same areas are auscultated with pressure applied)

TESTS
High fevers, abnormal urine studies not reproducible if the patient is directly observed. (Patients may surreptitiously heat their thermometers or contaminate urine specimens.)

Lab
- Skin infection (abscesses, IV sites, Foley sites): Culture shows infection via *E. coli*, presumably a patient's own fecal material (4)[B].
- Lab results fail to show the expected markers of the disease suggested by the patient's reported symptoms.
- Lab results may reveal the ingestion of agents that could mimic disease states (insulin, to produce hypoglycemia; thyroxine or cytomel to produce hyperthyroidism; laxative and diuretic abuse, to produce hypokalemia; self-injection of epinephrine or isoproterenol hydrochloride, to mimic Cushing disease; warfarin, to produce bleeding; quinidine, to produce purpura; alkylating agents, to produce pancytopenia) (5)[B].

Diagnostic Procedures/Surgery
Invasive diagnostic procedures and surgeries are often welcomed by the patient. Clinicians should avoid these, if possible, in patients with factitious disorders. However, reports that patients have often undergone several such procedures before the psychological nature of their illness was discovered.

DIFFERENTIAL DIAGNOSIS
- For factitious disorder with predominantly physical signs and symptoms, also consider
  – Somatization disorders: A chronic psychiatric disease in which a patient's unconscious need to be cared for leads him to experience recurrent physical symptoms, such as GI, sexual, pain, and neurologic symptoms (see "Conversion Disorder," below), and these symptoms cannot be explained fully by any evident physical disorder.
  – Conversion disorder: A psychological conflict is unconsciously transformed into physical symptoms that resemble a neurologic disorder.
  – Malingering: Reporting symptoms that do not exist (or are the result of self-inflicted injury) as part of a conscious decision to attain a financial goal or to avoid a responsibility.
  – Cultural differences in expressing pain and experiencing illness.
  – Occult medical illness (early stages of disease when blood tests may still show negative results)
  – Unusual presentations of disease
  – False negative lab results
- For factitious disorder with predominantly psychological signs and symptoms, in addition to psychiatric illnesses that can have true psychotic symptoms, also consider medical etiologies, such as
  – Drugs, ingested as prescribed or abused, such as benzodiazepines, cocaine, PCP, steroids
  – Poisoning (alcohol, lead, manganese, mercury)
  – Stroke
  – Traumatic brain injury
  – Cultural differences, especially in mourning ("seeing" the deceased as if he or she were alive) or in times of extreme stress (having the "devil" telling the patient to make certain choice)
- For the combined disorder, also consider
  – Infection (especially sepsis)
  – Postsurgical anesthesia/ metabolic/ psychological causes.
  – Pneumonia (especially in older patients)
  – Urinary tract infection (especially in older patients)
  – Thiamine deficiency/Wernicke encephalopathy

ALERT

Münchhausen by proxy: This is a form of child abuse. A parent will injure his child, then bring the child to doctors with a false history, stating the child is a patient needing treatment for a disease. The parent in this case may appear very involved and comfortable in the hospital setting, and not saddened or surprised by the child's illnesses. A child in this situation may end up very ill, have frequent hospitalizations (and may get more ill after the parent visits), and may die from these injuries. Steps must be taken to protect these children and their siblings.

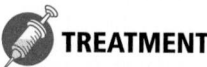 TREATMENT

INITIAL STABILIZATION

- Form an alliance with the patient, identifying their suffering.

- Seek, attempt to elicit, a detailed history of childhood events. Asking about the health history of parents and siblings may help reveal early traumas to the patient (6)[B].

GENERAL MEASURES

- Clinicians should seek access to patient's medical and mental health records (a mental health history is a comorbidity often initially denied by these patients) (6)[B].

- Patients with factitious disorder may accept a frank but empathetic assessment that their *actions* themselves constitute the disorder.

- Patients with Münchhausen syndrome generally respond angrily over clinician refusal to authorize the medical treatment they seek. They will often seek treatment from another provider at another hospital. They may accept referrals. Management may be limited to clinician recognition the disorder and making sure these patients are not offered unnecessary drugs, risky procedures, or surgeries (3)[B].

- Clinicians must remain aware of their own responses and feelings toward these patients, to avoid *countertransference*, and the unconscious failure to offer appropriate treatment. A clinician should consider consulting with a psychiatrist or psychologist (1)[B].

- Clinicians must acknowledge the uncertainty involved in treating suspected factitious disorder or Münchhausen patients, to help prevent the undertreatment of true medical issues (7)[B].

SPECIAL THERAPY

- Refer the patient to a specialist (psychiatrist, psychologist, social worker) to treat the underlying mood or anxiety disorder.
- "Contract conferences" with a psychiatrist, in which the patient is guided toward talking about painful feelings, rather than medical illness (8)[C]
- Cognitive behavioral therapy to deal with the obsessive nature of these syndromes

 MEDICATION (DRUGS)

Consider treating the underlying psychiatric disorder with appropriate drugs. Consult a psychiatrist for guidance.

SURGERY

Try to prevent unnecessary surgeries.

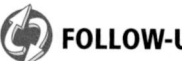 FOLLOW-UP

Admission Criteria

Factitious disorder or Münchhausen patients who appear resistant to treatment, and whose behavior threatens their own lives, may be considered for an emergency inpatient psychiatric commitment and evaluation (9)[C].

Issues for Referral

- Psychiatrist/psychologist/therapist: For underlying psychiatric disorders and treatment, or guidance on treatment
- Forensic psychiatrist: For the medico-legal issues surrounding treating such patients
- Neuropsychologist/neuropsychiatrist: For unexplained pain symptoms

PROGNOSIS

Fair to poor (especially if etiology underlying the disorder cannot be addressed)

COMPLICATIONS

Patient illness or death from self-harm and unnecessary medical interventions

REFERENCES

1. Ferenczi, S. Confusion of tongues between the adult and the child. *Int J Psychoanal* 1949;30: 225–230.
2. Turner MA. Factitious disorders: Reformulating the DSM-IV criteria. *Psychosomatics* 2006;47:23–32.
3. Beers MH, Berkow R, eds. Münchhausen syndrome. *The Merck Manual of Diagnosis and Therapy*, 17th ed. Merck and Company Inc. www.merck.com/mrkshared/CVMHighLight?file=/mrkshared/mmanual/section15/chapter 185/185d.jsp
4. Peebles R, Sabella C, Franco K, Goldfarb J. Factitious disorder and malingering in adolescent girls: Case series and literature review. *Clin Pediatr* 2005;44(3):237–243.
5. Wallach J. Laboratory diagnosis of factitious disorders. *Arch Intern Med* 1994;154(15): 1690–1696.
6. Binder LM, Campbell KA. Medically unexplained symptoms and neuropsychological assessment. *J Clin Experiment Neuropsychol* 2004;26(3): 369–392.
7. Bursztajn H, Feinbloom RI, Hamm RM, Brodsky A. Medical choices, medical chances: How patients, families and physicians can cope with uncertainty. New York: Delacorte/Lawrence, 1981.
8. Ritson B, Forrest A. The simulation of psychosis: A contemporary presentation. *Br J Med Psychol* 1970;43:31–37.
9. Johnson BR, Harrison JA. Suspected Münchhausen syndrome and civil commitment. *J Am Acad Psychiatry Law* 2000;28:74–76.

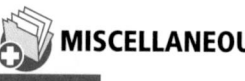 MISCELLANEOUS

CODES

ICD10

F68.1 Factitious disorder. (includes Münchhausen syndrome)

PATIENT TEACHING

Practitioners should try to enter into a therapeutic alliance with patients, telling patients that they want to help them understand how their suffering has come to be expressed in this way. Practitioners can try to reframe patients' false histories and self-imposed injuries as self-harm, rather than deceit.

F

FACTOR V LEIDEN

Marc Jeffrey Kahn, MD

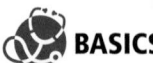 **BASICS**

DESCRIPTION
Factor V Leiden is a genetic disease that is the most common congenital cause of venous thrombosis. It leads to resistance to activated protein C.

- System(s) Affected: Cardiovascular; Gastrointestinal; Hemic/Lymphatic/Immunologic; Nervous; Pulmonary; Reproductive
- Synonym(s): Factor V Leiden thrombophilia; Factor V Leiden mutation

Pediatric Considerations
Thrombosis rare in this group, but has been described.

Pregnancy Considerations
Increases thrombosis risk in patients with factor V Leiden

GENERAL PREVENTION
Patients with factor V Leiden without thrombosis do not require prophylactic treatment.

EPIDEMIOLOGY
- Predominant age: Thrombosis typically occurs after the 2nd decade.
- Predominant sex: Male = Female

Incidence
- ~3–12% of whites are affected
  - The mutation is rare in other ethnic groups.
- ~15–20% of patients who present with thrombosis have factor V Leiden.

RISK FACTORS
- Oral contraceptives increase the risk of thrombosis
  - In homozygotes, the risk increases ~100-fold; in heterozygotes, ~35-fold.
  - The risk is halved when the patient uses desogestrel-containing oral contraceptives.
- Hormone replacement therapy (HRT) and selective estrogen receptor modulators (SERMs) both increase the risk of thrombosis, and in patients with factor V Leiden, that risk is increased substantially.
- Pregnancy and factor V Leiden increase the risk of thrombosis 7- to 16-fold during pregnancy and the puerperium. Other complications of pregnancy may be increased in patients with factor V Leiden.

Genetics
- Autosomal dominant
- Deep and superficial thrombosis of the venous system occurs with an odds ratio of 50:100 for homozygotes
  - The odds ratio is closer to 2.5 for heterozygotes.

PATHOPHYSIOLOGY
Point mutation causing substitution of arginine for glycine in residue 506 of factor V gene rendering it less susceptible to inactivation by activated protein C. Activated protein C is generated when protein C binds to its endothelial receptor, thrombomodulin. Activated protein C and its cofactor, protein S, lead to inactivation of factors V and VIII. Factor V Leiden is the most common cause of resistance to activated protein C.

ETIOLOGY
Genetic defect

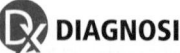 **DIAGNOSIS**

SIGNS AND SYMPTOMS
- Arterial thrombosis is rare in adults with factor V Leiden.
- Thrombosis in unusual locations such as the sagittal sinus, mesentery, and portal systems is less common in patients with factor V Leiden than in patients with deficiency of protein C or S.
- Obstetric complications and venous thrombosis are increased in patients with factor V Leiden, and in those taking oral contraceptives.

TESTS
Lab
- Factor V Leiden mutation analysis
- DNA-based test for factor V mutation
- Plasma-based coagulation assay using factor V–deficient plasma to which patient plasma is added along with purified activated protein C. The relative prolongation of the activated partial thromboplastin time (aPTT) is used to assay for the defect.

Imaging
Magnetic resonance angiography (MRA), venography, or arteriography to detect thrombosis

DIFFERENTIAL DIAGNOSIS
- Protein C deficiency
- Protein S deficiency
- Antithrombin deficiency
- Other causes of activated protein C resistance (e.g., antiphospholipid antibodies)
- Dysfibrinogenemia
- Dysplasminogenemia
- Homocysteinemia
- Prothrombin 20210 mutation
- Elevated factor VIII levels

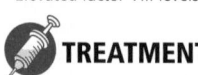 **TREATMENT**

GENERAL MEASURES
- Patients with factor V Leiden and a 1st thrombosis should be anticoagulated initially with heparin or low-molecular-weight heparin followed by oral anticoagulation with warfarin. (1)[A]
- Patients should be maintained on warfarin with an international normalized ratio (INR) of 2:3 for at least 6 months. (1)[A]
- Recurrent thrombosis requires indefinite anticoagulation. (1)[B]

Diet
No restrictions

Activity
No restrictions

 MEDICATION (DRUGS)

First Line
- Low-molecular-weight heparin (1)[A]
  - Enoxaparin (Lovenox): 1 mg/kg SC b.i.d. initially for at least 5 days or until INR is 2:3, at which time it can be stopped
  - Tinzaparin (Innohep): 175 anti-Xa IU/kg SC daily for 6 days and patient is adequately anticoagulated with Coumadin (INR of at least 2 for 2 consecutive days)
  - Dalteparin (Fragmin): 200 IU/kg SC daily
- Oral anticoagulant
  - Warfarin (Coumadin) 5 mg PO daily initially and adjusted to an INR of 2:3 (A)

- Contraindications
  - Active bleeding precludes anticoagulation. (1)[A]
  - Risk of bleeding is a relative contraindication to long-term anticoagulation. (1)[A]
  - Warfarin is contraindicated in patients with history of warfarin skin necrosis. (1)[A]

- Precautions
  - Observe patient for signs of embolization, further thrombosis, or bleeding.
  - Avoid IM injections. Periodically check stool and urine for occult blood; monitor CBCs including platelets.
  - Heparin: Thrombocytopenia and/or paradoxic thrombosis with thrombocytopenia
  - Warfarin: Necrotic skin lesions (typically breasts, thighs, or buttocks)
  - Low-molecular-weight heparin: Adjust dosage in renal insufficiency.
- Significant possible interactions
  - Agents that intensify the response to oral anticoagulants: Alcohol, allopurinol, amiodarone, anabolic steroids, androgens, many antimicrobials, cimetidine chloral hydrate, disulfiram, all NAIDs, sulfinpyrazone, tamoxifen, thyroid hormone, vitamin E, ranitidine, salicylates, and acetaminophen
  - Agents that diminish the response to anticoagulants: Aminoglutethimide, antacids, barbiturates, carbamazepine, cholestyramine, diuretics, griseofulvin, rifampin, and oral contraceptives

Second Line
- Heparin 80 mg/kg IV bolus followed by 18 μg/kg/h
- Adjust dose depending on aPTT.

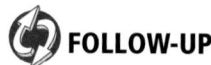 **FOLLOW-UP**

DISPOSITION
Outpatient care

PROGNOSIS
* Most patients heterozygous for factor V Leiden do not have thrombosis.
* Homozygotes have about a 50% incidence of thrombosis.
* Recurrence rates after a 1st thrombosis are not clear, with some investigators finding rates as high as 5% and others finding rates similar to the general population.
* Despite the increased risk for thrombosis, factor V Leiden does not increase overall mortality.

COMPLICATIONS
* Venous or arterial thrombosis
* Bleeding in anticoagulated patients

PATIENT MONITORING
Warfarin use requires periodic (~monthly after initial stabilization) INR measurements with a goal of 2:3 (1)[A]

REFERENCES
1. Kim RJ, Becker RC. Association between factor V Leiden, prothrombin G20210A, and methylenetetrahydrofolate reductase C677T mutations and events of the arterial circulatory system: A meta-analysis of published studies. *Am Heart J.* 2003;146:948.
2. Dahlback B. Resistance to activated protein C as risk factor for thrombosis; molecular mechanisms, laboratory investigation, and clinical management. *Semin Hematol.* 1997;34:217.
3. Greengard JS, et al. Variability of thrombosis among heterozygous siblings with resistance to activated protein C due to Arg Gln mutation in the gene for factor V. *N Engl J Med.* 1994;331:1559.

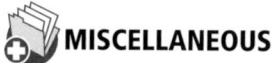 **MISCELLANEOUS**

See also: Thrombosis; deep vein (DVT)

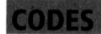 **CODES**

ICD9-CM
289.81 Primary hypercoagulable state

PATIENT TEACHING
* Patients should be educated about
  – Use of oral anticoagulant therapy
  – Avoidance of NSAIDs while on warfarin
* The role of family screening is unclear as most patients with this mutation do not have thrombosis. In a patient with a family history of factor V Leiden, consider screening during pregnancy or if considering oral contraceptive use.

 See Corresponding Diagnostic Algorithm

F

FAILURE TO THRIVE (FTT)

Garreth C. Biegun, MD
Frank J. Domino, MD

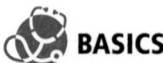

BASICS

DESCRIPTION
A symptom (rather than a disease) of interrupted growth characterized by failure to gain weight at an appropriate rate. Always due to "insufficient usable nutrition" (1)[C] either of caloric insufficiency or underutilization of ingested food.

May be caused by a wide variety of either organic or inorganic etiologies. In severe cases may lead to actual slowing of longitudinal growth or head circumferential growth.

This term is generally applied to the pediatric population, but may occasionally be used for geriatrics. The 2 entities are distinctly different, and this chapter refers to only the pediatric form.

- Definition (2)[C]
  - Weight <5th percentile for age and sex on >1 occasion
  - Weight <80% ideal body weight based on National Center for Health Statistics' Growth Charts
  - Depressed weight to height ratio
  - Weight that drops 2 or more major percentile lines on the standard growth charts
  - Rate of weight gain < expected for age
    - 0–3 months: 26–31 g/d
    - 3–6 months: 17–18 g/d
    - 6–9 months: 12–13 g/d
    - 9–12 months: 9 g/d
    - 1–3 years: 7–9 g/d

GENERAL PREVENTION
Stable home life with caring parents

EPIDEMIOLOGY
Incidence
- Poverty is the number 1 risk factor for FTT (3)[A]
- Predominant age: 6–12 months; almost all are <3–5 years of age
- Predominant sex: Male = Female

Prevalence
~1–5% of pediatric inpatient admissions are for evaluation of FTT. It is a common and difficult diagnostic problem.

RISK FACTORS
- Poverty
- Parent with psychosocial problems
- Premature or sick newborn
- Infant with physical deformity
- Unstable, disturbed family

Genetics
No consistent genetic pattern

PATHOPHYSIOLOGY
Many cases of FTT begin with some level of organic etiology. However, as the problem progresses, the caregivers and child begin to have interaction difficulties around feeding time. Thus, nearly all cases of FTT exist on a spectrum with organic and inorganic etiologies at opposite ends. Even if an organic etiology is found and corrected, the developed interpersonal problems will persist and also need to be treated.

ETIOLOGY
- Organic etiology: Usually GI or neurological. Includes some infants who were profoundly premature. Less commonly: Chronic infection, malignancy, cardiac, pulmonary, or renal
- Environmental deprivation: Many are simple educational problems, such as incorrect feeding
- Normal, small children: Not true FTT

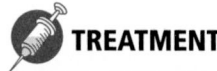

DIAGNOSIS

SIGNS AND SYMPTOMS
- Refer to definitions above
- Difficult personality, feeding and sleep problems
- Apathetic and withdrawn, or watchful and alert
- Poor hygiene
- Signs of inflicted trauma
- Primary caretaker characteristics: Psychosocial problems, often depressed
- Family characteristics: Unstable, disturbed

History
- Most important part of workup
- Elicit symptoms suggesting organic disease
- Take lots of time over multiple visits to gain trust of caregiver and obtain a complete unbiased nutritional history
  - Diarrhea, vomiting, regurgitation
  - Food or texture preferences
  - Fruit juice or other low-calorie liquids in diet
  - Food allergies
  - Family eating habits (together, TV, conflicts over feeding)

Physical Exam
Weight and height readings must be checked on >1 occasion, with great care for accuracy.

TESTS
Lab
- Routine laboratory workup should be kept to a minimum: It is rarely helpful in the diagnosis. Allow history and physical (H&P) to guide laboratory testing in the search for organic causes. Consider
  - CBC
  - Sedimentation rate
  - Urinalysis
  - Urine culture
  - Chemical profile including blood urea nitrogen, calcium, phosphorus, electrolytes, total protein, albumin, and bicarbonate
  - Blood glucose
  - Zinc, magnesium
  - Stool testing: Fat, ova and parasites tuberculosis
  - TB test
  - HIV Elisa
  - Sweat chloride test
- If suspicious of Turner or Down syndrome, a karyotype is indicated
- Other studies dictated by results of (H&P) examination, such as thyroid profile or pituitary studies
- Disorders that may alter lab results: Various blood chemistries may be altered by malnutrition regardless of cause.

Imaging
- Skeletal survey if there is suspicion or evidence of physical abuse
- Radiographs for bone age (wrist film)

Diagnostic Procedures/Surgery
- Evaluation by multidisciplinary team is key. May include pediatrician, specialist doctors, social worker, nursing, developmental specialist, nutritionist/dietician, psychiatry, physical therapy, occupation therapy, and others
- Observation of infant and his or her interaction with caretakers and environment essential
- Carefully plotted growth curves, including weight, height, and head circumference
- Consider sleep study and/or nasopharyngoscopy if upper airway obstruction is likely (e.g., snoring, sweating during sleep)

DIFFERENTIAL DIAGNOSIS
Any condition of sufficient severity can cause failure to gain weight adequately, including child abuse and/or neglect. Consider by system: Congenital, Metabolic, Immune, GI, Renal, Cardiopulmonary, Neurologic, Endocrine, or other (e.g., toxicity or malignant disease)

TREATMENT

GENERAL MEASURES
- Inpatient or outpatient treatment depending on severity and suspected etiology
- Maintain multidisciplinary treatment
- Use of few sympathetic primary caretakers in hospital
- Provision of stimulation, cuddling, affection as inpatient or outpatient

Diet
Goal is to allow "catch up" weight gain to recover correct body weight and size. Provision of balanced, calorically dense diet on both a scheduled and ad-libitum basis, that encourages (but does not force) the child to eat periodically but also allows the child to guide the total amount of increased intake. Usually 150–200% of caloric intake for a normal child of the same age. Nutrition consult must be obtained for assistance in designing an appropriate weight recovery diet.

Activity
No restrictions

SPECIAL THERAPY
Complementary and Alternative Medicine
Consider the presence of vegetarian or all-soy diets that may contribute to FTT. Safe vegetarian diets for children do exist, but must be chosen carefully.

MEDICATION (DRUGS)

Routine vitamin supplementation to include zinc and iron is important. Other vitamin or mineral deficiencies may develop as recovery growth occurs.

SURGERY
None

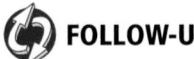

FOLLOW-UP

DISPOSITION
Admission Criteria
Severely malnourished children need admission for reseeding, given possibility of malnourished anorexia, refeeding-malabsorption, and electrolyte disturbances. Hospitalization is rarely helpful in the diagnostic workup.

PROGNOSIS
- Many children with FTT will remain small in height and weight even after full recovery.
- A significant proportion (1/3–1/2) will have long-term cognitive or behavioral abnormalities, but the etiology of this is unclear
  – Cognitive or behavioral problems may be the underlying cause of FTT.
  – Environmental factors causing FTT may also cause other problems.
  – FTT may stunt play and development during acute phase; this may never be completely recovered.
  – FTT may stunt neurologic development especially if head circumference is affected. Brain development and growth occur as much in year 1 as in all rest of life; FTT in this time may be particularly harmful.

PATIENT MONITORING
- When the etiology is organic, follow-up depends on the particular disease involved.
- Close long-term follow-up with frequent visits is important to create and maintain a healthy, supportive environment. Visiting nurses or social services are helpful for this purpose
  – If the family fails to comply, child protection authorities must be notified and foster care may be necessary.

REFERENCES

1. Perrin EC, et al. Criteria for determining disability in infants and children: Failure to thrive. Evidence Report: Technology Assessment (Summary). March 2003;(72):1–5.
2. Frank D. Failure to thrive. In: Darki S, Zuckeman B, Augustyn M, eds. *Behavioral and Developmental Pediatrics*, 2nd ed. Philadelphia, PA: Lippincott Williams & Wilkins; 2005:183.
3. Kane M. Pediatric failure to thrive. *Clinics in Family Practice*. June 2003;5(2).
4. Gartner B, Zitelli BJ, Carlton J Jr. *Common and Chronic Symptoms in Pediatrics: A Companion to the Atlas of Pediatric Physical Diagnosis*. St. Louis, MO: Mosby Year Book;1997.
5. Sills RH. Failure to thrive. In: Stockman JA, ed. *Difficult Diagnosis in Pediatrics*. Philadelphia, PA: WB Saunders;1990.
6. Stallings VA: Nutrition. In: Burg FD, ed. *Gellis and Kagan's Current Pediatric Therapy*. Philadelphia, PA: WB Saunders;1999.

MISCELLANEOUS

See also: Down syndrome; Turner syndrome; Inflammatory bowel disease

CODES

ICD9-CM
- 783.40 Lack of normal physiological development, unspecified
- 783.41 Failure to thrive, child
- 783.7 Failure to thrive, adult

PATIENT TEACHING

- Depends on etiology of FTT
- When environmental deprivation is established, attempting to re-educate in a nonpunitive way is essential.
- Nutrition must be engaged in teaching good feeding habits to the caregivers and choosing calorically dense foods (e.g., cookies made with half and half rather than milk).
- Treatment of underlying poverty and alertness to other risk factors by the primary care physician.

See Corresponding Diagnostic Algorithm

FATTY LIVER SYNDROME

Delores Burroughs-Biron, MD

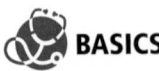 **BASICS**

DESCRIPTION
- Fatty liver
  - Liver biopsy diagnosis showing fatty deposits in >30% of liver cells. Fat is neutral and largely triglycerides.
  - No necrosis, no fibrosis
  - Alanine aminotransferase (ALT) and aspartate aminotransferase (AST) enzymes usually normal, but may be slightly elevated
  - Fatty liver is generally an asymptomatic and nonprogressive condition with essentially no adverse health consequences.
- Nonalcoholic steatohepatitis (NASH)
  - Liver biopsy diagnosis of fatty deposits in >50% of liver cells associated with acute and chronic inflammation and fibrosis
  - Asymptomatic in most patients
  - ALT and AST elevated
  - Disease may progress to cirrhosis; few long-term studies have been done to document this.
- Both diseases usually identified in the 40s and 50s, but may occur at any age
- Synonym(s): Steatosis, Steatonecrosis, Nonalcoholic fatty liver disease (NAFLD), Steatohepatitis, Nonalcoholic steatohepatitis (NASH)

ALERT
Pregnancy Considerations
- A severe complication of 3rd trimester is acute fatty liver of pregnancy
  - Abrupt onset of confusion and restlessness with possible jaundice and right upper quadrant pain
  - ALT and AST always elevated, usually <500
  - Emergency liver biopsy confirms
  - Prompt delivery corrects the liver disease. In most cases, fetus has an inborn error of lipid metabolism blocking same in mother
  - Recurrence rare in subsequent pregnancies

GENERAL PREVENTION
- Avoid excessive alcohol intake
- Maintain or attain appropriate body mass index (BMI)
- Avoid unessential medications including health food and over-the-counter (OTC) agents
- Obtain hepatitis A and B vaccination if not immune, particularly if other risk factors present
- Obtain Pneumovax and yearly influenza vaccination

EPIDEMIOLOGY
- Accounts for 10% of outpatient referrals to hepatologist
- Present in up to 2/3 of obese (BMI >30) and in 90% of morbidly obese (BMI >39%) (1)[C]
- Present in 5–10% type 2 diabetic patients
- NASH cirrhosis reason for liver transplantation in 518 recipients from January 1988–May 2006
- Alcoholic cirrhosis accounted for 9,506 recipients during same period; based on Organ Procurement and Transplant Network (OPTN) data as of August 4, 2006.**
- Candidates for transplant due to NASH cirrhosis and alcoholic cirrhosis were 342 and 2,610, respectively (OPTN data 8/4/06). **
- Predominant age: 40s–50s
- Predominant sex: Male = Female

RISK FACTORS
- Protein-calorie malnutrition
- Total parenteral nutrition >6 weeks
- Severe weight loss including starvation and bariatric surgery
- Hepatitis C
- Alcohol intake >30 g/d for men and >20 g/d for women. **Chronic alcoholism is most common cause in US
- HIV infection
- Organic solvent (chlorinated hydrocarbons, toluene) exposure
- Obesity; BMI >30 (2)[A]
- Diabetes mellitus type 2 (2)[A]
- Gene for hemochromatosis or other conditions with increased iron stores
- Small intestinal bacterial overgrowth
- Pituitary insufficiency
- Hyperlipidemia(2)[A]
- Drugs: Tetracycline, glucocorticoids, tamoxifen, methotrexate, valproic acid, fialuridine, most chemotherapy regimes, and nucleoside analogues
- Other toxins: Hypoglycin A (Jamaican vomiting sickness)

Pediatric Considerations
- Reyes syndrome: Fatty liver with encephalopathy characterized by
  - Vomiting with dehydration-usually postviral URI
  - Progressive CNS damage
  - Signs of hepatic injury: Liver morphologically shows extensive fatty vacuolization
  - Hypoglycemia
- Etiology unknown; viral agents and drugs, especially salicylates, are implicated.
- Mortality rate 50%
- TX-mannitol, IV glucose, and FFP

Genetics
Largely unknown; all types of obesity and diabetes; carriers of hemochromatosis gene are more likely to be affected

ETIOLOGY
- Fatty liver: Most commonly, an impaired ability of the liver to remove fatty acids
- In hyperinsulinemia, alcoholism, and a few other conditions, there is an increased production of fatty acids for the liver to store and dispose of.
- Nonalcoholic steatohepatitis
  - Almost always 2 factors occur simultaneously: A peripheral insulin resistance and increased hepatic oxidative stress from at least 1 of many different causes (2)[C].
  - Mitochondrial damage leading to impaired restoration of adenosine triphosphate stores, lipid peroxidation, and increased iron stores have each been found in 25–40% of the nonalcoholic steatohepatitis cases.

ASSOCIATED CONDITIONS
Preeclampsia, in pregnancy-related disease

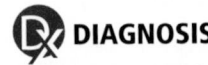 **DIAGNOSIS**

SIGNS AND SYMPTOMS
- Vast majority of patients are asymptomatic; however, presentation is related to time course of occurrence, degree of fat, and etiology. Disease is suspected by
  - Hepatomegaly: Incidentally observed enlarged liver or spleen on image
  - Unsuspected elevation of ALT or AST on screening biochemistry
- Most common signs and symptoms
  - Liver pain or tenderness
  - Mild to marked hepatomegaly
  - Splenomegaly
  - Fatigue
- Infrequent and limited to advanced cases
  - Abdominal collateral veins
  - Variceal hemorrhage
  - Ascites
  - Edema

TESTS
Lab
- Liver function tests (albumin, bilirubin, prothrombin time, alkaline phosphatase
  - γ-glutamyltranspeptidase) normal; but both ALT and AST elevated
  - Nonalcoholic ALT/AST >1
  - If alcohol-induced AST/ALT ≥2
- Level of liver enzyme elevation does not necessarily correlate with degree of fibrosis (3)[C].
- Lipids almost always abnormal. Cholesterol elevated 60%. 45% decreased high-density lipoprotein, 58% increased low-density lipoprotein. 50–80% elevated triglycerides.
- ~30–100% of the patients are diabetic with elevated insulin.
- Leptin is elevated more than expected in obese patients.
- Disorders that may alter lab results: Obesity, uncontrolled diabetes

Imaging
- Ultrasound often detects fatty infiltration; sensitivity 82–89% (1)
- CT scan is approximately equal to ultrasound in sensitivity (1) but better for detecting masses.
- Magnetic resonance spectroscopy is reportedly "sensitive, quantitative and noninvasive" (4).

Diagnostic Procedures/Surgery
Liver biopsy is the only reliable diagnostic method
- Liver biopsy separates benign fatty liver from nonalcoholic steatohepatitis. Biopsy is recommended in those patients with advanced liver disease or risk factors for same, and with AST/ALT persistently elevated despite treatment (1)[C].

Pathological Findings

Anatomic pathology

- Liver biopsy is the gold standard to differentiate fatty liver with good prognosis from nonalcoholic steatohepatitis (3)[C].
- In nonalcoholic steatohepatitis
  - Inflammation in the lobule with both an acute and chronic cellular response and fibrosis starting in the pericentral region are the major markers of a poor future prognosis.
  - Staging is based largely on the extent of fibrosis.
  - Mallory hyaline may be present.

DIFFERENTIAL DIAGNOSIS

- Viral hepatitis
- Drug- or toxin-induced hepatitis
- Occupational exposure
- Metabolic liver disease
- Autoimmune hepatitis

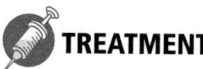 **TREATMENT**

Best evidence suggests that treatment focuses on medications (1)[C] and diet/weight loss (1)[C].

INITIAL STABILIZATION

Outpatient

GENERAL MEASURES

- Emerging data lend support to a recommendation for weight reduction and exercise therapy (5)[C].
- Diabetes should be tightly regulated.
- Other identified risk factors should be corrected, if possible, such as hyperalimentation, hemochromatosis, rapid weight loss.
- No studies to date have shown a reduction in morbidity or mortality for any intervention.
- All alcohol use should be discontinued permanently (2)[C].

Diet

- Control of weight, diabetes, and blood lipids are desirable goals.
- Regular visits to a dietitian are useful.
- Restriction of total calories, simple carbohydrates, and alcohol are required to control diabetes, weight, and lipids.

Activity

- No restrictions
- Daily exercise recommended

 MEDICATION (DRUGS)

No specific therapy currently exists, but several promising agents are under investigation, including (1)[C]

- Thiazolidinediones
- Ursodeoxycholic acid
- Gemfibrozil
- Vitamins E, C
- Betaine
- Metformin (6)[C]

ALERT

High-dose vitamin E ($\geq$400 IU/d) may increase all-cause mortality.

SURGERY

Newer bariatric procedures have been found to potentially ameliorate NASH (3).

 FOLLOW-UP

DISPOSITION

Issues for Referral

Individuals with persistent elevation of liver enzymes 2–3 times above the upper limit of normal or with fibrosis on liver biopsy should be seen by a hepatologist.

PROGNOSIS

Goals of treatment

- Fatty liver without NASH (no fibrosis, no hepatitis)
  - Nonprogressive disease
  - Treat to control symptoms
- Fatty liver with NASH
  - Potentially progressive disease
  - Treat to normalize ALT and AST and to diminish fat in liver(1)[C] as verified by yearly ultrasounds.
- NASH form of fatty liver
  - Slowly progressive
  - Normalization of ALT and AST with treatment slows progression, but does not stop it.
  - Diminution of fat demonstrated by serial images or biopsy slows progression but does not stop it.
  - Cirrhosis develops in 25% of patients >20–30 years.
  - Liver failure from cirrhosis occurs in 1–5%.
  - Transplantation is effective, but NASH may recur after transplantation (3)[C].

COMPLICATIONS

Limited to patients with NASH

- Progression of liver fibrosis to cirrhosis; believed to be the major cause of cryptogenic cirrhosis.
- Liver failure with ascites, encephalopathy, and bleeding varices
- Hepatocellular carcinoma

PATIENT MONITORING

- Repeat liver function tests every 2–4 months.
- Perform yearly ultrasound or CT scan to document diminution in fat
- Changes toward normal provide major motivation to continue lifestyle changes.
- Routine repeat liver biopsy is not recommended(3)[C].

REFERENCES

1. Bayard M, Holt J, and Boroughs E. Nonalcoholic fatty liver disease. *Am Fam Practice* 2006;73:1961-1968. (Review Article).
2. Choudhury J, Sanyal AJ. Insulin resistance and the pathogenesis of nonalcoholic fatty liver disease. *Clin Liver Dis* 2004;8:575–594.
3. Ghali P, Talwalkar JA. The spectrum of nonalcoholic fatty liver disease. *J Clin Outcomes Managem* 2005;12:585–593.
4. Szcepaniak LS, Nurenberg P, Leonard D, et al. Magnetic resonance spectroscopy to measure hepatic triglyceride content: Prevalence of hepatic steatosis in the general population. *Am J Physiol, Endocrinol Metabol* 2005;288:E462-468.
5. Ueno T, Sugawara H, Sujaku K, et al. Therapeutic effects of restricted diet and exercise in obese patients with fatty liver. *J Hepatology* 1997;27:103–107.
6. Bugianesi E, Gentilcore E, Manini R, et al. A randomized controlled trial of metformin versus vitamin E or prescriptive diet in nonalcoholic fatty liver disease. *Am J Gastroenterol* 2005;100:1082–1090.

 MISCELLANEOUS

See also: Alcohol use disorders; Cirrhosis of the liver; Diabetes mellitus, type 1; Diabetes mellitus, type 2; Disorders of pregnancy and pediatrics

CODES

ICD9-CM

- 331.81 Reye's syndrome
- 570 Acute and subacute
- 571.0 Alcoholic fatty liver
- 571.5 Cryptogenic cirrhosis
- 571.8 Other chronic nonalcoholic liver disease
- 646.70 Liver disorders in pregnancy, unspecified

PATIENT TEACHING

Planning for lifelong change in eating, exercise, and alcohol use is required. Thus, regular education and motivation sessions are of value.

F

FECAL IMPACTION

Felix B. Chang, MD
Elizabeth Gebhard, DO

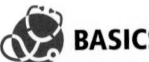 **BASICS**

DESCRIPTION
- Incomplete evacuation of feces, leading to formation of a large, firm, immovable mass of stool in the rectum (70%), sigmoid flexure (20%), or proximal colon (10%).
- System(s) Affected: Gastrointestinal
- Synonym(s): Terminal reservoir syndrome

GENERAL PREVENTION
- Establish regular, consistent toilet time by evoking gastrocolic reflex (1)[C].
- Maintain adequate hydration.
- Maintain high-fiber diet. (1)[C].
- Reinforce exercise (1)[B].
- Install user-friendly commodes.
- Use hydrophilic mucilloids (Metamucil: 2–6 capsules PO daily) or stool-wetting agents (Colace: 50–500 mg/d PO) as needed.
- Consider biofeedback; bowel training (2)[B].
- Use periodic enemas, if indicated.
- Use periodic polyethylene glycol powder (MiraLax), 1 heaping teaspoon in 8 oz (240 mL) water daily for 2 weeks.

EPIDEMIOLOGY
- Predominant age: >60 years
- Predominant sex
  – No sex preponderance in adults
  – Among children, 75% are boys

ALERT
Geriatric Considerations
- Much more likely to occur in patients >80 years.
- Megarectum may be present in physically and mentally impaired elderly.
- Constipation appears to correlate with decrease calories intake in the elderly.

Pediatric Considerations
- May develop megarectum
- Always rule out fecal impaction in chronic constipation in children.

Incidence
- General population: 1% (1,000/100,000)
- Children: 1.5%
- Nursing home residents: 30%
- Constipation more common in women, nonwhites, low income, <12 years of education

RISK FACTORS
- Institutionalization
- Psychogenic illness
- Immobility, inactivity
- Pica
- Chronic renal failure; renal transplant recipients
- Urinary incontinence
- Cognitive decline
- Constipation in
  – Diabetes mellitus
  – Hypothyroidism
  – Hypercalcemia
  – Heavy metal ingestion
- Poor toileting routines

Pediatric Considerations
- Habitual neglect of defecation urge, because of interference with play, may promote impaction.
- Fecal impaction has been reported to occur in >1/2 of all children with chronic constipation.

Genetics
Fecal impaction of the cecum may be seen in cystic fibrosis.

PATHOPHYSIOLOGY
- The rectosigmoid colon dilates to accommodate the mass, which, in turn, is not pliable enough to pass through the disproportionately small anal canal through the patient's weak defecation effort.
- Impacted stool may exist as a single mass (stercolith) or as a composite of small, rounded fecal particles (scybalum).

ETIOLOGY
- Diet lacking in fiber
- Drug side effects (1)[C]
  – Stimulant laxatives
  – Opiates
  – Benzodiazepines
  – Tricyclic antidepressants
  – Phenothiazines
  – Antihypertensives(calcium channel blockers)
  – Aluminum (sucralfate, antacids)
  – Iron
  – Antispasmodics
  – Vinca alkaloids
  – 5HT3 antagonist
- Painful rectal conditions inhibiting voluntary defecation (e.g., anal fissure, hemorrhoids, fistulas)
- Neoplastic or inflammatory obstructing lesions (e.g., rectal bezoars)
- Neurogenic disorders
  – Hirschsprung disease
  – Chagas disease
  – Diabetes mellitus
  – Autonomic neuropathy
  – Multiple sclerosis
  – Spinal cord injury
  – Cauda equine
  – Parkinson disease
- Non-neurogenic
  – Hypothyroidism
  – Hypokalemia
  – Hypercalcemia
  – Anorexia nervosa
  – Systemic sclerosis
  – Myotonic dystrophy
- Excess of gastrointestinal inhibitory hormones (prolactin, endorphins, glucagon, secretin)
- Severe idiopathic chronic constipation

- Irritable bowel syndrome
- Pelvic floor dysfunction
- Pelvic floor dyssynergia
- Encopresis

ASSOCIATED CONDITIONS
- Pulmonary aspiration
- Urinary tract obstruction
- Recurrent urinary tract infections
- Intestinal obstruction
- Spontaneous perforation of colon
- Stercoral ulceration
- Hernia
- Volvulus
- Megacolon
- Megarectum
- Rectal prolapse
- Pneumothorax
- Hypoxia
- Hypovolemic shock
- Iliac occlusion

Pregnancy Considerations
Impaction can produce dysfunctional labor, dystocia.

ALERT
In patients with constipation a more extensive workup should be consider if
- Hematochezia
- Weight loss of ≥10 pounds
- Family history of colon cancer
- Family history of bowel disease
- Anemia
- Positive occult blood test
- Acute onset of constipation in elderly persons
- A recent and persistent change in bowel habits

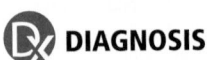 **DIAGNOSIS**

SIGNS AND SYMPTOMS
- Fecal incontinence, interpreted as diarrhea [C]
- Postprandial abdominal pain
- Tenesmus
- Colic
- Nausea
- Vomiting
- Anorexia
- Weight loss
- Dehydration
- Headache
- General malaise
- Agitation; confusion
- Fever to 39.4°C (103°F)
- Tachycardia
- Tachypnea
- Urinary frequency
- Urinary incontinence

Physical Exam
- The general physical examination is not helpful in most patients.
- Digital rectal examination
  – Identify fissures or hemorrhoids.
  – Sphincter tone: Neurologic disorders
- Large mass of stool palpable in lower left quadrant and rectal vault
- Fever may be present to 39.4°C (103°F)

TESTS

Lab
- Leukocytosis to 15,000 WBCs/mm^3
- Hyponatremia
- Hypokalemia
- Stool may be positive for occult blood.
- Anemia, owing to chronic blood loss
- Pediatrics
  - TSH
  - Antigliadin and antiendomysium antibodies for celiac disease
  - Lead

ALERT

Geriatric Considerations
Measure TSH, electrolyte activity, and BUN in elderly patients presenting with impaction.

Imaging
- Plain abdominal radiography may reveal stool or signs of obstruction if digital exam unrevealing.
- Stool retention is associated with megacolon.
- Barium enema can differentiate feces from tumor.

Diagnostic Procedures/Surgery
Sigmoidoscopy may be used to clarify the nature of a rectosigmoid mass.

DIFFERENTIAL DIAGNOSIS
- Irritable bowel syndrome
- Gastroenteritis, colitis
- Diverticulitis
- Appendicitis
- Carcinoma of the colon

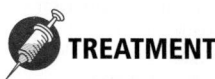 TREATMENT

GENERAL MEASURES
- Manual fragmentation and extraction of fecal mass (after lubrication with lidocaine jelly) may be attempted.
- Larger masses can be disimpacted with water jet directed through fiberoptic sigmoidoscope.
- Enemas containing 20% water-soluble contrast material (Hypaque) may help.
- If incomplete fragmentation
  - Suppositories or enemas with mineral oil, tap water, or sodium phosphate
- Ensure minimum fluid intake of 1.5–2.0 L/d.

Diet
- High fiber
- Home remedy: Mix 2 cups bran, 2 cups applesauce, and 1 cup unsweetened prune juice; refrigerate; take 2–3 tablespoons b.i.d.

Activity
Increased activity is important.

 MEDICATION (DRUGS)

First Line

- A daily 1-L bolus of polyethylene glycol-electrolyte (GoLYTELY,) solution given over 4–6 hours for up to 3 days (1)[B]

- Disimpaction in children, consider combination
  - Day 1: 1–2 phospho-soda enemas, 1 oz/ 10 kg–4.5 oz maximum
  - Day 2: Bisacodyl suppository per rectum daily or b.i.d.
  - Day 3: Bisacodyl tablet PO every day or b.i.d.
  - Repeat 3-day cycle if needed once or twice
- High-dose mineral oil: 15–30 mL PO per year of age per day to 8 oz max daily—b.i.d. for 3 days
- Enemas: 1–2 oz/10 kg to 4.5 oz maximum, daily—b.i.d. for 1–2 days

- Polyethylene 3350 (GoLYTELY) is safe and effective at of 1.5 g/kg/d for 3 days (3)[B].

- Precautions
  - Use magnesium citrate with caution in patients with renal insufficiency.
  - Be careful with lactulose; colonic distention can result from its bacterial fermentation.

SURGERY
- Laparotomy
  - Necessary only in extreme cases (1)[B]

- Electrohydraulic lithotripsy has been used to safely remove large calcified fecaliths.

 FOLLOW-UP

Admission Criteria
- Disimpaction usually is performed in outpatient setting.
- Hospitalization is necessary if several attempts of outpatient management have failed.
- Presence of complications

Issues for Referral
In the pediatric population, consultation with a pediatric gastroenterologist should be considered in children in whom oral or rectal medication are ineffective for disimpaction and in whom dietary changes and laxative therapy are ineffective.

PROGNOSIS
- Reimpaction likely if program is not followed.
- Prognosis is poor for perforation with peritonitis.
- Mortality with impaction and obstruction is highest in very young and very old (up to 16%).

COMPLICATIONS
- Sepsis
- Hypotension
- Instrumental perforation
- Bleeding
- Postoperative obstruction

PATIENT MONITORING
Less than 1 bowel movement every other day may lead to impaction.

REFERENCES
1. Hsieh E. Treatment of constipation in older adults. *Am Fam Physician.* 2005;72:2277–2284.
2. Tariq SH. Geriatric fecal incontinence. *Clin Geriatr Med.* 2004:20:571–587.
3. Torres M, McGregor T, Wilder I. What is the most effective way for relieving constipation in children aged >1 year? *J Fam Pract.* 2004;(9):744–746.
4. An evidence-based approach to the management of chronic constipation in North America. *Am J Gastroenterol.* 2005;100:S1 .

ADDITIONAL READING
- Higgins PD, Johanson JF. Epidemiology of constipation in North America: A systematic review. Am J Gastroenterol. 2004; 99:750
- Baker SS, Liptak GS, Colletti RB, et al. Constipation in infants and children; evaluation and treatment. A medical position statement of the North American Society for Pediatric Gastroenterology and Nutrition. J Pediatr Gastroenterol Nutr. 199; 29:612.
- Borowitz SM, Cox DJ, Kovatchev B, et al. Treatment of childhood constipation by primary care physicians: Efficacy and predictors of outcome. Pediatrics. 2005; 115:873.

 MISCELLANEOUS

See also: Constipation; Diarrhea, chronic; Encopresis

CODES

ICD9-CM
560.39 Impaction of intestine, other

PATIENT TEACHING
- Avoid catharsis.
- Comprehensive program, including use of laxative, behavior changes, dietary changes
- Effective education of the parents and child with regard to constipation is crucial in changing chronic behavior patterns.
- NOTE: No hot water, soap, or hydrogen peroxide enemas. They may burn or irritate rectal mucosa, causing bleeding.

F

FEVER OF UNKNOWN ORIGIN (FUO)

Benjamin L. Sapers, MD

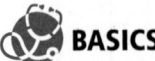 **BASICS**

DESCRIPTION
- The classic definition derived by Petersdorf and Beeson is
  - A fever >38.3°C on several occasions
  - Duration of fever for at least 3 weeks
  - Uncertain diagnosis after 1 week of study in the hospital.
- Modifications to the definition have been proposed, including eliminating the in-hospital evaluation requirement because of the improvements in outpatient evaluation.
- Some have suggested expansion of the definition to include nosocomial, neutropenic, and HIV-associated fevers that may not be prolonged.

ALERT
Geriatric Considerations
- Most common causes are acute leukemia, Hodgkin lymphoma, intra-abdominal infections, tuberculosis (TB), and temporal arteritis.
- Signs and symptoms in the elderly are more nonspecific.
- Coexisting diseases and numerous medications may cloud features.
- Mortality rates are higher in the elderly.

Pediatric Considerations
- Infections and collagen-vascular diseases are the most likely etiology.
- Inflammatory bowel disease is the common etiology in older children and adolescents.
- A better prognosis is noted than in nonpediatric cases.

Pregnancy Considerations
Fever is known to increase the risk of neural tube defects and trigger preterm labor.

EPIDEMIOLOGY
- Predominant age: None
- Predominant sex: Depends on cause

Incidence
No data on actual incidence

RISK FACTORS
- Recent travel
- Exposure to biologic or chemical agents
- Persons in AIDS risk group
- Elderly persons
- Drug abuse
- Immigrants
- Health care workers: Consider factitious fever
- HIV-infected patients with advanced disease
- Special attention should be paid to travel, occupational, sexual, and drug exposure.

ETIOLOGY
- >200 causes; each with a prevalence 5% or less.
- Infection
  - Abdominal abscesses
  - Mycobacterial infection (often with advanced HIV)
  - Cytomegalovirus
  - Endocarditis/pericarditis
  - Sinusitis
  - HIV (late stage)
  - Renal
  - Osteomyelitis
  - Catheter infections
  - Amebic hepatitis
  - Wound infections
  - Other miscellaneous infections
- Neoplasms
  - Lymphoma
  - Leukemia
  - Solid tumors (hypernephroma)
  - Hepatoma
  - Atrial myxoma
  - Colon cancer
- Collagen vascular disease
  - Giant cell arteritis
  - Polyarteritis nodosa
  - Rheumatic fever
  - Systemic lupus erythematosus
  - Rheumatoid arthritis
  - Polymyalgia rheumatica
- Other causes
  - Granulomatous diseases
  - Pulmonary emboli/deep vein thrombosis (DVT)
  - Drug fever
  - Thermoregulatory disorders
  - Endocrinologic diseases
  - Occupational causes
  - Periodic fever
  - Factitious/fraudulent fever
  - Cerebrovascular accident
  - Cirrhosis
  - Alcoholic hepatitis
  - Medication induced: Allopurinol, captopril, cimetidine, clofibrate, erythromycin, heparin, hydralazine, hydrochlorothiazide, isoniazid, meperidine, methyldopa, nifedipine, nitrofurantoin, penicillin, phenytoin, procainamide, and quinidine

DIAGNOSIS

SIGNS AND SYMPTOMS
- Fever does not present as the only manifestation of a disease.
- The type and pattern of fever is of little help in making the diagnosis.
- Constitutional symptoms that almost always accompany a fever
  - Headache
  - Myalgia
  - Malaise

Physical Exam
- Diagnostic clues often are not readily apparent.
- Repeated examination may be essential.
- Pay careful attention to the skin, mucous membranes, and lymphatic system.
- Palpate the abdomen for masses or organomegaly.

- Duke's clinical criteria can diagnose endocarditis (1)[A] with presence of 2 major criteria *or* 1 major and 3–5 minor
  - Major criteria
    - Positive blood cultures
    - Positive echocardiogram
    - New valvular regurgitation
  - Minor criteria
    - Predisposing heart condition or IV drug use
    - Fever (38°C)
    - Vascular phenomena: Major arterial emboli, septic pulmonary infarcts, mycotic aneurysm, intracranial hemorrhage, conjunctival hemorrhage, Janeway lesions
    - Immunologic phenomena: Osler nodes, glomerulonephritis, Roth spots, rheumatoid factor
    - Positive blood cultures not meeting major criteria or serologic evidence of active infection

TESTS

Lab (2)[B]
- CBC
- Liver function tests
- Blood cultures (not to exceed 6 sets)
- Urinalysis and urine culture
- Sputum and urine cultures for TB
- Tuberculin skin test: May not be helpful if anergic or acute infection; if test is negative, repeat in 2 weeks.
- C-reactive protein
- Sedimentation rate: Elevated
- Gastric washing for TB
- Serologic tests: Epstein-Barr, hepatitis, syphilis, Lyme disease, Q fever, cytomegalovirus, amebiasis/coccidioidomycosis
- HIV antibody test
- Serum protein electrophoresis
- Thyroid function tests
- Rheumatoid factor and antinuclear antibody test

Imaging
- Chest radiograph
- CT scan or MRI of abdomen and pelvis (plus directed biopsy, if indicated) (2)[C]
- Technetium-based scan: If infectious process or tumor suspected (2)[B]
- PET using the radiolabeled glucose analogue ^{18}F-fluorodeoxyglucose: If infectious process, inflammatory process, or tumor suspected
- Ultrasound of abdomen and pelvis (plus directed biopsy, if indicated): If mass lesions, renal obstruction or gallbladder/biliary tree pathology suspected
- Leg Doppler: If DVT/pulmonary embolism suspected
- ECG: If cardiac valve lesions, atrial myxomas, or pericardial effusion suspected (transthoracic vs. transesophageal)
- Ventilation/perfusion scan: If pulmonary emboli suspected
- Indium-labeled leukocyte scanning: If inflammatory process suspected
- Bone scan: If osteomyelitis or metastatic disease suspected

Diagnostic Procedures/Surgery
- Liver biopsy: If granulomatous disease suspected (2)[C]
- Temporal artery biopsy: Particularly in elderly (2)[B]
- Lymph node, muscle, or skin biopsy: If clinically indicated
- Spinal tap: If clinically indicated (see "Lab")
- Exploratory laparotomy: If otherwise unsuccessful in determining etiology

Pathological Findings
Depends on etiology

DIFFERENTIAL DIAGNOSIS
See "Etiology"

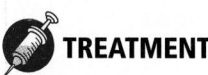

TREATMENT

GENERAL MEASURES
- Attempt to determine the etiology before initiating therapy.
- Avoid therapeutic trials unless as a last resort and only if therapy is reasonably specific.
- "Shotgun" approaches are condemned; they obscure the clinical picture, have untoward effects, and do not solve the problem (2)[C].

Diet
With temperature elevations, patients have increased caloric and fluid demands.

Activity
As tolerated

MEDICATION (DRUGS)

The proper medication to use depends on the diagnosis. In up to 1/5 of patients, the cause of the fever will not be identified despite a thorough workup. If the patient has symptoms with the fever or continues to decline, a therapeutic trial may be indicated.

- Antipyretics, such as acetaminophen or aspirin
- NSAIDs, such as indomethacin or naproxen
- Steroid trial based on patient's history
- Antibiotic trial based on patient's history
- Antituberculous therapy, if there is a high risk for granulomatous disease pending culture results
- Contraindications: Aspirin should be avoided in children, because of the risk of Reye syndrome.
- Precautions: If a steroid trial is initiated, the physician must be aware the patient may have a relapse after treatment or if certain conditions (such as TB) have been undiagnosed; the therapy may have deleterious effects.
- Significant possible interactions: Refer to the manufacturer's literature.

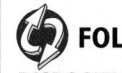

FOLLOW-UP

DISPOSITION
Admission Criteria
Hospitalization is reserved for the ill and debilitated and also in those in which factitious fever has been ruled out or an invasive procedure is indicated.

PROGNOSIS
Depends on etiology and age
- Patients with HIV have the highest mortality.
- 1-year survival rates reflecting deaths due to all causes

FUO 1-year survival rates (all causes)	
Age	**Survival**
<35	91%
35–64	82%
>64	67%

COMPLICATIONS
Depends on etiology

PATIENT MONITORING
If the etiology of the fever remains unknown, repeat the history and physical examination along with screening laboratory studies.

REFERENCES
1. Roth AR, Basello GM. Approach to the adult patient with fever of unknown origin. *Am Fam Physician*. 2003;68:2223–2228.
2. Mourad O, Palda V, Detsky AS. A comprehensive evidence-based approach to fever of unknown origin. *Arch Intern Med*. 2003;163:545–551.

ADDITIONAL READING
Davies GR, Finch RG. Fever of unknown origin. *Clin Med*. 2001;1:177–179.

MISCELLANEOUS

See also: Arthritis, juvenile rheumatoid; Colorectal malignancy; Cytomegalovirus inclusion disease; Endocarditis, infective; Giant cell arteritis; Hepatoma; HIV infection and AIDS; Leukemia; Osteomyelitis; Polyarteritis nodosa; Polymyalgia rheumatica; Pulmonary embolism; Rheumatic fever; Sinusitis; Stroke (brain attack); Systemic lupus erythematosus

CODES

ICD9-CM
- 659.20 Pyrexia of unknown origin during labor
- 672.0 Pyrexia of unknown origin during puerperium
- 778.4 Other disturbances of temperature regulation of newborn
- 780.6 Fever

PATIENT TEACHING
Maintain an open line of communication between physician and patient/family as the workup progresses; the extended time required in establishing a diagnosis can be frustrating.

 See Corresponding Diagnostic Algorithm

 See Patient Handout on CD

F

FIBROCYSTIC BREAST DISEASE

Cathryn Heath, MD
John C. Smulian, MD, MPH

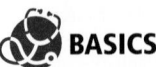 **BASICS**

DESCRIPTION

Fibrocystic changes of the breast (FCC) is a generalized term for benign breast disorders such as lumps and pain.

- Lumps
  - Physiologic nodularity: Lumps vary with the phase of the menstrual cycle, common in young women
  - Mastoplasia: A ropy, thickening of the breast tissue, most common in the upper outer quadrant, persists throughout the menstrual cycle
  - Cysts: Distended, fluid-filled masses caused by an imbalance between secretion and absorption in the breast lobule, common in 40–50-year-olds
  - Fibroadenoma: Benign solid tumor, smooth margins, mobile, most common tumor in teenagers and young women, may occur at any age after thelarche
  - Phyllodes tumors: Painless, solid, smooth, lobular, bulky; stromal hyperplasia; 17% are malignant, 7% borderline malignancy
- Nipple discharge
  - Although considered 1 of the warning signs for breast cancer, 90% of patients with nipple discharge have benign disease.
  - Bilateral galactorrhea: Consider prolactin secreting pituitary tumors (usually in association with amenorrhea); drugs (isoniazid, methyldopa, thiazides, reserpine, tricyclic antidepressants, birth control pills); hypothyroidism
  - Unilateral discharge from 1 duct; consider intraductal papilloma; ductal carcinoma; Paget disease
  - Discharge from multiple ducts consider FCC or ductal ectasia
- Pain
  - Cyclical mastodynia: Hormonal; an exaggeration of the normal premenstrual tenderness
  - Noncyclical: Sclerosing adenosis, cysts, trauma
- Inflammatory conditions
  - Fat necrosis: Solid lump with or without pain that can mimic carcinoma
  - Mastitis/abscess: Exquisite pain and tenderness; erythema (common); fever; not always a definite mass; common with lactation and squamous metaplasia of lactiferous ducts; Zuska disease [lactiferous fistulae], usually caused by staphylococcal organisms
- Growth disorders
  - Accessory nipples (polythelia)
  - Absence of the breast (amastia)
  - Absence of the nipple (athelia)
  - Hypoplasia (often associated with hypoplasia of the thorax and pectoral muscles and abnormalities of the hand [i.e., Poland syndrome])
  - Gigantomastia: Occurs during puberty and pregnancy
  - Gynecomastia: Occurs in men in association with puberty, senescence, liver disease, testicular tumors, and medications such as digoxin and cimetidine
- System(s) Affected: Skin/Exocrine
- Synonym(s): Chronic cystic mastitis; Adenosis; Benign breast disease

GENERAL PREVENTION

There are no general prevention strategies for FCC.

EPIDEMIOLOGY

- Predominant age
  - Symptoms tend to occur in menstruating women.
  - Cysts: Usually seen in women in their 40s
  - Cyclical mastodynia: Common in menstruating women
  - Noncyclical pain: Can occur at any age after breast development
- Predominant sex: Female > Male (almost exclusively)

Geriatric Considerations
Not as common in this age group

Prevalence
- Unknown
- It is estimated that up to 60% of women have FCC during their lifetime.

RISK FACTORS

- Unknown
- The effect of consumption of methylxanthine-containing substances (e.g., coffee, tea, cola, and chocolate) has not been found to be a contributing factor.

Genetics
Family history of cysts common

PATHOPHYSIOLOGY
See "Description."

ETIOLOGY

- Etiology unknown. Possible causes include the following
  - Estrogen likely a causative factor for many (1)[B]
  - BRCA1 and BRCA2 genes implicated [B]
  - Acquired genetic change: Loss of heterozygosity in DNA of lesions
  - Dietary fat intake

ASSOCIATED CONDITIONS
Breast carcinoma associated in those with specific pathology findings

DIAGNOSIS

SIGNS AND SYMPTOMS

- Asymptomatic
- Breast pain and tenderness
- Pain subsides after menses
- Smooth, tense, or fluctuant masses
- Bilateral masses
- Breast thickening
- Nipple discharge

TESTS
Lab
- Prolactin if galactorrhea
- Thyroid-stimulating hormone (TSH), if galactorrhea

Imaging
- Mammography
  - Signs of malignancy include irregular mass, clustered masses, calcifications, architectural distortion, and dilated duct.
  - May be normal in presence of malignancy
  - Difficult to interpret in women <35 years owing to dense breast tissue; ultrasound may be helpful
- Ultrasonography
  - Useful for differentiating cystic from solid lesions
- Thermography (available at a few institutions)

Diagnostic Procedures/Surgery
- Fine-needle aspiration and biopsy
  - Allows differentiation of cystic and solid lesion
  - Cells sent for cytology can reveal cancer with a relatively high degree of accuracy.
  - Low morbidity
  - If mass disappears, no further evaluation is necessary.
- Core needle biopsy
  - Usually not indicated for fibrocystic disease
  - Useful in diagnosis of cancer
- Excisional biopsy
  - Indicated for all solid lumps that are not clearly benign

ALERT
Pediatric Considerations
Biopsy in children should be avoided because a developing breast bud may be inadvertently removed.

Pathological Findings
- Atypia-relative risk 4:24
- Proliferative changes without atypia relative risk 1:88
- Nonproliferative changes relative risk of 1:27 (2)[B]

DIFFERENTIAL DIAGNOSIS
- Lumps
  - Breast cancer
  - Sebaceous cyst
- Skin changes
  - Breast cancer (peau d'orange: thickened skin similar to peel of an orange)
  - Eczema
- Pain
  - Costochondritis
  - Opectoralis muscle spasm
  - Neuralgia
  - Breast cancer
  - Angina pectoris
  - Gastroesophageal reflux
  - Superficial phlebitis of the thoracoepigastric vein (Mondor disease): Local tenderness and induration

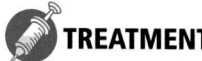 TREATMENT

GENERAL MEASURES

- Evaluate to be certain there is no malignancy by means of imaging and diagnostic procedures.
- Pain rarely severe or disabling
- Frequently resolves spontaneously
- Reassure patient there is no malignancy.
- Cold compresses may be helpful.
- Well-fitting, supportive brassiere (worn night and day)

Activity

No restrictions except to avoid activities that may cause trauma to the breasts

SPECIAL THERAPY

Complementary and Alternative Medicine

Evening primrose oil may result in symptomatic relief in 58% of cyclical mastalgia and 38% of noncyclical mastalgia: 1.5 g b.i.d.; usually responds within 1st 4 months. [3]

 MEDICATION (DRUGS)

First Line

- For cyclical pain and swelling
  - Nonsteroidal anti-inflammatories
- For more severe disease
  - Danazol (Danocrine): 100–400 mg/d in 2 divided doses
  - Bromocriptine: 2.5 mg b.i.d. for 3 months
  - Tamoxifen: 10 mg/day for 3–6 months
- Contraindications
  - Refer to the manufacturer's literature.
- Precautions
  - Refer to the manufacturer's literature.
- Significant possible interactions
  - Refer to the manufacturer's literature.

SURGERY

Possibly excision (under local anesthesia) of benign fibroadenoma or phyllode tumors and fat-necrosis lesions

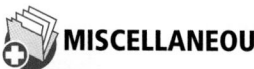 FOLLOW-UP

DISPOSITION

Issues for Referral

- ≤35 years: If discrete lesion, should be referred to surgeon.
- >35 years: Diagnostic mammography ± ultrasonography and then referred to surgeon (1)[C]

PROGNOSIS

Benign, chronic, recurring, intermittent

COMPLICATIONS

Fibrocystic change can make physical examination and mammograms difficult to interpret.

PATIENT MONITORING

- Patients need to be assessed with clinical examination, radiologic studies, and sometimes biopsy to be certain a lump is not malignant.
- Follow-up times are variable depending on the clinical situation
  - A young patient in whom physiologic nodularity is suspected should be observed through 1 menstrual cycle.
- Mammograms should be obtained at age 35 years, at least every 1–2 years after age 40 years, and yearly after age 50 years.
- Ultrasound is useful to differentiate cysts from solid lesions, but is not used for screening. May be helpful in women <35 for FCC
- Aspiration cytology is useful for diagnosis of cysts and solid lesions. The false-positive rate ranges from 0–5.8%, and the false-negative rate from 1.7–22%.
- When physical examination, mammography, and needle aspiration are used in combination, detection rates for breast cancer range from 93–100%.

REFERENCES

1. Santen RJ, Mansel R. Benign breast disorders. *N Engl J Med*. 2005;353:275–285.
2. Hartmann LC, et al. Benign breast disease and the risk of breast cancer. *N Engl J Med*. 2005; 353:229–237.
3. Townsend CM, Beauchamp RD, Evers BM, Mattok KL, eds. *Sabiston Textbook of Surgery*. 17th ed. Philadelphia, PA: WB Saunders Co; 2004.

 MISCELLANEOUS

CODES

ICD9-CM

- 610.0 Benign cyst of the breast
- 610.1 Fibrocystic disease of the breast
- 610.2 Adenofibrosis of the breast
- 611.6 Galactorrhea not associated with childbirth
- 771.5 Neonatal infective mastitis

PATIENT TEACHING

- American College of Obstetricians and Gynecologists 409 12th St. SW, Washington, DC 20024-2188; (800) 762-ACOG
- *Booklet on Breast Self-Examination from Primary Care and Cancer* (17 Prospect St., Huntington, NY 11743; 516-424-8900)
- National Cancer Institute 800 4-CANCER American Cancer Society, www.cancer.org/docroot/lrn/lrn_0.asp

 See Corresponding Diagnostic Algorithm

See Patient Handout on CD

F

FIBROMYALGIA

Bruce M. Rothschild, MD

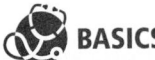 BASICS

DESCRIPTION
Common pain phenomenon occurring in a defined pattern, reproduced by pressure on "trigger points"
- Synonym(s): Fibrositis; Myofascial pain syndrome

ALERT
Geriatric Considerations
Common; polypharmacy may be part of the problem

Pediatric Considerations
Uncommon

Pregnancy Considerations
Limits therapeutic approach to physical therapy modalities

GENERAL PREVENTION
- Adequate sleep
- General conditioning exercises

EPIDEMIOLOGY
- Incidence/prevalence in US: 7–10%
- Predominant age: 18–70
- Predominant sex: Female > Male

RISK FACTORS (1–6)
- Sleep disturbance (e.g., sleep apnea)
- Trauma
- Depression
- Weather changes

ETIOLOGY
- Loss of nonrapid eye movement stage IV sleep
- Stress
- Trauma

ASSOCIATED CONDITIONS
- Restless legs syndrome
- Leg cramps
- Obesity

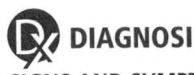 DIAGNOSIS

SIGNS AND SYMPTOMS (2–3,5–9)
- Pressure manually applied to specific sites, referred to as "trigger points" reproduce the patient's symptoms
  - Temporalis: Above the ear
  - Anterior to tragus of ear
  - Scalenus capitis
  - Sternocleidomastoid
  - Low anterior neck
  - Pectoralis minor
  - Manubriosternal
  - Anterior and posterior axillary folds
  - Trapezius ridge
  - Upper rhomboids
  - Lower rhomboids
  - Iliac crest
  - Mid-buttocks
  - Mid-rectus femoris
  - Mid-vastus lateralis
  - Quadriceps insertion—at the patella
  - Humeral epicondyles (many investigators would diagnose fibromyalgia, while some prefer epicondylitis) and negative tenderness at "neutral sites" (e.g., scapula, glabella)
  - Absence of neutral point tenderness
- Other signs and symptoms often of a chronic nature
  - Nonrestorative sleep with early morning awakening in an unrefreshed state
  - Typically insidious in onset
  - Pain is increased in the morning, with weather changes, anxiety, stress
  - Pain improved by mild physical activity or vacations (stress-relieving situations)
  - Abnormal nonrapid eye movement stage IV sleep
  - Generalized fatigue or tiredness
  - Anxiety
  - Chronic headache
  - Alternating diarrhea, constipation, and tenesmus
  - Subjective, nonconfirmable complaints of swelling or numbness, not associated with objective neurologic findings
  - Depression
  - Reduced physical endurance
  - Decreased social interaction

TESTS
Sleep study; rarely indicated, but consider if obstructive sleep apnea a consideration

Lab (10)
- Normal Westergren erythrocyte sedimentation rate
- Normal creatine phosphokinase and aldolase
- Normal thyroid-stimulating harmone
- Normal CBC, renal, and liver function
- Drugs that may alter lab results: Steroids

Diagnostic Procedures/Surgery
The clinical history and physical examination

DIFFERENTIAL DIAGNOSIS
- Hypothyroidism
- Psychogenic rheumatism
- Muscle strain/sprain
- Muscle disease (e.g., polymyositis)
- Polymyalgia rheumatica
- Temporal arthritis

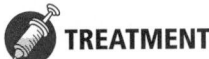 TREATMENT

INITIAL STABILIZATION
Outpatient

GENERAL MEASURES (11–15)
- Ultrasound, hot packs, strength training, aerobic conditioning, increasing social interactions, physical therapy
- Stress management (16,17)
- Transcutaneous electrical neural stimulation and the variant called muscular electrical neural stimulation have NO proven effect in treating fibromyalgia. (18,19)
- Low-intensity laser treatments under evaluation
- Conditioning exercises (4)

Diet
No restrictions

Activity
- Fully active; the pain of fibrositis may be so distracting as to reduce the patient's attentiveness, predisposing to error and accident
- Conditioning exercises as tolerated (20).

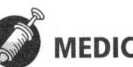 MEDICATION (DRUGS)

First Line (3,5,6,11,12)
- Sleep restorative without interfering with stage IV sleep
  - Zolpidem (Ambien): 5–10 mg at bedtime as required
  - Eszopiclone (Lunesta) 2 mg PO bedtime
  - Zaleplon (Sonata) 5–20 mg PO bedtime
  - Temazepam (Restoril): 15–30 mg bedtime as required (use as last resort as dependence may occur)
- Consider discontinuation of sleep restoratives if grogginess, aberrant behavior, memory loss, or thought process changes
- Psychological and/or physical dependence may occur. However, if the patient is nonfunctional without them, long-term use is reasonable.
- Contraindications: Zolpidem, temazepam, lidocaine (drug allergy, suicide potential)
- Significant possible interactions
  - NSAIDS: Refer to the manufacturer's literature.
  - Others: Digoxin, phenytoin, monoamine oxidase inhibitors

Second Line (3,5,6,21)
- Local injection of trigger points: Lidocaine 1% injectable, 0.5 cc
- Trazodone (Desyrel): 50 mg PO at bedtime as required
- Cyclobenzaprine (Flexeril): 10 mg b.i.d. as required (of lesser efficacy)
- Amitriptyline (Elavil): 20–50 mg at bedtime as required (of lesser efficacy)
- NSAIDS may provide nonnarcotic symptomatic pain relief (of lesser efficacy)
- Other: Benzodiazepine to assist with sleep (will induce dependence; use with extreme caution)

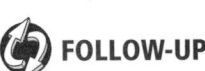 FOLLOW-UP

PROGNOSIS
- With resolution of sleep disturbance, may resolve totally
- Aggressive physical therapy is critical in those who do not respond
- ~5% of the patients do not respond to any form of therapeutic intervention. Hypnosis may be attempted in that group.

COMPLICATIONS
- Chronic pain, chronic loss of work
- Fibromyalgia is allegedly a greater source of work loss and dysfunction than rheumatoid arthritis.

PATIENT MONITORING
- For efficacy at 2–4 weeks
- For medication side effects every 3–6 months

REFERENCES

1. Desmeules JA, et al. Neurophysiologic evidence for a central sensitization in patients with fibromyalgia. *Arthritis Rheum*. 2003;48: 1420–1429.
2. Hsu ES. Myofascial pain syndrome and fibromyalgia. *Semin Anesth*. 2003;22:152–158.
3. Inanici F, Yunus MB. Fibromyalgia syndrome: Diagnosis and management. *Hosp Physician*. 2002;8:53–66.
4. Neumann L, et al. Outcome of post-traumatic fibromyalgia; a 3-year follow-up of 78 cases of cervical spine injuries. *Semin Arthritis Rheum*. 2003;32:320–325 [B]
5. Rothschild BM. Fibromyalgia: An explanation for the aches and pains of the 90's. *Compr Ther*. 1991;17:9–14.
6. Siceloff E, et al. Variability of fibromyalgia-like symptoms. *Compr Ther*. In press.
7. Graff-Radford SB, et al. Effects of transcutaneous electrical stimulation on myofascial pain and trigger point sensitivity. *Pain*. 1989;37:1–5.
8. Mease PJ, et al. OMERACT 7 workshop: Fibromyalgia syndrome. *J Rheumatol*. 2005; 53:724–731 [A]
9. Wolfe F, et al. The American College of Rheumatology criteria for the classification of fibromyalgia. *Arthritis Rheum*. 1990;33: 160–172.
10. Wallace DJ, et al. Cytokines play an aetiopathogenetic role in fibromyalgia: A hypothesis and pilot study. *Rheumatology*. 2001;40:743–749.
11. Cheng RS, Pomeranz B. Electroacupuncture analgesia could be mediated by at least two pain-relieving mechanisms: Endorphin and non-endorphin systems. *Life Sci*. 1979;25: 1957–1962.
12. Dai Y, et al. The effect of electroacupuncture on pain behaviors and noxious stimulus-evoked Fos expression in a rat model of neuropathic pain. *J Pain*. 2:151–159.
13. Ledergerber CP. Transcutaneous electroacupuncture and electroanalgesia. *Am J Acupunct*. 1979; 2:127–136.
14. Lehmann TR, Russell DW, Spratt KF. The impact of patients with nonorganic physical findings on a controlled trial of transcutaneous electrical nerve stimulation and electroacupuncture. *Spine*. 1983;6:625–634.
15. Leo KC. Use of electrical stimulation at acupuncture points for the treatment of reflex sympathetic dystrophy in a child. *Phys Ther*. 1983;63:957–959.
16. Thieme K, Gromnica-Ihle E, Flor H. Operant behavioral treatment of fibromyalgia: A controlled study. *Arthritis Rheum*. 2003;49:314–320.
17. Vu J, Rothschild BM. Retrospective assessment of fibromyalgia therapeusis. *Compr Ther*. 1994;20: 545–549.
18. Milne S, Welch V, Brosseau L. Transcutaneous electrical stimulation (TENS) for chronic low back pain. *Cochrane Database Syst Rev*. 2001;2: CD003008.
19. Sluka KA, Walsh D. Transcutaneous electric nerve stimulation: basic science mechanisms and clinical effectiveness. *J Pain*. 2003;4:109–121.
20. Dobkin PL, et al. Maintenance of exercise in women with fibromyalgia. *Arthri Care Res*. 2005;53:724–731 [A]
21. Sayar K, et al. Venlafaxine treatment of fibromyalgia. *Ann Pharmacother*. 2003;37: 1561–1565.
22. Dworkin RH, Fields HL, Levine JD. Is fibromyalgia a neuropathic pain syndrome? *J Rheumatol*. 32(Supp175):1–45 [B]
23. Sola AE. Myofascial trigger point therapy. *Resident Staff Physician*. 1981;8:38–46.

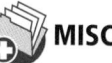 **MISCELLANEOUS**

- Other notes: Perhaps the most common cause of neck or back pain in this patient population and most common rheumatologic problem in general
- See also: Chronic fatigue syndrome; Insomnia, Irritable bowel syndrome; Restless legs syndrome

CODES

ICD9-CM
729.1 Myalgia and myositis, unspecified

PATIENT TEACHING

- Printed material
- Rothschild, B. Diagnosing and treating fibrositis and fibromyalgia. *Geriatr Arthritis Foundation Your Personal Guide to Living With Fibromyalgia. Atlanta, GA: Longstreet Press; 1997. Consult.* 1990;9: 26–28.
- *Your Personal Guide to Living with Fibromyalgia.* Arthritis Foundation, Atlanta, 1997.

 See Patient Handout on CD

F

FOLLICULITIS

Zainab Nawab, MD

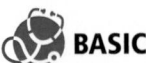 BASICS

DESCRIPTION
- Inflammation of hair follicle caused by infection, chemical irritation, or physical injury.
- It is divided into superficial and deep folliculitis.
- In HIV positive patients, a folliculitis can occur associated with an eosinophil shift of the WBC; this is theorized to be due to an altered immune system, and is called *eosinophilic pustular folliculitis* (EPS)
- System(s) Affected: Skin/Exocrine

ALERT
Pregnancy Considerations
Pruritic folliculitis of pregnancy is a rare disorder that resolves spontaneously after delivery.

GENERAL PREVENTION
- Practice good personal hygiene; avoid reinfection from contaminated clothing and washcloths.
- Minimize friction from clothing.
- Avoid shaving.

EPIDEMIOLOGY
- Predominant age: All ages
- Predominant sex: Male > Female

Incidence
Common

Prevalence
Common

RISK FACTORS
- Frequent shaving
- Pre-existing dermatoses
- Occlusive dressing
- Occlusive clothing
- Obesity
- Immunosuppression
- Long-term antibiotic use
- Use of hot tubs or saunas
- Diabetes mellitus

Genetics
No known genetic pattern

PATHOPHYSIOLOGY
Predisposing factors to folliculitis
- Nasal carriage of *S. aureus*
- Exposure to pools and hot tubs contaminated with *Pseudomonas aeruginosa* (may be due to inadequate chlorination)
- Candida folliculitis related to recent antibiotic or corticosteroid use

ETIOLOGY
- Superficial
  - Staphylococcal infection
  - Pseudofolliculitis
  - Superficial fungal infection
  - Cutaneous candidiasis
  - Acne vulgaris
  - Keratosis pilaris
- Deep
  - Furuncle and carbuncle
  - Sycosis barbae
  - Gram-negative acne
  - Pseudomonal folliculitis

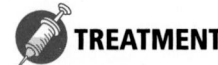 DIAGNOSIS

SIGNS AND SYMPTOMS
- Characteristic lesion: Multiple small papules and pustules with erythematous base pierced by a central hair.
- Most common is superficial form of infectious folliculitis known as *impetigo* caused by staphylococcus aureus.
- Uncommon form of superficial folliculitis is *tinea barbae* caused by dermatophytes.
- Gram-negative folliculitis occurs from long-term antibiotic therapy.
- Pseudomonal folliculitis occurs on exposure to contaminated water or wet suits.
- Pityrosporum folliculitis occurs more often in warm humid climates and more frequently in immunocompromised patients.
- Herpes folliculitis occurs from infection with herpes 1 and 2.

TESTS
Lab
In cases resistant to therapy
- Gram stain
- KOH preparation
  - Look for budding yeast or hyphae.
- Culture
- Biopsy
- Fasting blood sugar
- HIV status

Diagnostic Procedures/Surgery
Incision and drainage

Pathological Findings
- Superficial/Deep: Moderately intense infiltrate of inflammatory cells.
- Pseudofolliculitis: Perifollicular inflammatory infiltrate.
- Eosinophilic folliculitis: Collection of eosinophils within superficial follicle.

DIFFERENTIAL DIAGNOSIS
- Acne vulgaris
- Acneiform eruptions
- Cutaneous candidiasis
- Contact dermatitis
- Milia
- Miliaria
- Papular urticaria
- Insect bite

TREATMENT

GENERAL MEASURES
- Antibacterial soaps (Dial)
- Good hand-washing techniques
- Warm compresses
- Clean shaving instruments each day
- Change towels/washcloths and sheets daily
- Avoid nose picking

Diet
For obese individuals, weight reduction may be helpful.

Activity
Full activity

MEDICATION (DRUGS)

- Staphylococcal folliculitis
  - Mupirocin applied 2–5 times per day is drug of choice; oral agents are reserved for widespread disease.
  - Dicloxacillin: 250 mg q.i.d. PO for 14 days
  - Cephalosporin (Cephalexin): 250 mg q.i.d. or 1000 mg b.i.d. for 10 days
- For MRSA
  - Clindamycin 150–450 mg PO q6–8h for 10 d
  - Bactrim DS 1 b.i.d. for 10 days
  - Minocycline 100 mg PO b.i.d. for 10 days
- Pseudomonas folliculitis
  - Usually self-limited, no antibiotic indicated
  - If severe or persistent, adults can use ciprofloxacin 500 mg or ofloxacin 400 mg b.i.d. PO for 10 days.
- EPF
  - Topical corticosteroids
  - Itraconazole or fluconazole
- Herpetic folliculitis
  - Valacyclovir 500 b.i.d. for days
  - Famciclovir 125 mg b.i.d. for 5 days
  - Acyclovir 800 b.i.d. for 5 days

Second Line
Mupirocin (Bactroban) topical therapy to affected area t.i.d.

 FOLLOW-UP

DISPOSITION
Outpatient care

PROGNOSIS
- Usually resolves with treatment
- May recur in *Staphylococcus* carriers
  - Mupirocin may be required on nares of patient to treat carrier state.
  - Family carriers may also require treatment.
- Resistant or severe cases may warrant testing for diabetes mellitus or immunodeficiency.

COMPLICATIONS
May progress to become furuncles or abscesses

PATIENT MONITORING
- 1 return visit in 2 weeks if symptoms abate
- Resistant cases should be followed every 2 weeks until cleared.

REFERENCES

1. Sladden MJ, Johnston GA. More common skin infections in children. *Br Med J.* 2005;330(7501): 1194–1198.
2. Ratnam S, Hogan K, March SB, Butler RW. Whirlpool-associated folliculitis caused by *Pseudomonas aeruginosa. J Clin Microbiol.* 1986;23(3):655–659.
3. Böer A, Herder N, Winter K, Falk T. Herpes folliculitis: clinical, histopathological, and molecular pathologic observations. *Br J Dermatol.* 2006;154(4):743–746

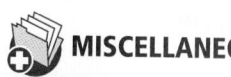 **MISCELLANEOUS**

ICD9-CM
704.8 Other specified diseases of hair and hair follicles

F

FOOD ALLERGY

Stanley Fineman, MD

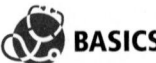 BASICS

DESCRIPTION
Hypersensitivity reaction that is caused by certain foods.

- System(s) Affected: Gastrointestinal (GI); Hemic/Lymphatic/Immunologic; Nervous; Pulmonary; Skin/Exocrine
- Synonym(s): Allergic bowel disease, Dietary protein-sensitivity syndrome

GENERAL PREVENTION
Avoidance of offending food

EPIDEMIOLOGY
- Predominant age: All ages, but more common in infants and children
- Predominant sex: Male > Female (2:1)

Incidence
- The incidence of IgE-mediated food allergy has been estimated to range from 1–7% of the population.
- In children up to 4 years of age, the incidence is between 8% and 6%. (1)[B]

Prevalence
Only ~3–4% of children >4 years have persisting food allergy; therefore, it is frequently a transient phenomenon. (2)[B]

RISK FACTORS
- Persons with allergic or atopic predisposition are at increased risk of hypersensitivity reaction to foods.
- Family members with a history of food hypersensitivity

Genetics
In family members with a history of food hypersensitivity, the probability of food allergy in subsequent siblings may be as high as 50%.

PATHOPHYSIOLOGY
Allergic response owing to immunologic mechanisms, such as the classic IgE allergic response or nonimmunologic-mediated mechanisms

ETIOLOGY
- Any food or ingested substance can cause allergic reactions
  - Most commonly implicated foods include cow's milk, egg whites, wheat, soy, peanuts, fish, tree nuts (walnut and pecan), shellfish, melons, sesame seeds, and sunflower seeds. (3)[A]
- Several food dyes and additives can elicit allergic-like reactions.

DIAGNOSIS

SIGNS AND SYMPTOMS
- GI (system usually affected)
  - More common: Nausea, vomiting, diarrhea, abdominal pain, occult bleeding, flatulence, and bloating
  - Less common: Malabsorption, protein-losing enteropathy, eosinophil-gastroenteritis, and colitis
- Dermatologic
  - More common: Urticaria/angioedema, atopic dermatitis, pallor, or flushing
  - Less common: Contact rashes
- Respiratory
  - More common: Allergic rhinitis, asthma and bronchospasm, cough, serous otitis media
  - Less common: Pulmonary infiltrates (Heiner syndrome), pulmonary hemosiderosis
- Neurologic
  - Less common: Hyperkinesis, tension-fatigue syndrome, migraine headaches, syncope
- Other symptoms
  - Systemic anaphylaxis, vasculitis
  - Suspected manifestations include enuresis, proteinuria, and arthropathy
  - Growth retardation

TESTS
Stool and mucus exam may show eosinophilia, but this is rarely done.

Lab
- Eosinophilia in blood or tissue suggests atopy
- Epicutaneous (prick or puncture) allergy skin tests are useful in documenting IgE-mediated immunologic hypersensitivity. In most clinical situations, the allergy skin tests are good for screening. Skin testing using the suspect food may be helpful. An oral challenge may be completed to accurately determine the clinical hypersensitivity. The overall agreement between allergy skin testing and oral food challenge is ~60% (i.e., a positive skin test showing a positive challenge reaction to a particular food). (4)[A]
- Radioallergosorbent test (RAST) can also detect specific IgE antibodies to offending foods
  - In certain laboratories, the RAST was almost as accurate as a skin test in predicting positive oral challenges.

- Leukocyte histamine release and assays for circulating immune complexes are predominantly research procedures and are of limited use in clinical practices
  - Assays for IgG and IgG 4 subclass antibodies are commercially available.
  - There are no convincing data that these tests are reliable for the diagnosis of food allergy. (3)[A]
- The provocative injection and sublingual provocative tests are both highly controversial and have been proven to be useless for the diagnosis of food allergy.
- The leukocytotoxic assay is an unproven diagnostic procedure and is not useful for the diagnosis of allergy.

Imaging
Upper GI series for gastric antral inflammation, in rare cases

Diagnostic Procedures/Surgery
Elimination and challenge test
- The best procedure for confirming food allergy
- 1st, the suspected food is eliminated from the diet for 1–2 weeks.
- The patient's symptoms are monitored. If the patient's symptoms disappear or substantially improve, an oral challenge with the suspected food should be performed under medical supervision.
- Optimally, this challenge should be performed in a double-blind, placebo-controlled manner.
- Patients with a history of anaphylaxis should not have an oral challenge unless lack of significant IgE sensitivity can be documented. (5)[B]
- Most allergic reactions will occur within 30 minutes to 2 hours after the challenge, although late reactions have also been described, which may occur from 12–24 hours.

Pathological Findings
Pathological findings are not common in food allergies; however, inflammatory changes can be seen in the gastrointestinal tract.

DIFFERENTIAL DIAGNOSIS
- A careful history is necessary to document a temporal relationship with the manifestations of suspected food hypersensitivity
- The GI, dermatologic, respiratory, neurologic, or other systemic manifestations may mimic a variety of clinical entities

TREATMENT

INITIAL STABILIZATION
Outpatient

GENERAL MEASURES
- Avoidance of the offending food is the most effective mode of treatment for patients with food allergies.
- Those patients with exquisite and severe allergy hypersensitivity to a food should be more cautious in their avoidance of that food. They should carry epinephrine for self-administration in the event that the offending food is ingested unknowingly and a subsequent immediate reaction develops.
- Immunotherapy or hyposensitization with food extracts by various routes, including subcutaneous immunotherapy or sublingual neutralization, are not recommended because the success with these methods have not been proven in controlled scientific studies.

Diet
As determined by tests

Activity
No restrictions

 MEDICATION (DRUGS)

First Line
- Patients with significant hypersensitivity should have epinephrine for auto-injection available.
- Symptomatic treatment for milder reactions (e.g., antihistamine)
- The use of cromolyn has been suggested, but is not practical for use in most patients with food allergy.
- Recent studies have suggested the use of ketotifen, which is a mast cell stabilizer
  − This drug is not available in the US.

 FOLLOW-UP

PROGNOSIS
- Most infants will outgrow their food hypersensitivity by 2–4 years. It may be possible to reintroduce the offending food cautiously into the diet (particularly helpful when the food is one that is difficult to avoid).
- Adults with food hypersensitivity (particularly to milk, fish, shellfish, or nuts) tend to maintain their allergy for many years.

COMPLICATIONS
- Anaphylaxis
- Angioedema
- Bronchial asthma
- Enterocolitis
- Eczematoid lesions

PATIENT MONITORING
As needed

REFERENCES

1. Chandra RK, Gill B, Kumari S. Food allergy and atopic disease. *Clin Rev Allergy Immunol*. 1995;13:293–314.
2. Sampson HA. Food allergy. *J Allergy Clin Immunol*. 2003;111(suppl):S540–S547.
3. Sichere SH, Teuber S. Current approach to the diagnosis and management of adverse reactions to foods. *J Allergy Clin Immunol*. 2004;114: 1146–1150.
4. Sampson HA. Utility of food-specific IgE concentrations in predicting symptomatic food allergy. *J Allergy Clin Immunol*. 2001;107: 891–896.
5. Sampson HA. Food allergy. Part 1: Immunopathogenesis and clinical disorders. *J Allergy Clin Immunol*. 1999;103(pt 1):717–728.
6. Fleischer DM, et al. The natural progression of peanut allergy: Resolution and the possibility of recurrence. *J Allergy Clin Immunol*. 2003;112: 183–189.
7. Ortolani C, et al. The oral allergy syndrome. *Ann Allergy*. 1988;61:47–52.

 MISCELLANEOUS

See also: Celiac disease; Epiglottitis; Irritable bowel syndrome; Pyloric stenosis

CODES

ICD9-CM
- 693.1 Dermatitis due to food taken internally
- 692.5 Contact dermatitis and other eczema due to food in contact with skin
- 995.60 Anaphylactic shock or reaction due to unspecified food

PATIENT TEACHING
- Patients should be counseled by a dietitian to be sure that they maintain a nutritionally sound diet in spite of avoiding those foods to which the patient is sensitive.
- Patient support: Food Allergy Network: 4744 Holly Ave., Fairfax, VA 22030-5647; 703-691-3179; Web site www.foodallergy.org
- Other information available at www.acaai.org and www.aaaai.org

 See Corresponding Diagnostic Algorithm

 See Patient Handout on CD

F

FOOD POISONING, BACTERIAL

Karl M. Schmitt, MD

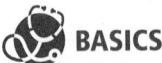 **BASICS**

DESCRIPTION
A variety of related illnesses resulting from ingestion of food contaminated with bacteria.
- May be produced by bacterial infection itself or by toxins produced by the bacteria
- Usually involves the large bowel, whereas viral etiologies generally involve the small intestine
- 80% of traveler's diarrhea is bacterial (1)

ALERT
Geriatric Considerations
- Nursing home outbreaks may occur
- Significant cause of mortality

Pediatric Considerations
- Day care center outbreaks may occur; perhaps at higher risk of complications from antiperistaltic drugs
- Newborns and infants are a high risk for mortality and complications.
- Shigellosis is a rare cause of chronic vaginal discharge in young girls.

Pregnancy Considerations
Perinatal salmonellosis, listeriosis, and campylobacteriosis may secondarily infect newborns causing sepsis and meningitis.

GENERAL PREVENTION
- Do not ingest raw or undercooked seafood, meats, or poultry.
- Avoid any unpasteurized dairy products, juices, or eggs.
- Thoroughly clean all food preparation areas.
- Ensure proper cold storage of any prepared foods not immediately consumed.
- Wash hands frequently and thoroughly when handling or preparing foods.
- Be wary of frozen fruit products from developing nations.
- In developing nations (e.g., Africa, S. Asia, Latin America, Middle East), avoid food from street vendors, "boil it, cook it, peel it, or forget it."[B]
- Bismuth subsalicylate: 2 tabs q.i.d. has some efficacy in prevention of traveler's diarrhea
- Probiotic Lactobacillus being studied (2)

EPIDEMIOLOGY
- Incidence/prevalence in the US
  – Poor reporting overall; ~6 million cases per year
- Predominant age: All ages
- Predominant sex: Male = Female

Incidence
- In the US *Campylobacter jejuni*, Salmonella, *Clostridium perfringens*, *Staphylococcus aureus*, account for 90% of the cases, totaling ~45,000 hospitalizations and 2,700 deaths US
- Approximate incidence is 2,500/100,000

Prevalence
One in 10 in US have food-borne diarrhea/year

RISK FACTORS
- Frequent associations with ingestion
  – *S. aureus*: High-protein foods: Egg salad, cream-filled pastries, poultry, ham
  – *Bacillus cereus*: Cereals, fried rice, dried foods and herbs, meats, vegetables

– *C. perfringens*: Meats, gravies, dried foods, vegetables.
– *C. jejuni*: Undercooked poultry, meat, raw dairy products, contaminated water, mushrooms
– *Yersinia enterocolitica*: Undercooked pork, other meat and dairy products
– *Escherichia coli*: Raw vegetables (especially sprouts), meats tainted fruit and juices, contaminated water and milk
– *Vibrio parahaemolyticus*: Raw and cooked seafood
– *Shigella*: Raw vegetables, egg salads, contaminated water
– *Salmonella*: Raw or undercooked eggs, poultry, dairy products, meat
– *Listeria monocytogenes*: Undercooked meat, dairy products, and many other foods
- Day-care contacts
- Lower gastric acidity (H₂ blocker, PPI): More susceptible to traveler's diarrhea
- Exposure to asymptomatic animals harboring infections and spreading them through feces and milk *E. coli, Listeria, Salmonella*

ETIOLOGY [3]
- Preformed enterotoxins
  – *S. aureus*
  – *B. cereus*
  – *C. perfringens* (enterotoxin elaborated in gut)
- Tissue invasion
  – *C. jejuni* #2 in US (#1 in Thailand)
  – *Y. enterocolitica*
  – *E. coli* #4 in US, #1 in Mexico (enterotoxigenic, verotoxigenic [hemorrhagic], and tissue invasive forms), including *E. coli* 0157:H7
  – *V. parahaemolyticus* (toxin elaboration, possibly invasion)
  – Shigella species #3 in US
  – Salmonella species: Most common in US
  – *L. monocytogenes*

 DIAGNOSIS

SIGNS AND SYMPTOMS
History
Food poisoning most often presents as gastroenteritis. Most cases of gastroenteritis have a viral etiology; some (Norwalk-like virus) can be foodborne. Suspect bacterial food poisoning when multiple persons become ill after eating the same meal. Timing and presentation can aid in establishing etiology.
- Fever more suggestive of invasive organisms (*Shigella, Salmonella, Campylobacter*)
- Nausea, vomiting 1–6 hours after meal (*S. aureus, B. cereus*)
- Cramps, diarrhea 8–16 hours after meal (*C. perfringens, B. cereus*)
- Fever, cramps, diarrhea 18–72 hours after meal (*C. jejuni, Y. enterocolitica, E. coli, V. parahaemolyticus, Shigella* and *Salmonella* species)
- Bloody diarrhea without fever 3–5 days after meal (verotoxigenic *E. coli*, occasionally *C. jejuni*)
- Pseudoappendicitis (*Y. enterocolitica*)

TESTS
Lab
- Culture of stool most reliable
- Routine cultures detect *Shigella, Salmonella, Campylobacter* and *E. coli* 0157:H7
- *Vibrio* and most *E. coli* species require specific media and orders to the laboratory.
- Drugs that may alter lab results: Prior or concomitant antibiotic therapy may eliminate pathogen from stool.

Diagnostic Procedures/Surgery
- Stool culture: Obtain if diarrhea is severe (patient is bedridden), temperature >101.5°F (38.5°C), persistently bloody stools, presence of fecal leukocytes, neurologic findings, severe abdominal pain
- Sigmoidoscopy in persistent and unresponsive cases
- Epidemiologic investigation
- Culture of suspected food source if available

Pathological Findings
Only present in invasive or colic syndromes

DIFFERENTIAL DIAGNOSIS
- Infectious gastroenteritis of any kind
- Inflammatory bowel disease
- Appendicitis and other acute surgical abdominal processes
- Hepatitis

TREATMENT

- Usually outpatient oral management sufficient in mild cases with attention to dehydration and electrolyte imbalances (1)[C]
- Hospitalization for septicemias or focal infections, severe electrolyte imbalance, or severe dehydration

GENERAL MEASURES
- Most are self-limited syndromes and do not require specific therapy
- Prescribe oral solutions for rehydration. Sport drinks and diluted fruit juices with broth and crackers are sufficient in mild cases. (1)[C]
- Avoid undiluted juices, soft drinks (1)[C]
- For moderate cases, consider 8 oz orange or apple juice plus 1/2 teaspoon honey and a pinch of salt followed by 8 oz water with 1/4 teaspoon baking soda.
- For infants or adults, rehydration products (e.g., Pedialyte) provide adequate fluid and electrolyte replacement. (4)[A] Don't use for >1–2 days without clinical reassessment of nutritional needs.

Diet
- Eliminate contaminated food.
- Reintroduction of bland or normal age-appropriate diets as soon as hydrated and able
- Generally, no dietary restrictions are broadly recommended.

Activity
Bed rest for comfort if needed during the acute phase

SPECIAL THERAPY

IV Fluids

- IV fluid or oral rehydration solutions containing 50–100 mEq Na/L and electrolyte replacement if necessary for more severe dehydration (particularly in the elderly) (1)[C]

 MEDICATION (DRUGS)

- Antibiotic use is controversial and often of limited benefit in US-acquired cases. (1)[C]
- For septicemias and focal infections, systemic antibiotic therapy may be indicated.

- Consider antibiotics in prolonged febrile state with fecal blood and/or leukocytes or moderate to severe traveler's diarrhea. (4)[A]
- *Shigella* or *Salmonella*: Trimethoprim-sulfamethoxazole 160 mg and 800 mg, respectively, b.i.d. for 5 days, or ciprofloxacin (Cipro) 500 mg b.i.d. for 10 days if acquired outside the US however, be aware that antibiotics may prolong carrier state in Salmonella (1)[A]

- *Campylobacter*: Erythromycin 250 mg q.i.d. for 5 days or ciprofloxacin (Cipro) 500 mg b.i.d. for 7 days
- *Yersinia*: Ceftriaxone 1 g IV/d
- Listeriosis: Ampicillin plus aminoglycoside

- Empiric treatment of traveler's diarrhea Azithromycin 10 mg/kg daily for 3 days in kids, or ciprofloxacin (Cipro) 500 mg b.i.d. for 3 days for adults (2)[A] Prophylaxis is not recommended by the Centers for Disease Control and Prevention (2)[C]

- Bismuth subsalicylate (Pepto Bismol) may have anti-inflammatory and bactericidal activity.
- Contraindications
  - In Shiga-toxin producing *E. Coli*, antibiotics may lead to prolonged bloody diarrhea and hemolytic urenic syndrome (HUS)
- Avoid antiperistaltic agents in colitic (bloody diarrhea) syndromes, may increase the chance of systemic dissemination if not given with antibiotics. (2)[C]
- Antiemetics may be given, but are usually unnecessary.
  - Significant possible interactions
  - Certain antibiotics have recognized drug-drug interactions.
  - Anticholinergics may have side effects in elderly or cardiac patients. *C. jejuni* and *Salmonella* antibiotic resistance is increasing

 FOLLOW-UP

PROGNOSIS

- Resolution of signs and symptoms over a few days in most cases
- Chronic sequelae include Guillain-Barré syndrome, reactive arthritis

COMPLICATIONS

- Cardiovascular collapse
- Arrhythmias from electrolyte disturbance
- Septicemias or other metastatic infections
- Hypoglycemic seizures or coma

PATIENT MONITORING

- Individualized based on degree of dehydration and electrolyte imbalance, or signs of sepsis
- Close medical follow-up and evaluation should be considered for persistence of symptoms unabated >48 hours, and in infants, elderly, and the immunocompromised.
- Serious disturbances require hospitalization, frequent vital signs, and strict recording of input and output with appropriate fluid replacement.

REFERENCES

1. Townes JM. Acute infectious gastroenteritis in adults. *Postgrad Med*. 2004;115(5):11–16.
2. Yates, J. Traveler's Diarrhea. *Am Fam Physician*. 2005;71(11):2095–2100.
3. *MMWR Recomm Rep*. 2005;54:352–6.
4. Infectious Diseases Society of America. Practice Guidelines for Management of Infectious Diarrhea. *Clin Infect Dis*. 2001;32(3):331–350.
5. Diagnosis and management of foodborne illnesses: A primer for physicians. *MMWR Recomm Rep*. 2001;50(RR-2):1–69.

 MISCELLANEOUS

- Health department reporting requirements: Anthrax, Botulism, Brucellosis, Cholera, Enterohemorrhagic *E. Coli*, Listeriosis, Salmonellosis, HUS
- Other notes: *C. jejuni* antimicrobial therapy resistance is increasing.
- See also: Appendicitis, acute; Botulism; Brucellosis; Dehydration; Diarrhea, acute; Eosinophilic gastroenteritis; Guillain-Barré syndrome; Hypokalemia; Intestinal parasites; *Salmonella* infection; Typhoid fever

CODES

ICD9-CM

- 003.0 *Salmonella* gastroenteritis
- 004.0 *Shigella* dysenteriae
- 004.9 Shigellosis, unspecified
- 005.0 Staphylococcal food poisoning
- 005.1 Botulism
- 005.9 Food poisoning, unspecified
- 008.00 Intestinal infection due to *Escherichia coli*, unspecified

PATIENT TEACHING

- Avoidance of raw or undercooked foods
- Proper food storage and preparation techniques such as refrigeration
- Instruction on prevention if patient traveling to foreign countries
- Avoid antidiarrheal drugs in most cases; they may prolong the carrier state.

F

FRAGILE X SYNDROME

Ruben Peralta, MD, FACS
Surah Guzofski, MD

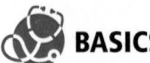 **BASICS**

DESCRIPTION

Fragile X syndrome (FXS) is the most common inherited form of mental retardation. Males are generally more severely affected.

EPIDEMIOLOGY

Prevalence

- Full mutation in 1:4000 males, 1:8000–9000 females (1)[B]
- Premutation in 1:800 males, 1:100–200 females (2)[B]

RISK FACTORS

- Transmitting males are intellectually normal and pass the affected chromosome to all their daughters, who may have affected sons.
- Affected females have a 50% chance of transmitting the affected chromosome to their offspring.

Genetics

- X-linked dominant with variable penetrance; however, this condition is seen in both sexes. Males are usually more severely affected than females.
- The gene for FXS is called FMR-1 (fragile X mental retardation-1). The condition received its name from the cytogenetic "fragile site," which is seen on the long arm of the X chromosome (Xq27.3).
- This is a trinucleotide repeat disorder, caused by abnormal expansion of CGG repeats in the FMR1 gene. The trinucleotide repeat expansion causes abnormal methylation of the FMR1 gene promotor region, silencing gene expression (1)[B], (3)[B].
- Premutation carriers have 61–200 repeats; with >200 repeats, the full syndrome is expressed (1)[B].

ETIOLOGY

Transmission of affected X chromosome

ASSOCIATED CONDITIONS

- Recurrent otitis media and sinusitis in childhood
- Mitral valve prolapse (develops in adolescence or adulthood)
- Seizure disorder
- 25% meet criteria for autism (1)[B]
- ADHD

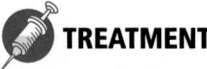 **DIAGNOSIS**

SIGNS AND SYMPTOMS

The signs and symptoms seen in the classic case of FXS may be diagnostic; however, the clinical presentation is extremely varied, age dependent, and sex influenced.

- Generally 1st detected when developmental milestones are missed, especially if there is a family history of mental retardation (2)[B]
- Newborns with FXS may have high birthweight and relative macrocephaly (4)[B].

History

- Family history of mental retardation
- Behaviors may include (1)[B]
  - Poor eye contact
  - Hand flapping or biting
  - Perseverative speech
  - Social avoidance, shyness, anxiety
- Cognitive functioning can range from borderline normal to severe mental retardation. Deficits in (1)[B]
  - Receptive language less impaired than expressive language
  - Abstraction
  - Quantitative skills
  - Short-term memory
  - Adaptive behaviors
  - Social skills
- Affected males almost always have mental retardation, most commonly moderate; ~1/3 of affected females will have MR ranging from mild to severe (2)[B].
- 50% of females who inherit the full mutation will be asymptomatic carriers (5)[B].

Physical Exam

Characteristic physical features (1, 4) [B]

- Macro-orchidism (postpuberty)
- Long, thin face
- Prominent jaw
- Large ears
- Midface hypoplasia
- Prominent forehead
- Hyperextensible metacarpophalangeal joints
- Mitral valve prolapse
- High arched palate

ALERT

Pregnancy Considerations

Prenatal diagnosis is available.

TESTS

Affected patients need educational and psychologic evaluation for the development of learning programs.

Lab

- Molecular genetic testing is the diagnostic test of choice.
- Full mutations, premutations, carriers can be identified.

DIFFERENTIAL DIAGNOSIS

- Pervasive developmental disorder
- Learning disability
- Autism
- Other causes of mental retardation

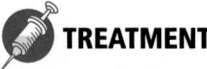 **TREATMENT**

GENERAL MEASURES

- Early detection allows initiation of preschool intervention programs.
- Early intervention with developmental stimulation and special education
- Speech therapy
- Behavioral therapy to address social skills, repetitive behaviors
- Occupational therapy

Diet

No special diet

Activity

Full activity

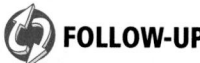 **FOLLOW-UP**

DISPOSITION
Issues for Referral
- Neuropsychologic testing may be helpful in developing an individualized learning plan.
- Psychiatric evaluation may be indicated for evaluation and treatment of ADHD, anxiety symptoms.

PROGNOSIS
Lifespan generally is not affected.

PATIENT MONITORING
General health maintenance

REFERENCES

1. Visootsak J, ST Warren, A Anido. Fragile X syndrome: An update an review for the primary pediatrician. *Clin Pediatr* 2005;44:371–381.
2. Wattendorf DJ, Muenke M. Diagnosis and management of fragile X syndrome. *Am Fam Physician* 2005;72:111–113.
3. Baba Y, RJ Uitti. Fragile X-associated tremor/ataxia syndrome and movement disorders. *Curr Opin Neurol* 2005;18:393–398.
4. Terracciano A, Chiurazzi P, Neri G. Fragile X syndrome. *Am J Med Genet Part C: Sem Med Genet* 2005;137C:32–37.
5. Wiesner GL, SB Cassidy, SJ Grimes. Clinical consult: Developmental delay/fragile X syndrome. *Prim Care Clin Office Pract* 2004;31:621–625.

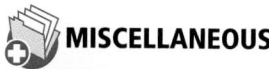 **MISCELLANEOUS**

CODES

ICD9-CM
759.83 Fragile X syndrome

PATIENT TEACHING
- The National Fragile X Foundation: www.fragilex.org
- FRAXA Research Foundation: www.fraxa.org

 See Corresponding Diagnostic Algorithm

F

FROSTBITE

Alan M. Ehrlich, MD

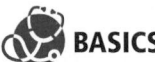 **BASICS**

DESCRIPTION
- A localized complication of exposure to cold, resulting in diminished blood flow to the affected part (especially hands, face, or feet).
- System(s) Affected: Endocrine/Metabolic; Skin/Exocrine
- Synonym(s): Dermatitis congelationis; Frostnip; Environmental injuries

GENERAL PREVENTION
- Dress in layers with appropriate cold-weather gear.
- Cover exposed areas and extremities appropriately.
- Prepare properly for trips to cold climates.
- Avoid alcohol.

EPIDEMIOLOGY
- Predominant age: All ages
- Predominant sex: Male = Female

RISK FACTORS
- Impaired cerebral function
- Under the effects of alcohol or drug abuse
- Underlying psychiatric disturbance
- Ambient temperature ≤17.8°C (0°F)
- Smoker
- Elderly
- Raynaud phenomenon

PATHOPHYSIOLOGY
- Dehydration, enzymatic destruction, and ultimately cell death occur.
- In severe cases, deep-tissue freezing may occur with damage to underlying blood vessels, muscles, and nerve tissue.

ETIOLOGY
- Prolonged exposure to cold
- Refreezing thawed extremities

ASSOCIATED CONDITIONS
Alcohol and/or drug abuse

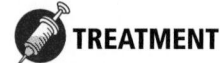 **DIAGNOSIS**

SIGNS AND SYMPTOMS
- Injured area 1st appears cold, hard, and white and is anesthetic to touch. It progresses to blotchy-red, swollen, and painful regions after rewarming.
- Loss of cutaneous sensation
- Numbness
- Throbbing pain
- Paresthesia
- Excessive sweating
- Joint pain
- Pallor
- Subcutaneous edema
- Hyperemia
- Blistering
- Blue discoloration
- Skin necrosis
- Gangrene

TESTS
ECG, with hypothermia
- Bradycardia
- Atrial fibrillation
- Atrial flutter
- Ventricular fibrillation
- Diffuse T-wave inversion
- Osborn waves (upward going "hump" just following S wave in the RS − T segment)

Lab
- Hemoconcentration
- Liver function tests for decreased hepatic function

Imaging
- Various imaging techniques such as thermography, angiography, digital plethysmography, and radioisotope vascular and bone scanning have been used to assess the degree of vascular injury.
- Helps surgeons make decisions, but no technique is entirely reliable during vascular instability, which lasts 2–3 weeks.

Pathological Findings
- Ice crystallization in the intravascular extracellular space
- Atrophy
- Fibroblastic proliferation
- Skin necrosis

DIFFERENTIAL DIAGNOSIS
- Frostnip, a superficial damp cold injury
- Chilblains (pernio)
- Immersion syndrome (trench foot)

TREATMENT

ALERT
Geriatric Considerations
- Associated disease states increase mortality
- Periarticular osteoporosis complicates
- More prone to hypothermia

Pediatric Considerations
Loss of epithelial growth centers

Pregnancy Considerations
Acidosis

INITIAL STABILIZATION
- Institute emergency measures for hypothermic patient without pulse or respiration. Such measures may include CPR and internal warming with warm IV fluids and warm oxygen (see "Hypothermia").
- Prevent refreezing.
- It may be necessary to keep the frostbitten part frozen until the patient can be transported to a care facility.
- Remove nonadherent wet clothing.
- Treat for hypothermia.
- Treat for pain
  - NSAIDs and/or narcotics if needed
- Do not rub areas to warm them; increased tissue damage may occur.

GENERAL MEASURES
- Cautious rewarming
  - May immerse frozen body part for several minutes in water no hotter than 40–42°C (104–108°F) (3)[B].
- After rewarming, injured parts should be covered with nonadhesive dressings, splinted, and elevated.
- Application of aloe vera and administration of NSAIDs are considered helpful in removal and inhibition of deleterious prostaglandins (e.g., ibuprofen 400–800 mg PO b.i.d. or a systemic anti-inflammatory given as early as possible).
- Keep the patient dry.
- If conscious, give the patient warm fluids with high sugar content.
- Amputation is not to be considered until it is definite that tissues are dead
  - May take ~3 weeks to know whether the tissue is permanently injured
- Prevent infection once treatment begins.
- Institute ongoing whirlpool therapy for cleansing and débridement.
- Prevent damage to other body parts.
- Maintenance
  - Gastric lavage, peritoneal dialysis, hemodialysis, and mediastinal lavage if needed (using warmed fluids)

Diet
- As tolerated
- Warm oral fluids

Activity
- As tolerated; protect injured body parts
- Initiate physical therapy once healing progresses sufficiently.

Special Therapy
Heated oxygen

IV Fluids
Warm IV fluids via central venous pressure line

MEDICATION (DRUGS)

First Line
- Tetanus toxoid
- For severe pain
  - Analgesics or narcotics
- Antibiotics may be required for infection.
- Contraindications: Refer to the manufacturer's profile of each drug.
- Precautions: Refer to the manufacturer's profile of each drug.
- Significant possible interactions: Refer to the manufacturer's profile of each drug.

Second Line
Consider nifedipine 10 mg PO t.i.d., nifedipine 30 mg XL PO daily, or pentoxifylline 400 mg PO t.i.d.

SURGERY
To remove necrotic tissue; often 1–3 months postinjury

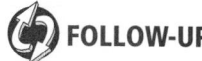 **FOLLOW-UP**

DISPOSITION
Outpatient or inpatient, depending on severity

PROGNOSIS
- Anesthesia and bullae may occur.
- The affected areas will heal or mummify without surgery
  - The process may take 6–12 months for healing.
- Patient may be sensitive to cold and experience burning and tingling.

COMPLICATIONS
- Hyperglycemia
- Acidosis
- Refractory arrhythmias
- Tissue loss
  - Distal parts of an extremity may undergo spontaneous amputation.
- Gangrene
- Death

PATIENT MONITORING
- Preferably electronic probe for temperature monitoring (rectal or vascular)
- Follow-up for physical therapy progress, infection, other complications

REFERENCES

1. Biem J, et al. Out of the cold: Management of hypothermia and frostbite. *CMAJ February* 2003.[B].
2. Murphy JV, et al. Frostbite: Pathogenesis and treatment. *J Trauma*. 2000;48(1):171–178. [B]
3. Reamy BV. Frostbite: Review and current concepts. *J Am Board Fam Pract*. 1998;11(1):34–40.

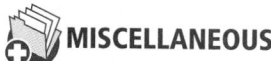 **MISCELLANEOUS**

See also: Hypothermia

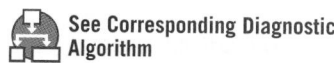 **CODES**

ICD9-CM
- 991.0 Frostbite of face
- 991.1 Frostbite of hand
- 991.2 Frostbite of foot
- 991.3 Frostbite of other and unspecified sites

PATIENT TEACHING

- Refer to local library for information.
- Provide education on
  - Exposure protection
  - Early signs and symptoms of frostbite

See Corresponding Diagnostic Algorithm

F

FROZEN SHOULDER

Vasilios Chrisostomidis, DO

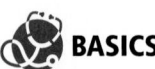 **BASICS**

DESCRIPTION
- Syndrome of painful restriction of active and passive range of motion (ROM) in 1 or both shoulders. Idiopathic adhesive capsulitis has 3 stages: Painful, adhesive, and recovery.
- System(s) Affected: Musculoskeletal
- Synonym(s): Pericapsulitis, Adherent bursitis; Obliterative bursitis; Adhesive capsulitis

GENERAL PREVENTION
- Early ROM exercises after injury
- Stretching, frequent physical activity

EPIDEMIOLOGY
- Predominant age: 40–70 years
- Predominant sex: Female > Male

ALERT
Geriatric Considerations
Common

Pediatric Considerations
Rare, but reported

Pregnancy Considerations
Primary (idiopathic): 2–3%

RISK FACTORS
- Systemic diseases (See "Etiology": Diseases and conditions associated with secondary adhesive capsulitis)
- Prolonged immobilization
- Age (more common in elderly)
- Diabetes

ETIOLOGY
- Idiopathic (primary)
- Diseases and conditions associated with secondary adhesive capsulitis
  - Trauma
  - Diabetes—most common
  - Postinflammatory
  - After coronary vascular accident
  - After myocardial infarction
  - After mastectomy (immobilization is the speculated cause)
  - Hypothyroidism/hyperthyroidism
  - Avascular necrosis
  - Tuberculosis
  - Scleroderma
  - Rheumatoid arthritis
  - Lung cancer or chronic lung disease

ASSOCIATED CONDITIONS
See "Etiology."

DIAGNOSIS

SIGNS AND SYMPTOMS
- Pain aggravated with movement and alleviated with rest
- Pain and tenderness to palpation of the shoulder
  - May interrupt sleep
- Preceding injury, illness, or immobilization (secondary adhesive capsulitis)
- Loss of active and passive ROM in all planes
- Loss of natural arm swing with gait
- Because of compensatory scapular elevation (to lift the arm), muscles may be painful and spastic.
- Muscle atrophy and weakness with time
- Inability to reach into a back pocket or fasten the back of a garment
- Stages of adhesive capsulitis
  - Painful stage (weeks to months):
    ○ Pain with movement
    ○ Generalized shoulder ache that is difficult to pinpoint
    ○ Muscle spasm
    ○ Increasing pain at night and at rest
  - Adhesive stage (up to 1 year)
    ○ Less pain
    ○ Increasing stiffness and restriction of movement
    ○ Decreasing pain at night and at rest
    ○ Discomfort felt at extreme ranges of movement
  - Recovery stage (weeks to months)
    ○ Decreased pain
    ○ Marked restriction with slow gradual increase in range of motion
    ○ Recovery is spontaneous, frequently incomplete.

History
- Subacute onset of shoulder pain and decreased ROM without trauma
- Night pain often interrupting sleep

Physical Exam
- Marked limitation of passive and active shoulder abduction, flexion, internal and external rotation
- Normal 5/5 strength in all planes
- No neurovascular deficits

TESTS
Lab
- No lab is diagnostic for frozen shoulder but may be required to rule out other disorders
- Rule out systemic/autoimmune disease
  - Thyroid-stimulating hormone
  - Erythrocyte sedimentation rate
  - Antinuclear antibody
  - CBC
  - Glucose level
- Disorders that may alter lab results
  - Systemic lupus erythematosus
  - Rheumatoid arthritis (RA)

Imaging
- Plain radiograph (anteroposterior [AP], axillary, supraspinatus outlet views) to rule out osteoarthritis, calcific tendinitis, avascular necrosis, osteomyelitis, fracture, dislocation, and tumor
  - AP: Check osteopenia, fractures, dislocations, and superior migration of humeral head
  - Axillary: Check subluxation or articular head damage (Bankart or Hills-Sachs lesions)
  - Supraspinatus outlet views: Check supraspinatus outlet narrowing to rule out acromial impingement
- Arthrography
  - Joint volume is reduced to 5–10 mL (normal, 20–30 mL).
  - Since this is invasive, arthrography is reserved for patients with uncertain diagnosis.
- Consider MRI to evaluate rotator cuff evaluating for thickening of the shoulder capsule and rule out other shoulder disorders.

Diagnostic Procedures/Surgery
- Joint aspiration if septic joint is suspected (rarely necessary)
- Arthroscopy to visualize fibrous bands in the joint space (rarely necessary)

Pathological Findings
- Fibrous bands traversing the glenohumeral joint space (occasional)
- Surgical findings of adherence of capsule to humeral head

DIFFERENTIAL DIAGNOSIS
- Rotator cuff strain/tear/impingement syndrome
- Bicipital/rotator/calcific tendinitis
- Septic arthritis
- Bursitis
- Glenohumeral or acromioclavicular joint osteoarthritis
- Cervical osteoarthritis
- Rheumatoid arthritis
- Bony neoplasm/metastases
- Dislocation
- Fracture (distal clavicle, proximal humerus)
- Avascular necrosis
- Fibromyalgia
- Myofascial pain syndrome

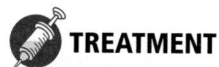 **TREATMENT**

INITIAL STABILIZATION
Outpatient care

GENERAL MEASURES
- Control of pain and preservation of mobility
- Avoid prolonged immobilization.
- Heat and/or ice
- Address underlying causes of secondary adhesive capsulitis (see "Differential Diagnosis").
- Physical therapy

Diet
No restrictions

Activity
- Encourage shoulder ROM
- Forceful shoulder exercises not recommended

SPECIAL THERAPY
Physical Therapy
- Avoid in the painful stage
- Focus on passive and active ROM exercises in the adhesive and recovery stages

Complementary and Alternative Medicine
Osteopathic Manipulative Technique may help decrease pain and increase shoulder range of motion

 MEDICATION (DRUGS)

Iontophoresis (electromotive drug administration) generally not recommended in this condition

First Line
- NSAIDs during painful stage
- Opioid analgesics (with physical therapy) if NSAIDs contraindicated
- Oral corticosteroids for a taper of 3–4 weeks (40 mg, 30 mg, 20 mg, 10 mg, then discontinue)
- Contraindications
  – NSAIDs: GI ulcer disease/bleeding
  – Renal disease: See the manufacturer's literature.
- Precautions
  – See the manufacturer's literature.
- Significant possible interactions
  – See the manufacturer's literature.

Second Line
- Low-dose tricyclic antidepressants (e.g., amitriptyline) may help with pain and sleep.
- Glenohumeral corticosteroid injection (e.g., triamcinolone, betamethasone)
  – Do not shorten recovery but may aid in decreasing discomfort with mobility exercises (controversial)
  – Systemic steroids not indicated

SURGERY
- Arthroscopic lysis of adhesions and manipulation under anesthesia are reserved for refractory cases (controversial).
- Capsular release

 FOLLOW-UP

PROGNOSIS
- Disorder is considered self-limiting
- Adhesive capsulitis may last from 6–9 months to as long as 1–3 years
  – Painful stage: 2–6 months
  – Adhesive stage: 4–6 months
  – Recovery stage: 1–3 months

COMPLICATIONS
- Long-term loss of some mobility (7–30%) or function (rare)
- Residual pain and stiffness

PATIENT MONITORING
Close monitoring and frequent encouragement usually needed for successful recovery

REFERENCES

1. Arslon S, et al. Comparison of the efficacy of local corticosteroid injection and physical therapy for the treatment of adhesive capsulitis. *Rheumatol Int.* 2001;21:20–3.
2. Butchbinder et al. Short course prednisolone for adhesive capsulitis (frozen shoulder or stiff painful shoulder): A randomized, double blind, placebo controlled trial. *Ann Rheum Dis.* 2004;63(11): 1460–1469.
3. Griggs, Sean M, et al. Idiopathic adhesive capsulitis: A prospective functional outcome study of non-operative treatment. *J Bone Joint Surg.* 2000;82:1398–1407.
4. Kivimacki J, et al. Manipulation under anesthesia for frozen shoulder with and without steroid injection. *Arch Phys Med Rehab.* 2001;82: 1188–1190.
5. Lee, Min Hee, et al. Adhesive capsulitis of the shoulder: Diagnosis using MR arthrography with arthroscopic findings as the standard. 2003;27(6):901–906.
6. Daigneault J, Cooney LM, Jr. Shoulder pain in older people. *J Am Geriatr Soc.* 1998;46:1145–1151.
7. Pearsall AW, Speer KP. Frozen shoulder syndrome: Diagnostic and treatment strategies in the primary care setting. *Med Sci Sports Exerc.* 1998; 30(suppl):S33–S39.
8. Siegel LB, Cohen NJ, Gall EP. Adhesive capsulitis: A sticky issue. *Am Fam Physician.* 1999;59: 1843–1851.
9. Woodward T, Best T. The painful shoulder. II: Acute and chronic disorders. *Am Fam Physician.* 2000;61:3291–3300.

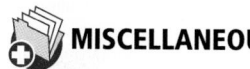 **MISCELLANEOUS**

 CODES

ICD9-CM
726.0 Adhesive capsulitis of shoulder

PATIENT TEACHING

Stretching exercises daily or b.i.d. during and after improvement

- Codman exercises: Sit sideways in a straight chair; rest armpit on the back of the chair; swing the arm slowly in circles. Start with smaller circles and then bigger circles (clockwise and counterclockwise).
- Climbing the wall: Put the hand flat on a wall in front of you; use the fingers to "climb" the wall; pause 30 seconds every few inches.
- Reaching: Put everyday objects on a high shelf so that reaching is done more often.

FURUNCULOSIS

W. Paul Slomiany, MD

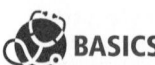 BASICS

DESCRIPTION
Acute abscess of a hair follicle due to bacterial infection (often *Staphylococcus aureus*)
- System(s) Affected: Skin/Exocrine
- Synonym(s): Boils

GENERAL PREVENTION
Patient education regarding self-care (See "General Measures": Treatment and prevention are interrelated.)

EPIDEMIOLOGY
- Predominant age
  – Adolescents and young adults
  – Clusters have been reported in teenagers living in crowded quarters, within families, or high school athletes. (1,2)
- Predominant sex: Male = Female

Incidence
Increase in frequency after puberty

Prevalence
Uncommon in young children unless immunodeficiency state present (e.g., can appear in young girls with hyperimmunoglobulin E–staphylococcal syndrome [Job syndrome])

RISK FACTORS
- Carriage of pathogenic strain of *Staphylococcus* species in nares, skin, axilla, and perineum
- Rarely, polymorphonuclear leukocyte defect or hyperimmunoglobulin E–*Staphylococcus* species abscess syndrome
- Diabetes mellitus, malnutrition, alcoholism, obesity
- Primary immunodeficiency disease (chronic granulomatous disease, Chediak-Higashi syndrome, C3 deficiency, C3 hypercatabolism, transient hypogammaglobulinemia of infancy, immunodeficiency with thymoma, Wiskott-Aldrich syndrome)
- Secondary immunodeficiency (leukemia, leukopenia, neutropenia, therapeutic immunosuppression)
- Medication use that impairs neutrophil function (e.g., omeprazole)

Genetics
Unknown

PATHOPHYSIOLOGY
Infection spreads away from hair follicle into surrounding dermis.

ETIOLOGY
Pathogenic strain of *S. aureus* (usually)

ASSOCIATED CONDITIONS
- Usually normal immune system
- Diabetes mellitus
- Polymorphonuclear leukocyte defect (rare)
- Hyperimmunoglobulin E–*Staphylococcal* abscess syndrome (rare)
- See "Risk Factors."

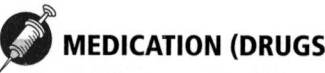 DIAGNOSIS

SIGNS AND SYMPTOMS
- Painful erythematous papules/nodules (1–5 cm) with central pustulation
- Located only in hirsute sites of body, especially areas prone to friction or minor trauma (e.g., underneath belt, anterior thighs, back of neck, buttocks)
- May be singular or multiple
- No fever or systemic symptoms
- Tender red perifollicular swelling, terminating in discharge of pus and necrotic plug
- Pus usually drains spontaneously.

TESTS
Lab
- Culture of abscess material
- Immunoglobulin levels in rare cases
- Culture of abscess material
- Drugs that may alter lab results
  – Antibiotics

Pathological Findings
Histopathology
- Perifollicular necrosis containing fibrinoid material and neutrophils
- At deep end of necrotic plug, in SC tissue, is a large abscess with a Gram stain positive for small collections of *S. aureus*.

DIFFERENTIAL DIAGNOSIS
- Folliculitis
- Pseudofolliculitis
- Carbuncles
- Ruptured epidermal cyst
- Myiasis (larva of botfly/tumbafly; C. or S. Amer) (3)
- Hidradenitis suppurativa
  – A particular form of furunculosis
- If abscess culture grows Gram-negative bacteria or fungus, then consider polymorphonuclear neutrophil leukocyte function defect.

TREATMENT

GENERAL MEASURES (4)
- Moist, warm compresses (provide comfort, encourage localization/pointing/drainage) 30 minutes q.i.d.
- If pointing or large, incise and drain.
- Consider packing to promote drainage.
- Routine culture not necessary for localized abscess in nondiabetic patients with normal immune system
- Systemic antibiotics usually unnecessary, unless extensive surrounding cellulitis or fever
- If recurrent, problem usually related to chronic skin carriage of particular strain of *Staphylococcus* organism in nares or on skin. Treatment goals are as follows (4)
  – Decrease or eliminate pathogenic strain *or*
  – Suppression of pathogenic strain
- Culture nares, skin, axilla, perineum (culture nares of family members)

- Apply mupirocin ointment to anterior nares b.i.d. ×5 days (patient and family carriers)
- Culture anterior nares every 3 months. If failure retreat with mupirocin or consider oral antibiotics. (5)[C]
- See "Medications, First Line, Suppression of Pathogenic Strain"
- Wash entire body and fingernails (with nailbrush) daily for 1–3 weeks with povidone–iodine (Betadine), hexachlorophene (Hibiclens), or pHisoHex soap (all can cause dry skin).
- Sanitary practices: Change towels, washcloths, and sheets daily; clean shaving instruments; avoid nose picking; change wound dressings frequently. (1,2)[C]

Diet
Unrestricted

Activity
Avoid contact sports (e.g., wrestling) if active lesions, otherwise no restrictions

MEDICATION (DRUGS)

First Line (6) [C]
- If abscesses multiple, if lesions have marked surrounding inflammation, cellulitis, systemic symptoms such as fever, or if immuno-compromised
  – Obtain culture and place on antibiotics directed at *S. aureus* for 10–14 days.
  – Dicloxacillin (Dynapen, Pathocil) 500 mg PO q.i.d., *or*
  – Cephalexin 250 mg PO q.i.d. or Clindamycin 150 mg q.i.d. if PEN allergic
- Suppression of pathogenic strain (if topical treatment fails) (4)
  – Dicloxacillin/cloxacillin 500 mg b.i.d. for 10–14 days
  – Cephalexin or clindamycin (if penicillin allergic)
  – If above fails, dicloxacillin/cloxacillin 500 mg plus rifampin 600 mg PO daily for 7–10 days or clindamycin 150 mg daily × 3 months. (7)[C]
- Contraindications
  – Cloxacillin and dicloxacillin: Penicillin allergy
  – Cephalexin: Cephalosporin allergy
  – Mupirocin: Hypersensitivity
- Precautions
  – Cloxacillin and dicloxacillin: Anaphylactic reaction

Second Line
- Resistant strains of *S. aureus* (Methicillin-resistant staphylococcus aureus): Clindamycin 300 mg q6h, or doxycycline 100 mg q12h, or TMP-SMX DS, 1 tab q8h. (6)
- If known or suspected impaired neutrophil function (e.g., impaired chemotaxis, phagocytosis, superoxide generation), add vitamin C 1,000 mg/d for 4–6 weeks (prevents oxidation of neutrophils).

- If fail with antibiotic regimens
  - May try oral pentoxifylline 400 mg t.i.d. for 2–6 months. (8)[C]
  - Contraindications: Recent cerebral and/or retinal hemorrhage; intolerance to methylxanthines (e.g., caffeine, theophylline)
  - Precautions: Prolonged prothrombin time (PT) and/or bleeding; if on warfarin, frequent monitoring of PT

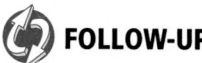 **FOLLOW-UP**

DISPOSITION
Outpatient care

PROGNOSIS
- Self-limited (usually drains pus spontaneously and will heal with or without scarring within several days)
- Recurrent/chronic lasting for months or years

COMPLICATIONS
- Scarring
- Bacteremia
- Metastatic seeding (e.g., septal/valve defect, arthritic joint)

PATIENT MONITORING
Instruct patient to see physician if compresses unsuccessful.

REFERENCES

1. Sosin DM, et al. An outbreak of furunculosis among high school athletes. *Amer J Sport Med*. 1989;17(6):828–832.
2. Zimakoff J, et al. Recurrent staphylococcus furunculosis in families. *Scand J Infect Diseases*. 1988;20(4):403–405.
3. Gerwirtzman A, et al. Botfly infestation (myiasis) masquerading as furunculosis. *Cutis*. 1999; 63:71.
4. Habif T. *Clinical Dermatology*. 4th ed. St. Louis, MO: Mosby; 2004.
5. Doebbeling BN, et al. Long Term Efficacy of Intranasal Mupirocin, A Prospective Cohort Study of Staphylococcal Aureus. *Arch Int Med*. 1994; 154:1505.
6. *Up To Date 2006*. Impetigo, Folliculitis, Furunculosis, and Carbuncles.
7. Klemper MS, Styrt B. Prevention of recurrent staphylococcal skin infections with low dose oral clindamycin therapy. *JAMA*. 1988;260:2682.
8. Wahba-Yahav AV. Intractable chronic furunculosis: Prevention of recurrence with pentoxifylline. *Acta Derm Venereol*. 1992; 72:461–462.
9. Winthropp KL, et al. An outbreak of mycobacterium furunculosis associated with footbaths at a nail salon. *N Engl J Med*. May 2002;346(18):1366–1371.
10. du Vivier A. *Dermatology in Practice*. Philadelphia, PA: JB Lippincott Co; 1990.
11. Levy R, et al. Vitamin C for the treatment of recurrent furunculosis in patients with impaired neutrophil function. *J Infect Dis*. 1996;173: 1502–1505.
12. Sams WM Jr, Lynch P. *Principles and Practice of Dermatology*. New York, NY: Churchill Livingstone; 1990.
13. West BC, et al. Furunculosis associated with repeated courses of omeprazole therapy. *Clin Infec Dis*. 1998;26:1234–1235.

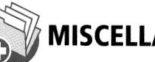 **MISCELLANEOUS**

See also: Folliculitis; Hidradenitis suppurativa

CODES

ICD9-CM
680.9 Carbuncle and furuncle, unspecified site

PATIENT TEACHING

Refer to Habif T. *Clinical Dermatology*. 3rd ed. St. Louis, MO: Mosby; 1996

F

GALACTORRHEA

Patricia Borman, MD

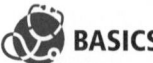 BASICS

DESCRIPTION
Milky nipple discharge not associated with gestation. Galactorrhea does not include serous, purulent, or bloody nipple discharge.
- System(s) Affected: Endocrine/Metabolic; Nervous; Reproductive
- Synonym(s): Disordered lactation; Nipple discharge

Pregnancy Considerations
- Adenomas can grow rapidly during pregnancy.
- Most cases of galactorrhea during pregnancy are physiologic.

GENERAL PREVENTION
Keep medication causes in mind.

EPIDEMIOLOGY
- Predominant age: 15–50 years (reproductive)
- Predominant sex: Female > Male (rare, 20% of patients with *MEN1* have prolactinomas)

Prevalence
One to fifty percent of nonpregnant reproductive-age women

PATHOPHYSIOLOGY
Disorders of lactation are associated with hyperprolactinemia from overproduction or loss of inhibitory regulation by dopamine.

ETIOLOGY
- Pituitary gland overproduction
  - Prolactinoma, acromegaly, empty sella, lymphocytic hypophysitis
- Hypothalamic region dysregulation
  - Craniopharyngiomas, meningiomas, dysgerminomas, tumors, sarcoid, irradiation, vascular insult, stalk disruption, or dissection
- Medications that suppress dopamine
  - Phenothiazines, atypical antipsychotics, selective serotonin reuptake inhibitors, tricyclic antidepressants, butyrophenones, cimetidine, ranitidine, reserpine, alpha methyl-dopa, verapamil, estrogens, isoniazid, opioids, stimulants, neuroleptics, metoclopramide, domperidone, protease inhibitors.
- Chest wall conditions
  - Zoster, fibrocystic breast disease, or surgical or other trauma
- Postoperative condition, especially oophorectomy
- Other causes
  - Primary hypothyroidism, cirrhosis, Cushing disease, ectopic prolactin secretion, renal failure, sarcoid, lupus, multiple sclerosis, polycystic ovary syndrome
- Physiologic with pregnancy or up to 6 months after stopping lactation
- Chiari-Frommel
  - Idiopathic galactorrhea >6 months postpartum
- Idiopathic
  - Normal prolactin levels

ASSOCIATED CONDITIONS
See "Etiology"

DIAGNOSIS

SIGNS AND SYMPTOMS
- Bilateral milky nipple discharge; other findings vary with causes
- Hypogonadism from hyperprolactinemia
  - Oligomenorrhea, amenorrhea
  - Inadequate luteal phase, anovulation, infertility
  - Decreased libido (especially in affected males)
- Mass effects from pituitary enlargement
  - Headache, cranial neuropathies
  - Bitemporal hemianopsia, amaurosis, scotomata
- Signs/symptoms of associated conditions
  - Adrenal insufficiency, acromegaly, hypothyroidism, chest wall conditions

TESTS
- Formal visual field testing if pituitary adenoma suspected
- Progesterone withdrawal bleed if amenorrheic

Lab
- Confirm microscopic of secretions is lipoid.
- Check prolactin level and thyroid-stimulating hormone.
- Check pregnancy test, liver and renal functions.
- Consider follicle-stimulating hormone and leuteinizing hormone if amenorrheic.
- Consider growth hormone levels if acromegaly suspected.
- Check adrenal steroids if signs of Cushing disease.
- Drugs that may alter lab results
  - See medications that can cause hyperprolactinemia.
- Disorders that may alter lab results:
  - See "Etiology"

Imaging
Pituitary MRI

Pathological Findings
- None unless pituitary resection required
- Gland can have woody fibrosis if patient took bromocriptine (Parlodel) for very long

DIFFERENTIAL DIAGNOSIS
- Primary hypothyroidism
- Nonmilky nipple discharge
  - Intraductal papilloma
  - Fibrocystic disease
- Purulent breast discharge
  - Mastitis
  - Breast abscess
  - Impetigo
  - Eczema
- Bloody breast discharge
  - Consider malignancy.

TREATMENT

GENERAL MEASURES
- Treat underlying cause if possible.
- Treat to manage symptoms, reduce patient anxiety, and restore fertility.
- Reduce tumor size or prevent progression to prevent neurologic sequelae.
- If microadenoma, watchful waiting can be appropriate, as 95% do not enlarge
- Treat asymptomatic tumors if >10 mm.
- Discontinue offending medications.

Diet
No restrictions

Activity
No restrictions

SPECIAL THERAPY

Radiotherapy (1)[B]
- Radiation is an alternate therapy
  - 20–30% success rate
  - 50% risk of panhypopituitarism after radiation
- Gamma knife is effective with high volume surgeons. (2)[B]

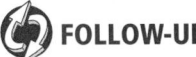 **MEDICATION (DRUGS)**

First Line (3)[B]

The dopamine antagonists work to reduce prolactin levels and shrink tumor size. Therapy is suppressive, not curative.

- Contraindications are similar for all and include
  - Uncontrolled hypertension
  - Sensitivity to ergot alkaloids
  - Pre-eclampsia
- Precautions
  - Nausea, vomiting, and drowsiness are common.
  - Orthostasis, light-headedness, or syncope
  - Hypertension, seizures, acute psychosis, and digital vasospasm are rare.
- Significant possible interactions
  - Phenothiazines, butyrophenones, other drugs listed under "Etiology"
  - Pergolide (Permax) (3)[B]
    - 0.05–0.15 mg PO once daily
    - Fewest side effects and less expensive
  - Cabergoline (Dostinex)
    - 0.25–1 mg PO weekly
    - Fewer side effects than bromocriptine
    - Convenient dosing

Second Line (3)[B]

Bromocriptine

- Start low 1.25 mg with food and increase to 2.5 mg PO t.i.d. Dosing as high as 30 mg/d may be required. Most expensive, worse side effects, and frequent dosing make this less desirable.
- Long-term treatment can cause woody fibrosis of the pituitary gland.

SURGERY

Macroadenomas need surgery if medical management does not halt growth if any neurologic symptoms, if >10 mm, or patient cannot tolerate medications

- Trans-sphenoidal pituitary resection
- 50% recurrence after surgery

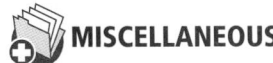 **FOLLOW-UP**

DISPOSITION

- Outpatient care unless pituitary resection required
- Bromocriptine patients need good hydration.

PROGNOSIS

- Depends on underlying cause
- Symptoms recur after discontinuation of medication.
- Surgery can have 50% recurrence.
- Prolactinomas <10 mm can resolve spontaneously.

COMPLICATIONS

- Depends on underlying cause
- If enlarging pituitary adenoma, risk of permanent visual field loss
- Panhypopituitarism can complicate radiation or surgical therapy.
- Osteoporosis if amenorrhea persists without estrogen replacement

PATIENT MONITORING

- Varies with cause; check prolactin levels every 6 weeks until normalized, then every 6–12 months.
- Monitor visual fields and MRI at least yearly; if clinical course is stable, then every 2–5 years.

REFERENCES

1. Nomikos P, Buchfelder M, Fahlbusch R. Current management of prolactinomas. *J Neurooncol*. 2001;54:139–150.
2. Molitch M. Medication-induced Hyperprolactinemia. *Mayo Clinic Proceeding Rochester*. 2005;80(8):1050–1058.
3. Verhelst J, Abs R. Hyperprolactinemia: Pathophysiology and management. (Therapy in Practice). *Treatments in Endocrinology*, 2003; 2(1):23–32.
4. Cho DY, Liau WR. Comparison of endonasal endoscopic surgery and sublabial microsurgery for prolactinomas. *Surg Neurol*. 2002;58:371–375; discussion 375–376.
5. Pena KS, Rosenfeld JA. Evaluation and treatment of galactorrhea. *Am Fam Physician*. 2001;63: 1763–1770.

MISCELLANEOUS

See also: Hyperprolactinemia

CODES

ICD9-CM

676.60 Galactorrhea associated with childbirth, unspecified

PATIENT TEACHING

- Warn about symptoms of mass enlargement in pituitary.
- Discuss treatment rationale and risks of treating or not.
- Patient education material available from Pituitary Tumor Network Association (16350 Ventura Blvd. #231, Encino, CA 91436; (805) 499-9973).

G

GASTRIC MALIGNANCY

Scott T. Henderson, MD

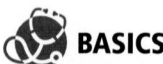 **BASICS**

DESCRIPTION
- May occur anywhere in the stomach
- Over the past 20 years, incidence of adenocarcinoma of the proximal stomach and the gastroesophageal junction has risen, whereas incidence of distal cancers has remained unchanged or decreased slightly.
- Infiltration to lymph nodes, omentum, lungs, and liver is rapid.
- Uncommon in US natives
- Synonym(s): Linitis plastica

Geriatric Considerations
Prevalence greater

Pediatric Considerations
Rare

Pregnancy Considerations
- Rarely diagnosed during pregnancy.
- Prognosis is poor if diagnosed.

GENERAL PREVENTION
- Insufficient data to establish that screening would decrease mortality in the US population.
- Screening may be of benefit in high-prevalence areas.
- Diets including 5–20 servings of both fruits and vegetables each week reduce the risk of gastric malignancy by ~1/2.

EPIDEMIOLOGY
- Predominant age: >55 (2/3 >65)
- Predominant sex: Male > Female (1.7:1)

Incidence
7/100,000; 21,860 new cases per year

RISK FACTORS
- *Helicobacter pylori* infection
- Diet rich in additives (e.g., smoked, pickled, or salted foods; highly spiced Asian foods)
- Achlorhydria
- Atrophic gastritis/intestinal metaplasia
- Pernicious anemia
- Prior gastric resection
- Smoking/tobacco abuse
- Ethnic background: Hispanic, Japanese, Chilean, Costa Rican. 1st-generation or 2nd-generation Japanese, Chilean, or Costa Rican in the United States.
- Family history: 2–4 times more common in 1st-degree relatives
- Patients in lower socioeconomic classes are at greater risk of developing gastric tumors.
- Polyps or dysplasia anywhere in alimentary canal
- Familial polyposis
- Barrett's esophagus
- Low consumption of fruits and vegetables
- Individuals with blood group A

Genetics
More common in people with blood group A

ETIOLOGY
Unknown

ASSOCIATED CONDITIONS
- Giant hypertrophic gastritis (Ménétrier disease)
- Intestinal metaplasia of the stomach
- Atrophic gastritis
- *H. pylori* infection

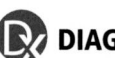 **DIAGNOSIS**

SIGNS AND SYMPTOMS
- Anorexia/Weight loss (70–80%)
- Chronic noncolicky abdominal pain (especially in epigastrium) ranging from postprandial fullness to severe steady pain (70%)
- Pain unrelieved by antacids
- Pain exacerbated by food
- Pain relieved by fasting
- Nausea and vomiting
- Change in bowel habits
- Cachexia
- Early satiety
- Gross gastrointestinal (GI) bleeding (10%)
- Dysphagia (rare)

History
Symptoms present late in course

Physical Exam
- Palpable left supraclavicular node (Virchow's)
- Sister Mary Joseph nodule at umbilicus

TESTS
Pentagastrin test—stomach pH <6.

Lab
- Positive stool guaiac for blood
- Hemoglobin <12 g/dL (1.86 mmol/L)
- Hematocrit <35 (0.35)
- Albumin <g/dL (30 g/L)
- Disorder that may alter lab results: Pernicious anemia may cause a false-positive pentagastrin test.

Imaging
Double contrast upper GI study—barium filling defect, endoscopy, endoscopic ultrasound, CT scan.

Diagnostic Procedures/Surgery
- Upper endoscopy for direct visualization, cytology, and biopsy
- Endoscopic ultrasound is most accurate preoperative staging tool

Pathological Findings
- Adenocarcinomas 90% (Types: Intestinal and diffuse [linitis plastica])
- Gastric lymphomas, sarcomas, and other rare types 10%

DIFFERENTIAL DIAGNOSIS
- Gastric lymphoma
- Peptic ulcer with or without hemorrhage
- Eosinophilic gastroenteritis
- Giant hypertrophic gastritis
- Carcinoma of the colon
- Functional dyspepsia
- Carcinoma of body or tail of the pancreas
- Angiodysplasia of the colon
- GI sarcoidosis
- Small intestinal lymphoma
- Crohn disease

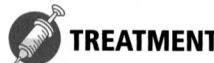 **TREATMENT**

Inpatient, although depending on stage at time of diagnosis, most of the following is often outpatient

GENERAL MEASURES
- Multidisciplinary treatment is mandatory.
- Surgical excision of the tumor is only potentially curative option
  - Extent of lymph nodes resection is debated (1)[B]
  - Even patients with incurable lesions should be offered an attempt at surgical reduction of the tumor, because it offers the best form of palliation and improves the likelihood of benefit if chemotherapy and/or radiation therapy is administered.
  - Endoscopic mucosal resection for early gastric cancer may be curative (2)[C]
- Adjuvant chemotherapy may provide benefit compared to surgery alone (3)[B].
- Radiation therapy
  - Of little benefit because of the radioresistance of gastric tumors
  - Does have use in the palliation of pain, bleeding, and obstruction
- Compared to best supportive care, chemotherapy significantly improves survival (4)[A]

Diet
Dependent on the surgical procedure

Activity
Adjusted to patient's ability

MEDICATION (DRUGS)

First Line

- Combination chemotherapy improves survival compared to single-agent 5-FU (4)[A]
  - Among the combination chemotherapy regimens studied, best survival results are achieved with regimens containing 5-FU, anthracyclines, and cisplatin.
    - In this category, epirubicin, cisplatin and continuous infusion 5-FU are tolerated best.

- Contraindications: Refer to the manufacturer's profile
- Precautions: Refer to the manufacturer's profile
- Significant possible interactions: Refer to the manufacturer's profile

Second Line

Ondansetron (Zofran), dronabinol (Marinol), metoclopramide (Reglan), and others for nausea control

SURGERY

- Radical subtotal gastrectomy with gastrojejunostomy or gastroduodenostomy is the usual treatment of choice
  - Large part of the stomach along with the greater and lesser omentum is removed en bloc
  - Splenectomy and distal pancreatectomy also sometimes performed
  - Direct extensions also excised
- Total gastrectomy indicated only if necessary to remove the local lesion
- Local excision or endoscopic laser therapy or electrocautery for palliation of incurable lesion by resection of bleeding area or area of obstruction

FOLLOW-UP

PROGNOSIS

- Because most lesions do not produce symptoms until late in course, gastric carcinomas are usually advanced at the time of diagnosis.
- Overall 5-year relative survival rate 23% (if local disease 58%, regional spread 23%, distant spread 3%)
- Early gastric cancers are usually detected as incidental findings or when screening endoscopy is performed in endemic areas. The 5-year survival rate is >40%, depending on specific staging and tumor differentiation.
- Primary gastric lymphoma is more treatable than gastric adenocarcinoma.
  - 5-year survival rate is 40–60% with subtotal gastrectomy followed by combination chemotherapy.

COMPLICATIONS

- Metastatic disease (especially hepatic, cerebral and pulmonary)
- Anemia (especially pernicious)
- Pyloric stenosis

PATIENT MONITORING

Routine, frequent follow-up is necessary to monitor disease state, assess treatments, monitor for recurrence/metastasis, and assess nutritional status.

REFERENCES

1. McCulloch P, et al. Extended versus limited lymph nodes dissection technique for adenocarcinoma of the stomach (Cochrane Review). In: *The Cochrane Library*, Issue 4, 2005. Chichester, UK: John Wiley and Sons, Ltd.
2. Wang YP, Bennett C, Pan T. Endoscopic mucosal resection for early gastric cancer. In: *The Cochrane Library*, Issue 1, 2006. Chichester, UK: John Wiley and Sons, Ltd.
3. Neri B, et al. Randomized trial of adjuvant chemotherapy versus control after curative resection for gastric cancer: 5-year follow-up. *Br J Cancer* 2001;84:878–880.
4. Wagner AD, et al. Chemotherapy for advanced gastric cancer (Cochrane Review). In: *The Cochrane Library*, Issue 4, 2005. Chichester, UK: John Wiley and Sons, Ltd.

ADDITIONAL READING

Layke JC, Lopez PP. Gastric cancer: Diagnosis and treatment options. *Am Fam Physician*. 2004; 69:1133–1140, 1145–1146.

MISCELLANEOUS

- See also: Esophageal tumors; Multiple endocrine neoplasia
- Other notes
  - Patients in lower socioeconomic classes are at greater risk of developing gastric tumors.
  - Migrants from high-incidence areas (e.g., Iceland, Chile, or Japan) to low-incidence areas maintain an increased risk, whereas their offspring have an occurrence rate that corresponds to that of the new location.

CODES

ICD9-CM

- 151.0 Malignant neoplasm of stomach, cardia
- 151.1 Malignant neoplasm of stomach, pylorus
- 151.2 Malignant neoplasm of stomach, pyloric antrum
- 151.3 Malignant neoplasm of fundus of stomach
- 151.4 Malignant neoplasm of body of stomach
- 151.5 Malignant neoplasm of lesser curvature of stomach, unspecified
- 151.6 Malignant neoplasm of greater curvature of stomach, unspecified
- 151.8 Malignant neoplasm of other specified sites of stomach
- 151.9 Malignant neoplasm of stomach, unspecified

PATIENT TEACHING

- Contact the local American Cancer Society.
- *Cancer Research Institute Helpbook: What to Do If Cancer Strikes*. FDR Station, Box 5199, New York, NY 10150–5199.

G

GASTRITIS

Michelle Whitehurst-Cook, MD

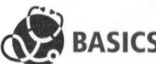 **BASICS**

DESCRIPTION

Inflammatory reaction in the stomach; typically involves the mucosa, seldom the full thickness of the stomach wall

- Patchy erythema of gastric mucosa: A common endoscopic finding; usually insignificant
- Erosive gastritis: A reaction to mucosal injury by a noxious chemical agent (e.g., drugs [especially NSAIDs] or alcohol)
- Reflux gastritis
  - A reaction to protracted reflux exposure to bile and pancreatic juice, usually associated with a defective pylorus
  - Typically limited to the prepyloric antrum
- Hemorrhagic gastritis (stress ulceration)
  - A reaction to hemodynamic disorder (e.g., hypovolemia or hypoxia [as in shock])
  - Also common in ICUs
- Infectious gastritis
  - Commonly associated with *Helicobacter pylori* (possibly causative, maybe opportunistic)
  - Viral infection, usually as a component of systemic infection, is common.
  - Significant infection by other specific microbes is rare.
- Gastric mucosal atrophy, sometimes called atrophic gastritis
  - Frequent, in varying degrees, in the elderly
  - Invariable in primary (pernicious) anemia
- Synonym(s): Erosive gastritis; Reflux gastritis; Hemorrhagic gastritis; Acute gastritis

ALERT

Geriatric Considerations
Persons >60 often harbor *H. pylori* infection

Pediatric Considerations
Gastritis rarely occurs in infants or children.

GENERAL PREVENTION

- Patients should be warned of known or potentially injurious drugs or chemical agents.
- Patients liable to hypovolemia or hypoxia (especially patients confined to an intensive care ward) should receive prophylactic therapy with antacids.
- H_2 receptor antagonists, prostaglandins, or sucralfate

EPIDEMIOLOGY

- Predominant age: All ages
- Predominant sex: Male = Female

RISK FACTORS

- Age >60
- Exposure to potentially noxious drugs or chemical agents
- Hypovolemia, hypoxia (shock)
- Candidal autoimmune

Genetics
Unknown

ETIOLOGY

- Alcohol
- Aspirin and other NSAIDs
- Bile reflux
- Pancreatic enzyme reflux
- Stress (hypovolemia or hypoxia)
- Radiation
- *Staphylococcus aureus* exotoxins
- Bacterial infection (e.g., *H. pylori*)
- Viral infection
- Pernicious anemia
- Gastric mucosal atrophy
- Portal hypertension gastropathy
- Emotional stress

ASSOCIATED CONDITIONS

- Gastric or duodenal peptic ulcer
- Primary (pernicious) anemia
- Portal hypertension

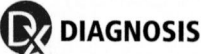 **DIAGNOSIS**

SIGNS AND SYMPTOMS

- Nondescript epigastric distress, often aggravated by eating
- Anorexia
- Nausea, with or without vomiting
- Significant bleeding is unusual except in hemorrhagic gastritis.
- Hiccups

TESTS
Special tests

- ^{13}C-urea breath test for *H. pylori* (not widely available)
- Serologic test available for *H. pylori* (office and clinical laboratory), inexpensive
- Gastric acid analysis may be abnormal, but is not a reliable indicator of gastritis.

Lab
Usually unremarkable, except when blood loss results in anemia

- Drugs that may alter lab results: Antibiotics or omeprazole may affect urea breath test for *H. pylori*.

Imaging
Nuclear scintigraphy is not done clinically.

Diagnostic Procedures/Surgery
Gastroscopy, usually with biopsy, is essential for a precise diagnosis. (It is recommended if there is a poor response to the initial treatment.)

Pathological Findings
Acute or chronic inflammatory infiltrate in gastric mucosa, often with distortion or erosion of adjacent epithelium. Presence of *H. pylori* may be confirmed.

DIFFERENTIAL DIAGNOSIS

- Functional gastrointestinal disorder
- Peptic ulcer disease
- Linitis plastica
- Viral gastroenteritis
- Pancreatic disease
- Gastric cancer (elderly)

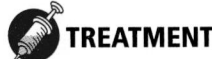 TREATMENT

INITIAL STABILIZATION
Outpatient, except for severe hemorrhagic gastritis

GENERAL MEASURES
- No specific therapy for gastritis (with the exception of *H. pylori* infection) (1)[C]
- Parenteral fluid and electrolyte supplements required if vomiting prevents food intake
- Consider discontinuing NSAIDs or adding misoprostol
- Encourage smoking cessation

Diet
Restrictions, if any, depend on the severity of the symptoms (e.g., light, soft foods); it is wise to avoid caffeine and spicy foods, as well as alcohol.

Activity
There are usually no restrictions.

 MEDICATION (DRUGS)

- Antacids: Best given in liquid form, 30 mL 1 hour after meals qhs; useful mainly as an emollient
- H_2 receptor antagonists (e.g., cimetidine [Tagamet]): "Priming" dose of 300 mg IV, then a steady infusion of 37.5–75 mg/h, dissolved in the running fluid; patients less severely ill: Oral cimetidine 300 mg q6h (or ranitidine [Zantac] or famotidine [Pepcid] or nizatidine [Axid]). Not shown to be clearly superior to antacids. (2)[C]
- Sucralfate (Carafate): 1 g q4–6h on an empty stomach; rationale uncertain, but empirically helpful
- Prostaglandins (e.g., misoprostol [Cytotec]): Can help allay gastric mucosal injury, suggested dosage of 100–200 μg q.i.d.
- To eradicate *H. pylori*
  - "Triple therapy" is advised: Bismuth (Pepto-Bismol) 30 mL liquid or 2 tablets q.i.d. for 4 weeks plus metronidazole 250 mg q.i.d. for the 1st week, plus tetracycline 250 mg q.i.d. or amoxicillin 250 mg t.i.d. for 2–4 weeks or
  - "Dual therapy" with omeprazole 20 mg b.i.d. plus amoxicillin 500 mg q.i.d. for 2 weeks
  - A short course therapy with 1 week of metronidazole, omeprazole, and clarithromycin b.i.d. is 90% effective.
- Contraindications: Hypersensitivity to the drug(s)
- Precautions
  - If bismuth is prescribed, warn the patient about the side effect of his or her stool becoming black.
  - Refer to the manufacturer's profile of each drug.
- Significant possible interactions: Refer to the manufacturer's profile of each drug.

 FOLLOW-UP

PROGNOSIS
- Most cases clear spontaneously when the cause has been identified and allayed.
- Recurrence of *H. pylori* infection may require a repeated course of treatment.

COMPLICATIONS
Bleeding from extensive mucosal erosion or ulceration

PATIENT MONITORING
- Gastroscopy should be repeated after 6 weeks if gastritis has been severe or if symptomatic response to treatment has not been achieved.
- Patients with chronic gastritis are at increased risk for gastric carcinoma.

REFERENCES

1. Graham DY, et al. Epidemiology of *Helicobacter pylori* in an asymptomatic population in the US. *Gastroenterology.* 1991;100:1495–1501.
2. Zinner MJ, et al. Misoprostol versus antacid titration for preventing stress ulcers in postoperative surgical ICU patients. *Ann Surg.* 1989;210:590–595.
3. Cutler AP. Testing for *Helicobacter pylori* in clinical practice. *Am J Med.* 1996;100:355–415.
4. Ofman JJ, et al. Management strategies for *Helicobacter pylori* seropositive patients with dyspepsia: Clinical and economic consequences. *Ann Intern Med.* 1997;126:280–291.
5. Richardson CT. Gastritis. In: Wyngaarden JB, Smith LH Jr, eds. *Cecil Textbook of Medicine.* Philadelphia, PA: WB Saunders; 1988:689–692.
6. Layka J, Lopez P, Gastric Cancer: Diagnosis and Treatment Opitons. *Am Fam Physicians.* 2004;69:1133–1140, 1145–1146.

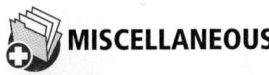 MISCELLANEOUS

CODES

ICD9-CM
535.50 Unspecified gastritis and gastroduodenitis without mention of hemorrhage

PATIENT TEACHING

- Explanation, reassurance
- Smoking cessation
- Dietary changes
- Relaxation therapy

 See Corresponding Diagnostic Algorithm

G

GASTROESOPHAGEAL REFLUX DISEASE (GERD)

Ruben Peralta, MD, FACS
Sarah Guzofski, MD

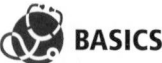 **BASICS**

DESCRIPTION
Reflux of gastroduodenal contents into the esophagus, larynx, or lungs with or without resultant esophageal inflammation

ALERT
Pregnancy Considerations
- Children affected: 1/300–1,000
- Reflux symptoms usually resolve by 18 months
- Symptoms: Vomiting, weight loss, failure to thrive
- Positional treatment: Use infant seat for 2–3 hours after meals; thickened feedings
- Drug treatment: Antacids or liquid histamine type 2 blockers, omeprazole, metoclopramide
- Surgery for severe symptoms (apnea, choking, persistent vomiting)

Pregnancy Considerations
Suggest small meals, avoiding lying down for 2–3 hours after meals, and elevating the head of the bed at night.

EPIDEMIOLOGY
Prevalence
- Prevalence of GERD: 10–20% in the US
- Prevalence of Barrett's esophagus: 1.5%
- 65% adults have had heartburn, 15% have weekly symptoms

RISK FACTORS
- Obesity
- Alcohol use
- Smoking
- Caffeine use

ETIOLOGY
- Occurs with loss of the normal pressure gradient between the lower esophageal sphincter (LES) and the stomach
- Most commonly due to inappropriate relaxation of LES
  - Idiopathic
  - Foods (high-fat, spicy, citrus, chocolate, peppermint, onions)
  - Medications (anticholinergic, smooth muscle relaxants such as calcium channel blockers and nitrates)
- Other contributing factors include
  - Pregnancy (progestational hormones decrease LES pressure)
  - Ineffective peristalsis
  - Scleroderma
  - Delayed gastric emptying
  - Positional: Recumbency, bending
  - Obesity

ASSOCIATED CONDITIONS
- Reflux esophagitis: Due to exposure to acid, pepsin; classified as erosive (mucosal damage apparent, ulcers, friability) or non-erosive
- Extraesophageal reflux
  - Asthma
  - Aspiration
  - Chronic cough
  - Laryngitis, vocal cord granuloma
  - Sinusitis
  - Otitis media
- Peptic stricture: In 10% with GERD
- Halitosis
- Hiatal hernia
- Barrett's esophagus
- Esophageal adenocarcinoma

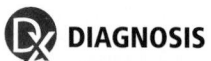 **DIAGNOSIS**

SIGNS AND SYMPTOMS
- Heartburn (70–85%)
- Regurgitation of digested food (60%)
- Anginalike chest pain (33%)
- Abdominal pain (29%)
- Hoarseness (21%)
- Dysphagia (for solids, if solids and liquids consider another cause) (20%)
- Bronchospasm (asthma) (15–20%)
- Aspiration (14%)
- Chronic cough
- Globus sensation
- Loss of dental enamel

History
- Heartburn: Retrosternal burning
- Regurgitation of undigested food, sour or acid taste in mouth
- Symptoms with bending or recumbency, often after meals
- Extra-esophageal symptoms such as cough, asthma
- Inquire about diet, alcohol, smoking, and caffeine
- Diagnosis often made based on history, often with a 1 week therapeutic trial with a proton pump inhibitor (PPI)

TESTS
- Treated empirically if no "Red Flags": Dysphagia odynophagia, weight loss, early satiety, anemia, new onset male >45 years
- 24-hour pH monitoring: Gold standard for diagnosis, records number of reflux episodes, number that occur supine or upright, can be correlated with symptom diary
- Esophageal manometry records pressure of LES and effectiveness of peristalsis

Lab
Check for anemia due to bleeding esophageal erosions or due to poor B_{12} absorption on PPI

Imaging
Barium swallow
- Presence of a sliding hiatal hernia appears to be a predictor of reflux esophagitis
- Mucosal irregularity due to inflammation and edema

Diagnostic Procedures/Surgery
- Endoscopy
  - Not part of initial work-up, unless anemia, unintentional weight low, progressive dysphagia, gastrointestinal bleeding, persistent vomiting, palpable epigastric mass, suspicion based on imaging study. (1)[B]
  - Recommended for patients >55 who continue to have symptoms after 4 weeks of treatment. (1)[B]
  - Confirm mucosal injury, look for Barrett's esophagus, biopsy for adenocarcinoma
  - ~50–70% of patients with heartburn have negative findings on endoscopy (nonerosive or endoscopy-negative reflux disease).
- Savary-Miller classification
  - For grading esophagitis based on endoscopic findings
    - Grade I: 1 or more non-confluent reddish spots, with or without exudate
    - Grade II: Erosive and exudative lesions in the distal esophagus; may be confluent, but not circumferential
    - Grade III: Circumferential erosions in the distal esophagus
    - Grade IV: Chronic complications such as deep ulcers, stenosis, or scarring with Barrett's metaplasia

Pathological Findings
- Acute inflammation (especially eosinophils)
- Hyperplasia of the basal zone of the epithelium seen in 85%
- Barrett's epithelial change: Gastric columnar epithelium replaces squamous epithelium in distal esophagus

DIFFERENTIAL DIAGNOSIS
- Infectious esophagitis (*Candida*, herpes, HIV, cytomegalovirus)
- Chemical esophagitis (lye ingestion)
- Pill-induced esophagitis
- Radiation injury
- Crohn disease
- Angina
- Stricture
- Esophageal carcinoma
- Achalasia
- Scleroderma
- Peptic ulcer disease

TREATMENT

GENERAL MEASURES

- Screen for symptoms concerning for esophageal cancer (rapidly progressive dysphagia and weight loss); if present, early endoscopy
- Lifestyle changes 1st intervention
- Stress reduction: Considered single most important to address
  - Elevate head of bed and avoid lying down soon after meals
  - Avoid stooping, bending, and tight-fitting garments
  - Avoid medications that relax the LES (anticholinergic, calcium channel blockers)
  - Lose weight
  - Stop smoking
  - Avoid alcohol

Diet
Avoid foods that make symptoms worse

Activity
Full activity, avoid recumbency after meals

MEDICATION (DRUGS)

First Line
- Stepped therapy
  - Phase I: Lifestyle and diet modifications plus H_2 blockers in prescription doses or PPIs
  - Phase II: Symptoms persist, consider endoscopic evaluation
  - Phase III: Surgery
- H_2 blockers in equipotent oral doses (e.g., cimetidine 800 mg b.i.d. or 400 mg q.i.d. or ranitidine 150 mg b.i.d. or famotidine 20 mg b.i.d. or nizatidine 150 mg b.i.d.
- PPIs: Irreversibly bind proton pump, onset of effect 4 days Include omeprazole 20 mg daily, lansoprazole 30 mg daily, pantoprazole 40 mg daily, rabeprazole 20 mg daily, esomeprazole 40 mg daily
- Erosive esophagitis: PPI given for 8 weeks will be effective for healing in 90%. PPI more effective than H_2 blocker for healing erosive esophagitis. (1)[B]

Second Line
- Antacids
- Metoclopramide: 5–10 mg before meals
- Precautions
  - Blood dyscrasias with PPIs and H_2 blockers
  - H_2 blockers must be renally dosed
  - Metoclopramide is a dopamine blocker; risk of dystonia and tardive dyskinesia
  - On PPI, monitor B_{12}, B_{12} absorption compromised on PPI
- Significant possible interactions
  - PPIs and H_2 blockers have multiple cytochrome P450 drug interactions; examples include warfarin, phenytoin, antifungals.

SURGERY
Open or laparoscopic Nissen or Toupet fundoplication
- Increase pressure gradient between stomach and esophagus by wrapping gastric fundus around distal esophagus, often circumferential (360° fundoplication)
- Indications: Evidence of severe esophageal injury, incomplete response to medical treatment, medication treatment that has been or is expected to be prolonged

- Rule out esophageal dysmotility prior to surgery. If motility problems, consider a partial (270°, Toupet) wrap.
- Open and laparoscopic procedures both produce >90% response, equally effective for symptom reduction, quality of life, decreased need for medications. (2)[A], (3)[B]
- Cost analysis has indicated that >10 years of PPI treatment, surgery may be more cost effective.

FOLLOW-UP

PROGNOSIS
- Symptoms and esophageal inflammation often return promptly when treatment is withdrawn; to prevent relapse of symptoms, patients should be treated with continued antisecretory therapy;
  - PPI maintenance therapy may improve quality of life better than H2 blocker maintenance. (4)[B]
  - Full dose PPIs more effective than 1/2 dose for maintenance (2)[A]
  - In erosive esophagitis, daily maintenance therapy with a PPI has been proven to prevent relapse; intermittent PPI therapy has not been proven effective. (5)[A]
- In terms of symptom reduction, medical and surgical therapy are equally effective. (2)[A]

- Anti-reflux surgery
  - 90–94% symptom response
  - 5% continued symptoms, should have anatomy evaluated by esophogram
  - Long-term follow-up shows some surgically treated patients may eventually require may require medical therapy
- Regression of Barrett's epithelium does not routinely occur despite aggressive medical or surgical therapy.

COMPLICATIONS
- Peptic stricture: 10–15%
- Barrett's esophagus: 10%
  - Adenocarcinoma from Barrett's epithelium (rate of cancer development 0.5% annually)
- Extraesophageal symptoms: 5–10% including asthma, hoarseness, aspiration including aspiration pneumonia
- Bleeding due to mucosal injury
- Noncardiac chest pain

ALERT
Geriatric Considerations
Complications more likely (e.g., aspiration pneumonia)

PATIENT MONITORING
- Follow symptomatically
- Repeat endoscopy at 4–8 weeks for poor symptomatic response to medical therapy, especially in older patients
- Current guideline is endoscopic surveillance every 2–5 years in patients with Barrett's if they would consider treatment if cancer was detected. (1)[B]

REFERENCES

1. Fox M, Forgacs I. Gastro-oesophageal reflux disease. *BMJ.* 2006;332:88–93.
2. Agency for Healthcare Research and Quality. Comparing effectiveness of management stategies for gastroesophageal reflux disease. 2005; available at: http://effectivehealthcare.ahrq.gov. Accessed June 2, 2006.
3. Bais JE, et al. Laparoscopic or conventional Nissen fundoplication for gastro-oesophageal reflux disease: Randomised clinical trial. The Netherlands Antireflux Surgery Study Group. *Lancet.* 2000;355: 170–174.
4. Hansen AN, et al. Long-term management of patients with symptoms of gastroesophageal reflux disease. *Int J Clin Pract.* 2006;60:15–22.
5. Zacny J, et al. Systematic review: the efficacy of intermittent and on-demand therapy with histamine H_2-receptor antagonists or proton pump inhibitors for gastro-oesophageal reflux disease patients. *Aliment Pharmacol Ther.* 2005;21:1299–1312.
6. Mine S, et al. Management of symptoms in step-down therapy of gastroesophageal reflux disease. *J Gastroenterol Hepatol.* 2005;20:1365–1370.

MISCELLANEOUS

CODES

ICD9-CM
- 530.81 Esophageal reflux
- 530.11 Reflux esophagitis
- 530.10 Esophagitis, unspecified
- 750.6 Congenital hiatus hernia
- 787.1 Heartburn

PATIENT TEACHING

Diet
- Chocolate, peppermint, citrus, onions, spicy foods and foods high in fat can make GERD symptoms worse.
- Avoid alcohol and caffeine.
- Eat small meals.
- Avoid lying down soon after meals.
- Elevate head of bed
- Lifestyle changes such as losing weight and smoking cessation

 See Corresponding Diagnostic Algorithm

 See Patient Handout on CD

G

GIANT CELL ARTERITIS

Eric P. Gall, MD

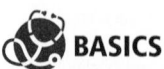 **BASICS**

DESCRIPTION (1)

A systemic granulomatous, predominantly large vessel arteritis, most commonly affecting the branches of the cranial arteries (but may involve other aortic branches), seen primarily in the elderly. Frequently associated with polymyalgia rheumatica (PMR)

- System(s) Affected: Cardiovascular; Hemic/Lymphatic/Immunologic; Musculoskeletal; Nervous
- Synonym(s): Temporal arteritis; Horton headache

EPIDEMIOLOGY

- Predominant age: >60 (very rare <50 years). Incidence increases with age.
- Predominant sex: Female > Male (2:1)

Pediatric Considerations

Does not occur in this age group

Incidence

- More common in northern latitudes (15–30/100,000 person >50 years per year) vs. southern latitudes (<2/100,000 in some series)
- Primarily white, Northern European descent

Geriatric Considerations

Incidence increases with age (twice as common in patients >80 years as it is in ages 50–59 years)

RISK FACTORS

- Age >50 years
- Presence of polymyalgia rheumatica

Genetics

May be important; several family clusters have been identified; Northern European ancestry

ETIOLOGY

- Unknown
- Possibly immunologic mechanism
- Cytokine L

ASSOCIATED CONDITIONS

Polymyalgia rheumatica

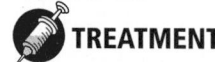 **DIAGNOSIS**

SIGNS AND SYMPTOMS (2)

- Onset may be abrupt or insidious over months.
- Local
  - Headache (usually unilateral temporal, may be generalized or occipital) seen in 2/3 of patients
  - Jaw/tongue "claudication" on mastication (fairly specific)
  - Visual disturbances: Early (amaurosis fugax, scotoma, diplopia) or late (ischemic optic neuritis, blindness)
  - Scalp tenderness
  - Swollen, red temporal artery (rare)
  - Decreased temporal artery pulse (may be increased early)
  - Sore throat, cough (10%)
  - Neurologic manifestations: Transient ischemic attack, stroke
- Systemic
  - Polymyalgia rheumatica: Seen in 40–60%
  - Fever (low grade): 15% with fever of unknown origin
  - Fatigue/malaise
  - Weight loss/anorexia
  - Arthralgias, myalgias, arthritis

Physical Exam

Tender temporal artery

TESTS

Lab

- Erythrocyte sedimentation rate (ESR; Westergren) usually >50 mm/h (may be >100 mm/h):
  - Westergren ESR is preferable. If other ESR used (e.g., Wintrobe), then cannot use the listed guidelines for abnormalities.
- ESR may be normal in <10% of patients.
- Elevated alkaline phosphatase >1.5 times normal (unusual)
- Elevated aspartate aminotransferase >1.5 times normal (unusual)
- Anemia
  - Mild to moderate
  - Normochromic/normocytic
- Mild leukocytosis
- Mild thrombocytosis
- Drugs that may alter lab results
  - Prednisone, methotrexate, other immunosuppressives
- Disorders that may alter lab results
  - Tumor, infection, and serum protein abnormalities all raise the ESR.
  - Congestive heart failure (CHF), microcytic anemia, and hemoglobinopathy may lower ESR.

Imaging

Temporal arteriography (in selected cases)

Diagnostic Procedures/Surgery

- Temporal artery biopsy
  - Minimum 2.5-cm segment of vessel with serial sections
  - Within 96 hours of starting steroids
  - If negative, must consider biopsy of contralateral artery (may increase yield up to 10–14%)

Pathological Findings

- Inflammatory infiltrate (either mononuclear cells or granulomas with giant multinucleated cells) seen in the intima and media of large vessels with resultant disruption of the internal elastic lamina. Lesions may be isolated (e.g., skip lesions).
- Biopsy may not show evidence of active arteritis. However, changes of healing arteritis or vasculitis support the diagnosis of giant cell arteritis. If it is a clinically active disease (headache, jaw claudication, elevated ESR), treat it as a giant cell arteritis and use high-dose steroids.

DIFFERENTIAL DIAGNOSIS

- Cerebral vasculitides
- Other causes of headache (tumor, other space-occupying lesions, sinusitis, cervical or temporomandibular joint arthritis)
- Cerebral vascular insufficiency
- Other connective tissue disease
- Retinal detachment or other causes of loss of vision
- Septic arteritis
- Embolic disease

TREATMENT

GENERAL MEASURES

Institute surveillance for corticosteroid side effects, including osteoporosis screening.

Diet

- Appropriate salt restriction
- Adequate calcium intake (1,500 mg/d)
- Watch serum glucose.

Activity

Ambulatory ad lib

MEDICATION (DRUGS)

First Line
- Prednisone—early
  - 60 mg prednisone per day; single morning dose (never use every-other-day steroids)
  - Begin slow taper after 6–8 weeks if asymptomatic and ESR decreased (occasionally patient may not normalize ESR).
- Prednisone—taper
  - Taper initially by 5 mg every 2 weeks to dose of 25 mg. Then slow taper by 2.5-mg decrements every 2–4 weeks to a dose of 10–15 mg if guidelines described in preceding sections are met (must be individualized).
  - Continue 10–15 mg daily for several months to a year, with periodic attempts to taper (e.g., every 3–6 months) by 1–2 mg.
  - Use symptoms and ESR to help guide taper.
  - Average time to disease remission: 3–4 years, range 1–10 years
- Contraindications
  - Systemic fungal infections, although physician must evaluate risks and benefits
  - Relative contraindications: Avoid, if possible, in patients with CHF, diabetes mellitus, systemic fungal or bacterial infection (must treat infection concurrently if steroids are necessary).
- Precautions
  - Long-term steroid use
    - Associated with several potentially severe adverse effects, including increased susceptibility to infection, glucose intolerance, adrenal suppression, muscle wasting, osteoporosis, peptic ulcer disease, sodium and water retention, cataracts, avascular necrosis, gastrointestinal bleeding, psychosis, weight gain
    - Use lowest possible dose
    - On discontinuing, if the patient has received long-term therapy, taper slowly to avoid addisonian crisis. May need temporary stress-dose steroids for surgical procedures, accidents, or severe infections
- Significant possible interactions
  - Refer to the manufacturer's literature.

Second Line
Methotrexate only if patient cannot use steroids (brittle diabetes mellitus, severe osteoporosis, CHF, etc.) or fails to respond to steroids. (3)

SURGERY
Temporal artery biopsy

 ## FOLLOW-UP

DISPOSITION
- Outpatient surgery (initially for temporal artery biopsy).
- With reasonable suspicion, immediately institute high-dose corticosteroid therapy while arranging temporal artery biopsy.

PROGNOSIS
- With early treatment, resolution of symptoms and preservation of vision
- Average length of disease 3–4 years
- With no treatment, high risks of blindness and stroke
- Occasionally ESR elevation is not related to giant cell arteritis activity and cannot be used to monitor and/or adjust treatment.

COMPLICATIONS
- Complications related to steroids
- Exacerbation of disease during therapy or taper
- Blindness
- Stroke

PATIENT MONITORING
- ESR
  - Repeat monthly initially and while tapering, then every 3 months.
- Follow visual/constitutional symptoms monthly initially, then as needed.

REFERENCES

1. Hellman DB, Hunder GG. Chapter 82: Giant cell arteritis and polymyalgia rheumatica. In: Harris ED, Budd RC, Firestein GS, et al., eds. *Textbook of Rheumatology.* 7th ed. Philadelphia, PA: WB Saunders; 2005:1343–1356. (Level 1,2,3)
2. Gonzales-Gay MA, et al. Giant cell arteritis: Disease patterns of clinical presentation in a series of 240 patients. *Medicine.* 2005;84:269.
3. Spiera RF, et al. A prospective, randomized, placebo contolled trial of methotrexate in the treatment of Giant Cell. *Arteritis Clin Exp Rheumatol.* 2001;19:495.
4. Hunder GG, et al. The American College of Rheumatology 1990 criteria for the classification of giant cell arteritis. *Arthritis Rheum.* 1990;33:1122–1128.

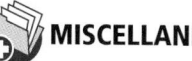 ## MISCELLANEOUS

See also: Depression; Fibromyalgia; Headache, cluster; Headache, Tension; Polymyalgia rheumatica; Polymyositis/Dermatomyositis

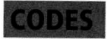 **CODES**

ICD9-CM
446.5 Giant cell arteritis

PATIENT TEACHING
- Precautions regarding steroid use, especially osteoporosis
- Exacerbation of disease with medication dose adjustment
- Adrenal suppression: Patients should wear a medical alert bracelet or neck tag.
- With CNS symptoms or headache, instruct patient to call physician immediately for adjustment of steroid dose.
- Excellent material available from Arthritis Foundation, http://www.arthritis.org
- If headache or visual changes recur on treatment, immediate action is required to increse therapy under a physicians guidance.

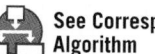 **See Corresponding Diagnostic Algorithm**

G

GIARDIASIS

Rodney D. Adam, MD

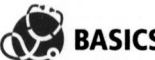 **BASICS**

DESCRIPTION

- Intestinal infection caused by the protozoan parasite *Giardia lamblia* (1,2)
- Infection results from ingestion of the cysts that excyst into trophozoites that colonize the small intestine and cause the symptoms.
- Cycle is continued when the trophozoites encyst in the small intestine and water, food, or hands are contaminated by feces of the infected person.
- Most infections result from fecal-oral transmission or ingestion of contaminated water and are less commonly the result of contaminated food.

ALERT

Pediatric Considerations
Most common in early childhood

Pregnancy Considerations
Concern for potential teratogenicity of medications; consult infectious disease specialist or gastroenterologist for symptomatic disease

GENERAL PREVENTION

- Good hand washing when caring for diapered children
- Water purification when camping and when traveling to developing countries

EPIDEMIOLOGY

- Predominant age: All ages, but most common in early childhood
- Predominant sex: Males > Females (slightly)

Prevalence
Five percent of patients with stools submitted for ova and parasite exams; overall prevalence is lower and variable

RISK FACTORS

- Day care centers
- Anal intercourse
- Wilderness camping
- Travel to developing countries

ETIOLOGY
Protozoan parasite (*G. lamblia*) infection acquired through fecal-oral transmission or ingestion of contaminated water, less commonly from contaminated food

ASSOCIATED CONDITIONS
Hypogammaglobulinemia and possibly IgA deficiency; diarrhea more severe and prolonged in these patients

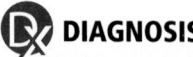 **DIAGNOSIS**

SIGNS AND SYMPTOMS

- ~25–50% of infected persons are symptomatic
- Chronic diarrhea (lasting >5–7 days and frequently weeks)
- Abdominal bloating
- Flatulence
- Loose, greasy, foul-smelling stools
- Weight loss
- Nausea
- Lactose intolerance

TESTS
String test (Entero-Test): A gelatin capsule on a string is swallowed and left in the duodenum for several hours or overnight.

Lab
- Stool for ova and parasites
  - Repeated 3 times if necessary
  - Cysts are seen in fixed or fresh stools, and, occasionally, trophozoites are found in fresh diarrheal stools.
- Fluorescent antibody (FA) and enzyme-linked immunosorbent assay (ELISA) tests of fecal specimens are available. A single FA or ELISA is at least as sensitive as 3 stools for ova and parasites.
- Drugs that may alter lab results: A number of drugs interfere with stool exams.

Diagnostic Procedures/Surgery
Esophagogastroduodenoscopy with biopsy and sample of small intestinal fluid

Pathological Findings
Intestinal biopsy shows flattened, mild lymphocytic infiltration and trophozoites on the surface

DIFFERENTIAL DIAGNOSIS

- Includes other etiologies of small intestinal diarrhea
- Infectious causes include cryptosporidiosis, isosporiasis, and cyclosporiasis.
- Other causes of malabsorption include celiac sprue, tropical sprue, bacterial overgrowth syndromes, and Crohn ileitis.
- Irritable bowel is suspected when diarrhea is not accompanied by weight loss.

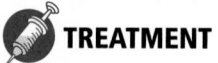 **TREATMENT**

Outpatient for mild cases, inpatient if symptoms are severe

GENERAL MEASURES

- Medical therapy for all infected individuals
- Fluid replacement if dehydrated

Diet
Good nutrition, low lactose, low fat

Activity
As tolerated

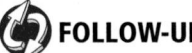 ## MEDICATION (DRUGS)

First Line (3)[A]

- Metronidazole (Flagyl): 250 mg t.i.d. for 5–7 days
- Tinidazole 2 g single dose (50 mg/kg up to 2 g for children)
- Contraindications: Relatively contraindicated in pregnancy, especially 1st trimester
- Precautions
  – Rare toxic psychosis with quinacrine
  – Theoretical risk of carcinogenesis with metronidazole
- Significant possible interactions: Occasional disulfiram reaction with metronidazole or tinidazole

Second Line

- Furazolidone: 8 mg/kg/d t.i.d. for 10 days (slightly less effective, but commonly used in pediatrics, because it is well tolerated)
- Paromomycin (Humatin): A nonabsorbable aminoglycoside that is probably less effective, but commonly recommended in pregnancy because of theoretical risk of teratogenicity of other agents
- Quinacrine: 100 mg t.i.d. for 5–7 days; was the treatment of choice for giardiasis, but is not available from most pharmacies in the US
- Albendazole: 400 mg/d for 5 days; Antihelminthic drug that may be as effective as metronidazole and better tolerated.
- Nitazoxanide suspension was approved by the Food and Drug Administration in 2003 for treatment of giardiasis in children ages 1–11. Children ages 1–4 receive 100 mg b.i.d. and ages 5–11 receive 200 mg b.i.d. for 3 days.

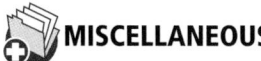 ## FOLLOW-UP

PROGNOSIS

- Untreated giardiasis lasts for weeks
- Patients usually (90%) respond to treatment within a few days.
- Most nonresponders or relapses respond to a 2nd course with the same or a different agent.

COMPLICATIONS

Malabsorption and weight loss

PATIENT MONITORING

Symptoms, weight, stool exams

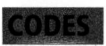 ## REFERENCES

1. Adam RD. The biology of *Giardia lamblia*. *Clin Microbiol Rev*. 2001;14:447–475.
2. Ortega I, Adam RD. Giardia: Overview and update. *Clin Infect Dis*. 1997;25:545–549.
3. Gardner TB, Hill DR. Treatment of giardiasis. *Clin Microbiol Rev*. 2001;14:114–128.

 ## MISCELLANEOUS

Other notes: *G. lamblia* is also called *G. duodenalis* and *G. intestinalis*.

CODES

ICD9-CM

007.1 Giardiasis

PATIENT TEACHING

See Corresponding Diagnostic Algorithm

G

GILBERT DISEASE

Robert A. Marlow, MD, MA

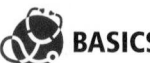 **BASICS**

DESCRIPTION
Mild chronic or intermittent unconjugated hyperbilirubinemia (not due to hemolysis) with otherwise normal liver function

ALERT
Pediatric Considerations
It is rare for the disorder to be diagnosed before puberty.

Pregnancy Considerations
The relative fasting that may occur with morning sickness can elevate the bilirubin level.

EPIDEMIOLOGY
- Predominant age: Present from birth, but most often presents in the 2nd or 3rd decade of life; heterozygous for single abnormal gene
- Predominant sex: Male > Female (2–7:1)

Prevalence
Prevalence in the US: About 7% of the population

RISK FACTORS
Male gender

Genetics
A gene defect resulting in reduced bilirubin uridine diphosphate–glucuronosyltransferase-1 appears to be necessary but not sufficient for Gilbert syndrome. (1)

ETIOLOGY
The hyperbilirubinemia results from impaired hepatic bilirubin clearance (~30% of normal). Hepatic bilirubin conjugation (glucuronidation) is reduced, although this is likely not the only defect.

ASSOCIATED CONDITIONS
Gilbert disease may be part of a spectrum of hereditary disorders that includes types I and II Crigler-Najjar syndrome.

 DIAGNOSIS

SIGNS AND SYMPTOMS
- No significant symptoms, although a variety of nonspecific symptoms have been described
- No abnormal physical findings other than occasional mild jaundice

TESTS
Lab
- Bilirubin: Elevated but <6 mg/dL (103 μmol/L) and usually <3 mg/dL (51 μmol/L), virtually all unconjugated (indirect)
- CBC with peripheral smear is normal.
- Reticulocyte count is normal.
- Liver function tests (aspartate aminotransferase [AST], alanine transaminase [ALT], alkaline phosphatase, γ-glutamyl transpeptidase [GGT] are normal.
- Fasting and postprandial serum bile acids are normal.
- Up to 60% of patients have clinically insignificant mild hemolysis that frequently can only be detected with sophisticated red cell survival studies.
- Drugs that may alter lab results: Bilirubin level may be raised by nicotinic acid and lowered by phenobarbital.
- Disorders that may alter lab results: Bilirubin levels increase during fasting and may increase during a febrile illness.

Diagnostic Procedures/Surgery
- A liver biopsy is not usually needed to exclude other diagnoses.
- Some clinicians recommend confirming the diagnosis by reducing daily caloric intake to 400 kcal for 48 hours, which results in a 2–3-fold increase in unconjugated bilirubin.
- After 12 hours of fasting, an increase of total bilirubin to >1.9 mg/dL 2 hours after an oral dose of rifampin 900 mg distinguishes patients with Gilbert disease with a sensitivity of 100% and a specificity of 100%. (4)

Pathological Findings
None

DIFFERENTIAL DIAGNOSIS
- Hemolysis
- Ineffective erythropoiesis (megaloblastic anemias, certain porphyrias, thalassemia major, sideroblastic anemia, severe lead poisoning, congenital dyserythropoietic anemias)
- Cirrhosis
- Chronic persistent hepatitis
- Pancreatitis
- Biliary tract disease

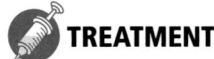 ## TREATMENT

Outpatient. The most important treatment is to make a positive diagnosis of Gilbert disease to reassure the patient and prevent further unnecessary procedures.

 ## FOLLOW-UP

PROGNOSIS
The disorder is benign with an excellent prognosis.

COMPLICATIONS
No known complications

PATIENT MONITORING
If history, physical examination, and laboratory tests are normal, see the patient on 2–3 further occasions during the ensuing 12–18 months. If the patient develops no symptoms, reticulocytosis or new liver function abnormalities, make the diagnosis of Gilbert disease.

REFERENCES

1. Bosma PJ, et al. The genetic basis of the reduced expression of bilirubin UDP-glucuronosyltransferase-1 in Gilbert's syndrome. *N Engl J Med*. 1995;333: 1171–1175.
2. Okolicsanyi L, et al. How should mild, isolated unconjugated hyperbilirubinemia be investigated? *Semin Liver Dis*. 1983;3:36–41.
3. Watson KJR, Gollan JL. Gilbert's syndrome. *Bailliere's Clin Gastroenterol*. 1989;3:337–355.
4. Murthy BD, et al. The utility of rifampin in diagnosing Gilbert's syndrome. *Am J Gastroenterol*. 2001;96:1150–1154.

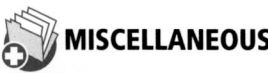 ## MISCELLANEOUS

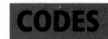 **CODES**

ICD9-CM
277.4 Disorders of bilirubin excretion

PATIENT TEACHING

Reassure the patient that the condition is benign with no known sequelae.

 See Corresponding Diagnostic Algorithm

G

GINGIVITIS

Hugh J. Silk, MD, FAAFP

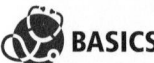 **BASICS**

DESCRIPTION

- A reversible form of Inflammation of the gingiva. A mild form of periodontal disease.
- Classification includes
  - Plaque induced
  - Not plaque induced (acute necrotizing gingivitis, denture related)
  - Modified by systemic factors (pregnancy, HIV, diabetes, leukemia)
  - Modified by medications (antihypertensives, antipsychotics, antiepileptics, hormones)
  - Modified by malnutrition (vitamin deficiencies)
- System(s) Affected: Gastrointestinal
- Synonym(s): Mild periodontal disease

ALERT

Geriatric Considerations
More frequent in this age group (owing more to lifelong accumulation than increased susceptibility)

Pediatric Considerations
Mild cases common in children (most common form of periodontal disease) and usually require no specific interventions

Pregnancy Considerations
Characteristics
- Hyperplasia
- Common; self-limited
- Pedunculated growths (pyogenic granuloma)

GENERAL PREVENTION
- Good oral hygiene, daily brushing and flossing (including correct size toothbrush, parental supervision for children)
- Cleaning by a dentist or hygienist every 6 months or sooner

EPIDEMIOLOGY
- Predominant age: >35 (but as young as 5)
- Predominant sex: Male = Female

Prevalence
- ~50% of children and adult population
- ~90% of adolescents

RISK FACTORS
- Poor dental hygiene
- Diabetes mellitus
- Malocclusion or dental crowding
- Smoking
- Mouth breathing
- Faulty dental restoration
- HIV positive; AIDS
- Pregnancy
- Stress
- Dental appliances (dentures, braces)

Genetics
Possible genetic link (up to 30% of population)

PATHOPHYSIOLOGY
Inflammation of gingiva that may progress to other sites

ETIOLOGY
- Noncontagious
- Inadequate plaque removal
- Blood dyscrasias (pregnancy)
- Reaction to oral contraceptives
- Allergic reactions
- Endocrine disturbances
  - → Pregnancy
  - Menses
  - Menarche
- Chronic debilitating disease
- Vincent disease
  - Fusiform bacillus or spirochete infection

ASSOCIATED CONDITIONS
- Periodontitis
- Glossitis

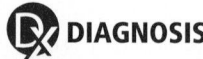 **DIAGNOSIS**

SIGNS AND SYMPTOMS
- Gum swelling and edema (usually painless)
- Gum redness
- Change of normal gum contours
- Plaque and calculus (not easily removed)
- Gum bleeding when flossing or brushing
- Edema of interdental papillae
- HIV gingivitis: Narrow band of bright red inflamed gum surrounding neck of tooth
- Mouth odor (especially in Vincent disease)
- Vincent disease
  - Ulcers
  - Fever
  - Malaise
  - Regional lymphadenopathy
  - Pain

TESTS

Lab
Possible smear or culture to identify causative agent (HIV gingivitis includes Gram-negative anaerobes, enteric strains, and *Candida*)

Pathological Findings
- Acute or chronic inflammation
- Hyperemic capillaries
- Polymorphonuclear infiltration
- Papillary projections in subepithelial tissue
- Fibroblasts

DIFFERENTIAL DIAGNOSIS
- Periodontitis (progression of gingivitis to connective tissue, ligaments, and alveolar bone)
- Glossitis
- Pericoronitis
- Specific forms of gingivitis: See "Description," including acute necrotizing ulcerative gingivitis (Vincent disease) and HIV gingivitis (linear gingival erythema)

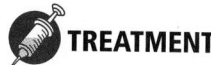 **TREATMENT**

GENERAL MEASURES
- Remove irritating factors (plaque, calculus, faulty dentures)
- Good oral hygiene
- Regular dental checkups
- No smoking
- Warm saline rinses b.i.d.
- Prophylaxis by dental hygienist
- Debridement for acute necrotizing ulcerative gingivitis

Diet
Ensure proper nutrition including adequate vitamins and minerals

Activity
No restrictions

 MEDICATION (DRUGS)

First Line
- Antibiotics indicated only for acute necrotizing ulcerative gingivitis (Vincent disease)
- Antibiotics
  - Penicillin V: Pediatric dose, 25–50 mg/kg/d divided q6h; adult dose 250–500 mg q6h, or
  - Erythromycin: Pediatric dose 30–40 mg/kg/d divided q6h; adult dose 250 mg q6h
- Topical corticosteroids
  - Triamcinolone (0.147 mg/g) in Orabase (spray), applied locally t.i.d., q.i.d.
- Contraindications
  - Allergy to antibiotics
- Precautions
  - Erythromycin frequently causes significant gastrointestinal issues.
- Significant possible interactions: Refer to the manufacturer's literature
- Chlorhexidine rinses may be used.

Second Line
Other antibiotics according to culture or smear

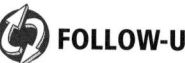 **FOLLOW-UP**

DISPOSITION
Outpatient

PROGNOSIS
- Usual course: Acute; relapsing; intermittent; chronic
- Prognosis: Generally favorable, responds well to appropriate treatment
- Left untreated, major cause of tooth loss

COMPLICATIONS
Severe periodontal disease

PATIENT MONITORING
Until clear; ensure dentist follow-up

REFERENCES
1. Obernesser MS. Gingivitis and periodontitis syndromes in adults. Updated 6/2005.
2. Genco RJ. Current view of risk factors for periodontal diseases. *J Periodontal.* 1996;67:1041.
3. Armitage GC. Development of a classification system for periodontal diseases and conditions. *Ann Periodontal.* 1999;4:1.
4. Griffen A. Overview of gingivitis in children and adolescents. *Up to Date.* Updated 3/2006.
5. Oliver RC, Brown LJ, Loe H. Periodontal disease in the United States population. *J Periodontal.* 1998;69:269.

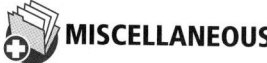 **MISCELLANEOUS**

See also: Glossitis

CODES

ICD9-CM
- 523.00 Acute gingivitis, plaque induced
- 523.01 Acute gingivitis, non–plaque induced
- 523.10 Chronic gingivitis, plaque induced
- 523.11 Chronic gingivitis, non–plaque induced

PATIENT TEACHING
Printable and viewable patient information available under "periodontal diseases" from the American Dental Association at www.ada.org; and the American Academy of Periodontology at www.perio.org

Diet
Well-balanced diet that includes fruits, vegetables, vitamin C

Prevention
- Regular brushing with fluoride toothpaste (parental supervision for children)
- Regular flossing
- Regular dental visits

 See Corresponding Diagnostic Algorithm

G

GLAUCOMA, PRIMARY ANGLE-CLOSURE

Nicole M. Nolan, PharmD

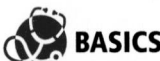 **BASICS**

DESCRIPTION
- Acute-angle closure*:
  - At least 2 of the following symptoms: Ocular pain; N/V; intermittent blurred vision with halos; *plus:*
  - At least 3 of the following signs: IOP >21 mm Hg; conjunctival injection; corneal epithelial edema; mid-dilated nonreactive pupil; shallower chamber in the presence of occlusion
- Primary angle closure*:
  - Occludable drainage angle *plus* signs that the peripheral iris has obstructed the trabecular meshwork (e.g.., elevated IOP, lens opacities)
- Chronic angle-closure glaucoma:
  - Refers to an eye with permanent closure of areas of the anterior chamber angle by peripheral anterior synechiae

* The term *glaucoma* is added when glaucomatous optic neuropathy is present.

ALERT
Geriatric Considerations
Increased risk with age and prior history of cataract or ocular surgery

Pediatric Considerations
Rare

Pregnancy Considerations
Medications used may cross the placenta and be excreted into breast milk

GENERAL PREVENTION
Routine eye exam for high-risk populations

EPIDEMIOLOGY
- 6th and 7th decade of life
- Female > Male
- Inuit and Asian > African and European

Incidence
10% of all glaucoma cases in the US

Prevalence
Acute angle closure glaucoma occurs in
- 1 in 1000 Caucasians
- 1 in 100 Asians
- 2–4 of 100 Eskimos

RISK FACTORS
- Small cornea
- Hyperopia
- Shallow peripheral anterior chamber
- Advancing age
- Female sex
- Cataract
- Iris and ciliary body cysts
- Medications that may induce angle-closure glaucoma
  - ACE inhibitors (rare)
  - Adrenergic agonists (albuterol)
  - Anticholinergics
  - Antihistamines
  - Antidepressants: SSRIs, TCAs
  - Cholinergic agents (pilocarpine)
  - Noncatecholamine adrenergic agonists
  - Sulfa-based drugs
  - Topiramate
  - Warfarin (rare)

Genetics
Polygenic inheritance: 1st-degree relatives have a 2–5% lifetime risk.

PATHOPHYSIOLOGY
- Obstruction of aqueous humor outflow through the trabecular meshwork by peripheral iris apposition to the cornea, which causes elevation in IOP.
- The underlying mechanism is pupillary block, in which aqueous egress through the pupil is limited, causing forward iris displacement.

ETIOLOGY
Predisposing ocular anatomy

ASSOCIATED CONDITIONS
- Cataract
- Microphthalmos
- Hyperopia

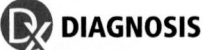 **DIAGNOSIS**

PRE HOSPITAL
- High index of suspicion of diagnosis
- Thorough ophthalmologic history and physical

SIGNS AND SYMPTOMS
- Acute
  - Ocular pain
  - Blurred vision
  - Lacrimation
  - Halos around lights
  - Frontal headache
  - Nausea and vomiting
  - Elevated intraocular pressure (usually 40–80 mm Hg)
  - Corneal microcystic edema
  - Lid edema, conjunctival hyperemia, and circumcorneal injection
  - Fixed mid-dilated pupil, often oval
  - Shallow anterior chamber, often with inflammatory reaction
- Chronic
  - May have symptoms of subacute form or may be asymptomatic
  - Multiple peripheral anterior synechiae
  - Normal or elevated intraocular pressure
  - Increased cup-to-disc ratio
  - Normal pupil

History
- Patient's previous medical and ophthalmologic history
- Family history of glaucoma
- Obtain history of Rx and OTC medications
- Review of symptoms

Physical Exam
Includes but not limited to the following, in the undilated eye (1)[C]
- Visual acuity
- Pupil size and reactivity
- External examination
- Slit-lamp biomicroscopy
- Determination of IOP
- Gonioscopy
- Visual field
- Evaluation of optic nerve head

TESTS
Lab
None
Imaging
None
Diagnostic Procedures/Surgery
Careful ophthalmic examination including indentation gonioscopy and tonometry (1)[C].
Pathological Findings
- Corneal stromal and epithelial edema
- Endothelial cell loss
- Iris stromal necrosis
- Anterior subcapsular cataract (glaukomflecken)
- Optic disc congestion, cupping
- Optic nerve atrophy

DIFFERENTIAL DIAGNOSIS
- Acute orbital compartment syndrome
- Conjunctivitis
- Corneal abrasion
- Glaucoma, malignant or neovascular
- Herpes zoster ophthalmicus
- Iritis and uveitis
- Orbital/periorbital infection
- Plateau iris syndrome
- Vitreous hemorrhage

 ## TREATMENT
- Obtain immediate ophthalmology consult
- Ocular goals of therapy through medical and surgical treatment
  - Reduce IOP to <35 mm Hg
  - Prevent damage to the optic nerve
  - Prevent or reverse angle closure

PRE HOSPITAL
- Initiate immediate emergency ophthalmologic treatment.
- Keep patient supine.
- Patch affected eye.

INITIAL STABILIZATION
- Initiate medical therapy first, using some or all of the following: (1)[C], (2)[B]
  - Systemic carbonic anhydrase inhibitor
  - Topical β-blocker
  - Topical α-agonist
  - Topical miotic
  - Systemic hyperosmotic agent
- Laser peripheral iridectomy per ophthalmology (1, 2)[B]

GENERAL MEASURES
For acute form
- Manage extraocular symptoms, such as nausea
Diet
Usual for patient
Activity
For acute form
- Maintain rest
Nursing
Implement emergency ophthalmic plan of care.

SPECIAL THERAPY
IV Fluids
IV access

 ## MEDICATION (DRUGS)
- Carbonic anhydrase inhibitors
  - Acetazolamide (Diamox) 500 mg IV plus/or 500 mg PO; dorzolamide 2% eyedrops, 1 drop in affected eye q8h
- β-Blockers
  - Timolol (Timoptic) 0.5% solution, levobunolol (Betagan) 0.5% solution, or betaxolol (Betoptic) 0.5% solution; 1 drop in affected eye q12h
- α-Agonist
  - Apraclonidine (Iopidine) 0.5–1% solution, 1 drop in affected eye q8h
- Miotics
  - Pilocarpine (2–4% solution, 1 drop in affected eye q6–8h
- Hyperosmotic agents
  - Glycerin, 1–2 g/kg PO, repeat q5h p.r.n.; Isosorbide, 1.5 g/kg PO; mannitol 20% solution, 1.5–2 g/kg over 30 minutes
- Precautions/contraindications
  - Carbonic anhydrase inhibitor: Caution in patient with metabolic acidosis
  - β-Blockers: Caution in patients with COPD, asthma, or cardiac history
  - Miotics: May paradoxically worsen the condition
  - Hyperosmotics
    ○ Glycerin: Caution in patients with CHF or diabetes
    ○ Mannitol: Caution in patients with CHF or renal failure

SURGERY
- Acute (1, 2)[B]
  - Laser peripheral iridectomy
  - Perform surgical iridectomy if laser is not possible
- Chronic: Goniosynechialysis

 ## FOLLOW-UP
DISPOSITION
- Schedule immediate ophthalmologic follow-up.
- Hospital admission if clinically warranted
Admission Criteria
- Patient requires metabolic ± electrolyte monitoring
- Maintain ophthalmology follow-up
Discharge Criteria
Patient is stable for outpatient follow-up
PROGNOSIS
- With adequate treatment, most patients recover lost vision
- Depends on
  - Time to treatment
  - Underlying eye disease
  - Ethnicity

COMPLICATIONS
- Chronic corneal edema
- Corneal fibrosis and vascularization
- Iris atrophy
- Cataract
- Lens subluxation
- Optic atrophy
- Malignant glaucoma
- Central retinal vein occlusion

PATIENT MONITORING
- Postsurgical follow-up
- Fellow eye evaluation
- Chronic monitoring post acute attack per ophthalmology

REFERENCES
1. American Academy of Ophthalmology. Primary angle closure preferred practice pattern. San Francisco: American Academy of Ophthalmology, 2005. Available at: www.aao.org.
2. Saw S, Gazzard G, Friedman DS. Interventions for angle-closure glaucoma: An evidence-based update. Ophthalmology. 2003;110:1869–1879.
3. Tripathi RC, Tripathi BJ, Haggerty C. Drug-induced glaucomas: Mechanism and mana gement. Drug Safety. 2003;26:749–767.

 ## MISCELLANEOUS
See also: Glaucoma, primary open-angle

CODES
ICD9-CM
- 365.22 Glaucoma, acute angle closure
- 365.23 Glaucoma, chronic angle closure

PATIENT TEACHING
- Advise patient to seek emergency medical attention if experiencing a change in visual acuity, blurred vision, eye pain, or headache.
- Medication education
- Proper eyedrop administration technique
- Patient education materials
  - Glaucoma Research Foundation at www.glaucoma.org
  - National Eye Institute at www.nei.nih.gov
Prevention
- Encourage good eye health
- Know family history

 See Corresponding Diagnostic Algorithm

See Patient Handout on CD

G

GLAUCOMA, PRIMARY OPEN-ANGLE (POAG)

Richard W. Allinson, MD

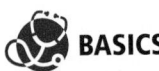 **BASICS**

DESCRIPTION
POAG is an optic neuropathy resulting in visual field loss frequently associated with increased intraocular pressure (IOP). Normal IOP is 10–22 mm Hg. However, glaucomatous optic nerve damage can also occur with normal IOP and as a secondary manifestation of other disorders, such as corticosteroid-induced glaucoma.
- System(s) Affected: Nervous
- Synonym(s): Chronic open-angle glaucoma

ALERT
Pregnancy Considerations
Prostaglandins should be avoided during pregnancy in the treatment of POAG

GENERAL PREVENTION
- Genetic testing may help screen for POAG.
- There may be a reduced risk of open-angle glaucoma with the long-term use of oral statins

EPIDEMIOLOGY
- Predominant age: Usually >40 years of age
- Predominant sex: Male = Female

Incidence
Increases with age

Prevalence
Prevalence of POAG in persons >40 years is ~1.8%.

Geriatric Considerations
Increasing prevalence with increasing age

RISK FACTORS
- Increased IOP
- African American
- Elderly
- Positive family history
- Myopia
- Diabetes mellitus
- Central corneal thickness <555 μm
- Larger vertical cup-to-disc ratio
- Larger horizontal cup-to-disc ratio
- Disc hemorrhage
- Prolonged use of topical, periocular, inhaled, or systemic corticosteroids

Genetics
A family history of glaucoma increases one's risk for developing glaucoma.

PATHOPHYSIOLOGY
Abnormal aqueous outflow resulting in increased IOP. Normally, aqueous is produced by the ciliary epithelium of the ciliary body and is secreted into the posterior chamber of the eye. Aqueous then flows through the pupil and enters the anterior chamber to be drained by the trabecular meshwork in the iridocorneal angle of the eye, into the Schlemm canal, and into the venous system of the episclera. 5–10% of the total aqueous outflow leaves via the uveoscleral pathway.

ETIOLOGY
- Impaired aqueous outflow through the trabecular meshwork
- Increased resistance within the aqueous drainage system

ASSOCIATED CONDITIONS
Diabetes mellitus

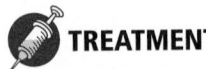 **DIAGNOSIS**

SIGNS AND SYMPTOMS
- Painless, slowly progressive visual loss. Patients are generally unaware of the visual loss until late in the disease, central visual acuity remains unaffected until late in the disease.
- Increased IOP
- Cup-to-disc ratio (C/D) >0.5
- Earliest visual field defects are paracentral scotomas and peripheral nasal steps.

TESTS
Lab
None

Imaging
Optical coherence tomography can be useful in the detection of glaucoma by measuring the thickness of the nerve fiber layer (NFL).
- NFL is thinner in patients with glaucoma.

Diagnostic Procedures/Surgery
- Visual field testing: Perimetry
- Tonometry to measure IOP
- Ophthalmoscopy to assess the optic nerve for glaucomatous damage

Pathological Findings
- Atrophy and cupping of the optic nerve
- Loss of retinal ganglion cells and their axons produces defects in the retinal nerve fiber layer.

DIFFERENTIAL DIAGNOSIS
- Normal-tension glaucoma
- Optic nerve pits
- Anterior ischemic optic neuropathy
- Compressive lesions of the optic nerve or chiasm
- Posthemorrhagic (shock optic neuropathy)

TREATMENT

INITIAL STABILIZATION
Outpatient care

GENERAL MEASURES
- The Early Manifest Glaucoma Trial showed the following
  - Early treatment delays progression
  - The magnitude of initial IOP reduction influences disease progression. (1)[A]
- The Ocular Hypertension Treatment Study showed the following
  - Patients who only had increased IOP in the range of 24–32 mm Hg were treated with topical ocular hypotensive medication.
  - Treatment produced ~20% reduction in IOP.
  - At 5 years, treatment reduced the incidence of POAG by >50%; that is, 9.5% in the observation group vs. 4.4% in the medication-treated group. (2)[A]
- The Collaborative Normal-Tension Glaucoma Study Group showed the following
  - Therapeutic intervention that resulted in a 30% decrease in IOP helped prevent progression of visual field loss. (3)[A]
- The Advanced Glaucoma Intervention Study showed the following
  - Eyes were randomized to laser trabeculoplasty or filtering surgery when medical therapy failed.
  - In follow-up, if the IOP was always <18 mm Hg, the visual fields tended to stabilize. When IOP was >17 mm Hg >1/2 the time, patients tended to have worsening of their visual fields. (4)[A]
  - Whites did better with trabeculectomy first, whereas African Americans did better with argon laser trabeculoplasty as the initial procedure.
- The Collaborative Initial Glaucoma Treatment Study showed the following
  - Both initial medical and surgical treatment achieved significant IOP reduction, and both had little visual field loss over time. (5)[A]

Diet
No restrictions

Activity
No limitations

MEDICATION (DRUGS)

First Line

More than 1 medication, with different mechanisms of action, may be needed. When ≥3 medications are required, compliance is difficult and surgery may be needed. Ocular hypotensive agent categories

- β-Adrenergic antagonists (nonselective and selective); decrease aqueous formation:
  – Timolol, 0.5%, 1 drop in affected eye, q12h
- Parasympathomimetics (miotic), including cholinergic (direct-acting) and anticholinesterase agents (indirect-acting parasympathomimetic), increase aqueous outflow
  – Pilocarpine 1–4%, 1 drop in affected eye, b.i.d.–q.i.d.: Cholinergic
  – Demecarium bromide 0.125%, 1 drop in affected eye b.i.d.: Antichlinesterase
- Carbonic anhydrase inhibitors (oral, topical): Decrease aqueous formation:
  – Acetazolamide 250 mg, PO q.i.d.
  – Dorzolamide 2%, 1 drop t.i.d.
- Adrenergic agonists (nonselective and selective α_2-agonists)
  – Epinephrine 0.5–2%, 1 drop b.i.d., and dipivefrin 0.1%, 1 drop b.i.d.: Nonselective agents that increase aqueous outflow through the trabecular meshwork and increase uveoscleral outflow
  – Brimonidine tartrate 0.15%, 1 drop t.i.d.: α_2-adrenergic agonist; decreases aqueous formation and increases uveoscleral outflow
- Prostaglandin analogues: Enhance uveoscleral outflow:
  – Latanoprost 0.005%, 1 drop at bedtime
- Hyperosmotic agents: Increase blood osmolality, drawing water from the vitreous cavity
  – Mannitol 20% solution, administered IV at 2 gm/kg of body weight
  – Glycerin 50% solution, administered orally. Dosage is usually 4–7 oz.
- Contraindications
  – Nonselective β-adrenergic antagonists: Avoid in asthma, chronic obstructive pulmonary disease, 2nd- and 3rd-degree atrioventricular block, and decompensated heart failure. Betaxolol is a selective β-antagonist and is safer in pulmonary disease
    ◦ Parasympathomimetics (miotic)
    ◦ Indirect-acting parasympathomimetic agents increase risk of ocular and systemic side effects and are rarely used.
  – Carbonic anhydrase inhibitors
    ◦ Do not use with sulfa drug allergies.
    ◦ Do not use with cirrhosis because of the risk of hepatic encephalopathy.
  – Adrenergic agonists: Caution recommended when using brimonidine and monoamine oxidase inhibitor or tricyclic antidepressant and in patients with vascular insufficiency
    ◦ Bormonidine can cause excessive sleepiness and lethargy in children.
  – Prostaglandin analogues: Caution with uveitis and avoided during pregnancy
  – Hyperosmotic agents
    ◦ Glycerin can produce hyperglycemia or ketoacidosis in diabetic patients.
    ◦ Can cause congestive heart failure
    ◦ Do not use in patients with anuria.

- Precautions
  – β-Adrenergic antagonists: Caution with obstructive pulmonary disease, heart failure, and diabetes
  – Parasympathomimetics (miotic) cause pupillary constriction and may cause decreased vision in patients with a cataract and may cause an eye ache or myopia owing to increased accommodation. All miotics break down the blood-aqueous barrier and may induce chronic iridocyclitis.
  – Adrenergic agonists (e.g., brimonidine): Caution with vascular insufficiency
  – Prostaglandin analogues may cause increased pigmentation of the iris and periorbital tissue (eyelid, eyelashes) and should be used with caution in active intraocular inflammation (iritis/uveitis). Caution is also advised in eyes with risk factors for herpes simplex, iritis, and cystoid macular edema. Macular edema may be a complication associated with treatment.
  – Hyperosmotic agents: Caution in diabetics, dehydrated patients, and those with cardiac, renal, and hepatic disease
- Significant possible interactions
  – β-Adrenergic antagonists: Caution in patients taking calcium antagonists because of possible atrioventricular conduction disturbances, left ventricular failure, or hypotension.
  – Parasympathomimetics (miotic): Indirect-acting parasympathomimetic agents, anticholinesterase eye drops, can reduce serum pseudocholinesterase levels. If succinylcholine is used for induction of general anesthesia, prolonged apnea may result.

SURGERY

- Argon laser trabeculoplasty (ALT)
  – Applied to 180° of the trabecular meshwork
  – Improves aqueous outflow
  – The Glaucoma Laser Trial Research Group showed, in newly diagnosed, previously untreated patients with POAG, that ALT was as effective as topical glaucoma medication within the 1st 2 years of follow-up.
  – Usually reserved for patients needing better IOP control while taking topical glaucoma drops
- Trabeculectomy (glaucoma filtering surgery)
  – Usually reserved for patients needing better IOP control after maximal medical therapy and who may have previously undergone an ALT
  – Mitomycin C can be applied at the time of surgery to increase the chances of a surgical success.
- Shunt surgery
  – For example, Molteno and Ahmed devices
  – Generally reserved for difficult glaucoma cases in which conventional filtering surgery has failed or is likely to fail.
- Ciliary body ablation
  – Indicated to lower IOP in patients with poor visual potential or those who are poor candidates for filtering or shunt procedures.

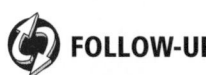 **FOLLOW-UP**

PROGNOSIS

- With standard glaucoma therapy, the rate of visual field loss in POAG is slow.
- Patients may still lose vision and develop blindness, even when treated appropriately
  – The rate of legal blindness from POAG over a follow-up of 22 years was 19%. (6)[B]

COMPLICATIONS
Blindness

PATIENT MONITORING

- Monitor vision and IOP every 3–6 months
- Visual field testing every 6–18 months
- Optic nerve evaluated every 3–18 months, depending on POAG control
- A worsening of the mean deviation by 2 decibels on the Humphrey Field Analyzer and confirmed by a single test after 6 months had a 72% probability of progression
- The IOP response to ocular hypotensive agents tends to be reduced in persons with thicker corneas

REFERENCES

1. Heijl A, et al. Early Manifest Glaucoma Trial Group. Reduction of intraocular pressure and glaucoma progression: Results from the Early Manifest Glaucoma Trial. *Arch Ophthalmol*. 2002;120: 1268–1279.
2. Kass MA, et al. The Ocular Hypertension Treatment Study: A randomized trial determines that topical ocular hypotensive medication delays or prevents the onset of primary open-angle glaucoma. *Arch Ophthalmol*. 2002;120:701–713.
3. Collaborative Normal-Tension Glaucoma Study Group. Comparison of glaucomatous progression between untreated patients with normal-tension glaucoma and patients with therapeutically reduced intraocular pressures. *Am J Ophthalmol*. 1998;126:487–497.
4. The AGIS Investigators. The Advanced Glaucoma Intervention Study (AGIS): 7. The relationship between control of intraocular pressure and visual field deterioration. *Am J Ophthalmol*. 2000;130:429–440.
5. Lichter PR, et al. CIGTS Study Group. Interim clinical outcomes in the Collaborative Initial Glaucoma Treatment Study comparing initial treatment randomized to medications or surgery. *Ophthalmology*. 2001;108:1943–1953.
6. Kwon YH, et al. Rate of visual field loss and long-term visual outcome in primary open-angle glaucoma. *Am J Ophthalmol*. 2001;132:47–56.

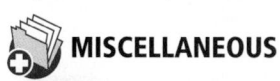 **MISCELLANEOUS**

CODES

ICD9-CM

- 365.00 Preglaucoma, unspecified
- 365.11 Primary open angle glaucoma
- 365.12 Low tension glaucoma
- 377.14 Glaucomatous atrophy (cupping) of optic disc

PATIENT TEACHING

POAG is a silent robber of vision, and patients may not appreciate the significance of their disease until much of their visual field is lost.

 See Corresponding Diagnostic Algorithm

 See Patient Handout on CD

G

GLOMERULONEPHRITIS, ACUTE

Watson C. Arnold, MD

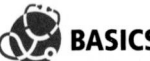 **BASICS**

DESCRIPTION
- An immunologic response to an infection (usually streptococcal) that damages the renal glomeruli
- Can be initiated by other bacterial and viral infections
- This is an immune complex, hypocomplementemic glomerulonephritis
- Most common in children
- Characterized by diffuse inflammatory changes in the glomeruli and clinically by the abrupt onset of hematuria with red blood cell casts and mild proteinuria.
- Accompanied in many cases by hypertension, edema, and azotemia
- Synonym(s): Acute nephritic syndrome; Postinfectious glomerulonephritis; Acute post-streptococcal glomerulonephritis

Pediatric Considerations
Common in children ages 2–16.

GENERAL PREVENTION
Treat streptococcal infections aggressively.

EPIDEMIOLOGY
- Incidence/prevalence in the United States: 20/100,000/year (1–2% of pyodermas and 8% of streptococcal infections in children; occurs with impetigo in the late summer and with streptococcal pharyngitis in the winter)
- Predominant age: 2–12 years old (60%); >40 years (10%)
- Predominant sex: Male > Female (60:40)

RISK FACTORS
- 15% occurrence rate after infection with nephritogenic strain of streptococcus
- Endemic with cyclic epidemics
- Subclinical cases 20 times more common
- Streptococcal infection (e.g., scarlet fever or erysipelas) can be associated with rheumatic fever or acute glomerulonephritis, rarely both

Genetics
No known genetic pattern

ETIOLOGY
- Follows group A beta-hemolytic *Streptococcus* infection
- "Nephritogenic" strains of strep: Groups 1, 4, 11, 12, 49 "Red Lake," 55, 60
- Unusual to have a 2nd attack: Protective immunity to nephritogenic antigen
- Cases of "postinfective" glomerulonephritis have also been reported from *Pneumococcus, Staphylococcus, Meningococcus,* chickenpox, and hepatitis
- Streptococcal infection precedes renal lesions by 1–3 weeks
- Pharyngitis precedes renal lesions by 1–2 weeks (types 1, 2, 4, 12)
- Impetigo (types 49, 55, 57) usually precedes throat or otitis media infection by 2–4 weeks

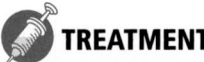 **DIAGNOSIS**

SIGNS AND SYMPTOMS
Classic findings of acute nephritis
- Hematuria: 100%
- Oliguria or anuria: 52%
- Edema: 85%
- Hypertension: 82%
- Hypocomplementemia (C3): 83%
- Gross hematuria: (30%), tea-colored urine
- Edema of face and eyes in the morning, feet and ankles in the afternoons and evenings
- Fever (rare)
  - Other signs and symptoms
    ○ Pharyngitis
    ○ Respiratory infection
    ○ Scarlet fever
    ○ Dark urine
    ○ Weight gain
    ○ Abdominal pain
    ○ Anorexia
    ○ Back pain
    ○ Pallor
    ○ Impetigo

TESTS
Lab
- Streptococcal tests (Streptozyme) that include many antigens are most sensitive (+ or −) for screening but not quantitative
- Antistreptolysin O—quantitative titer
  - Increased in 60–80% of cases
  - Increase begins 1–3 weeks, is highest 3–5 weeks, normal in 6 months
  - Unrelated to severity, duration or prognosis of renal disease
- RBCs casts on urinalysis
  - Destroyed by centrifugation
  - Disintegrate in urine, particularly alkaline urine
- Characteristically, RBCs from glomerular bleeding are distorted while those from lower urinary tract have normal morphology
- Urine protein/creatinine >40, decreased renin
- Culture throat and skin lesions for streptococcus
- C3 and C4 complements are best for evaluation
- Streptozyme
- Hypertriglyceridemia
- Proteinuria
- Decreased glomerular filtration rate
- Uremia
- Increased serum creatinine
- Anemia
- Antinuclear antibody to rule out systemic lupus erythematosus

Imaging
X-rays and/or ultrasound are not necessary to make the diagnosis.

Diagnostic Procedures/Surgery
- If progressive, consider renal biopsy
- Biopsy usually not indicated

Pathological Findings
On renal biopsy
- Diffuse proliferative and exudative glomerulonephritis
- Electron microscopy—subepithelial deposits
- Immunofluorescence—C3 in almost all cases, some with IgG and IgM

DIFFERENTIAL DIAGNOSIS
- Membranoproliferative glomerulonephritis
- Other postinfective glomerulonephritis
- Systemic lupus erythematosus
- IgA nephropathy
- Anaphylactoid purpura
- Rapidly progressive glomerulonephritis

TREATMENT

- Most patients can be safely followed as outpatients
- Inpatient usually until BP and creatinine normalized and edema begins to recede

GENERAL MEASURES
- Decrease salt: No-added-salt diet until edema and hypertension clear
- Decrease fluids to insensible losses plus 2/3 of the urine output until diuresis.
- Control hypertension with diuretics.
- Dialysis: Peritoneal dialysis or hemodialysis for symptomatic azotemia, unresponsive hyperkalemia, intractable acidosis, diuretic resistant pulmonary edema

Diet
- No-added-salt diet until edema, hypertension, and azotemia clear
- Restrict protein in presence of azotemia and metabolic acidosis
- Avoid high-potassium foods

Activity
- Can return to full activity after clinically improved
- May have increased hematuria after exercise for up to 2 years

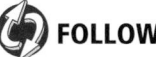 **MEDICATION (DRUGS)**

- Hyperkalemia
  - No potassium in IV fluids until hyperkalemia resolves
  - Sodium polystyrene sulfonate (Kayexalate) resin: 1 g/kg in 10% sorbitol, PR or PO
  - If acidosis present, treat as indicated below
  - Hypocalcemia with symptomatic hyperkalemia: 0.5 cc/kg 10% calcium gluconate IV over 30 minutes
  - Hypocalcemia with asymptomatic hyperkalemia: Oral calcium carbonate (Tums) 1–2 g calcium/day. (Tums have 650 mg calcium/tablet.)
- Pulmonary edema
  - Oxygen
  - Furosemide (Lasix)
  - Digitalization is not effective.
- Peripheral edema
  - Furosemide: 1–2 mg/kg per dose given b.i.d. or t.i.d. PO or IV
  - Treatment with diuretics decreases the duration and severity of edema and hypertension.
- Acidosis: Sodium bicarbonate 1–2 mEq/kg per dose (1–2 mmol/kg per dose) IV over 30 minutes to correct
- Strep infection
  - Give penicillin for 10 days (PO if possible)
  - Erythromycin in penicillin-allergic patients
- Hypertension: Control with diuretics (furosemide 0.5–1 mg/kg IV or 2 mg/kg PO b.i.d. or t.i.d.) and vasodilators (hydralazine [Apresoline] 0.25–1 mg/kg q.i.d. or nifedipine 0.25 mg/kg PO as needed or q.i.d.)

 FOLLOW-UP

PROGNOSIS

- Usually self-limited to 2–3 weeks
- Immediate mortality <0.5%
- Long-term: Excellent in children; almost all patients recover completely
- May have more morbidity in adults or in those with preexisting renal lesions
- Microscopic hematuria may persist for 24 months (or longer with complete recovery)
- Proteinuria persists for up to 3 months
- Symptoms can be exacerbated by a intercurrent illness but rarely after 12 months
- Urine may be darker (microscopic hematuria) after strenuous exercise

COMPLICATIONS

- Hypertensive retinopathy
- Hypertensive encephalopathy
- Rapidly progressive glomerulonephritis
- Abnormal urinalysis may persist for years (microhematuria)
- Chronic renal failure (rare)
- Nephrotic syndrome (~10%)
- Marked decline in glomerular filtration rate (rare)

PATIENT MONITORING

- Depends on severity of disease
- Urinalysis at 2, 4, and 8 weeks and 4, 6, and 12 months
- Stop follow-up when urinalysis is normal
- Monitor BP each visit
- Monitor serum creatinine at 2, 6, and 12 months
- C3 complement should be normal by 6 weeks

REFERENCES

1. Barratt T, Avner E, Harmon W, eds. *Pediatric Nephrology.* 4th ed. Baltimore, MD: Williams & Wilkins; 2000.
2. Brenner B, Rector F, eds. *The Kidney.* 6th ed. Philadelphia, PA: WB Saunders; 2000.

 MISCELLANEOUS

See also: Glomerulonephritis, membranous; Hyperkalemia; Hypertensive emergencies; Hypocalcemia; Renal failure, acute

CODES

ICD9-CM
580.9 Acute glomerulonephritis with unspecified pathological lesion in kidney

PATIENT TEACHING

- National Kidney Foundation, 30 E. 33rd Street, Suite 1100, New York, NY 10016; (212) 889-2210
- Web site: http://www.nlm.nih.gov/medlineplus/ency/article/000484.htm

See Corresponding Diagnostic Algorithm

G

GLOSSITIS

Karyn M. Sullivan, BSP, MPH, RPH
George Abraham, MD

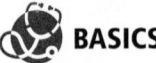 **BASICS**

DESCRIPTION
- An acute or chronic inflammation of the tongue either as primary disease or a symptom of systemic disease.
- System(s) Affected: Gastrointestinal
- Common forms
  - Atrophic glossitis (AG)
  - Benign migratory glossitis (BMG) or geographic tongue
  - Median rhomboid glossitis (MRG)
  - Herpetic geometric glossitis (HGG)

GENERAL PREVENTION
- Evaluation of nutritional status including B-vitamin deficiencies, anemias
- Cessation of tobacco use (including smokeless)
- Assess for irritation from teeth, dentures, or piercings

EPIDEMIOLOGY
- Predominant age: All ages
- Predominant sex
  - Male > Female (MRG)
  - Female > Male (BMG)

ALERT
Geriatric Considerations
Many patients with glossitis due to nutrition deficiencies are postmenopausal or elderly.

Prevalence
Varies; usual reported range: 1– 2.5%

RISK FACTORS
- Poor nutrition
- Dentures
- Piercings
- Allergic background (e.g., asthma, eczema, hay fever)
- Smoking, smokeless tobacco
- Alcoholism
- Anxiety, stress
- Depression
- Hormonal disturbances
- Advancing age
- Immunocompromised state

Genetics
Familial history may be present with BMG.

ETIOLOGY
- Systemic
  - Nutrition deficiencies (e.g., B_{12}, folic acid)
  - Anemia (pernicious, iron deficiency)
  - HIV (opportunistic infections such as candidiasis, herpes simplex virus [HSV]; or HIV-associated changes such as loss of papillae)
  - Broad-spectrum antibiotics
  - Topical or inhaled corticosteroids
  - Various other medications (e.g., captopril, clarithromycin, enalapril, lansoprazole, lithium, metronidazole, NSAIDs)
- Local
  - Infections (e.g., HSV, Epstein-Barr virus [EBV], candidiasis)
  - Trauma (ill-fitting dentures, piercings, burns, convulsive seizures)
  - Primary irritants (alcohol, tobacco, hot foods, spices, excessive peppermint, citrus)
  - Sensitization (chemical irritants, e.g., dyes, mouthwash, toothpaste, systemic drugs)
  - Malignancy (95% are squamous cell)

ASSOCIATED CONDITIONS
- Diabetes mellitus (rare)
- Psoriasis (rare)
- HIV infection (rare)
- Reiter syndrome (rare)
- Down syndrome (rare)
- Crohn disease (rare)

Pediatric Considerations
BMG has been associated with juvenile diabetes.

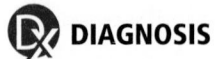 **DIAGNOSIS**

SIGNS AND SYMPTOMS
- Many are asymptomatic
- Oral discomfort
- Burning sensation on tongue
- Sensation of foreign body in the mouth
- Paroxysmal ear pain
- Swollen or painful submandibular lymph nodes

History
Symptoms tend to wax and wane (BMG).

Physical Exam
- AG
  - Smooth, red tongue (3)[B]
- BMG
  - Erythematous and white patches on the dorsum of tongue; lesions may lack papillae; irregular (map-like) and migratory lesions (4)[B]
- MRG
  - Rhomboid-shaped plaque in middle of tongue; hypertrophic or atrophic surface changes (4)[B]
- HGG
  - Linear fissures on dorsal tongue; geometric pattern is common; herpetic lesions usually are absent on other mucosal surfaces (4)[B]

TESTS
Lab
- AG
  - Test for B_{12}, folic acid, iron deficiency (3)[B]
- BMG
  - None (1, 4)[B]
- MRG
  - Viral culture, fungal smear (4)[B]
- HGG
  - Viral culture, Tzanck smear (4)[B]

Diagnostic Procedures/Surgery
- Biopsy solitary lesions that do not respond to treatment (1, 4)[B]
- 10% potassium hydroxide scrapings for suspected candidiasis (3)[B]

Pathological Findings
Vary according to underlying causes

DIFFERENTIAL DIAGNOSIS (1)[B]
- Psoriasis
- Candidiasis
- Reiter syndrome
- Lichen planus
- Leukoplakia
- systemic lupus erythematosus
- Herpes simplex virus
- Drug reaction

ALERT
Pediatric Considerations
Differential diagnosis includes local trauma and severe neutropenia (1)[B].

TREATMENT

INITIAL STABILIZATION
If glossitis is secondary to a severe primary condition, attend to any acute needs of the primary problem.

GENERAL MEASURES
- Outpatient
- Avoid any possible sensitizing irritants or agents (such as acidic or spicy foods and drinks).
- Analgesics when needed
- Request dental evaluation.
- Scrupulous oral hygiene

Diet
Bland or liquid diet

Activity
No restrictions unless systemic infection is present.

MEDICATION

First Line
- AG
  - Vitamin B$_{12}$, folic acid, iron (if deficient)
  - For candidiasis: Nystatin oral suspension 100,000 units/mL (4)[B] swish and spit 5 mL q.i.d. or clotrimazole 1–2 troches 4–5 times a day
- BMG
  - Usually no treatment
  - If lesions recur or no relief occurs with symptomatic treatment, then an antihistamine can be used such as diphenhydramine liquid: Rinse with 5–10 mL, holding it over the tongue for a few minutes and then swallowing, 3–4 times a day (5)[B] or Miracle Mouthwash swish and spit 5 mL, 3–4 times a day
- MRG
  - Usually no treatment
  - Topical antifungals (nystatin oral suspension or clotrimazole troches) may provide temporary improvement (4)[B].
- HGG
  - Oral antivirals such as acyclovir 200 mg 5 times daily (4)[B], (6)[C]

ALERT
Pediatric Considerations
- Diphenhydramine liquid: Rinse with 5–10 mL (depending on age and weight), holding it over the tongue for a few minutes and then swallowing, 3–4 times a day (5)[B]
- Topical antifungal/steroid agent: Triamcinolone acetonide 0.1% in nystatin suspension (7)[B]
- Alkaline saline mouth rinse (7)[B]
- Topical anesthetics/coating agents: 1-to-1 mixture of diphenhydramine liquid and Maalox (7)[B]

- Contraindications
  - Nystatin oral suspension: Hypersensitivity to nystatin products
  - Clotrimazole troche: Hypersensitivity to clotrimazole
  - Diphenhydramine
    - Hypersensitivity to diphenhydramine
    - Newborns or premature infants
    - Nursing mothers
  - Acyclovir (oral): Hypersensitivity to acyclovir or valacyclovir
- Precautions
  - Clotrimazole troche: Hepatic impairment
  - Diphenhydramine
    - May cause excitation in young children
    - Concurrent MAOI therapy
    - Concurrent use of CNS depressants
    - Decreases mental alertness and psychomotor performance
    - Older adults are more susceptible to side effects
    - Bladder neck obstruction
    - Symptomatic prostatic hypertrophy
    - Narrow-angle glaucoma
    - History of bronchial asthma, increased intraocular pressure, hyperthyroidism, cardiovascular disease, or hypertension
  - Acyclovir (oral)
    - Maintain adequate hydration
    - Geriatric patients (due to age-related decline in renal function)
    - Renal impairment
- Significant possible interactions
  - Diphenhydramine: Alcohol (increased sedation)
  - Acyclovir (oral): Meperidine (increased risk of CNS stimulation and seizures)
- Adverse effects
  - Clotrimazole troche
    - Nausea, vomiting, or diarrhea
    - Mild elevations in SGOT levels
  - Diphenhydramine
    - Sedation
    - Dizziness
    - Urinary retention
  - Acyclovir (oral)
    - Nausea, vomiting, and diarrhea
    - Myalgia
    - Transient renal impairment

 ## FOLLOW-UP

PROGNOSIS
Prompt improvement when cause can be identified and treated

COMPLICATIONS
- Recurrence
  - Evaluate for systemic etiology
- Chronicity
  - If not healing, biopsy is indicated

PATIENT MONITORING
- Revisit periodically when needed until healing occurs
- If lesions do not heal, biopsy is indicated.

REFERENCES
1. Assimakopoulos D, Patrikakos G, Fotika C, et al. Benign migratory glossitis or geographic tongue: An enigmatic oral lesion. Am J Med 2002;113: 751–755.
2. Pass B, Brown RS, Childers ELB. Geographic tongue: Literature review and case reports. Dent Today 2005;24 (8):54, 56–57.
3. Terai H, Shimahara M. Atrophic tongue associated with candida. J Oral Pathol Med 2005;34:397–400.
4. Byrd JA, Bruce AJ, Rogers RS 3rd. Glossitis and other tongue disorders. Dermatol Clin 2003;21: 123–134.
5. Sigal MJ, Mock D. Symptomatic benign migratory glossitis: Report of two case reports and literature review. Pediatr Dent 1992;14:392–96.
6. Grossman ME, Stevens AW, Cohen PR. Herpetic Geometric Glossitis. N Engl J Med 1993;329: 1859–1860.
7. Oh TJ, Wang HL. Periodontal diseases in the child and adolescent. J Clin Periodontol 2002;29: 400–410.

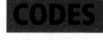 ## MISCELLANEOUS

- See also: Candidiasis; HIV infection and AIDS; Vitamin deficiency
- Other notes: Some symptoms of glossitis have no organic cause. Treat symptoms and reevaluate if no improvement.

CODES

ICD9-CM
529.0 Glossitis

PATIENT TEACHING

Diet
Educate on proper diet and nutrition

Activity
No restrictions

Prevention
Avoid sensitizing irritants

G

GONOCOCCAL INFECTIONS

Geoffrey R. Swain, MD, MPH

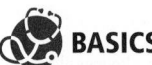 ## BASICS

DESCRIPTION
- Infection of urethra, endocervix, or almost any other mucous-membrane surfaces by *Neisseria gonorrhoeae*. Usually sexually transmitted.
- In women, salpingitis, local extension from endocervical canal to fallopian tubes, is common. Ovaries and surrounding pelvic cavity may be involved with abscess formation. Entire complex of upper genital tract infection is referred to as pelvic inflammatory disease (PID).
- In men, the epididymis may become infected with extension to testicle.
- Pharyngitis may occur in either sex.
- Hematogenous dissemination, while rare, may lead to fever, skin lesions, tendon or joint involvement, endocarditis, or rarely, meningitis.
- Asymptomatic carriers occur in both sexes.
- Gonococcal resistance to penicillins and tetracyclines is common; resistance to quinolones is also common in certain areas and among men who have sex with men (MSM)—consult your state or local health department for local data.
- System(s) Affected: Reproductive, Nervous, Cardiovascular, Musculoskeletal, Skin/Exocrine
- Synonym(s): GC, Clap

GENERAL PREVENTION
- Condoms offer substantial protection.
- Sexual contacts should be treated.

EPIDEMIOLOGY
- Predominant age: 15–29 years
- Predominant sex: Males more often symptomatic; females more often reported

Incidence
Estimated 600,000 new cases per year in US; age-specific rates are as high as 250–600 cases per 100,000 in 15–29 year olds.

RISK FACTORS
- Sexual exposure to an infected individual without barrier protection (condom)
- Multiple sexual partners
- Infants: Passage through infected birth canal
- Children: Sexual abuse by infected individual
- Autoinoculation (finger to eye)
- For PID: Use of intrauterine devices

Genetics
Individuals with congenital deficiency of late components of complement cascade (C7, 8, 9) are prone to dissemination of gonococcal infections.

ETIOLOGY
Neisseria gonorrhoeae (gonococcus)

ASSOCIATED CONDITIONS
Other STIs (chlamydia, syphilis, HIV, hepatitis B, herpes) and vaginal infections

DIAGNOSIS

SIGNS AND SYMPTOMS
- Adolescent and adult males
  - Scant to copious purulent urethral discharge usually present but often absent/subclinical
  - Dysuria or urethral stricture
  - Testicular pain
- Adolescent and adult females without PID
  - Cervical infection often asymptomatic
  - Endocervical discharge (on pelvic exam)
  - Vaginal discharge
  - Dysuria
  - Bartholin gland abscess
- Adolescent and adult females with PID
  - Fever
  - Dysmenorrhea or menometrorrhagia
  - Lower abdominal pain and tenderness
  - Cervical traction tenderness
  - Tender fallopian tubes and/or ovaries
  - Abdominal rebound tenderness
  - Infertility
  - Chronic pelvic pain
- Either sex, if receptive of anal intromission
  - Rectal discharge: Purulent or bloody
  - Tenesmus
  - Rectal burning or itching
  - Asymptomatic rectal infection
- Either sex, other syndromes
  - Pharyngeal infection: Most are asymptomatic; rare sore throat or exudative pharyngitis
  - Eye infection: Purulent discharge, eyelid edema, conjunctivitis, corneal ulceration
  - Disseminated syndromes: Fever, chills, arthralgias (small joints), synovial-sheath tenderness and swelling (hands and/or feet), painful skin lesions (pustular, red, tender), septic arthritis (usually asymmetric, polyarticular, and manifested by joint pain, swelling, and erythema)
  - Endocarditis: Rapid cardiac valve destruction, high fevers
  - Meningitis: Meningeal signs, headache, skin lesions, fever, altered mental status
- Infants and children
  - Eye infection (rare, because of routine ocular prophylaxis in US)
  - Pneumonia (of newborn): Fever, infiltrate on chest radiograph
  - Vulvovaginitis: Vaginal discharge
  - Rectal or pharyngeal infection
  - Endocarditis or meningitis
  - Other forms of disseminated infection similar to adults

TESTS
- Confirmation of isolate as gonococcus by standard bacterial culture, enzymatic tests, or DNA probes. Culture especially important in medico-legal situations such as rape or child abuse, because only culture is ~100% specific.
- Culture and sensitivity testing for antimicrobial susceptibility important in all cases of apparent therapy failure. Resistance to penicillins and tetracyclines is common; quinolone resistance is becoming more common.
- Concurrent testing of HIV and syphilis

Lab
- Nucleic acid amplification tests (NAAT, e.g., PCR, LCR, etc.) and other nucleic acid tests: Sensitivity >93% depending on population. NAAT specificity >99%; can replace culture confirmation in most cases of adult infection. Individual nucleic acid tests may not be approved for other than urethral or endocervical swab specimens.
- Gram stain of smear of exudate from infected mucosal surface showing pairs or clumps of gram-negative kidney-shaped diplococci associated with cytoplasm of polymorphonuclear leukocytes. Adjacent surfaces appear slightly concave. Gram stain specificity ~99%; a positive smear is presumptive evidence of infection. Urethral smear sensitivity in symptomatic male ~95%, but may be quite low in asymptomatic men may be quite low. Sensitivity of endocervical smear ~40%–60%.
- Culture of exudate on selective medium (e.g., modified Thayer-Martin) containing antibiotics to inhibit other microorganisms. Culture sensitivity ~50%, specificity ~100%. Culture should always be done in suspected cases in children.
- Sensitivity of blood culture in disseminated disease: ~50%. Sensitivity of joint fluid culture in septic arthritis: ~50%
- Drugs that may alter lab results: Prior administration of even small amounts of many antibiotics may render a culture falsely negative; NAATs may remain positive up to 4 weeks after antibiotic treatment.

Imaging
Pelvic ultrasound or CT scan may demonstrate thick, dilated fallopian tubes or abscess formation.

Diagnostic Procedures/Surgery
In PID, culdocentesis may demonstrate free purulent exudate and provide material for gram staining and culture. Gram-stained material from unroofed skin lesions may show typical organisms.

Pathological Findings
- Exudate of polymorphonuclear leukocytes is typical.
- In PID: Loss of ciliated columnar epithelium from fallopian tubes. Tubes, pelvic mesentery, and ovaries may be bound together with dense fibrosis and abscess formation.

DIFFERENTIAL DIAGNOSIS
Chlamydia infections (may mimic all aspects of gonococcal infections except disseminated syndromes), urinary tract infections, vaginitis caused by other infectious agents (yeast, trichomonas, bacterial vaginosis)

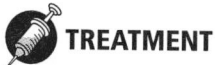
TREATMENT

INITIAL STABILIZATION
- Outpatient for uncomplicated infection, with contact notification and treatment
- Hospitalize for
  - Hematogenously disseminated infection
  - Pneumonia or eye infection in infants
  - PID: If pregnant, significant tubo-ovarian abscess, or unable to take oral medications
- Intensive care for hemodynamic instability or sepsis.

GENERAL MEASURES
- Due to high rate of coinfection, test all patients simultaneously and treat all patients presumptively for *Chlamydia* unless recent prior NAAT test for *Chlamydia* is negative.
- Serologic test for syphilis
- Encourage testing for HIV infection; however, treatment for gonorrhea is the same for HIV$^{+/-}$.

Diet
No special diet

Activity
- Sexual activity: Abstain until after full treatment, plus testing and treatment of partner(s).
- General: Fully active for uncomplicated disease

MEDICATION (DRUGS)

First Line
- Warning: Do not use quinolones for men who had sex with men (MSM), for persons with recent sexual exposure in Hawaii or Pacific coastal states or other areas with high resistance rates, or for others likely to be infected with a quinolone-resistant strain.
- Adults with uncomplicated gonococcal infection of urethra, cervix, or rectum
  - Recommended regimen
    - Single dose of ceftriaxone 125 mg IM *or* cefixime 400 mg PO *or* ciprofloxacin 500 mg PO *or* ofloxacin 400 mg PO *or* levofloxacin 250 mg PO *plus*
    - Agent active against chlamydia, e.g., doxycycline 100 mg PO b.i.d. for 7 days or azithromycin 1.0 g PO as single dose
  - Alternate regimens for gonorrhea include
    - Spectinomycin 2 g IM single dose.
    - Azithromycin 2 g in single dose is effective but often causes GI upset.
    - Other alternate cephalosporin and quinolone regimens are listed in CDC Treatment Guidelines.
  - Note: In pregnancy, ceftriaxone, another cephalosporin, or spectinomycin is treatment of choice.
- Other gonococcal infections in adults
  - Pharyngeal gonorrhea: Single dose of ceftriaxone 125 mg IM *or* ciprofloxacin 500 mg PO, *plus Chlamydia* treatment, is recommended. Spectinomycin is unreliable for treating pharyngeal infections.
  - Conjunctivitis: Ceftriaxone 1 g IM single dose
  - PID: See PID chapter of this text
  - Meningitis: Ceftriaxone 1–2 g IV q12h for 10–14 days
  - Endocarditis: Ceftriaxone 1–2 g IV q12h for 28 days

- Bacteremia and dermatitis/arthritis complex
  - Ceftriaxone 1 g IM or IV daily
  - Alternative regimens include cefotaxime 1 g IV q8h *or* ceftizoxime 1 g IV q8h *or* ciprofloxacin 400 mg IV q12h *or* ofloxacin 400 mg IV q12h *or* levofloxacin 250 mg IV daily *or* spectinomycin 2 g IM q12h.
  - With clinical improvement, complete 7–10 days of therapy with cefixime 400 mg PO b.i.d. *or* ciprofloxacin 500 mg PO b.i.d. or ofloxacin 400 mg b.i.d. *or* levofloxacin 500 mg PO daily, *or* other agents to which infecting organism has proven fully susceptible
- Treatment of Infants and children <45 kg (patients >45kg should receive full adult dose)
  - Uncomplicated genital, pharyngeal, rectal, or conjunctival infection; and infants born to mothers with untreated gonorrhea
    - Ceftriaxone 25–50 mg/kg IM or IV as a single dose, not to exceed 125 mg
    - Alternative: Spectinomycin 40 mg/kg up to 2 g as single IM dose
    - Test and treat also for *Chlamydia*, even in the case of ophthalmia neonatorum
  - Disseminated infections: Ceftriaxone 25–50 mg/kg IV or IM daily or cefotaxime 25 mg/kg IV or IM q12h
    - Bacteremia or dermatitis/arthritis complex: 7 days
    - Meningitis: 10–14 days
    - Endocarditis: 28 d
  - Ophthalmic neonatorum prophylaxis: Single application of
    - 0.5% erythromycin ophthalmic ointment, *or*
    - 1% tetracycline ophthalmic ointment
- Contraindications: Tetracyclines (including doxycycline) are contraindicated in pregnancy and in children. Quinolones are contraindicated in pregnancy and are not recommended for children under 16.
- Precautions and significant possible interactions: Refer to the manufacturer's profile of each drug.

Second Line
See alternatives listed in specific clinical situations above.

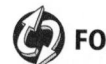
FOLLOW-UP

PROGNOSIS
With adequate, early therapy, complete cure with return to normal function is the rule. However, reinfection is common, particularly among adolescents and young adults.

COMPLICATIONS
- Men: Urethral stricture, epididymitis
- Women: Infertility, tubal ectopic pregnancy
- Corneal scarring after eye infections
- Destruction of joint articular surfaces, cardiac valves
- Death from congestive heart failure (CHF) or meningitis

ALERT
Pregnancy Considerations
PID may lead to infertility, premature labor and delivery, tubal ectopic pregnancy, or fetal loss.

PATIENT MONITORING
Retesting to document cure is not necessary if one of recommended regimens is used unless symptoms persist or concern exists about poor compliance with therapy. Reinfection is common, particularly in adolescents and young adults.

REFERENCES
1. Centers for Disease Control and Prevention (CDC). Sexually transmitted diseases treatment guidelines 2006. *MMWR Recomm Rep* 2006;55(RR11):1–94.
2. Warner L, Stone KM, Macaluso M, et al. Condom use and risk of gonorrhea and chlamydia: A systematic review of design and measurement factors assessed in epidemiologic studies. *Sexually Transmitted Dis* 2006;33(1):36–51.
3. http://www.cdc.gov/nchstp/dstd/Stats_Trends/Stats_and_Trends.htm (accessed August 14, 2006).
4. http://www.city.milwaukee.gov/display/router.asp?docid=15224 (accessed August 14, 2006).
5. Bozicevic I, Fenton KA, Martin IM, et al. Epidemiological correlates of asymptomatic gonorrhea. *Sexually Transmitted Dis* 2006;33(5): 289–295.

MISCELLANEOUS

See also: Chlamydial sexually transmitted diseases, Pelvic inflammatory disease (PID)

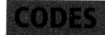
CODES

ICD9-CM
- 098.0 Acute gonococcal infection of lower genitourinary tract
- 614.9 Unspecified inflammatory disease of female pelvic organs and tissue

G

PATIENT TEACHING

Discuss HIV infection and risks; encourage patient and partner(s) to be tested.

See Corresponding Diagnostic Algorithm

GOUT
Bruce M. Rothschild, MD

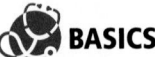 **BASICS**

DESCRIPTION
- Inflammatory reaction to urate crystals in joints, bones, and subcutaneous structures
- Hyperacute arthritis that may progress to a chronic arthritis. Rarely presents as chronic arthritis. Crystals in fluid is pathognomonic.
- Primary gout is the most common: Underexcretion or overproduction of uric acid
- Secondary gout is related to
  - Myeloproliferative diseases
  - Therapeutics inducing hyperuricemia
  - Renal failure
  - Renal tubular disorders
  - Lead poisoning
  - Hyperproliferative skin disorders
  - Enzymatic defects (glycogen storage diseases)

ALERT
Geriatric Considerations
Usually related to medications

Pediatric Considerations
Often inborn error of metabolism or disease

GENERAL PREVENTION
- Avoid exacerbating medications/diets/habits
- Maintain serum uric acid <7

EPIDEMIOLOGY
- Age <18: Rare
- Age 18–44: 3%
- Age 45–64: 21%
- Age >65: 35%
- Predominant age: 30–60
- Predominant sex: Male > Female (20:1)

Prevalence
100/100,000

RISK FACTORS
- Ethanol ingestion
- Family history
- Polynesian extraction (e.g., Samoan gout)
- Medications: Aminophylline, caffeine, corticosteroids, cytotoxic drugs (cyclosporine), diazepam, diphenhydramine, diuretics, L-dopa, dopamine, epinephrine, ethambutol, methaqualone, l-methyldopa, nicotinic acid, probenecid (low dose), pyrazinamide, salicylates, sulfinpyrazone (low dose), vitamins B_{12} and C
- Diuretics induces 20% of secondary gout
- Ketosis
- Surgery or trauma
- Obesity (50%)
- Hypertension (50%)
- Vascular disease
- Diabetes
- Renal failure
- Hypothyroidism
- Hyperparathyroidism; hypoparathyroidism
- Hyperlipidemia types II, IV, V
- Paget disease
- Hyperproliferative skin disorders (psoriasis)
- Lymphoproliferative disorders
- Calcium pyrophosphate deposition disease
- Sarcoidosis
- Hemolytic anemia
- Hemoglobinopathies
- Pernicious anemia
- Radiation treatment
- Type I glycogen storage disease
- Down syndrome
- Gut sterilization by antibiotics

ETIOLOGY
- Hyperuricemia
- Dietary excess (e.g., anchovies, sardines, sweetbreads, kidney, liver, and meat extracts)
- Inborn errors of metabolism
- Lead poisoning (moonshine)
- Kidney disease
- Hemoproliferative disorders
- Dehydration
- Low-dose aspirin

ASSOCIATED CONDITIONS
- Myeloproliferative disorders
- Lymphoproliferative disorders
- Alcoholism
- Hyperlipidemia
- Obesity
- Hypertension
- Diabetes
- Lesch-Nyhan syndrome

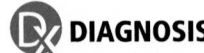 **DIAGNOSIS**

SIGNS AND SYMPTOMS
- Hyperacute onset (within 24 hours) of severe pain, swelling, redness, and warmth in 1 or 2 joints (75% are monoarticular)
- Soft tissue redness, swelling, warmth
- Exquisite tenderness
- Often 1st metatarsophalangeal joint, in 50% of initial attacks; eventually in 75%
- Acute untreated attacks last 2–21 days
- Repetitive attacks often separated by years
- Recurrent attacks last longer and occur more frequently with each recurrence.
- Between attacks, absence of inflammation (until the chronic or tophaceous phase occurs).
- Rarely polyarticular: Proximal interphalangeal, distal interphalangeal, metacarpal phalangeal, wrist, knee, ankle, midtarsal joints, heel
- Migratory polyarthritis is a rare presentation.
- 50% of untreated patients develop chronic arthritis
- Inflammatory synovial effusion
- Subcutaneous or intraosseous nodules (20%), referred to as tophi—may affect ears (antihelix), extensor aspects of peripheral joints (e.g., olecranon), rarely fingertips, cornea, aorta, spine or even intracranial (4)
- Subcutaneous nodules have urate discharge.
- Fever, chills
- Carpal tunnel syndrome
- Kidney stones

TESTS
- Synovial fluid WBC count is usually inflammatory (10,000–70,000 cells/dL), but may have as few as 1,000 WBC/dL.
- Wet mounts of synovial fluid reveal strongly negatively birefringent urate crystals on the polarizing exam.
- Gout crystals may be identified in asymptomatic joints.

Lab
- Hyperuricemia: Induced by drugs that reduce effective circulating blood volume (induced by low-dose aspirin, probenecid, or sulfinpyrazone)
- Cyclosporine-induced renal insufficiency
- Disorders that may alter lab results
  - Intra-articular steroids, alcoholism, sarcoidosis, lead poisoning, kidney failure, psoriasis, hemoglobinopathy

Imaging
- Radiograph is usually normal in the 1st year.
- Radiograph in chronic gout reveals "punched-out" erosions (lytic areas) often with periosteum overgrowing the erosion ("overhanging edge"). Also seen with amyloidosis, type IIa hyperlipoproteinemia, and by multicentric reticulohistiocytosis.
- Radiograph erosions with preservation of joint space; rarely reveals lytic areas (tophi).

Diagnostic Procedures/Surgery
- Arthrocentesis with polarizing optical examination
- Biopsy of synovial membrane or SC nodule, processing the specimen anhydrously (urate is water soluble)

Pathological Findings
- Urate crystals in synovial membrane (98% of specimens processed entirely anhydrously)
- Tophus in 29% with untreated gout of 5 years' duration, in 74% at 40 years' duration

DIFFERENTIAL DIAGNOSIS
- Infectious arthritis
- Pseudogout (calcium pyrophosphate deposition disease)
- Type IIa hyperproteinemia
- Amyloidosis
- Multicentric reticulohistiocytosis
- Hyperparathyroidism
- Spondyloarthropathy
- Rheumatoid arthritis (rarely)

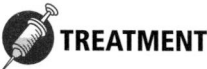 TREATMENT

GENERAL MEASURES
- Control the acute attack of gout.
- Address the underlying cause.

Diet
Reduce ingestion of fat, alcoholic beverages, sardines, anchovies, liver, and sweetbreads.

Activity
Affected joint(s) at rest until hyperacute phase is controlled

 MEDICATION (DRUGS)

First Line
- Acute attack
  – NSAID at full dosage for 2–5 days
  – Once attack is controlled, reduce dose by 1/2
- Chronic treatment
  – Initiate when acute attack controlled (unless kidneys at risk because of unusual uric acid load)
  – Use only if recurrent attacks or evidence of tophaceous or renal disease
  – Patient is tested for uric acid excretion (<600 mg/d while on purine-free diet or <800 mg/d on unrestricted diet implies hypoexcretor)
  – Hypoexcretor
    ○ Probenecid 500/d and increased by 500 mg/month, until uric acid is lowered to normal range or at least 2 mg/dL (0.12 mmol/L) less than the levels during which attacks are noted (maximum dose 2–3 g/d).
    ○ Febuxostat 80–120 mg/d (1)
  – Urinary alkalinization; drink large amounts of fluid as adjunct
- Hyperexcretor, tophaceous, or with renal disease
  – Allopurinol, initiated at 100 mg/d and increased by 100 mg weekly, to a maximum of 600 mg/d
  – Rasburicase (Elitek) 0.15 or 0.20 mg/kg IV infusion in 50 mL of 0.9% sterile sodium chloride over 30 minutes, daily for 5 days, but avoid in the presence of glucose-6 phosphate dehydrogenase deficiency or methemoglobinemia (12).
- Contraindications
  – NSAIDs
    ○ Peptic ulcer disease
    ○ Psychosis
    ○ Severe headache
    ○ Pregnancy
    ○ Concomitant anticoagulant use
    ○ Presence of a blood dyscrasia
    ○ Caution in renal insufficiency

  – Probenecid
    ○ Uric acid overproduction
    ○ Uric acid stones
    ○ Renal impairment
    ○ Concomitant salicylates
    ○ Tophi (relative)
  – Allopurinol
    ○ Bone marrow suppression
    ○ Liver disease
    ○ Concomitant cytotoxic drugs
    ○ Diuretics require increased dose of allopurinol
- Precautions
  – Probenecid and allopurinol may predispose to acute gouty attacks. Use low-dose NSAID for 6–24 months to reduce risk.
  – Reduce NSAID dosage in presence of renal or liver disease
  – Reduce cytotoxic drug dose in presence of allopurinol
  – With allopurinol, risk of skin rash
- Significant possible interactions
  – NSAIDs
    ○ Anticoagulants
    ○ Antidiabetic agents
    ○ Anticonvulsants
    ○ Lithium
  – Probenecid
    ○ Antibiotics
    ○ Antidiabetic agents
    ○ Thiopental
    ○ Ketamine
    ○ NSAIDs
    ○ Lorazepam
    ○ Rifampin
    ○ Antagonized by pyrazinamide, salicylates
  – Allopurinol
    ○ Mercaptopurine (requires reduction of chemotherapy dose to 1/3 of usual dose)
    ○ Azathioprine (requires reduction of chemotherapy dose to 1/3 of usual dose)
    ○ Methotrexate
    ○ Possibly cyclophosphamide
    ○ Anticoagulants
    ○ Antidiabetic agents

Second Line
- Related to control of the acute attack
  – Colchicine, a controversial toxic agent that must be taken within 24 hours of onset of the acute attack to be effective; preferred 2 mg IV, followed by 1 mg q6h for 2 doses; do not repeat in 1–3 days
  – Intra-articular long-acting corticosteroid (if infection definitely ruled out)
  – Adrenocorticotropic hormone 40–80 IU IM
- Related to control of the underlying hyperuricemia in the hypoexcretor
  – Sulfinpyrazone: Initiated at 400 mg/d
  – Fenofibrate: 160 mg/d; augments renal urate clearance (8,9)

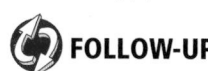 FOLLOW-UP

PROGNOSIS
- With early treatment, total control
- If recurrent attacks, successful uric acid adjustment (requiring lifelong use of uricosuric or allopurinol medication) usually effective
- During the 1st 6–24 months of uricosuric or allopurinol therapy, acute gout may occur

COMPLICATIONS
- Increased susceptibility to infection
- Urate nephropathy
- Uric acid nephropathy
- Renal stones
- Nerve/spinal cord impingement
- Recognition of urate crystals does not preclude concomitant infectious arthritis (10).

PATIENT MONITORING
- Related to medicinal control of the acute attack and suppressing attacks:
- CBC, renal, and LFTs, and urinalysis at 1 week, 6 weeks, and every 3 months

REFERENCES
1. Saag KG, Mikula TR. Recent advances in the epidemiology of gout. Curr Rheumatology Rep. 2005;7:235–241.
2. Kelley WN, Harris ED Jr, Ruddy S, et al. Textbook of Rheumatology. Philadelphia, PA: WB Saunders; 1997.
3. Yu TF. Gout. In: Katz W, ed. Diagnosis and Management of Rheumatic Diseases. Philadelphia: JB Lippincott, 1988.
4. Vazquez-Mellado J, et al. Intradermal tophi in gout. J Rheum. 1997;26:136–140.
5. Weniger FG, et al. Gouty flexor tenosynovitis of the digits: Report of three cases. J Hand Surg [Am]. 2003;28:669–672.
6. Liu SZ, et al. Isolated intraosseous gout in hallux sesamoid mimicking a bone tumor in a teenaged patient. Skeletal Radiol. 2003;32:647–650.
7. Becker MA, Schumacher HR, Wortmann RL, et al. A phase 3 study comparing the safety and efficacy of oral febuxostat and allopurinol in subjects with hyperuricemia and gout. Arthritis Rheum. 2004;50:4103–4104.
8. Hepburn AL, Kaye SA, Feher MD. Long-term remission from gout associated with fenofibrate therapy. Clin Rheumatol. 2003;22:73–76.
9. Takahashi S, et al. Effects of combination treatment using anti-hyperuricaemic agents with fenofibrate and/or losartan on uric acid metabolism. Ann Rheum Dis. 2003;62:572–575.

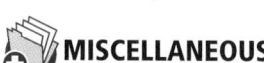 MISCELLANEOUS

See also: Alcohol use disorders; Anemia, sickle cell

CODES

ICD9-CM
- 274.0 Gouty arthropathy
- 274.10 Gouty nephropathy, unspecified
- 274.11 Uric acid nephrolithiasis
- 274.81 Gouty tophi of ear
- 984.9 Toxic effect of unspecified lead compound (including fumes)

PATIENT TEACHING
Arthritis Foundation
phttp://www.arthritis.org/conditions/diseasecenter/gout.asp

 See Corresponding Diagnostic Algorithm

 See Patient Handout on CD

G

GRANULOMA ANNULARE

Gary J. Silko, MD, MS

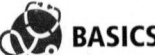 **BASICS**

DESCRIPTION
Chronic, self-limited inflammation of the skin exhibited by annularly arranged papules

- Forms
  - Localized: Most common form; consists of solitary group of flesh-colored papules that gradually involute centrally to form circles or semicircles
  - Disseminated: Occurs less often (≈15%) and usually consists of widespread lesions with same characteristics as localized type as well as infiltrated papules
  - Generalized perforating: Characterized by pinpoint umbilicated papules on extremities
  - Subcutaneous: Usually seen as painless subcutaneous nodule
- System(s) Affected: Skin/Exocrine

GENERAL PREVENTION
Patients with disseminated forms associated with light: Avoid sun exposure

EPIDEMIOLOGY
- Predominant age
  - Localized: Young adults
  - Disseminated: <10 years or >40 years (more common in geriatric patients)
  - Generalized perforating: Children and young adults
  - Subcutaneous: Children
- Predominant sex: Female > Male (2:1)

RISK FACTORS
- Diabetes mellitus
- Positive family history
- Rheumatoid arthritis (RA)
- HIV
- Herpes zoster

Genetics
Not specified, although a familial incidence has been noted among siblings, twins, and successive generations

ETIOLOGY
Unknown

ASSOCIATED CONDITIONS
- Diabetes mellitus is commonly associated with disseminated granuloma annulare; up to 20% of patients with disseminated granuloma annulare also have diabetes mellitus. Likewise, some patients with rheumatoid arthritis have developed granuloma annulare.
- Can be associated with other granulomatous disease, such as necrobiosis lipoidica, rheumatoid nodules, and sarcoidosis
- No definite relationship has been uncovered between granuloma annulare and presence of occult malignancies, but several cases have been reported. In older patients with skin lesions that histologically resemble classic granuloma annulare, investigation for lymphoma or other malignancy should be considered. (1)[B]

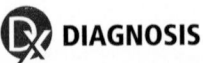 **DIAGNOSIS**

SIGNS AND SYMPTOMS
- Lesions
  - Papular
  - Flesh colored or slightly pink
  - Circular or semicircular
- Papules usually found on dorsal surface of hands, fingers, feet, extensor aspects of arms and legs, trunk
- Subcutaneous nodules seen on palms, legs, buttocks, scalp (usually the occiput)
- Papules can perforate.
- Lesions may be pruritic on rare occasions, but are usually asymptomatic

Physical Exam
Inspection of skin usually reveals diagnosis

TESTS
Lab
- If disseminated form, check blood sugar
- If symptoms of RA present, check rheumatoid factor

Diagnostic Procedures/Surgery
- Skin scraping to rule out fungi can be done.
- If diagnosis is in doubt, skin biopsy can be performed.

Pathological Findings
Palisading granuloma with histiocytes and epithelial cells surrounding a central zone of altered collagen in middle to upper dermis

DIFFERENTIAL DIAGNOSIS
- Papular lesions
  - Necrobiosis lipoidica
  - Cutaneous amyloidosis
  - Annular elastolytic granuloma
  - Papular sarcoid
  - Lichen planus
  - Tinea
  - Tuberculoid or borderline tuberculoid leprosy
  - Erythema migrans
  - Verruca plana
  - Majocchi granuloma
  - Appendageal hamartomas (e.g., eruptive syringomata)
- Subcutaneous nodules: Rheumatoid nodules

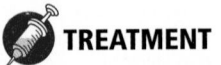 **TREATMENT**

INITIAL STABILIZATION
Outpatient

GENERAL MEASURES
Treatment not always satisfactory

Diet
American Diabetic Association guidelines when associated with diabetes

Activity
Full

MEDICATION (DRUGS)

First Line
- Localized form
  - Intralesional triamcinolone acetonide 5–10 mg/mL injected into elevated border only; use 30-gauge needle. May be repeated at monthly intervals
  - Topical steroids with occlusion or incorporated in tape are occasionally useful.
  - Superficial lesions respond to cryotherapy with liquid nitrogen, but atrophy is possible.
- Disseminated form:
  - Tetracylcine 500 mg b.i.d. plus nicotinamide 500 mg t.i.d. (2)[C]
- Precautions and significant possible interactions: See the manufacturer's profile of each drug.

Second Line
- Disseminated form
  - Isotretinoin 0.5–1 mg/kg
  - Dapsone 100 mg daily or b.i.d.
- Psoralen Ultra-violet A (PUVA) therapy used in more refractive cases
- Contraindictions: Dapsone should not be given to patients with G6PD deficiency.
- Potassium iodide or topical vitamin E have been reported to be effective.

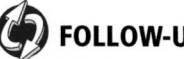 ## FOLLOW-UP

PROGNOSIS
- Lesions disappear without scarring in >1/2 of patients in 2 years.
- 40% of patients experience recurrences, often at original site. (3)[B]

COMPLICATIONS
Rarely, granuloma annulare may involve fascia and tendons, leading to sclerosis and deformity.

PATIENT MONITORING
Depends on nature of treatment; generally 2-week intervals while undergoing treatment

REFERENCES

1. Habif TP. *Clinical Dermatology*. 4th ed. New York, NY: Mosby; 2004:898–899.
2. James WD, Berger TG, Elston DM. *Andrews' Diseases of the Skin*. 10th ed. Philadelphia, PA: WB Saunders; 2006:703–705.
3. Freedberg IM, et al. *Fitzpatrick's Dermatology in General Medicine*. 6th ed. New York, NY: McGraw-Hill; 2003:980–984.
4. Li A, et al. Granuloma annulare and malignant neoplasms. *Am J Dermatopathol*. 2003;25: 113–116.

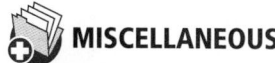 ## MISCELLANEOUS

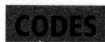 **CODES**

ICD9-CM
695.89 Other specified erythematous conditions, other

PATIENT TEACHING
If patient has disseminated form, papules may be accentuated by sun exposure.

 See Corresponding Diagnostic Algorithm

G

GRANULOMA INGUINALE

Omar A. Khan, MD, MHS

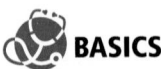 **BASICS**

DESCRIPTION
* Chronic bacterial infection, primarily STD, caused by Calymmatobacterium granulomatosis (Donovania granulomatis)
* Causative agent is an intracellular Gram-negative bacillus
* Organism similar to Klebsiella spp.
* Usually manifests as genital or anal lesions
* Sexual/anal intercourse thought to be main source
* Can also be acquired via fecal route, passage through an infected birth canal, or contact with laps of infected individuals (often a factor in children with the disease)
* Risk factor for acquiring HIV
* 4 varieties of skin lesions exist: Ulcerovegetative, nodular, cicatricial, and hypertrophic/verrucous types

GENERAL PREVENTION
* Safe sex practices: Latex condom use, avoid multiple sexual partners
* If infection likely, avoid sexual contact until evaluation by physician
* Notify all partners so that they may be medically evaluated

EPIDEMIOLOGY
* <100 cases annually in US, most from foreign travel
* Endemic in W. New Guinea, the Caribbean, W. Indies, S. India, S./C. Africa, SE Asia, Australia, and Brazil
* Incidence higher in blacks in US
* Males slightly more susceptible
* Highest incidence age 20–40 years, rarely seen in children or elderly

RISK FACTORS
* Residence in underdeveloped parts of tropical/subtropical countries
* Sexual contact with travelers to an endemic area
* Males having sex with males (MSM)
* Anal intercourse
* Low socioeconomic background
* HIV positivity

PATHOPHYSIOLOGY
* Modes via sexual contact or infected birth canal, fecal route
* Repeated exposure necessary for clinical infection to occur
* Communicable as long as the infected person remains untreated and bacteria from the lesion(s) is present.

ETIOLOGY
Infectious agent is Gram-negative pleomorphic bacillus, *Donovania granulomatis*

ASSOCIATED CONDITIONS
Can be associated with other sexually transmitted diseases including HIV

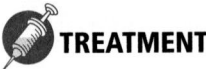 **DIAGNOSIS**

SIGNS AND SYMPTOMS
* Incubation 1–15 weeks
* Begins with subcutaneous nodules or superficial blisters in the genital area; may spread to inguinal folds and lead to surrounding depigmentation
* Blister becomes a slowly enlarging open sore
* 4 types; a common classification is
  – Ulcerovegetative (most common): Lesions develop from the nodular type and consist of large, usually painless spreading ulcers with a friable base, raised margins, beefy red appearance, and easy bleeding. Autoinoculation common, therefore local lesions can be seen on surrounding skin
  – Nodular: Soft, pruritic red nodules may ulcerate. Must be distinguished from buboes of other conditions.
  – Cicatricial: Dry ulcers develop into cicatricial plaque; may be associated with lymphedema
  – Hypertrophic/verrucous: Rare; proliferative reaction, forms large vegetative masses resembling warts

History
* Sexual contact ± genital lesions
* Possible recent travel
* History of HIV or other STDs

Physical Exam
* For types, see above
* Genital involvement in 90%, inguinal involvement in 10%
* In men, lesions occur on penis, scrotum, or glans
* Association with uncircumcised men if occurring in low-hygiene situations
* In women, lesions occur on the labia minora, mons veneris, fourchette, or cervix (in 10%)
* 10–50% infected men and women have lesions in the anal area
* Extragenital involvement (6%)
  – Lymph node enlargement due to secondary bacterial infection or pseudobuboes
  – Autoinoculation can lead to involvement of the oral cavity and GI tract
  – Hematogenous dissemination (usually associated with pregnancy and cervical infection) to spleen, lungs, liver, bones, orbits, can result in death

TESTS
* Mostly a clinical diagnosis as the organism is fastidious and most labs do not have culture available
* Consider testing for mimics and common coinfections
* Staining, biopsy, culture are also appropriate methods; however, difficult to access and not always accurate

Lab
* Isolation of organism difficult
* Culture beyond capabilities of most labs
* Most effective diagnostic method is direct visualization of the organisms within the macrophages, seen as safety pin–shaped intracytoplasmic inclusions (Donovan bodies)
* Tissue crush preparations from ulcer edge may be performed via punch biopsy specimen, curettage, or thin wedge of skin
  – Use Wright-Giemsa or Warthin-Starry stain to visualize Donovan bodies
* Polymerase chain reaction (PCR) currently used mostly for research but may soon be used clinically
* Indirect immunofluorescent technique not accurate enough for confirmatory diagnosis
* Papanicolaou smears may identify Donovan bodies on routine cervical cytological screening
* Testing for other STDs and HIV is warranted as multiple infections frequently coexist

Imaging
Consider radiographs if bony involvement is suspected

Diagnostic Procedures/Surgery
Surgical correction may be indicated; see "Treatment" section

DIFFERENTIAL DIAGNOSIS
* Lymphogranuloma venereum
* Condyloma lata of syphilis
* Chancroid
* HIV-associated herpetic ulcers
* Carcinoma of the penis, vulva, or cervix
* Tuberculosis of the cervix

TREATMENT

The evidence surrounding treatment guidelines is evolving. The first-line treatment now includes azithromycin as well as the previously recognized regimens of TMP/SMX and doxycycline.

PRE HOSPITAL
Can usually be treated in an outpatient setting, with appropriate antibiotics and clinical monitoring

INITIAL STABILIZATION
Usually not a concern unless patient presents with a surgical complication such as lymphatic or urethral obstruction.

GENERAL MEASURES
* Usually outpatient treatment with surgical involvement as necessary
* Empiric treatment should be comprehensive and cover all likely pathogens
* Antimicrobials should be given for at least 3 weeks and continued until re-epithelialization of the ulcer
* If the ulcer does not respond within the first few days of treatment, add an aminoglycoside IV
* Relapse may occur up to 18 months after treatment
* Tetracycline is no longer recommended due to bacterial resistance
* Care must be taken with pregnant and pediatric patients when choosing antimicrobials

Diet
As tolerated

Activity
As tolerated

Nursing
- Wound care as needed
- Monitoring for evidence of secondary bacterial infection, i.e. careful review of vital signs

SPECIAL THERAPY

IV Fluids
As clinically indicated. Usually not an issue unless surgical complications of widespread ulceration present.

 MEDICATION (DRUGS)

First Line
- All regimens to be administered for 3 weeks or until ulcer resolution)
- Azithromycin PO 1 g/d
- TMP/SMX DS PO b.i.d. (avoid in pregnancy)
- Doxycycline 100 mg PO b.i.d. (except in pregnancy)
- *Gentamicin* 1 mg/kg IM/IV t.i.d. in pregnancy or if other regimens not effective in 1st few days of treatment
- HIV-associated granuloma inguinale may take longer to heal; the addition of an aminoglycoside is highly recommended

Second Line
- Ciprofloxacin 750 mg PO b.i.d. for 3 weeks (avoid in pediatric and pregnant patients)
- Erythromycin base 500 mg PO q.i.d. for 3 weeks (use as 1st-line in pregnancy)
- Single-dose regimens of ciprofloxacin, azithromycin and ceftriaxone have been anecdotally reported

ALERT

Pediatric Considerations
Children born to mothers with untreated genital lesions of donovanosis are at risk of infection and a course of prophylactic antibiotics should be considered.

Pregnancy Considerations
- Use erythromycin 500 mg PO q.i.d. ± aminoglycoside.
- Doxycycline and ciprofloxacin are contraindicated in pregnancy.
- Sulfonamides are relatively contraindicated.

SURGERY
May need surgical correction for disfiguring genital lesions, abscess drainage, or correction of urethral/lymphatic obstruction

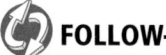 **FOLLOW-UP**

DISPOSITION
If treated in a timely manner, lesions usually resolve.

Admission Criteria
- Extensive, chronic or necrotizing lesions
- Hematogenous dissemination
- Need for inpatient consultative services such as urology or general surgery
- Patient compliance with outpatient regimen is a concern

Discharge Criteria
- Surgical clearance if surgical complications were part of reason for admission
- Ability to access and tolerate oral antimicrobials if needed
- Clinical improvement

Issues for Referral
- Surgical referral (e.g., urologic, gynecologic, colo-rectal surgery), based on complications
- Infectious disease consultation may be helpful if coexisting HIV or other STDs is present or suspected.

PROGNOSIS
- Goal of treatment is to reduce morbidity and prevent complications.
- Relapse may occur up to 18 months after treatment.
- If untreated, lesions may expand for years.

COMPLICATIONS
- Carcinoma (in 0.25%): Squamous cell carcinoma of the penis, vulva, or cervix
- After ulcer healing, fibrosis, stricture formation, phimosis, and scarring can occur, leading to deformity and functional disability.
- Balanitis and secondary infection of ulcers
- Elephantiasis of the genitals may occur secondary to lymphatic obstruction
- Extragenital involvement with potential fatal spread to the viscera
- Recurrent disease, even months–years after treatment (usually associated with HIV)

PATIENT MONITORING
- Monitor for hyperkalemia with extended TMP/SMX treatment
- Other monitoring varies per treatment regimen
- Monitor patient until resolution of symptoms

REFERENCES
1. Ndowa F. Granuloma inguinale. In: Heymann D, ed. Control of Communicable Diseases Manual, 18th ed. Washington DC: APHA Press, 2004.
2. 2002 National Guidelines for the management of donovanosis (granuloma inguinale). National Guidelines Clearinghouse. London: Association for Genitourinary Medicine (AGUM), Medical Society for the Study of Venereal Disease (MSSVD); 2002.
3. Cook GC, Zumla AI. Manson's Tropical Diseases, 21st ed. Philadelphia: Saunders, 2002.
4. O'Farrell N. Donovanosis. Tropical medicine series. Sex Transm Infect. 2002;78 (6): 452–457.
5. Cokonis CD. Granuloma inguinale (donovanosis). Emedicine.com. 11 Apr 2006.
6. CDC. Sexually transmitted diseases treatment guidelines. *MMWR* 2006;47(RR–1):1–118.

MISCELLANEOUS

Antibiotic resistance, patient compliance, need for long-term follow-up, cost, and coexistence of other STDs including HIV must be considered.

CODES

ICD9-CM
ICD-099.2

ICD10
A. 58

PATIENT TEACHING

Patient rapport is critical, because many patients will present late secondary to low self-esteem.

Diet
As tolerated

Activity
As tolerated

Prevention
- Prevention targeted to the mode of initial infection is of paramount importance.
- Examples of prevention may include use of barrier methods of contraception, avoidance of high-risk sexual activity, and appropriate gynecologic screening (including during the course of pregnancy).
- Sexual contacts within 60 days prior to symptom onset should be evaluated and offered treatment.

G

GRANULOMA, PYOGENIC

Jeffrey Mailhot, MD

 ## BASICS

DESCRIPTION
- Benign, solitary vascular mass that involves exposed areas such as distal extremities (especially the hands) and face as well as oral cavity (most frequently the gingiva)
- System(s) Affected: Gastrointestinal; Skin/Exocrine
- Synonym(s): Pregnancy tumor; Granuloma gravidum; Granuloma telangiectaticum

GENERAL PREVENTION
Good oral hygiene

EPIDEMIOLOGY
- Predominant age: Most frequent in children and young pregnant females
- Predominant sex: Slightly more common in females due to association with pregnancy

Incidence
- In children, accounts for <1% of all skin nodules
- 5% of pregnant women are affected in the US

Prevalence
Unknown

ALERT
Pregnancy Considerations
Lesion also occurs in pregnant women and is known as *pregnancy tumor* or pregnancy epulis when it is found on the gingiva (1)[C].

RISK FACTORS
- Pregnancy
- Intraoral trauma or surgery

ETIOLOGY
- Thought to be an aberrant healing response to minor trauma in many cases
- May be related to hormonal changes in pregnancy
- *Not* caused by bacterial infection, but associated with capillary proliferation
- *Not* considered a hemangioma or neoplasm
- Can be associated with isotretinoin therapy (2)[B] and indinavir therapy (3)[C].

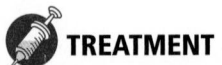 ## DIAGNOSIS

SIGNS AND SYMPTOMS
May be ulcerated, fragile, bleeding easily with any trauma

History
- Solitary lesion that develops rapidly from days to weeks after minor trauma and bleeds easily
- Grows early in pregnancy and partially regresses postpartum

Physical Exam
- Base of the lesion often has a fine collarette of scale
- Bright red, purple, yellow, or brown with moist and sometimes scaly appearing surface
- Ranges from a few millimeters to 2–3 cm in diameter (usually <1 cm)
- Sessile or pedunculated
- Granular, smooth, or slightly nodular
- Soft

Diagnostic Procedures/Surgery
Excisional biopsy

Pathological Findings
Micro
- Small, endothelial-lined vascular spaces
- Loose or dense connective tissue stroma
- Acute and chronic inflammatory cells
- No true granuloma formation
- Abundant mitotic activity

DIFFERENTIAL DIAGNOSIS
- Peripheral ossifying granuloma
- Giant-cell granuloma
- Odontogenic fibroma
- Kaposi sarcoma
- Malignant melanoma
- Angiolymphoid hyperplasia with eosinophilia
- Metastatic carcinoma
- In AIDS patients, bacillary angiomatosis, deep mycoses

TREATMENT

INITIAL STABILIZATION
Outpatient

GENERAL MEASURES
- Occasional spontaneous resolution without any treatment
- Good oral hygiene

Diet
As tolerated

Activity
As tolerated

MEDICATION (DRUGS)

None

SURGERY

- Electrosurgery (electrodesiccation and curettage)
- CO_2-laser destruction
- Surgical excision of lesion (with cleaning of adjacent teeth if lesion is gingival)
- Excision methods with local anesthesia: Punch, shave, and curettage with cauterization
- Excision must be adequate to avoid recurrence. Even a small fragment of tissue left behind may lead to recurrence.

 FOLLOW-UP

PROGNOSIS

- Some spontaneously resolve prior to excision (usually within 6 months).
- Complete resolution expected with adequate excision

COMPLICATIONS

Recurrence; after removal or destruction of solitary lesion, multiple satellite lesions can form around original treatment site.

PATIENT MONITORING

As needed

REFERENCES

1. Lewis CW, Winton GB. Dermatoses of pregnancy. *J Am Acad Dermatol*. 1982;6(6):977–998.
2. Exner JH, Jahod S, Pochi PE. Pyogenic granuloma-like acne lesions during isotretinoin therapy. *Arch Dermatol*. 1983;119(10):808–811.
3. Bouscarat F, Bouchard C, Bouhour D. Paronychia and pyogenic granuloma of the great toes in patients treated with indinavir [letter]. *N Engl J Med*. 1998;338(24):1776–1777.
4. Habif. *Clinical Dermatology* 4th ed. Chicago: Mosby, 2004.

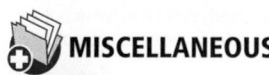 **MISCELLANEOUS**

CODES

ICD9-CM

- 522.6 Chronic apical periodontitis
- 528.9 Other and unspecified diseases of the oral soft tissues
- 686.1 Pyogenic granuloma

PATIENT TEACHING

Patient should avoid trauma to area following excision.

G

GROWTH HORMONE DEFICIENCY

Lee A. Mancini, MD
Brian D. Busconi, MD, CSCS

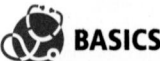 **BASICS**

DESCRIPTION

- Inadequate production of growth hormone (GH, also called *somatotropin*) in either adults or children.
- GH is a polypeptide hormone that stimulates growth and cell reproduction.
- *Hypopituitarism* is often used to describe GHD (growth hormone deficiency). However, hypopituitarism is actually defined as GH deficiency plus a deficiency in at least one other anterior pituitary hormone.
- *Panhypopituitarism* is defined as a deficiency in all the hormones produced in the pituitary gland.
- System(s) Affected: Endocrine; Musculoskeletal
- Synonym(s): Hypopituitarism

EPIDEMIOLOGY

- Most common cause of GHD in children is idiopathic.
- Most common cause of GHD in adults is a pituitary adenoma or treatment of the adenoma with surgery or radiotherapy.
  - 76% of patients with GHD had a pituitary tumor.
  - 13% had an extrapituitary tumor.
  - 8% the cause was unknown.
  - 1% had sarcoidosis.
  - 0.5% had Sheehan syndrome (1).

Prevalence

- In children, isolated GHD has been reported to affect 1 in 4000.
- Adult onset idiopathic GHD is extremely rare.

Genetics

A variety of congenital genetic cause GHD

- Transcription factor defects (PIT-1, PROP-1, LHX3/4, HESX-1, and PITX-2)
- GHRH receptor gene defects
- GH secretagogue receptor gene defects
- GH gene defects
- GH receptor/postreceptor defects
- Prader-Willi syndrome

PATHOPHYSIOLOGY

- GHD is caused by a complete lack of GH production or a decline in GH production. There are multiple causes.
- Hypothalamus secretes GH-releasing hormone (GHRH), which stimulates the pituitary to secrete GH. Somatostatin is secreted by the hypothalamus to inhibit GH secretion. When GH pulses are secreted into the blood, then insulinlike growth factor (IGF)-1 is released. GHD may result from disruption of the GH axis at numerous places; in the higher brain, the hypothalamus, or the pituitary gland.

ETIOLOGY

- Numerous causes for GHD
- Congenital
  - Genetic (see "Genetics")
  - Structural brain defects
    ○ Agenesis of corpus callosum
    ○ Septo-optic dysplasia
    ○ Empty sella syndrome
    ○ Holoprosencephaly
    ○ Encephalocele
    ○ Hydrocephalus
    ○ Arachnoid cyst
  - Associated midline facial defects
    ○ Single central incisor
    ○ Cleft lip/palate
- Acquired
  - Trauma
    ○ Perinatal
    ○ Postnatal
  - CNS infection
  - Tumors of hypothalamus or pituitary
    ○ Pituitary adenoma
    ○ Craniopharyngioma
    ○ Rathke cleft cyst
    ○ Glioma/astrocytoma
    ○ Germinoma
    ○ Metastatic
    ○ Other
  - Cranial irradiation
  - Surgery
  - Idiopathic

ASSOCIATED CONDITIONS

- Macroadenoma
- Sarcoidosis
- Sheehan syndrome

DIAGNOSIS

SIGNS AND SYMPTOMS

Adults

- Depression
- Social withdrawal
- Poor memory
- Loss of strength
- Loss of stamina
- Loss of muscle

History

- Adults
  - Fatigue
  - Weakness
- Children
  - Slower muscular development and delayed gross motor milestones such as standing, walking, and jumping
  - Important questions to ask are
    ○ Birth weight and length
    ○ Height of parents
    ○ Timing of puberty in parents
    ○ Previous growth points
    ○ Nutritional history
    ○ General health of child

Physical Exam

- Children with GHD
  - Most common presentation is short stature.
  - Newborns may present with hypoglycemia, jaundice, or micropenis.
  - Severe GHD children have maxillary hypoplasia and forehead prominence; "kewpie doll" appearance.
  - Accurately measure height and weight.
  - Assess pubertal status using Tanner staging system.
- Adults
  - Decreased lean body mass
  - Poor bone density

TESTS

- Testing for GHD by simple measurement of GH in a single blood sample is useless. This is because levels of GH are nearly undetectable for most of the day. In children, evaluate development along the growth curve.
- Low levels of IGF-1, IGF-2, and IGF binding protein (IGFBP)-3
- Multiple blood-sample testing for GH levels

Lab
- IGF-1, IGF-2, IGFBP-3
- Multiple GH levels
- TSH, thyroxine (hypothyroidism should be excluded as a cause)
- Serum electrolytes (low bicarbonate levels may indicate renal tubular acidosis)
- CBC and ESR
- Karyotype

Imaging
- Head CT or brain MRI to evaluate for a tumor may be ordered.
- Radiograph of left hand and wrist to determine skeletal age in children

Diagnostic Procedures/Surgery
- Provocative tests
  - Give a dose of an agent that in a normal person causes a surge in the release of GH.
  - After agent is given, GH serum levels are drawn every 15 minutes.
  - GH levels are checked for over 60 minutes.
  - Common agents used to stimulate GH release are argine, clonidine, glucagons, insulin, levodopa, and propranolol (3)[C].

DIFFERENTIAL DIAGNOSIS
- Turner syndrome
- Renal failure
- Small size for gestational age in newborns
- Prader-Willi syndrome
- Idiopathic short stature
- Noonan syndrome
- Russell-Silver syndrome
- Down syndrome

MEDICATION (DRUGS)

GHD is treated with GH replacement
- In 1985, GH was synthetically produced from recombinant DNA

First Line
- Several medications are approved for GHD treatment in children
  - Liquid solutions for SC injection. These are available in multidose pen devices. Daily therapy is more effective than 3-times-a-week therapy. The recommended dose is 0.04 mg/kg/d for children (4)[C].
  - Encapsulated GH in glycolide microspheres for deep SC administration. Either 1.5 mg/kg body weight once a month or 0.75 mg/kg twice a month.
  - Geref (sermorelin) has been removed from the market. It is a synthetic growth hormone-releasing hormone.
  - Several growth hormone-releasing peptides (GHRPs) or nonpeptide analogs are be evaluated in children and adults. It is too early to evaluate their long-term safety and efficacy.

FOLLOW-UP

- Children: Regular follow-up with a pediatric endocrinologist.
- Adults: Follow-up with an endocrinologist is recommended.

Issues for Referral
Patients with GHD should be referred to an endocrinologist.

PROGNOSIS
- In children, the prognosis for GHD is good. GH therapy is effective.
- 5 independent predictors of pubertal growth
  - Gender
  - Age at onset of puberty
  - Age at end of growth
  - Dose of growth hormone at onset of puberty
  - Deviation of target height from height at onset of puberty.

COMPLICATIONS
- In children
  - Slipped capital femoral epiphysis
  - Scoliosis
- In adults and children
  - Unmet expectations
  - Metabolic effects
  - Antibodies to growth hormone
  - Cancer: Lymphoma, tumor recurrence
  - Fluid retention: Pseudotumor cerebri, carpal tunnel syndrome, pancreatitis, and edema

PATIENT MONITORING
- Patients taking GH replacement therapy must be monitored.
- The dose of GH therapy is adjusted based on the response level of IGF-1. The goal is to achieve higher levels of IGF-1 (1.5—2 standard deviations above the age-matched mean).
- Initial starting dose for patients is 40 mcg/kg/d.
- Patient dosages of GH should be titrated and individualized based on IGF-1 levels. Adults are more susceptible to side effects of GH than children. Women require higher doses of GH than men. Older patients need less GH replacement doses than younger patients (5)[C].

REFERENCES

1. Bates AS, Hoff W, Vant Jones PJ, et al. The effect of hypopituitarism on life expectancy. *J Clin Endocrinol Metabol*. 1996;81:1169.
2. Rosenfield RG, Albertsson-Wikland K, Cassoria F, et al. Diagnostic controversy: the diagnosis of childhood growth hormone deficiency revisited. *J Clin Endocrinol Metabol*. 1995;80:1532.
3. Molich ME, Clemmons DR, Malozowski S, et al. Clinical practice guideline: Evaluation and treatment of adult growth hormone deficiency. An endocrine society clinical practice guideline. *J Clin Endocrinol Metabol*. 2006;91:1621–1634.
4. deMuink Keizer-Schrama SM, Rikken B, Wynne HJ, et al. Dose-response study of biosynthetic human growth hormone in GH-deficient children: Effects on axiological and biochemical parameters. *J Clin Endocrinol Metabol*. 1992;74:898.
5. Hoffman AR, Strasburger CJ, Zagar A, et al. Efficacy and tolerability of an individualized dosing regimen for adult growth hormone replacement therapy in comparison with fixed body weight-based dosing. *J Clin Endocrinol Metabol*. 2004;87:1974–1979.

G

GUILLAIN-BARRÉ SYNDROME

Mian Li, MD, PhD

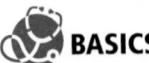 **BASICS**

DESCRIPTION
A group of predominately demyelinating diseases of the peripheral nerves causing acute progressive weakness, usually an ascending paralysis. Divided into 2 forms

- Demyelinating
  - Acute inflammatory demyelinating polyradiculoneuropathy: >90% of cases in Western countries; 30% of patients have nonspecific elevated anti-GM I antibodies
  - Miller-Fisher syndrome: Ophthalmoplegia,
  - Areflexia and ataxia of limbs with relatively preserved muscle strength; 90% of patients have elevated anti-GQ1b antibodies
- Axonal loss (poor prognosis)
  - Acute motor axonal neuropathy: 5% of cases
  - In Western countries, >50% in northern China; predominant motor involvement, recent *Campylobacter jejuni* gastroenteritis
  - Acute motor-sensory axonal neuropathy
- Occurs mostly in adults
- Synonym(s): Acute inflammatory demyelinating polyradiculopathy; Landry-Guillain-Barré-Strohl syndrome; Acute inflammatory neuropathy; Acute idiopathic polyneuritis; Acute immune-mediated polyneuritis; Landry ascending paralysis

ALERT
Thirty percent of the patients have respiratory paralysis requiring mechanical ventilation, but complete or substantial recovery is the rule.

Geriatric Considerations
Worse prognosis >60 years

Pediatric Considerations
Disease tends to be milder

GENERAL PREVENTION
None

EPIDEMIOLOGY
- Predominant age: All ages
- Predominant sex: Male > Female (1.5:1)

Incidence
In the US: 1–8/100,000; nonseasonal, nonepidemic

Prevalence
In the US: 3–10/100,000

RISK FACTORS
Diabetes mellitus, recent surgery, organ transplantation

Genetics
Presumed to be individual's idiosyncratic response to preceding infection, may have a genetic basis

ETIOLOGY
Autoimmune destruction of myelin and/or axon

ASSOCIATED CONDITIONS
- Vaccinations: Swine flu (but not other influenza vaccine) and rabies
- Malignancies, Hodgkin's lymphoma

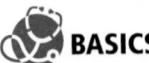 **DIAGNOSIS**

PRE HOSPITAL
- Neck muscle weakness, dysphagia, and dysarthria are predictors of respiratory failure.
- Monitoring respiratory rate

SIGNS AND SYMPTOMS
- Dysesthesias, paresthesias of feet and hands are usually the earliest symptoms
- Pain common, especially back, legs
- Autonomic neuropathy (50%): Labile BP, arrhythmias, ileus, urinary retention
- Respiratory muscle paralysis 30% in untreated cases
- Cranial nerve involvement <50%; usually facial weakness, 10–20% ophthalmoparesis

History
Upper respiratory or diarrheal within previous 1–3 weeks in 50–70%: *Campylobacter jejuni* (~40%), cytomegalovirus (13%), Epstein-Barr virus (10%), *Mycoplasma pneumoniae* (5%), HIV

Physical Exam
- Acute, symmetric, and usually ascending weakness of limbs within days of dysesthesias (1)[A]
- Areflexia and muscle weakness, decreased position, and vibratory sensation often present
- Gait disorder common in all age groups; most common presentation in children

TESTS
Special test: Serum anti-GM1 antibody titer in axonal variant (2)[A]

Lab
- Cerebrospinal fluid: Elevated protein and normal WBC (albuminocytological dissociation) is characteristic, except that in patients with HIV aseptic meningitis, cell counts may be high
- Blood
  - CBC/diff, thyroid-stimulating harmone, B_{12}/folate, liver and renal function, electrolytes, creatine kinase, electron spin resonance, HgA1C, anti-DNA antibodies
  - Others: When appropriate, rheumatoid factor, antineutrophil cytoplasmic antibodies, Sjögren syndrome A&B antibody, antiotensin converting enzyme (ACE) level, hepatitis B or C antigens, cryoglobulinemia, Institute of Professional Enviromental Practice, δ-aminolevulinic acid, and Lyme titer
- Urine: 24-hour urine for light chain for disimmune or amyloidosis
- Optional: Drug/toxin, heavy metal screen, HIV; in children, may check arylsulfatase A activity
- Disorders that may alter lab results
  - Demyelinating neuropathy of diabetes mellitus may have CSF similar to that of Guillain-Barré syndrome; however, Guillain-Barré syndrome usually has higher CSF protein (>0.4 g/dL).
- Protein normal in 50% in 1st week of illness

Imaging
- MRI of spinal cord if myelopathy or cord lesion
- Chest radiograph

Diagnostic Procedures/Surgery
- Nerve conduction studies: Most sensitive test
  - Initially, may show prolonged F-wave latency
  - Conduction block is common in Guillain-Barré syndrome, and characteristic of acquired demyelinating neuropathy
  - Prolonged distal latency and slowing of
- Conduction velocity in 2 nerves each in arms or legs confirms diagnosis
- Lumbar puncture: Elevated protein with normal cell counts

Pathological Findings
- Primary autoimmune attack involved in motor nerve roots and proximal nerve segments
- Sural nerve biopsy not indicated unless necessary to rule out vasculitis or amyloidosis; multifocal inflammatory cell infiltration with demyelination or axonal degeneration

DIFFERENTIAL DIAGNOSIS
- Brain
  - Acute cerebral vascular strokes
  - Encephalitis
- Spinal cord syndromes
  - Transverse myelitis: Similar early presentation
  - Cord compression
  - Cauda equina syndrome
  - B_{12} deficiency
  - Carcinomatous meningoradiculitis
- Motor neuron: Polio
- Peripheral neuropathy associated with
  - Vasculitis (polyarteritis nodosa, Wegner's, Churg-Strauss, nonsystemic vasculitis limited to peripheral nerve)
  - Connective tissue disorder, metabolic (diabetes mellitus, alcoholic, hypophosphatemia)
  - Disimmune process (paraneoplastic syndrome; polyneuropathy, organomegaly, endocrinopathy, monoclonal protein, and skin changes; angiofollicular lymphoma; monoclonal gammopathy; sarcoidosis; multifocal motor neuropathy w/conduction block)
  - Acute ICU neuromyopathy
  - Amyloidosis
  - Toxin (arsenic or thallium poisoning, vitamin B_6 overdose, glue sniffing, chemotherapeutics)
  - Infectious (tick paralysis, diphtheria, Lyme)
  - Flaring of hereditary/congenital neuropathy (porphyria, Fabry, mitochondria cytopathy)
- Neuromuscular junction
  - Myasthenia gravis
  - Eaton-Lambert
  - Toxins (botulism, organophosphates)
  - Hypermagnesemia
- Muscle
  - Polymyositis
  - Periodic paralysis
  - Toxic myopathy
- Psychiatric: Hysteria

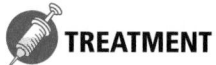 TREATMENT

PRE HOSPITAL
* Tachyarrhythmias: May not require treatment
* Bradyarrhythmias—atropine
* Sinus arrest and complete heart block—temporary pacemaker

INITIAL STABILIZATION
* Admitted to ICU; 50% of those need mechanical ventilation; 10–20% patients have mild disease without need of immune globulin IV or plasmapheresis (3)[A]
* Intubation for difficulty swallowing/aspiration from bulbar palsy
* Immune globulin IV or plasmaphoresis for all patients too weak to walk, rapid progression, or poor prognostic indicators

GENERAL MEASURES
* Serial forced vital capacity and oximetry; intubation for respiratory distress or forced vital capacity <20 mL/kg (<1 L in adults)
* Hypertension
  – Often does not need treatment
  – Avoid use beta-blockers or vasodilators; both could precipitate hypotension
  – In severe hypertension, use morphine bolus to prevent CHF
* Hypotension: Trendelenburg position and volume expansion (IV fluids)
* Pain common, can be severe and recalcitrant Analgesics including opioids; tricyclic antidepressants, carbamazepine, transcutaneous electrical nerve stimulation helpful adjuncts
* Constipation/ileus from autonomic neuropathy: Laxatives, enemas
* Urinary retention from autonomic neuropathy: Catheterization
* Prevent complications of immobilization (physical therapy) (e.g., pneumonia, decubitus ulcers, deep vein thrombosis (DVT), pulmonary embolism, contractures
* Depression: Frequent reminders that recovery is the rule; antidepressants

Diet
No special diet; enteral feedings if intubated

Activity
No limitation

Nursing
Respiratory care

SPECIAL THERAPY
Physical Therapy
Prevention of contractures and assist with weakness

IV Fluids
Regular

Complementary and Alternative Medicine
Analgesics for pain

 MEDICATION (DRUGS)

First Line
* Immune globulin has fewer adverse reactions but more expensive: 2 g/kg for 2–4 days or 400 mg/kg per day for 5 consecutive days
* Plasmapheresis/plasma exchange: 200–250 mL/kg in 3–5 sessions over 8–13 days
* Contraindications
  – Immune globulin: Risk of anaphylaxis (IgA deficiency)
  – Steroids not effective and possibly deleterious
* Precautions
  – Acute renal failure in elderly diabetics or preexisting renal disease, and hepatitis C
  – Headache and aseptic meningitis are frequent side effects of IV immune globulin; slowing the infusion rate will mitigate such events
  – Plasmapheresis: Hypotension, autonomic instability, sepsis

Second Line
* There is no advantage to using both IV immune globulin and plasmapheresis over using either 1 by itself.
* Investigative: IV monoclonal antibodies to adhesion molecules (e.g., integrin)

SURGERY
Tracheostomy for prolonged intubation

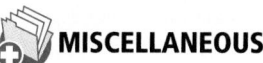 FOLLOW-UP

DISPOSITION
Admission Criteria
Any suspected case

Discharge Criteria
Neurologically stable

Issues for Referral
Emergency neurological consultation necessary

PROGNOSIS
* If untreated, 3 phases of illness
  – Initial progression phase 24 hours–3 weeks; >50% reach nadir before 14 days; highest risk of death and complications during this phase (4)[A]
  – Plateau phase same duration as initial phase
  – Recovery phase 1–6 months. In adults, no discernible improvement after 2 years.
* Mortality (most often from dysautonomia or complications): 2–5%, complete recovery: 50%, some residual disability: 45%, severe permanent disability: 5%
* Relapses may occur both before and after recovery; acute inflammatory demyelinating polyradiculoneuropathy as initial presentation of 2% of chronic inflammatory demyelinating polyradiculoneuropathy patients
* Poor prognostic signs
  – Rapid progression to severe disease (<7 days)
  – Mechanical ventilation;
  – Nerve conduction studies: Compound muscle action potential <10% or mean distal motor amplitude <20%
  – Acute motor axonal neuropathy (see "Differential Diagnosis")
  – Preceding *C. jejuni* infection
  – Age >60 years

COMPLICATIONS
* Paralysis, permanent residual weakness
* Respiratory failure, mechanical ventilation
* Hypotension, hypertension, labile BP
* Cardiac arrhythmias
* Ileus
* Urinary retention
* Aspiration, pneumonia, sepsis
* DVT, pulmonary embolism
* Psychiatric problems, including depression

PATIENT MONITORING
* Hospitalization with monitoring of respiratory function and elective intubation
* Intensive care monitoring for dysautonomia
* Cardiac monitoring for arrhythmias
* Forced vital capacity best measurement (oximetry/arterial blood gases normal until respiratory failure has occurred)

REFERENCES
1. Ruts L, van Koningsveld R, van Doorn PA. Distinguishing acute-onset CIDP from Guillain-Barré syndrome with treatment related fluctuations. *Neurology.* 2005;65:138–140.
2. Hiraga A, et al. Recovery patterns and long term prognosis for axonal Guillain-Barré syndrome. *J Neurol Neurosurg Psychiatry.* 2005;76:719–722.
3. Moussouttas M, Chandy D, Dyro F. Fulminant acute inflammatory demyelinating polyradiculopathy: Case report and literature review. *Neurocrit Care.* 2004;1:469–473.
4. Green DM, Ropper AH. Mild Guillain-Barré syndrome. *Arch Neurol.* 2001;58:1098.

 MISCELLANEOUS

See also: Botulism; Lead poisoning

CODES

ICD9-CM
357.0 Guillain-Barré disease or syndrome

PATIENT TEACHING

Activity
Important to emphasize on expectation of full/significant recovery

See Corresponding Diagnostic Algorithm

G

GYNECOMASTIA

Timothy L. Black, MD

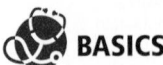 **BASICS**

DESCRIPTION
- Benign glandular enlargement of male breast that is generally bilateral (may be asymmetric or unilateral)
  - Type I: Benign adolescent hypertrophy: Physiologic discoid subacute mass
  - Type II: Physiologic gynecomastia: Generalized enlargement to greater degree
  - Type III: Simulated by obesity
  - Type IV: Pectoral muscle hypertrophy
- System(s) Affected: Endocrine/Metabolic; Skin/Exocrine
- Synonym(s): Male breast hypertrophy

GENERAL PREVENTION
In men taking estrogen for prostate cancer: Low-dose radiation prior to institution of diethylstilbestrol

EPIDEMIOLOGY
- Predominant age: Puberty, >65 years (especially with weight gain)
- Predominant sex: Male only

ALERT
Pediatric Considerations
Transient gynecomastia seen in neonatal boys

Geriatric Considerations
Drug-induced form more common

Prevalence
- 38–64% of pubertal males may have mild form. Usual onset is 11–12 years of age with resolution by age 16–17 years. (1)[C]
- Nonpubertal forms are rare except when drug induced

RISK FACTORS
- Klinefelter syndrome
- Obesity
- Testicular failure (enzymatic defects of testosterone production, androgen insensitivity)
- Testicular neoplasms (germ cell, Leydig cell, Sertoli cell tumors)
- Recovery from prolonged severe illness associated with malnutrition and weight loss (refeeding gynecomastia)
- Family history
- Peutz-Jeghers syndrome
- Male pseudohermaphroditism
- Hyperthyroidism
- Hypothyroidism
- Hepatic disease
- Prostate carcinoma
- Adrenal neoplasms (adenoma or carcinoma)
- Renal disease or dialysis
- True hermaphrodism
- Multiple therapeutic drugs

Genetics
Some instances of familial gynecomastia may be inherited as male-limited autosomal trait

ETIOLOGY
- Physiologic: Transient in neonatal boys and at puberty
- Exposure to high level of estrogen compared with testosterone concentration
- Tumors: Estrogen-secreting, gonadotropin-secreting, prolactin-secreting pituitary adenomas, hepatic fibrolamellar carcinoma
- Identifiable syndrome/cause found in 12% of pubertal boys (2)[C]
- Drugs: Hormones, marijuana, digitalis, spironolactone, cimetidine, ketoconazole, phenytoin, furosemide, verapamil, cytotoxic drugs, antihypertensives, sedatives, antidepressants, amphetamine
- Systemic disorders: Cirrhosis, thyrotoxicosis, renal failure
- Androgen production deficiency
- Androgen-insensitiivty syndromes
- Cirrhosis of the liver
- Idiopathic

ASSOCIATED CONDITIONS
Listed with "Etiology" and "Risk Factors"

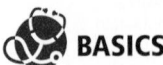 **DIAGNOSIS**

SIGNS AND SYMPTOMS
- Usually asymptomatic
- May be painful and tender if it has developed rapidly
- May involve 1 or both breasts
- Usually located concentrically beneath the nipple and areola

History
- To determine possible etiology
- Investigate concurrent drug treatments
- Investigate onset and duration of symptoms

Physical Exam
- Careful breast examination to evaluate characteristics of breast
- Careful testicular exam
- Abdominal exam
- Rectal exam

TESTS
Full endocrine investigations may be indicated.

Lab
- Laboratory evaluation rarely indicated
- Human chorionic gonadotropin (hCG) levels: High levels may indicate choriocarcinoma or other hCG-secreting tumor (1)[C]
- Plasma testosterone and luteinizing hormone measurements: Help diagnose hypogonadism (1)[C]
- Serum estradiol
- Serum prolactin
- Prostate-specific antigen
- Liver function tests
- Others if clinically indicated (e.g., thyroid function, chromosomal analysis)
- Disorders that may alter lab results
  - Cirrhosis
  - Thyrotoxicosis
  - Renal failure

Imaging
- CT chest and abdomen adrenal or extragonadal germ cell tumor suspected, testicular ultrasound (rarely indicated) (1)[C]

Diagnostic Procedures/Surgery
Biopsy, if suspicious

Pathological Findings
- Dense, periductal, hyaline, collagenous connective tissue
- Hyperplastic ductal lining
- Plasma cell infiltrate

DIFFERENTIAL DIAGNOSIS
- Obesity with increase in adipose tissue
- Carcinoma of male breast
- Lipomas
- Neurofibromas
- Cystic hygroma

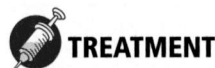 **TREATMENT**

GENERAL MEASURES
* Correct underlying disorder
* Withdrawal of causative drug (if feasible)
* Observation with reassurance that problem is transient

Diet
* No special diet
* If obesity a problem, weight-loss diet

Activity
No restrictions

 MEDICATION (DRUGS)

* Danazol and tamoxifen have been used (side effects may be significant) (1)[C]
* Testosterone
* Clomiphene

SURGERY
* Biopsy if suspicious for cancer
* Subcutaneous mastectomy for severe, painful, or persistent cases or for patients with psychologic concerns (3)[C]
* Usually performed as outpatient surgery
* General anesthesia required

 FOLLOW-UP

PROGNOSIS
* Type I: Resolves spontaneously
* Type II: Clears without treatment (may take up to 2 years)
* Type III: Little change without substantial weight loss
* Drug induced: Withdrawal cures
* Other causes: Outcome depends on etiology
* Good results with subcutaneous mastectomy

COMPLICATIONS
* Nipple inversion may occur following SC mastectomy
* Asymmetry of breasts
* Postoperative fluid collection
* Withdrawal behavior related to drugs
* Depression

PATIENT MONITORING
* Every 3–6 months for physiologic gynecomastia
* Until well for nonphysiologic gynecomastia

REFERENCES
1. Neuman JF. Evaluation and Treatment of Gynecomastia. *Am Fam Physician*. 1997;55: 1835–1844.
2. Sher ES, Migeon CJ, Berkovitz GD. Evaluation of boys with marked breast development at puberty. *Clin Ped*. 1998;37:367–372.
3. Gabra H, et al. Gynaecomastia in the adolescent: A surgically relevant condition. *European J Ped Surg*. 2004;14:3–6.

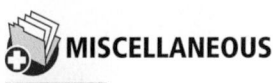 **MISCELLANEOUS**

 CODES

ICD9-CM
611.1 Hypertrophy of breast

PATIENT TEACHING

See Corresponding Diagnostic Algorithm

G

HEADACHE, CLUSTER

Roger K. Cady, MD

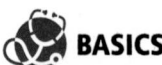 **BASICS**

DESCRIPTION (1)[C]

- Attacks of severe, unilateral headache typically localized in the periorbital area and temple associated with ipsilateral lacrimation, rhinorrhea, ptosis, miosis, and nasal congestion
- Individual attacks last 30–180 minutes and occur 1–6 times per day. 2 forms exist
  - Episodic: Attack phase lasts 4–16 weeks and is followed by a cluster-free interval of generally 6 months to >1 year
  - Chronic: Cluster-free interval of <1 week in a 12-month period
- System(s) Affected: Nervous
- Synonym(s): Migrainous neuralgia; Sphenopalatine neuralgia; Histamine cephalalgia; Horton headache

GENERAL PREVENTION

- Attacks may be induced by
  - Alcohol, nitroglycerin, and some foods
  - Disturbances in the sleep cycle (sleep cycle disruption is common because of anticipation and occurrence of nocturnal attacks)
  - Strong emotions, anger, excessive physical activity
- Tobacco may slow responsiveness to medication
- Narcotics may expedite transformation of episodic cluster to chronic cluster

EPIDEMIOLOGY

- Mean age of onset: 30 years in men, later in women
- Predominant sex: Male > Female (6:1)

Incidence

US adult population: 0.5–1%

ALERT

Pediatric Considerations

Reported pediatric cases very rare

Pregnancy Considerations

Very rare in pregnancy

RISK FACTORS

- Male gender
- Age >30 years
- Small amounts of vasodilators, e.g., alcohol, nitroglycerin
- Occasional relationship to previous head trauma or surgery

Genetics

Unknown

ETIOLOGY

Unknown; perhaps

- Disruption of circadian rhythm based on hypothalamus
- Disturbed autoregulation of cerebral arteries
- Disorder of serotonin metabolism or transmission in the CNS
- Disorder of histamine concentrations or receptors

ASSOCIATED CONDITIONS

- Significantly higher incidence of peptic ulcer and coronary heart disease (males with history of tobacco usage)
- Prior history of migraine (frequently in female patients)
- Increased risk of suicide

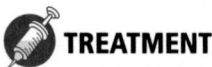 **DIAGNOSIS**

SIGNS AND SYMPTOMS

- Sudden onset of severe headache
- Headache reaches crescendo within 15 minutes, lasts <3 hours
- Pain is unilateral, oculotemporal, or oculofrontal; rare in other locations
- Severe, piercing, boring, exploding, penetrating (occasionally throbbing) pain
- Ipsilateral ptosis and miosis
- Lacrimation (84%)
- Injected conjunctiva (58%)
- Ptosis (57%)
- Nasal stuffiness (48%)
- Rhinorrhea (43%)
- Bradycardia (43%)
- Nausea (40%)
- Perspiration (26%)
- Restlessness and agitation during attacks
- Attacks may occur at same time for consecutive days; frequently an attack occurs within 90 minutes of falling asleep (corresponding to 1st REM sleep).

History

Diagnosis is generally made through careful history-taking.

Physical Exam

Characteristic appearance: "Leonine" face, thickened skin, above-average height; more likely to have hazel eye color and be heavy smokers; no evidence of specific psychologic type. Physical appearance may reflect use of tobacco.

TESTS

Lab

Not useful, except to rule out differential diagnosis

Imaging

Generally of little value, except in atypical presentations or those unresponsive to therapy

DIFFERENTIAL DIAGNOSIS

- Other head and neck pathology
- Migraine
- Trigeminal and other facial neuralgias
- Chronic paroxysmal hemicrania (probably a cluster variant)
- Temporal arteritis
- Pheochromocytoma

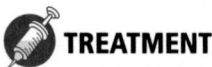 **TREATMENT**

INITIAL STABILIZATION

Outpatient treatment except in patient at risk for suicide

GENERAL MEASURES

- During cluster periods: Avoidance of alcohol, bright lights and glare, and excessive emotion and stress, as these may precipitate attacks
- Avoidance of narcotic analgesics, especially oral preparations
- Avoidance of tobacco (high predilection for tobacco use in this population); may make patient more refractory to therapy

Diet

- During cluster phase, alcohol, even in small amounts, frequently precipitates attacks.
- Rarely, specific foods may trigger attacks.

Activity

- Caution patient to avoid self-injury during bouts of excruciating pain.
- Vigorous physical activity at 1st symptom may abort attack in some patients.
- Compression of ipsilateral carotid or temporal artery may reduce pain in some patients. Exercise caution in recommending carotid massage in a patient at risk for occult carotid disease.

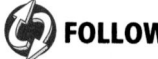 **MEDICATION (DRUGS)**

First Line (1)[C]
- General information
  - Prophylactic therapy is paramount.
  - Avoid pain therapy, especially narcotic analgesics, for acute attacks
  - Assess cardiovascular risk before instituting a vasoactive drug such as ergotamine or sumatriptan.
- For acute attacks
  - Oxygen 100% at least 7–10 L for 10–15 minutes, administered through a tight-fitting face mask with patient in sitting position and breathing at normal respiratory rate
  - Sumatriptan (Imitrex): 6 mg SC, maximum 12 mg/24 hours with at least 1 hour between injections (2)[A]
  - Dihydroergotamine mesylate (DHE 45): 1 mg IM or IV; may teach SC self-administration.
- Prophylaxis (to shorten cluster period or prevent expected attacks)
  - Verapamil up to 80 mg PO q.i.d., spaced evenly through waking hours (3)[B]
  - Lithium carbonate (Eskalith): 300 mg b.i.d to q.i.d.
  - Ergotamine timed to be at peak serum level during anticipated attack, e.g., 2 mg rectal or 1–2 mg PO 2 hours before; especially useful in preventing nocturnal attacks
  - Prednisone: various schedules, e.g., 60–80 mg PO for 7 days followed by rapid tapering over 6 days or 40 mg/d for 5 days tapered over 3 weeks. This therapy is initiated during the use of a long-term agent such as verapamil or lithium.
  - Other agents with small or inconclusive studies include sodium valproate, clonodine, Eletriptan, and topiramate.
- For contraindications, precautions, or possible drug interactions, refer to the manufacturers' literature.

Second Line
- Acute attack: Lidocaine intranasal instillation of 1 mL of 4% topical solution slowly on same side as symptoms. Position patient supine with head extended 45° and rotated 40° to the side of pain. May need to premedicate with 1–2 drops of intranasal 0.5% phenylephrine for nasal stuffiness. (3)[B]
- Prophylaxis
  - Indomethacin: up to 150 mg/d in divided doses; absolute responsiveness in chronic paroxysmal hemicrania and useful in female cluster patients
  - Nifedipine: 40–120 mg/d
  - Nimodipine: up to 240 mg/d
  - Combinations of verapamil and lithium with or without ergotamine may be useful when single drug therapy is ineffective.
  - Histamine desensitization is done at some major headache centers.

SURGERY
Radiofrequency trigeminal gangliolysis in carefully selected refractory patients with strictly unilateral attacks.

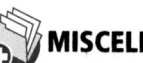 **FOLLOW-UP**

PROGNOSIS
- Recurrent attacks
- Prolonged remissions
- Possibility of transformation of episodic cluster to chronic cluster and occasionally chronic cluster to episodic cluster

COMPLICATIONS
- Self-injury during attack
- Side effects of medication, including unmasking of coronary heart disease
- Potential for drug abuse
- Problems with high-flow oxygen in patients with chronic obstructive pulmonary disease or in those who smoke

PATIENT MONITORING
- Anticipate cluster bouts and initiate early prophylaxis.
- Watch for adverse medication response and side effects.
- Watch for unmasking of underlying cardiovascular disorder.
- Educate patient and family.

REFERENCES

1. The International Classification of Headache Disorders 2nd Edition. *Cephalalgia.* 2004;24 (suppl 1):1–160.
2. Ekbom K, Monstad I, Prusinski A, Cole JA, Pilgram AJ, Noronha D. Subcutaneous sumatriptan in the acute treatment of Cluster headache: A dose comparison study. The Sumatriptan Cluster Headache Study Group. *Acta Neurol Scand.* 1993;88:63–69.
3. Blau JN, Engel HO. Individualizing treatment with verapimil for cluster headache patients. *Headache.* 2004;44:1013–1018.

ADDITIONAL READING

- Rozen TD. Cluster headache: Diagnosis and treatment. *Current Pain and Headache Reports.* 2005;9:135–140.
- Shapiro RE. Corticosteriod treatment in cluster headache: Evidence, rationale, and practice. *Current Pain and Headache Reports.* 2005;9:126–131.
- Adams SM, Standridge JB. Practical strategy for detecting and relieving cluster headaches. *J Fam Pract.* 2005;54(12):1035–1040.

 MISCELLANEOUS

See also: Headache, tension

CODES

ICD9-CM
- 346.20 Variants of migraine without mention of intractable migraine
- 346.21 Variants of migraine with intractable migraine, so stated
- 784.0 Headache

PATIENT TEACHING
- Focus on the validity, natural history, and pathology of the condition.
- Assist patient with learning self-treatment methods.
- Provide supportive relationship and follow-up.

 See Corresponding Diagnostic Algorithm

See Patient Handout on CD

H

HEADACHE, TENSION

Kaelen Dunican, RPh, PharmD

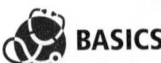 **BASICS**

DESCRIPTION
- Headache typically characterized by bilateral mild to moderate pain and pressure
- May be associated with pericranial tenderness
- 2 types
  - Episodic Tension-Type Headache (ETTH) divided into
    - Infrequent: <1 day per month
    - Frequent: ≥1 but <15 days per month
  - Chronic Tension-Type Headache (CTTH): ≥15 days per month for >3 months
- Synonym(s): Muscle contraction headache; Cephalgia; Stress headache

EPIDEMIOLOGY
Prevalence
- Most common type of primary headache
- Lifetime prevalence ranges from 30–78%
- More prevalent in female gender
- Prevalence of CTTH is 3%
- Prevalence of ETTH decreases with age, whereas the prevalence of CTTH increases with age.

RISK FACTORS
- Associated with triggers/precipitating factors
  - Stress
  - Change in sleep regimen
  - Skipping meals
  - Certain foods (caffeine, alcohol, chocolate)
  - Physical exertion
  - Environmental factors (sun glare, odors, smoke, noise, lighting)
  - Poor or sustained posture
  - Female hormonal changes
  - Medications (e.g., nitrates, SSRIs, antihypertensives)
  - Overuse of headache medication

Genetics
Genetic predisposition has been suggested by studies.

PATHOPHYSIOLOGY
- Debatable: Peripheral and/or central mechanisms
- Activation of peripheral nociceptors leads to muscle tenderness in ETTH
- Central sensitization associated with CTTH
  - Nitric oxide may have an important role in central sensitization
  - Debatable: Low platelet serotonin
- Peripheral may provoke the central mechanism leading from ETTH to CTTH

ETIOLOGY
Stress is most frequently reported precipitating factor.

ASSOCIATED CONDITIONS
- 83% of patients with migraine headaches also suffer from tension-type headaches.
- Debatable: Increased prevalence of comorbid anxiety and depression

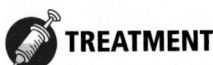 **DIAGNOSIS**

SIGNS AND SYMPTOMS
- Diagnostic criteria provided by the International Headache Society (IHS)
  - Headache lasting 30 minutes–7 days
  - At least 2 of the following
    - Bilateral location
    - Pressing/tightening (nonpulsating) quality
    - Mild or moderate intensity
    - Not aggravated by routine physical activity
  - Not associated with nausea or vomiting (chronic type may be associated with nausea)
  - No more than 1 of the following: Photophobia or phonophobia
  - Not attributed to another disorder
- Fronto-occipital or generalized pain
- Pain is usually described as dull, pressing, or bandlike
- Intensity varies throughout the day
- Often present on arising or shortly thereafter
- Associated symptoms
  - Fatigue
  - Irritability
  - Difficulty concentrating
  - Muscular tightness, tenderness or stiffness in neck, occipital and frontal regions

History
- Obtain a thorough headache history (to rule out other headache disorders) including
  - Severity, symptoms, onset, location and radiation of pain; quality of pain; concurrent medical conditions and medications; recent trauma or other procedures

Physical Exam
- General physical exam: Vital signs, funduscopic and cardiovascular assessment, and palpation of the head and neck
- Neurologic examination: Mental status, pupillary responses, motor strength testing, deep tendon reflexes, sensation, cerebellar function, gait testing, and signs of meningeal irritation

ALERT
Geriatric Considerations
Onset of new headache in patients >50 years is cause for careful study.

TESTS
Labs and neuro imagining (CT or MRI) are necessary when secondary cause is suspected.

DIFFERENTIAL DIAGNOSIS
- Migraine headache
- Cluster headache
- Head trauma
- Subarachnoid hemorrhage
- Subdural hematoma
- Unruptured vascular malformation
- Ischemic cerebrovascular disease
- Temporal arteritis
- Arterial hypertension
- Cerebral venous thrombosis
- Benign intracranial hypertension
- Intracranial neoplasm, infection, or meningitis
- Low cerebrospinal fluid pressure
- Medication (nonprescription analgesic dependency, nitrates)
- Caffeine dependency
- Metabolic disorders (hypoxia, hypercapnia, hypoglycemia)
- Toxic effects from drugs or fumes
- Temporomandibular joint syndrome
- Eyes: Glaucoma, refractive errors
- Sinusitis or middle-ear infection
- Cervical spondylosis
- Severe anemia or polycythemia
- Uremia and hepatic disorders
- Paget disease of bone

TREATMENT

- Acetaminophen (APAP) and aspirin (ASA) are effective for mild to moderate ETTH (1,2)[A].
- Nonsteroidal anti-inflammatory drugs (NSAIDs) are effective for moderate to severe ETTH (1,3)[A].
- Tricyclic antidepressants (TCAs) are effective prophylaxis of CTTH (1–3)[A].

INITIAL STABILIZATION
Outpatient treatment

GENERAL MEASURES
- Relief measures: Relaxation routines; rest in quiet, dark room; hot bath or shower; massage of back of neck and temples
- Biofeedback training

Activity
See "Physical Therapy"

Physical Therapy
- Heat, ice, ultrasound, or TENS
- Massage or cervical traction
- Injection of trigger points
- Stretching and strengthening neck exercises for cervical musculature

MEDICATION (DRUGS)

First Line
- For acute attack (ETTH): APAP, ASA, or NSAIDs
- APAP (Tylenol) 500–1000 mg may repeat q6h p.r.n. (maximum 4 g/d)
  - Adverse effects (rare): Rash, pancytopenia, liver damage
  - Precaution: Hepatic impairment, consumption of ≥3 alcoholic beverages per day
- Aspirin 500–1000 mg may repeat q6h p.r.n. (maximum 4 g/d)
  - Contraindication: ASA or NSAID allergy or bronchospasm, bleeding disorders
  - Drug interactions: Anticoagulants, antiplatelet drugs, ACE inhibitors, β-blockers, corticosteroids, NSAIDs, sulfonylureas
  - Adverse effects: GI irritation/ bleeding, thrombocytopenia
- NSAIDs
  - Ibuprofen (Motrin, Advil) 400–800 mg may repeat q8h p.r.n. (maximum 3.2 g/d)
  - Naproxen (Naprosyn) 375–500 mg or naproxen sodium (Aleve, Anaprox) 440–550 may repeat q8–12h p.r.n. (maximum 1250 mg naproxen base/d)
  - Ketoprofen (Orudis) 12.5–50 mg may repeat q6–8h p.r.n. (maximum 300 mg/d)
  - Diclofenac 50–100 mg may repeat q8h p.r.n. maximum 150 mg/d
  - Contraindications
    ○ ASA or NSAID allergy or bronchospasm
    ○ Advanced renal impairment
    ○ Bleeding disorders (peptic ulcer disease)
  - Precaution: Increased risk of cardiovascular events (MI, stroke, new onset or worsening of hypertension)
  - Drug interactions: Antihypertensives, anticoagulants, antiplatelet drugs, ASA, lithium, methotrexate
  - Adverse effects
    ○ Epigastric distress, peptic ulcer.
    ○ Rare: Thrombocytopenia, increased risk of cardiovascular events
- Prophylaxis for CTTH: TCAs
- Amitriptyline (Elavil): 10–75 mg/d
- Contraindications: Acute recovery phase of MI, use of monamine oxidase inhibitors (MAOIs) within 14 days
- Drug interactions: Clonidine, MAOIs, quinolone antibiotics, SSRIs, sympathomimetics, azole antifungals, valproic acid
- Adverse effects: Drowsiness, dry mouth, tachycardia, heart block, blurred vision, urinary retention, seizure

Second Line
- For acute attack (ETTH)
  - Caffeine combinations: 130 mg caffeine with 500 mg APAP and/or 500 mg ASA q6h p.r.n.
  - Isometheptene/dichloralphenazone/APAP (Midrin, Duradrin) 1–2 caps q4h (max 8/d)
  - Narcotic analgesics
  - Ketorolac 60 mg IM single dose

- For CTTH prophylaxis
  - Alternative TCAs
    ○ Desipramine (Norpramin) 50–100 mg/d
    ○ Imipramine (Tofranil) 50–100 mg/d
    ○ Nortriptyline (Pamelor) 25–50 mg/d
    ○ Protriptyline (Vivactil) 25 mg/d
  - Venlafaxine XR (Effexor XR) 37.5–300 mg/d
  - Tizanidine 2 mg daily increase up to 8 mg t.i.d.
  - Topiramate 25–100 mg/d

ALERT
Use of abortive agents >2 days per week may lead to *medication-overuse headaches*; must withdraw acute treatment to diagnose

Pediatric Considerations
ASA and antidepressants are contraindicated

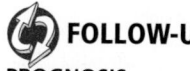 **FOLLOW-UP**

PROGNOSIS
- Usually follows a chronic course when life stressors are not changed.
- Most cases are intermittent.

COMPLICATIONS
- Loss days of work and productivity (>CTTH)
- Cost to health system
- Dependence/addiction to narcotic analgesics
- Gastrointestinal bleeding from NSAID use

REFERENCES
1. Ashina S, Ashina M. Current and potential future drug therapies for tension-type headache. *Curr Headache Rep*. 2003;2:466–474.
2. Moja PL, Cusi C, Sterzi RR, Canepari C. Selective serotonin re-uptake inhibitors (SSRIs) for preventing migraine and tension-type headaches. *Cochrane Database Systematic Rev*. 2006;3.
3. Zhao C, Stillman MJ. New developments in the pharmacotherapy of tension-type headaches. *Expert Opin Pharmacother*. 2003;4:2229–2237.
4. Clinch CR. Evaluation of acute headaches in adults. *Am Fam Physician*. 2001;63:685–692.
5. Headache Classification Subcommittee of the International Headache Society. The international classification of headache disorders: 2nd edition. *Cephalalgia*. 2004;24:1–151.
6. Mueller L. Tension-type, the forgotten headache: How to recognize this common but undertreated condition. *Postgrad Med*. 2002;111:25–50.
7. Lampl C, Marecek S, May A, Bendtsen L. A prospective, open-label, long-term study of the efficacy and tolerability of topiramate in the prophylaxis of chronic tension-type headache. *Cephalalgia*. 2006;26:1203–1208.

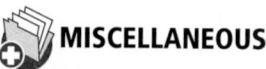 **MISCELLANEOUS**

CODES

ICD9-CM
307.81 Tension headache
ICD10
G44.2 Tension-Type Headache

PATIENT TEACHING
For additional information contact
- National Headache Foundation (888-643-5552, www.headaches.org)
- American Council for Headache Education (800-255-ACHE, www.achenet.org)

Diet
- Identification and avoidance of dietary triggers
- Regulate meal schedule

Activity
- Regulate sleep schedule
- Regular exercise

Prevention
- Identification and avoidance of triggers/ precipitating factors
- Minimize emotional stress, encourage relaxation techniques
  - Biofeedback, relaxation therapy, and physical therapy (as previously described)
  - Consider counseling/psychotherapy

 See Corresponding Diagnostic Algorithm

 See Patient Handout on CD

H

HEARING LOSS

Teresa V. Chan, MD
Daniel J. Lee, MD

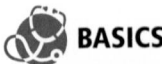 **BASICS**

DESCRIPTION
- Reduction in hearing thresholds manifested as decreased ability to detect or comprehend sound or speech
- May be conductive hearing loss (CHL), sensorineural hearing loss (SNHL), or both
- System(s) Affected: Auditory; Nervous

ALERT
- Any sudden SNHL is a medical emergency and should be referred to an otolaryngologist immediately.
- Treatment with high-dose steroids should begin ASAP, ideally within 10 days of onset.
- A simple 512-Hz tuning fork test lateralizes to unaffected ear in sudden SNHL.

GENERAL PREVENTION
- Limit noise exposure, use hearing protection when exposure cannot be avoided.
- Treat causes: Allergies, sinusitis, eustachian tube dysfunction, adenoid hypertrophy
- Limit ototoxic medications.

EPIDEMIOLOGY
- All ages affected, common in elderly
- Male = Female

Incidence
Hearing loss by age group
- 3 in 10 people >60
- 1 in 6 people ages 41–59
- 1 in 14 people ages 29–40
- At least 1.4 million children (18 or younger)

Prevalence
Hearing loss has doubled in the US during the past 30 years: 13.2 1971 to 28.2 million in 2000

Geriatric Considerations
- Aging and associated presbycusis are responsible for most of hearing loss in the US
- ~ 50% of people >85 years have hearing loss
- Hearing aids are underutilized
- Loss of communication is a source of emotional stress and a physical risk for elderly

Pediatric Considerations
Congenital hearing loss
- 1–3/1000 infants are born deaf
- Mandatory newborn screening
- NICU screening before discharge
- Audiologic testing after major intracranial infection (meningitis)

Pregnancy Considerations
Otosclerosis (a CHL).

RISK FACTORS
- Conductive
  - Allergy
  - Chronic sinusitis
  - Cigarette smoking, 2nd hand smoke
  - Sleep apnea with CPAP use
  - Adenoid hypertrophy
  - Nasopharyngeal mass
  - Eustachian tube dysfunction
  - Head trauma
  - Neuromuscular disease
  - Family history/Heredity
  - Altered immunity
  - Prematurity and low birth weight
  - Young age
  - Craniofacial abnormalities (e.g. cleft palate, Down syndrome)
- Sensorineural
  - Aging/older age
  - Loud noise/ acoustic trauma
  - Medications (aminoglycosides, loop diuretics, quinine, aspirin, chemotherapeutic agents)
  - Bacterial meningitis
  - Head trauma
  - Atherosclerosis
  - Vestibular schwannoma/skull base neoplasm
  - Previous ear surgery
- Sensorineural, pediatric-specific
  - Postnatal asphyxia
  - NICU hospitalization
  - Mechanical ventilation lasting ≥5 days
  - In utero infections (toxoplasmosis, rubella, cytomegalovirus, herpes simplex virus, syphilis)
  - Toxemia of pregnancy
  - Maternal diabetes
  - Rh incompatibility
  - Prematurity
  - Birth weight <1500 g
  - Hyperbilirubinemia; exchange transfusions
  - Measles
  - Encephalitis
  - Chicken pox
  - Influenza
  - Mumps

Genetics
- Connexin 26, (13q11–12)
- Mitochondrial mutations
  - May predispose to aminoglycoside ototoxicity
- Otosclerosis: Familial; no genetic cause
- Most common congenital syndromes
  - Hemifacial microsomia
  - Stickler syndrome
  - Congenital cytomegalovirus
  - Usher syndrome
  - Branchio-oto-renal syndrome
  - Pendred syndrome
  - CHARGE Association
  - Neurofibromatosis type II
  - Mitochondrial disorders
  - Waardenburg syndrome

PATHOPHYSIOLOGY
- CHL
  - Sound is conducted from the external ear, across the tympanic membrane (TM), amplified by the pressure difference and lever action of the ossicles onto the oval window to the inner ear.
  - Loss can result from middle ear effusion, obstruction of canal (canal stenosis, cerumen/foreign body, cholesteatoma, tumor), loss of continuity (ossicular discontinuity), stiffening of the components (myringosclerosis, tympanosclerosis otosclerosis), loss of the pressure differential across the TM (perforation).
- SNHL
  - Damage along the pathway from oval window, cochlea, auditory nerve, and brainstem. Examples include vascular insult (labyrinthine artery infarct), mass effect (cerebellopontine angle tumor), infection and inflammation (viral labyrinthitis, herpes zoster oticus), acoustic trauma (see below).
  - Noise-induced hearing loss is caused by acoustic insult that affects outer hair cells in organ of Corti causing them to be less stiff. Over time, severe damage occurs with fusion and loss of stereocilia. Eventually may progress to inner hair cells and auditory nerve as well.
- Vestibular aqueduct: A "third mobile window" shunts acoustic energy away from cochlea.

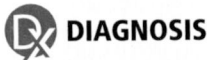 **DIAGNOSIS**

SIGNS AND SYMPTOMS
- Difficulty hearing
- Difficulty discriminating what is being said
- Tinnitus
- Otalgia
- Otorrhea
- Dizziness
- Ear fullness
- Facial nerve palsy
- Depression
- Anxiety

History
- Rapid vs. gradual decline: *Rapid* (<2 weeks' duration) is a *medical emergency* if suspect sudden SNHL
- Difficulty understanding in crowds
- Frequently having to ask speakers to repeat
- Friends/family complain of hearing loss
- TV, phone volume increasing
- History of ear infections or ear surgeries
- History of trauma or noise exposure
- Family history of hearing loss
- Tinnitus, bilateral or unilateral
- Dizziness
- Otalgia
- Otorrhea, clear or purulent
- Facial ticking or asymmetry
- History of recent viral infection
- Nasal obstruction
- Frequent epistaxis

Physical Exam

- 512-Hz tuning fork tests
  - Sensorineural loss
    - Placed on the forehead: Lateralizes to nonaffected (better hearing) ear (Weber test)
    - Placed on the mastoid and then in front of ear; fork is heard louder in front of the ear (Rinne test)
  - Conductive loss
    - Placed on the forehead or teeth lateralizes to affected or symptomatic ear
    - Placed on the mastoid and then in front of the ear; fork is heard louder behind the ear on the side of conductive deficit
- Otoscopy: Assess for deformity, canal patency, otorrhea, TM integrity/retraction/mobility with insufflation, canal or middle ear mass.
- Facial symmetry
- Cranial nerve exam
- Nasopharyngoscopy: Adenoid hypertrophy or nasopharyngeal mass (mandatory in adult patient with new unilateral serous effusion)
- Pediatric: Survey for syndromic anomalies

TESTS

- Audiometry
  - Including pure tone (air and bone), speech testing, and impedance (middle ear pressure) testing
  - Tympanometry: Type B or C tympanograms indicate fluid or retraction, respectively. Negative middle ear peak pressures seen even with normal (Type A) tympanograms.
- Other tests
  - Auditory brainstem response
  - Otoacoustic emissions: "Echo" of the cochlea
  - Behavioral (visual reinforcement) audiometry; used in children 6 months–5 years

Lab

Often labs are not needed; if indicated

- Pendred syndrome (goiter, mental retardation + SNHL) Perchlorate test, thyroid function tests
- Alport syndrome (nephritis + SNHL): Urinalysis, renal function tests
- Jervell and Lange-Nielsen syndrome (syncope, family history of sudden death + SNHL): EKG.
- Any pediatric patient with SNHL: Genetic testing for connexin 26, mitochondrial studies
- TORCH screening test
- RPR confirmed with FTA-ABS
- Lyme titer in endemic areas
- Sedimentation rate for autoimmune disease

Imaging

Often imaging is not required; if indicated

- Fine-cut CT temporal bones without contrast
- MRI of brain and brainstem with gadolinium

Diagnostic Procedures/Surgery

Myringotomy for aspiration of middle ear fluid is both diagnostic and therapeutic.

DIFFERENTIAL DIAGNOSIS

- Conductive
  - Cerumen impaction/foreign body
  - Perforation of tympanic membrane
  - Middle ear fluid (serous otitis media)
  - Acute otitis media
  - Adhesive otitis media
  - Cholesteatoma
  - Ossicular erosion (infection, cholesteatoma)
  - Myringosclerosis/Tympanosclerosis
  - Temporal bone fracture
  - Otosclerosis
  - Congenital malleus fixation
  - Glomus tumor
  - Congenital aural atresia
  - Osteogenesis imperfecta
  - Superior canal dehiscence
- Sensorineural
  - Presbycusis (hearing loss related to aging)
  - Noise induced (recreational, occupational)
  - Ménière disease
  - Ototoxicity (aspirin, quinine, aminoglycosides)
  - Viral labyrinthitis
  - Cerebellopontine angle tumor
  - Enlarged vestibular aqueduct syndrome
  - Syndromic hearing loss
  - Congenital cochlear malformation
  - Labyrinthine artery infarct
  - Idiopathic
  - Syphilis
  - CMV
  - Rubella
  - Temporal bone fracture
  - Metabolic (hyper/hypothyroid)
  - Paget disease
  - Perilymphatic (inner ear) fistula
  - Autoimmune disease

 ## TREATMENT

GENERAL MEASURES

- Early detection: If *sudden single-sided deafness* refer ASAP to otolaryngologist for hearing testing and prompt steroid therapy.
- Early hearing habilitation/rehabilitation (hearing aids or cochlear implants), especially in children, even if future interventions are planned

 ## MEDICATION (DRUGS)

Sudden SNHL: High-dose oral steroids: 1 mg/kg or 60–100 mg/d prednisone or 12–16 mg/d dexamethasone for 14 days, followed by a taper

SURGERY

- CHL often has surgical options for repair. Examples include
  - Tympanostomy and tube placement
  - Tympanoplasty
  - Mastoidectomy
  - Ossicular chain reconstruction
  - Stapedectomy/stapedotomy
- Those with profound bilateral SNHL may qualify for cochlear implantation.

Issues for Referral

Speech therapist, if speech delay or speech impediment is present

PROGNOSIS

SNHL is usually permanent and progressive.

COMPLICATIONS

Acute middle ear problems may become chronic (perforations, cholesteatoma).

PATIENT MONITORING

Audiogram and clinical examination are primary means of monitoring patient.

REFERENCES

1. National Institute on Deafness and Other Communication Disorders: http://www.nidcd.nih.gov/health/hearing/.
2. American Academy of Pediatrics Joint Committee on Infant Hearing: Joint Committee on Infant Hearing 1994 Position Statement. *Pediatrics*. 1995;95(1):152–156.
3. Tomaski SM, Grundfast KM. A stepwise approach to the diagnosis and treatment of hereditary hearing loss. *Pediatr Clin North Am*. 1999;46(1):35–48.
4. Brookhouser PE, Beauchaine KL, Osberger MJ. Management of the child with sensorineural hearing loss. Medical, surgical, hearing aids, cochlear implants. *Pediatr Clin North Am*. 1999;46(1):121–141.
5. Twefik TL, Teebi AS, Der Kaloustian VM. Syndromes and conditions associated with genetic deafness. In: Twefik TL, Der Kaloustian VM, eds. *Congenital Anomalies of the Ear, Nose, and Throat*. Oxford, England: Oxford University Press, 1997.
6. Seidman MD. Effects of dietary restriction and antioxidants on presbycusis. *Laryngoscope*. 2000;110(5 Pt 1):727–738.

ADDITIONAL READING

Sudden Deafness: www.suddendeafness.org

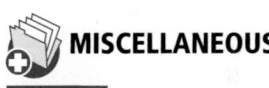 ## MISCELLANEOUS

CODES

ICD9-CM

- 389.9 Hearing deficit
- 389.00 Conductive hearing loss, NOS
- 389.10 Sensorineural hearing loss, NOS
- 389.8 Noise-induced hearing loss
- V53.2 Hearing aid

PATIENT TEACHING

 See Patient Handout on CD

H

537

HEAT EXHAUSTION AND HEAT STROKE

Scott A. Fields, MD

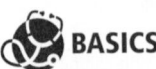 **BASICS**

DESCRIPTION

- A continuum of increasingly severe heat illnesses caused by dehydration, electrolyte losses, and failure of the body's thermoregulatory mechanisms
  - *Heat exhaustion* is an acute heat injury with hyperthermia owing to dehydration.
  - *Heat stroke* is extreme hyperthermia with thermoregulatory failure and profound central nervous system dysfunction.
- System(s) Affected: Endocrine/Metabolic; Nervous
- Synonym(s): Heat illness; Heat injury; Hyperthermia; Heat collapse; Heat prostration

ALERT

Geriatric Considerations
Elderly persons are more susceptible.

Pediatric Considerations
Children are more susceptible.

Pregnancy Considerations
May be more prone to volume depletion with heat stress

GENERAL PREVENTION

- Most important factor in preventing heat stress is adequate fluid replacement.
- Allow acclimatization to hot weather through proper conditioning and activity modification.
- Dress appropriately with loose-fitting, open-weave, light-colored clothing.

EPIDEMIOLOGY

- Predominant age: More likely in children or elderly
- Predominant sex: Male = Female

Prevalence
Dependent on predisposing conditions in combination with environmental factors

RISK FACTORS

- Poor acclimatization to heat or poor physical conditioning
- Salt or water depletion
- Obesity
- Acute febrile or gastrointestinal illnesses
- Chronic illnesses—uncontrolled diabetes or hypertension, cardiac disease
- Alcohol and other substance abuse
- High heat and humidity, poor air circulation in environment
- Heavy, restrictive clothing
- Nutritional supplementation that includes ephedra

ETIOLOGY

Failure of heat-dissipating mechanisms or an overwhelming heat stress leading to a rise in core temperature, dehydration, and salt depletion

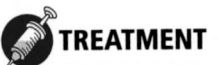 **DIAGNOSIS**

SIGNS AND SYMPTOMS

- Heat exhaustion
  - Fatigue and lethargy
  - Weakness
  - Dizziness
  - Nausea, vomiting
  - Myalgias
  - Headache
  - Profuse sweating
  - Tachycardia
  - Hypotension
  - Lack of coordination
  - Agitation
  - Intense thirst
  - Hyperventilation
  - Paresthesias
  - Core temperature elevated but <103°F (<39.4°C)
- Heat stroke
  - Exhaustion
  - Confusion, disorientation
  - Coma
  - Hot, flushed, dry skin
  - Core temperature >105°F (>40.5°C)

TESTS

Lab
- Used primarily to detect end organ damage
- Electrolytes, urinalysis
- Creatinine, blood urea nitrogen
- Liver enzymes
- CBC
- Increased urine specific gravity
- Results of above studies yield hypernatremia, hyperchloremia, and hemoconcentration.
- Drugs that may alter lab results: Diuretics

Diagnostic Procedures/Surgery
Rectal temperature monitoring

Pathological Findings
Only those associated with major organ system failure

DIFFERENTIAL DIAGNOSIS

Other causes of elevated temperature, dehydration, or circulatory collapse

- Febrile illnesses, sepsis
- Drug-induced fluid loss
- Cardiac arrhythmia or infarction
- Acute cocaine intoxication
- Malignant hyperthermia (an autosomally inherited disorder of skeletal and cardiac muscle in which patients have abnormal muscle metabolism on exposure to halothane or skeletal muscle reactants)

TREATMENT

INITIAL STABILIZATION
Emergency treatment—best in a hospital setting

- Rapid cooling—remove clothing, wet patient down, apply ice packs

GENERAL MEASURES
- Fluid and electrolyte replacement with hypotonic oral fluids or IV 0.5–1.0 L normal saline
- Consider central venous pressure monitoring.
- Body immersion in iced water (1,2)[C]
- Evaporative cooling: Spraying water over the patient and facilitating evaporation and convection with the use of fans (1,2)[C]
- Immersing the hands and forearms in cold water (1,2)[C]
- Use of ice or cold packs in the neck, groins, and axillae (8,9)

Diet (1,2)[C]
- Cool or cold clear liquids only (noncarbonated)
- Avoid caffeine.
- Unrestricted sodium

Activity
Rest with legs elevated (1,2)[C]

MEDICATION (DRUGS)

First Line
No medications are required in the initial management. Use isotonic saline solution to rehydrate. (1,2)[C]

Second Line
- Consider immunomodulators such as corticosteroids. (2)[C]
- Iced gastric, bladder, or peritoneal lavage (1,2)[C]
- Dantrolene 2–4 mg/kg for chemically assisted cooling (2)[C]
- In disseminated intravascular coagulation, consider appropriate replacement therapy.

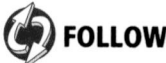 ## FOLLOW-UP

PROGNOSIS
- Good when mental function is not altered and when serum enzymes are not elevated. Recovery is within 24–48 hours in most cases.
- The mortality rate for heat stroke (10–80%) is directly related to the duration and intensity of hyperthermia as well as to the speed and effectiveness of diagnosis and treatment.

COMPLICATIONS
- May involve failure of any major organ system
- Cardiac arrhythmias or infarction
- Pulmonary edema, adult respiratory distress syndrome
- Coma, seizures
- Acute renal failure
- Rhabdomyolysis
- Disseminated intravascular coagulation
- Hepatocellular necrosis

PATIENT MONITORING
- Rectal temperature monitoring: Cooling may be discontinued when the core temperature drops to 102°F (38.9°C) and stabilizes.
- Heat stroke patients may require airway management, hemodynamic monitoring, and careful fluid and electrolyte administration and monitoring.
- Consider central venous pressure monitoring.

REFERENCES

1. Smith JE. Cooling methods used in the treatment of exertional heat illness. *Br J Sports Med*. 2005;39(8):503–507; discussion 507.
2. Yeo TP. Heat stroke: A comprehensive review. *AACN Clinical Issues*. 2004;15(2):280–293.
3. Bouchama A, Knochel JP. Heat stroke. *N Engl J Med*. 2002;346:1978–1988.
4. Bross MH, Nash BT, Carlton F. Heat emergencies. *Am Fam Physician*. 1994;50:389–396.
5. Charaton F. Ephedra supplement may have contributed to sportsman's death. *Br Med J*. 2003;326:464.
6. Graham BS. Features and outcomes of classic heat stroke. *Ann Intern Med*. 1999;130:613–614.
7. Griffin SL, Gardner JW, Flinn SD. Cooling methods for heat stroke victims. *Ann Intern Med*. 2000; 132:678.
8. Keatinge WR, Donaldson GC, Cordioli E, et al. Heat related mortality in warm and cold regions of Europe: Observational study. *Br Med J*. 2000; 321:670–673.
9. Khosla R, Guntupalli KK. Heat related illnesses. *Crit Care Clin*. 1999;15:251–263.

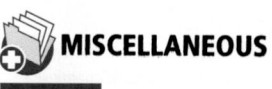 ## MISCELLANEOUS

CODES

ICD9-CM
- 992.5 Heat exhaustion, unspecified
- 992.0 Heat stroke and sun stroke

PATIENT TEACHING

- Stress the importance of proper conditioning and acclimatization.
- Instruct patients to recognize heat stress signs and symptoms.
- Maintain as much skin exposure as possible in hot, humid conditions, while using proper sun block protection.
- Avoid dehydration with proper fluids during activity or exercise—8 oz fluid intake for every 15 minutes of moderate exercise.
- Never leave children unattended in cars during hot weather.
- Try to gain access to air-conditioned environment during hot weather.

Prevention
The key to prevention is in proper hydration.

 See Patient Handout on CD

H

HEMATURIA

Brian Halstater, MD
Felix Horng, MD, MBA

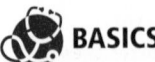 **BASICS**

DESCRIPTION
Blood or red blood cells in the urine
- May be
  - Gross or microscopic
  - Symptomatic or asymptomatic
  - At the beginning (initial), end (terminal), or throughout (total) the urine stream
- System(s) Affected: Renal/Urologic

GENERAL PREVENTION
Minimize indwelling catheterization; attempt to remove postoperative urinary catheters by postoperative day 3.

EPIDEMIOLOGY
- Predominant age: All ages
- Predominant Sex: Female > Male

Incidence
Up to 15% of general US population, though typically <1%

RISK FACTORS
- Smoking
- Occupational exposures (e.g., organic chemicals)
- Analgesic abuse (e.g., phenacetin)
- Medications (e.g., cyclophosphamide)
- Pelvic irradiation
- Chronic infection, especially with calculi
- Recent upper respiratory tract infection
- Positive family history of renal diseases (stones, glomerulonephritis)
- Underlying primary renal disorder

ETIOLOGY
- Trauma
  - Exercise induced (resolves with rest)
  - Abdominal trauma with renal, cystic, or ureteral injury
  - Pelvic fracture with bladder or urethral injury
  - Iatrogenic trauma after catheterization or abdominal or pelvic surgery
  - Foreign body, physical/sexual abuse
- Neoplasms
  - Malignancies of prostate, urethra, bladder, ureter, or kidney may present with hematuria (30% of patients with gross hematuria and 5% with microscopic hematuria will have a malignancy)
  - Benign tumors
  - Endometriosis of the urinary tract (suspect in females with cyclic hematuria)
- Inflammatory causes
  - Urinary tract infection (UTI): Probably the most common cause of hematuria in adults
  - Renal diseases: Glomerulonephritis, radiation nephritis, radiation cystitis, pyelonephritis
  - Endocarditis
- Metabolic causes
  - Calculus disease (85% of patients have hematuria)
  - Hypercalciuria with microcalculi or nephrocalcinosis: Most common cause of hematuria in children without UTI or glomerulonephritis
- Congenital causes
  - Cystic disease: Polycystic kidney disease, solitary renal cyst
  - Benign familial hematuria or thin basement membrane nephropathy
  - Alport syndrome (hematuria, proteinuria, hearing loss)
  - Renal tubular acidosis type 1, cystinuria, oxalosis
- Hematologic causes
  - Bleeding dyscrasias, e.g., hemophilia
  - Henoch-Schönlein purpura
  - Sickle cell anemia
- Vascular causes
  - Hemangioma
  - Arteriovenous malformations (rare)
  - "Nutcracker syndrome": Compression of left renal vein and subsequent renal parenchymal congestion
  - Renal vein thrombosis
  - Arterial emboli to kidney
- Chemical causes: Nephrotoxins—aminoglycosides, cyclosporine
- Obstruction
  - Hydronephrosis, from any cause
  - Benign prostatic hyperplasia: Rule out other causes of hematuria
- Idiopathic causes: Loin pain hematuria (most often in young women on oral contraceptives)

ASSOCIATED CONDITIONS
- Hypertension
- Nephrotic syndrome

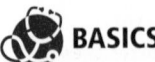 **DIAGNOSIS**

SIGNS AND SYMPTOMS
- Generally none
- Red or rose-colored urine with gross hematuria

ALERT
Geriatric Considerations
- Suspect UTI, sometimes occult
- More likely to have malignant etiology

Pediatric Considerations
- Isolated asymptomatic microscopic hematuria may not need full workup, must at least be watched (1)[B]

- Gross, or symptomatic hematuria needs a full workup.
- If eumorphic RBCs, consider bladder ultrasound (r/o stones, congenital abnormalities) and Urinary Ca/Urinary Cr ratio (hypercalcemia)
- If dysmorphic RBCs, consider renal consult
- Consider glomerulonephritis, child abuse; cystoscopy rarely needed, voiding cystourethrogram may be helpful

TESTS
- Consider nephrology evaluation to determine etiology of primary renal disease.
- Nonintrinsic renal parenchymal disease requires a urologic evaluation. Depth of evaluation depends on high-risk or low-risk status for the presence of the pathology
  - Upper urinary tract imaging adequate to determine presence or absence of abnormalities
  - Cystoscopy to evaluate lower urinary tract
  - Urine cytology for high risk of transitional cell carcinoma
  - Other modalities as needed to obtain detailed enough view of entire urinary system
- In pregnant women, consider vaginal source of bleeding

Lab
- Urine dipstick
  - False negatives: High-dose vitamin C; low urine pH (<5)
  - False positives: Oxidizers (povidone, bacterial peroxidases, bleach), myoglobin
  - Phenazopyridine may discolor the dipstick, making interpretation difficult
  - Not adequately reliable because specificity is only 65% (high sensitivity, however)
- Urinalysis to confirm dipstick findings and quantify RBCs
  - Normal urine contains ≤5 RBCs/high power field (hpf) on any single specimen and ≤3 RBCs/hpf on any 2 successive specimens on centrifuged specimens.
  - Red cell casts are pathognomonic of glomerular bleeding.
  - Proteinuria (large) suggests glomerular leak.
  - Dysmorphic RBCs most often are glomerular in origin.

– Criterion is based on a midstream, fresh, clean-catch voided urine sample. >3 RBCs/hpf on 2 of 3 successive urine specimens or >5 RBCs/hpf on any single specimen is considered abnormal. (See "Miscellaneous" for urine preparation.)

– Casts are best observed in *fresh* urine and may only be observed near the edges of the slide; delays in performing the urinalysis will decrease its usefulness as a diagnostic test, particularly for nephritis.

– Exclude benign, factitious, or nonurinary causes, such as menstruation, mild trauma, exercise, poor collection technique, chemical/drug causes, infection, and hematologic causes.

– Differentiate intrinsic renal parenchymal disease from other causes. Indicators of renal disease are significant proteinuria, red cell casts, and increased creatinine in the absence of an obstruction.

- Urine culture if pyuria is present
- Renal function tests: Blood urea nitrogen and creatinine
- Prothrombin time for patients on warfarin or suspected of abusing warfarin
- CBC
  – May show elevated WBCs
  – Anemia is unlikely from hematuria, although gross hematuria may produce significant blood loss.
  – Anemia and microscopic hematuria are usually secondary to chronic disease.
- Urine cytology: Although "atypical" cells can be seen with benign conditions; good for high-grade transitional cell carcinoma
- Urine calcium/urine creatine ratio >0.21 is suggestive of hypercalcuria in children with eumorphic RBCs.

Imaging
- IV pyelogram (IVP)
  – Overall best study; widely available, cost efficient
  – Limited sensitivity for small renal masses and for differentiating cystic from solid masses
  – Addition of tomography increases sensitivity
  – Potential reactions to IV iodine contrast media (especially in patients who are dehydrated, diabetic, or on metformin, and in preexistent renal insufficiency)
- Renal ultrasonography
  – Best for differentiating cystic from solid masses and finding radiolucent stones
  – Sensitive for hydronephrosis
  – No radiation or iodinated contrast exposure
  – Cost-efficient
  – Poor sensitivity for small renal masses
- Computed tomography (CT)
  – Obtain with/without IV contrast
  – Most sensitive test for evaluating renal masses and for perirenal pathology
  – Visualizes major renal vasculature
  – Satisfactory for stone detection but may misinterpret nonurologic calcifications
  – Visualization of ureters is discontinuous
  – Less cost-efficient
  – Potential reactions to IV iodine contrast media, identical to IVP
  – Need for oral contrast media to opacify bowel
- MRI
  – Similar to CT in sensitivity for renal masses
  – No radiation exposure
  – Least cost-efficient

Diagnostic Procedures/Surgery
- Renal biopsy
  – May be necessary to diagnosis glomerulonephritis
  – With gross hematuria and crescentic nephritis, urgent immunosuppressive therapy may be needed.
- Retrograde pyelogram: May be considered in patients with documented allergy to IV contrast
  – Sensitive for small lesions of supravesical collecting system
  – Valuable for patients with allergy or contraindication to iodine contrast because contrast is not absorbed in this test
  – Requires cystoscopy
- Cystoscopy
  – Best for evaluation of bladder pathology, especially small transitional carcinomas
  – Flexible cystoscopy is less painful and may have increased sensitivity
- Ureteroscopy/pyeloscopy
  – Best for visualization of suspected supravesical collecting system lesions
  – Biopsy, excision, fulguration, or extraction of lesions/stones possible
  – Requires anesthesia
  – Requires cystoscopy
  – Risk of injury to collecting system

Pathological Findings
Glomerulonephritis

DIFFERENTIAL DIAGNOSIS
- Artifactual discoloration of the urine (pseudohematuria)
  – Dehydration
  – Dyes, e.g., phenazopyridine (Pyridium), rifampin, food colorings
  – Precipitated urate crystals cause a pink or red urine color (e.g., in neonates).
- Vaginal bleeding (e.g., menses, dysfunctional uterine bleeding, vaginal trauma)
- Genital/perineal trauma
- Malingering/other secondary gain (urine obtained by catheterization will be helpful)

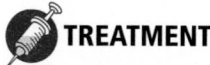

TREATMENT

INITIAL STABILIZATION
Outpatient treatment

GENERAL MEASURES
Diet
Not restricted; consider dye/drug ingestion in artifactual urine discoloration.

Activity
Not restricted, although trauma may necessitate inpatient care

MEDICATION (DRUGS)

None indicated for undiagnosed hematuria

SURGERY
- Gross hematuria: Clots may require continuous bladder irrigation with a large-bore Foley catheter (2-way or 3-way catheter may be helpful) to prevent clot retention.
- Trauma: The degree of hematuria is not well related to the degree of injury; additional imaging and surgical intervention may be required.

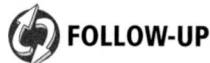

FOLLOW-UP

PROGNOSIS
- Generally excellent for common causes of hematuria
- Poorer for malignant tumors and certain types of nephritis

PATIENT MONITORING
- After initial workup, 35% of patients remain without a diagnosis.
- Follow-up of hematuria is unclear; some experts recommend "periodic" urinalysis and cytology, others suggest only symptomatic patients be reevaluated.
- Reevaluation is indicated for recurrence of gross hematuria, positive cytology, or significant symptoms; increasing proteinuria; presence of red cell casts; or worsening renal function.

REFERENCES
1. Bergstein J, Leiser J, Andreoli S. The clinical significance of asymptomatic gross and microscopic hematuria in children. *Archives of Pediatric and Adolescent Medicine.* 2005;159(4):353–355.
2. Grossfeld GD, Litwin MS, Wolf JS, et al. Evaluation of asymptomatic microscopic hematuria in adults: The American Urological Association best practice policy—part I: Definition, detection, prevalence, and etiology. *Urology.* 2001;57:599–603.
3. Sutton JM. Evaluation of hematuria in adults. *JAMA.* 1990;263:2475–2480.
4. Walsh PC, ed. *Campbell's Urology.* 7th ed. Philadelphia, PA: WB Saunders; 1998.

MISCELLANEOUS

- Preparation for routine urinalysis
  – Centrifuge ~10 mL of fresh, midstream, clean-catch voided urine
  – Discard the supernatant fluid
  – Place the spun sediment on a glass slide and cover with a coverslip
  – Observe with the 40-power microscope lens
- See also: Endocarditis, infective; Hemophilia, renal calculi; Renal cell carcinoma; UTI in females; UTI in males

CODES

ICD9-CM
599.7 Hematuria

PATIENT TEACHING

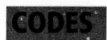
See Corresponding Diagnostic Algorithm

See Patient Handout on CD

H

HEMOCHROMATOSIS
Robert A. Marlow, MD, MA

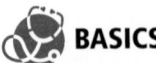 **BASICS**

DESCRIPTION
- A hereditary disorder in which the small intestine absorbs excessive iron (1)
- Because the body lacks any way to excrete iron, the excess is stored in glands and muscle, such as the liver, pancreas, and heart. Over the years, the involved organs begin to fail.
- System(s) Affected: Endocrine/Metabolic
- Synonym(s): Bronze diabetes; Troisier-Hanot-Chauffard syndrome

GENERAL PREVENTION
- Family members should be screened.
- Pregnant women should avoid iron supplements.

EPIDEMIOLOGY
- Predominant age: Present from birth, but symptoms usually present in the 5th and 6th decades.
- Predominant sex: Male = Female (clinical signs are more frequent in men [8:1 male/female ratio])

Prevalence
Three cases per 1,000 people (heterozygote frequency 1 in 10) (2); the most common abnormal gene in the US population
- Loss of blood, such as that which occurs during menstruation and pregnancy, delays the onset of symptoms.

ALERT
Pediatric Considerations
Although rare, iron overload may occur as early as 2 years of age. The disorder can be diagnosed before iron overload is clinically apparent.

RISK FACTORS
- The disease is a genetic disorder. Some variables influence the age of onset and severity of symptoms.
- Intake of iron, especially from vitamin supplements: May contain large amounts of iron as well as vitamin C, which enhances iron absorption.
- Alcohol increases the absorption of iron (as high as 41% of patients with symptomatic disease are alcoholic).

Genetics
Autosomal recessive; acquired; mutation in HFE gene. The phenotypic expression of the mutation is variable. A small proportion of homozygotes have no evidence of iron overload, indicating other influences, such as environmental factors.

PATHOPHYSIOLOGY
Etiology
- The mechanism for increased iron absorption in the face of excessive iron stores is not clear. Iron metabolism appears normal in this disease except for a higher level of circulating iron.
- Iron overload may be caused by thalassemia, sideroblastic anemia, liver disease, excess iron intake, or chronic transfusion.

ASSOCIATED CONDITIONS
See "Complications."

DIAGNOSIS

SIGNS AND SYMPTOMS
- Weakness (83%)
- Abdominal pain (58%)
- Arthralgia (43%)
- Loss of libido or potency (38%)
- Amenorrhea (22%)
- Dyspnea on exertion (15%)
- Neurologic symptoms (6%)
- Hepatomegaly (83%)
- Increased skin pigmentation (75%)
- Loss of body hair (20%)
- Splenomegaly (13%)
- Peripheral edema (12%)
- Jaundice (10%)
- Gynecomastia (8%)
- Ascites (6%)
- Testicular atrophy
- Hepatic tenderness
- Diabetes mellitus symptoms

TESTS
After the diagnosis is established, consider having the patient take an oral glucose tolerance test to rule out diabetes and echocardiogram to rule out cardiomyopathy.

Lab
- Transferrin saturation (serum iron concentration ÷ total iron-binding capacity × 100): >70% is virtually diagnostic of iron overload; 45% or higher warrants further evaluation. Iron supplements and transfusions may elevate serum iron.
- Serum ferritin: >300 μg/L for men and postmenopausal women and 200 μg/L for premenopausal women. (3) May be elevated by inflammatory reactions, other forms of liver disease, certain tumors (e.g., acute granulocytic leukemia), and rheumatoid arthritis.
- Urinary iron
- Increased urine hemosiderin
- Hyperglycemia
- Decreased follicle-stimulating hormone
- Decreased luteinizing hormone
- Decreased testosterone
- Increased serum glutamic-oxaloacetic transaminase
- Hypoalbuminemia

Imaging
Not indicated unless used to evaluate suspected liver disease

Diagnostic Procedures/Surgery
- Liver biopsy for stainable iron is the standard for diagnosis. Presence or absence of cirrhosis can also be ascertained. However, with the availability of genetic testing, liver biopsy is not frequently necessary to confirm the diagnosis. (3)
- DNA polymerase chain reaction testing for *HFE* gene mutations C282Y and H63D: Present in 85–90% of patients.
- Homozygosity for the C282Y mutation with biochemical evidence for iron overload can confirm the diagnosis.

Pathological Findings
- Increased hepatic parenchymal iron stores
- Hepatic fibrosis and cirrhosis with hepatomegaly
- Pancreatic enlargement
- Excess hemosiderin in liver, pancreas, myocardium, thyroid, parathyroid, joints, skin
- Cardiomegaly
- Joint deposition of iron

DIFFERENTIAL DIAGNOSIS
- Repeated transfusions
- Hereditary anemias with ineffective erythropoiesis
- Alcoholic cirrhosis
- Porphyria cutanea tarda
- Atransferrinemia
- Excessive ingestion of iron (rare)

TREATMENT

INITIAL STABILIZATION
Outpatient treatment

GENERAL MEASURES
- Removal of excess iron by repeated phlebotomy once or twice weekly to establish and maintain a mild anemia (hematocrit of 35–39%) (3)[C]
- When the patient finally becomes iron deficient, a lifelong maintenance program of 2–6 phlebotomies a year to keep storage iron normal—maintain serum ferritin ≤50 μg/L

Diet
- An iron-poor diet is not of significant benefit.
- Avoid alcohol, iron-fortified foods, iron-containing supplements, and uncooked shellfish.
- Restrict vitamin C to small doses between meals.
- Tea chelates iron and may be drunk with meals.

Activity
Full activity unless there is significant heart disease

MEDICATION (DRUGS)

None. Only when phlebotomy is not feasible or in the presence of severe heart disease should the iron-chelating agent deferoxamine (Desferal) be considered.

FOLLOW-UP

PROGNOSIS
- Patients diagnosed before cirrhosis develops and treated with phlebotomy have a normal life expectancy.
- Life expectancy is reduced in patients with cirrhosis and diabetes mellitus and those who require >18 months of phlebotomy therapy to return iron stores to normal.
- Patients with ferritin levels <1,000 μg/L are unlikely to have cirrhosis. (2)

COMPLICATIONS
- Cirrhosis
- Hepatoma (only in patients with cirrhosis)
- Diabetes mellitus
- Cardiomyopathy
- Arthritis
- Hypogonadism

PATIENT MONITORING
- Measure hematocrit before each phlebotomy; skip phlebotomy if hematocrit is <36%.
- Schedule an additional phlebotomy when hematocrit is >40%.
- When anemia becomes refractory, repeat transferrin saturation and serum ferritin to confirm depletion of iron stores.
- When iron stores are depleted, 2–6 phlebotomies a year should keep iron stores normal; maintain serum ferritin ≤50 μg/L.
- During maintenance therapy, measure transferrin saturation and serum ferritin yearly.

REFERENCES

1. Pietrangelo A. Hereditary hemochromatosis–a new look at an old disease. *N Engl J Med*. 2004;350: 2383–2397.
2. Brandhagen DJ, Fairbanks VF, Baldus W. Recognition and management of hereditary hemochromatosis. *Am Fam Physician*. 2002;65: 853–860.
3. Qaseem A, Aronson M, Fitterman N, et al. Screening for hereditary hemochromatosis: A clinical practice guideline from the American College of Physicians. *Ann Intern Med*. 2005;143: 517–521.
4. Barton JC, McDonnell SM, Adams PC, et al. Management of hemochromatosis. Hemochromatosis Management Working Group. *Ann Intern Med*. 1998;129:932–939.
5. Powell LW, George DK, McDonnell SM, Kowdley KV. Diagnosis of hemochromatosis. *Ann Intern Med*. 1998;129:925–931.

MISCELLANEOUS

Most patients with hemochromatosis go undiagnosed. Because treatment with phlebotomy will prevent all complications when begun early, physicians should consider the diagnosis of hemochromatosis much more frequently.

CODES

ICD9-CM
275.0 Disorders of iron metabolism

PATIENT TEACHING
- Iron Overload Diseases Association, Inc., PO Box 15857, West Palm Beach, FL 33416.
- American Hemochromatosis Society, Inc., 4044 W. Lake Mary Blvd., Unit #104, Lake Mary, FL 32746–2012.

See Corresponding Diagnostic Algorithm

See Patient Handout on CD

H

HEMOPHILIA

Ruben Peralta, MD, FACS
Sarah Guzofski, MD

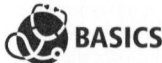 **BASICS**

DESCRIPTION

- Hemophilia A and hemophilia B are inherited bleeding disorders due to a deficiency of coagulant factor VIII (hemophilia A) or factor IX (hemophilia B, also called "Christmas" disease). They are clinically indistinguishable, but can be differentiated by assays that detect levels of factors VIII and IX.
- Disease severity is determined by the levels of the coagulant factor present
  - Severe: <2%
  - Moderate: 2–5%
  - Mild: >6–30%. Patients with >25% factor activity rarely bleed; however, bleeding after major surgery may occur in patients or carriers with factor VIII levels in the range of 25–35%.

EPIDEMIOLOGY

- Hemophilia A and B are congenital conditions.
- Females are generally asymptomatic carriers unless their factor level is <40%.

Incidence

- Estimated to affect 500,000 worldwide; 2/3 undiagnosed (1)[B].
- Incidence of hemophilia A is 1:5000 live male births; hemophilia B 1:30,000 live male births (2)[B].

RISK FACTORS

Genetics

Both hemophilia A and B are X-linked recessive.

30% of cases are due to spontaneous mutation (2)[B].

ETIOLOGY

When blood vessel walls are damaged, exposure of subendothelial tissue initiates the primary hemostatic response, with plasma proteins and platelets interacting with this tissue to generate the platelet plug. Vascular injury also activates the coagulation pathway, which generates thrombin, an element essential to the creation of the fibrin net that stabilizes the platelet plug.

Deficiencies in factor VIII or factor IX impair the coagulation pathway such that the platelet plug is inadequately stabilized, leading to excessive bleeding (3)[B].

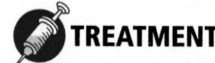 **DIAGNOSIS**

SIGNS AND SYMPTOMS

- Symptoms, usually pain, may precede objective evidence of bleeding. It may be days after trauma before bleeding becomes clinically apparent.
- Bleeding into soft tissue, muscle, and weight-bearing joints is the most common manifestation, but bleeding can occur in any organ.
- Compartment syndrome and ischemic nerve damage from large hematomas may occur, for example femoral nerve neuropathy due to undetected retroperitoneal hemorrhage.
- Repeated bleeding into a joint damages cartilage and subchondral bone. Progressive arthropathy with fixed joints and resultant muscle wasting may significantly impair mobility (1)[B].
- Hematuria
- Central nervous system (CNS) bleeding, usually posttraumatic
- Collections of blood may calcify; referred to as pseudotumor syndrome because can be mistaken for cancer

TESTS

Lab

- Hemophilia A: Diagnostic test is low factor VIII
- Hemophilia B: Diagnostic test is low factor IX
- Activated partial thromboplastin time (PTT) is prolonged, whereas platelet count and prothrombin time (PT) are normal.
- PTT is corrected when mixed with normal plasma.
- Bleeding time is prolonged in 15–20% of patients with hemophilia A.
- Recent aspirin use will increase bleeding time and can lead to confusion with von Willebrand disease.
- Inhibitors to factor VIII (see "Complications") are measured with the Bethesda assay, expressed as Bethesda units.

Diagnostic Procedures/Surgery

Prenatal diagnosis previously required sampling fetal blood for coagulant activity. Newer prenatal detection schemes detect an identifiable restriction fragment length polymorphism or a gene deletion or rearrangement in a sample of chorionic villus or from fluid obtained at amniocentesis.

Pathological Findings

In affected joints

- Synovial hemosiderosis
- Articular cartilage degeneration
- Thickening of periarticular tissues
- Bony hypertrophy

DIFFERENTIAL DIAGNOSIS

- von Willebrand disease
- Vitamin K deficiency (factor IX is vitamin K dependent)
- Other factor deficiencies, afibrinogenemia, dysfibrinogenemia, fibrinolytic defects, platelet disorders

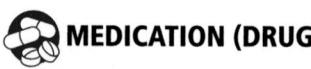 **TREATMENT**

GENERAL MEASURES

- Avoid aspirin or aspirin-containing drugs.
- Treat early; symptoms may occur before bleeding is clinically apparent.
- Mainstay of treatment is factor replacement, which can be plasma-derived or recombinant (2)[B].
- Plasma-derived factor replacement is treated to inactivate viruses, an important innovation because pooled plasma used previously carried high risk of HIV, hepatitis B and C transmission.
- Amount and duration of factor replacement depends on nature of the bleed; e.g., target raising factor level to 15–20% with an uncomplicated bleed and higher (e.g., >50%) with a life-threatening bleed. More significant bleeding requires treating for longer duration (e.g., 2 weeks after the event).
- If major surgery is undertaken, factor levels should be maintained at >50% for at least 2–3 weeks after the procedure.
- Those with frequent bleeds may require regular, scheduled prophylactic infusions.
- Hepatitis A and B vaccinations.
- The vast majority of females are asymptomatic carriers, although an occasional carrier will bleed at time of surgery. They require no specific treatment during pregnancy or delivery.

Diet

No special diet

Activity

Restrict activities in proportion to the degree of factor deficiency, with efforts to maintain a normal life and adequate physical condition.

MEDICATION (DRUGS)

First Line

- Hemophilia A

  - For mild hemophilia: Desmopressin (DDAVP) can raise factor VIII levels (4)[B].

  - Recombinant factor VIII is the treatment of choice. The target factor level depends on the indication for treatment (see "General Measures").
    - 1U of factor VIII (the amount in 1 mL of plasma)/kg body weight will raise the plasma level of the recipient by 2%.
    - Half-life of factor VIII is 8–12 hours; b.i.d. or t.i.d. dosing may be required.
- Hemophilia B
  - Recombinant factor IX exposure.
    - For moderate to severe hemorrhage and patients who are to undergo surgery: Factor IX concentrate 1 U/kg will raise levels 1%.

SURGERY

In selected patients

- Surgical or radionuclide synovectomy
- Joint replacement

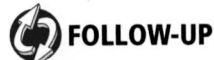 **FOLLOW-UP**

PROGNOSIS

- Repeated hemarthroses result in eventual deformity and progressive disability. Physical therapy may help maintain muscle strength and joint mobility.
- Survival is normal for those with mild disease; mortality is increased 2–6-fold in those with moderate to severe disease.
- At one time, AIDS surpassed intracranial hemorrhage as the leading cause of death in hemophilia (1)[B]. Risk for HIV infection has declined significantly due to development of recombinant and virus-inactivated factor replacement products.

COMPLICATIONS

- Until the mid-1980s, the risk of hepatitis was extremely high (nearly 100%) among those treated with pooled plasma products (4)[B]. Those with hepatitis B and C are at risk for cirrhosis and hepatocellular cancer.
- Some with hemophilia A will develop inhibitors to factor VIII (IgG antibodies), typically those with severe disease receiving multiple transfusions. Development of inhibitors is more common in those with hemophilia A (10–50% of patients compared to 1–3% in hemophilia B), and is especially common in those with severe disease. The highest risk for developing inhibitors is in the 1st 100 treatments. People with very low or no circulating factor VIII are at higher risk of developing antibodies, as are those exposed to exogenous factor VIII at <6 months of age (5)[B].

PATIENT MONITORING

Regular evaluations every 6–12 months, including a musculoskeletal evaluation, an inhibitor screen, liver tests, and tests for antibodies to hepatitis viruses and HIV.

REFERENCES

1. Bolton-Maggs PHB, Pasi KJ. Haemophilias A and B. *The Lancet* 2003;361:1801–1809.
2. Mannucci PM, Tuddenham EGD. The hemophilias—from royal genes to gene therapy. *N Engl J Med* 2001;344:1773–1779.
3. Dahlback B. Blood coagulation and its regulation by anticoagulant pathways: Genetic pathogenesis of bleeding and thrombotic disease. *J Int Med* 2005;257:209–223.
4. Bolton-Maggs PHB. Optimal haemophilia care versus reality. *BJH* 2006;132:671–682.
5. Leissinger CA. Prevention of bleeds in hemophilia patients with inhibitors: Emerging data and clinical direction. *Am J Hematol* 2004;77:187–193.

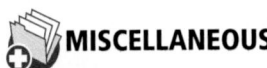 **MISCELLANEOUS**

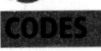 **CODES**

ICD9-CM

- 286.0 Congenital factor VIII disorder
- 286.1 Congenital factor IX disorder

PATIENT TEACHING

- National Hemophilia Foundation, www.hemophilia.org
- World Federation of Hemophilia, www.wfh.org

Prevention

Consider testing family members for carrier status. 1/3 will have factor levels low enough to cause clinically significant bleeding. Some may wish to use this information for reproductive decision-making (4)[B].

 See Corresponding Diagnostic Algorithm

H

HEMORRHOIDS

James T. McPhee, MD
Ruben Peralta, MD, FACS

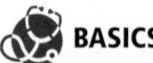 **BASICS**

DESCRIPTION
- Varicosities of the hemorrhoidal venous plexus
- External hemorrhoids are located below the dentate line and covered by squamous epithelium.
- Internal hemorrhoids are located above the dentate line.
- Classification of internal hemorrhoids
  - 1st degree: Hemorrhoids prolapse beyond dentate line with straining.
  - 2nd degree: Prolapse through the anus on straining but reduce spontaneously.
  - 3rd degree: Protrude and require digital reduction.
  - 4th degree: Cannot be reduced
- Hemorrhoids often progress from itching, bleeding stage to protrusion with easy reduction, then difficult reduction, and finally rectal prolapse. Thrombosis may occur at any protrusion stage.

ALERT
Geriatric Considerations
Common in elderly along with rectal prolapse

Pediatric Considerations
- Uncommon in infants and children. Look for underlying cause, e.g., venacaval or mesenteric obstruction, cirrhosis, portal hypertension.
- Occasionally, as in adults, hemorrhoids may result from chronic constipation, fecal impaction, and straining at stool. Surgery is rarely required in children.

Pregnancy Considerations
- Common in pregnancy
- Usually resolves after pregnancy
- No treatment required, unless extremely painful.

GENERAL PREVENTION
- Avoid constipation.
- Lose weight, if overweight.
- Avoid prolonged sitting on the toilet.

EPIDEMIOLOGY
- Predominant age: Adults
- Predominant sex: Male = Female

Incidence
Common

Prevalence
Common

RISK FACTORS
- Pregnancy
- Colon malignancy
- Liver disease
- Portal hypertension
- Constipation
- Occupations that require prolonged sitting
- Loss of muscle tone in old age, rectal surgery, episiotomy, anal intercourse
- Obesity
- Chronic diarrhea

Genetics
No known genetic pattern

ETIOLOGY
- Dilated veins of hemorrhoidal plexus
- Tight internal anal sphincter

ASSOCIATED CONDITIONS
- Liver disease
- Pregnancy
- Portal hypertension
- Constipation

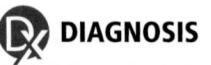 **DIAGNOSIS**

SIGNS AND SYMPTOMS
- All cases
  - Classically bright red blood per rectum. May be scanty blood on toilet paper, or copious in the toilet bowl.
  - Constipation or diarrhea
  - Straining with defecation
- Small or minimal external hemorrhoids: episodic bleeding on stool or toilet paper, pruritus
- More extensive internal hemorrhoids: Feeling of incomplete evacuation
- For protruding hemorrhoids: Mass, more prominent bleeding
- If not reducible, increased risk of strangulation and/or thrombosis with acute pain.
- External hemorrhoids cause pain, internal hemorrhoids generally do not.

TESTS
Diagnostic Procedures/Surgery
- Anorectal examination including anoscopy
- Sigmoidoscopy or colonoscopy depending on coexistent risk factors for malignancy
- Inspection following straining at stool

DIFFERENTIAL DIAGNOSIS
- Rectal or anal neoplasia
- Condyloma
- Skin tag
- Anal fistula, fissure, or abscess (1)[B]

 TREATMENT

All these treatments, except surgical, are outpatient with quick recovery time, usually <48 h.

GENERAL MEASURES
- Hemorrhoids are a recurrent disease, even after surgical excision; measures for prevention should be taken.
- For mild symptoms or prevention
  - Avoid prolonged sitting at stool.
  - Avoid straining.
  - Avoid constipation by eating a high-fiber diet or by taking fiber supplements; if necessary, take regular stool softeners.
  - Regular exercise
- For pain, sitz baths warm water, or hypertonic Epsom salts (1 cup per 2 quarts of water)
- Mild and minimal hemorrhoids respond to changed diet, relief of constipation, and brief stooling.
- Pruritus or mild discomfort after stooling responds to hydrocortisone ointment, anesthetic ointments or sprays.
- Constipation relief, anal hygiene, local ointments, and sitz baths are effective through the stage of easy reduction, but the more severe stages require rubber band ligation or rectal surgery.

Diet
High fiber, adequate fluids

Activity
- No restrictions
- Encourage physical fitness.
- Avoid prolonged sitting and straining on the toilet.

MEDICATION (DRUGS)

- Prevention
  - Fiber supplements
  - Stool softeners
- Pain
  - Hydrocortisone ointment (0.5–1.0%)
  - Analgesic sprays or ointments—benzocaine, dibucaine (Nupercainal)
  - Use sprays with caution as they may contain alcohol that can cause burning sensation when applied.
- Pruritus: Hydrocortisone (Anusol-HC, Cortifoam) ointment
- Bleeding
  - Astringent suppositories (Preparation H)
  - Hydrocortisone (Anusol; Cortifoam) ointment
- Treatment for special cases
  - Thrombosed external hemorrhoids: fairly common complication of hemorrhoidal disease. With severe acute pain, prompt excision should be performed under local anesthetic and the wound left open without packing.
  - Strangulated hemorrhoid: From irreducible 3rd- or 4th-degree hemorrhoid. If untreated, can progress to ulceration and thrombosis. Treatment requires urgent or emergent hemorrhoidectomy.
  - Acute hemorrhoidal bleeding associated with portal hypertension: Bleeding can be life-threatening. Treatment should be suture of the bleeding site with incorporation of the mucosa, submucosa, and internal sphincter. Coagulopathy should be corrected.

SURGERY

- Indications: Failure of medical and nonoperative therapy, symptomatic 3rd- or 4th-degree, symptoms in presence of a concomitant anorectal condition requiring surgery, or patient preference (1)[B]
- Incision of thrombosed hemorrhoid: For severe pain
- Severe protruding hemorrhoids
  - Rubber band ligation (internal hemorrhoids only)
  - Sclerotherapy: For small number of internal hemorrhoids
    - Cryotherapy no longer recommended due to high rate of complications (1)
  - Prolapsed rectum
    - Requires surgical correction
  - Surgical resection:
- Gold standard: Conventional hemorrhoidectomy should be considered for mixed internal and external, when prolapsed through anus, or when complicated by fissures, fistula, or extensive skin tags.
- Newer technique: Stapled hemorrhoidopexy, less painful than traditional surgery, lacks longer-term follow-up data. (2)[B] Also used for prolapsed hemorrhoids.

 FOLLOW-UP

PROGNOSIS
- Spontaneous resolution
- Recurrence

COMPLICATIONS
- Thrombosis
- Ulceration
- Anemia (rare)
- Incontinence
- Pelvic sepsis following hemorrhoidectomy (2)[B]

PATIENT MONITORING
As needed, depending on treatment

REFERENCES

1. American Gastroenterological Association Medical Position Statement: diagnosis and treatment of hemorrhoids. *Gastroenterology* 2004;126: 1461–1462.
2. Nisar PJ, et al. Stapled hemorrhoidopexy compared with conventional hemorrhoidectomy: systematic review of randomized, controlled trials. *Dis Colon Rectum* 2004;47:1837–1845.

 MISCELLANEOUS

See also: Colorectal malignancy, Portal hypertension

CODES

ICD9-CM
455.6 Unspecified hemorrhoids without mention of complication

PATIENT TEACHING

 See Corresponding Diagnostic Algorithm

 See Patient Handout on CD

H

HENOCH-SCHÖNLEIN PURPURA

Blaze Robert Gusic, MD
Bruce M. Rothschild, MD

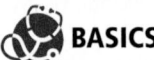 **BASICS**

DESCRIPTION
Henoch-Schönlein purpura (HSP) is an immunologically mediated, nonthrombocytopenic, purpuric, and systemic vasculitis involving the small blood vessels of the skin, gastrointestinal (GI) tract, joints, and kidneys.
- Defined by the presence of 2 of the following
  - Palpable purpura
  - Age of onset <20 years
  - Abdominal pain
  - Granulocytic infiltration of vessel walls
- In children, only palpable purpura with normal platelet count need be documented. Although most children do have purpura, colicky abdominal pain, and arthritis, up to one half may present with symptoms other than purpura.

EPIDEMIOLOGY
- Slightly more common in males
  - Male: Female ratio of 58:42 in 1 study
- Year-round occurrence, but more common in spring, winter, and fall
- Epidemics or clusters are rare.

Incidence
- Incidence of 13.5 cases per 100,000 school-aged children per year (90% of patients are <10 years old)
- Most common in whites, Japanese, and Native Americans. Low incidence in blacks, both in Africa and North America

RISK FACTORS
Genetics
- There is only anecdotal evidence of genetic predisposition.
- Familial history of IgA-related disorders or inherited defects in complement (C2, C4 deficiency) may predispose to HSP.

PATHOPHYSIOLOGY
- Capillaries, arterioles, and venules are affected in HSP as opposed to polyarteritis nodosa, Wegener and systemic lupus erythematosus (SLE), where small arteries are affected.
- Biopsy of skin lesions shows leukocytoclastic vasculitis with perivascular infiltration of small vessels with polymorphonuclear and mononuclear cells and eosinophils. Immunofluorescent microscopy shows granular deposits of IgA1, C3, and fibrin.
- Biopsy of the involved kidneys shows endocapillary proliferative glomerulonephritis involving endothelial and mesangial cells. Crescent formation may also be present. IgA, IgG, C3, and fibrin are commonly found in the mesangial regions.
- Considered to be an immune-mediated vasculitic disorder involving primarily IgA, specifically subclass IgA1. This is indirectly suggested by the elevation of serum IgA levels, circulating IgA immune complexes, IgA rheumatoid factor, IgA-fibronectin complexes, and immunoregulatory abnormalities involving IgA production.
- IgA from mucosal B cells interacts with IgG to form immune complexes that activate the alternate pathway of the complement system. Circulating IgA is deposited in the affected organs causing the inflammatory process.

- *O*-glycosylation abnormalities of IgA1 and the IgA receptor interactions that may be responsible for the findings in HSP are currently under investigation.

ETIOLOGY
- No single etiologic agent has been identified.
- Most cases associated with preceding upper respiratory infections, usually group A β-hemolytic streptococci. A recent study shows a significant association with *Bartonella henselae*. Also reported following infections with parvovirus, adenovirus, hepatitis A virus, *Helicobacter pylori*, and *Mycoplasma pneumoniae*. Parvovirus B19 previously proposed, but evidence is inconclusive.
- Also reported after drug ingestion (e.g., thiazides) and insect bites.

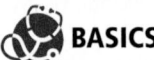 **DIAGNOSIS**

SIGNS AND SYMPTOMS
History
- Previous disease
  - Especially infections such as hepatitis, upper respiratory infection (URI), and streptococcal infections
- Abdominal pain
  - Pain is the most common GI tract symptom. Two thirds of children have GI tract symptoms. Emesis and melena are also reported.
- Transient, nondeforming, nonmigratory arthritis of knees, ankles, wrists, elbows, and digits
  - Frequent problem, most common in knees and ankles
- Presence of testicular pain or scrotal swelling, headache, cough, edema of the ankles or periorbital region, and hematuria
  - Vasculitic lesion in the associated system

Physical Exam
- Particular attention to BP
  - Hypertension is common.
- Low-grade fever is present in 50% of the cases.
- Rash that is petechial or purpuric in a pressure-dependent, symmetric distribution, usually around the lateral malleoli of the ankles, on the ventral surfaces of the feet, and on the buttocks
  - Purpura may be briefly preceded by maculopapular or urticarial lesions.
- Joints should be examined for swelling and limitation of motion
  - Redness and warmth are not common. Symptoms precede the rash by up to 2 weeks in 25% of patients.
- Nonpitting subcutaneous edema of the scalp, periorbital region, hands, and feet is often noted
  - Generalized edema is more common in children younger than 3 years. May lead to acute hemorrhagic edema, now considered to be a variant of HSP
  - Abdomen is often tender to palpation, but without rebound tenderness. Hepatosplenomegaly may be found. Because intussusception and appendicitis are possible complications, serial examinations may be necessary to determine if radiographic studies are indicated.
  - Abdominal symptoms may precede the rash by up to 2 weeks.

- Orchiitis, where affected testicle may be tender and swollen. Swelling and bruising may be noted on the scrotum
  - Testicular torsion has also been reported in HSP and may mimic orchitis.
- Neurologic changes
  - Central nervous system (CNS) involvement may present with headaches, seizures, or behavioral changes.

TESTS
There are no definitive tests to confirm the diagnosis of HSP.

Lab
- Complete blood count (CBC)
  - Normal platelet count differentiates from thrombocytopenic purpura. Hemoglobin is usually normal; leukocytosis; eosinophilia especially, may be present.
- Erythrocyte sedimentation rate (ESR)
  - Normal or elevated
- Prothrombin (PT) and partial thromboplastin time (PTT)
  - Normal
- IgA
  - Often elevated in the acute phase of illness, with normal or increased IgG and IgM
- C3
  - Normal (decreased in poststreptococcal glomerulonephritis and SLE)
- Antinuclear antibody
  - Negative (elevated in SLE)
- Throat swab for group A β-hemolytic streptococci
  - Positive in up to 75% of cases
- Serum basic/comprehensive chemistries
  - Elevated blood urea nitrogen (BUN) and creatinine levels and decreased protein and albumin are seen with renal involvement.
- Urinalysis
  - Gross hematuria and proteinuria are present in many patients. Proteinuria alone is rare. Microscopic blood, red blood cells (RBCs), white blood cells (WBCs), and casts suggest glomerulonephritis.
- Stool guaiac
  - GI tract involvement may present as guaiac-positive stools, bloody stools, or melena. Important to have a low suspicion for intussusception, which is a known complication of HSP

Imaging
- Chest radiograph
  - May show interstitial lung disease
- Abdominal ultrasound
  - Barium enemas are *not* indicated for suspected intussusception. They will not reduce the ilioileal intussusception common to HSP (idiopathic intussusception is usually iliocolic in location) and may damage or perforate the inflamed bowel.

Diagnostic Procedure/Surgery
- Renal biopsy
  - With severe renal failure, a biopsy should be performed to determine the extent of disease.
- Skin biopsy (optional)
  - Direct Immunofluorescence for IgA helpful in confirming the diagnosis

DIAGNOSIS

- Petechial and purpuric rashes seen in thrombocytopenia from
  - Idiopathic thrombocytopenic purpura (ITP)
  - Sepsis/infection: Meningococcemia, Rocky Mountain spotted fever
  - Leukemia
  - Hemolytic uremic syndrome (HUS)
  - Coagulopathies
- Vasculitic rashes may result from primary and secondary vasculitides
  - Polyarteritis nodosa
  - Wegener granulomatosis
  - Infection related
  - Connective tissue diseases (e.g., SLE), Berger disease (IgA nephropathy): glomerulonephritis similar to HSP both clinically and immunologically, but not associated with the skin, GI tract, or joint manifestations of HSP streptococcal glomerulonephritis
  - Infantile acute hemorrhagic edema: vasculitis that presents with urticarial or maculopapular rash that then becomes purpuric. It is differentiated from HSP in that it usually affects children from 4 months to 2 years of age, is more common in the winter, and is not associated with systemic symptoms. On biopsy, IgA deposits are not a consistent finding as they are with HSP.
  - Rheumatoid arthritis
  - Rheumatic fever

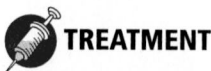

TREATMENT

GENERAL MEASURES

HSP usually resolves spontaneously without specific therapy

- Analgesics and nonsteroidal anti-inflammatory drugs (NSAIDs) may be used for control of joint pain and inflammation, but salicylates and other agents that affect platelet function should be avoided if GI tract bleeding is present.
- Steroids are used for painful cutaneous edema, arthritis, and abdominal pain (2 mg/kg/d of prednisone until clinical resolution); however, steroids have not been shown to affect purpura or to decrease duration of disease or frequency of recurrences.
- No consensus on management of GI and renal involvement. Oral prednisone at 2 mg/kg/d has shown faster resolution of abdominal pain, whereas other studies indicate the symptoms will resolve similarly without intervention.
- In nephritis, immediate treatment with steroids may prevent more serious renal disease; however, most will improve spontaneously. Treatment should be considered for children at high risk for chronic renal insufficiency or failure (those presenting with nephrotic syndrome or renal insufficiency).
- More than 50% crescentic glomerulonephritis on renal biopsy has a greater risk of future renal failure. Such cases should be considered for aggressive therapy with pulse or oral steroids and/or immunosuppressants (azathioprine, cyclophosphamide, cyclosporine) or plasmapheresis, intravenous immunoglobin (IVIG), danazol, or fish oil.
- Treatment of hypertension may delay or prevent progression of renal disease in patients with glomerulonephritis.

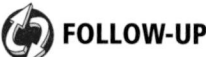

FOLLOW-UP

PROGNOSIS

- Generally excellent: Most (>60%) children are better within 4 weeks of the onset.
- Better prognosis associated with younger age
- Recurrence within the 1st 6 weeks in up to 33%
- Most have only 1–3 episodes of purpura; however, a few will continue to experience symptoms for months or years. These patients have a poor prognosis and are more likely to develop severe nephritis.
- GI tract disease accounts for the most significant morbidity in the short term.
- Renal involvement is the cause of the most serious long-term morbidity. Microscopic hematuria alone or with mild proteinuria generally has a good outcome. A nephritic and nephrotic combination is more guarded, and those patients with a high percentage of crescent formation do less well.

COMPLICATIONS

- Persistent hypertension
- End-stage kidney disease (acute or as a late sequela)
- Intussusception (most common GI tract complication; affecting 1–5% of patients)
- Protein-losing enteropathy
- Hemorrhagic pancreatitis
- Hydrops of the gallbladder
- Strictures of the esophagus and ileus
- Bowel perforations, ischemia, and infarctions
- Pseudomembranous colitis
- Appendicitis
- Skin necrosis
- Subarachnoid, subdural, and cortical hemorrhage and infarction
- Peripheral mononeuropathies and polyneuropathies (Guillain-Barré syndrome)
- Pulmonary hemorrhage (uncommon, but may result in death)
- Torsion of the testis and appendix testes, and priapism
- Scrotal swelling and pain

PATIENT MONITORING

- Patients should be seen weekly during the acute illness. Visits should include history and physical exam, along with blood pressure measurement and urinalysis.
- All patients, even those who did not present with renal involvement, should have urine checked for blood weekly for 6 months and then monthly for 3 years because deterioration or renal function has been observed years after presentation in some patients.
- Women with a history of HSP should be monitored for proteinuria and hypertension during pregnancy.

REFERENCES

1. Ayoub EM, McBride J, Schmiedere M, et al. Role of *Bartonella henselae* in the etiology of Henoch-Schönlein purpura. *Pediatr Infect Dis J.* 2002; 21:28–31.
2. Davin JC, Weening JJ. Henoch Schönlein purpura nephritis: an update. *Eur J Pediatr.* 2001;160: 689–695.
3. Dillon MJ. Henoch-Schönlein purpura (treatment and outcome). *Cleve Clin J Med.* 2002;69(suppl 2):SII121–123.
4. Heegaard ED, Taaning EB. Parvovirus B19 and parvovirus V9 are not associated with Henoch-Schönlein purpura in children. *Pediatr Infect Dis J.* 2002;21:31–34.
5. Kraft DM, McKee M, Scott C. Henoch-Schönlein purpura: a review. *Am Fam Physician.* 1999;58:405–408.
6. Piette WW. What is Schönlein-Henoch purpura, and why should we care? *Arch Dermatol.* 1997;133:515–518.
7. Saulsbury FT. Epidemiology of Henoch-Schönlein purpura. *Cleve Clin J Med.* 2002;69(suppl 2): SII87–89.
8. Saulsbury FT. Henoch-Schönlein purpura. *Curr Opin Rheumatol.* 2001;13:35–40.

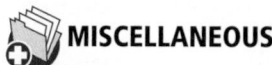

MISCELLANEOUS

CODES

ICD9-CM
287.0 Henoch-Schönlein purpura

PATIENT TEACHING

 See Corresponding Diagnostic Algorithm

H

HEPARIN INDUCED THROMBOCYTOPENIA

Ruben Peralta, MD, FACS
Sarah Guzofski, MD

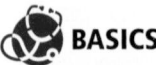 **BASICS**

DESCRIPTION

- Unexpected decrease in platelet count to below baseline in patient treated with heparin
- Most significant adverse effect of heparin other than bleeding
- Most common drug-induced thrombocytopenia
- Idiosyncratic reaction
- 2 types
  - Heparin Associated Thrombocytopenia or HIT type I: onset 1–4 days after starting heparin, mild thrombocytopenia (>100,000), few complications
  - Heparin Induced Thrombocytopenia or HIT type II: less common, onset 5–10 days after exposure to heparin. Thrombocytopenia often <100,000 but usually >20,000

GENERAL PREVENTION

- Inquire about history of prior HIT.
- Proper documentation of past HIT reaction in chart
- Lower, but still some risk of developing 1st episode of HIT with low-molecular-weight heparin (LMWH); after a patient has developed HIT, however, LMWH may not be used.

EPIDEMIOLOGY

Incidence

- 10–15% of heparin-treated patients will experience decrease in platelet count
- 0.3–3% will develop HIT II

RISK FACTORS

Recent surgery causing endothelial injury (releases additional platelet factor 4)

PATHOPHYSIOLOGY

- HIT I: Due to a direct interaction between heparin and platelets; not an antibody-mediated reaction
- HIT II: Antibodies to the complex of heparin and platelet factor 4 cause platelet activation. The activated platelets aggregate and may be destroyed causing thrombocytopenia, or may cause thrombosis.
- In HIT II, the precise mechanism for thrombosis is not clear, but is thought to be related to prothrombotic agents released from activated platelets.

ASSOCIATED CONDITIONS

- Venous or arterial thrombosis
- Skin necrosis

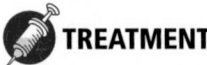 **DIAGNOSIS**

SIGNS AND SYMPTOMS

- HIT I: Asymptomatic drop in platelet count
- HIT II
  - Venous thrombosis
    - Local skin reaction
    - Deep vein thrombosis
    - Pulmonary embolism
    - Cerebral venous thrombosis
    - Venous catheter thrombosis
  - Arterial thrombosis
    - Limb ischemia/infarction
    - Stroke
    - Renal, splenic mesenteric ischemia
  - Spontaneous bleeding possible but unusual given platelet count generally >20,000

History

- Previous exposure to heparin, including heparin flushes, heparin-coated catheter
- In patients being treated with heparin for thrombosis, if there is recurrence of thrombosis during heparin treatment, consider HIT as potential cause; check platelet count.

Physical Exam

- Ischemic changes (signs of limb, renal, splenic, mesenteric ischemia)
- Signs of venous thrombosis
- Skin necrosis (begins with erythema, progressing to ecchymosis and necrosis)
- Bleeding (less common)

TESTS

Lab

- Serial platelet counts in patients receiving heparin; suspect if low count or 50% decrease from baseline. Check at baseline, 24 hours, then every other day for 1st 14 days (1)[B]

- Often a clinical diagnosis given time required to obtain confirmatory lab results
- ELISA assay for HIT II antibodies >90% sensitive
- Platelet aggregation: Patient plasma added to donor platelet and platelet aggregation with addition of heparin is measured; 50–80% sensitive
- Serotonin release assay: Donor platelets with radiolabeled serotonin; patient plasma added. Test is positive if serotonin released with addition of therapeutic amount of heparin; 90% sensitive with high specificity

DIFFERENTIAL DIAGNOSIS

- HIT: Platelet nadir <50,000, thrombosis common, bleeding rarely
- Other drug-induced immune thrombocytopenia with nadir <10,000, bleeding, uncommon thrombosis

TREATMENT

GENERAL MEASURES

- Discontinue all heparin products (including flushes and heparin-coated catheters).
- HIT I generally resolves when heparin is stopped.
- Avoid platelet transfusions.
- Adverse reaction to heparin should be clearly documented in medical record with instruction to "avoid all heparin products."

Nursing

- Avoid heparin flushes.
- Avoid platelet transfusion (can precipitate thrombosis).
- Clearly document in all charts to avoid use of heparin.

MEDICATION (DRUGS)

- Most patients will require anticoagulation either because of
  - Risk of thrombosis in 1st 30 days after HIT; consider prophylaxis with anticoagulation over 1st months after HIT (2)[B] *or*
  - Pre-existing thrombosis
- Dosing of anticoagulation will depend on indication (prophylaxis vs. treatment)
- Direct thrombin inhibitors (1)[A]
  - Reduce risk of thrombosis by ~30% (3)[B]
  - Hirudin: Avoid if abnormal renal function, monitor PTT
  - Argatroban: Monitor dosing in hepatic failure, monitor PTT
- Fondaparinux: Reports of its use, theorized to be useful and additional studies being pursued; platelet factor Xa inhibitor, monitored with "heparin assay" (anti-factor Xa assay), avoid if renal dysfunction (3)[B]
- Warfarin
  - Must anticoagulate with another agent before starting warfarin; use of warfarin without other anticoagulation should be avoided as it can cause thrombosis (2)[B]
  - Should begin use of warfarin after platelet count >100,000; INR should be >2 before other anticoagulation discontinued. Note that direct thrombin inhibitors prolong INR
- Although LMWH has a lower risk of initiating an HIT reaction, it should not be used when antibodies are already present. These antibodies can cross react with the LMWH and can induce thrombosis and thrombocytopenia. (1)[A]
- See manufacturer's information for specific risk and side effect information.

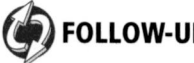 **FOLLOW-UP**

- Depending on clinical presentation
- Patient at highest risk for thrombosis in 1st 30 days following HIT

PROGNOSIS
- Platelet counts normalize within weeks after stopping heparin.
- Risk of thrombosis, especially 1st 30 days. Thrombosis in HIT has mortality 20–30% with additional morbidity from stroke and limb ischemia.

COMPLICATIONS
Thrombosis after platelet count decreases by 30–50%; risk of thrombosis for up to 30 days after heparin discontinued

PATIENT MONITORING
- Serial platelet counts
- Monitor PTT or INR as determined by the anticoagulation agent.

REFERENCES
1. Warkentin TE, Greinacher A. Heparin-induced thrombocytopenia: Recognition, treatment and prevention. *Chest*. 2004;126:311S–337S.
2. Dager WE, White RH. Treatment of heparin-induced thrombocytopenia. *Ann Pharmacother*. 2002;36: 489–503.
3. Spinler SA. New concepts in heparin-induced thrombocytopenia: Diagnosis and management. *J Thromb Thrombolysis*. 2006;21:17–21.

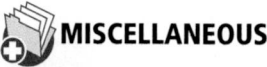 **MISCELLANEOUS**

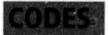 **CODES**

ICD9-CM
287.4 Thrombocytopenia due to drugs

PATIENT TEACHING
Patient should inform all health care providers of his or her adverse reaction to heparin.

H

HEPATIC ENCEPHALOPATHY

Walter M. Kim, AB
Jyoti Ramakrishna, MD

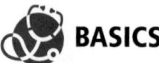 **BASICS**

DESCRIPTION

- Altered mental and neuromotor functioning associated with acute or chronic liver disease and/or portal systemic shunting of blood
- The prominent features are confusion, impaired arousability, and a "flapping tremor" (asterixis).
- System(s) Affected: Gastrointestinal (GI); Nervous
- Synonym(s): HE; Hepatic coma; Liver coma; Portosystemic encephalopathy

GENERAL PREVENTION

- Recognition of early signs and seeking of prompt treatment
- Avoidance of nonessential medications, particularly opiates and sedatives

EPIDEMIOLOGY

Predominant sex: Male = Female (reflecting underlying liver disease)

Prevalence

- Occurs in 1/3 of cirrhosis cases
- Occurs in all cases of fulminant hepatic failure
- Present in nearly 1/2 of patients who require transplantation
- Parallels the age predominance of fulminant liver disease: Peaks in the 40s; cirrhosis peaks in the late 50s; may occur at any age

RISK FACTORS

In patients with underlying liver disease

- Infection (overt or occult, including spontaneous bacterial peritonitis)
- GI hemorrhage
- Use of sedative or opiate drugs
- Electrolyte disturbance (K^+, Mg^{2+}, or other electrolyte depletion)

Genetics

- Unknown
- Conditions such as cystic fibrosis, α-1 antitrypsin deficiency, and Wilson disease can contribute to HE.

PATHOPHYSIOLOGY

- Failure of liver to detoxify agents noxious to the central nervous system, e.g., ammonia, mercaptans, fatty acids
- Increased aromatic and reduced branched chain amino acids in blood
- These act as false neurotransmitters, supposedly interacting with the GABA receptor.

ETIOLOGY

- Shunting of intestinal blood through the severely diseased liver without the intervention of viable liver cells
- Most common in long-standing cirrhosis of the liver with spontaneous shunting of intestinal blood through collaterals
- Shunting of such blood through collateral circulation or surgically constructed portacaval shunts
- Transjugular intrahepatic portacaval shunt, a widely used radiologically inserted shunt to lower portal pressure, produces liver encephalopathy.
- Acute onset of HE: Search for risk factors (see above)

ASSOCIATED CONDITIONS

- Liver disease—100%
- Occurs rarely with portacaval shunt with normal liver function
- May occur as a complication of acute fatty liver of pregnancy

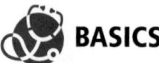 **DIAGNOSIS**

SIGNS AND SYMPTOMS

- Ages 10–60 years
  - Prominent signs of underlying liver disease (50%); jaundice most common, ascites 2nd most common
  - GI hemorrhage with hematemesis or melena (20%)
  - Systemic infection, urinary tract or pulmonary (20%)
  - 4 stages of confusion and obtundity described
    - (1) Forgetfulness, disturbance in nocturnal sleep, daytime drowsiness
    - (2) Mild confusion, drowsy but arousable
    - (3) Patient arousable, markedly confused, with limited orientation and inability to follow commands
    - (4) Patient is unable to be aroused and exhibits extensive posturing
  - Handwriting and hand coordination deteriorated in Stages 1 and 2
  - Asterixis prominent in Stage 2
  - Reflexes symmetrically hyperactive in Stage 3
  - Psychotic thoughts infrequent
  - Mental and neurologic signs change rapidly (over 6–12 hours)
- Age >60
  - Signs of underlying liver disease diminished (25%)
  - Confusion more prominent
  - Precipitating GI hemorrhage or infection less often identified
  - Remains in Stage 1 or 2 for many days
  - Progression slower
- Age <10
  - Signs of underlying liver disease prominent; usually fulminant hepatic failure or extremely advanced cirrhosis
  - Progression through the stages very rapid, often 6–12 hours
  - Wilson disease can imitate HE

History

Pre-existing liver disease

Physical Exam

- Vital signs
  - Bradycardia
  - Increased BP suggestive of increased intracranial pressure
- Jaundice, ascites, and other correlates of liver disease
- CNS exam pertaining to stage of HE—assess short-term memory and presence of asterixis

TESTS

- The clinical setting and findings are adequate in 80% of the cases.
- The treatment response often confirms the diagnosis
- Electroencephalogram: Shows symmetric slowing of basic (alpha) rhythm common with other forms of metabolic encephalopathy (1)[A]; useful to a limited extent
- Visual evoked potential: Specific in Stages 2, 3, and 4
- Number connection test (NCT), line drawing test, and other psychometric tests may be used to assess for minimal HE. (2)[A]

Lab

- Liver tests, including SGOT, SGPT, and serum albumin to evaluate severity of underlying liver disease
- Prothrombin time elevated in liver failure
- Venous ammonia helpful in patients with chronic liver disease when the clinical findings are confusing
- CBC to identify anemia and signs of infection
- Standard biochemistry profile to identify hypokalemia, bilirubinemia, altered calcium status, hypomagnesemia, urea, hypoglycemia
- Blood, sputum, and urine cultures to identify infection
- Arterial blood gases
- Toxicology screen for illicit drugs
- Elevated ammonia often present (3)[A]; levels affected by
  - Infusion of amino acid solutions
  - Opiate administration producing severe constipation
  - Uremia
  - Rapid and severe tissue breakdown, massive burns, trauma, or infection

Imaging

- Useful only to rule out other diagnoses
- CT scan of the head is most useful. (4)[A]

Diagnostic Procedures/Surgery

EEG has typical rhythm (see above).

Pathological Findings

- Brain edema in 100% of fatal cases
- Glial hypertrophy in chronic encephalopathy

DIFFERENTIAL DIAGNOSIS

- Head trauma, concussion, subdural hematoma
- Alcohol withdrawal syndrome
- Alcohol intoxication
- Toxic confusion due to medication
- Toxic confusion due to illicit drug use
- Meningitis
- Metabolic encephalopathy related to anoxia, hypoglycemia, hypokalemia, hypocalcemia or hypercalcemia, or uremia
- Wilson disease
- Reye syndrome

 TREATMENT

INITIAL STABILIZATION

- Monitor closely in Stages 1 and 2 when diagnosis is clear and watch for progression.
- Inpatient management for Stages 3 and 4
- Stages 3 or 4 in fulminant hepatic failure is a strong indication for evaluation for liver transplantation; transfer to a transplant center should be considered.

GENERAL MEASURES

- Identify and vigorously treat precipitating causes: GI bleeding, infection, sedative drugs, and electrolyte imbalance are most common.
- Stage 2 or higher: Insure adequate fluid intake and at least 1,000 kcal (4.19 megajoules [MJ]) daily; avoid hypoglycemia.
- Give initial enema to all patients without diarrhea.
- If clumsiness and poor judgment are prominent, be sure the patient has the care needed to avoid falls, smoking burns, and machinery/auto accidents.
- Avoid sedative or opiate medications. Benzodiazepine sedatives and opiate derivatives, such as diphenoxylate/atropine, have caused liver coma.
- Stage 4: Protect the airway, as aspiration is common (tracheal intubation is often used); feed IV or with jejunal feeding tube.

Diet

- Integrate with needs of underlying liver disease
- Lower total protein (0.8–1.2 g/kg/d); vegetable protein diets are better tolerated than animal protein diets; special IV/enteral formulations with increased branched chain amino acids are available.
- Stage 3 and 4 patients need parenteral nutrition or jejunal feeds.
- As coma improves, increase dietary protein as tolerated.

Activity

- As tolerated
- Avoid driving or operating machinery.

 MEDICATION (DRUGS)

First Line

- Lactulose syrup: 30–60 mL of 50% solution q.i.d. Diminish to 15–30 mL b.i.d. when 3 or more bowel movements occur daily
- If worsening occurs, or there is no improvement in 2 days, add antibiotics.
  - Neomycin: 1 to g/d in 4 divided doses, if renal status is good
  - Metronidazole is an alternative antibiotic.
  - Rifaximin is an alternative treatment. (5)[A]; nonabsorbable antibiotic
- Antacids as needed
- Contraindications
  - Total ileus
  - Hypersensitivity reaction
- Precautions
  - Potassium depletion
  - Electrolyte imbalance
  - Renal failure
- For significant possible interactions, refer to manufacturer's profile of each drug.

Second Line

Flumazenil

SURGERY

- Artificial liver perfusion devices have proven useful in fulminant hepatic failure to bridge the patient until a donor liver is available for transplantation.
- Stage 3 and 4 patients should be considered for liver transplantation.

 FOLLOW-UP

Issues for Referral

Refer early to a transplant center.

PROGNOSIS

- Acute or fulminant disease: With adequate aggressive treatment, disappears without residue or recurrence
- Chronic disease
  - Coma returns
  - With each recurrence, becomes more and more difficult to treat
  - Plateau of maximum improvement shows a decrement over several years such that the degree of improvement with treatment is less and less; the mortality rate is 80%.

COMPLICATIONS

- Recurrence
- Stable, chronic, impaired status
- With many recurrences, permanent basal ganglion injury (non-Wilsonian hepatolenticular degeneration)
- Hepatorenal syndrome
- Acute tubular necrosis
- Bleeding
- Disseminated intravascular coagulation
- Bacteremia
- Shock

PATIENT MONITORING

- To optimize treatment, a trail-making test should be followed. Apply to Stage 1 and Stage 2 patients to determine how much maintenance treatment is needed and what diet is appropriate. The test should be run daily at 1st and then at each visit when changes in drugs and diet are made.
- Patients with changed findings should be seen twice weekly.
- Stable patients should be seen monthly.
- Trail-making test at each office visit
- In cirrhosis, evaluate for transplantation for death likely in 24 months

REFERENCES

1. Saxena N, Bhatia M, Joshi YK, et al. Electrophysiological and neuropsychological tests for the diagnosis of subclinical hepatic encephalopathy and prediction of overt encephalopathy. *Liver*. 2002;22:190–197.
2. Wessenborn K, Ennen JC, Schomerus H, et al. Neuropsychological characterization of hepatic encephalopathy. *J Hepatol* 2001;34:768–773.
3. Ong JP, Aggarwal A, Krieger D, et al. Correlation between ammonia levels and the severity of hepatic encephalopathy. *Am J Med*. 2003;114:188–193.
4. Guillen JCQ, Gutierrez JMH. Diagnostic methods in hepatic encephalopathy. *Clin Chim Acta*. 2006; 365:1–8.
5. Zeneroli ML, Avallone R, Corsi L, et al. Management of hepatic encephalopathy: Role of rifaximin. *Chemotherapy*. 2005;90–95.
6. Blei AT, Cordoba J; Practice Parameters Committee of the American College of Gastroenterology. Hepatic encephalopathy. *Am J Gastroenterol*. 2001;96:1968–1976.
7. Als-Nielsen B, Gluud LL, Gluud C. Non-absorbable disaccharides for hepatic encephalopathy: Systematic review of randomised trials. *BMJ*. 2004;328:1046–1511.

 MISCELLANEOUS

CODES

ICD9-CM
572.2 Hepatic coma

PATIENT TEACHING

Pamphlets suitable for patient and family are available from the American Association for the Study of Liver Diseases, 1729 King Street, Suite 200, Alexandria, Virginia 22314; (703) 299–9766; aasld@aasld.org.

Diet

Have dietitian instruct patient in eating lower-protein diet.

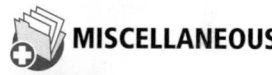 **See Corresponding Diagnostic Algorithm**

H

HEPATITIS A

Rajiv R. Varma, MD
Kia Saeian, MD

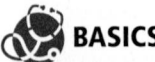 **BASICS**

DESCRIPTION
- A systemic viral infection primarily involving the liver
- System(s) Affected: Gastrointestinal

GENERAL PREVENTION
- Good sanitation, hygiene
- Hand washing, particularly food handlers, health care and day care workers
- Washing and covering of cuts and bruises
- Hepatitis A virus (HAV) vaccine (Havrix, Vaqta)
  - 0.5 mL IM for children >2 years, 1 mL IM for adults; second dose 6–12 months later for those age >8 years
  - Separate syringe site from immune globulin
  - Use for travelers, day care staff/children, custodial facility employees, sewage workers, military, homosexual men, food handlers, Native Americans, Alaskan natives
- Immune globulin (passive immunization): 0.02 mL/kg IM (given 1–2 weeks after exposure prevents illness in 80–90%)
  - With prolonged exposure, give every 5 months
  - Also use for close contacts, day care staff/children (if case occurs), institutions with multiple cases, and travelers to areas of high prevalence (with 3-week lead time, use vaccine).
- Blood exposure is rare.

EPIDEMIOLOGY
- Predominant age: HAV is rare in infants; severity increases with age
- Predominant sex: Male = Female

Incidence
Infections per year: 125,000–200,000, 70% symptomatic; declining incidence with vaccination

Prevalence
Antibodies in 33% of the US population

RISK FACTORS
- Employment in health care/other high risk occupations
- Household exposure
- Intimate exposure
- Recent body piercing; tattoos less likely, role controversial

Genetics
Some predisposition to immunologic manifestations; DR4—positive increase with concurrent immunologic disease

ETIOLOGY
- Multiple viruses possible as coinfection
- Hepatitis A and E viruses are transmitted enterically (fecal–oral); parenteral route is rare
- Maximum infectivity 2 weeks before jaundice
- May be endemic in institutions; in day care centers
- No chronicity in HAV

ASSOCIATED CONDITIONS
- Arthritis
- Urticaria
- Immune complex nephritis (particularly membranous glomerulopathy)
- Anemias (including aplastic anemia)

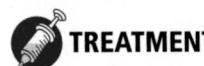 **DIAGNOSIS**

SIGNS AND SYMPTOMS
- Fever (60%)
- Malaise (67%)
- Nausea and vomiting
- Anorexia (54%)
- Jaundice (in adults, 62%)
- Hepatomegaly
- Dark urine (84%)
- Pale stools, usually transient
- Abdominal/right upper quadrant pain
- Fatigue
- Meningismus (occasional)
- Vast majority of patients are minimally symptomatic or asymptomatic, especially children

History
Exposure source

Physical Exam
- Tenderness over the liver may be hepatomegaly.
- Jaundice often is not present.

Pediatric Considerations
Disease is milder, usually anicteric; may be unrecognized.

TESTS
Lab
- Aspartate aminotransferase (AST)/alanine aminotransferase (ALT): Marked elevation (acute hepatitis, particularly ALT, 400 to several 1,000 units per liter). Serum liver function tests are often elevated before bilirubin increases; measure aminotransferases in acute illnesses when there is no evident cause.
- Alkaline phosphatase: Mild elevation
- Bilirubin: Normal to markedly elevated; with elevation, conjugated and unconjugated fractions usually increased
- Serum biochemical markers for each virus are diagnostic in 90% of patients.
- For severe hepatitis
  - Prothrombin time and partial thromboplastin time, albumin, electrolytes, and glucose
  - CBC
- Drugs that may alter lab results: Corticosteroids, other immunosuppressive drugs
- Disorders that may alter lab results: Leukopenia; may exacerbate viral replication

Imaging
Usually not needed

Diagnostic Procedures/Surgery
Liver biopsy usually is not needed.

Pathological Findings
- Features of acute hepatocellular injury with variable inflammation and necrosis
- Lymphoid aggregates are uncommon.
- Chronic liver disease or cirrhosis does not occur.

Positive Serum Markers in Hepatitis A

Status	Marker
A, R	Anti-HAV (total) and IgM both positive
P	Anti-HAV total positive, Anti-HAV IgM negative

Infection status: A, acute; R, recent; P, previous; HAV, hepatitis A virus; IgM, immunoglobulin M.

DIFFERENTIAL DIAGNOSIS
- Other hepatitis viruses
- Infectious mononucleosis
- Primary or secondary hepatic malignancy
- Ischemic hepatitis
- Drug-induced hepatitis
- Alcoholic hepatitis
- Autoimmune hepatitis
- Wilson disease
- Rheumatic and skin manifestation may suggest immunologic disorder.

TREATMENT

INITIAL STABILIZATION
- Treatment is usually outpatient; severe cases need to be admitted.
- Segregation of food handlers with HAV is helpful.

GENERAL MEASURES
- Monitor coagulation defects, fluid and electrolytes, acid–base imbalance, hypoglycemia, and impairment of renal function.
- Report acute cases to public health department.

Diet
Adequate calories; balanced nutrition

Activity
As tolerated

MEDICATION (DRUGS)

Antiviral therapy is not indicated in acute HAV infections, as spontaneous resolution occurs in almost all patients. Corticosteroids may add to morbidity and increase mortality.

SURGERY

Liver transplantation in fulminant hepatic failure

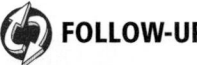 **FOLLOW-UP**

DISPOSITION

Issues for Referral
Fulminant hepatic failure

PROGNOSIS
- Mild disease usual; often no jaundice
- No chronic liver disease
- Mortality <1%
- Lifetime immunity usual with recovery

COMPLICATIONS
- Icteric disease
- 3 rare variants: relapsing, cholestatic, fulminant
- Liver failure

PATIENT MONITORING
- Serial measurement of serum AST/ALT, PT, bilirubin, albumin
- Appropriate serum viral markers are useful for evaluation of recovery or progression.
- Liver biopsies in acute cases if diagnosis remains in doubt
- Monitor for metabolic complications.

 MISCELLANEOUS

See also: Hepatitis B; Hepatitis C; Immunizations

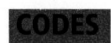 **CODES**

ICD9-CM
070.1 Viral hepatitis

PATIENT TEACHING

 See Corresponding Diagnostic Algorithm

H

HEPATITIS B

Rajiv R. Varma, MD
Kia Saeian, MD

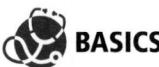 **BASICS**

DESCRIPTION
- A systemic viral infection primarily involving the liver
- System(s) Affected: Gastrointestinal

Pediatric Considerations
More acute, less prolonged, with fewer complications, but may become chronic

GENERAL PREVENTION
- Screen blood products.
- Proper use and disposal of needles
- Good sanitation; proper hygiene, especially by food handlers
- Not sharing razors, toothbrushes, or nail clippers
- Washing and covering cuts and bruises
- Maximum infectivity 2 weeks before jaundice
- May be endemic in institutions, day care centers; vaccinate for hepatitis B virus (HBV)
- HBV transmitted sexually, perinatally, occupationally, and via parenteral drug use (e.g., shared needles); also enterically
- Hepatitis B vaccine: New vaccine to include pres and S2 antigens will be available soon; more effective, especially in nonresponders
- HBV is present in saliva and vaginal secretions; vaccination of sexual partner and household contacts against hepatitis A and B viruses
- High-risk groups: Hepatitis B human immune globulin within 24 hours of exposure (0.06 mL/kg IM)

Pregnancy Considerations
- HBV screening in pregnant women; vaccinate all infants at birth
- Test, in later gestation, for HBsAg
- HBV transmitted vertically (<10%) as well as perinatally and produces carrier state in 30%. Give infant HBIg 0.5 mL and HBV vaccine (Recombivax HB; separate sites) within 12 hours of birth, followed by HBV vaccine 0.5 mL IM at ages 1 and 6 months. Check HBsAg and HBsAb at age 12 months.
- Vertical transmission is increased in HIV co-infection.

EPIDEMIOLOGY
- Predominant age: All ages
- Predominant sex: Fulminant HBV: Male > Female (2:1)

Incidence
Infections per year in the US: 140,000–320,000

Prevalence
- 1–1.25 million people in the US are chronically infected.
- Posttransfusion hepatitis B is rare.
- 350 million carriers worldwide

RISK FACTORS
- Health care worker/other occupational risks
- Hemodialysis
- Recipient of blood and/or blood products (especially before 1992)
- IV drug use: Accounts for 60–70% of new infections
- Sexually active homosexual male
- Household exposure
- Intimate exposure
- Positive needlestick
- Transplanted organs
- Snorting cocaine

- Recent body piercing; tattoos less likely, role controversial
- Perinatal transmission to neonate of hepatitis B-infected mother, rare with hepatitis C virus (HCV) unless mother is HIV positive

ETIOLOGY
HBV

ASSOCIATED CONDITIONS
- Arthritis
- Urticaria
- Immune complex nephritis (particularly membranous glomerulopathy)
- Anemias (including aplastic anemia)
- Dermatitis
- Cardiomyopathy (usually with HBV, rare with HCV)

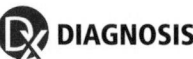 **DIAGNOSIS**

SIGNS AND SYMPTOMS
- Fever (60%)
- Malaise (67%)
- Nausea and vomiting
- Anorexia (54%)
- Jaundice (in adults, 62%)
- Hepatomegaly
- Dark urine (84%)
- Pale stools, usually transient
- Abdominal/right upper quadrant pain
- Fatigue
- Meningismus (occasional)
- Arthralgia/arthritis
- Vast majority are minimally symptomatic or asymptomatic

History
Exposure source

Physical Exam
- Tenderness over the liver may be hepatomegaly.
- Jaundice may not be present in most patients.

TESTS
Lab
- AST/ALT: Marked elevation (acute hepatitis, particularly ALT, 400 to several 1,000 U/L). Serum liver function tests are often elevated before bilirubin increases; measure aminotransferases in acute illnesses when there is no evident cause.
- Alkaline phosphatase: Mild elevation
- Bilirubin: Normal to markedly elevated; with elevation, conjugated and unconjugated fractions are usually increased
- Serum biochemical markers: Diagnostic in 90% of the patients
- Alcohol abuse is a major factor for chronic liver disease. Measure viral biochemical markers in patients with alcoholic liver disease (especially anti-HCV).
- For severe hepatitis
  - Measure PT and PTT, albumin, electrolytes, glucose, and CBC.
- If HBV is chronic, test HBV DNA titer.

Positive Serum Markers in Hepatitis B

Status	Marker
HBV	Anti HBc should be included in hepatitis B panel as it may be the only abnormality indicative of HBV infection. In window period neither HBsAG nor Anti-HBs may be detected
A, E	HBsAg and ± (anti-HBc IgM, window period)
Rcv	Anitbodies to HBe, HBs and HBc antigens detected.
C	HBsAg, HBeAg Markers of replications: HBeAg and anti-HBe and HBV DNA
V	Anti-HBs ± anti-HBc

Infection status: A, acute; R, recent; C, chronic; P, previous; Rcv, recovered; V, vaccinated; E, early/carrier state

- Patients with severe HBV infection should be tested for coinfection or superinfection with hepatitis D virus (HDV). Testing for HDV is also indicated in sexually active homosexual men and in those with a history of IV drug abuse.
- Hepatitis Be antigen (HBeAg) indicates higher infectivity. Hepatitis B virus DNA (HBV DNA) at higher levels (HBV DNA $\geq 10^5$ copies/mL) and HBeAg positivity. Signify active viral replication, which may require antiviral therapy. HBV precore mutations have undetectable HBeAg despite active viral replication which can be measured by HBV DNA levels. Antibody to hepatitis antigen (Anti HBe) is detectable in precore mutations. Risk of hepatocellular carcinoma rises with viral replication, even in the absence of cirrhosis.
- Persistence >6 months indicates probable chronic liver disease.
- Drugs that may alter lab results: Corticosteroids, other immunosuppressive drugs
- Disorders that may alter lab results: Leukopenia: May exacerbate viral replication

Imaging
- Usually helpful
- Ultrasound may demonstrate ascites or exclude obstruction; helpful when cancer is suspected
- CT with IV contrast and MRI in selected cases
- Early cirrhosis usually is not detected by imaging studies; a liver biopsy is needed.

Diagnostic Procedures/Surgery
A liver biopsy is usually needed to determine the type and extent of the liver injury in persistent disease and to exclude other diseases. Also, it is usually necessary before starting antiviral treatment.

Pathological Findings
- Liver biopsy in persistent or chronic disease shows wide range of histologic changes (variable inflammation and/or necrosis, cholestasis, fibrosis, cirrhosis, or chronic active hepatitis).
- Clinical course may not predict severity of histopathologic changes.
- Microvesicular steatosis and lymphoid aggregates suggest hepatitis C infection.

DIFFERENTIAL DIAGNOSIS
- Infectious mononucleosis
- Other hepatitis viruses
- Primary or secondary hepatic malignancy
- Ischemic hepatitis
- Drug-induced hepatitis
- Alcoholic hepatitis
- Autoimmune hepatitis
- Wilson disease
- Rheumatic and skin manifestation may suggest immunologic disorder.

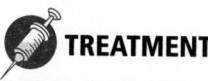

TREATMENT

INITIAL STABILIZATION
Treatment is usually outpatient; severe cases need inpatient care.

GENERAL MEASURES
- Monitor coagulation defects, fluid and electrolytes, acid–base imbalance, hypoglycemia, and impairment of renal function.
- Report acute cases to public health department.
- Use a multidisciplinary approach, especially in those with cirrhosis. Familiarity with risks, side effects, and monitoring for liver cancer and mutations of hepatitis B is essential.

Diet
Adequate calories, balanced nutrition

Activity
As tolerated

Chronic Hepatitis B Therapy

HBeAg	HBV-DNA	ALT*	Rx
+	+	+	IFN, ADV, or LAM
−	−	Normal	Monitor
+/−	+	CC	LAM or ADV
+/−	+	DC	LAM or ADV; Liver transplant
+/−	−	CC	Monitor
+/−	−	DC	Liver transplant

*ALT + when >2x normal; CC, compensated cirrhosis; DC, decompensated cirrhosis; IFN, interferon alpha; ADV, adefovir.

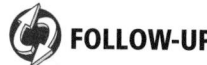

MEDICATION (DRUGS)

First Line
- Acute hepatitis B: Antiviral therapy is not indicated, because spontaneous resolution occurs in ~95% of the patients; others need close monitoring for chronicity or fulminant hepatic failure.
- Chronic hepatitis B: Persistent hepatitis B surface antigenemia >6 months
  - 5 agents are currently licensed: Adefovir, entecavir, lamivudine, peg interferon alfa 2a, and interferon alfa 2b. 1st 3 are oral agents and are usually taken for prolonged periods. Interferons are generally administered for 24 weeks. Interferons are contraindicated in patients with hepatic decompensation; oral agents in these carefully selected cases is safer. Dose adjustments are needed in those patients with elevated serum creatinine.
  - Goals of therapy: Decrease in HBV DNA to undetectable level; loss of HBeAg and appearance of anti-HBe; loss of HBsAg from serum—seldom achieved but ideal
- Contraindications
  - Interferon: Platelet count <50,000
  - Mouse immunoglobulin, egg protein, or neomycin allergy
  - Corticosteroids may add to morbidity/increased mortality.
- Precautions
  - Other disorders of coagulation, myelosuppression, seizures, depression (especially suicide ideation), pregnancy, fertile age group, lactation
  - Increased serum triglycerides may occur during IFN therapy; may cause abnormal ALT
  - Psychiatric evaluation may be prudent prior to IFN treatment.
  - Lamivudine-resistant mutations may be present.
- Significant possible interactions: Refer to the manufacturer's profile of each drug.

Second Line
- Famciclovir (Famvir): 500 mg 2 b.i.d. for chronic hepatitis
- Tenofovir may be available soon.

SURGERY
Consider a liver transplantation in fulminant acute hepatitis/end-stage liver disease (HCV) and in early stages of primary liver cancer. Refer the patient to a tertiary care center with liver and other organ transplant facilities.

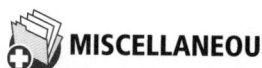 FOLLOW-UP

PROGNOSIS
- Recovery from acute infection in 95% of patients
- Severity of hepatic encephalopathy best predictor of poor survival in hepatic failure
- HBV (mortality 1%) and HDV (with icterus, mortality 2–20%) more severe symptoms; often lead to persistent/chronic liver disease, cirrhosis, liver failure, hepatocellular carcinoma; more severe problems if impaired immune function. Follow treatment with HBV DNA levels.

COMPLICATIONS
- Acute or subacute necrosis
- Chronic active or chronic hepatitis
- Cirrhosis
- Hepatic failure
- Hepatocellular carcinoma (HBV, HCV)

PATIENT MONITORING
- Serial measurement of serum AST/ALT
- Appropriate serum viral markers: Useful for evaluation of recovery or progression
- Liver biopsies in chronic disease; in acute cases if diagnosis remains in doubt
- Monitoring for metabolic complications
- White blood cells, platelets with INF-α therapy
- Chronic HBV: HBV DNA valuable for predicting favorable response to IFN. High pretreatment ALT and low pretreatment HBV DNA associated with favorable response
- Monitoring for hepatic decompensation (e.g., ascites, hepatic encephalopathy, spontaneous bacterial peritonitis) in cirrhotics

REFERENCES
1. Lok ASF, McMahon BJ. Chronic hepatitis B. Practice guidelines on chronic hepatitis B. *Hepatology*. 2004;39:857–861.
2. Proceedings from the roundtable: A cross disciplinary discussion on chronic hepatitis B., Wright TL, ed. *Am J Gastroenterol*. 2006;101(1 Suppl)S1–S39.

 MISCELLANEOUS

See also: Hepatitis A; Hepatitis C; Immunizations

CODES

ICD9-CM
070.30 Viral hepatitis

PATIENT TEACHING

See Corresponding Diagnostic Algorithm

HEPATITIS C

Gennine M. Zinner, RNCS, ANP

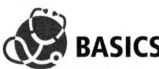 **BASICS**

DESCRIPTION
- A systemic viral infection primarily involving the liver. Can result in both acute and chronic disease.
- System(s) Affected: Gastrointestinal

ALERT
Pediatric Considerations
Uncommon

GENERAL PREVENTION
- Avoid sharing razors, toothbrushes, and nail clippers.
- Wash and cover cuts and bruises.
- Use and dispose of needles properly.
- Observe proper hygiene, particularly when handling food.
- Sexual transmission is low, but does occur.
- Maximum infectivity occurs 2 weeks before jaundice.
- Vertical transmission is increased in pregnant women with HIV.

EPIDEMIOLOGY
- Predominant age: Affects all ages.
- Predominant sex: Male = Female

Incidence
- 16% of sporadic hepatitis
- 40,000 new cases per year in the US
- 8,000–13,000 US deaths per year due to chronic infection
- Donor blood screening has reduced risk.

Prevalence
In the US, 3 million people are chronically infected (60–80% of those infected). Most common cause of chronic liver disease and most frequent reason for liver transplantation in US.

RISK FACTORS
- Health care worker/other occupational risks
- Hepatitis C virus (HCV) is transmitted through blood or its products; in 40%, mode is unknown.
- Hemodialysis
- Recipient of blood and/or blood products (especially before 1992)
- IV drug use: 60–70% of new infections
- Sexually active homosexual male (much more likely with hepatitis B than with C)
- Household exposure
- Intimate exposure
- Positive needlestick
- Transplanted organs
- Inhaled cocaine
- Controversial: Body piercing; tattoos
- HIV positively increases risk of hepatitis B and C virus infection.
- Perinatal transmission of HCV to neonate of hepatitis C–infected mother is rare unless mother is HIV positive.

Genetics
Some predisposition to immunologic manifestations; DR4-positive increase with concurrent immunologic disease

ETIOLOGY
HCV

ASSOCIATED CONDITIONS
- Arthritis
- Urticaria
- Diabetes mellitus
- Autoimmune disorders: Thyroiditis, immune complex nephritis (particularly membranous glomerulopathy)
- Hematologic diseases: Anemias (including aplastic anemia), lymphoma
- Dermatitis
- Cardiomyopathy (rare)
- HCV implicated in sporadic form of idiopathic mixed cryoglobulinemia, porphyria cutaneous tarda, polyarteritis nodosa
- Hepatocellular carcinoma
- HIV–HCV: More severe course

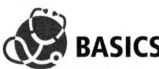 **DIAGNOSIS**

SIGNS AND SYMPTOMS
- Fever (60%)
- Malaise (67%)
- Nausea and vomiting
- Anorexia (54%)
- Jaundice (<25%)
- Hepatomegaly
- Dark urine (84%)
- Pale stools, usually transient
- Pruritus
- Abdominal/right upper quadrant pain
- Fatigue (major complaint)
- Meningismus (occasional)
- Arthralgia/arthritis
- Vast majority of cases are minimally symptomatic or asymptomatic. If acute symptoms occur, usually last for 2–12 weeks.

History
Exposure source; exclude drugs, both prescription and OTC, and herbs. Substance-use history (past and current) should be explored.

Physical Exam
- Tenderness over the liver/hepatomegaly.
- Jaundice may not be present in most cases.

TESTS
Lab
- Aspartate aminotransferase (AST)/alanine aminotransferase (ALT)
  - Marked elevation (acute hepatitis, particularly ALT, 400 to several thousand units per liter)
  - ALT may be normal (up to 1/3 of chronic cases have normal ALT)
  - AST/ALT ratio ≥ 1 is associated with cirrhosis in chronic HCV
- Alkaline phosphatase: Mild elevation
- Serum liver function tests often are elevated before bilirubin increases; measure aminotransferases in acute illnesses when no cause is evident. On the average, these become elevated 6–12 weeks after exposure.
- Bilirubin: Normal to markedly elevated; with elevation, conjugated and unconjugated fractions usually are increased.
- Acute, ongoing HCV: Confirm by other markers—radioimmune-binding assay (RIBA) or enzyme-linked immunosorbent assay (ELISA), HCV-RNA (for chronic HCV); higher viral counts, genotypes 1, 2, 3, and 4
- In early acute HCV infection, anti-HCV may be negative; becomes positive as early as 8 weeks following exposure.
- HCV RNA becomes positive early in acute cases (within days–8 weeks following exposure).

Positive Serum Markers in Hepatitis C

Status	Marker
A, C	Anti-HCV ELISA III or RIBA HCV RNA: (qualitative and quantitative) Genotypes 1–4

Infection status: A, acute; C, chronic; HCV, hepatitis C virus; ELISA, enzyme-linked immunosorbent assay; RIBA, radioimmune-binding assay.

- HCV genotypes may be useful. Genotypes with favorable prognosis: 2a, 2b, 3a; less favorable: 1a, 1b
- Serum biochemical markers for each virus are diagnostic in 90% of patients.
- Alcohol abuse is a major factor in chronic liver disease from HCV. Measure viral biochemical markers in patients with alcoholic liver disease (especially anti-HCV).
- For severe hepatitis:
  - Prothrombin and partial thromboplastin time, albumin, electrolytes, and glucose
  - CBC
- Persistence for >6 months indicates probable chronic liver disease.
- Check alpha-fetoprotein (AFP) periodically in those with chronic infection (especially cirrhotics) to screen for possible hepatocellular carcinoma.
- Drugs that may alter lab results Corticosteroids, immunosuppressive drugs
- Disorders that may alter lab results Leukopenia may exacerbate viral replication

Imaging
- Ultrasound may demonstrate ascites or exclude obstruction; helpful when cancer is suspected.
- CT with IV contrast and MRI may be used in selected cases.
- Early cirrhosis is usually not detected by imaging studies; a liver biopsy is needed.

Diagnostic Procedures/Surgery
A liver biopsy usually is needed to determine the type and extent of the liver injury in persistent disease and to exclude other diseases. Also, it is usually necessary before starting antiviral treatment such as interferon (INF)-α.

Pathological Findings
- Liver biopsy in persistent or chronic disease shows wide range of histologic changes (variable inflammation and/or necrosis, cholestasis, lymphoid aggregate, steatosis, fibrosis, cirrhosis, or chronic active hepatitis).
- Clinical course may not predict severity of histopathologic changes.
- Microvesicular steatosis and lymphoid aggregates suggest hepatitis C infection.

DIFFERENTIAL DIAGNOSIS
- Infectious mononucleosis
- Other viral hepatitides
- Primary or secondary hepatic malignancy
- Ischemic hepatitis
- Drug-induced hepatitis
- Alcoholic hepatitis
- Autoimmune hepatitis
- Wilson disease

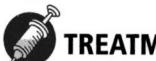 TREATMENT

INITIAL STABILIZATION
Outpatient, unless symptoms are severe

GENERAL MEASURES
- Monitor coagulation defects, fluid and electrolytes, acid–base imbalance, hypoglycemia, and impairment of renal function.
- Report acute cases to Dept. of Public Health.
- Use multidisciplinary approach led by experienced physician-led team.
- Careful patient selection is essential.

Diet
Adequate calories, balanced nutrition

 MEDICATION (DRUGS)

- Better outcomes of treatment more likely with age ≤40, absence of cirrhosis/bridging fibrosis, HCV RNAS ≤2 million copies/mL, genotypes 2 and 3, lighter body weight, absence of HIV, shorter duration of infection.
- Acute hepatitis C: Antiviral therapy is highly effective for acute infections.
  - Pegylated interferon (Peg-I) for 12–24 weeks.
  - Other options: Peg-IFN + Ribavirin; IFN
- Chronic hepatitis C: Peg-IFN + Ribavirin
  - Peg-IFN alfa-2b 1.5 mcg/kg SC per week
  - Peg-IFN alfa-2a 180 mcg SC per week
  - Ribavirin: 400–600 mg PO b.i.d (dose based on patient's weight and type of interferon used. With Peg-IFN, use 400 mg b.i.d.)
  - Other options: Peg-IFN monotherapy, IFN/Ribavirin; IFN-β.
  - Duration of therapy: 24 weeks–1 year, depending on drug combination, genotype, and response (measured at 12 and 24 weeks with quantitative HCV-RNA)
- Contraindications
  - IFN: Platelet count <50,000
  - Mouse immunoglobulin, egg protein, or neomycin allergy
  - Corticosteroids may add to morbidity/increased mortality
- Precautions
  - Other disorders of coagulation, myelosuppression, seizures, depression (especially suicidal ideation), pregnancy, fertile age group, lactation
  - Ribavirin may induce hemolytic anemia (hemoglobin 2 g/dL below pretreatment level is common); avoid in pregnancy.
  - Increased serum triglycerides may occur during IFN therapy; may cause abnormal ALT. Measure HCV RNA to assess response in such patients.
  - A psychiatric evaluation may be prudent prior to an IFN treatment due to depression being a potential adverse effect.
- Significant possible interactions: Refer to the manufacturer's profile of each drug.

SURGERY
Consider liver transplantation in fulminant acute hepatitis/end-stage liver disease and in early stages of primary liver cancer. Refer to tertiary care center with liver/organ transplant facilities.

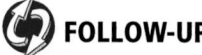 FOLLOW-UP

PROGNOSIS
- Severity of hepatic encephalopathy is the best predictor of poor survival in hepatic failure.
- Regardless of severity
  - 60–80% progress to chronic hepatitis
  - ~20–30% progress to cirrhosis and some to liver failure
  - Typically slow progression: 10–30 years
  - May progress to hepatocellular carcinoma, but IFN may decrease risk
  - Associated with type II autoimmune hepatitis
  - Chronic HCV is unlikely to clear HCV RNA spontaneously.
  - HCV after needlestick is usually a sustained IFN response.
  - Final-phase HCV is a rare cause of fulminant hepatic failure, but may be more common in those coinfected with hepatitis B virus.
- Alcohol increases severity of chronic HCV, possible even with relatively low intake.

COMPLICATIONS
- Acute or subacute necrosis, chronic hepatitis, hepatic failure
- Primary liver cancer risk
- HCV-associated cirrhosis: 1–3% per year; lifetime risk 20–30%. Cirrhosis patients need surveillance for hepatocellular carcinoma.

PATIENT MONITORING
- Serial measurement of serum AST/ALT
- Appropriate serum viral markers are useful for evaluation of recovery or progression.
- Liver biopsies in chronic disease; in acute cases if diagnosis remains in doubt
- Monitoring for metabolic complications
- White blood cells, platelets with IFN-α therapy
- Undetectable HCV RNA (quantitative serum HCV RNA) at 12 weeks is associated with a sustained response. Persistently positive HCV RNA at 24 weeks indicates lack of response; prolonged course is unlikely to be beneficial.
- Monitoring for hepatic decompensation (e.g., ascites, hepatic encephalopathy, spontaneous bacterial peritonitis) in cirrhotics
- Goal of therapy is eradication of HCV; HCV RNA test should become persistently undetectable.
- Early virologic response is ≥2 log decrease in HCV RNA level after 12 weeks of treatment.
- In patients with cirrhosis, the risk of hepatic cellular carcinoma is high (20% lifetime risk). Monitor for hypervascular lesions by imaging (ultrasound, helical CT) every 6 months.

REFERENCES
1. Alter MJ, Kruszan-Moran D, Naiman OV, et al. The prevalence of hepatitis C virus infection in the United States. *N Engl J Med*. 1999;341:556–562.
2. Gane E, Portmann B, Naouniov N, et al. Long-term outcome of hepatitis C infection after liver transplantation. *N Engl J Med*. 1996;334:815–820.
3. Jaeckel E, Cornberg M, Wedemeyer H, et al. Treatment of acute hepatitis C with interferon alfa-2b. *N Engl J Med*. 2001;345:1452–1457.
4. Lauer GM, Walker BD. Hepatitis C virus infection. Medical progress. *N Engl J Med*. 2001;345:41–52.
5. Manns MP, McHutchison JG, Gordon SC, et al. Peg-interferon alfa 2b plus ribavirin compared with interferon alfa 2b plus ribavirin for initial treatment of chronic hepatitis C: A randomized controlled trial. *Lancet*. 2001;358:958–965.
6. Seeff LB. Emerging and reemerging issues, infections diseases: hepatitis C: A meeting ground for the generalist and the specialist. *Am J Med*. 1999;107(Suppl 6B):1–100.
7. Dienstag JL, Mchutchison JG. American Gastroenterological Association technical review on the management of hepatitis C. *Gastroenterology*. 2006;130:231–264.

 MISCELLANEOUS

See also: Hepatitis A; Hepatitis B; Immunizations

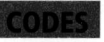 CODES

ICD9-CM
070.51 Viral hepatitis

PATIENT TEACHING

 See Corresponding Diagnostic Algorithm

H

HEPATITIS, AUTOIMMUNE

Nicholas Miller, MD

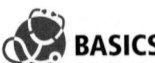 **BASICS**

DESCRIPTION

Autoimmune hepatitis (AIH) is a chronic inflammatory disorder of the liver, of unknown etiology, characterized by interface hepatitis, hypogammaglobinemia, and autoantibodies.

- Type I (classic)
  - Most common type
  - Effects all age groups
- Type II (ALKM-1)
  - Primarily affects young females
- Type III is clinically identical to type I, but with different antibody profile.
  - Least well established type

EPIDEMIOLOGY

Predominant sex: Women > Men

- Type II generally affects children

Incidence

1.9 per 100,000 per year

Prevalence

16.9 per 100,000

RISK FACTORS

- Female sex
- Young age
- HLA DR3 or DR4
- Associated autoimmune conditions (see Associated Conditions)

Genetics

- Type I associated with HLA DR3 (DRB1*0301) and DR4 (DRB1*401). Those with DRB1*0301 tend to be younger and have poorer outcomes.
- Type II associated with DRB1*0701, HLA B14, DR3, and C4A-QO.

PATHOPHYSIOLOGY

Inflammation of the liver leading to fibrosis and cirrhosis in advanced cases

- Cell-mediated and antibody-dependent cytotoxicity have been implicated.

ETIOLOGY

Unknown

ASSOCIATED CONDITIONS

- Type I diabetes mellitus
- Thyroiditis
- Hemolytic anemia
- Idiopathic thrombocytic purpura
- Celiac sprue
- Ulcerative colitis
- Vitiligo
- Synovitis
- Primary biliary cirrhosis and primary sclerosing cholangitis occasionally overlap with AIH (1)

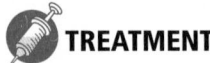 **DIAGNOSIS**

SIGNS AND SYMPTOMS

- Often asymptomatic, but may present as fulminant hepatitis
- RUQ pain, fatigue, anorexia, weakness, nausea, jaundice, pruritus, arthralgia

History

- 40% of cases abrupt in onset
- Often history of other autoimmune disorder especially in type II AIH
- History of previous episode of AIH (relapse common)
- History of drug use or heavy alcohol consumption make diagnosis less likely

Physical Exam

Physical examination often normal, however possible findings include

- Hepatomegaly
- Splenomegaly
- Stigmata of chronic liver disease
- Jaundice

TESTS

Lab

- Alkaline phosphatase, AST, ALT
  - Alk phos:AST (or ALT) ratio of <1.5 suggest AIH (2)[C]
- Serum globulins or IgG >1.0 suggests AIH (2)[C]
- Autoantibodies with titers >1:40 suggest AIH, including (2)[C]
  - Antinuclear antibodies (ANA)
  - Antismooth muscle antibodies (ASMA)
  - Antibodies to liver/kidney microsomes (ALKM-1) (suggests type II AIH)
- Antimitochondrial antibodies (presence makes AIH less likely)
- HLA-DR3 or HLA-DR4 positive (2)[C]

Diagnostic Procedures/Surgery

Liver biopsy

Pathological Findings

- Interface hepatitis characteristic of AIH; plasma cell infiltrate and rosettes also common (2)[C]
- Portal mononuclear cell infiltrate (3)[C]
- Eosinophils frequently present (3)[C]
- Biliary tree generally spared (3)[C]
- Fibrosis usually present with bridging in advanced cases (3)[C]

DIFFERENTIAL DIAGNOSIS

- AIH is a diagnosis of exclusion; hereditary, viral, and drug-induced causes must be ruled out.
- Primary biliary cirrhosis
- Primary sclerosing cholangitis
- Acute or chronic viral hepatitis
- Steatohepatitis (alcoholic or nonalcoholic)
- Systemic lupus erythematosus
- Wilson disease
- Hemochromatosis
- α-1-Antitrypsin deficiency
- Drug-induced hepatitis (e.g., minocycline, isoniazid, α-methyldopa hydrazine, nitrofurantoin)

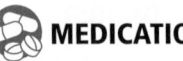 **TREATMENT**

GENERAL MEASURES

Keep patient comfortable, with analgesics as necessary.

Diet

As tolerated

Activity

As tolerated

SPECIAL THERAPY

IV-Fluids

If significant nausea or vomiting occurs, replace fluid losses.

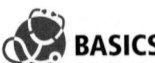 **MEDICATION (DRUGS)**

Treatment indicated in following conditions

- AST >10 times normal (4)[C]
- AST >5 times normal with serum gamma globulin >2 times normal (4)[C]
- Histologic features of bridging necrosis or multiacinar necrosis (4)[C]
- Treatment generally indicated in pediatric patients (4)[C]

First Line

- Prednisone 30 mg (taper down to 10 mg) with azathioprine 50 mg (3–5)[B]
  - Preferred therapy
- Prednisone 60 mg (taper down to 20 mg) alone (3–5)[B]

- Relative contraindications to use of prednisone
  - Osteoporosis
  - Postmenopause
  - Diabetes
  - Hypertension
  - Obesity
  - Acne
  - Emotional lability
- Relative contraindications to use of azathioprine
  - TPMT deficiency (can be screened for)
  - Cytopenia
  - Pregnancy

Second Line

- 6-Mercaptopurine may be substituted for azathioprine (4,5)[C]
- Cyclosporine may be used in children who do not tolerate prednisone (4,5)[C]
- Cyclophosphamide, mycophenolate mofetil, deflazacort, tacrolimus have shown some benefit in small trials (5)[C]

ALERT
Geriatric Considerations
Use corticosteroids with caution in the elderly.

Pediatric Considerations
AIH often more advanced in children, and treatment is generally advised.

Pregnancy Considerations
- AIH associated with increased risk of low birth weight, prematurity, and fetal demise. Pregnancy is not a contraindication to treatment.
- Azathioprine is relatively, but not absolutely contraindicated in pregnancy.

SURGERY
Liver transplant for liver failure
- AIH may reoccur after transplant.

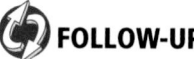 **FOLLOW-UP**

- Although resolution of clinical and laboratory findings usually occurs within 2 weeks, treatment should be continued for 3–6 months after this, because histological improvement lags behind clinical improvement (3,4)[C].
  - Liver biopsy may be helpful before discontinuing or reducing maintenance dose (4)[C].
    - Liver biopsy also may be helpful for monitoring. One author suggests biopsying 1 year after normalization of laboratory values and/or 2 years after initial presentation (3)[C].
- Relapse is common after discontinuation of therapy, especially within the 1st year; characterized by AST level 3 times normal (4)[C].
  - Monitor AST regularly after discontinuing therapy. May decrease frequency of monitoring if no relapse occurs.
  - Relapse treated same as initial AIH.
  - Long-term low-dose therapy may be indicated after multiple relapses.

DISPOSITION
Emergency or outpatient evaluation with admission to hospital for moderate to severe cases or those sudden in onset

Admission Criteria
None; use clinical judgment. Severe cases should be admitted and treated promptly to prevent fulminant hepatitis. Children tend to present at more advanced stages of the disease and may also warrant hospitalization.

PROGNOSIS
- In severe cases, without treatment, 10-year survival only 10%
- With treatment survival >80% at 20 years (no statistical difference from general population)
  - Despite treatment, 40% develop cirrhosis within 10 years. However, this does not impact immediate prognosis

COMPLICATIONS
- Secondary to cirrhosis and liver failure or to drug side effects
- Hepatocellular cancer is a rare complication in those with cirrhosis for at least 5 years

PATIENT MONITORING
- As above
- Consider screening for hepatocellular cancer in patients with cirrhosis every 6–12 months with ultrasound and α-fetoprotein (no benefit established)

REFERENCES
1. Ben-Ari Z, Czaja AJ. Autoimmune hepatitis and its variant syndromes. *Gut* 2001;49(4):589–594.
2. Alvrez F, et al. International Autoimmune Hepatitis Group Report: Review of criteria for diagnosis of autoimmune hepatitis. *J Hepatol* 1999;31:929–938.
3. Krawitt EL. Autoimmune hepatitis. *NEJM* 2006;354:54–66.
4. Ah-Khalidi JA, Czaja AJ. Current concepts in the diagnosis, pathogenesis, and treatment of autoimmune hepatitis. *Mayo Clin Proc* 2001;76(12):1237–1252.
5. Manns MP, Vogel A. Autoimmune hepatitis, from mechanism to therapy. *Hepatology* 2006;43(2):S123–144.

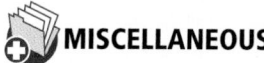 **MISCELLANEOUS**

PATIENT TEACHING
Avoid alcohol and tobacco products.

Diet
- Dieting to control weight and lipids is advised.
- Supplementary vitamin K, D, as well as calcium

Activity
Regular exercise is advised.

 See Corresponding Diagnostic Algorithm

H

HEPATOMA

Ruben Peralta, MD, FACS
Venu G. Pillarisetty, MD

BASICS

DESCRIPTION
Primary malignant tumor of the liver arising from hepatic parenchymal cells (hepatocytes), blood vessels, or cholangioles within the liver, excluding gallbladder and biliary passages. With the exception of the rare fibrolamellar type, 85% are associated with an underlying liver disease, usually cirrhosis.

GENERAL PREVENTION
- Prevent hepatitis B virus (HBV) and hepatitis C virus (HCV) infection/cirrhosis: Safe sexual practices, avoid shared drug paraphernalia, HBV vaccination in high-risk individuals and all children
- Treat HBV and HCV with α-interferon to avoid cirrhosis
- Avoid excessive alcohol use.
- Screening in at-risk individuals
  - AFP has highly variable sensitivity and specificity
  - Ultrasound (US) frequently used to screen high-risk individuals
  - MRI has the highest sensitivity (81%) and moderately high specificity (85%)
  - Patients exposed to ≥ 10 years of vinyl chloride should have sonography every 6 months. New nodules should be promptly biopsied.

EPIDEMIOLOGY
Incidence
- 5th most common malignancy worldwide; most common hepatic malignancy worldwide
- 1–5 new cases per 100,000 of the US population per year
- Among known cirrhotics, 2–5 cases per 100 per year

Prevalence
- Asians > Whites > Blacks > Hispanics > Native Americans
- Predominant age: Mean age 55–62 in West, 2–3 decades earlier in Asia and Africa
- Male > Female (3–4:1)

ALERT
Pediatric Considerations
Extremely rare in children; may be seen in children with Hepatitis B and/or cirrhosis.

RISK FACTORS
- For hepatocellular carcinoma
  - All forms of cirrhosis: Hepatitis B and C, alcoholism, hemochromatosis, nonalcoholic steatohepatitis, α_1-antitrypsin deficiency, biliary cirrhosis
  - Long-term use of oral contraceptives or hormone replacement
  - Repeated ingestion of fungus-infected food
  - Choledochal cysts
  - Clonorchiasis
- For fibrolamellar type: Risk factors unknown
- For angiosarcoma: Vinyl polymer

Genetics
No known genetic pattern

ETIOLOGY
- Cirrhosis accounts for 60–80% HCC
  - Alcoholic cirrhosis most important in Western world. Reported risk of hepatoma in alcoholic cirrhosis is 3–10% with micronodular pattern
- HBV and HCV independent and synergistic risk factors for HCC
  - Associated with >70% of cases worldwide
  - Most important factor in Africa and Asia
- Chronic alcohol use
- Chronic smoking
- Mycotoxins (aflatoxins)
  - Metabolite of the fungus *Aspergillus flavus* that contaminates foods
- Vinyl polymer, but not the finished product, produces angiosarcoma.

ASSOCIATED CONDITIONS
- Infections
  - Viral hepatitis B, C, D
  - Clonorchiasis
  - Schistosomiasis
- Alcoholic cirrhosis
- Primary liver diseases
  - Primary biliary cirrhosis
- Metabolic diseases
  - α_1-Antitrypsin deficiency
  - Hemochromatosis
  - Tyrosinemia

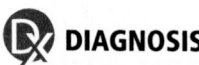
DIAGNOSIS

SIGNS AND SYMPTOMS
- In children
  - Feminization, precocious puberty
  - Palpable nodule on liver
  - In ages 2–6 years, abdominal mass in liver, abdominal pain, irregular hepatomegaly
- In adults
  - Known cirrhosis or prominent clinical signs of cirrhosis: 80%
  - Abdominal pain: 80%; right upper quadrant, dull ache to severe
  - Hepatomegaly: 80–90%; irregular, nodular, firm to hard, tender
  - Weight loss: 30%
  - Hepatic arterial bruit: 20%
  - Friction rub: Rare, more common in metastatic liver disease
  - Nausea, vomiting
  - Paraneoplastic syndrome: Hypertrophic osteoarthropathy, carcinoid syndrome, feminization, polycythemia
  - Hemoperitoneum: Most common tumor cause
  - Unexplained deterioration of stable cirrhosis
  - Budd-Chiari syndrome

TESTS
Lab
- Liver function test abnormalities
- Rare paraneoplastic syndrome: Erythrocytosis, elevated calcium, low glucose
- Tumor markers
  - AFP: Single most important lab test for screening and diagnosis of hepatoma: most useful test for hepatocellular carcinoma Level >400 ng/mL (>400 μg/L) is diagnostic; level does not correlate with prognosis, useful in monitoring for recurrence
- Disorders that may alter lab results (all cause slight elevation of AFP)
  - Acute or chronic hepatitis
  - Germ-cell tumors
  - Pregnancy

Imaging
- Ultrasound
  - Capable of detecting tumor >1 cm
  - May be positive when AFP is normal
  - Has been useful in serially following cases of cirrhosis to identify hepatocellular cancer when <2 cm and curable
  - May also be used to guide percutaneous liver biopsy and to guide other percutaneous guided therapy (injection or ablation)
- CT scan
  - Can detect tumors at 1 cm
  - Valuable in determining extrahepatic spread of the disease
- PET/PET-CT improves CT detection rates
- MRI: More sensitive than helical CT for early detection of hepatocellular carcinoma, and may help differentiate benign from malignant tumors. Helpful in delineating the details of tumor and the invasion of vessels
- Hepatic arteriography: Less commonly used as MRI technology improves, used to define vascular anatomy for resection or embolization

Diagnostic Procedures/Surgery
- Tissue diagnosis must be made for appropriate treatment.
- Liver biopsy: Usually ultrasound-guided or CT-guided when nodules are not palpable
- Laparoscopy occasionally used to evaluate extent in cirrhosis

Pathological Findings
- Nodular: 75%; usually in cirrhotic liver
- Massive: Common in children and noncirrhotic livers; more prone to rupture
- Diffuse: Rare; a large part of liver is involved
- Hepatocellular origin
  - Most commonly multicentric, well differentiated; usually superimposed on underlying cirrhosis

DIFFERENTIAL DIAGNOSIS

- Early asymptomatic tumor: Underlying liver conditions
  - Cirrhosis
  - Chronic hepatitis
  - Benign liver nodules
  - Hamartoma
  - Hemangioma
  - Metastatic adenocarcinoma
  - Gallstones
  - Gallbladder polyp
- Late symptomatic tumor with hepatomegaly
  - Hepatic cyst
  - Adenoma
  - Hemangioma
  - Abscess
  - Metastatic malignancy of liver
  - Cirrhosis
  - Thrombosis of hepatic veins, portal vein, or inferior vena cava
  - Active viral hepatitis or alcoholic hepatitis
- Ruptured tumor
  - All causes of acute abdomen
  - Traumatic hemoperitoneum

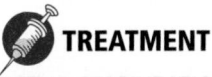 **TREATMENT**

INITIAL STABILIZATION
Inpatient treatment

GENERAL MEASURES
Precautions to avoid falls

Diet
Attention to nutrition: High-calorie, low-protein

Activity
As tolerated

 MEDICATION (DRUGS)

- Chemotherapy has no survival benefit
- Treatment of hepatoma in patients with hepatitis C with pegylated interferon-α and ribavirin prolongs survival and improves quality of life.

SURGERY
- Surgical resection is the only cure.
  - Should be considered in children, and may include up to a lobe of the liver.
  - High cure rate when ≤3 or fewer nodules, each <5 cm
- Radiography-guided radiofrequency ablation (or the less-effective alcohol injection) is effective palliation and may make surgery possible.
- Embolization of the tumor-supplying artery with chemotherapy, under radiographic guidance, is effective palliation and may make surgery possible.
- The presence of small tumors (no more than 3, each <5 cm) increases the priority for transplantation if it is otherwise indicated.
- Fibrolamellar variant should be treated by surgical resection, and yields excellent survival.

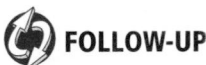 **FOLLOW-UP**

PROGNOSIS
- Unresectable symptomatic tumors: Grave; patients seldom live >6 months.
- Resectable asymptomatic tumors
  - Surgery is curative in >70% of children, 40% of adults
  - Surgery is curative in >80% of tumors <3 cm in cirrhosis
- Transplantation: Same survival as that for tumorfree patients when hepatoma is incidentally discovered or is <2 cm in diameter; only slight reduction in survival with up to 3 tumor nodules <5 cm
- Fibrolamellar has better prognosis.

COMPLICATIONS
- Rupture
- Hemoperitoneum
- Liver failure
- Cachexia
- Metastases to other organs
- Thrombosis of portal, hepatic, renal veins

PATIENT MONITORING
- After successful resection, a high risk for recurrence
- Check AFP every 3 months.
- Ultrasound every 4–6 months

REFERENCES

1. Colli A, Fraquelli M, Casazza G, et al. Accuracy of ultrasonography, spiral CT, magnetic resonance, and alpha-fetoprotein in diagnosing hepatocellular carcinoma: A systematic review. *Am J Gastroenterol.* 2006;101:513–523.
2. Stipa F, Yoon SS, Liau KH, et al. Outcome of patients with fibrolamellar hepatocellular carcinoma. *Cancer.* 2006;106(6):1331–1338.
3. Thomas MB, Abbruzzese JL. Opportunities for targeted therapies in hepatocellular carcinoma. *J Clin Oncol.* 2005;23(31):8093–8108.

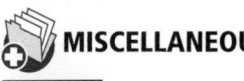 **MISCELLANEOUS**

CODES

ICD9-CM
155.0 Malignant neoplasm of liver, primary

PATIENT TEACHING

Emphasize preventive measures; Hep B vaccine

 See Corresponding Diagnostic Algorithm

H

HEPATORENAL SYNDROME

Michael M. Van Ness, MD

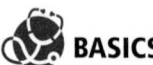

BASICS

DESCRIPTION
- An acute, functional, and progressive reduction in renal blood flow and glomerular filtration rate (GFR) secondary to intense renal cortical vasoconstriction in the setting of decompensated cirrhosis
- Other etiologies for renal failure in cirrhosis must be absent to diagnose hepatorenal syndrome (HRS). HRS may be classified as
  - Type I— rapidly progressive decline in GFR (<2 weeks)
  - Type II—not as rapidly progressive (>2 weeks)
- System(s) Affected: Endocrine/Metabolic; Gastrointestinal; Hemic/Lymphatic/Immunologic; Nervous; Renal/urologic
- Synonym(s): Renal failure of cirrhosis; Functional renal failure of cirrhosis; Hepatic nephropathy; Heyd syndrome; Oliguric renal failure of cirrhosis; Hemodynamic renal failure of cirrhosis

GENERAL PREVENTION
See "Risk Factors."

EPIDEMIOLOGY
- Unknown (clear-cut differentiation between HRS and acute tubular necrosis [ATN] or prerenal state not always made)
  - Estimate: 32–41/100 admitted to the hospital for cirrhosis with ascites develop HRS at 2 and 5 years
  - 1 other study in patients with cirrhosis and ascites: 18% and 39% (of HRS) at 1 and 5 years
- Predominant age: Usually after 4th decade (increased incidence of alcoholic cirrhosis), but may occur at any age
- Predominant sex: Male > Female (increased incidence and prevalence of alcoholic cirrhosis)

RISK FACTORS
Any reduction of effective blood volume in cirrhosis, including
- Excessive diuresis and GI blood loss (e.g., variceal bleeding)
- Excessive diarrhea (lactulose-induced)
- Bacteremia
- Reduction in venous return with tense ascites
- Vomiting, GI bleeding
- Protein-calorie malnutrition, especially with alcoholic cirrhosis

Genetics
Not important except as risk for liver disease (e.g., infantile or autosomal recessive polycystic kidney disease or α_1-antitrypsin deficiency)

ETIOLOGY
- End-stage liver disease from alcohol or toxins
- Viral hepatitis
- Fulminant hepatic failure
- Malignancy
- Any other injury that leads to cirrhosis (e.g., *Schistosoma*) with accompanying risk factors

ASSOCIATED CONDITIONS
- See "Etiology" and "Differential Diagnosis"
- Pregnancy may be associated with HRS if liver failure occurs during pregnancy.

DIAGNOSIS

SIGNS AND SYMPTOMS
- Oliguria in the setting of cirrhosis
- Jaundice, ascites, encephalopathy
- GI bleeding
- Poor nutritional status
- Splenomegaly
- Spider angioma
- Peripheral vasodilatation
- Tachycardia and bounding pulse often present with HRS (almost always develop during a hospitalization, not on admission).

TESTS
Lab
- Azotemia in the setting of cirrhosis with appropriate spot urine values (consistent with tubular function)
  - Sodium <10 mEq/L (10 mmol/L)
  - Fractional excretion of sodium <1%
  - Urine/plasma creatinine >30:1
  - Osmolality: Mild to moderate reduction in concentrating ability (400–600 mOsm/kg/water)
  - All reversible causes should be ruled out (e.g., prerenal azotemia, obstruction)
- Urinalysis: Absence of ATN casts; <500 mg/dL protein
- Lack of improvement in renal function following diuretic withdrawal and expansion of plasma volume with 1.5 L of normal saline
- Minor criteria
  - Urine volume <500 mL/d
  - Urine red blood cells <50/high-power field
  - Serum sodium <130 mcg/L
- Other
  - Prolonged prothrombin time
  - Decreased serum albumin concentration
  - Elevated bilirubin

Imaging
- Renal ultrasound shows normal kidneys without obstruction
- Xenon-133 washout curves show a profound reduction in renal cortical perfusion (historic interest)
- Though experimental presently, renal duplex Doppler ultrasonography appears to have predictive value in separating cirrhotics who will develop HRS from those who will not based on resistive index.

Pathological Findings
- Liver: Cirrhosis or acute fulminant failure
- Kidneys: Would function if transplanted into hosts without liver disease; a functional renal derangement only

DIFFERENTIAL DIAGNOSIS
For abrupt onset of oliguria in cirrhosis
- Volume contraction
- Cardiac failure (possibly alcoholic cardiomyopathy)
- Acute vasomotor nephropathy
- Obstruction
- Interstitial nephritis (drug-induced)

TREATMENT

INITIAL STABILIZATION
Maintenance of volume status in cirrhosis

GENERAL MEASURES
- Supportive
  - Avoid iatrogenic events that precipitate HRS.
  - Diagnose and treat correctable causes of azotemia in cirrhosis: Try volume expanders (100 g of albumin in 500 mL of normal saline) possible; maximize left ventricular function if possible; relieve urinary obstruction when present.
- Other
  - Large-volume paracentesis
  - Dialysis: Indicated only as ancillary support for patients awaiting liver transplant or in patients with acute, potentially reversible liver failure
  - Head-out water immersion and LeVeen shunts: Of dubious value
  - Acute liver failure with HRS may reverse if the liver regenerates.

Activity
Bed rest

MEDICATION (DRUGS)

First Line
- Low-dose dopamine may provide temporary benefit. Not curative or proven in clinical studies
- Avoid NSAIDs, demeclocycline, aminoglycosides, or other nephrotoxins.
- Judicious use of loop diuretics
- Avoid iatrogenic volume contraction in cirrhotic inpatients.
- Significant possible interactions: Refer to the manufacturer's literature.

Second Line
Vasopressin analogues (terlipressin and ornipressin) combined with plasma volume expansion demonstrate some effect on the short-term reversibility of renal dysfunction and may act as a bridge to liver transplantation. Questions over efficacy however.

SURGERY
Liver transplantation when feasible is the only curative treatment. The observed 3-month to estimated 6-month to 1-year survival in patients with transjugular intrahepatic portosystemic stent-shunts is improved. LeVeen shunt may provide similar benefit.

 ## FOLLOW-UP

PROGNOSIS
- Grave without liver transplant in chronic cirrhosis or without regeneration of the liver in acute fulminant failure
- If liver transplantation is performed, actuarial patient survival afterward is lower in patients with preceding HRS.
- The patient may be supported with hemodialysis, continuous arteriovenous hemofiltration, or continuous arteriovenous hemodialysis and transjugular portosystemic stent-shunt prior to organ availability for transplantation.

COMPLICATIONS
Death

REFERENCES

1. Arroyo V, Gines P, Gerbes AL, et al. Definition and diagnostic criteria of refractory ascites and hepatorenal syndrome in cirrhosis. *Hepatology*. 1996;23:164–176.
2. Bateller R, Sort P, Gines P, Arroyo V. Hepatorenal syndrome: Definition, pathophysiology, clinical features and management. *Kidney Int*. 1998;53 (suppl 66):47–53.
3. Brensing KA, Textor J, Strunk H, et al. Transjugular intrahepatic portosystemic stent-shunt for hepatorenal syndrome. *Lancet*. 1997;349: 697–698.
4. Celeb H, Dondy E, Celikes H. Renal blood flow detection with Doppler ultrasonography in patients with hepatic cirrhosis. *Arch Int Med*. 1997;157: 564–566.
5. Epstein M. Hepatorenal syndrome: Emerging perspectives. *Semin Nephrol*. 1997;17:563–575.
6. Gines P, Arroyo V, Rodes J. Ascites and hepatorenal syndrome: Pathogenesis and treatment strategies. *Adv Intern Med*. 1998;43:99–143.
7. Roberts LR, Kamath PS. Ascites and hepatorenal syndrome; pathophysiology and management. *Mayo Clin Proc*. 1996;71:874–881.
8. Sussman NL, Lake JR. Treatment of hepatic failure-1996: Current concepts and progress toward liver dialysis. *Am J Kidney Dis*. 1996;27:605–621.
9. Van Roey G, Moore K. The hepatorenal syndrome. *Pediatr Nephrol*. 1996;10:100–107.

 ## MISCELLANEOUS

See also: Acetaminophen poisoning; Cirrhosis of the liver; Hepatitis A; Hepatitis B; Hepatitis C; Renal failure, acute (ARF); Schistosomiasis of the liver, chronic

 CODES

ICD9-CM
- 572.4 Hepatorenal syndrome
- 997.4 Digestive system complications, NEC

PATIENT TEACHING

In alcoholic cirrhosis, abstention from alcohol is essential and may prevent further deterioration of cirrhosis.

H

HEREDITARY NEUROPATHY

Terence S. Edgar, MD

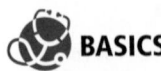 **BASICS**

DESCRIPTION
Inherited, symmetric distal polyneuropathy with mixed motor and sensory manifestations Includes several forms

- Demyelinating neuropathy
  - Charcot-Marie-Tooth disease (CMT)1 (A–D)
    - Hereditary neuropathy with liability to pressure palsies (HNPP)
    - CMTX
  - CMT3
    - Dejerine-Sottas disease (DSD)
    - Congenital Hypomyelinating Neuropathy (CHN)
  - CMT4
- Axonal neuropathy
  - CMT2
  - Giant Axonal Neuropathy (GAN)
- Hereditary Sensory and Autonomic Neuropathies (HSAN)—rare
  - HSAN1
  - HSAN3
  - HSAN4

GENERAL PREVENTION
Test and counsel at-risk individuals and their families.

EPIDEMIOLOGY
CMT1A accounts for 60% of autosomal dominant neuropathies and CMT2 ~22%. CMTX ~16%

Prevalence
CMT: 30/100,000

Genetics
- Autosomal Dominant (AD)
  - CMT1
    - HNPP
  - CMT2
  - CMT3
  - HSAN1
- Autosomal Recessive (AR)
  - CMT4
  - GAN
  - HSAN3
  - HSAN4
- X-linked
  - CMTX (XD/XR)

ETIOLOGY
- Peripheral Myelin Protein 22 (PMP22)
  - Chromosome 17p11.2
  - Duplication with 3 copies of the gene (increased PMP dosage) results in the CMT1 phenotype. Most common mutation causing CMT1 phenotype
  - 4 copies of the gene presents as DSD
  - Deletion (1 copy of the gene) results in the HNPP phenotype
- Myelin Protein Zero (MPZ or P0)
  - Functions to compact myelin
  - Chromosome 1q22
  - Mutations present as different phenotypes (CMT1B, DSD, CHN, and CMT2)
- Early Response Growth Gene 2 (ERG2)
  - Zinc finger transcription factor
  - Chromosome 10q21. Mutation leads to disruption of Schwann cell differentiation
  - Severe demyelinating phenotype (CMT1, DSD, CHN)
- Connexin 32 (CMTX)
  - Gap junction protein: Xq13.1

ASSOCIATED CONDITIONS
- Hearing loss, optic atrophy, retinopathy, scoliosis, contractures
- CMT2C: Vocal cord and phrenic nerve involvement
- Sleep apnea: With pharyngeal nerve involvement

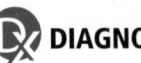 **DIAGNOSIS**

SIGNS AND SYMPTOMS
History
- Delayed motor milestones, clumsiness, weakness, frequent falls, and loss of fine motor control
- Positive family history of foot deformities or gait difficulties

Physical Exam
- Signs are those of distal muscle wasting and weakness, with pes cavus and foot drop.
- Loss of tendon reflexes
- Difficulty heel walking
- Thickened nerves
- Shortened Achilles tendon

- Abnormalities of vibration sense, proprioception, and 2 point discrimination can usually be demonstrated in the older child.
- Pelvic girdle weakness in 10% (late teens)
- Postural tremor in 1/4 of patients
- HNPP: Recurrent peripheral nerve palsies due to mechanical compression of nerve trunks. (Peroneal, ulnar, radial, median, and brachial plexus)
- HSAN (rare): Present with altered pain perception

TESTS
Lab
- Confirm by nerve conduction studies (NCS) and EMG.
- Demyelination (slow nerve conductions)
  - Autosomal dominant or X-linked
    - Gene test: PMP22, MPZ, ERG2, other....
  - Autosomal recessive
    - Gene test: ERG2, other.....
- Axonal (evidence for denervation, NCS may be normal)
  - Gene test: MPZ, other....
- Indeterminate
  - Consider a nerve biopsy

Pathological Findings
- Demyelinating neuropathies: Loss of large myelinated fibers with demyelinated and remyelinated segments and "onion bulb" formation
- May show evidence for axonal swelling

DIFFERENTIAL DIAGNOSIS
- Exclude an acquired neuropathy, especially if family history is negative. In acquired neuropathies the NCS will show evidence for scattered demyelination with conduction block. With hereditary neuropathies the demyelination is uniform and symmetric.
- Predominantly motor neuropathy
  - Guillain-Barre syndrome, lead, porphyria
- Predominantly sensory neuropathy
  - Amyloidosis, diabetes, leprosy, Lyme, malignancy, Vitamin B_{12} deficiency
- Painful neuropathy
  - Diabetes, Fabry, Krabbe, Lyme, vasculitis

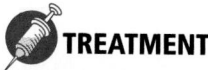 **TREATMENT**

GENERAL MEASURES
There are 3 principle reasons for decreased motion in patients with neuropathies: Pain, contracture, and weakness.

* Pain
  - Uncommon feature of hereditary neuropathy.
  - Consider gabapentin, nortriptyline, and carbamazepine.
* Contracture and weakness
  - Exercises to preserve strength and range of motion
  - Prevent contractures with daily passive range of motion, optimal positioning, and splinting in a functional position.
  - Orthotic devices to compensate for weak dorsiflexors, subtalar instability, plantar flexor weakness, and knee instability

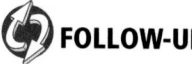 **FOLLOW-UP**

PROGNOSIS
* With rare exceptions, the patient's life span is generally not altered. The degree of disability is highly variable and difficult to predict.
* Disability in 44% and depression in 18%

COMPLICATIONS
Neurotoxic drugs may exacerbate the underlying neuropathy.

REFERENCES
1. Kuhlenbaumer G, Young P, Humermund G, et al. Clinical features and molecular genetics of hereditary peripheral neuropathies. *J Neurol*. 2003;249:1629–1650.
2. Young P, Sutter U. The causes of Charcot-Marie-Tooth disease. *Cell Mol Life Sci*. 2003;60:2547–2560.

ADDITIONAL READING
* Online Mendelian Inheritance in Man
* http://www.ncbi.nlm.nih.gov/omim/
* The National Neuropathy Association
Lennox Hill Post Office
P.O Box 2055
New York, NY 10021
Phone: (800) 247–6069
www.neuropathy.org

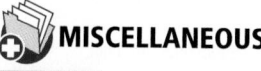 **MISCELLANEOUS**

 CODES

ICD9-CM
356.0 Neuropathy, peripheral hereditary

H

HERPANGINA

Aamir Siddiqi, MD

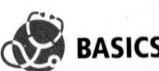 **BASICS**

DESCRIPTION
- Infectious disease caused by coxsackievirus group A
- Characteristics
  - Fever of short duration
  - Typical vesicular or ulcerated lesions in the posterior pharynx or on the soft palate
- Usual course—acute
- System(s) Affected: Endocrine/Metabolic; Gastrointestinal

GENERAL PREVENTION
Avoid contact with infected individual.

EPIDEMIOLOGY
- Predominant age: 3 months to 16 years
- Predominant sex: Male = Female

Incidence
Year round in tropical climate; summer and fall in temperate climate. (1)[B]

RISK FACTORS
Contact with infected person

ETIOLOGY
- Common: Coxsackievirus A—types 1–10, 16, and 22 (2)[B]
- Infrequent
  - Coxsackievirus B—types 1–5
  - Echovirus—types 6, 9, 11, 17, 22, and 25
  - Other enterovirus (3)[B]

DIAGNOSIS

SIGNS AND SYMPTOMS
- Anorexia
- Drooling
- Sore throat
- Fever
- Malaise
- Irritability
- Listlessness
- Local pain
- Emesis
- Backache
- Headache
- Coryza
- Diarrhea
- Bilateral discrete vesicles, gray base
- Erythematous patches
- Vesicles may rupture to form ulcers.
- Posterior pharynx location—pharynx, tonsils, soft palate, little involvement of anterior 2/3 of mouth

History
The patient may have low or high grade fever, general malaise, sore throat, and characteristic oro-pharyngeal lesions.

Physical Exam
Oro-pharyngeal lesions in the form of vesicles with erythromatous edges

TESTS
- Complement fixation
- Hemagglutinin inhibition tests
- Serum antibodies to coxsackievirus—titers should show a 4-fold rise in serial samples.

Lab
- Slight leukocytosis
- Positive viral culture—mouth washings, stool

DIFFERENTIAL DIAGNOSIS
- Herpes simplex
  - Multiple ulcers on lips and anterior mouth
  - Diagnose with herpes culture.
- Drug reactions—cutaneous lesions often present (urticaria, erythema multiforme).
- Recurrent aphthous stomatitis
  - Buccal, labial, alveolar, mucosal ulcers
  - Recurrent crops
  - Few systemic symptoms
- Lichen planus—painful ulcer, white lacy pattern on mucosa or may have cutaneous lesions that are purple and pruritic
- Hand, foot, and mouth disease—classic distribution of vesicular rash on hands, buttocks, feet, and mouth

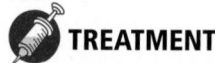 **TREATMENT**

INITIAL STABILIZATION
Outpatient

GENERAL MEASURES
- Self-limited
- Palliative and supportive
- Hydration

Diet
Clear liquids

Activity
No restrictions

 MEDICATION (DRUGS)

- Analgesics—acetaminophen, NSAIDs
- Topical anesthetics
- Mouthwash—aqueous solution of 1% dyclonine and 1% diphenhydramine (Benadryl) in 50% attapulgite (Kaopectate)
- 2% viscous lidocaine solution

 FOLLOW-UP

PROGNOSIS
Complete recovery

COMPLICATIONS
Complications are rare
- Exanthem
- Aseptic meningitis
- Myocarditis
- Encephalitis

PATIENT MONITORING
Hydration

REFERENCES

1. Ho M, Chen ER, Hsu KH, et al. An epidemic of enterovirus 71 infection in Taiwan. Taiwan Enterovirus Epidemic Working Group. *N Engl J Med*. 1999;341:929–935.
2. Melnick JL. Enteroviruses: Polioviruses, Coxsackieviruses, echoviruses, and newer enteroviruses. In: *Field's Virology*. 1990:549–598.
3. Chang LY, Tsao KC, Hsia SH, et al. Transmission and clinical features of enterovirus 71 infections in household contacts in Taiwan. *JAMA*. 2004;291(2):222–227.

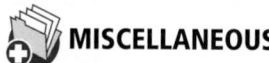 **MISCELLANEOUS**

See also: Herpes simplex

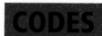 **CODES**

ICD9-CM
074.0 Herpangina

PATIENT TEACHING

Activity
As tolerated with no limitations

Prevention
- Because the mode of transfer is feco-oral, general hygiene as hand washing should be suggested.
- Benign and self-limiting course of the disease should be explained to the patient.

H

HERPES EYE INFECTIONS

Thomas W. Hejkal, MD, PhD

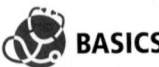 **BASICS**

DESCRIPTION

- Eye infections caused by herpes simplex virus (HSV) types 1 and 2 or varicella-zoster virus (VZV)
- Can cause conjunctivitis, keratitis, or uveitis; retinitis or optic neuritis are also possible.
- HSV classically causes a dendritic keratitis.
- Reactivation of latent infection most common
- Primary HSV keratitis, when it occurs, is more common in children.
- System(s) Affected: Eye; Skin
- Synonym(s): HSV keratitis; Herpes zoster ophthalmicus

GENERAL PREVENTION

- Contact precautions with active lesions
- VZV can be spread to individuals who have not had chickenpox.
- Avoid precipitating factors for reactivation.
- Antiviral prophylaxis while on topical steroids
- Varicella vaccination prior to infection
- Oral acyclovir 400 mg b.i.d.

  - Reduces recurrence rate of HSV keratitis by 50% (1,2)[A]

  - May not be cost effective (3)

ALERT
Pregnancy Considerations
- Pregnant women who have not had chickenpox should especially avoid contact with patients with active zoster.
- Pregnancy increases risk of recurrence.

EPIDEMIOLOGY
- Predominant age: HSV may affect any age; Zoster usually affects older people.
- Predominant sex: Male = Female

Incidence
- HSV: 500,000 cases per year; 1/10,000 infants born with neonatal HSV
- Zoster: 300,000 new cases per year

Prevalence
149 per 100,000 person-years

RISK FACTORS
- HSV history or close contacts with HSV
- History of varicella infection
- Reactivating factors
  - Ultraviolet light
  - Illness, stress, menstruation
  - Local trauma
  - Immunosuppression

Genetics
No genetic pattern

ETIOLOGY
- Primary infections
  - Neonatal usually HSV- 2
  - Primary ocular HSV usually HSV- 1
- Recurrent infections
  - Reactivation from trigeminal ganglion
  - HSV-1, HSV-2, or VZV

ALERT
Immunosuppression, AIDS, malignancy (Consider immunodeficiency in all zoster patients <40 years of age.)

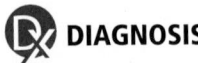 **DIAGNOSIS**

SIGNS AND SYMPTOMS
Varies according to the virus and the ocular structures involved

ALERT
- Dendritic corneal lesions are characteristic.
- Corneal scarring may be present.
- Eye pain
- Red eye (usually unilateral)
- Photophobia
- Tearing
- Decreased vision
- Anterior chamber cells if uveitis present
- Vesicular skin/eyelid rash
  - Unilateral and follows dermatome in VZV
  - Primary HSV
- Fever (VZV or systemic HSV)
- Malaise (VZV or systemic HSV)

History
Recurrent eye infections

Physical Exam
- Conjunctival injection
- Dendritic corneal lesions

TESTS
Special tests
- Fluorescein staining of cornea—HSV
- Rose bengal staining—HSV and VZV
- Corneal sensation—usually decreased
- Slit-lamp exam
- Intraocular pressure
- Dilated fundus exam
- Evaluate zoster patients <age 40 years for immunodeficiency.

Lab
Corneal swab for HSV DNA by PCR (PPV = 96%)

DIFFERENTIAL DIAGNOSIS
- Bacterial, fungal, allergic, or other viral conjunctivitis
- Corneal abrasion
- Recurrent corneal erosion
- Toxic conjunctivitis
- Iritis or scleritis

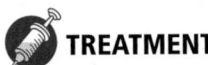 **TREATMENT**

INITIAL STABILIZATION
- Outpatient
- Hospitalize and initiate IV therapy if severe systemic spread or known immunodeficiency

GENERAL MEASURES
Gentle débridement of corneal epithelial lesions (optional)

Diet
Regular

Activity
As tolerated

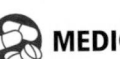 **MEDICATION (DRUGS)**

First Line
- Skin and eyelid lesions
  - Bacitracin or erythromycin b.i.d.
  - Eyelid margin involvement
    ○ Trifluorothymidine (Viroptic) 1% drops or vidarabine 3% ointment 5 times per day

  - Zoster—acyclovir 800 mg PO 5 times per day for 10 days or famciclovir 500 mg PO t.i.d. for 7 days if started within 7 days of onset and active lesions are present [A]

  - Severe or persistent zoster—acyclovir 5–10 mg/kg IV q8h for 5–10 days; hospitalize if indicated for systemic disease
  - Options for postherpetic neuralgia
    ○ Prednisone 60 mg PO for 3–7 days and taper over 1–2 weeks (H_2-blocker while on prednisone)
    ○ Amitriptyline 25 mg PO t.i.d.
- HSV corneal epithelial disease

  - Trifluorothymidine 1% drops 9 times per day or vidarabine 3% ointment 5 times per day; taper over 10–21 days based on response (1,4)[A]

- Stromal keratitis or uveitis (without epithelial disease)
  - Cycloplegia with scopolamine 0.25% or cyclopentolate 1% drops t.i.d.
  - Prednisolone acetate 1% drops q.i.d. (4)[A]
  - Trifluorothymidine 1% drops q.i.d. for prophylaxis while on topical steroids [C]
- HZV optic neuritis, chorioretinitis, or cranial nerve involvement
  - Acyclovir 5–10 mg/kg IV q8h for 1 week
  - Prednisone 60 mg PO for 3–7 days and taper over the next 1–2 weeks

Contraindications:
Pregnancy Considerations
- Systemic steroids and acyclovir are contraindicated in pregnancy.
- Prednisone should not be used in immunocompromised patients.

ALERT
Topical steroids are contraindicated with active corneal epithelial disease.

Precautions
- Topical antiviral agents are toxic to corneal epithelium.
- Topical steroids can raise intraocular pressure.
- Acyclovir dosage should be reduced in renal insufficiency.

Second Line
- Idoxuridine 0.5% ointment or 0.1% drops 5 times per day (1)[A]
- Nonsteroidal anti-inflammatory agents PO for scleritis associated with zoster Oral acyclovir 2 g/d in divided doses over 10 days in patients intolerant of topical antivirals (1,3)[A]
- Oral valacyclovir 500–1,000 mg b.i.d. as an alternative to acyclovir.

SURGERY
Corneal transplant for severe scarring or perforation

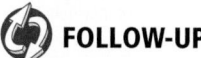

FOLLOW-UP

DISPOSITION
Admission Criteria
- Severe systemic VZV disease
- Systemic HSV in children

Discharge Criteria
Resolution of systemic disease

Issues for Referral
Follow up with ophthalmology at a frequency according to severity of disease.

PROGNOSIS
ALERT
Pediatric Considerations
- Neonatal primary HSV often disseminated with high mortality rate; 37% have vision worse than 20/200.
- Pediatric cases more likely to be bilateral (26%); recurrent (48% in 15 months) and may cause amblyopia
- Recurrent ocular HSV
  - HSV epithelial disease—without treatment, 40% resolve without sequelae; with treatment, 90–95% resolve without complication.
  - HSV stromal keratitis usually resolves in weeks to months with some scarring.

- Herpes zoster ophthalmicus
  - Dermatitis 8–14 days acute phase with subsequent scarring possible
  - 2/3 of patients develop keratitis and decreased corneal sensation.
  - Uveitis occurs in ~40%.
  - Neurotrophic keratitis occurs in 1/2; most recover sensation in 2–3 months.
  - Secondary glaucoma occurs in 10%.
  - Postherpetic neuralgia in 20–40%; usually longer lasting in older patients
- Recurrence common for HSV and herpes zoster ophthalmicus

COMPLICATIONS
- Corneal neovascularization and scarring resulting in poor vision
- Neurotrophic ulcer with perforation
- Secondary bacterial or fungal infection
- Secondary glaucoma
- Necrotizing interstitial keratitis
- Postherpetic neuralgia with zoster
- Vision loss from optic neuritis or chorioretinitis

Pediatric Considerations
- Neonatal HSV often systemic and life-threatening
- Amblyopia may occur in children.

PATIENT MONITORING
- Monitor with slit-lamp exam every 1–2 days until improvement, then every 3–4 days until epithelial defect resolves.
- Weekly after epithelial disease resolves until off of topical antivirals

REFERENCES
1. Wilhelmus KR. Interventions for herpes simplex virus epithelial keratitis. *The Cochrane Database Reviews.* 2003, Issue 2;CD002898.
2. Choa VB, Rezendo RA, Carrasco MA, et al. Long-term acyclovir use to prevent recurrent ocular herpes simplex virus infection. *Arch Ophthalmol.* 2003;121:1702–1704.
3. Lairson DR, Begley CE, Reynolds TE, et al. Prevention of herpes simplex virus eye disease: A cost-effectiveness analysis. *Arch Ophthalmol.* 2003;121:115–116.
4. Tullo A. Pathogenesis and management of herpes simplex virus keratitis. *Eye.* 2003;17:919–922.

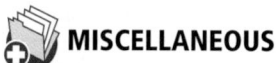

MISCELLANEOUS

ICD9-CM
- 054.40 Herpes simplex with unspecified ophthalmic complication
- 053.29 Herpes zoster (HZV) with ophthalmic complications, other

PATIENT TEACHING
Diet
No restrictions

Activity
No restrictions

Prevention
Report eye pain, redness, or decreased vision to physician.

H

HERPES GESTATIONIS

Gary Mendese, MD
Jeremy S. Bordeaux, MD, MPH

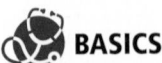

BASICS

DESCRIPTION
- Often called pemphigoid gestationis, herpes gestationis is a rare dermatopathic, immune-mediated, and self-limited eruption most often occurring during midpregnancy.
- Onset is in 2nd trimester of pregnancy, with remission after delivery except for some postpartum flares; it may recur in subsequent pregnancies.
- Characterized by pruritic polymorphous vesicles, papules, and/or bullae often located in periumbilical or other truncal areas. May affect the buttocks, forearms, palms, or soles; less frequently scalp and face may be involved. Clustered vesicles may coalesce to form bullae, rupture to form crusts, then heal with hyperpigmentation.
- Mucous membranes are spared, but intestinal mucosa may have celiac-like lesions without significant clinical malabsorption.
- System(s) Affected: Reproductive; Skin/exocrine
- Synonym(s): Dermatitis gestationis; Pemphigoid gestationis

ALERT
Pediatric Considerations
- Has been associated with preterm birth (22%) and stillbirth (<10%)
- Rare cases of transient neonatal herpes gestationis are usually mild and resolve spontaneously; these are probably from passive transfer of anti–basement membrane antibodies and herpes gestationis factor.

Pregnancy Considerations
By definition, a condition of pregnancy and puerperium; rarely seen also with hydatidiform moles and choriocarcinoma.

GENERAL PREVENTION
- Avoid other people with infections, because there is susceptibility of open skin lesions and decreased resistance secondary to corticosteroids.
- Some authorities recommend Caesarean section when mother is known to be infected.
- Avoid scalp monitors if disease involves maternal genitalia.
- Use of estrogens or progesterone may trigger flare-up.

EPIDEMIOLOGY
- Predominant age: Child-bearing years
- Predominant sex: Female only

Incidence
Rare: 1 per 50,000 pregnancies; mainly whites

RISK FACTORS
- Episode in prior pregnancy
- Herpes simplex does not increase risk.

Genetics
Genetic predisposition is possible, suggested by increased HLA-A1, -B8, and -DR3 antigens in affected women.

ETIOLOGY
- Unknown, but immune alterations suspected
- Higher association with HLA-DR3 and HLA-DR4
- Possible role of major histocompatibility complexes (MHC) class II antigen
- Not caused by herpes virus

ASSOCIATED CONDITIONS
- Pregnancy
- Hydatidiform mole
- Choriocarcinoma

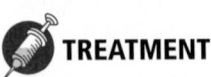

DIAGNOSIS

SIGNS AND SYMPTOMS
Intensely pruritic papules and/or vesicles, occurring 1st in periumbilical area and spreading more generally

History
History of current or recent pregnancy

Physical Exam
Pruritus associated with pruritic vesicles, papules and/or bullae primarily on the trunk in a pregnant female. Lesions may also be present on buttocks, forearms, palms and soles. Typically spares the scalp and face, although these areas can rarely become involved.

TESTS
Special tests

- Biopsy with direct immunofluorescence shows intense deposition of C3 (100%) and less intense IgG (25–40%) along basement membrane (1)[A].

- Serum may have circulating IgG anti–basement membrane autoantibodies (20–60%) by indirect immunofluorescence, but when coupled with complement, 90% of patients are shown to have autoantibodies present (2)[C].

Lab
- Tzanck smear negative
- Herpes simplex virus culture negative
- Peripheral eosinophilia may be present.

Diagnostic Procedures/Surgery
Biopsy

Pathological Findings
- Subepidermal vesicle often with eosinophils and edema of dermal papillae
- Acantholysis is rare.
- Inflammation surrounds superficial and deep dermal vessels.

DIFFERENTIAL DIAGNOSIS
- Other pruritic conditions of pregnancy
  - Besnier prurigo gestationis with excoriated papules and no vesicles; usually limited to extensor surface of extremities
  - Papular urticarial papules and plaques of pregnancy (PUPPP) syndrome, which has urticarial plaques and small papules with a narrow, pale halo and no vesicles; usually in primigravidas near term

  - Impetigo herpetiformis has sterile pustules, not vesicles, and may involve mucous membranes, groin, and inner thighs.
  - Papular dermatitis of pregnancy
- Nonpregnancy conditions to consider
  - Dermatitis herpetiformis (much more chronic and more often in middle-aged males)
  - Bullous pemphigoid
  - Toxic drug eruption including erythema multiforme

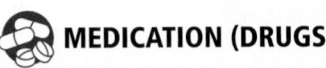

TREATMENT

Outpatient

GENERAL MEASURES
- Differentiate from herpes virus infection.
- Relieve pruritus.
- Prevent secondary infection.
- Soothing compresses such as with aluminum acetate (Burow solution, Domeboro) may help relieve itching.

Diet
No special diet

Activity
As tolerated

Nursing
Apply and change soothing compresses

MEDICATION (DRUGS)

First Line
- Topical steroids and oral antihistamines for mild pruritus

- May use topical corticosteroids for early urticarial lesions (3)[C]. Most will require systemic corticosteroids in doses of 20–40 mg/d (at the minimum effective dose) through 1st month postpartum (1)[A]. Often able to taper off before delivery, and then increase in the postpartum period as needed.

- Contraindications: Weigh risk of aggravating hyperglycemia, potential effects on maternal and fetal bone, increased susceptibility to infections versus benefit of relieving pruritus and resolving the lesions.
- Precautions
  - Use prednisone cautiously in patients with immune impairment, diabetes, or thrombophlebitis.
  - If prednisone has been used over several weeks, taper when discontinuing to prevent cortisol deficiency.
- Significant possible interactions Methylprednisolone may enhance toxicity of erythromycin.

Second Line
Pyridoxine, cyclophosphamide, gold, methotrexate for refractory cases (1)[A].

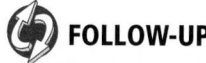 **FOLLOW-UP**

PROGNOSIS

- Spreads during 2nd–3rd trimester
- Remits after delivery within weeks
- Often flares in puerperium, especially with oral contraceptives
- Tends to recur in subsequent pregnancies, and when it recurs, it is likely to begin earlier and be more severe.
- Systemic steroids may suppress new lesions, relieve pruritus, and dampen course, but fetal outcome may be worsened..
- Duration observed less in breast-feeding women

COMPLICATIONS

- Secondary bacterial infection
- Excess systemic medication in pregnancy
- Fetal deaths
- Premature births
- Fetal growth retardation
- Conjunctivitis
- Keratitis
- Cataracts
- Shock
- Transient herpes gestationis in the neonate

PATIENT MONITORING

Watch for secondary bacterial infection.

REFERENCES

1. Kroumpouzos G, Cohen L. Specific dermatoses of pregnancy: An evidence-based systematic review. *Am J Obstet Gynecol* 2003;188:1083–1092.
2. Fabbri P, Caproni M, Berti S. The role of T lymphocytes and cytokines in the pathogenesis of pemphigoid gestationis. *Br J Dermatol*. 2003;148(6):1141–1148.
3. Kroumpouzos G, Cohen. Dermatoses of pregnancy. *J Am Acad Dermatol* 2001;45:1–19.

 MISCELLANEOUS

Other notes: Uncommon intrauterine infections are associated with microcephaly, intracranial calcification, and chorioretinitis.

CODES

ICD9-CM

- 646.80 Other specified complications of pregnancy, unspecified
- 646.83 Other specified complications of pregnancy, antepartum condition or complication

PATIENT TEACHING

- Educate about difference between this and herpes virus infection.
- Inform of possible fetal risks and possibility of limited disease in newborn.

See Corresponding Diagnostic Algorithm

H

HERPES SIMPLEX

Michelle Whitehurst-Cook, MD

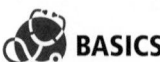 **BASICS**

DESCRIPTION
- Viral disease with many manifestations
- Usually seen as painful vesicles that often occur in clusters on skin, cornea, or mucous membranes
- May occur as encephalitis, pneumonia, or disseminated infection, and/or skin lesions

EPIDEMIOLOGY
- Predominant age: Affects all ages
- Predominant sex: Male = Female

Incidence
29.2/100,000 office visits per year

Prevalence
- Widespread; 0.65–20% of adults may be excreting herpes simplex virus type 1 or 2 (HSV-1, HSV-2) at any given time
- Prevalence of antibodies varies from 30% in higher socioeconomic strata to 100% in lower socioeconomic strata; 20,000–70,000/100,000

RISK FACTORS
- Immune compromise (brief, as with occurrence of other illness or stress; or more chronic, as with chemotherapy, malignancy, or AIDS)
- Newborns: If exposed to actively infected mother via birth canal or if exposed to case in nursery (insufficient maternal passive antibody transfer); risk greatest for neonate of mother with active primary herpes simplex infection
- Prior HSV infection
- Sexual intercourse with infected person (condoms may help prevent HSV, but location of lesions may limit effectiveness)
- Occupational exposure (medical/dental risk more for HSV-1 whitlow and general community for HSV-2 whitlow)

ALERT

Pregnancy Considerations
- Caesarian section and/or acyclovir indicated if any active genital lesions (or prodrome) present at the time of delivery; consider if primary genital herpes occurred within 4 weeks of expected delivery (2,3)[C]. Avoid fetal scalp electrodes if mother has history of genital HSV.
- Risk of viral shedding at delivery from asymptomatic recurrent genital HSV is low (~1.6%); not predicted by monitoring cultures

Geriatric Considerations
Decreased immunologic competence of old age may increase risk.

ETIOLOGY
HSV, a DNA virus of 2 major types: HSV-1 and HSV-2. Most often, HSV-1 is associated with oral lesions and HSV-2 with genital lesions, but reverse also occurs.

ASSOCIATED CONDITIONS
Erythema multiforme

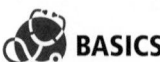 **DIAGNOSIS**

SIGNS AND SYMPTOMS
- Vesicles: Usually cluster and open as painful ulcerated lesions, often with erythematous base
- Herpetic whitlow: Localized primary infection on a finger with intense itching and pain, followed by vesicles that may coalesce with swelling and erythema, and may mimic pyogenic paronychia; neuralgia and axillary adenopathy sometimes occur; heals over 2–3 weeks without incision. Primary inoculation of other abraded skin may occur (e.g., herpes gladiatorum in wrestlers).
- Primary herpetic gingivostomatitis and pharyngitis: 1st infection with HSV-1 usually in early childhood; incubation from 2–12 days, then fever, sore throat, pharyngeal edema, and erythema; small vesicles develop on pharyngeal and oral mucosa, rapidly ulcerate, and increase in number to involve soft palate, buccal mucosa, tongue, floor of mouth, and often lips and cheeks; tender gums may bleed; fetid breath, cervical adenopathy, fever, general toxicity, poor oral intake, and drooling contribute to dehydration; autoinoculation of other sites may occur; resolves in 10–14 days with slower resolution of adenopathy
- Primary genital herpes: See "Herpes, Genital"
- Primary herpes keratoconjunctivitis: By HSV-1 usually; may present as unilateral conjunctivitis with regional adenopathy, as blepharitis with vesicles on lid margin, as keratitis with dendritic lesions, or with punctate opacities; lasts 2–3 weeks, but systemic involvement prolongs process
- Eczema herpeticum: Diffuse pox-like eruption complicating atopic dermatitis; 1 cause of Kaposi varicelliform eruption; sudden appearance of lesions in typical atopic areas (upper trunk, neck, head); high fever, local edema, adenopathy, umbilicated vesicles develop hemorrhagic crust or become pustular; vesicles appear in crops for up to a week; significant fluid or blood loss and secondary bacterial infections may cause fatality; similar serious inoculations may occur in severe burn patients and go unrecognized under the eschar
- Neonatal herpes simplex: Perinatal primary infection is life-threatening and usually acquired by vaginal birth of infected mother; fetal risk and neonatal risk are greater in mothers with primary genital herpes infection because shedding is more prolonged and the inoculum is greater; incubation from 5–7 days usually (rarely 4 weeks); cutaneous, mucous membrane, or ocular signs in only 70%; congenital infection via prenatal transplacental virus transfer may present with jaundice, hepatosplenomegaly, disseminated intravascular coagulation, encephalitis, seizures, temperature instability, chorioretinitis, and/or conjunctivitis with or without skin vesicles; neurologic morbidity worse with HSV-2 than with HSV-1 in neonates; fatal hepatic or adrenal necrosis may occur

- Recurrent diseases from endogenous reactivation include
  - Herpes labialis: recurrent lesions on lips with HSV-1; usually <1 recurrence per 6 months, but 5–25% may have >1 attack per month; precipitating events may be sunlight, fever, trauma, menses, stress; prodrome of pain, burning, itching may last 6–48 hours before vesicles appear, often at vermilion border, with increased pain; vesicles ulcerate and crust within 48 hours; heals within 8–10 days generally; may have local adenopathy
  - Ocular herpes: May recur as keratitis, blepharitis, or keratoconjunctivitis; patients may have dendritic ulcers, decreased corneal sensation, less visual acuity; uveitis may cause permanent visual loss
  - Recurrent genital herpes (herpes progenitalis): See "Herpes, Genital"

TESTS
Screen for other sexually transmitted diseases with primary genital herpes.

Lab
- Tzanck smear shows multinucleated giant cells with 12–15 nuclei, often with eosinophilic intranuclear inclusions (scrape material from lesion onto slide, fix with ethanol or methanol, stain with Giemsa or Wright preparation; alternatively, spray slide with cytologic fixative and stain as for Pap smear); varicella (herpes zoster) has identical findings
- HSV culture: Only 1/2 of true positives available in 2 days; rest may take 6 days or longer to be positive; not reliable near delivery
- Antibody tests do not reliably distinguish between HSV-1 and HSV-2, but primary infection is ruled out with initially high titers or <4-fold rise of titers between acute and convalescent sera
- Immunoglobulin M HSV antibodies may appear in 1st 4 weeks of life in infected infants.

Diagnostic Procedures/Surgery
Occasionally a biopsy is needed.

Pathological Findings
- See Tzanck prep above.
- Intraepithelial edema (ballooning degeneration) and intracellular edema
- A brain biopsy (in encephalitis) has hemorrhagic necrosis of gray and white matter with acute and chronic inflammation, thrombosis and fibrinoid necrosis of parenchymal vessels, and intranuclear inclusions in astrocytes, oligodendroglia, and neurons.

DIFFERENTIAL DIAGNOSIS
- Impetigo: Straw-colored vesicles that crust
- Aphthous stomatitis: Grayish, shallow erosions with ring of hyperemia, usually only anterior in mouth and lips
- Herpes zoster: Unilateral dermatome distribution
- Syphilitic chancre: Usually painless ulcer
- Herpangina: Vesicles predominate on anterior tonsillar pillars, soft palate, uvula, and oropharynx but not more anteriorly on lips or gums (usually caused by group A coxsackievirus)
- Stevens-Johnson syndrome
- Other causes of Kaposi varicelliform eruption are varicella and coxsackievirus A16.

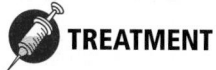

TREATMENT

ALERT

Pediatric Considerations
Neonates with possible exposure to HSV at birth or later with signs of infection: Lethargy, poor feeding, fever, lesions: Culture (urine, stool, cerebrospinal fluid [CSF], eyes, throat; treat immediately with IV acyclovir if HSV illness suspected (2)[C]

INITIAL STABILIZATION
Outpatient treatment

GENERAL MEASURES
- Limited skin lesions (as in recurrent herpes labialis) may benefit from early unroofing of vesicles and application of Campho-Phenique.
- Intermittent cool moist dressings with Domeboro or Burow solution
- Inability to void due to painful lesions is helped by pouring a cup of warm water over genitals while urinating or by sitting in a warm bath while urinating.
- Children with gingivostomatitis or extensive skin disease (eczema herpeticum) may require intravenous hydration and volume replacement.
- In pregnant women: Caesarean section and/or acyclovir indicated if any active genital lesions (or prodrome) present at time of delivery; consider if primary genital herpes occurred within 4 weeks of expected delivery (2,3)[C]

Diet
Avoid acidic foods with gingivostomatitis.

Activity
No restrictions

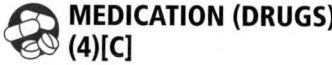

MEDICATION (DRUGS) (4)[C]

First Line
- Acyclovir short half-life and poor bioavailablity requiring a frequent dosing schedule
  - Primary herpes labialis: 15 mg/kg (up to 200 mg) PO × 5 doses daily for 10 days
  - Primary genital herpes: 400 mg PO t.i.d. or 200 mg PO × 5 doses daily for 7–10 days
  - Recurrent genital herpes: 800 mg PO b.i.d. or 200 mg PO × 5 doses daily for 7–10 days; for chronic suppression in persons with frequent recurrences, 400 mg b.i.d.
  - Neonatal herpes simplex or encephalitis: 20 mg/kg IV over 1 hour q8h for 14–21 days
  - Primary herpes gingivostomatitis, recurrent herpes labialis, and other HSV skin infections: 200 mg PO q4h × 5 doses daily for 10 days
  - In pregnancy: May give orally for 1st episode of genital herpes or severe recurrent herpes. Give IV for severe or complicated disease.

- Penciclovir (Denavir): Oroherpes recurrence: 1% cream q2h while awake for 4 days
- Valacyclovir (Valtrex): Better bioavailability orally than acyclovir; is converted to acyclovir
  - Primary genital herpes: 1 g PO b.i.d. for 10 days
  - Recurrent genital herpes: 500 mg PO b.i.d. for 3 days; chronic suppression, 1 g PO daily (10 or more recurrences per year) or 500 mg PO daily (9 or fewer recurrences per year)
- Famciclovir (Famvir): Converted to penciclovir, with longer intracellular half-life and higher levels than those of acyclovir
  - Primary genital herpes: 250 mg PO t.i.d. for 7–10 days
  - Recurrent genital herpes: 125 mg PO b.i.d. for 5 days; chronic suppression, 250 mg PO b.i.d.
- Contraindications for acyclovir, valacyclovir, and famciclovir: Hypersensitivity or intolerance
- Precautions
  - Reduce dosage in renal insufficiency for acyclovir, valacyclovir, and famciclovir.
  - Acyclovir may produce encephalopathic reactions, particularly in the elderly.
  - Valacyclovir: Thrombotic thrombocytopenia purpura/hemolytic uremic syndrome reported in some immunocompromised persons in trials on high doses (8 g daily) for cytomegalovirus suppression
- Significant possible interactions: Probenecid with intravenous acyclovir and possibly probenecid with valacyclovir may reduce renal clearance and elevate antiviral drug levels.

Second Line (4)[C]
- Foscarnet: Drug of choice for acyclovir resistance in immunocompromised persons with systemic HSV
  - 40 mg/kg IV q8h (assume valacyclovir and famciclovir resistance also if acyclovir resistance occurs)
- Other topicals: Ophthalmic preparations for herpes keratoconjunctivitis—acyclovir, vidarabine (Vira-A), idoxuridine, and trifluorothymidine; refer to ophthalmologist

FOLLOW-UP

PROGNOSIS
- Good for treatment of recurrent episodes; expect frequent recurrences
- The usual course of the primary disease is 2 weeks.
- The duration of the recurrence varies.
- Viral shedding in recurrence is briefer than with the primary disease.
- Newborns or immunocompromised individuals are at risk for major morbidity or mortality.

COMPLICATIONS
- Herpes encephalitis: A brain biopsy may be needed for diagnosis
- Herpes pneumonia
- Aseptic meningitis
- Herpes viremia

PATIENT MONITORING
Observe for disappearance of lesions and resolution of systemic manifestations.

REFERENCES
1. Amir J, Harel L, Smetana Z, Varsano I. Treatment of herpes simplex gingivostomatitis with acyclovir in children: A randomised double blind placebo controlled study. *BMJ*. 1997;314:1800–1803.
2. Rudneck C, Hoekzema GS. Neonatal herpes simplex virus infection. *Am Fam Physicians*. 2002;65:1138–1142,1143.
3. Dwyer DE, Cunningham AL. Herpes simplex virus infection in pregnancy. *Baillieres Clin Obstet Gynaecol*. 1993;7:75–105.
4. Centers for Disease Control and Prevention. Sexually transmitted diseases treatment guidelines 2002. *MMWR Recomm Rep*. 2002;51(RR-6): 12–17.
5. Hirsch MS. Herpes simples virus. In: Mandell GL, Bennett JE, Dolin R, eds. *Principles and Practice of Infectious Diseases*. New York, NY: Churchill Livingstone; 1990.
6. Beauman JG. Genital herpes: A review. *Am Fam Physician*. 2005;72:1527–1534, 1541–1542.

MISCELLANEOUS

See also: Herpes, genital

CODES

ICD9-CM
- 054.0 Eczema herpeticum
- 054.9 Herpes simplex without mention of complication
- 771.2 Other congenital infections

PATIENT TEACHING
Reassure and reduce stigma.

Prevention
- Avoid contact with immunocompromised people.
- Wash hands often.
- Genital herpes: Avoid sexual contact while disease is active; discuss condom benefits and limits and reinforce benefits of mutually monogamous sexual relations.
- Sexual abstinence only sure way to not acquire disease

 See Corresponding Diagnostic Algorithm

 See Patient Handout on CD

H

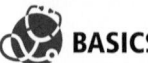# HERPES ZOSTER
Robert Hyde, MD, EMT-P

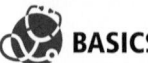 BASICS

DESCRIPTION
- Usually presents as a painful unilateral vesicular eruption within a dermatone
- Results from reactivation of varicella zoster virus (human herpes virus type 3)
- Postherpetic neuralgia (PHN) is usually defined as pain persisting at least 1 month after rash has healed. Because of variable definitions of PHN used in research, the term *zoster-associated pain* may be more clinically useful.
- System(s) Affected: Nervous; Integumentary; Exocrine
- Synonym(s): Shingles

GENERAL PREVENTION
- Varicella vaccines currently available will theoretically reduce zoster incidence in the future.
- Vaccines are being tested for prevention of herpes zoster in individuals previously infected with wild varicella-zoster virus.
- Zoster patients may transmit virus-causing varicella (chickenpox) to susceptible persons.

EPIDEMIOLOGY
Predominant sex: Male = Female

Incidence
- 215/100,000/year; incidence is increasing as population ages.
- Active herpes zoster: 23.9/100,000
- PHN: 86/100,000
- Increases with age: 80% of cases occur in persons >20 years (2.2–3.4 per 1000 age 20–50; 10 per 1,000 >80 years).
- PHN increases dramatically with age (4% age 30–50; 50% >80 years).

Prevalence
Occurs in 10–20% of the population at some time

ALERT
Pregnancy Considerations
May occur during pregnancy

Geriatric Considerations
- Increased incidence
- Increased incidence of PHN

Pediatric Considerations
- Occurs less frequently in children
- Has been reported in newborns primarily infected in utero

RISK FACTORS
- The vast majority of persons affected have no underlying illness.
- Increasing age
- Reduced immunity associated with some malignancies (lymphoma, etc.)
- Treatment of malignancy (chemotherapy or radiotherapy)
- HIV infection
- Use of immunosuppressant drugs after organ transplant surgery or for disease management
- Spinal surgery

ETIOLOGY
Reactivation of varicella zoster virus (human herpes virus type 3) from dorsal root or cranial nerve ganglia

ASSOCIATED CONDITIONS
Immunocompromised individuals, including HIV infection, posttransplantation, immunosuppressive drugs, and malignancy

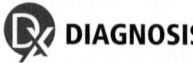 DIAGNOSIS

SIGNS AND SYMPTOMS
- Prodromal phase (sensations over involved dermatome prior to rash)
  - Tingling
  - Itching
  - Boring or knifelike pain
- Acute phase
  - Constitutional symptoms variable (fatigue, malaise, headache, low-grade fever)
  - Dermatomal rash
  - Weakness (1% may have weakness in distribution of rash)
  - Initially erythematous and maculopapular, evolves rapidly to grouped vesicles
  - Vesicles become pustular and/or hemorrhagic in 3–4 days.
  - Resolution of rash, with crusts separating by 14–21 days
- Possible sine herpete (zoster without rash) and other chronic disorders associated with varicella-zoster virus without the typical rash
- Chronic phase
  - PHN (15% overall; increases with age)
  - A small percentage (1–5%) may affect the motor nerves, causing weakness (called zoster motoricus), e.g., facial nerve (Ramsay Hunt syndrome), spinal motor radiculopathies

TESTS
Lab
- Rarely necessary as clinical appearance is usually sufficiently distinctive
- Viral culture
- Tzanck smear (does not distinguish from herpes simplex, and false negatives occur)
- Polymerase chain reaction analysis
- Immunofluorescent antigen staining
- Varicella zoster specific immunoglobulin M

Pathological Findings
- Multinucleated giant cells with intralesional inclusion
- Lymphatic infiltration of sensory ganglia with focal hemorrhage and nerve cell destruction

DIFFERENTIAL DIAGNOSIS
- Rash
  - Herpes simplex virus
  - Coxsackievirus
  - Contact dermatitis
  - Superficial pyoderma
- Pain
  - Cholecystitis
  - Appendicitis
  - Nephrolithiasis
  - Pleuritis
  - Myocardial infarction
  - Diabetic neuropathy

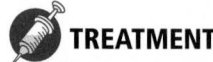 TREATMENT

INITIAL STABILIZATION
Outpatient treatment unless disseminated or occurring as complication of serious underlying disease requiring hospitalization

GENERAL MEASURES
- Treatment should be directed to control acute symptoms and prevent complications.
- Antiviral therapy decreases viral replication, lessens nerve damage and inflammation, and reduces the severity and duration of long-term pain syndromes. (1)[A]
- Prompt analgesic control of pain may shorten the duration of zoster-associated pain.
- Lotions such as calamine and colloidal oatmeal may reduce itching and burning sensation.

Diet
No special diet

Activity
No restrictions

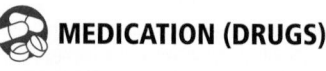 MEDICATION (DRUGS)

First Line
- Acute treatment
  - Antiviral agents initiated within 72 hours of rash may relieve symptoms, speed resolution of rash, and prevent and/or ameliorate PHN. (1)[A]
  - Valacyclovir 1,000 mg t.i.d. for 7 days
  - Famciclovir 500 mg t.i.d. for 7 days
    ○ Acyclovir 800 mg q4h (5 doses daily) for 7 days
    ○ Analgesics (acetaminophen, NSAIDs, opioids)
    ○ Corticosteroids to prevent postherpetic neuralgia; may help acute symptoms but theoretically may increase risk of dissemination. If used, should be in combination with antiviral therapy.
- Treatment of complications: Secondary bacterial skin infections—silver sulfadiazine topically and/or systemic antibiotics
- PHN and zoster-associated pain (1)
  - Tricyclic antidepressants (TCAs; amitriptyline 25 mg at bedtime and other low-dose TCAs) relieve pain acutely and may reduce pain duration.
  - Lidocaine (Lidoderm) patch 5% applied after skin rash closure over painful areas (limit 3 patches simultaneously or trim a single patch) for up to 12 hours was reported effective in 1 limited trial.
  - Gabapentin: 100–600 mg t.i.d. for pain and other quality-of-life indicators; limited by adverse effects
  - Opioids, capsaicin cream and other analgesics may be useful adjuncts.
  - Pregabalin: 50–100 mg t.i.d. reduces pain, but usefulness is limited by side effects
- Prevention of PHN and zoster-associated pain: No treatment has been shown to prevent PHN completely, but treatment may shorten duration and/or reduce severity of symptoms. (4)
  - Antiviral therapy with valacyclovir, famciclovir, or acyclovir given during acute skin eruption may be effective in limiting the duration of pain.

– Low-dose amitriptyline in the same dosage as for treatment of PHN but started within 72 hours of rash onset and continued for 90 days may reduce PHN incidence or duration.

– Corticosteroids do not reduce incidence, severity, or duration of PHN. (5)

• Contraindications: Refer to the manufacturer's profile of each drug.
• Precautions
  – Assess renal function prior to using valacyclovir, famciclovir, or acyclovir.
  – Valacyclovir, famciclovir, acyclovir: Pregnancy category B
  – Refer to the manufacturer's profile of each drug.
• Significant possible interactions: Refer to the manufacturer's profile of each drug.

Second Line
>40 have been advocated (but no good supporting evidence has been published).

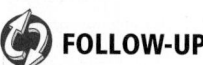 FOLLOW-UP

PROGNOSIS
• Immunocompetent individuals should experience spontaneous and complete recovery within a few weeks.
• Resolution of acute rash within 14–21 days
• PHN may occur in patients age >50 years despite treatment with antiviral medications.

COMPLICATIONS
• PHN
• Ophthalmic herpes zoster (10–20%)
• Superinfection of skin lesions
  – Meningoencephalitis
  – Cutaneous dissemination
  – Hepatitis
  – Pneumonitis
  – Myelitis
  – Cranial and peripheral nerve palsies
  – Acute retinal necrosis

PATIENT MONITORING
Depends on symptoms

REFERENCES
1. Mounsey AL, et al. Herpes zoster and postherpetic neuralgia: Prevention and management. *Am Fam Physician*. 2005;72(6):1075–1080.
2. Opstelten W, Zaal MJW. Managing ophthalmic herpes zoster in primary care. *BMJ*. 2005;331: 147–151.
3. Johnson RW, Dworkin RH. Treatment of herpes zoster and postherpetic neuralgia. *BMJ*. 2003;326: 748–750.
4. Weinberg JM, et al. Skin infections in the elderly. *Dermatol Clin*. 2004;22:51–61.
5. Gnann JW, Whitley RJ. Herpes zoster. *N Engl J Med*. 2002;347(5):340–346.

 ## ADDITIONAL READING
• Oxman MN, et al. A Vaccine to prevent herpes zoster and postherpetic neuralgia in Older Adults. *N Engl J Med*. 2005;352(22):2271–2284.
• Gnann JW. Varicallea-zoster virus: Atypical presentations and unusual complications. *J Infect Dis*. 2002;186(suppl 1):S91–S98.
• Johnson RW. Consequences and management of pain in herpes zoster. *J Infect Dis*. 2002;186 (suppl 1):S83–S90.
• Wood M. Understanding pain in herpes zoster: An essential for optimizing treatment. *J Infect Dis*. 2002;186(suppl 1):S78–S82.
• Gilden DH, et al. Neurologic complications of the reactivation of varicella-zoster virus. *N Engl J Med*. 2000;342(9):635–645.
• www.IHMF.org
• www.vzvfoundation.org

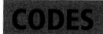 MISCELLANEOUS

See also: Bell palsy; Chickenpox; Herpes eye infections; Herpes simplex

 CODES

ICD9-CM
053.9 Herpes zoster without mention of complication

PATIENT TEACHING
• Inform patient that the duration of rash is 2–3 weeks.
• Encourage good hygiene and proper skin care.
• Warn of potential for dissemination (dissemination must be suspected with constitutional illness signs and/or spreading rash).
• Warn of potential PHN.
• Warn of potential risk of transmitting illness (chickenpox) to susceptible persons.

 See Corresponding Diagnostic Algorithm

See Patient Handout on CD

H

HERPES, GENITAL

Theresa N. Grabo, PhD, APRN, BC, FNP

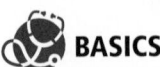 **BASICS**

DESCRIPTION
- Herpes (from Greek "to creep or crawl") simplex virus infection involving the genitals
- Primary genital herpes: Genital herpes due to herpes simplex virus HSV-1 or HSV-2 with no antibody to HSV-1 or HSV-2 at time of infection
- Nonprimary 1st episode genital herpes: Genital herpes due to HSV-2 with existing antibody to HSV-1 or genital herpes due to HSV-1 with existing antibody to HSV-2
- Recurrent genital herpes: Reactivation of latent genital herpes with existing antibody to the same HSV type recovered from the lesion
- Synonym(s): Herpes genitalis

GENERAL PREVENTION
- Sexual abstinence is the only option to provide complete prevention.
- Condoms in sexual activity reduce transmission by >60%.
- Avoid multiple sexual partners.
- Pregnant women without evidence of HSV antibody should avoid unprotected sex in late pregnancy.

EPIDEMIOLOGY
- Predominant age: 18–40 years
- Predominant sex: Female > Male

Incidence
50–200/100,000 (300,000–900,000 cases)

Prevalence
10,000–30,000/100,000 people (45–50 million)

RISK FACTORS
- Primary inoculation
  - Increasing age, lower socioeconomic status, African American race, number of lifetime partners, and past history of sexually transmitted diseases (STDs)
  - Fomites: Wet towels (rare)
- Transmission
  - Incubation period: 1–45 days (mean 5.8)
  - Annual risk for susceptible female acquiring disease from an infected male partner is 10–30%; for susceptible male from infected female, ~5%
  - Patients without HSV-1 antibody are at greater risk for acquiring HSV-2 infection.
  - >70% of new cases result from transmission during asymptomatic or clinically unrecognized shedding.
  - Risk of asymptomatic shedding is highest within 1 year of 1st occurrence.
  - Acyclovir and valacyclovir (LOE = 1b) daily suppresses shedding and reduces transmission of HSV-2 to partners.
- Triggers (recurrent): Genital trauma, menses, intercurrent infection, emotional stress, ultraviolet light; recurrences more common in men

ALERT
Pediatric Considerations
Neonatal infection occurs in 10–20/100,000 live births. Most infections result from asymptomatic maternal viral shedding.

PATHOPHYSIOLOGY
Pathologic stages
- Primary mucocutaneous infection
- Acute sacral ganglionic infection
- Establishment of latency
- Ganglionic reactivation

ETIOLOGY
- HSV: A double-stranded DNA, Alphaherpesvirinae virus subfamily
- HSV-1: 10–30% (increasing incidence); is now greater than HSV-2 in some clinical settings
- HSV-2: 70–90%

ASSOCIATED CONDITIONS
- Herpes labialis
- Syphilis
- Gonorrhea
- Nongonococcal urethritis/cervicitis
- Genital warts (human papilloma virus)
- AIDS (HIV)
- Trichomoniasis

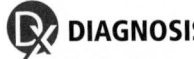 **DIAGNOSIS**

SIGNS AND SYMPTOMS
- Difficult to differentiate among primary, 1st episode nonprimary, and recurrent disease on the basis of symptoms and clinical findings
- 60–70% of HS2 are asymptomatic or do not recognize clinical manifestations of the disease.
- Primary genital herpes
  - Fever, headache, malaise, myalgia (40–60%)
  - Burning genital pain
  - Dysuria (female)
  - Dyspareunia
  - Sacral paresthesia
  - Inguinal adenopathy
  - Aseptic meningitis in 30%
  - Occasional urinary retention
  - Vesicles, on an erythematous base, that ulcerate, crust over, and resolve spontaneously within 21 days
  - Bilateral lesions, primarily affecting the external genitalia
    ○ Female: Labia majora/minora, inner thighs, vaginal mucosa, cervix, perianal skin
    ○ Male: Penile glans, penile shaft, urethra
- Nonprimary–1st episode
  - Burning genital pain
  - Vesicles resolve within 14–17 days
- Nonprimary—recurrent
  - Prodromal symptoms: Burning, numbness, tingling, paresthesia of genitals at site of previous lesions that occurs ~24 hours before new vesicles erupt
  - Vesicles resolve within 7–10 days
  - Unilateral lesions

ALERT
Pediatric Considerations
Genital lesions child suggest sexual abuse.

Physical Exam
- Female: Pelvic examination of internal reproductive organs; external genitalia, vagina, cervix.
- Male: Penis and scrotum
- Male and female: Rectum, thighs, buttocks, pubic hair area, mouth, inguinal lymph nodes.

Herpes Simplex Serology

Lesion*	Serology†	Stage‡
HSV-1	Negative	P HSV-1
HSV-2	Negative	P HSV-2
HSV-1	HSV-2	NP HSV-1
HSV-2	HSV-1	NP HSV-2
HSV-1	HSV-1 ± HSV-2	R HSV-1
HSV-2	HSV-2 ± HSV-1	R HSV-2

*Culture, EIA, or PCR
†Type-specific antibody
‡P, primary; R, recurrent; NP, nonprimary first episode.

TESTS
Lab
- Viral detection from lesion
  - Swab vesicle fluid or ulcer; viral culture, enzyme immunoassay, DNA detection by PCR (2–3 times more sensitive than culture)
  - Use Dacron-tipped swabs.
- Tzanck test: Sensitivity 40–50% compared with culture; multinucleated giant cells
- Pap smear: Sensitivity 60–70%
- Type-specific serologic assays (TSST)
  - Immunodot, Western blot (gold standard), and monoclonal antibody (glycoprotein-G) to discriminate between HSV-1 and HSV-2.
- Commercially available tests include Herpes Select-1 & 2 (ELISA), Herpes Select 1/2 (immunoblot), and POCkit-HSV-2 (point-of-care).
- Potential indications for obtaining type-specific herpes virus serology
  - Evaluate asymptomatic long-term sexual partner of infected individual.
  - Recurrent undiagnosed genital ulcers
  - Screen pregnant women with infected partners.
  - Differentiate primary from nonprimary genital infection.

Pathological Findings
- Histopathologic–cytopathic changes
- Intracellular edema of epithelial cells
- Nuclear margination of chromatin
- Formation of Cowdry type A intranuclear inclusion bodies
- Cell fusion into multinucleated giant cells

DIFFERENTIAL DIAGNOSIS
- Primary syphilis
- Chancroid
- Lymphogranuloma venereum
- Herpes zoster
- Trauma
- Inflammatory bowel disease
- Behçet syndrome
- Stevens-Johnson syndrome
- Ulcerative balanitis
- Granuloma inguinale
- Neoplasia

TREATMENT

GENERAL MEASURES
- Cool compresses of aluminum acetate (Burow solution) 4–6 times a day
- Ice packs to perineum
- Sitz baths
- Topical anesthetic
- Analgesics, NSAIDs

Activity
- Avoid intercourse with symptomatic lesions.
- Rest if systemic manifestations are present

 MEDICATION (DRUGS)

First Line
- Acyclovir (Zovirax)
  - Primary episode: 400 mg PO t.i.d. for 10 days or 200 mg PO 5 times a day for 7–10 days; 5 days for recurrent episodes
  - Severe local or disseminated disease: 5–10 mg/kg IV q8h for 5–7 days
  - Recurrent: 200 mg PO 5 times a day for 5 days (or 400 mg t.i.d. for 5 days, or 800 mg b.i.d. for 5 days, or 800 mg t.i.d. for 2 days)
  - Chronic suppression: Recommended for frequent (≥6 per year) or clinical/psychological disabling recurrences: 400 mg PO b.i.d. (or 200 mg PO 3–5 times a day)
  - HIV infection: 400 mg PO 3–5 times a day until clinical resolution attained
- Precautions
  - Pregnancy: Not FDA-approved for routine use (category C). Studies have demonstrated safety of use.
  - Drug is excreted in breast milk.
  - Modify dose in patients with significant renal insufficiency.
  - Acyclovir resistance (also famciclovir and valacyclovir resistance): Mostly in HIV-infected patients (5–10%)
  - Obtain viral isolates for sensitivity testing if lesions persist or recur after adequate antiviral therapy.
- ACOG Clinical Management Guidelines
  - Primary HSV during pregnancy, or lesions near/at term, should receive therapy.
  - Women with 1st episode nonprimary genital herpes at risk for recurrence at or beyond 36 weeks, consider antiviral therapy; may reduce Caesarean section rate, clinical HSV, and HSV shedding; should continue until delivery; acyclovir 400 mg t.i.d. (LOE = 1a) or valacyclovir 500 mg b.i.d.
  - Pregnant women on acyclovir: Report to CDC/Wellcome (800) 722–9292, ×38465.
- Significant possible interactions
  - Methotrexate
  - Interferon
  - Probenecid will decrease renal excretion and increase serum concentration.
- Use with caution in combination with nephrotoxic agents.
- Valacyclovir (Valtrex)
  - May cause TTP/hemolytic uremic syndrome in some immunocompromised patients
  - Pregnancy category B
  - 1st episode: 1 g PO b.i.d. for 7–10 days
  - Recurrent: 500 mg PO b.i.d. for 3–5 days
  - Chronic suppression: 250 mg b.i.d. or 500 mg PO daily or 1000 mg/d (LOE = 1b)

- Famciclovir (Famvir)
  - Activity/side effects similar to acyclovir; greater bioavailability than acyclovir
  - Pregnancy category B
  - 1st episode: 250 mg PO t.i.d. for 7–10 days
  - Recurrent: 125 mg PO b.i.d. for 5 days
  - Chronic suppression: 250 mg PO b.i.d.

Second Line
- Acyclovir topical: Less effective; do not use
- Foscarnet: 40 mg/kg IV q8h in severe disease with proven or suspected acyclovir-resistant strains
- Vidarabine: 10 mg/kg/d infused over 10 hours; benefits HIV patients with HSV-1 infection failing acyclovir and foscarnet therapy
- Cidofovir (Vistide) topical: 0.1–0.3% gel for 5 days, for progressive/resistant lesions
- Trifluridine (Viroptic) ophthalmic solution, for mucocutaneous lesions resistant to acyclovir

ALERT
Pediatric Considerations
- High-risk infant: Acyclovir 30 mg/kg/d IV q8h for 10–14 days
- Low-risk infant, asymptomatic: Culture eyes, nose and mouth at 24–36 hours and observe

 FOLLOW-UP

PROGNOSIS
- Resolution of signs/symptoms
  - Primary in 14–21 days
  - 1st episode nonprimary in 14–17 days
  - Recurrent in 7–10 days
- Latent infection: Recurrences in 80% of patients within 1 year of initial HSV-2 infection; immunocompetent average 3–4 a year
- HSV infection in immunocompromised (AIDS) patient: More severe, difficult to treat
- Treatment with antiviral agents does not eliminate virus from body.

ALERT
Pediatric Considerations
Neonatal infection survival rates: Localized, >95%; CNS, 85%; systemic, 30%

COMPLICATIONS
- Vaginal discharge
- Secondary bacterial infection
- Urinary retention
- Aseptic meningitis
- Transmission to neonate; spontaneous abortion, preterm birth, low-birth-weight infants
- Increased risk for HIV infection (2–3 times)
- Lowered self-esteem, guilt, anger, depression, fear of rejection, fear of transmission to partner
- In pregnancy
  - Primary/1st episode: Spontaneous abortion (45%); preterm labor (35%)
  - Greatest risk for neonatal infection with primary (50% transmission rate) or nonprimary 1st episode (30%) infected mother at delivery; enhanced by prolonged rupture of membranes, fetal scalp electrode, cervical lesions, and prematurity
  - Low risk: Recurrent asymptomatic HSV shedding in mother (3%); mothers with high titer of neutralizing antibodies
  - Caesarean section is indicated if herpetic genital lesions are present during labor.

PATIENT MONITORING
- Acute episode: Follow-up if complications
- Latent infection: Check pregnant women at prenatal visits and onset of labor.
- Consider testing for other sexually transmitted diseases in setting of initial HSV infection.
- Reassess suppression therapy yearly.

REFERENCES
1. Beauman JG. Genital herpes: a review. Am Fam Physician. 2005;72:1527–1534.
2. Reitano M, Tyring S, Lang W. Valacyclovir for the suppression of recurrent genital herpes simplex infection: A large dose range-finding study. J Infect Dis. 1998;178:603–610.
3. Sheffield JS, Hollier LM, Hill JB, et al. Acyclovir prophylaxis to prevent herpes simplex virus recurrence at delivery: A systematic review. Obstet Gynecol. 2003;102:1396–1403.
4. Corey L, Wald A, Patel R. Once daily valacyclovir to reduce the risk of transmission of genital herpes. N Engl J Med. 2004;350:11–20. [A] (1)
5. Wald A, Langenberg AG, Link K, et al. Effect of condoms on reducing the transmission of herpes simplex virus type 2 from men to women. JAMA. 2001;285:3100–3106. [B] (2).
6. Leone P. Reducing the risk of transmitting genital herpes: Advances in understanding and therapy. Curr Med Res Opin. 2005;21:1577–1582. [C] (3).
7. Centers for Disease Control and Prevention. Diseases characterized by genital ulcers. Sexually transmitted diseases treatment guidelines 2006. MMWR Recomm Rep. 2006;55(RR-11):1–94. [C] (3).

ADDITIONAL READING
- Patel R. Managing patients with genital herpes and their sexual partners. Infect Dis Clin North Am. 2005;19(2):427–438.
- Hill J. Herpes simplex virus in pregnancy: New concepts in prevention and management. Clin Perinatol. 2005;32(3):657–670.

 MISCELLANEOUS

- See also: Herpes simplex
- Selected web sites:
  - http://www.ashastd.org
  - http://www.ihmf.org
  - http://www.niaid.nih.gov

CODES

ICD9-CM
054.10 Genital herpes, unspecified

PATIENT TEACHING
- Herpes Resource Center Hotline: (919) 361–8488
- Toll free herpes hotline: (888) 411-4347

Prevention
- Avoid sex if lesions or prodromal symptoms present and for 2 days after resolved
- Correct and consistent use of male latex condoms

See Patient Handout on CD

H

HICCUPS

James H. Lewis, MD

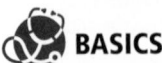 BASICS

DESCRIPTION
- Sudden involuntary contraction of the inspiratory muscles (predominantly the diaphragm) terminated by abrupt closure of the glottis stopping the inflow of air and producing the characteristic sound
- System(s) Affected: Nervous; Pulmonary
- Synonym(s): Hiccoughs; Singultus

ALERT
Geriatric Considerations
Can be a serious problem among the elderly

Pregnancy Considerations
- Fetal hiccups noted as rhythmic fetal movements (confirmed sonographically) that can be confused with contractions
- Fetal hiccups often recur in subsequent pregnancies.

GENERAL PREVENTION
- Identify and correct underlying cause.

EPIDEMIOLOGY
- Predominant age: All ages (including fetus)
- Predominant sex: Male > Female (4:1)

Prevalence
Self-limited hiccups are extremely common, as are intra- and postoperative hiccups; intractable hiccups are rare.

RISK FACTORS
- General anesthesia; conscious sedation
- Postoperative state
- Genitourinary disorders
- Irritation of the vagus nerve branches
- Structural, vascular, infectious, neoplastic, or traumatic CNS lesions

ETIOLOGY
- Pathophysiologic significance is unknown; may be a vestigial reflex; hiccups have been associated with >100 underlying disorders.
- Results from stimulation of 1 or more limbs of the hiccup reflux arc (vagus and phrenic nerves) with a "hiccup center" located in the upper spinal cord
- In men >90% have an organic basis, whereas in women a psychogenic cause may be more likely.
- Specific underlying causes include
  - Alcoholism
  - CNS lesions (brainstem tumors, vascular lesions, Parkinson disease)
  - Diaphragmatic irritation (tumors, pericarditis, eventration, splenomegaly, hepatomegaly, peritonitis)
  - Hair, insect, or foreign body irritating tympanic membrane
  - Pharyngitis, laryngitis

- Mediastinal and other thoracic lesions (pneumonia, aortic aneurysm, tuberculosis, myocardial infarction, lung cancer, rib exostoses)
- Esophageal lesions (reflux esophagitis, achalasia, Candida esophagitis, carcinoma, obstruction)
- Gastric lesions (ulcer, distention, cancer)
- Hepatic lesions (hepatitis, hepatoma)
- Pancreatic lesions (pancreatitis, pseudocysts, cancer)
- Inflammatory bowel disease
- Cholelithiasis, cholecystitis
- Prostatic disorders
- Appendicitis
- Postoperative, abdominal procedures
- Toxic metabolic causes (uremia, hyponatremia, gout, diabetes)
- Drug induced (dexamethasone, methylprednisolone, anabolic steroids, benzodiazepines, alpha methyldopa)
- Psychogenic causes (hysterical neurosis, grief, malingering)
- Idiopathic

ASSOCIATED CONDITIONS
See "Etiology."

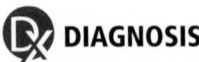 DIAGNOSIS

SIGNS AND SYMPTOMS
- Hiccup attacks usually occur at brief intervals and last only a few seconds or minutes. Bouts lasting >48 hours often imply an underlying physical or metabolic disorder.
- Intractable hiccups may occur continuously for months or years.
- Hiccups usually occur with a frequency of 4–60 per minute.

History
Recent surgery (especially genitourinary), general anesthesia; medications; alcoholism; GI, cardiac or pulmonary disorders (see "Etiology")

Physical Exam
(See "Etiology" for specific findings to look for); examine ear canal for foreign bodies

TESTS
Lab
Routine CBC, metabolic panel

Imaging
Fluoroscopy is useful to determine if 1 hemidiaphragm is dominant.

Diagnostic Procedures/Surgery
- Upper endoscopy, colonoscopy, CT scan (or other imaging) of brain, thorax, abdomen, and pelvis looking for etiological causes; exploratory laparoscopy or laparotomy for peritoneal lesions (carcinomatosis, etc.); GYN pathology, etc.
- The extent of the workup is often in proportion to the duration and severity of the hiccups.

DIFFERENTIAL DIAGNOSIS
See "Etiology" (burping [eructation] may be confused with hiccups).

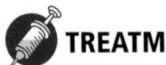 TREATMENT

- Outpatient (usually)
- Inpatient (if elderly, debilitated, or intractable hiccups)

GENERAL MEASURES
- Treat any specific underlying cause when identified
  - Dilate esophageal stricture or obstruction.
  - Treat ulcers or reflux disease.
  - Remove hair or foreign body from ear canal.
  - Angostura bitters for alcohol-induced hiccups
  - Catheter stimulation of pharynx for operative and postoperative hiccups
  - Antifungal treatment for *Candida* esophagitis
  - Correct electrolyte imbalance.
- Medical measures
  - Relief of gastric distention (gastric lavage, nasogastric aspiration, induced vomiting)
  - Counterirritation of the vagus nerve (supraorbital pressure, carotid sinus massage, digital rectal massage), to be used with caution
  - Respiratory center stimulants (breathing 5% carbon dioxide)
  - Psychiatric (hypnosis, behavioral modification)
  - Phrenic nerve block or electrical stimulation (or pacing) of the dominant hemidiaphragm
  - Miscellaneous (cardioversion)

Activity
As tolerated

SPECIAL THERAPY
Complementary and Alternative Medicine
Acupuncture is increasingly being used to manage persistent hiccups.

- Simple home remedies
  - Swallowing a spoonful of sugar
  - Sucking on a hard candy or swallowing peanut butter
  - Holding breath and increasing pressure on diaphragm (Valsalva maneuver)
  - Tongue traction
  - Lifting the uvula with a cold spoon
  - Drinking from the far side of a glass
  - Inducing fright
  - Smelling salts
  - Rebreathing into a paper (not plastic) bag
  - Sipping ice water

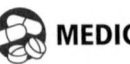 MEDICATION (DRUGS)

First Line
Possible drug remedies
- Baclofen, a GABA analog, 5–10 mg t.i.d. (best choice)
- Chlorpromazine 25–50 mg IV
- Haloperidol 2–12 mg IM
- Phenytoin 200 mg IV, then 100 mg q.i.d.
- Metoclopramide 5–10 mg q.i.d.
- Nifedipine 10–20 mg daily to t.i.d.

- Amitriptyline 10 mg t.i.d.
- Lidocaine 1.5 mg/kg IV infusion followed by 0.75 mg/kg on subsequent days
- Gabapentin (Neurontin) up to 1,800 mg/d in divided doses
- Contraindications: Refer to manufacturer's literature. (Baclofen is not recommended in patients with stroke or other cerebral lesions.)
- Precautions: Refer to manufacturer's literature. (Abrupt withdrawal of baclofen should be avoided.)
- Significant possible interactions: Refer to manufacturer's literature.
- Maintenance drug therapy (e.g., baclofen 5–10 mg t.i.d.; phenytoin 100 mg q.i.d.; valproic acid 15 mg/kg undivided doses; nifedipine 10–20 mg daily to t.i.d.; metoclopramide 10 mg q.i.d.); gabapentin up to 1800 mg in divided doses (see "Medications")

Second Line
- Amantadine, carbidopa-levodopa in Parkinson disease
- Steroid replacement in Addison disease
- Antifungal agent in *Candida* esophagitis
- Ondansetron in carcinomatosis with vomiting
- Nefopam (a nonopioid analgesic with antishivering properties related to antihistamines and antiparkinsonian drugs) is available outside the United States in both IV and oral formulations.

SURGERY
- Phrenic nerve crush or transection of the dominant diaphragmatic leaflet
- Resection of rib exostoses

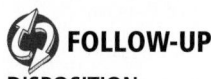 **FOLLOW-UP**

DISPOSITION
Admission Criteria
Most patients can be managed as outpatients; those with severe intractable hiccups may require rehydration, pain control, IV medications, or surgery.

Issues for Referral
For acupuncture or phrenic nerve crush, block, or electrostimulation

PROGNOSIS
- Hiccups often cease during sleep.
- Most acute benign hiccups resolve with home remedies or spontaneously.
- Intractable hiccups may last for years and decades.
- Hiccups have persisted despite bilateral phrenic nerve transection.

COMPLICATIONS
- Inability to eat
- Weight loss
- Exhaustion, debility
- Insomnia
- Cardiac arrhythmias
- Wound dehiscence
- Death (rare)

PATIENT MONITORING
Until hiccups cease

REFERENCES
1. Lewis JH. Hiccups and their cures. *Clin Perspect Gastroenterol*. 2000;3:277–283.
2. Okuda Y. Use of a nerve stimulator for phrenic nerve block in treatment of hiccups. *Anesthesiology*. 1998;88:525–527.
3. Porzio G, Aielli F, Narducci F, et al. Hiccup in patients with advanced cancer successfully treated with gabapentin: Report of three cases. *N Z Med J*. 2003;116:U605.
4. Ramirez FC, Graham DY. Treatment of intractable hiccup with baclofen: Results of a double-blind randomized, controlled, cross-over study. *Am J Gastroenterol*. 1992;87:1789–1791.
5. Schiff E, River Y, Oliven A, et al. Acupuncture therapy for persistent hiccups. *Am J Med Sci*. 2002;323:166–168.
6. Kranke P, Eberhart LH, Morin AM, et al. Treatment of hiccup during general anesthesia or sedation: A qualitative systematic review. *Eur J Anaesthesiol*. 2003;20:239–244.
7. Bilotta F, Rosa G. Nefopam for severe hiccups. *N Engl J Med*. 2000;343:1973–1974.

ADDITIONAL READING
- Dickerman RD, Jaikumar S. The hiccup reflex arc and persistent hiccups with high-dose anabolic steroids: Is the brainstem the steroid-responsive locus? *Clin Neuropharmacol*. 2001;24:62–64.
- Bagheri H, Cismondo S, Montastruc JL. Drug-induced hiccup: A review of the French pharmacologic vigilance database. *Therapie*. 1999;54:35–39.
- Smith HS, Busracamwongs A. Management of hiccups in the palliative care population. *Am J Hosp Palliat Care*. 2003;20:149–154.

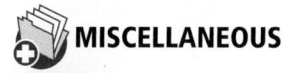 **MISCELLANEOUS**

CODES

ICD9-CM
786.8 Hiccough

PATIENT TEACHING
See "General Measures."

Diet
Avoid gastric distension from overeating, carbonated beverages, and aerophagia.

Activity
As tolerated

Prevention
- Avoid gastric distention
- Seek medical attention for frequent bouts or persistent hiccups
- Acupuncture appears to be as or more efficacious than chronic drug therapy to control hiccups.

 See Corresponding Diagnostic Algorithm

 See Patient Handout on CD

H

HIDRADENITIS SUPPURATIVA

Jeffrey Mailhot, MD

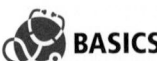 **BASICS**

DESCRIPTION

- Acute, tender, cystlike abscesses in apocrine gland–bearing skin (axillae, anogenital area, pubes, areolae, also apocrine glands scattered around umbilicus, scalp, trunk, and face); often a chronic condition
- Over time, fibrotic sinus tracts develop with intermittent drainage and periodic acute abscesses.
- Common from late puberty through 40 years
- System(s) Affected: Skin/Exocrine
- Synonym(s): Apocrinitis, Hidradenitis axillaris, Acne inversa

ALERT

Geriatric Considerations
Rare after menopause

Pediatric Considerations
Rarely occurs before puberty (1 case reported in a 2-year-old)

Pregnancy Considerations
No isotretinoin (Accutane) treatment during pregnancy

GENERAL PREVENTION

- Minimize heat exposure and sweating.
- Lose weight if overweight.
- Avoid constrictive clothing/frictional trauma.
- Avoid underarm antiperspirants and deodorants.

EPIDEMIOLOGY

- Predominant age: Peak onset age 11–30 years, commonly 30–40 years; rare before puberty
- Predominant sex: Female (perianal) > Male (axillary)

Prevalence
0.3–4%

RISK FACTORS

- Obesity
- Female
- Acne
- Diabetes mellitus
- Hypercholesterolemia
- Low basal metabolic rate
- Smoking possibly

Genetics
Unknown; possibly single gene transmission (autosomal dominant), possibly polygenic

ETIOLOGY

- Traditionally considered a disorder of apocrine glands, but now believed to be caused by occlusion of terminal follicular epithelium (hair follicles) within apocrine gland–bearing skin. Bacterial involvement is not a primary pathogenic event, but secondary.
- Historically part of follicular occlusive triad: Acne conglobata, dissecting cellulitis of scalp, hidradenitis suppurativa. Pilonidal sinus was later added to form a tetrad.
- Sebum excretion not an important factor (7).
- Smoking may be a major triggering factor.

ASSOCIATED CONDITIONS

- Acne
- Perifolliculitis capitis abscedens et suffodiens (dissecting cellulitis of scalp)
- Obesity with associated diabetes mellitus, atopy, acanthosis nigricans

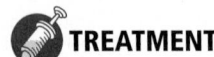 **DIAGNOSIS**

SIGNS AND SYMPTOMS

- Early signs of pruritus, erythema, and local hyperhidrosis
- Multiple recurrences at the same site
- Healing sites accompanied by scarring and sinus tracts
- Associated arthritis (rare)

Physical Exam
- Comedones may be present.
- Distribution is over the area of apocrine glands, with axillae and groin being most common.
- Papules (dome-shaped) 1–3 cm in size are present.
- Nodules (dome-shaped) 1–3 cm in size are present.
- Large lesions often are fluctuant.

TESTS
Culture discharge from lesion(s).

Lab
- Culture of exudate from lesion: staphylococci, streptococci, *Escherichia coli*, *Proteus* with chronic condition, usually not anaerobes.
- Increasing antibiotic resistance
- Possibly increased ESR, leukocytosis, decreased serum iron, normocytic anemia, and changes in serum electrophoresis pattern, probably owing to chronic inflammatory process

Diagnostic Procedures/Surgery
- Incision and drainage of lesion(s) with biopsy
- Clinical criteria for early diagnosis (proposed by Mortimer)
  - Recurrent deep boils >6 months in flexural sites
  - Onset after puberty
  - Poor response to conventional antibiotics
  - Strong tendency toward relapse or recurrence
  - Comedones in apocrine gland–bearing skin
  - Routine culture of pus from boils; no pathogens
  - Personal or family history of acne or pilonidal sinuses and exacerbation of boils premenstrually in women

Pathological Findings
- Acute and chronic inflammation
- Multiple comedones
- Sinus tracts when recurrent

DIFFERENTIAL DIAGNOSIS

- Furunculosis. Differentiate by specific culture and also by the response to specific antibiotics.
- Carbuncles, granulomatous disease, infected epidermoid cysts, tuberculosis cutis, actinomycosis, tularemia, and carcinoma. With inguinal involvement: Granuloma inguinale and lymphogranuloma venereum
- Inflammatory bowel disease with anogenital fistula (may also coexist with hidradenitis suppurativa or be mistaken for it)

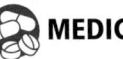 **TREATMENT**

INITIAL STABILIZATION
Generally outpatient

GENERAL MEASURES

- Symptomatic treatment acute lesions
- Prevention of new lesions
- Local cleansing (germicidal soap)
- Improve environmental factors that cause follicular blockage.

Diet
No restrictions

Activity
Fully active

MEDICATION (DRUGS)

- Antibiotics (not curative; relapse almost always inevitable once medication is stopped); treatment sometimes for ≥2 months
  - Clindamycin 2% lotion or neomycin cream topically to control odor and pain. Topical clindamycin as effective as systemic tetracyclines for stage 1 or 2 disease. Oral clindamycin also is effective.
  - Tetracycline 250 mg PO q.i.d. or 500 mg PO t.i.d.
  - Minocycline (Minocin) 100 mg PO b.i.d.
  - Erythromycin 1–1.5 g PO daily
  - Doxycycline 100 mg PO b.i.d. 7–14 days
  - Other antibiotics depending on culture
- Consider oral retinoids
  - Isotretinoin (Accutane) 40–80 mg/d PO for 4 months
  - No Accutane during pregnancy (highly teratogenic)
  - Equivocal results, still frequent recurrences
- Birth control pills (female only), if antibiotic therapy fails. Low-dose progesterone birth control pills (e.g., Norinyl, Ortho-Novum, Enovid)
- Anti-TNF-α (Etanercept) SQ has been used minimally in some resistant cases (3).
- Consider steroids
  - Injection of lesions with depot-type steroids (e.g., triamcinolone)
  - Consider brief course of systemic corticosteroids.
  - Antiandrogen therapy is controversial.
- Contraindications: Tetracycline: Pregnancy, children <8 years
- Precautions
  - Tetracycline: Use sunscreen (SPF 15 or better) to avoid phototoxicity.
  - Review professional literature before prescribing birth control pills or Accutane.

SURGERY

- Wide excision with healing by granulation (considered more efficacious than drug treatment), but medical treatment is tried 1st because of extensive nature of surgery treatment.
- Incision and drainage of lesions
  - Remove sinus tracts.
  - Exteriorization with curettage and electrodesiccation
- Treatment for severe, intractable cases: Excision of all apocrine glands and skin graft
- Radical surgery best for preventing recurrence of axillary and perianal HS, least effective (50%) for submammary (5).
- CO_2 laser stripping with healing by secondary intention

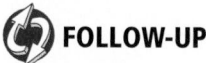 **FOLLOW-UP**

PROGNOSIS

- Individual lesions (with or without drainage) heal slowly in 10–30 days.
- Recurrences may last for several years.
- Rare spontaneous resolution
- Relentlessly progressive scarring and sinus tracts

COMPLICATIONS

- Contracture formation at the sites of lesions
- Restricted limb mobility
- Squamous cell carcinoma may develop in indolent sinus tracts (usually anogenital).
- Disseminated infection septicemia (unusual)
- Lymphedema
- Urethral/rectal fistula
- Anemia
- Arthritis
  - Asymmetrical pauciarticular to symmetrical polyarthritis/polyarthralgia in larger joints.
- Amyloidosis
- Renal failure
- Interstitial keratitis

PATIENT MONITORING

Revisits monthly, or more often if needed

REFERENCES

1. Bell BA, Ellis H. Hidradenitis suppurativa. *J R Soc Med.* 1978;71:511–515.
2. Brown TJ, Rosen T. Hidradenitis suppurativa. *South Med J.* 1998;91:1107–1114.
3. Buckley C, Cusack C. Etanercept: effective in the management of hidradenitis suppurativa. *Br J Dermatol.* 2006;154(4):726–729.
4. Clemmensen OJ. Topical treatment of hidradenitis suppurativa with topical clindamycin. *Int J Dermatol.* 1983;22(5):325–328.
5. Harrison BJ, Hughes LE, Mudge M. Recurrence after surgical treatment of hidradenitis suppurativa. *Br Med J.* 1987;294(6570):487–489.
6. Jemec GB, Wendelboe P. Topical clindamycin versus systemic tetracycline in the treatment of hidradenitis suppurativa. *J Am Acad Dermatol.* 1998;39(6):971–974.
7. Jemec GB, Gniadecka M. Sebum excretion in hidradenitis suppurativa. *Dermatology.* 1997;194(4):325–328.
8. Konig A. Cigarette smoking as a triggering factor of hidradenitis suppurativa. *Dermatology.* 1999;198:261–264.
9. Krahl D, Sellheyer K. "Hidradenitis suppurativa" is acne inversa! An appeal to (finally) abandon a misnomer. *Int J Dermatol.* 2005;44(7):535–540.
10. Lapins J, Marcusson JA, Emtestam L. Surgical treatment of chronic hidradenitis suppurativa: CO_2 laser stripping-secondary intention technique. *Br J Dermatol.* 1994;131:551–556.
11. Morgan WP, Harding KG, Hughes LE. A comparison of skin grafting and healing by granulation, following axillary excision for hidradenitis suppurativa. *Ann R Coll Surg Engl.* 1983;65(4):235–236.
12. Mortimer PS et al. A double-blind controlled cross-over trial of cyproterone acetate in females with hidradenitis suppurativa. *Br J Dermatol.* 1986;155(3):263–268.

 MISCELLANEOUS

- See also: Folliculitis, furunculosis
- Other notes
  - Some patients develop only 2 or 3 papules per year. Others develop new lesions and drain as rapidly as old ones resolve.
  - Although 50% of patients receiving Accutane, in doses similar to those for acne, obtain appreciable improvement, relapse occurs quickly on discontinuing.
  - Fox-Fordyce disease presents in anatomic locations similar to HS; however it primarily affects apocrine glands and does not progress to abscess formation or suppuration.
  - Hidradenitis suppurativa is considered a misnomer by many. *Acne inversa* is the more accepted terminology.

CODES

ICD9-CM
705.83 Hidradenitis

PATIENT TEACHING

- Minimize heat exposure and sweating.
- Reduce weight if obese.
- Avoid constrictive clothing (i.e., tight-fitting underwear and T-shirts).
- Explain medication precautions.

 See Patient Handout on CD

H

HIP FRACTURE

Brian Busconi, MD
Adam Harder, MD

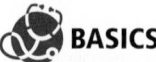 **BASICS**

DESCRIPTION
- Hip fractures are common injuries, most frequently affecting elderly individuals.
- Different types of hip fractures exist, and they are treated in different ways.
  - Femoral neck fractures occur just before the femoral head.
  - Intertrochanteric hip fractures occur in the region between the greater and lesser trochanters, below the lever of femoral neck fractures.

GENERAL PREVENTION
- Ensure adequate calcium and vitamin D intake.
- Remain active, with particular emphasis on weightbearing exercises.
- Avoid smoking and excessive alcohol use.
- Institute adequate screening and medical treatment of osteoporosis.

EPIDEMIOLOGY
- In 2003, there were 345,000 hospitalizations for hip fractures in the US.
- The average age of patients with hip fractures is 77 years for women and 72 years for men
- Nearly 80% occur in women

Incidence
- 63.3 per 100,000 person-years for women in the US.
- 27.7 per 100,000 person-years for men in the US.

RISK FACTORS
- Osteoporosis: Bones are weakened by decreased amounts of calcium and other minerals
- Increased age: Bone density decreases with age
- Female sex
  - Women are 2–3 times more likely than men to sustain a hip fracture.
  - They lose bone density faster than men do, particularly following menopause.
- Caucasian and Asian race
- Chronic medical conditions
  - Endocrine disorders
    - Diabetes mellitus
    - Hypogonadism
  - Gastrointestinal disorders
    - Interfere with calcium and vitamin D absorption
  - Rheumatoid disorders
  - Parkinson disease
  - Multiple sclerosis
  - Dementia
  - Depression
- Limited physical activity
- Poor nutrition: Lack of calcium and vitamin D lowers peak bone mass and increases risk of fracture later in life
- Tobacco and alcohol use interfere with bone metabolism and remodeling, leading to faster bone loss with age.
- Medications
  - Corticosteroids
  - Anticonvulsants
  - Thyroid medications
  - Some diuretics and anticoagulants

Genetics
Genetic factors influence bone size, bone mass, and bone density.

PATHOPHYSIOLOGY
- With aging, bones become less dense as they slowly lose minerals.
- Gradual loss of density weakens bones and makes them more susceptible to a hip fracture.

ETIOLOGY
- Most commonly caused by a fall in elderly patients.
- In younger patients, more common causes include high-energy injuries such as car accidents.
- Pathologic fractures may occur through bone weakened by tumor or infection.

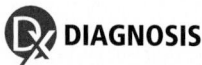 **DIAGNOSIS**

SIGNS AND SYMPTOMS
- Severe pain in hip or groin
- Inability to bear weight
- Stiffness, bruising, and swelling around the hip

History
- Elderly patients will typically present with hip pain after suffering a fall.
- Obtaining a history of loss of consciousness, prior syncopal episodes, chest pain, prior hip pain, and preinjury ambulatory status is essential.
- Younger patients will complain of pain after suffering a much higher-energy injury, such as a high-speed motor vehicle accident or a fall from a significant height.
- Cyclical loading stress fractures can be seen in athletes, military recruits, and ballet dancers.

Physical Exam
- Shortened and externally rotated lower extremity
- Pain with passive range of motion of the affected extremity
- Tenderness to palpation of the groin
- A careful neurovascular exam should be performed
- Rule out other fractures or injuries with a comprehensive musculoskeletal examination

TESTS
- CBC, chemistry, coagulation studies, and a type and screen should be obtained preoperatively.
- UA is recommended given the high incidence of urinary tract infections in the elderly population.

Imaging
- Plain radiographs
  - Fractures are visible in all but 1% of cases
  - An internal rotation view of the hip taken with the lower extremity internally rotated ~15 degrees will permit better visualization of the entire femoral neck.

- CT
  - May be performed if plain radiographs are inconclusive, suspicion is high, and MRI is contraindicated or unavailable.
  - A negative CT does not rule out the possibility of an occult fracture.
- MRI
  - The investigation of choice in situations in which plain radiographs are inconclusive or suspicion is high.
- Bone scan
  - Maybe useful if MRI is contraindicated
  - Results may be normal for up to 72 hours after the injury.

DIFFERENTIAL DIAGNOSIS
- Avascular necrosis
- Pelvic or acetabular fracture
- Osteoarthritis
- Inflammatory arthritis
- Septic arthritis
- Metastatic disease
- Muscle contusion
- Bursitis
- Lumbar disc disease

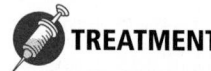 **TREATMENT**

GENERAL MEASURES
- The treatment of hip fractures is largely surgical.
- The type of surgery performed depends on the type of hip fracture.
- The goal of treatment is to stabilize the fracture to achieve better pain control and allow early ambulation.
- Nonoperative treatment is largely reserved for individuals who have severe medical problems that preclude surgery or in some certain types of stress fractures.
  - Much higher complication rate is associated with the prolonged immobilization required for fractures to heal with nonoperative measures.

Diet
- NPO prior to surgery
- Postoperatively, the diet can be advanced as tolerated.

Activity
- Patients must be on bed rest and nonweightbearing on the affected extremity prior to surgery.
- Weightbearing postoperatively varies depending on the type of fracture and type of fixation utilized.
- Patients should be mobilized beginning on the 1st postoperative day.

Nursing
- A catheter should be placed at the time of admission.
- Neurovascular checks should be performed on the affected extremity.
- 5 pounds of Buck's traction may be applied to help with comfort prior to surgery.
- Provide adequate analgesia.

Physical Therapy
All patients should work with physical therapy beginning on the 1st postoperative day.

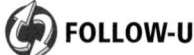 MEDICATION (DRUGS)

- Medical treatment of osteoporosis may help with the prevention of hip fractures
  - Bisphosphonates
  - Selective estrogen receptor modulators
  - Calcitonin
- Perioperative antibiotics
  - Initiated within 2 hours of surgery and continued for 24–48 hours
  - 1st generation cephalosporins are the treatment of choice.
- Thromboembolic prophylaxis
  - Pneumatic compression devices preoperatively
  - Chemical prophylaxis postoperatively for 10–14 days

SURGERY

- Early surgery within 24–48 hours of admission should be the goal unless more time is absolutely required for stabilization.
  - Lower 1-year mortality
  - Lower incidence of pressure sores
  - Decreased confusion
  - Lower risk of fatal pulmonary embolism
- Femoral head fractures
  - Cannulated screws
    - Indicated for nondisplaced or minimally displaced fractures in which the blood supply to the femoral head is not disrupted
    - Also indicated for displaced fractures in younger patients in which every attempt is made to avoid the use of prostheses and to preserve the femoral head
  - Hip hemiarthroplasty
    - Indicated for displaced fractures in which the blood supply to the femoral head is thought to be disrupted.
  - Total hip arthroplasty
    - Indicated for displaced fractures in patients who have underlying hip arthritis with involvement of the acetabulum
- Intertrochanteric hip fractures
  - Open reduction and internal fixation with some type of hardware depending on the exact fracture type is the treatment of choice

FOLLOW-UP

DISPOSITION

- Hospital stays after surgery typically last less than a week.
- Many patients will require placement in a rehab facility prior to returning home.

PROGNOSIS

- Only 25% of patients who sustain a hip fracture will return to their preinjury level of activity.
- Mortality rates in the 1st year following a hip fracture are ~25%.

COMPLICATIONS

- Many complications are secondary to any prolonged immobilization
  - Blood clots
  - Pulmonary embolism
  - Pneumonia
  - Urinary tract infections
  - Decubitus ulcers
- Any patient who sustains a hip fracture is at higher risk of sustaining fractures in the future.
- Delirium
- Avascular necrosis (AVN)
  - Occurs in 5% of nondisplaced fractures and up to 25% of displaced fractures of the femoral neck
  - Occurs in <2% of intertrochanteric hip fractures

REFERENCES

1. Parker M, Johansen A. Hip fracture. *Br Med J.* 2006;333:27–30.
2. Koval KJ, Zuckerman JD. Hip fractures I: Overview and evaluation and treatment of femoral-neck fractures. *JAAOS.* 1994;2:141–149.
3. Koval KJ, Zuckerman JD. Hip fractures II: Evaluation and treatment of intertrochanteric fractures. *JAAOS.* 1994;150–156.

ADDITIONAL READING

Rao SS, Cherukuri M. Management of hip fracture: The family physician's role. AAFP. 2006;17:2195–2200.

MISCELLANEOUS

CODES

ICD9-CM

- 820.0 Transcervical fracture, closed
- 820.1 Transcervical fracture, open
- 820.2 Petrochanteric fracture, closed
- 820.3 Petrochanteric fracture, open
- 820.8 Unspecified part of neck of femur, open
- 820.9 Unspecified part of neck of femur, closed

PATIENT TEACHING

Prevention of fractures can be optimized by having discussions with elderly patients regarding fall prevention and aggressive medical management of osteoporosis. Many patients are not aware of the risks associated with sustaining hip fractures. Providing them with this knowledge can help protect them against sustaining falls and fractures.

See Patient Handout on CD

H

HIRSUTISM

Laura L. Novak, MD

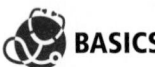

BASICS

DESCRIPTION
- Presence of excessive body and facial hair, in a male pattern, in women
- May be present in normal adults as an ethnic characteristic or may develop as a result of androgen excess
- Often accompanied by menstrual irregularities
- System(s) affected: Dermatologic; Endocrine/Metabolic; Reproductive
- Synonym(s): Excessive hair

ALERT
Pregnancy Considerations
- May have related infertility. Offer intervention if desired.
- As hormone balance improves, fertility may increase; provide contraception as needed.
- Several medications used for treatment are contraindicated in pregnancy.

GENERAL PREVENTION
- There is an increased incidence of diabetes and insulin resistance in polycystic ovarian disease that can increase risk of heart disease.
- Prolonged amenorrhea may, over time, put the patient at risk for endometrial hyperplasia or carcinoma.
- Women with late-onset congenital adrenal hyperplasia may be carriers for the severe early-onset childhood disease—counsel.
- Avoid quackery and unlicensed electrolysis.

EPIDEMIOLOGY
Prevalence
Eight percent of adult women

RISK FACTORS
- Family history
- Anovulation

Genetics
Multifactorial

ETIOLOGY
Hirsutism is due to increased androgenic (male) hormones-either from increased peripheral binding (idiopathic) or increased production from the ovaries, adrenals, or fat. Exogenous medications can also be associated with hirsutism.

ASSOCIATED CONDITIONS
- Polycystic ovary syndrome (PCOS): The most common cause of hirsutism accompanied by menstrual irregularity of amenorhea. Often associated with acne, obesity, and multicystic ovaries, but up to 50% of cases are atypical.
- Hypothyroidism: When associated with anovulation
- Hyperprolactinoma: When accompanied by galactorrhea (milk production)
- Late-onset congenital adrenal hyperplasia (LOCAH): A genetic enzyme deficiency associated with more severe and earlier onset hirsutism. Present in <2% of hirsute, amenorrheic patients.
- Tumor: Rare (<0.2%); Ovarian or adrenal; associated with rapid onset, extreme changes; virilization; cliteromegaly, balding, deepening voice.
- Cushing syndrome: Rare; central obesity, moon facies, striae, hypertension

DIAGNOSIS

SIGNS AND SYMPTOMS
- The Ferriman-Gallway scale (an instrument that rates hair growth in 9 areas on a scale of 0–4 with >8 being positive) is used for diagnosis, but underrates localized hirsutism
- Onset is usually gradual.
- Irregular menses may indicate PCOS
- Increased androgens are associated with acne, obesity, insulin resistance, and hyperlipidemia.
- Virilization: Deep voice, balding, clitoromegaly can indicate risk of tumor.

History
- Onset, duration of symptoms
- Menstrual and fertility history
- Medication history: Valproic acid, testosterone, danazole, athletic performance drugs

Physical Exam
Acanthosis nigricans: Velvety black skin in the axilla, neck and under the breast; associated with insulin resistance. (HAIR-AN syndrome; hyperandrogenic insulin resistance; acanthosis nigricans)

TESTS
Diagnosis is clinical. Lab testing is to rule out associated conditions or diseases. The recommendations for workup range from a minimal work-up (testosterone and thyroid level—ACOG practice bulletin) (1)[C] to a complete endocrinologic workup. (2)[C] As hirsutism is common and serious underlying disease is rare, clinical judgment can be applied.

- Testosterone level: Random level vs. free morning testosterone. Random testosterone is less sensitive, but will not miss significant disease. (3,4)[A] A level >200 ng/dL may indicate ovarian tumor.

- Insulin resistance testing: Results vary with age and ethnicity. Fasting insulin level >20 or fasting glucose/insulin ratio <4.5 may indicate resistance.

- Dehydroepiandrostenedione sulfate (DHEA-S) elevation can indicate an adrenal source. Used much less commonly. (3,4)[A] Levels >700 may indicate adrenal tumor.

- 17-Hydroxyprogesterone (17-HP): Elevations (>300) can indicate late-onset congenital adrenal hyperplasia. Rare (<2%). Consider in patients with onset in early adolescence. Elevated levels require additional testing.

Lab
- Lab testing is performed to rule out underlying tumor and pituitary disease, which are rare. Empiric treatment without lab workup is an acceptable option.
- Basic workup: Total testosterone, thyroid-stimulating hormone, if clinically suspicious, insulin resistance workup (as above)
- Prolactin level if galactorrhea

Imaging
- If testosterone is >200 or dehydroepiandrosterone sulfate is >700, get CT of ovaries or adrenals.
- Ovarian ultrasound can help in the diagnosis of PCOS.

DIFFERENTIAL DIAGNOSIS
Hirsutism is associated with a number of different conditions (see "Etiology").

TREATMENT

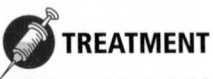

INITIAL STABILIZATION
Outpatient

GENERAL MEASURES
- Treatment is slow and often lifelong.
- If patient desires pregnancy, induction of ovulation may be necessary.
- Provide contraception as needed.
- Encourage patient to maintain ideal weight.
- Treat accompanying acne.

Diet
No special diet

Activity
No special activity

Complementary and Alternative Medicine
Serenoa repens (saw palmetto): In small studies decreases hair growth via blocking 5-α-reductase activity in the skin.

MEDICATION (DRUGS)

First Line

Treatment goal is to decrease new hair growth and improve metabolic disorders.

- Oral contraceptives take 6–12 months to show effect; any brand is effective
- Eflornithine (Vaniqa) HCl cream: Apply b.i.d.; reduces facial hair in 40% of women (with long-term use)

Second Line

- Insulin sensitizers (metformin, thioglitazoles) decrease insulin resistance, improving hormone binding proteins and decreasing androgens. Effective, but less potent than oral contraceptives.
- Antiandrogenic drugs (used in combination with oral contraceptives to prevent menorrhagia and potential fetal toxicity) will further reduce hirsutism 15–25%.
  – Spironolactone: 25–200 mg/d—onset of action is slow; side effects include menorrhagia, hyperkalemia; contraindicated in pregnancy
  – Ketoconazole: 400 mg/d—avoid with astemizole, triazolam
  – Finasteride: 5 mg/d decreases androgen binding; not FDA approved

 FOLLOW-UP

PROGNOSIS

- Good (with long-term therapy) for halting further hair growth
- Moderate to poor for reversing current hair growth

COMPLICATIONS

- Dysfunctional uterine bleeding and anemia
- Anovulation may increase uterine cancer risk.
- Androgenic excess may adversely affect lipid status, cardiac risk, and bone density.
- Poor self-image/shame

PATIENT MONITORING

Monitor for known side effects of medications.

REFERENCES

1. ACOG (American College of Obstetrics and Gynecology) Clinical Practice Guidelines on the diagnosis and management of Polycystic Ovarian Syndrome. #41. Dec 2002
2. AACE (American Academy of Clinical Endocrinology) Medical Guidelines for clinical practice for the diagnosis and treatment of hyperandrogenic disorders. *Endocr Pract*. 2001;7(2):120–134.
3. Azzir R. The evaluation and management of hirsutism. *Obstet Gynecol*. 2003;101:995–1006.
4. Rosenfeld RL. Hirsutism. *N Eng J Med*. 2005; 353(24):2578–2588.

 MISCELLANEOUS

See also: Acne vulgaris; Infertility; Polycystic ovarian syndrome (PCOS)

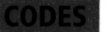

ICD9-CM

704.1 Hirsutism

PATIENT TEACHING

- Hormonal treatment stops further hair growth, but will not usually reverse present hair.
- Treatment takes 6–24 months and may be lifelong.
- Cosmetic measures include plucking, bleaching, shaving, electrolysis, laser hair removal, and cover-up cosmetics.
- Electrolysis should be by a licensed professional.

 See Patient Handout on CD

H

HISTOPLASMOSIS

Robert P. Baughman, MD

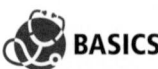

BASICS

DESCRIPTION
Fungal infection with *Histoplasma capsulatum*, a dimorphic soil-dwelling saprophyte that has multiple clinical manifestations

- Initial infection is often asymptomatic.
- Other manifestations include a self-limited flu-like syndrome, mediastinal fibrosis, scar tissue residual, chronic cavitary disease in those with obstructive lung disease, and disseminated histoplasmosis, which is more frequent in the immunocompromised host and infants.
- Histoplasma capsulatum
  - Worldwide distribution: Most endemic region in North America is central US
  - Exists in mycelial form in nature and in yeast phase when exposed to mammalian temperatures
  - Spores may remain active for up to 10 years
  - Exposure to bird or bat excrement promotes growth of the fungus for unexplained reasons.
- Chronic pulmonary histoplasmosis: Usually occurs in white males with obstructive lung disease and apical bullous lung pathology. These patients exhibit evidence of an indolent infectious process.
- Disseminated histoplasmosis infection in the immunocompromised is a rare opportunistic infection, which may mimic sepsis syndrome and progress to multiple organ system failure.
- System(s) Affected: Gastrointestinal; Hemic/ Lymphatic/Immunologic; Pulmonary; Skin/Exocrine

ALERT
Geriatric Considerations
Increased incidence of disseminated histoplasmosis in males during 6th and 7th decades

Pediatric Considerations
One third of cases of disseminated histoplasmosis occur in infants <1 year old

GENERAL PREVENTION
Maintenance therapy is required in AIDS.

EPIDEMIOLOGY
Predominant sex: Acute histoplasmosis: Male = Female
Disseminated histoplasmosis: Male > Female (5–10:1)

Incidence
- Infection in endemic areas is virtually 100%.
- Few patients develop active disease.
- ~500,000 new infections in the US each year
- Occurrence in AIDS patients is 2–5%.
- Disseminated histoplasmosis occurs in <0.05% of infections.

Prevalence
Disseminated histoplasmosis
- Infants <1 year old are at higher risk for disseminated histoplasmosis (1/3 of all occurances).
- In adults there is an increased prevalence with age >60 years.

RISK FACTORS
- Spelunking
- Cleaning chicken coops
- Excavation near bird roosts
- Demolition or remodeling of old buildings
- Exposure to decayed wood or dead trees
- Performing routine activities in areas with high accumulation of bird droppings
- Immunosuppression

ETIOLOGY
Dimorphic fungus Histoplasma capsulatum

ASSOCIATED CONDITIONS
- Disseminated histoplasmosis is an opportunistic infection in the immunocompromised host
- HIV infection

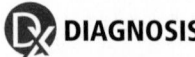

DIAGNOSIS

SIGNS AND SYMPTOMS
- Primary infection is usually asymptomatic
- 1% immunocompetent individuals with low-level exposure develop symptoms
- 99% subclinical infection
- Arthralgia—erythema nodosum—erythema multiforme is associated with acute infection
- Low-grade fever, anorexia, weight loss, night sweats, and productive cough are associated with chronic infections

TESTS
- Determine the presence of urinary *H. capsulatum* antigen.
- Bronchoscopy
- Liver and bone marrow biopsies

Lab
- For disseminated histoplasma antigen in AIDS patients, urinary and blood histoplasmosis
- Polysaccharide antigen detection is a rapid test for diagnosis and for monitoring relapse.
- Complement fixation may be negative in ~30% in acute histoplasmosis and 50% in disseminated histoplasmosis
- Immunodiffusion test may be negative in ~50% of patients with acute histoplasmosis. Maximum positivity of test occurs 4–6 weeks after exposure.

- Complement fixation antibodies at titers 1:8 or 1:16 are presumptive for diagnosis, >1:32 is strongly supportive as is an acute 4-fold titer rise. Determining the presence of H and M bands may be helpful.
- For chronic histoplasmosis and disseminated disease, cultures of sputum, bronchoalveolar lavage, bone marrow, lymph nodes, blood, liver, and cerebrospinal fluid may be positive. Demonstration of characteristic organisms by silver stain on biopsy and bronchoalveolar lavage and bronchial washing specimens is diagnostic.
- Disorders that may alter lab results
  - Serologic tests may be falsely negative early in infection or in the immunocompromised.
  - False-positive results may occur with tuberculosis and other fungal diseases.
  - Slow clearance of antibodies may identify patients with past histoplasmosis infection who now present with a different disease.
  - False-positive complement fixation titers may occur after histoplasmin skin antigen testing.
  - False-positive *H. capsulatum* polysaccharide antigen test may occur with patients with disseminated blastomycosis and coccidioidomycosis.

Imaging
- Routine CXR may reveal focal mid-lung field infiltrates (27%), hilar or mediastinal adenopathy (25%) or both (30%). May see miliary or diffuse pattern with disseminated disease following large antigen load.
- If indicated, chest CT scan to differentiate mediastinal fibrosis from mediastinal granuloma

Diagnostic Procedures/Surgery
- Serologic blood work
- Bronchoscopy with bronchoalveolar lavage and transbronchial biopsy
- Liver and bone marrow biopsies for suspected disseminated disease
- Mediastinoscopy for lymph node biopsy

Pathological Findings
Poorly formed caseating granulomas on biopsy or bronchoscopy specimens with identification of characteristic yeast forms by methenamine silver stain

DIFFERENTIAL DIAGNOSIS
- Atypical pneumonia and viral pneumonitis
- Other fungal diseases such as blastomycosis, coccidioidomycosis
- Other granulomatous diseases such as M. tuberculosis
- Sarcoidosis
- Pneumoconiosis
- Lymphoma
- Malignancies associated with hilar lymphadenopathy

TREATMENT

GENERAL MEASURES

- Appropriate health care: Usually outpatient
- Disseminated histoplasmosis requires hospitalization for initial treatment.
- 99% of acute primary histoplasmosis resolve spontaneously; symptomatic treatment only

Activity
Avoid high-risk exposures.

MEDICATION (DRUGS)

First Line
- Disseminated histoplasmosis
  - Amphotericin B: Test dose is 1mg followed by 0.25 mg/kg per dose, which may be slowly increased to 0.5 mg/kg per dose; cumulative dose to 1–2 g (at least 35 mg/kg is indicated).
  - Itraconazole (induction therapy with 200 mg b.i.d. for 3 days, then 200 mg once or b.i.d.) for mild disease
  - Ketoconazole (induction therapy with 400 mg/d for 3 days, then maintenance therapy 200 mg or 400 mg/d) for mild disease
- AIDS patients
  - Itraconazole for mild disease: Induction therapy with 600 mg/d for 3 days, then 400 mg/d; drug of choice for primary and maintenance therapy is itraconazole; Ketoconazole is not effective in AIDS-related histoplasmosis; maintenance therapy with itraconazole 400 mg/d or amphotericin B 50–100 mg weekly (1 mg/kg)
- Chronic cavitary histoplasmosis
  - Amphotericin B: For severe or moderately severe disease, 2.0–2.5 g cumulative
  - Itraconazole (induction therapy with 200 mg b.i.d. for 3 days, then 200 mg once or b.i.d.) for mild disease
  - Ketoconazole (induction therapy with 400 mg/d for 3 days, then maintenance therapy 200 mg or 400 mg/d) for mild disease
- Acute pulmonary histoplasmosis
  - Amphotericin B for severe or moderately severe disease; test dose is 1 mg followed by 0.25 mg/kg per dose, which may be slowly increased to 0.5 mg/kg per dose; cumulative dose at least 35 mg/kg
  - Ketoconazole (induction therapy with 400 mg/d for 3 days, then maintenance therapy 200 mg or 400 mg/d), or Itraconazole (induction therapy with 200 mg b.i.d. for 3 days, then 200 mg once or b.i.d.) for mild disease
- Duration of treatment
  - Optimal duration of treatment with antifungals has not been established
  - Disseminated histoplasmosis: 6 months course
  - Chronic cavitary histoplasmosis: At least 12-months course with stable CXR findings over 3–6 months
  - Acute pulmonary histoplasmosis: 2–3 month course
  - AIDS-related or relapsed: Chronic, life-long, maintenance therapy

- Mediastinal granuloma
  - Can mimic fibrosing mediastinitis, may respond to treatment with amphotericin B
- Fibrosing mediastinitis
  - Has no active infection present and is not treatable
- No contraindications to treatment in patients with progressive cavitary disease or disseminated histoplasmosis. The latter has a mortality rate of 80%, if untreated.
- Precautions
  - Amphotericin B: Dosage probably does not need to be adjusted for creatinine clearance. It is nephrotoxic. Renal function must be monitored closely. Monitor electrolytes, especially potassium and magnesium. Rigors can be prevented by pre-infusion meperidine. Fever and chills can be diminished by pre-infusion dose of acetaminophen plus diphenhydramine.
  - Ketoconazole: Associated with gastrointestinal upset; may inhibit testosterone synthesis and should be used with caution in patients with underlying hepatic dysfunction.
- Significant possible interactions
  - Expected benefits outweigh possible risks.
  - Ketoconazole: Requires an acid environment for dissolution. If the patient requires antacid or H_2 blockade, administer at least 2 hours after dose of ketoconazole. This may increase cyclosporine levels and decrease Rifampin and INH levels, as well as ketoconazole levels. Phenytoin levels may also be increased.
  - Itraconazole: Rifampin levels may decrease itraconazole to undetectable levels. May increase digoxin levels; questionable effect on cyclosporine levels
  - Fluconazole: May increase cyclosporine levels; may increase warfarin effect

Second Line
- Fluconazole has not been approved for histoplasmosis therapy.
  - Fluconazole is undergoing investigational studies in its use for chronic pulmonary and disseminated histoplasmosis.
  - Preliminarily, fluconazole doses of 400 mg/d or higher may be necessary for therapeutic outcome.
- Liposomal amphotericin may be used if amphotericin nephrotoxicity is encountered.
  - Questionable effect of rifampin on fluconazole

FOLLOW-UP

PROGNOSIS
- Primary histoplasmosis: 99% resolve spontaneously
- The prognosis for chronic cavitary pulmonary histoplasmosis is determined by the loss of lung parenchyma and pulmonary function
- Treatment of disseminated disease in AIDS/non-AIDS cases does improve outcome with ketoconazole having >80% success rate and amphotericin B being 60–100% successful. Despite maintenance therapy, AIDS patients have a 10–50% relapse rate.

COMPLICATIONS
- Bronchial, tracheal or esophageal obstruction secondary to adenopathy, broncholithiasis
- Pulmonary, splenic and hepatic calcifications, rarely pericarditis, pleurisy, or effusion
- CNS histoplasmosis (rare): Chronic meningitis or intracranial histoplasmosis
- Endocarditis involving aortic or mitral valves
- Pericardial effusions (sterile exudates) not thought to be secondary to hematogenous spread
- Fibrosing mediastinitis can cause stenosis of vascular and bronchial structures within the mediastinum causing pulmonary hypertension, superior vena cava syndrome, and bronchial obstruction.
- Acute renal failure and hepatic dysfunction secondary to medications
- Amphotericin-induced hypokalemia
- Relapse occurring in the immunocompromised or inadequately treated patient with disseminated histoplasmosis

PATIENT MONITORING
- Renal function and liver chemistries every 1–2 months for chronic therapy patients
- Chest x-ray to evaluate therapy response at regular intervals

REFERENCES
1. Dismukes WE, Cloud G, Bowles C, et al. Treatment of blastomycosis and histoplasmosis with ketoconazole. *Ann Intern Med*. 1985;103: 861–872.
2. Como JA, Dismukes WE. Oral azole drugs as systemic antifungal therapy. *N Engl J Med*. 1994;330:263–272.
3. Wheat JL, Connolly-Stringfield P, Kohler RB, et al. Histoplasma capsulatum polysaccharide antigen detection in diagnosis and management of disseminated histoplasmosis in patients with acquired immunodeficiency syndrome. *Am J Med*. 1989;87:396–400.
4. Wheat JL, Conces D, Allen SD, Blue-Hnidy D, Loyd J. Pulmonary histoplasmosis syndromes: recognition, diagnosis, and management. Se, *Resp Crit Care Med*. 2004;25:129–144.
5. Wheat J. Histoplasmosis: recognition and treatment. *Clin Infect Dis*. 1994;1(Suppl):S19–S27.

MISCELLANEOUS

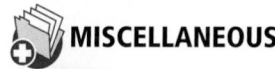

ICD9-CM
- 115.90 Histoplasmosis, unspecified without mention of manifestation
- 115.99 Histoplasmosis, unspecified other

PATIENT TEACHING

Extended treatment needs in chronic cavitary histoplasmosis; maintenance therapy in AIDS

 See Corresponding Diagnostic Algorithm

HISTRIONIC PERSONALITY DISORDER

Melissa E. Arthur, LCSW, MA

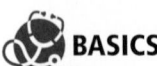 **BASICS**

DESCRIPTION

- A condition characterized by persistent patterns of dysfunctional behavior (excessive emotionality and attention seeking) deviating from one's culture and social environment that lead to functional impairment and distress to the individual and those who have regular interaction with the individual.
- Behaviors are perceived by the patient to be "normal" and "right" and patients have little insight as to their responsibility for these behaviors.
- Condition is classified based on the predominant symptoms and their severity.
- Cluster B Personality Disorder (inclusive of antisocial, borderline, histrionic, and narcissistic personality disorders) characterized by a pervasive pattern of excessive emotionality and attention seeking, present in a variety of contexts (5 or more symptom patterns to diagnose) (1)[C]
  - Shows self-dramatization, theatricality, and exaggerated expressions of emotion
  - Is suggestible, i.e., easily influenced by others or circumstances
  - Uncomfortable when not center of attention
  - Interaction with others is often characterized by inappropriate sexually seductive behavior
  - Rapidly shifting and shallow expression of emotion
  - Draws attention through physical appearance
  - Has a style of speech that is excessively impressionistic and lacks detail
  - Considers relationships more intimate than they are (1)[C]

Incidence

Starts in adolescence and early 20s and persists throughout one's life in the absence of treatment. (1)[C]

Prevalence

- 2–3% general population (1)[C]
- Tends to be identified more frequently in females (1)[C]

RISK FACTORS

Genetics

- Major character traits may be inherited
- Other character traits due to a combination of genetics and environment including adverse childhood experiences

ETIOLOGY

Environmental and genetic factors including adverse childhood experiences including lack of parental attention.

ASSOCIATED CONDITIONS

- Depression
- Anxiety disorders
- Panic disorder
- Somatization disorders
- Body dysmorphic disorder (strong emphasized on physical appearance)
- Anorexia
- Post traumatic stress disorder including dissociative disorders
- Substance abuse
- Other psychiatric disorders in patient and family members

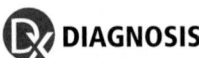 **DIAGNOSIS**

DSM IV CRITERIA

Diagnostic Code: 301.50

SIGNS AND SYMPTOMS

- Distress, excessive emotionality (2)[C]
- Impairment of social and/or occupational functioning (2)[C]
- Not due to direct physiological effects of substance abuse, drug abuse, medication use or general medical conditions

History

- Comprehensive interview and mental status examination
- Family session to assess persistent pattern of behavior

TESTS

Psychological testing, e.g., MMPI-II

Lab

TSH, VDRL, CBC, CMP, HIV

Imaging

CT scan and MRI of the brain may be necessary in newly developed symptoms in the absence of a triggering event to rule out the rare instance of organic brain disease.

DIFFERENTIAL DIAGNOSIS

- Narcissistic Personality Disorder
- Somatization Disorder
- Borderline Personality Disorder
- Substance Abuse
- Can co-occur with Borderline, Narcissistic, Antisocial, and Dependent Personality disorders

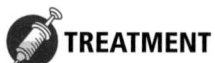

TREATMENT

PRE HOSPITAL
In patients who have attempted overdose, transport all appropriate pill bottles to hospital.

INITIAL STABILIZATION
Appropriate psychiatric security measures should be in place to prevent lethality.

GENERAL MEASURES
Diet
Emphasize importance of basic nutritional guidelines. No known special diet

Activity
Exercise as a means of reducing stress.

SPECIAL THERAPY
Complementary and Alternative Therapies
- Biofeedback
- Meditation

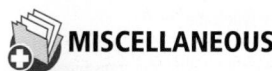

MEDICATION (DRUGS)

No known drug to treat personality disorder, however, medications can reduce symptoms (3)[C] associated with the Axis I Disorders such as Mood disorders (Antidepressants: SSRIs) and Anxiety disorders (Anxiolytics: Benzodiazepines, buspirone, and the SSRIs) (3)[C]

FOLLOW-UP

COMPLICATIONS
- Unstable relationships with family, friends and coworkers
- May be characterized by separations and divorces
- Disruptive work patterns (e.g., absenteeism, frequent job changes, and decreased productivity)
- Increased demand for outpatient medical visits due to psychological condition and attention-seeking behavior

PATIENT MONITORING
- If the patient is on a pharmacological regime, initial monitoring should be frequent (every 2 weeks) to evaluate the effectiveness, potential side effects of medication, and suicidal ideation.
- In the absence of pharmacological treatment, frequent regular visits (every 4–6 weeks) will help prevent attention-seeking phone calls/visits.

REFERENCES

1. American Psychiatric Association. *Diagnostic and Statistical Manual of Mental Disorders*. 4th ed. Washington DC: American Psychiatric Association; 1994.
2. Kraus G, Reynolds DJ. The A-B-C's of the cluster B's: Identifying, understanding and treating cluster B personality disorders. *Clin Psychol Rev*. 2001;21(3):345–373.
3. Ward RK. Assessment and management of personality disorders. *Am Fam Phys*. 2004;70(8): 1505–1512.

ADDITIONAL READING

Horowitz MJ. Psychotherapy for histrionic personality disorders. J Psychother Practice Res 1997;6:93–107.

MISCELLANEOUS

CODES
ICD9-CM
301.5 Histrionic personality disorder

H

HIV INFECTION AND AIDS

Ligia Peralta, MD
Ruben Peralta, MD, FACS

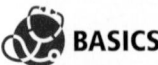 **BASICS**

DESCRIPTION

- Immunodeficiency virus (HIV) is a retrovirus that integrates into CD4 T lymphocytes, causing cell death and resulting in severe immunodeficiency, opportunistic infections (OI) and malignancies.
- Due to treatment advances, HIV is now a chronic disease.
- The natural history of untreated HIV infection includes: Viral transmission, acute retroviral syndrome, recovery and seroconversion, asymptomatic chronic HIV infection and symptomatic HIV infection or acquired immunodeficiency syndrome (AIDS).
- Without antiretroviral treatment, the average patient develops AIDS about 10 years after transmission.
- All HIV infected persons with CD4 <200 cells/mm^3 are categorized as having AIDS.

ALERT

Geriatric Considerations
Progresses more rapidly in age >50.

Pediatric Considerations
Progresses more rapidly in infants.

GENERAL PREVENTION
- Avoid unprotected sexual intercourse
- Use condoms
- Avoid injection drug abuse
- Needle exchange for active IDUs
- Avoid unscreened blood products

EPIDEMIOLOGY

Incidence
- 40,000 new infections every year
- 900,000 persons living with HIV/AIDS
- Ethnic and racial minorities make up a disproportionate number of new AIDS cases.

Prevalence
- Predominantly young adults: 25–44
- Male > Female
- Younger women and girls are particularly vulnerable.

RISK FACTORS
- Sexual activity (70% of world transmission)
- Injection drug use
- Children of HIV-infected women
  - Maternal HIV-1 RNA level is the best predictor of transmission risk.
  - HIV testing of pregnant women and the use of antiretroviral drugs in pregnant women and their newborns has reduced the incidence of HIV perinatal transmission by ~70% (from 25–29% without treatment to 8% with; demonstrated in Pediatric AIDS Clinical Trials Group Protocol 076) (1). Pregnant women should be treated until viral load is undetectable.
  - Can be transmitted through breast-feeding.
- Recipients of blood products, especially hemophiliacs who received pooled plasma between 1975 and March 1985
- Occupational exposure

Genetics
People who lack CCR5, a cell surface protein and primary coreceptor used by HIV to infect cells, are highly resistant to HIV infection (2).

ETIOLOGY
Human immunodeficiency virus (HIV); a retrovirus

ASSOCIATED CONDITIONS
- Syphilis may be more aggressive in HIV-infected persons.
- Tuberculosis is coepidemic with HIV; test all persons with TB for HIV. Patients dually infected with HIV and TB have a 100 times greater risk of developing active TB disease compared with non–HIV-infected people. They also have higher rates of multidrug-resistant TB.
- Hepatitis C coinfected patients have more rapid progression to cirrhosis.

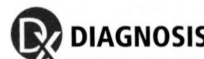 **DIAGNOSIS**

SIGNS AND SYMPTOMS
- Acute retroviral syndrome: Precipitous decline in CD4 lymphocyte count and increased viremia, about 6–8 weeks after infection.
- Mononucleosis-like syndrome. Symptoms include
  - Fever
  - Adenopathy
  - Pharyngitis
  - Rash
  - Myalgias
  - Less commonly: Headache, diarrhea, nausea, vomiting, hepatosplenomegaly, weight loss, thrush, and neurologic symptoms.
- Asymptomatic infection: Variable duration. Persistent lymphadenopathy: >1 cm in ≥2 extra inguinal sites, persists >3 months.
- Symptomatic conditions (B symptoms)
  - Constitutional: Fever or diarrhea >1 month, bacillary angiomatosis, thrush, persistent candidal vulvovaginitis, cervical dysplasia or carcinoma in situ, oral hairy leukoplakia, herpes zoster, idiopathic thrombocytopenic purpura, pelvic inflammatory disease, peripheral neuropathy or myelopathy.
- Other symptoms and conditions
  - Secondary cancers: Kaposi sarcoma Hodgkin, non-Hodgkin, and primary brain lymphoma; and invasive cervical cancer
  - Cardiac: Myopathy, pericarditis
  - Renal: HIV nephropathy
  - Other conditions: Seborrheic dermatitis, severe chronic fatigue, chronic lymphoid interstitial pneumonitis, extra-intestinal strongyloides, listeriosis, nocardioses
- AIDS-defining opportunistic infections: Candidiasis, coccidioidomycosis, cryptococcus, cryptosporidiosis, cytomegalovirus, herpes simplex, histoplasmosis, isosporiasis, mycobacterium avium complex, *M. kansasii, M. tuberculosis,* other mycobacterium, *P jiroveci, bacterial pneumonias (>2/yr), recurrent salmonella septicemia, toxoplasmosis of brain*
- Malignancy: Invasive cervical cancer, Kaposi sarcoma, Burkitt lymphoma, immunoblastic lymphoma, primary brain lymphoma,
- HIV encephalopathy/dementia
- Progressive multifocal leukoencephalopathy
- HIV wasting syndrome (>10% weight loss)

History
- Past medical history, including STDs and TB
- Complete review of systems focusing on fever, chills, night sweats, diarrhea, weight loss, fatigue, adenopathy, oral sores, odynophagia (esophageal candidiasis), cough, shortness of breath and dyspnea on exertion (early *P. carinii* pneumonia), visual changes (CMV retinitis <200 CD4), skin rash, neurologic symptoms (CNS infection, malignancy, or dementia), sinusitis
- Social history, transmission risks, adherence
- Immunization review

Physical Exam
Focus on weight, skin, retinal examination, oropharynx; lymph nodes; liver, spleen, mental status, sensation, genital and rectal examinations.

TESTS

Lab
- Screening: ELISA, reported as reactive or nonreactive; sensitivity and specificity >98%
  - New testing strategies: Rapid and use oral fluid
- Confirmatory: Western blot
  - Results positive, negative, or indeterminate
  - Per CDC: Positive test is reaction with 2 of these 3 bands: P24, gp41, and gp 120/160. If indeterminate, repeat test in 3–6 months.
- CBC with differential
- CD4 cell count and %
- HIV-RNA viral load
- Serum chemistry
- Serologies: Hepatitis A, B, C, syphilis, CMV, toxoplasma
- Urine screen for sexually transmitted infections (*N. gonorrhoeae, C. trachomatis*)
- Cervical or anal cytology (for MSMs)
- PPD
- Glucose-6-Phosphate (G-6PD) levels
- At baseline and during highly active antiretroviral therapy (HAART): Fasting blood and lipids
- Genotypic and phenotypic tests for resistance to antiretrovirals; indicated if virologic failure on HAART or before initiation of therapy
- Imaging: Chest radiograph

DIFFERENTIAL DIAGNOSIS
- Screen for HIV infection when there is prolonged illness without ready explanation.
- Screen in the presence of syphilis or TB.

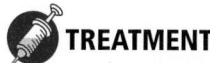 **TREATMENT**

GENERAL MEASURES (3–5)

- Current standard of care requires HAART, with 3–4 drugs that block separate enzymes used for replication.
- Main goal of HAART is to reduce the viral load and delay immune suppression.
- Other goals include preventing HIV-associated complications, short and long-term HAART adverse drug reactions, HIV transmission, HIV drug resistance, and preservation of HIV treatment options.
- Standard initial regimen include
  - 2 nucleosides with a non-nucleoside reverse transcriptase inhibitor (NNRTI)
  - 2 nucleosides and a protease inhibitor (PI) or a ritonavir-boosted PI
  - 3 nucleosides are not as effective.
- Starting HAART
  - According to US Department of Health and Human Services (4,5), begin when CD4 count <200 or AIDS-defining illness and symptoms are present.
  - For other categories: Some debate about when to begin HAART; benefits must outweigh risks, such as side effects and medication resistance (if nonadherent).
- Side effects can lead to nonadherence.
- With prolonged use of HAART, virus may mutate; medication will be less effective, but resistant strains have more difficulty reproducing. (Medication less effective than in a nonresistant patient.)
- Occupational exposure: Postexposure treatment in conjunction with expert consultation
- Prophylactic antimicrobial agents and vaccines (6)
  - *P jiroveci (former Pneumocystis carinii):* TMP-SMX 1 DS/day or 1 SS/day indicated if CD4 <200/mm³, prior PCP, thrush, or unexplained fever for >2 weeks
  - *M. tuberculosis:* Treat if PPD >5 mm induration without prior prophylaxis or treatment, recent TB contact, or history of inadequately treated TB that healed. Confirmed by culture. Treatment is based on susceptibility.
  - *Toxoplasma gondii:* 33% per year risk of infection in untreated patients with CD4 <100/mm³. Prophylaxis: TMP-SMX DS/day.
  - *M. avium complex (MAC):* 20–40% risk with CD4 <50 and no HAART. Preferred prophylaxis is clarithromycin 500 mg PO b.i.d. or azithromycin 1200 mg PO weekly.
  - *Varicella (VZV):* Seronegative and unexposed are at risk if exposed to chickenpox or shingles. Preferred regimen is VZIG 5 vials within 96 hours, preferably within 48 hours.
  - *S. pneumoniae:* 50–100 times increased risk of invasive infection compared with general population; Pneumovax every 5 years.
  - *Influenza* vaccine each fall.
  - Hepatitis A and B vaccines for at-risk patients
  - *Tetanus:* dT vaccine in adults.
  - Polio: Use *IPV,* not OPV in children.

Diet

- Encourage good nutrition, multivitamins.
- Avoid raw eggs, unpasteurized milk. Severely immunocompromised should boil tap water to prevent *Cryptosporidium.*

Activity

Encourage regular exercise.

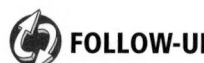 **MEDICATION (DRUGS)**

First Line

- Nucleoside reverse transcriptase inhibitors: Abacavir (ABC, Ziagen), Didanosine (ddl, Videx), Emtricitabine (FTC, Emtriva), Lamivudine (3TC, Epivir), Stavudine (d4T, Zerit), Tenofovir (Viread), Zalcitabine (ddC, Hivid), Zidovudine (AZT, Retrovir), Zidovudine + lamivudine (Combivir), Zidovudine + lamivudine + abacavir (Trizivir), Tenofovir + emtricitabine (Truvada)
- Non-nucleoside reverse transcriptase inhibitors: Delavirdine (Rescriptor), Efavirenz (Sustiva), Nevirapine (Viramune)
- Protease inhibitors: Amprenavir (Agenerase), Atazanavir (Reyataz), Fosamprenavir (Lexiva), Indinavir (Crixivan), Lopinavir-ritonavir (Kaletra), Nelfinavir (Viracept), Ritonavir (Norvir), Saquinavir (Fortovase, Invirase), Tipranavir (Aptivus)
- Fusion inhibitors: Enfuvirtide (Fuzeon)
- Drug failure: Before selecting regimen, review clinical symptoms, history of HAART, and adherence. Perform resistance testing.
- Protease inhibitors can cause metabolic syndrome (lipodystrophy, decreased HDL, increased triglycerides, high blood pressure, and hyperglycemia)
- Entry inhibitors.
- HAART, especially the protease inhibitors have potentially life-threatening interactions.

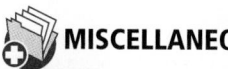 **FOLLOW-UP**

PROGNOSIS

- When untreated HIV infection leads to AIDS, the life expectancy is 3.7 years.
- AIDS-defining opportunistic infections usually do not develop until CD4 <200.
- In HIV untreated infection, CD4 counts decline at a rate of 50 to 80/year, with more rapid decline as counts drop <200.

COMPLICATIONS

- Immunodeficiency
- Opportunistic infections
- Malignancy including cervical or anal cancer

PATIENT MONITORING

- Determined by the patient's clinical status.
- Every 3–4 months, perform careful physical exam, complete review of systems, CD4 counts, viral load; Pap every 6 months in female patients.

REFERENCES

1. US Public Health Service Task Force Recommendations for Use of Antiretroviral Drugs in Pregnant HIV-1 Infected Women for Maternal Health Interventions to Reduce Perinatal HIV-1 Transmission in the US *MMWR.* 2002;51:138.
2. Berger EA, Murphy PM, Farber JM. Chemokine receptors as HIV-1 coreceptors: Roles in viral entry, tropism and disease. *Annu Rev Immunol.* 1999;17:657700.
3. Yeni PG, Hammer SM, Hirsch MS, et al. Treatment for adult HIV infection: 2004 recommendations. *JAMA.* 2004;292:251265.
4. A Guide to Primary Care of People with HIV/AIDS. US Dept of Health and Human Services, Health Resources and Services Administration, HIV/AIDS Bureau, 2004.
5. Guide for the Use of Antiretroviral Agents in HIV-1 Infected Adults and Adolescents. US Dept of Health and Human Services. http://aidsinfo.nih.gov/guidelines/adult/AA`040705.
6. Guidelines for preventing opportunistic infections among HIV-infected persons—2002. *MMWR.* 2002;51.

 MISCELLANEOUS

CODES

ICD9
042 Human immunodeficiency virus disease

PATIENT TEACHING

- Provide nonjudgmental prevention counseling, reviewing routes and behaviors leading to transmission to others and acquisition of super infection with resistant strains.
- Counsel on importance of adherence to HAART and prevention of resistance.
- National AIDS Hotline: (800) 342-2437 [Spanish (800) 342-7432].
- National Institute of Health AIDS Clinical Trials Group: (800) 874-2572.
- American Foundation for AIDS Research: (212) 719-0033 (new treatments and research).

See Corresponding Diagnostic Algorithm

See Patient Handout on CD

H

HODGKIN DISEASE

Mark Steenbergen, DO

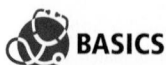 **BASICS**

DESCRIPTION
- A malignant disease of lymphoid tissue, probably caused by clonal proliferation of transformed B cells in the majority of cases, or rarely may involve T cells.
- Reed-Sternberg (RS) cells are pathognomonic.
- Disease spreads to contiguous lymphoid tissue and eventually to nonlymphoid tissue.
- Rye classification-based on pathologic findings
  - Lymphocyte predominant: 2–10%
  - Mixed cellularity: 20–40%
  - Lymphocyte depleted: 2–15%
  - Nodular sclerosis: 40–80%
- System(s) Affected: Hemic/Lymphatic/Immunologic
- Synonym(s): Malignant lymphoma

ALERT
Geriatric Considerations
Usually presents in more advanced stage and shows unfavorable histology

Pediatric Considerations
- Increased risk for males
- Young females (>20) who are treated with thoracic radiation are at high risk for breast cancer.

Pregnancy Considerations
- Pregnancy is not known to affect course of disease.
- Not known to affect pregnancy or fetus if therapy can be postponed until delivery.
- Normal pregnancy can occur after treatment, if fertility is maintained.
- Risk of disease progression during pregnancy is variable; management must be individualized.

GENERAL PREVENTION
- Pneumococcal vaccine, if splenectomy is planned for staging.
- Consider vaccines for *Haemophilus* and *Neisseria* species as well.

EPIDEMIOLOGY
Predominant sex: Male > Female (1.4:1)

Incidence
- 3.1/100,000
- ~7,000 new cases expected yearly
- Incidence is lower in underdeveloped countries.

Prevalence
- Bimodal age distribution
  - Early peak in mid to late 20s
  - Later peak around 60–70
- Rare under age 5

RISK FACTORS
- Immunodeficiency (inherited or acquired)
- Autoimmune disorders
- HIV infection

Genetics
- 1st degree relatives: 3 times risk
- Siblings of younger patients: 7 times risk

ETIOLOGY
- Unknown
- EB virus may play a role.

ASSOCIATED CONDITIONS
- T lymphocyte defects, which persist after successful treatment
- Patients with HIV tend to present with more advanced disease.

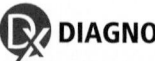 **DIAGNOSIS**

SIGNS AND SYMPTOMS
- Asymptomatic lymphadenopathy (usually cervical or supraclavicular)
- Fever (Pel-Epstein pattern)
- Night sweats
- Weight loss
- Fatigue
- Anorexia
- Alcohol-induced pain
- Unexplained itching

TESTS
Lab
- CBC
- Chemistry profile
- ESR
- Liver function tests
- Renal function tests
- HIV (if risk factors present)
- Hepatitis serology (if risk factors present)
- Drugs that may alter lab results: Phenytoin may produce pseudolymphoma.

Imaging
- Chest radiograph
- Thoracic CT scan
- Abdominal and pelvic CT scan (or possibly MR scan)
- PET scan (exact role is under investigation)
- Lymphangiography
- Bone scan, gallium scan, abdominal ultrasound (used infrequently)

Diagnostic Procedures/Surgery
- Excisional lymph node biopsy (needle biopsy not sufficient)
- Exploratory laparotomy with splenectomy; this procedure is becoming uncommon
- Bone marrow biopsy, especially with systemic symptoms
- Liver biopsy (in selected cases)

Pathological Findings
- RS cell
  - Abundant cytoplasm
  - 2 or more nuclei or nuclear lobes, each with a prominent nucleoli
- Background infiltrate of lymphocytes, histiocytes, granulocytes, plasma cells, and fibroblasts

DIFFERENTIAL DIAGNOSIS
- Non-Hodgkin lymphoma
- Infectious lymphadenopathy
- Other solid tumor metastases
- Sarcoidosis
- Autoimmune disease
- AIDS/HIV infection
- Drug reaction

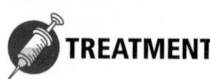 **TREATMENT**

- Initial staging is critical to therapy.
- Cotswold classification
  - Stage I: Single lymph node group
  - Stage II: 2 or more node groups on same side of diaphragm
  - Stage III: Node groups on both sides of diaphragm
  - Stage IV: Dissemination involving extranodal organs (not the spleen, which is considered lymphoid tissue)
  - Subclass designations: A = no symptoms; B = systemic symptoms (fever, night sweats, weight loss >10% body weight); X = bulky disease (widened mediastinum, >1/3 intrathoracic diameter, or >10 cm nodal mass); E = single extranodal site involvement in proximity with known nodal site

GENERAL MEASURES
- Treatment is aimed for cure with minimum toxicity, including treatment-induced late mortality.
- Treatment can be radiation therapy (RT), chemotherapy, or combined radiation and chemotherapy (CMT), based on stage and tumor burden.
  - Early stages (favorable prognosis): Low amount (2–3 cycles) chemotherapy plus involved field RT or extended field RT
  - Early stages (unfavorable prognosis): Moderate chemotherapy (<4 cycles) plus RT
  - Advanced stages: Extensive chemotherapy (<8 cycles) with or without RT
- Autologous bone marrow transplant for selected patients who fail conventional therapy

Activity
As tolerated

MEDICATION (DRUGS)

First Line
ABVD chemotherapy, 4-week cycles
- Doxorubicin (Adriamycin): 25 mg/m^2 IV days 1 and 15
- Bleomycin: 10 mg/m^2 IV days 1 and 15
- Vinblastine: 6.0 mg/m^2 IV days 1 and 15
- Dacarbazine: 375 mg/m^2 IV days 1 and 15

ALERT
- Must be monitored by experienced oncologist
- Contraindications: As in general for chemotherapy
- Precautions: Chemotherapy toxicity, bone marrow suppression
- Significant possible interactions: Refer to the manufacturer's literature.

Second Line
- MOPP chemotherapy, 4-week cycles
  - Mechlorethamine (nitrogen mustard): 6 mg/m^2 IV days 1 and 8
  - Vincristine (Oncovin): 1.4 mg/m^2 IV days 1 and 8
  - Procarbazine: 100 mg/m^2 PO days 1–14 (avoid vanilla, cheese, and wine)
  - Prednisone: 40 mg/m^2 PO days 1–14 during cycles 1 and 4
- Alternate cycles with MOPP/ABVD to minimize toxicity
- BEACOPP (bleomycin, etoposide, doxorubicin, cyclophosphamide, vincristine, procarbazine, prednisone)
- Stanford V regimen (nitrogen mustard, doxorubicin, vinblastine, vincristine, bleomycin, etoposide, prednisone)

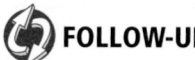 **FOLLOW-UP**

PROGNOSIS
- Overall 5-year survival: 83%
- Long-term survival: 75%
- 10-year survival rates correlate with stage at diagnosis
  - Stage IA, IB, IIA non-bulky: 85–95%
  - Stage IIA bulky: IIB 80–85%
  - Stage IIIA: 75–90%
  - Stage IIIB: 60–65%
  - Stage IV: 55–60%
- Unfavorable prognostic factors in advanced disease
  - Sed rate >70
  - Age >45
  - Male gender
  - Albumin <4 g/dL
  - Hemoglobin <10.5 g/dL
  - Lymphopenia <600 cells/L
  - Leukocyte count ≥15,000 cells/L

COMPLICATIONS
- Secondary malignancies following therapy
- Sterility, gonadal dysfunction
- Hypothyroidism
- Bone marrow suppression
- Immunosuppressed infections, including herpes zoster
- Anemia
- ITP, TTP
- Coronary artery disease, cardiomyopathy
- Radiation pneumonitis, pulmonary fibrosis
- Transient radiation myelopathy (Lhermitte sign)

PATIENT MONITORING
- CBC, nutrition, and hydration during therapy
- Posttreatment monitoring (at least yearly)
  - CBC, ESR
  - TSH, if RT to the neck
  - Chest radiograph

REFERENCES

1. Fung HC, Nademanee AP. Approach to Hodgkin's lymphoma in the new millennium. *Hematol Oncol*. 2002;20:1–15.
2. Horwitz SM, Horning SJ. Advances in the treatment of Hodgkin's lymphoma. *Curr Opin Hematol*. 2000;7(4):235–240.
3. Tesch H, Sieber M, Diehl V. Treatment of advanced stage Hodgkin's disease. *Oncology*. 2001;60(2):101–109.
4. National Comprehensive Cancer Network. NCCN practice guidelines for Hodgkin's disease. *Oncology (Huntingt)*. 1999;13:78–110.
5. Urba WJ, Longo DL. Hodgkin's disease. *New Engl J Med*. 1992;326:678–687.

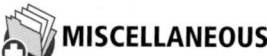 **MISCELLANEOUS**

See also: Lymphoma, non-Hodgkin

CODES

ICD9-CM
201.90 Hodgkin disease, unspecified, unspecified site, extranodal and solid organ sites

PATIENT TEACHING
- Reproductive impact
  - Spermatogenesis often impaired prior to therapy
  - Gonadal side effects of therapy
  - Sperm banking option for males
  - Oophoropexy in premenopausal female if pelvic RT contemplated
- Risks of secondary malignancy
- Careful oral and dental care during therapy
- Leukemia Society of America, 733 3rd Avenue, New York, NY 10017

 See Corresponding Diagnostic Algorithm

H

HOMELESSNESS

Erik Garcia, MD

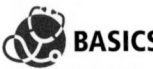 BASICS

DESCRIPTION

- Homelessness is a societal illness wherein affected individuals may reside on the streets, in abandoned buildings, vehicles or encampments, in shelters, missions, or rooming houses, or live doubled up with others.
- The instability of living arrangements faced by a homeless person has a profound effect on his health and access to health care.
- 2/3 of homeless patients suffer from alcohol, drug, or mental health problems.
- Homelessness increases risk of exposure to HIV, hepatitis C, tuberculosis, infestations (scabies, head lice), and to sexual, physical, and emotional trauma.

EPIDEMIOLOGY

- 43% of homeless are single men; 33% families with children; 17% single women.
- 64% of homeless clients seeking health care are from racial or ethnic minorities.

Prevalence

- 2.3–3.5 million people in the US are homeless at some point during the year.
- Each day, ~800,000 homeless people live in the US, including 200,000 children in homeless families (1).

RISK FACTORS

- Poverty and rising housing costs are most closely linked to homelessness.
- Displacement from housing or support network by choice (immigration) or necessity (financial hardship, natural disaster)
- Substance abuse
- Un/under treated mental illness
- Domestic violence (2)

ASSOCIATED CONDITIONS

- Delusional disorders (schizophrenia, bipolar disorder, substance abuse)
- Malnutrition
- Exposure: Hypothermia, frostbite, sunburn, dehydration, heatstroke
- MRSA skin infections
- Infestations: Scabies, head lice
- Trauma/violence
- Seizure disorder
- COPD
- Poor dental health

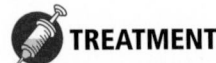 DIAGNOSIS

SIGNS AND SYMPTOMS

- Erratic utilization of health care: May only present in crisis or extremis
- Frequent ER visits with poor follow-up
- Evidence of active substance abuse with physical/social sequelae
- Homelessness is usually not identified in patients who are doubled up or living in a sober or family shelter.

History

- Determine and address patients' immediate concerns.
- Assess strengths, resources, and available support system.
- Assess health risks and risk behaviors based on living arrangement, active substance abuse, health care utilization to date.
- Determine barriers to health care, such as transportation, office hours, health insurance. or access to prescriptions at local free clinics/community health centers.

Physical Exam

- Be sensitive to possible trauma/abuse history: Ask permission to perform exam.
- Genital/breast examination may be deferred as comfort level allows unless specifically indicated.
- Document weight; assess oral, skin, and podiatric health; include assessment of lymph nodes, liver, and spleen and evidence of trauma or infection in addition to problem; perform a focused exam.

TESTS

- Depression scale such as the Patient Health Questionnaire (PHQ)
- Drug and alcohol screening

Lab

With concern of drug and/or alcohol abuse assess

- AST/ALT, albumin, bilirubin
- Serologic testing for HIV, hepatitis B and C
- RPR
- Toxicology screening is not useful unless it is part of the treatment plan or medically indicated (e.g. assessment of mental status changes)

TREATMENT

GENERAL MEASURES

- Initial treatment goal is geared toward establishing a rapport sensitive to negative prior health care/authority interactions
  - Nonjudgmental history
  - Be respectful and attentive
  - Validate experiences and concerns
  - Be flexible (e.g., unscheduled/late visits)
  - Keep goals and expectations realistic
- Enlist available resources for comprehensive care
  - Case management
  - Mental health, substance abuse programs
  - Regional health care for the homeless program
  - Free care clinic/resources
- Request and update emergency contact information.
- Assess and update adult/childhood immunizations.
  - Adults: Hep A, hep B, Td, Pneumovax, influenza, pertussis
- Minimize language/cultural barriers
  - On site/phone interpreters
  - Bi/multilingual signs, instructions

MEDICATION (DRUGS)

- Assess ability to obtain prescriptions.
- Simplify dosing.
- Avoid medications that require specialized storage.
- When prescribing, be aware food, water, and bathroom availability may be limited.
- Avoid sedating medications.
- Use addictive medications with caution.
- Keep instructions clear, including safety with alcohol, opiates.

 FOLLOW-UP

Patients should receive follow-up appointment soon after initial evaluation with instructions that permit easy access for missed appointments or urgent visits.

PROGNOSIS
- Availability of local and regional resources greatly influences outcomes.
- Individuals who are temporarily homeless tend to have best outcomes.
- Transient and unstable nature makes outcome measurement difficult.
- Poor prognostic indicators include
  – Active and refractory substance abuse
  – Comorbid illness: Diabetes, COPD, CAD

COMPLICATIONS
- Sequelae of untreated diabetes, hypertension, hyperlipidemia, exposure to elements
- Depression
- Patients with substance abuse
  – Viral hepatitis B and C
  – HIV
  – Cirrhosis
  – Traumatic brain injury
  – Seizure
  – MRSA/abscess, cellulitis
  – Endocarditis
  – Osteomyelitis
- Death

REFERENCES

1. Montauk SL. The homeless in America: Adapting Your Practice. *AAFP*. 2006;74(7):1132–1138.
2. O'Connell J, eds. The healthcare of homeless persons. Boston: Guthrie Nixon Smith, 2004.
3. Hwang SW. Homelessness and HEALTH. *CMAJ*. 2001;164(2):229–233.

 MISCELLANEOUS

See also Substance use disorders, Alcohol use disorders, Hypothermia, frostbite

 CODES

V60.0 Housing problem/Homeless

HORDEOLUM (STYE)

Konstantinos Deligiannidis, MD, MPH
Alexandra Schultes, MD

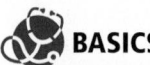 **BASICS**

DESCRIPTION
- An acute inflammation or infection of the eyelid margin involving the sebaceous gland of an eyelash (external hordeolum) or of a meibomian gland (internal hordeolum)
- System(s) Affected: Skin/Exocrine
- Synonym(s): Internal hordeolum, External hordeolum, Zeisian stye, Meibomian stye, Stye

GENERAL PREVENTION
Eyelid hygiene

EPIDEMIOLOGY
- Predominant age: None
- Predominant sex: Male = Female

Incidence
Unknown

Prevalence
Common

RISK FACTORS
- Poor eyelid hygiene
- Contact lens wearers
- Application of makeup
- Predisposing blepharitis (low-grade infections of the eyelid margin)

Genetics
No known genetic pattern

PATHOPHYSIOLOGY
Bacterial infection of sebaceous or meibomian glands, causing an acute inflammatory reaction

ETIOLOGY
- Most commonly caused by *Staphylococcus aureus*, or *S. epidermidis*.
- Seborrhea can predispose to infections of the eyelid.

ASSOCIATED CONDITIONS
- Acne
- Seborrhea

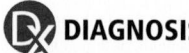 **DIAGNOSIS**

SIGNS AND SYMPTOMS
- Localized inflammation of the eyelashes
- Itching or scaling of the eyelids, collection of discharge, redness, and irritation, leading to localized tenderness and pain

History
- Localized inflammation (versus involvement of the entire eyelid or surrounding skin)
- Prior episodes are common.

Physical Exam
Localized swelling and tenderness on the internal or external aspect of the eyelid with an opening to either side

TESTS
Lab
Culture of the eyelid margins usually is not necessary.

Diagnostic Procedures/Surgery
History and eye examination

Pathological Findings
Bacterial contamination and white cells in eyelid discharge

DIFFERENTIAL DIAGNOSIS
- Blepharitis
- Eyelid neoplasms
- Chalazion
- Periorbital cellulitis

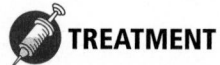 **TREATMENT**

INITIAL STABILIZATION
Outpatient

GENERAL MEASURES
- The hordeolum should not be expressed.
- Warm compresses to the area of inflammation can help increase blood supply and encourage spontaneous drainage.
- Application of an antibiotic ointment (such as erythromycin) to the margin of the eyelid after proper cleansing (except in children <12 years old, in whom there is a risk of blurred vision and amblyopia) helps reduce bacterial proliferation.
- Good personal hygiene with attention to cleansing the eyelids on a daily basis to prevent recurrent infections.

Diet
No special diet

Activity
No restrictions

MEDICATION (DRUGS)

- Erythromycin ophthalmic ointment
- Occasionally, use of an aminoglycoside ophthalmic ointment, such as gentamicin or tobramycin, may be necessary if condition is refractory to simpler treatment.
- Oral dicloxacillin or cephalexin for 2 weeks if refractory to topical antibiotics
- Treat underlying dry eye with artificial tears.

SURGERY

- If the infection becomes localized to a single gland, incision, drainage, and curettage sometimes is necessary. This is an in-office procedure with a local anesthetic. The use of combined antibiotic ointment (neomycin sulfate, polymyxin B sulfate, and gramicidin) after surgery was not shown to have any statistically significant difference to artificial tears (1)[B].

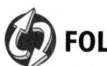 **FOLLOW-UP**

PROGNOSIS

Responds well to treatment, but tends to recur in some patients.

COMPLICATIONS

An internal hordeolum, if untreated, may lead to generalized cellulitis of the lid.

PATIENT MONITORING

The patient should be seen within several weeks to assess the effectiveness of therapy, or at least call the physician's office with progress report.

REFERENCES

1. Hirunwiwatkul P. Effectiveness of combined antibiotic ophthalmic solution in the treatment of hordeolum after incision and curettage: a randomized, placebo-controlled trial: a pilot study. *J Med Assoc Thai* 2005;88(5):647–650.

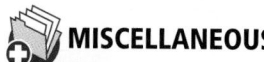 **MISCELLANEOUS**

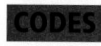 **CODES**

ICD9-CM

- 373.11 Hordeolum externum
- 373.00 Blepharitis, unspecified

PATIENT TEACHING

- The patient should be instructed in proper cleansing of the eyelids using a solution of tap water and baby shampoo or a commercially prepared hypoallergenic cleanser.
- The stye should not be squeezed or incised.

 See Patient Handout on CD

H

HORNER SYNDROME

Felix B. Chang, MD

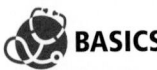 **BASICS**

DESCRIPTION

- Horner syndrome is caused by interruptions of the sympathetic nerve supply to the eye, and results in miosis, ptosis, enophthalmos (sometimes), and absence or decrease of sweating of the ipsilateral face and neck (hypohidrosis).
- Droopy eye, pupil size disparity
  - Peripheral lesion (complete syndrome) is distal to superior cervical ganglion.
  - Central lesion (incomplete syndrome) is proximal to superior cervical ganglion.
- System(s) Affected: Nervous; Skin/Exocrine
- Synonym(s): Bernard-Horner syndrome; Bernard syndrome; Cervical sympathetic syndrome; Oculosympathetic syndrome, oculosympathetic paralysis, oculosympathetic deficiency

GENERAL PREVENTION
None known

EPIDEMIOLOGY
- Predominant age: May occur at any age
- Predominant sex: Male = Female

Prevalence
Unknown

ALERT
In children, Horner syndrome may be the 1st manifestation of neuroblastoma.

Geriatric Considerations
Horner syndrome in the presence of acute-onset, ipsilateral facial or neck pain may indicate carotid artery dissection.

RISK FACTORS
- Apical bronchogenic carcinoma (Pancoast tumor)
- Aneurysm of the carotid or subclavian artery
- Injuries to the carotid artery high in the neck
- Congenital Horner syndrome
- Dissection of the carotid arteries
- Cluster headaches
  - ~20% have an accompanying ipsilateral Horner syndrome
  - The syndrome may outlast the headaches.
- Carotid artery occlusion
  - ~15% of patients with carotid artery occlusion develop ipsilateral Horner syndrome.
  - May occur without evidence of cerebral ischemia, neck injuries, or operative procedures
- Syringomyelia
- Inflammatory process
- Cervical nerve root avulsion

Genetics
Some autosomal dominant familial incidence

PATHOPHYSIOLOGY
Constellation of signs produced when sympathetic innervation to the eye is interrupted

ETIOLOGY
- Interruption of the sympathetic nerve fibers that originate in the hypothalamus and travel down to the lateral part of the brainstem to exit in the thoracic area. These fibers synapse in the cervical sympathetic ganglia, and the postganglionic fibers travel to the eye along the wall of the carotid and ophthalmic arteries.
- Idiopathic
- 1st-order neuron
  - Arnold-Chiari malformation
  - Basal meningitis (e.g., syphilis)
  - Basal skull tumors
  - Cerebral vascular accident (CVA)
    ○ Wallenberg syndrome
  - Demyelinating disease (multiple sclerosis)
  - Intrapontine hemorrhage
  - Neck trauma
  - Pituitary tumor
  - Syringomyelia
- 2nd-order neuron
  - Pancoast tumor
  - Birth trauma with injury to lower brachial plexus
  - Cervical rib
  - Aneurysm/dissection of aorta
  - Subclavian or common carotid artery
  - Central venous catheterization
  - Trauma/surgical injury
  - Chest tubes
  - Lymphadenopathy (Hodgkin, leukemia, TB, mediastinal tumors)
  - Mandibular tooth abscess
  - Lesions of the middle ear (Acute otitis media)
  - Neuroblastoma
- 3rd-order neuron lesions
  - Internal carotid artery dissection
  - Raeder syndrome (paratrigeminal syndrome)
  - Carotid cavernous fistula
  - Cluster/migraine headaches
  - Herpes zoster
- Drugs
  - Acetophenazine, alseroxylon, bupivacaine, butaperazine, carphenazine, chloroprocaine, deserpidine, diacetylmorphine, diethazine, ethopropazine, etidocaine, guanethidine, influenza virus vaccine, levodopa, lidocaine, mepivacaine, mesoridazine, methdilazine, methotrimeprazine, oral contraceptives, perazine, prilocaine, procaine, prochlorperazine, promazine, propoxycine, reserpine, thioproperazine, thioridazine, trifluoperazine.

ASSOCIATED CONDITIONS
- Wallenberg syndrome
- Pancoast tumor
- C8 radiculopathy

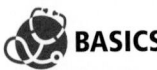 **DIAGNOSIS**

SIGNS AND SYMPTOMS
- Ptosis (drooping of the eyelid)
- Miosis (narrowing of the pupil of the eye)
- Anhidrosis or hypohidrosis
  - Ipsilateral side of the body: Central (1st-order neuron)
  - Ipsilateral face: (2nd-order neuron)
  - Absent or limited to an area above the ipsilateral brow: Postganglionic lesions after vasomotor and sudomotor fiber have branched off
- Enophthalmos is sometimes found.
- In congenital Horner, long standing Horner syndrome, or Horner syndrome that occurs in children <2 years: Iris has reduced pigmentation, blue-gray, mottling of the affected eye (heterochromia iridis)
- Loss of ciliospinal reflex. Pinching skin of neck normally produces ipsilateral pupil dilation.
- Ipsilaterally impaired flushing may be found.

History
- 1st-order neuron may be associated with dysarthria, dysphagia, ataxia, vertigo and nystagmus.
- 2nd-order neuron presents history of previous trauma, neck, axillary, shoulder or arm pain, cough, hemoptysis, history of thoracic or neck surgery, history of chest tube or central venous catheter, or neck swelling.
- 3rd-order neuron presents with diplopia, numbness in the distribution of the first and second division of the trigeminal nerve.
- The presence, absence, and/or location of anhydrosis is an important sign elicited from the history.

Physical Exam
- Measurement of papillary diameter in dim and bright light and their reactivity to light and accommodation
- Examination of the upper lids for ptosis
- Examination of the lower lids for upside-down ptosis
- Extraocular movements
- Biomicroscopic examination of the papillary margin and iris structure and color
- Confrontational visual field testing and testing of facial sensation
- Observation of the presence of nystagmus, facial swelling, lymphadenopathy, or vesicular eruptions

TESTS

- A normal pupil will dilate in response to instillation of 10% cocaine. The miotic pupil in Horner will not dilate, or will dilate poorly, because of the absence of norepinephrine at the nerve endings.
- To distinguish a 3rd-order neuron disorder from a 1st- and 2nd-order neuron disorder, 1% hydroxyamphetamine or 5% (Pholedrine) can be instilled 48 hours later. In a 1st- or 2nd-neuron lesion, dilation will take place. Failure of the Horner pupil to dilate, or poor dilatation, indicates a 3rd-order neuron lesion.

Lab

- CBC
- FTA
- VDRL
- PPD
- Vanillylmandelic acid (VMA), homovanillic acid (HVA) to rule out neuroblastoma in pediatrics

Imaging
CT/MRI/MRA of the brain, chest, spinal cord

Diagnostic Procedures/Surgery
Spinal tap is occasionally indicated in addition to tests

Pathological Findings

- Brainstem lesion
- Massive hemisphere lesion
- Cervical cord lesion
- Root lesion
- Sympathetic chain lesion

DIFFERENTIAL DIAGNOSIS

- Neurologic diseases
- 3rd nerve palsy
- Unilateral use of miotics
- Unilateral use of mydriatics
- Adie pupil
- Iris sphincter muscle damage
- Anisocoria

 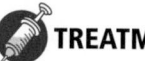

TREATMENT

Inpatient or outpatient, depending on cause

GENERAL MEASURES

- Search for tumor or other compressive lesion is indicated for any patient who develops Horner syndrome.
- Horner syndrome in itself does not produce any disability or require treatment.
- Treatment is management of the underlying condition.

Diet
Disease dependent

Activity
Disease dependent

SPECIAL THERAPY
Radiotherapy
Upon the particular etiology

MEDICATION (DRUGS)

Therapy appropriate for the underlying disease

SURGERY
Surgical care depends on the particular etiology.

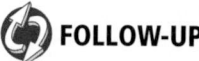

FOLLOW-UP

Issues for Referral

- Neurologic or neuro-ophthalmic consultation may be considered.
- Vascular surgery is interventional in cases of suspected carotid artery dissection or aneurysm.
- Surgical oncology, oncology, or radiotherapy consultation depends on the particular etiology.

PROGNOSIS
Variable with cause

COMPLICATIONS
Chronic pupillary constriction

PATIENT MONITORING
Disease dependent

ALERT
Special Consideration

- Horner syndrome in the presence of pain merits special consideration.
- Horner syndrome in the presence of axial, shoulder, scapula, arm, or hand pain may be related to apical (Pancoast) lung tumor.
- Acute-onset, ipsilateral facial or neck pain may suggest carotid artery dissection.

REFERENCES

1. Bardorf CM, Van Stavern GP, Garcia Valenzuela E, et al. *Horner Syndrome.*
2. Freedman KA, Brown SM. Topical apraclonidine in the diagnosis of suspected Horner syndrome 2005;Un;25(2):83–85.
3. Mokhtari F, Massin P, Paques M, et al. Central retinal artery occlusion associated with spontaneous internal carotid artery dissection. *Am J Ophthalmol.* 2000;129(1):108–109.

ADDITIONAL READING
www.emedicine.com/oph/topic336.htm

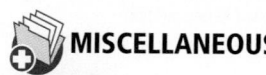

MISCELLANEOUS

CODES

ICD9-CM
337.9 Unspecified disorder of autonomic nervous system

PATIENT TEACHING

See Corresponding Diagnostic Algorithm

HOT FLUSHES

Jennifer W. McCaul, MD
Sandra M. Sulik, MD

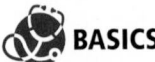 ## BASICS

DESCRIPTION
- Sensation of heat experienced by the patient accompanied by perspiration, flushing, anxiety, and palpitations
  - Lasting 4–10 minutes
  - Followed by a drop in core temperature with or without shivering
  - May be experienced as night sweats
  - Can occur several times per hour to several times per week
- System(s) Affected: Thermoregulatory; Psychiatric; Cutaneous; Cardiovascular

GENERAL PREVENTION
Unknown

EPIDEMIOLOGY
- Less common in Asian women
- More common in African American and Caucasian women
- Predominant Age: Menopausal and perimenopausal women; younger women and males can be affected if surgically or chemically induced.

Incidence
90% after surgical menopause.

Prevalence
Thirty percent to 80% of menopausal women; 10–20% find them intolerable.

RISK FACTORS
- Low circulating estradiol or estrone concentration in menopausal women
- Abrupt menopause: Surgical, chemotherapy, radiation, drug-induced
- Underweight, lack of exercise, smokers
- Menopause at a younger age

PATHOPHYSIOLOGY
Inappropriate peripheral vasodilation with increased cutaneous blood flow and perspiration
- Results in decreased core temperature, causing shivering

ETIOLOGY
Currently unknown, theories include
- Decreased circulating estrogen or increased circulating gonadotropins causing alteration in hypothalamic thermoregulatory set point
- Decreased estrogen causes decline in serotonin, increasing sensitivity of hypothalamic serotonin receptors involved in thermoregulation
- Endogenous opiod peptide withdrawal associated with estrogen deficiency

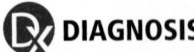 ## DIAGNOSIS

SIGNS AND SYMPTOMS
Subjective sensation of heat accompanied by perspiration, palpitations, flushing, and anxiety
- May be followed by shivering
- Frequency and severity vary by individual.
- Other symptoms of menopause include joint pain, sleep problems, fatigue, forgetfulness, and urinary incontinence.

History
Menstrual irregularity, vaginal dryness, and above symptoms can help confirm diagnosis.
- Symptoms may appear after surgical menopause or after treatment for breast or prostate cancer.

Physical Exam
Signs of menopause include skin thinning, vaginal atrophy, hirsutism, and central adiposity.

Lab
Not usually necessary however
- Can check FSH and estradiol in patients <40 or who have regular menses
- Can check FSH and estradiol in older patients on oral contraceptives who wish to stop
- FSH >40 mIU/mL or Estradiol <30 pg/mL helps confirm menopause.

DIFFERENTIAL DIAGNOSIS
Other causes are rare but include (1)
- Diseases: Carcinoid, mastocytosis, anxiety, carcinomas (pancreatic, renal cell, medullary thyroid), pheochromocytoma, dumping syndrome, migraine, brain or spinal cord lesion
- Drugs: Alcohol, opiates, calcium channel blockers, cholinergics, cephalosporins, azoles, aromatase inhibitors
- Additives: MSG, sodium nitrate, sulfites

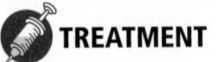 ## TREATMENT

GENERAL MEASURES
Avoid or reduce cigarette smoking.

Activity
No restrictions

Complementary and Alternative Therapies
- Herbal remedies
  - Black Cohosh (Remifemin) decreased hot flushes in several short studies, but no long term safety information is available. (2)[B]
  - Dong Quai, Ginseng, Red Clover, Chaste Tree Berry, and Evening Primrose oil have all shown no benefit over placebo. (2)[B]
  - Wild yam/Progesterone cream—1 trial showed significant improvement in symptoms but also induced worrisome postmenopausal bleeding in some patients. (2)[B]
- Dietary Phytoestrogens decreased symptoms in multiple studies, but effects are modest and lasted <6 weeks. (20)[B] Soy foods are assumed safe; however, no safety information is available for high dose extracts.
- Vitamin E has shown no significant improvement over placebo. (2)[B]
- Acupuncture and Paced Respiration, behavioral therapy, have shown some benefit in frequency of hot flushes. Studies are limited. (2)[B]

MEDICATION (DRUGS)

First Line
Estrogen or combined estrogen/progesterone

- Various treatment regimens resulted in a 75% mean reduction in frequency of hot flushes and a significant reduction in severity when compared with placebo. (3)[A]
  - Of note, there was a 58% reduction in hot flush frequency in the placebo group at the end of the study. (3)[A]
- Common regimens include
  - Premarin 0.625 mg + Provera 2.5 mg daily
  - Premarin 0.625 mg daily + Provera 5 mg during the last 14 days or the month.
  - Can increase premarin to 1.25 mg/d for refractory cases. However, lowest dose possible should always be used.
  - Combination therapies—Prempro, Premphase.
  - Transdermal estradiol can also be used for estrogen component. (0.05–0.1 mg/d patch applied once or twice weekly
  - Vaginal conjucated estrogen creams give unpredictable blood levels and should not be used for hot flush treatment.
- With an intact uterus, progestins must always be used to protect against endometrial hyperplasia.
- Contraindications: Hormone-dependent cancers (Breast, Uterine), history of DVT, Liver dysfunction or undiagnosed vaginal bleeding.
- Side effects include nausea, breast pain, vaginal bleeding, headache, libido change.
- Serious adverse effects of long term use

  - Increased risk of cardiac event in years 1–4 of combined therapy (no significant risk seen after 5 years. (4)[A] RR 1.37 (95% CI 1.05–1.79) to 1.74 (95% CI 1.05–2.89).
  - Increased risk of stroke after 3 or more years of therapy. (4)[A] RR 1.37 (95% CI 1.1.08–1.73) to 1.47 (95% CI 1.02–2.11).
  - Increased risk of venous thromboembolism with >1 year of therapy. (4)[A] RR 2.09 (95% CI 1.60–2.74) to 3.59 (95% CI 1.95–6.61).
  - Increased risk of dementia in combined HT, RR 1.97 (95% CI 1.16–3.33). (4)[A]

  - No statistically significant risks for TIA.
  - Breast cancer risk may be increased with >5 years use of combined therapy.

  - No Increase in colorectal cancer, endometrial cancer, or death from any cause were found. (4)[A]

  - The majority of data for these risks was obtained from the WHI study, only enrolling women >65.These risks may or may not be present for younger women with shorter courses of HT.
- Therapy should be discontinued gradually or slowly tapered to prevent recurrence of symptoms.
- There may be a decreased risk of hip fracture with long term HT; however, studies conflict.

Second Line
- Selective serotonin reuptake inhibitors

  - Have been found to decrease hot flush frequency by 50–60% in RCTs (placebo resulted in 20–36% decrease). (1)[B]

  - Studied medications include Venlafaxine, Fluoxetine and Paroxetine.
  - Represent a reasonable alternative for women in whom HT is contraindicated
  - Adverse effects are rare and include GI symptoms, sexual dysfunction and SIADH.
  - The dose of SSRI helpful for hot flushes may be less than that for depression. It is appropriate to start at the lowest dose. Additionally, improvement is usually seen sooner than when used for depression.
- Neurontin (Gabapentin) has been shown to be more effective than placebo in limited studies, more research is needed.
- Clonidine (0.1 mg PO b.i.d.) has been shown to be moderately more effective then placebo for mild to moderate hot flush relief. Studies are limited. (1)[B]

  - Side effects such as dry mouth, constipation, and orthostatic hypotension limit use.
- Tibolone is a synthetic steroid widely used in Europe known to increase bone density. There is a possible increase in breast cancer in a large observational study. (1)[C]

- Testosterone: Adding testosterone to a HT regimen has been shown to increase sexual function and libido. It also had the effect of lowering HDL; the amount of decrease varied with dosing regimen. (5)[A]

Complementary and Alternative Medicine
Some positive evidence exists for the use of soy isoflavones and black cohosh, though better quality studies are needed (6,7).

FOLLOW-UP

DISPOSITION
May consider further workup looking for atypical causes or specialist referral for symptoms with no response to conventional hormone therapy

Issues for Referral
Usually only necessary if no response to conventional hormone therapy

PROGNOSIS
- Hot flushes resolve spontaneously within 5–6 years in 80–90% of patients.
- Some may continue up to 15 years.
- Most patients will experience at least some relief in frequency or severity of hot flushes with therapy.

PATIENT MONITORING
Due to nature of symptoms and risks involved in therapy, patients should be seen frequently and medications adjusted until symptoms are managed.
- Decisions regarding treatment should be made collaboratively with patient awareness of risks and benefits.

REFERENCES

1. Stearns V, Ullmer L, et al. Hot Flushes. *Lancet.* 2002;360:1851–1861.
2. Kronenberg F, Fugh-Berman A. Complementary and alternative medicine for menopausal symptoms: A review of randomized controlled trials. *Ann Intern Med.* 2002;137:805–813.
3. McLennan AH, Broadbent JL, et al. Oral oestrogen and combined oestrogen/progestogen therapy versus placebo for hot flushes. *The Cochrane Database of Systemic Reviews* 2004, Issue 4. Art. No.: CD002978. pub2. DOI:10. 1002/14651858. CD002978.pub2.
4. Farquhar CM, Marjoribanks J, et al. Long term hormone therapy for perimenopausal and postmenopausal women. *The Cochrane Database of Systemic Reviews* 2005, Issue 3. Art. No.: CD004143.pub2. DOI: 10.1002/14651858.CD004143.pub2.
5. Somboonporn W, Davis S, et al. Testosterone for peri- and postmenopausal women. *The Cochrane. Database of Systematic Reviews* 2005, Issue 4. Art. No.: CD004509.pub2.DOI: 10.1002/14651858.CD004509.pub2.
6. Upmalls DH, Lobo R, Bradley L, et al. Vasomotor symptom relief by soy isoflavone extract tablets in postmenopausal women: a multicenter, double-blind, randomized, placebo-controlled study. *Menopause.* 2000;7(4):236–242.
7. Pockaj BA, Gallagher JG, Loprinzi CL, et al. Phase III double-blind, randomized, placebo-controlled crossover trial of black cohosh in the management of hot flashes. *J Clin Oncol.* 2006 Jun 20;24(18):2836–41.

MISCELLANEOUS

CODES

ICD9-CM
- 627.2 Symptomatic menopausal or female climacteric states
- 627.4 Symptomatic states associated with artificial menopause

PATIENT TEACHING

Diet
Apart from possibly adding more soy based foods, patients may also try to avoid hot beverages, as these act as a trigger for many women.

Activity
Patients can maintain their usual activity level; however, they should be cautioned to wear light clothing and keep core body temperature low to prevent triggering hot flushes.

 See Patient Handout on CD

H

HUNTINGTON DISEASE

Richard Viken, MD

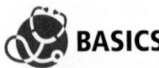

BASICS

DESCRIPTION
- An inherited disease characterized by dementia and chorea that has a gradual onset and slow progression
  - Symptoms usually don't develop until >30 years of age.
  - By the time of diagnosis the patient has usually reproduced and passed the disease to another generation.
- System(s) Affected: Nervous
- Synonym(s): Chronic progressive hereditary chorea; Huntington chorea

ALERT
Geriatric Considerations
Usually fatal before geriatric age group; but onset is after age 50 in 20%.

Pediatric Considerations
- Juvenile form, defined by onset before age 21, occurs in 7% of cases.
- Characteristics
  - Transmission from affected father
  - Large numbers of cytosine-adenine-guanine (CAG) repeats
  - More severe neuropathological involvement, including rigidity and seizures

GENERAL PREVENTION
Genetic counseling

EPIDEMIOLOGY
- Predominant age: Young adult: 16–40; Middle age: 40–75
- Predominant sex: Male = Female

Incidence
In the US: 4–8 cases/100,000 people

RISK FACTORS
Family history is a definite risk factor, although a small percent of patients with DNA-proven Huntington disease will have a negative family history.

Genetics
- Autosomal dominant
- Genetic marker on chromosome 4
- ~20% of relatives at 1-in-2 risk of inheriting Huntington disease from an affected parent now accept the offer of presymptomatic testing.

ETIOLOGY
Associated with a CAG trinucleotide repeat expansion in a large gene on the short arm of chromosome 4. The gene encodes the protein huntingtin, which selectively accumulates in clumps within brain cells. These cells appear sensitive to damage by the aggregated, toxic levels of Huntington.

ASSOCIATED CONDITIONS
- A lower incidence of cancer among patients with Huntington disease seems to be related to intrinsic biologic factors.
- An autosomal dominant disorder arising from a different CAG expansion mutation, termed "Huntington disease-like 2," has clinical and MRI features indistinguishable from Huntington disease.

DIAGNOSIS

SIGNS AND SYMPTOMS
- Early (1)[C]
  - Anxiety
  - Emotional lability
  - Impaired problem solving
  - Depression
  - Hypotonia
  - Abnormal eye movements
  - Facial twitching
  - Bradykinesia
  - Impulsiveness
  - Hostility
  - Agitation
  - Impaired odor recognition and discriminability
- Late (1)[C]
  - Chorea
  - Dysphagia
  - Dysarthria
  - Bladder and bowel incontinence
  - Gait disturbance
  - Postural instability
  - Hyperkinesia
  - Dementia
  - Rigidity
  - Hypertonia
  - Clonus
  - Primitive reflexes
- Variable
  - Weight loss
  - Aggressiveness, including sexual
  - Mania
  - Hallucinations
  - Paranoia

TESTS
Lab
- Decreased endogenous gamma-aminobutyric acid (GABA)
- Decreased glutamic acid decarboxylase
- Decreased choline-acetyltransferase
- Special tests
  - Presymptomatic detection of the disease via genetic linkage analysis is possible, but widespread testing awaits the resolution of social and ethical considerations.

Imaging
- CT or MRI: Cerebral atrophy and atrophy of basal ganglia
- Positron emission tomography (PET): Reduced glucose utilization, lowered dopamine receptor binding
- Head CT: Enlarged lateral ventricle

Diagnostic Procedures/Surgery
Neuropsychological testing measures may capture early striatal neuron loss by demonstrating impairment 2 years before development of motor disease.

Pathological Findings
- Gross
  - Cerebral atrophy
  - Atrophic caudate nucleus
  - Atrophic putamen
  - Ventricular enlargement
  - Atrophic globus pallidus
  - Atrophic frontal lobes
  - Atrophic parietal lobes
  - Cortical atrophy
- Micro
  - Loss of small neurons of striatum with fibrillary gliosis
  - Loss of small neurons with fibrillary gliosis in ventrolateral thalamic nucleus
  - Loss of small neurons with fibrillary gliosis in substantia nigra
- Electron microscopy
  - Membranous whorls
  - Increased numbers of dense synaptic vesicles in presynaptic nerve terminals

DIFFERENTIAL DIAGNOSIS
- Movement disorder: Hereditary
  - Huntington disease
  - Hereditary nonprogressive chorea
  - Neuroacanthocytosis
  - Wilson disease
  - Ataxia-telangiectasia
  - Lesch-Nyhan syndrome
  - Hallervorden-Spatz disease
  - Fahr disease
- Movement disorder: Secondary
  - Infections/Immunologic: Sydenham chorea, encephalitis, systemic lupus erythematosus, tertiary syphilis
  - Drug induced: Levodopa, anticonvulsants, anticholinergics, cimetidine, isoniazid
  - Metabolic and endocrine: Chorea gravidarum, hyperthyroidism, birth control pills, hyperglycemic nonketotic encephalopathy
  - Vascular: Hemichorea/hemiballism with subthalamic nucleus lesion, periarteritis nodosa
- Movement disorder: Unknown etiology
  - Senile chorea
  - Essential chorea
  - Parkinson disease
- Dementia
  - Alzheimer disease
  - Creutzfeldt-Jakob
  - Pick disease
- Emotional and perceptual disorders
  - Bipolar disorder
  - Schizophrenia
- Abnormal behavior
  - Alcoholism
  - Antisocial personality disorder

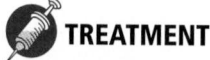 **TREATMENT**

INITIAL STABILIZATION
Outpatient

GENERAL MEASURES
- ~7–8% of Huntington disease patients are in nursing homes
  - Women outnumber men.
  - The most robust predictor of placement is advanced motor impairment (marked chorea, bradykinesia, impaired gait and balance). (2)[B]
- Genetic counseling
- Consider electroconvulsive therapy (ECT) for drug-resistant depression.
- Speech and occupational therapy
- Smoking cessation in late (choreiform) stage

Diet
Soft diet with liquid supplements may be needed.

Activity
Full activity as long as possible

 MEDICATION (DRUGS)

First Line
- Behavioral problems: (3)[B]
  - Risperadone (Risperdal), start at 1 mg b.i.d., slowly increase to usual effective dose of 4–8 mg/d in 2 divided doses
- Choreoathetosis: (3)[B]
  - Riluzole (Rilutek) 50 mg q12h
  - Olanzapine (Zyprexa), start with 5 mg/d; may work up to maximum of 20 mg/d
  - Amantadine (Symmetrel) 100 mg b.i.d.
- Rigidity
  - Baclofen (Lioresal), start at 10 mg/d, increase slowly to 120 mg maximum in a divided dose
  - May combine with clonazepam (Klonopin), start at 0.5 mg at bedtime, increasing over several months to 9 mg maximum in a divided daily dose
- Depression: (3)[B]
  - Fluoxetine (Prozac), start at 10 mg/d, increase by 10 mg increments to 60 mg/d maximum
  - Mirtazapine, start at 15 mg/d; may work up to 45 mg/d
- Contraindications: Refer to manufacturer's literature
- Precautions
  - Extrapyramidal reactions, tardive dyskinesia may occur
  - Can be treated with anticholinergic medication

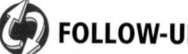 **FOLLOW-UP**

PROGNOSIS
- Poor, progressive impairment
- Fatal outcome within 20 years, usually from pneumonia

COMPLICATIONS
- Choking
- Subdural hematoma
- Personality changes
- Suicide

PATIENT MONITORING
- Periodically for behavioral changes
- Effect of drug therapy may be monitored using the Unified Huntington Disease Rating Scale, a protocol by which patients are evaluated on a series of motor, behavioral and functional criteria.

REFERENCES
1. Anderson K. Huntington's disease and related disorders. *Psychiatr Clin N Am*. 2005;28:275–290.
2. Wleelock VL, Tempkin T, Marder K, Nance M, et al. Predictors of nursing home placement in Huntington disease. *Neurology*. 2003;60: 998–1001.
3. Bonelli RM, Wenning GK, Kapfhammer HP. Huntington's disease: Present treatments and future therapeutic modalities. *Int Clin Psychopharmacol*. 2004;19:51–62.

ADDITIONAL READING
Medical historians may be interested in the following article: Innes Am, Chudley AE. Genetic landmarks through philately: Woodrow Wilson 'Woody' Guthrie and Huntington disease. *Clin Genet*. 2002;61: 263–267.

 MISCELLANEOUS

Experiments using a mouse model of Huntington disease suggest that intracerebroventricular administration of a caspase inhibitor delays disease progression and activity. The caspases are a family of proteases, active in the brains of mice and humans with Huntington disease, which regulate apoptosis.

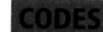 **CODES**

ICD9-CM
333.4 Huntington disease

PATIENT TEACHING
- Counseling for offspring
- Newsletter and printed information available from: Huntington Disease Society of America, 140 W. 22nd St, 6th Floor, New York, NY 10011-2420; (212) 242-1968; fax (212) 243-2443; www.hdsa.org.
- Website: www.stanford.edu/group/hopes.

H

HYDROCELE

Timothy L. Black, MD
James P. Miller, MD

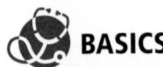 **BASICS**

DESCRIPTION
Hydrocele is a collection of fluid within the scrotum.

- Communicating hydrocele
  - Associated with a patent processus vaginalis
  - Has associated indirect inguinal hernia
- Noncommunicating hydrocele
  - Infantile type—Frequent spontaneous resolution
  - Adult type—Infrequent resolution
- Hydrocele of the cord: Distal portion of processus vaginalis has closed, midportion patent and fluid filled, proximal portion may be open or closed
- Acute hydrocele: Acute fluid collection resulting from an acute process within the tunica vaginalis
- System(s) Affected: Reproductive

ALERT
Pediatric Considerations
In communicating hydrocele, consider contralateral inguinal exploration.

EPIDEMIOLOGY
- Predominant age: Childhood
- Predominant sex: Male only

Prevalence
- 1,000 per 100,000
- Estimated to be 1% of adult males

RISK FACTORS
- Ventriculoperitoneal shunt
- Exstrophy of the bladder
- Ehlers-Danlos syndrome
- Peritoneal dialysis

Genetics
Unknown

ETIOLOGY
- Closure of processus vaginalis trapping peritoneal fluid (noncommunicating)
- Closure of distal processus, trapping fluid in midportion of processus vaginalis (hydrocele of cord)
- Failure of closure of processus vaginalis (communicating hydrocele)
- Infection
- Tumors
- Trauma
- Ipsilateral renal transplantation

ASSOCIATED CONDITIONS
- Testicular tumors
- Trauma
- Ventriculo-peritoneal shunt
- Nephrotic syndrome
- Renal failure with peritoneal dialysis

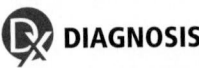 **DIAGNOSIS**

SIGNS AND SYMPTOMS
- Swelling in scrotum or inguinal canal
- Demonstrated fluctuation in size (communicating hydrocele)
- Usually not painful
- Sensation of heaviness in scrotum
- Pain radiating to back (occasionally)
- Fluid collection in scrotum that transilluminates

History
- Acute or subacute onset of scrotal swelling
- Frequent changes in size of the hydrocele (indicative of a communication)

Physical Exam
Scrotal mass, usually fluctuant

TESTS
Imaging
- Abdominal radiograph—may be useful to distinguish incarcerated hernias from hydroceles (rarely needed)
- Inguinoscrotal ultrasound—can demonstrate presence of bowel, e.g., distinguish incarcerated hernia from a hydrocele of the cord as well as the presence of testicular torsion.
- Testicular nuclear scan or Doppler ultrasound—to distinguish testicular torsion

Diagnostic Procedures/Surgery
Aspiration of hydrocele should be discouraged

Pathological Findings
Patent processus vaginalis in communicating hydroceles

DIFFERENTIAL DIAGNOSIS
- Indirect inguinal hernia
- Orchitis
- Epididymitis
- Traumatic injury to testicle
- Torsion of testicle or torsion of appendix testes

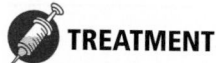 **TREATMENT**

INITIAL STABILIZATION
- Outpatient surgery
- Observation in early infancy until definite communication demonstrated or until 1 year of age

GENERAL MEASURES
Diet
Regular

Activity
Full activity after surgery

SURGERY
- In adults no therapy is needed unless hydrocele causes discomfort or unless there is a significant underlying cause such as tumor
- Inguinal approach with ligation of processus vaginalis and excision, or distal splitting, or drainage of hydrocele sac in children. (In hydrocele of cord, sac can be completely removed.) (1)[B]
- Scrotal approach with internal drainage of hydrocele in adults (highest recurrence rate) (2)[C]
- Scrotal approach with resection of hydrocele (highest complication rate, lowest recurrence rate). (2)[C]
- Jaboulay-Winkelmann procedure (for thick hydrocele sac)—hydrocele sac wrapped posteriorly around cord structures (2)[C] (3)[A]
- Lord procedure (for thin hydrocele sac)—radial sutures used to gather hydrocele sac posterior to testis and epididymis (2)[C] (3)[A]
- Aspiration of the hydrocele with instillation of sclerosing agent (talc is best) has been successfully used in adults (4)[B]

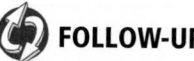 **FOLLOW-UP**

PROGNOSIS
Recovery should be rapid and complete.

COMPLICATIONS
- Postoperative traumatic hydrocele common. Usually resolves spontaneously
- Injury to vas deferens or spermatic vessels
- Suture granuloma
- Hematoma
- Wound infection
- Recurrence of hydrocele

PATIENT MONITORING
- Follow at 3-month intervals until decision for/against surgery made.
- Postoperative, follow-up at 2–4 weeks and then at 2–3-month intervals until resolution of any postoperative (traumatic) hydrocele.

REFERENCES
1. Gahukamble DB, Khamage AS. Prospective randomized controlled study of excision versus distal splitting of hernial sac and processus vaginalis in the repair of inguinal hernias and communicating hydroceles. *J Ped Surg.* 1995; 30:624–625.
2. Ku JH, Kim ME, Lee NK, et al. The excisional placation and internal drainage techniques: A comparison of the results for idiopathic hydrocele. *BJU.* 2001;87:82–84.
3. Miroglu C, Tokuc R, Saporta L. Comparison of an extrusion procedure and eversion procedures in the treatment of hydrocele. *Int Urol Nephrol.* 1994; 26:673–679.
4. Yilmaz U, Ekmekcioglu O, Tatlisen A, et al. Does pleurodesis for pleural effusions give bright ideas about the agents for hydrocele sclerotherapy? *Int Urol Nephrology.* 2000;32:89–92.

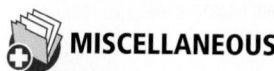 **MISCELLANEOUS**

CODES

ICD9-CM
603.9 Hydrocele, unspecified

H

HYDROCEPHALUS, NORMAL PRESSURE

Dennis E. Hughes, DO

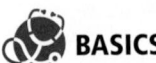 **BASICS**

DESCRIPTION
- Normal pressure hydrocephalus (NPH) is a clinical triad of gait instability, incontinence, and dementia. Originally described by Hakim and Adams is 1965, it occurs rarely, but is potentially treatable.
- Idiopathic
- Secondary to subarachnoid hemorrhage, head injury, or infection

ALERT
Geriatric Considerations
Idiopathic NPH primarily affects persons >60 years.

EPIDEMIOLOGY
- No formal epidemiologic data exist regarding NPH because of the lack of consensus-derived diagnostic criteria. The natural history of untreated NPH has not been studied. (1,2).
- Idiopathic form primarily affects elderly.
- Secondary can occur at any age.
- Affects both genders equally.

Incidence
Estimated to be the cause of dementia in ≤5% of affected individuals (3).

RISK FACTORS
- Idiopathic risk is unknown.
- Secondary form is due to head trauma, subarachnoid hemorrhage, meningitis, or encephalitis.

Genetics
None identified

PATHOPHYSIOLOGY
- This is a communicating hydrocephalus; a disorder is of decreased CSF absorption. The subarachnoid granulations fail to maintain their baseline removal of CSF as a result of scarring or fibrosis.
- The result is a pressure gradient between the subarachnoid space and the ventricular system.
- CSF production decreases in the face of an increased pressure set point.
- Elevated pressure distends ventricles and compresses the brain parenchyma.
- As a result of compression, ischemic changes occur in the parenchymal vasculature (3).

ETIOLOGY
- Some believe that the idiopathic form is a result of persistently insufficient removal of CSF by immature subarachnoid granulations from childhood (3).
- Secondary NPH may result from
  - Subarachnoid hemorrhage
  - Head trauma
  - Resolved acute meningitis
  - Chronic meningitis(TB, syphilis)
  - Paget disease of the skull

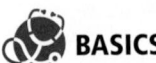 **DIAGNOSIS**

SIGNS AND SYMPTOMS
- Insidious and usually progressive, gait instability usually manifests initially, followed by changes in mentation, and eventually urinary incontinence.
- Difficulty with initiation of movement: Feet appear "glued to the floor." Gait is wide-based, shuffling, and turning appears "en bloc."
- Inattention, forgetfulness, and lack of spontaneity often are seen with the subcortical dementia of NPH.
- Urinary urgency initially, followed by lack of inhibition and then frank incontinence.
- Behavioral changes have been reported to include depression, mania, and psychotic features (1).

History
- A minimum duration of at least 3–6 months of symptoms and progression over time.
- A remote trauma or infection suggests secondary vs. the idiopathic form.
- A lack of psychiatric, neurologic, or other medical conditions to explain the symptoms.
- Because memory impairment may be present, it is important to include a knowledgeable informant who is familiar with the patient's premorbid state (2).

Physical Exam
Features observed on clinical testing
- Decreased step height and length
- Reduced speed of walking (cadence)
- Widened standing base
- Swaying of trunk during walking
- Decreased fine motor speed and accuracy
- Recall impaired for recent events
- Impaired ability to do multistep tasks or interpret abstractions

TESTS
Formal neuropsychological testing and video filming of movement can be helpful for documentation of response to therapy.

Lab
To establish no other reversible etiology exists
- TSH
- Syphilis serology
- CBC
- Serum B_{12}, folate
- Metabolic profile
- Blood alcohol, analysis for drugs of abuse
- Urinalysis

Imaging
- Imaging is essential to the diagnosis. Either CT or MRI show the ventriculomegaly with preservation of the cerebral parenchyma (as opposed to ventricular enlargement seen in other forms of dementia where brain atrophy is present).
- MRI can allow detection of other features such as signs of altered brain water content and callosal angles. However, these supportive findings are not independently diagnostic of NPH (1,2).

Diagnostic Procedures/Surgery
- A number of studies can be used to assess patients for NPH and the potential response to therapy.
- Lumbar puncture (opening pressure in the left lateral recumbent position is 150 mm H_2O [±45 mm H_2O] and glucose, protein are normal)
- High volume LP (removal of 30–60 mL CSF) with symptom comparison before and after.
- Prolonged lumbar drainage (3–5 days), with ongoing assessment of patient's condition, may predict response to therapy.
- Intracranial pressure monitoring to assess for CSF pressure spikes often seen in NPH.
- CSF outflow studies with intracranial saline infusion (2–4).

DIFFERENTIAL DIAGNOSIS
- Alzheimer disease
- Parkinson disease
- Chronic alcoholism
- Intracranial infection
- Multi-infarct dementia
- Subdural hematoma
- Carcinomatous meningitis
- Collagen vascular disorders
- Depression
- Syphilis
- B_{12} deficiency
- Urologic disorders
- Other hydrocephalus disorders

TREATMENT

Most recent review of the available evidence failed to indicate whether placement of an intraventricular shunt is effective in the management of NPH. A recognized difficulty has been in selecting those patients who might benefit from shunting. To date, there are no high-quality, blinded studies of the natural history of the disorder vs. the current surgical treatment (4).

INITIAL STABILIZATION
Evaluation can be done as an outpatient. If infection or other systemic illness identified, treatment per accepted standards.

GENERAL MEASURES
- Assessment and modification of environment for fall risks.
- Evaluation for ability to operate a motor vehicle safely (if driving).

Diet
No special diet

Activity
No limitations, unless physically unable to ambulate independently

Physical Therapy
Gait training and use of ambulation assist devices as indicated

 MEDICATION (DRUGS)

- No medication is significantly helpful.
- Use of carbonic anhydrase inhibitors (Acetazolamide) with repeat lumbar punctures has provided mild and transient relief.
- Lack of response to normal medication used to treat Parkinson should prompt physician to search for other etiology (of dementia, gait disturbance) (3).

SURGERY
- Current therapy is limited to placement of ventriculoperitoneal or ventriculoatrial shunt from a lateral ventricle tunneled subcutaneously and drained into the peritoneal cavity (or right atrium).
- Success depends on appropriate patient selection. No specific test accurately identifies who will benefit from the CSF diversion.
- Studies show persistent improvement in symptoms and quality of life ranging from 29–72%.
- Patients whose symptoms have been present for a shorter period (<2 years) have a greater chance of improvement with shunting. However, improvement has been seen in patients with symptoms present for a long time (3,4).

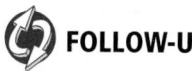 **FOLLOW-UP**

Issues for Referral
Neurology or neurosurgical consultation in suspected cases when other reversible medical conditions are ruled out.

PROGNOSIS
Poor, given the variable response to surgical treatment. The natural history is one of progressive deterioration. Patient's axial skeletal stability worsens with inability to walk, stand, sit, or turn over in bed.

COMPLICATIONS
- In patients treated surgically, cerebral infarcts, hemorrhage, infection, and seizures (in addition to the usual surgical risks)
- Shunt malfunction (especially when symptoms recur after successful shunt placement)
- Falls due to gait instability
- Urinary tract infection
- Skin breakdown, pressure ulcers, infections as movement dysfunction progresses

PATIENT MONITORING
Repeat neuropsychological testing to evaluate the status of the dementia after treatment. Improvement in the incontinence and walking speed can also be objectively measured.

REFERENCES

1. Relkin N, et al. Diagnosing idiopathic normal-pressure hydrocephalus. *Neurosurgery.* 2005;57(3Suppl):4–16.
2. Verrees M, Selman WR. Management of normal pressure hydrocephalus. *Amer Fam Phy.* 2004;70(6):1071–1078.
3. Bradley WG. Normal pressure hydrocephalus: new concepts on etiology and diagnosis. *Am Jour Neuro Rad.* 2000;21:1586–1591.
4. Esmond T, Cooke S. Shunting for normal pressure hydrocephalus. *Cochran Database Sys Rev.* 2006;4.

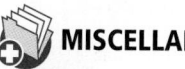 **MISCELLANEOUS**

CODES

ICD9-CM
333.1 Communicating hydrocephalus

PATIENT TEACHING
Information at: emedicinehealth/
normalpressurehydrocepalus.com

H

HYDRONEPHROSIS

Alison H. Blatt, MD

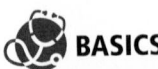 **BASICS**

DESCRIPTION
- "Hydronephrosis" describes a renal pelvi-calyceal collecting system dilated with urine
  - This may be obstructive, physiological, or secondary to reflux.
  - Presentation ranges from severe pain to an incidental finding.
- "Obstructive uropathy" refers to the damage to renal parenchyma resulting from obstruction. This term should not be used interchangeably with "hydronephrosis."

EPIDEMIOLOGY
- Hydronephrosis is found in 3% of autopsy specimens.
- Acute unilateral obstruction is more common than bilateral.

PATHOPHYSIOLOGY
- Hydronephrosis is a compensating mechanism designed to protect the kidney from high pressures and renal damage.
- Obstruction of outflow results in increased intrapelvic pressure resulting in pyelolymphatic and pyelovenous urine backflow as well as possible calyceal fornix rupture and extravasation.
- Coexistence of infection with obstruction results in direct movement of bacteria into the renal vascular tree, resulting in potentially life-threatening sepsis.

ETIOLOGY
- Obstruction: May be acute/chronic, partial/complete, uni/bilateral:
  - Intramural: Calculi, sloughed renal papillae, blood clot
  - Transmural: Transitional cell cancer, benign prostatic hypertrophy, prostate cancer, congenital Pelvi-Ureteric Junction (PUJ) obstruction, ureterocoele, neurogenic bladder (functional obstruction), urethral stricture, tuberculosis
  - Extramural: Extraurinary malignancy (lymphoma, colon, cervix), aortic/iliac aneurysm, retroperitoneal fibrosis, uterine prolapse (15% affected), endometriosis
- Vesico-Ureteric Reflux (VUR) resulting in varying degrees of hydroureteronephrosis
- Physiological hydronephrosis of pregnancy
- Hydronephrosis due to excessive diuresis, e.g., diabetes insipidus, psychogenic polydipsia
- Hydronephrosis of infection: Due to bacterial toxins inhibiting smooth muscle contraction of the renal pelvis and ureter

ALERT
Pediatric Considerations
- Antenatal and childhood hydronephrosis requires complete evaluation.
- Hydronephrosis is the most common cause of abdominal mass in the neonate.
- The spectrum of causes in children differs significantly from adult causes
  - The most common childhood causes of hydronephrosis are VUR, congenital PUJ obstruction, neurogenic bladder, and posterior urethral valve.

- Pediatric diagnostic algorithm differs due to different spectrum of causes as well as tailoring investigations to suitability for children.

Pregnancy Considerations
- Physiological hydronephrosis of pregnancy is seen increasingly as gestation progresses.
  - Dilatation caused by a combination of relaxing hormones and compression of ureter (usually right side) by gravid uterus
- It affects 90% by the 3rd trimester, although most are asymptomatic and go unnoticed.
- If symptomatic and refractory to medical management, ureteric calculus should be considered and urinary infection must be excluded.

DIAGNOSIS

SIGNS AND SYMPTOMS
Urinary tract obstruction symptoms vary according to cause, chronicity, completeness of obstruction, and bilateralism.

History
- Pain may range from typical severe renal colic of acute obstruction (loin to groin) to vague intermittent or chronic pains.
- Dietl crisis: Intermittent flank pain occurring during periods of forced diuresis, such as after consumption of alcohol, associated with unilateral chronic partial obstruction
- Nausea, vomiting, chills associated with severe pain
- High fevers if coexisting infection
- Polyuria may occur due to poor renal concentrating ability in partial obstruction
- Anuria if complete bilateral obstruction
- Chronic renal failure symptoms if gradual bilateral obstruction: Anorexia, malaise, weight gain, edema, shortness of breath, mental state changes, tremors, gastrointestinal bleeding
- Lower urinary tract symptoms which may relate to cause, i.e., bladder outlet obstruction: Weak urine stream, nocturia, straining to pass, overflow incontinence, urgency
- General medical and surgical history: Malignancy (extrinsic compression), radiotherapy (ureteric stricture/fibrosis), surgery (iatrogenic obstruction), trauma (hematoma or fibrosis), gynecological disease (endometriosis, ovarian masses, uterine prolapse), smoking (urothelial cancer), drugs (idiopathic retroperitoneal fibrosis)

Physical Exam
- General signs
  - Volume overload (edema, respiratory crackles, hypertension)
  - Diaphoresis, tachycardia, tachypnoea with pain
  - High-grade fever if infection
- Abdominal exam: Palpable abdominal mass, (rarely visible, particularly in thin children); tender flank if acute, painful obstruction
- Pelvic exam: Pelvic mass, uterine prolapse, palpable enlarged prostate (cancer or benign), urethral meatal stenosis, phimosis

TESTS
Lab
- Dipstick urinalysis: Hematuria, proteinuria, crystalluria, pyuria
- Mid-stream urine, microscopy, culture, and sensitivity: Exclude infection or hematuria
- Creatinine, urea and electrolytes: May demonstrate rising creatinine, urea, potassium, and decreased bicarbonate consistent with acidosis
- CBC: Anemia of renal failure, leukocytosis if infection, platelet count prior to considering intervention
- PSA in adult males >50 or with abnormal digital rectal examination, or outlet obstruction signs or symptoms
- Urine cytology for malignant cells
- Note: CA 19-9 is elevated in benign hydronephrosis and not a useful marker for malignancy in these patients.

Imaging
- Ultrasound: Often makes the initial diagnosis of hydronephrosis
  - Poor sensitivity for detecting cause and level of obstruction
  - Accurate measure of renal parenchymal disease (thinning, cysts)
  - Safe in pregnancy, contrast allergy or renal failure
  - The degree of hydronephrosis does not correlate with the duration or severity of the obstruction.
  - False positives: Normal extrarenal pelvis, parapelvic cysts, VUR, excessive diuresis
  - False negatives: Dehydration; renal cortical cysts actually representing intrarenal calyceal dilatation; at immediate onset of acute obstruction before dilatation has occurred
- IVP: Both functional and anatomical assessment of site, severity and cause of obstruction
  - Typically demonstrates a delayed nephrogram, as well as delayed filling of the collecting system; dilated collecting system; enlarged kidney; extravasation of urine if ruptured fornix; thinned renal cortex or small kidney in the case of chronic onstruction
- Radionuclide scan (diuretic renogram)
  - Useful in determining presence of obstruction as well as total and separate (R vs. L) renal function
  - Advantages: Less radiation than IVP; safe in contrast allergic patients
  - Most common agents are DTPA and MAG-3
  - After 20 minutes, furosemide is given; the t1/2 for the clearance of tracer from the system is measured.
  - T1/2 <10 minutes is unobstructed, >20 minutes is obstructed, and 10–20 minutes is equivocal; some experts consider <15 minutes normal.
  - False positives occur in patients with reduced creatinine clearance due to delayed excretion, and in massive dilatation causing a water-reservoir effect of delayed excretion without obstruction.
  - False negatives occur in dehydrated patients or inadequate diuretic challenges.

- Computer tomography ± contrast
  - Noncontrast helical CT of the abdomen and pelvis is the investigation of choice for acute flank pain suspicious of renal colic.
    - Stone is most commonly found at levels of ureteric luminal narrowing: PUJ, pelvic brim, and the vesico-ureteric junction
    - If the obstruction is acute, proximal ureter and renal pelvis is dilated to the level of obstruction and perinephric "stranding" is seen as well as renal swelling.
    - If chronic, renal atrophy may be noted.
  - Multiphase contrast-enhanced CT
    - Nonenhanced phase detects stones and swelling
    - Parenchymal phase demonstrates decreased density of renal parenchyma of acutely obstructed kidney; extraurinary causes of obstruction; can also be used to determine the relative GFR of each kidney with equal accuracy to diuretic renography
    - Delayed phase allows visualization of the collecting system and soft tissue filling defects (e.g., urothelial cancer).
- If contrast is contraindicated (creatinine >2 ng/dL), Magnetic Resonance Urography (MRU) is superior to noncontrast CT in diagnosing soft-tissue causes including strictures.
  - MRU disadvantages: Insensitive for stone detection (only 70%); increased expense; less availablility; increased acquisition time compared to CT (35 minutes vs. 5 minutes)
  - MRU is also described in pregnancy, although it rarely alters management decisions.
- Duplex Doppler ultrasound to determine the Resistive Index (RI); controversial role in diagnosis of obstruction with variable accuracy reported in the literature
- Whitaker Test: The gold standard test for obstruction, measuring renal pressure via a percutaneous nephrostomy and bladder pressure via an indwelling catheter; highly invasive and rarely performed
- Voiding Cysto-Urethrogram as part of diagnostic algorithm in VUR

Diagnostic Procedures/Surgery
Cystoscopy, retrograde pyelogram ± ureteroscopy, biopsy are occasionally required in order to make a diagnosis (e.g., small urothelial cancer missed on imaging) or to confirm a normal distal ureter prior to pyeloplasty

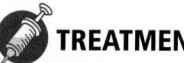 TREATMENT

INITIAL STABILIZATION
Obstruction coexisting with infection (pyonephrosis) is a true urologic emergency requiring urgent drainage.

GENERAL MEASURES
- Treatment of hydronephrosis depends on cause (obstructed or nonobstructed), complications (atrophy, pain, renal failure, infection), and level of obstruction.
- Relief of obstruction
  - Bladder outlet obstruction: Urethral or suprapubic catheter
  - Ureteric obstruction: Retrograde (cystoscopic) or antegrade (percutaneous) stenting
- Correction of fluid and electrolyte abnormalities
- Analgesia depending on cause and severity of pain: NSAIDs and acetaminophen-codeine for renal colic, followed by IV morphine if required
- Antibiotics as an adjunct to drainage if infection present
- VUR is often managed conservatively with antibiotics; surgical management is required in severe cases in children or women of child-bearing age.

SURGERY
- Hydronephrosis due to obstruction
  - Congenital PUJO: Pyeloplasty (open or laparoscopic), minimally invasive stricture incision (accusize, laser)
  - Stone obstruction: Stent, ESWL, lithotripsy, PCNL
  - Transitional cell cancer: Nephroureterectomy
  - Idiopathic retroperitoneal fibrosis: Ureterolysis (frees ureters from inflammatory mass)
  - Prostate disorders: Various treatment modalities including TURP and radical prostatectomy
- Nonobstructed hydronephrosis
  - VUR: Ureteric reimplantation

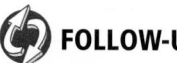 FOLLOW-UP

PROGNOSIS
- After relief of obstruction, renal function is usually recovered.
- Determinants of reversibility of renal damage
  - Renal perfusion prior to relief of obstruction
  - GFR prior to relief of obstruction
    - >10 mL/min/1.73m^2: Kidney should stabilize or improve
    - <10 mL/min/1.73m^2: Kidney is irreversibly damaged

COMPLICATIONS
- Urine stasis: Increased risk of infection and calculus formation
- Back pressure causes progressive cortical atrophy of kidney with irreversible loss of renal function.
  - Tubules lose ability to concentrate urine, conserve sodium, or excrete H$^+$.
  - Glomerular damage decreases GFR.
- Spontaneous rupture of a calyx may occur with urine extravasation in the perinephric space. This occasionally requires separate drainage.
- Postobstructive diruesis: Marked polyuria after relief of bilateral obstruction or obstructed solitary kidney
  - Caused mostly by fluid and solute overload, but may be exacerbated by impaired renal tubular concentrating ability
  - Monitor all patients for an output >200 mL/h and replace losses with IV normal saline, monitoring electrolytes.

REFERENCES
1. Abo El-Ghar ME, Shokeir AA, El-Diasty TA, Refaie HF, Gad HM, Shehab El-Dein AB. Contrast enhanced spiral computerized tomography in patients with chronic obstructive uropathy and normal serum creatinine: A single session for anatomical and functional assessment. *J Urol*. 2004;172(3):985–988.
2. Khalaf IM, Shokeir AA, El-Gyoushi FI, Amr HS, Amin MM. Recoverability of renal function after treatment of adult patients with unilateral obstructive uropathy and normal contralateral kidney: A prospective study. *Urology*. 2004;64(4): 664–668.
3. Worster A, Preyra I, Weaver B, Haines T. The accuracy of noncontrast helical computed tomography versus intravenous pyelography in the diagnosis of suspected acute urolithiasis: A meta-analysis. *Ann Emerg Med*. 2002;40(3): 280–286.

 MISCELLANEOUS

CODES

ICD9-CM
- 753.20 Unspecified obstructive defect of renal pelvis and ureter
- 591 Hydronephrosis

H

HYPERCALCEMIA ASSOCIATED WITH MALIGNANCY

Ruben Peralta, MD, FACS
Jacqueline J. Wu, MD

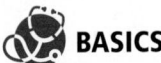 **BASICS**

DESCRIPTION
- Hypercalcemia associated with malignancy is the most common cause of severe hypercalcemia diagnosed in a hospital setting.
- Often a very poor prognostic sign

GENERAL PREVENTION
Encourage adequate hydration and activity, especially in multiple myeloma.

EPIDEMIOLOGY
Incidence
Occurs in ~10–20% of cancer patients

RISK FACTORS
- Dehydration
- Immobilization

ETIOLOGY
- Normally, calcium is regulated by parathyroid hormone, calcitriol, and calcitonin.
- Main mechanisms of hypercalcemia in malignancy
  - Ectopic production of parathyroid related protein (PTH-rP). PTH-rP increases bone resorption by osteoclasts. Associated with
    - Squamous cell lung carcinoma.
    - Other squamous cell cancers
    - Breast cancer
    - Renal cell carcinoma
    - Prostate cancer
    - Melanoma
  - Calcitriol production
    - Lymphoma
  - Bone resorption by osteoclasts, activated by PTH-rp or other factors such as TNF, interleukins generated by solid-tumor metastasis or multiple myeloma. (In multiple myeloma, impaired renal function and calcium excretion)

DIAGNOSIS

SIGNS AND SYMPTOMS
- The severity of symptoms depends on calcium level, rapidity of onset of hypercalcemia, state of hydration, and underlying malignancy.
- Early symptoms often include nausea, vomiting, anorexia.
- Cardiovascular
  - Arrhythmias, bradycardia
  - QT shortening
  - Calcium increases vascular tone.
- Genitourinary
  - Nephrolithiasis, especially in the elderly
  - Polyuria because of impaired concentrating ability
- Gastrointestinal
  - Peptic ulcers
  - Pancreatitis
  - Constipation
  - Anorexia
  - Nausea, vomiting
- Musculoskeletal
  - Weakness, hypotonia
  - Hyporeflexia
  - Osteopenia, fractures
- Neuropsychiatric
  - Depression, lethargy
  - Obtundation, coma
  - Memory impairment, confusion
  - Psychosis
  - Headache
  - Seizures

TESTS
Lab
- Serum calcium: Either ionized (gold standard), or must also check albumin and correct:
  $Ca(adj) = Ca(tot) - 0.8x (albumin - 4)$
- Electrolytes including magnesium and phosphate (If hypercalcemia due to PTH-rP expect low phosphate, hyperchloremia, mild alkalosis)
- Renal function
- Urine calcium will be elevated
- PTH-related peptide
  - Most commonly elevated in breast and lung cancer
- If underlying malignancy unknown, commence workup, for example, serum and urine electrophoresis for multiple myeloma.

ALERT
- Lithium, thiazide diuretics, and vitamin D preparations can all increase serum calcium.
- Special tests: Staging techniques as necessary to determine extent of malignancy

Imaging
None indicated for the immediate management of hypercalcemia, but studies such as bone scan may be helpful for underlying condition.

DIFFERENTIAL DIAGNOSIS
- Hyperparathyroidism
- Immobilization
- Calcium administration
- Renal causes
  - Chronic or acute renal failure
  - Post renal transplantation
- Hypocalciuric hypercalcemias
  - Familial
  - Hypothyroidism
  - Adrenal insufficiency
  - Bartter syndrome
- Granulomatous disease
  - Sarcoidosis
  - Histoplasmosis
  - Coccidioidomycosis
  - Tuberculosis
- Hyperthyroidism
- AIDS
- Hypophosphatemia
- Pheochromocytoma
- Acromegaly
- Drugs
  - Calcium
  - Lithium
  - Theophylline
  - Thiazides
  - Vitamin A or D toxicity

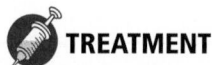 TREATMENT

GENERAL MEASURES
- Treatment of underlying malignancy
- Hemodialysis can be utilized when saline diuresis and medications fail.

Activity
Avoid bed rest or immobilization as much as possible.

 MEDICATION (DRUGS)

First Line
- Hydration: The initial therapy of choice because many symptoms are due to dehydration.
  - Vomiting and renal losses can cause profound dehydration.
  - Volume expansion with intravenous normal saline
  - If congestive heart failure a concern, loop diuretics may be helpful after hydration.
- Increase renal calcium excretion
  - Use only after adequate hydration.
  - Monitor for possible hypokalemia and hypomagnesemia.
  - Loop diuretics (furosemide): Increases renal calcium excretion but only after adequate hydration. Works by suppressing proximal sodium and calcium reabsorption and enhances kaliuresis. If diuretics are used before dehydration is corrected and glomerular filtration rate restored, renal clearance of calcium is further impaired and hypercalcemia may worsen.
  - Calcitonin: Also requires adequate rehydration; inhibits calcium reabsorption in the distal tubule. Rapid onset of action (within 6–24 hours); side effects include nausea, vomiting, abdominal cramps, rash, flushing, diarrhea, tachyphylaxis.

Second Line
- Given that most hypercalcemia of malignancy is due to bone reabsorption, some therapy is aimed at reducing calcium release from bone.
- Bisphosphonates by inhibiting osteoclasts
  - Zoledronic acid (Zometa)
    - Duration of action is 30 days
    - Nephrotoxic potential, especially in myeloma patients receiving thalidomide
  - Pamidronate (Aredia)
    - Normalizes calcium up to 3 weeks
- Plicamycin (previously mithramycin)
  - May work via direct toxic effect on osteoclasts. Reserved for patients who do not respond to bisphosphonates, but can induce normocalcemia in 80% of those who receive it.
  - Side effects limit its use (nausea, vomiting, cellulitis at infusion site, cytopenias, hepatic toxicity, nephrotoxicity, platelet inhibition). Can have rapid rebound hypercalcemia.
  - Onset of action within 12 hours, with maximal effect seen in 24–48 hours
- Gallium nitrate
  - Onset of action 48–72 hours
  - Side effects: Nausea, vomiting, nephrotoxicity, hypophosphatemia, anemia, hypotension
- Inorganic phosphates
  - Potentially lethal side effects limit the use to patients with life-threatening hypercalcemia; IV use no longer supported.
  - Side effects: Precipitation of calcium into tissues of the lung, heart, kidneys, blood vessels can lead to organ damage, hypotension, and death.
  - Oral and rectal routes safer than IV
- Glucocorticoids
  - Direct effects in treating hypercalcemia of malignancy are unclear.
  - Has direct tumoricidal effects on hematologic cancers such as multiple myeloma, lymphoma, and leukemias

 FOLLOW-UP

PROGNOSIS
Median survival after diagnosis of tumoral hypercalcemia depends on type and extent of the malignancy, but usually indicates a poor prognosis.

PATIENT MONITORING
Frequent serum calcium and electrolyte determinations; expect relapse

REFERENCES
1. Deftos LJ. Hypercalcemia in malignancy and inflammatory diseases. *Endocrinol Metab Clin North Am.* 2002;31:141–158.
2. Stewart AF. Hypercalcemia associated with cancer. *N Engl J Med.* 2005;352(4):373–379.
3. Lipton A. Management of metastatic bone disease and hypercalcemia of malignancy. *Am J Cancer.* 2003;2(6):427–438.
4. Pecherstorfer M, Breener K, Zojer N. Current management strategies for hypercalcemia. *Treat Endocrinol.* 2003;2(4):273–292.

 MISCELLANEOUS

See also: Addison disease; HIV infection and AIDS; Hyperparathyroidism; Hyperthyroidism; Milk-alkali syndrome; Rhabdomyolysis; Sarcoidosis; Tuberculosis

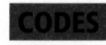 CODES

ICD9-CM
- 275.40 Unspecified disorder of calcium metabolism
- 275.42 Hypercalcemia

H

HYPERCHOLESTEROLEMIA

James L. Young, MD
Peter Libby, MD

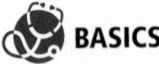 **BASICS**

DESCRIPTION
- Serum cholesterol >200 mg/dL (5.18 mmol/L)
  - Due mainly to lifestyle habits in westernized countries; however, rule out genetic and secondary causes.
- Lipoprotein subpopulations are commonly used clinically to augment risk prediction, favoring the term *dyslipidemia* which encompasses
  - High density lipoprotein fraction of cholesterol (HDL)—Atheroprotective
  - Low density lipoprotein (LDL)—Atherogenic
  - Triglycerides
- Genetic etiologies may skew increases in specific lipoprotein fractions.
- System(s) Affected: Cardiovascular; Endocrine/Metabolic

ALERT
Though very low cholesterol readings are associated with higher mortality (J-Curve Phenomenon), this trend may be confounded by other disease processes, such as cancer and liver disease. Clinical trials have yet to determine a lower limit of benefit afforded by cholesterol-lowering treatments.

Pregnancy Considerations
- Fetal nutritional demands may alter diet and drug treatment.
- Statins contraindicated

GENERAL PREVENTION
Prudent diet, frequent exercise, and weight control for all

EPIDEMIOLOGY
- Predominant age: Increases with age
- Predominant sex: Male = Female

Prevalence
- 100 million people in US with cholesterol ≥200 mg/dL (5.18 mmol/L)
- 34.5 million people in US with ≥240 mg/dL (6.22 mmol/L)

RISK FACTORS
- Obesity (BMI >30 kg/m^2)
- Physical inactivity
- Diet rich in saturated fat and cholesterol
- Heredity

Genetics
Familial hypercholesterolemia has autosomal codominant inheritance.
- Most prevalent lipoprotein disorder (1 in 500 cases)

PATHOPHYSIOLOGY
Atherosclerotic disease
- Coronary artery disease
- Cerebrovascular disease
- Peripheral vascular disease
- Renal artery stenosis
- Abdominal aneurysm

ETIOLOGY
- Primary
  - Diet/Sedentary lifestyle/Obesity
  - Heredity
- Secondary
  - Hypothyroidism
  - Diabetes mellitus
  - Glycogen storage disorders
  - Nephrotic syndrome
  - Chronic renal failure
  - Obstructive liver disease
  - Cirrhosis
  - Progestins
  - Estrogens
  - Anabolic steroids
  - Corticosteroids
  - Retinoic acid derivatives
  - Diuretics except indapamide (Lozol)
  - Beta-blockers except those with intrinsic sympathomimetic activity (ISA)
  - Some immunosuppressants (e.g., cyclosporine)

ASSOCIATED CONDITIONS
- Atherosclerotic disease
- Hypertension
- Obesity
- Diabetes mellitus

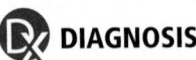 **DIAGNOSIS**

SIGNS AND SYMPTOMS
- Few direct symptoms, most secondary to atherosclerotic disease
  - Angina pectoris
  - Stroke
  - Myocardial infarction (MI)
  - Arterial bruits
  - Claudication
- Genetic familial hypercholesterolemia
  - Corneal arcus age <50 years
  - Xanthomata
  - Xanthelasma

TESTS
Lab
- Lipoprotein panel: Total cholesterol, HDL, LDL, triglycerides
  - LDL is typically a calculated value and is accurate under fasting conditions and if triglycerides <350 mg/dL (<4.0 mmol/L).
    - Direct LDL measurement may be available in specialty labs.
- Thyroid-stimulating hormone (TSH) to assess hypothyroidism

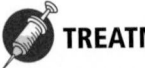 **TREATMENT**

INITIAL STABILIZATION
Outpatient, except for complicating emergencies (e.g., myocardial infarction)

GENERAL MEASURES
Diet
- National Cholesterol Education Program (NCEP) Therapeutic Lifestyle Changes (TLC) Diet
  - Dietary fats: 25–35% of total calories
    - Saturated: 7% of total calories
    - Polyunsaturated: 10% of total calories
    - Monounsaturated: 20% of total calories
  - Cholesterol <200 mg/d
  - Carbohydrates: 50–60% of total calories
    - Mainly complex carbohydrates from whole grain, fruits, and vegetables
- Olive oil should be preferentially used.
- Omega-3-fatty acids and fish oil may be used.
- Minimal daily alcohol use may increase HDL.
- Dietary adherence generally may be expected to result in a 10% LDL reduction.

Activity
Walking or other sustained cardiovascular exercise for 30 minutes, 3–4 times per week
- Important for increasing HDL, lowering total cholesterol, and losing weight.

 MEDICATION (DRUGS)

- Treatment initiation depends on LDL, HDL, and triglyceride levels as modified by risk factors and history of previous coronary heart disease (CHD) or risk equivalents (1,2)[A]
  - Risk factors
    - Cigarette smoking
    - Hypertension (BP >140/90)
    - Age (Male >45 years, Female >55 years)
    - HDL <40 mg/dL
    - MI or stroke in 1st-degree relative (male <55 years or female <65 years)
  - CHD or CHD risk equivalent (Major coronary events ≥20% per 10 years)
    - Coronary, carotid, aortic, or peripheral vascular disease
    - Diabetes mellitus
- Primary goal: LDL lowering for patients refractory to exercise, diet treatment (1,2)[A]
  - CHD or CHD risk equivalent: <100 mg/dL
  - 2+ Risk factors: <130 mg/dL
  - 0–2 Risk factors: <160 mg/dL
    - An optional goal of LDL <70 mg/dL for very high-risk patients is supported by clinical trial evidence. (3,4)[A]
- Secondary goal: In patients with triglycerides >200 mg/dL, non-HDL cholesterol (total cholesterol-HDL) <130 mg/dL (1,2)[A]
- Pharmacologic measures to increase HDL are not supported by current clinical trials. (1,2)

First Line
- HMG-CoA reductase inhibitors (statins)
  - Fluvastatin (Lescol), lovastatin (Mevacor), or pravastatin (Pravachol): 20–80 mg/d Effects: 20–40% LDL decrease, increased HDL, and lower triglycerides
  - Simvastatin (Zocor): 10–80 mg may decrease LDL 50% increase HDL, and lower triglycerides.
  - Atorvastatin (Lipitor): 10–80 mg may decrease LDL 55% and lower triglycerides.
  - Rosuvastatin (Crestor): 10–40 mg may decrease LDL 55%, lower triglycerides, and increase HDL.
- Contraindications
  - HMG-CoA reductase inhibitors: Active liver disease, pregnancy
- Precautions:
  - Liver function tests 6–12 weeks after initiation of therapy, then every 6 months for 1 year, then periodically
  - Myositis with markedly elevated creatine kinase (CK) may occur.
- Significant possible interactions
  - Concomitant gemfibrozil, niacin, cyclosporine, azole antifungals, or macrolide antibiotics may increase possibility of myositis.

ALERT
- Avoid taking statins with grapefruit juice.
- Take statins late in day as majority of liver cholesterol synthesis occurs at night.
  - Exception: Atorvastatin and Rosuvastatin

Second Line
- Cholestyramine (Questran) or colestipol (Colestid) bile acid–binding resins: 1–6 packets per day taken b.i.d. or t.i.d. or colesevelam (WelChol) 6 tablets daily
  - Effect: 15–20% fall in LDL
- Niacin (nicotinic acid): 500 mg to 3 g taken 1–3 times daily with meals in timed release formulation, or Niaspan at bedtime
  - Effect: 15–30% LDL lowering, decreases triglycerides, increases HDL
  - Hepatic dysfunction more common in patients who take immediate release niacin than in those who take sustained release form
- Ezetimibe (Zetia): 10 mg/d
  - Selectively inhibits intestinal absorption of cholesterol and related phytosterols
  - Effect: 18–25% LDL lowering either when used primarily or added to a statin
- Fibric acid derivative (Fibrates)
  - Gemfibrozil (Lopid) effective for reducing triglycerides with modest elevation of HDL and variable effect on LDL

- Contraindications
  - Cholestyramine: Complete biliary obstruction, triglycerides >200
  - Nicotinic acid: Hepatic dysfunction, acute peptic ulcer, diabetes mellitus, hyperuricemia
- Precautions
  - Cholestyramine: Gradually increase dose on weekly basis to minimize GI side effects (particularly constipation, flatulence).
  - Nicotinic acid: Titrate dose to minimize side effects (e.g., cutaneous flushing)
- Significant possible interactions
  - Cholestyramine: Other drugs taken <1 hour before or within 6 hours after may be bound and not absorbed as well. Fat-soluble vitamins A, D, E, and K absorption may be impeded.
  - Nicotinic acid: Concomitant gemfibrozil, niacin, or immunosuppressives increase possibility of myositis.
  - Fibric acid derivatives: May potentiate effects of warfarin and oral hypoglycemic agents

Complementary and Alternative Medicine
Beta-sitosterols and red yeast rice can reduce total cholesterol and LDL. Niacin and policosanol can reduce total cholesterol and LDL while increasing HDL. (5,6,7,8)

 ## FOLLOW-UP

PROGNOSIS
1% decrease in cholesterol results in 2% decreased risk of CHD.

COMPLICATIONS
- Atherosclerotic disease
  - Coronary artery disease
  - Cerebrovascular disease
  - Peripheral vascular disease
  - Renal artery stenosis
  - Abdominal aneurysm
- Generalized arteriosclerosis

PATIENT MONITORING
- While on medication, monitor cholesterol, HDL, LDL, triglycerides, liver enzymes (on statins, niacin) every 6–12 weeks until goal LDL reached, then every 6–12 months
- All adults 20 and over: Lipoprotein panel every 5 years

REFERENCES

1. Expert Panel on Detection, Evaluation, and Treatment of High Blood Cholesterol in Adults. Executive Summary of The Third Report of The National Cholesterol Education Program (NCEP) Expert Panel on Detection, Evaluation, And Treatment of High Blood Cholesterol In Adults (Adult Treatment Panel III). *JAMA*. 2001; 285:2486–2497.
2. Gibbons RJ, Abrams J, Chatterjee K, et al. ACC/AHA 2002 Guideline Update for the Management of Patients with Chronic Stable Angina: A Report of the American College of Cardiology/American Heart Association Task Force on Practice Guidelines. Available at www.acc.org/clinical/guidelines/stable/stable.pdf.
3. Cannon CP, Braunwald E, McCabe CH, et al. Comparison of intensive and moderate lipid lowering with statins after acute coronary syndromes. *N Engl J Med.* 2004;350:1495–1504.
4. LaRosa JC, Grundy SM, Waters DD, et al. Intensive Lipid Lowering with Atorvastatin in Patients with Stable Coronary Disease. *N Engl J Med.* 2005; 352:1425–1435.
5. Nguyen TT, Dale LC, von Bergmann K, and Croghan IT. Cholesterol-lowering effect of stanol ester in a US population of mildly hypercholesterolemic men and women: A randomized controlled trial. *Mayo Clin Proc* 1999;74(12):1198–1206.
6. Schectman G, Hiatt J. Dose-response characteristics of cholesterol-lowering drug therapies: Implications for treatment. *Ann Intern Med* 1996;125(12): 990–1000.
7. Chen JT, Wesley R, Shamburek RD, et al. Meta-analysis of natural therapies for hyperlipidemia: Plant sterols and stanols versus policosanol. *Pharmacotherapy* 2005;25(2): 171–183.
8. Thompson Coon JS and Ernst E. Herbs for serum cholesterol reduction: A systematic view. *J Fam Pract.* 2003;52(6):468–478.

 ## MISCELLANEOUS

See also: Atherosclerosis; Atherosclerotic occlusive disease; Hypothyroidism, adult

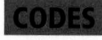 **CODES**

ICD9-CM
272.0 Pure hypercholesterolemia

PATIENT TEACHING
American Heart Association publications

 See Corresponding Diagnostic Algorithm

 See Patient Handout on CD

H

HYPERCOAGULABLE STATES

David D. Henderson, MD

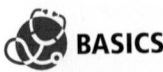 **BASICS**

DESCRIPTION
- Venous thromboembolic disease represents a spectrum of disease that includes
  - Deep venous thrombosis (DVT)—most often involving the lower extremities
  - Pulmonary Embolus (PE)
- System(s) Affected: Cardiovascular

EPIDEMIOLOGY
Increased incidence with increasing age

Incidence
First time thromboembolism
- 100/100,000 per year in general population
- <5/100,000 in those <15 years old
- 500/100,000 in 80-year-olds

Prevalence
40–70% in lower extremity orthopedic procedures without prophylaxis

RISK FACTORS
- Immobilization
- Advanced age (>60 years old)
- Malignancy
- Trauma
- Obesity (BMI >30)
- Recent surgery
- Pregnancy (especially the postpartum period)
- Oral contraceptives (OCP)/Estrogen therapy
- CHF
- Hyperviscosity (Sickle cell, Polycythemia)
- Hyperhomocystinemia
- Inherited thrombophilias
- Risk stratification
  - Low risk: Age <40, laproscopic surgery, obesity
  - Moderate risk: Age >40, major surgery, MI, CHF, OCP, thrombophilia, prior history
  - High risk: Malignancy, lower extremity orthopedic surgery, hip or pelvic fracture

PATHOPHYSIOLOGY
Virchow Triad
- Venous trauma, Venous stasis, and Hypercoagulability

ETIOLOGY
- See "Risk Factors" above
- Upper extremity DVT: Venous catheters and young athletes (Paget–Schroetter Syndrome)

HYPERCOAGULABLE CONDITIONS
- Factor V Leiden – activated Protein C (aPC) Resistance
  - aPC does not cleave Factor Va and Thrombin formation continues
  - 5–8% prevalence in whites, rare in African Americans, Asians
  - Heterozygotes 90% of aPC resistance
  - OCPs, smoking, obesity are synergistic
- Protein C deficiency
  - Autosomal dominant
  - Homozygotes and heterozygotes are hypercoagulable
  - Vitamin K dependent, produced in the liver
  - Inactivates Va and VIIa
  - Protein S increases its activity
  - Acquired deficiency in liver disease, sepsis, DIC, ARDS

- Protein S deficiency
  - Autosomal dominant
  - Homozygotes and heterozygotes are hypercoagulable
  - Vitamin K dependent, produced in the liver
  - Cofactor for Protein C
  - Acquired deficiency in OCP use, pregnancy, liver disease, sepsis, DIC, HIV, nephrosis
- Prothrombin gene mutation
  - Prevalence 6% among Europeans
  - Heterozygotes are hypercoagulable
  - Associated with high prothrombin levels
  - Vitamin K dependent, produced in the liver
- Antithrombin deficiency
  - Autosomal dominant
  - Deactivated thrombin
  - Produced in the liver
  - Acquired deficiency in DIC, sepsis liver disease
- Hyperhomocysteinemia
  - 5–6% in general population
  - Increases risk of CAD/MI, CVA, DVT/PE
  - Seen in folate, B_{12}, and B_6 deficiencies
  - Fibrates, niacin, smoking raise levels
- Other conditions include lupus anticoagulant and antiphospholipid syndrome.

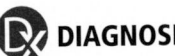 **DIAGNOSIS**

SIGNS AND SYMPTOMS
History
- DVT: Calf pain, swelling, erythema, edema
- PE: Chest pain, shortness of breath

Physical Exam
- DVT: Unilateral calf tenderness, erythema, edema
- PE: Dyspnea, hypoxia, hemoptysis

DIFFERENTIAL DIAGNOSIS
- DVT: Superficial phlebitis, ruptured Baker cyst, muscle tear, compartment syndrome
- PE: Myocardial infarction, pneumonia, pneumothorax, pericardial tamponade, pulmonary edema

TESTS
Lab
- The evaluation proceeds from the assessment of risk/probability of having DVT/PE. Wells criteria for risk assessment follows.
- Routine lab tests include
  - CBC including platelet count
  - PT/INR, APTT
  - Electrolytes, BUN, creatinine
  - Hepatic panel
  - EKG (common findings: Sinus tachycardia, atrial fibrillation, $S_1Q_3T_3$)
  - Set aside blood prior to treatment (Protein S and C assays, antithrombin III assay are inaccurate once on anticoagulant therapy)
- Thrombophilia risk stratification
  - 1st episode, transient risk factor and no family history—no evaluation needed
  - Age >50, idiopathic 1st episode of DVT and no family history—consider genetic test for Factor 5 Leiden, prothrombin gene mutation, lupus anticoagulant, antiphospholipid antibodies, homocysteine level
  - Age <50 *or*
  - Family History of thromboembolism, *or*

Wells Criteria for DVT

	Points
Lower limb trauma/surgery/casting	+1
Immobilization/surgery within 4 wk	+1
Tenderness popliteal/femoral veins	+1
Swelling of entire limb	+1
>3 cm difference in calf size	+1
Unilateral pitting edema	+1
Dilated collateral veins	+1
Malignancy (treated in prior 6 mo)	+1
Alternative diagnosis as/more likely	−2
Total score ≥3	**High Probability**
Total score 1–2	**Moderate Probability**
Total score <1	**Low Probability**

Wells Criteria for DVT

	Points
Clinical symptoms of DVT	3
Other diagnosis less likely than PE	1
Previous DVT/PE	1.5
Heart Rate >100 bpm	1.5
Immobilization/surgery within 4 wk	1.5
Malignancy	1
Hemoptysis	1
Total score >6	**High Probability**
Total score 2–6	**Moderate Probability**
Total score <2	**Low Probability**

  - Recurrent thrombolism—check Factor 5 Leiden, prothrombin gene mutation, lupus anticoagulant, antiphospholipid antibodies, homocysteine level, Protein S and C assays, antithrombin III assay

Diagnostic Procedures
- DVT: Low probability
  - Negative D-dimer (by ELISA) rules out DVT
  - Positive D-dimer warrants ultrasound (US)
- DVT: Moderate or high probability
  - Positive US establishes diagnosis
  - Negative US should be followed by D-dimer
  - Positive US and negative D-dimer should be followed by repeat US in 1 week
  - Negative US and negative D-dimer rules out DVT
- PE: Low probability
  - Negative D-dimer rules out DVT
  - Positive D-dimer-V/Q scan or CT angiography
- PE: Moderate or high probability
  - CT angiography or V/Q scan
  - Negative study rules out PE
  - Non-diagnostic studies—D-dimer and US

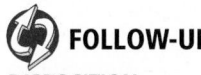 **TREATMENT**

PRE HOSPITAL
- Support ABCs
- Initiate O_2, IV, monitor throughout transport

INITIAL STABILIZATION
Initial priority is stability of patient
- Hemodynamically stable
  - ABC support, IV hydration
- Hemodynamically unstable (e.g., massive PE with respiratory distress, hypoxemia, or hypotension or massive iliofemoral DVT)
  - ABC support, ICU
  - Consider emergent systemic thrombolytic therapy. Local delivery via pulmonary artery cathetization not recommended

GENERAL MEASURES
- Identify risk factors.
- Consider empiric anticoagulant therapy with high clinical suspicion or if unstable.
- Elevation of lower extremity
- NPO until hemodynamically stable
- Limit activity initially.

OVERVIEW OF DRUG THERAPY
- Unfractionated Heparin (UFH)
  - Usually IV as a continuous drip, but can be used SC
  - IV bolus 80 units/kg then infusion at 18 units/kg/h (use of protocol advisable)
  - Goal to maintain PTT 1.5–2.5 × normal
  - Complication thrombocytopenia and bleeding
- Low Molecular Weight Heparin (LMWH)
  - Administered SC once or twice daily
  - Predictable pharmokinetics and improved bioavailability compared to UFH
  - Monitoring of PTT is not routinely warranted.
  - Less likely to cause thrombocytopenia
  - Can be administered at home
- Warfarin
  - May be started concurrently with heparin
  - Appropriate long-term treatment of VTE (except in pregnancy, malignancy)
  - Not appropriate for initial therapy of VTE
  - Initiation to 10 mg daily shortens time to adequate anticoagulation (INR >2)
  - Careful monitoring with serial PT/INR

DVT/PE

Acute Therapy
- All have the following: Contraindications: Hypersensitivity, active bleeding, recent surgery, lumbar puncture, pregnancy, advanced liver disease
- Precautions: Use with caution in patients with uncontrolled hypertension, renal disease, vitamin K deficiency
- Low molecular weight heparin recommended as initial therapy (4 choices) (3)
  - Enoxaparin (Lovenox)
    - Dose: Acute VTE
    - 1 mg/kg b.i.d. or 1.5 mg/kg/d
    - Prophylaxis: 30 mg (SQ) b.i.d. or 40 mg/d
  - Interactions: Aspirin, NSAIDs, clopidogrel, some cephalosporins and penicillins
  - Adverse reactions: Thrombocytpenia, bleeding, hyperkalemia
  - Pregnancy Risk Factor B

  - Fondaparinux (Arixta) should be started in conjunction with warfarin
    - Dose: Acute VTE
    - Weight <50 kg: 5 mg SC daily
    - Weight 50–100 kg: 7.5 mg SC daily
    - Weight >100 kg: 10 mg SC daily
    - Prophylaxis: 2.5 mg SC daily
  - Dalteparin (approved for DVT prophylaxis/long-term therapy)
    - Dose: 200 IU/kg/d for 1 month, then 150 IU/kg/d
  - Tinzaparin (approved for DVT prophylaxis/long-term therapy)
    - Dose: 175 IU/kg/d
- UFH IV (or SC b.i.d.) is also an appropriate alternative
  - Dose: Acute VTE
    - Dose (SC): IV bolus 5000 IU followed by 17,500 b.i.d. for 1st 24 hours. Check PTT 6 hours after the morning SC dose.
    - IV bolus 80 units/kg, then infusion at 18 units/kg/h (use of protocol advisable)
  - Dose: Prophylaxis
    - 5000 units SC q12h
  - Interactions: See LMWH
  - Adverse reactions: Thrombocytopenia, fever, skin necrosis, hyperkalemia, elevated AST/ALT. 2% risk immune-mediated heparin-induced thrombocytopenia
- Warfarin
  - May be started concurrently with heparin
  - Initiation to 10 mg/d shortens time to adequate anticoagulation (INR >2)
  - Therapeutic range: 2–3
  - Contraindications: Hypersensitivity, active bleeding, recent surgery, lumbar puncture, pregnancy, advanced liver disease
  - Precautions: Uncontrolled hypertension, renal disease, vitamin K deficiency
  - Interactions: Too numerous to mention here.
  - Adverse reactions: Bleeding, fever, elevated AST/ALT, gangrene, skin necrosis, "purple toes syndrome"
- Continue therapy with LMWH or UFH for 5 days and until INR is stable at >2.

Long-Term Therapy
- For 1st episode DVT/PE reversible risk factor
  - Therapy for 3 months usually with warfarin (3)
- For 1st episode of idiopathic DVT/PE
  - Therapy for 6–12 months usually with warfarin, consider of indefinite therapy (3)
- For patients with DVT/PE and cancer
  - Therapy with LMWH for at least 3–6 months, until cancer is cured, or indefinitely (3)
- For 1st episode of DVT/PE, antiphospholipid antibodies or 2 or more thrombophilias
  - Therapy with LMWH for 12 months with consideration of indefinite therapy (3)
- For 1st episode of DVT/PE and thrombophilia other than antiphospholipid antibodies
  - Therapy with LMWH for 6–12 months with consideration of indefinite therapy (3)
- For 2 or more episodes of DVT/PE
  - Indefinite therapy recommended (3)

Other Therapies
Nonmedical
- Elastic stockings
  - Postthrombotic syndrome (PTS)
    - Pressure 30–40 mm Hg at the ankle
- Pneumatic compression stockings for PTS
  - Appropriate for severe leg edema
- Inferior vena cava filter
  - If contraindication to anticoagulation
  - Recurrent DVT despite anticoagulation

SURGERY
Catheter extraction/Surgical thrombectomy: Only in extreme emergencies (e.g., massive PE where thrombolysis is not feasible)

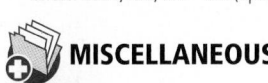 **FOLLOW-UP**

DISPOSITION

Admission Criteria
- Outpatient treatment of proximal DVT if
  - PE is absent, patient can inject self
  - Close follow-up of PT/INR can be assured.
- All patients with PE should be admitted.

Discharge Criteria
- Hemodynamically stable and INR >2 on warfarin
- Or if stable on LMWH and warfarin (3)

PROGNOSIS
Despite adequate anticoagulation VTE has a recurrence rate of 7% at 6 months. Death occurs in 6% of cases of DVT and 12% of cases of PE within 1 month of diagnosis (1)

COMPLICATIONS
- Acute cardiopulmonary failure
- Postthrombotic syndrome
- Pulmonary hypertension

REFERENCES
1. Blann AD, Yip GY. Venous thromboembolism. *BMJ*. 2006;332;215–219.
2. Ramzi DW, Leeper KI. DVT and pulmonary embolism: Diagnosis. *AAFP*. 2006;69(12).
3. Antithrombotic therapy. The VII ACCP Conference on Antithrombotic and Thrombolytic Therapy, *Chest*. 2004;126;401–428 (updated Feb, 2006).

 MISCELLANEOUS

CODES

ICD9-CM
- 451.1 DVT
- 453.9 PE

PATIENT TEACHING

See Corresponding Diagnostic Algorithm

H

HYPEREMESIS GRAVIDARUM

Scott A. Fields, MD

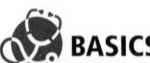 **BASICS**

DESCRIPTION
- Persistent vomiting in a pregnant woman that interferes with fluid and electrolyte balance, as well as nutrition
- Usually associated with the 1st 8–20 weeks of pregnancy
- Believed to have biomedical and behavioral aspects
- Associated with high estrogen levels
- Symptoms usually begin ~2 weeks after 1st missed period.
- System(s) Affected: Endocrine/Metabolic; Gastrointestinal; Reproductive
- Synonym(s): Morning sickness

ALERT
Pregnancy Considerations
Problem is confined to early pregnancy.

GENERAL PREVENTION
Anticipatory guidance in 1st and 2nd trimesters regarding dietary habits, in hopes of avoiding volume and nutritional depletion

EPIDEMIOLOGY
- Predominant age: Childbearing age
- Predominant sex: Female only

Pregnancy Considerations
- 2% of pregnancies have electrolyte disturbances.
- 50% of pregnancies have at least some gastrointestinal disturbance.

RISK FACTORS
- Trophoblastic activity
- Gonadotropin production stimulated
- Altered gastrointestinal function
- Various odors
- Taste or sight of food
- Hyperthyroidism
- Hyperparathyroidism
- Obesity
- Multiple gestations
- Nulliparity
- Liver dysfunction

Genetics
Unknown

ETIOLOGY
- Unknown
- Possible psychologic factors
- Hyperthyroidism
- Hyperparathyroidism
- Gestational hormones
- Liver dysfunction
- Autonomic nervous system dysfunction

ASSOCIATED CONDITIONS
Hyperthyroidism

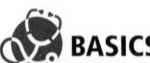 **DIAGNOSIS**

SIGNS AND SYMPTOMS
- Hypersensitivity to smell
- Alteration in taste
- Nausea
- Vomiting with retching
- Acidosis
- Decreased urine output
- Volume depletion
- Fatigue
- Starvation

TESTS
- TSH, T4
- Electrolytes, BUN, creatinine
- Calcium

Lab
- Electrolytes decreased
- Urinalysis—glucosuria, albuminuria, granular casts, and hematuria (rare); ketosis more common
- Increased uric acid
- Reduced protein
- Drugs unlikely to alter lab results
- If hypercalcemia, consider PTH for hyperparathyroidism.

Imaging
No imaging is indicated for the diagnosis of hyperemesis gravidarum.

Diagnostic Procedures/Surgery
Indicated only if it is necessary to rule out other diagnoses as listed below

Pathological Findings
- Fatty degeneration of the liver
- Renal tubular damage
- Heart damage in pregnant patient
- Petechial brain hemorrhages in pregnant patient

DIFFERENTIAL DIAGNOSIS
Other common causes of vomiting must be considered
- Gastroenteritis
- Gastritis
- Reflux esophagitis
- Peptic ulcer disease
- Cholelithiasis
- Cholecystitis
- Pyelonephritis
- Anxiety
- Hyperparathyroidism

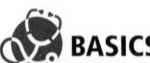 **TREATMENT**

INITIAL STABILIZATION
- Outpatient therapy
- In some severe cases, inpatient parenteral or enteral volume and nutrition repletion may be indicated.

GENERAL MEASURES (1–3)[C]
- Patient reassurance
- Bed rest
- If dehydrated, IV fluids. Repeat if there is a recurrence of symptoms following initial improvement.

Diet (2)[C]
- NPO for 1st 24 hours if patient is ill enough to require hospitalization
- For outpatient: A diet rich in carbohydrates and protein, such as fruit, cheese, cottage cheese, eggs, beef, poultry, vegetables, toast, crackers, rice. Limit intake of butter. Patients should avoid spicy meals and high-fat foods.

Activity
As tolerated after improvement (1–3)[C]

MEDICATION (DRUGS) (4)[A]

- Pyridoxine 10–30 mg IV daily
- Antihistamines (e.g., diphenhydramine [25–50 mg q4–6h] or dimenhydrinate, or doxylamine)
- Phenothiazines (e.g., promethazine or prochlorperazine)
- Meclizine 25 mg q6h
- Methylprednisolone 16 mg PO × daily for 3 days, then taper over 2 weeks
- Ginger 350 mg PO t.i.d. may help (see "References").
- Contraindications: All medications taken during pregnancy should balance the risks and benefits both to the mother and the fetus. Avoid all drugs if possible.
- Precautions: Phenothiazines associated with prolonged jaundice, extrapyramidal effects, hyper- or hyporeflexia in newborns
- Significant possible interactions: Refer to manufacturer's profile for each drug.

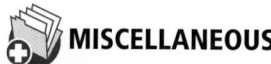 **FOLLOW-UP**

PROGNOSIS

- Self-limited illness with good prognosis if patient's weight is maintained at >95% of prepregnancy weight
- With complication of hemorrhagic retinitis, mortality rate of pregnant patient is 50%.

COMPLICATIONS

- Patients with >5% weight loss are associated with intrauterine growth retardation and fetal anomalies.
- Hemorrhagic retinitis
- Liver damage
- CNS deterioration, sometimes to coma

PATIENT MONITORING

- In severe cases, follow-up on a daily basis for weight monitoring.
- Special attention should be given to monitoring for ketosis, hypokalemia, or acid–base disturbances due to hyperemesis.

REFERENCES

1. Cowan MJ. Hyperemesis gravidarum: Implications for home cure and infusion therapies. *J Intraven Nurs*. 1996;19:46–58.
2. Eliakim R, Abulafia O, Sherer DM. Hyperemesis gravidarum: A current review. *Am J Perinatol*. 2000;17:207–218.
3. Goodwin TM. Hyperemesis gravidarum. *Clin Obstet Gynecol*. 1998;41:597–605.
4. Jewell D, Young G. Interventions for nausea and vomiting in early pregnancy. Cochrane Pregnancy and Childbirth Group Cochrane Database of Systematic Reviews. 1, 2006.
5. Yost NP, McIntire DD, Wians FH, Ramin SM, Balko JA, Leveno KJ. A randomized, placebo-controlled trial of corticosteroids for hyperemesis due to pregnancy. *Obstet Gynecol*. 2003;102:1250–1254.
6. Borrelli F, Capasso R, Aviello G, Pittler MH, Izzo AA. Effectiveness and safety of ginger in the treatment of pregnancy-induced nausea and vomiting. *Obstet Gynecol*. 2005;105(4):849–856.
7. Trogstad LI, Stoltenberg C, Magnus P, Skjaerven R, Irgens LM. Recurrence risk in hyperemesis gravidarum. BJOG: An International Journal of Obstetrics & Gynaecology. 2005;112(12): 1641–1645.

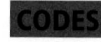 **MISCELLANEOUS**

CODES

ICD9-CM

- 643.00 Mild hyperemesis gravidarum, unspecified
- 643.1 Hyperemesis gravidarum with metabolic disturbance, unspecified

PATIENT TEACHING

- Attention should be given to psychosocial issues such as possible ambivalence about the pregnancy.
- Patients should be instructed to take small amounts of fluid frequently to avoid volume depletion.

Diet

- Avoidance of individual foods known to be irritating to the patient
- Wet-to-dry nutrients (sherbet, broth, gelatin, to dry crackers, toast)
- Pyridoxine (vitamin B_6)

H

HYPERKALEMIA

Jacqueline J. Wu, MD
Ruben Peralta, MD, FACS

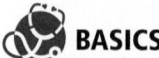 **BASICS**

DESCRIPTION
- A common electrolyte disorder with plasma potassium (K) concentration >5.5 mEq/L (>5.0 mmol/L). Can be life-threatening.
- 4 major causes
  - Increased load: Either endogenous from tissue release or exogenous from a high intake, which is usually in association with impaired excretion
  - Decreased excretion: Due to decreased glomerular filtration rate
  - Cellular redistribution: Shifting of intracellular (which is the major store of K) to extracellular space
  - Pseudohyperkalemia: Related to improper collection or transport of blood sample
- Synonym(s): Hyperpotassemia

ALERT
Geriatric Considerations
Increased risk for hyperkalemia due to decreases in renin and aldosterone as well as increased number of comorbid conditions.

Pediatric Considerations
Rare congenital abnormalities.

GENERAL PREVENTION
Diet and oral supplement compliance

EPIDEMIOLOGY
Incidence
Common

Prevalence
Male = Female

RISK FACTORS
- Impaired renal function is the major risk factor
- Acidemia
- Massive cell breakdown
- Use of K-sparing diuretics
- Excess K supplementation

Genetics
Rare, autosomal dominant skeletal muscle sodium channel defect causing hyperkalemic paralysis

ETIOLOGY
- Pseudohyperkalemia
  - Hemolysis (most common)
  - Thrombolysis
  - Leukocytosis
  - Thrombocytosis
  - Hereditary spherocytosis
  - Infectious mononucleosis
- Familial
- Traumatic venipuncture or fist clenching during phlebotomy
- Transcellular shift (Redistribution)
  - Metabolic acidosis
  - Insulin deficiency
  - Hyperglycemia
  - Nonselective β-blockade
  - Digitalis intoxication
  - Succinylcholine
  - Arginine hydrochloride/lysine hydrochloride
  - Fluoride intoxication
  - Exercise with heavy sweating
  - Mannitol
  - Somatostatin
  - Intravenous amino acids
- Increased endogenous K load
  - Hemolysis
  - Exercise
  - Rhabdomyolysis
  - GI bleeding
  - Acute tumor lysis
  - Catabolic states
- Increased exogenous K load
  - Parenteral administration
  - High-K food
  - Salt substitutes
  - K penicillin G
  - Stored blood
  - Overdose of K supplements
- Decreased renal K excretion
  - Decreased glomerular filtration rate
    ○ Chronic renal failure
    ○ Acute renal failure
  - Impairment of distal renal tubular system
    ○ Renal tubular acidosis II and IV
    ○ Systemic lupus erythematosus
    ○ Sickle cell disease
    ○ Obstructive uropathy
    ○ Post kidney transplantation
    ○ Amyloidosis
    ○ Tubulointerstitial nephritis
  - Alterations of rennin-angiotensin-aldosterone system
    ○ ACE inhibitor
    ○ Angiotensin receptor blocker
    ○ NSAIDs
    ○ Calcineurin inhibitors (tacrolimus, cyclosporine)
    ○ Heparin
    ○ Lithium
    ○ Aldosterone antagonist (spironolactone, eplerenone)
  - Primary hypoaldosteronism

ASSOCIATED CONDITIONS
- Renal failure
- Mineralocorticoid deficiency

DIAGNOSIS

SIGNS AND SYMPTOMS
- Cardiac: Most important, and frequent symptoms
  - Peaked T wave
  - Flattened P wave
  - Prolonged PR interval
  - Widened QRS complex
  - Sine wave
  - Ventricular fibrillation
  - Cardiac arrest
- Neuromuscular
  - Diarrhea
  - Abdominal pain
  - Myalgias
  - Numbness
  - Weakness
  - Decreased deep tender reflexes
  - Flaccid paralysis of extremities

TESTS
Lab
- K >5.5 mEq/L (5.0 mmol/L)
- Disorders that may alter lab results
  - Acidemia: K shifts from the intracellular to extracellular space in an effort to buffer the acid load. Once acidemia is corrected, the K may return to normal or even become decreased.
  - Insulin deficiency
- Special tests
  - ECG changes usually evolve as K rises above 6.0mEq/L
  - Cortisol and aldosterone levels to check for mineralocorticoid deficiency when other causes are ruled out

DIFFERENTIAL DIAGNOSIS
- Cardiac arrhythmias
- Hypocalcemia

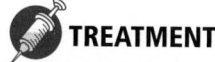 ## TREATMENT

INITIAL STABILIZATION
Inpatient with cardiac monitoring if ECG changes are present or K is >6.0 mEq/L (6.0 mmol/L)

GENERAL MEASURES
- If hyperkalemia is severe, treat 1st, then do diagnostic investigations.
- Discontinue any K-sparing drugs or dietary K.
- Major goal is to find the cause of hyperkalemia

Diet
80 mEq (80 mmol) or less of K per 24 hours

Activity
Bed rest

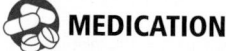 ## MEDICATION (DRUGS)

First Line
- Discontinue any medications that may increase K (e.g., K-sparing diuretics, exogenous K).
- Dextrose: (1 ampule of D50) and insulin (10 units of regular subcutaneous)
  – Temporarily shifts K intracellularly; takes effect in the 1st 30 minutes and only lasts a short time
- β-Adrenergic agonists (epinephrine, albuterol, terbutaline, salbutamol, salmeterol)
  – Can be administered IV or via nebulizer
- Sodium polystyrene sulfonate (Kayexalate): 30–60 g PO or rectally
  – This is effective in 1–4 hours and is a definitive treatment. This may be repeated q6h, if necessary.
- Diuretics (loop and thiazides)
- Calcium gluconate: 1 ampule is cardioprotective only and should only be used when ECG changes are present.
- Hemodialysis is an option when other measures are not effective.

ALERT
- Kayexalate provides a sodium load that may exacerbate fluid overload in cardiac or renal failure patients.
- Rapid administration of calcium in patients with suspected digitalis toxicity may result in a fatal dysrhythmia.
- Calcium and dextrose/insulin are only temporizing measures and do not actually lower total body K levels.
- Sodium bicarbonate is no longer recommended to lower K, although it may be appropriate in patients with severe metabolic acidosis.

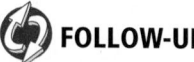 ## FOLLOW-UP

PROGNOSIS
- Full resolution with correction of the underlying cause
- Reduction of plasma K should begin within the 1st hour of initiation of treatment.

COMPLICATIONS
- Life-threatening cardiac arrhythmias
- Hypokalemia

PATIENT MONITORING
- Serum K levels should be rechecked every 2–4 hours until the patient has stabilized and recurrent hyperkalemia is no longer a threat.
- Identification and elimination of possible causes and risk factors for hyperkalemia is essential.

REFERENCES
1. Evans KJ, Greenberg A. Hyperkalemia: a review. *J Intensive Care Med*. 2005;20:272–290.
2. Hollander-Rodriguez JC, Calvert JF Jr. Hyperkalemia. *Amer Family Phys*. 2006(73)2:283–290.
3. Schaefer TJ, Wolford RW. Disorders of potassium. *Emerg Med Clin North Amer*. 2005;23:723–747.

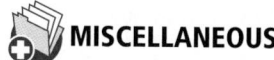 ## MISCELLANEOUS

See also: Addison disease, Hypokalemia

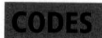 **CODES**

ICD9-CM
276.7 Hyperpotassemia

PATIENT TEACHING
Consult with dietitian about a low-K diet.

 See Corresponding Diagnostic Algorithm

H

HYPERNATREMIA

Fae Gwen B. Ganiron, BS, PharmD
Joshua M. V. Mammen, MD

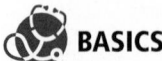 **BASICS**

DESCRIPTION
- Serum sodium (Na) concentration level >145 mEq/L and usually represents a state of hyperosmolality. Hypernatremia results from primary Na + gain or water deficit.
- Hypernatremia may exist with hypo-, hyper-, or euvolemia.
- Hypovolemic hypernatremia: Most common type; occurs with a decrease in total body water (TBW) and a lesser decrease in total body Na.
- Euvolemic hypernatremia: Increase in TBW with normal total body Na.
- Hypervolemic hypernatremia: Increase in total body Na and a lesser increase in TBW.

ALERT
Geriatric Considerations
- More common in the hospitalized patient, resulting in a higher morbidity or mortality.
- Hypernatremia may be caused by dehydration due to administration of loop diuretics.
- Increased risk occurs because of impaired renal function and decline in thirst mechanism.
- Chronically ill patients are at higher risk due to consumption of high-solute formulas.

Pediatric Considerations
- May occur in low-birth-weight newborns.
- May result from improper preparation of infant formula or high concentration of Na in breast milk.

GENERAL PREVENTION
- Treatment or prevention of underlying cause
- Avoid preparing infant formula at home, and never add salt to any commercial infant formula.
- Keep well hydrated.

EPIDEMIOLOGY
Incidence
- Common in elderly, infants, and children
- Gastroenteritis with diarrhea is the most common cause of hypernatremia in infants.

Prevalence
Females are at an increased risk due to their decreased TBW.

RISK FACTORS
- Children
- Elderly
- Patients who are intubated or have altered mental status

Genetics
Some diabetes insipidus may be hereditary.

ETIOLOGY
- Excess Na (increase in total body Na) resulting from
  - Incorrect infant formulary preparation
  - Salt given as punishment or as a prank
  - Sea water ingestion
  - Excessive use of $NaHCO_3$ as an antacid
  - IV NaCl or $NaHCO_3$ during cardiopulmonary resuscitation, metabolic acidosis, or hyperkalemia
  - Intrauterine NaCl for abortion
  - Excessive Na in dialysate solutions
  - Disorders of the adrenal axis (Cushing syndrome, Conn syndrome, congenital adrenal hyperplasia)
- Water deficit (total body Na normal) resulting from
  - Adipsia (e.g., impaired thirst regulation, decreased access to water)
  - Increased urine water loss (e.g., diabetes insipidus)
  - Increased insensible water loss (e.g., fever, hyperventilation, hypermetabolic state, sweat, severe burns, heat exposure, newborns under radiant warmers)
- Hypotonic fluid loss (total body Na decreased) resulting from
  - Loss of fluid containing Na without adequate water replacement
- Urinary loss
  - Osmotic diuretics
  - Diabetes mellitus
  - Diuresis from acute tubular necrosis (ATN) or from relief of acute urinary obstruction
- GI loss
  - Diarrhea, especially in children

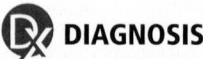 **DIAGNOSIS**

SIGNS AND SYMPTOMS
- Varies with the underlying disorder and extent of hypernatremia
- Cardiovascular: Sinus tachycardia, hypotension, orthostatic hypotension
- Dermatologic: Decreased skin turgor, cool skin, dry sticky mucous membranes, gray skin, fever
- GI: Excessive thirst, nausea and vomiting (common in infants and children), diarrhea
- Musculoskeletal: Muscle cramps and weakness
- Neurologic: Altered mental status, restlessness, mania, irritability, lethargy, coma, hemiparesis, seizures (symptomatic when Na >160 mEq/L), hyperreflexia, high-pitched cry, chorea, muscle twitching
- Ophthalmic: Sunken eyes
- Respiratory: Dyspnea
- Urologic: Oliguria or anuria, polyuria (suspect diabetes insipidus in the absence of osmotic diuresis)

History
- Obtain list of current and recent medications.
- Obtain history of recent illnesses and activities.

TESTS
- Serum Na and osmolality
- Urine Na and osmolality
- Urinalysis
- Serum glucose
- Special tests
  - Water deprivation (with diabetes insipidus, urine osmolality does not increase when hypernatremic)
  - Antidiuretic hormone (ADH) stimulation (with nephrogenic diabetes insipidus, urine osmolality does not increase after ADH or DDAVP)

Lab

- Serum Na >150–170 mEq/L (>150–170 mmol/L): Usually dehydration
- Serum Na >170 mEq/L (>170 mmol/L): Usually diabetes insipidus
- Serum Na >190 mEq/L (>190 mmol/L): Usually chronic salt ingestion
- Diabetes insipidus
  - Urine osmolality less than serum osmolality
  - Urine Na usually low
  - Polyuria
  - Neurogenic vs. nephrogenic diabetes insipidus
- Hyperosmolar coma
  - Blood sugar elevated
  - Decreased urine output
  - Increased urine osmolality
- Salt ingestion
  - Increased urine Na
  - Increased urine osmolality
- Hypertonic dehydration
  - Decreased urine Na
  - Increased urine osmolality

ALERT
A variety of medications may raise or lower Na levels. Refer to a laboratory test reference.

Imaging
CT or MRI in diabetes insipidus to rule out craniopharyngioma, tumor, or median cleft syndrome

Diagnostic Procedures/Surgery
History, physical, laboratory studies, family history for neurogenic diabetes insipidus

DIFFERENTIAL DIAGNOSIS

- Diabetes insipidus
- Hyperosmotic coma
- Salt ingestion
- Hypertonic dehydration

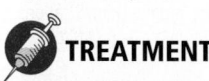

TREATMENT

GENERAL MEASURES

- Appropriate healthcare: Inpatient (many patients are already hospitalized, and hypernatremia develops after admission)
- Treat hypovolemia 1st, then treat hypernatremia.
- Water replacement orally, if patient is conscious
- Restore intravascular volume with IV fluids to normalize serum Na levels
- Calculated water deficit (liters) = $[(0.6 \times wt) \times (Na - 140)] \div 140$
  - Note: wt = weight in kilograms; Na = current serum Na.
- Dialysis: Especially with serum Na >200 mEq/L (200 mmol/L)
- Speed of correction depends on severity of symptoms or rate of development of hypernatremia.

Diet

- Ensure proper nutrition during acute phase.
- After resolution of acute phase, may want to consider Na-restricted diet for patient
- Severe salt restriction in nephrogenic diabetes insipidus

Activity
Bed rest until stable or underlying condition resolved or controlled

MEDICATION (DRUGS)

First Line

- Hypovolemia
  - Isotonic saline (normal saline or Ringer's lactate): 10–20 mL/kg IV over 1–2 hours. May repeat if ≥10% dehydration
  - Isotonic fluids: 5% dextrose with half-normal saline until urine output established
- Hypernatremia
  - Hypotonic fluids (NaCl or dextrose 5% in water)
  - Decrease serum Na by 0.5 mEq/L/hr (0.5 mmol/L/hr) or by no more than 20 mEq/L/d (20 mmol/L/d). Allows idiogenic osmoles to resolve (mostly taurine in brain cell water)
  - Hypocalcemia may occur during correction of hypernatremia. Add calcium (50 mg/kg 10% calcium gluconate) to IV fluids.
  - Acidosis often is present in severely dehydrated patients. Add sodium bicarbonate, 50 mEq/L, to IV fluids. If both acidosis and hypocalcemia are present simultaneously, correct the calcium deficit 1st.
  - Potassium and phosphate, if needed
- Neurogenic diabetes insipidus (DI)
  - Desmopressin (DDAVP) acetate: Adults 10–40 μg intranasally in 1–3 divided doses; children 5–30 μg in a single evening dose or in 2 divided doses. Oral DDAVP now available, dosage varies
  - May use 2.5% dextrose in water if giving large volumes of water in diabetes insipidus or neurogenic diabetes insipidus to avoid glycosuria
- Nephrogenic diabetes insipidus (NDI)
  - Chlorothiazide: 10 mg/kg per dose given b.i.d.
  - Chlorpropamide: 100–250 mg each morning
- Contraindications: Refer to manufacturer's literature.
- Precautions
  - Rapid correction of hypernatremia can cause cerebral or pulmonary edema, seizures, or death. Hypocalcemia often occurs during correction.
  - Diabetes insipidus: High rates of dextrose 5% in water can cause hyperglycemia and glucose-induced diuresis.
- Significant possible interactions: Refer to manufacturer's literature.

Second Line
Consider NSAIDs in nephrogenic diabetes insipidus.

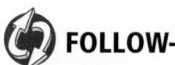

FOLLOW-UP

DISPOSITION
Admission Criteria
Symptomatic patient with serum Na >155 mEq/L requires IV fluid therapy.

Discharge Criteria
Stabilization of serum Na level and symptoms are minimal.

Issues for Referral

- Children should be referred to a pediatrician.
- Underlying renal involvement associated with hypernatremia should be seen by a nephrologist.
- Follow-up with primary care physician is essential.

PROGNOSIS
Most recover, but rate of neurologic impairment is high.

COMPLICATIONS

- Central nervous system (CNS) thrombosis or hemorrhage
- Seizures
- Mental retardation
- Hyperactivity
- Chronic hypernatremia: >2 days' duration has higher mortality.
- Serum Na >180 mEq/L (>180 mmol/L): Often results in residual CNS damage

PATIENT MONITORING

- Frequent re-examinations in an acute setting
- Frequent electrolytes
- Urine osmolality and urine output in diabetes insipidus
- Ensure adequate ingestion of calories, because patients may ingest so much water that they feel full and do not eat.
- Daily weights

REFERENCES

1. Adrogue HJ, Madias NE. Hypernatremia. *N Engl J Med*. 2000;342:1493–99.
2. Barratt T, Avner E, Harmon W, eds. Pediatric Nephrology, 4th ed. Baltimore: Williams & Wilkins; 2000.
3. Kokko J, Tannen R, eds. Fluid and Electrolytes, 3rd ed. Philadelphia: WB Saunders; 1996.
4. Kraft MD, Btaiche IF, Sachs GS, et al. Treatment of electrolyte disorders in adult patients in the intensive care unit. *Am J Health-System Pharm.*, 2005;62:166382.
5. Kugler JP, Hustead T. Hyponatremia and hypernatremia in the elderly. *Am Fam Physician*. 2000;61:3623–3630.

MISCELLANEOUS

See also: Diabetes insipidus

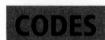 CODES

ICD9-CM
270.6 Disorders of urea cycle metabolism

PATIENT TEACHING
Patients with nephrogenic diabetes insipidus must avoid salt and drink large amounts of water.

 See Corresponding Diagnostic Algorithm

H

HYPERPARATHYROIDISM

Matthew P. Hill, MD

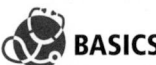 **BASICS**

DESCRIPTION
Hyperparathyroidism represents an acute or chronic dysfunction of the body's normal regulatory feedback mechanism on the parathyroid glands, resulting in gland hyperfunction and abnormal calcium metabolism.

- Primary hyperparathyroidism
  - Intrinsic gland dysfunction causing inappropriate parathyroid hormone (PTH) secretion
- Secondary hyperparathyroidism
  - Gland hyperactivity induced by extrinsic factors causing hypocalcemia
- Tertiary hyperparathyroidism
  - Gland hyperactivity autonomous from normal negative feedback mechanisms
- System(s) Affected: Endocrine/Metabolic

ALERT
Geriatric Considerations
- More likely to have a secondary disease
- May cause confusion and be interpreted as senile dementia

Pregnancy Considerations
Untreated can cause fetal complications: Intrauterine growth retardation, low birth weight, preterm delivery, intrauterine fetal demise, postpartum neonatal tetany, permanent hypoparathyroidism

EPIDEMIOLOGY
- Predominant age
  - More common in persons >50 years
  - Male adults >60 years: 100 cases per 100,000
  - Female adults >60 years: 300–400 cases per 100,000
  - All-age adjusted incidence: 42 cases per 100,000
- Predominant sex: Females > Male (4:1)

Prevalence
Prevalence (all ages): 250 cases per 100,000 population

RISK FACTORS
- Age: >50 years
- Female
- Chronic lithium therapy
- History of neck irradiation

ETIOLOGY
- Primary hyperparathyroidism: Unregulated increase of PTH production and release, causing increase in serum calcium
  - Solitary adenoma (85%)
  - Diffuse hyperplasia (15%) caused by
    - Multiple adenomas, multiple endocrine neoplasia types I and II, familial hypocalciuric hypercalcemia
  - Parathyroid carcinoma (<1%)
- Secondary hyperparathyroidism: Adaptive parathyroid gland hyperplasia and hyperfunction
  - Chronic renal disease resulting in
    - Renal parenchymal loss causing hyperphosphatemia
    - Impaired calcitriol production causing hypocalcemia
  - General skeletal and renal resistance to PTH.

- Tertiary hyperparathyroidism: Hyperplasia resulting in autonomous PTH oversecretion
  - Chronic kidney disease

ASSOCIATED CONDITIONS
Multiple endocrine neoplasia (MEN) syndromes

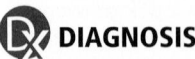 **DIAGNOSIS**

SIGNS AND SYMPTOMS
- Painful bones, renal stones, abdominal groans, and psychic moans. You must think of it to diagnose it.
- Renal: Nephrolithiasis, nephrocalcinosis, reduced glomerular filtration rate, thirst, polydipsia, polyuria
- Gastrointestinal: Abdominal distress, gastroduodenal ulcer, pancreatitis, pancreatic calcification, constipation, vomiting, anorexia, weight loss
- Skeletal: Bone pain, cystic bone lesions, skeletal demineralization, spontaneous fracture, vertebral collapse, osteoporosis
- Mental: Fatigue, apathy, anxiety, depression, psychosis
- Neurologic: Somnolence, coma, diffuse EEG changes
- Neuromuscular: Muscle fatigue, weakness, hypotonia
- Cardiovascular: Hypertension, short QT interval
- Articular/periarticular: Arthralgia, gout, pseudogout, periarticular calcification
- Ocular: Band keratopathy, conjunctivitis, conjuctival calcium deposits

TESTS
Immunoassay directed against intact PTH molecule

Lab
- Elevated corrected serum calcium >10.2 mg/dL (2.55 mmol/L) on 2 occasions
- Elevated serum immunoreactive PTH levels >3.0 pmol/L (30 ng/L)
  - Value in upper 1/2 of reference range in the presence of elevated calcium is highly suggestive. (1)[B]
- Low serum phosphate levels, <2.5 mg/dL (0.81 mmol/L)
- Elevated serum chloride levels
- Decreased serum CO_2
- Hyperchloremic metabolic acidosis
- Increase in urinary cyclic adenosine monophosphate (AMP)
- Obtain 24-hour urinary collection for calcium and creatinine excretion (to assess calcium/creatinine ratio: >0.02 suggestive of primary hyperparathyroidism) (2)[C]
- Drugs that may alter test results: Thiazides, lithium
- Disorders that may alter lab results: Hypoalbuminemia

Imaging
- Neck ultrasonography
- Thallium technetium (Tc) scanning
- Magnetic resonance imaging
- Computed tomography (CT) scanning with and without contrast
- Tc 99m sestamibi scan with single photon emission CT
  - Greatest accuracy for primary hyperparathyroidism. (1)[B]
  - Sensitivity 90.7%, Specificity 98.8%. (1)[B]
- Obtain bone mineral density (DXA). (2)[C]

Diagnostic Procedures/Surgery
- Percutaneous needle biopsy aspiration for cytology and PTH determination
- Open surgical removal with frozen section diagnosis

Pathological Findings
- Parathyroid hyperplasia: All parathyroid glands with cellular changes
- Parathyroid adenoma: Only 1 gland usually with cellular changes
- Parathyroid carcinoma: Cellular changes consistent with malignancy (i.e., atypia, lymph node changes)

DIFFERENTIAL DIAGNOSIS
- Other causes of elevated serum calcium level must be excluded.
- Increased PTH
  - Ectopic hyperparathyroidism
- Nonparathyroid causes
  - Malignancy: Lung (squamous cell) carcinoma, breast carcinoma, multiple myeloma, lymphoma, leukemia, prostate cancer, Paget disease
  - Granulomatous disease: Sarcoidosis, tuberculosis, berylliosis, histoplasmosis, coccidioidomycosis
  - Drugs: Thiazide diuretics, vitamin D intoxication, vitamin A excess, lithium, milk alkali syndrome, exogenous calcium intake
  - Endocrine: Hyperthyroidism, acute adrenal insufficiency
  - Familial: Hypocalciuric hypercalcemia
  - Immobilization

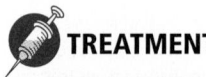 **TREATMENT**

GENERAL MEASURES
- A few patients with mild asymptomatic hypercalcemia owing to hyperparathyroidism may not be candidates for surgery and may be managed conservatively.
- Avoiding dehydration is the most important treatment.
  - Initiate IV fluid therapy with normal saline.

Diet
As indicated by condition of patient
- Pay attention to calcium consumption.

Activity
As tolerated

SPECIAL THERAPY
IV Fluids
For symptomatic hypercalcemia
- Normal saline to expand extracellular volume and promote calcium excretion

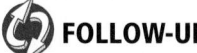 MEDICATION (DRUGS)

First Line
- Loop diuretics (i.e., furosemide).
  - Useful in well-hydrated hypercalcemic patients
  - Avoid in hypocalcemia.
- Bisphosphonates, specifically alendronate. (3)[A]
  - Reduces bone turnover and helps maintain bone density
  - Avoid in kidney disease.
- Calcimimetics (i.e., cinacalcet) (4)[A]
  - Mimics calcium and binds to calcium sensing receptor (CaR)
  - Shown to decrease calcium and PTH levels in primary hyperparathyroidism, secondary hyperparathyroidism, and in association with chronic kidney disease
- Hormone replacement therapy with estrogens and SERM therapy (i.e., raloxifene). (5)[B]
  - Use in postmenopausal women who do not undergo or refuse surgery
  - Must weigh benefit with risks of known systemic effects
- Contraindications: Refer to manufacturer's literature.
- Precautions: Refer to manufacturer's literature.
- Significant possible interactions: Refer to manufacturer's literature.
- Cost information: Refer to manufacturer's literature.

SURGERY
- Surgical removal of diseased gland is only proven curative therapy for hyperparathyroidism.
- Indications for surgery in asymptomatic primary hyperparathyroidism. (4)[C]
  - Serum Ca 1.0 mg/dL above normal, >400 mg 24 hour urinary Ca, creatinine clearance reduced by 30%, BMD T-score <−2.5 (any site), age <50 years
- Bilateral open neck exploration is procedure of choice.
  - Success rate of 95–98%. (1)[C]
- Minimally invasive parathyroidectomy using intraoperative adenoma localization may be indicated for some.
- Removal of obviously diseased gland with biopsies of other glands to make sure physiologically viable
- Total resection of all four glands with transplantation of normal gland to forearm advocated by some
- Special attention must be paid during exploration and removal of parathyroid glands to ectopic gland in the neck area.
- Postoperative course needs special attention paid to serum calcium level, bleeding, and risk of airway compromise.
  - Injectable calcium and seizure precautions maintained at bedside
- Monitor renal functions closely.

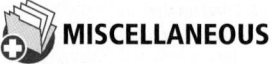 FOLLOW-UP

PROGNOSIS
- Postoperative course requires following of serum calcium to make sure hyperparathyroid state does not redevelop.
- Prognosis is excellent in primary hyperparathyroidism with resolution of many of the preoperative symptoms.
- Secondary hyperparathyroidism carries a poor prognosis because of the primary disease state of chronic renal failure.

COMPLICATIONS
- Skeletal damage (pathologic fractures)
- Renal damage
- Urinary tract infections
- "Parathyroid poisoning"
- Hypertension
- Surgery
  - Hypoparathyroidism
  - Recurrent laryngeal nerve damage
  - Bleeding
  - Infection
  - Unsuccessful surgery (5%)

PATIENT MONITORING
- Monitoring for asymptomatic primary hyperparathyroidism who do not undergo surgery (4)[C]
  - Serum calcium (semi-annually), serum creatinine (annually), bone density (annually)
  - Initial measurements of 24-hour urinary calcium, creatinine clearance, abdominal x-ray
- Postoperatively
  - Monitor renal function closely.
  - Potential precipitous fall in serum calcium resulting in development of transient tetany

REFERENCES

1. Davies M, Fraser WD, Hosking DJ. The management of primary hyperparathyroidism. *Clin Endocrinol*. 2002;57:145–155.
2. AACE/AAES Task Force on Primary Hyperparathyroidism. The American Association of Clinical Endocrinologists and the American Association of Endocrine Surgeons position statement on the diagnosis and management of primary hyperparathyroidism. *Endocr Pract*. 2005;11(1):49–54.
3. Bilezikian JP, Brandi ML, Rubin M, Silverberg SJ. Primary hyperparathyroidism: New concepts in clinical densitometric and biochemical features. *J Intern Med*. 2005;257:6–17.
4. Joy MS, Kshirsagar AV, Franceschini N. Calcimimetics and the treatment of primary and secondary hyperparathyroidism. *Ann Pharmacol*. 2004;38:1871–1880.
5. Arnaud CD. The parathyroid glands, hypercalcemia, and hypocalcemia. In: Wyngaarden JB, Smith LH, eds. *Cecil Textbook of Medicine*. 18th ed. Philadelphia: WB Saunders; 1988.
6. Clark O, Quan-Yank D. Primary hyperparathyroidism: A surgical perspective. *Endocrinol Metab Clin North Am*. 1989; 18:701–715.
7. Taniegra TD. Hyperparathyroidism. *Am Fam Physician*. 2004;69(2):333–339.

 MISCELLANEOUS

See also: Multiple endocrine neoplasia (MEN)

CODES

ICD9-CM
- 252.0 Hyperparathyroidism
- 259.3 Ectopic hormone secretion, NEC
- 588.8 Other specified disorder resulting from impaired renal function

PATIENT TEACHING
- Medications
- Importance of periodic lab exams

See Corresponding Diagnostic Algorithm

H

HYPERPROLACTINEMIA

Ruben Peratta, MD, FACS

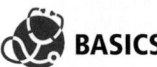 **BASICS**

DESCRIPTION
Hyperprolactinemia is an abnormal elevation in the serum prolactin with multiple possible etiologies.

EPIDEMIOLOGY
Prevalence
- Reproductive age
- Female > Male
- More readily detected in females because slight elevation in prolactin causes changes in menstruation and galactorrhea.

ETIOLOGY
- Prolactin, which is produced by lactotrophs in the anterior pituitary, is regulated by
  - Inhibitory factors, primarily dopamine, produced in the hypothalamus and delivered via the hypothalamic/pituitary vessels in the pituitary stalk
  - Stimulatory factors, primarily thyrotropin-releasing hormone
- Causes of hyperprolactinemia include
  - Physiologic
    ○ Pregnancy
    ○ Breast feeding
    ○ Nipple stimulation
    ○ Stress, including postoperative state
  - Medications (1)[B]
    ○ Dopamine (D_2) blockers: Antipsychotics, metoclopramide
    ○ Dopamine depleters: α-Methyldopa, reserpine
    ○ Opiates
    ○ Verapamil (but no other calcium-channel blockers; thought to decrease hypothalamic synthesis of dopamine)
    ○ Possibly antidepressants (minimal data)
  - Hypothyroidism (due to elevated TRH)
  - Chest wall conditions
    ○ Herpes zoster
    ○ Post thoracotomy
    ○ Trauma
  - Prolactin-secreting adenoma, categorized as
    ○ Microadenoma: 1 cm or less
    ○ Macroadenoma: >1 cm
  - Pituitary stalk compression/disruption
    ○ Craniopharyngioma
    ○ Rathke cleft cyst
    ○ Meningioma
    ○ Astrocytoma
    ○ Metastases
    ○ Head trauma
    ○ Infiltrative/inflammatory disorders
  - Diminished prolactin clearance
    ○ Renal failure
    ○ Cirrhosis
  - Cocaine

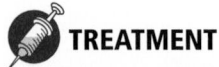 **DIAGNOSIS**

SIGNS AND SYMPTOMS
- Galactorrhea
- Amenorrhea
- Oligomenorrhea
- Infertility
- Osteoporosis/osteopenia
- Decreased libido
- Impotence in males
- Weight gain
- May also have signs and symptoms of pituitary enlargement
  - Headache
  - Visual field impairment (bitemporal hemianopsia)
  - Hypopituitarism (secondary to tumor pressure on surrounding structures)
- May also have signs and symptoms of associated conditions
  - Hypothyroidism
  - Cushing disease
  - Acromegaly

Physical Exam
- Visual field testing
- Cranial nerve exam

TESTS
Lab
- Serum prolactin (most accurate results if checked fasting, in morning)
- Pregnancy test
- Thyroid function tests
- LH/FSH if amenorrheic
- Chemistry, renal function
- Liver function tests
- Special tests: Formal visual field testing if pituitary adenoma suspected

Imaging
- MRI (even if prolactin is minimally elevated, to rule out hypothalamic tumors that may compress the pituitary stalk and thereby decrease delivery of prolactin inhibitory hormone with subsequent rise in prolactin)
- CT if MRI contraindicated

DIFFERENTIAL DIAGNOSIS
Macroprolactinemia: Macroprolactin, a polymer of several units of prolactin, is detected by immunologically based lab tests but is not biologically active. If patient is asymptomatic, but found to have elevated PRL, consider this diagnosis and notify lab. No treatment required (2)[B].

TREATMENT

GENERAL MEASURES
- Discontinue offending medications, if any.
- Treat underlying causes.
- For asymptomatic patients with mild PRL elevations, observation alone may be considered (3)[B].
- Medications indicated for (4)[B]
  - Symptoms of hypogonadism, such as decreased libido
  - Galactorrhea (if bothersome to patient)
  - Restoration of fertility
  - Pituitary adenoma
  - Prevention of osteoporosis

SPECIAL THERAPY
Radiotherapy
- Radiation therapy and stereotactic radiosurgery sometimes are considered in medically unresponsive, surgically unresectable tumors; PRL normalizes in 20–30%, with a high risk of hypopituitarism (3)[B].

MEDICATION (DRUGS)

First Line

- Dopamine agonists
  - Bromocriptine (Parlodel): Often, 1st-line treatment given this has longest clinical history. Dosed b.i.d.
  - Cabergoline (Dostinex): Dosed twice weekly; may be better tolerated; some consider this 1st-line; indicated with bromocriptine failure or resistance (3)[B]
  - Both are effective for reducing tumor size and improving symptoms (4, 5)[B]
- Adverse effects (better tolerated if start with low dose, slow titration, given at night with food)
  - Nausea/vomiting
  - Headache
  - Dizziness
  - Fatigue
  - Lightheadedness
  - Postural hypotension
- Pergolide (Permax), also a dopamine agonist, is less commonly used.

SURGERY

- For adenomas, medical treatment will be successful in 80–90% of patients, but in some cases, surgery is indicated (5)[B].
- Indications (4, 5) [B]
  - Intolerance or resistance to medical treatment
  - Headache
  - Visual field loss
  - CSF leak due to tumor apoplexy or shrinkage
  - Cranial nerve deficit
- Risks
  - High recurrence rate (up to 40%) (4)[B]
  - CSF leakage
  - Meningitis
  - Pituitary insufficiency

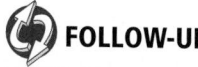 **FOLLOW-UP**

PROGNOSIS

- Tends to recur after discontinuation of medical therapy
- Over 10 years, 7% chance of progression of prolactin-secreting microadenoma (2)[B]

COMPLICATIONS

- Depends on underlying cause
- If pituitary adenoma, risk of permanent visual field loss

PATIENT MONITORING

- Depends on etiology
- Consider
  - Prolactin level every 6–12 months
  - Formal visual field testing yearly
  - Serial MRIs if clinically indicated

ALERT

Pregnancy Considerations

If pregnancy is desired in a woman with hyperprolactinemia (3)[B]

- With microprolactinoma: Treat with bromocriptine; monthly pregnancy tests; discontinue bromocriptine when pregnancy confirmed.
- With macroprolactinomas: Treat with bromocriptine at least until optic system no longer compromised, then attempt pregnancy
- Careful monitoring of visual field testing and PRL levels during pregnancy is advised.

REFERENCES

1. Molitch ME. Medication-Induced Hyperprolactinemia. *Mayo Clin Pro.* 2005;80:1050–1057.
2. Serri O, Chik CL, Ehud U. Diagnosis and management of hyperprolactinemia. *Can Med J* 2003;169.
3. Pickett CA. Diagnosis and management of pituitary tumors: recent advances. *Prim Care Clin Office Pract* 2003;30:765–789.
4. Jackson J, Safranek S. What is the recommended evaluation and treatment for elevated serum prolactin? *JFP* 2006;54:897–899.
5. Hamilton DK, Vince ML, Boulos PT, et al. Surgical Outcomes in hyporesponsive prolactinomas: Analysis of patients with resistance or intolerance to dopamine agonists. *Pituitary* 8:53–60.
6. Pinzone JJ, Katznelson L, Danila DC. Primary medical therapy of micro- and macroprolactinomas in men. *J Clin Endocrinol Metabol* 2002;85: 3053–3057.

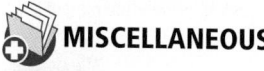 **MISCELLANEOUS**

CODES

ICD9-CM

- 611.6 Galactorrhea not associated with childbirth
- 259.9 Unspecified endocrine disorder

PATIENT TEACHING

Discussion of risks of untreated hyperprolactinemia:

- Headache
- Visual field loss
- Decreased bone density
- Infertility

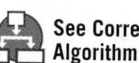 **See Corresponding Diagnostic Algorithm**

H

HYPERSENSITIVITY PNEUMONITIS

Sarah A. Tapyrik, MD
Muhanned Abu-Hijleh, MD, FCCP

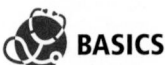 **BASICS**

DESCRIPTION
- Hypersensitivity pneumonitis (extrinsic allergic alveolitis) is a diffuse inflammatory disease of the lung caused by repeated inhalation of dust constituted of animal proteins, plant proteins, or reactive inorganic compounds.
- Common features (regardless of the etiologic inhalant)
  - Involvement of peripheral airways, alveoli, and interstitium
  - Mononuclear cell infiltration of interstitium with granuloma formation and increased alveolar macrophage activity
  - Precipitating antibodies against offending dust without complement activation
  - Normal IgE and eosinophil levels are present in a chronic form. The patient may present as either acute or subacute to chronic progressive pneumonitis.
- System(s) Affected: Pulmonary
- Synonym(s): Extrinsic allergic alveolitis; Allergic interstitial pneumonia

ALERT
Pregnancy Considerations
- Avoidance of antigen in early pregnancy
- Avoidance of antigen and medication in later pregnancy

GENERAL PREVENTION
Antigens must be avoided to stop the process.

EPIDEMIOLOGY
- Predominant age: Tends to occur in adults because of occupation-related exposure
- Predominant sex: Male = Female

Incidence
- National prevalence unknown
- 1–8% of farmers and 6–15% of pigeon breeders develop related pneumonitis.

RISK FACTORS
- Intensity of exposure
- Size (1–5-micron particles reach deep into lung)
- Smokers at lower risk than nonsmokers

Genetics
Not related to atopic predisposition, blood type or HLA type

ETIOLOGY
Exposure to dust capable of inciting immune response
- Farmer lung (*Thermophilic actinomycetes*)
- Air conditioner lung (*T. actinomycetes*)
- Bagassosis (*T. actinomycetes*)
- Bird breeder lung (avian protein and blood)
- Rat handler lung (rat urine and protein)
- Isocyanate lung (toluene diisocyanate [TDI], methylene diisocyanate [MDI] exposure)
- Washing powder lung (*Bacillus subtilis* enzymes)

DIAGNOSIS

SIGNS AND SYMPTOMS
- Acute hypersensitivity pneumonitis: Occurs within 6 hours of exposure to the offending antigen; may mimic an acute infectious pneumonia.
  - Fever up to 40°C
  - Cough
  - Dyspnea
  - Malaise
  - Body aches
  - Rare hemoptysis or sputum production
  - Hypoxia
  - Fine, mid-inspiratory to end-inspiratory crackles in chest
- Chronic hypersensitivity pneumonitis: Chronic progressive condition without acute exacerbation
  - Chronic cough
  - Dyspnea and exercise limitation
  - Anorexia and weight loss
  - Fatigue
  - Progressive hypoxia and cyanosis
  - Clubbing
  - Fine, mid-inspiratory to end-inspiratory crackles in chest
  - Cor pulmonale with right heart failure

TESTS
Lab
- Leukocytosis with polymorphonuclear predominance in acute form
- Nonspecific elevation of immunoglobulins and ESR
- Positive rheumatoid test and mononucleosis spot test
- Negative blood, sputum, throat cultures

ALERT
- Bronchodilators alter lung function
- Asthma or atopy may lead to eosinophilia or increased IgE levels and confuse picture.
- Special tests
  - Serum IgG precipitating antibodies to offending agent
  - Note: 40–50% of nonhypersensitive individuals with high exposure have positive precipitating antibodies.
  - Skin testing: Standardized agents poorly available and of limited use
  - Inhalation challenge testing can cause severe reactions and, therefore, is usually not performed except in specialized, in-hospital units.
  - Pulmonary function studies demonstrate
    - Reduced lung volume; impaired gas transfer; forced expiratory volume (FEV) 1, forced vital capacity (FVC), and FEV1/FVC ratio may be normal early on and then drop with the development of chronic airway obstruction; forced expiratory flow (FEF) 25–75 and flows near residual volume may be reduced; decreased lung compliance
- Bronchoalveolar lavage (BAL)
  - Acute form with neutrophils and lymphocytes
  - Chronic form with high lymphocytes (60%) mostly T cells of CD-8 type
  - Differentiate from sarcoid which has mostly T cells of CD-4 type

Imaging
- Acute hypersensitivity pneumonitis on chest radiograph (CXR)
  - Abnormal CXR: 30–40%
  - Diffuse interstitial infiltrate with hazy background
  - Fine nodular shadows from 1–3 mm in size
  - Linear striated shadows
  - Occasional lower lobe consolidation
  - Resolution between attacks
- Chronic hypersensitivity pneumonitis on CXR
  - Reticulonodular pattern
  - Linear shadows and nodules change from fine to coarse pattern with progression of disease
  - No hilar adenopathy, pleural effusion, or pneumothorax
  - Upper lobe predominance in 40–50% of cases with ring shadows and bronchiectasis
- The role of a CT scan is unclear.

Diagnostic Procedures/Surgery
A lung biopsy is rarely needed if treatment and avoidance of exposure results in improvement (see "Pathological Findings").

Pathological Findings
- Acute hypersensitivity pneumonitis
  - Alveolar walls are infiltrated by polymorphs, lymphocytes, macrophages, and plasma cells.
  - Eosinophils are rare.
  - Alveolar space contains proteinaceous exudate and edema.
  - Alveolar capillaries contain fibrin/platelet thrombi, but no vasculitis.
- Chronic hypersensitivity pneumonitis
  - Alveolitis and interstitial inflammation with lymphocytes, plasma cells, and histiocytes with noncaseating granulomas
  - Focal granulomatous inflammation of bronchioles
  - Interstitial fibrosis and honeycombing in severe cases

DIFFERENTIAL DIAGNOSIS
- Acute hypersensitivity pneumonia
  - Acute infectious pneumonia
  - Influenza
  - Adenovirus
  - Mycoplasma
  - Pyogenic bacteria
  - *Pneumocystis carinii* pneumonia
  - Fungus
- Chronic hypersensitivity pneumonia
  - Tuberculosis
  - Sarcoidosis
  - Pneumoconiosis
  - Scleroderma
  - Rheumatoid lung
  - Lupus erythematosus
  - Eosinophilic granuloma
  - Lymphangitic carcinomatosis
  - Fungal infections
  - *Pneumocystis carinii* pneumonia
  - Drug reactions
  - Hemosiderosis
  - Idiopathic pulmonary fibrosis

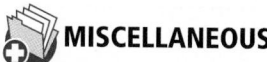

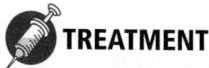 **TREATMENT**

GENERAL MEASURES
- Appropriate health care: Outpatient except for acute pneumonitis cases and admission for workup (BAL, lung biopsy, challenge studies)
- Avoidance of offending antigen

Activity
Full activity, unless advanced disease

 MEDICATION (DRUGS)

First Line
- Avoidance is primary therapy.
- Corticosteroids
  - Prednisone, 2 mg/kg/d or 60 mg/m^2/d, or other comparable corticosteroids
  - Initial course of 1–2 weeks with progressive withdrawal of medication
  - Alternate-day therapy may help, if the exposure cannot be discontinued. The progression may not be prevented, however.
- Contraindications: Refer to the manufacturer's literature.
- Precautions: Observation for side effects
  - Immunosuppression
  - Salt and water retention
  - Osteoporosis
  - Acne
  - Hirsutism
  - Behavioral changes
  - Weight gain/appetite increase
- Significant possible interactions: In patients with renal or cardiovascular disease, a corticosteroid with minimal sodium retention should be chosen.

Second Line
- Bronchodilators may symptomatically improve patients.
- Oxygen may be needed in advanced cases.

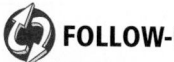 **FOLLOW-UP**

PROGNOSIS
- Excellent prognosis with reversal of pathologic findings with effective treatment of early disease.
- Stabilization of severe, advanced disease with avoidance and anti-inflammatory medication.

COMPLICATIONS
- Progressive interstitial fibrosis with end-stage lung disease
- Cor pulmonale and right heart failure

PATIENT MONITORING
Initial follow-up should be weekly–monthly, depending upon severity and course.

REFERENCES
1. Sharma OP. Hypersensitivity pneumonitis. *Dis Mon*. 1991;37:409–471.
2. Krumpe PE, Lum CCQ, Cross CE. Approach to the patient with diffuse lung disease. *Med Clin North Am*. 1988;72:1225–1246.

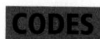 **MISCELLANEOUS**

In the acute form, consider other toxic, nonhypersensitivity-related conditions, such as silo-filler lung.

CODES

ICD9-CM
495.9 Unspecified allergic alveolitis and pneumonitis

PATIENT TEACHING
- Stress pathogenesis and critical importance of allergen avoidance.
- Stress risk of irreversible lung damage with continued exposure.
- Note that chronic exposure may lead to a loss of acute symptoms with exposure (i.e., patient may lose awareness of exposure–symptom relationship).
- American Lung Association, 1740 Broadway, New York, NY 10019;(212)315–8700.

H

HYPERTENSION, ESSENTIAL

David E. Burtner, MD

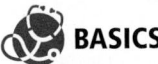 **BASICS**

DESCRIPTION
Hypertension is defined as 2 or more elevated BP (systolic BP of 140 mm Hg or greater and/or diastolic BP of 90 mm Hg or greater) at 2 or more visits. Operationally is any BP at which drug treatment results in a net benefit.

- Hypertension is a strong risk factor for cardiovascular disease.
- Prehypertension: Systolic pressure 120–139 mm Hg or diastolic 80–89 mm Hg
- System(s) Affected: Cardiovascular
- Synonym(s): Benign hypertension; Idiopathic hypertension; Familial hypertension; High BP; Chronic hypertension; Genetic hypertension

ALERT
Geriatric Considerations
- Isolated systolic hypertension is more common.
- Therapy has been shown to be effective and beneficial at preventing stroke, although adverse reactions to medications are more frequent. (4)[A]

Pediatric Considerations
BP should be measured during routine examinations.

Pregnancy Considerations
- Elevated BP during pregnancy may be either chronic hypertension or pregnancy-induced preeclampsia.
- Maternal and fetal mortality benefit from treatment. (See: "Preeclampsia")

GENERAL PREVENTION
- Diet
- Exercise
- Reduce stress
- Avoid tobacco use
- Little or no alcohol

EPIDEMIOLOGY
- Predominant age: Usually onset in the 20s–30s.
- Predominant sex: Males tend to run higher than females, but more importantly have a significantly higher risk of cardiovascular disease at any given BP.

Incidence
- 50 million (1988–1991 NHANES III); 20% of the US population
- Lifetime risk for men and women age 55 or 65 by age 80–85 is >90%

RISK FACTORS
- Family history
- Obesity
- Alcohol
- Excess dietary sodium
- Stress
- Physical inactivity

Genetics
BP levels are strongly familial, but there is no clear genetic pattern. The strong familial risk for cardiovascular diseases should be considered.

ETIOLOGY
Over 90% of hypertension has no identified cause.
- Secondary causes of hypertension
  - Renal parenchymal: Glomerulonephritis, pyelonephritis, polycystic kidneys
  - Endocrine: Primary hyperaldosteronism, pheochromocytoma, hyperthyroidism, Cushing syndrome
  - Vascular: Coarctation (of the aorta), renal artery stenosis
  - Chemical: Oral contraceptives, NSAIDs, decongestants, antidepressants, sympathomimetics, many industrial chemicals, corticosteroids, ergotamine alkaloids, lithium, cyclosporine
  - Sleep apnea

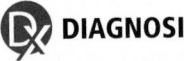 **DIAGNOSIS**

SIGNS AND SYMPTOMS
- Hypertension should be considered asymptomatic except in extreme cases or after related cardiovascular complications develop.
- Headache can be seen especially with higher BP, often present on awakening and occipital in nature.
- Retinopathy: Narrowed arteries, AV nicking, copper or silver wiring of retinal arterioles
- Increased A2 heart sound

TESTS
- ECG
- Special tests (only if history, physical, or lab indicates)
  - Arteriogram, aortogram
  - Numerous drugs and foods interfere with these measurements.

Lab
- CBC
- Complete urinalysis (sometimes reveals proteinuria)
- Potassium, calcium, and creatinine
- Cholesterol (total and HDL)
- Fasting blood glucose
- Uric acid
- If indicated: Plasma catecholamines and renin; urinary metanephrines/VMA

Imaging
If history or physical indicate
- EKG
- Chest x-ray
- Ultrasonography
- IVP
- Provocative renal nuclear scans (e.g., captopril renogram)
- Digital subtraction arteriography
- Gadolinium-enhanced magnetic resonance angiography (MRA)
- Angiogram

Diagnostic Procedures/Surgery
- Renal biopsy if renal parenchymal disease is suspected
- A presumptive diagnosis of hypertension can be made if the average of at least 2 BP measurements exceeds either 140 mm Hg systolic or 90 mm Hg diastolic, assuming proper resting conditions, cuff size, and application are maintained.
- The JNC (3) recommends emphasis on
  - Family or personal history of hypertension, cardiovascular, cerebrovascular, renal disease as well as diabetes
  - Previous elevated BP
  - Previous treatments
  - History of weight gain, exercise activities, sodium intake, fat intake, and alcohol use
  - Symptoms suggesting secondary hypertension
  - Psychosocial and environmental factors affecting BP and risk for cardiovascular disease
  - Other cardiovascular risk factors such as obesity, smoking, hyperlipidemia, and diabetes
  - Funduscopic exam for arteriolar narrowing, arteriovenous compression, hemorrhages, exudates, and papilledema
  - Body mass index
  - Waist circumference
  - BP in both arms
  - Complete cardiac and peripheral pulse exam: Compare radial and femoral pulse for differences in volume and timing, auscultation for carotid and femoral bruits.
  - Abdominal exam for masses and bruits: Listen high in the flanks over the kidneys.
  - Neurological assessment

Pathological Findings
Late complications include
- Stroke
- Retinal vascular narrowing, hemorrhages, exudates, papilledema
- Left ventricular hypertrophy
- CHF
- Ischemic heart disease
- Proteinuria and nephrosclerosis

DIFFERENTIAL DIAGNOSIS
Secondary hypertension (because of the low incidence of reversible secondary hypertension, special tests should be considered only if the history, physical, or basic laboratory evaluation indicates the possibility)

TREATMENT

GENERAL MEASURES

- Stage 1 hypertension (140–159/90–99): Begin thiazide diuretics for most patients.
- Stage 2 hypertension (>160/>100): Consider starting 2 drugs or a thiazide-containing combination.
- Individualize goal BPs based on risk factors, but generally treat to systolic <140 mm Hg (<21.3 kPa) and diastolic <90 mm Hg (<12 kPa)
- Aerobic exercise
- Weight reduction if overweight.
- Smoking cessation is an important part of a cardiovascular risk reduction program.
- Biofeedback and relaxation exercise: Risk stratification affects the treatment.
  - Prehypertension (120–139/80–89): Drug therapy for chronic renal disease or diabetes
- Primary focus is achieving systolic BP goal

Diet

- ~20% of patients will respond to reduced salt diet (<100 mmol/d; <6 g NaCl or <2.4 g Na).
- Limit alcohol consumption to <1 oz/d.
- Decrease saturated fats and increase monounsaturated fats.
- Consider increasing potassium and calcium levels, although absolute effect uncertain

Activity

Encourage regular aerobic activity: 30 minutes per day

MEDICATION (DRUGS)

- Thiazide diuretics have the most proven benefits.
- Beta blockers have been strongly recommended until recent metanalysis. (5)[B]
- ACE inhibitors should be used in patients with diabetes or CHF.
- Alpha adrenergic agents might benefit males with BPH.
- Beta blockers might benefit patients with ischemic heart disease, CHF, or migraine.
- Calcium channel blockers could be considered in patients with migraine or asthma.
- Combination products are available and may improve compliance with multidrug regimens.

First Line

- Thiazide diuretics
  - Hydrochlorothiazide: 6.25–50 mg/d
  - Chlorthalidone: 12.5–50 mg/d
  - Indapamide: 1.25–5 mg/d
- ACE inhibitors:
  - Captopril: 25–450 mg b.i.d.
  - Enalapril: 2.5–40 mg/d
  - Fosinopril: 10–80 mg/d
  - Lisinopril: 5–40 mg/d
  - Ramipril: 2.5–20 mg/d
  - Quinapril: 10–80 mg/d
  - Enazepril: 10–40 mg/d

- Angiotensin II receptor blocker
  - Losartan: 25–100 mg in 1 or 2 doses
  - Valsartan: 80–320 mg/d
  - Irbesartan: 75–300 mg/d
  - Candesartan: 4–32 mg/d
  - Telmisartan: 40–80 mg/d
- Calcium channel blockers
  - Diltiazem: CD, 180–360 mg/d
  - Felodipine: 5–20 mg/d
  - Nicardipine: 20–40 mg t.i.d.
  - Nifedipine (sustained release): 30–120 mg/d
  - Verapamil (sustained release): 120–480 mg/d
  - Amlodipine: 2.5–10 mg/d
- Beta blockers
  - Acebutolol: 400–800 mg/d
  - Atenolol: 25–100 mg/d
  - Metoprolol: 50–200 mg/d
  - Nadolol: 40–320 mg/d
  - Pindolol: 5–30 mg b.i.d.
  - Propranolol: 20–120 mg b.i.d.
  - Timolol: 5–20 mg b.i.d.
  - Betaxolol: 5–40 mg/d
  - Bisoprolol: 2.5–20 mg/d
- Contraindications
  - Diuretics may worsen gout and diabetes.
  - Beta blockers (relatively) in reactive airway disease, heart block, diabetes, and peripheral vascular disease
  - Diltiazem or verapamil: Caution with heart failure or block
  - ACE inhibitors can worsen bilateral renovascular disease.
- For precautions and possible interactions, see the manufacturer's profile of each drug.

Second Line

- Many may be combined.
- Centrally acting adrenergic inhibitors
  - Clonidine: 0.1–1.2 mg b.i.d.or weekly patch 0.1 mg/d to 0.3 mg/d
  - Guanabenz: 4–32 mg b.i.d.
  - Guanfacine: 1–3 mg/d
  - Methyldopa: 250–2,000 mg b.i.d.
- Alpha adrenergic agents
  - Prazosin: 1–10 mg b.i.d.
  - Terazosin: 1–20 mg/d
  - Doxazosin: 1–16 mg/d
- Peripherally acting adrenergic inhibitors
  - Guanadrel: 2.5–37.5 mg b.i.d.
  - Guanethidine: 10–50 mg/d
  - Reserpine: 0.1–0.25 mg/d
  - Labetalol: 100–900 mg b.i.d.
- Vasodilators
  - Hydralazine: 25–150 mg b.i.d.
  - Minoxidil: Rarely used due to adverse effects
- Loop diuretics (for patients with volume overload)
  - Furosemide: 20–320 mg/d
  - Bumetanide: 0.5–2 mg/d
  - Ethacrynic acid: 25–100 mg/d
- Potassium sparing diuretics, in patients with hypokalemia while taking thiazides
  - Amiloride: 5–10 mg/d
  - Spironolactone: 25–100 mg/d
  - Triamterene: 50–150 mg/d

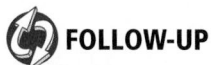

FOLLOW-UP

PROGNOSIS

Good with adequate control

COMPLICATIONS

- CHF
- Renal failure
- Myocardial infarction
- Stroke
- Hypertensive heart disease

PATIENT MONITORING

- Re-evaluate patients every 3–6 months.
- Review compliance, effectiveness, and adverse reactions.
- Quality-of-life issues, including sexual function, should be considered.
- Annual (at least) evaluation of urinalysis, creatinine, and potassium as part of a screening laboratory panel.

REFERENCES

1. Kaplan NM. *Clinical Hypertension.* 8th ed. Baltimore, MD: Lippincott Williams & Wilkins; 2002.
2. National High Blood Pressure Education Program Working Group on High Blood Pressure in Children and Adolescents. The fourth report on the diagnosis, evaluation, and treatment of high blood pressure in children and adolescents. *Pediatrics.* 2004;114:555–576.
3. Chobanian AV, Bakris GL, Black AR, et al. The seventh report of the joint national committee on prevention, detection, evaluation, and treatment of high blood pressure: The JNC 7 report. *JAMA.* 2003;289:2560–2572.
4. SHEP Cooperative Research Group. Prevention of stroke by anti-hypertensive drug treatment in older persons with isolated systolic hypertension. Final results of the Systolic Hypertension in the Elderly Program (SHEP). *JAMA.* 1991;265:3255–3264.
5. Lindholm LH, Carlberg B, Samuelsson O. Should beta blockers remain first choice in the treatment of primary hypertension? A meta-analysis. *Lancet.* 2005;366(9496):1545–1553.

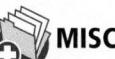

MISCELLANEOUS

See also: Hypertensive emergencies; Polycystic kidney disease

CODES

ICD9-CM

401.1 Essential hypertension, benign

PATIENT TEACHING

- Emphasize the asymptomatic nature of hypertension and the importance of lifetime treatment.
- Review risk factors for cardiovascular disease.
- Printed Aids for High BP Education: http://www.nhlbi.nih.gov/health/public/heart/index.htm#hbp

 See Corresponding Diagnostic Algorithm

 See Patient Handout on CD

H

HYPERTENSIVE EMERGENCIES

John Guisto, MD
Arthur Sanders, MD

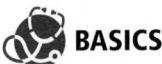 **BASICS**

DESCRIPTION

Terminology is confusing as numerous terms can be used in the literature and often overlap (see "Synonyms"). Some definitions include a specific diastolic or systolic BP reading, whereas others emphasize an acute change in the BP or the presence of specific clinical syndromes.

- Severe hypertension is defined as a diastolic BP of 115 mm Hg (15.3 kPa) or greater. Patients with severe hypertension may or may not have a hypertensive emergency.
- A hypertensive emergency occurs only when an acute elevation of BP causes rapid and progressive end-organ damage, particularly in the cardiovascular, renal, and central nervous systems.
- System(s) Affected: Cardiovascular; Nervous; Pulmonary; Renal
- Synonym(s): Hypertensive crisis; Severe hypertension; Malignant hypertension; Accelerated hypertension; Hypertensive emergency

ALERT

Pediatric Considerations
- Usually associated with renal disease
- May present with abdominal pain

Pregnancy Considerations
- Hydralazine is drug of choice because nitroprusside decreases placental blood flow and cyanide metabolite crosses the placenta; may result in fetal toxicity with prolonged exposure.
- Treat pre-eclampsia.

GENERAL PREVENTION

Counsel the patient on the importance of compliance with antihypertensive treatment and the dangers of stopping the medications abruptly.

EPIDEMIOLOGY

- Predominant age: Young or middle-aged patients with known hypertensive disease
- Predominant sex: Male > Female

Incidence
<1% of patients with hypertension

RISK FACTORS
- History of hypertension
- Drug abuse
- Noncompliance with medications

ETIOLOGY
- Medications
  - Selective serotonin reuptake inhibitors
  - Decongestants
  - Appetite suppressants
  - Steroids (including oral contraceptives)
  - Monoamine oxidase inhibitors in combination with certain foods or drugs
  - Drugs of abuse such as cocaine or amphetamine

- Withdrawal from antihypertensives, especially clonidine (Catapres)
- Withdrawal from CNS depressants
- Eclampsia/preeclampsia
- Thrombotic thrombocytopenic purpura (TTP)
- Pheochromocytoma
- Idiopathic hypertension
- Renal disease
- Severe burns
- Postoperative hypertension

ASSOCIATED CONDITIONS
- Chronic renal failure
- Renovascular hypertension
- Acute glomerulonephritis
- Renal vasculitis

 **DIAGNOSIS**

SIGNS AND SYMPTOMS
Clinical presentation will vary depending on organ system affected.

History
- Headache
- Nausea, vomiting
- Neurologic disturbance
- Shortness of breath, dyspnea, orthopnea
- Chest pain
- Abdominal pain

Physical Exam
- Hypertension
- Focal neurologic deficits, stupor, coma
- Retinopathy
- Pulmonary edema
- Hemorrhage, thrombosis, embolus
- Acute renal failure

TESTS
- ECG may reveal ischemia or left ventricular hypertrophy.
- The funduscopic examination may reveal papilledema, exudates, or hemorrhages.

Lab
- Urinalysis and renal function tests (red cell casts, hematuria, proteinuria are all common)
- Urine drug screen in selected patients
- Blood count and smear may indicate microangiopathic hemolytic anemia or thrombocytopenia.
- Serum electrolytes, which may indicate hypokalemic alkalosis
- Calcium, glucose, uric acid, and lipid profiles
- Subsequent work-up for renal artery stenosis or pheochromocytoma in selected patients

Imaging
- Chest radiographs
  - May show pulmonary edema and cardiomegaly due to CHF
  - Mediastinal widening and blunting of the aortic knob consistent with a dissecting aneurysm
- Head CT
  - Assess the patient with CNS symptoms for intracranial bleeding.

Diagnostic Procedures/Surgery
The BP should be measured with an appropriately sized cuff, and 2 or more readings from both arms; BP averaged before the BP is accepted as elevated

Pathological Findings
Extreme BP elevations can overwhelm the autoregulatory mechanisms for organ blood flow resulting in damage to the arteriolar and capillary beds. This process produces organ hemorrhages and edema.

DIFFERENTIAL DIAGNOSIS
- Myocardial infarction or angina pectoris
- Aortic dissection
- CHF
- Stroke
- Other CNS pathology
- Acute pulmonary edema

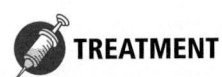 **TREATMENT**

INITIAL STABILIZATION
Intensive care unit

GENERAL MEASURES
- Comfortable environment, which may lower the BP
- The general goal is to lower the mean arterial pressure by ~20–25% or reduce the diastolic pressure to 100–110 mm Hg (13.3–14.6 kPa) over 1 hour.
- If ongoing end-organ damage is thought to be secondary to the hypertensive state, prompt treatment with IV medication is indicated. Monitor patient closely so that a rapid fall in BP can be avoided. A reasonable target is to reduce mean arterial pressure by 20–25%.
- Optimally, an arterial catheter is used to monitor BP.
- IV infusion pump
- The mean arterial pressure is ~1/3 of the sum of twice the diastolic pressure plus the systolic pressure.

Diet
Low sodium when tolerated

Activity
Bed rest

SPECIAL THERAPY
IV Fluids
Fluid restriction may be appropriate for associated pathology such as pulmonary edema.

MEDICATION (DRUGS)

First Line
- IV (unless otherwise indicated)
  - Nitroprusside (Nipride, Nitropress): Infusion 0.5–10 μg/kg per minute; contraindicated in pregnancy
  - Fenoldopam (Corlopam): 0.1 mcg/kg/min IV initial dose. Increase by 0.1 mcg/kg/min q15min to desired effect. Maximum dose 1.6 mcg/kg/min.
  - Hydralazine: Bolus 5–15 mg; preferred in pregnancy
  - Labetalol (Normodyne, Trandate): Bolus 20–80 mg q10–15 minutes; infusion 0.5–2.0 mg/min
  - Nitroglycerin (NTG): Infusion 5–100 μg/min
  - NTG: 0.4 mg SL tablet. Repeat q5min if needed. Consider IV infusion after 3 doses.
  - Phentolamine (Regitine): Bolus 5–10 mg q5–15min
  - Esmolol: 0.05–0.3 mg/kg/min
  - Enalaprilat: 0.625–1.25 mg
  - Nicardipine: 4–15 mg/h
- The drug(s) used depends on the end organs affected and the patient's clinical status.
  - Hypertensive encephalopathy: Nitroprusside infusion; or labetalol or enalaprilat
  - CNS events: Nitroprusside infusion (treat only if diastolic pressure >130 mm Hg [>17.3 kPa])
  - Myocardial ischemia: Nitroglycerin infusion; or labetalol, esmolol, or enalaprilat
  - CHF: Nitroprusside infusion; or nitroglycerin infusion; or enalaprilat or nicardipine
  - Aortic dissection: Nitroprusside or Esmolol infusion
  - Renal failure: Nitroprusside infusion; or labetalol
  - Pheochromocytoma: Phentolamine; or labetalol; or nitroprusside infusion
  - Antihypertensive withdrawal: Labetalol; or phentolamine
  - Interactions between monoamine oxidase inhibitors and foods or drugs: Phentolamine; or labetalol
  - Eclampsia/preeclampsia: Hydralazine
- Severe hypertension (hypertensive urgencies) without evidence of acute end-organ damage: Treatment is controversial. No emergent treatment recommended
- Contraindications
  - Labetalol: Not recommended for patients with asthma, chronic obstructive lung disease, CHF, heart block, cardiogenic shock, or severe bradycardia (due to its beta-blockade property)
  - Nitroprusside: Not recommended in pregnancy

- Precautions
  - Nitroprusside: When nitroprusside is continued IV for >48–72 hours or the patient has compromised renal function, plasma thiocyanate levels should be monitored. Use with clonidine has caused myocardial infarction.
  - Hydralazine: May produce reflex tachycardia with increased myocardial oxygen consumption, which can be prevented by pretreatment with IV beta blocker. Use with caution in suspected myocardial infarction.
  - Topical clonidine: Slow onset of action and is generally not useful in hypertensive emergencies
  - Oral/SL nifedipine (Adalat, Procardia): May cause serious adverse effects such as cerebral vascular ischemia, stroke, or severe hypotension, and should not be used for hypertensive emergencies.

Second Line
- Oral clonidine: Oral loading dose of 0.2 mg followed by 0.1 mg/h until BP has been lowered or a total dose of 0.8 mg has been administered
- Trimethaphan (Arfonad): Infusion 0.5–5 mg/min

FOLLOW-UP

DISPOSITION
Admission Criteria
- All patients who present with hypertensive emergencies should be hospitalized.
- Associated end-organ effects may require specific treatment, e.g., acute myocardial infarction.

PROGNOSIS
BP should return to acceptable levels within 24 hours.

COMPLICATIONS
- Abrupt or excessive lowering of BP may result in inadequate cerebral or cardiac blood flow, leading to stroke or myocardial ischemia.
- Authorities have questioned whether the benefits of aggressive treatment outweigh the risks in patients with severe hypertension but no end-organ damage. No studies have proven that aggressive treatment reduces the risk of long-term morbidity or mortality from hypertensive urgencies.

PATIENT MONITORING
- Monitor the patient closely to avoid a rapid fall in BP.
- Begin oral therapy as soon as possible after BP control has been achieved with IV medications.

REFERENCES

1. Murphy C. Hypertensive emergencies. *Emerg Med Clin North Am.* 1995;13:973–1007.
2. Shayne PH, Pitts SR. Severely increased blood pressure in the emergency department. *Ann Emerg Med.* 2003;41:513–529.
3. Clinical policy: Critical issues in the evaluation and management of adult patients with asymptomatic hypertension in the emergency department. *Ann Emerg Med.* 2006;47:237–249.
4. Fenoldopam, a dopamine agonist, for hypertensive emergency: A multicenter randomized trial. *Acad Emerg Med.* 2000;7:653–662.
5. Abdelwahab W, Frishman W, Landau A. Management of hypertensive urgencies and emergencies. *J Clin Pharmacol.* 1995;35:747–762.
6. Management of patients with hypertensive urgencies and emergencies: A systematic review of the literature. *JGIM.* 2002;17:937–945.

ADDITIONAL READING

Joint National Committee on Prevention, Detection, Evaluation, and Treatment of High Blood Pressure. The Seventh Report of the Joint National Committee on Prevention, Detection, Evaluation, and Treatment of High Blood Pressure: the JNC 7 report. *JAMA.* 2003;289:2560–2572.

MISCELLANEOUS

See also: Aortic dissection; Eclampsia (Toxemia of Pregnancy); Hypertension, essential; Pheochromocytoma; Preeclampsia

CODES

ICD9-CM
- 401.0 Essential hypertension, malignant
- 405.01 Secondary malignant renovascular hypertension
- 437.2 Hypertensive encephalopathy
- 642.90 Unspecified hypertension complicating pregnancy, childbirth, or the puerperium, unspecified

PATIENT TEACHING

Diet
Salt intake may affect risk in susceptible patients.

Prevention
- Importance of medication compliance
- Lack of symptoms with hypertension until organ damage occurs

See Corresponding Diagnostic Algorithm

H

HYPERTHYROIDISM

Matthew P. Hill, MD

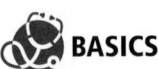 **BASICS**

DESCRIPTION
- Reaction to excess thyroid hormone
- Graves disease (GD): The most common form; an autoimmune disease
  - Thyroid-stimulating hormone (TSH) receptor autoantibodies (TSH-R Ab) bind and stimulate the thyrotropin (TSH) receptor. This mimics the action of TSH and causes excess secretion of thyroxine (T4) and triiodothyronine (T3). Goiter and ophthalmopathy are common characteristics. Pretibial myxedema is rare.
- Toxic multinodular goiter: Occurs later in life
  - Nodules are insidious and almost never malignant.
  - No ophthalmopathy or localized myxedema is present.
- Toxic uninodular goiter: Solitary nodule with autonomous function; almost always benign
- Iodine-induced hyperthyroidism
- Other rare causes include TSH-secreting pituitary tumors, surreptitious ingestion of thyroxine or triiodothyronine, functioning trophoblastic tumors.
- Subclinical hyperthyroidism: Suppressed TSH with normal T4
- System(s) Affected: Endocrine/Metabolic
- Synonym(s): Thyrotoxicosis

ALERT
Geriatric Considerations
- Characteristic symptoms and signs may be absent ("apathetic hyperthyroidism"); may mimic depression or malignancy
- Atrial fibrillation is common in patients >60.

Pediatric Considerations
Neonates and children are treated with antithyroids for 2–3 months.

Pregnancy Considerations
- Treat with lowest effective dose of propylthiouracil or methimazole due to increased risk of spontaneous abortion and premature delivery in hyperthyroid pregnant women.
- Avoid treatment-induced hypothyroidism.
- Autoimmune thyrotoxicosis often improves during pregnancy and relapses at postpartum.
- Radioiodine therapy is absolutely contraindicated.

EPIDEMIOLOGY
- Predominant age: 3rd and 4th decades
- Predominant sex: Female > Male

Incidence
- Female: 1:1,000
- Male: 1:3,000

RISK FACTORS
- Positive family history
- Female
- Other autoimmune disorders
- Iodide repletion after iodide deprivation

ETIOLOGY
- GD: Autoimmune disease
- Toxic multinodular goiter: Iodine deprivation followed by iodine repletion
- Toxic uninodular goiter: Unknown
- Hashimoto disease: Autoimmune

ASSOCIATED CONDITIONS
- Other autoimmune diseases
- Down syndrome

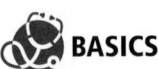 **DIAGNOSIS**

SIGNS AND SYMPTOMS
- Adults
  - Nervousness (85%)
  - Increased sweating (70%)
  - Heat intolerance (70%)
  - Palpitations and tachycardia (75%)
  - Dyspnea (75%)
  - Fatigue and weakness (60%)
  - Weight loss (52%)
  - Increased appetite (40%)
  - Exophthalmos (34%)
  - Goiter (87%)
  - Tremor (65%)
  - Warm and moist skin (72%)
  - Emotional lability
  - Subclinical; may present with atrial fibrillation, cardiomegaly, skeletal demineralization with low thyroid-stimulating hormone
- Children
  - Linear growth acceleration
  - Ophthalmic abnormalities more common

History
Onset of symptoms and signs listed above

Physical Exam
See list above

TESTS
Lab
- TSH for diagnosis; repeat with T3, T4, T3RU and CBC if TSH is undetectable
- T3: Triiodothyronine: Total triiodothyronine by immunometric assay >200 ng/mL
- T4: Thyroxine: By immunometric assay >12.5 g/dL (161 nmol/L)
- Free thyroxine index: >12
- Free thyroxine: >1.5 ng/dL
- TSH: Thyroid stimulating hormone: Below normal, often undetectable
- T3RU: Radioiodine uptake: High in overproduction states (GD, toxic nodules); low in thyroiditis, iodide-induced and thyroid hormone-induced hyperthyroidism
- TSH Autoantibodies rarely needed
- FTI: Free Thyroxine Index: T4 times T3RU is an estimate of free Thyroxine
- Elevated TSH with high T4 suspicious for pituitary tumor
- Drugs that may alter lab results
  - Anabolic steroids
  - Androgens
  - Estrogens
  - Heparin
  - Iodine containing compounds (especially amiodarone)
  - Phenytoin
  - Rifampin
  - Salicylates
  - Thyroxine
  - Triiodothyronine
- A variety of nonthyroidal illnesses can alter thyroxine and triiodothyronine with little effect on thyroid-stimulating hormone
- Free thyroxine index permits correction of misleading results caused by pregnancy and estrogens.

Imaging
- Thyroid scans I 123: Interpretation: Diffuse uptake in GD, focal in toxic nodules
- Ultrasonography with fine needle aspiration to investigate suspicious nodules

Pathological Findings
- GD: Hyperplasia
- Toxic nodules: Nodule formation

DIFFERENTIAL DIAGNOSIS
- Anxiety
- Malignancy
- Diabetes
- Pregnancy
- Menopause
- Pheochromocytoma

TREATMENT

GENERAL MEASURES
- Appropriate health care: Outpatient except for thyroid storm, a rare life-threatening condition, which may cause heart failure, fever, and mania
- Antithyroid drugs, therapeutic radioiodine for underlying disease, beta blockers for symptomatic control, and NSAIDs for thyroiditis(1)[B]
- Obtain CBC and LFT's prior to initiation of medication; they may cause agranulocytosis and may be hepatotoxic
- Symptomatic treatment for subclinical hyperthyroidism due to thyroiditis; consider treatment for TSH <0.1mLU/L if due to GD or multinodular goiter. (2)[B]

Diet
Sufficient calories to prevent weight loss and adequate B vitamins

Activity
Modify activity according to the disease severity.

MEDICATION (DRUGS)

First Line
- Initial treatment
  – Methimazole (Tapazole): Adults (15–60 mg/d PO given once daily); children age 6–10, 0.4 mg/kg/d PO once daily
  – Propylthiouracil: Adults (preferred in elderly, those with cardiac disease, thyroid storm, and pregnant and lactating women) 100–900 mg/d PO t.i.d.; no more than 200 mg/d during pregnancy
  – Ablation with I 131 is often the 1st choice for adults and children age >10, 5, 10 or 15 mCi; often induces resultant hypothyroidism
- Maintenance with antithyroids
  – Methimazole: Adults, 5–30 mg/d PO given once daily; no more than 20 mg/d during pregnancy; children, 0.2 mg/kg/d PO given daily
  – Propylthiouracil: Adults, 50–600 mg/d PO b.i.d.; children, 50 mg b.i.d. PO (or 1/2–2/3 of initial dose)
- Thyrotoxic crisis
  – Propylthiouracil: Adults 15–20 mg PO q4h during the 1st day (as an adjunct to other therapies); neonates 10 mg/kg/d PO q4h; adjust doses by following clinical status, free thyroxine (or free thyroxine index) and, when appropriate, thyroid-stimulating hormone; saturated solution of potassium iodide (SSKI) 5 drops q6h for 24–72 hours until improvement
- Additional therapies
  – Radioiodine therapy: Sodium iodide I-131 (Iodotope–Beta blocker: Propranolol (Inderal) 40–240 mg PO daily

- Contraindications
  – Radioiodine therapy: Pregnancy and nursing
  – Propranolol: CHF, asthma, chronic bronchitis, pregnancy, hypoglycemia
- Precautions
  – Propylthiouracil and methimazole: May cause dermatitis, agranulocytosis, or hepatotoxicity; measure TSH and LFT's every 2–3 months
  – Radioiodine therapy: Often causes permanent hypothyroidism and may cause fetal hypothyroidism or malformation if administered during pregnancy
- Significant possible interactions: Oral anticoagulants may be potentiated by propylthiouracil.

Second Line
Ipodate sodium (Oragrafin): 0.5 g q.i.d. PO

SURGERY
Thyroidectomy for compressive symptoms, masses, concern of thyroid malignancy and may be used in 2nd trimester of pregnancy.

FOLLOW-UP

DISPOSITION
Graves ophthalmopathy should be referred to experienced ophthalmologist.

PROGNOSIS
Good (with precise diagnosis and adequate treatment)

COMPLICATIONS
- Hypoparathyroidism, recurrent laryngeal nerve damage, and hypothyroidism with subtotal thyroidectomy
- Development of hypothyroidism after radioiodine treatment
- Relapse of Graves highest with antithyroid drug as primary therapy.
- Visual loss or diplopia due to severe ophthalmopathy
- Localized pretibial myxedema at any time
- Cardiac failure in the elderly with underlying heart disease
- Atrial fibrillation
- Muscle wasting; proximal muscle weakness

PATIENT MONITORING
- Repeat thyroid tests once a year
- CBC and liver function tests when appropriate
- Therapy with antithyroids continues 12–18 months (3)[A]
- After radioiodine therapy, thyroid function tests at 6 weeks, 12 weeks, 6 months, and annually thereafter if euthyroid. TSH may remain undetectable for months after patient euthyroid; follow T3 and T4. (1)[B]

REFERENCES
1. Woeber KA. Update on the management of hyperthyroidism and hypothyroidism. *Arch Intern Med*. 2000;160:1067–1071.
2. Surks MI, Ortiz E, Daniels GH, et al. Subclinical thyroid disease. Scientific review and guidelines for diagnosis and management. *JAMA* 2004;291(2): 228–238.
3. Abraham P, Avenell A, Watson WA, et al. A systematic review of drug therapy for Graves' hyperthyroidism. In: *The Cochrane Database of Systematic Reviews*, 2, 2005.

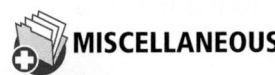 **MISCELLANEOUS**

 CODES

ICD9-CM
- 242.00 Toxic diffuse goiter without mention of thyrotoxic crisis or storm
- 242.01 Toxic diffuse goiter with mention of thyrotoxic crisis or storm
- 242.90 Thyrotoxicosis without mention of goiter or other cause without mention of thyrotoxic crisis or storm
- 242.91 Thyrotoxicosis without mention of goiter or other cause with mention of thyrotoxic crisis or storm

PATIENT TEACHING
Importance of compliance with drug therapy and surveillance for hypothyroidism

See Corresponding Diagnostic Algorithm

See Patient Handout on CD

H

HYPERTRIGLYCERIDEMIA

Reza Moattari, MD

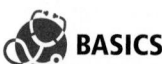 **BASICS**

DESCRIPTION

- Triglycerides: Fatty molecules of long-chain fatty acids and glycerol
- Hypertriglyceridemias: Heterogeneous family of disorders owing to disturbances in synthesis and/or degradation of triglyceride-rich plasma lipoprotein
- Normal triglyceride level
  - Children: <100 mg/dL (1.13 mmol/L)
  - Adults: <150 mg/dL (1.70 mmol/L)
- Abnormal hypertriglyceridemia: 150–500 mg/dL (1.7–5.65 mmol/L)
- Distinct hypertriglyceridemia: >500 mg/dL (5.65 mmol/L)
- Physiology: Major triglycerides containing lipoproteins
  - Chylomicron: In postprandial state, from absorption of dietary fat from gut
  - Very low density lipoprotein (VLDL): In fasting state, endogenous synthesis from carbohydrates and fatty acid in liver
  - Intermediate-density lipoprotein (IDL): From degradation of chylomicrons and VLDL
- Classification (based on lipoprotein pattern)
  - Type I: Markedly elevated chylomicrons. Presents with high triglyceridemia and minimally elevated cholesterol. Usually presents in childhood. Clinically associated with abdominal pain owing to pancreatitis, eruptive xanthoma, hepatosplenomegaly, and lipemia retinalis. Risk for atherosclerosis not increased. Causes are either primary (autosomal recessive owing to lipoprotein lipase or apo-C deficiency) or secondary, that is, systemic lupus erythematosus (SLE) and dysgammaglobulinemia.
  - Type II-A: Elevated LDL. Presents with high cholesterol
  - Type II-B: Elevated LDL and VLDL. Presents with high cholesterol and high triglycerides. Strong risk for atherosclerosis. Primary causes include several genetic disorders. Secondary causes include hypothyroidism, liver and kidney disease, porphyria, multiple myeloma
  - Type III: Elevated IDL (dysbetalipoproteinemia). Presents with high cholesterol and triglycerides. Most patients with primary disorder are homozygous for apoprotein E2. Secondary causes: Hypothyroidism and dysgammaglobulinemia
  - Type IV: Elevated VLDL. Presents with high triglycerides and minimally elevated cholesterol. In some, increased risk for atherosclerosis
  - Type V: Elevated chylomicrons and VLDL. Presents with very high triglycerides and high cholesterol. Genetic form is autosomal recessive owing to LPL or apo-C deficiency. Increased risk of atherosclerosis

Note: Above classification is only descriptive and provides little insight into genetics and mechanism of disorder. Plasma lipoprotein changes with time in any individual, a phenomenon to be expected because of precursor–product relationship in metabolism of VLDL and LDL and effect of diet on VLDL. Single disease state can lead to several different lipoprotein patterns, and single lipoprotein phenotype can be caused by multiple disease states.

- System(s) Affected: Cardiovascular; Endocrine/Metabolic; Gastrointestinal
- Synonym(s): Hyperlipidemia; Chylomicronemia syndrome

GENERAL PREVENTION
See "Patient Teaching Section."

EPIDEMIOLOGY
Predominant sex: Male > Female

Prevalence
- Familial combined hyperlipidemia: 1–2%
- Familial hypertriglyceridemia: 1–2%
- Familial dyslipoproteinemia: 1/10,000

RISK FACTORS
- Genetic susceptibility
- Obesity
- Diabetes
- Alcoholism
- Certain drugs
- Medical illness may exacerbate condition (see secondary causes).

Genetics
- Familial hypercholesterolemia: Autosomal dominant
- Polygenic hypercholesterolemia: Polygenic
- Familial hypertriglyceridemia: Autosomal dominant
- Familial combined hyperlipidemia: Autosomal dominant
- Familial dysbetalipoproteinemia: Autosomal recessive
- LPL and apo-C deficiency: Autosomal recessive

ETIOLOGY
- Primary
  - Sporadic
  - Genetic
- Secondary
  - Conditions associated with hypertriglyceridemia: Obesity, metabolic syndrome, diabetes mellitus, pregnancy, uremia/dialysis, hypothyroidism, nephrotic syndrome, acromegaly, Cushing syndrome, systemic lupus erythematosus, dysgammaglobulinemias, glycogen storage Type I, lipodystrophy
  - Drugs associated with hypertriglyceridemia: Alcohol, estrogen, tamoxifen, birth control pills, beta-blockers, diuretics, glucocorticoids, isotretinoin/retinoid, HIV antiretrovirals, and protease inhibitors; bile acid–binding resins cause a modest (<10%) elevation in some patients with Type II hyperlipidemia.

ASSOCIATED CONDITIONS
- Mostly associated with
  - Low HDL cholesterol
  - Dense LDL particle (Type B)
- May be associated with hypercholesterolemia
- Metabolic syndrome (3 of following)
  - Abdominal obesity (Male waist >40 in., Female waist >35 in.)
  - Triglycerides >150 mg/dL
  - HDL cholesterol (Male <40, Female <50)
  - BP >130/85
  - Fasting glucose >100–125 mg/dL

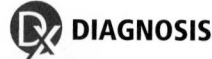 **DIAGNOSIS**

SIGNS AND SYMPTOMS
- Pancreatitis (triglycerides >1,000)
- Chylomicronemia syndrome (triglycerides >2,000)
  - Memory loss/dementia
  - Dyspnea
  - Headache/vertigo
  - Eruptive xanthoma
  - Lipemia retinalis
  - Hepatosplenomegaly
  - Lymphadenopathy
  - Peripheral neuropathy/paresthesia
- Atherosclerosis

TESTS
Lab
- Serum: Turbid and milky
- Fasting plasma lipid profile
- Triglycerides, after 12–14-hour fast in
  - Any individual with total cholesterol level of ≥240 mg/dL (6.22 mmol/L)
  - Men with HDL-C <40 mg/dL, women with HDL-C <50 mg/dL
  - Patients with acute pancreatitis, signs and symptoms of chylomicronemia syndrome or lactescence plasma
  - Individuals with past and present history of atherosclerosis, family history of premature arteriosclerosis
  - Individuals with 2 or more coronary heart disease (CHD) risk factors, a disease or medications that raise triglycerides
  - Diabetic patients: Elevated fasting glucose
  - Hypertensive patients (BP ≥130/85 mm Hg)
  - Patients with abdominal obesity waist circumference: Men >40 in., women >35 in.
- HDL cholesterol (inversely related to triglycerides)
- Apoprotein B measurement (may define a subset of mild hypertriglyceridemia in patients at excess risk for CHD)
- LDL fractionation (Type B or dense LDL seen with atherogenic hypertriglyceridemia)
- Genetic testing for apoprotein E2
- Disorders that may alter lab results
  - In triglyceride-induced pancreatitis, both serum and urinary amylase concentration may be normal owing to interference of plasma lipids or some other inhibitor with assay.
  - Triglycerides may interfere with hemoglobin measurement; bilirubin may be artificially elevated.
  - Pseudohyponatremia may result from very high triglycerides.

Imaging
- Pancreatitis: CT of pancreas
- Atherosclerosis: Doppler, angiography, ultrafast CT of heart

Pathological Findings
- Atherosclerosis
- Pancreatitis
- In chylomicronemia syndrome: Lipid-laden macrophage (foam cell) infiltration of visceral organs, bone marrow, and skin

DIFFERENTIAL DIAGNOSIS
Primary versus secondary hypertriglyceridemia

TREATMENT

GENERAL MEASURES

- Usually outpatient
- Inpatient if underlying disorder warrants
- Search thoroughly for correctable secondary causes; treat underlying illness or remove incriminated drug.
- Primary hypertriglyceridemia: Screen other family members.
- Distinct hypertriglyceridemia: Treatment indicated to prevent acute pancreatitis
- Mild hypertriglyceridemia: Treatment indicated to prevent coronary artery disease (CAD) in patients with high risk, that is, strong family or personal history of atherosclerosis
- Severe hypertriglyceridemia associated with pancreatitis: Hospitalize, eliminate dietary fat; if diabetic, continuous IV infusion of insulin.

Diet

- Weight reduction to ideal body weight with American Heart Association (AHA) Step I Diet (50–55% carbohydrate, <30% fat)
- Pediatric: In severe cases only, AHA Step I Diet is recommended.
- Activity: Usually no restrictions
- Exercise is important.

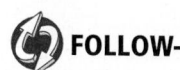

MEDICATION (DRUGS)

First Line

- Fibrates: Fenofibrate (Tricor) 54–160 mg/d gemfibrozil (Lopid) 600 mg b.i.d.
  - Reduce triglycerides 20–70%
  - Decrease hepatic VLDL synthesis.
  - Increase VLDL metabolism.
- Niacin (Niaspan): 1–3 g/d
  - Reduces triglycerides by 20–50%
  - Inhibits hepatic VLDL synthesis
- Contraindications: Refer to manufacturer's literature.
- Precautions
- Gemfibrozil and fenofibrate
  - Side effects: Upper and lower GI side effects (usually mild; most frequent adverse effects), cholelithiasis, myalgia, hepatotoxicity
  - May increase incidence of myopathy/rhabdomyolysis if given with HMG-CoA reductase inhibitors

- Nicotinic acid
  - Side effects
    - Flushing and pruritus (prostaglandin mediated and alleviated by aspirin)
    - Upper GI discomfort and peptic ulcer disease
    - Hepatotoxicity (more with sustained-release preparation)
    - Hyperuricemia and gout, hyperglycemia, toxic amblyopia
    - Flushing less with extended-release forms
    - Fulminant hepatic necrosis reported with extended-release forms
- Significant possible interactions: Gemfibrozil with warfarin
  - Enhanced anticoagulation effect
  - Monitor PT closely following addition or withdrawal of gemfibrozil.

Second Line

- HMG-CoA reductase inhibitors: Lower triglycerides 10–30%
  - Lovastatin (Mevacor, Altocor)
  - Pravastatin (Pravachol)
  - Simvastatin (Zocor)
  - Fluvastatin (Lescol)
  - Atorvastatin (Lipitor)
  - Rosuvastatin (Crestor)
- Fish oil
- Glitazones: Pioglitazone and rosiglitazone
- Clofibrate (Atromid-S)

ALERT

Pregnancy Considerations

All drugs contraindicated during pregnancy

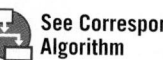

FOLLOW-UP

PROGNOSIS

- Primary disorder: May need lifelong treatment
- Secondary disorder: Good if underlying causes are eliminated

COMPLICATIONS

- Acute pancreatitis
- Atherosclerosis

PATIENT MONITORING

- Fasting lipid profile
- Liver function test
- Creatine kinase
- CBC with differential count
- Target triglyceride levels
  - Pancreatitis: <500 mg/dL (<5.65 mmol/L)
  - CHD, diabetes, and 2 or more risk factors: <150 mg/dL (<1.7 mmol/L)

REFERENCES

1. Grundy SM. Hypertriglyceridemia, insulin resistance, and the metabolic syndrome. *Am J Cardiol*. 1999;83(9B):25F–29F.
2. Miller M. Current perspectives on the management of hypertriglyceridemia. *Am Heart J*. 2000;140:232–240.
3. The National Cholesterol Education Program (NCEP) expert panel on detection, evaluation, and treatment of high blood cholesterol in adults (Adult Treatment Panel III). *JAMA*. 2001;285:2486–2497.

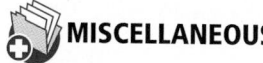

MISCELLANEOUS

See also: Hypercholesterolemia.

CODES

ICD9-CM

- 272.0 Pure hypercholesterolemia
- 272.1 Pure hypertriglyceridemia
- 272.2 Mixed hyperlipidemia
- 272.3 Hyperchylomicronemia
- 272.4 Other and unspecified hyperlipidemia

PATIENT TEACHING

Smoking cessation

Diet

Elimination of alcohol

See Corresponding Diagnostic Algorithm

H

HYPOCHONDRIASIS

Sarah Guzofski, MD
Ruben Peralta, MD

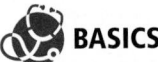 **BASICS**

DESCRIPTION

- Hypochondriasis is a psychiatric disorder characterized by at least 6 months of the fear of having or the belief that one has a serious illness based on misinterpretation somatic symptoms or sensations. The person is generally convinced that he or she has a serious illness. (1C)
- Synonym(s): Hypochondriacal neurosis, Hypochondria

EPIDEMIOLOGY

- Predominant sex: Men = women
- Predominant age: Most common onset in 3rd or 4th decade.

Prevalence

In the US
- 1-4.5% of the community population.
- 4-6% of medical outpatients meet criteria for hypochondriasis.
- 12% of primary care patients report a physical symptom that will not have a clear medical explanation (2C)

RISK FACTORS

Exposure to life-threatening medical conditions and procedures in one's childhood, adolescence, or in adult life

Genetics

Some studies show an increased prevalence of hypochondriasis in families, especially among identical twins and first-degree relatives.

ETIOLOGY

- Biologic: There is some evidence suggesting that patients with hypochondriasis may be born with a tendency to amplify somatic sensations and that they have lower threshold and a lower tolerance of physical discomfort
- Childhood events: The experience of numerous or serious actual medical illnesses during one's childhood may predispose the individual to hypochondriasis later on in life.
- Cognitive: Patients with hypochondriasis over-estimate their risk of developing a serious illness. (3B)

ASSOCIATED CONDITIONS

- Depressive disorders in as many as 40%
- Anxiety disorders
- Obsessive Compulsive Disorder

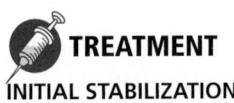 **DIAGNOSIS**

SIGNS AND SYMPTOMS

- Diagnostic criteria include (DSM IV-TR, 1C)
- Preoccupation with fears of having, or the idea that one has, a serious disease based on the person's misinterpretation of bodily symptoms
- The preoccupation persists despite appropriate medical evaluation and reassurance.
- The belief is not of delusional intensity (as in delusional disorder, somatic type) and is not restricted to a circumscribed concern about appearance (as in body dysmorphic disorder).
- The preoccupation causes clinically significant distress impairment in social, occupational, or other important areas of functioning.
- The duration of the disturbance is at least 6 months.
- The preoccupation is not better accounted for by generalized anxiety disorder, obsessive-compulsive disorder, panic disorder, a major depressive episode, separation anxiety, or another somatoform disorder.
- Concern with the illness often becomes a central feature of the person's identity.
- Despite significant concern about health, do not tend to have particularly healthy habits.
- Often believe they are not getting good medical care; common to have multiple changes in health care providers.

History

- Patient may report the following common concerns
  - Worry about sensations associated with normal body function, such as heartbeat or diaphoresis
  - Minor physical abnormalities, such as a small rash, rare cough.
  - Vague physical sensations.
- Attributes symptoms to a disease of concern.
- May focus on multiple systems or a single disease.

TESTS

Lab

Lab tests are used to rule out organic diseases.

Diagnostic Procedures/Surgery

Care to avoid non-essential tests. Do not perform tests solely to provide reassurance because the reassurance is likely to be short-lived. (Barsky A)

DIFFERENTIAL DIAGNOSIS

- Any patient suffering from hypochondriasis, as with any other psychiatric disorder, is not immune from developing a medical/organic disease. Such organic diseases as those affecting many organ systems such as connective tissue diseases, autoimmune diseases, as well as more focused single-organ type diseases, must always be considered as a possibility in these patients.
- Underlying depressive disorders
- Schizophrenia
- Delusional disorders
- Conversion disorder
- Anxiety disorder
- Panic disorder
- Obsessive-compulsive disorder
- Factitious disorder with physical symptoms
- Somatization disorder
- Chronic pain disorder
- Body dysmorphic disorder
- Malingering
- Munchausen syndrome

TREATMENT

INITIAL STABILIZATION

Outpatient

GENERAL MEASURES

- Treatment should focus on careful history and physical exam with clear and straightforward explanation of any findings.
- Regular medical appointments with clear goals with repeated reassurance and adequate explanation.
- May see referral to a psychiatrist as dismissing their concerns.
- Some evidence suggests cognitive behavioral therapy (CBT) is helpful to improve hypochondriacal concerns and overall functioning. (2C, 3B)
  - Explains that focusing on a symptom tends to increase its intensity.
  - Describes anxiety and depression as worsening physical symptoms.
  - Teach distraction techniques.
- Group therapy using a CBT model can help reduce hypochondriacal concerns as well as anxiety for at least a year after treatment. (Lidbeck B)
- A good doctor-patient relationship is essential.

Diet

Good nutrition

Activity

Regular exercise in moderation

MEDICATION (DRUGS)

First Line
- No specific medications have been proven effective for hypochondriasis. (Barsky C)
- Antidepressants and antianxiety medications are most successful in patients who have a preponderance of anxiety and depressive symptoms. (Creed B)
- Selective serotonin reuptake inhibitors are commonly used. (Barsky B)

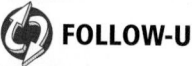 **FOLLOW-UP**

PROGNOSIS
The natural history of this condition is usually chronic. 50–70% will continue to meet diagnostic criteria after one year.

COMPLICATIONS
Risks of repeated and unnecessary lab and diagnostic procedures

PATIENT MONITORING
- Patients should be seen on a regular basis in the primary care physician's office or with a psychotherapist.
- Appointments should be scheduled regardless of whether the patient has new symptoms or not.
- Avoid the use of long hospitalizations and unnecessary lab workups.

REFERENCES
1. American Psychiatric Association (APA). *Diagnostic and Statistical Manual Fourth Edition Text Revision*. 2000. American Psychiatric Association Press.
2. Lamberg L. New Mind/Body Tactics Target Medically Unexplained Physical Symptoms and Fears. *JAMA* 2005;294:2152–2154.
3. Barsky AJ, Ahern DK, Bailey ED. Hypochondriacal Patient's Appraisal of Health and Physical Risks. *Am J Psychiatry* 2001;158:783–787.
4. Creed F, Barsky A. A systematic review of the epidemiology of somatisation disorder and hypochondriasis. *J Psychosom Res.* 2004;56(Apr): 391–408.
5. Barsky AJ. Clinical Practice: The patient with Hypochondriasis. *NEJM* 2001;345:1359–9.
6. Barsky AJ, Ahern DK. Cognitive behavioral therapy for hypochondriasis: A randomized controlled trial. *JAMA* 2004;291:1464–70.
7. Lidbeck J. Group therapy for somatization disorders. *Acta Psychiatr Scand.* 2003;107:449–456.

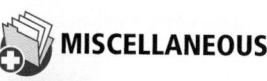 **MISCELLANEOUS**

CODES

ICD9-CM
300.7 Hypochondriasis

PATIENT TEACHING
Clear explanations of all test results.

H

HYPOGLYCEMIA, DIABETIC

Joseph A. Florence, MD

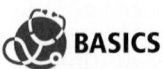 **BASICS**

DESCRIPTION
- Abnormally low concentration of glucose in circulating blood of diabetic. Often referred to as an *insulin reaction*
- Classification includes (1)
  - Severe hypoglycemia: An event requiring assistance of another person to actively administer treatment
  - Documented symptomatic hypoglycemia: An event during which typical symptoms are accompanied by a measured plasma glucose concentration of ≤70 mg/dL (3.9 mmol/L)
  - Asymptomatic hypoglycemia: An event not accompanied by typical symptoms, but with a measured glucose of ≤70 mg/dL (3.9 mmol/L)
  - Probable symptomatic hypoglycemia: An event with symptoms of hypoglycemia, but glucose not tested
  - Relative hypoglycemia: An event with typical symptoms, but measured plasma glucose >70 mg/dL (3.9 mmol/L)
- Hypoglycemia is the leading limiting factor in the glycemic management of Type 1 and Type 2 diabetes. (2)
- System(s) Affected: Endocrine/Metabolic

ALERT
- Hypoglycemic unawareness
  - Major risk factor for severe hypoglycemic reactions
  - Most commonly found in patients with long-standing Type 1 diabetes and children <7 years of age
- Can be reversed by
  - Meticulous prevention of hypoglycemia
  - Avoidance of iatrogenic hypoglycemia

GENERAL PREVENTION
- Maintaining a routine schedule of diet, medication, and exercise
- Stabilize daily carbohydrate intake
- Regular blood glucose testing
  - 3 or more times daily testing if multiple injections of insulin
- Intensive therapy for diabetes should be adjusted to minimize occurrence of severe hypoglycemia; the tighter the diabetic control, the greater the importance of home glucose monitoring.
- Patients who experience recurrent hypoglycemic episodes should be individually evaluated, and when appropriate, the employment position should be modified if contributing to frequent insulin reactions.
- Severe or frequent hypoglycemia indicates a need to modify glycemic goals and treatment regimens.

EPIDEMIOLOGY
- Predominant age: All ages
- Predominant sex: Males = Females

Prevalence
- Hypoglycemia most common in Type 1 diabetics
- Type 1 diabetics
  - Most experience hypoglycemia.
  - If tightly controlled: Experience hypoglycemia 2–3 times more frequently, often weekly (3)
- Type 2 diabetics
  - If treated with diet and exercise alone: Experience hypoglycemia much less frequently than do Type 1 diabetics: Uncommon
  - If treated with insulin and/or insulin secretagogues: Common

RISK FACTORS
- Nearly 3/4 of severe hypoglycemic episodes occur during sleep.
- Autonomic neuropathy
- Illness, stress, and unplanned life events
- Duration of diabetes >5 years
- Advanced age
- Renal, liver disease
- CHF
- Hypothyroidism
- Hypoadrenalism
- Gastroenteritis
- Starvation or prolonged fasting
- Alcoholism
- Oral hypoglycemics with long duration and high potency have greater hypoglycemic risks.
- α-Glucosidase inhibitors, biguanides, and thiazolidinediones when used in combination with insulin and/or sulfonylureas or meglitinides

ETIOLOGY
- Loss of hormonal counter-regulatory mechanism in glucose metabolism
- Diet
  - Too little food (skipping meal)
  - Decreased carbohydrate intake
- Medication: Too much insulin or oral hypoglycemic agent (improper dose or timing)
- Erratic absorption of insulin or oral hypoglycemics
- Adverse reaction from other medications
- Exercise: Unplanned or excessive
- Alcohol consumption
- Vomiting or diarrhea
- Gastroparesis

ASSOCIATED CONDITIONS
- Autonomic dysfunction
- Neuropathies
- Cardiomyopathies

DIAGNOSIS

SIGNS AND SYMPTOMS
History

Symptoms are idiosyncratic and vary considerably between individuals. (4)[A]

Gather detailed history.

- Adrenergic hypoglycemia symptoms include
  - Hunger, trembling, pallor
  - Sweating, shaking, pounding heart, anxiety
- Neuroglycopenic hypoglycemia symptoms include
  - Dizziness, poor concentration, drowsiness, weakness, confusion, lightheadedness, slurred speech, blurred vision, double vision, unsteadiness, poor coordination
- Behavioral hypoglycemia symptoms include
  - Tearfulness, confusion, fatigue, irritability, aggressiveness

Physical Exam
Document

- General: Confusion, lethargy
- HEENT Diplopia
- Cor: Tachycardia
- Neuro: Tremulousness, weakness, paresthesias, stupor, seizure, or coma
- Mental status: Irritability, inability to concentrate, or short-term memory loss
- Skin: Pale, diaphoresis
- End organ damage—microvascular, macrovascular, ophthalmologic, neurologic, renal

TESTS
Lab
- Plasma or whole-blood glucose <70 mg/dL
- Suspect hypoglycemic unawareness in asymptomatic Type 1 diabetes with low or normal HgbA1c.
- Chronic hypoglycemia is indicated by low glycohemoglobin level.
- Disorders that may alter lab results: Hemoglobinopathies may alter HgbA1c results.

Diagnostic Procedures/Surgery
- History and physical exam
- Plasma, or whole blood glucose

DIFFERENTIAL DIAGNOSIS
- Aspirin induces hypoglycemia in some children.
- Hypoglycemia is well documented in chronic alcoholics and binge drinkers.
- Gastrointestinal dysfunction causing postprandial hypoglycemia or alimentary reactive hypoglycemia
- Hormonal deficiency states (hormonal reactive hypoglycemia)
- Idiopathic reactive hypoglycemia (reactive hypoglycemia, a popular diagnosis 20 years ago, is actually quite rare)
- Hypoglycemia of sepsis
- Islet cell tumors
- Factitious hypoglycemia from surreptitious injection of insulin
- Hypoglycemia may be found in nondiabetics under certain conditions such as early pregnancy, prolonged fasting, long periods of strenuous exercise, heart failure, malignancy, and renal or liver disease.

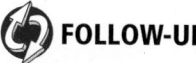 **TREATMENT**

PRE HOSPITAL
Treatment should be managed by the patient whenever possible.

GENERAL MEASURES
- Blood glucose targets should be individualized.
- Glucose: Preferred treatment; however, any form of carbohydrate that contains glucose should be effective (5)[A]
- Any sugar-containing food or beverage that can be rapidly absorbed, for example, juice (4–6 ounces), candy (5–6 pieces of hard candy), or nondiet soda
- OTC glucose tablets or gels
- Glucagon: People in close contact with people with diabetes should be instructed in using an emergency glucagons kit. (5)[A]

Diet
- If alcohol consumed, combine with food to reduce risk of hypoglycemia
- Protein does not slow absorption of carbohydrates.
- Fats may slow absorption of carbohydrates and may retard and then prolong the actue glycemic response. (6)[B]

Activity
Rest until glucose is normal.

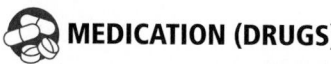 **MEDICATION (DRUGS)**

First Line
- General
  - Glucose
    - Oral administration of small-molecule sugars (saccharose/glucose): glucose preferred
    - ~60–90 calories (15–20 g glucose) repeated every 15 minutes until blood sugar is ≥100 mg/dL (5.55 mmol/L)
    - Takes ~15 minutes for carbohydrates to be digested and enter blood stream as glucose
- In patients with loss of consciousness at home
  - Administer glucagon IM or SC in the deltoid or anterior thigh.
    - <5 years old: 0.25–0.50 mg
    - 5–10 years old: 0.50–1 mg
    - >10 years: 1 mg
- In unconscious patients, if emergency medical personnel are present or patient hospitalized
  - Give 1/2 ampule 50% dextrose every 5–10 minutes until patient awakens.
  - Then feed orally and/or administer 5% dextrose IV at level that will maintain blood glucose >100 mg/dL.
  - Patients with hypoglycemia secondary to oral hypoglycemics should be monitored for 24–48 hours, because hypoglycemia may recur after apparent clinical recovery.

- Contraindications: None
- Significant possible interactions
  - Treatment may cause hyperglycemia (called *Somogyi phenomenon*).
  - Clearance of certain oral hypoglycemics from plasma may be prolonged in persons with liver disease.

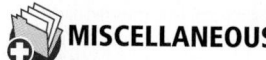 **FOLLOW-UP**

DISPOSITION
Admission Criteria
Admit patient if
- Any doubt of cause
- Expectation of prolonged hypoglycemia (e.g., caused by sulfonylurea drug)
- Inability of patient to drink
- Treatment has not resulted in prompt recovery of sensorium
- Seizures, coma, or altered behavior (e.g., ataxia, disorientation, unstable motor coordination, dysphasia) secondary to documented or suspected hypoglycemia

Discharge Criteria
Patient has normoglycemia and risk of severe hypoglycemia is negligible.

Issues for Referral
- Frequent, recurring, or episodes which do not readily respond to treatment
- Unresolved dysfunction after treatment

PROGNOSIS
Full recovery usually depends on rapidity of diagnosis and treatment.

COMPLICATIONS
- Coma, seizure
- Prolonged or severe hypoglycemia may cause permanent neurological damage and/or cognitive impairment.
- Evaluation of neuropsychologic shows no evidence of significant cognitive deterioration associated with repeated episodes of severe hypoglycemia. Repeated episodes of severe hypoglycemia not necessarily associated with cognitive dysfunction (3)[A]
- Myocardial infarction, stroke, especially in elderly

PATIENT MONITORING
Self-monitoring of blood glucose

REFERENCES

1. American Diabetes Asosociation, Workgroup on Hypoglycemia. Defining and reporting hypoglycemia in diabetes. *Diabetes Care*. 2005;28(5):1245–1249.
2. Cryer PE. Hypoglycaemia: The limiting factor in the glycemic management of type I and type II diabetes. *Diabetologia*. 2002;45:937–948.
3. Diabetes Control and Complications Trial (DCCT). Adverse events and their association with treatment regimens in the Diabetes Control and Complications Trial. *Diabetes Care*. 1995;18:1415–1427.
4. McAulay V, Deary IJ, Frier BM. Symptoms of hypoglycaemia in people with diabetes. *Diabetes UK, Diabetic Medicine*. 2001;18:690–705.
5. American Diabetes Association. Clinical practice recommendations. *Diabetes Care*. 2006;Suppl 1.
6. Gannon MC, Nuttal FZ. Protein and diabetes. In: Franz MJ, Bantle JP, eds. *American Diabetes Association Guide to Medical Nutrition Therapy for Diabetes*. Alexandria, VA: American Diabetes Association; 1999: 107–125.

MISCELLANEOUS

CODES

ICD9-CM
- 250.81 Diabetes with other specified manifestations, Type 1, not stated as uncontrolled
- 250.82 Diabetes with other specified manifestations, Type 2 or unspecified type, uncontrolled
- 250.83 Diabetes with other specified manifestations, Type 1, uncontrolled
- 300.19 Other and unspecified factitious illness
- 579.3 Other and unspecified postsurgical nonabsorption
- 775.0 Syndrome of "infant of a diabetic mother"
- 775.6 Neonatal hypoglycemia
- 962.3 Poisoning by insulins and antidiabetic agents

PATIENT TEACHING

Diet
Always keep some type of quick-acting carbohydrate close by.

Activity
For patients taking insulin
- For planned exercise, consider a reduced insulin dosage.
- Additional carbohydrates may be needed for unplanned exercise.
- Moderate-intensity exercise increases glucose uptake by 2–3 mg/kg/min above usual requirements (70-kg person needs ≈10–15 g carbohydrates per hour of moderate physical activity).

Prevention
- See "General Prevention"
- Educate patients and their relatives, close friends, teachers, and supervisors.
  - Blood glucose testing should be available at school or workplace.
    - Personnel should be aware of diabetes diagnosis and signs/symptoms of hypoglycemia and treatment.
- Teach self-monitoring of blood glucose and self-adjustment for insulin therapy, diet control, and exercise regimen.
- Patient should wear medical alert identification bracelet or necklace.

H

HYPOGLYCEMIA, NONDIABETIC

F. David Schneider, MD, MSPH

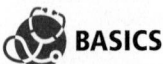 **BASICS**

DESCRIPTION

- Hypoglycemia defined by Whipple triad
  - Low plasma glucose level
  - Symptoms (see list below)
  - Symptoms relieved with correction of low blood sugar
- Occurs often in diabetic patients (covered under separate topic); less common in nondiabetic patients
- Reactive hypoglycemia
  - Occurs in response to meal, specific nutrients, or drugs
  - May occur within 2–3 hours after a meal, or later
  - Generally occur when serum glucose ≤60 mg/dL
  - Also seen after gastrointestinal surgery (in association with dumping syndrome in some patients)
- Spontaneous (fasting) hypoglycemia
  - May be associated with a primary condition, for example, hypopituitarism, Addison disease, myxedema, or in disorders related to hepatic malfunction or renal failure
  - If hypoglycemia presents as a primary manifestation, other disorders to consider include hyperinsulinism and extrapancreatic tumors.
- Types based on cause
  - Postprandial hypoglycemia
  - Functional hypoglycemia
  - Idiopathic hypoglycemia
  - Alimentary hypoglycemia
  - Postgastrectomy hypoglycemia
  - Alcohol-induced hypoglycemia
  - Factitious hypoglycemia
  - Iatrogenic hypoglycemia
  - Exogenous hypoglycemia
- System(s) Affected: Endocrine/Metabolic

GENERAL PREVENTION

- Follow dietary and exercise guidelines.
- Patient recognition of early symptoms and taking corrective action

EPIDEMIOLOGY

- Predominant age: Older adult
- Predominant sex: Female > Male

Incidence
Unknown

Prevalence
Unknown

RISK FACTORS
Listed with "Etiology"

Genetics
Some aspects may involve genetics (e.g., hereditary fructose intolerance).

ETIOLOGY

- Reactive: Postprandial
  - Alimentary hyperinsulinism
  - Meals high in refined carbohydrates
  - Certain nutrients, for example, fructose, galactose, leucine
  - Glucose intolerance (prediabetic)
  - Gastrointestinal surgery
  - Idiopathic (unknown)
- Spontaneous
  - Fasting
  - Drugs or alcohol (insulin or sulfonylureas, beta blockers, salicylates, quinine, fluoroquinones, disopyramide, or pentamidine)
  - Surreptitious drug use (self-injection of insulin or ingestion of oral hypoglycemic in nondiabetic patients)
  - Hepatic disease
  - Islet cell hyperplasia or tumor
  - Catecholamine deficiency
  - Glucagon deficiency
  - Eating disorders
  - Extrapancreatic tumor
  - Exercise
  - Fever
  - Pregnancy
  - Renal glycosuria
  - Large tumor
  - Ketotic hypoglycemia of childhood
  - Adrenal insufficiency
  - Hypopituitarism
  - Enzyme deficiencies or defects
  - Severe malnutrition
  - Sepsis
  - Total parenteral nutrition therapy

ALERT

Geriatric Considerations
More likely to have underlying disorders or be using causative drugs

Pediatric Considerations
Usually divided into 2 syndromes
- Transient neonatal hypoglycemia
- Hypoglycemia of infancy and childhood

ASSOCIATED CONDITIONS

- Insulinoma
- Severe liver disease
- Alcoholism
- Adrenocortical insufficiency
- Myxedema
- Malnutrition (patients with renal failure)
- Gastrointestinal surgery
- Panhypopituitarism
- Addison disease

DIAGNOSIS

SIGNS AND SYMPTOMS

- CNS (neuroglycopenic) symptoms: Predominate if glucose dropping gradually
  - Headache
  - Confusion
  - Lightheadedness
  - Fatigue and weakness
  - Visual disturbances
  - Changes in personality
  - Convulsions
  - Coma
  - Heart
  - Palpitations
  - Hypotension
- Gastrointestinal symptoms
  - Hunger
  - Nausea
  - Belching
- Adrenergic symptoms: More prominent in acute drop in glucose (as in insulin reaction)
  - Anxiety
  - Tremulousness
  - Dizziness
  - Diaphoresis
  - Warmth/flushing
  - Palpitations
  - Nervousness

History
Symptoms as noted above

Physical Exam
Generally normal

TESTS

Lab

- Blood sugar ≤45 mg/dL when patient is symptomatic followed by symptom resolution upon feeding
- Plasma glucose overnight fasting: <60 mg/dL (<3.33 mmol/L)
- Plasma glucose 72-hour fasting: <45 mg/dL (<2.5 mmol/L) for females; <55 mg/dL (<3.05 mmol/L) for males; fast may be ended when Whipple's triad is achieved or hypoglucermia and symptoms are demonstrated
- Oral glucose tolerance
  - <50 mg/dL (<2.78 mmol/L)
  - Misinterpretation of glucose tolerance tests may lead to misdiagnosis of hypoglycemia; >1/3 of normal patients have hypoglycemia with or without symptoms during 4-hour glucose tolerance test. However, these individuals may be at risk for developing Type 2 diabetes mellitus.
- C-peptide measurement
- Check liver studies, serum insulin, and cortisol.
- Insulin radioimmunoassay: Elevated insulin levels if islet cell tumor present
- Drugs that may alter lab results: Many drugs can affect levels; refer to drug or laboratory reference.

Imaging
Abdominal CT to rule out abdominal tumor

Diagnostic Procedures/Surgery
For definitive diagnosis, patient should have

- Documented occurrence of low blood glucose levels
- Symptoms that occur when blood glucose low
- Evidence that symptoms are relieved specifically by ingestion of sugar or other food
- Identification of the particular type of hypoglycemia

DIFFERENTIAL DIAGNOSIS
- CNS disorders
- Psychogenic
- Pseudohypoglycemia: Symptoms of hypoglycemia or self-diagnosis in patients in whom low blood sugars may not be detectable and who may be impossible to convince that they do not suffer from hypoglycemia after all tests are found to be normal

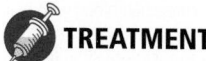 ## TREATMENT

GENERAL MEASURES
- Outpatient except for severe cases; may also be inpatient for testing
- Oral carbohydrate for alert patient without drug overdose (2–3 tablespoons sugar in glass of water or fruit juice, 1–2 cups milk, piece of fruit, soda cracker)
- If patient unable to swallow, glucagon IM or SC
- If caused by drugs or certain nutrients: Avoid or control causative agents.
- If following meals: Try high-protein diet with restricted carbohydrates.
- Nonhypoglycemic hypoglycemia or pseudohypoglycemia
  - Many patients (often females, ages 20–45) present with diagnosis of reactive hypoglycemia (self-diagnosed or misinterpretation of tests).
  - Symptoms usually pertain to chronic fatigue and somatic complaints (stress often has a role in these symptoms).
  - Management difficult; listening important. Dietary changes, for example, 120 g carbohydrate diet, low in simple sugars, can be recommended.
  - Counseling: May be useful for stress or other problems.

Diet
- High protein, low carbohydrate
- Frequent small feedings 6 instead of 2 to 3 larger meals
- Avoid fasting.

Activity
May need to revise exercise routine

 ## MEDICATION (DRUGS)

First Line
- Once diagnosis established, drug therapy appropriate to underlying disorder
- In patient unable to swallow: Glucagon IM or SC. If no response, give IV glucose. For serious hypoglycemia, give IV bolus of 25–50 g of 50% glucose solution followed by constant infusion of glucose until patient can take by mouth.
- Insulinoma: See separate topic.
- Postsurgical gastrectomy patients unresponsive to diet changes may benefit from propantheline, which delays gastric emptying.
- Contraindications, precautions, significant possible interactions: Refer to manufacturer's literature.

SURGERY
If islet cell tumor (insulinoma): Surgery is treatment of choice. If inoperable, drug therapy may relieve symptoms.

 ## FOLLOW-UP

DISPOSITION
Admission Criteria
Hypoglycemia unresponsive to oral intake

PROGNOSIS
Favorable, with recognition and appropriate treatment

COMPLICATIONS
- In insulinoma: If tumor removed, some surgical risk involved
- Organic Brain Syndrome—from prolonged hypoglycemia

PATIENT MONITORING
- Depends on type and severity of symptoms and treatment of underlying cause
- Hypoglycemia from sulfonylurea can last for days.

REFERENCES
1. Carroll MF, Burge MR, Schade DS. Severe hypoglycemia in adults. *Rev Endocr Meta Dis*. 2003;4(2):149–157.
2. Service FJ. Classification of hypoglycemic disorders. *Endocrinol Metab Clin North Am*. 1999;28:501–517.

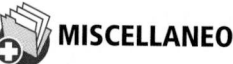 ## MISCELLANEOUS

See also: Hypoglycemia, diabetic; Insulinoma

 ## CODES

ICD9-CM
- 251.0 Hypoglycemic coma
- 251.1 Other specified hypoglycemia
- 251.2 Hypoglycemia, unspecified

PATIENT TEACHING
- Instructions about fasting tests and interpretations of results
- Dietary instruction
- Counseling for stress, if appropriate
- Recognition of early symptoms of hypoglycemia and how to take corrective action

See Corresponding Diagnostic Algorithm

H

HYPOKALEMIA

Ruben Peralta, MD, FACS
Jacqueline J. Wu, MD

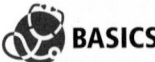 **BASICS**

DESCRIPTION
Occurs when serum potassium concentration is below 3.5 mEq/L. (Normal range: 3.5– 5.0 mEq/L)

GENERAL PREVENTION
Patients being started on diuretics, especially loop diuretics and thiazide diuretics, should be advised to increase their dietary potassium intake (see "Diet").

EPIDEMIOLOGY
Predominant sex: Male = Female

Incidence
- Most commonly encountered electrolyte abnormality in clinical practice (1)[B]
- Found in >20% of hospitalized patients (when defined as potassium <3.6 mEq/L)

Prevalence
Not common in pediatric population, but may occur in chronic gastrointestinal loss or secondary to hyperadrenalism

RISK FACTORS
Any disorder or medication regimen requiring potassium supplementation

Genetics
Some familial disorders are rare causes of hypokalemia
- Familial hypokalemic periodic paralysis
- Congenital adrenogenital syndromes
- Liddle syndrome
- Familial interstitial nephritis

ETIOLOGY
- General causes
  - Decreased intake (uncommon): Anorexia nervosa, deficient diet in alcoholics and elderly
  - Gastrointestinal loss: Vomiting, diarrhea, losses from nasogastric tubes, laxative abuse, fistulas, villous adenoma, ureterosigmoidostomy, malabsorption, chemotherapy, radiation enteropathy
  - Intracellular shift of potassium: Metabolic alkalosis, insulin excess, β-adrenergic catecholamine excess (acute stress, intake of B_2 agonists), hypokalemic periodic paralysis, intoxications (theophylline, barium, toluene)
- Renal potassium loss
  - Drugs: Diuretics (especially loop and thiazides), amphotericin B
  - Mineralocorticoid-excess states: Primary hyperaldosteronism, secondary hyperaldosteronism (CHF, cirrhosis, nephrotic syndrome, malignant hypertension, renin-producing tumors), renovascular hypertension, Bartter syndrome, Gitelman syndrome, congenital adrenogenital syndromes, exogenous mineralocorticoids (glycyrrhizic acid in licorice, carbenoxolone, steroids in nasal sprays), Liddle syndrome, vasculitis
  - Glucocorticoid-excess states: Cushing syndrome, exogenous steroids, ectopic ACTH production, II B hydroxysteroid dehydrogenase deficiency
  - Renal tubular acidosis (type I and II)
  - Leukemia
  - Magnesium depletion
  - Thyrotoxic hypokalemic paralysis

ALERT
Geriatric Considerations
Diuretic therapy, diarrhea, and chronic laxative abuse are most common causes. The elderly, especially those living alone or with disabilities, are more likely to have a potassium-poor diet.

ASSOCIATED CONDITIONS
Acute GI illnesses with severe vomiting or diarrhea

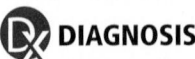 **DIAGNOSIS**

SIGNS AND SYMPTOMS
- Patients with hypokalemia often have no symptoms, especially if the hypokalemia is mild (serum potassium 3.0–3.5 mEq/L).
- Neuromuscular (most prominent manifestations)
  - Skeletal muscle weakness (proximal > distal muscles) may range from mild weakness to total paralysis, including respiratory muscles; may lead to rhabdomyolysis in severe cases.
  - Smooth muscle involvement may lead to gastrointestinal hypomotility, producing ileus and constipation.
- Cardiovascular (rare in patients without pre-existing heart disease)
  - Ventricular arrhythmias
  - Hypotension
  - Cardiac arrest
- Renal: Polyuria, polydipsia, nocturia owing to impaired concentrating ability
- Metabolic: Hyperglycemia

TESTS
- ECG (2)[B]
  - Hypokalemia increases the myocyte resting potential, which increases the refractory period; this can lead to arrhythmias.
  - Flattening or inversion of T waves
  - Increased prominence of U waves (small positive deflection after T wave, best seen in V2 and V3)
  - Depression of ST segment
  - Ventricular ectopia
- Workup for cause
  - Excessive renal potassium loss present when urinary potassium is >20 mEq/d in presence of hypokalemia
  - In patient with excessive renal potassium loss and hypertension, plasma renin and aldosterone levels should be determined to differentiate adrenal from nonadrenal causes of hyperaldosteronism.
  - If hypertension is absent and patient is acidotic, renal tubular acidosis should be considered.
  - If hypertension is absent and serum pH is normal to alkalotic, high urine chloride (>10.mEq/d [>10.mmol/d]) suggests hypokalemia secondary to diuretics or Bartter syndrome; low urine chloride (<10 mEq/d [<10 mmol/d]) suggests vomiting as probable cause.

Lab
- Serum potassium <3.5 mEq/L (<3.5 mmol/L)
- Drugs that may alter lab results: Diuretics
- Disorders that may alter lab results: Leukemia and other conditions with high WBC

Imaging
CT scan of adrenal glands, if evidence of mineralocorticoid excess (see "Special Tests")

Pathological Findings
- Vacuolization of proximal and distal renal tubular cells
- In severe hypokalemia, necrosis of cardiac and skeletal muscle

DIFFERENTIAL DIAGNOSIS
- Spurious hypokalemia: Occurs when blood with high WBC count (>100,000/mm^3) is allowed to stand at room temperature (WBCs extract potassium from plasma)
- Thyrotoxicosis

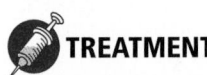 **TREATMENT**

GENERAL MEASURES
- For asymptomatic patients being treated with oral replacement, outpatient follow-up is sufficient.
- Patients with cardiac manifestations require intravenous replacement with cardiac monitoring in an intensive-care setting.
- Mild hypokalemia: Treat underlying cause.
- Severe hypokalemia: Potassium replacement is necessary.

ALERT
Geriatric Considerations
May need to correct magnesium depletion

Diet
Mild hypokalemia (potassium 3.0–3.5 mEq/L [3.0–3.5 mmol/L]) not caused by GI losses: Dietary supplementation may be sufficient; potassium-rich foods include oranges, bananas, cantaloupes, prunes, raisins, dried beans, dried apricots, and squash.

Activity
No restrictions

MEDICATION (DRUGS)

First Line

- Nonemergent conditions (serum potassium >2.5 mEq/L [>2.5 mmol/L], no cardiac manifestations)
  - Oral therapy preferred; doses of 40–120 mEq/d (40–120 mmol/d) usually adequate
  - IV potassium should be given only when oral administration is not feasible (e.g., vomiting, postoperative state). Rate should not exceed 10 mEq/h, and concentration should not exceed 40 mEq/L. Up to 40 mEq in 100 mL over 1 hour can be safely given through a central venous line. Patient's cardiac rhythm should be closely monitored.
  - Potassium chloride is suitable for all forms of hypokalemia.
  - Other potassium salts may be indicated if coexisting disorder is present: Potassium bicarbonate or bicarbonate precursor (gluconate, acetate, or citrate) in metabolic acidosis or phosphate in phosphate deficiency.
- Emergent situations (serum potassium <2.5 mEq/L [<2.5 mmol/L], arrhythmias): IV replacement
  - Rate of administration should not exceed 20 mEq/h (20 mmol/h); maximum recommended concentration 60 mEq/L (60 mmol/L) of saline for peripheral administration. Administration through central venous lines may allow for greater concentrations.
- Precautions
  - Any form of potassium replacement carries risk of hyperkalemia.
  - Serum potassium should be checked more frequently in groups at higher risk: Elderly, diabetic patients, and patients with renal insufficiency.
  - Patients receiving digitalis and patients with diabetic ketoacidosis in whom intracellular shift in potassium is expected after insulin therapy is initiated must have more aggressive replacement.
- Significant possible interactions: Concomitant administration of potassium-sparing diuretics (spironolactone, triamterene, amiloride ACE inhibitors) magnifies risk of hyperkalemia.

 FOLLOW-UP

PROGNOSIS

Ease of correction of hypokalemia and need for prolonged treatment rests on primary cause; if it can be eliminated (e.g., resolution of diarrhea, discontinuation of diuretics, removal of adrenal tumor), hypokalemia can be expected to resolve and no further treatment is indicated.

COMPLICATIONS

Hyperkalemia can occur in the course of treatment.

PATIENT MONITORING

- Patients receiving IV therapy should have serum potassium level checked frequently (q4–6h).
- Patients requiring potassium supplements should have serum potassium studied at intervals dictated by clinical judgment and patient compliance.

REFERENCES

1. Schaefer T, Wolford R. Disorders of potassium. *Emerg Med Clin North Am* 2005;723–747.
2. Webster A, Brady W, Morris F. Recognising signs of danger: ECG changes resulting from abnormal serum potassium concentration. *Emerg Med J* 2002;19:74–77.
3. Gennari FJ. Disorders of potassium homeostasis. Hypokalemia and hyperkalemia. *Crit Care Clin* 2002;18:273–288.

 MISCELLANEOUS

See also: Hyperkalemia

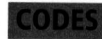 **CODES**

ICD9-CM
276.8 Hypopotassemia

PATIENT TEACHING

- Instructions for diet
- If potassium supplementation necessary, stress need for compliance

 See Corresponding Diagnostic Algorithm

H

HYPOKALEMIC PERIODIC PARALYSIS

Frank J. Domino, MD

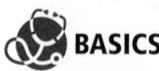 **BASICS**

DESCRIPTION
- Episodic weakness associated with low serum potassium (K) levels
- 2 forms
  - Familial hypokalemic periodic paralysis (FHPP)
  - Hypokalemic periodic paralysis with thyrotoxicosis (thyrotoxic hypokalemic periodic paralysis or THPP)
- System(s) Affected: Endocrine/Metabolic; Musculoskeletal; Nervous
- Synonym(s): Paroxysmal myoplegia

GENERAL PREVENTION
See "Medication" (prevention of attacks) and "Diet"

EPIDEMIOLOGY
- Predominant age: Onset of disease in late childhood or adolescence (FHPP), early adulthood (THPP). Onset >35 years of age extremely rare.
- Age of onset depends on type of genetic mutation.
- Predominant sex
  - FHPP: Male > Female (3:1)
  - THPPs: Male > Female (20:1). Usually affects Asian males

Prevalence
- 1 in 100,000 (estimated)
- FHPP more common than THPP

RISK FACTORS
- Male
- Age <35
- Family history (familial hypokalemic periodic paralysis)
- Asian (thyrotoxic hypokalemic periodic paralysis)

Genetics
Familial hypokalemic periodic paralysis: Autosomal dominant; incomplete penetrance in females in certain genetic mutations

PATHOPHYSIOLOGY
- Abnormality is in muscle membrane.
- Hypokalemia is caused by intracellular shift of K.
- Total body K is normal (i.e., hypokalemia not a result of K loss).
- Muscle fibers are chronically depolarized by 10–15 mV, but membrane conductance normal between attacks.

ETIOLOGY
- Exact pathogenesis unknown.
- Several mutations in either calcium (Ca) transport channels (type 1 familial hypokalemic periodic paralysis) or sodium (Na) transport channels (type 2 familial hypokalemic periodic paralysis) have been identified (α-1 subunit of ion channel protein).
- Both Ca and Na channel mutations show incomplete phenotypic penetrance in females.
- Very rare form of familial hypokalemic periodic paralysis owing to K channel mutation was recently reported.
- Ca channel mutation may induce familial hypokalemic periodic paralysis by changing behavior or expression of other ion channels in muscle.
- Contractile apparatus is normal.
- Pathogenesis of familial hypokalemic periodic paralysis and thyrotoxic hypokalemic periodic paralysis may be different because thyroid hormone doesn't worsen familial hypokalemic periodic paralysis.
- Acetazolamide may precipitate attacks in patients with type 2 familial hypokalemic periodic paralysis caused by Na-channel mutation.

ASSOCIATED CONDITIONS
Thyrotoxic hypokalemic periodic paralysis: Hyperthyroidism

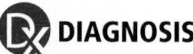 **DIAGNOSIS**

SIGNS AND SYMPTOMS
- Episodic attacks of limb muscle weakness that last from a few hours to several days
- Typical attack comes on during sleep that was preceded by strenuous exercise.
- Attacks also are provoked by high-carbohydrate or high-Na meals.
- Cold, stress, alcohol, diuretics, insulin, or epinephrine also may exacerbate attack.
- Attacks are more common in summer and fall (THPP).
- Strength between attacks usually is normal.
- After years of prolonged, frequent attacks, patient may develop persistent proximal weakness.
- Myalgias are present.
- Muscles of the eyes, face, tongue, pharynx, larynx, diaphragm, and sphincters rarely are involved.
- Deep-tendon reflexes are hypoactive.
- Sensation is preserved.
- Patients with thyrotoxic hypokalemic periodic paralysis may manifest signs of hyperthyroidism (especially systolic hypertension and tachycardia).

TESTS
- Mild hypokalemia: ECG may show S-T depression, flattened T waves, or presence of U waves.
- Severe hypokalemia: ECG may show peaked P waves, prolonged P-R interval, or widened QRS.
- Electromyography not helpful (usually normal between attacks)
- Genetic testing (DNA sequencing) to differentiate type 1 from type 2 familial hypokalemic periodic paralysis (Ca channel vs. Na channel mutations)

Lab
- Low serum K (as low as 1.3 mEq/L [1.3 mmol/L]) is Hallmark.
- Low serum phosphorous and low serum magnesium also found
- Urine K normal
- Elevated T3, T4, free thyroid index, and decreased thyroid-stimulating hormone (TSH; thyrotoxic hypokalemic periodic paralysis only)
- Serum creatine kinase (CK) level normal or slightly increased
- Acid–base balance normal
- Urine K/creatinine ratio low (<2)

Imaging
Thyroid scans using radioiodine (thyrotoxic hypokalemic periodic paralysis only)

Diagnostic Procedures/Surgery
Provocative testing (50–100 g of oral glucose with 2–4 g of oral Na followed by exercise, or 50–100 g of oral glucose with 10–20 units SC regular or fast-acting insulin may be required); monitor closely for insulin-precipitated hypoglycemia. Patient should have cardiac monitoring during testing.

Pathological Findings
- Muscle biopsy may show atrophy, centrally placed vacuoles of sarcoplasm.
- Electromicroscopy studies show vacuoles are a result of progressive dilatation of sarcoplasmic reticulum.

DIFFERENTIAL DIAGNOSIS
- Hyperkalemic periodic paralysis (adynamia episodica)
- Myotonia congenita
- Paramyotonia congenita
- Normokalemic periodic paralysis
- Barium poisoning
- Hyperventilation
- Secondary hypokalemia (laxative or diuretic use, diarrhea, vomiting, renal or adrenal disease, clay ingestion)
- Myasthenia gravis
- Guillain-Barré syndrome
- Tick paralysis
- Cataplexy
- Sleep paralysis
- Presyncope
- Drop attacks
- Akinetic epilepsy
- Andersen syndrome (episodic paralysis, ventricular dysthymias, and dysmorphic features)
- Episodic ataxia

TREATMENT

GENERAL MEASURES
- Severe hypokalemia or weakness: Inpatient with cardiac monitoring
- Mild hypokalemia or weakness: Outpatient with close follow-up
- May rarely need respiratory support

Diet
- Avoid high-carbohydrate, high-Na foods.
- K-rich foods are of dubious benefit.

Activity
As tolerated

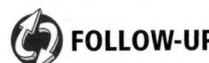 **MEDICATION (DRUGS)**

First Line
- Acute attack
  - Oral potassium chloride (KCl): 0.2–0.4 mEq/kg (0.2–0.4 mmol/kg), repeated every 15–30 minutes depending on response of ECG, serum K+, muscle strength (usual total dose: 40 mEq [40 mmol])
  - In life-threatening situation or if vomiting, give IV KCl in mannitol (5% glucose or normal saline IV may worsen situation). Bolus 0.1 mEq/kg (0.1 mmol/kg) q5–10min; monitor ECG, serum K. (Usual dose: 15 mEq [15 mmol] over 15 minutes, then 10 mEq/hr [10 mmol/hr] if peripheral IV, up to 60 mEq/hr [60 mmol/hr] if central IV and cardiac monitoring)
  - IV propranolol (thyrotoxic hypokalemic periodic paralysis only)
- Prevention of attacks in familial hypokalemic periodic paralysis
  - Oral KCl
  - Acetazolamide (Diamox): 125–1,000 mg/d divided per day to b.i.d. (type 1 familial hypokalemic periodic paralysis only)
- Prevention of attacks in thyrotoxic hypokalemic periodic paralysis
  - Treat underlying thyrotoxicosis with β-adrenergic blocking agents (propranolol [Inderal] and others)
  - Acetazolamide contraindicated
- Contraindications
  - Acetazolamide: Marked hepatic or renal dysfunction, hypersensitivity, adrenal failure, hyperchloremic acidosis, low serum sodium, K (type 2 familial hypokalemic periodic paralysis, thyrotoxic hypokalemic periodic paralysis)
  - Propranolol: Cardiogenic shock, sinus bradycardia, 2nd- or 3rd-degree atrioventricular (AV) block, CHF, bronchial asthma
- Precautions
  - Infusion of IV KCl must be monitored to avoid inadvertent infusion of large and potentially fatal doses.
  - Peripheral IV KCl infusion rates >10 mEq/h (10 mmol/h) may be painful.
  - Rebound hyperkalemia may occur in patients who receive >90 mEq KCl in 24 hours and in patients with thyrotoxic hypokalemic periodic paralysis who receive KCl and propranolol.
  - Acetazolamide: Drowsiness or paresthesias at high doses. May precipitate or worsen paralysis in patients with type 2 familial hypokalemic periodic paralysis
  - Propranolol: Impaired hepatic or renal function

- Significant possible interactions
  - Acetazolamide: High-dose aspirin
  - Propranolol: Reserpine, verapamil, aluminum hydroxide, phenytoin, rifampin, chlorpromazine, cimetidine, theophylline

Second Line
- Acute attack: None
- Prevention of attacks in familial hypokalemic periodic paralysis
  - Triamterene (Dyrenium): 25–100 mg/d
  - Spironolactone (Aldactone): 25–200 mg/d
- Prevention of attacks in thyrotoxic hypokalemic periodic paralysis: Propylthiouracil, radioactive ablation of thyroid

 FOLLOW-UP

PROGNOSIS
- Frequency of attacks usually lessens with age.
- After years of prolonged, frequent attacks, patient may develop persistent proximal weakness.

COMPLICATIONS
- Cardiac arrhythmias
- Respiratory collapse

PATIENT MONITORING
- Follow serum K and electrolytes (if on acetazolamide).
- Follow thyroid function tests (if on propranolol or propylthiouracil).

REFERENCES

1. Antes LM, Kujuba DA, Fernandez PC. Hypokalemia and the pathology of ion transport molecules. *Semin Nephrol*. 1998;18:31–45.
2. Cannon SC. An expanding view for the molecular basis of familial periodic paralysis. *Neuromuscul Disord*. 2002;12:533–543.
3. Dias da Silva MR, Cerutti JM, Tengan CH, et al. Mutations linked to familial hypokalaemic periodic paralysis in the calcium channel alpha1 subunit gene (Cav1.1) are not associated with thyrotoxic hypokalaemic periodic paralysis. *Clin Endocrinol (Oxf)*. 2002;56:367–375.
4. Gutmann L. Periodic paralyses. *Neurol Clin*. 2000;18:195–202.
5. Hoffman EP. Voltage-gated ion channelopathies: Inherited disorders caused by abnormal sodium, chloride, and calcium regulation in skeletal muscle. *Annu Rev Med*. 1995;46:431–441.
6. Ko GTC, Chow CC, Yeung HHL, et al. Thyrotoxic periodic paralysis in a Chinese population. *Q J Med*. 1996;89:463–468.
7. Lehmann-Horn F, Jurkat-Rott K, Rüdel R. Periodic paralysis: Understanding channelopathies. *Curr Neurol Neurosci Rep*. 2002;2:61–69.
8. Lehmann-Horn F, Rüdel R. Channelopathies: The nondystrophic myotonias and periodic paralyses. *Semin Pediatr Neurol*. 1996;3:122–139.
9. Lin S, Chiu J, Hsu C, et al. A simple and rapid approach to hypokalemic paralysis. *Am J Emerg Med*. 2003;21:487–491.
10. Lin S, Lin Y. Propranolol rapidly reverses paralysis, hypokalemia, and hypophosphatemia in thyrotoxic periodic paralysis. *Am J Kid Dis*. 2001;37:620–623.
11. Lin Y, Wu C, Pei D, et al. Diagnosing thyrotoxic periodic paralysis in the ED. *Am J Emerg Med*. 2003;21:339–342.
12. Magsino CH, Ryan AJ. Thyrotoxic periodic paralysis. *South Med J*. 2000;93:996–1003.
13. Manoukian MA, Foote JA, Crapo LM. Clinical and metabolic features of thyrotoxic periodic paralysis in 24 episodes. *Arch Int Med*. 1999;159:601–606.
14. Ober KP. Thyrotoxic periodic paralysis in the United States: Report of 7 cases and review of the literature. *Medicine*. 1992;71:109–120.
15. Ptacek L. The familial periodic paralyses and nondystrophic myotonias. *Am J Med*. 1998;104:58–70.
16. Renner DR, Ptacek LJ. Periodic paralyses and nondystrophic myotonias. *Adv Neurol*. 2002;88:235–252.
17. Ruff RL. Insulin acts in hypokalemic periodic paralysis by reducing inward rectifier K+ current. *Neurology*. 1999;53:1556–1563.
18. Ruff RL. Skeletal muscle sodium current is reduced in hypokalemic periodic paralysis. *Proc Natl Acad Sci U.S.A*. 2000;97:9832–9833.
19. Stedwell R, Allen KM, Binder LS. Hypokalemic paralysis: a review of the etiologies, pathophysiology, presentation, and therapy. *Am J Emerg Med*. 1992;10:143–148.
20. Sternberg D, Maisonobe T, Jurkat-Rott K. Hypokalemic periodic paralysis Type 2 caused by mutations at codon 672 in the muscle sodium channel gene SCN4A. *Brain*. 2001;124:1091–1099.
21. Tassone H, Moulin A, Henderson S. The pitfalls of potassium replacement in thyrotoxic periodic paralysis: A case report and review of the literature. *J Emerg Med*. 2004;2:157–161.

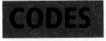 **MISCELLANEOUS**

See also: Guillain-Barré syndrome; Hyperthyroidism; Hypokalemia; Myasthenia gravis

CODES

ICD9-CM
359.3 Familial periodic paralysis

PATIENT TEACHING

Familial hypokalemic periodic paralysis: Genetic counseling; 50% risk of transmitting abnormal gene to offspring and ~50% chance of affected siblings

H

HYPONATREMIA

Peter Kozisek, MD

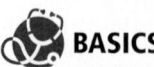 **BASICS**

DESCRIPTION
Plasma sodium concentration <135 mEq/L (<135 mmol/L)
- System(s) Affected: Endocrine/Metabolic

GENERAL PREVENTION
Dependent on underlying condition

ALERT
Rapid correction of severe symptomatic hyponatremia has been associated with central pontine myelinolysis (CPM), a neurologic disorder that induces loss of myelin and supportive structures in pons and occasionally in other areas of the brain. CPM is seen one to several days after rapid correction of serum sodium and is characterized by gradual neurologic deterioration.

EPIDEMIOLOGY
- Predominant age: All ages
- Predominant sex: Male = Female
- Most common electrolyte disorder seen in general hospital population
- Incidence/prevalence below based on recent study of hospitalized patients

Incidence
1%

Prevalence
2.5%

RISK FACTORS
Excessive fluid intake

PATHOPHYSIOLOGY
- Hypovolemic hyponatremia: decrease in total body water and greater decrease in total body sodium. Decreased extracellular fluid volume. Orthostatic hypotension and other changes consistent with hypovolemia are present.
- Euvolemic hyponatremia: Increase in total body water with normal total body sodium. Extracellular fluid volume is minimally to moderately increased, but no edema
- Hypervolemic hyponatremia: Increase in total body sodium and greater increase in total body water. Extracellular fluid increased markedly; edema present
- Redistributive hyponatremia: Shift of water from intracellular compartment to extracellular compartment with resultant dilution of sodium. Total body water and total body sodium unchanged. Occurs with hyperglycemia
- Pseudohyponatremia: Dilution of aqueous phase by excessive proteins, glucose or lipids. Total body water and total body sodium unchanged. Occurs in hypertriglyceridemia or multiple myeloma

ETIOLOGY
- Hypovolemic hyponatremia: Extrarenal loss of sodium
  - Gastrointestinal loss: Vomiting, diarrhea
  - Third spacing: Peritonitis, pancreatitis, burns, rhabdomyolysis
  - Skin loss: Burns, sweating, cystic fibrosis
  - Lung loss: Bronchorrhea
- Hypovolemic hyponatremia: renal loss of sodium:
  - Salt-losing nephritis
  - Mineralocorticoid deficiency
  - Diuretic
  - Bicarbonaturia: Renal tubular acidosis, metabolic alkalosis
  - Ketonuria or anion gap acidosis
  - Partial urinary tract obstruction
  - Osmotic diuresis
- Euvolemic hyponatremia
  - Hypothyroidism
  - Pure glucocorticoid deficiency
  - Drugs
  - Stress
  - Psychiatric, primary polydipsia
  - Syndrome of inappropriate antidiuretic hormone release: Causes include pulmonary and central nervous system disorders.
- Hypervolemic hyponatremia
  - Nephrotic syndrome
  - Cirrhosis
  - Congestive heart failure (CHF)
  - Renal failure
- Redistributive hyponatremia
  - Hyperglycemia
  - Mannitol infusion
- Pseudohyponatremia
  - Hypertriglyceridemia
  - Multiple myeloma, hyperglycemia

ASSOCIATED CONDITIONS
- Hypothyroidism
- Hypopituitarism
- Adrenocortical hormone deficiency
- Malignancy, most commonly small cell lung cancer

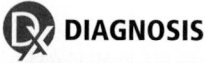 **DIAGNOSIS**

SIGNS AND SYMPTOMS
- Lethargy
- Disorientation
- Generalized weakness
- Muscle cramps
- Anorexia
- Hiccups
- Nausea and vomiting
- Agitation or delirium
- Stupor
- Coma
- Depressed deep-tendon reflexes
- Hypothermia
- Positive Babinski responses
- Cheyne-Stokes respiration
- Pseudobulbar palsy
- Seizures
- Orthostatic hypotension
- Cranial nerve palsies

TESTS
Lab
- Serum sodium <135 mEq/L (<135 mmol/L)
- Plasma osmolality
- Urine sodium
- BUN
- Creatinine
- Hypovolemic hyponatremia
  - Plasma osmolality low
  - BUN/creatinine ratio >20:1
  - Urine sodium >20 mEq/L (>20 mmol/L): Renal loss
  - Urine sodium <10 mEq/L (<10 mmol/L): Extrarenal loss
  - Serum potassium >5.0 mEq/L (>5 mmol/L): Consider mineralocorticoid deficiency.
- Euvolemic hyponatremia
  - Plasma osmolality low
  - BUN/creatinine ratio <20:1
  - Urine sodium >20 mEq/L (>20 mmol/L)
  - Thyroid-stimulating hormone test to rule out hypothyroidism
  - 1-hour cosyntropin-stimulation test to rule out adrenal insufficiency
- Hypervolemic hyponatremia
  - Plasma osmolality low
  - Urine sodium <10 mEq/L (<10 mmol/L) in nephrotic syndrome, CHF, cirrhosis
  - Urine sodium >20 mEq/L (>20 mmol/L) in acute and chronic renal failure
- Redistributive hyponatremia
  - Plasma osmolality normal or high
  - Glucose or mannitol levels elevated
- Pseudohyponatremia
  - Plasma osmolality normal
  - Triglyceride, glucose or protein levels elevated

Imaging
- CT of head if pituitary problem suspected or if syndrome of inappropriate antidiuretic hormone secretion from CNS problem suspected
- Chest radiograph to rule out pulmonary pathology if syndrome of inappropriate antidiuretic hormone secretion diagnosed

DIFFERENTIAL DIAGNOSIS
See "Etiology".

TREATMENT

GENERAL MEASURES

- Inpatient treatment mandatory if acute hyponatremia or symptomatic
- Inpatient treatment advised if asymptomatic and serum sodium <125 mEq/dL
- Assess all medications patient is taking.
- Institute seizure precautions.

Diet

- Euvolemic hyponatremia: Water restriction to 1,000 cc per day
- Hypervolemic hyponatremia: Water and sodium restriction
- Hypovolemic hyponatremia: Isotonic saline
- Redistributive or pseudohyponatremia: Treat underlying cause.

Activity

Varies according to patient mental status

 MEDICATION (DRUGS)

First Line

- Severe symptomatic hyponatremia: hypertonic saline (3%): 1 cc/kg/h
  - Use clearly indicated only in patients who are both severely symptomatic and have sodium concentrations <120 mEq/L (<120 mmol/L)
  - Will raise serum sodium level by ~1 mEq/L per hr (1 mmol/L/h)
  - Hypertonic saline infusion should continue only until serum sodium of 120 mEq/L (120 mmol/L) reached or patient becomes asymptomatic.
  - Avoid correction by >12 mEq/L/d (>12 mmol/d).
  - Precaution: Rapid correction of severe symptomatic hyponatremia has been associated with central pontine myelinolysis (CPM), a neurologic disorder that induces loss of myelin and supportive structures in pons and occasionally in other areas of the brain. CPM is seen one to several days after rapid correction of serum sodium and is characterized by gradual neurologic deterioration.
- Chronic hyponatremia: Demeclocycline
  - Consider if hyponatremia does not improve with fluid restriction or other appropriate treatment.
  - Contraindication: Can cause nephrotoxicity in patients with liver disease
  - Precaution: Photosensitivity and nausea can occur.
  - In doses of 600–1,200 mg/d, drug produces a nephrogenic diabetes insipidus.
  - Significant possible interactions: Oral anticoagulants, oral contraceptives, penicillin
- Maintenance: Clinical judgment

 FOLLOW-UP

PROGNOSIS

- Dependent on underlying condition
- With recognition and proper treatment, return to normal serum sodium and resolution of neurologic symptoms expected

COMPLICATIONS

- Occult tumor may present with syndrome of inappropriate antidiuretic hormone secretion.
- Hypervolemia if saline used
- CPM

PATIENT MONITORING

- Monitor serum sodium level when clinically indicated; if 3% saline used, check sodium level hourly.
- If 3% or 0.9% saline used, monitor volume status.

REFERENCES

1. Rose BD, Post TW. *Clinical Physiology of Acid-Base and Electrolyte Disorders*. 5th ed. New York: McGraw-Hill; 2001.
2. Schrier RW. *Renal and Electrolyte Disorders*. 6th ed. Boston: Little Brown & Co; 2002.

 MISCELLANEOUS

CODES

ICD9-CM
276.1 Hyposmolality and/or hyponatremia

See Corresponding Diagnostic Algorithm

H

HYPOPARATHYROIDISM

Carol Lynn Touma, MD
Robert Dobrzynski, MD

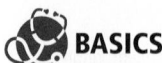 BASICS

DESCRIPTION

- Deficiency of parathyroid hormone from disease, injury, or congenital absence or malfunction of parathyroid glands. Manifested as hypocalcemia, producing neuromuscular symptoms ranging from paresthesia to tetany.
- Classifications
  - Acquired hypoparathyroidism: Follows accidental removal or damage to parathyroid glands during surgery, by irradiation, or by infiltrative diseases; may be transient or permanent
  - Idiopathic hypoparathyroidism: Autoimmune or congenital
- System(s) Affected: Endocrine/Metabolic; Musculoskeletal; Nervous
- Synonym(s): Parathyroid tetany

ALERT

Pediatric Considerations
- May occur in premature infants
- Congenital absence of parathyroids
- May appear later in childhood as idiopathic

Geriatric Considerations
Hypocalcemia is fairly common in the elderly, however it is rarely secondary to hypoparathyroidism (1)[B].

GENERAL PREVENTION
Care in any surgical procedure that may damage parathyroid glands

EPIDEMIOLOGY
- Predominant age: All ages
- Predominant sex: Male = Female

Incidence
Secondary hypoparathyroidism is most commonly due to a postsurgical complication.

Prevalence
All forms are rare.

RISK FACTORS
- Neck surgery, especially thyroid
- Neck trauma
- Head and neck malignancies

Genetics
Familial hypoparathyroidism is most commonly seen with mutations in CaSR (calcium sensing receptor) GATA3 genes (2).

ETIOLOGY
- Idiopathic
  - DiGeorge syndrome
  - Congenital absence
  - Late onset, autoimmune
- Postsurgical (may be transient)
- Infiltrative: Metastatic carcinoma and others
- Irradiation
- Hypomagnesemia
- Alcohol

ASSOCIATED CONDITIONS
- DiGeorge syndrome
- Addison disease
- Mucocutaneous candidiasis

DIAGNOSIS

SIGNS AND SYMPTOMS
- Chronic hypocalcemia may be asymptomatic.
- Perioral numbness
- Neuromuscular excitability as carpopedal spasm
- Increased deep-tendon reflexes
- Chvostek sign: Hyperirritability of facial nerve when tapped
- Trousseau sign: Carpal spasm within 2 minutes of inflating BP cuff over systolic pressure
- Dysphagia
- Organic brain syndrome
- Psychosis
- Mental deficiency (children)
- Tetany (paresthesias, pain, difficulty walking, laryngospasm, stridor, cyanosis, seizures)
- Dry hair
- Brittle fingernails
- Dry, scaly skin
- Cataracts
- Cardiac arrhythmias (2)[B]

History
- Neck trauma
- Head and neck irradiation

Physical Exam
Slit lamp: May show early posterior lenticular cataract formation

TESTS
ECG: Increased Q-T and S-T intervals (owing to hypocalcemia)

Lab
- Serum total and ionized calcium: Decreased
- Serum phosphorus: Increased (>5.4 mg/dL [>1.74 mmol/L])
- Parathyroid hormone (by immunometric assay): Decreased
- Serum β-carotene (normal)
- Stool fat (72-hour)
- Drugs that may alter lab results: Corticosteroids
- Disorders that may alter lab results: Other hormonal disorders; hypoalbuminemia

Imaging
Radiographs
- Increased bone density
- Tooth roots absent
- Calcification of cerebellum, choroid plexus, cerebral basal ganglia

Pathological Findings
- Parathyroid gland parenchymal tissue completely or almost completely replaced by fat
- Brain blood vessels calcified

DIFFERENTIAL DIAGNOSIS
- Rickets and osteomalacia (vitamin D deficiency)
- Polyglandular autoimmune (PGA) syndrome type I (candidiasis, hypoparathyroidism, adrenal insufficiency)
- Pseudohypoparathyroidism (no deficiency in parathyroid hormone, but target organs do not respond to its action)
- Addison disease
- Pernicious anemia
- Hypocalcemia of severe illness

TREATMENT

INITIAL STABILIZATION
- Outpatient unless severe
- Inpatient for tetany and laryngospasm (3)[A]
- Transient forms of hypoparathyroidism may not require treatment.

GENERAL MEASURES
- Acute-attack hypoparathyroid tetany
  - Life-threatening; requires immediate IV calcium treatment to raise calcium levels
  - Verify presence of adequate airway.
  - If patient is awake, breathing into paper bag can help raise serum ionized-calcium levels.
  - Seizure precaution
  - May require tracheostomy
- Maintenance
  - Lifelong calcitriol and calcium
  - Maintain serum calcium in low normal range: 8.5–9 mg/dL (2.12–2.25 mmol/L)
  - Skin softeners for scaly skin
  - Adequate control requires careful attention to avoid over- or undertreatment.

Diet
No special diet

Activity
As tolerated

Nursing
Monitoring for hypocalcemic symptoms

MEDICATION (DRUGS)

First Line
- For tetany
  - Immediate IV calcium gluconate: 10% solution 10–20 mL given slowly until tetany ceases
  - Calcium salts: PO as soon as possible, 1–2 g/d
  - Oral vitamin D (calcitriol in US): 0.5–2 mcg/d (dose to be titrated to normalized serum ionized calcium)
  - Calcitriol: Pediatric dose: 0.04–0.08 g/kg/24h. Adult dose: 0.25 g per 24 hours, then 0.25 g every other day. Adjust based on calcium and phosphorus levels.
- Maintenance
  - Calcium: 1–2 g/d in divided doses
  - Oral vitamin D and calcitriol
  - If associated endocrinopathies: Appropriate hormone replacement
  - Thiazide diuretic: For some patients to increase phosphate excretion and decrease calcium excretion
- Contraindications: Refer to manufacturer's literature.
- Precautions: Refer to manufacturer's literature.
- Significant possible interactions: Refer to manufacturer's literature.

Second Line
Oral vitamin D (ergocalciferol: 500 IU/d)

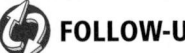 **FOLLOW-UP**

DISPOSITION
- Periodic measurement of serum calcium and phosphorous.
- Ophthalmologic referral for cataracts

Admission Criteria
- Laryngospasm
- Seizures
- Tetany

Discharge Criteria
Discharge is appropriate once tetany/laryngospasm resolved and patient is stable.

PROGNOSIS
- Hypoparathyroidism following neck surgery: Often transient
- Good outlook with diagnosis and treatment

COMPLICATIONS
- Neuromuscular symptoms (reversible)
- Cataracts
- Basal ganglia calcifications
- If condition starts early in childhood: Stunting of growth, malformation of teeth, mental retardation
- Hypothyroidism
- Parkinsonian symptoms
- Ossification of paravertebral ligaments
- Complications of over- or undertreatment
- Institutionalization owing to permanent mental damage

PATIENT MONITORING
- Outpatient after tetany corrected
- Periodic blood chemistry evaluations

REFERENCES
1. Agus ZS. Etiology of Hypocalcemia in Adults. Wellesley, MA: UpToDate, 2006.
2. Chiu WY. Identification of three novel mutations in the gata3 gene responsible for familial hypoparathyroidism and deafness in the Chinese population. *J Clin Endocrinol Metab*. 2006;91(11):4587–4592.
3. Potts JT. Starling review. *J Endocr*. 2005;187: 311–325.
4. Becker KL, ed. Principles and Practice of Endocrinology and Metabolism, 3rd ed. Philadelphia: Lippincott Williams & Wilkins; 2001:588–597.

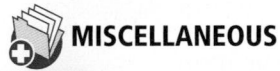 **MISCELLANEOUS**

CODES

ICD9-CM
252.1 Hypoparathyroidism

PATIENT TEACHING
- Provide careful and detailed instructions about maintenance therapy.
- Explain importance of periodic blood chemistry evaluations.
- Instruct patient to watch for signs and symptoms of over- and undertreatment.

 See Corresponding Diagnostic Algorithm

H

HYPOPITUITARISM

Michele Roberts, MD

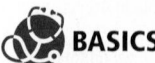 **BASICS**

DESCRIPTION
- Generalized condition caused by partial or total failure of pituitary gland's vital hormones: Adrenocorticotropic hormone (ACTH), thyroid-stimulating hormone (TSH), luteinizing hormone (LH), follicle-stimulating hormone (FSH), growth hormone (GH), prolactin
- System(s) Affected: Endocrine/metabolic; Gastrointestinal; Musculoskeletal; Nervous; Reproductive; Skin/Exocrine
- Synonym(s): Pituitary cachexia; Hypopituitarism syndrome; Simmonds syndrome; Panhypopituitarism

GENERAL PREVENTION
None

EPIDEMIOLOGY
- Predominant age: Occurs in adults and children. In children it causes dwarfism and pubertal delay.
- Predominant sex: Male = Female

Prevalence
Relatively rare

RISK FACTORS
- Trauma
- Pregnancy and delivery

Genetics
Some pituitary defects are congenital.

ETIOLOGY
- Lesions or tumors of anterior pituitary gland (intrasellar or extrasellar)
- Congenital defects
- Pituitary apoplexy
- Hypophysectomy
- Infiltrative diseases (e.g., sarcoidosis, histiocytosis X)
- Sometimes idiopathic
- Lymphocytic hypophysitis
- Irradiation
- Accidental or surgical trauma
- Hypothalamic disease
- Severe postpartum hemorrhage

ASSOCIATED CONDITIONS
- Childhood hypopituitarism
- Sheehan syndrome
- Hypothyroidism
- Kallmann syndrome

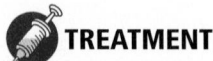 **DIAGNOSIS**

SIGNS AND SYMPTOMS
- Usually starts with hypogonadism or gonadotropin failure (decreased FSH and LH)
- Signs of hypofunction of target glands
- Secondary amenorrhea
- Impotence
- Infertility
- Decreased libido
- Diabetes insipidus (rare)
- Lethargy
- Tiredness
- Sensitivity to cold
- Anorexia
- Nausea
- Abdominal pain
- Lactation failure
- Retarded growth
- Failure of secondary sexual characteristics to develop
- Mental aberrations
- Headache
- Visual field defects
- Blindness

TESTS
Lab
- Confirm hormonal deficiencies.
- Radioimmunoassay of pituitary and target gland hormones
- Provocative tests
- Drugs that may alter lab results: Any hormone
- Disorders that may alter lab results
  - Cushing syndrome
  - Addison disease
  - Hyperthyroidism
  - Hypothyroidism

Imaging
- Radiographs: Chest, skull, hands, wrists (for bone age)
- Pituitary CT or MRI

Pathological Findings
- Destruction of anterior pituitary
- Atrophy of adrenal cortex, thyroid, gonads

DIFFERENTIAL DIAGNOSIS
- Primary hypothyroidism
- Anorexia nervosa
- Chronic liver disease
- Myotonia dystrophica
- Addison disease
- Primary psychosis
- Primary hypogonadism

ALERT
Geriatric Considerations
More difficult to diagnose in elderly

TREATMENT

GENERAL MEASURES
- Outpatient
- Inpatient for surgery when hypopituitarism is a result of pituitary tumor
- Hormonal replacement
- Exercise program for rehabilitation

Diet
High-calorie, high-protein diet

Activity
Encourage active physical exercise program.

MEDICATION (DRUGS)

First Line

- Replacement of hormones secreted by target glands
  - Hydrocortisone
  - Thyroxine
  - Androgen or cyclic estrogen
  - Human growth hormone (for treating dwarfism and in selected adult patients)
  - Dosages and administration schedule vary according to age and sex; refer to manufacturer's literature.
- Refer to manufacturer's literature for contraindications, precautions, and significant possible interactions.

SURGERY

For pituitary tumor

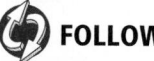 **FOLLOW-UP**

PROGNOSIS

- Variable, but guardedly favorable with replacement therapy
- If a result of postpartum necrosis, may have complete or partial recovery

COMPLICATIONS

- Blindness
- Adrenal crisis

PATIENT MONITORING

- 3- and 12-month evaluations for posttreatment hormonal status
- Patients with pituitary tumors: Include visual fields, thyroid and adrenal function, and sellar computerized imaging.

REFERENCES

1. Sheehan H, Summers VK. The syndrome of hypopituitarism. *Q J Med*. 1949;42:319–378.
2. Vance M. Hypopituitarism. *N Engl J Med*. 1994;330:1651–1662. Erratum in: *N Engl J Med*. 1994;331:487.

 ALERT

Pediatric Considerations

Hypopituitarism in this age group leads to dwarfism owing to lack of growth hormone.

Pregnancy Considerations

Lymphocytic hypophysitis may be triggered by pregnancy.

 MISCELLANEOUS

CODES

ICD9-CM

253.2 Panhypopituitarism

PATIENT TEACHING

- Wear medical identification bracelet or necklace.
- In patient with documented ACTH deficiency, stress need for additional cortisone at time of any major physical stress (e.g., fever above 101°F [38.3°C]; acute illness).

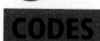 **See Corresponding Diagnostic Algorithm**

H

HYPOTHERMIA

Scott T. Henderson, MD

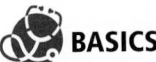 **BASICS**

DESCRIPTION
- A core temperature of <35°C (95°F)
- May take several hours to days to develop
- Patients with cold water immersion can appear to be dead but can still be resuscitated.
- System(s) Affected: All body systems
- Synonym(s): Accidental hypothermia

ALERT
Geriatric Considerations
- Mortality rates increase with increasing age.
- More common due to lower metabolic rate, impaired ability to maintain normal body temperature, and impared ability to detect temperature changes.

Pediatric Considerations
- A child's body temperature drops faster than an adult's when immersed in cold water. This may increase tolerance of cardiac arrhythmias.
- Infants may present with bright red, cold skin and very low energy.

Pregnancy Considerations
Controlled hypothermia in the operating suite is safe, especially with cerebrovascular surgery.

GENERAL PREVENTION
- Appropriate clothing with particular attention to head, feet, and hands
- For outdoor activities, carry survival bags with space blankets for use if stranded or injured.
- Avoid alcohol.
- Alertness to early symptoms and initiating preventive steps (e.g., drinking warm fluids)
- Identify medications that may predispose to hypothermia (e.g., neuroleptics, sedatives, hypnotics, tranquilizers).

EPIDEMIOLOGY
- Predominant age: Very young and the elderly
- Predominant sex: Male > Female

Prevalence
Estimates vary widely due to lack of pathologic evidence, and it is usually considered a secondary cause in diagnosing disorders.

RISK FACTORS
- Malnutrition
- Cold water immersion
- Exposure to high winds
- Homelessness
- Vehicle breakdown
- Outdoor work
- Trauma (especially head)
- Alcohol consumption
- Mental illness; Alzheimer disease
- Drug intoxication
- Endocrinopathies
- Hypothalamic and CNS dysfunction
- Sepsis
- Cardiovascular disease
- Bronchopneumonia
- Hepatic failure
- Uremia
- Extensive skin disease (psoriasis dermatitis)
- Excessive fluid loss

ETIOLOGY
- Decreased heat production
- Increased heat loss
- Impaired thermoregulation

ASSOCIATED CONDITIONS
- CHF
- Hypothyroidism
- Hypopituitarism
- Uremia
- Addison disease
- Ketoacidosis
- Pulmonary infection
- Sepsis
- Brain injury, tumor
- Diabetes

DIAGNOSIS

SIGNS AND SYMPTOMS
- Mild (32–35°C)
  - Lethargy and mild confusion
  - Shivering
  - Tachypnea
  - Loss of fine motor coordination
  - Increased pulse and blood pressure
  - Peripheral vasoconstriction
- Moderate (28–32°C)
  - Delirium
  - Bradycardia
  - Hypotension
  - Hypoventilation
  - Cyanosis
  - Arrhythmias
  - Semicoma and coma
  - Muscular rigidity
  - Generalized edema
  - Slowed reflexes
- Severe (<28°C)
  - Very cold skin
  - Rigidity
  - Apnea
  - No pulse: Ventricular fibrillation or asystole
  - Areflexia
  - Unresponsive
  - Fixed pupils

ALERT
History of prolonged exposure to cold may make the diagnosis obvious, but hypothermia may be overlooked, especially in comatose patients.

Physical Exam
Use special thermometers that can record low temperatures and measure core temperatures.

TESTS
Lab
- Arterial blood gases (reported in the uncorrected form)
- CBC and platelet count
- Toxicology screen
- Serum electrolytes
- Urinalysis
- Prothrombin time
- Partial thromboplastin time
- Fibrinogen levels
- Blood culture
- BUN/creatinine
- Glucose
- Amylase
- Liver function studies
- Thyroid function tests
- Serum cortisol
- Cardiac enzymes
- Special tests
  - ECG
  - Thyroid and pituitary function tests
- Drugs that may alter lab results: Refer to laboratory test reference.
- Disorders that may alter lab results: Refer to laboratory test reference.

Imaging
Cervical spine, chest, abdomen, if appropriate

Pathological Findings
- Moderate dilation of right heart
- Pulmonary edema

DIFFERENTIAL DIAGNOSIS
- Cerebrovascular accidents
- Intoxication
- Drug overdose
- Complications of diabetes, hypothyroidism, hypopituitarism

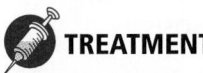 TREATMENT

GENERAL MEASURES
- ABCs of basic life support. Give warm humidified oxygen. Correct metabolic acidosis.
- Remove wet garments.
- Protect against heat loss and wind chill.
- Rewarming
  - Dependent on severity of hypothermia
  - Warm center of body 1st.
  - Rewarming at rate of 0.5–2°C per hour
- Monitor core temperature and cardiac rhythm.
- Evaluate for frostbite and other trauma.
- Mild hypothermia
  - Passive rewarming
  - Administration of heated (43°C) IV solutions (D$_5$NS)
  - Warm fluids may be given if fully alert.
- Moderate hypothermia
  - Active external rewarming with forced warm air systems. (1)[B]
- Severe hypothermia
  - Active internal (core) rewarming
    - Peritoneal dialysis
    - Gastrointestinal, colonic, or bladder lavage with warm fluids (43°C)
    - Heated IV fluids
    - Heated humidified oxygen
    - Thoracic cavity lavage (43°C)
    - Extracorporeal blood rewarming (1)[B]
- Cardiac arrhythmias
  - Atrial fibrillation and sinus bradycardia are common, but patients usually convert to normal sinus rhythm with rewarming.
  - Do not treat transient ventricular arrhythmias.
  - If cardiac pacing required, preferable to use external noninvasive pacemaker

Diet
Warm fluids only, if alert and able to swallow

Activity
Bed rest. Because of the cold, heart is irritable and susceptible to arrhythmias. Take special care in moving and transporting.

 MEDICATION (DRUGS)

First Line
- For sepsis or bacterial infections: Antibiotics based on site and etiology
- If ventricular fibrillation requires treatment, bretylium, 5 mg/kg, or magnesium sulfate, 100 mg/kg
- For hypoglycemia, D$_{50}$W at a dose of 1 mg/kg
- Thiamine, 100 mg, if alcoholic or cachectic
- Naloxone, 2.0 mg
- Levothyroxine 150–500 μg for myxedema
- For severe acidosis: Sodium bicarbonate
- Contraindications
  - Medications, including epinephrine, lidocaine, and procainamide, can accumulate to toxic levels if used repeatedly.
  - Routine use of steroids or antibiotics has not been shown to increase survival or decrease postresuscitative damage.
- Precautions
  - If no response to the initial 3 defibrillation attempts or initial drug therapy, subsequent defibrillations or medication should be avoided until core temperature is >30°C
    - When temperature reaches >30°C, IV medications are indicated, but at longer than the standard intervals.
  - Avoid vasopressors due to arrhythmogenic potential and delayed metabolism.
  - Avoid fluid overload.
  - Avoid lactated Ringer solution because of decreased lactate metabolism.
- Significant possible interactions
  - Use all drugs cautiously due to impaired metabolism and renal elimination.
  - Once rewarming has occurred, there is mobilization of depot stores.

 FOLLOW-UP

PROGNOSIS
- Mortality rates are decreasing due to increased recognition and advanced therapy.
- Mortality usually dependent on the severity of underlying cause of hypothermia
- In previously healthy individuals, recovery is usually complete.
- Mortality rate in healthy patients is <5%.
- Mortality rate in patients with coexisting illness is >50%.

COMPLICATIONS
- Cardiac arrhythmias
- Hypotension
- Hyperkalemia
- Hypoglycemia
- Rhabdomyolysis
- Bladder atony
- Pneumonia (aspiration and broncho)
- Pulmonary edema
- Acute respiratory distress syndrome (ARDS)
- Pancreatitis
- Peritonitis
- Gastrointestinal bleeding
- Acute tubular necrosis
- Intravascular thromboses
- Metabolic acidosis
- Gangrene of extremities
- Compartment syndromes

PATIENT MONITORING
- During acute episode
  - Monitor electrolytes and glucose frequently.
  - Monitor urinary output.
  - Follow blood gases.
- Following acute episode
  - Continued therapy for any underlying disorder

REFERENCES
1. McCullough L, Atora S. Diagnosis and treatment of hypothermia. *Am Fam Physician*. 2004;70: 2325–2332.
2. Biem J, Koehncke N, Dosman J. Out of the cold: Management of hypothermia and frostbite. *CMAJ*. 2003;168:305–311.

 MISCELLANEOUS

See also: Frostbite; Near drowning

CODES

ICD9-CM
- 778.2 Cold injury syndrome of newborn
- 778.3 Other hypothermia of newborn
- 780.99 Hypothermia not associated with low environmental temperature
- 991.6 Hypothermia
- 995.89 Other specified adverse effects, NEC, Other

PATIENT TEACHING

Activity
Urge persons with cardiovascular disease to avoid outdoor exercise in cold weather.

Prevention
Referral to social service agency for help with adequate housing, heat, or clothing

 See Corresponding Diagnostic Algorithm

H

HYPOTHYROIDISM, ADULT

Barbara A. Majeroni, MD

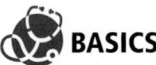 **BASICS**

DESCRIPTION

Clinical state resulting from decreased circulating levels of free thyroid hormone or from resistance to hormone action

- System(s) Affected: Endocrine/Metabolic
- Synonym(s): Myxedema

EPIDEMIOLOGY

- Predominant age: >40
- Predominant sex: Female > Male, 5:1 to 10:1

Prevalence

- 5–10/1000 in general population
- Common in elderly
- >65 years of age, increases to 6–10% of women, 2–3% of men

RISK FACTORS

- Increasing age
- Autoimmune diseases
- Previous postpartum thyroiditis
- Previous head or neck irradiation

Genetics

- No known genetic pattern for idiopathic primary hypothyroidism
- May be associated with Type II autoimmune polyglandular syndrome, which is associated with HLA-DR3, DR4
- Secondary hypothyroidism frequently results from treatment for Graves disease, which may be familial.

ETIOLOGY

- Postablative: Follows radioactive iodine therapy or thyroid surgery. Delayed hypothyroidism may develop in patients treated with thioamide drugs (propylthiouracil, methimazole) 4–25 years later.
- Primary: May develop as result of autoimmune thyroiditis or be idiopathic
- With goiter: Most commonly a result of autoimmune disease, such as Hashimoto thyroiditis. Other causes: Heritable biosynthetic defects, iodine deficiency (rare in US), or drugs (iodides, lithium, phenylbutazone, aminosalicylic acid, amiodarone, aminoglutethimide, and interferon alpha)
- Central or secondary: May be owing to deficiency of thyroid-releasing hormone (TRH) from hypothalamus or thyroid-stimulating hormone (TSH) from pituitary
- Transient: May result from silent thyroiditis (most common in postpartum period) and subacute granulomatous thyroiditis

ASSOCIATED CONDITIONS

- Hyponatremia
- Anemia
- Idiopathic adrenocorticoid deficiency
- Diabetes mellitus
- Hypoparathyroidism
- Myasthenia gravis
- Vitiligo
- Hypercholesterolemia
- Mitral valve prolapse
- Depression
- Rapid-cycling bipolar disorder
- Ischemic heart disease

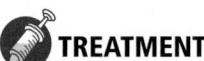 **DIAGNOSIS**

SIGNS AND SYMPTOMS

- Symptoms
  - Onset may be insidious, subtle
  - Weakness, fatigue, lethargy
  - Cold intolerance
  - Decreased memory
  - Hearing impairment
  - Constipation
  - Muscle cramps
  - Arthralgias
  - Paresthesias
  - Modest weight gain (10 lb [4.5 kg])
  - Decreased sweating
  - Menorrhagia
  - Depression
  - Hoarseness
  - Carpal tunnel syndrome
- Signs
  - Dry, coarse skin
  - Dull facial expression
  - Coarsening or huskiness of voice
  - Periorbital puffiness
  - Swelling of hands and feet
  - Bradycardia
  - Hypothermia
  - Reduced systolic BP
  - Increased diastolic BP
  - Reduced body and scalp hair
  - Delayed relaxation of deep-tendon reflexes
  - Macroglossia
  - Euvolemic hyponatremia
  - Anemia (usually normochromic, normocytic)
  - Enlarged heart on chest radiograph (often owing to pericardial effusion)

ALERT

Geriatric Considerations

Characteristic signs and symptoms frequently changed or absent. Diagnosis based on laboratory criteria

TESTS

Lab

- Primary hypothyroidism (1)[C]
  - TSH elevated
  - Serum free thyroxine (T4) decreased
- Central hypothyroidism
  - TSH low
  - Serum free T4 decreased
  - Impaired TSH response to TRH
- Severe hypothyroidism
  - Anemia
  - Elevated cholesterol
  - Elevated CPK, LDH, AST
  - Hyponatremia
- Subclinical hypothyroidism
  - TSH elevated
  - Serum free T4 normal
- Drugs that may alter lab results
  - Thyroid supplement
  - Cortisone
  - Dopamine
  - Phenytoin
  - Estrogen or androgen therapy in excess of replacement
  - Amiodarone
  - Salicylates

- Disorders that may alter lab results
  - Any severe illness
  - Pregnancy
  - Chronic protein malnutrition
  - Hepatic failure
  - Nephrotic syndrome

Imaging

None necessary

Pathological Findings

Thyroid may be small, atrophic, or enlarged.

DIFFERENTIAL DIAGNOSIS

- Nephrotic syndrome
- Chronic nephritis
- Neurasthenia
- Depression
- Euthyroid sick syndrome
- CHF
- Primary amyloidosis
- Dementia from other causes

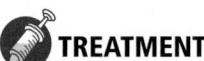 **TREATMENT**

GENERAL MEASURES

- Outpatient, except for complicating emergencies (e.g., coma, hypothermia)
- Treatment goals: Restore and maintain euthyroid state.

ALERT

Pregnancy Considerations

- Replacement therapy may need adjustment. TSH levels should be monitored monthly during 1st trimester. (2)[C]
- Postpartum: Check TSH levels at ~6 weeks.
- Painless subacute thyroiditis may occur in postpartum period leading to transient hypothyroidism lasting ~3 months. Treatment with replacement therapy may be warranted. Up to 30% of these individuals develop permanent hypothyroidism.

Diet

High-bulk diet may be helpful to avoid constipation.

Activity

As tolerated

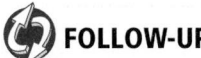 MEDICATION (DRUGS)

First Line
- Levothyroxine (Synthroid, Levothroid)
  - 1.6 μg/kg/d; increase by 25 μg/d every 4–6 weeks until TSH in normal range (3)[A]
  - Dosage requirements may vary with age, sex, residual secretory capacity of thyroid gland, other drugs being taken by patient, intestinal function
  - Elderly patients may require ~2/3 of dose used in young adults because clearance is decreased.
- Contraindications
  - Thyrotoxic heart disease
  - Uncorrected adrenocorticoid insufficiency
- Precautions
  - Start with lower doses in elderly and in patients with heart disease.
  - Diabetic patients may need readjustment of hypoglycemic agents with institution of thyroxine.
  - Dosage of oral anticoagulants may need adjustment; monitor prothrombin time while initiating treatment.
- Significant possible interactions
  - Oral anticoagulants
  - Insulin
  - Oral hypoglycemics
  - Estrogen
  - Oral contraceptives
  - Cholestyramine
  - Ferrous sulfate, calcium carbonate, and cholestyramine may decrease absorption when taken concomitantly.

Second Line
None currently recommended

SURGERY
- Hypothyroid patients (mild to moderate) tolerate surgery with mortality and complications similar to euthyroid states.
- If surgery is elective, render patient euthyroid prior to procedure.
- If surgery is urgent, proceed with procedure with individualized replacement therapy preoperatively and postoperatively.

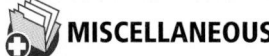 FOLLOW-UP

DISPOSITION
Admission Criteria
Myxedema coma, hypothermia

PROGNOSIS
- Return to normal state is the rule.
- Relapses will occur if treatment is interrupted.
- If untreated, may progress to myxedema coma

COMPLICATIONS
- Treatment-induced CHF in people with coronary artery disease
- Myxedema coma: Life threatening
- Increased susceptibility to infection
- Megacolon
- Organic psychosis with paranoia
- Adrenal crisis with vigorous treatment of hypothyroidism, especially in patients with undiagnosed polyendocrine syndromes
- Infertility
- Hypersensitivity to opiates
- Overtreatment over long periods can lead to bone demineralization.
- Subclinical hypothyroidism is associated with increased ischemic heart disease and increased all-cause mortality in men, but not in women. It is not clear whether treatment changes that risk.

PATIENT MONITORING
- Every 6 weeks until stabilized, then every 6 months
- Follow cardiac status closely in older patients.

REFERENCES

1. Supit EJ, Peiris AN. Interpretation of laboratory thyroid function tests for the primary care physician. *South Med J.* 2002;95:481–485.
2. Alexander EK, Marquese E, Lawrence J, et al. Timing and management of increases in levothyroxine requirements during pregnancy in women with hypothyroidism. *N Engl J Med.* 2004;351:241–249.
3. Roos A, Linn-Rasker SP, van Domburg RT, Tijssen JP, Berghout A. The starting dose of levothyroxine in primary hypothyroidism treatment: A prospective, randomized, double-blind trial. *Arch Int Med.* 2005;165:1714–1720.

ADDITIONAL READING

Roberts CG, Ladenson PW. Hypothyroidism. *Lancet.* 2004;363:793–803.

MISCELLANEOUS

See also: Hyperthyroidism; Thyroiditis

CODES

ICD9-CM
- 244.0 Postsurgical hypothyroidism
- 244.1 Other postablative hypothyroidism
- 244.2 Iodine hypothyroidism
- 244.8 Other specified acquired hypothyroidism
- 244.9 Unspecified hypothyroidism

PATIENT TEACHING
- Stress importance of compliance with thyroid replacement therapy.
- Explain need for lifelong treatment.
- Instruct to report to physician any signs of infection or heart problems.
- Describe signs of thyrotoxicity.

Diet
High fiber, low fat diet

See Corresponding Diagnostic Algorithm

H

ID REACTION

Jeremy Golding, MD

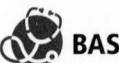 **BASICS**

DESCRIPTION
- A cutaneous eruption ("autoeczematization") associated with, but distant to, the main lesion of the disease.
- *Id* is a word termination often combined with a root reflecting the causative factor, i.e., bacterid, syphilid, and tuberculid.
- The dermatophytid is the most frequently referenced id reaction in dermatology. A dermatophytid is an autosensitization reaction in which a secondary cutaneous reaction occurs at a site distant to a primary fungal infection. The eruption begins typically within 1–2 weeks of the onset of the main lesion, or following exacerbation of the main lesion.
- System(s) Affected: Skin/Exocrine
- Synonym(s): Dermatophytid; Trichophytid

GENERAL PREVENTION
- Minimize factors for developing fungal infections.
- Promptly treat any developing fungal infection.

EPIDEMIOLOGY
- Predominant age: All ages
- Predominant sex: Male = Female

Prevalence
In the US: Not infrequent

RISK FACTORS
- Fungal infection of the skin.
- Stasis dermatitis.

ETIOLOGY
Precise pathophysiology is uncertain. Circulating antigens may react with antibodies at sensitized areas of the skin, or abnormal immune recognition of autologous skin antigens may occur

ASSOCIATED CONDITIONS
- Primary fungal infection.
- Stasis dermatitis.

 **DIAGNOSIS**

SIGNS AND SYMPTOMS
- Usual
  - Symmetric, pruritic vesicles on the hands
  - Tinea infection on the feet, contact or other eczematous dermatosis, or bacterial, fungal, or viral infection of the skin
  - Generalized reactions can occur.
- Less common
  - Papules
  - Lichenoid eruption
  - Eczematoid eruption

TESTS
Lab
- Fungal infection at the primary site proven by potassium hydroxide (KOH) or fungal culture
- No fungal demonstrable at the site of the presumed id reaction
- Special tests: Skin shows a positive trichophyton reaction.

Pathological Findings
- Vesicles in the upper dermis
- Superficial perivascular lymphohistiocytic infiltrate
- Small numbers of eosinophils
- Moderate acanthosis
- Increased granular cell layer
- No infectious agents present in biopsy specimen

DIFFERENTIAL DIAGNOSIS
- Pompholyx (dyshidrotic eczema)
- Contact dermatitis
- Drug eruptions
- Pustular psoriasis
- Folliculitis
- Scabies

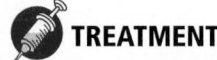 **TREATMENT**

GENERAL MEASURES
- Appropriate health care: Outpatient
- Treatment of the underlying infection or eczematous dermatitis
- Symptomatic treatment of pruritus with antihistamines and/or topical steroids if needed
- Treatment for secondary bacterial infection

Diet
No special diet

Activity
As tolerated

MEDICATION (DRUGS)

First Line

- Antifungals: Topical and/or systemic
- Contraindications: Refer to manufacturer's profile of each drug.
- Precautions: Refer to manufacturer's profile of each drug.
- Significant possible interactions: Refer to manufacturer's profile of each drug.

Second Line

- Topical or systemic antibiotics for any secondary infection
- Antihistamines for any pruritus
- Topical steroids for pruritus
- Systemic steroids only if reaction is florid or generalized nature

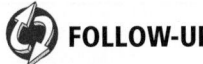 **FOLLOW-UP**

PROGNOSIS

After appropriate treatment, virtual resolution in a few days to 2 weeks

COMPLICATIONS

Secondary bacterial infection (cellulitis)

REFERENCES

1. Habif T. Clinical Dermatology, 4th ed. St. Louis: Mosby, 2004.
2. Evans M, Bronson D. Id reaction (autoeczematization). E-Medicine; Oct 2005.

 MISCELLANEOUS

See also: Tinea corporis; Tinea pedis

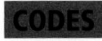

ICD9-CM

692.89 Contact dermatitis and other eczema due to other specified agents, other

PATIENT TEACHING

- Avoid hot, humid conditions that promote fungal growth.
- Aerate susceptible body areas (e.g., wear sandals or open footwear).
- If possible, wear boxer shorts or loose fitting clothing, dry off wet skin after bathing, use powders and antiperspirants to make the environment less conducive to fungal growth.
- Treat primary dermatitis promptly.

I

IDIOPATHIC HYPERTROPHIC SUBAORTIC STENOSIS

Peter Kozisek, MD

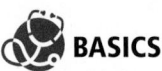 BASICS

DESCRIPTION

First-known form of the hypertrophic cardiomyopathies with characteristic finding of inappropriate (disproportionate to hemodynamic load) myocardial hypertrophy

- System(s) Affected: Cardiovascular
- Synonym(s): Hypertrophic obstructive cardiomyopathy; Muscular subaortic stenosis

GENERAL PREVENTION

- Avoid strenuous exercise, especially competitive sports.
- Avoid rapid standing.
- Avoid inotropic drugs and diuretics.
- Use antitussives for infections accompanied by cough.

EPIDEMIOLOGY

- Predominant age: Most commonly presents in 3rd decade (disease of young adulthood), but occurs from newborns to elderly
- Predominant sex: Male = Female

ALERT

Geriatric Considerations

- Occurrence more frequent with increasing age
- Female prevalence greater in this age group

Prevalence

Uncommon

RISK FACTORS

Family history of hypertrophic cardiomyopathy

Genetics

- Autosomal dominant with >50% penetrance
- Evidence of disease (usually milder) found in 25% of 1st-degree relatives. Relatives usually do not have outflow obstruction, exhibit only localized hypertrophy, and are asymptomatic.

PATHOPHYSIOLOGY

- Etiology characterized by dynamic pressure gradient in subaortic area leading clinically to
  - Diastolic dysfunction with impaired ventricular filling and elevated atrial filling pressures producing dyspnea *and*
  - Systolic dysfunction with limitation of cardiac output response to exercise, exertional syncope, and secondary left ventricular (LV) hypertrophy
- Diagnosis usually made by recognition of signs associated with outflow obstruction, but symptoms are predominantly characterized by diastolic dysfunction
  - Thickened septum impinging on anterior mitral-valve leaflet during systole, causing outflow obstruction

ASSOCIATED CONDITIONS

- Mitral regurgitation
- Essential hypertension
- Mitral valve prolapse
- Angina pectoris

DIAGNOSIS

SIGNS AND SYMPTOMS

- Dyspnea: Mainly result of diastolic dysfunction; onset initially exertional (50–90%)
- Angina pectoris (50–90%)
- Syncope: Exertional (50–90%)
- Presyncope: Exertional (50–90%)
- Fatigue (50–90%)
- Palpitations (50–90%)
- Paroxysmal nocturnal dyspnea (50%)
- Double apical impulse owing to prominent atrial system
- Point of maximal impulse displaced laterally
- Rapidly rising bifid carotid pulse
- Prominent S4
- S2 variable splitting (depending on degree of outflow obstruction)
- Harsh systolic crescendo/decrescendo murmur best heard between apex and left sternal border
- Murmur: Increases and lengthens with Valsalva maneuver, standing, amyl nitrite; decreases with sudden squatting, lying down, passive leg raising, isometric handgrip

ALERT

Pediatric Considerations

- Idiopathic hypertrophic subaortic stenosis being recognized with increasing frequency
- Children may be asymptomatic. Evaluation of a heart murmur may disclose idiopathic hypertrophic subaortic stenosis.

TESTS

- Electrocardiogram: Common findings (50–90%)
  - Nonspecific ST-T wave abnormalities
  - LV hypertrophy
- Electrocardiogram: Less common findings (<50%):
  - Prominent and abnormal Q waves in anterior precordial and lateral limbs lead, simulating myocardial infarction
  - P-wave abnormalities indicating left atrial enlargement
  - Short PR interval with QRS morphology suggesting pre-excitation without clear evidence of pre-excitation (rare)
  - Holter findings: Frequent ventricular arrhythmias with up to 25% revealing ventricular tachycardia
  - Atrial fibrillation: Late finding, sign of poor prognosis

Imaging

- Chest radiograph: Variable findings, from normal cardiac size to cardiomegaly, none of which is pathognomonic
- Echocardiography
  - Asymmetric septal hypertrophy with septal to free-wall ratio >1.3:1
  - Abnormal systolic anterior leaflet motion of mitral valve
  - LV hypertrophy
  - Left atrial enlargement
  - Small ventricular chamber size with increased contractility
  - Partial systolic closure of aortic valve in midsystole
  - Mitral valve prolapse
  - Mitral regurgitation by Doppler
  - Decreased midaortic flow coincident with systolic anterior leaflet motion of mitral valve by Doppler
- Radionuclide: Thallium scintigraphy with stress at times reveals positive defects in setting of arteriographically normal coronary arteries.
- Cardiac catheterization and angiocardiography
  - Hemodynamic measurement documents degree and lability of outflow obstruction, and diastolic characteristics of LV.
  - Angiocardiography documents LV and RV anatomy and coronary arterial anatomy.

Pathological Findings

- Distinctive pattern of LV hypertrophy: Localized, disproportionate hypertrophy of LV septum with ratio of septal to free-wall thickness >1.3:1 without anatomic evidence of pressure overload
- Dilated atria
- Increased LV mass and small chamber sizes
- Mural plaque of LV outflow tract
- Mitral valve thickening
- Anatomic variants
  - Apical form; not associated with intraventricular gradients
  - Localized midventricular obstructive form
- Disorganization and disarray septal muscle bundles
- Abnormal intramural coronary arteries

DIFFERENTIAL DIAGNOSIS

Fixed-outflow obstruction such as aortic stenosis

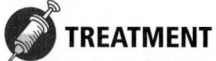 **TREATMENT**

GENERAL MEASURES

- Outpatient usually
- Inpatient for studies and/or surgery
- Therapy based on pathophysiology, namely interventions to reduce ventricular contractility or increase ventricular volume, ventricular compliance, and outflow-tract dimensions
- Pacemaker therapy: AV sequential pacing is frequently helpful in symptomatic patients with an outflow obstruction who do not respond to medical therapy.

Diet

No special diet, but may need to reduce caloric intake owing to reduced activity

Activity

- Strenuous exercise, especially competitive sports, should not be undertaken because of high risk of sudden death. Younger patients with little or no functional impairment have greatest risk of sudden death.
- Sports participation not permitted if any of following are present
  - Marked LV hypertrophy
  - Significant outflow gradient
  - Significant supraventricular and/or ventricular arrhythmias
  - History of sudden death in relative(s) with hypertrophic cardiomyopathy

 MEDICATION (DRUGS)

First Line

- Beta-blockers (e.g., propranolol, metoprolol)
  - May decrease outflow obstruction: Some evidence suggests they may increase ventricular compliance. No clear evidence that they reduce incidence of sudden death
  - 1/3 to 2/3 of patients experience symptomatic improvement.
  - May titrate up to 320 mg/d of propranolol equivalent to obtain clinical effect, provided patient tolerates dose
- Calcium-channel blockers (primarily verapamil)
  - Alternative to propranolol
  - May have better effect on exercise performance
  - Decreases outflow gradient owing to depression of cardiac contractility
  - Improves diastolic filling by improved diastolic relaxation
- Amiodarone (Cordarone)
  - Limited use in treating ventricular arrhythmias because of documented proarrhythmic effects in hypertrophic cardiomyopathy
  - Use only in patients with ventricular tachycardia associated with hemodynamic compromise. Use of drug is to be guided by initial and follow-up electrophysiologic studies.
- Contraindications: Verapamil
  - Major side effects include depression of impulse formation and A-V block, negative inotropism, and vasodilatation—all of which can result in hypotension, shock, pulmonary edema, and death.
  - Therefore, relatively contraindicated for use in patients with increased LV end diastolic pressure, paroxysmal nocturnal dyspnea, orthopnea, and/or sinus node disease and A-V block (unless there is an appropriate pacing device)
  - Digitalis glycosides contraindicated except for atrial fibrillation with uncontrolled response
  - Nitrates and sympathomimetic amines (e.g., isoproterenol) contraindicated except with concomitant coronary heart disease
  - Diuretics relatively contraindicated because of their effect on ventricular volume and LV myotomy
- Precautions: Refer to manufacturer's literature.
- Significant possible interactions: Refer to manufacturer's literature.

Second Line

- Diltiazem
- Disopyramide

SURGERY

LV myomectomy

- Only in setting of severe symptoms refractory to medical therapy or sequential pacing in those patients with outflow gradient >50 mm Hg (<6.65 kPa), either at rest or with provocation
- 95% successful in abolishing gradient, with 70% of patients having marked symptomatic improvement for ≥5 years

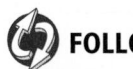 **FOLLOW-UP**

PROGNOSIS

- Annual mortality rate: 4% a year (sudden death most common reason)
- Chronic illness with restricted lifestyle

COMPLICATIONS

- Sudden death
- CHF
- Arrhythmia
- Atrial fibrillation with mural thrombosis formation
- Infective mitral endocarditis

PATIENT MONITORING

Yearly when symptoms and pharmacologic regimens become stable

REFERENCES

1. Braunwald E, ed. *Heart Disease:* A Textbook of Cardiovascular Medicine. 6th ed. Philadelphia: WB Saunders; 2001.
2. Goldman L, Braunwald E, eds. Primary Cardiology. 2nd ed. Philadelphia: WB Saunders; 2003.
3. Maron BJ, Robert WC, Epstein SE. Sudden death in hypertrophic cardiomyopathy: a profile of 78 patients. *Circulation.* 1982;65:1388–1394.

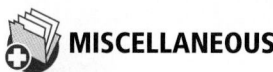 **MISCELLANEOUS**

CODES

ICD9-CM
425.1 Hypertrophic obstructive cardiomyopathy

PATIENT TEACHING

- Refer for psychosocial counseling if appropriate. (Patient and family may suffer from problems associated with restricted lifestyle and chronic disease.)
- Recommend family learn cardiopulmonary resuscitation methods
- Genetic counseling may be appropriate.

Activity

Restrictions (see "Treatment")

 See Corresponding Diagnostic Algorithm

IDIOPATHIC THROMBOCYTOPENIC PURPURA (ITP)

Jeffery T. Kirchner, DO

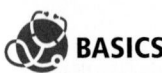 **BASICS**

DESCRIPTION (1,2)
- Decrease in circulating number of platelets (<100,00/mL) in the absence of toxic exposure or disease associated with low platelet count
- Occurs as secondary effect of peripheral platelet destruction as well as decreased platelet production
- Diagnosis of exclusion
- Acute ITP: Relatively common disease of childhood that often follows acute infection and has spontaneous resolution within 2 months; platelet counts <20,000
- Chronic ITP: Persists after 6 months without a specific cause; usually seen in adults and persists for months to years; platelet count typically 30,000–80,000
- System(s) Affected: Heme/Lymphatic/Immunologic
- Synonym(s): Post infectious thrombocytopenia; Immune thrombocytopenic purpura; Werlhof disease

GENERAL PREVENTION
The patient should avoid medications (when feasible) that inhibit platelet function (such as aspirin) or those that suppress bone marrow.

EPIDEMIOLOGY
- Predominant age
  - Acute ITP (primarily a childhood disease): 2–6 years old
  - Chronic ITP: >50 years
  - Uncommon in geriatric population; look for other cause of low platelet count
- Predominant sex:
  - Acute ITP: Male = Female
  - Chronic ITP: Female > Male (2:1)

Prevalence
1 in 10,000

RISK FACTORS
- Acute infection
- Age (see "Epidemiology" listed previously)
- Cardiopulmonary bypass
- Hypersplenism
- Antiphospholipid antibody syndrome
- Preeclampsia
- HIV infection

Genetics
No known genetic pattern

ETIOLOGY
IgG autoantibodies on platelet surface that are bound to and destroyed by reticuloendothelial phagocytes

ASSOCIATED CONDITIONS
- Acute ITP
  - Varicella
  - Other viral infections (EBV, CMV)
- Chronic ITP
  - HIV
  - *Helicobacter pylori*
  - Graves disease
  - Hashimoto thyroiditis
  - Sarcoidosis
  - Systemic lupus erythematosus
  - Autoimmune hemolytic anemia (Evans syndrome)

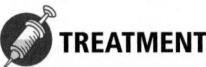 **DIAGNOSIS**

SIGNS AND SYMPTOMS
- Posttraumatic bleeding at 40,000–60,000 platelet count
- Petechial hemorrhages
- Purpura
- Bruising tendency
- Gingival bleeding
- Gastrointestinal bleeding
- Mucocutaneous hemorrhages
- Menometrorrhagia
- Menorrhagia
- Recurrent epistaxis
- Neurological symptoms secondary to intracerebral bleeding
- Nonpalpable spleen (absence of splenomegaly is essential diagnostic criterion)
- Spontaneous bleeding occurs with platelet count <20,000.

TESTS
Lab
- Decreased platelet count: 5,000–75,000
- Relative lymphocytosis and slight eosinophilia
- Prolonged bleeding time (not useful in presence of thrombocytopenia)
- Anemia
- PT, PTT normal
- Platelet associated antibody (PA-IgG)
  - Optional bound and unbound test available
  - Bound is superior: Sensitivity 49–66%, specificity 78–92%

Imaging
Head CT to rule out intracranial bleeding if clinically indicated

Diagnostic Procedures/Surgery
Bone marrow aspiration/biopsy (consider in refractory cases)
- Does not need to be done before giving gamma globulin
- Not needed in patients <60 who have typical clinical and lab presentation
- Rarely indicated in children, but preferred by some hematologists if steroids will be used in treatment

Pathological Findings
- Peripheral smear
  - Routinely recommended
  - Shows normal red and white cells with diminished but large platelets
  - Helps rule out pseudothrombocytopenia
- Marrow reveals abundant megakaryocytes with normal erythroid and myeloid precursors

DIFFERENTIAL DIAGNOSIS
- Drug-induced immune thrombocytopenia; >150 drugs have been implicated
- Infections
- Acute leukemia
- Thrombotic thrombocytopenia purpura
- Hemolytic uremic syndrome
- Factitious: "Platelet clumping on the peripheral smear"
- Thrombocytopenia secondary to sepsis
- Myelodysplastic syndrome, particularly in older patients
- Decreased production in marrow: Malignancy, drugs, viruses, megaloblastic anemia
- Post transfusion
- Isoimmune neonatal purpura
- Disseminated intravascular coagulation
- Alcohol-induced thrombocytopenic purpura

TREATMENT

GENERAL MEASURES
- Outpatient management unless patient at risk for bleeding (platelet count <20,000)
- Admit patients with active bleeding.
- Children do not require treatment with
  - Platelet count >30,000 and asymptomatic
  - Minor purpura
- Treat adults with
  - Platelet count <20,000
  - Platelet count <50,000 with symptoms or risks for bleeding, such as HTN or peptic ulcers
- Specific treatment usually not necessary unless count <100,000; possibly <30,000 with chronic ITP
- Platelet transfusions for significant bleeding

ALERT
Pregnancy Considerations
- Only if <50,000 platelet count: May consider Caesarean section
- A patient in labor should receive IV gamma globulin due to the risk to the infant.
- Platelet autoantibodies cross the placenta and may cause neonatal thrombocytopenia. Consider prednisone 10–20 mg/d for 10–14 days prior to delivery.
- Preeclampsia or gestational thrombocytopenia may cause thrombocytopenia unrelated to ITP.

Diet
No special diet

Activity
- Minimal activity to prevent injury or bruising
- Avoid contact sports.

SPECIAL THERAPY
- Plasmapheresis
- Autologous hematopoietic stem cell transplantation
- Investigational or experimental therapies
- Autologous bone marrow transplant: Investigational/experimental

MEDICATION (DRUGS)

First Line (2,3)
- Acute ITP: Oral Prednisone 1–2 mg/kg/d for 2–4 weeks, then taper
- Chronic ITP
  - Oral prednisone 1–2 mg/kg/d with tapers over 4–6 weeks; most responses occur within 1st week of treatment (2,3)[B]
  - For patients who do not respond, consider IV immune globulin 0.4 g/kg/d for 5 days, *or* anti-D, 50 μg/kg once (repeat as necessary), *or* dexamethasone 20–40 mg/d for 4 days (2,3)[C]
  - If no response to these therapies, consider splenectomy
  - Also limited data to screen for and eradicate *Helicobacter pylori*
- Emergency treatment of patients with internal or mucocutaneous bleeding or who need emergent surgery treatment should include (3)[C]
  - IV immune globulin 1 g/kg/d for 2 days
  - IV methylprednisolone 1 g/d for 3 days
  - Platelet transfusions (5 U q4–6h or 2 U/h)
- Contraindications: Do not administer gamma globulin if patient has IgA deficiency.
- Precautions: Refer to the manufacturer's literature.
- Significant possible interactions: Anaphylaxis in patients with IgA deficiency who have IgA autoantibodies

Second Line (3,4)
- Acute ITP: IV immune globulin (gamma globulin):
  - Single dose (1–2 g/kg) or 400 mg/kg/d for 5 days (3,4)[C]
  - Minor adverse reactions: Chills, nausea, headache, and joint pain may occur in 2–7% of the patients. If so, slow the rate of infusion.
  - Gamma globulin may be effective alone or as pretreatment to facilitate platelet transfusion. This treatment may delay the need for a splenectomy.
- Chronic ITP: High doses of IV gamma globulin in emergencies
- Anti-Rho(D) immune globulin 250 IU (50–75 μg/kg) as single dose or in 2 divided doses given over 2 days; indications for use
  - Children with acute or chronic ITP
  - Adults with chronic ITP who are Rh D-positive
  - ITP secondary to HIV infection
- Azathioprine: 1–4 mg/kg/d modified according to WBC
- Cyclophosphamide: 1–2 mg/kg/d
- Vincristine or vinblastine
- Danazol: 400–800 mg/d
- Cyclosporin A: 3 mg/kg/d
- Rituximab, campath-1H, mycophenolate mofetil
- Investigational or experimental therapies
  - Monoclonal antibodies against CD20 and CD154
  - Immune globulin IV (1 g/kg for 2–3 days), if platelets <5,000 despite several days of steroids
  - Thrombopoietin
  - Etanercept
  - Monoclonal antibody to Fcγ RI receptor
  - Monoclonal antibody to CD40 ligand

SURGERY (5)
Splenectomy
- In-patients who fail medical therapy
- Consider Hib and meningococcal vaccine
- Be sure to administer the pneumococcal vaccine at least 2 weeks prior
- Criteria remain poorly defined; decision based on response, severity, and patient preference regarding risks/benefits of surgery.
- Splenectomy considered if after 3–6 months patient needs prednisone >10–20 mg/d to keep platelets above 30,000/mm^3 of (5)[C]

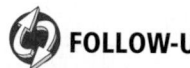 **FOLLOW-UP**

PROGNOSIS
- Acute ITP
  - ~80–85% of the patients completely recover within 2 months.
  - 15% proceed to chronic ITP.
- Chronic ITP
  - ~10–20% of the patients recover spontaneously.
  - Remainder with diminished platelets for months to years
  - May see spontaneous remissions (5%) and relapses

ALERT
Pediatric Considerations
Better prognosis in children than adults

COMPLICATIONS
- 1% mortality due to intracranial hemorrhage
- Severe blood loss
- Corticosteroid adverse effects
- Pneumococcal infections if patient must have splenectomy. Use pneumococcal vaccine.

PATIENT MONITORING
- Frequent platelet counts, daily to weekly, depending on severity and treatment
- Follow clinical status of hemostasis.

REFERENCES
1. Cines DB. Thrombocytopenic purpura. *N Engl J Med*. 2002;346:995–1008.
2. Di Paola JA, Buchanan GR. Immune thrombocytopenic purpura. *Pediatric Clin North Am*. 2002;49:911–928.
3. Stasi R, Provan R. Management of ITP in adults. *Mayo Clin Proc*. 2004;79:504–522.
4. McMillan R. Classical management of refractory adult immune (idiopathic) thrombocytopenic purpura. *Blood Rev*. 2002;16:51–55.
5. Kojouri K. Systematic review of splenectomy for ITP. *Blood*. 2004;104:2623–2634.

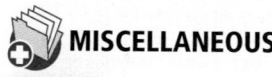 **MISCELLANEOUS**

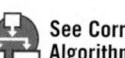 **CODES**

ICD9-CM
287.3 Primary thrombocytopenia

PATIENT TEACHING
- Avoidance of ASA and other platelet-inhibiting drugs
- No data on immunizations, strictly recommendations

See Corresponding Diagnostic Algorithm

IMMUNIZATIONS

Richard Kent Zimmerman, MD, MPH
Richard D. Clover, MD

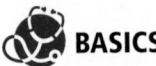 **BASICS**

DESCRIPTION

For the prevention of certain diseases. Specific indications include

- Hepatitis B:
  - Infants
  - Health care workers
  - Laboratory personnel who might be exposed to the virus
  - IV drug users
  - Male homosexuals
  - Patients with a sexually transmitted disease
- Pneumococcal polysaccharide
  - All persons age ≥65 years (once)
  - All patients prior to splenectomy
  - Patients with chronic liver, heart, lung, or renal disease
  - Patients with diabetes mellitus, HIV, asplenia
- Influenza inactivated (annually)
  - All persons age ≥50 years
  - Health care workers
  - Patients with chronic heart, lung, or renal neumomsucluar, disease diabetes mellitus, HIV, pregnancy
  - Healthy children age 6–59 months including household contacts of these children and out-of-home
  - Caregivers
  - Contacts of high-risk persons
- Live, attenuated influenza vaccine (LAIV) for healthy persons 5–49 years old who wish to be vaccinated
- Pediatric diphtheria and tetanus toxoids and acellular pertussis vaccine (DTaP)
  - All children starting at age 2 months
  - May be given up to the 7th birthday
- Diphtheria and tetanus (pediatric) toxoids
  - Children <7 years who cannot take DTaP
- Tdap (adult)
  - Tdap at ages 11–12 and may be given as catch-up in 2 years after a previous Td.
  - Td is recommended every 10 years.
  - Among adults Tdap replaces one of the decennial Td doses; Tdap not licensed past 64 years yet
  - Tdap is recommended for health care workers.
- Measles, mumps, and rubella (MMR)
  - Children at age 12–15 months and again between 4 and 6 years
  - Adults (especially medical personnel and day care workers) born after 1956 without prior immunization or uncertain immunizations
  - International travelers
  - College students: 2 doses total if not previously vaccinated
- Varicella
  - Children at age 12–18 months (1 dose)
  - Catch-up vaccination for children 18 months to 12 years (1 dose) without history of chickenpox
  - Susceptible persons ≥13 years without history of chickenpox (2 doses)
  - Health care workers without a previous history of chickenpox
  - Varicella vaccine may be given within 3–5 days for postexposure prophylaxis

- Polio: All inactivated poliovirus vaccine (IPV) schedule
  - All children starting at 2 months of age
  - Adults previously immunized who will travel to areas where polio is prevalent
  - 4 doses of IPV now recommended
  - For school entry, 4 doses of polio vaccine (IPV and/or trivalent oral poliovirus vaccine) needed
- *Haemophilus influenzae* Type b (Hib)
  - All children starting at 2 months of age
- Hepatitis A
  - All 12- to 23-months-olds should receive 2 doses
  - Travelers to higher risk countries
  - Patients with chronic liver disease
  - Certain high-risk communities, states, and ethnic groups, e.g., Native American/Alaskan
  - Homosexual males
  - Street drug users
  - Laboratory personnel who might be exposed
- Pneumococcal conjugate vaccine
  - Infants at 2, 4, 6, 12, to 15 months
  - Catch-up children 24–59 months who are high-risk, including chronic illness, African American, Native American, sickle cell disease
- Meningococcal conjugate vaccine (MCV4)
  - Age 11–12, catch-up about 15, college freshman in dormatories
- Oral Ritavurys vaccube (Rota Teq)
  - 3 doses at 2, 4, 6 months of age; finish by 32 weeks
- Human papilloma virus (HPV)
  - 3 doses beginning at age 11–12
  - 2nd dose 2 months after 1st, and 3rd dose 6 months after 1st
  - Best given prior to onset of sexual activity. Recommended for women up to age 26 even if sexually active already
- Varicella zoster vaccine
  - Single dose recommended for adults ≥60 years of age regardless of whether they have had an episode of herpes zoster before or not.
- Synonym(s): Vaccinations; Inoculations

ALERT

Geriatric Considerations
Pneumococcal polysaccharide, influenza, and adult diphtheria and tetanus toxoids (Td) are needed in older age groups.

Pediatric Considerations
- Most vaccines are given before entry into school.
- Do not delay DTaP immunization of the preterm infant unless specific contraindications exist.

Pregnancy Considerations
- MMR and varicella should not be routinely given to pregnant women or women who are planning pregnancy within 28 days, but given to susceptibles in the post-partum period
- Pregnancy is a high-risk indication for Tdap vaccination; ensure proper vaccination within last 10 years.

 TREATMENT

GENERAL MEASURES

- Informed patient consent should discuss consequences of specific diseases and risks of immunizations: Vaccine Information Statements should be given prior to vaccination.
- Antipyretics (e.g., acetaminophen) are useful for the fever that may accompany certain immunizations.

Diet
No specific restrictions after immunization

Activity
No restrictions after immunization

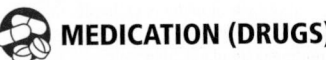 **MEDICATION (DRUGS)**

- Immunization administration guide: Wounds and immunization recommendations
- Tetanus immune globulin (TIG)
  - ≥3 doses of Td given in past: TIG not needed
  - <3 doses of Td given in past: Give TIG, except in patients with a clean (minor) wound.
- Td
  - Give Td if patient not immunized within 10 years
  - Give Td if patient not immunized within 5 years and wound is dirty (contaminated with dirt, feces, or saliva), puncture (penetration beyond epidermis), or major (burn, frostbite, crush injury).
- Contraindications
  - Anaphylaxis to thimerosal: See manufacturer's insert. Thimerosal has been removed from almost all childhood vaccines.
  - Anaphylaxis to neomycin: MMR, DTP, conjugated *Haemophilus influenzae* Type b vaccine, varicella zoster, inactivated (Hib), IPV, varicella contraindicated
  - Anaphylaxis to streptomycin: IPV contraindicated
  - Anaphylaxis to previous dose
  - Encephalopathy within 7 days after DTP: Give pediatric diphtheria and tetanus toxoids for next dose(s).
  - Pregnancy: MMR, varicella, varicella zoster
  - Known active, untreated tuberculosis: Varicella contraindicated
  - Anaphylaxis to eggs: Influenza (inactivated and LAIV)
  - Immunocompromised patients should, in general, not receive live viral vaccines (MMR, LAIV, rotavirus, varicella, and varicella zoster), although patients with HIV may receive MMR if not severely immunocompromised. Varicella vaccine is generally contraindicated, but may be given to some specified groups: See ACIP recommendations for details (i.e., certain HIV-infected children and humoral immunodeficiencies).
  - Varicella zoster vaccine contraindications include pregnancy, any immunodeficiency state, active untreated tuberculosis, or anaphylaxis to neomycin or gelatin

- Precautions: DTaP
  - Suspected neurologic disease: Delay immunization until clarified.
  - Fever of ≥40.5°C (105°F) within 48 hours after previous DTP/DTaP
  - Collapse or shocklike state (hypotonic-hyporesponsive episode) within 48 hours after DTP/DTaP
  - Seizure within 3 days after DTP/DTaP
  - Persistent, inconsolable crying lasting ≥3 hours within 48 hours after DTP/DTaP
  - The following are *not* contraindications and DTaP may be given if present
    - Family history of convulsions (pretreat with acetaminophen and after DTaP q4h for 24 hours)
    - Family history of sudden infant death syndrome (SIDS)
    - Family history of adverse event following DTaP/DTP
    - Temperature <40.5°C (105°F) following a prior DTaP/DTP
- Varicella, LAIV
  - Avoid salicylates for 6 weeks.
- Varicella zoster vaccine
  - Extensive vaccine-associated rash or disseminated disease may occur if the vaccine is given to immunocompromised individuals
- Significant possible interactions
  - Avoid MMR and varicella vaccine within 3–11 months after gamma globulin (see ACIP).
  - Give MMR and varicella either together or separated by 1 month.

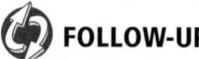

FOLLOW-UP

PROGNOSIS
Most patients develop antibodies.

COMPLICATIONS
- Fever, malaise, local reactions (redness, pain) are most common
- Rarely, allergic reactions
- Febrile seizures rarely occur after DTaP.

PATIENT MONITORING
- None routinely needed
- Hepatitis: Measure antibody (anti-HBs) response after hepatitis B vaccine for health care workers, immunocompromised persons, and offspring of hepatitis B carriers.

REFERENCES

1. Advisory Committee on Immunization Practices (ACIP).
2. American Academy of Pediatrics. *Red Book 2006: Report of the Committee on Infectious Diseases.* American Academy of Pediatrics; 2006.
3. Shots 2006. [PDA software] Version 6.0. Society for Teachers of Family Medicine: 2006. (Available at www.immunizationed.org).
4. American Academy of Family Physicians.
5. 2007 Immunization Supplement to Journal of Family Practice.

MISCELLANEOUS

- See also: Chickenpox; Diphtheria; Hepatitis A; Hepatitis B; Influenza; Measles; Rubella; Measles; Rubeola; Meningococcus; Mumps; Pertussis; Pneumonia, bacterial; Poliomyelitis; Tetanus
- Other notes
  - Purified protein derivative may be given at same time as MMR, or wait 4 weeks after immunization to do skin test.
  - Culture-proven pertussis provides immunity; use pediatric diphtheria and tetanus toxoids instead of DTaP.
  - *Haemophilus* disease: Immunity not provided when child younger than 2 years; administer Hib as if no disease has occurred.
  - Combination vaccines are available.
- Recommended immunizations and appropriate schedules can be downloaded as tables, brochures, or in PDA format from: www.cdc.gov/nip/home-hcp.htm

CODES

ICD9-CM
V05.9 Need for prophylactic vaccination and inoculation against unspecified single disease

PATIENT TEACHING

Report adverse events promptly. Minor redness, swelling, and or soreness at the site of injections can be expected; ice packs and acetaminophen may be helpful. Report serious reactions to VAERS at 800-822-7967.

IMMUNODEFICIENCY DISEASES

Weily Soong, MD

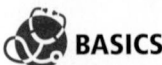 **BASICS**

DESCRIPTION
Disorders associated with the disruption of the integrity of immune system which results in increased susceptibility to infections

- Primary: An intrinsic defect in the immune mechanism
  - Humoral immunodeficiencies: Defects in antibody production
    - Agammaglobulinemia: X-linked (absent immunoglobulins; mutation in Bruton Tyrosine Kinase gene) and autosomal recessive (absent immunoglobulins; defect in B-cell development)
    - IgA deficiency (most common primary immunodeficiency; very low or absent IgA; defect unknown)
    - Common variable immunodeficiency (decreased levels of IgG, IgA, and/or IgM and poor responses to vaccinations; usually adult onset; unknown defects but likely not a single abnormality)
    - IgG subclass deficiency (decrease in IgG subclasses; defect unknown)
    - Specific antibody deficiency (poor antibody response to specific antigens; defect unknown)
    - Transient hypogammaglobulinemia of infancy (temporary decrease in IgG and IgA due to delayed maturation of the humoral system; unknown cause)
    - Others (includes Ig kappa chain defects; Ig heavy chain gene deletions; defects in UNG and ICOS genes; NEMO)
  - Combined immunodeficiencies: Defects in the cellular effector (T- and B-lymphocytes and NK cells) and humoral mechanisms
    - Severe combined immunodeficiency-SCID (all forms have absent T cells, and depending on the genetic mutation, may or may not have B cells and NK-cells; X-linked or autosomal recessive; includes mutations in adenosine deaminase deficiency gene, common interleukin g chain, Jak3, CD45, RAG1 and 2 genes)
    - Hyper-IgM syndrome (normal to high IgM with low IgG and IgA; X-linked-defect in CD40 ligand with features of combined immunodeficiency; autosomal recessive–defect in AID gene)
    - Wiskott-Aldrich syndrome (WAS) (X-linked; eczema, thrombocytopenia, repeated infections, decrease in T cells)
    - Ataxia telangiectasia (A-T) (cerebellar ataxia, oculocutaneous telangiectasia, and cellular and humoral immunodeficiency; autosomal recessive)
    - Omenn syndrome (erythroderma, eosinophilia, hepatosplenomegaly, increased IgE; autosomal recessive)
    - Purine nucleoside phosphorylase (PNP) deficiency (severe lymphopenia, especially T cells; hemolytic anemia; neurologic abnormalities; autosomal recessive)
    - Others (includes ZAP70 and CD40 defects)

- Phagocytic immunodeficiencies
  - Chronic granulomatous disease (mutations in the oxidation mechanism; X-linked and autosomal recessive)
  - Chediak-Higashi syndrome (mutations in lysosomal transport protein; albinism and neurological symptoms; autosomal recessive)
  - Leukocyte adhesion deficiency (defects in leukocyte endothelial adherence and chemotaxis; autosomal recessive)
  - Other (cyclic neutropenia, G-6PD deficiency, myeloperoxidase deficiency)
- Complement deficiencies: Usually autosomal recessive
  - Early complement (C1q, C1r, C2, C4): Cause autoimmune diseases, like lupus
  - Late complement (C5–C9): Susceptible to recurrent Neisserial infections and autoimmune diseases
  - C3 and mannose binding lectin deficiency: Susceptible to recurrent pyogenic infections
- Pure cellular deficiencies and other well-defined syndromes
  - DiGeorge syndrome (thymic hypoplasia; decrease in T cells; associated with 22q11.2 chromosome deletions; de novo mutation or autosomal dominant)
  - X-linked lymphoproliferative syndrome (causes fatal infectious mononucleosis)
  - Chronic mucocutaneous candidiasis or Autoimmune Polyglandular Syndrome Type 1 (mutations in the autoimmune regulator AIRE gene; causes autoimmune responses to endocrine tissues; autosomal recessive)
  - Hyper-IgE syndrome (high IgE, chronic dermatitis, and recurrent infections)
  - Autoinflammatory disorders: Recurrent fevers (Familial Mediterranean Fever, Muckle-Wells, Familial Cold Urticaria; autosomal recessive or dominant)
  - WHIM syndrome: Associated with warts, hypogammaglobulinemia, infection, myelokathexis (retention of leukocytes in the bone marrow); autosomal dominant
  - Autoimmune lymphoproliferative syndrome (defects in apoptosis; adenopathy, autoimmune cytopenias; autosomal recessive)
- Secondary: A result of a secondary process, like another illness, age, injury, or treatment
  - Premature and newborn
  - Hereditary and metabolic diseases
    - Chromosomal abnormalities (Down syndrome) and Sickle Cell disease
    - Diabetes mellitus
    - Uremia and nephrotic syndrome
    - Malnutrition, vitamin, and mineral deficiencies; Protein-losing enteropathies
  - Medications (immunosuppressive drugs, such as corticosteroids, immune modulators, radiation, chemotherapy; phenytoin)
  - Infections (includes HIV and mononucleosis)
  - Infiltrative and hematological diseases (includes sacoidosis, leukemias, lymphomas, myeloma, aplastic anemia)
  - Surgery and trauma (burns, splenectomy)
  - Other (lupus and other autoimmune diseases, chronic hepatitis, cirrhosis, aging, thymoma, chronic stress)

GENERAL PREVENTION
- For primary deficiencies: Goal is to avert microbial infection by identification of at-risk newborns using genetic screening/counseling and prenatal diagnostic tests.
- For secondary deficiencies: Depends on the etiology

EPIDEMIOLOGY
- Secondary immunodeficiencies are more common than primary.
- Children are most likely to present with primary immunodeficiencies.
- Primary immunodeficiencies occur from 1 in 10,000 births to 1 in 2000 births.
  - Relative distribution: (65% humoral deficiencies, 15% combined deficiencies, 10% phagocytic deficiencies, 5% cellular deficiencies, 5% complement deficiencies
- Infectious complications with primary humoral disorders usually appear >6 months of age.
- IgA deficiency is the most common primary immunodeficiency (about 1 in every 500 people)
- Common variable immunodeficiency affects 1 in 30,000–50,000 people and appears usually in early adulthood.

Genetics
Primary: Inherited genetic defect. See "Description".

ETIOLOGY
- Primary immunodeficiency diseases
  - Defects in genes and gene products resulting in inherited defects of the immune system
  - Manifested by infections after birth, but may not be expressed clinically until later in life
- Secondary immunodeficiency diseases:
  - Multiple possible etiologies

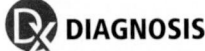 **DIAGNOSIS**

SIGNS AND SYMPTOMS
- 10 warning signs of primary immunodeficiency from the Modell Foundation
  - 8 or more new ear infections within 1 year
  - 2 or more serious sinus infections within 1 year
  - 2 or more months on antibiotics with little effect
  - 2 or more pneumonias within 1 year
  - Failure of an infant to gain weight or grow normally
  - Recurrent, deep skin or organ abscesses
  - Persistent thrush in mouth or elsewhere on skin, > age 1
  - Need for IV antibiotics to clear infections
  - 2 or more deep-seated infections
  - A family history of primary immunodeficiency
- Unusual susceptibility to infection. Type of infection might help determine the type of immunodeficiency
  - Humoral deficiencies
    - Associated with bacterial and protozoan infections (e.g., chronic sinusitis, recurrent respiratory infection, chronic diarrheal disease)
    - Infections include *S. pneumoniae*, *H. influenzae*, *S. aureus*, *P. aeruginosa*, mycoplasm, enteroviruses, Giardia
  - Combined deficiencies
    - Associated with severe fungal, bacterial, protozoan, and viral infections
    - Infections include all viral infections; bacterial infections found in humoral deficiencies plus Listeria and Salmonella, enteric flora; mycobacteria; Candida; Pneumocystis; Toxoplasma; Cryptococcus

- Cellular deficiencies
  - Associated with severe viral, mycobacterial, and fungal infections
  - Infections include salmonella, mycobacteria, and Candida
- Phagocytic defects—infections include *S. aureus*, enteric flora, Serraia, Nocardia, *P. aeruginosa*, *S. typhi*, *A. fumigatus*, *C. albicans*, Pneumocystis; mycobacteria
- Complement deficiencies infections include bacterial infections found in humoral deficiencies, especially *N. meningitidis*
- Also associated with autoimmune disorders and malignancies, especially lymphoreticular

History
A thorough history and family history will direct the proper search for a differential diagnosis.

Physical Exam
A careful physical exam will direct the proper search for a differential diagnosis.

TESTS
Lab
- High percentage of immunodeficiencies will be discovered by
  - CBC with differential smear
  - Immunoglobulin levels, including IgG, IgA, IgM, and IgE; include IgG subclasses
  - Antibody reponses to previous vaccines (tetanus, Pneumococcus, *H. influenzae*, diphtheria)
  - Classical Complement Pathway Test—CH50
  - Infection evaluation, such as ESR, C-reactive protein, microbiology cultures
- Flow cytometry looking at lymphocyte subsets (CD4, CD8, CD3, CD19, CD20)
- Delayed Hypersensitivity Skin Tests (Anergy panel to mumps, Candida, tetanus, Trichophyton)
- Lymphocyte proliferation responses to mitogens and antigens
- Specific complement levels
- Phagocyte function: NBT test, dihydrorhodamine reductase test
- Specific cytokine function tests
- Genetic analysis
- Additional specific tests for suspected acquired causes for immunodeficiencies

Imaging
- Chest x-ray of a newborn infant to look for an absence of a thymic shadow in SCID or DiGeorge
- Depends on the suspected etiology and infection

TREATMENT
GENERAL MEASURES
- Depend on the complexity of the immune deficiency
- If newborn has been identified as being at risk, prior planning needs to be done, such as cord blood storage for stem cell transplants, appropriate labs and genetic tests, and potential need for isolation in sterile environment.
- If patient with cellular or combined defects has to be transfused, must use irradiated and CMV-negative blood products.
- Avoid all live attenuated viral vaccines in patients with severe cellular or antibody immunodeficiencies (varicella, oral polio, measles, mumps, rubella, smallpox, BCG)
- Bone-marrow, stem-cell, or thymic transplant for certain immunodeficiencies (e.g., SCID and DiGeorge); best done at referral research centers

MEDICATION (DRUGS)
- Antibiotics with appropriate spectra for infecting organism(s)
  - May be used acutely, chronically, or prophylactically
- Antiviral therapy for HIV, varicella, herpes, influenza, and RSV
- Antifungal agents for specific fungal infections
- Intravenous immunoglobulin (IVIG)
  - For diseases deficient in IgG, such as agammaglobulinemias, common variable, hyper-IgM, WAS, and A-T (1)[A]
- Enzyme replacement therapy for adenosine deaminase deficiency
- For secondary immunodeficiencies, treatment depends on the specific etiology

FOLLOW-UP
DISPOSITION
Issues for Referral
- Primary immunodeficiency patients should be referred to a physician specializing in Allergy and Clinical Immunology for working-up and managing immunodeficiency diseases.
- Referral for secondary immunodeficiency patients depends on the specific etiology.

PROGNOSIS
- Short-term prognosis is related closely to the severity of the infectious complication.
- Long-term prognosis is related to the nature of the immune defect and the type and degree of immunodeficiency.

COMPLICATIONS
- Autoimmune disorders
- Reactions to gamma globulin treatment
- Malignancies, especially lymphoreticular
- Overwhelming infection
- Fatal Graft-versus-Host disease following blood transfusions in patients with SCID

PATIENT MONITORING
- Monitor for infections and their complications.
- Infection control precautions: Depends on the situation and includes frequent hand washing, gloves, gowns, masks, safe water supply
- Monitor and maintain IgG levels in common variable hypogammaglobulinemia.

REFERENCES
1. Ballow M. Primary immunodeficiency disorders: Antibody deficiency. *J Allergy Clin Immunol*. 2002;109:581–591.
2. Bonilla FA, Geha RS. Primary immunodeficiency diseases. *J Allergy Clin Immunol*. 2003;111: S571–S581.
3. Buckley RH. Primary cellular immunodeficiencies. *J Allergy Clin Immunol*. 2002;109:747–757.
4. Conley ME, Notarangelo LD, Etzioni A. Diagnostic criteria for primary immunodeficiencies. *Clin Immunol*. 1999;93:190–197.
5. Immune Deficiency Foundation. The Clinical Presentation of the Primary Immunodeficiency Diseases (Physician's Primer). 1992. www.primaryimmune.org.
6. The Jeffrey Modell Foundation. www.info4pi.org and www.jmfworld.com.
7. Notarangelo L, et al. Primary immunodeficiency diseases: An update. *J Allergy Clin Immunol*. 2004;114:677–687.
8. Simonte SJ, Cunningham-Rundles C. Update on primary immunodeficiency: Defects on lymphocytes. *Clin Immunol*. 2003;109:109–118.
9. Stiehm ER, Ochs HD, Winkelstein JA. *Immunologic Disorders in Infants and Children*. 5th ed. Philadelphia, PA: Elsevier; 2004.

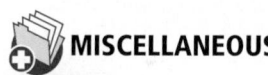

MISCELLANEOUS
CODES
ICD9-CM
- 279.0 Deficiency of humoral immunity
- 279.1 Deficiency of cell-mediated immunity
- 279.2 Combined immunity deficiency
- 279.3 Unspecified immunity deficiency
- 288.1 Functional disorders of polymorphonuclear neutrophils

PATIENT TEACHING
Patient information available from
- Immune Deficiency Foundation, 25 West Chesapeake Ave. Room 206, Towson, MD 21204. Tel: 800-296-4433. www.primaryimmune.org.
- Jeffrey Modell Foundation, 747 Third Avenue, New York, NY 10017. Tel: 212-819-0200. www.info4pi.org and www.jmfworld.com.

IMPETIGO

Elizabeth L. Backer, MD

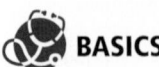

BASICS

DESCRIPTION
- A superficial, intraepidermal infection occurring prominently on exposed areas of the face and the extremities. Affected patients usually have multiple lesions. Cultures now give >80% with *Staphylococcus aureus* alone or combined with group A β-hemolytic streptococci. Change over past 20 years to predominately *S. aureus*.
- Nonbullous impetigo: Formation of vesiculopustules, which rupture, leading to crusting with a characteristic golden appearance. Local lymphadenopathy may occur.
- Bullous impetigo: Staphylococci impetigo that progress rapidly to small to large flaccid bulla (newborns/young children) caused by epidermolytic toxin release. Less lymphadenopathy; <30% of cases
- Folliculitis: Considered by some to be *S. aureus* impetigo of hair follicle
- Ecthyma: A deeper, ulcerated, impetigo infection often with lymphadenitis
  - Poststreptococcal glomerulonephritis may follow impetigo (in young children).
- System(s) Affected: Skin/Exocrine
- Synonym(s): Pyoderma; Impetigo contagiosa; Impetigo vulgaris; Fox impetigo

ALERT
Pediatric Considerations
Impetigo neonatorum may occur by nursery contamination.

GENERAL PREVENTION
Close attention to family hygiene, particularly hand washing. Avoid crowding. Treat atopic dermatitis.

EPIDEMIOLOGY
- Predominant sex: Male = Female
- Predominant age: 2–5 years

Prevalence
In the US: Unreported

RISK FACTORS
- Warm, humid environment
- Tropical or subtropical climate
- Summer or fall season
- Minor trauma, insect bites
- Poor hygiene, poverty, crowding, epidemics, during war
- Familial spread
- Poor health with anemia and malnutrition
- Complication to pediculosis, scabies, chickenpox, eczema
- Contact dermatitis (Rhus)
- Burns
- Atopic dermatitis
- Contact sports
- Children in day care
- Possibly tobacco exposure
- Carriage of group A streptococcus and *S. aureus* predisposes to impetigo. (1)[C]

ETIOLOGY
- Coagulase positive staphylococci: Pure culture ~50–90%. More contagious via contact
- β-Hemolytic streptococci: Pure culture only ~10% of the time
- Mixed infections of streptococci and staphylococci common (3)[A], (4)[C]. Data suggest increasing importance of staphylococci over past 20 years.
- Direct contact or insect vector
- Can be contamination at trauma site
- Regional lymphadenopathy

ASSOCIATED CONDITIONS
- Malnutrition and anemia
- Crowded living conditions
- Poor hygiene
- Neglected minor trauma
- Any chronic dermatitis

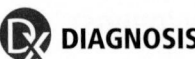

DIAGNOSIS

SIGNS AND SYMPTOMS
- May be slow and indolent or rapidly spreading
- Tender red macule or papule as early lesion
- Thin roofed vesicle to bullae: Usually nontender
- Pustules
- Weeping shallow red ulcer
- Honey-colored crusts
- Most frequent on face around mouth and nose or at site of trauma
- Satellite lesions
- Often multiple sites
- Bullae on buttocks, trunk, face

TESTS
Lab
- None usually required
  - Culture: Taken from the base of lesion after removal of crust. Blood agar grows both staphylococci and group A streptococci (not usually done).
  - ASO titer: Can be weak positive for streptococci (not usually done)
  - Streptozyme: Positive for streptococci (not usually done)
- Disorders that may alter lab results
  - Streptococci pharyngitis will alter streptococci enzyme tests.

DIFFERENTIAL DIAGNOSIS
- Nonbullous
  - Chickenpox
  - Herpes
  - Folliculitis
  - Erysipelas
  - Insect bites
  - Severe eczematous dermatitis
  - Scabies
  - Tinea corporis
- Bullous
  - Burns
  - Pemphigus vulgaris
  - Bullous pemphigoid
  - Stevens-Johnson syndrome

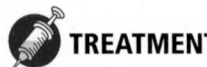

TREATMENT

GENERAL MEASURES
- Prevention with Mupirocin or triple antibiotic ointment t.i.d. to sites of minor skin trauma
- Removal of crusts, cleanliness with gentle washing 2–3 times daily. Clean with antibacterial soap, chlorhexidine, or betadine.
- Washing of entire body may prevent recurrence at distant sites.

Diet
No special diet

Activity
- Athletes restricted from contact sports
- School and day care contagious restrictions

MEDICATION (DRUGS)

First Line

Note: The 2005 Infectious Disease Society of America (IDSA) recommends topical treatment for limited lesions and oral medication when the disease is more severe/extensive (8)[C]. Optimal treatment is unclear due to limited quality of evidence (9,10)[A]. Penicillin no longer recommended. Erythromycin, Cephalexin, Dicloxacillin, topical mupirocin, and fucidic acid effective unless local staphylococcal strains are resistant. Consult the local hospital or health department for microbial resistance information.

- Nonbullous (minor spread, treat 7 days; widespread, treat 10 days); bullous (treat 10 days)
  - Mupirocin (Bactroban) topical ointment applied t.i.d., 7–10 days (nonbullous only). Not as effective on scalp as around mouth
  - Erythromycin base: Adults 1 g/d divided doses q6h in adults (Pediatric: 30–40 mg/kg/d q6h)
  - Dicloxacillin: adult 250 mg PO q.i.d. Pediatric 12–25 mg/kg/d divided q6h
- Contraindications: Drug allergy
- Precautions: Refer to manufacturer's profile of each drug.
- Significant possible interactions
  - Erythromycin with theophyllines, astemizole, and other drugs
  - Refer to manufacturer's profile of each drug.

Second Line

Note: Oral doses
- 1st generation cephalosporins: Children
  - Cephalexin: 25–50 mg/kg/d divided q6h
  - Cefaclor: 20–40 mg/kg/d divided q8h
  - Cephradine: 25–50 mg/kg/d divided q6h–q12h
  - Cefadroxil: 30 mg/kg per 24 hours divided b.i.d.
- 1st generation cephalosporins: Adults
  - Cephalexin: 250 mg q.i.d.
  - Cefaclor: 250 mg t.i.d.
  - Cephradine: 500 mg b.i.d.
  - Cefadroxil: 1 g/d in divided doses
- Amoxicillin–clavulanate acid
  - Adult: 250 mg t.i.d.
  - Pediatric: 20–40 mg/kg/d of amoxicillin divided q8h
- Azithromycin:
  - Adult 500 mg on day 1 followed by 250 mg/d for days 2–5
  - Pediatric 10 mg/kg on day 1 followed by 5 mg/kg days 2–5
- Clarithromycin
  - Adult 250 mg b.i.d.
  - Pediatric 15 mg/kg/d divided b.i.d.
- Vancomycin
- Clindamycin
- Ciprofloxacin plus rifampin (rifampicin)
- Severe bullous disease may require IV therapy such as nafcillin or cefazolin.

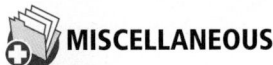 **FOLLOW-UP**

PROGNOSIS
- Complete resolution in 7–10 days with treatment
- Antibiotic treatment will not prevent or halt glomerulonephritis as it will with rheumatic fever.
- If not clear within 7–10 days, culture is necessary to find resistant organism.
- Recurrent impetigo: Evaluate for carriage of *S. aureus* in nares (also perineum, axillae, toe web). Apply Mupirocin ointment to nares b.i.d. for 5 days for clearance.

COMPLICATIONS
- Ecthyma
- Erysipelas
- Poststreptococcal acute glomerulonephritis
- Cellulitis
- Bacteremia
- Osteomyelitis
- Septic arthritis
- Pneumonia
- Lymphadenitis

PATIENT MONITORING
If not clear within 7–10 days, culture the lesions.

REFERENCES

1. Dajani AS, et al. Natural history of impetigo. II. Etiologic agents and bacterial interactions. *J Clin Invest*. 1972;51:2863–2871.
2. www.uptodate.com
3. Baddour LM. Primary skin infections in primary Care: An update. *Infect Med*. 1993;10:42.
4. Britton JW, et al. Comparison of mupirocin and erythromycin in the treatment of impetigo. *J Pediatr*. 1990;117:827–829.
5. Dagan R. Impetigo in childhood: Changing epidemiology and new treatments. *Pediatr Ann*. 1993;22:235–240.
6. Isselbacher KJ, Braunwald E, Wilson JD, et al., eds. *Harrison's Principles of Internal Medicine*. 13th ed. New York: McGraw-Hill; 1994.
7. Ko WT, Adal KA, Tomecki KJ. Infectious diseases. *Med Clin North Am*. 1998;82:1001–1031.
8. Stevens DL, et al. Practice guidelines for the diagnosis and management of skin and soft-tissue infections. *Clin Infect Dis*. 2005;41:1373–1406.
9. Konig S, et al. Interventions for impetigo. *Cochrane Database Syst Rev*. 2004;2:CD003261.
10. George, A, et al. A systematic review and meta-analysis of treatments for impetigo. *Br J Gen Pract*. 2003;53:480–487.
11. Peters G, ed. *Red Book*. New York: American Academy of Pediatrics; 1997.
12. Rakel RE, ed. *1997 Conn's Current Therapy*. Philadelphia: WB Saunders; 1997.
13. Rhody C. Bacterial infections of the skin. *Prim Care*. 2000;27:459–473.

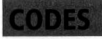 **MISCELLANEOUS**

CODES

ICD9-CM
684 Impetigo

PATIENT TEACHING

 See Corresponding Diagnostic Algorithm

 See Patient Handout on CD

I

INFERTILITY

Eric S. Miller, MD

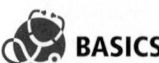 **BASICS**

DESCRIPTION
Failure to conceive >1 year of unprotected intercourse
- 35–40 years: Initiate workup after 6 months of unprotected intercourse; over 40 years: Initiate workup immediately.

GENERAL PREVENTION
- Maintain normal body mass index
  - Loss of just 5–10% may be beneficial
- Prevention of sexually transmitted disease and subsequent PID
- Treat endometriosis when diagnosis is made
  - Chronic condition
  - Birth control pills until fertility desired

EPIDEMIOLOGY
Increases with age: Ages 30–34 years: 14%; ages 35–39 years: 20%; ages 40–45 years: 25%

Incidence
Increasing as 20% of women are delaying childbearing until after age 35

Prevalence
10–15% of all couples

RISK FACTORS
Life style
- Cigarette smoking: OR for infertility 1.60 (95%, CI 1.34–1.91), Augood,1998
- Obesity: BMI >27 kg/m^2 relative risk ovulatory infertility 3.1 (95%, CI 2.2–4.4)
- Alcohol: >8 drinks/week associated with ovulatory infertility
- Caffeine: >2 cups/d associated with a slight decrease in fertility

Genetics
- Higher prevalence of karyotype abnormalities than the general population (1)[C]
- Possibly genetic defects
  - Klinefelter syndrome (XXY)
  - Y chromosomal defects
  - Turner syndrome (mosaics)
- Polycystic ovarian disease (PCO)
  - Hyperandrogenic chronic anovulation, exclude secondary causes
  - Clusters in families
  - 4–6% women
  - Main theory: Intraovarian androgen production overly sensitive to insulin (insulin gene polymorphism)

ETIOLOGY
Most couples have more than 1 factor
- Male factors 30–40%
- Ovulation factors 15%
- Cervical/uterine factors 10%
- Tubal/peritoneal factors including endometriosis 40%
- Immunologic factors 5%
- Psychogenic/nutritional/metabolic factors 5%
- Unexplained infertility 10–20%

ASSOCIATED CONDITIONS
- Intrauterine device (IUD) use and nonmonogamous sex increases risk of infection.
- Also small risk at insertion of IUD

 DIAGNOSIS

SIGNS AND SYMPTOMS
- Genital/pelvic infection (e.g., PID often associated with an obstruction of reproductive tract)
- Endocrine dysfunction (e.g., hypothyroidism, hypogonadism, abnormal puberty) often associated with abnormalities of ovulation or spermatogenesis
- Sexual dysfunction (e.g., premature ejaculation) may contribute to the problem.
- Anovulatory cycles are frequently irregular, without premenstrual symptoms or dysmenorrhea.
- Some patients may have features (e.g., hirsutism, obesity, acne) suggestive of PCO.
- Endometriosis is often associated with cyclic premenstrual pain, secondary dysmenorrhea, and dyspareunia.

History
Thorough history for each partner

Physical Exam
- Thorough physical exam for each partner
- Increasing anovulation with increasing age
- Increased disease burden with age from diseases such as endometriosis and cumulative exposure to environmental/occupational hazards
- Unruptured luteinized follicle
  - To prevent this complication, one should avoid nonsteroidal anti-inflammatory drugs (NSAIDs) while trying to get pregnant.

TESTS
Most of the tests of spermatogenesis and ovulation should be repeated at least once if abnormal.
- Basal body temperature charting
  - Assesses ovulation and adequacy of the luteal phase.
  - Morning temperature should rise about 1°F at the time of ovulation and remain elevated for 13–14 days (<11 days is abnormal).

Lab
- Semen analysis; normal values are as follows (modified strict Krueger)
  - Volume: 2–6 mL
  - Ph: 7–8
  - Viscosity: Liquefies within 1 hour
  - Count: ≥20 million/mL
  - Motility: ≥50%
  - Morphology: ≥14% normal morphology

- Multiple tests (e.g., hamster egg penetration assay to assess sperm's ability to fertilize) are available to study specific aspects of reproduction, but are used only by fertility specialists and available only in specialized labs. Also the hemizona assay and immunobead-binding test. Tests are now bypassed by intracytoplasmic sperm injection (ICSI)
- Serum progesterone
  - Assesses ovulation and corpus luteum function
  - A level of 3–10 mg/mL or greater correlates with ovulation.
  - Should be obtained on ~ days 21–23 of a 28-day menstrual cycle
- Assessment of ovarian reserve: Day-3 FSH if <15 mIU/ml-adequate reserve (good in vitro fertilization [IVF] candidate). If >15 mIU/mL—poor reserve
- The following tests are useful to evaluate underlying causes of anovulation or low sperm counts
  - Thyroid stimulating hormone
  - Prolactin: >20 ng/mL
  - Testosterone: Decreased in primary male gonadal failure; increased in female hyperandrogenism, PCO
  - FSH and luteinizing hormone (LH) level (elevated in primary gonadal failure, decreased in hypopituitarism); LH/FSH ratio >2.5 consistent with PCO
  - Karyotype (elevated FSH/LH), e.g., Klinefelter syndrome, Turner syndrome (mosaic)
  - Late-onset congenital adrenal hyperplasia: 17 OH progesterone
  - Adrenal disease: DHEAS
- Postcoital test (not that useful; historic value)
  - Evaluates sperm/cervical mucus interaction
  - Midcycle cervical mucus assessed for ferning, elasticity, >20 forward moving sperm

Imaging
- Hysterosalpingogram (HSG)
  - Evaluates tubal patency and uterine contour.
  - This procedure may have some therapeutic benefit. (2)[A]
  - Avoid if history suggests an infection.
- Pelvic ultrasound
  - Fibroids
  - Ovarian pathology
  - Endometriomas
  - Subcortical ovarian cysts (PCO)
  - Müllerian defects
- Magnetic resonance imaging (MRI)
  - Müllerian defects

Diagnostic Procedures/Surgery
- Endometrial biopsy (confirms short luteal phase <11 days, luteal phase defect)
  - Assesses ovulation, function of the corpus luteum (historic value)
- Laparoscopy
  - Should be deferred until basic evaluation is complete
  - Can be diagnostic and therapeutic (e.g., chromotubation, simultaneous hysteroscopy, and operative laparoscopy)
  - May be bypassed for intrauterine insemination/clomiphene trial
  - Ovarian drilling in clomiphene-resistant PCO decreases testosterone load (can cause adhesions).

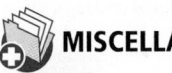

TREATMENT

GENERAL MEASURES

- Dispel myths and provide accurate information.
- Simultaneously evaluate and counsel both partners without blame!
- Find and correct causes of infertility.
- Provide information on adoption.
- Consider donor insemination or intrauterine insemination for refractory abnormalities of semen analysis
  - ICSI available for oligospermia, antisperm antibodies, poor cervical mucus, or poor capacitation
- Discontinue smoking, excessive alcohol, and/or illicit drugs. Avoid toxins.
- Consider IVF
  - Severe tubal disease: need for donor eggs, sperm manipulation (ICSI)
  - IVF is indicated >2 years of unexplained infertility, >1 year of treatment for a particular defect, or >1 year of donor insemination or ovulation induction.
- Unexplained infertility
  - Intrauterine insemination (IUI) and clomiphene trial increases fertility rate 3 times compared with that of placebo.
  - Clomiphene alone — or 2.5 per clomiphene treatment cycle (95% CI, 1.35-4.62) (3)[A]
  - Consider oocyte donation with older couples or those with poor ovarian reserve.

Activity

- Males with low sperm counts should avoid hot tubs/saunas (decreased spermatogenesis)
- If the male has low sperm counts, intercourse should be timed to occur ~q24–36h during the fertile period. Start 5–6 days before expected ovulation and continue for 2 days afterward. Highest probability for conception 1–2 days before ovulation. (4)[B]
- Regular intercourse 2–3 times a week for most couples
- Abstaining to "save up" not proven

MEDICATION (DRUGS)

First Line

- Clomiphene (Clomid)
  - Indicated for induction of ovulation
  - Typical dose: 25–50 mg/d for 5 days on days 3–7 of cycle
  - If 1st course of therapy does not result in ovulation (day 23 progesterone level), then try second course of 100 mg PO/d for 5 days. Possibly increase to 150 mg.
  - This estrogen antagonist binds to receptors in the hypothalamus and stimulates increased release of gonadotropin releasing hormone (GnRH), leading to increased secretion of FSH and LH from the pituitary.
- Metformin
  - Several studies have advocated metformin after failed clomiphene therapy.
  - Some start with metformin, a recent prospective randomized study showed a higher pregnancy rate in the metformin group, 15.1% vs 7.2%, p = .009. (9)[B]
    - Gradually increase to the treatment dose of 500 mg t.i.d. or 850 mg b.i.d.
- Bromocriptine/cabergoline
  - Indicated for treatment of anovulation associated with galactorrhea, hyperprolactinemia, or pituitary microadenomas
- Precautions
  - Clomiphene: Hyperstimulation syndrome, multiple pregnancy, hot flashes. Pelvic exams are useful to rule out ovarian enlargement. Cervical mucus may be scant and require estrogen supplementation.
  - Bromocriptine/cabergoline: headaches, nausea, lightheadedness
  - Metformin: GI side effects, lactic acidosis, stop once pregnancy diagnosed.

Second Line

- IUI
  - Oligospermia
  - Cervical factors (LEEP)
  - Coital problems
- Luteal phase defect
  - Clomiphene
  - Supplemental progesterone
- Adrenal component (elevated DHEAS)
  - Glucocorticoids
- Fertility specialists with access to specialized lab
  - Human menopausal gonadotropin (FSH, LH) or urofollitropin (FSH)
  - GnRH analogs: hypogonadotrophic hypogonadism

SURGERY

- Laparoscopy if workup suspicious for tubal blockage/endometriosis
  - Destruction of endometriosis in mild to moderate disease helpful (Marcoux, 1997)
- Operative hysteroscopy
  - Correction of Müllerian defects
  - Removal of polyps, submucous fibroids (only after other factors ruled out)
  - If large may prevent implantation or block tubal ostia
- Male infertility
  - Vasovasostomy—previous vasectomy
  - Vasoepididymostomy—anatomic problems
  - Testicular sperm extraction procedure—blocked/absent vas deferens
  - Varicocele repair for abnormal semen analysis (controversial, refuted by scientific trials)

PROGNOSIS

- About 1/2 of couples conceive during the 2nd year of unprotected intercourse.
- If the couple has been infertile for ≥4 years, the prognosis tends to be poor.
- Encourage initiation of adoption process.

COMPLICATIONS

- Plural gestation with ovulation induction: <10%
- Ectopic pregnancy following tubal reanastomosis: 15% risk
- Risk of ovarian cancer with 11 cycles or more of clomiphene has been discounted. ACOG recommends limit to 12 or fewer cycles.

REFERENCES

1. Clementini E, Palka C, Iezzi I, et al. Prevalence of chromosomal abnormalities in 2078 infertile couples referred for assisted reproductive techniques. *Human Reprod.* 2005;20:437–442.
2. Johnson N, Vandekerckhove P, Watson A, et al. Tubal flushing for subfertility. *Cochrane Database Syst Rev.* 2002;cd003718
3. Hughes E, Collins J, Vandekerckhove P. Clomiphene citrate for unexplained subfertility in women. *Cochrane Database Syst Rev.* 2000;cd000057
4. Stanford JB, White GL, Hatasaka H. Timing intercourse to achieve pregnancy: current evidence. *Obstet Gynecol.* 2002;100:1333–1341.
5. Palomba S, Orio F, Falbo A, et al. Prospective parallel randomized, double-blind, double-dummy controlled clinical trial comparing clomiphene citrate and metformin as the first-line treatment for ovulation induction in nonobese anovulatory women with polycystic ovary syndrome. *J Clin Endocr Metabol.* 2005;90:4068–4074.

MISCELLANEOUS

CODES

ICD9-CM
- 606.9 Male infertility, unspecified
- 628.9 Female infertility of unspecified origin

PATIENT TEACHING

- http://www.resolve.org
- http://www.endometriosis.org
- http://familydoctor.org

See Patient Handout on CD

INFLUENZA

Richard Kent Zimmerman, MD, MPH

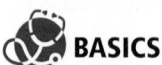 **BASICS**

DESCRIPTION
- Acute, usually self-limited, viral, febrile, infection caused by influenza virus Types A and B
- Marked by inflammation of nasal mucosa, pharynx, conjunctiva, and respiratory tract
- Outbreaks occur almost every winter with varying degrees of severity.
- Influenza virus rarely displays antigenic shift (variation), which leads to strains of virus to which little immunologic resistance exists in population and may result in pandemics. Displays minor antigenic variation called drift.
- System(s) Affected: Pulmonary
- Synonym(s): Flu; Grip; Acute catarrhal fever

GENERAL PREVENTION
- Incubation: 1–4 days; infected persons most contagious during peak symptoms
- Trivalent influenza vaccine
  - Recommended for all adults age ≥50
  - Recommended for high-risk individuals: Chronic pulmonary disease, cardiovascular disease, immunosuppression, neuromuscular diseases that impair respiratory function, hemoglobinopathies, renal diseases, metabolic disease, diabetes, HIV, long-term aspirin therapy, asplenia, alcoholism, and pregnancy
  - Recommended for health care providers, home care providers, staff, and residents of nursing homes and other chronic care facilities, homeless, public safety workers, and close contacts of high-risk individuals
  - Vaccination of healthy 6–59-month-olds, their household contacts, and out-of-home caregivers is recommended.
  - Should be administered in fall prior to influenza season
  - Protection occurs 1–2 weeks after immunization.
  - Some side effects possible, e.g., fever and mild, local reaction at vaccination site
  - Dose: ≥3 years old: 0.5 mL IM; children 6–35 months old: 0.25 mL
  - Single dose/year except for children <9 years old, who should receive 2 doses (1 month apart) 1st year they receive vaccine
  - Vaccine contraindications: Anaphylaxis to eggs (do skin testing first)
- Live attenuated influenza vaccine
  - For healthy persons 5–49 years old
  - Contraindications: Anaphylaxis to eggs, immunocompromising conditions, pregnancy, high-risk conditions, history of Guillain-Barré syndrome

ALERT
Pediatric Considerations
Vaccinate 6–59-month-olds with inactivated vaccine.

Pregnancy Considerations
- Women at risk for influenza complications should receive inactivated influenza vaccine regardless of trimester.
- Advisory Committee on Immunization Practices recommends vaccinating all women who will be pregnant during influenza season.
- Antiviral prophylaxis, Amantadine, and rimantadine no longer recommended. Prophylaxis with oseltamivir (75 mg/d for Types A and B): Take for duration of outbreak if no vaccine given; discontinue after 14 days if used in addition to vaccine. May be used prophylactically
  - In high-risk groups (that have not been vaccinated or need additional control measures) during epidemics. Should not be considered as substitute for vaccination unless vaccine contraindicated
  - During influenza season for those with contraindications to vaccine
  - For staff and residents in nursing home outbreaks
  - For immune-deficient persons who are expected not to respond to vaccination

EPIDEMIOLOGY
- Predominant age
  - Incidence: Highest in young and school-aged children (3 months to 16 years); young adults (16–40 years)
  - Morbidity: Highest in elderly (>75 years) and those with concurrent medical illnesses, such as lung disease. Also higher in young children
  - Hospitalization rates also higher in infants
- Predominant sex: Male = Female

Incidence
- Cases per year: 95 million
- Attack rates in healthy children: 10–40% each year

RISK FACTORS
- For contracting disease
  - Patients in semi-closed environments such as nursing homes
  - Students, prisoners
  - Crowded, close environments during epidemics
- For complications
  - Chronic pulmonary diseases
  - Cardiovascular diseases including valvular problems and CHF
  - Metabolic diseases
  - Hemoglobinopathies
  - Malignancies
  - Pregnancy, especially in 3rd trimester
  - Neonates, infants, elderly
  - Immunosuppression
  - Neuromuscular diseases that limit respiratory function and secretion handling

ETIOLOGY
Orthomyxovirus (influenza antigenic Types A and B); transmitted person-to-person, often by airborne route

ASSOCIATED CONDITIONS
Bacterial pneumonia

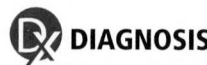 **DIAGNOSIS**

SIGNS AND SYMPTOMS
Sudden onset of
- High fever
- Myalgia (sometimes severe and lasting for days)
- Sore throat/pharyngitis
- Nonproductive cough
- Headache
- Chills
- Nasal congestion
- Malaise
- Rhinorrhea
- Sinusitis
- Sneezing

History
Close attention to epidemiology (e.g., current outbreak in community). Contact www.cdc.gov/flu/weekly/fluactivity.htm or health department to determine type or do testing.

Physical Exam
See "History"

TESTS
Lab
- PCR is best test influenza as back in 24 hours and accurate
- Lymphopenia
- Leukocytosis may signal complications.
- Tissue culture of nasopharyngeal swab or aspirate—takes time for results
- Rapid ELISA antigen test. Some rapid tests diagnose influenza A, while others diagnose influenza A and B. Sensitivity and specificity varies

Imaging
Chest x-ray
- Usually normal unless secondary infection
- Basilar streaking

Pathological Findings
Inflammation of respiratory tract

DIFFERENTIAL DIAGNOSIS
- Respiratory viral infections including RSV, parainfluenza, adenovirus, enterovirus
- Atypical *Mycoplasma pneumonia*
- Q fever
- Viral or streptococcal tonsillitis
- Infectious mononucleosis
- Coxsackievirus infections
- *Chlamydia pneumoniae*

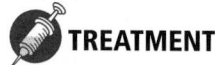 TREATMENT

INITIAL STABILIZATION
Outpatient except for treatment of severe complications or treatment of those in high-risk groups

GENERAL MEASURES
- Symptomatic treatment (saline nasal spray, analgesic gargle)
- Cool-mist, ultrasonic humidifier to increase moisture of inspired air
- Modified respiratory isolation techniques
- Hospitalized patients may require oxygen or ventilatory support.
- Avoid smoking.

Diet
Increase fluid intake.

Activity
As tolerated

 MEDICATION (DRUGS)

First Line
Antivirals effective if administered within 1st 48 hours
- Amantadine and rimantadine no longer recommended due to resistance I to H3N2 in 2005–2006.
- Zanamivir and Oseltamivir must be given within the 1st 24–30 hours of symptom onset and in patients with fever at presentation to be effective.
- Effect is reduction of symptoms by 24 hours.
- Zanamivir and oseltamivir effective for influenza Types A and B
  - Shorten duration by 1 day
  - Oseltamivir also reduces complications of influenza
  - Zanamivir dose: 2 inhalations b.i.d. for 5 days (age ≥7 years)
  - Oseltamivir dose: 75 mg PO b.i.d. for 5 days (age ≥13 years). If severe renal impairment, 75 mg PO once per day. Children: if <15 kg, then 30 mg b.i.d. if >15–23 kg, then 45 mg b.i.d., if >23–40 kg, then 60 mg b.i.d., if >40 kg, then 75 mg b.i.d.
- Antipyretics
  - Acetaminophen: In children
  - Aspirin: Should not be used in children <16 years due to risk of Reye syndrome, a rare and severe complication associated with aspirin use.
  - Contraindications: Just allergy to a product
- Precautions
  - Zanamivir may cause bronchospasm; the patient should have a bronchodilator available.
  - Oseltamivir
    - May cause nausea and vomiting; may be less severe if taken with food
    - Decrease dose if renal failure creatinine clearance <30 mL/min

Second Line
Ibuprofen or other NSAIDs for symptomatic relief (no aspirin in children)

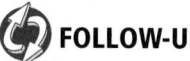 FOLLOW-UP

PROGNOSIS
Favorable

COMPLICATIONS
- Otitis media
- Pneumonia
- Reye syndrome
- Rhabdomyolysis
- Post-influenza asthenia
- Acute sinusitis
- Croup
- Apnea in neonates
- Bronchitis
- Death
- Exacerbation of CHF

ALERT
Geriatric Considerations
Complications more likely in elderly

PATIENT MONITORING
- Mild cases: Usually no follow-up required
- Moderate or severe cases: Follow until symptoms resolved and any complications treated effectively

REFERENCES
1. Report of the Committee on Infectious Diseases, 2006.Elk Grove Village, IL: American Academy of Pediatrics; 2006.
2. Harper SA, et al. Prevention and control of influenza. Recommendations of the Immunization Practices Advisory Committee (ACIP). *MMWR.* 2005;54:1–40.
3. Mandell GL, ed. *Principles and Practice of Infectious Diseases.* 5th ed. New York, NY: Churchill Livingstone; 2000.

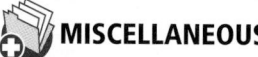 MISCELLANEOUS

Persons with HIV infection should get annual influenza vaccination; however, antibody response to vaccine may be low in persons with advanced HIV-related illnesses.

CODES
ICD9-CM
- 487.0 Influenza with pneumonia
- 487.1 Influenza with other respiratory manifestations

PATIENT TEACHING
For a listing of sources for patient education materials favorably reviewed on this topic, physicians may contact: American Academy of Family Physicians Foundation, P.O. Box 8418, Kansas City, MO 64114, (800) 274-2237, ext. 4400.

Prevention
Educate high-risk patients about prevention and strict hand-washing procedures.

 See Patient Handout on CD

I

INSECT BITES AND STINGS

Hans House, MD

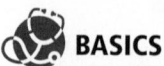 **BASICS**

DESCRIPTION

Arthropods affect man by being pests, inoculating poison, invading tissue, or transmitting disease. Inoculation of poison may occur as either a bite or a sting. This discussion is limited to the irritative, poisonous, and allergic effects of these pests.

- Harmful arthropods of the US include
  - Bees: Bumblebees, honeybees
  - Wasps: Hornets, wasps
  - Ants: Fire ants, harvester ants
  - Brown recluse spiders
  - Black widow spiders
  - Hobo spiders
  - Scorpions
  - Mosquitoes
  - Flies: Deer, horse, black, stable, and biting midges
  - Lice: Body, head, pubic
  - Bugs: Kissing, bed, wheel
  - Fleas: Human, cat, dog
  - Mites: Itch mite (scabies), red bugs (chiggers)
  - Ticks
  - Caterpillars: Puss, browntail, buck, moth saddleback
  - Centipedes
- Characteristic reactions include
  - Local tissue irritation, inflammation, and destruction
  - Systemic effects related to inoculated poisons
  - Allergic reactions: Immediate or delayed
- System(s) Affected: Skin/Exocrine

ALERT

Geriatric Considerations
More at risk

Pediatric Considerations
More at risk

Pregnancy Considerations
Not a contraindication to appropriate management

GENERAL PREVENTION

- Avoid re-exposure in known hypersensitive individuals.
- Prescribe anaphylactic (ANA kit) or EpiPen, if indicated.
- Educate on risks of increasing anamnestic responses in future.
- Consider desensitization with immunotherapy in severe cases.
- DEET or other proven insect repellants
- Permethrin applied to clothes is better against ticks than DEET. (1)[B]

EPIDEMIOLOGY

Prevalence
Widespread (seasonal and regional variance)

RISK FACTORS

- Living environment
- Climate
- Season
- Clothing
- Lack of protective measures
- Perfumes, colognes
- Previous sensitization
- Young or elderly at more risk

ETIOLOGY

- Local tissue inflammation and destruction from poison
- Allergic reaction from previous sensitization
- Toxic reaction from large inoculation of poison

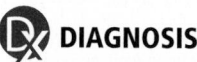 **DIAGNOSIS**

SIGNS AND SYMPTOMS

- Local reactions
  - Erythema
  - Pain
  - Heat
  - Induration
  - Itching
  - Blisters
  - Secondary infection: Cellulitis, abscess
  - Necrosis
  - Ulceration
  - Drainage
- Toxic reactions: Nonantigenic
  - Nausea
  - Vomiting
  - Headache
  - Fever
  - Diarrhea
  - Light-headedness
  - Syncope
  - Drowsiness
  - Muscle spasms
  - Edema
  - Convulsions
- Systemic reactions: Allergic
  - Itching eyes
  - Facial flushing
  - Generalized urticaria
  - Dry cough
  - Chest/throat constriction
  - Wheezing
  - Dyspnea
  - Cyanosis
  - Abdominal cramps
  - Diarrhea
  - Nausea
  - Vomiting
  - Vertigo
  - Chills/fever
  - Stridor
  - Shock
  - Loss of consciousness
  - Involuntary bowel/bladder action
  - Frothy sputum
  - Respiratory failure
  - Cardiovascular collapse
  - Death

- Delayed reaction
  - Serum sickness–like reactions
  - Fever
  - Malaise
  - Headache
  - Urticaria
  - Lymphadenopathy
  - Polyarthritis
- Unusual reactions
  - Encephalopathy
  - Neuritis
  - Vasculitis
  - Nephrosis
  - Extreme fear/anxiety

Physical Exam
In the case of tick paralysis, finding the attached tick is an essential step in management. [C]

TESTS

Lab
- Leukocytosis, thrombocytopenia, hypofibrinogenemia, abnormal coagulation, DIC, proteinuria, hemoglobinemia, hemoglobinuria, myoglobinemia, myoglobinuria, and azotemia are uncommon but possible manifestations in severe reactions.

Pathological Findings
- Inflammation
- Ulceration
- Vesiculation
- Pustulation
- Rupture
- Eschar
- Swelling

DIFFERENTIAL DIAGNOSIS

- Local reaction: Infection, cellulitis, dermatoses, punctures, foreign bodies
- Toxic reaction: Chemical exposure/ingestion, medications, IV drug abuse, environmental, plants
- Allergic reaction: Medications, illicit drugs, foods, topical products, environmental, plants, chemicals

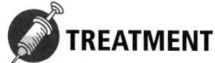
TREATMENT

INITIAL STABILIZATION
- Outpatient or inpatient, depending on individual response to injury
- Hospitalize for severe systemic reactions with threatened airway obstruction, bronchospasm, hypotension, severe angiodermatitis, or pain.

GENERAL MEASURES
- First aid measures, local treatment, activate emergency services in severe reactions. If history of allergy or large envenomations, do not wait to seek emergency care.
- Use ANA kit and OTC antihistamines, if available and required. (2)[C]
- Local (depending on severity)
  - Remove stinger (scrape it out, do not squeeze with tweezers).
  - Remove attached ticks by mechanical extraction, rather than applied chemicals or heat. (3)[B]
  - Cleanse wound.
  - Ice packs to bite or sting site, ASA paste does not reduce the duration of pain or swelling, and may prolong the redness. (4)[B]
  - Elevation of affected part
  - Rest the affected area.
  - Débride ulcers.
  - Drain abscesses.
- Systemic (depending on severity, and type of reaction)
  - Home use: EpiPen
  - Adequate airway (intubation, tracheostomy): If needed to bypass obstruction
  - Oxygen if needed for respiratory distress
  - Hospitalize and observe 24–48 hours.

Diet
No special diet; NPO if severe systemic reaction

Activity
Rest to limit spread of poison.

MEDICATION (DRUGS)

First Line
- Local (depending on severity)
  - Analgesics
  - Antihistamines: Diphenhydramine (Benadryl) 25–50 mg q.i.d.
  - Steroids topical or oral: Prednisone 20–40 mg/d
  - Antibiotics
- Systemic (depending on severity and reaction type)
  - Epinephrine (1:1000) IM or SC to combat urticaria, wheezing, angioedema (child 0.01 mL/kg, adult 0.3–0.5 mL). IM route may be faster than SC. (2)[B] Epinephrine (1:10,000) IV should be reserved for severe cases with cardiovascular collapse. (2)[C]
  - Diphenhydramine: To combat urticaria, wheezing, angioedema, 25–50 mg IV or IM
  - IV fluids (Ringer lactate): If needed for hypotension, hypovolemia
  - Dopamine: To correct vascular collapse, 200 mg in 250 mL at 5 μg/kg/min. Titrate to maintain systemic BP >90 mm Hg.
  - Hydrocortisone: If needed for severe urticaria or spider bite, 100–250 mg IV

- Tetanus prophylaxis and antibiotics: If indicated
- Diazepam (Valium): If needed for severe muscle spasms, 5–10 mg
- Morphine or meperidine (Demerol): If needed for pain
- Antivenins (e.g., black widow spider, scorpion) are available and appropriate in certain cases based on availability and identification of organism.
- Topical insecticides
  - Lice: 1% permethrin (Nix, Elimite) is drug of choice, but 0.5% malathion (Ovide) or pyrethrin (Rid) is effective. (5)[B] Lindane (Kwell) has fallen out of favor for the treatment of lice due to growing resistance and reported cases of neurotoxicity.
  - Scabies: 5% permethrin is drug of choice, but 10% crotamiton (Eurax) or lindane is effective. (5)[B]
- Contraindications: Refer to manufacturer's literature.
- Precautions
  - Dosing appropriate to age
  - If severe reaction, do not delay treatment.
  - Severe vascular collapse may require central pressure monitor.
- Significant possible interactions: Refer to manufacturer's literature.

Second Line
- Other antihistamines, e.g., loratadine (Claritin), fexofenadine (Allegra). (6)[B]
- Oral ivermectin (Mectizan) appears effective for lice and scabies (7)[B], but is not FDA approved for this purpose. It is administered in a dose of 200 μg/kg once, followed by a 2nd dose of equal size 1–2 weeks later.

SURGERY
Optimal treatment of necrotic spider bites is not well defined. Surgical repair may be required of severe ulcerative lesions, but not until primary necrotizing process is complete.

FOLLOW-UP

PROGNOSIS
- Minor reactions: Excellent
- Severe reactions: Excellent with early, appropriate treatment

COMPLICATIONS
- Infection
  - Bacterial
  - Arthropod-associated diseases with tick, fly, bug, and mosquito bites, (e.g., *Lyme borreliosis*, West Nile Fever, rickettsial disease [Rocky Mountain spotted fever], ehrlichiosis, arboviral encephalitis, malaria, leishmaniasis, trypanosomiasis, dengue)
- Scarring
- Drug reactions
- Multisystem failure
- Death

PATIENT MONITORING
Follow-up wound care.

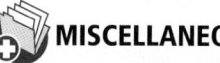
REFERENCES

1. Evans SR, Korch GW Jr, Lawson MA. Comparative field evaluation of permethrin and deet-treated military uniforms for personal protection against ticks (Acari). *J Med Entomol.* 1990;27(5): 829–834.
2. McLean-Tooke APC, Bethune CA, Fay AC, Spickett GP. Adrenaline in the treatment of anaphylaxis: What is the evidence? *BMJ.* 2003;327:1332–1335.
3. De Boer R, van den Bogaard AE. Removal of attached nymphs and adults of Ixodes ricinus (Acari: Ixodidae). *J Med Entomol.* 1993;30(4): 748–752.
4. Balit CR, Isbister GK, Buckley NA. Randomized controlled trial of topical aspirin in the treatment of bee and wasp stings. *J Toxicol Clin Toxicol.* 2003;41(6):801–808.
5. Walker GJA, Johnstone PW. Interventions for treating scabies. *The Cochrane Database of Systematic Reviews.* Volume (4), 2005.
6. Muller U, Mosbech H, Blaauw P, et al. Emergency treatment of allergic reactions to Hymenoptera stings. *Clin Exp Allergy.* 1991;21(3):281–288.
7. Drugs for parasitic infections. *Med Lett Drugs Ther.* 1998;40(2):1–12.
8. Usha V, Gopalakrishnan Nair TV. A comparative study of oral ivermectin and topical permethrin cream in the treatment of scabies. *J Am Acad Dermatol.* 2000;42(2P1):236–240.
9. Necrotic arachnidism—Pacific Northwest, 1988–1996. *MMWR Morb Mortal Wkly Rep.* 1996;45(31):433–436.
10. Mosquitoes and mosquito repellants: A clinician's guide. *Ann Intern Med.* 1198;128:931–940.

MISCELLANEOUS
- Other notes: Imported fire ants and Africanized bees in endemic areas of the southern US pose increased risks to persons living in these areas.
- See also: Pediculosis; Scabies

CODES

ICD9-CM
- 989.5 Toxic effect of venom
- 910.8 Other and unspecified superficial injury of face, neck, and scalp except eye, without mention of infection

PATIENT TEACHING

See Corresponding Diagnostic Algorithm

See Patient Handout on CD

I

INSOMNIA

L. Cassandra Vawter, MD
Sheldon Benjamin, MD

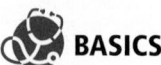 **BASICS**

DESCRIPTION
Insomnia: Difficulty initiating or maintaining sleep, early morning awakening, nonrestful sleep, or a combination, leading to consequences such as daytime tiredness, low energy, irritability, or difficulty concentrating
- Transient: Secondary to life crises, bereavement, change in environment or concomitant illness
- Chronic: Associated with medical and psychiatric conditions, drug intake, and maladaptive behavioral patterns

ALERT
Associated with MVAs, psychiatric disorder, impaired role function, cognitive dysfunction, increased medical utilization

Geriatric Considerations
- Caution when prescribing benzodiazepines or other sedative-hypnotics to the elderly—use short-acting nonbenzodiazepine benzodiazepine agonists or melatonin agonist if absolutely necessary for short-term treatment of sleep onset insomnia.
- Increased risk of falls and confusion

Pregnancy Considerations
Transient insomnia occurs secondary to change of sleep position, nocturia, gastritis, back pain, anxiety

GENERAL PREVENTION
- Avoid or treat known etiologies.
- Practice consistent sleep hygiene.

EPIDEMIOLOGY
- Predominant age: Increases with age
- Predominant sex: Female > Male (1.5:1)

Prevalence
Chronic insomnia: 10% middle-aged adults; 1/3 of people over 65

RISK FACTORS
- Chronic illness
- Age
- Polypharmacy
- Obesity
- Depression/Anxiety

ETIOLOGY
- Transient/Intermittent
  - Stress/Excitement/Bereavement
  - Shift work
  - Medical illness
  - High altitude
- Chronic
  - Medical: GERD, COPD, Asthma, Fibromyalgia
  - Primary sleep disorder: Idiopathic (primary), breathing related, restless leg syndrome, sleep state misperception, parasomnias
  - Circadian Rhythm disorder: Irregular pattern, jet lag, delayed/advanced sleep phase, shift work
  - Environmental: Light (LCD clocks), noise (snoring, household, traffic) movements: Partner/pets
  - Neurological: Dementia, stroke, Parkinson's/extrapyramidal dysfunction, epilepsy, headache/pain, myotonic dystrophy, traumatic brain injury
  - Behavioral: Poor sleep hygiene, psychophysiologic, adjustment sleep disorder
  - Substance-induced
  - Mood and anxiety disorders

ASSOCIATED CONDITIONS
- Obstructive sleep apnea
- Restless leg syndrome
- Drug or alcohol addiction/dependence
- Psychiatric disorders

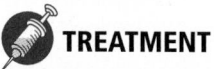 **DIAGNOSIS**

SIGNS AND SYMPTOMS
- Perceived reduction in sleep time
- Initial insomnia: Difficulty initiating sleep at usual time
- Middle insomnia: Wakefulness during the usual sleep cycle, tossing and turning
- Terminal insomnia: Early awakening
- Daytime sleepiness and napping
- Unintended sleep episodes (driving, working)
- Tiredness
- Anticipatory anxiety

History
- Sleep hygiene: Bedtime/wakening time, physical environment of sleep area—clocks/TV/lighting/noise, nighttime eating
- Related: Medical conditions such as pain, stressors, mood issues, medications/timing of administration
- History from partner/family: Snoring, irregular breathing, sleep movements, length of sleep, mood/performance changes
- Insomnia history: Duration, time of problem: Difficulty falling asleep, onset of sleep, difficulty maintaining sleep (repeated awakening ± "mind racing" thoughts), early AM awakening, or nonrestorative sleep
- Hypersomnia history: Daytime naps, drowsiness, situation/location of daytime sleep
- Narcolepsy symptoms: Excessive daytime sleepiness, cataplexy, hypnagogic/hypnopompic hallucinations, sleep paralysis

TESTS
Polysomnography for evaluation of sleep apnea, restless legs, parasomnia, or when sleep history does not provide diagnosis

DSM Criteria
- Primary insomnia
  - c/o 1 month: Difficulty initiating/maintaining sleep, or nonrestorative sleep
  - Impairment in social, occupational, or other important areas of functioning
  - Does not occur exclusively during Narcolepsy, Breathing-related Sleep Disorder, Circadian Rhythm Sleep Disorder, or Parasomnia
  - Does not occur exclusively during Major Depressive Disorder, Generalized Anxiety Disorder, Delirium, etc.
  - Is not secondary to physiological effects of substance or General Medical Condition
  - Sleep disturbance (or resultant daytime fatigue) causes clinically significant distress
- Secondary insomnia
  - Due to substance abuse, medication induced (diuretics, stimulants, etc.), primary depressive disorder, generalized anxiety disorder or phobias, acute situational stress, PTSD, pain, etc.

DIFFERENTIAL DIAGNOSIS
Transient stress, substance abuse, mood and anxiety disorders, Primary sleep disorders (insomnia, hypersomnia, parasomnia), insomnia due to medical or neurological disorder, pain, depression, anxiety

TREATMENT

GENERAL MEASURES
- Appropriate health care: Outpatient
- Transient insomnia
  - Lasts <4 weeks
  - May use medications for short term only
- Chronic insomnia
  - Rule out secondary causes (MDD, GAD, medications, substance abuse, etc.)
  - Thorough sleep history, drug/caffeine intake, diet, and exercise pattern may uncover correctable causes
  - Cognitive behavioral therapy is 1st line treatment for chronic insomnia.
  - Address underlying causes: e.g., pain, drugs/alcohol, depression, etc.
  - Avoid daytime napping; develop bedtime rituals conducive to sleep.
  - Refrain from using bed for anything besides sleeping or sex (no eating, work, reading, T.V.)
  - Remove large or bright clocks from bedroom to prevent focusing on how little sleeping is accomplished as well as light stimulus

Diet
- Avoid caffeine.
- Avoid heavy late night snacks (light snack at bedtime may help).
- Avoid alcohol after 5 PM or within 6 hours of retiring.

Activity
- A daily exercise routine improves quality of sleep.
- Avoid exercise within 3 hours of bedtime.

Nursing
- No vitals when asleep unless needed
- Schedule medications in manner conducive to sleep.

MEDICATION (DRUGS)

Best reserved for transient insomnia such as with jet lag, stress reactions, transient medical conditions

- Nonbenzodiazepine benzodiazepine receptor agonists (all may induce dependence)
  – Zaleplon (Sonata) 5–20 mg; half-life 1–1.5h
  – Zolpidem (Ambien) 2.5–10 mg; half-life 1.5–4h
  – Zolpidem ER 1–3 mg; half-life 5–7h
  – Eszopiclone (Lunesta) 1–3 mg; half-life 5–7h
- Benzodiazepine hypnotics
  – Intermediate acting
    ○ Temazepam 7.5–30 mg; half-life 8–12h
    ○ Oxazepam 10–30 mg; half-life 5–15h
  – Long acting
    ○ Alprazolam 0.25–1 mg; half-life 12–20h
    ○ Lorazepam 0.5–2 mg; half-life 10–22h
    ○ Clonazepam 0.5–2 mg; half-life 22–38h
    ○ Diazepam 2.5–10 mg; half-life 20–50h
- Contraindications/Precautions
  – Not indicated for long-term treatment of chronic insomnia due to risks of tolerance, dependency, daytime attention and concentration compromise, incoordination, rebound insomnia
  – Avoid in elderly, pregnant or breast-feeding, substance abusers, patients with suicidal or parasuicidal behaviors
  – Avoid in patients with untreated obstructive apnea and chronic pulmonary disease.
- Melatonin receptor agonist
  – Ramelteon 8 mg; half-life 1–2.6h
- Serotonergic antidepressants
  – Trazodone 25–200 mg; half-life 3–9h
  – Doxepin 25–150 mg; half-life 6–8h
  – Amitriptyline 25–150 mg; half-life 10–50h
  – Mertazapine 15–60 mg; half-life 20–40h
- Gamma-hydroxy butyrate
  – Sodium oxybate 4.5–9 mg; half-life 40 min (only for insomnia due to narcolepsy)

Complementary and Alternative Medicine
- Melatonin can decrease sleep latency in the elderly when taken 30–120 minutes prior to bedtime, however, effects of long-term use are unknown (9).
- Inclusive evidence exists for the use of valerian (10).

SURGERY
Pharyngoplasty may be useful for sleep apnea, though weight loss can also help.

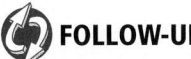 FOLLOW-UP

Issues for Referral
- Referral to psychiatrist may be indicated if psychiatric disturbance is suspected.
- Referral to sleep lab if sleep history does not reveal cause of insomnia, for breathing-related sleep disorders, parasomnias, or insomnia unresponsive to treatment

PROGNOSIS
- Situational insomnia should resolve with time.
- Treatment of underlying etiology is key, as is consistent sleep hygiene.

COMPLICATIONS
- Transient insomnia can become chronic.
- Daytime sleepiness, cognitive dysfunction
- Pulmonary hypertension if chronic sleep apnea left untreated
- Sleep apnea may lead to hypertension, stroke, cardiac ischemia

PATIENT MONITORING
- Reassess need for medications periodically—avoid standing prescriptions.
- Caution patients that nonbenzodiazepine benzodiazepine agonists (zolpidem, zaleplon, eszopiclone) as well as benzodiazepines, can be habit-forming.

REFERENCES

1. *Diagnostic and Statistical Manual of Mental Disorders*, DSM-IV-TR, 4th ed., Washington, DC: American Psychiatric Press, Inc.; 2000.
2. *International Classification of Sleep Disorders: Diagnostic and Coding Manual*. 2nd ed. Westchester, IL: American Academy of Sleep Medicine; 2005.
3. Kushida C, Littner M, Morgenthaler T, et al. Practice parameters for the indications for polysomnography and related procedures: An update for 2005. *Sleep*. 2005;28(4):499–521.
4. Glass J, Lanstot K, Herrmann N, et al. Sedative hypnotics in older people with insomnia: Meta-analysis of risks and benefits. *Br Med J*. 2005;331:1169–1173.
5. Hillman DR, Murphy AS, Pezzulo L. The economic cost of sleep disorders. *Sleep*. 2006;29(3): 299–305.
6. Buscemi N, et al. Efficacy and safety of exogenous melatonin for secondary sleep disorders and sleep disorders accompanying sleep restriction: Meta-analysis. *Br Med J*. 2006;332(7538): 385–393.
7. American Academy of Sleep Medicine. Practice parameters for the evaluation of chronic insomnia. *Sleep*. 2000;23(2):237–241.
8. Edinger J, et al. Cognitive behavioral therapy for treatment of chronic primary insomnia. *JAMA*. 2001;285(14):1856–1864.
9. Hughes RJ, Sack RL, Lewy AJ. The role of melatonin and circadian phase in age-related sleep-maintenance insomnia: Assessment in a clinical trial of melatonin replacement. *Sleep*. 1998;21(1):52–68.
10. Stevinson C, Ernst E. Valerian for insomnia: Systematic review of randomized clinical trials. *Sleep Med*. 2000;1:91–99.

MISCELLANEOUS

See also: Anxiety/Depression; Fibromyalgia; Sleep apnea, obstructive

CODES

ICD9-CM
- 780.50 Sleep disturbance, unspecified
- 780.51 Insomnia with sleep apnea
- 780.52 Other insomnia

PATIENT TEACHING

Describe limitations and noxious effects of drugs used for insomnia.

Diet
Light carbohydrate-rich snack before bed may be helpful; avoid large protein-rich meals.

Activity
- Develop a daily exercise routine.
- No exercise <3 hours before bedtime

Prevention
- Sleep hygiene
- Establish regular sleep–wake schedule on weekdays; use same on weekends.
- Sleep in cool, dark, quiet environment.
- No activities or stimuli in bedroom associated with anything but sleep or sex
- Institute a 30-minute wind-down time before sleep.
- If >30 minutes spent in bed worrying about sleep, move to another environment and engage in quiet activity until sleepiness sets in
- Limit caffeine intake to mornings.
- Do not use alcohol as sleep aid.
- No excessive alcohol or smoking in evenings

 See Corresponding Diagnostic Algorithm

I

INSULINOMA

Frederico Milla, MD
Ruben Peralta, MD, FACS

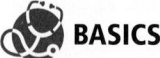 **BASICS**

DESCRIPTION
- Most common functional tumor of the pancreas.
- Tumors of the pancreatic β-cells of the islets of Langerhans. Pancreatic β-cells secrete both insulin and C-peptide.
- Whipple's triad is the basis for the clinical diagnosis of insulinomas
  - Symptomatic fasting or postexercise hypoglycemia
  - Low blood glucose levels <50 mg/dL (2.78 mmol/L) during symptoms
  - Resolution of symptoms when treated with PO or IV glucose
- Usually very small, with 70% measuring <1.5 cm
- Usually single and benign; only 10–15% malignant, only 10% multiple tumors
- The malignant potential is not as clinically important as the functional ability to secrete insulin, which leads to symptomatic hypoglycemia.
- Symptomatic hypoglycemia secondary to persistent, absolute, or relative hyperinsulinemia that is unresponsive to normal feedback mechanisms.
- Hypoglycemic episodes are irregular, recurrent, and tend to increase in frequency and severity over time.
- Hypoglycemic episodes are especially likely to occur when fasting or after exercise.
- Awareness is key to early diagnosis
- Synonym(s): β-Cell tumor, β-Cell adenoma, Nesidioblastoma

EPIDEMIOLOGY
- Predominant age
  - Rare: <20 years old
  - 20% of the cases are adults <40 years.
  - 40% of the cases are 40–60 years.
  - 40% of the cases are >60 years old.
- Predominant sex: Females > Male (60%)

Incidence
1 in 1.25 million annually

RISK FACTORS
- Age >40
- Multiple endocrine neoplasia (MEN)-1 syndrome

Genetics
No known genetic pattern, unless part of MEN 1 syndrome.

ETIOLOGY
Unknown

ASSOCIATED CONDITIONS
MEN 1 syndrome

DIAGNOSIS

SIGNS AND SYMPTOMS
- Due to hypoglycemia or catecholamine compensatory release
- Neurologic
  - Apathy, irritability
  - Confusion, disorientation
  - Delirium, hallucinations
  - Coma
  - Convulsions
  - Diplopia, blurred vision
  - Inarticulate speech
  - Tremor
  - Dizziness, vertigo
- Cardiovascular
  - Palpitations
  - Tachycardia
  - Angina
  - Diaphoresis
- Gastrointestinal
  - Hunger
  - Abdominal discomfort
  - Nausea
  - Vomiting
  - Weight gain

TESTS
- Fast for 72 hours or until symptoms develop. When symptomatic, determine insulin, C-peptide, and glucose levels. Document high insulin/glucose ratio.
- Provocative testing
  - IV calcium gluconate (15 mg/kg of elemental calcium) over 4 hours to determine insulin and glucose levels
  - Tolbutamide bolus (1 g after overnight fast); determine insulin and glucose levels at 150 minutes
  - C-peptide suppression with 0.1 U/kg of regular insulin; determine C-peptide and glucose levels

Lab
- Document low blood sugar during symptoms.
- Laboratory diagnosis is based on inappropriately high serum insulin and C-peptides during periods of low blood glucose (shows over-secretion and endogenous origin).
- Malignant tumors may secrete β-hCG

Imaging
- After the diagnosis is confirmed by lab results, attempts are made to localize the tumor, usually by CT and endoscopic ultrasound.
- Endoscopic ultrasound is particularly helpful in localization.
- High-quality spiral CT is the initial imaging study of choice.
- Selective mesenteric arteriography can be used with portovenous sampling and/or intra-arterial calcium stimulation, a complex technique.
- MRI (sensitivity ~90%) reserved for cases in which the tumor is not localized by less expensive tests.
- Somatostatin analogue I123 labeled TyR 3-octreotide scintigraphy

Diagnostic Procedures/Surgery
Intraoperative tumor localization includes intraoperative palpation and intraoperative ultrasound (sensitivity up to 95%) to confirm preoperative localization and to look for multiple small tumors.

Pathological Findings
- Usually small and single
- Malignant tumors tend to be larger and multiple.
- Metastases found in liver or regional lymph nodes (distant metastases rare)
- Tumors are evenly distributed throughout pancreas (1/3 in head, 1/3 in body, 1/3 in tail).

DIFFERENTIAL DIAGNOSIS
- Medications
  - Surreptitious insulin or oral hypoglycemic use
  - β-Blockers
  - Salicylates
  - Quinine
- Very rare causes
  - Nesidioblastosis
  - Large sarcomas
  - Hepatocellular carcinoma
- Reactive hypoglycemia
- Functional hypoglycemia
- Adrenocortical insufficiency
- Hypopituitarism
- Significant liver disease

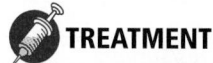 **TREATMENT**

GENERAL MEASURES
- Treatment is primarily surgical; medical treatment is available for surgically incurable lesions.
- Observe closely for severe hypoglycemic symptoms.
- Attempt to increase glucose levels.
- Attempt to decrease insulin levels.
- Keep a ready glucose source available.

Diet
Frequent high-carbohydrate meals and snacks

Activity
Avoid exercise

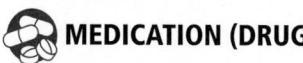 **MEDICATION (DRUGS)**

First Line
- To decrease insulin secretion
  - Diazoxide inhibits the release of stored insulin, 100–150 mg PO q8h (3–8 mg/kg/d in 2 or 3 divided doses)
  - Octreotide acetate (long-acting analog of somatostatin); 50–100 mcg SQ b.i.d.; increase as needed to control symptoms; effective in <30% of patients; insulinomas often do not express somatostatin receptors.
- To increase glucose levels
  - PO or IV glucose
  - IM or SC glucagon
- For metastatic disease
  - Streptozocin plus doxorubicin
  - Fluorouracil

Second Line
- Dacarbazine (DTIC, 5-dimethyltriazenoimidazole-4-carboxamine): For metastatic disease
- To increase glucose levels
  - Corticosteroids
  - Propranolol
  - Phenytoin

SURGERY
- Surgical resection is the treatment of choice.
- Enucleation for small lesions
- Deep-seated or invasive tumor: Partial pancreatectomy
- Cure rates of 75–98% after surgery
- Mechanical ablative techniques (hepatic arterial embolization for refractory metastases)

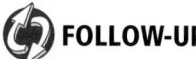 **FOLLOW-UP**

PROGNOSIS
Excellent, if tumor is solitary, benign, and completely resected.

COMPLICATIONS
From surgery
- Pancreatitis
- Pancreatic leaks
- Fistulae
- Peritonitis
- Abscess
- Pseudocysts

PATIENT MONITORING
Watch for recurrence of hypoglycemic symptoms.

REFERENCES
1. Brentjens R, Saltz L. Islet cell tumors of the pancreas: The medical oncologist's perspective. *Surg Clin North Am.* 2001;81:527–542.
2. Burns AR, Dackiw AP. Insulinoma. *Curr Treat Options Oncol.* 2003;4:309–317.
3. Grant CS. Insulinoma. *Surg Oncol Clin NA.* 1998;7:819–844.
4. Pereira PL, Wiskirchen J. Morphological and functional investigations of neuroendocrine tumors of the pancreas. *Eur Radiol.* 2003;13:2133–2146.
5. McAuley G, Delaney Colville J, et al. Multimodality preoperative imaging of pancreatic insulinomas. *Clin Radiol.* 2005;60(10):1039–1050.
6. Modlin IM, Lewis JJ, Ahlman H, Bilchik AJ, Kumar RR. Management of unresectable malignant endocrine tumors of the pancreas. *Surg Gynecol & Obstet.* 1993;176:507–518.
7. Tucker ON, Crotty PL, Conlon KC. The management of insulinoma. *Br J Surg.* 2006;93(3):264–275.

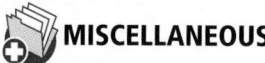 **MISCELLANEOUS**

- 80% of patients with MEN 1 syndrome have insulinomas.
- Insulinomas associated with MEN 1 syndrome tend to be multiple tumors and present at an earlier age.
- See also: Multiple endocrine neoplasia (MEN)

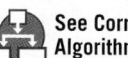 **CODES**

ICD9-CM
- 157.4 Malignant neoplasm of Islets of Langerhans
- 211.7 Benign neoplasm of Islets of Langerhans

PATIENT TEACHING

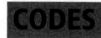 **See Corresponding Diagnostic Algorithm**

I

INTERSTITIAL CYSTITIS

Montiel T. Rosenthal, MD

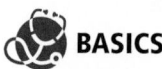 **BASICS**

DESCRIPTION

A disease of unknown cause probably representing a final common pathway from several etiologies. Likely pathogenesis is disruption of urothelium, impaired lower urinary tract defenses, and loss of bladder muscular wall elasticity. The symptoms in many patients are insidious, and the disease progresses over years before the diagnosis is established.

- Mild: Normal bladder capacity under anesthesia. Ulceration, cracking, or glomerulation of mucosa (or not) with bladder distention under anesthesia. No incontinence. Symptoms wax and wane and may not progress. A bladder sensory problem
- Severe: Progressive bladder fibrosis. Small true bladder capacity under anesthesia. Poor bladder wall compliance. Often ulcer present at cystoscopy. May have overflow incontinence and/or chronic bacteriuria that is unresponsive to antibiotics.
- System(s) Affected: Renal/Urologic
- Synonym(s): Urgency frequency syndrome; Painful bladder syndrome

ALERT

Pregnancy Considerations

Unpredictable symptom improvement or exacerbation during pregnancy. No known fetal effects from interstitial cystitis. Usual problems of unknown effect on fetus with medications taken during pregnancy.

EPIDEMIOLOGY

- Caucasians predominant
- Predominant age: 20s–40s for mild; 20s–70s for severe
- Predominant sex: Female > Male (10:1)

Pediatric Considerations

- <10 years old and again at 13–17
- Daytime enuresis, dysuria without infection

Prevalence

In the US

- Up to 500,000 affected. Many cases likely unreported
- 0.052%, but may be higher—up to 10% (1)[C]

RISK FACTORS

Unknown

Genetics

Probably not an inherited disease

ETIOLOGY

- Unknown. Not primarily psychosomatic
- Possible causes
  - Subclinical urinary infection
  - Damage to glycosaminoglycan mucus layer increasing bladder wall permeability to irritants such as urea
  - Autoimmune
  - Mast cell histamine release
  - Neurologic upregulation/stimulation

ASSOCIATED CONDITIONS

- Fibromyalgia
- Allergies
- Chronic Fatigue Syndrome
- Depression
- Chronic Prostatitis
- Chronic Pelvic Pain
- Irritable Bowel Syndrome

DIAGNOSIS

SIGNS AND SYMPTOMS

- Frequent, urgent, relentless urination day and night, >8 voids/24h
- Pain with full bladder that resolves with bladder emptying (except if bacteriuria present)
- Urge urinary incontinence if bladder capacity is small.
- Sleep disturbance
- Dyspareunia especially with full bladder
- Secondary symptoms from chronic pain and sleeplessness, especially depression

History

- Pelvic Pain and Urgency/Frequency (PUF) Symptom Scale: Self reporting questionnaire for screening potential interstitial cystitis patients (2)[B]
- Frequent UTIs, vaginitis, or symptoms in week before menses

Physical Exam

- Perineal/prostatic pain in males
- Anterior vaginal wall pain in females

TESTS

Lab

- Urinalysis: Normal except with chronic bacteriuria (rare)
- Urine culture from catheterized specimen: Normal except with chronic bacteriuria (rare) or partial antibiotic treatment
- Urine cytology: Normal
  - Reserve for men >40 and women with hematuria

Diagnostic Procedures/Surgery

- Cystoscopy (especially in men >40 or women w/hematuria)
  - Bladder wall visualization
  - Hydraulic distention: No improved diagnostic certainty over history and physical exam alone (3)[C]
- No role for urodynamic testing
- K^+ Sensitivity test (2)[B]
  - Insert catheter, empty bladder, instill 40 mL of H_2O over 2–3 min, rank urgency at 0–5 in intensity, rank pain at 0–5 in intensity, drain bladder, instill 40 mL of KCl 0.4 mol/L solution
    - If immediate pain, flush bladder w/60 mL of H_2O and treat (*See "Medications: Bladder Instillations")
    - If no immediate pain, wait 5 min and rate urgency and pain
  - If urgency or pain >2 on pain scale, treat by flushing bladder with 60 mL of H_2O and treat with (see "Medications: Bladder Instillations")
  - Test considered positive for Interstitial Cystitis if pain or urgency scores rank >2 and no history of radiation exposure or findings of acute bacterial cystitis

Pathological Findings

- Nonspecific chronic inflammation on bladder biopsies
- Urine cytology negative for dysplasia and neoplasia
- Possible mast cell proliferation in mucosa

DIFFERENTIAL DIAGNOSIS

- Uninhibited bladder (urgency, frequency, urge incontinence, less pain, symptoms usually decrease when asleep)
- Urinary infection: Cystitis, prostatitis
- Bladder neoplasm
- Bladder stone
- Neurologic bladder disease
- Nonurinary pelvic disease (sexually transmitted diseases, endometriosis, pelvic relaxation)

TREATMENT

GENERAL MEASURES

- Appropriate health care: Outpatient
- Eliminate foods and liquids that exacerbate symptoms on individual basis.
- Biofeedback bladder retraining

Diet

- Variable effects from person to person
- Common irritants include caffeine, chocolate, citrus, tomatoes, carbonated beverages, K$^+$-rich foods, spicy foods, acidic foods, and alcohol.

Complementary and Alternative Medicine

Intravesical dimethyl sulfoxide (DMSO) may be useful in patients who have not responded to other therapies (6).

SPECIAL THERAPY

Physical Therapy

Modified Thiele Massage—transvaginal of pelvic floor muscles (4)[C]

 MEDICATION (DRUGS)

First Line

- Oxybutynin, hyoscyamine, and other anticholinergic medications decrease frequency.
- Doxepin decreases frequency.
- NSAIDs for pain and any inflammatory component
- Pentosan polysulfate (Elmiron) 100 mg t.i.d. May take several months to become effective (only FDA-approved treatment for interstitial cystitis)
- Triple drug therapy: 6 months of pentosan, hydroxyzine, doxepin
- Antibacterials for bacteriuria
- Prednisone (used for ulcerative lesions)
- Monteleukast
- Hydroxyzine
- Amitripyline
- Bladder instillations:
  - *Lidocaine, *sodium bicarbonate, and *heparin or pentosan polysulfate sodium (5)[C]
  - Dimethyl sulfoxide (DMSO) every 1–2 weeks for 3–6 weeks, then as needed
  - Heparin sometimes added to DMSO
  - Other agents: Steroids, silver nitrate, oxychlorosene (Clorpactin)
- Contraindications: No anticholinergics with patients having closed-angle glaucoma
- Significant possible interactions: Refer to manufacturer's profile of each drug.

Second Line

Note that phenazopyridine, a local bladder mucosal anesthetic, is usually not very effective.

SURGERY

- Hydraulic distention of bladder under anesthesia: Symptomatic but transient relief
- Cauterization of bladder ulcer
- Augmentation cystoplasty to increase bladder capacity and decrease pressure, with or without partial cystectomy. Expected results in severe cases: Much improved, 75%; with residual discomfort, 20%; unchanged, 5%
- Urinary diversion with total cystectomy only if disease completely refractory to medical therapy

 FOLLOW-UP

PROGNOSIS

- Mild: Exacerbations and remissions of symptoms. May not be progressive. Does not predispose to other diseases.
- Severe: Progressive problems that usually require surgery to control symptoms

COMPLICATIONS

Severe with long-term continuous high bladder pressure could be associated with renal damage.

PATIENT MONITORING

Not specifically needed unless symptoms unresponsive to treatment

REFERENCES

1. Parsons CL, Tatsis V. Prevalence of interstitial cystitis in young women. *Urology*. 2004;64:866–870.
2. Parsons CL, Dell J, et al. Increased prevalence of interstitial cystitis; previously unrecognized urologic and gynecological cases identified using a new symptom questionnaire and intravesical potassium sensitivity. *Urology*. 2002;60:573–578.
3. Ottem DP, Teichman JM. What is the value of cystoscopy with hydrodistention for interstitial cystitis? *Urology*. 2005;66:494–499.
4. Ozama IA, Rejba A, et al. Modified Thiele massage as therapeutic intervention for female patients with interstitial cystitis and high-tone pelvic floor dysfunction. *Urology*. 2004;64:862–865.
5. Parsons CL Current strategies for managing interstitial cystitis. *Exp Opin Pharmacother*. 2004;5:287–293.
6. Peeker R, Haghsheno MA, Holmang S, et al. Intravesical bacillus Calmette-Guerin and dimethyl sulfoxide for treatment of classic and nonulcer interstitial cystitis: A prospective, randomized double-blind study. *J Urol*. 2000;164(6): 1912–1915.

 MISCELLANEOUS

See also: Urinary tract infection in females

CODES

ICD9-CM

595.1 Chronic interstitial cystitis

PATIENT TEACHING

Interstitial Cystitis Association,110 Wash. St. Suite 340, Rockville, MD 20850; 1(800) HELPICA; www.ichelp.org

See Corresponding Diagnostic Algorithm

INTERSTITIAL NEPHRITIS

Tyeese Gaines-Reed, DO, MA

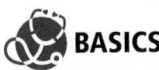 **BASICS**

DESCRIPTION
- Inflammatory response of the kidney involving interstitial edema and, at times, tubular cell damage. It may be an acute reaction or a result of long-term damage
- System(s) Affected: Renal/Urologic; Endocrine/Metabolic; Immunologic
- Synonym(s): Tubulointerstitial nephritis (TIN); Acute interstitial allergic nephritis

GENERAL PREVENTION
Avoid offending agents (see "Etiology").

EPIDEMIOLOGY
Incidence
Interstitial nephritis accounts for 10–15% of kidney disease in the US
- Children exposed to lead poisoning more likely to develop nephritis as a young adult.
- TIN with uveitis presents in adolescent females.
- Analgesic-induced nephritis 5–6 times more common in women.
  - Peak incidence in women 60–70 years
- Atherosclerotic or ischemic nephritis more common in the elderly

RISK FACTORS
See "Etiology"

ALERT
Geriatric Considerations
Elderly have more severe disease and increased risk of permanent damage.

PATHOPHYSIOLOGY
- Acute interstitial nephritis
  - Delayed hypersensitivity reaction, usually due to drugs
  - May cause acute renal insufficiency
- Chronic interstitial nephritis
  - Follows long-term exposure to offending agents
  - Often found on routine labs or evaluation for hypertension
- TIN is sometimes associated with uveitis

ETIOLOGY
- Acute interstitial nephritis
  - Hypersensitivity to drugs (70%)
    - Antibiotics: PCN, cephalosporins, sulfonamides, rifampin
    - NSAIDs/analgesics
    - Sulfa-containing diuretics
    - Phenytoin
    - Allopurinol
  - Infectious
  - Acute transplant rejection
  - Immunologic
    - SLE, Sjögren syndrome, sarcoidosis, cryoglobulinemia
  - Idiopathic (isolated or with uveitis)

- Chronic interstitial nephritis
  - Drugs
    - Analgesics, lithium, antineoplastics, antibiotics, anticonvulsants, antihypertensives, immunosuppressants, diuretics, Chinese herbal medicine
  - Heavy metals
    - Lead, cadmium
  - Obstruction
    - Stones, neoplasm, prostatic hypertrophy
  - Metabolic
    - Hypercalcemia, hyperoxaluria, chronic hypokalemia, cystinosis
  - Vascular changes
    - Cholesterol emboli, HTN, sickle hemoglobinopathy, radiation
  - Other
    - Balkan-endemic nephropathy, Ebstein-Barr virus

ASSOCIATED CONDITIONS
- Alport disease
- Medullary cystic disease
- Inflammatory bowel disease
- Multiple myeloma
- Primary biliary cirrhosis

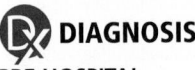 **DIAGNOSIS**

PRE HOSPITAL
ABCs, IV, oxygen

SIGNS AND SYMPTOMS
- Acute interstitial nephritis
  - Fever (80%)
  - Transient maculopapular rash (25–50%)
  - Acute renal insufficiency
    - Decreased urine output (50%)
    - Signs of fluid overload or depletion
    - Altered mental status
    - Nausea, vomiting
- Chronic interstitial nephritis
  - HTN
  - Decreased urine output or polyuria
  - Inability to concentrate urine
  - Polydipsia
  - Acidosis
  - Anemia
  - Fanconi syndrome

History
- Medications
- Alcohol and illicit drug use
- Exposure to heavy metals
- Tobacco use
- Dyslipidemia/atherosclerosis
- Cancer
- HTN

Physical Exam
- Increased BP
- Altered mental status
- Pericardial rub if uremic pericarditis
- Lung crackles if fluid overload
- Extremity swelling
- Weight gain from fluid retention

TESTS
EKG

Lab
- CBC
  - Eosinophilia (80%):
    - Not seen in NSAID-induced AIN
  - Anemia
- Chemistry
  - Acidosis
  - Hypokalemia/hyperkalemia
  - Increased BUN and creatinine
- Urinalysis
  - Hematuria (95%)
  - Mild proteinuria
  - Specific gravity
  - Pyuria, WBC casts
- Serologic testing for immunologic disease
  - Sarcoidosis, Sjögren syndrome, Wegener granulomatosis, Behçet
- Lead level
  - Not useful in chronic lead exposure
    - >90% of lead resides in bone

Imaging
- Ultrasound
- KUB
- IVP
- Gallium scan

Diagnostic Procedures/Surgery
Renal biopsy (Gold standard)

Pathological Findings
- Acute
  - Cellular infiltration with eosinophilia
- Chronic
  - Cellular infiltration with mononuclear cells

DIFFERENTIAL DIAGNOSIS
- Acute renal failure
- Urinary tract obstruction

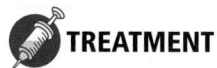 **TREATMENT**

For acute interstitial nephritis, corticosteroids have not been shown to improve outcomes (1)[B].

PRE HOSPITAL
ABCs, EKG

INITIAL STABILIZATION
ABCs, EKG

GENERAL MEASURES
- Discontinue offending agent.
- Reduce exposure to other nephrotoxic agents.
- Supportive measures
- Control BP and anemia.
- Correct electrolyte imbalances.
- Dialysis if criteria met

Diet
- Low-fat/low-cholesterol
- Low-protein (2)[A]
- Low-sodium
- Low-potassium

Activity
No restrictions

Nursing
- Ensure patient comfort.
- Adhere to medical orders.
- Patient education about nephrotoxic agents

SPECIAL THERAPY
IV Fluids
IV fluid repletion if normal urine production

 MEDICATION (DRUGS)

If renal failure persists after removing agent, attempt medication therapy.

First Line
- Prednisone 0.5–2 mg/kg/d PO for 1–2 weeks, followed by a taper
  - Studies support steroid use in chronic interstitial nephritis, not acute (1)[B], (3, 4)[C], (5)[A].
  - Continue corticosteroids for 6 months in patients with sarcoidosis (3)[C].

Second Line
- Lead toxicity: Repeated chelation therapy may improve renal function (6)[A].
  - Succimer 10 mg/kg PO q8h for 5 days, then q12h for 14 days, or
  - EDTA 2 g IV/IM. If IM, use with 2% lidocaine
- SLE nephritis
  - Steroids plus cyclophosphamide or azathioprine (5)[A]
- Urate nephropathy
  - Allopurinol to decrease urate level (3)[C]
  - Use with caution, because allopurinol is nephrotoxic.
- Lithium-induced nephritis
  - Use amiloride as adjunct (3)[C].
- Cidofovir-induced nephritis
  - Use probenecid as adjunct (3)[C].

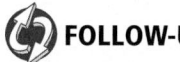 **FOLLOW-UP**

DISPOSITION
Admission Criteria
- Oliguria or anuria persists
- Severe electrolyte abnormalities
- EKG changes

Discharge Criteria
- Stable vitals, labs, and EKG
- Normal urine production

Issues for Referral
- Request early nephrology consult.
- Refer to nephrology as outpatient if symptoms persist.

PROGNOSIS
- Renal biopsy reveals extent of damage
- Acute interstitial nephritis
  - Recovery within weeks–months
  - Acute dialysis needed for 1/3 of patients before resolution
  - Rarely progresses to ESRD
- Chronic interstitial nephritis
  - Can persist to ESRD
- TIN with uveitis
  - Renal disease remits in 1 year if untreated.
  - Uveitis has relapsing course, requiring systemic corticosteroids.
- Untreated acute renal failure has a 45–70% mortality

COMPLICATIONS
- ESRD
- Papillary necrosis
- Analgesics increase risk of transitional cell cancers of uroepithelium.

PATIENT MONITORING
If patients must remain on nephrotoxic medications, frequently measure renal function, electrolytes, and phosphorus.

REFERENCES

1. Clarkson MR, Giblin L, Fionnuala PO, et al. Acute interstitial nephritis: Clinical features and response to corticosteroid therapy. *Nephrol Dialysis Transplant.* 2004;19:2778–2783.
2. Fougue D, Laville M, Boissel, JP. Low-protein diets for chronic kidney disease in nondiabetic adults. *Cochrane Database of Systematic Reviews.* 3, 2006.
3. Braden GL, O'Shea MH, Mulhern JG. Tubulointerstitial diseases. *Am J Kidney Dis.* 2005; 46:560–572.
4. Markowitz GS, Perazella MA. Drug-induced renal failure: A focus on tubulointerstitial disease. *Clinica Chimica Acta.* 2005;351:31–47.
5. Flanc RS, Roberts MA, Strippoli GFM, et al. Treatment for lupus nephritis. *Cochrane Database of Systemic Reviews* 2004,1:CD002922.
6. Lin JL, Lin-Tan D, Hsu H, et al. Environment lead exposure and progression of chronic renal diseases in patients without diabetes. *N Engl J Med.* 2003;348:277–286.

ADDITIONAL READING
- Internet references
  - Emedicine at www.emedicine.com
  - Atlas of Diseases of the Kidney at http://www.kidneyatlas.org
- Lum GM. Chapter 22. Kidney and urinary tract. Current Pediatric Diagnosis and Treatment, 17th ed.
- Watnick S, Morrison G. Chapter 22. Kidney. Current Medical Diagnosis and Treatment, 45th ed.
- Feinfeld DA, Anthony VL. Chapter 27. Renal principles. Goldfrank's Toxicologic Emergencies, 8th ed. 2006

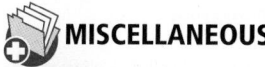 **MISCELLANEOUS**

CODES

ICD9-CM
- 580.89 Acute interstitial nephritis
- 582.89 Chronic interstitial nephritis
- 583.89 Interstitial nephritis (diffuse, focal)
- 403.9 Atherosclerotic or hypertensive kidney

PATIENT TEACHING
Printed materials for patients: National Kidney Disease Education Program, (866) 4-KIDNEY, www.nkdep.nih.gov

Prevention
- Early recognition and prompt discontinuation of offending agents
- Remove all sources of heavy metals, including ceramics.
- Avoid further nephrotoxicity.

 See Corresponding Diagnostic Algorithm

INTESTINAL OBSTRUCTION

Abdulrazak Abyad, MD, PhD, MBA, MPH

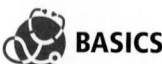 **BASICS**

DESCRIPTION

Intestinal obstruction exists where there is a failure, reversal, or impairment of the normal transit of intestinal contents. Obstructions may be partial or complete and are manifested by abdominal pain, emesis, and obstipation.

- System(s) Affected: Gastrointestinal

ALERT

Geriatric Considerations

- Colon neoplasms more common
- Chronic constipation/impactions more common

Pediatric Considerations

Different etiologies of obstruction in childhood

- Duodenal malformations
- Jejunoileal atresia
- Malrotation and midgut volvulus
- Meconium ileus
- Necrotizing enterocolitis
- Hirschsprung disease
- Intussusception
- Duplications
- Meckel diverticulum
- Imperforate anus

EPIDEMIOLOGY

Predominant sex: Male = Female

Prevalence

In the US: Accounts for ~20% of all admissions for acute abdominal conditions

RISK FACTORS

- Previous abdominal and/or pelvic surgery
- Hernia
- Chronic constipation
- Cholelithiasis
- Inflammatory bowel disease
- Ingested foreign bodies: Pica, enteric potassium tablets, etc.
- Diverticular disease

Genetics

Unknown

ETIOLOGY

- Luminal lesions
  - Impactions
  - Gallstones
  - Meconium in newborns
  - Intussusception in infants
- Intrinsic lesions
  - Congenital (e.g., atresia and stenosis, imperforate anus, duplications, Meckel diverticulum)
  - Trauma
  - Inflammatory (e.g., Crohn disease, diverticulitis, ulcerative colitis, radiation, toxic [ingestions])
  - Neoplastic (most common cause of colon obstruction in adults)
  - Miscellaneous (e.g., endometriosis)
- Extrinsic lesions
  - Adhesions (most common cause of small bowel obstruction)
  - Hernia and wound dehiscence
  - Masses (e.g., annular pancreas, anomalous vasculature, abscess and hematoma, neoplasms)
  - Volvulus
  - Neuromuscular defect (e.g., megacolon, neuro/myopathic motility disorders)

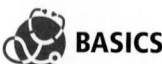 **DIAGNOSIS**

SIGNS AND SYMPTOMS

- Abdominal pain: Diffuse, poorly localized abdominal cramping at intervals of 5–15 minutes
- Emesis: Usually occurs immediately after obstruction of bowel. More frequent in proximal obstruction. Unusual in colon obstruction until small bowel distention occurs
- Obstipation: Common symptom. May pass contents distal to obstruction especially in high intestinal obstruction. Pain followed by explosive diarrhea often seen in partial obstruction
- Inspection: With or without distention (a late finding), less likely in proximal obstructions
- Auscultation: High-pitched bowel sounds, peristaltic rushes
- Palpation: Tenderness, mass, presence of peritoneal signs (these suggest strangulation)
- Rectal examination: May reveal fecal impaction. Occult blood may suggest colon malignancy.

TESTS

Lab

- White blood cell count: Slight rise (15,000/mm^3). Significant increases associated with strangulation
- Hematocrit: Moderate rise associated with extracellular fluid loss
- Renal: Urine specific gravity 1.025–1.030 and increase in blood urea nitrogen and creatinine owing to extracellular volume loss
- Amylase: May be elevated. Unreliable as an indicator of obstruction or strangulation
- Blood gases: May be normal. Late changes are those of acidosis
- No single or series of laboratory studies are useful in diagnosis of intestinal strangulation.

Imaging

- Abdominal and chest radiographs
  - Distention of small bowel or colon
  - Air–fluid levels (may be seen in ileus, gastroenteritis, constipation)
  - Lack of colon gas
  - Free intraperitoneal air (strangulation with perforation)
  - "Bird beak" lesion in colonic volvulus
  - Foreign body visualization
- Contrast studies
  - Barium enema is useful for diagnosis of colonic obstruction and may be therapeutic in intussusception.
  - Barium or gastrografin orally may differentiate obstruction from ileus.
  - Enteroclysis may identify site of small bowel obstruction.

Diagnostic Procedures/Surgery

- Rigid proctoscopy. May be therapeutic in sigmoid volvulus
- Flexible sigmoidoscopy

Pathological Findings

- Edema of mucosa
- Hypersecretion
- Necrosis

DIFFERENTIAL DIAGNOSIS

Adynamic ileus

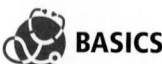 **TREATMENT**

INITIAL STABILIZATION

- Inpatient
- Treatment directed at early gastrointestinal decompression, correction of fluid and electrolyte abnormalities, timely operative intervention, surgical/GI consultation required

GENERAL MEASURES

- Nasogastric suction
- Foley catheter
- Swan-Ganz catheter or other central monitor, if required
- IV fluids: Normal saline/Ringer solution with potassium supplementation as required
- Antibiotic use controversial in absence of sepsis, but prophylactic antibiotics probably appropriate

Diet

NPO

Activity

Bed rest

MEDICATION (DRUGS)

Surgeon's choice for prophylaxis

SURGERY

- Timing of operative intervention critical; must correct electrolytes, volume quickly prior to surgery
- Surgical procedures
  - Closed bowel procedures: Lysis of adhesions, reduction of intussusception, reduction of volvulus, reduction of incarcerated hernia
  - Enterotomy for removal of bezoars, foreign bodies, gallstones
  - Resection of bowel for obstructing lesions, strangulated bowel
  - Bypasses of intestine around obstruction
  - Enterocutaneous fistulae proximal to obstruction: Colostomy, cecostomy

 FOLLOW-UP

PROGNOSIS

Usually excellent prognosis. In general, mortality from intestinal obstruction ranges from <1 to >20% depending on etiology, bowel viability, comorbidities.

COMPLICATIONS

- Slow return of bowel function
- Higher risk of subsequent obstruction
- Sepsis

PATIENT MONITORING

Follow weekly postoperatively for 2–8 weeks.

REFERENCES

1. Sleisenger MH, Fordtran JS, eds. *Gastrointestinal and Liver Disease: Pathophysiology, Diagnosis, Management*. 6th ed. Philadelphia: WB Saunders; 1998.

 MISCELLANEOUS

Other notes

- Rectal examination showing occult blood may represent colon malignancy as cause of the obstruction.

 CODES

ICD9-CM

- 560.0 Intussusception
- 560.3 Impaction of intestine, unspecified
- 560.9 Unspecified intestinal obstruction

PATIENT TEACHING

 See Corresponding Diagnostic Algorithm

INTESTINAL PARASITES

D. W. MacPherson, MD, MSc (CTM), FRCPC

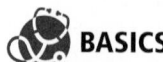 **BASICS**

DESCRIPTION

- The class of infectious agents called parasites is divided into 2 parts
  - Protozoa are single-cell animals that characteristically divide and multiply within the host, are usually direct fecal-oral in transmission, and do not cause an eosinophilia.
  - Helminths (worms) are multicellular animals and, with rare exceptions (i.e., *Strongyloides stercoralis, Hymenolepis nana*), do not multiply within the host and are often associated with some degree of eosinophilia. The level of eosinophilia is associated with the degree of mucosal invasiveness. The worms have a limited life span within the host, and without reinfection would eventually die on their own.
- Not all of the bowel parasites remain in the bowel. Some are invasive, and some do not release their infective forms into the bowel. This latter group (i.e., *Toxoplasma gondii, Echinococcus, Trichinella*) won't be covered here.
- Most worms require either a prolonged incubation period outside the host before being infectious or need a specific vector for transmission. An exception to this rule is *Enterobius vermicularis* (pinworm); their eggs are infectious shortly after being passed, so autoinfection occurs readily.
- Direct person-to-person transmission of worms is uncommon, except for pinworm.
- The likelihood of acquiring an intestinal parasite depends on the presence of the infectious agent, an appropriate vector or mode of transmission, and a susceptible host. The worldwide distribution of parasites is determined by geographic factors, socioeconomic factors, age, and crowding, with poor food preparation and a break in the standard of water and personal sanitation being the major factors.
- System(s) Affected: Gastrointestinal

ALERT

Geriatric Considerations
Illness may cause more severe debilitation.

Pediatric Considerations
Most common age group affected

Pregnancy Considerations
Many of the treatments are contraindicated.

EPIDEMIOLOGY
Usually involves matters of personal, food, and/or water sanitation

- Predominant sex: Male = Female
- Predominant age: Pediatric

Prevalence
In the US
- From laboratory statistics: 5–30% of general population
- From day care surveys: Asymptomatic 20–30%; symptomatic 50–80%
- Intestinal protozoa account for most parasitologic findings in North America.
- In a random sampling, at least 1 parasite would be found in the stools of 5–10% of all people. If *Blastocystis hominis* were included in this accounting, 20–30% of specimens examined would be positive. *B. hominis* is probably a commensal enteric fungus and of no clinical significance.

- Helminths account for <10% of parasites; their presence is highly dependent on population demographics and prior geographic exposure risk factors.

RISK FACTORS
- Age (children)
- Low socioeconomic status
- Poor sanitation: Personal, food, water
- International travel
- Crowding: Day care centers, institutional care
- Multiple medical conditions, pregnancy, gastric hypoacidity, immunosuppression (AIDS)

Genetics
Genetic factors play a minor role in the acquisition, pathogenesis, and clearance of these infections.

ETIOLOGY
- Protozoan pathogens
  - *Giardia lamblia*
  - *Entamoeba histolytica*
  - *Cryptosporidium* sp.
  - *Isospora belli*
  - *Balantidium coli*
  - *Cyclospora cayetanensis*
  - Microsporida
- Possible protozoan pathogens
  - *Dientamoeba fragilis*
- Probable nonpathogenic protozoa
  - All other *Entamoeba* species
  - *Endolimax nana*
  - All other intestinal flagellates
- Helminthic pathogens: Nematodes (roundworms)
  - *Enterobius vermicularis*
  - *Trichuris trichiura*
  - *Ascaris lumbricoides*
  - Hookworm (*Necator americanus, Ancylostoma duodenale*)
  - *Strongyloides stercoralis*
  - *Capillaria philippinensis*
  - *Trichostrongylus* sp.
- Helminthic pathogens: Trematodes (flukes)
  - *Fasciolopsis buski*
  - *Clonorchis sinensis*
  - *Opisthorchis viverrini*
  - *Heterophyes heterophyes*
  - *Fasciola hepatica*
  - *Paragonimus westermani*
  - *Schistosoma mansoni*
  - *S. japonicum*
  - *S. hematobium*
  - *S. mekongi*
- Helminthic pathogens: Cestodes (tapeworms)
  - *Taenia saginata*
  - *Taenia solium*
  - *Diphyllobothrium latum*
  - *Hymenolepis nana*
  - *Hymenolepis diminuta*
  - *Dipylidium caninum*

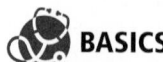 **DIAGNOSIS**

SIGNS AND SYMPTOMS
- Diarrhea
- Abdominal pain/tenderness
- Excessive gas: Bloating, eructation, flatulence, borborygmi
- Nausea or vomiting
- Weight loss and anorexia
- Dysentery, i.e., bleeding (rare, but associated with *Entamoeba histolytica, Balantidium coli*)
- Pruritus ani (*E. vermicularis, Trichuris trichiura, S. stercoralis*, tapeworms)
- Passing a worm or a worm segment
- Increased bowel sounds
- Perirectal or vulvar rash

TESTS
- Special techniques for the detection of *Cryptosporidium, Isospora belli, Cyclospora*, and *microsporidia* often require that the laboratory be informed of the risk profile of the patient before these tests will be done.
- Pinworm paddles provide a greater diagnostic yield when *Enterobius vermicularis* is being considered. Multiple tests (5) may be needed to exclude the diagnosis of pinworms.
- Parasite culture is possible for a few organisms— *Giardia lamblia, Entamoeba histolytica, Strongyloides stercoralis*—but are rarely indicated and are usually available only in referral laboratories.
- Rarely, a biopsy will demonstrate the presence of an invasive helminth on tissue section.

Lab
- Examination of a single stool specimen collected into a preservative (i.e., sodium acetate formalin [SAF]), well mixed to fix and preserve all elements, will provide an accurate diagnosis in 90% of patients. Additional specimens will need to be examined for greater diagnostic accuracy.
- Newer techniques of lab exam of stool specimens (such as monoclonal antibodies, other antigen detection techniques, DNA detection) are exciting developments, but currently provide little advantage over routine techniques.
- Serology: Useful if parasite does not produce a patent infection in the bowel (not found in stool samples), or if low numbers of parasites; available only through referral centers
- Drugs that may alter lab results
  - Use of antibiotics, oil-based laxatives, and barium in the stool may make a parasitologic diagnosis difficult.

Imaging
Diagnostic radiology is rarely needed. Exception is for invasive infections such as amebiasis where colitis, amebomas, and liver abscesses may be demonstrated.

Diagnostic Procedures/Surgery
- Invasive diagnostic procedures are rarely needed or indicated.
- With hemorrhagic colitis and a possible diagnosis of invasive amebiasis, sigmoidoscopy will reveal a mucopurulent colitis with ulceration. A scraping from an ulcer, promptly examined by microscopy, will reveal the motile hematophagous trophozoites of *E. histolytica*.
- Upper intestinal endoscopy can yield fluid to be examined for *Giardia lamblia* and *Strongyloides stercoralis*.

Pathological Findings
- Most intestinal parasites are not invasive and produce no or nonspecific changes in the histology of the bowel.
- Invasive amebiasis of the bowel produces a classic endoscopic and histologic picture of ulceration and inflammation in the colon.
- Protozoa and helminths may be seen in bowel biopsies.

DIFFERENTIAL DIAGNOSIS
- Other intestinal infections
- Food poisoning
- Malabsorption; lactose, gluten; sprue
- Inflammatory and irritable bowel diseases
- Hemorrhoids
- Rectal fissures

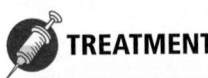 TREATMENT

INITIAL STABILIZATION
Outpatient except for rare surgery

GENERAL MEASURES
- Therapy must be assessed in the best interest of the patient. Not all patients need to be treated with drugs.
- Symptomatic treatment is indicated for patient comfort once specific therapy has been initiated.
- Bowel-paralyzing drugs, for diarrhea caused by invasive organisms, are relatively contraindicated.

Diet
- Nutritional support may be required.
- Many patients during and following bowel infections, especially when infected with *Giardia lamblia*, experience irritable bowel syndrome and/or lactose intolerance.

Activity
As tolerated

 MEDICATION (DRUGS)

- Protozoa
  - *Entamoeba histolytica* asymptomatic needs individual assessment.
  - *Entamoeba histolytica* symptomatic intestinal: Iodoquinol or diloxanide furoate
  - *Entamoeba histolytica* invasive disease: Iodoquinol or diloxanide furoate. Plus metronidazole alone or dehydroemetine or emetine plus chloroquine phosphate
  - *Giardia lamblia*: Metronidazole or tinidazole or furazolidone or quinacrine. Note: Albendazole, available in US only from manufacturer, may have activity against *G. lamblia*.
  - *Cryptosporidium*: None proven effective
  - *Isospora belli* protozoa: Trimethoprim-sulfamethoxazole
  - *Balantidium coli*: Tetracycline or iodoquinol or metronidazole
  - *Cyclospora*: Sulfamethoxazole-trimethoprim
  - *Microsporidia*: Albendazole (some species)
- Helminths
  - Nematodes (except *Strongyloides* and *Trichostrongylus*): Mebendazole or pyrantel pamoate or piperazine citrate or albendazole (available in US only from manufacturer)
  - *Strongyloides* and *Trichostrongylus*: Thiabendazole or albendazole (available in US only from manufacturer)
  - Cestodes: Praziquantel or niclosamide
  - Trematodes: Niclosamide or praziquantel
- Contraindications: Refer to manufacturer's profile of each drug.
- Precautions: Refer to manufacturer's profile of each drug.
- Significant possible interactions: Refer to manufacturer's profile of each drug.

SURGERY
- Surgical procedures play little role in treatment except when amebic liver abscesses need to be drained, especially left lobe abscesses. Drainage can be accomplished by directed catheter placement in radiology, with surgical backup as required.
- Surgery may be required if bowel or other organ obstruction occurs, as can be seen with *Ascaris lumbricoides* migration or for severe or complicated amebic colitis.

 FOLLOW-UP

DISPOSITION
Admission Criteria
Admission is rarely required except for intestinal obstruction, dystentry, or systemic invasion.

PROGNOSIS
See specific text on individual parasite.

COMPLICATIONS
Chronic persistent diarrhea, irritable bowel syndromes, chronic malabsorption

PATIENT MONITORING
Repeat examination, to ensure clearance, should be timed taking into account the life cycle of the parasite and the risk of reinfection.

REFERENCES
1. Abramowicz M, ed. Drugs for parasitic infections. In: *The Medical Letter*. New York: The Medical Letter; August 2004.
2. CDC. Division of Parasitic Diseases. *Parasitic Disease Information. Alphabetical Listing*. Available at: http://www.cdc.gov/ncidod/dpd/parasites/listing.htm.
3. Senay H, MacPherson DW. Parasitology: Diagnostic yield of stool examination. *Can Med Assoc J*. 1989;140:1329–1331.
4. Senay H, MacPherson DW. Blastocystis hominis: Epidemiology and natural history. *J Infect Dis*. 1990;162:987–990.

 MISCELLANEOUS

CODES

ICD9-CM
129 Intestinal parasitism, unspecified

PATIENT TEACHING
- Educating the patient is important to reduce the risk of reinfection or transmission.
- Education will depend on the parasite, host characteristics, and the environment in which the 2 interact.

I

INTUSSUSCEPTION

Timothy L. Black, MD
James P. Miller, MD

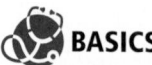 **BASICS**

DESCRIPTION
Invagination of a portion of intestine into itself (may involve any part of small intestine, ileocolic [95%] or colocolic)

- System(s) Affected: Gastrointestinal

ALERT

Geriatric Considerations
90% have lead point (1)[C]

Pediatric Considerations
- Usually no identified "lead point" (site of initiation of event); lead point present in 2–12% of children, >90% in adults
- Represents the most common abdominal emergency in infancy (2)[C]
- Postoperative intussusception (1–24 days postoperatively) is virtually always in small bowel and only rarely can be reduced hydrostatically.

EPIDEMIOLOGY
- Predominant age
  - 5–10 months (65% are <1 year of age)
  - Only 10–25% of cases occur >1 year of age
- Predominant sex: Male > Female (3:2): Male preponderance is more obvious in older infants.

Incidence
In the US
- 1.5–4/1,000 live births
- 0.5% after laparotomy

RISK FACTORS
- Henoch-Schönlein purpura
- Leukemia
- Lymphoma
- Cystic fibrosis
- Recent upper respiratory infection (21%)
- Recent operation (1–24 days previously)
- Recent viral gastrointestinal illness
- Meckel diverticulum
- Recent rotavirus vaccine administration (3)[C]

ETIOLOGY
- Children
  - Marked hypertrophy of Peyer patches (92–98%)
  - Lead point in 2–12% (polyp, Meckel diverticulum, duplication cyst, ectopic pancreas, lymphoma, Henoch-Schönlein purpura, lipoma, carcinoma)
  - Allergic reactions, diet changes, and changes in intestinal activity may be other causes.
  - Possible adenovirus or rotavirus infection
  - Rotavirus vaccine (3)[C]
    - Vaccine administered 3–14 days before onset of current symptoms
    - Infants usually older than 3 months
  - Recent operative procedure
- Adults
  - Virtually always associated with lead point

ASSOCIATED CONDITIONS
- Henoch-Schönlein purpura
- Cystic fibrosis

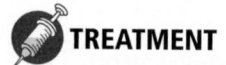 **DIAGNOSIS**

SIGNS AND SYMPTOMS
- Vomiting (80–100%)
- Blood per rectum: Currant-jelly stools (65–95%), highest percentage in infants
- Intermittent, colicky abdominal pain (almost all children)
- Lethargy (22%): More pronounced with longer duration of illness
- Palpable mass (16–41%)
- Diarrhea (7%)
- Prolapse of intussusception through anus (3%)
- Fever
- Extreme pallor in some
- In postoperative patients, usually present as small bowel obstruction (5)[C]

History
- History of intermittent abdominal pain with episodes lasting 5–10 minutes, frequently with completely asymptomatic period separating the episodes.
- History of bloody stool

Physical Exam
- Abdominal distension sometimes marked, depending on the duration of symptoms
- Bowel sounds hyperactive initially, may be absent later

TESTS

Lab
- Electrolytes
- Complete blood count
- Urinalysis
- Stool guaiac

Imaging
- Ultrasound is diagnostic (2)[C], (4)[B]

- Transient small bowel intussusception is frequently seen in patients with gastroenteritis; these usually resolve spontaneously without additional treatment.
- Plain film: Flat and upright abdominal films may suggest the diagnosis.
- CT scan may occasionally be helpful.

Diagnostic Procedures/Surgery
- Contrast enema (barium, water-soluble contrast, or air)
- Abdominal ultrasound

Pathological Findings
- Hyperplasia of Peyer lymphatic patches of terminal ileum (92%) with or without mesenteric lymphadenopathy
- Recognizable lead point, 2–12% (see list in "Etiology")

DIFFERENTIAL DIAGNOSIS
- Adhesive band small bowel obstruction
- Appendicitis
- Gastroenteritis
- Rectal prolapse (if intussuscepted bowel protrudes from anus)

TREATMENT

INITIAL STABILIZATION
Inpatient until resolved

GENERAL MEASURES
- IV fluid resuscitation
- Foley catheter (if child severely dehydrated)
- Nasogastric tube
- Antibiotics useful only if necrotic bowel present

- Nonoperative care (2)[C], (4)[B]
  - Hydrostatic/pneumatic reduction of intussusception (50–80% success)
  - Barium column should be 40–42 inches high.
  - Enema continued as long as progress is made. Contrast may be drained and the enema repeated up to 3 times.
  - Pneumatic reduction pressure should not exceed 120–140 mm Hg (16–18.6 kPa).

Diet
Liquids started after abdominal distension resolves and bowel function returns

Activity
As tolerated after reduction

SURGERY
- Right lower quadrant incision
- Gentle manipulation by pushing intussusception (not pulling)
- If unable to reduce or nonviable bowel, segmental resection with reanastomosis
- Enterotomy if lead point suspected
- Incidental appendectomy commonly done
- Postoperative intussusception usually requires laparotomy and operative reduction. (5)[C]
- In adults, segmental bowel resection usually required

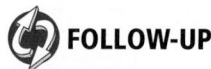 **FOLLOW-UP**

DISPOSITION

Admission Criteria
Infants are admitted for overnight observation after nonoperative reduction, due to high incidence of recurrence in 1st 24 hours.

Discharge Criteria
Normal bowel function

PROGNOSIS
- Mortality should not exceed 1–2%.
- Possible recurrence (5–13%) after hydrostatic reduction
- Possible recurrence (3%) after operative reduction

COMPLICATIONS
- Bowel perforation during attempted reduction (in 0.16–2.8% of patients with pneumatic reduction)
- Prolonged ileus
- Adhesions with intestinal obstruction
- Incisional hernia
- Ischemic intestine requiring 2nd operation
- Electrolyte abnormality
- Anemia
- Pleural effusion
- Sepsis
- Recurrence

PATIENT MONITORING
Office visit 1–2 weeks after discharge

REFERENCES
1. Pang C. Intussusception revisited: Clinicopathologic analysis of 261 cases, with emphasis on pathogenesis. *South Med J*. 1989;82:215–228.
2. Sorantin E, Lindbichler F. Management of intussusception. *Eur Radiol*. 2004;14:L146–L154.
3. Bines JE. Rotavirus vaccines and intussusception risk. *Curr Opin Gastroenterol*. 2005;21:20–25.
4. Applegate KE. Clinically suspected intussusception in children: Evidence-based review and self assessment module. *AJR Am J Roentgenol*. 2005;185:S175–S183.
5. Holcomb GW, Ross AJ, O'Neill JA. Postoperative intussusception: Increasing frequency or increasing awareness? *South Med J*. 1991;84:1334–1339.

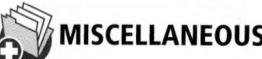 **MISCELLANEOUS**

See also: Cystic fibrosis; Henoch-Schönlein purpura; Intestinal obstruction

 CODES

ICD9-CM
560.0 Intussusception

PATIENT TEACHING
- Instruct family on possibility of recurrence (5–13%).
- Most recurrences occur in 1st 24 hours postreduction.

IRON TOXICITY, ACUTE

John J. Santos, MD

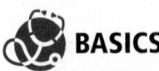 **BASICS**

DESCRIPTION
- Acute iron overload owing to accidental or intentional ingestion.
- Accidental ingestion is not uncommon since iron-containing compounds are readily available, brightly colored, and are often sugar coated.
- Acute symptoms are characterized by vomiting, diarrhea, mild lethargy, upper abdominal pain, pallor, and hyperglycemia with more severe clinical findings including cyanosis, stupor, acidosis, hematemesis, shock, and coma.
- System(s) Affected: Cardiovascular; Gastrointestinal; Hemic/Lymphatic/Immunologic
- Synonym(s): Iron poisoning

ALERT
Pediatric Considerations
For a 2-year-old, the average lethal dose of elemental iron is 3 g.

GENERAL PREVENTION
- Keep prescription and over-the-counter iron products/vitamins out of reach of children.
- Unit-dose packaging of iron supplements has resulted in a reduction of iron poisoning in children and should be recommended as the preferred packaging to patients (1)[A].

EPIDEMIOLOGY
Predominant age
- Children most frequently involved (in 2004 >25,000 iron exposures reported to Poison Control Centers with most exposures in children <6 years of age)
- Frequency of exposure calls involving iron has declined from 2.99 to 1.91 per 1000 calls, and death attributable to iron decreased from 29 during 1988–1997 to 1 death from 1998–2002.

Incidence
In 2002, 2,197 cases of iron poisoning were reported in the US.

Prevalence
- Iron poisoning is a common cause of unintentional poisoning death in children (2)[C].
- From 1988–1992, ~17% of children's deaths reported to Poison Control Centers in the US were iron poisonings.
- From 1983–1990 unintentional iron poisoning was the single most frequent cause of unintentional pharmaceutical ingestion fatality in children <6 years.
- In 1991, there were 11 deaths from accidental iron ingestion accounting for 65% of unintentional pediatric overdoses.

RISK FACTORS
- Access to iron products by children resulting in accidental ingestion
- The birth of a sibling within 6 months was identified as a risk factor for children <3 years old, likely due to the presence of prenatal vitamins.

ETIOLOGY
- Excessive iron ingestion: The average human lethal dose is 200–250 mg of elemental iron per kg of body weight (equivalent to about 230 ferrous sulfate based on 60 mg of elemental iron per tablet).
- Toxicity is likely following 60 mg/kg of elemental iron ingestion.

DIAGNOSIS

SIGNS AND SYMPTOMS
Typically 5 phases (these phases do not occur in all patients. For example, in massive overdose, patients may present in shock)
- I: From 0.5–6 hours: GI symptoms predominate including vomiting, hematemesis, abdominal pain, diarrhea
- II: From 4–12 hours: Apparent recovery may contribute to a false sense of security after initial ingestion; observe patient closely for hypoperfusion and acidosis.
- III: From 6–72 hours: Profound shock, severe acidosis, cyanosis, and fever. Potential recurrence of GI bleeding and vomiting.
- IV: From 12–96 hours: Hepatotoxicity and necrosis may occur leading to coma, coagulopathy, and jaundice. Symptoms may recur and can include pulmonary edema, shock, acidosis, convulsions, anuria, hyperthermia, and death (3). These symptoms occur in only a small minority of patients (4)[C].
- From 2–6 weeks: If patient survives, pyloric or antral stenosis resulting from stricture formation, hepatic cirrhosis, and central nervous system (CNS) damage can be seen.

TESTS
Lab
- CBC
- Electrolytes and glucose
- Measurement of serum iron and total iron binding capacity (TIBC) at least 4 hours after ingestion; serial measures may not be helpful
- Prothrombin time/international normalized ratio (PT/INR) and activated partial thromboplastin time (aPTT)
- Serum bicarbonate
- Liver function tests in severe overdose
- Amylase and lipase
- ABG to detect anion gap metabolic acidosis
- Drugs that may alter lab results: Deferoxamine can falsely lower serum iron unless a reducing agent is added to the specimen. Should obtain a free iron concentration
- Disorders that may alter lab results: TIBC rises factitiously in the presence of high iron levels.

Imaging
Abdominal and chest radiographs to evaluate for tablets in the gut

DIFFERENTIAL DIAGNOSIS
- If unknown iron ingestion
  - Gastritis
  - Small bowel obstruction
  - Drug intolerance/overdose
  - Alcohol toxicity
  - Viral illness
  - Diabetic ketoacidosis
  - Metabolic acidosis
- Other poisonings including aspirin, theophylline, organophosphates, carbamates, other metals and metalloids, paraquat, colchicines, and mushrooms

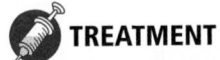 TREATMENT

INITIAL STABILIZATION
- Emergency room for acute ingestion
- Inpatient for severe ingestion
- Supportive treatment

GENERAL MEASURES
- Consult with a Poison Control Center (1-800-222-1222).
- Maintain proper airway, respiration, and circulation.
- Assess the amount of iron ingested.
- Remove iron from the GI tract.
- Hemodialysis, peritoneal dialysis, and exchange transfusion have also be used in lethal overdoses.
- Maintain electrolyte balance; treat shock, hypotension, and hyperglycemia.
- Explore psychologic issues if an intentional ingestion.

 MEDICATION (DRUGS)

- Decontamination with syrup of ipecac PO (1–12 years, 15 mL; adult, 30 mL) if a patient has recent iron ingestion and is a candidate for emesis.
- Contraindications are signs of oral pharyngeal/esophageal irritation, a depressed gag reflex, or CNS excitation/depression.
- Controversy exists as to whether to give ipecac to children <6 months of age. Of great concern is the administration of syrup of ipecac in the home without the advice of a health care professional (5)[C].
- Criteria for emesis/lavage
  - <20 mg/kg ingested
  - Symptomatic
  - Adults
- Gastric lavage, using tepid water, may be indicated in patients who are comatose or at risk for convulsing. Use if >20 mg/kg or unknown amount of iron has been ingested (3,6)[A].
- Whole bowel irrigation with a solution containing polyethylene glycol (Colyte, GoLYTELY) electrolyte lavage gives rapid diarrhea with relatively little fluid and electrolyte imbalance (children, 25 mL/kg/h; adults, 1.5–2 L/h)
  - Indicated when radiographic evidence of iron past the pylorus or if tablets persist in the GI tract after other attempts of decontamination
  - End point: Clear rectal effluent, disappearance of radiopacities
- Large clumps of coalesced iron tablets persist in stomach or duodenum: Can lead to perforation, so may need removal by gastroscopy or gastrotomy
- If serum iron exceeds TIBC or peak serum iron is >300 g/dL, administer IV deferoxamine, 15 mg/kg/h, for not more than 24 hours to chelate iron and prevent it from entering into chemical reactions. Serum iron levels drop usually within 12–48 hours (6)[C], (7)[B].
- Contraindications: Deferoxamine is relatively contraindicated in patients with severe renal disease or anuria, primary hemochromatosis.
- Precautions: Deferoxamine may cause flushing of skin, urticaria, hypotension, and shock with rapid IV injections.

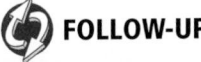 FOLLOW-UP

DISPOSITION
Admission Criteria
All known overdoses

PROGNOSIS
Depends on amount ingested and length of time patient exposed

COMPLICATIONS
Two to 4 weeks after severe ingestion has resulted in pyloric or antral stenosis, hepatic cirrhosis, and CNS damage may occur.

PATIENT MONITORING
- Kidney, urine, and bladder (KUB) until no pills are seen
- Serum iron concentration
- CBC, electrolytes, serum bicarbonate, blood glucose, serum iron, and TIBC
- Some patients' urine will turn a characteristic vin rosé color after treatment with deferoxamine; previously this was used as a diagnostic test of significant iron poisoning.

REFERENCES
1. Tenenbein M. Unit-dose packaging of iron supplements and reduction of iron poisoning in young children. *Arch Pediatr Adolesc Med*. 2005;159:557–560.
2. Cheyney K, Gumbiner C, Benson B, Tenenbein M. Survival after a severe iron poisoning treated with intermittent infusions of deferoxamine. *J Toxicol Clin Toxicol*. 1995;33:61–66.
3. Thomson Editorial Staff. Iron: Micromedex POISINDEX®System v 127. Thomson Micromedex, Greenwood Village, CO. (Edition expires 3/2006).
4. Proudfoot AT, Simpson T, Dyson EH. Management of acute iron poisoning. *Med Toxicol*. 1986;1:83–100.
5. American Academy of Pediatrics, Committee on Injury, Violence, and Poison Prevention. *Pediatrics*. 2003;112:1182–1185.
6. Ioannides AS, Panisello JM. Acute respiratory distress syndrome in children with acute iron poisoning: The role of intravenous desferrioxamine. *Eur J Pediat*. 2000;159:158–159.
7. Singhi SC, Baranwal AK, Hayashree M. Acute iron poisoning: Clinical picture, intensive care needs and outcomes. *Indian Pediatr*. 2003;40:1177–1182.

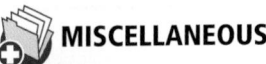 MISCELLANEOUS

CODES

ICD9
964.0 Poisoning by iron and its compounds

PATIENT TEACHING
- Undertake prevention counseling on proper storage of iron products out of the reach of children.
- Encourage purchase of iron supplements in unit-dose packaging.
- Educational material from Poison Control Centers may be available to use.
- An informative poster is available, at no charge, from the Department of Health and Human Services, 5600 Fishers Lane (HFI-40), Rockville, MD 20857.

I

IRRITABLE BOWEL SYNDROME

Kelly J. O'Callahan, MD

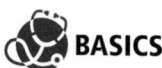 **BASICS**

DESCRIPTION

A condition characterized by a chronic abdominal pain associated with alteration in bowel habits in the absence of organic pathology. May be characterized as diarrhea predominant or constipation predominant or may alternate between diarrhea and constipation

- Synonym(s): Mucous colitis; Spastic colon; Irritable colon

GENERAL PREVENTION

See "Diet"

EPIDEMIOLOGY

Incidence

- Estimated to be ~15% of the population of North America; however, only 15% of these patients actually seek medical attention.
- IBS accounts for up to 50% of gastrointestinal visits in some practices and is 2nd to upper respiratory infection as cause for lost workdays.

Prevalence

- Predominant age
  - Late 20s, rarely in late teens
  - If over age 50, consider other diagnoses.
- Predominant sex: In the US: Female > Male (2:1)

RISK FACTORS

- Other members of the family with similar gastrointestinal disorder
- History of childhood sexual abuse
- Sexual or domestic abuse in women
- Depression

ALERT

Pregnancy Considerations

No risk to mother or fetus.

Genetics

Unknown, but more common in families of IBS patients

ETIOLOGY

The etiology is unknown, but patients demonstrate intestinal motility abnormalities with enhanced visceral perception and pain. The stimulus may be luminal or environmental.

ASSOCIATED CONDITIONS

- Migraine
- Urinary frequency and urgency
- Nocturia
- Fibromyalgia
- Dyspareunia
- Depression

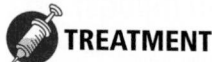 **DIAGNOSIS**

SIGNS AND SYMPTOMS

- Rome II criteria: 12 weeks or more in past 12 months of abdominal pain or discomfort that has 2 of 3 features
  - Relieved by defecation
  - Onset associated with change in frequency of stool
  - Onset associated with change in form of stool
- Symtoms can also include
  - Mucus in stools
  - Constipation
  - Diarrhea
  - Abdominal distention
  - Upper abdominal discomfort after eating
  - Straining for normal consistency stools
  - Urgency of defecation
  - Feelings of incomplete evacuation
  - Abnormal stool form
  - Nausea, vomiting (rarely)

History

- As above, but also may have history of abuse or depression
- Patient may note worsening of symptoms with stress or around menses.
- IBS is unlikely in patients with a history of weight loss, bleeding, nocturnal diarrhea, fever, or anemia.

Physical Exam

Generally normal, with perhaps some abdominal tenderness to palpation.

TESTS

In the setting of a good history and the lack of warning signs such as anemia, weight loss, etc., it is reasonable to obtain baseline labs as discussed below and begin treatment. In those who do not respond to treatment, further evaluation with imaging studies and endoscopy is warranted to exclude organic pathology.

Lab

As needed to rule out other pathology specific to the patient's symptoms

- Diarrhea predominant: ESR, CBC, tissue transglutaminase, TSH and stool for ova and parasite
- Constipation predominant: CBC, TSH, electrolytes
- Abdominal pain: LFTs and amylase

Imaging

- Abdominal CT scan or abdominal ultrasound to evaluate pain is generally normal.
- Small bowel series to rule out Crohn disease of small intestine may be considered, but also normal.
- Sitzmarker study to evaluate colon transit in patients with constipation

Diagnostic Procedures/Surgery

Sigmoidoscopy/Colonoscopy may be used to rule out inflammatory bowel disease or microscopic colitis but is normal. Should be performed in all persons >50 years of age for colorectal cancer screening.

Pathological Findings

None

DIFFERENTIAL DIAGNOSIS

- Inflammatory bowel disease
- Lactose intolerance
- Infections (*Giardia lamblia, Entamoeba histolytica, Salmonella, Campylobacter, Yersinia, Clostridium difficile*)
- Microscopic colitis
- Cathartic use
- Magnesium-containing antacids
- Celiac sprue
- Hypo/hyperthyroidism
- Pancreatic insufficiency
- Depression
- Somatization
- Villous adenoma
- Endocrine tumors
- Diabetes mellitus
- Radiation damage to colon or small bowel

TREATMENT

GENERAL MEASURES

Outpatient evaluation as outlined above with focus on explaining mechanism of disease and reassurance. Biofeedback and stress reduction can help.

Diet

- Increase fiber slowly to avoid increased intestinal gas production.
- During initial evaluation may wish to try 2 weeks of lactosefree diet to rule out lactose intolerance as etiology of symptoms.
- Avoid large meals, fatty foods, and caffeine, which can often exacerbate symptoms.

MEDICATION (DRUGS)

First Line

- For patients with alternating diarrhea and constipation, fiber supplements, such as Metamucil or Citrucel 1–2 tbsp per day work well. (1)[B] Synthetic agents such as Citrucel tend to be less gas producing, which may be an issue in some patients.

- Constipation predominant
  – Fiber as above

  – Teagaserod (Zelnorm) 5-HT-4 receptor agonist, 6 mg b.i.d. (approved for women only). (2)[A]

- Diarrhea predominant
  – Fiber as above
  – Loperamide (Imodium) 4 mg initial dose, then 2 mg after each unformed stool or diphenoxylate-atropine (Lomotil) 2.5–5.0 mg (1–2 tablets) after each unformed stool
  – Antispasmodics: Dicyclomine (Bentyl) 10–20 mg b.i.d. or q.i.d.; chlordiazepoxide-clidinium (Librax) 1 or 2 before meals and every night at bedtime; hyoscyamine (Levbid) 0.375 mg b.i.d.; phenobarbital-scopolamine-hyoscyamine-atropine (Donnatal) 1 or 2 tablets before meals and at bedtime. (3)[B]
  – Antidepressants: Tricyclic antidepressants such as elavil 25–50 mg at bedtime are effective in decreasing neuropathic pain and may slow gut transit. (4)[B] SSRIs and other antidepressants may be of use if depression is a factor.

  – Antiflatulents: Simethicone (Mylicon) 2–4 tablets after meals and at bed time, Beano
- Lactose intolerance: Lactase (Lactaid) capsules or tablets; 1–2 tablets prior to ingesting milk products

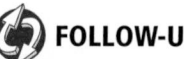 ## FOLLOW-UP

DISPOSITION

Issues for Referral
Possible psychiatric referral for those with depression

PROGNOSIS
- There is no progression to cancer or inflammatory disease.
- One should expect recurrences, when under stress, throughout life.

PATIENT MONITORING
As needed for symptoms

REFERENCES

1. Quartero AO, Meineshe-Schmidt V, Muris J, et al. Bulking agents, antispasmodic and antidepressant medication for the treatment of irritable bowel syndrome. *Cochrane Database Syst Rev.* 2005;2: CD0003460.
2. Tack J, Muller-Lissner S, Bytzer P, et al. A randomized controlled trial assessing the efficacy and safety of repeated tegaserod therapy in women with irritable bowel syndrome with constipation. *Gut.* 2005;54:1707–1713.
3. Poynard T, Regimbeau C, Benhamou U. Meta-analysis of smooth muscle relaxants in the treatment of irritable bowel syndrome. *Aliment Pharmacol Ther.* 2001;15:355–361.
4. Jackson JL, O'Malley PG, Tomkins G, et al. Treatment of functional gastrointestinal disorders with anti-depressant medications: A meta-analysis. *Am J Med.* 2000;108:65–72.

 ## MISCELLANEOUS

Patients should not be given the impression that this is a psychiatric illness.

 ## CODES

ICD9-CM
564.1 Irritable bowel syndrome

PATIENT TEACHING

 See Corresponding Diagnostic Algorithm

See Patient Handout on CD

KAPOSI SARCOMA

Felix B. Chang, MD
Aaron W. Way, DO

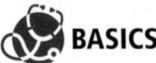

BASICS

DESCRIPTION

- A malignant multifocal neoplasm characterized by vascular tumors of skin and viscera in several different forms
  - Indolent (classic) Kaposi sarcoma (KS)
    - Older men of Mediterranean and Jewish descent
  - African (endemic) KS
    - Equatorial, sub-Saharan Africa
  - AIDS-related (epidemic) KS
    - HIV-infected patients and with AIDS
  - Form associated with immunosuppressive medications
    - Organ transplant–associated
- Human herpes virus 8 (HHV-8) has been identified by PCR in all 4 types of Kaposi sarcoma
- System(s) Affected: Hemolytic/Lymphatic/Immunologic; Skin/Exocrine
- Synonym(s): Endotheliosarcoma; Multiple idiopathic hemorrhagic sarcoma; Human herpes virus 8

ALERT
Geriatric Considerations
The indolent form is most likely to occur in men.

Pediatric Considerations
In eastern and southern Africa, KS represents 25–50% of all the soft-tissue sarcomas.

Pregnancy Considerations
Maternal–infant HIV transmission may occur.

GENERAL PREVENTION
- Safe sex practices
- Possible prophylaxis with antiviral medications
- Avoid needle sharing
- Avoid deep kissing
- Careful screening of organs transplant

EPIDEMIOLOGY
- Predominant age: 16–75
- Predominant sex: Classic and AIDS-related forms Male > Female (15:1)
- KS Endemic: Children = Adults
- AIDS-related or epidemic KS (1)
  - KS is the most common tumor arising in HIV-infected persons and is an AIDS-defining illness
  - Most common in homosexual or bisexual men
  - >20,000 times more common in AIDS patients than in the general population
  - 300 times more common in AIDS than in other immunosuppressed host
  - Homosexual men: 20–30%
  - Heterosexual injection drug users: 3%
  - Transfusion recipients: 3%
  - Women or children: 3%
  - Hemophiliacs: 1%

Incidence
- Indolent/lymphadenopathy: Rare
- In AIDS patients: Common
- Male homosexual with AIDS most affected
- The incidence of KS after transplantation is estimated to be 0.4 % in the US.
- KS represent 5.7% of malignancies after transplantation (excluding skin cancer)

RISK FACTORS
- HIV infection
- Living in endemic area (especially Zaire or Uganda)
- Immunosuppressant medications
- Transplantation and chemotherapy
- Sexual activity
- Maternal–fetal transmission
- Maternal–child transmission
- Injection drug use
- Exposure to infectious saliva
- Possible association with trauma in susceptible host
- An unknown route transmits many cases.
- A herpes virus designated "KS herpes virus" (KSHV) or human herpes virus type 8 (HHV8) is required for the development of KS.
- Samples from KS lesions have been found to contain DNA sequences identical with HHV8, and HHV8 can be propagated from skin lesions of patients with KS.
- Immunosuppression of the host is an important cofactor in development of KS.
- HHV-8 may be transmitted by blood transfusion.
- High risk for KS
  - Increasing anti-HHV-8 antibody titers
  - The presence of HHV-8 viremia
  - HIV seropositivity
  - Reduced levels of neutralizing antibodies

ETIOLOGY
Kaposi sarcoma is a low-grade vascular tumor associated with HHV-8, also know as the KS-associated herpesvirus (KSHV)

ASSOCIATED CONDITIONS
- AIDS
- HIV infection
- Lymphoma

DIAGNOSIS

SIGNS AND SYMPTOMS
- Indolent Kaposi
  - Multicentric red–blue violaceous tumors on the skin
  - Tender skin tumors
  - Pruritic skin tumors
  - In older men, lesions appear 1st on toes or legs.
- African (endemic) Kaposi
  - Usually involves skin, viscera, lymph nodes and bones
  - It is not typically associated with immunodeficiency.
  - More aggressive than classical KS
- KS associated with HIV infection (epidemic)
  - Skin lesions widely disseminated on the face, arms, and trunk
  - Lesions on mucous membranes
  - Lesions in lymph nodes
  - Lesions in viscera
- Immunosuppression-associated Kaposi
  - Tends to be aggressive
  - High amount of lymph node involvement
  - Visceral organs involved in 1/2

TESTS
Special tests: Tissue examination

Lab
- Specific HHV8 antibodies present in 70–90%
- Southern blot hybridization assay of KS lesions for HHV8
- Polymerase chain reaction (PCR) assay

Imaging
CT or MRI scan (chest, abdomen) may assess visceral involvement.

Diagnostic Procedures/Surgery
- Biopsy of skin or lymph node
- Bronchoscopy with biopsy
- Liver biopsy

Pathological Findings
- Neovascularization with aberrant proliferation of small vessels
- Spindle-shaped cell with leukocytic infiltration
- Angiogenesis
- Proliferation of atypical spindle cells
- Proliferation of vascular channels
- Large hyperchromic nuclei
- Spindle-shaped perivascular cells
- Hemosiderin laden macrophages

DIFFERENTIAL DIAGNOSIS
- Bacillary angiomatosis
- Granuloma faciale
- Vascular proliferation
- Purpuric lesions
- Dermatofibrosarcoma protuberans

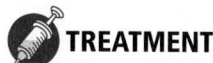 **TREATMENT**

GENERAL MEASURES
- Appropriate health care
  - Outpatient
  - Outpatient surgery
- If KS is due to immunosuppressant medications, eliminate or reduce medication dosage.
- If KS is HIV-related, optimize anti-HIV therapy to reduce HIV viral load.
- Treatment is otherwise determined by the extent and location of the disease.
- Observation
- Radiotherapy (electron beam) or x-ray therapy 1,000–2,000 rads
- Systemic chemotherapy, immunotherapy, or antiviral therapy

Activity
Remain active as long as possible.

 MEDICATION (DRUGS)

First Line
- Chemotherapy
  - Doxorubicin
  - Bleomycin
  - Vinblastine
  - Vincristine: Parenteral or intralesional
  - Daunorubicin
  - Paclitaxel
  - Interleukins
  - Thalidomide
  - Interferon: Parenteral or intralesional
  - Alitretinoin gel
- Note: Both doxorubicin and daunorubicin are available and approved for use in liposomal forms. These liposomal formulations offer improved outcome with less toxicity.
- Contraindications: Refer to manufacturer's literature.
- Precautions: Refer to manufacturer's literature. Myelosuppression with chemotherapy
- Significant possible interactions: Refer to manufacturer's literature.

Second Line
- Several studies have reported that some individuals have responded to antiviral medications such as foscarnet (Foscavir), ganciclovir (Cytovene), and cidofovir (Vistide).
- Photodynamic therapy

SURGERY
- Cryotherapy
- Intralesional chemotherapy or immunotherapy
- Surgical excision
- CO_2 laser

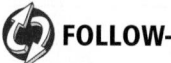 **FOLLOW-UP**

PROGNOSIS
- Improved HIV treatments and antiviral drugs may result in improved HIV-related KS survival.
- Indolent form: 10-year survival

COMPLICATIONS
- Extensive pulmonary involvement may lead to hypoxemia.
- Extensive lymphatic involvement may lead to severe edema.

PATIENT MONITORING
In HIV patients with KS, other opportunistic infections must be aggressively treated.

REFERENCES
1. Beral V, Peterman TA, Berkelman RL, et al. KS among persons with AIDS: A sexually transmitted infection? *Lancet*. 1990;335:123.
2. Dedicoat M, Vaithilingum M, Newton R. Treatment of Kaposi's sarcoma in HIV-1 infected individuals with emphasis on resource-poor settings. *Cochrane Database Sys Rev*. 2003;3:CD003256,DOI, 1002/14651858.CD003256.
3. Litte RF, Wyvill KM, Pluda JM, et al. Activity of thalidomide in AIDS-related Kaposi's sarcoma. *J Clin Oncol*. 2000;18:2593.
4. Webster-Cyriaque J. Development of Kaposi's sarcoma in surgical wound. *N Engl J Med*. 2002;346:1207–1212.

 MISCELLANEOUS

See also: HIV infection and AIDS

CODES

ICD9-CM
- 176.0 Kaposi sarcoma of skin
- 176.1 Kaposi's sarcoma, soft tissue
- 176.2 Kaposi's sarcoma, palate
- 176.3 Kaposi's sarcoma, gastrointestinal sites
- 176.4 Kaposi's sarcoma, lung
- 176.5 Kaposi's sarcoma, lymph nodes
- 176.8 Kaposi's sarcoma, other specified sites

ICD10
- C46.0 Kaposi's sarcoma of skin
- C46.1 Kaposi's sarcoma of soft tissue
- C46.2 Kaposi's sarcoma of palate
- C46.3 kaposi's sarcoma of lymph nodes
- C46.7 kaposi's sarcoma of other sites

PATIENT TEACHING
- HIV risk prevention
- Injection drug rehabilitation

K

KAWASAKI SYNDROME

Kiran V. Raman, BA, MSIV

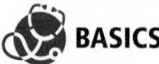 **BASICS**

DESCRIPTION

- An acute, distinct, self-limited, exanthematous febrile disease of young children, notable for its cardiac sequelae. Vasculitis affecting the coronary arteries can result in aneurysms or ectasia, further leading to myocardial infarction/ischemia or sudden death.
- System(s) Affected: Cardiovascular; Gastrointestinal; Hemic/Lymphatic/Immunologic; Musculoskeletal; Nervous; Pulmonary; Renal/Urologic; Skin/Exocrine
- Synonym(s): Mucocutaneous lymph node syndrome

ALERT
Kawasaki syndrome should be considered in any child with extended high fever unresponsive to antibiotics or antipyretics, rash, and nonexudative conjunctivitis.

Pediatric Considerations
Incomplete or atypical cases that exhibit <4 clinical criteria often occur in infants ≤6 months, or older children/adolescents. The frequency of coronary aneurysms is often higher in this subset of patients due to missed diagnosis. In these cases, elevated CRP or ESR, suggesting systemic inflammation, and echo, may be helpful.

EPIDEMIOLOGY
Leading cause of acquired heart disease in kids

- Predominant age
  - 1–5 years (peak age in the US: 18–24 months; Japan: 6–11 months)
  - 76% of the children are <5 years old and 50% are <2 years old.
- Predominant sex: Males > Females (1.6:1 in US, 1.35:1 in Japan)

Incidence
- Worldwide, affects all races but most prevalent in Japan. In the US, the annual incidence rate among children <5 years is 9–16/100,000 for non-Asians, and 33/100,000 for Asian Americans.
- The incidence in Japan is ~112/100,000 in children <5 years of age.

Prevalence
- Highest to lowest prevalence: Asians > Blacks > Hispanics > Caucasians
- Seasonal variation: Increased in winter and early spring and outbreaks at 2–3-year intervals

Genetics
- Increased incidence of HLA types B54, Bw15, Bw35, and Bw22 in Japanese patients; In US, Caucasians, HLA types Bw51, B5, B44 are increased; In Israelis, HLA type Bw51
- Siblings of cases in Japan have been found to have a 10-fold relative risk.

PATHOPHYSIOLOGY
Acute Kawasaki syndrome causes marked cytokine cascade activation and proteinase elevation, which may play a role in vasculitis and aneurysmal formation secondary to weakened vessel walls. Intimal thickening due to extensive remodeling may result in progressive stenosis.

ETIOLOGY
- Unknown
- An infectious cause is favored due to the acute, self-limited nature of Kawasaki syndrome. Community-wide outbreaks and seasonality point to a transmissable childhood disease.

 **DIAGNOSIS**

ALERT
Prolonged fever presenting without rash and treated with antibiotics may cause clinicians to believe that later rash development is due to a drug reaction.

SIGNS AND SYMPTOMS
- Fever for ≥5 days
  - Fever is high (103–105°F [39.4–40.5°C]) and unresponsive to antibiotics
  - May be prolonged (2–3 weeks with average duration of 11 days)
- Extensive polymorphous rash
  - May be maculopapular, scarletiniform, morbilliform, erythema multiforme, or rarely micropustular
  - Perineal desquamation
- Bilateral nonpurulent conjunctival injection
- Changes of lips and oral cavity
  - Reddening of lips in the acute stage which crack, fissure, and bleed in the subacute phase
  - Strawberry or erythematous tongue
  - Diffuse injection of oral and pharyngeal mucosa without exudate
- Acute, unilateral cervical lymphadenopathy
  - Lymph nodes >1.5 cm and nontender
  - Generalized lymphadenopathy usually absent
- Extremity changes
  - Reddened palms and soles on days 3–5
  - Edema of hands and feet on days 4–7
  - Periungual desquamation of fingers and toes at 2–3 weeks
- Other organ system involvement
  - Cardiovascular: Myocarditis; pericarditis (often subclinical) coronary artery and other medium-sized arterial aneurysms
  - Gastrointestinal: Anorexia; vomiting or diarrhea; acute gallbladder hydrops
  - Renal: Nephritis, urethritis
  - Respiratory: Pneumonitis, atelectasis, or pleural effusion; cough
  - Joints: Polyarthritis of small joints in acute phase; weight-bearing joints affected in 3rd week
  - Neurologic: Irritability; aseptic meningitis; peripheral neuropathy

Physical Exam
- Cardiac exam: Tachycardia, gallop rhythms hyperdynamic precordium, innocent flow murmurs
- Skin exam: Rash involving both trunk and extremities, erthema/induration at BCG vaccination site, if applicable

ALERT
ESR can be artificially high after IVIG therapy

- Anemia (normochromic, normocytic)

TESTS

Lab
- Leukocytosis (12,000–40,000 cells/mm^3) with immature forms and neutrophilia
- Elevated CRP, ESR, and alpha 1-antitrypsin concentrations
- Platelet counts rise after week 1 and peak in convalescent at 750,000–1,500,000.
- Mildly elevated AST, ALT, GGT, and bilirubin
- Decreased albumin
- Abnormal plasma lipids: Decreased cholesterol, HDL, and apo-AI
- CSF pleocytosis may be seen.
- Hyponatremia
- Sterile urethral pyuria (in 33% of patients)

Imaging
- ECG may show arrythmias, prolonged PR interval, and ST/T wave changes.
- Echocardiogram may show perivascular brightening, ectasia, decreased LV contractility, pericardial effusion, or aneurysms.
- CXR for baseline; may show pleural effusion, atelectasis, and CHF.
- MRI and MRA for aneurysms in both coronary and peripheral arteries

Diagnostic Procedures/Surgery
- No laboratory study proves diagnosis; the diagnosis rests on clinical features and exclusion of other illnesses in differential diagnosis.
- Symptoms may not all occur at once.
- Coronary angiography can be used to detect stenosis/thrombosis if echo suggests the diagnosis.

Pathological Findings
- 7–9 days after onset, neutrophilic infiltrates involve the pericardium, myocardium, endocardium, and vascular endothelium.
- Necrosis may develop and result in aneurysmal dilatation of medium-sized arteries.
- Mononuclear infiltration predominates in the 2nd week of illness, gradually resolving with or without fibrosis.
- In addition to cardiac involvement, arteritis may also develop in lungs, kidneys, gastrointestinal tract, and other organs.

DIFFERENTIAL DIAGNOSIS
- Staphylococcal scalded skin syndrome
- Toxic shock syndrome
- Stevens-Johnson syndrome
- Viral syndromes (i.e., measles, adenovirus)
- Scarlet fever
- Juvenile rheumatoid arthritis
- Reiter syndrome
- Epstein-Barr virus infections
- Mycoplasma infection
- Lyme disease
- Rocky Mountain Spotted Fever
- Toxoplasmosis
- Acrodynia (Mercury Hypersensitivity)
- Drug reactions
- Other vasculitides

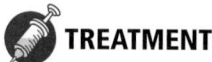 **TREATMENT**

GENERAL MEASURES

- When seen acutely, most children are hospitalized for diagnostic evaluation and supportive care.
- Antibiotics are given until bacterial etiologies are excluded.
- Once Kawasaki syndrome is suspected, all patients need a cardiac evaluation, including electrocardiogram and echocardiogram.

Activity
Should be limited in acute phase; longer with cardiac involvement. In patients with giant or multiple aneurysms, contact and high-risk sports should be avoided.

IV Fluids
- NS for rehydration in cardiogenic shock
- 1/2 NS for maintenance therapy

 MEDICATION (DRUGS)

First Line

- Immune globulin (IVIG): 2 g/kg IV over 12 hours at the time diagnosis is made (preferably within the 1st 10 days of the illness) lowers the risk of coronary artery aneurysms and may shorten the duration. (1)[A] Retreatment is advised if clinical response is incomplete, or if fever persists or returns 48 hours after start of IVIG treatment.
- Aspirin: 80–100 mg/kg/d in 4 doses beginning with IVIG administration. (1)[A] Switch to low-dose aspirin (3–5 mg/kg/d) when child has been afebrile 48–72 hours, or after 2 weeks, depending on the institution. Maintain this dose for 6–8 weeks for antithrombotic effects until follow-up echo is normal. Continue regimen in children with coronary abnormalities long-term or until documented regression of aneurym. (1)[B]
- Contraindications
  - IVIG-documented hypersensitivity, IgA deficiency, anti-IgE/IgG antibodies, severe thrombocytopenia, or coagulation disorders
  - Aspirin-vitamin K deficiency, bleeding disorders, liver damage, documented hypersensitivity, hypoprothrombinemia
- Precautions
  - Brands of IVIG prepared with β-propriolactone or enzyme digestion may be less effective. (3)[C]
  - High-dose aspirin therapy can result in tinnitus and transient decrease of renal function.
- Significant possible interactions
  - Aspirin therapy is associated with Reye syndrome in children who develop viral infections, especially influenza B and varicella. Yearly influenza vaccination is thus recommended for children requiring long-term treatment with aspirin.

Second Line

- Clopidogrel: 1 mg/kg/d or dipyridamole 2–6 mg/kg/d t.i.d. is used for prevention of thrombosis in patients with enlarged coronaries.
- Fibrinolytic agents (urokinase IV, streptokinase IV) for treatment of coronary thrombosis. (1)[C]
- Corticosteroids for Kawasaki syndrome resistant to IVIG: Methylprednisone 30 mg/kg/d IV over 2–3 hours for 1–3 days (1)[C]
- Anti-TNF agents (i.e., Infliximab) and plasmapheresis have been used for refractory Kawasaki syndrome.
- Warfarin 0.1 mg/kg/d adjusted to keep INR between 2.0 and 2.5, used in conjunction with aspirin long term. (4)[C]

SURGERY

- CABG for severe obstruction (>75%) of LCA or high-grade obstructions in 2 of 3 coronary arteries. Younger patients have higher mortality rate.
- Coronary revascularization via percutaneous coronary intervention (PCI) for patients with evidence of ischemia upon stress testing. (4)[C] PCI carries a risk of neoaneurysm formation.

 FOLLOW-UP

DISPOSITION

Admission Criteria
Any child with suspected Kawasaki syndrome should be admitted for further work-up.

Discharge Criteria
Although each case should be treated individually, children are usually discharged after 24–48 hours of remaining afebrile postIVIG treatment. Children should then be closely followed by specialists or PCP in order to monitor for reoccurence of symptoms.

Issues for Referral
- Referral to pediatric cardiologist if coronary abnormalities suspected on echo.
- Referral to pediatric cardiac surgeon if extensive stenosis/pathology is suspected.

PROGNOSIS
- Usually self-limited
- Possible permanent cardiovascular sequelae
- Sudden death is possible in early adulthood
- Moderate sized aneurysms usually regress in 1–2 years, resolving in 50–66% of cases.

COMPLICATIONS
- 15–25% of untreated patients develop coronary artery aneurysms in convalescent phase.
- 2–7% of treated patients develop aneurysms
- Risk factors for aneurysm
  - Male sex, age <1 year old, high ESR >4 weeks
  - Fever >2 weeks, in treated patients, fever >48 hours after IVIG treatment
- Mortality 0.08–0.17%, related to cardiovascular sequelae

PATIENT MONITORING
- Patient must be closely followed after discharge by PCP and/or pediatric cardiologist depending on their cardiac profile. Children who have little/no cardiac abnormalities on f/u echo should have a cardiology exam every 3–5 years.
- Repeat ECG and echo at 6–8 weeks. If abnormal, repeat echo at 6–12 months, otherwise this is unnecessary. (6)[C]

REFERENCES

1. Newburger JW, et al. Diagnosis, treatment, and long-term management of Kawasaki disease: A statement for health-care professionals. *Pediatrics.* 2004;114(6):1708–1733.
2. Simonini G, et al. Diagnosing Kawasaki syndrome: The need for a new clinical tool. *Rheumatology.* 2005;44(8):959–961.
3. Tsai MH, et al. Clinical responses of patients to different brands of intravenous immunoglobulin. *J Pediatr.* 2006;148:38–43.
4. Levy DM, et al. Long term outcomes in patients with giant aneurysms secondary to Kawasaki disease. *J Rheumatol.* 2005;32:928–934.
5. Falcini F. Kawasaki disease. *Curr Opin Rheumatol.* 2006;18(1):33–38.
6. Tuohy AMM, et al. How many echocardiograms are necessary for follow-up evaluation of patients with Kawasaki disease? *Am J Cardiol.* 2001;88(3):328–330.

 MISCELLANEOUS

CODES

ICD9-CM
446.1 Acute febrile mucocutaneous lymph node syndrome [MCLS]

K

KELOIDS

Ronald E. Pust, MD

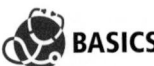 **BASICS**

DESCRIPTION

- Abnormally large overgrowth of fibrous tissue (scar) occurring as a result of trauma or irritation that does not subside with time
- System(s) Affected: Skin/Exocrine
- Synonym(s): Razor bumps

ALERT

Pediatric Considerations
Keloid formation is more common during adolescence.

Pregnancy Considerations
Keloid formation is more likely during pregnancy.

GENERAL PREVENTION

- Primary prevention: Avoid elective surgery or body piercing in high-risk patients.
- When feasible, laparoscopic approaches are preferred in keloid formers.
- Compressive pressure dressings may be useful in high-risk (e.g., burn) patients. Local steroid injection postoperatively in high-risk patients is also effective.

EPIDEMIOLOGY

Predominant sex: Male = Female

Prevalence
4–16% of the black and hispanic population

RISK FACTORS

- Family history of keloids
- Dark skin pigment
- Certain locations on the body (e.g., deltoids, chest, earlobes)
- Pregnancy
- Adolescence

Genetics
- More common in blacks and Asians (5–15 times) than in whites. In all races, more darkly pigmented individuals are at higher risk.
- Both autosomal dominant and autosomal recessive familial inheritance have been reported.

ETIOLOGY

- Wounds: Traumatic, surgical, body piercing
- Burn injury
- Other injuries
  - Insect bite
  - Folliculitis barbae and nuchae
  - Acne

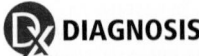 **DIAGNOSIS**

SIGNS AND SYMPTOMS

History
- Pain
- Tenderness
- Hyperesthesia
- Pruritus (occasional)

Physical Exam
- Firm, smooth, elevated scar with sharply demarcated borders
- Initially may be pale or mildly erythematous
- Older lesion hypopigmented or hyperpigmented
- Scar extends beyond margins of the initial wound.
- Over period of years, keloids may continue to grow and may develop clawlike projections.

TESTS

Diagnostic Procedures/Surgery
Biopsy, only if unable to differentiate from carcinoma or infectious disease, because a biopsy may increase the keloid's size. If possible, use a 2-mm punch biopsy to minimize trauma.

Pathological Findings
Histology shows whorllike arrangements of hyalinized collagen bundles with pressure thinning of papillary dermis and minimal elastic tissue.

DIFFERENTIAL DIAGNOSIS

- Hypertrophic scar (usually spontaneously regresses; does not cross wound margins)
- Dermatofibroma
- Infiltrating basal cell carcinoma
- Sclerosing metastatic malignancies
- Desmoplastic melanoma
- Sarcoidosis
- Leprosy (nodular LL type)
- Other fibronodular skin diseases, e.g., neurofibromatosis, post-kala-azar dermal leishmaniasis

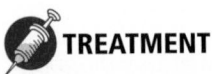 **TREATMENT**

GENERAL MEASURES

- Appropriate health care: Outpatient
- Intralesional corticosteroid injection causes atrophy and is the most successful therapy. (1)[A]
- Pressure bandages must maintain 24 mm Hg, and should be worn for 6–12 months. (1)[C] Bandages should not be removed for >30 minutes/day. Pressure clips (Zimmer splints) are useful for earlobes. Designer splints look like fashion earrings.
- Radiation or laser: No advantage over other methods; therefore, use only if other methods fail, and then use in conjunction with them. (1)[C]
- Cryotherapy: May be useful for small keloids, e.g., acne scars (1)[C]
- Topical agents: No evidence to support efficacy (e.g., retinoic acid, Vitamin E, allantoin, onion extract) (1)

Diet
No special diet

Activity
Full activity

Nursing
No specific nursing

SPECIAL THERAPY

Radiotherapy
See above

Physical Therapy
May be useful if contractures associated

Complementary and Alternative Medicine
None proven (1)

MEDICATION (DRUGS)

First Line
- 2 treatments are backed by RCTs

Triamcinolone (Kenalog) suspension 10 mg/mL (1)[A]
- Use 27–30-gauge needle and a TB syringe (total dose 20–30 mg of triamcinolone). May inject 3 lesions at a time, using 10 mg/lesion
- Advance needle while injecting to distribute medication evenly.
- Early keloids are more responsive to this therapy than are older lesions.
- Reinject every 4 weeks until keloid shrinks to near skin surface.
- If no response to 10 mg/mL triamcinolone suspension, may try 40 mg/mL suspension
- May mix dilute triamcinolone (5–10 mg/mL) with local anesthetic for excision of keloids. Postoperative steroid injections at 2–4 weeks and then monthly for 6 months helps prevent recurrences.

- Contraindications: None are absolute.
- Precautions
  - Systemic absorption with adrenal suppression (reversible)
  - Local effects: Skin atrophy, ulceration, depigmentation, telangiectasias
  - Both types of side effects more common with 40 mg/mL triamcinolone suspension
- Significant possible interactions: Rare interactions (only with very large doses of corticosteroids and systemic absorption); silica gel sheeting (1)[A], (2)

Second Line
- Verapamil locally may be helpful. 1 study (3) supports repeated intralesional injections of 2.5 mg/mL of verapamil at repeated intervals as an adjuvant following excision and topical silicone. (1)[C]
- Interferon-alfa 2b may be helpful after excision. (1)[C]
- Intralesional 5-fluorouracil (1)[C], (4)
- Intralesional bleomycin (1)[C], (5)
- See also "General Measures."

SURGERY
- Surgery: High recurrence rate (45–100%), therefore used only for debulking of large keloids or if a lesion is unresponsive to steroid injections or other therapy
- Laser surgery: No definitive evidence of efficacy; no advantage over other methods; therefore, use only if other methods fail, and then use in conjunction with them. (1)[C]

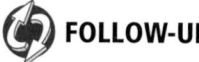 **FOLLOW-UP**

Issues for Referral
When intralesional steroids fail, referral may be indicated.

PROGNOSIS
When treatment is successful, lesions gradually diminish with therapy over a 6–18-month period, leaving a flat, shiny scar.

COMPLICATIONS
Skin atrophy, ulceration, depigmentation, and telangiectasias can occur as a result of local steroid injections.

PATIENT MONITORING
Monthly visits up to a year, for evaluation and possible steroid reinjections

REFERENCES

1. Mustoe TA, Cooter RD, Gold MH, et al. International Advisory Panel on Scar Management. International clinical recommendations on scar management. *Plast Reconstr Surg*. 2002;110: 560–571. (also in German: Ziegler UE [International Clinical recommendations on scar management. *Zentralblatt Chirurgie*. 2004;129: 296–306.])
2. Poston J. The use of silicone gel sheeting in the management of hypertrophic and keloid scars. *J Wound Care*. 2000;9:10–16.
3. D'Andrea F, Brongo S, Ferraro G, et al. Prevention and treatment of keloids with intralesional verapamil. *Dermatology*. 2002;204(1):60–62.
4. Gupta S, Kalra A. Efficacy and safety of intralesional 5-fluorouracil in the treatment of keloids. *Dermatology*. 2002;204(2):130–132.
5. Russell R, Horlock N, Gault D. Zimmer splintage: A simple effective treatment for keloids following ear-piercing. *Br J Plast Surg*. 2001;54:509–510.

ADDITIONAL READING

Stanford textbooks of dermatology and plastic surgery

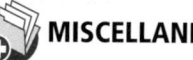 **MISCELLANEOUS**

See also: Animal bites; Burns; Warts; Leprosy and other diagnoses listed in "Differential"

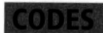 **CODES**

ICD9-CM
701.4 Keloid scar

PATIENT TEACHING
- Stress possibility of recurrence despite appropriate treatment.
- May require many months of treatment with combined modalities

Prevention
In those with risk factors or previous keloids, caution against activities or procedures that may entail dermal disruption, and early treatment of any such events.

K

KERATOSIS, ACTINIC

John R. Person, MD

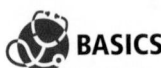

BASICS

DESCRIPTION
- Common, usually multiple premalignant skin lesions of sun-exposed areas. There has been recent philosophical debate about the real nature of these lesions, ranging from frank malignancy to an initiated tumor that does not become malignant unless tumor promotion occurs.
  - Most common indicator of excessive cumulative ultraviolet light exposure
  - The risk of transformation to squamous carcinoma is quite low: 0.25% risk of malignant transformation per lesion per year
- System(s) Affected: Skin/Exocrine

ALERT
Geriatric Considerations
Frequent problem

Pediatric Considerations
Rare

GENERAL PREVENTION
Sun protective techniques (see "Patient Education")

EPIDEMIOLOGY
- Predominant age: ≥40; progressive with age (if child, look for freckling and other stigmata of xeroderma pigmentosum)
- Predominant sex: Male > Female (from occupational sun exposure)

Incidence
Common in those with blonde and red hair; rare in African Americans

RISK FACTORS
- Equatorial latitudes
- High elevations
- Outdoor occupation (farmers, sailors, ranchers)
- Outdoor athletics
- Sun worshippers
- Accompanying heat, wind, humidity augment carcinogenic effect
- Occupational exposure (i.e., petroleum products)
- Immunosuppression, especially organ transplantation

Genetics
Relates to complexion

ETIOLOGY
- Short-wave ultraviolet light (UVB)
- Possibly UVA
- Bowen disease can be caused by the carcinogenic types of human papilloma virus and arsenic exposure.

ASSOCIATED CONDITIONS
Squamous cell carcinoma

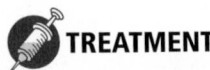

DIAGNOSIS

SIGNS AND SYMPTOMS
- Lesions usually fairly flat, red, and rough to palpitation; can be lichenoid (i.e., resembling lichen, a flat papule or aggregate of papules)
- Mild hyperesthesia common over lesions
- Hypertrophic verrucous lesions (called *cutaneous horns* if extreme) may be impossible to differentiate from squamous cell carcinoma clinically.
- A brown, pigmented variant also exists.
- Actinic cheilitis usually involves lower lip.
- Only photo-exposed areas involved, often with other stigmata of chronic actinic damage: Lentigines, actinic elastosis, atrophy

TESTS
Diagnostic Procedures/Surgery
Biopsy

Pathological Findings
The diagnosis is usually made clinically except where there is a suspicion of carcinoma.
- Malignant cells sparse except in Bowenoid variety
- Hyperkeratosis
- Hypertrophic, atrophic, Bowenoid, acantholytic, and pigmented varieties show the corresponding epidermal findings.
- Usually a sparse lymphocytic and plasma cell infiltrate

DIFFERENTIAL DIAGNOSIS
- Squamous cell carcinoma (hypertrophic type)
- Verruca vulgaris (hypertrophic type)
- Seborrheic dermatitis or psoriasis (near hairline)
- Lentigo maligna (pigmented type)
- Lupus erythematosus

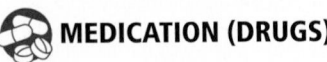

TREATMENT

GENERAL MEASURES
- Appropriate healthcare: Outpatient
- Sun-protective techniques (see "Patient Education")

MEDICATION (DRUGS)

First Line
- Topical fluorouracil (Efudex, Carac, Fluoroplex cream, Fluoroplex solution) destroys even subclinical lesions, also nonscarring; usually applied b.i.d. for 3–4 weeks (for larger number of lesions)

Second Line
- 3% diclofenac (Solaraze) gel b.i.d. for 3 months
- Topical imiquimod (Aldara) 5% cream, an interferon-inducer. Apply twice weekly for 16 weeks to small (<25 cm^2) areas of involvement.
- Topical tretinoin (Retin-A) or tazarotene (Tazorac) may be used to enhance the efficacy of topical fluorouracil.
- Photodynamic therapy with aminolevulinic acid and blue light

SURGERY
- Cryosurgery
- For extensive lesions (medical treatment usually preferred)
  - Medium-depth peels, i.e., 35% trichloroacetic acid
  - CO$_2$ laser therapy
  - Dermabrasion

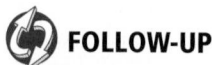 **FOLLOW-UP**

PROGNOSIS
Excellent, if prevention taken by patient

COMPLICATIONS
Actinic keratosis is a premalignant lesion and may undergo carcinomatous proliferation to become squamous cell carcinoma.

PATIENT MONITORING
Dependent on associated malignancy and frequency with which new actinic keratoses appear

REFERENCES

1. Nelson C, et al. Phase IV, open label assessment of the treatment of actinic keratoses with 3.0% diclofenac sodium topical gel [Solaraze]. *J Drugs Dermatol.* 2004;3:401–407.
2. Jury CS, et al. A randomized trial of topical 5-fluorouracil in the treatment of actinic keratoses comparing daily with weekly treatment. *Br J Dermatol.* 2005;153:808–810.
3. Heaphy MR Jr, Ackerman AB. The nature of solar keratosis: A critical review in historic perspective. *J Am Acad Dermatol.* 2000;43:138–150.
4. Person JR. An actinic keratosis is neither malignant nor premalignant: It is an initiated tumor. *J Am Acad Dermatol.* 2003;48:637–638.

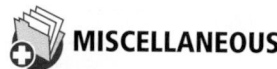 **MISCELLANEOUS**

See also: Dermatitis, seborrheic

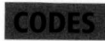 **CODES**

ICD9-CM
702.0 Actinic keratosis

PATIENT TEACHING

- Teach sun-protective techniques.
- Transfer hobbies and other outdoor activities to early morning or late afternoon.
- Wear protective clothing and hats.
- Daily use of topically applied sunscreens with SPF >15; preferably containing titanium dioxide or avobenzone (Parsol-1789) to afford protection in the UVA range also
- Teach self-examination for cutaneous carcinoma (melanoma, squamous cell, basal cell).

K

LABYRINTHITIS

Teresa V. Chan, MD
Daniel J. Lee, MD

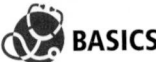 **BASICS**

DESCRIPTION
Inflammation of the vestibular labyrinth (a system of intercommunicating cavities and canals in the inner ear). There are many possible causes (see "Differential Diagnosis"). The most constant and pervasive symptom is vertigo.
- System(s) Affected: Nervous
- Synonym(s): Acute peripheral vestibulopathy; Vestibular neuronitis; Vestibular neuritis

ALERT
Geriatric Considerations
- Very common in this age group, especially benign positional vertigo
- Avoid scopolamine or use with extreme caution in this age group.

Pediatric Considerations
Unusual in this age group

Pregnancy Considerations
Avoid medications.

GENERAL PREVENTION
No preventive measures

EPIDEMIOLOGY
- Predominant age: All ages beyond infancy
- Predominant sex: Male = Female

Prevalence
In the US
- 2nd most common cause of dizziness owing to peripheral vestibular condition (9%) after benign positional vertigo (16%)

RISK FACTORS
- Trauma
- Stress
- Drug ingestion
- Predisposing virus infection
- Cardiovascular disease
- Cerebrovascular disease

Genetics
No known genetic pattern

ETIOLOGY
- Pathologic: Imbalance in the vestibular system caused by a lesion within vestibular pathways (inner ear to cerebral cortex)
- Infections (especially viral, such as mumps)
- Tumors
- Vasculitis
- Infarction
- Ototoxic drugs, especially aminoglycosides
- Head injury
- Neuronitis

ASSOCIATED CONDITIONS
- Ménière disease
- Head injury

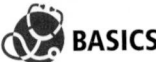 **DIAGNOSIS**

SIGNS AND SYMPTOMS
- Vertigo
- Dizziness
- Hearing loss, fluctuating
- Nausea and vomiting
- Tinnitus
- Perspiration
- Increased salivation
- Generalized malaise
- Hypercapnia
- Nystagmus
- Ataxia

TESTS
Lab
- Routine laboratory studies not helpful
- Special tests
  - Electronystagmography
  - Caloric test
  - Doll's eye test
  - Forced voluntary hyperventilation for 1–3 minutes to mimic symptoms if cause is physiologic or emotional
- Drugs that may alter lab results
  - All drugs with potential ototoxicity

Imaging
Computed tomography or magnetic resonance imaging for suspected lesions involving the 8th cranial nerve

Diagnostic Procedures/Surgery
History and physical

DIFFERENTIAL DIAGNOSIS
- Acute viral labyrinthitis
- Benign paroxysmal positional vertigo (BPPV)
- Ménière syndrome
- Postconcussive syndrome
- Chronic bacterial otomastoiditis
- Drug-induced damage to vestibular labyrinth
- Vascular insufficiency
- Cerebellopontine-angle tumors, such as acoustic neuroma
- Multiple sclerosis
- Parainfectious encephalomyelitis
- Parainfectious cranial polyneuritis
- Ramsay Hunt syndrome
- Cerebral or systemic vasculitis
- Temporal lobe epilepsy
- HIV infection
- Perilymphatic fistula

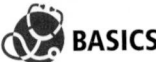 **TREATMENT**

GENERAL MEASURES
- Appropriate health care: Outpatient
- Treat underlying disorder when possible.
- Symptomatic treatment to accompany specific treatment
- Visual–vestibular exercises for prolonged cases

Diet
Reduced sodium

Activity
- Lie still with eyes closed in darkened room during acute attacks. Otherwise, activity as tolerated
- Minimize head movement.

MEDICATION (DRUGS)

- Meclizine (Antivert) 25 mg q.i.d. PO
- Diazepam (Valium) 5 mg q.i.d. PO
- Promethazine (Phenergan) 25 mg q.i.d. PO or PR
- Prochlorperazine (Compazine) suppositories 25 mg, for vomiting
- Scopolamine transdermal where available
- Contraindications
  – Refer to the manufacturer's literature.
- Precautions
  – All the listed medications have significant adverse reactions. Use with caution. Avoid scopolamine in the elderly.
- Significant possible interactions
  – Refer to the manufacturer's literature.

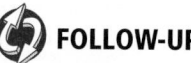 FOLLOW-UP

PROGNOSIS
Depends on cause.

COMPLICATIONS
Permanent hearing loss

PATIENT MONITORING
As needed

REFERENCES

1. Baloh RW, Honrobia V. *Clinical Neurology of the Vestibular System*. 2nd ed. Philadelphia, PA: FA Davis; 1990.
2. Goetz CG. *Textbook of Clinical Neurology*. Philadelphia: WB Saunders; 1999.
3. Kroenke K, et al. How common are various causes of dizziness? A critical review. *South Med J*. 2000;93:160–167.
4. Noble J. *Textbook of Primary Care Medicine*. 3rd ed. St. Louis, MO: Mosby; 2001.
5. Rakel RE, ed. *Conn's Current Therapy*. 54th ed. Philadelphia, PA: WB Saunders; 2002.

 MISCELLANEOUS

See also: Ménière disease; Postconcussive syndrome; Tinnitus

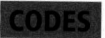 **CODES**

ICD9-CM
386.30 Labyrinthitis, unspecified

PATIENT TEACHING

 See Corresponding Diagnostic Algorithm

 See Patient Handout on CD

L

LACRIMAL DISORDERS

Robert M. Kershner, MD

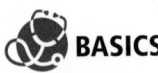 **BASICS**

DESCRIPTION
- Diseases and abnormalities of tear production and tear film
- The most common lacrimal disorder is dry eye.
- Lacrimal duct disorders, seen in the pediatric age group, often result in overflow tearing.
- System(s) Affected: Skin/Exocrine
- Synonym(s): Epiphora (excessive tearing)

GENERAL PREVENTION
- Prevent exposure to eye irritants from pollution, cigarette smoke, and sun exposure.
- Ensure adequate vitamin A intake in the diet or as a supplement.

EPIDEMIOLOGY
- Predominant age: Dry eye symptoms increase with age. Most common in the elderly
- Predominant sex: Female > Male

Prevalence
Very common in the US; more often seen in arid climates of the desert Southwest

ALERT
Geriatric Considerations
Most common in this age group

RISK FACTORS
Individuals who live in arid regions, are on diuretics, or have a history of collagen vascular diseases such as rheumatoid arthritis, Sjögren syndrome, Bell palsy, eyelid abnormalities, and thyroid disease are most at risk.

ETIOLOGY
Poor tear production and/or rapid evaporation of the tears

ASSOCIATED CONDITIONS
- Sjögren syndrome and age-related factors are more commonly seen in the geriatric population.
- Dry eyes can frequently be associated with pregnancy in an otherwise healthy individual. Vitamin A intake should not exceed 6,000 IU/d.

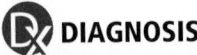 **DIAGNOSIS**

SIGNS AND SYMPTOMS
- Gritty sensation in the eyes
- Visual blurring
- Redness
- Excessive tearing and mucus production
- Inadequate tears on the ocular surface

ALERT
Pediatric Considerations
May find lacrimal duct blockage in infants

TESTS
Lab
Tear production can be measured using a Schirmer filter strip after instillation of topical anesthetic. Wetting of <10 mm of the slip >5 minutes is indicative of insufficient tear production.

Diagnostic Procedures/Surgery
Staining of the ocular surface with fluorescein will show areas of abnormal uptake and patches of drying. Rose bengal will be taken up by dead or dying epithelial cells and may be a more sensitive test.

Pathological Findings
In Sjögren syndrome, infiltration of the lacrimal gland with inflammatory cells may be evident.

DIFFERENTIAL DIAGNOSIS
- Lacrimal disorders must be differentiated from ocular infections and allergy.
- An important consideration is the variety of anticholinergic-affecting drugs that decrease tear production.
- Symptoms of dry eye are most often overlooked by practitioners when considering conjunctivitis (pink eye) and allergic disorders.

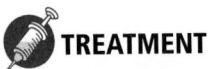 **TREATMENT**

INITIAL STABILIZATION
Outpatient care

GENERAL MEASURES
- Those with systemic illnesses predisposed to dry eye should be informed and instructed in the appropriate use of artificial tear supplements.
- Cool mist vaporizer and home humidification are helpful.

Diet
No special diet

Activity
No restrictions

MEDICATION (DRUGS)

- Artificial tear drops, excluding those that have preservatives; the dosage of the drop varies depending on the severity of the symptoms. Usually 1 drop in each eye several times throughout the day can prevent ocular discomfort.
- The use of a bland ophthalmic ointment at bedtime between the eyelid and the eye can help prevent drying of the eye at night.
- Vitamin A supplements
- Dry eye has been identified as having an inflammatory component that responds in refractory cases to topical immunosuppressives, such as cyclosporine (Restasis) 0.05%, 1 drop to each eye b.i.d. Patients on cyclosporine should be monitored at the slit lamp by an ophthalmologist at least weekly.

 FOLLOW-UP

PROGNOSIS
Lacrimal disorders can be adequately managed with artificial tear supplements. Blocked tear ducts can be managed with probing and punctal dilation and/or dacryocystorhinostomy procedures in more severe cases.

COMPLICATIONS
Severe dry eye may lead to corneal breakdown, secondary invasion by bacteria, and eye infections.

PATIENT MONITORING
Monitor early to determine the effectiveness of treatment. Occasionally, the use of more viscous drops or increased frequency of tear supplements may be required.

REFERENCES

1. Orbit, Eyelids, and Lacrimal System, Basic and Clinical Course. San Francisco: American Academy of Ophthalmology, 2001.

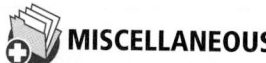 **MISCELLANEOUS**

See also: Sjögren syndrome

CODES

ICD9-CM
- 375.11 Dacryops
- 375.15 Tear film insufficiency, unspecified

PATIENT TEACHING

All individuals with systemic illnesses predisposed to dry eye, menopausal women, and those residing in arid climates or >60 years should be instructed in the use of artificial tear supplements to combat dry eye symptoms.

 See Patient Handout on CD

L

LACTOSE INTOLERANCE

Jennifer E. Cyrkler, MD

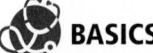 **BASICS**

DESCRIPTION

- Inability to digest lactose (the primary sugar in milk) into its constituents, glucose and galactose, due to low levels of the lactase enzyme in the brush border of the duodenum.
  - Congenital lactose intolerance: Very rare
  - Primary lactose intolerance is common in adults in whom a low level of lactase has developed after childhood.
  - Symptoms are experienced after consumption of milk and milk-containing products. Intolerance varies with amount of lactose consumed and rate of gastric emptying.
  - Secondary lactose intolerance is the inability to digest lactose caused by any condition injuring the intestinal mucosa (e.g., diarrhea) or a reduction of available mucosal surface (e.g., resection). This is usually transient, with the duration of the intolerance determined by the nature and course of the primary condition.
  - Infants with induced acute or chronic diarrhea may develop lactose intolerance, especially with rotavirus disease. Lactose intolerance is also fairly common with giardiasis and ascariasis, inflammatory bowel disease, tropical and nontropical sprue, and the AIDS malabsorption syndrome.
  - Lactose malabsorption is defined as the inability to absorb lactose. This does not necessarily parallel lactose intolerance.
- System(s) Affected: Endocrine/Metabolic; Gastrointestinal
- Synonym(s): Lactase deficiency

ALERT

Geriatric Considerations
No increase in lactose intolerance in this age group.

Pediatric Considerations
- Primary lactose intolerance occurs after weaning, which usually begins in late childhood.
- Breast milk contains a large quantity of lactose, but does not seem to worsen diarrhea associated with viral or bacterial diseases.
- Lactosefree formulas are available.
- Exclude a milk protein allergy.

Pregnancy Considerations
44% of lactose-intolerant women will be able to tolerate lactose while pregnant.

GENERAL PREVENTION
Avoidance of lactose in large quantities will relieve symptoms. Patients can learn what level of lactose is tolerable in their diet.

EPIDEMIOLOGY

Incidence
- Primary lactose intolerance varies according to race
  - American Indians, Blacks, Asians, Mediterranean descent, and Jews: 75–90%
  - <5% of descendants of Northern and Central Europeans
- Secondary lactose intolerance
  - ≥50% of infants with acute or chronic diarrheal disease have lactose intolerance, especially with rotavirus disease.
  - Lactose intolerance also is fairly common with giardiasis and ascariasis, inflammatory bowel disease, tropical and nontropical sprue, and the AIDS malabsorptive syndrome.

Prevalence
- Predominant age
  - Primary: Teenage and adult
  - Secondary: Depends on the underlying condition
- Secondary lactose intolerance can begin at any age.
- Predominant sex: Male = Female

RISK FACTORS
- Race
- Age

ETIOLOGY
- Primary lactose intolerance: Normal decline in the lactase activity in the intestinal mucosa after weaning; this is genetically controlled and permanent.
- Secondary lactose intolerance: Associated with gastroenteritis in children
- Also: Nontropical and tropical sprue, regional enteritis, abetalipoproteinemia, cystic fibrosis, ulcerative colitis, immunoglobulin deficiencies in both adults and children

ASSOCIATED CONDITIONS
- Tropical or nontropical sprue
- Giardiasis
- Immunoglobulin deficiencies
- Crohn disease
- Cystic fibrosis

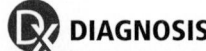 **DIAGNOSIS**

SIGNS AND SYMPTOMS
- Bloating
- Cramping
- Abdominal discomfort
- Diarrhea or loose stools
- Flatulence
- Rumbling (borborygmi)
- Only 1/3–1/5 of the people with lactose malabsorption will develop symptoms. The degree of the symptoms varies with the lactose load and with other foods consumed at the same time.
- In children vomiting is common, as well as frothy, acid stools; malnutrition can occur.

History
Symptoms may arise 30 minutes to 2 hours after consumption of products containing lactose and may be distinguished from IBS with a trial of a lactosefree diet.

TESTS
- Lactose breath hydrogen test (especially in children)
- Lactose absorption test: Alternative to lactose breath hydrogen test in adults (more invasive and equivalent sensitivity and specificity as breath test)

Lab
- Low fecal pH and reducing substances are only valid when stools are collected fresh and assayed immediately.
- Fairly insensitive

Diagnostic Procedures/Surgery
Small bowel biopsy for assay of lactase activity: May be normal if deficiency is focal or patchy (not readily available and usually not necessary)

Pathological Findings
Lactase deficiency in intestinal mucosa might be patchy or focal. Rarely used in clinical practice.

DIFFERENTIAL DIAGNOSIS
- Sucrase deficiency
- Diseases listed under secondary lactose intolerance
- Irritable bowel syndrome

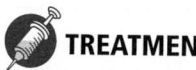 **TREATMENT**

INITIAL STABILIZATION
Outpatient, except in severe cases of malnutrition

GENERAL MEASURES
Diet
- Reduce or restrict dietary lactose to control symptoms.
- Yogurt and fermented products, such as hard cheese, are tolerated better than milk.
- Supplement calcium in the form of calcium carbonate.
- Commercially available "lactase" preparations (Lactaid or Lactrase) are effective in reducing symptoms in many people.
- Prehydrolyzed milk (Lactaid) is available and effective.

Activity
Full activity

Complementary and Alternative Medicine
Certain probiotic formulations taken with meals may alleviate some of the symptoms of lactose intolerance in select patients (1)[B].

 MEDICATION (DRUGS)

First Line
- Lactase (Lactaid, Lactrase) tablets
  - Take 1–2 capsules or tablets prior to ingesting milk products. These vary in effectiveness at preventing symptoms.
  - Can add tablets or contents of capsules to milk before drinking.
  - Also available in milk in some areas.
- Not effective for all people with lactose intolerance.

 FOLLOW-UP

PROGNOSIS
- Normal life expectancy
- Symptoms can be controlled

COMPLICATIONS
Calcium deficiency

REFERENCES
1. Levri KM, Ketvertis K, Deramo M, et al. Do probiotics reduce adult lactose intolerance? A systematic review. *J Fam Pract* 2005;54:613.
2. Savaiano DA, Boushey CJ, McCabe GP. Lactose intolerance symptoms assessed by meta-analysis; a grain of truth that leads to exaggeration. *J Nutr* 2006;136:1107–1113.

 MISCELLANEOUS

CODES

ICD9-CM
271.3 Intestinal disaccharidase deficiencies and disaccharide malabsorption

PATIENT TEACHING
- Patients must read labels on commercial products because milk-sugar is used in many products and may cause symptoms.
- Lactose intolerant patients may tolerate whole milk or chocolate milk better than skim.
- Lactose consumed with other food products is better tolerated than when it is consumed alone.
- Primary lactase deficiency is permanent; secondary lactose intolerance is usually temporary, although it may persist for several months after the inciting disease has been cured.
- 20% of the prescription drugs and 6% of over-the-counter medicines use lactose as a base.

Diet
- Keeping a food diary, with symptomatic episodes documented, can help identify food sources that may be more problematic.
- Patients should read ingredient labels to look for milk or lactose but also for ingredients such as whey and curd, which indicate the presence of lactose.
- Patients must maintain adequate calcium intake, especially if dairy products are not included in their daily diet.

 See Patient Handout on CD

L

LARYNGEAL CANCER

Monica Lee, MD

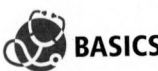 **BASICS**

DESCRIPTION
- <1% of all malignant lesions. Squamous cell carcinomas constitute 5–98% of all malignant neoplasms of the larynx.
- <2% of all carcinomas
- At the time of diagnosis, 62% will have local disease, 26% regional disease, and 8% distant disease in the lungs, liver, and/or bone.
- No racial predilection
- System(s) Affected: Pulmonary
- Synonym(s): Cancer of larynx

GENERAL PREVENTION
- Indirect laryngoscopy for patients with persistent hoarseness lasting beyond 1–2 weeks
- Cessation of smoking and/or alcohol abuse

EPIDEMIOLOGY
- Predominant age
  - Median age of occurrence in the 6th and 7th decades
  - <1% of laryngeal cancers arise in patients <30 years of age.
  - Very rare in young patients, in general
- Predominant sex: Male > Female (5:1); however, increasing incidence in women who smoke

Incidence
5 in 100,000 (12,500 new cases per year)

RISK FACTORS
See "Etiology"

Genetics
Unknown

ETIOLOGY
- Smoking
- Alcohol abuse

ASSOCIATED CONDITIONS
<10% of patients may have a synchronous squamous cell carcinoma in the lower or upper aerodigestive tract, most notably in the esophagus or lungs.

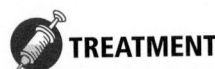 **DIAGNOSIS**

SIGNS AND SYMPTOMS
- Persistent hoarseness in an elderly or middle-aged cigarette smoker
- Dyspnea and stridor
- Ipsilateral otalgia
- Dysphagia
- Odynophagia
- Chronic cough
- Hemoptysis
- Weight loss owing to poor nutrition
- Halitosis owing to tumor necrosis
- Mass in the neck from metastatic lymph node
- Laryngeal tenderness owing to tumor necrosis or suppuration
- Lump in the neck
- Broadening of the larynx on palpation with loss of crepitation
- Tenderness of the larynx
- Fullness of the cricothyroid membrane

TESTS
Lab
Liver function tests (LFTs) to rule out metastatic disease

Imaging
- CT or MRI if chest and liver or brain metastasis suspected
- Bone scan if bone metastasis suspected
- Screening chest radiograph to rule out metastatic disease

Diagnostic Procedures/Surgery
- Laryngoscopy: Fungating, friable tumor with heaped-up edges and granular appearance, with multiple areas of central necrosis and exudate surrounding areas of hyperemia
- Indirect and/or direct laryngoscopy and biopsy to determine stage of disease as well as histologic confirmation

DIFFERENTIAL DIAGNOSIS
- Acute or chronic laryngitis
- Benign vocal cord lesions such as polyps, nodules, and papillomas
- Tuberculosis or fungal infection of the larynx

TREATMENT

INITIAL STABILIZATION
Primarily outpatient care

GENERAL MEASURES
- Tracheotomy care, when applicable
- In pregnancy
  - Natural history of disease and treatment side effects have to be weighed against the possibilities of continuing on to delivery.

Diet
- Nasogastric or gastrostomy feeding may be necessary if tumor involves esophageal inlet.
- No special diet otherwise

Activity
Patient may remain fully active unless debilitated from more advanced disease and/or greater degree of surgery.

MEDICATION (DRUGS)

- Narcotics may be necessary for pain control during treatment for mucositis secondary to radiation therapy.
- Nystatin mouth rinses for oral thrush

SURGERY

- Tracheotomy may be necessary if tumor is large enough to cause upper airway obstruction.
- Early disease may be treatable by either radiation therapy or laser cordectomy on an outpatient basis. 90% cure rates are the rule.
- More advanced disease needs inpatient care necessitating partial or total laryngectomy and postoperative radiation therapy 4–5 weeks after surgery, depending on the stage of disease.

 ## FOLLOW-UP

PROGNOSIS

Early disease is expected to have >90% cure.

COMPLICATIONS

- Temporary odynophagia or dysphagia secondary to mucositis and/or thrush during radiation therapy
- Persistent hoarseness despite adequate treatment, necessitating further adjunctive procedures and/or speech therapy
- Tracheostomal stenosis requiring stenting with laryngectomy tubes or further surgery
- Dysphagia secondary to upper esophageal stricture after total laryngectomy, necessitating dilatation
- Aspiration after partial laryngectomy, necessitating complete laryngectomy or tracheotomy
- Inability to decannulate after partial laryngectomy because of laryngeal stenosis and/or aspiration
- Radiation-induced chondronecrosis, which mimics tumor recurrence
- Radiation edema, necessitating emergent tracheotomy

PATIENT MONITORING

- Repeat indirect laryngoscopy and complete head and neck examinations for at least 5 years after treatment to detect early recurrence or second primary
- Yearly chest radiographs and LFT
- Patients with dysphagia should undergo barium swallow and/or esophageal endoscopy to rule out 2nd tumor in the esophagus.
- Patients with unexplained pain should have appropriate radiologic or nuclear medicine, bone scans
- Mental status change indicates CT scan of the brain to rule out brain metastases.

REFERENCES

1. Ariyan S. Cancer of the Head and Neck. St. Louis, MO: Mosby, 1987.
2. Cummings CW, et al., eds. Otolaryngology Head and Neck Surgery, Vol. 3, 3rd ed. New York: Mosby, 1998.
3. Suen JY, Myers EN. Cancer of the Head and Neck, 3rd ed. Philadelphia: WB Saunders, 1996.

 ## MISCELLANEOUS

CODES

ICD9-CM
161.9 Malignant neoplasm of larynx, unspecified

PATIENT TEACHING

Material is available from local cancer society.

L

LARYNGITIS

Rohit Uppal, MD
Bruce T. Vanderhoff, MD

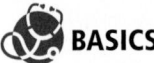 **BASICS**

DESCRIPTION
- Inflammation, erythema, and edema of the mucosa of the larynx
- Most cases are acute and are associated with viral URI or acute vocal strain.
- System(s) Affected: Pulmonary
- Synonym(s): Acute laryngitis; Chronic laryngitis

ALERT
Geriatric Considerations
May be sicker and slower to heal.

Pediatric Considerations
- Common in this age group
- Consider congenital causes.

GENERAL PREVENTION
- Avoid overuse of voice.
- Influenza virus vaccine is suggested for high-risk individuals.
- Quit smoking.
- Avoid alcohol and caffeine.
- Maintain proper hydration status.

EPIDEMIOLOGY
- Predominant age: All ages
- Predominant sex: Male = Female

Incidence
Common

RISK FACTORS
- Acute
  - Upper respiratory tract infection
  - Pneumonia
  - Influenza
  - Pertussis/Measles/Diphtheria
  - Immunocompromised
- Chronic
  - Allergy
  - Chronic rhinitis/sinusitis
  - Voice abuse
  - GERD
  - Smoking/alcohol abuse
  - Constant exposure to dust or other irritants
  - Previous endotracheal intubation

ETIOLOGY
- Virus infections: Influenza A, B, parainfluenza, adenovirus, coronavirus, rhinovirus, HPV, CMV, VZV, HSV, RSV, and Coxsackie
- Bacterial infections: Beta-hemolytic streptococcus, *Streptococcus pneumoniae*, *H. influenza*, tuberculosis, leprosy, and Moraxella catarrhalis, *Mycoplasma pneumoniae*, *Chlamydia pneumoniae*, TB
- Misuse or abuse of voice
- Inhaling irritating substances (e.g., air pollution)
- Aspiration of caustic chemical
- Aging changes: Muscle atrophy, loss of moisture in larynx, and bowing of vocal cords
- GERD
- Fungal infections: Histoplasmosis, blastomycosis, coccidioides, cryptococcus, and candida
- Allergic
- Idiopathic
- Vocal cord nodules/polyps ("singer's nodes")
- Injury or compression of recurrent laryngeal nerve
- Retropharyngeal abscess
- Tumor
- Neuromuscular disorder (myasthenia)
- Trauma (e.g., endotracheal intubation)

ASSOCIATED CONDITIONS
- Viral pharyngitis
- Croup
- Bronchitis
- Pneumonitis
- GERD

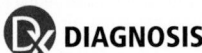 **DIAGNOSIS**

SIGNS AND SYMPTOMS
- Hoarseness
- Abnormal sounding voice
- Aphonia
- Throat tickling
- Feeling of throat rawness
- Constant urge to clear the throat
- Fever
- Malaise
- Dysphagia/Odynophagia
- Cough
- Regional lymphadenopathy
- Stridor in children
- Referred otalgia

TESTS
Lab
- Rarely needed
- WBC elevated in bacterial laryngitis
- Viral culture (seldom necessary)

Imaging
Only if needed for differential diagnosis

Diagnostic Procedures/Surgery
- Fiberoptic or indirect laryngoscopy: Red, inflamed and occasionally hemorrhagic vocal cords, with rounded edges, and exudate (Reinke's edema)
- Consider otolaryngologic evaluation and biopsy: Laryngitis of >2 weeks in adults with history of smoking or alcohol abuse to rule out malignancy
- Consider 24-hour pH probe: Chronic laryngitis in adults with gastroesophageal reflux
- Strobovideo laryngoscopy for diagnosis of subtle lesions

DIFFERENTIAL DIAGNOSIS
- Croup
- Measles
- Diphtheria
- Vocal nodules or polyps
- Laryngeal malignancy
- Thyroid malignancy
- Gastroesophageal reflux
- Epiglottitis

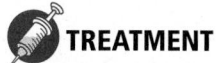 **TREATMENT**

INITIAL STABILIZATION
Outpatient

GENERAL MEASURES
- Acute
  - Usually a self-limited illness and not severe
  - Avoid excessive voice use
  - Steam inhalations or cool-mist humidifier
  - Increase fluid intake.
  - Analgesics
  - Avoid smoking (or second hand exposure).
- Chronic
  - Symptomatic treatment as above
  - Voice therapy (for patients with intermittent dysphagia and vocal abuse)
  - Stop smoking.
  - Reduce alcohol intake.
  - Occupational change or modification, if exposure
  - Consider discontinuing inhaled corticosteroids.
  - Reflux laryngitis: Elevate head of bed, other antireflux management
- Consider otolaryngology consultation
  - Hoarseness >2–3 weeks
  - Hoarseness associated with hemoptysis, difficulty swallowing or breathing, or a lump in neck
  - Loss or severe voice change for more than a few days
  - Professional singer

Activity
Rest until fever subsides.

 MEDICATION (DRUGS)

First Line
- Usually none
- Analgesics
- Antipyretics
- Cough suppressants
- Little or no benefit from antibiotics
- Prescribe antacids, H_2 blockers, or proton pump inhibitors for GERD; the dosage may have to be doubled in cases with symptoms suggestive of pharyngeal or laryngeal reflux disease.
- Consider empiric proton pump inhibitor for chronic laryngitis without obvious reflux symptoms.
- For contraindications, precautions, and significant possible interactions, refer to the manufacturer's literature.

SURGERY
- Vocal cord biopsy of hyperplastic mucosa and areas of leukoplakia if cancer or TB is suspected
- Removal of nodules or polyps if voice therapy fails

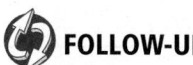 **FOLLOW-UP**

DISPOSITION
Issues for Referral
ENT consultation should be considered if hoarseness persists >2 weeks.

PROGNOSIS
Complete clearing of the inflammation without sequelae

COMPLICATIONS
Chronic hoarseness

REFERENCES

1. Avila M, et al. Viral etiology in acute respiratory infections. *Am Rev Respir Dis*. 1998;104:634.
2. Reveiz L, et al. Antibiotics for acute laryngitis in adults. *Cochrane Database Syst Rev*. 2005;(1): CD004783.
3. Vaezi M , Sensitivity and specificity of reflux-attributed laryngeal lesions: Experimental and clinical evidence. *Am J Med*. 2003;115.
4. Banfiels G, Tandon F, Solomons N. Hoarse voice: An early symptom of many conditions. *Practitioner*. 2000;244:267–271.
5. Braunwald E, et al., eds. *Harrison's Principles of Internal Medicine*. 15th ed. New York, NY: McGraw-Hill; 2001.
6. El-Serag HB, et al. Lansoprazole treatment of patients with chronic idiopathic laryngitis: A placebo-controlled trial. *Am J Gastroenterol*. 2001;96:979–983.
7. Neuenschwander MC, et al. Laryngeal candidiasis. *Ear Nose Throat J*. 2001;80:138–139.
8. Rosen CA, Anderson D, Murry T. Evaluating hoarseness: Keeping your patient's voice healthy. *Am Fam Physician*. 1998;57:2775–2782.

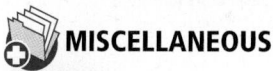 **MISCELLANEOUS**

CODES

ICD9-CM
- 464.00 Acute laryngitis without mention of obstruction
- 464.01 Acute laryngitis with obstruction
- 476.0 Chronic laryngitis

PATIENT TEACHING
- Educate on the importance of voice rest.
- Provide assistance with smoking cessation.
- Help the patient with modification of other predisposing habits or occupational hazards.

L

LARYNGOTRACHEOBRONCHITIS

Garreth C. Biegun, MD
Frank J. Domino, MD

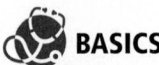 **BASICS**

DESCRIPTION
Subacute viral illness characterized by barking cough, stridor, and fever

- Most common cause of upper airway obstruction or stridor in children
- Spasmodic croup: Non-infectious form
  - Croupy cough with sudden night-time onset
  - No fever or radiographic changes
  - In spectrum, must be initially treated as croup
  - Usually self-limited and resolves with mist therapy at home
  - May recur in same night or within 2–3 nights
- System(s) Affected: Pulmonary
- Synonym(s): Croup; Infectious croup; Viral croup; LTB

EPIDEMIOLOGY
- Predominant age
  - Common 6 months to 3 years
  - Most common in 2nd year of life
  - Rare >6 years
- Predominant sex: Male > Female (1.4:1)
- Timing
  - Follows parainfluenza type 1
  - Any time of year possible but most common in late summer and early fall

Incidence
- 6 cases of croup per 100 children
- 1.5–6% require hospitalization
- 1–5% of those require intubation
- Decreasing incidence in US

RISK FACTORS
- Past history of croup
- Recurrent upper respiratory infections

Genetics
Unknown

PATHOPHYSIOLOGY
- Small children have a small airway with more compliant walls.
- The subglottic region/larynx is entirely encircled by the cricoid cartilage.
- Inflammatory edema and subglottic mucous production decrease airway radius.
- Negative pressure inspiration pulls airway walls closer together.
- Small decrease in airway radius leads to significant decrease of air flow area.

ETIOLOGY
- Parainfluenza virus
  - Most common pathogen ~75% of cases of croup
  - Type 1 is most common, causes 18% of all cases of croup
  - Type 2, 3, and 4 are also common.
  - Type 3 may cause a particularly severe illness.
- *Paramyxovirus*
- Influenza virus type A or B
- Respiratory syncytial virus
- Other viruses
  - Adenovirus
  - Rhinovirus
  - Enterovirus
  - Coxsackievirus
  - Echovirus
  - Reovirus
  - Measles virus
- Haemophilus influenza type B
  - Now rare with routine immunization
- *Mycoplasma pneumoniae*: New and rare cause

ASSOCIATED CONDITIONS
If recurrent (>2 episodes in a year) or in 1st 90 days of life, consider host factors

- Underlying anatomic abnormality (e.g., subglottic stenosis)
- Foreign body
- Paradoxical vocal cord dysfunction
- GERD
- Prolonged neonatal intubation

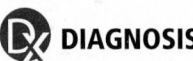 **DIAGNOSIS**

- This is a clinical diagnosis; labs and imaging serve only ancillary purposes.
- Westley Croup Scale: ≤2 mild; 3–7 moderate; ≥ 8 severe
  - Level of consciousness: Normal, including sleep = 0; disoriented = 5
  - Cyanosis: None = 0; with agitation = 4; at rest = 5
  - Stridor: None = 0; with agitation = 1; at rest = 2
  - Air entry: Normal = 0; decreased = 1; markedly decreased = 2
  - Retractions: None = 0; mild = 1; moderate = 2; severe = 3

SIGNS AND SYMPTOMS
- Barking, spasmodic cough
- Biphasic stridor
- Low-grade to moderate fever
- Upper respiratory infection prodrome lasting 1–7 days
- Hypoxia/cyanosis
- Fatigue
- Non–toxic-appearing child
- Normal voice, no drooling
- No change in stridor with positioning
- Nontender larynx
- Inflamed subglottic region
- Normal-appearing supraglottic region

History
- 2–3 days nonspecific prodromal syndrome
- Low-grade fever, coryza, rhinorrhea
- Lack of prodrome indicates spasmodic croup

Physical Exam
- Overall appearance: Child comfortable or struggling?
- Work of breathing: Labored or comfortable?
- Sound of breathing and voice: Hoarse, stridor, inspiratory wheezing, short sentences?
- Observed/subjective tidal volume: Sufficient for child size?

TESTS
Lab
- No laboratory abnormality is diagnostic.
- WBC may be low, normal, or elevated.
- Lymphocytosis expected but not required.
- Rapid antigen or viral culture tests are available in some centers.
  - Guide isolation precautions not management
- Pulse oximetry often is normal because there is no disturbance of alveolar gas exchange.

Imaging
- Posteroanterior and lateral neck films show funnel-shaped subglottic region with normal epiglottis— "steeple," "hour glass," or "pencil point" sign (present in 40–60% of children with laryngotracheobronchitis).
- CT may be more sensitive for defining etiology of obstruction in a confusing clinical picture.
- Patient should be monitored during imaging— progression of airway obstruction may be rapid.

Pathological Findings
- Inflammatory reaction of respiratory mucosa
- Loss of epithelial cells
- Thick mucoid secretions

DIFFERENTIAL DIAGNOSIS
- Epiglottitis—currently rare
- Foreign body aspiration
- Subglottic stenosis (congenital or acquired)
- Bacterial tracheitis
- Simple upper respiratory infection
- Subglottic hemangioma
- Retropharyngeal or peritonsillar abscess
- Trauma
- Allergic reaction (acute angioneurotic edema)

TREATMENT

INITIAL STABILIZATION
- Outpatient care in mild cases
- Intensive care unit (ICU) for patients with tachypnea, tachycardia, hypoxia, cyanosis, reactions, pneumonia, or CHF
- In most cases, ED observation after medical management is sufficient.

GENERAL MEASURES
- Minimize labs, imaging, and other procedures that upset the child; agitation that worsens tachypnea is more detrimental than accepting a clinical diagnosis.
- Frequent checks are more sensitive to worsening disease than pulse-oximetry.
- IV fluids
- ECG monitoring and pulse oximetry

Diet
- NPO and IV fluids for severe cases
- Frequent small feedings with increased fluids for mild cases

Activity
Must keep patient quiet; crying may exacerbate symptoms

SPECIAL THERAPY
Complementary and Alternative Medicine
Mist therapy not proven to work but may be beneficial. Cool temperature misters are preferable to high temperature (e.g., tea kettles).
- Some children respond well to cold dry air
- Avoids the risk of burns

 MEDICATION (DRUGS)

First Line
- Immediate: Racemic or L-epinephrine (Vaponefrin): 0.05 mL/kg/dose (max 0.5 mL) of 2.25% racemic epinephrine delivered in 3 mL of normal saline nebulized (1)[A], (2)[B]
  – Onset in 10–30 minutes, duration ~2 hours
  – Repeat as necessary if side-effects tolerated
- Dexamethasone 0.15–0.6 mg/kg once IM/PO have proven equal efficacy. (3)[A]
  – Nebulized Budesonide also proven effective (4)[B]
- Antibiotics NOT indicated in this viral illness
  – Antecedent or subsequent bacterial infection is uncommon.
- Oxygen as needed
- Contraindications
  – Refer to the manufacturer's literature.
- Precautions
  – Avoid oversedation.
- Significant possible interactions
  – Refer to the manufacturer's literature.

Second Line
Amantadine for influenza A: 100 mg PO b.i.d. for 3–5 days

SURGERY
- Intubation required in 1–6% for 3–5 days; use smallest tube possible
  – After trial of medical management, intubation is for fatigue due to work of breathing or beginning total obstruction; not secondary to low oxygen saturation
  – Direct laryngoscopy if child is not in acute distress
  – Fiberoptic laryngoscopy is the procedure of choice when available.
- Tracheotomy—rarely

 FOLLOW-UP

DISPOSITION
Most patients will be seen in ED or PCP office setting. Some will be overnight by telephone.

Admission Criteria
Minor cases need no visit to hospital or PCP.
- No stridor at rest, no difficulty breathing
- Child able to tolerate PO liquids
- No underlying medical condition
- Caretakers able to assess changes to clinical picture and re-access medical care

Discharge Criteria
Patients who maintain a good response to medical therapy for 3–4 hours (after epi dose) may be safely discharged as long as they have reliable caretakers and good access to medical services if symptoms return. (5)[C]

PROGNOSIS
- Up to 1/3 of patients will have recurrence.
- If required, intubation is maintained for 3–5 days.
- If required, tracheotomy is maintained for 3–7 days.
- Recovery is usually full and without lasting effects.

COMPLICATIONS
- Rare
- Subglottic stenosis in intubated patients
- Bacterial tracheitis
- Cardiopulmonary arrest
- Pneumonia

PATIENT MONITORING
Severe cases require ICU care with respiratory monitoring for hypoxemia and hypercapnia.

REFERENCES
1. Westley CR, Cotton EK, Brooks JG. Nebulized racemic epinephrine by IPPB for the treatment of croup: A double-blind study. *Am J Dis Child*. 1978;132(5):484–487.
2. Wasiman Y, et al. Prospective randomized double-blind study comparing L-epinephrine and racemic epinephrine aerosols in the treatment of laryngotracheitis (croup). *Pediatrics*. 1992;89(2): 302–306.
3. Geelhoed GC, Turner J, MacDonald WB. Efficacy of a small single dose of oral dexamethasone for outpatient croup: A double-blind placebo controlled cinical trial. *Br Med J*. 1996;313(7050):140–142.
4. Cetinkaya F, Tufekci BS, Kutluk G. A comparison of nebulized budesonide, and intramuscular, and oral dexamethasone for treatment of croup. *Int J Pediatr Otorhinolaryngol*. 2004;68(4):453–456.
5. Klassen TP. Croup: A current perspective. *Pediatr Clin North Am*. 1999;46:1167–1178.

MISCELLANEOUS

See also: Bronchiolitis; Common cold; Epiglottitis; tracheitis, bacterial

CODES

ICD9-CM
- 464.20 Acute laryngotracheitis without mention of obstruction
- 464.21 Acute laryngotracheitis with obstruction
- 464.4 Croup Syndrome
- 476.1 Chronic laryngotracheitis

L

PATIENT TEACHING
- Educate parents about when to seek emergency care if mild cases progress.
- Emotional support and reassurance for the patient

LAXATIVE ABUSE

Duane C. Roe, MD

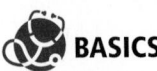 **BASICS**

DESCRIPTION
Diarrhea caused by self-medication or by a patient simulating diarrhea by the addition of fluid (e.g., urine) to the stool.

- System(s) Affected: Gastrointestinal, Nervous, Psychiatric
- Synonym(s): Factitious diarrhea, Cathartic colon

GENERAL PREVENTION
- Suspicion in patients with unsolved chronic diarrhea
- Monitor "doctor hopping."
- Avoid exploratory surgery.
- Avoid repeated testing for diagnosis.

EPIDEMIOLOGY
- Predominant age
  - 18–40 years with bulimia nervosa
  - 40–60 years without bulimia
- Predominant sex: Female > Male

ALERT
Geriatric Considerations
Unusual to start age >60 years

Incidence
Unknown

ETIOLOGY
- Ingestion of any laxative agent
- Psychologic factors
  - Bulimia nervosa
  - Secondary gain of attention
  - Hysterical behavior
  - Multiple personality disorders
  - Inappropriate perception of "normal" bowel habits
- Chronic constipation

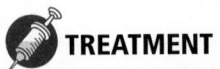 **DIAGNOSIS**

SIGNS AND SYMPTOMS
- Diarrhea
- Additional symptoms: Abdominal pain, rectal pain, nausea, vomiting, weight loss, muscle weakness, bone pain
- Additional signs: Hypokalemia, skin pigmentation, finger clubbing, cyclic edema, kidney stones, melanosis coli
- The signs and symptoms will persist in spite of years of investigation and re-evaluation.

TESTS
Lab
- Serum test—hypokalemia, metabolic alkalosis
- Urinalysis may be abnormal.
- Stool sodium, potassium
- Stool pH (alkalinization suggests presence of phenolphthalein)
- Stool for laxative titers
- Urine volume and electrolytes

Imaging
Barium enema—cathartic colon

Diagnostic Procedures/Surgery
- Carefully selected when needed to rule out other diseases
- Try not to repeat prior evaluations.
- Sigmoidoscopy
- High index of suspicion

Pathological Findings
- Melanosis coli
- "Cathartic colon"—refers to dilation and ahaustral appearance on barium enema

DIFFERENTIAL DIAGNOSIS
Include any diarrhea of secretory or osmotic source.

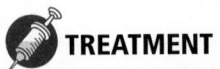 **TREATMENT**

INITIAL STABILIZATION
Hospitalization may be needed (hypokalemia, malnutrition).

GENERAL MEASURES
- Psychologic support is essential.
- Confront the patient, gently and with support and understanding
- Discontinue laxative use.
- Long-term laxative abuse requires weaning.
- Treat constipation.

Diet
Ensure good nutritional habits.
- Increase fiber intake.
- Adequate calories, especially with bulimia

Activity
Physical exercise program

MEDICATION (DRUGS)

- Based on psychologic assessment
- Nonstimulant laxatives if needed
  - Senna best during pregnancy and lactation
  - Lactulose
  - Fiber
- Contraindications
  - Danthron—hepatotoxic
- Precautions
  - Patients will be manipulative in attempts to hide problem and often large quantities of laxatives.
- Significant possible interactions
  - Increased rate of intestinal flow may affect rate of absorption of medications, e.g., antibiotics, hormones.
  - Docusate sodium may potentiate hepatotoxicity of other drugs.

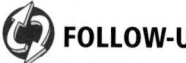 **FOLLOW-UP**

DISPOSITION
Admission Criteria
- Persistant diarrhea
- Electrolyte/Metabolic complications

Discharge Criteria
- Psychologic support
- Diet and bowel programs

PROGNOSIS
- Protracted course
- Prognosis related to psychologic response

COMPLICATIONS
- Risk of multiple tests, procedures, and surgeries
- Malnutrition
- Electrolyte imbalances (hypokalemia)
- Renal failure
- Fatalities, especially in children given laxatives by parents
- Renal calculi

ALERT
Pediatric Considerations
- Death
- Lifelong laxative dependence

PATIENT MONITORING
- Careful psychologic counseling
- Careful medical support. Show concern by frequent visits as needed.
- Assess serum electrolytes.

REFERENCES

1. Kovacs D, Palmer RL. The association between laxative abuse and other symptoms among adults with anorexia nervosa. *Int J Eat Disord*. 2004;36(2): 224–228.
2. Duncan A, Forrest JA. Surreptitious abuse of magnesium laxatives as a cause of chronic diarrhea. *Eur J Gastroenterol Hepatol*. 2001;13(5):599–601.
3. Baker EH, Sandle GI. Complications of laxative abuse. *Ann Rev Med*. 1996;47:127–134.

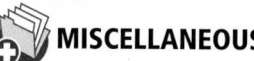 **MISCELLANEOUS**

See also: Bulimia nervosa; Constipation; Hypokalemia; Renal calculi; Renal failure, Acute (ARF); Renal failure, chronic

 CODES

ICD9-CM
305.90 Other, mixed, or unspecified drug abuse, unspecified

PATIENT TEACHING

See "General Measures."

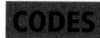 **See Corresponding Diagnostic Algorithm**

L

LEAD POISONING

Jason Chao, MD, MS

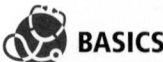 **BASICS**

DESCRIPTION
Consequence of a high body burden of lead (Pb), an element with no known physiologic value
- Synonym(s): Lead poisoning, inorganic

GENERAL PREVENTION
Family should receive counseling on potential sources of lead and methods to decrease lead exposure. Children at high risk should receive blood Pb screening. (1)[C]

EPIDEMIOLOGY
- Predominant age: 1–5 years old; adult workers
- Predominant sex: Adult Male > Adult Female
  – Gender ratio: 1:1 in childhood

Incidence
New York state 1999: 34 per 1000 pediatric cases with blood Pb level ≥20 µg/dL; a dramatic decrease from 1980

Prevalence
- 1999–2000, CDC estimated 2.2% of US children 1–5 years old had blood Pb levels >10 µg/dL, but levels are variable among communities and populations
- Sporadic cases in adults

RISK FACTORS
- Children with pica, or with iron deficiency anemia
- Residence or frequent visitor in deteriorating, pre-1960 housing with leaded-paint surfaces
- Children with hyperkinetic or autistic behavior
- Sibling or playmate with lead poisoning
- Dust from clothing of lead worker
- Lead dissolved in water from lead or lead-soldered plumbing
- Lead-glazed ceramics, especially with acidic food or drink
- Soil/dust near lead industries and roads
- Folk remedies
  – Mexican: Azarcon, greta
  – Dominican Republic : Litargirio, a topical agent
  – Asian: Chuifong tokuwan, pay-loo-ah, ghasard, bali goli, kandu, Ayurvedic herbal medicine from South Asia
  – Middle Eastern: Alkohl, surma, saoott, cebagin
- Hobbies: Glazed pottery making, target shooting at firing ranges, lead soldering, painting, preparing lead shot or fishing sinkers, stained-glass making, car or boat repair, home remodeling
- Occupational exposure: Plumbers, pipe fitters, lead miners, auto repairers, glass manufacturers, shipbuilders, printers, plastic manufacturers, lead smelters and refiners, steel welders or cutters, construction workers, rubber product manufacturers, battery manufacturers, bridge reconstruction workers
- Dietary: Zinc or calcium deficiency

ALERT
Pediatric Considerations
- Children are at increased risk because of incomplete development of the blood–brain barrier <3 years, allowing more lead into the central nervous system; ingested lead has 40% bioavailability in children compared with 10% in adults
- Common childhood behaviors such as frequent hand-to-mouth activity and pica (repeated ingestion of nonfood products) greatly increase the risk of ingesting lead.

PATHOPHYSIOLOGY
Pb replaces calcium in bones. Pb interferes with heme synthesis; causes interstitial nephritis; interferes with neurotransmitters, especially glutamine; high levels affect blood–brain barrier leading to encephalopathy, seizures, and coma

ETIOLOGY
Inhalation of lead dust or fumes, or ingestion of lead

ASSOCIATED CONDITIONS
Iron deficiency anemia

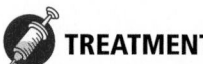 **DIAGNOSIS**

SIGNS AND SYMPTOMS
History
- Often asymptomatic
- Mild to moderate toxicity
  – May cause myalgia or paresthesia, fatigue, irritability, lethargy
  – Abdominal discomfort, arthralgia, difficulty concentrating, headache, tremor, vomiting, weight loss, muscular exhaustibility
- Severe toxicity: Leads to 3 major clinical syndromes
  – Alimentary type: Anorexia, metallic taste, constipation, severe abdominal cramps owing to intestinal spasm and sometimes associated with rigidity of the abdominal wall
  – Neuromuscular type (characteristic of adult plumbism): Peripheral neuritis, usually painless and limited to extensor muscles
  – Cerebral type or lead encephalopathy (more common in children): Seizures; coma; long-term sequelae including neurologic defects, retarded mental development, and chronic hyperactivity
- Chronic exposure may cause renal failure.

Physical Exam
Often normal; abdominal tenderness may be severe; neurologic exam may reveal neuropathy or encephalopathy

TESTS
Lab
- Blood lead (Pb) >10 µg/dL (0.48 µmol/L), collected with lead-free container

CDC Lead Poisoning Classification

Class	Lead (µg/dL)
I	<10
II	10–19
III	20–44
IV	45–69
V	>70

µg/dL = 0.04826 µmol/L, e.g., 70 µg/dL = 3.38 µmol/dL

- Screening capillary lead levels >10 µg/dL (0.48 µmol/L) should be confirmed with a venous sample.
- Hemoglobin and hematocrit slightly low. Eosinophilia or basophilic stippling on peripheral smear may be seen, but is not diagnostic of lead toxicity.
- Renal function decreased in late stages

Imaging
- Abdominal radiograph for lead particles in gut if recent ingestion is suspected
- Radiograph of long bones may show lines of increased density in the metaphyseal plate resulting from growth arrest, but does not usually alter management.

DIFFERENTIAL DIAGNOSIS
- Alimentary type may be confused with acute abdomen
- Neuromuscular type may be confused with other polyneuropathies
- Cerebral type may be confused with attention deficit disorder, mental retardation, autism, dementia, other causes of seizures
- Elevated erythrocyte protoporphyrin may be caused by iron deficiency anemia or less commonly, hemolytic anemia. Erythropoietic protoporphyria produces a very high erythrocyte protoporphyrin.

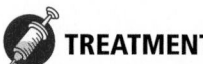 **TREATMENT**

INITIAL STABILIZATION
Outpatient care unless parenteral chelation is required

GENERAL MEASURES
- Case report to local health department for classes III to V. Complete inspection of home or workplace to determine source of Pb. Screen all family members. (1)[C]
- Consider oral chelation for class IV. Chelation (preferably parenteral) for class V or symptomatic class III or IV (1)[C]
- Do not begin chelation until Pb particles present in gut are cleared. (2)[C]
- Remove patient from potential source of Pb for class IV or V until complete home inspection is performed. (3)[C]

Diet
- If symptomatic, avoidance of excessive fluids
- Avoidance of pica
- Adequate calcium, iron, and vitamin C to reduce absorption and retention of lead (1)[C]

Activity
Avoid visit to any site of potential contamination.

MEDICATION (DRUGS)

First Line
- Oral chelation: Succimer (Chemet, dimercaptosuccinic acid, DMSA) 10 mg/kg q8h for 5 days, then 10 mg/kg q12h for 2 weeks. May be repeated after 2 weeks off if Pb levels are not stabilized below 15 μg/dL (<0.72 μmol/L). (2)[C]
- Parenteral chelation (begin after establishment of adequate urine output) (2)[C]
  - Class V or symptomatic: Dimercaprol (British antilewisite, BAL) 75 mg/m^2 given deep IM, then BAL 450 mg/m^2/d divided q4h for 5 days plus Ca EDTA (edetate calcium disodium) 1,500 mg/m^2/d continuous IV infusion for 5 days. If rebound lead level $\geq$45 μg/dL ($\geq$2.17 μmol/L), chelation may be repeated after 2-day interval if symptomatic, after 5-day interval if asymptomatic.
  - Class IV asymptomatic: Ca EDTA 1,000 mg/m^2/d for 5 days. May be repeated after 5–7 days
- Diazepam for initial control of seizures; further control maintained with paraldehyde
- Contraindications
  - BAL should not be given to patients allergic to peanuts (the drug solution contains peanut oil).
- Precautions
  - Succimer: Gastrointestinal upset, rash, nasal congestion, muscle pains, elevated liver function tests
  - Ca EDTA: Renal failure, increased excretion of zinc, copper, and iron
  - BAL: Nausea, vomiting, fever, headache, transient hypertension, hepatocellular damage
- Significant possible interactions
  - Vitamins should not be given concurrently with oral chelation.
  - BAL may precipitate hemolytic crisis in a patient with glucose-6-phosphate dehydrogenase deficiency.

Second Line
Oral chelation with penicillamine (D-penicillamine, Depen, Cuprimine)
- Penicillin-allergic patient should not receive D-penicillamine (cross-sensitivity is common).
- 10–20 mg/kg b.i.d. mixed in apple juice/sauce on empty stomach (not Food and Drug Administration approved)
- D-Penicillamine may cause gastrointestinal upset, renal failure, granulocytopenia, liver dysfunction, iron deficiency, drug-induced lupuslike syndrome

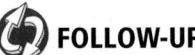 ## FOLLOW-UP

DISPOSITION
Admission Criteria
- Blood lead level >70 μg/dL
- Blood lead level >35 μg/dL and symptomatic

Discharge Criteria
If the source is in the home, the patient must reside elsewhere until the abatement process is completed.

Issues for Referral
Consider consultation if parenteral chelation is required.

PROGNOSIS
- Symptomatic lead poisoning without encephalopathy generally improves with chelation, but subtle central nervous system toxicity may be long lasting or permanent.
- If encephalopathy occurs, permanent sequelae (mental retardation, seizure disorder, blindness, hemiparesis) in 25–50%

COMPLICATIONS
- Central nervous system toxicity may be long lasting or permanent.
- Long-term lead exposure may cause chronic renal failure (Fanconi-like syndrome); gout; lead line (blue-black) on gingival tissue.
- Lead exposure in pregnancy is associated with reduced birth weight and premature birth.
- Lead is an animal teratogen.

PATIENT MONITORING
- After chelation, check for rebound Pb level in 7–10 days. Follow with regular monitoring, initially biweekly or monthly.
- Correct iron deficiency or any other nutritional deficiencies present.
- For class II or higher, repeat testing every 3 months until class I level achieved.

REFERENCES
1. American Academy of Pediatrics Committee on Environmental Health. Lead exposure in children: Prevention, detection, and management. *Pediatrics*. 2005;116:1036–1046.
2. American Academy of Pediatrics Committee on Drugs. Treatment guidelines for lead exposure in children. *Pediatrics*. 1995;96:155–160.
3. Centers for Disease Control and Prevention. *Managing Elevated Blood Lead Levels among Young Children: Recommendations from the Advisory Committee on Childhood Lead Poisoning Prevention*. Atlanta, GA: Centers for Disease Control and Prevention; 2002.
4. Dietrich KN, et al. Effect of chelation therapy on the neuropsychological and behavioral development of lead-exposed children after school entry. *Pediatrics*. 2004;114:19–26.

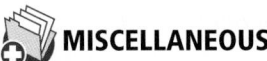 ## MISCELLANEOUS

See also: Iron deficiency anemia

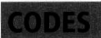 ### CODES

ICD9-CM
984.9 Toxic effect of unspecified lead compound (including fumes)

PATIENT TEACHING
- Needleman HL, Landrigan PJ. *Raising Children Toxic Free: How to Keep Your Child Safe From Lead, Asbestos, Pesticides, and Other Environmental Hazards*. New York, NY: Avon Books; 1995.
- National Lead Information Center, 422 South Clinton Avenue, Rochester, NY 14620; (800) 424-5323; http://www.epa.gov/lead/pubs/nlic.htm
- Alliance to End Childhood Lead Poisoning, 227 Massachusetts Ave NE, Suite 200, Washington, DC 20002; (202) 543-1147; http://www.aeclp.org
- National Safety Council, 1121 Spring Lake Dr., Itasca, IL 60143-3201; (800) 621-7619; http://www.nsc.org/issues/lead/

Prevention
Wet mopping and dusting with a high phosphate solution (e.g. powdered automatic dishwasher detergent with 1/4 cup per gallon water) will help control lead-bearing dust.

 See Corresponding Diagnostic Algorithm

LEGG-CALVÉ-PERTHES DISEASE

Francisco G. Valencia, MD
Patrick C. Henderson, MD

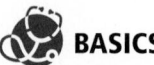 **BASICS**

DESCRIPTION
- Idiopathic necrosis of capital femoral epiphysis of the femoral head.
- 10–20% of cases are bilateral.
- Occurs in pediatric patients.
- System(s) Affected: Musculoskeletal

GENERAL PREVENTION
Because etiology is not clearly understood, prevention is not possible.

EPIDEMIOLOGY
- Predominant age: Susceptible age is 2–12 years. However, ~80% occur between the ages of 4–9.
- Predominant sex: Males > Females (4:1). In bilateral cases, males predominate 7:1. However, females seem to have more severe involvement.

Incidence
15:100,000

Prevalence
75:100,000

RISK FACTORS
Increased incidence in children with low birth weight and delayed physical maturation

Genetics
No known genetic pattern identified

ETIOLOGY
- Unclear
- Related to interruption of blood flow to femoral epiphysis

ASSOCIATED CONDITIONS
- Short stature
- Delayed bone age.
- Possible association with hypercoagulable states.

DIAGNOSIS

SIGNS AND SYMPTOMS
- Primarily hip or groin pain, although referred pain to the knee and thigh is not uncommon.
- May present with a limp.
- Bilateral cases usually do not become symptomatic at the same time.

Physical Exam
- Range of motion (ROM) is limited, especially in internal rotation and abduction.
- Atrophy of thigh musculature owing to disuse
- Leg length discrepancy secondary to collapse of the femoral head
- Short stature is common.

TESTS
Lab
- CBC (to rule out infection, if suspected)
- Sedimentation rate (to rule out infection, if suspected)

Imaging
- Serial radiographs, anteroposterior and frog lateral of the pelvis, are crucial for determining the extent of involvement and progression of healing.
- Full extent of involvement may not be evident for several months, because radiographic findings lag symptoms.
- MRI is most sensitive test; facilitates early diagnosis of necrosis and visualization of articular surface.
- Dynamic arthrography is used to assess congruency of femoral head.
- Technetium[99] bone scan may be helpful in delineating the extent of avascular changes.
- Delayed bone age is present in up to 90% of cases.

Diagnostic Procedures/Surgery
Hip aspiration to rule out septic arthritis if clinical suspicion of infection exists.

Pathological Findings
- Early (necrosis, resorption) stage: Necrosis of bone with subchondral bone fracture and subsequent collapse of subchondral bone
- Late (healing) stage: Revascularization by creeping substitution of necrotic bone

DIFFERENTIAL DIAGNOSIS
- Unilateral
  - Septic arthritis
  - Toxic synovitis
  - Juvenile rheumatoid arthritis
- Bilateral
  - Spondyloepiphyseal dysplasia
  - Metaphyseal dysplasia
  - Hypothyroidism

TREATMENT

INITIAL STABILIZATION
- Pediatric orthopaedic consultation
- Ambulatory treatment is usual; however, some patients may require inpatient traction or surgical procedures.

GENERAL MEASURES
Goals of treatment
- Relieve weightbearing across affected hip, thus reducing irritability of the hip.
- Obtain and maintain hip ROM (1)[B].
- Maximize regeneration and spherical development of the femoral head by containing the femoral epiphysis within the acetabulum (1)[B].

Diet
No special diet

Activity
- Ambulatory status depends on extent/stage of disease.
- Limit weightbearing in cases of hip irritation.

SPECIAL THERAPY
Physical Therapy
May be prescribed by pediatric orthopaedist to maintain hip motion.

MEDICATION (DRUGS)

First Line
Ibuprofen 10 mg/kg PO t.i.d.–q.i.d. to decrease inflammation and pain
- Contraindications: Allergy to ibuprofen
- Precautions: Gastrointestinal irritation

Second Line
Acetaminophen as needed for pain relief.

SURGERY
- Surgical outcome depends on age at presentation and severity of disease at the time of surgery (2)[A].
- Adductor tenotomy may be used to help restore ROM secondary to adductor contracture. (3)[B].
- Femoral and/or pelvic osteotomy may be used to help contain femoral epiphysis within the confines of the acetabulum (in older children or in cases of hip subluxation) (3)[B].

 ## FOLLOW-UP

DISPOSITION
Admission Criteria
No admission necessary unless the patient undergoes surgery.

Issues for Referral
Baseline pediatric orthopaedic surgery referral is recommended.

PROGNOSIS
- Most patients have a favorable outcome.
- Outcome depends on patient's age at the time of diagnosis (the younger, the better).
- Prognosis also is related to the degree of involvement of the femoral head (as determined by radiography).

COMPLICATIONS
- Permanent distortion of the femoral head
- Distorted joint susceptible to early degenerative joint disease
- Limb-length discrepancy

PATIENT MONITORING
- Initially, close pediatric orthopaedic follow-up including radiographic evaluation is needed to determine extent of necrosis.
- Once healing phase is entered, follow-up can be every 6 months.
- Long-term follow-up is necessary to determine final outcome.

REFERENCES
1. Thompson GH, Price CT, Roy D, et al. Legg-Calve-Perthes disease: Current concepts. *Instr Course Lect*. 2002;51:367–384.
2. Grzegorzewski A, Kozlowski P, Szymczak W, et al. Leg length discrepancy in Legg-Calve-Perthes disease. *J Pediatr Orthop*. 2005;2005:206–209.
3. Herring JA. The treatment of Legg-Calve-Perthes disease. A critical review of the literature. *J Bone Joint Surg Am*. 1998;73A:448–458.
4. Herring JA, Kim HT, Browne R. Legg-Calve-Perthes Disease. Part II: Prospective multicenter study on the effect of treatment on outcome. *J Bone Joint Surg Am*. 2004;86A:2121–2134.

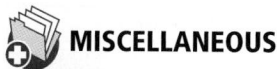 ## MISCELLANEOUS

 CODES

ICD9-CM
732.1 Juvenile osteochondrosis of hip and pelvis

PATIENT TEACHING
- Legg-calve-Perthes disease is a self-limited disease with revascularization occurring within 3 years.
- Treatment is directed at maintaining an appropriate ROM and maximizing containment of the femoral head.

Activity
As indicated by pediatric orthopaedic surgeon.

 See Corresponding Diagnostic Algorithm

L

LEGIONNAIRES DISEASE

Ramesh Nathan, MD

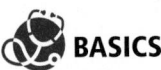 **BASICS**

DESCRIPTION

Legionnaires disease was coined for an epidemic of lower respiratory tract disease occurring in Philadelphia in 1976, in war veterans. The causative bacterium was identified and named *Legionella pneumophila*; it may cause pneumonia or flu-like illness.

- Ranks among the 3 most common pneumonias in the clinical setting
- System(s) Affected: Gastrointestinal; Pulmonary
- Synonym(s): Legionella pneumonia; Legionellosis

ALERT

Geriatric Considerations
Increased incidence >50

Pediatric Considerations
Less common

GENERAL PREVENTION

- Heating water to 60–70°C may help prevent water contamination.
- Ultraviolet light or copper-silver ionization are bactericidal.

EPIDEMIOLOGY

Incidence
- True incidence is not well known.
- Only 2–10% of cases are probably reported.
- May increase with the rise in population density in some urban areas, certain travel and leisure activities, and more complex infrastructures
- Outbreaks occur most often at the end of the summer and early fall.

Prevalence
- Predominant age: 15 months–84 years; increased after age 50
- Predominant sex: Male > Female

RISK FACTORS

- Smoking
- Alcohol abuse
- Immunosuppression/HIV
- Chronic cardiopulmonary disease
- Surgery
- Advanced age
- Renal failure
- Fever >39°C
- Hyponatremia
- Liver dysfunction
- Creatine kinase elevation

ETIOLOGY

- *Legionella pneumophila*, a weak gram-negative organism, is a saprophytic water bacterium, which is widely distributed in soil and water. Serogroups 1, 2, and 6 account for most of the cases. The optimum temperature for growth is 40–45°C. It can also be associated with organic material in sediment.

- Mode of transmission
  - Aerosolization
  - Aspiration
  - Direct instillation into the lungs by equipment (such as respiratory equipment)
  - Most important mode: Aerosolization and airborne dissemination of contaminated water
  - Patients may acquire by inhaling organisms while showering.
  - Recently, community outbreaks have been associated with whirlpools, spas, and fountains.

ASSOCIATED CONDITIONS

Pontiac fever: Self-limited flulike illness with pneumonia

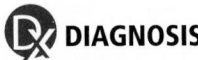 **DIAGNOSIS**

SIGNS AND SYMPTOMS

- Range of illness from asymptomatic seroconversion, mild febrile illness, to severe pneumonia
- Incubation 2–10 days
- Fever, chills
- Malaise, weakness, lethargy
- Anorexia
- Myalgia
- Headache
- Watery diarrhea in up to 50%
- Nausea and vomiting in 10–20%
- Dry cough which may become productive
- Pleuritic chest pain in up to 33%
- Relative bradycardia in up to 67% of patients
- Neuropsychiatric symptoms of confusion, disorientation, obtundation, depression, hallucinations, insomnia, seizures in up to 25%
- Blood-streaked sputum; gross hemoptysis rare
- Hyponatremia
- Hypophosphatemia
- Elevated serum transaminases
- Elevated creatine kinase
- ~50% of hospitalized patients present with PO_2 <60 mm Hg
- Hypotension (17%)
- Wound infections with *Legionella* have been reported.

History
- Elicit immunosuppression risk factors.
- Elicit characteristics about cough (may not be productive).
- Chest pain with hemoptysis can occur.
- Gastrointestinal symptoms with diarrhea and nausea are frequent.

Physical Exam
Rales with signs of consolidation. Fever is usually present.

TESTS

Lab
- Disorders that may alter lab results: Direct immunofluorescence can cross-react with *Pseudomonas* and *Bacteroides* sp., *E. coli*, and *Haemophilus*.
- Special tests: Silver and Gimenez stains for lung tissue/specimens
- Nonspecific abnormalities may include renal and hepatic dysfunction, thrombocytopenia, hyponatremia, and hematuria
- Gold standard is sputum culture for *Legionella*. Alert lab about possible diagnosis (buffered charcoal yeast extract agar)
- Urinary antigen detects serogroup 1 (which causes most human disease)
- The combination of respiratory specimen cultures and urine *Legionella* antigen testing is optimal for diagnosis.

Imaging
Chest radiograph

- Not specific for *Legionella*
- Commonly with lower lobe patchy alveolar infiltrate with consolidation, usually unilateral
- Cavitation or abscess, especially in immunocompromised
- Pleural effusion in up to 50%
- May take from 1–4 months for the radiograph to return to normal. Progression of infiltrate may be seen despite antibiotic therapy.

Diagnostic Procedures/Surgery
Transtracheal aspiration or bronchoscopy for sputum/lung samples

Pathological Findings
- Multifocal pneumonia with alveolitis and bronchiolitis, with fibrinous pleuritis; may have serous or serosanguineous pleural effusion
- Abscess formation occurs in up to 20% of patients.
- Progression of infiltrates, despite appropriate therapy, may be suggestive of Legionnaires' disease. Also, improvement on radiograph may not correlate with clinical findings (longer lag times on radiographic findings).

DIFFERENTIAL DIAGNOSIS

- Other bacterial pneumonias
- Atypical pneumonias with *Mycoplasma* and *Chlamydia*
- Viral pneumonias

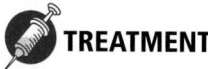 TREATMENT

GENERAL MEASURES
- Appropriate health care: The severity of the illness and the support available in the outpatient setting will dictate the appropriate site for care.
- Supportive care
- Maintaining oxygenation, hydration, and electrolyte balance while providing antibiotic therapy

 MEDICATION (DRUGS)

First Line
- Antibiotics that achieve high intracellular concentrations are most effective (macrolides, rifampin, tetracyclines, and quinolones)
- Levofloxacin may be preferred agent
- Levofloxacin 500 mg IV/d (switch to PO when patient is afebrile) times 10–14 days
- Azithromycin 500 mg IV/PO q24 times 7–10 days
- Addition of rifampin: 600 mg q12h PO or IV; this should be provided along with the above recommendations in very ill patients.
- Contraindications: Hypersensitivity reactions
- Precautions: Liver disease
- Significant possible interactions
  – Can increase theophylline, carbamazepine, and digoxin levels; can increase activity of oral anticoagulants.
  – May decrease the effectiveness of oral anticoagulants, steroids, digoxin, quinidine, oral contraceptives, and hypoglycemic agents.

Second Line
- Erythromycin 30–60 mg/kg/d PO or IV, divided into 4 doses for 10–21 days
- May be used along with rifampin
  – 100 mg q12h IV for 2 doses, then 100 mg b.i.d. or PO 200 mg for 1 dose, then 100 mg b.i.d.
  – 100 mg IV or PO q12h
- Sulfamethoxazole IV or PO: 5 mg/kg TMP q8h

 FOLLOW-UP

DISPOSITION
Admission Criteria
- Inability to tolerate oral antibiotics
- Hypoxemia

Discharge Criteria
- Afebrile
- Able to tolerate oral antibiotics

PROGNOSIS
- Recovery is variable; some patients experience rapid improvement with defervescence in 3–5 days and recovery is complete in 6–10 days, whereas others may have a much more protracted course despite treatment.
- Mortality rate can approach 50% with nosocomial infections.

COMPLICATIONS
- Dehydration
- Hyponatremia
- Respiratory insufficiency requiring ventilator support
- Endocarditis (most common extrapulmonary site)
- Disseminated intravascular coagulation
- Renal failure
- Multiple organ dysfunction syndrome (MODS)
- Coma
- Death occurs in 10% of the treated nonimmunocompromised patients and in up to 80% of the untreated immunocompromised patients.
- Bacteremia or abscess formation occurs in the immunocompromised.

PATIENT MONITORING
- Respiratory status, hydration, and electrolyte status should be monitored closely.
- A chest radiograph is not useful to monitor the clinical response.

ADDITIONAL READING
- Mulazimoglu L, Yu VL. Can Legionnaires disease be diagnosed by clinical criteria? *A critical review.* Chest. 2001;120:1049.
- Tan MJ, Tan JS, Hamor RH, et al. The radiologic manifestations of Legionnaire's disease. The Ohio Community-Based Pneumonia Incidence Study Group. *Chest.* 2000;117:398.
- Fields BS, Benson RF, Besser RE. Legionella and Legionnaires' disease: 25 years of investigation. *Clin Microbiol Rev.* 2002;15:506.
- Blazquez RM, Espinosa FJ, Martinez-Toldos CM, et al. Sensitivity of urinary antigen test in relation to clinical severity in a large outbreak of Legionella pneumonia in Spain. *Eur J Clin Microbiol Infect Dis.* 2005;24:488.

 MISCELLANEOUS

- See also: Pneumonia, bacterial
- Extrapulmonary disease can occur in the form of
  – Encephalitis
  – Cellulitis
  – Sinusitis
  – Pancreatitis
  – Pyelonephritis
  – Endocarditis
  – Pericarditis
  – Perirectal abscess

CODES

ICD9-CM
- 482.83 Pneumonia due to other gram-negative bacteria
- 482.84 Legionnaires disease

PATIENT TEACHING
- Educate patients regarding prevention/avoidance measures, lowering their risk status and if infected already, about the expected course of the disease.
- Disease prevention: Elimination of the pathogens from water supplies
- Person-to-person transmission has not been observed.

L

LEISHMANIASIS

Ryung Suh, MD, MPP, MBA, MPH
Brent R. Gibson, MD, MPH

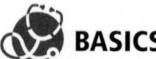 **BASICS**

DESCRIPTION

- An infective condition caused by several species of the protozoan *Leishmania*. The vector for the disease is the sandfly; the leishmaniasis parasite infects the host's leukocytes via inoculation with the promastigote form of the organism.
- 4 major clinical syndromes are recognized
  - Visceral leishmaniasis (kala azar, black fever) may be endemic, epidemic, or sporadic. Different forms are
    - African kala azar: Found in eastern 1/2 of Africa from Sahara in the north to Equator. Disease of older children and young adults (ages 10–25 years); Males > Females.
    - Mediterranean or infantile kala azar: Seen primarily in the Mediterranean area, China, and Latin America. Dogs, jackals, foxes, and rats are potential reservoirs. The strains responsible for the Mediterranean and American disease are sometimes referred to as *Leishmania infantum* and *Leishmania chagasi*, respectively.
    - Indian kala azar: Age and sex distribution similar to that of African kala azar. Humans are the only known reservoir; transmission is by anthropophilic sandflies.
  - Cutaneous leishmaniasis of the Old and New Worlds: Characterized by 1 or more localized lesions on exposed areas. These ulcerate centrally and spread centrifugally. Spontaneous healing is less common in New World disease. Satellite lesions and lymphadenopathy may or may not occur.
  - Mucocutaneous leishmaniasis (espundia): 1 or more lesions on the legs that may ulcerate. In 2–5% of patients, metastatic lesions appear in the nasopharynx after months or years, and may result in painful, mutilating erosions of soft tissue. Lesions may occur rarely in perineum.
- Diffuse cutaneous leishmaniasis: Extensive skin lesions but no visceral lesions. Clinical picture may be similar to that of lepromatous leprosy.
- System(s) Affected: Gastrointestinal; Hemic/lymphatic/immunologic; Pulmonary; Skin/exocrine
- Several notable emerging issues with this increasingly widespread disease (2)
  - Northward spread of disease (*L. infantum*) from endemic areas of Italy
  - Canine leishmaniasis in North America
  - Occurrence of unusual species in known endemic areas
  - Identification of cats and horses as new animal reservoirs
  - Decline of HIV-leishmaniasis infection in certain areas
- Synonym(s): Visceral leishmaniasis; Kala azar; Black fever; Dumdum fever

GENERAL PREVENTION

- Use of pesticides, especially synthetic pyrethroids, against sandflies. Resistance to DDT is high in many areas.
- Insect repellants for travelers
- Permethrin-coated fine netting for travelers
- Early diagnosis and treatment of human cases
- Elimination of animal reservoirs

- Deltamethrin-treated collars fitted to dogs have reduced incidence of the disease in children in the treated areas.
- Currently no vaccine other than for *L. major* (discontinued because of poor tolerability), but vaccine development appears feasible and promising.

EPIDEMIOLOGY

- Predominant age
  - Children and young adults (10–25 years). Mediterranean or infantile kala azar, usually <4 years of age
- Predominant sex
  - African kala azar, Indian kala aza: Male > Female
- The disease is widely distributed and found in 88 nations, the majority of which are in the developing world (1).
- The distribution of cutaneous and visceral forms of leishmaniasis are distinct but overlapping. The majority of VL is found in Bangladesh, India, Nepal, Sudan, and Brazil, whereas the majority of CL is found in Afghanistan, Algeria, Brazil, Iran, Peru, Saudi Arabia, and Syria (1).

Incidence

- According to World Health Organization (WHO), annual worldwide incidence of cutaneous leishmaniasis (CL) is 1–1.5 million; that of visceral leishmaniasis (VL) is 12 million. The overall prevalence is 350 million (1).
- 2 confirmed cases of visceral leishmaniasis have been reported in US military personnel who returned to the US after serving in Afghanistan from 2002–2004.

ALERT

Pediatric Considerations

- Pediatric Mediterranean or infantile kala azar is usually a disease of children <4 years of age.
- African or Indian kala azar is usually a disease of children and young adults (10–25 years).

RISK FACTORS

- In endemic areas, children are affected more than young adults.
- Malnutrition
- AIDS (coinfection is a recognized entity)
- Incomplete therapy of initial disease
- Nonimmune people migrating to or working in endemic areas (military deployments, seasonal migration, urbanization, etc.).

ETIOLOGY

Several species of *Leishmania*, including *L. donovani* (kala-azar), *L. infantum*, *L. chagasi* (Mediterranean and American forms), *L. tropica* (cutaneous form), *L. major* (in Middle East, Afghanistan, and India), *L. mexicana*, *L. braziliensis*, and others. Organisms are transmitted by female sandflies of the genus *Phlebotomus* in the Old World and *Lutzomyia* in the New World.

ASSOCIATED CONDITIONS

Fulminant kala azar has been described in association with AIDS and malnutrition.

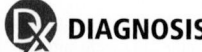 **DIAGNOSIS**

SIGNS AND SYMPTOMS

- Incubation period: ~3 months for the visceral form and 2–24 months for others
- Onset: Insidious/abrupt
- Malabsorption; failure to thrive in infants and children
- Fever: Nocturnal, no signs of toxemia
- Cough
- Diarrhea, gastrointestinal bleeding
- Lymphadenopathy
- Splenomegaly
- Moderate hepatomegaly
- Cirrhosis, portal hypertension (in 10% of patients)
- Anemia, pancytopenia
- Cutaneous lesions: May ulcerate and heal spontaneously
- Nasal stuffiness
- Epistaxis
- Edema, cachexia, and hyperpigmentation in late stages
- Hypoalbuminemia
- Hypergammaglobulinemia

TESTS

- Leishmanin skin test: Positive 6–8 weeks after recovery in cutaneous forms but not in diffuse leishmaniasis. Negative in visceral leishmaniasis.
- Monoclonal antibodies or hybridization of tissue touch blots with labeled kinetoplast DNA probes: Used for identification of different strains of *Leishmania*
- ELISA is sensitive and specific in visceral disease.
- Montenegro skin test: Nonstandardized and used only in epidemiologic studies. Negative in visceral leishmaniasis.
- Immunochromatographic strip test for rapid detection of antibodies to leishmania antigen rK39

Lab

- Demonstration of parasites in
  - Splenic aspirate: Most sensitive
  - Bone marrow aspirate
  - Lymph node aspirate or biopsy
  - Biopsy material from suspicious skin lesions after cleaning with alcohol to reduce bacterial contamination
- The intracellular amastigote form in the macrophages, formerly known as the Leishman-Donovan (LD) body, has a characteristic pear-shaped body with a dark circular nucleus and short rod-shaped kinetoplasts.
- Hypergammaglobulinemia
- Direct agglutination test detects IgM antibody, which indicates acute disease.

Diagnostic Procedures/Surgery

- Demonstration of the organism by smear or culture from aspirate or biopsy material. Novy-MacNeal-Nicolle medium or other liquid media used for cultures are maintained at 22–28°C for 21 days. Motile promastigotes can be observed microscopically.
- Speciation using monoclonal antibody or labeled DNA probes is unlikely to be cost effective.

Pathological Findings
- Marked lymphocytic infiltration
- Ulcerating lesions in the skin and mucosa of nasopharynx

DIFFERENTIAL DIAGNOSIS
- Malaria
- Brucellosis
- Tuberculosis
- Typhoid
- Hepatic abscess
- Lepromatous leprosy for diffuse leishmaniasis: Post–kala azar dermal lesion (PKDL) must be differentiated from leprosy, syphilis, and yaws.

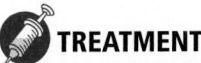 TREATMENT

INITIAL STABILIZATION
Inpatient care for blood transfusions and complicating superinfections. Outpatient care once the condition stabilizes.

GENERAL MEASURES
- Bed rest, oral hygiene, and good nutrition are important.
- Transfusions for anemia and antibacterial chemotherapy for bacterial complications must supplement specific therapy.
- Periodic electrocardiographic monitoring during prolonged therapy with pentavalent antimonials

Diet
Rich in nutritients

Activity
Bed rest during acute stages. Level of activity depends on severity of disease and organ systems involved.

 MEDICATION (DRUGS)

First Line
- Sodium antimony (Sb5 +) gluconate (Pentostam) 100 mg Sb5 + /mL IV/IM; single daily dose of 20 mg/kg for 20–30 days.
- Meglumine antimonate (Glucantime) 85 mg Sb5 + /mL; same dose and duration of treatment as above may also be used
- In the U.S., these drugs are available only from the Centers for Disease Control and Prevention, Atlanta, GA 30333; emergency telephone (404) 639-2888 (www.cdc.gov).
- Relapses and incomplete responses should be treated with the same regimen for 40–60 days. Addition of oral allopurinol (Zyloprim) 20–30 mg/kg/d in 3 divided doses has been effective.
- According to some experts, Miltefosine is effective in treating visceral leishmaniasis. Approved for use in India, Germany, and Colombia. Administered in a 28-day course, and currently has very high efficacy. The dosing schedule in India for visceral leishmaniasis is 2.5 mg/kg (100 mg/d) for 28 days (94% cure rate). Effective in the cutaneous form at 133 mg and 150 mg daily (3, 4)[B].
- Contraindications: Refer to manufacturer's profile for each drug.
- Precautions: Refer to manufacturer's profile for each drug. Periodic ECG monitoring is recommended during prolonged therapy.
- Significant possible interactions: Refer to manufacturer's profile for each drug.

Second Line
- Relapses with drug-resistant organisms are usually treated with:
  - Amphotericin B (Fungizone) 0.5–1 mg/kg IV on alternate days
  - Liposomal amphotericin B: excellent for visceral leishmaniasis. It has been administered IV at a total dose of 21 mg/kg given at 3 mg/kg/d on days 1–5, 7, and 14.
- Or
  - Pentamidine (Pentam) 3–4 mg/kg IV 3 times a week for 5–25 weeks
  - In patients with concomitant HIV, the disease is resistant to all current drugs.
  - Paromomycin ointment has been shown to be effective for the cutaneous form.

SURGERY
- Adjunctive splenectomy
- Reconstructive surgery for tissue damage

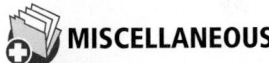 FOLLOW-UP

PROGNOSIS
With early treatment, cure rate is >90%, although in advanced cases, mortality remains at 15–25%. In untreated cases, death occurs in 3–20 months in up to 95% of adults and 85% of children.

COMPLICATIONS
- Edema, cachexia, hyperpigmentation in late stages
- Superinfections and gastrointestinal bleeding may cause death in untreated patients with visceral disease (kala azar).
- 3–10% of treated cases develop PKDL, characterized by depigmented macules and wartlike nodules over the face and extensor surfaces of the limbs.
- Metastatic lesions in the nasopharynx, with tissue destruction in patients with mucocutaneous leishmaniasis

PATIENT MONITORING
- Follow-up at 3 and 12 months to detect relapses
- PKDL should be treated in the same fashion as the initial illness.
- Periodic monitoring of electrocardiogram, liver function, and renal function during prolonged therapy

REFERENCES
1. Desjeux, P. Leishmaniasis: current situation and new perspectives. *Comp Imunol Microbiol infec Dis*. 2004;27:305–318.
2. Gramiccia M, Gradoni L. The current status of zoonotic leishmaniasis and approaches to disease control. *Int J Parasito*. 35:1169–1180.
3. Murray HW, Berman JD, Davies OR, Saravia NG. Advances in leishmaniasis. *Lancet*. 2005;366: 1561–1577.
4. Sundar S, Jha TK, Thakur CP, et al. Oral miltefosine for Indian visceral leishmaniasis. *N Engl J Med*. 2002;347:1739–1746.

MISCELLANEOUS

CODES

ICD9-CM
- 085.0 Leishmaniasis, visceral (kala azar)
- 085.9 Leishmaniasis, unspecified

PATIENT TEACHING
- Explain prevention measures.
- Help for patients: www.cdc.gov/ncidod/dpd/parasites/leishmania

L

LEPROSY

Jane Y. Yu, MD

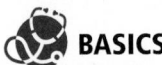 **BASICS**

DESCRIPTION
- A chronic granulomatous infection caused by *Mycobacterium leprae*, an acid-fast bacillus preferentially affecting cooler regions of the body (e.g., skin, mucous membranes, peripheral nerves)
- Classification (World Health Organization [WHO] system most frequently used)
  - Paucibacillary (PB): No more than 5 skin lesions; no detectable bacilli on skin smears
  - Multibacillary (MB): 6 or more lesions; may be skin-smear positive
- Classification (Ridley-Jopling) based on skin/neurologic changes and biopsy
  - Indeterminate (I), tuberculoid (TT), borderline tuberculoid (BT), mid-borderline (MB), borderline lepromatous (BL), lepromatous (LL)
- System(s) Affected: Endocrine/Metabolic, Hemic/Lymphatic/Immunologic, Musculoskeletal, Nervous, Pulmonary, Reproductive, Skin/Exocrine
- Synonym(s): Hansen disease

GENERAL PREVENTION
- Early case finding to suppress infectiousness and control spread
- Antileprosy prophylaxis not recommended by WHO

EPIDEMIOLOGY
- In recent decades, multidrug therapy (MDT) and WHO's efforts at eliminating leprosy have had a great impact on leprosy control (>10 million patients cured in last 15 years).
- Highest rates of endemic disease in India, Brazil, Madagascar, Mozambique, Myanmar, and Nepal
- May present at any age, although cases in infants <1 year are extremely rare
- Male : Female = 1.5:1

Incidence
Rare in the US: 118 cases in 1999, mostly among immigrants

ALERT
Pediatric Considerations
Rare in infants <1 year

Prevalence
- Prevalence rate has dropped from 21 per 10 K in 1985 to 2.8 in 2000
- 641,091 registered cases worldwide in 2000

RISK FACTORS
- Close family contacts of untreated leprosy patients have 8-fold increased risk.
- Impaired cell-mediated immunity
- Poor socioeconomic status

Genetics
Specific HLA-associated genes may be linked to different classes of disease

PATHOPHYSIOLOGY
- Spread via respiratory transmission, possibly via broken skin
- Widespread dissemination once respiratory tract is infected

ETIOLOGY
M. leprae: Incubation period is frequently 3–5 years, although a range of 6 months to several decades has been seen.

ASSOCIATED CONDITIONS
HIV-positive patients with early or subclinical leprosy more likely to develop overt disease. Concurrent leprosy may accelerate HIV disease course.

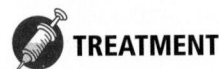 **DIAGNOSIS**

SIGNS AND SYMPTOMS
- Consider diagnosis in patient with skin lesions or enlarged nerves with sensory loss
- Sensory loss in typical skin patch or ulnar nerve thickening may aid in diagnosis (1)[C].

History
Known or suspected contact with patient with leprosy

Physical Exam
- Indeterminate leprosy
  - 1 or more hypopigmented or hyperpigmented macules
  - Anesthetic patches, although sensation is preserved in early stages
- TT
  - Initial hypopigmented, hypesthetic macules with sharp demarcations
  - Nerve involvement occurs early: Ulnar, peroneal (foot drop), and greater auricular nerves may be palpably and visibly enlarged; neuritic pain; muscle atrophy—small muscles of the hand; facial nerve involvement leads to lagophthalmos, keratitis, and corneal ulceration.
- LL
  - More generalized, sometimes nondistinct lesions
  - Nerve involvement occurs later; affects distal extremities initially

TESTS
Lab
- Demonstration of acid-fast bacilli in skin smears made by scraped-incision method
- Histologic involvement of peripheral nerves pathognomonic
- Mild anemia, elevated ESR, hyperglobulinemia
- Serodiagnostic assay: Detects antibody to phenolic glycolipid 1; sensitivity of >95% in LL and ~30% in TT
- Detection of *M. leprae* in tissue by polymerase chain reaction

Diagnostic Procedures/Surgery
Skin biopsy

Pathological Findings
- TT: Noncaseating granulomas containing lymphocytes, epithelioid cells, and perhaps giant cells; bacilli difficult to demonstrate
- LL: Granulomas comprising macrophages, large foam cells, and many intracellular bacilli frequently in spheroidal masses
- Borderline leprosy: Granulomas change from epithelioid cell predominance in BT to a macrophage predominance as the lepromatous pole is approached.

DIFFERENTIAL DIAGNOSIS
- Lupus erythematosus
- Lupus vulgaris
- Sarcoidosis
- Yaws
- Dermal leishmaniasis
- Other skin conditions
- Peripheral neuropathy
- Syringomyelia

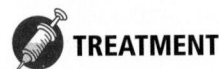 **TREATMENT**

Multidrug therapy (MDT) for fixed durations has been associated with a decline in the prevalence of leprosy (1)[A].

INITIAL STABILIZATION
Outpatient care usually; except in reactional states, in which inpatient care is called for

GENERAL MEASURES
- Multidisciplinary approach including orthopedic surgery, ophthalmology, and physical therapy in addition to specific drugs
- Rigid-soled footwear or walking plaster casts to prevent plantar ulcers
- Physical therapy and casts prevent hand contractures
- Vocational retraining and rehabilitation along with psychologic support
- Immediate recognition and treatment of eye problems are essential.
- Manage mild reactional states such as reversal reaction and erythema nodosum leprosum (ENL) with bed rest, analgesics, and sedatives. Severe reactions require corticosteroids, thalidomide, or clofazimine. Specific therapy must be continued without interruption.

Diet
Nutritious, balanced diet

Activity
Depends on severity of disease

MEDICATION (DRUGS)

First Line
- Multidrug therapy (MDT) standard for treatment
- In US (where patients are considered to have more active disease)
  - PB: Rifampin 600 mg PO daily + dapsone 100 mg PO daily; treat for 1 year
  - MB: Rifampin 600 mg PO daily + dapsone 100 mg PO daily + clofazimine 50 mg PO daily; treat for 2 years
- Outside US (WHO regimen)
  - PB: Rifampin 600 mg PO monthly + dapsone 100 mg PO daily; treat for 6 months
  - MB: Rifampin 600 mg PO monthly + clofazimine 300 mg PO monthly + dapsone 100 mg PO daily + clofazimine 50 mg PO daily; treat for 1 year
- Contraindications
  - Clofazimine and minocycline: Pregnancy
  - Ofloxacin: Relative contraindication in children and adolescents
  - Minocycline in pregnancy, during lactation, and in children up to 5 years old
- Precautions
  - Hemolysis and methemoglobinemia are common untoward reactions to dapsone.
  - Screen for glucose 6-phosphate dehydrogenase deficiency to prevent drug-induced hemolysis.
  - Reactionary states should be anticipated and treated aggressively.
  - Dapsone: Gastrointestinal upset, headaches, pruritus, agranulocytosis, fever, rash
  - Clofazimine: Gastrointestinal upset and skin pigmentation
  - Minocycline: Reduce dosage in renal damage

Second Line
Weak evidence for shorter regimens or newer drug combinations (2)[A]

ALERT
Clofazimine and minocycline contraindicated during pregnancy; dapsone may be used.

Pediatric Considerations
Minocycline is contraindicated in children <5 years.

SURGERY
- Reconstructive surgery: Nerve and tendon transplants, release of contractures, and other cosmetic procedures may give more functional mobility and social acceptance.
- Tarsorrhaphy or horizontal lid shortening for lagophthalmos with lid gap >5 mm or even lesser degree in patients with 1 eye. Cataract surgery with posterior chamber intraocular lens implantation to avoid glasses in patients with nasal bridge collapse.

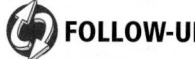 **FOLLOW-UP**

PROGNOSIS
- Generally indolent, but may be interrupted by ENL and type 1 lepra reaction. Prognosis is good with early detection and therapy, especially with ROM.
- May show gradual clearing of skin lesions within 1st year

COMPLICATIONS
- Crippling of the hand and foot
- Trauma and secondary infection leading to loss of digits and extremities
- Corneal opacities and uveitis may lead to blindness.
- Cataracts
- Lucio phenomenon—arteritis
- Secondary amyloidosis
- ENL: Therapy with thalidomide 200 mg b.i.d., tapering to 50–100 mg/d in chronic patients
- Severe reversal reaction: Prednisolone 40–60 mg/d, tapering slowly

PATIENT MONITORING
- Frequent follow-up visits until therapy course is stabilized, then monthly supervision
- Drug toxicity uncommon after 1st year of treatment
- Periodic complete blood count, renal and hepatic function
- Yearly skin scrapings from most active sites if possible

REFERENCES
1. Saunderson P, Groenen G. Which physical signs help most in the diagnosis of leprosy? *Lepr Rev.* 2000;71:34–42.
2. Britton WJ, Lockwood DN. Leprosy. *Lancet.* 2004; 363:1209–1219.
3. Lockwood DN, Kumar B. Treatment of leprosy. *BMJ.* 2004;328:1447.

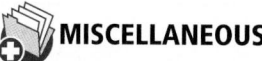 **MISCELLANEOUS**

The National Hansen's Disease Programs (NHDP) Baton Rouge, LA (800) 642-2477 provides consultation for physicians.

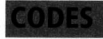 **CODES**

ICD9-CM
030.9 Leprosy, unspecified

PATIENT TEACHING
- Educate about the indolent course of the disease and importance of therapeutic completion.
- Information pamphlets and awareness to ease psychologic trauma and stigma, emphasizing that a cure is possible with newer drug regimen
- Encourage case reporting, because early treatment may prevent/reduce tissue damage and deformities.

L

LEUKEMIA

Mark R. Dambro, MD

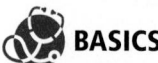 **BASICS**

DESCRIPTION

- Proliferation and accumulation of abnormal immature blood cell progenitors (blasts) in the bone marrow and other tissues. The outstanding characteristic is the development of marrow failure. Intracerebral leukostasis may develop if the blood blast count becomes greatly elevated.
- Classified according to the type of blast and according to the course, if untreated
  - Acute lymphoblastic leukemia (ALL)
  - Acute nonlymphoblastic leukemia (ANLL)
  - Chronic myelocytic leukemia (CML)
  - Chronic lymphocytic leukemia (CLL)
- System(s) Affected: Hemic/Lymphatic/Immunologic

ALERT

Geriatric Considerations

- Older patients do not tolerate allogenic bone marrow transplant. Age 50 is usual cutoff for transplant.
- Autologous transplant may be tried in patients >50, if no organ failure is present and performance status is good.
- Adding granulocyte-macrophage colony stimulating factor (GM-CSF) to induction for ANLL patients ≥60 years significantly reduced toxicity and made induction a feasible option in this patient profile.

Pediatric Considerations

Tolerate intense treatments better.

Pregnancy Considerations

Chemotherapy is a viable option in the 2nd and 3rd trimesters.

EPIDEMIOLOGY

- Predominant age
  - 70% occurs in adults, mostly CLL and ANLL
  - 30% in children, mostly ALL
  - With the current cure rate especially good for childhood ALL, it is estimated that, by the year 2010, 1 in 1,000 young adults (15–45 years of age) in the U.S. will be a childhood ALL survivor.
- Predominant sex: Males > females

Incidence

- Male: 13.2:100,000
- Female: 7.7:100,000

RISK FACTORS

- Genetic and chromosomal abnormalities (e.g., trisomy 21, breakage and translocation, especially t9,22. Also AML, MLL, genes)
- MLL gene for mixed lineage leukemia located on chromosome 11q23. Its abnormalities and rearrangements are easier detected with fluorescent in situ hybridization (FISH) or polymerase chain reaction (PCR). Most rearrangements in this gene result in aggressive AML, secondary AML (after chemotherapy), and infant leukemia. Example: t(11;19)(q23;p13) (MLL-ENL).
- t(12;21)(p13,q22) detected by FISH and by screening for TEL/AML1 rearrangement by PCR is now known to be the most common rearrangement in childhood ALL and carries a favorable prognosis.
- Radiation exposure
- Immunodeficiency states
- Chemical and drug exposure (nitrogen mustard and benzene)
- Preleukemia
- Cigarette smoking

Genetics

Unknown, some are familial

ETIOLOGY

Precise causes unknown

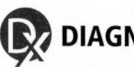 **DIAGNOSIS**

SIGNS AND SYMPTOMS

- Mostly nonspecific and related to marrow failure or infiltration
  - Fever
  - Bleeding (e.g., petechiae, purpura, easy bruising, or oozing)
  - Bone pain, pallor, fatigue
  - Splenomegaly
  - Hepatosplenomegaly
  - Lymphadenopathy
- If CNS is involved, symptoms of increased intracranial pressure can be present
- Gingival swelling

TESTS

Lab

- CBC, differential, platelets show subnormal RBC, neutrophils, and possibly subnormal platelets
- In some types, no circulating leukemic blasts need be present to establish the diagnosis. If 2 of the 3 above parameters are affected, or only 1 profoundly decreased, bone marrow failure should be ruled out.
- Reticulocyte count <0.5
- ESR usually elevated
- LDH and uric acid can be elevated.
- Immunoglobulin (IG) can be low or rarely elevated.
- Coagulation profile can be normal or prolonged, especially in promyelocytic leukemia (ANLL subtype).
- Drugs that may alter lab results: Chemotherapy agents, especially corticosteroids. Don't prescribe these before finalizing the bone marrow studies. Some leukemic blasts are very sensitive and can have massive cell kill from as little as 1 dose of corticosteroids.
- Special tests: Spinal tap may reveal fluid with leukemic cells.

Imaging

- Chest radiograph may reveal a large mediastinal mass.
- Ultrasonography or CT scan of the abdomen may discover organomegaly.

Diagnostic Procedures/Surgery

- Bone marrow studies are necessary to make the final diagnosis.
- Aspirates are stained with a buffered Wright's stain and provide good resolution for cell morphology.
- Biopsies are demineralized, sectioned, and stained with hematoxylin-eosin (H&E) stain. They provide valuable information for cellularity, architecture, and megakaryocytic series.
- Marrow cell suspension used for
  - Cytochemistries (e.g., myeloperoxidase and Sudan black are positive in myeloblasts)
  - Immunophenotyping especially useful for lymphoid leukemia and can indicate whether it is monoclonal or polyclonal, B lymphocytes or T lymphocytes, early, or late, etc.
  - Chromosome studies will show the ploidy and/or the presence of a translocation, which is of prognostic value.
  - Immunofluorescent stain for terminal deoxyribonucleotide transferase (TdT), another marker that differentiates between myeloid and lymphoid blasts

Pathological Findings

- The marrow will be hypercellular and the normal architecture effaced.
- The percentage of leukemic cells compared to the remainder of the cell population is usually >30%.
- The liver, spleen, and kidneys can be enlarged and infiltrated with leukemic cells.

DIFFERENTIAL DIAGNOSIS

- Viral induced cytopenia, lymphadenopathy, and organomegaly
- Immune cytopenias
- Drug 2-induced cytopenias
- Other marrow failure and infiltrative diseases: Aplastic, hypoblastic, and refractory anemias; paroxysmal nocturnal hemoglobinuria; myelodysplastic syndromes, Gaucher disease

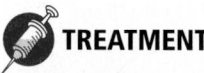 **TREATMENT**

INITIAL STABILIZATION

- Consult with a chemotherapist.
- Induction for acute leukemia treatment requires inpatient care.

GENERAL MEASURES

- Assessment of liver, heart, and kidney functions and performance status
- In acute leukemia induction, establish good hydration and urine flow (especially in ALL patients).
- Give platelet transfusion if platelet count is <20,000 or if patient is having bleeding symptoms.
- Avoid aspirin products.
- Give packed red blood cell transfusion if patient is symptomatic from the anemia (e.g., orthostatic hypotension, dizziness, fatigue, hyperactive precordium) or if a cerebral or a cardiopulmonary problem is present.

- If the absolute neutrophil count (ANC) <1,000, exert close temperature monitoring. (ANC = WBC × (percentage of Polys + Bands) ÷ 100). If patient becomes febrile (even low-grade fever), appropriate cultures should be taken and patient placed on broad-spectrum IV antibiotics covering *Pseudomonas* and gram-positive bacteria.
- Isolation (when the absolute neutrophil count is low) has no value, because the majority of the infecting agents in this situation are the patient's own normal flora of the skin, mouth, or gut.
- In promyelocytic leukemia (ANLL subtype), patients are especially at risk for DIC when treatment is started. Heparinization is indicated with close follow-up of coagulation parameters.

Diet
- Ensure adequately balanced calorie/vitamin intake.
- Follow weight closely.

Activity
Ambulatory as tolerated; no intense or contact sports; no aspirin due to low platelets

MEDICATION (DRUGS)

First Line
- Medical treatment changes frequently as a result of research.
- ALL
  – Induction: Vincristine plus prednisone plus asparaginase with or without doxorubicin or daunorubicin. CNS prophylaxis, intrathecal methotrexate with or without cranial irradiation. Add cyclophosphamide for adult ALL.
  – Maintenance: Vincristine, prednisone, mercaptopurine (6-mercaptopurine) daily and methotrexate weekly for 2–3 years
  – Intensification with IV methotrexate without rescue for children or with IV cyclophosphamide, cytarabine, 6-mercaptopurine, 6-thioguanine with or without 3 weeks of induction-like regimen is used for both adult and children with ALL.
- ANLL
  – Induction: Cytarabine plus daunorubicin, cytarabine plus idarubicin, or cytarabine plus mitoxantrone. Idarubicin seems to be superior to daunorubicin in the treatment of ANLL. Yeast-derived GM-CSF and granulocyte colony stimulating factor (G-CSF) do not stimulate leukemia cell growth, but help in the resolution of marrow hypoplasia associated with chemotherapy.
  – Maintenance: Combined agents and high-dose cytarabine (ARA-C) with timed sequence
- Promyelocytic leukemia
  – All-*trans*-retinoic acid (ATRA) promotes maturation to normal granulocyte and provides remissions with lower toxicity.
  – Arsenic is showing success in relapse.
- CLL: An anti-CD33 monoclonal antibody has the potential for eradicating minimal residual disease.
  – Chlorambucil with or without prednisone used only if symptomatic or cytopenic. Fludarabine and cladribine (2-CDA) are showing great promise in refractory CLL. Fludarabine as a first-line therapy was effective with 81% response rate, and 2-CDA in a small study showed 85% response rate. New agents, such as somatostatin analog, cyclosporine, and theophylline, have significant activity in CLL.
  – Added measurements for CLL management can include splenectomy, leukophoresis, radiation therapy, pentostatin, and 2'-deoxycoformycin.

- Hairy cell leukemia: Interferon
- CML
  – In the chronic phase, an allogenic bone marrow transplantation is recommended; if not possible, busulfan, hydroxyurea, or interferon-α can prolong survival.
  – In the acute phase, daunorubicin plus cytarabine plus vincristine plus prednisone with or without thioguanine, or
  – STI571, a specific inhibitor of the BCR-ABL (oncogene) tyrosine kinase, has substantial activity in both chronic and blast crises in CML and in Philadelphia chromosome-positive ALL.
  – High dose cytarabine with or without daunorubicin
- Contraindications: No absolute contraindications
- Precautions
  – Administration of chemotherapy agents should be by skilled and specifically trained individuals. IV vincristine, daunorubicin, and doxorubicin may lead to chemical burns in the event of extravasation.
  – If liver injury, the toxicity of vincristine, anthracyclines, and antimetabolites can be pronounced. If liver injury is advanced and hyperbilirubinemia is present, avoid those medications or reduce dosage.
  – Avoid anthracyclines if patient has a pre-existing cardiac problem.
  – Close monitoring of the WBCs, polys, RBC, and platelets is required especially in CML (chronic phase or ALL maintenance in order not to induce profound myelotoxicity).
  – Patients will be immunosuppressed during treatment. Avoid live vaccines. Administer varicella-zoster or measles immunoglobulin as soon as exposure of a patient at risk becomes known.
- Significant possible interactions: Allopurinol accentuates the toxicity of 6-mercaptopurine.

SURGERY
- Bone marrow transplant
  – Allogenic bone marrow transplantation in 1st remission for ANLL is advocated if a matched sibling is available. Autologous bone marrow transplant is also acceptable in 1st remission.
  – Allogenic or autologous bone marrow transplant is acceptable in 1st remission in high-risk ALL, especially in adults. They are acceptable in 2nd remission for childhood ALL.
  – Early studies using an allogenic nonrelated matched donor seem to be promising and might replace the autologous route when a full sibling match is not available.

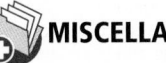

FOLLOW-UP

PROGNOSIS
- ALL remission rate is very good. In children, long-term survival is the rule.
- AML remission rate is 60–80%, with only 20–40% long-term survival
- CML invariably transforms into the acute phase within 2 years (median of 45 months). Afterward, survival rate is poor.
- CLL usually is asymptomatic for several years, especially Rai, stages 0–II. In Rai series the mean interval (in stages 0–II) is 5.3 years from diagnosis until therapy was needed. Median overall survival in CLL is thought to be 9 years.

COMPLICATIONS
- Side effects of chemotherapy
- Rarely in lymphoid leukemia, acute tumor lysis syndrome may develop leading to hyperuricemia, hyperkalemia, hyperphosphatemia, hypocalcemia, and/or uric acid nephropathy.
- Late-onset cardiomyopathy has been described in children treated with standard-dose anthracyclines.

PATIENT MONITORING
- Repeat bone marrow studies every week or every other week during induction of acute leukemia. Less frequently later. Also perform if a relapse is suspected.
- Follow uric acid level and urinary function.
- Physical evaluation, including weight and blood pressure, should be done with every treatment and as frequently as once a week.

REFERENCES

1. Devita VT Jr, Helman S, Rosenberg SA, eds. Cancer: Principles & Practice of Oncology, 3rd ed. Philadelphia: J.B. Lippincott, 1989.
2. The Medical Letter on Drugs and Therapeutics: Drugs of Choice for Cancer Chemotherapy. 1991; 33:840.
3. Yearbook of Hematology, 1997. St. Louis: Mosby, 1997.

MISCELLANEOUS

See also: Leukemia, acute lymphoblastic in adults (ALL)

CODES

ICD9-CM
- 202.40 Leukemic reticuloendotheliosis, unspecified site, extranodal and solid organ sites
- 204.00 Acute lymphoid leukemia without mention of remission
- 204.10 Chronic lymphoid leukemia
- 205.00 Acute myeloid leukemia without mention of remission
- 205.10 Chronic myeloid leukemia without mention of remission
- 206.00 Acute monocytic leukemia without mention of remission

PATIENT TEACHING
- Prognosis and treatment toxicity
- Leukemia Society of America: 33 Third Ave., New York, NY 10017, (212) 573-8484.
- NCI (Bethesda, Maryland) has pamphlets and telephone education.
- "You and Leukemia: A Day at a Time," by Dr. Lynn S. Baker, W. B. Saunders Co.

See Corresponding Diagnostic Algorithm

L

LEUKEMIA, ACUTE LYMPHOBLASTIC IN ADULTS (ALL)

Richard A. Larson, MD

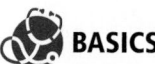 **BASICS**

DESCRIPTION
- A malignant proliferation and accumulation of immature lymphocytes
- System(s) Affected: Hemic/Lymphatic/Immunologic
- Synonym(s): Acute lymphocytic leukemia

ALERT
Pregnancy Considerations
Many chemotherapy drugs are teratogenic.

EPIDEMIOLOGY
- Predominant age: Median age is 35–40 years but incidence increases with age
- Predominant sex: Male > Female (slightly)

Incidence
In the US 1,000 adult cases/year

RISK FACTORS
- Age >60
- Incidence appears increased following exposure to chemical agents such as benzene or to radiation (but acute myeloid leukemia [AML] is more common).
- May follow aplastic anemia

Genetics
- Increased incidence in children with Down syndrome or in rare familial diseases such as ataxia-telangiectasia, Bloom syndrome, Fanconi anemia, Klinefelter syndrome, and neurofibromatosis
- Can rarely occur in adult identical twins

ETIOLOGY
Unknown. Epstein-Barr virus is implicated in Burkitt leukemia/lymphoma.

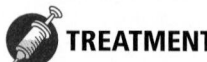 **DIAGNOSIS**

SIGNS AND SYMPTOMS
- Anemia: Fatigue, shortness of breath, lightheadedness, angina, headache
- Thrombocytopenia: Petechiae, ecchymoses, epistaxis, retinal hemorrhages
- Granulocytopenia: Fever, infection
- Lymphocytosis: Lymphadenopathy, hepato/splenomegaly, bone pain
- Immunosuppression
- Metabolic abnormalities: Hyperuricemia, renal failure, increased lactate dehydrogenase (LDH)
- Central nervous system: Cranial nerve palsies, confusion

TESTS
Lab
- Anemia: Normochromic, normocytic
- Thrombocytopenia
- Peripheral blood lymphoblasts
- Elevated LDH
- Elevated uric acid
- Special tests
  - Immunophenotyping of marrow/blood lymphoblasts: B-lineage (CD19, CD20, CD24): T-lineage (CD2, CD5, CD7); CALLA ([common ALL antigen], CD10); human leukocyte antigen (HLA)-DR; terminal deoxynucleotidyl transferase (TdT); aberrant myeloid antigens (CD13, CD33); stem cell antigen (CD34)
  - Cytochemical stains: Myeloperoxidase negative; Sudan black B usually negative; TdT positive; nonspecific esterase +/−; periodic acid Schiff (PAS) +/−
  - Cytogenetics: Specific recurring chromosomal abnormalities have independent diagnostic and prognostic significance (hyperdiploidy >50 chromosomes is favorable; the Philadelphia chromosome, t[9;22], t[4;11], −7, and +8 are unfavorable)
  - HLA typing of patient and siblings for marrow transplantation

Imaging
- Chest radiograph to evaluate for mediastinal mass or hilar adenopathy and for pulmonary infiltrates suggestive of infection
- Ultrasound exam to assess splenomegaly or renal enlargement suggestive of leukemic infiltration

Diagnostic Procedures/Surgery
- Bone marrow examination with aspiration, biopsy, immunophenotyping, cytochemistry, and cytogenetics
- Lymph node biopsy is rarely necessary but can be diagnostic.
- Lumbar puncture should be done if neurological symptoms or signs are present. Repeat lumbar puncture after bone marrow remission is achieved to evaluate occult CNS involvement.

Pathological Findings
Diffuse replacement of marrow and lymph node architecture by sheets of malignant lymphoblasts

DIFFERENTIAL DIAGNOSIS
- Malignant disorders: Other leukemias, especially AML; prolymphocytic leukemia; malignant lymphomas; multiple myeloma; bone marrow metastases from solid tumors (breast, prostate, lung, renal); myelodysplastic syndromes (1)[A]
- Nonmalignant disorders: Aplastic anemia; myelofibrosis; autoimmune diseases (Felty syndrome, lupus); infectious mononucleosis; autoimmune thrombocytopenic purpura; leukemoid reaction to infection

TREATMENT

GENERAL MEASURES
- Appropriate health care
  - Inpatient care during remission induction chemotherapy
  - Postremission therapy is usually outpatient.
  - Access to the resources and expertise of a major oncology center is important for appropriate support.
- Protective isolation from infection

Diet
- Nutritional support including IV hyperalimentation, if necessary
- Avoid alcohol.

Activity
Ambulatory as tolerated

SPECIAL THERAPY
Complementary and Alternative Medicine
Unproven and may result in dangerous drug interactions with chemotherapy

MEDICATION (DRUGS)

First Line

Optimal therapy is not yet known (2,3)[A]. All treatment regimens are still investigational, although clearly effective for some fraction of patients. CALGB protocol 9111 is an example of therapy (4)[A]

- Remission induction
  - Cyclophosphamide: 1,200 mg/m² on day 1 (800 mg/m² if > 60 years old)
  - Daunorubicin: 45 mg/m² on days 1, 2, and 3 (30 mg/m² if > 60 years old)
  - Vincristine: 2 mg on days 1, 8, 15, and 22
  - Asparaginase (L-asparaginase): 6,000 units/m² on days 5, 8, 11, 15, 18, and 22
  - Prednisone: 60 mg/m² on days 1–21 (days 1–7 if > 60 years old)
  - Filgrastim, G-CSF: 5 μg/kg per day SQ starting on day 4 has been shown to shorten the duration of neutropenia and improve the CR rate, especially in older patients
  - Imatinib mesylate: 600–800 mg/d is effective alone and in combination with chemotherapy for Philadelphia chromosome positive ALL
- Consolidation (repeat twice in 8 weeks)
  - Cyclophosphamide: 1,000 mg/m² on day 1
  - Intrathecal (IT) methotrexate: 15 mg with hydrocortisone 50 mg on day 1
  - Mercaptopurine (6-mercaptopurine): 60 mg/m² on days 1–14
  - Cytarabine: 75 mg/m² SC on days 1–4 and 8–11
  - Vincristine: 2 mg on days 15 and 22
  - Asparaginase: 6,000 units/m² on days 15, 18, 22, and 25
- CNS prophylaxis and interim maintenance—2400 cGy cranial irradiation
  - IT-methotrexate: 15 mg with hydrocortisone 50 mg on days 1, 8, 15, 22, and 29
  - Mercaptopurine (6-mercaptopurine): 60 mg/m² on days 1–70, taken in the evening
  - Oral methotrexate: 20 mg/m² on days 36, 43, 50, 57, and 64
- Late intensification
  - Doxorubicin: 30 mg/m² on days 1, 8, and 15
  - Vincristine: 2 mg on days 1, 8, and 15
  - Dexamethasone: 10 mg/m² on days 1–14
  - Cyclophosphamide: 1,000 mg/m² on day 29
  - Thioguanine (6-thioguanine): 60 mg/m² on days 29–42
  - Cytarabine: 75 mg/m² SC on days 29–32 and 36–39
- Prolonged maintenance
  - Vincristine: 2 mg/month for 16 months
  - Prednisone: 60 mg/m² for 5 days with the vincristine
  - Mercaptopurine (6-mercaptopurine): 60 mg/m² a day for 16 months, taken in the evening
  - Oral methotrexate: 20 mg/m²/wk for 16 months
  - **Philadelphia chromosome-positive ALL**
    - Imatinib mesylate (400–800 mg/d) is effective alone and in combination with chemotherapy.
  - Contraindications: Doses and schedule may need to be altered for older patients and for concurrent infection and organ toxicity.

- Precautions
  - Tumor lysis syndrome (elevated uric acid, potassium, and phosphate with decreased calcium leading to renal failure, disseminated intravascular coagulation, and cardiac arrhythmias) may be prevented by administering allopurinol 300 mg/d. Begin 2 days before chemotherapy begins. Reduce doses if used with mercaptopurine or azathioprine. Give increased fluids; IV urate oxidase (Rasburicase) can be used to treat hyperuricemia rapidly.
  - Oral sulfamethoxazole-trimethoprim or aerosolized pentamidine is given for *Pneumocystis carinii* prophylaxis.
  - Profound immunosuppression: Take appropriate precautions when patient is neutropenic.
  - High dose cyclophosphamide causes severe nausea and vomiting. Use appropriate antiemetic regimen to prevent.
  - Neurotoxicity, ileus with vincristine
  - Asparaginase may cause severe allergic reactions as well as impaired pancreatic and liver function. Monitor serum glucose concentrations frequently and carefully. Pancreatitis or thrombosis may occur.

Second Line

Other anthracyclines, investigational chemotherapy agents. Allogeneic hematopoietic stem cell transplantation is recommended for any patient with relapsed ALL.

SURGERY

Surgical placement of a percutaneous silastic double-lumen central venous catheter

FOLLOW-UP

PROGNOSIS

- ~80–95% of patients <60 years old will achieve a complete remission, and 35–60% will remain free of disease at 5 years. (5,6)[A]

- Older patients (>60 years) do less well, but still 80% may achieve a complete remission.
- Patients with unfavorable cytogenetic subtypes (especially t[9;22] and t[4:11]) should undergo allogeneic stem cell transplantation in 1st remission if an HLA-identical donor were available.

COMPLICATIONS

- Infections (*pneumocystis carinii* pneumonia, bacterial pneumonia or sepsis, fungal pneumonia)
- Bleeding
- Need for transfusions
- Sterility from treatment
- Arachnoiditis and CNS effects from intrathecal chemotherapy and irradiation
- Pancreatitis and liver dysfunction from chemotherapy
- Relapse of ALL in marrow or extramedullary sites (CNS, testis)

PATIENT MONITORING

- Daily during induction chemotherapy for metabolic and infectious complications
- Weekly during remission consolidation chemotherapy
- Monthly during maintenance therapy
- Every 3 months thereafter

REFERENCES

1. Hoffman R, et al., eds. *Hematology: Basic Principles and Practice.* 3rd ed. New York, NY: Churchill Livingstone; 2000.
2. Laport GF, Larson RA. Treatment of adult acute lymphoblastic leukemia. *Semin Oncol.* 1997;24:70–82.
3. Finiewicz KJ, Larson RA. Dose-intensive therapy for adult acute lymphoblastic leukemia. *Semin Oncol.* 1999;26:6–20.
4. Larson RA, et al. A randomized controlled trial of filgrastim during remission induction and consolidation chemotherapy for adults with acute lymphoblastic leukemia. *Blood.* 1998;92:1556–1564.
5. Kantajian H, Hoelzer D, Larson RA, eds. Advances in the treatment of adult acute lymphocytic leukemia, Parts I and II. *Hematol Oncol Clin North Am.* 2000 and 2001.
6. Pui CH, Relling MV, Downing JR. Acute lymphoblastic leukemia. *N Engl J Med.* 2004;350:1535–1548.

MISCELLANEOUS

Other notes

- Burkitt leukemia/lymphoma (ALL-L3)
  - The outcome is clearly better if high dose methotrexate and alkylating agents are used for initial therapy.
  - Only 18 weeks of treatment is required.

CODES

ICD9-CM

- 204.00 Acute lymphoid leukemia without mention of remission
- 204.01 Acute lymphoid leukemia in remission

PATIENT TEACHING

- Risks of infection, transfusion, chemotherapy
- Stop smoking.

L

LEUKEMIA, CHRONIC MYELOGENOUS (CML)

Krista Johansen, MD
Liberto Pechet, MD

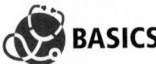 **BASICS**

DESCRIPTION
- Triphasic clonal stem cell disorder characterized by the proliferation of myeloid cells, CML is a myeloproliferative disorder (MPD)
- The 3 phases, consist of a chronic phase, an accelerated phase, and transformation into an acute leukemia (blastic) phase.

GENERAL PREVENTION
None currently identified

EPIDEMIOLOGY
- Most common in middle-aged patients, median age is 53 years
- Slight male predominance

Incidence
In Western countries, 1–2 per 100,000 per year

Prevalence
Accounts for 15–20% of adult leukemias

RISK FACTORS
Ionizing radiation exposure (uncommon)

Genetics
Not inherited; acquired genomic changes

PATHOPHYSIOLOGY
Genetic mutation in hematologic stem cells characterized by the translocation between BCR (on chromosome 22) and ABL (on chromosome 9) genes, results in abnormal clone of bone marrow cells. They have proliferative advantage over normal hematopoietic cells, due to the fusion protein (BCR-ABL) that is a constitutively active tyrosine kinase and resistant to apoptosis (cell death).

ASSOCIATED CONDITIONS
None

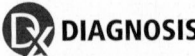 **DIAGNOSIS**

PRE HOSPITAL
85–90% present in the chronic phase

SIGNS AND SYMPTOMS
History
- Common: Fatigue, weight loss, night sweats, abdominal fullness due to enlarged spleen
- Less common: Left upper quadrant abdominal pain occasionally referred to the left shoulder (due to splenic infarction or rupture), extramedullary tumors, sternal pain (due to expanding bone marrow) and gouty arthritis
- Up to 30% of cases can be asymptomatic.

Physical Exam
- Common: Splenomegaly (60–70%), hepatomegaly (30%)
- Less common: Splenic friction rub, lymphadenopathy

TESTS
Lab
- CBC
  - Hematocrit: May be normal or slightly increased or decreased.
  - WBC: Markedly increased (50–100 K), with granulocytes in all stages of development, including occasional blasts, basophilia, eosinophilia
  - Platelets: Normal, elevated (34%), or occasionally low
  - In accelerated phase: Anemia, >20% blasts, >20% basophils, thrombocytopenia
- Low or absent leukocyte alkaline phosphatase (LAP) in neutrophils
  - Gold standard: Demonstration of the Philadelphia chromosome, t(9,22, by cytogenetic techniques, or by FISH
    - Additional cytogenetic abnormalities occur in the accelerated and blast phases (trisomy 8, Philadelphia chromosome duplication, isochromosome 17q).
    - Some patients are Philadelphia chromosome negative by cytogenetic analysis (15%) but have BCR-ABL within multiple translocations.
    - Elevated uric acid

Imaging
Abdominal ultrasound or CT scan shows splenomegaly; not mandatory

Diagnostic Procedures/Surgery
Bone marrow aspirate and biopsy: Myelocytic hyperplasia, increased reticulin fibrosis, hypervascularity of marrow tissue

DIFFERENTIAL DIAGNOSIS
Acute myelogenous leukemia (AML), chronic myelomonocytic leukemia (CMML), chronic neutrophilic leukemia, chronic eosinophilic leukemia, juvenile myelomonocytic leukemia (JMML), infectious mononucleosis, leukemoid reaction, polycythemia vera, treatment with granulocyte stimulating factors

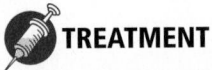 **TREATMENT**

INITIAL STABILIZATION
Hydroxyurea to rapidly reduce the white cell count; allopurinol to prevent tumor lysis syndrome, in cases with very high counts; to be administered before chemotherapy is instituted; probably not necessary when Gleevec is used

GENERAL MEASURES
Activity
Avoid contact sports, trauma to abdomen

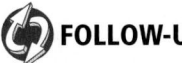 **MEDICATION (DRUGS)**

- Medications are not curative but can provide control of the disease.
- The response to medication is categorized as follows
  - Complete hematologic response
    - No leukemic cells are identified in peripheral blood smear.
  - Cytogenetic response (complete, incomplete, or absent)
  - Molecular response by PCR, (complete or incomplete; to be performed only in cases of complete cytogenetic response)

First Line
- Gleevec (Imatinib mesylate), an oral tyrosine kinase inhibitor 400 mg PO b.i.d., 6–800 mg
- Side effects: Nausea, rash, leukopenia, thrombocytopenia, fever, abdominal pain
- 2nd-generation tyrosine kinase inhibitors are currently being investigated with good results reported in some patients resistant to Gleevec.

Second Line
- Interferon alpha, 3 MI Units, IM, daily for 5 days per week
  - Side effects: Fever, flulike symptoms
- Hydroxyurea, 2–8 g/d in patients resistant to imatinib, or to rapidly decrease very elevated counts
- Side-effects: Pancytopenia

SURGERY
Bone marrow transplant

- Is only known cure
- Most effective in patients <50 who are in the chronic phase
- Initial mortality is higher than medical management but provides higher rates of survival
- Matched related donors have a better prognosis than matched unrelated donors for allogeneic donation.

FOLLOW-UP

Frequency depends on stage at presentation, response to 1st line therapy

Admission Criteria
Acute abdominal symptoms (infarcted or ruptured spleen); acute lysis syndrome due to initial therapy; complications of bone marrow transplantation

Discharge Criteria
Abatement of acute symptoms

Issues for Referral
All patients with CML should be referred to a hematologist.

PROGNOSIS
- Without treatment: CML will invariably progress to accelerated phase within 2–5 years and blast phase within several months of the accelerated phase.
- Poor prognosis: Patients presenting in accelerated or acute leukemia or presenting with very large spleen size, platelets >700,000, and patients resistant to current therapies

COMPLICATIONS
- Splenic infarct or rupture
- Progression to accelerated or blast phase
- Thrombotic events due to elevated platelets
- Bleeding due to low or dysfunctional platelets
- Sequelae of anemia

PATIENT MONITORING
- Weekly during initial treatment until stabilized on medication, then 1–2 times per month
- Monitoring should assess for response to drug and for side effects, and progression of disease.
- Cytogenetic and molecular studies should be repeated after stabilization to assess response.

REFERENCES
1. Savage DG, Szydlo RM, Goldman JM. Clinical features at diagnosis in 430 patients with chronic myeloid leukemia seen at a referral center over a 16-year period. *Br H Haematol*. 1997;96:111–116.
2. Goldman JM, ed. Management decisions in chronic myeloid leukemia. In: *Semin Hematol*. 2003;40(1): 97–103.
3. Calabretta B, Perrotti D. The biology of CML blast crisis. *Blood*. 2004;103:4010–4022.

ADDITIONAL READING
Blood, Principles and Practice of Hematology 2nd edition, 2003. Handin RI, Lux SE, Stossel TP, editors, Lippincot, Williams and Wilkins, publishers, Chronic Myelogenous Leukemia, pp. 433–454

L

LEUKOPLAKIA, ORAL

Jeremy Golding, MD
Fady Faddoul, MD

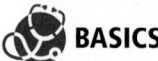 **BASICS**

DESCRIPTION
- A nonspecific clinical term used to describe a white patch in the oral mucosa that remains despite attempts to rub it off. It does not correlate with any specific microscopic findings and may be related to a variety of lesions, from benign hyperkeratosis to squamous cell carcinoma.
- System(s) Affected: Gastrointestinal

GENERAL PREVENTION
- Avoid tobacco, alcohol, habitual biting.
- Provide well-fitting dental prosthesis.
- Regular dental checkups to avoid bad restorations
- Diet rich in fresh fruits and vegetables may help prevent cancer

EPIDEMIOLOGY
- Predominant age: 90% of lesions found in patients >40 years
- Predominant sex: Male > Female
  - Some studies show no gender difference.

Prevalence
- 1–3% of the adult population is affected, usually men >40 years.
- Rare before age 40

ALERT
Geriatric Considerations
More common in older patients

RISK FACTORS
- Age >40 years
- Tobacco or alcohol use
- Repeated or chronic trauma or irritation to oral regions

ETIOLOGY
- Tobacco use in any form
- Alcohol consumption
- Oral infections
- *Candida albicans*
- Human papilloma virus, types 11 and 15
- Sunlight
- Vitamin deficiency
- Syphilis
- Dental restorations
- Prosthetic dental appliances
- Alcoholism
- Estrogen therapy
- Chronic trauma or irritation

ASSOCIATED CONDITIONS
- Leukokeratosis nicotina palati is rarely malignant.
- HIV infection is closely associated with hairy leukoplakia.
- Erythroplakia in association with leukoplakia is a marker for underlying dysplasia.

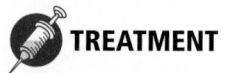 **DIAGNOSIS**

SIGNS AND SYMPTOMS
- Usually asymptomatic
- Location
  - 50% on tongue, mandibular alveolar ridge, and buccal mucosa
  - Also seen on maxillary alveolar ridge, palate, and lower lip
  - Infrequently seen on floor of the mouth and retromolar areas
- Appearance
  - Varies from nonpalpable, faintly translucent white areas to thick, fissured, papillomatous, indurated lesions
  - May feel rough or leathery
  - Color may be white, gray, yellowish-white, or brownish-gray, although mixed white and red ("speckled leukoplakia") more likely to be dysplastic or malignant
  - Cannot be wiped off
  - Macular or plaquelike
  - Nodular and verrucous variants more likely to be malignant.

Diagnostic Procedures/Surgery
- Biopsy is necessary to rule out carcinoma if lesion is persistent or unexplained.
- Brush biopsy and analysis of cells with a special neural network–based image-processing system allows detection of as few as 1 or 2 abnormal individual cells in several hundred thousand cells. Patients with such cells on a simple brush specimen should undergo more formal biopsy..

Pathological Findings
- Biopsy specimens range from hyperkeratosis to invasive carcinoma.
- At initial biopsy, 6% are invasive carcinoma.
- 4% subsequently undergo malignant transformation.
- Location is important: 60% on floor of mouth or lateral border of tongue are cancerous, rarely so on buccal mucosa.

DIFFERENTIAL DIAGNOSIS
- White oral lesions that can be wiped away
  - Candidiasis
  - Aspirin burn
- White oral lesions that cannot be rubbed off
  - Traumatic or frictional keratosis (e.g., linea alba)
  - Leukoedema
  - Galvanic keratosis
  - Lichen planus
  - Verrucous carcinoma
  - Lupus
  - Squamous cell carcinoma
  - Oral hairy leukoplakia, commonly on the lateral border of the tongue with a bilateral distribution
  - Leukokeratosis nicotina palati

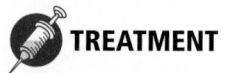 **TREATMENT**

INITIAL STABILIZATION
- Eliminate etiologic factors.
- Re-evaluate in 7–14 days.
- Biopsy if lesion is persistent.

GENERAL MEASURES
- Eliminate habitual lip biting.
- Correct ill-fitting dental appliances, bad restorations, or sharp teeth.
- Stop smoking and using alcohol.
- If dysplasia is evident, remove lesion. Consider otolaryngologist or oral surgery referral.
- Some small lesions may respond to cryosurgery.
- β-Carotene may cause partial regression (experimental).
- For hairy tongue: Tongue brushing

Diet
Regular

Activity
Full

MEDICATION (DRUGS)

- Generally none needed
- Hairy leukoplakia
  – Acyclovir 2–4 g/d PO systemically is effective, but the lesions recur when the treatment is stopped.
  – Topical retinoids
  – Topical podophyllin 25% resin applied twice, 1 week between applications; however, the bad taste is poorly tolerated.
- Leukoplakia: Isotretinoin (Accutane) 1–2 mg/kg/d PO may lead to temporary remission, but side effects are poorly tolerated.

SURGERY
Excision is the treatment of choice for lesions exhibiting dysplasia or malignant transformation.

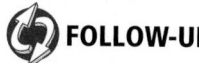 **FOLLOW-UP**

PROGNOSIS
- Curable if detected early
- 4–6% of initially benign lesions subsequently develop into cancer.
- More likely to be cancerous if on floor of mouth or lateral border of tongue

COMPLICATIONS
- Carcinoma
- New lesions may develop after treatment.

PATIENT MONITORING
Regular, close follow-up, even after successful treatment. Biopsy as needed.

REFERENCES
1. Scully C. Leukoplakia, Oral in E-medicine. 2006.
2. Fitzpatrick T, et al. Color Atlas and Synopsis of Clinical Dermatology, 2nd ed. New York: McGraw-Hill, 1992.
3. Regezi JA, Sciubba JJ, Pogrel MA. Atlas of Oral and Maxillofacial Pathology. Philadelphia: WB Saunders, 2000.
4. Yeats D, Burn J. Common oral mucosal lesions in adults. *Am Fam Physician*. 1991;44:2043–2050.

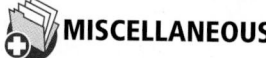 **MISCELLANEOUS**

- See also: Epstein-Barr virus infections; HIV infection and AIDS
- Other notes
  – Uncommonly found on other mucosal surfaces (e.g., vaginal, anal)
  – Linea alba: A white line on the buccal mucosa along the occlusal plane

 CODES

ICD9-CM
528.6 Leukoplakia of oral mucosa, including tongue

PATIENT TEACHING
- If biopsy is negative, stress importance of periodic and careful follow-up.
- Initiate a dental referral to eliminate dental factors.
- Stress importance of stopping tobacco and alcohol use.
- Encourage participation in smoking cessation program.

L

LICHEN PLANUS

Herbert P. Goodheart, MD

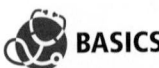 **BASICS**

DESCRIPTION
A relatively uncommon cutaneous inflammatory disorder. Besides the skin and mucous membranes, hair and nails may also be affected.

Classic (Idiopathic) Lichen Planus
- Characterized by small flat, angular, red to violaceous, shiny, pruritic papules on the skin and by fine, white lacy patches or erosions of the oral mucosa
- Course unpredictable. Onset is abrupt or gradual.
- May resolve spontaneously, recur intermittently, or be chronic for many years

Drug or Chemically Induced Lichenoid Eruptions
- Clinical and histopathologic findings may mimic those of classic lichen planus. Usually lack Wickham striae (see below)
- There is generally a latent period of several months from drug introduction before lesions appear.
- Lesions resolve when inciting agent is discontinued, often after a prolonged period of time.
- System(s) Affected: Skin/Exocrine
- Synonym(s): Lichenoid eruptions

GENERAL PREVENTION
N/A

EPIDEMIOLOGY
- Predominant age: 30–60 years; rare in children and the geriatric population
- Predominant sex: Female > Male

Prevalence
In the US, 450 in 100,000

RISK FACTORS
Exposure to certain drugs or chemicals
- Thiazides, furosemide, beta-blockers, sulfonylureas, antimalarials, penicillamine, gold salts, and angiotensin-converting enzyme inhibitors.
- Rarely: Photo-developing chemicals, dental materials, tattoo pigments

ETIOLOGY
A cell-mediated immune response of unknown origin

ASSOCIATED CONDITIONS
- An association has been noted between lichen planus and hepatitis C virus infection (more common in Japan and Italy), chronic active hepatitis, lichen nitidus, and primary biliary cirrhosis.
- Lichen planus has also infrequently been reported to be found in association with other diseases of altered immunity than would be expected by chance; these conditions include
  - Bullous pemphigoid
  - Alopecia areata
  - Myasthenia gravis
  - Vitiligo
  - Ulcerative colitis
  - Graft versus host reaction
  - Lupus erythematosus (lupus erythematosus-lichen planus overlap syndrome)
  - Morphea and lichen sclerosus et atrophicus

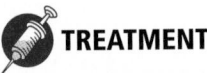 **DIAGNOSIS**

SIGNS AND SYMPTOMS
- Skin
  - Pruritus: Often severe
  - Papules: 1–10 mm, shiny, flat-topped (planar) lesions that occur in crops
  - Evidence of scratching, i.e., crusts and excoriations, are usually absent.
  - Color: Violaceous, with white lacelike pattern (Wickham striae) on surface of papules. Wickham striae are best seen after topical application of mineral oil, and if present, are virtually pathognomonic for lichen planus.
  - Shape: Polygonal or oval shaped. Annular lesions may appear on trunk and mucous membranes. Various shapes and sizes may be noted (polymorphic).
  - Arrangement: May be grouped, linear, or scattered individual lesions
  - Köebner phenomenon (*isomorphic response*): New lesions may be noted at sites of minor injuries such as scratches or burns.
  - Distribution: Ventral surface of wrists and forearms, dorsa hands, glans penis, dorsa feet, groin, sacrum, shins, and scalp. Hypertrophic (verrucous) lesions may occur on lower legs. May be generalized.
  - Postinflammatory hyperpigmentation–lesions typically heal leaving darkly pigmented macules in their wake.
- Mucous membranes
  - Seen in 40–60% of patients with skin lesions; 20% of patients have mucous membrane lesions only.
  - Most commonly asymptomatic, nonerosive, milky-white lines with an elegant, lacy net-like, streaked pattern
  - Usually seen on buccal mucosa, but may appear on tongue, gingiva, palate, or lips
  - May be erosive, rarely bullous
  - Painful, especially if ulcers present
  - Lesions may develop into squamous cell carcinoma (1–3%)
  - Glans penis and labia minora may be involved.
- Hair and nails
  - Scalp: Atrophic scalp skin and destruction of hair follicles. May result in permanent patchy, scarring alopecia *(lichen planopilaris)*
  - Nails (10%): Involvement of nail matrix may cause proximal to distal linear grooves and partial or complete destruction of nail bed with pterygium formation

TESTS
Lab
If suggested by history
- Serology for hepatitis B and C
- Liver function tests

Diagnostic Procedures/Surgery
- Skin biopsy
- Direct immunofluorescence helps distinguish lichen planus from discoid lupus erythematosus

Pathological Findings
- Vacuolar degeneration of the basal layer
- Hyperkeratosis and irregular acanthosis. Increased granular layer
- Basement membrane thinning with "sawtoothing"
- Degenerative keratinocytes, known as colloid or Civatte bodies, are found in the lower epidermis.
- Dense, bandlike lymphocytic infiltrate of the upper dermis
- Melanin pigment in macrophages

DIFFERENTIAL DIAGNOSIS
- Skin
  - Lichen simplex chronicus
  - Eczematous dermatitis
  - Psoriasis
  - Other lichenoid eruptions (those that resemble lichen planus)
  - Pityriasis rosea
  - Lichen nitidus
- Oral mucous membranes
  - Leukoplakia
  - Oral hairy leukoplakia
  - Candidiasis
  - Squamous cell carcinoma (particularly in ulcerative lesions)
  - Aphthous ulcers
  - Herpetic stomatitis
  - Secondary syphilis
- Genital mucous membranes
  - Psoriasis (penis and labia)
  - Fixed drug eruption (penis)
  - Candidiasis (penis and labia)
  - Pemphigus vulgaris, bullous pemphigoid, and Behçet disease (all rare)
- Hair and scalp
  - Scarring alopecia (pseudopelade)

TREATMENT

INITIAL STABILIZATION
Outpatient care

GENERAL MEASURES
- Goal is to relieve itching and resolve lesions.
- Asymptomatic oral lesions require no treatment.

Diet
No special diet

Activity
Full

MEDICATION (DRUGS)

First Line

- Skin
  - Superpotent topical steroids (e.g., 0.05% clobetasol propionate) b.i.d. for 2 weeks
  - Potent topical steroids such as triamcinolone acetonide 0.1% or fluocinonide 0.05% under occlusion
  - Intralesional corticosteroids (e.g., triamcinolone [Kenalog] 5–10 mg/mL) for recalcitrant and hypertrophic lesions
  - Antihistamine (e.g., hydroxyzine 25 mg PO q6h) if needed for itching
- Mucous membranes
  - Topical corticosteroids (0.1% triamcinolone [Kenalog] in Orabase) or 0.05% clobetasol propionate ointment b.i.d.
  - Intralesional corticosteroids for erosive, painful lichen planus
  - Topical 1% tacrolimus ointment b.i.d.
  - Topical retinoids (e.g., 0.05% tretinoin [retinoic acid] in Orabase)

Second Line

- Oral prednisone: Used only for a short course (e.g., 30–60 mg daily for 2–4 weeks). Patients with history of hypersensitivity to corticosteroids or any of the above medications
  - Precautions with systemic steroids
  - Systemic absorption of steroids may result in hypothalamic-pituitary-adrenal axis suppression, Cushing syndrome, hyperglycemia, or glucosuria
  - Increased risk with high potency topical steroids —i.e., use over large surface area, prolonged use, occlusive dressings
  - In pregnancy—Usually safe but benefits must outweigh the risks
- Children may absorb a proportionally larger amount of topical steroid because of larger skin surface-to-weight ratio
  - Oral retinoids: Isotretinoin, acitretin
- Oral metronidazole
- Cyclosporine may be used in severe cases, but cost and potential toxicity limit its use. Topical use for severe oral involvement refractory to other treatments
- Thalidomide
- PUVA or narrow-band UVB
- Griseofulvin
- Azathioprine
- Mycophenolate mofetil

ALERT

Avoid retinoids during pregnancy.

 FOLLOW-UP

PROGNOSIS

- Spontaneous resolution in weeks is possible, but disease may persist for years, especially oral lesions and hypertrophic lesions on the shins.
- There is a tendency toward relapse
- Recurrence in 12–20%, especially in those with generalized involvement

COMPLICATIONS

- Alopecia
- Nail destruction
- Squamous cell carcinoma of the mouth

PATIENT MONITORING

Serial oral examinations for erosive/ulcerative lesions

REFERENCES

1. Eisen D. The clinical features, malignant potential, and systemic associations of oral lichen planus: A study of 723 patients. *J Am Acad Dermatol*. 2002;46:207–214.
2. Morrison L, Kratochvil J, Gorman A. An open trial of topical tacrolimus for erosive oral lichen planus. *J Am Acad Dermatol*. 2002;47:617–620.
3. Camisa C, Popovsky JL. Effective treatment of oral erosive lichen planus with thalidomide. *Arch Dermatol*. 2000;136(12):1442–1443.

 MISCELLANEOUS

Other notes: Remember the 7 *P*'s of lichen planus: **p**urple, **p**lanar, **p**olygonal, **p**olymorphic, **p**ruritic, **p**apules, that heal with **p**ostinflammatory hyperpigmentation

 CODES

ICD9-CM

697.0 Lichen planus

PATIENT TEACHING

Diet

Oral, erosive or ulcerative lichen planus: Annual follow-up to screen for malignancy

- Avoid spicy foods, cigarettes, excessive alcohol
- Avoid crispy foods such as corn chips, pretzels, and toast.

 See Corresponding Diagnostic Algorithm

L

LICHEN SIMPLEX CHRONICUS

Amy Y. Wang, MD

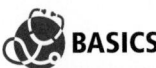 BASICS

DESCRIPTION
- A chronic dermatitis resulting from continued, repeated rubbing or scratching part of the skin
- System(s) Affected: Skin/Exocrine
- Synonym(s): Lichen simplex, Neurodermatitis, Neurodermatitis circumscripta

ALERT

Geriatric Considerations
Common in those >60 years

Pediatric Considerations
Rare in preadolescents

GENERAL PREVENTION
Avoid irritants and other known causative agents

EPIDEMIOLOGY
- Predominant age: Mainly adults, less common in children
- Predominant sex: Female > Male

Incidence
- Common
- Peak incidence between 30 and 50 years of age

Prevalence
Common

RISK FACTORS
- Any pre-existing pruritic dermatosis can result in the development of lichen simplex chronicus.
- Exposure to irritants is a risk factor.

Genetics
None known

PATHOPHYSIOLOGY
- Repeated scratching or rubbing of an area of skin causes inflammation and pruritus.
- Pruritus results in to continued scratching.
- Scratching may become a conditioned response to anxiety.
- Habitual scratching and scratch-itch cycle result in a chronic dermatosis.

ETIOLOGY
- Idiopathic in many instances
- Some causes of apparent idiopathic disease may be secondary to a previously unrecognized dermatosis.
- Secondary forms may begin as another pruritic skin disease that evolves into neurodermatitis after resolution of the primary dermatitis.
- Primary dermatoses from which neurodermatitis may develop include lichen planus, stasis dermatitis, atopic dermatitis, contact dermatitis, psoriasis, tinea corporis, seborrheic dermatitis, xerosis, eczema, and herpes zoster.
- Anxiety and emotional stress may play a role.

ASSOCIATED CONDITIONS
- Prurigo nodularis is a nodular variety of the same disease process.
- Atopic dermatitis

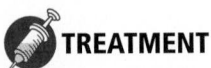 DIAGNOSIS

SIGNS AND SYMPTOMS

History
- Gradual onset
- Begins as a localized area of pruritus
- Most commonly involves easily accessible areas, including nape of neck, lower legs, ankles, wrists, extensor surfaces of forearms, scalp, external ear, and anogenital region
- Pruritus out of proportion to the appearance of the lesion is typically paroxysmal and worse at night and may occur during sleep.
- Nuchal and suboccipital regions are more commonly affected in women.
- Anxiety and obsessive disorders are commonly associated with this condition.
- The perineal region is more commonly affected in men.

Physical Exam
- Lichenified, excoriated pruritic patches of skin
- Nonerythematous
- Accentuation of normal skin lines
- Verrucous thickening and changes in pigmentation
- Vesicles or weeping are rare.
- Moist scale, serum crusting, or pustules suggest the presence of infection.
- Scarring may be present following serious secondary infections.

TESTS

Lab
- None diagnostic
- Appropriate tests to evaluate for other conditions, such as potassium hydroxide preparation or culture

Diagnostic Procedures/Surgery
Skin biopsy to evaluate for other conditions if no response to treatment

Pathological Findings
- Hyperkeratosis
- Acanthosis
- Lengthening of rete ridges
- Hyperplasia of all components of epidermis
- Chronic inflammatory infiltrate of dermis

DIFFERENTIAL DIAGNOSIS
- Atopic dermatitis
- Contact dermatitis
- Cutaneous T-cell lymphoma
- Drug reaction
- Lichen planus
- Lichenified psoriasis
- Photodermatitis
- Stasis dermatitis
- Cutaneous amyloidosis
- Fungal infection
- Seborrheic dermatitis
- Lupus vulgaris (cutaneous tuberculosis)

TREATMENT

INITIAL STABILIZATION
Outpatient management

GENERAL MEASURES
- Patient education
- Treat pruritus to interrupt the scratch–itch cycle.
- Treat underlying pruritic skin conditions.
- Lubricating lotions and creams
- Nail trimming

Diet
Regular

Activity
- As tolerated
- Encourage exercise in those cases in which stress may play a role.

SPECIAL THERAPY

Complementary and Alternative Medicine
- Cognitive-behavioral treatment focusing on thoughts leading to and awareness of itching and substitution of other activities has been shown to be helpful.
- Hypnosis focusing on nonscratching behavior and lessening the sensations of pruritus has been beneficial.

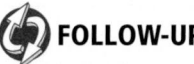 **MEDICATION (DRUGS)**

First Line
- Standard topical antipruritic agents
  - Menthol preparations (e.g., Sarna)
  - Pramoxine (e.g., PrameGel)
  - Calamine lotion—for weeping lesions only
- Topical doxepin cream 5% is an effective antipruritic agent.
- Topical capsaicin cream can be helpful.
- Topical steroids are 1st-line agents for treating lichen simplex chronicus.
  - High-potency steroids alone, such as 0.05% betamethasone dipropionate cream or 0.05% clobetasol propionate cream, can be used initially, but should not be used on the face, anogenital region, or intertriginous areas. They should be used on small areas only, and for no longer than 2 weeks.
  - Switch to intermediate- or low-potency steroids alone as response allows.
  - An intermediate-potency steroid, such as 0.025% or 0.1% triamcinolone cream, may be used for initial treatment of the face and intertriginous areas and for maintenance treatment of other areas. A low-potency steroid, such as 1% hydrocortisone cream, should be used for maintenance treatment of the face and intertriginous areas.
  - Steroid tape, flurandrenolide (e.g., Cordran)
    - Optimized penetration
    - Provides a barrier to further trauma
- Contraindications
  - High-potency topical steroids should not be used on the face or intertriginous areas.
- Precautions
  - Topical and intralesional steroid therapy can cause epidermal and dermal atrophy as well as hypopigmentation.
  - Oral anxiolytics may be beneficial in patients with an anxiety component.

Second Line
- Cold Burow solution compresses
  - One packet of Domeboro powder in 1 qt of ice-cold water applied with a cloth for 15 minutes as needed
- Coal tar preparations are useful but cosmetically less appealing.
- Oral antihistamines can be used for their antipruritic and sedative effects.
- Unna boot for barrier protection
- For resistant cases, consider a course of prednisone 40 mg/d for 2 weeks.
- Intralesional corticosteroids
- Topical aspirin has been shown to be helpful in treating neurodermatitis. [A]
- Topical pimecrolimus has been shown to decrease the symptoms of vulvar lichen simplex chronicus. [B]
- Botulinum toxin A injected intradermally has been reported to improve symptoms in patients with recalcitrant pruritus. [C]
- Oral antibiotics for secondary infections

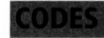 **FOLLOW-UP**

DISPOSITION
Issues for Referral
- No response to treatment
- Worsening of symptoms
- Presence of signs and symptoms suggestive of a systemic cause of pruritus

PROGNOSIS
- Often chronic and recurrent
- The prognosis is good for those patients in whom the scratch–itch cycle can be broken.
- After healing, the skin should have a normal appearance unless secondary infection has occurred, which can cause scarring.

COMPLICATIONS
- Secondary infection
- Rare scarring due to secondary infection
- Complications related to therapy, as mentioned in medication precautions

PATIENT MONITORING
Patients should be followed closely and regularly for response to therapy, complications from therapy, and secondary infections.

REFERENCES
1. Brunner N, Yawalkar S. A double-blind, multicenter, parallel-group trial with 0.05% halobetasol prionate ointment versus 0.1% diflucortolone valerate ointment in patients with severe, chronic atopic dermatitis or lichen simplex chronicus. *J Am Acad Dermatol*. 1991;25(6 Pt 2):1160–1163.
2. Drake LA, Millikan LE. The antipruritic effect of 5% doxepin cream in patients with eczematous dermatitis. *Arch Dermatol*. 1995;131(12): 1403–1408.
3. Datz B, Yawalkar S. A double-blind, multicenter trial of 0.05% halobetasol propionate ointment and 0.05% clobetasol 17-propionate ointment in the treatment of patients with chronic, localized atopic dermatitis or lichen simplex chronicus. *J Am Acad Dermatol*. 1991;25(6 Pt 2):1157–1160.
4. Goldstein AT, Parneix-Spake A. Pimecrolimus cream 1% for treatment of vulvar lichen simplex chronicus: An open label trial. *Obstet Gynecol*. 2006;107(4 Suppl):54S–55S.
5. Heckmann M, et al. Botulinum toxin type A injection in the treatment of lichen simplex: An open pilot study. *J Am Acad Dermatol*. 2002;46: 617–619.
6. Kantor GR, Resnik KS. Treatment of lichen simplex chronicus with topical capsaicin cream. *Acta Derm Venereol*. 1996;76(2):161.
7. Lynch PJ. Lichen simplex chronicus (atopic/neurodermatitis) of the anogenital region. *Dermato Ther*. 2004;17:8–19.
8. Moses S. Pruritus. *Am Fam Physician*. 2003;68(6): 1135–1142.
9. Shenefelt PD. Biofeedback, cognitive-behavioral methods, and hypnosis in dermatology: Is it all in your mind? *Dermatol Ther*. 2003;16:114–122.
10. Yosipovitch G, et al. The effect of topically applied aspirin on localized circumscribed neurodermatitis. *J Am Acad Dermatol*. 2001;45: 910–913.

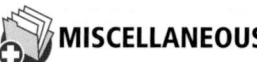 **MISCELLANEOUS**

See also: Dermatitis, atopic; Dermatitis, contact; Dermatitis, seborrheic; Dermatitis, stasis; Pruritus ani; Pruritus vulvae

CODES

ICD9-CM
698.3 Lichenification and lichen simplex chronicus

PATIENT TEACHING
Patients should understand the cause of this disease and their role in helping resolve the condition.

Activity
- Stress reduction techniques can be helpful in those patients in whom stress plays role.
- Emphasize that scratching and rubbing must stop for lesions to heal.

Prevention
Avoid exposure to known irritants.

L

LIPOMA

Joseph R. Stenger, MD

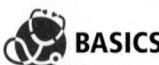 **BASICS**

DESCRIPTION

- Lipomas are soft-tissue tumors composed of normal adipose tissue. They are slow growing, often asymptomatic, and usually diagnosed by palpation.
- Lipomas are soft, homogeneous, oval, nontender, and the overlying skin is mobile over them. They are commonly from 1–6 cm diameter.
- They are usually subcutaneous and often found in the upper trunk, especially the shoulders, back, neck, and head, but can be anywhere on the body.
- Individuals can have single lesions or a few. In ~5% of cases, patients have multiple lesions.
- On surgical approach, they often have a thin enveloping membrane or capsule.
- Lipomas have been reported in anatomic locations as varied as cardiac, intrathoracic, endobronchial, retroperitoneal, breast, intermuscular, calf, thigh, scapular, intraosseous, fingers, palmar, toe, epidural, spinal, intraarticular (knee), parapharyngeal, nasopharyngeal, adrenal, inguinal, bladder, scrotal, ovarian, intracranial, intraneural, and in the GI tract (most often in the ileum).
- They are reported to occur after trauma.
- Lipomas rarely, if ever, become malignant.

GENERAL PREVENTION

None

EPIDEMIOLOGY

They can occur from infancy to old age, but are most common in middle-aged adults, peaking in the 40–60 year age group. They are rare <20 years of age.

RISK FACTORS

None

Genetics

Unknown

PATHOPHYSIOLOGY

Lipomas can result in compressive neuropathy in locations such as the forearm or ankle.

ETIOLOGY

They are reported to occur after trauma or after steroid injection, but most are idiopathic.

ASSOCIATED CONDITIONS

- Admixture of other tissue types leads to fibrolipomas, angiolipomas, and myolipomas.
- Unusual syndromes include the giant variety, hereditary multiple lipomatosis, adiposis dolorosa (multiple tender diffuse lesions), and Madelung disease (numerous, symmetrically distributed lipomas of the upper trunk).
- Liposarcomas rarely develop from benign lipomas. They can occur anywhere in the body, mostly in deep structures.

 DIAGNOSIS

SIGNS AND SYMPTOMS

- Lipomas can cause pain, pressure, or neuropathic symptoms if compression occurs.
- Most often, patients show them to physicians for explanation and reassurance.
- Occasionally, they are first noted by physicians on a physical exam.

History

Generally slow-growing, without definite date when 1st noticed.

Physical Exam

Lipomas are soft, homogeneous, oval, nontender, and the overlying skin is mobile over them. They are commonly from 1–6 cm in diameter.

TESTS

If diagnosis is uncertain, excisional biopsy is the preferred assessment tool.

Lab

None relevant.

Imaging

MRI has been used to differentiate lipomas from liposarcomas.

Diagnostic Procedures/Surgery

See "Surgery"

Pathological Findings

Lipomas are composed of adipose tissue, with varying amounts of a network of connective tissue.

DIFFERENTIAL DIAGNOSIS

Benign lipomas must be differentiated from liposarcomas. Rapid growth and pain should prompt consideration of malignancy.

TREATMENT

Most lipomas can be observed without treatment. They need excision if there is diagnostic uncertainty, rapid growth, associated pain, or cosmetic concern. Treatment is excision, but steroid injection or liposuction can be useful in certain locations (such as facial).

SURGERY

- Careful planning of the incision to fit along skin lines, if possible, is advantageous.
- After anesthesia, the incision is carried out down to the level of the capsule.
- Blunt and sharp dissection is used as needed to free up 1 end of the tumor and to separate it from the inferior normal tissue.
- As the lobule is lifted, the dissection is continued to free up the entire tumor.
- Care is needed to obtain good hemostasis.
- The dead space should be closed with deep absorbable sutures and then the skin is closed.
- If there is excessive skin remains after the deep layer is closed, some trimming may be needed to avoid redundancy.

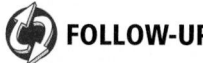 **FOLLOW-UP**

- Usual surgical follow-up is needed, with treatment of any hematoma formation or infection.
- Occasionally a bilobar lipoma may be missed, resulting in "recurrence."

DISPOSITION

Issues for Referral
Lipomas in anatomic areas that are technically difficult may require referral.

PROGNOSIS
Most lipomas grow very slowly or remain stable.

COMPLICATIONS
- Surgical complications. as noted above.
- Lipomas that grow rapidly or become painful or nodular must be evaluated for liposarcoma.

REFERENCES
1. Dale D. ACP Medicine. *WebMD* 2006;2, XI, 12 and 12, XIII, 3–4.
2. Salam GA. Lipoma excision. *Am Fam Physician*. 2002;65:901–905.
3. Springfield D. Liposarcoma. *Clin Orthopaed Rel Res*. 1993;(289):50–57.

ADDITIONAL READING
- Kenawi MM. "Squeeze delivery" excision of subcutaneous lipoma related to anatomic site. *Br J Surg*. 1995;82:1649–1650.
- Blount JP, Elton S. Spinal lipomas. *Neurosurg Foc*. 2001;10(1):e3.

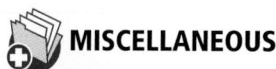 **MISCELLANEOUS**

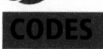

ICD9-CM
214.9 Lipoma

PATIENT TEACHING
Handout:
http://www.aafp.org/afp/20020301/905ph.html

L

LISTERIOSIS

Ramesh Nathan, MD, MPH

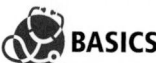

BASICS

DESCRIPTION
- Infection caused by the ubiquitous, weakly hemolytic, Gram-positive bacillus *Listeria monocytogenes*; pathogenic to many species.
- Occurs most often in fetuses (disseminated infantile listeriosis), neonates, and immunosuppressed patients
- Most adult patients have pre-existing disease (cirrhosis, lymphomas, solid tumors, AIDS, cancer therapy, organ transplant recipients) or are on corticosteroid therapy.
- Usual course: Acute
- In 2002, 46 culture-confirmed cases, 7 deaths, and 3 miscarriages were linked to eating sliceable turkey deli meat.
- System(s) Affected: Endocrine/Metabolic; Gastrointestinal; Hemic/Lymphatic/Immunologic; Nervous; Pulmonary; Renal/Urologic
- Synonym(s): *Listeria monocytogenes*; Listerial disease

GENERAL PREVENTION
- For pregnant, older, or immune-compromised patients: Check US Department of Agriculture Web site for recalled foods.
- Avoid handling livestock.
- Avoid contaminated silage.
- Avoid contaminated sewage.
- Avoid raw, unpasteurized, or milk products.
- Avoid soft cheeses (Mexican and feta).
- Wash all raw vegetables carefully.
- Separate uncooked meats from vegetables.
- Wash hands after handling uncooked foods.
- Avoid foods from deli counter.
- Cook leftovers, hot dogs, cold cuts, and deli meats until steaming hot before eating.

EPIDEMIOLOGY
- Predominant age: Neonates, elderly
- Predominant sex: Male > Female

Prevalence
- Pregnancy ~20 times more likely
- In AIDS, infection ~300 times more likely.

Incidence
In the US: 2500 serious illnesses, 500 deaths per year

RISK FACTORS
- Age: Fetus, neonate, elderly
- Metastatic malignant disease
- HIV infection
- Alcoholism
- Renal hemodialysis
- Immunosuppression (including corticosteroid therapy)
- Exposure to infected animals (e.g., by veterinarians, butchers). Animal-to-human transmission is rare.
- Ingesting contaminated food or drink (e.g., soft Mexican-style cheese or feta cheese)

ALERT
Pregnancy Considerations
- Pregnant women are more susceptible to infection with *L. monocytogenes*; transmission to fetuses and neonates occurs with high mortality.
- Requires prompt and vigorous treatment to prevent transfer of disease to fetus (pregnant patient's symptoms may begin as a flulike illness or be absent)

Genetics
No known genetic pattern

ETIOLOGY
L. monocytogenes, a small Gram-positive bacillus; infection with other species of *Listeria* is rare. Illnesses may begin 2–8 weeks after eating contaminated food.

ASSOCIATED CONDITIONS
- Cirrhosis
- Lymphomas
- Solid tumors
- Immunodeficiencies
- Pregnancy
- Organ transplant recipients
- Hemochromatosis and iron overload

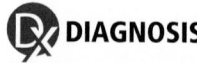

DIAGNOSIS

SIGNS AND SYMPTOMS
- Asymptomatic
- Abdominal pain
- Adult respiratory distress syndrome
- Cervical lymphadenopathy
- Chills
- Conjunctivitis
- Decreased fetal movement
- Diarrhea
- Dysuria
- Fatigue
- Fever
- Hepatosplenomegaly
- Malaise
- Myalgia
- Nausea
- Vomiting
- Findings suggestive of meningitis
  - Fever
  - Headache
  - Nausea and vomiting
  - Stiff neck
  - Delirium
  - Coma
- Findings suggestive of sepsis
  - High fever and generalized severe illness without evidence of localization (in patients with alcoholism, malignancies, immunosuppression, AIDS)

History
- Identify patients with risk factors (see "Associated Conditions").
- Ask about ingestion of meat or soft cheese products.

Physical Exam
Nonspecific, but may find signs of meningitis

TESTS
Lab
- Cerebrospinal fluid (CSF)
  - Gram stain: Small Gram-positive rods or coccobacillary forms with tumbling motility. (Sometimes are difficult to identify, because organisms not present in large numbers.)
  - Cell count: The predominant cell type is the neutrophil; however, mononuclear cells may predominate. RBCs frequently seen.
  - Protein concentration: WNL to 735 mg/dL
  - Glucose: WNL to undetectable
  - CSF culture: Demonstrates β-hemolysis (*L. monocytogenes* grows well on 5% sheep's blood or chocolate agar). Need at least 10 mL of spinal fluid for culture.
  - Counterimmunoelectrophoresis latex agglutination
- Other tests
  - Blood cultures should be done.
  - CBC may show an elevated neutrophil count and/or left shift.
  - Other cultures in newborn: Cervical vaginal secretions and lochia from the mother; cord blood; grossly abnormal portions of the placenta, meconium, and exudate expressed from an incised skin papule of the neonate
- Drugs that may alter lab results: Antibiotics
- Disorders that may alter lab results: Cultures may be confusing in patients with mixed infections.
- Specimens for serologic testing should be submitted to the local public health laboratory. In outbreaks, serotyping may be desirable.
- Notify laboratory at time of sending any specimen that listeriosis is a possibility.
- Specimens must be sent to laboratory promptly (few organisms more difficult to culture).

Imaging
MRI for any patient with CNS symptoms

Diagnostic Procedures/Surgery
Lumbar puncture

Pathological Findings
- Gross: Multiorgan miliary granulomatosis
- Microscopic
  - Nodular focal abscess
  - Necrotic amorphous basophilic debris
  - Increased tissue macrophages
  - Gram-positive bacilli
- Motile bacilli with "tumbling motility" seen
- Chinese-letter aggregates

DIFFERENTIAL DIAGNOSIS
- Other infections: *Staphylococcus*, Gram-negative *Klebsiella*, *Candida*, *Cryptococcus*, viruses
- Infantile listeriosis, *Escherichia coli* infection, group B streptococci infection
- Infectious mononucleosis

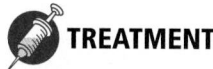

TREATMENT

INITIAL STABILIZATION
Inpatient care during acute phase

GENERAL MEASURES
- Bed rest
- Isolation if patient is immunosuppressed
- Secretion precautions
- Respiratory assistance (if patient has apnea or central nervous system depression)

Diet
- For acute cases: Total parenteral nutrition, nasogastric tube, or softer diet if tolerated
- Avoid eating raw or partially cooked foods and soft cheeses.
- An updated list of recalled food products can be found at the U.S. Dept. of Agriculture Web site: www.fsis.usda.gov/OA/recalls/rec_intr.htm.

Activity
Bed rest

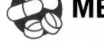

MEDICATION (DRUGS)

First Line
- Neonates: IV treatment for 14–21 days
  - Meningitis in infants >1 month old: Ampicillin 300–400 mg/kg/d
  - Meningitis in neonates <2000 g: In patients <1 week old, ampicillin 50 mg/kg q12h; in patients >1 week, ampicillin 50 mg/kg q8h plus gentamicin 7.5 mg/kg/d for 14 days. Discontinue gentamicin when cerebrospinal fluid is sterile.
  - Alternate therapy for neonates: G 100,000–200,000 u/kg/d for 14–21 days plus gentamicin as above
  - Bacteremia or pneumonia: 100–150 mg/kg/d ampicillin (or penicillin G 200,000 units/kg/d) plus gentamicin 5.0 mg/kg/d. Discontinue gentamicin when blood cultures become negative.
- Pregnant women: Ampicillin 2 g IV q4h for 14–21 days plus gentamicin 120 mg IV q8h. Adjust for peak 5–6 μg/mL.
- Immunocompromised/older patients: Ampicillin 2 g IV q4h plus ceftriaxone 2 g IV q12h or cefotaxime 2 g IV q6h plus vancomycin 500 mg IV q6h and dexamethasone 0.4 mg/kg IV q12h for 2 days; give 1st dose with 1st dose of antibiotic
- For endocarditis and typhoidal listeriosis: Penicillin G 75,000–100,000 units/kg IV q4h, and continue for 14 days after defervescence, plus tobramycin 2 mg/kg load, then adjust based on levels. Aim for peak at 5–6 μg/mL; continue for 4 weeks after defervescence.
- For oculoglandular listeriosis: 30 mg/kg/d as 4 equal doses q6h; continue for 1 week after defervescence.
- Contraindications: Allergy to penicillins
- Precautions: Cephalosporins are not adequate treatment. Refer to manufacturer's literature.

Second Line
Sulfamethoxazole may be most effective for adults. Total dose 10 mg/kg IV (based on trimethoprim component) in divided doses

PROGNOSIS
High mortality if symptomatic

ALERT
Pediatric Considerations
- Infected fetuses are usually stillborn or premature.
- 50% mortality in treated neonates

Geriatric Considerations
Greater morbidity and mortality

COMPLICATIONS
- Premature delivery
- Amnionitis
- Meningitis
- Septicemia
- Pulmonary abscess
- Hepatic abscess
- Placental abscess
- Splenic abscess
- Lymph node abscess
- Endocarditis
- Peritonitis
- Abortion
- Stillbirth
- Neonatal death

PATIENT MONITORING
- Arterial blood gases during acute phase
- Repeat lumbar puncture at 24–48 hours and at the end of treatment.

REFERENCES

1. Lorber B. *Listeria monocytogenes*. In: Mandell GL, Bennett JE, Dolin R (eds.), Principles and practice of infectious diseases, 6th ed. Philadelphia: Churchill Livingstone; 2005:2478.
2. Mylonakis E, Paliou M, Hohmann EL, et al. Listeriosis during pregnancy: A case series and review of 222 cases. Medicine (Baltimore). 2002;81:260.
3. Ooi ST, Lorber B. Gastroenteritis due to *Listeria monocytogenes*. *Clin Infect Dis*. 2005;40:1327.
4. CDC website: http://www.cdc.gov/ncidod/dbmd/diseaseinfo/listeriosis.

MISCELLANEOUS

Listeria is the most common cause of bacterial meningitis in patients with underlying neoplastic disease, especially lymphomas, in organ transplant recipients, or in those receiving corticosteroids for any reason.
Other notes
- Reportable disease: Contact Centers for Disease Control and Prevention at (404) 639-2215 or www.fsis.usda.gov/OA/recalls/reactv.htm.
- For questions regarding safety of deli meat: U.S. Department of Agriculture (800) 535-4555
- www.cdc.gov/foodnet

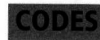 **CODES**

ICD9-CM
027.0 Listeriosis

PATIENT TEACHING

Centers for Disease Control and Prevention, National Center for Infectious Diseases; www.cdc.gov/ncidod/ncid.htm/

 See Corresponding Diagnostic Algorithm

L

LOW BACK PAIN

Michele Matthews, PharmD
Ambareen Ali, MD

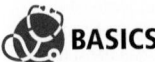 **BASICS**

DESCRIPTION

- Mechanical low back pain is a diagnosis of exclusion. It is generally a benign and self-limiting condition responsive to conservative measures that include maintaining activity while utilizing short-term pharmacologic therapy.
- Patients typically present with pain, muscle tension, or stiffness at the posterior belt line with occasional referred pain to the buttocks and/or posterior thighs. These symptoms are often the result of the mechanical stresses and functional demands placed on the low back area by everyday activities.
- For most patients, pain is of short duration, and complete recovery is expected within 6 weeks.
- The primary goal is to rule out red-flag symptoms that indicate possible underlying spinal pathology or nerve root problems (see "Neotory"). When such symptoms are absent, the patient is considered to have nonspecific low back pain.
- System(s) Affected: Musculoskeletal; Nervous
- Synonym(s): Low back syndrome; Lumbar strain/sprain; Lumbago

ALERT
Geriatric Considerations
Tumors, degenerative conditions, fractures, and stenosis are more common.

Pediatric Considerations
The presence of low back pain is considered a red-flag symptom. A thorough workup is imperative.

Pregnancy Considerations
Pregnancy is commonly associated with low back pain and/or sciatica; treatment is conservative.

GENERAL PREVENTION
- Maintaining physical fitness
- Weight loss
- Smoking cessation
- Stress reduction
- Avoidance of aggravating tasks (e.g., heavy lifting, bending, twisting, sudden unexpected movements, or any combination of these tasks)

EPIDEMIOLOGY
Incidence
- 90% of Americans experience mechanical low back pain sometime in their life.
- Low back pain is 1 of the most common complaints heard during primary care visits.
- Repetitive episodes are common.

Prevalence
- Predominant age: ≥25 years
- Predominant sex: Male = Female

RISK FACTORS
- Age
- Activity (e.g., heavy lifting, bending, twisting)
- Smoking
- Obesity
- Vibration (e.g., driving motor vehicles)
- Sedentary lifestyle
- Psychosocial factors such as increased stress, anxiety or depressed mood

ETIOLOGY
- Normal aging process of musculoskeletal system aggravates an acute event.
- Degenerative joint disease of LS spine

ASSOCIATED CONDITIONS
- Deconditioning
- Obesity
- Psychosocial disease
- Compression fracture

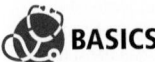 **DIAGNOSIS**

SIGNS AND SYMPTOMS
History
- Onset of low back pain begins either suddenly after injury or gradually over the next 24 hours.
- Occasional radiation of pain to buttocks and/or posterior thighs stopping at knees
- Pain pattern is referred rather than radicular.
- Back pain is worse than leg pain.
- Pain is aggravated by back motion, sitting, standing, lifting, bending, and twisting.
- Pain is relieved by rest.
- Bowel and bladder function are preserved.
- Psychosocial stressors at work and/or home may be present.
- Medical history and previous injuries should be noted
- Red flags (requiring lab evaluation):
- Age >50 or <20 (neoplastic)
- History of cancer (carcinoma recurrence)
- Night sweats or weight loss (neoplasm, rheumatologic)
- Incontinence or saddle anesthesia (nerve compromise/cauda equina syndrome)
- Recent bacterial infection (infectious)
- Pain worse when supine (rheumatologic, nerve compromise)
- History of trauma (fracture)

Physical Exam
- Observation reveals preferred posture, facial expressions, and pain behaviors.
- Normal motor, sensory, and reflex examinations
- Decreased lumbar range of motion, paraspinous musculature tenderness, and spasm
- Nerve root stretch tests are often negative.
- Straight-leg raise (causing spinal motion) may increase low back pain, but not leg pain.

TESTS
Lab
- Not typically indicated upon initial presentation (1)
- For those with red flags, pain that worsens, persists for more than 6 weeks, and/or is recalcitrant to conservative treatment measures, consider the following
- screening laboratory studies
- CBC with differential
- Erythrocyte sedimentation rate

- Alkaline and acid phosphatase
- Serum calcium
- Serum protein electrophoresis
- Special tests: System-directed investigation

Imaging
- Plain radiographs
- Not recommended with no red flags (2)[B]
- Indicated for persistent symptoms (>6 weeks), age >50, systemic symptoms, presence of neurologic deficits, trauma, history of cancer, use of immunosuppressants, IV drug abuse, or if abnormalities such as ankylosing spondylitis are suspected
- Anteroposterior, lateral, spot lateral of L5–S1 and oblique films are included in routine lumbo-sacral series
- Bone scan (scintigraphy)
- Technetium^{99m}-labeled phosphorus to rule out fractures, infections, or metastases

Diagnostic Procedures/Surgery
MRI, CT only indicated for persistent symptoms, neurologic deficits, and/or suspected infection or malignancy.
- MRI is useful for visualization of soft tissue.
- CT is useful for visualization of bony anatomy.

DIFFERENTIAL DIAGNOSIS
- Structural
- Acute lumbar back pain
- Chronic lumbar back pain
- Lumbar strain/sprain
- Herniated lumbar intervertebral disc
- Degenerative disc disease
- Degenerative segmental instability
- Spinal stenosis
- Spondylolisthesis
- Congenital disease: Severe kyphosis, severe scoliosis
- Fractures
- Inflammatory
- Ankylosing spondylitis and related inflammatory spondylopathies
- Infection: Vertebral osteomyelitis
- Rheumatoid arthritis
- Neoplastic
- Primary tumors
- Metastases
- Referred pain
- Orthopaedic: Osteoarthritis of hip
- Sacroiliac joint disease
- Gastrointestinal: Duodenal ulcer, chronic pancreatitis, cholecystitis, irritable bowel syndrome, diverticulitis
- Genitourinary: Pyelonephritis, nephrolithiasis, prostatism
- Gynecological: Pregnancy, endometriosis, ovarian cystic disease, PID
- Cardiovascular: Abdominal aortic aneurysm, vascular claudication

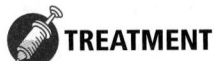 TREATMENT

GENERAL MEASURES

- Outpatient management is appropriate
- Activity modification as appropriate
- Short-term nonopioid analgesics at fixed time intervals
  - NSAIDs
  - Muscle relaxants
- Short-acting combination opioid analgesic products (e.g., Vicodin) associated with inducing chronic LBP; avoid
- Spinal manipulation (short course)

Diet

Weight reduction, if appropriate

Activity

- Bed rest is *not* recommended (1)[A]
- Restricted activities for 3–6 weeks
- Back-specific exercises should be avoided.
- Activities of daily living should be resumed as soon as possible. (1)[A]

Complementary and Alternative Medicine

- Chiropractic manipulation (1)[B]
- Devil's claw, white willow bark, and capsaicin have demonstrated efficacy versus placebo for acute episodes of chronic low back pain (3)[B].

 MEDICATION (DRUGS)

First Line

- NSAIDs
  - Agents are considered equally effective (4)[A]
    - Ibuprofen: 800 mg PO q6h for 10 days then as needed (max 3200 mg/d)
    - Naproxen: 500 mg PO b.i.d. for 10 days then as needed (max 1500 mg/d)
  - Adverse reactions
    - Common: Fluid retention, rash, GI discomfort, dizziness
    - Serious: GI bleeding, acute renal failure
  - Contraindications: Treatment of perioperative pain in the setting of CABG; aspirin allergy
  - Precautions: High risk of cardiovascular event, high risk of GI bleeding, history of ulcer disease, elderly, renal disease
  - Possible interactions: Antiplatelets, ACE inhibitors, lithium, LMWH
- Muscle relaxants
  - Use with caution (avoid alcohol, no driving or operating heavy machinery); comparative efficacy to NSAIDs is unknown (5)[A].
    - Cyclobenzaprine (Flexeril): 10 mg PO at bedtime or q8h (max 60 mg/d)
    - Carisoprodol (Soma): 350 mg PO t.i.d. and at bedtime
    - Metaxalone (Skelaxin): 800 mg PO t.i.d.–q.i.d.
  - Adverse reactions: Common; sedation, N/V, dizziness
  - Contraindications
    - Cyclobenzaprine: Arrhythmias, CHF, hyperthyroidism, concomitant MAOIs
    - Carisoprodol: Acute intermittent porphyria
    - Metaxalone: Anemia, renal or hepatic impairment
  - Precautions: Concomitant use of CNS depressants, history of substance abuse
  - Possible interactions: CNS depressants

Second Line

Short-acting combination opioid analgesic products should only be considered for moderate to severe pain not controlled with NSAIDs and/or muscle relaxants alone (1)[B].

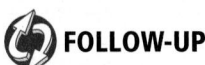 FOLLOW-UP

PROGNOSIS

- Usually self-limiting; recovery is expected within 6 weeks in 90% of cases (5).
- Symptoms can recur in 50–80% of patients within the 1st year.

COMPLICATIONS

- Incorrect diagnosis
- Chronic low back pain
- Persistent psychosocial impairment

PATIENT MONITORING

Estimated duration of care is 1–6 weeks

- Assess the following at each follow-up visit: pain, functional status, and medication-related adverse effects

REFERENCES

1. Koes BW, van Tulder MW, Thomas S. Diagnosis and treatment of low back pain. *BMJ*. 2006;332: 1430–1434.
2. Jarvik JG, Deyo RA. Diagnostic evaluation of low back pain with emphasis on imaging. *Ann Intern Med*. 2002;137:586–597.
3. Gagnier JJ, van Tulder MW, Berman B, Bombardier C. Herbal medicine for low back pain. *Cochrane Database Syst Rev*. 2006;Apr 19(2).
4. van Tulder MW, Scholten RJPM, Koes BW, Deyo RA. Non-steroidal anti-inflammatory drugs for low back pain. *Cochrane Database Syst Rev*. 2006; Feb 3(3).
5. van Tulder MW, Touray T, Furlan AD, Solway S, Bouter LM. Muscle relaxants for non-specific low back pain. *Cochrane Database of Syst Rev*. 2006; Nov 11(3).

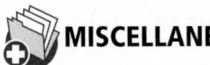 MISCELLANEOUS

- Adverse psychosocial factors to resolving back pain
  - Pending litigation or compensation
  - Prolonged use of habit-forming medications or alcohol
  - Depressed or hostile patient
- See also: Lumbar (intervertebral) disk disorders

CODES

ICD9-CM

- 722.2 Displacement of intervertebral disc, site unspecified, without myelopathy
- 722.6 Degeneration of intervertebral disc, site unspecified
- 724.2 Lumbago
- 724.5 Backache, unspecified

PATIENT TEACHING

- Educate the patient about the condition and inform him that he must play an active role in the management.
- Advise the patient to stay active.
- Advise the patient to use medication exactly as prescribed and discuss adverse drug effects.

 See Corresponding Diagnostic Algorithm

 See Patient Handout on CD

L

LUMBAR (INTERVERTEBRAL) DISK DISORDERS

Scott Kinkade, MD, MSPH

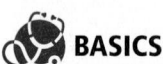 **BASICS**

DESCRIPTION

- Many patients with low back pain have lumbar disk disease and involvement of surrounding spinal ligaments, muscles, and skeleton.
- Over time may progress to disk degeneration, disk herniation, spinal narrowing, and arthritic proliferation of the facet joint
- Management is based on symptoms and disability because the distinction between the normal aging of the spine and pathological findings is hard to distinguish.
- Nonradicular low back pain (acute and chronic): The low back pain remains near the belt-line and is caused by soft tissue or disk injury.
- Radicular low back pain (acute and chronic): The neuropathic pain is greater in the buttocks, hips, or legs rather than the back.
- There may or may not be signs of weakness, numbness, or loss of reflex.
- In younger patients, the source of the pain is likely to be mechanical compression or chemical irritation of a nerve root.
- Spinal stenosis is more likely to be the etiology of radicular pain in patients >55 years.
- System(s) Affected: Musculoskeletal; Nervous
- Synonym(s): Degenerative disk disease; Intervertebral disk dislocation

ALERT

Geriatric Considerations
Usually multifactorial lesions of spine; degenerative spondylolisthesis, spinal stenosis, with neurogenic claudication, and osteoporosis are more likely

Pediatric Considerations
Scoliosis, onset age 10 years, rarely symptomatic

Pregnancy Considerations
Increased incidence of low back pain and/or sciatica; conservative treatment

GENERAL PREVENTION
- Modification of jobs to reduce exposure to known risk factors
- Selection of workers for certain jobs by such means as strength testing
- Avoid smoking.
- Lessen obesity.

EPIDEMIOLOGY
- Predominant age: 20–40 years old, infrequent <20 or >65
- Predominant sex: Male = Female

Incidence
- 1 of the most frequent complaints for which adults seek medical attention and 2nd to the common cold for the most time off work.
- The incidence rate is 5% annually. Among patients with acute back pain, only 4% of them have nerve root symptoms due to a herniated disk.
- 95% of herniations are at the L4-5 disk or L5-S1 disk. 5% of herniated discs occur at L3-L4. Other lumbar disk herniations are rare.
- <2% of the patients with low back pain have infections, neoplasms, or inflammatory spondyloarthropathies.

Prevalence
Lifetime prevalence of low back pain is 60–90%.

RISK FACTORS
- Normal aging process >20 years of age
- Cigarette smoking
- Stress, muscle tension
- Obesity

ETIOLOGY
- Trauma, major or minor
- Frequent lifting of heavy objects, especially bending at the waist and twisting movements
- Vibration (e.g., driving motor vehicles)

ASSOCIATED CONDITIONS
- Poor physical conditioning/posture
- Obesity
- Osteoarthritis
- Osteoporosis
- Depression, other psychiatric disorders

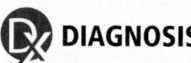 **DIAGNOSIS**

SIGNS AND SYMPTOMS
- Variable pain; usually dull, originating in back, extending below knee
- The pain may radiate (often unilaterally) in the nerve root distribution.
- Back pain decreases at night. Bed rest usually improves symptoms at least temporarily.
- Pain may increase with sitting or standing
- Constitutional symptoms absent
- Sciatica can occur without back pain.
- Often sensory aberrations in extremities, paresthesias, and numbness
- Occasionally muscle group weakness
- Most disk ruptures are posterolateral and press upon the lumbar nerve root with radiating pain.
- Lumbar scoliosis possible, trunk tilted toward or away from affected side, depending on location of extrusion
- Paraspinal muscle spasm

History
- Assess location, onset, aggravating and relieving factors, and associated symptoms.
- **Red flag conditions** that may be associated with a more serious etiology include age >50, fevers, weight loss, night pain, recent infection, history of cancer, immunosuppression, IV drug use, progressive neurological deficits, or failure to improve after 4–6 weeks of conservative treatment.

Physical Exam
- Assess range of motion.
- Assess motor strength in both lower extremities. Brief screening tests include raising heels off ground and walking on toes and raising toes off ground and walking on heels.
- Assess deep tendon reflexes in the Achilles and patellar tendons.
- Straight leg raise test (SLR): In supine position, elevation of affected leg between 30° and 60° degrees elicits pain (sens = 0.80, spec = 0.40)
- Crossed SLR test: in supine position, elevation of the leg opposite the side of pain between 30° and 60° degrees elicits pain (sens = 0.25, spec = 0.90)

TESTS
Lab
ESR or C-reactive protein; only indicated if Red Flags are present (elevation may signify infection, autoimmune arthropathy, or cancer)

Imaging
- Lumbosacral plain films: Rarely indicated, may identify tumor, vertebral compression facture, osteoarthritis, sponylolisthesis
- Magnetic resonance preferred over CT scan and myelogram (for surgical candidate evaluation or to help rule out more serious etiology such as tumor, infection, fracture). Note: In asymptomatic adults getting MRI of the lumbar spine, disk herniation is found in ~1/3 of the patients and disk bulging is found in more than 1/2 of the patients.

Diagnostic Procedures
- Myelograms not commonly used
- Electromyography useful to distinguish peripheral neuropathy from cord or nerve root impairment. May confirm level of lesion

Pathological Findings
It is difficult to distinguish the normal aging process of disk degeneration from specific lesions causing low back pain and sciatica.

DIFFERENTIAL DIAGNOSIS
- Acute or chronic lumbosacral strain
- Spondylosis
- Spondylolisthesis
- Spinal arthritis
- Fibrositis
- Compression fracture
- Metastatic and primary tumors
- Vertebral infection
- Pain referred from hip, retroperitoneum, aneurysms, or pelvis, neurogenic claudication
- Cauda equina syndrome: Signs include perineal (saddle) anesthesia, bowel or bladder dysfunction, and severe lower extremity neurological impairment (often bilateral)

TREATMENT

INITIAL STABILIZATION
Outpatient for majority; inpatient for severe disability and/or surgery

GENERAL MEASURES
- Conservative treatment is recommended for the 1st 4–6 weeks. Most herniated disks improve with time. For persistent or severe pain and neurological deficits, consider evaluating the patient for surgery.
- Emergent surgical referral for cauda equina syndrome
- Initial: Minimize bed rest, ordinary activities as tolerated, local heat, analgesics, muscle relaxants, physical therapy (∼75% respond)
- Manipulation therapy: Safety and efficacy are unclear in patients with sciatica
- For chronic nonradicular pain: Improve physical fitness with low impact aerobic exercise. Manipulation and physical therapy have been shown to be beneficial.
- Transcutaneous electrical nerve stimulation (TENS), acupuncture: Very short-term benefit

Diet
Weight reduction if appropriate

Activity
- After pain is controlled (2–4 days), begin progressive walking program. Short walks initially 4 times a day and lengthen as tolerated
- Return to work as soon as possible with avoidance of high-risk activities (e.g., heavy lifting, vibration, smoking).

MEDICATION (DRUGS)

First Line
- Analgesia with NSAIDs; may require short-term opioids for severe pain
- Muscle relaxants
- Precautions: Elderly, hypertension, prior peptic ulcer disease or bleeding, renal disease, liver disease, cardiac dysfunction, addiction
- Contraindications/Significant possible interactions: Refer to the manufacturer's profile of each drug.

Second Line: Invasive Treatments
- Injections
  - Epidural steroid injections may benefit some patients, but the evidence is not strong.
- Chemonucleolysis using chymopapain is more effective than placebo, but less effective than surgical discectomy.
- Surgical discectomy
  - Techniques include open and microsurgical discectomy; percutaneous laser, percutaneous suction, and arthoscopic discectomies are newer techniques.
  - Spinal fusion (arthrodesis): Indicated for spinal instability
- Absolute indications for discectomy
  - Cauda equina syndrome
  - Progressive neurological deficit despite conservative treatment
- Relative indications for discectomy
  - Intolerable pain
  - Multiple episodes of radiculopathy

- Persistent dysfunctional pain: These patients have been reported to improve more rapidly postoperatively, but long-term results show little difference from nonoperative treatment.
- Static neurological deficit: No reported difference between operative or nonoperative treatment for the improvement in weakness or sensory disturbance.

FOLLOW-UP

DISPOSITION
Issues for Referral
- Progressive or severe neurologic deficit
- Cauda equine syndrome
- Persistent sciatica for at least 1 month with corresponding clinical and imaging findings
- Persistent neurological deficit despite 4–6 weeks of conservative therapy

PROGNOSIS
- Acute low back pain (90%) and/or radiculopathy (75–90%) can be expected to recover spontaneously with conservative therapy.
- Chronic nonradicular low back pain: Most patients respond to conservative management such as manipulation, fitness, weight reduction, and education regarding back care.
- Chronic radicular pain: Good selection of surgical candidates have found satisfactory results (85% in long-term studies).

COMPLICATIONS
- Foot drop with weakness of anterior tibial, posterior tibial, and peroneal muscles
- Loss of ankle jerk
- Bladder and rectal sphincter weakness with retention or incontinence
- Limitation of movement and restricted activity
- Narcotic addiction

PATIENT MONITORING
Outpatient
- Return visit ∼10 days following initial visit, should be improving
- Thereafter monitor every 2 weeks until fully functional.
- Follow pain history and neurological status.
- Monitor exercise program.

REFERENCES
1. Atlas SJ, Nardi RA. Evaluation and treatment of low back pain: An evidence-based approach to clinical care. *Muscle Nerve*. 2003;27:265–284.
2. Atlas SJ, et al. Long-term outcomes of surgical and nonsurgical management of sciatica secondary to a lumbar disc herniations: 10 year results from the Maine lumbar spine study. *Spine*. 2005;30:927–935.
3. Smeal WL, Tyburski M, Alleva J. Discogenic/radicular pain. *Dis Mon*. 2004;50:636–669.
4. van Tulder MW, et al. Outcome of invasive treatment modalities on back pain and sciatica: An evidence-based review. *Eur Spine J*. 2005;15 Suppl 1:S82–S92.
5. Jarvik JG, Deyo RA. Diagnostic evaluation of low back pain with emphasis on imaging. *Ann Intern Med*. 2002;137:586–597.

MISCELLANEOUS

- See also: "Low back pain"
- Features that predict best surgical outcome
  - Definable neurological deficit
  - Pathology in imaging which correlates with deficit
  - Positive nerve root tension signs
  - Leg pain > back pain
  - No response to nonsurgical therapy for 4–6 weeks
- Adverse psychosocial factors to resolving back pain
  - Pending litigation or compensation
  - Depressed or hostile patient
  - Low IQ or poorly educated may not be able to participate in assessment or decision
  - Prolonged use of narcotics or alcohol

CODES

ICD9-CM
- 722.10 Displacement of lumbar intervertebral disk without myelopathy
- 722.52 Degeneration of lumbar or lumbosacral intervertebral disk

PATIENT TEACHING
Good posture, proper body mechanics, physical fitness, physical therapy, if appropriate

 See Corresponding Diagnostic Algorithm

 See Patient Handout on CD

L

LUNG ABSCESS

Federico Milla, MD
Ruben Peralta, MD, FACS

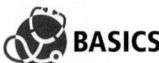 **BASICS**

DESCRIPTION

A localized collection cavity of necrotic lung tissue and pus resulting from severe lung infection

- Presentation may be acute or chronic (symptoms for >4 weeks).
- Usual course is subacute progression of symptoms.
- Synonym(s): Pulmonary abscess

GENERAL PREVENTION

- Treatment of predisposing diseases
- Aspiration precautions
- Treatment of periodontal diseases

EPIDEMIOLOGY

- Predominant age: Mainly 4th–6th decades
- Predominant sex: Male > Female (4:1)

Prevalence

Unknown; relatively rare since advent of antibiotics

ALERT

Pediatric Considerations

Occurs in children; *Staphylococcus* most common organism

RISK FACTORS

- Risk for aspiration
  - Periodontal disease (gingivitis), dental abscess, dental surgery
  - Substance abuse
  - Epilepsy
  - Cerebrovascular accident with oropharyngeal dysfunction
  - Sinusitis
  - General anesthesia with surgery
  - Dysphagia
  - Tracheal/nasogastric tube
  - Severe gastroesophageal reflux disease
  - Cerebral palsy
- Large bacterial burden
  - Necrotizing pneumonia
  - Bacteremia (especially *Staphylococcus*)
  - Septic embolism (especially in endocarditis)
  - Disseminated septic phlebitis
- Airway obstruction
  - Bronchial stenosis
  - Pulmonary embolism
  - Cavitary infarction
  - Lung neoplasia
  - Enlarged lymph node
  - Foreign body
- Immunocompromise
  - Diabetes mellitus
  - HIV
  - Chronic steroid use
- Amebic lung abscess: Most often from direct extension from liver abscess, through the diaphragm to the right lower lobe

Genetics

No known genetic pattern

ETIOLOGY

- May be due to aspiration of anaerobic oral flora (most common) or less commonly, septic emboli from endocarditis.
- Oral flora anaerobes (60–75% of cases)
  - *Peptostreptococcus*
  - *Prevotella*
  - *Fusobacterium*
  - *Bacteroides* sp.
- Aerobes (10–20% of cases)
  - *Staphylococcus aureus*
  - *Streptococcus pyogenes*
  - *Klebsiella* sp.
  - *Pseudomonas aeruginosa*
  - *Streptococcus milleri*
- Atypical aerobes
  - *Legionella*
  - *Nocardia*
  - *Actinomyces*

ASSOCIATED CONDITIONS

- Pneumonia
- Alcoholism
- Empyema
- Tuberculosis
- Immunocompromise

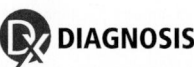 **DIAGNOSIS**

SIGNS AND SYMPTOMS

- Cough with purulent, foul-smelling, putrid, sour-tasting sputum
- Fever
- Malaise
- Night sweats
- Weight loss
- Chest pain/pleurisy
- Dyspnea
- Diaphoresis
- Anorexia
- Hemoptysis

Physical Exam

- Vital signs: Tachypnea, tachycardia
- Lung exam
  - Crackles
  - Wheezing
  - Dullness to percussion
  - Consolidation by auscultation
  - Cavernous breath sounds
  - Decreased breath sounds
- Clubbing of digits

TESTS

Lab

- Leukocytosis
- Anemia
- Hypoalbuminemia
- Sputum smear: Neutrophils, mixed bacteria
- Sputum culture: Often grow normal respiratory flora; may help in atypical presentations.
- Blood culture: Often negative in anaerobic abscess
- Drugs that may alter lab results: Prior antibiotics

Imaging

- Chest radiography
  - Lung cavity with air-fluid level
  - Consolidation with radiolucency, infiltrates, pleural effusion, mediastinal adenopathy
- CT
  - Defines location and extent (typical location depends on segments such as posterior segments of upper lobes or superior segments of lower lobes)
  - May detect obstructing lesion

Diagnostic Procedures/Surgery

- Bronchoscopy if obstruction is suspected
- Bronchoscopic brushing
- Bronchoalveolar lavage
- Transthoracic needle aspiration (rarely done)

Pathological Findings

- Solitary abscess
- Multiple abscesses
- Cavitation with necrosis
- Effusion/empyema

DIFFERENTIAL DIAGNOSIS

- Bronchogenic carcinoma
- Bronchiectasis
- Empyema with bronchopulmonary fistula
- Tuberculosis
- Mycotic lung infections
- Vasculitis
- Parasitic lung infections
- Infected pulmonary bulla
- Wegener granulomatosis
- Pulmonary sequestration
- Subphrenic or hepatic abscess with perforation into a bronchus
- Bronchogenic or parenchymal cyst
- Aspirated foreign body

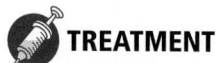 TREATMENT

INITIAL STABILIZATION
Inpatient care for monitoring and treatment

GENERAL MEASURES
- Postural drainage
- Nasotracheal suctioning if needed
- Prolonged course of antibiotics
- Pulmonary physiotherapy
- Bronchoscopy with selective therapeutic lavage (rarely done)

Diet
No restrictions

Activity
Reduced until radiographic evidence of clearing

MEDICATION (DRUGS)

First Line
Antibiotics according to culture and sensitivity results. For presumed anaerobes, clindamycin 600 mg q6h IV followed by 300 mg q6h PO for 4 weeks

Second Line
- Standard therapy had historically been penicillin G 1 million–2 million units IV q4h until improvement, followed by 1.2 million units (750 mg) PO q6h for 3–4 weeks; now many relevant pathogens produce β-lactamase.
- Cefoxitin 2.0 g IV q8h
- Piperacillin-tazobactam 3.375 g IV q6h
- Ticarcillin-clavulanate 3.1 g IV q6h
- Metronidazole has not proven as effective as clindamycin, but often is recommended for use as an adjunctive therapy (500 mg IV q6h).
- Full course of therapy may be needed for 8 weeks.

SURGERY
- Antibiotic treatment successful in the majority of cases; surgical options are considered when medical therapy fails (1)[B].
- Tube thoracostomy with medical failure or prohibitive operative risk (2)[B].
- Pulmonary resection only if complications occur or patient fails therapy (Mortality 11–16%)

FOLLOW-UP

PROGNOSIS
- Clinical improvement with decrease in fever expected 3–4 days after starting antibiotics
- Defervescence expected in 7–10 days
- Overall mortality 15–20%
- Prognosis depends on the underlying disease or immunosuppression.
- Patients with primary abscess (otherwise healthy, typical aspiration) have cure rate of 90–95%.
- Patients with secondary abscess (underlying neoplasm, obstruction, HIV) have 75% mortality.
- Certain factors tend to have worse prognosis
  - Large abscess (>6 cm)
  - Anatomic obstruction
  - Right lower lobe location
  - Certain bacteriologic species: *S. aureus*, *Klebsiella*, *Pseudomonas*

ALERT
Geriatric Considerations
Mortality higher in this age group

COMPLICATIONS
- Extension
- Empyema
- Massive hemoptysis
- Pneumothorax
- Brain abscess

PATIENT MONITORING
Serial radiographs until resolution of cavity

REFERENCES
1. Mansharamani N, Koziel H. Chronic lung sepsis: Lung abscess, bronchiectasis, and empyema. *Curr Opin Pulmon Med* 2003;9:181–185.
2. Wali SO, Shugaeri A, Samman YS, Abdelaziz M. Percutaneous drainage of pyogenic lung abscess. *Scand J Infect Dis* 2002;34:673–679.
3. Herth F, Ernst A, Becker HD. Endoscopic drainage of lung abscesses: Technique and outcome. *Chest* 2005;127:1378–1381.
4. Chirinos JA, Garcia J, Alcaide ML. Septic thrombophlebitis: Diagnosis and management. *Am J Cardiovasc Drugs* 2006;6:9–14.

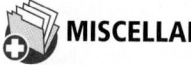 MISCELLANEOUS

See also: Pneumonia, bacterial

CODES

ICD9-CM
513.0 Abscess of lung

PATIENT TEACHING
Pulmonary physiotherapy techniques

 See Corresponding Diagnostic Algorithm

L

LUNG, PRIMARY MALIGNANCIES

Federico Milla, MD
Ruben Peralta, MD, FACS

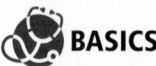 **BASICS**

DESCRIPTION

- Leading cause of cancer death in men and women in the US (28% of all cancer deaths)
- The most common (bronchogenic carcinoma) may be divided into 2 broad categories.
- Non-small cell cancer (NSCLC)
  - Adenocarcinoma 40%: From bronchial epithelium (mucus-producing cells), metastasizes earlier than squamous cell. Bronchoalveolar, a sub-type of adenocarcinoma has better prognosis.
  - Squamous cell cancer 20–30%: 2/3 centrally located, may compress bronchus, may have cavitation and necrosis
  - Other histologic types 30%
- Small cell cancer (SCLC) 20%: 80% centrally located; early metastases
- Other less common primary thoracic malignancies include mesothelioma, carcinoid tumor, sarcoma, melanoma.
- NSCLC tumors are staged for treatment and prognostic purposes from stages 0–IV. The definitions of each stage depend on the primary tumor (T), lymph node status (N), and presence of metastasis (M).
- SCLC tumors are staged on location of disease: Limited to ipsilateral hemithorax (stages I–IIIB); or extensive if metastatic beyond hemithorax (stages IIIB and IV).
- Tumor locations: Upper 60%, lower 30%, middle 5%, overlapping and mainstem 5%
- May spread by local extension to involve chest wall, diaphragm, pulmonary vessels, vena cava, phrenic nerve, esophagus, pericardium.
- Most commonly metastasize to lymph nodes (pulmonary, mediastinal), then liver, adrenal, bone (osteolytic), renal, brain

ALERT
Geriatric Considerations
More common >75 years

GENERAL PREVENTION
- No cost-effective screening measure available. Prevention via aggressive smoking cessation counseling and therapy. A 20–30% risk reduction occurs within 5 years of cessation.
- Per American Cancer Society: 175,000 cancer deaths annually are attributable to tobacco use.

EPIDEMIOLOGY
Incidence
- 175,000 new cases per year
- 70/100,000 population
- Most common cancer worldwide (17.6% of cancers in men)

Prevalence
- 87% of the new cases are NSCLC, and 50% are metastatic at diagnosis.
- Predominant age: 50–70 years
- Predominant sex: Male > Female

RISK FACTORS
- Smoking (attributable in 87% of cases)
- Second hand smoke exposure
- Chronic obstructive pulmonary disease
- Preexisting lung disease (pulmonary fibrosis)
- Environmental; occupational exposure
  - Asbestos exposure
  - Ionizing radiation
  - Atmospheric pollution
  - Gases: Halogen ethers, radon, mustard gas, aromatic hydrocarbons
  - Metals: Inorganic arsenic, chromium, nickel
- Possibly HIV (adenocarcinoma)

Genetics
1.5–3 times increased risk in 1st-degree relatives

ETIOLOGY
Multifactorial; see "Risk Factors"

ASSOCIATED CONDITIONS
- Paraneoplastic syndromes (hypertrophic pulmonary osteoarthropathy, Eaton-Lambert syndrome, Cushing syndrome)
- Pancoast syndrome
- Superior vena cava syndrome

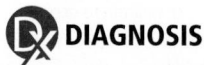 **DIAGNOSIS**

SIGNS AND SYMPTOMS
- May be asymptomatic for majority of course
- Pulmonary
  - Cough (new or change in chronic cough)
  - Wheezing
  - Dyspnea
  - Hemoptysis
  - Pneumonia
- Constitutional
  - Bone pain
  - Excess fatigue
  - Weight loss
  - Fever
  - Anemia
  - Clubbing of digits
- Other presentations
  - Chest pain
  - Shoulder/arm pain (Pancoast tumors)
  - Dysphagia
  - Plethora (swelling of face or neck)
  - Hoarseness
  - Horner syndrome

Physical Exam
- HEENT: Horner syndrome, dysphonia, stridor, scleral icterus
- Neck: Supraclavicular lymph nodes, mass
- Lungs: Effusion, wheezing
- Abdomen/groin: Masses or lymphadenopathy

TESTS
Lab
- CBC: Anemia
- Liver enzymes, alk phos
- Calcium
- Special tests
  - Pulmonary function studies
  - Quality of life assessments: Karnofsky Performance Scale (KPS), Eastern Cooperative Oncology Group (ECOG)
  - Bone marrow aspirate (small cell)

Imaging
- Chest radiograph (compare with old films)
  - Nodule or mass, especially if calcified
  - Persistent infiltrate
  - Atelectasis
  - Mediastinal widening
  - Hilar enlargement
  - Pleural effusion
- CT scan of chest (with IV contrast)
  - Nodule or mass (central or peripheral)
  - Lymphadenopathy
  - Defines relationship of tumor to mediastinal structures
- Other CT scans to look for metastatic disease
  - Brain: Lesions may be necrotic, bleeding
  - Abdomen: Hepatic, adrenal, renal masses
- MRI: May help in evaluating involvement of mediastinal structures.
- PET scan: Evaluate metastasis (1)[A]
- Bone scan: If advanced disease, if complaints of bone pain

Diagnostic Procedures/Surgery
- Enlarged mediastinal lymph nodes necessitate staging, which may be done by mediastinoscopy, video-assisted thoracoscopy, fine-needle aspiration
- Trans-bronchial biopsy (Wang Needle)
- Bronchoscopy before resection (for surgical planning)

Pathological Findings
Pathologic changes from smoking are progressive: Basal cell proliferation, development of atypical nuclei, stratification, metaplasia of squamous cells, carcinoma in situ, then invasive disease

DIFFERENTIAL DIAGNOSIS
- Consider both pulmonary and extrapulmonary causes for symptoms.
- Pulmonary
  - Chronic bronchitis
  - Granulomatous diseases (tuberculosis, sarcoidosis)
- Cardiac
  - CHF
  - Cardiomyopathy

TREATMENT

GENERAL MEASURES

- Surgery should be undertaken for localized disease. Chemotherapy is treatment for metastatic disease.
- Stages I and II are surgically resectable and may be treated by surgery alone, Stage III includes locally advanced disease with lymph node or mediastinal spread; surgery does not treat likely micrometastases but may be undertaken for local control. Stage IV is metastatic and not amenable to surgery.
- NSCLC: Surgical resection, chemotherapy, radiation therapy
- SCLC: Chemotherapy generally treatment of choice given likelihood of aggressive metastases; 30% have complete response. Radiation used for palliation and may enhance chemotherapy effect. Surgery rarely performed.
- Discussions with patient and family about wishes for end-of-life care

Diet
No restrictions; good nutrition is important during treatment.

Activity
No limitations; per patient tolerance

SPECIAL THERAPY
Radiotherapy
- Radiation may be used in combination with chemotherapy and may improve response.
- Postoperative radiation may help with local control, but does not have proven survival benefit if resection was complete and there is no evidence of lymph node metastases. May reduce local recurrence.
- Palliative for brain or bone metastases.
- Radiopharmaceuticals such as strontium[89] and samarium[153] seem to be helpful in reducing pain and need for opiate medications (2)[B].

 ## MEDICATION (DRUGS)

First Line
- Chemotherapy is the mainstay of treatment for SCLC and may be used in advanced NSCLC. Survival rates may be further improved by addition of radiation to chemotherapy treatment.
- Effective regimens include
  – Cisplatin (Platinol) and cisplatin-based regimens are standard, although response rates with cisplatin alone are <20% in stage IIIB–IV disease with a 3-year survival rate of 8%. Combination regimens can improve survival an average of 2 months with a 5-year survival rate improved by about 10% in stage III disease.
  – Etoposide (Toposar): Beneficial in combination with cisplatin and radiation (becoming standard)
- Palliative measures
  – Analgesics
  – Dyspnea: oxygen, morphine, benzodiazepines

SURGERY
- Resection for non-small cell cancer, for stages I, II, and IIIa if medically fit to undergo surgery
- Resection of isolated, distant metastases has been achieved and may improve survival.
- Resection involves lobectomy in 71%, wedge in 16%, and complete pneumonectomy in 18% (3)[B]
- Resection should be accompanied by lymph node dissection for pathologic staging.

 ## FOLLOW-UP

PROGNOSIS
- Perioperative mortality 5.2%
- For combined, all types and stages, 5-year survival 15%, varies by stage
  – Localized disease (stages I and II): 50%
  – Regional disease: 20%
  – Distant metastatic disease: 2%
- SCLC: 5-year survival 5%

COMPLICATIONS
- Development of metastatic disease to brain, bones, and liver
- Local recurrence of disease
- Postsurgical complications
- Side effects of chemotherapy or radiation
  – Dysphagia (radiation-induced, fungal)
  – Infections
  – Bleeding
  – Radiation pneumonitis
- Superior vena cava syndrome
- Atelectasis
- Spinal cord compression
- Pulmonary abscess
- Horner syndrome
- Hypercalcemia (ectopic parathyroid hormone)
- Syndrome of inappropriate antidiuretic hormone (SIADH)
- Hypercoagulable state
- Terminal restlessness (anorexia, dyspnea)

PATIENT MONITORING
- Depends on clinical history, but in general, postoperative visits every 3–6 months in the year after surgery with physical and chest radiograph
- Follow-up CT scans as indicated

REFERENCES

1. Kieninger AN, Welsh R, Bendick PJ, et al. Positron-emission tomography as a prognostic tool for early-stage lung cancer. *Am J Surg* 2006;191: 433–436.
2. Bauman G, Charette M, Reid R. Radiopharmaceuticals for the palliation of painful bone metastasis—a systematic review. *Radiother Oncol* 2005;75:258–270.
3. Little AG, Rusch VW, Bonner JA, et al. Patterns of surgical care of lung cancer patients. *Ann Thorac Surg* 2005;80:2051–2056.

 ## MISCELLANEOUS

Controversial subjects

- Surgical resection for oligometastatic disease
- Extended lymphadenectomy during surgical resection

 CODES

ICD9-CM
162.9 Malignant neoplasm of bronchus and lung, unspecified

PATIENT TEACHING
- www.lungcanceronline.org
- www.cancer.about.com

 See Corresponding Diagnostic Algorithm

L

LUPUS ERYTHEMATOSUS, DISCOID

Gary J. Silko, MD, MS

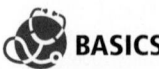 BASICS

DESCRIPTION

Discoid lupus erythematosus (DLE) is the most common form of chronic cutaneous lupus. It is a chronic skin disease characterized by sharply marginated dull, red macules with adherent scales extending into areas of atrophy, telangiectasias, or follicular plugging.

- Localized DLE: More common form with lesions occurring on the face, especially the malar areas, bridge of nose, lower lip, lower eyelids, and ears
- Generalized DLE: Lesions seen on upper extremities and thorax most often, along with usual sites for localized DLE
- System(s) Affected: Skin/Exocrine
- Synonym(s): Chronic cutaneous lupus erythematosus; Subacute cutaneous lupus erythematosus (SCLE)

ALERT
Pediatric Considerations
Neonatal lupus erythematosus is a syndrome of cutaneous lupus and/or congenital heart block. It is caused by transplacental passage of 1 of several maternal antibodies.

Pregnancy Considerations
Be aware if systemic retinoids used, pregnancy category X

GENERAL PREVENTION
Avoid sun exposure or excessive heat, cold, or skin trauma.

EPIDEMIOLOGY
- Predominant age: 25–45
- Predominant sex:
  - Localized DLE: Female > Male (3:1)
  - Generalized DLE: Female > Male (9:1)

Incidence
- White females: 3/100,000; African American Females: 8/100,000
- 100/100,000

RISK FACTORS
Systemic lupus erythematosus (SLE)

ASSOCIATED CONDITIONS
- SLE
- Mixed connective tissue disease (MCTD)
- Antiphospholipid syndrome

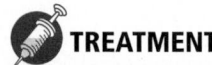 DIAGNOSIS

SIGNS AND SYMPTOMS
- Red plaquelike lesions on face, thorax, or extensor aspect of upper extremities; rare below waist
- Older lesions atrophy and appear as smooth white or hyperpigmented scars with telangiectasias.
- Scarring alopecia with scalp lesions
- "Carpet tack" appearance of skin when scale removed
- Lesions occasionally slightly pruritic or stinging
- Oral ulceration in 15% of the patients
- Photosensitivity
- Koebner response (precipitation by cutaneous trauma)

TESTS
Lab
- Localized DLE: Positive ANA in low titer (30%)
- Generalized DLE: May find increased sedimentation rate, positive ANA (60–80%), positive SS-A (80%), positive SS-B (40%) autoantibodies, positive dsDNA (<5%), leukopenia, hematuria, and albuminuria if concomitant SLE
- Special tests: Immunofluorescent staining of skin biopsies (lupus band test)
- Disorders that may alter lab results: Concomitant SLE

Diagnostic Procedures/Surgery
Skin biopsy

Pathological Findings
- Hyperkeratosis and parakeratosis
- Focal epidermal atrophy
- Hydropic degeneration of basal cell layer
- Edema, mucin, and inflammation of dermis
- Follicular plugging
- Basement zone thickened with strong periodic acid-Schiff reaction staining

DIFFERENTIAL DIAGNOSIS
- Actinic keratoses
- Polymorphous light eruption
- Drug eruptions
- Sarcoid
- Cutaneous leishmaniasis
- Lupus vulgaris
- Seborrheic dermatitis
- Lichen planus
- Plaque psoriasis
- Rosacea
- Pemphigus erythematosus
- Tinea faciei
- Jessner-Kanof disease
- Granuloma faciale

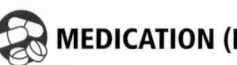 TREATMENT

INITIAL STABILIZATION
Outpatient

GENERAL MEASURES
Avoid sun exposure, excessive heat, cold, or trauma.

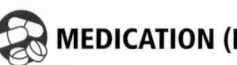 MEDICATION (DRUGS)

First Line
- Localized DLE
  - Low to medium potency topical corticosteroid (e.g., triamcinolone 0.1% b.i.d.) on all active lesions
  - If no response in 2–3 weeks, move to higher potency topical corticosteroid applied t.i.d. (e.g., betamethasone) with or without occlusion.
  - Intralesional corticosteroid (e.g., triamcinolone 2.5–5 mg/mL for the face or 5–10 mg/mL elsewhere) for resistant lesions. Use 0.5 mL per 1 cm plaque.
  - Superpotent topical steroids (e.g., clobetaso) applied b.i.d. for 2 weeks followed by a 2-week rest period. (1)[C]
- Generalized DLE
  - Hydroxychloroquine: 6.5 mg/kg/d. If no response after 3 months, switch to chloroquine 250 mg/d.
  - Short-term (1–2 weeks) of topical corticosteroids is helpful at the same time antimalarials are being started.
- Contraindications: Antimalarials, such as hydroxychloroquine, may have to be avoided in patients with pre-existing retinal or hepatic disease. Do not give to individuals with G6PD deficiency. Quinacrine rarely causes hematologic cytopenia.
- Precautions
  - Observe the patient for skin atrophy with topical steroids, especially when used on the face.
  - Patients on antimalarials should have an eye examination by an ophthalmologist at the start of the treatment and at 6-month intervals to monitor signs of retinal damage.

Second Line
- Localized DLE
  - Intralesional triamcinolone: 2.5 mg/cc injected at monthly intervals
  - Prednisone: 15 mg b.i.d., then tapered after response
- Generalized DLE
  - Quinacrine: 100 mg/d
  - Dapsone: 100 mg/d
  - Azathioprine: 100 mg/d
  - Systemic retinoid (e.g., etretinate 1 mg/kg)
  - Thalidomide 50–300 mg/d is also effective. (1)[C]
    - Dapsone is useful in patients who also have vasculitis. It is the treatment of choice for patients with bullous LE.

FOLLOW-UP

DISPOSITION

Issues for Referral
Given the scarring nature of this illness, dermatology referral is frequently indicated. Also the treatment consists of medications less commonly used by primary care providers.

PROGNOSIS
- 40% of the patients remit completely; 1–5% may develop systemic lupus (these patients usually have generalized DLE).
- Not life-threatening unless it turns into systemic type

COMPLICATIONS
Hypertrophic scarring, hypopigmentation (especially in African Americans)

PATIENT MONITORING
- Recheck patients once or twice per month.
- Ophthalmology follow-up at 6-month intervals, if patient on antimalarial
- If lesions subside, reduce dosage of antimalarials over 2–3 months, then discontinue.

 REFERENCES

1. James WD, Berger TG, Elston DM. *Andrews' Diseases of the Skin*. 10th ed. Philadelphia, PA: WB Saunders; 2006: 157–165.
2. Freedberg IM, et al. *Fitzpatrick's Dermatology in General Medicine*. 6th ed. New York, NY: McGraw-Hill; 2003: 1682–1693.
3. Habif TP. *Clinical Dermatology*. 4th ed. New York, NY: Mosby; 2004;593–606.
4. Lebwohl MG, et al. eds. *Treatment of Skin Disease*. 1st ed. New York, NY: Mosby; 2002.

 MISCELLANEOUS

See also: Systemic lupus erythematosus

 CODES

ICD9-CM
695.4 Lupus erythematosus

PATIENT TEACHING
- Teach patients proper use of sunscreens and other measures to prevent sun exposure (e.g., wide-brimmed hats, long sleeves).
- Advise the patient about symptoms of SLE for which they should watch.
- *Griffith's Instructions for Patients*, Elsevier, Philadelphia, PA.

See Corresponding Diagnostic Algorithm

L

LYME DISEASE

Barbara A. Majeroni, MD

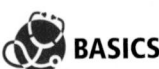 BASICS

DESCRIPTION

A multisystem infection caused by the spirochete *Borrelia burgdorferi*, which is transmitted primarily by Ixodid ticks.

- Stage 1, early localized Lyme disease, includes a characteristic expanding skin rash (erythema migrans) and constitutional flulike symptoms
- Stage 2, early disseminated Lyme disease, may present with involvement of 1 or more organ systems. Neurologic (15%) and cardiac (8%) disease are most common.
- Stage 3, chronic Lyme disease involves arthritis (50%) and chronic neurological syndromes.
- System(s) Affected: Hemic/Lymphatic/Immunologic; Musculoskeletal; Skin/Exocrine
- Synonym(s): Lyme arthritis

ALERT

Pediatric Considerations
- The drug of choice in pediatrics is amoxicillin.
- Tetracyclines are contraindicated.

Pregnancy Considerations
- Because *B. burgdorferi* can cross the placenta, pregnant patients with active disease should receive parenteral antibiotics.
- Doxycycline should not be used in pregnancy.

GENERAL PREVENTION
- Awareness of the disease, protective clothing, and careful skin inspection with timely removal of ticks may reduce the incidence of disease.
- A 3-dose vaccine, LYMErix, is no longer available.
- Prophylactic treatment with one dose of 200 mg of doxycycline within 72 hours of a tick bite in endemic areas has been suggested.

EPIDEMIOLOGY
- Predominant age: Can occur in all ages, but most common in children ages 5–14 and in the 50–59-year age group.
- Predominant sex: Male > Female

Incidence
Overall incidence: 8.2/100,000

Prevalence
Cases have been reported in all states except Hawaii, Montana, and Oklahoma. Most prevalent in the northeastern, middle Atlantic, and north central states (1).

RISK FACTORS
- Exposure to tick-infested area; most common in May to September
- Ixodid ticks are commonly found on deer. Hunters may be at an increased risk.

Genetics
HLA: Haplotype DR4 or DR2 may be more susceptible to prolonged arthritis

ETIOLOGY
Infection with spirochete *B. burgdorferi*, transmitted by the bite of Ixodid ticks.

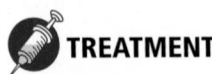 DIAGNOSIS

SIGNS AND SYMPTOMS
- Stage 1
  - Erythema migrans (60–80%)
  - Fever
  - Headache
  - Myalgias
  - Arthralgias
  - Some patients may be asymptomatic.
- Stage 2 (Involvement of 1 or more organ systems)
  - Multiple erythema migrans
  - Facial palsies or other cranial neuropathies
  - Aseptic meningitis
  - Heart block
  - Pericarditis
  - Orchitis, hepatitis, or iritis
  - Arthritis (usually large joint monarthritis)
- Stage 3
  - Recurrent synovitis
  - Recurrent tendinitis and bursitis
  - Controversial: Neuropsychiatric symptoms may include psychotic behavior, memory loss, dementia, depression, sleep disorders
  - Encephalopathic symptoms: Headache, decreased memory, difficulty concentrating, confusion, fatigue (clinical overlap with fibromyalgia)
  - Symptoms mimicking other CNS diseases: Multiple sclerosis-like syndromes, stroke-like symptoms, vestibular neuronitis, transverse myelitis, parkinsonian symptoms
  - Peripheral neuropathic symptoms: Carpal tunnel syndrome, motor, sensory, or autonomic neuropathies
  - Ophthalmic manifestations: Iritis, keratitis, retinal vasculitis, optic neuritis
- In Europe, borrelia lymphocytoma and acrodermatitis chronica are manifestations of Lyme borreliosis, but are rarely seen in the US.

ALERT
- Transmission does not occur if tick attachment is <48 hours, and only ~25% transmission for attachments of <72 hours.
- Infection is preceded by a tick bite, although patient may be unaware of tick attachment.
- History of a tick bite followed by illness with erythema migrans is the key to diagnosis. (2)[C]

TESTS

Lab
- Testing and treatment not indicated if tick attachment is <48 hours.
- Diagnosis is based mainly on clinical findings in endemic areas.
- ELISA for IgM and IgG *B. burgdorferi* antibodies (usually detectable 4–6 weeks after the initial infection), followed by a Western blot test if positive or equivocal (3)[A]
- Culture of CSF for *B. burgdorferi*
- Drugs that may alter lab results: Late-stage disease with negative serology may be seen in patients who received early antibiotic treatment.
- Disorders that may alter lab results: False-positive response has been seen with Rocky Mountain spotted fever, syphilis, systemic lupus erythematosus, and rheumatoid arthritis.

Diagnostic Procedures/Surgery
- Diagnosis is based on clinical features with exposure to a tick bite in an endemic area.
- Lumbar puncture when neurologic findings are present, with ELISA of CSF for *B. burgdorferi* antibodies

Pathological Findings
Culture of *B. burgdorferi* from blood or skin biopsy specimens has a very low yield.

DIFFERENTIAL DIAGNOSIS
- Juvenile rheumatoid arthritis
- Viral syndromes
- Later stages may mimic many other diseases (see "Signs and Symptoms").

TREATMENT

GENERAL MEASURES
Appropriate health care
- Stage 1: Clinical diagnosis; can be treated as an outpatient
- Stage 2 and 3: May require more intensive treatment, based on symptoms
- Prevention of the infection is possible by careful examination of skin for ticks after outdoor activities.
- The prompt removal of ticks may limit transmission.
- Clothing that covers the ankles should be worn in endemic areas, and the use of insect repellants is recommended.

MEDICATION (DRUGS)

First Line

Cefuroxime (Ceftin) axetil: 500 mg b.i.d. for 14–21 days (4)[A]

- Stage 1
  - Doxycycline (Vibramycin): 100 mg PO b.i.d. for 14–21 days (do not use in children under 12 or in pregnancy); *or*
  - Amoxicillin: 500 mg PO t.i.d. for 14–21 days, (pediatric dose 25–100 mg/kg/d) *or*
- Stage 2
  - Normal CSF, treat for 14–21 days: Doxycycline 100 mg PO b.i.d. or Amoxicillin 500 mg PO t.i.d.
  - With abnormal CSF, treat for 14–21 days Ceftriaxone (Rocephin) 2 g IV daily
- Stage 3
  - Oral treatment for 28 days with doxycycline 100 mg b.i.d. or amoxicillin 500 mg t.i.d.
  - If oral treatment fails, begin an IV treatment for 2–3 weeks with ceftriaxone 2 g daily; or cefotaxime 2 g q8h; or 150 mg/kg/d in 3–4 doses for children.
- Contraindications
  - Allergy to agent
  - Doxycycline is contraindicated in children and in women who are pregnant or breast-feeding.
- Precautions: Refer to the manufacturer's profile of each drug.
- Significant possible interactions
  - If the patient is taking oral anticoagulants, it may be necessary to reduce the dose.
  - Oral contraceptives may be less effective.

Second Line

Cefuroxime (Ceftin): 500 mg b.i.d. for Stage 1 disease, or t.i.d. for Stage 2 or 3 of the disease

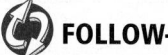 **FOLLOW-UP**

PROGNOSIS

- Early treatment with antibiotics can shorten the duration of the symptoms and prevent later disease.
- Response of late-stage disease is variable.

COMPLICATIONS

- Recurrent synovitis, tendonitis, bursitis
- Chronic neurological symptoms
- Peripheral neuropathies
- See "Signs and Symptoms" (Stage 3)

PATIENT MONITORING

Based on the severity of the symptoms, patients with Stage 2 or 3 of the disease require careful monitoring over a period of months to years.

REFERENCES

1. CDC. Lyme Disease—United States 2001–2002. *MMWR*. 2004;53:365–367.
2. Tick-borne diseases. *Med Clin North Am*. 2002;86: 205–349.
3. CDC. Notice to readers: Caution regarding testing for Lyme disease. *MMWR*. 2005;54:125.
4. Treatment of Lyme disease. *The Medical Letter*. 2005;47:41–43.

ADDITIONAL READING

Stanek G, Strle F. Lyme borreliosis. *Lancet*. 2003;362: 1639–1647.

 MISCELLANEOUS

- Cases of Lyme disease should be reported to the health department.
- Ixodid ticks require white-footed mice to complete their life cycle.
- Investigators have had some success in eradicating the ticks by providing permethrin-laced cotton in areas where the mice forage for bedding material.

 CODES

ICD9-CM

088.81 Lyme disease

PATIENT TEACHING

- In endemic areas, patients should be advised to protect themselves against tick exposure.
- American Lyme Disease Foundation, 293 Route 100, Suite 204, Somers, NY 10589.

 See Corresponding Diagnostic Algorithm

 See Patient Handout on CD

L

LYMPHANGITIS

Tyeese Gaines-Reid, DO, MA

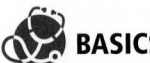 **BASICS**

DESCRIPTION
- Local inflammation of lymphatic vessels; can be acute or chronic
- Usually due to trauma and/or infection of the nearby skin

GENERAL PREVENTION
Proper wound care (1)[A]

RISK FACTORS
- Diabetes Mellitus
- Chronic steroid use
- Varicella infection
- Immunocompromise
- Human, animal or insect bites
- Fungal skin infections
- Any trauma to the skin

ETIOLOGY
- Acute or chronic infection of the skin causing inflammation of lymphatic channels
- Acute infection
  - Usually caused by *Streptococcus pyogenes*
  - Uncommonly caused by
    - *Staphylococcus aureus*
    - *Pasteurella multocida*
    - *Spirillum minus* (rat-bite disease)
    - *Pseudomonas*
    - Other strep species
- Chronic infection
  - Caused by parasites (filariasis) or fungi (sporotrichosis)
- Immunocompromised patients can be infected with Gram-negative rods, Gram-negative bacilli or fungi
- In freshwater, think *Aeromonas hydrophila*
- Worldwide, *Wuchereria bancrofti* is most common causative agent

ASSOCIATED CONDITIONS
- Lymphedema
- Lymph node dissection
- Athlete's foot
- Sporotrichosis
- Cellulitis
- Erysipelas (often coexists)
- Filarial infection

 DIAGNOSIS

SIGNS AND SYMPTOMS
- Local symptoms
  - Red macular linear streaks from site of infection toward the regional draining lymph node
  - Tenderness and warmth over affected skin
  - May have lymph node involvement
  - May have blistering of affected skin
- Systemic symptoms
  - Malaise
  - Fever and chills
  - Loss of appetite
  - Headache
  - Muscle aches

History
History of trauma to skin, cut, abrasion, or fungal infection (like athlete's foot)

Physical Exam
- Look for abscess.
- May have lymph node tenderness

TESTS
Lab
- CBC may show leukocytosis
- Blood cultures

Imaging
Plain radiology unnecessary

Diagnostic Procedures/Surgery
Aspirate and culture any pus
- Use sensitivity to guide antibiotic treatment

DIFFERENTIAL DIAGNOSIS
- Septic thrombophlebitis (2)[C]
- Superficial thrombophlebitis (2)[C]
  - Feel for induration over the vein
- Contact dermatitis (2)[C]
- Allergic reaction (2)[C]
  - Less likely to be allergic if >24 hours after exposure (i.e., insect bite)

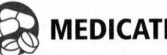 **TREATMENT**

Antifilarial medication does not help the lymphangitis associated with filariasis. (1)[A]

INITIAL STABILIZATION
- ABCs
- Fluids if in hypotensive shock

GENERAL MEASURES
- Hot, moist compresses to affected area
- If lymphedema is involved, compression garments and weight loss may help

Activity
Elevate affected area when at rest, if possible (3)[C].

MEDICATION (DRUGS)

- If nontoxic and >3 years, treat as an outpatient with oral antibiotics
- If no improvement after 48 hours of oral antibiotics, change to IV antibiotics
- If systemic involvement, start IV antibiotics immediately
- If Group A β-hemolytic streptococcus is suspected, treat aggressively

First Line
- Antibiotics (1)[A]
  - Dicloxacillin
    - Adults: 500 mg PO q6h
    - Children: 50 mg/kg/d divided into q.i.d. dosing
  - Nafcillin
    - Adults: 2 g IV q4h
    - Children: 150 mg/kg/d divided into q.i.d. dosing
  - Cephalexin
    - Adults: 500 mg PO q6h
    - Children: 50 mg/kg/d PO divided into q.i.d. dosing
  - Clindamycin (if PCN or cephalosporin allergy)
    - Adults: 150–300 mg PO q6–8h or 600 mg IV q8h
    - Children: 8–20 mg/kg/d PO divided into t.i.d. or q.i.d. dosing; 20–40 mg/kg/d IV/IM divided into t.i.d. or q.i.d. dosing

- Tylenol or Motrin for pain and fever

Second Line
- Bactrim (Good for areas with high rates of MRSA)
  - Adults: 160 mg TMP/800 mg PO q12h for 10–14 days
  - Children >2 months: 10–20 mg/kg/d PO or IM divided into t.i.d. or q.i.d. doses for 14 days

SURGERY
Incision and drainage of abscessed areas

FOLLOW-UP

48-hour follow-up to ensure proper antibiotic coverage (if outpatient)

DISPOSITION

Admission Criteria
• If patient requires IV antibiotic therapy
• If symptoms are severe (3)[C], (4)[C]
  – High fever
  – Rigor
  – Systemic toxicity
  – Shock
  – Altered mental status

Discharge Criteria
Patient can be discharged on oral antibiotics once systemic symptoms resolve.

PROGNOSIS
• Good prognosis for uncomplicated lymphangitis
• Antimicrobial therapy is effective in 90% of cases.
• Untreated, can spread rapidly, especially Group A streptococcus

COMPLICATIONS
• Sepsis
• Bacteremia
• Cellulitis extending from vessels

PATIENT MONITORING
Close follow-up to ensure decreasing inflammation

REFERENCES

1. Badger C, Preston N, Seers K, et al. Antibiotics/ anti-inflammatories for reducing acute inflammatory episodes in lymphoedema of the limbs (Cochrane Review). In: *The Cochrane Library.* 2006;1. Oxford: Update Software.
2. Falagas ME, Bliziotis IA, Kapaskelis AM. Red streaks on the Leg. *Am Fam Phys.* 2006;73(6):1061–1062.
3. Bonnetblanc JM, Bedane C. Erysipelas: recognition and management. *Am J Clin Dermatol.* 2003;4(3): 157–163.
4. Edlich RF, Winters KL, Britt LD. Bacterial diseases of the skin. J Long-Term Effects Med Implants. 2005; 15(5):499–510.

ADDITIONAL READING

Internet references:
Emedicine
www.emedicine.com
MedlinePlus Medical Encyclopedia
http://www.medlineplus.gov

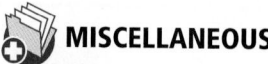 **MISCELLANEOUS**

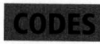

ICD9-CM
457.2 Lymphangitis

PATIENT TEACHING

Instruct patients on proper wound care (and foot care, if applicable).

 See Corresponding Diagnostic Algorithm

L

LYMPHOGRANULOMA VENEREUM

Grant C. Fowler, MD

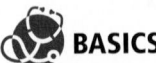 **BASICS**

DESCRIPTION

A rare systemic sexually transmitted disease caused by the 3 most virulent strains or serovars of *Chlamydia trachomatis*, the same organism responsible for chlamydial urethritis

- Tender inguinal and/or femoral lymphadenopathy, usually unilateral, painless vesicular or ulcerative lesions on the external genitalia may be seen in early disease, and severe anogenital inflammation and scarring may result from untreated disease.
- Usually a disease of the tropics, especially Africa, but also seen in the Caribbean (Haiti and Jamaica), South America, East Asia, and Indonesia.
- System(s) Affected: Gastrointestinal; Hemic/Lymphatic/Immunologic; Reproductive
- Synonym(s): Tropical bubo; Climatic bubo; Strumous bubo; Poradenitis inguinalis; Durand-Nicolas-Favre disease; Lymphogranuloma inguinale; 4th or 5th or 6th venereal disease

ALERT
Pregnancy Considerations
Congenital transmission does not occur, but may be acquired through an infected birth canal.

GENERAL PREVENTION
- Treat sexual contact(s).
- Condoms should be worn with sexual activity outside of long term monogamous relationships.
- Condoms may provide protection against genital-anogenital transmission, but have no impact on transmission between other sites.

EPIDEMIOLOGY
- Predominant age: 3rd decade; corresponds with average age of peak sexual activity
- Predominant sex: Male > Female (5:1)

Incidence
In the US, ~300 cases reported each year.

Prevalence
Anorectal lymphogranuloma venereum (LGV): Prevalence is increasing in the United States in homosexual males.

RISK FACTORS
- Unprotected intercourse
- Anal intercourse
- Residing in tropical or developing countries
- Prostitution

ETIOLOGY
Three of 15 known strains of *C. trachomatis*, described as serovars L1, L2, and L3, are responsible for LGV. Although the strains of Chlamydia that cause urethritis appear to infect only squamocolumnar cells, LGV strains are more invasive and capable of replication in macrophages.

ASSOCIATED CONDITIONS
Any of the sexually transmitted diseases. Screening should be done for syphilis and HIV.

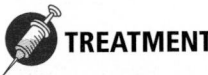 **DIAGNOSIS**

SIGNS AND SYMPTOMS
Three stages

- Primary: Superficial lesions such as papules, vesicles, ulcers, or erosions appear on the external genitalia 3–30 days after exposure. Lesions are painless and disappear in a few days, leaving no scar. This stage often escapes notice.
- Secondary: The inguinal syndrome (bubonic stage) or hemorrhagic proctitis following rectal intercourse
  - Predominantly in men (male-to-female ratio >10:1)
  - Fever, chills, headache, myalgias
  - Inguinal syndrome: Regional lymphadenopathy occurring a week to months after the primary stage. Buboes begin as a mass of firm, tender, enlarged, matted lymph nodes, often unilateral and eventually involving the overlying skin with erythema and adhesions. As the buboes enlarge, the patient experiences severe groin pain and often walks with a limp. Within 1–2 weeks, the buboes may become fluctuant and rupture, relieving the pain, leaving fistulas to drain or involute and form firm inguinal masses.
  - Proctitis: Anal pruritus and a mucous rectal discharge, multiple discrete superficial ulcerations with irregular borders, rectal pain, and tenesmus
- Tertiary: Anogenital stage
  - Lymphatic obstruction or scarring
  - Genitalia or anorectal canal inflammation
  - Predominantly women and homosexual men.
  - Lymphatic obstruction may produce either perianal growths or lymphoid tissue resembling hemorrhoids.
  - Perirectal abscesses, ischiorectal and rectovaginal fistulas, anal fistulas, and rectal strictures or stenosis may occur.

History
Recent unprotected intercourse with a prostitute or homosexual male, especially anal intercourse or intercourse with someone recently visting or from the tropics such as Africa, the Caribbean, South America, East Asia, or Indonesia may increase the likelihood of LGV.

Physical Exam
In the primary stage, painless, superficial papules, vesicles, ulcers, or erosions near the area of exposure may be all that is noted. In the secondary stage, swollen, tender lymph glands, often unilateral, are the most common finding. These glands may become fluctuant within 1–2 weeks. Patients with LGV practicing anal intercourse may have a mucous rectal discharge and hemorrhagic proctitis on anoscopy.

TESTS
- Immunoglobulin M microimmunofluorescence (MIF) is a test that may be used for LGV.
- Antibody levels to L1, L2, and L3 serovars of *C. trachomatis* can also be measured with complement fixation, although cross-reactivity with other chlamydial organisms is possible.
- A fourfold rise in MIF titer to LGV antigen or a complement fixation titer >1:64, with the proper clinical scenario is probably LGV. Complement levels >1:128 confirm the LGV diagnosis.
- MIF titers are more sensitive and specific than the complement fixation test.
- Polymerase chain reaction (PCR) testing—recently developed to diagnose LGV

Lab
- Leukocytosis with lymphocytosis or monocytosis
- Elevated erythrocyte sedimentation rate
- VDRL/rapid plasma regain, HIV, herpes simplex virus (HSV) testing
- Drugs that may alter lab results: Antibiotics
- Disorders that may alter lab results: Chlamydial urethritis

Imaging
- Computerized tomography for retroperitoneal adenitis
- Barium enema may reveal the characteristic elongated stricture of rectal LGV.

Diagnostic Procedures/Surgery
Aspiration or drainage of bubo for culture

DIFFERENTIAL DIAGNOSIS
- Inguinal adenitis
  - Chancroid, granuloma inguinale (donovanosis), genital herpes, or syphilis
  - Inguinal adenitis includes catscratch disease, lymphoma, HIV, and reactive adenopathy.
  - Less common: Lymphoproliferative buboes
- Buboes or suppurative adenitis: Chancroid, donovanosis, plague, tularemia, sporotrichosis, actinomycosis, or tuberculosis
- Retroperitoneal adenitis
- Proctitis: Gonococcal and non-LGV chlamydial proctitis, inflammatory bowel disease
- Lymphatic obstruction: Schistosomiasis or malignancy.

TREATMENT

INITIAL STABILIZATION
Outpatient care except for rare complications, such as severe pain or for surgical repair of complications

GENERAL MEASURES
Diet
No special diet unless tetracyclines are used

SPECIAL THERAPY
IV Fluids
Only necessary for severe pain control, for surgery if complications occur, or for patients unable to tolerate oral medications

MEDICATION (DRUGS)

First Line
- For acute cases: Doxycycline 100 mg PO b.i.d. for 21 days (strength of evidence B)
- For chronic or relapsing cases: Consider longer course of therapy.
- Contraindications: Tetracycline allergy or sensitivity
- Precautions: Antibiotic-induced diarrhea may ensue.

ALERT

Pregnancy Considerations
Treat pregnant and lactating women with an erythromycin regimen. Doxycycline is contraindicated in pregnancy.

Second Line
- Erythromycin base 500 mg PO q.i.d. for 21 days or azithromycin 1.0 g PO once weekly for 3 weeks (data are lacking).
- Sulfisoxazole 500 mg PO q.i.d. for 21 days or equivalent sulfonamide course
- Chloramphenicol and rifampin may be used.

SURGERY
In the acute bubonic stage, nodes should be aspirated or incised and drained.

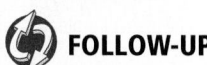

FOLLOW-UP

DISPOSITION

Admission Criteria
Patient unable to tolerate oral antibiotics, unable to ambulate or perform self-care due to pain or other complications, or patients preparing to undergo surgery.

Discharge Criteria
If the patient lives alone, they can be discharged when they are able to perform self-care. If unable to perform self-care, the patient can be discharged when the family is capable of providing care, or the patient can be discharged to a nursing home or other step-down care facility.

Issues for Referral
If at all possible, surgery for complications should be delayed until antibiotic therapy has been administered for at least a few days and any fever has resolved. Referral should be considered for patients with probable LGV failing to respond to 14 days of antibiotics or those getting worse after 7 days of antibiotics. Referral should also be considered for patients in which the diagnosis is uncertain or for those likely to experience complications during or following treatment.

PROGNOSIS
- Improved by early treatment
- Complete resolution of symptoms is usual if treatment is undertaken before scarring.
- Reinfection and/or inadequate treatment may result in relapse.

COMPLICATIONS
- Scarring, including possible ureteral or bowel obstruction, persistent rectovaginal fistula, or gross destruction of the anal canal, anal sphincter, or perineum. Repair of such complications as well as plastic repair of some of the complications of lymphatic obstruction, such as genital elephantiasis, are the more common surgical indications. Surgery should be performed only after antibiotic treatment.
- Mild rectal strictures can occasionally be dilated on an outpatient basis.
- Squamous cell carcinoma has been associated with LGV.

PATIENT MONITORING
- Fever and bubo pain usually abate within 1–2 days after starting antibiotics. For persistent fever or malaise, monitor closely for complications such as abscesses or superinfections.
- Treatment has no effect on existing scar tissue; therefore, monitor for surgical complications.
- Dual infections with other sexually transmitted diseases are common; appropriate monitoring should be performed, especially for syphilis and HIV.
- Patients should be observed until signs and symptoms resolve.

REFERENCES

1. Mabey D, Peeling RW. Lymphogranuloma venereum. *Sex Transm Infect.* 2002;78(2): 90–92. Available from http://sti.bmjjournals.com/cgi/content/full/78/2/90
2. Centers for Disease Control and Prevention. Sexually transmitted diseases treatment guidelines 2002. *MMWR Recomm Rep.* 2002;51(RR-6):1–78. Available from http://www.cdc.gov/std/chlamydia/default.htm
3. Spaargaren J, Schachter J, Moncada J, et al. Slow epidemic of lymphogranuloma venereum L2b strain. *Emerg Infect Dis* [serial on the Internet]. 2005 Nov [date cited]. Available from http://www.cdc.gov/ncidod/EID/vol11no11/05-0821.htm
4. World Health Organization. Guidelines for the management of sexually transmitted infections. Geneva: WHO; 2003. Available from http://www.who.int/reproductive-health/publications/rhr_01_10_mngt_stis/index.html

MISCELLANEOUS
- Other notes: HIV-infected patients with LGV should be treated with usual LGV regimen, but may require longer therapy.
- See also: Chancroid; Chlamydial sexually transmitted diseases; Herpes, genital; Syphilis

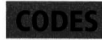

CODES

ICD9-CM
099.1 Lymphogranuloma venereum

PATIENT TEACHING
- LGV is a sexually transmitted disease. The patient should be counseled about other sexually transmitted diseases and safe sex practices.
- Sexual partner(s) should be treated, especially those with contact within 30 days before onset of symptoms.
- Offer HIV and syphilis counseling and testing.

Diet
Dietary restrictions are only needed for patients taking tetracyclines, and these should be taken on an empty stomach except for doxycycline which can be taken with food. Patients taking antibiotics for prolonged periods should seek medical care for persistent diarrhea, especially if it is associated with a fever.

Activity
Patients should abstain from intercourse or other sexual contact until treatment is complete. Patients taking tetracyclines should either avoid the sun or use sunscreens to minimize the risk of photosensitization. Otherwise, activities are only limited by symptoms.

Prevention
Patients should be counseled about other sexually transmitted diseases, and sexual contacts should be treated. Sexual abstinence or sexual activity restricted to a diseasefree, mutually monogamous relationship are the only methods of preventing LGV. Sexual activity with prostitutes, anal intercourse, and sexual activity with homosexual men increase the risk of acquiring LGV.

See Corresponding Diagnostic Algorithm

L

LYMPHOMA, BURKITT

Jeremy Golding, MD

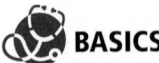 **BASICS**

DESCRIPTION

- Highly aggressive B-cell lymphoma
- Most rapidly growing of all lymphomas
- Primarily involves the lymphatic and hematologic systems, but may involve sites other than lymph nodes or reticuloendothelial system, particularly ileocecal region, ovaries, kidneys, breasts, and central nervous system (CNS). At diagnosis, bone marrow involvement is present in 20% of patients.
- 1st tumor to be etiologically associated with a virus (Epstein-Barr [EBV]), and a specific chromosome translocation [t(8;14)].
- 3 distinct forms, differing in epidemiology, clinical presentation, and genetics
  - Endemic, or African
  - Sporadic, nonendemic, or American
  - Immunodeficiency-related, or HIV/AIDS-related
- 3 morphologic variants are defined
  - Classic
  - Atypical
  - Burkitt lymphoma with plasmacytoid differentiation
- System(s) Affected: Hematologic; Lymphatic; Immunologic
- Synonym(s): Undifferentiated lymphoma, Burkitt and non-Burkitt type (modified Rappaport classification); Malignant lymphoma, small noncleaved cell, Burkitt type (Working Formulation); Burkitt lymphoma and high-grade B-cell lymphoma, Burkitt-like (REAL Classification); Acute lymphoblastic leukemia, L3 type (FAB Classification)

ALERT

Pediatric Considerations
Common age group for this disorder

Geriatric Considerations
Unusual in this age group

Pregnancy Considerations
Described in pregnancy. With aggressive treatment, good maternal and fetal outcome.

GENERAL PREVENTION
Tumor is associated with EBV infection, immunodeficiency, and malaria.

EPIDEMIOLOGY

- Predominant age: 3 months–16 years
- WHO describes 3 clinical settings: Endemic (central Africa), sporadic, and HIV-associated
- In endemic regions, Burkitt lymphoma is the most common tumor of childhood, most frequently occurring in 4–7-year-old children
- Male > Female (2:1)
- More common in children and immunosuppressed adults than in healthy adults.
- HIV- associated Burkitt occurs mainly in adults.

Incidence
- Rare in US
- One of the most common tumors associated with HIV
- Most common tumor of children in endemic region; incidence 50-fold higher than in the US.
- Accounts for 30–40% of lymphomas in children in the US and western Europe
- Comprises <1% of adult NHL

Prevalence
Burkitt lymphoma is highly aggressive, with high mortality in untreated patients.

RISK FACTORS
- In endemic areas, children with early acquisition of EBV infection are at increased risk.
- Association with EBV: 95% in endemic regions, 15–20% in sporadic cases
- Immunodeficiency, especially HIV-related, more commonly in patients with CD4 counts >200 cells μ/L.
- In patients with malaria, a 100-fold increase in incidence of Burkitt lymphoma, entirely EBV-positive disease

Genetics
- Reciprocal chromosome translocation involving *c-myc* and immunoglobulin heavy chain (IgH) gene [t(8;14)] (80%)
- Reciprocal chromosome translocation involving *c-myc* and κ or λ light chain (IgL) gene t(2;8) or t (8;22)] (20%)

ETIOLOGY
- Deregulation of *c-myc* is the defining biologic feature, resulting in unabated cell proliferation. Translocation of *c-myc* to immunoglobulin coding regions results in constitutive expression of this oncogene.
- High association with EBV. Any condition resulting in an increase in the number of EBV-infected cells that are recruited into germinal-center reactions may increase the risk of chromosomal translocation.
- In malaria: T-cell suppression and antigenic stimulation result in increased activation of EBV-infected B cells
- In AIDS patients with persistent generalized lymphadenopathy and polyclonal B-cell activation, poorly regulated proliferation of genetically unstable B cells increases the chance of translocations involving *c-myc*.

ASSOCIATED CONDITIONS
- EBV infection
- Immunodeficiency, especially AIDS
- Malaria

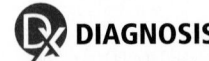 **DIAGNOSIS**

SIGNS AND SYMPTOMS
- Endemic (African)
  - Jaw or facial bone tumor, which may present as mouth pain, loose teeth, or jaw mass
  - Anemia
  - Spread to extranodal sites including mesentery, ovary, testis, kidney, breast, bone marrow, meninges
- Nonendemic (American): Extranodal disease, abdominal presentation typical
  - Bulky disease, ascites, tumor involving distal ileum, stomach, cecum, mesentery, kidney, testis, ovary, breast, bone marrow, CNS
  - Abdominal pain, nausea, vomiting, bowel obstruction, gastrointestinal bleeding, symptoms mimicking acute appendicitis or intussusception.
- Immunodeficiency-associated lymphoma may involve lymph nodes, bone marrow, and extranodal sites, usually abdominal.

TESTS

Lab
- Diagnosis is suggested by cellular morphology on histologic examination of bone marrow aspirate or lymph node biopsy. Histologic impression is supported by immunophenotypic data and cytogenetic studies. Burkitt-like lymphoma is a problematic entity with little reproducibility of diagnosis, and may be confused with diffuse large B cell lymphoma (DLBCL).
- Immunologic studies: Cells express surface IgM and B-associated antigens. According to the Revised European-American Lymphoma classification (REAL), Burkitt lymphoma cells are positive for CD10, CD19, CD20, and are negative for CD5 and CD23.
- Cytogenic studies to visualize chromosomal translocation:[t(8;14), t(2;8), or t (8;22)]; fluorescence in situ hybridization (FISH) or long-segment polymerase chain reaction may be necessary to identify translocation. Translocation is characteristic of, although not specific for, Burkitt.
- CBC: Anemia
- Elevated serum lactate dehydrogenase and uric acid levels as measures of tumor load

Imaging
- Chest radiograph
- CT scan of chest and abdomen

Diagnostic Procedures/Surgery
- Bone marrow biopsy and aspiration
- Lumbar puncture for CSF cytology
- Lymph node biopsy
- Diagnostic laparotomy, resection of localized disease.

Pathological Findings
- Histology shows a monotonous diffuse infiltrate of medium-size round cells, with round or oval nuclei, several prominent nucleoli, and coarse chromatin. Cytoplasm is moderately abundant.
- Mitotic rate is high; 100% of viable cells should be actively engaged in cell cycle, and therefore should express Ki-67.
- Spontaneous apoptosis gives rise to the "starry sky" histologic appearance resulting from the presence of tingible body macrophages. Starry sky pattern is characteristic, although not pathognomonic for Burkitt lymphoma.
- Although usually diffuse, early lesions may show selective involvement of germinal centers.

DIFFERENTIAL DIAGNOSIS
- Burkitt-like lymphoma: Immunophenotype and molecular characteristics differ from those of classic Burkitt lymphoma; may appear intermediate between Burkitt and DLBCL
- DLBCL: Large, irregular cells, often with BCL rearrangement
- Precursor B-lymphocytic lymphoma
- Precursor T-lymphocytic lymphoma
- Mantle cell lymphoma, blastoid variant
- Florid follicular hyperplasia

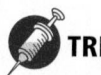 TREATMENT

INITIAL STABILIZATION
- Burkitt lymphomas have high growth fractions and short doubling times. Reduction of tumor burden may be necessary to manage abdominal complications.
- Because of the high rate of tumor growth, rapid initiation of definitive chemotherapy is essential.

GENERAL MEASURES
- Chemotherapy should be initiated without delay.
- Physical encroachment of tumor may become life-threatening.
- Patients with Burkitt lymphoma are particularly at risk for tumor lysis syndrome.

Radiotherapy
Radiotherapy has no role in the treatment of Burkitt lymphoma.

IV Fluids
Manage tumor lysis syndrome.

MEDICATION (DRUGS)
- Treatment is with multiagent chemotherapeutic programs, over a short period of time.
- Chemotherapeutic agents include cyclophosphamide, methotrexate, vincristine, prednisone, high-dose methotrexate, high-dose cytarabine, etoposide, isophosphamide.
- CNS prophylaxis is warranted in most patients except in the case of limited disease remote from the CNS.
- Intrathecal methotrexate with or without IV methotrexate and cytarabine may be used for CNS prophylaxis.
- Chemotherapy may be of short duration, but subsequent cycles should be initiated as soon as hematologic recovery permits.
- Tumor has high proliferative rate; delay of chemotherapy may result in regrowth of resistant tumor between cycles.
- High-dose chemotherapy with hematopoietic stem cell transplantation is also described.
- Type and extent of therapy depend on stage of disease.

SURGERY
Surgery for biopsy and staging

FOLLOW-UP

Detection of recurrence.

Issues for Referral
Refer to hematologist/oncologist.

PROGNOSIS
- Overall mortality for endemic Burkitt lymphoma remains high where access to health care is limited.
- Tumor burden may be the most important variable affecting prognosis.
- In localized disease, 5-year disease-free survival exceeds 90%.
- Aggressive treatment of advanced disease yields >80% 5-year disease-free survival.
- Recurrent disease tends to be highly resistant to therapy.
- Prognosis is poor for immunocompromised patients.
- Without treatment, prognosis is grave.

COMPLICATIONS
- Complications of extensive abdominal disease include obstructive jaundice and pancreatitis, bowel obstruction, or intestinal perforation.
- Tumor lysis syndrome with renal failure (uric acid nephropathy) secondary to high tumor burden and rapid cell turnover may occur prior to and especially following initiation of chemotherapy.
- Other complications of chemotherapy include neurotoxicity from chemotherapeutic agents, myelosuppression, alopecia, and mucositis.

REFERENCES
1. Blum KA, et al. Adult Burkitt leukemia and lymphoma. *Blood*. 2004;3009–3020.
2. Ferry J. Burkitt's lymphoma: Clinicopathologic features and differential diagnosis. *Oncologist*. 2006;11:375–383.
3. Freedman AS, Harris NL. Clinical and pathological features of Burkitt's lymphoma. UpToDate; 2006.
4. Koniaris LG et al. Management of gastrointestinal lymphoma. *J Am Coll Surg*. 2003;197127–197141.
5. Okebe JU, et al. Therapeutic interventions for Burkitt's lymphoma in children. *Cochrane Database Sys Rev*. 2006.
6. Song KW, et al. Hematopoietic stem cell transplantation as primary therapy of sporadic adult Burkitt lymphoma. *Br J Hematol*. 2006;133:634–637.
7. Rizzieri DA, et al. Intensive chemotherapy with and without cranial radiation for Burkitt leukemia and lymphoma. *Cancer*. 2004;1001438–1001448.

MISCELLANEOUS

CODES

ICD9-CM
200.20 Burkitt tumor or lymphoma, unspecified site, extranodal and solid organ sites level list item

PATIENT TEACHING
Educational materials are available from the Leukemia Society of America. 733 3rd Ave., New York, NY 10017; (800) 955-4572(212) 573-8424.

 See Corresponding Diagnostic Algorithm

L

MACULAR DEGENERATION, AGE-RELATED (ARMD)

Richard W. Allinson, MD

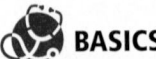 **BASICS**

DESCRIPTION
- Pigmentary changes in the macula or typical drusen associated with visual loss to the 20/30 level or worse, not caused by cataract or other eye disease, in individuals >50 years
- Some definitions exclude age or visual-acuity criteria.
- Leading cause of irreversible, severe visual loss in persons >65 years
- Stages
  - Atrophic/nonexudative
  - Neovascular/exudative
- System(s) Affected: Nervous
- Synonym(s): Senile macular degeneration; Subretinal neovascularization; ARMD

GENERAL PREVENTION
- UV protection for eyes
- Routine ophthalmologic visits
  - Every 2–4 years for patients 40–64 years
  - Every 1–2 years after age 65
- Daily Amsler grid testing
- Patients who take statin drugs, which modify lipid profiles, may have a reduced risk.

EPIDEMIOLOGY
- Neovascular/exudative form is rare in blacks and more common in whites.
- Predominant sex: Female

Incidence
- In the Framingham Eye Study (FES) drusen were noted in 25% of all participants who were ≥52 years old. ARMD-associated visual loss was noted in 5.7%.
- Atrophic/nonexudative stage accounts for 20% of cases of severe visual loss.
- Neovascular/exudative stage accounts for 80% of cases of severe visual loss.

Prevalence
- Per FES study
  - People 52–64 years of age: 1.6%
  - People 65–74 years of age: 11%
  - People ≥75 years of age: 27.9%
- Increases with age
  - >75 years: 1/4 of men and 1/3 of women will have evidence of ARMD.

RISK FACTORS
- Obesity (increased BMI)
- Ethnicity: Non-Hispanic whites
- Low educational level
- Cigarette smoking
- Chlamydophila pneumoniae infection
- Family history
- Conflicting data exist for the following
  - Excess sunlight exposure
  - Blue or light iris color
  - Hyperopia
  - Diets lacking vitamin E and beta carotene
  - History of cardiovascular disease (hypertension, circulatory problems)
  - Short height

Genetics
Genetic susceptibility may be a factor in ARMD.
- ~1/4 genetically determined

PATHOPHYSIOLOGY
- Breaks in Bruch membrane allows choroidal neovascular membranes (CNVMs) to invade the retinal pigment epithelium (RPE) and grow into the subretinal space.
- Atrophic/nonexudative: Drusen and/or pigmentary changes in the macula
- Neovascular/exudative: Growth of blood vessels underneath the retina

ETIOLOGY
- Visible light can result in the formation and accumulation of metabolic byproducts in the RPE, a pigment layer underneath the retina that normally helps remove metabolic byproducts from the retina. Excess accumulation of these metabolic byproducts interferes with the normal metabolic activity of the RPE and can lead to the formation of drusen.
- Neovascular stage generally arises from the atrophic stage.
- Most patients do not progress beyond the atrophic/nonexudative stage; however, those who do are at a greater risk of developing severe visual loss.

ASSOCIATED CONDITIONS
- Presumed ocular histoplasmosis syndrome
- Exudative retinal detachment
- Vitreous hemorrhage
- Other causes of CNVMs

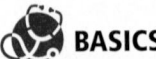 **DIAGNOSIS**

SIGNS AND SYMPTOMS
- Atrophic/nonexudative stage
  - Drusen
  - Small yellowish-white lesions
  - Can be subdivided into types such as hard drusen and soft drusen
  - Atrophy of the retinal pigment epithelium
- Neovascular/exudative stage
  - Blood vessels growing underneath the retina from the choroid are called CNVMs or subretinal neovascularization (SRN). The choroid is the vascular layer underneath the retinal pigment epithelium.
  - Subretinal fluid
  - Exudates
  - Subretinal hemorrhage
  - Patients frequently notice distortion of central vision. On Amsler grid testing the horizontal or vertical lines may become broken, distorted, or missing. Patients may notice straight lines appear crooked (e.g., telephone poles).
  - Disciform scar: An advanced stage resulting in a fibrovascular scar

TESTS

Diagnostic Procedures/Surgery
- Daily Amsler grid testing
- Eye examination with dilated fundus examination
- Fluorescein angiography
  - Detection of choroidal neovascular membranes
  - Differentiate between atrophic and neovascular ARMD
- Indocyanine green videoangiography: Identify occult or hidden CNVMs
- Optical coherence tomography (OCT) may be useful in identifying CNVMs.

Pathological Findings
Drusen: Deposits of hyaline material between the RPE and Bruch membrane (the limiting membrane between the RPE and the choroid)

DIFFERENTIAL DIAGNOSIS
- Idiopathic SRN
- Presumed ocular histoplasmosis syndrome
- Diabetic retinopathy
- Hypertensive retinopathy

TREATMENT

GENERAL MEASURES
- Atrophic/nonexudative macular degeneration
  - Free radical formation in the retina, induced by visible light, may play a role in cellular damage that results in ARMD.
  - Vitamins A, E, and C and beta-carotene may be useful in preventing cellular damage.
  - Oral zinc may retard visual loss.
  - Laser photocoagulation to treat drusen is being investigated.
- Neovascular/exudative macular degeneration
  - The Macular Photocoagulation Study (MPS) demonstrated a treatment benefit for laser treatment of CNVMs that were 200 μm (200 μm = 0.2 mm) or greater from the center of the macula.
  - The MPS showed that the benefits of argon laser photocoagulation were greatest 1 year after treatment. At that time, the proportion of eyes with severe visual loss was reduced 51% by treatment, from 43% in untreated eyes to 21% in treated eyes. The deterioration in treatment effect in the MPS is primarily due to recurrent CNVMs growing toward the center of the macula.
  - Fluorescein angiogram usually can determine whether a CNVM is present, if it is well defined, and if it is in a treatable position.
- Treatment of CNVMs 1–199 μm from the center of the macula has been studied by the Age-Related Macular Degeneration Study-Krypton Laser (ARMDS-K). The benefit of laser treatment was greatest among patients without evidence of hypertension. No benefit was observed among patients who had highly elevated BP and/or used antihypertensive medication.
- Vitrectomy has been used to remove choroidal neovascular membranes, but this is generally not recommended.
  - CNVMs can bleed spontaneously leaving blood underneath the retina. Vitrectomy to remove subretinal blood may be of benefit and should be performed within 7 days of the bleed. Tissue plasminogen activator (tPA) instilled into the eye may help remove a subretinal hemorrhage. In some cases, intravitreal gas with or without tPA may displace submacular blood.
- Macular translocation involves intentionally creating a retinal detachment and attempting to shift the macula away from the CNVM. Laser is then applied to the CNVM after the retina is translocated. This procedure is associated with potential serious surgical risks.
- Photodynamic therapy (PDT) with verteporfin reduces vision loss in patients with ~50% "classic" subfoveal CNVMs. Verteporfin is administered IV, and a diode laser at 689 nm is applied to the CNVM.
  - After 24 months of follow-up in patients who underwent PDT to treat predominantly classic subfoveal CNVM, 59% of the verteporfin-treated eyes versus 31% of the placebo-treated eyes lost fewer than 15 letters from baseline. (1)[A]
  - In occult subfoveal CNVMs with no classic component, PDT significantly reduces the risk of moderate and severe vision loss.

  - PDT treatment benefit may not only depend on lesion type, but also on lesion size and presenting visual acuity. The treatment benefit may be related to smaller lesion size and worse presenting visual acuity.
  - Patients should be informed that there is about a 4% risk of acute, severe vision loss after PDT.
  - Intravitreal triamcinolone combined with PDT may result in improved visual acuity for patients with CNVMs. (2)[B]
- Low-vision aids may be helpful.

Diet
- High in vitamins A, E, C, and beta-carotene along with zinc may be of benefit
- Eating dark green, leafy vegetables (spinach or collard greens), which are rich in carotinoids, may decrease the risk of developing the neovascular/exudative stage.

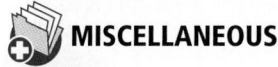

MEDICATION (DRUGS)

First Line
Zinc and antioxidants may be of benefit.

- Age-Related Eye Disease Study (AREDS) found that a high-dose regimen of vitamin and mineral supplements reduces progression of ARMD in some cases. (3)[A]
  - Recommended daily doses: Vitamin C 500 mg, vitamin E 400 IU, beta-carotene 15 mg, zinc oxide 80 mg, and cupric oxide 2 mg
  - Exercise caution with beta-carotene use in smokers due to potential link to lung cancer.

Second Line
- Anecortave acetate is being tested in the treatment of exudative ARMD.
  - Injected next to the eye, via a posterior juxtascleral injection
- Pegaptanib sodium (Macugen) is a compound that binds to and neutralizes VEGF. The usual dose is 0.3 mg injected intravitreally every 6 weeks as needed for the treatment of neovascular ARMD. (4)[A]
- Ranibizumab (Lucentis) is another promising anti-VEGF compound being tested in the treatment of exudative ARMD. This is administered intravitreally every 4 weeks.
- Bevacizumab (Avastin) is another anti-VEGF compounded administered systemically and intravitreally which is being evaluated in the treatment of neovascular ARMD.

SURGERY
See "General Measures."

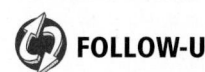

FOLLOW-UP

- Outpatient care for laser treatment
- Inpatient or outpatient care for vitrectomy surgery

PROGNOSIS
- Patients with bilateral soft drusen and pigmentary changes in the macula, but no evidences of exudation, have an increased likelihood of developing CNVMs and subsequent visual loss.
- Patients with bilateral drusen carry a cumulative risk of 14.7% over 5 years of suffering significant visual loss in 1 eye from the neovascular stage of ARMD.

- Patients with neovascular stage in 1 eye and drusen in the opposite eye are at an annual risk of 5–14% of developing the neovascular stage in opposite eye with drusen.
- High incidence of recurrence after thermal laser treatment for CNVMs.

COMPLICATIONS
Blindness

PATIENT MONITORING
- Laser-treated patients should be reexamined promptly if new visual symptoms occur.
- Amsler grid can aid in discovering visual disturbances.
- Patients with soft drusen or pigmentary changes in the macula are at an increased risk of visual loss. They should be instructed that it is important to monitor their vision, such as by Amsler grid testing and subjective measures of visual acuity, such as reading vision and image clarity. If there are no new symptoms, follow-up examination in 6–12 months.

REFERENCES

1. Bressler NM. Photodynamic therapy of subfoveal choroidal neovascularization in age-related macular degeneration with verteporfin: Two-year results of two randomized clinical trials—Tap Report 2. *Arch Ophthalmol*. 2001;119:198–207.
2. Augustin AJ, Schmidt-Erfurth U. Verteporfin therapy combined with intravitreal Triamcinolone in all types of choroidal neovascularization due to age-related macular degeneration. *Ophthalmology*. 2006;113:14–22.
3. Age-Related Eye Disease Study Research Group. A randomized, placebo-controlled, clinical trial of high-dose supplementation with vitamins C and E, beta carotene, and zinc for age-related macular degeneration and vision loss: AREDS Report No.8. *Arch Ophthalmol*. 2001;119:1417–1436.
4. Gragoudas ES, et al. Pegaptanib for neovascular age-related macular degeneration. *N Engl J Med*. 2004;351:2805–2816.

MISCELLANEOUS

CODES

ICD9-CM
- 362.51 Nonexudative senile macular degeneration
- 362.52 Exudative senile macular degeneration
- 362.57 Drusen (degenerative)

PATIENT TEACHING
Instruct visually impaired patients to check with the local low-vision center for aids.

 See Patient Handout on CD

M

MALARIA

Maryellen Antonetti, MPH, PA-C, RN

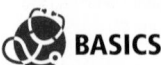 **BASICS**

DESCRIPTION
- An acute and chronic protozoan infection transmitted to humans by *Anopheles* spp. mosquitoes.
- 4 species of *Plasmodium* cause human infection, *P. falciparum, P. vivax, P. ovale,* and *P. malariae*.
- Most morbidity and mortality is caused by *P. falciparum*; it is responsible for >1.5 million deaths annually, the majority of which occur in children <5 years in sub-Saharan Africa.
- System(s) Affected: Primarily Hemic/Lymphatic/Immunologic

GENERAL PREVENTION
- Use malarial chemoprophylaxis when in endemic area. A retrospective study investigating all malaria-related deaths in the US over the last several decades determined >80% were preventable.
- Oral chemoprophylaxis is available.
- Mefloquine (begin 1 week before arrival and continue for 4 weeks after leaving area). Adults, 250 mg (1 tablet) weekly; children <15 kg, 5 mg/kg; children 15–19 kg, 1/4 tablet weekly; children 20–30 kg, 1/2 tablet weekly; children 31–45 kg, 3/4 tablet weekly; children >45 kg, 1 tablet weekly
- Malarone (begin 1–2 days before arrival and continue for 1 week after leaving area). Adults, 250 mg/100 mg/d (1 adult tablet); children 11–20 kg, 62.5 mg/25 mg/d (1 pediatric tablet); children 21–30 kg, 2 pediatric tablets daily; children 31–40 kg, 3 pediatric tablets daily; children >40 kg, 1 adult tablet daily
- Doxycycline (begin 1–2 days before arrival and continue for 4 weeks after leaving area). Adults, 100 mg/d; children, 2 mg/kg/d, up to 100 mg/d (not for children <8 years old)
- Oral chemoprophylaxis for areas with chloroquine-sensitive *Plasmodium* species: Chloroquine phosphate (begin 1–2 weeks before arrival and continue for 4 weeks after leaving area). Adults, 300 mg base (500 mg salt) weekly; children, 5 mg base/kg weekly up to 300 mg
- Primaquine may also be a 2nd-line agent but only be so in consultation with expert or CDC.
- Personal measures (variable efficacy)
  – DEET-containing insect repellent
  – Clothing that covers most of the body
  – Mosquito nets sprayed with permethrin
  – Air conditioning

EPIDEMIOLOGY
- Predominant age: All ages
- Predominant sex: Male = Female

Incidence
- Most cases (>99%) are imported. Very rare endemic spread in the US.
- Causes of all reported cases in the US in 2002
  – *P. falciparum*: 52%
  – *P. vivax*: 25%
  – *P. malariae*: 3%
  – *P. ovale*: 3%

RISK FACTORS
- Traveling and/or migration from an area where malaria is endemic (most cases, particularly *P. falciparum*, originate in sub-Saharan Africa)
- Rarely, blood transfusion, mother-to-fetus transmission and autocanthous transmission (3)[A]

Genetics
No known specific genetic predilection but inherited conditions may affect disease severity and susceptibility (i.e., glucose-6-phosphate deficiency [G6PD], sickle cell disease or trait, and hereditary ovalocytosis probably help protect against severe *P. falciparum* infection).

PATHOPHYSIOLOGY
P. falciparum induces human RBCs to secrete a protein on their surface (histidine-rich protein). This makes RBCs stick to the intravascular surface of small blood vessels, causing obstruction and end-organ ischemia. All species, including *P. falciparum*, cause release of cytokines and TNF-α.

ETIOLOGY
P. falciparum, P. malariae, P. vivax, P. ovale

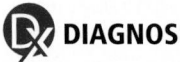 **DIAGNOSIS**

SIGNS AND SYMPTOMS
- 1st symptoms of malaria are nonspecific
  – Fever
  – Malaise
  – Myalgias
  – Chills
  – Headache
  – Nausea
  – Splenomegaly (with chronic infection)
  – Hypotension
- *P. falciparum* (aka *malignant tertian malaria*)
  – Incubation period is usually 12–14 days, with fevers within 2 months of infection.
  – Large parasitemia: Anemia, jaundice, thrombocytopenia, and vascular collapse
  – Other complications include gastroenteritis, central nervous system impairment, renal failure, and pulmonary edema.
- *P. vivax* (benign tertian malaria) and *P. ovale*
  – Incubation period up to 12 months (occasionally longer), presents with fevers
  – Dormant parasites may remain in liver and reactivate years after initial infection.
- *P. malariae* (benign quartan malaria)
  – Incubation period ~35 days, with high fevers every 72 hours
  – May become chronic; untreated can persist asymptomatically in human host for years

Physical Exam
- Often not specific (elevated temperature, perspiration, fatigue)
- In severe malaria (by *P. falciparum*), clinical findings (confusion, coma, neurologic signs, anemia, respiratory difficulties) are possible.

TESTS
- Malarial smear thick and thin preparations obtained every 6–12 hours for 3 samplings. Microscopy to evaluate for parasite forms (best to obtain blood during or right after fever spike)
- Other tests: Species-specific polymerase chain reaction (PCR) and indirect fluorescent antibody

Lab
- In uncomplicated infection
  – Elevated liver function tests and lactate dehydrogenase (>50% of cases)
  – Thrombocytopenia (40%)
  – Anemia (25%)
  – Leukopenia (25%)
- Drugs that may alter lab results: Antimalarial agents may reduce parasitemia.

Diagnostic Procedures/Surgery
- Malarial peripheral blood smears (blood film). Also, rapid antigen tests are available outside the US. PCR is available from research and some government laboratories (mostly used for confirmation and speciation of infection).
- A low to low-normal platelet count or a slightly high bilirubin is typical and should alert the clinician to malaria exposure.

Pathological Findings
- Malaria causes hemolysis.
- With severe infection, hemolysis of parasitized RBCs activates cytokines, causing sludging within microcirculation, causing necrosis.
- Edema, hemorrhage, and the presence of malarial pigments are frequent findings.

DIFFERENTIAL DIAGNOSIS
- Infections (extensive)
  – Localized (abscess)
  – Viral (mononucleosis)
  – Gastroenteritis (in children)
  – Typhoid/paratyphoid (other bacteremias)
  – Rickettsial
  – Mycobacterial
  – Collagen vascular diseases:
  – Systemic lupus erythematosus
  – Primary vasculitides
  – Mixed connective tissue diseases
- Neoplasms
  – Lymphoma
  – Leukemia
  – Other causes of tropical splenomegaly and blood dyscrasias
- Severe *P. falciparum* infection may mimic hepatitis, hemolytic anemia, pneumonia, stroke.

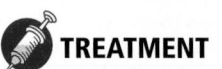 **TREATMENT**

INITIAL STABILIZATION
Inpatient care for all cases of *P. falciparum* malaria in nonimmune patients; outpatient care for others

GENERAL MEASURES
- Antiemetics and antipyretics are recommended.
- Avoid use of aspirin in children.
- In severe cases, watch for complications such as severe anemia and renal failure.

Activity
May resume as tolerated once fever is under control. Avoid contact and exercise if splenomegaly is present.

SPECIAL THERAPY
If severe, exchange transfusions

IV Fluids
Maintenance IV fluids are recommended for those unable to tolerate fluids or medications by mouth.

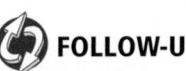

MEDICATION (DRUGS)

First Line
- Oral therapy for chloroquine-resistant *P. falciparum*
- Drug of choice for mild to moderate
  - Atovaquone-proguanil (Malarone) 250 mg/100 mg. Adults: 4 tablets per day for 3 days. Children 11–20 kg: 1 adult tablet per day. Children 21–30 kg: 2 adult tablets per day. Children 31–40 kg: 3 adult tablets per day. Dose may be b.i.d. for better tolerance.
- Alternatives
  - Quinine sulfate plus doxycycline or clindamycin. Adults: Quinine sulfate 650 mg salt t.i.d. for 3–7 days plus doxycycline 100 mg b.i.d. for 7 days or plus clindamycin 900 mg t.i.d. for 5 days. Children: Quinine sulfate 10 mg salt/kg (maximum 650 mg salt) t.i.d. for 3–7 days plus doxycycline (not for those <8 years of age) 2 mg/kg b.i.d. for 7 days or plus clindamycin 20–40 mg/kg/d divided into 3 doses for 5 days.
- Oral therapy for *P. ovale*, *P. malariae*, chloroquine-sensitive *P. falciparum* (rare), and chloroquine-sensitive *P. vivax* (New Guinea has some resistance but most are CQ sensitive)
  - Chloroquine phosphate. Adults: 600 mg base (1 g salt) followed by 300 mg at 6, 24, and 48 hours. Children: 10 mg base/kg (maximum of 600 mg), then 5 mg/kg at 6, 24, and 48 hours.
  - Primaquine phosphate (must be added to chloroquine therapy for cure of dormant forms of *P. vivax* and *P. ovale*). Adults: 30 mg base (52.6 mg) daily for 2 weeks or 45 mg base (79 mg) weekly for 8 weeks. Children: 0.6 mg base/kg daily for 2 weeks. See "Precautions."
- Oral therapy for chloroquine-resistant *P. vivax*
  - Atovaquone/Proguanil or quinine sulfate plus doxycycline: Dosages above. Must follow with primaquine for liver-dormant forms.
  - Mefloquine. Adults: 1,250 mg once (usually divided as 750 mg, then 500 mg 8 hours later). Children: 15 mg/kg, then 10 mg/kg 8 hours later (high GI adverse event profile)
- Severe infection is characterized by
  - Clinical features
    - Impaired level of consciousness (LOC)
    - Respiratory distress, Jaundice
    - Repeated convulsions, shock
  - Laboratory features
    - Hypoglycemia (glucose <40 mg/dL)
    - Elevated bilirubin (total >2.5 mg/dL)
    - Acidosis (plasma bicarbonate <15 mmol/L)
    - Lactic acidosis (serum lactate >45 mg/dL)
    - Elevated aminotransferase (>3 times)
    - Serum creatinine >3 mg/dL
- Parenteral therapy: Quinidine gluconate. Adults and children: 10 mg/kg in normal saline over 1–2 hours followed by 0.02 mg/kg/min continuous infusion, or repeat initial dose q8h until oral therapy can be started. When IV quinidine is not immediately available, IV clindamycin and/or oral quinidine should be immediately instituted until IV quinidine is obtained (may obtain from Eli Lilly Company 1-800-821-0538). Intensive care monitoring is necessary. Assistance via CDC: 404-770-7100; speak to the Malaria Branch.

- Precautions
  - Primaquine may cause hemolysis in patients with G6PD; screen if suspected.
  - Avoid Malarone in breast-feeding women and in patients with severe renal impairment (creatinine clearance <30 mL/min).
  - Avoid mefloquine in patients with seizure, psychiatric illness, or cardiac abnormalities.
- Significant possible interactions: Refer to the manufacturer's literature for each drug.

ALERT
Pregnancy Considerations
- Chloroquine is safe in low doses, but contraindicated during breast-feeding; FDA Category C.
- Mefloquine is probably safe, FDA Category C, particularly during 2nd and 3rd trimesters, and is recommended if no effective alternative is available.
- Malarone has not been studied in pregnant women; it has not been shown to cause birth defects or other problems in animal studies; FDA Category C.
- No primaquine, tetracyclines, quinine, and quinidine during pregnancy or breast-feeding.

Second Line
- Mefloquine: Oral therapy regardless of *Plasmodium* species although for *P. vivax* and *ovale*, it should be followed by primaquine.
  - Adults: 1,250 mg once (may divide as 750 mg and 500 mg over 12 hours)
  - Children: 15 mg/kg then 10 mg/kg at 12 hours
  - Nausea and vomiting are common.

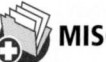

FOLLOW-UP

DISPOSITION
Admission Criteria
Any nonimmune patient with suspected or proven *P. falciparum* malaria or signs of severe disease (see "Signs and Symptoms"). Nonimmune with *P. falciparum* may die within 12 hours of onset of symptoms.

Discharge Criteria
Clinical improvement, ability to tolerate oral medications and fluids, with documented decreasing parasitemia levels

Issues for Referral
All severely ill patients must have a malaria expert involved in clinical management.

PROGNOSIS
Only *P. falciparum* infection carries a poor prognosis, with high mortality if untreated. However, if diagnosed early and treated appropriately, the prognosis is excellent.

ALERT
Geriatric Considerations
Potentially serious outcomes in this age group

COMPLICATIONS
- *P. falciparum*: If not treated early, may cause cerebral malaria, acute renal failure, acute gastroenteritis, pulmonary edema, and massive hemolysis. In chronic malaria, splenomegaly is common and may lead to splenic rupture. Death from malaria is virtually limited to *P. falciparum* infection or infection with other species in a patient with other underlying illness.
- *P. malariae*: Nephrotic syndrome may develop in patients with chronic infection.

- Other complications: Seizures, anuria, delirium, coma, dysentery, algid malaria, blackwater fever, hyperpyrexia

REFERENCES

1. Shetty A, Woods C. Prevention of malaria in children. *Pediatr Infect Dis J*. 2006;25(12):1173.
2. Centers for Disease Control and Prevention: Malaria surveillance—United States, 2002. *MMWR Surveill Summ*. 2006;55:23–37. Available at: www.cdc.gov.
3. Centers for Disease Control and Prevention. Treatment of Malaria (Guidelines for clinicians). August 23, 2005. Available at http://www.cdc.gov/malaria/pdf/treatmenttable.pdf
4. Chen LH, Keystone JS. New strategies for the prevention of malaria in travelers. *Infect Dis Clin North Am*. 2005;19(1):185–210.
5. Newman RD, et al. Malaria-related deaths among U.S. travelers, 1962–2001. *Ann Intern Med*. 2004;141(7):547–555.
6. http://www.who.int/malaria/docs/TreatmentGuidelines2006.pdf.

MISCELLANEOUS

- Most areas of the world have chloroquine-resistant *P. falciparum* (the form of malaria most prevalent worldwide). Some multidrug-resistant strains of *P. falciparum* and *P. vivax* are present in Southeast Asia.
- Current information regarding malaria treatment and prophylaxis is always available from the Centers for Disease Control and Prevention (www.cdc.gov).

CODES

ICD9-CM
- 084.0 Falciparum malaria (malignant tertian)
- 084.1 Vivax malaria (benign tertian)
- 084.2 Quartan malaria
- 084.3 Ovale malaria
- 084.5 Mixed malaria
- 084.6 Malaria, unspecified
- 084.8 Blackwater fever
- 084.9 Other pernicious complications of malaria
- 573.2 Hepatitis in other infectious diseases classified elsewhere
- 771.2 Other congenital infections

PATIENT TEACHING

Prevention
- Prophylaxis
- Repellants
- Insecticide-treated bed nets (ITNs)
- Protective clothing
- Indoor residual spraying (IRS)
- Intermittent preventative therapy (IPT)
- Avoid travel to endemic areas

See Corresponding Diagnostic Algorithm

M

MALNUTRITION, PROTEIN-CALORIE

Jonathan Spector, BSc, MBBS

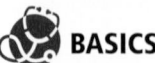 BASICS

DESCRIPTION

- Protein-calorie malnutrition (PCM) is present when sufficient energy and/or protein is not available to meet metabolic demands, leading to impairment in normal physiologic processes.
- Often includes elements of both macronutrient and micronutrient deficiency
- Affects all age groups. Children are particularly vulnerable, but certain adult and elderly populations are also at high risk.
- Malnutrition in children is a major underlying factor in ~5 million preventable deaths annually (1).
- Classified in children according to phenotypic appearance and degree of severity. 2 distinct phenotypes exist: Marasmus and kwashiorkor
- Marasmus is a wasting condition resulting from deficiency of calories and protein. Weight is decreased relative to that expected for the patient's height/length. 3 categories of severity are recognized
  - Mild: Characterized by a weight-for-height ratio (W:H) 80–90% of normal
  - Moderate: W:H between 70–79%.
  - Severe: W:H <70% (3 standard deviations below the mean)
- Kwashiorkor is distinguished by generalized edema. In the past, thought to develop from relative protein deficiency, but this hypothesis has been called into question. Weight is normal or elevated due to increased body fluid.
- Adult and elderly malnutrition occurs from inadequate intake, including that which occurs in famine settings, or secondary to other disease.
- Malnutrition compromises posttransplantation survival. Pretransplantation nutritional assessment and support may improve transplantation outcomes.
- System(s) Affected: Immunologic; Gastrointestinal; Endocrine/Metabolic; Hematologic; Musculoskeletal; Neurologic

GENERAL PREVENTION

- Emphasis on food security and nutritional education
- In children, routine record of anthropomorphic measurements and developmental milestones
- Observation and recording of patients' nutritional intake
- Early recognition of increased nutritional requirements during stress, infection, and other medical illness
- Frequent interactions among physician, nurse, and dietitian to assess nutritional needs
- Avoidance of risk factors when possible

EPIDEMIOLOGY

- Predominant age: Young children are especially susceptible to PCM due to significant energy requirements for growth and reliance on others for food distribution.
- Elderly with physical impairments, poor cognitive function, and depression are at high risk.
- Malnutrition may be common, but difficult to recognize, in hospital populations (2).
- Predominant sex: Male = Female

Prevalence

- Worldwide, over 70 million children suffer from moderate and severe acute malnutrition (1)
- Prevalence ranges 11–61% in hospitalized adults and elderly (3)

RISK FACTORS

- Nutritional
  - Prolonged and severe reduction of intake
  - Anorexia nervosa
- Underlying illnesses
  - Fever, infection, trauma, burns, and other hypercatabolic states
  - Malabsorptive and maldigestive states
  - Protein-losing enteropathy, nephrotic syndrome, enteric fistulas
  - Metabolic disorders (diabetes, hyperthyroidism)
  - Chronic cardiac disease
- Physiologic states in which requirements are increased
  - Pregnancy and lactation
  - Growth and development during infancy, childhood, and adolescence

ETIOLOGY

- Inadequate dietary intake
- Increased metabolic demands
- Increased nutrient losses

ASSOCIATED CONDITIONS

- Weakens immune system, predisposing to bacterial, viral, and parasitic infections
- Electrolyte disturbance results from poor maintenance of cell walls, diminished cellular pump activity, and altered renal function.
- Hypoglycemia develops from decreased glycogen stores (muscle loss, liver damage) and increased glucose utilization (infection, poor thermoregulation).
- Micronutrient deficiency
- Malabsorptive and maldigestive states

DIAGNOSIS

SIGNS AND SYMPTOMS

- Children
  - Weight loss, stunted growth, subcutaneous fat and muscle wasting, delayed puberty, diminished cognitive and psychosocial development
- Adults and elderly
  - Weight loss, muscle wasting, reduction of subcutaneous fat
  - Decreased hand grip strength
  - Delayed wound healing and recovery
  - Lethargy, early satiety, vomiting, and constipation
  - Subnormal heart rate, blood pressure, and core body temperature
  - Impaired work capacity

History

- Quantity and quality of nutritional intake
- Vomiting and diarrhea
- Urine output (assess for dehydration)
- Chronic medical illness

Physical Exam

- Anthropomorphic measurements
  - Weight and height. In children, measure W:H. In adults, BMI is <18.5 kg/ m² in PCM (3)
  - Mid-upper arm circumference (MUAC) is a simple, inexpensive, rapid screening tool for PCM. In children 1–5 years of age MUAC >125 mm is normal; 110–125 corresponds to a state of mild or moderate malnutrition; <110 mm corresponds to severe malnutrition. In adults, MUAC <200 is suggestive of PCM.
  - Triceps skin-fold thickness
  - Midarm muscle area: $[M ? \pi(T)]^2 - \div 4\pi$, where M is midarm circumference (mm), T is triceps skin fold (mm), and π is 3.1415
- Marasmic children are thin and have little subcutaneous fat. Wasting is especially evident at the shoulders, buttocks, arms, and thighs.
- Children with kwashiorkor are irritable, with bilateral pedal edema and anasarca. Hair is sparse, brittle, and reddish. Rash commonly referred to as "flaky paint" dermatosis is characterized by blackish discoloration and excoriation. Hepatomegaly from fatty infiltration may be present.
- Adults with decreased subcutaneous tissue

ALERT

- Commonly utilized markers of dehydration (dry mucous membranes, lack of tears, skin testing) are not valid in PCM. Oliguria and sunken fontanelle are more reliable indicators.
- Poor immune function may make identification of superimposed infection difficult: Fevers, swelling, and redness are often absent.

TESTS

Lab

- Where PCM is endemic, laboratory resources are scarce; thus malnutrition is a clinical diagnosis.
- Serum chemistries: Hypernatremia, hypokalemia, hypocalcemia, hypophosphatemia, hypomagnesemia
- Hypoglycemia
- Anemia, decreased lymphocyte count
- Plasma albumin: Decreased
- Blood urea: Decreased
- Plasma transferrin: Decreased
- Plasma essential amino acids: Decreased
- Plasma β-lipoprotein: Decreased
- Plasma cortisol, growth hormone: Increased, but insulin is low

Imaging

Chest radiography: Evaluate for pneumonia, tuberculosis, and cardiomegaly (suggestive of cardiac failure; may result from marked anemia)

DIFFERENTIAL DIAGNOSIS

- Secondary growth failure owing to malabsorption, congenital defects, or deprivation
- Pellagra (niacin deficiency)
- Nephritis or nephrosis
- Cardiac failure
- Disorders of glycogen metabolism
- Cystic fibrosis

TREATMENT

INITIAL STABILIZATION
- Aggressive identification and treatment of potentially life-threatening conditions associated with PCM: Dehydration, superimposed infection (including bacteremia, pneumonia, cellulitis, UTI), electrolyte imbalance, hypoglycemia, hypothermia, anemia, and cardiac failure
- Stable patients may be treated on an outpatient basis

GENERAL MEASURES
- Slowly restore and maintain fluid and electrolyte balance.
- Consider administration of empiric antibiotics, because infection may be difficult to diagnose.
- Oral iron and folate supplements (begin iron therapy ~2 weeks after initiation of dietary treatment to avoid bacterial infection)
- Blood transfusion if severe anemia is present (hemoglobin <4–6 g/dL)
- Ensure immunizations are up to date (PCM is not a contraindication to vaccination).

Diet
- For children, initially provide 100 kcal/kg/d with 3 g/kg/d of protein. When tolerated, advance to at least 200 kcal/kg/d with 5 g/kg/d of protein.
- Small, frequent feedings are preferred.
- Consider low-lactose formulas to decrease diarrhea from to disaccharidase deficiency.
- Target growth: 10–15 g/kg/d
- Supplement with vitamins and micronutrients, especially vitamin A and zinc.
- Refeeding of adults should occur slowly and, if possible, in consultation with a nutritionist.

Activity
As tolerated

Nursing
Maintain thermoregulation

 MEDICATION (DRUGS)

Antibiotics when indicated to treat concurrent infections

 FOLLOW-UP

DISPOSITION
Discharge Criteria
- Children are discharged from a nutritional rehabilitation program when W:H is >85%, at least 1 week of consistent weight gain has been achieved, and all disease conditions associated with PCM have been addressed.
- Adults should obtain a BMI of 18.5 kg/m^2.

PROGNOSIS
- Excellent when PCM is identified early and managed aggressively
- Mortality varies between 15% and 40%
- Compromised immune function returns to normalcy with recovery.
- Behavioral and mental issues may persist following treatment of severe cases.

COMPLICATIONS
Fatalities in the early days of treatment usually result from electrolyte imbalance, infection, hypothermia, or circulatory failure. Lethargy, anorexia, stupor, and petechiae are ominous signs.

ALERT
Pregnancy Considerations
Pregnant women with PCM are at risk of delivering a growth-restricted infant.

PATIENT MONITORING
Following discharge, close follow-up is critical to ensure continued appropriate nutritional intake.

REFERENCES
1. Collins S, Dent N, Binns P, et al. Management of severe acute malnutrition in children. *Lancet*. In press. Available online September 27, 2006.
2. van Bokhorst de van der Schueren M, Klinkenbers M, Thijs A. Profile of the malnourished patient. *Eur J Clin Nutrit*. 2005;59:1129–1131.
3. Hickson M. Malnutrition and ageing. *Postgrad Med J*. 2006;82:2–8.

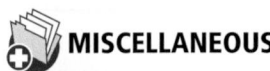 MISCELLANEOUS

CODES
ICD9-CM
- 260 Kwashiorkor
- 261 Nutritional marasmus
- 263.9 Unspecified protein-calorie malnutrition

PATIENT TEACHING

Emphasis on nutrition education

See Corresponding Diagnostic Algorithm

M

MARFAN SYNDROME

Timothy R. McCurry, MD

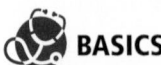 BASICS

DESCRIPTION

An autosomally dominant inherited disorder of connective tissue (i.e., elastic fibers) primarily affecting the musculoskeletal and cardiovascular systems and the eye

- System(s) Affected: Endocrine/Metabolic; Musculoskeletal

ALERT

Pediatric Considerations

Early medical or surgical intervention may reduce the degree of scoliosis.

Pregnancy Considerations

Pregnant women with Marfan syndrome need to be managed as high-risk patients, preferably with the involvement of a cardiologist. The outcomes of these patients are usually excellent.

GENERAL PREVENTION

- Because of incomplete penetrance and variable phenotypic expression, no genetic screening is being done, but presymptomatic diagnosis of family members of affected individuals may be possible at some research centers.
- Antibiotic prophylaxis for endocarditis should be prescribed for all patients with Marfan syndrome with either a heart murmur or echocardiographic evidence of valvular or aortic root abnormalities.
- Athletes who are especially tall should be screened for aortic root dilation.

EPIDEMIOLOGY

- Predominant age: Congenital, disorder is present from birth. However, clinical manifestations do not usually become apparent until adolescence or young adulthood.
- Predominant sex: No gender, ethnic, or racial predilection

Prevalence

1 in 10,000–20,000 (estimated 1 in 15,000)

RISK FACTORS

Advanced paternal age gives rise to a slightly increased risk only in those cases that are not clearly familial.

Genetics

- Each child has a 50% chance of inheriting the disorder from an affected parent. Clinical manifestations vary, however, so children may be more or less severely affected.
- Autosomal dominant with high but variable penetrance; 15–25% spontaneous mutation
- Associated mutations have been found on the FBN1 or TGFBR2 genes. (1)[C]

ETIOLOGY

Genetic; at least 5% of cases are obviously familial, the rest result from apparent spontaneous mutations.

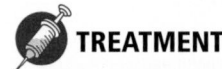 DIAGNOSIS

SIGNS AND SYMPTOMS

- Musculoskeletal
  - Tall stature
  - Thin, gangly body habitus so that limb length is out of proportion to trunk
  - Arachnodactyly (i.e., long, thin fingers)
  - Pectus deformity
  - High arched palate
  - Hyperextensible joints
  - Kyphoscoliosis
  - Joint laxity
- Cardiovascular
  - Aortic root dilatation
  - Aortic regurgitation
  - Aortic dissection
  - Mitral valve prolapse
  - Mitral regurgitation
- Ocular
  - Subluxation of lens, usually upward
  - Myopia
  - Retinal detachment (uncommon)
- Other
- Dura ectasia (2)[B]
  - Easy bruising (uncommon)
  - Excessive bleeding (uncommon)
  - Sleep apnea
  - Uterine prolapse or urinary incontinence

TESTS

Lab

- No specific laboratory abnormalities are associated with Marfan syndrome.
- Suspected patients should have urinary homocystine measured to rule out homocystinuria.

Imaging

- Plain radiographs of spine are necessary during growth years to detect and quantify scoliosis.
- Annual screening echocardiograms are recommended beginning in adolescence to detect presymptomatic aortic root dilatation or valvular degeneration.

Diagnostic Procedures/Surgery

Slit-lamp examination is necessary to detect lens subluxation.

Pathological Findings

- Cystic medial necrosis of the aorta
- Myxomatous degeneration of the cardiac valves
- FBN1 gene on chromosome 15 codes for fibrillin, a large glycoprotein constituent of microfibrils. Mutations in this gene have been found in >90% of patients with Marfan syndrome, when tested.

DIFFERENTIAL DIAGNOSIS

Various rare conditions, all clearly distinguishable from Marfan syndrome

- Homocystinuria
- Contractural arachnodactyly
- Ehlers-Danlos syndrome
- Shprintzen-Goldberg syndrome
- Trisomy

TREATMENT

INITIAL STABILIZATION

Outpatient

GENERAL MEASURES

Multidisciplinary approach including primary care physician, cardiologist, ophthalmologist, and possibly orthopedic surgeon. A clinical geneticist, if available, would be ideal as primary care physician.

Diet

No special diet

Activity

- Several highly trained athletes with Marfan syndrome have suffered sudden death during competition, leading to some concern that people with Marfan syndrome should be discouraged from participating in sports.
- Sports and physical education that can increase chances of aortic root enlargement or pneumothorax including weightlifting and acceleration/deceleration sports should be avoided. Examples of low-risk sports include bowling, golf, skating (but not ice hockey), snorkeling, brisk walking, treadmill walking, or stationary biking, modest hiking, and doubles tennis. (3)[C]
- See "Prognosis."

MEDICATION (DRUGS)

- No specific medical therapy is available; however, drugs are used to try to prevent some complications.
- Propranolol or other β-adrenergic blocking drugs are used to decrease the force of cardiac contraction, in the hope of delaying development or progression of aortic root dilatation. The dosage of these drugs is adjusted to target heart rate (i.e., resting rate of 60 beats per minute, with an increase to no more than 80 beats per minute after moderate exertion).
- Calcium channel blockers have also been shown to retard aortic growth in children and adolescents.
- Estrogen combined with progestogen has been used to induce puberty in preadolescent girls in an attempt to shorten the growth spurt, thereby mitigating scoliosis and preventing excessively tall stature. Do this only under the supervision of an endocrinologist.
- Contraindications
  - CHF, asthma, diabetes for the β-adrenergic blocking drugs
  - Thromboembolic disease in the case of estrogen/progestogen therapy
- Precautions: Refer to manufacturer's profile of each drug.
- Significant possible interactions: Amphetamines, antihistamines, antidiabetics, and oral contraceptives

SURGERY

Many, if not most, affected patients will ultimately require reconstructive cardiovascular surgery.

- Aorta and aortic valve replacement
- Mitral valve replacement

FOLLOW-UP

PROGNOSIS

- Life-threatening complications involve cardiovascular dysfunction. Before routine corrective surgery was available, most Marfan syndrome patients died before reaching the age of 35 years.
- With appropriate surgical intervention, most patients' life span will be normal.

COMPLICATIONS

- Bacterial endocarditis
- Aortic dissection
- Aortic or mitral valve insufficiency
- Dilated cardiomyopathy
- Retinal detachment

PATIENT MONITORING

- Frequent examinations (at least twice a year) while patient is still growing, with particular attention to cardiovascular system and to scoliosis
- When cardiac symptoms develop or aortic root diameter equals or exceeds 50 mm, surgical intervention should be considered.
- When lens subluxation is detected, surgical correction is possible. However, incidence of glaucoma is high, so surgery should be offered only to those whose condition cannot be treated with corrective lenses.

REFERENCES

1. Mizuguchi T, et al. Heterozygous TGFBR2 mutations in Marfan syndrome. *Nat Genet.* 2004;36(8):855–860. Epub 2004 Jul 4.
2. Fattori R, et al. Importance of dural ectasia in phenotypic assessment of Marfan's syndrome. *Lancet.* 1999;354(9182):910–913.
3. Maron BJ, et al. Recommendations for physical activity and recreational sports participation for young patients with genetic cardiovascular diseases. *Circulation.* 2004;109(22):2807–2816.
4. Carley ME, et al. Urinary incontinence and pelvic organ prolapse in women with Marfan's syndrome. *Am J Obstet Gynecol.* 2000;182:1021–1023.
5. Cistulli PA, et al. Relationship between craniofacial abnormalities and sleep disturbed breathing in Marfan's syndrome. *Chest.* 2001;120:1455–1460.
6. Gott VL, et al. Replacement of the aortic root in patients with Marfan's syndrome. *N Engl J Med.* 1999;340:1307–1313.
7. Kinoshita N, et al. Aortic root dilation among young competitive athletes. *Am Heart J.* 2000;139:723–728.
8. Rossi-Foulkes R, et al. Phenotypic features and impact of beta-blocker or calcium channel antagonist therapy on aortic root lumen size in Marfan's syndrome. *Am J Cardiol.* 1999;83:1364–1368.

MISCELLANEOUS

- Future trends suggest that successful gene therapy in the mouse model may lead to development of a human therapy.
- See also: Topic on Multiple endocrine neoplasia (MEN).

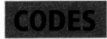
CODES

ICD9-CM
759.82 Marfan syndrome

PATIENT TEACHING

Information available from the National Marfan Foundation, 382 Main St., Port Washington, NY 11959; 800-8MARFAN

See Corresponding Diagnostic Algorithm

M

MASTALGIA

Anya S. Koutras, MD

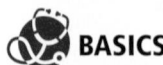 BASICS

DESCRIPTION
- Painful breast tissue that can be cyclic (1) and usually associated with hormonal changes related to menses, hormones, pregnancy, or menopause.
- Noncyclical pain can be constant or intermittent.
- Pain is often bilateral.
- System(s) Affected: Skin/Exocrine
- Synonym(s): Mastodynia, Breast pain

GENERAL PREVENTION
See "Risk Factors."

EPIDEMIOLOGY
- Predominant age
  - Generally adolescence through menopause
- Predominant sex
  - Most common in women, rarely men
  - May occur in adolescent males during puberty

Incidence
Most mild, but 11% report mild to severe pain (2)

RISK FACTORS
- Diet high in saturated fats
- Cigarette smoking
- Recent weight gain
- Pregnancy
- Large pendulous breasts (caused by stretching of Cooper's ligament)
- Caffeine has *not* been shown to be a risk factor (3)

Genetics
Familial tendency

ETIOLOGY
- Hormonal influences (i.e., hormone replacement therapy, OCPs, pregnancy, menses, puberty, menopause)
- Benign breast disorders (i.e., fibrocystic changes)
- Lactation problems (engorgement, mastitis, breast abscess)
- Extramammary tissue
- Hidradenitis suppurativa
- Breast masses, including breast cancer
- Postthoracotomy syndrome
- Spinal and paraspinal disorders
- Potential side effects of medications
- Postradiation effects
- Costochondritis (Tietze syndrome)
- Trauma (including sexual abuse/assault)

ASSOCIATED CONDITIONS
- Premenstrual syndrome
- Pregnancy

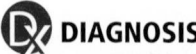 DIAGNOSIS

SIGNS AND SYMPTOMS
- Breasts aching, heavy, or tender
- Breasts enlarged

History
- Duration, frequency, associated symptoms, related activities
- Past medical history with focus on Gyn/OB history
- Diet/smoking
- Family history (especially of breast cancer)

Physical Exam
Examine for nipple discharge, skin changes, lymphadenopathy, breast mass

TESTS
- Possibly thyroid-stimulating hormone test
- Prolactin test if galactorrhea is found
- Papanicolaou test of discharge, if any present

Lab
No relevant findings

Imaging
Mammography and/or ultrasound (if <35 years) to rule out cancer

Diagnostic Procedures/Surgery
- Cysts may need to be aspirated to relieve symptoms and verify diagnosis.
- Biopsies may be indicated based on results of examination or mammography.

Pathological Findings
- Normal breast tissue
- Benign (fibrocystic changes, duct ectasia, solitary papillomas, simple fibroadenomas)
- Small increased risk of breast cancer (ductal hyperplasia without atypia, sclerosing adenosis, diffuse papillomatosis, complex fibroadenomas)
- Moderate increased risk (atypical ductal hyperplasia, atypical lobular hyperplasia)
- Breast cancer

DIFFERENTIAL DIAGNOSIS
- The major alternate disease to consider is breast cancer, particularly if pain is localized.
- Manipulation or trauma can also worsen symptoms.
- Chest-wall pain or referred pain resulting from splenomegaly must also be differentiated from mastalgia.
- Sometimes flare-up is concurrent with PMS.
- Ductal ectasia of the breast

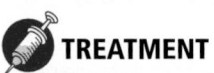 TREATMENT

INITIAL STABILIZATION
Outpatient

GENERAL MEASURES
- Stop or modify current hormonal therapy.
- Repeat examination may help establish any cyclic nodularity pattern.
- Wear properly fitted support bra (may be fitted by a professional).
- Reassurance (sufficient for most patients)
- Weight loss for obese patients
- Smoking cessation
- Relaxation training

Diet
Decrease fat intake to 20% of total calories.

Activity
No restrictions

Nursing
Correct any breastfeeding difficulties; treat underlying mastitis or breast abscess

SPECIAL THERAPY
Complementary and Alternative Medicine
Vitamin E and evening primrose oil has *not* been found to be of benefit for chronic mastalgia. (6)[B]

MEDICATION (DRUGS)

First Line
- No drugs are needed unless required by severity of symptoms.
- Reassurance, acetaminophen, ibuprofen, or topical NSAIDs (4)[B].

Second Line
- Frequently used agents (limited evidence to support their effectiveness)
  - Diuretics (usually spironolactone) before 5 days prior to menses
  - Oral contraceptives may help some patients.
  - If on oral contraceptive, switch to one that has a slightly higher progesterone component.
  - Oral progesterone
- Other possibilities for patients with refractory symptoms, used infrequently because of potential side effects
  - Danazol: 100 mg b.i.d. (possibly lower doses). May be the most effective. Major adverse effects: Menstrual irregularities, weight gain, acne, hirsutism, and voice change. *May be used during luteal phase only.* Approved by FDA for this indication.
  - Bromocriptine: 2.5–5.0 mg/d. Major adverse effects: Nausea, dizziness, orthostatic hypotension
  - Tamoxifen: 10 mg/d. Major adverse effects: Cataracts, hepatocellular carcinoma, endometrial carcinoma. *May be used during luteal phase only.*
  - Toremifene (8)[B]
  - Gonadotropin-releasing hormone agonists: Induces menopause

SURGERY
Patient may need reduction mammoplasty if cause is macromastia.

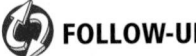 **FOLLOW-UP**

PROGNOSIS
- Premenstrual mastalgia increases with age, then generally stops at menopause unless patient is receiving hormone replacement therapy.
- Most patients can control symptoms without receiving hormone treatment.
- Several months of hormone treatment may provide several more months of relief, but mastalgia may recur.
- Cyclic mastalgia responds better than noncyclic mastalgia to treatment.
- Effects of long-term hormonal treatment are unknown.
- If other treatment fails, a final possibility is subcutaneous mastectomy (used rarely).
- Oophorectomy is drastic, but may also provide relief for some patients.

PATIENT MONITORING
- As needed for patients not receiving pharmacotherapy
- Time of follow-up will vary by type of pharmacotherapy and patient's particular problems.

REFERENCES

1. Davies EL, Gateley CA, Miers M, Mansel RE. The long-term course of mastalgia. *J R Soc Med*. 1998;91:462.
2. Ader DN, Shriver CD. Cyclical mastalgia: Prevalence and impact in an outpatient breast clinic sample. *J Am Coll Surg*. 1997;185:466.
3. Levinson W, Dunn PM. Nonassociation of caffeine and fibrocystic breast disease. *Arch Intern Med*. 1986;146:1773.
4. Colak et al. Efficacy of topical nonsteroidal antiinflammatory drugs in mastalgia treatment. *J Am Coll Surg*. 2003;196:525.
5. Bespalov et al. [Study of an antioxidant dietary supplement "Karinat" in patients with benign breast disease]. *Voprosy onkologii*. 2004;50:467.
6. Blommers et al. Evening primrose oil and fish oil for severe chronic mastalgia: A randomized, double-blind, controlled trial. *Am J Obstet Gynecol*. 2002;187:1389.
7. McFadyen et al. A randomized double blind-cross over trial of soya protein for the treatment of cyclical breast pain. *Breast*. 2000;9:271.
8. Gong C, Song E, Jia W, et al. A double-blind randomized controlled trial of toremifene therapy for mastalgia. *Arch Surg*. 2006;141(1):43–47.

ADDITIONAL READING

Love S, Lindsey K, Williams M. Dr. Susan Love's Breast Book, 4th ed. 2005.

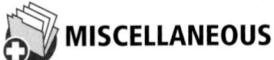 **MISCELLANEOUS**

See also: Premenstrual syndrome (PMS)

CODES

ICD9-CM
611.71 Mastodynia

M

MASTITIS

Montiel T. Rosenthal, MD

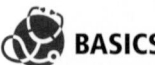 **BASICS**

DESCRIPTION
- Inflammation of the breast parenchyma and possibly associated tissues (areola, nipple, subcutaneous fat) usually associated with bacterial infection (and milk stasis in the postpartum mother).
- Usually an acute condition, but can become chronic cystic mastitis.

GENERAL PREVENTION
Regular emptying of both breasts and nipple care to prevent fissures among breast-feeding women

EPIDEMIOLOGY
- Predominantly affects females
- Mostly in the puerperium
- Neonatal form
- Posttraumatic
  - Ornamental nipple piercing increases risk of transmission of bacteria to deeper breast structures
    - *Staphylococcus aureus* predominant organism
- Epidemic form rare in the age of reduced hospital stays for mothers and newborns

Incidence
- 2.5% of breast-feeding mothers develop nonepidemic mastitis
- Greatest incidence among breast-feeding mothers 2–3 weeks postpartum
- Neonatal form
  - 1–5 weeks of age with equal gender risk and unilateral presentation
- Pediatric form
  - Around or after puberty
  - 82% of cases in girls

RISK FACTORS
- Milk stasis
  - Inadequate emptying of breast
    - Scarring of breast due to prior mastitis
    - Scarring due to previous breast surgery
  - Breast engorgement
    - Interruption of breast-feeding
- Ornamental nipple piercing increases risk of transmission of bacteria to deeper breast structures.
  - *S. aureus* predominant organism
- Neonatal colonization with epidemic staphylococcus
- Mother's breast-feeding
- Neonatal
  - Bottle-fed babies
  - Manual expression of "witch's milk"
  - Can predispose to lethal necrotizing fasciitis
- Maternal diabetes
- Maternal HIV
- Maternal vitamin A deficiency

ALERT

Pediatric Considerations
TMP/SMZ given to breast-feeding mothers with mastitis can potentiate jaundice for neonates.

PATHOPHYSIOLOGY
- Micro abscesses along milk ducts and surrounding tissues
- Inflammatory cell infiltration of breast parenchyma and surrounding tissues
- Nonpuerperal (infectious)
  - *S. aureus, Bacteroides* sp., *Peptostreptococcus, Staphylococcus* (coagulase neg.), *Enterococcus faecalis*
  - *Histoplasma capsulatum*
- Puerperal (infectious)
  - *S. aureus, Streptococcus pyogenes* (Group A or B), *Corynebacterium* sp., *Bacteroides* sp., *Staphylococcus* (coagulase neg.), *Escherichia coli, Salmonella* sp.
  - MRSA (1)[C]
- Rare secondary site for tuberculosis in endemic areas (1% of mastitis cases in these areas)
  - Single breast nodule with mastalgia
- *Corynebacterium sp.* associated with greater risk for development of chronic cystic mastitis
- Granulomatous mastitis
  - Idiopathic
  - *Histoplasma capsulatum*

ETIOLOGY
- Puerperal
  - Retrograde migration of surface bacteria up milk ducts
  - Bacterial migration from nipple fissures up breast lymphatics
  - Secondary monilial infection in the face of recurrent mastitis and/or diabetes (2)
  - Seeding from mother to neonate in cyclical fashion
- Nonpuerperal
  - Ductal ectasia
  - Breast carcinoma
  - Inflammatory cysts
  - Chronic recurring subcutaneous or subareolar infections
  - Parasitic infections: *Echinococcus; Filariasis;* Guinea worm in endemic areas
  - Herpes simplex (3)[C]
  - Cat-scratch disease

ASSOCIATED CONDITIONS
Breast abscess

DIAGNOSIS

DISPOSITION
Most patients evaluated and treated entirely as outpatients

SIGNS AND SYMPTOMS
- Fever
- Malaise
- Nausea ± vomiting
- Localized breast tenderness
- Localized breast heat and redness
- Possible breast mass

History
- Breast tenderness
- "Hot cords burning in chest wall"
  - Consider monilial infection in lactating mother, especially if mastitis is recurrent

Physical Exam
- Localized breast induration, redness, and warmth
- Peau d'orange appearance to overlying skin

TESTS
- Mother can check if she produces salty milk from affected side (higher Na and Cl concentrations) as compared with unaffected side.

Lab
Rarely needed except for patients ill enough to be hospitalized
- CBC
- Blood culture
- In epidemic puerperal mastitis
  - Milk leukocyte count
  - Milk culture
  - Neonatal nasal culture

Imaging
- Mammography for women with nonpuerperal mastitis
- Breast ultrasound to rule out abscess formation in women
  - Special consideration for this in women with breast implants who have mastitis

Diagnostic Procedures/Surgery
Options if further progression to abscess formation
- Needle aspiration
- I & D
- Excisional biopsy

DIFFERENTIAL DIAGNOSIS
- Abscess
- Tumor
- Ductal cyst

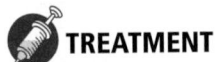 **TREATMENT**

PRE HOSPITAL
- Oral antibiotics
- Frequent emptying of breasts if breast-feeding
- Analgesics for pain
  - Acetaminophen
  - NSAIDs

GENERAL MEASURES
Diet
- Encourage oral fluids
- Multivitamin including vitamin A

Activity
Bed rest for lactating mothers, up to bathroom

Nursing
- Breast-feeding/pumping of breasts encouraged
- Start infant with feedings on affected side
- Abscess drainage is not a contraindication for breast-feeding

SPECIAL THERAPY
- The use of a breast pump may aid in breast emptying, especially if the infant is unable to assist in doing this.
- Wear supporting bra that is not too tight

Physical Therapy
Warm packs (or ice packs) to affected breast for comfort

 MEDICATION (DRUGS) (4)[B]
- Prioritized on the basis of likelihood of MRSA as etiologic factor and clinical severity of condition
- Treat for 10–14 days

- Prednisone for granulomatous mastitis (5)[C]

First Line
- Outpatient
  - Dicloxacillin 500 mg q.i.d.
  - Cephalexin 500 mg q.i.d.
  - TMP/SMX –DS BID (MRSA possible)
- Inpatient
  - Nafcillin 2 g q4h
  - Oxacillin 2 g q4h
  - Vancomycin 1 g q12h (MRSA possible)
- Breast-feeding beyond 1 month
  - PCN, ampicillin, or erythromycin

Second Line
- If mastitis is odoriferous and localized under areola add metronidazole 500 mg t.i.d. IV or PO
- Topical, oral, and neonatal nystatin if yeast is suspected in recurrent mastitis

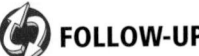 **FOLLOW-UP**

DISPOSITION
Admission Criteria
- Failure of outpatient/oral therapy
- Patient unable to keep down oral therapy
- Patient noncompliant with oral therapy
- Neonatal mastitis

Discharge Criteria
- Afebrile
- Tolerating oral antibiotics well

Issues for Referral
- Abscess formation
- Need for breast biopsy

PROGNOSIS
Puerperal
- Good with prompt (within 24 hours of symptom onset) antibiotic treatment and breast emptying—96% success rate
- 11% risk of abscess if left untreated with antibiotics
- Antibodies develop in breast glands within first few days of infection, which may provide protection against infection or reinfection
- Rare risk of abscess formation beyond 6 weeks postpartum if no recurrent mastitis

COMPLICATIONS
- Breast abscess
- Recurrent mastitis with resumption of breast-feeding or with breast-feeding after next pregnancy
- Bacteremia
- Sepsis

REFERENCES

1. Gastelum DT, Dassy D, Mascola L, Yasuda LM. Transmission of community-associated MRSA from breast milk in the neonatal intensive care unit *Ped Inf Dis J* 2005;24(12):1122–1124.
2. Lawrence R. *Breast-feeding: A guide for the medical profession*. Chicago: Mosby-Yearbook; 1994, 265.
3. Soo MS, Ghate S. Herpes simplex virus mastitis. *Amer J Roentgenol* 2000;174:1087–1088.
4. Gilbert D. et al. *The Sanford guide to antibiotic therapy*. 2005; 3.
5. Goldberg J, Baute L, Storey L, Park P. Granulomatous mastitis in pregnancy *Obstet Gynecol* 2000;96(5pt2):813–815.

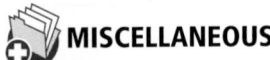 **MISCELLANEOUS**

CODES

ICD9-CM
- Puerperal
  - 675.21 Non-Purulent mastitis, delivered w/ or w/o ante partum condition
  - 675.22 Non-Purulent mastitis, delivered w/ post-partum condition
  - 675.23 Non-Purulent mastitis, delivered w/ ante partum condition or complication
  - 675.24 Non-Purulent mastitis, delivered w/ post-partum condition or complication
  - 675.8 Other specified infections of breast
  - 675.94 Unspecified infection of the breast and nipple; lactation
- Nonpuerperal
  - 611.0 Mastitis, NOS
  - 610.1 Chronic Cystic Mastitis
- 771.5 Neonatal Infectious Mastitis

PATIENT TEACHING

Diet
Encourage oral fluids

Activity
Rest essential

Prevention
- Regular emptying of both breasts with breast-feeding
- Nipple care to prevent fissures

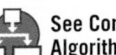 **See Corresponding Diagnostic Algorithm**

M

MASTOIDITIS

John J. Santos, MD

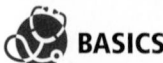 **BASICS**

DESCRIPTION
- Inflammatory process in the mastoid air cells
- Acute mastoiditis: Sudden-onset suppurative inflammatory process, typically after acute otitis media. It is the most common complication of acute otitis media.
- Chronic mastoiditis: Usually associated with cholesteatoma and chronic ear disease
- Masked mastoiditis: Indolent process with minimal signs and symptoms
- System(s) Affected: Pulmonary, Auditory

GENERAL PREVENTION
- Adequate antibiotic treatment for acute otitis media
- Treatment of chronic eustachian tube dysfunction (i.e., pressure equalization tubes)
- Early identification of cholesteatoma

EPIDEMIOLOGY
- Predominant age: Children, mainly <2 years
- Predominant sex: Male = Female

Incidence
1–4 cases per 100,000 person years

Prevalence
Unknown

RISK FACTORS
- Cholesteatoma
- Recurrent acute otitis media
- Immunocompromised host
- Native American descent

Genetics
No known genetic pattern

ETIOLOGY
- Acute otitis media
- Inadequately treated suppurative otitis media
- Cholesteatoma
- Blockage of outflow tract of mastoid air cells (i.e., aditus to mastoid antrum)
- *Streptococcus pneumoniae* infection

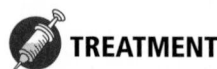 **DIAGNOSIS**

SIGNS AND SYMPTOMS
- Otalgia
- Bulging erythematous tympanic membrane
- Postauricular or supra-auricular edema, erythema, or tenderness.
- Protrusion of auricle
- Fever
- Increased leukocyte count
- Possible otorrhea if tympanic membrane is perforated
- Subperiosteal abscess
- Hearing loss
- Headache
- Outward and upward displacement of pinna
- Sagging of posterosuperior wall of external auditory canal
- Tympanic membrane can be normal in 10% of patients: Suspicious when symptoms of acute otitis media persist >2 weeks

TESTS
Lab
CBC with differential: Increased leukocyte count

Imaging
- Plain radiographs of mastoid area: Clouding of mastoid air cells; can be negative finding, however. Coalescence of air cells; diagnostic but rare
- CT scan if complications suspected. Clouding of air cells: Loss of bony septation of the air cell system
- Technetium 99 bone scan: More sensitive to osteolytic changes than CT
- MRI or CT with contrast if venous thrombosis is suspected as a complication

Diagnostic Procedures/Surgery
- Myringotomy (also therapeutic)
- Consider audiography in cases of suspected hearing loss.
- Culture material obtained at myringotomy.
- Obtain CSF if suspect intracranial extension
- Biopsy if tissue protruding through TM or tympanostomy tube

Pathological Findings
- Inflammatory tissue in air cell system
- Granulation tissue
- Osteitis

DIFFERENTIAL DIAGNOSIS
- Postauricular inflammatory adenopathy
- Severe external otitis
- Postauricular cellulitis
- Benign neoplasm: Aneurysmal bone cyst, fibrous dysplasia
- Malignant neoplasm: Rhabdomyosarcoma, neuroblastoma
- HIV infection
- Furuncle of meatus of ear
- Parotitis
- Local trauma to auricula or mastoid

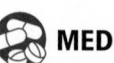 **TREATMENT**

INITIAL STABILIZATION
Inpatient care during acute phase

GENERAL MEASURES
Keep affected ear dry.

MEDICATION (DRUGS)

First Line
- IV antibiotics
  - Directed against most common organisms: Group A β-hemolytic streptococcus, *Streptococcus pneumoniae, and Staphylococcus aureus*
  - In patients with cholesteatoma, consider *Pseudomonas organisms* and, less commonly, enteric gram-negative rods or *Staphylococcus aureus*..
  - IV antibiotics for adult: Ampicillin, 1–2 g q6h or ampicillin-sulbactam (Unasyn) or cefuroxime, 750 mg q8h, to ensure coverage against β-lactamase-producing organisms
  - IV antibiotics for children: Ampicillin, 100 200 mg/kg/d divided q6h or cefuroxime, 150 mg/kg/d divided q8h or oxacillin plus cefotaxime or ceftriaxone
- Topical/oral antibiotics
  - Topical drops: Ofloxacin otic solution (0.3%) for chronic mastoiditis
  - Oral antibiotic: Amoxicillin-clavulanate (Augmentin) or clindamycin plus 3rd-generation cephalosporin
- Contraindications: Refer to the manufacturer's literature.
- Precautions: Refer to the manufacturer's literature.
- Significant possible interactions: Refer to the manufacturer's literature.

Second Line
Other antibiotics depending on sensitivity or refractoriness of pathogen

SURGERY
- Myringotomy; placement of pressure equalization tube
- Frequent cleaning of ear canal under microscope to ensure pressure-equalization tube patency and adequate drainage of middle ear
- Topical antibiotic drops are also usually used after insertion of pressure-equalization tube.
- If subperiosteal abscess is present, it should be aspirated. If aspiration is not sufficient, incision and drainage should be performed.
- Mastoidectomy is reserved for those patients whose condition fails to improve despite these measures within 18–72 hours or those with meningeal or intracranial complications.

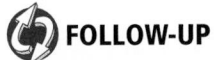 **FOLLOW-UP**

PROGNOSIS
- Depends on severity of disease
- Conductive hearing loss may require reconstructive surgery.
- Expect to avoid complications with early treatment.

COMPLICATIONS
- Subperiosteal abscess
- Gradenigo syndrome (palsy of the 6th cranial nerve, draining ear, and retro-orbital pain)
- Bezold abscess (abscess of sternocleidomastoid muscle)
- Sigmoid sinus thrombosis
- Meningitis
- Intracranial abscess epidural/subdural/intraparenchymal
- Periosteitis
- Osteitis
- Central venous sinus thrombosis
- Suppurative labyrinthitis (resulting in deafness)
- Citelli abscess (osteomyelitis of the calvaria)
- Facial nerve paralysis

PATIENT MONITORING
- Postoperative: Audiogram after acute flare-up has subsided
- After surgery, IV antibiotics to cover the most common pathogenic organisms
- Frequent cleansing of ear canal is needed to keep the pressure-equalization tube patent.
- Oral antibiotics for 3 weeks following satisfactory course of IV antibiotics
- For chronic mastoiditis, consider antimicrobial prophylaxis with amoxicillin for several months.

REFERENCES

1. Behrman RE, Kliegman M, eds. Nelson Textbook of Pediatrics, 17th ed. Philadelphia: WB Saunders, 2004.
2. Mandell GL, ed. Principles and Practice of Infectious Diseases, 6th ed. New York: Churchill Livingstone, 2005.
3. Marx J, et al. Rosen's Emergency Medicine: Concepts and Clinical Practice, 6th ed. St. Louis: Mosby, 2006.
4. Cummings. Otolaryngology: Head and Neck Surgery, 4th ed. St.Louis: Mosby, 2005.
5. Long. Principles and Practice of Pediatric Infectious Diseases, 2nd ed. New York: Churchill Livingston, 2003.

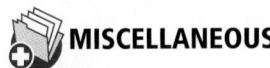 **MISCELLANEOUS**

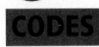

ICD9-CM
- 383.00 Acute mastoiditis without complications
- 383.01 Subperiosteal abscess of mastoid
- 383.02 Acute mastoiditis with other complications
- 383.1 Chronic mastoiditis
- 383.9 Unspecified mastoiditis

PATIENT TEACHING

Diet
No special diet

Activity
Precautions about getting ear(s) wet

M

MEASLES (RUBEOLA)

Ryung Suh, MD, MPP, MBA, MPH
Brent R. Gibson, MD, MPH

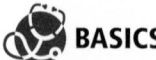 **BASICS**

DESCRIPTION
- Measles is an acute epidemic viral exanthem that classically presents as a confluent erythematous maculopapular rash that begins on and about the head and spreads inferiorly to involve the trunk and extremities. The rash is preceded by the triad of cough, coryza, and conjunctivitis plus a pathognomonic enanthem (Koplik spots).
- Measles continues to be a major public health problem in the developing world, where it causes significant morbidity and mortality (see below).
- System(s) Affected: Hemic/Lymphatic/Immunologic; Pulmonary; Skin/Exocrine
- Synonym(s): Rubeola

ALERT
Pediatric Considerations
Infants have a higher rate of complications than do older children.

Pregnancy Considerations
- Increased fetal morbidity and mortality with infection during pregnancy
- Live vaccine is considered contraindicated in pregnant women.

GENERAL PREVENTION
- The Centers for Disease Control and Prevention defines an outbreak of measles as a single case. Once identified, all efforts must be taken to prevent this disease from spreading.
- General populations should be vaccinated. Persons not requiring vaccination include individuals with laboratory confirmed immunity to measles, mumps, and rubella; men born before 1957; women born before 1957 who will not have more children, already had rubella vaccine, or have a positive rubella test; individuals who have had 2 doses of MMR or 1 dose of MMR plus a 2nd dose of measles vaccine; individuals who have had 1 dose of MMR and are not at high risk of measles exposure (3)[C].
- Postexposure prophylaxis
  - Vaccine use: Protective if given within 72 hours postexposure
- Passive immunization
  - Immune globulin: Prevents/modifies illness if given within 6 days postexposure. Dose: Usually 0.25 mL/kg IM (for immunocompromised children, 0.5 mL/kg IM), not to exceed 15 mL. Indicated for the following susceptible household contacts
    ○ Infants <1 year old, pregnant women, and immunocompromised people.
    ○ All HIV-infected children and adolescents, regardless of prior measles immunization status; if exposed, should receive IV immune globulin (400 mg/kg) or immune globulin prophylaxis (0.5 mL/kg) unless receiving monthly IV immune globulin (last dose within the previous 3 weeks).
- Active immunization
  - Live further-attenuated strain vaccine: Only currently licensed vaccine, available as monovalent vaccine or in combination with prophylaxis for mumps and rubella (i.e., measles and rubella [MR]; measles, mumps, and rubella [MMR])
- Indications
  - According to the 2006 Childhood and Adolescent Immunization Schedule, primary vaccination consists of 2 doses of the vaccine. The 1st MMR inoculation is given at 12–15 months of age, second dose SC at school age (4–6 years old). It may be given at any time, provided that 4 weeks have elapsed since the 1st dose. The 2-dose vaccination schedule mandated by need to compensate for primary vaccine failures and global efforts to eradicate measles. During outbreaks, monovalent measles vaccine may be given to infants >6 months old. These children must be vaccinated with MMR vaccine as already suggested here. For a comprehensive discussion of the complete use and control of measles outbreaks, see the reference section citation of the *Red Book*.
  - HIV-infected children should be vaccinated while asymptomatic and before they develop profound immunosuppression. The 2nd dose of vaccine may be given as early as 1 month after the 1st dose.
- Adverse events associated with vaccination in 5–15% of susceptible patients who were vaccinated
  - Fever (7–12 days after vaccination)
  - Transient rashes in 5% of those vaccinated
  - Convulsions (most likely febrile)
  - Children with egg allergy are at low risk for anaphylactic reactions to MMR vaccination.
  - Recent epidemiologic evidence has not substantiated any link between MMR vaccine and autism.

EPIDEMIOLOGY
- Predominant age: Between 1985 and 1994, children ≤2 years constituted largest proportion of cases (≥90% of these unvaccinated). During a 7-week period in 1997, no indigenous cases were reported, suggesting an interruption of measles transmission.
- Predominant sex: Male = Female

Incidence
- In 2000, in the developing world, an estimated 30–40 million cases of measles, which resulted in 777,000 deaths (5).
- Number of cases in the U.S peaked during 1990 at 27,786, followed by marked decline. By 2003, number of new cases was 56 (2).
- Attack rate (number of cases/100,000): 1991, 3.82; 1992, 0.87; 1993, 0.12; 1994, 0.37

RISK FACTORS
- Not being vaccinated
- Infants and adults are at higher risk of death than children.
- Pregnant women

ETIOLOGY
Single antigenic type of a RNA Morbillivirus in the paramyxovirus family

ASSOCIATED CONDITIONS
- Primary measles in an immunosuppressed patient with leukemia or symptomatic HIV-1 infection may present with or without a rash and giant cell pneumonitis.
- Giant cell pneumonitis
- Increased mortality with malnutrition
- Possible reactivation of latent tuberculosis secondary to measles

DIAGNOSIS

SIGNS AND SYMPTOMS
- Incubation period
  - 10–14 days from exposure to symptoms
  - 14 days average to onset of rash (range, 7–18 days)
  - Patients contagious from 1–2 days before symptoms (3–5 days before appearance of rash) to 4 days after onset of rash; immunocompromised patients remain contagious for duration of illness.
- Prodromal period
  - Lasts 31 days
  - Classic triad (i.e., brassy cough, coryza, conjunctivitis)
  - Fever
  - Malaise
  - Photophobia
  - Exanthem (Koplik spots): Minute, whitish spots over buccal/labial mucosa; number rapidly increases and these coalesce. Underlying mucosa bright red and granular; spots appear 2 days before rash and resolve within 3 days after rash onset.
- Exanthem period
  - Appearance begins behind ears and at hairline.
  - Spread is centrifugal from head to feet.
  - Red, morbilliform, blanching rash appears.
  - Discrete lesions become confluent.
  - Confluence more prominent over upper body.
  - Clearing begins after 3–4 days.
  - Rash becomes coppery and nonblanching.
  - Fever resolves 2–3 days after onset of rash.
  - Pharyngitis
  - Lymphadenopathy
  - Croup, vomiting, and diarrhea (in young children)
  - Patients are contagious from 2 days before symptoms to 4 days after onset of rash

History
Patients often present with a cough, rhinorrhea, and high fever (103–105°F or 39.4–40.6°C); a minority present with rash.

TESTS
Lab
- Viral isolation in tissue culture
- Detection of measles antigen in exfoliative cells by immunofluorescence
- Demonstration of measles-specific IgM or substantial rise in IgG tilers between acute and convalescent sera
- Recent work has demonstrated that ELISA used to detect antibodies from whole blood samples deposited on filter paper is as effective as traditional methods in diagnosing measles (4)[B].
- Drugs that may alter lab results: Immunosuppressive agents that may impair rise in specific antibody titers
- Disorders that may alter lab results
  - Primary immune deficiencies (e.g., severe combined immunodeficiency [SCID])
  - Acquired immune deficiencies (e.g., HIV-1 infection, cancer chemotherapy)

Pathological Findings
Multinucleated giant cells

- Reticuloendothelial types (Warthin-Finkeldey cells) in lymphoid tissues
- Epithelial syncytial giant cells in skin and respiratory mucosa
- Damaged respiratory ciliated epithelium

DIFFERENTIAL DIAGNOSIS
- Typical measles
  – Any erythematous maculopapular rash
- Exanthems secondary to
  – Drug eruptions
  – Infectious mononucleosis
  – *Mycoplasma pneumoniae* infection
  – Rubella
  – Erythema infectiosum
  – Roseola
  – Enteroviruses
- Atypical measles
  – Rocky Mountain spotted fever
  – Drug eruptions
  – Anaphylactoid purpura
  – *Mycoplasma pneumoniae* infection

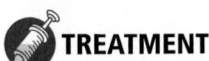 ## TREATMENT

INITIAL STABILIZATION
Outpatient except when complications develop (e.g., encephalitis, pneumonitis)

GENERAL MEASURES
- Symptomatic therapy (i.e., antipyretics, antitussives, humidification, increased consumption oral fluids)
- Control
  – All patients with the disease should be placed in respiratory isolation until 4 days after the onset of the exanthem; immunocompromised patients should be isolated for the entire illness.
  – Notify public health officials of suspected cases.
  – Initiate preventive measures for all exposed susceptible patients or those at high risk for severe infection (i.e., symptomatic HIV infection, children <12 months old)
  – Live measles vaccine can provide protection to susceptible patients if given within 72 hours postexposure.
  – Immune globulin (Ig) given within 6 days postexposure can prevent or modify measles infection (0.25 mL/kg, maximum dose 15 mL; 0.5 mL/kg for immunocompromised patients).
  – Patients with symptomatic HIV infection should receive immune globulin regardless of prior immunization.
  – Immune globulin also is indicated for susceptible household contacts of measles patient and all pregnant women.

Diet
As tolerated

Activity
Restricted during febrile phase

 ## MEDICATION (DRUGS)

First Line
- No proven specifically antiviral agent is available.
- Following onset of infection, immune globulin has no significant effect on symptoms or duration of illness.
- Antibiotics should be reserved as therapy for *bacterial* superinfection.

Second Line
- Vitamin A
  – A single randomized clinical trial has demonstrated the effectiveness of 200,000 IU given once each day for 2 days to children with measles improved outcomes (1)[B].
  – 200,000 IU/d PO for 2 days (100,000 IU for infants between 6 and 12 months old) has been shown to decrease mortality and morbidity of severe measles in areas where vitamin A deficiency exists and mortality related to measles is ≥1%; efficacy in non–life-threatening infections not established.
  – Vitamin A is currently recommended for the following patients
    ○ Children ages 6–24 months hospitalized with complications of measles
    ○ Children <6 months old with immunodeficiency, malabsorption, moderate to severe malnutrition, ophthalmologic evidence of vitamin A deficiency, or recent immigration from areas with vitamin A deficiency
- Ribavirin
  – Virus is susceptible in vitro to ribavirin.
  – Immunosuppressed children with severe measles have been treated with IV or aerosolized ribavirin, but no controlled data exist and this use has not been approved by the U.S. Food and Drug Administration (FDA).

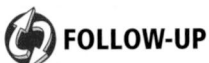 ## FOLLOW-UP

PROGNOSIS
Self-limited; prognosis good

COMPLICATIONS
- Otitis media (most common)
- Laryngotracheitis
- Bronchopneumonia: Viral (Hecht or giant cell pneumonitis) or bacterial in origin
- Encephalitis (incidence 1/1,000)
- Hemorrhagic lesions ("black measles") of skin and bowel
- Thrombocytopenic purpura
- Myocarditis and pericarditis
- Subacute sclerosing panencephalitis: Secondary to persistent infection following natural disease; disappearing as a result of mass vaccination

PATIENT MONITORING
Not required unless complications develop

REFERENCES
1. Centers for Disease Control and Prevention. 2001. Measles—What you need to know. National Immunization Program. www.cdc.gov/nip/diseases/measles/vac-chart.htm
2. Perry RT, Halsey NA. 2004. The clinical significance of measles: a review. *J Infect Dis.* 189:Suppl 1.
3. Centers for Disease Control and Prevention. 2006. Measles. National Center for Health Statistics. http://www.cdc.gov/nchc/faststs/measles.htm
4. Chakravarti A, Rawat D, Yadav S. 2003. Whole blood samples as an alternative to serum for detection of immunity to measles virus by ELISA. *Diagn Microbiol Infect Dis.* 47:563–567.
5. Barclay AJ, Foster A, Sommer A. 1987. Vitamin A supplements and mortality related to measles: A randomized clinical trial.

 ## MISCELLANEOUS

See also: Measles, rubella

CODES

ICD9-CM
055.9 Measles without mention of complication

PATIENT TEACHING
Avoid exposure to other children and potential secondary bacterial pathogens until respiratory symptoms resolve.

M

MEASLES, GERMAN (RUBELLA)

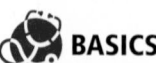

Richard Viken, MD

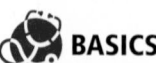 BASICS

DESCRIPTION
An endemic and epidemic viral exanthematous infection of children and adults, worldwide in distribution. Many infections are subclinical, but this virus can cause fetal infection with resultant birth defects.
- System(s) Affected: Hemic/Lymphatic/Immunologic; Nervous; Pulmonary; Skin/Exocrine
- Synonym(s): German measles; 3-day measles

ALERT
Pediatric Considerations
Postnatal rubella is a milder disease in children than in adults.

Pregnancy Considerations
- Women vaccinated against rubella are advised not to become pregnant for at least 1 month. The vaccine-type virus can cross the placenta. However, no case of congenital rubella has occurred after inadvertent vaccination. (1)[C]
- If a pregnant woman is exposed to rubella (i.e., native disease, not vaccine associated), obtain an antibody titer. Presence of antibody implies immunity and no risk. If antibody is not detectable, obtain a 2nd titer in 3 weeks. If antibody is present in the 2nd specimen, infection has occurred. If antibody is again not isolated in result, obtain a 3rd titer in 3 more weeks (6 weeks after exposure). At this time, a negative test result means that infection has not occurred; a positive test result means that infection *did* occur, and the fetus is at risk for congenital rubella.
- Congenital rubella can result in spontaneous abortion and IUGR, and will ultimately lead to birth defects in live fetuses in >60% of pregnancies; these include audiologic, ophthalmologic, and cardiac defects.
- A reliable (87–100% sensitive) polymerase chain reaction–based method of detecting viral RNA in amniotic fluid allows rapid diagnosis of fetal infection, if performed after 15 weeks gestation. (1)[B]
- The single most effective policy for prevention of congenital rubella syndrome is screening pregnant women for rubella immunity and immunizing nonimmune women postpartum. (2)[C]

GENERAL PREVENTION
- Rubella vaccine
  - A 2-dose schedule in combination with measles–mumps vaccine (MMR) is recommended for those born after 1956. The 1st dose is recommended at age 12–15 months; the 2nd dose is recommended either at 4–6 years of age or at 11–12 years of age. Children with HIV should receive MMR vaccine at 12 months of age if no contraindications exist.
  - Recommended for susceptible people in the following groups: Prepubertal boys and girls, premarital or postpartum women, college students, day care personnel, health care workers, and military personnel

  - It is contraindicated in pregnancy, immunodeficiency or immunocompromised state (except HIV), receipt within the last 3 months of immunoglobulin (Ig) or blood, severe febrile illness, or hypersensitivity to vaccine components. (1)[C]
- Patients who receive rubella vaccine do not transmit rubella to others, although the virus can be isolated from the pharynx.
- During outbreaks of rubella, serologic screening before vaccination is not recommended, because rapid mass vaccination is necessary to stop the spread of the disease. (3)[A]
- Strong evidence exists against the hypothesis that MMR vaccination causes autism. (3)[A]

EPIDEMIOLOGY
- Predominant age: Children 5–9 years of age
- Predominant sex: Male = Female

Incidence
In 2005, incidence of postnatal rubella was 0.005 cases/100,000 population, with 1 case of congenital rubella syndrome. At present, the source of most rubella cases is infected people from countries where rubella is not included in routine immunization, was only recently introduced in worldwide distribution, or was administered in mass campaigns. (2)[C]

RISK FACTORS
- Inadequate immunization
- Immunodeficiency states
- Immunosuppressive therapy
- Pregnancy
- Crowded living conditions
- School, day care facility
- Late winter and spring are most likely seasons for transmission and outbreak.
- International travel on commercial airplanes and cruise ships

Genetics
Children with congenital rubella syndrome and children with insulin-dependent diabetes mellitus share a high frequency of HLA-DR3 histocompatibility antigen and a high prevalence of islet cell antibodies. (1)[B]

ETIOLOGY
Rubella virus is a single-stranded RNA virus in the Togavirus family. The virus replicates in the nasopharynx and regional lymph nodes during a 16–18-day incubation period. After invading the bloodstream, it may spread to skin and other distal organs or, transplacentally, to the developing fetus. Organogenesis occurs 2–6 weeks postconception, so that infection is the greater hazard (40–80% risk) to heart and eyes at that time. During the 2nd trimester, the fetus increases in immunologic competence, making the fetus less susceptible (e.g., a 10% risk). (1)[C]

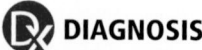 DIAGNOSIS

SIGNS AND SYMPTOMS
- Postnatal rubella
  - Adenopathy: Posterior auricular, posterior cervical, suboccipital
  - Low-grade fever
  - Exanthem: Descending, maculopapular, may desquamate
  - Enanthem: Soft palate petechiae
  - Conjunctivitis
  - Splenomegaly (rare)
  - Coryza
  - Malaise
  - Headache
  - Polyarthralgia/polyarthritis, especially in young women
  - Asymptomatic (25–50%)
- Congenital rubella: (T, transient; P, permanent; D, developmental) (1)[C]
  - Cataracts (P)
  - Microphthalmia (P)
  - Chorioretinitis (P)
  - Patent ductus arteriosus (P)
  - Pulmonic stenosis (P, D)
  - Atrial and ventricular septal defects (P)
  - Sensorineural deafness (P, D)
  - Microcephaly (P)
  - Meningoencephalitis (T)
  - Mental retardation (P, D)
  - Low birth weight (T)
  - Purpuric (so-called blueberry muffin) skin lesions (T)
  - Radiolucent bone disease (T)
  - Hepatosplenomegaly (T)
  - Large anterior fontanelle (T)
  - Language and behavior disorders (P, D)
  - Cryptorchidism (P)
  - Inguinal hernia (P)

TESTS
Cell-mediated immune responses are selectively impaired in children with congenital rubella.

ALERT
See "Pregnancy Considerations" for testing of pregnant women who are exposed to Rubella.

Lab
- Postnatal rubella
  - Mild leukopenia with relative lymphocytosis
  - Fourfold rise in serum levels of antibody to Rubella
  - Pharynx, nose, and blood culture positivity to rubella virus
- Congenital rubella
  - Presence of rubella-specific IgM antibody in serum up to 1 year of age, at which time IgG becomes the dominant antibody
  - Isolation of rubella virus from pharynx, blood, urine, cerebrospinal fluid
- Disorders that may alter lab results
  - After re-exposure to rubella, a person with a low level of antibody from past infection or vaccination may experience an acute rise in antibody levels. This is not associated with a high incidence of contagion to others or of fetal risk.

Diagnostic Procedures/Surgery
Congenital rubella has been diagnosed by placental biopsy at 12 weeks.

Pathological Findings
- Inhibition of cellular growth after infection
- Fetal vasculitis
- Placental angiopathy
- Tissue necrosis

DIFFERENTIAL DIAGNOSIS
- Postnatal rubella
  - Measles virus (rubeola)
  - Scarlet fever
  - Infectious mononucleosis
  - Toxoplasmosis
  - Roseola infantum (i.e., exanthem subitum)
  - Erythema infectiosum (Fifth disease)
  - Drug eruptions
  - Other exanthematous enteroviral infections
- Congenital rubella
  - Cytomegalovirus
  - Varicella-zoster virus
  - Picornaviruses (Coxsackievirus, Echovirus)
  - Poliovirus
  - Herpes simplex virus
  - Western equine virus
  - Measles virus (rubeola)
  - Hepatitis B virus
  - Mumps virus
  - Influenza virus
  - Toxoplasmosis
  - Congenital syphilis
  - Malaria

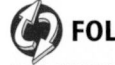 **TREATMENT**

INITIAL STABILIZATION
Outpatient usually

GENERAL MEASURES
- Postnatal rubella: Mild and self-limited. Treat for symptomatic relief.
- Congenital rubella: Supportive care, unless neurologic or hemorrhagic complications develop

Diet
No special diet

Activity
- For postnatal rubella: Contact isolation for 7 days after onset of rash; bed rest is not necessary.
- Contact isolation of congenitally infected infants for 1 year, unless nasopharyngeal and urine cultures after 3 months of age test negative for rubella virus

 MEDICATION (DRUGS)

First Line
Acetaminophen for fever q4h if needed: 10–15 mg/kg/dose

Second Line
None

 FOLLOW-UP

PROGNOSIS
- Postnatal rubella
  - Fever, 1–2 days
  - Rash, 3 days
  - Coryza, 5 days
  - Lymphadenopathy, 1 week
  - Arthralgia (when present), 2 weeks
  - Complete and full recovery without sequelae is the rule.
- Congenital rubella
  - Varied and unpredictable spectrum of consequences, ranging from stillbirth to completely normal infancy and childhood
  - Disease is characterized by chronic infection; infants may remain contagious for months after birth.
  - Detectable levels of hemagglutination-inhibiting antibody (IgG) persist for years, then may decline. By age 5, 20% have no detectable antibody.
  - Overall mortality 10%; greatest during 1st 6 months
  - 70% of those with encephalitis develop residual neuromotor defects, including an autistic syndrome.
  - Prognosis is excellent when only minor defects are present.

COMPLICATIONS
- Postnatal rubella (1)[C]
  - Postinfectious encephalitis (1/5,000 cases)
  - Thrombocytopenic purpura (1/3,000 cases)
  - Arthritis/arthralgias
- Congenital rubella
  - Spontaneous abortion
  - Stillbirth
  - Premature delivery
  - Progressive rubella panencephalitis
  - Endocrine disturbances (e.g., diabetes mellitus, thyrotoxicosis, hypothyroidism)

- Rubella vaccine
  - Lymphadenopathy
  - Fever
  - Rash
  - Arthritis/arthralgia (older girls, women) (1)[C]
  - Polyneuropathy
  - Idiopathic thrombocytopenic purpura (ITP)

PATIENT MONITORING
- People immune to rubella via natural infection or vaccine may be reinfected when re-exposed; such infection is usually asymptomatic and detectable only by serologic means.
- In congenital rubella, it is extremely important to detect auditory and visual impairment early, so that adequate education and counseling can begin.
- 2/3 of internationally adopted children entering the US have no written records of overseas immunizations.

REFERENCES
1. Banatvala JE, Brown DWG. Rubella. *Lancet*. 2004;363:1127–1137.
2. Muchowski K, Paladine H. An ounce of prevention: The evidence supporting periconception health care. *J Fam Pract*. 2004;53:126–133.
3. Demicheli V, Jefferson T, Rivetti A, Price D. Vaccines for measles, mumps and rubella in children. *The Cochrane Database of Systematic Reviews* 2005, Issue 4. Art. No.:CD004407.DOI:10.1002/14651858.CD004407.pub2.

MISCELLANEOUS
- Other notes: Rubella vaccine is currently the only vaccine designed for the purpose of protecting someone other than the vaccine recipient.
- See also: Measles, rubeola

CODES

ICD9-CM
- 056.9 Rubella without mention of complication
- 771.0 Congenital rubella

PATIENT TEACHING
- Make every effort to avoid exposing infected patient to pregnant women.
- JAMA Patient Page on Rubella located at www.jama.com; go to Patient Page Index. Click on Previous Topics, Rubella (1/23–30/2002).

See Corresponding Diagnostic Algorithm

M

MELANOMA

David P. Sealy, MD

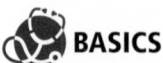 BASICS

DESCRIPTION
- Malignant degeneration of cells from the melanocytic system
  - Most arise in the skin, but may also present as primary lesion in any tissue pigmentation.
  - Metastatic spread to any region in the body
- Variants
  - Lentigo maligna
  - Cutaneous lesion: Slowest growing malignant melanoma with least tendency to metastasize
  - Occurs most often on the face, beginning as a circumscribed macular patch of mottled pigmentation showing shades of dark brown, tan, or black, mostly in the elderly
  - Ocular
  - Malignant progressive lesion of the eye
- System(s) Affected: Skin/Exocrine

ALERT
Geriatric Considerations
Lentigo maligna is most commonly seen in elderly patients who have had a slowly enlarging pigmented lesion, and is usually found on the face.

Pediatric Considerations
- Congenital large nevi (>5 cm) are risk factors and should be followed.
- Blistering sunburns in childhood increase adult risk.

Pregnancy Considerations
- Because melanocyte-stimulating hormone (MSH) levels are markedly increased during pregnancy and melanoma is 1 of the few carcinomas that can spread to the placenta, concern has been that pregnancy exacerbates melanoma. This has not been proven.
- Many authors suggest waiting 1–2 years if further pregnancy is desired for patients with recent melanomas.
- If invasion extends into the lymphatic structures, further pregnancy is probably contraindicated.

GENERAL PREVENTION
- Avoidance of prolonged and high-altitude solar exposures
- Use of sunscreen when exposure unavoidable.
- High-risk individuals should avoid sunburn especially during the adolescent years.

EPIDEMIOLOGY
- Predominant age
  - Median age: 57 years
  - >50% of all individuals with melanoma are between 20 and 40 years.
- Predominant sex: Male = Female

Incidence
- 2005 (est.)
  - 59,580 new cases
  - 7,770 deaths
- 2000
  - 1:74 in US
  - 6th most common cancer in US
- Highest annual incidence rate of any cancer in whites between the ages of 25 and 29 years and in white males between 35 and 39 years old

Prevalence
- >24/100,000 white males and 16/100,000 white females
- 2% of all cancer deaths

RISK FACTORS
- Heavy UVA and UVB exposure
- Previous pigmented lesions (especially dysplastic or melanocytic nevi)
- Fair complexion, freckling, blue eyes, and blond hair
- Those with increased numbers of nevi
- Family history of melanoma
- Tanning bed use before age 30 years (controversial)
- Changing nevus
- Large (>5 cm) congenital nevi
- Other skin cancers
- Immunosuppression
- Blistering sunburns in childhood

Genetics
- Familial dysplastic nevus syndrome
- Lighter pigmented individuals
- Chromosomes 1, 6, 7, 9, 10 most common affected
- Changes in oncogenes, suppressor genes growth factors, and receptors

ETIOLOGY
- Under investigation
- Probably radiation in the UVA and UVB range

DIAGNOSIS

SIGNS AND SYMPTOMS
Change in a pigmented lesion
- Hypo- or hyperpigmentation
- Bleeding
- Scaling
- Size change
- Texture change
- Follow the ABCDE mnemonic: Asymmetry; Border irregularity; Color variegation; Diameter >6 mm with the location on whites being primarily back and lower leg, and on blacks being hands, feet, and nails; and Elevation above skin surface

TESTS
Those designed to follow metastatic disease

Lab
Imaging
Imaging studies are of benefit only in detecting metastatic disease, which is usually to the brain, lymph nodes, and lungs.

Diagnostic Procedures/Surgery
Surgical biopsy is the only form of appropriate diagnostic procedure.
- Any suspicious nevus or pigmented lesion should be fully excised.
- A full-thickness total excisional biopsy must be sent for pathologic examination.
- Lesions should never be curetted, electrodesiccated, or shaved.
- Any irregularly pigmented lesion >2 cm in a preadolescent individual should be considered for excision.

Pathological Findings
- Gross pathologic features include 4 clinical types
  - Superficial spreading melanoma: 70%
  - Nodular: 15%
  - Acral lentiginous: 2–8%
  - Lentigo maligna: 4–10%; a small percentage are amelanotic
- Nodular melanoma is primarily vertical growth, whereas the other 3 types are horizontal.

DIFFERENTIAL DIAGNOSIS
- Dysplastic and blue nevi
- Vascular skin tumor
- Actinic keratosis
- Traumatic hematoma
- Lentigo
- Pigmented squamous cell and basal cell carcinomas, seborrheic keratoses, other changing nevi

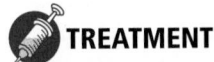 **TREATMENT**

INITIAL STABILIZATION
Outpatient or inpatient surgery

GENERAL MEASURES
Diet
No restrictions

Activity
- No restrictions
- Avoid sun exposure.

 MEDICATION (DRUGS)

First Line
- No 1 chemotherapeutic agent has shown unequivocal benefit. (1,2) [B]
- Early benefit with vaccines has not stood the test of time. (1,2) [B]
- Interferon alfa-2b has shown mild increased benefit in diseasefree time and overall survival. (2)[B]

Second Line
Many have been tried.

SURGERY
- Appropriate health care for melanoma is surgical excision.
- Extent of excision margins is controversial. Generally, achieve margins of 0.5–1 cm if the lesion is <1 mm thick. If thicker, extend margins to 2 cm. (1,3,4) [B]
- Sentinel lymph node biopsy for lesions of 1–4 mm depth has become standard of care. However, increased survival has not been clearly demonstrated.

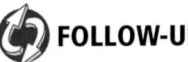 **FOLLOW-UP**

PROGNOSIS
Prognosis is based on staging of the initial lesion.
- Staging (falls into 3 categories)
  - Breslow: 70% 5-year survival of patients without local or distant lymphatic spread
  - Clark staging depends on depth of invasion by skin layer. The best prognosis is for those lesions that are <0.85 mm (especially if restricted to the stratum granulosum or higher), which carry 95–100% 5-year survival. Spread to lymphatics or regional lymph nodes carries <5% 5-year survival.
  - AJCC: Stage 0 in situ and lentigo maligna, Stage I and II localized to skin, Stage III regional LN or satellite lesions, Stage IV distant metasteses (5)
- Women have a better prognosis than men.
- Truncal lesions have a poorer prognosis.
- With distant metastases, disease is uniformly lethal.
- Lesions with ulceration at the time of presentation have a significantly poorer prognosis.

COMPLICATIONS
- Metastatic spread
- Unsatisfactory cosmetic results following the primary surgery

PATIENT MONITORING
- Key to cure is prevention.
- Skin exams every 3–6 months
- Those with 1 melanoma diagnosed are at much greater risk for subsequent new primary melanomas
- Thorough self skin exams weekly
- Only chest radiographs on an annual basis have been shown to be of any benefit: 6% of recurrences were detected, though does not alter prognosis

REFERENCES

1. Rager EL, Bridgefort EP, Ollila DW. Cutaneous melanoma: Update on prevention, screening, diagnosis and treatment. *Am Fam Phys*. 2005;72:269–276.
2. Verma S, et al. Systematic review of systemic adjuvant therapy for patients at high risk for recurrent melanoma. *Cancer*. 2006;106(7): 1431–1442.
3. Sladden MJ, et al. Surgical excision margins for localized cutaneous melanoma. *The Cochrane Database of Systematic Reviews* 2004, Issue 3. Art. No.: CD004835. DOI: 10.1002/14651858. CD004835.
4. Thomas JM, et al. Excision margins in high-risk malignant melanoma. *N Engl J Med*. 2004;350(8): 757–766.
5. Balch CM, et al. Final version of the American Joint Committee on Cancer staging system for cutaneous melanoma. *J Clin Oncol*. 2001;19:3635–3648.
6. *Cancer Facts and Figures 2005*. Atlanta GA: American Cancer Society; 2005. www.cancer.org/ downloads

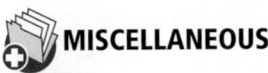 **MISCELLANEOUS**

CODES

ICD9-CM
172.9 Melanoma of skin, site unspecified

PATIENT TEACHING
- Patients with a history of melanoma or dysplastic nevi syndrome must have frequent total body examinations for any abnormal-appearing or changing nevi.
- Educational materials available at the National Cancer Institute, Department of Health And Human Services, Public Inquiries Section, Office of Cancer Communications, Building 31, Room 101-18, 9000 Rockville Pike, Bethesda, MD 20892; (301) 496-5583.

 See Corresponding Diagnostic Algorithm

 See Patient Handout on CD

M

MÉNIÈRE DISEASE

John F. Sullivan, MD
Sheldon Benjamin, MD

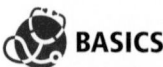 BASICS

DESCRIPTION

An inner ear (labyrinthine) disorder in which volume and pressure of the fluid of the inner ear (endolymph) increase, resulting in recurrent attacks of hearing loss, tinnitus, vertigo, and sensations of aural fullness.

- Usually unilateral at outset, but 45% of cases later involve the contralateral ear
- Severity and frequency may diminish over the years, but with increasing loss of hearing.
- Usually idiopathic (Ménière disease), but may be secondary to another condition causing endolymphatic hydrops (Ménière syndrome)
- System(s) Affected: Nervous
- Synonym(s): Ménière syndrome; Endolymphatic hydrops

ALERT

Geriatric Considerations
Less likely to occur in elderly. Patients exposed to loud noise levels over many years are, however, more susceptible.

Pediatric Considerations
Unusual, but when found is most often related to congenital malformation. Dizziness in children is more likely to result from central nervous system disease.

Pregnancy Considerations
Not a common problem, but difficult to treat because of risk of the medication's producing fetal abnormalities

GENERAL PREVENTION
- Reduce stress.
- Reduce salt intake.
- Do not smoke.
- Avoid significant noise exposure or use ear protectors.
- Avoid use of ototoxic medications (e.g., aspirin, quinine, kanamycin, and many others).

EPIDEMIOLOGY
- Predominant age: Peak age of onset: 40–60 years old
- Predominant sex: Female > Male (1.3:1)

Incidence
Estimates of incidence and prevalence vary widely, and no reliable comprehensive figures are available. Based on a report from the Mayo Clinic in 1980, incidence in the US is ~15 cases per 100,000 per year.

Prevalence
Estimated prevalence is 200/100,000.

RISK FACTORS
- Stress
- Allergy
- Increased salt intake
- Chronic exposure to loud noise

Genetics
Some families show increased incidence but genetic versus environmental components are not understood.

ETIOLOGY
Unknown. Likely caused by decreased resorption of endolymph. Numerous theories suggest this is caused by a variety of injuries (e.g., reduced middle ear pressure, allergy, endocrine disease, lipid disorders, vascular, viral, syphilis, auto-immune).

ASSOCIATED CONDITIONS
- Cochlear hydrops (hearing problem only)
- Vestibular hydrops (balance problem only)
- Drop attacks

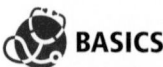 DIAGNOSIS

SIGNS AND SYMPTOMS
- Hearing loss: Low frequency, fluctuating
- Vertigo: Horizontal-rotational
- Ear fullness
- Tinnitus
- Occurs as attacks, duration: 20 minutes to several hours, with intervening remission
- During severe attacks
  - Pallor
  - Sweating
  - Nausea and vomiting
  - Falling
  - Prostration
  - All symptoms are exacerbated by motion.
  - Between attacks, affected patients may experience motion-related imbalance without vertigo.

History
- Attacks are typically spontaneous, but may be preceded by an aura of increasing fullness in the ear and tinnitus.
- Attacks may occur in clusters with long symptom-free periods between.

Physical Exam
- Horizontal nystagmus seen during attacks.
- Otoscopy typically normal.
- Triggering of attacks in the office with Dix-Hallpike maneuver suggests diagnosis of benign paroxysmal positional vertigo, not Ménière. (Positive if nystagmus with the following: Patient sitting, neck extended and turned to one side; patient is then moved to supine, so that head hangs over edge of the bed; patient is observed for nystagmus; patient is then moved upright and observed again for nystagmus; repeat test with head turned to the other side)

TESTS
- Auditory
  - Audiometry using pure tone and speech to show low frequency sensorineural (nerve) loss and impaired speech discrimination
  - Tuning fork tests (i.e., Weber and Rinne) will confirm validity of audiometry.
  - Auditory brainstem response audiometry (ABR) to rule out acoustic neuroma
  - Electrocochleography (ECOG) may be useful to confirm etiology.
- Vestibular:
  - Caloric testing: Electronystagmography (ENG) may show reduced caloric response. Can obtain reasonably comparable information with use of 0.8 mL of ice water instilled in ear canal, then noting duration and frequency of resulting nystagmus with 40-diopter lenses in place. Reduced activity on either side is consistent with Ménière diagnosis but is not itself diagnostic.

Lab
- Lab studies must be done to rule out other conditions and disorders.
- Serologic tests specific for *Treponema pallidum*: Microhemagglutination (MHA), fluorescent treponemal antibody (FTA), *Treponema* immobilization test (TPI)
- Thyroid studies
- Lipid studies
- Drugs that may alter lab results
  - Any medication that produces a significant degree of sedation is likely to affect vestibular testing and thus invalidate such testing.
- Disorders that may alter lab results
  - Many conditions may produce auditory and vestibular findings identical to those associated with Ménière disease.

Imaging
MRI to rule out acoustic tumor, which can produce identical symptoms and findings

Pathological Findings
Autopsy only. Shows dilation of inner ear fluid system (endolymph).

DIFFERENTIAL DIAGNOSIS
- Acoustic tumor
- Syphilis
- Perilymphatic fistula
- Multiple sclerosis
- Viral labyrinthitis
- Vertebrobasilar disease
- Other labyrinthine disorders that produce similar symptoms (e.g., Cogan syndrome, benign positional vertigo, temporal bone trauma)

TREATMENT

INITIAL STABILIZATION
Can usually be managed in outpatient setting. Inpatient for surgery.

GENERAL MEASURES
- There is a paucity of evidence-based guidelines regarding treatment for Ménière disease, therefore there is no "gold standard" treatment.
- Medications are given primarily for symptomatic relief of vertigo and nausea. No medication is currently available that affects the disease process itself.
- During attacks, bed rest with eyes closed and protection from falling. Attacks rarely last >4 hours.
- Some physicians prescribe betahistine, a histamine agonist, which is not commercially available in the US but may be obtained via a "compounding pharmacist." A Cochrane review found insufficient evidence to determine its effectiveness. (1)

Diet
Limit total intake during attacks because of nausea. Otherwise, diet is usually not a factor unless attacks are brought on by certain foods. A restricted salt diet may be useful in some cases.

Activity
- Limit activity during attacks.
- Between attacks patient may be fully active, but this may be limited by fear of impending attack, unsteadiness following attacks, ear fullness or tinnitus, or hearing loss in involved ear that may severely limit the patient's ability to perform work duties or to participate in social life.

MEDICATION (DRUGS)

First Line
- Acute attack: For severe episodes, 1 of the following agents may be used (adult dosages are indicated here)
  – Atropine: 0.2–0.4 mg IV
  – Diazepam (Valium): 5–10 mg IV
  – Transdermal scopolamine: 1 patch, or smaller segment of patch, applied to skin surface and not replaced before 3 days have passed.
- Maintenance (titrate doses to avoid sedation)
  – Meclizine (Antivert, Bonine): 25–100 mg orally, either at bedtime or in divided doses
  – Diazepam (Valium): 2 mg (or less) t.i.d.
  – Diuretics are frequently used as they may reduce endolymphatic volume.
    ○ Hydrochlorothiazide/Triamterene (Diazide, Maxzide): 25/37.5 mg/d
    ○ Acetazolamide (Diamox) 250–500 mg b.i.d.
- Contraindications
  – Atropine: Cardiac disease, especially SVT and other arrhythmias
  – Scopolamine: Children and elderly
  – Diuretics: Electrolyte abnormalities, renal disease

- Precautions
  – Sedating drugs should be used with caution, particularly in the elderly. The need to lower the dosage is common. Patients should be cautioned not to operate motor vehicles when taking these drugs because of the sedative effect.
  – Atropine and scopolamine should be used with particular caution.
  – Diuretics: Monitor electrolytes. Use with caution in patients with sulfa allergy.
- Significant possible interactions
  – Transdermal scopolamine: Anticholinergics, belladonna products, antihistamines, tricyclic antidepressants, among others

Second Line
- Acute attack
  – Droperidol: 1.5–2.5 mg IV push slowly administered (in hospital setting)
  – Promethazine (Phenergan): 12.5–25 mg IV push slowly administered
  – Diphenhydramine (Benadryl): 50 mg IV push slowly administered
- Maintenance
  – Dimenhydrinate (Dramamine): 50 mg PO q4–6h
  – Promethazine (Phenergan): 12.5–25 mg PO q4–6h
  – Diphenhydramine (Benadryl): 25–50 mg PO q6–8h (maximum, 100 mg/24h)
  – Addition of Prednisone 30 mg/day to diuretic treatment reduced severity and frequency of tinnitus and vertigo in one pilot study. (2)[C]

SURGERY
- Interventions that preserve hearing
  – Endolymphatic sac surgery, either decompression or drainage of endolymph into mastoid or subarachnoid space
  – Alternative procedure is to cut the vestibular nerve (intracranial procedure).
  – Intratympanic infusion of gentamicin has been found to improve vertigo symptoms in patients who have failed medical management. (3)[B]
  – Another newer procedure is to place a ventilation tube through a myringotomy, and then use a pressure-producing instrument called a Meniett device so as to apply intermittent pressure to the inner ear several times a day. This has been found helpful for the relief of dizziness, but not to reduce frequency of attacks or hearing loss. (4)[B]
  – A pilot study of intratympanic corticosteroid infusion demonstrated symptomatic improvement. (5)[B]
- If patient has lost all hearing on affected side: Labyrinthectomy

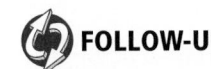 FOLLOW-UP

PROGNOSIS
- Alternating attacks and remission
- 1/2 of cases resolve spontaneously within 2–3 years, but can last >20 years. Severity and frequency of attacks diminish, but hearing loss is progressive.
- Most patients can be managed successfully with medication. ~5–10% of patients require surgery for incapacitating vertigo.
- Clinicians must not overlook possibility of acoustic tumor, which produces an identical clinical picture.

COMPLICATIONS
- Failure to diagnose acoustic neuroma
- Loss of hearing
- Injury during attack
- Inability to work

PATIENT MONITORING
The most common complaint by patients with Ménière disease is that the primary care physician did not take the condition seriously and did not seem interested in providing ongoing care. Because of the emotional impact alone, these patients need close follow-up care. It is important to monitor the status of their hearing, and to continue to consider the possibility of a more serious underlying problem (e.g., acoustic tumor).

REFERENCES
1. James AL, Burton MJ. Betahistine for Ménière's disease or syndrome. Cochrane Ear, Nose and Throat Disorders Group, *Cochrane Database of Systematic Reviews*. 1, 2006.
2. Morales-Luckie E, et al. Oral administration of prednisone to control refractory vertigo in Ménière's disease: A pilot study. *Otol Neurotol*. 2005;26(5):1022–1026.
3. Stokroos R, Kingma H. Selective vestibular ablation by intratympanic gentamicin in patients with unilateral active Ménière's disease: A prospective, double-blind, placebo-controlled, randomized clinical trial. *Acta Otolaryngol*. 2004;124(2):172–175.
4. Thomsen J, Sass K. Local overpressure treatment reduces vestibular symptoms in patients with Ménière's disease: A clinical, randomized, multicenter, double-blind, placebo-controlled study. *Otol Neurotol*. 2005;26(1):68–73.
5. Garduno-Anaya MA, et al. Dexamethasone inner ear perfusion by intratympanic injection in unilateral Meniere's disease: A two-year prospective, placebo-controlled, double-blind, randomized trial. *Otolaryngol Head Neck Surg*. 2005;133(2):285–294.

 MISCELLANEOUS

See also: Labyrinthitis; Tinnitus; Hearing loss

CODES

ICD9-CM
386.00 Ménière disease, unspecified

PATIENT TEACHING
Patient information, including support group contacts, is available from the Vestibular Disorders Association: www.vestibular.org.

 See Corresponding Diagnostic Algorithm

 See Patient Handout on CD

M

MENINGITIS, BACTERIAL

Paul R. Gordon, MD, MPH

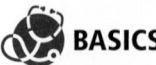 **BASICS**

DESCRIPTION
- Inflammation of the pia-arachnoid and its fluid and the fluid of the ventricles; always cerebrospinal
- System(s) Affected: Nervous

ALERT
Bacterial meningitis is a medical, neurological, and sometimes neurosurgical emergency. Community-acquired meningitis caused by *Streptococcus pneumoniae* has a case fatality rates from 19–37% in adults.

Geriatric Considerations
Several signs and symptoms may be less evident in elderly patients with other disorders, such as CHF and pneumonia.

GENERAL PREVENTION
- Prompt medical treatment for infections
- Strict aseptic techniques when treating patients with head wounds or skull fractures
- Look for evidence of cerebrospinal fluid fistula in patients with recurrent meningitis.

EPIDEMIOLOGY
- Predominant age: Neonates, infants, and elderly
- Predominant sex: Male = Female

Incidence
3–10 cases per 100,000 population

RISK FACTORS
- Immunocompromised host
- Alcoholism
- Neurosurgical procedure or head injury
- Abdominal surgery at risk for gram-negative infection

Genetics
Individuals of Navajo Indian or American Eskimo descent may have genetic or acquired vulnerability to invasive disease.

PATHOPHYSIOLOGY
Bacterial infection causes inflammation of the pia-arachnoid and its fluid and the fluid of the ventricles.

ETIOLOGY
Bacteria are divided into age groups to guide empiric therapy (percentages indicate relative incidence). Any organism can cause meningitis in any age group; therapy should be guided by culture whenever possible.

- Neonates (0–4 weeks)
  – Group B or D *Streptococcus* organisms: 70%
  – *Listeria monocytogenes*: 20%
  – *S. pneumoniae*: 10%
  – *Escherichia coli*
  – Non–group B *Streptococcus* organisms
- Infants (4–12 weeks)
  – *Neisseria meningitides*: 55%
  – *S. pneumoniae*: 40%
  – *Haemophilus influenzae*: 5%
  – Group B *Streptococcus* organisms
  – *L. monocytogenes*
  – *E. coli*

- Children (3 months to 18 years)
  – *N. meningitides*: 55%
  – *S. pneumoniae*: 30%
  – *H. influenzae*: 10%
- Adults (>18 years)
  – *S. pneumoniae:* 30–50%
  – *N. meningitides*: 10–35%
  – Staphylococci: 5–15%
  – Gram-negative bacilli (e.g., *E. coli, H. influenzae)*: 1–10%)
  – Streptococci: 5%
  – *Listeria* species: 5%
  – *H. influenzae*: 1–3%

ASSOCIATED CONDITIONS
The following conditions worsen prognosis
- Coma
- Seizures
- Alcoholism
- Old age
- Infancy
- Diabetes mellitus
- Multiple myeloma
- Head trauma

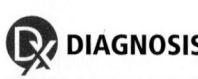 **DIAGNOSIS**

SIGNS AND SYMPTOMS
The triad of fever, neck stiffness, and altered mental status has low sensitivity (44%). However, almost all patients present with at least 2 of 4 symptoms: Headache, fever, neck stiffness, and altered mental status.

History
- Antecedent upper respiratory infection
- Fever
- Headache
- Vomiting
- Photophobia
- Seizures
- Nausea
- Rigors
- Profuse sweats
- Weakness
- Elderly: Subtle findings commonly including confusion

Physical Exam
- Meningismus
- Signs of cerebral dysfunction
- Altered mental status
- Focal neurologic deficits
- Meningococcemia
- Rash: Macular and erythematous at 1st, then petechial or purpuric

TESTS
Lab
- Cerebrospinal fluid (CSF) analysis: (Turbid)
- Neonates
  – >10 WBCs in CSF
  – CSF: Blood glucose ratio <0.6
  – CSF protein >150 mg/dL
- Infants/children
  – >5 WBCs in CSF
  – CSF: Blood glucose ratio <0.6
  – CSF protein >50 mg/dL
- Adults
  – 1,000–100,000 WBCs in CSF
  – CSF: Blood glucose ratio <0.4
  – CSF protein above 45 mg/dL (usually 150–400 mg/dL)
  – Suspect ruptured brain abscess when WBC count is unusually high (>100,000)
- In all age groups
  – CSF opening pressure above 180 mm H_2O (1.77 kPa) (kilopascal)
  – CSF gram stain positive in 75% of untreated patients
  – CSF culture positive: 70–80% of cases
  – Bacterial testing using PCR (particularly in those with negative cultures). (*Not yet routinely recommended.*)
- Serum WBCs
- Serum blood cultures
  – Blood culture positive: 40–60% of cases

Imaging
- CT scan of head if concern for increased intracranial pressure, or warning signs of space-occupying lesion (new-onset seizure, evolving signs of brain tissue shift or papilledema)
- Chest radiograph may reveal silent area of pneumonitis or abscess.
- Sinus/skull radiographs may reveal cranial osteomyelitis, paranasal sinusitis, or skull fracture.
- Later in course, head CT scan, if hydrocephalus, brain abscess, subdural effusions, or subdural empyema are considered or in those patients who have not responded clinically after 48 hours of appropriate antibiotics

Diagnostic Procedures/Surgery
Lumbar puncture

Pathological Findings
Pleocytosis in CSF

DIFFERENTIAL DIAGNOSIS
- Bacteremia
- Sepsis
- Brain abscess
- Seizures
- Other nonbacterial meningitides

TREATMENT

GENERAL MEASURES
- Appropriate antibiotic therapy
- Vigorous supportive care with constant nursing to ensure prompt recognition of seizures and prevention of aspiration
- Therapy for coexisting conditions
- Measures to prevent hypothermia and dehydration

Diet
Regular as tolerated, except when SIADH (syndrome of inappropriate secretion of antidiuretic hormone) complicates course

Activity
As tolerated in hospital and on discharge

Nursing
- ICU monitoring may be needed to recognize changes in the patient's consciousness and the development of new neurologic signs, subtle seizures, and to treat severe agitation effectively.
- Patients with suspected meningococcal infection require respiratory isolation for 24 hours.

SPECIAL THERAPY
IV Fluids
There is no evidence to support other than maintenance fluid therapy (5)[A]

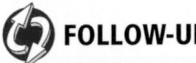 MEDICATION (DRUGS)

Empiric IV therapy until culture results available:
- Consider local patterns of bacterial sensitivity.
- See "Etiology" for age definitions and likely organisms.

First Line
The following regimens are somewhat simplified but will adequately treat all patients pending culture results. Additional subgroupings may simplify treatment in some patients. Penicillin-allergic patients present a special challenge not covered here.

- Antibiotics: 2 IV regimens are presented; the 1st is usual therapy and the 2nd is provided as an alternative (6)[A]
  - Ceftriaxone: 100 mg/kg/d q12–24h (maximum, 2 g q12h) or cefotaxime 200 mg/kg/d q4–6h
  - Ampicillin: 300–400 mg/kg/d q4h (maximum, 2 g q3–4h)
  - Vancomycin: 10–15 mg/kg q12h (maximum, 1,500 mg q12h) or
- Neonates (give both) (1)[B]
  - Ampicillin: 100–400 mg/kg/d divided q6–12h
  - Tobramycin: 7.5 mg/kg/d q6–8h (premature or <1 week of age, 2.5 mg/kg q12h)

- Infants >4 weeks of age (give both)
  - Ampicillin: 300–400 mg/kg/d divided q4–6h (maximum 2 g q3–4h)
  - Chloramphenicol: 75–100 mg/kg/d divided q6h

- Adults (3,7)[A]
  - Vancomycin: 1 g IV q12h
  - Ceftriaxone: 1–2 g IV q12–24h (maximum, 2 g q12h) or cefotaxime 2 g IV q4–6h

- Precaution: Ototoxicity from aminoglycoside
- Contraindications: Allergies to specific antibiotic

- Treatment duration (3)[A]
  - N. meningitides, H. influenzae: 7–10 days
  - S. pneumoniae: 10–14 days
  - Group B Streptococcus organisms, E. coli, L. monocytogenes: 14–21 days
  - Neonates: 12–21 days or at least 14 days after a repeated culture is sterile
- Corticosteroids (2,4)[B],(6)[A]
  - Early treatment with dexamethasone decreases mortality and morbidity for pediatric patients older than 1 month and in adults with acute bacterial meningitis, and does not increase the risk of gastrointestinal bleeding.
  - Dexamethasone: 0.15 mg/kg q6h, or 10 mg for adults, started 15–20 minutes before or with the antibiotic for 4 days.

Second Line
- Antipseudomonal penicillins
- Aztreonam
- Quinolones (e.g., ciprofloxacin)
- Meropenem

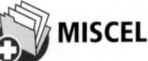 FOLLOW-UP

DISPOSITION
- If diagnosis is suspected, lumbar puncture should be done in office with antimicrobial therapy begun before transfer to hospital.
- Inpatient care: ICU often required

Admission Criteria
Meningitis requires hospitalization.

Discharge Criteria
May consider home therapy for completion of IV antibiotic course once patient is clinically stable and culture and sensitivity results are known.

Issues for Referral
Consultation from intensive care specialist

PROGNOSIS
Overall case fatality 14%
- H. Influenzae: 5%
- N. meningitidis: 10%
- S. pneumoniae: 19–37%

COMPLICATIONS
- Seizures: 20–30%
- Focal neurologic deficit
- Cranial nerve palsies (III, VI, VII, VIII)
  - Comprises 10–20% of the cases
  - Usually disappear within a few weeks
- Sensorineural hearing loss: 10% in children
- Neurodevelopmental sequelae: 30% subtle learning deficits
- Obstructive hydrocephalus
- Subdural effusions
- Decline in consciousness which may be due to meningoencephalitis

PATIENT MONITORING
Brainstem auditory evoked response (BAER) test should be done on infants before hospital discharge.
- Further follow-up will depend on its results and course of meningitis while in hospital.

REFERENCES
1. Anonymous. Therapy for children with invasive pneumococcal infections: American Academy of Pediatrics Committee on Infectious Diseases. Pediatrics. 1997;99:289–299.
2. de Gans J, van de Beek D. European Dexamethasone in Adulthood Bacterial Meningitis Study Investigators. Dexamethasone in adults with bacterial meningitis. N Engl J Med. 2002; 347:1549–1556.
3. van de Beek, D, de Gans J, Tunkel AR, Wijdicks EFM. Community-acquired bacterial meningitis in adults. N Engl J Med. 2006;354:44–53.
4. Odio CM, et al. The beneficial effects of early dexamethasone administration in infants and children with bacterial meningitis. N Engl J Med. 1991;324:1525–1531.
5. Oates-Whitehead RM, Maconochie I, Baumer H, Stewart MER. Fluid therapy for acute bacterial meningitis. The Cochrane Library, The Cochrane Collaboration Volume (4), 2005.
6. van de Beek D, et al. Corticosteroids in acute bacterial meningitis [comment appears in ACP J Club 2004;140:34]. Cochrane Database Syst Rev. 2003;3:CD004305.
7. Prasad K, Singhal T, Jain N, Gupta PK. Third generation cephalosporins versus conventional antibiotics for treating acute bacterial meningitis. The Cochrane Library, The Cochrane Collaboration Volume (4), 2005.

 MISCELLANEOUS

See also: Meningitis, viral; Meningococcemia

CODES

ICD9-CM
320.9 Meningitis due to unspecified bacterium

PATIENT TEACHING
Available at the AAP, 141 Northwest Point Blvd., P.O. Box 927, Elk Grove Village, IL 60009-0927; (800) 433-9016.

Prevention
- Meningitis caused by Haemophilus influenza has been nearly eliminated due to routine vaccination.
- Conjugate vaccines against S. pneumoniae may reduce the burden of disease in childhood and may produce herd immunity among adults.
- Persons with close contact to patients with meningococcal meningitis must receive chemoprophylaxix to eradicate carriage.

See Corresponding Diagnostic Algorithm

M

MENINGITIS, VIRAL

Eric S. Grajkowski, DO

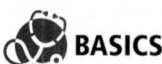 **BASICS**

DESCRIPTION
- Viral infection of the meninges and spinal fluid, with negative cerebrospinal fluid (CSF) bacterial cultures
- System(s) Affected: Nervous
- Synonym(s): Abacterial meningitis; Aseptic meningitis

ALERT
Geriatric Considerations
- Rarely seen in the elderly
- Consider alternative diagnosis (e.g., carcinomatous meningitis)

Pediatric Considerations
PMN predominance may occur in the majority of cases with viral meningitis, especially within the 1st 24 hours. (3)

EPIDEMIOLOGY
- Predominant age: Affects all ages, but most common in young adults
- Predominant sex: Male = Female

Incidence
- Peaks in summer
  - Enteroviruses and arthropod-borne viruses predominate in warm months.
  - Mumps usually occurs in the winter and spring, often in epidemics.
- >10,000 reported cases per year in the US, estimated 11 per 100,000 worldwide; probably many more unreported

Prevalence
With the short course of viral meningitis, the incidence is greater than the prevalence.

RISK FACTORS
- Unknown
- Immunocompromised hosts may be more susceptible to cytomegalovirus (CMV) and adenovirus.

ETIOLOGY
Usual cause is acute and may be relapsing.
- Coxsackie A, B
- ECHO virus (enteroviruses 70–75% of all cases)
- Poliovirus
- Lymphocytic choriomeningitis (LCM)
- Mumps
- Herpes (simplex and zoster)
- Recurrent (Mollaret) meningitis (80% of cases due to Herpes)
- Epstein-Barr virus (EBV)
- Arthropod-borne viruses
- CMV
- Adenovirus
- HIV
- West Nile virus, St. Louis encephalitis virus, and California encephalitis virus

ASSOCIATED CONDITIONS
Encephalitis

DIAGNOSIS

PRE HOSPITAL
Pretreatment with antibiotics may result in "partially treated" bacterial meningitis that mimics viral meningitis.

SIGNS AND SYMPTOMS
- Fever
- Headache, often severe
- Stiff neck
- Nausea and vomiting
- Photophobia
- Generalized aches and pains
- Occasional rash

History
- Travel and exposure history
- Sexual activity (HSV, HIV, etc.)
- Camping (lyme)
- Rodent exposure (LCM)

Physical Exam
- Presence of at least 1 of the following: Fever, neck stiffness, and change in mental status had a sensitivity of 99% in immunocompetent adults.
- Absence of all 3 virtually rules out meningitis. (4)[A]

TESTS
- CSF analysis
  - CSF pleocytosis: Usually predominantly mononuclear but may show more polys early on
  - CSF white blood cell count up to 3,000–4,000, but usually 50–200
  - CSF: Increased pressure
  - CSF: Serum antiviral antibody
  - Elevated CSF protein, but usually <150 mg/dL (<1,500 mg/L)
  - CSF glucose level usually normal (exceptions: Herpes, mumps)
  - Negative CSF gram stain and culture for bacteria
  - Negative CSF latex agglutination or counter immunoelectrophoresis for bacterial antigens
  - Polymerase chain reaction (PCR) has a sensitivity of 95–100% for HSV type 1, EBV, and enterovirus allowing for earlier hospital discharge and less intervention. (6)[A]
- Disorders that may alter lab results include the following
  - Diabetes: Alteration in CSF glucose level
  - Preexisting neurologic diseases (e.g., brain tumor, demyelinating disease)
- Electroencephalogram (EEG) in some cases, especially if encephalitis is a consideration

Lab
- CBC: Normal or mildly elevated WBC
- Viral cultures and/or antibody titers
- Culture CSF for enteroviruses, HSV-2, mumps; throat for enteroviruses, mumps; stool for enteroviruses.
  - Seldom helpful
  - CSF PCR for HSV, West Nile virus, or enteroviruses
  - Serology for Epstein-Barr, HIV, mumps

Imaging
CT scan or MRI scan of the brain, if the patient presents with abnormal neurologic signs
- Usually performed before lumbar puncture

Diagnostic Procedures/Surgery
Lumbar puncture

Pathological Findings
Lymphocyte infiltration of meninges and ventricles

DIFFERENTIAL DIAGNOSIS
- Bacterial meningitis
- Encephalitis
- Acute encephalopathy
- Postinfectious encephalomyelitis
- Parameningeal infections (e.g., subdural empyema)
- Carcinomatous meningitis
- Meningeal leukemia
- Migraine headache
- Viral syndrome (e.g., influenza)
- Chemical meningitis
- Brain abscess
- Other infectious agents
  - Tuberculosis
  - Syphilis
  - Ameba
  - Leptospirosis

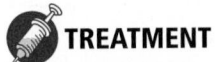 TREATMENT

GENERAL MEASURES
- Fever control
- IV fluids if oral intake is poor or vomiting is present

Diet
Determined by symptoms
- May need to NPO due to nausea or vomiting
- Advance to clear fluids and regular diet as tolerated.

Activity
Activity as tolerated, especially if other causes of meningitis are ruled out

Nursing
Contact precautions until bacterial meningitis is ruled out

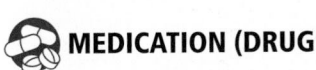 MEDICATION (DRUGS)

First Line
- Analgesics (adult doses)
  - Morphine: 2–5 mg IV q3h
  - Nalbuphine (Nubain): 10 mg IM
  - Acetaminophen-codeine or acetaminophen-oxycodone (Percocet): 1–2 tablets PO q3h as needed
- Antiemetics
  - Promethazine (Phenergan): 12.5–25 mg IV q4h
  - Prochlorperazine (Compazine): 10 mg IM q4h
  - Ondansetron (Zofran) 4–8 mg IV q8h
- Antipyretics
  - Acetaminophen (Tylenol): 650 mg PO or rectal suppository q4h (pediatric dose: ~60 mg per year of age in children or 10–15 mg/kg per dose)
- Antiviral agents
  - Not indicated, unless there is a possibility of viral encephalitis or meningoencephalitis where one can start Acyclovir 10 mg/kg q8h
- Antibiotics
  - Not indicated for treatment of viral meningitis
  - Often initiated until a diagnosis is firmly established
  - If parameters suggest a viral etiology, treat symptomatically and follow the patient closely in the hospital setting.
  - If in doubt, initiate IV broad-spectrum antibiotic with good CSF penetration. The choice may be dictated by local sensitivities, as well as a consideration of age-related pathogens.
- Precautions
  - Aspirin should be avoided in children and adolescents due to a possible association with Reye syndrome.
  - Phenothiazines may produce a dystonic reaction, especially in adolescents.

Second Line
Symptomatic relief may be provided by a variety of antiemetics and analgesics (e.g., NSAIDs).

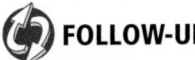 FOLLOW-UP

DISPOSITION
Usually inpatient, depending on severity of symptoms
- Private room indicated with moderate sterile precautions
- Stress hand washing.

PROGNOSIS
- Complete recovery in 2–7 days
- Headaches and other uncomfortable symptoms may persist intermittently for 1–2 weeks.

COMPLICATIONS
- Deafness
- Fatigue
- Irritability
- Muscle weakness
- Seizures (rare)

PATIENT MONITORING
- Once the acute illness begins resolving, follow at least once within 7–10 days.
- Repeated lumbar puncture not necessary unless the clinical course is atypical

REFERENCES
1. Krugman S, et al. *Infectious Diseases of Children*. 9th ed. New York, NY: C.V. Mosby; 1990.
2. Mandell G, Douglas RG Jr, Bennett JE. *Principles and Practice of Infectious Diseases*. 4th ed. New York, NY: Churchill Livingstone; 1995.
3. Negrini B, et al. Cerebrospinal fluid findings in aseptic versus bacterial meningitis. *Pediatrics*. 2000;105(2):316–319.
4. Parrino T. Review: The physical examination can exclude diagnosis of meningitis in low-risk adults. *Evid Based Med*. 2000;5:28.
5. Rotbart HA. Enteroviral infections in the central nervous system. *Clin Infect Dis*. 1995;20:971–981.
6. Seehusen DA, et al. Cerebrospinal fluid analysis. *Am Fam Physician*. 2003;68.
7. Vokshoor A, et al. Viral meningitis. Available at: www.emedicine.com/neuro/topic607.htm

 MISCELLANEOUS

See also: Encephalitis, viral; Meningitis, bacterial

 CODES

ICD9-CM
047.9 Unspecified viral meningitis

PATIENT TEACHING
- Discuss possibility, but low probability, of transmission to contacts.
- Expected duration of illness (2–7 days)
- For patient education materials, contact the American Academy of Pediatrics, 141 Northwest Point Blvd., P.O. Box 927, Elk Grove Village, IL 60009-0927; (800) 433-9016.

See Corresponding Diagnostic Algorithm

M

MENINGOCOCCEMIA

Hans House, MD

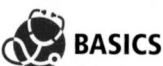 **BASICS**

DESCRIPTION

Neisseria meningitidis in the blood, which results in a broad spectrum of clinical manifestations

- Bacteremia without sepsis: Patient has upper respiratory symptoms only and recovers spontaneously without antibiotic.
- Bacteremia without meningitis: Patient is acutely ill, and may have skin manifestations (rashes, petechiae, ecchymosis) and hypotension.
- Bacteremia with meningitis
  - Predominant clinical picture of meningitis: Headache, decreased sensorium, and neck rigidity
  - Skin manifestations and hypotension may also be present.
- Bacteremia with acute arthritis dermatitis syndrome: Patient may have tenosynovitis typical of gonococcal etiology.
- System(s) Affected: Cardiovascular; Endocrine/Metabolic; Hemic/Lymphatic/ Immunologic; Musculoskeletal; Nervous; Renal/Urologic; Skin/Exocrine
- Synonym(s): Spinal meningitis

ALERT

Geriatric Considerations
Less common

Pediatric Considerations
Highest risk in those aged 3 months to 1 year

GENERAL PREVENTION

Vaccine containing polysaccharides of groups A, C, Y, and W-135 is available for the following

- Persons with late complement deficiency or anatomic or functional asplenia
- Travelers to the Haj in Saudi Arabia and other areas with epidemic meningococcal disease (e.g., West Africa)
- Recommended for children at age 11, 12, teens entering high school, and freshmen college students living in dormitories 1[C]

EPIDEMIOLOGY

- Predominant age
  - Infants ages 3 months to 1 year
  - May affect all ages
- Predominant sex: Male = Female

Incidence
0.5–5/100,000 worldwide

RISK FACTORS

- Age: 3 months to 1 year
- Late complement component deficiency (C5, C6, C7, C8, or C9)
- Household contacts
- Contacts in nurseries and day care centers
- Close quarters (e.g., dormitories, campus bars, and military barracks)

Genetics
Late complement component deficiency has an autosomal recessive inheritance.

ETIOLOGY

Neisseria meningitidis, a gram-negative diplococcus with at least 13 serotypes

- Major serogroups: A, B, C, Y, and W-135
  - Serogroup A may cause epidemics in many parts of the developing world.
  - Serogroup B is predominant cause of meningococcemia in children <1 year of age.
  - Serogroup C has caused recent outbreaks in the US.
  - Serogroup Y is becoming more common in the US.

 DIAGNOSIS

SIGNS AND SYMPTOMS

- Malaise
- Fever
- Chills, rigor
- Sore throat
- Cough
- Headache
- Changes in mental status
  - Restlessness
  - Agitation
  - Confusion
  - Delirium
  - Lethargy
  - Stupor
  - Coma
- Myalgia
- Vomiting
- Convulsions
- Stiff neck
- Focal neurologic signs
- Tachycardia
- Tachypnea
- Hypotension
- Cyanosis
- Maculopapular rash
- Petechiae
- Ecchymosis, purpura
- Arthritis
- Tenosynovitis

Physical Exam
Look for skin findings: Maculopapular rash, petechiae, ecchymosis, and purpura.

TESTS

Prior antibiotic administration may render blood and/or cerebrospinal fluid (CSF) culture negative within 2 hours.

Lab

- Leukocytosis or leukopenia
- Left shift of leukocytes, toxic granulation
- Thrombocytopenia
- Lactic acidosis
- Prolonged prothrombin time
- Prolonged partial thromboplastin time
- Low fibrinogen
- Elevated fibrin degradation products
- Blood culture growing *N. meningitidis*
- CSF
  - Cloudy
  - Increased WBCs with polymorphonuclear cells predominant
  - Gram stain showing gram-negative diplococci
  - Glucose-to-blood glucose ratio <0.4
  - Protein >45 mg/dL
  - Positive for *N. meningitidis* antigen (MAT or PCR) (2)[B]
  - Culture positive for *N. meningitidis*

Imaging
CT scan of head if concern for space-occupying lesions

Diagnostic Procedures/Surgery

- Blood culture
- Lumbar puncture
  - After a brief history and physical examination suggest meningitis, initiate antibiotics and proceed with lumbar puncture within 1 hour. (2)[C]

Pathological Findings

- Disseminated intravascular coagulation
- Exudates on meninges
- Polymorphonuclear infiltration of meninges
- Hemorrhage of adrenal glands

DIFFERENTIAL DIAGNOSIS

- Septicemia due to other microorganism
- Meningitis due to other pyogenic bacteria
- Gonococcemia
- Acute bacterial endocarditis
- Rocky Mountain spotted fever
- Hemolytic uremic syndrome
- Gonococcal arthritis dermatitis syndrome
- Influenza

TREATMENT

INITIAL STABILIZATION

- If meningitis suspected, initiate antibiotics and then proceed to immediate lumbar puncture. (2)[C], (3)[B]
- Admit patient to ICU if severe sepsis or meningitis is suspected.
- Droplet isolation for 24 hours from the beginning of antibiotic therapy.

GENERAL MEASURES

- Appropriate antibiotic
- Supportive care
  - IV fluids
  - Oxygen when needed
- Close monitoring of patient for seizure activity
- Treat complications
  - Disseminated intravascular coagulation
  - Adult respiratory distress syndrome
  - Renal failure
  - Adrenal failure

Diet

As tolerated, depending on clinical condition

Activity

As tolerated, depending on clinical condition

SPECIAL THERAPY

IV Fluids

Replace volume as needed.

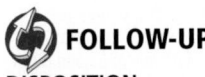 ## MEDICATION (DRUGS)

First Line

- In patients strongly suspected of having meningitis, consider administering dexamethasone 0.15 mg/kg q6h for 16 doses, starting 15 minutes before 1st dose of antibiotic. (4)[B]
- Treatment for suspected meningococcal meningitis must begin as soon as possible and so coverage for other possible causes of meningitis must be included until a definitive diagnosis is made.

- Age influences etiologic organism.
- Age <4 weeks: Ampicillin plus cefotaxime or ceftriaxone
- Age 4–12 weeks: Ampicillin plus cefotaxime or Ceftriaxone plus Vancomycin
- Age 12 weeks to adulthood: cefotaxiime or ceftriaxone plus vancomycin
- When treating an adult patient with suspected meningitis, initiate early therapy as above. Once *N. meningitidis* is identified, the drug of choice remains penicillin. (2,5)[C]
- For meningitis
  - Penicillin G 4 million units IV q4h (pediatric dose: 0.25 mU/kg IV q4-6h) or ampicillin 2 g IV q4h (pediatric dose: 200–300 mg/kg IV q6h)
  - Use alternate drugs if patient allergic to penicillin
- For other infections: Use 1/2 the dose for meningitis.
- Duration of treatment 7–10 days

- Chemoprophylaxis for close contacts (household members and personnel in nurseries, day care centers, nursing homes, dormitories, and other closed institutions). No chemoprophylaxis is needed for casual contacts, health care personnel (except persons giving mouth-to-mouth resuscitation), schoolmates, and office co-workers.
  - Rifampin 600 mg (pediatric dose: 10 mg/kg) PO q12h for 2 days or (for adults only) 1 dose of ciprofloxacin 750 mg PO (6)[B]
- Precautions
  - Adjust dosage of both medications in patients with severe renal dysfunction.
  - Rifampin ingestion causes orange urine.

Second Line

- For meningitis
  - Chloramphenicol 1 g IV q6h (pediatric dose: 75–100 mg/kg q6h) or ceftriaxone 2 g IV q12h (pediatric dose: 80–100 mg/kg q12–24h)
- Precautions
  - Ceftriaxone should not be used in patients with history of anaphylactic reactions to penicillin (e.g. hypotension, laryngeal edema, wheezing, hives)
  - Chloramphenicol may cause aplastic anemia.
- For other infections
  - Ceftriaxone 1 g (pediatric dose: 40 mg/kg) IV q24h

 ## FOLLOW-UP

DISPOSITION

Before discharge, to eradicate carriage, give patient a prescription for rifampin 600 mg (children 10 mg/kg) PO q12h for 2 days or, for adults only, 1 dose of ciprofloxacin 500–750 mg PO. (6)[B]

Issues for Referral

In patients with neurologic deficits, follow-up with a neurologist may be needed.

PROGNOSIS

Overall mortality 10%

COMPLICATIONS

- Disseminated intravascular coagulation
- Acute tubular necrosis
- Seizures
- Focal neurologic deficit
- Cranial nerve palsies
- Sensorineural hearing loss
- Obstructive hydrocephalus
- Subdural effusions
- Acute adrenal hemorrhage
- Waterhouse-Friderichsen syndrome

REFERENCES

1. Recommended Childhood and Adolescent Immunization Schedule—United States, 2006. *MMWR Morb Mortal Wkly Rep.* 2006;54(52); Q1–Q4.
2. van de Beek D, de Gans J, Tunkel AR, Wijdicks EF. Community-acquired bacterial meningitis in adults.
3. Kanegaye JT, Soliemanzadeh P, Bradley JS. Lumbar puncture in pediatric bacterial meningitis: Defining the time interval for recovery of cerebrospinal fluid pathogens after parenteral antibiotic pretreatment. *Pediatrics.* 2001;108(5):1169–1174.
4. de Gans J, van de Beek D. Dexamethasone in adults with bacterial meningitis.
5. Sinner SW, Tunkel AR. Antimicrobial agents in the treatment of bacterial meningitis.
6. Fraser A, Gafter-Gvili A, Paul M, Leibovici L. Antibiotics for preventing meningococcal infections. *Cochrane Database of Systematic Reviews.* 2005;(1):CD004785.
7. Diaz PS. The epidemiology and control of invasive meningococcal disease. *Pediatr Infect Dis J.* 1999;18:633–634.
8. Rosenstein NE, et al. Meningococcal disease. *N Engl J Med.* 2001;344:1378–1388.

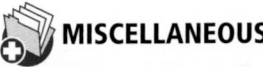 ## MISCELLANEOUS

See also: Meningitis, bacterial; Sepsis

CODES

ICD9-CM

- 036.2 Meningococcemia
- 036.0 Meningococcal meningitis

PATIENT TEACHING

- Educate family and close contacts regarding risk of contracting meningococcal infections.
- Educate health care personnel who are not at risk of contracting meningococcal infections.

See Corresponding Diagnostic Algorithm

M

MENINGOMYELOCELE

David J. Donahue, MD

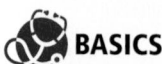 **BASICS**

DESCRIPTION

- Meningomyelocele is the most common nonlethal malformation in the spectrum of neural-tube deficits.
- Incomplete closure of the vertebral column during embryogenesis, thus exposing meninges and spinal cord
- Always associated with the constellation of findings known as the Chiari II malformation, which include small posterior fossa, hindbrain herniation into the upper cervical spinal canal, dysgenesis or agenesis of the corpus callosum, neuronal migration disorders of varying degree, and hydrocephalus
- Chiari II abnormality is associated with meningomyelocele, anencephaly, and encephalocele, all of which belong to a group of disorders known as neural tube defects. These serious congenital anomalies of the nervous system, which occur during the 1st 4 weeks of gestation, result from faulty formation of the neural tube.
- Postneurulation defects develop after 25 days of intrauterine life, that is, after neurulation is complete.
  - Lesions include simple meningocele, lipomeningomyelocele, diastematomyelia, myelocystocele, neurenteric cyst, and intraspinal and pelvic meningoceles.
  - Characterized by intact skin over the underlying lesion
- System(s) Affected: Musculoskeletal; Nervous; Renal/Urologic; Skin/Exocrine
- Synonym(s): Myelomeningocele; Spinal dysraphism; Spina bifida; Open neural tube defect

ALERT

Pediatric Considerations
Congenital defect

Pregnancy Considerations
Ultrasound is the key investigative modality for intrauterine diagnosis of this condition.

GENERAL PREVENTION

- Adequate folate intake (0.4 mg/d) by sexually active women before pregnancy and through 1st trimester
- For women with prior pregnancy of child with neural tube defect: 4 mg/d of folate before conception and through 1st trimester
- Fetal surgery places both the mother and fetus at risk for complications, including a high risk of preterm delivery. (1)
- Intrauterine repair (which remains an experimental procedure) has been shown to decrease the severity of hindbrain herniation and reduce the incidence of shunt-dependent hydrocephalus, but does not appear to improve lower extremity function. (2)
- Although intrauterine meningomyelocele repair may reduce the incidence of shunt-dependent hydrocephalus, even this group remains at significant risk of developing hydrocephalus. (3)

EPIDEMIOLOGY

- Predominant age: Congenital anomaly, apparent at birth
- Predominant sex: Male = Female

Incidence

- In whites: Neural tube defects (also referred to as spina bifida) incidence is 1:700 live births.
- In African Americans: <1:3,000

Prevalence
RISK FACTORS

- Use of valproic acid and derivatives (valproate sodium) during the 1st gestational trimester
- High-risk pregnancy: Previous children with spina bifida
- Insufficient maternal levels of folic acid
- >90% of spina bifida infants are the product of low-risk pregnancies.

Genetics

- Meningomyelocele and other neural tube defects (e.g., anencephaly, encephalocele) represent examples of multifactorial inheritance.
- Parents of an affected infant have a 1:30 chance of producing a 2nd affected child. An affected patient, if able to have children, has a 3–4% chance of having an affected child. Parents with 2 affected children run a 7–8% risk of having a 3rd child so affected. 2nd-degree relatives of an affected person (e.g., nephews, nieces) have a 1:100 risk; the risk for 1st cousins is 1:200.

PATHOPHYSIOLOGY ETIOLOGY

- Maternal folic acid deficiency is an environmental factor that is strongly associated with neural tube defects. Serum from women with pregnancy complicated by a neural tube defect contains autoantibodies that bind folate receptors and block the cellular uptake of folate. Further study is warranted to assess whether the observed association between maternal antibodies against folate receptors and neural tube defects reflects a causal relationship.
- The ultimate cause of spinal dysraphism is unclear.
- Dysraphic malformations probably occur when environmental agents affect underlying hereditary risk factors.

ASSOCIATED CONDITIONS
Infants with a so-called simple meningocele may have associated intraspinal abnormalities requiring treatment.

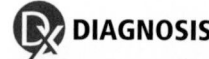 **DIAGNOSIS**

SIGNS AND SYMPTOMS
Neonate

- Meningomyelocele is usually apparent on physical examination.
- The meningomyelocele is usually single and involves the lumbosacral spine.
- Neonate
  - Neurologic examination, including pinprick examination of trunk, legs, and perineum. Functional integrity present if stimulus causes purposeful limb movements, arousal, crying, or anal wink.
- Hydrocephalus requiring cerebrospinal fluid diversion occurs in >80% of infants with the Chiari II abnormality and meningomyelocele.

TESTS
Prenatal diagnosis

- Amniocentesis: > α-fetoprotein in amniotic fluid (by 14 weeks' gestation) suggests open neural tube defects.
- Ultrasound: Hydrocephalus usually diagnosed readily. Other signs associated with Chiari II anomaly may be discernible (e.g., banana sign, callosal anomalies, megachoroid plexus).

Lab

- Prenatal: Maternal serum α-fetoprotein levels. Elevated α-fetoprotein level at 16–18 weeks suggests fetal open neural tube defects, indicating further prenatal evaluation and genetic counseling.
- Newborn: No specific lab studies are indicated.

Imaging
Neonate: Cranial ultrasound is the most efficient way to assess ventricular size promptly; may demonstrate associated anomalies (e.g., callosal agenesis)

Diagnostic Procedures/Surgery

- Direct laryngoscopy is indicated for infants with stridor, an ominous sign suggesting the need for urgent CSF diversion and/or posterior fossa decompression.
- Cranial ultrasound at birth assesses the presence and severity of hydrocephalus and the need for prompt CSF diversion.

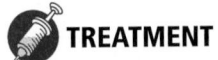 **TREATMENT**

INITIAL STABILIZATION
Inpatient

GENERAL MEASURES
- Multidisciplinary approach: Pediatric neurosurgery, orthopedics, urology, nursing, social services, pediatrics, and physical therapy
- Most patients with meningomyelocele have neurogenic bladder, necessitating intermittent catheterization to prevent severe secondary urologic disorders.

Diet
- Obesity is a major cause of morbidity in patients with meningomyelocele.
- Modified as needed to facilitate bowel and bladder training

Activity
- Determined by level of the lesion
- Optimized by physical therapists and multidisciplinary team

SURGERY
- The Chiari II malformation (i.e., hindbrain herniation into the upper cervical spinal canal) requires surgical decompression in some affected children.
  - If symptomatic, it can impair cranial nerve control of swallowing/respiration and, less frequently, cause pyramidal signs.
  - Syringomyelia, cystic expansion of the central spinal canal, is often present.
  - Surgical hindbrain decompression, if done promptly after onset of symptoms of hindbrain compression, may reverse or arrest these symptoms (e.g., stridor, respiratory difficulties, laryngomalacia), but the latter syndromes are often confused with respiratory infections, thus delaying treatment.
- Meningomyelocele repair, ideally within 24–48 hours of birth.
- CSF diversion (usually ventriculoperitoneal shunt) usually required at birth or shortly thereafter
- Orthopedic correction of extremity and spinal deformities is more elective but requires early evaluation.
- Infants with clinical evidence of hindbrain compression despite adequate CSF diversion require prompt posterior fossa decompression.
- Prenatal (fetal) surgery to close meningomyelocele defects is being tested in several institutions, but this remains an investigative procedure.
- In most authors' opinion, *neonatal* hydrocephalus associated with meningomyelocele seems more effectively addressed by CSF shunting procedures than by endoscopic 3rd ventriculostomy.

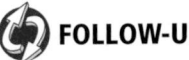 **FOLLOW-UP**

PROGNOSIS
- >80% of treated patients with open neural tube defects have normal IQ.
- Since the 1970s, management techniques have improved as a result of the creation of multidisciplinary spina bifida clinics.
- Shunt infection and malfunction are less common but remain major causes of morbidity.
- Generally, early prediction of motor and intellectual outcome in neonates with Chiari II and meningomyelocele is doubtful.
- Infants with head circumference >50 cm at birth (e.g., severe hydrocephalus) have dismal cognitive prognosis.

COMPLICATIONS
- Late neurologic deterioration due to tethering of spinal cord
- Shunt obstruction: Headache, nausea and vomiting, visual disturbances, cognitive difficulty; the latter 2 problems may be chronic, unaccompanied by headache or vomiting.
- Shunt obstruction may result in hydromyelia, which may manifest only with intrinsic muscle weakness of the hands.
- Inadequate bladder hygiene can result in hydronephrosis progressing to renal failure.
- Seizures may result from cortical migration disorders or herald shunt malfunction.
- Meningomyelocele patients are at risk for latex allergy. Take precautions in latex use.

PATIENT MONITORING
- Regular follow-up in spina bifida clinic, with multidisciplinary assessment including pediatrics, neurosurgery, orthopedics, and urology.
- Symptomatic spinal cord tethering develops in 3–15% of children with myelomingocele. (4)

REFERENCES

1. Jobe AH. Fetal surgery for myelomeningocele: Perspective. *N Engl J Med*. 2002;347:230–231.
2. Tubbs RS. Late gestational intrauterine myelomeningocele repair does not improve lower extremity function. *Pediatr Neurosurg*. 2003;38:128–132.
3. Tulipan N, et al. The effect of intrauterine myelomeningocele repair on the incidence of shunt-dependent hydrocephalus. *Pediatr Neurosurg*. 2003;38:27–33.
4. Phuong LK, Schoeberl K, Raffel C. Natural history of tethered cord in patients with meningomyelocele. *Neurosurgery*. 2002;50:989–995.
5. American Academy of Pediatrics. Folic acid for the prevention of neural tube defects. Committee on Genetics. *Pediatrics*. 1999;104:325–327.
6. Beuls E, et al. The Arnold-Chiari type II malformation at midgestation. *Pediatr Neurosurg*. 2003;39:149–158.
7. Czeizel AE, Dudas I. Prevention of the first occurrence of neural-tube defects by periconceptional vitamin supplementation.
8. McLone DG, Knepper PA. The cause of Chiari II malformation: A unified theory. *Pediatr Neurosci*. 1989;15:1–12.
9. Rothenberg SP, et al. Autoantibodies against folate receptors in women with a pregnancy complicated by a neural-tube defect. *N Engl J Med*. 2004;350:134–142.
10. van Zalen-Sprock RM, van Vugt JM, van Geijn HP. First and early second trimester diagnosis of anomalies of the central nervous system. *J Ultrasound Med*. 1995;14:603–610.

 MISCELLANEOUS

Other notes: Decisions about performing operative procedures or letting the disorder "take its natural course" in severely affected infants presents serious ethical problems; usually, the more aggressive course is best.

CODES

ICD9-CM
- 741.00 Spina bifida with hydrocephalus, unspecified region
- 741.90 Spina bifida without mention of hydrocephalus, unspecified region

PATIENT TEACHING
- Genetic counseling
- Signs and symptoms of shunt malfunction
- Bowel/bladder care
- Patient resources: Spina Bifida Association of America, 4590 MacArthur Blvd, Suite 250, Washington, DC 20007-4226; (800) 621-3141; e-mail sbaa@sbaa.org

M

MENOPAUSE

Sarah Guzofski, MD
Ruben Peralta, MD, FACS

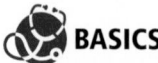

BASICS

DESCRIPTION
- Menopause is said to have occurred when 12 menstrual cycles have been missed.
- Perimenopause: Period from the onset of menstrual changes through the 1st year after menopause
  - Average length of perimenopause is 4 years.
- Postmenopause: Period after menopause, usually accounting for more than 1/3 of a woman's life
  - Premature menopause: Occurs before age 30 and may be associated with sex chromosome abnormalities

EPIDEMIOLOGY
Average age for onset of perimenopause is 47.5. Mean age for onset of menopause is between ages 51–52.

Incidence
In the US, 1.3 million women reach menopause annually.

RISK FACTORS
- Increasing age
- Oophorectomy
- Sex chromosome abnormalities (e.g., Turner syndrome)

ETIOLOGY
- Physiologic
  - As women age, the number of ovarian follicles decreases. Ovarian production of estrogen and inhibin decreases, and leuteinizing and follicle stimulating hormone production increases. Without estrogen, a failure of endometrial development occurs and menstrual cycles become irregular then cease.
- Surgical
  - Removal of functioning ovaries because of disease or incidental to hysterectomy
- Medical
  - Treatment of endometriosis
  - Treatment of breast cancer (antiestrogens). This cause is reversible.
  - May occur after cancer chemotherapy and be permanent or reversible

ASSOCIATED CONDITIONS
- Osteoporosis
- Sleep disorders

DIAGNOSIS

SIGNS AND SYMPTOMS
- Cessation of menses
  - Generally preceded by a period of irregular cycles and/or diminished bleeding
- Vasomotor symptoms
  - Hot flashes, sweating (85%)
  - Hot flashes last ~3–4 minutes, occur at unpredictable intervals
  - The frequency generally declines over the years following menopause.
- Depression (20%)
- Insomnia (40–50%)
- Urogenital atrophy
  - Dyspareunia due to atrophic vaginitis
  - Urge urinary incontinence
- Osteoporosis
- Breast tenderness
- Change in intensity and severity of migraines

TESTS
Lab
- Usually none is required because patient's age and symptoms readily establish the diagnosis. Symptoms may precede changes in laboratory parameters.
- If laboratory confirmation is desired
  - Elevated serum follicle stimulating hormone (FSH) level indicates ovarian failure (FSH >40 mIU/mL).
- Drugs that may alter lab results: Estrogens, androgens, hormonal contraceptives
- Luteinizing Hormone (LH) is not useful in diagnosing menopause

Imaging
- None for physiologic menopause
- Brain MRI if pituitary tumor suspected
- Bone density determination of hip/spine
- If history is concerning for endometrial cancer, abnormal vaginal bleeding may be evaluated by vaginal sonography or endometrial biopsy.
  - If the double-wall thickness of the endometrial stripe is <5 mm, endometrial carcinoma is unlikely.

Diagnostic Procedures/Surgery
- Pap smear
- Bimanual pelvic examination
- Endometrial biopsy and/or dilatation and curettage if diagnosis of endometrial cancer is in differential

DIFFERENTIAL DIAGNOSIS
- Pregnancy
- Polycystic ovarian disease
- Microadenoma of pituitary
- Hypothalamic dysfunction
- Asherman syndrome
- Obstruction of uterine outflow tract
- Sheehan syndrome

TREATMENT

GENERAL MEASURES
To retard development of osteoporosis:
- Weight-bearing exercise
- Avoid smoking
- Avoid excessive alcohol or caffeine intake

Diet
For protection against osteoporosis:
- Increased calcium intake (500 mg t.i.d. for those not treated with estrogen, 400 mg t.i.d. with estrogen therapy)
- Adequate vitamin D (6800 IU daily)
- Limit caffeine and alcohol intake

Activity
Active, weight-bearing exercise

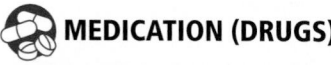

MEDICATION (DRUGS)

First Line
- Hormone replacement therapy

  - Combination estrogen-progestin therapy is effective treatment for menopausal symptoms, including insomnia, urogenital atrophy, and vasomotor symptoms. It is also useful for prevention of osteoporotic fractures and may help with mood symptoms (1)[A], (2)[B] (3)[A].
  - Patterns for prescribing hormone replacement therapy changed when the Women's Health Initiative study found those treated with combination estrogen-progestin therapy had an increased risk of invasive breast cancer, coronary heart disease, stroke, and pulmonary embolism at 5 years of use (1)[A].

  - Current recommendations for use of estrogen-progestin therapy is for the treatment of menopausal symptoms in women who do not have a history of or high risk for coronary heart disease, stroke, thromboembolism, or stroke. If these conditions are present, or if the woman is asymptomatic, alternative treatments to prevent bone loss should be considered.
  - If hormone replacement therapy is selected, estrogen should be given in combination with progestin for women with an intact uterus. Unopposed estrogen carries the risk of endometrial cancer. Most data available are for continuous treatment (as opposed to cyclical) with combined conjugated estrogen 0.625 mg and medroxyprogesterone acetate 2.5 mg.
  - Contraindications
    ○ Estrogen-dependent malignancies
    ○ Unexplained abnormal uterine bleeding
    ○ History of thromboembolism
    ○ Coronary heart disease
    ○ History of stroke
    ○ Active liver disease

– Precautions
  ○ Women on cyclic therapy may bleed normally only during those days when no therapy is given. Any other bleeding must be evaluated for the possibility of endometrial cancer.
  ○ Higher doses of estrogen can cause hypercoagulability, breast tenderness, gallbladder disease, and hypertension.
• For osteoporosis prevention in women who do not have menopausal symptoms or who elect to avoid hormone replacement
  – Bisphosphonates: Slow the rate of bone resorption and reduce risk of osteoporotic fractures
    ○ Alendronate: 10 mg/d or 70 mg every week PO
    ○ Risedronate: 5 mg/d or 30 mg every week PO
  – Raloxifene: Acts as an estrogen agonist in some tissue (including bone) and an antagonist at other tissue sites. 60 mg/d prevents bone loss and is shown to decrease vertebral fracture.
  – Calcium: 1,000–1,500 mg elemental calcium PO every day
  – Vitamin D: 800 IU PO every day
• For atrophic vaginitis
  – Topical estrogen: Conjugated estrogens (Premarin cream); best for local therapy of atrophic vaginitis only; blood levels are unpredictable; applied to vaginal mucosa

Second Line
For vasomotor symptoms, generally less effective than estrogen, but helpful when wish to avoid hormone replacement:

• Clonidine, oral or transdermal (4, 5)[B]
• Antidepressants: SSRI paroxetine and the serotonin-norepinephrine reuptake inhibitor venlafaxine ER have been shown to have some benefit in reducing vasomotor symptoms (2, 4–6)[B].
• Gabapentin (4)[B]

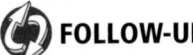 FOLLOW-UP

PROGNOSIS
• If untreated
  – Ultimate disappearance of vasomotor symptoms; usually takes several years
  – Osteoporosis: Possible fractures especially of the hip, vertebrae, and wrists.
• If treated
  – Minimal effects of estrogen deprivation
  – Slower bone loss

COMPLICATIONS
• Osteoporosis: 1–2% annual decrease in bone density (for Caucasian and Asian women). Increased risk of fracture among those not receiving estrogen replacement. Smoking cessation, physical activity, and calcium supplementation should be encouraged to decrease risk of osteoporosis.
• Arteriosclerosis
• Urge urinary incontinence

PATIENT MONITORING
• Annual Pap smear, pelvic and breast examinations
• Monthly breast self-examination
• Annual mammography
• Endometrial sampling in patients with abnormal bleeding

REFERENCES

1. Nelson HD, Humphrey LL, Nygren P. Postmenopausal hormone replacement therapy: Scientific review. *JAMA* 2002;288:872–881.(A)
2. NIH State of the Science Panel. National Institutes of Health state-of-the-science conference statement: Management of menopause-related symptoms. *Ann Intern Med* 2005;142:1003–1013.(B)
3. US Preventive Services Task Force: http://www.ahrq.gov/clinic/epcsums/menosum.pdf. (A)
4. Nelson HD, Vesco KK, Haney E. Nonhormonal therapies for menopausal hot flashes: Systematic review and meta-analysis. *JAMA* 2006;295:2057–2071.(B)
5. Stearns V, Beebe KL, Iyengar M, et al. Paroxetine controlled release in the treatment of menopausal hot flashes: A randomized controlled trial. *JAMA* 2003;289:2827–2834.(B)
6. Carroll DG. Nonhormonal therapies for hot flashes in menopause. *Am Fam Physician* 2006;73:457–464. (B)

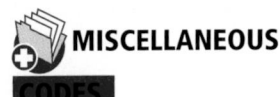 MISCELLANEOUS

CODES

ICD9-CM
• 627.0 Premenopausal menorrhagia
• 627.2 Symptomatic menopausal or female climacteric states
• 627.4 Symptomatic states associated with artificial menopause
• 716.30 Climacteric arthritis, site unspecified

PATIENT TEACHING
Educational materials are available at the American College of Obstetricians and Gynecologists, ACOG; 409 12th St. S.W., Washington, D.C. 20024; (800) 673-8444; www.acog.com.

 See Corresponding Diagnostic Algorithm

 See Patient Handout on CD

M

MENORRHAGIA

Donald A. F. Nelson, MD

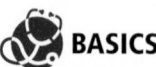 **BASICS**

DESCRIPTION

Excessive amount or duration of menstrual flow, at more or less regular intervals. Flow ≥ 80 mL per cycle, compared to normal average 30–40 mL. (1,2)

- Distinguishable from but may overlap with
  - Metrorrhagia: Irregular or frequent flow, noncyclic
  - Menometrorrhagia: Frequent, excessive, irregular flow (menorrhagia plus metrorrhagia)
  - Polymenorrhea: Frequent flow, cycles of 21 days or fewer
  - Intermenstrual bleeding: Bleeding between regular menses
  - Dysfunctional uterine bleeding (DUB): Abnormal endometrial bleeding of hormonal cause and related to anovulation
- System(s) Affected: Reproductive

ALERT

Geriatric Considerations

True menorrhagia cannot occur after menopause. However, genital atrophy as well as uterine and ovarian cancers may be associated with vaginal bleeding in the elderly.

Pediatric Considerations

Genital bleeding before puberty can result from trauma, foreign bodies, vaginal infection, or exogenous hormone administration.

Pregnancy Considerations

Bleeding in pregnancy is not menorrhagia. Complications of pregnancy or cervical/vaginal lesions should be considered.

GENERAL PREVENTION

Periodic Pap smears and pelvic examinations at appropriate intervals based on age and risk factors.

EPIDEMIOLOGY

- Predominant age
  - Menarche to menopause; ~50% of cases occur in patients >40 years of age
  - Dysfunctional bleeding is fairly common in adolescence and near menopause.
  - In adolescence, irregular bleeding owing to anovulation and immaturity of the hypothalamic-pituitary-ovarian axis is common.
- Predominant sex: Female only

Prevalence

~30% of women complain of excessive bleeding at some point. (1)

RISK FACTORS

- Obesity
- Anovulation
- Estrogen administration (± progestin)
- Prior treatment with progestational agents or oral contraceptives increases risk of endometrial atrophy, but decreases risk of endometrial hyperplasia or neoplasia.

ETIOLOGY

- Hypothyroidism
- Endometrial proliferation/excess/hyperplasia
  - Anovulation, oligoovulation
  - Ovarian tumor
  - Prolonged estrogen, progestin, or oral contraceptive administration
  - Polycystic ovarian syndrome
- Local factors
  - Endometrial atrophy, postmenopause
  - Abnormal endometrial prostaglandin levels
  - Endometrial polyps
  - Endometrial neoplasia
  - Adenomyosis/endometriosis
  - Uterine myomata (fibroids)
  - Intrauterine device (IUD)
  - Uterine sarcoma
- Coagulation disorders
  - Thrombocytopenia, platelet disorders
  - von Willebrand disease, factor deficiencies
  - Leukemia
  - Ingestion of aspirin/acetylsalicylic acid or anticoagulants
  - Renal failure/dialysis

ASSOCIATED CONDITIONS

Metrorrhagia, menometrorrhagia, androgenic disorders

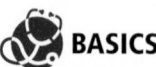 **DIAGNOSIS**

SIGNS AND SYMPTOMS

History

- Excessive menstrual flow is defined subjectively and varies greatly from woman to woman.
- Useful features
  - Bleeding substantially heavier than usual flow
  - Bleeding lasting >7 days
  - Flow associated with significant clots
  - Anemia
- Symptoms that suggest cycles are ovulatory
  - Regular menstrual interval
  - Midcycle pain (mittelschmerz)
  - Dysmenorrhea
  - Premenstrual symptoms: Breast soreness/tenderness, mood changes
- Abdominal pain or cramps at other times of the cycle may be associated with structural causes
  - Myomas
  - Polyps
  - Ovarian tumors

Physical Exam

Hirsutism, acne, obesity may accompany chronic anovulation

TESTS

- Exclude pregnancy 1st.
- Endometrial biopsy detects hyperplasia, dysplasia, or atrophy. If done before expected menses, it may also help confirm the diagnosis of anovulation or luteal phase defect.
- After age 35–40 endometrial carcinoma is significant cause of bleeding. Obtain endometrial sampling before attempting hormonal treatment. (3)[C]

Lab

- Pregnancy test
- CBC to assess severity of blood loss and to rule out thrombocytopenia and leukemia. (2)
- In selected cases
  - TSH test
  - Coagulation screen, with follow-up testing if screen is abnormal
  - Creatinine, BUN
  - Serum progesterone: 5–20 ng/mL (15.9–63.6 nmol/L) in luteal phase, <1 ng/mL (<3.18 nmol/L) in follicular phase or anovulatory cycle
- Drugs that may alter lab results
  - Progestins used before endometrial biopsy may cause decidualization and obscure correct diagnosis.

Imaging

- Transvaginal ultrasonography can help distinguish bleeding owing to atrophy from bleeding caused by hyperplasia, polyps, or myomas.
- Ultrasonography to evaluate adnexal masses or myomas suspected from pelvic exam
- CT is used in investigation of potentially malignant pelvic masses.

Diagnostic Procedures/Surgery

- Pelvic and rectal examination
- Pap smear
- Endometrial biopsy
- Diagnostic dilatation and curettage
- Hysteroscopy

Pathological Findings

Vary with etiology. In ~50% of cases, no uterine pathology is found. (1)

DIFFERENTIAL DIAGNOSIS

- Pregnancy complications
  - Threatened abortion
  - Incomplete abortion
  - Ectopic pregnancy
- Nonuterine bleeding
  - Cervical ectropion/erosion
  - Cervical neoplasia/polyp
  - Cervical or vaginal trauma/foreign body
  - Condylomata
  - Atrophic vaginitis
- Pelvic inflammatory disease (PID)
  - Endometritis
  - Tuberculosis

TREATMENT

INITIAL STABILIZATION
- Most cases can be managed as outpatient in office or emergency department.
- Inpatient care required for bleeding accompanied by orthostatic hypotension or hematocrit <25%

GENERAL MEASURES
- Rule out pregnancy complications and nonuterine bleeding.
- Treat severe or life-threatening bleeding acutely
  - IV estrogen
  - Curettage if necessary
  - Hysterectomy in extreme case
- Proceed to identify underlying cause of bleeding and treat to prevent recurrence
  - Hormonal therapy
  - Dilatation and curettage for cases that fail to respond to hormone therapy
  - Consider endometrial ablation or hysterectomy in persistent cases in which fertility is not a concern.
  - Specific treatment for neoplasia, polyps, systemic disease
  - Patients in whom fertility is a consideration may also need appropriate treatment for anovulation, endometriosis, and myomas.

Diet
Iron supplementation may help correct for increased blood loss.

Activity
As tolerated

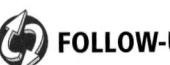 **MEDICATION (DRUGS)**

First Line
- For acute control of severe bleeding
  - Estrogen, conjugated (Premarin): 25 mg IV q4h up to 6 doses or 10–20 mg/d PO in 4 divided doses until bleeding abates. (3)[C]
- For less severe bleeding or after control of acute bleeding has been achieved
  - Medroxyprogesterone acetate (Provera): 10–30 mg/d for 5–10 days
  - Any combination oral contraceptive (i.e., usually a high-dose oral contraceptive) 1 tablet q.i.d. for 5–7 days
- To prevent heavy bleeding in subsequent cycles
  - Medroxyprogesterone acetate: 5–30 mg/d for 10 days per month
  - Usual cyclic dose of a combination oral contraceptive. (3)[C]
- Contraindications to estrogen, oral contraceptives, or progestins
  - Pregnancy
  - Breast or endometrial cancer
  - Thromboembolic disease, past or present
  - Impaired liver function
- Precautions
  - Nausea and vomiting are common from IV estrogen; antiemetics are helpful.
  - Estrogen may precipitate acute intermittent porphyria or cholestatic jaundice in susceptible patients.
- Significant possible interactions: Refer to the manufacturer's profile of each drug.

Second Line
- Nonsteroidal prostaglandin-synthetase inhibitors (e.g., naproxen, mefenamic acid, ibuprofen) can reduce blood loss ~25% with ovulatory cycles and reduce dysmenorrhea. (4)[B]

- Norethindrone acetate (Aygestin): 2.5–10 mg/d for 10–21 days per month.

- Levonorgestrel intrauterine system (Mirena) can reduce blood loss >90%. (4)[B]

- Danazol and GnRH agonists are also effective therapies, but more likely to have adverse side effects. Mifepristone (RU-486) has been used experimentally. (1)

SURGERY
- Hysterectomy when indicated to treat coexisting conditions (myomas, endometrial dysplasia) or for bleeding unresponsive to other measures. (1)

- Endometrial ablation by laser, electrosurgical, microwave, or thermal means is a conservative alternative to hysterectomy, but long-term control of bleeding and patient satisfaction are lower than with hysterectomy. (1)[A]

 FOLLOW-UP

PROGNOSIS
- Varies with cause of bleeding
- Most patients whose condition results from hormonal causes will respond to hormonal manipulation.

COMPLICATIONS
Anemia

PATIENT MONITORING
- Varies with cause of bleeding
- Medical treatment of hyperplastic/dysplastic endometrium should be followed by repeat biopsy to confirm that histologic structure has returned to normal.

REFERENCES
1. Oehler MK, Rees MCP. Menorrhagia: An update. *Acta Obstet Gynecol Scand*. 2003;82:405–422.
2. Siegel JE. Abnormalities of hemostasis and abnormal uterine bleeding.
3. Management of anovulatory bleeding. ACOG Practice Bulletin 14, March 2000.
4. Reid PC, Virtanen-Kari S. Randomised comparative trial of levonorgestrel intrauterine system and mefenamic acid for the treatment of idiopathic menorrhagia.

 MISCELLANEOUS

See also: Amenorrhea; Cervical dysplasia; Cervical malignancy; Cervical polyps; Cervicitis; Cervicitis, ectropion, and true erosion; Dysmenorrhea; Menopause; Polycystic ovarian disease; Uterine myomas

CODES

ICD9-CM
- 626.2 Excessive or frequent menstruation
- 626.3 Menorrhagia, pubertal
- 626.4 Irregular menstruation
- 626.6 Metrorrhagia
- 626.8 Menstrual disorder, NEC
- 626.9 Menstrual disorder, NOS

PATIENT TEACHING
Information about side effects of medications should be provided.

See Corresponding Diagnostic Algorithm

M

MENTAL RETARDATION

Sarah Guzofski, MD
Ruben Peralta, MD, FACS

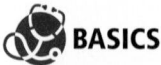 **BASICS**

DESCRIPTION
- Mental retardation (MR) is defined as an IQ <70 along with limitations in 2 or more of the following areas of adaptive functioning
  - Communication
  - Self-care
  - Home living
  - Social skills
  - Community use
  - Self-direction
  - Health and safety
- Cognitive and adaptive behavior deficits are manifested before age 18.
- Mental retardation is subdivided into the following groups
  - Mild: IQ 55–69 (85%)
  - Moderate: IQ 40–54 (10%)
  - Severe: IQ 25–39 (5%)
  - Profound: IQ 0–24 (<1%)
- Synonym(s): Mental deficiency

ALERT
Pregnancy Considerations
For some causes of mental retardation, prenatal testing is available.

GENERAL PREVENTION
- Public health efforts to reduce alcohol and drug use by pregnant women
- Increase use of prenatal folic acid supplementation

EPIDEMIOLOGY
- Predominant age: By definition, mental retardation begins in childhood.
- Predominant sex: Male > Female 2:1 for mild MR, 1.5:1 for severe MR

Incidence
In the US, 125,000 births per year by the American Association on Mental Retardation

Prevalence
- In US, 1–2.5% of the population
- 85% with MR have mild MR

RISK FACTORS
- Maternal substance use during pregnancy
- Maternal infection during pregnancy
- For some causes, family history is a risk factor.
- Mild MR is more common in children of women who did not complete high school; likely related to genetic and socioeconomic factors (e.g., undernutrition, poverty).

ETIOLOGY
- Mild MR is most likely to be associated with environmental causes, and severe MR is more likely to have a genetic or other biologic cause.
- The cause of mild MR is identified in less than half of cases. The cause of severe MR is identified in >75% of cases.
- Causes include
  - Maternal substance abuse (e.g., alcohol use/abuse). Fetal alcohol syndrome is a leading environmental cause of mental retardation.
  - Maternal infections: All TORCH viruses (e.g., toxoplasmosis, other infections, rubella, cytomegalovirus, and herpes simplex)
  - Trisomy: e.g., Down syndrome, which is trisomy 21
  - Sex chromosome abnormalities: Fragile X, Turner syndrome, Klinefelter syndrome
- Autosomal dominant conditions
  - Neurocutaneous syndromes (e.g., neurofibromatosis, tuberous sclerosis)
- Autosomal recessive conditions
  - Amino acid metabolism (e.g., phenylketonuria, maple syrup urine disease)
  - Carbohydrate metabolism (e.g., galactosemia, fructosuria)
  - Lipid metabolism
  - Tay-Sachs disease
  - Gaucher disease
  - Niemann-Pick disease (e.g., mucopolysaccharidosis)
  - Purine metabolism (e.g., Lesch-Nyhan disease)
  - Other (e.g., Wilson disease)
- Maternal use of prescription medications (e.g., Accutane, Dilantin)
- Perinatal factors
  - Prematurity
  - Birth injuries
  - Perinatal anoxia
- Postnatal factors
  - Childhood diseases (e.g., meningitis, encephalitis, hypothyroidism)
  - Trauma (e.g., accidents, physical abuse)
  - Marked deprivation
  - Poisoning (e.g., lead, carbon monoxide, household products)

ASSOCIATED CONDITIONS
- Seizures
- Slightly higher risk of mood disorders, ADHD
- Down syndrome associated with (1)[B]
  - Congenital heart defects
  - Cataracts, strabismus
  - Hypothyroidism
  - Leukemia
  - Atlanto-axial subluxation
  - Early onset Alzheimer disease

DIAGNOSIS
SIGNS AND SYMPTOMS
- Profoundly and severely retarded children frequently are diagnosed at the time of birth or during the newborn period. Children with profound or severe retardation are more likely to have dysmorphic features.
- Children with mild or moderate MR are more likely to come to clinical attention when they fail to meet motor or language milestones.
- Mild MR: May progress to 6th grade educational level, thinking tends to be concrete. Often able to maintain employment and live independently or with some supervisions.
- Moderate MR: Verbal, but with problems reading and writing (often no more than 2nd grade level). Concrete thinking often focused on own immediate needs.
- Severe MR: Limited speech, require supervision for activities of daily living.
- Profound MR: Require supervision to meet basic needs, limited vocalizations.
- With more significant degrees of MR, higher incidence of stereotypies and self-injurious behaviors.

Physical Exam
Careful examination for morphologic features suggestive of MR (for example, microcephaly) (2)[B]

TESTS
- Visual and hearing tests to rule out these etiologies as cause of impairment and because children with MR are more likely to have problems with hearing and vision
- Formal testing of intelligence and adaptive functioning; test selection depends on patient age
- Commonly used intelligence tests: Bayley Scales of Infant Development, Stanford-Binet Intelligence Scale, Weschler Intelligence Scales.
- Most common test of adaptive functioning is the Vineland Adaptive Behavior Scale, which tests communication, social skills, activities of daily living, and motor skills

Lab
- Consider karyotyping if family history of MR or multiple physical anomalies
- Fragile X screening if family history, suggestive morphologic characteristics
- If progressive neurologic changes, metabolic workup (blood lactate, serum, and urine amino acids)

Imaging
- Consider depending on clinical presentation (for example with rapid or focal neurologic changes)
- MRI may show mild cerebral abnormalities but is unlikely to establish etiology of MR (2)[B]

Diagnostic Procedures/Surgery
See "Tests."

Pathological Findings
Pathology of brains of people with MR show nonspecific changes that correlate poorly with the degree of impairment.

DIFFERENTIAL DIAGNOSIS

- Brain tumors
- Hearing and/or speech impairment
- Autism (in autism, language and social skills more affected than other cognitive abilities)
- Cerebral palsy
- Emotional disturbance
- Lack of environmental opportunities for appropriate development

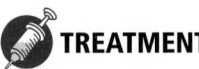 TREATMENT

- Individualized family support plan for early intervention services
- Individualized education program and, depending on level of impairment, social skills and behavioral plans
- Behavioral interventions (such as positive reinforcement for behavioral modification) to increase desirable behaviors
- Medication may be appropriate for comorbid conditions, for example anxiety, ADHD, depression
- Careful attention to changes in behavior as an indication of pain or illness

GENERAL MEASURES

Diet
No restrictions, except in case of metabolic and storage disorders (i.e., phenylketonuria).

Activity
Many adults and children with MR have poor physical fitness. Preliminary studies suggest that structured exercise programs are effective to engage this population in healthy activities (3)[A].

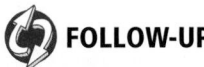 FOLLOW-UP

PROGNOSIS
Lifelong, generally not progressive

PATIENT MONITORING
Primary care with attention to associated medical conditions

REFERENCES

1. Tyler C, Edman JC. Down syndrome, Turner syndrome, and Klinefelter syndrome: Primary care throughout the lifespan. *Prim Care Clin Office Pract* 2004;31:627–648.
2. van Karnebeek CDM, Jansweijer MCE, Offringa M. Diagnostic investigations in individuals with mental retardation: A systematic literature review of their usefulness. *Eur J Human Genet.* 2005;13:6–25.
3. Heller T, Hsieh K, Rimmer JH. Attitudinal and psychological outcomes of a fitness and health education program on adults with Down syndrome. *Am J Ment Retard* 2004;109:175–185.
4. Aman MG, De Smedt GD, Derivan A. Double-blind, placebo-controlled study of risperidone for the treatment of disruptive behaviors in children with subaverage intelligence. *Am J Psychiatry* 2002;159:1337–1346.

 MISCELLANEOUS

See also: Attention deficit/hyperactivity disorder, Cerebral palsy, Down syndrome, Fragile X syndrome, Lead poisoning, Williams syndrome

CODES

ICD9-CM
- 317 Mild mental retardation
- 318.0 Moderate mental retardation
- 318.1 Severe mental retardation
- 318.2 Profound mental retardation
- 319 Unspecified mental retardation

PATIENT TEACHING

- Families should be referred to the local Association for Retarded Citizens; web site www.thearc.org.
- Additional information available from the American Association on Mental Retardation. http://www.aamr.org/

 See Corresponding Diagnostic Algorithm

M

METABOLIC SYNDROME

Simone Stromer, MD, MBBS

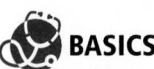

BASICS

DESCRIPTION
- A common metabolic disorder, also known as Syndrome X, resulting largely from obesity-related insulin resistance
- Involves a cluster of metabolic abnormalities
  - Abdominal obesity
  - Dyslipidaemia
  - Hypertension
  - Insulin resistance with or without impaired glucose tolerance
- The co-occurrence of these metabolic abnormalities leads to an increased risk of type 2 diabetes mellitus and cardiovascular disease.

GENERAL PREVENTION
- Effective weight loss and maintenance of normal body weight
- Regular and sustained physical activity

EPIDEMIOLOGY
- Predominant age: >60 years old
- Predominant sex: Male = Female

Prevalence
- Affects 25% of US adults
- Data vary among populations because there is no standardized international definition for the metabolic syndrome.

ALERT
Pediatric Considerations
Obese children and adolescents are at high risk of the metabolic syndrome, and the risk increases with the severity of the obesity.

RISK FACTORS
- Older age
- Ethnicity
- Family history
- Central obesity

Genetics
Genetic factors may account for up to 50% of syndrome traits.

PATHOPHYSIOLOGY
Insulin resistance and an excess of adipose tissue underpin pathogenesis.

ETIOLOGY
The main etiological factors are
- Obesity (particularly abdominal) and excess adipose tissue
- Insulin resistance
- Other contributing factors
  - Advancing age
  - Proinflammatory state
  - Genetics
  - Endocrine, e.g., postmenopausal state

ASSOCIATED CONDITIONS
- Polycystic ovary syndrome
- Fatty liver (nonalcoholic steatohepatitis)
- Chronic renal disease
- Obstructive sleep apnea
- Gallstones (cholesterol)

DIAGNOSIS

Based on the National Cholesterol Education Program's Adult Treatment Panel III (ATP III) report, a diagnosis of metabolic syndrome can be made when 3 or more of the following 5 characteristics are present (1)[C]

- Abdominal obesity: Men >102 cm, Women >88 cm (different waist circumference criteria are used for non-Europeans)
- Blood pressure ≥130/85 mm Hg
- Triglycerides ≥150 mg/dL
- HDL: Men <40 mg/dL, Women <50 mg/dL
- Fasting glucose ≥100 mg/dL

SIGNS AND SYMPTOMS
- Obesity: Fatigue, poor exercise tolerance, aches and pains
- Dyslipidaemia: Xanthomata, xanthelasma, etc.
- Hypertension: Symptoms of cardiac failure, headaches, dizziness, vertigo, etc.
- Insulin resistance: Difficulty losing weight, infertility in women, etc.
- Type 2 diabetes mellitus: Polyuria, polydypsia
- Cardiovascular disease: Angina

History
- Family history of metabolic syndrome
- Comprehensive lifestyle history
  - Diet including intake of saturated fats
  - Exercise regimen
  - Alcohol intake
  - Cigarette smoking

Physical Exam
See ATP III diagnostic criteria above.

TESTS
Laboratory tests are required for diagnosis as per ATP III diagnostic criteria.

Lab
- Fasting lipids (particularly triglycerides and HDL)
- Fasting glucose

Imaging
None necessary to diagnose metabolic syndrome

Diagnostic Procedures/Surgery
- May require 24-hour blood pressure monitoring (rules out white coat hypertension)
- ECG, stress test, coronary angiography may be used for diagnosis of cardiovascular disease arising as a complication of the syndrome

Pathological Findings
- Microalbuminuria
- Increased white blood cell count
- Increased C-reactive protein
- Increased fibrinogen
- Increased pro-inflammatory cytokines, e. g., tumor necrosis factor alpha
- Increased uric acid
- Increased homocysteine
- Type 2 diabetes
- Fatty liver (complicated by end-stage liver disease and hepatocellular carcinoma)
- Hypertensive and/or diabetic eye disease
- Renal impairment/failure
- Peripheral vascular disease
- Coronary artery disease
- Cerebrovascular disease

DIFFERENTIAL DIAGNOSIS
Diagnosis is dependent on fulfilling the ATP III diagnostic criteria.

TREATMENT

PRE HOSPITAL
- Reduce weight.
- Treat dyslipidemia.
- Treat hypertension.
- Reduce risk of progression to diabetes from insulin resistance/impaired fasting glucose (IFG)/impaired glucose tolerance (IGT).
- Treat prothrombotic state.

INITIAL STABILIZATION
Involves management of complications such as acute coronary syndrome

GENERAL MEASURES
- Avoid or stop smoking.
- Avoid excess alcohol intake.

Diet
- Weight reduction to correct abdominal obesity is a primary goal.
- Can be achieved by reduction of energy intake and increased physical activity (2)[C]
- Reduction by 500 calories/day will usually achieve a weight loss of 0.5 kg/wk.
- A Mediterranean diet and 1 that is low in glycemic index is beneficial.
- Other beneficial dietary principles are
  - Low intake of saturated fats, trans fats, and cholesterol (3)[A]
  - High intake of fruit, vegetables, fiber, and whole grains
  - 2–3 fish meals per week to lower cholesterol
  - Low salt intake

Activity
- Regular exercise will improve all components of the metabolic syndrome.
- 30 minutes of moderate-intensity exercise daily is recommended as a minimum.
- Encourage changing of sedentary activity choices (e.g., driving car, taking elevator, etc.) to more active ones (e.g., walking, cycling, etc.).

Nursing
Education about and encouragement to comply with recommended diet and physical activity regimens

SPECIAL THERAPY
- Dietitian
- Exercise physiologist
- Endocrinologist
- Counseling programs for smoking cessation

Complementary and Alternative Therapies
Fish oils and plant sterol esters can be used to lower cholesterol levels.

 MEDICATION (DRUGS)

- Daily treatment with aspirin is recommended for patients with cardiovascular disease.
- Medication may be required for the treatment of obesity, dyslipidamia, hypertension, and/or IGT.

First Line
- Obesity: It should be emphasized that lifestyle changes are the cornerstone of treatment.
- Orlistat: 120 mg t.i.d. with meals (4A)
- Dyslipidaemia: Drug therapy can be commenced after 6 weeks of lifestyle modification therapy.
  - Statin if predominantly high LDL, e.g., atorvastatin 10 mg/d
  - Fibrate if predominantly high triglycerides, e.g., gemfibrozil 600 mg b.i.d.
- Hypertension
  - Angiotensin-converting enzyme (ACE) inhibitor, e.g., ramipril 10 mg/d (decreases progression to type II diabetes mellitus in both normotensive and hypertensive patients)
- Impaired glucose tolerance
  - It must be emphasized that current guidelines state that treatment should be with diet and exercise as described earlier in this chapter.
  - Metformin 500 mg–1 g 1–3 times daily in combination with the above, may be considered.

Second Line
- Obesity: Sibutramine 10–15 mg/d
- Dyslipidaemia
  - Cholestyramine 12–16 g/d in 2–3 divided doses if predominantly high LDL
  - Fish oils alone or in combination with fibrate if predominantly high triglycerides
- Hypertension: Angiotensin II receptor blocker, e.g., losartan 50 mg/d if intolerant of ACE I inhibitor

SURGERY
Bariatric surgery to treat obesity

 FOLLOW-UP

Referral to an endocrinologist and/or cardiologist may be required.

DISPOSITION
Management of the metabolic syndrome does not usually require hospital admission.

Admission and Discharge Criteria
- Serious complications, e.g., acute coronary syndrome, hypertensive crisis, diabetic coma, etc.
- Indications for discharge of patients with complications of metabolic syndrome are beyond the scope of this chapter.

Issues for Referral
Complications require frequent and close follow-up.

PROGNOSIS
- Increased risk of both type 2 diabetes mellitus and cardiovascular disease
- The degree to which the syndrome can predict future risk of all-cause mortality, cardiovascular disease, and diabetes is not known.

COMPLICATIONS
Long-term complications described previously in this chapter

PATIENT MONITORING
- Regular monitoring of weight and abdominal circumference measurements, BP, fasting lipids, and sugar.
- Lipids can be reviewed weekly during initial treatment phase.
- Fasting sugar should be checked at least yearly in those whose levels are normal.

REFERENCES
1. Adult Treatment Panel III. Third report of the National Cholesterol Education Program (NCEP) expert panel on detection, evaluation, and treatment of high blood cholesterol in adults. Final Report. *Circulation*. 2002;106:3143–3421.
2. National Institutes of Health. Clinical Guidelines on the Identification, Evaluation, and Treatment of Overweight and Obesity in Adults—The Evidence Report. *Obes Res*. 1998;6(suppl 2):51S–209S.
3. Hooper L, et al. Dietary fat intake and prevention of cardiovascular disease: Systematic review. *BMJ*. 2001;322:757–763.
4. O'Meara S, et al. A systematic review of the clinical effectiveness of orlistat used for the management of obesity. *Obes Rev*. 2004;5:51–68.

 MISCELLANEOUS

See also: Diabetes mellitus, Type 2; Obesity; Hypertension; Polycystic ovarian disease

CODES

ICD9-CM
277.7 Metabolic Syndrome

PATIENT TEACHING
Education on diet and physical activity

Prevention
Maintenance of normal body weight

 See Corresponding Diagnostic Algorithm

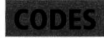 **See Patient Handout on CD**

M

METATARSALGIA

Daniel Casto, MD

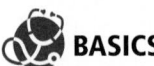

BASICS

DESCRIPTION
General term for pain of the plantar surface of the forefoot in the metatarsal head region
- System(s) Affected: Musculoskeletal

ALERT

Geriatric Considerations
- Arthritis should be ruled out early.
- More frequent in older athletes
- Symptoms are more pronounced in older people.

Pediatric Considerations
- Muscle imbalance disorders (e.g., Duchenne muscular dystrophy) are a cause of foot deformities in children.
- In adolescent girls, consider Freiberg infraction (i.e., aseptic necrosis of the metatarsal head usually in adolescents who jump or sprint).

Pregnancy Considerations
- Forefoot pain during pregnancy usually results from change in gait, increased weight, and joint laxity.
- Properly fitted low-heeled shoes are especially important in this group of patients.

GENERAL PREVENTION
- Wear properly fitted shoes with good padding.
- Start weight-bearing exercise programs gradually.

EPIDEMIOLOGY
Predominant sex: Female > Male

Incidence
Common especially in athletes with high impact sports (running, jumping, etc).

Prevalence
Common

RISK FACTORS
- Obesity
- High heels or narrow shoes
- Competitive athletes for weight-bearing sports (e.g., ballet, basketball, running)
- Foot deformities (e.g., pes planus, pes cavus, tight Achilles, tarsal tunnel syndrome)

ETIOLOGY
- Abnormal pressure distribution plantar to the metatarsal heads
- General
  - Excessive or repetitive stress: Wearers of high heels, ballet dancers, competitive athletes
  - Soft tissue dysfunction: Intrinsic muscle weakness, laxity in the Lisfranc ligament
  - Abnormal foot posture: Forefoot varus or valgus, cavus or equinus deformities, loss of the metatarsal arch, splay foot, pronated foot
  - Dermatologic: Warts, calluses
- Great toe
  - Hallux valgus (bunion), either varus or rigidus
- Lesser metatarsals
  - Freiberg infraction (i.e., aseptic necrosis of the metatarsal head usually seen in adolescents who jump or sprint)
  - Hammertoe or claw toe
  - Morton syndrome (i.e., long second metatarsal)

ASSOCIATED CONDITIONS
See "Etiology".

DIAGNOSIS

SIGNS AND SYMPTOMS
- Acute, chronic, or recurrent symptoms located in the region of the metatarsal heads usually on the plantar surface
- Pain: Often described as seeming like walking with a pebble in the shoe
- Swelling
- Tenderness of the metatarsal head(s) with pressure applied between the examiner and finger
- Calluses
- Erythema (occasionally)

History
Gradual chronic onset is more common than acute presentation.

Physical Exam
- Point tenderness over metatarsal heads
- Pain in the interdigital space or a positive metatarsal squeeze test suggests Morton neuroma.

TESTS

Lab
Only if diagnosis is in question: Erythrocyte sedimentation rate, rheumatoid factor, HLA antigen, venereal disease research laboratories test, uric acid, glucose, complete blood chemistry with differential
- Disorders that may alter lab results: Acute infections

Imaging
- Weight-bearing radiographs: Anteroposterior, lateral, and oblique views. Occasionally metatarsal or sesamoid axial films (to rule out sesamoid fracture) or skyline view of the metatarsal heads: Obtained with the metatarsophalangeal joints in dorsiflexion (to evaluate alignment)
- Increasing use of sonograpy and MRI, but still no benefit over clinical assessment.
- Bone scan if high index of suspicion of stress fracture exists

Pathological Findings
Because of its 2 sesamoid bones, the 1st metatarsal head usually carries about 30% of the weight when walking. A normal metatarsal arch also ensures this balance. The 1st metatarsal head has adequate padding to accommodate it. A pronated splayfoot disturbs this balance, causing equal weight bearing on all metatarsal heads. Any foot deformity also changes distribution of weight to areas of the foot that do not have sufficient padding.

DIFFERENTIAL DIAGNOSIS
- Stress fracture (most commonly 2nd metatarsal)
- Morton neuroma (i.e., interdigital neuroma)
- Sesamoiditis or sesamoid fracture
- Arthritis (e.g., gouty, rheumatoid, inflammatory, osteoarthritis, septic)
- Infection (e.g., cellulitis, diabetic foot, Lyme disease, leprosy)
- Bone tumors (rare)
- Ganglion cyst
- Foreign body
- Vasculitis (diabetes)

TREATMENT

INITIAL STABILIZATION
Outpatient

GENERAL MEASURES
- Relieve pain.
  - Rest: Temporary alteration of weight-bearing activity; use of cane or crutch. For more physically active patients, suggest an alternative exercise or cross-training.
  - Ice initially
  - Moist heat later
  - Taping or Gelcast
  - Stiff-soled shoes will act as a splint.
- Relieve the pressure beneath the area of maximal pain with
  - Weight loss
  - Low-heeled wide-toe-box shoes
  - Metatarsal pads and arch supports
  - Orthotics/rockerbar
  - Thick-soled shoes
- Improve flexibility and strength of the muscles of the foot with
  - Exercises (e.g., towel grasps, pencil curls)
  - Physical therapy to maintain ROM.

Activity
- Alteration of weight-bearing exercises may be temporarily necessary.
- Use cross-training principles (i.e., bicycle or swimming instead of running for the acute phase).
- Gradual return to previous level of activities with arch support in running shoes

Complementary and Alternative Medicine
Magnetic insoles are not beneficial.

MEDICATION (DRUGS)

First Line
- NSAIDs (ibuprofen 800 mg t.i.d. 7–14 days or naproxen 500 b.i.d. 7–14 days)
- Contraindications: Gastrointestinal bleeding or ulcer
- Precautions in patients with
  – Renal disease
  – Hepatic disease
  – Coagulation disorders
- Significant possible interactions
  – Anticoagulants
  – Digoxin
  – Lithium
  – Methotrexate
  – Cyclosporin

Second Line
COX 2 inhibitors

SURGERY
- If no improvement with conservative therapy for 3 months, referral to foot/ankle ortho or surgical podiatrist may be necessary.
- If a correctable anatomic abnormality exists: Bunionectomy, partial ostectomy, osteotomy, or surgical fusion. Success rates vary depending on procedure.

 FOLLOW-UP

DISPOSITION
Issues for Referral
Athletes may warrant early podiatric evaluation.

PROGNOSIS
Outcome depends on the severity of the problem and whether surgery is required to correct it.

COMPLICATIONS
Back, knee, and hip pain owing to change in gait

PATIENT MONITORING
Follow-up visit at 2 weeks if condition not improved or has worsened. If stress fracture has been ruled out and patient's condition has not improved >3 months of conservative treatment, consider surgical evaluation.

REFERENCES

1. Winemiller MH, et al. Effect of magnetic vs sham-magnetic insoles on nonspecific foot pain in the workplace: A randomized, double-blind, placebo-controlled trial. *Mayo Clin Proc*. 2005; 80(9):1138–1145.
2. Thomson CE, Gibson JN, Martin D. Interventions for the treatment of Morton's neuroma. *Cochrane Database Systematic Review*. 2004;(3):CD003118.
3. Sharp RJ, et al. The role of MRI and ultrasound imaging in Morton's neuroma and the effect of size of lesion on symptoms. *J Bone Joint Surg*. 2003; 85(7):999–1005.
4. Iagnocco A, et al. Sonograpy in the study of metatarsalgia. *J Rheumatol*. 2001;28(6): 1338–1340.
5. Wu K. Morton neuroma and metatarsalgia. *Curr Opin Rheumatol*. 2000;12:131–142.

ADDITIONAL READING

- Birrer R. *Common Foot Problems in Primary Care*. 2nd ed. Philadelphia, PA: Hanley & Belfus; 1998:67–73.
- van Wyngarden TM. The painful foot. Part I: Common forefoot deformities. *Am Fam Physician*. 1997;55:1866–1876.
- Merril DPM. *Medical and Surgical Therapeutics of the Foot and Ankle. Part 4: Metatarsalgia*. Baltimore, MD: Williams & Wilkins; 1992:384–390.
- Cailliet R. *Foot and Ankle Pain*. 3rd ed. Philadelphia, PA: FA Davis; 1997:141–147.

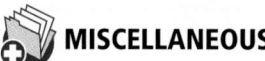 **MISCELLANEOUS**

See also: Morton neuroma (interdigital neuroma)

 CODES

ICD9-CM
726.70 Enthesopathy of ankle and tarsus, unspecified

PATIENT TEACHING

Instruct about wearing proper sort of shoes and gradual return to activity.

M

METHANOL POISONING

Ruben Peralta, MD, FACS

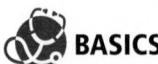 BASICS

DESCRIPTION
- Methanol is a clear, colorless solvent found in many commercial and industrial fluids (e.g., antifreeze, cleaning solutions, gasoline additives, paint, paint thinner, liquid fuel) (1)[C].
- Methanol ingestion most commonly occurs in those with alcohol dependence; methanol is less expensive than ethanol and may be more readily obtained in restricted environments (i.e., prison).
- Less commonly, intoxication is secondary to methanol-contaminated grain alcohol, accidental ingestion, or suicide attempt.

ALERT
Pregnancy Considerations
Avoid ethanol therapy as treatment for methanol poisoning during first trimester of pregnancy. May substitute fomepizole, which is a Category C drug.

GENERAL PREVENTION
Proper storage of methanol-containing products

EPIDEMIOLOGY
- Predominant age: Usually >18 years
- Predominant sex: Male > Female

Prevalence
In the US, 2,418 methanol exposures were reported in 2000 (2)[C].

RISK FACTORS
- Alcoholism
- Epidemics may occur in institutionalized settings where ethyl alcohol is unavailable (i.e., prisons).

ETIOLOGY
- Fatal dose is 15–240 mL, depending on concentration.
- Peak blood levels occur 30– 60 minutes after ingestion (1)[C].
- Methanol itself is minimally toxic, but it is hepatically metabolized, 1st (by alcohol dehydrogenase) to formaldehyde, which is then very rapidly oxidized to formic acid (by formaldehyde dehydrogenase). Formic acid is the metabolite responsible for toxicity. It can be metabolized to carbon dioxide and water in the presence of tetrahydrofolate (1)[C].
- Acidosis due to methanol poisoning is likely due to formic acid, as well as the systemic effects of toxicity, which cause accumulation of lactic acid (1)[C].

ASSOCIATED CONDITIONS
Alcoholism

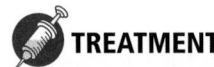 DIAGNOSIS

SIGNS AND SYMPTOMS
- Latent period after ingestion of between 12–24 hours before onset of symptoms
- Initial CNS depression or inebriation, depending on coingestion of ethyl alcohol. Coingestion of ethyl alcohol may delay onset of symptoms by up to 24 hours (1)[C].
- Visual disturbance, ranging from mild blurring to complete blindness
- Other CNS symptoms include headache, vertigo, lethargy, confusion. Severely intoxicated patients can present with coma and convulsions.
- Gastrointestinal symptoms may include nausea, vomiting, and marked abdominal pain.
- Dyspnea

Physical Exam
Funduscopic exam reveals retinal edema, hyperemia, or loss of physiologic disc cupping. Other ocular findings include visual field defects and loss of pupillary reactions.

TESTS
Lab
- Serum methanol and ethanol concentrations
- Electrolytes, calcium, BUN, creatinine, serum osmolarity
- Liver function tests,
- Amylase
- Creatinine kinase
- Urinalysis
- Arterial blood gas
- Toxicologic screens if coingestants are suspected (e.g., aspirin, acetaminophen in suicide attempt, drugs of abuse)
- Anion-gap metabolic acidosis
- In cases of acute intoxication, serum methanol concentrations >20 mg/dL are associated with CNS effects; >100 mg/dL are associated with visual defects; >200 mg/dL are associated with death in untreated patients.
- Serum methanol concentrations are less useful for treatment or prognosis decisions after the latency period because toxicity is determined by serum formic acid concentration, which cannot be inferred from methanol concentration once metabolism is underway.

Imaging
CT or MRI scan of the brain if indicated by results of neurologic exam. Brain imaging may reveal hypodensities in the putamen or caudate nucleus, cerebral edema, or cerebral hemorrhage (1)[C].

DIFFERENTIAL DIAGNOSIS
- Ingestion of other alcohols, including ethyl alcohol, benzyl alcohol, or isopropyl alcohol
- Other toxic ingestions, including ethylene glycol, paraldehyde, and formaldehyde
- Increased anion-gap metabolic acidosis caused by renal failure, diabetic ketoacidosis, and lactic acidosis

TREATMENT

INITIAL STABILIZATION
Standard emergency management of airway, breathing, and circulation

GENERAL MEASURES
- Management priorities depend on the timing of presentation in relationship to ingestion or exposure.
- Determine amount ingested and inhibit methanol metabolism in any case when ingestion suspected. Initial management is directed toward preventing metabolic acidosis and ophthalmologic complications.
- Obtain IV access and administer isotonic fluids to maintain adequate urine output.
- Gastric decontamination with induced emesis, charcoal, or gastric lavage is *not* indicated unless a concomitant ingestion is known (1)[C].
- 2 methods for inhibiting methanol metabolism: Ethanol and fomepizole
  – Ethanol has a higher affinity for alcohol dehydrogenase than methanol, so it competitively inhibits its metabolism to toxic metabolites.
  – Fomepizole also inhibits alcohol dehydrogenase.
- Sodium bicarbonate should be administered if serum pH <7.2 to maintain pH >7.3.
- Folinic acid (leucovorin) or folic acid may be administered.
- Consider urgent hemodialysis when significant acidosis (pH <7.2) unresponsive to therapy, deteriorating vital signs despite intensive support, renal failure, electrolyte imbalance, or serum methanol concentration >50 mg/dL.

Diet
No special diet; thiamine supplementation in patients with long-term alcoholism

Activity
Restricted if patient is inebriated, has altered level of consciousness, or visual impairments

SPECIAL THERAPY
IV Fluids
Isotonic IV fluid to maintain urine output

MEDICATION (DRUGS)

- Ethanol: Dose based on protocol with IV loading dose, then maintenance dosing based on hourly serum ethanol levels. Target therapeutic ethanol level is 100–150 mg/dL. Treat until serum methanol <20 mg/dL (1)[C]. Side effects include phlebitis and volume overload (3)[C].
- Fomepizole: IV loading dose, then dosed q12h until serum methanol <20 mg/dL (1)[C]. Induces P450 enzymes, so protocol includes higher doses as treatment progresses (4)[C].
- Folinic acid (leucovorin) or folate: May enhance formic acid metabolism
- Avoid ethanol therapy with CNS depressants

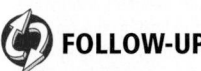 ## FOLLOW-UP

DISPOSITION

Issues for Referral

- For patients with substance abuse, referral to detox, rehabilitation, and/or AA/NA
- Ophthalmology follow-up for patients with visual disturbances

PROGNOSIS

- Outcome varies depending on time to presentation and quantity of methanol ingested.
- Outcome is related to degree of acidosis, coma, or seizures at time of presentation. Diagnostic and treatment delays are correlated with poor outcome (5)[C]

COMPLICATIONS

- Blindness and other visual disturbances
- Myoglobinuric renal failure
- Pancreatitis
- Parkinsonian syndrome

REFERENCES

1. Barceloux DG. American Academy of Clinical Toxicology practice guidelines on the treatment of methanol poisoning. *Clin Toxicol* 2002;40: 415–446.
2. Litovitz TL, Klein-Schwartz W, White S, et al. Annual report of the American Association of Poison Control Centers Toxic Exposure Surveillance System. *Am J Emerg Med* 2001;19:337–395.
3. Chu J, RY Wang, NS Hill. Update in clinical toxicology. *AM J Respir Care Med* 166:9–15.
4. Megarbane B, SW Borron, FJ Baud. Current recommendations for treatment of severe toxic alcohol poisonings. *Intensive Care Med* 2005;31: 189–195.
5. Hovda KE, OH Hunderi, O Dunlop. Methanol outbreak in Norway 2002–2004. *J Int Med* 2003;258:181–190.

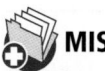 ## MISCELLANEOUS

CODES

ICD9-CM

- 980.1 Methanol poisoning
- E860.2 Accidental methanol poisoning
- E950.9 Suicide attempt by solid or liquid substances
- E980.9 Poisoning by solid or liquid substances, undetermined whether accidentally or purposefully inflicted

PATIENT TEACHING

- Anticipatory guidance for parents regarding storage of hazardous chemicals
- Motivational interviewing for those with substance dependence and referral for additional treatment
- American Academy of Clinical Toxicology www.clintox.org

 See Corresponding Diagnostic Algorithm

M

MIGRAINE

Roger K. Cady, MD

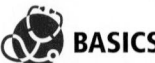

BASICS

DESCRIPTION
Recurrent paroxysms of headache capable of altering daily function that last from 4–72 hours. Exists in both episodic and chronic form: Episodic: <15 days of migraine/month, return to normal neurological function between attacks; Chronic >15 days of migraine per month for >6 months. (1)[C] Preheadache symptoms are nonspecific, may occur hours to days before headache. Most frequent subtypes are as follows

- Without aura: Common migraine defining >80% of attacks
- With aura: Classic migraine characterized by focal disruption of neurologic function begining and ending prior to headache onset
- Variants of migraine include
  - Transformed migraine: Chronic headache pattern evolving from episodic migraine. Migraine-like attacks are superimposed on a daily or near-daily headache pattern (e.g., tension headache).
  - Basilar migraine: Occipital headache, with aura symptoms of dysarthria, vertigo, tinnitus, ataxia, and bilateral paresis or bilateral paresthesias
  - Hemiplegic migraine: Aura consisting of hemiplegia and/or hemiparesis
  - Ophthalmoplegic: Palsy of the ipsilateral 3rd cranial nerve during the headache phase. May be cranial neuralgia rather than migraine.
  - Retinal: Symptoms of retinal vascular involvement during headache
  - Childhood periodic syndromes (migraine equivalents): Recurrent often cyclic episodes of symptoms
  - Status migrainosus: Persistent migraine that does not resolve spontaneously
  - Migrainous stroke: Persistent or permanent neurologic deficits persisting beyond migraine attack usually with neuroimaging changes
- System(s) Affected: Gastrointestinal; Musculoskeletal; Nervous

ALERT
Geriatric Considerations
- Rare onset of noncephalalgic migraine (aura without subsequent headache) >40 years of age. Possible relationship to transient global amnesia.
- Late onset of migraine requires diagnostic evaluation.

Pediatric Considerations
- Recurrent abdominal pain and cyclic vomiting may predominate; attacks may be of shorter duration.
- Headache description by younger children may appear atypical and shorter in duration.

Pregnancy Considerations
- May decrease in 2nd and 3rd trimesters.
- No treatment drug has US Food and Drug Administration approval during pregnancy.
  - Ergotamines are contraindicated.
  - Early data for sumatriptan suggest no increase in birth defect to date. (2)[B]
  - Sumatriptan and zolmitriptan recommended "pump and dump" of milk (3)[B]

GENERAL PREVENTION
- Avoid precipitants of attacks.
- Biofeedback and psychological intervention
- Prophylactic therapy
  - If attacks interfere with lifestyle or are not controlled by acute interventions, prophylactic therapy may be appropriate.
- Regularly scheduled follow-up is mandatory.

EPIDEMIOLOGY
Predominant sex
- Male ≥ Female in childhood
- Female > Male (3:1) menarche to adult
- Female > Male (2:1) postmenopausal women

Prevalence
- Adults: Women, 18%; Men, 6%
- Childhood: Unknown

RISK FACTORS
- Foods, alcohol, missing meals, menstrual cycle, excessive sleep, fatigue, emotional stress, let down (relief of stress)
- Medications
  - Cyclic estrogen replacement
  - Birth control pills
  - Vasodilators
- Family history of migraine
- Female gender
- Young age
- History of childhood cyclic vomiting, cyclic abdominal pain, motion sickness

Genetics
- >80% of patients have positive family history.
- Chromosomal abnormality confirmed in familial hemiplegic migraine

ETIOLOGY
Etiology unknown; may be a genetically-linked, neuronal disease; serotonin, dopamine, glutamate, and norepinephrine may have role

ASSOCIATED CONDITIONS
- Depression
- Panic disorder
- Sleep disturbance
- Cerebral vascular disease
- Myocardial disease
- Peripheral vascular disease
- Seizure
- Irritable bowel syndrome

DIAGNOSIS

SIGNS AND SYMPTOMS
There are 5 phases of a migraine. Symptoms vary from patient to patient or from attack to attack within the same individual.
- Premonitory symptoms (50–80% of patients)
  - A variety of "warnings" precede migraine, frequently characterized by mood disruptions (e.g., euphoria, irritability, depression), fatigue, muscle tension, food craving, bloating, yawning, or subtle disruption of sensory processing.
- Aura
  - Visual disruptions are most common, including scotoma, hemianopsia, fortification spectra, geometric visual patterns, and occasionally hallucinations.
  - Somatosensory disruption in face or arms
  - Headache typically begins within 1 hour of aura.
- Headache
  - Headache usually begins with mild pain that escalates into a unilateral (30–40% bilateral), throbbing (40% nonthrobbing) pain of 4–72 hours duration.
  - Intensified by movement and associated with systemic manifestations: Nausea (87%), vomiting (56%), diarrhea (16%), photophobia (82%), phonophobia (78%), muscle tenderness (65%), lightheadedness (72%), vertigo (33%)
- Headache termination
  - Untreated, usually occurs with sleep
  - Occasionally, vomiting or strong emotional experiences abort headache.
- Postdrome
  - Headache pain resolved but other manifestations linger on, such as food intolerance, impaired concentration, fatigue, muscle soreness

TESTS
To rule out underlying pathology
Lab
To rule out secondary causes of headache

Imaging
Required (CT or MRI equally effective)
- New-onset in patient >50 years of age
- Change in established headache pattern
- Atypical pattern or symptoms
- Prolonged or bizarre aura
- Progressive headache
- Unremitting/progressive neurological symptoms

Diagnostic Procedures/Surgery
Based on careful history and physical findings

Pathological Findings
- Changes in blood serotonin levels and serotonin metabolites in the urine
- Changes in regional blood flow
- Changes visible in sophisticated imaging studies

DIFFERENTIAL DIAGNOSIS
- Other primary headache disorders
- Secondary headaches, such as tumor, infection, vascular pathology, or prescription or illicit drug (e.g., cocaine) use
- Drug-seeking patients
- Psychiatric disease
- Rarely, atypical forms of epilepsy

TREATMENT

GENERAL MEASURES
- Cold compresses to area of pain
- Rest with pillows comfortably supporting head or neck in area devoid of sensory stimulation, including light, sound, and odors.
- Withdrawal from stressful surroundings
- Sleep is desirable.
- Most patients manage attacks with self-care.

Diet
- Maintain fluid intake.
- Avoid dietary precipitants of migraine.

Activity
In bed in a dark quiet environment

Complementary and Alternative Medicine
- Riboflavin 400 mg/d possibly effective as preventative agent
- Feverfew is no more effective than placebo for the prevention of migraines (7)

MEDICATION (DRUGS)

First Line
- Combination drugs
- Combination of acetaminophen, aspirin, and caffeine (Excedrin, others); as effective as other agents with fewer adverse events
  - Isometheptene-dichloralphenazone-acetaminophen (Midrin): 2 at onset then 1 per hour if needed; maximum, 5 in 12 hours
- 5-HT-1 agonists (triptans) intervention during the mild phase of headache, but many adverse events and contraindications (4)[A]
- 5-HT-1 agonists recommended if combinations fail for migraine. (5)[A]
  - Oral tablets more effective in early mild headache phase.
  - Sumatriptan (Imitrex), 6 mg self-administered injection with efficacy of 70–85%. If initial injection fails to relieve migraine after 1 hour, do not repeat injection. 20-mg, or 25-mg, 50-mg, and 100-mg tablets with efficacy of 65%. If headache returns, may repeat, nasal spray, or oral tablets.
  - Zolmitriptan (Zomig, Zomig-ZMT): 2.5 mg tablet at onset of migraine; 5 mg tablet available; efficacy ~65%
  - Naratriptan (Amerge): 2.5 mg initially; 1 mg tablet available, both oral; slower to act than other triptans, but fewer adverse effects
  - Rizatriptan (Maxalt) tablet and orally disintegrating tablet: Initial dose 10 mg. Efficacy similar to other triptans
  - Almotriptan: Oral tablets (6.25 or 12.5 mg); efficacy similar to other triptans
  - Frovatriptan (Frova): 2.5 mg at onset; up to 3 oral doses in 24-hour period
  - Eletriptan (Relpax): Oral tablets (20 mg and 40 mg); similar efficacy to other triptans
  - Avoid eletriptan within 72 hours of ketoconazole, itraconazole, nefazodone, troleandomycin, or clarithromycin.

- Ergotamines
  - Dihydroergotamine (DHE): Drug of choice in status migrainosus
  - Most effective ergotamine; available as IV, IM, or SC injection. Also available as nasal spray (Migranal).
  - Dose: 0.5–1 mg with up to 3 mg IM or 2 mg IV in 24 hours
  - Maximum weekly doses of 4–6 mg
  - Use antiemetic, such as metoclopramide or prochlorperazine 5–10 mg IM or IV prior to DHE administration.
  - Dihydroergotamine (Migranal) nasal spray 2 mg intranasal (0.5 mg in each nostril repeated in 15 minutes)
  - Ergotamine tartrate
  - Oral preparations contain 1 mg of ergotamine and 100 mg of caffeine. 2 tablets at onset of symptoms. Repeat after 30 minutes up to maximum dose of 6 mg every day. Avoid chronic daily or near-daily use.
- Nonsteroidal anti-inflammatories (NSAIDs): No clear superiority in efficacy established for any particular agent; early administration improves efficacy.
- Contraindications
  - Avoid 5-HT-1 agonists (triptans) in coronary heart disease, peripheral vascular disease, uncontrolled hypertension, and complex migraine, such as basilar or hemiplegic migraine.
  - 5-HT-1 agonists (triptans) should not be used within 24 hours of an ergot derivative or other 5-HT-1 agonists.
  - Selective 5-HT-1 agonists (triptans) are pregnancy category C. Ergotamines are pregnancy category X.
  - Avoid NSAIDs if danger of gastric erosion or renal or hepatic disease.
  - Avoid narcotics or butalbital in addiction-prone patients.
  - Avoid vasoconstrictors in uncontrolled hypertension, coronary heart disease, and peripheral vascular disease.
  - Avoid sumatriptan, zolmitriptan, and rizatriptan within 2 weeks of MAOI usage.
- Precautions
  - Administer ergotamines and triptans early.
  - Frequent use of acute-treatment drugs may lead to increase in migraine patterns.
- Significant possible interactions
  - Other sedatives, analgesics, alcohol, and vasoconstrictors (including decongestants)
  - Ergotamine and macrolide antibiotics

Second Line
- Any analgesic, antiemetic, or sedative.
- Narcotics including butorphanol (Stadol) are reserved for rescue therapy.
- In emergency department: Sumatriptan, DHE, adequate analgesics, antiemetic (chlorpromazine or prochlorperazine), and fluid replacement
- Prophylactic therapy: If attacks significantly interfere with lifestyle or are not adequately controlled by appropriate acute interventions, daily prophylactic therapy may be appropriate. Prophylaxis includes the following (6)
  - Propranolol (Inderal): 80–320 mg/d
  - Atenolol (Tenormin): 50–100 mg/d
  - Nadolol (Corgard): 40–80 mg/d
  - Timolol (Blocadren): 10–20 mg/d
  - Metoprolol (Lopressor): 100–450 mg/d
  - Amitriptyline (Elavil): 10–150 mg/d
  - Nortriptyline (Pamelor): 10–150 mg/d

  - Verapamil (Calan, Isoptin): 80–120 mg/d
  - Valproic acid (Depakene) or divalproex (Depakote): 250–1,500 mg/d
  - Cyproheptadine (Periactin): 4–16 mg/d
  - Topiramate: 100–200 mg/d

Issues for Referral
- Obscure diagnosis, concomitant medical conditions, significant psychopathology
- Unresponsive to usual treatment
- Analgesic-dependent headache patterns

PROGNOSIS
- With age, reduction in severity, frequency, and disability of attacks
- Most attacks subside within 72 hours.

COMPLICATIONS
- Rare
  - Status migrainosus
  - Cerebral ischemic events
- Iatrogenic effects of treatment

PATIENT MONITORING
- Early intervention to assist management
- Monitor frequency of attacks, pain behaviors, and medication usage.
- Encourage lifestyle modifications.
- Regularly scheduled follow-up is mandatory.

REFERENCES

1. The International Classification of Headache Disorders. 2nd ed. *Cephalalgia*. 2004; 24(suppl 1):1–160.
2. The Sumatriptan and Naratriptan Pregnancy Registry: Data from GlaxoSmithKline.
3. Hale TW. *Medications and Mother's Milk*. 11th ed. Amarillo, TX: Pharmasoft Pub.; 2004.
4. Brandes JL, Kudrow D, Cady R. Eletriptan in migraine. *Cephalalgia*. 2005;25:735.
5. Matchar DB, et al. Evidence-based guidelines for migraine headache in the primary care setting: AAN Headache Guidelines. *Am Acad Neurol* 2000.
6. Ramadan NM, et al. Evidence-based guidelines for migraine headache. 2006.
7. Pittler MH, Ernst E. Feverfew for preventing migraine. Cochrane Pain, Palliative and supportive Care Group Cochrane Database of Systematic Reviews. 4, 2006.

MISCELLANEOUS

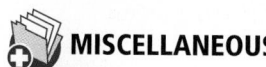

ICD9-CM
- 346.00 Classical migraine without mention of intractable migraine
- 346.21 Variants of migraine with intractable migraine, so stated
- 346.90 Migraine, unspecified without mention of intractable migraine
- 784.0 Headache

See Corresponding Diagnostic Algorithm

See Patient Handout on CD

M

MILIARIA RUBRA

Aamir Siddiqi, MD

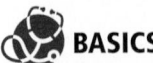 **BASICS**

DESCRIPTION
Miliaria rubra or prickly heat is a papulovesicular eruption of eccrine sweat glands that often occurs in high heat and humidity.
- System(s) Affected: Skin/Exocrine

GENERAL PREVENTION
- Acclimatize slowly to hot weather.
- See "General Measures".

EPIDEMIOLOGY
- Predominant age: Common in infants, less common in adults
- Predominant sex: Male = Female

Incidence
May be present in up to 4% of neonates with a mean age of the neonate being 1–14 days

ALERT
Geriatric Considerations
- Less common
- Backs of hospitalized patients

Pediatric Considerations
More common in this age group

RISK FACTORS
- Hot humid environment
- Occlusive bandages
- Plastic sheets
- High fever

ETIOLOGY
Keratinous plugging of the sweat ducts as a result of toxins produced by resident bacteria, leading to rupture of sweat duct producing sweat-retention vesicle

ASSOCIATED CONDITIONS
Exposure to hot and humid conditions

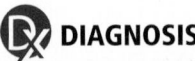 **DIAGNOSIS**

SIGNS AND SYMPTOMS
- Fine papules and vesicles on an erythematous base (1)[B]
- May become inflamed pustules (miliaria pustulosa) (2)[B]
- Prevalent in areas of friction caused by clothing and in areas of flexure
- In infants: Trunk, diaper area, neck, groin, axilla, face
- Pilosebaceous follicles, palms, and soles are spared.
- Lesions appear after person has been in a hot humid environment that causes sweating.
- Pruritus or prickly, mildly stinging sensation in affected body areas

TESTS
Diagnostic Procedures/Surgery
Miliaria rubra is a clinical diagnosis.

Pathological Findings
- Keratinous plugging of sweat ducts
- Sweat-retention vesicle

DIFFERENTIAL DIAGNOSIS
- Acne
- Folliculitis
- Viral exanthems
- Drug eruptions
- Erythema toxicum
- Yeast infections
- Pyogenic infections
- Syringomas (3)[B]

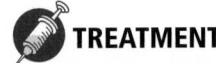 **TREATMENT**

INITIAL STABILIZATION
Outpatient

GENERAL MEASURES
- Avoid wearing heavy, tight clothing or garments that may cause friction.
- Avoid plastic or occlusive dressings/garments in hot environments.
- Avoid excessive use of soap and contact with irritants.
- Frequent cool baths with Aveeno colloidal, oatmeal, or cornstarch mixtures
- Provide cool, dry environment for 8–10 hours per day.
- Topical applications of lotions containing lanolin, calamine, boric acid, and menthol

Diet
No special diet

Activity
Avoid vigorous activity that causes excessive sweating.

Complementary and Alternative Medicine
Use of Tannic acid has not been shown to be effective.

MEDICATION (DRUGS)

First Line

- Topical steroids to relieve pruritus: 0.1% betamethasone (Valisone) b.i.d. for 3 days
- Systemic antibiotics in cases of bacterial secondary infection: Antibiotic effective against staphylococci (e.g., dicloxacillin 250 mg q.i.d. for 10 days unless strain is resistant to agent)
- If sweating is owing to fever, antipyretic drugs may be useful.
- Precautions: Care should be taken with fluorinated steroid application in children. These agents may cause systemic effects.

Second Line

Over-the-counter preparations with menthol, camphor for pruritus: Hydrocortisone (Sarna) or pramoxine (Prax)

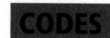 ## FOLLOW-UP

DISPOSITION
As needed; routine follow-up not needed.

PROGNOSIS
- Benign: Responds to cooling
- Avoiding causative agents is key.

COMPLICATIONS
- Secondary bacterial infections
- Miliaria profunda secondary to repeated miliaria rubra can cause anhidrosis.

PATIENT MONITORING
As needed for persistence of symptoms

REFERENCES

1. Bondi J, Jegasothy B, Lazarus G. *Dermatology, Diagnosis and Therapy*. Norwalk, CT: McGraw-Hill/Appleton & Lange; 1992.
2. Gan VN, Hoang MP. Generalized vesicular eruption in a newborn. [Case Reports. Clinical Conference. Journal Article] *Pediatr Dermatol*. 2004;21(2): 171–173.
3. Wilkinson TM, Mizelle CB, Morrell DS. Multiple milia-like dermal papules. [Case Reports. Journal Article] *Pediatr Dermatol*. 2004;21(3):269–271.

 ## MISCELLANEOUS

CODES

ICD9-CM
705.1 Prickly heat

PATIENT TEACHING

- Cause of eruption/avoidance
- General measures for home care

Diet
No specific diet

Activity
As tolerated with no limitiations

Prevention
- Avoid hot and humid conditions.
- Dress appropriately for warm environmental conditions.
- Understand the self-limiting nature of the disease.

See Corresponding Diagnostic Algorithm

 M

MILK-ALKALI SYNDROME

Stanley G. Smith, MA, MB

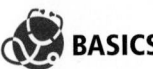 ## BASICS

DESCRIPTION

A condition resulting from ingestion of excessive amounts of calcium and absorbable alkali (e.g., sodium bicarbonate and calcium carbonate) usually during self-treatment for indigestion, peptic ulcer, or gastroesophageal reflux disease, or as part of osteoporosis prevention

- System(s) Affected: Endocrine/Metabolic; Gastrointestinal; Renal/Urologic
- Synonym(s): Burnett syndrome; Milk poisoning; Milk drinker syndrome

ALERT
Geriatric Considerations
Occurs predominantly in this age group

GENERAL PREVENTION
Avoid excess milk and/or absorbable antacids.

EPIDEMIOLOGY
- Predominant age: 40–75 years
- Predominant sex: Male = Female; female risk is rising due to osteoporosis prevention

Incidence
Infrequent

Prevalence
Infrequent

RISK FACTORS
- Peptic ulcer
- Hiatal hernia
- Malignancies

Genetics
Unknown

PATHOPHYSIOLOGY
Exact mechanism unclear
- Increased calcium absorption may lead to suppression of parathyroid hormone, which leads to the kidneys retaining increased bicarbonate. This eventually leads to alkalosis, which also causes increased calcium resorption in the kidneys.

ETIOLOGY
Excess intake of milk and alkali as therapy for gastrointestinal problems accompanied with gastric hyperacidity (e.g., peptic ulcer, esophageal reflux)

ASSOCIATED CONDITIONS
- Peptic ulcer disease
- Hiatal hernia
- Gastroesophageal reflux
- Hyperparathyroidism
- Hypercalcemia of malignancy

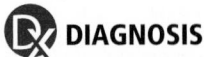 ## DIAGNOSIS

SIGNS AND SYMPTOMS
- Anorexia
- Band keratopathy
- Constipation
- Dehydration
- Depression
- Dizziness
- Food distaste
- Headache
- Irritability
- Mental status changes
- Myalgias
- Nausea
- Periarticular calcinosis
- Polydipsia
- Polyuria
- Vomiting
- Weakness

TESTS
Lab
- Mild alkalosis
- Hypercalcemia
- Normocalciuria
- Decreased urine phosphate
- Increased BUN and serum creatinine levels
- Normal alkaline phosphatase level

Pathological Findings
- Nephrocalcinosis
- Ectopic calcification

DIFFERENTIAL DIAGNOSIS
Other causes of hypercalcemia
- Excessive osteolysis with malignant disease
- Vitamin intoxication
- Thyroid disease
- Sarcoidosis
- Thiazide diuretic treatment
- Hyperparathyroidism

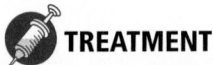 ## TREATMENT

INITIAL STABILIZATION
Inpatient treatment

GENERAL MEASURES
- Withdraw milk and alkali.
- Treat hypercalcemia.
- IV treatment to cause calcinosis (usually with sodium chloride solution)
- Goal of treatment: Maintain urine volume of 3 L/d
- Renal dialysis for significant renal insufficiency

Diet
Increased fluid intake

Activity
Bed rest during active treatment

MEDICATION (DRUGS)

First Line

- To treat hypercalcemia
  – Isotonic sodium chloride: 0.9% IV when serum calcium exceeds 15 mg/dL (3.75 mmol/L) (see "Hypercalcemia"), plus
  – Furosemide: 80–100 mg IV q2h for 24 hours after volume depletion has been corrected
- Precautions: Replace sodium and potassium losses associated with furosemide use.

Second Line

- Biphosphonates inhibit bone resorption.
- Dialysis is occasionally indicated.

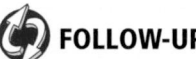 **FOLLOW-UP**

PROGNOSIS
Favorable with appropriate therapy

COMPLICATIONS
- Renal failure
- Nephrocalcinosis

PATIENT MONITORING
- Kidney function
- Fluid intake and output
- Urine electrolytes

REFERENCES

1. Labhart A. *Clinical Endocrinology: Theory & Practice*. 2nd ed. Springhouse, PA: Springer-Verlag; 1987.
2. Wilson JD, Foster DW, eds. *Williams' Textbook of Endocrinology*, 8th ed. Philadelphia, PA: WB Saunders; 1992.

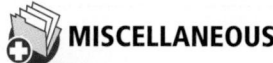 **MISCELLANEOUS**

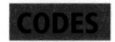 **CODES**

ICD9-CM
999.9 Other and unspecified complications of medical care, NEC

PATIENT TEACHING

Provide education on prevention of syndrome.

 See Corresponding Diagnostic Algorithm

M

MITRAL REGURGITATION

Kerry J. Murphy, MD

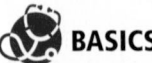 **BASICS**

DESCRIPTION

- Disorder of the mitral valve due to structural abnormalities of the mitral annulus, mitral valve leaflets, chordae tendinea, or papillary muscles.
- Part of left ventricular (LV) stroke volume is pumped into the left atrium (LA); as a result, reducing cardiac output and increasing LA volume and pressure.
- Types of mitral regurgitation (MR)
  - Acute MR
  - Chronic MR
  - Ischemic MR
- System(s) Affected: Cardiac; Pulmonary

GENERAL PREVENTION

- Antibiotic prophylaxis to prevent rheumatic heart disease following streptococcal pharyngitis
- Antibiotic prophylaxis to prevent endocarditis
  - Prosthetic heart valve
  - Previous endocarditis
  - Acquired MR
  - MV Prolapse (MVP) with MR (1)[C]
- Prevention of CAD by controlling risk factors

EPIDEMIOLOGY
Prevalence
- Mild MR: 19.1% in women; 19% in men
- Moderate MR: 1.9%
- Severe MR : 0.2%

ALERT
Geriatric Considerations
Consider medical therapy alone for patients >75 with MR due to increased operative mortality and decreased survival (compared with those with AS), especially with preexisting CAD or need for MV replacement (1)[B]

Pregnancy Considerations
- MR with NYHA Functional Class III-IV at high risk for maternal and/or fetal risk during pregnancy
- Avoid vasodilators in pregnant patients unless concomitant systemic hypertension (1)[C]

RISK FACTORS
- Age
- Hypertension
- Rheumatic heart disease
- Endocarditis
- Anorectic drugs

PATHOPHYSIOLOGY
- Acute MR
  - Acute damage to mitral valve leads to sudden LV volume overload and increased LV preload. Without time for development of compensatory LV hypertrophy, cardiac output is impaired, leading to pulmonary congestion and possible shock.
- Chronic MR
  - Chronic mitral valve damage leads to eccentric LV hypertrophy and subsequent compensatory increase in LV end diastolic volume and stroke volume. This maintains cardiac output and reduces symptoms of pulmonary congestion.
- Ischemic MR
  - Papillary muscle rupture or ischemia during acute MI causing acute MR
  - Functional MR due to incomplete coaptation of valve leaflets or restricted valve movement due to ischemia.

ETIOLOGY
- Acute MR
  - Ruptured chordae tendinea
  - Papillary muscle dysfunction due to acute MI or ischemia
  - Infective endocarditis
  - Flail leaflet
- Chronic MR
  - Mitral valve prolapse (MVP)
  - Rheumatic heart disease
  - CAD
  - Connective tissue disorder
  - Infective endocarditis
  - HOCM
  - Congenital AV cushion defect
  - Anorectic drugs

ASSOCIATED CONDITIONS
MVP with MR common in Marfan syndrome

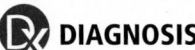 **DIAGNOSIS**

SIGNS AND SYMPTOMS
- Acute MR
  - Dyspnea
  - Orthopnea
  - Paroxysmal nocturnal dyspnea
  - Fatigue
- Chronic MR
  - Fatigue
  - Weakness
  - Atrial fibrillation

History
- Baseline exercise tolerance
- Rheumatic heart disease
- Prior MI
- Connective tissue disorder

Physical Exam
- Acute MR
  - Systolic murmur at left sternal border and base
    - Early, mid or holosystolic murmur
    - Often soft, low-pitched, decrescendo murmur
  - S3 and S4 (if in sinus rhythm)
  - Tachycardia
  - Tachypnea
  - Rales
- Chronic MR
  - Holosystolic murmur at apex that radiates to axilla
  - Left displaced LV apical impulse
  - Soft S1 and widely split S2
  - Loud P2 (if pulmonary hypertension)
  - S3
  - Brisk upstroke of arterial pulse
  - Ankle edema, JVD, ascites if development of right heart failure

TESTS
Imaging
- Chest radiograph
  - Acute MR
    - Pulmonary edema
    - Normal heart size
  - Chronic MR:
    - LA and LV enlargement
- EKG
  - Acute MR: No EKG abnormalities
  - Chronic MR
    - P mitrale from LA enlargement
    - LV hypertrophy
    - Q waves due to prior MI
    - Atrial fibrillation

Diagnostic Procedures/Surgery
- EKG
- Transthoracic Echocardiogram (TTE) with MV Doppler interrogation.
  - Indications for TTE
    - Baseline evaluation to quantify severity of MR and LV function
    - Evaluation of mechanism of MR
    - Surveillance of LV function
    - Evaluation after surgery to assess status
  - Acute MR findings
    - Evidence of etiology such as flail leaflet or infective vegetations
    - Normal LA and LV size
  - Chronic MR findings
    - Enlarged LA
    - LV enlargement with progression
- Transesophageal Echocardiogram (TEE)
  - Intraoperatively to define severity/cause of MR and/or LV function
  - Nondiagnostic TTE
  - Evaluation of prosthetic heart valves (2)[C]

DIFFERENTIAL DIAGNOSIS
Other systolic murmurs

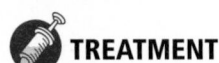 **TREATMENT**

PRE HOSPITAL
- Acute MR
  - Stabilize ABCs
  - IV, O$_2$, and monitor
  - Sit patient upright to lessen symptoms of pulmonary congestion
  - Oxygen

INITIAL STABILIZATION
- Acute MR
  - Treat underlying cause (e.g., MI)
  - Treat acute pulmonary edema:
    - Lasix
    - Morphine
    - Nitrates
    - Intra-aortic balloon pump to maintain cardiac output (1)[C].

GENERAL MEASURES
Activity
- Competitive athletes with MR
  - Asymptomatic with normal LV function: No restrictions
- Mildly symptomatic patients and those with LV dilatation
  - Activities with low to moderate dynamic and static cardiac demand allowed
- Post MV repair
  - Avoid sports with risk for bodily contact or trauma
  - Low-intensity competitive sports allowed
- Atrial fibrillation and anticoagulation
  - No contact sports (3)[C]

MEDICATION (DRUGS)

- Acute MR
  - Nitroprusside (+ dobutamine if hypotensive) (1)[C]
- Chronic MR
  - Asymptomatic: No medications necessary
- Symptomatic MR
  - Due to increased preload: Quinapril may reduce LV volume and mass and improved functional class in patients with NYHA Class I–III (1)[C].
- With atrial fibrillation and preserved LV function
  - Rate control with
    - Digitalis, calcium channel blockers, or β-blockers (1)[A])
  - Anticoagulation

SURGERY
- Symptomatic MR
  - Normal LV function (EF >60% and end-systolic dimension ESD <45 mm)
    - 1st line: MV repair if feasible
    - Second line: Mitral valve replacement (MVR) w/chordal preservation
  - LV dysfunction (EF <60% and ESD >45 mm)
    - 1st line: MV repair
    - Second line: MV replacement
  - LV dysfunction with EF <30%
    - Medical therapy alone (1, 4)[A]
- Asymptomatic MR
  - Normal LV function
    - Newly acquired severe MR or recent onset of episodic or chronic atrial fibrillation: MV repair
    - Others: No surgery recommended
  - LV dysfunction (EF<60% and ESD >45 mm)
    - 1st line: MV repair
    - 2nd line: MV replacement (1)[C])
- Ischemic MR
  - Early percutaneous revascularization is treatment for MR due to ischemia.
  - MV repair is treatment for papillary muscle rupture or flail leaflet (1)[A].

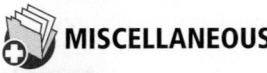 ## FOLLOW-UP

- Chronic MR
  - Asymptomatic
    - Mild MR: Annual clinical evaluation to assess symptom progression
    - Moderate MR: Annual clinical evaluation and echo to assess LV function
    - Severe MR: Annual clinical evaluation and echo every 6–12 months
    - Consider serial chest radiographs and EKGs.
    - Consider exercise stress test if exercise capacity is in question.
- Post MV repair
  - Early follow-up to assess efficacy of repair necessary as failures occur soon after procedure
- Post MV replacement
  - Anticoagulation is necessary with mechanical prosthesis.
    - Follow PT/INR (1)[C]

PROGNOSIS
- Acute severe MR
  - Mortality risk with surgery 50%
  - Mortality risk with medical therapy alone 75% in 1st 24 hours; 95% at 2 weeks
- Chronic
  - Asymptomatic severe MR with normal LVEF
    - 10% yearly rate of progression to symptoms and subnormal resting LVEF
  - Symptomatic severe MR
    - 8-year survival rate 33% without surgery
    - Mortality rate 5% yearly
  - MV repair vs. replacement
    - Operative mortality 2–4% versus 5–10% respectively
  - MV prolapse: Repair vs. replacement
    - Survival rate 80–94% versus 40–60% at 5–10 years

COMPLICATIONS
- Acute pulmonary edema
- CHF
- Atrial fibrillation
- Bleeding risk with anticoagulation
- Endocarditis

PATIENT MONITORING
See "Follow-Up"

REFERENCES

1. Bonow RO, Carabello B, de Leon AC Jr., et al. ACC/AHA guidelines for the management of patients with valvular heart disease: A report of the American College of Cardiology/American Heart Association Task Force on Practice Guidelines (Committee on Management of Patients with Valvular Heart Disease). *J Am Coll Cardiol.* 1998;32:1486–1588.
2. Irvine T, Li XK, Sahn DJ, Kenny A. Assessment of mitral regurgitation. *Heart.* 2002;88(Suppl IV):iv11–iv19.
3. Bonow BO, Cheitlin MD, Crawford MH, Douglas PS. Task Force 3: Valvular heart disease. *JACC.* 2005;45:1334–1340.
4. Borer JS, Bonow RO. Contemporary approach to aortic and mitral regurgitation. *Circulation.* 2003;108:2432–2438.

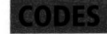 ## MISCELLANEOUS

CODES

ICD9-CM
396.3 Mitral valve/Aortic regurgitation

PATIENT TEACHING

 See Corresponding Diagnostic Algorithm

M

MITRAL STENOSIS

Matthew P. Hill, MD

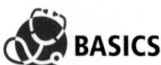 **BASICS**

DESCRIPTION
- Resistance to diastolic filling of the left ventricle due to mitral valve narrowing
- The mitral valve is the valve most commonly affected by rheumatic heart disease.
- System(s) Affected: Cardiovascular

ALERT
Geriatric Considerations
- Atrial fibrillation and complicating arterial embolism are more common.
- Anticoagulation therapy recommended despite bleeding risk (unless specifically contraindicated) due to high risk of clot formation in the left atrial appendage with systemic embolism and valve thrombosis (especially if atrial fibrillation present)

Pregnancy Considerations
- Increased cardiac output causes increased transmitral gradient and increased left atrial pressure, producing marked cardiac deterioration.
  - General rule: Symptomatic status will increase by 1 New York Heart Association class. (1)[C]
- Congenital mitral stenosis is a rare congenital malformation, manifested in only 0.42% of children with congenital heart disease.
- May cause worsened pulmonary congestion and increased pulmonary hypertension.

GENERAL PREVENTION
- Bacterial endocarditis prophylaxis for dental and invasive procedures continued for life
- Appropriate treatment of strep throat (group A streptococcal infection)
- Rheumatic fever prophylaxis when indicated (see "General Measures")

EPIDEMIOLOGY
- Predominant age: Symptoms primarily occur in middle age (40–70 years)
- Predominant sex: Female > Male (2–3:1)

Incidence
Overall incidence of rheumatic heart disease is decreasing, causing decrease in mitral stenosis.

Prevalence
Rough index of severe disease: ~1500 valvotomies per year

RISK FACTORS
History of rheumatic fever

PATHOPHYSIOLOGY
Scarring of the leaflets with fibrosis restricting valve mobility
- Mitral stenosis → pressure gradient between left atrium (LA) and ventricle (LV) → increased LA pressure → LA enlargement → pulmonary congestion → decreased LV output → pulmonary hypertension → right heart failure

ETIOLOGY
- In adults, mitral stenosis is usually secondary to rheumatic heart disease.
- Congenital (rare)

ASSOCIATED CONDITIONS
CHF

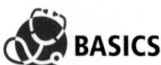 **DIAGNOSIS**

SIGNS AND SYMPTOMS
- Most common
  - Effort-induced dyspnea
  - Palpitations
  - Effort fatigue
  - Hemoptysis (late)
  - Apical early diastolic low-pitched rumble often with presystolic accentuation (listen with bell of stethoscope in left lateral decubitus position)
  - Loud S_1 (early in disease; as the valve becomes more stenotic and less mobile, this is less common)
  - Opening snap after S_2 (may also diminish in intensity with increasing stenosis)
  - Right ventricle enlargement
- Others
  - Paroxysmal nocturnal dyspnea
  - Orthopnea
  - Recumbent cough
  - Hoarseness
  - Digital clubbing
  - Chest pain
  - Peripheral edema
  - Systemic embolization
  - Rales, atrial fibrillation, malar rash (rare)
  - Holosystolic murmur of mitral regurgitation may accompany the valvular deformity of mitral stenosis
  - If pulmonary hypertension is present: Right ventricular lift, increased pulmonic 2nd sound, high-pitched decrescendo diastolic murmur of pulmonic insufficiency (Graham Steell murmur)
  - If right ventricular failure has developed: Increased jugular venous distention, holosystolic murmur of tricuspid regurgitation at left sternal border, hepatomegaly, and peripheral edema
  - May also find associated aortic, or less commonly, tricuspid murmurs (due to aortic or tricuspid valve involvement with rheumatic heart disease)

History
- History of murmur
- History of rheumatic fever
- History of pulmonary edema with pregnancy, exercise, infection, or arrhythmia (commonly atrial fibrillation)

TESTS
ECG (indicative, not diagnostic)
- Left atrial enlargement (manifested by broad, notched P waves in lead II with a negative terminal deflection of the P wave in lead V_1)
- Atrial fibrillation common
- With right ventricular hypertrophy, right axis deviation and a large R wave in V_1 may be noted

Imaging
Chest radiograph (indicative, not diagnostic)
- Left atrial enlargement with straightening of the left heart border, a "double density," and elevation of the left mainstem bronchus
- Pulmonary venous pattern changes with redistribution of flow toward apices
- Prominent pulmonary arteries at the hilum with rapid tapering
- Right ventricular enlargement
- Kerley B lines
- Pulmonary edema pattern (late)

Diagnostic Procedures/Surgery
- 2D echocardiography with doppler: An accepted minimally invasive technique. (1)[C]
  - Establishes anatomy showing "hockey stick appearance."
  - Severity determined by the following (1)[C]
    ○ Valve area by planimetry (decreased)
    ○ Doppler interrogation of transvalvular pressure gradient
    ○ Valve area by pressure half-time technique
  - Evaluates other valves, as well as pulmonary arterial pressure and LV function.
- Cardiac catheterization: Necessary after equivocal noninvasive investigations. (1)[C]
  - Calculates valve area using cardiac output and transvalvular gradients (Gorlin Formula)
  - Pulmonary capillary wedge pressure substituted for left atrial pressure (increased)
  - Can find additional cardiovascular disease

Pathological Findings
- Scarring of the mitral valve leaflets with fibrosis
  - Leaflet thickening, commissural fusion, chordal shortening and fusion
- Left atrial dilatation/thrombi, right ventricular hypertrophy, pulmonary arterial thickening

DIFFERENTIAL DIAGNOSIS
- Uncommon atrial myxoma or vegetation due to endocarditis obstructing left ventricle inflow
- Diastolic flow murmurs can be heard in the absence of true stenosis due to the increased flow across a normal valve. These murmurs are generally limited to early diastole and may be associated with anemia, thyrotoxicosis, shunts, and significant mitral regurgitation.

TREATMENT

GENERAL MEASURES
- Mitral stenosis is generally a progressive disease.
- Asymptomatic patients with noncritical mitral stenosis can be followed with appropriate evaluation.
- Patients should avoid unusual stresses (emotional and physical).
- Mitral stenosis is a moderate risk factor for bacterial endocarditis.
  - All patients require endocarditis prophylaxis for various dental, respiratory, GI, and GU procedures. (2)[C]
- Patients with a documented history of rheumatic fever require rheumatic fever propylaxis.
  - With carditis: Continue for 10 years or until age 25. (2)[C]
  - Without carditis: Continue 5 years or until age 18. (2)[C]
- Mitral stenosis requiring anticoagulation (3)[C]
  - Rheumatic valve disease plus afib/systemic embolism: Oral anticoagulation (warfarin)
  - Rheumatic valve disease in sinus rhythm: Oral anticoagulation if LA diameter >5.5 cm (unclear benefit)
  - Mitral valvuloplasty: Oral anticoagulation 3 weeks prior to and 4 weeks after procedure
- Atrial fibrillation accompanying mitral stenosis impairs left ventricular filling, especially with a rapid ventricular response.
  - Rate control is necessary with beta or calcium channel blockers.
  - Cardioversion is indicated for medical failure or if patient is unstable.

Diet
Low salt

Activity
Adequate rest and reasonable physical activity

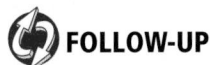

MEDICATION (DRUGS)

First Line
- Judicious addition of diuretics if symptoms indicate
- Atrial fibrillation
  - Acute with rapid ventricular response
    ○ Beta blockers or calcium channel blockers to achieve rate control
    ○ Cardioversion if medications fail
  - Chronic rate control
    ○ Beta blockers and rate altering calcium channel blockers
    ○ May add digoxin (rate control only)
- Antithrombotic therapy (3)[C]
  - Oral anticoagulation with warfarin to achieve INR of 2.5 (range 2.0–3.0)
- Rheumatic fever prophylaxis (2)[C]
  - Benzanthine penicillin G, 1.2 mU IM every 3–4 weeks or
  - Penicillin V 250 mg PO b.i.d.
  - If penicillin-allergic, consider erythromycin stearate 250 mg PO b.i.d.
- Bacterial endocarditis prophylaxis
  - Procedure dependent
  - Dental, oral, respiratory, esophageal, GI, GU: Amoxocillin—adults 2 g; children 50 mg/kg PO 1 hour before procedure. (2)[C]
  - Presence of prosthesis requires more aggressive prophylaxis.
  - Contraindications: Penicillin allergy
- Significant possible interactions
  - Many when using the combination of warfarin and digoxin
  - Use caution when adding new medications.
  - Refer to the manufacturer's profile of each drug.

Second Line
- Erythromycin: 250 mg PO b.i.d. for rheumatic fever prophylaxis (penicillin-allergic patients). (2)[C]
- Clindamycin: Adults 600 mg; children 20 mg/kg PO 1 hour before procedure for bacterial endocarditis prophylaxis: Dental, oral, respiratory, esophageal (penicillin-allergic patients). (2)[C]
- Vancomycin: Adults 1 g IV over 1–2 hours; children 20 mg/kg IV over 1–2 hours for bacterial endocarditis prophylaxis: GU/GI (except esophageal) (penicillin-allergic patients). (2)[C]

SURGERY
- Open commissurotomy vs. balloon valvuloplasty
  - Significant increase in valve area and decrease in gradient in both at 24 months. (4)[B]
  - Marked improvement in symptoms at 24 months by New York Heart Association class. (4)[B]
  - No difference in occurrence of mitral regurgitation. (4)[B]
  - Balloon valvuloplasty less invasive alternative
  - Onset of more than mild symptoms is reasonable indication for surgery.
- Mitral valve prosthesis
  - Indicated when other procedures fail or rheumatic involvement precludes valve conservation

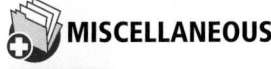

FOLLOW-UP

DISPOSITION
Outpatient except for complications or surgery

PROGNOSIS
- Although a milder course is now seen in North America, the classic mitral stenosis history is 10 years from the episode of rheumatic fever to the development of a murmur, another 10 years until symptomatic, and another 10 years for the patient to develop serious disability.
- Operative mortality 1–2% for mitral commissurotomy; 2–5% for mitral valve replacement

COMPLICATIONS
- Thromboembolism from mitral stenosis is a major potential complication (anticoagulation therapy has lessened this risk substantially).
- Recurrent rheumatic fever
- Bacterial endocarditis
- Pulmonary hypertension
- Pulmonary edema

PATIENT MONITORING
Close regular visits for assessment of the gradually progressive symptoms

REFERENCES
1. Carabello BA. Modern management of mitral stenosis. *Circulation*. 2005;112:432–437.
2. Gilbert DN, Moellering RC, Eliopoulos GM, Sande MA. *The Sanford Guide to Antimicrobial Therapy*. 35th ed. Hyde Park, VT: Antimicrobial Therapy, Inc.; 2005.
3. Salem DM, et al. Antithrombotic therapy in valvular heart disease—native and prosthetic: The Seventh ACCP Conference on Antithrombotic and Thrombolytic Therapy. *Chest*. 2004;126(3): 457S–482S.
4. Cardoso LF, et al. Comparison between percutaneous balloon valvuloplasty and open commissurotomy for mitral stenosis. *Cardiology*. 2002;98:186–190.
5. Dalen JE, Alpert JS. *Valvular Heart Disease*, 2nd ed. New York, NY: Little Brown; 1987.
6. Hurst JW, et al. *The Heart*. 8th ed. New York, NY: McGraw-Hill; 1994.

MISCELLANEOUS

CODES

ICD9-CM
394.0 Mitral stenosis

PATIENT TEACHING
Educate the patient about symptoms of mitral stenosis and necessity of reporting them should they occur.

See Corresponding Diagnostic Algorithm

M

MITRAL VALVE PROLAPSE

Lisa S. Gussak, MD

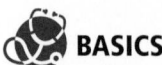 **BASICS**

DESCRIPTION

Mitral valve prolapse (MVP) is exaggerated billowing of the mitral valve leaflets into the left atrium (LA) during systole without valve coaptation, resulting in mitral regurgitation (MR).
Synonym(s): Systolic click-murmur syndrome; Barlow syndrome; Billowing mitral cusp syndrome; Myxomatous mitral valve; Floppy-valve syndrome; Redundant cusp syndrome

EPIDEMIOLOGY

- Age: MVP has been described in all groups, but is most common in young women.
- Sex: Female > Male (2:1)

Prevalence

One of the most prevalent cardiovascular abnormalities, affecting ~2% of the general population

RISK FACTORS

- MVP generally is a primary cardiovascular disorder. Several conditions may be associated with it (see below).
- MVP tends to be more common in patients with asthenic body habitus, straight backs, shallow chest wall, and pectus excavatum.

Genetics

MVP syndrome is thought to be at least partly heritable, with an autosomal-dominant mode of transmission with variable penetrance.

PATHOPHYSIOLOGY

Severe MVP is associated with MR. Severe MR may lead to heart failure symptoms.

ETIOLOGY

Myxomatous degeneration of the mitral valve apparatus; likely due to a connective tissue abnormality

ASSOCIATED CONDITIONS

- Hyperthyroidism
- Marfan syndrome
- Ehlers-Danlos syndrome
- Pseudoxanthoma elasticum
- Periarteritis nodosa
- Osteogenesis imperfecta
- Myotonic dystrophy
- Von Willebrand disease

DIAGNOSIS

SIGNS AND SYMPTOMS

- The majority of patients with MVP are asymptomatic.
- However, many patients have increased anxiety, fatigue, palpitations, orthostatic hypotension, and evidence of autonomic dysfunction, although it has not been confirmed that these symptoms occur more frequently than in the general population.
- Chest pain is a frequent complaint, although it is generally atypical with regard to angina.
- The chest pain with MVP usually occurs at rest and is sharp in character.
  - Thought to be due to abnormal tension on papillary muscles
  - Palpitations are common and can represent both benign atrial and malignant ventricular tachyarrhythmias. An increased associated of Wolf-Parkinson-White syndrome is noted in patients with MVP.

Physical Exam

- Auscultatory examination shows a systolic click at least 0.14 seconds after the 1st heart sound, occurring just after the carotid upstroke, which helps differentiate the click of MVP from an ejection click.
- The prolapse is a volume-dependent phenomenon; at low ventricular volumes more stress is placed on the abnormal mitral apparatus, and the valve may prolapse earlier or more so than in a volume-overloaded condition.
- The ejection click is best heard with the stethoscope diaphragm at the left sternal border and is followed by a mid to late crescendo systolic murmur lasting until the 2nd heart sound.
- Occasionally, only the ejection click or the murmur alone is present.
- The duration of the murmur corresponds with the severity of MR.
- Arterial vasodilation, augmented contractility, and decreased venous return cause the click and murmur to move toward S1.
- Dynamic auscultation with amyl nitrate, early Valsalva, or upright posture causes the click and murmur to move toward S1.
- Squatting, leg raise, and isometric exercise delays the click and murmur toward S2.

TESTS

Cardiac catheterization can visualize the mitral valve leaflets prolapsing into the atrium as well as a scalloped appearance of the leaflets consistent with redundant tissue; should be considered in patients with chest pain and abnormal noninvasive ischemia test results.

Imaging

- The ECG is usually normal in asymptomatic patients. However, biphasic T-waves and nonspecific ST-segment abnormalities, perhaps secondary to papillary muscle ischemia, may be noted in leads II, III, and aVF.
- Paroxysmal supraventricular tachycardia is the most frequent arrhythmia noted with MVP, although premature atrial beats, ventricular beats, and sinus node dysfunction with bradyarrhythmias are also common.
- In patients with dizziness, syncope, or QT prolongation, consider 24-hr ECG monitoring if no clear explanation for these symptoms exists.
- M-mode echocardiography shows posterior movement of the mitral valve leaflets in mid-systole.
- On 2-D echocardiography, the valve leaflets are thickened and redundant and prolapse back into the atrium during systole.
- The parasternal view is the most specific for the diagnosis of MVP.
- Color-flow Doppler usually shows a mitral regurgitant jet.

Diagnostic Procedures/Surgery

- MVP was previously grossly overdiagnosed before more stringent clinical and echocardiographic criteria were accepted.
- For diagnosis, patients must have of 1 of the following
  - Mid to late systolic click with late murmur or whoop
  - Marked superior displacement of the mitral valve leaflets($\geq$2 mm) above the annulus
  - Mild to moderate superior displacement of the MV leaflets above the annulus, along with other supportive findings on echo or physical exam (classic click, murmur in a young patient, or whoop)

Pathological Findings

- Myxomatous proliferation of the middle layer (spongiosa) of the valve, resulting in increased mucopolysaccharide deposition and myxomatous degeneration
- By electron microscopy, the collagen fibers in the valve leaflets are disorganized and fragmented.
- With increased stroma deposition, the valve leaflets enlarge and become redundant.
- The endothelium is usually noncontiguous and a frequent site for thrombus or infective vegetation.

DIFFERENTIAL DIAGNOSIS

- Mitral regurgitation
- Tricuspid regurgitation
- Tricuspid valve prolapse
- Papillary muscle dysfunction
- Hypertrophic cardiomyopathy

TREATMENT

GENERAL MEASURES
- Reassurance is necessary with the asymptomatic patient.
- Patients with a documented focal neurologic event should be considered for aspirin or anticoagulation therapy.
- Patients with significant MR should be treated with afterload reduction or considered for mitral valve repair or replacement.
- Patients with arrhythmias or long QT syndromes should have 24-hour ECG monitoring.
- Electrophysiologic studies may be considered in symptomatic patients because of the rare association of MVP and sudden cardiac death.
- Endocarditis prophylaxis is recommended for patients with systolic click and murmur of MR and in those with the systolic click and echo findings of prolapse. No prophylaxis is recommended for an isolated systolic click.

MEDICATION (DRUGS)

First Line
- β-Blockers are drug of choice for patients with MVP and palpitations.
- Chest pain syndromes are also best treated with β-blockers.
- Angiotensin-converting enzyme (ACE) inhibitors and angiotensin receptor blockers may be used to reduce blood pressure and regurgitation in the appropriate clinical setting, but should not be used in the presence of severe MR and left ventricular remodeling without consideration of mitral valve repair.

Second Line
Hydralazine and nitrates in combination for afterload reduction

SURGERY
Indications are the same as for MR.

PROGNOSIS
- For asymptomatic patients, prognosis is excellent.
- For patients with severe MR or reduced ejection fraction, the prognosis is similar to nonischemic MR.

COMPLICATIONS
- Sudden cardiac death (very rare)
- Chordae rupture with acute mitral insufficiency
- Endocarditis
- Fibrin emboli
- Heart failure with progressive MR

PATIENT MONITORING
- Asymptomatic patients should be followed with transthoracic echocardiogram every 3–5 years.
- Patients with more severe MR should be followed annually.

REFERENCES
1. Hayek E, Gring CN, Griffin BP. Mitral valve prolapse. *Lancet* 2005;365:507–518.
2. Maron BJ, Ackerman MJ, Nishimura RA, et al. Task Force 4: HCM and other cardiomyopathies, mitral valve prolapse, myocarditis, and Marfan syndrome. *J Am Coll Cardiol* 2005;45:1340–1345.
3. Wu WC, Aziz GF, Sadaniantz A. The use of stress echocardiography in the assessment of mitral valvular disease. *Echocardiography* 2004;21:451–458.

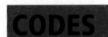 MISCELLANEOUS

See also: Mitral regurgitation

CODES

ICD9-CM
354.9

PATIENT TEACHING
Patient education on avoidance of alcohol, caffeine, stimulants, and nicotine may be sufficient to control symptoms in some instances.

Diet
Sodium and water restriction should be encouraged if the MR is severe enough to affect left ventricular function.

Activity
No limitations unless heart failure or anginal symptoms predominate

Prevention
- Endocarditis prophylaxis is recommended for patients with both the mid-systolic click and mitral regurgitant murmur, with click and echo findings, or with typical echo findings (see above).
- Women under the age of 45 with the systolic click only may not require prophylaxis unless undergoing upper respiratory or genitourinary procedures.

See Corresponding Diagnostic Algorithm

M

MOLLUSCUM CONTAGIOSUM

Cecilia M. Kipnis, MD

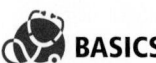 **BASICS**

DESCRIPTION

Molluscum contagiosum is a common, benign, viral skin disorder characterized by small, firm papules with a central umbilication. Papules are flesh or pearl colored and become red when inflamed. It is spread by skin-to-skin contact and fomites. Host requires a functioning immune system (T cells) to resolve infection. Molluscum contagiosum is a self-limited disorder in the immunocompetent host, but is difficult to treat and can be disfiguring in the immunocompromised host.

- Giant molluscum is a variation in which the lesions are up to 3 cm in size.
- System(s) Affected: Skin/Exocrine

GENERAL PREVENTION

Avoid skin-to-skin contact (this includes contact sports such as wrestling) with infected individuals. Avoid scratching to prevent autoinoculation. The sharing of towels, baths, and pools has been implicated in the transmission of molluscum contagiosum. Sexually active patients should refrain from intercourse (condoms only decrease risk of transmission) and refer their partners for exam/treatment.

EPIDEMIOLOGY

- Predominant age: Can occur at any age, but predominantly in children <15 years of age, the sexually active (it is considered an STD), and the immunocompromised (especially those with HIV/AIDS).
- Predominant sex: Male = Female (1:1)

Incidence
- 20% worldwide
- 30% in HIV/AIDS patients with a CD4 count <100

Prevalence
- Occurs worldwide, but is more prevalent in tropical areas
- 5–18% in the HIV/AIDS population

RISK FACTORS

Skin-to-skin contact with infected people

- Contact sports; sexual contact; sharing baths, towels, or pools

PATHOPHYSIOLOGY

Virions invade and replicate in the cytoplasm of epidermal cells and cause abnormal cell proliferation. The genome encodes for proteins that inhibit host inflammatory and immune responses. Molluscum contagiosum is limited to the epidermis and is not associated with malignancy.

ETIOLOGY

DNA virus of the poxviridae family. 4 genetically subdivided, but clinically indistinguishable viral types. Incubation period in the human host is 2–7 weeks. The virus cannot be grown in cell cultures and lacks the ability to cross-hybridize with or be reactivated by other poxviruses.

ASSOCIATED CONDITIONS

- Advanced HIV/AIDS
- Immunosuppression with corticosteroids or chemotherapy
- Atopic dermatitis

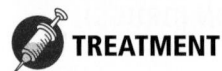 **DIAGNOSIS**

SIGNS AND SYMPTOMS

- Diagnosis is based on clinical findings. Lesions may be asymptomatic or can be painful and itchy. Immunocompetent hosts have an average of 11–20 lesions, 2–5 mm (range = 1 mm to 1 cm) in diameter. Hosts with HIV/AIDS can have hundreds of widespread lesions.
- The papules can be found on any part of the skin and mucosa (rarely oral mucosa). When seen in children, lesions generally appear on the trunk, extremities, and face. In sexually active patients, lesions appear on the inner thighs and anogenital area. Lesions are more commonly found on the face and trunk in patients with HIV/AIDS.

History
May report history of contact with person infected with molluscum contagiosum. Inquire about participation in sports and if sexually active.

Physical Exam
- Lesions are discrete, firm papules with central umbilication (this may be difficult to appreciate in small children). Beneath umbilicated center is a white curd-like core. Lesions are flesh, pearl, or red in color and can have an area of surrounding erythema or dermatitis.
- Perform thorough skin exam including conjunctiva and anogenital area. If molluscum contagiosum was contracted as an STD, consider testing for other STDs, including HIV.

TESTS

Lab
- Virus cannot be cultured.
- Tzank preparation from scraping of lesion demonstrates molluscum bodies.
- Culture and sensitivities from lesion if concerned about secondary infection

Diagnostic Procedures/Surgery
Biopsy if diagnosis cannot be made on clinical findings

Pathological Findings
- Histological examination reveals keratinocytes containing eosinophilic cytoplasmic inclusion bodies (molluscum bodies).
- Electromicroscopy reveals brick-shaped poxvirus particles.

DIFFERENTIAL DIAGNOSIS

- Dermatofibroma
- Basal cell carcinoma
- Benign appendageal tumors
- Verruca vulgaris
- Keratoacanthoma
- Etopic/hyperplastic sebaceous glands
- Folliculitis/furunculosis
- Trichoepithelioma
- Vesicular skin disorders
- Condyloma
- Chalazion (if on conjunctiva)
- In HIV/AIDS patients
  – Cryptococcosis
  – Histoplasmosis
  – Coccidiomycosis

ALERT

Pediatric Considerations
Consider immunodeficient state or alternative diagnosis if child is febrile and has >50 lesions.

TREATMENT

Diet
No restrictions

Activity
No restrictions

Complementary and Alternative Medicine
Apply duct tape to strip lesions daily for 10–20 cycles. (5)[C]

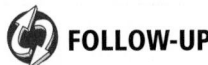 **MEDICATION (DRUGS)**

Many treatment modalities exist for molluscum contagiosum. The following recommendations are based on expert opinion or clinical experience. In addition to these treatments, consider topical corticosteroids or antihistamines for pruritis.

First Line
- Cimetidine 40 mg/kg/d divided in 2 doses until lesions resolve (1,5)
  - Pregnancy category B
  - Adverse effects: Headache, diarrhea, gynecomastia
  - Precautions: Not recommended for use while nursing
- Cantharidin solution 0.7%–0.9%: Apply to lesions 1 time per week until lesions resolve (in office treatment) (1,5)
  - Adverse effects: Blistering, erythema, pain
  - Precautions: Do not use on face; apply sparingly.
- Imiquimod cream 5%: Apply to lesions once daily 3 times a week until lesions resolve, up to 16 weeks (1,3,4)
  - Adverse effects: Erythema, edema, pruritis, postinflammatory pigment changes
  - Contraindications: Do not use in pregnancy.
- Podofilox cream 0.5%: Apply to lesions once daily for 3 days, then do not treat for 4 days; may repeat this cycle 4–6 times (4,5)
  - Adverse effects: Erythema, edema, pain
  - Contraindications: Do not use in pregnancy.
- Podophyllin 25%: Apply to lesions 1 time per week for 4–6 weeks (in office treatment) (4,5)
  - Adverse effects: Erythema, edema, pain
  - Contraindications: Do not use in pregnancy, infants, children, or on oral mucosa.

Second Line
- Potassium hydroxide 5–10%: Apply to lesions b.i.d. for up to 6 weeks (1,5)
  - Adverse effects: Erythema, edema, pain, scarring, postinflammatory pigment changes
- Tretinoin cream/gel 0.05–0.1%: Apply to lesions up to b.i.d. for 4–6 weeks (1,4,5)
  - Adverse effects: Erythema, dry skin
  - Contraindications: Do not use in pregnancy
- Trichloroacetic acid peel performed at 2-week intervals (in office treatment) (4)
  - Adverse effects: Erythema, edema, pain, scarring
- For HIV/AIDS patients with refractory lesions consider
  - Starting or maximizing HAART therapy (5)
  - IV or topical cidofovir (1,4,5)

SURGERY
Based on expert opinion or clinical experience. Options include
- Cryotherapy: 5–10 seconds with 1–2 mm margins. Repeat every 3–4 weeks as needed until lesions disappear (1,4,5)
  - Adverse effects: Erythema, edema, pain, blistering
  - Contraindications: Cryoglobulinemia, Raynaud disease
- Curettage (± electrodessication) under local or topical anesthesia (1,5)
  - Adverse effects: Pain, scarring
- Incision and expression of central particle (1,5)
- CO_2 (4,5) or pulsed dye (1,5) lasers (for recalcitrant lesions)
  - Adverse effects: Pain, edema, scarring

ALERT
Pediatric Considerations
Surgical interventions tend to be 2nd line in small children because of the pain associated with them. May pretreat small children with topical lidocaine or EMLA before surgical treatment to decrease discomfort. (NOTE: Methylhemoglobinemia and CNS toxicity may occur when using lidocaine or EMLA over a large body surface area in small children. Please refer to manufacturer's recommendations on dosing and use in children.)

Pregnancy Considerations
Curettage, cryotherapy, incision, and expression are safe treatments during pregnancy. Do not use podophyllin, podofiliox, tretinoin, or imiquimod because they may cause serious harm to the fetus.

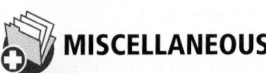 **FOLLOW-UP**

PROGNOSIS
- In immunocompetent hosts, molluscum contagiosum is self-limited and resolves on average in 3–12 months (range = 2 months–4 years)
- Lesions are difficult to treat in immunocompromised hosts and may persist for years.

COMPLICATIONS
- Secondary infection
- Scarring, hyper/hypopigmentation

PATIENT MONITORING
Dependant on choice of treatment

REFERENCES
1. Brown J, et al. Childhood molluscum contagiosum. *Int J Dermatol*. 2006;45:93–99.
2. Dohil MA, et al. The epidemiology of molluscum contagiosum in children. *J Am Acad Dermatol*. 2006;54:47–54.
3. Stulberg DL, Hutchinson AG. Molluscum contagiosum and warts. *Am Fam Physician*. 2003;67:1233–1240.
4. Ting PT, Dytoc MT. Therapy of external anogenital warts and molluscum contagiosum: A literature review. *Dermatol Ther*. 2004;17:68–101.
5. Valentine CL, Diven D. Treatment modalities for molluscum contagiosum. *Dermatol Ther*. 2000;13:285–289.

MISCELLANEOUS

CODES

ICD9-CM
078.0 Molluscum contagiosum

PATIENT TEACHING

Prevention
Molluscum contagiosum is spread by direct skin-to-skin contact. It can also be spread to others by sharing baths, towels, and pools. Avoid scratching to prevent autoinoculation. If you are sexually active and have lesions in the groin or genital area you can reduce the likelihood of spreading the rash to your partner by refraining from sexual contact or by using condoms.

M

MONONUCLEOSIS

W. Franklin Sease, Jr., MD

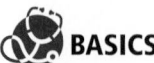

BASICS

DESCRIPTION
- Infectious mononucleosis, the classic triad of fever, lymphadenopathy, and pharyngitis, is caused by the Epstein-Barr virus (EBV) in ~80% of cases. Most other cases are due to cytomegalovirus (CMV) infection.
- Symptoms result from effects on the lymphoreticular system.
- Transmission via oropharyngeal secretions and saliva is often attributed to kissing.
- Incubation period is 30–50 days, with the Epstein-Barr virus replicating in nasopharyngeal epithelial cells.
- System(s) Affected: Cardiovascular; Gastrointestinal; Hematologic/Lymphatic/Immunologic; Nervous; Pulmonary
- Synonym(s): Mono; Infectious mononucleosis (IM)

ALERT
Pediatric Considerations
- Children have subclinical or mild infections.
- Most adolescents have clinically apparent infections.

Pregnancy Considerations
Mono-like syndromes can occur with toxoplasmosis, acute HIV, and CMV and have potential pregnancy complications.

GENERAL PREVENTION
- Avoid saliva of infected people.
- DNA vaccine research in progress
- No blood donation for at least 6 months

EPIDEMIOLOGY
- Predominant age: Ages 10–19; female patients 2 years earlier than male
- Predominant sex: Male = Female

Incidence
- Ages 10–30, up to 8 cases per 1,000 persons per year
- By young adult life, up to 95% of people are seropositive.
- No clear seasonal pattern.

RISK FACTORS
- High school and college students
- Kissing
- Blood transfusion ("post pump perfusion syndrome"), due to Cytomegalovirus transmission

Genetics
Unknown; possibly related to severity of illness

ETIOLOGY
Epstein-Barr virus: A double-stranded DNA herpes virus (~80%); others due to Cytomegalovirus

ASSOCIATED CONDITIONS
Streptococcal pharyngitis often present (30%); finding does not rule out mononucleosis and deserves appropriate treatment.

DIAGNOSIS

SIGNS AND SYMPTOMS
- In most cases, the clinical triad of sore throat (the most frequent complaint), fever, and lymphadenopathy (the most frequent finding) is present.
- Lymphadenopathy (94%)
- Pharyngitis (84%)
- Sore throat (82%)
- Fever (76%)
- Malaise (57%)
- Splenomegaly (52%)
- Headache (51%)
- Anorexia (21%)
- Myalgias (20%)
- Chills (16%)
- Nausea, hepatomegaly, palatal exanthem, rash, jaundice, abdominal discomfort, cough, vomiting, arthralgias (all <15%)

History
Classically the worst sore throat of the patient's life

Physical Exam
Lymphadenopathy, pharyngitis, and fever are most common.

TESTS
- Heterophil antibody tests (Monospot or differential absorption): 40% of cases are positive in 1st week, 90% of cases are positive in 3rd week. Not helpful in children < age 5. May remain positive for 2 years in up to 20% of infected individuals.
- Specific Epstein-Barr virus titers (use in heterophil negative or complications): Elevated in >90% of cases at the onset of the disease
  - Viral capsid antigen (VCA): IgG and IgM peak at 3–4 weeks. IgG then declines, but persists for life. IgM declines rapidly and is undetectable by 3 months. High persisting IgG suggests remote infection, systemic lupus, chronic renal failure, Burkitt lymphoma, nasopharyngeal cancer, leukemia, sarcoidosis, cancer, AIDS, Hodgkin lymphoma, rheumatoid arthritis, and other immunodeficient states.
  - Early antigen (EA): Occurs in 70–90%, persists for 2–3 months. May persist in up to 20% of remote infections. High persisting titers might suggest pregnancy, immunodeficient states, Hodgkin lymphoma, lymphoma, leukemia, AIDS, Burkitt lymphoma, or nasopharyngeal carcinoma.
  - Epstein-Barr nuclear antigen (EBNA): Develops after 2 months and persists indefinitely. E antigen in mononucleosis primarily. K antigen in nasopharyngeal carcinoma primarily. Absence suggests immunodeficiency.

Lab
- Complete blood chemistry and LFTs
  - Relative lymphocytosis (>50%)
  - Atypical lymphocytosis (10–20% or more) Atypical monocytosis (90%)
  - Thrombocytopenia (50%)
- Elevated liver function test results (90%)

Imaging
- Ultrasound if clinically important to diagnose or follow splenomegaly
- CT best if splenic injury is suspected

Diagnostic Procedures/Surgery
Laparotomy with unstable patient with splenic or hepatic concerns

Pathological Findings
- B-cell lymphocytes infected
- Polyclonal proliferation of B cells
- Strong T-cell response

DIFFERENTIAL DIAGNOSIS
- Cytomegalovirus
- Toxoplasmosis
- Rubella
- Adenovirus
- Herpes viruses
- Drug adverse effects
- Streptococcal pharyngitis
- Viral tonsillitis
- Diphtheria
- Viral hepatitis
- Lymphoma or leukemia
- Human herpesvirus-6
- Roseola
- Mumps
- Primary HIV infection

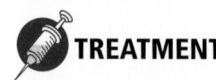

TREATMENT

INITIAL STABILIZATION
Outpatient usually; 95% of patients recover uneventfully without specific treatment.

GENERAL MEASURES
- No specific treatment
- Quarantine not indicated
- General supportive measures
- Gargles/Lozenges
- Avoid vigorous splenic palpation.

Diet
Liquids then soft as tolerated

Activity
Rest (bed rest possibly during acute phase)

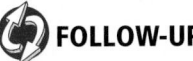 ## MEDICATION (DRUGS)

First Line
- Analgesics
  - Acetaminophen (Tylenol)
  - Codeine
- Consider stool softeners to avoid constipation and its associated intra-abdominal pressure.

Second Line
- Antibiotics for secondary infections only (1)[C]
- Steroids may be indicated in certain complications only: Prednisone, 40–80 mg/d (1–2 mg/kg), taper over 5–7 days. Consider in threatened airway obstruction, hemolytic anemia, and thrombocytopenia. No evidence that steroids will decrease splenomegaly (2)[C]
- Specific antiviral therapy is of no benefit to lessen symptoms; only decreases oral shedding of the virus during time of administration. (3)[B]
- Contraindications: Aspirin/acetylsalicylic acid (associated with Reye syndrome)
- Precautions: Refer to the manufacturer's profile for each drug.
- Significant possible interactions: Refer to the manufacturer's profile for each drug.

SURGERY
- Splenic rupture: Inpatient observation, with the ability to perform splenectomy if indicated
- Airway compromise: Tonsillectomy or tracheostomy where clinically necessary

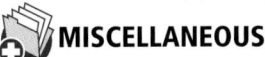 ## FOLLOW-UP

PROGNOSIS
- Fever subsides in ~10 days.
- Adenopathy and splenomegaly subside in ~4 weeks.
- Children should be able to return to school when signs of infection have decreased, appetite returns, and alertness, strength, and sense of well-being allow.
- Return to sports is recommended after 4 weeks if noncontact or 7 weeks if splenic enlargement is suspected or contact sports. Because identification of splenomegaly is unreliable on physical exam, ultrasound should be considered to assist in determining when someone may return to activity.
- Spontaneous splenic rupture typically occurs within the 1st 3 weeks of illness.
- Death is uncommon (splenic rupture, blood dyscrasias, hypersplenism, or encephalitis).
- Potential role in some malignancies, especially in context of immune suppression.

COMPLICATIONS
- Chronic Epstein-Barr virus infections (i.e., chronic fatigue syndrome, which diagnosis remains highly controversial)
- Splenic rupture (rare, 0.1–0.5% of patients with proven mononucleosis)
- Hemolytic anemia (mild)
- Thrombocytopenia
- Hemolytic-uremic syndrome
- Seizures and other neurologic abnormalities
- Nerve palsies
- Meningoencephalitis
- Reye syndrome
- Myocarditis/electrocardiographic changes
- Airway obstruction
- Acute interstitial nephritis

PATIENT MONITORING
- Reevaluate as needed based on clinical findings
  - Airway concerns
  - Splenomegaly
- Preferable documentation of resolution of splenomegaly before resuming contact sports

REFERENCES

1. Wick MJ, Woronzoff-Dashkoff KP, McGlennen RC. The molecular characterization of fatal infectious mononucleosis. *Am J Clin Pathol*. 2002;117: 582–588.
2. Ebell MH. Epstein-Barr infectious Mononucleosis. *Am Fam Phys*. 2004;70:1279–1287.
3. Torre D, Tambini R. Acyclovir for treatment of infectious mononucleosis: A meta-analysis. *Scand J Infect Dis*. 1999;31:543–547.
4. Maki DG, Reich RM. Infectious mononucleosis in the athlete. Diagnosis, complications, and management. *Ame J Sports Med*. 1982;10: 162–173.
5. Waniger K, Harcke T. Determination of safe return to play for athletes recovering from infectious mononucleosis: A review of the literature. *Clin J Sports Med*. 2005;15:410–416.

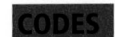 ## MISCELLANEOUS

- 70–90% shed virus 2–6 months after initial infection.
- 20–30% of affected people shed virus after 6 months.
- 10–20% culture rate from the oropharynx of normal adults and 50% from renal transplant and HIV-positive patients
- See also: Epstein-Barr virus infections

CODES

ICD9-CM
075 Infectious mononucleosis

PATIENT TEACHING
- Convalescence may take several weeks.
- Avoid stress.
- Discuss feasibility of continuing with school or work.
- Emphasize risk of splenic rupture from contact sports.

Diet
To ease throat discomfort, patient may want to drink milk shakes, fruit juices, and consume soft foods.

Activity
- Avoid contact sports, heavy lifting, and strenuous athletics as long as splenomegaly persists. (4)[C]
- Return to vigorous activity before 3 weeks from onset of symptoms should have documented resolution of splenomegaly (difficult because spleen sizes are variable).
- Because the majority of splenic ruptures have occurred between 3 and 21 days, most clinicians feel comfortable with return to activity as tolerated after 4 weeks. (5)[C]

 See Corresponding Diagnostic Algorithm

 See Patient Handout on CD

M

MORTON NEUROMA (INTERDIGITAL NEUROMA)

Matthew J. Plante, MD

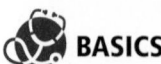 BASICS

DESCRIPTION
- Perineal fibrosis of the common digital nerve as it passes between metatarsals. The most common site is the interspace between the 3rd and 4th metatarsals. The interspace between the 3rd and 2nd metatarsals is the 2nd most common site.
- System(s) Affected: Musculoskeletal; Nervous
- Synonym(s): Plantar digital neuritis

GENERAL PREVENTION
- Wear proper fitting shoes.
- Avoid high heels and narrow toe boxes.

EPIDEMIOLOGY
- Mean age: 45–50 years
- Predominant sex: Female > Male (8:1)

Incidence
Unknown

Prevalence
Unknown

RISK FACTORS
- High-heeled shoes: Cause more weight to be transferred to the front of the foot
- Tight-toed shoes (tight toe boxes): Cause lateral compression
- Pes planus (flat feet): Causes nerve to be pulled more medially, which increases irritation
- Obesity
- Ballet dancing, basketball, aerobics, tennis, running, and similar stressful activity

PATHOPHYSIOLOGY
- Lateral plantar nerve combines with part of medial plantar nerve. The 2 nerves combine, creating a nerve with larger diameter than nerves going to other digits.
- Nerve lies in subcutaneous tissue, deep to the fat pad of foot, just superficial to the digital artery and vein.
- Overlying the nerve is the strong, deep transverse metatarsal ligament, which holds the metatarsal bones together.
- With each step the patient takes, the inflamed nerve becomes compressed between the ground and the deep transverse metatarsal ligament.

ETIOLOGY
- Excessive stress of the forefoot
- Repetitive trauma
- Congenitally enlarged plantar digital nerve

DIAGNOSIS

SIGNS AND SYMPTOMS
- Most common complaint is pain localized to interspace between 3rd and 4th toes
- Pain is less severe when nonweightbearing
- Pain, cramping, or numbness of the forefoot with weightbearing or immediately after strenuous foot exertion
- Radiation of pain to the toes
- Pain is relieved by removing the shoe and massaging the foot.
- Patients often state: "Feels like I am walking on a marble."

Physical Exam
- A palpable nodule in the metatarsal interspace is an occasional finding.
- Positive Mulder sign: See "Diagnostic Procedures."
- Intense pain on pressure between metatarsal heads.
- Assess midfoot motion and digital motion to determine if arthritis or synovitis.
- Palpate along metatarsal shafts to assess for metatarsalgia or stress fractures.

TESTS
Imaging
- Radiographs may help rule out osseous pathology if diagnosis is in question, but films are usually normal in patients with a Morton neuroma.
- Ultrasound shows hypoechoic nodule between the metatarsal interspace. Ultrasound had a 65% specificity and a 98% sensitivity for Morton neuromas. Ultrasound is not good at assessing the size of the lesion (1)[C].
- MRI is used to ensure that compression is not caused by a malignant tumor in the foot. MRI is helpful in determining how much of the nerve to surgically resect. MRI has a sensitivity of 83% and a specificity of 99% (1)[C].

Diagnostic Procedures/Surgery
- Mulder sign: A "click" and pain produced by squeezing the metatarsal heads together and simultaneously compressing the neuroma between the thumb and index finger of the other hand
- Corticosteroid injection can significantly reduce symptoms. Inject 1–2 mL of lidocaine and 0.5–1 mL of dexamethasone just proximal to the metatarsal heads. More that 1 injection is often needed, usually once a week for 3 weeks (2).

Pathological Findings
Chronic fibrosis and thickening of the digital nerve

DIFFERENTIAL DIAGNOSIS
- Stress fracture
- Hammer toe
- Metatarsophalangeal synovitis
- Metatarsalgia
- Arthritis
- Bursitis
- Foreign body

TREATMENT

INITIAL STABILIZATION
Outpatient

GENERAL MEASURES
- Flat shoes with a roomy toe box (3)[C]
- Metatarsal pads placed immediately proximal to the two involved metatarsal heads (3)[C]
- Corticosteroid injection into the dorsal part of the foot with medium- or long-acting steroid (e.g., betamethasone, methylprednisolone) mixed with local anesthetic (e.g., lidocaine) (3)[C]
- If patient has pes planus, an arch support is used (3)[C].
- Literature suggests wide variability in success rate (50–98%) (3).

Diet
No restrictions

Activity
Modifying, shortening, or temporarily discontinuing activities involving standing, walking, or running

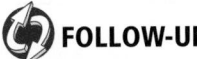 **MEDICATION (DRUGS)**

First Line
- Injectable steroids (e.g., betamethasone phosphate/acetate or methylprednisolone): Use if conservative measures fail (2,4)[C].
- Contraindications: Refer to the manufacturer's literature.
- Precautions: Refer to the manufacturer's literature.
- Significant possible interactions: Refer to the manufacturer's literature.

Second Line
- NSAIDs for temporary symptom relief (1,2)[C].
- Precautions: Refer to the manufacturer's literature.

SURGERY
Surgical removal of the neuroma in refractory cases; excision under local anesthesia (5,6)[C]

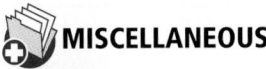 **FOLLOW-UP**

DISPOSITION
Issues for Referral
Continued pain despite conservative treatments and injections

PROGNOSIS
- 40–50% improve after 3 months of conservative treatment
- 45–50% improve after steroid injection
- 96% improve after surgery

COMPLICATIONS
Knee and hip pain related to a change in gait

PATIENT MONITORING
If no improvement after 3 months of conservative treatment, consider corticosteroid injection. Repeat injection if no improvement after 2–4 weeks.

REFERENCES

1. Sharp RJ, et al. The role of MRI and ultrasound imaging in Morton's neuroma and the effect of size of lesion on symptoms. *Br J Bone Joint Surg.* 2003;85:999–1005.
2. Tallia AF, Cardone DA. Diagnostic and therapeutic injection of the ankle and foot. *Am Fam Physician.* 2003;68:1356–1362.
3. Thompson CE, Gibson JNA, Martin D. Interventions for the treatment of Morton's neuroma. *Cochrane Database Sys Rev.* 2005.
4. Wu KK. Morton's interdigital neuroma: A clinical review of its etiology, treatment, and results. *J Foot Ankle Surg.* 1996;35:112–119.
5. Hirschberg GG. A simple cure for Morton's neuralgia. *J Am Podiatr Med Assoc.* 2000;90:100–101.

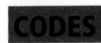 **MISCELLANEOUS**

 CODES

ICD9-CM
355.6 Lesion of plantar nerve

PATIENT TEACHING
Wearing of properly fitted comfortable shoes

See Patient Handout on CD

M

MOTION SICKNESS

Courtney Jarvis, PharmD

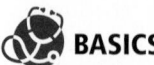 BASICS

DESCRIPTION
- Not a true sickness, but a normal response to an abnormal situation in which sensory conflict about body motion exists among visual receptors, vestibular receptors, and body proprioceptors. Can also be induced when patterns of motion differ from those previously experienced.
- System(s) Affected: Nervous
- Synonym(s): Car sickness; Sea sickness; Air sickness; Space sickness; Physiologic vertigo

GENERAL PREVENTION
See "General Measures"

ALERT
Pediatric Considerations
- Rare in children <2 years
- Incidence peaks between age 3 and 12 years
- Antihistamines may cause excitation in children

Geriatric Considerations
- Age confers some resistance to motion sickness.
- Elderly at increased risk of anticholinergic side effects from treatment

Pregnancy Considerations
- Pregnant patients more likely to experience motion sickness
- Treat with medications thought to be safe during morning sickness (meclizine, dimenhydrinate)

Prevalence
Females > Males

RISK FACTORS
- Motion (auto, plane, boat, amusement rides)
- Travel
- Visual stimuli (i.e., moving horizon)
- Poor ventilation (fumes, smoke, carbon monoxide)
- Emotions (fear, anxiety)
- Zero gravity
- Pregnancy, menstruation, oral contraceptive use
- History of migraine headaches
- Other illness or poor health

ETIOLOGY
- Precise etiology unknown; thought to be due to a mismatch of vestibular and visual sensations.
- Nausea and vomiting occur as a result of increased levels of dopamine and acetylcholine, which stimulate chemoreceptor trigger zone and vomiting center in CNS.

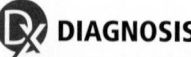 DIAGNOSIS

SIGNS AND SYMPTOMS
- Nausea
- Vomiting
- Diaphoresis
- Pallor
- Hypersalivation
- Yawning
- Hyperventilation
- Anxiety
- Panic
- Malaise
- Fatigue
- Weakness
- Confusion
- Dizziness

DIFFERENTIAL DIAGNOSIS
- Mountain sickness
- Vestibular disease
- Gastroenteritis
- Metabolic disorders
- Toxin exposure

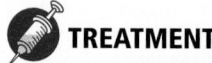 TREATMENT

- Following guidelines under general prevention category to prevent motion sickness (1)[C]
  - Premedicate prior to travel with either antidopaminergic, anticholinergic, or antihistamine agent (1)[A]
  - For extended travel, consider treatment with scopolamine transdermal patch (2)[A]
  - 2nd generation (nonsedating) antihistamines are not effective at preventing motion sickness (3)[B]
- Conflicting data exists on the efficacy of acupressure for nausea vomiting associated with motion sickness (4)[B]

GENERAL MEASURES
- Minimize exposure (seat in middle of plane or boat).
- Improve ventilation, avoid noxious stimuli.
- Semirecumbent seating
- Fix vision on horizon, avoid fixation on moving objects, keep eyes fixed on still, distant objects.
- Avoid reading while actively traveling.
- Minimize food intake prior to travel, avoid alcohol.
- Increase air flow around face.
- Acupressure on point PC6 shown to reduce feelings of nausea, but not incidence of vomiting, during pregnancy, after surgery, and in cancer chemotherapy. However, conflicting evidence of efficacy found for motion sickness. Point PC6 (Neiguan on pericardium meridian): 2 cm proximal from transverse crease of palmar side of wrist, between tendons of m. palmaris longus and m. flexor radialis.

Diet
- Decrease oral intake or take frequent small feedings.
- Avoid alcohol.

Activity
- Semirecumbent seating
- Avoid reading while actively traveling.

SPECIAL THERAPY
Complementary and Alternative Medicine
Ginger: 940 mg or 1 g; take 4 hours before travel (evidence controversial)

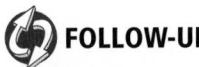 **MEDICATION (DRUGS)**

First Line

- Scopolamine transdermal patch: Apply 2.5 cm² (4 mg) patch behind ear at least 4 hours (preferably 6–12 hours) before travel and replace every 3 days
- Dimenhydrinate (Dramamine): Take 0.5–1 hour before travel
  - Adults and adolescents: 50–100 mg q4–6h, maximum 400 mg/d
  - Children 6–12 years old: 25–50 mg q6–8h, maximum 150 mg/d
  - Children 2–6 years old: 12.5–25 mg q6–8h, maximum 75 mg/d
- Meclizine (Antivert): Take 0.5–1 hour before travel
  - Adults and adolescents >12 years: 12.5–25 mg q12–24h
- Cyclizine (Marezine): Take 0.5–1 hour before travel
  - Adults and adolescents: 50 mg q4–6h, maximum 200 mg/d
  - Children 6–12 years old: 25 mg up to t.i.d.
- Promethazine (Phenergan): Take 0.5–1 hour before travel
  - Adults and adolescents: 25 mg q12h
    - 25–50 mg IM if already developed severe motion sickness
  - Children 2–12 years old: 0.5 mg/kg q12h (maximum 25 mg b.i.d.)
- Contraindications: Patients at risk for acute angle closure glaucoma
- Precautions
  - Young children
  - Elderly
  - Pregnancy
  - Urinary obstruction
  - Pyloric-duodenal obstruction
- Adverse reactions
  - Drowsiness
  - Dry mouth
  - Blurred vision
  - Confusion
  - Headache
  - Urinary retention
- Significant possible interactions
  - Sedatives (antihistamines, alcohol, antidepressants)
  - Anticholinergics (belladonna alkaloids)

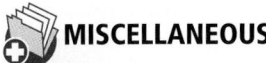 **FOLLOW-UP**

PROGNOSIS

- Symptoms should resolve when motion exposure ends.
- Resistance to motion sickness seems to increase with age.

COMPLICATIONS

- Hypotension
- Dehydration
- Depression
- Panic
- Syncope

REFERENCES

1. Committee to advise on tropical medicine and travel. Statement on motion sickness. *CCDR*. 2003;29:1–12.
2. Spinks AB, Wasiak J, Villanueva EV, Bernath V. Scopolamine for preventing and treating motion sickness. *Cochrane Database of Systematic Rev*. 2006;3: No pages.
3. Cheung BS, Heskin R, Hofer KD. Failure of cetirizine and fexofenadine to prevent motion sickness. *Ann Pharmacother*. 2003;37:173–177.
4. Streitberger K, Ezzo J, Schneider A. Acupuncture for nausea and vomiting: An update of clinical and experimental studies. *Auton Neuro*. 2006;129:107–117.

MISCELLANEOUS

CODES

ICD9-CM
994.6 Motion sickness

M

MRSA SKIN INFECTIONS

Stephen A. Martin, MD, EdM
Paul Belliveau, PharmD, RPh

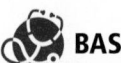 **BASICS**

DESCRIPTION

- Community-associated methicillin-resistant *Staphylococcus aureus* (CA-MRSA) has properties that allow it to create skin and soft-tissue infections (SSTIs), often in otherwise healthy hosts. It has a different virulence and disease pattern from hospital-acquired MRSA (HA-MRSA).
- MRSA infections acquired by persons who have not been recently (<1 year) hospitalized or had a medical procedure (e.g., dialysis, surgery, catheters) are known as CA-MRSA infections.
- The prevalence of CA-MRSA is rapidly increasing in the US
- CA-MRSA typically causes mild-to-moderate SSTIs, particularly abscesses, furuncles, and carbuncles. Severe disease from CA-MRSA is less frequent, but can include necrotizing pneumonia with abscesses, necrotizing fasciitis, septic thrombophlebitis, and sepsis.
- Although much less frequent, HA-MRSA can still cause SSTIs in the community, and clinicians should be alert to this possibility. 1 study showed no significant difference in hospitalization rates among CA-MRSA, HA-MRSA, and MSSA.
- System(s) Affected: Skin; Soft Tissue

GENERAL PREVENTION

- Prior research has established colonization, particularly of the anterior nares, as a risk factor for subsequent *S. aureus* infection. It is not yet clear whether this is also the case for CA-MRSA.
- Research for a vaccine is underway.

EPIDEMIOLOGY

- Predominant age: All ages, generally younger
- Predominant sex: Female > Male

Incidence
18.0–26/100,000/year (2001–02)

Prevalence
- Still significantly affected by local epidemiology.
- 25–30% of US population is colonized with *S. aureus*; 1% is colonized with MRSA.
- CA-MRSA was isolated in 59% of skin and soft tissue infections presenting to 11 emergency departments (range 15–74%).
- Accounts for up to 75% of all community staphylococcal infections in children.

RISK FACTORS

- Although several factors are associated with CA-MRSA, their presence or absence cannot reliably predict CA-MRSA itself; in one study, almost 1/2 the patients with CA-MRSA had no established risk factor.
- Any antibiotic use in past month
- Presence of an abscess
- Reported spider bite
- History of MRSA infection
- Close contact with a similar infection
- Children, particularly in day care centers
- Competitive athletes
- Incarceration
- High prevalence in the community
- Hospitalization in the past 12 months

ETIOLOGY

First noted in 1980, CA-MRSA's current US epidemic began in 1999. The USA 300 clone is predominant. CA-MRSA is currently distinguished from HA-MRSA by

- Lack of a multidrug-resistant phenotype.
- Presence of exotoxin virulence factors
- Type IV staphylococcus cassette cartridge (contains the methicillin-resistance gene *mecA*)

ASSOCIATED CONDITIONS
Many patients are otherwise healthy.

 DIAGNOSIS

SIGNS AND SYMPTOMS

- Erythema
- Increased warmth
- Tenderness
- Swelling
- Fluctuance
- Infected wound
- Folliculitis, pustular lesions
- Appearance like an insect or spider bite
- Tissue necrosis

History
- Potential risk factors
- Complaint of "spider bite"

Physical Exam
Examination consistent with a furuncle/carbuncle (boils) or abscess. An isolated cellulitis is also possible, although less common with *S. aureus*.

TESTS

Lab
- Wound cultures are essential for diagnosis.
- Susceptibility testing; many labs use oxacillin instead of methicillin.
- A "D-zone disk-diffusion test" evaluates for inducible clindamycin resistance in CA-MRSA resistant to erythromycin.

Imaging
- In unclear cases, ultrasound may help delineate an abscess.
- Although CT or MRI may show fascial plane edema in necrotizing fasciitis, they should not delay intervention.

Diagnostic Procedures/Surgery
Purulent lesions should be incised and drained (I&D), cultured, and tested for susceptibilities.

DIFFERENTIAL DIAGNOSIS
Skin and soft-tissue infections due to another cause.

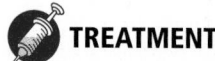 **TREATMENT**

Evidence for the treatment of CA-MRSA SSTIs has not been systematically evaluated in randomized controlled trials. Recommendations are based on results of small case series, anecdotal reports, and anticipated susceptibility profiles (1)[C].

- To date, studies do not support use of agents to eliminate MRSA colonization for patients with infection or their close contacts (2)[B].

INITIAL STABILIZATION

- Most CA-MRSA infections are localized SSTI that do not require hospitalization or vancomycin therapy.
- Initial empirical antibiotic coverage should be based on local CA-MRSA prevalence and individual patient risk factors (3)[C].

GENERAL MEASURES

- For purulent infections, basic principles include surgical drainage and debulking, wound culture, and narrow-spectrum antimicrobials. Successful I&D may have more of an effect than antibiotics in mild cases for both adults and children and is important in general. Moist heat may work for small furuncles.
- Modify therapy as necessary based on culture and susceptibility testing.
- Determine if household or other close contacts have SSTI or other infections, and facilitate evaluation.
- Treat underlying condition (e.g., tinea pedis).

Activity
- Restrict contact if wound cannot be covered
- Elevation of the affected area

Nursing
Contact precautions

MEDICATION (DRUGS)

ALERT

- CA-MRSA is resistant to β-lactams (including oral cephalosporins and antistaphylococcal penicillins) and often macrolides/azalides.
- Although most CA-MRSA isolates are susceptible to rifampin, this drug should never be used as a single agent because of concerns for rapid emergence of resistance. The role of combination therapy with rifampin in CA-MRSA SSTIs is not clearly defined.
- Older fluoroquinolones (ciprofloxacin) possess unreliable activity against CA-MRSA isolates; susceptible isolates may rapidly develop resistance. Although newer fluoroquinolones possess better activity against gram-positive organisms, resistance concerns preclude routine use of such agents for CA-MRSA SSTIs.
- Although CA-MRSA isolates are susceptible to vancomycin, oral vancomycin cannot be used for CA-MRSA SSTIs because this drug has negligible enteral absorption.
- Tetracyclines and TMP-SMX do not cover Group A *streptococcus* (GAS)

First Line

CA-MRSA SSTIs: Treat with a 7–14 day course of one of the following agents (duration of therapy depends on severity and clinical response)

- Clindamycin: 300–450 mg PO t.i.d. (10–20 mg/kg/d PO in 3 divided doses for children), taken with full glass of water. Check D-zone test (avoid if positive).
- Doxycycline or minocycline: 100 mg PO b.i.d. (children >8 years and <45 kg; 2–5 mg/kg/d PO in 1–2 divided doses, not to exceed 200 mg/d; children >8 years and >45 kg: use adult dosing), taken with a full glass of water
- Trimethoprim/sulfamethoxazole: DS (160 mg TMP and 800 mg of SMX) 1 tablet PO b.i.d. daily (8–12 mg/kg/d of trimethoprim component in 2 divided doses for children)

Pediatric Considerations

- Tetracyclines not recommended <8 years
- TMP-SMX not recommended <2 months

Pregnancy Considerations

- Tetracyclines are contraindicated
- TMP-SMX not recommended in 3rd trimester.

ALERT

- The above medication options are *not sufficient* for treatment of severe CA-MRSA SSTIs requiring hospitalization or for HA-MRSA SSTIs. For such infections, consider one of the following (4)[A]

- Vancomycin: Generally 1 g IV q12h [30 mg/kg/d IV in 2 divided doses] (children: 40 mg/kg/d IV in 4 divided doses)
- Linezolid: 600 mg IV/PO b.i.d. (children <5 years of age, 30 mg/kg/d in 3 divided doses; 20 mg/kg/d IV/PO in 2 divided doses for children 5–11 years of age; children >11 years of age, use adult dosing)
- Daptomycin: 4 mg/kg/d IV (safety/efficacy not established in patients <18 years of age) if no pulmonary involvement

SURGERY

Progression to serious SSTIs, including necrotizing fasciitis, is possible and mandates prompt surgical evaluation.

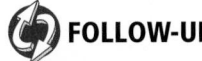 FOLLOW-UP

DISPOSITION

Depends on severity of SSTI, presence of SSTI complications (sepsis, necrotizing fasciitis), and comorbidities

Admission Criteria

Consider admission in patients either

- Systemically ill (e.g., febrile) with stable comorbidities, or
- Systemically well with comorbidities that may delay or complicate resolution of their SSTI

Discharge Criteria

If admitted for IV therapy

- Afebrile for 24 hours
- Clinically improved
- Able to take oral medication
- Has adequate social support and available for outpatient follow-up

Issues for Referral

In addition to inpatient concerns, consider consultation with an infectious disease specialist in cases of

- Refractory CA-MRSA infection
- Plan to eradicate colonization

PROGNOSIS

- In outpatients, improvement should occur within 48 hours.
- Data are limited as to risk of recurrence.

COMPLICATIONS

- Necrotizing pneumonia or empyema (after an influenzalike illness)
- Necrotizing fasciitis
- Sepsis syndrome
- Pyomyositis and osteomyelitis
- Purpura fulminans
- Disseminated septic emboli
- Endocarditis

PATIENT MONITORING

For outpatients

- Return promptly if patient develops systemic symptoms, worsening local symptoms, or does not improve within 48 hours.
- Consider a follow-up within 48 hours of initial visit to assess response and review culture.

REFERENCES

1. Rybak MJ, LaPlante KL. Community-associated methicillin-resistant *Staphylococcus aureus*: A review. *Phamacotherapy*. 2005;25(1):74–85.
2. Loeb M, Main C, Walker-Dilks C, Eady A. Antimicrobial drugs for treating methicillin-resistant *Staphylococcus aureus* colonization. *Cochrane Database Syst Rev*. 2003(4):CD003340.
3. Kowalski TJ, Berbari EF, Osmon DR. Epidemiology, treatment, and prevention of community-acquired methicillin-resistant *Staphylococcus aureus* infections. *Mayo Clin Proc*. 2005;80(9): 1201–1207.
4. Stevens DL, Bisno AL, Chambers HF, et al. Practice guidelines for the diagnosis and management of skin and soft-tissue infections. *Clin Infect Dis*. 2005;41(10):1373–1406.
5. Grayson ML. The treatment triangle for staphylococcal infections. *N Engl J Med*. 2006; 355(7):724–727.
6. Weller T. MRSA (Treatment). *Clin Evid*. Epub 01 June 2006 (based on July 2005 search).

ADDITIONAL READING

- Gorwitz RJ et al. Strategies for clinical management of MRSA in the community: Summary of an experts' meeting convened by the Centers for Disease Control and Prevention. 2006. Available at
- http://www.cdc.gov/ncidod/dhqp/ar_mrsa_ca.html.

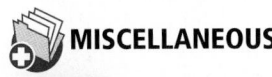 MISCELLANEOUS

CODES

ICD9-CM

- 682.9 Cellulitis/Abscess
- 680.9 Furuncle
- 041.11 Infection, *S. aureus*
- 10060 Incision and drainage

PATIENT TEACHING

- Keep wounds that are draining covered with clean, dry, bandages.
- Clean hands regularly with soap and water or alcohol-based gel. Hot shower daily with soap.
- Do not share items that may be contaminated.

M

MULTIPLE ENDOCRINE NEOPLASIA (MEN)

Caroline K. Buckway, MD

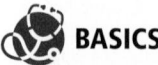 **BASICS**

DESCRIPTION

- 3 subtypes are identified
  - MEN1: Parathyroid glands (hyperparathyroidism: 90% by age 40), pancreatic islets (gastrinoma, insulinoma, glucagonoma, VIPoma, or pancreatic polypeptide-producing tumor), and anterior pituitary (most commonly prolactinoma and GH-secreting tumors)
  - MEN2A: Medullary thyroid carcinoma (90%), pheochromocytoma (50%), and hyperparathyroidism 20–30%)
  - MEN2B: Medullary thyroid carcinoma (90%) and pheochromocytoma, marfanoid habitus, and mucosal and intestinal ganglioneuromatosis
- System(s) Affected: Endocrine/Metabolic; Gastrointestinal
- Synonym(s): Multiple endocrine adenomatosis (MEA); Wermer syndrome (MEN 1); Sipple syndrome (MEN 2); Wagenmann-Froboese syndrome

GENERAL PREVENTION

- No prevention except for prophylactic thyroidectomy in children with MEN2A by age 5 and with MEN2B by age 1
- Monitor for tumor expression (see "Lab").

EPIDEMIOLOGY

Predominant sex: Male > Female (2:1)

Prevalence

- Adults: 0.02–0.2 per 1000
- Children: Data not available

ALERT

Pediatric Considerations

- MEN1 onset typically < age 4
- In MEN2, medullary thyroid carcinoma presents in childhood.
  - MEN2A mutation testing of RET by age 5 years. If positive, prophylactic thyroidectomy with lymph node dissection.
  - MEN2B, thyroidectomy should be done by age 1 year.

Geriatric Considerations

Present < age 40

Pregnancy Considerations

May occur in patients after treatment of prolactinoma

RISK FACTORS

- Significant family history. Screen for MEN2 in all medullary thyroid carcinoma.
- Most hyperparathyroidism, pituitary tumors, and pancreatic islet cell tumors are sporadic, rarely related to MEN1.

Genetics

- Autosomal dominant
- Gene responsible for MEN1: Tumor-suppressor gene located on chromosome 11q13 encoding the protein menin. Patients have germline mutations and develop tumors when a 2nd hit to other allele occurs; 10% of mutations arise de novo; 10–20% of mutations are not identifiable.
- Gene responsible for MEN2: Protooncogene RET on chromosome 10q11.2. De novo mutations in 5% of MEN 2A and 50% of MEN 2B. No mutation identified in 2–5%
- Degree of penetrance of MEN1 at age 20 is ~43%.
- MEN2A diagnosed by mutation testing for RET by age 5 years and by age 1 year in MEN2B

ETIOLOGY

- MEN1: Lack of functional menin
- MEN2: RET mutation

ASSOCIATED CONDITIONS

- MEN1: Tumors of skin, adipose tissue, adrenal gland, and thymus
- MEN2A: Cutaneous lichen amyloidosis and Hirschsprung's disease

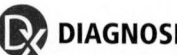 **DIAGNOSIS**

SIGNS AND SYMPTOMS

- Hypercalcemia in hyperparathyroidism
- Hypoglycemia in insulinomas
- Abdominal pain in gastrinomas

TESTS

Lab

Investigations of the different tumor expression patterns: (1)

- MEN1
  - Beginning at age 5: Annual fasting glucose, insulin, prolactin, and insulin-like growth factor 1
  - Beginning at age 8: Annual calcium, parathyroid hormone
  - Beginning at age 20: Annual gastrin, chromogranin-A, glucagon, proinsulin
- MEN2
  - Calcitonin, plasma metanephrines
  - *Or* 24-hour urinary catecholamines
  - *Or* metanephrines, calcium, and parathyroid hormone

Imaging

MEN1: Every 3 years

- Abdominal CT scan (beginning at age 20)
- Brain MRI (beginning at age 5)

Diagnostic Procedures/Surgery

Biopsy as indicated

Pathological Findings

- Hyperplasia of parathyroid glands
- Pancreatic microadenomas (mostly in pancreatic tail)
- Duodenal tumors most often are gastrinomas staining positive for gastrin.
- Diffuse hyperplasia of enterochromaffin-like cells is found in stomach.
- Pituitary tumors are generally single in anterior part of gland.
- Medullary thyroid carcinoma
- Unilateral or bilateral pheochromocytoma

DIFFERENTIAL DIAGNOSIS

Isolated tumors versus MEN syndromes

 TREATMENT

GENERAL MEASURES

- Outpatient, with the exception of inpatient stays for surgery
- Gastrinoma: Proton pump inhibitors to reduce acid hypersecretion. Surgery is controversial.
- Insulinoma: Unresectable tumors are treated with diazoxide.
- VIPoma: In unresectable tumors, octreotide may control diarrhea.
- Prolactinoma: Dopamine agonists, such as bromocriptine or cabergoline
- Growth hormone–producing pituitary tumor: Transsphenoidal surgery or therapy with a growth hormone–receptor antagonist

MEDICATION (DRUGS)

- Omeprazole (Prilosec) or other proton pump inhibitors to reduce gastric acid secretion in gastrinomas
- Diazoxide (Hyperstat) to increase blood glucose in insulinomas
- Octreotide (Sandostatin) to decrease diarrhea in VIPomas
- Bromocriptine (Parlodel) or cabergoline (Dostinex) to treat prolactinomas
- Contraindications
  – See the manufacturer's literature for each drug.
- Precautions
  – See the manufacturer's literature for each drug.
- Significant possible interactions
  – See the manufacturer's literature for each drug.

SURGERY

- Parathyroidectomy in hyperparathyroidism
- Thyroidectomy in medullary thyroid carcinoma. Prophylactic thyroidectomy in children with MEN2A by age 5 and with MEN2B by age 1
- Partial pancreatectomy for tumors such as insulinomas, glucagonomas, VIPomas
- Pheochromocytoma requires surgical excision under α-adrenergic blockade starting 7–10 days prior to surgery
- Transsphenoidal pituitary surgery in some cases of pituitary tumors

 FOLLOW-UP

PROGNOSIS

Screening for tumors may reduce mortality, but there is no cure or prevention.

COMPLICATIONS

- Morbidity from development of tumors including nephrocalcinosis, osteoporosis, Zollinger-Ellison syndrome
- Complications from medullary thyroid carcinoma

PATIENT MONITORING

Annual screening, lifelong

REFERENCES

1. Brandi ML, et al. Guidelines for diagnosis and therapy of MEN type 1 and type 2. *J Clin Endocrinol Metab*. 2001;86:5658–5671.
2. Carney JA. Familial multiple endocrine neoplasia: The first 100 years. *Am J Surg Pathol*. 2005;29(2): 254–274.
3. Carling T. Multiple endocrine neoplasia syndrome: Genetic basis for clinical management. *Curr Opin Oncol*. 2005;17(1):7–12.

 MISCELLANEOUS

See also: Gastric malignancy; Hyperparathyroidism; Insulinoma; Marfan syndrome; Pheochromocytoma; Prolactinoma; Thyroid malignant neoplasia

 CODES

ICD9-CM
258.0 Polyglandular activity in multiple endocrine adenomatosis

PATIENT TEACHING

- Counseling re: Inheritance pattern: 50% chance in siblings (unless de novo mutation) and children
- Importance of routine screening for tumor expression

 See Corresponding Diagnostic Algorithm

M

MULTIPLE MYELOMA

Mark C. Leeson, MD

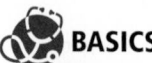 **BASICS**

DESCRIPTION

Multiple myeloma (malignant tumor of plasma cells) is the most common primary malignancy of bone. The disease process encompasses a spectrum of localized and disseminated disease forms.

- System(s) Affected: Hematologic; Lymphatic; Immunologic; Musculoskeletal; Nervous
- Synonym(s): Myeloma; Plasma cell

ALERT

Geriatric Considerations
More common in older adults

EPIDEMIOLOGY

- Predominant age: Ages 40–80 (with a peak incidence in the 70s)
- Predominant sex: Male = Female

Prevalence
~1% of all types of malignant disease and slightly >10% of hematologic malignancies.

Genetics
Occasional familial occurrence, indicating recessive heredity

PATHOPHYSIOLOGY

- Monoclonal tumor cell proliferation that usually reveals monoclonal protein in the serum or urine of >90% of patients.
- Tumor cells characteristic of plasma cells arising from bone marrow

ETIOLOGY
Unknown

ASSOCIATED CONDITIONS

Multiple myeloma has an association with systemic amyloidosis in which the amyloid is derived from immunoglobulin light chains. In 1 autopsy series, 15% of the patients had generalized amyloidosis with deposits in the kidneys, spleen, adrenal bodies, and liver. Kidney involvement often leads to azotemia and secondary renal failure.

DIAGNOSIS

SIGNS AND SYMPTOMS

- Bone pain (65%)
  - Pathologic fracture occurs in ~1/3 of these patients
- Weakness and fatigue
- Bleeding (nose, gums), often evidenced by purpura or epistaxis, may occur in the presence of thrombocytopenia or secondary amyloidosis.
- Recurrent infections
- Renal insufficiency or renal failure
- Swelling on ribs, skull, sternum, vertebrae, clavicles, shoulder, pelvis
- Weight loss
- Hyperviscosity syndrome

TESTS

Lab

- Anemia is present in 70% of the patients at the time of diagnosis.
  - Nearly all patients will develop anemia as the disease progresses.
- Peripheral blood smear
  - Rouleaux formation
- Serum protein electrophoresis
  - Usually shows a spike or a localized band (M spike in ~80% of patients). Of these, 50% are IgG protein, 20% IgA, and 17% free monoclonal light chains (Bence Jones protein).
- Urine electrophoresis
  - Positive ~70% of the time for light chains, but inconsistencies hinder diagnosis
- Hypercalcemia
- Decreased platelets
- Elevated sedimentation rate
- Elevated creatinine and BUN levels

Imaging

- Skeletal radiographs
  - When the long bones are involved, they often show a radiolucent or a lytic lesion.
  - Skull often shows punched-out lytic lesions with no sclerotic or reactive border.
  - Periosteal reaction is uncommon.
  - Vertebral compression fractures, with occasional extraosseous or extradural cord compression, are commonly seen.
- Although technetium-99 bone scans have often been described as cold, they will actually show some slight uptake increase in involved skeletal regions, particularly in the presence of fracture; however, the amount of uptake is far less than that demonstrated in other malignancies of bone.
- MRI scans can be extremely valuable in determining the extent of marrow involvement as well as the difference between benign compression fractures and multiple myeloma lesions.

Diagnostic Procedures/Surgery
Bone marrow biopsy

- Test most likely to yield definitive diagnosis.
- Bone marrow will contain increased numbers of plasma cells at various stages of maturation.

Pathological Findings
- Secondary amyloidosis
- Myeloma kidney

DIFFERENTIAL DIAGNOSIS
- Metastatic carcinoma
- Primary malignancy of bone (sarcoma, lymphoma)
- Metabolic bone disease
- Monoclonal gammopathy of undetermined significance (MGUS)

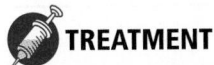 # TREATMENT

GENERAL MEASURES

- Radiation therapy is limited to patients with intractable bone pain (failing chemotherapy).
- Patients with impending or pathologic fractures should have those fractures rigidly stabilized along with removal of the tumor, if possible. Patients with impending paraplegia secondary to spinal cord involvement should undergo immediate radiation therapy and bracing and/or surgical decompression and stabilization.

Diet
No special diet

Activity
As tolerated

SPECIAL THERAPY
Radiotherapy
See "General Measures."

 # MEDICATION (DRUGS)

First Line
Chemotherapy is the primary treatment for symptomatic multiple myeloma, but the ideal chemotherapy is unknown. The most common initial protocol management includes the oral administration of melphalan (Alkeran) and prednisone. This protocol produces an objective response in 50–60% of the patients. It is usually given in oral doses of 0.25 mg/kg/d for 4 days, along with 50 mg of prednisone b.i.d. for the same period. The dosage should be repeated every 6 weeks with leukocyte and platelet counts evaluated at 3-week intervals.

- Contraindications
  - Refer to the manufacturer's profile of each drug.
- Precautions
  - Melphalan: Myelosuppression is the major dose-limiting toxicity of this drug (mainly leukopenia, thrombocytopenia). Monitor CBC and platelet counts every 3 weeks.
  - Prednisone: Usual hazards of long-term corticosteroid administration. Refer to the manufacturer's literature.

Second Line
In the event of failure of the 1st-line regimen, alternate protocols include the following:

- Cyclophosphamide, carmustine (BCNU), vincristine, and prednisone
- VAD: Combination of vincristine, doxorubicin (Adriamycin), and dexamethasone

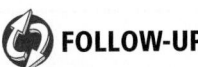 # FOLLOW-UP

DISPOSITION
Outpatient care, except during intensive chemotherapy periods

PROGNOSIS
- Average survival time varies considerably.
  - Median survival ~24 months. A significantly large number of patients survive for much longer periods with evidence of disease present.
- Occasional temporary remissions with therapy
- Bone marrow transplantation should be considered in younger patients.

COMPLICATIONS
- Skeletal destruction
- Spontaneous fractures
- Secondary amyloidosis
- Renal insufficiency
- Recurrent infections (e.g., *Streptococcus pneumoniae*, *Haemophilus influenzae*)
- Hyperviscosity syndrome

PATIENT MONITORING
CBC and platelet count every 6 weeks

REFERENCES
1. DeVita VT, Hellman S, Rosenberg SA. *Cancer: Principles and Practices of Oncology.* 6th ed. Philadelphia, PA: Lippincott Williams & Wilkins; 2001.

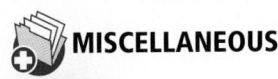 ## MISCELLANEOUS

CODES

ICD9-CM
203.00 Multiple myeloma without mention of remission

PATIENT TEACHING

Educational materials are available through the American Cancer Society.

 See Corresponding Diagnostic Algorithm

M

MULTIPLE SCLEROSIS

Stanley G. Smith, MA, MB

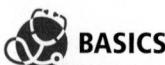 **BASICS**

DESCRIPTION

- Multiple sclerosis (MS) is a recurrent (occasionally progressive) inflammatory demyelinization of the white matter of the brain and spinal cord resulting in multiple and varied neurologic symptoms and signs.
- Usual course: Intermittent, progressive, and relapsing
  – Acute or slowly progressive course
- A major cause of disability in young adults
- System(s) Affected: Nervous
- Synonym(s): Disseminated sclerosis; Insular sclerosis; Neuromyelitis optica; Devic disease

ALERT

Geriatric Considerations
Remissions less frequent in this age group

Pediatric Considerations
Unlikely before puberty

Pregnancy Considerations
A triggering factor for multiple sclerosis in some cases

GENERAL PREVENTION

- No known preventive measures
- Avoid factors that may precipitate an attack, particularly stress from hot weather.

EPIDEMIOLOGY

- Predominant age: Young adult (16–40 years)
- Predominant sex: Female > Male

Incidence
There are 25,000 new cases each year.

RISK FACTORS

- Living in temperate zone
- Northern European descent
- Family history of the disease

Genetics
Appears to be a strong genetic component in determining susceptibility to the disease

ETIOLOGY
Unknown: Various theories

- Autoimmune theory: Supported by HLA linkage, hereditary pattern, immunocytes in plaques, changes in peripheral blood immunocytes
- Viral theory: Supported by increasing incidence of disease at higher latitudes, clusters of cases with families, geographic clusters of cases, animal studies of infectious diseases of myelin
- Combined theory: Autoimmune disorder triggered by environmental exposure to toxin or virus early in life

DIAGNOSIS

SIGNS AND SYMPTOMS

- Ataxia
- Babinski sign
- Blurred, double, or loss of vision in a single eye; often triggered by retrobulbar neuritis and its visual sequelae; 30–40% of the patients with optic neuritis alone eventually develop other signs.
- Clonus
- Clumsiness
- Dysarthria
- Emotional lability
- Fatigue
- Genital anesthesia
- Hand paralysis
- Hemiparesis
- Hyperactive deep tendon reflexes
- Hyperesthesia
- Incoordination
- Loss of position sense
- Loss of vibration sense
- Monoparesis
- Ocular paralysis
- Paresthesias
- Sexual impotence in men
- Urinary frequency, hesitancy, incontinence
- Trigeminal neuralgia

TESTS

- Visual evoked response (VER): Abnormal in 75–97% of definite MS cases
- Somatosensory evoked potentials: Abnormal in 72–96% of cases
- Brainstem auditory evoked responses: Abnormal in 57–65% of cases
- Cerebrospinal fluid (CSF)
  – Oligoclonal bands
  – Increased IgG

Lab

- CSF
  – Abnormal colloidal gold curve
  – Gammaglobulin IgG elevated
  – Mild mononuclear pleocytosis (<40 cells/mL)
  – Myelin debris
  – Protein normal or slightly elevated 50–100 mg/100 mL (50–100 mg/dL [500–1,000 mg/L])
- Tests to exclude other disorders
  – Serology for syphilis (CSF and serum)
  – Fluorescent treponemal antibody absorption (FTA-ABS)
  – Sedimentation rate
  – Screens for clinically suspected vasculitic disorders
  – Human T-lymphotropic virus-1 (HTLV-I) serology

Imaging

- MRI (more sensitive than CT): May show many plaques
- CT scan (double-dose, delayed): Plaques

Diagnostic Procedures/Surgery

- No test specific to diagnose MS
- History, physical, CSF analysis, MRI, evoked potential studies, repeated observations over a period of time
- Surgery not indicated

Pathological Findings

- Destruction of myelin sheaths of nerve fibers and axis cylinders, sparing axons, glia, and other structures
- Atrophy of optic nerves and cerebral hemispheric white matter
- T-cell lymphocytes about venules

DIFFERENTIAL DIAGNOSIS

- Amyotrophic lateral sclerosis
- Behçet disease
- Brainstem tumor
- Central nervous system infection
- Cerebellar tumor
- Friedreich ataxia
- Hereditary ataxia
- Leukodystrophy
- Neurofibromatosis
- Pernicious anemia
- Progressive multifocal leukoencephalopathy
- Ruptured intervertebral disk
- Small cerebral infarcts
- Sarcoidosis
- Spinal cord tumor
- Syphilis
- Syringomyelia
- Systemic lupus erythematosus
- Vasculitides

TREATMENT

GENERAL MEASURES
- Remissions occur spontaneously and make treatment evaluations difficult.
- Emotional support, encouragement
- Occupational therapy
- Urologic evaluation including any sexual dysfunction problems (impotence common in male patients)
- Self-catheterizations for inadequate bladder emptying (indwelling catheter may be necessary in a few patients)
- Custodial care, if patient cognitively impaired

Diet
If constipation a problem, high fluid intake, plus a high-fiber diet

Activity
- Maintain activity; avoid overwork and fatigue.
- Rest during periods of acute relapse.

SPECIAL THERAPY
Physical Therapy
Physiotherapy to maintain range of movement and strength and to avoid contractures

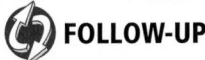 **MEDICATION (DRUGS)**

First Line
Drug therapy directed toward relieving symptoms

- Methylprednisolone: 1,000 mg/d IV for 5 days followed by tapered oral prednisone for acute attacks, especially retrobulbar neuritis (recommended by some clinicians)
- Spasticity
  - Baclofen: Low dosage to start, 5 mg PO 1–3 times a day, increase as needed, or diazepam PO 2–5 mg at bedtime
- Constipation
  - Stool softeners, bulk-producing agents, laxative suppositories
- Urinary problems
  - Propantheline: 7.5 mg PO q3–4h to start, increase to 15 mg t.i.d. to q.i.d. plus 15–30 mg at bedtime; or oxybutynin chloride PO 5 mg t.i.d.–q.i.d.
  - Prophylactic antibiotics for urinary infections
- Incoordination or tremors
  - No ideal therapy; may try beta-blockers (if not contraindicated), primidone, or clonazepam
- Depression and emotional lability
  - Amitriptyline: 10–25 mg PO at bedtime to start, increase as tolerated
- Paranoia or mania
  - Haloperidol or lithium
- Musculoskeletal pain or discomfort
  - NSAIDs
- Hemifacial and dysesthesias
  - Carbamazepine: 100–200 mg PO once or twice a day to start; increase to total daily dosage of 600–1,600 mg t.i.d.–q.i.d.
  - Must monitor serum levels
- Immunosuppressive agents (e.g., azathioprine, ACTH (adrenocorticotropic hormone), methylprednisolone, cyclophosphamide, interferons, cyclosporine) still investigational

Second Line
- Oral steroids: Poor evidence for use alone
- Chronic fatigue: Amantadine 200–300 mg/d PO (no specific evidence that this works)
- Spasticity: Baclofen 40–80 mg/d PO in divided doses
- Interferon-beta approved for relapsing MS: 0.25 mg SC every other day
- Copolymer-1(Glatiramer acetate)
  - Approved for relapsing MS
  - Mitoxantrone
  - Shown to be moderately effective
  - IV immunoglobulins also promising

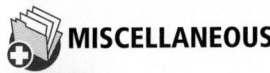 **FOLLOW-UP**

DISPOSITION
- Outpatient care as long as possible
- Long-term care facility for physical therapy or complications such as pyelonephritis

PROGNOSIS
- Highly variable and unpredictable
- ~70% of patients lead active, productive lives with prolonged remissions.
- May disable the patient by early adulthood or cause death within months of onset
- Average duration exceeds 25 years.
- 30% relapse in 1 year, 20% in 5–9 years, and 10% in 10–30 years.

COMPLICATIONS
- Coma
- Delirium
- Emotional lability
- Nystagmus
- Optic nerve atrophy
- Paraplegia
- Sexual impotence (men)
- Urinary tract infections

PATIENT MONITORING
Requires patient follow-up at regular intervals

REFERENCES
1. Adams RD, Victor M. *Principles of Neurology.*, 5th ed. New York, NY: McGraw-Hill; 1993.
2. Beck RW, et al. The effect of corticosteroids for acute optic neuritis on the subsequent development of multiple sclerosis. *N Engl J Med*. 1994;329:1764–1769.
3. Matthews WB, Compston A, Allen IV. *McAlpine's Multiple Sclerosis*. 2nd ed. New York, NY: Churchill Livingstone; 1991.
4. Rowlan LP, ed. *Merritt's Textbook of Neurology*. 9th ed. Philadelphia, PA: Williams & Wilkins; 1995.
5. The Cochrane Database of Systemic Reviews 2006.
6. Sibley WA. *Therapeutic Claims in Multiple Sclerosis*. 2nd ed. New York, NY: Demos; 1988.

 MISCELLANEOUS

CODES

ICD9-CM
340 Multiple sclerosis

PATIENT TEACHING
- Because the course is highly variable and unpredictable, avoid a hopeless outlook.
- For patient education materials favorably reviewed on this topic, contact the National Multiple Sclerosis Society, 205E 42nd St., New York, NY 10017; (800) 624-8236.

See Corresponding Diagnostic Algorithm

M

MUMPS

Maryellen Antonetti, MPH, PA-C, RN

BASICS

DESCRIPTION
- Acute, generalized paramyxovirus infection usually presenting with unilateral or bilateral parotitis, lasting 2 days, without apparent cause
- Epidemics in late winter and spring with transmission by respiratory secretions.
- Incubation ~14–24 days
- System(s) Affected: Hemic/Lymphatic/Immunologic; Reproductive; Skin/Exocrine
- Synonym(s): Epidemic parotitis; Infectious parotitis

GENERAL PREVENTION
- Vaccination
  - 2 doses of live mumps vaccine or measles–mumps–rubella (MMR) recommended at 12–15 months and 4–6 years of age
  - 95% effective
  - Adverse effects: Most common proven effect is ITP, with incidence of 3.3 per 100,000 doses
- Immune globulin not effective in prevention
- Postexposure vaccination does not protect from recent exposure.
- Isolate hospitalized patients until 9 days past onset.

ALERT
- Cases of mumps are reportable through the National Notifiable Diseases Surveillance System (NNDSS) http://www.cdc.gov/epo/dphsi/nndsshis.htm
- For children aged 1–12 years, MMRV vaccine can be considered if varicella vaccine is indicated

Pregnancy Considerations
No proven complications of vaccine, but theoretically should not vaccinate in pregnancy

EPIDEMIOLOGY
- Geriatric population: Most are immune
- Acute epidemic mumps
  - Most cases occur in children aged 5–15 years.
  - Unusual in children <2 years old
  - Most infants <1 year old are immune.
- Predominant age: 85% occur <15 years, but more severe in adults
- Predominant sex: Male = Female

Incidence
0.09/100,000 (231 per year in 2003)

Prevalence
- 0.0064/100,000
- 90% of adults are seropositive even without history.

ETIOLOGY
- Mumps paramyxovirus
- Other viruses, such as Coxsackie (rare)

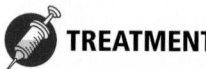 DIAGNOSIS

SIGNS AND SYMPTOMS
- Parotid pain and swelling in 1 or both glands
- Rare prodrome of fever, neck muscle ache, malaise
- Parotitis: Unilateral >bilateral, ~10–20%; rarely results in infertility
- Meningeal signs in 15%, encephalitis in 0.5%
- Rarely arthritis, orchitis, thyroiditis, mastitis, pancreatitis
- Rare maculopapular, erythematous rash
- Up to 50% of cases may be asymptomatic.

History
- Initial parotid swelling just behind jaw
- Swelling peaks in 1–3 days, lasts 3–7 days.
- Sour foods cause pain in parotid gland region.
- Fever, usually not above 104°F (40°C). High fever associated with complications

Physical Exam
- Obscures angle of mandible
- Elevates earlobe
- Erythema at Stensen duct but no pus
- Sternal swelling is rare, but pathognomonic of mumps

TESTS
Lab
- Special tests are rarely necessary.
- Viral isolation from throat washings, urine, blood, or spinal fluid
- Serum amylase elevated
- Rise in paired antibodies: Anti-S antibodies peak early and may be seen at time of presentation.
- Cerebrospinal fluid: Leukocytosis
- Leukopenia
- Easier salivary test for IgM is pending.

Imaging
Testicular ultrasound may be useful to differentiate mumps orchitis from testicular torsion.

Pathological Findings
Periductal edema and lymphocytic infiltration

DIFFERENTIAL DIAGNOSIS
- Parainfluenza parotitis, other viruses
- Suppurative parotitis: Often associated with *Staphylococcus aureus* (presence of Wharton duct pus on massaging parotid gland nearly excludes diagnosis of mumps)
- Recurrent allergic parotitis
- Salivary calculus with intermittent swelling
- Lymphadenitis from any cause, even HIV
- Cytomegalovirus parotitis in immunocompromised patients
- Mikulicz syndrome: Chronic, painless parotid- and lacrimal-gland swelling of unknown cause that occurs in tuberculosis, sarcoidosis, lupus, leukemia, and lymphosarcoma.
- Malignant or benign salivary gland tumors
- Drug-related parotid enlargement (iodides, guanethidine)
- Other causes of the complications of mumps (meningoencephalitis, orchitis, oophoritis, pancreatitis, polyarthritis, nephritis, myocarditis, prostatitis)
- Mumps orchitis must be differentiated from testicular torsion and from chlamydial or bacterial orchitis. (Testicular sonogram can be useful.)

TREATMENT

INITIAL STABILIZATION
Outpatient supportive care, if no complications

GENERAL MEASURES
- High fever and testicular pain: May hospitalize for steroids or interferon
- Orchitis
  - Ice packs to scrotum can help relieve pain.
  - Scrotal support with adhesive bridge while recumbent and/or athletic supporter while ambulatory

Diet
Liquid diet if unable to chew

Activity
Mumps orchitis: Bed rest and local supportive clothing (e.g., 2 pairs of briefs) or adhesive-tape bridge

IV Fluids
If severe nausea or vomiting accompanies pancreatitis

MEDICATION (DRUGS)

First Line
- Corticosteroids or a NSAID may diminish pain and swelling in acute orchitis and arthritis mumps, but is usually not necessary.
- May use acetaminophen for fever and/or pain
- Contraindications: Refer to the manufacturer's profile for each drug.
- Precautions: Avoid aspirin for pain in children. Aspirin use in children with viral infection has been associated with Reye syndrome.
- Significant possible interactions: Refer to the manufacturer's profile for each drug

Second Line
- Mumps arthritis may improve with corticosteroids or a NSAID.
- Interferon-γ 2b for 7 days has been used experimentally in severe bilateral orchitis to prevent infertility.

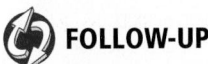 FOLLOW-UP

DISPOSITION
Admission Criteria
If CNS symptoms occur, hospitalize.

PROGNOSIS
- Complete recovery is usual; immunity is permanent.
- Transient sensorineural hearing loss in 4% of adults
- Rare recurrence >2 weeks may be recurrent nonepidemic parotitis.

COMPLICATIONS
- May precede, accompany, or follow salivary gland involvement, and may occur (rarely) without primary involvement of the parotid gland.
- Orchitis is common (30%) in postpubertal boys; it starts within 8 days after parotitis. Fever; swollen testis of 4-day's duration; impaired fertility in 13%, but absolute sterility is rare.
- Meningitis or encephalitis may present 10 days after 1st symptoms of illness. Aseptic meningitis is typically mild, but meningoencephalitis may lead to seizures, paralysis, hydrocephalus, or, in 2% of cases, death.
- Acute cerebellar ataxia has been reported after mumps infections; self-resolving in 2–3 weeks.
- Cerebrospinal fluid pleocytosis, usually lymphocytes, are found in 65% of cases with parotitis.
- Oophoritis in 7% of postpubertal females causes no decreased fertility.
- Pancreatitis, usually mild
- Nephritis, thyroiditis, or arthralgias are rare.
- Myocarditis: Usually mild, but may depress ST segment, may be linked to endocardial fibroelastosis
- Deafness: 1/15,000 unilateral nerve deafness; may not be permanent
- Inflammation about the eye (rare)
- Dacryoadenitis, optic neuritis

ALERT
Pediatric Considerations
- Orchitis is more common in adolescents.
- Young children are less likely to develop complications.
- Most complications occur in postpubertal group.
- Avoid aspirin use in children with viral symptoms.

Pregnancy Considerations
Disease may increase rate of spontaneous abortion in 1st trimester.

PATIENT MONITORING
Most cases will be mild. Monitor hydration status.

REFERENCES
1. Madsen KM. A population based study of MMR vaccine and autism. *N Engl J Med*. 2002;347:1477.
2. Centers for Disease Control. Update: Multistate Outbreak of Mumps—United States, January 1–May 2, 2006. *MMWR*. 2006;55:559–563
3. Dale DC, Federman DD, eds. Scientific American Medicine. New York: WebMD, 2001.
4. Nussinovitch M, et al. Post-infectious acute cerebellar ataxia in children. *Clin Pediatr (Phila)*. 2003;42:581–584.
5. Peltola H, et al. Mumps and rubella eliminated from Finland. *JAMA*. 2000;284:2643–2647.

 MISCELLANEOUS

- Up to 20% of those infected with mumps virus have no parotid swelling and a clinically inapparent infection.
- Highly contagious; 90% transmission rate for nonimmune household contacts
- Urban epidemics, nonvaccinated population
- Usual communicable period is 24 hours before to 72 hours after onset of parotitis.
- Incubation period usually is 18 days.

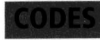 CODES

ICD9-CM
072.9 Mumps without mention of complication

PATIENT TEACHING
Orchitis is common in older children, but rarely results in sterility.

Activity
Must be out of school until no longer contagious, about 9 days after onset of pain

Prevention
- Immunization of family may protect against later exposures but not the present case.
- No relationship between autism and MMR.

M

MUSCULAR DYSTROPHY

Terence S. Edgar, MD

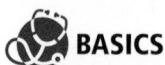 **BASICS**

DESCRIPTION

- Inherited progressive diseases of muscle with wide ranges of clinical expression. Includes several forms
- Congenital muscular dystrophy (CMD):
  - Extracelluar matrix protein defects
    - Laminin α2-deficient
    - Ulrich CMD
  - Glycosyltransferases (abnormal 0-glycosylation of α-dystroglycan)
    - Walker-Warburg syndrome
    - Muscle Eye Brain disease
    - Fukuyama CMD
    - CMD + secondary laminin deficiency
    - CMD + mental retardation + pachygyria
  - Proteins of the endoplasmic reticulum
    - Rigid Spine Syndrome (RSD)
- Myotonic dystrophy
- Dystrophinopathies
  - Duchenne muscular dystrophy (DMD)
  - Becker muscular dystrophy (BMD)
- Limb-girdle muscular dystrophy (LGMD)
- Emory-Dreifuss muscular dystrophy (EDMD)
- Fascioscapulohumeral muscular dystrophy (FSHD)
- System(s) Affected: Musculoskeletal; Nervous; Cardiac

GENERAL PREVENTION

- Maternal carrier evaluation by creatine kinase in DMD (80% sensitive) and BMD (60% sensitive)
- DNA probes for carrier status determination and antenatal diagnosis in DMD and BMD
- Polymerase chain reaction (PCR) technology available for antenatal diagnosis of myotonic dystrophy due to myotonin mutation
- EDMD: Emerin determination in skin biopsies can be useful in identifying female carriers. Carriers at risk of cardiac conduction defects

EPIDEMIOLOGY

- Predominant age
  - Birth to infancy: CMD
  - Infancy to early childhood
    - DMD, BMD, FSHD, EDMD
    - LGMD2
  - Late childhood to adolescence
    - BMD, LGMD 1 and 2, FSHD
    - Myotonic dystrophy
- Predominant sex: Male > Female

Incidence

- DMD: 1 in 3,300 live male births
- BMD: 1 in 18,000 live male births
- CMD: 5 per 100,000 births
- Congenital myotonic dystrophy: 1 per 10,000

Prevalence

FSHD: 1 in 20,000

RISK FACTORS

- X-linked forms: Affected male on maternal side of family (female carriers may rarely be symptomatic)
- Autosomal dominant forms: Affected parent; myotonic dystrophy more severe if mother is affected parent

Genetics

- Xq28 recessive: EDMD 1 (encoding emerin)
- Autosomal dominant
  - LGMD 1 (A-E)
  - Myotonic dystrophy (3q and 19q13)
  - EDMD 2 (1q21 encoding laminin A/C)
  - FSHD (4q35)
- Autosomal recessive
  - LGMD 2 (A-J), CMD (laminin α2: 6q22)
  - EDMD 1 (rare)
- Xp21 recessive
  - DMD, BMD

ETIOLOGY

- CMD: Ulrich CMD (Collagen VI gene mutation), RSD (deficiency of selenoprotein N). A subgroup represents disorders of 0-glycosylation.
- Myotonic dystrophy
  - Chromosome 19. CTG expansion affecting a protein kinase. Repeat size ranges from 50 to >2,000. The larger the repeat, the earlier the presentation.
  - Anticipation in successive generations may occur.
- Dystrophinopathies
  - DMD: 96% with frame-shift mutation, 30% with new mutation
  - BMD: 70% with in-frame mutation
- LGMD: Most common LGMDs in childhood due to disruption of sarcolemmal proteins; part of a complex linking extracellular collagen with intracellular matrix proteins
- EDMD
  - EDMD 1: Chromosome Xq28. Most are nonsense mutations causing complete loss of emerin (nuclear membrane protein).
  - EDMD 2: Chromosome 1q21. Encodes laminin A/C (nuclear membrane protein). (Mutations within laminin A/C gene can also present as LGMD 1B and cardiomyopathy with conduction block.)
- FSHD: Primary mechanism unknown. All patients have decreased number of tandem repeats, of sequence D4Z4. Normal patients have >10 copies of this repeat. Patients with FSHD have 1–8 copies. Links to chromosome 4q35

ASSOCIATED CONDITIONS

- Mental retardation: DMD (25%), myotonic dystrophy with early onset
- Malignant hyperthermia seen in DMD
- Cardiomyopathy

ALERT

Pregnancy Considerations

Maternal myotonic dystrophy: Increased risk for polyhydramnios, breech, preterm labor

DIAGNOSIS

SIGNS AND SYMPTOMS

- CMD and congenital myotonic dystrophy
  - Marked hypotonia and weakness, with feeding and respiratory difficulties; neonatal arthrogryposis; cardiac function generally normal. Seizures in up to 30%.
- DMD and BMD
  - Normal milestones until child begins to walk
  - Progressive symmetric muscle weakness, proximal > distal, with inability to jump or climb stairs. Difficulty in rising to standing position: Gower sign. Lumbar lordosis
  - Pseudohypertrophy of calf muscles with heel-cord contractures, toe walking, waddling gait, and frequent falls
  - Inability to flex neck when lying supine helps to distinguish DMD from BMD.
- LGMD
  - LGMD 2: Presents as DMD or BMD
  - LGMD 1: Older onset, slower progression Exceptions are LGMD 1C (caveolin mutations) and LGMD 1B (laminin A/C mutations), which may present in childhood.
- EDMD
  - Presents < age 5 with toe walking
  - Contractures develop early (flexors of arms and legs and cervical extensor muscles).
  - Muscle weakness initially involves the humeral and peroneal muscles.
  - Cardiac conduction abnormalities, usually in 3rd decade
- FSHD
  - Facial/eye weakness and perioral muscles
  - Shoulder and proximal arm weakness with relative sparing of biceps ("Popeye" arms). Inability to perform push-ups, scapula winging, forward-sloping shoulders
  - Muscle involvement typically asymmetrical
  - Retinal vasculopathy and sensorineural hearing loss present in some patients
- Myotonic dystrophy
  - Weakness of face, eyes, forearms, and hands (Proximal weakness seen in a later-onset form: Proximal myotonic myopathy)
  - High forehead; receding hairline; open, triangular mouth; and droopy eyelids
  - Sustained muscle contraction with percussion of thenar eminence
  - Difficulty in letting go (myotonia) after handshake. Myotonia worsened by cold
  - Cataracts, cardiac conduction defects, gonadal dysfunction, personality changes

TESTS

Lab

- Creatine kinase
  - Marked elevation (>10 times normal value): DMD, BMD, LGMD
  - Mild to normal: CMD, myotonic dystrophy, FSHD, EDMD
- Drugs that may alter lab results
  - Opiates (codeine, heroin, meperidine, morphine)
  - Dexamethasone, ethanol, digoxin
  - Furosemide, aminocaproic acid, halothane
  - Imipramine, phenobarbital, lithium, clofibrate
- Disorders that may alter lab results
  - Polymyositis/dermatomyositis
  - Muscle trauma: Exercise, seizures, IM injections, needle electromyelogram
  - Hypothyroidism, hyperthyroidism
  - Myocardial infarction, stroke, sepsis, shock

Imaging

Brain MRI in CMD may show periventricular white-matter changes, focal cortical dysplasias, agyria, and pontocerebellar hypoplasia.

Diagnostic Procedures/Surgery

- EMG
  - Typically shows low amplitude, short duration motor unit potentials with early recruitment.
  - In myotonic dystrophy, high-frequency repetitive, waxing and waning discharges
- Muscle biopsy
  - Biopsy weak muscle (vastus lateralis, triceps) not studied by needle EMG
  - Immunostaining: Determines where the protein is present or absent. Useful in DMD, BMD, LGMD, CMD
  - Western blot analysis: In DMD, dystrophin content is <3% of normal; in BMD dystrophin content is <20% of normal.
- Prenatal diagnosis
  - DMD/BMD: Dystrophin studies in chorionic villous sampling and amniocytes; analysis of fetal RBC in maternal blood
  - CMD: Direct mutation analysis of chorionic villous material or direct trophoblast staining for laminin α2 chain
- Commercially available DNA testing: DMD/BMD, EDMD, FSHD, myotonic dystrophy

Pathological Findings

- Muscle biopsy
  - DMD/CMD: (Dystrophic muscle changes) fiber splitting, centralized nuclei, necrosis, and growth with increased connective tissue
  - LGMD: Nonspecific, or may show dystrophic changes as with DMD
  - FSMD: Highest yield in supraspinatus. Variability in fiber size, with cellular infiltrates and small, round, atrophic fibers
  - EDMD: Changes, with type 1 fiber atrophy

DIFFERENTIAL DIAGNOSIS

- Onset from birth to early infancy
  - Encephalopathy, spinal muscular atrophy, infantile botulism, myasthenia gravis, congenital myopathies, metabolic myopathies, chromosomal disorders
- Onset from infancy to early childhood
  - Mitochondrial myopathies, carnitine deficiency, acid-maltase deficiency, spinal muscular atrophy, channelopathies
- Onset from childhood to adolescence
  - Inflammatory myopathies, mitochondrial myopathies, spinal muscular atrophy, congenital and metabolic myopathies, channelopathies, myasthenia gravis

 TREATMENT

INITIAL STABILIZATION

Outpatient with team approach: Neurologist, orthopedic surgeon, primary care provider, physical and occupational therapists, social worker, and orthotist

GENERAL MEASURES

- Broad goal of management: Lessen impairments that result from disease and deter functional limitations and concomitant disability
  - Prevent contractures: Stretching, physical therapy, positioning, splinting.
  - Maintain muscle strength.
  - Promote cardiopulmonary endurance.
  - Maintain mobility: Bracing and walking aids.
  - Monitor pulmonary and cardiac function.
  - Influenza and pneumococcal vaccines if wheelchair bound or on steroids

Diet

Weight control essential. Obesity adversely affects physical performance and respiratory function.

Activity

Moderate exercise. Excessive demand can damage dystrophic muscle.

 MEDICATION (DRUGS)

- Phenytoin for symptomatic relief of myotonia
- Prednisone 0.75 mg/kg/d improves muscle strength in boys with DMD.
- Precautions: Monitor for side effects of long-term steroid use.

SURGERY

- Surgical release of contractures
- Stabilization of spine for scoliosis decreases the frequency of pneumonia and improves wheelchair comfort.

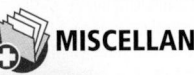 **FOLLOW-UP**

PROGNOSIS

- DMD and BMD
  - Progressive weakness, contractures, inability to walk
  - Kyphoscoliosis and progressive decline in vital capacity
  - Early death (Duchenne 16 $\pm$ 4 years; Becker 42 $\pm$ 16 years)
- CMD with brain involvement and congenital myotonic dystrophy
  - Progressive hypotonia and weakness
  - Respiratory failure and early death
- Other types: Slow progression and near-normal life span

COMPLICATIONS

- Cardiac arrhythmias or myopathy
  - EDMD
  - BMD
  - DMD
  - Myotonic dystrophy
- Hypertension: FSHD
- Dysphagia or acute gastric dilation
  - DMD
  - Myotonic dystrophy
- Malignant hyperthermia: DMD
- Respiratory failure and early death
  - CMD (15%)
  - Congenital myotonic dystrophy (>50%)
- Endocrinopathies: Myotonic dystrophy
- Cataracts: Myotonic dystrophy
- Sensorineural hearing loss: FSHD
- Seizures and cerebral dysplasia: CMD with cerebral involvement
- Increase in fetal breech presentation: Female carriers of DMD

PATIENT MONITORING

- DMD: After age 11, yearly pulmonary function tests, EKG, CXR, A/P, and lateral spine films
- EDMD: Detection of cardiac conduction defects and use of pacemaker can be lifesaving.

REFERENCES

1. Finder JD, et al. Respiratory care of the patient with Duchenne muscular dystrophy. American Thoracic Society consensus statement. *Am J Respir Crit Care Med*. 2004;170:456–465.
2. Moxley RT 3rd, et al. Practice parameter: Corticosteroid treatment of Duchenne dystrophy: Report of the Quality Standards Subcommittee of the American Academy of Neurology and the Practice Committee of the Child Neurology Society. *Neurology*. 2005;64:13–20.
3. Mathews K. Muscular dystrophy overview: Genetics and diagnosis. *Neurol Clin*. 2003;21:795–816.

 MISCELLANEOUS

CODES

ICD9-CM

- 359 Muscular dystrophies and other myopathies
- 359.0 Congenital hereditary muscular dystrophy
- 359.1 Hereditary progressive muscular dystrophy
- 359.2 Myotonic disorders

PATIENT TEACHING

Printed material and clinical services available through the Muscular Dystrophy Association, 3561 E. Sunrise Dr., Tucson, AZ 85718; (800) 221–1142; www.mdausa.org

Prevention

Genetic counseling

See Corresponding Diagnostic Algorithm

M

MYASTHENIA GRAVIS

Brian D. Petroni, MD

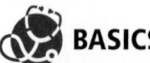 BASICS

DESCRIPTION
Most common primary disorder of the neuromuscular junction, resulting in a pure motor syndrome characterized by fluctuating skeletal muscle weakness, particularly of the extraocular, pharyngeal, facial, and respiratory musculature.

- 2 clinical forms: Ocular and generalized
- Ocular MG (15%): Weakness limited to eyelids and extraocular muscles
- Generalized MG (85%): Commonly affects ocular as well as a variable combination of bulbar, proximal limb, and respiratory muscles
- 50% of patients present with ptosis or diplopia.
- 50% of patients who 1st present with ocular symptoms develop generalized MG within 2 years.
- Onset may be sudden and severe, but is typically mild and intermittent over many years.
- System(s) Affected: Hematologic/Lymphatic/Immunologic; Musculoskeletal

EPIDEMIOLOGY
- Occurs at any age, but a bimodal distribution to the age of onset
  - 20–40 (female predominance)
  - 60–80 (male predominance)
- Overall, Male = Female

Incidence
10–20 per million per year

Prevalence
10–20 per 100,000 in the US

RISK FACTORS
- Familial MG
- Other autoimmune diseases

Genetics
- Transient neonatal MG is seen in 10–20% of infants born to myasthenic mothers due to the transplacental passage of acetylcholine receptor antibodies. The condition resolves in weeks to months, and these infants do not have an increased risk for the long-term or future development of MG.
- Congenital MG syndrome describes a collection of rare hereditary disorders. This condition is not immune-mediated, but instead results from the mutation of a component of the neuromuscular junction. Onset is usually at birth or in early childhood, and inheritance is typically autosomal recessive.
- Familial predisposition seen in 5% of cases.

ETIOLOGY
Humoral, antibody-mediated, T-cell–dependent attack of the acetylcholine receptors or receptor-associated proteins at the postsynaptic membrane of the neuromuscular junction

ASSOCIATED CONDITIONS
- Thymic hyperplasia (60–70% of MG patients)
- Thymoma (10–15% of MG patients)
- Autoimmune thyroid disease (3–8% of MG patients)
- Other autoimmune diseases

DIAGNOSIS

SIGNS AND SYMPTOMS
- Ptosis
- Diplopia
- Dysphagia
- Dysarthria
- Fatigable chewing
- Facial weakness
- Dysphonia
- Neck weakness
- Proximal limb weakness (arm > leg)
- Respiratory weakness

ALERT
Myasthenic crisis: Respiratory muscle weakness producing respiratory insufficiency and pending respiratory failure

History
- Severity of weakness fluctuates during the day; least severe in the morning and worse as the day progresses.
- Weakness typically worse after prolonged use of affected muscles and improves with rest.
- Early in MG, symptoms are transient, with asymptomatic periods lasting days or weeks.
- With progression of MG, asymptomatic periods shorten or are lost entirely, at which point constant symptoms fluctuate from mild to severe.

Physical Exam
- Ptosis may worsen with propping of opposite eyelid (curtain sign) or sustained upward gaze.
- "Myasthenic sneer," in which the mid-lip rises, but corners of mouth do not move.
- In addition to proximal muscles, wrist extensors, finger extensors, and foot dorsiflexors also are commonly involved.
- Pupillary sparing

TESTS
- Bedside tests
  - Tensilon (Edrophonium) test:
    - Initial dose 2 mg IV, can be followed by another 2 mg every 60 seconds up to a maximum dose of 10 mg.
    - A positive test shows improvement of strength within 30 seconds of administration.
    - Sensitivity 80–90%
    - Cardiac disease and bronchial asthma are relative contraindications, especially in elderly
    - Atropine 0.4–0.6 mg IV may rarely be required as antidote; must be available.
  - Ice pack test
    - Can be used in patients with ptosis in whom Tensilon test is contraindicated
    - Ice pack applied to closed eyelid for 60 seconds, then removed; extent of ptosis immediately assessed
    - Ice will decrease the ptosis induced by myasthenia gravis
    - Sensitivity 80% in patients with prominent ptosis

- Electromyography
  - Repetitive nerve stimulation (RNS):
    - Widely available, most frequently used
    - Moderately sensitive for both generalized MG (75%) and ocular MG (50%).
    - Positive test shows a decremental response (>10%) at 3Hz.
  - Single-fiber EMG (SFEMG)
    - Assesses temporal variability between 2 muscle fibers within same motor unit (jitter).
    - Highly sensitive (90–95%), but less specific.
    - Technically difficult to perform; limited availability.

Lab
- Acetylcholine receptor (AChR) antibody
  - 80–85% of all MG patients are seropositive:
    - Generalized myasthenia: 75–85%
    - Ocular myasthenia: 50%
    - MG and thymoma: 98–100%
  - Poor correlation between antibody titer and disease severity
- MuSK (muscle specific tyrosine kinase) antibody
  - Used if MG suspected, patient seronegative
  - Present in 40–50% of seronegative patients with generalized MG; absent in ocular MG
- Thyroid function tests

Imaging
CT or MRI scan of anterior mediastinum
- Thymoma

Pathological Findings
- Muscle electron microscopy
  - Receptor infolding and synaptic cleft widening
- Immunofluorescence
  - IgG antibodies and complement on receptor membranes

DIFFERENTIAL DIAGNOSIS
- Thyroid ophthalmopathy
- Oculopharyngeal muscular dystrophy
- Myotonic dystrophy
- Kearns-Sayre syndrome
- Chronic progressive external ophthalmoplegia
- Brainstem and motor cranial nerve lesions
- Botulism
- Motor neuron disease (e.g., ALS)
- Lambert-Eaton myasthenic syndrome (LEMS)
- Drug-induced myasthenia
- Congenital myasthenic syndrome
- Depression

TREATMENT

INITIAL STABILIZATION
Typically outpatient care

GENERAL MEASURES
- Management of MG is difficult and should be carried out by a neurologist.
- Treatment must be tailored for each patient based on several factors including age, gender, severity of disease, and progression of disease.
- 3 basic approaches to treatment: Symptomatic, immunosuppressive, and supportive. Few patients (if any) should receive a single therapeutic modality.
  - Symptomatic therapy
    - Consists of reversal of weakness with an acetylcholinesterase inhibitor
    - Does not stop the ongoing immunologically mediated damage to the muscle receptor
    - Overdose of these agents may induce severe weakness known as a "cholinergic crisis."
    - Suspect cholinergic crisis if other signs of cholinergic overactivity (excessive secretions, diarrhea, bradycardia) present.
  - Immunomodulatory therapy
    - Usually necessary in some form.
    - Acute: Plasmapheresis, IV immune globulin
    - Chronic: Corticosteroids, other immunosuppressive drugs
    - Surgical: Thymectomy
  - Supportive therapy
    - May be required intermittently or continually
    - May include intubation, tracheostomy, artificial ventilation, respiratory therapy, administration of antibiotics, nasogastric tube, and/or gastrostomy.

Diet
As tolerated

Activity
- As tolerated
- Heat and exercise can exacerbate symptoms

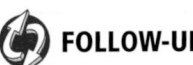

MEDICATION (DRUGS)

First Line
- Anticholinesterases
  - Pyridostigmine bromide (Mestinon)
    - Available as 60-mg tablet, 180-mg sustained-release tablet, or 60-mg/5 mL syrup.
    - Starting dose of 30 mg PO t.i.d.
    - Increase dose in 30 mg increments as needed
    - Maximum dose: 120 mg q3–4h
  - Neostigmine methylsulfate (Prostigmin)
    - Available in 0.25-, 0.5-, and 1-mg/mL concentrations.
    - Starting dose of 0.5 mg subcutaneously or IM q3h.
    - Titrate dosage to clinical need.

Second Line
- Immunosuppressants
  - Prednisone
    - Should be initiated on an inpatient basis
    - Start with a 60–80 mg/d PO; taper the dosage every 3 days.
    - Switch to alternate day regimen within 2 weeks.
    - Taper very slowly to establish the minimum dosage necessary to maintain remission.
  - Mycophenolate: 1 g PO or IV b.i.d.
  - Azathioprine: 100–200 mg/d PO
  - Cyclophosphamide
    - Adults: 1–5 mg/kg/d PO
    - Children: 2–8 mg/kg/d PO
  - Cyclosporine
  - Immune globulin: 2 g/kg IV over 2–5 days
- Contraindications: Refer to the manufacturer's literature.
- Precautions: Numerous
  - Avoid aminoglycosides and other drugs with potential for neuromuscular blockade, which may precipitate weakness.
  - Refer to the manufacturer's literature.
- Significant possible interactions: Numerous; refer to the manufacturer's literature.

SURGERY
Thymectomy
- Recommended for most MG patients,
- Especially helpful for young patients, early onset
- No clear clinical benefit if onset at ≥60 years unless thymoma present

ALERT
Pediatric Considerations
- Infants with severe weakness from transient neonatal myasthenia may be treated with oral pyridostigmine and whatever degree of general support (mechanical respiratory ventilation, for example) is necessary until the condition clears.
- Corticosteroids limited only to severe disease

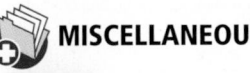

FOLLOW-UP

Admission Criteria
- Plasmapheresis
- Intravenous γ-globulin
- Management of pulmonary infections
- Myasthenic or cholinergic crises

PROGNOSIS
- Overall good, but highly variable.
- Many patients achieve sustained remission.
- Myasthenic crisis associated with substantial morbidity and 4% mortality

COMPLICATIONS
- Acute respiratory arrest
- Chronic respiratory insufficiency
- Atelectasis, aspiration, pneumonia

PATIENT MONITORING
- ICU during myasthenic or cholinergic crises
- Inpatient for initiation of corticosteroids
- Outpatient follow-up every 3 months with stable patients

REFERENCES
1. Keesey JC. Clinical evaluation and management of MG. *Muscle Nerve*. 2004;29:484.
2. McConville J, Farrugia ME, Beeson D, et al. Detection and characterization of MuSK antibodies in seronegative MG. *Ann Neurol*. 2004;55:580.
3. Merriggioli MN, Sanders DB. Myasthenia gravis: diagnosis. *Semin Neurol*. 2004;24:31.
4. Saperstein DS, Barohn RJ. Management of MG. *Semin Neurol*. 2004;24:41.

MISCELLANEOUS

CODES

ICD9-CM
- 358.00 MG without acute exacerbation
- 358.01 MG with acute exacerbation

PATIENT TEACHING
Printed materials, reference lists, and other forms of patient and family support available from the following
- MG Foundation of America (MGFA), 1821 University Ave. West, Suite S256, St. Paul, MN 55104; (800) 541-5454 or (651) 917-6256; www.myasthenia.org
- Muscular Dystrophy Association (MDA), 3300 E. Sunrise Dr., Tucson, AZ 85718; (800) 344-4863; www.mdausa.org

See Corresponding Diagnostic Algorithm

M

MYELODYSPLASTIC SYNDROMES (MDS)

Richard A. Larson, MD

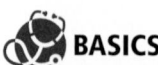 **BASICS**

DESCRIPTION

Heterogeneous group of acquired hematopoietic stem cell disorders characterized by cytologic dysplasia in the bone marrow and blood and by various combinations of anemia, neutropenia, and thrombocytopenia

- There is a natural progression of disease between categories as cellular maturation becomes more arrested and blast cells accumulate. There is a great deal of overlap between arbitrary diagnostic subgroups.

World Health Organization Classification (1)[A]

- Refractory anemia (RA)
  – <5% blasts in marrow; <1% blasts in blood
- Refractory anemia with ringed sideroblasts (RARS)
  – <5% blasts in marrow; >15% ringed sideroblasts; <1% blasts in blood
  – Also known as acquired idiopathic sideroblastic anemia (AISA)
- Refractory cytopenia with multilineage dysplasia (RCMD)
  – Marked trilineage dysplasia but without excess blasts
- Refractory cytopenia with multilineage dysplasia and ringed sideroblasts (RCMD-RS)
- Refractory anemia with excess blasts – 1 (RAEB-1)
  – ~5–9% blasts in marrow; <5% blasts in blood
- Refractory anemia with excess blasts – 2 (RAEB-2)
  – ~10–19% blasts in marrow; 5–19% blasts in blood; +/– Auer rods
- Refractory anemia with isolated del(5q) syndrome
  – RA with erythroid hyperplasia, mono- or biloculated megakaryocyte nuclei, and normal or increased platelets
- Acute MDS with sclerosis
  – RAEB with marked myelosclerosis
- Chronic myelomonocytic leukemia (CMMoL) is now grouped with MDS/myeloproliferative disorders.
  – ~1–20% blasts in marrow; <5% blasts in blood with >1,000 monocytes/μL
  – Refractory anemia with excess of blasts in transformation (RAEBT) is now considered acute myeloid leukemia (AML).
  – ~20–30% blasts in marrow; >20% blasts in blood
  – Incidence: 2:1 (Female > Male)
  – Characteristic interstitial deletion on the long arm of chromosome 5
- Therapy-related (t-MDS) (2)[A]
  – Seen 3–7 years after treatment with alkylating agents and/or radiation therapy
  – Evolves to acute myeloid leukemia (AML) over ~6 months
- System(s) Affected: Hematologic/Lymphatic/Immunologic
- Synonym(s): Dysmyelopoietic Syndrome; Hemopoietic dysplasia; Preleukemia; Smoldering or subacute myeloid leukemia; CMMoL; Chronic myelomonocytic leukemia; CMML; Chronic myelomonocytic leukemia

ALERT
Pediatric Considerations
Pediatric presentations of MDS
- Monosomy 7 syndrome
- Juvenile chronic myelogenous leukemia

EPIDEMIOLOGY
- Predominant age
  – Median age: >65 years
  – Uncommon in children and young adults
- Predominant sex: Male = Female

Incidence
Apparent increased incidence (1–2/100,000/year) in recent years may be due to improved diagnosis.

RISK FACTORS
- Primary MDS is associated with occupational exposure to petroleum solvents (benzene, gasoline).
- Secondary (therapy-related) MDS is associated with prior treatment with alkylating agents or radiation therapy.

Genetics
- Most are clearly clonal neoplasms by cytogenetics, G6PD isoenzyme analysis, or RFLP analysis.
- Mutations in RAS oncogene have been reported.

ETIOLOGY
Unknown

 **DIAGNOSIS**

SIGNS AND SYMPTOMS
- Anemia
  – Fatigue
  – Shortness of breath
  – Lightheadedness
  – Angina
- Leukopenia
  – Fever
  – Infection
- Thrombocytopenia
  – Ecchymoses
  – Petechiae
  – Epistaxis
  – Purpura
- Splenomegaly (uncommon)
  – Mild to moderate enlargement may be encountered, particularly in CMMoL
- Skin infiltrates

TESTS

- Cytogenetics (3)[A]
  – At least 1/2 of patients with primary MDS and nearly all with therapy-related MDS have clonal chromosomal abnormalities (+8,−7,−5, del(5q), del(7q), del(20q), iso(17), and complex karyotypes).
  – Detection of clonal abnormality establishes a diagnosis of neoplasm and rules out a nutritional, toxic, or autoimmune cause.
- Granulocyte function tests: Abnormal in 1/2 (decreased myeloperoxidase activity, phagocytosis, chemotaxis, and adhesion)
- Platelet function tests: Impaired aggregation

- Marrow colony assays in vitro
  – Results variable and correlate poorly with clinical course.
  – Poor clonal growth may suggest more rapid evolution to AML.
- Immunophenotyping
  – Nonspecific myeloid markers are present.
  – Occasionally, evidence can be found for concomitant lymphoproliferative disorder.
  – Loss of CD59 expression suggests PNH.

Lab
- Anemia: Often macrocytic; occasional poikilocytosis, anisocytosis; variable reticulocytosis
- Granulocytopenia: Hypogranular or agranular neutrophils with poorly condensed chromatin. Pelger-Huet anomaly with hyposegmented nuclei
- Thrombocytopenia: Occasionally giant platelets or hypogranular platelets
- Fetal hemoglobin: > in 70%
- Flow cytometry to detect loss of CD59 on RBC, CD16 on granulocytes, and CD14 on monocytes; typical of PNH
- Direct antiglobulin (Coombs) test: Positive in some
- Paraprotein: Present in some
- Erythropoietin: Usually normal or physiologically compensated levels unless renal failure is present
- Increased serum and tissue iron, especially if anemia has been long-standing

Imaging
Liver/spleen scan or CT, although rarely necessary, may disclose occult splenomegaly or lymphadenopathy.

Diagnostic Procedures/Surgery
- Bone marrow aspiration, biopsy, and cytogenetics
- Review peripheral blood smear.

Pathological Findings
- Ineffective hematopoiesis with dysplasia in 1 or more cell lineages dominates the bone marrow picture in MDS.
- Marrow cellularity is usually normal or increased for the patient's age but may be hypoplastic in ~10%.
- Reticulin fibrosis is usually minimal except in therapy-related MDS.
- Myeloblasts may be clustered in the intertrabecular spaces with abnormal localization of immature precursors (ALIP).

DIFFERENTIAL DIAGNOSIS
- Other malignant disorders
  – Evolving AML or erythroleukemia
  – Chronic myeloproliferative disorders (CML)
  – Polycythemia vera
  – Myeloid metaplasia with myelofibrosis
  – Malignant lymphoma
  – Metastatic carcinoma
- Nonmalignant disorders
  – Aplastic anemia
  – Autoimmune disorders (Felty syndrome, lupus)
  – Nutritional deficiencies (pyridoxine, vitamin B_{12}, protein malnutrition)
  – Heavy metal intoxication
  – Alcoholism
  – Chronic liver disease
  – Hypersplenism
  – Chronic inflammation
  – Recent cytotoxic therapy or irradiation
  – HIV infection
  – Paroxysmal nocturnal hemoglobinuria (PNH)

TREATMENT

GENERAL MEASURES

- Immunize for pneumococcal pneumonia and influenza and hepatitis B.
- RBC transfusions to alleviate symptoms
- Platelet transfusions only for bleeding or prior to surgery to avoid alloimmunization
- Early use of antibiotics for fever, even while culture results are pending, due to quantitative and qualitative granulocyte disorder
- Iron chelation therapy to avoid iron overload from chronic transfusions

Diet

- Reduce alcohol use.
- Reduce iron intake.

Activity

As tolerated

MEDICATION (DRUGS)

First Line

- Only 5-azacitidine has been proven more effective for these heterogeneous disorders than supportive care with antibiotics and transfusions as needed. Vitamins, iron, corticosteroids, androgens, or thyroid hormone are rarely helpful unless evidence of a specific deficiency exists.
- Clinical trials with 5-azacitidine, 75 mg/m^2 SC for 7 days; repeated every 28 days, decreases RBC transfusion requirements and yields longer times to AML or death and improvements in quality of life. (4)[A]
- Lenalidomide 10 mg PO daily for 21 days every 4 weeks has yielded complete remissions in patients with MDS and del(5q). (5)[B]
- Intensive chemotherapy
  - Younger patients with MDS may benefit from AML chemotherapy, especially if Auer rods are present, but toxicity may be severe for older patients.
  - Remission durations are variable (median, ~1 year).
- Allogeneic bone marrow transplantation
  - Recommended for younger patients with HLA-matched donors to eradicate the malignant clone and resupply normal hematopoietic stem cells
- Aminocaproic acid (epsilon-aminocaproic acid, EACA) or tranexamic acid may benefit patients with chronic, severe thrombocytopenia and bleeding.
- Contraindications: Cytotoxicity of chemotherapy may increase the risk of bleeding and infection and the need for transfusion support.
- Precautions: Aspirin, salicylates, and NSAIDs should be avoided.

Second Line

- Possible differentiating agents, such as tretinoin (all-*trans* retinoic acid), homoharringtonine, arsenic trioxide, thalidomide, and other hematopoietic growth factors, are under investigation.
- Danazol or prednisone may benefit concomitant autoimmune thrombocytopenia.
- Investigational agents
  - Low doses of cytarabine or decitabine, 13-*cis* retinoic acid, interferon, cyclosporine, granulocyte macrophage–colony-stimulating factor (GM-CSF), or granulocyte colony-stimulating factor (G-CSF), interleukin-3 (IL-3)
  - Agents, such as thalidomide, that inhibit production of tumor necrosis factor in the marrow
- Amifostine may stimulate proliferation of normal hematopoiesis.

FOLLOW-UP

DISPOSITION

Usually outpatient except when necessary to hospitalize for treatment of infection, blood transfusions, or intensive chemotherapy

PROGNOSIS

- Median survival for RA and RARS is 5 years but may extend much longer.
- Refractory anemia with del(5q) syndrome is quite favorable.
- Median survival for RAEB, RCMD, and CMMoL is ~1 year with 1/2 of the patients evolving to AML and the other 1/2 dying of infection or bleeding.

COMPLICATIONS

- Infection
- Bleeding
- Complications of anemia and transfusions

PATIENT MONITORING

- At least monthly during supportive care
- More frequently if receiving treatment

REFERENCES

1. Jaffe ES, Harris NL, Stein H, Vardiman JW, eds. *WHO Classification of Tumours. Pathology and Genetics of Tumours of Haematopoietic and Lymphoid Tissues.* Lyon, France: IARC Press: 2001.
2. Thirman MJ, Larson RA. Therapy-related myeloid leukemia. *Hematol Oncol Clin North Am.* 1996;10:293–320.
3. Greenberg P, et al. International scoring system for evaluating prognosis in myelodysplastic syndromes. *Blood.* 1997;89:2079–2088.
4. Silverman LR, et al. Randomized controlled trial of azacitidine in patients with the myelodysplastic syndrome: A study of the cancer and leukemia group B. *J Clin Oncol.* 2002;20:2429–2440.
5. List A, et al. Efficacy of lenalidomide in myelodysplastic syndromes. *N Engl J Med.* 2005;352:549–557.

MISCELLANEOUS

CODES

ICD9-CM
238.7 Neoplasm of uncertain behavior of other lymphatic and hematopoietic tissues

PATIENT TEACHING

- Stop smoking.
- Seek early medical attention for fever, bleeding, or symptoms of anemia.
- Advise about the risks of chronic transfusion therapy.

See Corresponding Diagnostic Algorithm

M

MYELOPROLIFERATIVE DISORDERS

Javed M. Gilani, MD, FACP, FRCP

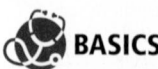 **BASICS**

DESCRIPTION

- Neoplasms of the pluripotent hematopoietic stem cell, including chronic myelogenous leukemia (CML), polycythemia vera (PV), chronic idiopathic myelofibrosis (CIMF; also known as agnogenic myeloid metaplasia or myelofibrosis with myeloid metaplasia), and essential thrombocytosis (ET). PV is discussed in another chapter.
- With each disorder, the proliferation of 1 particular cell line tends to dominate. Variable tendency for reactive proliferation of the bone marrow fibroblast, which is not a part of the malignant clone, resulting in myelofibrosis, and a variable tendency for termination in an acute leukemic phase. These disorders can mimic one another closely; CML is the only 1 that is readily distinguished from the others by the presence of the Philadelphia chromosome.
- CML
  - Characterized by splenomegaly and increased granulocytes, particularly neutrophils
  - Runs a mild course until it transforms to a frankly leukemic (blastic) phase
- CIMF
  - Characterized by extramedullary hematopoiesis in the spleen or multiple other organs, and myelofibrosis
  - Myelofibrosis appears to be a reaction to the presence of the abnormal, proliferating hematopoietic clone
- ET: Dominated clinically by a markedly elevated platelet count
- System(s) Affected: Hematologic/Lymphatic/ Immunologic

EPIDEMIOLOGY

- Predominant age
  - CML: Median age at diagnosis 50–60 years
  - CIMF, ET: Median age at diagnosis 60 years; a distinct 2nd peak incidence of ET occurs in younger patients, usually women, at ~30 years of age.
  - All these disorders are rare in the young; more often found in middle and later years.
- Predominant sex
  - CML: Male > Female (1.4:1)
  - CIMF: Male = Female
  - ET: Female > Male (1.3:1)

Incidence

- CML: 1–2/100,000/year; increases with age
- CIMF: 0.5–1.5/100,000/year
- ET: 1–2.5/100,000/year

RISK FACTORS

- Family history of similar disorder (rare)
- CML: Increased incidence in atomic bomb survivors and following radiation treatment of ankylosing spondylitis and cervical cancer

Genetics

- CML: No genetic predisposition known
- CIMF: Rare familial occurrence
- ET: May be familial
- CML: >95% of patients are Philadelphia chromosome positive (shortened chromosome 22 due to a reciprocal translocation between chromosomes 9 and 22). This results in a fusion of the *ABL* gene on chromosome 9 to the *BCR* gene on chromosome 22.

ETIOLOGY

Unknown; may be familial for some types

ASSOCIATED CONDITIONS

CIMF: Immunologic abnormalities have been reported, including presence of antinuclear antibodies, elevated rheumatoid factor titers, presence of lupus anticoagulants, direct Coombs positivity, hypocomplementemia

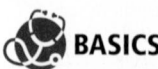 **DIAGNOSIS**

SIGNS AND SYMPTOMS

- General
  - Most are asymptomatic at the time of diagnosis.
  - Vague constitutional symptoms
  - Hypermetabolic state (fever, sweating)
  - Acute gouty arthritis
  - Left upper quadrant abdominal pain or fullness from splenomegaly
- CML: Splenomegaly (palpable 90% of time)
- CIMF
  - Splenomegaly in virtually all patients; may be massive
  - Hepatomegaly: 50%
  - Lymph node enlargement: 10%
  - Jaundice, edema, and ascites: 10–20%
  - Petechiae: up to 25%
- ET
  - May be asymptomatic in >50%
  - Easy bruising, unusual bleeding after minor dental procedures, large-vessel bleeding in the absence of trauma
  - Transient ischemic attacks, or even frank strokes, may occur in patients with markedly elevated platelet counts.

TESTS

Lab

- CML
  - Marked leukocytosis consisting of mature polymorphonuclear neutrophils and myelocytes or metamyelocytes
  - Chronic phase typically presents with <2% myeloblasts in peripheral blood and <5% blasts in the bone marrow.
  - The blast crisis is defined when ≥20% blast cells are present in the bone marrow and/or peripheral blood.
  - Basophilia
  - Elevated serum vitamin B_{12} level
  - Hyperuricemia
  - Markedly decreased LAP (absent in 5–10%)
- CIMF
  - Mild anemia: >50% at time of diagnosis; eventually in almost all patients; progressive
  - Leukocytosis: 30%
  - Leukoerythroblastic blood picture: >90%
  - Leukopenia: 25%
  - Thrombocytopenia: 30%
  - Marked thrombocytosis (>800,000 platelets/L): 12%
  - Occasional RBC autoantibodies
- ET: World Health Organization criteria
- Thrombocytosis persistently >600,000 platelets/L in the absence of an identifiable cause

- Bone marrow biopsy showing increased numbers of enlarged, mature megakaryocytes
  - No evidence of PV (normal total RBC mass)
  - Presence of iron in the bone marrow, normal ferritin, or normal mean corpuscular volume
  - Absence of collagen fibrosis; minimal or absent reticulin fibrosis in bone marrow
  - Absence of the Philadelphia chromosome
  - No evidence of myelodysplastic syndrome (MDS)
  - No evidence of reactive thrombocytosis
- Disorders that may alter lab results
  - In CML, LAP rises during infection, glucocorticoid use, or successful therapy
  - False-positive hyperkalemia may be seen in ET as a result of release of platelet potassium upon blood clotting.

Imaging

CIMF: Radiographic osteosclerosis in 25–66% of patients, particularly in the axial skeleton and proximal long bones

Diagnostic Procedures/Surgery

- Peripheral blood smear
- Bone marrow aspiration and core biopsy
- Cytogenetic studies
- Molecular studies (reverse-transcriptase polymerase chain reaction to detect the *BCR-ABL* fusion gene)

Pathological Findings

CIMF

- Foci of extramedullary hematopoiesis may be seen in multiple organs, including spleen, liver, kidneys, lymph nodes, adrenal glands, lungs, and spinal column.
- Bone marrow megakaryocytic hyperplasia and atypia, reticulin and/or collagen fibrosis, osteosclerosis (new bone formation). Bone marrow cellularity is variable depending on the degree of fibrosis.

DIFFERENTIAL DIAGNOSIS

- CML
  - Leukemoid reaction
  - Chronic myelomonocytic leukemia that has features of both myeloproliferative and myelodysplastic syndromes
  - Low or absent leukocyte alkaline phosphatase (LAP) also is seen in paroxysmal nocturnal hemoglobinuria.
- CIMF
  - Spent PV (late stage of PV)
  - CML
  - MDS with fibrosis
  - Secondary myelofibrosis
- ET
  - Secondary thrombocytosis (including inflammation, iron deficiency, and neoplasia)
  - PV
  - CML

TREATMENT

INITIAL STABILIZATION
Treat to relieve symptoms and prevent infections

GENERAL MEASURES
- Splenectomy has no impact on mortality, but is occasionally done for symptomatic relief. Extreme thrombocytosis, progressive and massive liver enlargement may ensue.
- CML
  - Molecularly targeted therapy (with imatinib mesylate)
  - Chemotherapy (for advanced disease)
  - Bone marrow transplantation is only known curative option; disease-free survival 50–70%; offer to young patients with human lymphocyte antigen-matched donors
- CIMF
  - No standard therapy
  - Rule out other treatable causes for anemia.
  - Radiotherapy for symptomatic extramedullary hematopoietic tumors or symptomatic splenomegaly
  - Successful bone marrow transplantation leads to the reversal of established fibrosis; only known potential cure
- ET
  - Young, asymptomatic patients with platelet count <1,500,000/L usually not treated.
  - Lower the platelet count in those >60 years, with a history of thrombosis or with other cardiovascular risk factors, or if platelet count >1,500,000/L.

MEDICATION (DRUGS)

First Line
- CML
  - Imatinib mesylate (Gleevec), a potent inhibitor of the Abl tyrosine kinase, produces complete hematologic remissions in 95% and major cytogenetic remissions in 87% of newly diagnosed patients in chronic phase. Dosage: 400 mg/d in chronic phase CML, 600–800 mg/d in accelerated/blast-phase disease.
  - Interferon-α produces 55% complete hematologic remissions and 35% major cytogenetic remissions; it has largely been replaced by imatinib as the treatment of choice for most patients.
  - Hydroxyurea may be useful for controlling the excessive myelopoiesis at the initial diagnosis in the chronic-phase of the disease in conjunction with imatinib.
  - Allopurinol to control hyperuricemia: Begin prior to hydroxyurea therapy
  - Accelerated phase and blast crises are usually treated with regimens designed for treatment of acute leukemia. Imatinib mesylate induces hematologic remissions in 50% of patients with myeloid blast crises, and major cytogenetic remissions in 16%. This response is transient in duration.
  - Severe congenital defects have been reported with busulfan. Interferon-α is safe in pregnancy for myeloproliferation.

- ET
  - Hydroxyurea is generally favored over alkylating agents for control of thrombocytosis because it has little to no known leukemogenic potential.
  - Anagrelide also may be used to control thrombocytosis, particularly in younger patients with ET. Interferon is also useful for cytoreduction and is safe in pregnancy.
  - Caution: Prolonged use of platelet-antiaggregating agents may increase the risk of gastrointestinal hemorrhage.
- CIMF
  - Anemia is treated with transfusions as required. Androgenic steroids: Fluoxymesterone (Halotestin) 10 mg b.i.d. and prednisone 0.5 mg/kg/d may be useful for anemia. Erythropoietin (in patients with endogenous EPO levels of <100 IU/mL) and Danocrine (Danazol) have also been used for treatment of anemia.
  - Hydroxyurea is useful for control of splenomegaly, thrombocytosis, and leukocytosis.
  - Investigational drug therapy should be considered because there is no standard therapy that significantly impacts mortality.

Second Line
- CIMF
  - Androgens and glucocorticoids for anemia.
  - Corticosteroids for autoimmune hemolysis
- ET
  - Aspirin, with or without dipyridamole, may prove useful in preventing thrombotic or ischemic symptoms in some patients.
  - Erythromelalgia (described under Complications) responds to rapid reduction of the platelet count or to administration of NSAIDs.

FOLLOW-UP

PROGNOSIS
- CML
  - Median survival >5 years from time of diagnosis, ~12–18 months after development of accelerated phase, and 3–6 months after blast crisis.
  - Adverse prognostic factors include advanced age, degree of splenomegaly, elevated platelet count, degree of leukocytosis, presence of blasts or large numbers of eosinophils or basophils, percentage of immature cells in the marrow, and clonal evolution.
  - 85% will die in blast crisis
  - Pregnancy does not affect the course of the disease.
  - >95% of mothers survive to delivery, with >80% fetal survival rate through gestation
- CIMF
  - Progressive splenomegaly, anemia, and thrombocytopenia
  - Median survival is 5 years from diagnosis.
  - Patients usually die from hemorrhagic or thrombotic complications and infections; 10–20% of the cases terminate in a rapidly progressive form of acute leukemia.
  - Adverse prognostic factors: Hemoglobin <10 g/dL, leukocytosis (>30,000/L) or leukopenia (<10,000/L), circulating blasts, complex cytogenetic abnormalities, and hypercatabolic symptoms
- ET
  - Overall life expectancy is only slightly shortened. Some studies indicate no significant difference in survival between patients and age/sex-matched controls.

COMPLICATIONS
- Transformation to acute leukemia
- Gout due to hyperuricemia
- Uric acid nephropathy
- CIMF
  - Portal hypertension
  - Splenic infarcts
  - Budd-Chiari syndrome
  - Pulmonary hypertension
  - Pleural or peritoneal effusions due to extramedullary hematopoiesis (EMH)
  - Paraspinal/epidural EMH
- ET
  - Thrombohemorrhagic complications in 1/3
  - Erythromelalgia (vaso-occlusive syndrome with pain, burning, and warmth of distal extremities); may progress to gangrene
  - Increased risk of 1st-trimester abortion

REFERENCES
1. Doll DC, Gabrail NY, List AF, eds. Myeloproliferative disorders. *Semin Oncol*. 1995;22:305–411.
2. Jaffe ES, et al., eds. World Health Organization Classification of Tumours. Pathology and Genetics of Tumours of Haematopoietic and Lymphoid *Tissues*. Lyon, France: IARC Press, 2001.
3. O'Brien SG, et al. Imatinib compared with interferon and low dose cytarabine for newly diagnosed chronic-phase chronic myeloid leukemia. *N Engl J Med*. 2003;348:1048–1050.
4. Tefferi A. Myelofibrosis with myeloid metaplasia. *N Engl J Med*. 2000;342:1255–1265.

MISCELLANEOUS

See also: Leukemia; Polycythemia vera

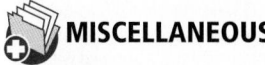

ICD9-CM
- 205.10 Chronic myeloid leukemia without mention of remission
- 205.11 Chronic myeloid leukemia in remission
- 238.7 Neoplasm of uncertain behavior of other lymphatic and hematopoietic tissues
- 289.89 Other specified diseases of blood and blood-forming organs

PATIENT TEACHING
- Explain the disorder, treatment protocols, lab studies, and prognosis.
- Advise the patient on symptoms of recurrence to watch for.
- Stress the importance of follow-up examinations.

M

MYOCARDIAL INFARCTION

Felix B. Chang, MD
Rajneesh S. Hazarika, MD, MS

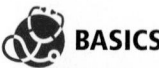 **BASICS**

DESCRIPTION

- Acute myocardial infarction (MI) is the rapid development of myocardial necrosis resulting from a sustained and complete absense of blood flow to a portion of the myocardium, produced by a superimposed thrombosis, and generated by a ruptured atherosclerotic plaque.
- Criteria for acute, evolving or recent MI
- Either typical rise and fall of biochemical markers of myocardial necrosis (gradual increase of troponin, or more rapid rise and fall for CK-MB) and at least 1 of
  – Ischemic symptoms
  – Development of pathologic Q waves on ECG
  – ECG changes indicative of ischemia (ST segment elevation or depression)
  – Coronary artery intervention
  – Or pathologic finders of acute MI
- Criteria for establish MI: Either of the following
  – Development of new pathologic Q waves on serial ECGs
  – Pathologic findings of healed or healing MI
- Clinical consequences depend on size and location of infarct and rapidity with which blood flow can be restored by pharmacologic or mechanical modalities.
- After occlusion, myocardial necrosis is complete in 4–6 hours. Flow to ischemic area must remain >40% of preocclusion levels for area to survive.
- Infarctions can be divided into Q wave and non-Q wave categories: Q wave-transmural is associated with a totally obstructed infarct-related artery; non–Q wave-nontransmural is associated with patent but narrowed infarct-related artery.
- Total occlusion of the left main coronary artery, which supplies 70% of left ventricle, is catastrophic and results in death in minutes.
- Location of infarction
  – Anterior: Left anterior descending coronary artery
  – Septal MI: Left anterior descending coronary artery
  – Lateral: Left circumflex coronary artery
  – Posterior: Right coronary artery
  – Interior MI: Right coronary artery
- System(s) Affected: Cardiovascular
- Synonym(s): Coronary thrombosis; Coronary occlusion; Heart attack

EPIDEMIOLOGY

- Predominant age: >40 years
- Predominant sex:
  – Age 40–70: Male > Female
  – Age >70: Male = Female

Incidence

- Leading cause of death in Western society
- Up to 1,500,000 Americans have an attack each year, with about 1/3 mortality; 600/100,000.

RISK FACTORS

- Dyslipidemia (decreased high-density lipoprotein; increased low-density lipoprotein)
- Family history of premature (age <55 years for men, age <65 years of women) onset of coronary disease
- Tobacco abuse
- Diabetes mellitus (DM is considered CHD Risk Equivalent)
- Hypertension or on a hypertensive medication
- Age >45 (male) or >55 (female)
- Secondary risk factors
  – Obesity/sedentary lifestyle

ETIOLOGY

- Atherosclerotic coronary artery disease
  – Acute coronary thrombosis superimposed on atherosclerotic plaque
  – Sudden thrombotic occlusion at site of fissured or rupture atherosclerotic plaque embolizing coronary arteries
- Nonatherosclerotic
  – Emboli
    ○ Thrombi from left ventricle (acute MI, cardiomyopathy), left atrium (mitral stenosis, catheters during angiography)
    ○ Air emboli (coronary angiography)
    ○ Infectious endocarditis
    ○ Atrial myxoma
  – Mechanical obstruction
    ○ Chest trauma
    ○ Dissection or aorta
    ○ Dissection of coronary arteries (postpartum, post-PTCA, angiography)
  – Increase vasomotor tone; variant angina
  – Arteritis
    ○ Collagen vascular disease (PAN,SLE,RA)
    ○ Takayasu disease
    ○ Kawasaki syndrome
    ○ Luetic aortitis (syphilis)
  – Others
    ○ Hematologic (DIC)
    ○ Aortic stenosis
    ○ Hypertrophic cardiomyopathy
    ○ Cocaine, prolonged hypotension
    ○ Electrical burn
    ○ Tay-Sachs disease, amyloidosis

ASSOCIATED CONDITIONS

- Abdominal aortic aneurysm
- Extracranial cerebrovascular disease
- Atherosclerotic peripheral vascular disease

℞ DIAGNOSIS

SIGNS AND SYMPTOMS

- Pain—arm, back, jaw, epigastrium, neck, chest
- Anxiety
- Lightheadedness, pallor, weakness, syncope
- Nausea, vomiting, diaphoresis
- Chest heaviness, tightness
- Cough, diaphoresis, dyspnea, rales, wheezing
- S_4 heart sound

- Arrhythmias
- Hypertension, hypotension
- Jugular venous distention
- Cannon jugular venous A waves (in presence of heart block or right ventricular failure)

TESTS

- Electrocardiography (ECG)
  – ST segment elevation in a regional pattern: Typical of acute transmural ischemia
  – ST segment depression with T wave inversions: Typical of subendocardial ischemia
  – New or presumably new bundle branch block
  – ST segment changes are findings of ischemia; transmural infarction may show normal ECG.
  – Q waves representing transmural myocardial necrosis appear within 24–48 hours.

Lab

- Troponin I is a specific indicator of MI; appears 3–6 hours after MI, peaks at 16 hours, and decreases in 9–10 days.
- Creatine kinase (CK): Rises following infarction within 4–8 hours; peaks 18–24 hours; and subsides over 3–4 days. Specific indicator for myocardial necrosis; has 15% false-positive rate
- CK isoenzymes: BB in brain and kidney, and MB in cardiac muscle
- Lactate dehydrogenase: Rises within 24 hours, peaks within 3–6 days, and returns to baseline within 8–12 days
- ESR: Rises within 3 days and may remain elevated for several weeks
- Leukocytes: Rise within several hours after MI, peak in 2–4 days, and normal within 1 week

Imaging

- ECG
  – 2-dimensional and M-mode echocardiography are useful in evaluating wall motion in MI and left ventricular function.
  – Useful in assessing mechanical complications (e.g., mitral valve rupture or VSD) and mural thrombus
- Chest radiography to evaluate for CHF.
- Radionuclide studies: Thallium scanning: Accumulates in viable myocardium

Diagnostic Procedures/Surgery

- Angiography to reestablish coronary perfusion is preferable to thrombolytics during the 1st 12 hours. Early intervention shown to be safe.
- Procedural coronary intervention (PCI) with tirofiban or abciximab prior to catheterization: Recommended for suspected non-Q wave infarction (new ST segment depression or T wave inversion and initial cardiac enzyme elevation)

Pathological Findings

- Myocardial necrosis
- Atherosclerosis, if etiologic
- Thrombosis; not usually seen because spontaneous thrombolysis occurs within 24 hours

DIFFERENTIAL DIAGNOSIS

- Unstable angina pectoris: Serial ECG and enzymes to differentiate
- Aortic dissection
- Pulmonary embolism
- Pleuropericarditis: Differentiated by history of postural improvement of pain and pleuritic component, plus friction rub and upward concave diffuse ST segment elevation on ECG
- Esophageal spasm: No ECG or enzyme change
- Pancreatitis and biliary tract disease
- Hyperventilation syndrome

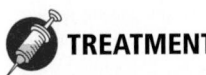 TREATMENT

INITIAL STABILIZATION
Inpatient treatment in coronary care unit

GENERAL MEASURES
- Analgesia
- Limitation of infarct size/salvage myocardium
- Arrhythmias
  - Ventricular tachycardia: Direct-current (DC) countershock, lidocaine, or IV amiodarone (Cordarone)
  - Ventricular fibrillation: DC countershock and cardiopulmonary resuscitation (CPR), IV amiodarone (Cordarone)
  - Atrial flutter and fibrillation: Digitalis or IV diltiazem (Cardizem) or verapamil. If hemodynamic compromise, DC countershock or rapid atrial pacing. May also use IV amiodarone (Cordarone)
  - Sinus bradycardia: No treatment unless hypotension or hemodynamic compromise; treat with atropine and, if ineffective, perform electrical pacing
  - Atrioventricular block: In inferior infarction, transvenous pacing if patient is hemodynamically compromised. In anterior infarction, pacing is usually required because escape rhythm is unstable, with ventricular asystole occurring quite suddenly.
  - Cardiac catheterization followed by percutaneous transluminal coronary angioplasty (P/stent) or coronary artery bypass grafting (CABG). Use clopidogrel as pretreatment; abciximab plus unfractionated heparin when clinically indicated. Door-to-balloon time should be <90 minutes.

Diet
NPO until stable; later, low-fat, low-salt diet

Activity
- Bed rest for 1st 24 hours; bedside commode
- Medically supervised rehabilitation plan

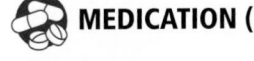 MEDICATION (DRUGS)

First Line
- Coronary reperfusion
  - Aspirin : 325 mg PO acutely
  - (Alteplase); tissue plasminogen activator: 15 mg IV bolus, 50 mg over 30 minutes, then 35 mg over 60 minutes
  - Heparin by protocol or low-molecular-weight heparin; enoxaparin (Lovenox) 1 mg/kg q12h SC (preferred)
- Acute MI, general
  - Nitrates: 5 μg/min IV, increase slowly. Do not lower arterial blood pressure beyond 90 mm Hg. Change to oral or topical when stable.
  - Oxygen: 2–4 L/min

- Morphine: 2–6 mg IV q2–4h as needed for pain relief/sedation
- Metoprolol (Lopressor): 5 mg IV × 3, 5 minutes apart, followed by 50 mg PO q6h starting 15 minutes after last IV dose
- Stool softeners: Docusate sodium (dioctyl sodium sulfosuccinate) 100 mg 2 b.i.d.
- Lidocaine: 1–2 mg/kg IV once, then 1–4 mg/min IV drip. Use for ventricular arrhythmias only, not for prophylaxis
- Post MI
  - β-Blockers reduce mortality.
  - Nitrates may be needed for angina.
  - ACE inhibitors may assist with remodeling.
- Contraindications
  - β-Blockers are relatively contraindicated in acute heart failure and bronchospasm; may use IV esmolol (short-acting) safely.
  - IV thrombolysis is contraindicated in patients with active internal hemorrhage; recent head trauma, intracranial neoplasm, or hemorrhagic cerebrovascular accident; pregnancy; persistent hypertension (>200/120 mm Hg); prolonged (>10 minutes) or traumatic CPR; hemorrhagic retinopathy; trauma or major surgery within 2 weeks; or advanced age (>80 years). Relatively contraindicated with peptic ulcer or heme-positive stools, bleeding disorders, anticoagulation, prior exposure to streptokinase or streptococcal infection in past 6 months, minor trauma or major surgery within 2 months.

Second Line
- Thrombolytics: Tenecteplase or reteplase
- β-Blockers for acute arrhythmia: Atenolol 5 mg IV over 5 minutes; 2nd dose 10 minutes later; followed by 50 mg PO 10 minutes after 2nd IV dose; then q12h for at least 7 days

SURGERY
- Coronary reperfusion
  - Emergency stenting is a mechanical form of coronary reperfusion. It is considered superior to IV thrombolysis if within 1st 12 hours.
  - Can be accomplished with low mortality.
- Pump failure: Intra-aortic balloon pump

 FOLLOW-UP

DISPOSITION
- No evidence supports bed rest >12 hours after uncomplicated MI (2).
- Hospitalization >72 hours after thrombolysis of uncomplicated MI is not cost-effective in decision analysis.

PROGNOSIS
Overall mortality rate is 10% during the hospital phase, with an additional 10% mortality rate during the year post MI. More than 60% of the deaths occur within 1 hour of the onset of the event.

COMPLICATIONS
- CHF
- Cardiogenic shock
- Myocardial rupture
  - Ventricular free wall rupture
  - Papillary muscle rupture
- Left ventricular aneurysm
- Left ventricular and peripheral embolism
- DVT and pulmonary embolism
- Pericarditis
- Dysrhythmias
- Mitral regurgitation
- Ventricular septal defect
- Dressler syndrome
- Cardiac arrest
- Severe depression
- Death
  - Prehospital deaths are related to arrhythmias (VF). Most occur during 1st 4 hours after symptom onset; about 50% of total acute MI mortality
  - In-hospital death due to low cardiac output (CHF, cardiogenic shock) in first 48 hours.

ALERT
Geriatric Considerations
Incidence of all complications is higher.

PATIENT MONITORING
Early intervention: Recurrent chest pain, CHF, hemodynamic instability, sustained V. tachycardia

REFERENCES
1. Braunwald E, et al. American College of Cardiology/American Heart Association Task Force on Practice Guidelines. ACC/AHA guideline update for the management of patients with unstable angina and non-ST-segment elevation myocardial infarction. *Circulation*. 2002;106:1893–1900.
2. Cannon CP, Weintraub WS, Demopoulos LA. TACTICS Comparison of early invasive and conservative strategies in patients with unstable coronary syndromes treated with the glycoprotein IIb/IIIa inhibitor tirofiban. *N Engl J Med*. 2001;344.

ADDITIONAL READING
- Printed patient information is available from the American Heart Association, 7320 Greenville Avenue, Dallas, TX 75231;(214)373-6300
- American Heart Association/American College of Cardiology (AHA/ACC) 2004 guidelines on ST myocardial infarction (STEMI) can be found at http://www.acc.org/clinical/guidelines/stemi/index.htm.

 MISCELLANEOUS

See also: CHF

PATIENT TEACHING

 See Corresponding Diagnostic Algorithm

See Patient Handout on CD

M

NARCISSISTIC PERSONALITY DISORDER (NPD)

Lawrence E. Udom, MD, MPH

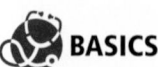 BASICS

DESCRIPTION
Narcissism is characterized as a Cluster B Personality Disorder. It is defined as an enduring pattern of inflexible and maladaptive behaviors/traits that cause either significant impairment in social or occupational functioning or subjective distress. The features of NPD are a pervasive pattern of grandiosity (in fantasy or behavior), need for admiration, and lack of empathy, beginning by early adulthood and present in a variety of contexts (see "Diagnosis").

ALERT
Geriatric Considerations
Exacerbated by aging due to the inability to adapt to the physical, mental, and occupational restrictions it imposes, leading to depression.

GENERAL PREVENTION
No known prevention for NPD

EPIDEMIOLOGY
- Predominant age: Occurs in early adulthood.
- Predominant sex: Male > Female (50–75%)

Prevalence
The lifetime prevalence rate of NPD is ~0.5–1% among the general population; however, the estimated prevalence in clinical settings is ~2–16%. (1)

RISK FACTORS
Genetics
No definitive data indicates a genetic basis for NPD.

ASSOCIATED CONDITIONS
- Bipolar disorder
- Depression
- Obsessive compulsive disorder

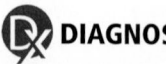 DIAGNOSIS

SIGNS AND SYMPTOMS
Several articles have attempted to characterize the diagnosis criteria for NPD; the essential features are
- Superiority: Grandiose sense of self-importance
  - These individuals exaggerate achievements and talents to the point of lying; they demand to be recognized as superior without commensurate achievements
- Grandiose fantasies, and preoccupation with beauty, brilliance, ideal love, power, or unlimited success
- Uniqueness: Possess the belief of being special and unique and can only be understood, or can only associate with people of high status
- Requires excessive admiration
- Sense of entitlement: Possess unreasonable expectation of being treated with favor or expecting an automatic compliance to their wishes. They will use others to achieve their goals
- Lack of empathy: These individuals are unable or unwilling to identify with or acknowledge the feelings and needs of others
- Envy: These individuals believe others are envious of them or are envious of others
- Exhibit arrogant or haughty attitudes/behaviors
- High achievement, these patients often have periods of success (e.g., academic, employment, or social), which may only serve to verify their sense of superiority. (1,2)

History
- Must rule out other general medical conditions, or other psychiatric illnesses
- See "Signs and Symptoms."

TESTS
Patients can be evaluated for NPD using the Diagnostic Interview for Narcissism. (3)[A]

DIFFERENTIAL DIAGNOSIS
- Other personality disorders are often confused with NPD due to their common features (1)
  - Histrionic, antisocial, and borderline personality disorders also possess the indifferent, callous, and oftentimes needy characteristics. NPD can be distinguished by the grandiosity characteristic.
  - The relative stability of self-image as well as the relative lack of self-destructiveness, impulsivity, and abandonment concerns also help distinguish NPD from borderline personality disorder
  - Borderline, histrionic, and NPD patients require attention; however, NPD individuals require that attention to be admiring.
  - Individuals with antisocial and NPD tend to be self-centered, superficial, exploitative, and un-empathic. However, NPD does not necessarily include characteristics of impulsivity, aggression, and deceit, and usually do not give the same history of conduct disorder or criminal behavior.
  - Both NPD and obsessive-compulsive personality disorder have a goal of perfectionism and believe that others cannot do things as well. But NPD individuals often believe that they have achieved perfection.
  - NPD individuals may exhibit suspiciousness and social withdrawal similar to schizotypal or paranoid personality disorder; however, when present with NPD, these emotions are usually derived from fears of having their imperfections or flaws revealed.
- Traumatic brain injury
- CNS tumor/infection
- Dementia
- Delirium
- Substance abuse
  - NPD must also be distinguished from symptoms that may develop in association with chronic substance use (e.g., cocaine-related disorder).

TREATMENT

GENERAL MEASURES

- Individual and group psychotherapy are offered for NPD, with only anecdotal reports of success. [A]

- Individuals with NPD usually come for therapy with presenting issues other than the aforementioned diagnostic features—most often for depression and anxiety. (4) They often see the difficulties that they have with others as external and independent of their behavior. Their depression is often precipitated by situations that challenge the narcissistic grandiosity and reflects the discrepancy between NPD expectations or fantasies and reality.

- Individuals with NPD may have trouble entering treatment because they associate needing help as demeaning and unacceptable. If the situation becomes sever enough, however, they will seek treatment in order to re-establish feelings of superiority and achievement.

- Therapy is often complicated by narcissists' view of themselves. Their past, their current situation, and what they need from treatment will all be distorted by their need for acknowledgement of their superiority. They will resist feedback and may reject treatment if they are not sufficiently affirmed
  - Complication to treatment is that NPDs chronically devalue those around them and demonstrate little empathy, thereby setting up potential countertransference situations with health care providers.
  - Another complication is that the return to comfort for individuals with NPD may be all that they are seeking and they will leave treatment prematurely.
  - Treatment can also be complicated by concomitant depression diagnosis.

- Treatment can fail in terms of psychotherapy, when consideration of possible substance abuse is ignored.

 ## MEDICATION (DRUGS)

NPDs are vulnerable to severe depression, particularly when their superiority is challenged or with maladaptation to the effects of aging. Antidepressant medication may be needed, selective seratonin reuptake inhibitors have been used to reduce target symptoms of interpersonal reactivity. (5)[B]

PROGNOSIS

The prognosis for an adult suffering from NPD is poor, though their adaptation to situations and relationships can improve with treatment

COMPLICATIONS

- Family and relationship dysfunction
- Alcohol and other substance abuse. There is no single pattern of substance use or abuse that can be identified for NPD; however, cocaine, as a high-status drug, is particularly attractive to the narcissist. (6)
- Major depressive disorder
- Dysthymia
- Obsessive-compulsive behaviors
- Eating disorders (particularly in young women) (7)

REFERENCES

1. American Psychiatric Association. *DSM-IV-TR 2000: Diagnostic & Statistical Manual of Mental Disorders*. 4th ed. Washington, DC: American Psychiatric Publishing. Inc; 2000.
2. Ronningstam E, Gunderson JR. Identifying criteria for narcissistic personality disorder. *Am J Psychiatry*. 1990;147:918–922.
3. Gunderson JR: The diagnostic interview for narcissistic patients. *Arch Gen Psychiatry*. 1990;47(7):676–680.
4. Beck AT, Freeman A. *Cognitive therapy of personality disorders*. New York, NY: Guilford Press; 1990.
5. Sperry L. *Handbook of Diagnosis and Treatment of the DSM-IV Personality Disorders*. New York, NY: Brunner/Mazel; 1995.
6. Beck AT, et al. *Cognitive Therapy of Substance Abuse*. New York, NY: The Guilford Press; 1993.
7. Brunton JN, et al. Narcissism and eating characteristics in young nonclinical women. *J Nerv Ment Dis*. 2005;193(2):140–143.

MISCELLANEOUS

CODES

ICD9-CM
301.81

N

NARCOLEPSY

Jeffrey F. Minteer, MD

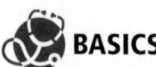

BASICS

DESCRIPTION
Disorder of unknown etiology characterized by excessive sleepiness typically associated with cataplexy and other REM sleep phenomena, such as sleep paralysis and hypnagogic hallucinations. Commonly misconceived as representing low intelligence and/or poor motivation. Syndrome frequently overlooked, with an average of 15 years of symptoms prior to diagnosis. Onset usually in teenage years.
- System(s) Affected: Nervous

EPIDEMIOLOGY
- Predominant age: Mean age at onset 18, 50% >40 years
- Predominant sex: Male = Female

ALERT
Pediatric Considerations
Uncommon in childhood

Prevalence
One in 3,000 diagnosed

RISK FACTORS
- Head trauma
- CNS infectious disease
- Anesthesia
- Family history

Genetics
- Autosomal recessive
- Increased incidence in families with positive history
- Incidence in 1st-degree relative of index case is 1–2% (vs. 0.02% general population)
- Biologic marker HLA-DR2 allele on short arm of chromosome 6 in 100% of white patients; 1/3 normal subjects are also positive. African American narcoleptic patients: 30% are non-DR 2, but all with HLA-Dw1.

ETIOLOGY
- Unknown; associated with loss of the neurotransmitter hypocretin-1 in CNS
- Possible involvement of immune system
- 75% of narcoleptic patients: No detectable hypocretin in CSF

ASSOCIATED CONDITIONS
Obstructive sleep apnea

DIAGNOSIS

REM periods during Multiple Sleep Latency Test (MSLT)
- Diagnostic criteria according to International Classification of Sleep Disorders
- Minimal criteria is B plus C, or A plus D plus E plus G
  - A. Excessive sleepiness
  - B. Recurrent lapses into sleep daily for ≥3 months
  - C. Cataplexy
  - D. Associated features: Sleep paralysis, hypnagogic hallucinations, disrupted sleep
  - E. MSLT abnormalities as described
  - F. Biologic markers (see "Genetics")
  - G. Absence of medical or psychiatric disorder
  - H. CSF hypocretin-1 level low: 99% specificity, 87% sensitivity; useful in children unable to do MSLT

SIGNS AND SYMPTOMS
- Tetrad: 10–20% with all symptoms
  - Excessive daytime sleepiness, cataplexy, sleep paralysis, hypnagogic hallucinations (4 most common symptoms)
- Excessive daytime sleepiness and sleep attacks: Primary symptom, most severe form of narcolepsy
  - Instantaneous, irresistible REM sleep
  - 1st and most disabling symptom
  - Tendency to take naps lasting 5–10 minutes
  - Episodes last minutes to hours
  - 1–8 naps per day, 24-hour duration of sleep normal
  - Increased in monotonous environment, warm environment, after a large meal, or with strong emotions
  - 20–25% of all patients with excessive somnolence
- Cataplexy: Auxiliary symptom (70%)
  - Sudden bilateral weakness of skeletal muscles
  - Provocation by sudden strong wave of emotion
  - Lack of impairment of consciousness and memory
  - Short duration (less than a few minutes)
  - Responsiveness to treatment with clomipramine and imipramine)
  - Can be limited to a particular muscle group (e.g., jaw droop with inability to speak; arm, neck, or leg weakness
- Sleep paralysis: Auxiliary symptom (50%)
  - When falling asleep or on awakening, patient wants to move but cannot
  - Brain wakes from sleep while body remains in REM sleep
  - Lasts seconds to minutes
  - Patients are aware of events around them, but cannot open eyes or move
  - Can be preceded by hallucinatory phenomena
  - 50% of normal population have 1 or more episodes (nonspecific)
- Hypnagogic hallucinations: Auxiliary symptom (60%)
  - Vivid, frightening auditory or visual illusions or hallucinations at onset of sleep
  - Dreamlike experiences that occur during wakefulness or suddenly at sleep onset
  - Characteristic hallucinations include seeing human or animal faces or feeling that someone else is in the room.

- Disturbed nocturnal sleep (66%)
  - Normal total sleep with decreased sleep efficiency
  - More frequent transitions from wakefulness to sleep
  - Retrograde amnesic and automatic behavior lasting minutes to hours
  - Increased periodic leg movements (50%)

TESTS
Lab
HLA-DR2

Diagnostic Procedures/Surgery
- Nighttime polysomnography: Monitoring of patients in sleep laboratory will usually document fragmented sleep with normal amount of REM sleep but a pattern of sleep-onset REM. Polysomnography rules out other causes of excessive daytime sleepiness including sleep apnea syndromes and nocturnal myoclonus.
- Multiple sleep latency test: Begins ≥90 minutes after nighttime test. Patient monitored during 4–5 naps taken at 2-hour intervals. Rapidity of sleep onset and type of sleep pattern are documented. Supportive test includes mean sleep latency (time to fall asleep) of ≤5 minutes and 1 or more sleep-onset REM periods. Sensitivity 77%, specificity 97%, positive predictive value 73%.
- Human leukocyte antigen typing in ambiguous cases

DIFFERENTIAL DIAGNOSIS
Excessive daytime sleepiness present in 4% of population; most are not narcolepsy; causes include
- Sleep apnea syndromes: 40–50% of those with excessive somnolence
- Epileptic seizures and syncope
- Idiopathic CNS hypersomnolence: 5–10% of those with excessive somnolence
- Nocturnal myoclonus
- Psychomotor seizures
- Abuse of sedative drugs
- Clinical diagnosis possible if cataplexy present

TREATMENT

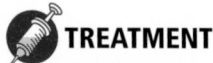

GENERAL MEASURES
- Inpatient for sleep-laboratory analysis, outpatient for follow-up
- Usually managed with medication
- Regularly scheduled time for naps may help in mild cases.
- Regular sleep-wake schedule

Diet
No special diet; avoid alcohol

Activity
Exercise can sometimes decrease number of sleep attacks; seek to achieve optimal physical fitness

MEDICATION (DRUGS)

First Line
- Excessive daytime sleepiness
  - Nonamphetamines
    - ○ Modafinil (Provigil): Structurally distinct from amphetamines; 200–400 mg/d; start with 100 mg and increase over 3–4 days [A]
    - ○ Selegiline: Selective MAO-B inhibitor; anticataplectic and effective for excessive daytime sleepiness; 20–40 mg/d divided a.m. and noon [B]
  - Amphetamines
    - ○ Methylphenidate (Ritalin): Initial dose 30 mg/d divided b.i.d. or t.i.d.; maximum dose 100 mg/d [B]
    - ○ Dextroamphetamine: 5–30 mg b.i.d.
    - ○ Pemoline (Cylert): Longer half-life (than methylphenidate), 8–10 hours. Initial dose 37.5 mg/d divided a.m. and noon; maximum dose 150 mg/d. Monitor liver function studies 4 weeks after start and then once a year. No longer routinely used due to hepatotoxicity. [B]
    - ○ Dextroamphetamine: Initial dose 15 mg/d divided b.i.d. or t.i.d.; maximum dose 100 mg/d [B]
    - ○ Combination of long and short acting: Pemoline plus single or multiple doses of methylphenidate
- Auxiliary symptoms (cataplexy, hypnagogic hallucination, sleep paralysis): Antidepressants suppress REM sleep
  - Imipramine 75–150 mg/d
  - Protriptyline 10–40 mg/d
  - Clomipramine 150–250 mg/d
  - Fluoxetine 20–60 mg/d
  - Venlafaxine: 75–150 mg b.i.d.
  - Sodium oxybate (Xyrem): 2.5–4.5 g qhs, may take 3 months to achieve full response, "date-rape" drug with abuse potential
- Contraindications: Stimulants in hypertensive patients
- Precautions
  - Amphetamines
    - ○ If patient develops tolerance to stimulants, switch drugs rather than increase dose—little cross-tolerance
    - ○ Headaches, irritability, hypertension, psychosis, anorexia, habituation, rebound hypersomnia
    - ○ Pemoline: Fewer cardiovascular side effects, longer acting, liver toxicity, little abuse potential
  - Other
    - ○ Imipramine: Dry mouth, sedation, urinary retention, impotence
    - ○ Modafinil: Less rebound hypersomnia; may become drug of choice; does not affect BP; tolerance limited, best if initial treatment; does not treat cataplexy; main side effect, headache
    - ○ Selegiline: Doses >20 mg require low-tyramine diet because drug begins to lose selectivity
    - ○ Patient may develop tolerance to anticataplectic effect of tricyclic antidepressants (TACs) and can get a rebound in cataplexy when withdrawn
- Significant possible interactions: Combination of TACs and stimulants can lead to significant hypertension

Second Line
- Excessive daytime sleepiness
  - Propranolol 280–480 mg/d, good for patients during withdrawal from stimulants or patients with hypertension
  - Dextroamphetamines 5–60 mg/d
  - L-Tyrosine 64–120 mg/d
- Ancillary symptoms
  - Codeine 150 mg/d
  - Triazolam 0.25 mg improves nocturnal sleep quality.

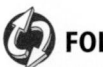 **FOLLOW-UP**

PROGNOSIS
- Lifelong disease
- Symptoms can worsen with aging.
- In women, symptoms can improve after menopause.

PATIENT MONITORING
- Frequent BP checks
- Follow-up every 6 months

REFERENCES

1. Chaudhary B, Husain I. Narcolepsy. *J Fam Pract*. 1993;36:207–213.
2. Feldman NT. Narcolepsy. *South Med J*. 2003;96: 277–282.
3. Green P, Stillman M. Signs, symptoms, differential diagnosis, and management of narcolepsy. *Arch Fam Med*. 1998;7:472–478.
4. Mitler M, et al. Narcolepsy. *J Clin Neurophysiol*. 1990;7:93–118.
5. Nahmias J, Karetzky M. Current concepts in narcolepsy. *N J Med*. 1989;86:617–622.
6. Nishino S, Mignot E. Drug treatment of patients with insomnia and excessive daytime sleepiness. *Clin Pharmacokinet*. 1999;37:305–330.
7. Parkes JD, Clift SJ, Dahlitz MJ. The narcoleptic syndrome. *J Psychiatry*. 1995;59:221–224.
8. Scharf M, Fletcher K, Jennings SW. Current pharmacologic management of narcolepsy. *Am Fam Physician*. 1988;38:143–148.
9. Standards of Practice Committee of the American Sleep Disorders Association. Practice parameters for the use of stimulants in the treatment of narcolepsy. *Sleep*. 1994;17:348–351.

 MISCELLANEOUS

See also: Sleep apnea, Obstructive

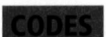 **CODES**

ICD9-CM
347 Cataplexy and narcolepsy

PATIENT TEACHING
- Symptoms can spontaneously improve or worsen.
- The American Narcolepsy Association, P.O. Box 1187, San Carlos, CA 94070; (800) 327-6085
- Narcolepsy Sleep Disorder Association: Online newsletter at www.narcolepsy.com

N

NEAR DROWNING

Alan J. Cropp, MD, FCCP

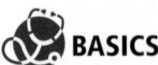 ## BASICS

DESCRIPTION
Multisystem, potentially fatal disease, resulting from near suffocation secondary to submersion of a person's face or head. A form of acute respiratory distress syndrome (ARDS) with neurologic complications. Most near-drowning victims do not aspirate large volumes of fluid.
- System(s) Affected: Cardiovascular; Nervous; Pulmonary; Renal

GENERAL PREVENTION
- Proper adult supervision of children
- Knowledge of water safety guidelines
- Mandatory pool fencing
- Avoidance of alcohol or recreational drugs around water
- Swimming instruction at an early age
- Boating safety knowledge
- Personal flotation device (life preserver if necessary)

ALERT
Pediatric Considerations
Children frequently do not swim well.

EPIDEMIOLOGY
- Leading cause of injury-related death in children <5 years
- Predominant age: Teenagers and toddlers
- Predominant sex: Male > Female

Incidence
- 6,000–8,000 deaths yearly (1)
- 90,000 near-drowning victims

Prevalence
- Drowning is the 3rd leading cause of accidental death in the US. (1)
- ~2 cases/100,000 population

RISK FACTORS
- Low socioeconomic class
- Alcohol
- Seizure disorder
- Inability to swim
- Improper pool fencing
- Inadequate adult supervision of children
- Cardiac arrhythmias
- Living in sunbelt states
- Adolescents: May be intoxicated or using drugs
- Adults: Most near drownings are associated with boating accidents with or without alcohol.

PATHOPHYSIOLOGY
Hypoximia and acidosis cause most of the physiologic problems.

ETIOLOGY
- Swimming accidents, scuba diving, water sports
- Hyperventilation before underwater swimming
- Boating mishaps
- Motor vehicle accidents (e.g., automobile submerged in water)
- Suicide
- Drug overdose (including alcohol)
- Bathtub drowning in children <1 year
- Head trauma while swimming

ASSOCIATED CONDITIONS
- Cardiopulmonary arrest before submersion
- Trauma, especially to the head, causing altered mental status
- Seizure disorder
- Alcohol or drug overdose
- Hypothermia

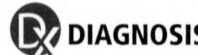 ## DIAGNOSIS

SIGNS AND SYMPTOMS
- Altered level of consciousness or comatose
- Cough
- Abdominal distention

History
Victim found in or near water
- Water temperature may be important
- Distinguish between fresh and salt water

Physical Exam
- Absent or thready pulse
- Tachypnea or agonal respirations
- Cyanosis
- Wheezing
- Hypothermia
- Poorly reactive, dilated, and fixed pupils
- Poor peripheral perfusion

TESTS
- Central venous pressure monitoring
- ECG
- Electroencephalogram

Lab
- Salt water
  - Hypoxemia
  - Hypercarbia
  - Hypokalemia with significant aspiration
  - Mixed acidosis
  - Slight increase in serum sodium
  - Normal or minimally increased hemoglobin
  - Rare albuminuria
  - Rare oliguria
  - Rare hemoglobinuria
  - Hypovolemia possibly, or hypervolemia
- Fresh water
  - Hypoxemia
  - Hypercarbia
  - Hypokalemia with significant aspiration
  - Mixed acidosis
  - Slight decrease in serum sodium
  - Normal or slightly decreased hemoglobin
  - Albuminuria rarely
  - Oliguria rarely
  - Rare hemoglobinuria
  - Evidence of hemolysis
- Disorders that may alter lab results
  - Any underlying condition that may alter normal fluid and electrolyte balance (e.g., CHF) or alter normal pulmonary function (e.g., emphysema)

Imaging
Chest radiograph may show pulmonary edema, consolidation from aspiration, atelectasis, or pneumothorax

Pathological Findings
- "Dry lungs"
  - ~10% of victims drown without aspiration.
  - Accomplished swimmers may drown by hyperventilation before prolonged underwater swimming or by becoming fatigued following a particularly strenuous or long swim.
- Loss of normal pulmonary architecture (fresh water)
  - Loss of surfactant (1)
  - Alveolar consolidations, collapse, hyaline membrane formation, intrapulmonary shunting
- Increased lung weight and intra-alveolar hemorrhages (salt water)
- Lung hyperexpansion
- Pneumonia, abscess, and ARDS in those who survive only a few hours or days
- Renal: Acute tubular necrosis
- Neurologic: Cerebral edema

DIFFERENTIAL DIAGNOSIS
The submersion may have resulted from loss of consciousness and accidentally falling into water because of another medical condition (e.g., head trauma, arrhythmia, seizure, etc.) (2)

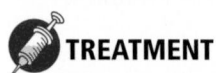 ## TREATMENT

INITIAL STABILIZATION
- Begin resuscitation at the scene. [A]
  - Initiate mouth to mouth resuscitation while still in water if possible
- Remove from water quickly and place in normal CPR position. [A]
- Support neck in case of spinal cord injury. [A]
- Supplemental oxygen [A]

GENERAL MEASURES
- Positive end-expiratory pressure or continuous positive airway pressure for persistent hypoxia B
- Avoid abdominal thrust unless airway obstruction is present. (1)[B]
- Monitor pH and adjust bicarbonate administration accordingly. [C]
- Monitor arterial oxygenation. [A]
- Avoid steroids. [C]
- Avoid prophylactic antibiotics.
- Hyperventilate patient (keep $PaCO_2$ 25–30 mm Hg) [C]
- Warm hypothermic patients. (3)[B]

Diet
NPO until mental status normalizes

Activity
Bed rest for at least the initial 24 hours

Nursing
Careful monitoring of neurologic status

SPECIAL THERAPY
Oxygen for all patients

IV Fluids
To maintain adequate intravascular volume [C]

Complementary and Alternative Medicine
Core warming with gastric or bladder lavage and/or providing warmed air through a ventilator may be necessary

MEDICATION (DRUGS)

First Line

- Unconscious patient without known pH
  - Sodium bicarbonate: 1.0 mEq/kg [C]
- For bronchospasm: aerosolized bronchodilator [C]
  - Albuterol (Proventil, Ventolin) 3 mL of 0.083% solution *or*
  - 0.5 mL of 0.5% solution diluted in 3 mL saline
- Patients who develop pneumonia [A]
  - Appropriate antibiotic based on sputum or endotracheal lavage culture
- Fresh water drowning patients with hemolysis
  - Transfusion may be necessary.
- Prophylactic antibiotics and steroids are not helpful. [C]
- Contraindications: Refer to the manufacturer's profile of each drug.
- Precautions: Refer to the manufacturer's profile of each drug.
- Significant possible interactions: Refer to the manufacturer's profile of each drug.

Second Line

For bronchospasm

- Aerosolized bronchodilator: Metaproterenol (Alupent) 0.3 mL in 3 mL normal saline or levalbuterol (Xopenex) 0.63 mg or 1.25 mg
- Aminophylline

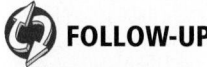 **FOLLOW-UP**

DISPOSITION

Admission Criteria

- Hospitalize all patients initially. [B]
- Monitor patients in an intensive care setting, except for those few who present to the ED in an alert condition without evidence of respiratory compromise [B]
- The incidence of delayed drowning is 5%; therefore, all patients who have had a significant submersion accident should be hospitalized at least 24–48 hours. [C]

Discharge Criteria

- Mental status back to normal [C]
- Improved physiologic parameters [C]

Issues for Referral

Refer severe cases to an intensivist or a trauma specialist.

PROGNOSIS

- Patients who are alert or mildly obtunded at the time they present to the hospital have an excellent chance for a full recovery.
- Patients who are comatose or receiving CPR at the time of presentation or who have dilated and fixed pupils and no spontaneous respiratory activity have a more guarded and often poor prognosis.
- Secondary drowning from neurogenic pulmonary edema may occur within 48 hours of initial presentation.

COMPLICATIONS

- Early
  - Bronchospasm
  - Vomiting/aspiration
  - Hypoglycemia
  - Hypothermia
  - Seizure
  - Hypovolemia
  - Electrolyte abnormalities
  - Arrhythmia from hypoxia or hypothermia (rarely from electrolyte imbalance)
  - Hypotension
- Late
  - Adult respiratory distress syndrome
  - Anoxic encephalopathy
  - Pneumonia
  - Lung abscess/empyema
  - Renal failure
  - Coagulopathy
  - Sepsis
  - Barotrauma
  - Seizure

PATIENT MONITORING

- Frequent check of vital signs/O_2 saturation [C]
- Arterial blood gas monitoring [B]
- Pulmonary artery catheter may be needed for hemodynamic monitoring [C]
- Intracranial pressure monitoring in selected patients [C]
- Serial chest radiographs [C]
- Serum electrolyte determinations [B]

REFERENCES

1. Harries M. Near drowning. *BMJ*. 2003; 327:1336–1338.
2. Sachdeva RC. Near drowning. *Crit Care Med*. 2002;15:281–296.
3. Weinstein MD, Krieger BP. Near-drowning: Epidemiology, pathophysiology, and initial treatment. *J Emerg Med*. 1996;14:461–467.

 MISCELLANEOUS

CODES

ICD9-CM

- 518.5 Pulmonary insufficiency following trauma and surgery
- 994.1 Drowning and nonfatal submersion

PATIENT TEACHING

Proper water safety techniques may help to avoid this problem.

N

NEPHROPATHY, URATE

Douglas Hunt, MD

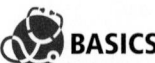**BASICS**

DESCRIPTION
- Renal parenchymal damage and dysfunction associated with disordered uric acid metabolism.
- Affects the renal/urologic system. Several syndromes may present
  - Hyperuricemic acute renal failure: Precipitated by distal tubular obstruction resulting from acute massive elevation of serum uric acid, often due to cell lysis during induction chemotherapy or radiation.
  - Uric acid nephrolithiasis: Most commonly seen in patients with underlying hyperuricemia or gout who have abnormally low urine pH due to low ammonia excretion. Frequency of stone formation increases with increasing serum uric acid levels and urinary uric acid excretion rates. ~20% of patients with gout will form uric acid stones.
  - Hyperuricemia of chronic renal failure: An early result of chronic renal failure due to retention of uric acid resulting from decreased tubular secretion or altered postsecretory reabsorption, or both. Secondary gout occurs in <1% of all cases.
  - Chronic urate nephropathy: Renal insufficiency attributed to parenchymal damage secondary to medullary urate deposition. Effect of hyperuricemia on development and progression of chronic renal disease in humans is largely unknown. Studies in animals have shown an association between hyperuricemia and intrarenal vascular disease. (1)

GENERAL PREVENTION
- Appropriate pretreatment prior to chemotherapy of leukemia or lymphoma
- Avoidance of factors that can cause abrupt or persistent increases of serum uric acid or urinary uric acid excretion

EPIDEMIOLOGY
- Predominant age: Adults
- Predominant sex: Male > Female

Incidence
1 of every 114 patients newly diagnosed with gout develop uric acid stones per year.

Prevalence
Gout 1%, hyperuricemia 5–10%, uric acid nephrolithiasis 0.1% in the US

RISK FACTORS
- Hyperuricemic acute renal failure (2)
  - Sudden increase in uric acid load
  - Volume depletion
  - Pre-existing acute or chronic renal insufficiency
  - Large tumor burden
  - LDH >1500 IU
  - Extensive bone marrow involvement
  - Elevated tumor sensitivity to chemotherapeutic agents
- Uric acid nephrolithiasis (3)
  - Decreased urine pH
  - Diminished urinary volume
  - Excessive urinary uric acid
  - Acute diarrheal states and inflammatory bowel disease
  - Diabetes mellitus
  - Metabolic syndrome
  - Probenecid and aspirin use

ETIOLOGY
- Hyperuricemic acute renal failure
  - Endogenous uric acid overproduction: Rapid cell turnover/destruction due to malignancy or rhabdomyolysis, enzymatic/metabolic abnormalities, inappropriate high dose of uricosuric agent in hyperuricemic individual
  - Exogenous uric acid overproduction: Excessive dietary purine ingestion
- Uric acid nephrolithiasis
  - Idiopathic: Sporadic
  - Familial (primary hyperuricemia)
    ○ Congenital gout, hypertension, and hyperuricemia (autosomal dominant)
    ○ Congenital hypoxanthine-guanine phosphoribosyltransferase (HGPRT) deficiency (X-linked recessive)
    ○ Congenital phosphoribosyl pyrophosphate (PRPP) overactivity (X-linked recessive)
    ○ Congenital glycogen storage disease, type I
  - Secondary hyperuricemia
    ○ Lead intoxication
    ○ Diuretics
    ○ Cytotoxic chemotherapy or radiation in leukemia or lymphoma
    ○ Heat stress and exercise
    ○ Diabetic ketoacidosis
    ○ Starvation ketosis
    ○ Chronic myeloproliferative disease
    ○ Psoriasis
  - Secondary hyperuricosuria: Primary gout, excessive purine intake, tubular reabsorptive defect, uricosuric drugs (probenecid, phenylbutazone, salicylates, radiocontrast)
  - Dehydration: GI or skin loss

ALERT
Pediatric Considerations
Gout and uric acid nephrolithiasis may have onset in infancy or childhood with familial causes of hyperuricemia.

ASSOCIATED CONDITIONS
- Gout (4)
- Hypertension (1)
- Myocardial infarction (1)
- Stroke (1)
- IgA nephropathy—worse prognosis with elevated uric acid levels (1)

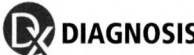**DIAGNOSIS**

SIGNS AND SYMPTOMS
- Hyperuricemic acute renal failure (2)
  - Precipitated by chemotherapy for leukemia or lymphoma or some solid tumor malignancies
  - Hyperkalemia: Weakness, paresthesias, muscle cramps, nausea, vomiting, diarrhea, anorexia
  - Hyperphosphatemia: Acute nephrocalcinosis
  - Hypocalcemia: Muscle cramps, tetany, cardiac arrhythmia, seizures
  - Oliguria
  - Anuria
  - Anorexia, nausea, vomiting, encephalopathy, and other manifestations of uremia
  - Hypertension
  - Dehydration

- Uric acid nephrolithiasis
  - Flank pain
  - Groin pain
  - Microscopic or gross hematuria
  - Anorexia
  - Nausea, vomiting
  - Ureteral obstruction
  - UTI
  - Dehydration
- Hyperuricemia of chronic renal failure
  - Established chronic renal failure with glomerular filtration rate (GFR) <15–20 mL/min
  - Serum uric acid 7–10 mg/dL chronically
  - Acute onset of uremic symptoms

TESTS
Lab
- Hyperuricemic acute renal failure
  - Serum uric acid >15–20 mg/dL (0.88–1.18 mmol/L)
  - Rising blood urea nitrogen (BUN) and creatinine
  - Urinary uric acid-to-creatinine ratio >1; ratio of 0.6–0.75 suggests another cause of renal failure (2)[C]
  - Uric acid crystals in urine
- Uric acid nephrolithiasis
  - Urine pH <6 (Nitrazine paper) (3)[A]
  - Uric acid crystals in urine
  - 24-hour urinalysis: Urinary uric acid often >4800 μmol/d in men and >4400 μmol/d in women or uric acid:creatinine ratio >530 μmol/mmol (hyperuricosuria) (5)[A]
  - Measure serum uric acid, calcium, and creatinine: Serum uric acid often normal, especially with low urine pH <6.2 (3)[A]
  - Hematuria
  - Stone analysis: Uric acid or mixed uric acid with calcium oxalate or calcium phosphate
- Hyperuricemia of chronic renal failure
  - Serum uric acid usually 7–10 mg/dL and is rarely >10 mg/dL due to compensatory increase in GI secretion of uric acid (1)[A]
  - Serum uric acid remains normal until GFR <20 mL/min (6)[C]

Imaging
- IV pyelography: Filling defects (3)
- Nonenhanced CT: Lower density than calcium stones (3)[A]

Diagnostic Procedures/Surgery
- Cystoscopy and retrograde pyelography (3)
- Renal biopsy

Pathological Findings
- Hyperuricemic acute renal failure: Uric acid crystals in collecting ducts, eventually obstructing nephrons (2)
- Uric acid nephrolithiasis: Radiolucent, often orange or red stones that can occlude ureters or entire renal collecting system (3)
- Chronic urate nephropathy: Birefringent, needlelike crystals in the tubular lumen or in the interstitium with surrounding inflammatory cells and fibrosis (5)

DIFFERENTIAL DIAGNOSIS

- Hyperuricemic acute renal failure: Prerenal failure, contrast nephropathy, ATN, tumor infiltration of kidneys, obstruction
- Uric acid nephrolithiasis: Calcium oxalate, calcium phosphate, struvite, cystine stones
  - 20% of patients with calcium nephrolithiasis have hyperuricemia (3)
- Chronic urate nephropathy: Other causes of chronic renal failure, including diabetes, hypertension, and glomerular disease are more likely

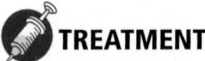 ## TREATMENT

INITIAL STABILIZATION

Outpatient treatment except for complicated nephrolithiasis and hyperuricemic acute renal failure

GENERAL MEASURES

- Hyperuricemic acute renal failure
  - IV hydration
  - Hemodialysis in severe cases
- Uric acid nephrolithiasis
  - Hydration to increase urine output
  - Normalize renal uric acid excretion
  - Normalize urine pH
  - Antibiotic treatment of urinary tract infection

Diet

- Moderation of purine intake (5)[C]
- For nephrolithiasis, ensure fluid intake adequate to produce urine output at least 2 L per day, unless urine output is limited by acute or chronic renal failure. (5)[A]
- In renal failure, restrict sodium for hypertension and potassium for hyperkalemia.

Activity

No restrictions

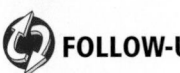 ## MEDICATION (DRUGS)

First Line

- Hyperuricemic acute renal failure: Prevent by pretreating with allopurinol or rasburicase and hydrating patient prior to administration of chemotherapeutic agents for leukemia or lymphoma (2)[A]
  - Begin hydration 2 days prior and continue for 2 days after induction chemotherapy (2)[A]
  - Allopurinol 200–600 mg/d (adult) (2)[A] and 10 mg/kg q8h (pediatric) (7)[A]
  - Rasburicase 0.2 mg/kg IV daily during initial chemo for pediatric patients with advanced stage lymphoma or high tumor burden leukemia (7)[B]
  - Promptly correct metabolic abnormalities (2)[A]
  - Dialyze when renal failure fails to resolve with conservative management or when life-threatening electrolyte or volume-overload disorders are present. (2)[A]
- Uric acid nephrolithiasis
  - Encourage hydration to obtain urine output 1.5–2.0 L. (5)[A]
  - Alkali to maintain urine pH 6.0–7.0. Give potassium alkali 20–30 mEq b.i.d. to t.i.d. (3,5)[A]
  - If hyperuricosuric and urinary alkalinization is unsuccessful, give allopurinol starting at 100–300 mg/d. (5)[B]
- Hyperuricemia of chronic renal failure
  - Consider allopurinol only in patients with prior history of gout or nephrolithiasis. (6)[C]
- Asymptomatic hyperuricemia: There is insufficient evidence to indicate treatment of asymptomatic hyperuricemia. (1)[A]
- Precautions
  - In patients with renal impairment, dosing for allopurinol, which is cleared renally, must be adjusted. (2)[A]
  - Avoid abrupt decreases or increases in serum uric acid, which may precipitate acute gouty arthritis.
- Significant possible interactions of allopurinol
  - Inhibits metabolism of mercaptopurine and azathioprine
  - Ethanol decreases its effects.
  - Increases likelihood of skin rash when used with amoxicillin or ampicillin
  - Risk of nephrolithiasis with excess vitamin C.

SURGERY

Uric acid nephrolithiasis resistant to conservative management: Lithotripsy, cystoscopic stenting, percutaneous nephrostomy (3)[A]

 ## FOLLOW-UP

PROGNOSIS

- With effective drug therapy and general management, prognosis is excellent in patients with hyperuricemic acute renal failure (2) and nephrolithiasis (3).
- Development of progressive renal insufficiency in patients with gout or hyperuricemia is unlikely to occur unless caused by underlying renal disease or associated medical conditions with adverse renal effects (4).

COMPLICATIONS

- Gout and asymptomatic hyperuricemia: No renal complications proven in humans (1)
- Hyperuricemic acute renal failure (2)
  - Irreversible renal failure (end-stage renal disease)
  - Residual renal insufficiency
  - Persistent renal tubular functional defects
- Uric acid nephrolithiasis (4)
  - Urinary obstruction
  - Urinary tract infection, pyelonephritis
  - Renal insufficiency
- Hyperuricemia of chronic renal failure: Progression to end-stage renal failure

ALERT

Geriatric Considerations

Renal insufficiency more likely because of age and associated medical conditions

REFERENCES

1. Kanellis J, Feig DI, Johnson RJ. Does asymptomatic hyperuricaemia contribute to development of renal and cardiovascular disease? *An old controversy renewed. Nephrology* 2004;9(6):394–399.
2. Davidson MB, Thakkar S, Hix JX, et al. Pathophysiology, clinical consequences, and treatment of tumor lysis syndrome. *Am J Med* 2004;1116(8):546–554.
3. Coe FL, Evan A, Worcester E. Kidney stone disease. *J Clin Invest* 2005;115:2598–2608.
4. Nakagawa T, Marilda M, Kang DH, et al. Uric acid—a uremic toxin? *Blood Purification* 2006; 24:67–70.
5. Reynolds TM. Best Practice No 181. Chemical pathology clinical investigation and management of nephrolithiasis. *J Clin Pathol* 2005;58:134–140.
6. Snaith ML. ABC of rheumatology: Gout, hyperuricemia, and crystal arthritis. *BMJ* 1995;310: 521–524.
7. Goldman SC, Holcenberg JS, Finklestein JZ, et al. A randomized comparison between rasburicase and allopurinol in children with lymphoma or leukemia at high risk for tumor lysis. *Blood* 2001;97(10): 2998–3003.

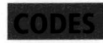 ## MISCELLANEOUS

 ### CODES

ICD9-CM

- 274.10 Gouty nephropathy, unspecified
- 274.11 Uric acid nephrolithiasis

PATIENT TEACHING

 See Corresponding Diagnostic Algorithm

See Patient Handout on CD

N

NEPHROTIC SYNDROME

Saritha Dhruvakumar, MD

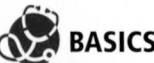 **BASICS**

DESCRIPTION

A syndrome composed of glomerular proteinuria (3.5 g/1.73 m^2 body surface area/day), hypoalbuminemia, hypercholesterolemia, and edema as a result of a primary renal disease or secondary to another disease process

- System(s) Affected: Endocrine/Metabolic; Renal/Urologic

EPIDEMIOLOGY

- Predominant age
  - Children: 1.5–6 years—minimal change disease (MCD)
  - Adults: All ages—MCD, focal segmental glomerulosclerosis (FGS), membranous nephropathy, membranous glomerulonephritis (MGN) more common in the US; IgG-IgA worldwide
- Predominant sex: Male = Female

Incidence

- Children: 2/100,000 new cases/year
- Adults: 3/100,000 new cases/year

RISK FACTORS

- Any of the disorders listed in Etiology
- Drug addiction (e.g., heroin [FGS])
- Hepatitis B and C, HIV, other infections
- Immunosuppression
- Nephrotoxic drugs
- Vesicoureteral reflux (FGS)
- Cancer (usually MGN, may be MCD)
- Chronic analgesic use/abuse
- Preeclampsia

Genetics

- 2–8% of cases familial
- Finnish type congenital nephrotic syndrome inherited in an autosomal recessive fashion
  - Associated with NPHS1 and NPHS2 genes

PATHOPHYSIOLOGY

- Altered permeability of glomerular basement membrane due to primary or secondary renal disease leads to proteinuria and hypoalbuminemia
- Edema likely result of primary renal salt retention in addition to arterial underfilling from decreased plasma oncotic pressure
- Hyperlipidemia thought to be a consequence of increased hepatic synthesis resulting from low oncotic pressure and urinary loss of regulatory proteins
- Hypercoagulable state likely due to loss of antithrombin III in urine

ETIOLOGY

- Primary renal disease
  - Fibrillary glomerulopathy (primary)
  - Focal glomerulonephritis
  - FGS
  - IgA nephropathy
  - Membranoproliferative glomerulonephritis
  - MGN
  - Mesangial proliferative glomerulonephritis
  - MCD
  - Rapidly progressive glomerulonephritis (RPGN)
  - Congenital nephrotic syndrome

- Secondary renal disease. Associated primary renal disease shown in brackets
  - Allergens (snake venoms, antitoxins, poison ivy, insect stings)
  - Amyloidosis
  - Carcinoma (bronchogenic, breast, colon, stomach, kidney) (MGN and others)
  - Diabetes mellitus (most common)
  - Erythema multiforme
  - Fibrillary glomerulopathy; secondary: Amyloid, cryoglobulins, multiple myeloma, chronic lymphocytic leukemia
  - Henoch-Schönlein purpura
  - Heredofamilial (Alport syndrome, Fabry disease)
  - Infections: Ventriculoatrial shunt infection, bacterial endocarditis, HIV, hepatitis B and C viruses (HBV, HCV), schistosomiasis, tuberculosis, leprosy, poststreptococcal glomerulonephritis (20% are nephrotic)
  - Leukemias
  - Lymphoma (Hodgkin [MCD], non-Hodgkin [MGN])
  - Focal glomerulosclerosis (reflux nephropathy, heroin abuse, nephron ablation, extensive glomerular scarring in acute glomerulonephritis, chronic renal allograft rejection, end-stage kidney disease, morbid obesity, thromboembolism)
  - Malignant hypertension
  - Melanoma
  - Nephrotoxins and drugs (gold, penicillamine, mercury [MGN], NSAIDs [MCD], and interstitial nephritis)
  - Polyarteritis nodosa
  - Preeclampsia
  - Sarcoid
  - Serum sickness
  - Sjögren syndrome
  - Systemic lupus erythematosus (SLE) [MGN, FGS, focal, mesangial, diffuse, proliferative]
  - Preeclampsia

ASSOCIATED CONDITIONS

See "Etiology."

DIAGNOSIS

SIGNS AND SYMPTOMS

- Fluid retention: Abdominal distention, ascites, edema, puffy eyelids, scrotal swelling, weight gain, shortness of breath
- Anorexia
- Hypertension
- Oliguria
- Orthostatic hypotension
- Retinal sheen
- Skin striae
- Foamy urine

History

- Systemic renal disease in 1/3 of patients
- Assess for risk factors

Physical Exam

See "Signs and Symptoms"

TESTS

Lab

- Complement levels
- Antinuclear antibody, anti–double-stranded DNA
- Serum protein electrophoresis
- Urine immune electrophoresis
- Blood cultures
- Diabetic testing
- HBV, HCV, HIV, rapid plasma reagent
- Serum albumin
- Lipid panel
- Serum blood urea nitrogen/Creatinine
- Urinalysis
  - Proteinuria (>3 g/24 hours)
    - Spot urine protein: Creatinine or 24 hour
  - Glycosuria
  - Hematuria
  - Aminoaciduria
  - Granular casts
  - Hyaline casts
  - Fatty casts
  - Foamy appearance
  - Lipiduria (may see Maltese Crosses under polarized light)
- Drugs that may alter lab results: See "Etiology"

Imaging

- Radiography
- Ultrasound
- CT
- MRI or venography for renal vein thrombosis
- Fluorescein angiography (for retinopathy)

Diagnostic Procedures/Surgery

- Fat pad biopsy
- Renal biopsy
  - Not usually indicated for systemic disease, unless it may affect management
  - Controversial in idiopathic cases

Pathological Findings

- Light microscopy
  - May see nothing (e.g., MCD)
  - Disease specific: Sclerosis (e.g., FGS in diabetes)
- Immunofluorescence: Mesangial IgA (Henoch-Schönlein, IgG-IgA nephropathy; others specific for disease).
- Electron microscopy (specific for disease as in subepithelial deposits of IgG in MGN)

DIFFERENTIAL DIAGNOSIS

- See "Etiology."
- Edema: CHF, cirrhosis, hypothyroidism

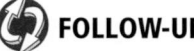 TREATMENT

PRE HOSPITAL
Most patients can be managed as outpatient; inpatient admission for complications

GENERAL MEASURES
- Treatment of underlying disease
- Vigorous treatment of infections (especially bacteriuria, endocarditis, peritonitis)
- Vaccines: Pneumococcal, influenza, and *Haemophilus influenzae*
- Avoidance of excess sunlight
- Avoidance of nephrotoxic drugs
- Consultation with nephrologist often required

Diet
- Normal protein (1 g/kg/d)
  - 0.6 g/kg/d for patients with glomerularfiltration rate <25, prior to dialysis
- Low fat (cholesterol)
- Reduced sodium
- Liberal potassium (unless hyperkalemic)
- Supplemental multivitamins and minerals, especially D and iron
- Fluid restriction if hyponatremic
- Caloric restriction if obese or diabetic

Activity
As tolerated

Nursing
Strict input/output daily weights

MEDICATION (DRUGS)

First Line
- For edema–salt restriction most important, then judicious use of thiazide, loop diuretics
  - If resistant, a combination of loop and distal diluting segment diuretics (e.g., metolazone) is synergistic
- Statins have been shown to improve both endothelial function (1)[B] as well as decreasing proteinuria (2)[A]
- Angiotension-converting enzyme inhibitors or angiotensin II receptor blockers thought to reduce proteinuria, hyperlipidemia, and thrombotic tendencies, progression of renal failure (3)[B] and to control hypertension if present.
- For steroid-responsive disease (MCD and FGS), steroids dosed in consultation with nephrologist
- Other nephrotic renal diseases: Frequently relapsing MCD, RPGN, MGN, SLE
  - Bolus steroids and/or immune suppression (cyclophosphamide, mycophenolate mofetil, chlorambucil, cyclosporine)

Second Line
- Prescribe anticoagulants for thrombotic events. There are data to suggest prophylactic oral anticoagulation in all cases of membranous glomerulonephritis.
- Hypocalcemia from vitamin D loss should be treated with oral vitamin D (dihydrotachysterol) 0.2 mg/d
- MGN patients with a poor prognosis: Probably benefit from cytotoxic therapy (chlorambucil or cyclophosphamide).

FOLLOW-UP

DISPOSITION
Admission Criteria
Respiratory distress, sepsis/severe infection, thromboses, renal failure, hypertension, or other complications

Discharge Criteria
Hemodynamically stable patients without complications may be managed as outpatients.

Issues for Referral
Consultation with nephrologist for renal biopsy, nephrotic syndrome not caused by systemic renal disease, cytotoxic therapy

PROGNOSIS
Varies with specific causes. Complete remission is expected if the basic disease is treatable (infection, malignancy, drug induced); otherwise, It may progress to dialysis dependence (e.g., diabetic glomerulosclerosis).

COMPLICATIONS
- Hypercoagulability, especially renal vein thrombosis
- Pulmonary emboli
- Pleural effusion
- Ascites
- Hyperlipidemia, cardiovascular disease
- Acute renal failure, progressive renal failure
- Protein malnutrition
- Infection
- Iron deficiency (uncommon)

PATIENT MONITORING
Frequent monitoring for azotemia, hypertension, edema, nephrotoxicity, cholesterol, and weight. Acute flank pain and hematuria may suggest renal vein thrombosis

REFERENCES
1. Dogra GK, et al. Statin therapy improves brachial artery endothelial function in nephrotic syndrome. *Kidney Int*. 2002; 62:550–557.
2. Fried LF, et al. Effect of lipid reduction on the progression of renal disease: A meta-analysis. *Kidney Int*. 2001;59:260–269.
3. Nakao N, et al. Combination treatment of angiotensin II receptor blocker and angiotensin-converting-enzyme inhibitor in non-diabetic renal disease (COOPERATE): A randomized controlled trial. *Lancet*. 2003; 361:117–124.
4. Madaio MP, Harrington JT. The diagnosis of glomerular diseases: Acute glomerulonephritis and the nephrotic syndrome. *Arch Intern Med*. 2001; 161:25–34.
5. Remuzzi G, Schieppati A, Ruggenenti P. Clinical practice. Nephropathy in patients with type 2 diabetes. *N Engl J Med*. 2002;346:1145–1151.
6. Schwarz A. New aspects of the treatment of nephrotic syndrome. *J Am Soc Nephrol*. 2001; 12(Suppl 17):S44–S47.

MISCELLANEOUS

See also: Amyloidosis; Diabetes mellitus; Glomerulonephritis, acute; HIV infection and AIDS; Multiple myeloma; Renal failure, acute (ARF); Renal failure, chronic; Systemic lupus erythematosus (SLE)

CODES

ICD9-CM
581.9 Nephrotic syndrome with unspecified pathological lesion in kidney

PATIENT TEACHING
- Printed material for patients: National Kidney Foundation, 30 E. 33rd Street, Suite 1100, New York, NY 10016; (800) 622-9010.
  - Childhood Nephrotic Syndrome (order #02-23NN)
  - Diabetes and Kidney Disease (order #02-09CP)
  - Focal Glomerulosclerosis (order #02-28NN)
- Normal protein, reduced sodium, reduced fat diet recommended for most patients.
- Avoid causative factors whenever possible.
- Detect and treat infections vigorously.

See Corresponding Diagnostic Algorithm

See Patient Handout on CD

N

NEUROBLASTOMA

Timothy L. Black, MD

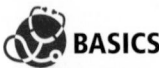**BASICS**

DESCRIPTION
- A neoplasm of neural crest origin that may arise anywhere along the sympathetic ganglion chain or in the adrenal medulla
- Staging
  - Stage 1: Localized tumor with complete resection, with or without microscopic residual disease
  - Stage 2A: Localized tumor with incomplete gross excision, ipsilateral lymph node negative
  - Stage 2B: Localized tumor with or without complete excision, ipsilateral lymph nodes positive; contralateral lymph nodes negative
  - Stage 3: Unresectable tumor extending across midline, or localized tumor with positive contralateral lymph nodes, or midline tumor with bilateral extension unresectable
  - Stage 4: Any primary tumor with distant metastases
  - Stage 4S: Localized primary tumor with dissemination limited to skin, liver, and/or bone marrow in infants <1 year of age
    - Amplification of n-myc oncogene (poor prognosis)
    - Normal DNA ploidy: Worse prognosis than hyperploidy
- Sites of disease (1)[C]
  - Adrenal medulla 40–60%
  - Retroperitoneal sites 20%
  - Mediastinum 10%
  - Pelvis 2–6%
  - Neck 2%
- System(s) Affected: Endocrine/Metabolic; Nervous

EPIDEMIOLOGY
- The most common tumor in infants <1 year of age in the US
- Accounts for 6–10% of all childhood cancers
- 4th most common pediatric malignancy
- Predominant age (1)[C]
  - 90% occur in 1st 8 years of life.
  - 30% occur in children in the 1st year of life
  - 50% occur between ages 1 and 4 years
  - Most common intra-abdominal malignancy in the newborn
- Predominant sex: Males > Females (1.2:1)

Incidence
- 27.8 cases/million children/year for 1st 5 years of life in the US
- 8.7 cases/million in children/year for 1st 15 years of life in the US
- Denmark: 1/12,000–14,000 live births
- Japan: 1/15,000–18,749 infants
- 1/7000 live births in the US and the UK (2)[C]

RISK FACTORS
- Beckwith-Wiedemann syndrome
- Pancreatic islet cell dysplasia
- Maternal phenytoin treatment
- Fetal alcohol syndrome
- Hirschsprung disease

Genetics
- Familial cases reported (1–2%)
- Genetic abnormalities in 80%
- Deletions in short arm of chromosome 1p36
- Amplification of n-myc oncogene occurs on chromosome 2 (poor prognostic sign, present in ~20–25%)
- Many other chromosomal abnormalities have also been described (1)[C]
- Cellular DNA ploidy (hyperdiploidy in infants <1 year of age is associated with excellent long-term survival, diploidy in the same age group is associated with treatment failure) (2)[C]

ETIOLOGY
Genetic abnormalities in 80% of cases

ASSOCIATED CONDITIONS
See "Risk Factors."

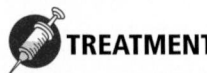**DIAGNOSIS**

SIGNS AND SYMPTOMS
- 50–60% present with metastatic disease
- Abdominal mass (50–75%)
- Weight loss
- Anemia
- Failure to thrive
- Abdominal pain and distension
- Bone pain
- Fever
- Diarrhea
- Hypertension (25%)
- Horner syndrome (ptosis, miosis, enophthalmos, heterochromia of iris)
- Orbital ecchymosis (panda eyes)
- Respiratory distress
- Dysphagia
- Paraplegia
- Cauda equina syndrome
- Flushing, sweating, irritability
- Cerebellar ataxia (chaotic nystagmus): Dancing eye syndrome

TESTS
Lab
- CBC and platelet count
- Liver function studies
- Renal function studies
- Urinary catecholamines (85% secrete catecholamine metabolites) (1)[C]
- Uric acid level
- Creatinine level
- Magnesium level
- Calcium level
- Lactate dehydrogenase (LDH) level
- Electrolytes
- Bilirubin, aspartate aminotransferase, and alanine aminotransferase levels
- Gd2 monoclonal antibody levels
- Serum neuron-specific enolase
- Serum ferritin
- Bone marrow aspiration
- Assay for vasoactive intestinal polypeptide

Imaging
- Chest radiograph
- Skeletal survey (including orbital views)
- Bone scan
- CT or MRI of neck, chest, abdomen, or pelvis (depending on location of tumor) (also to evaluate for metastatic disease)
- Myelogram for neurologic symptoms

Diagnostic Procedures/Surgery
- Myelogram if needed
- Bone marrow aspiration

Pathological Findings
- Small, dark, round cells
- Immature tumors tend to be large, red, lobular soft, friable
- Mature tumors are fibrous, contain calcification, hemorrhage, necrosis, cysts, rosettes, and nerve filaments
- May be neuroblastoma, ganglioneuroblastoma, or benign neuroblastoma (depends on cell maturity)
- Favorable histology:
  - Stroma-rich, well-differentiated and intermixed tumors
- Unfavorable histology
  - Stroma-rich nodular and stroma-poor, undifferentiated tumors

DIFFERENTIAL DIAGNOSIS
- Rhabdomyosarcoma
- Wilms tumors
- Other tumors of neck, chest, abdomen, and pelvis
- Hydronephrosis

TREATMENT

GENERAL MEASURES
- Radiation therapy in children >1 year of age with stage III disease
- Chemotherapy for stage II and greater

Diet
No special diet

Activity
As tolerated

Radiotherapy
See "General Measures."

MEDICATION (DRUGS)

First Line
- Cyclophosphamide
- Melphalan
- Vincristine
- Dacarbazine
- Teniposide
- Etoposide
- Doxorubicin (Adriamycin)
- Cisplatin
- Peptichemio
- Carboplatin
- Ifosfamide (with mesna to protect against hemorrhagic cystitis)
- Topotecan
- Contraindications: See the manufacturer's information for each drug.
- Precautions: See the manufacturer's information for each drug.
- Significant possible interactions: See the manufacturer's information for each drug.

Second Line
- By protocol
- Ondansetron (Zofran), dronabinol (Marinol), metoclopramide (Reglan), and others for nausea control

SURGERY
- Surgical resection may be complete, incomplete, or biopsy only: For stage I, excision only
- If resection incomplete or biopsy, chemotherapy followed by 2nd-look operation
- Dumbbell extension through vertebral foramina, chemotherapy alone vs. laminectomy and decompression
- Stages IV–S: Resection of primary tumor and chemotherapy
- Bone marrow transplantation considered in stages III and IV
- Current Children's Oncology Group risk stratification (2)[C]
  – Low-risk disease treated with surgery alone
    ○ Includes Stage 1, 2a, 2b with favorable histology, and 4S with normal NMYC and favorable histology
  – Intermediate-risk disease treated with chemotherapy, surgery, and local radiation
    ○ Includes Stage 3 with normal NMYC amplification and favorable histology, stage 4 with normal NMYC, and stage 4S with unfavorable histology
  – High-risk disease treated with chemotherapy, surgery, and bone marrow transplant or stem cell rescue
    ○ Includes Stage 2b with unfavorable histology, Stage 3 with amplified NMYC and unfavorable histology, Stage 4 with amplified NMYC and >1 year of age, and stage 4S with amplified NMYC

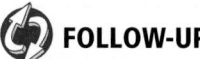 FOLLOW-UP

DISPOSITION
Admission Criteria
Inpatient workup and treatment until stable and induction chemotherapy completed

PROGNOSIS
- Overall survival 58% (3)[C]
  – Stage I: Expected survival ~100%
  – Stage II: Survival 75%
  – Stage III: Survival 43%
  – Stage IV: Survival 15%
  – Stage IV-S: Survival 70–80%
- Normal DNA ploidy, NMYC amplifications, and/or unfavorable histology indicates worse than usual prognosis for same tumor
- Infants <1 year of age have better outcome
- Patients with cervical, pelvic, and mediastinal tumors have better prognosis than those with retroperitoneal, paraspinal, or adrenal tumors
- Survival for those presenting with opsoclonus and nystagmus is nearly 90% (seen especially in mediastinal tumors in infants <1 year of age)
- Neuron-specific enolase level >100 ng/mL correlates with advanced disease and reduced survival
- Serum LDH level <1,500 IU/mL may indicate improved survival rate

COMPLICATIONS
- Nausea
- Vomiting
- Alopecia
- Bone marrow suppression
- Immunosuppression
- Hemorrhagic cystitis
- Azotemia
- Diarrhea
- Antidiuretic hormone secretion
- Local tissue necrosis
- Myocardiopathy
- Renal toxicity
- Hearing loss
- Hypocalcemia
- Hypomagnesemia

PATIENT MONITORING
- Multiagent chemotherapy every 3–4 weeks for 4 courses, then reevaluate with bone marrow or 2nd-look operation
- Follow every 3 months for 1st year, every 4 months for 2nd year, every 6 months for 3rd year, then at least yearly
- Follow with CT or MRI every 3–6 months initially, then yearly

REFERENCES

1. Ashcraft KW, Holcomb GW, Murphy JP, eds. *Pediatric Surgery*, 4th ed. Philadelphia, PA: WB Saunders, 2005.
2. Weinstein JL, Katzenstein HM, Cohn SL. Advances in the diagnosis and treatment of neuroblastoma. *The Oncologist*. 2003;8:278–292.
3. Grosfeld JL, et al. Neuroblastoma in the 1st year of life: Clinical and biologic factors influencing outcome. *Sem Pediatr Surg*. 1993;2:37–46.
4. Matthay KK. Neuroblastoma: A clinical challenge and biological puzzle. *CA Cancer J Clin*. 1995; 45:179–182.
5. O'Neill JA, et al. *Pediatric Surgery*, 5th ed. St Louis, MO: Mosby; 1998.

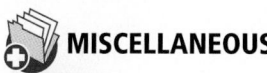 MISCELLANEOUS

CODES

ICD9-CM
- 71.8 Malignant neoplasm of other specified sites of connective and other soft tissue
- 194.0 Malignant neoplasm of adrenal gland
- 195.1 Malignant neoplasm of thorax

PATIENT TEACHING
- Patient and family teaching regarding long-term outlook
- Possibility of 2nd malignancy
- Side effects of treatment

N

NEUROFIBROMATOSIS (TYPES 1 AND 2)

Nuhad D. Dinno, MD

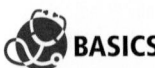 **BASICS**

DESCRIPTION

The most common disease of the neurocutaneous syndromes (phakomatoses [1], which includes neurofibromatosis type 1 (1/3,000) and neurofibromatosis type 2 (1/50,000). Although they are named similarly and both are autosomal dominant disorders, they are 2 distinctly different conditions with genes now identified on 2 separate chromosomes.

- Type 1 (NF1) is also known as von Recklinghausen disease.
- Type 2 (NF2) is also known as bilateral acoustic neurofibromatosis.
- System(s) Affected: Musculoskeletal; Nervous; Skin/Exocrine
- Synonym(s): von Recklinghausen disease (NF1); Bilateral acoustic neurofibromatosis (NF2)

GENERAL PREVENTION

Genetic counseling

EPIDEMIOLOGY

Predominant sex: Male = Female

Prevalence

- NF1: 1/3,000
- NF2: 1/50,000

RISK FACTORS

Family history

Genetics

- NF1: Autosomal dominant inheritance. Nearly 50% of cases are attributed to new mutations. The NF1 gene is mapped to chromosome 17. Prenatal diagnosis is possible. (2)
- NF2: Autosomal dominant inheritance. The NF2 gene is mapped on chromosome 22. (2)

ETIOLOGY

Congenital

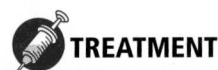 **DIAGNOSIS**

SIGNS AND SYMPTOMS

- NF1: 2 or more of the following (3,4)
  - 6 or more café-au-lait macules measuring 5 mm or more in prepubertal individuals or ≥15 mm in adults (97%)
  - 2 or more neurofibromata or plexiform neurofibroma (15%)
  - Axillary or inguinal freckling (91%)
  - 2 or more Lisch nodules (30%)
  - Optic glioma (11–15% using MRI)
  - Characteristic osseous lesions such as sphenoid dysplasia, long bone cortical thinning, ribbon ribs, angular scoliosis (6%)
  - 1st-degree relative with NF1, according to above criteria
  - A recent European study concludes that NF1 can be diagnosed by routine physical examination by age 6, with attention to the disease associated skin stigmata (5)
- NF2: When 1 or more present, diagnosis is likely (3)
  - Bilateral vestibular schwannomas
  - Family history of NF2, plus unilateral 8th nerve mass or family history and any 2 of the following: Neurofibroma, meningioma, glioma, schwannoma, and juvenile posterior subcapsular lenticular opacity

ALERT

Geriatric Considerations

Cutaneous lesions and tumors increase in size and number with age

Pediatric Considerations

External stigmata subtle or absent in young children

TESTS

- NF1
  - Dictated by findings and clinical evaluation
  - Slit lamp ocular exam
  - Radiology of skull and spine
  - Psychological testing
  - Characteristic radiographic findings, such as sphenoid dysplasia, long bone cortical thinning, ribbon ribs, and angular scoliosis (6%)
- NF2
  - Clinical examination—skin, eyes, and hearing
  - Audiologic evaluation—brainstem-evoked response
  - Radiologic examination—MRI of head
  - When 1 or more of the following are present, the diagnosis of NF2 is likely: Bilateral vestibular schwannomas; family history of NF2, plus unilateral 8th nerve mass or family history and any 2 of the following—neurofibroma, meningioma, glioma, schwannoma, and juvenile posterior subcapsular lenticular opacity

Imaging

See above

Pathological Findings

NF1: Generalized disorder of cells of neural crest origin

DIFFERENTIAL DIAGNOSIS

- NF1: Familial café-au-lait spots (autosomal dominant)—no other NF1 features
- NF2: Solitary acoustic neuroma (develops later in life and is not hereditary)

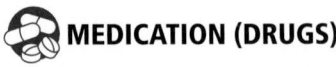 **TREATMENT**

INITIAL STABILIZATION

Outpatient treatment

GENERAL MEASURES

- Access to patient support groups
- Referral of patient to National Neurofibromatosis Organization, local and state chapters
- NF1 (1)
  - General outpatient follow-up of symptomatic patients for early identification of complications
  - Periodic exams with particular attention to central nervous system findings and close attention to any masses or focally arising "new" pain
  - Referral for psychosocial issues of family and affected individuals
  - Educational intervention for children with learning disabilities or attention deficit hyperactivity disorder (ADHD; 40%)
- NF2 (1)
  - Annual neurologic examination
  - Annual ophthalmologic exam
  - Annual hearing examination, or more frequently as necessitated
  - Hearing augmentation as needed
  - Speech therapy as needed
  - Counseling and education regarding insidious problems associated with hearing loss, balance, or sense of direction
  - Genetic counseling for pregnant patients

Diet

No restrictions

Activity

NF2: Caution advised in swimming, diving, or climbing heights

MEDICATION (DRUGS)

First Line

NF1

- Anticonvulsants for seizure control
- Stimulant (or nonstimulant atomoxetine) medications for ADHD
- Significant possible interactions: Caution necessary with these classes of drugs. Refer to the manufacturers' profiles.

Second Line

Multiple clinical trials are recruiting patients with NF and progressive plexiform neurofibromas for experimental treatment with pharmaceutical agents (for more information, see http://www.clinicaltrials.gov)

SURGERY

- NF1: Surgical treatment if indicated for scoliosis, plexiform neurofibromata, or malignancy
- NF2: Excision of tumor as indicated

FOLLOW-UP

PROGNOSIS
- NF1: Variable; most patients have a mild expression and lead normal lives
- NF2: Variable

COMPLICATIONS
NF1
- Disfigurement: Skin neurofibromata develop primarily on exposed areas
- Scoliosis: Common; most cases mild
- CNS: A large head is common but rarely associated with hydrocephalus. Optic glioma or other CNS tumors arise usually during childhood (5–10%).
- Learning disability: Common; often diagnosed upon entering school. May be associated with ADHD
- Rare complications
  - Mental retardation
  - Epilepsy
  - Hypertension
  - Variable onset of puberty
  - Slightly higher risk for malignancy (e.g., Wilms tumor, leukemia, rhabdosarcoma)

PATIENT MONITORING
Annual evaluation and periodic assessment for at-risk individuals

REFERENCES

1. Gutmann DH, et al. The diagnostic evaluation and multidisciplinary management of neurofibromatosis 1 and neurofibromatosis 2. *JAMA*. 1997;278: 51–57.
2. North K. Neurofibromatosis type 1. *Am J Med Genet*. 2000;97:119–127.
3. Martuza RL, Eldridge R. Neurofibromatosis 2. *N Engl J Med*. 1988;318:684–688.
4. Listernick R, Charrow J. Neurofibromatosis type 1 in childhood. *J Pediatr*. 1990;116:845–853.
5. Marga L, et al. Prevalence of Neurofibromatosis 1 in German Children at Elementary School Enrollment. *Arch Dermatol*. 2005;141:71–73.
6. Evans DG, Sainio M, Baser ME. Neurofibromatosis type 2. *J Med Genet*. 2000;37:897–904.

 MISCELLANEOUS

See also: Ataxia-telangiectasia; Tuberous sclerosis complex; von Hippel-Lindau disease

CODES

ICD9-CM
237.70 Neurofibromatosis, unspecified

PATIENT TEACHING
- Genetic counseling and patient education regarding future complications and decisions about family planning
- The National Neurofibromatosis Foundation has been incorporated in the Childrens Tumor Foundation, but many state chapters have elected to remain independent, concentrating only on Neurofibromatosis. Contact individual state chapters to learn which direction they have chosen and what resources are available. The Childrens Tumor Foundation is located at www.CTF.org.

 See Corresponding Diagnostic Algorithm

 See Patient Handout on CD

N

NEUROPATHIC PAIN

Jill D. Mahoney, MD

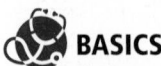 **BASICS**

DESCRIPTION

- Neuropathic pain is defined as pain in association with nerve injury or dysfunction.
- It may be triggered by numerous insults including direct nerve injury, infection, metabolic dysfunction, autoimmune disease, neoplasm, drugs, and neurovascular disorders.
- It may reflect the pathologic operation of a dysfunctional nervous system rather than a manifestation of any underlying pathology itself (i.e., phantom limb pain, complex regional pain syndrome). Patients may paradoxically experience pain and hypersensitivity in an area of denervation.
- System(s) Affected: Nervous; Musculoskeletal

EPIDEMIOLOGY

- Epidemiologic data are limited.
- Difficult to estimate precisely the incidence, prevalence, and sex differences given the number of disease-specific indications for neuropathic pain

Prevalence
Estimated at 1.5% of population

RISK FACTORS

- Diabetes mellitus
- Alcohol abuse
- Trauma
- Nutritional deficiencies (B_{12}, folate)
- Medications (AIDS medications DDC and DDI, antibiotics metronidazole and isoniazid, some chemotherapeutics, amiodarone, hydralazine, phenytoin, nitrofurantoin)

PATHOPHYSIOLOGY
Not well understood. Multiple complex mechanisms likely involved in peripheral and central nervous system dysfunction

ETIOLOGY

- Typically associated with a predisposing factor
- In addition to possible etiologies listed as "Risk Factors" above, others include
  - Demyelinating disorders (multiple sclerosis, Guillain-Barré)
  - Infections (HIV/AIDS, herpes zoster)
  - Neoplasm (primary or metastatic)
  - Neurovascular (central post stroke syndrome, trigeminal neuralgia)
  - Autoimmune disease (Sjögren syndrome, polyarteritis nodosa)
  - Structural disease (herniated disc disease)
- Neuropathic pain of the lower back represents over 1/2 of all those with neuropathic pain.

ASSOCIATED CONDITIONS

- Depression
- Anxiety
- Sleep disturbance

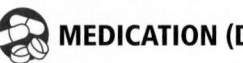 **DIAGNOSIS**

SIGNS AND SYMPTOMS

- Both positive and negative signs and symptoms
- Motor symptoms may be subtle

History

- Patients may have a history of nervous system insult; however, absence of such a history does not exclude the diagnosis of neuropathic pain.
- Pain described as burning, shock-like, tingling, numbing, intensely hot or cold.
- Motor symptoms include weakness, fatigability, decreased range of motion, joint stiffness, spontaneous muscle spasm.

Physical Exam

- Aberrant perception of pain
  - Hyperalgesia: An exaggerated pain response to a noxious stimulus
  - Allodynia: A pain response to a stimulus that does not typically produce pain; may include exaggerated pain response to gentle mechanical pressure, light pinprick, hot or cold stimuli, vibration
  - Negative signs and symptoms also may be present, including reduced sensation to touch, pinprick, temperature, or vibration.
- Motor signs may include hypotonia, tremor, dystonia, ataxia, or motor neglect.

TESTS

- No specific diagnostic test are available for neuropathic pain.
- Labs and studies, when clinically indicated, are intended to exclude underlying causes and direct the provider to disease-specific treatments.
- Studies may include nerve conduction studies, electromyography, evoked potentials, quantitative sensory testing, thermography

Imaging

- PET and SPECT scans, standard MRI and functional MRI all have been used to map synaptic activity in the thalamus and somatosensory cortex.
- Initial studies using these imaging techniques have suggested maladaptive reorganization of the thalamus and somatosensory cortex.

Diagnostic Procedures/Surgery

- Sympathetic nerve blocks
- Epidural steroids
- Trigger point injections

DIFFERENTIAL DIAGNOSIS
See "Etiology"

TREATMENT

SPECIAL THERAPY

- A multidisciplinary approach is widely recommended, combining pharmacologic treatment with adjuncts including physical therapy, complementary medicine (i.e., acupuncture, massage, meditation, hypnosis, biofeedback), psychoeducational interventions (i.e., cognitive behavioral therapy, counseling). Surgical therapy is a last resort.
- Overall, a lack of clear data support clinical efficacy of adjunctive therapy.

MEDICATION (DRUGS)

First Line

- Gabapentin
  - Has the broadest evidence for efficacy against neuropathic pain, FDA approved for its treatment (1)[A]
  - Evidence supports efficacy in treatment of painful diabetic neuropathy (PDN), post herpetic neuralgia (PHN), phantom limb pain, Guillain-Barré syndrome, acute and chronic pain from spinal cord injury, and complex regional pain syndrome type 1 (1)[A]
  - Start 300 mg daily, increase gradually; dosing up to 600 mg t.i.d. is suggested; max dose of 3,600 mg/d in divided doses; adjust dose in renal insufficiency
  - Interactions: No major drug–drug interactions
  - Adverse effects: Dizziness, somnolence, gastrointestinal symptoms, peripheral edema
- Tricyclic antidepressants
  - Among the group of antidepressants, these have the most evidence supporting their role in neuropathic pain. (1)[A]
  - Dosing: Start at 10–25 mg, titrate up to antidepressant drug levels.
  - Secondary amines nortriptyline and desipramine are safer than amitriptyline and imipramine.
  - Precautions: Small therapeutic-to-toxic window; use caution in prescribing to those with cardiac risk factors, glaucoma, urinary retention; suicide; absolute contraindication with MAOIs
  - Interactions: Numerous possible drug–drug interactions (type 1C antiarrhythmics, SSRIs, anticholinergics, sympathomimetics, CNS depressants)
  - Adverse effects: QT interval abnormalities, arrhythmias, sedation, dry mouth, constipation, sexual dysfunction, weight gain, postural hypotension

- Tramadol (2)[A]
  - Dosage: 250 mg/d in divided doses, max 400 mg/d
  - Precautions: Avoid in those with seizure history
  - Interactions: Increased seizure risk in those taking SSRIs, TCAs, MAOIs, neuroleptics concomitantly; increased risk of serotonergic symptoms if used with SSRIs, MAOIs; adjust dose for renal insufficiency, hepatic disease
  - Adverse effects: Dizziness, nausea, constipation, somnolence, orthostatic hypotension
- 5% Lidocaine patch (2)[A]
  - FDA approved for treatment of postherpetic neuralgia but has been used for other focal neuropathic pain syndromes.
  - Dosage: Up to 3 patches for 12 hours daily
  - Interactions: No significant drug–drug interactions
  - Adverse effects: Mild skin reactions
- Carbamazepine
  - FDA approved for the treatment of trigeminal neuralgia with well established efficacy. (2)[A]
  - Dosage: Start 100 mg b.i.d., max 1200 mg/d
  - Precautions: Rare severe, dermatologic reactions (Steven Johnsons syndrome), pregnancy category D, risk of blood dyscrasias, liver dysfunction
  - Interactions: Numerous drug–drug interactions including CYP 3A4 inhibitors and inducers
  - Adverse effects: Dizziness, drowsiness, unsteadiness, nausea, vomiting
- Pregabalin
  - FDA approved for treatment of neuropathic pain secondary to postherpetic neuralgia and diabetic polyneuropathy. (3)[A]
  - Dosage: Start at 75 mg b.i.d., maximum dose 300 mg b.i.d.
  - Interactions: No major drug–drug interactions
- Opioids (2)[A]
  - According to World Health Organization, should be used in "ladder" fashion, added to nonopioid agents if they are insufficient.
  - Controlled-release opioids recommended (controlled release oxycodone, morphine, transdermal fentanyl, methadone)
  - Dosage: Start with short-acting analgesic equivalent to oral morphine sulfate 5–15 mg q4h; after 1–2 weeks of treatment, calculate equivalent dose of long-acting agent and use short-acting opioids for breakthrough.
  - No clear maximum dosage, but trials do not show benefits at doses higher than 180 mg/d of morphine.
  - Precaution: Avoid in those with history of substance abuse, use with caution in the elderly, may cause respiratory depression
  - Interactions: Additive effects with CNS depressants, increased risk of serotonin syndrome with serotonergic agents
  - Adverse effects: Constipation, sedation, nausea, lightheadedness
  - Consider adjuvant therapies with opioids to treat nausea/vomiting, constipation, sedation, pruritus, etc.

Second Line
Some limited data support the efficacy of numerous other medications for the treatment of neuropathic pain including

- Other antidepressants: Paroxetine, venlafaxine, duloxetine, bupropion, citalopram
- Other anticonvulsants: Lamotrigine
- Antiarrhythmics: Mexiletine
- NMDA receptor antagonists: Ketamine, dextromethorphan
- Other agents: Baclofen, clonidine, capsaicin (3,4)[B]

SURGERY
Nerve destructive procedures
- Sympathomectomy
- Dorsal root entry zone lesion (dorsal rhizotomy)
- Lateral cordotomy
- Trigeminal nerve ganglion ablation

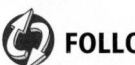 ## FOLLOW-UP

DISPOSITION
Issues for Referral
Referral to pain clinic, neurosurgery in refractory cases

PROGNOSIS
Chronic course of pain symptoms often requires management with numerous medications and adjunctive therapies.

REFERENCES

1. Irving G. Contemporary assessment and management of neuropathic pain. *Neurology* 2005;64(12):S21–S27.
2. Dworken et al. Advances in neuropathic pain. *Arch Neurol* 2003;60(11):1524–1534.
3. Finnerup et al. Algorithm for Neuropathic Pain Treatment: An evidenced based proposal. *Pain* 2005;118(3):289–305.
4. Gorman et al. When is spinal pain neuropathic? *Orthop Clin N Am* 2004;35(1):73–84.

ADDITIONAL READING

- Belgrade M. Following the clues to neuropathic pain. Postgrad Med 1999;106(6):127–140.
- Taylor R. Epidemiology of refractory neuropathic pain. Pain Practice 2006;6(2):22–26.

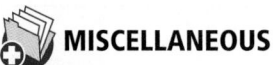 **MISCELLANEOUS**

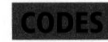 **CODES**

ICD9-CM
- 357.9 Neuropathy, unspecified
- 729.2 Neuralgia, NOS

PATIENT TEACHING

 See Corresponding Diagnostic Algorithm

N

NICOTINE ADDICTION

Brett White, MD

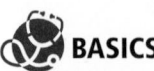 **BASICS**

DESCRIPTION
Habit of nicotine use characterized by signs of dependence

GENERAL PREVENTION
• School-based smoking prevention education
• Physician advice to quit smoking

EPIDEMIOLOGY
Incidence
20–25% of US population smokes.

Prevalence
70.3 million Americans ≥12 years reported current use of tobacco (59.9 million were cigarette smokers, 13.7 million smoked cigars, 7.2 million used smokeless tobacco, 1.8 million smoked pipes). (1)

ALERT
Pediatric Considerations
In the past month, 4 million American adolescents have used a tobacco product. (1)

RISK FACTORS
• Mental Illness (including depression, PTSD, bipolar, and schizophrenia)
• Low SES
• Low educational status

Genetics
• Mutation in the α4 subunit of nicotinic acetylcholine receptors (nAChRs) expressed by neurons lowers the threshold for the induction of nicotine dependence. (2)
• "T" variant gene associated with decreased activity of CYP2B6 (enzyme that breaks down nicotine in the brain) may lead to increased craving during smoking cessation, these patients are also 1.5 times more likely to resume smoking during treatment. (3)

PATHOPHYSIOLOGY
• Mechanism by which nicotine binds to nAChR and how this leads to dependence is still poorly understood.
• Brains from smokers exhibit an upregulation of high-affinity nicotine binding sites.
• Nicotine has both stimulating and depressing effects within the CNS; relaxing and euphoric effects may contribute to psychological dependence.

Pregnancy Considerations
• Carbon monoxide and nicotine may interfere with oxygen supply to the fetus, resulting in fetal growth restriction and decreased birth weight.
• Newborns can also demonstrate signs of drug withdrawal.
• Smoking may increase the incidence of spontaneous abortion, SIDS, and learning or behavioral problems in children. (1)

ETIOLOGY
• Exposure to tobacco products
• Polymorphisms in neuronal nicotinic receptor genes could be associated with increased susceptibility to tobacco dependence. (2)

ASSOCIATED CONDITIONS
• COPD (emphysema and chronic bronchitis)
• Cancers (lung, oral/pharyngeal, kidney, bladder, cervical, anal)
• Coronary artery disease
• Periodontal disease

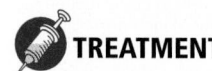 **DIAGNOSIS**

PRE HOSPITAL
Nicotine toxicity may present with nausea, vomiting, sweating, diarrhea, headaches, abdominal pain, weakness, and confusion.

SIGNS AND SYMPTOMS
• Aroma of cigarette smoke often present on breath or clothing
• Nicotine withdrawal can be diagnosed in a patient who has been smoking for several weeks and has ≥4 of the following symptoms after abrupt cessation
  – Depressed mood
  – Insomnia
  – Irritability
  – Anxiety
  – Decreased concentration
  – Restlessness
  – Decreased heart rate
  – Increased appetite/weight gain

History
Nicotine dependence identified as ≥3 of the following within 12 months (DSM-IV-TR criteria)
• Tolerance (need for increased amount of nicotine or diminished effect with continued use)
• Withdrawal (symptoms may be less apparent with nicotine)
• Using nicotine over longer periods or in greater quantities than intended
• Desire to cut down (often with unsuccessful attempts to discontinue use)
• Spend a great deal of time obtaining or using nicotine
• Social or recreational activities reduced because of nicotine use
• Continues to use nicotine despite harm to self (4)

Physical Exam
• Pulmonary
  – Tachypnea
  – Diminished breath sounds if COPD present
• Cardiac
  – Tachycardia
  – Elevated BP

TESTS
Spirometry
• Decreased FEV1 (may be present in COPD)

Lab
ABG
• Hypoxia (may be present in COPD)
• Hypercapnia (may be present in COPD)

Imaging
Chest radiograph or CT scan if clinically indicated

Diagnostic Procedures/Surgery
Thoracentesis/bronchoscopy/surgery if clinically indicated

Pathological Findings
Destruction of alveolar septae or excessive mucous secretion may be found in COPD

DIFFERENTIAL DIAGNOSIS
• Depression
• COPD
• α-1-Antitrypsin deficiency
• Asthma
• CHF
• Respiratory infections
• Lung cancer
• Cystic fibrosis

TREATMENT

PRE HOSPITAL
For nicotine toxicity: Initiate IV, oxygen, and monitor

INITIAL STABILIZATION
Avoid continued nicotine exposure

GENERAL MEASURES
Develop a plan to quit smoking
• Make a commitment to quit
• Set a date for quitting
• Obtain support of family and friends
• Remove all tobacco paraphernalia
• Quit smoking
• Utilize medications to reduce withdrawal symptoms
• Avoid locations and circumstances where nicotine use is common (bars, long car rides, etc.)

Diet
Weight gain possible after smoking cessation, therefore helpful to recommend a healthy diet.

Activity
Encourage routine exercise as a component of smoking cessation treatment.

IV Fluids
As needed for toxic exposure.

Complementary and Alternative Medicine
• Acupuncture: No consistent evidence that acupuncture is effective for smoking cessation (5)[A]

• Hypnotherapy

MEDICATION (DRUGS)

First Line
- Nicotine replacement (must discontinue smoking at initiation of treatment)
  - Nicotine gum (Nicorette): For >25 cigarettes/d habit, 4 mg gum q1–2h for 6 weeks; for <25 cigarettes/d habit, 2 mg gum q1–2h for 6 weeks; decrease dosing by q1–2h for 3 weeks; chew, then tuck between cheek and gingiva.
  - Nicotine transdermal (NicoDerm CQ): For >10 cigarettes/d habit 21 mg patch per day for 6 weeks, then 14 mg patch per day for 2 weeks, then 7 mg patch per day for 2 weeks; for <10 cigarettes/d habit 14 mg patch per day for 6 weeks, then 7 mg patch per day for 2 weeks.
  - Nicotine lozenge (Commit): For patients who have 1st cigarette within 30 min after waking, 4 mg lozenge PO q1–2h for 6 weeks; 1st cigarette >30 min after waking, 2 mg lozenge PO q1–2h for 6 weeks; decrease dosing by q1–2h for 3 weeks.
  - Nicotine nasal (Nicotrol NS): 1–2 sprays (0.5 mg/spray) each nostril q1h for 8 weeks then taper; maximum 10 sprays/h and 80 sprays/d.
  - Nicotine inhaled (Nicotrol Inhaler): 6–16 cartridges inhaled (4 mg/cartridge) per day for 6–12 weeks then taper.
- Medications
  - Bupropion (Zyban): An antidepressant; start 150 mg/d PO for 3 days; then 150 mg PO b.i.d.; stop smoking 5–7 days after starting treatment; continue 7–12 weeks.
  - Varenicline (Chantix): Blocks nicotinic acetylcholine receptors; start 0.5 mg/d PO for 3 days; then 0.5 mg PO b.i.d.; stop smoking 7 days after starting treatment; may continue for 12 weeks
- Counseling

  - A strong dose–response relationship exists between the intensity of tobacco dependence counseling and its effectiveness. Treatments involving person-to-person contact (via individual, group, or proactive telephone counseling) are consistently effective, and their effectiveness increases with treatment intensity (e.g., minutes of contact). (6)[A]

Second Line
Medications

- Nortriptyline: Tricyclic antidepressant; start 25 mg/d, gradually increase to target dose of 75–100 mg/d; stop smoking 2–4 weeks after starting treatment; continue for 12 weeks.
  - Contraindications: Narrow-angle glaucoma or heart disease (AMI, AV or bundle branch block, QT prolongation)
  - Caution: Pregnancy category D
- Clonidine: 0.1 mg patch per week, increase dose as needed; continue for 3–10 weeks
  - Caution: Must monitor BP closely and taper when discontinuing
- Benzodiazepines: Although this class of drug has not improved rates of abstinence from smoking, patients with a high level of anxiety could possibly benefit from anxiolytics as a smoking cessation intervention. (7)[C]

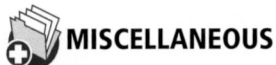 FOLLOW-UP

Patients motivated to quit smoking and who have initiated therapy should follow-up routinely with the physician to monitor response to treatment and observe for any medication side effects.

DISPOSITION
Admission Criteria
For severe nicotine toxicity, as clinically indicated.

Discharge Criteria
Routine

PROGNOSIS
Within 6 months, 75–80% of people who try to quit smoking relapse. (1)

PATIENT MONITORING
For medication side effects

REFERENCES

1. National Institute on Drug Abuse. Tobacco Addiction. National Institute of Health; 2006 July. *NIH Publication Number* 06–4342.
2. Hogg RC, Bertrand D. What genes tell us about nicotine addiction. *Science* 2004;306:983–985.
3. Lerman C, et al. Pharmacogenetic investigation of smoking cessation treatment. *Pharmacogenetics* 2002;12:627–634.
4. American Psychiatric Association: Diagnostic and Statistical Manual of Mental Disorders, 4th ed., Text Revision. Washington, DC: American Psychiatric Association, 2000;192–195.
5. White AR, Rampes H, Campbell JL. Acupuncture and related interventions for smoking cessation. Cochrane Database of Systematic Reviews 2006, Issue 1. Art. No.: CD000009. DOI: 10.1002/14651858.CD000009.pub2.
6. Fiore MC, Bailey WC, Cohen SJ, et. al. Treating tobacco use and dependence. Quick Reference Guide for Clinicians. Rockville, MD: U.S. Department of Health and Human Services. Public Health Service, 2000.
7. Jain A. Treating nicotine addiction. *BMJ* 2003;327: 1394–1395.
8. Glover ED, et al. Treating nicotine dependence. *Am J Med Sci* 2003;326:183–186.

ADDITIONAL READING

- The Agency for Health Care Policy and Research Smoking Cessation Clinical Practice Guideline [Consensus Statement]. JAMA 1996; 275: 1270–1280.
- United States Department of Health and Human Services website for health care professionals: http://www.surgeongeneral.gov/tobacco/
- CDC MMWR, "Cigarette Smoking Among Adults- United States, 2002," at: http://www.cdc.gov/ tobacco/research data/adults prev/MM52804.pdf

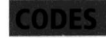 MISCELLANEOUS

CODES

ICD9-CM
- V15.82 Personal history of tobacco use, presenting hazards to health
- 989.84 Toxic effect of tobacco

PATIENT TEACHING
- http://www.smokefree.gov/
- http://www.nicotine-anonymous.org/
- http://quitnet.com/

Diet
Regular

Activity
Routine

Prevention
- Smoking cessation programs
- Self-help materials

N

NOCARDIOSIS

Brock D. Lutz, MD
Ronald A. Greenfield, MD

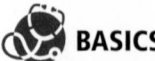 **BASICS**

DESCRIPTION
- An acute, subacute, or chronic infection occurring primarily in cutaneous, pulmonary, and disseminated forms occurring in patients who are immunocompromised or have chronic pulmonary disease. Nocardiosis produces suppurative necrosis and abscess formation at sites of infection.
- Primary cutaneous nocardiosis presents as cutaneous infection (cellulitis or abscess), lymphocutaneous infection (similar to sporotrichosis), or SC infection (actinomycetoma).
- Pulmonary infection presents as an acute, subacute, or chronic pneumonitis.
- Disseminated nocardiosis may involve any organ (lesions in the brain or meninges are most frequent).
- System(s) Affected: Nervous; Pulmonary; Renal/Urologic; Skin/Exocrine

EPIDEMIOLOGY
- Predominant age: All ages are susceptible; mean age at diagnosis is the 4th decade of life.
- Predominant sex: Males > Female (3:1)

Incidence
- 0.4 cases/100,000 person years overall
- 53 cases/100,000 person years among individuals with AIDS
- 128 cases/100,000 person years among bone marrow transplant recipients
- 1,122 cases/100,000 person years among solid organ transplant recipients
- It is estimated that 500–1,000 new cases occur per year in the US.

RISK FACTORS
- Most cases occur as opportunistic infection of immunocompromised hosts or hosts with predisposing pulmonary abnormalities.
- Solid organ transplantation, chronic granulomatous disease of childhood, dysgammaglobulinemias, pemphigus, Cushing's disease, hemochromatosis, cirrhosis, bronchiectasis, tuberculosis (TB), sarcoidosis, anthracosilicosis, pulmonary alveolar proteinosis, lymphoma, leukemia, glucocorticoid and cytotoxic therapy, solid malignancies, and AIDS
- Immunologically normal individuals may develop primary cutaneous disease days to weeks after receiving a wound contaminated with soil.

ALERT
Pediatric Considerations
An association has been reported between chronic granulomatous disease of childhood and nocardiosis.

PATHOPHYSIOLOGY
Nocardiosis is an acute suppurative bacterial infection.

ETIOLOGY
Inhalation or traumatic inoculation of Nocardia species bacteria (predominantly *N. asteroides*, but also *N. brasiliensis*, *N. caviae*, *N. farcinica*, *N. transvalensis*, *N. otitidiscaviarum*, and *N. nova*, although a host of new species continue to be described) from soil.

ASSOCIATED CONDITIONS
See "Risk Factors."

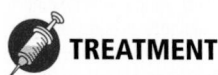 **DIAGNOSIS**

SIGNS AND SYMPTOMS
- Pulmonary nocardiosis
  - Fever (70%)
  - Cough (52%)
  - Pleuritic chest pain (32%)
  - Dyspnea (16%)
  - Anorexia
  - Weight loss
  - Hemoptysis
  - Tachypnea
  - Rales
  - CNS dysfunction in those with CNS involvement
  - Other focal infections in those with disseminated infection
- Cutaneous nocardiosis
  - Abscesses
  - Lymphadenopathy
- Disseminated nocardiosis
  - Confusion
  - Disorientation
  - Dizziness
  - Headache
  - Nausea and/or vomiting
  - Seizures
  - Shortness of breath

TESTS
Lab
- The diagnosis is established by observing the characteristic microscopic appearance of the organism in Gram-stained and modified acid-fast-stained preparations of sputum or pus or histopathologic samples. Confirmation is by culture of these same specimens.
- When attempting recovery of Nocardia from sputum, clinical microbiology laboratory should be so advised because of the organism's slow growth and propensity to be overgrown by oral flora
- Blood cultures should be obtained in all cases of suspected nocardiosis.

Imaging
- Radiography
  - Confluent bronchopneumonia with or without cavitation
  - Pleural effusion is common (up to 50%).
  - Other chest radiographic presentations include masses, nodules, cavities, and interstitial infiltrates.
- CT or MRI of the brain may reveal single or multiple intracranial abscesses and is indicated in all patients with pulmonary or disseminated nocardiosis.
- Other sites of focal infection may be identified by imaging in disseminated disease.

Diagnostic Procedures/Surgery
- If evaluation of sputum is nondiagnostic, bronchoscopy for bronchoalveolar lavage and transbronchial lung biopsy may prove valuable for diagnosis.
- Percutaneous aspiration of lung lesion is often useful.

Pathological Findings
Histopathology reveals a suppurative lesion with acute necrosis and abscess formation and the microorganism, which may stain positive on modified acid-fast stains.

DIFFERENTIAL DIAGNOSIS
Includes other causes of acute, subacute, or chronic pneumonitis, particularly those occurring principally in immunocompromised hosts
- TB
- Histoplasmosis
- Polymicrobial bacterial lung abscess
- Carcinoma

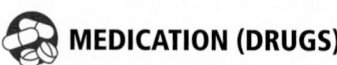 **TREATMENT**

INITIAL STABILIZATION
Patients with moderate or severe illness generally require hospitalization.

GENERAL MEASURES
Respiratory support is often necessary in such hospitalized patients.

Diet
No special diet

Activity
Acute phase usually requires bed rest; increase activity as condition improves

MEDICATION (DRUGS)

First Line
- Survival may be improved if a sulfa-containing regimen is used. (2)[B] Some prefer sulfadiazine because of possibly better CNS penetration (2)[B]; should be given as 4–8 g/d PO in 4 divided doses. Dosage should be adjusted to maintain sulfonamide serum levels in the range of 8–16 mg/dL.
- Some prefer to use trimethoprim-sulfamethoxazole. (2)[B] This agent must be used if parenteral sulfonamide therapy is required. Initial dose based on trimethoprim component: 640 mg trimethoprim daily. Base subsequent doses on sulfamethoxazole level. Dosage should provide sulfonamide dosing and levels equivalent to those of sulfonamide when used alone.
- Duration of therapy is usually 3 months for immunocompetent hosts and 6 months for those who are immunocompromised.
- Contraindications
  - Sulfonamides—during the last month of pregnancy (should be used only when the potential benefits outweigh the risks).
  - All antimicrobial agents above are contraindicated in the presence of known hypersensitivity to the agent.
- Precautions: With the use of high-dose sulfadiazine, high urine flow should be maintained to minimize risk of crystalluria. Generally, patients should be advised to drink 2–3 L/d.

- Significant possible interactions
  - Sulfonamides may increase the therapeutic effects of oral anticoagulants, phenytoin, sulfonylurea hypoglycemic agents, methotrexate, and thiopental.
  - Decreased absorption of digoxin may be encountered.

Second Line
- Alternatives for sulfonamide-allergic patients include doxycycline or minocycline, ampicillin plus erythromycin, amikacin, meropenem, β-lactam/β-lactamase inhibitor combinations, cefotaxime or ceftriaxone, and linezolid. (6)[B] Clinical experience with these alternative regimens is limited.

- Species-specific trends in susceptibility have been identified; therefore, therapy should be guided by *in vitro* antimicrobial susceptibility.
- Empiric therapy for the acutely ill patient:
  - Ceftriaxone 2 g IV q12h or meropenem 1 g IV q8h plus amikacin 15 mg/kg IV daily.

SURGERY
Surgical drainage of abscesses other than intrapulmonary abscesses is generally indicated if technically feasible.

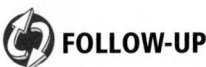 FOLLOW-UP

PROGNOSIS
- Overall modern mortality is 7–44%.
- Mortality in renal transplant recipients
  - 25% overall
  - 0% with isolated cutaneous involvement
  - 29% with localized pleuropulmonary disease
  - 42% with CNS involvement
- In patients with AIDS, mortality is 30%.

COMPLICATIONS
- CNS infection (brain abscess or meningitis; 16%)
- Secondary cutaneous nocardiosis (13%)
- Septic arthritis (2%)
- Hematogenous osteomyelitis (1%)
- Other focal manifestations of disseminated infection (13%)

PATIENT MONITORING
Patients on high-dose sulfonamide therapy should have a CBC and assessment of hepatic and renal function at least every other week.

REFERENCES
1. Filice GA. Nocardiosis in persons with HIV infection, transplant recipients, and large, geographically defined populations. *J Lab Clin Med*. 2005;145:156–162.
2. Lerner PI. Nocardiosis. *Clin Infect Dis*. 1996;22: 891–902.
3. Mamelak AN, et al. Nocardial brain abscess: Treatment strategies and factors influencing outcome. *Neurosurgery*. 1994;35:622–631.
4. Marrie TJ. Pneumonia caused by Nocardia species. *Semin Respir Infect*. 1994;9:207–213.
5. Marquez-Diaz F, Soto-Ramirez LE, Sifuentes-Osornio J. Nocardiosis in patients with HIV infection. *AIDS Patient Care STDS*. 1998;12: 825–832.
6. Saubolle MA, Sussland D. Nocardiosis: Review of clinical and laboratory experience. *J Clin Microbiol*. 2003;41:4497–4501.

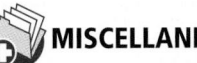 MISCELLANEOUS

Unusual nocardial infections
- Keratoconjunctivitis associated with contact lenses or penetrating injury or ophthalmological surgery
- Peritonitis in patients on continuous ambulatory peritoneal dialysis
- Upper respiratory and digestive tract infections
- Pericarditis and cardiac tamponade
- Hematogenous endophthalmitis
- Prosthetic joint infections
- Natural or prosthetic valve endocarditis
- Infections of the male genitourinary tract
- Intravascular access device–related infection

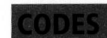 CODES

ICD9-CM
039.9 Actinomycotic infections of unspecified site

PATIENT TEACHING
- Not a contagious disease
- Advise patients of the need for long-term antimicrobial therapy to reduce the likelihood of relapse and inform patients of potential adverse reactions.

N

NOSOCOMIAL INFECTIONS

Theodore R. Hartenstein, MD

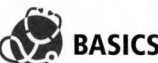 **BASICS**

DESCRIPTION
- Also known as health care–associated infections (HAI)
- 2 sub-types
  - Infections acquired by patient while in a health care facility
  - Infections acquired by health care providers or visitors to health care facilities
- Centers for Disease Control and Prevention categories
  - Urinary tract infection (UTI)
  - Surgical site infection
    - Superficial incisional site infection
    - Deep incisional site infection
    - Organ/space infection
  - Pneumonia
  - Bloodstream infection
  - Bone and joint infection
  - CNS infection
  - Cardiovascular system infection
  - Ear, eye, nose throat, or mouth infection
  - Gastrointestinal system infection
  - Lower respiratory system infection (excluding pneumonia)
  - Reproductive tract infection
  - Skin and soft tissue infection
  - Systemic infection

GENERAL PREVENTION
- Hand hygiene
  - Alcohol-based product
    - When hands not visibly soiled (1)[A]
    - Most effective way to remove microbes (2)
    - Rub hands together until dry (1)[B]
  - Soap and water
    - After eating (1)[B]
    - After using bathroom (1)[B]
    - When visibly soiled (1)[A]
- Hospital-based surveillance programs
  - Estimated to reduce overall infection rate by 32% (3)
- Establishment of multidisciplinary infection control (IC) teams
- Careful and regular review of IC policies
- Employee education on nosocomial infections
- Active employee health department
- Minimize invasive procedures
- Judicious use of antibiotics
- Isolation of known pathogen carriers
  - Contact precautions
    - Pathogens spread by direct contact
    - Includes methicillin-resistant *Staphylococcus Aureus*, Vancomycin-resistant enterococcus, *Clostridium difficile*
  - Droplet precautions
    - Infectious particles measure >5 μm
    - Shed via coughing, sneezing, mucosal shedding, airway suctioning
    - Includes *Neisseria meningitis*, influenza, *Haemophilus influenzae*, diphtheria
  - Airborne precautions
    - Infectious particles measure <5 μm
    - Shed via coughing
    - Includes tuberculosis, varicella zoster virus measles

- Infection-specific measures
  - UTI
    - Placement of catheter with sterile technique (2)
    - Closed urine collection system (2)
    - Use of catheter only as necessary (2)
    - Removal of catheter as early as possible (2)
  - Pneumonia
    - Intubation only as necessary (4)[C]
    - Avoidance of nasotracheal intubation (4)[B]
    - In-line suctioning (4)[C]
    - Head elevation of 30–45° (4)[C]
  - Bloodstream infection
    - Placement of catheter with sterile technique (5)[A]
    - Removal of catheter as early as possible (5)[A]
    - Proper hand hygiene (5)[A]
    - Regular monitoring of catheter site (5)[B]
  - Surgical site infection
    - Proper surgical hand hygiene (6)[B]
    - Prophylactic antibiotic therapy (6)[A]
    - Elimination of underlying infections before surgery (6)[A]
    - Adequate post-operative blood sugar control (6)[B]

EPIDEMIOLOGY
- General
  - Up to 10% of all hospitalized patients in US (2)
  - Up to 50% of patients in ICU (7)
  - Estimated cost in 2001 was $7.5 billion (7)
- Infection-specific
  - UTI
    - Hospital stay increased by 1–3 days (8)
    - Cost up to $600 per infection (8)
  - Pneumonia
    - Hospital stay increased by 5–9 days (7)
    - Cost up to $5,000 per infection (8)
  - Bloodstream infection
    - Hospital stay increased by 7–20 days (8)
    - Cost up to $39,000 per infection (2)
  - Surgical site infection
    - Hospital stay increased 7.3 days (6)
    - Cost >$3,000 per infection (6)

Incidence
- Incidence of resistant *S. aureus* and Vancomycin resistant enterococcus increasing dramatically in last 15 years.
- >2 million HAI per year (2)
- Majority of affected have single-site infection
- UTI 28% of HAI (3)
  - >900,000 cases per year in US (8)
  - 2.39 per 100 admissions (8)
- Pneumonia: 25% of HAI (3)
  - >225,000 cases per year in US (8)
  - 0.60 per 100 admissions (8)
- Bloodstream infection: 12% of HAI (3)
  - >100,000 cases per year in US (8)
  - 0.27 per 100 admissions (8)
- Surgical site infection: 11% of HAI (3)
  - >500,000 cases per year in US (8)
  - 2.79 cases per 100 surgeries (8)
- Soft tissue and skin infection: 7% of HAI (3)
- Others: 17% of HAI (3)

RISK FACTORS
- Extremes of age
- Immunodeficiency
- Chronic disease
- Anesthesia
- Malnutrition
- Medications
  - Antibiotics
  - Antacids
  - Sedatives
- Breakdown of mucosal or cutaneous barriers
- Colonization with pathogenic strains of flora

Genetics
No known role

PATHOPHYSIOLOGY
- Endogenous spread (majority of cases)
  - Patient's own normal flora causes invasive disease
- Exogenous route
  - Flora from within health care facility causes invasive disease

ETIOLOGY
- UTI
  - *Pseudomonas aeruginosa*
  - *Escherichia coli*
  - Enterococcus species
  - *Candida albicans*
- Surgical site infection
  - *S. aureus*
  - Gram-negative bacilli
- Pneumonia
  - Enteric Gram-negative bacilli
  - *S. aureus*
  - *Pseudomonas aeruginosa*
- Bloodstream infection
  - Staphylococcal species

DIAGNOSIS

SIGNS AND SYMPTOMS
Consistent with nature of infection

History
- Exposure to health care facility
- Recent surgery
- History of invasive procedure
  - Urinary catheter placement
  - In-dwelling vascular catheter
- Recent intubation/mechanical ventilation
- Past infections

Physical Exam
Consistent with nature of infection

TESTS
As appropriate for suspected infection

Lab
As appropriate for suspected infection

Imaging
As appropriate for suspected infection

Diagnostic Procedures/Surgery
As appropriate for suspected infection

Pathological Findings
Consistent with underlying infection

DIFFERENTIAL DIAGNOSIS
- Community-acquired infection
- Non-infectious process

 **TREATMENT**

INITIAL STABILIZATION
As appropriate for suspected infection

GENERAL MEASURES
Treat the underlying infection as indicated

Diet
No restrictions

Activity
As tolerated

Nursing
As applicable

SPECIAL THERAPY
IV Fluids
As needed

Complementary and Alternative Therapies
As appropriate for specific infection

 MEDICATION (DRUGS)

First Line
As appropriate for specific nature of infection

Second Line
As appropriate for specific nature of infection

SURGERY
As appropriate for specific nature of infection

 FOLLOW-UP

As appropriate for specific nature of infection

DISPOSITION
When infection resolved or patient stable

Admission Criteria
When infection resolved or patient stable

Issues for Referral
As appropriate

PROGNOSIS
- Responsible for 88,000 deaths per year in US (7)
- Increases risk of death by 100% (7)
- Bloodstream infection mortality: 25–50% (7)
- Nosocomial pneumonia mortality: 7–27% (7)

COMPLICATIONS
Related to specific nature of infection

PATIENT MONITORING
As appropriate for specific type of infection

REFERENCES

1. Boyce JM, Pittet D. Guideline for hand hygiene in health-care settings: Recommendations of the healthcare infection control practices advisory committee and the HICPAC/SHEA/APIC/IDSA hand hygiene task force. *MMWR Recommendations and Reports.* 2002;51:1–56.
2. Coffin SE, Zaoutis TE. Infection control, hospital epidemiology, and patient safety. *Infect Dis Clin North Am.* 2005;19: 647–665.
3. Sax H, et al. Variation in nosocomial infection prevalence according to patient care setting: A hospital-wide survey. *J Hosp Infect.* 2001;48: 27–32.
4. Tablan OC, et al. 2004. Guidelines for preventing health-care associated pneumonia, 2003: Recommendations of CDC and the healthcare infection control practices advisory committee. *MMWR Recommendations and Reports.* 2004; 53:1–40.
5. O'Grady NP, et al. Guidelines for the prevention of intravascular catheter-related infections. *Pediatrics.* 2002; 110:e51.
6. Mangram AJ, et al. Guideline for prevention of surgical site infection, 1999. *Am J Infect Control.* 1999;27:97–134.
7. Cohen J, et al. *Infectious diseases.* 2nd ed. Edinburgh, U.K.: Mosby; 2004.
8. Jarvis WR. Selected aspects of the socioeconomic impact of nosocomial infections: Morbidity, mortality, cost, and prevention. *Infect Control Hosp Epidemiol.* 1996;17:552–557.

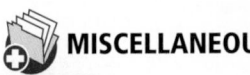 **MISCELLANEOUS**

CODES

ICD9-CM
See specific infection headings for code

PATIENT TEACHING

N

OBESITY

Maya Roberts, BA
Jeremy Golding, MD

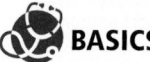 **BASICS**

DESCRIPTION
- Excess adipose tissue associated long-term health problems
- Body-mass index (BMI)
  - >25 is overweight
  - >30 is obese
  - >40 is severely obese
- Android obesity (male pattern or abdominal obesity) is associated with a higher risk for increased morbidity and mortality than gynecoid obesity (typical female pattern or gluteal obesity).
- System(s) Affected: Endocrine/Metabolic; Cardiac; Respiratory; Gastrointestinal; Musculoskeletal
- Synonym(s): Overweight; Adiposis; Adiposity

ALERT
Geriatric Considerations
The BMI associated with the lowest risk of mortality increases with advanced age.

GENERAL PREVENTION
- Encourage routine exercise and moderation in diet with follow-up for children/young adults, and if there is a family history of obesity or diabetes mellitus.
- Emphasize avoiding calorie-dense and nutrient-poor foods like soda and fruit-flavored drinks.

EPIDEMIOLOGY
- Predominant age: All ages
- Predominant sex: Female > Male

Prevalence
- Mean prevalence of obesity is 32.2% in the US.
- Overweight: 40% of men and 25% of women
- Obese: 20% of men and 25% of women

Pediatric Considerations
- Prepuberty and young adulthood are sensitive periods for the onset of obesity.
- The prevalence of obesity is increasing in the pediatric population.
- Decreased physical activity, increased consumption of sweetened beverages, and increased television viewing have been implicated, among other factors.

RISK FACTORS
- Parental obesity
- Sedentary lifestyle
- High-fat diet
- Pregnancy
- Low socioeconomic status
- Ethnic variations

Genetics
- Rare genetic syndromes such as Prader-Willi and Bardet-Biedel syndrome
- Studies are inconclusive regarding specific genetic predictors of obesity.

ETIOLOGY
- Obesity is caused by an imbalance between food intake and energy expenditure.
- Rare causes include insulinoma, hypothalamic disorders, hypothyroidism, and Cushing syndrome
- Menopause and smoking cessation are associated with significant weight gain secondary to changes in metabolic rate.
- Some medications are associated with significant weight gain, including corticosteroids, neuroepileptics (particularly the "atypical" antipsychotics), and antidepressants.

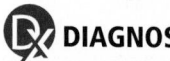 **DIAGNOSIS**

SIGNS AND SYMPTOMS
Elevated BMI and increased adipose tissue

History
- Any prior attempts at weight loss
- Reported readiness to change lifestyle
- Diet and exercise habits
- Associated risk factors: Diabetes mellitus, hypertension, hyperlipidemia, sleep apnea
- Symptoms suggesting hypothyroidism, Cushing syndrome, genetic syndromes

Physical Exam
- BMI = body weight (kg) / (body height (m))^2
  - Overweight is BMI = 25–29.9 kg/m^2
  - Obesity is BMI $\geq$30 kg/m^2
  - Morbidly obese is $\geq$40 kg/m^2

BMI Obesity Threshold by Height

Height		BMI = 25 Weight (lb/kg)	BMI = 27 Weight (lb/kg)	BMI = 30 Weight (lb/kg)
5′	0	128/58	138/63	153/70
5′	2″	136/61	147/67	164/74
5′	4″	145/66	157/71	174/79
5′	6″	155/70	167/76	186/84
5′	8″	164/74	177/81	197/89
5′	10″	174/79	188/85	209/95
6′	0″	184/83	199/90	221/100
6′	2″	194/88	210/95	233/106
6′	4″	205/92	221/101	246/112

- Fat distribution pattern
  - Waist circumference is measured around the abdomen, at the umbilicus:
  - >40 inches (102 cm) for men and >35 inches (88 cm) for women is associated with increased risk for most obesity-related medical conditions. (1)[C]

TESTS
Lab
- Used to determine the presence of and to monitor associated risk factors and conditions
- Serum lipid panel and fasting glucose
- Consider thyroid-stimulating hormone (TSH)
- Hypothyroidism may alter other lab results

Pathological Findings
- Hypertrophy and/or hyperplasia of adipocytes
- Cardiomegaly
- Hepatomegaly

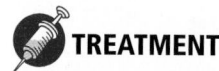 **TREATMENT**

GENERAL MEASURES
- Primary-care physician should perform the following assessments
  - Degree of health risk from BMI and waist circumference (1)[C] (see "Diagnosis")
  - Motivation to lose weight (1)[C]
  - Patient-specific goals of therapy
  - Necessary counseling or referral to a dietitian for diet, exercise, and behavior modification (1)[B]
  - Appropriate long-term follow-up (1)[C]
- An appropriate goal for therapy is to achieve and sustain weight loss up to 10% of body weight for overweight and obese patients. (1)[A]
- Behavior therapy and cognitive-behavioral methods can result in modest weight loss, but are most effective when combined with dietary and exercise treatments. (2)[A]
- Effective commercial and community-based programs include those diets meeting the US recommended daily allowance (RDA) for nutrients, exercise, behavior modification, and provision for maintenance of ideal weight and eating habits.

ALERT
Pregnancy Considerations
- Weight loss is not appropriate for most pregnant or lactating women. (1)[C]
- During pregnancy, obese women should gain <25 pounds recommended for nonobese women.

Diet
- Long-term studies suggest that net calorie reduction of 500–1,000 kcal/d and ease of adherence are more important than diet composition for long-term results.
  - A reduction of 500 kcal/d intake results in ~1 lb (0.45 kg) weight loss per week. (1)[A]
  - Low-fat, high-complex carbohydrate, and high-fiber diets are most commonly recommended. (1)[A]
  - Portion-controlled servings are recommended.
- Very-low-calorie diets (VLCDs)
  - 400–800 kcal/d can result in more rapid weight loss than higher-calorie diets, but have less effective long-term results.
  - Complications include dehydration, orthostatic hypotension, fatigue, muscle cramps, constipation, headache, cold intolerance, and relapse after discontinuation.
  - Contraindications include recent myocardial infarction or cerebrovascular accident, renal or hepatic disease, cancer, pregnancy, insulin-dependent diabetes mellitus, and some psychiatric disturbances.

Activity

- Exercise may improve long-term results of treatment and should be an integral part of any weightloss program. However, it alone rarely results in significant weight loss. (1)[A]

- Exercise regimens should involve 30–90 minutes, 5–7 times per week.

- Combination of weight training and aerobic activity is preferred over aerobic activity alone.

- Increasing calories expended in daily activities is also important.

 MEDICATION (DRUGS)

National Institutes of Health (NIH) guidelines suggest

- Nonpharmacologic treatment for 6 months
- Medication treatment for unsatisfactory weight loss in those with a BMI >30 or with a BMI >27 combined with associated risk factors (coronary heart disease, diabetes, sleep apnea, hypertension, hyperlipidemia).

- Diet, exercise, and behavior therapy must be included in pharmacologic treatment. (1)[B]

First Line

- Medications produce modest weight loss (3)[A].

- The appetite suppressant Sibutramine is a serotonin and norepinephrine reuptake inhibitor.
  - Dose: 10–15 mg PO daily (10 mg starting dose)
- The lipase inhibitor Orlistat decreases the absorption of dietary fat.
  - Dose: 120 mg PO t.i.d. with meals. Patients must avoid fat-soluble vitamin supplements within 2 hours of taking orlistat.
- Contraindications
  - Sibutramine: Uncontrolled hypertension, severe renal or hepatic dysfunction, narrow-angle glaucoma, history of substance abuse, symptomatic cardiovascular disease, CHF, arrhythmias, stroke, use of monoamine oxidase inhibitor within 2 weeks
  - Orlistat: Chronic malabsorption syndromes, cholestasis
- Precautions: Relapse after discontinuation of drug
- Significant possible interactions
  - Pulse and BP elevations possible with Sibutramine.
  - Concurrent use with general anesthetics may cause arrhythmias.
  - Serotonergic agents may cause "serotonin syndrome" in combination with sibutramine.

Second Line

- Appetite suppressants recommended for short-term treatment (several weeks)
- Schedule IV drugs
  - Diethylpropion
  - Phentermine
- Schedule II drugs
  - Phendimetrazine
  - Benzphetamine

SURGERY

Patients meeting criteria (including severe obesity [BMI >40 kg/m²]) can be treated with gastric bypass procedures

- Malabsorptive surgery reduces the length of the small intestine
- Restrictive surgery reduces the size of the stomach's capacity
  - This requires complex presurgical evaluation, surgery and follow-up in a skilled treatment center. (1)[C]
  - Lifelong medical surveillance is necessary after obesity surgery. (1)[C]
  - Surgical treatment is the most effective long-term weight loss treatment available for morbid obesity. (4)[B]

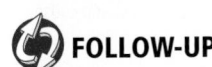 **FOLLOW-UP**

DISPOSITION
Outpatient care

PROGNOSIS

- Lowest mortality associated with a BMI of 22.
- Long-term maintenance of weight loss is extremely difficult.
- A motivated patient is most likely to achieve successful weight loss.
- There have been several controversial studies suggesting that a BMI in the overweight range is associated with a decreased risk or mortality relative to a BMI in the underweight or obese range.

COMPLICATIONS

- Cardiovascular disease
- Stroke (in men)
- Thromboembolism
- Heart failure
- Hypertension
- Increased mortality (largely due to cardiovascular disease)
- Premature death
- Hypoventilation and sleep apnea syndromes
- Higher death rates from cancer: Colon, breast, prostate, endometrial, gallbladder, liver, kidney
- Diabetes mellitus
- Skin changes
- Hyperlipidemia
- Gallbladder disease
- Cholelithiasis
- Osteoarthritis
- Gout
- Poor self-esteem
- Discrimination
- Increased sick leave

PATIENT MONITORING
Long-term routine follow-up is crucial to prevent further weight gain or relapse after weight loss.

REFERENCES

1. Bray G. Clinical evaluation of the overweight adult: Overview of therapy for obesity in adults: surgical management of severe obesity, and health hazards for associated with obesity in adults. UpToDate. 2006.
2. Colquitt J, et al. Surgery for morbid obesity (Cochrane Review). *The Cochrane Library*, Issue 4. Chichester, U.K.: John Wiley & Sons, Ltd., 2005.
3. Institute of Medicine, Food and Nutrition Board, Committee on Nutritional Status during Pregnancy, part I: Nutritional Status and Weight Gain. Washington, DC: National Academy Press, 1990.
4. Flegal K, Graubard B, Williamson D, Gail M. Excess deaths associated with underweight, overweight, and obesity. *JAMA*. 2005;20:293(15):1861–1867.
5. National Institutes of Health Clinical guidelines on the identification, evaluation, and treatment of overweight and obesity in adults: The evidence report. NIH Publication No. 98-4083, 1998.
6. Padwal R, Li SK, Lau DCW. Long-term pharmacotherapy for obesity and overweight (Cochrane Review). *The Cochrane Library*, Issue 4. Chichester, U.K.: John Wiley & Sons, Ltd., 2005.
7. Shaw K, et al. Psychological interventions for overweight and obesity (Cochrane Review). *The Cochrane Library*, Issue 4. Chichester, U.K.: John Wiley & Sons, Ltd., 2005.

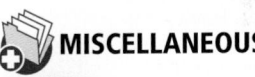 **MISCELLANEOUS**

CODES

ICD9-CM

- 278.00 Obesity, unspecified
- 278.01 Morbid obesity

PATIENT TEACHING

- Emphasize the value of a healthy BMI.
- Recommended web sites
  - http://www.shapeup.org for general information and specific resources
  - www.gastro.org for the American Gastroenterological Association
  - http://www.nal.usda.gov/fnic/foodcomp/search for the FDA nutritional content in common foods.

 See Corresponding Diagnostic Algorithm

 See Patient Handout on CD

O

OBSESSIVE COMPULSIVE DISORDER

Anna K. Morin, PharmD

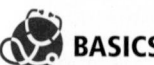 **BASICS**

DESCRIPTION

- Obsessive compulsive disorder (OCD) is a psychiatric condition classified as an anxiety disorder in *DSM-IV-R* and characterized by obsessions (recurrent, intrusive thoughts, ideas, or images) and compulsions (repetitive, ritualistic behaviors or mental acts).
- System(s) Affected: Nervous
- Synonym(s): Obsessive compulsive neurosis

ALERT
Not to be confused with obsessive compulsive personality disorder

Geriatric Considerations
- Diagnosis rarely is made after age 50 years.
- Consider neurologic disorders in new-onset OCD in elderly patients.

Pregnancy Considerations
- Onset of OCD has been noted during postpartum period.
- Safety of medications has not been established during pregnancy or lactation.

Pediatric Considerations
- Child/adolescent onset in 33% of cases
- At this age, Males > Females (3:1)
- Insidious onset; consider brain insult in acute presentation of childhood OCD

EPIDEMIOLOGY
- Predominant age
  – Mean age 22–36 years
  – 1/3 of cases present by age 15 years
  – 85% of cases present before age 35 years
  – New cases rare after age 50 years
- Predominant sex
  – Male = Female (males present at younger age)

Incidence
- 1.5–2.1% 1-year prevalence in adults
- 0.7% 1-year prevalence in children and adolescents

Prevalence
- 2.5% lifetime prevalence in adults
- 1–2.3% prevalence in children and adolescents

RISK FACTORS
Genetics
- Greater concordance in monozygotic twins
- Positive family history in ~20% of cases
- Evidence of a dominant or codominant mode of transmission

PATHOPHYSIOLOGY
See "Etiology."

ETIOLOGY
- Dysregulation of neurotransmitter, serotonin
- Pediatric autoimmune neuropsychiatric disorder associated with streptococcal infections

ASSOCIATED CONDITIONS
- Depression
- Panic disorder
- Social phobia
- Phobia
- Tourette syndrome
- Substance abuse
- Eating disorder
- Body dysmorphic disorder

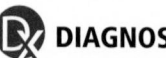 **DIAGNOSIS**

SIGNS AND SYMPTOMS
- Obsessions and compulsions cause marked distress, are time consuming (>1 hour per day) and cause significant occupational/social impairment.
- Patients know obsessions come from their own minds and are not imposed from outside (as in thought insertion).
- Compulsions are designed to relieve the anxiety of obsessions; they are not inherently enjoyable ("ego dynastic") and do not result in completion of a useful task.
- Common obsessive themes
  – Harm (i.e., being responsible for an accident)
  – Doubt (i.e., whether doors or windows locked or iron turned off)
  – Blasphemous thoughts (i.e., in a devoutly religious person)
  – Contamination, dirt, or disease
  – Symmetry or orderliness
- Common rituals or compulsions
  – Hand washing, cleaning
  – Checking
  – Counting
  – Hoarding
  – Ordering, arranging
  – Repeating
- Neither obsessions nor compulsions are related to another mental disorder (i.e., thoughts of food in presence of eating disorder).
- 80–90% of patients with OCD have obsessions and compulsions.
- 10–19% of patients are pure obsessional.

Physical Exam
Dermatologic problems caused by excessive washing may be observed.

TESTS
- Yale Brown obsessive-compulsive scale (Y-BOCS)
- Maudsley obsessive-compulsive inventory (MOCI)
- Children's Yale Brown obsessive-compulsive scale (CY-BOCS)

Lab
No diagnostic laboratory findings identified

Imaging
Positron emission tomography (PET) scan
- Abnormal metabolism in frontal cortex and caudate nuclei (not generally available other than in research centers)

Diagnostic Procedures/Surgery
Psychiatric interview

DIFFERENTIAL DIAGNOSIS
- Not to be confused with obsessive compulsive personality disorder (see "Differential Diagnosis")
- Impulse control disorders
  – Compulsive gambling, sex, or substance abuse: The "compulsive" behavior is not in response to obsessive thoughts, and patient derives pleasure from the activity.
- Depression
- Brooding, but ideas not as senseless as OCD
- Schizophrenia
  – Patient perceives thought to be true and coming from an external source.
- Obsessive compulsive *personality* disorder
  – In personality disorder, traits are "ego syntonic." Traits include perfectionism, preoccupation with detail, trivia, or procedure and regulation. Patient tends to be rigid, moralistic, and stingy. Often rewarded in patient's job as desirable traits.
- Generalized anxiety, phobic disorders, separation anxiety
  – Similar response of heightened anxiety, but presence of obsessions or rituals clarifies OCD diagnosis.
- Anxiety disorder due to general medical condition
  – It may be that obsessions or compulsions are assessed to be a direct physiologic consequence of a general medical condition.

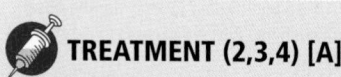 **TREATMENT (2,3,4) [A]**

GENERAL MEASURES
- Combined medications and cognitive behavior therapy (CBT) is most effective
- Psychiatric referral for CBT (in vivo exposure and prevention of compulsions)
- Family psychoeducation
- Parent behavior management training if patient with OCD is a child or adolescent

MEDICATION (DRUGS) (2,3,4) [A]

First Line
- Adequate trial at least 10–12 weeks
- Optimal doses may exceed typical doses for depression
- Selective serotonin reuptake inhibitor (SSRI), fluoxetine (Prozac)
  - Adults: Begin 20 mg/d every morning and increase every 4–6 weeks to obtain maximal response. Dose range: 20–80 mg/d.
  - Children: Begin with 10 mg/d every morning and increase every 4–6 weeks to obtain maximal response. Dose range: 20–60 mg/d.
- SSRI, sertraline (Zoloft)
  - Adults: Begin with 50 mg/d and increase every 4–7 days until response. Dose range: 50–200 mg/d; may divide if above 100 mg/d.
  - Children: Begin with 25 mg/d; increase in 25-mg increments until clinical response. Dose range: 50–200 mg/d.
- SSRI, paroxetine (Paxil)
  - Adults: Begin with 20 mg/d; increase every 4–7 days in 10-mg increments until maximal clinical response. Dose range: 40–60 mg/d.
  - Children: Safety and efficacy have not been established for OCD.
- SSRI, fluvoxamine (Luvox)
  - Adult: Begin with 100 mg/d and increase every 4–7 days in 50-mg increments until clinical response. Dose range: 200–300 mg/d.
  - Children (8–17 years): Begin with 25 mg/d; increase every 4–7 days in 25–50 mg increments until clinical response. Dose range: 50–200 mg/d.

Second Line
- Try switch to another SSRI
- Tricyclic, clomipramine (Anafranil)
  - Adults: Begin with 25 mg/d; increase gradually to 100 mg over 1st 2 weeks, then to 250 mg (maximum dose) over next several weeks, as tolerated.
  - Children: Begin with 25 mg/d over 1st 2 weeks as in adults, then titrate, as tolerated, up to 3 mg/kg or 200 mg/d (whichever is smaller) over the next several weeks.
- Contraindications
  - Suicidal ideation and behavior or worsening depression; increased risk, particularly in children and adolescents, during 1st few months of therapy with antidepressants
  - Absolute SSRI contraindications
    - Hypersensitivity to the selective serotonin reuptake inhibitors
    - Within 14 days of monoamine oxidase (MAO) inhibitor
  - Relative SSRI contraindications
    - Severe liver impairment
    - Seizure disorders (lowers seizure threshold)
  - All SSRIs pregnancy category C, except paroxetine, which is pregnancy category D

- Clomipramine is a tricyclic antidepressant and carries the same contraindications as drugs in that class
  - Tricyclic class of antidepressants dangerous in overdose.
- Absolute clomipramine contraindications
  - Within 6 months of myocardial infarction
  - Narrow-angle glaucoma
  - 3rd-degree atrioventricular (AV) block
  - Within 14 days of MAO inhibitor
- Relative clomipramine contraindications
  - Prostatic hypertrophy (urinary retention)
  - Seizure disorder (lowers seizure threshold)
  - 1st- or 2nd-degree AV block, bundle branch block, and CHF (proarrhythmic effect)
  - Pregnancy category C
- Precautions
  - A drug should to be taken for a minimum of 10 weeks before considering it a treatment failure; could be several months before peak efficacy is seen.
  - Because patients with OCD may have concomitant depression, suicide potential must be assessed.
  - Long 1/2-life of fluoxetine (>7 days) may be troublesome if patient has an adverse reaction.
  - May cause drowsiness and dizziness when therapy is initiated. Warn patients about driving and heavy-equipment hazards.
- Significant possible interactions
  - Clomipramine
    - Not yet fully elucidated
    - May interfere with guanethidine, clonidine
    - Serum level increased if used concomitantly with haloperidol
    - Probable plasma increase if used with cimetidine, fluoxetine, methylphenidate
    - Increases serum level of phenobarbital
  - Fluoxetine and sertraline cause increased concentrations of warfarin, phenytoin, carbamazepine, diazepam, tricyclic antidepressants, and neuroleptics

SURGERY
Neurosurgery (last resort)

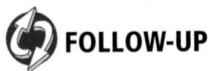

FOLLOW-UP

DISPOSITION
Outpatient care

PROGNOSIS
- Chronic waxing and waning course in majority
- 24–33% fluctuating course
- 11–14% phasic with periods of remission
- 54–61% chronic progressive course
- Early onset a poor outcome predictor

COMPLICATIONS
- Depression in 1/3 of patients with OCD
- Avoidant behavior (phobic avoidance)
  - Children may drop out of education
  - Adults may become home-bound
- Anxiety and paniclike episodes associated with obsessions

PATIENT MONITORING
- Y-BOCS
- MOCI

REFERENCES
1. Diagnostic and Statistical Manual of Mental Disorders DSM-IV (Text Revision), 4th ed. Washington, DC: American Psychiatric Association, 2000.
2. Kaplan HI, Sadock BJ, eds. Comprehensive Textbook of Psychiatry, 8th ed. Baltimore: Williams & Wilkins, 2004.
3. Jenike MA. Clinical practice: Obsessive-compulsive disorder. *N Engl J Med*. 2004;350:259–265.
4. Heyman I, Mataix D, Fineberg NA. Clinical review: Obsessive-compulsive disorder. *Br Med J*. 2006; 333:424–429.

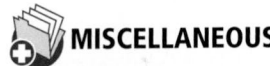 MISCELLANEOUS

See also: Anxiety, depression

 CODES

ICD9-CM
300.3 Obsessive-compulsive disorders

PATIENT TEACHING
- Obsessive-Compulsive Foundation (P.O. Box 70, Milford, CT 06460-0070; (203) 878-5669 or (203) 874-3843 for recorded information); http://www.ocfoundation.org
- Printed patient information available from Obsessive Compulsive Anonymous (P.O. Box 215, New Hyde Park, NY 11040; (516) 741-4901).

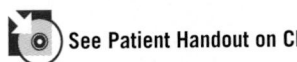 See Patient Handout on CD

O

OCULAR CHEMICAL BURNS

Nicholas Miller, MD

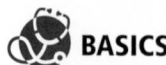 **BASICS**

DESCRIPTION

- Chemical exposure to the eye can result in rapid, devastating, and permanent damage and is one of the true emergencies in ophthalmology.
- Separate alkaline from acid chemical exposure
  - Alkaline burns: More severe—alkali penetrates and saponifies tissues easily, may produce injury to lids, conjunctiva, cornea, sclera, iris, lens, and retina
  - Acid burns: Acid usually does not damage internal structures, because protein coagulation limits acid penetration (hydrofluoric and to a lesser extent sulfurous acids are an exception to this rule). Injury often limited to lids, conjunctiva, and cornea
- System(s) Affected: Nervous; Skin/Exocrine
- Synonym(s): Chemical ocular injuries

ALERT

Geriatric Considerations

- Compromised ocular surface from keratitis sicca or other disease is associated with poorer prognosis.
- Compromised corneal endothelium or preexisting glaucoma may also complicate clinical management.

GENERAL PREVENTION

Safety glasses to safeguard uninvolved eye

EPIDEMIOLOGY

- Predominant age: Can occur at any age, peak from 16–25 years of age
- Predominant sex: Male > Female

Incidence

Estimated 300/100,000 per year

- Alkali burns twice as common as acid burns

RISK FACTORS

- Construction work (plaster, cement, whitewash)
- Use of cleaning agents (drain cleaners, ammonia)
- Automobile battery explosions (sulfuric acid)
- Industrial work (many possible agents)
- Alcoholism
- Any risk factor for assault (~10% or injuries due to deliberate assault)

PATHOPHYSIOLOGY

- Precipitation of glycosaminoglycans causes corneal opacification.
- Saponification of cell membranes causes cell death.
- Cation binding to collagen results in hydration, thickening, and shortening of collagen fibrils. This can mechanically elevate intraocular pressure.

ETIOLOGY

- Alkali
  - Ammonia (NH_3)
  - Lye (NaOH)
  - Magnesium hydroxide [$Mg(OH)_2$]
  - Potassium hydroxide (KOH)
  - Lime [$Ca(OH)_2$]
- Acids
  - Hydrochloric (HCl)
  - Hydrofluoric (HF)
  - Acetic (CH_3COOH)
  - Nitrous (HNO_2)
  - Sulfuric (H_2SO_4)
  - Sulfurous (H_2SO_3)

ASSOCIATED CONDITIONS

Facial cutaneous chemical or thermal burns

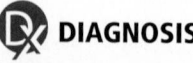 **DIAGNOSIS**

SIGNS AND SYMPTOMS

- Mild burns
  - Pain and blurred vision
  - Eyelid skin erythema and edema
  - Corneal epithelial defects or superficial punctate keratitis
  - Conjunctival chemosis, hyperemia, and hemorrhages without perilimbal ischemia
  - Mild anterior chamber reaction
- Moderate to severe burns
  - Severe pain and markedly reduced vision
  - 2nd- and 3rd-degree burns of eyelid skin
  - Corneal edema and opacification
  - Corneal epithelial defects
  - Marked conjunctival chemosis and perilimbal blanching
  - Moderate anterior chamber reaction
  - Increased intraocular pressure
  - Local necrotic retinopathy
  - In alkaline burns, can have initial pain that later diminishes

TESTS

- Measure pH of tear film with litmus paper or electronic probe (irrigating fluid with nonneutral pH [e.g., normal saline has pH of 4.5] may alter results).
- Careful slit lamp examination, fundus ophthalmoscopy, tonometry, and measurement of visual acuity
- Full extent of damage from alkaline burns may not be apparent until 48–72 hours after exposure.

Imaging

Not necessary unless suspicion of intraocular or orbital foreign body is present

DIFFERENTIAL DIAGNOSIS

- Thermal burns
- Ocular cicatricial pemphigoid
- Other causes of corneal opacification
- Ultraviolet radiation keratitis

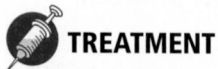 **TREATMENT**

GENERAL MEASURES

- Copious irrigation and removal of corneal or conjunctival foreign bodies are always the initial treatment. (1, 2)[A]

  - Passively open patient's eyelid and have them look in all directions while irrigating.
  - Be sure to remove all reservoirs of chemical from the eyes.
  - Continue irrigation until the tear film and superior/inferior cul-de-sac is of neutral pH and pH is stable. (2)[C]
    - Severe burns should be irrigated for at least 15 minutes to as much as 2–4 hours; this irrigation should not be interrupted during transportation to hospital. (2)[C]
    - It is impossible to overirrigate.
  - Use whatever nontoxic fluid is available for irrigation on scene. In hospital sterile water, normal saline, lactated Ringer's solution may be used.
    - Some experts suggest using higher osmolarity fluids, such as lactated Ringer's. (2)[C]
  - Sweep the conjunctival fornices every 12–24 hours to prevent adhesions. (2)[C]

Diet

Usual for patient

Activity

Ambulatory

MEDICATION (DRUGS)

First Line

- Further treatment (depending on severity and associated conditions)
  - Topical prophylactic antibiotics: Any broad-spectrum agent, e.g., bacitracin–polymyxin B (Polysporin) ointment q2–4h, ciprofloxacin (Ciloxan) drops q2–4h, chloramphenicol (Chloroptic) ointment q2–4h (1)[C]
    - Some experts suggest that systemic tetracycline derivatives (especially doxycycline) may be beneficial because studies performed in animals have shown an additional anti-inflammatory effect (by inhibiting metalloproteinases) and improved corneal healing in alkali burns. (1,2)[C]
  - Tear substitutes: Hydroxypropyl methylcellulose (HypoTears PF, Refresh Plus) drops q4h, carboxymethylcellulose (Refresh PM) ointment at bedtime. (1)[C]
    - Most beneficial in those with impaired tear production (elderly patients)
  - Cycloplegics for photophobia and/or uveitis: Cyclopentolate 1% t.i.d., or scopolamine 1/4% b.i.d. (1)[C]
  - Antiglaucoma for elevated intraocular pressure (IOP): latanoprost (Xalatan) 0.005% q24h, or timolol (Timoptic) 0.5% b.i.d., or levobunolol (Betagan) 0.5% b.i.d., and/or acetazolamide (Diamox) 125–250 mg PO q6h, or methazolamide (Neptazane) 25 to 50 mg PO b.i.d., and/or IV mannitol 20% 1 to 2 g/kg as needed. (1)[C]
  - Corticosteroids for intraocular inflammation: Prednisolone (Pred-Forte) 1% or equivalent q1–4h for 7–10 days; if severe, prednisone 20–60 mg PO daily for 5–7 days. Taper rapidly if epithelium is intact by this time. (1)[C]
    - Use of corticosteroids past 10 days may do harm by inhibiting repair. (1)[C]
  - Consider vitamin C (ascorbic acid) 500 mg PO q.i.d. and/or acetylcysteine (Mucomyst) 10–20% topically q4h if corneal melting occurs. (1)[C]
- Precautions
  - Timolol and levobunolol: History of CHF or chronic obstructive pulmonary disease
  - Acetazolamide and methazolamide: History of nephrolithiasis or metabolic acidosis
  - Mannitol: History of CHF or renal failure
  - Scopolamine: History of urinary retention
  - Topical corticosteroids must be used with caution in the presence of damaged corneal epithelium, because iatrogenic infection can occur. Daily follow-up or consultation with an ophthalmologist is recommended.
- Significant possible interactions: Refer to manufacturer's literature for each drug.

Second Line

Where available, topical fibronectin, epidermal growth factor, prokinase inhibitors. (1)[C]

SURGERY

- Débridement of necrotic tissue (1)[C]
- Conjunctival/Tenon's advancement (tenoplasty) to restore vascularity in severe burns (1)[C]
- Tissue adhesive (e.g., isobutyl cyanoacrylate) for impending or actual corneal perforation of <1 mm (1)[C]
  - Tectonic keratoplasty for acute perforation >1 mm (1)[C]
- Limbal autograft transplantation for epithelial stem cell restoration (1)[C]
- Conjunctival or mucosal membrane transplant to restore ocular surface in severe injury (1)[C]
- Lamellar or penetrating keratoplasty for tectonic stabilization or visual rehabilitation (1)[C]

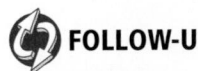 **FOLLOW-UP**

DISPOSITION

Emergency department evaluation with inpatient admission and ophthalmology consultation, depending on severity

Issues for Referral

See "Medication, Drugs."

PROGNOSIS

- Depends on severity of initial injury
- Increasing amounts of limbal ischemia and corneal opacification correlate with poorer prognosis.
- For mildly injured eyes, complete recovery is the norm.
- For severely injured eyes, permanent loss of vision is not uncommon.
- Autologous cultivated corneal epithelium has been used for long-term restoration of vision.
- Autologous nasal mucosal transplantation also has been employed successfully.

COMPLICATIONS

- Persistent epitheliopathy
- Fibrovascular pannus
- Corneal ulcer/perforation
- Progressive symblepharon and entropion
- Neurotrophic keratitis
- Glaucoma
- Cataract
- Hypotony
- Phthisis bulbi
- Blindness

PATIENT MONITORING

- Depending on severity of ocular injury
  - From daily to weekly visits initially
- May be inpatient
- If on mannitol or prednisone, consider frequent serum electrolytes

REFERENCES

1. Wagoner MD. Chemical injuries of the eye: Current concepts in pathophysiology and therapy. *Survey Ophthalmol* 1997;41:275–313.
2. Kuckelkorn R, Schrage N, Keller G, Redbrake C. Emergency treatment of chemical and thermal eye burns. *Acta Ophthalmol Scand* 2002;80:4–10.

 MISCELLANEOUS

See also: Burns

 CODES

ICD9-CM

- 940.2 Alkaline chemical burn of cornea and conjunctival sac
- 940.3 Acid chemical burn of cornea and conjunctival sac

PATIENT TEACHING

- Safety glasses
- Need for immediate ocular irrigation with any available water following chemical exposure to the eyes

O

ONYCHOMYCOSIS

Konstantinos Deligiannidis, MD, MPH
Stephen T. Earls, MD

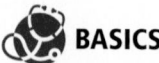 **BASICS**

DESCRIPTION
- Infection of nail by fungi (mostly dermatophytes; also *Candida*, molds)
- System Affected: Skin/Exocrine
- Synonym(s): Tinea unguium; Ringworm of the nail

EPIDEMIOLOGY
- Predominant age: Dermatophytes common in adults; molds in older adults
- Predominant sex: Candidal: Adult women

Prevalence
In US, 22–130 cases per 1,000

ALERT
Geriatric Considerations
Mold onychomycosis more common

Pediatric Considerations
Rare before puberty

RISK FACTORS
- Dermatophytes
  - Warmth, moisture, hyperhidrosis
  - Tight-fitting shoes, rubber shoes
  - Peripheral vascular disease
  - Immunodeficiency
  - Indirect contamination
- Candidal
  - Direct contamination: Anovular, perirectal pruritus
  - Chemical or mechanical damage to cuticle
  - Maceration or occlusion
  - Contact with substances containing sugar
  - Hyperhidrosis
  - Chilblain
  - Cold hands (Raynaud phenomenon)
  - Psoriatic onycholysis
  - Diabetes mellitus
  - Hyperparathyroidism
  - Addison disease
  - Malnutrition
  - Malabsorption
  - Dyscrasias
  - Malignancies
  - Postoperative conditions
  - Immunodeficiency
- Molds
  - Soil contamination
  - Peripheral vascular disease
  - Overlapping toes
  - Onychogryphosis (deforming overgrowth of nails resulting in hooked or curved state)

Geriatric Considerations
- Predisposing diseases are more common.
- Hepatic/renal reserve is limited.

ETIOLOGY
- Dermatophytes (invade normal keratin)
  - *Trichophyton rubrum:* Most common
  - *Trichophyton mentagrophytes* var. interdigitale: 25% as common as *T. rubrum* (most common pathogen for white superficial onychomycosis)
  - *Epidermophyton floccosum, Trichophyton violaceum, Microsporum* species less common

- *Candida*
  - *C. albicans*, 70%
  - *C. parapsilosis, C. tropicalis, C. krusei* (less common)
- Molds (invade altered keratin): *Scopulariopsis brevicaulis, Hendersonula toruloidea, Aspergillus* species, *Alternaria tenuis, Cephalosporium, Scytalidium hyalinum*

ASSOCIATED CONDITIONS
Immunodeficiency or chronic metabolic disease

 DIAGNOSIS

SIGNS AND SYMPTOMS
- Dermatophytes: Commonly preceded by dermatophyte infection at another site; 80% involve toenails, especially hallux; simultaneous infection of fingernails and toenails rare. Four clinical forms occur
  - Distal subungual onychomycosis: Spreads from hyponychium to nail bed to nail plate; subungual hyperkeratosis; subungual paronychia; onycholysis; nail dystrophy; discoloration—yellow-brown; bois vermoulu ("worm-eaten wood"); onychomadesis
  - Lateral onychomycosis (common): Yellowish discoloration of lateral nail groove; onycholysis, proximal or distal
  - Proximal onychomycosis (rare): Hands or feet; leukonychia—begins under posterior nail groove, spreading to nail plate and lunula; seen with immunodeficiency
  - White superficial onychomycosis (rare): Hallux preferentially affected; infection of upper part of nail plate; opaque white spots on nail plate eventually merge to involve entire surface of the nail
- Candidal
  - Hands, 70%, especially dominant hand
  - Middle finger most common
  - Pain mild, unless secondarily infected
  - Increases on prolonged contact with water
  - Primarily affects tissue surrounding nail
  - Begins with cuticle detachment
  - Dark yellowish to blackish-brown zone along lateral border of nail
  - Secondary ungual changes: Convex, irregular, striated nail plate with dull, rough surface
  - Onycholysis, especially on hands
  - Distal subungual onychomycosis may occur
  - Primary involvement of the nail plate is uncommon (thin, crumbly, opaque, brownish nail plate deformed by transverse grooves).
  - Periungual edema/erythema may occur (club-shaped, bulbous fingertips).
  - Superficial white onychomycosis: Young children
- Molds
  - More common in those age >60 years
  - More common in nails of hallux
  - Resembles distal and lateral onychomycosis

ALERT
Pediatric Considerations
Candidal infection presents more commonly as superficial white onychomycosis

TESTS
Lab
- Potassium hydroxide (KOH) preparation
  - Clip or file away some of nail plate as needed.
  - Collect scales from stratum corneum of most proximal area (beneath nail or crumbling nail itself) with 1 mm curette.
  - KOH (5%) plus gentle heat
  - 100% sensitive if >2 preparations examined
- Cultures: Negative in 30% (secondary to loss of dermatophyte viability; improved by immediate culture on Sabouraud cell culture media)
- Histologic examination; punch biopsy: Proximal lesions with periodic acid-Schiff stain
- Discontinue all topical medication several days before obtaining sample.

Pathological Findings
Pathogens within the nail keratin

DIFFERENTIAL DIAGNOSIS
- Herpetic whitlow
- Eczema
- Pustular psoriasis
- Tumor
- Darier disease
- Pityriasis rubra pilaris
- Trophic changes, peripheral vascular disease
- Immunodeficiency
- Drugs; chemicals
- Trauma
- Alopecia areata
- Lichen planus
- Yellow nail syndrome (icterus, carotenemia, lymphedema, amyloidosis)
- White acquired nail disease (trauma, acute infection, chronic disease, thallium or arsenic poisoning, hepatic cirrhosis, chronic hypoalbuminemia)
- Brown-black pigment (melanotic, hematoma)
- Green dyschromia (*Pseudomonas aeruginosa;* molds, e.g., *Penicillium*)
- Connective tissue disorders: Dermatomyositis, scleroderma, Reiter disease

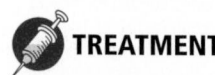 **TREATMENT**

INITIAL STABILIZATION
Outpatient treatment unless secondary cellulitis/osteomyelitis

GENERAL MEASURES
- Avoid factors that promote fungal growth (heat, moisture).
- Treat underlying disease risk factors.
- Treat secondary infections.

Diet
No special diet

Activity
Restrictions based on promoting factors, underlying disease, or secondary infection

MEDICATION (DRUGS)

First Line

- Dermatophytes—local: Cheaper, but less effective than systemic; apply under occlusive dressing; may mix with keratinolytic chemicals
  - Allylamines: Terbinafine (Lamisil), Naftifine (Naftin); may be slightly more effective, but are more expensive than imidazoles. Recommended if imidazoles or undecylenic acid are not working. (1)[B]
  - Imidazoles: Clotrimazole (Lotrimin, Mycelex), miconazole (Monistat), butoconazole, tioconazole, econazole (Spectazole), ketoconazole (Nizoral), sulconazole (Exelderm), oxiconazole (Oxistat); should be tried before allylamines for topical treatment. (1)[B]
  - Unsaturated fatty acid derivatives: Propionic acid, undecylenic acid, tolnaftate (Tinactin); should be tried before allylamines for topical treatment. (1)[B]
- Dermatophytes—systemic
  - Terbinafine (Lamisil): 250 mg PO daily for 3 months; fewer drug–drug interactions, and fewer contraindications than imidazoles; terbinafine may be slightly more effective than itraconazole. (2,3)[A]
  - Itraconazole (Sporanox): 200 mg PO 2 times a week for 1 week per month for 2 months for fingernails and 3–4 months for toenails (pulse therapy)
  - Fluconazole (Diflucan): 300 mg PO weekly for 6 months (pulse therapy); overall, better tolerated than ketoconazole; expensive; reserve for extreme cases (disseminated disease, immunocompromised patient)
- *Candida*
  - Imidazole derivative
  - If bacterial infection is present, use antibacterial plus anticandidal; for example, nystatin (Mycostatin), topical amphotericin B (Fungizone), or itraconazole (Sporanox) 200 mg PO daily for 3 months, or fluconazole 300 mg PO weekly for 6 months
- Mold: 1% iodinated alcohol, benzoic acid (Whitfield ointment), silver nitrate, glutaraldehyde, imidazole derivatives, itraconazole
- Contraindications
  - Griseofulvin: Porphyria, hepatocellular failure, serious side effects (leukopenia, persistent anemia), pregnancy
  - Ketoconazole: Hepatocellular disease, pregnancy
  - Fluconazole: Hepatocellular failure, pregnancy
- Precautions
  - Topical agents: Use with caution on broken skin or in vascular compromise or decreased sensation.
  - Griseofulvin: Monitor for hepatic, renal, hematopoietic side effects; photosensitivity; lupuslike symptoms; or exacerbation. Take with meals to enhance absorption.
  - Ketoconazole: Hepatotoxicity (may be severe or fatal); anaphylaxis may (rarely) occur with 1st dose; decreased testosterone levels
  - Fluconazole: Decrease dose in renal failure, hepatotoxicity.
- Significant possible interactions
  - Griseofulvin: Warfarin, barbiturates, alcohol, oral contraceptives
  - Ketoconazole: Warfarin, rifampin, cyclosporine, phenytoin, terfenadine

- Fluconazole: Phenytoin (Dilantin), cyclosporine, oral hypoglycemics, oral anticoagulants, rifampin, hydrochlorothiazide
- Itraconazole and ketoconazole require gastric acid for absorption; effectiveness reduced with antacids, H₂ blockers, and proton-pump inhibitors.
- Drug choices are limited in pregnancy.

Second Line

- Dermatophytes—local
  - Ciclopirox (Loprox, Penlac): 8% topical lacquer for patients without lunula involvement
  - Amorolfine (Loceryl): 5% lacquer
  - Butenafine with tea tree oil
  - Cationic surfactants, for example, benzalkonium chloride (Cetylcide), cetrimide, cetylpyridinium chloride (Ony-Clear, Fungoid)
  - Halogenated/chlorinated/iodinated derivatives (chloramine, tincture of iodine)
  - Dyes (malachite green, crystal violet)
  - Mercury derivatives (thimerosal)
  - Phenols
  - Glutaraldehyde

- Dermatophytes—systemic: Griseofulvin (Fulvicin, Gris-PEG, Grisactin) ultramicrosize; usual adult dose is 250–500 mg b.i.d. with meals for 6–12 months; however, terbinafine 250 mg PO daily was statistically significantly more effective for 4–6 weeks. (3)[A]

ALERT

Geriatric Considerations

Decreased ability for topical self-treatment

SURGERY

Nail removal to remove infected keratin

- Mechanical: Soften with occlusive dressing with 40% urea gel; detach from nail bed with tweezers or file with abrasive stone.
- Chemical: Protect peripheral tissue with adhesive strips; apply ointment of 30% salicylic acid, 40% urea, or 50% potassium iodide under occlusive dressing.
- Surgical avulsion: For involvement of a few nails

 FOLLOW-UP

PROGNOSIS

- Relapse is common; prognosis is poor if 1 hand, 2 feet, or multiple nails are involved.
- 20–40% of nails fail to respond.
- 40–70% of patients show long-term relapse.

COMPLICATIONS

Secondary infections with progression to cellulitis/osteomyelitis

PATIENT MONITORING

- Topical agents: Slow response expected; visits every 6–12 weeks
- Griseofulvin: CBC and liver function tests initially, then every 3 months
- Ketoconazole: Liver function tests every 3 weeks for the 1st 3 months, then monthly
- Itraconazole and fluconazole: Liver function tests at start and at 4 weeks
- Terbinafine: Liver function and hematologic tests at start and at 4 weeks
- Treatment duration (months): Fingernails (6–9), toenails (9–12), great toenail (12–24)

REFERENCES

1. Crawford F, Hart R, Bell-Syer S, Torgerson D, et al. Topical treatments for fungal infections of the skin and nails of the foot. [Systematic Review] Cochrane Skin Group. *Cochrane Database of Systematic Reviews.* 1, 2006.
2. De Keyser P, De Backer M, Massart DL, Westerlinck KJ. Two week oral treatment of tinea pedis, comparing terbinafine (250mg/day) with itraconazole (100mg/day): A double blind multicentre study. *Br J Dermatol.* 1994;130(Suppl 43):22–25.
3. Bell-Syer SEM, Hart R, Crawford F, et al. Oral treatments for fungal infections of the skin of the foot. [Systematic Review] Cochrane Skin Group. *Cochrane Database of Systematic Reviews.* 1, 2006.

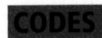 **MISCELLANEOUS**

- Definitions
  - Onycholysis: Detachment of nail plate from nail bed
  - Dystrophy: Thickening, deformation, crumbling
  - Onychomadesis: Shedding of nail
  - Leukonychia: Yellowish white spots
- See also: HIV infection and AIDS

CODES

ICD9-CM

- 110.1 Dermatophytosis of nail
- 112.3 Candidiasis of skin and nails

PATIENT TEACHING

Advise patient to

- Keep affected area clean and dry.
- Avoid rubber or other occlusive footwear.
- Avoid tight or ill-fitting footwear.
- Wear absorbent cotton socks; avoid wool or synthetic fibers.
- Change clothing and towels frequently and launder them in hot water.

 See Corresponding Diagnostic Algorithm

 See Patient Handout on CD

O

OPTIC ATROPHY

Tyeese Gaines-Reid, DO, MA

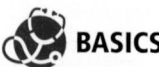 BASICS

DESCRIPTION
- The loss of the ganglion cell axons that form the optic nerve
- Primary optic atrophies (genetic defect)
  - Leber hereditary optic neuropathy
  - Autosomal dominant optic atrophy with and without cataracts
  - Autosomal recessive atrophies (rare)
- Primary optic atrophies accompanied by neurologic symptoms
- Secondary (metabolic) optic atrophies
- Mitochondrial disorders
- Peroxisomal disorders
  - Lysosomal storage diseases (Tay-Sachs, Niemann-Pick, mucopolysaccharide diseases)
  - Other (amino acid metabolism disorders, hereditary ataxias)
  - System(s) Affected: Nervous, Metabolic
  - Synonym(s): Leber hereditary optic neuropathy; Optic neuropathy

ALERT
Pediatric Considerations
Optic atrophy in small children is difficult to recognize because disks normally have a pale appearance.

GENERAL PREVENTION
Regular ophthalmologic exam in high-risk groups

EPIDEMIOLOGY
- Predominant age: Inherited forms occur from shortly after birth to the 3rd decade; acquired forms tend to occur later.
- Predominant sex: Male > Female (inherited forms)
- Leber hereditary optic neuropathy: Predominately 20–30-year-old males (1)

Incidence
Unknown

Prevalence
Unknown

RISK FACTORS
- Hereditary
  - Family history of visual loss
  - Inborn errors of metabolism
- Acquired
  - Diabetes mellitus
  - Hypertension
  - Radiation exposure
  - Alcoholism
  - Renal failure
  - Arteriosclerosis

Genetics
- Inherited forms may be autosomally recessive, autosomally dominant, or X-linked recessive. (2)[C]
- Several studies show a mitochondrial link. (3)[C]

ETIOLOGY
- Compression of the nerve
  - Glaucoma
    - Chronic papilledema
    - Tumor
    - Aneurysm
  - Hydrocephalus
- Inflammation
  - Graves disease
- Chronic optic neuritis
- Trauma
- Syphilis
- Ischemic optic neuropathy
- Central retinal artery or vein occlusion
- Retinal degeneration
- Congenital optic atrophy
  - Possibly due to lack of oxygen during pregnancy, labor, or early days life
- Radiation neuropathy
- Drugs
  - Amiodarone
  - Chloroquine
  - Ethambutol
  - Oral contraceptives
  - Streptomycin
  - Vincristine
- Nutritional deficiencies
  - Vitamin B_{12}
  - Folic acid
  - Thiamine
- Demyelinating disorders
- Toxins/poisons
  - Cyanide
  - Lead
  - Methanol

ASSOCIATED CONDITIONS
- Inherited neurodegenerative conditions
  - Hereditary ataxia
  - Charcot-Marie-Tooth disease
  - Storage diseases
  - Leukodystrophies
- Multiple sclerosis
- Menkes syndrome

DIAGNOSIS

SIGNS AND SYMPTOMS
- Painless loss of visual acuity
  - Can be simultaneously bilateral or sequential
  - In primary optic atrophies, often the only clinical feature
- Abnormalities in color vision and contrast sensitivity
- Pallor of the optic disk
- Loss of pupillary reactions
- Visual field defects

History
- Family history of visual loss
- Congenital disorders

Physical Exam
Funduscopic exam
- Small pale optic disk is classic
- Enlarged peripapillary atrophy if glaucoma is the cause (4)[B]
- Unilateral disk swelling points toward nerve compression

TESTS
- Automated visual field test (e.g., Humphrey)
- Color vision testing
- Visual evoked potentials
- Fluorescein angiography

Lab
- CBC
- Electrolytes
- Antinuclear antibody test (ANA)
- ESR
- Fluorescent treponemal antibody absorption test (FTA-ABS)
- Serologic test for syphilis
- Heavy-metal screen
- Genetic testing if high suspicion for Leber hereditary optic neuropathy

Imaging
CT or MRI of head

Diagnostic Procedures/Surgery
- Carotid Doppler (adult-acquired optic atrophy)
- Complete ophthalmologic exam including dilated evaluation of retina

DIFFERENTIAL DIAGNOSIS
- Myopia
- Postoperative cataract extraction (no natural yellow color from the human lens)

TREATMENT

GENERAL MEASURES

- Optic nerve damage is usually permanent, so early detection is best. (2)[C]
- Treat the underlying cause.
- Correction of an underlying nutritional deficiency or discontinuation of the causative drug may halt progression.
- Optic nerve pressure may be relieved by neurosurgery.

Diet
No special diet

Activity
No restriction

 MEDICATION (DRUGS)

First Line
None

Second Line

- Corticosteroids may briefly improve vision acuity when optic neuritis present.
- Long-term benefits are unproven.

 FOLLOW-UP

DISPOSITION
Outpatient care

PROGNOSIS

- Visual loss occurs over weeks to months.
- Correction of an underlying nutritional deficiency or discontinuation of the causative drug may halt progression.

PATIENT MONITORING
Annual evaluations if stable

REFERENCES

1. Teive HAG, Troiano AR, Raskin S, et al. *Sao Paulo Med J*. 2004;122(6):
2. Huizing M, Brooks BP, Anikster Y, et al. Optic atrophies in metabolic disorders. *Mol Genet Metabol*. 2005;86:51–60.
3. Howell N. LHON and other optic nerve atrophies: The mitochondrial connection. *Dev Ophthalmol*. 2003;37:94–108.
4. Jonas JB. Clinical implications of peripapillary atrophy in glaucoma. *Curr Opin Ophthalmol*. 2005;16(2):84–88.

ADDITIONAL READING

University of Michigan Kellogg Eye Center
www.kellogg.umich.edu

 MISCELLANEOUS

CODES

ICD9-CM
377.10 Optic atrophy, unspecified

PATIENT TEACHING

- Low-vision counseling
- Genetic counseling if inherited
- Glaucoma education
- For patient education materials favorably reviewed on this topic, contact the National Eye Institute, Information Officer, Department of Health and Human Services, 9000 Rockville Pike, Bethesda, MD 20892; (301) 496-5248
- American Council of the Blind, (800) 424-8666

 See Corresponding Diagnostic Algorithm

OPTIC NEURITIS

Brian D. Petroni, MD

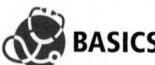

BASICS

DESCRIPTION
- Primary inflammation of the optic nerve
- Most common form is acute demyelinating optic neuritis, but can also be associated with a variety of systemic autoimmune disorders.
- Optic disc may either be spared (retrobulbar optic neuritis) (70%) or swollen (papillitis) (30%).
- Key features
  - Abrupt visual loss
  - Periorbital pain (90%)
  - Dyschromatopsia
  - Afferent pupillary defect
- Usually unilateral in adults; bilateral disease more common in children
- System(s) Affected: Nervous
- Synonym(s): Papillitis; Retrobulbar neuritis

GENERAL PREVENTION
Prevention of viral upper respiratory infections

EPIDEMIOLOGY
- More common in northern latitudes
- Predominant age: Typically 20–50 years
- Predominant sex: Female > Male

Incidence
One to 5 per 100,000 per year

Prevalence
Twenty to 100 per 100,000

PATHOPHYSIOLOGY
Primary idiopathic inflammatory demyelination of the optic nerve

ETIOLOGY
- Idiopathic
- Multiple sclerosis (MS)
- Viral infections of childhood (measles, mumps, chickenpox, coxsackie)
- Other viral infections (adenovirus, herpes zoster, hepatitis A, CMV, HIV_1)
- Bacterial infections (syphilis, tuberculosis, meningococcus, strep B, Bartonella, Lyme disease)
- Contiguous inflammation of the meninges, orbit, or sinuses
- Intraocular inflammations
- Lead toxicity
- Chronic high-dose chloramphenicol
- Posterior uveitis
- Vascular lesions of optic nerve
- Tumors
- Fungal infections

ASSOCIATED CONDITIONS
- MS (common)
- Devic disease (neuromyelitis optica)

DIAGNOSIS

SIGNS AND SYMPTOMS
- Decreased visual acuity, deteriorating in hours to days, usually reaching lowest level in 1 week
- Tenderness of the globe, deep orbital pain or brow ache, especially with eye movement due to traction of superior and medial recti on optic nerve sheath
- Retro-orbital pain may precede visual loss
- Central, cecocentral, or arcuate visual field deficits
- Decreased color vision (dull or faded colors)
- Apparent dimness of light intensities
- Impairment of depth perception (80%), worse with moving objects (Pulfrich phenomenon)
- Transient increase in visual symptoms with increased body temperature and exercise (Uhthoff phenomenon)

Physical Exam
- Funduscopic exam often normal (60%), but may show papillitis (20%) or peripheral hemorrhage (20–40%)
- Relative afferent pupillary defect (Marcus Gunn pupil), unless disease is bilateral

TESTS
- Visual acuity
- Visual fields (preferably automated Humphrey or octopus)
  - Central scotoma classic, but loss varies and may be either diffuse or focal
  - 70% of patients also have defects in contralateral eye.
- Color vision testing
- Contrast sensitivity

ALERT
Pediatric Considerations
Optic disk swelling and bilateral disease are more common in children, as is severe loss of visual acuity (20/200 or worse).

Lab
- CSF analysis
- CBC
- Antinuclear antibody (ANA) test
- ESR
- Rapid plasma reagin (RPR) test
- Fluorescent treponemal antibody absorption (FTA-ABS) test
- Serologic test for syphilis

Imaging
- Brain MRI for detection of possible MS lesions
- Chest radiograph to rule out sarcoid
- MRI of orbits with Gd shows enlargement and enhancement of optic nerve.

Diagnostic Procedures/Surgery
- Complete ophthalmologic exam including pupillary assessment, color vision evaluation with color plates, dilated retinal examination with optic nerve assessment
- Full neurologic exam
- Check BP
- Lumbar puncture (to rule out MS)
- Patients with atypical features of optic neuritis (absence of orbital pain, failure to recover vision within 1 month, severe papillitis) should undergo a more aggressive workup including serologies and orbital MRI.

DIFFERENTIAL DIAGNOSIS
- Demyelinating disease (especially MS)
- Acute papilledema
- Anterior ischemic optic neuropathy (AION)
- Toxic/nutritional optic neuropathy
- Orbital tumor compressing the optic nerve
- Intracranial tumor pressing on the afferent visual pathway
- Leber hereditary optic neuropathy (LHON)
- Temporal arteritis and other vasculitides
- Inflammation or infection contiguous with optic nerve

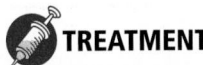

TREATMENT

GENERAL MEASURES
Referral to an ophthalmologist

Diet
As tolerated

Activity
As tolerated

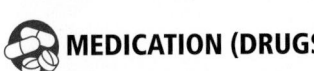

MEDICATION (DRUGS)

First Line
For significant vision loss, corticosteroids may be indicated. These should be administered in conjunction with a neurology consult.

Second Line
- Pulse steroids
  - IV methylprednisolone 250 mg q6h for 12 doses in the hospital followed by prednisone 1 mg/kg/d PO for 11 days, taper over 1–2 weeks.
  - IV methylprednisolone hastens recovery of visual function, but does not affect long-term visual outcome.
- Antiulcer medication is given with steroids.

ALERT
Oral prednisone alone may increase the risk for recurrent optic neuritis and should be avoided.

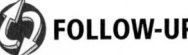

FOLLOW-UP

PROGNOSIS
- Orbital pain resolves within 1 week
- Visual acuity
  - Begins to improve 2–3 weeks after onset, and this continues for several months.
  - Often returns to normal or near-normal levels (20/40 or better) within 1 year (90–95%).
  - Complete recovery common, even after near blindness.
- Other visual disturbances (e.g., contrast sensitivity, stereopsis) often persist after acuity returns to normal.
- Recurrence risk of 35% within 10 years
  - 14% in affected eye
  - 12% in contralateral eye
  - 9% bilaterally
  - Twice as high in MS patients (48% vs. 24%)
- Patients with poor vision who receive IV steroids often recover faster.
- When baseline vision is good, IV steroids have no beneficial effect.
- Children with bilateral visual loss have better prognosis than adults.
- Poor prognostic factors
  - Absence of pain
  - Low initial visual acuity
  - Involvement of intracanalicular optic nerve
- >50% of adult patients with optic neuritis will eventually develop MS.

COMPLICATIONS
Permanent loss of vision

PATIENT MONITORING
Monthly follow-up to monitor visual changes

REFERENCES

1. Balcer LJ. Optic Neuritis. *N Engl J Med*. 2006; 354:1273–1280.
2. Jacobs DA, Galetta SL. Multiple Sclerosis and the visual system. *Ophthalmol Clin N Am* 2004; 17(3):265–273, v.
3. Lee AG, Brazis PW. Systemic infections of neuro-ophthalmologic significance. *Ophthalmol Clin N Am*. 2004;17(3):397–425, vii.

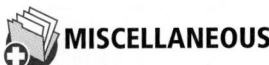

MISCELLANEOUS

See also: Multiple sclerosis

CODES

ICD9-CM
377.30 Optic neuritis, unspecified

PATIENT TEACHING
- Provide reassurance about recovery of vision.
- If the disease is believed to be secondary to demyelinating disease, patient should be informed of the risk of developing MS.
- For patient education materials favorably reviewed on this topic, contact the National Eye Institute, Information Officer, Department of Health and Human Services (9000 Rockville Pike, Bethesda, MD 20892; 301-496-5248).

See Corresponding Diagnostic Algorithm

ORAL CAVITY NEOPLASMS

Roy R. Casiano, MD

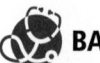 **BASICS**

DESCRIPTION

- Malignant tumors affecting the lip, tongue, floor of the mouth, salivary glands, inside of cheeks, gums, and palate
- System(s) Affected: Gastrointestinal

GENERAL PREVENTION

- Avoid smoking or the use of smokeless tobacco.
- Avoid alcohol use.

EPIDEMIOLOGY

- Predominant age: >50 years, now being seen increasingly in younger age groups with the use of smokeless tobacco
- Predominant sex: Male > Female

Incidence

- 12/100,000 (30,300 new cases a year)
- 5,000 persons die of this disease annually.
- High incidence in Asia, related to the habit of chewing betel nut, fresh betel leaf, and habitual reverse smoking (lighted end held within the oral cavity)

ALERT

Geriatric Considerations

Greater incidence >50 years of age

Prevalence

Oral cavity neoplasms account for 4% of all cancers occurring in men and 2% in women.

PATHOPHYSIOLOGY

Of neoplasms 90% are squamous cell carcinomas; the others are lymphomas, melanomas, and adenocarcinomas from minor salivary gland origin, and sarcomas

ETIOLOGY

- Use of tobacco (smokeless or smoked)
- Use of snuff
- Excessive alcohol consumption
- Exposure to ultraviolet light in the instances of lip carcinoma
- Riboflavin or iron deficiency anemia, and Plummer-Vinson syndrome associated with oral cancers
- Betel nut or betel leaf chewing

ASSOCIATED CONDITIONS

Leukoplakias or erythroplasias should be biopsied because they are considered premalignant and are associated with carcinoma at least 10% of the time.

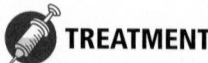 **DIAGNOSIS**

SIGNS AND SYMPTOMS

- Dysphagia
- Odynophagia
- Problems articulating
- Regurgitation of liquids secondary to nasopharyngeal incompetence from the tumor
- Ipsilateral otalgia from referred pain
- Friable granular exophytic and/or infiltrative mass or ulcer that frequently is tender and confused with infection
  - Usually has hard, indurated margins by palpation that extend beyond the confines of the ulcer itself
- Hard neck mass suggesting metastatic disease in the nodal chain along the internal jugular vein

TESTS

Lab

- Liver function tests to rule out metastasis to the liver
- Disorders that may alter lab results
  - Alcoholism
  - Hepatitis

Imaging

- Chest radiograph to rule out metastasis to the lungs
- Imaging bone scans if there is pain in the bones suggesting bone metastasis
- CT or MRI if clinical suggestion of intracranial or liver metastasis

Diagnostic Procedures/Surgery

Transoral biopsy as an outpatient makes the definitive diagnosis.

Pathological Findings

Malignant changes characteristic of cell types

DIFFERENTIAL DIAGNOSIS

- Exudative tonsillitis (usually bilateral involvement)
- Stomatitis or glossitis secondary to infectious etiology, most commonly candidiasis
- Benign tumors of the oral cavity (slow growing and usually not erosive or ulcerative)
- Kaposi sarcoma
- Mycosis fungoides
- Premalignant lesions such as leukoplakia or erythroplasia
- Lichen planus

 TREATMENT

GENERAL MEASURES

- Treatment varies depending on location (e.g., tongue, buccal wall, pharynx, palate, lip).
- Unresectable lesions usually are treated with radiation therapy and/or chemotherapy for palliation.

Diet

- Depends on the extent of disease and whether the patient is able to chew or swallow
- Usually early lesions can be managed with a regular diet. As disease progresses, a soft diet is necessary.
- Nutrition is of prime importance for normal wound healing, should patient require surgery. Patients may need nasogastric and/or gastrostomy feedings if they are orally disabled.

Activity

As tolerated by patient's nutritional and physical status

MEDICATION (DRUGS)

Narcotics for pain relief

SURGERY

- Wide resection with or without radiation therapy and/or chemotherapy is the treatment of choice.
- Tracheotomy may be necessary if the patient has problems handling secretions or difficulty breathing.

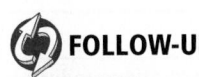 **FOLLOW-UP**

DISPOSITION
Inpatient for surgery

PROGNOSIS
Early lesions with adequate treatment leads to a >80% cure.

COMPLICATIONS
- Functional and/or cosmetic disabilities proportional to the degree of surgery and stage of tumor
- Stomatitis with or without candidiasis secondary to radiation therapy or chemotherapy
- Persistent dysphagia secondary to surgery or radiation therapy
- Persistent problems with articulation or deglutition depending on the amount of tongue resection

PATIENT MONITORING
Routine periodic head and neck exams to detect possible 2nd primary or recurrence in the upper respiratory and digestive tract

REFERENCES
1. Cumming CW, et al., eds. *Otolaryngology Head and Neck Surgery*, Vol. 2. New York, NY: Mosby; 1998.

 MISCELLANEOUS

CODES

ICD9-CM
- 145.9 Malignant neoplasm of mouth, unspecified
- 198.89 Secondary malignant neoplasm of other specified sites, other
- 210.4 Benign neoplasm of other and unspecified parts of mouth
- 230.0 Carcinoma in situ of lip, oral cavity, and pharynx
- 235.1 Neoplasm of uncertain behavior of lip, oral cavity, and pharynx

PATIENT TEACHING
Literature is available from the American Cancer Society.

O

ORAL REHYDRATION

William A. Primack, MD

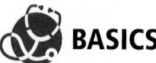 **BASICS**

DESCRIPTION

- Dehydration and ongoing fluid losses from infectious gastroenteritis (GE) can be treated effectively with oral rehydration solutions (ORSs) except in the most severe cases, in which initial parenteral fluid resuscitation is required. (1,4)[B],(2,3)[A]
- ORSs for rehydration should have a sodium content of about 75 mEq/L (75 mmol/L). Maintenance ORSs, with a sodium content of 40–50 mEq/L (40–50 mmol/L), are useful for repair of mild dehydration and treatment of ongoing losses with relatively low sodium content (e.g., rotavirus). (1)[B]
- High-sodium diarrheal losses such as occur with cholera may require higher-sodium-content ORSs (World Health Organization [WHO] solution = 90 mEq/L [90 mmol/L] Na). In 2002, WHO reduced the sodium content of its ORS from 90 mEq/L to 75 mEq/L, and in 2003, the Centers for Disease Control and Prevention (CDC) endorsed this approach. (2)[A]

- System(s) Affected: Endocrine/Metabolic; Gastrointestinal

EPIDEMIOLOGY
- Predominant age: Primarily infants and children Effective for all ages
- Predominant sex: Male = Female

PATHOPHYSIOLOGY
This therapy takes advantage of the coupled transport of sodium and glucose in the small intestine even during a course of GE. Water follows osmotically after sodium entry. Potassium is passively absorbed via solvent drag. A glucose concentration of 2% allows maximal sodium absorption.

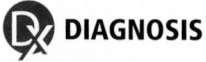 **DIAGNOSIS**

SIGNS AND SYMPTOMS
- Frequency and volume of urination
- Constipation
- Vomiting
- Fever
- Weight loss
- Travel
- Exposure to others with GE
- Recent antibiotic use

Physical Exam
- Level of consciousness
- Capillary refill (abnormal if >2 seconds)
- Mucous membranes: Dry, cracked
- Tears: Decreased
- Heart rate: Increased
- Respiratory rate: Increased
- BP: Orthostasis
- Pulse: Faint
- Skin turgor: Tenting
- Eyes: Sunken
- Urine output: Decreased

TESTS
Lab
If moderate to severe, obtain sodium, potassium, bicarbonate, chloride, glucose, BUN, creatinine

---

TREATMENT

GENERAL MEASURES
- In developed countries, most diarrheal losses are low sodium. Consequently, maintenance ORSs can be used for rehydration.
- Estimate replacement at 60 mL/kg for mild dehydration and 80–100 mL/kg for moderate dehydration over the 1st 4–8 hours.
  - Very important to replace any ongoing losses and add maintenance fluids.
- Replace ongoing stool losses with an ORS. In infant, estimate 5–10 mL/kg per stool or weigh diapers.
- Add maintenance requirements to replacement
  - Estimate
    ○ 0–10 kg: 4 mL/kg/h
    ○ Plus 10–20 kg: 2 mL/kg/h
    ○ Plus >20 kg: 1 mL/kg/h
  - Use a maintenance ORS.
  - Traditional clear fluids (e.g., fruit juice, soda) are inappropriate for oral rehydration therapy.
- If the patient has hypertonic dehydration, oral rehydration should be planned for 12–24 hours.
- If vomiting occurs, small amounts of ORS given frequently are usually effective.
- If the patient is not vomiting and is alert, the patient's thirst is an excellent indicator of fluid needs.
- ORS is not to be diluted
- A maintenance oral rehydration therapy begins when the deficit is replaced and provides for ongoing losses
  - Maintenance ORS or a combination of ORS and water or other clear liquids can be used.
- Effective at all ages
  - If child refuses because of taste, flavor with a commercial artificially sweetened flavoring such as Nutrasweet flavored Kool-Aid and use ~1/4 tsp to 4 oz ORS.
  - Prepackaged, ORS-flavored freeze pops (often well accepted)
- If necessary, rehydration by nasogastric tube is appropriate
- Begin feeding as soon as rehydration is achieved.

Diet
- For breast-feeding infants, mother should continue nursing.
- For bottle-fed babies, early institution of formulas. Lactose-free formulas rarely are required.
- Age appropriate
  - Complex carbohydrate-rich (e.g., rice, bread, potato, cereal), low-fat foods should be offered as soon as the dehydration deficit is replaced.
  - Cow's milk can be added to diet after several days.

Activity
As tolerated

SPECIAL THERAPY
IV Fluids
To be used for initial resuscitation in very severe cases only

---

Comparison of oral rehydration products

Solution	Type†	Na+	K+	COH
WHO (1975)	R	90	20	20
WHO (2002)	R	75	20	13.5
Rehydralyte	R	75	20	25
Pedialyte	M	45	20	25
Enfalyte	M	50	25	30

†R = rehydration
M = maintenance
Na+ = sodium (mEq/L or mmol/L)
K+ = potassium (mmol/L)
COH = carbohydrate (g/L)

MEDICATION (DRUGS)

- Many premixed ORSs commercially available in liquid (Pedialyte) and powder forms (Liqulyte)
- Typical formulation
- Na 45 mEd/L, K 20 mEq/L, Cl 35 mEq/L
- Rehydrate Na = 75 mEq/L—use for rehydration, not maintainence
- Contraindications
  - Conditions predisposing to risk of aspiration: Altered consciousness, seizure activity, severe hypotension, shock
  - Persistent vomiting (as in pyloric stenosis)
  - Absent bowel sounds
- Precautions
  - The ingredients should be provided in premixed packets in order to avoid iatrogenic errors in mixing.
  - If water safety is questionable, it should be boiled or treated for purification.
  - Discard the solution after 12 hours if held at room temperature, or 24 hours if refrigerated.
  - After rehydration is complete, ORSs should not be used as the only fluid intake because the high sodium content may lead to hypernatremia.

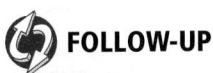 **FOLLOW-UP**

DISPOSITION
- Primarily outpatient
- Designed to be administered by family members

Admission Criteria
Failure of oral therapy

PROGNOSIS
- Rapid clinical improvement despite continuing diarrhea is the usual course.
- The overall complication rate for oral rehydration is the same as that for parenteral rehydration in cases of mild and moderate dehydration. (4)[B]

COMPLICATIONS
Change to IV hydration if the patient has increasing weight loss (fluid deficit), clinical deterioration, or intractable vomiting.

PATIENT MONITORING
The patient needs to be evaluated frequently to ensure establishment of an improving clinical status and an adequate urine output.

REFERENCES
1. Duggan C, Fontaine O, Pierce NF, et al. Scientific rationale for a change in the composition of oral rehydration solution. *JAMA*. 2004;291: 2628–2631.
2. Hahn S, Kim S, Garner P. Reduced osmolarity oral rehydration solution for treating dehydration caused by acute diarrhoea in children. *Cochrane Database Syst Rev*. 2002;(1):CD002847.
3. Fonseca BK, Holdgate A, Craig JC. Enteral vs IV rehydration therapy for children with GE: A meta-analysis of randomized controlled trials. *Arch Pediatr Adolesc Med*. 2004;158:483–490.
4. Spandorfer PR, et al. Oral vs IV rehydration of moderately dehydrated children: A randomized controlled trial. *Pediatrics*. 2005;115: 295–301.
5. Fontaine O, Gore S, Pierce N. Rice-based ORS for treating diarrhea. In: *Cochrane Library*, Issue I. Oxford: Update Software; 2002.
6. Ramakrishna BS, et al. Amylase-resistant starch plus oral rehydration solution for cholera. *N Engl J Med*. 2000;342:308–313.
7. Nalin DR, et al. Clinical concerns about reduced-osmolarity oral rehydration solution. *JAMA*. 2004;291:2632–2635.

 MISCELLANEOUS

- See also: Cholera; Dehydration; Diarrhea, acute
- Other notes: Advantages of oral rehydration over IV rehydration include a much lower cost, minimal storage requirements (for powder forms), and no need for sterile conditions.

PATIENT TEACHING
- Awareness and availability of ORS markedly diminishes morbidity from GE.
- Travelers concerned with severe diarrhea should carry ORS packets on trips.

O

OSGOOD-SCHLATTER DISEASE

David P. Sealy, MD

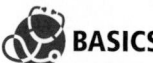 **BASICS**

DESCRIPTION
- A syndrome associated with traction apophysitis in adolescent boys and girls, consisting of pain of the tibial tubercle with swelling
- System(s) Affected: Musculoskeletal

GENERAL PREVENTION
- Avoidance of those sports involving heavy quadriceps loading
- Patients may compete if the pain is minimal.
- Increase hamstring and quadriceps flexibility.

EPIDEMIOLOGY
- Predominant age: Girls: 10–16 years old; Boys: 11–18 years old
- Predominant sex: Male > Female

ALERT
Pediatric Considerations
Seen in skeletally mature boys and girls, with boys more frequently affected than girls

Prevalence
- Not known, but common (13% of athletes in 1 Finnish study)
- Incidence in girls increasing

RISK FACTORS
- Age between 11–18 years
- Male sex
- Rapid skeletal growth
- Involvement in repetitive jumping sports like football, volleyball, basketball, hockey, soccer, skating, gymnastics, and ballet
- Sports involving heavy quadriceps activity

Genetics
Unknown

ETIOLOGY
- Basic etiology unknown, but clearly exacerbated by exercise
  - Jumping and pivoting sports are the worst: Repetitive trauma the most likely source
- Possible association with tight hip flexors, quadriceps, and hamstring muscle groups

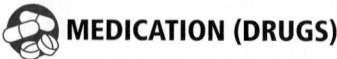 **DIAGNOSIS**

SIGNS AND SYMPTOMS
- Unilateral or bilateral (30%) tibial tuberosity pain
- Pain exacerbated by exercise, especially jumping and landing after jumping
- Tibial tuberosity swelling
- Pain increased with knee extension against resistance or kneeling
- Knee pain with squatting or crouching
- Absence of effusion or condyle tenderness
- Erythema of tibial tuberosity

TESTS
Lab
No blood tests indicated unless other diagnostic considerations are entertained

Imaging
- Radiographic imaging of the proximal tibia and knee may show heterotopic calcification in the patellar tendon
  - X-rays are rarely diagnostic.
  - Calcified thickening of the tibial tuberosity with irregular ossification at insertion of tendon to tibial tubercle
- Bone scan may show increased uptake in the area of the tibial tuberosity; will have increased uptake in apophysis in any child, but may be more than opposite side
- Ultrasound is becoming an excellent alternative, with characteristic findings and classifications. (1)[C]

Pathological Findings
- Osteochondritis of the tibial tubercle
- Heterotopic bone formation at insertion of the patellar tendon
- Bony fusion of the tibial metaphysis
- Inflammatory infiltrate of the epiphysis in severe cases
- Complete avulsion of the tibial tubercle with nonunion of the tubercle with the tibia—possible complication (extremely rare)

DIFFERENTIAL DIAGNOSIS
- Stress fracture of the proximal tibia
- Pes anserinus bursitis
- Quadriceps tendon avulsion
- Patellofemoral stress syndrome
- Chondromalacia patellae
- Proximal tibial neoplasm
- Osteomyelitis of the proximal tibia
- Tibial plateau fracture
- Sinding-Larsen-Johansson syndrome (patellar apophysitis
- Patellar fracture
- Infrapatellar bursitis
- Patellar tendinitis

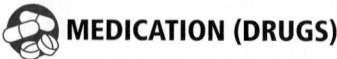 **TREATMENT**

GENERAL MEASURES
- Frequent ice applications after exercise with pain
- Rest
- Knee immobilization in extension (severe cases)
- In more severe cases, avoidance of activities that increase pain or swelling
- Quadriceps isometric strengthening, hip extensions, adductor strengthening, and hamstring and quadriceps stretching exercises
- Patients with marked pronation may benefit from orthotics.
- Open and closed chain, eccentric quadriceps strengthening

Activity
Restricted to those activities that do not cause pain

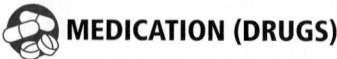 **MEDICATION (DRUGS)**

First Line
None in particular, but all analgesics may be considered. NSAIDs are of minimal benefit; however, narcotics are not recommended. (2)[B]

Second Line
- More potent analgesics such as narcotics may be considered for short-term use or in extreme situations.
- Injectable corticosteroids universally not recommended due to reports of subcutaneous atrophy. (2)[C]

SURGERY
- Débridement of a thickened cosmetically unsatisfactory tibial tubercle (rare) or removal of heterotopic bone
- Surgical excision of a painful tibial tubercal rarely needed (<5%), but most return to sport painfree. (2)[C]

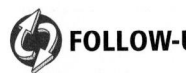 FOLLOW-UP

DISPOSITION
Outpatient treatment

PROGNOSIS
Except in rare complicated cases, this is a self-limiting illness that resolves within 2 years after full skeletal maturation. However, up to 60% of adults with prior Osgood-Schlatter disease will still report occasional symptoms and have pain with kneeling.

COMPLICATIONS
- Nonunion of the tubercle to the tibia
- Upriding of the patella
- Patellar tendon avulsion
- Patellofemoral degenerative arthritis
- Patella alta
- Chondromalacia

PATIENT MONITORING
Follow-up on an as-needed basis for management of pain and disability.

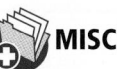 REFERENCES

1. Zaid AA, et al. "The Immature Athlete" *Clin Sports Med*. 2002;21:3.
2. Bloom OJ, Mackler L. What is the best treatment for Osgood Schlatter disease? *J Fam Prac*. 2004; 53(2):153–156.
3. Hogan KA, Gross RH. Overuse injuries in pediatric athletes. *Ortho Clin N Amer*. 2003;34:3.

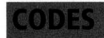 MISCELLANEOUS

See also: Tendinitis

CODES

ICD9-CM
732.4 Juvenile osteochondrosis of lower extremity, excluding foot

PATIENT TEACHING
- Consider avoidance of jumping sports. Assure family that symptoms and findings will diminish with time and rest.
- Can play sport with mild pain
- www.kidskneepain.com

 See Corresponding Diagnostic Algorithm

O

OSTEITIS DEFORMANS (PAGET'S DISEASE OF BONE)

Mark R. Dambro, MD

BASICS

DESCRIPTION
- Inflammatory focal or generalized condition of the skeleton characterized by rapid, chaotic bone resorption followed by equally chaotic and excessive bone formation. Leads to enlarged but weakened and highly vascularized bone, which is painful, easily deformed, and subject to fractures with minimal trauma. Cranial and vertebral involvement can also cause neurologic deficits.
- System(s) Affected: Musculoskeletal
- Synonym(s): Paget disease of bone

GENERAL PREVENTION
Avoid excessive mechanical stress on afflicted bones, to reduce chance of fractures and other complications.

EPIDEMIOLOGY
- Predominant age: >50 years; occasional cases ages 20–50 years
- Predominant sex: Male = Female

Prevalence
- 3% of white individuals >50 years have at least 1 focus.
- More prevalent if ancestry white, especially United Kingdom, Northern Europe (excluding Scandinavia), Italy, Australia, and New Zealand
- Rare in African Americans and Asians

ALERT
Geriatric Considerations
Common

RISK FACTORS
None known

Genetics
- 15–50% of patients have 1 or more involved 1st-order relatives with osteitis deformans.
- Recent data suggest an 18q locus is involved, but other chromosomal sites may also confer susceptibility.

ETIOLOGY
Unknown; best evidence to date is for slow virus infection in genetically susceptible individuals

ASSOCIATED CONDITIONS
- Hyperparathyroidism
- Gouty diathesis
- Secondary osteoarthritis
- Angioid streaks
- Mottled retinal degeneration
- Bone sarcoma (rare)
- Peyronie disease

DIAGNOSIS

SIGNS AND SYMPTOMS
- Frequently asymptomatic
- Bone pain
- Skeletal deformities
- Bowing of extremities
- Acetabular protrusion
- Headaches
- Head enlargement
- Fractures
- Secondary osteoarthritis
- Vertebral compression
- Neurologic deficits
- Osteoporosis circumscripta
- High-output CHF (rare)
- Hypercalcemia (rare)
- Renal calculi (calcium, uric acid)
- Peyronie syndrome
- Angioid streaks (rare)
- Mottled retinal degeneration (rare)
- Increased skin temperature over affected areas
- Bone sarcomas (rare)
- Peripheral neuropathies
- Carpal/tarsal tunnel syndromes
- Valvular/endocardial calcification
- Accelerated atherosclerosis
- Gouty diathesis
- Hyperparathyroidism
- Sensorineural hearing loss
- Conductive hearing loss

TESTS
- Neurologic examination
- Audiogram, if skull involvement
- Visual field study, if skull involvement

Lab
- Serum calcium level
  – Usually normal
  – Rarely increased
- Serum alkaline phosphatase (total or bone specific): Usually increased
- Serum gamma glutamyl transpeptidase: Normal
- Serum osteocalcin (binary ghost-pulse constraint): Usually increased
- Urinary pyridinoline collagen crosslinks: Usually increased
- N- and C-telopeptide (collagen crosslinks): Usually increased in serum and urine
- Drugs that may alter lab results
  – Vitamin D and its metabolites
  – Hepatotoxic drugs
- Disorders that may alter lab results
  – See "Differential Diagnosis."
  – Osteomalacia
  – Liver disorders
  – Traumatic fractures

Imaging
- X-rays show irregular pattern of alternating bone formation and resorption in enlarged deformed bones and resorptive fronts at advancing edge.
- Bone scans show intense uptake in focal pattern.
- CT and MRI show extra-bony extension if sarcomatous degeneration occurs.

Diagnostic Procedures/Surgery
Bone biopsy needed only in confusing cases (rare)

Pathological Findings
Chaotic bone resorption at advancing edge of disease
- Osteoclasts are large, contain 10–100 nuclei, and have abnormal configuration.
  – Electron photomicroscopy shows that nuclei and cytoplasm contain myriad inclusion bodies resembling viral nucleocapsids.
  – Later, excessive osteoblastic bone formation predominates, with sclerotic bone–containing cement lines forming mosaic pattern.

DIFFERENTIAL DIAGNOSIS
- Polyostotic fibrous dysplasia
- Osteitis fibrosis cystica (skeletal hyperparathyroidism)
- Primary bone neoplasms
- Osteolytic, osteoblastic metastases

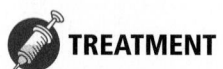

TREATMENT

GENERAL MEASURES
- Rarely, splints for severely resorbed areas with high risk of fracture
- Hearing aids for severe deafness: Of some (but not great) value in sensorineural deafness

Diet
- No special diet

Activity
- Full activity to maintain function
- Avoid excessive mechanical stress on involved bones.

MEDICATION (DRUGS)

First Line

Add NSAIDs to the following drugs for secondary osteoarthritis. COX-2 inhibitors may be substituted.

- Synthetic injectable salmon calcitonin (Miacalcin): 50 IU SC/IM 3 times weekly to 100 IU SC/IM daily, courses 1.5–3 years; or
- Etidronate (Didronel), 5 mg/kg PO daily (~400 mg; taken on an empty stomach) for 6 months. Rarely, 20 mg/kg/d for 1 month. Courses may be repeated after a 3–6-month rest period; or
- Alendronate (Fosamax) 40 mg PO daily (taken on an empty stomach) for 6 months; or
- Risedronate (Actonel) 30 mg PO daily (taken on an empty stomach) for 2 months; or
- Pamidronate (Aredia) 60 mg/d by 4–6 hour infusions for 2–3 days. Alternately, 30 mg/d by 4–6 hour infusions once a week for 6 weeks. May be repeated several months later if effect wears off.
- Contraindications
  - History of allergy or hypersensitivity
  - For alendronate and risedronate, esophageal dysfunction, severe upper gastrointestinal tract symptoms, gastroesophageal reflux disease, etc.
- Precautions
  - Adverse side effects may require ameliorative measures or temporary dose reduction.
  - Salmon calcitonin: Nausea, vomiting, anorexia, flushing, rash, including urticaria (rare)
  - Etidronate disodium: Nausea, vomiting, diarrhea, increased bone pain
  - Alendronate and risedronate: Heartburn, epigastric pain, and musculoskeletal pain. Take on an empty stomach with copious water. No food, beverages, or other medications for 30–60 minutes. Remain upright for 1 hour.
  - Pamidronate disodium: Transient fever, leukopenia, hypocalcemia, headache, malaise, loss of appetite
- Significant possible interactions: None

Second Line

NSAIDs or COX-2 inhibitors for mildly symptomatic disease in nonstrategic areas

SURGERY

- Joint replacement (hip, knee) sometimes needed
- Osteotomy procedures for extreme deformity
- Decompression procedures (skull, spinal column) for acute neurologic deficits (rarely needed)
- Bone biopsy (rarely needed)
- Extirpative surgery for sarcomatous complications
- Open reduction of fractures

 FOLLOW-UP

DISPOSITION

Outpatient, except when IV treatment is used

PROGNOSIS

- Depends on severity, often asymptomatic
- Slow progression if untreated
- Significant amelioration with treatment (85% or greater)
- Poor prognosis if bone sarcoma develops

COMPLICATIONS

- Fractures
- Severe deformities
- Head enlargement
- Acetabular protrusion
- Carpal/tarsal tunnel syndromes
- Neurologic deficits
- Deafness
- Visual impairment
- CHF (high output)
- Renal calculi
- Peyronie syndrome
- Sarcomatous degeneration

PATIENT MONITORING

- Follow-up visits every 2–4 months during drug therapy; yearly if drugs not being used
  - Alkaline phosphatase level (total or bone specific) before each visit
- Repeat x-rays and bone scan every 3–5 years or as needed.

REFERENCES

1. Ankrom MA, Shapiro JR. Paget's disease of bone (osteitis deformans). *J Amer Geriatr Soc.* 1998;46: 1025–1033.
2. Delmas PD, Meunier PJ. The management of Paget's disease of bone. *N Engl J Med.* 1997;336: 558–566.
3. Hadjipavlou A, et al. Malignant transformation in Paget's disease of bone. *Cancer.* 1992;70: 2802–2808.
4. Morales-Piga AA, et al. Frequency and characteristics of familial aggregation of Paget's disease of bone. *J Bone Miner Res.* 1995;10: 663–670.
5. Noor M, Shoback D. Paget's disease of bone: Diagnosis and treatment update. *Curr Rheumatol Rep.* 2000;2:67–73.
6. Rothschild BM. Paget's disease of the elderly. *Compr Ther.* 2000;26:251–254.
7. Siris ES. Paget's disease of bone. *J Bone Miner Res.* 1998;13:1061.
8. Wallach S. Identifying and controlling Paget's disease. *J Musculoskel Med.* 1997;14:66–82.

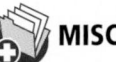 **MISCELLANEOUS**

See also: Arthritis, osteo; Bone tumor, primary malignant; Hyperparathyroidism

CODES

ICD9-CM

731.0 Osteitis deformans without mention of bone tumor

PATIENT TEACHING

Paget Foundation, 120 Wall St., Suite 1602, New York, NY 10005; tel. (212) 509-5335; fax (212)-509-8492; e-mail: pagetfdn@aol.com

O

OSTEOCHONDRITIS DISSECANS

Phyllis Montellese, MD

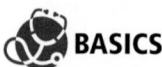

BASICS

DESCRIPTION
Condition in which a segment of subchondral bone of any diarthrodial joint becomes separated from surrounding bone, which can progress to include the cartilage and eventually to formation of a loose body in the affected joint
- System(s) Affected: Musculoskeletal

ALERT
Pediatric Considerations
Multisport athletics, especially gymnastics and overhead sports participation increase risk

GENERAL PREVENTION
No clear way to avoid its development

EPIDEMIOLOGY
- Predominant age: Young adults in their 2nd–4th decades of life and juvenile type (JOCD), which includes children and adolescents prior to physeal closure
- Predominant sex: Male > Female (3:1)

Incidence
Unknown

Prevalence
Unknown

RISK FACTORS
- Seen in active children and adults
- Multisport athletics, especially gymnastics and overhead sports participation

Genetics
No distinct genetic pattern known, but bilateral lesions have been noted in up to 30% of patients

PATHOPHYSIOLOGY
- Primary change in the bone
- Necrosis occurs in a focal area.
- Overlying cartilage changes are secondary to the bony changes.
- Loss of subchondral bone support leads to degenerative cartilage changes: Softening and fibromatous fissuring.
- Fragment may detach and become loose body within the affected joint.
- Cartilage itself is without a vascular supply.
- Healing occurs by vascular supply to bone, which stimulates inflammation, repair, and remodeling.
- It is difficult to predict which lesions will go on to heal and remodel.

ETIOLOGY
- Etiology unclear, but most often associated with trauma or repetitive microtrauma
- Most commonly affected joints are the knee, ankle, and elbow
  - Knee: Overuse and with patellar dislocation and with injury to the anterior cruciate ligament
  - Elbow: Overuse injury in overhead throwers and in female gymnasts
  - Ankle: Frequently associated with history of previous ankle sprain
- Possible theories include vulnerability secondary to fragile blood supply of the physeal line

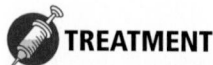

DIAGNOSIS

SIGNS AND SYMPTOMS
History
- Insidious or posttraumatic onset of pain, which improves with rest
- Pain may be associated with clicking, swelling, locking, and stiffness
- Locking may be experienced if fragment detaches
- Pain usually defined as a deep ache

Physical Exam
May be associated with secondary muscle atrophy, effusion, and decreased range of motion (ROM)

TESTS
Lab
No specific tests

Imaging
- Plain x-rays are frequently normal
  - Knee: Anteroposterior (AP), lateral, and "tunnel" views (most likely location for abnormality is in the lateral portion of the medial condyle)
  - Elbow: Routine elbow series (common involvement of the humeral capitellum)
  - Ankle: AP, lateral, oblique, and mortise views (lesions most commonly involve the posteromedial or anterolateral talus)
  - MRI: Can delineate the bony lesion, involvement of cartilage, and any fluid behind the fragment
- CT scan
  - Provides architectural description of bone lesion
  - Provides less information than MRI
- Technetium-99 bone scan: May be useful in evaluation of healing potential, but this is controversial

DIFFERENTIAL DIAGNOSIS
- In the knee
  - Meniscal tear
  - Patella-femoral pain syndrome
- Stress fracture
- Tendinopathy

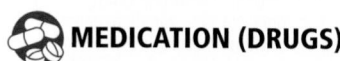

TREATMENT

GENERAL MEASURES
- Goals of treatment
  - Maintain smooth congruous joint surface
  - Alleviate pain
  - Prevent degenerative joint disease
  - Promote revascularization of necrotic fragment and regeneration of affected cartilage
- There are no randomized controlled trials, however, in JOCD, nonsurgical treatment initially is the norm. [B]
- Treatment options include a spectrum of alternatives from relative rest (removal from sport) to crutches (partial or non–weight-bearing) to cylindrical casting and splinting. [C]

Diet
No specific diet recommended

Activity
Non–weight-bearing, immobilization with intermittent maintenance of ROM
- Follow closely for 12 weeks for healing
- Casting is used for 6-week intervals, especially with JOCD, due to issues of compliance

MEDICATION (DRUGS)

NSAIDs or acetaminophen

SURGERY
- Surgical treatment is used when
  - Conservative measures have failed
  - Physeal closure is approaching, which carries a worse prognosis for healing (adult form)
  - Fragment separation has occurred
- Surgical treatment includes drilling to increase blood supply, screw fixation of fragment, and/or allograft insertion and requires an orthopedic consultation [B]

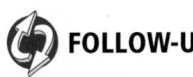 **FOLLOW-UP**

DISPOSITION
- Outpatient care usually
- Inpatient for surgery

PROGNOSIS
- Patient age and degree of physeal closure have a significant effect on healing potential.
- An incongruous joint surface may lead to degenerative changes in the future.
- Clinical improvement may precede radiologic healing.
- Fragment displacement may occur, in which case arthroscopy is indicated.

COMPLICATIONS
- Failure to revascularize and heal
- Displacement of fragment becoming loose body within a joint

PATIENT MONITORING
- Initially should be followed every 6 weeks with serial x-rays to check for healing and possible displacement.
- Expect healing in 4–6 months.
- In JOCD, x-rays at 1 year may show no residual abnormality.

REFERENCES

1. Birk GT, DeLee JC. Osteochondral injuries: Clinical findings. *Clin Sports Med*. 2001;20:279–286.
2. Bucholz R, ed. *Rockwood and Green: Fractures in Adults and Fractures in Children*, 4th ed. Philadelphia, PA: Lippincott-Raven; 1996:289–293.
3. Cahill BR, Ahten SM. Osteochondral injuries of the knee. *Clin Sports Med*. 2001;20:287–298.
4. Delee JD, Drez D, eds. *Orthopedic Sports Medicine: Principles and Practice*. 2nd ed. Philadelphia, PA: WB Saunders; 2003:1273–1279.
5. Rockwood CA, ed. *Fractures in Children*, 4th ed. Philadelphia, PA: Lippincott-Raven; 1996: 1290–1294.
6. Wall E, Von Stein D. Juvenile osteochondritis dissecans. *Orthop Clin North Amer*. 2003;34: 341–353.
7. Cahill B. Osteochondritis dissecans of the knee: Treatment of juvenile and adult forms. *J Am Acad Orthop Surg*. 1995;237–247.
8. Wasiak J, Villanueva E. Autologous cartilage implantation for full thickness articular cartilage defects of the knee; Cochran Database of systematic reviews. 2005;5.

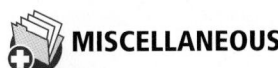 **MISCELLANEOUS**

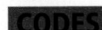 **CODES**

ICD9-CM
732.7 Osteochondritis dissecans

PATIENT TEACHING
- Compliance with immobilization and possibility of further trauma should be emphasized, especially with younger athletes.
- Many lesions heal without surgical intervention.

 See Corresponding Diagnostic Algorithm

O

OSTEOMALACIA AND RICKETS

Mark C. Leeson, MD

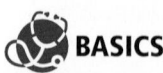 **BASICS**

DESCRIPTION
An excess organic bone matrix secondary to defective or inadequate bone mineralization
- System(s) Affected: Musculoskeletal
- Synonym(s): Rickets

GENERAL PREVENTION
- Adequate dietary intake of vitamin D
- Adequate sunlight exposure
- Fortified cow's milk

EPIDEMIOLOGY
- Predominant age: All ages; in adults, osteomalacia is usually a disease of the older population (50–80 years old).
- Predominant sex: Female > Male (slightly)

ALERT
Geriatric Considerations
Studies have suggested that vitamin D deficiency osteomalacia is a relatively common condition in the acutely ill elderly population, with an estimated prevalence of ~3–5%; however, it often goes undiagnosed.

RISK FACTORS
- Poverty
- Inadequate nutrition and sunlight exposure

PATHOPHYSIOLOGY
- Defective calcification of growing bone
- Hypertrophy of epiphyseal cartilages

ETIOLOGY
- Can be caused by a wide variety of pathogenic processes, including, but not limited to, vitamin D deficiency (reduced exposure to sunlight, poor nutrition, malabsorption syndromes)
- Defective metabolism of parent vitamin D to active metabolites (drug-induced e.g., anticonvulsants such as phenytoin [Dilantin], chronic renal failure), hypophosphatemia (renal tubular acidosis, hypophosphatemic syndrome), miscellaneous (long-term hemodialysis, malnutrition, vitamin D–dependent rickets)

ASSOCIATED CONDITIONS
- Chronic renal disease
- Epilepsy
- Malnutrition
- Previous gastric surgery
- Pregnancy nutritional factors

DIAGNOSIS

SIGNS AND SYMPTOMS
- Bone pain, tenderness, muscle weakness
- Bone pain is dull and tends to be poorly localized, usually affecting the ribs and upper thighs
- Muscle weakness is usually proximal.
- Other symptoms of malnutrition or an underlying problem such as chronic renal disease may also be clinically evident.
- Weight loss
- Anorexia
- Tetany
- In young children: Restlessness, poor sleep patterns, craniotabes, costochondral beading, bowlegs, kyphoscoliosis

TESTS
Lab
- Alkaline phosphatase level: Increased
- Serum calcium: Low or normal (never high)
- Hypophosphatemia
- Aminoaciduria
- Acidosis
- Glucosuria
- Hypouricemia

Imaging
Radiographic changes are nonspecific
- Earliest manifestation is thinning of cortical bone.
- In long-term osteomalacia: Bone softening (protrusio acetabuli), looser lines, stress fractures, and pathologic fractures

Diagnostic Procedures/Surgery
Bone biopsy and subsequent histopathologic evaluation
- Deliver the most accurate diagnosis of osteomalacia
- Biopsy usually taken from the iliac crest, and calcified and noncalcified studies and special stains (including von Kossa stain) are helpful.

DIFFERENTIAL DIAGNOSIS
- Osteoporosis
- Metastatic bone disease
- Primary bone malignancies (lymphoma, myeloma)

TREATMENT

GENERAL MEASURES
- Treatment of osteomalacia depends on the cause (e.g., gastrointestinal, renal, or nutritional).
- For nutritional osteomalacia, calcium and vitamin D have been shown to correct the disease process.
- Treatment can be monitored by observing simple bone biochemistry.
- Treatment results depend on identifying and correcting the cause.

Diet
- Ensure adequate vitamin D intake.
- Provide instructions for a high-calcium diet and information about calcium supplements, if appropriate.

Activity
Full activity is encouraged, including a neuro-conditioning program.

MEDICATION (DRUGS)

First Line
For adults and uncomplicated rickets: Vitamin D (ergocalciferol) 2,000–4,800 IU once a day for 1 month, then reduce dose gradually

Second Line
- IV calcium salts if tetany complicate single IM dose of 100,000 IU in adolescents each fall
- Alfacalcidol
- Calcitriol

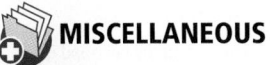 **FOLLOW-UP**

DISPOSITION
Can be managed on an outpatient basis, except for complicating emergencies/fractures

PROGNOSIS
Variable

COMPLICATIONS
- Fractures
- Osteomyelitis
- Renal failure
- Renal tubular acidosis
- Seizures
- Growth deformity; bowing long bones in children

PATIENT MONITORING
Office visits every 6 months

REFERENCES
1. Mare GM, McKenna MJ, Frame B. Osteomalacia. *Bone Mineral Res*. 1986;4:335.

 MISCELLANEOUS

CODES

ICD9-CM
268.2 Osteomalacia, unspecified

PATIENT TEACHING
Educate family and patient on nutrition.

See Corresponding Diagnostic Algorithm

OSTEOMYELITIS

Jeffery T. Kirchner, DO

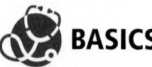 **BASICS**

DESCRIPTION
An acute or chronic infection of the bone and its structures caused most commonly by bacteria and rarely by other micro-organisms. This infection may be acquired either by hematogenous, contiguous, or direct inoculation such as trauma or surgery.
- System(s) Affected: Musculoskeletal

EPIDEMIOLOGY
- Predominant age: Commonly seen in older adults; hematogenous inoculation is bimodal; also seen in infants and children; higher incidence in diabetics
- Predominant sex: Male > Female

ALERT
Geriatric Considerations
- Vertebral osteomyelitis more common
- Contiguous focus of infection more common

Pediatric Considerations
Occurs most often in 5–14 age group and more frequently in boys

RISK FACTORS
- Diabetes mellitus
- Sickle cell disease
- Other conditions that predispose to bone infarcts
- IV drug use
- Hemodialysis
- Local trauma
- Open fractures
- Presence of prosthetic orthopedic implant
- Vascular insufficiency
- Neuropathy

Genetics
No known genetic predisposition

ETIOLOGY (1)
- Acute hematogenous osteomyelitis
  - *Staphylococcus aureus* (most common)
  - *Streptococcus*, coagulase-negative *Staphylococcus*, *Haemophilus influenzae*, and Gram-negative organisms (less common)
- Vertebral osteomyelitis
  - *S. aureus* and Gram-negative enteric organisms (common)
  - Other micro-organisms to consider include *Mycobacterium tuberculosis* and fungi
- Contiguous focus osteomyelitis and vascular insufficiency osteomyelitis: Mixed aerobic/anaerobic micro-organisms are frequently found.
- Prosthetic device infection
  - Coagulase-negative *Staphylococcus*, and *S. aureus* (most common)
  - Diphtheroids, and Gram-negative bacteria (less common)

Geriatric Considerations
Vascular insufficiency is the most common cause of osteomyelitis in the 50–70 age group (usually as a result of the presence of associated conditions).

ASSOCIATED CONDITIONS
See "Etiology."

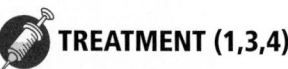 **DIAGNOSIS**

SIGNS AND SYMPTOMS (1,4)
- Hematogenous long bone infection (in children with hematogenous osteomyelitis)
  - Abrupt onset of high fever
  - Irritability
  - Malaise
  - Restriction of movement of the involved extremity
  - Signs of localized inflammation
- Hematogenous vertebral infection (in adults with vertebral osteomyelitis)
  - Illness is insidious and behaves more like a chronic infection.
  - History of an acute bacteremic episode associated with infection of a specific organ may be found in some patients.
- Contiguous and vascular insufficiency–associated infection
  - Acute constitutional manifestations are seldom seen.
  - Localized signs and symptoms of inflammation with or without drainage frequently found
- Chronic osteomyelitis
  - Nonhealing ulcer or draining sinus
  - Constitutional symptoms: When present, indicate acute suppurative condition in the bone or surrounding tissues
- Prosthetic device-associated infection
  - Infection may be acquired either by hematogenous route or by contiguous foci such as local infection, operative contamination, or postoperative infection.
  - Acute postoperative infection may present as fever, localized swelling, tenderness, and drainage.
  - Chronic infection is characterized by joint discomfort, swelling, erythema, and joint dysfunction.

TESTS
Lab
- Definitive diagnosis is made by needle aspiration or bone biopsy and demonstration of the micro-organism by culture or histology.
- Blood culture may be positive in ~50% of younger patients with acute hematogenous disease.
- Leukocyte count is usually elevated in the acute cases but not in the chronic cases.
- Sedimentation rate or C-reactive protein is usually elevated but nonspecific. CRP helpful for follow-up of treatment response.
- Drugs that may alter lab results: Antimicrobial agents given before bone culture
- Disorders that may alter lab results
  - Cultures from the sinus tract are unreliable because of frequent contamination.
  - Superficial cultures are helpful only in identifying methicillin-resistant *S. aureus*.

Imaging (2)
- No technique can absolutely confirm or exclude osteomyelitis.
- Routine radiography (findings on plain radiograph are often delayed for 10–14 days in acute infection)
- Radionuclide scanning (technetium, indium, or gallium) is also useful but is limited by low specificity.
- CT with good resolution; artifact may decrease specificity.
- MRI is excellent but more expensive than other radiologic tests. It is also not helpful for follow-up due to persistence of bony edema.

Diagnostic Procedures/Surgery (3)
Needle biopsy or open bone biopsy for bacterial culture (gold standard); however, antibiotic therapy within the past 2–4 weeks may prevent isolation of a specific pathogen.

Pathological Findings
Inflammatory process of the bone with pyogenic bacteria

DIFFERENTIAL DIAGNOSIS
- Systemic infection from other source
- Aseptic bone infarction
- Localized inflammation or infection of overlying skin and soft tissues
- Neuropathic joint disease
- Fractures
- Gout

TREATMENT (1,3,4)

INITIAL STABILIZATION
Hospitalize the patient with suspected acute osteomyelitis for diagnostic workup and initial treatment.

GENERAL MEASURES
Symptomatic treatment of pain

Diet
No restriction

Activity
Bed rest and immobilization of the involved bone and joint

MEDICATION (DRUGS)

First Line (6,7)[B]
These are essentially choices. Antimicrobial agent(s) based on susceptibility testing and known clinical efficacy. The duration of therapy for acute osteomyelitis should be at least 4–6 weeks. In chronic osteomyelitis, longer duration of therapy may be needed.

- Empiric antibioitic choices (6)[B]
  - Age <15 years
    - Penicillinase-resistant synthetic penicillin and 3rd-generation cephalosporin. Alternatives include vancomycin or clindamycin plus a 3rd-generation cephalosporin.
  - Adults
    - Same as above; ciprofloxacin and rifampin.
  - Diabetes
    - "Mild infections" (oral route) dicloxacillin, clindamycin, cephalexin, trimethoprin/sulfamethoxazole amoxicillin/clavulanate, levofloxacin.
    - "Moderate infections" (oral or parenteral based on clinical situation and agent selected). TMP/SMX, amoxicillin/clavulanate, levofloxacin, ceftriaxone, ticarcillin/clavulanate; levofloxacin or ciprofloxacin with clindamycin.
    - "Severe infections" Piperacillin/tazobactam; levofloxacin or ciprofloxacin with clindamycin; imipenem-cilastatin; vancomycin and ceftazidime.
  - Puncture wound
    - Ceftazidime; cefepime; ciprofloxacin.
  - Trauma
    - Nafcillin and ciprofloxacin; vancomycin and 3rd-generation cephalosporin with antipseudomonal activity.
- *S. aureus* and coagulase-negative *Staphylococcus*: Nafcillin 2 g IV q4–6h. Vancomycin 1 g q12h for methicillin-resistant *Staphylococcus* or linezolid (Zyvox) 600 mg PO b.i.d. or IV b.i.d.
- *Streptococcus* spp.: Penicillin G 2–4 million units IV q4h
- Enteric Gram-negative bacilli and *Pseudomonas aeruginosa*: Piperacillin 4 g IV q4–6h, plus aminoglycoside
- Mixed aerobic/anaerobic infection (diabetic foot, bite wound): β-lactamase inhibitor combination (ticarcillin/clavulanate 3.1 g IV q6h; ampicillin/sulbactam 3 g IV q6h); piperacillin/tazobactam 3.375 g IV q6h
- Contraindications: Allergy
- Precautions: In patients with renal or hepatic insufficiency, antimicrobial dose may need adjustment.
- Significant possible interactions: Refer to the manufacturer's literature.

Second Line (1)[B], (4)[C]
- *S. aureus* and coagulase-negative *Staphylococcus*: Clindamycin 600 mg IV q6h, nafcillin 2 g IV q4h, cefazolin 1 g q8h, or vancomycin 1 g IV q12h
- *Streptococcus* spp.: Penicillin G 2 million units q4h, cefazolin 1 g IV q8h, or clindamycin 600 mg IV q6h
- Enteric Gram-negative bacilli and *P. aeruginosa*: Ceftazidime 1 g IV q8h or ciprofloxacin (or other quinolone) 750 mg PO q12h
- Mixed aerobic/anaerobic infection (diabetic foot, bite wound): Clindamycin plus 3rd-generation cephalosporin or quinolone
- Home therapy often used; consider a simplified antibiotic regimen for outpatient use or oral therapy.
- Some published studies recommend use of hyperbaric oxygen, but none is a randomized, controlled trial.

 ## SURGERY
- Surgical drainage and removal of necrotic tissues are of utmost importance to effect cure.
- In patients with vascular insufficiency or severe gangrenous infection, amputation may be the only effective treatment.
- Revascularization may be an option for some patients.

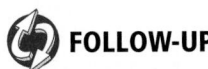 ## FOLLOW-UP

PROGNOSIS
- Cure of osteomyelitis with medical treatment is notoriously unpredictable, especially when not accompanied by surgical débridement.
- In patients with acute hematogenous osteomyelitis, the prognosis is usually good even without surgery. Cure takes ~6 weeks; radiographic improvement may take 3–6 months.
- The prognosis is improved if all infected bone has been removed.

COMPLICATIONS
- Abscess formation
- Bacteremia
- Fracture
- Loosening of the prosthetic implant
- Postoperative infection

PATIENT MONITORING
Blood level of antimicrobial agents, serum antibacterial titers, sedimentation rate, and repeat plain radiography, CT, or MRI to confirm healing

REFERENCES
1. Lew DP, Waldvogel FA. *Osteomyelitis Lancet*. 2004;364:369–379.
2. Santiago Restrepo C, Gimenez CR, McCarthy K. Imaging of osteomyelitis and musculoskeletal soft tissue infections: Current concepts. *Rheum Dis Clin North Am*. 2003;29:89–109.
3. Zuluaga A, et al. Etilogic diagnosis of chronic osteomyelitis. *Arch Intern Med*. 2006;166:95–100.
4. Danville T, Jacobs RF. Management of acute hematogenous osteomyelitis in children. *Pediatr Infect Dis J*. 2004;23:255–257.
5. Lipsky BA. Medical treatment of diabetic foot infections. *Clin Infect Dis*. 2004;39 (Suppl 2): S104–S114.
6. Lipsky BA. Diagnosis and treatment of diabetic foot infections. (IDSA Guidelines) *Clin Infect Dis*. 2004; 39:885–910.
7. King RW. Osteomyelitis. Available at: www.emedcine.com. Accessed June 2, 2006.

 ## MISCELLANEOUS

CODES

ICD9-CM
- 376.03 Orbital osteomyelitis
- 526.4 Inflammatory conditions of jaws
- 730.00 Acute osteomyelitis, site unspecified
- 730.10 Chronic osteomyelitis, site unspecified

PATIENT TEACHING
- Stress need for long-term treatment and follow-up.
- Advise patient to avoid further stress and weight bearing until healing

See Corresponding Diagnostic Algorithm

OSTEONECROSIS

Richard Viken, MD

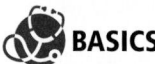 **BASICS**

DESCRIPTION
- Death of the cellular components of bony tissue due to compromise in blood flow
- Accounts for 10% of total joint replacement procedures performed annually in US (1)[C]
- System(s) Affected: Musculoskeletal
- Synonym(s): Idiopathic osteonecrosis, Avascular necrosis; Lunatomalacia; Kienböck disease; Subchondral fracture

GENERAL PREVENTION
Early diagnosis and treatment of underlying disease

EPIDEMIOLOGY
- Predominant age: 3rd–6th decade
- Predominant sex: Male > Female

Incidence
In the US: Dependent on the underlying condition

RISK FACTORS
- Gaucher disease: Especially likely as a postoperative infection
- Diabetes mellitus
- Alcoholism: The most frequent cause
- Type II or IV hyperlipemia
- Cortisone therapy (may be seen with Cushing disease)
- Obesity
- Oral contraceptives
- Organ transplant, especially kidney
- Pregnancy
- Decompression sickness ("bends")
- Chronic pancreatitis
- Crohn disease
- Myeloproliferative disorders
- Radiation treatment
- Rheumatoid arthritis (RA)
- Sickle cell anemia
- Systemic lupus erythematosis

ALERT
Pregnancy Considerations
Pregnancy is a risk factor.

Genetics
The underlying conditions of hemoglobinopathies, especially sickle cell disease, diabetes, and type II or IV hyperlipemia, are inheritable and associated with a high incidence of osteonecrosis. Other forms have no proven genetic relationship.

ETIOLOGY
Idiopathic (i.e., multifactorial)

TESTS
Lab
Bone scan shows decreased bone uptake (sometimes increased uptake, depending on the stage). Later, the uptake increases as reparative processes begin within the bone.

Imaging
- Plain films of the epiphyseal region show arc like subchondral radiolucent lesions, patchy lucent areas and sclerosis, osseous collapse, and preservation of the joint space. However, these abnormalities do not appear for several months after the onset of symptoms; therefore, they are not a sensitive indicator of early disease. Further, the initial features of osteonecrosis may simulate the aggressive pattern of bone destruction that accompanies malignancy or osteomyelitis. (3)[C]

- MRI will show a decreased signal intensity of the involved bone and is the most sensitive diagnostic exam. (1)[B]

Diagnostic Procedures/Surgery
The presence of a crescent sign is practically diagnostic (see "Differential Diagnosis"). It is caused by a subchondral fracture.

Pathological Findings
The subchondral fracture occurs during bone repair as necrotic bone is resorbed. Later, a collapse of the bone occurs with subsequent irregularities at the joint surface. This will eventually produce osteoarthritic changes.

DIFFERENTIAL DIAGNOSIS
- RA
- Osteoarthritis
- Femoral neck fracture
- Lumbar disk disease
- Muscle strain
- Groin injury
- Septic arthritis
- Secondary hyperparathyroidism

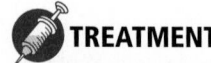 **TREATMENT**

GENERAL MEASURES
- Appropriate health care: Outpatient normally; inpatient if surgery indicated
- The following conditions are ones that are amenable to treatment in order to decrease the accompanying incidence of osteonecrosis
  - Alcoholism: Abstinence
  - Dysbarism: New tables of decompression, if followed, will lower osteonecrosis incidence of divers
  - Transplant patients: Decreased doses of cortisone and regulation of calcium and phosphorous metabolism
  - Sickle cell disease: Treat a crisis vigorously with hydration, possible exchange transfusion and oxygenation, especially hyperbaric oxygen

Diet
No special diet

Activity
As tolerated

MEDICATION (DRUGS)

First Line
- NSAIDs consistent with the underlying disease may be used for painful episodes.
- Acetaminophen: 500 mg q.i.d. can alleviate symptoms.
- Biosphosphonates
  - Alendronate (Fosamax): 10 mg/d or 70 mg weekly
  - Risedronate (Actonel): 5 mg/d or 35 mg weekly
  - Calcium supplementation: 500–1,000 mg/d
  - Vitamin D supplementation: 400–800 IU/d
- Contraindications
  - See the manufacturer's profile for each drug.
- Precautions
  - NSAIDs: If history of peptic ulcer is present, the use of ranitidine (Zantac) 150 mg b.i.d. or 300 mg at bedtime can be given. Misoprostol (Cytotec) 100 μg b.i.d. will usually prevent gastritis (not needed with acetaminophen)
- Significant possible interactions: See the manufacturer's profile for each drug.

Second Line
Other H$_2$-receptor antagonists in patients with a history of peptic ulcer disease

SURGERY
- Core decompression, bone grafts, joint reconstruction, allografts, and arthrodesis may be used, depending on the joint involved.
- Hip is amenable to resurfacing arthroplasty (2)[B]
  - Advantages
    - Bone conservation
    - Preservation of joint mechanics
    - More physiologic loading of bone
    - Lower incidence of postoperative complications
    - Easier conversion to secondary procedure in case of failure
  - Disadvantages
    - High rate of femoral and acetabular loosening
    - Femoral neck fractures
    - Loss of acetabular bone stock, making secondary revision more difficult

 FOLLOW-UP

PROGNOSIS
Gaucher disease is associated with a high risk of infection following surgery.

ALERT
Pediatric Considerations
Légg-Calvé-Pérthes occurs in the 6–12-year-old age group. Prognosis is better in younger patients.

COMPLICATIONS
- Latrogenic, secondary to surgical induced trauma. (1)[C]
- Progression of disease: Leads to osteoarthritis of the involved joint to a varying degree. Arthroplasty of the hip carries a much poorer prognosis than osteoarthritis alone. It should be postponed as long as possible.

PATIENT MONITORING
X-rays should be made every 12–18 months, more frequently if symptoms become more severe.

REFERENCES
1. Assuoline-Dayan Y, et al. Pathogenesis and natural history of osteonecrosis. *Semin Arthritis Rheum*. 2002;32(2):94–124.
2. Grecula MJ. Resurfacing arthroplasty in osteonecrosis of the hip. *Orthop Clin North Am*. 2005;36:231–242.
3. Steinberg ME, Steinberg DR. Classification systems for osteonecrosis: An overview. *Orthop Clin North Am*. 2004;35:273–283.

 MISCELLANEOUS

See also: Arthritis, osteo; Légg-Calvé-Pérthes disease

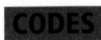 **CODES**

ICD9-CM
730.10 Chronic osteomyelitis, site unspecified

PATIENT TEACHING
The patient should be instructed in the use of crutches and/or canes when the lower extremity is involved. Proper use of a walking cane can decrease the pressure on the femoral head 20–30% when walking.

 See Corresponding Diagnostic Algorithm

O

OSTEOPOROSIS

Anirudh Sridharan, MD

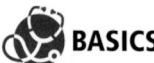 **BASICS**

DESCRIPTION

A multifactorial skeletal disease characterized by severe bone loss, disruption of skeletal microarchitecture, disturbed bone strength and bone quality sufficient to predispose to atraumatic fractures of the vertebral column, upper femur, distal radius, proximal humerus, pubic rami, and ribs

GENERAL PREVENTION

- Osteoporosis is a preventable disease
  - Exercise (weightbearing/aerobic and strength training)
  - Calcium (500 mg t.i.d.)
  - Vitamin D (minimally 800 IU/d)
  - Smoking cessation
- The US Preventive Services Task Force recommends routine screening for all women ≥65 years and in women 60 and older who are at high risk for fracture. (1)[B]
- There are no clear screening guidelines for men.
- Correct treatable medical conditions and other risk factors.

EPIDEMIOLOGY

- Predominant age: Elderly
- Predominant sex: Female > Male

Prevalence
- 24% in women >50
- 7.5% in men >50

RISK FACTORS

- Increasing age and female gender
- Dietary: Lean body habitus, low body weight, inadequate calcium or vitamin D; excessive phosphate/protein
- Physical: Immobilization, sedentary lifestyle
- Social: >2 alcohol drinks per day, current smoking, high caffeine intake
- Medical: Chronic diseases, malabsorption, endocrinopathies (see also "Secondary Osteoporosis" in "Etiology" section)
- Iatrogenic: Corticosteroids (>3 months use), excess thyroid hormone replacement, medroxyprogesterone acetate, chronic heparin or antiseizure medication (phenytoin, phenobarbital) use, chemotherapy, tamoxifen (premenopausal), lithium, radiation therapy
- Genetic/familial: Suboptimal bone mass at maturity, familial "fast bone losers," nulliparity

Genetics
Familial predisposition: More common in whites and Asians than in African American and Latino ethnic groups

ETIOLOGY

- Postmenopausal: Hypoestrogenemia
- Secondary causes: Chronic liver disease, corticosteroid excess, eating disorders, elite athletes/ballet dancers with hypoestrogenism, gastrectomy, hemochromatosis, hyperparathyroidism, hyperthyroidism, hypogonadism, inflammatory bowel disease, malabsorption syndromes, mastocytosis, medications (see "Iatrogenic" section under "Risk Factors"), multiple myeloma, multiple sclerosis, osteomalacia, pernicious anemia, rheumatoid arthritis, sprue, thalassemia

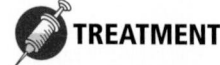 **DIAGNOSIS**

SIGNS AND SYMPTOMS

- Backache/pain, acute/chronic
- Kyphosis/scoliosis, height loss >1.5 inches
- Atraumatic fractures

TESTS

Lab
Serum lab tests to evaluate secondary causes
- 25 hydroxy vitamin D: Vitamin D deficiency
- PTH, ionized calcium: Hyperparathyroidism
- TSH: Hyperthyroidism
- Testosterone: Hypogonadism in men
- CBC, serum and urine protein electrophoresis, Cushing syndrome
- Urinary free cortisol: Multiple myeloma
- Vitamin B_{12} level and intrinsic factor antibody: Pernicious anemia
- IgA anti-endomysial antibodies: Celiac sprue
- Osteomalacia: 25 hydroxy-vitamin D, serum and urine calcium, alkaline phosphatase, serum phosphate

Imaging
- Central dual-energy x-ray absorptiometry (DXA) of the lumbar spine/hip is the gold standard for measuring bone mineral density (BMD).
- Ultrasound densitometry is used to measure BMD at the calcaneus (heel). It requires lower cost and no radiation exposure. Is not as accurate as DXA.
- Only DXA is accurate enough to be used to serially measure changes in BMD. (DXA does not always correlate with decreased fracture risk.)
- Plain radiographs lack sensitivity to diagnose osteoporosis, but changes should prompt evaluation of bone density if abnormalities are seen (e.g., widened intervertebral spaces, rib fractures, vertebral compression fractures, etc.).
- BMD is expressed in terms of T scores.
- The T score is the number of standard deviations (SD) a patient's BMD deviates from the mean for young normal (age 25–40) controls of the same sex and, in some cases, ethnic group.
- The WHO defines normal BMD as a T score of −1 and above; osteopenia is defined as a T score between −1 and −2.5; and osteoporosis is defined as a T score at or below −2.5.

Diagnostic Procedures/Surgery
Bone biopsy rarely is needed to rule out neoplasms and other metabolic bone diseases. Sometimes it is used to quantitate bone loss.

Pathological Findings
- Reduced skeletal mass, trabecular bone thinned or lost more so than cortical bone
- Osteoclast and osteoblast number variable
- No evidence of other metabolic bone diseases and no increase in unmineralized osteoid
- Marrow normal or atrophic

DIFFERENTIAL DIAGNOSIS
- Multiple myeloma or other neoplasms
- Osteomalacia
- Type I collagen mutations
- Osteogenesis imperfecta

TREATMENT

INITIAL STABILIZATION
- Usually outpatient care
- Inpatient care for acute back pain, especially for new vertebral fractures and for acute treatment of upper femoral and pelvic fractures
- Nursing home or home care may be needed following peripheral fractures.

GENERAL MEASURES
- As required by pain and disability (e.g., heat, analgesics, physical therapy)
- Decrease falls.
- Avoid psychotropic effects of drugs.

Diet
- Diet to maintain normal body weight.
- Intake of 1,500 mg of calcium daily.
- Intake of 800 IU vitamin D daily
- Avoidance of excess phosphoric acid–containing beverages and excess protein intake

Activity
Weightbearing exercises such as walking, jogging, stair climbing, and tai-chi should be encouraged. These activities may moderately increase bone density and have been shown to decrease falls.

MEDICATION (DRUGS)

Treat patients with T-score of −2.5 or less at the hip with no risk factors; patients with T-score of −1.5 or less at the hip with 1 or more risk factors; patients with a prior history of fracture at the spine or hip.

First Line
- Bisphosphonates (alendronate, risedronate, and ibandronate)
  - Become incorporated into skeletal tissue, where they inhibit the resorption of bone tissue by osteoclasts
  - Only effective if given with calcium, Vitamin D, and weightbearing exercise
  - Have been shown to provide a relative risk reduction of vertebral, hip, and wrist fractures by 40–50% over 3 years in patients with osteoporosis [NNT = 91] (2)[B]

Second Line
- Calcitonin
  - Acts by reducing the number of osteoclasts and therefore decreasing bone turnover
  - Calcitonin has been shown to increase BMD, but no studies have conclusively shown a reduction in the occurrence of fractures.
- Raloxifene
  - A selective estrogen receptor modulator with positive effects on BMD and fracture risk but no stimulatory action on the breasts or uterus
  - It has been shown to decrease the incidence of vertebral fractures by ∼50%, but studies have failed to show it reduces the incidence of hip or wrist fractures.
- Teriparatide
  - A recombinant formulation of parathyroid hormone (PTH). When given daily it promotes new bone formation.
  - Studies have shown a reduction in the incidence of vertebral fractures by 65%. (3)[B]
  - No data exists on its safety and efficacy >2 years of use.
  - Primarily indicated for those with worsening osteoporosis despite bisphosphonate therapy
- Hormone replacement therapy (HRT)
  - Effective in prevention and treatment of osteoporosis (35% reduction in the incidence of hip and vertebral fractures after 5 years of use), but the risks (increased rates of myocardial infarction, stroke, breast cancer, pulmonary embolus, and deep vein thrombosis) must be weighed against benefits. (4,5)[B]

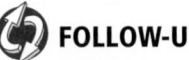 **FOLLOW-UP**

PROGNOSIS
- With treatment, 80% of patients stabilize skeletal manifestations, increase bone mass, increase mobility, and have reduced pain.
- 15% of vertebral and 20–40% of hip fractures may lead to chronic care and/or premature death.

COMPLICATIONS
- Severe, disabling pain
- Dorsal/lumbar neurologic deficits secondary to vertebral fracture (rare)

PATIENT MONITORING
- Bimonthly initially, then every 6 months
- Periodic multiphasic screening; annual gynecologic exam, breast exam, and mammography
- Annual or every-2-year BMD with same test
- Radiographs for acute pain, suspected fractures

REFERENCES

1. Nelson HD, Helfand. Screening for postmenopausal osteoporosis. United States Preventive Services Task Force, September 2002.
2. Cummings SR, Black DM, Thompson DE, et al. Effects of alendronate on risk of fracture in women with low bone density but without vertebral fractures: Results from the Fracture Intervention Trial. *JAMA*. 1998;280:2077–2082.
3. Neer RM, Arnaud, CD, Zanchetta JR, et al. Effect of parathyroid hormone (1-34) on fractures and bone mineral density in postmenopausal women with osteoporosis. *N Engl J Med*. 2001;344:1434–1441.
4. Cauley JA, Robbins J, Chen Z, et al. Effects of estrogen plus progestin on risk of fracture and bone mineral density. *JAMA*. 2003;290(13):1729–1738.
5. Rossow JE, Anderson GL, Prentice RL, et al. Risks and benefits of estrogen plus progestin in healthy postmenopausal women. *JAMA*. 2002;288: 321–333.

 MISCELLANEOUS

CODES

ICD9-CM
733.00 Osteoporosis, generalized

PATIENT TEACHING

National Osteoporosis Foundation: www.nof.org

 See Patient Handout on CD

O

OTITIS EXTERNA
Douglas S. Parks, MD

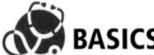 BASICS

DESCRIPTION
Inflammation of the external auditory canal
- Acute diffuse otitis externa: The most common form; an infectious process, usually bacterial, occasionally fungal (10%)
- Acute circumscribed otitis externa: Synonymous with furuncle; associated with infection of the hair follicle
- Chronic otitis externa: Same as acute diffuse but of longer duration (>6 weeks)
- Eczematous otitis externa: May accompany typical atopic eczema or other primary skin conditions
- Necrotizing malignant otitis externa: An infection that extends into the deeper tissues adjacent to the canal; may include osteomyelitis and cellulitis; rare in children
- System(s) Affected: Skin/Exocrine
- Synonym(s): Swimmer's ear

GENERAL PREVENTION
- Avoid prolonged exposure to moisture.
- Use preventive antiseptics: Acidifying solutions with 2% acetic acid diluted 50/50 with water or isopropyl alcohol or 2% acetic acid with aluminum acetate (less irritating) after swimming
- Treat predisposing skin conditions.
- Eliminate self-inflicted trauma to canal with cotton swabs and other foreign objects.
- Diagnose and treat underlying systemic conditions.
- Use ear plugs when swimming.

EPIDEMIOLOGY
- Predominant age: All ages
- Predominant sex: Male = Female

Incidence
Unknown; higher in the summer months and warm, wet climates

Prevalence
- Acute, chronic, and eczematous: Common
- Necrotizing: Uncommon

RISK FACTORS
- Acute and chronic otitis externa
  - Traumatization of external canal
  - Swimming
  - Hot, humid weather
  - Hearing aid use
- Eczematous: Primary skin disorder
- Necrotizing otitis externa in adults
  - Advanced age
  - Diabetes mellitus
  - Debilitating disease
  - AIDS
- Necrotizing otitis externa in children (rare)
  - Leukopenia
  - Malnutrition
  - Diabetes mellitus
  - Diabetes insipidus

ETIOLOGY
- Acute diffuse otitis externa
  - Traumatized external canal (e.g., from use of cotton swab)
  - Bacterial infection (90%): *Pseudomonas* (67% cases), *Staphylococcus*, *Streptococcus*, Gram-negative rods
  - Fungal infection (10%): *Aspergillus* (90% cases), *Candida, Phycomycetes, Rhizopus, Actinomyces, Penicillium*

- Chronic otitis externa: Bacterial infection: *Pseudomonas*
- Eczematous otitis externa (associated with primary skin disorder)
  - Eczema
  - Seborrhea
  - Psoriasis
  - Neurodermatitis
  - Contact dermatitis
  - Purulent otitis media
  - Sensitivity to topical medications
- Necrotizing otitis externa
  - Invasive bacterial infection: *Pseudomonas*
  - Associated with immunosuppression

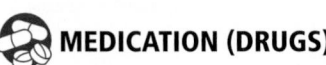 DIAGNOSIS

SIGNS AND SYMPTOMS
- Itching
- Plugging of the ear
- Otalgia
- Periauricular adenitis
- Erythemetous canal
- Purulent discharge
- Eczema of pinna
- Cranial nerve (VII, IX–XII) involvement (rare)

History
Variable length history of itching, plugging of ear, ear pain and discharge from ear

Physical Exam
- Ear canal red, containing discharge and debris
- Pain on manipulation of the pinnae
- Possible periauricular adenitis

TESTS
Lab
- Gram stain and culture of canal discharge (occasionally helpful)
- Antibiotic pretreatment may affect results.

Imaging
Radiologic evaluation of deep tissues in necrotizing otitis externa with high-resolution CT, MRI, gallium scan, and bone scan

Pathological Findings
- Acute and chronic otitis externa: Desquamation of superficial epithelium of external canal with infection
- Eczematous otitis externa: Pathologic findings consistent with primary skin disorder; secondary infection on occasion
- Necrotizing otitis externa: Vasculitis, thrombosis, and necrosis of involved tissues; osteomyelitis

DIFFERENTIAL DIAGNOSIS
- Idiopathic ear pain
- Hearing loss
- Cranial nerve (VII, IX–XII) palsy with necrotizing otitis externa
- Wisdom tooth eruption
- Basal cell or squamous cell carcinoma

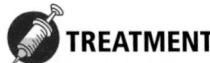 TREATMENT

Outpatient treatment, except for resistant cases and necrotizing otitis externa

GENERAL MEASURES
- Cleansing of external canal may facilitate recovery
- Analgesics as appropriate for pain
- Antipruritic and antihistamines (eczematous form)
- Ear wick (Pope) for nearly occluded ear canal

Diet
No restrictions

Activity
No restrictions

Complementary and Alternative Medicine
- Tea tree oil in various concentrations has been used as an antiseptic. Ototoxicity reported in animal studies at very high doses.
- Grapefruit seed extract in various concentrations has been described as useful.

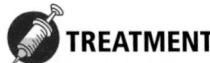 MEDICATION (DRUGS)

First Line
- Acute bacterial and chronic otitis externa
  - Neomycin/polymyxin B/hydrocortisone (Cortisporin) 5 drops q.i.d.—if the tympanic membrane is ruptured, use the suspension; otherwise, the solution may be used. May be ototoxic and resistance developing in *Staph* and *Strep* species. (2)[B]
  - Betamethazone 0.05% solution was more effective than a polymyxin B combination without risk of ototoxicity or antibiotic resistance. (3)[A]
  - 2% acetic acid with 1% hydrocortisone (VoSoL HC) 3–5 drops q4–8h ×7d. May cause local stinging. As effective as neomycin/polymyxin B. (4)[B] Inexpensive. May be option for 3rd-world settings.
  - A wick may be helpful in severe cases by keeping the canal open and keeping antibiotic solution in contact with infected skin. (5)[C]
  - Oral antibiotics are indicated only if there is associated otitis media or cellulitis of the outer ear.
  - Analgesics as needed, narcotics may be necessary
- Fungal otitis externa
  - Topical therapy, antiyeast for *Candida* or yeast: 2% acetic acid 3–4 drops q.i.d.; clotrimazole 1% solution; itraconazole oral
  - Parenteral antifungal therapy: Amphotericin B
  - Patients with Ramsay Hunt syndrome: Acyclovir IV
- Eczematous otitis externa: Topical therapy
  - Acetic acid 2% in aluminum acetate
  - Aluminum acetate (5%; Burow solution)
  - Steroid cream, lotion, ointment (e.g., triamcinolone 0.1% solution)
  - Antibacterial, if superinfected

- Necrotizing otitis externa
  - Parenteral antibiotics: Antistaphylococcal and antipseudomonal
  - 4–6 weeks of therapy
  - Quinolones PO for 2–4 weeks
- Contraindications
  - Hypersensitivity to topical or parenteral therapy
  - Renal or hepatic failure when using amphotericin B
- Precautions
  - Dosage adjustment for amphotericin B in patients with renal or hepatic dysfunction
  - Sensitivity with neomycin
- Significant possible interactions
  - Hypokalemia associated with amphotericin B may lead to digitalis toxicity.
  - Concurrent administration of nonabsorbable anions, such as carbenicillin, may exacerbate hypokalemia.

Second Line

- Ciprofloxacin (Ciprodex) 0.3% and dexamethisone 0.1% suspension 3–4 drops b.i.d. × 7d (1)[B]
- Ciprofloxacin (Cipro HC) 0.2% and hydrocortisone 1% suspension 3–4 drops b.i.d. × 7d.
- Ofloxacin (Floxin Otic) 0.3% solution 10 drops once a day
- Azole antifungals for fungal otitis externa

SURGERY

For necrotizing otitis externa or furuncle

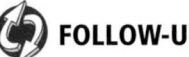 **FOLLOW-UP**

DISPOSITION

Admission Criteria

Necrotizing otitis media requiring parenteral antipsuedomonal antibiotics

Discharge Criteria

Resolution of infection

Issues for Referral

Resistant cases or those requiring surgical intervention

PROGNOSIS

- Acute otitis externa: Rapid response to therapy with total resolution
- Chronic otitis externa: With repeated cleansing and antibiotic therapy, most cases will resolve. Occasionally, surgical intervention is required for resistant cases.
- Eczematous otitis externa: Resolution will occur with control of the primary skin condition.
- Necrotizing otitis externa: Can usually be managed with débridement and antipseudomonal antibiotics. Recurrence rate is 100% when treatment is inadequate. Surgical intervention may be necessary in resistant cases or if there is cranial nerve involvement. Mortality rate is significant, probably secondary to the underlying disease.

COMPLICATIONS

- Mainly a problem with necrotizing otitis externa; may spread to infect contiguous bone and CNS structures
- Acute otitis externa may spread to pinna, causing chondritis.

PATIENT MONITORING

- Acute otitis externa
  - 48 hours after therapy instituted to assess improvement
  - At the end of treatment
- Chronic otitis externa
  - Every 2–3 weeks for repeated cleansing of canal
  - May require alterations in topical medication, including antibiotics and steroids
- Necrotizing otitis externa
  - Daily monitoring in hospital for extension of infection
  - Baseline auditory and vestibular testing at beginning and end of therapy

REFERENCES

1. Roland P, et al. Efficacy and safety of topical ciprofloxacin/dexamethasone versus neomycin/polymixin B/hydrocortisone for otitis externa. *Curr Med Res Opin*. 2004;20(8): 1175–1183.
2. Cantrell H, et al. Declining susceptibility to Neomycin and Polymixin B of pathogens recovered in otitis externa clinical trials. *South Med J*. 2004;97(5): 465–471.
3. Emgard P, Hellstrom S. A group III steroid solution without antibiotic components: An effective cure for otitis media. *J Laryngol Otol*. 2005;119:342–347.
4. van Balen F, et al. Clinical efficacy of 3 common treatments in acute otitis externa in primary care: Randomized controlled trial. *Brit Med J*. 2003; 327:1201–1203.
5. Block S. Otitis externa: Providing relief while avoiding complications. *J Fam Pract*. 2005;54(8): 669–676.

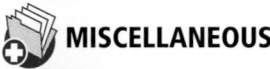 **MISCELLANEOUS**

CODES

ICD9-CM
380.10 Infective otitis externa, unspecified

PATIENT TEACHING

Prevention
- Avoid trauma to ear canal such as by cotton swabs.
- Ear plugs for swimming or drying agents such as alcohol and acetic acid solutions after swimming

 See Corresponding Diagnostic Algorithm

 See Patient Handout on CD

O

OTITIS MEDIA

Mohammad Alhabbal, MD

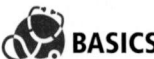

BASICS

DESCRIPTION
- Infection or inflammation of the middle ear
- Acute otitis media (AOM): Infection of the middle ear following a viral upper respiratory infection (URI); rapid onset of signs and symptoms
- Recurrent AOM: ≥3 episodes in 6 months, or ≥4 episodes in 1 year
- Otitis media with effusion (OME): Persistent inflammation manifested as asymptomatic middle ear fluid that follows AOM or arises without prior AOM
- Chronic otitis media with or without cholesteatoma
- System(s) Affected: Nervous
- Synonym(s): Secretory otitis media; Serous otitis media

ALERT
Pediatric Considerations
Primarily a pediatric disease

GENERAL PREVENTION
- Breast-feeding decreases incidence of AOM.
- Eliminate cigarette smoking in the household.
- The heptavalent pneumococcal conjugate vaccine (with nontoxic diphtheria-toxin analog carrier protein, CRM197) is safe, decreases AOM caused by the *S. pneumoniae* serotypes included in the vaccine, and has slightly decreased the overall incidence of disease.

EPIDEMIOLOGY
- Predominant age: Peak incidence age 6–18 months; declines >7 years; rare in adults. 80–90% percent of children have at least 1 episode by age 3.
- Predominant sex: Male > Female (for AOM and recurrent AOM)
- Placement of tympanostomy tubes is 2nd only to circumcision as the most frequent surgical procedure in infants.

Incidence
By age 7 years, 93% of children have had 1 or more episodes of AOM; 39% have had 6 or more episodes. After AOM, 10–20% still have OME 3 months later.

RISK FACTORS
- Bottle feeding while supine
- Day care attendance
- Formula feeding/pacifier
- Smoking in household
- Male gender
- Family history of middle ear disease
- AOM in 1st year of life is a risk factor for recurrent AOM.
- Sibling history of otitis media
- Underlying disease (e.g., cleft palate, Down syndrome, allergic rhinitis)

Genetics
May be influenced by skull configuration or immunologic defects

ETIOLOGY
- AOM, bacterial: A preceding viral URI produces eustachian tube dysfunction that may increase risk of infection:
  - Pneumococci: 40%
  - *Haemophilus influenzae*: 20–25%; 40% of these produce β-lactamases that hydrolyze amoxicillin and some cephalosporins.
  - *Moraxella (Branhamella) catarrhalis*: 10–15%; 90% of these produce β-lactamases that hydrolyze amoxicillin and some cephalosporins.
  - Group A streptococci: 3%
  - *Staphylococcus aureus*: 12%
  - Sterile/nonpathogens: 25–30%
- AOM, viral
  - ~15% of AOM infections are caused primarily by viruses (respiratory syncytial virus, parainfluenza, influenza, enteroviruses, adenovirus).
- OME
  - 20–40% silent bacterial infection
  - Eustachian tube dysfunction thought important
  - Allergic causes rarely substantiated

ASSOCIATED CONDITIONS
- URI
- Bacteremia
- Meningitis
- Allergies

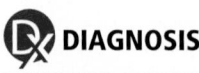

DIAGNOSIS

SIGNS AND SYMPTOMS
- AOM: Acute history, signs and symptoms of middle ear inflammation, and middle ear effusion
  - Earache
  - Fever, although more often afebrile
  - Accompanying URI symptoms
  - Decreased hearing
  - Otorrhea if eardrum is perforated
  - Unusual irritability
  - Difficulty in sleeping
  - Tugging at the ear
  - Loss of balance
  - Decreased eardrum mobility (as observed by pneumatic otoscopy)
  - Eardrum bulging, opaque, often yellowish or inflamed. Redness alone is not a reliable sign.
- AOM in infants
  - May cause no symptoms in the 1st few months of life
  - Irritability is sometimes the only indication of earache.
  - Eardrum bulging, opaque, often yellowish or inflamed. Redness alone is not a reliable sign.
- OME
  - Usually asymptomatic
  - Decreased hearing probably universal but not always measurable, and rarely appreciated by parents
  - Eardrum often dull, but not bulging
  - Decreased eardrum mobility (as observed by pneumatic otoscopy)

TESTS
- To document the presence of middle ear fluid: Tympanometry, acoustic reflex measurement, or acoustic reflectometry
- Hearing testing helpful to assess the need for early surgical intervention in OME
- Nasopharyngoscopy

Lab
WBC count is higher in bacterial AOM than in sterile AOM.

Diagnostic Procedures/Surgery
Tympanocentesis for microbiologic diagnosis recommended for treatment failures; may be followed by myringotomy

DIFFERENTIAL DIAGNOSIS
- Tympanosclerosis
- Redness because of crying
- Earache with a normal ear examination may be caused by referred pain from the jaw or teeth.

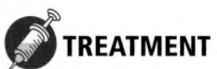

TREATMENT

INITIAL STABILIZATION
Outpatient treatment except when surgery is indicated

GENERAL MEASURES
- AOM: Outpatient except for febrile infants <2 months old
- The American Academy of Pediatrics/American Association of Family Physicians guideline committee recommends the following criteria for observation vs. antibacterial therapy
  - Antibacterial therapy should be administered to any child <6 months of age, regardless of the degree of diagnostic certainty. (3)[B]
  - Children 6 months–2 years: Antibacterial therapy is recommended when the diagnosis of AOM is certain or the illness is severe (moderate to severe otalgia or fever ≥39°C in the previous 24 hours). [A]
  - Children >2 years: Antibacterial therapy is recommended if the diagnosis is certain and the illness is severe. Observation is an option when the diagnosis is certain but illness is not severe, and the patient is with uncertain diagnosis. (3)[B]
- OME: Presence of effusion without signs or symptoms of acute infection does not require antibiotics for initial treatment.
- Antihistamine/decongestant preparations offer no added benefit to resolution of symptoms.

Diet
No special diet

Activity
No restrictions

MEDICATION (DRUGS)

Eighty-one percent of patients >2 years of age resolve without the use of antibiotics.

First Line

- AOM: Amoxicillin ()[B] 40–45 mg/kg b.i.d. in children >2 years old, 5–7 day course with no complications, 10-day course for children <2 years old [C]; probably the most effective of penicillins/cephalosporins against relatively resistant (but not highly resistant) pneumococci

- If Penicillin allergic: Azithromycin (10 mg/kg/d [maximum dose 500 mg/d] as a single dose on day 1 and 5 mg/kg/d [maximum dose 250 mg/d] for days 2–5)

- Recurrent AOM: Consider antibiotic prophylaxis only for recurrent AOM (>3 distinct, well-documented episodes in 6 months)—amoxicillin 20 mg/kg/d for 3–6 months or until summer

- OME: Antihistamines and decongestants are ineffective. (3)[B] Indications for steroids are not defined.
  - Promotes resolution in 10–15%, but effect is usually transitory—not recommended; no long-term benefit.

- NOTE: If patient does not appear toxic and is >2 years, you may choose to treat with antipyrine/benzocaine drops and acetaminophen as long as close follow-up is available.
- Contraindications: Allergy to penicillins
- Precautions: Refer to the manufacturer's profile of each drug.
- Significant possible interactions: Refer to the manufacturer's profile of each drug.

Second Line

- Alternative drugs are indicated for the following AOM patients with
  - Allergy
  - Persistent symptoms after 48–72 hours of amoxicillin
  - AOM within 1 month of amoxicillin therapy
  - Severe earache
  - Age <6 months, with high fever
  - Immunocompromised
  - AOM caused by *Chlamydia trachomatis*—will respond to macrolides and sulfonamides
  - AOM caused by *Mycoplasma pneumoniae*—will respond to macrolides
- For AOM (treat for 10 days)
  - Amoxicillin/clavulanate [B] 40 mg/kg/d of amoxicillin component t.i.d.: Effective against resistant *H. influenzae* and *M. catarrhalis*; amoxicillin component effective against relatively resistant pneumococci
    - 40 mg/kg/d b.i.d.–t.i.d.: Less effective than other alternatives
    - 8 mg/kg/d b.i.d. or single daily dose: Effective against resistant *H. influenzae* and *M. catarrhalis*; less effective than amoxicillin for pneumococci
    - 10 mg/kg/d b.i.d.: Less effective in vivo against *H. influenzae* than are other drugs
    - 50 mg/kg IM single dose: Effective against major pathogens but expensive and painful, so reserved for sick infants

- 10 mg/kg (max 500 mg/d) on day 1, then 5 mg/kg × 4 days (5-day course)
- 15 mg/kg/d b.i.d.: Not effective in vivo against *H. influenzae*
  - TMP/sulfamethoxazole 8 mg TMP/kg/d b.i.d.: Up to 30% of pneumococci are resistant
  - Sulfisoxazole 40 mg erythromycin component/kg/d q.i.d.: Some strains of pneumococci are resistant.
- Recurrent AOM: 75 mg/kg in single daily dose for penicillin-allergic patients
- Analgesics and antipyretics as needed

SURGERY

- OME: Referral for surgery if: >4–6 months bilateral OME, and/or >6 months unilateral OME, and/or hearing loss >25 decibels
- Recurrent AOM: Referral for surgery if >2 or 3 AOM episodes occur while on chemoprophylaxis. Tympanostomy tubes and adenoidectomy/adenotonsillectomy are effective surgical procedures for OME and recurrent AOM, but not in all cases.

 FOLLOW-UP

PROGNOSIS

- Children treated immediately with antibiotics usually have <1 day of symptoms.
- Symptoms of AOM (mostly otalgia) spontaneously resolve in 2/3 of children by 24 hours and in 80% at 2–7 days (number needed to treat = 17)
- AOM: Symptoms usually improve in 48–72 hours; OME following AOM resolves in 90% by 3 months.
- OME: ~50% resolve after 8 weeks of observation.
- Recurrent AOM and OME: Usually subsides in school-age children; only a small percentage have complications.

COMPLICATIONS

- AOM
  - Perforation/otorrhea
  - Acute mastoiditis
  - Facial nerve paralysis
  - Otitic hydrocephalus
  - Meningitis
  - Hearing impairment
- OME
  - Hearing loss
  - Speech and language disabilities may occur with hearing impairment.
- Recurrent AOM and OME
  - Atrophy and scarring of eardrum
  - Chronic perforation and otorrhea
  - Cholesteatoma
  - Permanent hearing loss
  - Chronic mastoiditis
  - Brain abscess
  - Other intracranial suppurative complications

PATIENT MONITORING

- AOM: Otoscopic examination 4 weeks after diagnosis
- OME: Monthly otoscopic or tympanometric exams as long as OME persists

REFERENCES

1. Eskola J, et al. Efficacy of pneumococcal conjugate vaccine against acute otitis media. *N Engl J Med.* 2001;344:403–409.
2. Bluestone CD, Klein JO, eds. Otitis Media in Infants and Children, 3rd ed., Philadelphia: WB Saunders, 2001.
3. McConaghy JR. The evaluation and treatment of children with acute otitis media. *J Fam Pract.* 2001;50:457–457, 463–465.
4. Flyn C, Griffin G, Schultz J. Decongestants and antihistamines for acute otitis media in children. *Cochrane Database Sys Rev.* 2004;3:CD001727.
5. Turner D, et al. Acute otitis media in infants younger than 2 months of age: Microbiology, clinical presentation and therapeutic approach. *Pediatr Infect Dis J.* 2002;21:669.

 MISCELLANEOUS

CODES

ICD9-CM

- 381.00 Acute nonsuppurative otitis media, unspecified
- 382.00 Acute suppurative otitis media without spontaneous rupture of eardrum
- 382.9 Unspecified otitis media

PATIENT TEACHING

 See Corresponding Diagnostic Algorithm

 See Patient Handout on CD

O

OTOSCLEROSIS (OTOSPONGIOSIS)

Jeffrey D. Wolfrey, BA

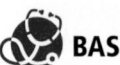 **BASICS**

DESCRIPTION
- A primary bone dyscrasia involving the otic capsule. It is the leading cause of conductive hearing loss in adults.
- Histologic otosclerosis: Asymptomatic form in which abnormal bone spares vital structures of the ear
- Clinical otosclerosis: Abnormal spongy bone involves ossicular chain or other structures, leading to altered physiology
- System(s) Affected: Nervous

EPIDEMIOLOGY
- Predominant age
  - Clinical onset usually in early 20s.
  - Peak incidence in 4th and 5th decades
- Predominant sex: Female > Male (2:1)

Prevalence
- 4–8% among whites; 1% among African Americans (histologic form)
- Whites: 5000/100,000; African Americans: 1000/100,000 (histologic form)

RISK FACTORS
Unknown

Genetics
- 60% of those affected give positive family history
- Appears to be transmitted by autosomal dominant gene with variable penetrance

ETIOLOGY
- Unknown
- Some authorities believe that fluoride metabolism plays a role.

ASSOCIATED CONDITIONS
- Van der Hoeve syndrome (rare triad of osteogenesis imperfecta, blue sclera, and otospongiosis)
- Tinnitus
- Vertigo

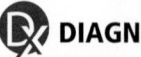 **DIAGNOSIS**

SIGNS AND SYMPTOMS
- Progressive conductive hearing loss, usually with well-preserved speech discrimination
- May have sensorineural hearing loss with cochlear involvement
- Carhart notch: A dip in bone conductive threshold at 2,000 Hz on audiometric testing
- Schwartze sign: Reddish hue on promontory at otoscopic examination
- Patients often soft spoken and aware they seem to hear better in noisy environments

ALERT
Pregnancy Considerations
Progression may accelerate during pregnancy. Some women 1st notice hearing loss at this time.

TESTS
Tuning fork and audiometric testing for conductive and/or sensorineural hearing loss
- Will lateralize to more impaired ear with Weber test

Imaging
Coaxial or CT sometimes helpful

Pathological Findings
- Gross
  - Off-white to reddish bone formation, most often located anterior to the oval window and extending to involve the stapedial footplate. Sometimes covers entire oval window (obliterative). May be found anywhere in otic capsule
  - Bilateral in 75% of cases
- Micro
  - Spongy-appearing bone with increased vascular spaces
  - Osteoblasts and osteoclasts are plentiful.

DIFFERENTIAL DIAGNOSIS
- Chronic suppurative otitis media
- Serous otitis media
- External auditory canal occlusion
- Ossicular chain disruption
- Congenital fixation of stapes
- Presbycusis
- Advanced otosclerosis mimics sensorineural deafness

ALERT
- Important differential diagnosis for presbycusis
- Surgical results similar in older vs. younger patient cohorts (1)[A]

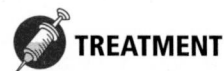 **TREATMENT**

GENERAL MEASURES
Hearing aids

Diet
No special diet

Activity
No restrictions

MEDICATION (DRUGS)

- No specific drug therapy, but sodium fluoride, vitamin D, and calcium gluconate have been tried, especially in cases of predominantly sensorineural hearing loss
- Contraindications: Refer to the manufacturer's literature for each drug.
- Precautions: Refer to the manufacturer's literature for each drug.
- Significant possible interactions: Refer to the manufacturer's literature for each drug.

SURGERY
- Surgical correction (stapedectomy)
  - Usually involves mobilization or removal of the stapedial foot plate with placement of a stapes prosthesis
  - Recent procedural innovations have involved use of lasers.
  - Cochlear implantation may achieve better results in advanced cases. (2)[B]
- Relative indications for surgery include negative Rinne test (air-bone audiometric gap at least 20 dB) or bilateral involvement

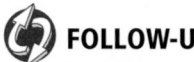 **FOLLOW-UP**

DISPOSITION
- Inpatient for surgery
- Outpatient if surgery not feasible

PROGNOSIS
- Progressive hearing loss if not treated
- Surgery improves hearing by at least 15 dB in 90% of cases

COMPLICATIONS
Surgical risks include chorda tympani nerve injury, tympanic membrane laceration, ossicular chain disruption, otitis media and externa, labyrinthitis, granuloma formation, perilymph fistulae, and total deafness ("dead ear")

PATIENT MONITORING
Interval audiometric testing

REFERENCES

1. Meyer TA, Lambert PR. Primary and revision stapedectomy in elderly patients. *Curr Opin Otolaryngol Head Neck Surg.* 2004;12(5):387–392.
2. Berrettini S, et al. Far advanced otosclerosis: Stapes surgery or cochlear implantation? *J Otolaryngol.* 2004;33(3):165–171.
3. Lee KJ: *Essential Otolaryngology: Head & Neck Surgery.* 4th ed. New Hyde Park, NY: Medical Examination Publishing; 1987.
4. Weber PC, Klein AJ. Hearing loss. *Med Clin North Amer.* 1999;83:125–137.

 MISCELLANEOUS

See also: Hearing loss

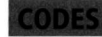 **CODES**

ICD9-CM
387.9 Otosclerosis, unspecified

PATIENT TEACHING
- Because speech discrimination is usually preserved, patients should be advised of the possible benefit from hearing aids (as an alternative or adjunct to surgery).
- Mayo Foundation for Medical Education and Research, Section of Patient and Health Education, Sieber Subway, Rochester, MN 55905; (507) 284-8140.

O

OVARIAN CANCER

Laura J. Sacco, MD

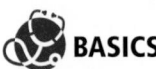 **BASICS**

DESCRIPTION
A variety of malignancies that arise from the epithelium (85–90%), stromal cells, or germ cells, or are metastatic to the ovary. These include:

- Epithelial
  - Serous (fallopian tubelike epithelium)
  - Mucinous (cervical and gastrointestinal mucinous epithelium)
  - Endometrioid (endometrial epithelium)
  - Clear cell (mesonephroid)
  - Brenner (transitional cell epithelium)
  - Carcinosarcoma and mixed mesodermal
- Stromal
  - Granulosa cell tumor
  - Theca cell tumor
  - Sertoli-Leydig cell tumors
  - Gynandroblastoma
  - Lipid cell tumor
- Germ cell
  - Teratoma (mature [e.g., dermoid cyst] and immature)
  - Dysgerminoma
  - Embryonal carcinoma
  - Gonadoblastoma
  - Endodermal sinus tumor
  - Embryonal carcinoma
  - Choriocarcinoma
- Metastatic disease from
  - Breast
  - Endometrium
  - Lymphoma
  - Gastrointestinal tract (Krukenberg tumor)
- System(s) Affected: Endocrine/Metabolic; Gastrointestinal; Reproductive

ALERT
Pregnancy Considerations
Dermoid cyst and serous cystadenoma most common

GENERAL PREVENTION
For epithelial cancer, frequency of ovulation appears to be important. The following factors are protective
- Use of oral contraceptives
- Multiparity
- Late menarche
- Early menopause
  - Premenopausal women without contraindications should be encouraged to use oral contraceptive pills (OCPs). The progestin component of OCPs may protect against ovarian cancer by regulating apoptosis of the ovarian epithelium.
  - Recent studies have shown that no clear association exists between ovarian cancer and use of ovulation induction agents such as Clomiphene, however more long-term studies are necessary. (1)[B]
  - Oral contraceptives, NSAIDs and acetaminophen use have been shown to reduce risk of ovarian cancer. (2)[B]
  - Women with family histories of ovarian cancer (2 or more 1st-degree relatives) should be counseled concerning cancer risk. (3)[B]

- Patients with hereditary ovarian cancer syndromes should be counseled about prophylactic oophorectomy after childbearing is completed or by age 35. (3)[B] Even after oophorectomy, a small risk exists of developing intra-abdominal carcinomatosis histologically identical to ovarian carcinoma.

- Screening: No adequate or cost-effective screening measures are available for ovarian cancer.
  - The routine use of CA-125 and transvaginal ultrasound for screening is currently discouraged. Annual pelvic examinations are recommended, particularly in postmenopausal women. An adnexal mass in a premenarchal female or a palpable adnexa in a postmenopausal female warrants immediate further evaluation.
  - Women with a family history of a hereditary ovarian cancer syndrome should undergo pelvic examinations, CA-125, and transvaginal ultrasonography every 6–12 months.

EPIDEMIOLOGY
Predominant age
- Epithelial: 40–75 years
- Germ cell malignancies: Usually observed in patients age <20 years

Incidence
In the US
- Per year: 26,500 new cases; 14,500 deaths per year
- Leading cause of gynecologic cancer death in women. Mortality of ovarian cancer has not decreased significantly during the last 6 decades.

Prevalence
One in 70 women develop disease.

RISK FACTORS
- Family history
  - Multiple genetic factors.
- Environmental factors as yet undefined.
- Infertile patients are at a higher risk for ovarian cancer than the general population

Genetics
- For a woman who has a 1st-degree relative with a history of ovarian cancer, her risk for disease increases from 1.4–5%. With 2 or more such relatives, lifetime risk is 7%
- Hereditary ovarian cancer syndromes
  - Risk of developing ovarian cancer increases to 40–50%
  - Breast/ovarian cancer syndrome: Early onset breast or ovarian cancer, autosomal-dominant transmission, usually associated with BRCA-1 mutation
  - Lynch II syndrome: Autosomal dominant inheritance, increased risk for colorectal, endometrial, stomach, small bowel, breast, pancreas, and ovarian cancers. Defect in mismatch repair genes
- In women diagnosed with breast cancer prior to the age of 40, the risk for ovarian cancer increases by 60%. If this same woman has a family history of either breast or ovarian cancer in a 1st-degree relative, then her risk for ovarian cancer increases 17-fold more than a woman without breast cancer. Consequently, women with onset of breast cancer prior to age 40 should be monitored for ovarian cancer.

ETIOLOGY
Unknown

ASSOCIATED CONDITIONS
- Ascites
- Pleural effusion
- Decrease of serum albumin
- Breast carcinoma
- Bowel obstruction

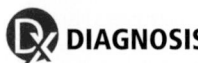 **DIAGNOSIS**

SIGNS AND SYMPTOMS
- Often vague and nonspecific; often relate to pressure on surrounding abdominopelvic organs
- Vague gastrointestinal symptoms, such as early satiety
- Bloating and dyspepsia
- Sense of abdominal fullness
- Abdominopelvic cramping
- Occasional vaginal discharge
- Irregular vaginal bleeding
- Urinary frequency in absence of infection
- Fatigue
- Dyspareunia
- Weight loss/loss of appetite
- Severe pain secondary to ovarian rupture or torsion; seen with germ-cell tumors
- Precocious puberty (choriocarcinoma, embryonal carcinoma)

Physical Exam
- Increased abdominal girth
- Ascites
- Cul-de-sac and/or pelvic nodularity
- Pelvic mass
- Hirsutism in androgen-secreting germ cell tumors

TESTS
Lab
- CA-125 (normal <35 u/mL); not to be used as a screening test
- Liver function tests (LFTs) to rule out hepatic involvement
- CBC
- Urinalysis
- Carcinoembryonic antigen (CEA) if gastrointestinal primary suspected
- Chorionic gonadotropin (β-hCG [dysgerminoma, choriocarcinoma, embryonal carcinoma]), α-fetoprotein (endodermal sinus tumor, embryonal carcinoma), LDH (dysgerminoma), or inhibin (granulosa cell tumor)
- Disorders that may alter lab results: CA-125 may be elevated with gynecologic disease (endometriosis, peritonitis, myomas, pelvic inflammatory disease, Meigs syndrome) and with CHF, pancreatitis, systemic lupus erythematosus, or liver disease.

Imaging
- Pelvic ultrasound
- Chest radiograph
- Mammogram
- Abdominopelvic CT scan with contrast
- IV pyelograph (IVP)
- Barium enema only as warranted.

Diagnostic Procedures/Surgery
- Surgery is definitive.
- Paracentesis for cytology is not advised.
- Endometrial biopsy if menstrual abnormalities

Pathological Findings
At surgery, most common: Epithelial ovarian cancer

DIFFERENTIAL DIAGNOSIS
- Gastrointestinal or gynecologic malignancies
- Irritable bowel syndrome
- Colitis
- Hepatic failure with ascites
- Diverticulitis
- Tubo-ovarian abscess
- Uterine fibroids
- Pelvic kidney

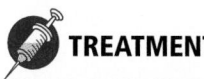 TREATMENT

INITIAL STABILIZATION
Inpatient

GENERAL MEASURES
Diet
- High-protein diet
- Follow serum protein with significant ascites.

Activity
As tolerated

 MEDICATION (DRUGS)

First Line
- Chemotherapy: Women with stage 1a grade 1 and most 1b grade 1 tumors do not require adjuvant therapy. Patients with clear cell carcinomas, grade 3 tumors, or tumors staged at 1c or worse require adjuvant therapy. Patients should be encouraged to participate in clinical trials whenever possible.
- Paclitaxel (Taxol) is recommended in combination therapy with platinum as the 1st-line treatment of epithelial ovarian cancer. (4)[A]
- Carboplatin is the platinum drug of choice in both single and combination therapy. (4)[A]
- Doxorubicin with disease progression within 6 months of therapy with 1st-line chemotherapeutic agents such as Taxol and Carboplatin
- Intraperitoneal (IP) chemotherapy in combination with IV chemotherapy shown to increase survival with advanced ovarian cancer. (5)[A] IP chemotherapy was associated with more adverse effects during treatment.
- Contraindications: Patient too ill to receive chemotherapy, excessive toxicity, hypersensitivity
- Precautions: All regimens cause bone marrow suppression. Cisplatin associated with ototoxicity, renal toxicity, and peripheral neuropathy. Taxol can cause neutropenia and neuropathy.
- Significant possible interactions: Refer to manufacturer's literature.

Second Line
- Etoposide
- 5-Fluorouracil
- Doxorubicin (Adriamycin)
- Cyclophosphamide
- Tamoxifen may be used in recurrent disease when chemotherapy is not appropriate. (6)[C]
- Other members of the alkylating agent family (melphalan, hexamethylmelamine, ifosfamide [with mesna to protect against hemorrhagic cystitis], thiotepa)

- Ondansetron (Zofran), dronabinol (Marinol), metoclopramide (Reglan), prochlorperazine (Compazine), promethazine (Phenergan)

SURGERY
- Surgical staging and optimal debulking are critical. Maximal cytoreduction of tumor burden enhances effectiveness of adjuvant therapy; associated with longer survival.
- For epithelial malignancies staging, tumor excision/debulking includes
  - Peritoneal fluid (or washings from peritoneal lavage) is aspirated and cytology evaluated.
  - Omentum is biopsied or excised
  - Peritoneal surfaces inspected and palpated
  - Cytologic smear of right hemidiaphragmatic
  - Biopsy of adhesions
  - Biopsy of paracolic recesses, pelvic side walls, and bladder cul-de-sac
  - Pelvic and para-aortic lymph node biopsy
  - Total abdominal hysterectomy–bilateral salpingo-oophorectomy (TAH-BSO) and extirpation of any masses as feasible
- Germ-cell cancers (less likely to be bilateral)
  - Salpingo-oophorectomy (unilateral if only 1 ovary involved) in young patient
  - Careful staging, including lymph node dissection, may be adequate

 FOLLOW-UP

PROGNOSIS
- 5-year survival rates for ovarian cancer based on FIGO data

Stage I:	a 84%,	b 79%,	c 73%
Stage II:	a 65%,	b 54%,	c 51%
Stage III:	a 52%,	b 29%,	c 18%
Stage IV:	14%		

- In germ-cell and stromal tumors, outcome is related to histologic cell type in addition to clinical stage and histologic grade.
- In epithelial cell cancers, prognosis is determined by stage, histologic grade, and the amount of residual disease rather than the histologic cell type.

ALERT
Geriatric Considerations
Poorer prognosis compared with younger patients

COMPLICATIONS
- Pleural effusion
- Pseudomyxoma peritonei
- Ascites
- Radiotherapy and chemotherapy adverse reactions
- Bowel obstruction
- Malnutrition
- Electrolyte disturbances
- Fistula formation

PATIENT MONITORING
- A sevenfold fall in CA-125 suggests a good response, but normal values correlate poorly (<50%) with absence of disease. Persistent elevations reflect a poor response to therapy.
- A rise in CA-125 usually requires a change in therapy, whereas an inadequate drop after 3 courses of chemotherapy may require a change.
- In germ-cell cancers, serum markers should fall to normal range.
- Regular pelvic exams and Pap smears

REFERENCES
1. Brinton LA, Lamb EJ, Moghissi KS, et al. Ovarian cancer risk after the use of ovulation-stimulating drugs. *Obstet Gynecol.* 2004;103(6): 1194–203.
2. Schildkraut JM, Moorman PG, Halabi S, et al. Analgesic drug use and risk of ovarian cancer. *Epidemiology.* 2006;17(1):104–107.
3. Genetic Risk Assessment and BRCA mutation testing for breast and ovarian cancer susceptibility: Recommendation statement. *ACP Journal Club.* 2006;144(2):37.
4. Scottish Intercollegiate Guidelines Network (SIGN). Epithelial ovarian cancer. A national clinical guideline. Scottish Intercollegiate Guidelines Network (SIGN) 2003;75:36.
5. Jaaback K, Johnson N. Intraperitoneal chemotherapy for the initial management of primary epithelial ovarian cancer. *Cochrane Database of Systematic Reviews.* 2006;1.
6. Williams CJ, Simera I. Tamoxifen for relapse of ovarian cancer. *Cochrane Database of Systematic Reviews.* 2006;1.

 MISCELLANEOUS

Patients <65 years have a better prognosis because they present in earlier stage.

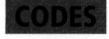 CODES

ICD9-CM
183.0 Malignant neoplasm of ovary

PATIENT TEACHING
What You Need to Know About Ovarian Cancer and Chemotherapy and You: A Guide to Self-Help During Treatment. National Institutes of Health pamphlets

 See Corresponding Diagnostic Algorithm

OVARIAN HYPERSTIMULATION SYNDROME (OHSS)

Kimberly E. Liu, MD
Ellen Greenblatt, MD

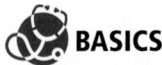 **BASICS**

DESCRIPTION

OHSS is an iatrogenic physiologic complication of controlled ovarian hyperstimulation (most often related to treatment for infertility). This results in ovarian enlargement, increased vascular permeability with resultant 3rd space loss and intravascular fluid depletion, electrolyte imbalance, hemoconcentration and ascites.

- Symptom(s): Onset during the luteal phase or early pregnancy during a cycle of controlled ovarian hyperstimulation (COH) or assisted reproduction.
- System(s) Affected: Reproductive; Hemic/Lymphatic/Immunologic; Renal/Urologic

GENERAL PREVENTION

If a patient is noted to be at high risk of OHSS, the stimulation and monitoring protocol may be modified to reflect this risk. In some circumstances, consideration should be given to canceling the stimulation by withholding the preovulatory injection of human chorionic gonadotropins (hCG). (1)[B]

EPIDEMIOLOGY

- Predominant age: Women of reproductive age
- Predominant sex: Female

Incidence

With in-vitro fertilization

- Mild OHSS: 20–33% of cycles
- Moderate OHSS: 3–6% of cycles
- Severe OHSS: 0.1–2% of cycles

RISK FACTORS

- Previous history of OHSS
- Young age
- Low body weight
- High doses of gonadotropins
- Large number of intermediate sized follicles
- Number of oocytes retrieved
- Rapidly rising estradiol levels
- High estradiol levels
- Use of hCG for luteal support
- Polycystic ovarian syndrome (PCOS) or polycystic ovaries on ultrasound
- Achievement of a pregnancy
- Multiple pregnancy

Genetics

None

PATHOPHYSIOLOGY

- Ovarian hyperstimulation leads to increased capillary permeability and intravascular fluid shifts
- Fluid shifts can lead to ascites and pleural effusions
- Intravascular volume depletion can lead to hemoconcentration, decreased renal perfusion and thrombosis.
- The ovarian renin-angiotensin system, cytokines, prostaglandins and other inflammatory mediators may play a role in the pathophysiology of OHSS.

ETIOLOGY

- OHSS is an iatrogenic syndrome which occurs during COH for infertility treatment.
- Generally, OHSS is associated with the use of exogenous gonadotrophins such as purified luteinizing hormone and follicle stimulating hormone.

ASSOCIATED CONDITIONS

- Infertility
- PCOS
- Assisted reproductive technologies

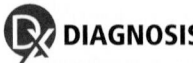 **DIAGNOSIS**

SIGNS AND SYMPTOMS

- Abdominal discomfort/bloating
- Nausea, vomiting, diarrhea
- Loss of appetite
- Lethargy
- Shortness of breath
- Rapid weight gain
- Oliguria/anuria
- Hemoconcentration
- Leukocytosis
- Hypovolemia
- Hyponatremia
- Hyperkalemia
- Ascites
- Pleural effusions
- Pericardial effusions
- Hypercoagulability
- Thrombotic events
- Adult respiratory distress syndrome
- Multiple organ failure

History

- Details of stimulation cycle
  - Medications used
  - Date of oocyte retrieval and embryo transfer
- Symptoms of dehydration
- Abdominal pain and distention
- Weight changes
- Fluid intake
- Shortness of breath

Physical Exam

- Vital signs
- Weight
- Chest and cardiovascular exam

ALERT

Pelvic and abdominal exams are contraindicated to avoid ovarian hemorrhage or rupture.

TESTS

OHSS is a clinical diagnosis based on history, physical examination, ultrasound findings, and laboratory results.

Lab

- Hemoconcentration (hematocrit >50% indicates severe disease)
- Leukocytosis
- Hyponatremia
- Hyperkalemia
- Decreased renal function
- Increased liver enzymes

Imaging

- Abdominal/pelvic ultrasound to assess ovarian size, ovarian torsion or rupture, and abdominal ascites
- Chest x-ray to evaluate pleural effusion in presence of shortness of breath

Diagnostic Procedures/Surgery

- None

Pathological Findings

- Ovarian enlargement
- Decreased renal perfusion
- Thromboembolism
- Abdominal ascites
- Pleural effusions
- Pericardial effusions

DIFFERENTIAL DIAGNOSIS

- Hemorrhagic ovarian cyst
- Ovarian torsion

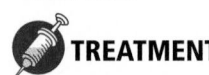 **TREATMENT**

- Mild OHSS
  - Oral fluid intake at least 1 L/d
  - Daily weight
  - Avoid physical exertion or abdominal trauma
  - Monitor for development of further symptoms
  - Self-limiting
  - Frequent follow-up required
- Moderate or severe OHSS
  - Admit to hospital for further management

INITIAL STABILIZATION

Vital signs and O₂ saturation

GENERAL MEASURES

- Daily body weight determination
- Frequent monitoring of vital signs
- Strict monitoring of input and output
- Monitoring of hemotocrit, hemoglobin and leukocyte count, creatinine, and electrolytes and liver enzymes
- Intensive monitoring may be required for pulmonary support in cases of acute respiratory distress syndrome or for renal failure
- Anticoagulation prophylaxis (2)[C]

Diet

- Outpatient management
  - Oral intake of 1.0–1.5 L daily of balanced salt solution (sports drink) is recommended.
  - Record daily weight and urine output.
- Inpatient management
  - In the initial phase of hospitalization, patients may feel too nauseated to eat or drink. Once 3rd-space edema re-enters the intravascular space, hemoconcentration reverses, and the patient begins to spontaneously diurese. Fluid restriction at this point may prevent hemodilution.

Activity

Bed rest or reduced activity. The enlarged ovaries are at risk of torsion and ovarian hemorrhage spontaneously, or from injury or trauma.

SPECIAL THERAPY

- Ascites should not be treated with diuretics because of the risk of intravascular fluid depletion
- Paracentesis/Thoracentesis may be required for symptomatic control and for pulmonary and/or renal compromise. A transvaginal ultrasound–guided approach is recommended to avoid the enlarged ovaries.

IV Fluids
- Hypovolemia requires fluid resuscitation with crystalloid solutions.
- Patients who cannot sustain adequate urine output with crystalloids may need 25% albumin.

Complementary and Alternative Therapies
None

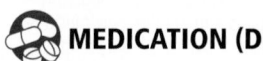 ## MEDICATION (DRUGS)

First Line
Heparin 5,000 U SC q8–12h. Hospitalized patients should be on anticoagulation prophylaxis to prevent thrombotic events. (2)[C]

SURGERY
Surgery should be avoided whenever possible in these patients. In a situation of ovarian torsion, surgery may be performed to attempt to revascularize the ovary by unwinding the adnexa. When ovarian hemorrhage is suspected, surgery may be necessary. The goal should be hemostasis, and the ovaries should be conserved when possible.

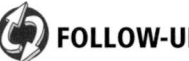 ## FOLLOW-UP

Once discharged from hospital, patients should continue to be followed closely with readmission to hospital as clinically indicated.

Admission Criteria
- Abdominal pain suspicious of torsion or hemorrhage
- Intolerance of food or liquids
- Hypotension
- Abdominal ascites or plural effusions
- Hemoconcentration
  - Hct >50%, WBC >25,000
- Hyponatremia (Na <135 mEq/L)
- Hyperkalemia (K >5.0 mEq/L)

Discharge Criteria
- Tolerating oral liquids and diet
- Resolution of hemoconcentration and electrolyte imbalances
- Adequate urine output

Issues for Referral
Should be referred and followed by a reproductive endocrinology specialist until resolution of symptoms

PROGNOSIS
OHSS is a self-limiting disease that will run its course over 10–14 days in the absence of an ensuing pregnancy, and may persist for weeks in the pregnant patient. Supportive treatment is initiated to prevent further deterioration of the patient's condition.

COMPLICATIONS
- Ovarian hemorrhage
- Ovarian torsion
- Arterial and venous thrombosis
- Adult respiratory distress syndrome
- Liver failure
- Renal failure

PATIENT MONITORING
- Patients discharged from the hospital should be followed with frequent health care provider contact until symptom resolution.
- Patients who have conceived should have an early ultrasound to confirm pregnancy and rule out multiple gestations, and then routine antenatal care as indicated by their pregnancy

ALERT
Pregnancy Considerations
- Patients who conceive a multiple gestation are at higher risk of OHSS.

- Several studies have shown an increased risk of spontaneous abortion, prematurity, low birth weight, pregnancy-induced hypertension, and gestational diabetes in women who had severe OHSS. (3)[B]

REFERENCES
1. Delvigne A, Rozenberg S. Epidemiology and prevention of ovarian hyperstimulation syndrome (OHSS): A review. *Hum Reprod Update*. 2002; 8:559–577.
2. Whelan J, Vlahos N. The ovarian hyperstimulation syndrome. *Fertil Steril*. 2000;73:883–896.
3. Abramov Y, Elchalal U, Schenker J. Obstetric outcome of in vitro fertilization pregnancies complicated by severe ovarian hyperstimulation syndrome: A multicenter study. *Fertil Steril*. 1998;70:1070–1076.

 ## MISCELLANEOUS

See also: Polycystic Ovarian Disease; Ovarian Tumor, Benign

CODES

ICD9-CM
256.1 Other ovarian hyperfunction

PATIENT TEACHING
- OHSS is a self-limiting disease. Patients who have conceived may have a longer course; however, the disease will often resolve within 2 weeks. Supportive measures are the only treatment until the disease runs its course.
- Patients who have had OHSS are more at risk for OHSS in the future, and this should be taken into consideration in their next treatment cycles
- Consume 1.0–1.5 L/d of a balanced salt solution such as a sports drink.
- Monitor their oral intake and urinary output
- Reduced activity or bed rest to avoid abdominal trauma or impact
- Patients need to inform their health care providers of a history of OHSS when considering further assisted reproductive technology treatment.

O

OVARIAN TUMOR (BENIGN)

Mary Anne Condon, NP, PhD

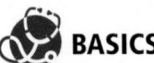 BASICS

DESCRIPTION
- The ovaries are a source of many tumor types (benign and malignant) because of the histologic variety of their constituent cells.
- Benign ovarian tumors create difficulties in differential diagnosis because of the need to identify malignancy and discriminate a tumor from cysts, infectious lesions, ectopic pregnancy, and endometriomas.
- The tumors are often clinically silent until well developed; they may be solid, cystic, or mixed; and they may be functional (producing sex steroids, as with arrhenoblastomas and gynandroblastomas) or nonfunctional.
- System(s) Affected: Endocrine/Metabolic; Reproductive

ALERT
Geriatric Considerations
Because incidence of malignancy increases with age, postmenopausal patients warrant comprehensive evaluation and follow-up.

Pediatric Considerations
Malignancy must be ruled out in premenarchal patients. Early neonatal cysts are rare.

GENERAL PREVENTION
- Although oral contraceptives do not appear to increase rates of cyst resorption, they do decrease risk for forming new ovarian cysts.
- A large British cohort of 5,479 women demonstrated that the resection of benign cysts has no impact on future risk for ovarian cancer.

EPIDEMIOLOGY
Predominant age: Premenopausal; concern for malignancy greater in premenarchal girls and postmenopausal women

Incidence
- 30% of regularly cycling females
- 50% of women without regular cycles

RISK FACTORS
- As yet poorly characterized for benign tumors. Cigarette smoking increases the relative risk for developing functional ovarian cysts 2-fold.
- Possible contributory factors are early menarche, obesity, infertility, and hypothyroidism.

ETIOLOGY
- Endometriosis with localized, repeated ovarian hemorrhage
- Physiologic cysts
- Tumorigenesis, with genetics as yet poorly defined

DIAGNOSIS

SIGNS AND SYMPTOMS
- Usually asymptomatic
- Pain related to torsion, endometriosis, or rupture
- Increased abdominal girth
- Bowel pressure or bladder pressure sensations
- Menstrual irregularities
- Hirsutism or sexual precocity
- Early satiety
- Dyspepsia/bloating
- Severe acne
- Deepening of the voice
- Dyspareunia
- Virilization

History
Careful history is important

Physical Exam
Pelvic exam is single most important diagnostic approach

TESTS
Lab
- CBC
- Pregnancy test
- Urinalysis
- Endometrial biopsy or dilatation/curettage if mass accompanied by menstrual abnormality
- Pap smear
- Erythrocyte sedimentation rate
- Guaiac stool testing
- Serum tumor markers as indicated
  - Cancer antigen 125
  - α-Fetoprotein
  - Chorionic gonadotropin (hCG)
  - Serum lactate dehydrogenase
  - Serum estrogens and androgens
- Disorders that may alter lab results
  - CA 125: Endometriosis, peritonitis, pelvic inflammatory disease (PID), Meigs syndrome, uterine fibroids, hepatitis, pancreatitis, systemic lupus erythematosus, diverticulitis
  - hCG: Pregnancy, hydatidiform mole
  - Lactate dehydrogenase: Liver disease, drug-induced hepatotoxicity
  - α-Fetoprotein: Hepatocellular carcinoma, hepatic cirrhosis, acute or chronic hepatitis

Imaging
- Cystoscopy if hematuria is present in the absence of infection or if IV pyelogram reveals intravesical surface irregularity
- Cystometry if urinary symptoms are not explained by extrinsic compression
- Transabdominal or transvaginal ultrasonography may differentiate tumors from other pelvic lesions and identify features that place the patient at greater risk for malignancy (solid component, papillations, multiple septations, ascites, bilaterality, fixed and irregular, rapidly enlarging, accompanied by cul-de-sac nodules).
- Sonography may be the best means to determine the architecture of an ovarian cyst or mass.
- Color flow Doppler evaluation may also be helpful.
- Abdominopelvic CT scan with contrast
- Barium enema, colonoscopy, or IV pyelogram as indicated
- MRI with ADC mapping (apparent diffusion coefficient values) may be useful in the differential diagnosis of cystic masses.

Diagnostic Procedures/Surgery
Exploratory laparoscopy or laparotomy

Pathological Findings
- Follicular (fluid distention of atretic follicle) and corpus luteum cysts (corpus luteum hematoma)
- Endometrioma
- Pregnancy luteoma (composed of hyperplastic stromal theca-lutein cells)
- Serous and mucinous cystadenomas and mixed serous/mucinous cystadenomas
- Granulosa cell tumors
- Benign connective tissue tumors (thecomas, fibromas, Brenner tumors)
- Cystic teratoma (dermoid cyst)
- Germinal inclusion cyst (regarded by some as the precursor for epithelial ovarian cancer)

ALERT
Pregnancy Considerations
- The majority of cysts discovered during pregnancy are corpus luteum or follicular cysts.
- The 2 most commonly encountered tumors during pregnancy are cystadenomas (serous or mucinous) and dermoid cysts.

DIFFERENTIAL DIAGNOSIS
- Ovarian malignancies
- Endometrioma
- Uterine leiomyoma
- Appendicular cysts
- Diverticulitis or bowel abscess
- PID with tubo-ovarian abscess
- Distended urinary bladder
- Ectopic pregnancy
- Hydrosalpinx
- Functional cysts (follicular and corpus luteum cysts)
- Polycystic ovaries

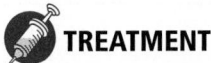 **TREATMENT**

GENERAL MEASURES
- In premenopausal patients with cystic lesions <10 cm in diameter, simple observation for 4–6 weeks is acceptable. No evidence suggests that use of a contraceptive pill is more effective than time alone in facilitating ovarian cyst resorption.
- If the cyst remains unchanged after 4–6 weeks of observation, then surgical exploration is indicated.
- Appropriate health care: Inpatient if surgery necessary

Diet
No special diet

Activity
As tolerated

 MEDICATION (DRUGS)

- Oral contraceptives decrease risk for forming new ovarian cysts.
- Contraindications: Those established for oral contraceptive pills (e.g., hypercoagulable state or history of DVT, ischemic heart disease, history of cerebrovascular accident, hypertension, hepatic adenoma, smoking after the age of 35 years)

SURGERY
- Cystectomy or wedge resection for cyst with benign features
- Surgical removal of tumor to establish diagnosis when
  – Premenopausal cysts >5 cm that persist >6–8 weeks
  – Mass that is solid
  – Mass >10 cm
  – Mass in a premenarchal or postmenopausal female
  – Suspicion of torsion or rupture
  – Postmenopausal cysts
  – Cysts with worrisome ultrasound features (e.g., papillations)

 FOLLOW-UP

PROGNOSIS
Complete cure

COMPLICATIONS
Complications of untreated dermoid and mucinous cysts may include rupture and pseudomyxoma peritonei.

PATIENT MONITORING
- Most require only yearly exams
- Varies by diagnosis

REFERENCES

1. Benacerrif BR, et al. Sonographic accuracy in the diagnosis of ovarian masses. *J Reprod Med*. 1990;35:491–495.
2. Bird C, et al. Benign neoplasms of the ovary. In: Sciarra J, Droegemueller W, eds. Clinical Gynecology. Philadelphia: JB Lippincott, 1990.
3. Crayford TJB, et al. Benign ovarian cysts and ovarian cancer: A cohort study with implications for screening. *Lancet*. 2000;355:1060–1063.
4. DiSaia PJ, Creasman WT. *Clinical Gynecologic Oncology*, 5th ed. St Louis: Mosby, 1997.
5. Drake J. Diagnosis and management of the adnexal mass. *Am Fam Physician*. 1998; 57:2471–2476.
6. Hillard PA. Benign diseases of the female reproductive tract: Symptoms and signs. In: Berek JS, Adashi EY, Hillard PA, eds. Novak's Gynecology, 12th ed. Baltimore: Williams & Wilkins, 1996.
7. Jones HW. Ovarian cysts and tumors. In: Jones HW, Wentz AC, Burnett LS, eds. Novak's Textbook of Gynecology, 11th ed. Baltimore: Williams & Wilkins, 1988.
8. Mishell DR. Noncontraceptive benefits of oral contraceptives. *J Reprod Med*. 1993;38: 1021–1029.
9. Steinkampt MP, Hammond KR, Blackwell RE. Hormonal treatment of functional ovarian cysts: A randomized, prospective study. *Fertil Steril*. 1990;54:775–777.
10. Turan C, et al. Expectant management of functional ovarian cysts: An alternative to hormonal therapy. *Int J Gynaecol Obstet*. 1994; 47:257–260.
11. Nakayama T, Yoshimitsu K, Irie H, et al. Diffusion-weighted echo-planar MR imaging and ADC mapping in the differential diagnosis ovarian cystic masses: Usefulness of detecting keratinoid substances in mature cystic teratomas. *J Magn Reson Imag*. 2005;22(2):271–278.
12. Holt V, Crushing-Haugen K, Daling J. Oral contraceptives, tubal sterilization, and functional ovarian cyst risk. *Obstet Gynecol*. 2003;102(2): 252–258.

ADDITIONAL READING

- Labarge PY, Levesque S. 2006. Short-term morbidity and long-term recurrence rate of ovarian dermoid cysts treated by laparoscopy versus laparotomy. *J Obstet Gynecol Can*. 2006;28(9):789–793. [B]
- Borgfeldt C, Andolf E. Cancer risk after hospital discharge diagnosis of benign ovarian cysts and endometriosis. *Acta Obstet Gynecol Scand*. 2004; 83(4):395. [B]

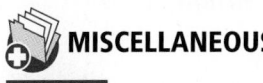 **MISCELLANEOUS**

CODES

ICD9-CM
220 Benign neoplasm of ovary

PATIENT TEACHING
A variety of excellent patient education materials (e.g., "Ovarian Cyst") can be downloaded from the American Association of Family Physicians and American College of Obstetricians and Gynecologists Internet sites, available at http://www.aafp.org/afp and http://www.acog.com.

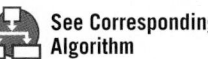 **See Corresponding Diagnostic Algorithm**

O

PAGET DISEASE OF THE BREAST

Mark C. Horattas, MD

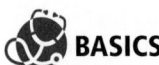 **BASICS**

DESCRIPTION
Rare type of carcinoma that appears unilaterally as dermatitis of the nipple, representing an extension to the epidermis of an underlying carcinoma of a mammary duct
System(s) Affected: Skin/Exocrine

GENERAL PREVENTION
None known

EPIDEMIOLOGY
- Predominant age: 40–75 years old
- Predominant sex: Female

Incidence
In the US
- 1,000–4,000 new cases each year
- ~1–2% of all cases of breast cancer

RISK FACTORS
Same as for nonheritable breast carcinoma
- Early menarche
- Late menopause
- Nulliparity
- 1st birth >30 years
- Family history of breast cancer
- History of radiation exposure
- History of alcohol use
- Proliferative benign breast disease

Genetics
No known genetic pattern

ETIOLOGY
The cause is unknown, but certain women seem to be at a higher risk of developing any type of breast cancer.

ASSOCIATED CONDITIONS
Underlying carcinoma

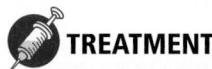 **DIAGNOSIS**

SIGNS AND SYMPTOMS
- Nipple skin changes that do not respond to conservative treatment
- Nipple itching
- Nipple burning
- Nipple oozing
- Nipple bleeding
- Eczematoid nipple changes
- Breast mass
- Nipple fissures
- Nipple ulceration
- Local hyperemia
- Local edema

TESTS
Imaging
Mammography: Useful, but cannot exclude malignancy without clinicopathologic correlation

Diagnostic Procedures/Surgery
Any chronic or nonhealing nipple lesion should be biopsied.

Pathological Findings
- Micro: Malignant cell invasion of the epidermis with large pale staining cells
- Underlying ductal adenocarcinoma

DIFFERENTIAL DIAGNOSIS
- Eczema
- Psoriasis
- Skin tumors (e.g., Bowen disease)
- Squamous cell carcinoma
- Basal cell carcinoma

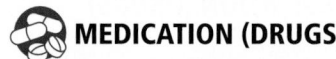 **TREATMENT**

GENERAL MEASURES
- Appropriate health care
  - Treatment of the underlying breast cancer with surgery. Additional adjuvant chemotherapy and/or radiation therapy dependent on cancer histology, size, and stage
- Radiotherapy
- Chemotherapy
- Hormonal manipulation

Diet
No special diet

Activity
Full activity

MEDICATION (DRUGS)

- Chemotherapy per oncology study protocols
  - Doxorubicin (Adriamycin)-based regimen
  - Cyclophosphamide, methotrexate, 5-fluorouracil (CMF)
  - Tamoxifen
  - Paclitaxel (Taxol)
- Contraindications: Refer to the manufacturer's literature for each drug.
- Precautions: Refer to the manufacturer's literature for each drug.
- Significant possible interactions: Refer to the manufacturer's literature for each drug.

SURGERY
To be determined by specific situation

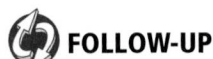 **FOLLOW-UP**

PROGNOSIS
Dependent on stage of underlying breast carcinoma; see Table 1

Table 1

Stage	10 yr*
1 <2-cm tumor; − nodes	70–95%
2 >2-cm tumor or + nodes	40–45%
3 >5-cm tumor; + nodes or fixed nodes	10–15%
4 Metastatic disease	<5%

*10-year disease-free survival

COMPLICATIONS
Metastases

PATIENT MONITORING
Routine screening for women >40 years
- Annual mammogram
- Monthly self-exams
- Annual physician exams

REFERENCES
1. Bland KI, Copeland EM, eds. *The Breast*. Philadelphia, PA: WB Saunders; 1998.
2. DeVita VT Jr, Hellman S, Rosenberg A, eds. *Cancer: Principles and Practices of Oncology*. 5th ed. Philadelphia, PA: JB Lippincott; 1997.
3. Fitzpatrick TB, et al., eds. *Dermatology in General Medicine*. 5th ed. New York, NY: McGraw-Hill; 1999.

 MISCELLANEOUS
- See also: Breast cancer
- Other notes: Extramammary Paget disease can also occur.

CODES

ICD9-CM
- 174.0 Malignant neoplasm of female breast, nipple and areola
- 174.9 Malignant neoplasm of female breast, unspecified

PATIENT TEACHING
National Cancer Institute, Department of Health and Human Services, Public Inquiries Section, Office of Cancer Communications, Building 31, Room 101-18, 9000 Rockville Pike, Bethesda, MD 20892; (301) 496-5583

See Corresponding Diagnostic Algorithm

PANCREATIC CANCER

Venu G. Pillarisetty, MD
Ruben Peralta, MD, FACS

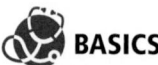 **BASICS**

DESCRIPTION
- Pancreatic malignancies represent only 2% of all cancers, but are the 4th leading cause of cancer deaths in the US (SEER A); 90% of all pancreatic tumors are adenocarcinomas; 5-year survival for pancreatic adenocarcinoma is 4%.
- Pancreatic cancers include exocrine tumors (adenocarcinoma, cystadenocarcinoma, and acinar cell carcinoma) and endocrine/islet cell tumors (insulinoma, gastrinoma, and other secretory tumors).
- Exocrine tumors are divided into 2 broad categories
  - Periampullary lesions: Most commonly adenocarcinoma of the head of the pancreas. Of lesser frequency are malignant lesions of the ampulla, duodenum, and common bile duct. Lesions in these areas are characterized by jaundice, weight loss, and abdominal pain.
  - Lesions of the body and tail account for 25% of adenocarcinomas of the pancreas. Because of their retroperitoneal location and distance from the common bile duct, lesions are usually large at diagnosis. Common symptoms are weight loss and pain.
- Endocrine tumors are rare; 85% secrete biologically active substances, resulting in specific clinical syndromes.

GENERAL PREVENTION
Smoking, diabetes, and obesity are risk factors.

EPIDEMIOLOGY
- Mean age: 80% occur between ages 60 and 80
- Sex: Male < Female (1.5:1–2:1)

Incidence
~32,000 new cases diagnosed per year in the US

Prevalence
Highest in African Americans and Hawaiians

ALERT
Geriatric Considerations
More common in this age group, especially men

RISK FACTORS
- Probable
  - Race
  - Diabetes mellitus
  - Tobacco use
- Possible
  - Environmental/occupational exposures
  - Dietary lipids
  - Genetic predisposition in individuals with chronic familial pancreatitis, Peutz-Jeghers syndrome, and familial polyposis

Genetics
Research suggests pancreatic cancer could be due to mismatch repair genes, tumor suppressors, and oncogenes.

ETIOLOGY
- Not known, although many associations exist
- Association with chronic pancreatitis is controversial.

ASSOCIATED CONDITIONS
- Diabetes
- Other findings associated with metastases, for example, superior vena cava syndrome, Horner syndrome

DIAGNOSIS

SIGNS AND SYMPTOMS
- Weight loss
- Abdominal or back pain, often worse in supine position
- Anorexia
- Diabetes mellitus
- Malnutrition
- Hepatomegaly
- Palpable gallbladder
- Abdominal tenderness
- Mass
- Ascites
- For tumors in the head of the pancreas obstructing the bile duct: Jaundice, pruritus, dark urine, acholic stools.

TESTS
Lab
- Bilirubin level mean of 15 mg/dL (256.5 μmol/L); higher than in benign diseases
- Recent onset of jaundice, bilirubin > 10 mg/dL (171.0 μmol/L); consider neoplastic obstruction of common bile duct until proven otherwise.
- Alkaline phosphatase: Mean of 550 U/L not significantly different from level in patients with bile duct obstruction from benign disease
- Anemia in ~60% of patients
- Stool occult blood present in ~90% of patients with periampullary tumors
- Elevated amylase found in <5% of patients
- Gastrin, insulin may be elevated when endocrine/islet cell is tumor present
- Tumor markers: No definitive screening
  - CA 19-9 is the primary marker used at present. ~80% of patients with pancreatic cancer have serum CA 19-9 levels >37 mcg/mL. Also elevated in acute pancreatitis (30%), chronic pancreatitis (10%), biliary tract disease (20%), and chronic liver disease (20%).
  - Carcinoembryonic antigen (CEA) is elevated in ~50% of patients, most of whom are nonresectable for cure.
- Anemia, prolonged prothrombin time given malnutrition and malabsorption of fat-soluble vitamins.

Imaging
- Some controversy as to best imaging option because accuracy varies with site and size of tumor
- Helical CT scan is considered most useful imaging technique, with sensitivity of 90% and specificity of 95%; provides the ability to determine resectability based on the relationship of tumor to the superior mesenteric vein and artery.
- Abdominal ultrasound is useful initial screen in patients presenting with jaundice. It is falling out of favor because it is not useful for staging and accuracy, is operator dependent, and limited by overlying bowel.
- Endoscopic retrograde cholangiopancreatography (ERCP): Patients with suspected cancer in whom CT or ultrasound does not reveal a mass lesion within the pancreas and in those in whom the differential diagnosis includes chronic pancreatitis. Allows for biopsy

- MRI/magnetic resonance cholangiopancreatography: Sensitivity/specificity similar to ERCP
- Endoscopic ultrasonography (EUS): Increasingly studied as diagnostic tool. Appears useful in diagnosis of small tumors (<2–3 cm in diameter) and allows for fine-needle aspiration of tissue during exam. Operator dependent

Diagnostic Procedures/Surgery
- Pancreatic secretions for cytology and CEA, CA 19-9 assays
- Biopsy
  - CT-guided percutaneous needle aspiration has sensitivity of 85% with specificity of ~100% in pancreatic adenocarcinoma. Few complications and extremely low risk of tract seeding
  - EUS-guided fine-needle biopsy is gaining popularity for diagnosis/staging.
  - Pseudocyst aspiration can differentiate benign pseudocysts from cystadenocarcinoma. Fluid in cystadenocarcinoma has low amylase and high CEA and lactate dehydrogenase levels; malignant cells usually are present.
  - Liver biopsy may be useful in patients with hepatic metastases.
  - Laparoscopy with ultrasonography and biopsy is becoming a popular staging technique.

Pathological Findings
- Review of resected ductal pancreatic cancer reveals pancreatic intra-epithelial neoplasia (PanIN) in the ducts and ductules, likely a precursor lesion to invasive cancer (1)[B]
- Adenocarcinoma (90%)
- Acinar cell carcinoma (1.2%)
- Other (0.8%)
- Uncertain (9.2%)

DIFFERENTIAL DIAGNOSIS
- Choledocholithiasis
- Pancreatitis
- Pancreatic pseudocyst
- Cholangiocarcinoma
- Carcinoma of the ampulla of Vater
- Duodenal neoplasms
- Endocrine tumors of pancreas
- Miscellaneous malignancies with extrinsic bile duct compression
- Biliary tract stricture
- Choledochal cyst

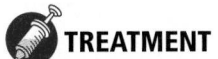 **TREATMENT**

INITIAL STABILIZATION
Inpatient treatment for testing, preliminary therapy, surgery, or other protocols

GENERAL MEASURES
- Management is highly variable and influenced by the overall health of the patient, presence of metastases, and location and size of tumor.
- Analgesia
- Management of pruritus
- Control of diabetes (usually brittle) if total pancreatectomy performed
- Nonoperative procedures
  - Biliary decompression by use of endoprostheses, transhepatic drainage catheters
  - Celiac blockade and epidural catheter placement for analgesia
  - Chemotherapy: Multiple protocols
  - Radiation therapy: External beam (intraoperative, largely investigational)
  - Duodenal endoprosthesis for malignant duodenal obstruction

Diet
As tolerated; small, frequent meals

Activity
As tolerated

 MEDICATION (DRUGS)

- Analgesics
- Antacids
- Agents to manage pruritus, for example, phenothiazines, cholestyramine
- Chemotherapy: Multiple protocols (2)[B]
  - Typically either gemcitabine monotherapy or in combination with 5-FU or cisplatin
  - Pancreatic enzymes
- Diabetes control

SURGERY
- Surgery is the definitive treatment, but only 10–20% of tumors are considered resectable at time of diagnosis given metastases, invasion of inferior vena cava, aorta, celiac axis, or superior mesenteric artery. (3)[B]
- Preoperative staging most often uses spiral CT with oral and intravenous contrast.
- Possible surgical procedures include
  - Pancreaticoduodenectomy (Whipple procedure)
  - Total pancreatectomy
  - Regional pancreatectomy: Resection of pancreas, portal vein, regional nodes; subtotal gastrectomy
  - Biliary decompression for unresectable disease: T-tube, bilioenteric anastomoses
  - Gastrojejunostomy for gastric outlet obstruction in unresectable disease

 FOLLOW-UP

PROGNOSIS
- Overall 5-year survival rate is <5% given high likelihood of metastasis at time of diagnosis and is <1% if tumor is nonresectable at time of diagnosis.
- Only treatment modality with potential for cure is surgical resection.

COMPLICATIONS
- Pain
- Jaundice
- Malnutrition
- Diabetes, especially in patients undergoing total pancreatectomy
- Operative mortality varies from 10–40%

PATIENT MONITORING
Variable

REFERENCES
1. Wilentz RE, Hruban RH. Pathology of cancer of the pancreas. *Surg Oncol Clin North Amer*. 1998;7:43.
2. Willett CG, Clark JW. Update on combined-modality treatment options for pancreatic cancer. *Oncology*. 2003;17:29–36.
3. Freelove R, Walling AD. Pancreatic cancer: Diagnosis and management. *Am Fam Phys*. 2006;73:485–492.
4. Surveillance, epidemiology, and end results (SEER) program (www.seer.cancer.gov)
5. El-Rayes BF, Philip PA. A review of systemic therapy for advanced pancreatic cancer. *Clin Adv Hematol Oncol*. 2003;1(7):430–434.
6. American Gastroenterological Association technical review on the epidemiology, diagnosis, and treatment of pancreatic ductal adenocarcinoma. *Gastroenterology*. 1999;117:1463–1464.

 MISCELLANEOUS

See also: Pancreatitis

CODES

ICD9-CM
- 157.0 Malignant neoplasm of head of pancreas
- 157.9 Malignant neoplasm of pancreas, part unspecified

PATIENT TEACHING
Printed patient information is available from the National Cancer Institute, Department of Health and Human Services, Public Inquiries Section, Office of Cancer Communications, Building 31, Room 101-18, 9000 Rockville Pike, Bethesda, MD 20892; (301) 496-5583.

See Corresponding Diagnostic Algorithm

PANCREATITIS

Frank J. Domino, MD

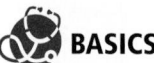 **BASICS**

DESCRIPTION
- Acute pancreatitis: An acute inflammatory process of the pancreas with variable involvement of regional or remote tissues
  - Inflammatory episode with symptoms related to intrapancreatic activation of enzymes with pain, nausea, and vomiting, and associated intestinal ileus
  - Varies widely in severity, complications, and prognosis
- Chronic pancreatitis: Irreversible
  - Progressive destruction of the pancreas
  - Results in both exocrine and endocrine deficiencies
  - Pain, maldigestion, and diabetes mellitus are the major features.
- System(s) Affected: Gastrointestinal

GENERAL PREVENTION
- Avoidance of alcohol
- Correction of underlying causes, for example, hyperlipidemia, drug use, adult respiratory distress syndrome, gallstones

EPIDEMIOLOGY
- Predominant age
  - Acute pancreatitis: None
  - Chronic pancreatitis: 35–45 years (usually related to alcohol)
- Predominant sex: Male = Female

Incidence
One to 5 per 10,000

Prevalence
- Acute: 19/10,000
- Chronic: 8.3/10,000

RISK FACTORS
See "Etiology."

Genetics
Hereditary pancreatitis is a rare condition with an autosomally dominant inheritance pattern.

PATHOPHYSIOLOGY
- Acute pancreatitis: Autodigestion of the pancreas, interstitial edema, hemorrhage, cell and fat necrosis
- Chronic pancreatitis: Calcification, fibrosis

ETIOLOGY
- Gallstones/microlithiasis
- Alcohol
- Trauma/surgery
- Acute discontinuation of medications for diabetes or hyperlipidemia
- Following endoscopic retrograde cholangiopancreatography (ERCP)
- Medications
  - AIDS therapy
  - Antimicrobials
  - Diuretics
  - Therapy for inflammatory bowel disease
  - Immunosuppressants
  - Neuropsychiatric therapies
  - Others
- Metabolic causes
  - Hypertriglyceridemia
  - Hypercalcemia
  - Renal failure

- Hereditary causes
- Systemic lupus erythematosus
- Infections
  - Mumps
  - Coxsackie B
  - Hepatitis A and B
  - Ascariasis
  - Salmonellosis
- Penetrating peptic ulcer (rare)
- Cystic fibrosis and CFTR gene mutations
- Tumors (e.g., ampullary)
- Idiopathic
- Pancreas divisum
- Scorpion venom
- Sphincter of Oddi dysfunction
- Vascular disease
- Acute fatty liver of pregnancy

ALERT

Geriatric Considerations
Vascular disease is possible

Pediatric Considerations
Mumps are sometimes complicated by pancreatitis.

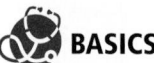 **DIAGNOSIS**

SIGNS AND SYMPTOMS
- Similar to an acute abdomen of any cause
- Abdominal pain: Epigastric; may radiate into back
- Nausea and/or vomiting
- Other
  - Fever
  - Hypotension/shock
  - Jaundice
  - Ileus
  - Pleural effusion
- Special (rare)
  - Flank discoloration (Grey Turner sign)
  - Umbilical discoloration (Cullen sign)

History
- Acute pancreatitis
  - Alcohol use
  - Family history of gallstones
  - Medication use
- Chronic pancreatitis
  - Alcohol use
  - Signs of steatorrhea
  - Signs of hyperglycemia

TESTS

Lab
- No test is 100% sensitive or specific.
- Acute pancreatitis
  - Elevated serum amylase (amylase P)
  - Elevated serum lipase
  - Elevated (mild) alanine aminotransferase and/or aspartate aminotransferase, when associated with alcoholic hepatitis or choledocholithiasis
  - Elevated alkaline phosphatase (mild), when associated with alcoholic hepatitis or choledocholithiasis
  - Hyperbilirubinemia, when associated with alcoholic hepatitis or choledocholithiasis
  - Glucose increased, in severe disease
  - Calcium decreased, in severe disease
  - WBCs: 10,000–25,000/L

- Chronic pancreatitis
  - Tests sometimes normal
  - Hyperglycemia
  - Steatorrhea
  - Flare-ups may mimic acute pancreatitis
  - Elevated alkaline phosphatase, bilirubin
- Drugs that may alter results: Insulin and corticosteroids
- Disorders that may alter results
  - Biliary tract disease
  - Penetrating peptic ulcer
  - Intestinal obstruction
  - Intestinal ischemia/infarction
  - Ruptured ectopic pregnancy
  - Renal insufficiency
  - Burns
  - Macroamylasemia, macrolipasemia

Imaging
- Acute pancreatitis
  - Plain film of abdomen: Signs of ileus
  - Chest radiograph: Pleural effusion
  - Ultrasound/CT scan of abdomen/MRI
  - ERCP
- Chronic pancreatitis
  - Radiograph of abdomen: Pancreatic calcification
  - Ultrasound and/or CT scan of abdomen: Pseudocyst formation/calcification
  - ERCP/magnetic resonance cholangiopancreatography: Ductal deformity, retained common bile duct stone, pancreatic duct stones and strictures
  - Endoscopic ultrasound

Diagnostic Procedures/Surgery
- Acute pancreatitis
  - CT-guided aspiration of necrotic areas
  - ERCP for common duct stone removal
- Chronic pancreatitis (tests of endocrine function)
  - Secretin stimulation test
  - Secretin/chymotrypsin
  - Stool fat

DIFFERENTIAL DIAGNOSIS
- Acute pancreatitis
  - Penetrating or perforated peptic ulcer
  - Acute cholecystitis
  - Choledocholithiasis
  - Macroamylasemia, macrolipasemia
  - Mesenteric vascular obstruction and/or infarction
  - Perforation of a viscus
  - Intestinal obstruction
  - Aortic aneurysm
- Chronic pancreatitis
  - Pancreatic cancer
  - Other malabsorptive processes
  - Other cause of biliary obstruction

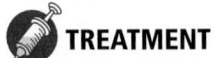 TREATMENT

INITIAL STABILIZATION

- Acute pancreatitis: Hospitalization, unless very mild and patient can maintain oral intake
- Chronic pancreatitis: Outpatient treatment except for complications

GENERAL MEASURES

- Acute pancreatitis
  - P—pain control: Meperidine
  - A—arrest shock: IV fluids
  - N—nasogastric tube for vomiting
  - C—calcium monitoring
  - R—renal evaluation
  - E—ensure pulmonary function
  - A—antibiotics
  - S—surgery or special procedures in selected cases
- Chronic pancreatitis
  - Pain: Alcohol abstinence, analgesia (avoid narcotics if possible), celiac ganglion block, surgery, pancreatic enzyme preparations
  - Maldigestion: Pancreatic enzyme supplements, histamine (H$_2$)-blockers
  - Diabetes mellitus: Insulin

Diet

- Acute pancreatitis: Begin diet after pain, tenderness, and ileus have resolved; small amounts of high-carbohydrate, low-fat, and low-protein foods. Advance as tolerated. Nothing by mouth or nasogastric tube if patient is vomiting.
- Total parenteral nutrition if oral is not tolerated (no lipids if triglycerides are increased)
- Chronic pancreatitis: Small meals high in protein. Adjust if diabetes mellitus is present.

Activity

- Acute pancreatitis: Usually bed rest, although sitting in a chair may be more comfortable
- Chronic pancreatitis: Not restricted

 MEDICATION (DRUGS)

- Acute pancreatitis: Meperidine (Demerol) 50–100 mg IM/IV q3–4h
- Antibiotics
- Somatostatin
- Chronic pancreatitis
  - Analgesics: Acetaminophen (Tylenol), acetaminophen/oxycodone (Tylox), acetaminophen-hydrocodone (Vicodin), propoxyphene napsylate
  - Pancreatic enzyme supplements (Pancrease MT, Creon)
  - H$_2$-blockers (reducing gastric acid increases availability of pancreatic enzymes)
- Contraindications
  - Normeperidine, a metabolite of meperidine, may accumulate following several days of around-the-clock dosing. May cause mental status changes or seizures.
  - Antibiotic allergy
- Precautions: Narcotic addiction
- Significant possible interactions: Refer to the manufacturer's profile of each drug.

SURGERY

- Acute pancreatitis—infected necrosis: Peritoneal lavage
- Chronic pancreatitis—pain: Pseudocyst drainage

 FOLLOW-UP

DISPOSITION

Admission Criteria

- Acute pancreatitis
  - Abdominal pain
  - Nausea/Vomiting
  - Ileus
  - Shock
- Chronic pancreatitis
  - Uncontrolled pain
  - Malnutrition

Discharge Criteria

- Acute pancreatitis:
  - Pain control
  - Diet tolerance
  - Etiology determined
  - Alcohol rehab, if needed

PROGNOSIS

- Acute pancreatitis: 85–90% resolve spontaneously; 3–5% mortality. APACHE II scoring is most accurate but difficult to apply; Ranson Criteria (see below) has a sensitivity of ~40%:
  - On admission: Age >55 years, WBCs >16,000/mm, blood glucose >200 mg/dL (11.1 mmol/L), serum lactate dehydrogenase >350 IU/L, serum glutamic-oxaloacetic transaminase (AST) >250 IU/L
  - Within 48 hours: Hematocrit decrease >10%, serum calcium <8 mg/dL, blood urea nitrogen increase >8 mg/dL, arterial PO$_2$ <60 mm Hg, base deficit >4 mEq/L, fluid retention >6 L
  - Ranson scoring
    - Ranson score of 0–2: Minimal mortality
    - Ranson score of 3–5: 10–20% mortality
    - Ranson score of >5: >50% mortality
- Chronic pancreatitis: Patient may have recurrent episodes of acute pancreatitis; slow progression; may "burn out" with resolution of symptoms. Narcotic addiction frequently occurs.

COMPLICATIONS

- Acute pancreatitis
  - Infection
  - Pseudocyst
  - Abscess
  - Systemic: Encephalopathy, fat necrosis, splenic hematuria
- Chronic pancreatitis
  - Pseudocyst/abscess
  - Duodenal/biliary stenosis
  - Fistulae
  - Cancer (4% lifetime risk)
  - Diabetes
  - Splenic vein thrombosis

PATIENT MONITORING

- Ensure alcohol abstinence.
- Follow-up and correct any etiologic cause, such as hypertriglyceridemia, choledocholithiasis.
- Persistent elevation of amylase weeks after acute pancreatitis suggests possibility of pseudocyst; perform imaging study.

REFERENCES

1. Anderson MA. Severity assessment in acute pancreatitis. *Evidence-Based Gastro*. 2001; 2(1):34–35.
2. Tenner S. Initial management of acute pancreatitis: Critical issues during the first 72 hours. *Am J Gastro*. 2004;99:2489–2494.
3. Stevens T, Conwell DL, Zuccaro G. Pathogenesis of chronic pancreatitis: an evidence-based review of past theories and recent developments. *Am J Gastro*. 2004;99:2256–2270.
4. DiMagno MJ, DiMagno EP. Chronic pancreatitis. *Curr Opin Gastro*. 2003;19(5):451–457.

 MISCELLANEOUS

- See also: Alcohol use disorders; Choledocholithiasis; Peptic ulcer disease; Systemic lupus erythematosus (SLE)

CODES

ICD9-CM

- 577.0 Acute pancreatitis
- 577.1 Chronic pancreatitis

PATIENT TEACHING

- For patient education materials favorably reviewed on this topic, contact the National Digestive Diseases Information Clearinghouse, Box NDDIC, Bethesda, MD 20892; (301) 468-6344.

See Corresponding Diagnostic Algorithm

PANIC DISORDER

Katherine L. Margo, MD
Geoffrey M. Margo, MD, PhD

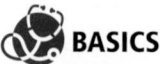 **BASICS**

DESCRIPTION

Panic disorder is a condition of repeated panic attacks of quick onset and lasting usually <1 hour; in some patients the attacks have no obvious precipitant, while in others they have situational precipitants in which the person feels trapped in a setting where escape is difficult (e.g., driving on a bridge, riding in a bus, train, or plane) or embarrassing (e.g., church service, public events, or shopping lines). This second type, panic disorder with agoraphobia, often keeps people stuck at home, forced to only frequent places that feel safe, or dependent on "safe people" who must accompany them on all activities.

The symptoms of the attacks are intense, can simulate a medical emergency, and cause enormous distress to the extent that the patient has anticipatory anxiety that significantly affects everyday and work functioning even in the absence of an actual panic attack.

GENERAL PREVENTION
None

EPIDEMIOLOGY
- Predominant age: All ages including children.
  - In school age children, it can be confused with conduct disorder and school avoidance.
  - Peak age of onset is in the 3rd decade of life.
- Predominant sex: Males > Females.

Prevalence
- Lifetime prevalence 1–3%
- ~8% in a primary care practice population.
- 25% of patients presenting with chest pain in the ER have panic disorder. Chest pain more likely due to panic if atypical chest pain, younger age, women, higher acknowledged problems with anxiety.

RISK FACTORS
- Life stressors of any kind can precipitate panic disorder. However, there is no clear relationship between life stress and panic disorder
- Cigarette smoking is risk factor.
- Cocaine, pseudoephedrine, and caffeine may provoke attacks.

Genetics
- Twin and family studies support a genetic predisposition in some patients.
- The genetic contribution to the development of panic disorder is estimated at 0.48, with the remaining contribution coming from life events.
- Monozygotic twins have a higher concordance rate than dizygotic twins.

PATHOPHYSIOLOGY
Although the neurophysiological mechanisms are not yet elucidated, the final common pathway in panic attacks is intense, sudden sympathetic stimulation. Current neurobiological research is focusing on abnormal responses to anxiety-producing stimuli in the hypocampus, amygdala and pre-frontal cortex. For example, there appears to be impairment in the ability to learn from experience, so that an original frightening experience dominates future responses even when subsequent exposures are not objectively threatening.

ETIOLOGY
- Unknown
- Biological theories focus on limbic system malfunction in dealing with anxiety-evoking stimuli.
- Psychological theories speak of deficits in managing strong affects such as fear and anger.

ASSOCIATED CONDITIONS
- Significant overlap found with several psychiatric conditions: >70% have some combination with 1 or more of agoraphobia, depression, other anxiety disorders, substance abuse disorders.
- Common for depression and panic disorder to develop in close temporal relation.
- Panic disorder is more common in some medical conditions vs. controls, such as irritable bowel syndrome, mitral valve prolapse, hypertension, interstitial cystitis.

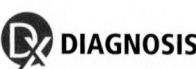 **DIAGNOSIS**

Diagnosis based on DSM-IVR criteria
- Recurrent, unexpected panic attacks (defined below), and at least 1 is followed by a month or more of persistent concern about having further attacks, worry about the implication of the attack (heart attack, going crazy, etc.) or significant behavior change as a result.
- Agoraphobia may be present.
- Symptoms are not related to substance abuse or another medical condition.
- The attacks are not better accounted for by conditions in the differential diagnosis.

SIGNS AND SYMPTOMS
Panic attacks consist of a period of intense fear or discomfort in which 4 or more of the following symptoms develop abruptly and peak in about 10 minutes
- Palpitations, pounding heart, increase heart rate
- Sweating
- Trembling, shaking
- Shortness of breath, feeling smothered
- Feeling of choking
- Chest pain or discomfort
- Nausea or abdominal distress
- Dizziness, unsteady, lightheaded, faint
- Derealization or depersonaliztion
- Fear of losing control or going crazy
- Fear of dying
- Paresthesias
- Chills or hot flashes

History
Panic attacks are not subtle. There is frequent inter-episode story of anticipatory anxiety, or the marked limitations in daily activities with agoraphobia. However, obtaining a clear history, especially with a new patient, is difficult for 2 reasons: 1st, in the throes of a panic attack many patients are convinced that the disorder is physical (after all the symptoms are physical, frighteningly so); 2nd, patients are often deeply embarrassed by their problem, which they see as a personal failure. Consequently, the physician should have a high suspicion for panic disorder with the pattern of symptoms noted above, their abrupt onset, and their recurrent nature. Tactful, nonjudgmental questioning is called for after the worst of the attack is over.

Physical Exam
During an attack the autonomic hyperactivity will be seen in tachycardia, hyperventilation, and sweating.

TESTS

Lab
No specific lab tests except to rule out conditions in the differential diagnosis. Minimally, thyroid-stimulating hormone hematocrit, electrolye panel, and EKG in those with cardiac symptoms.

Imaging
ECG for mitral valve prolapse, if indicated.

Diagnostic Procedures/Surgery
None specific to panic disorder, but if a medical cause of anxiety is strongly suspected, the workup appropriate to that condition should be done.

Pathological Findings
None

DIFFERENTIAL DIAGNOSIS
- Psychiatric conditions that have overlapping symptomatology include the anxiety disorders such as generalized anxiety disorder, obsessive-compulsive disorder and posttraumatic stress disorder.
- Co-occurring disorders include depression and other affective disorders, substance abuse, and phobias.
- Somatization disorder is also an illness of multiple unexplained medical symptoms, but the presenting picture is usually one of chronic symptoms rather than the acute, dramatic onset of a panic attack.
- Medical conditions with physical symptoms similar to those in panic, such as myocardial infarction, asthma, paroxysmal supraventricular tachycardia, pulmonary embolus, seizure disorder, transient ischemic attacks, carcinoid syndrome, Cushing's disease, hyperthyroidism, and pheochromocytoma

TREATMENT

PRE HOSPITAL
- Education and support are essential features of inter-episode management. It is helpful for patients to know about the physiology of anxiety so that the dramatic symptoms of an attack can be understood, and hence become less frightening.
- Techniques such as controlled breathing and progressive relaxation can be learned and used in an acute attack.

INITIAL STABILIZATION
- At the time of severe attack, a quick-acting benzodiazepine such as lorazepam or alprazolam may be used, in addition to active support and assurance of safety.
- Rebreathing from a paper bag is a useful way to reduce the hypocapnea of hyperventilation.

GENERAL MEASURES
Diet
No restriction

Activity
Exercise reduces general anxiety levels.

SPECIAL THERAPY
Psychotherapy
- Psychotherapy is effective in the treatment of panic disorder.
- Cognitive-behavioral therapy, tailored for panic disorder consists of several steps: Education, changing cognitions about the attack and the illness, relaxation and controlled breathing techniques, and, if appropriate, exposure to anxiety-provoking conditions coupled with in vivo relaxation exercises.
- Psychodynamic psychotherapy has been shown effective in helping patients understand their illness and themselves in the context of current psychological stresses. Length of remission is considerably improved over medication-only treatments.

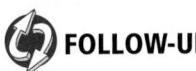 MEDICATION (DRUGS)

Medication management is indicated if psychotherapy is not successful or may be initiated together with psychotherapy. Often patient preference plays a big part in this decision. Medications should be maintained for at least 6 months after symptom control.

First Line
- Selective seratonin reuptake inhibitor (SSRI) antidepressants are effective in preventing or reducing the frequency and intensity of panic attacks. Fluoxetine is considered to cause more initial nervousness than the others. Paroxetine and sertraline have specific indications for panic disorder. Dosing is started at a lower level than the usual antidepressant dose and raised slowly, to avoid side effects of agitation, anxiety.
- Clonazepam, lorazepam, and alprazolam are useful in acute panic attacks
- Chronic benzodiazepines may be considered if SSRIs are insufficient and the the severity of the illness outweighs the risk of dependence. In this situation, clonazepam is less likely to cause withdrawal problems but must still be tapered down slowly.

Second Line
- Tricyclic antidepressants, particularly imipramine, are useful. It is considered 2nd line because of somewhat more difficulty in dosing and greater risk in overdose compared to the SSRIs.
- Venlafaxine has been found to reduce panic attack occurrence and severity in recent studies.

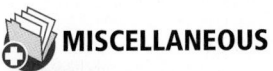 FOLLOW-UP

Regular follow-up following an acute panic attack is important for several reasons: To provide support and education, to initiate or make a referral for psychotherapy, and to monitor and adjust medications

DISPOSITION
Patients with panic disorder are usually managed as outpatients.

Admission Criteria
- Rarely a medical or psychiatric admission is required. If the emergency physician is not satisfied with the rule out of life-threatening medical conditions, such as a myocardial infarction or pulmonary embolus, a medical admission is justified to complete the work up.
- If a panic disorder patient is suicidal, a psychiatric admission is indicated.

Issues for Referral
Panic disorder should be managed by a psychiatrist or primary care physician to assess the overlap of symptoms with medical illness and to manage medication. Psychotherapy should be handled by a competent therapist knowledgeable about the disorder. A new model of collaborative care has shown good results. The model has several components, including primary care physician management with psychiatric consultation, psycho-education and telephone-based follow-up and support provided by a trained non-professional worker with structured feedback to the physician.

PROGNOSIS
~50% of patients recover with treatment although the duration of episodic illness can extend over decades. Even recovered patients are at risk for future recurrences. Panic disorder must be thought of as a chronic condition with an emphasis on long-term support and a renewal of active treatment when needed.

COMPLICATIONS
Suicide in ~7%, up to 20% in patients with other co-occurring psychiatric disorders.

PATIENT MONITORING
Regular follow up important for medication and tracking the activity of the illness.

REFERENCES
1. Ham P, et al. Treatment of panic disorder. *Am Fam Physician.* 2005;71:733–740.
2. Roy-Byrne PP, Wagner AW, Schraufnagel TJ. Understanding and treating panic disorder in the primary care setting. *J Clin Psychiatry.* 2005;66(suppl 4):16–22.
3. Simon NM, Fischmann D. The implications of medical and psychiatric comorbidity with panic disorder. *J Clin Psychiatry.* 2005;66(suppl 4):8–15.

ADDITIONAL READING
Roy-Byrne P, et al. Pharmacotherapy of panic disorder: proposed guidelines for the family physician. *J Am Board Fam Pract.* 1998;11:282–90.

 MISCELLANEOUS

CODES

ICD9-CM
- 300.01 Panic disorder
- 300.21 Agoraphobia with panic attacks

PATIENT TEACHING
Patient information handouts in *Am Fam Physician* 2005;71:740 and 2002;66:1293.

 See Corresponding Diagnostic Algorithm

See Patient Handout on CD

PARANOID PERSONALITY DISORDER

Margo Lauterbach, MD
Patrick Smallwood, MD

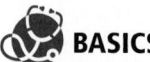 ## BASICS

DESCRIPTION
- Paranoid personality disorder is a maladaptive persistent pattern of behavior characterized by suspiciousness, inappropriate mistrust of people, and hostility toward others, who are often perceived as malicious. Consequently, patients avoid intimate relationships, bear grudges, and expect to be exploited by others.
- Paranoid personality disorder is one of the Cluster A personality disorders.

EPIDEMIOLOGY
- 1st manifests in childhood or adolescence
- More commonly diagnosed in males

Incidence
Increased in families with delusional disorder (persecutory type) and chronic schizophrenia

Prevalence
- 0.5–2.5% of the general population
- 2–10 % of psychiatric outpatients
- 10–30% of psychiatric inpatients

RISK FACTORS
- Positive family history
- Childhood abuse/neglect

Genetics
Genetic predisposition may play a role (see "Incidence")

PATHOPHYSIOLOGY
Paranoid sense of mistrust can result from childhood abuse/neglect and/or genetic predisposition to paranoia

ETIOLOGY
Specific causes unknown

ASSOCIATED CONDITIONS
- May develop major depressive disorder and may be at increased risk for obsessive-compulsive disorder and agoraphobia
- At risk for alcohol or other substance abuse or dependence

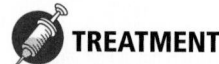 ## DIAGNOSIS

SIGNS AND SYMPTOMS
- Diagnosis is based on fulfilling 4/7 DSM-IV criteria for the disorder
  - Suspects exploitation, harm, or deceit by others
  - Unjustified doubt of others' loyalty or trustworthiness
  - Fears malicious retaliation if confides in others, thus avoids doing so
  - Believes benign remarks or situations are threatening or demeaning
  - Unforgiving; hypersensitive to slights
  - Unjustifiably perceives attacks on character/reputation and may become hostile or counterattack
  - Suspects infidelity or spouse/sexual partner
- Associated features include
  - Strong sense of autonomy
  - Stubborn
  - Litigious
  - Can be perceived as fanatics
  - May form closed groups or cults
  - Can foster fear in others

History
- Thorough psychiatric history and mental status examination
- Collateral history to establish pervasive pattern of behavior

TESTS
Psychological testing (e.g., MMPI-II)

Imaging
Brain imaging may rule out organic disease for those with emerging symptoms.

DIFFERENTIAL DIAGNOSIS
- Although brief psychotic states can result from significant stressors, primary psychotic disorders including paranoid schizophrenia, delusional disorder (paranoid type), and mood disorder with psychotic features must be ruled out.
- Schizoid personality disorder; avoidant personality disorder
- Medical disorders (e.g., temporal lobe epilepsy) with behavioral changes
- Culturally appropriate behavior, sometimes marked by defensiveness or guardedness, must not be mistaken for paranoia. Minorities, immigrants, and refugees also can present similarly, but may be plagued by unfamiliarity.
- Paranoid traits can develop in the face of physical handicaps, such as hearing impairment.

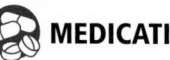 ## TREATMENT

GENERAL MEASURES
- Treatment is difficult and often avoided by the patient.
- Supportive psychotherapy, a form of therapy that is predictable, respectful, and straightforward, is preferred. Overly warm and empathetic styles can be regarded as intrusive.
- Mistrust issues can undermine group therapy and behavioral therapy.
- Family therapy may be helpful.

MEDICATION (DRUGS)

- Although little evidence suggests that the core personality features of paranoid personality disorder respond to psychopharmacologic treatment, psychotic paranoid ideation, acute hostility, anxiety, or psychosis can respond to low-dose antipsychotics or short-term benzodiazepines.
- Short-term benzodiazepines, such as diazepam, can be useful in treating acute agitation, hostility, or anxiety.
- Acute psychotic states and delusional thinking can respond to low-dose antipsychotics, such as haloperidol.
- Taking medications can be interpreted by the patient as powerlessness and loss of autonomy.

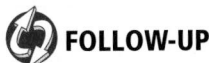 **FOLLOW-UP**

Admission Criteria

Patients who become suicidal or homicidal may require psychiatric hospitalization for safety stabilization. Patients with acute psychotic states also may require hospitalization if the patient is unable to care for himself or poses a risk to others.

Discharge Criteria

A hospitalized patient is usually discharged after appropriate therapeutic interventions and discharge planning has taken place. Suicidal ideation, homicidal ideation, and/or acute psychotic states must be resolved.

Issues for Referral

Patient should be referred for individual psychotherapy and psychiatric follow-up if psychiatric medication(s) are indicated.

PROGNOSIS

- Good for those with good ego strength and strong support system
- Poor prognosis for those with poor insight, lack of primary support system, or comorbid Axis I psychiatric diagnosis

COMPLICATIONS

Significant impairment in work and interpersonal relationships

REFERENCES

1. American Psychiatric Association. Diagnostic and statistical manual of mental disorders (4th ed., Text Revision). Washington, DC: American Psychiatric Press, 2000.
2. Bender S, Dolan T, Skodol E, et al. Treatment utilization by patients with personality disorders. *Am J Psychiatry*. 2001;158(2):295–302.
3. Meissner SJ. Paranoid personality disorder. In: Gabbard GO, Treatments of Psychiatric Disorders (3rd ed.). Washington, D.C.: American Psychiatric Press.; 2227–2236.
4. Svrakic DM, Cloninger CR. Paranoid personality disorder. In: Sadock BJ, Sadock VA (eds.), Kaplan & Sadock's Comprehensive Textbook of Psychiatry (8th ed.). Philadelphia: Lippincott, Williams & Wilkins, 2005; 2081.
5. Smallwood P. (2004). Personality disorders. In: Stern TA, Herman JB (eds.), Massachusetts General Hospital Psychiatry Update and Board Preparation (2nd ed., pp. 188–189).

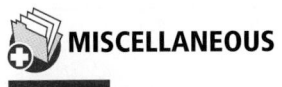 **MISCELLANEOUS**

CODES

ICD9-CM
301.0 Paranoid Personality Disorder

PARKINSON DISEASE

Jeffrey F. Minteer, MD

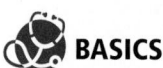 **BASICS**

DESCRIPTION

An adult-onset neurodegenerative disorder of the extrapyramidal system characterized by a combination of tremor at rest, rigidity, and bradykinesia

- Diagnosis requires therapeutic response to levodopa, which implies normal striatal neurons
- Only neurodegenerative disease treatable long term
- System(s) Affected: Musculoskeletal; Nervous
- Synonym(s): Paralysis agitans; Shaking palsy

EPIDEMIOLOGY

- Predominant age: 60 years, with 5% between the ages of 21–39
- Predominant sex: Male > Female (1.4:1)

Incidence

In the US: 50,000 new cases per year

Prevalence

- In ages 55–64, 0.3%
- In ages 65–74, 1%
- In ages 75–84, 3.1%
- In ages 85–94, 4.3%

ALERT

Geriatric Considerations

Common among elderly

Pediatric Considerations

May occur as secondary parkinsonism in this age group

RISK FACTORS

- Unknown in the idiopathic disease
- Association between smoking and increased caffeine intake and reduced risk for Parkinson disease has been reported.

Genetics

May be a genetic role, with risk 2.95-fold in patients with positive family history in late-onset disease, 7.76-fold increase in early-onset disease (age <50 years)

ETIOLOGY

- Unknown
- Loss of dopaminergic neurons in the substantia nigra, with rate of loss 1% per year in patients with Parkinson vs. 0.5% in normal aging
- No clear environmental causes identified
- Known toxins: MPTP, pesticides. Other nondopaminergic neurons may be affected.

ASSOCIATED CONDITIONS

- Psychosis
- Depression

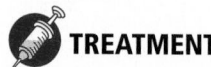 **DIAGNOSIS**

SIGNS AND SYMPTOMS

- Cardinal signs
  - Tremor (4–8 Hz) in repose: Diagnostic, but not required; relieved with activity, concentration, and sleep; increases with stress; 10% of patients present with only tremor, 30% present without; most begin with unilateral tremor
  - Bradykinesia: Required for diagnosis; most disabling symptom; movement initiation difficult, causes the gait and postural abnormalities; fine, repetitive movements affected more than large
  - Rigidity: Lead-pipe type; cogwheel with tremor
- Common presentation
  - Asymmetric tremor
  - Clumsy or weak limb: Early sign of bradykinesia
  - Stiff or uncomfortable limb: Early rigidity
  - Gait disorder: Asymmetric slowness, shuffling, reduced arm movement or imbalance
- Other associated signs and symptoms
  - Speech is poorly enunciated, low volume, clipped
  - Ocular abnormalities: Decreased blinking, blepharospasm, impaired upward gaze
  - Seborrhea
  - Dysautonomia with constipation, incontinence, sexual dysfunction
  - Depression in 2/3 of patients
  - Dementia in 20% of patients mild to moderate
  - Gait disturbances including no arm swing, en mass turning, problems getting up from chair, festination, freezing
  - Leaning posture
  - Propulsion or retropulsion
  - Micrographia
  - Mask faces
  - Neglect of swallowing with drooling
- Hoehn and Yahr scale of disability
  - Stage 1: Unilateral, minimal functional impairment
  - Stage 2: Bilateral, without impairment of balance
  - Stage 3: Bilateral, positive instability; patient is physically independent
  - Stage 4: Severe disability; patient can walk or stand without assistance, but is markedly incapacitated
  - Stage 5: Patient is wheelchair bound or bedridden unless aided

Physical Exam

Diagnostic criteria

- Clinically definite if any 3 of the following are present or any 2 of the 1st 3 display asymmetry
  - Rest tremor
  - Rigidity
  - Bradykinesia
  - Impaired postural reflexes

TESTS

Imaging

- CT or MRI to help rule out other disorders
- Positron emission tomography scanning

Pathological Findings

Lewy bodies

DIFFERENTIAL DIAGNOSIS

- Parkinsonism: Bradykinesia with little or no response to levodopa, indicating that the striatal neurons are also degenerated
  - Progressive supranuclear palsy
  - Multisystem atrophy
  - Alzheimer with extrapyramidal features
  - Side effects of neuroleptic medications
  - Infectious—postencephalitic
  - Vascular—lacunar state
  - Toxins
  - Metabolic—Wilson disease: Onset at age <40
- Benign essential tremor: Positive family history and relief with alcohol
- Consider other conditions if
  - Falls or early dementia
  - Symmetric Parkinsonism
  - Wide-based gait
  - Abnormal eye movements
  - Orthostatic hypotension
  - Babinski sign
  - Urinary retention
  - Rapid progression

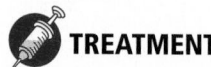 **TREATMENT**

INITIAL STABILIZATION

Outpatient treatment

GENERAL MEASURES

- Drugs have therapeutic and toxic effects.
- Acute worsening may indicate depression, noncompliance, or supervening illness.
- Course is progressive with or without drugs. Lifelong therapy directed toward symptom control—treat disability
- Investigate for drug-induced cause; if found, discontinue drug. Symptom resolution may take weeks to months.

Diet

- Small, frequent meals if difficulty in eating
- High liquid intake important; high-bulk foods
- Reduced-protein diet is unnecessary

Activity

Maintain activity at whatever level possible; use cane for walking

SPECIAL THERAPY

New approaches to treatment are undergoing study

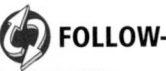 **MEDICATION (DRUGS)**

First Line

- Levodopa/carbidopa (Sinemet): Most effective and the initial drug of choice in older patients with more severe symptoms, speech disorders and falls are resistant to levodopa
  - Sinemet 25/100 1/2 tablet t.i.d. after food. Increase by 100 mg levodopa per day until desired effect or side effects occur. Usual dose 1–2 tabs t.i.d., increase to 1,000 mg/d or until response
  - If switching to the SR, increase daily dose by 25%.
  - Add agonist if wear off or dyskinesia appears or when 500–1,000 mg levodopa per day is being taken.
- Dopamine agonists slightly less effective; long half-life; reduces wearing-off effects of levodopa. Add when levodopa >500 mg/d. Early monotherapy may reduce levodopa use and long-term side effects. May be initial drug of choice in younger patients with milder symptoms. Usually need addition of levodopa in 1st 5 years of monotherapy. Avoid with dementia
- Non-ergot–preferred due to less side effects
  - Pramipexole (Mirapex): 0.125 mg t.i.d., maximum 4.5 mg/d; useful for drug-resistant tremor
  - Ropinirole (ReQuip): 0.25 mg t.i.d., maximum 24 mg/d
- Ergot derivatives
  - Bromocriptine: Start with 1.25 mg/d or b.i.d.
  - Pergolide (Permax): 0.05 mg/d for 2 days and increase by 0.1 mg/d every 3 days for 12 days. Mean dose is 3 mg.
  - Titrate the levodopa/carbidopa combination downward as these agents are added

Second Line

- Monoamine oxidase (MAO) inhibitors: Block metabolism of dopamine; may be neuroprotective; added to levodopa to diminish motor fluctuations
  - selegiline 5 mg; start with 1/2 tablet every morning and 1/2 tablet every noon; increase to 5 mg b.i.d.; if added to levodopa/carbidopa, lower dosage 20%.
- Anticholinergics: For tremor and rigidity in early stages or as an adjunct (30% improvement in 50% of patients). Not recommended for patients >65 years.
  - Trihexyphenidyl (Artane): 1 mg/d; increase by 2 mg every 3 days until 6–10 mg/d
  - Benztropine (Cogentin): 1–2 mg/d. Start with 0.5 mg/d and increase slowly by 0.5 mg every 6 days. Maximum 6 mg/d
- Amantadine: N-Methyl-D-Aspartate antagonist (100–200)
  - Similar to anticholinergics; improves bradykinesia and rigidity; short-term effectiveness
- Catechol-O-methyltransferase (COMT) inhibitors
  - Reduce peripheral metabolism of levodopa, useful as levodopa extender: Decrease motor fluctuation in late-stage disease and reduce early wearing off of levodopa
  - Tolcapone (Tasmar): 100 mg t.i.d., maximum 1,200 mg/d
  - Entacapone (Comtan): 200 mg t.i.d., maximum 1,600 mg/d, also formulated in pill with sinemet (Stalevo)

- Levodopa/carbidopa may cause late effects
  - Time-related dosage problems occur in 50% of patients in 4–5 years.
  - Dyskinesias, probably secondary to receptor hypersensitivity; limb choreoathetosis and grimacing; change to sustained release; reduce levodopa dose plus add agonist or clozapine 100–200 mg. Diphasic dyskinesia; "Off" period dyskinesia: May begin as early-morning dystonia (foot); reduce interdose interval or switch to sustained release or agonist.
  - Wear-off phenomenon: 3–4 hours after last dose. 1st sign of drug-response problems caused by increased severity of nigral degeneration. Use sustained-release form with an agonist or selegiline.
  - On/off phenomenon: 15–20% of patients. Slow-release preparations, can decrease dose until on/off disappears and then restart drug. COMT inhibitors increase "on" time and reduce "off" time.
  - Psychiatric side effects: Confusion, hallucinations (well-formed visual or auditory), paranoia, nightmares. If mainly at night, reduce last evening dose or try clozapine.
- Agonists
  - Somnolence (27%), nausea, nightmares, agitation, orthostatic hypertension, hallucinations (17%), edema (14%)
  - Raynaud phenomenon in doses >30 mg/d, edema, hypertension, worsening congestive heart failure
  - If stopped abruptly, may result in a syndrome resembling neuroleptic malignant syndrome
  - Ergot derivatives rarely cause fibrosis and pergolide associated thickening of cardiac valves
- MAO inhibitors anxiety/sleep disturbance
- Anticholinergics confusion, constipation, urinary retention, dry mouth, and glaucoma.
- COMT: Hepatotoxicity

Adjuvant Drugs

- Tricyclic antidepressants for nighttime sedation and associated depression (50% of patients with Parkinson)
- Antioxidants or vitamin E have shown no definite benefit.
- Apomorphine as agonist or for freezing (use limited by adverse effects [vomiting] and need for parenteral administration)
- Clozapine: 70–200 mg suppress frequency of dyskinesia and increase "on" time; also useful for hallucinations (<50 mg/d). Side effects include sedation, sialorrhea, and agranulocytosis.
- Donepezil: 5 mg; cognitive impairment
- Modafinil: 100–200 mg excessive daytime sleepiness

SURGERY

- Adrenal medullary transplants—unproven
- Thalamotomy—akinesia
- Stereotactic pallidotomy—akinesia
- Deep brain stimulation of subthalamic nucleus—dyskinesia, tremor response 88%; may worsen pre-existing psychiatric disorders; fewer "off" problems, fewer "on" dyskinesias, and 50% reduction of medications

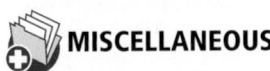 **FOLLOW-UP**

PROGNOSIS

- More rapid progression: Older at disease onset; dementia
- Milder disease: Predominant feature is tremor

COMPLICATIONS

- Aspiration pneumonia
- Falls
- Associated with a 2-fold increase in risk of death

PATIENT MONITORING

Lifelong

REFERENCES

1. Koller WC, Calne DB, eds. Strategies for treating complications of levodopa therapy. *Neurology.* 1994;44(suppl 16).
2. Krauss JK, Jankovic J. Surgical treatment of Parkinson's disease. *Am Fam Physician.* 1996;54:1621–1628.
3. Nutt J, Wooten GF. Diagnosis abd initial management of Parkinson's disease. *NEJM.* 2005;353(10):1021–1027.
4. Siderowf A, Stern M. Update on Parkinson disease. *Ann Intern Med.* 2003;138:651–658.
5. Stacy M. Pharmacotherapy for advanced Parkinson's. *Pharmacotherapy.* 2000;20:85–165.

 MISCELLANEOUS

See also: Dementia; Depression

CODES

ICD9-CM

332.0 Paralysis agitans

PATIENT TEACHING

- Local support groups
- United Parkinson Foundation, 360 W. Superior St., Chicago, IL 60610; (312) 664–2344
- American Parkinson Disease Foundation, 1250 Hyland Blvd., Staten Island, NY 10305; (800) 223–2732
- Avoid drugs known to cause tardive dyskinesia, such as fluphenazine, perphenazine, prochlorperazine, thiopropazate, trifluoperazine, promazine, thioridazine, haloperidol, droperidol, benperidol, fluspirilene, pimozide, trifluperidol, chlorprothixene, clopenthixol, and thiothixene.

See Corresponding Diagnostic Algorithm

PARONYCHIA

Jeffrey B. Kreher, MD

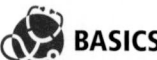 **BASICS**

DESCRIPTION
- Infectious or eczematous inflammation of the folds of skin surrounding the fingernail or toenail. May be acute or chronic.
  - Acutely, it often appears 2–5 days posttrauma.
- System(s) Affected: Skin/Exocrine
- Synonym(s): Eponychia; Perionychia

ALERT
Pediatric Considerations
Thumb/finger sucking is a risk factor (anaerobes and *E. coli* may be present).

GENERAL PREVENTION
- Chronic: Avoid allergens and frequent wetting of hands; wear rubber gloves with cloth liner.
- Good diabetic control
- Expectant treatment for candidiasis

EPIDEMIOLOGY
- Predominant age: All ages
- Predominant sex: Female > Male (3:1)

Incidence
Common in the US

RISK FACTORS
- Acute: Trauma to skin surrounding nail, ingrown nails, manicured/sculptured nails, diabetes mellitus
- Chronic: Frequent immersion of hands in water (cooks, chefs, bartenders, housekeepers, swimmers), diabetes mellitus, immunosuppressed

Genetics
No known genetic pattern

PATHOPHYSIOLOGY
- A paronychial infection usually starts in the lateral nail fold.
- Occasionally, the infection includes the complete margin of skin around the nail plate:
  - It results from mechanical separation of the nail plate from the perionychium.
- Early in the course of this disease process (<24 hours), cellulitis alone may be present
  - An abscess can form if the infection does not resolve quickly.
- Chronic infections most likely represent eczematous reaction with secondary infection.

ETIOLOGY
- Acute: *Staphylococcus aureus* and *Streptococcus pyogenes*. Less frequently streptococci and pseudomonas
- Chronic: Eczematous reaction with secondary *Candida albicans* (~95%). Less frequent: Dermatophytes and, occasionally, molds (*Scytalidium Fusarium*)

ASSOCIATED CONDITIONS
- Diabetes mellitus
- If chronic, eczema or atrophic dermatitis
- Certain medications: Cetuximab, paclitaxel, antiretroviral therapy (especially protease inhibitors and lamivudine, with toes more commonly involved)
- If multiple, consider pemphigus vulgaris (rare).

DIAGNOSIS

SIGNS AND SYMPTOMS
- Separation of nail fold from nail plate
- Red, painful swelling of skin around nail plate
- Purulent
- Secondary changes of nail plate
- Green changes in nail (pseudomonas)

History
- Localized pain and tenderness
- Previous trauma (bite nails, ingrown nails, manicured)
- Contact with herpes infections
- Contact with allergens or irritants (frequent water immersion, latex)

Physical Exam
- Acute: Red, hot, tender, tense nailfold +/– abscess
- Chronic: Swollen, tender, boggy nailfold +/– abscess
- Occasional elevation of nail bed

TESTS
Lab
- None required unless condition is resistant to treatment, then
  - Gram stain
- Culture and sensitivity
  - Potassium hydroxide wet mount plus fungal culture
- Drugs that may alter lab results: Use of OTC antimicrobials or antifungals

Diagnostic Procedures/Surgery
- Scraping for wet mount and culture in chronic cases
- Incision and drainage for suppurative or cases not responding to conservative management

DIFFERENTIAL DIAGNOSIS
- Herpetic whitlow (similar in appearance, very painful, often associated with vesicles)
- Felon (abscess of fingertip pulp; urgent diagnosis required)
- Allergic contact dermatitis (latex, acrylic)
- Reiter disease
- Psoriasis

TREATMENT

GENERAL MEASURES
- Outpatient care is appropriate.
- Acute: Water or vinegar/water (1:1) soaks (t.i.d.—q.i.d.), warm compresses, elevation
- Chronic: Keep fingers dry.

Diet
No special diet

Activity
Full activity

Nursing
Ensure proper education about disease etiology and treatment.

MEDICATION (DRUGS)

First Line
- Tetanus booster when appropriate
- No evidence that antibiotics are better or worse than incision and drainage (5)
- Acute (if anaerobes or *E. Coli* are suspected)
  - Clindamycin (Cleocin) 300 mg q.i.d.
  - Pediatric: 10 mg/kg/dose q8h
  - Amoxicillin-clavulanate potassium (Augmentin): 875 mg q12h
  - Pediatric: 45 mg/kg/dose q12h (for <40 kg)
- Acute (if diabetic, suppurative or more severe cases)
  - Dicloxacillin 250 mg t.i.d.
  - Erythromycin 333 mg t.i.d.
  - Cephalexin (Keflex) 500 mg b.i.d.–t.i.d.
- Chronic
  - Topical steroids: Potent Class II–III (4)
- Contraindications: Allergy to antibiotic
- Precautions: Erythromycin may cause significant gastrointestinal upset.
- Significant possible interactions
  - Erythromycin affects levels of theophylline and effects of carbamazepine, digoxin, and corticosteroids. Cardiac toxicity with terfenadine or astemizole is possible.
  - Ketoconazole, astemizole, itraconazole, fluconazole: Terfenadine, statin drugs

Second Line
Acute
- Bacterial: Mupirocin (Bactroban) (Centany)
- Yeast or dermatophyte: Topical imidazoles (econazole, ketoconazole, terbinafine)
- Systemic antifungals (rarely needed):
  - Itraconazole (Sporanox) 200 mg/d for 90 days (may have longer action because it is incorporated in nail plate). Pulse therapy may be useful (200 mg b.i.d. for 7 days, repeated monthly for 2 months)
  - Terbinafine (Lamisil) 250 mg/d for 6 weeks (fingernails) or 12 weeks (toenails)
  - Fluconazole (Diflucan) 150 mg/wk for 4–6 months
- Antipseudomonal drugs (e.g., 3rd-generation cephalosporin, aminoglycosides)

SURGERY
- Incision and drainage of abscess, if present.
- If a subungual abscess or ingrown nail is present, it will require partial or complete removal of nail.

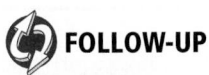 **FOLLOW-UP**

DISPOSITION

Issues for Referral
Uncertainty of diagnosis or failure to respond to treatment

PROGNOSIS
- With adequate treatment and prevention, healing can be expected.
- If no response in chronic lesions, rarely benign or malignant neoplasm may be present and referral should be considered.

COMPLICATIONS
- Acute: Subungual abscess
- Chronic: Secondary ridging, thickening, and discoloration of nail, nail loss

PATIENT MONITORING
Routine follow-up until healed

REFERENCES
1. Baran R, Dawber RPR, eds. Diseases of the nail and their management, 2nd ed. Boston: Blackwell Scientific; 1994.
2. Fitzpatrick TB, et al., eds. Dermatology in general medicine, 5th ed. New York: McGraw-Hill; 1999.
3. Moschella SC, Hurley HJ, eds. Dermatology, 3rd ed. Philadelphia: WB Saunders; 1992.
4. Tosti A, Piraccini BM, Ghetti E, Colombo MD. Topical steroids versus systemic antifungals in the treatment of chronic paronychia: An open, randomized double-blind and double dummy study. *J Am Acad Dermatol*. 47:73,2002. (B)
5. Shaw, Body. Best evidence topic report. Incision and drainage preferable to oral antibiotics in acute paronychial nail infection? *Emerg Med J*. 2005;22:813. (B)

ADDITIONAL READING
Rockwell PG. Acute and chronic paronychia. *Am Fam Physician*. 2001;63:1113.

 MISCELLANEOUS

- May be considered work-related in bartenders, waitresses, nurses, and others who often wet their hands
- See also: Onychomycosis

CODES

ICD9-CM
- 112.3 Candidiasis of skin and nails
- 681.02 Paronychia, finger
- 681.11 Paronychia, toe

CPT
- 10060 Incision and drainage, simple or single
- 10061 incision and drainage, complicated or multiple

PATIENT TEACHING

Diet
If diabetic, institute appropriate dietary changes for better control.

Activity
Chronic: Avoid frequent immersion, triggers, allergens.

Prevention
Chronic: Keep fingers dry, avoid allergens.

 See Corresponding Diagnostic Algorithm

PARVOVIRUS B19 INFECTION

Benjamin Barankin, MD

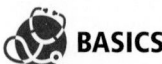 **BASICS**

DESCRIPTION

- Human parvovirus B19 is the primary cause of erythema infectiosum (EI, or fifth disease). It also causes aplastic anemia in patients with increased red blood count turnover (e.g., sickle cell anemia), chronic anemia in immunodeficient individuals, and arthritis and arthralgias in normal hosts. There is also the potential for intrauterine infection after maternal parvovirus B19 infection.
- System(s) Affected: Hemic/Lymphatic/Immunologic; Musculoskeletal; Renal/Urologic; Skin/Exocrine
- Synonym(s): Fifth disease; Erythema infectiosum

ALERT

Geriatric Considerations
None known

Pregnancy Considerations
See "General Prevention."

GENERAL PREVENTION

- Standard hygienic practices can minimize spread.
- Because EI is so common, it is not possible to avoid exposure completely. Also, period of contagion is before clinical illness (rash) appears
- Pregnant health care workers should avoid caring for patients with aplastic crises.
- Pregnant child care workers are at some increased risk; however, exclusion from the workplace will not eliminate this risk, and therefore is not recommended.

EPIDEMIOLOGY

- Predominant age
  - Infection is common in childhood; ~2–11% of children <11 years of age are parvovirus B19 seropositive.
  - Peak age for EI is 4 to 12 years old
- Predominant sex: Male = Female

Prevalence

- In the US: Extremely common; 50% of adults have evidence of prior infection. Most common as community epidemics in winter and spring in nontropical regions.
- Antibody prevalence (age and percent):
  - 1–5 years, 2–15%
  - 6–9 years, 20–40%
  - 11–19 years, 35–60%
  - >50 years, >75%

RISK FACTORS

- Aplastic crisis: Increased RBC turnover (e.g., sickle cell anemia)
- Chronic anemia: Immunodeficient individuals
- Intrauterine infection: Pregnant, nonimmune woman
- School-related epidemic and nonimmune household contacts have a secondary attack rate of 50%.
- Health care workers have a secondary attack rate of 35%, with the highest rate being among nurses exposed to children with aplastic crises.

Genetics

Erythrocyte P antigen-negative individuals are resistant to infection.

ETIOLOGY

- Small (20–25 mm), nonenveloped, single-stranded DNA virus. It is the only known parvovirus to infect humans and belongs to the family Parvoviridae.
- In EI, the period of viral shedding precedes the development of the rash, suggesting that the pathogenesis of the rash is immune related.
- In fetal infection, maternal viremia with transplacental passage is the source of infection. Respiratory secretions and rarely blood products are sources of human spread of virus.

DIAGNOSIS

SIGNS AND SYMPTOMS

- In adults, asymptomatic infection or unrecognized illness is the most common manifestation.
- EI
  - Incubation period 4–14 days
  - Epidemics often occur in late spring every 2–4 years
  - No preclinical symptoms most commonly. Fever is absent or low grade.
  - Onset of rash noted 1st on the face ("slapped-cheek appearance") with diffuse erythema of the face followed 1–4 days later by a 2nd stage of a lacy reticular rash on the trunk and limbs
  - A 3rd stage of the rash is characterized by marked evanescence and recrudescence, sometimes associated with bathing, exercise, or sun exposure.
  - Pruritus and mild arthralgia may occur.
  - Headache, pharyngitis, coryza, myalgia, arthralgias, arthritis, and gastrointestinal disturbances are more frequent and severe in adults.
- Joint disease
  - In adults, 80% of patients may manifest arthritis and/or arthralgia.
  - In children, joint symptoms are less common.
  - Knees, hands, and ankles (frequently symmetrical) are most commonly involved.
  - Joint symptoms usually subside within 3 weeks, but may persist for months and may be associated with the onset of juvenile rheumatoid arthritis. Joint destruction generally not seen
- Transient aplastic crisis
  - Seen in patients with chronic hemolysis, such as sickle cell anemia, spherocytosis, thalassemia, and pyruvate kinase deficiency
  - Aplastic event is self-limited, with reticulocytes reappearing in 7–10 days and full recovery in 2–3 weeks
  - In those children with sickle cell hemoglobinopathies and heredity spherocytosis, fever is the most common symptom (73%), and rash is highly unlikely.
- Chronic anemia
  - Seen in immunodeficient individuals
  - No manifestations of fever, rash, or joint symptoms usually
- Fetal/neonatal infection
  - Risk of transplacental spread of virus ~33% in infected mothers
  - Clinical manifestations range from asymptomatic seroconversion (most commonly), no seroconversion, 2nd-trimester fetal death, or stillbirth secondary to severe anemia and the development of fetal hydrops

- B19 infection should always be suspected in cases of nonimmune hydrops.
- The principal organ involved in the fetus is the bone marrow: RBC survival is shortened and profound anemia can result from B19-induced erythroid bone marrow aplasia.
- A pregnant woman with a new rash or arthralgia should be tested for parvovirus B19.
- Risk of fetal loss in pregnancy is highest in 1st-trimester B19 infection (9%).
- Anemia is the most common manifestation of later infection.
- In 1 study, 84% of B19-infected pregnant women who carried to term delivered normal infants.
- No known long-term developmental problems in infant survivors
- Glove-sock syndrome: Severe petechial and ecchymotic rash in hand–foot distribution with associated febrile tonsillopharyngitis

TESTS

- Antigen detection in tissue or fluids by nucleic acid hybridization or polymerase chain reaction is available on an investigational basis in many academic centers.
- B19 cannot be grown in traditional tissue culture systems, but can be detected by enzyme immunoassays, immune fluorescence, and Western blot assays.

Lab

- Anemia with reticulocytopenia
- Serum IgM antibody to B19 is usual method of confirming diagnosis. During acute infection, B19 IgM persists for 1–2 months (less in neonates).
- To exclude congenital B19 in infants with negative B19 IgM, one must follow an infant's B19 IgG serology in the 1st year of life.
- Maternal serum α-fetoprotein may be increased in fetuses with hydrops fetalis.

Imaging
Maternal infection: Fetal ultrasound

Diagnostic Procedures/Surgery
Amniotic fluid and chorionic villus sampling may be useful diagnostically in investigation of some maternal infections

Pathological Findings

- Skin biopsy usually normal or mild inflammation, usually consisting of perivascular infiltrations of mononuclear cells
- In hydrops fetalis, may see intranuclear inclusions in nucleated RBCs
- In stillbirths, virus can be detected in all tissues.

DIFFERENTIAL DIAGNOSIS

- Rubella
- Enteroviral disease
- Systemic lupus erythematosus
- Drug reaction
- Lyme disease
- Rheumatoid arthritis

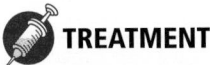 **TREATMENT**

INITIAL STABILIZATION
- Outpatient management for EI
- Inpatient for aplastic crisis, other severe manifestations

GENERAL MEASURES
Diet
No special diet

Activity
- Unrestricted for EI
- Arthritis patients may require physical therapy/exercise program

 MEDICATION (DRUGS)

- No therapy needed usually
- Immune globulinl IV has been used successfully for refractory anemias, especially with AIDS.
- Cessation of immunosuppressive therapy has allowed some patients to clear chronic infections.
- RBC transfusions may be required for aplastic crisis.
- Anti-inflammatory agents may alleviate arthritic symptoms.
- Precautions
  - Contact and respiratory isolation for patients hospitalized with aplastic crisis
  - EI not contagious once rash has appeared

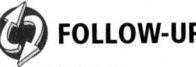 **FOLLOW-UP**

PROGNOSIS
- Usually self-limited
- Joint symptoms subside in weeks (often by 2 weeks)
- ~20% of infections result in delayed virus elimination and viremia persisting for several months to years
- Full recovery from aplastic crisis in 2–3 weeks

COMPLICATIONS
Rare, but more commonly seen in adults than children
- Arthritis
- Persistent anemia
- Hemophagocytic syndrome
- Pneumonitis
- Encephalopathy
- Stroke
- Reports of congenital anomalies and chronic fatigue syndrome, but no clear-cut association
- Glomerulonephritis and other renal diseases have been reported in both immunocompromised and immunocompetent patients.
- Nephrotic syndrome
- Hepatitis
- Neuropathies
- Rarely associated temporally in Henoch-Schonlein purpura or vasculitis diseases in children
- Myocarditis/pericarditis

PATIENT MONITORING
Periodic blood counts for anemic patients

REFERENCES

1. Al-Khan A, Caligiuri A, Apuzzio J. Parvovirus B-19 infection during pregnancy. *Infect Dis Obstet Gynecol*. 2003;11(3):175–179.
2. Harris JW. Parvovirus B19 for the hematologist. *Amer J Hematol*. 1992;39:119.
3. Katta R. Parvovirus B19: A review. *Dermatol Clin*. 2002;20(2):333–342.
4. Kellermayer R, Faden H, Grossi M. Clinical presentation of parvovirus B19 infection in children with aplastic crisis. *Pediatr Infect Dis J*. 2003; 22(12):1100–1101.
5. Manaresi E, et al. Humoral immune response to parvovirus B19 and serological diagnosis of B19 infection. *Clin Lab*. 2002;48(3–4):201–205.
6. Seishima M, Oyama Z, Yamamura M. Two-year follow-up study after human parvovirus B19 infection. *Dermatology*. 2003;206(3):192–196.
7. Taylor G, Drachenberg C, Faris-Young S. Renal involvement of human parvovirus B19 in an immunocompetent host. *Clin Infect Dis*. 2001;32(1):167–169.
8. van Elsacker-Niele AM, Kroes AC. Human parvovirus B19: Relevance in internal medicine. *Neth J Med*. 1999;54(6):221–230.

 MISCELLANEOUS

See also: Abortion, spontaneous; Anemia, sickle cell; Arthritis, rheumatoid, (RA); Henoch-Schönlein purpura; systemic lupus erythematosus (SLE)

 CODES

ICD9-CM
057.0 Erythema infectiosum (fifth disease)

PATIENT TEACHING

- Patients with chronic hemolytic diseases should be aware of risks for aplastic crisis if exposed to EI.
- Pregnant women should avoid exposure to patients with active or chronic infections. However, most adults have already had inapparent infection and are therefore not at risk. Exclusion of pregnant women from the workplace where EI is occurring is not recommended.
- Children with symptoms are not infectious and may attend child care or school (e.g., transmission of virus occurs in the asymptomatic interval between infection and symptom expression).
- Immunocompromised patients (e.g., receiving chemotherapy) are at increased risk of infection.

PATENT DUCTUS ARTERIOSUS (PDA)

Ryan Johnson, MD
Brent J. Barber, MD

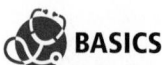 **BASICS**

DESCRIPTION
PDA is the failure of the ductus arteriosus to close after birth. 75% of time occurs as isolated defect.
- System(s) Affected: Cardiovascular
- Synonym(s): Aorticopulmonary shunt; Aorticopulmonary communication

ALERT
Geriatric Considerations
Good results expected with repair age 50–70 years.

Pediatric Considerations
- Symptoms and signs depend largely on size of shunt.
- Some infants with coexisting cardiac anomalies benefit temporarily from a patent ductus to provide shunting to the lungs (right heart obstructions) or periphery (coarctation of the aorta). This benefit is short lived, so definitive treatment should proceed as soon as feasible.
- Moderate to large shunts usually diagnosed in infancy or childhood. Small shunts occasionally diagnosed in adults

Pregnancy Considerations
- Women with small- to moderate-sized ductus and left-to-right shunt can expect an uncomplicated pregnancy.
- High risk in those with high pulmonary resistance and right-to-left shunt

EPIDEMIOLOGY
- Predominant age: Infancy
- Predominant sex: Female > Male (2–3:1)

Prevalence
In the US: 8/1,000 live births

RISK FACTORS
- Premature birth
- High altitudes
- Maternal rubella
- Coexisting cardiac anomalies
- Any condition resulting in hypoxia (pulmonary, hematologic, etc.)

Genetics
Classically thought to be multifactorial–non Mendelian inheritance. However, recent reports of autosomal dominant and autosomal recessive transmission. (1)[A]

PATHOPHYSIOLOGY
The main features of the natural history include spontaneous ductal closure, bacterial endocarditis, late CHF, and the development of pulmonary vascular obstructive disease.

ETIOLOGY
- Prematurity
- Congenital
- Hypoxia
- Prostaglandins

ASSOCIATED CONDITIONS
- Coarctation of the aorta
- Pulmonary valve stenosis or atresia
- Peripheral pulmonary stenosis (maternal rubella)
- Aortic stenosis
- Ventricular septal defect
- Necrotizing enterocolitis
- Club feet, cataracts, blindness, systemic arterial stenosis (associated with maternal rubella)

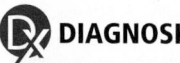 **DIAGNOSIS**

SIGNS AND SYMPTOMS
- Children
  - Failure to grow
  - Recurrent respiratory infections
  - Easy fatigability
  - Dyspnea on exertion
- Adult
  - Leg fatigue
  - Fatigue
  - Shortness of breath
  - Angina
  - Syncope
- Signs (left-to-right shunt)
  - Rough systolic murmur
  - Continuous "machinery" murmur
  - Thrill at left upper sternal border
  - Bounding pulse with wide pulse pressure
  - Prominent, displaced apical impulse
  - Systolic ejection click
  - Diastolic flow murmur (across mitral valve)
  - Excessive sweating
  - Tachypnea, tachycardia, rales if failure ensues
- Signs (right-to-left shunt)
  - Cyanosis, especially lower extremities
  - Clubbing
  - Diastolic Graham-Steell murmur (high-velocity pulmonic insufficiency secondary to pulmonary hypertension)
  - Right ventricular heave
  - Polycythemia

TESTS
Lab
- Arterial blood gas
- Special tests
  - ECG in children and adults may show left ventricle and left atrial hypertrophy.
  - ECG in infants usually normal

Imaging
- Echocardiography/Doppler
- Contrast echocardiography
- Radionuclide angiography
- MRI
- Chest radiograph usually normal in infants
- Chest radiograph in children and adults (shunt vascularity, calcifications, left ventricle and left atrial enlargement, dilated ascending aorta, dilated pulmonary arteries)

Diagnostic Procedures/Surgery
- Cardiac catheterization and angiography: Will demonstrate the shunt and determine the degree of shunting, pulmonary pressures, and other coexisting cardiac abnormalities
- Echocardiography: Identify size of patent ductus, evaluate for left atrial and left ventricular enlargement.
- Doppler: Displays direction and velocity of shunt. May be useful to estimate pulmonary artery pressure.

Pathological Findings
- Left ventricular and atrial enlargement
- Patent ductus may have abnormal intima (maternal rubella).

DIFFERENTIAL DIAGNOSIS
- Venous hum
- Total anomalous pulmonary venous return
- Ruptured sinus of Valsalva
- Arteriovenous communications
- Anomalous origin of left coronary artery from pulmonary artery
- Absence or atresia of pulmonary valve
- Aortic insufficiency with ventricular septal defect
- Peripheral pulmonary stenosis (maternal rubella)
- Truncus arteriosus
- Aortopulmonary fenestration
- Coronary artery fistula

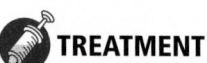 **TREATMENT**

GENERAL MEASURES
- Appropriate health care: Inpatient surgery
- Small, asymptomatic shunts may not need closure
- Pulmonary support
- Oxygen to correct hypoxia
- Sodium and fluid restriction
- Correction of anemia (hematocrit >45)

Diet
No special diet

Activity
As tolerated

MEDICATION (DRUGS)

First Line

- Indomethacin 0.2–0.25 mg/kg per dose IV preferred. Repeat every 12–24 hours for 3 doses. (Decreased efficacy in term infants; not effective in children or adults) (2)[A] *or*
- Ibuprofen 10 mg/kg on day 3 of life, 5 mg/kg/d for 2 days. Not commercially available in IV preparation.
- Oxygen
- Diuretics
- Antibiotic prophylaxis if not surgically repaired
- Contraindications: To treatment with indomethacin:
  – Renal dysfunction
  – Overt bleeding
  – Shock
  – Necrotizing enterocolitis
  – Myocardial ischemia
- Precautions: With indomethacin treatment, oliguria, hyponatremia; can have significant adverse effects on renal, gastrointestinal and cerebrovascular blood flow
- Significant possible interactions: Refer to the manufacturer's profile of each drug.
- Alprostadil (Prostaglandin E1) treatment to maintain patency of duct in ductal dependent lesions

SURGERY

- Surgical transection and ligation for moderate/large shunts best option in premature infants when medical treatment has failed or is contraindicated (3)[A]
- Transfemoral catheter technique to occlude PDA withcoil embolization, wire mesh, or double umbrella for larger ducts (4,5)[A]; Option for larger infants and children.

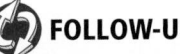

FOLLOW-UP

PROGNOSIS

- Spontaneous closure after 3 months is rare.
- Before 3 months, closure in premature infants is 75%.
- Before 3 months, closure in term infants is 40%.
- Best postoperative results if closed before age 3 years
- Increased pulmonary vascular resistance and pulmonary hypertension more common if closed after age 3 years
- No firm statistics but decreased survival for large shunts

COMPLICATIONS

- Left heart failure
- Pulmonary hypertension
- Right heart hypertrophy and failure
- Eisenmenger physiology
- Bacterial endarditis
- Myocardial ischemia
- Necrotizing enterocolitis

PATIENT MONITORING

- Annual routine follow-up after closure
- Shunts that have not been closed should be followed more closely.

REFERENCES

1. Gelb BD. Genetic basis of congenital heart disease. *Curr Opin Cardiol*. 2004;19:110–115.
2. Van Overneire B, et al. A comparison of ibuprofen and indomethacin for closure of patent ductus arteriosus. *N Engl J Med*. 2000;343:674–681.
3. Malviya M, Ohlsson A, Shah S. Surgical versus medical treatment with cyclooxygenase inhibitors for symptomatic patent ductus arteriosus in preterm infants. *The Cochrane Database of Systematic Reviews* 2006 Issue 1.
4. Gray DT, et al. Transcatheter occlusion of native persistent ductus arteriosus using conventional Gianturco coils. *Am J Cardiol*. 1997;79:1430–1432.
5. Pass RH, et al. Multicenter USA Amplatzer PDA occlusion device trial: Initial and mid-term results. *Circulation*. 2002;106:II486.
6. Adams FH, Emmanouilides GC, Riemenschneider TA. *Moss' Heart Disease in Infants, Children and Adolescents*. 5th ed. Baltimore, MD: Williams & Wilkins; 1995.
7. Braunwald E, ed. *Heart Disease: A Textbook of Cardiovascular Medicine*. 5th ed. Philadelphia, PA: WB Saunders; 1996.
8. Makowitz JS, et al. Transcatheter versus surgical closure of patent ductus arteriosus. *N Engl J Med*. 1994;330;1014.

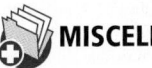

MISCELLANEOUS

Other notes: No need for antibiotic prophylaxis after surgical repair

 CODES

ICD9-CM
747.0 Patent ductus arteriosus

PATIENT TEACHING

Discuss prematurity and explain different treatments of premature infants and full-term infants.

PEDICULOSIS (LICE)

George E. Kikano, MD

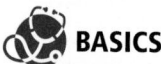

BASICS

DESCRIPTION

- Pediculosis is an infestation by lice.
- Characteristics of lice
  - Feed solely on human blood, by piercing the skin, injecting saliva, and then sucking blood
  - Move quickly
  - A mature adult female lays 3–6 eggs (nits) a day. Nits are 0.8 mm long, white, and appear cemented to the base of the hair.
  - Nits may survive 3 weeks when removed from host.
- 2 species of lice infest humans
  - *Pediculus humanus* has two subspecies, the head louse (capitis) and the body louse (corporis). Both species are smaller than 2 mm, flat, wingless, and have 3 pairs of legs that attach closely behind the head.
  - *Phthirus pubis* (pubic or crab louse): Resembles a sea crab and has widespread claws on the 2nd and 3rd legs.
- System(s) Affected: Skin/Exocrine
- Synonym(s): Lice; Crabs

GENERAL PREVENTION

- Proper hygiene
- Careful follow-up in schools by public health nurses may help prevent recurrence and spread of head lice.
- Washing combs, brushes, hats, coats, collars, sheets, pillow cases, etc., will help to prevent reinfestation by head lice.
- Safe sex (pubic lice)

EPIDEMIOLOGY

- Predominant age
  - Pubic lice: Most common in adults
  - Head lice: Most common in children 3–10 years old
- Predominant sex: Female > Male

Incidence

In the US: 6–12 million new cases per year

RISK FACTORS

- Overcrowded sleeping quarters (*Pediculosis capitus* and *corporis*)
- Sexual contact (*Phthirus pubis*)
- Immunosuppression
- Sharing combs, hats, clothing, and bed linen
- Close personal contact
- Poor personal hygiene (not a risk factor for *P. capitus*)

Genetics

No genetic pattern

ETIOLOGY

Infestation by lice

ASSOCIATED CONDITIONS

- Pubic lice are readily transmitted by sexual contact, with a 90% transmission rate. Up to 1/3 of patients have at least 1 concomitant sexually transmitted disease (STD).
- Eyelash infestation on a child may be a sign of sexual abuse.

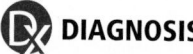

DIAGNOSIS

SIGNS AND SYMPTOMS

- *Pediculosis capitis* (head lice)
  - Found most often on the back of the head and neck and behind the ears (warmer areas of the hair)
  - Nits are white spheres found on the hair shaft. They cannot be moved.
  - Pruritis common, mostly at night
  - Scratching can cause inflammation and secondary bacterial infection.
  - Eyelashes may be involved.
  - Lymphadenopathy in severe infestation
- *P. corporis* (body louse)
  - Poor hygiene
  - Adult lice and nits in the seams of clothing
  - Pruritus
  - Secondary infection
  - Uninfected bites present as red papules, 2–4 mm in diameter, with an erythematous base.
- *P. pubis* (pubic louse)
  - Anogenital pruritus
  - May have no symptoms during 30-day incubation period
  - Nits are present at the base of hair shafts.
  - Delay in treatment may lead to development of groin infection and regional adenopathy.
  - Pubic hair most common site
  - Lice may spread to hair around anus, abdomen, axillae, chest, beard, eyebrows, and eyelashes.
  - Infested adult patients may spread lice to eyelashes of children. This may induce blepharitis.

TESTS

Lab

Special tests

- Careful examination of hair shafts under the microscope
- Lice and nits can easily be seen under a microscope. Nits cannot be moved from hair shaft.
- On Wood's lamp exam, live nits fluoresce white, empty nits fluoresce gray.
- Examination of the seams of clothing reveals body lice and their eggs.

Diagnostic Procedures/Surgery

- History and physical exam
- Microscopic exam

DIFFERENTIAL DIAGNOSIS

- Scabies and other mite species that can cause cutaneous reactions in humans
- Dandruff can sometimes look like head lice.

TREATMENT

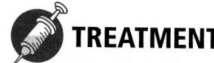

GENERAL MEASURES

Nit removal

- After treatment with shampoo or lotion, nits remain in scalp or pubic hair.
- Nits are best removed with a very fine comb (nit comb). Removal may be made easier by soaking the hair in a solution of equal parts water and white vinegar and wrapping wet scalp in a towel for at least 15 minutes.
- Repeat treatment periodically as needed for stubborn nits.
- All family contacts possibly infested with head lice should be treated concomitantly.
- Discard the clothes or wash them in hot water.
- Evaluate for other STD (if diagnosed with pubic lice).

Diet

No special diet

Activity

No restrictions

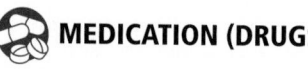

MEDICATION (DRUGS)

First Line

- Head lice: Many topical preparations are effective (1% lindane may be used but may have to be repeated in 1 week; 1% permethrin or pyrethrin is effective). They should be applied and washed off after 10 minutes.
- Pubic lice: Treatments available include synergized pyrethrins, or permethrin. These can be used either as the shampoo left on for 10 minutes or the lotion, which can be left on for several hours for best results.
- Body lice: Best treated with synergized pyrethrins lotion applied once and left on for several hours
- Eyelash infestation: Treated by careful manual removal of lice and nits, or by application of petroleum jelly t.i.d.–q.i.d. for 5 days
- In rare cases, oral trimethoprim/sulfamethoxazole can be used.
- Contraindications: Avoid lindane in premature infants, infants, and pregnant women
- Precautions
  - Pediculicides should never be used to treat eyelash infections.
  - Accidental ingestion and gross overuse of lindane may be associated with central nervous system toxicity. Use carefully in immunocompromised patients.
  - Lindane: Use properly to avoid neurotoxicity.

Second Line

For resistant head lice, shaving the head or oral antibiotics may be indicated.

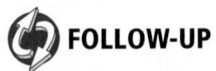 **FOLLOW-UP**

PROGNOSIS
- With appropriate treatment, >90% cure rate
- Recurrence common, mainly from reinfection, failure to comply with treatment

COMPLICATIONS
- Persistent itching may be caused by too-frequent use of the pediculicide.
- Secondary bacterial infections

PATIENT MONITORING
As needed

REFERENCES
1. Habif T. *Clinical Dermatology*. 4th ed. St. Louis, MO: Mosby; 2004.

 MISCELLANEOUS

- See also: HIV Infection and AIDS; Typhus Fevers
- Other notes: Typhus, relapsing fever, and trench fever are spread by body lice during wartime and in underdeveloped countries.

CODES

ICD9-CM
132.9 Pediculosis, unspecified

PATIENT TEACHING
- Poor hygiene is not a risk factor in acquiring *P. capitis*.
- Printed patient information is available from Mayo Foundation for Medical Education and Research, Section of Patient and Health Education, Sieber Subway, Rochester, MN 55905; (507) 284–8140

 See Patient Handout on CD

PELVIC INFLAMMATORY DISEASE (PID)

Mary Anne Condon, NP, PhD

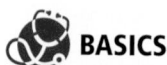 **BASICS**

DESCRIPTION
- Clinical syndrome caused by the ascent of microorganisms from the vagina and endocervix to the endometrium, fallopian tubes, ovaries, and contiguous structures.
- PID is a broad term that includes a variety of upper genital tract infections unrelated to pregnancy or surgical procedures, such as salpingitis, salpingo-oophoritis, endometritis, tubo-ovarian inflammatory masses, and pelvic or diffuse peritonitis.
- System(s) Affected: Reproductive
- Synonym(s): Salpingitis; Salpingo-oophoritis; Adnexitis; Pyosalpinx; Tubo-ovarian abscess; Pelvic peritonitis; Upper genital tract infection

GENERAL PREVENTION
- Educational programs about safer sex practices
- Education, particularly for those who have had an episode of PID
- Intrauterine device (IUD) is contraindicated in women with a history of PID or lifestyle associated with sexually transmitted diseases (STD).
- Oral contraceptives appear to decrease risk of PID in cases with cervicitis; the PID cases that do occur are generally less severe.
- Barrier contraceptives, especially condoms, and spermicidal creams or sponges provide protection, the extent of which is not well documented.
- Evaluation and treatment of sex partners
- Compliance with management instructions
- Early medical care when genital lesions or discharge appear
- Routine check-ups for STD for those in non–mutually monogamous relationship(s)

EPIDEMIOLOGY
- Predominant age: 1/3 of patients are <20 years, 2/3 are <25 years.
- Predominant sex: Female only
- Rare during pregnancy but occurs occasionally, and the possibility must be kept in mind.
- PID in pregnancy may run a more virulent course that may require aggressive antibiotic therapy.
- HIV-infected women may have a more virulent or complicated course of PID.

Incidence
In the US, ~1 million women are treated each year.

Prevalence
100–200/100,000

ALERT
Geriatric Considerations
PID is rare after menopause, although postmenopausal adnexal abscess is a well-documented entity.

Pediatric Considerations
- Rare before puberty
- Adolescents are highly vulnerable to STDs, including PID. Early vigorous therapy to prevent infertility is especially important in this age group.

Pregnancy Considerations
- In pregnant women with PID there is an increased risk of premature rupture of membranes and preterm labor.
- Tetracyclines use is contraindicated in pregnancy.

RISK FACTORS
- Sexually active, reproductive age peak 15–24 age group
- Most common in adolescents
- Multiple sexual partners
- Use of an IUD; greatest risk in 1st few months after insertion
- Previous history of PID; 20–25% will have a recurrence
- Chlamydial or gonococcal cervicitis; 8–10% will develop PID
- Gonococcal salpingitis occurs commonly within 7 days of onset of menses.
- Condoms and vaginal spermicides lessen the risks of developing PID.

PATHOPHYSIOLOGY
The precise mechanism by which microorganisms ascend from the lower genital tract is not known:
- 1 possibility is that chlamydial or gonococcal endocervicitis alters the defense mechanisms of the cervix, allowing ascent of the vaginal flora with or without the original pathogen.
- Other possibilities suggest that polymicrobial infection can occur without *Neisseria gonorrhoeae* or *Chlamydia trachomatis*.
- Factors that predispose to the ascent of bacteria include the use of an IUD and the hormonal and physical changes associated with menstruation.

ETIOLOGY
- Bacteriology: Multiple organisms act as etiologic agents in PID, and most cases are polymicrobial
  - *C. trachomatis, N. gonorrhoeae,* and a wide variety of aerobic and anaerobic bacteria are recognized as etiologic agents.
  - *Mycoplasmas* have also been implicated, but their role is less clear.
  - The proportion of cases infected with chlamydia or gonorrhea varies widely depending on the population studied.
  - The most common anaerobes include *Bacteroides, Peptostreptococcus,* and *Peptococcus* species.
  - The organisms involved in bacterial vaginosis are similar to the nongonococcal, nonchlamydial bacteria often found in the upper genital tract of women with PID, but the relationship between these conditions is unclear.

ASSOCIATED CONDITIONS
- In PID patients with an IUD in situ, especially if an adnexal abscess is present, the possibility of actinomyces infection requiring penicillin treatment must be kept in mind.
- The IUD is contraindicated in women with a previous episode of PID.
- Rupture of an adnexal abscess is rare but life threatening. Early surgical exploration is mandatory.
- Chlamydial or gonococcal perihepatitis may occur with PID. This combination is called the Fitz-Hugh and Curtis syndrome and characterized by severe pleuritic right-upper quadrant pain.

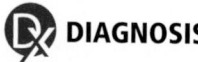 **DIAGNOSIS**

SIGNS AND SYMPTOMS
- May be asymptomatic
- Lower abdominal pain
- Fever and malaise
- Vaginal discharge
- Irregular bleeding
- Urinary discomfort, proctitis
- Nausea and vomiting
- Abdominal tenderness
- Tenderness with cervical motion
- Adnexal tenderness
- Unilateral or bilateral tender adnexal mass

TESTS
- PID diagnosis is elusive, and even asymptomatic patients are at risk for sequelae. Diagnosis is incorrect in up to 1/3 of women. Laparoscopic diagnosis is best, but impractical as routine and generally reserved for problem situations. It is wiser to overtreat a lower-tract genital infection than to miss an upper-tract infection.
- Criteria for diagnosis (for empiric treatment)
  - Uterine/adnexal tenderness, or
  - Cervical motion tenderness
- Additional criteria
  - Temperature ≥38.3°C
  - WBC count ≥10,500/mm³
  - Purulent material by culdocentesis
  - Adnexal mass
  - ESR >15 mm/h
  - Laboratory evidence of gonorrhea or chlamydia
  - Elevated C-reactive protein
  - Presence of WBCs on wet mount
- Definitive criteria
  - Histopathologic endometritis on biopsy
  - Adnexal abscess on sonography
  - Laparoscopic evidence of PID
  - CDC recommends diagnosis on only 1 of the following manifestations
    ○ Adnexal
    ○ Cervical motion
    ○ Uterine tenderness

Lab
- Pregnancy test
- Leukocyte count > 10,000 cells/mm^3
- Endocervical Gram stain for Gram-negative intracellular diplococci
- ESR ≥ 15 mm/h
- Endocervical culture or antigen test for gonorrhea and chlamydia
- Plasma cell endometritis on biopsy
- Saline microscopy of vaginal fluid with increased WBCs

Imaging
- Pelvic ultrasound
- CT
- MRI

Diagnostic Procedures/Surgery
- Culdocentesis with culture
- Diagnostic laparoscopy with culture of fallopian tubes
- Endometrial biopsy reveals endometritis

DIFFERENTIAL DIAGNOSIS
- Appendicitis
- Ectopic pregnancy
- Ovarian torsion
- Hemorrhagic or ruptured ovarian cyst
- Endometriosis
- Irritable bowel syndrome
- Somatization disorder

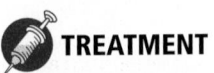 TREATMENT

INITIAL STABILIZATION
- Outpatient treatment, normally
- Hospitalization recommended in the following
  – Uncertain diagnosis
  – Surgical emergencies cannot be excluded (e.g., appendicitis)
  – Suspected pelvic abscess
  – Pregnancy
  – Adolescent patient with uncertain compliance with therapy
  – Severe illness
  – Intolerance to outpatient regimen
  – Failure to respond to outpatient therapy
  – Inability to arrange clinical follow-up within 72 hours of starting antibiotics
  – HIV infection

GENERAL MEASURES
- Patient should avoid sex until treatment is completed.
- Refer of sex partners for appropriate evaluation and treatment. Partners should be treated, irrespective of evaluation, with regimens effective against chlamydia and gonorrhea.

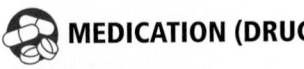 MEDICATION (DRUGS)

First Line
Several antibiotic regimens are highly effective, with no single regimen of choice, but coverage should include chlamydia, gonorrhea, anaerobes, Gram-negative rods, and streptococci. The Centers for Disease Control and Prevention (CDC) regimens that follow are recommendations, and the specific antibiotics named are examples.
- Parenteral; regimen A
  – Cefoxitin 2 g IV q6h or cefotetan 2 g IV q12h (or other cephalosporins, such as ceftizoxime, cefotaxime, and ceftriaxone) plus doxycycline 100 mg PO or IV q12h
  – Parenteral therapy for 24 hours after clinical improvement; continue doxycycline after discharge for a total of 10–14 days
- Parenteral; regimen B
  – Clindamycin 900 mg IV q8h plus gentamicin loading dose IV or IM (2 mg/kg of body weight) followed by a maintenance dose (1.5 mg/kg) q8h
  – Parenteral therapy for 24 hours after clinical improvement; continue doxycycline after discharge as above, or clindamycin 450 mg PO q.i.d. for a total of 14 days
- Outpatient treatment; regimen A
  – Ofloxacin 400 mg PO b.i.d. for 14 days or levofloxacin 500 mg PO once daily for 14 days with or without metronidazole 500 mg PO b.i.d. for 14 days
- Outpatient treatment; regimen B
  – Cefoxitin 2 g IM plus probenecid 1 g PO concurrently or ceftriaxone 250 mg IM or equivalent cephalosporin plus doxycycline 100 mg PO b.i.d. for 10–14 days with or without metronidazole 500 mg PO b.i.d. for 14 days
- Contraindications, precautions, and possible drug interactions: Refer to the manufacturer's profile of each drug.

Second Line
Many other antibiotic regimens have been proposed and used with success, for example, tobramycin in place of gentamicin, tetracycline in place of doxycycline (see "References–MMWR").

SURGERY
- Reserved for failures of medical treatment and for suspected ruptured adnexal abscess with resulting acute surgical abdomen
- Conservative surgery preferred; allows a 10–15% postoperative fertility rate
- Hysterectomy and adnexectomy for older patients with completed childbirth
- Failure of medical therapy is associated with adnexal abscess, which may be amenable to transabdominal or transvaginal drainage under guidance by ultrasonography, CT, or laparoscopy.

 FOLLOW-UP

PROGNOSIS
- Wide variation with good prognosis if early, effective therapy is instituted and further infection is avoided
- Poor prognosis related to late therapy and continued unsafe lifestyle

COMPLICATIONS
- A tubo-ovarian abscess will develop in ~7–16% of patients.
- Recurrent infection occurs in 20–25% of patients.
- Risk of ectopic pregnancy increased 7–10-fold to ~8% of women who have had PID
- Tubal infertility in 15%, 35%, and 55% of women after 1, 2, and 3 episodes of PID, respectively
- Chronic pelvic pain in 20% related to adhesion formation, chronic salpingitis, or recurrent infection

PATIENT MONITORING
- Close observation of clinical status, particularly for fever, symptoms, level of peritonitis, WBC
- Follow adnexal abscess size and position with ultrasonography.

REFERENCES
1. Pelvic inflammatory disease: Guidelines for prevention and management. *MMWR Recomm Rep.* 1991;40(RR-5):1–25.
2. Sexually transmitted diseases treatment guidelines 2002. *MMWR Recomm Rep.* 2002;51(RR-6):1–78.
3. Barrett S, Taylor C. A review on pelvic inflammatory disease. *Int J STD AIDS.* 2005;16(11):715–21.
4. Ness RB, et al. Effectiveness of treatment strategies of some women with pelvic inflammatory disease. *Obstet Gynecol.* 2005;106:573–80. [A]
5. Risser W, Cromwell P, Bortot A, Risser J. Impact of new diagnostic criteria on the prevalence and incidence of pelvic inflammatory disease. *J Pediatr Adolesc Gynecol.* 2004;17(1):39–44. [B] (2)
6. Sheeder J, Stevens-Simon C, Lezotte D, et al. Cervicitis; To treat or not to treat? The role of the patient preferences and decision analysis. *J Adolesc Health.* 2006;39(6):887–892. [C] (2).
7. Ness R, Hillier S, Kip K, et al. Bacterial vaginosis and risk of pelvic inflammatory disease. *Obstet Gynecol.* 2004;104:761–769. [B] (2)

ADDITIONAL READING
Yeh J, Hook E, Goldie S. A refined estimate of average lifetime cost of pelvic inflammatory disease. Sex Trans Dis. 2003;30(5):. B (2)

 MISCELLANEOUS

See also: Chlamydial sexually transmitted diseases; Gonococcal infections; Syphilis

 CODES

ICD9-CM
614.9 Unspecified inflammatory disease of female pelvic organs and tissue

PATIENT TEACHING

 See Corresponding Diagnostic Algorithm

 See Patient Handout on CD

PEMPHIGOID, BULLOUS

Nicole R. Leboeuf, MD

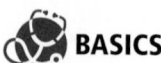 **BASICS**

DESCRIPTION
- Chronic, benign, autoimmune bullous eruption presenting primarily >60 years of age.
- System(s) Affected: Dermatologic; Hematologic/Lymphatic/Immunologic; Exocrine
- Synonym(s): Pemphigoid

ALERT
Geriatric Considerations
Older patients with pemphigoid have a higher rate of malignancy than do age-matched controls.

Pediatric Considerations
Rare in children and infants

EPIDEMIOLOGY
Incidence
Most common autoimmune bullous disease; incidence in the US estimated at 10 per million; incidence ranges from 2–30 per million in various parts of Europe

RISK FACTORS
- Age >60
- Possible drug associations: Furosemide, penicillamine, sulfasalazine, nalidixic acid, enalapril, captopril, phenacetin, some penicillins

ETIOLOGY
- Autoimmune disorder
- Autoantibodies against protein component in hemidesmosome of basal keratinocytes leads to complement activation, cellular invasion, and release of inflammatory mediators; lamina lucida splits.

ASSOCIATED CONDITIONS
May occur with various malignancies, although paraneoplastic significance remains unclear

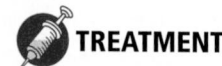 **DIAGNOSIS**

SIGNS AND SYMPTOMS
- Prodrome of pruritic papules and urticaria
- After weeks or months of prodrome, sudden eruption of bullae, which are often tender
- Bullae generally range in size from 0.5–7 cm. May arise from normal or erythematous, inflamed skin and may be local or generalized.
- Bullae remain intact for many days, collapse, crust over, and heal with post-inflammatory hyperpigmentation changes.
- Common sites include axillae, groin, flexor surfaces of arms, legs, and abdomen.
- Occasionally located on the scalp, palms, and soles; mucous membranes (10–35%)
- Intact blisters outnumber erosions, the reverse of what is seen in pemphigus vulgaris.
- Bullae may contain serous or serosanguineous fluid.
- Some patients are asymptomatic.

History
Full history recommended

Physical Exam
Complete physical exam is required

TESTS
Lab
- Circulating antibasement membrane autoantibodies in 70% (via indirect immunofluorescence)
- Demonstration of antibodies directed toward bullous pemphigoid antigens BP230 (BPAG1e) and BP180 (BPAG2)
- Eosinophilia may be present.

Pathological Findings
- Light microscopy classically reveals subepidermal blister with perilesional inflammation containing many eosinophils, neutrophils, and mononuclear cells; eosinophilic spongiosis.
- Direct immunofluorescent studies: Deposition of C3 (100%) and linear IgG (65–90%) in lamina lucida
- If no circulating antibodies are detected, direct immunoelectron microscopy or laser scanning confocal microscopy can localize IgG in patient's skin for diagnosis. (1)[C]

DIFFERENTIAL DIAGNOSIS
- Pemphigus
- Bullous erythema multiforme
- Dermatitis herpetiformis
- Drug eruptions
- Epidermolysis bullosa acquisita
- Porphyria cutanea tarda
- Bullosis diabeticorum
- Linear IgA dermatosis
- Paraneoplastic pemphigus (almost all affected patients have a malignant tumor; most commonly lymphoma)

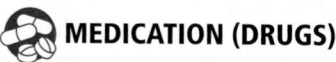 **TREATMENT**

INITIAL STABILIZATION
Outpatient, except in patients with significant complications

GENERAL MEASURES
- Soak active lesions to débride and remove crusts.
- Analgesic mouth washes (see "Medications")

Diet
Liquid for mucosal involvement; resume regular diet when tolerated

Activity
As tolerated, depending on severity of symptoms

MEDICATION (DRUGS)

First Line
- Topical very potent (class I) corticosteroid (0.05% clobetasol propionate cream 20 g to affected body surface b.i.d. until 2 weeks after disease is controlled. Then decrease to 20 g daily for 1 month, 10 g daily for 2 months, 10 g every other day for 2 months, 10 g twice weekly for 4 months (2)[B]

- If no significant or promising response occurs to topical therapy after 3 weeks, institute one of the following systemic therapies

  – Prednisone: 0.5–0.75 mg/kg/d. Start gradual taper 2 weeks after disease is controlled. Decrease dose by 15% every 3 weeks. (3)[B] Attempt a switch to alternate days based on patient response.

  – Tetracycline: 2 g/d divided q.i.d. plus nicotinamide 1.5 g/d divided t.i.d. Treat for 2 months then decrease tetracycline dose by 500 mg each month and stop, based on patient response. (4)[C]
  – Dapsone: 100 mg/d (check G6PD level before therapy); may have limited effect. Best if used in patients with neutrophil rich infiltrate. (5)[C]
  – Azathioprine (Imuran): May be used rarely as monotherapy in patients with no response to tetracycline or Dapsone who cannot tolerate steroids. Also used as adjuvant therapy with prednisone. Check thiopurine-methyl-transferase (TPMT) levels (6)[C]
    ○ <5.0 U/mL RBCs do not use this drug
    ○ 5–13.7 U/mL RBCs dose 0.5 mg/kg
    ○ 13.7–19.0 U/mL RBCs use 1.5 mg/kg
    ○ >19.0 U/mL RBCs use 2.5 mg/kg
- Intralesional corticosteroids may be used in patients with localized disease.
- Hydroxyzine 10–50 mg q4h as needed for pruritus
- Oral analgesics for mucosal involvement
  – Elixir of diphenhydramine (Benadryl) for oral ulcers
  – Lidocaine (Xylocaine) viscous
  – Dyclonine solution
- Contraindications: Refer to manufacturer's literature.
- Precautions: Avoid systemic treatment when possible. Patients who have only occasional lesions may be managed without the need for internal medication and their adverse effects.
- Significant possible interactions: Refer to manufacturer's literature.

Second Line
- Plasmapheresis can be considered and may allow lower corticosteroid dose, but it is not effective enough to use as standard therapy. (7)[C]
- Methotrexate (10–25 mg/wk) and Mycophenolate mofetil (500–1,000 mg b.i.d.) can be used as alternative adjuncts or as monotherapy.
- Pulsed cyclophosphamide, cyclosporine, intravenous immune globulin or pulsed intravenous steroids may be tried in resistant cases. (6)[C]

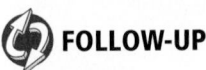 FOLLOW-UP

PROGNOSIS
- A chronic disease of unpredictable duration and frequency of relapse
- Often lasts months to years with complete remission in most patients by 5 years
- Old lesions heal rapidly as new lesions appear.
- Accompanying debilitation usually is not as great as with pemphigus vulgaris.
- Older age (>75), poor general medical condition, antibodies against BPAG2, and extensive disease are risk factors for poor prognosis
- Mortality at 1 year is 6–12% in US, 19–41% in Europe

COMPLICATIONS
- Superimposed infection; may result in death in elderly, debilitated patients
- Complications of steroid therapy
- Rare associated malignancy
- Untreated severe disease can be fatal
- Mortality most commonly secondary to sepsis and cardiovascular disease, often related to treatment

PATIENT MONITORING
- Dapsone (G6PD, methemoglobinemia, methemoglobinuria, complete blood chemistry, platelets, alanine transaminase, and alkaline phosphatase)
- Methotrexate (liver and renal function and complete blood chemistry)
- Mofetil (complete blood chemistry and gastrointestinal intolerance test)
- Cyclosporine (BP, blood urea nitrogen, creatinine, uric acid, and magnesium)

REFERENCES
1. Wozniak K, Kazama T, Kowalewski C. A practical technique for differentiation of subepidermal bullous diseases. *Arch Dermatol* 2003;139:1007–1011.
2. Joly P, et al. A comparison of oral and topical corticosteroids in patients with bullous pemphigoid. *N Engl J Med* 2002;346:321–327.
3. Khumalo NP, et al. A systematic review of treatments for bullous pemphigoid. *Arch Dermatol* 2002;138:385–389.
4. Fivenson DP, Breneman DL, Rosen GB, et al. Nicotinamide and tetracycline therapy of bullous pemphigoid. *Arch Dermatol* 1994;130:753–758.
5. Bouscarat F, et al. Treatment of bullous pemphigoid with dapsone: Retrospective study of thirty-six cases. *J Am Acad Dermatol* 1996;34:683.
6. Korman NJ. Bullous pemphigoid, the latest in diagnosis, prognosis, and therapy. *Arch Dermatol* 1998;134:1137–1141.
7. Guillaume JC, et al. Controlled trial of azathioprine and plasma exchange in addition to prednisolone in the treatment of bullous pemphigoid. *Arch Dermatol* 1993;129:49–53.

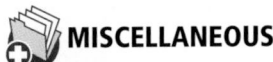 MISCELLANEOUS

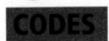

ICD9-CM
694.5 Pemphigoid

PATIENT TEACHING
- Advise patient on use of oral analgesics.
- Advise about side effects and possible adverse reactions to steroid therapy.

Prevention
Scratching and UV exposure may lead to new bullae formation and worsen existing lesions. Scratching also may increase infection risk.

PEMPHIGUS VULGARIS

Amit Garg, MD

 BASICS

DESCRIPTION
- Rare, debilitating, potentially fatal autoimmune blistering disease characterized by painful intraepidermal bullae that appear on normal-looking skin without surrounding inflammation, often starting in the mouth.
- System(s) Affected: Gastrointestinal; Exocrine; Skin

EPIDEMIOLOGY
- Occurs in people 30–70 years of age
- No gender predilection

Incidence
Rare.

Prevalence
Per year: 0.75–5 cases per million

RISK FACTORS
- Increased incidence in Ashkenazi Jews
- Medications (particularly penicillamine)

Genetics
High incidence of human leukocyte antigen DR4, and the DRB1*0402 haplotype among Ashkenazi Jews

ETIOLOGY
The reason or stimulus for antibody formation is unknown. A few cases have been associated with therapy with captopril, penicillamine, piroxicam, phenobarbital, and from abuse of heroin.

PATHOPHYSIOLOGY
Pathogenic IgG antibodies directed against desmoglein, a keratinocyte adhesion molecule, result in intraepidermal blister formation. With limited mucosal disease, antibodies to desmoglein-3 predominate. With extensive cutaneous disease, autoantibodies to both desmoglein-3 and -1 are present.

ASSOCIATED CONDITIONS
- Thymomas
- Other internal malignancies
- Other autoimmune diseases

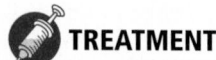 **DIAGNOSIS**

SIGNS AND SYMPTOMS
- Oral mucous membrane lesions (particularly in the back of the mouth) often precede the cutaneous lesions (sometimes by several weeks or months). Virtually all patients have oropharyngeal disease during the course of their disease.
- On skin, predilection for scalp, face, trunk, axillae, and groin
- Bullae arise from normal-appearing skin.
- Blisters are flaccid and rupture easily.
- Crusted erosions, more often than blisters, are present at the time of exam. Intact bullae are found only on the 1st 1–2 days of their existence.
- After blister roof breaks, a bright red or crusted shallow erosion ensues; it requires weeks or months to heal.
- Nikolsky sign is typically present.
- Lesions are painful.
- Lesions do not heal without therapy.

TESTS
Lab
- Indirect immunofluorescence on a serum specimen identifies circulating autoantibodies to desmogleins in 80–90%
- IIF titers often correlate with disease activity and may also be used to titrate therapy.

Diagnostic Procedures/Surgery
Biopsy of lesional and perilesional skin

Pathological Findings
- Light microscopy: Suprabasal cleft formation and acantholysis. There is no disruption of the basement membrane.
- Direct immunofluorescence of perilesional skin reveals IgG deposition in the epidermal intercellular space.
- Causative antigens (desmogleins) are located on the exterior surface of the cytoplasmic membrane of epithelial cells.

DIFFERENTIAL DIAGNOSIS
- For oral mucosal lesions
  – Aphthous ulcers, herpes simplex virus, erythema multiforme, erosive lichen planus
- For cutaneous disease
  – Paraneoplastic pemphigus, bullous pemphigoid, dermatitis herpetiformis, Hailey-Hailey disease, erythema multiforme, drug eruptions, bullous impetigo, varicella-zoster, herpes simplex virus

TREATMENT

GENERAL MEASURES
- Long-term care with a dermatologist. Patients require years to life-long immunosuppression to achieve the primary goal of reducing autoantibody formation.
- Topical treatments have no influence on the overall course of disease.
- Topical antibiotic treatment to crusted erosions: Roofs of ruptured blisters act as a biologic dressing and need not be débrided unless pyoderma is present.
- Ruptured bullae require weeks to heal.
- Analgesic mouth washes (see "Medications")
- Rare incidence of the disease prohibits large randomized controlled trials that evaluate potential treatments.

Diet
Liquids or soft-food diet for patients with active oral lesions. Resume regular diet as tolerated.

Activity
As dictated by severity of disease and patient's medical status.

MEDICATION (DRUGS)

First Line
- Oral analgesics as needed, choose 1
  - Diphenhydramine (Benadryl) elixir
  - Lidocaine (Xylocaine) viscous
  - Dyclonine solution or lozenges
- Prednisone, initially at 1 mg/kg/d to reduce antibody formation. (2,3)[C] Duration at this dose will vary, but control of disease should be attained in 2–3 months. Prednisone is tapered over 6–9 months to an ideal maintenance dose of 5 mg every other day Maintenance therapy may be continued for years.
- Adjuvant immunosuppression is indicated if blister formation is not controlled on lower doses of prednisone. Steroid-sparing agents include azathioprine (4 mg/kg/d), cyclophosphamide (2–3 mg/kg/d), mycophenolate mofetil, and cyclosporine.
- Contraindications: Refer to the manufacturer's literature.
- Precautions: Refer to the manufacturer's literature.
- Significant possible interactions: Refer to the manufacturer's literature.

Second Line
- Mycophenolate mofetil (4)[C]
- Cyclophosphamide (2–3 mg/kg/d). Extremely effective, but also potentially very toxic.
- Azathioprine (4 mg/kg/d), as concomitant therapy with corticosteroids
- Immune globulin IV for cases in which adjunctive therapy not effective with prednisone, or significant side effects from systemic corticosteroids (e.g., prednisone) are present. It has been effective as monotherapy; however, it is costly.
- Rituximab, a chimeric anti-CD 20 monoclonal antibody, for refractory cases (5)[C]
- Plasmapheresis physically removes pathogenic autoantibodies from circulation.
- Chlorambucil
- Tetracycline with niacinamide (worth a trial in mild cases)

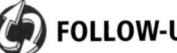 **FOLLOW-UP**

PROGNOSIS
- Chronic; Inevitably fatal if not treated
- ~10% of patients achieve remission
- Mortality rate with corticosteroid and immunosuppressive therapy is ~5% and mostly related to iatrogenic complications.

COMPLICATIONS
- Iatrogenic complications, such as sepsis, lead to morbidity and mortality.
- Inadequate nutrition and debilitation owing to pain associated with oral lesions
- Sepsis/death in untreated or poorly controlled cases

PATIENT MONITORING
Close follow-up is required for acute phases and over the long-term for adverse effects associated with corticosteroid and other immunosuppressant use.

REFERENCES

1. Bystryn JC, Rudolph JL. Pemphigus. *Lancet*. 2005;366:61.
2. Rosenberg FR, Sanders S, Nelson CT. Pemphigus: A 20-year review of 107 patients treated with corticosteroids. *Arch Dermatol*. 1976;112:962–970.
3. Scully C, Paes D, Almeida O, et al. Pemphigus vulgaris: the manifestations and long-term management of 55 patients with oral lesions. *Br J Dermatol*. 1999;140:84.
4. Mimouni D, Anhalt GJ, Cummins DL, et al. Treatment of pemphigus vulgaris and foliaceus with mycophenolate mofetil. *Arch Dermatol*. 2003;139:739–742.
5. Dupuy A, Viguier M, Bedane C, et al. Treatment of refractory pemphigus vulgaris with rituximab (anti-CD20 monoclonal antibody). *Arch Dermatol*. 2004;140:91–96.

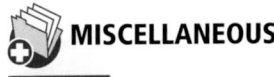 **MISCELLANEOUS**

CODES

ICD9-CM
694.4 Pemphigus

PATIENT TEACHING

Patients should be made aware of the chronic course of disease and the need for long-term immunosuppression. Patients should be familiar with signs and symptoms of infections that may result as complications to immunosuppression.

PEPTIC ULCER DISEASE

Cindy L. Lee, MD
Felix Horng, MD, MBA

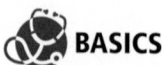 BASICS

DESCRIPTION

- Duodenal ulcer: Most common form of peptic ulcers. Usually located in the duodenal bulb. Multiple ulcers common, and if distal to the bulb, raises possibility of Zollinger-Ellison syndrome
- Gastric ulcer: Much less common than duodenal ulcer in absence of NSAIDs. Commonly located along lesser curvature of the antrum near the incisura and in the antepyloric area
- Esophageal ulcers: Located in the distal esophagus and may be part of a Barrett epithelial change.
- Ectopic gastric mucosal ulceration: May develop in patients with Meckel diverticula or other sites of ectopic gastric mucosa

ALERT

Pediatric Considerations

- Uncommon before puberty, but hemorrhage and perforation are more common.
- Positive family history in 50% of early-onset duodenal ulcer patients <20 years old
- May account for chronic abdominal pain
- Consider pyloric stenosis in those with gastric outlet obstruction

GENERAL PREVENTION

- NSAID–ulcers: Avoid salicylates and NSAIDs
  - If NSAIDs 3 are needed, add misoprostol (Cytotec) or proton pump inhibitor (PPI) or double dose H_2 blockers
  - To reduce ulcer risk, eradicate Helicobacter pylori before starting therapy with NSAIDs.
  - Use of selective COX-2 inhibitors (e.g. celecoxib) at time of publication is controversial due to potential safety risks.
- Maintenance antisecretory therapy with PPIs or H_2 blockers is indicated for patients with a history of ulcer complications, frequent ulcer recurrences, refractory H. pylori positive ulcers, or H. pylori negative ulcers.
- H. pylori eradication reduces gastric cancer risk.

EPIDEMIOLOGY

- Peptic ulcer: No predilection by gender
- 70% of ulcers occur between ages 25–64
- Ulcer incidence increases with age

Incidence

- Peptic ulcer: ~500,000 cases/year
- Recurrence: 4 million/year

Prevalence

- Peptic ulcer: 1.8% in the US
- Lifetime prevalence is 8–14%

RISK FACTORS

- NSAID use
- Smoking cigarettes
- Family history of ulcers
- Zollinger-Ellison syndrome (gastrinoma)
- Possibly associated: Corticosteroids (high dose and/or prolonged therapy); blood group O; HLA-B12, B5, Bw35 phenotypes; stress; poverty; manual labor

PATHOPHYSIOLOGY

Imbalance between aggressive factors (e.g., gastric acid, pepsin, bile salts, pancreatic enzymes) and defensive factors maintaining mucosal integrity (e.g., mucus, bicarbonate, blood flow, prostaglandins, growth factors, cell turnover).

ETIOLOGY

- Etiology of peptic ulcers may be multifactorial.
- H. pylori infection: Associated with 90% of duodenal ulcers and 70–90% of gastric ulcer
  - Lifetime risk for peptic ulcer disease in H. pylori-infected people is 15%.
  - Annual risk of developing duodenal ulcer in H. pylori-infected people is ≤1%.
- Ulcerogenic drugs (e.g., NSAIDs)
- Hypersecretory syndromes: (e.g., Zollinger-Ellison syndrome).
- Retained gastric antrum
- Less common: Crohn disease, vascular insufficiency, radiation therapy, cancer chemotherapy

ASSOCIATED CONDITIONS

- Zollinger-Ellison syndrome (gastrinoma)
- Systemic mastocytosis
- Multiple endocrine neoplasia type 1
- Chronic obstructive pulmonary disease, chronic renal failure, cirrhosis, hyperparathyroidism, carcinoid syndrome, polycythemia rubra vera, basophilic leukemia, porphyria cutanea tarda

DIAGNOSIS

SIGNS AND SYMPTOMS

- Peptic ulcer disease can present with a variety of symptoms or be asymptomatic prior to complications.
- NSAID-induced ulcers often silent; perforation or bleeding may be initial presentation.
- Duodenal ulcer in adults
  - Gnawing or burning epigastric pain 1–3 hours after meals
  - Relieved by food, antacids, or antisecretory agents.
  - Nocturnal pain
  - Epigastric pain in 60–90%
  - Nonspecific dyspeptic complaints (e.g., belching, bloating, abdominal distention, food intolerance) in 40–70%
  - Intermittent periods of symptoms
  - Some seasonal occurrence (e.g., spring and fall)
- Gastric ulcer in adults
  - Symptom complex similar to duodenal ulcers
  - Weight loss
- Complications of Peptic ulcers
  - Hemorrhage: Dizziness, syncope, hematemesis, or melena
  - Perforation: Sudden, severe midepigastric pain radiating to right shoulder, peritoneal signs, free peritoneal air.
  - Obstruction: Early satiety, nausea, vomiting, anorexia, and weight loss

TESTS

Lab

- Indications for H. pylori testing: New onset peptic ulcer disease, history of peptic ulcer disease, persistent symptoms after empiric antisecretory therapy, use of maintenance antisecretory therapy, gastric mucosa-associated lymphoid tissue lymphoma, uninvestigated dyspepsia.
- H. pylori diagnostic tests
  - Histology: Steiner stain of gastric biopsy for direct visualization of organism
  - Rapid urease test: Conducted on gastric biopsies
  - Serology antibody: Most commonly used for of testing in primary care but cannot be used to identify persistent infection
  - Urea breath test: Used for posttreatment testing
  - Stool antigen: Can be used for screening and post-treatment testing
- False negative results can occur with antisecretory medication.
- Other lab tests
  - CBC: Rule out anemia
  - Fecal occult blood test
  - Elevated serum gastrin or secretin stimulation test: Rule out Zollinger-Ellison syndrome
  - Gastric analysisrule out achlorhydria, acid hypersecretion

Imaging

Upper GI with barium: Radiographic features of benign gastric ulcer include ulcer projecting beyond the lumen, radiolucent band (Hampton line) paralleling ulcer base, radiating folds.

Diagnostic Procedures/Surgery

- Current recommendations for diagnosing H. pylori in peptic ulcer disease
- Known peptic ulcer disease without complications
  - Serology antibody test (1)[A]
- Dyspepsia with a history of untreated peptic ulcer disease
  - Serology antibody test (1)[A]
- Dyspepsia with a history of peptic ulcer disease treated for H. pylori
  - Stool antigen or urea breath test
  - If positive, treat with a different regimen
  - Confirm negative H. pylori by urea breath test or stool antigen 2–4 weeks later (1)[B]
- Persistence after antisecretory therapy
  - Serology antibody test
  - If negative, discontinue therapy and consider endoscopy or GI consult

DIFFERENTIAL DIAGNOSIS

- Dyspepsia not related to ulcer
- Gastric carcinoma
- Gastritis
- Gastroesophageal reflux disease
- Crohn disease (gastroduodenal)
- Pancreatitis
- Variant angina pectoris
- Cholelithiasis syndrome

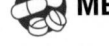 **TREATMENT**

INITIAL STABILIZATION
- A noninvasive "test and treat" strategy for *H. pylori* results in an equivalent outcome compared with prompt endoscopy (1)[C]
- Empiric treatment with H_2 blockers and PPIs for young healthy patients with dyspepsia (1)[C]
- Immediate endoscopy for patients with complicated ulcers or >45 year with alarm symptoms (weight loss, melena, anemia, dysphagia, abdominal mass, jaundice, family history of gastric cancer) (1)[A]
- Patients with nonulcer dyspepsia are unlikely to benefit from *H. pylori* therapy.
- Emergency endoscopy and hospitalization for suspected ulcer-related bleeding

GENERAL MEASURES
- Eliminate NSAIDs and psychologic stress.
- Avoid or eliminate cigarette smoking.

Diet
Regular meals but avoidance of dietary spices, alcohol, caffeine, or acetaminophen (1)[C]

Activity
Fully active in uncomplicated cases

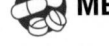 **MEDICATION (DRUGS)**

First Line
- Acid suppression
  - H_2 blockers
    - Ranitidine or nizatidine 150 mg PO b.i.d. or 300 mg PO q.h.s. Cimetidine 400 mg PO b.i.d. or 800 mg PO q.h.s. Famotidine 150 mg PO b.i.d. or 300 mg PO q.h.s.
  - PPI
    - Omeprazole 20 mg PO daily; Lansoprazole 30 mg PO daily; Rabeprazole 20 mg PO daily; Esomeprazole 40 mg PO daily; Pantoprazole 40 mg PO daily.
    - Administer PPIs before breakfast.
  - Treat duodenal ulcers for 4 weeks and gastric ulcers for 8 weeks.
  - PPIs heal peptic ulcers more rapidly and should not be taken with H_2 blockers.
- Optimal *H. pylori* eradication regimens (2)[A]
  - Triple therapy: 2 antibiotics plus a PPI for 14 days
    - Omeprazole 20 mg PO b.i.d. or Lansoprazole 30 mg PO b.i.d. *plus*
    - Metronidazole 500 mg PO b.i.d. or Amoxicillin 1 g PO b.i.d. *plus*
    - Clarithromycin 500 mg PO b.i.d.
  - Alternative triple therapy regimen:
    - Ranitidine bismuth citrate 400 mg PO b.i.d. *plus*
    - Clarithromycin 500 mg PO b.i.d. or Metronidazole 500 mg PO b.i.d. *plus*
    - Tetracycline 500 mg PO b.i.d. or Amoxicillin 1 g PO b.i.d.
- Bacterial resistance: Clarithromycin 10%, amoxicillin 1.4%, metronidazole 37%

- 2nd-line for treatment failures (2)[A]
  - Bismuth quadruple therapy for 14 days
    - Bismuth subsalicylate 525 mg PO t.i.d. *plus*
    - Metronidazole 250 mg PO t.i.d. *plus*
    - Tetracycline 500 mg PO t.i.d.
    - H_2 blocker for 28 days or PPI for 14 days
  - Alternative 2nd-line therapy
    - Levofloxacin 250 mg PO b.i.d. *plus*
    - Amoxicillin 1,000 mg PO b.i.d. *plus*
    - PPI PO b.i.d.
  - Another alternative salvage therapy
    - Rifabutin 300 mg PO daily *plus*
    - Amoxicillin 1,000 mg PO b.i.d. *plus*
    - PPI PO b.i.d.
- Consider culture and sensitivity after 2 treatment failures.
- Other
  - Treatment of *H. pylori*–negative ulcers
    - Usually due to NSAIDs–discontinue.
    - Treat acutely with PPIs for 4–12 weeks.

Second Line
- Alternative ulcer healing drugs
  - Sucralfate 1 g PO t.i.d. or 2 g PO b.i.d. × 4–8 weeks
  - Antacids can be taken 1–3 hours after meals (4–7 doses daily).
- Contraindications
  - Renal insufficiency
    - Reduce H_2 blocker dosage by 50%
    - Avoid magnesium-containing antacids.
- Significant possible interactions
  - Cimetidine inhibits cytochrome P-450 isozymes (avoid with theophylline, warfarin, phenytoin, and lidocaine).
  - Ranitidine and famotidine rarely associated with increased theophylline levels
  - Omeprazole may prolong elimination of diazepam, warfarin, and phenytoin.
  - Sulcrafate reduces absorption of tetracycline, norfloxacin, ciprofloxacin, and theophylline, leading to subtherapeutic levels.

ALERT
Pregnancy Considerations
- Peptic ulcer disease unusual in gestation
- H_2 blockers and proton pump inhibitors:
  - Cimetidine, famotidine, ranitidine, and nizatidine–Class B
  - Lansoprazole, esomeprazole, pantoprazole, and rabeprazole–Class B
  - Omeprazole–Class C
- Sucralfate–Class B
- Antacids are generally accepted as safe.

SURGERY
Selective vagotomy used in cases of complications of bleeding, obstruction, or perforation

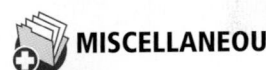 **FOLLOW-UP**

PROGNOSIS
After *H. pylori* eradication:
- Low ulcer relapse rate. If relapse, suspect surreptitious use of NSAIDs.
- Reinfection rates <1% per year
- Low risk of rebleeding
- Decreased NSAID ulcer reoccurrence

COMPLICATIONS
- Hemorrhage: Up to 25% of cases (initial presentation in 10%)
- Perforation <5% of cases
- Gastric outlet obstruction: Up to 5% of duodenal or pyloric channel ulcers. Male predilection found.
- Risk of gastric adenocarcinoma increased up to 9-fold in *H. pylori*–infected patients

PATIENT MONITORING
- Eradication of *H. pylori*: Expected in >90% (with double antibiotic regimen):
  - Confirm eradication by urea breath test or stool antigen in patients who remain symptomatic or experience relapse.
- Acute duodenal ulcer: Monitor clinically
- Acute gastric ulcer: Confirm healing via endoscopy after 6–12 weeks.
- Removal of malignancy of unhealed ulcer via biopsy
- Symptom response does not rule out malignancy

REFERENCES
1. Meuer L, Bower D. Management of Helicobacter pylori infection. *Am Fam Physician.* 2002;65:1327–1336.
2. Saad R, Chey W. A clinician's guide to managing Helicobacter pylori infection. *Cleve Clin J Med.* 2005;72:109–124.
3. Suerbaum S, Michetti P. *Helicobacter pylori* infection. *N Engl J Med.* 2002;347:1175–1186.

 MISCELLANEOUS

CODES

ICD9-CM
- 531.90 Duodenal ulcer, unspecified as acute or chronic, without mention of hemorrhage, perforation, or obstruction
- 532.90 Gastric ulcer, unspecified as acute or chronic, without mention of hemorrhage, perforation, or obstruction

 See Corresponding Diagnostic Algorithm

See Patient Handout on CD

PERICARDITIS

Christopher P. Ruisi, MD

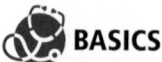 **BASICS**

DESCRIPTION
- Inflammatory process of the pericardium with or without associated pericardial effusion; a broad spectrum of etiologies with most common causes viral or idiopathic.
- System(s) Affected: Cardiovascular
- Synonym(s): Acute suppurative pericarditis

RISK FACTORS
Genetics
Unknown

Incidence
- 1–6% in postmortem studies
- Diagnosed in 0.1% of hospitalized patients and 5% patients evaluated in emergency room for chest pain without myocardial infarction (MI).

ETIOLOGY
- Idiopathic
- Viral: Coxsackievirus, Echovirus, Adenovirus, Epstein-Barr virus, Cytomegalovirus, Hepatitis C, Parvo B 19, Influenza, HIV, Rubella, Mumps, etc.
- Bacterial: *Haemophilus* sp. (especially children), *Staphylococcus* sp., *Pneumococcus* sp., *Salmonella* sp., *Meningococcus* sp., *Gonococcus* sp., *Legionella* sp., *Mycoplasma* sp., *Treponema pallidum*, Borreliosis
- Fungal: Candidal, histoplasmosis, *Aspergillus*, *Nocardia*
- Mycobacterial: *Mycobacterium tuberculosis*
- Parasites, protozoans
- Vaccination (smallpox)
- Neoplastic: Breast, lung, lymphoma, mesothelioma, sarcoma
- Drug-induced: Hydralazine, bleomycin, phenytoin, minoxidil, mesalamine, and others
- Connective tissue disease: Systemic lupus erythematosus, rheumatoid arthritis, scleroderma, acute rheumatic fever
- Radiation
- MI, Dressler syndrome
- Postpericardiotomy
- Uremia
- Trauma
- Myxedema
- Cholesterol pericarditis
- Aortic dissection
- Sarcoidosis
- Pancreatitis
- Inflammatory bowel disease
- Gaucher disease
- Gout
- Chylopericardium
- Familial

ASSOCIATED CONDITIONS
Depends on etiology

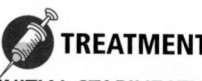 **DIAGNOSIS**

Should document at least 2 of the following features with or without pericardial effusion
- Chest pain
- Pericardial friction rub
- Widespread saddle-shaped or concave up ST segment elevation on ECG

SIGNS AND SYMPTOMS
- Prodrome may involve anorexia, malaise, and myalgias.
- Fever or other features of sepsis can accompany viral or bacterial pericarditis.
- Substernal chest pain, typically sharp, and usually with radiation to the trapezoid line
- Pain often is sudden in onset, worse with inspiration.
- Pain may be reduced by leaning forward and sitting up.
- Arrhythmias are uncommon and usually occur in patients with underlying cardiac disease.

Physical Exam
- Heart rate is usually rapid and regular.
- Pericardial friction rub
  - Highly specific for diagnosis and present in up to 85% patients
  - High-pitched sound best heard during end expiration at left sternal border with patient leaning forward
  - May be transient and mono-, bi-, or triphasic
- New S3 may suggest perimyocarditis
- Cardiac tamponade suggested by the presence of
  - Systemic arterial hypotension
  - Elevated jugular venous pressure
  - Pulsus paradoxus (inspiratory fall in arterial pressure of at least 10 mm Hg)

TESTS
Lab
- Leukocytosis, increased ESR or c-reactive protein
- May observe elevated creatine kinase, troponin, lactate dehydrogenase, or aspartate transaminase
  - Elevated troponins associated with younger age, male gender, pericardial effusion at presentation, and ST segment elevation on ECG (1)[B]
  - Adverse outcomes not predicted by elevated troponin (1,2)[B]
- Additional testing includes tuberculin skin test, rheumatoid factor, antinuclear antibody, and HIV serology if clinically appropriate. (3)[C]
- Viral cultures and antibody titers rarely clinically useful

Imaging
- ECG findings include widespread upward concave ST-segment elevation and PR-segment depression that may evolve through 4 stages:
  - Stage 1: Diffuse ST segment elevation and PR-segment depression
  - Stage 2: Normalization of the ST and PR segments
  - Stage 3: Widespread T-wave inversions
  - Stage 4: Normalization of T waves
- ECG may demonstrate low voltage and electrical alternans with tamponade.
- Chest radiograph is performed to rule out pulmonary/mediastinal pathology. (2)[B]
  - Enlarged cardiac silhouette suggests large pericardial effusion.

- Transthoracic echocardiogram recommended to evaluate for presence of pericardial effusion to support diagnosis of pericarditis. (4)[B]
- Echocardiographic evidence of tamponade indicates need for pericardiocentesis.
- CT and MRI permit visualization of pericardium to assess for complications (2,3)[B]

Diagnostic Procedures/Surgery
- Pericardiocentesis indicated for cardiac tamponade and for suspected purulent, tuberculous, or neoplastic pericarditis (2,3)[B]
- Pericardiocentesis considered for large effusions and persistent symptoms (2)[B]
- Pericardial biopsy considered for evaluation of malignant or granulomatous causes of pericarditis
- Surgical drainage preferred for traumatic hemopericardium and documented purulent pericarditis

Pathological Findings
- Microscopic examination reveals hyperemia, leukocyte accumulation, and fibrin deposition
- Pericardial fluid typically dominated by neutrophils in bacterial pericarditis
- Lymphocytic predominance in viral, tuberculous, and neoplastic pericarditis
- Hemorrhagic effusions more common in tuberculous, neoplastic, or traumatic pericarditis

DIFFERENTIAL DIAGNOSIS
- Acute MI
- Pneumonia with pleurisy
- Pulmonary emboli
- Aortic dissection
- Pneumothorax
- Mediastinal emphysema
- Cholecystitis
- Pancreatitis
- Esophageal inflammation, perforation, or rupture

TREATMENT

INITIAL STABILIZATION
Outpatient therapy reported successful in 87% patients with low-risk features (4)[B]

GENERAL MEASURES
- Specific therapy directed toward underlying disorder for patients with identified cause other than viral or idiopathic disease
- Therapy aimed at symptomatic relief for idiopathic pericarditis and not demonstrated to prevent tamponade or constrictive pericarditis

Diet
No restrictions, but suggest weight-loss program in overweight patients

Activity
Physical activity may exacerbate accompanying myocarditis.

MEDICATION (DRUGS)

First Line

- NSAIDs are considered mainstay of therapy; dosage is tapered to reduce recurrence rate. (2,3)[B]
  - Ibuprofen 300–800 mg q6–8h, to be continued for days or weeks as needed
  - Aspirin 800 mg q6–8h preferable for patients with recent MI, because other NSAIDs impair scar formation in animal studies
  - Gastrointestinal protection should be provided.
- Colchicine (1–2 mg 1st day, with maintenance dose 0.5–1 mg/d) effective as monotherapy or as adjunct to an NSAID for initial attack and prevention of recurrences (2,5)[B]

- Contraindications: Hypersensitivity to aspirin or NSAID, active peptic ulcer or gastrointestinal bleeding
- Precautions: Use with caution in patients with asthma, 3rd-trimester pregnancy, coagulopathy, renal or hepatic dysfunction

Second Line

- Indomethacin 25–50 mg q6–8h is effective alternative; avoid use in patients with CAD, given concerns about reduction of coronary flow. (3)[C]

- Systemic glucocorticoid treatment (prednisone, 1.1.5 mg/kg/d) indicated in connective tissue disease, uremic or, tuberculous pericarditis or severe recurrent symptoms unresponsive to NSAIDs or colchicine (2,3)[B]
- Intrapericardial administration of steroids may be effective and limits systemic side effects. (2)[B]

SURGERY

Pericardiectomy considered for frequent and highly symptomatic recurrences resistant to medical therapy (2,3)[B]

 ## FOLLOW-UP

DISPOSITION
Admission Criteria

- Inpatient therapy recommended for pericarditis associated with high-risk features (4)[B]
  - Fever >38°C
  - Subacute onset of symptoms
  - Immunosuppressed state
  - Trauma
  - Oral anticoagulant therapy
  - Myopericarditis
  - Cardiac tamponade or large pericardial effusion that does not decrease with therapy
  - Failure to respond to NSAID therapy

PROGNOSIS
Most patients experience complete resolution of pain and symptoms within 2 weeks of therapy.

COMPLICATIONS
- Recurrent pericarditis
  - Occurs in up to 30% patients; thought to represent autoimmune process
  - Symptoms recur at variable times after initial attack but 1st recurrence usually within 18–20 months of initial presentation.
  - Rarely associated with tamponade or constriction
- Cardiac tamponade
  - Rare complication with increased incidence in neoplastic, purulent, and tuberculous pericarditis
- Constrictive pericarditis
  - Rare complication in which rigid pericardium produces abnormal diastolic filling with elevated filling pressures.
  - Pericardiectomy remains definitive therapy.

PATIENT MONITORING
Follow-up evaluation is not required for patients with small effusion unless symptoms recur or new symptoms develop.

REFERENCES

1. Imazio M, Demichelis B, Cecchi E, et al. Cardiac troponin i in acute pericarditis. *J Am Coll Cardiol.* 2003;42:2144–2148.
2. Maisch B, Seferovic PM, Ristic AD, et al. Guidelines on the diagnosis and management of pericardial diseases of the European Society of Cardiology. *Eur Heart J.* 2004;25:587–610.
3. Troughton RW, Asher CR, Klein AL. Pericarditis. *Lancet.* 2004;363:717–727.
4. Imazio M, Demichelis B, Parrini I, et al. Day-hospital treatment of acute pericarditis: a management program for outpatient therapy. *J Am Coll Cardiol.* 2004;43:1042–1046.
5. Imazio M, Bobbio M, Cecchih E, et al. Colchicine in addition to conventional therapy for acute pericarditis: Results of the Colchicine for acute Pericarditis (COPE) Trial. *Circulation.* 2005;112: 2012–2016.

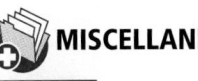 ## MISCELLANEOUS

CODES

ICD9-CM
- 420.91 Acute idiopathic pericarditis
- 420.99 Other acute pericarditis

PATIENT TEACHING

Primary-care physicians must educate patients about the possible return of symptoms and necessary follow-up visits.

 See Corresponding Diagnostic Algorithm

PERIODIC LIMB MOVEMENT DISORDER (PLMD)

Donald E. Watenpaugh, PhD
John R. Burk, MD

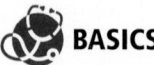 **BASICS**

DESCRIPTION

PLMD is a sleep-related movement disorder with the following features (1,2)[A]

- Consists of episodes of stereotyped, periodic limb movements (PLMs) during sleep.
- Movements usually involve bilateral ankle and toe dorsiflexion sometimes accompanied by knee and hip flexion.
- Arm or more generalized involvement occurs less commonly and in severe cases.
- The movements commonly produce brief sleep disturbances (microarousals) unbeknownst to the patient.
- Associated with complaints of insomnia, unrestorative sleep, daytime fatigue, and/or somnolence.
- Bed partner commonly complains of movements.
- Another primary sleep disorder (e.g., obstructive sleep apnea) does not cause the PLMs.
- System(s) Affected: Musculoskeletal; Nervous systems
- Synonym(s): Nocturnal myoclonus; Sleep myoclonus; Periodic leg movements of sleep

EPIDEMIOLOGY

- Predominant age: All ages; incidence increases with age.
- Predominant sex: Male = Female

Incidence

- PLMs are common and increase with age: ~1/3 of patients age >60 exhibit PLMs.
- However, PLMs meeting all criteria above, thus constituting PLMD, are much less common.
- PLMs occur in ~15% of insomnia patients.
- A common associate of PLMs, restless legs syndrome (RLS) occurs about twice as often in parous women than in men.

Prevalence

Prevalence and severity increase with age.

ALERT

Geriatric Considerations

May cause or exacerbate circadian disruption and sundowning

Pediatric Considerations

- Association with RLS more common in children.
- Associated with ADHD. (3,4)[B]

Pregnancy Considerations

- PLMs usually subside after delivery
- Most severe in 3rd trimester
- May be secondary to iron and/or folate deficiency

RISK FACTORS

- RLS (~85% exhibit PLMs)
- REM sleep behavior disorder (~70% exhibit PLMs)
- Narcolepsy (~55% exhibit PLMs)
- Iron deficiency and conditions associated with iron insufficiency (pregnancy, gastric surgery, end-stage renal disease).
- ADHD
- Aging
- Peripheral neuropathy (as with diabetes) and other sources of chronic limb pain or discomfort.

Genetics

Unstudied, but RLS has a susceptibility locus on chromosome 12q.

ETIOLOGY

Primary PLMD: Evidence suggests central nervous dopaminergic impairment, which itself may be secondary to chronic iron deficiency.

- PLMD may occur secondary to
  - Iron deficiency
  - Peripheral neuropathy (as from diabetes)
  - Arthritis
  - Renal failure
  - Synucleinopathies such as multiple system atrophy
  - Spinal cord injury
  - Pregnancy
- Medications that may precipitate or worsen PLMD include
  - Most antidepressants (exception: Bupropion)
  - Dopamine antagonists such as metoclopramide
  - Antihistamines

ASSOCIATED CONDITIONS

- RLS
- REM sleep behavior disorder
- Narcolepsy
- Iron deficiency
- CNS dopaminergic dysfunction
- Renal failure
- Gastric surgery
- Pregnancy
- Arthritis
- Synucleinopathies such as multiple system atrophy
- Spinal cord injury
- Peripheral neuropathy
- Insomnia, insufficient sleep
- ADHD
- Depression
- Sundowning

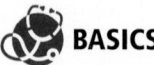 **DIAGNOSIS**

SIGNS AND SYMPTOMS

- Insomnia: Difficulty going to or maintaining sleep
- Unrestorative sleep and other common hallmarks of poor or insufficient sleep: Fatigue, oppositional behaviors, depression, and memory impairment
- Daytime somnolence
- ADHD (3,4)[B]

TESTS

Electromyography and nerve conduction studies may be indicated to check for peripheral neuropathy and radiculopathy.

Lab

In addition to complaints of disturbed or unrestorative sleep, PLMD diagnosis requires polysomnographic finding of repetitive, stereotyped limb movements defined as (2)[A]

- Pre-tibial electromyographic activity lasting 0.5–5.0 s
- Amplitude equals at least 25% of that elicited by conscious ankle dorsiflexion
- Movements occur in a sequence of 4 or more at intervals of 5–90 s
- An index of 5 or more movements per hour in children or 15 in adults
- Commonly associated with heart rate variability from autonomic arousals during sleep
- Most PLM episodes occur in the 1st hours of sleep
- Measure serum ferritin to exclude iron deficiency.

Lab

Diagnostic Procedures/Surgery

- Clinical history (patient and bedpartner)
- Polysomnography

DIFFERENTIAL DIAGNOSIS

- Obstructive sleep apnea: PLMs occur during microarousals from breathing disturbance; successful treatment of sleep apnea eliminates PLMs (1)[A]
- Sleep starts (hypnic jerks): Nonperiodic, occur only during transition from wake to sleep, and shorter in duration (20: 100 ms).
- Sleep-related leg cramps: Isolated painful events leading to full wakefulness.
- Fragmentary myoclonus: EMG activity of 75–150 ms with little associated movement and no periodicity.
- Nocturnal seizures: Epileptiform EEG activity not seen with PLMD; motor pattern not seen with PLMD.
- Fasciculations and tremor: No association with sleep.
- Sleep-related rhythmic movement disorder: Voluntary movement during wake–sleep transition; higher frequency than PLMs.
- When PLMs occur along with RLS, REM sleep behavior disorder, or narcolepsy, those disorders are diagnosed as "with PLMs," and PLMD is not diagnosed separately (1)[A]

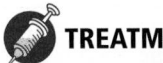

TREATMENT

GENERAL MEASURES
Appropriate health care: Outpatient
- Daily physical activity
- Warming the legs with long socks, leg warmers, or an electric blanket
- Hot bath

Diet
- Avoid caffeine, alcohol, tobacco, and antihistamines, especially late in the day.
- Supplements to correct deficiencies in iron, folate, and magnesium

Activity
Regular exercise is helpful.

MEDICATION (DRUGS)

Dosing prior to bedtime. 4 classes of drugs apply, in usual order of preference (5,6)[A]
- Dopamine agonists
  – Ropinirole (Requip): 0.25–4.0 mg 1 hour before bed; increase by 0.25 mg every 3 days to determine optimal dose.
  – Pramipexole (Mirapex): Same protocol as above but start at 0.125 mg and increase by 0.125 mg steps; usual maximum dose 1.5 mg.
  – Augmentation of symptoms (increased PLMs and sleep disturbance, emergence of RLS) can occur with prolonged use of dopamine agonists. Augmentation requires reduction of dopaminergic agent and addition of adjunct medication. Symptoms may rebound with reduction or withdrawal of dopaminergic therapy.
- Anticonvulsants
  – Gabapentin (Neurontin): 300–1,800 mg per night; particularly useful for PLMD associated with pain or neuropathy
- Benzodiazepines and agonists: Particularly useful for patients with major complaint of insomnia
  – Clonazepam (Klonopin): 0.5–3.0 mg per night
  – Other potentially useful benzodiazepines include temazepam, triazolam, alprazolam, zaleplon, zolpidem, and diazepam.
- Opioids: Low risk for dose escalation and dependence in patients without substance abuse history
  – Hydrocodone: 5–20 mg per night
  – Oxycodone: 2.5–20 mg per night
  – Almost any hypnotic may be helpful as add-on treatment.
- Severe cases and augmentation require combination therapy.

- Most of the above medications can cause daytime sleepiness as a side effect, although this is unusual with the doses and timing employed for PLMD.
- Risks, side-effects, and interactions of medications must be considered individually (e.g., benzodiazepine use in elderly). Refer to literature.

Second Line
- Iron supplementation: 200–300 mg ferrous sulfate with 200 mg vitamin C, t.i.d. between meals, to facilitate absorption. Monitor for side effects including hemochromotosis. It may take months for iron repletion, during which PLMD usually continues without other treatment. (5,6)[B]

- Vitamin and mineral supplements, including magnesium, B_{12}, and folate (5,6)[C]
- Quinine
- Clonidine: 0.1–0.7 mg/d

FOLLOW-UP

PROGNOSIS
- Primary PLMD: A lifelong condition with no current cure
- Secondary PLMD: May partially or completely subside with resolution of precipitating factors
- PLMD progresses with age.
- Current therapies usually control the problem.
- PLMD commonly precedes and predicts emergence of RLS.

COMPLICATIONS
- Tolerance to medications requiring increased dose or alternatives
- Augmentation of symptoms in response to dopaminergic therapy
- Medication side effects and interactions, including from iron and other vitamin/mineral supplementation

PATIENT MONITORING
- At monthly intervals until stable.
- Annual and follow-up thereafter as needed

REFERENCES
1. Periodic Limb Movement Disorder. In: *International Classification of Sleep Disorders Diagnostic & Coding Manual*, 2nd ed. Editor: MJ Sateia. Westchester, IL: American Academy of Sleep Medicine; 2005;182–186.
2. Recording and scoring leg movements. The Atlas Task Force. *Sleep.* 1993;16:748–759.

3. Cortese S, et al. Restless legs syndrome and attention-deficit/hyperactivity disorder: A review of the literature. *Sleep.* 2005;28(8):1007–1013.
4. Crabtree VM, et al. Periodic limb movement disorder of sleep in children. *J Sleep Res.* 2003;12(1):73–81.
5. Hening WA, et al. An update on the dopaminergic treatment of restless legs syndrome and periodic limb movement disorder. *Sleep.* 2004;27(3):560–583.
6. Silber MH, et al. An algorithm for the management of restless legs syndrome. *Mayo Clinic Proceedings.* 2004;79(7):916–922.

MISCELLANEOUS

Other notes
- Wide variation in night-to-night PLM activity.

- In adults and children, PLMs and ADHD commonly coexist. Accumulating data indicate sleep disturbance, including that from PLMs, causes or exacerbates ADHD. (3,4)[B]

CODES

ICD9-CM
327.51

PATIENT TEACHING
- Wilson V. *Sleep Thief.* Orange Park, FL: Glaxy Books; 1996.
- National Sleep Foundation; 1522 K Street NW, Suite 500; Washington, DC 20005; nsf@sleepfoundation.org; http://www.sleepfoundation.org; tel: (202) 347-3471; fax: (202) 347-3472
- WE MOVE (Worldwide Education & Awareness for Movement Disorders); 204 West 84th Street; New York, NY 10024; wemove@wemove.org; http://www.wemove.org; tel: (212) 875-8312; fax: (212) 875-8389

PERIPHERAL ARTERIAL DISEASE (PAD)

Zhen Lu, MD

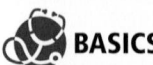 **BASICS**

DESCRIPTION
PAD is a manifestation of systemic atherosclerosis in which there is partial or total blockage in the arteries, exclusive of the coronary and cerebral vessels.

- Objectively, PAD is defined as a resting ankle-brachial index of >0.90.

EPIDEMIOLOGY
Highly prevalent syndrome that affects ~8–12 million individuals in the US

- Predominant age: >40
- Predominant sex: Male > Female (2:1) based on the Framingham study
- Patients with symptomatic PAD have a 5-year mortality rate of ~30%

Incidence
Population per year overall: 1.0–2.7/1,000

Prevalence
- US prevalence: 2.7–4.1%
- Age-adjusted prevalence of PAD is close to 12%.
- Up to 29% among patients in primary care practices

RISK FACTORS
- Age >40 years
- Cigarette smoking
- Diabetes mellitus
- Obesity
- Hypertension
- Hyperlipidemia
- Hyperhomocysteinemia

Genetics
Current National Institutes of Health–funded research focuses on single nucleotide polymorphisms in candidate genes that are regulated in the vasculature, in an attempt to explore genetic factors responsible for PAD.

PATHOPHYSIOLOGY
In patients with peripheral arterial disease, arterial stenoses cause inadequate blood flow in distal limbs, and fail to meet the metabolic demand during exertion.

- The degree of ischemia is proportional to the size and proximity of the occlusion to the end organ.
- The acidic products of anaerobic metabolism build up within the muscle and result in claudication clinically.
- Arterial occlusion also causes significantly diminished distal pressure in patients with PAD due to the atherosclerotic lesions.

ETIOLOGY
The most common cause of arterial stenoses is atherosclerosis.

ASSOCIATED CONDITIONS
- See "Risk Factors."
- Associated with other common complications of atherosclerosis, including myocardial infarction, transient ischemic attack, stroke, and limb amputation
- Occurs in ~40% of patients with cardiovascular disease

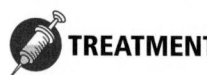 **DIAGNOSIS**

SIGNS AND SYMPTOMS
History
- ~1/2 of the patients with PAD are asymptomatic.
- Intermittent claudication (symptoms typically resolve within 2–5 minutes of rest)
- Rest leg pain (especially in a supine position)
- Skin ulceration
- Gangrene
- Impotence

Physical Exam
- Reduced or absent extremity pulses
- Skin pallor with leg elevation above the level of the heart
- Dependent rubor
- Dry and scaly skin
- Poor nail growth
- Hair loss

TESTS
Lab
- Fasting lipid profile is indicated for risk assessment of hyperlipidemia
- Serum glucose is recommended for screening diabetes mellitus.

Imaging
- Magnetic resonance angiography, coupled with 3-D reconstruction, is highly sensitive and specific for the localization of occluded lesions.
- CT has limited role in evaluating PAD
- Duplex ultrasonography and Doppler color-flow imaging are useful in detecting stenosed segments and assessing lesion severity
- Angiography remains the gold standard in the diagnosis of PAD.

Diagnostic Procedures/Surgery
- Doppler ankle-brachial index (ABI) measures the ratio of (1) the higher systolic BPs between the dorsalis pedis and the posterior tibial artery to (2) the higher of the systolic BPs in the 2 brachial arteries.
  - ABI<0.4: Severe ischemia
  - 0.4<ABI<0.9: Moderate peripheral arterial obstruction
  - 0.9<ABI<1.3: Reduction of ABI by 20% after exercise is suggestive of PAD; otherwise, normal
  - Pathological ABI >1.3: Calcified vessel and additional diagnostic studies are needed
- Segmental limb pressures: Usually obtained if abnormal ABI measurement is identified. A 20 mm Hg or greater reduction in pressure is considered significant for PAD
- Treadmill exercise test assesses the severity of claudication and the response to treatment
- Segmental volume plethysmogrphy: Often used in conjunction with segmental limb pressures to measure the volume change in an organ or limb. The study is indicated for calcified vessel when ABI cannot be applied diagnostically.

DIFFERENTIAL DIAGNOSIS
- Arterial embolism
- Deep venous thrombosis
- Thromboangitis obliterans (Buerger disease)
- Osteoarthritis
- Restless legs syndrome
- Peripheral neuropathy
- Spinal stenoses (pseudoclaudication
- Intervertebral disc prolapse

TREATMENT

GENERAL MEASURES
- Claudication exercise rehabilitation program; patient to walk until develops symptoms, then rest and start again, for a total of 30 minutes initially; walking is then increased by 5 minutes until 50 minutes of intermittent walking is achieved.
- Modification of risk factors including smoking, diabetes mellitus, hypertension, and hyperlipidemia
  - Weight loss is associated with decrease in risk of cardiovascular disease, but has not been shown to improve PAD. (1)[C]
  - Simvastatin (20–40 mg/d) has been shown to reduce the incidence of new intermittent claudication from 3.6–2.3% in patients with coronary arterial disease. (2)[A]
  - Beta-adrenergic antagonists should be used with caution in individuals with severe PAD. (1)[B]
  - Smoking cessation, by use of nicotine replacement therapy and bupropion, is likely to reduce the severity of claudication. (1)[C]

Diet
Low-fat cardiac diet is recommended

Activity
Exercise training program composed of walking or bicycle riding improves maximal treadmill walking distance and therefore enhances functional capacity. (2)[A]

SPECIAL THERAPY
Complementary and Alternative Therapies
Acupuncture, biofeedback, chelation therapy, and supplements such as Ginkgo biloba, omega-3 fatty acids, and Vitamin E have been studied.

- Ginko baloba modestly improves symptoms of intermittent claudication (120 mg/d for up to 6 months) and can be considered as an adjunct to exercise therapy. Inconclusive evidence exists for the use of vitamin E. (5,6)

MEDICATION (DRUGS)

Antiplatelet therapy is the mainstay treatment to prevent ischemic events in patients with PAD.

- Although the effect of aspirin on the risk reduction of overall ischemic events is inconclusive, it has been shown to delay disease progression and reduce the need for surgical intervention, and should be recommended for patients with PAD. (1)[A]
- Low-dose aspirin (75–150 mg/d) is as effective as higher doses of Aspirin (1)
- Ticlopidine (250 mg b.i.d.) reduces the risks of myocardial infarction, stroke, and death by 1/3 in patients with PAD, but has complication of thrombocytopenia in 2–3% of patients (1)[A]
- Clopidogrel (dose: 75 mg/d) is Food and Drug Administration–approved for the secondary prevention of atherosclerotic events in patients with PAD (2)[A]
- Neither vasodilators nor anticoagulant therapy (e.g., heparin, low-molecular-weight heparin or oral anticoagulant) have any clinically proven efficacy for the treatment of claudication. (1)[B]

- Other medications that may improve claudication include Pentoxifylline (1.2 g/d), Cilostazol (100 mg b.i.d.), Nafitdrofuryl (600 mg/d), and Prostaglandins (120 mcg/d).

SURGERY

Surgical interventions, such as revascularization, are warranted for those individuals who have debilitating intermittent claudication, ischemic rest pain, or tissue loss.

- Transluminal balloon angioplasty is a percutaneous method of dilating arterial stenoses or recanalizing occluded vessels with or without stents (reserved for short, isolated, and hemodynamically significant lesion of the iliac or proximal superficial femoral artery).
- Bypass surgery is the standard operative treatment for lower extremity peripheral occlusive disease

 FOLLOW-UP

PROGNOSIS

Among patients with intermittent claudication, 15–20% will experience worsening claudication, 5–10% will undergo lower extremity bypass surgery, and 2–5% will need primary amputation. (Rates for smokers and diabetics are much higher).

- 30,000–50,000 people in the US undergo amputations annually due to PAD.

REFERENCES

1. Hankey GJ, et al. Medical treatment of peripheral arterial disease. *JAMA*. 2006;295(5):547–553.
2. Gey DC, et al. Management of peripheral arterial disease. *Am Fam Physician*. 2004;69(3):525–532.
3. Hiatt WR, et al. Medical treatment of peripheral arterial disease and claudication. *NEJM*. 2001; 344:1608–1621.
4. Burns P, et al. Management of peripheral arterial disease in primary care. *BMJ*. 2003;326:584–588.
5. Pittler MH, Ernst E. Ginkgo biloba extract for the treatment of intermittent claudication: A meta-analysis of randomized trials. *Am J. Med* 2000, 108(4):276–281.
6. Kleijnen I, MacKerras D. Vitamin E for intermittent claudication. Cochrane Peripheral Vascular Diseases Group Cochrane Database of Systematic Reviews. 4, 2006.

 MISCELLANEOUS

CODES

ICD9-CM

- 440.21 Atherosclerosis of the extremities with intermittent claudication
- 440.22 Atherosclerosis of the extremities with rest pain

PATIENT TEACHING

- Weight reduction, smoking cessation, and BP control are essential in treating claudication.
- A walking program should include at least 3 times per week for 30–60 minutes each time, and has been shown to improve quality of life
- A healthy diet high in complex carbohydrates (such as whole grains and pastas), fruits, and vegetables, and low in salt and animal fats

 See Corresponding Diagnostic Algorithm

 See Patient Handout on CD

PERITONITIS, ACUTE

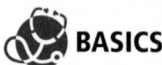

Ramothea L. Webster, PhD

BASICS

DESCRIPTION
- An acute inflammation of the visceral and parietal peritoneum
- 3 types are recognized
  - Spontaneous bacterial (SBP) abscess
  - Persistent
  - Recurrent peritonitis (from previously treated disease, often seen in chronic liver disease)
- System(s) Affected: Cardiovascular; Endocrine/metabolic; Gastrointestinal
- Spontaneous Bacterial Peritonitis (SBP) implies an intraabdominal bacterial infection without a surgically treatable source.
- Secondary Bacterial Peritonitis (2BP) is an intraabdominal infection with a surgically treatable source.

ALERT
Geriatric Considerations
Mortality is greater in this age group. Symptoms may be muted.

GENERAL PREVENTION
- Prophylactic antibiotics during abdominal surgery
- Prophylactic antibiotics for patients with cirrhosis and/or gastrointestinal bleeding and in high-risk patients who have recurrent peritonitis or low ascitic fluid total protein levels

EPIDEMIOLOGY
- Predominant age: None
- Predominant sex: Male > Female

Incidence
Recurrence rates of SBP within 6 months as high as 43%; within 1 year 69%

Prevalence
- SBP: 3.5% in asymptomatic outpatients with cirrhosis and ascites
- SBP: 10–30% of hospitalized patients with cirrhosis and ascites
- SBP is the cause of 1/3 of all bacterial infections seen in patients with cirrhosis.

RISK FACTORS
- Cirrhosis with ascites
- Low ascitic fluid total protein level
- Upper GI bleeding
- Ischemia–reperfusion of the gut
- Prior episode of SBP
- Indwelling IV and urinary bladder catheters

Genetics
No known genetic pattern

PATHOPHYSIOLOGY
- SBP: Cirrhosis predisposes patients to develop bacterial overgrowth probably secondary to altered small intestinal motility. This leads to intestinal bacterial translocation (Gram negative > Gram positive) into mesenteric lymph nodes, which rupture because of induced by high pressures associated with portal hypertension. The result is bacteremia, producing seeding of the liver, and consequent seeding of the ascitic fluid.
- Other modes of bacterial seeding are urinary tract infections, pneumococcal sepsis, cellulitis, pharyngitis, and dental infections.
- 2nd-degree BP: Ruptured peritoneal organ or tissue, or abscess seeding the peritoneum with bacteria causing a surgical abdomen.

ETIOLOGY
- Primary: SBP
  - Ascites associated with cirrhosis, and rarely associated with cardiac, nephrotic, or malignancy-related ascites, and alcohol or viral hepatitis
- Secondary: 2nd-degree BP
  - Perforation of bowel
  - Peritoneal abscess
  - Abdominal trauma
  - Continuous ambulatory peritoneal dialysis
  - Appendicitis
  - Colitis: Infectious, inflammatory
  - Peptic ulcer perforation
  - Gangrene of the bowel
  - Diverticulitis
  - Pancreatitis
  - Postoperative (intra-abdominal surgery)
  - Acute cholecystitis

ASSOCIATED CONDITIONS
SBP has a strong correlation with liver cirrhosis.

DIAGNOSIS

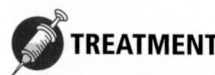

SIGNS AND SYMPTOMS
- Acute abdominal pain $+/-$ exacerbation with motion, $+/-$ rebound tenderness, $+/-$ rigidity
- Abdominal distention
- Ascites
- Fever ($>37.8°C/100°F$)
  - Note: Patients with advanced cirrhosis are usually mildly hypothermic
- Nausea/vomiting, Chills
- Change in GI motility
- Decrease in renal function
- Dyspnea
- Altered mental status (54% of cirrhosis patients either due to infection or hepatic dysfunction) (1)[B]

Physical Exam
Abdominal pain with tenderness is a classical sign, but this sign may be diminished in SBP patients because ascites separates the visceral from the parietal peritoneal surfaces, thus preventing abdominal tenderness and/or rigidity. (1)[B]

TESTS
Lab
- Basic metabolic panel
- CBC with differential
- Blood culture
- Liver function test with amylase/lipase
- Ascitic fluid analysis: (1)[B]
  - Check cell count with differential, culture, Gram stain, total protein, lactate dehydrogenase, glucose, amylase, and albumin
  - SBP analysis shows absolute polymorphonuclear (PMN) count ≥250 cells/mm^3, and culture grows typically 1 organism.
  - 2nd-degree BP analysis shows absolute PMN count ≥250 cells/mm^3, and culture typically grows multiple organisms.
- Urine analysis and culture
- Drugs that may alter lab results: Antibiotics prior to blood studies

Imaging
- Flat and upright abdominal film: Free air in peritoneal cavity, large bowel dilatation, small bowel dilatation, intestinal wall edema, or extravasation of water-soluble gut contrast
- Chest radiograph: Elevated diaphragm
- CT: Intra-abdominal mass, ascites
- Sonograph: Intra-abdominal mass, ascites

Diagnostic Procedures/Surgery
- Ascites: Abdominal paracentesis
- Diagnostic laparotomy, unless contraindicated
- Colonoscopy may be useful, particularly in patients >65 years with diffuse symptoms

Pathological Findings
Predominant PMN infiltration noted in ascitic fluid

DIFFERENTIAL DIAGNOSIS
- Abscess formation (subdiaphragmatic, subhepatic, peritoneal, pelvic)
- Ileus (volvulus, intussusception)
- Mesenteric adenitis
- Appendicitis
- Pancreatitis
- PID
- Cholecystitis
- Pyelonephritis
- Ruptured ectopic pregnancy
- Tubo-ovarian cyst

TREATMENT

GENERAL MEASURES
- Treat paralytic ileus (nasogastric decompression).
- Treat dehydration (IV fluids usually indicated).
- Antibiotics are started empirically to cover a broad spectrum of organisms once infection is suspected, with an ascitic fluid PMN count of ≥250 cells/mm^3. The choice of antibiotic may be altered after culture and sensitivity results are obtained.
- Respiratory support if needed
- Blood transfusions (occasionally)

Diet
- IV fluids and electrolytes
- Oral feedings only after return of bowel sounds and passage of flatus and/or feces
- Total parenteral nutrition may be necessary

Activity
Bed rest until infection is under control

MEDICATION (DRUGS)

First Line

- SBP
  - Cefotaxime 2 g IV t.i.d. for 5 days, then reassess
    - Excellent penetration into ascites with no nephrotoxicity; common side effect is rash.
  - Amoxicillin-clavulanic acid 1 g IV q6h for 2 days, then 500 mg/125 mg PO t.i.d. for 6–12 days
    - Highly nephrotoxic, avoid usage (2,3) [A]

- Secondary bacterial peritonitis
  - Must cover against anaerobic organisms and gram-negative aerobic/facilitative organisms
  - Agents active against anaerobic organisms include cefoxitin, cefotetan, ticarcillin-clavulanate, piperacillin–tazobactam, ampicillin–sulbactam, imipenem

- Associated with chronic ambulatory peritoneal dialysis
  - Vancomycin plus gentamicin instilled in peritoneal cavity

- Recommended dose is 1.5 g/kg IV albumin on day 1 and 1 g/kg on day 3 to hospitalized SBP patients. (3)[A]

- Prevention of SBP in patients with cirrhosis and gastrointestinal bleeding
  - Norfloxacin 400 mg PO b.i.d. or trimethoprim/sulfamethoxazole (T/S) 1 double-strength tablet b.i.d. for 7 days (2–4)[A]

- Recurrent peritonitis
  - Use long-term daily prophylactic treatment; norfloxacin 400 mg PO once a day or T/S 1 double-strength tablet PO once a day (less expensive) (4)[A]

- Patients with ascitic fluid total protein levels <1 g/dL
  - Give prophylactic therapy during hospitalization only, or give long-term (1)[B]

- Once on prophylactic therapy, breakthrough infections should be treated with cefotaxime ± gram-positive coverage, depending on culture results. (1)[B]

Second Line

- Ofloxacin 400 mg PO b.i.d. for 8 days
  - Benefits only a selected population of SBP patients (3)[A]

- Diuretic therapy decrease ascitic fluid, resulting in an increased total protein level in ascitic fluid, and therefore decreasing risk of infection.

SURGERY
Treat underlying condition(s) and infection (by surgery if necessary)

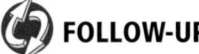 **FOLLOW-UP**

DISPOSITION
Admission Criteria
Totally subjective: If a cirrhosis patient looks sick, admit: if not, treat with outpatient antibiotics.

PROGNOSIS
- Mortality rate for SBP is 10–30% with 1/2 of deaths caused by GI bleed, renal failure, or liver failure.
- Presence of renal insufficiency is the strongest independent prognostic indicator for mortality. (1)[B]
- Other indicators: Peripheral leukocytosis, older age, ileus, or high Child-Pugh score
- Survival is unlikely in patients with SBP who go into shock prior to receiving empiric antibiotics.
- Patients with hospital-acquired versus community-acquired SBP have a greater risk of mortality. (4)[A]

COMPLICATIONS
- Hypovolemic consequences
- Septicemia
- Septic shock
- Acute renal failure
- Acute respiratory insufficiency
- Liver failure
- Abscess formation

PATIENT MONITORING
Frequent monitoring acutely

REFERENCES

1. Sheer TA, Runyon BA. Spontaneous bacterial peritonitis. *Dig Dis*. 2005;23(1):39–46.
2. Runyon BA. Management of adult patients with ascites due to cirrhosis. *Hepatology*. 2004;39(3):841–856.
3. Parsi MA, Atreja A, Zein NN. Spontaneous bacterial peritonitis: Recent data on incidence and treatment. *Cleve Clin J Med*. 2004;71(7):569–576.
4. Frazee LA, Marinos AE, Rybarczyk AM, and Fulton SA. Long-term prophylaxis of spontaneous bacterial peritonitis in patients with cirrhosis. *Ann Pharmacother*. 2005;39:908–912.

 MISCELLANEOUS

- SBP develops in pre-existing ascites; it does not cause ascites.
- Mortality of SBP is ~80% if a patient unnecessarily receives an exploratory laparotomy.
- Mortality of 2nd-degree BP approaches 100% if treated only with antibiotics and no surgical intervention.
- An ascitic fluid culture growing multiple organisms, but with a PMN count of <250 cells/mm^3 on analysis is most likely polymicrobial bacterascites secondary to bowel puncture with paracentesis needle. This is rare: <0.6% of all paracenteses. (1)[B]
- See also: Appendicitis, acute, Crohn disease, Diverticular disease, Ectopic pregnancy, Pancreatitis

CODES

ICD9-CM
- 567.2 Other suppurative peritonitis
- 567.9 Unspecified peritonitis

 See Corresponding Diagnostic Algorithm

PERITONSILLAR ABSCESS

Matthew R. Leibowitz, MD

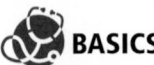 **BASICS**

DESCRIPTION
Infection with abscess formation and collection of pus in the space between the anterior and posterior tonsillar pillars and the superior pharyngeal constrictor muscle. Usually follows an episode of acute pharyngitis or tonsillitis.
- System(s) Affected: Gastrointestinal; Pulmonary
- Synonym(s): Quinsy

EPIDEMIOLOGY
- Predominant age: All age groups, with greatest incidence in adolescents and young adults 15–30 years of age
- Predominant sex: Male = Female

Incidence
In the US: Estimated 45,000 new cases yearly (30/100,000 person years)

RISK FACTORS
- Prior episodes of tonsillitis
- Age (young are more susceptible)

ETIOLOGY
- Polymicrobial infection is the rule in peritonsillar abscess, and multiple bacteria will likely be grown from cultures of drained pus. *Streptococcus* species are the most common pathogens.
- Aerobic bacteria
  - *Streptococcus pyogenes*
  - *Streptococcus milleri* group
  - *Haemophilus influenzae*
  - *Viridans streptococci*
  - Neisseria species
  - *Staphylococcus aureus*
- Anaerobic bacteria
  - Fusobacterium
  - Peptostreptococcus
  - Porphyromonas
  - Prevotella
  - Bacteroides

ASSOCIATED CONDITIONS
- Pharyngitis
- Tonsillitis
- Peritonsillar cellulitis
- Retrophrayngeal abscess
- Lateral space abscess
- Septic jugular vein thrombophlebitis (Lemierre syndrome)

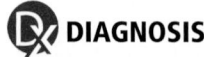 **DIAGNOSIS**

SIGNS AND SYMPTOMS
History
- Extreme sore throat or neck pain
- Odynophagia
- Dysphagia

Physical Exam
- Fever >38°C
- Trismus
- "Hot potato voice" (thickened, muffled voice)
- Drooling and pooling of saliva in the mouth
- Tonsillar exudates seen uncommonly
- Erythematous, edematous tonsil
- Asymmetry of the oropharynx with inferior and medial displacement of the infected tonsil often with contralateral deviation of the uvula
- Cervical adenopathy

TESTS
Lab
- Leukocytosis
- Culture of pathogens from aspirated or drained pus to identify organism(s)

Imaging
- Intraoral ultrasonography will often show a discrete abscess cavity if present
- CT, best performed with contrast, will also show a discrete abscess cavity if present. Edema of the surrounding tissues can also be seen on CT scan.

Diagnostic Procedures/Surgery
Incision and drainage of pus, via needle aspiration or an operative procedure under general anesthesia or conscious sedation

DIFFERENTIAL DIAGNOSIS
- Peritonsillar cellulitis
- Tonsillar abscess
- Retropharyngeal abscess
- Lateral space abscess
- Infectious mononucleosis (Epstein-Barr virus infection)
- Aspiration of foreign body
- Dental infection
- Salivary gland infection
- Cervical adenitis
- Mastoiditis
- Internal carotid artery aneurysm

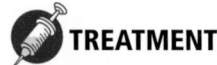 **TREATMENT**

GENERAL MEASURES
- Appropriate health care: Inpatient. Same-day surgery is possible in some cases with outpatient management.
- IV rehydration
- Pain control

Diet
No restrictions; liquid diet may be tolerated best until pain improves

Activity
As tolerated

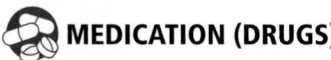 **MEDICATION (DRUGS)**

First Line
- Penicillin remains the standard antimicrobial therapy, with initial therapy delivered parenterally. Tailor therapy to cultured pathogens as possible. If organisms other than oral *Streptococci* are suspected, expanded therapy may be indicated. With growing concern for β-lactamase–producing organisms, antibiotics with β-lactamase inhibitors or cephalosporins may be preferred. If Fusobacterium or Bacteroides are implicated, additional anaerobic therapy with metronidazole may be indicated with increasing resistance to penicillin among these pathogens. (1,2)[C]
  - Penicillin G 1–4 million units IV q4h; *or*
  - Benzathine penicillin G 1.2 million units IM 1 time; *or*
  - Benzathine penicillin G 900,000 units and procaine penicillin G 300,000 units IM 1 time; *followed by*
  - Penicillin V 500 mg (25–50 mg/kg for children) PO t.i.d. to complete 10–14 days of total therapy
- For penicillin-allergic patients
  - Erythromycin ethyl succinate 300–400 mg PO t.i.d.; *or*
  - Cephalexin 250 to 500 mg PO t.i.d.
- If resistant organisms (including oral anaerobes) are suspected, add to the above oral therapy
  - Metronidazole 500 mg PO t.i.d.–q.i.d.; *or*
  - Clindamycin 150–450 mg PO t.i.d.–q.i.d.
- Alternatively
  - Ampicillin-Sulbactam (Unasyn) 3 g IV q6h; *or* Ticarcillin-Clavulanate (Ticar) 3–4 g IV q4–6h; *or*
  - Amoxicillin-Clavulanate (Augmentin) 500 mg PO t.i.d. or 875 mg PO b.i.d.; *or*
  - Cefuroxime 500 mg PO b.i.d. (or other 2nd- or 3rd-generation cephalosporin) and metronidazole 500 mg PO t.i.d.–q.i.d.

- Contraindications: Allergy to specific antibiotic
- Precautions: Refer to the manufacturer's profile for each drug.
- Significant possible interactions: Refer to the manufacturer's profile for each drug.

Second Line

The role of adjunctive corticosteroids in the treatment of peritonsillar abscess is controversial. (3) A recent small randomized study suggests that a single high dose of methylprednisolone (2–3 mg/kg up to 250 mg) administered after needle drainage and before antimicrobial therapy may improve a patient's ability to open the mouth and drink water earlier, speed resolution of fever, and decrease length of hospital stay. (4)[C]

SURGERY

- Small studies indicate that rates of success are equivalent between needle aspiration and operative incision and drainage. (3)[C]
  – Needle aspiration with intraoral ultrasound or CT guidance
  – Operative incision and drainage when needle aspiration is too difficult due to trismus or lack of patient cooperation

- Immediate tonsillectomy at the time of incision and drainage (known as quinsy tonsillectomy) has decreased in favor, due to increased risk of hemorrhage and overall low rates of abscess recurrence without tonsillectomy. (3,5)[C]
- Delayed tonsillectomy (known as interval tonsillectomy) is also less commonly performed, due to the low rates of recurrent abscess. (1,3)[C]

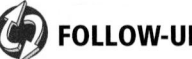 **FOLLOW-UP**

PROGNOSIS

- Symptoms will improve rapidly after incision and drainage and appropriate antibiotics.
- Pain and inflammation may persist for up to a week after treatment.
- Recurrent peritonsillar abscess does occur, but is rare

COMPLICATIONS

- Airway obstruction
- Spread to parapharyngeal (lateral) or retropharyngeal spaces
- Septic jugular vein thrombosis
- Brain abscess
- Sepsis
- Possible complications of incision and drainage
  – Pulmonary aspiration of blood and pus with bronchopneumonia
  – Tonsillar hemorrhage
  – Perforation of the carotid artery

PATIENT MONITORING

- Follow-up to ensure resolution of symptoms and tonsillar inflammation
- Lack of improvement may indicate antibiotic-resistant pathogens or residual abscess necessitating repeat drainage.

REFERENCES

1. Schraff S, et al. Peritonsillar abscess in children: A 10-year review of diagnosis and management. *Int J Pediatr Otorhinolaryngol*. 2001;57(3):213–218.
2. Steyer TE. Peritonsillar abscess: diagnosis and treatment. *Am Fam Physician*. 2002;65(1):93–96.
3. Johnson RJ, et al. An evidence-based review of the treatment of peritonsillar abscess. *Otolaryngol Head Neck Surg*. 2003;128:332–343.
4. Ozbek C, et al. Use of steroids in the treatment of peritonsillar abscess. *J Laryngol Otol*. 2004;118(6):439–42.
5. Dunne AA, et al. Peritonsillar abscess—critical analysis of abscess tonsillectomy. *Clin Otolaryngol*. 2003;28(5):420–424.

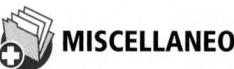 **MISCELLANEOUS**

See also: Epiglottitis; Pharyngitis

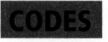 **CODES**

ICD9-CM
475 Peritonsillar abscess

PATIENT TEACHING

Important to complete course of antibiotics

 See Corresponding Diagnostic Algorithm

PERSONALITY DISORDERS (PD)

Moshe S. Torem, MD, FAPA

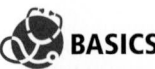 **BASICS**

DESCRIPTION

A group of conditions, with onset at or before adolescence, characterized by enduring patterns of maladaptive and dysfunctional behavior that deviate markedly from one's culture and social environment, leading to functional impairment and distress to the individual, coworkers, and the family.

- These behaviors are perceived by patients to be "normal" and "right," and they have little insight as to their responsibility for these behaviors.
- These conditions are classified based on the predominant symptoms and their severity.
- System(s) Affected: Nervous/Psychiatric
- Synonym(s): Character disorders; Character pathology

ALERT

Geriatric Considerations
Coping with stresses of elderly life difficult

Pediatric Considerations
History of childhood neglect, abuse, and trauma are not uncommon.

Pregnancy Considerations
Adds pressure in coping with the activities of daily living (ADLs)

EPIDEMIOLOGY

- Predominant age: Starts in adolescence and early 20s and persists throughout patient's life
- Predominant sex: Male = Female; some personality disorders are more common in females and others are more common in males.

Prevalence
- In the US: 12%
- In male prisoners, the prevalence of antisocial personality disorder is ~60%.

RISK FACTORS

- Positive family history
- Pregnancy risk factors
  - Nutritional deprivation
  - Use of alcohol or drugs
  - Viral and bacterial Infections
- Dysfunctional family with child abuse and neglect

Genetics
Major character traits inherited; others result from a combination of genetics and environment

ETIOLOGY
Environmental and genetic factors

ASSOCIATED CONDITIONS
Depression, other psychiatric disorders in patient and family members

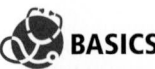 **DIAGNOSIS**

SIGNS AND SYMPTOMS

- Criteria for a personality disorder include an enduring pattern of
  - Inner experience and behavior manifesting in 2 or more of the following areas: Cognition, affectivity, interpersonal functioning, or impulse control
  - Inflexibility and pervasiveness across a broad range of personal and social situations
  - Significant distress or impairment in social, occupational, or other important areas of functioning
  - Onset can be traced to adolescence or early adulthood.
  - Not better accounted for as a manifestation or consequence of another mental disorder
  - Not due to the direct physiologic effects of a substance, such as a drug of abuse, or a medication, or a general medical condition, such as a head trauma
- PDs are classified into 3 major clusters
  - Cluster A: Eccentricism and oddness. Paranoid PD (unwarranted suspiciousness and distrust of others, defensive, guarded, and overly sensitive). Schizoid PD (emotional, cold, or detached, apathetic to criticism or praise, socially isolated). Schizotypal PD (eccentric behavior, odd belief system, perceptions and speech, social isolation, and general suspiciousness).
  - Cluster B: Dramatic, emotional, or erratic behavioral patterns. Antisocial PD (aggressive, impulsive, irritable, irresponsible, dishonest, deceitful, and at times reckless disregard for safety of self or others). Borderline PD (pervasive pattern of unstable interpersonal relationships, self-image, with high impulsivity from early adulthood. Intense fear of abandonment, mood swings, poor self-esteem, chronic boredom, and feelings of inner emptiness). Histrionic PD (excessive emotionality and attention seeking in a variety of contexts. Needs to be the center of attention, with self-dramatizing behaviors; suggestive with flowing and impressionistic speech). Narcissistic PD (grandiosity, a need for affirmation and for admiration from others. Lack of empathy for other people's pain or discomfort. Grandiose sense of self-importance and preoccupation with fantasies of success, power, brilliance, beauty, or ideal love. Belief that the individual is special, unique, and deserves special treatment. At times may show arrogance, haughty behaviors, or attitudes.)
  - Cluster C: Anxiety, excessive worry, fear, and different patterns to cope with these emotions. Avoidant PD (social inhibition, feelings of inadequacy, and hypersensitivity to negative evaluation; avoidance of occupational and interpersonal activities that involve the risk of criticism by others; avoids taking chances and

risks involving significant interpersonal contact, preoccupied with fears of being criticized and rejected, and view self as socially inept, and personally unappealing or inferior to others). Dependent PD (excessive need to be taken care of, leading to submissive, clinging behavior, and fears of separation; needs constant and repeated reassurance and guidance by others; difficulties making decisions with ADLs; avoids expressing disagreements with others due to fear of losing support and approval; usually seeks out strong and confident people as friends or spouses and feels more secure in such relationships). Obsessive-compulsive PD (preoccupation with cleanliness, orderliness, perfectionism, and control of events and people at the expense of flexibility, openness, and efficiency preoccupation with excessive details, rules, lists, order, organization, and schedules to the extent that the major point of the activity is lost; exhibits perfectionism that interferes with task completion; indecisive, overconscientious, scrupulous, and rigid about matters of morality, ethics, or values; reluctant to delegate tasks at work or home and sometimes unable to discard worn-out or worthless objects (even if they have no sentimental value). PD, not otherwise specified (a mixture of characteristics from other PDs without a predominant pattern compatible with above categories); it can also be used for specific personality disorders not mentioned in the American Psychological Association classification [*DSM-IV-TR*] such as depressive PD, masochistic PD, passive-aggressive PD, and others).

History
- Comprehensive interview and mental status examination
- Interview of relatives and friends helpful in establishing an enduring pattern of behavior

TESTS

Lab
- Thyroid-stimulating hormone (TSH), Venereal Disease Research Laboratory syphilis test (VDRL) or rapid plasma reagin (RPR), comprehensive metabolic panel, CBC, HIV
- Psychological testing (e.g., MMPI-II)

Imaging
CT scan and MRI of the brain may be necessary in newly developed symptoms to rule out organic brain disease (e.g., frontal lobe tumor).

DIFFERENTIAL DIAGNOSIS

- Medical disorders (e.g., brain diseases) with behavioral changes
- Other psychiatric disorders, with similar symptoms, have a specific time of onset, signifying a change from a previously different pattern of behavior, or have a difference in self-perception
  - In obsessive compulsive disorder (OCD), symptoms are ego-dystonic (i.e., perceived as foreign and unwanted). In addition, OCD has a pattern of relapse and perhaps remission.
  - In obsessive compulsive personality disorder (OCPD), symptoms are perceived as desirable behaviors (ego-syntonic) that the patient feels proud of and wants others to emulate. In addition, OCPD has a life-long pattern (i.e., without significant relapse or remission).

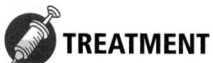
TREATMENT

INITIAL STABILIZATION
Outpatient individual psychotherapy and group therapy

GENERAL MEASURES
- Long-term psychotherapy and cognitive behavior therapy
- Group therapy is helpful in the utilization of therapeutic confrontation and increasing one's awareness and insight regarding the damaging effects of dysfunctional behavior patterns.

Diet
Emphasize variety of healthy foods; avoid obesity

Activity
Regular physical exercise helps in coping with stress and the ADLs.

MEDICATION (DRUGS)

First Line
- No specific drugs treat PDs; however, specific medications can reduce the intensity, frequency, and dysfunctionality of certain behaviors, thoughts, and feelings.
- Symptom management
  – Minipsychosis (associated with paranoid, schizoid, and schizotypal PDs). Atypical antipsychotics: Clozapine (Clozaril), risperidone (Risperdal), quetiapine (Seroquel), olanzapine (Zyprexa), ziprasidone (Geodon), and aripiprazole (Abilify). Start with a low dose, gradually adjusting to the patient's needs.
  – Anxiety. Anxiolytics (benzodiazepines, buspirone, and the selective serotonin reuptake inhibitors [SSRIs])
  – Depressed mood. Antidepressants (SSRIs)
  – Many patients with borderline PD respond well to small doses of atypical neuroleptics and mood stabilizers
- Contraindications: Refer to the manufacturer's profile for each drug.
- Precautions: Risperidone and ziprasidone may be associated with hyperglycemia and ketoacidosis.
- Significant possible interactions: Refer to the manufacturer's profile for each drug.

Second Line
Mood stabilizers (e.g., lithium carbonate, divalproex [Depakote]) and antiepileptic drugs may be helpful.

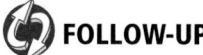
FOLLOW-UP

PROGNOSIS
PDs are enduring patterns of behavior throughout one's lifetime and are not easily responsive to treatment.

COMPLICATIONS
- Disruptive family life with frequent divorces and separations, alcoholism, substance abuse, and drug addiction
- Disruptive behaviors in the workplace may cause absenteeism, loss of productivity, and loss of self-support
- Violation of the law and disregard for the concerns and rights of others

PATIENT MONITORING
- If substance abuse is suspected, check drug screens
- Infrequent sessions, with relative or friends, helpful in monitoring progress and behavior changes

REFERENCES

1. Bajaj P, Tyrer P. Managing mood disorders and comorbid personality disorders. *Curr Opin Psychiatr.* 2005;18(1);27–31.
2. Widiger TA. A dimensional model of personality disorder. *Curr Opin Psychiatr.* 2005;18(1)41–43.
3. Pfohl B. Personality Disorders. UpToDate Online 2004. Available at: www.uptodate.com. Accessed June 2, 2006.
4. Potter NN. Perplexing issues in personality disorders. *Curr Opin Psychiatr.* 2004; 17(6):487–492.
5. Shelder J, Westen D. Refining personality disorder diagnosis: Integrating science and practice. *Am J Psychiatr.* 2004;161(8):1350–1365.
6. Bienvenu OJ, Stein MB. Personality and anxiety disorders: A review. *J Personal Discord.* 2003;17(2):139–151.
7. Coid J. Epidemiology, public health and the problem of personality disorder. *Brit J Psychiatry.* Suppl 2003;44:S3–S10.
8. Cloninger CR. *Personality and Psychopathology.* Washington, DC: American Psychiatric Press; 1999.
9. Ekselius L, et al. Personality disorders in the general population: DSM-IV and ICD-10 defined prevalence as related to sociodemograhpic profile. *Pers Individ Dif.* 2001;30(2):320–331.
10. Endler NS, Kocovski NL. Personality disorders at the crossroads. *J Personal Disord.* 2002;16(6):487–502.
11. Jablensky A. The classification of personality disorders: Critical review and need for rethinking. *Psychopathology.* 2002;35(2–3):112–116.
12. Kendell RE. The distinction between personality disorder and mental illness. *Brit J Psychiatry.* 2002;180:110–115.
13. Links PS, Boggild A, Sarin N. Psychopharmacology of personality disorders: Review and emerging issues. *Curr Psychiatry Rep.* 2001;3(1):70–76.
14. Moran P. The epidemiology of antisocial personality disorder. *Soc Psychiatry Psychiatr Epidemiol.* 1999; 34(5):231–242.
15. Newton Howes G, Tyrer P. Pharmacotherapy for personality disorders. *Expert Opin Pharmacother.* 2003;4(10):1643–1649.
16. Ogrodniczuk JS, Piper WE. Day treatment for personality disorders: A review of research findings. *Harv Rev Psychiatry.* 2001;9(3):105–117.
17. Parker G, et al. Defining disordered personality functioning. *J Personal Disord.* 2002;16(6):503–522.
18. Piper WE, Ogrodniczuk JS. Psychotherapy of personality disorders. *Curr Psychiatry Rep.* 2001;3(1):59–63.
19. Rizvi SL, Linehan MM. Dialectical behavior therapy for personality disorders. *Curr Psychiatry Rep.* 2001;3(1):64–69.
20. Sater N, et al. Epidemiology of personality disorders. *Curr Psychiatry Rep.* 2001;3(1):41–45.
21. Torgersen S, Kringlen E, Cramer V. The prevalence of personality disorders in a community sample. *Arch Gen Psychiatry.* 2001;58(6):590–596.
22. Widiger TA, Chaynes K. Current issues in the assessment of personality disorders. *Curr Psychiatry Rep.* 2003;5(1):28–35.
23. American Psychiatric Association. *Diagnostic and Statistical Manual of Mental Disorders: Text Revision.* 4th ed. Washington, DC: American Psychiatric Press. 2000.

MISCELLANEOUS

See also: Obsessive-compulsive disorder

CODES

ICD9-CM
- 300.3 Obsessive-compulsive disorders
- 301.0 Paranoid personality disorder
- 301.20 Schizoid personality disorder, unspecified
- 301.22 Schizotypal personality
- 301.50 Histrionic personality disorder, unspecified
- 301.6 Dependent personality disorder
- 301.7 Antisocial personality disorder
- 301.81 Narcissistic personality
- 301.82 Avoidant personality disorder
- 301.83 Borderline personality
- 301.9 Unspecified personality disorder

PATIENT TEACHING
- Bibliotherapy and writing therapy, specific assignments, and watching certain movies to better understand the nature and origin of one's specific condition are helpful.
- The movie *As Good As It Gets* illustrates someone with obsessive-compulsive behaviors and its impact on ADLs and relationships with family and friends
- The movie series *The Godfather* includes several characters with antisocial PD and shows how this affects their interpersonal relationships and their own physical and mental health.

See Corresponding Diagnostic Algorithm

PERTUSSIS

Mary Cataletto, MD

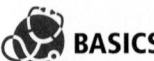 **BASICS**

DESCRIPTION

- Pertussis or whooping cough is a highly communicable, respiratory bacterial infection. Characteristically, it produces a paroxysmal spasmodic cough, ending in prolonged high-pitched inspiratory whoop.
- Worldwide
- Mostly endemic; epidemic cycles of 3–5 years
- Affects all age groups
- Transmission is by close contact with aerosolized droplets from infected person; untreated patients are contagious for ~3 weeks. Incubation period averages 7–10 days (up to 21 days) postexposure.
- Usual course: Generally lasts 6–10 weeks and has 3 stages: Catarrhal, paroxysmal, and convalescent
- Neither infection nor immunization confers lifelong immunity.
- System(s) Affected: Pulmonary
- Synonym(s): Whooping cough

ALERT

Geriatric Considerations
May be more serious in this age group, especially with neuromuscular disorders.

Pediatric Considerations
- Most serious and highest mortality in infants >6 months of age, particularly if unimmunized or preterm birth (death usually due to complications)
- Mortality rate between 1% and 3% in affected neonates

GENERAL PREVENTION

- Early reporting to appropriate public health agency
- Respiratory Isolation: Quarantine inadequately immunized household contacts >7 years for 3 weeks following exposure or until cases and contacts have been treated, whichever comes first.
- Protection of contacts
  - Immediately immunize all close unimmunized and underimmunized contacts >7 years.
  - Tdap vaccine should be given to children age 11–18 if they have not previously received Tdap.
  - Chemoprophylaxis of close contacts: All household contacts and other close contacts, including those in child care
  - Observe all contacts for symptoms for 21 days after exposure.

EPIDEMIOLOGY

- Predominant age: 3 months–6 years old (infants comprise about half of cases)
- Predominant sex: Female > Male, but only in older age groups

Incidence
In US

- Infants <1 year (2001–03): 55.2 cases/100,000
- Children age 10–19 years (2003): 10.9 cases/100,000
- In 2004, 25,827 cases were reported in the US.
  - Attack rates up to 100% in susceptible individuals

RISK FACTORS

- Unimmunized and underimmunized children
- Young infants (<6 months)
- Contact with an infected person
- Immunodeficiency
- Pregnancy

PATHOPHYSIOLOGY
Infectious process with predilection for ciliated respiratory epithelium

ETIOLOGY
- *Bordetella pertussis* (responsible for ~95% cases)
- *Bordetella parapertussis*
- Pneumonia
- Otitis media
- Seizures
- Apnea in young infants
- Encephalopathy

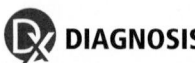 **DIAGNOSIS**

SIGNS AND SYMPTOMS
- Catarrhal stage: Rhinorrhea, mild cough, low-grade fever
- Paroxysmal stage: Cough becomes paroxysmal, worsening in both frequency and severity; posttussive whoop and vomiting may occur. Between paroxysms, patients may appear normal. Attacks may be more frequent at night.
- Convalescent stage: Lasts ~1–2 weeks, with decreasing severity and frequency of coughing paroxysms

History
Infants with pertussis may present with apnea.

Physical Exam
See "Signs and Symptoms." Infants <6 months, as well as adolescents and adults, may not have characteristic whoop.

TESTS
Lab
- WBC: Elevated (15,000–60,000), with marked lymphocytosis in infants and young children; not always present in teens
- *B. pertussis* culture is gold standard diagnostic test (takes ~10 days)
  - A negative culture does not exclude diagnosis.
  - Lacks sensitivity in previously immunized patients
- Direct fluorescent antibody (DFA) has variable sensitivity and low specificity; not recommended for confirmation of diagnosis.
- Polymerase chain reaction (PCR) assay is rapid, with improved sensitivity.
- Culture and PCR are negative after 4 weeks of illness.

Imaging
Chest radiograph may be normal or show signs of hyperinflation, with increased AP diameter and flattened diaphragms; focal atelectasis, peribronchial cuffing, or pneumonia also may be present.

Diagnostic Procedures/Surgery
Nasopharyngeal aspirate or Dacron or calcium alginate swab

Pathological Findings
- Focal emphysema
- Mucopurulent exudate
- Patchy ulceration of respiratory epithelium

DIFFERENTIAL DIAGNOSIS
- Other infectious airway disease
- Sinusitis
- Airway foreign body

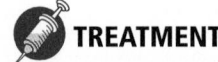 **TREATMENT**

GENERAL MEASURES
- Initiate treatment in anyone at risk of exposure and symptoms <21 days in duration (treatment only during catarrhal stage no longer required).
- Hospitalization for seriously ill infants
- Outpatient for milder cases
- General supportive, skilled nursing care
- Standard precautions
- Droplet precautions for 5 days after initiation of effective therapy in hospitalized cases
- IV fluid therapy if needed
- Oxygen as needed
- Careful observation for apnea in young infants; avoid stimuli that trigger paroxysms
- Mechanical ventilation if necessary

Diet
- May need to provide frequent small meals to assure adequate nutrition
- Infants may require tube feeding.
- Correct dehydration.

Activity
Rest during active phase in quiet environment

Nursing
- Standard precautions
- Isolation of hospitalized patients with respiratory precautions for 5 days after the initiation of effective antibiotic treatment; for 3 weeks after onset of paroxysms if antibiotics are not used
- Gentle suctioning of nasal secretions
- Avoid triggers that trigger paroxysms

SPECIAL THERAPY
IV Fluids
Indicated for dehydration and when oral fluids are either not indicated or poorly tolerated

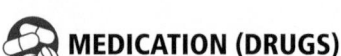 **MEDICATION (DRUGS)**

First Line
- Antibiotic dosing for age ≥6 months, children
  - Azithromycin: 10 mg/kg as a single dose on day 1 (maximum 500 mg); then 5 mg/kg/d as a single dose on days 2–5 (maximum 250 mg/d);
  - Clarithromycin: 15 mg/kg/d in 2 divided doses for 7 days (maximum 1 g/d)
  - Erythromycin: 40–50 mg/kg/d in 4 divided doses for 14 days (maximum 2 g/d)
- Antibiotic dosing for adolescents and adults
  - Azithromycin: 500 mg as single dose on day 1, then 250 mg/d on days 2–5
  - Clarithromycin: 1 g/d in 2 divided doses for 7 days
  - Erythromycin: 2 g/d in 4 divided doses for 14 days
- Contraindications: Refer to manufacturer's literature
  - Antibiotics during catarrhal stage may ameliorate symptoms but afterwards are recommended to limit disease spread.
  - Insufficient data to establish efficacy of azithromycin or clarithromycin in infants <1 month of age. Azithromycin and clarithromycin have not been approved by the FDA for use in infants <6 months of age with pertussis. See Red Book and consider pediatric infectious disease consultation in this high-risk age group.

Second Line

- Trimethoprim–sulfamethoxazole (TMP–SMX) is an alternative for those patients with macrolide-resistant strains and who cannot tolerate macrolides. TMP-SMX is contraindicated in infants <2 months of age.
- Short acting β_2-agonists and corticosteroids: Controlled, prospective data are unavailable.

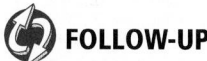 **FOLLOW-UP**

DISPOSITION

Admission Criteria

Consider for

- Infants <6 months of age, especially preterms
- Unimmunized and underimmunized infants
- Infants with apnea, hypoxia, feeding difficulty
- Any patient with serious complications
- Patients with underlying disease, especially neuromuscular disorders
- For supportive care or accelerating symptoms

Discharge Criteria

- Clinically stable
- Resolution of above needs

Issues for Referral

- Apnea or seizures at time of illness may be associated with subsequent impairment. Consultation with a pediatric neurologist or neurodevelopmental pediatrician may be indicated.
- Infants <1 month of age

PROGNOSIS

- Complete recovery in majority of cases
- Most severe morbidity and highest mortality in affected infants <6 months of age
- Infants <1 month of age who receive treatment with a macrolide antibiotic should be monitored for 1 month for idiopathic hypertrophic pyloric stenosis.

COMPLICATIONS

- Pneumonia
- Encephalopathy
- Seizures
- Hernia
- Death

PATIENT MONITORING

- ICU may be necessary for severely ill infants.
- Older children and adults with mild cases do not need to be confined to bed or admitted to hospital.

REFERENCES

1. Feigin RD, Cherry JD, Demmier GJ, Kaplan SL. *Textbook of Pediatric Infectious Diseases*, 5th ed., Vol. 1. Philadelphia: Saunders, 2004.
2. Tiwari T, Murphy T, Moran J. Recommended antimicrobial agents for the treatment and postexposure prophylaxis of pertussis. *MMWR* Dec 9, 2005;54(RR14):1–16.
3. Pickering LK, Baker CJ, Long SS, McMillan JA, eds. *Red Book: 2006 Report of the Committee on Infectious Diseases*, 27th edition. Elk Grove Village, IL:
4. http://www.cdc.gov/nip/publications/pertussis/guide.htm
5. http://www.aap.org

 MISCELLANEOUS

- Do not use cough suppressants.
- Reporting of selected adverse reactions with certain vaccines is required by the National Childhood Vaccine Injury Act of 1986. Toll-free information number: (800) 822-7967.
- MedWatch (telephone: 1 800 FDA-1088): Cases of pyloric stenosis in infants treated with macrolides should be reported.
- See also: Adenovirus infections; Bronchiolitis; Common cold; Cystic fibrosis; Failure to thrive (FTT); Immunizations; Influenza; Otitis media; Pneumonia, bacterial; Tuberculosis

 CODES

ICD9-CM

033.9 Whooping cough, unspecified organism

PATIENT TEACHING

- For patient education materials favorably reviewed on this topic, contact: American Academy of Pediatrics, 141 Northwest Point Blvd., P.O. Box 927, Elk Grove Village, IL 60009-0927. (800) 433-9016.
- http://www.cdc.gov is another helpful resource for further information on pertussis.

Prevention

Readers are referred to immunization guidelines in the AAP Red Book and CDC website.

 See Corresponding Diagnostic Algorithm

PHARYNGITIS

David E. Burtner, MD

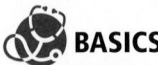 **BASICS**

DESCRIPTION

Inflammation of the pharynx most commonly caused by acute viral infection. Group A streptococcus is a focus of diagnosis owing to its potential for preventable rheumatic sequelae. Chronic low-grade symptoms usually related to reflux disease or vocal abuse. Also called sore throat, tonsillitis, and streptococcal throat

- System(s) Affected: Respiratory

GENERAL PREVENTION

Avoid contact with infected people.

EPIDEMIOLOGY

- Estimated 30 million cases are diagnosed yearly.
- 12–25% of all sore throats are thought to require visits to physicians.
- Predominant age: All age groups.
- Predominant sex: Male = Female

Incidence

Incidence of rheumatic fever is decreasing with estimate of 64/100,000.

ALERT

Pediatric Considerations

Streptococcal infection has greatest incidence in patients 5–18 years of age.

Prevalence

Eleven percent of all school-age children visit a physician annually because of pharyngitis.

RISK FACTORS

- Group A beta-hemolytic streptococcal epidemics occur.
- Age (i.e., young people are more susceptible)
- Family history
- Close quarters, such as in new military recruits
- Immunosuppression
- Fatigue
- Smoking
- Excess alcohol consumption
- Receptive oral sex
- Diabetes mellitus
- Recent illness

Genetics

Patients with a positive family history of rheumatic fever have a higher risk of rheumatic sequelae following an untreated group A beta-hemolytic streptococcal infection.

ETIOLOGY

- Acute: Bacterial
  - Group A beta-hemolytic streptococci
  - *Neisseria gonorrhoeae*
  - *Corynebacterium diphtheriae* (diphtheria)
  - *Haemophilus influenzae*
  - *Moraxella (Branhamella) catarrhalis*
  - Groups C and G streptococcus, rarely
- Acute: Viral
  - Rhinovirus
  - Adenovirus
  - Parainfluenza virus
  - Coxsackievirus
  - Coronavirus
  - Echovirus
  - Herpes simplex virus
  - Epstein-Barr virus (EBV) (mononucleosis)
  - Cytomegalovirus
- Chronic
  - More likely noninfectious
  - Irritation from postnasal discharge of chronic allergic rhinitis or reflux
  - Chemical irritation or smoking
  - Neoplasms and vasculitides

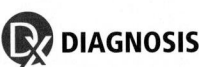 **DIAGNOSIS**

Clinical Prediction Rule: Centor Criteria

- Tonsilar exudates (for streptococcal etiology)
- Tender anterior chain cervical adenopathy
- Fever by history
- Absence of cough
- If 3 out of 4 present, Positive Predictive Value of ~50%
- If 3 or 4 not present, Negative Predictive Value of ~80% (6)[C]

SIGNS AND SYMPTOMS

- Sore throat
- Enlarged tonsils
- Pharyngeal erythema
- Tonsillar exudates
- Soft palate petechiae
- Cervical adenopathy
- Absence of cough, hoarseness, or lower respiratory symptoms
- Fever >102.5°F (39.1°C).
- Scarlet fever rash: Punctate erythematous macules with reddened flexor creases and circumoral pallor (streptococcal pharyngitis)
- Gray pseudomembrane found in diphtheria and occasionally, mononucleosis
- Characteristic erythematous-based clear vesicles are found in herpes stomatitis.
- Anorexia
- Chills
- Malaise
- Headache
- Conjunctivitis, more commonly with adenovirus infections

Physical Exam

Examination to evaluate for signs as above

TESTS

Lab

- Blood agar throat culture from swab. Bacitracin disc sensitivity of hemolytic colonies suggest group A streptococci. Specific antibody identification is available.
- Rapid screening for streptococci can be done from throat swab with antigen agglutination kits. 5–10% false negatives lead some clinicians to suggest routine backup of all negatives with blood agar culture. Newer optic immunoassay tests are more sensitive.
- Special tests usually done only if history is suggestive of a different diagnosis
- Screening for gonococcal infection requires warm Thayer-Martin plate.
- Viruses can be cultured in special media.
- Mono spot test for EBV
- Gram stain can be helpful.
- Streptococcal isolates can be immunologically typed.

Pathological Findings
Culture of pathogens will help identify which causative

DIFFERENTIAL DIAGNOSIS
- See "Causes."
- Sore throat may be seen in association with leukopenia.

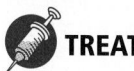 TREATMENT

Outpatient

GENERAL MEASURES
- Salt water gargles
- Acetaminophen
- Dyclonine lozenges
- Cool-mist humidifier

Diet
As tolerated; encourage consumption fluids.

Activity
As tolerated

 MEDICATION (DRUGS)

First Line

For streptococcal pharyngitis, penicillin is the standard therapy. Only penicillin has been proven to prevent rheumatic fever. Penicillin courses <10 days are not as effective. (1)[A] Other anitibiotics use streptococcal eradiction as proxy of effectiveness due to the low incidence of RF and the ethics of further controlled studies.
- Penicillin V 250 mg PO t.i.d. (25–50 mg/kg/d) (1)[A], *or*
- For patients allergic to penicillin, erythromycin ethylsuccinate 300–400 mg PO t.i.d. (30 mg/kg/d) [B], *or*

- Cephalexin 250 mg PO t.i.d. (30 mg/kg/d) [C]
- Contraindications: Allergy to specific antibiotic
- Precautions: Refer to the manufacturer's profile of each drug.
- Significant possible interactions: Refer to the manufacturer's profile of each drug.

Second Line
- Treatment of carrier state is difficult, usually requiring addition of rifampin to penicillin regimen.
- Penicillin is the treatment most documented to prevent rheumatic sequelae, but cephalosporins have lower rate of bacteriologic failure.
- Bacterial eradication rates of 10 or more days' therapy with penicillin have been achieved with 6 days of amoxicillin and 5 days with various cephalosporins.
- The newer macrolides, azithromycin and clarithromycin, are also effective against streptococcal pharyngitis, but more expensive. The chief advantage of azithromycin is its 5-day course with 10-day effective duration.
- Other cephalosporins are generally effective for streptococcal pharyngitis, but more expensive than cephalexin.

 FOLLOW-UP

- Patient must complete 10-day course of antibiotics regardless of system's response.
- Patients may consider themselves noninfectious after 24 hours of antibiotic therapy.
- No follow-up culture is recommended.

PROGNOSIS
- Streptococcal pharyngeal infection runs a 5–7-day course with peak of fever at 2–3 days.
- Symptoms will resolve spontaneously without treatment, but rheumatic complications are still possible.
- Suppurative complications (e.g., peritonsillar abscess) require surgical intervention.

COMPLICATIONS
- Rheumatic fever (carditis, valve disease, arthritis, etc.)
- Poststreptococcal glomerulonephritis
- Peritonsillar abscess
- Systemic infection
- Otitis media
- Mastoiditis
- Septicemia
- Rhinitis
- Sinusitis
- Pneumonia

REFERENCES
1. Denny FW, et al. Prevention of rheumatic fever. Treatment of the preceding streptococcic infection. *JAMA* 1950;143:151–153.
2. Bisno AL, et al. Diagnosis and management of group A streptococcal pharyngitis: A practice guideline. Infectious Diseases Society of America. *Clin Infect Dis*. 1997;25:574–583.
3. Goldman L, Ausiello D, eds. *Cecil Textbook of Medicine*. 22nd ed. Philadelphia, PA: WB Saunders; 2004.
4. Pichichero ME. Controversies in the treatment of streptococcal pharyngitis. *Am Fam Physician*. 1990;42:1558–1560.
5. Pichichero ME, Cohen R. Shortened course of antibiotic therapy for acute otitis media, sinusitis and tonsillopharyngitis. *Pediatr Infect Dis*. 1997;16:680–695.
6. Cooper, RJ, et al. Principles of appropriate antibiotic use for acute pharyngitis in adults. *Ann Intern Med*. 2001;134(6):509–517.

 MISCELLANEOUS

See also: Herpes simplex; Mononucleosis; Rheumatic fever

CODES

ICD9-CM
- 034.0 Streptococcal sore throat
- 034.1 Scarlet fever
- 462 Acute pharyngitis
- 463 Acute tonsillitis
- 472.1 Chronic pharyngitis
- 474.00 Chronic tonsillitis

PATIENT TEACHING

See Corresponding Diagnostic Algorithm

PHEOCHROMOCYTOMA

Mark C. Horattas, MD

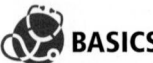

BASICS

DESCRIPTION
- Catecholamine-producing tumor. In 90% of cases, the tumors are found in the adrenal medulla, but they may also be found in other tissues derived from neural crest cells.
- Systems affected: Endocrine/Metabolic; Cardiovascular (secondary effects from catecholamines)

ALERT
Pregnancy Considerations
Consult with endocrinologist during pregnancy

EPIDEMIOLOGY
- Affects all ages, but peaks in patients between 30 and 60 years old
- No gender predilection

Incidence
0.1–1% of people with hypertension

Prevalence
1–2 per 100,00 adults

RISK FACTORS
- Familial pheochromocytoma
- Multiple endocrine neoplasia types IIA and B
- Neurofibromatosis type 1
- Von Hippel-Lindau syndrome
- Familial paraganglioma

Genetics
80–90% of cases are sporadic, 10% familial

ETIOLOGY
Catecholamine-producing tumor: Rule of 10
- 10% are extra-adrenal.
- 10% are multiple or bilateral.
- 10% are malignant.
- 10% recur after surgical removal.
- 10% occur in children.
- 10% or more are familial.
- 10% present as adrenal incidentalomas. (1)[A]

ASSOCIATED CONDITIONS
- Multiple endocrine neoplasia type IIA (medullary thyroid carcinoma and primary hyperparathyroidism)
- Multiple endocrine neoplasia type IIB (medullary thyroid carcinoma and mucosal neuromas)
- Neurofibromatosis type 1
- Von Hippel-Lindau syndrome (retinal angiomatosis and cerebellar hemangioblastoma)
- Familial paraganglioma
- Ataxia-telangiectasia
- Tuberous sclerosis
- Sturge-Weber syndrome
- Renal artery stenosis

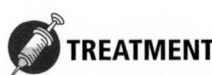

DIAGNOSIS

SIGNS AND SYMPTOMS
- Paroxysmal spells, remember mnemonic (the 5 Ps)
  - Pressure: Sudden increase in BP
  - Pain: Headache, chest, and abdominal pain
  - Perspiration
  - Palpitation
  - Pallor
- Additional symptoms
  - Constipation
  - Tremor
  - Weight loss
  - Anxiety
- Signs
  - Hypertension: Paroxysmal in 1/2 of affected patients
  - Orthostatic hypotension
  - Neurofibromatosis
  - Café au lait spots
  - Tachyarrhythmias
  - Cardiomyopathy
  - Grade II–IV retinopathy
  - Fever
  - Hyperglycemia
  - Hypercalcemia
  - Erythrocytosis
  - 10% of patients are asymptomatic.

History
Patients with paroxysmal spells and hypertension or those with hypertension that is refractory to control should be screened to rule out pheochromocytoma. Exclude multiple endocrine neoplasia (MEN) syndrome.

Physical Exam
Screen all refractory hypertensive patients (see "History").

TESTS
Lab (2)A
- Elevated 24-hour urine metanephrine
- Elevated 24-hour urine or plasma catecholamines
- Elevated 24-hour VMA
- Elevated fractionated plasma metanephrines
- If results are equivocal or normal, repeat 24-hour urine collection when a paroxysmal spell occurs.
- Drugs that may alter lab results
  - Increased by
    - Amphetamines
    - Tricyclic antidepressants
    - Clonidine or other drug withdrawal
    - Labetalol
    - Ethanol
    - Methyldopa
    - Sotalol
    - Levodopa
  - Decreased by
    - Central α_2 agonists
    - Reserpine
- Disorders that may alter lab results: Major physical stress (e.g., surgery, stroke)

Imaging
- Abdominal image; MRI is preferable to CT
- I^{123}: I-metaiodobenzylguanidine scan
- In^{111}: pentetreotide scan

Diagnostic Procedures/Surgery
- Clonidine suppression test
- Suppression/provocation tests

Pathological Findings
A catecholamine-producing tumor in the adrenal medulla, para-aortic sympathetic chain, wall of the urinary bladder, or sympathetic chain in the neck of mediastinum

DIFFERENTIAL DIAGNOSIS
- Labile essential hypertension
- Anxiety and panic attacks
- Paroxysmal cardiac arrhythmia
- Thyrotoxicosis
- Menopausal syndrome
- Hypoglycemia
- Mastocytosis
- Withdrawal of adrenergic-inhibiting medications
- Angina
- Hyperventilation
- Migraine headache
- Amphetamine or cocaine use
- Sympathomimetic ingestion

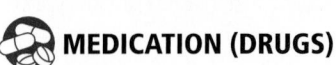

TREATMENT

GENERAL MEASURES
- Combined α-blockade and β-blockade
- Cardiovascular and hemodynamic variables must be closely monitored.

Diet
Preoperatively, follow a high-salt diet to increase blood volume.

MEDICATION (DRUGS)

First Line
- Combined α-adrenergic and β-adrenergic blockade required preoperatively
- Initiate α-blockade first: Phenoxybenzamine (Dibenzyline) 10 mg PO daily and increase by 10–20 mg every 2 days as needed to control BP and paroxysmal spells (average dose is 0.5–1.0 mg/kg/d)
- β-Blockade after α-blockade can follow α-blockade: Propranolol (Inderal) 10 mg q6h initially and increase as necessary to control tachycardia
- Acute hypertensive crises should be treated with phentolamine (Regitine) or nitroprusside administered intravenously.
- Contraindications
  - β-Adrenergic blockade in patients with asthma, sinus bradycardia, and >1st-degree block, or CHF.
  - Avoid β-blockers with intrinsic sympathomimetic activity.
- Precautions
  - β-Adrenergic blockade alone may result in more severe hypertension owing to the unopposed α-adrenergic stimulation; patients should be cautioned about postural hypotension.
  - β-Adrenergic blockade is initiated at low doses using a short-acting agent owing to the possible side effect of pulmonary edema in the patient with catecholamine myocardiopathy.
- Significant possible interactions: For β-adrenergic blockade: Verapamil, phenytoin, phenobarbitone, rifampin, chlorpromazine, and cimetidine

Second Line
- α-Adrenergic blocking agents: Prazosin (Minipress), terazosin (Hytrin), doxazosin (Cardura)
- β-Adrenergic blocking agents: Nadolol (Corgard), atenolol (Tenormin), metoprolol (Lopressor)
- Combined β-adrenergic and α-adrenergic blocker: Labetalol (Normodyne, Trandate)
- Catecholamine synthesis inhibitor: Metyrosine (Demser) (3)[A]

SURGERY
High-risk surgical procedure requires an experienced surgeon, anesthetist, and clinical team. It Is often amenable to laparoscopic adrenalectomy.

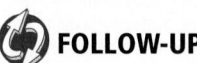

FOLLOW-UP

PROGNOSIS
- The survival rate after removal of a benign pheochromocytoma is nearly that of controls when matched for age and gender.
- For malignant pheochromocytoma, the 5-year survival rate is <50%.

COMPLICATIONS
- When diagnosed at autopsy, 75% of patients died from MI or CVA.
- 1/3 of sudden deaths occurred after unrelated minor operative procedures.
- Postural hypotension with α-adrenergic blockade
- Pulmonary edema with β-adrenergic blockade
- Intraoperative hypertensive crisis

PATIENT MONITORING
- Daily BP monitoring before surgery
- Intraoperative hemodynamic monitoring
- 2 weeks postoperatively: 24-hour urine for measurement of catecholamines and metanephrines; if normal, recheck annually, for indefinite period (4)[B]

REFERENCES

1. Clark OH, Duh QY. *Textbook of Endocrine Surgery*. Philadelphia: WB Saunders, 2005.
2. DeQuattro V, Lee D. Pheochromocytoma. Best Practice of Medicine. October 1999; at http://praxis.md/index.cfm?page=bpm`brief&chapter=CPM02EN314&search`cpm=yes&hilight=pheochromocytoma.
3. Federman DD. *The Adrenal Medulla. Pheochromocytoma. Update 2*. New York: Scientific American Medicine, 2000;1:15.
4. Young WF. Pheochromocytoma: 1926–1993: *Trends Endocrinol Metab*. 1993;4:122–127.

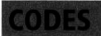 **MISCELLANEOUS**

See also: Hypertension, essential; Multiple endocrine neoplasia (MEN).

 CODES

ICD9-CM
- 194.0 Malignant neoplasm of adrenal gland
- 227.0 Benign neoplasm of adrenal gland

PATIENT TEACHING

Patient educational materials from National Adrenal Disease Foundation (NADF), 505 Northern Blvd., Great Neck, NY 11021; 516-407-4992; e-mail: nadfmail@aol.com.

See Corresponding Diagnostic Algorithm

PHIMOSIS AND PARAPHIMOSIS

Michail Wollin, MD

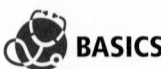 **BASICS**

DESCRIPTION
- Phimosis: Tightness of the penile foreskin that prevents it from being drawn back from over the glans
- Paraphimosis: Constriction of glans penis by proximally placed phimotic foreskin
- System(s) Affected: Renal/Urologic; Reproductive; Skin/Exocrine

ALERT
Geriatric Considerations
Recurrent infection and irritations (condom catheters) can lead to phimosis.

Pediatric Considerations
- Recurrent balanitis, either chemical or infectious, can lead to an acquired phimosis.
- Forced reduction of a physiologic foreskin can lead to chronic scarring and acquired phimosis.

GENERAL PREVENTION
Good patient and parental education

EPIDEMIOLOGY
- Predominant age: Infancy and adolescence
- Predominant sex: Male only

Prevalence
In the US: 1% of males >16 years of age

RISK FACTORS
- Phimosis
  - Poor hygiene
  - Diabetes
  - Frequent diaper rash in infant
- Paraphimosis
  - Presence of foreskin
  - Inexperienced health care provider (e.g., leaving foreskin retracted after catheter placement)

ETIOLOGY
- Phimosis
  - Physiologic: Present at birth and resolves spontaneously during the 1st 2–3 years of life through nocturnal erections, which slowly dilate the phimotic ring.
  - Congenital: Unresolved physiologic phimosis
  - Acquired: Recurrent infection, irritation, or traumatic from forced reduction of infants "physiologic" phimosis
    ○ Paraphimosis
  - Foreskin not pulled back over the glans after cleaning, cystoscopy, or catheter insertion

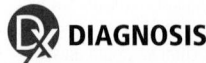 **DIAGNOSIS**

SIGNS AND SYMPTOMS
History
- Phimosis
  - Painful erections
  - Recurrent balanitis
  - Foreskin balloons with voiding
- Paraphimosis
  - Uncircumcised by history
  - Pain
  - Drainage

Physical Exam
- Phimosis
  - Foreskin cannot retract
  - Secondary balanitis
- Paraphimosis
  - Edema
  - Drainage
  - Ulceration

DIFFERENTIAL DIAGNOSIS
- Penile lymphedema, which can be related to insect bites, trauma, or allergic reactions
- Penile tourniquet syndrome: Foreign body around penis, most commonly a hair

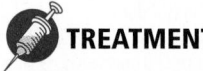 **TREATMENT**

GENERAL MEASURES
- Phimosis
  - 0.05% Betamethasone b.i.d. with gradual traction placed on foreskin. Over 4–6 weeks the phimotic ring should open. (1)[C]
- Paraphimosis
  - Manual reduction if possible (should be done with the patient sedated). Place the middle and index fingers of both hands on the engorged skin proximal to the glans. Place both thumbs on glans and, with gentle pressure, push on the glans and pull on foreskin to attempt reduction. If unsuccessful, a dorsal slit will be necessary with eventual circumcision after the edema resolves.
  - Osmotic agents: Granulated sugar placed on edematous tissue for several hours to reduce edema (2)[C]
  - Puncture technique. Multiple punctures of foreskin with a 21 gauge needle will allow edematous fluid to escape, and thus allow reduction (3)[C]
- Appropriate health care: Outpatient except for complications
- Pain control

Diet
No limitations

Activity
No sexual activity following circumcision until healing is complete

SURGERY
- Phimosis: Circumcision
- Paraphimosis
  - Dorsal slit with delayed circumcision, if reduction is not possible
  - Operative exploration if the possibility of penile tourniquet syndrome can not be eliminated. Hair removal cream can be applied if a hair is seen as the etiology of the tourniquet.

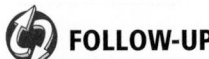 **FOLLOW-UP**

DISPOSITION
Admission Criteria
Tissue loss with paraphimosis

Issues for Referral
Consider circumcision for recurrent balanitis and paraphimosis.

PROGNOSIS
Complete resolution if treatment is carried out effectively

COMPLICATIONS
- Unreduced paraphimosis can lead to gangrene of the glans.
- Posthitis (inflammation of the prepuce)

PATIENT MONITORING
Monitor for 1 week after reduction of paraphimosis and for 1–2 weeks after a circumcision.

REFERENCES

1. Orsola A, Caffaratti J, Garat JM. Conservative treatment of phimosis in children using a topical steroid. *Urology*. 2000;56:307–310.
2. Cahill D, Rome A. Reduction of paraphimosis with granulated sugar. *BJU Int*. 1999;83:362.
3. Reynard JM, Barua JM. Reduction of paraphimosis the simple way—the Dundee technique. *BJU Int*. 1999;83:859–860.

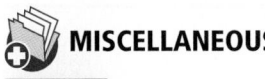 **MISCELLANEOUS**

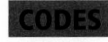

ICD9-CM
605 Redundant prepuce and phimosis

PATIENT TEACHING

Prevention
If the patient is uncircumcised, appropriate hygiene and care of the foreskin is necessary to prevent phimosis and paraphimosis.

PHOBIAS

Cheryl A. Wehler, MD

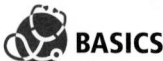 **BASICS**

DESCRIPTION
- A persistent and excessive or unreasonable fear of a specific object, activity, place, or situation that results in a compelling desire to avoid the perceived fear. When forced to endure the phobic stimulus, it is done so with dread.
- Psychiatric conditions classified in *DSM-IV-R* as anxiety disorders. (1)
  - When confronted with the phobic stimulus, patient reacts with intense anxiety, adults usually realize the fear is excessive or unreasonable.
  - When a fear causes significant distress, or it interferes with normal functions of life, then it is considered a psychiatric disorder.
- Agoraphobia: Fear of being trapped in a place or situation where escape is difficult or embarrassing, or in which help is not available if paniclike symptoms develop. Agoraphobic fears involve: (a) fear of being alone, (b) fear of being away from home, and (c) fear of being in a place from which escape is difficult (seen most often in association with panic disorder).
- Specific phobia: Fear of clearly discernible, circumscribed objects or situations such as animals, insects, heights, flying, closed spaces (claustrophobia), blood-injury phobia (syncope related to the sight of blood)
- Social phobia: Fear of social or performance situations in which embarrassment or humiliation may occur under scrutiny by others (e.g., performance anxiety, speaking in public, or eating in public)
- System(s) Affected: Nervous/Psychiatric

ALERT
Pediatric Considerations
Anxiety may be expressed by crying, tantrums, freezing, or clinging. Fears of animals and other objects in natural environment are common and usually transitory in childhood.

EPIDEMIOLOGY
- Predominant age: Median (50th percentile) age of onset (2)
- Agoraphobia: 20 years
- Social phobia: 13 years
- Predominant sex: Female > Male

Prevalence
The 12-month prevalence in the general U.S. population of specific phobias is 8.7% social phobia, 6.8% and agoraphobia without panic, 0.8% (3).

RISK FACTORS
- An increased risk of phobias is noted in 1st-degree biologic relatives with the disorder compared with the general population.
- Transmission unknown.
- Twin studies have not fully differentiated the role of genetic versus environmental factors.

Genetics
No consistent genetic pattern

ETIOLOGY
- Evidence suggests a complex interplay among genetic vulnerability, development neurobiology, and environment.
- Vulnerability may lead to persistence or exaggeration of learned response, perhaps learned initially as a protective mechanism (such as avoidance of large dogs by small children).

ASSOCIATED CONDITIONS
- For all phobias: Other anxiety disorders, depression, and drug use disorders
- Social and agoraphobia: Panic attacks or panic disorder

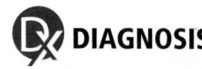 **DIAGNOSIS**

SIGNS AND SYMPTOMS
- Extreme anxiety when exposed to phobic stimulus
- Tremors
- Palpitations
- Sweating
- Blushing
- Dyspnea
- Dizziness
- Associated nausea

History
- Careful history and observation of the patient
- Description of the behavior by patient, family, or friends
- Psychiatric examination

TESTS
Lab
No specific tests for detection, although thyroid stimulating hormone and ECG is warranted in those >40 years.

DIFFERENTIAL DIAGNOSIS
- For agoraphobia
  - Panic disorder with agoraphobia
  - Social phobia
  - Specific phobia
  - Major depressive disorder
  - Avoidance in delusional disorder
  - Avoidance in obsessive-compulsive disorder
  - Separation anxiety disorder
  - Avoidance that results from realistic concerns associated with a general medical condition
- For specific phobia
  - Panic disorder with agoraphobia
  - Social phobia
  - Avoidance in posttraumatic stress disorder
  - Avoidance in obsessive-compulsive disorder
  - Avoidance in separation anxiety disorder
  - Avoidance in psychotic disorders
  - Nonpathological avoidance of circumscribed objects or situations
- For social phobia
  - Panic disorder with agoraphobia
  - Agoraphobia without history of panic disorder, generalized anxiety disorder, specific phobia
  - Separation anxiety disorder
  - Pervasive developmental disorder, schizoid personality disorder
  - Avoidant personality disorder
  - Social anxiety and avoidance associated with other mental disorders
  - Nonpathologic performance anxiety, stage fright, or shyness

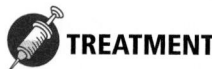 **TREATMENT**

Outpatient

GENERAL MEASURES
- Agoraphobia
  - Cognitive behavioral treatment (CBT) including exposure, cognitive restructuring, and relaxation techniques
  - Pharmacologic treatment required when agoraphobia is associated with panic disorder.
- Specific phobia
  - Behavior modification techniques of systemic desensitization or in vivo exposure
  - Fear of flying specifically: Short-acting benzodiazepine
- Social phobia
  - CBT including exposure, cognitive restructuring, and relaxation techniques (4)[A]
  - Social skills training
  - Performance anxiety or situations where patient in a circumscribed setting: β-Blocker

Diet
- Consider restriction of stimulants such as caffeine, nicotine, xanthines, and sympathomimetics, which can overdrive anxiety.
- If taking phenelzine or other monoamine oxidase (MAO) inhibitors, a tyramine-free diet must be followed to decrease the risk of hypertensive crisis.

Activity
No restriction

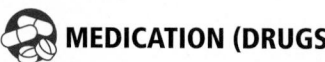 **MEDICATION (DRUGS)**

First Line
- Agoraphobia: selective serotonin reuptake inhibitors (SSRIs) (paroxetine (10–50 mg/d) and sertraline (50–200 mg/d); FDA approved, others used off-label) (5)[A]
- Specific phobia: None recommended, except for fear of flying. A short-acting benzodiazepine, such as alprazolam, may be helpful. Initial dose as low as 0.25 mg, titrated upward as needed.
- Social phobia (acute): β-Blocker (e.g., propranolol [Inderal]) 20–40 mg, 45–60 minutes before anticipated performance
- Social phobia (generalized)
  - Strongest evidence of treatment efficacy observed in SSRIs (6)[A]
  - Venlafaxine ER (75–225 mg/d) equally efficacious and well tolerated (7,8)[A]

Second Line

- Agoraphobia

  - High-potency benzodiazepines, reversible MAO inhibitors, and tricyclic antidepressants also have antipanic efficacy (9)[A]; comparative studies have shown that TCAs and SSRIs are equally effective but the latter are better tolerated. (10)[A]

- Social phobia (generalized): Phenelzine (a monoamine oxidase [MAO] inhibitor), clonazepam, or gabapentin also are effective, but less well tolerated. (11)[A]

- Contraindications

  - β-Blocker: Asthma or bronchospasm, CHF, bradycardia
  - Phenelzine: Not with other antidepressants, tyramine in diet, decongestants, diet pills, meperidine (Demerol), dextromethorphan, levodopa, and sympathomimetics

- Precautions

  - Do not discontinue alprazolam abruptly, because of potential for withdrawal seizures.
  - Monitor BP in patients taking β-blockers.
  - Consult drug information before using phenelzine.

- Significant possible interactions

  - Phenelzine: Significant dietary restrictions, due to potential for hypertensive crisis; avoid sympathomimetics, tricyclic antidepressants (TCAs), fluoxetine, other SSRIs, central nervous system depressants.
  - Consult drug information sources before adding new medications in patients.

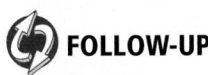 FOLLOW-UP

PROGNOSIS

- Agoraphobia: Usually associated with panic disorder; chronic. Often patient becomes increasingly home-bound as condition continues.
- Simple phobia: Some remit spontaneously as person ages (as in some simple phobias of childhood); alternatively, some become chronic. Impairment can be minimal if object can be avoided (such as snakes). Although improvement occurs with in vivo exposure, phobia can recur after successful treatment.
- Social phobia: Chronic course

COMPLICATIONS

- Avoidance behavior
- Episodic alcohol, barbiturate, and anxiolytic abuse/overuse and dependence as patients try to self-medicate to ameliorate symptoms
- Development of mild depression

PATIENT MONITORING

Outpatient as needed

REFERENCES

1. American Psychiatric Association. Diagnostic and Statistical Manual of Mental Disorders (DSM-IV-R), 4th ed. Washington, DC: American Psychiatric Association, 2000.
2. Kessler RC, et al. Lifetime prevalence and age-of-onset distributions of DSM-IV disorders in the National Comorbidity Survey Replication. *Arch Gen Psychiatr.* 2005;62(6):593–768.
3. Kessler RC, et al. Prevalence, severity, and comorbidity of 12-month DSM-IV disorders in the National Comorbidity Survey Replication. *Arch Gen Psychiatr.* 2005;62(6):617–627.
4. Rodebaugh TL, et al. The treatment of social anxiety disorder. *Clin Psychol Rev.* 2004;24(7): 883–908.
5. Ham P, et al. Treatment of panic disorder. *Am Fam Phys.* 2005;71:733–739.
6. Stein DJ, et al. *Cochrane Database Sys Rev.* 2004;(4):CD001206.
7. Liebowitz MR, et al. A randomized controlled trial of venlafaxine extended release in generalized social anxiety disorder. *J Clin Psychiatr.* 2005;66(2):238–247.
8. Liebowitz MR, et al. Venlafaxine extended release vs placebo and paroxetine in social anxiety disorder. *Arch Gen Psychiatr.* 2005;62(2): 190–198.
9. Pollack MH, et al. WCA recommendations for the long-term treatment of panic disorder. *CNS Spectrums.* 2003;8(8 Suppl 1):17–30.
10. Bakker A, et al. SSRIs vs. TCAs in the treatment of panic disorder: A meta-analysis. *Acta Psychiatr Scand.* 2002;106(3):163–167.
11. Blanco C, et al. Pharmacological treatment of social anxiety disorder: A meta-analysis. *Depression Anxiety.* 2003;18(1):29–40.

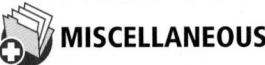 MISCELLANEOUS

See also: Anxiety and depression; Dissociative disorders; Obsessive-compulsive disorder; Posttraumatic stress disorder (PTSD); Schizophrenia

CODES

ICD9-CM

- 300.20 Phobia, unspecified
- 300.21 Agoraphobia with panic attacks
- 300.22 Agoraphobia without mention of panic attacks
- 300.23 Social phobia
- 300.29 Other isolated or simple phobias

PATIENT TEACHING

- Cognitive therapy
- Phobia clinic or group therapy, if available
- Anxiety Disorders of America, http://www.adaa.org

 See Corresponding Diagnostic Algorithm

PHOTODERMATITIS

Aamir Siddiqi, MD

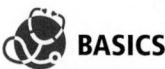 **BASICS**

DESCRIPTION
- Light-induced eruptions seen in a pattern of photodistribution
  - Phototoxic reactions: Result of the acute toxic effect on skin of UV light alone (sunburn) or together with a photosensitizing substance (nonallergic)
  - Photoallergic eruptions: A form of allergic dermatitis resulting from combined effects of a photosensitizing substance (drugs or chemical) plus UV light (immunologic/delayed hypersensitivity)
  - Polymorphous light eruption (PLE): Chronic, intermittent light-induced eruption with erythematous papules, urticaria, or vesicles on areas exposed to sunlight
- System(s) Affected: Skin/Exocrine
- Synonym(s): Sun poisoning; Sun allergy

GENERAL PREVENTION
- Sunlight avoidance/protective clothing
- Identification and avoidance of causative drugs (see "Etiology")
- Sunscreens: Apply before exposure.
  - Zinc oxide: Opaque, cosmetically less acceptable
  - Chemical: Use sun-protective factor >30 for maximum protection; substantively resistant to sweat and swimming; cosmetically more acceptable (2)[C]

EPIDEMIOLOGY
- Predominant age: All ages
- Predominant sex: Male = Female

RISK FACTORS
- Job-related exposure to sunlight
- Light and fair-colored skin

Genetics
Predisposition occurs in inbred populations (e.g., Pima Indians)

ETIOLOGY
- Sunlight
- Phenothiazines
- Diuretics
- Tetracyclines
- Sulfonamides
- Oral contraceptives
- Topicals: Psoralens, coal tars, photoactive dyes (eosin, acridine orange)
- 5-Fluorouracil
- Quinine
- Sunscreens containing para-aminobenzoic acid (PABA)
- In the US: ~115 chemical agents used topically are known to cause photodermatitis.

ASSOCIATED CONDITIONS
- Sunlight aggravation of systemic lupus
- Persistent light reactivity
- Actinic reticuloid

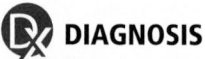 **DIAGNOSIS**

SIGNS AND SYMPTOMS
- Phototoxic
  - Erythema
  - With increasing severity: Vesicles and bullae
  - Classic example: Sunburn
  - Nails may exhibit onycholysis.
  - Chronic: Epidermal thickening, elastosis, telangiectasia, and pigmentary changes
  - Sharp lines of demarcation between involved and uninvolved skin (sunlight exposure)
  - Phototoxic eruption due to topicals: Area of application
  - Usually develops shortly after sun exposure
  - Hyperpigmentation may follow resolution
  - Pain

- Photoallergic (2)[C]
  - Papules with erythema and occasionally vesicles
  - Area exposed to light with less distinct borders
  - Usually delayed 24 hours or more after exposure
  - May spread to unexposed areas
  - Pruritus
- PLE
  - Erythematous papules
  - Occasionally urticaria or vesicles
  - Scattered over sun-exposed areas with normal skin in between
  - Can spread to nonexposed areas
  - Often flares in spring or early summer
  - Desensitization affect (less over the course of the summer)
  - Burning or pruritus may precede lesions

TESTS
Lab
- Antinuclear antibody (ANA) to rule out systemic lupus erythematosus
- Photo-testing: Exposing patient to UV light
- Photopatch testing: Applying suspected agents and chemicals to patient's skin
- Skin biopsy: To rule out other disorders

Diagnostic Procedures/Surgery
Physical examination and medical history

Pathological Findings
Nonspecific

DIFFERENTIAL DIAGNOSIS
Systemic lupus erythematosus

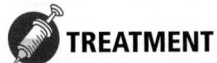 **TREATMENT**

GENERAL MEASURES
- Appropriate health care: Outpatient
- Avoid sunlight/limit exposure.
- Protective clothing/sunscreens
- Ice packs/cold water compresses

Diet
No special diet

Activity
Avoid sunlight

Complementary and Alternative Medicine
Taking beta-carotene orally seems to modestly reduce the risk of sunburn in individuals who are sensitive to sun exposure.

 MEDICATION (DRUGS)

First Line
- Topical corticosteroids (betamethasone valerate 0.1% cream)
- NSAIDs (indomethacin 25 mg PO t.i.d.; aspirin; others)
- Prednisone for severe reactions (0.5–1 mg/kg PO daily) for 3–10 days
- Antihistamines for pruritus (hydroxyzine 25–50 mg PO q.i.d.)
- Sunscreens (>30 SPF) for prevention. Use broad-spectrum sunscreen to block both UVA and UVB. PABA may aggravate photodermatitis in sensitized patients (due to the sulfa moiety). (2)[C]
- Contraindications: Refer to the manufacturer's profile for each drug.
- Precautions: Refer to the manufacturer's profile for each drug.
- Significant possible interactions: Refer to the manufacturer's profile for each drug.

ALERT
Geriatric Considerations
More likely to experience adverse reactions to causative drugs

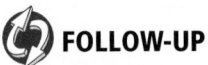 **FOLLOW-UP**

DISPOSITION
- Follow-up as needed
- Treated as outpatient only

PROGNOSIS
Good with avoidance/protection measures

COMPLICATIONS
Rare (secondary bacterial infection)

PATIENT MONITORING
As necessary for persistence or recurrence

REFERENCES

1. Bondi J, Jegasothy B, Lazarus G. *Dermatology, Diagnosis and Therapy*. Norwalk, CT: McGraw-Hill/Appleton and Lange; 1992.
2. Deleo V. Sunscreen use in photodermatoses. *Dermatologic Clinics*. 2006;24(1):27–33.
3. Morison WL. Clinical practice. Photosensitivity. *N Engl J Med*. 2004;350(11):1111–1117.

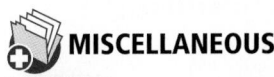 **MISCELLANEOUS**

CODES

ICD9-CM
- 692.79 Other dermatitis due to solar radiation
- 692.9 Contact dermatitis and other eczema due to unspecified cause

PATIENT TEACHING
- Avoidance of sunlight
- Avoidance of photosensitizing drugs
- Protective clothing (e.g., hats, long sleeves)
- Sunscreens >15 SPF

Diet
None specific

Activity
No restriction

Prevention
- Avoid direct sun exposure.
- Regular use of sunscreen lotions
- Wear appropriate gear to avoid sunlight exposure.

PILONIDAL DISEASE

Michael Rousse, MD, MPH

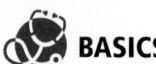 **BASICS**

DESCRIPTION
A cyst, abscess, or sinus tract that develops in the upper part of the natal cleft
- Synonym(s): Jeep disease

GENERAL PREVENTION
Remove excess hair from gluteal cleft in the region of any congenital dimpling

EPIDEMIOLOGY
- Predominant sex: Male > Female (3–4:1)
- Predominant age: Usually 3rd decade, rare >45 years old
- Ethnic consideration: Whites > African Americans > Asians

Incidence
No true incidence numbers available; most cases treated as outpatients

Prevalence
No true prevalence numbers available

RISK FACTORS
- Sedentary/prolonged sitting
- Excessive body hair
- Obesity
- Congenital natal dimple

Genetics
Congenital dimple in the natal cleft

PATHOPHYSIOLOGY
Pilonidal = nest of hair, excoriation by hair in the natal cleft allows hair to be drawn into the deeper tissues via negative pressure caused by movement of the buttocks (1)[C]

ETIOLOGY
Infection of subcutaneous tissues
- Polymicrobial, likely from enteric pathogens given proximity to ano-rectal contamination

ASSOCIATED CONDITIONS
None

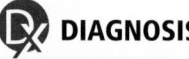 **DIAGNOSIS**

PRE HOSPITAL
3 distinct clinical presentations (2)[C]
- Asymptomatic: Painless cyst or sinus
- Acute abscess: Severe pain, swelling, discharge
- Chronic abscess: Persistent drainage from a sinus tract

SIGNS AND SYMPTOMS
Pain, swelling, redness, and drainage

History
- Common: Patient presents with an acutely inflamed cystic mass at the top of the gluteal cleft that may or may not have drained spontaneously
- Less common: Patient is found, on routine exam, to have a sinus that may have drained in the past with or without symptoms

Physical Exam
- Common: Inflamed cystic mass with limited surrounding erythema, +/− drainage or a sinus tract
- Less common: Significant cellulitis

TESTS
Lab
CBC and wound culture if significant cellulitis

Imaging
MRI could be used to differentiate between peri-rectal abscess and pilonidal disease

Pathological Findings
Inflammation and granulation tissue

DIFFERENTIAL DIAGNOSIS
- Furunculosis
- Hydradenitis suppurativa
- Anal fistula
- Peri-rectal abscess

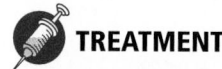 **TREATMENT**

PRE HOSPITAL
- Shave area, remove hair from crypts
- Depiliators

INITIAL STABILIZATION
Incision and drainage (I&D)

GENERAL MEASURES
- Weight loss
- Trim hair in/around gluteal cleft

Diet
No restrictions

Activity
Decrease sitting

MEDICATION (DRUGS)

- Antibiotics not indicated unless there is significant cellulitis
- If antibiotics are needed, a culture to direct therapy might be useful.

First Line
Cefazolin and metronidazole

SURGERY
Five levels of care based on severity or recurrence of disease (3)[C]

- I&D, remove hair, curette granulation tissue
- Excision of midline "pits," allow drainage of lateral sinus tracts
- Pilonidal cystotomy: Insert probe into sinus tract, excise overlying skin, close wound
- Marsupialization: Excise overlying skin and roof of cyst, suture skin edges to cyst floor
- Excision: Use of flap closure

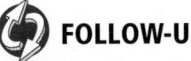 **FOLLOW-UP**

DISPOSITION
Admission Criteria
Degree of cellulitis

Issues for Referral
- Patients who cannot comply with frequent dressing changes required after I&D
- Patients who have recurrence after I&D
- Patients who have complex disease with multiple sinus tracts

PROGNOSIS
- Simple I&D has a 55% failure rate, median time to healing 5 weeks
- More extensive surgical excisions involve hospital stays and longer time to heal

COMPLICATIONS
Malignant degeneration is a rare complication of untreated chronic pilonidal disease.

PATIENT MONITORING
Postsurgical weekly wound checks are essential because of a high recurrence rate.

REFERENCES
1. MacLeod, J. *A Method of Proctology*. New York, NY: Harper & Row
2. Hull TL, Wu J. Pilonidal diseases. *Surg Clin North Am*, 2002;82(6):1169–1185.
3. Sullivan DJ. Pilonidal disease. *UpToDate [database]*. Dated October 23, 2003. Waltham, MA: UpToDate; 2003.

 MISCELLANEOUS

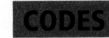 **CODES**

ICD9-CM
685 Pilonidal cyst

PATIENT TEACHING
- Wash area briskly with washcloth daily
- No prolonged sitting

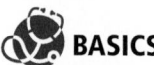

PINWORMS

Linda M. Spooner, PharmD, BCPS
Edward Liu, MD

BASICS

DESCRIPTION
- Intestinal infection with *Enterobius vermicularis*, characterized by perineal and perianal itching, usually worse at night
- System(s) Affected: Gastrointestinal; Skin/Exocrine
- Synonym(s): Enterobiasis

ALERT
Pediatric Considerations
More common in children, who are more likely to become reinfected.

GENERAL PREVENTION
- Careful hand washing, especially after bowel movements; clip and maintain short fingernails
- Wash anus and genitals at least once a day, preferably during a shower.
- Do not scratch anus or put fingers near nose or mouth.

EPIDEMIOLOGY
Predominant age: 5–14 years
Prevalence
- Most common helminthic infection in the US, with 20–42 million people harboring the parasite.
- ~30% of children are infected throughout the world.

RISK FACTORS
- Institutionalization
- Crowded living conditions
- Poor hygiene
- Warm climate

PATHOPHYSIOLOGY
- Small white worms (2–13 mm) inhabit the cecum, appendix, and adjacent portions of the ascending colon following ingestion.
- Female worms migrate to the perianal and perineal areas at night, depositing ~11,000 eggs, resulting in irritation and itching of the perianal area.
- Scratching of the perianal and perineal areas followed by touching of the mouth can lead to ingestion of the eggs and continuation of pinworm's life cycle in the host.

ETIOLOGY
Infestation by the intestinal nematode *Enterobius (Oxyuris) vermicularis*

ASSOCIATED CONDITIONS
Pruritus ani

DIAGNOSIS

SIGNS AND SYMPTOMS
- Many patients are asymptomatic
- Perianal itching
- Perineal itching
- Vulvovaginitis
- Dysuria
- Abdominal pain (rare)
- Insomnia
- Restless sleep

Physical Exam
Perineal and perianal exam

TESTS
- Adhesive tape test: A piece of transparent cellophane tape is stuck to the perianal skin in the early morning before bathing and then affixed to a microscope slide after removal. This procedure must be performed at least 3 times to achieve 90% sensitivity. Alternatively, anal swabs or a pinworm paddle coated with adhesive material can also be useful. (1,2)[C]
- Digital rectal examination with saline slide preparation of stool on gloved finger (1)[C]

Pathological Findings
- Identification of ova on low-power microscopy or direct visualization of the female worm (10 mm long). Ova are asymmetric, flattened on 1 side, and measure 56 × 27 μm.

DIFFERENTIAL DIAGNOSIS
- Idiopathic pruritus ani
- Atopic dermatitis
- Contact dermatitis
- Psoriasis
- Lichen planus
- Infection with human papillomavirus
- Herpes simplex
- Fungal infections
- Erythrasma
- Scabies
- Vaginitis
- Hemorrhoids

TREATMENT

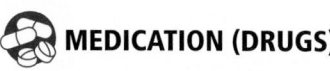

- Treatment for pinworms includes use of either mebendazole, albendazole, or pyrantel pamoate. (1)[A]
- Close contacts should be treated as well.
- Retreatment after 2 weeks is recommended by many experts due to the difficulty eradicating this parasite. (1)[C]

INITIAL STABILIZATION
Outpatient

GENERAL MEASURES
- All symptomatic family members should be treated simultaneously. (1)[C]
- Bedclothes and underwear of patients should be washed in hot water at the time of treatment. (1)[C]
- Meticulous hand washing can help prevent fecal–oral transmission. (1)[C]
- Practice good hygiene (i.e., showers, nail clipping). (1)[C]

Diet
No restrictions

Activity
No restrictions

MEDICATION (DRUGS)

Pregnancy Considerations
- Drug therapy should be avoided in pregnancy. Treatment should be delayed until after delivery. (4)[C]
- Some clinicians recommend repeat treatment after 2 weeks due to the high frequency of reinfection and autoinfection. Occasionally, refractory cases may require retreatment every 2 weeks for 4–6 cycles. Treatment options include any of the following (1,3)[A], (5)[C]
  - Mebendazole (Vermox): Chewable tablet 100 mg as a single dose in adults and children >2 years. Use with caution in children <2 years *or*
  - Albendazole: 400 mg PO tablets as a single dose in adults and children >2 years; 200 mg PO tablet as a single dose in children ≤2 years *or*
  - Pyrantel pamoate (Pin-X, Reese's Pinworm Medicine): Oral liquid or tablet 11 mg/kg as a single dose in adults and children >2 years. Maximum dose 1 g. Use with caution in children <2 years.
- Contraindications: Hypersensitivity to the agent
- Precautions
  - All family members should be treated.
  - Take medicine with food.
  - May cause diarrhea, nausea, and abdominal discomfort.
- Significant possible interactions
  - Phenytoin and carbamazepine reduce the effectiveness of mebendazole.
  - Refer to product labeling for additional information.

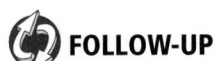 **FOLLOW-UP**

PROGNOSIS
- Asymptomatic carriers are common.
- Symptomatic infections are cured >90% of the time by pharmacotherapy.
- Reinfection is common, especially among children.

COMPLICATIONS
- Perianal scratching may lead to bacterial superinfection.
- Females: Vulvovaginitis, urethritis, endometritis, salpingitis
- Urinary tract infections
- Rarely, ectopic disease involving granulomas of the pelvis, urinary tract, female genitourinary tract, and appendix.

PATIENT MONITORING
Unnecessary unless symptoms do not abate following drug therapy.

REFERENCES

1. Jones JE. Pinworms. *Am Fam Phys*. 1988;38: 159–164.
2. Cram EB. Studies on oxyuriasis, 28. Summary and conclusions. *Am J Dis Child*. 1943;65:46–59.
3. Hamblin J, Connor PD. Pinworms in pregnancy. *J Amer Board Fam Practice*. 1995;8:321–324.
4. Kucik CJ, Martin GL, Sortor BV. Common intestinal parasites. *Am Fam Phys*. 2004;69:1161–1168.
5. Drugs for parasitic infections. *Med Lett Drugs Ther*. August 2004, 1–12.

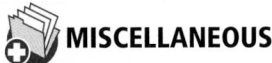 **MISCELLANEOUS**

See also: Pruritis ani

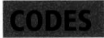 **CODES**

ICD9-CM
127.4 Enterobiasis

ICD10
B80 Enterobiasis

PATIENT TEACHING

For patient education materials on this topic: Centers for Disease Control, http://www.cdc.gov/ncidod/dpd/parasites/pinworm/factsht_pinworm.htm

Prevention
- Practice good hygiene.
- Encourage frequent and careful handwashing.
- Clip fingernails short.

 See Patient Handout on CD

PITUITARY ADENOMA

Jacob R. Brodsky, MD

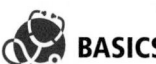 **BASICS**

DESCRIPTION
- Most common tumor of the pituitary gland
- May secrete hormones or cause mass effect
- Defined as microadenoma <10 mm and macroadenoma ≥10 mm
- Subtypes (Hormone): Prolactinoma (PRL), Corticotropinoma (Adrenocorticosteroid hormone [ACTH]), Thyrotropinoma (thyroid-stimulating hormone [TSH]), Somatotropinoma (growth hormone [GH]), Gonadotropinoma (Luteinizing hormone/follicle-stimulating hormone [LH/FSH]), Null Cell, Mixed
- System(s) Affected: Endocrine; Neurologic

EPIDEMIOLOGY
- Predominant age: Age increases incidence
- Predominant sex: Female > Male (3:2) for microadenomas (often delayed diagnosis in men)

Incidence
1.5/100,000 annually (symptomatic)

Prevalence
0.02% (symptomatic); 16.7% (autopsy)

RISK FACTORS
- Multiple Endocrine Neoplasia I: Autosomal dominant; pituitary, parathyroid, islet cell tumors
- McCune-Albright syndrome: Somatic mutation; Polyostotic fibrous dysplasia, skin lesions, and functional pituitary adenomas
- Carney complex: Autosomal dominant; primary nodular adrenal disease, nevi, sertoli cell testicular tumors, melanocytic schwannomas, cardiac myxomas, and somatotropinomas

Genetics
- Most due to monoclonal loss-of-function mutation, though specific mechanisms unclear
- See "Risk Factors" for syndromes.

PATHOPHYSIOLOGY
- Monoclonal adenohypophysial cell growth
- Hormonal effects typical of microadenomas, prompting diagnosis before mass effect
- PRL increased by functional prolactinomas or inhibition of dopaminergic suppression of PRL by macroadenoma mass effect

ETIOLOGY
See "Risk Factors" and "Genetics."

ASSOCIATED CONDITIONS
See "Risk Factors."

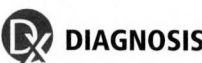 **DIAGNOSIS**

SIGNS AND SYMPTOMS
History
- Common
  - Hyperprolactinemia: Infertility, amenorrhea, galactorrhea, gynecomastia, impotence
  - Headache (sellar expansion)
  - Visual disturbances: Bitemporal hemianopsia
- Less common
  - Hypersomatotropinemia: Acromegaly (coarse features, hand/foot swelling, sweating)
  - Hyposomatotropinemia: Failure-to-thrive (FTT) (children), asymptomatic (adults)

- Intracranial pressure (ICP) elevation: Headache, nausea, seizures
- Hypercoticotropinemia: Cushing disease (buffalo hump, moon face, hirsutism, acne)
- Rare
  - Apoplexy: Headache, sudden collapse
  - Secondary hyperthyroidism: Palpitations, diaphoresis, heat intolerance, diarrhea
  - Secondary adrenal insufficiency: Weakness, irritability, anorexia, nausea/vomiting
  - Hypothalamic compression: Temperature, thirst/appetite disorders

Physical Exam
- Common
  - Visual disturbances: Bitemporal hemianopsia
  - Hyperprolactinemia: Hypogonadism, galactorrhea, gynecomastia
  - Hypersomatotropinemia: Acromegaly (coarse features, hand/foot swelling, diaphoresis)
  - Hyposomatotropinemia: FTT (children), none (adults)
- Less common
  - ICP elevation: Papilledema, dementia
  - Cushing disease: Centripetal obesity, buffalo hump, moon face, hirsutism, acne
- Rare
  - Apoplexy: Hypotension, tachycardia, oliguria
  - Secondary hyperthyroidism: Tachycardia, tachypnea, diaphoresis, warm/moist skin
  - Adrenal crisis: Orthostatic hypotension
  - Hypothalamic compression: Temperature dysregulation, obesity, increased urination

TESTS
Lab
- Select based on dysfunction(s) suspected
  - Hyperprolactinemia: Serum PRL >20ng/mL
  - Acromegaly/Hypersomatotropinemia: Serum IGF-1 elevated; Oral Glucose Tolerance Test with GH given at 0, 30, and 60 minutes (Normally suppresses GH to <1 μg/L)
  - Hyposomatotropinemia: Low GHRH response
  - Cushing disease/hypercorticotropinemia
    - 24-hour urinary free cortisol >50 μg
    - Overnight low-dose dexamethasone suppression test (DMST): Fasting plasma cortisol (FPC) >3 μg/dL at 8 a.m. (after 1 mg given at 11 p.m. on night prior)
    - ACTH level assay (If DMST results abnormal): <20 pg/mL = Adrenal tumor; ≥20 pg/mL = Ectopic/Pituitary source
  - Hypocorticotropinemia/Secondary glucocorticoid deficiency
    - High-dose Corticotropin Stimulation Test: FPC >18 μg/dL 1 hour after 250 μg given
    - Metyrapone test: 11-deoxycortisol <150 ng/L; after 2 g given (Prepare to give steroids as test may worsen insufficiency)
  - Hypogonadotropism: Gonadotropin-releasing hormone stimulation of LH/FSH blunted in pituitary hypergonadism, but increased in primary hypogonadism
  - Hyper/Hypothyroidism: TSH and free T4 both increased for pituitary hyperthyroidism and both decreased for pituitary hypothyroidism

- A typical panel for asymptomatic tumors includes PRL, IGF-1, 24-hr urinary-free cortisol or overnight DMST, α-subunit FSH, LH, TSH, T4

Imaging
- MRI preferred (>90% sensitivity/specificity)
- Octreotide scintigraphy is useful in identifying tumors with somatostatin receptors

Diagnostic Procedures/Surgery
Petrosal sinus sampling: ACTH sampled from inferior petrosal sinuses to distinguish Cushing disease (pituitary source) from ectopic ACTH

Pathological Findings
- Cell types identified by immunohistochemistry
- Light microscope: Eosinophilic (GH, PRL), Basophilic (FSH/LH, TSH, ACTH), Chromophobic

DIFFERENTIAL DIAGNOSIS
- Pituitary hyperplasia (e.g., pregnancy)
- Rathke's cleft cyst
- Granulomatous disease (e.g., Tuberculosis, Sarcoidosis)
- Lymphocytic hypophysitis
- Metastatic tumor
- Germinoma
- Craniopharyngioma

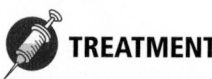 **TREATMENT**

INITIAL STABILIZATION
Pituitary apoplexy (see "Complications"): Must treat immediately to prevent death
- Support airways, breathing, circulation initiate IV, O$_2$, and monitor
- Maintain BP with fluids and/or pressor agents
- Contact neurosurgery

GENERAL MEASURES
Diet
No restrictions

Activity
No restrictions

Nursing
- Adrenal crisis: Monitor BP and input/outputs (I/Os)
- Pituitary apoplexy: Strict I/Os, central venous pressure (CVP), ICP monitoring, and frequent neurological checks

SPECIAL THERAPY
Radiotherapy
- Fractionated radiotherapy: Often effective as adjunctive when surgery inadequate (1)[A]
- Stereotactic radiosurgery: Alternative to surgery in high-risk patients or as adjunct (1)[B]

IV Fluids
- Diabetes Insipidus: Hyposmolar IV fluids
- Adrenal Crisis: Normal saline

MEDICATION (DRUGS)

Medical therapy is primary therapy for prolactinomas and adjunct for other tumors (2–4)[A]

First Line
- Hyperprolactinemia: Dopaminergic agonists increase dopaminergic suppression of PRL
  - Cabergoline (Dostinex): D_2 receptor-specific
    - Initial dose: 0.25 mg PO twice weekly
    - Maintenance dose: Increase q4wk by 0.25 mg 2x/wk per PRL (Max 2 mg/wk)
    - Contraindications: Hypersensitivity (ergots), high blood pressure (HTN), pregnancy-induced HTN
    - Precautions: Caution with liver impairment
    - Interactions: May be inhibited by tricyclic antidepressants, phenothiazines, opiates
    - Adverse reactions: Orthostatic hypotension, vertigo, dyspepsia, hot flashes
- Somatotropinemia: GH suppressants
  - Octreotide (Sandostatin): Long-acting analog of somatostatin:
    - Initial dose: 50 mcg SC/IV t.i.d., then titrate to GH (Max 1,500 mcg/d)
    - Contraindications: Hypersensitivity
    - Precautions: Caution with biliary, thyroid, cardiac, liver, or kidney disease
    - Interactions: Pimozide increases risk of QT prolongation; variable effects with beta-blockers, diuretics, oral glycemic agents
    - Adverse reactions: Ascending cholangitis, arrhythmias, congestive heart failure, glycemic instability
    - More effective as adjuvant than as primary treatment for somatotropinomas (2)[A]
- Corticotropinemia: Peripheral inhibitors
  - Mitotane (Lysodren)
    - Initial dose: 2–6 g PO t.i.d. (Max: 19 g/d)
    - Maintenance dose: 2–16 g t.i.d.
    - Contraindications: Hypersensitivity
    - Precautions: Caution with liver dysfunction and brain damage
    - Interactions: Contraindicated with rotavirus vaccine; caution with other vaccines
    - Adverse reactions: HTN, orthostatic hypotension, hemorrhagic cystitis, rash
- Gonadotropinemia
  - Bromocriptine: See above
    - Dosing: Start at 1.25–2.5 mg PO qhs; increase 1.25–2.5 mg q3–7d up to 20–30 mg daily (100 mg/d max)
- Thyrotropinemia
  - Octreotide: See above

Second Line
- Hyperprolactinemia: Dopaminergic agonists
  - Bromocriptine (Parlodel)
    - Initial dose: 1.25–5 mg PO daily
    - Maintenance dose: Increase 2.5 mg/d q2–7d up to 2.5–15 mg daily

- Pediatric dose: Same as adult with max 10 mg if age <15 years. Not for age <11 years.
- Contraindications: Hypersensitivity (ergots), HTN, coronary artery disease, PVD, Pregnancy
- Precautions: Caution with liver/renal impairment, HTN, Pulmonary disease, psychosis, myocardial infarction (MI) hx
- Interactions: May cause seizures, HTN and V-tach when used with decongestants, antihistamines, or pseudoephedrine
- Adverse reactions: Hypotension, seizures, stroke, HTN, MI, arrythmias, psychosis
- Corticotropinemia: Peripheral inhibitors
  - Metyrapone
    - Dose: 250–600 mg PO daily
    - Contraindications: Porphyria
    - Precautions: Caution in liver/thyroid disease
    - Interactions: Dilantin increases metabolism
    - Adverse reactions: Nausea, hypotension
- Gonadotropinemia
  - Octreotide: See above

SURGERY
- Most now done transphenoidally through nose
- Indications: Symptoms or treatment-resistant (3)
- Follow-up: Serial neuro/hormonal evaluations to evaluate complications (Diabetes Insipidus, CNS damage) and need for more treatment (3)
- Remission rates: 72–87% for microadenoma, but only 50–56% for macroadenomas (3)

 FOLLOW-UP

DISPOSITION
Admission Criteria
- Outpatient management unless apoplexy (see "Complications") or adrenal crisis (hypotension, hyponatremia, hyperkalemia)
- Keep as inpatients post-op until diabetes insipidus and/or adrenal insufficiency managed

Discharge Criteria
See "Admission Criteria".

Issues for Referral
- Endocrinologist referral if symptomatic
- Neurosurgery consultation as soon as tumor with symptoms identified (except for prolactinoma)
- Ophthalmologist evaluation prior to surgery

PROGNOSIS
- Depends on type, size, symptoms, and therapy
- Acromegaly's 10-year life expectancy reduction prevented if posttherapy GH <2.5 μg/L (4)

COMPLICATIONS
- Postoperative diabetes insipidus and/or hypogonadism (usually transient/common)
- Pituitary apopexy (acute/uncommon): Acute hemorrhagic pituitary infarction; adrenal crisis with severe headache; surgical decompression required to prevent shock, coma, and death
- Nelson syndrome (subacute/uncommon): Rapid adenoma growth post-adrenalectomy
- Pituitary hormone insufficiency (chronic/uncommon): Often years after treatment
- Optic nerve neuropathy and brain necrosis: May occur after >60 Gy radiotherapy (chronic/rare)

PATIENT MONITORING
- Typically outpatient treatment
- Follow-up MRI at 6 and 12 months
- Involved hormone(s) followed post-operatively, especially post-radiation, because hypopituitarism may develop many years later (2)

REFERENCES
1. Mondok A, et al. Treatment of pituitary tumors: Radiation. *Endocrine*. 2005;28:77–85.
2. Tichomirowa MA, Daly AF, Beckers A. Treatment of pituitary tumors: Somatostatin. *Endocrine*. 2005;28:93–99.
3. Buchfelder M. Treatment of pituitary tumors: Surgery. *Endocrine*. 2005;28:67–75.
4. Drange MR, et al. Pituitary tumor registry: A novel clinical resource. *J Clin Endo Met*. 2000;85: 168–174.

 MISCELLANEOUS

See also: Acromegaly; Cushing disease and syndrome; Galactorrhea

CODES

ICD9-CM
227.3 Benign Neoplasms of the Pituitary Gland and Craniopharyngeal Duct (Pouch)

See Corresponding Diagnostic Algorithm

PITYRIASIS ALBA

Mitchell S. King, MD
Jasmine Chao, DO

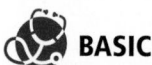

BASICS

DESCRIPTION
- A chronic skin disorder characterized by 1 or more groups of poorly marginated, pale pink or tan/white patches and plaques that appear on the cheeks, neck, and lateral arms of children and young adults
- System(s) Affected: Skin/Exocrine
- Synonym(s): Pityriasis streptogenes; Pityriasis simplex; Pityriasis sicca faciei; Erythema streptogenes; Furfuraceous impetigo

ALERT
Geriatric Considerations
Rare in this age group

Pediatric Considerations
More common in children aged 3–10 years

GENERAL PREVENTION
No known preventive measures

EPIDEMIOLOGY
- Predominant age: 90% of affected patients are ages 6–12 years. Rare >25 years.
- Predominant sex: Male = Female

Incidence
Common, exact incidence unknown, but frequently seen in people with dark skin in sunnier climates

RISK FACTORS
Children with a genetic predisposition to atopic disease

Genetics
Unknown, but condition is seen primarily in children with a genetic predisposition to atopic disease

ETIOLOGY
- Unknown; may be part of an atopic diathesis
- Possibly defects in melanin production or transfer

ASSOCIATED CONDITIONS
Atopic dermatitis

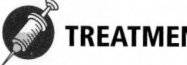

DIAGNOSIS

SIGNS AND SYMPTOMS
- Description: Small, ill-defined pale pink or tan/white patches 0.5–3 cm
- Rash evolves from pink patch to white macule with fine scale to smooth hypopigmented macule.
- Location: Cheeks and lateral arms
- Number: 1–12 or more patches
- Palpation: Smooth or slightly rough, but dry
- Appearance: Pinpoint white papules (representing accentuation and keratinization of follicular orifices)
- Scale is either invisible or fine and light.
- More common in dark-skinned people
- Usually asymptomatic
- Pruritis (rare)
- More apparent in summertime in light-skinned people
- Lesions do not tan in summer.
- Even a small amount of sunlight exposure causes lesions to redden.
- History and physical exam: Atopic diathesis is of diagnostic significance.

TESTS
Negative finding on potassium hydroxide skin scraping

Pathological Findings
Irregular melanin pigmentation of basal layer, follicular plugging, follicular spongiosis, and atrophic sebaceous glands

DIFFERENTIAL DIAGNOSIS
- Pityriasis versicolor
- Vitiligo
- Milia
- Keratosis pilaris
- Indeterminate or uncharacteristic leprosy

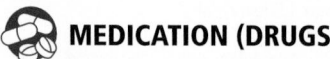

TREATMENT

INITIAL STABILIZATION
Outpatient

GENERAL MEASURES
- No truly effective therapy is available. Lubricating cream application may palliate roughness and/or dryness.
- Sun exposure may promote repigmentation

Diet
No special diet

Activity
No restrictions

Nursing
SPECIAL THERAPY
Phototherapy (e.g., UVB light) for extensive involvements in adults only

MEDICATION (DRUGS)

First Line
- Topical steroids if needed to reduce redness due to sunburn or spontaneous inflammation
- Anecdotal evidence supports use of topical corticosteroids, but not Food and Drug Administration (FDA) approved for use in this condition

Second Line
- Coal tar preparations (e.g., alphosyl, estar, balneta): Applied topically once daily or b.i.d.; treatment is not mandatory
- NOTE: Neither coal tar nor corticosteroids will change the pigmentation, but may improve pruritus, roughness, and/or dryness, if the lubricating cream is not sufficient.
- Tacrolimus or picrolimus have been used off label for pityriasis alba, but currently not FDA approved.
- Precautions:
  – Refer to the manufacturer's literature for each drug.

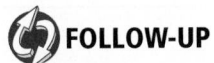 **FOLLOW-UP**

PROGNOSIS
Permanent resolution during 2nd or 3rd decade of life

COMPLICATIONS
None expected

PATIENT MONITORING
As needed, only if lesions become symptomatic

REFERENCES

1. Arnold KL, Odom RB, James WD. *Andrews' Diseases of the Skin*. 9th ed. Philadelphia, PA: WB Saunders; 2000.
2. Fitzpatrick TB, et al., eds. *Dermatology in General Medicine*. 5th ed. New York, NY: McGraw-Hill; 1999.
3. Galen EB. Pityriasis alba. *Cutis*. 1998;61:11–13.
4. Habif T. *Clinical Dermatology*. 4th ed. St. Louis, MO: Mosby; 2004.
5. Halder RM, Nandedkar MA, Neal KW. Pigmentary disorders in ethnic skin. *Dermatol Clin*. 2003;21:617–628.
6. Sams WM, Lynch PJ, eds. *Principles and Practices of Dermatology*. 2nd ed. New York, NY: Churchill Livingstone; 1996.
7. Miller DC Pigmentation disorders in adults *Clinics in Family Practice*. 2003;5(3):691.

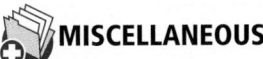**MISCELLANEOUS**

See also: Keratosis, Actinic; Tinea Versicolor; Vitiligo

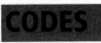

ICD9-CM
696.5 Other and unspecified pityriasis

PATIENT TEACHING

Stress long-term chronicity and permanent resolution of condition in 2nd or 3rd decade of life

PITYRIASIS ROSEA

Kristyn Fagerberg, MD

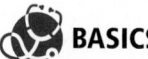 BASICS

DESCRIPTION
- An idiopathic, self-limited skin eruption characterized by widespread papulosquamous lesions
- System(s) Affected: Skin/Exocrine

ALERT
Pediatric Considerations
Face and distal extremities are more often involved in children, and lesions may be more papular.

EPIDEMIOLOGY
- Predominant age: 10–35 years, but occurs in all age groups
- Predominant sex: Male = Female, some studies have shown a slight female preponderance. (1,2)
- No racial predominance

Incidence
Relatively common, but exact frequency is unknown.

RISK FACTORS
Genetics
<5% of those affected give a positive family history.

ETIOLOGY
Unknown; may be a viral agent or an autoimmune disorder. Several studies have implicated the human herpes viruses, most commonly HHV-7, but other research has not confirmed this association. (1–8)[B]

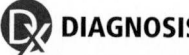 DIAGNOSIS

SIGNS AND SYMPTOMS
- The most common initial sign is a 2–10 cm salmon-colored patch or plaque known as the *herald patch*. The herald patch is present 40–76% of the time. (1)
- The more widespread rash begins 7–14 days after the onset of the herald patch, although it may appear up to 3 months later.
- Salmon to light brown oval plaques with fine scales centrally and so-called collarette of loose scales along borders
- Lesions average 1–2 cm in diameter and usually spare face, hands, and feet in adults
- Lesions frequently oriented along skin cleavage lines in Christmas tree pattern
- Mild pruritus, rarely severe
- Fever, malaise, headache, gastrointestinal discomfort, and arthralgias are rare
- Variant forms include purpuric, urticarial, and vesicular lesions.

TESTS
Potassium hydroxide preparation to distinguish disease from tinea corporis

Lab
No specific lab markers. Consider serology to rule out syphilis.

Pathological Findings
Chronic inflammation with cytolytic degeneration of keratinocytes adjacent to Langerhans cells

DIFFERENTIAL DIAGNOSIS
- Secondary syphilis
- Viral exanthems
- Drug rashes
- Psoriasis
- Parapsoriasis
- Eczema
- Lichen planus
- Tinea corporis

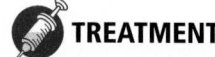 TREATMENT

INITIAL STABILIZATION
Outpatient

GENERAL MEASURES
- Symptomatic treatment
- Topical antipruritics as needed
- UV therapy has been used, but a controlled study found minimal benefit. (9)[B]
- Lukewarm oatmeal baths (*not* hot, because heat can intensify itching)

Diet
Normal

Activity
Full activity with good skin hygiene to prevent secondary infection

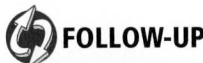 **MEDICATION (DRUGS)**

First Line
- Topical steroids to reduce itching, if needed
  – Triamcinolone 0.1% cream
- Oral antihistamines
  – Diphenhydramine (Benadryl) 25 mg t.i.d.
  – Chlorpheniramine 8 mg t.i.d.

Second Line
Erythromycin showed apparent benefit in 1 trial although azithromycin failed to show significant benefit in another trial. (8,10)[B]

High-dose acyclovir (800 mg 5 times a day for 7 days) used early in the disease course, also showed benefit. (11)

FOLLOW-UP

PROGNOSIS
Gradual resolution in 1–14 weeks (usually 2–6 weeks)

COMPLICATIONS
Secondary infection (e.g., impetigo)

PATIENT MONITORING
- Check syphilis serology
- Return visit for re-evaluation, if lesions persist >8–10 weeks

REFERENCES

1. Chuh A, et al. Pityriasis rosea—an update. *Indian J Dermatol Venereol Leprol*. 2005;71:311–315.
2. Gonzalez L, et al. Pityriasis rosea: An important papulosquamous disorder. *International J Derm*. 2005;44:757–764.
3. Drago F, et al. Human herpesvirus 7 in patients with pityriasis rosea. Electron microscopy investigations and polymerase chain reaction in mononuclear cells, plasma and skin. *Dermatology*. 1997;195:374–378.
4. Kempf W, et al. Pityriasis rosea is not associated with human herpesvirus 7. *Arch Dermatol*. 1999;135:1070–1072.
5. Chuh A, Chan H, Zawar V. Pityriasis rosea-evidence for and against an infectious aetiology. *Epidemiol Infect*. 2004;132(3):381–390.
6. Chuh A, Kempf W. The identification of primary human herpesvirus 7 infection in young adults with pityriasis rosea by investigating avidity of antibodies. *J Eur Acad Dermatol Venereol*. 2006;20(5):629–630.
7. Broccolo F, et al. Additional evidence that pityriasis rosea is associated with reactivation of human herpesvirus-6 and -7. *J Investigative Derm*. 2005;124:1234–1240.
8. Amer A, Fischer H. Azithromycin does not cure pityriasis rosea. *Pediatrics*. 2006;117:1702–1705.
9. Leenutaphong V, Jiamton S. UVB phototherapy for pityriasis rosea: A bilateral comparison study. *J Amer Acad Dermatol*. 1995;33:996–999.
10. Sharma PK, et al. Erythromycin in pityriasis rosea: a double-blind, placebo-controlled clinical trial. *J Amer Acad Dermatol*. 2000;42:241–244.
11. Drago F, Vecchio F, Rebora A. Use of high-dose acyclovir in pityriasis rosea. *J Amer Acad Derm*. 2006;54(1):82–85.
12. Cheong WK, Wong KS. Pityriasis rosea. *Singapore Med J*. 1989.
13. Habif T. *Clinical Dermatology*, 4th ed. St. Louis: Mosby, 2004.

 MISCELLANEOUS

See also: Dermatitis, exfoliative; Pityriasis alba; Tinea versicolor

 CODES

ICD9-CM
696.3 Pityriasis rosea

PATIENT TEACHING
- Reassure patient about self-limited nature of condition.
- Printed patient information available from: American Academy of Dermatology, (708) 330-0230

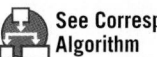 **See Corresponding Diagnostic Algorithm**

PLACENTA PREVIA

Frank J. Domino, MD

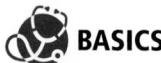

BASICS

DESCRIPTION
- Placental implantation in the lower uterine segment in advance of the presenting fetal part
  - Total previa: Placenta covers entire cervical os.
  - Partial previa: Placenta covers part of the cervical os.
  - Marginal previa: Placental edge just reaches cervical os.
  - Low-lying placenta: Placental edge is in the lower uterine segment but does not encroach on the cervical os.
- System(s) Affected: Cardiovascular; Reproductive

GENERAL PREVENTION
- Decrease physical activity to avoid bleeding or rebleeding.
- All vaginal exams, sexual intercourse, douching, or other vaginal manipulation may cause rebleeding.

EPIDEMIOLOGY
- Predominant age: Childbearing
- Predominant sex: Female

Prevalence
- 0.5–0.8% of all pregnancies at time of delivery, ~4/1,000 births
- <10% of low-lying placentas seen in early pregnancy persist to term (follow with ultrasound to confirm resolution prior to delivery). (1)[A]

RISK FACTORS
- Prior history of placenta previa (4–8%)
- Multiparity (5% in grand multiparous patient)
- Advanced maternal age
- Multiple gestation
- Smoking
- Cocaine use
- Male fetus
- C-section primipara with 1 cesarean section: Odds ratio OR = 1.28 (95% confidence interval, 0.82–1.99)
  - Multipara with 4 or more deliveries and 1 cesarean section: OR = 1.72 (95% confidence interval, 1.12–2.64)
  - Multipara with >4 deliveries and >4 cesarean sections: OR = 8.76 (95% confidence interval, 1.58–48.53) (2)[C]
- Induced abortion:
  - Sharp curettage: 3 or more cesarean sections: OR = 2.9 (95% confidence interval, 1.0–8.5).
  - Vacuum aspiration: Not associated with increased risk of placenta previa (3)[C]

ETIOLOGY
Prior uterine insult or injury or other uterine factors

ASSOCIATED CONDITIONS
- Abnormal presentations (e.g., oblique and/or transverse lie)
- Persistent high fetal station
- Postpartum hemorrhage
- Increased incidence of small-for-gestational-age babies with previas

DIAGNOSIS

SIGNS AND SYMPTOMS
- Typically painless bright red bleeding in 2nd or 3rd trimester
- Average time of 1st bleed is between 27 and 32 weeks.
- Contractions are variably present
- 1st bleed usually is self-limited.
- Maternal hemodynamic status is consistent with clinical blood loss estimate
- Cases of complete placenta previa may bleed earlier and not "migrate."

Physical Exam
- Careful vaginal speculum exam
- Not contraindicated
  - Check for cervical or vaginal source of bleeding.
  - Check ferning and Nitrazine testing.
  - Perform cultures: Gonorrhea, chlamydia, group B strep.
- Do not perform cervical digital exam

TESTS
- Betke-Kleihauer test if concerned about fetal-maternal transfusion
- Bedside clot test (use red-top tube): Draw blood from mother and observe for clot quality at 7–10 minutes. If there is no clot or if clot is friable, result may indicate disseminated intravascular coagulation.

Lab
- Maternal blood type and Rh
- Hemoglobin and hematocrit
- Platelet count
- Prothrombin time, partial thromboplastin time, fibrinogen
- Type and cross-match packed erythrocytes (at least 3 units)
- Wright stain applied to a slide smear of vaginal blood, looking for nucleated erythrocytes, which are usually from cord blood and not adult blood
- Lecithin: Sphingomyelin ratio for fetal maturity if needed

Imaging
- External sector sonography with moderately full and empty bladder
- Vaginal probe sonography may be done if active bleeding is not present. Place the probe just inside vaginal os and use 5- or 6.5-MHz transducers.
- MRI is accurate, but more expensive, less widely available, and more time-consuming.

Diagnostic Procedures/Surgery
If placental location is unknown and sonography is not available, a double-setup bimanual vaginal exam may be done in the OR with complete cesarean section readiness.

Pathological Findings
- Normocytic, normochromic anemia with acute bleed
- Coagulopathy rare, but may occur
- Positive Betke-Kleihauer sign if fetal/maternal transfusion

DIFFERENTIAL DIAGNOSIS
- Abruptio placentae
- Vasa previa
- Vaginal and cervical causes, including marked "bloody show"
- Infections

TREATMENT

INITIAL STABILIZATION
- Inpatient observation and bed rest initially; after becoming stable, preterm patient may be observed on an outpatient basis without difference in outcome (4)[A]
- May consider transfer to high-risk birthing center based on condition and local services

GENERAL MEASURES
- Optimizing maternal stability while delaying delivery to term, if possible, to improve perinatal outcome
- Amniocentesis for lecithin: Sphingomyelin ratio for maturity as needed
- Cesarean section indicated for partial or complete previa if fetus is mature or if the situation is urgent and the fetus is immature.
- A trial of labor may be considered with anterior marginal previa, including oxytocin (Pitocin) augmentation IV.
- IV fluid support, oxygen, transfusions of packed erythrocytes, platelets, and fresh frozen plasma if needed
- External fetal and labor monitoring
- Other intervention or observation based on maternal condition
- DIC risk is low unless massive bleeding is present. Follow coagulation studies and give fresh frozen plasma (FFP), platelets as needed, or cryoprecipitate if fibrinogen <100–150 mg/dL (<1.0–1.5 g/L).
- Transfuse platelets at <20,000 (or <50,000 prior to surgery).
- Blood volume increased in pregnancy; the patient can lose >30% maternal blood volume before shock may be considered as confirmed.
- Central line placement only after checking coagulation studies
- May use sector probe with condom at introitus if vaginal probe is unavailable
- With significant hemorrhage, Rh-negative women should receive Rho(D) immune globulin (RhoGAM) with each instance of bleeding.

Diet
NPO initially, then based on delivery decisions

Activity
- Bed rest
- Pelvic rest; intercourse abstinence, avoidance of douching

MEDICATION (DRUGS)

First Line

- For IV fluids: lactated Ringer's or normal saline solution
- Oxygen for all affected patients, because oxygen consumption is increased 20% in pregnancy and fetus is more prone to hypoxia
- FFP and platelets as needed
- Cryoprecipitate and fibrinogen if measures suggested here prove unsuccessful
- Tocolytics may have role in certain preterm patients, but tachycardia with β-agonists (e.g., terbutaline) and risk of placental hypoperfusion with calcium channel blockers may make magnesium sulfate the drug of choice. For magnesium sulfate, use 4 g IV load and 1–4 g/h as indicated.
- Contraindications: Avoid tocolytics with term infant or unstable mother.
- Precautions
  - β-Agonists and calcium channel blockers may complicate clinical picture.
  - Cryoprecipitate and fibrinogen may increase infection transmission risk.
- Significant possible interactions: Refer to the manufacturer's profile for each drug.

Second Line

Ritodrine (Yutopar) IV may be an alternate β-agonist, but carries same concerns as terbutaline (i.e., tachycardia, palpitations, or tremor, which may complicate clinical evaluation of hypovolemia and hypoxia).

SURGERY

Cervical cerclage may reduce risk of delivery before 34 weeks (rate ratio = 0.45 [95% confidence interval, 0.23–0.87]) or birth weight <2 kg, rate ratio = 0.34 (confidence interval, 0.14–0.83) or low 5-minute Apgar score rate ratio = 0.19 (confidence interval, 0.04–1.00). (4)[A]

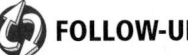 **FOLLOW-UP**

PROGNOSIS

- If term and complete or partial: Cesarean delivery
- If term and anterior marginal: Trial of labor may be acceptable course (must have emergent cesarean delivery capability during entire labor process)
- If preterm and maternal and fetal status stable: Observe and delay delivery

COMPLICATIONS

- Maternal mortality is rare with cesarean section available. Greatest fetal risk is preterm delivery.
- History of prior cesarean section and/or general anesthesia increases risk for need of transfusion.
- Attempted tocolysis may compromise maternal status.
- Rebleeding risk may be greater than that associated with delivery and management.
- If placenta previa is present after 30 weeks, there is greater risk of persisting placenta previa.
- Low-lying posterior marginal previa is associated with dystocia and greater need for cesarean section.
- Placental accreta is strongly associated with placenta previa (up to 15% of patients). Higher incidence in women with placenta previa and multiple prior cesarean sections.
- Vasa previa
- Intrauterine growth restriction: 16% incidence
- Congenital anomalies: Most common major anomalies of the central nervous system, cardiovascular system, and the respiratory and gastrointestinal tracts
- Fetal anemia and Rh isoimmunization

PATIENT MONITORING

- Inpatient follow-up
- Outpatient care with frequent visits

REFERENCES

1. Faiz AS, Ananth CV. Etiology and risk factors for placenta previa: An overview and meta-analysis of observational studies. *J Matern Fetal Neonatal Med*. 2003;13:175–190.
2. Gilliam M, Rosenberg D, Davis F. The likelihood of placenta previa with greater number of cesarean deliveries and higher parity. *Obstet Gynecol*. 2002;99:976–980.
3. Johnson L, Mueller B, Daling J. The relationship of placenta previa and history of induced abortion. *Int J Gynaecol Obstet*. 2003;81:191–198.
4. Neilson JP. Interventions for suspected placenta praevia (Cochrane Review). In: The Cochrane Library, Issue 2, 2002. Oxford, UK: Update Software.

 MISCELLANEOUS

See also: Abruptio placentae

CODES

ICD9-CM

- 641.00 Placenta previa without hemorrhage, unspecified
- 641.10 Hemorrhage from placenta previa, unspecified
- 641.20 Premature separation of placenta, unspecified
- 762.1 Premature separation of placenta (when causing newborn complications)

PATIENT TEACHING

- 1st bleed is rarely fatal.
- Rebleed risk with activity or cervical stimulation is common; therefore, pelvic rest is important, including abstaining from vaginal intercourse, no douching.
- Greatest cause of perinatal mortality is prematurity.

 See Corresponding Diagnostic Algorithm

PLAGUE

D. W. MacPherson, MD, MSc(CTM), FRCPC

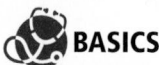

BASICS

DESCRIPTION
- Acute infection due to *Yersinia pestis*
- Sporadic limited geographic distribution, especially in developing nations and Southwestern United States
- Epidemics associated with war, famine, and disaster
- Disease of rats and other small vertebrates
- Transmitted to humans by rat flea or human flea
- Occasional transmission to humans who handle infected tissues
- Occasional human-human transmission by pulmonary secretions
- Recently shown that infected cats may transmit disease to humans by biting, licking, or scratching
- *Yersinia pestis*, the infective pathogen, has been described as a bioweapon.
- System(s) Affected: Hematologic/Lymphatic/Immunologic; Pulmonary; Skin/Exocrine
- Synonym(s): Black death

GENERAL PREVENTION
- Avoid contact with vectors, infected tissue, or aerosol droplets (e.g., confirmed pneumonic plague case)
- Killed vaccine for people at high risk to reduce risk and/or severity; tetracycline prophylaxis. Vaccine available from US Centers for Disease Control and Prevention, Atlanta, GA.

EPIDEMIOLOGY
Predominant sex: Male = Female

Incidence
Few cases annually in US; Southwest, usually spring, summer, fall

RISK FACTORS
- Exposure to rats and fleas
- Close contact with infected cat
- Close contact with pneumonic plague patient
- Plague bacillus in laboratory
- Hunters who skin wild animals
- Potential agent of bioterrorism
- Occupational risk: Field workers, animal researchers, and others exposed in endemic regions

ETIOLOGY
- *Yersinia pestis*, transmitted by bite of a flea from an infected rodent; secondary contact through other infected animal or human
- Untreated bubonic plague may progress to secondary pneumonic strain, which can be transmitted by contaminated respiratory droplets.

DIAGNOSIS

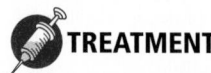

SIGNS AND SYMPTOMS
- Bubonic plague
  - Acute onset after 2–8 days' incubation
  - Fever
  - Chills
  - Weakness
  - Headache
  - Bubo: Painful, tender enlargement of regional lymph node(s) that drain inoculation site. Overlying edema. Typically, absence of overlying skin lesion, ascending lymphangitis
  - Skin lesions: Pustules, vesicles, eschars in area of flea bite(s), purpura
- Septicemic plague
  - Features of bubonic plague
  - Occasional occurrence without bubo
  - Hypotension
  - Hepatosplenomegaly
  - Delirium
  - Seizures in children
  - Shock
- Secondary pneumonic plague
  - Features of bubonic and septicemic plague
  - Cough
  - Chest pain
  - Hemoptysis
- Primary pneumonic plague
  - Acute onset within hours to 1 day after inhalation of infective bacteria
  - Fever
  - Chills
  - Cough
  - Chest pain
  - Dyspnea
  - Hemoptysis
  - Lethargy
  - Hypotension
  - Shock

TESTS

Lab
- Elevated leukocyte count, predominantly mature and immature neutrophils; sometimes leukemoid reaction
- Measure platelets: With low platelet number, evidence of disseminated intravascular coagulation may be seen.
- Stained smears of aspirate of bubo, sputum, and peripheral blood reveal Gram-negative coccobacilli with bipolar staining, so-called safety pin appearance
- Aspirate, blood, sputum cultures (e.g., infusion broth, blood and MacConkey agar) grow typical bacteria. Public health authorities arrange definitive identification and serologic follow-up.
- Drugs that may alter lab results
  - Antibiotics: Prior use

Imaging
Chest x-ray: Patchy or confluent pulmonary consolidation in pneumonic plague

Pathological Findings
Acute lymphadenitis with inflammation dominated by neutrophils, necrosis, masses of plague bacilli, seropurulent pericarditis

DIFFERENTIAL DIAGNOSIS
Other causes of fulminant bacteremia, pneumococcal sepsis, meningococcemia; other causes of acute suppurative lymphadenitis (bubo), or rapidly progressive pneumonitis

TREATMENT

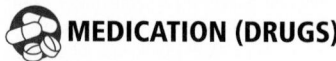

INITIAL STABILIZATION
- Hospitalization. For suspected pneumonic plague, respiratory isolation until 48 hours after initial effective therapy or after sputum test provides negative result.
- Notify public health authorities.

GENERAL MEASURES
- Do not create aerosol droplets.
- Handle blood and bubo aspirate with gloves.
- Notify laboratory to take precautions.
- Hot, moist compresses for buboes

Diet
As tolerated during recovery

Activity
Bed rest until convalescent

SPECIAL THERAPY
As required

MEDICATION (DRUGS)

First Line
- Aminoglycoside: gentamicin 5.1 mg/kg/d or streptomycin 15 mg/kg IV
- If condition allows, oral medication: Tetracycline 25–50 mg/kg/d, equally divided, q6h, for 10 days
- For meningitis: IV chloramphenicol 25 mg/kg loading dose, followed by 60 mg/kg/d divided doses q6h for 10 days
- Fluoroquinolones (e.g., levofloxacin, ofloxacin) and 3rd-generation cephalosporins (e.g., cefotaxime) may also be effective.
- Contraindications:
  - Tetracyclines: Contraindicated in pregnancy and patients <8 years old
- Precautions:
  - Reduce dose of aminoglycoside with finding of renal impairment.
  - Pregnant women and those with hearing disorders (e.g., aminoglycosides)
  - Chloramphenicol associated with hematologic toxicity

Second Line
No other drugs have been demonstrated to be as effective or any less toxic.

FOLLOW-UP

PROGNOSIS

• Untreated plague mortality >50%; 100% in primary pneumonic plague
• Plague may be fulminant (e.g., exposure, 1st symptoms, and death in 1 day in primary pneumonic plague). Must *not* delay treatment of suspected cases until laboratory-confirmed diagnosis. Delay of initial therapy beyond 24 hours after onset of primary pneumonic plague regularly leads to death.

COMPLICATIONS

• Progression of bubonic form to septicemic and pneumonic forms
• Necrosis of bubo may require aspiration or incision and drainage.
• Pericarditis
• Adult respiratory distress syndrome
• Meningitis
• Death

PATIENT MONITORING

• Complete blood chemistry for hematologic toxicity of chloramphenicol
• Aminoglycoside blood levels, if indicated
• Clinical testing for antibiotic toxicity, if indicated

REFERENCES

1. Anonymous. Human plague in 1995. *Wkly Epidemiol Rec*. 1997;S72:344–347.
2. Centers for Disease Control and Prevention. Plague Information. Available at: http://www.bt.cdc.gov/agent/plague/#fact. Accessed June 3, 2006.
3. Dennis DT, Chow CC. *Pediatr Infect Dis J*. 2004; 23:69–71.
4. Frean JA, et al. In vitro activities of 14 antibiotics against 100 human isolates of *Yersinia pestis* from a southern African plague focus. *Antimicrob Agents Chemother*. 1996;40:2646–2647.
5. Gratz NG. Emerging and re-surging vector-borne diseases. *Annu Rev Entomol*. 1999;44:51–75.
6. Inglesby TV, et al. Plague as a biological weapon: Medical and public health management. Working Group on Civilian Biodefense. *JAMA*. 2000;283: 2281–2290.
7. Kilonzo BS. Plague epidemiology and control in eastern and southern Africa during the period 1978–1997. *Central Afr J Med*. 1999;45:70–76.
8. Kohler W, Kohler M. Plague and rats, the "plague of the Philistines," and: What did our ancestors know about the role of rats in plague. *Int J Med Microbiol*. 2003;293:333–340.
9. Leggiadro RJ. The threat of biological terrorism: A public health and infection control reality. *Infect Control Hosp Epidemiol*. 2000;21:53–56.
10. Perry RD, Fetherston JD. *Yersinia pestis*: Etiologic agent of plague. *Clin Microbiol Rev*. 1997;10: 35–36.
11. Titball RW, Leary SE. Plague. *Brit Med Bull*. 1998;54:625–633.

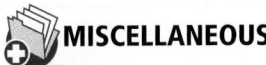

MISCELLANEOUS

CODES

ICD9-CM

• 020.0 Bubonic plague
• 020.2 Septicemic plague
• 020.5 Unspecified pneumonic plague
• 020.3 Primary pneumonic plague
• 020.4 Secondary pneumonic plague

PATIENT TEACHING

• Avoid contact with wild animals.
• Reduce rat and flea population in immediate human environment.

PLANTAR FASCIITIS

Warren J. Ferguson, MD

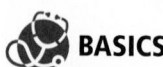 **BASICS**

DESCRIPTION
Inflammation of plantar fascia at origin from plantar tuberosity of calcaneum

- Pain on plantar surface on weight-bearing, especially in morning

GENERAL PREVENTION
- Maintain normal body weight:
  - Higher prevalence with body-mass index (BMI) >30 (1)
- Avoid prolonged barefoot or slippers

EPIDEMIOLOGY
Prevalence
Lifetime = 10% of population

- Data suggests persistence with BMI >30
- Condition is self-limiting, most resolve within 10 months

RISK FACTORS
- Dancers, runners, aerobic exercisers
- Obesity
- Pes planus (flat feet)
- Systemic connective tissue disorders

PATHOPHYSIOLOGY
- Repetitive partial tearing of plantar fascia
- Chronic inflammation of plantar fascia at insertion on medial tubercle of calcaneus

ETIOLOGY
Excessive pronation

ASSOCIATED CONDITIONS
- Usually isolated
- Heel spurs common but not marker of severity
- Posterior tibial neuropathy

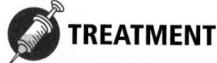 **DIAGNOSIS**

History
- Pain on plantar surface of calcaneus
  - Worst when arising out of bed; after prolonged sitting
  - Described as "pebble in shoe"
- Pain with prolonged ambulation or standing
- Limp with excessive toe walking
- Numbness and burning medial hindfoot with posterior tibial nerve compression

Physical Exam
- Point tenderness on calcaneus at insertion of plantar fascia
- Pain along plantar fascia with foot dorsiflexion
- Spasm in foot muscles that compensate for injury

TESTS
Imaging
- 2 radiographic views of foot to removal of (r/o) bone pain
- Ultrasound: Signs of inflammation at insertion
- MRI for r/o complex conditions

DIFFERENTIAL DIAGNOSIS
- Calcaneal stress fracture
- Pain from neoplasm or infection
- Posterior tibial nerve compression
- Painful or atrophic heel pad
- Tendonitis of posterior tibialis
- Spondyloarthropathy
- In association with connective tissue disorder
  - Rheumatoid arthritis
  - Polymyositis

TREATMENT

Limited evidence on which to base clinical practice (2)

GENERAL MEASURES
- Wear supportive footwear, particularly rigid shoes to help avoid excess pronation
- Ice (frozen juice can roll)
- Massage (golf ball roll)
- Weight reduction

Activity
- Modified rest may help
- Stretching exercises
  - See "Patient Teaching"

SPECIAL THERAPY
- Steroid injection (3)
  - Only short-term improvement proven
- Extra corporeal shock wave therapy (4)
  - Pain improvement at 12 weeks
  - Uncomfortable to patients
- Night splints in dorsiflexion
  - RTC demonstrated no benefit (5)
  - Some evidence that forefoot dorsiflexion may produce better results
- Custom or flexible orthotics
  - Some evidence that flexible commercial orthotics provide better outcome
- Some orthopedic surgeons prefer casting in severe cases

Physical Therapy
Stretching and physical therapy may be more effective than other modalities (6)

- Corticosteroid iontophoresis proven not effective as component of physical therapy

Complementary and Alternative Therapies
Heel cup with magnet proven ineffective

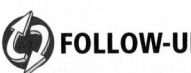 **MEDICATION (DRUGS)**

First Line
NSAIDs for 3 weeks and as needed
• No controlled studies that speed recovery

SURGERY
In small percentage of patients necessary
• Calcaneal spur resection
• More likely in severely obese

FOLLOW-UP

• Following 6 weeks of conservative treatment
  – See "Patient Teaching"
• Consider formal physical therapy program if conservative measures don't show improvement

DISPOSITION
Issues for Referral
Podiatry may be helpful
• Orthotics
• Corticosteroid injection

PROGNOSIS
Excellent prognosis, as condition is self-limiting in 90% of cases

COMPLICATIONS
Rupture of plantar fascia

REFERENCES

1. Rano JA, Fallat LM, Savoy-More RT. Correlation of heel pain with body mass index and other characteristics of heel pain. *J Foot Ankl Surg.* 2001;40(6):351–6.
2. Crawford F, Thomson C. Interventions for treating plantar heel pain. *The Cochrane Database of Systematic Reviews.* 2006;1.
3. Crawford F, et al. Steroid injection for the treatment of plantar fasciitis: Evidence of short term effectiveness. A randomized, double-blind, placebo controlled study. *The Am J Sports Med.* 1997;25(3):312–316.
4. Rompe JD, et al. Effectiveness of low energy extracorporeal shock waves for chronic plantar fasciitis. *Foot and Ankle Surgery.* 1996;2:215–221.
5. Probe RA, et al. Night splint treatment for plantar fasciitis: A prospective randomized study. *Clin Orthop Relat Res.* 1999;368:190–195.
6. Digiovanni BF, et al. Tissue-specific plantar fascia stretching exercise enhances outcomes in patients with chronic heel pain: A prospective, randomized study. *J Bone Joint Surg.* 2003;85-A(7):1270–7.

 MISCELLANEOUS

CODES

ICD9-CM
• 729.4 Fasciitis
• 728.71 Plantar

PATIENT TEACHING

• Weight reduction
• Keep supportive footwear at bedside
• Gently arise from sitting to standing upon arising from bed or prolonged sitting
• Ice using frozen juice can, rolling foot over can for 10 minutes in morning and after work
• Massage plantar fascia by rolling foot over golf ball
• Grab cloth or carpet by plantar flexing toes
• Stretch plantar fascia by pulling toes into dorsiflexion
• For athletes, back off on repetitive stress
• Taping may help athletes

Prevention
• Weight reduction
• Avoidance of excess walking barefoot, in slippers or sandals that don't offer arch support

 See Corresponding Diagnostic Algorithm

 See Patient Handout on CD

PLEURAL EFFUSION

Felix B. Chang, MD

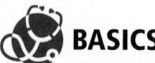

BASICS

DESCRIPTION
- Pleural effusion is an abnormal accumulation of fluid in the pleural space. The pleural cavity contains a small volume of lubricating serous fluid, formed primarily by transudation from the parietal pleura and absorbed primarily by the capillaries and lymphatics.
- Pleural effusion develops when
- The balance between formation and removal of fluid may be compromised by any disorder that
  - Increase the venous pressure
  - Lowers the plasma oncotic pressure
  - Increase capillary permeability
  - Or obstruct the lymphatic circulation
- Effusions are classified as: Transudates or exudates.
  - Transudates are caused by
    - Decrease plasma oncotic pressure
    - Nephrotic syndrome
    - Cirrhosis
    - Hypoalbuminemia
  - Increased hydrostatic pressure
    - CHF
    - Superior vena cava obstruction
  - Exudates are caused by increased permeability of the pleural surface or by obstruction of the lymphatics.
  - Malignancy (bronchogenic carcinoma, lymphoma, metastatic tumor)
  - Inflammatory process
    - Infections: Pneumonia, tuberculosis
    - Pulmonary embolism
    - Collagen vascular disease (e.g., rheumatoid arthritis)
    - Subdiaphragmatic process
    - Asbestosis
    - Pancreatitis
    - Hypothyroidism
  - Trauma
- System(s) Affected: Cardiovascular; Pulmonary

EPIDEMIOLOGY
May occur at any age; no gender predilection.

Incidence
Unknown

Prevalence
Unknown

ETIOLOGY
- In CHF, effusion usually is bilateral; if unilateral, it is right to left.
- Hypoalbuminemic states (e.g., cirrhosis, nephrotic syndrome)
- Constrictive pericarditis
- Dressler syndrome with pericardial effusion
- Infection: Parapneumonic effusion or empyema.
  - Etiologic pathogens include bacteria (e.g., *Mycoplasma, Mycobacterium tuberculosis*), viruses, fungi, and parasites.
  - Empyema usually is caused by polymicrobial anaerobic infection (e.g., *Pseudomonas, Staphylococcus aureus, Escherichia coli*, and occasionally *Streptococcus pneumoniae*).

- Pulmonary embolism/infarction
- Neoplastic processes: Mesothelioma from asbestos exposure, bronchogenic carcinoma, breast carcinoma, lymphoma, leukemia, metastatic disease
- Rheumatologic disease (e.g., systemic lupus erythematosus, rheumatoid arthritis)
- Pancreatitis (left-sided exudate with high amylase concentration)
- Esophageal rupture
- Drug reaction, possibly accompanied by eosinophilia
- Uremia
- Atelectasis
- Meigs syndrome
- Subdiaphragmatic abscess
- Cirrhosis with ascites
- Chylous or pseudochylous effusion (e.g., thoracic duct injury)
- Trauma leading to intrapleural hemorrhage
- Idiopathic

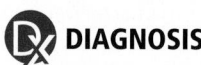

DIAGNOSIS

SIGNS AND SYMPTOMS
- None in small-volume effusion
- Pleuritic chest pain and referred abdominal or shoulder pain
- Cough, may be productive or nonproductive, depending on cause
- Chest wall splinting
- Dyspnea
- Tachypnea, particularly with lung compression or more severe infections
- Diminished chest wall excursion
- Decreased tactile fremitus
- Bronchial breathing and or egophony
- Dullness to percussion over effusion
- Diminished or absent breath sounds
- Friction rub
- Chills
- Mediastinal shift (on chest radiograph)
- Weight loss
- Night sweats
- Hemoptysis
- Anorexia
- General malaise

Physical Exam
The mediastinum shifts away from the side of a large effusion unless it is fixed by a tumor on the affected side, if it has become completely atelectatic.

TESTS
Lab
- Leukocytosis with bandemia
  - PMN predominance: Pneumonia, PE, pancreatitis, early tuberculosis (TB), abdominal abscess
  - Mononuclear predominance: Tumor, TB
  - Eosinophil predominance (40% of idiopathic effusions): Blood or air in the pleural space, asbestos, drugs, paragonimiasis
  - Eosinophil predominance reduces likelihood of TB (10x) and malignancy (2x)

- Anemia
  - Pleurocrit/hematocrit >0.5 hemothorax
- Hypoalbuminemia
- Antinuclear antibody titer >1:160 or > serum level: Suggests SLE effusion
- Rheumatoid factor >1:320 or > serum level: Suggests rheumatoid arthritis
- Pancreatic enzymes
- Cancer antigen 125
- Cancer antigen 19-9
- Creatinine/blood urea nitrogen
- Aerobic/anaerobic blood/pleural fluid cultures
- Evaluation of pleural fluid withdrawn by thoracentesis. A transudate has none of the following characteristics; however, an exudate must meet one of the following criteria
  - Pleural fluid protein/serum protein >0.5
  - Serum albumin-pleural albumin <1.2 g/dL
  - Pleural fluid lactate dehydrogenase/serum lactate dehydrogenase >0.6
  - Pleural fluid lactate dehydrogenase exceeds 2/3 upper limit of that in serum
- All exudates must be evaluated for
  - Differential cell count
  - Amylase level: Elevated in esophageal perforation, pancreatic disease, malignancy
  - Glucose level
    - <60 mg/dL: Parapneumonic (<40 mg/dL –chest tube), neoplasia, TB, hemothorax, paragonimiasis, Churg-Strauss
    - <30 mg/dL: Rheumatoid arthritis
    - <60 mg/dL and pH <7.3 is highly suggestive of malignancy.
  - Comprehensive microbiologic culturing and Gram staining: If infection is suspected, the effusion should be evaluated for aerobic and anaerobic bacteria, mycobacteria, protozoa, fungi, and parasites, as appropriate. TB effusions may be associated with elevations in lysozyme and adenosine deaminase.
  - Cytology: Mesothelial cells is nonspecific, but >2–3% excludes diagnosis of TB.
  - Triglyceride levels >110 mg/dL is consistent with chylothorax, excluded if <50 mg/dL.
- Additional studies: pH, erythrocyte count (if hemorrhagic effusion is >100,000/mL, consider trauma as cause for effusion)
- In the absence of a known primary tumor and/or in the presence of a high index of suspicion for malignancy, the cells harvested from an effusion can be evaluated for a variety of tumor markers (e.g., VIM, CD-15, CA-19-9, CA-125, cancer antigen, hierarchical block-motion estimation-I).
- Transudative or exudative: PE (35% trans), malignancy (10% trans), sarcoidosis, diuretic-treated CHF

Imaging
- Chest radiography (CXR)
  - Anteroposterior
    - ~75 mL to obliterate the posterior costophrenic sulcus
    - ~175 mL to obscure the lateral costophrenic sulcus (upright CXR)
    - ~500 mL will obscure the diaphragmatic contour if reaches the level of the 4th anterior rib; close to 1,000 mL are present

- Lateral view
  - Small effusion: Thinner than 1.5 cm
  - Moderate: 1.5–4.5 cm thick
  - Effusion thicker than 1 cm is usually large enough for sampling by thoracocentesis, at least 200 mL.
- Thoracic ultrasound
- CT scan

Diagnostic Procedures/Surgery

- Pleural biopsy if suspicion of TB or neoplasm
- Diagnostic thorancentesis is not required in small pleural effusion with secure clinical diagnosis, or in patient with obvious CHF.
  - Consider in suspected CHF in the following situations
    - Unilateral effusion is present, particularly if it is left-sided
    - Bilateral effusions, but of disparate sizes
    - Evidence of pleurisy
    - Febrile patient
    - Cardiac silhouette appears normal
    - Alveolar–arterial oxygen gradient is widened out of proportion of the clinical setting
  - Contraindications for thoracentesis:
    - Anticoagulation, bleeding diathesis, Pt or PTT > x2 normal, platelets <25,000/mm^3
    - Creatinine >6 mg/dL
    - Small pleural effusion
    - Mechanical ventilation; risk of persistent air leak (bronchopleural fistula) if pneumothorax does occur
- Thoracoscopy (provides direct view of both parietal and visceral aspects of pleura)

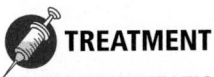

TREATMENT

INITIAL STABILIZATION
Inpatient care is required with this condition.

GENERAL MEASURES
- Supportive care
  - Supplemental oxygen
  - IV fluid hydration
  - Chest physiotherapy
  - Therapeutic/diagnostic thorancentesis
- Antibiotics
  - Empirically by age/social circumstances and modified by blood and pleural effusion fluid culture results
- Empyema
  - Consider antibiotics alone with close monitoring in children.
  - Antibiotics with chest tube drainage in adults
  - Pleurectomy in cases of trapped lung

- Pleural fluid loculation
  - May inject 250,000 units of streptokinase or 100,000 units of urokinase intrapleurally to dissolve fibrin meshes creating loculation. If unsuccessful, then either thoracoscopic adhesiolysis or decortication via thoracotomy is indicated.
- Malignancy
  - Consider treatment of primary source. However, most malignancies accompanied by malignant pleural effusions are advanced and cure is unlikely with chemotherapeutic intervention.
  - If effusion is causing dyspnea, perform therapeutic thorancentesis and, if fluid reaccumulates rapidly, place chest tube for continuous drainage.
  - Other therapeutic interventions include placement of a pleuroperitoneal shunt and chemical pleurodesis.
- Chylothorax
  - Radiation therapy if from malignant cause or surgical repair of thoracic duct trauma
- Hemothorax
  - Usually caused by trauma or rupture of a tumor. Drainage through tube thoracostomy indicated. If bleeding persists or is of high volume, emergency thoracotomy is indicated.

MEDICATION (DRUGS)

First Line
- Antimicrobial therapy according to pathogens and associated sensitivities if necessary
- Recurrent pleural effusion: Chemical pleurodesis with doxycycline 500 mg, bleomycin 60 units, or talc in a slurry, as indicated. The patient should be provided IV narcotic analgesia, because this procedure can cause considerable pain. Pleurodesis can be extremely effective therapy for preventing nonmalignant recurrent effusions. If pleurodesis fails, the patient may be offered pleural abrasion, although this is not commonly performed.
- Chemotherapy according to current oncologic protocols
- Steroids and NSAIDs for rheumatologic and inflammatory causes
- Diuresis as appropriate for effusions secondary to CHF and ascites

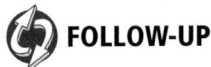

FOLLOW-UP

PROGNOSIS
Mortality rate is ~20% for exudative effusions; worse for elderly patients or those with serious underlying conditions.

COMPLICATIONS
- Chronic empyema
- Drainage through chest wall: Pleurocutaneous fistula
- Bronchopleural fistula
- Toxic shock syndrome

PATIENT MONITORING
- Serial CXR, with frequency/interval determined by patient status/diagnosis
- Pulmonary function testing as indicated
- Serum studies, echocardiography, renal/hepatic function tests as indicated to monitor for stability/progression of nonmalignant/noninfectious factors precipitating effusions

REFERENCES

1. Light RW. Pleural effusion. *N Engl J Med*. 2002;346:1971–1977.
2. Sallach SM, Sallach JA, Vasquez E, et al. Volume of pleural fluid required for diagnosis of pleural malignancy. *Chest*. 2002;122:1913.
3. Cameron R, Davies HR. Intra-pleural fibrinolytic therapy versus conservative management in the treatment of parapneumonic effusions and empyema. *Cochrane Database Sys Rev*. 2004;1:CD002312. DOI10.1002/14651858.CD002312.pub2.

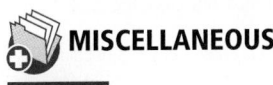

MISCELLANEOUS

CODES

ICD9-CM
- 511.9 Unspecified pleural effusion
- 511.1 Pleurisy with effusion, with mention of a bacterial cause other than tuberculosis
- 197.2 Secondary malignant neoplasm of pleura

PATIENT TEACHING
Patient oriented literature and support from American Lung Association, 1740 Broadway, New York, New York 10038

See Corresponding Diagnostic Algorithm

PNEUMONIA, ASPIRATION

Bevin Kenney, MD

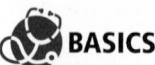 **BASICS**

DESCRIPTION

Aspiration pneumonia is pneumonia due to inhalation of microorganisms from the oral cavity or nasopharynx.

- In contrast to community-acquired pneumonia, which occurs by direct inhalation of infectious particles, from air
- Results from impaired mechanical, humoral, or cellular immunity, such as impaired cough reflex or glottic closure, that protect lower airways
- System(s) Affected: Pulmonary

EPIDEMIOLOGY

Age affected: Risk is 6 times higher if ≥75 years of age

Prevalence

- Silent aspiration is common even in normal individuals
  - Occurs in 2–25% of acute stroke patients
  - Up to 50% of normal adults aspirate during sleep
- Up to 20% of severe community-acquired pneumonia requiring hospitalization are polymicrobial, suggesting aspiration, but specific bacteria are not isolated in a majority of cases (see "Etiology").
- Pneumonia is 2nd most common infection in hospitalized patients

RISK FACTORS

- Reduced consciousness, alcoholism, dementia, uremia, and poor nutritional status
- Mechanical ventilation, bronchoscopy, upper endoscopy
- Pulmonary diseases: Chronic obstructive pulmonary disease (COPD)
- Gastrointestinal diseases: Gastroesophageal reflux disease, esophageal disease
- Dysphagia: Due to stroke, neuromuscular diseases, radiation to the neck or oropharynx
- Enteral feeding tubes, nasogastric tube feeding
- Immunosuppressed patients: Solid organ transplantation, steroid use >20 mg/d for more than 2 weeks, HIV

PATHOPHYSIOLOGY

- Must contrast to chemical pneumonitis which is due to aspiration of contents toxic to lung parenchyma independent of bacterial involvement, (e.g., gastric acid)
  - Abrupt onset of symptoms and prominent dyspnea
  - Chest x-ray changes within 2 hours

- Role of immunosuppression
  - Normal oropharynx is colonized by mixed flora of low virulence
  - Increased colonization of Gram-negative bacilli in malnutrition, alcoholism, diabetes, COPD, etc.
  - Interaction of virulence and quantity of aspirated bacteria and integrity of defenses determine development of pneumonia
- Aspiration pneumonia shows bronchopneumonia pattern
  - Usually caused by and *Staphylococcus aureus, Pseudomonas* aeruginosa and Gram negatives
  - Leads to consolidation of lung segments and subsegments

ETIOLOGY

- Pathogens vary according to setting (1,2)
  - Community-acquired aspiration pneumonia: Gram positives and some Gram negatives, (e.g., *Streptococcus) pneumonia, S. aureus, Haemophilus* influenza and enterobacteria
  - Hospital-acquired: Gram positives, mostly Gram-negative bacilli including *P. aeruginosa,* anaerobes including *Bacteriodes fragilis* and *S. aureus*
- Specific bacteria identified in minority of cases
- Most cases associated with predisposing factors (see "Risk Factors")

ASSOCIATED CONDITIONS

See "Risk Factors."

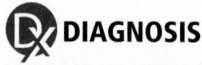 **DIAGNOSIS**

SIGNS AND SYMPTOMS

US Preventive Task Force showed that a full bedside examination including a detailed history, physical exam of mouth and throat, and observing the patient swallow various liquids and solids, was capable of diagnosing 80% of aspirations.

History

- Common
  - Productive cough with putrid sputum
  - Delirium, change in mental status
  - Indolent course
  - Fever
  - Dyspnea
  - Pleuritic chest pain
- Less common
  - Rigors
  - Weight loss

Physical Exam

- Common
  - Altered mental status
  - Periodontal disease, poor oral hygiene
  - Rhonchi
  - Decreased resonance on percussion, bronchovesicular breath sounds showing consolidation
- Less common
  - Wheezes
  - Crackles
  - Severe dyspnea or acute respiratory failure

TESTS

Lab

- O_2 monitoring
  - O_2 saturation to determine need for supplemental O_2
- Leukocytosis: WBC >12,000
- Sputum culture
  - Anaerobic oral flora notoriously difficult to culture, not uncommon to lack results
- Arterial blood gas if suspect acidosis
- Anemia of chronic disease occasionally present

Imaging

- Chest x-ray, postero anterior and lateral:
  - Involvement of lower lobes favors aspiration as cause
  - Chest x-ray may be normal in early infection
- Chest CT
  - More sensitive detection of infiltrates, but should be used only if clinically indicated

Diagnostic Procedures/Surgery

- Bronchoscopy
  - Bronchoscopic brush cultures show improved sensitivity of etiologic diagnosis, but affected by pre-procedural administration of antibiotics
  - Commonly used for ventilator-associated pneumonia, but controversial in clinical practice
- Swallowing evaluation, including possible videofluoroscopic evaluation used in patients with suspected dysphagia

DIFFERENTIAL DIAGNOSIS

- Aspiration pneumonitis
- Lung abscess
- Viral pneumonia
- Fungal pneumonia
- Foreign body aspiration
- Lung cancer

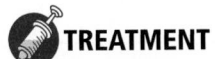 **TREATMENT**

INITIAL STABILIZATION
- Support airways, breathing circulation (ABCs)
- Assess for signs of sepsis, hemodynamic instability
- IVF if necessary

GENERAL MEASURES
Diet
- NPO if reduced consciousness, sepsis
- Soft diet, encourage smaller bites, frequent swallowing
- Tube feeding: Usually reserved for continued aspiration despite other preventive measures, though this remains controversial

Nursing
- Aggressive oral hygiene and pulmonary toileting
- Elevate head of bed, semirecumbent position: 30–45°

SPECIAL THERAPY
IV Fluids
IV fluid (IVF) if sepsis, hemodynamic instability, NPO

 MEDICATION (DRUGS)

If at all possible, antibiotics should be started empirically after obtaining cultures

First Line
Clindamycin 600 mg IV b.i.d. or 300 mg PO q.i.d. (3,4)[B]
- Covers *S. pneumonia*, methicillin-sensitive *S. aureus* (MSSA) and anaerobes like *B. fragilis*
- Recent randomized controlled trials showed clindamycin alone to be equally effective to ampicillin/sulbactam, with or without the addition of 2nd- or 3rd-generation cephalosporin
- Clindamycin is low cost and not associated with increase in adverse events
- Lower rates of methicillin-resistant *S. aureus* (MRSA) after use

Second Line
- Ampicillin/sulbactam 3 gm IV b.i.d.
- Amoxicillin/clavulanate 875 mg PO b.i.d.
- Piperacillin/tazobactam 3.375 gm IV q6h
- Ticarcillin/clavulanate 3.1 g IV q6h
  - All of the above cover *S. pneumonia*, MSSA, many Gram-negative bacteria (including Klebsiella) and anaerobes (including *B. fragilis*)
  - Pip/tazo and Tic/clav cover *P. aeruginosa*
- Metronidazole 500 mg IV or PO t.i.d. plus Penicillin G 1–2 million units IV q4–6h *or* amoxicillin 500 mg PO t.i.d.
  - Metronidazole not as effective in putrid lung abscess as clindamycin
  - Penicillin G has historically been effective alone, but Gram positives show increasing resistance

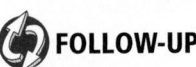 **FOLLOW-UP**

DISPOSITION
Admission Criteria
Admission recommended for anyone with signs of sepsis, immunosuppression, significant cormorbid illness, poor functional or nutritional status

Issues for Referral
If patient without dysphagia fails appropriate therapy or aspiration recurs, consider bronchoscopy to rule out neoplasm

PROGNOSIS
- Increased mortality with pneumonia due to gram-negative bacilli
  - *P. aeruginosa* mortality 28% in recent study (5)
- Age, poor functional and nutritional status, and significant comorbid illness are independent predictors of increased mortality

COMPLICATIONS
- Early complications
  - Sepsis
  - Acute respiratory distress syndrome
- Late complications
  - Lung abscess
  - Necrotizing pneumonia
  - Empyema

REFERENCES
1. El-Solh AA, et al. Microbiology of severe aspiration pneumonia in institutionalized elderly. *Am J Respir Crit Care Med*. 2003;167:1650–1654.
2. Marik PE, Kaplan D. Aspiration pneumonia and dysphagia in the elderly. *Chest*. 2003;124: 328–336.
3. Kadowaki M, et al. Reappraisal of clindamycin IV monotherapy for treatment of mild-to-moderate aspiration pneumonia in elderly patients. *Chest*. 2005;127:1276–1282.
4. Allewelt M, et al. Ampicllin + sulbactam vs. clindamycin +/−cephalosporin for the treatment of aspiration pneumonia and primary lung abscess. *Clinical microbiology and infection*. 2004;10: 163–170.
5. Arancibia F, et al. Community-acquired pneumonia due to gram negative bacteria and Pseudomonas aeruginosa. *Arch Intern Med*. 2002;162: 1849–1858.

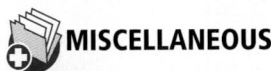 **MISCELLANEOUS**

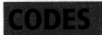 **CODES**

ICD9-CM
507.0

PATIENT TEACHING
- Encourage soft diet, smaller bites
- Mechanical strategies
  - Elevated head 30–45° when eating; Especially important if enteral feeding
- Aggressive oral hygiene

PNEUMONIA, BACTERIAL

Bhanu Sud, MD
Ronald A. Greenfield, MD

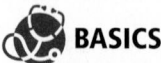 **BASICS**

DESCRIPTION
- An acute, bacterial infection of the lung parenchyma and pulmonary system.
- Infection may be community-acquired or health care–associated
  - Most commonly, community-acquired bacterial pneumonia is caused by *Streptococcus pneumoniae, Haemophilus influenzae* (particularly in cigarette smokers), or *Mycoplasma pneumoniae.*
  - Hospital-acquired pneumonia is usually caused by Gram-negative bacilli 60% (*e.g., Pseudomonas/ Enterobacter*) or *Staphylococcus aureus* (30%).
- Polymicrobial infection involving both aerobes and anaerobes is common in patients with aspiration of oropharyngeal contents.
- Synonym(s): Lobar pneumonia; Classic pneumococcal pneumonia

ALERT
Geriatric Considerations
Morbidity and mortality high in patients >70, especially with comorbidity or mechanical ventilation.

Pediatric Considerations
Morbidity and mortality high in children <1 year of age.

GENERAL PREVENTION
- Eliminate or reduce risk factors where possible, particularly cigarette smoking.
- Bedridden and postoperative patients
  - Deep breathing and coughing exercises, incentive spirometry, prevent aspiration during nasogastric tube feedings, use antacid therapies only as needed.
- Avoid indiscriminate use of antibiotics for minor viral upper respiratory infections (URI).
- Annual influenza vaccine
- Pneumococcal vaccine for all adults >50 or with comorbid conditions and children >2 years

EPIDEMIOLOGY
Incidence
- Community-acquired: 1,200 cases per 100,000 persons per year
- Nosocomial: 800 cases per 100,000 admissions annually

RISK FACTORS
- Tobacco smoking
- Recent/concurrent viral URI or influenza
- Hospitalization, particularly with mechanical ventilation, antecedent antibiotics, nasogastric tubes
- Age extremes
- Alcoholism
- AIDS or other immunocompromising condition or immunosuppressive therapy
- Renal failure
- Cardiovascular disease
- Functional asplenia
- Chronic obstructive pulmonary disease (COPD)
- Diabetes mellitus
- Malnutrition
- Malignancy
- Altered level of consciousness or gag reflex (e.g., seizures, stroke, neuromuscular disease)
- Occupational exposure
- Poorly implemented infection control practices (e.g., poor handwashing)
- Postoperative atelectasis

ETIOLOGY
- Sources
  - Aspiration from the oropharynx
  - Inhalation
  - Hematogenous spread
- Bacterial pathogens
  - *S. pneumoniae* (pneumococcus)
  - *H. influenzae*
  - *M. pneumoniae*
  - *S. aureus*
  - *Legionella pneumophila*
  - *Chlamydophila pneumoniae, C. psittaci*
  - *Moraxella catarrhalis*
  - *Pseudomonas aeruginosa*
  - *Klebsiella pneumoniae* (and other Gram-negative rod-shaped pathogens)
  - Anaerobes

ASSOCIATED CONDITIONS
See "Risk Factors."

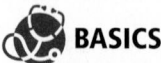 **DIAGNOSIS**

SIGNS AND SYMPTOMS
- Cardinal signs and symptoms
  - Cough and fever
  - Chest pain (pleuritic or nonpleuritic)
  - Chill, with sudden onset
  - Dark, thick, bloody or rusty sputum. In patients with COPD: Change in quantity and character of sputum.
- Respiratory signs of consolidation
  - Tubular breath sounds
  - Crackles
  - Egophony
- Signs of pleural involvement
  - Decreased breath sounds
  - Dullness to percussion
  - Friction rub
- Signs of respiratory distress
  - Tachypnea
  - Tachycardia or bradycardia
  - Cyanosis
- CNS
  - Mentation changes to include anxiety, confusion, and restlessness
- Gastrointestinal
  - Abdominal pain
  - Anorexia
  - Diarrhea

Lab
- Blood cultures: 2 set minimum if possible
  - Positive in 10–20% of adult patients and 7% of pediatric patients with community-acquired pneumonia (partially because many have been pretreated with antibiotics) and 8–20% of those with nosocomial pneumonia.
- CBC
  - Usually leukocytosis with an shift to immature forms, also may have leukopenia
- Chemistry
  - Hyponatremia
  - Renal insufficiency
  - Hyperbilirubinemia
- Arterial blood gases
  - Hypoxemia
  - Hypocapnia initially, then hypercapnia
- Consider urine testing for Legionella antigen.
- Consider urine testing for pneumococcal antigen.

Imaging

Chest radiograph for all patients being evaluated for hospitalization, with lateral decubitus views if pleural effusion present:

- Lobar or segmental consolidation (air bronchogram)
- Bronchopneumonia
- Interstitial infiltrate
- Pleural effusion (free-flowing or loculated as discerned by ultrasound or CT)

Diagnostic Procedures/Surgery

- Tuberculin skin test (purified protein derivative): For hilar adenopathy or cavitary lesions
- Gram stain and culture of respiratory secretions (of limited value in evaluation and treatment)
  - Induced sputum if necessary
  - Nasotracheal or endotracheal suctioning for culture
  - Bronchoscopy with bronchoalveolar lavage or protected telescoping catheter brushing for culture
- Thoracentesis for pleural fluid studies

Pathological Findings

Lung

- Segmental, lobar, or multifocal peribronchial consolidation
- Positive tissue Gram stain for bacteria

DIFFERENTIAL DIAGNOSIS

- Other causes of infectious pneumonitis
  - Viruses (human metapneumovirus, severe acute respiratory syndrome–associated coronavirus, respiratory syncytial virus, adenovirus, cytomegalovirus, parainfluenzavirus, influenzae A and B viruses, varicella virus, measles virus, rubella virus, hantavirus)
  - *Nocardia* (a special type of bacterial pneumonia)
  - Various fungi (*Blastomyces, Cryptococcus, Aspergillus, Histoplasma, Coccidioides, Pneumocystis jeroveci* [*P. carinii*])
  - Protozoans (*Toxoplasma*)
  - *Rickettsia* (*Coxiella burnetii*: Q fever)
  - Tuberculosis (TB) or atypical mycobacterial infection (special types of bacterial pneumonia)
- Pulmonary embolism with infarction
- Bronchiolitis obliterans with organizing pneumonia
- Pulmonary contusion
- Pulmonary vasculitis
- Sarcoidosis
- Hypersensitivity pneumonitis
- Acute respiratory distress syndrome (ARDS)
- Pneumothorax

 TREATMENT

Admission Criteria

- Community-acquired
  - Assessment of comorbid conditions, calculation of pneumonia severity index, and clinical judgment should be deployed to determine whom to admit.
- Nosocomial: Patients already hospitalized.

GENERAL MEASURES

- Oxygen supplementation for patients with cyanosis, hypoxia, dyspnea, circulatory disturbances, or delirium
- Mechanical ventilation for respiratory failure
- Hydration
- Analgesia for pain
- Electrolyte correction
- Respiratory isolation if TB is a possibility

Diet

- NPO if incipient respiratory failure present
- Consider soft, easy-to-eat foods

Activity

Bed rest and/or reduced activity during acute phase

 MEDICATION (DRUGS)

First Line

Initial therapy

- Usually empiric for most likely pathogens given clinical situation: If specific cause is identified, adjust antimicrobial therapy based on results of cultures and *in vitro* susceptibility testing.
- Community-acquired
  - Outpatient, no comorbidities, no recent antibiotic therapy: Macrolide (clarithromycin or azithromycin) or doxycycline (3)[A]
  - Outpatient, no comorbidities, antibiotics in previous 3 months: Avoid previously used class and use respiratory fluoroquinolone (levofloxacin or moxifloxacin) or macrolide plus high dose (4 g/d) amoxicillin ± clavulanate (3)[A]
  - Outpatient with comorbidities: Fluoroquinolone ormacrolide (3)[A]
  - Outpatient with comorbidites + previous antibiotic therapy: Alternate class and use fluoroquinolone or β-lactam agent + macrolide (3)[A]
  - Inpatient: Fluoroquinolone or β-lactam agent + macrolide. If patient has received an agent from these classes in previous 3 months use the alternative regimen (3)[A]

  - ○ ICU, Pseudomonas is not an issue: Cefotaxime or ceftriaxone or ampicillin/sulbactam or ertapenem plus either a macrolide or a fluoroquinolone (3)[A]; if penicillin allergic: Fluoroquinolone ± clindamycin.
  - ○ ICU, Pseudomonas is an issue: An Antipseudomonal β-lactam agent plus either a fluoroquinolone or a macrolide (3)[A]

  - Health care–associated

  - ○ No known risk factors for multidrug-resistant pathogens and onset within 5 days of hospitalization: Ceftriaxone or fluoroquinolone or ampicillin/sulbactam or ertapenem (1)[A]

  - ○ Risk factors for multidrug-resistant pathogens and/or late onset: Antipseudomonal cephalosporin (ceftazidime or cefepime) or antipseudomonal carbapenem (imipenem or meropenem) or piperacillin/tazobactam plus antipseudomonal fluoroquinolone (ciprofloxacin or levofloxacin) or aminoglycose plus linezolid or vancomycin (1)[A]

REFERENCES

1. Anonymous. Guidelines for the management of adults with hospital-acquired, ventilator-associated and healthcare-associated pneumonia. *Am J Resp Crit Care Med*. 2005;171:388–416.
2. Aujesky D, et al. Prospective comparison of three validated prediction rules for prognosis in community-acquired pneumonia. *Am J Med*. 2005;118:384–392.
3. Mandell LA, et al. Update of practice guidelines for the management of community-acquired pneumonia in immunocompetent adults. *Clin Infect Dis*. 2003;37:1405–1433.

 MISCELLANEOUS

See also: Pneumonia, mycoplasma; Pneumonia, viral

CODES

ICD9-CM

- 481 Pneumococcal pneumonia [*Streptococcus pneumoniae* pneumonia]
- 486 Pneumonia, organism unspecified

PATIENT TEACHING

See Corresponding Diagnostic Algorithm

PNEUMONIA, MYCOPLASMA

George R. Bergus, MD

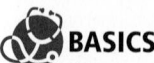 **BASICS**

DESCRIPTION
- Interstitial pneumonia caused by extensive infection of the lungs and bronchi, particularly the lower lobes of the lungs, by *Mycoplasma pneumoniae*. Usual course is acute. Incubation period is about 18–21 days and includes prodromal symptoms. Little seasonal variation of incidence; therefore, a greater percentage of pneumonia in summer and fall is from *Mycoplasma*. Epidemics in communities tend to be prolonged, sometimes over many months, and occur every 4–5 years.
- Synonym(s): Primary atypical pneumonia (PAP); Eaton agent pneumonia; Cold agglutinin-positive pneumonia

ALERT
Geriatric Considerations
Unusual finding in this age group

Pediatric Considerations
- Unusual in infants
- *M. pneumoniae* is associated with increased incidence of asthma attacks in older children.

Pregnancy Considerations
Tetracycline therapy contraindicated in pregnant patients

GENERAL PREVENTION
Highly contagious, *M. pneumoniae* is carried in respiratory droplets. Consider isolation of active cases in closed communities (schools, camps, military bases). Azithromycin prophylaxis (standard 5-day course) may lower attack rate.

EPIDEMIOLOGY
- Predominant age: 5–15, but may occur at any
- Predominant sex: Male

Incidence
130 cases per 100,000 people

Prevalence
Estimated to be most common cause of pneumonia in school children and young adults (without chronic underlying condition). The incidence varies considerably each year. Major outbreaks are repeated every 3–5 years.

RISK FACTORS
- Close community living (e.g., hospitals, prisons, military bases, fraternity houses). Some of largest outbreaks have been in army recruits.
- Family exposure
- Immunocompromised patients

ETIOLOGY
Infection by *M. pneumoniae*

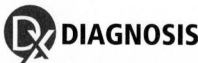 **DIAGNOSIS**

SIGNS AND SYMPTOMS
- Gradual onset with upper respiratory infection symptoms that progress
- Most will develop fever, cough, headache, sore throat, rales, and wheeze.
- Many will develop myalgias, nasal congestion, chest pain.
- Some patients will develop pleural effusion, pleural friction rub, cervical adenopathy, bullous myringitis, and skin rash.

TESTS
Lab
- Positive cold agglutinins (titer of 1:1024 or greater; or rising 4-fold) in 50% of infections
- *M. pneumoniae* culture (requires 7–10 days)
- Complement fixation serologic assay shows 4fold rise in titer at 2–4 weeks after symptom onset.
- IgM antibody to *M. pneumoniae* in 80% of patients after 1–2 weeks of illness (enzyme immunoassay)
- Detection of *M. pneumoniae* DNA by polymerase chain reaction testing of nasopharyngeal aspirate

Imaging
Chest radiograph: Diffuse interstitial infiltrates; small bilateral pleural effusion present in 25% of cases

Pathological Findings
Absence of bacterial pathogens on Gram stain and culture of sputum or transtracheal aspirate. Mycoplasma is a fastidious and slow-growing organism.

DIFFERENTIAL DIAGNOSIS
- Viral pneumonia
- Bacterial pneumonia (including plague and tularemia in severe cases)
- Fungal pneumonias
- *Pneumocystis jerovici* (formerly *P. carinii*)
- *Chlamydia pneumoniae*, TWAR, or *C. psittaci*
- *Legionella pneumophila*
- Tuberculosis

TREATMENT

INITIAL STABILIZATION
Inpatient for cases with severe symptoms

GENERAL MEASURES
Diet
Patients ought to consume plenty of fluids.

Activity
Rest during acute phase of illness

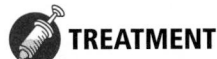 **MEDICATION (DRUGS)**

First Line
- Erythromycin: Children 30–50 mg/kg/d PO for 10–14 days; adults 500 mg PO q6h for 10–14 days
- Clarithromycin: Children 15 mg/kg/d PO for 10–14 days; adults 500 mg PO b.i.d. for 10–14 days
- Azithromycin: Children 10 mg/kg PO 1st day, 5 mg/kg PO for days 2–5; adults 500 mg PO 1st day, then 250 mg PO every day for 4 days
- Consider 3 weeks of therapy if patient has persistent cough or airway reactivity.
- Penicillins are ineffective against *M. pneumoniae*.
- Contraindications: Refer to the manufacturer's literature.
- Precautions: Refer to the manufacturer's literature.
- Significant possible interactions: Erythromycin and other macrolides inhibit the cytochrome P-450 microsomal enzyme system and can reduce elimination of other drugs such as carbamazepine, phenytoin, lovastatin, and theophylline. Prolongation of the QT interval and ventricular tachycardia have occurred in some patients receiving astemizole or terfenadine concomitantly with erythromycin.

Second Line
- Doxycycline: 100 mg PO b.i.d. if >9 years
- Levofloxacin shows good activity against *M. pneumoniae*.
- Adjunctive drugs: Albuterol inhaler, 2 puffs q.i.d. for wheezing
- Children >9 years: Doxycycline 100 mg PO b.i.d.

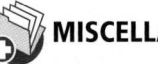 **FOLLOW-UP**

PROGNOSIS
- Mycoplasma infection symptoms usually resolve in ~2 weeks.
- Some constitutional symptoms may persist for several weeks.
- With correct therapy, even most severe cases can expect complete recovery.

COMPLICATIONS
NOTE: All complications are rare except reactive airway disease, hemolytic anemia, and erythema multiforme:
- Reactive airway disease
- Hemolytic anemia
- Erythema multiforme
- Meningoencephalitis
- Polyneuritis
- Polyarthritis
- Stevens-Johnson syndrome
- Pericarditis
- Myocarditis
- Respiratory distress syndrome
- Cerebral ataxia
- Thromboembolic phenomena
- Pleural effusion
- Nephritis

PATIENT MONITORING
- Follow up either in person or by telephone.
- Clearing of condition of chest radiograph should be documented in patients >50 years. In smokers, document a clear radiograph in 6–8 weeks.

REFERENCES
1. Bartlett JG, et al. Practice guidelines for the management of community-acquired pneumonia in adults. Infectious Diseases Society of America. *Clin Infect Dis*. 2000;31:347–382.
2. Hyde TB, et al. Azithromycin prophylaxis during a hospital outbreak of *Mycoplasma pneumoniae* pneumonia. *J Infect Dis*. 2001;183:907–912.
3. Neher JO, et al. Clinical inquiries. What is the best macrolide for atypical pneumonia? *J Fam Pract*. 2004 March;53(3):229–30.
4. O'Handley JG, Gray LD. The incidence of *Mycoplasma pneumoniae*. *J Am Board Fam Pract*. 1997;10:425–429.

 MISCELLANEOUS

- See also: Pneumonia, bacterial; Pneumonia, *Pneumonia carinii* (PCP); Pneumonia, viral

CODES

ICD9-CM
483.0 *Mycoplasma pneumoniae*

PATIENT TEACHING
Printed patient information is available from the American Lung Association, 1740 Broadway, New York, NY 10019; (212) 315-8700; www.lungusa.org

See Corresponding Diagnostic Algorithm

PNEUMONIA, PNEUMOCYSTIS JIROVECI

Cynthia Gail Carmichael, MD

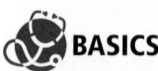 **BASICS**

DESCRIPTION

A form of pneumonia arising in immunosuppressed patients caused by *Pneumocystis jiroveci*. This is one of the most common opportunistic infections occurring in patients infected with HIV.

Pneumocystis infection can cause organ involvement and disseminated disease as well as pneumonia.

- Synonym(s): Pneumocystis, Pulmonary pneumocystosis, Interstitial plasma cell pneumonia, *Pneumocystis carinii* pneumonia

ALERT

Pediatric Considerations

- Early onset (5 months of age) and high mortality (median survival 1 month)
- Important to distinguish from lymphoid interstitial pneumonitis, because treatment and prognosis differ

GENERAL PREVENTION

- All AIDS patients with a history of pneumocystis pneumonia (or CD4 cells <200 or evidence of immunodeficiency such as oral candida) require prophylaxis with daily trimethoprim/sulfamethoxazole (double-strength) PO, daily dapsone (100 mg) PO, or monthly aerosolized pentamidine (300 mg). In patients intolerant of trimethoprim/sulfamethoxazole, consider a rechallenge or desensitization with trimethoprim/sulfamethoxazole; various protocols exist.
- Prophylaxis may be discontinued in patients on antiretroviral therapy with CD4 cell counts >200 for a 3-month period:
  - Restart Pneumocystic cacinil pneumonia (PCP) prophylaxis is CD4 cell count decreases <200.

Pediatric Considerations

All babies born to HIV-infected mothers must receive prophylaxis after 4–6 weeksof life. Drug of choice is trimethoprim/sulfamethoxazole; 150 mg/m^2/d PO (trimethoprim component) 3 times weekly (on consecutive days). This should be continued until the baby has a negative test result for HIV or for the 1st year of life, after which the CD4 cell count itself may be used to guide prophylaxis.

EPIDEMIOLOGY

- Predominant age
  - In HIV-infected children not taking prophylaxis, median age of onset is 5 months of age
  - In HIV-infected adults, PCP may occur at any age
- Predominant sex: Male > Female

Incidence

- Pneumocystis pneumonia is the AIDS indicator disease in 43% of patients.
- Because of more effective prophylaxis and antiretroviral therapy, its incidence is decreasing.

RISK FACTORS

- Immunodeficiency (e.g., premature infants, neoplasia, congenital, acquired or drug-induced immunodeficiency states, CD4 counts <200 in adults)
- Patients with a history of previous pneumocystis pneumonia

ETIOLOGY

The ubiquitous *P. jiroveci* may cause infection in normal hosts (2/3 of young children have positive serology), but will rarely cause symptoms in immunocompetent people. Studies suggest person-to-person transmission possible.

ASSOCIATED CONDITIONS

- AIDS
- HIV infection

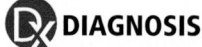 **DIAGNOSIS**

SIGNS AND SYMPTOMS

- Usually insidious but occasionally abrupt in onset
- Dyspnea on exertion progressing to continuous dyspnea
- Weakness, fatigue, malaise
- Fever, chills
- Cough: Nonproductive or productive of scant white or clear sputum
- Tachypnea
- Extrapulmonary pneumocystis may occur (e.g., visceral, cutaneous, ocular), particularly in patients receiving therapy with aerosolized pentamidine for prophylaxis.

TESTS

Lab

- Arterial blood gases reveal hypoxemia and increased alveolar-arterial gradient (varies with severity of disease).
- Levels of serum lactate dehydrogenase frequently (non-specific)
- CD$_4$ cell count is generally <200 in HIV-infected patients with pneumocystis pneumonia.
- Drugs that may alter lab results: Inhaled pentamidine used to prevent pneumocystis pneumonia may change radiographic picture to infiltrates in predominantly upper lobe distribution.
- Sputum induced with inhaled 3–5% hypertonic saline may reveal pneumocystis on cytologic evaluation using various stains. An immunofluorescence technique is also available. Sensitivity may be as high as 90% in labs with personnel experienced in the technical procedures involved.

Imaging

- Chest radiograph
  - Shows bilateral diffuse interstitial or perihilar infiltrate in 75% of cases
  - May also be normal or show unilateral disease, pleural effusions, abscesses or cavitations, pneumothorax, or lobar consolidations.
  - Upper lobe infiltrates may be present in patients receiving pentamidine for prophylaxis.
- Gallium scanning of the lungs is highly sensitive for pneumocystis pneumonia, but is not specific. May be useful when sputum studies are inconclusive and bronchoscopy is not available

Diagnostic Procedures/Surgery

- Fiberoptic bronchoscopy with bronchoalveolar lavage or transbronchial biopsy (90–100% sensitive) is the preferred method of diagnosis when sputum test results are negative.
- Open lung biopsy is rarely required.
- A test for pneumocystis based on polymerase chain reaction may be useful in the future on sputum, bronchoalveolar fluid.

Pathological Findings

Pneumonitis caused by presence of organism and inflammatory response

DIFFERENTIAL DIAGNOSIS

- Tuberculosis
- Mycobacterium avium intracellulare
- Viral pneumonias
- Fungal pneumonias
- Lymphoid interstitial pneumonitis (in children)
- Bacterial pneumonia
- Cytomegalovirus pneumonia

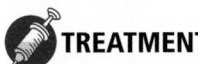 **TREATMENT**

INITIAL STABILIZATION

Outpatient for mild cases, otherwise in patient

GENERAL MEASURES

Oxygen therapy is often necessary.

Diet

No special diet needed

Activity

As tolerated

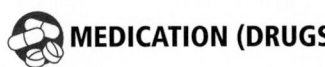 **MEDICATION (DRUGS)**

ALERT

Pediatric Considerations

Pneumocystis pneumonia prophylaxis with trimethoprim/sulfamethoxazole, dapsone, or pentamidine for all HIV-positive children <1 year old is recommended. For older HIV-positive children, prophylaxis therapy should be individualized based on CD4 counts (see "Prevention").

Pregnancy Considerations

Trimethoprim/Sulfamethoxazole (TMP/SMX) (or dapsone as alternative) has been used for treatment and prophylaxis in pregnant patients.

First Line

- TMP/SMX (Bactrim, Septra): 15–20 mg/kg/d PO of trimethoprim component in 3 divided doses or IV for 21 days. (or TMP/SMX DS2 PO t.i.d.). Reduce dose of TMP/SMX in patients with renal failure.
- Adjunctive corticosteroid (prednisone or methyl prednisolone) therapy begun within 72 hours of diagnosis decreases mortality in AIDS patients (adults and children) with moderate to severe pneumocystis pneumonia (those with PO_2 <70 mm Hg). Prednisone dose: 40 mg b.i.d. days 1–5; 40 mg daily days 6–10; 20 mg daily days 1–21.
- Contraindications: Use with care in pregnant patient and infants <2 months.

- Precautions
  - History of sulfa allergy
  - A high percentage of patients with AIDS will develop intolerance to TMP/SMX. Especially common are dermatologic reactions, hematologic toxicity, or fever.
  - Patients receiving this therapy must avoid direct sunlight.
- Significant possible interactions: Phenytoin, oral anticoagulants, oral sulfonylureas, digitalis

Second Line

- Pentamidine: 4 mg/kg/d IV over 60 minutes for 21 days
- Dapsone: 100 mg PO daily plus trimethoprim 15 mg/kg/d divided t.i.d. or q.i.d. Check glucose 6-phosphate dehydrogenase level before beginning dapsone, because hemolysis may result.
- Clindamycin: 300–400 mg PO t.i.d.–q.i.d. plus primaquine 30 mg PO daily for 21 days
- Atovaquone suspension: 750 mg b.i.d. PO for 21 days

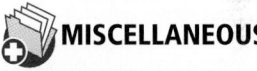 **FOLLOW-UP**

All patients with PCP require secondary prophylaxis for life (after adequate treatment for PCP) unless CD4 cell count increases. (See "General Prevention.")

PROGNOSIS

- Mortality from 1st episode pneumocystis pneumonia is 10–15%. With prophylactic therapy, mean survival has increased.
- 40% of patients with pneumocystis pneumonia will have a recurrence unless prophylaxis is given.

COMPLICATIONS

- Respiratory failure
- Pneumothorax (even after successful treatment)
- Extrapulmonary pneumocystis (especially in patients on inhaled pentamidine prophylaxis)

PATIENT MONITORING

Serum lactate dehydrogenase levels, pulmonary function test results, and arterial blood gases measurements generally normalize with treatment.

REFERENCES

1. Centers for Disease Control and Prevention. Guidelines for preventing opportunistic infections among HIV-infected persons-2002 recommendations of the US Public Health Service and the Infectious Disease Society of America. *MMWR*. 2002;51(No. rr-8).
2. Centers for Disease Control and Prevention. Treating opportunistic infections among HIV-infected adults and adolescents: Recommendations from CDC, the National Institutes of Health, and the HIV Medicine Association/Infectious Disease Society of America. *MMWR*. 2004;53(No. RR15)
3. Dohn MN, et al. Geographic clustering of *Pneumocystis carinii* pneumonia in patients with HIV infection. *Am J Respir Crit Care Med*. 2000;162:1617–1621.
4. Furrer H, et al. Discontinuation of primary prophylaxis against *Pneumocystis carinii* pneumonia in HIV-1-infected adults treated with combination antiretroviral therapy. *N Engl J Med*. 199;340:1301–6.
5. Stringer JR, et al. A new name (*Pneumocystis jiroveci*) for Pneumocystis from humans. *Emerg Infect Dis*. 2002;8:891–896.

 MISCELLANEOUS

- See also: HIV infection and AIDS

CODES

ICD9-CM

136.3 Pneumocystosis

PATIENT TEACHING

See Corresponding Diagnostic Algorithm

PNEUMONIA, VIRAL

Kathleen Doyle, MD

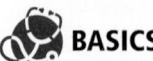 BASICS

DESCRIPTION
- Inflammatory disease of the lungs; affects pulmonary system.
- Most viral pneumonia results from exposure of a susceptible nonimmune person to infection in the form of aerosolized secretions.

ALERT
Geriatric Considerations
Greatest rates of morbidity and mortality

Pediatric Considerations
Adenoviral infections in children are serious. More serious respiratory virus infections are almost always seen in infants and in immunocompromised patients.

Pregnancy Considerations
Pregnant patients should avoid contact with anyone who has a viral infection. Consider vaccination if patient will be >3 months pregnant during the influenza season.

GENERAL PREVENTION
- Influenza A and B vaccine: Use in patients with chronic cardiovascular lung disease, residents of long-term care facilities, medical personnel with extensive contact with high-risk patients, people >50 years of age or those with chronic diseases, immunosuppressed patients (including all those with HIV), health care workers, and people in frequent contact with any high-risk person.
- For those patients who are unable to receive influenza vaccine (e.g., with egg allergy or other) and are at high risk because of age, comorbid illness, or other risk factor, amantadine, rimantadine, or oseltamivir can be given throughout the infectious season if tolerated.
- For those who did not receive the vaccine and have been exposed to influenza, or in geographic areas where an influenza A outbreak has been documented, amantadine, rimantadine, or oseltamivir may also be taken for 2 weeks until vaccination has produced immunity.
- Health care workers who are pregnant must take proper precautions to avoid infectious patients.
- Measles vaccine
- Varicella vaccine

EPIDEMIOLOGY
- Predominant age: Children
- Predominant sex: Male = Female

Prevalence
- Prevalence is unknown, and varies with seasonal outbreaks, but disease is more common during winter months.
- ~90% of all cases of childhood pneumonia have viral cause.

RISK FACTORS
- Immunocompromised state
- Living in close quarters
- Seasonal: Epidemic upper respiratory illness
- Elderly patients
- Cardiac disease
- Chronic pulmonary disease
- Recent upper respiratory infection
- Travel to endemic area (Hantavirus and severe acute respiratory virus)
- Nonvaccinated person

Genetics
No known genetic pattern has been recognized.

PATHOPHYSIOLOGY
ETIOLOGY
- Influenza A, B, and C
- Parainfluenza 1, 2, 3, and 4
- Respiratory syncytial virus (especially in young children)
- Adenovirus
- Cytomegalovirus, particularly in immunocompromised patients
- Varicella (chickenpox)
- Herpes simplex
- Enterovirus
- Coronavirus
- Rubeola (measles)
- Epstein-Barr virus
- Hantavirus
- Human metapneumovirus
- Avian influenza A (H5N1)
- Mixed infection with bacterial pathogens common
- Between 4% and 39% of diagnosed pneumonia in adults has been ascribed to viral cause in different published series.

ASSOCIATED CONDITIONS
- Bacterial forms of pneumonia
- Fungal infection and *Pneumocystis jerovici* pneumonia/pneumocystic pneumonia in immunocompromised patients

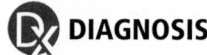 DIAGNOSIS

SIGNS AND SYMPTOMS
- Fever
- Chills
- Cough (with or without purulent sputum production)
- Dyspnea
- Pulmonary rales and rhonchi
- Altered breath sounds
- Pleurisy
- Friction rub
- Headache
- Myalgias
- Malaise
- Gastrointestinal symptoms

History
Avian flu is currently not a risk for persons in the US, but is a risk for those with poultry (chicken, duck, and turkey) contact in Asia, Europe, and the UK.

TESTS
Lab
- Sputum Gram stain and culture to identify bacterial copathogens if present
- Appropriate direct fluorescent antibody or enzyme immunoassay from throat nasopharyngeal washings (children) or swab (adults), tracheal aspirate, or bronchoalveolar lavage specimens (herpes simplex virus, varicella-zoster virus, influenza viruses A and B, respiratory syncytial virus, adenovirus)
- Viral culture
- Cytopathology (cytomegalovirus, herpes simplex virus, measles virus)
- Normal or near normal granulocyte count, occasionally leukopenic with increased lymphocyte percentage
- Hypoxemia with severe disease
- Hemoconcentration (hantavirus)
- Serology (4-fold rise in acute compared with convalescent titers)
- Polymerase chain reaction detection if modality available
- Disorders that may alter lab results: Coronavirus antibody or reverse-transcriptase polymerase chain reaction if severe acute respiratory virus infection is suspected

Imaging
Chest radiograph: Interstitial or alveolar infiltrates, peribronchial thickening, pleural effusion

Diagnostic Procedures/Surgery
- Nasopharyngeal throat swab
- Bronchoscopy with bronchoalveolar lavage
- Serologic testing for hantavirus; enzyme immunoassay if available from health departments

Pathological Findings
- Heavy lungs
- Enlarged regional lymph nodes
- Cytoplasmic inclusion bodies (cytomegalovirus [CMV])
- Intranuclear inclusion bodies (adenovirus, CMV, herpesvirus, varicellovirus)
- Intense inflammatory reaction with mononuclear cells
- Multinucleated giant cells (parainfluenza virus, measles virus, herpes simplex virus, varicellovirus)

DIFFERENTIAL DIAGNOSIS
- Bacterial pneumonia (especially atypical etiologies: *Chlamydophilia pneumoniae* and *C. psittaci*, *Mycoplasma pneumoniae*, *Legionella pneumophila*)
- Pulmonary edema
- Pneumocystis pneumonia/*Pneumocystis jiroveci* pneumonia
- Aspiration pneumonia
- Hypersensitivity pneumonitis
- Bronchiolitis obliterans with organizing pneumonia
- Pulmonary embolus/infarction
- Cystic fibrosis (in infants)
- Severe acute respiratory syndrome or severe acute respiratory syndrome–associated Coronavirus

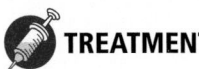 TREATMENT

Outpatient for most cases. Inpatient for infants <4 months of age or older people, or for any patient with diffuse, severe infection (e.g., hypoxemia, hypercarbia, hypotension or shock, adult respiratory distress syndrome) or significant comorbidity (e.g., CHF, coronary artery disease, chronic obstructive pulmonary disease)

GENERAL MEASURES
- Encourage coughing and deep breathing exercises to clear secretions.
- Careful disposal of secretions/universal precautions
- Hydration
- Respiratory isolation for varicella virus, which is highly contagious (i.e., negative pressure)

Diet
Increase fluids; provide high-calorie, high-protein, soft diet

Activity
Rest

 MEDICATION (DRUGS)

First Line
- Oseltamivir (Tamiflu): Influenza virus A and B
  – Patients >18: 75 mg PO q12h for 5 days; dosage adjusted to 75 mg PO q24h in cases where creatinine clearance rate is <30 mL/min. (Due to resistance development, this was drug of choice for influenza during the 2005–2006 season).
  – Rimantadine (Flumadine), an amantadine analog, is equally effective as amantadine and has fewer adverse effects. Useful for Influenza A. Effective only in 1st 24–48 hours. Preferable to amantadine due to lower side effects.
- Acyclovir (Zovirax): Pulmonary infections involving herpes simplex virus, herpes zoster, or varicella virus
  – Adults: 5 mg/kg IV q8h for pneumonia caused by herpes simplex virus and 10 mg/kg IV q8h for pneumonia caused by varicellovirus
  – Children: 250 mg/m^2 IV q8h
- Ganciclovir (Cytovene): Infection owing to cytomegalovirus or herpes simplex virus
  – 5 mg/kg IV q12h

- Ribavirin (Virazole): Respiratory syncytial virus, possibly Hantavirus and influenza B virus (20 mg/mL via continuous aerosol administration for 12–18 hours per day for 3–7 days). Indicated only in severe respiratory syncytial virus infections, given via small-particle aerosol generator
- Zanamivir (Relenza): Influenza virus A and B
  – Patients <12: 10 mg (2 inhalations) inhaled PO q12h for 5 days
- Contraindications: Refer the to manufacturer's literature.
- Precautions
  – Amantadine should be used cautiously in patients with liver disease, epilepsy, renal disease, eczematoid rash, and those with a history of psychotic illness.
  – Ribavirin is teratogenic and should not be administered by pregnant health care personnel; its cost is high and benefits are marginal.
- Significant possible interactions: Refer to the manufacturer's literature.

Second Line
- Amantadine (Symmetrel): Influenza A (not effective for influenza B): Effective only in 1st 24–48 hours
  – Patients <10 years: 4–8 mg/kg/d PO in 2 divided doses. Not to exceed 150 mg/d PO.
  – Patients aged 10–65 years: 100 mg PO q12h. Adults may be given a loading dose of 200 mg PO initially.
- Patients >65: 100 mg PO once a day
- Antibiotics for superimposed bacterial infections
- Foscarnet (Foscavir) for cytomegalovirus, herpes simplex virus, varicellovirus infections, 60 mg/kg IV q8h
- Immune globulin: IV may increase response in non-AIDS, immunosuppressed patients with cytomegalovirus pneumonia. Dose and dosage regimen are not well established, but 500 mg/kg IV daily for 10 doses may be beneficial.
- Amantadine and rimantadine not effective for avian flu, but oseltamivir and zanamivir probably are.

 FOLLOW-UP

PROGNOSIS
Usually favorable prognosis, with illness lasting several days to a week. Postviral fatigue is common. However, death can occur, especially in pediatric or bone marrow transplant patients with adenovirus infections or in older people with influenza.

COMPLICATIONS
- Superimposed bacterial infections such as *Streptococcus pneumoniae*, *Staphylococcus aureus*, *Haemophilus influenzae*, and others
- Respiratory failure requiring mechanical ventilation
- Adult respiratory distress syndrome
- Reye syndrome after influenza in children

PATIENT MONITORING
- Physical examinations
- Chest radiograph
- Oxygenation if illness severe enough for hospitalization

REFERENCES
1. Mandell GL, ed. *Principles and Practice of Infectious Diseases*, 6th ed. Philadelphia: Churchill Livingstone, 2005.
2. de Roux A, et al. A. Viral community-acquired pneumonia in nonimmunocompromised adults. *Chest*. 2004;125(4):1343–1351.
3. Fields BN, Knipe DM, Chanock RM, eds. *Virology*, 2nd ed. New York: Raven, 1990.
4. Gorbach SL, Bartlett JG, Blacklow NR, eds. *Infectious Diseases*. Philadelphia: WB Saunders, 1998.

ADDITIONAL READING
- www.cdc.gov/flu/pandemic
- www.idsociety.org

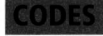 MISCELLANEOUS

- See also: Bronchiolitis obliterans; Severe acute respiratory syndrome.
- Information on severe acute respiratory syndrome for clinicians is available at cdc.gov/ncidod/sars/clinicians.htm.

CODES

ICD9-CM
480.9 Viral pneumonia, unspecified

PATIENT TEACHING
For patient education materials on this topic, contact American Lung Association, 1740 Broadway, New York, NY 100919;(800) LUNG-USA.

 See Corresponding Diagnostic Algorithm

PNEUMOTHORAX

Felix B. Chang, MD
Alfonso Tafur, MD

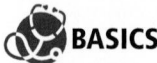 **BASICS**

DESCRIPTION
- Accumulation of air or gas between the parietal and visceral pleurae
- Spontaneous pneumothorax (SP) may be primary (PSP) or secondary (SSP).
- PSP is found in patients who are in their early 20s but otherwise healthy; rarely seen in patients >40.
- SSP is a complication to underlying lung disease (e.g., chronic obstructive pulmonary disease [COPD], cystic fibrosis, AIDS, tuberculosis [TB])
- Traumatic pneumothorax, both closed and open, may exist in tandem with hemothorax.
- Tension pneumothorax: Inspired air accumulates into the pleural space with no means of escape, like a check valve mechanism. More air increases lung compression and causes hypoxia and hemodynamic compromise.
- Occult pneumothorax (OP) describes pneumothorax that is not suspected on the basis of clinical examination or plain radiography but is ultimately detected with thoracoabdominal CT.
- System(s) Affected: Pulmonary; Cardiovascular

ALERT
Geriatric Considerations
Higher rates of morbidity and mortality

Pediatric Considerations
Unusual in this age group except after trauma; can be found in neonates with respiratory distress syndrome and aspiration of meconium

Pregnancy Considerations
A known but unusual complication of labor and delivery. It should be suspected in the pregnant patient with dyspnea and chest pain.

GENERAL PREVENTION
No preventive measures known, but patients may avoid some risk factors (e.g., exposure to high altitudes, flying in nonpressurized aircraft, scuba diving, smoking).

EPIDEMIOLOGY
- >20,000 new SP cases occur each year in the US, at a cost of more than $130 million
- Predominant sex: Male > Female
- Predominant age: Adults 20–40 years

Incidence
One to 2% otherwise healthy newborns at birth (asymptomatic)

Prevalence
- 7.4/100,000 in men
- 2.1/100,000 in women

RISK FACTORS
- Trauma (broken rib, ruptured bronchus, perforated esophagus)
- Rupture of superficial lung bulla after coughing or blowing into a musical instrument
- Strenuous activity
- Flying when pressurization lost
- Scuba diving (ascension or decompression)
- Pneumoconioses
- TB
- Pneumonia: *Mycobacterium tuberculosis*, *Klebsiella* sp., *Staphylococcus aureus*
- Subpleural pneumocystic pneumonia (e.g., in AIDS patients receiving prophylaxis via pentamidine aerosol)
- Bronchial obstruction
- COPD, particularly emphysema
- Asthma
- Neoplasms
- In the ICU setting, body weight <80 kg
- History of adult immunodeficiency syndrome, ARDS, use of inotropic agents during the 1st 24 hours have been found to be a risk
- Endometriosis (during menstruation)
- Marfan or Ehlers-Danlos syndromes (rare)
- Rupture of an infected abscess
- Lymphangioleiomyomatosis
- Cystic fibrosis
- Cigarette smoking
- Procedures including intubation, central line placement, liver biopsy, mechanical ventilation, thoracentesis, and acupuncture
- Iatrogenic pneumothorax is a life-threatening complication seen in 3% of ICU patients.

Genetics
- Possible predisposition exists in tall, thin young men, especially those with marfanoid habitus.
- An X-linked recessive pattern of disease also is reported; episodes of PSP per patient are seen more commonly in the autosomal dominant form with incomplete penetrance.
- FBN1 gene mutation may be causative, as well as certain causative HLA haplotypes, and an autosomal recessive inheritance pattern.

PATHOPHYSIOLOGY
Loss of negative intrapleural pressure, collapse lung

ETIOLOGY
- Perforation of the visceral pleura and entry of gas from the lung
- Gas generated by microorganisms in an empyema
- Penetration of the chest wall, diaphragm, mediastinum, or esophagus
- Blunt trauma to thorax

ASSOCIATED CONDITIONS
See "Etiology."

DIAGNOSIS

SIGNS AND SYMPTOMS
- Finding of chest pain may simulate myocardial infarction or acute abdomen.
- Pleuritic chest pain
- Cough
- Dyspnea
- Cyanosis
- Moderate to severe: Profound respiratory distress, shock, circulatory collapse
- Asymmetry of respirations
- Diminished breath sounds on affected side
- Referred pain to shoulder
- Tachycardia
- Rapid, shallow breathing
- Decrease fremitus
- Absent egophony and bronchophony on affected side
- Variable findings on chest expansion
- Hyper-resonance to percussion
- Subcutaneous emphysema/crepitus over chest wall and neck
- Tension pneumothorax: Weak, rapid pulse; pallor; neck vein distention; anxiety; tracheal deviation, hypotension, altered mental status
- Consider with sudden onset of tachycardia and hypotension in patient on ventilator.

History
Careful history and physical are mandated.

Physical Exam
The physical findings depend on size of pneumothorax.

TESTS
Lab
Arterial blood gases in significant pneumothorax
- pH <7.35
- PO_2 <80 mm Hg (10.6 kPa)
- PCO_2 >45 mm Hg (6.0 kPa)

Imaging
- Chest radiographs (CXRs) in inspiration and expiratory views
  - Air without lung markings peripherally, mediastinal shift to contralateral side
  - Small pneumothorax may be evident only with expiratory or lateral decubitus film.
  - Upright chest radiograph: As little as 50 mL of pleural gas can be visible.
  - Lateral decubitus view: As little as 5 mL of pleural gas is visible.
  - Supine chest radiograph: 500 mL of pleural gas is needed for definitive diagnosis.
  - Tension pneumothorax: Can see mediastinal shift to opposite side
- Ultrasound: Helpful in major trauma patients in whom possibility of chest radiograph may be limited (in early stages of use).
- CT scan for poorly visualized pneumothoraces

DIFFERENTIAL DIAGNOSIS
- Pleurisy
- Pericarditis
- Myocardial infarction
- Pulmonary embolism
- Diaphragmatic hernia
- Stomach herniation through diaphragm
- Dissecting aneurysm
- Flail chest
- Hemothorax
- Angina pectoris
- Asthma
- Exacerbation of COPD

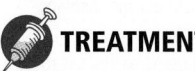 TREATMENT

INITIAL STABILIZATION
- Outpatient: Lung collapse <30%, no dyspnea, no signs of tension pneumothorax, no underlying lung disease
- Inpatient: If >30% collapse, tension pneumothorax, or underlying lung disease
- Tension pneumothorax is a medical emergency. Decompress as soon as possible.

GENERAL MEASURES
- Outpatient: Bed rest
- Inpatient
  – Monitor BP, pulse rate, respirations.
  – Institute oxygen at high concentration; it may accelerate rate of absorption.
  – Treat any underlying condition.
- Serial radiographs to document improvement
- Open pneumothorax: Place dressing over wound. Secure only on 3 sides to avoid tension pneumothorax.

Activity
- Bed rest until chest and lung have re-expanded
- No air travel until radiographs are normal
- Athletes with pneumothorax may return to sports activity after 2–3 weeks of rest as symptoms permit; athletes who require inpatient care should have a follow-up CXR before resuming sport activity.
- A 25% pneumothorax takes ~20 days to reabsorb spontaneously

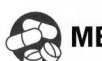 MEDICATION (DRUGS)

- Pleurodesis for recurrent pneumothorax
  – Intrapleural doxycycline: 5 mg/kg in a total volume of 50 mL. Intrapleural doxycycline therapy is painful, so premedicate patient with short-acting benzodiazepine and give 4 mg/kg lidocaine in a total volume of 50 mL intrapleurally before doxycycline is injected.
  – Intrapleural talc: 5 g in 250 mL isotonic saline; talc more effective than tetracycline derivatives, but safety concerns exist.

- Contraindications: If patient is a possible candidate for future lung transplant, do not try sclerosing pleurodesis (sclerosing agents increase risk of bleeding at surgery, making patients ineligible for transplant).
- Precautions
  – Procedure has precipitated respiratory distress syndrome in 2 reports.
  – Pain at time of intrapleural instillation and postprocedure is the most common side effect. Premedicate patient with benzodiazepine and/or narcotic.
- Significant possible interactions: Refer to the manufacturer's literature.

SURGERY
- Simple aspiration: 1st step for primary spontaneous pneumothorax unless unstable. Insert 16 F cannula into 2nd anterior intercostal space at midclavicular line and attach a 3-way stopcock and 60-mL syringe. Withdraw air manually until no more can be aspirated. Close stopcock and repeat chest radiograph after 4 hours. Remove if lung re-expanded. Observe patient 2 more hours.
- Thoracostomy tube (16–22 F): Usually 1st step for secondary spontaneous pneumothorax. Insert in 4ht, 5th, or 6th intercostal pace at midaxillary line and connect underwater seal. Clamp after 12 hours if no bubbles have appeared.
- Tension pneumothorax: Immediate decompression. Insert 19 F or larger needle into the 2nd intercostal space at midclavicular line over superior aspect of rib to avoid vessels, and attach a 3-way stopcock. Use a large syringe to withdraw air. Follow with a chest tube.
- Recurrent pneumothorax (more often occurs with larger pneumothoraces)
  – Consider chemical pleurodesis
  – Consider thoracoscopy or video-assisted thoracoscopy (VAT) following
    ○ 2 or more spontaneous pneumothoraces
    ○ If lungs not expanded after 7 days
    ○ Persistent bronchopleural fistula
  – Consider surgical correction for occupation or avocation that would put person at risk if pneumothorax recurs (e.g., pilot, diver).
  – Open thoracotomy in patients who fail the VAT procedure
- The mini-drain is a satisfactory option in patients with uncomplicated pneumothorax, but cases with pleural fluid should be avoided.

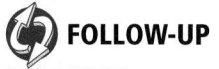 FOLLOW-UP

PROGNOSIS
- Air is reabsorbed from small spontaneous pneumothorax in a few days.
- Air is reabsorbed from larger air space in 2–4 weeks.
- Risk of recurrence is 30–50%.

COMPLICATIONS
- Re-expansion pulmonary edema following suction
- Bronchopleural fistulae requiring repair
- Surgery indicated following 2 spontaneous pneumothoraces on the same side
- Myocardial infarction
- Respiratory arrest

PATIENT MONITORING
- Outpatient management should include follow-up CXR to document resolution of pneumothorax, typically in several days.
- Blood pressure, respiratory rate, arterial blood gases, for hospitalized patients
- After simple aspiration: Clamp chest tube for 24 hours, then remove if no recurrence on radiograph. If lung is not fully re-expanded after 7 days, consider persistent air leak/bronchopleural fistula.

REFERENCES
1. Baumann MH. Management of spontaneous pneumothorax. *Clin Chest Med*. 2006;27:369–381.
2. Henry M, Arnold T, Harvey JE. BTS guidelines for the management of spontaneous pneumothorax. *Thorax*. 2003;58(Suppl II):39–52.
3. De Lassence A, Timsit JF, Tafflet M. et al. Pneumothorax in the intensive care unit: Incidence, risk factors and outcomes. *Anesthesiology*. 2006;104(1):5–13.

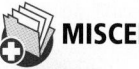 MISCELLANEOUS

 CODES

ICD9-CM
- 512.0 Spontaneous tension pneumothorax
- 512.1 Iatrogenic pneumothorax
- 512.8 Other spontaneous pneumothorax

PATIENT TEACHING
Counsel patient to stop smoking

See Corresponding Diagnostic Algorithm

POLIOMYELITIS

Omar A. Khan, MD, MHS

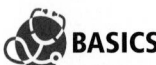 **BASICS**

DESCRIPTION

- Poliomyelitis describes the acute illness: The majority of patients contracting the poliovirus are asymptomatic; ~5% develop symptoms, and 0.1% develop the paralytic form of poliomyelitis.
- Symptomatic cases may present with diarrhea.
- A subset will develop neurologic disease.
- Illness is biphasic; paralysis occurs in 2nd phase. Paralytic disease occurs with rapid onset.
- Spread by direct fecal-oral contact; more common in warm months.
- Virus secreted for weeks in stool.
  - Poliomyelitis syndromes: Encephalitic; bulbar (which produces cranial nerve paralysis), spinal (causing weakness in the extremities, particularly the legs).
  - Post-polio syndrome (PPS) is a distinct entity, affecting those previously diagnosed with poliomyelitis. Involves atrophy of muscle groups unaffected by original illness.
- System(s) Affected: Nervous; Musculoskeletal
- Synonym(s): Infantile paralysis; Acute anterior poliomyelitis; Acute lateral poliomyelitis

ALERT

Geriatric Considerations
Extremely rare; primary vaccination not recommended (except if travel to endemic areas)

Pediatric Considerations
Most common in this age group. Infection is extremely rare in the US since introduction of effective vaccines (see also "Immunizations").

Pregnancy Considerations
A risk factor for developing polio (incidence and severity of polio are increased in pregnant women)

GENERAL PREVENTION

- Poliovirus vaccination via the inactivated poliovirus vaccine (IPV) is recommended in the US and other developed settings. Oral poliovirus vaccine (OPV) is administered in countries considered to be endemic or at-risk for polio.
- The U.S. vaccination schedule calls for IPV to be administered 4 times: At ages 2, 4, between 6 and 18 months and 4–6 years of age.
- In developing countries, safe water treatment to avoid contaminated water and food sources is preventive.

EPIDEMIOLOGY

- 3 months–16 years; rarely adults
- Predominant sex: Male = Female
- PPS can manifest years to decades after initial infection

Incidence
Now rare; present in (a) endemic settings, (b) small outbreaks in areas where polio eradication has occurred and, (c) rarely as vaccine-associated paralytic polio (VAPP) cases.

Prevalence
- 1,593 cases in 2006; 1,486 cases in 2005.
- Endemic countries: Afghanistan, India, Nigeria and Pakistan

RISK FACTORS

- Poor sanitation and hygiene
- Poverty
- Unimmunized status, especially if <5 years

Genetics
No genetic susceptibility has been identified.

PATHOPHYSIOLOGY

- Poliovirus initially infects the gastrointestinal tract. It may spread to lymph nodes and rarely to central nervous system.
- Pharyngeal spread is less common, but is the prevalent mode of transmission in areas of good hygiene.
- Person-to-person spread is the most common means of transmission, followed by contaminated water and sewage.

ETIOLOGY

- 3 serotypes of poliovirus (genus *Enterovirus*)
- Type 1 most frequently associated with epidemics; Types 2 and 3 usually associated with vaccine-associated paralytic polio (VAPP)

ASSOCIATED CONDITIONS

- Intramuscular injections or trauma during the prodrome of paralytic polio can precipitate paralysis.
- Tonsillectomy is considered a risk factor for bulbar paralysis.

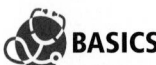 **DIAGNOSIS**

PRE HOSPITAL

- Isolation of virus from samples of stool, oral secretions or CSF
- Antibody response useful for ruling out rather than ruling in polio, since immunization also may provoke such a response.

SIGNS AND SYMPTOMS

- Although the majority of polio infection is asymptomatic, ~10% will show signs and symptoms of a minor gastrointestinal illness, including fever, malaise, nausea, and vomiting.
- A minority of these cases will progress to the major illness, which includes asymmetric paralysis of extremities (usually lower).
- Aseptic meningitis occurs in a minority of cases with the major illness.

History
- Factors relating to poor hygiene, fecal-oral transmission risk, and unvaccinated status
- If the affected person is from a nonendemic country, travel history is important.

Physical Exam
- Significant motor loss on affected side or limb
- Meningeal signs may be present in minor illness or early phases of paralytic polio.
- Decreases deep tendon reflexes
- Muscle atrophy affected areas

TESTS
Spinal fluid and pharynx virus isolation (early in disease) and/or feces (early and late in disease)

Lab
- Increased CSF protein
- Lymphocytosis, especially of CSF
- Normal CSF glucose
- Serology
- Virus culture from stool or pharynx

Imaging
MRI may be helpful to evaluate involvement of anterior horn of the spinal cord or other findings.

Diagnostic Procedures/Surgery
- Electromyelogram may be useful to assess progress of paralysis and of PPS.
- Viral culture of cerebrospinal fluid, stool, and pharyngeal secretions

Pathological Findings
Spinal cord: Perivascular cuffing, abnormal motor nuclei, chromatolysis of motor neurons, intermediate & posterior column inflammation

DIFFERENTIAL DIAGNOSIS

- For acute flaccid paralysis and paralytic polio
  - Guillain-Barré syndrome
  - Transverse myelitis
  - Acute motor axonal neuropathy ("China paralytic syndrome")
  - Traumatic neuritis
  - Myasthenia gravis
  - Polymyositis
  - Periodic paralysis
  - Trichinosis
  - Aseptic, bacterial and tuberculous meningitis/encephalitis
  - Toxic encephalopathies
  - Tick paralysis
- For nonparalytic acute polio infection
  - Enteroviruses, echoviruses, and coxsackievirus

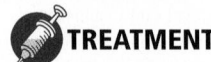 **TREATMENT**

The European Federation of Neurological Societies (EFNS) has guidelines on PPS describing muscular training, targeted physical therapy, and assistive devices as needed.

INITIAL STABILIZATION
Inpatient for acute phase or if concern for respiratory/bulbar paralysis exists; outpatient or rehabilitation facility for therapy.

GENERAL MEASURES
- Mechanical ventilation, if required
- Public health: With all suspected cases, report immediately to local health authority such as public health department (in the US) or WHO affiliate in developing countries.
- Any case of polio is considered an emergency

Diet
May require tube feedings if paralysed.

Activity
Bed rest during active phase of disease

Nursing

The main concerns relate to mobilization to regain function, assurance of hygiene if bowel/bladder are incontinent, appropriate skin care if mobility is severely restricted, and pain control in case of contractures.

- Provide bed that has firm mattress, footboard, foam rubber pads, or sandbags. Change patient's positions frequently. Ensure good skin care.
- Management of fecal impaction and urinary retention. Catheterization may be necessary.
- Hot, moist packs

Physical Therapy

- Early physical therapy in acute paralytic polio may help child regain function and develop adaptations.
- With paralysis (acute or post-polio), extended physical therapy may be required.
- Long-term rehabilitation plan: Using physical therapy, braces, special shoes, possibly orthopedic surgery; team effort with doctors, physical and occupational therapists, and social worker or psychiatrist, if necessary

 ## MEDICATION (DRUGS)

- Aspirin or other nonnarcotic analgesics
- Antibiotics, if intercurrent infection develops
- Parasympathomimetic pharmacotherapy (e.g., bethanechol) for urinary retention, 10–50 mg PO b.i.d.–q.i.d. Up to 100 mg q.i.d. may be required.
- Preliminary investigations suggest IV immunoglobulin (IVIG) may improve quality of life for PPS patients.
- Small studies on lamotrigine, modafinil, amantadine, and pyridostigmine suggest benefit but no conclusive evidence is available to recommend this as therapy.
- Contraindications and precautions: Refer to the manufacturer's literature.
- Significant possible interactions: Refer to the manufacturer's literature.

SURGERY

- Tracheostomy for respiratory paralysis.
- Surgery may be required in the case of muscle contractures or to relieve severe deformity resulting from muscle atrophy and paralysis.

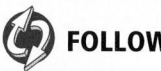 ## FOLLOW-UP

DISPOSITION

- Physical therapy is essential in paralytic polio.
- Counseling for the patient, caregivers, and family is useful in managing lifetime sequelae.

Admission Criteria

- New-onset neurologic symptoms such as stiff neck, seizures, paralysis
- Once diagnosed, cases of paralytic polio may need admission to observe for bulbar paralysis.
- Surgical admissions for sequelae of polio or PPS
- Dehydration resulting from the minor illness

Discharge Criteria

- In case of minor illness, self-limited resolution
- In case of major illness, criteria include a plan for outpatient follow-up by the family physician, specialist, and physical therapist.

Issues for Referral

- Referral to a neurologist is indicated in the case of major illness.
- Infectious disease referral is warranted at the time of diagnosis.
- After discharge, referral to physical therapy, neurology, or physical medicine and rehabilitation is indicated, especially for PPS.
- Psychiatry or clinical psychology referral can be helpful for patient and caregivers.

PROGNOSIS

- Often irreversible paralysis; <5% mortality during acute disease
- Increased mortality in patients >40 years
- Poor recovery for totally paralyzed muscle groups; good recovery for partially paralyzed muscle groups
- Variable recovery for PPS; can be facilitated with appropriate physical therapy

COMPLICATIONS

- Urinary tract infection
- Skin ulcers
- Traumatic injuries to affected limb(s)
- Atelectasis
- Pneumonia
- Myocarditis
- Postpoliomyelitis progressive muscular atrophy: Progressive weakness 30 years or more after an attack of poliomyelitis. Adult survivors of childhood polio now suffer late complications.
- Postpoliomyelitis motor neuron disease: Occurs years after acute poliomyelitis; less common than postpoliomyelitis progressive muscular atrophy.
- Vaccine-associated paralytic poliomyelitis is a rare complication of oral poliovirus vaccine.

REFERENCES

1. Aylward RB. Poliomyelitis. In Heymann DL (ed). Control of Communicable Diseases Manual. Washington, DC: APHA Press, 2004.
2. Farbu E, Gilhus N, Barnes M, et al. EFNS guideline on diagnosis and management of post-polio syndrome. Eur J Neurol. 2006;13:795–801.
3. Gonzalez H, Stibrant S, Sjoberg I, et al. Intravenous immunoglobulin for post-polio syndrome: A randomised controlled trial. Lancet Neurol. 2006;5(6):493–500.

ADDITIONAL READING

- Oshinsky DM. Polio: An American Story. Oxford University Press, 2006.
- Brookes T, Khan OA. The End of Polio? APHA Press, 2006.
- Seytre B, Shaffer M. The death of a Disease: A History of the Eradication of Poliomyelitis. Rutgers University Press, 2005.

 ## MISCELLANEOUS

Wild-type polio no longer exists in the US. Polio remains in wild-type strains in 4 countries in Asia and Africa. The WHO has a goal to eradicate the disease by the end of 2006.

 CODES

ICD9-CM
045.1 Acute poliomyelitis

ICD10
A80 Poliomyelitis

PATIENT TEACHING

For patient education materials favorably reviewed on this topic, contact

- International Polio Network, 4502 Maryland Avenue, St. Louis, MO 63108; (314) 361-0475
- Educational presentation on polio from the CDC: http://www.cdc.gov/nip/ed/slides/polio8p.ppt
- PPS patient materials via Post-Polio Health International: http://www.post-polio.org/
- The Global Polio Eradication Initiative, coordinated by the WHO: www.polioeradication.org
- CDC FAQ on Polio: http://www.cdc.gov/nip/vaccine/Polio/polio-faqs-hcp.htm
- WHO information on global polio eradication: http://www.polioeradication.org/features/qa/def_questions.asp#questions

POLYARTERITIS NODOSA

Eric P. Gall, MD

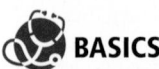 **BASICS**

DESCRIPTION

Polyarteritis nodosa presents pathologically as an ongoing segmental inflammatory, necrotizing vasculitis response within the media of small and medium-sized muscular arteries

- Organ involvement: Kidney, gastrointestinal (GI) tract, skin, muscles, joints, genitourinary tract, peripheral and central nervous systems, heart, testes, epididymis, and ovaries
- 1 of the vasculitic syndromes that vary in involvement from mild, self-limited skin lesions to severe systemic isolated and combined multiorgan dysfunction and death
- Although heterogeneity and overlap manifestations abound, polyarteritis nodosa is classified as a systemic necrotizing vasculitis.
- System(s) Affected: Cardiovascular; GI; Musculoskeletal; Nervous; Renal/Urologic; Skin/Exocrine
- Synonym(s): Periarteritis; Panarteritis; Necrotizing arteritis

ALERT
Pregnancy Considerations
One case report suggests that if a patient attains remission before becoming pregnant, the chance of successful delivery remains reasonable.

EPIDEMIOLOGY
- Predominant age: All ages, children through older people. Mean age is 50 years.
- Predominant sex: Male > Female (2.5:1)

Incidence
917/100,000

RISK FACTORS
Genetics
Unknown

ETIOLOGY
Unclear. Evidence suggests immunologic involvement
- Endothelial COH antibodies
- Antineutrophilic cytoplasmic antibody
- Tissue deposition of immune complexes
- Hepatitis B antigenemia in 30% of cases
- Hepatitis B antigen in circulating immune complexes
- Hepatitis B antigen, complement, and IgM demonstrated in vascular walls
- Hepatitis C association

ASSOCIATED CONDITIONS
- Churg-Strauss syndrome
- Benign cutaneous periarteritis nodosa (bears watching and investigating because not necessarily benign)
- Hepatitis B
- Hepatitis C

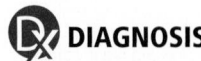 **DIAGNOSIS**

SIGNS AND SYMPTOMS (1–3)
- General (often nonspecific): Multisystemic involvement
  - Fever
  - Weakness
  - Weight loss
  - Malaise
  - Myalgia
  - Livedo reticularis
  - Headache
  - Abdominal pain and vague discomfort
- Related to organ system involved (may dominate clinical picture and course)
  - Renal: Hypertension, hematuria (usually microscopic), proteinuria, progressive renal failure
  - Musculoskeletal: Myalgia, migratory arthralgia, and arthritis
  - Skin: Purpura, urticaria, SC hemorrhages, polymorphic rashes, SC nodules (uncommon but characteristic), persistent livedo reticularis and Raynaud phenomenon (rare)
  - GI: Recurrent and severe pain, hepatomegaly, nausea, vomiting, and bleeding; cholecystitis, acute abdomen
  - Lung: Hilar adenopathy, patchy infiltrates, reticular or nodular lesions, often fleeting
  - CNS: Seizures, cerebrovascular stroke, headache, papillitis, altered mental states
  - Peripheral nervous system: Mononeuritis multiplex
  - Cardiac: Pericarditis, CHF associated with hypertension and/or myocardial infarction
  - Genitourinary: Usually asymptomatic but may have testicular, epididymal, ovarian pain. Neurogenic bladder reported, glomerulonephritis

TESTS (1–3)
Lab
- Nonspecific
  - Abnormal urine sediment
  - Rheumatoid factor
  - Endothelial cell antibodies
  - High neutrophil count
  - Eosinophilia rare, suggests granulomatous involvement when present
  - Anemia of chronic disease
  - Elevated sedimentation rate and C-reactive protein
  - Hypergammaglobulinemia
  - Hepatitis B surface antigen positive in 10–50% of cases (strong circumstantial evidence)
  - Hepatitis C antibody or hepatitis C virus RNA
- Specific
  - Mainly based on pathologic findings of biopsy material from involved organs
  - Necrotizing arteritis
  - Careful examinations of biopsies from acute abdomen, especially in males between the 2nd and 4th decades
  - Antineutrophil cytoplasm antibodies; rare
  - Drugs that may alter lab results: Corticosteroids, cytotoxic agents
  - Disorders that may alter lab results: Allergic reactions and other immunologic disorders

Imaging
Angiography: Mesenteric artery aneurysm, renal aneurysm, hepatic aneurysm, intestinal aneurysm

Diagnostic Procedures/Surgery
- Angiographic demonstration of aneurysmal changes of small and medium-sized arteries involving renal hepatic and mesenteric arteries represents strong evidence supporting the diagnosis.
- Arterial or organ biopsy

Pathological Findings
- Necrotizing inflammation with fibrinoid necrosis, in various stages, of small and medium muscular arteries. Segmental in distribution, it is often seen at bifurcations and branchings. Involvement of venules not seen in classic polyarteritis nodosa.
- Acute lesions show infiltration of polymorphonuclear cells through vessel wall and perivascular area
- Subsequent proliferation, degeneration, appearance of monocytes, necrosis with thrombosis, and infarction of the involved tissue. Aneurysmal dilatations are characteristic.
- Aortic dissection reported attributed to necrotizing vasculitis of the vasa vasorum
- Peripheral nerves positive 50–70%
- GI vessels 50% (at autopsy)
- Gallbladder and appendix 10%
- Muscle vessels 50%
- Testicular vasculature often positive when males are symptomatic

DIFFERENTIAL DIAGNOSIS

- Systemic lupus erythematosus
- Multiple sclerosis
- Atrial myxoma
- Dissecting aneurysm
- Cryoglobulinemia
- Subacute endocarditis
- Trichinosis
- Some rickettsial diseases
- Microscopic polyangiitis
- Other vasculitis
- The key differences from other necrotizing vasculitides are lack of granuloma formation and sparing of veins and pulmonary arteries.

 ## TREATMENT

INITIAL STABILIZATION
Depends on extent and involvement of specific organs

GENERAL MEASURES
Same as those needed for patients in treatment with steroids (e.g., high risk of infection), cytotoxic agents, and plasmapheresis. Biologic agents are under study.

Diet
Low salt if patient has attendant hypertension

Activity
As tolerated

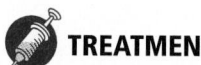 ## MEDICATION (DRUGS)

First Line
- Favorable results reported with prednisone and cyclophosphamide. Reports differ as to the benefits of adding plasmapheresis.
- Other immunosuppressive agents: Azathioprine (Imuran)
- Plasma exchange (efficacy not established)
- High-dose IV pulse steroids
- Hepatitis B vaccine may be considered for the amelioration of any subsequent development of life-threatening complications of hepatitis B virus–associated polyarteritis nodosa.
- Contraindications: Refer to the manufacturer's profile of each drug.
- Precautions: Refer to the manufacturer's profile of each drug.
- Significant possible interactions: Refer to the manufacturer's profile of each drug.

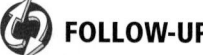 ## FOLLOW-UP

PROGNOSIS (4)
- Expected course of untreated polyarteritis nodosa is poor.
- 5-year survival rate: 13%
- Steroid and cytotoxic therapy treatment may increase percentage of survival rate significantly. (5,6)
- Renal and GI signs are most serious prognostic factors
- Patients with microscopic polyangiitis have worse prognosis

COMPLICATIONS
- Glomerulonephritis
- Renal failure
- Thrombosis
- Infarction
- Tissue/organ necrosis
- Stroke
- Myocardial infarct
- Mononeuritis multiplex

PATIENT MONITORING
- Complete blood chemistry, urinalysis, and renal and hepatic profiles
- Careful monitoring for infection
- Delayed appearance of neoplasms
- Angiographic changes may improve rapidly with combination steroid/cyclophosphamide therapy.
- Acute phase reactants such as interleukin-6 and C-reactive protein may be useful in diagnosis and monitoring activity level during treatment and follow-up.

REFERENCES

1. Braunwald E, et al., eds. *Harrison's Principles of Internal Medicine*. 15th ed. New York, NY: McGraw-Hill; 2001.
2. Goldman L, Bennett JC, eds. *Cecil Textbook of Medicine*. 21st ed. Philadelphia, PA: WB Saunders; 2001.
3. Soto O, Conn DL. Polyarteritis nodosa and microscopic polyangiitis. In: Hochberg MC, et al., eds. *Rheumatology*. 3rd ed. St. Louis, MO: Mosby; 2003:1611–1621.
4. Bourgarit A, et al. Deaths occurring during the first year after treatment onset for Poyarteritis nodosua, microscopic poyangiitis, & Churg-Strauss syndrome: A retrospective analysis of causes & factors predictive of mortality based on 595 patients. *Medicine*. 2005;84:323.
5. Gayraud M, et al., and the French Vasculitis Study Group. Long-term followup of polyarteritis nodosa, microscopic polyangiitis, and Churg-Strauss syndrome: Analysis of four prospective trials including 278 patients. *Arthritis Rheum*. 2001;44:666–675.
6. Guillevin L, et al. Prognostic factors in polyarteritis nodosa and Churg-Strauss syndrome. A prospective study in 342 patients. *Medicine (Baltimore)*. 1996;75:17–28.
7. Garanger TA, et al. Anti-neutrophil cytoplasmic antibodies in patients with the American College of Rheumatology criteria for pain. *Autoimmunity*. 1995;20:33–37.
8. Lightfoot RW Jr, et al. The American College of Rheumatology 1990 criteria for the classification of polyarteritis nodosa. *Arthritis Rheum*. 1990; 33:1088–1093.
9. Iino T, et al. Polyarteritis nodosa. *J Rheumatol*. 1992;19:1632–1636.
10. Nakayama H. Distinct response interleukin-6 and other laboratory parameters to treatment in a patient with polyarteritis nodosa. *Angiology*. 1992;43:512–516.

ADDITIONAL READING

Jennette JC, Falk RJ. Small vessel vasculitis. *N Engl J Med*. 1997;337:1512–1523.

 ## MISCELLANEOUS

See also: Hepatitis B; Hepatitis C

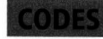 **CODES**

ICD9-CM
446.0 Polyarteritis nodosa

PATIENT TEACHING

Advise patient materials are available from Arthritis Foundation, 1314 Spring St, N.W., Atlanta, GA 30309; (800) 283-7800.

POLYCYSTIC KIDNEY DISEASE (PKD)

Eric Nelson, MD
Leonard G. Gomella, MD

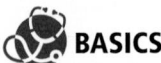 **BASICS**

DESCRIPTION

There are 15 cystic diseases of the kidney, with the primary distinction between genetic and nongenetic disease. Polycystic kidney disease is in the genetic disease spectrum and further subdivided into Autosomal Recessive ("Infantile") Polycystic Kidney Disease (ARPKD) and Autosomal Dominant ("Adult") Polycystic Kidney Disease (ADPKD) and are characterized by bilateral renal cyst development and account for 5–10% of patients with end stage renal disease (ESRD).

- System(s) Affected: Renal/Urologic; Cardiovascular; Hepatobilliary

ALERT

Geriatric Considerations
Renal insufficiency affects 50% of patients by age 70; accounts for 5–10% of patients receiving dialysis

Pregnancy Considerations
Higher frequency of new onset hypertension than in women without polycystic kidney disease. No adverse effect on the course of the polycystic kidney disease in asymptomatic patients. Patients with hypertension, proteinuria, or renal insufficiency are at increased risk of complications

Pediatric Considerations
Most often ARPKD; usually diagnosed in neonates, but sometimes in adolescents and young adults. Most severe forms of disease are seen earliest in life. All patients have varying degrees of congenital hepatic fibrosis.

GENERAL PREVENTION
Genetic counseling

EPIDEMIOLOGY
- Predominant age: Most cases identified between 30–50 years of age in ADPKD; ARPKD is most severe earliest in life, and 50% newborns die in first few hours or days of life. If not apparent at birth, will usually be diagnosed before age 13. All subjects will eventually manifest disease if they live long enough.
- Predominant sex: Male = Female

Incidence
ARPKD affects 1/40,000 live births; ADPKD affects 1/500–1/1,000 live births. Found on all continents and in all races.

Prevalence
Prevalence in US: ~600,000

RISK FACTORS
- Dialysis
- A more rapid clinical course increased by hypertension, renal hemorrhage, multiple pregnancies, male gender, PKD1 disease genotype

Genetics
- ARPKD
  - Autosomal recessive inheritance
  - Siblings have 1:4 chance of being affected
  - Genetic defect on chromosome 6

- ADPKD
  - Autosomal dominant inheritance
  - 50% of children of an affected adult affected
  - 100% penetrance; genetic imprinting and genetic anticipation seen as well
  - 2 genes isolated: PKD1 on chromosome 16 (85–90% of cases); PKD2 on chromosome 4 (5–10% of cases); there is a presumed PKD3, although not yet identified

PATHOPHYSIOLOGY
- 5 theories for etiology of cyst development
  - Defect in basement membrane of renal tubules
  - Epithelial hyperplasia leads to obstruction and weakening of the tubular wall
  - Defect in protein of extracellular connective tissue matrix
  - Apical position of Sodium-Potassium ATP-ase in cystic epithelium rather than basal position
  - Abnormality in ciliary structure or function
- Expansion of cysts mediated by epidermal growth factor (EGF), and patients with ADPKD are unusually responsive to the stimulus of EGF

ETIOLOGY
- Inherited autosomal dominant abnormality linked to chromosome 16. 90% penetrance by age 90 in gene carriers. A 2nd gene on chromosome 4 recently identified. Rare autosomal recessive form exists in neonates. Children of affected people have a 50% chance of acquiring disease. Can be detected in amniocentesis.
- Acquired polycystic kidney disease: Found in 50% of patients on dialysis >3 years

ASSOCIATED CONDITIONS
- Cerebral aneurysms in 10–40% of patients
- Colonic diverticula in 80%
- Liver cysts in approximately 50%
- Pancreatic and ovarian cysts
- Mitral valve prolapse in 26%

DIAGNOSIS

SIGNS AND SYMPTOMS
- Flank pain
- Hypertension (principle form of presentation and seen in up to 80% of patients)
- Increased abdominal girth
- Kidney stones (30%)
- Renal colic (secondary to clots or stone)
- Microscopic or gross hematuria (50% of patients); presenting symptom in 19–35%; caused by rupture of cyst into pelvis of kidney, stones, infections, or tumor
- Neonates: Stillbirth, respiratory distress in severe disease
- Nocturia
- Urinary tract infection (UTI) (usually women)/pyelonephritis

- ARPKD
  - The earlier the disease identified, the more severe the disease
  - All patients have liver involvement (hepatic fibrosis +/− biliary ectasia and periportal fibrosis)
  - Usually enormous flank masses
  - Oligohydramnios, Potter's facies, limb deformities
- ADPKD specific
  - Hepatic cysts and fibrosis
  - Berry aneurysms (10–40%)
  - Intracranial hemorrhages
  - Mitral valve prolapse
  - Colonic diverticulosis

TESTS

Lab
- Hematocrit level: Elevated in 5% of cases
- Urinalysis: May confirm hematuria and mild proteinuria
- Serum creatinine level: May be elevated
- Kidney stones: Usually calcium oxalate

Imaging
- 85% of patients can be detected by age 25.
- ARPKD
  - Ultrasound
    - Can make diagnosis with in utero ultrasound
    - Enlarged, homogeneously hyperechogenic kidneys, especially when compared with the liver; may have no apparent macrocysts
    - Hyperechogenic renal pyramids
  - CT: Is more sensitive if diagnosis is in doubt
  - IV urography: May see radial or medullary streaking (sunburst pattern); persist for 48 hours after the study
- ADPKD
  - Ultrasound
    - Bilateral cysts (echo-free areas) as well as cysts in other organs
    - Sometimes appears similar to ARPKD
  - IV urography
    - Usually see bilateral renal enlargement, calyceal and collecting system distortion, and a bubble or Swiss cheese appearance in the nephrogram phase
    - Calyces may be stretched by cysts
    - Medullary streaking of contrast (see above)
  - CT
    - Useful when ultrasonography equivocal
    - Helpful in identifying cysts in other organs
    - Can diagnose hemorrhage within cysts (higher density: 50–90 Hounsfield units)
    - Valuable for prognosis for renal function
  - MRI
    - Useful with compromised renal function
    - T2 weighted especially sensitive for small cysts and early stages of disease
  - Presumptive diagnosis can be made with evidence of bilateral renal cysts, and 2 of the following criteria
    - Bilateral renal enlargement
    - >2 hepatic cysts
    - Cerebral aneurysm
    - Solitary cyst of the arachnoid, pineal gland, pancreas, or spleen

Diagnostic Procedures/Surgery
- Genetic evaluation and linkage studies appropriate if ARPKD/ADPKD suspected
- Children of parents with ADPKD should be examined by ultrasound

Pathological Findings
- Kidneys are diffusely cystic and, although enlarged, retain their general shape
- Renal cysts range from a few millimeters to a few centimeters
- Cysts appear throughout cortex and medulla
- Papillae and pyramids become less distinguishable as disease progresses
- 1 kidney may be larger than the other
- Cysts originate from renal tubules and are less differentiated as disease progresses
- Will see arteriosclerosis in patients with worsening renal function

DIFFERENTIAL DIAGNOSIS
- Genetic
  - Juvenile nephronophthisis (medullary cystic disease complex)
  - Juvenile nephronophthisis (autosomal recessive)
  - Medullary cystic disease (autosomal dominant)
  - Congenital nephrosis (familial nephritic syndrome) (autosomal recessive)
  - Familial hypoplastic glomerulocystic disease (autosomal dominant)
  - Multiple malformation syndromes with renal cysts (e.g., tuberous sclerosis, von Hippel-Lindau disease)
- Nongenetic
  - Simple cysts
  - Multicystic dysplastic kidney
  - Benign multilocular cyst (cystic nephroma)
  - Medullary sponge kidney
  - Sporadic glomerulocystic kidney disease
  - Acquired renal cystic disease
  - Calyceal diverticulum (pyelogenic cyst)

TREATMENT

INITIAL STABILIZATION
Outpatient except for cases involving complicating emergencies (infected cysts require 2 weeks IV antibiotics, then long-term oral antibiotics)

GENERAL MEASURES
- Outpatient except for complicating emergencies (e.g., infected cysts)
- Hypertension: Moderate sodium restriction, weight control, and regular exercise
- Medications: Angiotensin converting enzyme (ACE) inhibitors; angiotensin receptor blocker. Diuretics are helpful for hypertension and stones, but cause hypokalemia, which can increase cyst growth and development.
- Pain: Narcotics and other analgesics; bed rest; limit NSAIDs (worsen renal function). Chronic pain: Transcutaneous opiate patches, perinephric injections of local anesthetics, transcutaneous nerve stimulation, hypnotherapy, and transcendental meditation.
- Urolithiasis: Treated with alkalinization of urine and hydration therapy; surgery as needed

- UTIs/Infections of cysts lipid-soluble antibiotics more effective (e.g., trimethoprim-sulfamethoxazole and chloramphenicol); fluoroquinalones also useful
- Dialysis for end-stage renal disease patients
- Hematuria: Reduced physical activity or bedrest; desmopressin acetate and aprotinin may be of benefit in controlling severe bleeding. Transcatheter arterial infarction for recurrent hemorrhage.

Diet
Low-protein diet may retard renal insufficiency

Activity
None in early stages of the disease; avoid vigorous activity if disease advanced. Recurrent gross hematuria is secondary to trauma associated with faster decline of renal function.

SPECIAL THERAPY
Complementary and Alternative Medicine
See "General Measures: Pain."

 ## MEDICATION (DRUGS)

First Line
- No drug therapy available for polycystic kidney disease
- Hypertension: ACE inhibitors; avoid diuretics (possible adverse effects with cyst formation)
- An EGF-tyrosine kinase inhibitor is now in Phase I and II clinical trials.
- Chemotherapeutic agents have been used experimentally in mice.

SURGERY
- Indications for surgical intervention
  - Uncontrollable hypertension
  - Severe back and loin pain, abdominal fullness
  - Renal deterioration due to enlarging cysts
  - Hematuria/hemorrhage or recurrent UTI
- Open and laparascopic cyst unroofing: May decrease pain and narcotics requirements; has not been proven to prevent renal failure or to prolong current renal function
- Percutaneous cyst aspiration +/− injection of sclerosing agent: Not usually performed secondary to recurrent fluid accumulation
- Renal transplant for ESRD

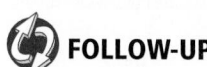 ## FOLLOW-UP

Monitoring of BP and renal function

DISPOSITION
Admission Criteria
Severe pain, gross hematuria with clots

Issues for Referral
- Nephrologist primary management
- Urologic consultation for management of symptomatic/infected cysts
- Genetic counseling is critical.

PROGNOSIS
- Slowly progressive
- Renal failure in 2% by age 40 years, 23% by age 50, 48% by age 73
- ADPKD accounts for 10–15% of dialysis patients
- Patients with PKD2 mutations have slower progression of disease and longer life expectancy. If patient has both PKD1 and PKD2 mutations, more severe clinical course seen.
- Incidence of renal cell carcinoma no higher than general population

COMPLICATIONS
- Cyst rupture, infection or hemorrhage
- Progression to renal failure
- Renal calculi

PATIENT MONITORING
- Avoid nephrotoxic drugs.
- Creatinine and blood pressure monitoring at least twice a year; more often as needed

REFERENCES
1. Brenner BM. *Brenner & Rector's The Kidney*, 7th ed. 2004. Elsevier. 1745–1757.
2. Ketan BK, et al. Autosomal dominant polycystic kidney disease and pain—A review of the disease from aetiology, evaluation, past surgical treatment options to current practice. *Journal of Postgraduate Medicine*. 2004;50(3):222–226.
3. Wilson, PD. Mechanisms of disease: Polycystic kidney disease. *N Eng J Med*. 2004.350(2); 151–164.

 ## MISCELLANEOUS

See also: Renal Calculi; Renal Failure; Chronic

CODES
ICD9-CM
- 753.12 Polycystic kidney, unspecified type
- 753.13 Polycystic kidney, autosomal dominant
- 753.14 Polycystic kidney, autosomal recessive

PATIENT TEACHING
- http://kidney.niddk.nih.gov: A kidney disease site sponsored by the NIH
- http://patients.uptodate.com: The patient version of the well-respected *UpTodate* database
- Avoid contact sports
- For women, UTI frequency can be decreased by tub baths rather than showers, frequent voiding, voiding immediately after intercourse, good perineal hygiene

 See Corresponding Diagnostic Algorithm

POLYCYSTIC OVARIAN DISEASE (PCOD)

Nicholas J. Spirtos, DO

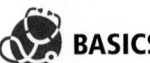 **BASICS**

DESCRIPTION
PCOD is characterized by a state of chronic oligo-ovulation alone or combined with anovulation that culminates in either oligomenorrhea or amenorrhea.

- System(s) Affected: Reproductive; Endocrine/Metabolic; Skin/Exocrine
- Synonym(s): Stein-Leventhal syndrome; Polycystic ovary syndrome

ALERT
- Condition may begin at puberty.
- Pregnancy does not resolve the syndrome.

GENERAL PREVENTION
Avoid endometrial and breast carcinoma.

EPIDEMIOLOGY
- Predominant age: Reproductive age
- Predominant sex: Females only

Prevalence
Premenopausal females: 6%

RISK FACTORS
- Endometrial hyperplasia
- Endometrial carcinoma
- Obesity
- Hypertension
- Diabetes mellitus
- Breast cancer
- Infertility

Genetics
Probably transmitted genetically, especially if associated with 21-hydroxylase deficiency or that of other enzymes

ETIOLOGY
Disruption of hypothalamic-pituitary-ovarian axis (high-normal luteinizing hormone (LH) and low-normal follicle-stimulating hormone (FSH) leading to ovarian hyperandrogenism and follicular atresia and anovulation) or secondary to increased levels of insulin or increased sensitivity to normal levels of insulin

ASSOCIATED CONDITIONS
- Obesity
- Hypertension
- Endometrial hyperplasia and/or carcinoma
- Breast carcinoma
- Diabetes mellitus
- Hyperandrogenism, insulin resistance, acanthosis nigricans (HAIRAN) syndrome
- Infertility
- Hyperthecosis

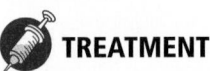 **DIAGNOSIS**

SIGNS AND SYMPTOMS
- Amenorrhea
- Oligomenorrhea
- Obesity
- Hirsutism
- Acne
- Dysfunctional uterine bleeding
- Infertility
- Acanthosis nigricans
- Hypertension
- Virilism
- Enlarged ovaries
- Enlarged clitoris
- Deep voice
- Seborrhea

History
Take complete patient history.

Physical Exam
Conduct physical exam.

TESTS
Lab
- LH/FSH level $\geq$ 2.5–3.0/1
- Testosterone increased, but < 200 ng/dL (6.94 nmol/L)
- Dehydroepiandrosterone sulfate level increased, but < 800 μg/dL (20.8 μmol/L)
- Dehydroepiandrosterone level increased
- 17-OH progesterone level increased
- Estrone level increased
- Androstenedione level increased
- Sex hormone binding globulin level decreased
- Prolactin level increased slightly
- Increased fasting insulin levels and possibly elevation in fasting glucose; plasminogen activator inhibitor-1
- Drugs that may alter lab results
  - Oral contraceptives
  - Steroids
  - Antidepressants

Imaging
Pelvic ultrasound revealing enlarged ovaries with multiple small follicular cysts

Diagnostic Procedures/Surgery
- Fasting serum glucose, insulin level, and plasminogen level to rule out insulin resistance and glucose intolerance
- Overnight dexamethasone suppression test (Decadron 1 mg PO at 11:00 p.m. and fasting serum cortisol at 8:00 a.m. the next morning) to rule out Cushing syndrome
- Endometrial biopsy to rule out hyperplasia and/or carcinoma

Pathological Findings
- Ovary usually enlarged with a smooth white glistening capsule
- Ovarian cortex lined with follicles in all stages of development but most atretic
- Thecal cell proliferation with an increase in the stromal compartment

DIFFERENTIAL DIAGNOSIS
- Cushing syndrome
- HAIRAN syndrome
- Testosterone-producing ovarian or adrenal tumor
- Prolactin-producing pituitary adenoma
- Hyperthecosis
- Adult-onset adrenal hyperplasia
- Partial congenital adrenal hyperplasia (21-hydroxylase deficiency)
- Endometrial hyperplasia
- Endometrial carcinoma
- 11 β-hydroxylase deficiency
- 17β-hydroxysteroid dehydrogenase deficiency
- Acromegaly
- Drug-induced hirsutism, oligo-ovulation (e.g., danazol, steroids)

TREATMENT

INITIAL STABILIZATION
- Outpatient
- Inpatient, if surgery for wedge resection has been recommended (rare).
- Laser drilling, which is controversial because it may cause adhesions.

GENERAL MEASURES
No ideal treatment exists. Therapy must be individualized according to the needs and desires of each patient.

Diet
Regular diet, but recommend weight loss if the patient is overweight.

Activity
Full activity

MEDICATION (DRUGS)

First Line
- Drug costs related to this condition are high.
- If pregnancy not desired
  - Cyclic withdrawal bleeding with medroxyprogesterone (Provera) 10 mg PO for 12–14 days per month *or*
  - Low-dose oral contraceptives
- If pregnancy desired
  - Ovulation induction with clomiphene (Clomid, Serophene) *or*
  - Human menopausal gonadotropins: Menotropins (Pergonal, Humegon, Repronex) *or*
  - Pure FSH (Follistim, Gonal-F) with or without the addition of gonadotropin-releasing hormone (GnRH) agonist: Leuprolide (Lupron) or nafarelin (Synarel), or in a combination with GnRH antagonist: Cetrorelix (Cetrotide) or ganirelix (Antagon)
  - Metformin (Glucophage): 500–2,000 mg PO daily has been shown to improve hyperandrogenism and restore ovulation. Use from cycle Day 1 and stop with ovulation. Many times the drug is continued throughout the 1st trimester or the entire pregnancy if there is a history of spontaneous abortion or glucose intolerance. Refer to a perinatologist for opinion in high-risk patient.
- Contraindications: None, but if using oral contraceptive agents to prevent sequelae of anovulation, be aware of contraindications.
- Precautions
  - Risk of multiple fetuses with clomiphene citrate is 8%.
  - Risk of multiple fetuses with human menopausal gonadotropin, FSH is 25%.
  - Risk of severe ovarian hyperstimulation syndrome is <1%.
  - Diarrhea and gastrointestinal symptoms occur with metformin.
  - Check liver function monthly with troglitazone
- Significant possible interactions: Refer to the manufacturer's profile of each drug.

Second Line
- Bromocriptine if prolactin level is elevated
- Prednisone or dexamethasone (Decadron) if dehydro epiardrosterone sulfate level is elevated

SURGERY
Ovarian wedge resection and laparoscopic laser drilling are controversial and rarely used today.

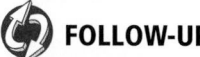 **FOLLOW-UP**

PROGNOSIS
- Prognosis for fertility is excellent depending on other fertility factors.
- Proper treatment and follow-up of chronic anovulation can prevent endometrial hyperplasia or carcinoma.

COMPLICATIONS
- Multiple pregnancies
- Ovarian hyperstimulation syndrome
- Oral contraceptives are not taken without risk.

PATIENT MONITORING
- Counsel patient about the risk of endometrial and breast carcinoma, insulin resistance, and diabetes, as well as obesity and its role in infertility.
- See patient frequently throughout the menstrual cycle, depending on which drug combination is used to induce ovulation.
- Make patient aware that costs of monitoring are high.

REFERENCES
1. Danforth DM, et al., eds. *Obstetrics and Gynecology*. 9th ed. Philadelphia, PA: Lippincott Williams & Wilkins; 2003.

 MISCELLANEOUS

- See also: Amenorrhea; Fertility Problems

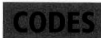 CODES

ICD9-CM
- 256.4 Polycystic ovaries
- 628.0 Female infertility associated with anovulation

PATIENT TEACHING

 See Corresponding Diagnostic Algorithm

 See Patient Handout on CD

POLYCYTHEMIA VERA

Rimini Varghese, MD

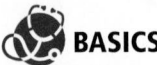 **BASICS**

DESCRIPTION

- Clonal cell hematologic malignant disorder hallmarked by increased red cell mass with excessive erythroid, myeloid, and megakaryocytic elements in the bone marrow
- One of a group of myeloproliferative disorders
- System(s) Affected: Hemic/Lymphatic/Immunologic
- Synonym(s): Primary polycythemia; Vaquez disease; Polycythemia, splenomegalic; Vaquez-Osler disease

GENERAL PREVENTION

No known preventive measures

EPIDEMIOLOGY

Incidence

- Predominant age: Middle to late years; mean is 60 years (range 15–90)
- Predominant sex: Male > Female (slightly)

Prevalence

Incidence/prevalence in US: 1.9/100,000 person years (3)

RISK FACTORS

- Ashkenazi Jewish ancestry (may have increased frequency)
- Familial history (rare)

Genetics

JAK2 V617F (tyrosine kinase) mutation has recently been identified in multiple studies to be strongly associated with PV with possible causal influence. (4,5)[A]

ETIOLOGY

Unknown; all 3 hematopoietic cell lines originate in a single clone.

ASSOCIATED CONDITIONS

- May present as thrombosis in any organ, as in Budd-Chiari syndrome
- Mesenteric artery thrombosis
- Myocardial infarction (MI)
- CVA
- DVT/PE

DIAGNOSIS

SIGNS AND SYMPTOMS

- Early stages may produce no symptoms.
- Erythromelalgia
- Pathognomonic
- Burning pain of feet or hands, occasionally with erythema, pallor, cyanosis, or acral paresthesias
- Headaches
- Tinnitus
- Vertigo
- Blurred vision
- Epistaxis
- Increased blood viscosity
- Spontaneous bruising
- Upper gastrointestinal (GI) bleeding
- Peptic ulcer disease
- Arterial and venous occlusive events
- Pruritus
- Sweating
- Weight loss
- Plethora (face, hands, feet)
- Splenomegaly
- Hepatomegaly
- Hyperhistaminemia
- Bone pain (ribs and sternum)
- Bone tenderness (ribs and sternum)

TESTS

- Bone marrow aspiration (red cell hyperplasia, panmyelosis, clustering/clumping of pleomorphic megakaryocytes, absent iron stores, no pronounced inflammatory reaction)
  – Cytogenetic testing (JAK2 V617F)
- Biopsy: Fibrosis during spent phase of the disease (characterized by increased presence of reticulin)

Lab

- PV Study Group (PVSG) (1960s) major (A) and minor criteria (B)
  – A1: Increased RBC mass: Female ≥32 mL/kg, male ≥36 mL/kg
  – A2: Normal arterial oxygen saturation (≥92%)
  – A3: Splenomegaly
  – B1: Thrombocytosis platelet count >400,000/L
  – B2: Leukocytosis >12,000/L
  – B3: Leukocyte alkaline phosphatase increased
  – B4: Increased serum vitamin B_{12} or increased unsaturated vitamin B_{12} binding capacity
- PVSG diagnosis acceptable with following combinations
  – A1 + A2 + A3
  – A1 + A2 + any 2 from B category (splenomegaly absent in ~25% of patients)
- Recent advances have prompted development of other diagnostic models, namely the discovery of JAK2 V617 and improved assays for EPO measurement.

- Other clinical and pathologic characteristics that support the diagnosis as described in European Clinical and Path (ECP) Criteria + WHO Bone Marrow Criteria
  – Clinical
    ○ Generally RCM is optional when Hb>18.5/ >16.5g/dL male/female HCT>51/>48% male/female
    ○ Early of latent stage PV HCT: 0.45–0.51 male and 0.43–0.48 female
    ○ Platelet-mediated microvascular ischemic, thrombotic complications
    ○ Typical PV signs and symptoms of hypervolemia
    ○ Itching, fatigue, upper abdominal pain
    ○ Absence of any secondary cause of erythrocytosis
  – Pathologic
    ○ BM pathology (see "Tests")
    ○ BM Biopsy: Spontaneous endogenous erythroid colony (EEC) formation
- Some authors feel that diagnosis can be reliably made based on clinical symptoms, presence of JAK2 V617 mutation and low EPO. (6)[B]
- Other lab findings
  – Hyperuricemia
  – Hypercholesterolemia
  – Elevated blood histamine level
- Drugs that may alter lab results: Diuretics may cause a spurious polycythemia.
- Disorders that may alter lab results: Excessive use of alcohol or tobacco

Imaging

CT splenomegaly (if not palpable)

Diagnostic Procedures/Surgery

Bone marrow aspiration and biopsy

Pathological Findings

- Plethoric congestion in all organs and tissues
- Major vessels contain thick, viscous blood.
- Sinuses of spleen packed with RBCs

DIFFERENTIAL DIAGNOSIS

- Secondary polycythemias
- Hemoglobinopathy
- Spurious polycythemia

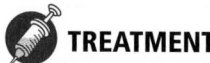

TREATMENT

Outpatient

GENERAL MEASURES
- Individualized management necessary
- Dependent on many factors: Age, disease duration, disease phenotype, complications, disease activity
- Currently, phlebotomy is the mainstay of therapy. Beyond that, differences exist among authorities about use and effectiveness of myelosuppressives.
- Phlebotomy
  - To reduce hematocrit to ~45%
  - Performed as often as every 2–3 days until normal hematocrit reached. Phlebotomies of 250–500 m/L. Reduce to 250–350 m/L in elderly patients or patients with cardiovascular disease.
  - Concomitant therapy possibilities; for example, some form of myelosuppression, radioactive phosphorus (in elderly patients), hydroxyurea
  - Phlebotomy repeated as necessary for maintenance
  - If patient cannot tolerate phlebotomy, then chemotherapy (hydroxyurea is the least mutagenic agent) or radiation therapy
- Other therapy
  - Maintain hydration.
  - Pruritus therapy
  - Manage thrombotic or hemorrhagic complications the same as with nonpolycythemic patient.
  - Uric acid reduction therapy

Diet
Avoid iron supplements

Activity
No restrictions

MEDICATION (DRUGS)

First Line
- Myelosuppression

  - Low-dose aspirin (81 mg PO) has been demonstrated in 1 study to reduce the risk of thrombotic events without increasing bleeding complications when used in conjunction with phlebotomy. (7)[B]

  - Hydroxyurea if unable to maintain on phlebotomy alone or if at high risk for thrombosis (start 15–20 mg/kg/d)
  - Radioactive phosphorous in selected cases when life expectancy <10 years given mutagenic potential
  - Note: Refer to hematologist/oncologist for further dosing and instructions.
- Symptomatic/adjunctive
  - Allopurinol: 300 mg/d PO for uric acid reduction
  - Cyproheptadine: 4–16 mg PO as needed for pruritus
  - H₂-receptor blockers or antacids for GI hyperacidity; cimetidine is also used for pruritus
  - Other pruritus therapy: Interferon-α and, most recently, SSRIs have shown some efficacy in controlling pruritus in setting of PV. (8)[B]

Second Line
- Myelosuppression: Chlorambucil; some authors believe contraindicated.
- Interferon-α may be an effective alternative to present forms of treatment and is under investigation.

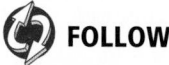

FOLLOW-UP

PROGNOSIS
Currently, survival is >9 years with treatment.

COMPLICATIONS
- Uric acid stones
- Secondary gout
- Vascular thromboses (major cause of death)
- Transformation to leukemia
- Transformation to myelofibrosis
- Hemorrhage
- Peptic ulcer
- Increased risk for complications and mortality from surgery procedures. Assess risk–benefits and ensure optimal control of disorder before any elective surgery.

PATIENT MONITORING
- Frequent monitoring during early treatment until satisfactory hematocrit is reached
- Monitor hematocrit often and phlebotomize when needed.

REFERENCES

1. Beutler E, et al., eds. *Williams Hematology*, 6th ed. New York: McGraw-Hill, 2000.
2. Conley CL. Polycythemia vera, diagnosis and treatment. *Hosp Practice*. 1987;22:107.
3. Ania BJ, Suman VJ, Sobell JL, et al. Trends in the incidence of polycythemia vera among Olmsted county, Minnesota residents, 1935–1989. *Am J Hematol*. 1994;47:89.
4. James C, Ugo V, Le Couedic JP, et al. A unique clonal JAK2 mutation leading to constitutive signalling causes polycythaemia vera. *Nature*. 2005;434:1144.
5. Michiels JJ, De Raeve H, Berneman Z, et al. The 2001 World Health Organization and updated European clinical and pathological criteria for the diagnosis, classification, and staging of the Philadelphia chromosome-negative chronic myeloproliferative disorders. *Semin Thromb Hemost*. 2006;32:307.
6. Tefferi A. The diagnosis of polycythemia vera: New tests and old dictums. *Best Prac Res Clin Haematol*. 2006;19:455.
7. Landolfi R, Marchioli R, Kutti J, et al. Efficacy and safety of low-dose aspirin in polycythemia vera. *N Engl J Med*. 2004;350:114.
8. Tefferi A, Fonseca R. Selective serotonin reuptake inhibitors are effective in the treatment of polycythemia vera-associated pruritus. *Blood*. 2002;99:2627.

MISCELLANEOUS

See also: Myeloproliferative disorders

CODES

ICD9-CM
238.4 Polycythemia vera

PATIENT TEACHING
- Stress importance of lifelong maintenance.
- Alert patients to complications to watch for.

 See Corresponding Diagnostic Algorithm

POLYMYALGIA RHEUMATICA

Eric P. Gall, MD

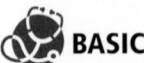

BASICS

DESCRIPTION
Clinical syndrome characterized by aching and stiffness of the shoulder and hip girdle muscles affecting older patients, associated with an elevated erythrocyte sedimentation rate, lasting >1 month, and responsive to low-dose steroids

- System(s) Affected: Hemic/Lymphatic/Immunologic; Musculoskeletal
- Synonym(s): Senile rheumatic disease; Forestier-Certonciny syndrome; Polymyalgia rheumatica syndrome; Rhizomelic pseudoarthrosis

ALERT
Geriatric Considerations
Incidence increases with age.

Pediatric Considerations
Does not occur in this age group

EPIDEMIOLOGY
Incidence (1)
- Predominant age: 60 years or older. Incidence increases with age (rare <50 years old).
- Predominant sex: Female > Male (2:1)

Prevalence
Approximate US prevalence: 50/100,000 patients >50 years

RISK FACTORS
- Age >50 years
- Presence of giant-cell arteritis

Genetics
Associated with human leukocyte antigen determinants

ETIOLOGY
Unknown

ASSOCIATED CONDITIONS
- Giant-cell arteritis
- Temporal arteritis

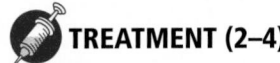

DIAGNOSIS (2–4)

SIGNS AND SYMPTOMS
- Onset—abrupt or insidious
- Pain and stiffness at shoulder and hip girdle
- Usually symmetrical
- Symptoms more common in the morning
- Gel phenomena (stiffness after prolonged inactivity)
- Constitutional symptoms—fatigue, malaise, depression, weight loss, low-grade fever
- Arthralgias/arthritis (noninflammatory)
- No weakness (pain may limit strength)
- Muscle tenderness mild to moderate
- No muscle atrophy
- Decreased range-of-motion (ROM) of joints usually because of pain
- May have signs and symptoms of giant-cell arteritis (seen in 15% of patients)
- Mild synovitis, hands and wrists

TESTS (2)
Temporal artery biopsy if symptoms of giant-cell arteritis

Lab
- Erythrocyte sedimentation rate (Westergren) elevation >50
  - Westergren erythrocyte sedimentation rate is the preferred laboratory technique. If other types of erythrocyte sedimentation rate studies are used (e.g., Wintrobe), the guidelines for abnormal levels are different.
- Anemia—normochromic/normocytic
- Creatine phosphokinase—normal
- Rheumatoid factor—negative (5–10% patients age >60 years will have positive rheumatoid factor without rheumatoid arthritis [RA])
- Mild elevations in liver function tests
- Drugs that may alter lab results: Prednisone
- Disorders that may alter lab results: Disorders causing acute phase reactants can elevate erythrocyte sedimentation rate (e.g., infection, neoplasm, renal failure).

Diagnostic Procedures/Surgery
In patients with symptoms suggesting giant-cell arteritis, a temporal artery biopsy may be indicated.

Pathological Findings
- Muscle biopsy: Either none or type II fiber atrophy without inflammation
- Mild nonspecific synovitis

DIFFERENTIAL DIAGNOSIS
- RA
- Other connective tissue disease
- Fibromyalgia
- Giant-cell arteritis
- Depression
- polymyositis-dermatomyositis (check creatine phosphokinase, aldolase)
- Thyroid disease
- Viral myalgia
- Osteoarthritis
- Occult infection
- Occult malignancy (extensive search usually not necessary)
- Myopathy (steroid, alcohol, electrolyte depletion)

TREATMENT (2–4)

INITIAL STABILIZATION
Outpatient

GENERAL MEASURES
Physical therapy for ROM exercises if necessary

Diet
- Adequate calcium (1,500 mg/d) and electrolyte intake
- Regular diet

Activity
Do not exercise excessively to cause exertion.

MEDICATION (DRUGS) (2,5)

First Line
Prednisone

- 10 mg/d PO initially (average initial effective dose 10–15 mg/d) (5)
- Usually dramatic (diagnostic) response
- May increase to 20 mg if no immediate response
- Begin slow taper at 4–6 weeks by only 1 mg every 1–4 weeks to a dose of 5–7.5 mg. (5) Continue at this dose for 18 months to 2 years, if no recurrence of symptoms.
- After 18–24 months of treatment, attempt to taper by 1 mg every 2–4 weeks until drug discontinued. Patient may, however, require steroids for ≥3 years.
- Increase prednisone for recurrence of symptoms (relapse common).
- Contraindications
  - Use steroids with caution in patients with chronic heart failure, diabetes mellitus, systemic fungal or bacterial infection
  - Must treat infections concurrently if steroids are absolutely necessary.
- Precautions
  - Long-term steroid use associated with several significant adverse effects, including sodium and water retention, exacerbation of chronic heart failure, hypokalemia, increased susceptibility to infection, osteoporosis, cataracts, avascular necrosis
  - Patients may develop temporal arteritis while on low-dose corticosteroid treatment for polymyalgia. This requires immediate increase in dose to 60 mg.
  - Alternate-day steroids not effective
- Significant possible interactions: Refer to the manufacturer's literature.

Second Line
NSAIDs have been used; rarely successful.

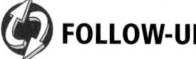 **FOLLOW-UP**

PROGNOSIS
- Average length disease is 3 years (range 1–10 years)
- Exacerbation if steroids tapered too fast
- Prognosis very good if treated (may gradually remit even if no treatment)
- Relapse common

COMPLICATIONS
- Medication—complications related to steroid use
- Disease—exacerbation of disease with taper of steroids; development of giant-cell arteritis (may occur when polymyalgia rheumatica is being adequately treated)

PATIENT MONITORING (2–4)
- Follow monthly initially and during taper of medication, every 3 months otherwise.
- Follow erythrocyte sedimentation rate as steroids tapered.
- Follow up with patient for symptoms of giant-cell arteritis. Educate patient to report such symptoms immediately (e.g., headache, visual and neurologic)

REFERENCES

1. Cimmino, MA, Zaccaria, An epidemiology of polymyalgia rheumatica. *Clin Ecp Rheum*. 2000;18:S9.
2. Hellman, DB, Hunder GG. Chapter 82: Giant cell arteritis and polymyalgia rheumatica. In: Harris ED, Budd, RC, Firestein, GS, et al, eds. *Textbook of Rheumatology*. 7th ed. Philadelphia, PA: WB Saunders; 2005:1343–1356.
3. Hazelman BL. Polymyalgia rheumatica and giant cell arteritis. In: Hochberg MC, Silman AJ, Smolen JS, et al, eds. *Rheumatology*. 3rd ed. Edinburgh, U.K.: Mosby; 2003:1623–1633.
4. Weyland CM, Goronzy JJ. Polymyalgia rheumatica and giant cell arteritis. In: Koopman WJ, ed. *Arthritis and Allied Disorders*. 14th ed. Philadelphia, PA: Lippincott Williams & Wilkins; 2001.
5. Kremers HM, Reinalda MS, Crawson CS, et al. Relapse in population based cohort of patients with polymyalgia rheumatica. *J Rheumatol*. 2005;32:65.

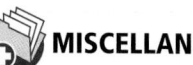 **MISCELLANEOUS**

See also: Arthritis, osteo; Arthritis, rheumatoid; Depression; Fibromyalgia; Giant-cell arteritis; polymyositis-dermatomyositis

CODES

ICD9-CM
725 Polymyalgia rheumatica

PATIENT TEACHING
- Precautions regarding steroid use
- Instruct the patient about symptoms of giant-cell arteritis and to report them immediately.
- For a listing of sources for patient education materials favorably reviewed on this topic, physicians may contact: American Academy of Family Physicians Foundation, P.O. Box 8418, Kansas City, MO 64114; (800) 274-2237, ext. 4400
- Excellent materials also available from Arthritis Foundation, http://www.arthritis.org/

POLYMYOSITIS/DERMATOMYOSITIS

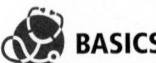

Christopher M. Wise, MD

BASICS

DESCRIPTION
Systemic connective tissue disease characterized by inflammatory and degenerative changes in proximal muscles, sometimes accompanied by characteristic skin rash

- If skin manifestations (Grotton Sign: Symmetric, scaly, violaceous erythematous eruption over the extensor surfaces of the metacarpophalangeal and interphalangeal joints of the fingers; Heliotrope: Reddish-violaceous eruption on the upper eyelids), are present, it is designated as dermatomyositis.
- Different types of myositis include
  - Idiopathic polymyositis
  - Idiopathic dermatomyositis
  - Polymyositis/dermatomyositis as an overlap
  - HIV-associated myopathy
  - Primary idiopathic dermatomyositis
  - Primary polymyositis
- System(s) Affected: Cardiovascular; Musculoskeletal; Pulmonary; Skin/Exocrine
- Synonym(s): Myositis

ALERT
Geriatric Considerations
Elderly patients with myositis or dermatomyositis at increased risk of neoplasm

Pediatric Considerations
Childhood dermatomyositis likely a separate entity, associated with cutaneous vasculitis and muscle calcifications

EPIDEMIOLOGY
- Predominant age: 5–15 years, 40–60 years, peak incidence in mid-40s
- Predominant sex: Female > Male (2:1)

Incidence
Estimated at 0.5–0.8/100,000

Prevalence
1–2 patients 100,000

RISK FACTORS
Family history of autoimmune disease or vasculitis

Genetics
Mild association with human leukocyte antigen (HLA) DR3, HLA-DRw52

ETIOLOGY
Unknown; potential factors
- Inciting viral infection
- T-cell activation
- Cytokine release
- Immune-mediate muscle destruction
- Human T-cell lymphocytotrophic virus I

ASSOCIATED CONDITIONS
- Malignancy (in 15–25%)
- Progressive systemic sclerosis
- Vasculitis
- Systemic lupus erythematosus

DIAGNOSIS

SIGNS AND SYMPTOMS
- Symmetrical proximal muscle weakness causing difficulty
  - Arising from sitting or lying positions
  - Kneeling
  - Climbing stairs
  - Descending stairs
  - Raising arms
- Joint pain/swelling
- Dysphagia
- Respiratory impairment
- Decreased deep tendon reflexes of proximal muscle groups
- Muscle swelling, stiffness, induration
- Rash over face (eyelids, nasolabial folds), upper chest, dorsal hands (especially knuckle pads), fingers ("mechanic's hands")
- Periorbital edema
- Calcinosis cutis (childhood cases)
- Mesenteric arterial insufficiency/infarction (childhood cases)
- Cardiac impairment; arrhythmia, failure

TESTS
Special tests
- ECG: Arrhythmias, conduction disturbances
- Electromyography: Muscle irritability, low-amplitude potentials, polyphasic action potentials, fibrillations
- Muscle biopsy (deltoid or quadriceps femoris)

Lab
- Increased creatine kinase
- Increased aldolase
- Increased serum glutamic-oxaloacetic transaminase/aspartate aminotransferase
- Increased lactate dehydrogenase
- Myoglobinuria
- Increased erythrocyte sedimentation rate
- Positive rheumatoid factor (<50% of patients)
- Positive antinuclear antibody (>50% of patients)
- Leukocytosis (<50% of patients)
- Anemia (<50% of patients)
- Hyperglobulinemia (<50% of patients)
- Increased creatinine (<50% of patients)
- Myositis-specific antibodies have been described in a minority of patients
  - Anti-Jo-1 is the most common and has been found in <20% of patients.
  - Associated with an increased incidence of interstitial lung disease
- Disorders that may alter lab results: Liver disease and hemolysis may cause increased serum glutamic-oxaloacetic transaminase/aspartate aminotransferase, lactate dehydrogenase. Creatine phosphokinase (CPK) and aldolase elevated in other myopathies

Imaging
- Chest radiograph: Interstitial disease
- MRI to assess muscle edema and inflammation

Diagnostic Procedures/Surgery
- Diagnosis usually relies on four findings (1,2)[C]
  - Weakness
  - Creatine phosphokinase elevation
  - Abnormal electromyogram
  - Findings on muscle biopsy
- Presence of skin rash of dermatomyositis

Pathological Findings
- Microscopic findings
  - Muscle fiber degeneration
  - Phagocytosis of muscle debris
  - Perifascicular muscle fiber atrophy
  - Inflammatory cell infiltrates in adult form
  - Via electron microscopy—inclusion bodies (inclusion body myositis only)
  - Sarcoplasmic basophilia
- Muscle fiber increased in size
- Vasculopathy (childhood polymyositis/dermatomyositis)

DIFFERENTIAL DIAGNOSIS
- Vasculitis
- Progressive systemic sclerosis
- Systemic lupus erythematosus
- Rheumatoid arthritis
- Muscular dystrophy
- Eaton-Lambert syndrome
- Sarcoidosis
- Amyotrophic lateral sclerosis
- Endocrine disorders
  - Thyroid disease
  - Cushing syndrome
- Infectious myositis (viral, bacterial, parasitic)
- Drug-induced myopathies
  - Cholesterol-lowering agents
  - Colchicine
  - Corticosteroids
  - Ethanol
  - Chloroquine
  - Zidovudine
- Electrolyte disorders (magnesium, calcium, potassium)
- Heritable metabolic myopathies

TREATMENT

Outpatient

GENERAL MEASURES
- Search for malignancy in all adults.
- Follow serum muscle enzymes carefully.

Diet
No special diet

Activity
Curtailed until after inflammation subsides

Physical Therapy
Range-of-motion exercises to prevent contractures

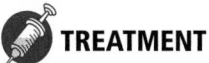 **MEDICATION (DRUGS)**

- Contraindications
  - Refer to the manufacturer's literature.
  - Methotrexate contraindicated with previous liver disease, alcohol use, pregnancy
- Precautions
  - Prednisone: Adverse effects associated with long-term steroid use include adrenal suppression, sodium, water retention, hypokalemia, osteoporosis, cataracts, increased susceptibility to infection
  - Azathioprine: Adverse effects include bone marrow suppression, increased liver function tests, increased risk of infection
  - Methotrexate: Adverse effects include stomatitis, bone marrow suppression, pneumonitis, and risk of liver fibrosis and cirrhosis with prolonged use.
- Significant possible interactions: Refer to the manufacturer's literature.

First Line
- Prednisone (3)[B]
  - 40–80 mg/d PO in divided doses
  - Consolidate doses and reduce prednisone slowly when enzyme levels are normal.
  - Probably need to continue 5–10 mg/d for maintenance in most patients
- For steroid-refractory or dependent cases (3)[B]
  - Azathioprine: 1.0 mg/kg PO (arthritis dose) once daily or b.i.d. Maintain at lowest possible dose.
  - Methotrexate: 10–25 mg PO weekly, useful in most steroid-resistant cases
- Rash of dermatomyositis may require topical steroids, oral hydroxychloroquine.

Second Line
- Other immunosuppressant drugs such as cyclophosphamide, chlorambucil, cyclosporine, and mycophenolate can be added to steroids.
- Combination methotrexate and azathioprine may also be useful in refractory cases (3)[B]

 FOLLOW-UP

PROGNOSIS (4)[B]
(Ponyi)
- Residual weakness 30%
- Persistent active disease 20%
- 5-year survival 75%
- Survival worse for women and African Americans, and patients with associated cancer
- Most patients improve with therapy.
- 50% have full recovery.

COMPLICATIONS
- Pneumonia
- Infection
- Myocardial infarction
- Carcinoma (especially breast, lung)
- Severe dysphagia
- Respiratory impairment owing to muscle weakness, interstitial lung disease
- Aspiration pneumonitis
- Steroid myopathy
- Steroid-induced diabetes, hypertension, hypokalemia, osteoporosis

PATIENT MONITORING
- Serial serum muscle enzyme testing
- Any adult should be studied for malignancy.
- Monitor for steroid-induced complications (hypokalemia, hypertension, hyperglycemia).
- Bone densitometry and consideration of calcium, vitamin D, and bisphosphonate therapy
- If azathioprine, methotrexate, or other immunosuppressant is used, appropriate laboratory monitoring should be done periodically (e.g., hematology, liver enzymes, creatinine)

REFERENCES
1. Dalakas MC. Inflammatory disorders of muscle: Progress in polymyositis, dermatomyositis, and inclusion body myositis. *Curr Opin Neurol*. 2004;17:561–567 (C).
2. Mastaglia FL, Phillips BA. Idiopathic inflammatory myopathies: Epidemiology, classificaion, and diagnostic criteria. *Rheum Dis Clin North Am*. 2002;28:723–741 (C).
3. Choy EH, et al. Immunosuppressant and immunomodulatory treatment for dermatomyositis and polymyositis. *Cochrane Database Syst Rev*. 2005;CD003643 (B).
4. Ponyi A, et al. Functional outcome and quality of life in adult patients with idiopathic inflammatory myositis. *Rheumatology (Oxford)*. 2005;44:83–88 (B).

 MISCELLANEOUS

See also: Osteoporosis

CODES

ICD9-CM
- 710.3 Dermatomyositis
- 710.4 Polymyositis

PATIENT TEACHING

Muscular Dystrophy Association, 3561 E. Sunrise Dr., Tucson, AZ 85718; (800) 221-1142
- Avoid caloric excess due to risk of weight gain with steroid therapy
- Avoid alcohol.
- Initial emphasis on range of motion, stretching, avoid resistance or aerobic exercise while muscle inflammation (elevated CPK)
- Once inflammation is controlled, gradual resumption of aerobic exercises

PORPHYRIA

Jeremy Golding, MD

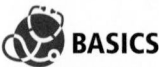 **BASICS**

DESCRIPTION

- Several heme synthesis pathway enzyme deficiencies with overproduction and accumulation of intermediate metabolic products and resultant neuropsychiatric-abdominal or dermatologic symptoms and syndromes
  - Porphyria cutanea tarda: Dermatologic
  - Acute intermittent porphyria: Pyrroloporphyria; neuropsychiatric-abdominal
  - Protoporphyria: Erythropoietic or hepatoerythropoietic; mild dermatologic
  - Variegate porphyria: South African porphyria, prevalence in South Africa is 1/400
  - Hereditary coproporphyria: Neuropsychiatric, occasionally dermatologic
  - Porphobilinogen synthetase deficiency: δ-Aminolevulinic aciduria; neuropsychiatric-abdominal
  - Congenital erythropoietic porphyria: Günther disease; severe dermatologic
  - Other rare genetic variants reported
- System(s) Affected: Gastrointestinal; Skin/Exocrine; Hematologic/Lymphatic/Immunologic; Nervous
- Synonym(s): δ-Aminolevulinic aciduria; Erythropoietic porphyria; Günther disease; Hepatoerythropoietic porphyria; Pyrroloporphyria; South African porphyria

ALERT

Unpredictable disease activity

GENERAL PREVENTION

- Avoid precipitating drugs
  - Alcohol
  - Barbiturates
  - Carbamazepine
  - Chlorpropamide
  - Danazol
  - Ergots
  - Estrogens and progestins
  - Ethchlorvynol
  - Glutethimide
  - Griseofulvin
  - Mephenytoin
  - Meprobamate
  - Methotrexate
  - Methyprylon
  - Metoclopramide
  - Phenytoin
  - Pyrazolones
  - Succinimides
  - Sulfonamide antibiotics
  - Valproic acid
- Eat a diet with high-carbohydrate intake.

EPIDEMIOLOGY

- Predominant age
  - Congenital erythropoietic porphyria: Early childhood
  - Protoporphyria: Older childhood
  - Acute intermittent porphyria, variegate porphyria, hereditary coproporphyria, porphobilinogen synthetase deficiency: Young adult
  - Porphyria cutanea tarda: Middle age
- Predominant sex
  - Protoporphyria, congenital erythropoietic porphyria: Male = Female
  - Porphyria cutanea tarda: Male > Female
  - Acute intermittent porphyria, variegate porphyria, hereditary coproporphyria, porphobilinogen synthetase deficiency: Female > Male

Incidence

- Porphyria cutanea tarda: 1/10,000; most common of the porphyrias in US and Europe
- Acute intermittent porphyria, protoporphyria, variegate porphyria: 1/10,000–100,000
- Hereditary coproporphyria: <1/100,000
- Porphobilinogen synthetase deficiency, congenital erythropoietic porphyria—very rare

Prevalence

All more common in whites than in African Americans or Asians

RISK FACTORS

- Multiple precipitating factors, especially acute intermittent porphyria, variegate porphyria, hereditary coproporphyria
- Drugs (e.g., barbiturates and sulfas in acute intermittent porphyria)
- Estrogens, especially oral contraceptives
- Steroids
- Liver disease
- Menstrual cycles
- Infection
- Fasting
- Heavy alcohol use
- Hexachlorobenzene exposure

Genetics

- Autosomal dominant: Porphyria cutanea tarda (<20% of cases), acute intermittent porphyria, protoporphyria, variegate porphyria, hereditary coproporphyria
- Autosomal recessive: Porphobilinogen synthetase deficiency, congenital erythropoietic porphyria
- Latency common with variable expression, many asymptomatic or minimally symptomatic carriers
- Porphyria cutanea tarda also sporadic and acquired (>80% of cases)
- The pathogenesis of the inherited porphyrias has been defined at the molecular level. It is clear that a great deal of genetic heterogeneity is present in each porphyria.

ETIOLOGY

- Genetic enzyme deficiencies
  - Porphyria cutanea tarda: Uroporphyrinogen decarboxylase
  - Acute intermittent porphyria: Porphobilinogen deaminase
  - Protoporphyria ferrochelatase
  - Variegate porphyria: Protoporphyrinogen oxidase
  - Hereditary coproporphyria: Coproporphyrinogen oxidase
  - Porphobilinogen synthetase deficiency: Porphobilinogen synthetase
  - Congenital erythropoietic porphyria: Uroporphyrinogen III synthetase (cosynthetase)
- Causes of acquired porphyria cutanea tarda:
  - Hepatitis C virus (strong association)
  - Heavy alcohol use
  - Decreased enzyme associated with steroids and hormones
  - Specific exposure to polyhalogenated hydrocarbons (e.g., hexachlorobenzene)
  - Lead poisoning may alter pathways.
  - HIV
  - Possibly ascorbic acid deficiency

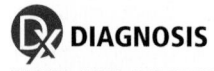 **DIAGNOSIS**

SIGNS AND SYMPTOMS

- All usually reversible, lasting days to weeks
- May be permanent
- Urine may turn dark red or brown on standing (*porphyria* is from the Greek *porphyra*, "purple").
- Abdominal
  - Rather severe abdominal pain, occasionally in back and extremities
  - Generalized more often than localized
  - Often colicky
  - Can mimic acute abdomen
  - Fever not usually present
  - Chronic constipation common
  - Severity of symptoms often out of proportion to physical findings
- Neurologic
  - Essentially any neurologic picture may be seen
  - Includes sensory and motor systems
  - Includes autonomic nervous system
  - May include seizures
  - May lead to quadriplegia and/or respiratory paralysis with death
- Psychiatric
  - Essentially any psychiatric disorder may be mimicked
  - Psychosis most common
  - Visual hallucinations common
  - Disorientation frequent
  - Chronic depression frequent
- Dermatologic
  - Photosensitivity (common)
  - Scrapes, ulcerations, blisters with minimal trauma
  - Hyperpigmentation, especially hands and face
  - Scarring frequent
  - Facial hypertrichosis

- Congenital erythropoietic porphyria (mutilating, with hemolysis, erythrodontia, splenomegaly)
- Protoporphyria (occasional hepatic disease, including hepatic failure)

TESTS
Genetic studies when applicable

Lab
- Urine for porphyrins during acute attack. Urine may be normal at other times.
- Individual enzyme activity in erythrocytes or other body cells/tissues
- Stool for porphyrins in protoporphyria, variegate porphyria, hereditary coproporphyria, congenital erythropoietic porphyria
- Bile for porphyrin in variegate porphyria
- Plasma for fluorescence emission spectroscopy in variegate porphyria
- Saliva for porphyria in porphyria cutanea tarda
- Erythrocyte uroporphyrin in congenital erythropoietic porphyria
- Protoporphyria exception urine unremarkable; test erythrocyte protoporphyrin.
- Ferritin typically elevated in porphyria cutanea tarda due to increased iron stores
- Drugs that may alter lab results: Unknown
- Disorders that may alter lab results:
  - Numerous conditions may cause slight increase in porphyrinuria, but patients are asymptomatic
    ○ Acute liver disease
    ○ Hepatoma
    ○ Hodgkin lymphoma
    ○ Multiple neurologic diseases

DIFFERENTIAL DIAGNOSIS
- Vast and protean
- Pseudoporphyria is a rare syndrome, indistinguishable from porphyria cutanea tarda, owing to some NSAIDs (e.g., nabumetone and naproxen) and flutamide.

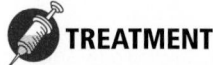 **TREATMENT**

Outpatient, except for crises

GENERAL MEASURES
- Neuropsychiatric-abdominal: Avoid drugs, alcohol, known toxins
- Dermatologic: Shade, protective clothing; avoid skin trauma; porphyria cutanea tarda phlebotomy weekly to monthly may help prevent.
- Congenital erythropoietic porphyria: Consider bone marrow transplantation.

Diet
Neuropsychiatric: Large quantities of carbohydrates have been reported to help.

Activity
Normal, except avoid sun exposure

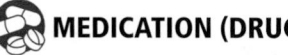 **MEDICATION (DRUGS)**

First Line
- Neuropsychiatric-abdominal
  - IV glucose 400 g/d for 1–2 days
  - Hematin (ferriprotoporphyrin IX, hemin [Panhematin]) IV 1–4 mg/kg/d over 10–15 minutes for 3–14 days
  - Seizures: Consider clonazepam or gabapentin.
  - Depression: Consider selective serotonin reuptake inhibitors.
- Dermatologic: Oral carotenoids (e.g., β-carotene [Solatene], 30 mg, 1–10 capsules per day)
- Contraindications: Known sensitivity to drug
- Precautions: Hematin phlebitis at IV site, reduced clotting ability
- Significant possible interactions: None

Second Line
- Porphyria cutanea tarda
  - Chloroquine 125 mg twice weekly, or hydroxychloroquine 250 mg t.i.d., in conjunction with phlebotomy
  - With hepatitis C virus: Interferon beneficial for both congenital erythropoietic porphyria and plumboporphyria.
  - In vitro gene therapy has been successful.
- Acute intermittent porphyria
  - Luteinizing hormone-releasing hormone (LHRH) analogs being studied
  - Antioxidants ineffective
  - Menstruating women: Hematin premenstrual; cycle suppressors (e.g., LHRH analogues)
  - Autonomic manifestations: β-Blockers
  - Other symptoms: Treat symptomatically

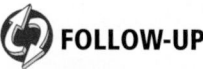 **FOLLOW-UP**

PROGNOSIS
- In all porphyrias
  - Patients who are asymptomatic or minimally symptomatic: Unaffected longevity
  - Patients who are more symptomatic: Treatable and do well
  - Neurologic complications (e.g., peripheral neuropathy, neurosis, or hemiplegia), at times permanent
- In acute intermittent porphyria
  - Acute attacks have 25% mortality.
  - Increased risk of hepatocellular carcinoma
- Acquired porphyria cutanea tarda
  - HIV
  - Hepatitis C virus
  - Hepatic malignancies

REFERENCES
1. Dombeck TA. *Emerg Med Clin North Am.* 2005;23(3):885–899.
2. Goldman. *Cecil Textbook of Medicine,* 22nd ed. Philadelphia: WB Saunders, 2004.
3. Braunwald E, Fauci et al., eds. *Harrison's Principles of Internal Medicine,* 15th ed. New York: McGraw-Hill; 2001:2261–2267.
4. Kelly WN, Dupont HL, eds. *Textbook of Internal Medicine,* 3rd ed. New York: Lippincott-Raven; 1997:880–882.

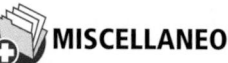 **MISCELLANEOUS**

Some drugs considered safe
- Acetaminophen
- Amiodarone
- Aspirin
- Atropine
- Bromides
- Chlorpromazine
- Diazepam (in small doses)
- Dicumarol
- Digoxin
- Diphenhydramine
- Ether
- Glucocorticoids
- Guanethidine
- Heparin
- Insulin
- Lithium
- Magnesium
- Neostigmine
- Nitrous oxide
- Penicillin and derivatives
- Phenothiazines
- Promethazine
- Narcotic analgesics
- Propranolol
- Streptomycin
- Succinylcholine
- Thiazides

 CODES

ICD9-CM
277.1 Disorders of porphyrin metabolism

PATIENT TEACHING
Porphyria Foundation, P.O. Box 22712, Houston, TX 77227; (713) 266-9617.

PORTAL HYPERTENSION

Venu G. Pillarisetty, MD
Ruben Peralta, MD, FACS

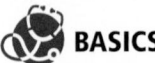 **BASICS**

DESCRIPTION
- Increased portal venous pressure >10 mm Hg that occurs in association with splanchnic vasodilatation, portosystemic collateral formation, and a hyperdynamic circulation.
- Most commonly secondary to elevated hepatic venous pressure gradient (the gradient between the portal and central venous pressures)
- Course is generally progressive, with risk of complications including acute variceal bleeding, encephalopathy, ascites, and hepatorenal syndrome.

ALERT
Geriatric Considerations
Mortality and complication rates are increased.

Pediatric Considerations
Uncommon. Generally etiology is different from adults.

GENERAL PREVENTION
- Abstinence from alcohol
- Adequate and appropriate nutrition

EPIDEMIOLOGY
- Incidence/prevalence in US unknown.
- Predominant age: Adult
- Predominant sex: Male > Female

RISK FACTORS
See "Etiology."

Genetics
No known genetic patterns except those associated with specific hepatic diseases that cause portal hypertension

ETIOLOGY
- Causes generally classified as
  - Prehepatic (portal vein thrombosis or obstruction)
  - Intrahepatic (cirrhosis most common)
  - Posthepatic (right sided heart failure, Budd Chiari syndrome)
- Adult: May be intrahepatic or extrahepatic
  - Cirrhosis accounts for ~85% of cases, may be due to
    - Alcoholism
    - Viral (hepatitis B, hepatitis C, hepatitis D)
    - Wilson disease
    - Hemochromatosis
    - Primary biliary cirrhosis
    - Schistosomiasis
    - May also occur without cirrhosis, as with portal vein thrombosis
- In children, portal vein thrombosis is most common cause; intrahepatic causes are more likely to be biliary atresia, viral hepatitis, metabolic liver disease; extrahepatic causes may be due to congenital anomalies of the portal vein.

ASSOCIATED CONDITIONS
As described under "Signs and Symptoms"

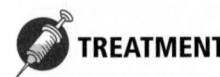 **DIAGNOSIS**

SIGNS AND SYMPTOMS
- May be general or related to specific complications
- General
  - Splenomegaly
  - Caput medusa
  - Umbilical bruit
  - Hemorrhoids
  - Spider angiomata
  - Gynecomastia
  - Testicular atrophy
  - Digital clubbing
  - Palmar erythema
- Gastroesophageal varices
  - Hematemesis
  - Melena
  - Anemia
  - Hypotension
  - Tachycardia
- Ascites
  - Distended abdomen
  - Fluid wave
  - Shifting dullness with percussion.
- Hepatic encephalopathy
  - Confusion
  - Asterixis
  - Hyper-reflexia
- Hepatorenal syndrome
  - Oliguria

TESTS
Specific to underlying disease

Lab
Nonspecific changes associated with underlying disease
- Hypersplenism
  - Anemia (may also be due to malnutrition or bleeding), leukopenia, thrombocytopenia
- Hepatic dysfunction
  - Hypoalbuminemia
  - Hyperbilirubinemia
  - Elevated alkaline phosphatase
  - Elevated liver enzymes
  - Abnormal clotting (PT, PTT)
- Gastrointestinal bleeding
  - Iron-deficiency anemia
  - Elevated serum ammonia
- Hepatorenal syndrome
  - Elevated serum creatinine, blood urea nitrogen
  - Urine Na <5 mEq/L (<20 mmol/L)

Imaging
- Upper GI series may outline varices in esophagus and stomach
- CT scan and ultrasound may detect cirrhosis, splenomegaly, ascites, and varices
- Duplex-Doppler (ultrasound)
  - Can determine presence and direction of flow in portal and hepatic veins
  - Useful in diagnosing portal vein and/or shunt thrombosis
- Angiography
  - Demonstrates corkscrewing of intrahepatic vessels (cirrhosis)
  - Can identify varices and vascular anomalies

Diagnostic Procedures/Surgery
- Endoscopy can diagnose esophageal and gastric varices and portal hypertensive gastropathy or can directly visualize other bleeding sites (peptic ulcers, gastritis, Mallory-Weiss tears)
- Hepatic venous wedge pressure
  - Correlates with portal pressure
  - Risk of variceal bleeding is increased if hepatic venous pressure gradient >12 mm Hg.

Pathological Findings
Specific for underlying disease

DIFFERENTIAL DIAGNOSIS
- Usually related to specific complications/presentations
- Gastroesophageal varices with hemorrhage
  - Portal hypertensive gastropathy
  - Hemorrhagic gastritis
  - Peptic ulcer disease
  - Mallory-Weiss tear
- Ascites
  - Spontaneous bacterial peritonitis
  - Pancreatic ascites
  - Peritoneal carcinomatosis
  - Tuberculous peritonitis
  - Nephrotic syndrome
  - Fluid overload from heart failure
- Hepatic encephalopathy
  - Delirium tremens
  - Intracranial hemorrhage
  - Sedative abuse
  - Uremia
- Hepatorenal syndrome
  - Drug nephrotoxicity
  - Renal tubular necrosis

TREATMENT

GENERAL MEASURES
- If acute variceal bleeding: Type and cross; initial resuscitation with isotonic fluid until PRBCs available. Correct coagulopathy. Endoscopy as soon as the patient is stabilized (for diagnosis and treatment).
- Avoid sedatives, which may precipitate encephalopathy.
- Limit sodium administration; cirrhotic patients avidly retain sodium.

Diet
Restrict sodium and protein.

Activity
Bed rest for acute complications (bleeding, encephalopathy, or hepatorenal syndrome)

MEDICATION (DRUGS)

First Line

- Prophylaxis against variceal bleeding (because 1/3 with known varices will eventually bleed)
  – Nonselective β-blockade (1)[B]
- Therapy for acute variceal hemorrhage
  – Management directed at acute complications as well as longer-term symptom management.
- Therapy for acute variceal hemorrhage: IV vasopressin, somatostatin, or octreotide traditionally used. Terlipressin (Glypressin) is a more selective splanchnic vasoconstrictor and may be associated with fewer complications. (1)[B]
- For prevention of recurrence and for overall reduction of mortality: Propranolol or nadolol reduce portal venous blood inflow by blocking the adrenergic dilatation of mesenteric arterioles.
- Nitrates similarly reduce portal pressures and bleeding rates, and have been show to reduce mortality.
- Therapy for encephalopathy
  – Correct precipitating event: GI Bleed, hypovolemia, electrolyte abnormalities, infection, medication side effect
  – Lactulose: Induces diarrhea and traps intracolonic ammonia
  – Neomycin: Reduces bacterial production of nitrogenous substances in colon
- Therapy for ascites
  – Furosemide (Lasix)
  – Spironolactone

SURGERY

- Liver transplantation considered for patients with advanced disease (2)[B]
- Other less aggressive approaches are available for specific complications of portal hypertension (in addition to or if refractory to medications) (3)[B]
  – Gastroesophageal varices with hemorrhage
    ○ Endoscopic variceal sclerosis or banding: The 1st-line treatment in many cases for acute hemorrhage.
    ○ Portacaval shunting
    ○ Transjugular intrahepatic portosystemic shunt
  – Ascites refractory to medical management:
    ○ Large-volume paracentesis
    ○ Peritoneovenous shunt
    ○ Transjugular intrahepatic portosystemic shunt

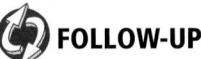 **FOLLOW-UP**

PROGNOSIS

- Hepatic reserve defined by Child-Pugh classification: Rating based on encephalopathy, ascites, bilirubin, albumin, prothrombin
- Variceal bleeding: 50% rebleed, usually within 2 years unless portal pressure is reduced by surgical or transjugular intrahepatic portosystemic shunt procedure
- Ascites and encephalopathy often recurrent

COMPLICATIONS

As described under "Signs and Symptoms"

PATIENT MONITORING

- Acute complications of portal hypertension require intensive monitoring of vital signs and organ function.
- Long-term management includes regular follow-up of all affected organ systems.

REFERENCES

1. Samonakis DN, Triantos CK, Thalheimer U, et al. Management of portal hypertension. *Postgrad Med* 2004;80:634–641.
2. Abraldes JG, Angermayr B, Bosch J. The management of portal hypertension. *Clin Liver Dis* 2005;9:685–713.
3. Wright AS, Rikkers LF. Current management of portal hypertension. *J Gastrointest Surg* 2005;9:992–1005.

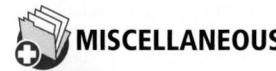 **MISCELLANEOUS**

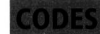 **CODES**

ICD9-CM
572.3 Portal hypertension

POSTCONCUSSIVE SYNDROME

Dana Collaguazo, MD

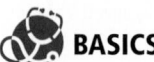 **BASICS**

DESCRIPTION

- Concussion is defined as an acute alteration in mental status that occurs after minor head injury with or without initial loss of consciousness.
- Primary cause is diffuse axonal and small vessel injury resulting from shearing forces caused by rapid deceleration, flexion-extension injury, and rotatory injury. Neuronal injury continues for 6–12 hours secondary to free-radical formation and other factors.
- By definition, these patients have an initial Glasgow Coma Scale rating of 13–15.
- Concussion grading is controversial and changing based on recent research, however, it does give some assistance in guiding return to play (RTP)
- American Academy of Neurology formed the following guidelines (1)[C]
- Concussion grades
  – 1: No loss of consciousness, symptoms <15 minutes
  – 2: No loss of consciousness, symptoms >15 minutes
  – 3: Any loss of consciousness
- System(s) Affected: Nervous

ALERT

Geriatric Considerations
- Slower improvement, prolonged symptoms
- Those >55 years are more likely to have permanent deficits.

Pediatric Considerations
- May have longer recovery
- Should manage with stricter RTP guidelines because almost all reported cases of 2nd impact syndrome are in younger patients (2)[B]

GENERAL PREVENTION
- Seatbelt/helmet use
- No driving under the influence of drugs and alcohol

EPIDEMIOLOGY
- Predominant age: 15–24 years
- Predominant sex: Female > Male

Incidence
Occurs in up to 50% of patients with mild traumatic brain injury

Prevalence
Occurs in 180/100,000 persons, with 27/100,000 being persistent

RISK FACTORS
- People predisposed to falls, motor vehicle collisions (MVC), and mishaps involving drugs and alcohol
- Some association with litigation, female gender, preexisting headaches, and low socioeconomic status

ETIOLOGY
Falls, MVCs, assaults, and other violent incidents

ASSOCIATED CONDITIONS
See "Risk Factors."

DIAGNOSIS

SIGNS AND SYMPTOMS

History
- Report of a fall, MVC, assault, or other violent incident
- Obtain details pertaining to concussion grade (e.g., loss of consciousness, duration of confusion)
- Chronic headache; some may be severe.
- Chronic neck pain
- Dizziness or vertigo
- Poor concentration
- Memory deficits
- Personality changes
- Irritability, depression, anxiety
- Decrease in ability to smell or taste (5%)
- Sleep-wake disturbances
- Other cognitive disturbances

Physical Exam
Positive result to Dix-Hallpike test (nystagmus and/or vertigo induction with certain head motions) in traumatic vestibulopathy

TESTS
Neuropsychological testing may demonstrate subtle abnormalities not otherwise detected; however, none have met criteria supporting a clinical application, and thus should not be part of routine standard of care. (3)[C]

Glascow Coma Score

Best Eye Response (E)
1 No eye opening
2 Eye opening to pain
3 Eye opening to verbal command
4 Eyes open spontaneously

Best Verbal Response (V)
1 No verbal response
2 Incomprehensible words
3 Inappropriate words
4 Confused
5 Oriented

Best Motor Response (M)
1 No motor response
2 Extension to pain
3 Flexion to pain
4 Withdrawal from pain
5 Localizing pain
6 Obeys commands

---

(1) Score on Glasgow Coma Scale with components (e.g., E2V3M4 = GCS 9)
(2) Interpretation: >12 mild brain injury; 9–12 moderate injury; <9 severe injury

Imaging
- CT scan usually produces normal findings.
- MRI may show small petechial hemorrhages or focal cortical contusions.
- Single-photon emission CT may show small areas of focal edema.
- Because rapid diagnosis and treatment of Diffuse Axonal Injury may decrease acute effects of concussion and prevent neurodegenerative diseases; these new modalities hold promise; however, need further study (4)[C]

Pathological Findings
Diffuse axonal injury on postmortem.

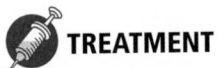 **TREATMENT**

GENERAL MEASURES

Many cases can be handled solely by the patient's primary care physician with involvement of a neurologist and/or psychologist as appropriate.

- Address the patient's symptoms (e.g., neck pain, headaches, depression) using standard measures.
- Involvement of vocational rehabilitation may be necessary.
- Behavioral therapy and similar modalities may be tried.

Diet

As tolerated

Activity

- Sports and other active pursuits should be limited based on degree of injury.
- A 2nd injury may be mild alone, but may have cumulative effects with the 1st and may be fatal.
- Activity limitation guidelines have been designed to minimize the chances of a 2nd impact syndrome phenomenon from occurring. One common set of guidelines, published by the American Academy of Neurology, is below (1)[C]
  - Grade 1 concussion: Athlete removed from sports activity, examined immediately and at 5-minute intervals. Allowed to RTP if symptoms resolve within 15 minutes. If a 2nd Grade 1 concussion occurs on the same day, remove from activity until asymptomatic for 1 week.
  - Grade 2 concussion: Remove from activity and examine frequently, with more extensive diagnostic evaluation if symptoms worsen or persist for >1 week. RTP after asymptomatic for 1 week. If a Grade 2 concussion occurs after having sustained a Grade 1 concussion on the same day, remove from activity until asymptomatic for 2 weeks.
  - Grade 3 concussion: Remove from activity for 1 week without symptoms if loss of consciousness (LOC) brief or 2 weeks without symptoms if LOC prolonged. If patient remains unconscious or if abnormal neurologic signs, transport to nearest emergency department. An athlete with a Grade 3 concussion after a Grade 1, should be removed from activity until asymptomatic for 1 month. If abnormal CT or MRI, remove from activities for the season and discourage from future participation in contact sports.
- National Trainers' Association (2) has made its own recommendations on RTC [C]
  - Serial assessments every 5 minutes until improved with monitoring for a few days to detect delayed signs/symptoms
  - Concussion severity determined by severity and persistence of all signs and symptoms using a symptom checklist
  - Formal cognitive and postural stability testing to assist in defining severity and RTP
  - Once symptom free, RTP after incremental increase in activity

 MEDICATION (DRUGS)

- Sleep disorders/depression/headache
  - Tricyclic antidepressants
  - Selective serotonin reuptake inhibitors (SSRIs) are less well studied
  - Benzodiazepines should be avoided.
- Neck pain/headache
  - NSAIDs
  - Avoid narcotics.
- Contraindications
  - Allergy to medication
- Precautions
  - NSAIDs may cause ulcer disease, elevated blood pressure, renal dysfunction, and bleeding.
  - Tricyclics can cause arrhythmias and should not be used in a suicidal patient; tricyclics can also cause anticholinergic side effects (urinary retention, constipation, etc.)
- Significant possible interactions
  - NSAIDs: Warfarin, angiotension-converting enzyme inhibitors, and lithium
  - Ibuprofen-oral hypoglycemics: Hypoglycemia
  - Tricyclics: Multiple drug interactions including cimetidine and monoamine oxidase inhibitors (MAOI).
  - MAOIs: Should never be given together; risk of serotonin syndrome. These may also cause tricyclic toxicity when used together.

 FOLLOW-UP

PROGNOSIS

- Most patients recover within 12 weeks, but 15% with minor traumatic brain injury will be symptomatic at 1 year, and some never become asymptomatic.
- Patients whose condition has not improved after 1 year will probably not get better.
- Resolution of litigation does not generally result in improvement of this disorder.
- Outcome correlates better with length of posttraumatic amnesia than GCS scoring.

COMPLICATIONS

Loss of source of income and resulting problems

PATIENT MONITORING

- As needed. Each case is individualized.
- Consider a repeat head CT within the 1st couple of weeks if symptoms persist. The symptoms of postconcussive syndrome can also be due to subdural hemorrhages.

REFERENCES

1. Practice parameter: The management of concussion in sports. *Neurology*. 1997;48: 581–585.
2. Guskiewicz KM, et al. National Athletic Trainers' Association position statement: Management of sport-related concussion. *J Athl Training*. 2004; 39:280–297.
3. Randolph C, McCrea M, Barr WB. Is neuropsychological testing useful in the anagement of sport-related concussion. *J Ath Training*. 2005; 40(3):139–154.
4. Bazarian JJ, Blyth B, Cimpello L. Bench to bedside: Evidence for brain injury after concussion-looking beyond the computed tomography scan. *Acad Emer Med*. 2006;13:199–214.
5. Alexander MP. Mild traumatic brain injury: Pathophysiology, natural history, and clinical management. *Neurology*. 1995;45:1253–1260.
6. Rees PM. Contemporary issues in mild traumatic brain injury. *Arch Phys Med Rehabil*. 2003;84: 1885–1894.

 MISCELLANEOUS

See also: Brain injury, traumatic; Cervical spine injury; Depression; Migraine

 CODES

ICD9-CM
310.2 Postconcussion syndrome

PATIENT TEACHING

 See Corresponding Diagnostic Algorithm

POSTPARTUM DEPRESSION

Nancy Byatt, DO, MBA
Rebecca Lundquist, MD

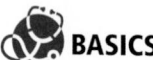 **BASICS**

DESCRIPTION

Postpartum depression, postpartum blues, and postpartum psychosis are the 3 main behavioral conditions that may occur after the delivery. Any recurring psychiatric condition may also reoccur or have it's onset in the postpartum. (1)[C]

- System(s) Affected: Nervous
- Synonym(s): Postnatal depression; Postgestational depression

GENERAL PREVENTION

- Routinely assess women in the 3rd trimester to diagnose depression and risk factors for depression and begin treatment before or immediately after delivery. (2)[A]
- Edinburgh Postnatal Depression Scale should be used as a screening tool (2–4)[A]

EPIDEMIOLOGY

- Predominant age: Women of reproductive age. It has been also described in mothers adopting a baby. (1)[C]
- Predominant sex: Female only

Prevalence

Of new mothers, 10–19% develop postpartum depression. 1–2 woman per 1,000 normal births develop postpartum psychosis, which is a psychiatric emergency. (5)[B]

RISK FACTORS

- Previous episodes of postpartum depression
- Previous episodes of depression
- History of depression during pregnancy
- Family history of depression
- Early childhood losses
- Growing up with alcoholic dysfunctional parents
- Unwanted pregnancy
- Socioenconomic stress
- Lack of social and family support system (6,7)[C]

ETIOLOGY

Unknown. Perhaps multifactorial, including biologic-genetic predisposition in terms of brain chemistry, sudden drop in estrogen and progesterone levels at delivery, and psychosocial stressors.

ASSOCIATED CONDITIONS

- Bipolar mood disorder
- Depressive disorder not otherwise specified
- Dysthymic disorder
- Cyclothymic disorder
- Recurrent major depressive disorder (6,8)[C]

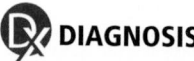 **DIAGNOSIS**

SIGNS AND SYMPTOMS

- Sleep increase/decrease
- Interest in formerly compelling or pleasurable activities diminished
- Guilt, low self-esteem
- Energy poor
- Concentration poor
- Appetite increase/decrease
- Psychomotor agitation or retardation
- Suicidal ideation

TESTS

Lab

Thyroid-stimulating hormone test (8)[A]

Imaging

Head CT/MRI rarely needed

Diagnostic Procedures/Surgery

- Edinburgh Postnatal Depression Scale is primary screening tool
- Beck, Hamilton, and Zung depression inventories may provide information about the severity of the depression and suicidal risks. (2–4)[A]

DIFFERENTIAL DIAGNOSIS

- Baby blues: Mood lability, not a psychiatric disorder, resolves within a couple of weeks
- Postpartum psychosis: A psychiatric emergency
- Postpartum anxiety/panic disorder
- Postpartum obsessive-compulsive disorder
- Hypothyroidism
- Sleep apnea
- Postpartum thyroiditis can occur in up to 7.5 % of patients and can present as depression (9)[A]

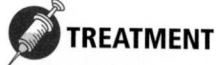 **TREATMENT**

INITIAL STABILIZATION

- Most patients respond to outpatient-basis individual psychotherapy in combination with pharmacotherapy.
- Support/therapy groups may be helpful.
- Assess patients for homicidal and suicidal ideation and any thoughts of harming baby (9)[A]
- Visiting nurse services can provide direct observations of the mother about safety issues and mother-child bonding (7)[A]
- Obtain psychiatric consultation for patients with psychotic symptoms: If psychotic delusions or hallucinations are present, immediate hospitalization is mandatory. The psychotic mother should *not* be left alone with the baby. (1,8,10)[A]

GENERAL MEASURES

- Proper sleep and rest for the new mother are important for stable mood (7)[C]
- Patient education and providing reading material for the patient and her family may be helpful and valuable. (7)[C]
- Psychotherapy treatment: Interpersonal psychotherapy and cognitive behavior therapy shown to be effective (11,12)[C]
- Bright light therapy may be helpful. (13)

Diet

- Good nutrition and hydration
- The addition of a multivitamin with minerals may be helpful.

Activity

Based on patient's physical condition

SPECIAL THERAPY

Physical Therapy

Occupational therapy consultation may be useful.

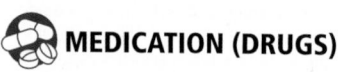 **MEDICATION (DRUGS)**

First Line

- Selective serotonin reuptake inhibitors (SSRIs) are generally effective and safe. (14)[A]
  - Fluoxetine (Prozac): 20–80 mg/d PO (most activating of all SSRIs); less expensive (14)[A]
  - Sertraline (Zoloft): 50–200 mg/d PO (sedating) (14)[A]
  - Paroxetine (Paxil): 20–60 mg/d PO (sedating) (15)[A]
  - Citalopram (Celexa): 20–60 mg/d PO (10)[C]
- Tricyclic antidepressants are effective and less expensive. They are lethal in overdose and have unfavorable side effects. (16)[A]
- Bupropion (Wellbutrin): 150–450 mg/d PO in patients with depression plus psychomotor retardation, hypersomnia, and with weight gain. Bupropion is less likely to cause weight gain or sexual dysfunction. It is highly activating. (17)[A]

- Mirtazapine (Remeron): 15–45 mg/d PO qhs. This antidepressant (not an SSRI) helps with sleep restoration and weight gain; no sexual dysfunction (18)[A]
- Venlafaxine (Effexor XR): A dual-action antidepressant that blocks the reuptake of serotonin in doses of up to 150 mg/d and then blocks the reuptake of norepinephrine in doses of 150–450 mg/d PO (18)[A]

- Contraindications to treatment with antidepressants
  – Known drug allergy

  – Some antidepressants are excreted in breastmilk. Consult with the infants' pediatrician. (1)[D], (13,19)[A]

- Precautions
  – Bipolarity requires treatment with mood stabilizer
  – Antidepressants generally compatible with lactation. Must consult with pediatrician. For further info see book, *Medications and Mothers Milk* by Thomas Hale, PhD.

  – Avoid tricyclic antidepressants in mothers with a known history of suicide attempts. (19)[A]

- Significant possible drug interactions

  – Do not use any previously mentioned antidepressants with any agent in the monoamine oxidase inhibitor class. (9,19)[A]

Second Line
Electroconvulsive therapy (ECT): Some patients who cannot tolerate the antidepressant medication or who are actively engaged in suicidal self-destructive behaviors or who have a previous history of responding favorably to ECT, should be seriously considered for such treatment. (10)[C]

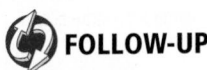 **FOLLOW-UP**

DISPOSITION
Admission Criteria
Presence of suicidal or homicidal ideation and/or psychotic symptoms and/or thoughts of harming baby (1,8,10)[C]

Discharge Criteria
Absence of suicidal or homicidal ideation and/or psychotic symptoms and/or thoughts of harming baby (8,10)[C]

Issues for Referral
Patient and family should be referred for psychotherapy. Referral for psychiatric follow-up if psychiatric medications are indicated. (20)[C]

PROGNOSIS
Generally good. Improvement is expected within a few months to a year. Some patients, particularly those with undertreated or undiagnosed depression, may develop chronic depression requiring long-term treatment. (12)[C]

COMPLICATIONS
- Suicide
- Self-injurious behavior
- Psychosis
- Neglect of baby
- Harm to the baby (1,8,10)[A]

PATIENT MONITORING
Observe quality and safety of mother's interaction with baby. Home observation and monitoring are helpful. (7)[A]

REFERENCES

1. Seyfried LS, Marcus SM. Postpartum mood disorders. *Int Rev Psychiatry*. 2003;15:231–242.
2. Georgiopoulos AM, et al. Routine screening for postpartum depression. *J Fam Pract*. February 2001;50:117–122.
3. Austin MP, Lumley J. Antenatal screening for postnatal depression: A systematic review. *Acta Psychiatr Scand*. 2003;107:10–17.
4. Holden JM. Postnatal depression: Its nature, effects and identification using the Edinburgh Postnatal Depression Scale. *Birth*. 1991;18:211–221.
5. Gavin NI, et al. Perinatal depression: A systematic review of prevalence and incidence. *Obstet Gynecol*. 2005;106:1071–1083.
6. Henshaw C. Mood disturbance in the early puerperium: A review. *Arch Women Ment Health*. 2003;6(suppl 2):S33–S42.
7. Ogrodniczuk JS, Piper WE. Preventing postnatal depression: A review of research findings. *Harvard Rev Psychiatry*. 2003;11:291–307.
8. Wisner KL, Parry BL, Piontek CM. Postpartum depression. *N Engl J Med*. 2002;347:194–199.
9. Stagnaro-Green A. Postpartum thyroiditis. *Best Pract Res Clin Endocrinol Metab*. 2004 Jun;18(2):303–316.
10. Marcus SM, et al. Treatment guidelines for depression in pregnancy. *Int J Gynaecol Obstet*. January 2001;72:61–70.
11. O'Hara MW, et al. Efficacy of interpersonal therapy for postpartum depression. *Gen Psychiatry*. 2000;57:1039–1045.
12. Steinberg SI, Bellavance F. Characteristics and treatment of women with postpartum depression. *Int J Psychiatry Med*. 1999;20:209–233.
13. Corral MK, Dernetra AK. Bright light therapy's effect on postpartum depression. *Am J Psychiatry*. 2000;157:303–304.
14. Kulin NA, et al. Pregnancy outcome following maternal use of the new selective serotonin reuptake inhibitors: A prospective controlled multicenter study. *J Am Med Assoc*. 1996;279:609–61.
15. Patuszak A, et al. Pregnancy outcome following first-trimester. *J Am Med Assoc*. 1993;269:2246–2248.
16. Stowe ZN, et al. Sertraline and desmethylsertraline in human breast milk and nursing infants. *Am J Psychiatry*. 1997;269:1255–1260.
17. Kendell RE, Chalmers JC, Platz C. Epidemiology of puerpereal psychoses. *Br J Psychiatry*. 1987;150:662–673.
18. *Glaxo Wellcome. Bupropion pregnancy registry interim report*. Research Triangle Park, NC: Glaxo Wellcome; 1999.
19. American Psychiatric Association. Practice guideline for the treatment of patients with major depressive disorder (revision). *Am J Psychiatry*. 2000;157:1–45
20. Tammentie T, et al. Family dynamics and postnatal depression. *J Psychiatr Ment Health Nursing*. 2004;11:141–149.

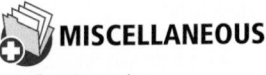 **MISCELLANEOUS**

See also: Depression

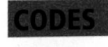 **CODES**

ICD9-CM
648.44 Mental postartum condition or complication

PATIENT TEACHING
- Patient and family education helpful
- Encourage the patient to read, for example:
  – *That Isn't What I Expected: Overcoming Postpartum Depression*, by Karen R. Kleinman and Valerie Davis Radkin
  – *Sleepless Days: One Woman's Journey Through Postpartum Depression*, by Susan Kushner Resnick
  – *A Mother's Tears: Understanding the Mood Swings that Follow Childbirth*, by Arlene M. Huysman
  – *Overcoming Postpartum Depression and Anxiety*, by Linda Sebastian, 1998
  – *Down Came the Rain: My Journey Through Postpartum Depression*, by Brooke Shields, 2005
  – *Behind the Smile: My Journey Out of Postpartum Depression*, by Marie Osmond, Marcie Wilkie, and Judith Morre, 2001
  – *Medication and Mothers Milk*, by Thomas Hale, 2004
- Web Resources:
  – Postpartum support international: www.postpartum.net
  – Depression After Delivery, Inc: www.depressionafterdelivery.com
  – La Leche League: www.lalecheleague.org

 See Corresponding Diagnostic Algorithm

POST TRAUMATIC STRESS DISORDER (PTSD)

Sarah Guzofski, MD
Ruben Peralta, MD, FACS

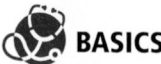 BASICS

DESCRIPTION
In response to a highly traumatic event, a set of physical and emotional symptoms including
- Re-experiencing the trauma (nightmares, flashbacks)
- Avoidance, dissociation, emotional numbing
- Persistent increased physical arousal (hypervigilance, insomnia)

GENERAL PREVENTION
Survivors of trauma are at risk for future trauma and may benefit from counseling about high-risk behaviors.

EPIDEMIOLOGY
- Late adolescence highest risk time for trauma exposure
- Inconsistent findings about racial differences
- 60% males, 50% females experience trauma
- 9% who experience trauma develop PTSD
- PTSD twice as common in females

Prevalence
Lifetime prevalence in US, 8%
- Estimated lifetime prevalence 5% males, 10% females

RISK FACTORS
- Exposure to trauma
  - Some traumas yield higher rates of PTSD: Rape, military combat, captivity, surviving genocide, longer duration of trauma.
- Risk of developing PTSD
  - Female > Male, because of the types of trauma experienced, higher rate mood disorders
  - Mood disorder increases rate of developing PTSD after trauma
  - Previous trauma
  - Refugees have high risk of developing PTSD

ETIOLOGY
- 50% are exposed to traumatic events over lifetime; minority develop PTSD
- Interplay of genetic predisposition, early life events (e.g., prior trauma) and nature of traumatic event itself
- Theory that those with PTSD continue to perceive threat based on their prior traumatic experience, that memory of the trauma is not fully addressed because of avoidance symptoms. (McCleery C)
- With PTSD, develop dysfunction in the hypothalamic-pituitary-adrenal (HPA) axis

ASSOCIATED CONDITIONS
- Mood disorders
- Substance abuse/dependence
- Anxiety: Generalized, panic, agoraphobia
- Obsessive-compulsive disorder
- Social phobia, specific phobia
- Somatoform disorder
- Eating disorders (in women)

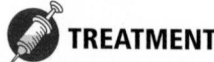 DIAGNOSIS

SIGNS AND SYMPTOMS
- After acute trauma
  - In days immediately following traumatic event may have increased anger, arousal, fear; may feel numb or dissociate. Request detailed history of traumatic event only as is needed for other acute medical care.
- Re-experiencing the trauma (flashbacks, nightmares), emotional numbing or dissociation, hyper-arousal (see "DSM Criteria")
- Exaggerated startle response, sensitivity to physical contact, anxiety may be apparent

History
- Some, but not all, who go on to have PTSD, 1st experience Acute Stress Disorder (ASD). Includes dissociative symptoms during or immediately after the trauma, plus re-experiencing and increased arousal, lasts <1 month.
- Allow patient to determine level of detail they disclose about past trauma
- Ask about suicidal and self-harmful thoughts and behaviors. Increased risk of self-cutting, burning, starvation, suicide attempts with PTSD.

TESTS
Lab
None for diagnosis; changes in HPA axis noted in research studies

Imaging
- None for diagnosis; some research findings
- Hippocampus: Smaller volume in chronic PTSD
- Increased amygdala response and decreased anterior cingulated responses by functional MRI (Osuch C)

DSM Criteria
- A. Exposure to a traumatic event in which
  - Experienced, witnessed, or was confronted with actual or threatened death, serious injury, threat to physical integrity of self or others
  - Emotional reaction was intense fear, horror, or helplessness
- B. Traumatic event is re-experienced in at least 1 of the following ways
  - Recurrent, intrusive, distressing recollections of the event, including images, thoughts, or perceptions
  - Recurrent distressing dreams of the event
  - Acting or feeling as if the event was recurring (sense of reliving the experience, illusions, hallucinations, flashbacks)
  - Intense psychological distress at exposure to internal or external cues that symbolize or resemble the event
  - Physiologic reactivity at exposure to internal or external cues that symbolize or resemble the event
- C. Persistent avoidance of stimuli associated with the trauma and numbing of general responsiveness (3 or more of the following)
  - Efforts to avoid thoughts, feelings, or conversations associated with the trauma
  - Efforts to avoid activities, places, or people who arouse memories of the trauma
  - Inability to recall an important aspect of the trauma
  - Markedly diminished interest or participation in significant activities
  - Feeling of detachment or estrangement from others
  - Restricted affect
  - Sense of foreshortened future
- D. Persistent symptoms of increased arousal (2 or more of the following)
  - Difficulty falling or staying asleep
  - Difficulty concentrating
  - Hypervigilance
  - Exaggerated startle response
- E. Duration of symptoms >1 month
- F. Causes significant social impairment
- Specify
- Acute: Symptoms last <3 months
- Chronic: symptoms last >3 months
- With delayed onset: Begins 6 months after trauma

DIFFERENTIAL DIAGNOSIS
- ASD: If symptoms <1 month; must include dissociative symptoms
- Adjustment disorder: With less severe stressor, without avoidance, re-experiencing, increased arousal
- Psychotic disorder: Distinguish flashbacks from hallucinations; in PTSD no thought disorder
- Major depression: Shares features of avoidance, diminished pleasure, insomnia

TREATMENT

INITIAL STABILIZATION
- Critical incident debriefing: A counselor-led detailed re-telling of the trauma, has not been proven helpful to prevent the development of PTSD and may increase symptoms. (Ursano C, Boris C)
- After acute trauma, focus on immediate safety, comfort, and symptoms, not therapy or processing of traumatic event

GENERAL MEASURES
- Combination of medication management and therapy most effective
  - Treat comorbid mental illness, substance abuse
- Cognitive behavioral therapy (Bradley A)
  - Effective in acute and chronic phases
  - Recall the trauma in detail, focus on hyper-arousal and anxiety; teach relaxation
- Psychodynamic psychotherapy (Ursano C)

Diet
No restriction unless treated with MAOI

MEDICATION (DRUGS)

Antidepressants are the standard treatment. They reduce symptoms, especially when combined with therapy. (Ursano C)

- Initial treatment should be 12 months with longer courses if needed. Many will relapse with medication discontinuation. (Cooper B)
- Benzodiazepines are not recommended; no proven benefit for PTSD-specific symptoms (numbing, re-experiencing) and carry risk of dependence, withdrawal, and rebound anxiety (Ursano C)

First Line
Selective Serotonin Reuptake Inhibitors (SSRIs) (Ursano C, Stein, A)

- Improvement in all symptom groups (re-experiencing, avoidance, hyperarousal)
- Also appropriate for frequently comorbid depression, panic, borderline personality disorder, impulsiveness
- Equal efficacy, choose based on pharmacokinetics, interactions, side effects
- SSRIs include citalopram 20–60 mg/d, escitalopram 10–20 mg/d, fluoxetine 20–60 mg/d, fluvoxamine 50–150 mg b.i.d., paroxetine 20–50 mg/d, sertraline 50–200 mg/d
- 4–6 weeks for effect
- Side effects: Nausea, diarrhea, headache, insomnia, anxiety, anorexia, dizziness, tremor, sweating, sexual dysfunction
- Monitor for serotonin syndrome, especially with rapid dose escalation; symptoms: Confusion, autonomic instability, hyperreflexia, myoclonus
- Monitor for increase in suicidal thoughts when starting SSRI.

ALERT
Pediatric Considerations
Black box warning for pediatric patients that SSRIs can increase suicidality. If decision to treat with SSRI, close monitoring required.

Second Line
- Limited evidence for tricyclic antidepressants; more dangerous in overdose, more side effects
- Limited evidence for MAOLs; more dangerous in overdose, more side effects, strict diet
- Limited/mixed effects in small studies of divalproex, topiramate, carbamazepine (Ursano C)
- Preliminary studies suggest propranolol given within 6 hours of hospital admission for acute trauma, continued for 10 days found to decrease PTSD symptoms at 1 and 2 months; additional study needed (Pitman B, Vaiva B)
- Atypical antipsychotics are commonly used to help with insomnia, hyperarousal (Budur C)

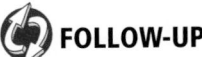 ## FOLLOW-UP

Outpatient psychopharmacology and therapy

DISPOSITION
Admission Criteria
Suicidal, homicidal, or unable to care for selves because of severe symptoms

Discharge Criteria
Not a danger to self or others; symptoms stabilized and outpatient treatment in place

Issues for Referral
Close coordination with primary care physician. Trauma history is associated with chronic gastrointestinal and pain syndromes, fibromyalgia, somatization disorder. (Ursano C)

PROGNOSIS
- 20% attempt suicide; 6x increased risk over general population
- Duration of symptoms varies; 1/2 have resolution within 3 months, 1/2 have a more chronic course
- Women have longer course of symptoms then men (48 month average vs. 12) (Seedat B)
- Exacerbations and relapses may begin with new trauma, anniversaries
- Substance abuse increases future trauma and must be treated.

REFERENCES
1. American Psychiatric Association. *Diagnostic and Statistical Manual IV-TR*. American Psychiatric Association; 2000.
2. Boris NW, Ou AC, Singh R. Preventing Post-traumatic stress disorder after mass exposure to violence. *Biosecurity and Bioterrorism.* 2005;3:154–163.
3. Bradley R, et al. A multidimensional meta-analysis of psychotherapy for PTSD. *Am J Psychiatry.* 2005;162:214–272.
4. Budur K, Falcone T, Franco K. Diagnosing and treating posttraumatic stress disorder. *Clev Clin J Med.* 2006;73:121–129.
5. Cook JM, O'Donnell C. Assessment and psychological treatment of posttraumatic stress disorder in older adults. *J Geriatr Psych Neur.* 2005;18:61–71
6. Cooper J, Carty J, Creamer M. Pharmacotherapy for posttraumatic stress disorder: Empirical review and clinical recommendations. *Aust NZ J Psychiat.* 2005;39:674–682.
7. McCleery JM, Harvey AG. Integration of psychological and biological approaches to trauma memory. *J Trauma.* 2004;27:485–496.
8. Osuch E, et al. Brain environment interactions: stress, posttraumatic stress disorder and need for a postmortem brain collection. *Psychiaty.* 2004;67:353–383.
9. Pitman PK, et al. Pilot study of secondary prevention with propranolol. *Biol Psychiatry.* 2003;51:189–192
10. Seedat S, Stein DJ, Carey PD. Post-traumatic stress disorder in women: Epidemiologic and treatment issues *CNS Drugs.* 2005;19:411–427.
11. Stein DJ, Ipser JC, Seedat S. Pharmacotherapy for post traumatic stress disorder. *Cochrane Database of Systematic Review, The Cochrane Collaboration.* 2006; 1
12. American Psychiatric Association. Practice guideline for the treatment of patients with acute stress disorder and posttraumatic stress disorder. Arlington, VA: American Psychiatric Association; 2004.
13. Vaiva G, et al. Immediate treatment with propranolol decreases posttraumatic stress disorder two months after trauma *Biol Psychiatry.* 2003;54:947–949.

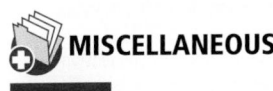 ## MISCELLANEOUS

CODES
ICD9-CM
309.81 Post traumatic stress disorder

PATIENT TEACHING
Prevention
- Review high-risk behaviors (abusive relationships, substance use)
- Identify triggers for symptoms (e.g., anniversary of sexual assault) and create plan to manage increased stress at that time.

 See Patient Handout on CD

PREECLAMPSIA

Irene C. Coletsos, MD
Frank J. Domino, MD

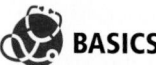 **BASICS**

DESCRIPTION

A disorder of pregnancy developing at the 20th week (or beyond), with hypertension, proteinurea, and/or edema with poor perfusion to vital organs, that may progress from mild to life-threatening in hours to days. The disease may include rapid weight gain and face and hand edema. The disorder is reversible by ending the pregnancy if at term or, if maternal or fetal health are in danger, a pre-term delivery.

- System(s) Affected: Cardiovascular; Renal; Reproductive; Feto-Placental; Central Nervous System; Hepatic
- Synonym(s): Pregnancy-induced hypertension; Toxemia of pregnancy

GENERAL PREVENTION

- Weight control
- Very small-scale studies support antioxidant therapy (1,000 mg vitamin C and 400 IU vitamin E) for prevention in females thought to be at risk. (1)[B]
- Low-dose aspirin may improve the pregnancy outcome for females with persistently abnormal uterine Doppler studies, but it is not recommended for patients with low risk. (2)[B]
- In some studies, Calcium supplements have reduced rates of preeclampsia in females considered to be high-risk, but not others. (3)[B]
- Neither aspirin nor nutritional supplements are recommended for patients at low risk of preeclampsia.

EPIDEMIOLOGY

Predominant age: Young, primigravid women; females >35 years old

Incidence

Older pregnant females (>35 years old) have increased incidence.

ALERT

Pediatric Considerations

Increased incidence in teenagers

Prevalence

~7% of 1st-time mothers and 3% in multiparous women, who had not had preeclampsia in earlier pregnancies.

RISK FACTORS

- Familial incidence
- Nulliparity
- Obesity
- Pre-pregnancy diabetes; vascular disease and (often undiagnosed) hypertension.
- Polycystic ovarian disease
- Pregnancy with multiple fetuses
- Molar pregnancy
- Fetal hydrops

Genetics

Thought to be multifactorial. Increased incidence in pregnant females whose mothers or sisters had the disease. Males born of preeclamptic or eclamptic pregnancies are more likely to father preeclamptic pregnancies.

ETIOLOGY

- Thought to be due to abnormal invasion of placental cells into uterine spiral arterioles, leading to:
- Maternal immune system hypersensitivity
- Vasospasm
- Abnormal placental production of increased thromboxane and decreased prostacyclin increased capillary permeability
- System-wide endothelial dysfunction
- Microthrombi
- Hypertension

ASSOCIATED CONDITIONS

- Abruptio placenta
- Placental insufficiency
- Fetal growth restriction
- Preterm delivery
- Fetal demise
- Maternal seizures (= eclampsia)
- Maternal pulmonary edema
- Maternal liver or kidney failure
- Maternal death

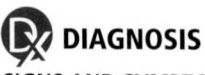 **DIAGNOSIS**

SIGNS AND SYMPTOMS

History

- May be asymptomatic
- In some cases: Rapid excessive weight gain (>5 lb/wk; 2.3 kg/wk)
- More severe cases are associated with
  – Epigastric pain
  – Headache
  – Altered mental status
  – Visual disturbance

Physical Exam

- Mild: Elevated BP ≥140 systolic or 90 diastolic, on 2 BP readings 6 hours apart
- Proteinuria (>300 mg/24 h or >1 g/L)
- Severe: Elevated BP ≥160 systolic or 110 diastolic, on 2 BP readings, 6 hours apart.
- Proteinuria (>5 g/24 h)
- Facial or hand edema
- Hyperreflexia
- Retinal arteriolar spasm
- Papilledema
- Epigastric/right upper quadrant (RUQ) pain
- Oliguria or anuria
- Petichiae, bruising, bleeding secondary to disseminated intravascular coagulation

TESTS

Lab

- 24-hour urine for proteinuria (see above); creatinine clearance: < 90 mL/min/1.73 m-squared
- Plasma urate: At 24–28 weeks, 4.03 mg/dL; at 33–36 weeks, 5.04 mg/dL
- Platelet count: Thrombocytopenia (<100,000 platelets)
- Coagulation profile/fibrin split products: Increased prothrombin time; increased fibrin degradation products; decreased fibrinogen. May reveal disseminated intravascular coagulation, a possible sequelae of preeclampsia.
- CBC: Increased blood urea nitrogen (>16 mg/dL [5.7 mmol/L]); increased hematocrit may be consistent with increased vasoconstriction; increased creatinine (>1.0 mg/dL) associated with worsening renal function.
- Liver function studies: Increased liver function tests (LFTs)
- Disorders that may alter lab results:
  – Chronic renal disease

Imaging/Monitoring

- Daily fetal movement monitoring by mother ("Kick Counts")
- Non-stress test at diagnosis, and then weekly, until delivery
- Ultrasound imaging for biophysical profile, estimation of fetal age, growth progress, amniotic fluid volume. Weekly for mild preeclampsia. Twice weekly in severe preeclampsia.

Diagnostic Procedures/Surgery

- Maternal: 24-hour urine test for protein
- Fetal: Amniocentesis for fetal pulmonary maturity such as lecithin/sphingomyelin ratio, a marker for lung maturity. >2.0 is associated with increased lung maturity and a decreased risk of respiratory distress syndrome. But meconium in amniotic fluid may lead to falsely high or low measures.

Pathological Findings

- Renal: Glomerular capillary endotheliosis, glomerular lesions.
- Hepatic: Hemorrhage into hepatic cellular columns; dislocation of hepatocytes. May progress to hepatic infarct and swelling of the hepatic capsule (leading to the epigastric or RUQ pain).
- CNS: Cerebral edemas
- Placental vascular abnormalities leading to placental infarcts

DIFFERENTIAL DIAGNOSIS

- Chronic hypertension: HTN prepregnancy; high blood pressure (HTN) before the 20th week; Diagnosis during pregnancy, but persisting beyond day 84 postpartum.
- Preeclampsia superimposed upon nongestational diabetes: HTN prior to the 20th week, followed by proteinurea; HTN and proteinurea prior to the 20th week.
- Gestational HTN: Increased BP 1st discovered during pregnancy, with no proteinurea. Normal BP by 12 weeks postpartum.
- Eclampsia: Preeclampsia with seizures (that cannot be explained by any other disorder).

- Thrombotic thrombocytopenic purpura: Fever, confusion, petechiae. Aggressive plasma replacement is necessary.
- Hemolytic uremic syndrome: Predominantly affects the kidneys; supportive treatment.

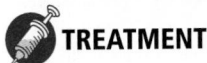 **TREATMENT**

- Mild
  - Outpatient care
  - Maternal: Daily home BP monitoring; daily weights. Weekly labs (24-hour protein; platelet count; creatinine; LFT.
  - Fetal: Patient-measured: Daily "kick counts,"Medical provider measured: Non-stress test; ultrasound biophysical profile (if gestational age <37 weeks, twice weekly non-stress test and a biophysical profile (BPP) every 3 weeks). (2)[B]

  Severe
- Inpatient care if patient condition deteriorates (BP ≥160/110; severe headache; visual changes–scotoma or "flashing lights"; impaired mentation; pulmonary edema; epigastric/RUQ pain; increasing LFTs; oligourea; thrombocytopenia) or if fetal status is deemed "non-reassuring."
- Maternal: Daily labs, adding coagulation tests; IV magnesium sulfate as anti-convulsive prophylaxis. IV labetolol and oral nifedipine antihypertensive therapy titrated to keep systolic BP <155 and diastolic BP <105. Keep diastolic >90 to avoid hypoperfusing the uterus.
- Fetal: Continuous heart monitoring. Daily ultrasound, with BPP, amniotic fluid levels, fetal growth assessment as deemed necessary.
- Management by gestational age of severe preeclampsia
- <23 weeks: Offer to terminate pregnancy.
- At 23–32 weeks: Antihypertensives; evaluate maternal-fetal condition; steroids to enhance fetal lung maturity; plan delivery at 34 weeks with magnesium sulfate prophylaxis or for worsening maternal or fetal jeopardy.
- At 33–34 weeks: Steroids, magnesium sulfate, and delivery.
- At 34 weeks +: Magnesium sulfate and delivery.
- Regardless of gestational age, delivery recommended within 2 days for pregnant women with severe hypertension that is resistant to antihypertensive therapy; or with cerebral disturbances despite magnesium sulfate therapy; or with elevated LFTs *and* epigastric/RUQ pain;or thrombocytopenia. (2)[B]

ALERT

Regardless of gestational age, emergent delivery is recommended if there are signs of maternal hypertensive crisis, abruptio placentae, uterine rupture, orfetal distress. (2)[B]

GENERAL MEASURES
Diet
Salt restriction is inadvisable because the patient is often experiencing intravascular hypovolemia.

Activity
- Mild: Restricted activity.
- Severe: Restricted activity, in-hospital
- Total bed rest is inadvisable, because there are no studies showing that it improves pregnancy outcome.

 MEDICATION (DRUGS)

- For seizure prophylaxis: Magnesium sulfate (MgSO$_4$) loading dose 4 g IV in 200-mL normal saline over 20–30 minutes. Maintenance dose 1–2 g/h IV. (4)[B]

- For hypertension
  - Nifedipine: (oral): 40–120 mg/d, plus
  - Labetalol (IV): 600–2,400 mg/d, both titrated to keep BP <155/105. Antihypertensives are inadvisable for mild hypertension/preeclampsia.
  - Avoid nitroprusside (decreased uterine blood flow plus possible lethal fetal cyanide levels).
- For seizures
  - Magnesium sulfate 4 g IV *slowly* to prevent further seizures
- Contraindications: Refer to the manufacturer's profile of each drug.
- Precautions
  - Therapeutic magnesium levels are 4–7 mEq/L.
  - Toxicity (e.g., flushing, sweating, hyporeflexia, flaccid paralysis, CNS depression, oliguria, decreased cardiac function)
  - Freqently recheck patient for signs of toxicity.
  - Continue for 24 hours postpartum.
  - Toxicity therapy with slow administration of 10% calcium gluconate, with supplementary oxygen
  - Give oxytocin (Pitocin) postpartum to prevent bleeding (60 U/L at 50 mL/h).
- Significant possible interactions
  - Refer to the manufacturer's profile of each drug.

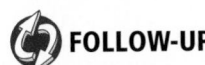 **FOLLOW-UP**

PROGNOSIS
- Prevention of seizures
- Delivery of viable fetus. Delivery date will depend on health of mother/measures of fetal health and lung maturity.
- Close monitoring of maternal and fetal health to prevent maternal or fetal mortality.

COMPLICATIONS
- Maternal
  - Eclampsia (seizures): 0–2%
  - Hypertensive crisis
  - Acute pyelonephritis
  - Acute fatty liver
  - Acute pulmonary edema
  - Severe preeclampsia involving hemolysis, elevated liver function, and low platelet syndrome (hemolysis elevated liver syndrome) (5–10%)
  - Maternal death
- Fetal
  - Intrauterine growth restriction
  - Hypoxemia
  - Perinatal mortality

PATIENT MONITORING
- Keep urine output >25 mL/h.
- Continue magnesium sulfate for 24 hours postpartum.
- Give oxytocin (pitocin) postpartum to prevent bleeding (60 U/L at 50 mL/h).
- Increased risk for pulmonary edema: Monitor IV fluids and blood products ("ins") against urinary output ("outs"); pulsoximetry, lung sounds.

REFERENCES
1. Rumbold A. et al. Antioxidants for preventing pre-eclampsia. *The Cochrane Database of Systemic Reviews*. 2006. Issue. 1 John Wiley & Sons Ltd.
2. Sibai BM. Diagnosis and Management of Gestational Hypertension and Preeclampsia. *Obstetrics & Gynecology*. 2003;102:181–192.
3. Atallah AN, et al. Calcium supplementation during pregnancy for preventing hypertensive disorders and related problems. *The Cochrane Database of Systemic Reviews*. 2006. Issue 1. John Wiley & Sons Ltd.
4. Duley L, Henderson-Smart D. Magnesium sulphate versus diazepam for eclampsia. *The Cochrane Database of Systemic Reviews*. 2006. Issue 1. John Wiley & Sons Ltd.
5. Abalos E, et al. Antihypertensive drug therapy for mild to moderate hypertension during pregnancy. *The Cochrane Database of Systemic Reviews*. 2006. Issue 1. John Wiley & Sons Ltd.
6. Churchil D, Duley L. 2006. Interventionist versus expectant care for severe pre-eclampsia before term. *The Cochrane Database of Systemic Reviews*. 2006. Issue 1. John Wiley & Sons Ltd.
7. Gifford RW, et al. The National High Blood Pressure Education Program Working Group on High Blood Pressure in Pregnancy. NIH publication #00-3029. Revised July 2000.
8. Yeast JD, et al. The risk of pulmonary edema and colloid osmotic pressure changes during magnesium sulfate infusion. *Am J Obstet Gynecol*. 1993;169(6):1566–71.

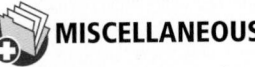 **MISCELLANEOUS**

See also: Eclampsia (toxemia of pregnancy).

CODES

ICD9-CM
- 642.40 Mild or unspecified pre-eclampsia, unspecified
- 642.50 Severe pre-eclampsia, unspecified
- 642.7 Pre-eclampsia or eclampsia superimposed on pre-existing hypertension

PATIENT TEACHING
- Avoid excessive weight gain (>25–30 lb [11.4–13.6 kg]) during pregnancy.
- Importance of prenatal care and frequent blood pressure checks.
- Recognition of the signs and symptoms (though mild forms are frequently asymptomatic).
- Preconception education, especially for patients with known risk factors.

PREMENSTRUAL DYSPHORIC DISORDER

Courtney Jarvis, PharmD

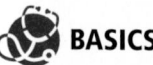 **BASICS**

DESCRIPTION
- Severe form of premenstrual syndrome (PMS) characterized by severe recurrent depressive and anxiety symptoms with premenstrual (luteal phase) onset that remit a few days after the start of menses.
- Symptoms are severe enough to disrupt social and occupational functioning.
- System(s) Affected: CNS
- Synonym(s): Late luteal phase dysphoric disorder (LLPDD)

EPIDEMIOLOGY
Incidence
Three percent to 8% of menstruating women

RISK FACTORS
- Age: Usually present in late 20s–mid 30s
- Past history of mood disorder (major depression, bipolar disorder), anxiety disorders, personality disorders, or substance abuse
- Family history
- Low parity
- Psychosocial stressors

Genetics
Role of genetic predisposition is controversial; however, twin studies suggest a genetic component.

PATHOPHYSIOLOGY
- Results from interaction of cyclic changes in ovarian steroids with central neurotransmitters (serotonin, β-endorphin, GABA), and the autonomic nervous system
- Inconclusive evidence regarding low levels of magnesium and calcium in women with PMDD

 DIAGNOSIS

SIGNS AND SYMPTOMS
- Anger
- Irritability/lability
- Internal tension
- Depressed mood
- Anxiety
- insomnia

History
- Determine regularity of the menstrual cycle using prospective patient record of symptoms for 2 months, The Daily Record of Severity of Problems (available online at http://www.pmdd.factsforhealth.org/drsp/drsp_month.pdf), or similar inventory
- DSM-IV Criteria
  - Symptoms occur 1 week before menses and resolve in the 1st few days after menses begin (over most menstrual cycles during the past year)
  - ≥5 of the follow (1 must be among the 1st 4)
    ○ Markedly depressed mood with feelings of hopelessness
    ○ Marked anxiety or tension
    ○ Marked affective lability
    ○ Irritability and anger
    ○ Decreased interested in usual activities and social withdrawal
    ○ Lack of energy
    ○ Appetite change
    ○ Change in sleeping pattern
    ○ Feeling out of control or overwhelmed

○ Difficulty concentrating
○ Somatic symptoms such as abdominal bloating, breast tenderness, headaches, or joint pain
- Symptoms must be severe enough to interfere with work, school, usual activities, etc.
- Symptoms may be superimposed on underlying psychiatric disorder but not be an exacerbation of another condition.
- Criteria must be confirmed by prospective daily charting for a minimum of 2 consecutive symptomatic menstrual cycles.

TESTS
Lab
- Therepetitive nature of symptoms precludes need for labs if a classic history is present.
- In the absence of such history, hemoglobin may behelpful to rule out anemia.
- Serum TSH

Imaging
Imaging to diagnose causes of pelvic painand dysmenorrhea may be appropriate.

DIFFERENTIAL DIAGNOSIS
- Premenstrual exacerbation of underlying psychiatric disorder
- Psychiatric disorders (especially bipolar disorder, major depression, anxiety)
- Thyroid disorders
- Perimenopause
- Premenstrual migraine
- Chronic fatigue syndrome
- Irritable bowel syndrome (painful sx)
- Seizures
- Anemia
- Endometriosis (painful sx)
- Drug or alcohol abuse

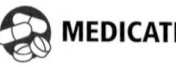 **TREATMENT**

- SSRIs (fluoxetine and sertraline most studied) are highly effective in the treatment of physical and behavioral symptoms of PMDD (mean difference in symptoms of −1.066 [95% CI −1.381 to −0.750], or of 6.91 [95% CI 3.9 to 12.2].) (1,2)[A]
  - Intermittent luteal phase dosing is as effective as full-cycle dosing, with fewer adverse effects (1,2)[A]
  - Higher doses are not correlated with increased response. (1,2)[A]
  - Other nonselective serotonergic agents (venlafaxine, clomipramine) may also be effective. (3)[C]
- Alternative therapies should be considered if no response to SSRI: Alprazolam, buspirone, GnRH agonists, danazol, bromocriptine, spironolactone, oral contraceptives, meclofenamate, progesterone (3)[C]
- Oral contraceptive pills (OCPs) may improve physical symptoms, but not mood. (3,4)[C]
  - OCPs can cause adverse effects similar to PMDD symptoms; monophasic preparations should be used continuously for PMDD. (3)[C]

- OCPs containing the progestin drospirenone (structurally similar to spironolactone) may improve physical symptoms and mood changes associated with PMDD. (4)[B]

- Calcium carbonate effectively reduces physical and emotional premenstrual symptoms. (5)[B]
- Vitamin B_6 may reduce severity of premenstrual symptoms. (6)[B]
- Cognitive behavioral therapy (CBT) is as effective as drug therapy, but there is no additional benefit of combining CBT and drug therapy. (7)[B]

GENERAL MEASURES
Diet
- Reduce consumption of salt, sugar, caffeine, dairy products, and alcohol (anecdotal reports)
- Eat small, frequent portions of food high in complex carbohydrates (limited data)

Activity
Aerobic exercise is helpful in decreasing premenstrual symptoms.

SPECIAL THERAPY
CBT

Complementary and Alternative Medicine
- Some data supports use of the following
  - Calcium: 600 mg b.i.d.
  - Vitamin B_6: 100 mg/d
  - Magnesium 200–400 mg/d
  - Vitamin E: 400 IU/d
  - Manganese: 1.8 mg/d
- Evidence supporting efficacy and/or safety of herbal products is lacking; the following products have *not* been found useful for PMS/PMDD
  - Evening primrose oil
  - Black current oil
  - Chaste tree extract
  - Black cohosh
  - Wild yam root
  - Dong quai
  - Kava kava
  - St. John's wort

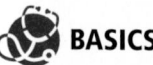 **MEDICATION (DRUGS)**

First Line
- Fluoxetine (Prozac, Sarafem) 20 mg/d every day, or 20 mg/d only during luteal phase, or 90 mg once a week for 2 weeks in luteal phase
- Sertraline (Zoloft) 50–150 mg/d every day, or 50–150 mg/d only during luteal phase
- Citalopram (Celexa) 10–30 mg/d every day, or 10–30 mg/d only during luteal phase
- Adverse effects
  - Gastrointestinal upset
  - Jitteriness
  - Headache
  - Sexual dysfunction
  - Insomnia
  - Fatigue
- Contraindications: Patients taking MAOIs
- Precautions
  - Increased risk of suicidal thinking and behavior in children and adolescents with depressive disorders
  - Bipolar disorder
  - Seizure disorder
  - Hepatic dysfunction
  - Renal dysfunction

- Possible interactions
  - MAOIs (phenelzine, isocarbazine, tranylcypromine, linezolid)
  - Selegiline
  - Pimizide
  - Thioridazine

Second Line

- Spironolactone (Aldactone): 50–100 mg/d for 7–10 days during luteal phase; helpful for fluid retention
  - Adverse reactions: Lethargy, headache, irregular menses, hyperkalemia)
- Oral contraceptives
  - Ethinyl estradiol/drospirenone (Yasmin/Yaz): 1 tablet/d; although unstudied, other OCPs may also be effective
- Alprazolam (Xanax) 0.25 mg t.i.d.–q.i.d. only during luteal phase, taper at onset of menses (other benzodiazepines not studied for PMDD)
  - Caution: Addictive potential
- GnRH agonists
  - Leuprolide (Lupron) depot 3.75 mg IM/m.
  - Precautions: Menopauselike side effects (osteoporosis, hot flashes, headaches, muscle aches, vaginal dryness, irritability) limit treatment to 6 months; if extended treatment is needed, supplement with estrogen and progesterone.
- Danazol (Danocrine): 300–400 mg b.i.d.
  - Adverse reactions: Androgenic and antiestrogenic effects (amenorrhea, weight gain, acne, fluid retention, hirsutism, hot flashes, vaginal dryness, emotional lability)

SURGERY

Bilateral oophorectomy, usually with concomitant hysterectomy, is option for rare, refractory cases with severe, disabling symptoms.

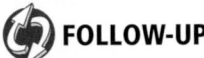 **FOLLOW-UP**

DISPOSITION

Issues for Referral

Referral to psychiatrist may be indicated for mood or anxiety disorder if patient has no symptomfree period.

REFERENCES

1. Wyatt KM, Dimmock PW, O'Brien PMS. Selective serotonin reuptake inhibitors for premenstrual syndrome. *Cochrane Database of Systematic Rev.* 2006;3:no pages. (Last updated 11/15/04).
2. Dimmock PW, Wyatt KM, Jones PW, O'Brien PMS. Efficacy of selective serotonin-reuptake inhibitors in premenstrual syndrome: A systematic review. *Lancet.* 2000;356:1131–1136.
3. Premenstrual dysphoric disorder: A review for the treating practitioner. *Clev Clin J Med.* 2004;71:303–321.
4. Douglas S. Premenstrual syndrome: Evidence-based treatment in family practice. *Can Fam Phys.* 2002;48:1789–1797.
5. Thys-Jacob S, Starkey P, Bernstein D, Tian J. Calcium carbonate and the premenstrual syndrome: Effects on premenstrual and menstrual symptoms. *Am J Obstet Gynecol.* 1998;179:444–452.
6. Wyatt KM, Dimmock PW, Jones PW, O'Brien PMS. Efficacy of vitamin B6 in the treatment of premenstrual syndrome: Systemic review. *BMJ.* 1999;318:1375–1381.
7. Hunter MS, Ussher JM, Browne SJ, et al. A randomized comparison of psychological (cognitive behavioral therapy), medical (fluoxetine) and combined treatment for women with premenstrual dysphoric disorder. *J Psychosom Obstret Gynaecol.* 2002;23:193–199.

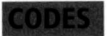 **CODES**

ICD9-CM
625.4

PATIENT TEACHING

- Counsel women that they are not "crazy." PMDD is a real disorder with a physiologic basis.
- Although incompletely understood, successful treatment is usually possible.

Diet
As addressed in "General Measures"

Activity
As addressed in general measures/activity

 See Corresponding Diagnostic Algorithm

 See Patient Handout on CD

PREMENSTRUAL SYNDROME (PMS)

Daphne J. Karel, MD

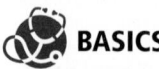 **BASICS**

DESCRIPTION

- Premenstrual syndrome is defined as a symptom complex severe enough to interfere with everyday life and occurring cyclically during the luteal phase of menses.
- The American Psychiatric Association's *DSM-MD IV* revised diagnosis is *premenstrual dysphoric disorder* when the dominant symptoms are emotional.
- System(s) Affected: Endocrine/Metabolic, Nervous, Reproductive
- Synonyms: Premenstrual dysphoric disorder, PMDD

GENERAL PREVENTION
Calcium with vitamin D (1,000–2,000mg elemental calcium) (1)[C]

EPIDEMIOLOGY
- Predominant age: Child-bearing years, increasing with age
- Predominant sex: Females only

Prevalence
Almost all women have some symptoms before menses (this is *not* premenstrual syndrome); ~5% have actual PMS.

RISK FACTORS
- High caffeine intake
- Stress may precipitate condition.
- Increasing age
- History of depression
- Tobacco use
- Family history

Genetics
Unknown; probably familial incidence

ETIOLOGY
Unknown; altered response to progesterone metabolites and serotonin are current theories.

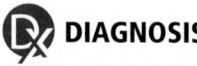 **DIAGNOSIS**

SIGNS AND SYMPTOMS
- Physiologic symptoms
  - Abdominal bloating/pain
  - Edema
  - Weight gain
  - Mastalgia/breast swelling
  - Fatigue
  - Headache
  - Sleep disturbance
  - Tension/muscle aches
  - Food cravings
- Psychologic/behavioral changes
  - Depressed mood/dysphoria
  - Mood swings/irritability
  - Anxiety
  - Sense of loss of control/poor coping
  - Poor concentration

History
Symptoms start in the week prior to menses, and the remainder of the month is symptom free.

Physical Exam
Unremarkable

TESTS
Lab
None, unless history indicates need to rule out other diagnosis.

Diagnostic Procedures/Surgery
- Prospective patient log of symptoms completed over a minimum of 2 months and showing luteal phase exacerbation of symptoms. (2)[A] Can include any of the following
  - Self diary (dates of menses and symptoms)
  - Standardized questionnaire completed throughout the follicular and luteal phases
    - COPE (Callender of Premenstrual Experiences)
    - PRISM (Prospective Record of the Impact and Severity of Menstruation)
    - VAS (Visual Analogue Scales)

DIFFERENTIAL DIAGNOSIS
- Diseases with symptom overlap
  - Thyroid disease
  - Adrenal disorders
  - Perimenopause
- Menstrual exacerbations of chronic illness
  - Asthma
  - Allergies
  - Seizure disorder
  - Migraines
  - Irritable bowel syndrome
  - Chronic fatigue syndrome
- Psychiatric disorders
  - Affective mood disorders
  - Panic disorder
  - Generalized anxiety disorder

 TREATMENT

INITIAL STABILIZATION
Outpatient

GENERAL MEASURES
- Increase daily exercise. (2)[C]
- Eat regular, balanced meals.
- Stop smoking.
- Get regular sleep.
- Use stress-reduction techniques.
- Try cognitive behavioral therapy.
- Join a support group.
- Try light-based therapy.

Diet
Low-salt; low-caffeine; low-fat; frequent, small meals high in complex carbohydrates (2)[B]

Activity
- No restrictions
- Exercise is recommended.

SPECIAL THERAPY
Complementary and Alternative Medicine

- Cognitive behavioral therapy (6 months of treatment provides improvement and maintenance of symptoms) (3)[B]
- Calcium with vitamin D (1,000–1,2000mg elemental calcium) (2)[B]
- Omega-3-fatty acids (2)[A]

- *Agnus castus* (Chaste tree) extract (1 tablet daily for 3 cycles) improved subjective symptoms.

- Vitamin E (400 IU for 5 days around menstrual period) for 2 cycles significantly reduced dysmenorrhea, analgesic need, and estimated blood loss. [B]

- Insufficient evidence to recommend black cohosh, dong quai, primrose oil, progestins, red clover, and soy extract.

 MEDICATION (DRUGS)

- No cure. Therapy is targeted at symptom control.
- Control of total symptom complex (physical and behavioral)
  - Selective serotonin reuptake inhibitors (SSRIs) with continuous or luteal phase dosing (4)[A]
    - Fluoxetine (Prozac, Sarafem)
    - Sertraline (Zoloft)
    - Escitalopram (Lexapro)
    - Citalopram (Celexa)
    - Venlafaxine (Effexor) (serotonin-norepinephrine reuptake inhibitor)
  - Some nutritional supplements may be minimally beneficial with little to no risk (2)[B]
    - Vitamin B_6 in modest doses (50 mg PO b.i.d; may be toxic in higher doses)
    - Magnesium 200–400 mg daily
    - Calcium with vitamin D (1,000–1,200 mg elemental calcium)
  - Drospirenone-containing oral contraceptives (2,5)[B]
  - Gonadotropin-releasing hormone (GnRH) agonists with or without hormone replacement (2)[B]

- Targeted symptom improvement
  - Cramping and pain: NSAIDs
  - Fluid retention: Spironolactone
  - Breast tenderness: Bromocriptine 2.5 mg t.i.d.
  - Depression: All non-SSRI antidepressants
  - Anxiety: Anxiolytics (buspirone, alprazolam)
- Contraindications: Refer to manufacturer's profile of each drug.
- Precautions
  - Effects of long-term hormonal treatment remain unknown.
  - Refer to manufacturer's profile of each drug.
- Significant possible interactions: Refer to manufacturer's profile of each drug.

First Line
- Lifestyle modification, calcium and vitamin E supplement (2)[C]
- Cognitive behavioral therapy (3)[B]
- Targeted symptom control

Second Line

- SSRIs (4)[A]
- GnRH agonists (2)[B]
- Surgical intervention (2)[B]

SURGERY

Bilateral oophorectomy provides relief in a limited subset of patients. Surgery may be offered to patients who fail 1st-line therapy and have a significant response to GnRH agonists over 3 months.

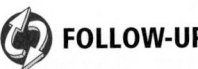 FOLLOW-UP

PROGNOSIS

- Many patients can have their symptoms adequately controlled. PMS disappears at menopause.
- PMS sometimes continues after hysterectomy.

PATIENT MONITORING

Provide general support and further patient education.

REFERENCES

1. Bertone-Johnson ER. *Arch Intern Med*. 2005;165(11):1246–1252.
2. Practice Bulletin. The American College of Obstetricians and Gynecologists. Management of premenstrual syndrome. *Clinical Management Guidelines No. 15*, April 2000.
3. Hunter MS, Ussher JM, Browne SJ, et al. A randomized comparison of psychological (cognitive behavior therapy), medical (fluoxetine) and combined treatment for women with premenstrual dysphoric disorder. *J Psychosom Obstet Gynaecol*. 2002;23:193–199.
4. Wyatt KM, Dimmock PW, O'Brien PM. Selective serotonin reuptake inhibitors for premenstrual syndrome. *Cochrane Database Sys Rev*. 2002;(4):CD001396.
5. Yonkers KA. Efficacy of a new low-dose oral contraceptive with drospirenone in premenstrual dysphoric disorder. *Obstet Gynecol*. 2005;106(3):492–501.
6. Ziaei S, Zakeri M, Kazemnejad A. A randomized controlled trial of vitamin E in the treatment of primary dysmenorrheal. *Br J Obstet Gynecol*. 2005;112:466–469.

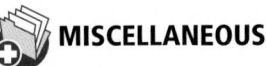 MISCELLANEOUS

See also: Mastalgia

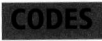 CODES

ICD9-CM

625.4 Premenstrual tension syndromes

PATIENT TEACHING

Explain PMS and treatment.

Diet

Balanced meals rich in calcium and omega-3 fatty acids and low in saturated fat and caffeine.

Activity

Increase aerobic exercise

Prevention

Calcium with vitamin D reduces the incidence of PMS.

 See Corresponding Diagnostic Algorithm

PRESSURE ULCER

Ruben Peralta, MD, FACS
Sarah Guzofski, MD

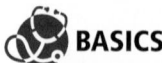 BASICS

DESCRIPTION
- Localized site of soft tissue breakdown when pressure between an external surface and a bony prominence causes local tissue ischemia and malnutrition.
- Common and serious complication affecting disabled, acutely ill, or immobile elderly patients, especially within long-term care settings
- Synonym(s): Decubitus ulcer; Bedsore; Trophic ulcer; Pressure sore

GENERAL PREVENTION
- Up to 95% of all pressure ulcers are preventable. Early identification of at-risk patients is essential, with early multidisciplinary care.
- Frequent patient repositioning if immobile, for example, every hour if wheelchair bound and every 2 hours if bedridden.
- Early mobilization when possible.
- Keep skin clean and dry by using mild soap, warm water, and moisturizer. Manage incontinence.
- Use mattress overlays, thick air seat cushions, and beds that reduce pressure on pressure points, especially for hospitalized patients.
- Aggressive glycemic control (1)[B]
- Assess nutrient status and provide required macronutrients and micronutrients by oral route, enteral, or parenteral if necessary.

EPIDEMIOLOGY
- Predominant age: 60–70% are >70; greatest risk >85
- Predominant sex: Female > Male (because of survival differential)

Incidence
- 2 million new patients each year
- Incidence is 43/100,000 population every year; 65% of elderly with femoral fractures; 33% of critical care patients, and over 60% prevalence among quadriplegic patients and orthopedic patients

Prevalence
Hospitalized adults 3–11%, long-term-care facilities 2.5–24%

RISK FACTORS
- Extended stay in hospital or nursing home, inadequate staffing (2)[B]
- Immobility (e.g., spinal cord injury, fracture, cerebrovascular accident)
- Malnutrition, recent weight loss, eating problems, hypoalbuminemia, vitamin C deficiency (2)[B]
- History of pressure ulcer
- Age-related skin changes
- Impairments of perfusion and oxygenation (anemia, low diastolic blood pressure, peripheral vascular disease)
- Immunocompromise (e.g., diabetes)
- Decreased sensation (e.g., neuropathy, spinal cord injury)

- Impaired awareness (e.g., dementia, delirium, over-sedation)
- Urinary or fecal incontinence
- For trauma and emergency patients, hard backboard should be removed as soon as possible after the secondary survey.
- Assessment scales for evaluating risk factors include Norton, Braden (Braden Q version for children), Waterlow, and Walsall.

ETIOLOGY
- Sustained pressure causes occlusion of blood and lymphatic vessels; this occlusion of the microcirculation can cause ischemia and necrosis. (3)[A] This occurs when the tissue pressure exceeds capillary filling (25 mm Hg).
- Skin is more resistant to pressure than is subcutaneous tissue.
- Moisture from incontinence or perspiration can increase the friction between two surfaces.

ASSOCIATED CONDITIONS
See "Risk Factors."

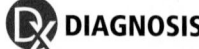 DIAGNOSIS

SIGNS AND SYMPTOMS
- 83% of hospitalized patients with decubitus ulcers develop them in 1st 5 days of hospitalization. (4)[B]
- National Pressure Ulcer Advisory Panel Classification
  - Stage I: Nonblanching erythema, warmth, induration
  - Stage II: May include dermis, appears as abrasion, blister, or superficial ulcer.
  - Stage III: Extends through subcutaneous tissues but not fascia. May appear necrotic with changes in pigmentation
  - Stage IV: Ulcers extend beyond deep fascia into muscle or bone, decayed area may be larger than visibly apparent wound, osteomyelitis or sepsis may be present, granulation tissue and epithelialization may be present at wound margins.

TESTS
Lab
- Culture of wound if evidence of infection (surrounding erythema, purulent drainage, foul odor)
- White blood cell count and differential, blood cultures if fever is present (>37°C)
- Erythrocyte sedimentation rate if osteomyelitis is suspected
- Nutritional assessment: Albumin, prealbumin, transferrin.

Imaging
Plain radiographs if bone involvement suspected

DIFFERENTIAL DIAGNOSIS
- Stasis or ischemic ulcers
- Vasculitides
- Cancers
- Radiation injury
- Pyoderma gangrenosum and other dermatologic conditions

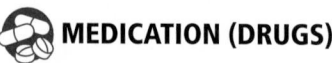 TREATMENT

Nutritional assessment to maximize protein, trace element, and vitamin intake, including selection of parenteral or enteral diet (1)[B]

GENERAL MEASURES
- Reduce pressure and prevent additional ulcers: Padding, frequent repositioning, mobilization if possible (4)[B]
  - Static surfaces for stage I and II ulcers: Air, foam, and water mattress overlays
  - Dynamic surfaces for stage III and IV ulcers: Alternating air overlays, low air loss beds
- Improve overall nutritional status (adequate protein intake, micronutrients).
- Wound management (4)[B]
  - Remove dead tissue (interferes with healing).
  - Dressing to manage drainage (e.g., Hydrocolloid, Hydrogel)
  - Dressing to protect from contamination, mechanical forces.
  - Chemical debridement may be indicated.
- Surgical debridement may be needed for stage III and IV wounds. Bone debridement may be necessary in deep ulcers.
- Vacuum-assisted closure is increasingly used for difficult wounds.
  - Negative pressure reduces wound edema and improves local tissue perfusion.
  - Removes necrotic debris and reduces bacterial load
  - Accelerates wound contraction (5)[B]

Diet
- Evaluation by a nutritionist to optimize oral or parenteral nutrition.
- Vitamin A to aid epithelialization and fibroblast stimulation
- Vitamin C (500 mg/d) to aid collagen synthesis and tensile strength
- Zinc (15 mg/d) for protein synthesis
- Copper for collagen production and cross-linking
- Manganese for collagen and ground substance

Activity
Perform passive range-of-motion exercises for patient or encourage patient to do active exercises if possible.

MEDICATION (DRUGS)

First Line
- For complications such as cellulitis, osteomyelitis, or sepsis, treat with systemic antibiotics. Regimen may be tailored based on culture and sensitivity.
- 2-week trial of topical antimicrobials for nonhealing ulcers, such as silver sulfadiazine or triple antibiotic ointment (6)[B]
- If cellulitis is suspected, osteomyelitis, tissue biopsy, and culture to determine antibiotic choice

SURGERY
May be considered for stage III and IV ulcers. Techniques include flap closure, direct closure, and skin grafts (6)[B]

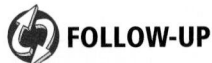 **FOLLOW-UP**

PROGNOSIS

Pressure ulcers are associated with increased rate of mortality, but with good medical care, most heal.

COMPLICATIONS

- Growth of resistant organisms if antibiotics used inappropriately
- Sepsis, cellulitis, septic arthritis, sinus tract or abscess, squamous cell carcinoma in ulcer
- Osteomyelitis in up to 25% of nonhealing ulcers
- Gangrene

PATIENT MONITORING

- Frequent evaluation of all patients with history of pressure sores, especially if limited mobility. Include nutritional status and dietary intervention.
- Early identification of areas of skin redness to prevent subsequent breakdown
- Skin cleansing as soon as soiled and at routine intervals

REFERENCES

1. Mechanick JI. Practical aspects of nutritional support for wound-healing patients. *Am J Surgery* 2004;188:525–565.
2. Horn SB, Bender SA, Ferguson ML. The National Pressure Ulcer Long-Term Study. *J Am Geriatric Soc* 2004;52:359–367.
3. Gray JE, Harding KG, Enoch S. Pressure ulcers. *BMJ* 2006;332:472–475.
4. Bansal C, Scott R, Stewart D. Decubitus ulcers: A review of the literature. *Int J Dermatol* 2005;44:805–810.
5. Moues CM, Vos MC, van den Bemd GJ, et al. Bacterial load in relation to vacuum-assisted closure wound therapy: A prospective randomized trial. *Wound Repair Regen* 2004;12:11–17.
6. Dharmarajan TS, Ahmed S. The growing problem of pressure ulcers. Evaluation and management for an aging population. *Postgrad Med* 2003;113:77–78,81–84,88–90.

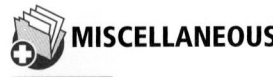 **MISCELLANEOUS**

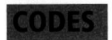 **CODES**

ICD9-CM
707.0 Decubitus ulcer

PATIENT TEACHING

 See Patient Handout on CD

PRETERM LABOR

John C. Smulian, MD, MPH
Cathryn Heath, MD

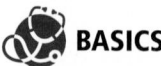 **BASICS**

DESCRIPTION
Labor occurring before completion of 36 weeks' gestation

ALERT
Pregnancy Considerations
By definition, a problem of pregnancy

GENERAL PREVENTION
- Patient education at each visit in 2nd and 3rd trimester for those at risk; for general population, periodically during 2nd and 3rd trimester
- Consider cerclage placement before 22 weeks' gestation for those at high risk because of an incompetent cervix or significant progressive cervical shortening. [B]
- Weekly injections of medroxyprogesterone from 16–32 weeks in at-risk pregnancies [A]

EPIDEMIOLOGY
- Predominant age: Child-bearing years
- Predominant sex: Female only
  - Race (increased in African Americans)

Incidence
Ten percent to 15% of pregnancies experience at least 1 episode of preterm labor

Prevalence
~12% of all births in the US

RISK FACTORS
- Prior preterm delivery (common)
- Multiple gestation
- Bacterial vaginosis (symptomatic)
- 3 or more 1st-trimester abortions
- Previous 2nd-trimester abortion
- Cervical incompetence
- Abdominal surgery/trauma during pregnancy
- Uterine or cervical anomalies
- Placenta previa
- Premature placental separation (abruption)
- Fetal abnormalities
- Polyhydramnios
- Serious maternal infections/diseases
- Vaginal bleeding during pregnancy
- Prepregnancy weight <45 kg (100 lb), body mass index <20
- Single parent
- No prenatal care
- Poverty
- Substance abuse (e.g., cocaine, tobacco)
- Intrauterine growth restriction

Genetics
Familial predisposition

ETIOLOGY
- Infections (urinary tract infection [UTI], pyelonephritis, pneumonia)
- Subclinical chorioamnionitis (e.g., intra-amniotic infections from aerobes, anaerobes, *Mycoplasma*; ureaplasma)
- Uterine abnormalities (e.g., incompetent cervix, leiomyomata; septa, diethylstilbestrol exposure)
- Overdistention (by multiple gestation or polyhydramnios)
- Premature rupture of membranes
- Trauma
- Iatrogenic
- Abruption of placenta
- Immunopathology (e.g., antiphospholipid antibodies)
- Placental hypoxia (preeclampsia and fetal growth restricton)

ASSOCIATED CONDITIONS
See "Risk Factors."

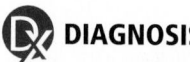 **DIAGNOSIS**

SIGNS AND SYMPTOMS
- Regular uterine contractions, with or without pain, continuing for 1 hour
- Dull low backache, pressure, or pain
- Intermittent lower abdominal or thigh pain
- Intestinal cramping, with or without diarrhea or indigestion
- Change in vaginal discharge
- Contractions every 5–10 minutes
- Dilatation of the cervix >1 cm
- Effacement of the cervix >50%
- Signs of ruptured membranes (continuous fluid leakage)

History
Address risk factors, especially etiologies of previous preterm birth

Physical Exam
- Uterine contraction monitoring
- Look for system infections
- Sterile speculum exam for membrane rupture evaluation, cultures, cervical inspection
- Check cervical dilation if intact membranes

TESTS
- Fetal fibronectin swabs, obtained from the posterior vaginal fornix after 22 weeks' gestation. If results are positive (≥50 ng/mL), patient is at increased risk of preterm birth (sensitivity 23%, specificity 97%). If negative, consider avoiding complicated or high-risk interventions. [A]
- Cervical sonography can identify women with a shortened cervix who are at higher risk for preterm birth. [A]
- Consider amniocentesis if ≥32 weeks' gestation for evaluation of lecithin:sphingomyelin (L:S) ratio and phosphatidalglyceral (PG). If L:S ratio is >2:1, and PG is present, hyaline membrane disease is unlikely. Also consider amniocentesis to evaluate for intra-amniotic infection (if cell count with differential; glucose; Gram stain; aerobic, anaerobic, mycoplasma, ureaplasma cultures. [C]

Lab
- Urinalysis and urine culture for evaluation of UTI
- Bacterial vaginosis evaluation
- Vaginal-rectal-perineal culture for group B *Streptococcus*
- Drug screen when appropriate
- CBC with differential
- Electrolytes, creatinine, and blood urea nitrogen to assess dehydration
- Nitrazine paper (blue color) and ferning test

Imaging
- Consider ultrasound to quantify gestational age, estimated fetal weight, multiple gestations, amount of amniotic fluid, and fetal growth [B]
- Transvaginal ultrasound to evaluate cervical length, funneling, and dynamic changes [B]

Diagnostic Procedures/Surgery
- Uterine monitoring for at least 2 hours or until contractions stop
- Speculum vaginal examination for signs of infection (e.g., purulent discharge, opaque membranes) and cultures
- pH and ferning testing for ruptured membranes

Pathological Findings
Placental inflammation; acute inflammation usually caused by infection; chronic inflammation caused by immunopathology; abruption.

DIFFERENTIAL DIAGNOSIS
- UTIs
- Round ligament pain
- Viral gastroenteritis
- Lumbosacral muscular back pain
- Vaginal infections
- Braxton-Hicks contractions/false labor
- Adnexal torsion
- Appendicitis
- Dehydration

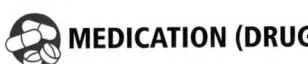

TREATMENT

GENERAL MEASURES

- Treat underlying risk factors with appropriate measures (e.g., antibiotics for infections, hydration for dehydration) [A]
- If delivery is inevitable, but not immediate, consider transport to a tertiary care center or hospital equipped with a neonatal ICU. [B]
- If mother is at 23–34 weeks' gestation and with no evidence of systemic infection, give glucocorticoids to decrease neonatal respiratory distress, intraventricular hemorrhage, and necrotizing enterocolitis. [A]

Diet
Liquids only or nothing by mouth if delivery imminent

Activity
- Pelvic rest (e.g., no douching or intercourse)
- Bed rest. Discontinue work and strenous physical activities.
- Hospitalization necessary if on IV tocolysis or if bed rest is impossible at home.

Nursing
Patient education about signs/symptoms of preterm labor

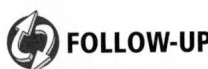

MEDICATION (DRUGS)

First Line
- Hydrate with 500-mL 5% dextrose normal saline solution or 5% dextrose lactated Ringer solution for 1st 1/2 hour.
- For tocolysis, protocols include
  – Magnesium sulfate solution of 40 g/1,000 mL of 5% dextrose normal saline solution. Bolus 4–6 g IV over 20 minutes, then begin infusion at 2 g/h, increasing by 0.5 g/h every 15–30 minutes to a maximum of 4 g/h; check reflexes and serum magnesium levels (therapeutic level is 6–8 mg/dL [2.47–3.29 mmol/L]). Stop when significant side effects found or if successful tocoysis for 6–12 hrs. Treat to allow steroid administration.
  – Nifedipine: 10 mg PO q10min up to 30 mg total; then 10–20 mg q6h×24h, then 10–20 mg PO q8h (do not use sublingual route). Check BP often and avoid hypotension. Concurrent use with magnesium sulfate is contraindicated.
- Antibiotics for group B Streptococcus prophylaxis pending cultures
- Glucocorticoids to decrease neonatal respiratory distress; protocols include
  – Betamethasone 12 mg IM 2 doses 24 hours apart or
  – Dexamethasone 6 mg IM b.i.d. for 4 doses or
  – Betamethasone 12 mg IM single dose can be repeated after 7 days as long as preterm delivery is likely; discontinue at 34 weeks' gestation.
- Tocolysis contraindications
  – Severe pre-eclampsia, hemorrhage, chorioamnionitis, advanced labor, intrauterine growth retardation, fetal heart decelerations, or lethal fetal abnormalities
  – Relative contraindications to terbutaline include maternal cardiac rhythm disturbance, poorly controlled diabetes or thyrotoxicosis.
  – Relative contraindications to magnesium sulfate are myasthenia gravis, hypocalcemia, renal failure, or concurrent use of calcium channel blockers.

- Precautions
  – Palpitations, nausea, intractable vomiting, pulse >140, decreased urine output
  – Long-term terbutaline may adversely affect glucose tolerance. Consider repeating glucose screen if using terbutaline >1 week.
- Significant possible interactions
  – Pulmonary edema from rehydration fluids and tocolytic agents, nifedipine, and magnesium sulfate

Second Line
- Terbutaline 0.25 mg SC q30min up to 3 doses until contractions stop. Then 0.25 SC q6h for 4 doses (optional). If contractions persist or pulse is >120, change to another tocolytic agent. (May be poorly tolerated by mothers).
- Indomethacin: 100 mg suppository per rectum q12h for 2 doses, then 25 mg q6–8h. Use for no longer than 72 hours owing to risk of premature closure of ductus arteriosus, oligohydramnios, and necrotizing enterocolitis.
- Oral maintenance therapy is controversial.
- Tebutaline infusion pumps potentially useful only in multiples or in very selected refractory or symptomatic cases

SURGERY
For malpresentation or fetal compromise, consider cesarean delivery if labor is progressing.

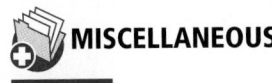

FOLLOW-UP

Based on symptoms

Admission Criteria
Suspected/threatened preterm labor

Discharge Criteria
Resolved regular contractions, no progressive contraction changes and able to follow decreased activity instructions at home

Issues for Referral
Consult maternal-fetal medicine specialist

PROGNOSIS
If membranes are ruptured and no infection is confirmed, delivery often occurs within 3–7 days. If membranes are intact, treat until 36–37 weeks' gestational age.

COMPLICATIONS
Labor resistant to tocolysis; pulmonary edema/fluid overload; other complications related to specific tocolytic used

PATIENT MONITORING
- Weekly office visits and cervical checks or cervical ultrasound for those at high risk for preterm labor [C]
- Ambulatory external tocodynamometry has not been proven effiective for preterm labor.

- Treating symptomatic bacterial vaginosis in 2nd trimester with metronidazole 250 mg PO t.i.d. for 7 days, erythromycin base 333 mg PO t.i.d. for 14 days; alternatively, using clindamycin 300 mg PO b.i.d. for 7 days may reduce risk of premature delivery. [B]
- Routine use of maintenance tocolysis has not been proven beneficial, especially with negative result to fetal fibronectin testing. [A]
- The role of cervicovaginal fetal fibronectin testing to assist risk assessment in asymptomatic women remains controversial. [C]

REFERENCES

1. Hollier LM. Preventing preterm birth: What works, what doesn't. *Obstet Gynecol Surv*. 2005;60(2): 124–31. [A]
2. Berghella V, et al. Cervical sonography in women with symptoms of preterm labor. *Obstet Gynecol Clin North Am*. 2005;32(3): 383–96. [A]
3. Berkman ND, et al. Tocolytic treatment for the management of preterm labor: A review of the evidence. *Am J Obstet Gynecol*. 2003;188(6):1648–1659. [A]

MISCELLANEOUS

CODES

ICD9-CM
- 644.03 Preterm labor (>22 weeks)
- 644.20 Early onset of delivery, unspecified as to episode of care or not applicable
- 644.21 Early onset of delivery, delivered with or without mention of antepartum condition

PATIENT TEACHING

Call physician or proceed to hospital whenever contractions last >1 hour, low back pain that comes and goes, change in vaginal discharge, "menstrual cramping," or intestinal cramping.

PRIAPISM

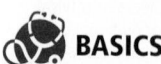

Bruce Block, MD

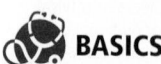

BASICS

DESCRIPTION
Painful and/or abnormally prolonged penile erection, either iatrogenic, pathologic, or idiopathic
- System(s) Affected: Reproductive

ALERT

Geriatric Considerations
Treatment is more difficult and is less likely to succeed in old people.

Pediatric Considerations
~85% likelihood of associated sickle cell anemia in affected African American children

GENERAL PREVENTION
- Avoid dehydration.
- Avoid excessive sexual stimulation.
- Avoid causative drugs (see "Causes") when possible.

EPIDEMIOLOGY
- Predominant age: Usually only young adults
- Predominant sex: Male only

Incidence
Unknown

Prevalence
Unknown

RISK FACTORS
Dehydration

ETIOLOGY
- Intracavernosal injections of vasoactive drugs for erectile dysfunction; most common cause
- Oral agents for erectile dysfunction
- Pelvic vascular thrombosis
- Prolonged sexual activity
- Sickle cell anemia
- Leukemia
- Other blood dyscrasias
- Pelvic hematoma or neoplasia
- Cerebrospinal tumors
- Tertiary syphilis
- Bladder calculus
- Injury to penis
- Urinary tract infections, especially prostatitis, urethritis, cystitis
- Several drugs suspected as causing priapism (e.g., chlorpromazine, prazosin, trazodone, and some corticosteroids, anticoagulants, and antihypertensives)
- Intracavernous fat emulsion

ASSOCIATED CONDITIONS
Sickle cell anemia

DIAGNOSIS

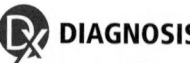

History
- Penile erection that is persistent, prolonged, painful, and tender
- Urination difficult during erection
- Loss of sexual function if treatment is not prompt and effective

Physical Exam
- Low-flow or ischemic priapism: Glans penis flaccid
- High-flow or arterial priapism: Glans penis rigid

TESTS

Lab
- Complete blood chemistry
- Sickling hemoglobin (Hgb) solubility test and Hgb electrophoresis
- Coagulation profile
- Platelet count
- Urinalysis

Imaging
Penile Doppler testing may be necessary to differentiate high-flow from low-flow priapism.

Diagnostic Procedures/Surgery
Physical examination is usually diagnostic.

Pathological Findings
- Pelvic vascular thrombosis
- Partial thrombosis of corpora cavernosa penis
- Corpus spongiosum, glans penis: No involvement
- Arterial priapism will show arteriocavernous fistula.

TREATMENT

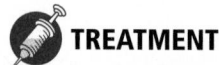

INITIAL STABILIZATION
Inpatient therapy required

GENERAL MEASURES
- Reassure patient about outcome if warranted.
- Continuous caudal or spinal anesthesia if etiology is neurogenic
- Treat any underlying cause.
- In sickle cell anemia: IV hydration; partial exchange or repeated transfusions to reduce percentage of sickle to <50%
- Relieve patient's pain.

Activity
Bed rest until condition resolves

MEDICATION (DRUGS)

- Narcotics for pain if needed
- Vasoconstrictors may be injected after dilution (e.g., metaraminol 1 mg into the penis)
- Contraindications
  - Refer to the manufacturer's literature.
- Precautions
  - Refer to the manufacturer's literature.
- Significant possible interactions
  - Refer to the manufacturer's literature.

SURGERY

- Introduction of 12- or 16-gauge needles into corpora cavernosa (best done by urologist if available) with aspiration of 20–30 mL of blood from corpus cavernosum penis. If caused by injected vasodilator, use intracavernous injection of 10–25 mg ephedrine sulfate or 5–10 μg epinephrine or 125–250 μg phenylephrine
  - May repeat 1 time in 20–30 minutes if no response
- Create fistula between glans and corpus cavernosum (with biopsy needle by urologist)
- Semipermanent diversion by saphenous shunt from one or both corpora
- Cavernosa-spongiosum shunt to permit re-establishment of pelvic circulation

 FOLLOW-UP

PROGNOSIS

- Even with excellent treatment, detumescence may require several weeks.
- Impotence is likely.

COMPLICATIONS

Erectile dysfunction (i.e., impotence)

PATIENT MONITORING

Close follow-up is required after surgery.

REFERENCES

1. Burnett AL. Pathophysiology of priapism: Dysregulatory erection physiology thesis. *J Urol*. 2003;170:26–34.
2. Harmon WJ, Nehra A. Priapism: Diagnosis and management. *Mayo Clin Proc*. 1997;12:350–355.
3. Pryor et al. Priapism. *J Sex Med*. 2004;1(1):200.
4. Smith DR. *General Urology*. 15th ed. Los Altos, CA: Lange Medical Publications; 2000.
5. Tanagho EA, McAninch JW, eds. *Smith's General Urology*. 12th ed. Norwalk, CT: Appleton & Lange; 1988.

 MISCELLANEOUS

See also: Anemia, Sickle Cell; Erectile Dysfunction

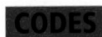

ICD9-CM
607.3 Priapism

PATIENT TEACHING

- Information about long-term outlook, referral for counseling
- Reduction of vasoactive drug therapy if responsible for priapism and elimination of offending drugs if causal

PROCTITIS

Felix B. Chang, MD

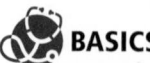 **BASICS**

DESCRIPTION
- An acute or chronic inflammation of the rectal mucosa
- System(s) Affected: Gastrointestinal

ALERT
Geriatric Considerations
Slower to heal, consider ischemia

Pediatric Considerations
- Not common, but if found, it is more apt to spread to full-blown disease in more proximal areas of the colon.
- Consider sexual abuse if gonorrheal infection is found on examination.

GENERAL PREVENTION
Practice techniques for safe sex, if sexually transmitted disease (STD) is causative.

EPIDEMIOLOGY
- Predominant age: Adult
- Predominant sex: Male > Female
- Radiation proctitis is usually encountered following treatment of cancers of the rectum, cervix, uterus, prostate, urinary bladder, and testes.

Incidence
0.5–3/100,000 (ulcerative proctitis)/10–30/100,000 (ulcerative proctitis)

RISK FACTORS
- Anal intercourse
- Radiation
- Rectal injury
- Rectal medications
- Jewish ancestry

Genetics
Higher incidence in Jews

ETIOLOGY
- Idiopathic
- Rectal gonorrhea
- Crohn disease
- Syphilis (usually secondary)
- Nonspecific sexually transmitted infection
- *Herpes simplex*
- *Chlamydia*
- Papillomavirus
- Amebiasis
- Lymphogranuloma venereum
- Ischemia
- Radiation therapy
- Toxins (e.g., hydrogen peroxide enemas)
- Vasculitis

ASSOCIATED CONDITIONS
- Syphilis
- Gonorrhea
- Other STD
- Prostate cancer (radiation therapy)

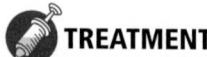 **DIAGNOSIS**

SIGNS AND SYMPTOMS
History
- Rectal and/or perianal discomfort
- Rectal bleeding and/or mucous discharge
- Diarrhea
- Tenesmus
- Urgency
- Constipation
- Fever
- Weight loss
- Rectal pain in radiation induce proctitis
- Radiation proctitis
  - Acute radiation injury occurs within 6 weeks of therapy
  - Chronic radiation proctitis: Delayed onset. The 1st sign most commonly occurs 9–14 month following radiation.

Physical Exam
- Radiation proctitis
  - Pale and friable mucosa, telangiectasias
- Proctosigmoidoscopy reveals friability, edema, and hyperemia of the mucosa. Ulceration and mucopurulent discharge may be present.

TESTS
Lab
- Serologic tests for syphilis, amebae, lymphogranuloma venereum
- Smear, culture from rectal wall
- Stool cultures
- If STD is suspected, check gonococcal and chlaymical culture and HIV.

Diagnostic Procedures/Surgery
- Flexible sigmoidoscopy
- Biopsy for histology, culture, viral studies, culture for *Chlamydia*
- Colonoscopy to exclude more proximal involvement

Pathological Findings
- Inflammation of rectal mucosa
- Ulceration
- Disruption of crypts

DIFFERENTIAL DIAGNOSIS
- Traumatic proctitis
- Radiation proctitis
- Ulcerative colitis
- Crohn disease
- Infections such as shigellosis or amebiasis
- Lymphogranuloma venereum
- Recurrent malignancies
- It is important to rule out: *Salmonella, Shigella, Campylobacter, E. coli, C. difficile* infection

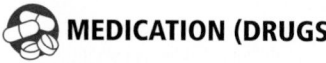 **TREATMENT**

INITIAL STABILIZATION
Outpatient, unless severe and refractory to usual measures

GENERAL MEASURES
- Treatment depends on the cause.
- Rectal Gram stains have a significant false-negative rate and, if clinician has strong suspicion of gonorrheal proctitis, empiric treatment is warranted while culture results are still pending.
- Avoid causative factors.
- Sitz baths may provide some relief.

Diet
No special diet

Activity
No restrictions

MEDICATION (DRUGS)

First Line
- Ulcerative proctitis
  - Topical 5-aminosalicylic acid (5-ASA) enemas and or suppositories for patient with mildly active proctitis (up to 8 bloody stools) low fever, mild abdominal pain (1)[B]
  - Topical steroids (e.g., hydrocortisone enemas or foam), mesalamine (Rowasa, 5-acetylsalicylic acid) enemas or suppositories; oral mesalamine (Asacol, Pentasa), olsalazine (Dipentum), sulfasalazine; systemic steroids are needed when condition is refractory to drugs mentioned here.
- Gonorrheal: 250 mg IM in a single dose plus doxycycline 100 mg PO b.i.d. for 7 days
- Herpetic: Oral acyclovir 200–400 mg 5 times a day for 10 days
- Chlamydial: 500 mg PO t.i.d. or doxycycline 100 mg PO b.i.d.
- Contraindications: Refer to the manufacturer's literature.
- Precautions: Refer to the manufacturer's literature.
- Significant possible interactions: Refer to the manufacturer's literature.
- Radiation proctitis
  - Topical butyrate enemas may accelerate healing in acute radiation injury.
  - Sucralfate enemas (20 mL of a 10% sucralfate suspension in water b.i.d.)
    ○ Sulfasalazine, aminosalicylates, hormonal therapy, hyperbaric oxygen, metronidazole, formaldehyde, vitamin A, argon plasma coagulation

Second Line
For gonorrheal proctitis: In patients unable to take ceftriaxone: 500 mg PO in a single dose. Perform culture 4–7 days after treatment to verify efficacy of treatment.

FOLLOW-UP

PROGNOSIS

- Satisfactory cure or control with appropriate treatment
- In patient with ulcerative proctitis, 10% of patients will not experience a recurrent attacks.
- Radiation proctitis may be associated with a significant decrease in health-related quality of life in up to 30% of patients.

COMPLICATIONS

- Chronic ulcerative colitis
- Fistula(e)/abscess formation
- Treatment failure (may be as high as 35% in gonorrheal proctitis)
- Perforation
- Radiation Injury: Fistulas, obstruction, associated urethral stenosis, cystitis
- Fecal incontinence, obstructed defecation in patient who develops fibrosis as a late complication of radiotherapy

PATIENT MONITORING

Follow until completely healed and monthly thereafter for 6 months.

REFERENCES

1. Denton A, Forbes A, Andreyev J, Maher EJ. Non surgical interventions for late radiation proctitis in patient who have received radical radiotherapy to the pelvis. Cochrane Database Sys Rev. *ISSN* 1464–780X.
2. Rompalo A. Diagnosis and treatment of sexually acquired proctitis and proctocolitis: An update. *Clin Infect Dis*. 1999;28(Suppl 1):S84–S90.
3. Cohen RD, Woseth DM, Thisted RA, Hanauer SB. A meta-analysis and overview of the literature on treatment options for left-sided ulcerative colitis and ulcerative proctitis. *Am J Gastroenterol*. 2000;95:1263.
4. Sutherland L, Roth D, Beck P, et al. Oral 5-aminosalicylic acid for maintaining remission in ulcerative colitis. *Cochrane Database Sys Rev*. 2000;Cdooo544.

 MISCELLANEOUS

See also: Crohn disease; Gonococcal infections; Herpes simplex; Lymphogranuloma venereum; Syphilis; Ulcerative colitis

CODES

ICD9-CM
569.49 Other specified disorders of rectum and anus, other

PATIENT TEACHING

Counsel about risk of HIV infection.

PROSTATIC CANCER

Drew A. Freilich, MD
Stephen Tosi, MD

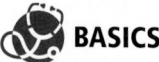

BASICS

DESCRIPTION

- The prostate is composed of acinar glands and their ducts arranged in a radial fashion with the stroma containing blood vessels, lymphatics, and nerves.
- 95% of prostate cancers are acinar adenocarcinomas.
- Staging: TNM Classification (AJCC 2002)
  - T1: Clinically inapparent tumor not palpable or visible by imaging.
  - T1a: Tumor incidental histological finding in ≤5% of tissue resected (by transurethral resection of prostate [TURP])
  - T1b: Tumor incidental histological finding in >5% of tissue resected (by TURP)
  - T1c: Tumor identified by needle biopsy (e.g., because of elevated PSA)
  - T2: Tumor confined within the prostate. (Note: Tumor found in 1 or both lobes by needle biopsy, but not palpable or visible by imaging, is classified as T1c).
  - T2a: Tumor involves ≤1/2 of 1 lobe.
  - T2b: Tumor involves >1/2 of 1 lobe, not both.
  - T2c: Tumor involves both lobes.
  - T3: Tumor extends through the prostatic capsule (Note: Invasion into the prostatic apex or into [but not beyond] the prostatic capsule is not classified as T3, but as T2).
  - T3a: Extracapsular extension (unilateral or bilateral)
  - T3b: Tumor invades seminal vesicle(s).
  - T4: Tumor is fixed or invades adjacent structures other than seminal vesicles; bladder neck, external sphincter, rectum, levator muscles, and/or pelvic wall.
- System(s) Affected: Reproductive; Urologic
- Synonym(s): Carcinoma of the prostate (CaP)

GENERAL PREVENTION
Data suggest a low/no-fat diet and/or a diet high in lycopene (i.e., tomatoes) may be preventative.

EPIDEMIOLOGY
- Predominant age: 6th or 7th decade; mean age at diagnosis is 71 years
- Most common cancer in men (~17% lifetime risk) and 2nd leading cancer cause of death in men (~3% of all CaP results in CaP-related death)

Incidence
In the US: 200/100,000 men per year

Prevalence
Most common malignancy in men. In the US, ~30% of 50-year-old men and 70% of 80-year-old men have pathologically discernible intraepithelial neoplasia of the prostate.

RISK FACTORS
- Age >50 years
- Positive family history
- Race (African Americans at increased risk)
- Endogenous hormonal influences
- Increased risk with vasectomy is unsupported

Genetics
Increased risk in patients with 1st-degree relatives with prostatic malignancy (~2X increased risk with 1st-degree relative affected at age <50)

PATHOPHYSIOLOGY
No gross functional changes in prostate

DIAGNOSIS

SIGNS AND SYMPTOMS
- May be asymptomatic early or late in disease course
- Induration/nodules on prostate on digital rectal examination (DRE)
- Symptoms of bladder outlet obstruction
- Hematospermia
- Weight loss
- Bone pain (with metastasis)
- Neurologic symptoms (with metastasis)

History
Ask about family history of CaP

Physical Exam
DRE to assess for prostatic masses/firmness

TESTS

Lab
- Total PSA: Elevated in most CaP
  - Total PSA ≥4.0 ng/mL (sensitivity ~80%, specificity ~65%) for CaP (1)
  - Rectal manipulation will not significantly increase PSA.
  - 5-α-Reductase inhibitors (i.e., Finasteride) decrease PSA ~50%. Double result to compare to premedication results
  - Prostatitis/BPH can cause PSA increase.
- Total PSA velocity ≥0.75 ng/mL/yr increases suspicion of CaP
- Alkaline phosphatase, elevated with metastasis
- Free PSA and age/race-adjusted PSA may be helpful in evaluating risk of CaP

Age/Race Adjusted "Normal" PSA Values (2)

Age	Asians	Blacks	Whites
40–49	0–2.0	0–2.0	0–2.5
50–59	0–3.0	0–4.0	0–3.5
60–69	0–4.0	0–4.5	0–4.5
70–79	0–5.0	0–5.5	0–6.5

PSA/Free PSA and Probability of Cancer (3)

PSA (ng/dl)	Cancer Rate	% Free PSA	Cancer Rate
0–2	1%	0–10%	56%
2–4	15%	10–15%	28%
4–10	25%	15–20%	20%
>10	>50%	20–25%	16%
		>25%	8%

- Patient-specific models to predict pathologic stage based on PSA, transrectal ultrasound (TRUS) biopsy results, and estimated clinical stage have been validated. (4)

Imaging
- Prostatic ultrasound, for biopsy guidance. TRUS alone for screening is not advocated.
- Bone scan: Positive with metastasis
  - Indication: PSA ≥20 ng/mL, Gleason ≥8, or bone pain (5).
- CT of pelvic lymph nodes, positive with metastasis
- MRI to assess extracapsular extension if cancer is confirmed.

Diagnostic Procedures/Surgery
- TRUS-guided biopsy
  - Indication: Abnormal DRE, elevated PSA
- Lymph node aspiration

Pathological Findings
- Small, closely packed glandular tissue
- Loss of basement membrane
- Perineural invasion

DIFFERENTIAL DIAGNOSIS
- Benign nodule prostate growth
- Prostatic intraepithelial neoplasia
- Prostate stones

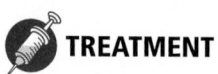

TREATMENT

Treatment selection recommendations
- T1a: Active surveillance may be appropriate.
- T1b, T1c: Candidate for prostatectomy, external beam radiation, brachytherapy (T1c only)
- T2a, T2b: Prostatectomy, external beam radiation, brachytherapy
- T3: Possible prostatectomy, possible radiation
- T4: Hormonal (androgen ablation) and/or chemotherapy

Diet
Low-fat diet, if strictly adhered to, may slow progression of prostate cancer.

SPECIAL THERAPY

Radiotherapy
- External beam radiation therapy
- Brachytherapy (radiation seed implantation)

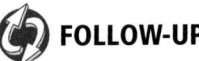

MEDICATION

First Line

- In androgen-dependent tumors, a reduction in serum testosterone is helpful in reducing tumor size, bone pain, and for improving survival. Orchiectomy (reduces serum testosterone ~90%) is the simplest androgen ablation method; however, medical castration can alternatively be utilized.
  – Indication: ≥T3a diagnosis, poor physical status, patient preference (5)
- GnRH agonists: Leuprolide, goserelin
- Contraindications: None
- Interactions possible: Refer to manufacturer's specific drug profile.
- Side effects
  – Osteoporosis
  – Gynecomastia
  – Erectile dysfunction/decreased libido
  – Flare phenomenon with metastatic disease
  – Fluid retention/weight gain
  – Hot flashes
  – Fatigue
  – Liver enzyme changes

Second Line

- Combined androgen blockade (GnRH agonist plus antiandrogen) often recommended, although some studies have shown no survival advantage over orchiectomy alone. Reduction in pain (54% vs. 37% in patients with orchiectomy alone) is significant.
- Antiandrogens: Bicalutamide, nilutamide, flutamide
  – Flutamide: No survival advantage over bicalutamide, and has increased diarrhea, Antabuse effects, and elevated LFTs
  – Nilutamide: Compared to bicalutamide has more side effects including diarrhea, interstitial pneumonitis, and light–dark adaptation problems.

Third Line

In addition to GnRH agonist and antiandrogen medications

- Chemotherapy: Mitoxantrone or docetaxel appears to improve survival, reduce pain in some patients. (6)
- Systematic androgen suppression: Ketoconazole: 30% response rate in those failing other antiandrogens by also suppressing adrenal androgens.

SURGERY

- Consider age and physical status
- Treatment options
  – Active surveillance (7)
  – Prostatectomy: (Retropubic, perineal, laparoscopic, robotic-assisted laparoscopic) +/− Intraoperative lymph node dissection:
    ○ Nerve sparing surgery possible if no extracapsular extension (ECE)
  – Brachytherapy
  – Cryoablation (1° for progression after external beam radiation therapy [EBRT])

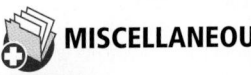

FOLLOW-UP

PROGNOSIS

- With early diagnosis and treatment, lesions should be curable.
- Advanced disease has a favorable prognosis if lesions are endocrine sensitive.
- Advanced unresponsive disease progresses in 18 months on average.

Prostate Cancer Survival by Stage

Stage	TNM	10-Year Survival
A	T1	NC
B	T2	75%
C	T3	55%
D	N1–2	(70% at 7 yr)
D	M1	15%

NC – No change from general population

- Postoperative nomograms to predict patient-specific CaP recurrence rates after prostatectomy and EBRT have been validated. (8)

PATIENT MONITORING

- Depends on treatment modality and patient-specific risk
- Prostatectomy: PSA/DRE every 6 months for 5 years, yearly thereafter
  – PSA >0.2 ng/mL after surgery is suggestive of recurrence.
- EBRT: PSA/DRE every 3 months for 1 year, every 3–6 months for 4 years, yearly thereafter
  – PSA ≥ 1.0 ng/mL or 3 consecutive PSA rises after EBRT is suggestive of recurrence
- CT/bone scans depend on PSA and symptoms

REFERENCES

1. Harris RP, Lohr KN, Beck R, et al. Screening for Prostate Cancer. Systematic Evidence Review No. 16. Rockville, MD: Agency for Healthcare Research and Quality. December 2001.
2. Oesterling JE, Jacobsen SJ, Chute CG. Serum prostate-specific antigen in a community-based population of healthy men. Establishment of age-specific reference ranges. JAMA. 1993;270(7):860–864.
3. Catalona WJ, Partin AW, Slawin KM, et al. Percentage of free PSA in black versus white men for detection and staging of prostate cancer: A prospective multicenter clinical trial. Urology. 2002;55(3): 372–376.
4. Partin AW, Kattan MW, Subong MS, et al. Combination of prostate specific antigen, clinical stage and Gleason score to predict pathological stage of localized prostate cancer: A multi-institutional update. JAMA. 1999;277:1445–1451.
5. National Comprehensive Cancer Network. Clinical practice guidelines: Prostate cancer. www.nccn.org. 2005.
6. Van Poppel H. Recent docetaxel studies establish a new standard of care in hormone refractory prostate cancer. Can J Urol. 2005;12(Suppl 1): 81–85.
7. Klotz L. Active surveillance versus radical treatment for favorable-risk localized prostate cancer. Curr Treat Options Onc. 2006;7(5):355–362.
8. Stephenson AJ, Sardino PT, Eastham JA, et al. Postoperative nomogram predicting the 10-year probability of prostate cancer recurrence after radical prostatectomy. J Clin Onc. 2005;22(29):7005–7012.
9. Rehabilitation therapy and urinary incontinence after radical retropubic prostatectomy: a critical review of the literature. Urologia Internationalis. 2006;76:193–198.

MISCELLANEOUS

CODES

ICD9-CM
185.0 Malignant neoplasm of prostate

PATIENT TEACHING

- "Prostate Cancer Awareness for Men"; American Urological Association. www.auanet.org
- American Cancer Society
- National Kidney and Urologic Diseases Information Clearinghouse (301) 468-6345

 See Corresponding Diagnostic Algorithm

See Patient Handout on CD

PROSTATIC HYPERPLASIA, BENIGN (BPH)

Ryan Frankel, MD
Pamela I. Ellsworth, MD

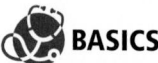 **BASICS**

DESCRIPTION
- Benign adenomatous increase of prostatic epithelial and stromal cells in the periurethral transition zone of the prostate leading to bladder outlet obstruction
- System(s) Affected: Renal/Urologic; Reproductive

GENERAL PREVENTION
Appears to be part of the aging process

EPIDEMIOLOGY
- Predominant age
  - Rarely seen in men <40
  - Seen in 50% of men >50; 80% of men >70
- Predominant sex: Male only

Incidence
- In US, universal pathologic phenomenon seen in older males
- No hard evidence suggesting racial predisposition

RISK FACTORS
- Intact testes (BPH rare in eunuchs)
- Aging (thus, rare in males <40 years old)
- No evidence of increased or decreased risk with smoking, alcohol, or any dietary factors
- Possible worsening of symptoms with abdominal obesity

Genetics
- Genetic factors may be involved.
- Males who had 1st degree relative with BPH are at increased risk

PATHOPHYSIOLOGY
Prostatic hyperplasia leading to bladder outlet obstruction, which may affect bladder function

ETIOLOGY
Primary causal factors involve androgens, growth factors, and genetics.

ASSOCIATED CONDITIONS
BPH symptoms are a strong and independent risk factor for sexual dysfunction including erectile dysfunction and ejaculatory disorders (1)[C]

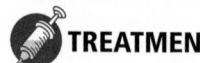 **DIAGNOSIS**

SIGNS AND SYMPTOMS
History
- Gross hematuria
- Obstructive symptoms
  - Decrease force or caliber of stream
  - Hesitancy
  - Postvoid dribbling
  - Sensation of incomplete bladder emptying
  - Overflow incontinence
  - Inability to voluntarily stop stream
  - Urinary retention
- Irritative symptoms
  - Frequency
  - Nocturia
  - Urgency
  - Urge incontinence
- Symptom scores such as American Urological Association (AUA) or International Prostate Symptom Score (IPSS) may be helpful in management

Physical Exam
- Distended bladder (>150 cc in order to detect by percussion)
- Digital rectal exam finding of enlarged prostate, but size does not always correlate with symptoms
- Clinical clues suggesting renal failure due to obstructive uropathy (edema, pallor, pruritus, ecchymoses, nutritional deficiencies)

TESTS
- Uroflow: Volume voided per unit time (Peak flow <10 mL/sec is abnormal)
- Post-void residual: Either with catheterization or bladder ultrasound (>100 mL demonstrates incomplete emptying)

Lab
- Urinalysis: Pyuria if stones or infection present, pH changes due to chronic residual urine
- Urine culture positive (sometimes due to chronic residual urine)
- Blood urea nitrogen and creatinine (if concerns for uremia)
- Prostate-specific antigen (PSA) may be elevated but usually <10 ng/mL (10 μg/L)
  - Acute urinary retention, prostatitis, urinary tract instrumentation, or prostatic infarction may elevate PSA

Imaging
- Transrectal ultrasound: Assessment of gland size
- Abdominal ultrasound: Can demonstrate increased post-void residual or hydronephrosis

Diagnostic Procedures/Surgery
- Pressure-flow studies (urine flow vs. voiding pressures): Best test to determine etiology of voiding symptoms
  - Obstructive pattern shows high voiding pressures with low flow rate
- Cystoscopy
  - Demonstrates presence, configuration, and site of obstructive tissue
  - Helps to show stricture, stones
  - May help determine best therapy option

Pathological Findings
Confirmation obtained by biopsy, resection, or surgical removal

DIFFERENTIAL DIAGNOSIS
- Obstructive
  - Prostate cancer
  - Urethral stricture or valves
  - Bladder neck contracture (usually secondary to prostate surgery)
  - Inability of bladder neck or external sphincter to relax appropriately during voiding
- Neurologic
  - Spinal cord injury
  - Stroke
  - Parkinsonism
  - Mutliple sclerosis
- Medical
  - Poorly controlled diabetes mellitus
  - Congestive heart failure
- Pharmacologic
  - Diuretics
  - Sympathomimetics (e.g., cold medications)
  - Anticholinergics
- Other
  - Bladder carcinoma
  - Prostatitis
  - Overactive bladder

TREATMENT

INITIAL STABILIZATION
Patients in urinary retention require bladder drainage
- If catheterization difficult, consider coude catheter or flexible cystoscopy
- Consider possible postobstructive diuresis; if present, monitor electrolytes

GENERAL MEASURES
- Avoid prolonged periods of not voiding.
- Avoid sympathomimetic or anticholinergic medications.

Diet
Avoid large boluses of oral or IV fluids or alcohol intake

Activity
Patient more likely to void after surgery or illness when ambulatory and able to stand over the toilet

Complementary and Alternative Medicine
- Phytotherapy

- Saw palmetto (*Serenoa repens*) has shown mild improvement of peak flow rates and appears to work by blocking 5-alpha-reductase (2)[A]

MEDICATION (DRUGS)

First Line
- Alpha-adrenergic antagonists
  - Terazosin (Hytrin): 1–10 mg/d PO (3)[A]
  - Doxazosin (Cardura): 1–8 mg/d PO
  - Tamsulosin (Flomax): 0.4 mg/d PO (4)[A]
  - Alfuzosin (Uroxatral): 10 mg/d PO
- 5-alpha-reductase inhibitors (better for larger prostates)
  - Finasteride (Proscar): 5 mg/d PO
  - Dutasteride (Avodart): 0.5 mg/d PO
  - Also useful in controlling prostatic bleeding
- Combination therapy of alpha blocker plus 5-alpha-reductase inhibitor is superior to monotherapy (5)[B]
- Contraindications
  - Alpha blockers can cause orthostatic hypotension; less risk with tamsulosin and alfuzosin
  - See specific recommendations for alpha blocker use with phosphodiesterase type 5 inhibitors (for erectile dysfunction)

ALERT
5-alpha-reductase inhibitors reduce PSA by 1/2, so PSA should be doubled for purposes of screening for prostate cancer

Geriatric Considerations
Drugs to be avoided include anticholinergics, antihistamines, sympathomimetics, tricyclic antidepressants, narcotics, and skeletal muscle relaxants when possible

SURGERY
- Indications for surgery
  - Urinary retention due to prostatic obstruction, recurrent
  - Intractable symptoms due to prostatic obstruction (AUA sx score >8 and bother)
  - Obstructive uropathy (renal insufficiency)
  - Recurrent or persistent urinary tract infections due to prostatic obstruction
  - Recurrent gross hematuria due to enlarged prostate
  - Bladder calculi
- Surgical procedures
  - Transurethral resection of the prostate: Gold standard
  - Open prostatectomy: Treatment of choice for patients with extremely large prostates (>100 g)
  - Transurethral incision of the prostate: Treatment of choice for men with obstruction and small prostates
  - Transurethral laser ablation: Holmium laser ablation of the tissue; useful in patients on anti-coagulant therapy
  - Transurethral needle ablation: Office-based minimally invasive approach usually used with small prostates
  - Transurethral microwave thermotherapy: Office-based minimally invasive approach usually used with small prostates
- Complications of TURP
  - Bleeding which can be significant
  - TUR syndrome: Hyponatremia secondary to absorption of hypotonic irrigant
  - Retrograde ejaculation

 FOLLOW-UP

PROGNOSIS
- Symptoms improve or stabilize in 70–80% of patients; 20–30% require treatment because of worsening symptoms.
- Of the men with BPH, 11–33% have occult prostate cancer.

COMPLICATIONS
- Urinary retention (acute or chronic)
- Bladder stones
- Prostatitis
- Renal failure
- Hematuria

PATIENT MONITORING
- Symptom index (IPSS) monitored every 3–12 months
- Digital rectal exam yearly
- PSA yearly: Should not be checked while patient is in retention, recently catheterized, or within a week of any surgical procedure to the prostate
- Consider monitoring pulmonary vascular resistance if elevated

REFERENCES
1. Rosen R, et al. Lower urinary tract symptoms and male sexual dysfunction: The multinational survey of the aging male. *European Urology.* 2003; 44:637–649.
2. Wilt T, Ishani A, MacDonald R. Seronoa repens for benign prostatic hyperplasia. *The Cochrane Database of Systematic Reviews.* 2005;4.
3. Wilt TJ, et al. Terazosin for benign prostatic hyperplasia. *The Cochrane Database of Systematic Reviews.* 2005;4.
4. Wilt TJ, MacDonald R, Rutks I. Tamsulosin for benign prostatic hyperplasia. *The Cochrane Database of Systematic Revews.* 2005;4.
5. McConnell JD, et al. Medical Therapy of Prostatic Symptoms Research Group. The long-term effect of doxazosin, finasteride, and combination therapy on the clinical progression of benign prostatic hyperplasia. *N Engl J Med.* 2003;349:2387–2398.
6. Hoffman RM, Macdonald R, Wilt TJ. Laser prostatectomy for benign prostatic obstruction. *The Cochrane Database of Systematic Reviews.* 2005;4.

 MISCELLANEOUS

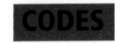 **CODES**

ICD9-CM
- 600.90 Hyperplasia of prostate, unspecified, without urinary obstruction
- 600.91 Hyperplasia of prostate, unspecified, with urinary obstruction

PATIENT TEACHING
- *The Prostate Book*, published by Krames Communications, 312 90th St, Daly City, CA 94015-1898.
- National Kidney and Urologic Diseases Information Clearinghouse, Box NKUDIC, Bethesda, MD 20893; (301) 468-6345.

 See Corresponding Diagnostic Algorithm

 See Patient Handout on CD

PROSTATITIS

Felix B. Chang, MD
Ximena M. Castro, MD

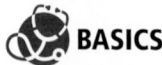 **BASICS**

DESCRIPTION
- 1 of several inflammatory or painful conditions affecting the prostate gland; National Institutes of Health's (NIH) prostatitis classification
- Acute bacterial prostatitis (NIH Class I): Generally associated with urinary tract infection (UTI), has characteristically abrupt onset
- Chronic bacterial prostatitis (NIH Class II): Cause of recurrent bacteriuria, less fulminant
- Chronic prostatitis (CP)/chronic pelvic pain syndrome (CPPS) (NIH Class III)
  - Inflammatory (NIH Class IIIa): Inflammatory cells in prostatic secretions, postprostatic massage urine or seminal fluid
  - Noninflammatory (NIH Class IIIb): Similar to chronic bacterial, but bacterial culture negative
- Asymptomatic inflammatory prostatitis (NIH Class IV): Incidental finding during prostate biopsy for infertility, cancer workup
- System(s) Affected: Renal/Urologic; Reproductive

NIH Classification of Prostatitis

Trad Class	-VB2- Cult	WBC	-EPS- Cult	WBC	NIH Class
ABP	+	+	+	+	I
CBP	+	+	+	+	II
NBP	0	0	0	+	IIIa
Pdyn[a]	0	0	0	0	IIIb
Asymt	+ −	+	+ −	−	IV

[a] pdyn, prostatodynia

GENERAL PREVENTION
Suppression therapy may benefit patients with chronic bacterial prostatitis.

EPIDEMIOLOGY
- Predominant age: 30–50, sexually active; chronic more common in ages >50
- Predominant sex: Male only
- Bacterial prostatitis occurs more frequently in patients with HIV than in the general population.

Incidence
Two million cases annually in US National Ambulatory Medical Care Surveys

Prevalence
Common

RISK FACTORS
- Male sex
- Age >50 years
- Prostatic calculi
- UTI
- Trauma (e.g., bicycle, horseback riding)
- Dehydration
- Sexual abstinence
- Chronic indwelling catheter
- Intermittent catheterization
- HIV positive
- Urethral stricture
- Cystoscopy
- Urethral dilatation
- Transurethral resection of the prostate (TURP)
- Transrectal biopsy

Genetics
No known genetic pattern

PATHOPHYSIOLOGY
- Extension of urinary tract infection
- May occur following manipulation of prostate or urethra

ETIOLOGY
- Bacterial
  - Ascending infection through urethra
  - Refluxing urine into prostate ducts
  - Direct extension or lymphatic spread from rectum
  - Hematogenous spread
  - Calculi serving as nidus for infection
  - Aerobic Gram-negative bacteria (*Escherichia coli, Pseudomonas, Klebsiella, Proteus*), *Neisseria gonorrhea, Enterobacteriaceae, Burkholderia pseudomallei*)
  - Miscellaneous: *Chlamydia trachomatis*
  - Gram-positive bacteria (*Streptococcus faecalis, Staphylococcus aureus*)
  - Organisms suspected, but unproven (*Staphylococcus epidermidis*, micrococci, non-group D *Streptococcus*, diphtheroids)
  - Uncommon: *Mycobacterium tuberculosis*, parasitic, mycoses (blastomycosis, coccidioidomycosis, cryptococcus, histoplasmosis, paracoccidiomycosis, candidiasis)
- Nonbacterial
  - Nonrelaxation (spasm) of the internal urinary sphincter and pelvic floor striated muscles leading to increased prostatic urethral pressure and intraprostatic urinary reflux; leading theory
  - *Ureaplasma, Trichomonas vaginalis*, and *Chlamydia* postulated, but not proven

ASSOCIATED CONDITIONS
- Prostatic hypertrophy
- Cystitis
- Urethritis
- Pyelonephritis

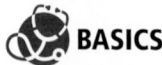 **DIAGNOSIS**

SIGNS AND SYMPTOMS
- Acute bacterial
  - Fever; chills, malaise
  - Tense, boggy, very tender and warm prostate
  - Low back pain, myalgias
  - Prostatodynia, perineal pain (Note: Prostatodynia, pain in the area of prostate, is sometimes inaccurately designated as a diagnosis)
  - Frequency
  - Urgency
  - Dysuria
  - Nocturia
  - Bladder outlet obstruction
- Chronic bacterial
  - Symptoms often absent
  - Prostatodynia, perineal pain
  - Dysuria, irritative voiding
  - Lower abdominal pain
  - Low back pain
  - Scrotal pain
  - Penile pain
  - Pain on ejaculation
  - Hematospermia

- Chronic prostatitis/chronic pelvic pain syndrome (inflammatory/noninflammatory)
  - Prostatodynia, perineal pain
  - Dysuria, irritative voiding
  - Lower abdominal pain
  - Low back pain
  - Scrotal pain
  - Penile pain
  - Pain on ejaculation
  - Hematospermia

ALERT
Avoid massage of the prostate in acute bacterial prostatitis; may induce iatrogenic bacteremia.

Geriatric Considerations
Consider prostatic hypertrophy and urinary retention more seriously.

Physical Exam
- Very tender boggy prostate on rectal exam
- Prostate may be warn, swollen, firm, irregular
- Prostatic massage is contraindicated.

TESTS
Lab
- Suspected acute prostatitis (NIH Class I)
  - Urinalysis, urine and blood cultures, urine Gram stain
  - CBC/differential
- Suspected chronic prostatitis/chronic pelvic pain (NIH Class III)
  - Urinalysis, urine culture, post-void residual (ultrasound or catheterization) if sensation of incomplete emptying of bladder. [C]
- Suspected chronic bacterial prostatitis (NIH Class II)
- Consider performing the fractional urine examination (4 glass test) specimen collection
  - VB1 (voided bladder 1): Initial 10 mL urine from urethra
  - VB2: Next 200 mL discarded, then midstream from bladder; expressed prostatic fluid (EPS), then expressed prostate secretion;
  - VB3: Urine after prostate massage
- Specimen handling
  - Urinalysis, culture, sensitivities, Gram stain on all samples
  - pH of EPS
  - Bacterial antigen-specific IgA and IgG levels in EPS
  - Wet mount of EPS
- Interpretation
  - 10–15 white cells per high-powered field suggest bacterial prostatitis.
  - Macrophages containing fat (oval bodies) suggest bacterial prostatitis.
  - A positive culture in EPS or VB3 but not VB1 or VB2 is diagnostic of bacterial prostatitis.
  - In acute bacterial prostatitis, serum and EPS fluid bacterial antigen-specific IgA and IgG can be detected immediately after the onset of the infection. Level declines over 6–12 months after successful antibiotic therapy.
  - Bacteria count is less in chronic prostatitis.
  - In chronic bacterial prostatitis, no serum IgG elevation is seen, whereas EPS fluid IgA and IgG levels are increased. With antibiotic therapy, IgG levels return to normal in several months, but IgA levels remain elevated for 2 years.

- Prostatic fluid is alkaline in chronic bacterial prostatitis.
- WBCs with a negative culture (although false-negative cultures are not uncommon) suggests nonbacterial prostatitis.
- No abnormal findings with chronic prostatitis without inflammation (this misnomer refers to patients with symptoms such as perineal pain, ejaculatory pain, and lower abdominal pain but not having inflammatory changes on lab studies)

- Prostate-specific antigen level is increased with acute prostatitis (do not order for PSA until at least 1 month after prostatitis is treated.) [B]

- Drugs that may alter lab results: Antibiotics

Imaging
- CT or ultrasound, if malignancy or abscess suspected
- Transrectal ultrasound (if prostatic calculi or abscess suspected)

Diagnostic Procedures/Surgery
- Needle biopsy or aspiration for culture
- Urodynamic testing (prostatodynia)
- Cystoscopy (in persistent nonbacterial prostatitis to rule out bladder cancer, interstitial cystitis)

Pathological Findings
Inflammatory changes (except prostatodynia)

DIFFERENTIAL DIAGNOSIS
- Cystitis (bacterial, interstitial)
- Urethritis
- Pyelonephritis
- Malignancy
- Obstructive calculus
- Foreign body
- Acute urinary retention

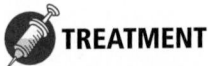 **TREATMENT**

INITIAL STABILIZATION
- Inpatient (proven or suspected abscess, urosepsis, immunocompromised)
- Outpatient, if nontoxic

GENERAL MEASURES
- Analgesics
- Antipyretics
- Stool softeners
- Hydration
- Sitz baths to relieve pain and spasm
- Suprapubic catheter for severe urinary retention
- Psychotherapy if sexual dysfunction
- Neuromodulation, acupuncture, heat therapy, antidepressants, antianxiolytics, analgesics

Activity
Bed rest in severe cases

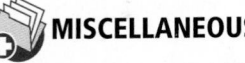 **MEDICATION (DRUGS)**

First Line
- Acute bacterial (outpatient)
  - If urine shows Gram-positive cocci, amoxicillin 500 mg PO t.i.d. for 30 days, otherwise, use
  - Trimethoprim-sulfamethoxazole, 1 DS tab b.i.d. PO for 30 days
- Acute bacterial (inpatient)
  - Ampicillin 1–3 g IV divided q6h plus aminoglycoside, gentamicin 2 mg/kg IV loading dose, 1.7 mg/kg IV q8h maintenance. Begin oral therapy after afebrile for 24–48 hours.
- Chronic bacterial
  - A fluoroquinolone (e.g., ofloxacin 300 mg b.i.d. PO, ciprofloxacin 500 mg 2 b.i.d. PO) for 4–12 weeks
- Chronic prostatitis/chronic pelvic pain syndrome without inflammation (3)[B]
  - α-Adrenergic blocking agents (e.g., terazosin, 1 mg PO qhs increased slowly to a maximum of 10 mg/d) may be useful (discontinue if no benefit after maximum of 6 months) (4)[A]

- Analgesics, NSAIDs
- Antipyretics
- Stool softeners
- Contraindications: Drug allergies
- Precautions
  - Renal disease
  - Hepatic disease
  - Elderly may not tolerate higher-dose benzodiazepines
  - G6PD deficiency may manifest with sulfonamides or NSAIDs
- Significant possible interactions Fluoroquinolones magnesium/aluminum antacids, theophylline, probenecid, NSAIDs, warfarin

Second Line
- Carbenicillin with aminoglycoside, erythromycin, tetracycline, cephalexin, fluoroquinolones, dicloxacillin, nafcillin IV, vancomycin IV

- Finasteride (in patients >45 years old, category IIIa inflammatory CP/CPPS, and enlarged prostate glands) (5)[A]
- Pentosan, 100 mg PO t.i.d., in patients with suprapubic discomfort associated with frequency and urgency (6)[B]

- Nonbacterial: May benefit from erythromycin, doxycycline, trimethoprim-sulfamethoxazole

SURGERY
- Surgical resection for intractable chronic disease, or to drain an abscess
- Transurethral microwave thermotherapy for chronic nonbacterial prostatitis

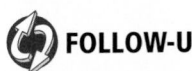 **FOLLOW-UP**

- Most improve with antibiotics for 3–4 weeks.
- No specific follow-up is necessary.
- Consider prostatic abscess in patients who do not respond well to therapy.

Issues for Referral
Urology referral for surgical drainage if an abscess is persistent after ≥1 week of therapy.

PROGNOSIS
- Often prolonged and difficult to cure; 55–97% cure rate depending on population and drug used.
- ~20% had reinfection or persistent infection.

COMPLICATIONS
- Prostatic abscess (common in HIV-infected)
- Gram-negative sepsis, bacteremia
- Urinary retention
- Epididymitis
- Chronic bacterial prostatitis (with acute prostatitis)
- Metastatic infection (spinal, sacroiliac)

PATIENT MONITORING
- Acute bacterial: Urinalysis and culture 30 days after initiating treatment
- Chronic bacterial: Urinalysis and culture every 30 days (may take several months)
- NIH-Chronic Prostatitis Symptom Index (NIH-CPSI) 13 items tabulated into 3 domain scores: (i) pain, (ii) urinary symptoms, and (iii) quality of life. Reference: http://www.niddk.nih.gov/fund/divisions/kuh/useful-tools/english-nih-cpsi.pdf.

REFERENCES
1. Schaeffer AJ. Etiology and management of chronic pelvic pain syndrome in men. *Urology.* 2004;63:75.
2. Game X, et al. Total Free serum prostate specific antigen levels during the first month of acute prostatitis. *Eur Urol.* 2003;43:702–705.
3. Nickle JC, et al. Failure of monotherapy strategy for difficult chronic prostatitis /chronic pain syndrome. *J Urol.* 2004;172:551–554.
4. Allopurinol for chronic prostatitis. Cochrane Database Sys Rev. *The Cochrane Library ISSN* 1464–780X.
5. McNaughton CM, Mac Donald R, Wilt T. Interventions for abacterial prostatitis. *Cochrane Database Sys Rev.* 2006;4.

 MISCELLANEOUS

See also: Prostatic cancer; Prostatic hyperplasia benign (BPH); Urinary tract infection

CODES

ICD9-CM
- 601.0 Acute prostatitis
- 601.1 Chronic prostatitis

PATIENT TEACHING
Printed patient information available from the National Kidney and Urologic Diseases Information Clearinghouse, Box NKUDIC, Bethesda, MD 20893; (301) 468-6345.

 See Corresponding Diagnostic Algorithm

See Patient Handout on CD

PROTEIN C DEFICIENCY

Marc Jeffrey Kahn, MD

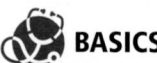 **BASICS**

DESCRIPTION

Protein C is a vitamin K–dependent factor made by the liver that becomes activated when thrombin binds to the endothelial receptor, thrombomodulin. Activated protein C, with protein S as a cofactor, inactivates factors Va and VIIIa. Patients with protein C deficiency have a thrombotic disorder that primarily affects the venous system.

- System(s) Affected: Cardiovascular, Hemic/Lymphatic/Immunologic, Pulmonary

GENERAL PREVENTION

Patients with protein C deficiency without thrombosis do not require prophylactic treatment

EPIDEMIOLOGY

- Predominant age: Mean age of first thrombosis is 45 years
- Predominant sex: Male = Female

Prevalence

- 0.3% of normal individuals
- 4–5% of persons with venous thrombosis

RISK FACTORS

- Oral contraceptives, pregnancy, and the use of hormone replacement therapy increase the risk of venous thrombosis in patients with protein C deficiency (1)[A]
- Patients with protein C deficiency and another prothrombotic state such as factor V Leiden have increased rates of thrombosis (1)[A]
- Patients heterozygous for protein C deficiency who are begun on warfarin without concomitant heparin can develop warfarin-induced skin necrosis because the half life of other vitamin K–dependent clotting factors, prothrombin, factor IX and factor X, are much longer than protein C (4–8 hours). These patients develop extremely low levels of protein C and develop necrosis of the skin over central areas of the body such as the breast, abdomen, buttocks, and genitalia. (1)[A]

ALERT

Pregnancy Considerations

Increases thrombotic risk in patients with protein C deficiency

Genetics

- Autosomal dominant. Heterozygotes have an odds ratio of venous thrombosis of 6.5:8.
- Arterial thrombosis is rare. Heterozygotes can have a fulminant thrombotic event in infancy, termed neonatal purpura fulminans.

ETIOLOGY

Polymorphisms in the promoter region of the protein C gene can affect antigen levels. At least 150 mutations have been described in the protein C gene that can lead to functional deficiency. Acquired protein C deficiency can occur with liver disease and rare patients can develop inhibitors to activated protein C. Neonates have lower levels of protein C than adults.

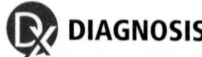 **DIAGNOSIS**

SIGNS AND SYMPTOMS

- Deep and superficial venous thrombosis, often spontaneous
- Up to 50% of homozygotes will have thrombosis
- Sites of thrombosis can be unusual, including the mesentery and cerebral veins.
- Arterial thrombosis is rare.

TESTS

Lab

- Protein C activity assay utilizing a snake venom protease to activate protein C
- Immunoassay for quantitative assessment of protein C level
- Drugs that may alter lab results
  – Oral contraceptives can raise protein C levels.
  – Warfarin reduces protein C levels
- Disorders that may alter lab results
  – Liver disease reduces protein C levels.
  – Acute thrombosis can lower protein C levels.

DIFFERENTIAL DIAGNOSIS

- Factor V Leiden
- Protein S deficiency
- Antithrombin deficiency
- Dysfi brinogenemia
- Dysplasminogenemia
- Homocysteinemia
- Prothrombin 20210 mutation
- Elevated factor VIII levels

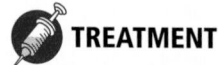 **TREATMENT**

INITIAL STABILIZATION
Outpatient

GENERAL MEASURES

- Routine anticoagulation for aymptomatic patients with protein C deficiency is not recommended (1)[A]

- Anticoagulation for 6–12 months is recommended for patients with protein C deficiency and a 1st thrombosis
- Some argue lifetime anticoagulation; data are limited
- Anticoagulation for life is indicated for patients with protein C deficiency and recurrent thrombosis

- The role of family screening for protein C deficiency is unclear because most patients with this mutation do not have thrombosis. Screening should be considered for woman considering using oral contraceptives or pregnancy with a family history of protein C deficiency. (2)[B]

Diet
No restrictions

Activity
No restrictions

MEDICATION (DRUGS)

First Line

- Low molecular weight heparin (LMWH) (1)[A]
  – Enoxaparin (Lovenox) 1 mg/kg SC b.i.d. Alternatively, 1.5 mg/kg/d SC. Initially for at least 5 days or until international normalized ratio (INR) is 2–3, at which time it can be stopped
  – Tinzaparin (Innohep) 175 anti-Xa IU/kg/d SQ
  – Dalteparin (Fragmin) 200 IU/kg/d
- Oral anticoagulant—warfarin (Coumadin) 5 mg/d PO initially and maintained on warfarin with an INR of 2–3 for at least 6 months (1)[A]

- Contraindications
  – Active bleeding precludes anticoagulation; risk of bleeding is a relative contraindication to long-term anticoagulation
  – Warfarin is contraindicated in patients with a prior history of warfarin-induced skin necrosis
- Precautions
  – Observe patient for signs of embolization, further thrombosis, or bleeding
  – Avoid IM injections.
  – Periodically check stool and urine for occult blood, monitor complete blood counts including platelets
  – Heparin—thrombocytopenia and/or paradoxical thrombosis with thrombocytopenia
  – Warfarin—necrotic skin lesions (typically breasts, thighs, and buttocks)
  – LMWH—adjust dose in renal insufficiency
- Significant possible interactions
  – Agents that intensify the response to oral anticoagulants: Alcohol, allopurinol, amiodarone, anabolic steroids, androgens, many antimicrobials, cimetidine, chloral hydrate, disulfiram, all NSAIDs, sulfinpyrazone, tamoxifen, thyroid hormone, vitamin E, ranitidine, salicylates, acetaminophen
  – Agents that diminish the response to oral anticoagulants: Aminoglutethimide, antacids, barbiturates, carbamazepine, cholestyramine, diuretics, griseofulvin, rifampin, oral contraceptives

Second Line
Heparin 80 mg/kg IV bolus followed by 18 mg/kg/hr Adjust dose depending on partial prothrombin time.

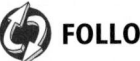 **FOLLOW-UP**

PROGNOSIS
- When compared to normal individuals, persons with protein C deficiency have normal life spans.
- By age 45, 1/2 of the people heterozygous for protein C deficiency will have venous thrombosis that is spontaneous 1/2 of the time

COMPLICATIONS
Recurrent thrombosis (requires indefinite anticoagulation)

PATIENT MONITORING
Warfarin requires periodic (monthly after initial stabilization) monitoring of the INR.

REFERENCES

1. Bick RL. Prothrombin G20210A mutation, antithrombin, heparin cofactor II, protein C, and protein S defects. *Hematol Oncol Clin North Am*. 2003;(1):9–36
2. Langlois NJ, Wells PS. Risk of venous thromboembolism in relatives of symptomatic probands with thrombophilia: A systematic review. *Thromb Haemost*. 2003;90(1):17–26
3. Thomas RH. Hypercoagulability syndromes. *Arch Intern Med*. 2001;161(20):2433–2439

 MISCELLANEOUS

See also: Protein S deficiency; Prothrombin 20210 (Mutation); Thrombosis, deep vein thrombophlebitis (DVT); Antithrombin deficiency; Factor V leiden

CODES

ICD9-CM
286.9 Other and unspecified coagulation defects

PATIENT TEACHING

Patients should be educated about use of oral anticoagulant therapy if taking such. Avoid NSAIDs while on warfarin.

PROTEIN S DEFICIENCY

Marc Jeffrey Kahn, MD

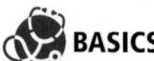 **BASICS**

DESCRIPTION

- Protein S is a vitamin K–dependent factor made principally by the liver that acts as a cofactor for protein C. Protein C becomes activated when thrombin binds to the endothelial receptor, thrombomodulin. Activated protein C, with protein S as a cofactor, inactivates factors Va and VIIIa. Protein S is also able to directly inhibit factors Va, VIIa and Xa independently of activated protein C. Patients with protein S deficiency have a thrombotic disorder that primarily affects the venous system.
- System(s) Affected: Cardiovascular; Hemic/Lymphatic/Immunologic; Pulmonary

GENERAL PREVENTION

Patients with protein S deficiency without thrombosis do not require prophylactic treatment (1)[A]

EPIDEMIOLOGY

- Predominant age: Mean age of 1st thrombosis is in the 2nd decade
- Predominant sex: Male = Female

Prevalence

- 0.3% of normal individuals
- Found in 3% of persons with venous thrombosis

RISK FACTORS

- Oral contraceptives, pregnancy, and the use of hormone replacement therapy increase the risk of venous thrombosis in patients with protein S deficiency (1)[A]
- Patients with protein S deficiency and another prothrombotic state such as factor V Leiden or the prothrombin 20210 mutation have increased rates of thrombosis (1)[A]
- Patients heterozygous for protein S deficiency who are begun on warfarin without concomitant heparin can develop warfarin-induced skin necrosis because the half life of prothrombin, another vitamin K–dependent clotting factor, is much longer than protein S (42 hours). These patients develop extremely low levels of protein S relative to prothrombin and develop necrosis of the skin over central areas of the body such as the breast, abdomen, buttocks, and genitalia. (2)[A]

ALERT

Pregnancy Considerations

Increases thrombotic risk in patients with protein S deficiency

Genetics

Autosomal dominant. Homozygotes have an odds ratio of venous thrombosis of 1.6:11.5. Arterial thrombosis is more frequent in patients with protein S deficiency who smoke. Homozygotes can have a fulminant thrombotic event in infancy, termed neonatal purpura fulminans.

ETIOLOGY

- Many mutations in the protein S gene have been described leading to an inherited protein S deficiency. Protein S reversibly binds to the C4b-binding protein. Only the free form acts as a cofactor for activated protein C. This leads to conditions where free protein S is low, but total protein S is normal. These individuals are prone to thrombosis.
- Acquired protein S deficiency from decreased free protein S can occur during pregnancy, in patients taking oral contraceptives or warfarin, in disseminated intravascular coagulation, liver disease, nephrotic syndrome, inflammation, and acute thrombosis
- Autoantibodies can develop to protein S in patients with acute varicella (2)[C]

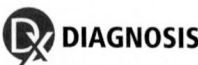 **DIAGNOSIS**

SIGNS AND SYMPTOMS

Deep and superficial venous thrombosis, often spontaneous. About half of thromboses are unprovoked.

TESTS

Lab

- Free protein S antigen can be measured by a monoclonal antibody technique
- Coagulation assay for protein S activity
- Drugs that may alter lab results
  – Oral contraceptives and oral anticoagulants can lower protein S levels
- Disorders that may alter lab results
  – Liver disease and pregnancy reduce protein S levels.
  – Acute thrombosis can lower protein S levels.

DIFFERENTIAL DIAGNOSIS

- Factor V Leiden
- Protein C deficiency
- Antithrombin deficiency
- Dysfibrinogenemia
- Dysplasminogenemia
- Homocysteinemia
- Prothrombin 20210 mutation
- Elevated factor VIII levels

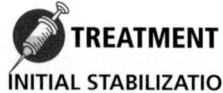 **TREATMENT**

INITIAL STABILIZATION

Outpatient

GENERAL MEASURES

- Routine anticoagulation for asymptomatic patients with protein S deficiency is not recommended. (1)[A]
- Patients with protein S deficiency and a first thrombosis should be anticoagulated for 6–12 months. (1)[A]

- Some data suggest lifetime anticoagulation to prevent recurrence.
- Lifetime anticoagulation is recommended for those patients with protein S deficieny and 2 or more thrombotic events.

- The role of family screening for protein S deficiency is unclear because most patients with this mutation do not have thrombosis. Screening should be considered for woman considering using oral contraceptives or pregnancy with a family history of factor protein S deficiency. (3)[B]

Diet

No restrictions

Activity

No restrictions

MEDICATION (DRUGS)

First Line

- Low molecular weight heparin (LMWH) (1)[A]
  - Enoxaparin (Lovenox). 1 mg/kg SC b.i.d. Alternatively, 1.5 mg/kg/d SC. Initially for at least 5 days or until international normalized ratio (INR) is 2–3, at which time it can be stopped.
  - Tinzaparin (Innohep) 175 anti-Xa IU/kg SC per day
  - Dalteparin (Fragmin) 200 IU/kg per day
- Oral anticoagulant—warfarin (Coumadin) 5 mg/d PO initially and adjusted to INR of 2–3. Patients should be maintained on warfarin for at least 6 months. (1)[A]

- Contraindications
  - Active bleeding precludes anticoagulation; risk of bleeding is a relative contraindication to long-term anticoagulation
  - Warfarin is contraindicated in patients with a prior history of warfarin-induced skin necrosis
- Precautions
  - Observe patient for signs of embolization, further thrombosis, or bleeding
  - Avoid IM injections
  - Periodically check stool and urine for occult blood, monitor CBCs, including platelets
  - Heparin: Thrombocytopenia and/or paradoxical thrombosis with thrombocytopenia
  - Warfarin: Necrotic skin lesions (typically breasts, thighs, and buttocks)
  - LMWH: Adjust dose in renal insufficiency
- Significant possible interactions
  - Agents that intensify the response to oral anticoagulants: Alcohol, allopurinol, amiodarone, anabolic steroids, androgens, many antimicrobials, cimetidine, chloral hydrate, disulfiram, all NSAIDs, sulfinpyrazone, tamoxifen, thyroid hormone, vitamin E, ranitidine, salicylates, acetaminophen
  - Agents that diminish the response to oral anticoagulants: Aminoglutethimide, antacids, barbiturates, carbamazepine, cholestyramine, diuretics, griseofulvin, rifampin, oral contraceptives

Second Line

Heparin 80 mg/kg IV bolus followed by 18 mg/kg/h. Adjust dose depending on partial prothrombin time.

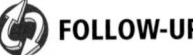 FOLLOW-UP

PROGNOSIS

- The odds ratio of thrombosis in a patient with protein S–deficiency is relatively low. However, families with protein S–deficiency have high rates of venous thromboembolism in protein S–deficient people as compared with unaffected family members.
- Smoking and obesity increase the thrombotic risk in protein S–deficient patients. (2)[B]

COMPLICATIONS

Recurrent thrombosis (requires indefinite anticoagulation). Recurrence rate is 3.5% per year.

PATIENT MONITORING

Warfarin requires periodic (monthly after initial stabilization) monitoring of the INR

REFERENCES

1. Thomas RH. Hypercoagulability syndromes. *Arch Intern Med*. 2001;161(20):2433–2439.
2. Nizzi FA Jr, Kaplan HS. Protein C and S deficiency. *Semin Thromb Hemost*. 1999;25(3):265–272.
3. Persson KE, Dahlback B, Hillarp A. Diagnosing protein S deficiency: Analytical considerations. *Clin Lab*. 2003;49(34):103–110.

 MISCELLANEOUS

See also: Protein C deficiency; Prothrombin 20210 (Mutation); Antithrombin deficiency; Thrombosis, deep vein thrombophlebitis (DVT); Factor V leiden

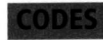 CODES

ICD9-CM

286.9 Other and unspecified coagulation defects

PATIENT TEACHING

Patients should be educated about use of oral anticoagulant therapy if taking such. Avoid NSAIDs while on warfarin.

PROTHROMBIN 20210 (MUTATION)

Marc Jeffrey Kahn, MD

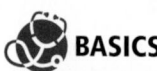 BASICS

DESCRIPTION

Polymorphism (replacement of G by A) in the 3'
untranslated end of the prothrombin gene causes
increased translation resulting in elevated synthesis
and secretion of prothrombin. This leads to an
increased risk for venous thrombosis.

- System(s) Affected: Cardiovascular;
  Hemic/Lymphatic/Immunologic; Nervous;
  Pulmonary; Reproductive
- Synonym(s): Prothrombin G20210A mutation;
  Prothrombin G20210 gene polymorphism;
  Prothrombin gene mutation

GENERAL PREVENTION

Patients with prothrombin 20210 without
thrombosis do not require prophylactic treatment.
(1)[A]

EPIDEMIOLOGY

- Found largely in Caucasian populations. Found in
  2–5% of European and Middle Eastern populations.
  Found in 4–8% of persons with venous
  thromboembolism and in up to 18% of patients
  with recurrent thrombosis.
- Predominant age: Mean age of 1st thrombosis is in
  the 2nd decade
- Predominant sex: Male = Female

Prevalence

Three percent to 5% of the population

RISK FACTORS

- Oral contraceptives, pregnancy, and the use of
  hormone replacement therapy increase the risk of
  venous thrombosis in patients with prothrombin
  20210. (2)[A]
- Patients with prothrombin 20210 and another
  prothrombotic state such as factor V Leiden have
  increased rates of thrombosis. (2)[A]

ALERT

Pregnancy Considerations

Increases thrombotic risk in patients with prothrombin
20210

Genetics

Autosomal dominant. Odds ratio for thrombosis in
affected individuals is 2:5.

ETIOLOGY

Replacement of G for A in the 3' untranslated region
of the prothrombin gene

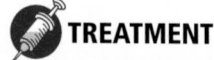 DIAGNOSIS

SIGNS AND SYMPTOMS

- Deep and superficial venous thrombosis, often
  spontaneous; sites of thrombosis can be unusual
  including the mesentery and cerebral veins
- Arterial thrombosis is rare.

Lab

- DNA analysis for mutation
- Although prothrombin levels are elevated, this is not
  a sensitive test to make the diagnosis.

DIFFERENTIAL DIAGNOSIS

- Factor V Leiden
- Protein S deficiency
- Antithrombin deficiency
- Dysfi brinogenemia
- Dysplasminogenemia
- Homocysteinemia
- Protein C deficiency
- Elevated factor VIII levels

TREATMENT

INITIAL STABILIZATION

Outpatient

GENERAL MEASURES

- Routine anticoagulation for asymptomatic patients
  with prothrombin 20210 is not recommended
  (1)[A]
- Patients with prothrombin 20210 and a 1st
  thrombosis should be anticoagulated for
  6–12 months. (2)[A]

- Patients with prothrombin 20210 and recurrent
  thrombosis should be treated indefinitely.

- The role of family screening for prothrombin 20210
  is unclear because most patients with this mutation
  do not have thrombosis. Screening should be
  considered for woman considering using oral
  contraceptives or pregnancy with a family history of
  prothrombin 20210. (1)[B]

Diet

No restrictions

Activity

No restrictions

MEDICATION (DRUGS)

First Line

- Low molecular weight heparin (LMWH) (2)[A]
  - Enoxaparin (Lovenox). 1 mg/kg SC b.i.d. Alternatively, 1.5 mg/kg/d SC. Initially for at least 5 days or until international normalized ratio (INR) is 2–3, at which time it can be stopped.
  - Tinzaparin (Innohep). 175 anti-Xa IU/kg/d SC
  - Dalteparin (Fragmin). 200 IU/kg/d
- Oral anticoagulant—warfarin (Coumadin) 5 mg PO per day initially and adjusted to INR of 2–3. Patients should be maintained on warfarin for at least 6 months. (2)[A]

- Contraindications: Active bleeding precludes anticoagulation; risk of bleeding is a relative contraindication to long-term anticoagulation.
- Precautions
  - Observe patient for signs of embolization, further thrombosis, or bleeding
  - Avoid IM injections
  - Periodically check stool and urine for occult blood, monitor CBCs including platelets
  - Heparin: Thrombocytopenia and/or paradoxical thrombosis with thrombocytopenia
  - LMWH: Adjust dose in renal insufficiency
- Significant possible interactions
  - Agents that intensify the response to oral anticoagulants: Alcohol, allopurinol, amiodarone, anabolic steroids, androgens, many antimicrobials, cimetidine, chloral hydrate, disulfi ram, all NSAIDs, sulfi npyrazone, tamoxifen, thyroid hormone, vitamin E, ranitidine, salicylates, acetaminophen
  - Agents that diminish the response to oral anticoagulants: Aminoglutethimide, antacids, barbiturates, carbamazepine, cholestyramine, diuretics, griseofulvin, rifampin, oral contraceptives

Second Line

Heparin 80 mg/kg IV bolus followed by 18 mg/kg/h. Adjust dose depending on partial prothrombin time.

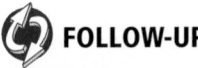 **FOLLOW-UP**

PROGNOSIS

When compared to normal individuals, persons with prothrombin 20210 have normal life spans.

COMPLICATIONS

Recurrent thrombosis (requires indefinite anticoagulation) (2)[B]

PATIENT MONITORING

Warfarin requires periodic (monthly after initial stabilization) monitoring of the INR

REFERENCES

1. Girolami A, et al. Homozygous patients with the 20210 G to A prothrombin polymorphism remain often asymptomatic in spite of the presence of associated risk factors. *Clin Appl Thromb Hemost*. 2001;7(2):122–125.
2. Girolami A, et al. Prothrombin and the prothrombin 20210 G to A polymorphism: Their relationship with hypercoagulability and thrombosis. *Blood Rev*. 1999;13(4):205–210.

 MISCELLANEOUS

See also: Protein C deficiency; Protein S deficiency; Antithrombin deficiency; Thrombosis, deep vein thrombophlebitis (DVT); Factor V leiden

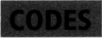 **CODES**

ICD9-CM
286.9 Other and unspecified coagulation defects

PATIENT TEACHING

Patients should be educated about use of oral anticoagulant therapy if taking such. Avoid NSAIDs while on warfarin.

PRURITUS ANI

Felix B. Chang, MD
Jeanette Lavasta, MD

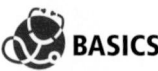 **BASICS**

DESCRIPTION
- Intense chronic itching in the anal and perianal skin. Usually acute. Chronic pruritus ani is a symptom, not a diagnosis or disease.
- Perianal dermatitis
- System(s) Affected: Skin/Exocrine

Pediatric Considerations
- Common in this age group
  - Commonly due to coarse or moist undergarments.
  - Nocturnal itching may be due to pinworms.
  - Also consider enterobiaisis and anal fissures.
- Exposure to sunlight or dry heat may be helpful for infants with inflamed anal area.

GENERAL PREVENTION
- Avoid topical agents.
- Avoid laxatives.
- Avoid tight underwear made of synthetic material.
- Practice good hygiene.
- Use talcum powder.
- Possibly *Lactobacillus acidophilus* (tablets or in milk); possibly malt soup extract
- Eat yogurt when taking broad-spectrum antibiotics.

EPIDEMIOLOGY
- Predominant age: All ages
- Predominant sex: Male > Female (4:1)
- Cases are under-reported

Incidence
Common

Prevalence
- Difficult to estimate since almost any anorectal discomfort is often attributed to symptomatic hemorrhoids.
- The prevalence in the general population is much higher than seen in clinical practice; the majority of patients do not seek medical attention.

RISK FACTORS
- Overweight
- Hairy, tendency to perspire a great deal
- Anxiety–itch–anxiety cycle

Genetics
No known genetic pattern

PATHOPHYSIOLOGY
Irritant in stool (excess alkalinity especially antibiotics, tomatoes, wine, ale, caffeine), citrus fruit, intermittent seepage, irritation on skin and mucosa

ETIOLOGY
- 20% idiopathic pruritus
- 75% Coexisting pathology in the colon or anorectum (hemorrhoids, anal fissures, rectal and anal cancer, adenomatous polyps)
- Fecal soilage in 50–75% patients

- Dermatologic disorders
  - Allergies (e.g., soap, topical anesthetics, oral antibiotics)
  - Fistulae
  - Fissures
  - Abscess
  - Neoplasms: Squamous cell cancer
  - Paget disease
  - Psoriasis
  - Eczema
  - Seborrheic dermatitis
  - Contact dermatitis
  - Atopic dermatitis
  - Hidradenitis suppurativa
- Infections
  - Pinworms and other worms
  - Scabies
  - Pediculosis
  - Candidiasis
  - Tinea
  - Sexually transmitted diseases (condyloma, herpes, syphilis, gonorrhea)
  - Bacterial infections: *Staphylococcus aureus*
- Other
  - Poor hygiene (e.g., fecal material allowed to dry on the skin)
  - Anatomic abnormalities making cleansing difficult (hemorrhoids)
  - Diabetes mellitus
  - Chronic liver disease
  - Diarrheic alkalotic irritation
  - Trauma from scented toilet paper
- Psychological causes
- Chemotherapy

ASSOCIATED CONDITIONS
- Diabetes mellitus
- Psoriasis
- Hyperhidrosis
- Parasitic infestations
- Hemorrhoids

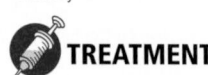 **DIAGNOSIS**

- Digital examination; suspicious anal lesions should be biopsied.
- Consider colonoscopy if history suggests colorectal pathology, heme in stool, if age >40, or a family history of colorectal cancer.

SIGNS AND SYMPTOMS
History
Rectal itching

Physical Exam
- Complete physical including digital rectal exam
- Evaluate internal sphincter tone
- Secondary infections with yeast, fungus, and/or bacteria are possible after prolonged scratching.
- Anal fissures
- Maceration
- Lichenification
- Excoriations

TESTS
- Blood sugar levels
- Cellophane tape applied to area may show pinworms
- Scraping with KOH prep for candidiasis
- Hemoccult testing of stool

Lab
- Glycosuria
- Hyperglycemia
- Skin scraping, for yeast
- Parasites
- Stool: Ova plus parasites
- Guaiac stools

Diagnostic Procedures/Surgery
- Inspection
- Anoscopy
- Biopsy to exclude neoplasia
- Colonoscopy

Pathological Findings
- Excoriation of epithelial layer of skin
- Lichenification

DIFFERENTIAL DIAGNOSIS
- Allergies
- Psoriasis
- Atopic dermatitis
- Fungus infection
- Bacterial infection
- Parasites
- Hyperhidrosis
- Diabetes mellitus
- Liver disease
- Neoplasia
- Anxiety

TREATMENT

Conservative treatment and reassurance are successful in ~90% of patients.

INITIAL STABILIZATION
Outpatient

GENERAL MEASURES
- Treat predisposing factors (e.g., parasites, diabetes, liver disease, cryptitis, scabies, pediculosis).
- Resist over use of soap and rubbing.
- Avoid tight clothing and underwear.
- Cleanse anal area after bowel movements with moistened absorbent cotton and plain water; baby wipes may be a convenient alternative.
- Dust area with nonmedicated talcum powder.
- If unable to completely empty rectum with defecation, use small plain water enema (infant bulb syringe) after each bowel movement. This may prevent postevacuation soilage and irritation.

Diet
If suspicious about food allergy, eliminate foods as a trial: Coffee, beer, cola, vitamin C tablets in excessive doses, spices, citrus fruits.

Activity
Avoid getting overheated.

MEDICATION (DRUGS)

- Specific treatment for allergies, microorganisms, bacterial and worm infestation
- For symptomatic treatment: Hydrocortisone cream 1% applied sparingly, usually at night. If severe, the patient may need to apply several times a day. Discontinue when itching subsides.
- Contraindications: Refer to the manufacturer's literature.
- Precautions: Not to be used >2 weeks: Skin atrophy – Refer to the manufacturer's literature.
- Significant possible interactions: Refer to the manufacturer's literature.
- Zinc oxide can be used in conjunction with steroids.
- Antihistamines may be useful until local measurers take effect.
- Topical salve
  – Combination of antipruritic, anti-inflammatory, and antifungal medication
  – 1/8% menthol, 1/8% camphor, hydrocortisone lotion 30 g, clotrimazole solution 30 mL, Nutraderm lotion to 90 mL. Apply sparingly to perianal area t.i.d–q.i.d for 2 weeks. Re-evaluate patient
- Topical capsaicin 0.0006% ointment 3 t.i.d. for 4 weeks
- Methylene blue injections may be used to destroy involved nerve endings in intractable cases. (1)

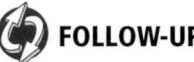 **FOLLOW-UP**

Issues for Referral
Intractable pruritus; consider referral to gastroenterology or dermatology

PROGNOSIS
- Conservative treatment and reassurance are successful in ~90% of patients.
- Depends on etiology; usually is good.
- Idiopathic form often is chronic, waxing and waning.
- Condition may be persistent and recurrent.
- Occasionally symptoms are intractable despite conservative measures.

COMPLICATIONS
- Secondary bacterial infection
- Chronicity
- Excoriation
- Lichenification
- Bleeding

PATIENT MONITORING
As needed

REFERENCES
1. Mentes BB, Akin M, Le Eventoglu S, et al. Intradermal methylene blue injection for the treatment of intractable idiopathic pruritus ani: Results of 30 cases. *Tech Coloproctol*. 2004;8:11.
2. Oztas MO, Oztas P, Onder M. Idiopathic perianal pruritus: Washing compared with topical corticosteroids. *Postgrad Med J*. 2004;80:295.
3. Zucatti G, Lotti T, et al. Pruritus ani. *Dermatolog Theory*. 2005;18(4):355–362.

ADDITIONAL READING
- Pfenninger J, Zanainea G. Common anorectal conditions. *Am Fam Phys*. 2001;63(12):2391–2398.
- Aus Fam Physician. 2004;33(7):510.
- Evidence-Based Medicine. 2004;9(3):86.

 MISCELLANEOUS

See also: Pinworms; Pruritus vulvae

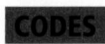 **CODES**

ICD9-CM
698.0 Pruritus ani

ICD10
L29.0 pruritus ani

PATIENT TEACHING
See "General Measures."

Diet
- Avoid foods and beverages known or suspected to exacerbate symptoms
  – Coffee, beer, cola, vitamin C tables in excessive does, spices, citrus fruits, chocolate, tea, tomatoes
- Foods or drugs that could be contributing to diarrhea or loose bowel movements should also be avoided or substituted.
- Fiber supplementation can help to bulk stools and prevent fecal leakage in patients who have fecal incontinence or partially formed stools

Activity
Avoid getting overheated

Prevention
- Appropriate anodermal care (2)
- Bathing after defecation is helpful.
- Premoistened pad or tissue can be used for wiping.
- Following bathing, the area should be dried using a soft towel with a dabbing motion, or with a hair drier.
- Unmedicated talcum powder may be used to keep the area clean.

PRURITIS VULVAE

Michael P. Hopkins, MD, MEd
William T. Schnettler, MD

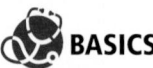 **BASICS**

DESCRIPTION

Pruritus vulvae is both a symptom and a pathologic process affecting the vulva. It is a symptom of an underlying disease in most patients. As a primary diagnosis, affected patients present with irritation and vulvar itching without an underlying pathologic etiology. Also called vulvar pruritus, vulvodynia, and burning vulva syndrome.

- System(s) Affected: Skin/Exocrine

ALERT
Geriatric Considerations
More frequently seen in this age group

GENERAL PREVENTION
- Irritants to the vulva, such as perfumes, soaps (use nonallergenic); perfumed douches must be avoided
- Only cotton underwear should be worn.
- No tight-fitting clothes or nylon pantyhose

EPIDEMIOLOGY
- Predominant age
  - Any age group can be affected.
  - In young girls, it is usually caused by infection.
  - Frequent in postmenopausal women
- Predominant sex: Female only

Incidence
Exact incidence is unknown, although most women complain of vulvar pruritus at some time during their lives

RISK FACTORS
Genetics
Unknown

ETIOLOGY
- Infectious causes: Vaginal yeast infections, *Gardnerella vaginalis*, other vaginal infections, and yeast dermatitis of the vulva itself
- Urinary tract infections produce vulvar burning on occasion.
- Vulvar vestibulitis (i.e., inflammation of the vestibular glands) produces constant burning with pruritus and dyspareunia.
- Human papillomavirus (HPV) has been associated with burning and itching of the vulva.
- Vulvar tissues are estrogen sensitive, so estrogen deprivation can produce burning and itching.
- A search for underlying malignancy should be paramount. Carcinoma in situ and invasive malignancy are often associated with pruritus.
- Changes in the epidermis, such as lichen sclerosis et atrophicus (thinning of the vulvar tissues and homogenization at the basement membrane) or hyperkeratosis of the vulva produce pruritus
- Anal incontinence with fecal soilage produces pruritus.
- Excessive heat produces symptoms due to sweat and irritation.
- Environmental and dietary irritants (e.g., nylon, soaps, perfumes, overzealous cleansing) can produce symptoms.
- Dietary irritants include methylxanthines (e.g., coffee, cola), tomatoes, and peanuts.

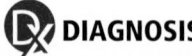 **DIAGNOSIS**

SIGNS AND SYMPTOMS
History
- Constant itching of the vulva
- Constant burning of the vulva

TESTS
Lab
- Vaginal secretions can be evaluated by wet mount (sodium chloride for *Trichomonas* or *Gardnerella* spp., and potassium hydroxide for yeast). Cultures are seldom required.
- Gram stain of the vagina is nondiagnostic because multiple organisms are present in the normal flora.

Diagnostic Procedures/Surgery
Whenever necessary, biopsy of the vulva should be used to establish the primary diagnosis. Areas for biopsy include ulcerations, discolorations, raised areas, macerated areas or in the area o f the most intense pruritus.

Pathological Findings
These are related to the underlying etiology. In primary vulvar pruritus, no changes will be noted. If HPV is present, these changes will be seen in the cornified layer of the squamous epithelium.

DIFFERENTIAL DIAGNOSIS
- Diagnosis of primary idiopathic vulvar pruritus must be made by exclusion.
- A search for infectious causes should be undertaken, with treatment of yeast and other manifestations of vaginitis.
- Biopsy any abnormal-appearing epithelium on the vulva to ensure that malignant changes are not present.
- Only when all other factors have been ruled out can the diagnosis of primary idiopathic vulvar pruritus be established.

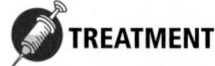 **TREATMENT**

INITIAL STABILIZATION
Outpatient

GENERAL MEASURES
- Treatment of any underlying cause must be undertaken.
- In cases of idiopathic primary vulvar pruritus, conservative measures include sitz baths, topical steroid creams, avoidance of chemical irritants, and dietary changes.
- When conservative measures fail, advanced cases can be treated with alcohol block or laser.

Diet
A trial of dietary alteration should be attempted for idiopathic pruritus. Coffee and caffeine-containing beverages should be avoided. Other foods to avoid include tomatoes and peanuts.

Activity
Unlimited

MEDICATION (DRUGS)

- Infectious sources should be treated with appropriate antimicrobials or antifungals.
- Lichen sclerosis is treated first with topical steroids then with 2% testosterone in petrolatum.
- Hyperkeratotic lesions are treated with topical steroids.
- Idiopathic primary vulvar pruritus can be treated with topical steroids such as triamcinolone (Kenalog) or desoximetasone (Topicort) cream.

SURGERY

Carcinoma in situ and premalignant changes are treated with excision or laser vaporization.

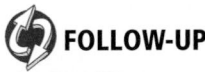 **FOLLOW-UP**

PROGNOSIS

- Vulvar pruritus can be kept under control with conservative measures and topical steroids.
- When it advances to uncontrollable symptoms, alcohol block or laser therapy may be necessary.

PATIENT MONITORING

Patients should be followed closely for the development of premalignant or malignant changes within the area of pruritus.

REFERENCES

1. Hopkins MP. Anatomy and pathology of the vulva and vagina. In Rebar R, Baker V, eds. *Gynecology & Obstetrics, an Integrated Approach*. New York, NY: Churchill Livingstone; 1993.
2. Hopkins MP. Benign and preinvasive lesions of the vulva and vagina. In Copeland LJ, ed. *Textbook of Gynecology*. 2nd ed. Philadelphia, PA: WB Saunders; 2000.
3. McKay M. Vulvodynia vs. pruritus vulvae. *Clin Obstet Gynecol*. 1985;28:123–133.
4. Smith L, Henricks D, McCullah R. Prospective studies on the etiology and treatment of pruritus ani. *Dis ColonRectum*. 1982;25:258–363.

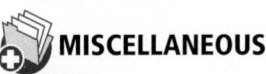 **MISCELLANEOUS**

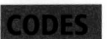 **CODES**

ICD9-CM
698.1 Pruritus of genital organs

 See Corresponding Diagnostic Algorithm

PSEUDOFOLLICULITIS BARBAE (PFB)

W. Paul Slomiany, MD

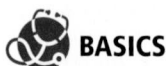 **BASICS**

DESCRIPTION
- Foreign body inflammatory reaction surrounding an ingrown hair (usually in beard area, especially in submandibular region, but may occur on scalp, axilla, or pubic area if these sites are shaved or plucked)
- Characterized by red papule/pustule at point of entry
- A mechanical problem
- System(s) Affected: Skin/Exocrine
- Synonym(s): Chronic sycosis barbae; Pili incarnate; Folliculitis barbae traumatica; Razor bumps

GENERAL PREVENTION (1)[C]
- Mild cases
  - Use tiny plastic hook to remove ingrown hairs before shaving.
  - Prior to shaving, rinse and compress face with warm water
  - Shave with either a manual adjustable razor at coarsest setting (avoids close shaves), a single-edge blade razor (Bump Fighter), a foil-guarded razor (PFB razor), electric triple "O-head" razor, or electric hair clipper with polyester skin-cleansing pad (Buf-Puf by Riker Laboratories).
  - Purchase Bump Fighter razor through the American Safety Razor Company (www.asrco.com).
  - Shave in direction of hair growth.
  - Do not stretch skin when shaving.
  - Use correct shaving cream/gel (Ef-Kay Shaving Gel, Edge Shaving Gel, Aveeno Therapeutic Shave Gel, Easy Shave Medicated Shaving Cream).
  - Consider 5% benzoyl peroxide after shaving and application of 1% hydrocortisone cream at bedtime (or LactiCare HC lotion after shaving).
  - Tretinoin cream 0.025% apply qhs
- Moderate cases:
  - Chemical depilatories (barium sulfide; Magic Shave powder)
  - Consider eflornithine HCl (Vaniqa) cream (but can cause PFB). (2)
- Severe cases
  - Laser therapy (3,4)[A]
  - Avoid shaving completely
- Use "collar extender" (JC Penney).

EPIDEMIOLOGY
- Predominant age: Postpubertal, middle age (40–75 years old)
- Predominant sex: Male > Female

Incidence
- Adult male African Americans: 50,000 in 100,000
- Adult male whites: 3,000–5,000 in 100,000
- 45% of African American soldiers who shave

Prevalence
Widespread

RISK FACTORS
- Curly hair
- Shaving too close with multiple razor strokes
- Plucking hairs
- Black and Hispanic races

Genetics
People with curly hair, especially African Americans and Hispanics. (1)

PATHOPHYSIOLOGY
- Because of its curvature, the advancing hair's sharp-tipped free end causes an epidermal invagination as it approaches the skin. This is accompanied by inflammation and often an intraepidermal abscess. (5)
- As the hair enters the dermis, more severe inflammation occurs, with downgrowth of the epidermis in an attempt to ensheath the hair.
- An abscess forms within the pseudofollicle, and a foreign body reaction forms at the tip of the invading hair.

ETIOLOGY
- Re-entry penetration of skin by external pointed tip of growing curved whisker; or sharp-tipped whisker may grow into follicular wall if shaved too close
- Plucking of hair may cause abnormal hair growth in injured follicles.

ASSOCIATED CONDITIONS
Keloidal folliculitis

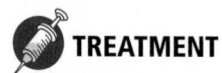 **DIAGNOSIS**

SIGNS AND SYMPTOMS
History
Pain on shaving; irritated "razor bumps"

Physical Exam
- Tender exudative, erythematous follicular papules or pustules in beard area (less commonly in scalp, axilla, pubic areas); range from 2–4 mm (1)
- Hyperpigmented "razor bumps" or "shave bumps"
- Alopecia
- Lusterless, brittle hair

TESTS
- Culture of pustules: Usually sterile; may show coagulase-negative staphylococcal epidermidis (normal skin flora)
- Clinical diagnosis

Pathological Findings
Follicular papules and pustules (5)

DIFFERENTIAL DIAGNOSIS (5)
- Bacterial folliculitis
- Impetigo
- Acne vulgaris
- Tinea barbae
- Sarcoidal papules

TREATMENT

Outpatient care

GENERAL MEASURES
Acute treatment
- Dislodge embedded hair with sterile needle
- Discontinue shaving until red papules have resolved (minimum 3–4 weeks; longer if moderate or severe)
- Massage beard area with washcloth, coarse sponge, or brush several times daily
- Systemic antibiotics if secondary infection is present

Diet
No restrictions

Activity
Unlimited

MEDICATION (DRUGS)

First Line
- Topical or systemic antibiotic for secondary infection
  - Application of clindamycin (Cleocin T) solution b.i.d or topical erythromycin if mild.
  - Low-dose erythromycin or tetracycline, 250–500 mg PO b.i.d if more severe inflammation. (6)
  - b.i.d. application of benzoyl peroxide (5%)/clindamycin (1%) gel (7)[C]
  - Administer until papule/pustule resolution
- Mild cases
  - Tretinoin cream 0.025% at bedtime (6)
- Moderate disease—chemical depilatories
  - Disrupt cross-linking of disulfide bonds of hair causing blunt hair tip
  - Apply no more frequently than every 3rd day: 2% barium sulfide (Magic Shave) or calcium thioglycolate (Surgex)
- Contraindications
  - Clindamycin—history of regional enteritis or ulcerative colitis; history of antibiotic-associated colitis
  - Erythromycin, tetracycline, tretinoin hypersensitivity only
- Precautions
  - Clindamycin: Colitis, eye burning and irritation, skin dryness; pregnancy category B
  - Erythromycin: Use cautiously in patients with impaired hepatic function; gastrointestinal side effects, especially abdominal cramping; pregnancy category B
  - Tetracycline: Permanent discoloration of teeth if given during last half of pregnancy
  - Tretinoin: Severe skin irritation; pregnancy category C
  - Benzoyl peroxide: Skin irritation and dryness, allergic contact dermatitis
  - Hydrocortisone cream: Local skin irritation, skin atrophy with prolonged use
- Significant possible interactions
  - Erythromycin: Increases theophylline and carbamazepine levels, decreases clearance of warfarin; cardiac toxicity with terfenadine and astemizole
  - Tetracycline: Depresses plasma prothrombin activity (therefore, warfarin dosage must be decreased)

Second Line
Topical application of glycolic acid lotion (8% buffered glycolic acid in a suitable carrier, either oil-in-water lotion or a nonlipid soap) b.i.d. This treatment may allow comfortable shaving every day. (8)[C]

ALERT
Pregnancy Considerations
Do not use tretinoin (Retin-A), tetracycline, or benzoyl peroxide.

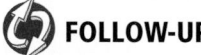 ## FOLLOW-UP

PROGNOSIS
- Course is recurrent if preventive measures are not followed.
- Prognosis is poor in presence of progressive scarring and foreign body granuloma formation

COMPLICATIONS
- Scarring (occasionally keloidal)
- Foreign-body granuloma formation
- Disfiguring postinflammatory hyperpigmentation
- Impetiginization of inflamed skin

PATIENT MONITORING
- As needed
- Educate patient on curative and preventive treatment

REFERENCES

1. Perry PK, et al. Defining pseudofolliculitis barbae in 2001: A review of the literature and current trends. *J Amer Acad Dermatol*. 2002;46(suppl 2): S113–S119.
2. Shenenberger DW, et al. Removal of Unwanted Facial Hair, *Amer Fam Phys*. 2002;66(10): 1907–1911.
3. Rogers CJ, Glaser DA. Treatment of pseudofolliculitis barbae using the q-switched Nd: YAG laser w/topical carbon suspension. *Dermatol* Surg. 2000;26(8):737–742.
4. Weaver SM 3rd, et al. Treatment of pseudofolliculitis barbae using the long-pulse Nd: YAG laser on skin types V–VI, *Dermatol Surg* 2003;29(12):1187–91.
5. Lever WF, Schaumburg-Lever G. *Histopathology of the Skin*. Philadelphia, PA: JB Lippincott; 1990.
6. *Up To Date 2006;* Pseudofolliculitis Barbae
7. Cook-Bolden FE, et al. Twice daily application of benzoyl peroxide 5% clindamycin 1% Gel versus vehicle in treatment of pseudofollicullitis barbae, *cutis*. 2004;73(6 suppl):13–24.
8. Perricone NV. Treatment of pseudofolliculitis barbae with topical glycolic acid: A report of two studies. *Cutis*. 1993;52:232–235.
9. Crutchfield CE 3d. The causes and treatment of pseudofolliculitis barbae. *Cutis*. 1998;61:351–356.
10. Dunn JF Jr. Pseudofolliculitis barbae. *Amer Fam Physician*. 1988;38:169–174.
11. Habif T. *Clinical Dermatology*. 4th ed. St. Louis, MD: Mosby; 2004.
12. Lewis CW, Coquilla BH. Management of pseudofolliculitis barbae. *Mil Med*. 1995;160:263–269.

 ## MISCELLANEOUS

See also: Folliculitis; Impetigo; Tinea barbae

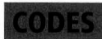 ### CODES

ICD9-CM
704.8 Other specified diseases of hair and hair follicles

PATIENT TEACHING
- Dunn JF Jr. Pseudofolliculitis barbae. *Amer Fam Physician*. 1988;38:170–172.
- Crutchfield CE 3d. The causes and treatment of pseudofolliculitis barbae. *Cutis*. 1998;61:355–356.

PSEUDOGOUT (CPPD)

Paul T. Cullen, MD

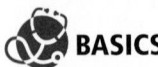 BASICS

DESCRIPTION
- Acute inflammatory arthritic disease usually involving large joint, primarily affecting the elderly and caused by calcium pyrophosphate dihydrate (CPPD) crystal deposition in joints; associated with chondrocalcinosis
  - CPPD crystal deposition may cause a progressive degenerative arthritis in numerous joints.
  - CPPD crystal deposition may cause a more insidious, smoldering, symmetrical polyarthritis similar to rheumatoid arthritis.
- System(s) Affected: Endocrine/Metabolic; Musculoskeletal
- Synonym(s): Calcium pyrophosphate deposition disease

GENERAL PREVENTION
Colchicine 0.6 mg b.i.d. may reduce frequency of episodes in recurrent monoarthritic CPPD (1)[C]

EPIDEMIOLOGY
- Predominant age: 80% of patients > age 60
- Predominant sex: Male = Female

Incidence
In United States: Not known; primarily a disease of the elderly; chondrocalcinosis present in 1:10 (ages 60–75) and 1:3 (age>80); only a small percentage develop pseudogout

RISK FACTORS
- Aging
- Trauma
- Pseudogout often occurs as a complication in patients hospitalized for other medical and surgical illnesses
- Metabolic diseases (≤10% of the cases).
  - Hyperparathyroidism
  - Hemochromatosis
  - Gout
  - Hypophosphatasia
  - Hypothyroidism
  - Ochronosis
  - Wilson disease
  - Amyloidosis
  - Hypomagnesemia

Genetics
- Uncommonly seen in familial pattern with autosomal dominant inheritance (<1% of cases)
- Most cases sporadic

ETIOLOGY
- Acute inflammatory reaction to CPPD crystals shed into synovial cavity
- Physical and chemical changes in aging cartilage that favor crystal growth

ASSOCIATED CONDITIONS
Consider in patients with pseudogout
- Hyperparathyroidism
- Hemochromatosis
- Gout
- Hypophosphatasia
- Hypothyroidism
- Ochronosis
- Wilson disease
- Amyloidosis
- Hypomagnesemia

DIAGNOSIS

SIGNS AND SYMPTOMS
- Acute pain and swelling of one or more joints; knee involved in 1/2 of all attacks; ankle, wrist, and shoulder also common
  - Inflammation, joint effusion, limitation of motion
  - 50% associated with fever
  - Any other synovial joint may be involved including first metatarsophalangeal
  - May develop after intra-articular injection of hyaluronic acid (Hyalgan, Synvisc) (2)[C]
  - May develop after partial/total joint replacement although infection should be first consideration (3)[C]
- Can present with a chronic progressive arthritis upon which acute inflammatory attacks are superimposed
- Progressive degenerative arthritis in numerous joints, including wrists, metacarpophalangeal, hips, shoulders, elbows, and ankles
- Low-grade inflammatory arthritis with multiple symmetrical joint involvement (mimics rheumatoid arthritis) <5% of cases

TESTS
- Synovial fluid analysis consistent with an inflammatory effusion
  - Cell count from 2,000–100,000 WBC/mL
  - Differential predominantly neutrophils (80–90%)
  - Wet prep with polarized microscopy may demonstrate small numbers of weakly positively birefringent crystals in the fluid and within neutrophils; false negative rate is high
- Metabolic studies. To exclude an underlying cause should always be obtained in patients age <50 and considered in the elderly
  - Serum calcium
  - Serum phosphorus
  - Serum alkaline phosphatase
  - Serum parathormone
  - Serum iron, total iron binding capacity, and serum ferritin
  - Serum magnesium
  - Serum and thyroid-stimulating hormone level

Lab
- Elevated sedimentation rate
- Leukocytosis with mild left shift

Imaging
X-rays of joints
- May demonstrate punctate and linear calcification in articular hyaline or fibrocartilage: Knees, hips, symphysis pubis, and wrists most often affected, may also be found in asymptomatic individuals
- In the chronic destructive indolent form of the disease: Subchondral cyst formation, fragmentation with formation of intra-articular radiodense bodies in joints not typically affected by degenerative joint disease

Diagnostic Procedures/Surgery
Aspiration of joint fluid with synovial fluid analysis required for proper confirmation of pseudogout; aspiration may relieve symptoms and speed resolution of inflammatory process

Pathological Findings
CPPD crystal deposition in articular cartilage, synovium, ligaments, and tendons

DIFFERENTIAL DIAGNOSIS
- Illnesses that may cause acute inflammatory arthritis in a single or multiple joint(s): Gout, septic arthritis, or trauma
- Other illnesses that may present with an acute inflammatory arthritis: Reiter syndrome, Lyme disease, acute rheumatoid arthritis

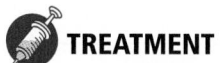

TREATMENT

INITIAL STABILIZATION
Appropriate health care
- If septic arthritis is considered possible, inpatient care may be required for empiric antibiotic therapy pending culture results.
- If the patient does not have an adequate support system, inpatient care may be required until the patient is able to walk.

GENERAL MEASURES
- Rest and elevate affected joint(s).
- Apply ice/cool compresses to affected joints.

Diet
No special diet

Activity
- Non-weight-bearing on affected joint while painful; use crutches or walker
- Isometric exercises to maintain muscle strength during the acute stage, (e.g., quadriceps isometric contractions and leg lifts), if knee affected
- Begin range of motion of joint as inflammation and pain subside
- Resume weight bearing when pain subsides

MEDICATION (DRUGS)

First Line
- NSAIDs: Choose 1 of the following
  - Indomethacin (Indocin): 50 mg PO t.i.d. with food
  - Naproxen (Naprosyn): 500 mg PO b.i.d. with food
  - Sulindac (Clinoril): 150–200 mg PO b.i.d. with food
  - Ibuprofen (Motrin): 600–800 mg PO t.i.d.–q.i.d. with food; maximum of 3.2 g daily
  - Other NSAIDs at anti-inflammatory doses are effective.
- Contraindications
  - History of hypersensitivity to NSAIDs or aspirin
  - Active peptic ulcer disease or history of recurrent upper gastrointestinal (GI) lesions
  - Avoid in renal insufficiency if serum creatinine >1.6 mg/dl
- Precautions
  - May interfere with platelet aggregation and prolong bleeding time; this effect is much shorter lived than with aspirin
  - May cause fluid retention and worsen congestive heart failure
  - Abnormal liver function tests may develop in ~15% of patients; discontinue use, if the findings worsen or systemic manifestations occur.
  - Serious GI bleeding can occur without warning; follow the patient carefully for internal bleeding. Administer proton pump inhibitor or misoprostol 200μg PO q.i.d. in patients with peptic ulcer disease history.
- Significant possible interactions
  - May elevate BP in treated hypertensives
  - May blunt antihypertensive effects of angiotensin-converting enzyme inhibitors
  - May prolong prothrombin time in patients taking oral anticoagulants
  - Avoid concomitant aspirin use.
  - May blunt diuretic effect of furosemide and hydrochlorothiazide
  - May increase plasma lithium level in patients taking lithium carbonate

Second Line
- Oral prednisone: Begin at 40–60 mg/d and taper over 10 days
- IM triamcinolone acetonide 60 mg may repeat in 1–4 days (4)[B]
- Intra-articular instillation of prednisolone sodium phosphate 4–20 mg or triamcinolone diacetate 2–40 mg with local anesthetic
- Oral colchicines 0.6 mg q.i.d. or 0.6 mg hourly until symptoms relieved or vomiting/diarrhea develop, maximum dose per attack 4–6 mg, avoid with significant renal insufficiency

FOLLOW-UP

PROGNOSIS
- Acute attack usually resolves in 10 days; prognosis for resolution of acute attack excellent
- Some patients experience progressive joint damage with functional limitation.

COMPLICATIONS
- Erosive destructive arthritis in a pattern of joints not usually affected by degenerative joint disease (e.g., metacarpophalangeal joints, wrists,
- Recurrences may occur

PATIENT MONITORING
Re-evaluate patient for response to therapy 48–72 hours after treatment instituted; reexamine 1 week later, then as needed

REFERENCES
1. Alvarellos A, Spilberg I. Colchicine prophylaxis in pseudogout. *J Rheumatol.* 89;13:804–805.
2. Hamburger MI, et al. Intra-articular hyaluronans: A review of product-specfic safety profiles. *Semin Arthritis Rheum.* 2003;32:296–309.
3. Kobayashi H, et al. Three cases of pseudogout complicated with unicondylar knee arthroplasty. *Arch Orthop Trauma Surg.* 2002;122:469–471.
4. Roane D, et al. Prospective use of intramuscular triamcinolone acetonide in pseudogout. *J Rheumatol.* 97;24:1168–1170.
5. Agudelo C, Wise C. Crystal-associated arthritis in the elderly. *Rheu Clin NA.* 2000;26:527–546.

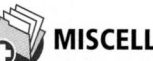

MISCELLANEOUS

See also: Gout; Osteoarthritis; Rheumatoid arthritis

CODES

ICD9-CM
- 712.10 Chondrocalcinosis due to dicalcium phosphate crystals, site unspecified
- 712.20 Chondrocalcinosis due to pyrophosphate crystals, site unspecified
- 712.30 Chondrocalcinosis, unspecified, site unspecified

PATIENT TEACHING

Activity
Specific instructions on exercise and activity

PSEUDOMEMBRANOUS COLITIS

Ruben Peralta, MD, FACS
Sarah Guzofski, MD

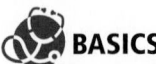 **BASICS**

DESCRIPTION

Diarrheal illness after antibiotic treatment. It ranges in severity from asymptomatic carrier state to fulminant disease and shock.

- Synonym(s): Antibiotic associated colitis; Pseudomembranous enterocolitis

GENERAL PREVENTION

- Judicious use of antimicrobial agents
- Appropriate handwashing and isolation procedures in hospital and chronic care facilities

EPIDEMIOLOGY

Prevalence

- Community: 1–5% asymptomatic colonization
- Hospital: 20% asymptomatic colonization
- Neonates: 40% colonized

ALERT

Geriatric Considerations

The elderly are at increased risk for exposure to and have a higher mortality rate from pseudomembranous colitis

RISK FACTORS

- Antibiotic exposure: All antibiotics associated with some risk; highest risk
  - 2nd/3rd generation cephalosporins
  - Penicillins
  - Clindamycin
- Increasing age
- Long duration of hospital stay
- Time spent in ICU
- Number of antibiotics received
- Long duration of antibiotic course
- Severe underlying disease
- Other gastrointestinal problems
- Immunosuppression

Genetics

No known factors

ETIOLOGY

- Colitis due to exotoxin of *Clostridium difficile* (anaerobic, Gram-positive bacillus)
- Forms heat-resistant spores
- Asymptomatic carriers are reservoirs
- Prior treatment with antibiotics alters intestinal flora. *C. difficile* spores ingested, germinate and in suitable host, colitis develops
- *C. difficile* secretes two exotoxins, A and B
- Toxin A causes inflammation, increased mucosal permeability and fluid secretion

ASSOCIATED CONDITIONS

- Infection requiring antibiotic treatment
- Can result in megacolon, ileus, perforation, sepsis

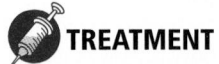 **DIAGNOSIS**

SIGNS AND SYMPTOMS

- Diarrhea (up to 20 watery stools daily, may be blood tinged, rarely grossly bloody, foul smelling)
- Lower abdominal pain, cramping
- Abdominal distension
- In severe cases, rebound tenderness
- Fever
- Dehydration

History

- Current antibiotic use
- Antibiotic use in past 3 months
- Recent/current hospitalization
- Resident of continuing care facility
- Patients with toxic megacolon may not have diarrhea

Physical Exam

- Abdominal tenderness
- Rebound tenderness in severe cases

TESTS

Lab

- *C. difficile* toxin: From stool, results in 24–48 hours
- Fecal leukocytosis (50% of cases)
- Elevated WBC
- Monitor for dehydration, electrolyte imbalance, hypoalbuminemia

Imaging

CT: Thickened or edematous colonic wall with pericolonic inflammation

Diagnostic Procedures/Surgery

Colonoscopy: In severe illness, when cannot wait for toxin test to return and need diagnostic information. Pseudomembrane may be visible; its absence does not rule of *C. difficile* colitis.

Pathological Findings

- Gross pathology: Yellow-white loosely adherent plaques on colonic and small intestinal mucosa
- Microscopic pathology: Necrosis, polymorphonuclear cells

DIFFERENTIAL DIAGNOSIS

- Other causes of watery diarrhea: Viral (Norwalk), bacterial (campylobacter), protozoan (giardia),
- Inflammatory bowel disease
- Malabsorption
- If severe illness, consider other causes of acute abdomen, shock

TREATMENT

GENERAL MEASURES

- Fluid and electrolyte repletion
- 15–25% cases resolve with stopping antibiotic. Mildest forms may not require further treatment (1)[A]
- Avoid anti-motility agents
- Do not treat asymptomatic carriers

Diet

NPO during fulminant phase

Activity

Bed rest during acute phase

SPECIAL THERAPY

IV Fluids

If unable to tolerate oral diet, IV fluid may be necessary to maintain adequate hydration and electrolyte balance

MEDICATION (DRUGS)

First Line
- Oral route most effective; >90% cases respond, usually in 2–4 days.
- Metronidazole: 250 mg PO q.i.d. or 500 mg t.i.d. for 10–14 days (2)[B]

- Contraindications
  – Refer to the manufacturer's literature.
- Significant possible interactions: Alcohol and metronidazole causes disulfiramlike reaction. Refer to the manufacturer's literature for other interactions.
- For severely ill patients, consider combination of metronidazole and vancomycin given by nasogastric or rectal tube (if unable to give orally; oral route is most effective)
- 10–20% relapse; usually not treatment failure, but due to germination of spores or reinfection. Can treat relapses with same regimen (2)[B]
- Avoid opiates and antiperistaltic drugs, such as diphenoxylate, atropine, and loperamide, to reduce the risk of toxic megacolon. (2)[B]

Second Line
- Vancomycin 500 mg PO t.i.d. for 10 days. (2)[B]

  Vancomycin is 2nd line, given emergence of vancomycin-resistant strains and greater expense.

- Probiotics are sometimes used for prevention and treatment but insufficient evidence to recommend for or against this (3)[B]

SURGERY
Emergent colectomy may be required in cases of impending perforation, severe ileus with megacolon, or sepsis.

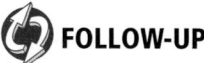 **FOLLOW-UP**

DISPOSITION
Admission Criteria
Consider severity of symptoms (acute abdomen, sepsis, ability to maintain oral intake), comorbidities, age (increased morbidity in older people

Discharge Criteria
- Able to tolerate oral diet
- Vital signs, hydration status, electrolytes adequately treated

PROGNOSIS
- If treated, most improve in 2–4 days, >90% recover
- 10–25% relapse
- Case mortality rate 1–2.5% (2)[B]
- In severely ill, colectomy sometimes required; 20–30% mortality with this degree of illness

COMPLICATIONS
- Hypoalbuminemia
- Ascites
- Dehydration, hypovolemia, shock
- Ileus
- Bowel perforation
- Toxic megacolon
- Sepsis
- Death

PATIENT MONITORING
Careful monitoring through fulminant phase

REFERENCES

1. Bricker E, et al. Antibiotic treatment for Clistridium difficile-associated diarrhea in adults. *Cochrane Database of Sytematic Reviews*. 2005.
2. Schroeder MS. Clostridium difficile-associated diarrhea. *Am Fam Physician*. 2005;71: 921–928.
3. Dendukuri N, et al. Probiotic therapy for the prevention and treatment of Clostridium difficile-associated diarrhea: A systematic review. *CMAJ*. 2005;173:167–170.
4. Starr J. Clostridium difficile associated diarrhea: Diagnosis and treatment. *BJM*. 2005;331: 498–501.

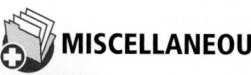 **MISCELLANEOUS**

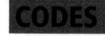

ICD9-CM
008.45 Intestinal infections due to *Clostridium difficile*

PATIENT TEACHING
Diet
Monitor hydration during acute episode.

Prevention
To prevent complications, do not use opiate or antidiarrheal medications during *C. difficile* colitis episode.

PSITTACOSIS

Ryung Suh, MD, MPP, MBA, MPH
Brent R. Gibson, MD, MPH

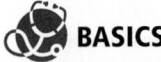 **BASICS**

DESCRIPTION
- A classic zoonotic disease, psittacosis is associated with bird handling and is also known as bird fancier's disease
  - Caused by *Chlamydphila (Chlamydia) psittaci*
  - First described in 1879 in Switzerland
  - Primarily affects the lung, where it causes a pneumonialike illness
  - May spread to other organs
- Infected birds may be asymptomatic
- Also known as ornithosis
- Synonym(s): Ornithosis; Bird-breeder's disease; Bird-fancier lung

GENERAL PREVENTION
- Avoidance of exposure
  - Maintain clean bird habitats
  - Avoid being with birds in confined spaces
- Infected birds should be treated
- When working outdoors in areas where there is contact with birds and their droppings, consider wearing protective equipment

EPIDEMIOLOGY
- Predominant age: Adults
- Predominant sex: Male = Female

Incidence
According to the Centers for Disease Control and Prevention, <50 cases have been reported annually in the US since 1996

Prevalence
In *bird* populations, prevalence of infection is estimated to be between 5% and 8%

ALERT
Pediatric Considerations
Uncommon in this age group

Geriatric Considerations
- Bird owners; especially those of parrots, parakeets, macaws, and cockatiels
- Poultry workers; especially those who handle turkeys and ducks
- Occasionally cows, goats, and sheep are the suspected reservoirs of disease
- For humans, strains transmitted from turkeys and psittacine birds (parrots and similar) appears to be the most virulent
- A recent study from Australia found the following risk factors in the studied population
  - Age of 50–64 years
  - Direct contact with wild birds
  - Mowing lawns without a grass catcher

Genetics
No known genetic predisposition

PATHOPHYSIOLOGY
- *C. psittaci* is an obligate intracellular organism
- In humans, the bacterium infects cells of the respiratory tract to include the pharynx, bronchi, and smaller airways
- If untreated, it can also infect other organs, to include
  - Pericardium
  - Heart
  - Liver
  - Kidneys
  - Joints
  - CNS

ETIOLOGY
- Humans are exposed through contact with dried secretions and excretions from infected birds
- Pet owners may be exposed through intimate contact with pets
- Human to human transmission is rare

ASSOCIATED CONDITIONS
There are numerous other diseases spread to humans from birds or by working with or around bird populations
- Avian influenza
- Viral encephalomyelitides (e.g., West Nile Virus)
- Salmonellosis
- Campylobacterosis
- Yersinosis
- *Mycopbacterium. avian* and *M. tuberculosis* infection
- Q fever
- Histoplasmosis
- Cryptococcosis
- Ectoparasite infections
  - *Dermanyssusgallinae* (chicken mites)
  - Schistosome dermatitis (Swimmers Itch)
- Newcastle disease

DIAGNOSIS (2)[C]

PRE HOSPITAL
Careful observations of 1st responders to identify association between patient and birds

SIGNS AND SYMPTOMS
- Incubation period of 1–4 weeks
- Multiple presentation variants
  - Non-specific viral: Fever and malaise
  - Mononucleosislike: Fever, pharyngitis, hepatosplenomegally and adenopathy
  - Typhoidal: Fever, bradycardia, malaise and splenomegaly
  - Atypical pneumonia: Nonproductive cough, fever, headache, and chest film abnormalities

History
- Insidious or abrupt onset
- Fever
- Chills
- Headache
- Malaise
- All followed by development of nonproductive cough and deteriorating condition

Physical Exam
- Fever without tachycardia
- Rales
- Other abnormal lung auscultation
- Enlarged spleen
- Rash

TESTS
- Culture requires special facilities and is rarely done
- Sera for serology should be collected 2–3 weeks apart (3–4 weeks for microimmunofluorescence, then a 2nd convalescent sera at 6–8 weeks if the pattern is uninterpretable)
- Complement fixation (CF) test—most common serologic test for psittacosis but is also positive with *Chlamydia pneumoniae* (a much more common respiratory pathogen) and *Chlamydia trachomatis* infections
  - A fourfold rise in CF titer is diagnostic of an acute infection with *Chlamydia*
  - A single or stable CF titer of >1:64 suggests a recent infection
- The species-specific microimmunofluorescence test for *C. psittaci* is preferred but is not as widely available as the CF test

Lab
- Leukocyte count is often normal or low
- Erythrocyte sedimentation rate is usually elevated
- Sputum is usually negative by Gram-stain and routine culture
- Proteinuria is possible during febrile period
- Liver enzymes may be elevated
- Increased IgG, IgM, IgA
- Leukocytes with left shift
- Hypoxemia
- Hypocapnia
- Eosinophilia
- Drugs that may alter lab results
  - Serologic response may be blunted by early treatment with tetracycline

Imaging
Chest radiography
- Often shows patchy alveolar infiltrates of interstitial pneumonitis and small nodular densities
- Lobar consolidation also common
- Hilar adenopathy
- Pleural effusion possible but usually scanty
- Radiographic abnormalities may persist for several months after successful treatment

Pathological Findings
- Characteristic gross findings
  - Inflamed trachea and bronchi
  - Rubbery, congested lungs
  - Mucous plugging
- Microscopic findings
  - Alveolar and interstitial exudates
    ○ Mononuclear cells predominate
  - Hyperplastic, proliferative alveolar lining cells
    ○ Basophilic intracytoplasmic inclusion

DIFFERENTIAL DIAGNOSIS
- Consider other common bacterial respiratory pathogens, including
  - *Streptococcus pneumoniae*
  - *Haemophilus influenzae*
  - *Klebsiella pneumoniae*
  - *C. pneumoniae*
  - *Mycoplasma pneumoniae*
  - *Legionella* species
- Typhoid fever, Q fever, brucellosis

TREATMENT

INITIAL STABILIZATION
- Outpatient care
- Patients with dyspnea, hypoxia, confusion, or other signs of severe disease should be hospitalized

GENERAL MEASURES
- History of avian exposure (particularly to a sick bird) is key to making early diagnosis
- Treatment depends primarily on severity of respiratory symptoms. Severely ill patients may require oxygen, IV fluids, and antibiotics
- Although human-to-human transmission is rare, sputum and respiratory secretion precautions should be observed

Diet
No special diet

Activity
Based on disease severity; no disease-specific restrictions

MEDICATION (DRUGS) (2)[C]

Treat for 10–21 days

First Line
- Oral tetracycline antibiotics
  - Doxycycline, 100 mg, q12h
  - Tetracycline, 500 mg, q6h
- IV antibiotics for severely ill
  - Doxycycline hyclate 4.4 mg/kg/d divided by into 2 infusions (up to 100 mg per dose)

Second Line
When tetracyclines are contraindicated, such as with children <9 or pregnant women, consider erythromycin or other macrolide.

FOLLOW-UP

In most states, this is a reportable disease. Contact state or local health authority

DISPOSITION
Issues for Referral
- Consult infectious disease service
- Consider investigating source of infection to identify other, undiagnosed, cases

PROGNOSIS
- Mortality rate is <1% with appropriate treatment.
- Patients usually respond within 24–48 hours following initiation of appropriate antibiotic therapy
- Full recovery may take weeks to months
- Relapse may occur, necessitating a second course of antibiotics
- Chest radiograph may not return to normal for up to 4 months

ALERT
Geriatric Considerations
Mortality rate may be higher in geriatric or debilitated patients.

COMPLICATIONS
- Meningitis and encephalitis
- Endocarditis, pericarditis, and myocarditis
- Renal failure
- Erythema nodosum
- Sinusitis
- Respiratory failure
- Hepatitis
- Reactive arthritis (rare)
- Disseminated intravascular coagulation (rare)
- Valvular heart disease (rare)
- Spontaneous abortion (rare): Has been reported with infection with some *C. psittaci* strains, primarily acquired from contact with sheep
- Thyroiditis (rare)
- Pancreatitis (rare)
- Transverse myelitis (rare)

PATIENT MONITORING
Determined by severity of illness in the acute period; no disease-specific monitoring

REFERENCES
1. Hullinger P, Chomel B. Bird zoonoses. California Department of Food and Agriculture. Division of Animal Industry, Animal Health Branch, Sacramento, CA. Available at: http://faculty.vetmed. ucdavis.edu/faculty/bbchomel/WHO`Zoonoses/PDF/ Avianzoo1. pdf.
2. Schlossberg D. *Chlamydophila (Chlamydia) psittaci* (Psittacosis). In: Mandell, Bennet, & Dolin: *Principles and Practice of Infectious Diseases*, 6th ed. New York, NY: Churchill Livingstone; 2005.
3. Smith K, et al. Compendium of measures to control *Chlamydophyla psittaci* (formerly *Chlamydia psittaci*) infection among humans (psittacosis) and pet birds (2006). National Association of State Public Health Veterinarians (NASPHV). Available at: http://www.avma.org/public_health/psittacosis.asp. 2006.
4. Telfar B, et al. Probable psittacosis outbreak linked to wild birds. *Emer Infect Dis*. 2005;11:391–391.
5. United States Centers for Disease Control and Prevention. Psittacosis. Available at: http://www.cdc.gov/ncidod/dbmd/diseaseinfo/ psittacosis_t.htm. Accessed June 5, 2006.

MISCELLANEOUS
- See also: *Chlamydia Pneumoniae*
- Other notes
  - Incubation period ranges from 5–40 days; usually 7–15 days
  - No persistent immunity to reinfection

CODES

ICD9-CM
- 073.9 Ornithosis, unspecified
- 495.8 Other specified allergic alveolitis and pneumonitis

PATIENT TEACHING
American Lung Association, 1740 Broadway, New York, NY 10019; (800) 586-4872

PSORIASIS

Atizazul Hassan Mansoor, MD

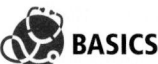 **BASICS**

DESCRIPTION
- T-cell mediated disorder of the skin leading to an epidermal proliferative rash characterized by well defined, brick red, papulosquamous plaques with a silvery scale (1,2)
- Characterized by flares and remissions
  - Flares may be related to systemic, emotional, and environmental factors
- Usual course: Acute; chronic; unpredictable
- Clinical forms (1–3)
  - Plaque psoriasis: Most common; patches appear on scalp, trunk and limbs (esp. extensor surfaces); nails may be pitted and/or thickened.
  - Guttate psoriasis: Presents most frequently age <20, numerous small papules over wide area of skin—greatest on trunk.
  - Inverse or flexural psoriasis: Affects intertriginous areas; lesions are moist and may be without scales.
  - Pustular psoriasis (von Zumbusch): A severe form of psoriasis characterized by widespread erythema, scaling, and pustule formation. Patient may appear toxic—a true emergency.
  - Erythrodermic psoriasis: Also a severe form. Patient's skin turns red. May present in the setting of chronic disease; may be precipitated by aggressive topical steroid use.
  - HIV-induced

GENERAL PREVENTION
- Avoid trauma/sunburns, irritating drugs, and alcoholic beverages.
- Limit stimulating drugs (Lithium; e.g., angiotensin converting enzyme inhibitors; beta-adrenergic blockers; tetracycline; NSAIDs; amiodarone; morphine; procaine; potassium iodide; salicylates; sulfapyridine; sulfonamides; and penicillin) (1)
  - Pustular flares may occur with steroid withdrawal. (1)
- Avoid antimalarial medications (aminoquinolone compounds)—not an absolute contraindication (1,2)

EPIDEMIOLOGY
Incidence
Old data: Based on 1980 study of a white-only population, the rate was 60.4/100,000 people (4)
- Weak evidence suggesting greater incidence among whites compared to African Americans (1,4)

Prevalence
- 0.6–4.8%
- Slight male predominance (4)
- Some evidence for a bimodal age distribution; more studies needed to confirm (1,4)

RISK FACTORS
- Family history
- Local trauma; local irritation
- Infection (Streptococcal pharyngitis can stimulate acute guttate psoriasis) (2)
- HIV
- Stress (physical and emotional)
- Withdrawal of Steroid Tx
- Medications (see "General Prevention")
- Alcohol use
- Smoking

Genetics
- Genetic predisposition (probably polygenic)
- 20–30% of psoriatics have 1st-degree relative with psoriasis (4)
- Type I psoriasis (onset age <40) theorized to have a strong familial pattern and more severe course as compared to Type 2 (onset age >40) (4,5)
- Increased incidence of specific Human Leukocyte Antigens (5)

ETIOLOGY
T-cell mediated: Triggered by some environmental antigen (e.g., trauma) or internal antigen (HIV) that promotes a cycle of cytokine production and cell proliferation (1,6)

ASSOCIATED CONDITIONS
- Depression/anxiety (1)
- Psoriatic arthritis (1)
- Crohn disease (6)
- Atopic dermatitis
- May be among 1st signs of AIDS (1,2)
- Nonmelanoma skin cancer (unclear whether related to disease process or treatment) (1)
- Sexual dysfunction (1)
- Hepatic abnormalities (pustular psoriasis) (3)

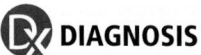 **DIAGNOSIS**

SIGNS AND SYMPTOMS
- Well-defined, red papules coalescing to plaques (1)[C]
- Silvery scales on red plaques (1)[C]
  - Auspitz sign: Underlying pinpoints of bleeding following scraping (1)[C]
- Knee-elbow-scalp distribution (1)[C]
- Pruritus (1)[C]
- Koebner phenomenon–psoriatic response in traumatic area (1)[C]
- Stippled nails and pitting

History
- History of present illness (trauma, previous treatments, pruritis)
- Family History

Physical Exam
Rash: Color, size, morphology, distribution, scale, Ausprtez sign?
- Special attention to scalp, umbilicus, intergluteal cleft, and nails (3)[C]

TESTS
Lab
- Diagnosis primarily by history and physical. Most labs will relate to treatment modality. (1)[C]
- Negative rheumatoid factor (7)[C]
- Increased erythrocyle sedimentation rate (7)[C]
- Elevated C-reactive protein (7)[C]
- Fungal studies may show a superimposed infection.

Diagnostic Procedures/Surgery
- Rarely, biopsy required to differentiate from differential diagnoses (1)[C]

Pathological Findings
- Epidermal hyperplasia (2,3,6)
- Parakeratotic scale (2,3,6)
- Loss of granular cell layer (6)
- Mitotic figures in basal cell layer (6)
- Elongation and thickening of rete ridges (6)
- Dilated tortuous capillary loops close to skin surface (3,6)
- Inflammatory infiltrate with T cells, neutrophils, mast cells, and macrophages (6)

DIFFERENTIAL DIAGNOSIS
- Scalp: Seborrheic dermatitis (1,3)
- Chronic/nummular eczema (1,3)
- Lichen simplex chronicus (1)
- Trunk: Pityriasis rosea, pityriasis rubra pilaris, tinea corporis

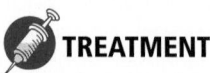 **TREATMENT**

GENERAL MEASURES
- Adequate topical hydration (emollients)
- Solar radiation (but avoid excessive exposure)
- Tar shampoos

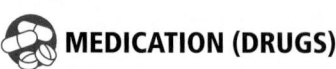 **MEDICATION (DRUGS)**

First Line
Mild to moderate disease
- Emollients b.i.d.: Most effective emollients include petrolatum or thick creams. (3,8)[C]

- Topical steroids (1,3,7,9)[A]
  - Tachyphylaxis develops over time. May alternate to prevent.
  - Side effects include skin thinning, hypopigmentation, and increased chance of local infection.
  - Occlusive dressing increases effectiveness, but also increases chance of side effects.
  - For scalp, use strong potency in alcohol base.
  - Low-potency corticosteroids on face and intertriginous areas and for infants Hydrocortisone 1% (3,8)[A]
  - Medium-potency corticosteroids (e.g., mometasone [Elocon] 0.1% or triamcinolone 0.1%) daily. (3,9)[A]
  - Strong-potency corticosteroids: Betamethasone 0.05%, fluocinonide 0.05% once daily. Good initial treatment for plaques. Alternate with medium/low potency for maintenance. (1,3,9)[A]
  - Super-potency corticosteroids: Clobetasol (Temovate), halobetasol (Ultravate). Limit use to 2 weeks; avoid occlusive dressings. Reserved for recalcitrant plaques (1,9)[A]
- Vitamin D analogs: Calcipotriene (Dovonex) ointment 0.005% b.i.d. shown to limit keritinocyte hyperproliferation. Improved results when used in concert with topical steroids. May be too irritating for face. Watch for hypercalcemia if large quantity used. Little or no tachyphylaxis. (1,3,7–9)[A]
- Topical retinoids: Tazarotene (Tazorac) 0.05% or 0.1% daily. Side effects include local irritation, and increased solar sensitivity. Minimal absorption; but still avoid in pregnant patients. (1,3,7,9)[A]

Moderate to severe disease

- May have to use combination therapy to appropriately control (9)[C]
- Light therapy: Natural sunlight is known to improve symptoms. Office administered light available as UVB (broadband or narrow band) versus PUVA (PO or bath Psoralen + UVA). Both shown to be effective. In some studies, narrowband UVB has been shown to be more effective than broadband. PUVA with higher risk of non-melanoma and melanoma skin cancers and genital squamous cell cancers in men. (1,3,7,9)[C]
  - Broadband UVB administered 3 times weekly with or without topical tar or anthralin, which may increase its effectiveness. After initial treatment period, can be at decreased rate (e.g. once weekly) to maintain remission. 1st-line treatment for children with moderate-severe disease. (3)[C]
  - PUVA administered within 2 hours of receiving psoralin; initially 3 times weekly for control, than twice or once weekly for maintenance. Generally contraindicated in children; may be used in certain difficult cases. Use bath Psoralen in pregnant females. (3,9)[C]

Systemic Therapies

- Methotrexate: Works by blocking DNA synthesis in rapidly dividing epithelial cells as well as suppressing T cells. Effectiveness established by long-term use, no clinical trials. Start 7.5–15 mg/wk, IV, PO, IM, or SC. Increase 2.5 mg every 2–3 weeks, up to 25 mg. (3,9,10)[C]
  - Side effects: Teratogenic; hepatotoxic; myelosuppression; malaise; nausea; stomitis; renal impairment. Folic acid, 1–5 mg/day, may lessen anemia, stomitis, and nausea. (1,3,9,10)[C]
  - Monitor liver function tests (LFT), renal functions, and CBC. May get liver biopsy when cumulative dose reaches 1.5 g. Strictly no alcohol, avoid Bactim, sulfamethoxazole, retinoids. (3,10)[C]
- Cyclosporine: Inhibits T cells. Start high dose, 5 mg/kg/d and taper. 0.5–1 mg/kg/d for maintenance. Pregnancy class C, so may consider in certain pregnant patients. (3,9,10)[B]
  - Side effects: Significant risk for renal toxicity; high blood pressure; flulike symptoms. Monitor renal functions, CBC with Mg^{2+} and K^+, and BP. Avoid aminoglycosides, bactrim, NSAIDs, and other potentially nephrotoxic agents. Consult drug index for interactions. (3,9,10)[C]
- Acitretin (Soriatane): Oral retinoid. For plaque psoriasis, only moderately effective as monotherapy; sometimes combined with PUVA. May be effective as monotherapy for pustular psoriasis; and for erythrodermic psoriasis when combined with emollients and topical steroids. Start 25–50 mg/d. (10)[C]
  - Fetotoxic: Pregnancy test before starting. Contraception needed 1 month before, during, and for at least 3 years after treatment. Ethanol may convert acitretin to etretinate, so strict avoidance. Women refrain from drinking alcohol for 2 months after the treatment is stopped. (10)[C] Check with the Food and Drug Administration for monitoring guidelines.
  - Side effects: Hepatotoxicity; hyperlipidemia; myalgias. Monitor LFTs, renal functions, CBC, creative phosphokinase (10)[C]
- Oral corticosteroids only for severe or life-threatening disease (risk of rebound). (8)[C]

Biologicals:

- Etanercept (Enbrel): Blocks TNF-a. Begin at 50 mg SC twice a week for 3 months, then maintenance of 50 mg/wk. (1,3,11)[B]
  - Side effects: Site reaction; upper respiratory infection; reactivation of tuberculoses; drug induced lupus; some concern of lymphoma; CNS demyelinating disorder (resolves on stopping med); very rarely heart failure (1,3,11)[C]
- Alefacept (Amevive): Interferes with CD2 on memory T-cells, inhibiting their activation. 7.5 mg IV weekly ×12 wks or 15 mg IM ×12 wks. Can give another round with 12-week rest between rounds. (1,3,11)[B]
  - Side effects: Lymphopenia; site reaction; flulike sxs.Check CD4 before each dose; discontinue if below 250/uL (1,3,11)[C]
- Efalizumab (Raptiva): Inhibits T-cells and their adhesion to endothelial cells. Initial dose of 0.7 mg/kg, then 1 mg/kg weekly, with a maximum single dose of 200 mg. 1 year cost (1,3,11)[B]
  - Side effects: Flulike symptoms; exacerbation of psoriasis; rarely thrombocytopenia. Monitor platelet counts every month for 3 months, and then every 3 months. (1,3,11)[C]
- Infliximab (Remicade): Like Etanercept, blocks TNF-a. 3–10 mg/kg IV at weeks 0, 2, 6, and 14. Maintenance can be 5 mg/kg at same schedule, then 5 mg/kg every 8 weeks. (1,3,11)[B]
  - Side effects: See "Etanercept." (1,3,11)[C]
- To increase efficacy and limit toxicity, combine, rotate, or use sequentially (9)[C]
- For contraindications, precautions, and significant possible interactions, please refer to the manufacturer's literature.

Second Line

- Topical Immunosuppressents: Tacrolimus (Prograf) or Pimecrolimus (Elidel). Consult dermatology and drug reference. (1)[C]
- Topicals: Salicylic acid; coal tar; anthralin. See dermatology reference. (1,3,8,9)[C]
- Consult dermatology reference for other, less used systemic agents. (1,10)[C]

 FOLLOW-UP

DISPOSITION

Admission Criteria

- Generalized pustular psoriasis-von Zumbusch
- Erythodermic psoriasis

Issues for Referral

- Psoriasis >20% of body (1)
- Difficult-to-treat psoriasis

PROGNOSIS

- Usually benign
- Life-threatening forms do occur.
- May be refractory to treatment

COMPLICATIONS

- Psoriatic arthritis
- Pustular psoriasis
- Erythodermic psoriasis
- See "Medications."

PATIENT MONITORING

See "Medications."

REFERENCES

1. Luba KM, Stulberg DL. Chronic Plaque Psoriasis. *Am Fam Physician.* 2006;73(4):636–644.
2. Habif T. *Clinical Dermatology.* 4th Ed. St. Louis, MO: CV Mosby; 2004.
3. Shaw JC. Overview of psoriasis. *UpToDate,* 2006. Available at: www.uptodate.com.
4. Naldi L. Epidemiology of psoriasis. *Curr Drug Targets Inflamm Allergy,* 2004;3:121–128.
5. Henseler T. Genetics of Psoriasis. *Arch Derm Res.* 1998;463–476.
6. Nickoloff BJ, Nestle FO. Recent insights into the immunopathogenesis of psoriasis proved new therapeutic opportuntities. *J Clin Ivest.* 2004;113(12):1664–1675.
7. Callen J, et al. AAD Consensus Statement on Psoriasis. *J Am Ac Derm.* 2003;49(5):897–899.
8. Greaves MW, Weinstein GD. Treatment of psoriasis. *N Eng J Med.* 1995;332:581–588.
9. Lebwohl M. A clinician's paradigm in the treatment of psoriasis. *J Am Acad Derm.* 2005;53(S1):559–569.
10. Yamauchi P, Rizk D, Kormeili T. Current systemic therapies for psoriasis: Where are we now? *J Am Acad Derm.* 2003;49(S2):S66–77.
11. Weinberg JM, et al. Biologic therapy for psoriasis: An update on the tumor necrosis factor inhibitors infliximab, etanercept, and adalimumab, and the T-cell-targeted therapies efalizumab and alefacept. *J Drugs Derm.* 2005;4(5):544–555.

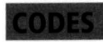 **MISCELLANEOUS**

See also: Psoriatic arthritis

CODES

ICD9-CM

- 696 Psoriasis and similar disorders
- 696.1 Other Psoriasis

PATIENT TEACHING

Patient Learning and Information

- American Academy of Family Physicians; (800) 274–2237, http://www.aafp.org/(click on Patients).
- National Psoriasis Foundation, (800) 723–9166; www.psoriasis.org.

 See Corresponding Diagnostic Algorithm

 See Patient Handout on CD

PSYCHOSIS

Sarah Guzofski, MD
Ruben Peralta, MD, FACS

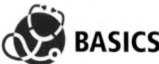 BASICS

DESCRIPTION

Syndrome seen with schizophrenia, schizoaffective disorders, mood disorders, substance use, medical problems, delirium, and dementia. Symptoms include

- Hallucinations (auditory, visual, tactile)
- Delusions (fixed, false beliefs that patient does not recognize as untrue)
- Disorganized speech or behavior

EPIDEMIOLOGY

- Predominant age: Men peak onset 18–25; women peak onset 25–35
- Predominant sex: Schizoaffective disorder and major depression, Female > Male; schizophrenia, Female = Male

Prevalence

- Schizophrenia: 1% of US population; thought to be similar worldwide
- Delusional disorder: 0.03%
- Major depression 5–9% of Females, 2–3% of males, prevalence of psychosis in depression not known and under-recognized
- Bipolar type I: 1% of population

RISK FACTORS

- Substance use
- Family history
- Schizophrenia is associated with lower socioeconomic status and urban setting

Genetics

- Genetic linkage studies underway
- Schizophrenia: 50% concordance for monozygotic twins

PATHOPHYSIOLOGY

- Increased dopamine in mesolimbic pathways causing delusions and hallucinations
- Dopamine deficiency in mesocortical pathways causes negative symptoms (apathy, withdrawal) seen in schizophrenia

ETIOLOGY

Postulated stress-diathesis model: Biologically at-risk people develop psychosis with a stressor

DIAGNOSIS

SIGNS AND SYMPTOMS

- Negative symptoms: Social withdrawal, flat affect, lack of initiative, poverty of thought
- Disorganized speech or behavior: Thought blocking, loose associations
- Delusions: Fixed false beliefs, in mood disorders, it is often mood congruent. Bizarre delusions more common in schizophrenia. Types
  - Persecutory: Being monitored, poisoned, tormented, spied on, or tricked
  - Bizarre: Impossible in real life
  - Somatic: Belief in having a serious illness
  - Believing own thoughts are being broadcast, thoughts put into or taken out of mind
  - Referential: Receiving messages from television or radio, thoughts or actions being manipulated by outside forces
  - Grandiose: Belief patient has special importance or powers
- Hallucinations: Auditory, visual, tactile
  - Auditory most common, voices commenting about patient, conversing, commands
- Mania, depression: Schizoaffective disorder, mania, depression with psychotic features

Physical Exam

- Screen for toxidromes of drugs of abuse
- Screen for medical causes of psychosis
- On antipsychotics, look for involuntary movements (AIMS exam), parkinsonism
- Look for catatonia: Extreme excitement, posturing, mutism, grimacing, waxy flexibility

TESTS

Lab

- Consider toxicology screen for drugs of abuse
- Screen thyroid function, rapid plasma reagin
- Prior to atypical antipsychotic treatment, fasting lipid profile, fasting blood sugar, liver function tests
- On atypical antipsychotic clozapine, frequent CBC and absolute neutrophil count as mandated by registry
- EKG: Antipsychotics can prolong corrected Q-T (QTC) interval

Imaging

- Schizophrenia: Enlarged lateral ventricles, decreased pre-frontal glucose metabolism by positron emission tomography, functional MRI less frontal activity during working memory task. (3)
- Depression: Functional imaging less blood flow, glucose hypometabolism in dorsolateral and dorsomedial pre-frontal cortex (3)

DSM IV-TR Criteria

- Psychotic disorders in the DSM IV-TR include
  - Schizophrenia, schizophreniform disorder
  - Schizoaffective disorder
  - Delusional disorder
  - Brief psychotic disorder
  - Substance–induced psychotic disorder
  - Psychosis due to a general medical condition
- Also an element for diagnosis of mania
- Course qualifier for major depression

DIFFERENTIAL DIAGNOSIS

- Schizophrenia
  - Combination of positive and negative symptoms, prodrome of social withdrawal
- Schizoaffective disorder
  - Mood disorder with hallucinations or delusions that persist when mood improves
- Mood disorder with psychotic features
  - Can occur in mania or depression
  - Delusions often mood congruent (e.g., somatic in depression, grandiose in mania)
  - Psychosis remits when mood improves
- Substance-induced psychosis: Establish timeline substance use vs. psychosis
  - Most common: Alcohol and benzodiazepine withdrawal, cocaine, PCP, cannabis, amphetamines, hallucinogens
  - May persist beyond acute intoxication
- Delusional disorder
  - Nonbizarre delusion (erotomanic, grandiose, jealous, persecutory, somatic), no other negative or mood symptoms
- Schizotypal personality disorder
  - No true psychosis, but discomfort in relationships and odd beliefs
- Psychosis due to general medical condition
  - Delirium, interictal, tumor, porphyria, syphilis, Wilson disease, thyroid, metachromatic leukodystrophy
- Medication-induced psychosis
  - Steroids, L-dopa
- Psychosis in dementia
  - Usually dementia evident prior to psychosis.
  - Visual hallucinations in Lewy Body dementia

 **TREATMENT**

INITIAL STABILIZATION

- Safety evaluation: Suicidality, homicidality, history of harm to self/others, severity, triggers. Use least-restrictive means to decrease risk (inpatient care, seclusion, restraint, medications)
- Treat agitation, if present
  - Consider etiology (substance use, psychosis, akithisia from antipsychotics) then treat; (often antipsychotics and/or benzodiazepines)

MEDICATION (DRUGS)

- Antipsychotics are the mainstay of treatment
  - Classified as typical vs. atypical
  - All are dopamine-2 (D2) receptor antagonists with varied affinity for the D2 receptor
  - Also block serotonin 5-HT2A receptors with varied affinity
  - Help positive symptoms more than negative
  - Nonspecific effect on agitation begins early; antipsychotic effect takes 3–6 weeks
- For mania with psychotic features, a mood stabilizer should be used (lithium, some anticonvulsants, atypical antipsychotic)
- For major depression with psychotic features, antidepressant (usually selective seratonin reuptake inhibitors) and antipsychotic better response rate than either medication alone
- In delirium, must treat underlying cause. High potency antipsychotic (e.g., haloperidol) often good choice for agitation/psychosis.
- Risks of antipsychotic medications include
  - Acute dystonia: Acute muscular rigidity; can cause laryngospasm—treat with IM/IV anticholinergics.
  - Parkinsonism: Masked facies, stooped posture, tremor, rigidity—lower dose, switch to atypical, or add anticholinergic agent
  - Akathisia: Intense restlessness, need to move, especially legs—lower dose or switch medication. Treat with beta blocker, anticholinergic, or benzodiazepine
  - Tardive dyskinesia: Variety of involuntary movements, 20% treated long term with typicals—try dose reduction, med change.
  - Neuroleptic malignant syndrome: Potentially fatal; rigidity, tremor, autonomic instability and mental status changes—stop neuroleptic, supportive care, may require ICU. No controlled studies; bromocriptine or dantrolene sometimes used.
  - Prolactinemia: D2 blockade decrease dopamine inhibition of prolactin, results in galactorrhea, amenorrhea, loss of libido

First Line

- Atypical antipsychotics recently considered the 1st line treatment for psychosis
- Benefits include less, but some, risk of extrapyramidal symptoms, such as tardive dyskinesia, possibly helps negative symptoms
- Compared to typicals, more risk of weight gain, new onset diabetes, and hyperlipidemia
- All atypical antipsychotics have same efficacy, except clozapine, which is the most efficacious, but 2nd line because risk of agranulocytosis.
- Olanzapine target dose of 10–20 mg/d, may cause more weight gain, hyperlipidemia, and hyperglycemia than other atypicals (6)[B]

- Quetiapine target dose of 400–800 mg/d b.i.d.–t.i.d.
- Risperidone target dose of 4–8 mg/d, higher risk of prolactinemia than other atypicals (6)[B]
- Ziprasidone target dose of 160 mg b.i.d., can prolong QTc, less likely to cause weight gain than other atypicals.
- Aripiprazole target dose 15 mg/d. Novel mechanism of action, partial D2 agonist.

ALERT
Geriatric Considerations

Some studies suggest increased risk of Cerebrovascular accident when atypicals used in elderly with dementia. Caution is advised in this population. (8)[A]

Second Line

- Clozapine: Despite being the most effective antipsychotic for reducing symptoms and preventing relapse, 2nd line given 1% risk of potentially fatal agranulocytosis
  - National registry for all patients on clozapine. Weekly or bi-weekly CBC with ANC required by registry to dispense clozapine
  - Long term treatment with clozapine reduces suicide risk. (5)[A]
- Typical antipsychotics
  - 2nd-line treatment due to extrapyramidal side effects and possibly less effective for negative symptoms.
  - Range from very potent D2 antagonists (e.g., haloperidol) with high extrapyramidal symptoms liability but lower anticholinergic side effects to low potency D2 antagonists with more anticholinergic properties (e.g., chlorpromazine). Equally efficacious, chosen by side effect profile.
- Depot preparations
  - Patients with chronic illness and history of noncompliance
  - Available for 2 typicals (haloperidol, fluphenazine), 1 atypical (risperidone); trial of oral meds first to assess tolerability

FOLLOW-UP

- Close follow-up in period immediately following discharge from inpatient unit (high-risk time for suicide)
- Risk for poor health; encourage primary care
- In early psychosis, cognitive behavioral therapy may help with adapting to symptoms (7)[B]

DISPOSITION
Admission Criteria

- At risk for harm to self or others or extreme functional impairment, unable to care for self
- New onset psychosis, for medication management and diagnostic workup.

Discharge Criteria

No longer a danger to self or others and adequate outpatient treatment in place.

Issues for Referral

- Encourage contact with advocacy groups (e.g., National Alliance for the Mentally Ill)
- Intensive case management
- Assertive Community Treatment, an outreach model of care for chronically ill
- Social and vocational rehab
- Substance abuse treatment, if indicated

PROGNOSIS

- Schizophrenia
  - Chronic illness with fluctuating course
  - 7% will die of suicide, 20–40% attempt; substance use, prior attempts, treatment compliance important factors. (4)
- Mood disorders with psychotic features
  - Episodic with good inter-episode recovery

PATIENT MONITORING

Medication noncompliance common cause of worsening symptoms. Some will benefit from supervised medication administration.

REFERENCES

1. *American Psychiatric Association Practice Guildeline for the Treatment of Patients with Schizophrenia,*2nd ed. Arlington, VA: American Psychiatric Association, 2004.
2. *American Psychiatric Association Diagnostic and Statistical Manual IV-TR*. Arlington, VA: American Psychiatric Association;2004.
3. Gupta A, Elheis M, Pansari K. Imaging in psychiatric illness. *Int J Clin Pract*. 2004;58:850–858.
4. Hawton K, et al. Schizophrenia and suicide: Systematic review of risk factors. *Br J Psychol*. 2005;187:9–20.
5. Hennen J, Baldessarinin RJ. Suicide risk during treatment with clozapine: A meta-analysis *Schizophr Res*. 2004;73:139–145.
6. Lieberman JA, Stroup TS, McEvoy JP. Effectiveness of antipsychotic drugs in patients with chronic schizophrenia. *N Eng J Med*. 2005;353: 1209–1223.
7. Penn DL, et al. Psychosocial treatment for first-episode psychosis: A research update. *Am J Psychiatry*. 2005;162:2220–2232.
8. Van Iersel MB, Zuidema SU, Koopmans R, Antipsychotics and psychological problems in elderly people with dementia: A systematic review of adverse events. *Drugs Aging*. 2005;22:845–858.

CODES

ICD9-CM
- 289.9 Unspecified psychosis
- 295.0 Schizophrenia
- 295.7 Schizoaffective disorder

PATIENT TEACHING

- National Alliance for the Mentally Ill, http://www.nami.org/
- Exercise program if on atypicals, given risk of weight gain

PUERPERAL INFECTION

Marcia L. Gasper, RNC, EdD

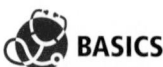 **BASICS**

DESCRIPTION
- Bacterial infection of the genital tract following delivery
- A complication of pregnancy
- Endometritis (infection of the endometrium) is the most common infection.
- Less common are infections of the myometrium and parametrial tissues, vaginal and cervical infections, perineal cellulitis, pelvic cellulitis, septic pelvic vein thrombophlebitis, and parametrial phlegmon.
- System(s) Affected: Reproductive
- Synonym(s): Postpartum infection; Endometritis; Endoparametritis; Endomyometritis; Myometritis; Endomyoparametritis; Metritis; Metritis with pelvic cellulitis

GENERAL PREVENTION
- Treat chorioamnionitis during labor.
- Treat prophylactically with cefazolin for cesarean section deliveries after the cord is clamped.
- Avoid unnecessary vaginal examinations.
- Avoid retained placental fragments or membranes.

EPIDEMIOLOGY
- Predominant age: Women of childbearing years
- Predominant sex: Female only

Prevalence
- Vaginal deliveries: <3%
- Cesarean sections: <10%
- Accounts for 7% of maternal deaths
- 4th leading cause of maternal mortality

RISK FACTORS
- Cesarean section
- Pre-existing chorioamnionitis
- Multiple vaginal examinations
- Indigent status
- Bacterial vaginosis or group B streptococcal colonization of genital tract
- Prolonged rupture of membranes, prolonged labor, and the use of internal fetal monitoring have been shown to be significant factors in univariate but not multivariate analysis.

ETIOLOGY
- The risk of endometritis increases 5–30-fold following cesarean delivery.
- Endometritis commonly follows chorioamnionitis.
- Other infections follow trauma to the perineum, vagina, cervix, and uterus.
- Infection is nearly always polymicrobial and involves organisms that have ascended from the lower genital tract
  - Aerobic isolates in 70%: *Streptococcus faecalis, S. agalactiae, S. viridans, Staphylococcus aureus, Escherichia coli, Klebsiella* sp., *Proteus* sp., *Gardnerella vaginalis*
  - Anaerobic isolates in 80%: *Peptococcus* sp., *Peptostreptococcus* sp., *Clostridium* sp., *Bacteroides bivius, B. fragilis, Fusobacterium* sp.

  - Other genital mycoplasmata; role in endometritis unclear
  - *Chlamydia trachomatis* responsible for some late (2–10 days) postpartum endometritis (see "Medication," "Drugs," "Second Line")
  - Range of number of isolates is 1–8.

ASSOCIATED CONDITIONS
Chorioamnionitis

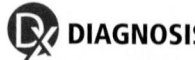 **DIAGNOSIS**

SIGNS AND SYMPTOMS
- Oral temperature >38.7°C (101.6°F) in 1st 24 hours postpartum or >38°C (100.4°F) in 2 of 1st 10 days postpartum (excluding 1st 24 hours)
- Uterine tenderness on examination
- Other localized tenderness on examination
- Ileus
- Tachycardia
- Chills, malaise, headache, anorexia
- Abdominal or localized pain
- Purulent or malodorous lochia
- Group A or B streptococcal bacteremia may have no localizing signs.

TESTS
Lab
- CBC: Interpret with care, because physiologic leukocytosis may be as high as 20,000 WBCs.
- Blood cultures if sepsis is suspected
- Amniotic fluid Gram stain: Usually polymicrobial
- Uterine tissue cultures: Difficult to obtain without contamination
- Genital tract cultures and rapid test for group B streptococci: May be done while patient is in labor
- Note: Diagnosis is usually made clinically.

Imaging
If patient is not responsive to antibiotics
- CT or MRI for pelvic vein thrombophlebitis
- Ultrasound, CT, or MRI for abscess, pelvic mass, or deep-seated wound infection

Diagnostic Procedures/Surgery
Paracentesis or culdocentesis with culture rarely is necessary.

Pathological Findings
- Microscopic sections of uterine lining show superficial layer of infected necrotic tissue.
- Thrombosis of any of the pelvic veins, including the vena cava
- Phlegmon on leaves of the broad ligament
- Abscess

DIFFERENTIAL DIAGNOSIS
Fever from other sources
- Urinary tract infection
- Viral syndrome
- Dehydration
- Pneumonia
- Wound infection
- Thrombophlebitis
- Thyroid storm
- Mastitis

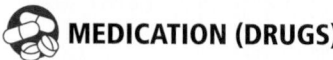 **TREATMENT**

INITIAL STABILIZATION
- Inpatient care for severe infection
- Low-grade endometritis may respond to outpatient treatment with oral antibiotics (see "Medication," "Drugs," "Second Line").
- Most infections (94%) occur after hospital discharge.

GENERAL MEASURES
- IV antibiotics and close observation for severe infections
- Open and drain infected wounds.
- Normalize fluid status.
- Note: Amnioinfusion during labor may decrease infections when membranes have been ruptured for >6 hours.

Diet
As tolerated, although may be limited by ileus

Activity
As tolerated

MEDICATION (DRUGS)

First Line
- Cefoxitin 2 g IV q6h. Add ampicillin 2 g IV q6h if clinical failure after 48 hours.
- Cefotetan 2 g IV q12h. Add ampicillin 2 g IV q6h if clinical failure after 48 hours.
- Piperacillin 4 g IV q6h
- Ampicillin–sulbactam (Unasyn) 1.5–3 g IM/IV q6h
- Clindamycin 600–900 mg IV q8h plus gentamicin 5 mg/kg IV q24h; traditional gold standard, but may cause nephrotoxicity, ototoxicity, pseudomembranous colitis, or diarrhea (in up to 6%) and may require gentamicin peak and trough levels.
- Note: Base therapy on cultures, sensitivities, and clinical response.
- Contraindications
  - Drug allergy
  - Renal failure (aminoglycosides)
  - Avoid chloramphenicol, sulfa, tetracyclines, and fluoroquinolones before delivery and if breast-feeding.
- Precautions
  - Chloramphenicol rarely causes bone marrow suppression.
  - Clindamycin and other antibiotics occasionally cause pseudomembranous colitis.
- Significant possible interactions: Refer to the manufacturer's literature for each drug.

Second Line
- Metronidazole 7.5 mg/kg IV q6h plus gentamicin 2 mg/kg IV once a day (see above)
- Amoxicillin–clavulanate (Augmentin) 500/125 mg PO t.i.d. for mild infections on an outpatient basis
- Clindamycin 300–450 mg PO q.i.d. for penicillin-allergic outpatients with mild infections
- Note: Consider adding a macrolide antibiotic (for chlamydia coverage) for infections occurring after 48 hours.
- Note: Heparin may be indicated for septic pelvic vein thrombophlebitis; requires 10 days at full anticoagulation.

SURGERY

- Curettage of retained products of conception
- Surgery to establish drainage of abscess
- Surgery to decompress the bowel
- Surgical drainage of a phlegmon is not advised unless it is suppurative.

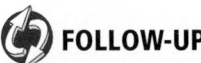 **FOLLOW-UP**

PROGNOSIS

- With supportive therapy and appropriate antibiotics, most patients improve within a few days.
- If no improvement occurs on antibiotics, consider retained placental fragments or membranes, abscess, wound infection, hematoma, cellulitis, phlegmon, or septic pelvic vein thrombosis.

COMPLICATIONS

- Resistant organisms
- Pelvic abscess
- Septic pelvic vein thrombosis
- Septic shock
- Death

PATIENT MONITORING

- Individualize according to severity
- IV antibiotics can be stopped when the patient is afebrile for 24–48 hours.
- Oral antibiotics on discharge are not necessary, except in cases of bacteremia.

REFERENCES

1. Casey BM, Cox SM. Chorioamnionitis and endometritis. *Infect Dis Clin North Amer*. 1997;11:203–222.
2. Creasy RK, Resnick R. Maternal-Fetal Medicine, 4th ed. Philadelphia: WB Saunders, 1999.
3. Deborah S, Yokoe et al. Epidemiology of and surveillance for postpartum infections. *Emerg Infect Dis*. 2001;7(5).
4. French LM, Smaill FM. Antibiotic regimens for endometritis after delivery. *Cochrane Database Sys Rev*. 2004;(4):CD00106.
5. Hamadeh G, Dedmon C, Mozley PD. Postpartum fever. *Am Fam Phys*. 1995;52:531–538.
6. Yokoe DS, et al. Epidemiology of and surveillance for postpartum infections. *Emerg Infect Dis*. 2001;7:837–841.

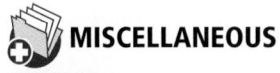 **MISCELLANEOUS**

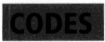

ICD9-CM

670.04 Major puerperal infection, postpartum condition or complication

PATIENT TEACHING

Advise patient to call her doctor if she has fever >38°C (100.4°F) postpartum or other symptoms of infection (see "Signs and Symptoms").

PULMONARY ARTERIAL HYPERTENSION, IDIOPATHIC

Jason Cross, PharmD
William T. McGee, MD, MHA

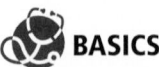

BASICS

DESCRIPTION
- Pulmonary arterial hypertension (PAH) is an elevation of pulmonary artery pressure. Can be idiopathic pulmonary arterial hypertension where no cause can be found, and/or secondary if cause is present.
  - Mean pulmonary arterial pressure (mPAP) ≥ 25 mm Hg
- 3 pathologic subtypes have been identified:
  - Thrombotic: 56%
  - Plexogenic: 28%
  - Veno-occlusive: 16%
- System(s) Affected: Pulmonary; Cardiovascular
- Synonym(s): Primary pulmonary vascular disease

EPIDEMIOLOGY
Incidence
In US
- ~1–2 cases/million
- 1% of all causes of cor pulmonale at autopsy
- ~0.5–2% of patients with portal hypertension or HIV

Prevalence
- Predominant age: Mean age 35 years 2nd incidence peak in males 50–59 years
- Predominant sex: Female > Male (3:1)

RISK FACTORS
Female sex

Genetics
Mutations in BMPR2 (autosomal dominant) carries a 10–20% lifetime risk of acquiring PAH.

ETIOLOGY
- Unknown; possible pulmonary arteriolar hyperactivity and vasoconstriction; occult thromboembolism; possibly autoimmune (high frequency of antinuclear antibodies)
- HIV$^+$ patients may have an increased incidence of PAH.
- Drug induced: Anorectic agents (fenfluramine and dexfenfluramine)

ASSOCIATED CONDITIONS
- Scleroderma
- Systemic lupus erythematosus
- Raynaud disease
- Portal hypertension
- HIV

DIAGNOSIS

SIGNS AND SYMPTOMS
- Loud P2: >80%
- Right ventricular lift: >80%
- Dyspnea: >75%
- Murmur of tricuspid insufficiency: 50–80%
- Increased jugular venous pressure: 50–80%
- Right ventricular S4: 50–80%
- Chest pain: >50%
- Fatigue: >50%
- Palpitations: <50%
- Syncope; dizziness: <50%
- Cough: <50%
- Hepatomegaly: <50%
- Pulmonic ejection click: <50%
- Right ventricular S3: <50%
- Murmur of pulmonic insufficiency: <50%
- Lower extremity edema: <50%

TESTS
- ECG: Right ventricular hypertrophy and right axis deviation
- Pulmonary function testing: Arterial hypoxemia, reduced diffusion capacity, hypocapnia
- Ventilation-perfusion ratio (V/Q) scan: Must rule out proximal pulmonary artery emboli
- Exercise test: Reduced maximal O_2 consumption, high minute ventilation, low anaerobic threshold, increased PO_2A-a (alveolar-arterial gradient). Correlation to severity of disease with 6-minute walk test

Lab
- Antinuclear antibody (ANA) positive (up to 40% of patients)
  - Collagen, vascular disease, lupus, scleroderma, CREST syndrome
  - Drugs that may alter lab results (positive ANA): Hydralazine, procainamide, isoniazid
- Liver function tests, portopulmonary hypertension
- HIV test (up to 0.5% of patients with HIV have PAH)

Imaging
- Chest radiograph
  - Enlarged central pulmonary arteries with pulmonary arterial branches attenuated
  - Right ventricular enlargement a late finding
  - If increased interstitial markings, consider lung parenchymal disease or veno-occlusive disease
- Echo-Doppler
  - Should be performed if suspicion of PAH is present (1)[C]
  - Most commonly used screening tool
    - Estimates mPAP and assesses cardiac structure and function
  - Right ventricular enlargement and overload
  - Important to rule out underlying cardiac disease, such as atrial septal defect with secondary pulmonary hypertension or mitral stenosis
- Ultra-fast CT
  - Sensitivity probably equal to pulmonary angiogram with lower contrast dose

Diagnostic Procedures/Surgery
- V/Q scan to rule out chronic thromboembolic pulmonary hypertension (CTEPH) (2)[B]
- Pulmonary angiography
  - Should be done if V/Q scan suggests CTEPH
  - Caution in pulmonary hypertension, because this can lead to hemodynamic collapse; use low osmolar agents, subselective angiograms
- Cardiac catheterization
  - Right heart catheterization necessary to measure pulmonary artery pressures and hemodynamics
  - Rule out underlying cardiac disease and response to vasodilator therapy
- Lung biopsy: Not recommended unless primary pulmonary parenchymal disease exists

Pathological Findings
- Microthromboemboli: 20–50%
- Veno-occlusive disease: 10–15%

DIFFERENTIAL DIAGNOSIS
Secondary pulmonary hypertension

- Pulmonary parenchymal disease (chronic obstructive pulmonary disease, asthma, pulmonary fibrosis, granulomatous disease, malignancy)
- Pulmonary vascular disease (pulmonary thromboembolism, collagen vascular disease, pulmonary arteritis, schistosomiasis, sickle cell disease)
- Cardiac disease: Pulmonary capillary wedge pressure (PCWP) ≥ 15 mmHg (cardiomyopathy, valvular heart disease, congenital heart disease, persistent fetal circulation, pulmonary venous hypertension)
- Other disorders of respiratory function (sleep apnea syndromes, neuromuscular diseases, pleural diseases, thoracic cage abnormalities)
- IV drug abuse

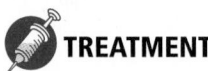

TREATMENT

Best evidence suggests that in patients with PAH, calcium channel blockers can be used if patient favorably responds to acute vasodilator test. (3)[C]

INITIAL STABILIZATION
Appropriate health care
- Medical therapy is first line and primarily palliative; health care is guided by clinical status.
- Hospitalization with invasive monitoring is needed to screen vasodilator responsiveness and initiate vasodilator therapy.
- National registry has been established by the National Heart, Lung, and Blood Institute

GENERAL MEASURES
- Primary modalities are oxygen supplementation, vasodilators, anticoagulants, and treatment of heart failure (e.g., diuretics).
- Oxygen supplementation is indicated for rest, exercise, or nocturnal hypoxemia.
- Acute response to vasodilators may improve survival.
- Treat underlying cause of secondary pulmonary hypertension.

Diet
Low-salt diet with heart failure

Activity
Restricted; exercise worsens pulmonary vascular resistance

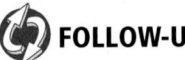 **MEDICATION (DRUGS)**

- Screening for responsiveness (acute vasodilator test)
  – IV epoprostenol
  – IV adenosine
  – Inhaled nitrous oxide
- Chronic vasodilator therapy
  – Positive response to acute vasodilator test: Lower pulmonary pressures while maintaining adequate systemic pressures
    ○ Calcium channel blocker (nifedipine, diltiazem, or amlodipine); ~1/3 will respond
    ○ Avoid verapamil, possesses significant negative inotropic effect
  – Negative response to acute vasodilator test or worsening on therapy (specific vasodilator choice is based on NYHA functional class; review treatment algorithm on p. 45S of referenced guideline (3)[C])
    ○ IV epoprostenol
    ○ Bosentan
    ○ IV treprostinil
    ○ Inhaled iloprost
    ○ Sildenafil
- Diuretic use is indicated in patients with peripheral edema and/or ascites.
  – Slow diuresis is recommended.
  – Monitor serum electrolytes and renal function.
- Digoxin use is controversial; not extensively studied in PAH.
  – Utilized in right ventricular failure and/or atrial dysrhythmias
  – Monitor drug levels and renal function.
- Anticoagulation
  – 2 small studies (3)[C] suggest prolonged survival. Warfarin with International Normalized Ratio ~2 (1.5–2.5).
  – Contraindications: Avoid warfarin in patients with syncope or significant hemoptysis.
  – Significant possible interactions: Refer to the manufacturer's literature.

SURGERY

- Patients with documented large vessel thromboembolic disease should be considered for pulmonary thrombectomy.
- Heart-lung or lung transplantation is an option for appropriate patients when medical therapy has failed.
- Atrial septostomy is considered when medical therapy has failed, and patient is not a candidate for transplantation.

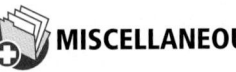 **FOLLOW-UP**

PROGNOSIS

- Mean survival 2–3 years from the time of the diagnosis, 75% mortality at 5 years, although survival is quite variable, as learned from the NIH registry
- Mode of death
  – Right heart failure: 63%
  – Pneumonia: 7%
  – Sudden death: 7%
  – Cardiac death: 5%
- Poor prognostic factors
  – PaO_2 <63%
  – RA pressure >20 mm Hg
  – Cardiac index <2 L/min/m^2
  – Mean pulmonary arterial pressure >85 mm Hg
  – New York Heart Assn. (NYHA) class 3 or 4
  – Raynaud phenomenon

COMPLICATIONS

- Thromboembolism
- Heart failure
- Sudden death

ALERT

Pregnancy Considerations
Pregnancy must be avoided; high mother and fetal wastage

PATIENT MONITORING
Frequent

REFERENCES

1. McGoon M, Gutterman D, Steen V, et al. Screening, early detection, and diagnosis of pulmonary arterial hypertension: ACCP evidence-based clinical practice guidelines. *Chest* 2004;126:14–34.
2. Worsley DF, Palevski HI, Alavi A. Ventilation-perfusion lung scanning in the evaluation of pulmonary hypertension. *J Nucl Med* 1994;35(5):793–796.
3. Badesch DB, Abman SH, Ahearn GS, et al. Medical therapy of pulmonary arterial hypertension: ACCP evidence-based clinical practice guidelines. *Chest* 2004;125:35–62.

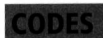 **MISCELLANEOUS**

See also: Cor pulmonale; Pulmonary embolism

CODES

ICD9-CM
416.0 Primary pulmonary hypertension

PATIENT TEACHING

- Discuss prognosis and options such as transplantation
- Avoidance of pregnancy

PULMONARY EDEMA

Peter Kozisek, MD

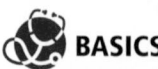 **BASICS**

DESCRIPTION
Pulmonary interstitial and/or alveolar fluid accumulation that results when the forces moving fluid out of the pulmonary capillary exceed the forces restraining that fluid
- System(s) Affected: Cardiovascular; Pulmonary

GENERAL PREVENTION
Compliance with medications and diet

EPIDEMIOLOGY
Incidence
In the US, ~150,000 persons per year are affected with noncardiogenic pulmonary edema.

Prevalence
- Predominant age: Middle age and elderly
- Predominant sex: Male = Female

RISK FACTORS
Dependent on etiology

Genetics
Multifactorial

ETIOLOGY
- Cardiogenic
  - Left heart failure
  - Ischemic heart disease
  - Acute myocardial infarction
  - Aortic and mitral valvular disease
  - Hypertensive heart disease
  - Cardiomyopathy
  - Volume overload
  - Arrhythmias
  - Endocarditis
  - Myocarditis
  - Congenital heart disease
  - Acute rheumatic fever and rheumatic heart disease
  - Septal defects
  - Cardiac tamponade
  - High cardiac output states (e.g., thyrotoxicosis, beriberi)
- Non-cardiogenic
  - Shock
  - Multiple trauma
  - Infection/sepsis (especially pneumonia)
  - Liquid aspiration (e.g., drowning, gastric contents)
  - Inhaled toxic gases
  - Pulmonary lymphatic obstruction
  - Drug overdose (especially narcotics)
  - High-altitude illness
  - Pancreatitis
  - Embolism (thrombus, fat, air, amniotic fluid)
  - Neurogenic
  - Hematologic and immunologic disorders
  - Disorders associated with high negative pleural pressure
  - Radiation pneumonitis
  - Disseminated intravascular coagulation
  - Eclampsia
  - Decreased plasma oncotic pressure (e.g., hypoalbuminemia)
  - After cardioversion, anesthesia, or cardiopulmonary bypass
  - Oxygen toxicity
  - Acute respiratory distress syndrome
  - Renal failure

ALERT
Usually secondary to lung immaturity, congenital heart disease, or associated with trauma

ASSOCIATED CONDITIONS
See "Etiology."

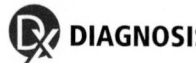 **DIAGNOSIS**

SIGNS AND SYMPTOMS
- Respiratory
  - Shortness of breath
  - Dyspnea with exertion
  - Orthopnea, paroxysmal nocturnal dyspnea
  - Cough, often accompanied by pink or blood-tinged and frothy sputum
  - Wheezing, rhonchi, gurgles
  - Moist, crepitant rales noted initially at bases and progressing to apices
  - Breathlessness, air hunger
  - Noisy respirations
  - Tachypnea
  - Dilated alae nasi
  - Inspiratory retraction of the intercostal spaces and/or supraventricular fossae
  - Cheyne-Stokes respirations
- Cardiovascular
  - Tachycardia
  - Elevated jugular venous pulse
  - Increased P2
  - S3
  - S4
  - Nocturnal angina
  - Pulsus alternans or presence of valvular heart disease
- General
  - Weakness, fatigue
  - Other symptoms depending on etiology
  - Anxiety
  - Diaphoretic, cold, ashen, or cyanotic skin
  - Lower-extremity edema

TESTS
Special tests
- Arterial blood gas
- ECG
- Pulmonary function tests
- Mixed venous oxygen saturation

Lab
- None specific for pulmonary edema; laboratory abnormalities (e.g., troponin, natriuretic peptide, amylase) may point to underlying etiology
- Hypoxemia
- Hypocarbia
- Respiratory alkalosis
- Increased A-a gradient
- Leukocytosis
- Drugs that may alter lab results
  - Administered oxygen may complicate arterial blood gas interpretation.
- Disorders that may alter lab results
  - Underlying pulmonary disease from an unrelated etiology may complicate arterial blood gas interpretation.

Imaging
- 2-dimensional echocardiography with Doppler may be useful in some cases of cardiogenic pulmonary edema (e.g., valvular heart disease, systolic vs. diastolic dysfunction)
- Chest radiograph (may be difficult or impossible to differentiate cardiogenic from noncardiogenic pulmonary edema)
  - Cardiogenic chest radiograph; interstitial edema, cardiomegaly, pulmonary venous redistribution, Kerley's B lines, alveolar edema (initially perihilar), pleural effusions (more common)
  - Non-cardiogenic chest radiograph; alveolar edema, cardiomegaly absent, pulmonary venous redistribution absent, pleural effusions less common

Diagnostic Procedures/Surgery
- Swan-Ganz catheter may help differentiate cardiogenic from noncardiogenic pulmonary edema
- Cardiac catheterization occasionally beneficial

Pathological Findings
- Cardiogenic
  - Heavy, wet, subcrepitant lungs
  - Intra-alveolar granular pink precipitate
  - Alveolar microhemorrhages and hemosiderin-laden macrophages
  - "Brown induration," chronic passive congestion
  - Hypostatic bronchopneumonia
- Noncardiogenic
  - Heavy, firm, red, and boggy lungs
  - Interstitial and intra-alveolar edema, inflammation, fibrin deposition, hemorrhage, and patchy atelectasis
  - Hyaline membrane formation
  - Interstitial and intra-alveolar fibrosis

DIFFERENTIAL DIAGNOSIS
Important to distinguish between cardiogenic and noncardiogenic pulmonary edema
- Pneumonia
- Asthma
- Chronic obstructive pulmonary disease exacerbation
- Pulmonary embolism
- Hyperventilation syndrome

TREATMENT

INITIAL STABILIZATION
Appropriate health care
- Generally inpatient or intensive care
- Outpatient for mildest forms

GENERAL MEASURES
- Treat underlying condition
- Patient sitting, with legs dangling
- Oxygen
- Rotating tourniquets or phlebotomy selectively
- Mechanical ventilation, often requiring positive end-expiratory pressure support
- Rapid reduction in altitude in cases of high-altitude pulmonary edema

Diet
Low-sodium diet

Activity
Bed rest in most cases

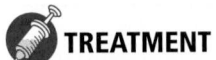 **MEDICATION (DRUGS)**

First Line
- Acute cardiogenic pulmonary edema
  – Morphine sulfate: 2–5 mg IV
  – Furosemide: 20–80 mg IV
  – Nitroglycerin paste: 1–2 inches
  – In selected cases: Nitroglycerin drip beginning at 5 μg/min and increasing by 5–10 μg/min every few minutes, titrating to BP. Nitroprusside IV drip beginning at 10-μg/min and increasing by 5–10-μg/min every few minutes, titrating to BP. Dobutamine 2 μg/kg/min IV titrating to BP, cardiac output, and pulmonary capillary wedge pressure.
- Chronic management of cardiogenic pulmonary edema:
  – Furosemide: 20–400 mg PO daily
  – Angiotensin converting enzyme (ACE) inhibitors (e.g., captopril 6.25–25 mg PO t.i.d., lisinopril 2.5–20 mg PO daily enalapril 2.5–15 mg PO b.i.d.)
  – Digoxin: 0.125–0.25 mg PO daily
  – Carvedilol: 3.125–25 mg PO 2 b.i.d.
  – Isosorbide dinitrate: 10–60 mg PO t.i.d.–q.i.d.
  – Thiazide diuretics (e.g., hydrochlorothiazide 25–50 mg PO daily)
  – Spironolactone: 25–200 mg PO daily
- Noncardiogenic pulmonary edema
  – Oxygen
  – Selected cardiovascular drugs to optimize tissue oxygen delivery
- Contraindications: Refer to the manufacturer's profile of each drug.
- Precautions
  – Avoid liberal IV fluids, especially normal saline or lactated Ringer.
  – Avoid use of carvedilol and other beta blockers in decompensated cardiac failure, bronchospastic disease, 2nd- or 3rd-degree atrio-ventricular block, sick sinus syndrome, and severe bradycardia.
  – Avoid calcium channel blockers and other negative inotropic agents in the setting of cardiogenic pulmonary edema.

– Avoid high forced inspiratory O_2 (FiO_2) >50% for prolonged periods of time, if possible
– Avoid prolonged administration of nitroprusside due to risk of cyanide toxicity. If nitroprusside is administered for >72 hours, obtain a thiocyanate level.
- Significant possible interactions: Additive hypotensive effects of nitrates, afterload reducers, diuretics

Second Line
- Chlorothiazide
- Metolazone
- Acetazolamide
- Bumetanide
- Potassium-sparing diuretics
- Other ACE inhibitors

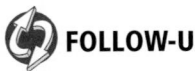 **FOLLOW-UP**

PROGNOSIS
- Dependent on underlying etiology
- Mortality ~50–60% for non-cardiogenic pulmonary edema and up–80% for cardiogenic shock

ALERT
Higher mortality

COMPLICATIONS
- Death
- Reversible or irreversible organ ischemia
- Pulmonary fibrosis, particularly with non-cardiogenic pulmonary edema

Clinical
Pulmonary edema may occur as a complication of tocolytic therapy with magnesium sulfate, terbutaline, or ritodrine.

PATIENT MONITORING
- Inpatient
  – Serial arterial blood gases or pulse oximetry, often in the ICU with 1 nursing
  – Strict measurement of intake and output
  – Attention to optimal fluid management
  – Attention to optimal ventilator settings
  – Serial chest radiographs
- Outpatient
  – Attention to clinical status
  – Serial weights to assess fluid accumulation

REFERENCES
1. Braunwald E, et al. *Harrison's Textbook of Internal Medicine*. 15th ed. New York, NY: McGraw-Hill; 2001.
2. Ingram RH, Braunwald E. Pulmonary edema. In: Braunwald E, ed. *Heart disease: A Textbook of Cardiovascular Medicine*. 7th ed. Philadelphia, PA: WB Saunders; 2005.
3. Fuster V, et al. Pulmonary edema. In: *The Heart*. 11th ed. New York NY: McGraw-Hill Inc; 2004
4. Kasper D, et al., *Harrison's Principles of Internal Medicine*. 16th ed. New York, NY: McGraw-Hill Inc; 2004.

 MISCELLANEOUS

See also: Altitude illness; Congestive heart failure; Respiratory distress syndrome, acute

 CODES

ICD9-CM
- 428.1 Left heart failure
- 518.4 Acute edema of lung, unspecified

PATIENT TEACHING

Diet
Low sodium, fluid restriction

Prevent
- Importance of medical compliance
- Symptoms and signs of pulmonary edema

See Corresponding Diagnostic Algorithm

PULMONARY EMBOLISM

Benjamin L. Sapers, MD

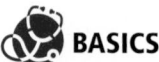 **BASICS**

DESCRIPTION

- Pulmonary embolism (PE) occurs when venous thrombi in the deep venous system dislodge and enter the pulmonary arterial circulation.
- Presentation ranges from the catastrophic to nearly asymptomatic and may include
  - Acute cor pulmonale: Obstructing >60–75% of the pulmonary circulation
  - Pulmonary infarction: With obstruction of a distal branch of the pulmonary circulation
  - Acute unexplained dyspnea, tachycardia, chest pain and/or syncope: In patients with submassive PE
- System(s) Affected: Pulmonary; Cardiovascular

ALERT
Geriatric Considerations
- Common and often fatal condition
- High risk for complications of anticoagulation
- With idiopathic venous thromboembolism (VTE), perform age-based cancer screening (1)[B]

Pediatric Considerations
- Rare in this age group
- Workup for hereditary clotting disorder

Pregnancy Considerations
- Increased risk in pregnancy and puerperium
- Incidence 0–13%
- Consider antiphospholipid antibody syndrome.
- Warfarin is teratogenic in 1st trimester
- Unfractionated heparin or low-molecular-weight heparin (LMWH) are drugs of choice.
- If VTE-positive during pregnancy, anticoagulation should be continued for 6 weeks postpartum.

GENERAL PREVENTION
- Prevention is paramount in patients with multiple risk factors for deep venous thrombosis (DVT).
- Prophylactic therapy includes low-dose heparin, warfarin, LMWH, graduated-compression stockings, or leg compression devices.

EPIDEMIOLOGY
- Rare in children; incidence increases with age
- Predominant sex: Male = Female

Incidence
One per 1,000 per year; for each 10-year increase in age, the incidence doubles.

Prevalence
- 600,000–700,000 cases yearly
- 100,000–300,000 deaths yearly

RISK FACTORS
- Prolonged immobility
- Advanced age
- CHF
- Myocardial infarction
- Malignancy
- Stroke
- Pregnancy and postpartum period
- Oral contraceptives
- Hormone replacement therapy
- Surgery/postoperative

- Trauma (especially spinal injuries)
- Chronic obstructive pulmonary disease (COPD)
- Previous thromboembolism
- Indwelling vascular devices
- Obesity
- Pulmonary hypertension

Genetics
Hypercoagulable states; protein C, protein S, antithrombin III deficiencies, activated protein C resistance, hyperhomocysteinemia, prothrombin gene mutation, antiphospholipid antibody syndrome, and lupus anticoagulant

ETIOLOGY
- Hypercoagulability
- DVT is responsible for 95% of cases of PE.

ASSOCIATED CONDITIONS
- DVT
- Occult cancer (e.g., lung, gastrointestinal tract, breast, uterus, brain, prostate)

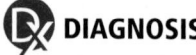 **DIAGNOSIS**

SIGNS AND SYMPTOMS
- Acute cor pulmonale
  - Syncope
  - Hypotension or cardiac arrest
  - Cyanosis
  - Pulmonary infarction
  - Pleuritic chest pain
  - Dyspnea
  - Cough
  - Hemoptysis possible
- Acute unexplained dyspnea
  - Dyspnea
  - Anxiety and apprehension possible
  - Tachycardia
  - Tachypnea
  - Signs of DVT are possible.

Physical Exam
- Distended neck veins/large A wave
- S3 gallop and increased P2 sound
- Lungs: Rales, wheezes, pleural effusion
- Signs of DVT may or may not be present.

ALERT
D-Dimer plus lung scanning (V/Q or spiral CT) provides adequate sensitivity with high specificity.

TESTS
- Before any diagnostic test is performed for VTE, the patient's pre-test probability should be estimated using an instrument like the Revised Geneva Score (2)[A]
  - Age >65: 1 point
  - Surgery with general anesthesia or lower limb fracture in the last month: 2 points
  - Active malignancy (or considered cured for <1 year): 2 points

- Previous VTE: 3 points
- Hemoptysis: 2 points
- Unilateral lower limb pain: 3 points
- Heart rate 75–94: 3 points
- >94; 5 points
- Pain on palpation of lower limb deep veins and edema: 4 points

- High Probability >10; Medium 4–10; Low 0–3

Lab
Blood
- Arterial blood gases (room air): Normal or decreased PO_2, decreased PCO_2
- D-Dimer: >500 NG/mL
- Check PT, PTT, CBC as baseline labs
- Consider stool guaiac

Imaging
- EKG
  - S1Q3T3 pattern,
  - T-wave inversions in V2 and V3
  - Incomplete right bundle branch block
- Chest radiograph
  - Usually nonspecific
  - May reveal parenchymal infiltrates, pleural effusion, atelectasis, consolidation, prominent central arteries, focal oligemia (Westermark sign), Hampton hump (wedge-shaped pleural density), and/or elevated hemidiaphragm
- Ventilation-perfusion (V/Q) scintigraphy (3)[A]
  - Normal V/Q = No PE
  - Intermediate probability = Intermediate (need another test)
  - High probability = + Pulmonary embolism
- CT angiogram (spiral CT) (4)[A]
  - Becoming test of choice
  - Fast
  - Identifies "other" causes
  - High sensitivity and specificity in the lobar pulmonary artery branches
- MRI
  - Limited experience
  - Can identify smaller clots
  - Time and limited availability
- Echocardiogram
  - Right ventricular strain and pulmonary hypertension
  - Tricuspid regurgitation
  - Septal flattening (reverse "D" sign)
  - May help in determining need for thrombolytic use
- Pulmonary angiogram
  - Invasive test (gold standard)
    - Morbidity risk: <1%
    - Mortality risk: <0.01%

DIFFERENTIAL DIAGNOSIS
- Pneumonia or bronchitis
- Myocardial infarction
- CHF
- Viral pleuritis
- Asthma
- Exacerbation of COPD
- Pulmonary edema
- Dissection of the aorta
- Rib fracture(s)
- Pneumothorax
- Musculoskeletal chest wall pain

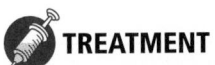 **TREATMENT**

INITIAL STABILIZATION
Hospitalization, ICU if patient hemodynamically unstable

GENERAL MEASURES
- Maintain cardiovascular and pulmonary function and to prevent recurrence of emboli.
- Oxygen therapy as needed
- Analgesic control

Diet
Limit foods and drugs that affect Coumadin (e.g., green leafy vegetables, proton pump inhibitors).

Activity
Bed rest until therapeutically anticoagulated, with frequent movement of legs

 MEDICATION (DRUGS)

First Line (4)[A]
- LMWH by SC injection daily (1.5 mg/kg) or b.i.d. (1 mg/kg) for at least 5 days *or*
- IV heparin by continuous infusion, at dose to prolong partial thromboplastin time to 1.5–2 times control for 5 days. Usual regimen requires beginning with 80 units/kg load followed by 18 unit/kg/h. Check partial thromboplastin time (PTT) q6h after beginning infusion, to keep the PTT in a range of 1.5–2.3 times mean normal. Check platelets count frequently to evaluate for heparin-induced thrombocytopenia (HIT).
- Continued dose should be adjusted according to results of PTT. Heparin nomograms for dose adjustment vary in each hospital; an example of a commonly used nomogram is shown (5)[A]

Weight-Based Heparin Dosing

aPTT	Bolus* (U/kg)	Hold†	Rate (/hr)	Repeat aPTT
Initial	80	NO	18	6 hrs
<35	80	NO	+4	6 hrs
35–45	40	NO	+2	6 hrs
46–70	None	NO	No change in AM	
71–90	None	NO	?2	6 hrs
91–120	None	60 min	?3	6 hrs

>120 Hold infusion and call physician
*Maximum heparin dose 7,500 units
†If bleeding, regardless of PTT results, hold heparin and evaluate patient;
NO, nitric oxide; aPTT activated partial thromboplastin time; PTT, partial thromboplastin time

- Warfarin, beginning day 1 or day 2 of hospitalization (5 mg or lower for the 1st dose). Warfarin should be continued for at least 6 months. The dose is adjusted to prolong PT to an international normalized ratio (INR) of 2–3. Warfarin should be continued for at least 6 months for unprovoked VTE.
- In the event of hypotension requiring vasopressors in a patient with documented PE, pulmonary embolectomy or IV thrombolytics should be considered.
- Contraindications: Refer to the manufacturer's profile of each drug.

- Precautions: Refer to the manufacturer's profile of each drug
  – The major complication of heparin therapy is hemorrhage. If the PTT is appropriately adjusted, the occurrence rate of a major hemorrhage should be low.
  – Unfractionated and LMW heparins are both associated with HIT. Check platelets frequently. If platelets fall <100,000, check HIT antibody (Platelet factor 4).
  – Use a lower initial dose of LMWH in obese patients or those with renal insufficiency. Use Xa levels to adjust dose further.
- Significant possible interactions: Refer to the manufacturer's profile of each drug.

Second Line (6)[B]
- Thrombolysis: 100 mg of tissue plasminogen activator infused over 2 hours; must continue other form of chronic anticoagulation

SURGERY
- Interruption of inferior vena cava may be indicated in patients who cannot take anticoagulants or those who have recurrent emboli despite adequate anticoagulant therapy.
- In patients with massive embolism who have persistent hypotension, pulmonary embolectomy may be life saving despite a mortality rate of ~30%. An alternative to embolectomy is thrombolytic therapy in patients without a contraindication.

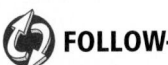 **FOLLOW-UP**

DISPOSITION
Admission Criteria
Currently all patients with PE should be admitted, although recent data suggest low-risk patients can be safely managed as outpatients; selected individuals with DVT who are otherwise clinically stable and have good follow-up and support can be treated as outpatient with LMWH.

Discharge Criteria
Stable patients with an INR between 2 and 3 on warfarin

Issues for Referral
Vascular surgery or interventional radiology evaluation if patient is appropriate for inferior vena caval filter.

PROGNOSIS
With appropriate therapy, hospital mortality is <5%. Long-term prognosis determined by comorbid disease.

COMPLICATIONS
- Pulmonary infarction
- Acute cor pulmonale
- Chronic pulmonary hypertension
- Recurrent DVT or PE, post phlebitic syndrome
- Treatment failure requiring surgical interruption
- Thrombolytics
  – Major hemorrhage associated with thrombolytics is 8%; incidence of intracerebral bleed is 2% and is fatal in 50% of cases.

PATIENT MONITORING
- After hospital discharge, INR should be kept between 2 and 3. Warfarin therapy should be continued for 6 months. In selected patients with continuous predisposition to DVT, cancer, or major thrombotic event, anticoagulation use should be considered indefinitely.
- If idiopathic VTE is noted, a thorough physical examination and symptoms-specific testing is recommended. At 2 years following idiopathic VTE, malignancy was found in 7%.

REFERENCES
1. Prandoni PF, Alanga A, Piccioli A. Cancer and venous thromboembolism. *Lancet Oncol.* 2005;6:401–410.
2. Le Gal G, et al. Prediction of pulmonary embolism in the emergency department: The revised Geneva score. *Ann Intern Med.* 2006;144:165–171.
3. The Prospective Investigation of Pulmonary Embolism Diagnosed Investigators. Value of the ventilation/perfusion scan in acute pulmonary embolism. Results of the prospective investigation of PE diagnosis (PIOPED). *JAMA.* 1990;263(20):2753–2759.
4. Buller HR, et al. Antithrombotic therapy for venous thromboembolic disease: The Seventh ACCP Conference on Antithrombotic and Thrombolytic Therapy. *Chest.* 2004;126(Suppl 3):401s–428s.
5. Raschke et al. The weight-based heparin-dosing nomogram compared with a "standard care" nomogram. *Ann Intern Med.* 1993;119:874–881.
6. Hyers TM, et al. Antithrombotic therapy for venous thromboembolic disease. *Chest.* 2001;119(Suppl 1):S176–S193.
7. Donkers-Van Rossum AB. Diagnostic strategies for suspected pulmonary embolism. *Eur Respr J.* 2001;18(3):589–597.

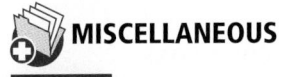 **MISCELLANEOUS**

 CODES

ICD9-CM
415.9 PE and infarction, other

PATIENT TEACHING
See Corresponding Diagnostic Algorithm

PULMONIC VALVULAR STENOSIS

Brent J. Barber, MD
Brad Friedman, MD

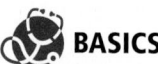 **BASICS**

DESCRIPTION
Congenital deformity that affects the cardiovascular system consisting of obstruction to right ventricular outflow at the level of the pulmonic valve; sometimes referred to as pulmonic stenosis

ALERT
Pediatric Considerations
This is a congenital disorder.

Pregnancy Considerations
In asymptomatic young women with mild-to-moderate pulmonic stenosis, pregnancy is generally well tolerated.

EPIDEMIOLOGY
Incidence
- Predominant age: Present in newborns, but often asymptomatic for years
- Predominant sex: Male = Female

Prevalence
- 10% of all cases of congenital heart disease
- In association with other lesions, may be as high as 25–30% of congenital heart disease

RISK FACTORS
Family history

Genetics
Genetic cause likely with numerous familial and syndromic cases. Associated with Noonan and LEOPARD syndromes and neurofibromatosis.

ETIOLOGY
Abnormal development of distal bulbus cordis secondary to
- Congenital/genetic
- Rubella embryopathy

ASSOCIATED CONDITIONS
Other cardiac abnormalities, such as ventricular and atrial septal defects.

DIAGNOSIS

SIGNS AND SYMPTOMS
- Acyanotic—unless septal defect allows right to left shunting.
- Usually asymptomatic. Exercise tolerance is excellent unless stenosis is severe.
- Dyspnea and fatigue are the most frequent symptoms.
- Occasionally dizziness or syncope occur, particularly exertional, due to low fixed cardiac output.
- Chest pain can occur.
- Myocardial infarction of the hypertrophied right ventricle has been noted.
- Prominent A wave of the jugular venous pulse
- Right ventricular heave
- Thrill—does not correlate with stenosis severity—often present in mild–moderate stenosis
- Pulmonic ejection sound/click: Louder during expiration; may be absent in patients with severe stenosis or dysplastic valve.
- Midsystolic murmur (increased duration and later peaking with increased severity). Heard best at left upper sternal border; may radiate throughout precordium and to left upper back.
- Delay in P2. P2 becomes softer in severe stenosis.

History
History of heart murmur since birth

TESTS
Imaging
- ECG: Tall peaked P waves (right atrial enlargement), rightward axis, right ventricular hypertrophy: Severity correlates with R:S ratio in lead V1 and V6. R in V1>30 mV correlates with severe stenosis. Abnormal t-waves in V1 (upright in children, inverted in adults) sign of right ventricular hypertrophy (RVH). Generally sinus rhythm, occasional supraventricular arrhythmias.
- X-ray: Poststenotic dilatation of the pulmonary trunk, prominence of right atrium and ventricle
- Echocardiography: Mobile, doming, thickened pulmonic valve. Post-stenotic dilatation of the pulmonary trunk (does not correlate with degree of stenosis)
- Continuous wave Doppler provides an estimate of the transvalvular gradient. (<40 mm Hg = mild; 40–70 mm Hg=moderate, >70 mm Hg = severe)
- Color flow Doppler: Delineation of areas of obstruction; assesses for pulmonary regurgitation

Diagnostic Procedures/Surgery
Cardiac catheterization
- Not indicated in mild pulmonic stenosis
- Essential in severe pulmonic stenosis for diagnosis and treatment. (1)[A]
- Used to assess morphology of the right ventricle, pulmonary outflow tract and the pulmonary arteries
- Also used to rule out associated lesions (e.g., atrial septal defect), although echocardiography may suffice

DIFFERENTIAL DIAGNOSIS
- Dysplastic pulmonic valve stenosis
- Discrete infundibular stenosis
- Subinfundibular obstruction
- Isolated pulmonary artery stenosis
- Supravalvar pulmonary stenosis
- Tetralogy of Fallot (Pink)

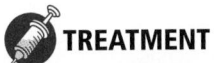 **TREATMENT**

INITIAL STABILIZATION
Usually outpatient, unless surgery is indicated

GENERAL MEASURES
- Although infective endocarditis is rare in pulmonary stenosis, prophylaxis for subacute bacterial endocarditis is currently recommended.
- Diagnostic treatment for critical pulmonary stenosis in newborns
- Intervention
  - None required for mild pulmonic stenosis
  - Intervention of asymptomatic patients with moderate pulmonic stenosis is controversial. At minimum, regular assessment is advisable.

Diet
No specific regimen is mandated.

Activity
No specific prescription, although a significant lesion will limit activity

 MEDICATION (DRUGS)

First Line
- No specific regimen in the absence of CHF
- Prophylaxis for endocarditis (2)[B]

- Contraindications: Refer to the manufacturer's literature.
- Precautions: Refer to the manufacturer's literature.
- Significant possible interactions: Refer to the manufacturer's literature.

SURGERY
- Balloon valvoplasty is the treatment of choice. (3)[A]
- Surgical pulmonic valvuloplasty in patients with obstruction that is unamendable to balloon valvuloplasty—most frequently supravalvar pulmonary stenosis or dysplastic pulmonary valve. (4)[B]

- Post-balloon or surgical repair, patients may manifest dynamic subvalvular gradient. This typically regresses with time.

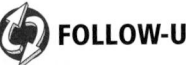 **FOLLOW-UP**

PROGNOSIS
Outcome after either balloon or surgical valvotomy is generally excellent.

COMPLICATIONS
- Up to 10% late mortality following valvotomy in critical pulmonary stenosis in neonates
- Slower recovery in those with chronic severe RVH
- Post valvotomy pulmonic regurgitation reported in up to 50% (variable severity)
- Residual atrial septal defect or patent foramen ovale
- Persistent repolarization abnormalities on electrocardiography associated with severe postoperative pulmonic regurgitation
- Late atrial arrhythmias

PATIENT MONITORING
- Postoperative (or after balloon valvotomy) Doppler ultrasound suggested at ~1 year after procedure
- After valvotomy, subacute bacterial endocarditis prophylaxis is still required.
- Regular follow-up assessment for patients not undergoing surgical correction

REFERENCES

1. Bonow et al. ACC/AHA task force report. *JACC*. 1198;(32):1486–1582.
2. Croft LB. Age-related prevalence of cardiac valvular abnormalities warranting infectious endocarditis prophylaxis. *Am J Cardiol*. 2004;94(3):386–389.
3. Sharieff S. Short and intermediate-term follow-up results of percutaneous transluminal balloon valvulopalsty in adolescents and young adults with congenital pulmonary valve stenosis. *J Invasive Cardiol*. 2003;15(9):484–487.
4. Perterson C. Comparative long-term results of surgery versus balloon valvuloplasty for pulmonary valve stenosis in infants and children. *Ann Thoracic Surg*. 2003;76:1078–1082.
5. Braunwald E, ed. *Heart Disease: Textbook of Cardiovascular Medicine*. 5th ed. Philadelphia, PA: W.B. Saunders; 1996.
6. Liberthson R. *Congenital Heart Disease: Diagnosis & Management in Children and Adults*. Boston, MA: Little-Brown; 1989.
7. Moller JH, Hoffman JIE. *Pediatric Cardiovascular Medicine*. 1st ed. Philadelphia, PA: W.B. Saunders; 2000.
8. Perloff J. *Clinical Recognition of Congenital Heart Disease*. 4th ed. Philadelphia, PA: W.B. Saunders; 1994.

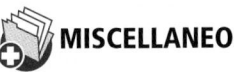 **MISCELLANEOUS**

See also: Tetralogy of fallot

CODES

ICD9-CM
- 424.3 Pulmonic valve disorders
- 746.02 Stenosis, congenital

PATIENT TEACHING

Information is available from the American Heart Association, 7320 Greenville Avenue, Dallas, TX 75231; (214) 373-630.0

PYELONEPHRITIS

Stephen A. Martin, MD, EdM

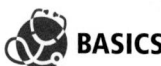 **BASICS**

DESCRIPTION

- Acute pyelonephritis is a syndrome caused by an infection of the renal parenchyma and renal pelvis, producing localized flank or back pain combined with systemic symptoms such as fever, chills, and nausea. It has a wide spectrum of presentation from mild illness to septic shock.
- Chronic pyelonephritis is the result of progressive inflammation of the renal interstitium and tubules, presumed to be caused by recurrent infection, vesicoureteral reflux, or both.
- Uncomplicated versus complicated
  - The presentation is considered uncomplicated if the infection is caused by a typical pathogen in an immunocompetent patient who has normal urinary tract anatomy and renal function.
- System(s) Affected: Renal; Urologic
- Synonym(s): Acute upper urinary tract infection (UTI)

ALERT
Geriatric Considerations
May present only as confusion; absence of fever is common in this age group.

Pregnancy Considerations
- The most common medical complication requiring hospitalization
- Affects 1–2% of all pregnancies
- Urine culture follow-up 1–2 weeks after therapy

Pediatric Considerations
- UTI is present in ~5% of 2 month–2-year-olds with fever and no source evident from H&P.
- The route for antibiotics and location of care should be based on the clinical situation.
- Delaying treatment >4 days may be associated with a greater risk of renal scarring.

EPIDEMIOLOGY
- Predominant age: All; increases >50 years of age
- Predominant sex: Females > Males

Incidence
- Community-acquired acute pyelonephritis: 28/10,000/yr.
- 250,000 total cases a year with 100,000 hospitalizations.

RISK FACTORS
- Underlying urinary tract abnormalities
- Indwelling catheter
- Recent urinary tract instrumentation
- Nephrolithiasis
- Immunocompromise, including diabetes
- Elderly, institutionalized women
- Prostatic enlargement
- Childhood UTI
- Acute pyelonephritis within the prior year
- Spermicide use
- Stress incontinence
- Pregnancy
- Hospital-acquired infection
- Symptoms >7 days at presentation

ETIOLOGY
- Infection with *Escherichia coli* (>80%)
- Other Gram-negative pathogens: *Proteus, Klebsiella, Serratia, Clostridium, Pseudomonas,* and *Enterobacter*
- *Enterococcus*
- *Staphylococcus*: *S. epidermis, S. saprophyticus* (#2 cause in young women), and *S. aureus*
- *Candida*

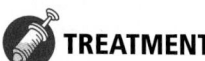 **DIAGNOSIS**

SIGNS AND SYMPTOMS
- In adults
  - Fever: ≥37.8°C (100°F)
  - Costovertebral angle tenderness
  - Malaise
  - Myalgia
  - Anorexia
  - Nausea +/– vomiting
  - Dysuria
  - Frequency
  - Urgency
  - Suprapubic discomfort
  - From no physical findings to septic shock
- In infants and children
  - Sepsis
  - Fever
  - Irritability
  - Poor skin perfusion
  - Inadequate weight gain or weight loss
  - Gastrointestinal symptoms
  - Jaundice to gray skin color

Physical Exam
A pelvic exam may be needed in female patients to assess for PID.

TESTS
Lab
- Urine culture (>10,000 colony-forming units [CFU]/mL) and sensitivities
- Urine Gram-stain
- UA: Pyuria with or without leukocyte casts, hematuria, and mild proteinuria
- Leukocyte esterase test in the urine
- Leukocytosis
- Blood culture(s): Indicated in diagnostic uncertainty, immunosuppression, or a suspected hematogenous source (1)[B]
- Drugs that may alter lab results: Antibiotics

Imaging
If patient's condition does not respond in >72 hours or if obstruction/anatomic abnormality suspected
- CT, abdomen and pelvis, with and without contrast
- Ultrasound, renal, with KUB
- IV pyelogram
- Cystoscopy with ureteral catheterization

Pathological Findings
- Acute: Abscess formation with neutrophils
- Chronic: Fibrosis with reduction in renal tissue

DIFFERENTIAL DIAGNOSIS
- Obstructive uropathy
- Acute bacterial pneumonia (lower lobe)
- Cholecystitis
- Acute pancreatitis
- Appendicitis
- Perforated viscus
- Aortic dissection
- Pelvic inflammatory disease
- Kidney stone
- Ectopic pregnancy
- Diverticulitis

TREATMENT

- Evidence for the treatment of pyelonephritis has not been fully evaluated in randomized controlled trials.
- For empiric oral therapy, a fluoroquinolone is recommended. For parenteral therapy, a fluoroquinolone, aminoglycoside ± ampicillin, or an extended-spectrum cephalosporin ± an aminoglycoside can be used. (2)[B]
- Total duration of antibiotics is usually 14 days, but must be guided by the clinical situation. (2)[A]
- IV antibiotics are indicated for inpatients. (5)[B]

INITIAL STABILIZATION
- Outpatient therapy if mild-to-moderate illness (not pregnant, no nausea or vomiting; fever and pain not severe), uncomplicated, and tolerating oral hydration and medications. Up to 70% of patients can be selected for outpatient management.
- Inpatient therapy for severe illness (e.g., high fevers, severe pain, marked debility, intractable vomiting, possible urosepsis), risk factors for complicated pyelonephritis, or extremes of age.

GENERAL MEASURES
- IV when needed
- Broad-spectrum antibiotics initially, tailoring therapy to culture and sensitivity results
- Analgesics and antipyretics
- Urinary analgesics (e.g., Phenazopyridine 200 mg t.i.d.) for severe dysuria

Diet
Encourage consumption of fluids.

Activity
As tolerated

MEDICATION (DRUGS)

First Line

- Severe illness: IV therapy until afebrile 24–48 hours and tolerating oral hydration and medications, then oral agents to complete 2 weeks. Adult doses:
- IV agents (assuming normal CrCl)
  – Ciprofloxacin: 400 mg q12h
  – Levofloxacin: 500 mg/d
  – Gatifloxacin: 400 mg/d
  – Cefotaxime: 1 g q8–12h up to 2 g q4h
  – Ceftriaxone: 1–2 g/d
  – Cefoxitin: 2 g q4–8h
  – Piperacillin-tazobactam: 3.375 g q6–8h
  – Ticarcillin-clavulanate: 3.1 g q4–6h
  – Gentamicin: 5–7 mg/kg of body weight daily (with or without ampicillin 2 g q6h for enterococcus)
- Oral agents
  – Ciprofloxacin: 500 mg q12h
  – Ciprofloxacin XR: 1000 mg/d
  – Levofloxacin: 500 mg/d
  – Norfloxacin: 400 mg q12h
  – Gatifloxacin: 400 mg/d
  – Trimethoprim-sulfamethoxazole (TMP-SMX) 160–800 mg q12h (Up to 30% *E. coli* strains are resistant to ampicillin and TMP-SMX in community-acquired infections.)
  – Cefixime 400 mg PO q12h
  – Cefpodoxime proxetil 200 mg q12h
  – Amoxicillin-clavulanate: 875/125 mg q12h or 500/125 mg t.i.d.
- Contraindications
  – Allergies to agents listed
  – Fluoroquinolones are contraindicated in adolescents, children, and pregnant women.
  – Nitrofurantoin does not achieve reliable tissue levels for pyelonephritis treatment.
- Precautions
  – Most antibiotics require adjustments in dosage in patients with renal insufficiency.
  – Observe for aminoglycoside levels and renal function.
  – If *Enterococcus* is suspected based on Gram stain, ampicillin plus low-dose once daily gentamicin is a reasonable empiric choice, unless patient is penicillin allergic, then use vancomycin. If outpatient, add amoxicillin to fluoroquinolone pending culture results and sensitivity. Do not use a 3rd-generation cephalosporin for suspect or proven enterococcal infection.

SURGERY

Perinephric abscess drainage as indicated

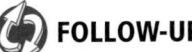 **FOLLOW-UP**

DISPOSITION
Issues for Referral
- Acute pyelonephritis unresponsive to therapy
- Chronic pyelonephritis

PROGNOSIS
Ninety-five percent of treated patients respond within 48 hours.

COMPLICATIONS
- Kidney abscess
- Metastatic infection: Skeletal system, endocardium, eye, meningitis with subsequent seizures
- Septic shock and death
- Acute or chronic renal failure
- Complications of antibiotics

PATIENT MONITORING
- Discharge on oral agent (see above) after patient is afebrile 24–48 hours to complete 2 weeks
- No response within 48 hours (5% of patients): Re-evaluate, review cultures; CT (spiral preferred), IV pyelogram or ultrasound; adjust therapy as needed; may need urologic consult. The 2 most common causes are a resistant organism and nephrolithiasis.
- Mild/moderate illness: Oral therapy for 2 weeks as outpatient
- Women: Routine follow-up cultures not recommended unless symptoms resolve but recur within 2 weeks; obtain urine culture, sensitivity, Gram stain, and CT or renal ultrasound. If symptoms resolve but recur after 2 weeks, treat as sporadic episode of pyelonephritis, unless 2 or more recurrences, then urologic evaluation necessary.
- Men, children, adolescents, patients with recurrent infections, patients with risk factors: Repeat cultures 1–2 weeks after completing therapy; urologic evaluation after 1st episode of pyelonephritis and with recurrences.

REFERENCES

1. Ramakrishnan K, Scheid D C. Diagnosis and management of acute pyelonephritis in adults. *Am Fam Physician*. 2005;71(5):933–942.
2. Warren JW, Abrutyn E, Hebel JR, et al. Guidelines for antimicrobial treatment of uncomplicated acute bacterial cystitis and acute pyelonephritis in women. Infectious Diseases Society of America (IDSA). *Clin Infect Dis*. 1999;29(4):745–758.
3. Sheffield JS, Cunningham FG. Urinary tract infection in women. *Obstet Gynecol*. 2005;106(5 Pt 1):1085–1092.
4. Larcombe J. Urinary tract infection in children. *Clin Evid*. 2005(14):429–440.
5. Neumann I, Fernanda Rojas M, Moore P. Pyelonephritis in non-pregnant women. *Clin Evid*. 2005(14):2352–2357.

 MISCELLANEOUS

See also: Urinary tract infection in females; Urinary tract infection in males

CODES

ICD9-CM
- 590.00 Chronic pyelonephritis without lesion of renal medullary necrosis
- 590.01 Chronic pyelonephritis with lesion of renal medullary necrosis
- 590.10 Acute pyelonephritis without lesion of renal medullary necrosis
- 590.11 Acute pyelonephritis with lesion of renal medullary necrosis
- 590.80 Pyelonephritis, unspecified

PATIENT TEACHING

 See Corresponding Diagnostic Algorithm

PYLORIC STENOSIS

Ruben Peralta, MD, FACS
Michael P. Hirsh, MD, FACS, FAAP

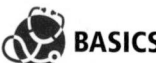 **BASICS**

DESCRIPTION
A progressive stenosis of the pyloric canal occurring in infancy

- Synonym(s): Infantile hypertrophic pyloric stenosis

EPIDEMIOLOGY
- Predominant age: Infancy; onset usually at 3–6 weeks of age, rarely in the newborn period or as late as 5 months of age
- Predominant sex: Male > Female (4:1)

Incidence
Among whites 2–5:1,000 less common among African American and Asian populations. (1)[B]

RISK FACTORS
- Incidence higher in 1stborn boys
- 40% of firstborns overall
- 5 times increased risk with affected 1st-degree relative (1)[B]

Genetics
No single gene locus identified

ETIOLOGY
Abnormal relaxation of the pyloric muscles leads to hypertrophy. Redundant mucosa fills the pyloric canal. Gastric outflow is obstructed, leading to gastric distension and vomiting.

ASSOCIATED CONDITIONS
- May be associated with tracheoesophageal fistula
- Hirschsprung disease

DIAGNOSIS

SIGNS AND SYMPTOMS
History
- Nonbilious projectile vomiting after feeding increasing frequency and severity
- Emesis may become blood tinged from vomiting-induced gastric irritation
- Hunger due to inadequate nutrition
- Diminished stools
- Weight loss

Physical Exam
- Palpable, firm, mobile mass ("olive"-like) in right upper quadrant
- Palpable 70–90% of the time.
- Epigastric distention
- Visible gastric peristalsis after feeding
- Rarely, jaundice when starvation leads to decreased glucuronyl transferase activity resulting in indirect hyperbilirubinemia. (1)[B]
- Late signs: Dehydration, weight loss

TESTS
Lab
- If prolonged vomiting
  - Hypokalemia
  - Hypochloremia
  - Metabolic alkalosis
- Elevated unconjugated bilirubin level (rare)
- Paradoxical aciduria: The kidney tubules excrete hydrogen to preserve potassium in face of hypokalemic alkalosis

Imaging
- Abdominal ultrasound is the study of choice; shows thickened and elongated pyloric muscle and redundant mucosa (1,2)[B]
- Upper gastrointestinal series reveals strong gastric contractions, elongated, narrow pyloric canal (string sign), parallel lines of barium in the narrow channel (double tract sign or railroad track sign). (2)[B]

Pathological Findings
Concentric hypertrophy of pyloric muscle

DIFFERENTIAL DIAGNOSIS
- Inexperienced or inappropriate feeding
- Gastroesophageal reflux
- Gastritis
- Congenital adrenal hyperplasia, salt-losing
- Pylorospasm
- Gastric volvulus
- Antral or gastric web

TREATMENT

INITIAL STABILIZATION
- Prompt treatment to avoid dehydration and malnutrition
- Correct acid-base and electrolyte disturbances
- Needs high concentration of potassium in preoperative fluids to correct alkalosis
- Patients need pre and post-op apnea monitoring. They have a tendency toward apnea to compensate with respiratory acidosis for their metabolic alkalosis. Surgery should be delayed until the alkalosis is corrected.

GENERAL MEASURES
Diet
- No preoperative feeding
- Initiate feeding 12–24 hours after surgery, goal of advancing to full oral feedings within 36–48 hours of surgery

SPECIAL THERAPY
IV Fluids
To correct dehydration and metabolic abnormalities

SURGERY
Ramstedt pyloromyotomy is curative
- Entire length of hypertrophied muscle is divided with preservation of the underlying mucosa.
- May be performed using open or laparoscopic techniques; no randomized controlled trials have compared these 2 approaches. (3)[C],(4)[B]

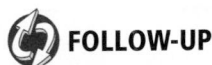 **FOLLOW-UP**

PROGNOSIS
Surgery is curative.

COMPLICATIONS
No long-term morbidity

PATIENT MONITORING
Routine pediatric health maintenance

REFERENCES

1. Hernanz-Schulman M. Infantile hypertrophic pyloric stenosis. *Radiology*. 2003;227:319–331.
2. Vasavada P. Ultrasound evaluation of acute abdominal emergencies in infants and children. *Radiol Clin N Amer*. 2004;42:445–456.
3. van der Bilt JDW, et al. Laparoscopic pyloromyotomy for hypertrophic pyloric stenosis. *Surg Endosc*. 2004;18:907–909.
4. Hall NJ, van der Zee J, Tan HL. Meta-analysis of laparoscopic versus open pyloromyotomy. *Ann Surg*. 2004;240:774–778.
5. Spevak MR, et al. Sonography of hypertrophic pyloric stenosis: Frequency and cause of nonuniform echogenicity of the thickened pylorus muscle. *AJR* 1992;158:129–132.

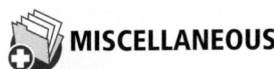 **MISCELLANEOUS**

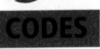

ICD9-CM
- 537.0 Acquired hypertrophic pyloric stenosis
- 750.5 Congenital hypertrophic pyloric stenosis

RABIES

Alan M. Ehrlich, MD

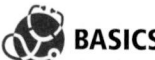 **BASICS**

DESCRIPTION

- A rapidly progressive infection of the CNS caused by an RNA virus and affecting mammals, including humans
- The disease is essentially 100% fatal once symptoms develop in the prodrome stage.
- Infection can be prevented by prompt, postexposure treatment of persons bitten by or otherwise exposed to animals known or suspected to be carrying the disease.
- System(s) Affected: Nervous
- Synonym(s): Hydrophobia

GENERAL PREVENTION

- Avoid wild and unknown domestic animals.
- Seek treatment promptly if bitten, scratched, or in contact with saliva.
- Thorough wound cleansing with soap is the 1st line of treatment.
- Undergo pre-exposure vaccination if at risk of unapparent or unrecognized exposure to rabies inside or outside the US.

EPIDEMIOLOGY

- Predominant age: Any
- Predominant sex: Male = Female

Incidence

8 human cases in 2004 in the US (most associated with bites of insectivorous bats, although patients rarely recall exposure); ~7,000 cases per year in animals (~37% raccoons, 27% skunks, 20% bats); about 30,000 postexposure treatments. In US citizens, rate of rabies is <0.001 in 100,000 per year.

RISK FACTORS

For exposure to rabies

- Professions or activities that may expose a person to wild or domestic animals (e.g., animal handlers, some lab workers, veterinarians, spelunkers [cave explorers])
- International travel to countries where canine rabies is endemic (most common risk factor)
- In the US, most cases appear to be caused by exposure to bats.
- Human-to-human transmission has occurred through cornea and other tissue transplants.

ETIOLOGY

Rabies virus, a neurotropic virus present in saliva of infected animals

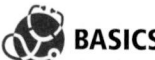 **DIAGNOSIS**

SIGNS AND SYMPTOMS

Usually proceed through 4 stages, although they may overlap

- Incubation period
  - The time between bite and 1st symptoms of disease: Between 1 and 3 months in 2/3 of cases. May be as short as 6 days or >6 years. It is shortest in patients with extensive bites about the head and trunk.
  - No symptoms except bite trauma
- Prodrome
  - Lasts 2–10 days
  - Pain or paresthesia at the bite site is the most specific symptom at this stage.
  - Symptoms are often extremely variable and nonspecific and include fever and headache.
  - May be referable to any of a number of organ systems
  - May suggest any of a number of common infections
- Acute neurologic period
  - Lasts 2–10 days
  - Symptoms referable to CNS dominate clinical picture
  - Generally takes 1 of 2 forms
  - Furious rabies: Episodes of hyperactivity last ~5 minutes and include hydrophobia, aerophobia, hyperventilation, hypersalivation, and autonomic instability interspersed with periods of normalcy.
  - Paralytic rabies: Paralysis dominates clinical picture; may be ascending (as in Guillain-Barré syndrome) or may affect 1 or more limbs differentially
- Coma
  - Lasts hours to days; with intensive care, may rarely last months
  - May evolve over a few days following acute neurologic period
  - May be sudden, with respiratory arrest
- Death
  - Usually occurs within 3 weeks of onset, as result of complications
  - Only 4 survivors reported in the world's literature

TESTS

- Available only at state and federal reference laboratories
- Rabies antibody titer should be obtained on serum and CSF
- Skin biopsy from nape of neck should be obtained for direct fluorescent antibody examination
- Saliva culture for rabies virus

Lab

- WBC count in CSF examination may be normal or show moderate pleocytosis.
- CSF protein may be normal or moderately elevated.
- Viral isolation from saliva or CSF
- Serum CSF for rabies antibody
- Corneal smear stains are positive by immunofluorescence in 50% of patients.
- Drugs that may alter lab results: Immunosuppressive agents

Imaging

Normal, or nonspecific findings consistent with encephalitis

Diagnostic Procedures/Surgery

- Spinal tap
- Skin biopsy to detect rabies antigen in hair follicles

Pathological Findings

Encephalitis may be found on brain biopsy, but abnormal findings may be confined to parts (brainstem, midbrain, cerebellum) examined only postmortem.

DIFFERENTIAL DIAGNOSIS

- Any rapidly progressive encephalitis; important to exclude treatable causes of encephalitis, especially herpes
- Diagnosis should be considered if there is a bite by an animal capable of transmitting the disease or travel to rabies-endemic country; however, most patients in the US do not recall exposure.

TREATMENT

INITIAL STABILIZATION
- If rabies encephalitis is suspected: Inpatient care with isolation
- If patient has been exposed to rabies: Inpatient care if wounds are serious; outpatient care for prophylactic treatment

GENERAL MEASURES
- Because there is no treatment for clinical rabies, this section is directed at prevention of disease following exposure to potentially rabid animals.
- People who observe abnormal behavior in any wildlife species should contact animal control or animal rescue agencies and should avoid approaching or handling these animals.
- Physicians should evaluate each possible exposure to rabies and consult local or state public health officials about the need for rabies prophylaxis
  - In the US, raccoons, skunks, bats, foxes, and coyotes are the animals most likely to be infected, but any carnivore can carry the disease.
  - Postexposure prophylaxis should be considered for any person who reports direct contact with bats, unless it is known that an exposure did not occur.
- Outside the US, dogs are a main reservoir, especially in developing countries.
- Before specific antirabies treatment is initiated, consider
  - Type of exposure (bite or nonbite)
  - Epidemiology of rabies in species involved
  - Circumstances of biting incident
  - Vaccination status of exposing animal

Diet
No restrictions

Activity
As tolerated

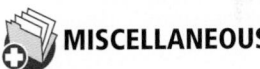 ## MEDICATION (DRUGS)

- Postexposure prophylaxis regimen (do all 3)
  - Local wound treatment: Immediate and thorough washing of all bite wounds and scratches with soap and water
  - Passive vaccination: Rabies immune globulin (RIG, Hyperab) administered once: 20 IU/kg body weight (formula is applicable for all ages). If anatomically feasible, all the RIG should be thoroughly infiltrated in the area around the wound. Any remaining RIG should be administered IM. RIG should never be administered in the same syringe or into the same anatomic site as vaccine.
  - Active vaccination: Rabies vaccine, human diploid cell (HDCV) or rabies vaccine adsorbed (RVA) or purified chick embryo cell vaccine IM in the deltoid. For children, the anterolateral aspect of the thigh is acceptable. Gluteal area should never be used for vaccine injections. Give the 1st dose, 1 mL, as soon as possible after exposure; 1 additional dose should be given on days 3, 7, 14, and 28.
- For previously vaccinated patients, 2 IM doses (1 mL each) of vaccine should be administered, 1 immediately and 1 dose 3 days later. RIG is not necessary in these patients.
- Pre-exposure vaccination: For people in high-risk groups, such as veterinarians, animal handlers, certain laboratory workers, and those spending time in foreign countries where rabies is enzootic
  - Primary pre-exposure: IM vaccination regimen consists of 3 1-mL injections of HDCV or RVA given in deltoid area, 1 each on days 1, 7, and 28. HDCV may also be given in intradermal doses, administered with a special syringe developed for that purpose (Imovax Rabies ID Vaccine); the 0.1-mL IM dose is administered in the deltoid area; follow the same schedule as for IM doses. Recently, the manufacturer discontinued production of Imovax Rabies ID.
  - Pre-exposure boosters: For people at frequent risk of exposure to rabies, serum should be tested every 2 years. A pre-exposure booster (1.0 mL IM) should be administered if this is less than acceptable level. If titer cannot be obtained, a booster can be administered instead.
- Contraindications: None for postexposure treatment
- Precautions: ~6% of people develop mild serum sickness reaction following HDCV boosters. Mild local and systemic reactions are common following vaccination. Mild reactions should not be a cause for interruption of immunization.
- Significant possible interactions: Antibody response may be suppressed by diseases that suppress the immune system.

 ## FOLLOW-UP

PROGNOSIS
No postexposure failures reported in the US since the 1970s.

COMPLICATIONS
None

PATIENT MONITORING
After primary vaccination, serologic testing is necessary only if the patient has disease or takes medications that may suppress the immune system.

REFERENCES

1. Bleck TP, Rupprecht CE. Rabies virus. In: Mandell GI, Bennett JE, Dolin R, et al. *Principles and Practice of Infectious Disease*, 5th ed. New York: Churchill Livingstone, 2000.
2. Fishbein DB. Rabies in humans. In: Baer G, ed. *Natural History of Rabies*, 2nd ed. Boca Raton, FL: CRC Press; 1991:519–549.
3. Rabies prevention–United States, 1999. *MMWR Recomm Rep.* 1999;48(RR-1):1–20.
4. Hankin DG, Rosekrans JA. Overview prevention and treatment of rabies. *Mayo Clin Proc.* 2004;79(5): 671–676.

ADDITIONAL READING
http://www.cdc.gov/ncidod/dvrd/rabies

MISCELLANEOUS
See also: Animal bites

CODES

ICD9-CM
- 071 Rabies
- V01.5 Rabies exposure
- V04.5 Need for prophylactic vaccination and inoculation against rabies

PATIENT TEACHING

Prevention
Homes should be secured from bats by using screens over ventilation areas in the roof.

See Patient Handout on CD

RADIATION SICKNESS

Brent R. Gibson, MD, MPH
Ryung Suh, MD, MPP, MBA, MPH

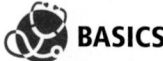 **BASICS**

DESCRIPTION
Any somatic or genetic disruption of function or form caused by electromagnetic waves or accelerated atomic particles

- Radiation illness may be classified as
  - Non-ionizing
    - Damage to exposed tissues from heating
    - Sources: Microwaves, infrared radiation
  - Ionizing
    - Damage to DNA
    - Sources include man-made: Nuclear warfare material and medical radiation; and natural: Radon and uranium
    - Examples: α particles, β particles, neutrons
- Units of measure
  - Absorbed dose: Radiation absorbed dose (Rad) or the SI unit, the Gray (Gy); 1 Gy = 100 rad.
  - Dose equivalent: Roentgen equivalent in man (Rem) or the SI unit Sievert (Sv); 1 Sv = 100 rem.
- Radiation includes
  - Electromagnetic emissions. Energy (hence, penetration) is inversely proportional to wavelength (e.g., x-rays, gamma rays).
  - Particles. α-particles are the nuclei of helium atoms, and β-particles are electrons. Both have low penetrance externally but are dangerous if ingested. Neutrons are damaging and penetrate well. Include electrons, protons, α-particles, neutrons, negative π-mesons, and heavy charged ions
- System(s) Affected: Cardiovascular; Gastrointestinal; Hemic/Lymphatic/Immunologic; Musculoskeletal; Nervous; Pulmonary; Renal/Urologic; Reproductive; Skin/Exocrine

ALERT
Pediatric Considerations
Infants and children are at increased risk for injury

Pregnancy Considerations
- Unborn children are at increased risk for injury
- Consult radiologist and health physicist for assistance in calculating fetal dose

GENERAL PREVENTION
- Avoidance of exposure
  - Exposure reduced by
    - Less exposure time
    - Distance
    - Shielding
- Pretreatment
  - In certain, situations, exposure of the thyroid may be reduced by pre-exposure consumption of radio-stable iodine
- Follow safety procedures.

EPIDEMIOLOGY
- Historically
  - In Japan, 120,000 individuals developed acute radiation syndrome as a result of nuclear explosions.
  - In the Marshall Islands, 7,266 people were exposed to radiation because of errors in judging winds after a nuclear test in the South Pacific.
  - In the Chernobyl accident in Ukraine in 1986, an estimated 50,000 individuals received at least 0.5 Sv of exposure.

- Most acute radiation injury is related to accidents or radiation therapy.
- Accidents are sporadic and usually involve small numbers of individuals
  - From 1944–2000 there have been 243 serious radiation accidents in the US
- Worldwide exposure (average/person/year)
  - Natural (gamma rays, radon, and others): 2.4 mSv
  - Occupational (from 6.5 M monitored workers): 1.8 mSv
  - Medical (330 examinations per 1,000 people): 0.4 mSv
  - Man-made environmental (atmospheric nuclear testing, Chernobyl accident, nuclear power production): 0.0072 mSv

Incidence
In the US, 400,000 patients per year receive radiation therapy for malignancies.

RISK FACTORS
- Young patients more susceptible than old
- Men more sensitive than women
- Patients who are debilitated are more susceptible than those who are healthy
- Natural: Residence in certain geographic regions
- Occupational
  - Medical professionals
  - Nuclear power workers
  - Industrial radiodiagnostic workers

Genetics
Females have greater tolerance than males. The exception is pregnant females, with risk of fetal injury at low dose.

PATHOPHYSIOLOGY
- Nonionizing radiation
  - Heating of tissues
    - Testes
    - Eye
- Ionizing radiation
  - Damage to cell DNA
  - Affects rapidly dividing cells most
    - Gastrointestinal (GI) mucosa
    - Bone marrow
    - Vascular endothelium
    - Reproductive organs

ETIOLOGY
- Routes of exposure
  - Irradiation
  - External contamination (clothing, skin)
  - Internal contamination (inhalation, ingestion)
- Acute radiation syndrome (ARS)
  - Results from whole body exposure
- Cutaneous syndrome (CS)
  - Damage to stem cells
  - Prolonged latency
  - Resembles thermal burns
  - Dry or moist desquamation

DIAGNOSIS

PRE HOSPITAL
- Strong index of suspicion and knowledge of radiation event
- Be prepared to triage if mass-casualty event (based on radiation exposure only) (1)[C]
  - Dose ≥10 Gy: Expectant
  - Dose 5–10 Gy: Immediate
  - Dose 3–5 Gy: Delayed
  - Dose ≤3 Gy: Minimal
- ARS
  - Non-specific
  - Nausea, vomiting, diarrhea, fever, or chills
- CS
  - Desquamation in absence of thermal or chemical burn, irritant or allergic dermatitis, or arthropod assault

SIGNS AND SYMPTOMS
- 4 distinct, sequential clinical phases to ARS (length of each differs by system and intensity of exposure)
  - Prodromal
  - Latency
  - Manifest Illness
  - Recovery (or death)
- 3 distinct clinical syndromes
  - Neurovascular
  - GI
  - Hematopoietic
- Acute radiation exposure is divided into several syndromes
  - Exposure of <200 rads = no disease. There may be some nausea >3 hours after the event. Most people involved in an accident of this type will complain of some nausea when questioned.
  - Exposure of 200–1,000 rads = hematopoietic syndrome. Acute nausea and vomiting within 3 hours. Acute granulocyte elevation, then lymphopenia, then thrombocytopenia and neutropenia, then anemia. Peak lowering of platelets and granulocytes at 3 weeks (resolving in 12 wks). Lymphopenia may last years. Survivors may have lung or kidney changes months later. Death rate is 0–80%, depending on dose received and treatment. Lethal dose for 1/2 the population of humans (LD_{50}) is 650 rads.
  - Exposure of 1,000–5,000 rads = GI syndrome. Nausea and vomiting 30–60 minutes postexposure. Loss of the villus structure of small bowel. Severe GI bleeding, diarrhea, and abdominal pain develop within 3 days after and precede the hematopoietic syndrome. Death due to blood loss or Gram-negative sepsis. Survivors usually die late of bone marrow suppression. Death rate is 80–100%.
  - Exposure of >5,000 rads = neurovascular syndrome or "Spock syndrome." After a 15–30 minute asymptomatic period, tremors, ataxia, vomiting, hypotension, seizures, and death. Death rate is 100%.

History
- Exposure to known source of radiation
  - Damaged radioisotope containing medical equipment
  - Industrial sources
  - Nuclear power plant
  - Research nuclear reactors
  - Terrorist event
    ○ Nuclear device or radioisotope-contaminated explosive device
    ○ Hidden source of radiation
- Generally, GI signs and symptoms occur 1st
- Symptoms
  - Nausea, vomiting, diarrhea
  - Anorexia
  - Fatigue
  - Abdominal pain, cramping
  - Headache
  - Pain and Itching of skin

Physical Exam
- Cognitive defects
- Erythema, blistering, ulceration, desquamation
- Hair loss, onycholysis
- Petechiae, bruising, spontaneous bleeding

TESTS
Total body dosimetry may suggest dose of compound ingested. Most radioisotopes are not excreted well.

Lab
- Lymphocyte count at 48 hours postevent
  - >1,500 = Trivial or no exposure
  - >1,000 = Survival without treatment
  - 500–1,000 = Survival with treatment
  - 100–400 = death without bone marrow transplant
  - <100 = certain death
- Drugs that may alter lab results
  - Chemotherapeutic agents cause bone marrow suppression identical to that seen in radiation exposure.

Pathological Findings
- Hypocellular marrow with the hematopoietic syndrome
- The GI syndrome with loss of villus margin and sloughing of villus structure
- Late cases with fibrosis of lung, liver, and kidney tissues
- Loss of hair indicates exposure of 350 rads and is complete at 700 rads.

DIFFERENTIAL DIAGNOSIS
Patient exposed to radiation
- Acute viral illness or anxiety (nausea)
- Blast or heat (skin redness)
- Chemical exposure (blistering and pain)

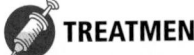 TREATMENT

INITIAL STABILIZATION
Inpatient care

GENERAL MEASURES
- Decontamination if external contamination
  - Precedence of decontamination depends on the nature of the situation and the professional judgment of the provider
- Treatment of collateral injuries, such as burns and lacerations, only after decontamination

Diet
As tolerated. Hyperalimentation for severe GI syndromes

Activity
Isolation techniques for immune system injury

SPECIAL THERAPY (2)[C]
- Pancytopenic patients may require reverse isolation
- Blood transfusion
- Platelet transfusion
- Stem cell transplantation
- Consider measures to estimate dose and specific radioisotope

 MEDICATION (DRUGS) (2)[C]
- Supportive therapy
  - Antiemetics
    ○ Promethazine or ondansetron
  - Antidiarrheals
    ○ Loperamide
  - Cytokine therapy
    ○ Granulocyte macrophage colony-stimulating factor
    ○ Granulocyte colony-stimulating factor (G-CSF) or pegylated G-CSF
- Infection prophylaxis
  - Antibiotics
    ○ Fluroquinolone
  - Antivirals
    ○ Acyclovir or gancyclovir
  - Antifungals
    ○ Fluconazole
  - Treat specific pathogens as identified
  - For exposure to radioactive iodine: Potassium iodide
  - For exposure to radioactive phosphorus: Parenteral magnesium sulfate
  - For nonspecific ingestions: Laxatives to increase gastrointestinal transit rate
- Contraindications: Refer to the manufacturer's literature for each drug.
- Precautions: Refer to the manufacturer's literature for each drug.
- Significant possible interactions: Refer to the manufacturer's literature for each drug.

SURGERY
- Débridement of all wounds to decontaminate
- All surgery within 2 days, before loss of white cell and platelet function
- Bone marrow transplant for severe exposure

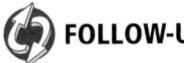 FOLLOW-UP

PROGNOSIS
- Patients surviving 12 weeks have excellent prognosis but should be monitored for long-term complications
- Hair growth usually resumes within 2 months

COMPLICATIONS
- Long-term fibrosis of kidneys, liver, and lung. Occurs within 6 months of acute exposure and with as little as 300 rads of exposure.
- Radiation exposure may induce malignancies.
- Increased long-term risk of leukemia (acute lymphocytic or chronic myelogenous)
- Multiple myeloma and cancers of the breast, esophagus, stomach, colon, lung, ovary, bladder, and thyroid
- Sterility
- In pregnancy: Injury to fetus likely

PATIENT MONITORING
- Daily CBC, platelet, granulocyte, and lymphocyte counts
- Stools for blood
- Vital signs q4h to look for sepsis

REFERENCES
1. Waselenko J, et al. Medical management of the acute radiation syndrome: Recommendations of the Strategic National Stockpile Radiation Working Group. *Ann Intern Med*.140:1037–1051.
2. Fong F, Schrader D, Fong S.Radiation. In: *Clinical Toxicology*, 1st ed. Philadelphia, PA: W.B. Saunders, 2001.
3. Burnham J, Franco J. Radiation. *Crit Care Clin*. 2005;21:785–813.
4. Ricks R, et al. REAC/TS radiation accident registry: Update of accidents on the United States. Unpublished. Oak Ridge Institute for Science and Education: Oak Ridge, TN;2000.
5. United Nations Scientific Committee on the Effects of Atomic Radiation. Report to the General Assembly. Volume I: Sources.2000.

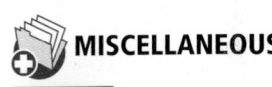 MISCELLANEOUS

CODES

ICD9-CM
990 Radiation effects, unspecified

PATIENT TEACHING
Recommend genetic counseling and screening to patients who have been exposed to significant amounts of radiation.

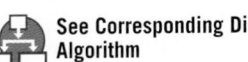 **See Corresponding Diagnostic Algorithm**

RAPE CRISIS SYNDROME

Christ G. Kyriakedes, DO, FACOEP, FACEP

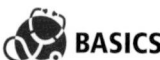 **BASICS**

DESCRIPTION

- Definitions (legal definitions may vary from state to state)
  - Sexual contact: Intentional touching of a person's intimate parts (including thighs) or the clothing covering such areas, if it is construed as being for the purpose of sexual gratification
  - Sexual conduct: Vaginal intercourse between a male and female, or anal intercourse, fellatio, or cunnilingus between persons, regardless of sex
  - Rape: Any sexual penetration, however slight, using force or coercion against the person's will
  - Sexual imposition: Similar to rape but without penetration or the use of force (i.e., nonconsenting sexual contact)
  - Gross sexual imposition: Nonconsensual sexual contact with the use of force
  - Corruption of a minor: Sexual conduct by an individual ≥ 18 years old with an individual < 16 years of age
- Most states have expanded rape statutes to include marital rape, date rape, shield laws
- System(s) Affected: Nervous; Reproductive
- Synonym(s): Sexual assault; Rape trauma

GENERAL PREVENTION

Scope of rape prevention is too complex and too broad to be discussed in detail. The public health approach should include prevention/avoidance of vulnerability factors and implementation of protective factors. Females may benefit from assertiveness training and self-defense training.

EPIDEMIOLOGY

- Predominant age
  - The incidence of sexual assault peaks in the 16–19 year age group with the mean occurring at 20 years of age.
  - Adolescent sexual assault has a greater frequency of anogenital injuries
  - For males, 75% of all rapes occur before age 18, and 48% occur before age 12
- Predominant sex: Female > Male

Incidence

- There were 198,850 rapes and sexual assaults measured in 2003 in the US
- Estimated that only 1:3–1:5 of adult cases reported. In 2003, 38.5% of rapes and sexual assaults were reported to the police.
- ~2/1,000 children in the US were confirmed by child protective agencies as having experienced sexual assault in 2003.
- Reported rape in 2003 by Bureau of Justice is 72,240. A decrease of nearly 23,000 from 2002.
- 1/7 males will be sexually assaulted during a lifetime.
- Between 20% and 25% of females will experience rape or attempted rape during their college years.
- Majority of rape victims either know or have some acquaintance with their attacker

RISK FACTORS

- Numerous and include multiple individual, relationship, community and societal factors.
- In general, adults are assaulted in their own homes, while adolescents are assaulted in their assailant's residence.

- Most perpetrators of sexual violence are males with all acts against females >90%, and most acts against males are >65% male perpetrators
- >32,000 pregnancies result from rape every year in the US.

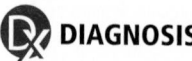 **DIAGNOSIS**

SIGNS AND SYMPTOMS

- In adults
  - History of sexual penetration
  - Sexual contact or sexual conduct without consent and/or with the use of force
- In children
  - Actual observation or suspicion of sexual penetration, sexual contact, or sexual conduct
  - Signs include evidence of the use of force and/or evidence of sexual contact (e.g., presence of semen and/or sperm).

History

- Avoid questioning that implies the patient is at fault.
- Record answers in patient's own words insofar as possible. Include date, approximate time, and general location as best as possible. Document physical abuse other than sexual. Describe all types of sexual contact, whether actual or attempted. Take history of alcohol and/or drugs before or after alleged incident.
- Document time of last activity that could possibly alter specimens (e.g., bath, shower, or douche). Thorough gynecologic history is mandatory, including last menstrual period, last consenting sexual contact, contraceptive practice, and prior gynecologic surgery.

Physical Exam

- Use of drawings and/or photographs is encouraged. Use UV light (Wood lamp) to detect seminal stains on clothing or skin. Document all signs of trauma or unusual marks. Document mental status/emotional state.
- Complete genital-rectal examination including evidence of trauma, secretions, or discharge. Use of a nonlubricated, water-moistened speculum is mandatory because commonly used lubricants may destroy evidence.

TESTS

Lab

- Record results of wet mount, noting the presence or absence of sperm and, if present, whether it is motile or immotile.
- If indicated, obtain a serum or urine pregnancy test and record the results.
- Drug/alcohol testing as indicated by history and/or physical findings
- Testing and/or specimen collection as indicated and in compliance with state requirements

DIFFERENTIAL DIAGNOSIS

Consenting sex among adults

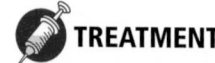 **TREATMENT**

INITIAL STABILIZATION

- Contact appropriate social services agency
- Majority of adult victims can be treated as outpatients, unless associated trauma (physical or mental) requires admission
- Majority of pediatric sexual assault/abuse victims will require admission or outside placement until appropriate social agency can evaluate home environment

GENERAL MEASURES

- Providing health care to victims of sexual assault/abuse requires special sensitivity and privacy.
- All such cases *must* be reported immediately to the appropriate law enforcement agency.
- With the victim's permission, enlist the help of personnel from local support agencies (e.g., Rape Crisis Center). When available, use of in-house social services is extremely helpful to victim and family.
- Give sedation and tetanus prophylaxis when indicated.
- Administer venereal disease prevention for gonorrhea/chlamydia.
- Discuss possible pregnancy and pregnancy termination with the victim. If hospital policy precludes such a discussion, then information about this option should be offered to the victim via follow-up mechanisms.
- Discuss suspected HIV and hepatitis B exposure and testing with the victim in accordance with hospital, regional, and state policies/protocols. The initial HIV test should be completed within 7 days of the suspected exposure.
- Sexual assault nurse examiner programs have been shown to be beneficial, especially in large cities and metropolitan areas with multiple emergency departments of varying capability and staff training/experience.

ALERT

Pregnancy Considerations

Conduct baseline pregnancy test; discuss pregnancy prevention with patient

Pediatric Considerations

Assure the child that he or she is a good person and was not the cause of the incident.

Diet

No restrictions

Activity

No restrictions

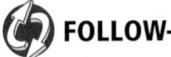 **MEDICATION (DRUGS)**

First Line

- Gonorrhea: Ceftriaxone 125 mg IM once or Ciprofloxin 500 mg PO or ofloxacin 400 mg PO or Levofloxin 250 mg PO. Chlamydia: Azithromycin (Zithromax) 1 g PO, single dose or doxycycline 100 mg PO b.i.d. × 7 days or erythromycin base 500 mg PO q.i.d. for 7 days or erythromycin ethylsuoccinate 800 mg PO q.i.d. for 7 days or ofloxacin 300 mg PO b.i.d. for 7 days or levofloxacin 300 mg PO b.i.d. for 7 days.
- Syphilis: Benzathine penicillin G 2–4 million units IM once or doxycycline 100 mg PO b.i.d. for 21 days. Trichomoniasis and bacterial vaginosis, if present. Metronidazole 500 mg PO b.i.d. for 7 days or metronidazole 2 g PO, single dose (considered less efficacious than 7-day therapy) or metronidazole gel 0.75% 1 full applicator (5 g) intravaginally, once a day for 5 days; or Clindamycin cream 2%, 1 full applicator (5 g) intravaginally at bedtime for 7 days (also less efficacious than metronidazole).
- If pregnancy prophylaxis is given, consider progestin plus estrogen: Ovral, 4 pills total; or Lo/Ovral, 8 pills total. 1/2 the total pills should be taken within 72 hours of alleged event, half the total pills 12 hours after the 1st dose.
- HIV: Currently, there is a low likelihood of HIV transmittance but the Centers for Disease Control and Prevention still recommends postexposure prophylaxis for victims of sexual assault. Regimen is lamivudine–zidovudine (Combivir) b.i.d. for 28 days or zidovudine 300 mg plus lamivudine 150 mg b.i.d. for 28 days.
- Hepatitis B: If prevalent in area or assailant known to be high risk—hepatitis B immune globulin 0.06 mL/kg IM, single dose, and initiate 3-dose hepatitis B virus immunization series.
- Note: Gonorrhea and chlamydia medications may be given concomitantly.
- Contraindications
  - Refer to the manufacturer's literature for each drug.
- Precautions
  - Refer to the manufacturer's literature for each drug.
- Significant possible interactions
  - Refer to the manufacturer's literature for each drug.

Second Line

Gonorrhea: Norfloxacin, ampicillin/probenecid, or amoxicillin/probenecid. NOTE: Be aware that drug resistance is on the rise in several major cities. In northeastern Ohio, a 20% resistance of gonorrhea to ciprofloxacin has been reported.

 FOLLOW-UP

PROGNOSIS

- Acute phase (usually 1–3 weeks following rape): Shaking, pain, wound healing, mood swings, appetite loss, crying. Also feelings of grief, shame, anger, fear, revenge, or guilt.
- Late or chronic phase: Female victim may develop fear of intercourse, fear of men, nightmares, sleep disorders, daytime flashbacks, fear of being alone, loss of self-esteem, anxiety, depression, posttraumatic stress syndrome.
- Recovery may be prolonged. Patients who are able to talk about their feelings seem to have a faster recovery.

COMPLICATIONS

- Sexually transmitted disease and subsequent treatment
- Pregnancy (with the possibility of abortion)
- Trauma (physical and mental)
- Posttraumatic stress disorder

PATIENT MONITORING

- The patient should be seen in 7–10 days for follow-up care including pregnancy testing and counseling by a gynecologist or appropriate gynecologic clinic
- Close examination for vaginitis, and treatment if necessary
- Follow-up test for syphilis and gonorrhea should occur in 5–6 weeks.
- Follow-up testing for HIV and hepatitis B should occur in 6 months.
- Provide telephone numbers of counseling agency(ies) that can provide counseling/legal services to the patient.
- Consider sexual assault nurse examiner, if available in area.

REFERENCES

1. Hogan TM, Uyenishi AA. Sexual assault: Medical and legal implications of the emergency care of adult victims. *Emerg Med Pract*. 2003;5.
2. A National Protocol for Sexual Assault Medical Forensic Examinations (Adults/Adolescents). U.S. Department of Justice, Office on Violence Against Women; September 2004.
3. Jones J, et al. Comparative analysis of adult versus adolescent sexual assault: Epidemiology and patterns of anogenital injury. *Acad Emerg Med*. 2003;10:872.
4. Bureau of Justice Statistics. National Center for Injury Prevention and Control. Sexual Violence: Fact Sheet and Rape and Sexual Assault National Crime Victim's Rights Week,2005.
5. Poirier M, Care of the female adolescent rape victim. *Pediatr Emerg Care*. 2002;18:53.

 MISCELLANEOUS

- Other notes
  - *Rape* is a legal term, and the examining physician is encouraged to use terminology such as *alleged rape* or *alleged sexual conduct*.
  - In majority of states, wife may now accuse husband of rape if they are estranged and living apart
  - Because "consent defense" is common, documentation of evidence supporting the use of force or the administration of drugs/alcohol is imperative
  - The use of a protocol is encouraged to assure every victim a uniform, comprehensive evaluation regardless of the expertise of the examining physician. The protocol must ensure that all evidence is properly collected and labeled, chain of custody is maintained, and the evidence is sent to the most appropriate forensic laboratory.
  - All medical records must be well documented and legible.
  - All medical personnel must be willing and able to testify on behalf of the patient.
- See also: Chlamydial Sexually Transmitted Diseases; Gonococcal Infections; Hepatitis B; Hepatitis C; HIV Infection and AIDS; Posttraumatic Stress Disorder (PTSD); Syphilis

CODES

ICD9-CM

- V71.5 Observation following alleged rape or seduction
- 959.9 Injury, unspecified site
- 959.19 Other injury of other sites of trunk

PATIENT TEACHING

- Information and help are available from local rape crisis support organizations.
- National Institute of Mental Health, Public Inquiries Branch, Office of Scientific Information, Department of Health and Human Services, Parklawn Bldg., Room 15C-05, 5600 Fishers Lane, Rockville, MD 20857; (301) 443-4513

 See Corresponding Diagnostic Algorithm

 See Patient Handout on CD

RAYNAUD PHENOMENON

Herbert L. Muncie Jr, MD

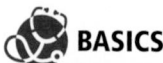 **BASICS**

DESCRIPTION
Idiopathic intermittent episodes of vasoconstriction of digital arteries, precapillary arterioles, and cutaneous arteriovenous shunts in response to cold temperatures or emotional stress

- Primary
  - Episodes are bilateral and non-progressive.
  - Manifested by extreme pallor, then cyanosis of the fingers (rarely, of the toes); with warming, vasodilatation and intense redness develop, followed by swelling, throbbing, paresthesias. Thumbs are rarely involved.
  - 80% of patients with Raynaud phenomenon have primary disease
  - Diagnose confirmed only if >2 years of symptoms no underlying associated disease develops.
- Secondary
  - Progressive and asymmetric
  - Spasm is more frequent and more severe with time. No gangrene; rarely ulceration; 13% may progress to atrophy of digital fat pads, ischemic ulcers of fingertips.
- System(s) Affected: Hemotologic; Lymphatic; Immunologic; Musculoskeletal; Dermatologic; Exocrine systems;

ALERT
Geriatric Considerations
Appearance of Raynaud phenomenon >40 years of age frequently indicates an underlying disease.

Pediatric Considerations
Associated with systemic lupus erythematosus and scleroderma

GENERAL PREVENTION
- Avoid exposure to cold.
- Stop smoking.
- Avoid trauma to fingertips.

EPIDEMIOLOGY
- Primary
  - Predominant age: 14 years; ~1/4 begin >40 years of age
  - Predominant sex: Female > Male (4:1)
- Secondary
  - Predominant age: >40 years of age
  - Predominant sex: No gender predilection

Prevalence
- Primary: ~3–16% of population (based on reporting of characteristic skin color changes, intolerance to cold)
- Secondary: Less common, only 3–9% of population

RISK FACTORS
- Smoking may reduce digital blood flow but is not associated with increased risk of Raynaud phenomenon.
- Existing autoimmune or connective tissue disorder

Genetics
Little information is available, but some studies suggest a dominant inheritance pattern. ~1/4 of primary patients have a 1st-degree relative with Raynaud phenomenon.

ETIOLOGY
Unknown. May involve increased sensitivity of α-2-adrenergic receptors in digital vessels in primary type. Serotonin receptors (5-HT2 type) may be involved in secondary Raynaud phenomenon. Platelet and blood viscosity abnormalities are also implicated.

ASSOCIATED CONDITIONS
- Lupus
- Rheumatoid arthritis (RA)
- Scleroderma
- Polymyositis
- Sjögren syndrome
- Occlusive vascular disease
- Cryoglobulinemia
- Use of vibrating tools

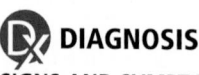 **DIAGNOSIS**

SIGNS AND SYMPTOMS
Pallor/whiteness of fingertips with cold exposure, followed by cyanosis, then redness and pain with warming

History
- Primary
  - Symmetric attacks
  - Absence of tissue necrosis, ulceration, or gangrene
  - Absence of secondary cause after history and general physical examination
  - If >2 years no abnormal clinical or laboratory signs have developed, secondary disease highly unlikely
- Secondary
  - Onset >40 years of age
  - Asymmetric episodes more intense and painful
  - Inquire regarding arthritis, myalgias, fever, dry membranes, rash, or cardiopulmonary symptoms
  - Inquire about past or current drug use
  - Any exposure to toxic agents
  - Any repetitive trauma

Primary and Secondary
- Ischemic attacks evidenced by demarcated or cyanotic skin limited to digits usually starts on one digit and spreads symmetrically to all fingers of both hands
- Beau lines: Transverse linear depressions in nail plate that can occur after exposure to cold temperature
- Primary
  - Normal general physical exam
  - Nail bed capillaries: Normal (place 1 drop grade B immersion oil on skin at base of fingernail and view capillaries with handheld ophthalmoscope at 10–40 diopters)

- Secondary
  - Clinical features suggestive of connective tissue disease (e.g., arthritis, abnormal lung function)
  - Ischemic skin lesions
    - Ulceration of finger pads, progressing to auto amputation in severe, prolonged cases
  - Nail bed capillaries distorted and anatomically abnormal

TESTS
Unnecessary to perform provocative test (e.g., immersion of patient's hand in ice water)

Lab
- Primary
  - Antinuclear antibody—negative
  - Erythrocyte sedimentation rate—normal
- Secondary
  - Tests for underlying secondary causes (complete blood chemistry, ESR)
  - Positive autoantibody has low positive predictive value for an associated connective tissue disease (30%)
  - Antibodies to specific autoantigens more suggestive of secondary disease (e.g., scleroderma with anticentromere or antitopoisomerase antibodies)

Imaging
Rarely necessary; cases may demonstrate osteolysis of distal metaphysial portions of phalanges, and with tapering and calcification of soft tissue

Diagnostic Procedures/Surgery
Diagnosis is determined by history.

DIFFERENTIAL DIAGNOSIS
- Thromboangiitis obliterans (Buerger disease): Primarily affects men; involves legs and feet; <5% have hand involvement; smoking related
- RA
- Progressive systemic sclerosis (scleroderma): Raynaud phenomenon may precede other symptoms by years.
- Systemic lupus
- Carpal tunnel syndrome
- Thoracic outlet syndrome
- Hypothyroidism
- CREST syndrome (calcinosis cutis, Raynaud phenomenon, esophageal dysmotility, sclerodactyly and telangiectasias)
- Cryoglobulinemias
- Waldenström macroglobulinemia
- Acrocyanosis
- Polycythemia
- Occupational (e.g., especially from vibrating tools, masonry work, exposure to polyvinyl chloride)
- Drugs (e.g., clonidine, ergotamine, methysergide, amphetamines, bromocriptine, bleomycin, vinblastine, cisplatin, cyclosporine)

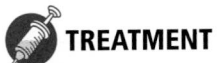 **TREATMENT**

GENERAL MEASURES
- Dress warmly, wear gloves, and avoid cold.
- Stop smoking.
- Avoid beta-blockers, amphetamines, ergot alkaloids, and sumatriptan.
- Temperature-related biofeedback may help patients increase hand temperature but at the 1-year follow-up no better than control
- Use finger guards over ulcerated fingertips.

Diet
No special diet

Activity
Avoid exposure to cold situations; avoid use of vibrating tools

Complementary and Alternative Medicine
Oral arginine no better than placebo

 MEDICATION (DRUGS)

First Line
- Nifedipine: 30–90 mg/d (sustained release form); may only be needed during winter; up to 75% experience improvement (1)[B]

- Symptomatic responses do not correlate with objective evidence of improvement.
- Contraindications: Allergy to drug, pregnancy, CHF
- Precautions: May cause headache, dizziness, lightheadedness, or hypotension
- Significant possible interactions
  – Increases serum level of digoxin: Monitor digoxin levels closely after nifedipine added.
  – May increase prothrombin time in patients taking warfarin

Second Line
- Amlodipine and nicardipine appear to be effective and may have fewer adverse effects.
- No data to support use of another calcium-channel blocker if initial one is ineffective
- Prazosin only well studied α_1-adrenergic-receptor blocker
- Small studies support benefit from losartan and fluoxetine
- Parenteral prostacyclin has offered subjective improvement, but the effect is short-lived and not statistically significant
  – Oral prostacyclin not proved useful
- Nitroglycerin patches may also be helpful, but use is limited by the incidence of severe headache.

SURGERY
Effect of cervical sympathectomy is transient; symptoms return in 1–2 years.

Acute Ischemic Crisis
- Short acting calcium-channel blocker such as nifedipine
- Aspirin
- Digital or wrist block with lidocaine or bupivacaine (without epinephrine)
- Short-term anticoagulation with heparin if persistent critical ischemia, evidence of large artery occlusive disease or both

 FOLLOW-UP

Issues for Referral
If an underlying disease is strongly suspected consider rheumatology consultation for evaluation and treatment

PROGNOSIS
- Attacks may last from several minutes to a few hours
- In cases of secondary Raynaud phenomenon, affected patients develop the hallmarks of underlying disease.
- ~13% of Raynaud phenomenon patients developed a secondary disorder, many of which were connective-tissue diseases

COMPLICATIONS
- Primary: Very rare
- Secondary: Gangrene; Autoamputation of fingertips

PATIENT MONITORING
Management of fingertip ulcers, including rapid treatment of infection

REFERENCES
1. Pope J: Raynaud's phenomenon (primary). *Clinical Evidence*. 2005;13:1–2.
2. Wigley FM. Raynaud's phenomenon. *N Engl J Med*. 2002;347:1001–1008.
3. Fawcett RS, Linford S, Stulberg DL. Nail abnormalities: Clues to systemic disease. *Am Fam Physician*. 2004;69:11417–24.

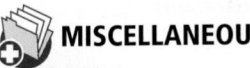 **MISCELLANEOUS**

 CODES

ICD9-CM
443.0 Raynaud (disease, syndrome, phenomenon, secondary)

PATIENT TEACHING
- Emphasize cessation of smoking.
- Discuss avoiding aggravating factors (e.g., trauma, vibration, cold).
- Dress warmly, wear gloves
- Warm hands when experiencing vasospasm

 See Corresponding Diagnostic Algorithm

 See Patient Handout on CD

RECTAL PROLAPSE

Timothy L. Black, MD
James P. Miller, MD

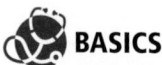 **BASICS**

DESCRIPTION
Protrusion of the rectum through the anus

- Partial prolapse: Involves only mucosa; frequently follows anal operative procedures (radial rectal folds prolapsed through anus)
- Complete prolapse: Involves the entire rectal wall (procidentia); occurs most commonly as a spontaneous event in children and as a complication of other disorders in the elderly (concentric rectal folds prolapsed through anus)
- System(s) Affected: Gastrointestinal

GENERAL PREVENTION
Avoid constipation and diarrhea.

EPIDEMIOLOGY
- Predominant age: <3 years in children, 5th decade in adults
- Predominant sex: Females represent 80–90% of adult patients; the male: female ratio represents an equal distribution in children [1](B)

Incidence
4.2/1,000 overall; 10/1,000 >65 years of age

ALERT
Geriatric Considerations
Common problem in the elderly

Pediatric Considerations
Idiopathic type most common in children

RISK FACTORS
- Myelomeningocele
- Exstrophy of the bladder
- Cystic fibrosis
- Chronic constipation or diarrhea
- Imperforate anus (2)[C]
- Multiple sclerosis
- Stroke/paralysis
- Mental retardation

Genetics
Unknown

ETIOLOGY
- Children
  - Idiopathic (most common)
  - Abnormal innervation of levator ani muscle complex or puborectalis or anal sphincter, or abnormal anatomic relationships of these muscle groups
- Adults
  - Diastasis of levator ani
  - Loose endopelvic fascia
  - Loss of normal horizontal position of rectum
  - Weak anal sphincter
  - Pudendal neuropathy
  - Redundant sigmoid colon
  - Loss of rectal-sacral attachments

ASSOCIATED CONDITIONS
- Cystic fibrosis
- Myelomeningocele
- Exstrophy of the bladder
- Chronic constipation or diarrhea
- Imperforate anus
- Paraplegia
- Stroke
- Incontinence
- Vaginal vault or uterine prolapse
- Mental retardation

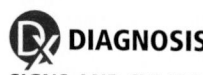 **DIAGNOSIS**

SIGNS AND SYMPTOMS
- Children
  - Sensation of anal mass
  - Pain
  - Rectal bleeding
  - Protruding mass
- Adults
  - Anorectal pain or discomfort during defecation if the patient has normal perineal sensation
  - Feeling of incomplete evacuation
  - Rectal and urinary incontinence (50–75% of adult patients)
  - Rectal bleeding or discharge

History
- History of visible mass
- History of rectal bleeding or soiling
- History of rectal pain
- History of prior anorectal surgery
- History of spinal cord injury or defect

Physical Exam
- Visible mass of rectal mucosa or full thickness of rectal wall
- Poor anal sphincter tone on rectal exam
- Reproduce prolapse with straining

TESTS
Lab
Evaluate for cystic fibrosis with genetic screening and sweat chloride evaluation

Imaging
Barium enema is useful in selected cases of recurrent rectal prolapse.

Diagnostic Procedures/Surgery
- Sigmoidoscopy is useful in recurrent prolapse to rule out rectal lesions.
- MRI of lumbosacral spine to evaluate for spinal canal defects if not already diagnosed
- Anal manometry
- Pudendal nerve terminal latencies

DIFFERENTIAL DIAGNOSIS
- Intussusception
- Rectal polyps
- Hemorrhoids

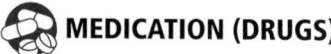 **TREATMENT**

INITIAL STABILIZATION
Outpatient care unless complications occur or surgical intervention is required

GENERAL MEASURES
For acute cases
- Prompt manual reduction of prolapse
- Treatment of diarrhea or constipation

Diet
- High fiber
- 100% bran granules

Activity
Full, when patient is able

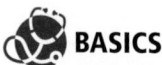 **MEDICATION (DRUGS)**

- Mineral oil
- Stool softeners
- Lactulose
- Polyethylene glycol (Miralax, Glycolax)

SURGERY
For recurrent cases
- Submucosal injection (sclerotherapy) of 5% phenol, 30% saline, or 25% glucose (or other sclerosants) in 4 quadrants under general anesthesia (outpatient)
- Linear electrocauterization (inpatient or outpatient)
- Transabdominal Ripstein procedure (suspension of rectum from sacrum by means of artificial material) (1)[B]
- Posterior sagittal rectal suspension and levator repair (3)[C]
- Ivalon sponge wrap procedure (rarely used in current era)
- Anterior resection of rectum (rarely used)
- Transabdominal proctopexy and may also be done laparoscopically (suture material, absorbable mesh, and non-absorbable mesh may be used) (1,4)[B]
- Perineal rectosigmoidectomy (1)[B]
- Thiersch wire (outpatient procedure; may be modified by using Marlex or Silastic strip or other strong suture material instead of wire); used more commonly in children, older patients, and poor-risk adults
- Gracilis sling procedure

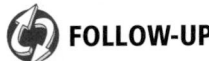 **FOLLOW-UP**

PROGNOSIS
- Spontaneous resolution is expected in most children.
- Recurrence rate is 5–10% for most procedures.
- Sclerotherapy frequently needs to be repeated
- Good prognosis with treatment

COMPLICATIONS
- Mucosal ulcerations
- Necrosis of rectal wall
- Persistent or recurrent prolapse
- Constipation in Thiersch wire is too tight
- Recurrence of rectal prolapse
- Fecal incontinence

PATIENT MONITORING
Monthly visits until possible need for surgery has been determined or until prolapse has resolved

REFERENCES
1. Madiba TE, Baig MK, Wexner SD. Surgical management of rectal prolapse. *Arch Surg.* 2005;140:63–73.
2. Belizon A, et al. Rectal prolapse following posterior sagittal anorectoplasty for anorectal malformations. *J Ped Surg.* 2005;40:192–196.
3. Ashcraft KW, et al. Rectal prolapse: 17 year experience with the posterior repair and suspension. *J Pediatr Surg.* 1990;25:992–995.
4. Brazzelli M, Bachoo P, Grant A. Surgery for complete rectal prolapse in adults (review). The Cochrane Database of Systematic Reviews,2006;1.

 MISCELLANEOUS

See also: Hemorrhoids; Intussusception

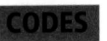 **CODES**

ICD9-CM
569.1 Rectal prolapse

PATIENT TEACHING
- Particular reassurance to parents of infants with prolapse regarding benign nature of problem and high rate of spontaneous resolution
- Diet instructions
- Teach measures to avoid constipation
- Teach family/patient to reduce prolapse

 See Corresponding Diagnostic Algorithm

R

REFRACTIVE ERRORS

Robert M. Kershner, MD

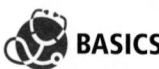 **BASICS**

DESCRIPTION

Inability of the eye to produce a focused image on the fovea or central part of the retina

- Emmetropia: When light rays are in perfect focus, the image being viewed is seen clearly.
- Ametropia: Any refractive error of the eye that prevents normal focusing of the image
- Hyperopia: When the cornea of the eye is too flat or the eye is too short, light rays fall in focus behind the retina, and the individual is "farsighted."
- Myopia: When the cornea is too steep or the length of the eyeball is too long, light rays fall short of the retina, and the individual is "nearsighted."
- Presbyopia: The natural tendency of the crystalline lens to harden or become sclerotic, limiting the focusing of the eye on near objects (accommodation). The human crystalline lens thickens with age. By the age of 40 years, most people do not have enough room within the eye to allow normal excursion of the lens and accommodation; viewing of near objects is blurred, and reading glasses are required.
- Astigmatism: When the cornea is steeper in 1 meridian more than the other or the globe is not round (i.e., is oval or almond shaped), visual blurriness occurs.
- System(s) Affected: Nervous

ALERT
Geriatric Considerations
Presbyopia occurs in later life.

Pediatric Considerations
Refractive errors can be detected early in life.

EPIDEMIOLOGY
- Predominant age: Refractive errors are present at birth but usually are not detected until puberty.
- Predominant sex: Male = Female
- Individuals >40 years of age are more likely to experience presbyopia or normal loss of accommodation that occurs with age, necessitating the use of reading glasses for close work.

Prevalence
Of the general US population 70% has some form of ametropia.

RISK FACTORS
Genetics
Inherited

ETIOLOGY
- Developmental (most common)
- Ocular trauma
- Iatrogenic (e.g., post-cataract removal)

ASSOCIATED CONDITIONS
Patients with diabetes mellitus have fluctuating myopia as a result of poorly controlled blood glucose and concomitant swelling of the crystalline lens.

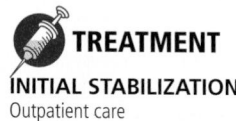 **DIAGNOSIS**

SIGNS AND SYMPTOMS
- Difficulty seeing objects at a distance
- Difficulty focusing on near objects
- Difficulty reading
- Squinting
- Headaches (from squinting)
- In children
  - Rubbing of the eyes
  - Sitting close to TV or computer screen
  - Problems in sports, particularly declining performance
  - Declining grades
  - Preference for front-row seating
  - Covering of an eye while reading

TESTS
Pinhole vision test: To distinguish a refractive error from an organic cause of visual blurring, have the patient look through a pinhole in a card without a corrective lens. Patients with a pure refractive error have improved vision because the pinhole blocks nonparallel and unfocusable rays of light.

Diagnostic Procedures/Surgery
- Methods
  - Objective streak retinoscopy may be used to measure the degree of refractive error in spherocylinder correction for the proper spectacle or contact lens
  - Antimuscarinic agents such as cyclopentolate (Cyclogyl) or tropicamide (Mydriacyl) applied topically paralyze the ciliary body, preventing accommodation. Cycloplegic refraction can then be performed.
- Age-related testing
  - Newborns should be examined for general eye health; ophthalmologic evaluation is indicated for any problems discovered.
  - Vision screening should occur at each well-child visit.
  - Visual acuity testing should be performed at ~3½ years of age.
  - Visual acuity and motility testing should be performed at age 5 years.
  - Visual acuity should be retested prior to obtaining a driver's license, at age 40 years, and every 2–4 years until age 65 years, when evaluations are recommended every 1–2 years.

DIFFERENTIAL DIAGNOSIS
- Corneal disease
- Cataract
- Retinal abnormalities
- Diseases of the optic nerve

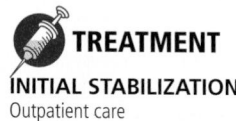 **TREATMENT**

INITIAL STABILIZATION
Outpatient care

GENERAL MEASURES
- Spectacle lenses (glasses)
- Soft or hard contact lenses

MEDICATION (DRUGS)

Precaution: Antimuscarinic agents may induce acute glaucoma via acute angle closure.

SURGERY

- Laser-assisted in-situ keratomileusis (LASIK), Food and Drug Administration (FDA) approved in 1997. A superficial corneal flap is created with the keratome, and the excimer laser removes a small amount of tissue, thus reshaping the cornea. Corrects all refractive errors. Healing is rapid because re-epithelialization is not needed. Considered an adjunctive procedure for use with the excimer laser
- Other modifications
  - Lasik and EPI Lasik involve removing just the superficial epithelium before laser application
  - Intralasik is a laser used to create the flap
  - Custom ablation: Wavefront maps of the cornea and eye for ablation
- Older methods now superseded by LASIK
  - Radial keratotomy: With topical anesthesia, using a surgical keratome, multiple (4–8) radial incisions are placed onto the surface of the peripheral cornea to flatten the central, optical zone. The length, depth, and proximity of the incision to the central optical zone determine its effect and degree of correction obtained. Radial keratotomy is safe and effective and corrects nearsightedness, astigmatism, or a combination of both, after the age of 18 years when the prescription has stabilized.
  - Photorefractive keratectomy: Surface corneal tissue is removed with the excimer laser to reshape the cornea, thus correcting nearsightedness, farsightedness, or astigmatism. Risks and disadvantages include pain, keratitis, and potential scarring. Healing requires 3 months with topical antibiotics and steroids, with associated risks of glaucoma, cataract, and chronic inflammation.
  - Automated lamellar keratoplasty: A microsurgical dermatome removes a layer of the superficial cornea to induce flattening; investigational.
- Excimer laser: The laser photoablates corneal tissue from the central visual axis, thus flattening it. Following the procedure, the cornea must re-epithelialize. Healing takes several months, during which there is a mild haze and blurring of vision. FDA approved October 1995.
- Implantable contact lens: A thin plastic lens is permanently implanted in the posterior chamber between the iris and the human crystalline lens. All refractive errors can be corrected. Risks include damage to the natural lens during surgery, cataract formation, and intraocular inflammation or infection; investigational anterior chamber Intraocular lens (FDA approved in 2005, VERISYES)
- Several scleral expansion procedures presently under investigation are methods to increase the space within the ciliary body by surgical means to restore lens movement and accommodation.
- Bifocal intraocular lenses
- Accommodative intraocular lenses (Crystalens).

 FOLLOW-UP

PROGNOSIS

- Good, if discovered early and corrected appropriately
- It is not unusual for refractive errors to be temporarily worsened during pregnancy because of hormonal changes in tear function and corneal swelling.

COMPLICATIONS

- Amblyopia
- Poor school performance

PATIENT MONITORING

- Routine annual adult eye examinations for individuals <40 years of age are not indicated.
- Individuals with risks need ocular examinations as indicated by their condition.

REFERENCES

1. *Frequency of Ocular Exams. Policy Statement #808.* San Francisco: American Academy of Ophthalmology; September 1990.
2. *Infant and Children's Vision Screening.* Policy Statement #812. San Francisco: American Academy of Ophthalmology; June 1991.
3. Kershner RM. *Lessons from the Practice: The Gift of Sight. A Guide to Understanding Your Eyes.* Thorofare, NJ: Slack; 1994.

 MISCELLANEOUS

Other notes

- Fax-on-Demand service of American Academy of Ophthalmology for policy statement and patient education materials: (908) 935-2761

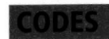 **CODES**

ICD9-CM

- 367.0 Hypermetropia
- 367.1 Myopia
- 367.4 Presbyopia
- 367.21 Regular astigmatism

PATIENT TEACHING

- All patients should have their eyes examined when starting school, and periodically thereafter.
- The options of eyeglasses, contact lenses, and permanent surgical correction of refractive errors should be considered.
- Encourage aggressive control of diabetes mellitus.

REITER SYNDROME

D. W. MacPherson, MD, MSc(CTM), FRCPC

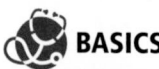 **BASICS**

DESCRIPTION

A classic triad of features including arthritis, conjunctivitis, and either urethritis or cervicitis

- The epidemiology is similar to other reactive arthritis syndromes characterized by sterile inflammation of joints associated with infections originating at nonarticular sites. A 4th feature may be buccal ulceration or balanitis. (Having only 2 features present does not rule out the diagnosis.)
- It has 2 forms: Sexually transmitted, in which symptoms generally emerge between 7–14 days after exposure during sexual intercourse, and postdysenteric.
- System(s) Affected: Musculoskeletal; Renal/Urologic; Dermatologic/Exocrine systems
- Synonym(s): Idiopathic blennorrheal arthritis; Arthritis urethritica; Urethrooculosynovial syndrome; Fiessinger-Leroy-Reiter disease

ALERT

Geriatric Considerations
Enteric etiology more likely than sexually transmitted infections related

Pediatric Considerations
Enteric etiology more likely than sexually transmitted

Pregnancy Considerations
No special considerations except as related to usual precautions concerning drugs

EPIDEMIOLOGY
Predominant age: 20–40 years
Predominant sex: Male > Female

Incidence
~0.24–1.5% incidence after epidemics of bacterial dysentery; complicates 1–2% of all cases of nongonococcal urethritis

RISK FACTORS
- Sexual intercourse 7–14 days before onset
- Food poisoning or bacterial dysentery

Genetics
HLA-B27 tissue antigen present in 60–80% of patients

ETIOLOGY
- *Chlamydia trachomatis* the usual causative organism of postvenereal variety
- Dysenteric form following enteric bacterial infection due to *Shigella, Salmonella, Yersinia,* and *Campylobacter* organisms. This form more likely in women, children, and old people.

ASSOCIATED CONDITIONS
- Earlier case of shigellosis
- Salmonellosis
- Infection with *Yersinia* sp.
- Infection with *Mycoplasma* or *Ureaplasma* spp.
- *Chlamydia* urethritis
- HIV infection

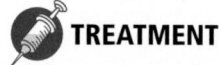 **DIAGNOSIS**

SIGNS AND SYMPTOMS
- Musculoskeletal
  - Asymmetric arthritis (especially knees, ankles, metararsophalangeal joints)
  - Enthesopathy (inflammation at tendinous insertion into bone, such as plantar fasciitis, digital periostitis, Achilles tendinitis)
  - Spondyloarthropathy (spine and sacroiliac joint involvement)
- Urogenital tract
  - Urethritis
  - Prostatitis
  - Occasionally cystitis
  - Balanitis
  - Cervicitis: Usually asymptomatic
- Eye
  - Conjunctivitis of 1 or both eyes
  - Occasionally scleritis, keratitis, corneal ulceration
  - Rarely uveitis and iritis
- Skin
  - Mucocutaneous lesions (small, painless, superficial ulcers on oral mucosa, tongue, glans penis)
  - Keratoderma blennorrhagica (hyperkeratotic skin lesions of palms and soles and around nails)
- Cardiovascular
  - Occasionally pericarditis, murmur, conduction defects, aortic incompetence
- Nervous system
  - Rarely peripheral neuropathy, cranial neuropathy, meningoencephalitis, neuropsychiatric changes
- Constitutional
  - Fever, malaise, anorexia, weight loss
  - Can appear seriously ill (e.g., fever, rigors, tachycardia, exquisitely tender joints)

History
Diarrhea or dysentery or urethritis or genital discharge and risk events for enteric or sexually acquired infections; including a travel history

Physical Exam
See "Signs and Symptoms."

TESTS
Lab
- Blood
  - Leukocyte count: 10,000–20,000
  - Neutrophilic leukocytosis
  - Elevated ESR
  - Moderate normochromic anemia
  - Hypergammaglobulinemia
- Synovial fluid
  - Leukocyte count: 1,000–8,000 cells/mm^3
  - Bacterial culture negative
- Collaborative tests
  - Cultures, antigens, or serology positive for *Chlamydia trachomatis,* or stool test positive for *Salmonella, Shigella, Yersinia,* or *Campylobacter* supports the diagnosis.
- Drugs that may alter lab results: Antibiotics may affect isolation of the bacterial pathogens

Imaging
X-ray
- Periosteal proliferation, thickening
- Spurs
- Erosions at articular margins
- Residual joint destruction
- Syndesmophytes (spine)
- Sacroiliitis

Diagnostic Procedures/Surgery
HLA-B27 histocompatibility antigen: Positive result in 60–80% of cases in non-HIV-related Reiter syndrome
Rheumatoid factor negative

Pathological Findings
- A seronegative spondyloarthropathy (similar to ankylosing spondylitis, enteric arthritis, and psoriatic arthritis)
- Villous formation in joints
- Joint hyperemia
- Joint inflammation
- Prostatitis
- Seminal vesiculitis
- Skin biopsy similar to psoriasis
- Nonspecific conjunctivitis

DIFFERENTIAL DIAGNOSIS
- For specific diagnosis, arthritis associated with urethritis for >1 month
- Rheumatoid arthritis
- Ankylosing spondylitis
- Arthritis associated with inflammatory bowel disease
- Psoriatic arthritis
- Juvenile rheumatoid arthritis
- Bacterial arthritis including gonococcal

TREATMENT

INITIAL STABILIZATION
Inpatient care may be needed during acute phase.

GENERAL MEASURES
- Treatment is determined by symptoms.
- Conjunctivitis does not require treatment.
- Iritis requires treatment.
- Mucocutaneous lesions do not require treatment.
- Physical therapy is needed during recovery.
- Arthritis may become prominent and disabling during the acute phase.

Diet
No special diet

Activity
Bed rest until joint inflammation subsides

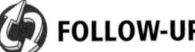 **MEDICATION (DRUGS)**

First Line
- Symptomatic management: NSAIDs including indomethacin, naproxen and others; intraarticular or systemic corticosteroids for refractory arthritis and enthesitis
- Specific treatment of pathogenic microorganism may be attempted if isolated
  - *C. trachomatis*: Doxycycline 100 mg PO b.i.d. 7–14 days (NOTE: all sexually transmited diseases should be treated whether associated with Reiter syndrome or not)
  - *Salmonella, Shigella, Yersinia,* and *Campylobacter* infections: Ciprofloxacin 500 mg PO b.i.d. for 5–10 days (NOTE: Emerging antimicrobial resistance may limit this agent's effectiveness in treatment and bacterial clearance). Antibiotic treatment does not improve gastrointestinal (GI) symptoms, duration of infection, or prevents carrier state)
- For GI upset: Antacids
- For iritis: Intraocular steroids
- For keratitis: Topical steroids
- Contraindications
  - GI bleeding
  - Patients with peptic ulcer, gastritis, ulcerative colitis
  - Renal insufficiency
- Precautions: Refer to the manufacturer's literature.
- Significant possible interactions: Refer to the manufacturer's literature.

Second Line
- Aspirin or other NSAIDs
- Sulfasalazine is promising, but not yet approved by the Food and Drug Administration.
- Methotrexate or azathioprine in severe cases (such usage still experimental and not approved nor agreed effective. Contraindicated, if patient suffers HIV-related Reiter syndrome).
- Consultation with specialist is recommended when considering immunomodulatory agents such as sulfasalazine, methotrexate, or azathioprine.
- Role of antibiotics under investigation and is unproven in effectiveness in sero-negative arthritis syndromes, but may be worth trying
- No published evidence confirms the effect of antibiotics on development and long-term outcomes in patients with Reiter syndrome.

 FOLLOW-UP

DISPOSITION
Admission Criteria
Severity, complications, and degree of disability

Issues for Referral
Joint and eye complications; complex management

PROGNOSIS
- Urethritis occurs 1–15 days after sexual exposure to causative agent
- Reiter syndrome onset within 10 to 30 days of either enteric or STD infection
- Mean duration of symptoms is 19 weeks
- Prognosis poor in cases involving heel, eye, or heart

COMPLICATIONS
- Chronic or recurrent disease in 5–50% of patients
- Ankylosing spondylitis develops in 30–50% of patients who test positive for HLA-B27 antigen
- Urethral strictures
- Cataracts and blindness
- Aortic root necrosis

PATIENT MONITORING
Monitor clinical response to medications. Observe for complications of therapy, sulfasalazine, and immunosupression.

REFERENCES
1. Mandell GL, Bennett JF, Dolin R, eds. *Principles and Practice of Infectious Diseases*. 6th ed. New York, NY: Churchill Livingstone; 2004.
2. Kataria RK, Brent LH. Spondyloarthropathies. *Am Fam Physician*. 2004;(5)69:2853–2860.
3. Amor B. Reiter's syndrome. Diagnosis and clinical features. *Rheum Dis Clin North Am*. 1998;24:677–695.
4. Banares A, et al. Eye involvement in the spondyloarthropathies. *Rheum Dis Clin North Am*. 1998;24:771–784.
5. Wollenhaupt J, Zeidler H. Undifferentiated arthritis and reactive arthritis. *Curr Opin Rheumatol*. 1998;10:306–313.
6. Olivieri I, et al. Clinical manifestations of seronegative spondyloarthropathies. *Euro J Radiol*. 1998;27(Suppl. 1):S3–S6.
7. Kean WF, MacPherson DW. Reiter's syndrome. In: Bellamy N, ed. *Prognosis in the Rheumatic Diseases*. London, UK: Kluwer Academic Publishers; 1991.
8. Mohana-Borges AV, Chung CB, Resnick D. Monoarticular arthritis. *Radiol Clin North Am*. 2004;42:135–149.
9. Hughes RA, Keat AC. Reiter's syndrome and reactive arthritis: A current view. *Semin Arthritis Rheumatism*. 1994;24:190–210.
10. Smieja M, et al. Randomised, blinded, placebo-controlled trial of doxycycline for chronic seronegative arthritis. *Ann Rheum Dis*. 2001;60:1088–1094.
11. Neumann S, et al. Reiter's syndrome as a manifestation of an immune reconstitution syndrome in an HIV-infected patient: Successful treatment with doxycycline. *Clin Infect Dis*. 2003;36:1628–1629.
12. Schneider JM, Matthews JH, Graham BS. Reiter's syndrome. *Cutis*. 2003;71:198–200.
13. Parker CT, Thomas D. Reiter's syndrome and reactive arthritis. *J Am Osteopath Assoc*. 2000;100:101–104.
14. Toivanen P, Toivanen A. Two forms of reactive arthritis? *Ann Rheum Dis*. 1999;58:737–741.
15. Kiss S, et al. Long-term progression, prognosis, and treatment of patients with recurrent ocular manifestations of Reiter's syndrome. *Ophthalmology*. 2003;110:1764–1769.

 MISCELLANEOUS

See also: Ankylosing Spondylitis; Arthritis, Psoriatic; Behçet Syndrome

CODES

ICD9-CM
099.3 Reiter disease

PATIENT TEACHING
- Educate on risk factors for exposure, occurrence, and recurrence
- Teach home physical therapy techniques.
- For a listing of sources for patient education materials favorably reviewed on this topic, physicians may contact: American Academy of Family Physicians Foundation, P.O. Box 8418, Kansas City, MO 64114; (800) 274-2237, ext. 4400.
- Arthritis Foundation, 1314 Spring Street N.W., Atlanta, GA 30309; (404) 872-7100.

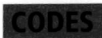 **See Corresponding Diagnostic Algorithm**

RENAL CELL CARCINOMA (RCC)

Marc Rucquoi, MD
Jonathan M. Firnhaber, MD

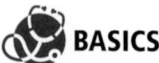 **BASICS**

DESCRIPTION

RCC represents 2–3% of all cancers and 2% of all cancer deaths; it is the 9th most common malignant tumor in men and the 13th most common malignant tumor in women. It is characterized by obscure and varied presentations, including paraneoplastic syndromes, vascular findings, and uncommon metastatic sites. Paraneoplastic and vascular syndromes do not indicate incurability or unresectability. Early, aggressive surgical management provides the best opportunity for cure.

• System(s) Affected: Renal/Urologic

ALERT

Geriatric Considerations
Condition most commonly presents in 5th–7th decades.

Pediatric Considerations
Condition is extremely rare in children

GENERAL PREVENTION
• Do not smoke; smoking may contribute to 1/3 of all cases.
• Take care around asbestos, cadmium, and petroleum distillates.

EPIDEMIOLOGY
• Predominant age: Patients in 5th–7th decades
• Predominant sex: Male > Female (2:1)

Incidence
• In the US: 30,000 new cases/year (1998); 11,600 deaths/year
• Males: 9.6 cases/100,000 population
• Females: 4.2/100,000

RISK FACTORS
• Smoking (doubles likelihood of RCC)
• Obesity (linear relationship in women)
• Increased risk in persons with acquired cystic disease of the kidney associated with end-stage renal disease
• Urban environment
• Cadmium
• Asbestos
• Petroleum byproducts
• Herpes simplex virus exposure
• Phenacetin or analgesic abuse for transitional cell of the renal pelvis

Genetics
• Oncogenes localized to the short arm of chromosome 3 may have etiologic implications. Chromosome 3p12–p26 are specific for clear cell RCC; 4% familial.
• The most common alteration with renal cell carcinoma is deletion of chromosome 3p. Recent evidence implicates gene p53 on chromosome 17p13.1 to be critical in RCC.
• People with human leukocyte antigen types Bw44 and DR8 are prone to develop renal cancer. These are rare familial renal carcinomas.

ETIOLOGY
Unknown

ASSOCIATED CONDITIONS
• Von Hippel-Lindau disease: 30–45% of these patients develop clear cell tumors

• Tuberous sclerosis: Associated primarily with angiomyolipoma and clear cell tumors
• Sickle cell trait: With few exceptions, renal medullary tumor is seen in young African American males with sickle cell trait
• Adult polycystic kidney disease
• Horseshoe kidney
• Acquired renal cystic disease from chronic renal failure

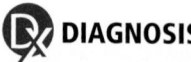 **DIAGNOSIS**

SIGNS AND SYMPTOMS
• Diverse and obscure presentations, "the internist's tumor"
• Solid renal masses, most 6–7 cm (incidentally discovered in asymptomatic patient due to increased use of CT and MRI)
• Classic triad of hematuria, abdominal mass, and flank pain in only 9% of cases
• Hematuria: 50–60%
• Elevated erythrocyte sedimentation rate: 50–60%
• Anemia: 21–41%
• Flank pain: 35–40%
• Palpable mass: 25%
• Hypertension: 22–38%
• Weight loss: 28–36%
• Pyrexia: 7–17%
• Nonmetastatic hepatic dysfunction (Stauffers' syndrome): 10–15%
• Hypercalcemia: 3–6%
• Erythrocytosis: 3–4%
• Neuromyopathy: 3%
• Scrotal varicoceles: 2–11% (most are left sided)
• Patients with vena cava thrombus present with lower extremity edema, new varicocele, dilated superficial abdominal veins, albuminuria, pulmonary emboli, right atrial mass, or nonfunction of the involved kidney.

TESTS
• Arteriography (rarely needed): For tumors larger than 10 cm, it may identify parasitic capsular vessels for early control.
• Cystoscopy: To rule out bladder cancer

Lab
• Increased ESR
• Hematuria
• Anemia (21–41% of patients)
• Polycythemia
• Alkaline phosphate may be elevated
• Urine: Neoplastic cells
• Hypercalcemia
• Increased renin
• Increased plasma fibrinogen

Imaging
• IV pyelography remains part of primary evaluation for hematuria. CT and ultrasound are the mainstays for evaluation of suspected renal mass.
• Ultrasonography: If mass appears using IV pyelography, it confirms the presence of a lesion and determines whether it is solid or cystic. Cystic lesions may either be merely observed or subjected to percutaneous cyst puncture.

• CT of abdomen and pelvis and, occasionally, arteriography: If solid or complex masses on ultrasonography require further evaluation. 3% of RCCs are bilateral by CT scan.
• MRI has not been shown to be superior to CT for tumors smaller than 8 cm; for larger tumors, it may have advantage in delineating the vena cava.
• Chest x-ray initially; chest CT if x-ray suggests metastatic disease
• Bone scan is indicated if the alkaline phosphatase level is elevated or the patient has bone pain.
• Brain CT is indicated if the patient has neurologic symptoms.

Diagnostic Procedures/Surgery
• Simple cyst need not be aspirated unless it is painful.
• Calcified cysts may contain renal cell cancer and therefore require open renal biopsy of the wall of the cyst or partial nephrectomy.
• Hemorrhagic cyst: Aspiration cytology may be helpful, but needle biopsy of solid masses is to be discouraged, particularly if the patient has a normal contralateral kidney.
• In solitary kidneys, open renal biopsy with wedge resection (not enucleation) can be performed if mass is 4 cm or smaller
• Doppler flow ultrasound of the renal veins or CT (thin cuts) that shows the renal vein entering the vena cava can be used to rule out tumor thrombus.

Pathological Findings
• Renal cell carcinoma tends to bulge out from the cortex producing a mass effect.
• 48% of RCCs measure <5 cm and are grossly yellow to yellow/orange due to high lipid content in the clear cell variety. Average renal cell size has been decreasing due to incidental discovery.
• Small tumors are homogenous.
• Large tumors may have areas of necrosis and hemorrhage.
• Tumor thrombi into the vena cava generally do not invade the vena caval wall.
• 5 distinct subtypes
  – Clear cell: 75–85%; proximal tubule; typically solitary
  – Papillary renal cell (previously termed chromophilic): 12–14%; proximal tubule; tumors tend to be bilateral and multifocal
  – Chromophobic: 4–6%; intercalated cells; tend to have a less aggressive course
  – Oncocytic: 2–4%; intercalated cells; rarely metastasize
  – Collecting duct tumors: <1%; medullary collecting duct; rare tumors, typically affect younger patients; most are at an advanced stage with metastases at time of diagnosis

DIFFERENTIAL DIAGNOSIS
• Any solid renal mass should be considered malignant until proven otherwise.
• Benign renal masses (e.g., renal hamartomas)
• Hydronephrosis
• Pyelonephritis
• Renal abscess
• Polycystic kidneys
• Renal tuberculosis
• Renal calculi
• Renal infarction
• Benign renal cyst

- Transitional cell carcinoma of the renal pelvis
- Wilms tumor
- Metastatic disease, especially melanoma

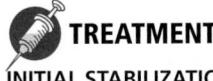

TREATMENT

INITIAL STABILIZATION
Inpatient

GENERAL MEASURES

Diet
Patients with proteinuria should follow a low-protein diet.

Activity
- No special preoperative limitations on activity.
- Postoperatively, activity as tolerated; resumption of full activity within 8 weeks

MEDICATION (DRUGS)

First Line
- For advanced renal cell carcinoma: Interleukin-2 and alpha-interferon result in 4% complete responders and 10–20% partial responders (1)[B]
- Metastatic RCC is typically refractory to standard cytotoxic chemotherapy regimens

Second Line
- Hormones-progesterone agents yield a 1–2% response rate
- Several molecular pathways involving vascular endothelial growth factor and platelet derived growth factor are implicated in RCC; small molecule inhibitors of the tyrosine kinase portion of vascular endothelial growth factor and polypeptide growth factor are under investigation (2)
- Phase I trials of IL-2/thalidomide combinations have shown 6% response (3)[C]

SURGERY
- Surgery is indicated. Cytotoxic drug therapy has been only erratically effective. Lesions are fairly resistant to radiation.
- Exploration wedge resection for solitary kidney or tumors <4 cm, otherwise radical nephrectomy in the face of a normal contralateral kidney is preferred.
- RCC (85% of renal parenchymal malignant tumors): CT solid mass >3 cm, radical nephrectomy if there is a normal contralateral kidney; <3 cm, wedge resection. Laparoscopic nephrectomy is still investigational.
- Angiomyolipoma (80% of tuberous sclerosis patients have these benign tumors): Classic CT findings; may be followed with serial CT
- Hemorrhage into a cyst: Aspiration cytology
- Complex cyst (calcified cyst wall or irregular wall): Open cyst wall biopsy if cytology is inconclusive
- Transitional cell carcinoma of the renal pelvis or calyces: Nephroureterectomy
- Oncocytoma: >3 cm, radical nephrectomy
- Sarcoma: Wide excision
- Wilms's tumor in adults: Radical nephrectomy for unilateral disease
- Cortical adenoma <3 cm (7–22% at autopsy): Wedge resection
- Surgical resection advised for pallation of solitary CNS metastases or for relief of spinal cord compression
- Image-guided radiofrequency ablation has been successful in limited studies for the treatment of small (average 2 cm) peripheral renal tumors (4)

FOLLOW-UP

COMPLICATIONS
- Paraplegia can result with little warning from spinal vertebral metastasis.
- Central nervous system metastases are not uncommon.
- ~30% of patients with RCC have metastatic disease when the diagnosis is established. The most common sites of metastasis are the lung (50–60%), bone (30–40%), regional nodes (15–30%), brain (10%), and adjacent organs (10%).

PATIENT MONITORING
- 1 CT scan of the abdomen and renal fossa can be done 3–6 months later, particularly if the capsule or lymph nodes are positive, to monitor recurrences and repeat resection if needed for flank pain or mass.
- For partial nephrectomy: Renal ultrasound every 6 months for 3 years, then annually.
- Chest x-rays to rule out pulmonary metastasis are performed quarterly for 2 years, then less often.
- Skeletal x-rays and bone scan can be useful in detecting skeletal metastasis but should only be obtained if patient complains of bone pain or if alkaline phosphatase is elevated.
- Postoperative follow up may be possible with plasma transcobalamin II or serum haptoglobin level to detect or monitor recurrences.

REFERENCES

1. Riglin RA. Renal cell carcinoma: Management of advanced disease. *J Urol*. 1999;16:381–387.
2. Rini BI. SU11248 and AG013736: Current data and future trials in renal cell carcinoma. *Clin Genitourin Cancer*. 2005;4(3):175–180.
3. Olencki T, et al. Phase I trial of thalidomide and Interleukin-2 in patients with metastatic renal cell carcinoma. *Invest New Drugs*. 2006;[Epub ahead of print].
4. Sabharwal R, Vladica P. Renal tumors: Technical success and early clinical experience with radiofrequency ablation of 18 tumors. *Cardiovasc Intervent Radiol*. 2006; [Epub ahead of print].
5. Resnick MY. *Current Therapy in Genitourinary Surgery*. 2nd ed. St. Louis, MO: Mosby-Year Book Publishers; 1992.
6. Franklin JR, Figlin R, Belldegrun A. Renal cell carcinoma: Basic biology and clinical behavior. *Semin Urol Oncol*. 1996;14:208–215, 230–243.
7. Brenner B, Rector F, eds. *Kidney*. 6th ed. Philadelphia, PA: W.B. Saunders; 2000.

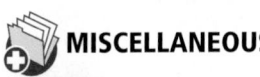

MISCELLANEOUS

CODES

ICD9-CM
189.0 Malignant neoplasm of kidney, except pelvis

PATIENT TEACHING
- Printed patient information available from: National Kidney & Urologic Diseases Information Clearinghouse, Box NKUDIC, Bethesda, MD 20893; (301) 468-6345.
- CancerNet (cancernet.nci.nih.gov).

See Corresponding Diagnostic Algorithm

RENAL FAILURE, ACUTE (ARF)

Eric Nelson, MD
Leonard G. Gomella, MD

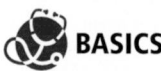 **BASICS**

DESCRIPTION
A syndrome of rapid reduction in renal function. May or may not be associated with oliguria; results in failure to excrete nitrogenous wastes and maintain normal volume and electrolyte homeostasis, with rising creatinine and blood urea nitrogen.

ALERT
Geriatric Considerations
- Elderly more susceptible to ARF (3.5 X more common); Creatinine clearance dependent on age
- 50% of ARF secondary to prerenal causes; 30% due to surgical complications
- Evolution to acute tubular necrosis more common

Pediatric Considerations
Congenital anomalies (e.g., nurethral valves, etc)

Pregnancy Considerations
- Infected uterus (e.g., Clostridium welchii clostridium perfringens)
- Toxemia and related obstetric complications
- Cortical necrosis
- Pregnant patients only group with a sharp drop in ARF mortality (1.7%)
- Intrinsic causes: Pre-eclampsia or eclampsia, ischemia, postpartum hemorrhage, abruptio placentae, amniotic fluid embolus, direct toxicity of illegal abortifacients, postpartum hemolytic uremic syndrome (HUS) or thrombotic thrombocytopenic purpose

GENERAL PREVENTION
- Early therapy and strict glycemic control shown to reduce mortality in the acutely ill patient
- Hydration beneficial, but optimum IV fluid choice controversial
- Minimize IV contrast toxicity: IV hydration, low osmolar agents, and oral N-acetylcysteine
- Minimize aminoglycoside toxicity: Single daily doses (effective as multiple doses), check levels
- Minimize chemotherapeutic toxicity, administer allopurinol prior

EPIDEMIOLOGY
- Predominant age: All ages (average age increasing)
- Predominant sex: Male = Female

Incidence
Five percent admitted to the hospital develop ARF; 10–15% of ICU patients; 2–7% open-heart patients develop ARF; 50% of hospital-acquired ARF is iatrogenic.

RISK FACTORS
- Advanced age
- Comorbid conditions (heart failure, liver or kidney failure, diabetes)
- Contrast exposure (dehydrated, diabetic)
- Nephrotoxic medications (aminoglycosides, NSAIDs, angiotensin converting enzyme inhibitors)
- Volume depletion (especially in diabetes)
- Rhabdomyolysis; surgery (cardiac surgery)

Genetics
No known genetic pattern

ETIOLOGY
- Prerenal (30–60% of all cases); potentially reversible (key point)
  - Volume depletion
    - Surgical: Hemorrhage, shock
    - Gastrointestinal (GI) losses: Vomiting, diarrhea, fistulas
    - Renal: Over-diuresis, salt-wasting disorders
  - Cardiac causes: Decrease in cardiac output:
    - Acute disorders: Myocardial infarction, arrhythmias, malignant hypertension, tamponade, endocarditis
    - Chronic disorders: Valvular diseases, chronic cardiomyopathy (ischemic heart disease hypertensive heart disease)
  - Redistribution of extracellular fluid
    - Hypoalbuminemic states: Nephritic syndrome, advanced liver disease, malnutrition
    - Physical cause: Peritonitis, burns, crush
    - Peripheral vasodilation: Sepsis, antihypertensive agents
    - Renal artery stenosis (bilateral)
- Postrenal (10% of all cases)
  - Ureteral obstruction: Bilateral or in a solitary kidney (calculi, neoplasm, clot, retroperitoneal fibrosis, iatrogenic)
  - Urethral obstruction: Prostatic hypertrophy, prostate cancer, prostatitis, clot, calculus, neoplasm, foreign object
  - Venous occlusion: Bilateral or a solitary kidney (renal vein thrombosis, neoplasm)
- Renal/Intrinsic causes
  - Glomerular and small vessel disease: Rapidly progressive glomerulonephritis (RPGN), subacute bacterial endocarditis, proliferative glomerulonephritis, vasculitides, progressive systemic sclerosis, malignant hypertension, HUS, cryoglobulinaemia, eclampsia, disseminated intravascular coagulation
  - Interstitial nephritis: Drug induced, infection, sarcoid, infiltrative
  - Tubular lesions: Post-ischemic, drugs pigment, light chain, hypercalcemia

ASSOCIATED CONDITIONS
- Hyperphosphatemia
- Hydronephrosis
- CHF, pericarditis
- Cirrhosis
- Malignant hypertension
- Vasculitis
- Bacterial infections
- Drug reactions
- Hypercalcemia, hyperuricemia
- Sepsis, severe trauma, burns
- Transfusion reactions
- Pericarditis
- Muscle injury, internal bleeding

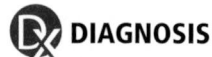 **DIAGNOSIS**

SIGNS AND SYMPTOMS
- General: Anorexia, fatigue, weakness, lethargy, somnolence
- Skin: Ecchymosis, petechiae, purpura (vasculitis), rash (acute interstitial nephritis)
- Cardiovascular: Dyspnea, edema, left ventricular failure, hypertension, tachycardia, tachypnea, pericarditis
- Respiratory: Hyperpnea, rales
- GI: Nausea, vomiting, diarrhea, GI hemorrhage
- Neurologic: Headache, coma, delirium, encephalopathy, seizures, asterixis, fasciculation, myoclonus
- Other: Back pain, muscle cramps, epistaxis, hiccups, oliguria, retinopathy, xerostomia, uriniferous odor

History
- Predisposing conditions (e.g., recent contrast administration, diabetes, malignancy)
- Medication history (NSAIDs, nephrotoxic antibiotics, chemotherapy)

Physical Exam
- Edema, rales, abdominal distension, palpable bladder
- Rectal exam (prostate consistency)

TESTS
Lab
- Creatinine (Cr) Clearance (Cl)
  - $CrCl = [140 - age]\,[kg]\,/[72]\,[Serum\ Cr]$
  - Decreasde clearance
  - Male < 97, Female < 88,
- Urinalysis: Proteinuria, hematuria,
- Urine sediment: Brown granular urinary casts, urinary renal tubular epithelial cells, coarse granular casts, renal tubular epithelial cells, eosinophils (acute interstitial nephritis) red cell or hemoglobin casts (RPGN), crystals (lithiasis, obstruction)
- Urine electrolytes/osmolality
  - Increased urine sodium (>20 mEq/L [>20 mmol/L]), increased fractional excretion of sodium (>3%) (e.g., renal). Fractional excretion of sodium = [(urine Na+/serum Na+)/(urine creatinine/serum Cr)] × 100
  - Urine isotonic to plasma
  - Low urine sodium <10 mEq/L (<10 mmol/L), low fractional excretion of sodium (≤1%), concentrate urine osmolality (≥500 mOsm/L) (e.g., prerenal)
- Other
  - Azotemia
  - Hyperphosphatemia
  - Hyperkalemia
  - Acidemia (increased anion gap), decreased serum bicarbonate
  - Decreased hemoglobin/hematocrit
  - Increased: Magnesium, uric acid, amylase, lipase
  - Hyponatremia
  - Hypocalcemia
  - Increased bleeding time

Imaging

- Ultrasound
  - Identifies kidney presence and size, hydronephrosis, nephrolithiasis
  - Doppler flow useful for renal artery stenosis and thrombosis
- Abdominal plain radiograph
  - Useful for identification of renal calculi
- Radionuclide renal scan
  - MAG3 more useful than dethylenetriainine tramine petaacetic acid in renal insufficiency
  - Evaluates both renal flow, renal function, and extravasation
- Angiography: Vascular disorders, including renal artery stenosis, systemic vasculitides
- MRI: An increase in T2-weighted signal may be seen in acute tubulointerstitial nephritis

Diagnostic Procedures/Surgery

- Cystoscopy with retrograde pyelogram—can be performed without worry of contrast toxicity; evaluates for obstruction and upper tract tumors/malformations
- Renal biopsy (ARF of unknown cause), diagnostic for SIN, rapidly progressive glomerulonephritis

Pathological Findings

Kidney biopsy

- Used when clinical, biochemical, and noninvasive imaging studies are insufficient for diagnosis
- Particularly useful for kidney transplant recipient or if clinical suspicion of rapidly progressive glomerulonephritis

DIFFERENTIAL DIAGNOSIS

See "Etiology."

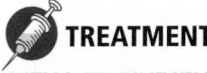 **TREATMENT**

INITIAL STABILIZATION

Inpatient and ICU

GENERAL MEASURES

- Prerenal: Restore BP and intravascular volume
- Postrenal: Urologic evaluation
- Intrinsic: Prevent hypotension and try to convert oliguira to nonoliguria; if edematous, try lasix; if nonedematous, try saline
- General
  - Discontinue/re-dose nephrotoxic drugs
  - Foley catheterization for accurate output
  - Daily weight, monitor BP, labs
  - Treat hyperkalemia
  - Hemodialysis: Refractory hyperkalemia, acidosis, mental status changes, electrolyte imbalances
  - Avoid peritoneal dialysis in acute setting
  - Hemofiltration for some critically ill patients
  - Correct easy bleeding with DDAVP, estrogen, and cryoprecipitate
  - Prednisone in acute interstitial nephritis may help
  - Decrease catabolism
  - Mannitol—alkaline diuresis in rhabdomyolysis
- Hyperkalemia: Severe (1 ampule Ca gluconate IV); other IV insulin + glucose, if acidosis also present (1 ampule NaHCO$_3$) Kayexalate PO 15–60 g/d if GI tract functions
- Mannitol: Alkaline diuresis in rhabdomyolysis

Diet

- Restrict fluids: Volume of urine output plus 500 mL/d
- Eliminate potassium if serum level increased

- Oral and IV amino acids
- Increase carbohydrates to decrease catabolism.
- Provide alimentation to decrease catabolism.

Activity

As tolerated

Nursing

Closely monitor weight, intake and output

SPECIAL THERAPY

IV Fluids

See "General Measures."

Complementary and Alternative Medicine

Many unregulated agents can be nephrotoxic ("Chinese herbal remedies")

 MEDICATION (DRUGS)

First Line

- Prior to fixed renal failure: IV expansion with normal saline followed by mannitol, and calcium channel blockers. Low-dose dopamine: No effect on survival. Volume expansion alone is beneficial in contrast injury.
- Precautions: All drugs used should be reviewed for appropriate adjustment.
- Potential interactions: Nonsteroidals plus other nephrotoxic drugs, male gender, increasing age, cardiovascular comorbidity, and recent hospitalization are synergistic in causing ARF.

SURGERY

- Relief of obstruction with retrograde ureteral catheters or percutaneous nephrostomy
- Hemodialysis acess

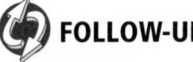 **FOLLOW-UP**

DISPOSITION

Admission Criteria

All patients with acute renal failure require urgent admission

Discharge Criteria

Stabilization of renal function and medical management while awaiting resolution

Issues for Referral

- Nephrology consultation: All cases
- Urology: Urinary obstruction

PROGNOSIS

- Potentially high mortality (5–80%) depending on cause, multi-organ involvement, and age
- Recovery in days to 6 weeks
- Good recovery expected in prerenal and postrenal failure, especially if dysfunction of short duration. Expect possible longer recovery if intrinsic etiology

COMPLICATIONS

- Death (50%)
- Sepsis infection (leading cause of mortality)
- Convulsions, paralysis
- Edema, pulmonary edema, CHF
- Hyperkalemia, uremia
- Arrhythmias, pericarditis/tamponade
- Bleeding, hypotension

PATIENT MONITORING

As needed

REFERENCES

1. Dagher PC. Newly developed techniques to study and diagnose acute renal failure. *J Am Soc Nephrol*. 2003;14:2188–2198.
2. Dudley C. Maximizing renal preservation in acute renal failure. *BJU International*. 2004;94:1202–1206.
3. Richie JP: In: Walsh PC, et al, eds. *Campbell's Urology* 2002:Philadelphia, PA: W.B. Saunders Co.
4. Venkatataraman R. Prevention of acute renal failure. *Critical Care Clinics*. 2005;21:281–289.

 MISCELLANEOUS

See also: Hepatorenal Syndrome; Hydronephrosis; Multiple Myeloma; Renal Failure, Chronic; Reye Syndrome; Rhabdomyolysis; Rocky Mountain Spotted Fever

CODES

ICD9-CM

584.9 Acute renal failure unspecified

PATIENT TEACHING

- http://www.nlm.nih.gov/medlineplus (sponsored Web site)
- National Kidney & Urologic Diseases Information Clearinghouse, Box NKUDIC, Bethesda, MD 20893; (301) 468-6345
- The National Kidney Foundation, Inc., 30 East 33rd Street, NY, NY 10016. "What Everyone Should Know About Kidneys and Kidney Disease" (Order #01-01BP - English), (Order #01-02BP -Spanish).
- Diet based on etiology
- Proper management of medication and glycemic control in diabetes mellitus

 See Corresponding Diagnostic Algorithm

 See Patient Handout on CD

RENAL FAILURE, CHRONIC

Atizazul Hassan Mansoor, MD

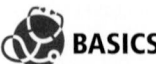 **BASICS**

DESCRIPTION
- Kidney damage >3 months as evident by structural or chemistry (blood/urine) abnormalities with or without a decreased glomorular filtration rate (GFR) *or* a decreased GFR of ≤60 mL/min/1.73 m² regardless of kidney damage (1)
- Classified into 5 stages by GFR (1)
  - Stage 1: Kidney damage with GFR >90 mL/min/1.73 m²
  - Stage 2: Kidney damage with GFR 60–89 mL/min/1.73 m²
  - Stage 3: GFR 30–59 mL/min/1.73 m²
  - Stage 4: GFR 15–29 mL/min/1.73 m²
  - Stage 5: GFR <15 mL/min/1.73 m² or dialysis
- System(s) Affected: Renal/Urinary; Cardiovascular; Skeletal; Endocrine; Metabolic; Hematologic; Lymphatic; Immune; Neurologic
- Synonym(s): Chronic kidney disease (CKD); Chronic renal insufficiency; End-stage renal disease (ESRD, Stage 5 CKD).

ALERT
Geriatric Considerations
- GFR normally decreases with age
  - Adjust renally cleared drugs for GFR
  - Use nephrotoxic agents with caution.
- Rule out such potentially reversible causes as urinary tract obstruction (particularly in men), renal arterial occlusion, hypercalcemia, use of nephrotoxic agents

Pediatric Considerations
Main causes in children include congenital renal and urinary tract malformations (signs appear <5 years of age), glomerular and hereditary renal diseases (appears between ages 5 and 15).

Pregnancy Considerations
Avoid angiotensin converting enzyme (ACE) Inhibitors and angiotensin receptor blockers (ARBs)—fetotoxic, teratogenic. Use other diuretics with caution.

GENERAL PREVENTION
- Limit nephrotoxic agents when possible (e.g., iodinated contrast; NSAIDs).
- Treat all disorders known to lead to/exacerbate CKD such as diabetes mellitus, high BP (HTN), or hyperlipidemia. (1,2)[A]
- In CKD, renally cleared drugs require dosage reduction to prevent toxicity.
- Avoid volume depletion.

EPIDEMIOLOGY
- Predominant age: All ages—more common in adults; increasing prevalence and incidence in the elderly
- Predominant sex: Male > Female (3)

Incidence
In 2003, 102,567 new patients initiated ESRD—an adjusted rate of 337.6/million. (3)
- African Americans had an adjusted rate for ESRD 2.95 times greater; 995.7 million; Native Americans and Latinos with high rates. (3)

Prevalence
- As of December 2003, a total of 452,957 patients with ESRD—an adjusted rate of 1496.2/million (3)
  - African Americans had an adjusted rate 3.15 times greater at 4712.3/mill; Native Americans and Latinos also had higher rates (3)
- Majority of people with CKD in stages 1–3 (1)

RISK FACTORS (1,4)
- Diabetes mellitus (common)
- HTN (common)
- Urinary tract obstruction (e.g., benign prostatic hyperslasia)
- Autoimmune disease/vasculitidies
- Urinary tract infections
- Family history
- Acute renal failure
- NSAID use
- IV contrast
- Smoking
- Increasing proteinuria correlates with faster progression of CKD

Genetics
- See "Incidence" and "Prevalence."
- Alport syndrome, Fabry disease, sickle cell anemia, and autosomal dominant polycystic kidney disease can lead to CKD. (4)

ETIOLOGY (4)
- Renal parenchymal/glomerular: Infections, toxins, autoimmune, neoplasia
  - Nephritic: Characterized by RBCs in urine
    ○ Membranoproliferative Glomerulonephritis; proliferative glomerulonephritis; crescentic glomerulonephritis.
  - Nephrotic: Characterized by proteinuria.
    ○ Minimal change disease, membranous nephropathy, focal segmental glomerulosclerosis
  - Mixed/Other: Diabetes mellitus (DM), amyloidosis, alport syndrome, connective tissue disease
- Vascular: HTN, thrombotic microangiopathies, vasculitidies
- Interstitial-tubular: Infections, obstruction, toxins, multiple myeloma, connective tissue disease, cystic disease, congenital
- Prerenal: Renal artery stenosis, cardiac compromise, hypotension, decreased effective volume, NSAIDs, contrast, shock
- Postrenal: Obstruction, see "Hydronephrosis"

ASSOCIATED CONDITIONS
See "Risk Factors" and "Genetics."

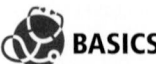 **DIAGNOSIS**

SIGNS AND SYMPTOMS (2)
- Oliguria; nocturia; polyuria
- Volume overload
- Hypertension
- Anemia (normochromic, normocytic)
- Hyperkalemia, hyperphosphatemia, hypocalcemia
- Bone disease, fatigue, depression
- Metabolic acidosis, pruritis
- Metallic taste in mouth, uremia (late)
  - Anorexia, nausea, vomiting, percarditis
  - CNS abnormalities (confusion, seizures, coma), neuropathy

History
Check for symptoms as in "Signs and Symptoms" and thorough review of system for renal/urinary, cardiovascular, and endocrine.

Physical Exam
Complete plus ophthalmic exam; assess volume status (e.g., BP with orthostatics; edema).

TESTS
Lab
- Calculate glomerular filtration rate (GFR) using one of available equations (e.g., Modification of diet in renal disease)—should use measurements from same laboratory for consistency (1)[A]
  - Pediatrics has its own set of equations. (5)
- Analyze urine
  - Electrolytes
  - Proteinuria/Albuminuria—dipstick (need special dipstick to detect albumin); quantitate positive result with a spot protein (or albumin) to creatinine ratio (a.m. sample better) (1)[A]
    ○ Monitor albumin in adults (1)[A]
    ○ Monitor total protein in children without diabetes (5)[A]
  - Urine analysis (WBCs, RBCs, casts) (1,5)[A]
- Blood (1)[A]
  - Normochromic, normocytic anemia
  - Thrombocytopenia
  - Increased bleeding time
- Chemistry (1)[A]
  - Elevated urea blood urea nitrogen (BUN)
  - Elevated ammonia
  - Increased parathyroid hormone
  - Decreased active vitamin D
  - Reduced calcium
  - Elevated phosphate
  - Elevated potassium
  - Hyperlipidemia
  - Elevated glucose; insulin resistance
- Drugs that may alter lab results (1)[C]
  - Cimetidine: Inhibits Cr secretion
  - Trimethoprim: Inhibits Cr secretion
  - Check for other medication interactions

Imaging
- Ultrasound: Decreased kidney size; signs of obstruction (e.g., hydronephrosis); cysts (1)[C]
- Doppler ultrasound to asses for thrombosis (1)[C]
- CT scan (non-contrast): Obstruction; calculi; cysts; neoplasm; rheumatoid arthritis stenosis (1)[C]
- MRI/magnetic resonance angiography for greater resolution.
- HIV and diabetic nephropathy may demonstrate normal-enlarged kidneys.

Diagnostic Procedures/Surgery
- Renal biopsy—if changes treatment plan (1)[C]
- Antinuclear antibody
- HIV testing

DIFFERENTIAL DIAGNOSIS
See "Etiology."

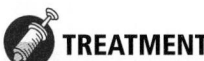 TREATMENT

GENERAL MEASURES
- Main goal is to slow progression.
- See "General Prevention" (1)[A]
  - If contrast needed, can try to limit damage with hydration; *N*-acetylcysteine use controversial (6)[A]
  - Treat anemia, see "Medications"
- Strict glycemic control in diabetics: Goal of HgA$_{1C}$ <7% (1,2)[A]
- HTN control: If proteinuria >1 g/d, goal <125/75; if less than 1 g/d, <130/80 (1,7)[A]
  - Use ACE inhibitors to slow progression, especially DM patients (1,7)[A]
  - Can tolerate up to 35% rise in serum Cr unless hyperkalemia develops (7)[A].
- Renal replacement: Prepare for dialysis or transplant for GFR <30 mL/min/1.73 m^2 (1)[A]
- Vaccines: Pneumococcal; influenza (8)[A]
- Treat dyslipidemia (goal LDL <100)
- Smoking cessation

Diet
- Nutrition consult for CKD diet (1)[C]
  - For GFR <60 mL/min/1.73 m^2 assess protein and energy intake; important to maintain adequate nutrition (1)[A]
  - Restricted intake of phosphates (1,2)[C]
  - Sodium restriction (2)[A]
  - Potassium restriction if hyperkalemic (2)[A]
- Restricted protein (1)[B]: Opinions differ.
- Water intake limited to maintain serum sodium concentration of 135–145 mEq/L

Activity
Restricted only by patient's condition

 MEDICATION (DRUGS)

First Line
- ACE-inhibitors for HTN control and decreased progression of proteinuria (e.g., CKD) (1)[A]
  - Potential for hyperkalemia
  - If goal not reached, add diuretic, followed by diltiazem or verapamil or a beta blocker. If goal still not reached, use ARB (2)[A]
- Non-aluminum, non-Mg, calcium-based phosphate binder with meals (2)[A]
- Oral calcium carbonate (without food) and Calcitriol to suppress parathyroid hormone (2)[A]
- Erythropoietin for anemia, ~10,000 units SC once weekly (2)[A]
  - Indication Hb <12.5 g/dL and no cause (1)[A]
- Statins for hyperlipidemia (2)[A]
- Uremic bleeding: Correct platelets preprocedures, correct anemia as above, may use desmopressin (dDAVP) (2)[B].

- Precautions
  - Monitor serum electrolytes carefully.
  - Monitor loop diuretic to avoid volume depletion.
  - Adjust all renally excreted medications.
- For contraindications/significant possible interactions: Refer to the manufacturers' literature.

Second Line
Renagel topically for phosphate control (2)[A]

SURGERY
Transplantation for ESRD

 FOLLOW-UP

DISPOSITION
Admission Criteria
- Acute decline evident by rise in serum Cr/BUN.

- Dialysis criteria (2)[B]
  - Indications include pericarditis, fluid overload unresponsive to diuretics, accelerated, unresponsive HTN; serum Cr >12 mg/dL or BUN >100 mg/dL.

  - May need to intervene earlier with peritoneal dialysis if GFR <10 mL/min/1.73 m^2 or evidence of malnutrition. (2)[C]
  - Need to anticipate (2)
    ○ Atro-ventricular fistulas can take up to 1 year to mature.
    ○ Peritoneal access can be used immediately.

Issues for Referral
Nephrology early (Cr >1.2) (1,2)[C]

PROGNOSIS
- Greatest morbidity is from cardiovascular disease (CVD) (1,2)
- Risk of death, especially from CVD, is greater than risk of progressing to dialysis (2)

COMPLICATIONS
- See "Signs and Symptoms."
- Dyslipidemia (common) (1,2,4)
- Infections (1,4)
- Malnutrition (1,2,4)
- Serositis
- Increased magnesium (2)
- Platelet dysfunction, bleeding (2)
- Pseudogout, gout
- Hypothyroidism (2)
- Metabolic calcification (4)
- Sexual dysfunction (2)
- Fractures

PATIENT MONITORING
- Monitor GFR yearly.
- Blood and urine chemistries and clinical status
- BP, volume monitored frequently

REFERENCES
1. National Kidney Foundation. K/DOQI clinical practice guidelines for chronic kidney disease: Evaluation, classification, and stratification. *Am J Kidney Dis*. 2002;39:S1.
2. Post T, Rose B. Overview of the management of chronic kidney disease in adults. *UpToDate*. 2006. www.UpToDate.com
3. U.S. Renal Data System, USRDS 2005 Annual Data Report: Atlas of End-Stage Renal Disease in the United States, National Institutes of Health, National Institute of Diabetes and Digestive and Kidney Diseases, Bethesda, MD, 2005.
4. Brenner B, *The Kidney*, 7th ed. Saunders. 2004.
5. Hogg RJ, Furth S, Lemley K, et al. National Kidney Foundation's kidney disease outcomes quality initiative for chronic kidney disease. *Pediatric*. 2003;111(6):1416–1421.
6. Barrett B, Parfrey P. Preventing nephropathy by contrast medium. *N Engl J Med*. 2006;354:379–86.
7. Chobanian A, et al. The seventh report of the Joint National Committee on Prevention, Detection, Evaluation, and Treatment of High Blood Pressure. *JAMA*. 2003;289(19):2560–2572.
8. Dinits-Pensy M, et al. The use of vaccines in adult patients with renal disease. *Am J Kidney Dis*. 2005;6(6):997–1011.

 MISCELLANEOUS

See also: Proteinuria; Hydronephrosis; Nephrotic Syndrome; Polycystic Kidney Disease; Renal Failure, Acute (ARF); HTN

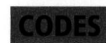 CODES

ICD9-CM
- 585 Chronic Kidney Disease
- www.kidney.org/professionals/tools

PATIENT TEACHING
- National Kidney Federation (NKF) patient Web site: www.kidney.org/patients
- Can order material from NKF: www.kidney.org/professionals/kdoqi/materials.cfm

 See Corresponding Diagnostic Algorithm

 See Patient Handout on CD

RENAL TUBULAR ACIDOSIS

Richard F. Salmon, DO
David E. Hall, MD

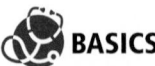 **BASICS**

DESCRIPTION

A group of disorders characterized by an abnormality of renal tubular acidification, which results in hyperchloremic acidosis and a normal anion gap. Several types have been identified

- Classic distal renal tubular acidosis (Type I): Usually secondary to impaired ability to secrete hydrogen ions into the distal tubule or collecting duct. Urine pH >5.5.
- Proximal renal tubular acidosis (Type II): Due to impaired bicarbonate reabsorption in the proximal tubule. Bicarbonate spills into the urine at lower than normal plasma bicarbonate concentrations. If the plasma bicarbonate level is low enough (typically between 15 and 18), the urine may be acidified (pH <5.5), in contrast to type I.
- Type III: No longer considered a distinct entity
- Distal hyperkalemic renal tubular acidosis (Type IV): Several subtypes are recognized, but all are characterized by aldosterone resistance or deficiency. This leads to hyperkalemia (not seen in Types I or II) along with acidosis. The urine pH may be <5.5.
- System(s) Affected: Endocrine/Metabolic; Renal/Urologic

GENERAL PREVENTION

Careful use or avoidance of agents listed as causative here

EPIDEMIOLOGY

- Predominant age: All ages
- Predominant sex: Male >Female (with regard to type II renal tubular acidosis with isolated defect in bicarbonate reabsorption)

RISK FACTORS

Genetics

- Type I renal tubular acidosis: Autosomal dominant or recessive. May occur in association with other genetic diseases (e.g., Ehlers-Danlos syndrome, hereditary elliptocytosis, or sickle cell nephropathy). The autosomal recessive form is associated with sensorineural deafness.
- Type II renal tubular acidosis: Autosomal dominant form is rare. Autosomal recessive form is associated with ophthalmologic abnormalities and mental retardation. Occurs in Fanconi syndrome, which is associated with several genetic diseases (e.g., cystinosis, Wilson disease, tyrosinemia, hereditary fructose intolerance, Lowe syndrome, galactosemia, glycogen storage disease, metachromatic leukodystrophy).
- Type IV renal tubular acidosis: Some cases familial, such as pseudohypoaldosteronism Type I (autosomal dominant)

ETIOLOGY

- Type I
  - Genetic: Autosomal dominant
  - Genetic: Autosomal recessive associated with sensorineural deafness
  - Sporadic
  - Ehlers-Danlos syndrome
  - Hematologic diseases: Sickle cell disease, hereditary elliptocytosis
  - Hypercalciuria
  - Vitamin D intoxication
  - Medullary cystic disease
  - Glycogenosis Type III
  - Autoimmune disease
  - Diseases causing nephrocalcinosis
  - Fabry disease
  - Wilson disease
  - Drug induced (amphotericin B, lithium, analgesics)
  - Toxin induced (toluene, glue)
  - Hypergammaglobulinemic syndrome
  - Obstructive uropathy
  - Chronic pyelonephritis
  - Chronic renal transplantation rejection
  - Leprosy
  - Hepatic cirrhosis
  - Malnutrition
- Type II
  - Diseases associated with Fanconi syndrome (see Genetics)
  - Sporadic
  - Multiple myeloma and other dysproteinemic states
  - Heavy metal poisoning (cadmium, lead, mercury)
  - Medications: Acetazolamide, sulfanilamide, ifosfamide, outdated tetracycline, topamax^{-4} [C]
  - Autoimmune disease
  - Amyloidosis
  - Interstitial renal disease
  - Nephrotic syndrome
  - Congenital heart disease
  - Defects in calcium metabolism (hyperparathyroidism)
- Type IV
  - Lupus nephropathy
  - Diabetic nephropathy
  - Obstructive nephropathy
  - Nephrosclerosis due to hypertension
  - Tubulointerstitial nephropathies
  - Addison disease
  - Acute adrenal insufficiency
  - Pseudohypoaldosteronism (end-organ resistance to aldosterone)
  - Gordon syndrome (2)[C]
  - Sickle cell nephropathy

ASSOCIATED CONDITIONS

- Type I in children: Hypercalciuria leading to rickets, nephrocalcinosis
- Type I in adults: Autoimmune diseases such as Sjögren disease
- Type II: Fanconi syndrome: A generalized tubular defect with bicarbonaturia, aminoaciduria, glycosuria, phosphaturia
- Type IV: Obstructive uropathy, renal insufficiency, diabetic nephropathy

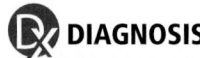 **DIAGNOSIS**

SIGNS AND SYMPTOMS

- Failure to thrive in children
- Anorexia, nausea
- Vomiting
- Weakness due to potassium loss
- Polyuria due to potassium loss
- Rickets in children
- Osteomalacia in adults
- Constipation
- Polydipsia

TESTS

Lab

- Electrolytes reveal hyperchloremic metabolic acidosis
- Plasma anion gap normal (anion gap = plasma Na−(Cl+CO2)). Normal values: Neonates <18; infants and children <16; adolescents and adults <14.
- Hypokalemia or normokalemia
  - Type I
  - Type II
- Hyperkalemia: Type IV
- Blood urea nitrogen and creatinine usually normal (rules out renal failure as cause of acidosis)
- Urine pH: Not acidified (pH >5.5) despite metabolic acidosis in type I
- Urine culture: Rule out urinary tract infection (UTI) with urea splitting organism (may elevate pH) and chronic infection
- Urine anion gap, an estimate of urine ammonium excretion (urine Na+K−Cl on random urine). Measure before treatment. Most useful if measured when patient is acidotic. Results tend to be
  - Negative in bicarbonate losses secondary to diarrhea
  - Negative in UTI due to urea splitting organism
  - Positive in Type I
  - Positive in Type IV (5)[C]
- Urine calcium
  - Typically normal in Type II
  - High in Type I
- Drugs that may alter lab results
  - Diuretics
  - Sodium bicarbonate
  - Cholestyramine

Imaging

Not needed except to rule out underlying conditions (e.g., nephrocalcinosis, complications)

Diagnostic Procedures/Surgery

- May be helpful to measure urine pH on fresh specimens with pH meter for increased accuracy instead of dipstick. Place oil over urine to avoid loss of carbon dioxide if pH cannot be measured quickly.
- Urine ammonium excretion (anion gap is indirect measurement of this, but is not as accurate)
- Ammonium chloride (NH4+) loading to evaluate acid excretion
- Bicarbonate titration curves

Pathological Findings
- Nephrocalcinosis
- Nephrolithiasis
- Rickets
- Osteomalacia
- Findings of an underlying disease causing renal tubular acidosis

DIFFERENTIAL DIAGNOSIS
- Anion gap should be normal. If not, look for causes of metabolic acidosis other than renal tubular acidosis. (MUDPILES: Metabolic disease or methanol ingestion, Uremia, Diabetic ketoacidosis, Paraldehyde ingestion, Iron or isoniazid ingestion, Lactic acidosis, Ethylene glycol ingestion, Salicylate ingestion)
- Diarrhea with bicarbonate loss in stools
- Acidosis of chronic renal failure
- Urinary diversion (e.g., ureterosigmoidostomy, ileal conduit)
- Ingestion of hydrochloric acid, ammonium chloride, lysine hydrogen chloride, excess calcium, or magnesium chloride
- Small bowel, pancreatic, or biliary fistulae (5)[C]

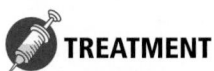

TREATMENT

INITIAL STABILIZATION
- Outpatient generally
- Inpatient if acidosis severe, patient unreliable, emesis persistent, infant with severe failure to thrive

GENERAL MEASURES
Treatment with appropriate medications to correct acidosis

Diet
Varies with type of acidosis

Activity
As tolerated

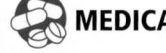

MEDICATION (DRUGS)

First Line
Provide oral alkali to raise serum bicarbonate to normal. Start at a low dose and increase until serum bicarbonate is normal. Give as sodium bicarbonate or citrate mixtures (1 mEq citrate = 1 mEq HCO3) such as Bicitra (1 mEq Na, 1 mEq citrate/mL, no K) or polycitra (1 mEq Na, 1 mEq K, 2 mEq citrate/mL) depending on need for potassium. Sodium bicarbonate tablets are available (7.7 mEq HCO3/tab). (1)[C]
- Type I: Typical doses 1–4 mEq/kg/d PO alkali divided t.i.d. or q.i.d., unless bicarbonate wasting present, in which case much larger doses required. May require potassium supplementation if serum potassium low. (3)[C]
- Type II: Typical doses 5–10 mEq/kg/d alkali. May be difficult to control and require 4–6 doses/d. May require potassium supplementation if serum potassium low.
- Type IV: 1–5 mEq/kg/d alkali b.i.d. or t.i.d. Avoid potassium. In some cases, furosemide used to lower potassium levels, but avoid if patient wastes salt. Fludrocortisone: 0.1–0.3 mg/d, if mineralocorticoid deficient.

- Contraindications: Refer to the manufacturer's literature.
- Precautions: Sodium bicarbonate may cause flatulence as carbon dioxide is formed, whereas citrate mixtures are metabolized to bicarbonate in the liver, thereby avoiding gas production.

Second Line
Hydrochlorothiazide: Use as an adjunct in Type II after maximal alkali replacement, but it may exacerbate already existing kaliuresis

SURGERY
If distal renal tubular acidosis is due to obstructive uropathy, surgical intervention may be required.

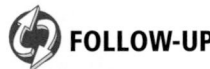

FOLLOW-UP

PROGNOSIS
- Depends on associated disease, otherwise good with therapy
- Transient forms of all types of renal tubular acidosis may occur.

COMPLICATIONS
- Nephrocalcinosis
- Hyperkalemia or hypokalemia
- Nephrolithiasis
- Rickets
- Osteomalacia
- Hypercalciuria

PATIENT MONITORING
- Varies with patient response. Suggested: Electrolytes every 2–4 weeks at onset of therapy, every 2 weeks for 1–2 months after bicarbonate concentration normal, then monthly for several months
- Monitor underlying disease as indicated.
- Poor compliance common due to t.i.d. or q.i.d. alkali dosing schedule

REFERENCES
1. Chan JC, Scheinman JI, Roth KD. Consultation with the specialist: Renal tubular acidosis. *Ped in Review*. 2001;22(8):277–287.
2. Rodriguez-Soriano J. New insights into the pathogenesis of renal tubular acidosis: From functional to molecular studies. *Pediatr Nephrol*. 2000;14:1121–1136.
3. Domrongkitchaiporn S, et al. Dosage of potassium citrate in the correction of urinary abnormalitites in pediatric distal renal tubular acidosis patients. *Am J Kidney Dis*. 2002;39(2):383–391.
4. Izzedine H, Launay-Vacher V, Deray G. Topiramate-induced renal tubular acidosis. *Am J Med*. 2004;116(4):281–282.
5. Casaletto J. Differential diagnosis of metabolic acidosis. *Emer Med Clin N Am*. 2005;23(3):771–87.

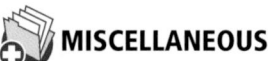

MISCELLANEOUS

See also: Hyperkalemia

CODES

ICD9-CM
- 270.0 Disturbances of amino acid transport
- 588.8 Other specified disorder resulting from impaired renal function

PATIENT TEACHING
- National Kidney & Urologic Diseases Information Clearinghouse, Box NKUDIC, Bethesda, MD 20893; (301) 468-6345; http://www.niddk.nih.gov/health/kidney/.
- National Kidney Foundation: http://www.kidney.org.

 See Corresponding Diagnostic Algorithm

RESPIRATORY DISTRESS SYNDROME, ACUTE

Kurt J. Wegner, MD

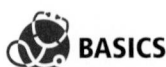 **BASICS**

DESCRIPTION

Acute respiratory distress syndrome is defined as the abrupt onset of respiratory distress accompanied by 3 components: Severe hypoxemia, bilateral pulmonary infiltrates on chest radiograph, and absence of clear evidence of heart failure or volume overload. Disease severity ranges from acute lung injury to full-blown adult respiratory distress syndrome. In addition, it is often progressive.

- System(s) Affected: Pulmonary; Cardiovascular
- Synonym(s): Shock lung, Wet lung, Noncardiac pulmonary edema

ALERT

Geriatric Considerations
Disease-related mortality increases directly with age.

EPIDEMIOLOGY
- Predominant age: Affects all ages
- Predominant sex: Male = Female

Prevalence
- Estimates range from 1.5–75 cases/100,000 population
- Pregnancy estimates are 16–70 cases/100,000 pregnancies

RISK FACTORS
- Severe infection (localized or systemic) accounts for 50% cases
- Multiple predisposing disorders increases risk
- Long-term alcohol abuse
- Chronic lung disease
- Low serum pH

Genetics
Flores and Pavlovic suggest that pulmonary surfactant and its components may provide markers to identify full-blown adult respiratory distress syndrome subgroups and provide a basis for identifying at-risk groups and for studying potential treatments

ETIOLOGY
- Recent studies have revealed that several mediators are involved in the initiation and perpetuation of adult respiratory distress syndrome
  - Cytokines (e.g., tumor necrosis factor, interleukin 1, interleukin 6)
  - Complement activation
  - Coagulation activation
  - Platelet-activating factor
  - Oxygen radicals
  - Lipoxygenase pathways (e.g., leukotrienes C4, D4, and E4)
  - Neutrophil proteases
  - Nitric oxide: May be deleterious or advantageous
  - Endotoxin
  - Cyclooxygenase pathway products (e.g., thromboxane A2, prostacyclin)
- Systemic inflammatory response with activation of the previous mediators can occur with direct or indirect injury to the lung
  - Direct
  - Aspiration
  - Pulmonary infections (e.g., bacterial, fungal, viral, and protozoan)
  - Air, fat, or amniotic fluid emboli (e.g., long bone fractures)
  - Near-drowning
  - Pulmonary contusion

- Inhalation of toxic gases (e.g., oxygen, smoke, NH_3, chlorine, plastics, phosgene, cadmium)
- Indirect
  - Sepsis (e.g., Gram-negative and Gram-positive organisms, fungi, tuberculous, pneumocystis pneumonia)
  - Shock (e.g., hemorrhagic, cardiogenic, septic, anaphylactic)
  - Transfusions
  - Trauma (e.g., head injury, burns)
  - Overdose
  - Pancreatitis, severe
  - Eclampsia
  - Carcinomatosis
  - Leukoagglutinin reaction

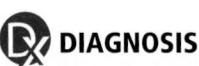 **DIAGNOSIS**

SIGNS AND SYMPTOMS
- Most patients demonstrate similar clinical and pathologic features regardless of the cause of the acute lung injury. There are 3 phases
  - Acute exudative phase characterized by profound hypoxia and associated with inflammation with infiltration of inflammatory and proinflammatory mediators and diffuse alveolar damage.
  - Fibrosing alveolitis phase coincides with recovery or after ~1–2 weeks. Patients continue to be hypoxic and have increased dead space and decreased compliance.
  - Resolution may require 6–12 months. Residual respiratory concerns are outlined after in Prognosis.
- Signs and symptoms
  - Tachypnea and tachycardia during the 1st 12–24 hours
  - Moist and cyanotic skin
  - Breathing difficulty with intercostal and accessory respiratory muscles
  - Dramatic increase in work of breathing
  - High-pitched end-expiratory crackles are heard throughout all lung fields
  - Increased agitation
  - Lethargy, then obtundation
  - Hypoxemia may be present long before clinical signs

TESTS
Lab
- Acute lung injury: $PaO_2/FiO_2 \leq 300$
- Adult respiratory distress syndrome: $PaO_2/FiO_2 \leq 200$
- Disorders that may alter lab results
  - Multiple pulmonary embli
  - Cardiogenic pulmonary edema
  - Severe chronic obstructive pulmonary disease
  - Severe pneumonia

Imaging
- Chest x-ray: Linear opacities, consistent with evolving fibrosis
- Chest CT: Diffuse interstitial opacities and bullae

Diagnostic Procedures/Surgery
- Invasive monitoring of vital signs, cardiac output, and pulmonary arterial wedge pressure
- Arterial blood gases
- Pulmonary artery catheterization to demonstrate
  - Normal pulmonary arterial occlusion pressure
  - NOTE: The main point of this study is to determine whether the pulmonary arterial occlusion pressure (PAOP) is inconsistent with cardiogenic pulmonary edema. A low PAOP with low serum albumin may lead to cardiogenic etiology. The patient with chronic congestive heart failure may have a high wedge, but still develop adult respiratory distress syndrome.

Pathological Findings
- Lungs show exudative, early proliferative, or late proliferative phases
- Interstitial and alveolar edema
- Inflammatory cells and erythrocytes spill into interstitium and the alveolus.
- Type I cells are destroyed, leaving a denuded basement membrane.
- Protein-rich fluid fills the alveoli.
- Type II alveolar cells initially appear unaltered.
- Type II cells begin to proliferate within 72 hours of initial insult.
- Type II cells cover the denuded basement membrane.
- Aggregates of plasma proteins, cellular debris, fibrin, and surfactant remnants form hyaline membranes.
- Over next 3–10 days, alveolar septum thickens by proliferating fibroblasts, leukocytes, and plasma cells.
- Capillary injury begins to occur
- Hyaline membranes begin to reorganize
- Fibrosis becomes apparent in respiratory ducts and bronchioles.

DIFFERENTIAL DIAGNOSIS
Cardiogenic pulmonary edema

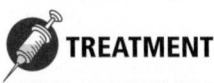 **TREATMENT**

INITIAL STABILIZATION
ICU

GENERAL MEASURES
- Treat underlying etiology (e.g., sepsis, pneumonia, shock) as appropriate
- Prevent complications (e.g., gastrointestinal bleeding, nosocomial infections, thromboembolus)
- Corticosteroids have not been shown to add benefit during the acute phase, but they may have value in patients with established full-blown adult respiratory distress syndrome.
- Support ventilation using lung protection strategies (e.g., low tidal volume and positive end-expiratory pressure).
- Consider paralyzing agents (to improve compliance and decrease barotrauma) if patient is fighting ventilator. Initiate anxiolytics when instituting treatment with paralytic agents.
- Maintain oxygen delivery and avoid supranormal oxygen delivery.

- Recruitment maneuvers may be helpful
  - High-level continuous positive end-expiratory pressure (PEEP).
  - Intermittent sighs
  - Intermittent and stepwise high PEEP and fixed pressure control maneuver
  - Prone positioning
- Measure cardiac output (CO) with each PEEP change. If CO decreases, give fluids to regain adequate CO and allow additional PEEP adjustments if necessary. A pulmonary artery catheter may be helpful in assessing left ventricular function, CO, oxygen delivery and consumption. It is necessary if high levels of PEEP are used.
- Fluid and hemodynamic management
  - Maintain intravascular volume at lowest level consistent with adequate perfusion (assessed by metabolic acid-base balance and renal function)
  - If perfusion is inadequate after restoration of intravascular volume (e.g., septic shock), vasopressor therapy is indicated.
  - Increase oxygen content with packed erythrocyte transfusions as necessary.
- Provide appropriate nutritional support.
- Extraordinary management
  - Extracorporeal membrane oxygenation
  - High-frequency ventilation
  - Pressure controlled inverse ratio ventilation
  - Extracorporeal CO_2 removal with low-frequency ventilation

Diet
Nutritional support

Activity
Bed rest

 MEDICATION (DRUGS)

First Line
No single or combination of drugs prevents or treats full-blown adult respiratory distress syndrome. Treatment is supportive while addressing the underlying cause.

- Inotropic agents: Dobutamine to maintain adequate cardiac output after appropriate fluid resuscitation fails to restore perfusion.
- Vasodilators: Nitroprusside, angiotensin-converting enzyme inhibitors, hydralazine (only if blood pressure adequate.)
- Anxiolytics (e.g., lorazepam)
- Deep vein thrombosis prophylaxis
- Ulcer prophylaxis
- Inhaled or systemic beta-agonists may be helpful during the resolution phase.
- Contraindications: See the manufacturer's profile of each drug.
- Precautions: See the manufacturer's profile of each drug.
- Significant possible interactions: See the manufacturer's profile of each drug.

Second Line
- Corticosteroids: Short-term use during the acute phase has not been shown to be effective. However, data suggest that sustained therapy in patients with established full-blown adult respiratory distress syndrome may be beneficial; therefore, a short course of high-dose glucocorticoids could be considered in a patient with severe, refractory disease.
- Atrial natriuretic polypeptide: Control trials have been done, and results are pending.
- Antioxidants (e.g., procysteine) have produced conflicting results in patients with full-blown adult respiratory distress syndrome.
- Pulmonary surfactant: Successful in infants with neonatal respiratory distress syndrome. However, data are insufficient to recommend its use in adults. Clinical trials continue.
- Vasodilators: Nitric oxide, sodium nitroprusside, hydralazine, alprostadil, and prostacyclin have not been found beneficial.
- Recombinant human activated protein C [drotrecogin alfa (Xigris)]. Published trials suggest benefit for patients with severe sepsis. Further trials are ongoing to determine appropriate patient selection.

 FOLLOW-UP

PROGNOSIS
There is a 35–60% mortality rate in the general population. Failure of lung function to improve in the 1st week of treatment portends a poor prognosis. Most survivors will regain normal or near-normal pulmonary function within 6–12 months. However, general health and respiratory-related quality of life and pulmonary function decrements may occur. Postpartum mortality rates are also high; neonatal outcomes associated with maternal acute respiratory distress syndrome are not well described. Residual impairment of respiratory mechanics includes mild restriction, mild obstruction, impaired carbon monoxide lung diffusion, or gas exchange abnormalities with exercise. Survivors who required prolonged ventilatory support as well as those with severe disease are more likely to have persistent respiratory abnormalities.

COMPLICATIONS
- Multiple organ dysfunction syndrome
- Death
- Permanent lung disease
- Oxygen toxicity
- Barotrauma
- Superinfection

PATIENT MONITORING
- Vital capacity and static lung compliance are important measures of mechanics.
- Daily labs are needed until no longer critical.
- Chest x-ray to assess: Endotracheal tube placement; the possible development of barotrauma; the presence of infiltrates; posteroanterior catheter migration
- Swan-Ganz catheter to help assess oxygen delivery and consumption; monitor cardiac output

REFERENCES
1. Cole D, et al. ARDS in pregnancy. *Crit Care Med*. 2005;33(10):S269–S278.
2. Piantadosi C, Schwartz D. The acute respiratory distress syndrome. *Ann Intern Med*. 2004;141: 460–470.
3. Ware LB, Matthay MA. Medical progress: The acute respiratory distress syndrome. *N Engl J Med*. 2000;342:1334–1349.
4. Petrucci N, Iacovelli W. Ventilation with lower tidal volumes versus traditional tidal volumes in adults for acute lung injury and acute respiratory distress syndrome, Cochrane Database of Systemic Reviews, Cochrane Library, Vol. 3,2003.
5. Hast AC, Hopkins CA. *ICD-9-CM Professional for Physicians, Vols. 1 & 2*, 6th ed. Salt Lake City, UT: Ingenix; 2003.
6. Kallet RH, Hass CF. Adult respiratory distress syndrome, Part 1. *Respir Clin North Am*. 2003;9.
7. Kallet RH, Hass CF. Adult respiratory distress syndrome, Part 2. *Respir Clin North Am*. 2003;9.
8. Flores J, Palovic J. Genetics of acute respiratory distress syndrome: Challenges, approaches, surfactant proteins as candidate genes. *Sem Resp Crit Care M*. 2003;24:161–168.
9. Bernard GR, et al. Extended Evaluation of Recombinant Human Activated Protein C United States Investigators. Extended evaluation of recombinant human activated protein C United States Trial (ENHANCE US): a single-arm, phase 3B, multicenter study of drotrecogin alfa (activated) in severe sepsis. *Chest*. 2004;125:2206–2216.

ADDITIONAL READING
Supportive care while identifying the underlying cause of acute respiratory distress syndrome continues to be important in the management of pregnant women with acute respiratory distress syndrome. However fetal wellbeing, possible need for delivery and physiologic changes associated with pregnancy need to be considered. Readers are referred reference 1.

 MISCELLANEOUS

See also: Congestive Heart Failure; Bacterial Pneumonia; Shock, Circulatory

CODES

ICD9-CM
- 518.5 Pulmonary insufficiency following trauma and surgery
- 518.82 Other pulmonary insufficiency, NEC
- 786.09 Dyspnea and respiratory abnormalities, other

PATIENT TEACHING

 See Corresponding Diagnostic Algorithm

RESPIRATORY DISTRESS SYNDROME, NEONATAL

Kurt J. Wegner, MD

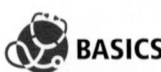 **BASICS**

DESCRIPTION

Serious disorder of prematurity, with clinical manifestation of respiratory distress. Pulmonary surfactants that are deficient at birth cause diffuse lung atelectasis. Must differentiate from pneumonia, sepsis, meconium aspiration.

- System(s) Affected: Pulmonary

ALERT

A disorder of the neonatal period

GENERAL PREVENTION

- Prevention of premature birth
- Systemic betamethasone given to mother when fetal lung profile is immature; at least 24 hours before delivery

EPIDEMIOLOGY

- Predominant age: Neonatal
- Predominant sex: Male = Female, although usually more severe in males

Incidence

Common

Prevalence

Common

RISK FACTORS

- Premature infants born <37 weeks, gestation
- Infants born of diabetic mothers
- More common and more severe with greater prematurity
- Fetal asphyxia
- Multiple births

Genetics

No known genetic pattern

ETIOLOGY

- Prematurity
- Deficient pulmonary surfactants in the neonatal period
- Possible pulmonary ischemia

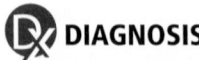 **DIAGNOSIS**

SIGNS AND SYMPTOMS

- Onset within few hours after birth
- Delayed, weak cry
- Expiratory grunt
- Frothing at lips
- Intercostal, sternal retractions
- Nasal flaring
- Rapid respiratory rate
- Respiratory excursions decreased
- Rales
- Cyanosis
- Peripheral edema
- Oliguria

TESTS

Lab

- Amniotic fluid
  - Lecithin: Sphingomyelin ratio (L:S ratio <2)
  - Absence of phosphatidyl glycerol
  - Surfactant production deficient
- Features of respiratory, metabolic acidosis
- Monitor arterial blood gases
  - Hypoxemia and hypercarbia
- Drugs that may alter lab results
  - Artificial or human surfactant; betamethasone

Imaging

Radiograph—reticulogranular appearance of lung fields demonstrating

- Diffuse atelectasis
- Air bronchograms

Pathological Findings

- Voluminous, noncrepitant, purplish-red lungs
- Dilatation right heart and vena cava
- Possible patent ductus
- Extensive resorptive atelectasis
- Hyaline membranes

DIFFERENTIAL DIAGNOSIS

- Early group B streptococcal pneumonia
- Transient tachypnea of newborn
- Meconium aspiration pneumonia
- Sepsis with group B streptococcus pneumonia

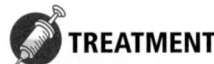 **TREATMENT**

PRE HOSPITAL

Inpatient intensive care

GENERAL MEASURES

- Warm, humidified, oxygen-enriched gases by hood
- Continuous positive airway pressure
- Positive pressure ventilation per endotracheal (ET) tube
- Monitor respiratory and circulatory status carefully.
- Umbilical artery catheter placed for monitoring BP and sampling arterial blood gases
- Transcutaneous monitors to measure O_2 and CO_2 tension
- Pulse oximetry
- Radiant infant warmer
- Tube feedings or hyperalimentation
- High-frequency ventilation. Choices include conventional ventilation at faster-than-normal rates, high-frequency jet ventilation, and high-frequency oscillation.
- Relationship between using surfactant and high-frequency ventilation still being studied
- Extracorporeal membrane oxygenation measure of last resort. Its use is still uncommon, and there are risks associated. Not available for infants <2 kg.

Diet

Special premature formula or parenteral alimentation

Activity

None; may require sedation or paralysis while on ventilator

MEDICATION (DRUGS)

- Beractant (Survanta): Bovine surfactant. Dose: 2.6–8.0 mL depending on patient's weight (see the manufacturer's dosing table). Other surfactant preparations available. Prophylaxis: As soon as possible after birth. Therapeutic: When signs and symptoms of respiratory distress syndrome appear
- Contraindications
  - Refer to the manufacturer's literature.
- Precautions
  - Do not administer beractant into a mainstem bronchus. Check ET tube placement before administration. Be prepared for rapidly changing lung compliance; peak ventilator pressures may need to be reduced immediately.
- Significant possible interactions
  - Refer to the manufacturer's literature.

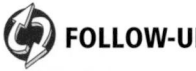 **FOLLOW-UP**

PROGNOSIS
- Course
  - Acute, possibly fatal within 48 hours in 20–30%, increasing with lower birth weights, especially <1,000 gs.
  - In larger premature neonates, course may be brief and uncomplicated, with recovery in 1 week.
- Prognosis
  - Successful outcome expected in tertiary care centers in children >28 weeks' gestation
  - Chronic lung disease, bronchopulmonary dysplasia (BPD), frequent in severe cases, especially after prolonged artificial ventilation
  - Careful postdischarge follow-up needed, including monitoring of oxygen saturation, growth, and development

COMPLICATIONS
- Intraventricular hemorrhage
- Intracranial pathology
- Tension pneumothorax
- Retinopathy of prematurity
- Apnea
- Chronic lung disease—BPD—5–20%

PATIENT MONITORING
- Continuous monitoring in an intensive care nursery
- Should have stable vital signs and pulse oximetry before discharge

REFERENCES
1. Avery GB, Fletcher MA, MacDonald MG, eds. *Neonatology: Pathophysiology and Management of the Newborn*. 5th ed. Philadelphia, PA: Lippincott Williams & Wilkins; 1999.
2. Hageman JR. The Pediatric Clinics of North America. *Neonatology Update*. Philadelphia, PA: WB Saunders; 1998.

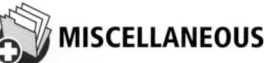 **MISCELLANEOUS**

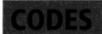 **CODES**

ICD9-CM
770.89 Other respiratory problems after birth

PATIENT TEACHING
For patient education materials favorably reviewed on this topic, contact: American Lung Association, 1740 Broadway, New York, NY 10019; (212) 315-8700.

RESPIRATORY SYNCYTIAL VIRUS (RSV) INFECTION

John P. Haran, MD
Frank J. Domino, MD

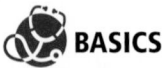 **BASICS**

DESCRIPTION
- Cause of respiratory illness
- Adults: Upper respiratory infections
- Infants and children: Bronchitis, bronchiolitis, pneumonia
- Premature infants are at increased risk for severe acute RSV infection
- Leading cause of pediatric admissions for respiratory illness
- System(s) Affected: Pulmonary

GENERAL PREVENTION
- Avoid exposure to those ill with RSV.
- Good hand-washing practices (given that hand-nose and hand-eye transmission is common)
- Avoid rubbing the eyes (common RSV inoculation route)
- Palivizumab (Synagis): Recommended for
  - Infants and children <2 years of age with chronic lung disease who have required medical therapy < 6 months prior to RSV season (fall, winter, spring).
  - Premature infants <32 weeks old
  - Premature infants 32–35 weeks old may benefit from prophylaxis.
  - Dosage: 15 mg/kg of body weight IM, monthly. (2,3)[A]

EPIDEMIOLOGY
- Predominant age: Birth to age 2 years
- Predominant sex: Outpatients: Males = Females; (Outpatient); Males > Females inpatients 2:1

Incidence
Common in winter

Prevalence
Almost everyone is infected 1 or more times during his or her lifetime.

ALERT
Pediatric Considerations
Most common <2 years old

RISK FACTORS
- Impaired immunity
  - AIDS
  - Chemotherapy
  - Other types of impaired immunity
- Occupational exposure
  - Day care workers
  - Pediatric hospital staff
  - Schoolteachers
- Neonatal/congenital conditions
  - Congenital heart disease
  - Respiratory distress syndrome
  - Chronic lung disease
  - Premature birth
- Low socioeconomic status
- More common in urban versus rural areas

Genetics
Two major strains are A and B

ETIOLOGY
Infection with RSV

ASSOCIATED CONDITIONS
- Asthma is worse with RSV, and vice versa
- Sudden infant death syndrome may be a sequela of RSV

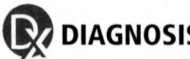 **DIAGNOSIS**

SIGNS AND SYMPTOMS
- Cold signs and symptoms (mild disease)
  - Fever
  - Cough
  - Coryza
  - Congestion
  - Malaise
- Bronchitis/bronchiolitis/pneumonia
  - Cough
  - Chest congestion
  - Wheezing
  - Dyspnea
  - Hypoxia
  - Cyanosis
- Vomiting

Physical Exam
- Fever
- Wheezing
- Rales/rhonchi
- Retractions
- Signs of hypoxia
- Dry mucus membranes, poor skin tugor

TESTS
Lab
- WBCs may be normal to elevated.
- Positive RSV antigen test on nasal washings
- Serology is of limited utility.

Imaging
Chest radiography
- Hyperinflation—most common, characteristic finding
- Peribronchiolar thickening
- Atelectasis—occasionally seen
- Interstitial infiltrates—fairly common
- Segmental or lobar consolidation in pneumonia
- Pleural fluid—rare

Diagnostic Procedures/Surgery
None

Pathological Findings
Lymphocytic peribronchiolar infiltrates (autopsy)

DIFFERENTIAL DIAGNOSIS
- Mild illness/upper respiratory tract
  - Colds (non-RSV)
  - Allergic rhinitis
  - Sinusitis
  - Croup
- Severe illness/lower respiratory tract
  - Asthma
  - Bronchitis
  - Bronchiolitis
  - Pneumonia
- Foreign body aspiration

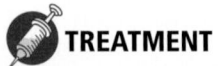 **TREATMENT**

INITIAL STABILIZATION
Outpatient care for mild cases; inpatient for severe disease or for those with underlying disorders. Illness may last from days to several weeks.

GENERAL MEASURES
- Outpatient
  - Rest/supportive care
  - Bronchodilators—albuterol nebulizer/inhaler
  - Monitor oxygenation—pulse oximeter
- Inpatient
  - Oxygen
  - Bronchodilators—albuterol or racemic epinephrine nebulizer q4h
  - Contact precautions
  - Ribavirin
  - Antibiotics for secondary bacterial pneumonia
  - Monitor arterial blood gases/pulse oximeter
  - Use of steroids is controversial; may help in some cases
- Avoid exposing others
  - Remove from day care/school until well
  - Good hand-washing practices
  - Respiratory isolation in hospital

Diet
- Maintain nutrition
- Avoid overhydration (may increase lung congestion)

Activity
Decreased household activity; rest

MEDICATION (DRUGS)

First Line

- Ribavirin 20 mg/mL mist 12–18 h/d for 3–7 days (may shorten the duration of mechanical ventilation and reduce days of hospitalization in addition to decreasing the long-term incidence of recurrent wheezing) (4)[A]
- Bronchodilators produce modest short-term improvement in clinical scores (5)[A]

Second Line

- Antibiotic appropriate for identified or suspected bacterial pathogen
- Theophylline use is acceptable but not recommended.

ALERT
Pregnancy Considerations

- Avoid ribavirin therapy during pregnancy.
- Health care workers who may be pregnant should avoid exposure to ribavirin.
- Bronchodilators: Albuterol nebulizer q4h (dose appropriate for age)
- Antibiotics for secondary bacterial infections/pneumonia
  – Appropriate to particular pathogen
  – Prophylactic use of antibiotics is controversial.
- Potential use of RSV immune globulin in high-risk infants
- Contraindications
  – See specific drug-related information.
- Precautions
  – Avoid exposure of pregnant or potentially pregnant women to ribavirin.
- Significant possible interactions
  – See specific drug-related information.

 FOLLOW-UP

PROGNOSIS

- Usually resolves within 2 weeks without sequelae
- Hospitalization rate of children ill with RSV varies from 1/50–1/200 (children <2 years old)
- Increasing immunity with subsequent infections by RSV usually results in less serious illness.

COMPLICATIONS

- Pneumonia
- Sudden infant death
- Death from severe lower respiratory tract infections
- Possible residual lung damage

PATIENT MONITORING

- Uneventful resolution is the norm.
- No special monitoring is needed as illness resolves.
- Educate parents about sudden infant death syndrome: Avoid prone sleeping in infants.

REFERENCES

1. Greenough A, Broughton S. Chronic manifestations of respiratory syncytial virus infection in premature infants. *Pediatr Infect Dis J*. 2005;24(11 Suppl):S184–7, discussion S187–8.
2. Centre for Reviews and Dissemination. A systematic review of the effectiveness and cost-effectiveness of palivizumab (Synagis) in the prevention of respiratory syncytial virus (RSV) infection in infants at high risk of infection. Database of Abstracts of Reviews of Effectiveness. Issue2006;1.
3. Wang EEL, Tang NK. Immunoglobulin for preventing respiratory syncytial virus infection. *Cochrane Database of Systematic Reviews*. 2006;1.
4. Ventre K, Randolph AG. Ribavirin for respiratory syncytial virus infection of the lower respiratory tract in infants and young children. *Cochrane Database of Systematic Reviews*.2006;1.
5. Kellner JD, et al. Bronchodilators for bronchiolitis. *Cochrane Database of Systematic Reviews*. 2006;1.

 MISCELLANEOUS

See also: Bronchiolitis; Bronchitis, Acute; Pneumonia, Bacterial; Pneumonia, Viral;

CODES

ICD9-CM

- 466.11 Bronchiolitis due to respiratory syncytial virus
- 466.19 Bronchiolitis (acute) (infectious) (subacute)
- 480.1 Pneumonia due to respiratory syncytial virus

PATIENT TEACHING

- Printed patient information available from ICN Pharmaceuticals, Inc., ICN Plaza, 3300 Hyland Ave., Costa Mesa, CA 92626; *All about RSV: A Guide for Parents*.
- RSV Information Center: http://www.rsvinfo.com

RESTLESS LEGS SYNDROME (RLS)

Sarita S. Warrier, MD
Geoffrey R. Hamilton, MD

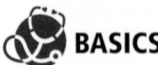 **BASICS**

DESCRIPTION

- Restless Legs Syndrome (RLS) is a sensorimotor disorder defined by the following 4 criteria in adults (1)[A]
  - A strong urge to move the legs is present, usually accompanied by an uncomfortable sensation.
  - The urge to move or discomfort occurs during periods of rest or inactivity (seated or lying).
  - The urge is relieved immediately by movement such as walking or stretching; relief continues as long as movement continues.
  - The condition is worse in the evening/night than in daytime.
- Patients may also complain of involuntary jerking of legs while sitting or lying awake.
- Primary RLS starts earlier and usually progresses slowly.
- Secondary RLS is precipitated by other conditions/disorders or medications, and resolves when the disorder is treated or the medication is withdrawn; tends to progress rapidly.
- System(s) Affected: Musculoskeletal; Nervous
- Synonym(s): Ekbom syndrome; Leg akathisia

EPIDEMIOLOGY

- Predominant age: Onset at any age; prevalence increases as age increases.
- Predominant sex: Male = Female (nulliparous); Female (parous) > Male

Incidence
Incidence increases with age.

Prevalence
- Estimated at 5–15% of US/Europe adults
- Prevalence <3% where studied in Asia

ALERT

Pediatric Considerations
- Young children may find symptoms difficult to describe. If they fail to meet all 4 criteria above, diagnose with the 1st 3 along with 2 of (1)[A]
  - Sleep disturbance
  - RLS in immediate family member
  - Periodic limb movements during sleep
- Can be misdiagnosed as growing pains or attention deficit hyperactivity disorder (ADHD).

Pregnancy Considerations
- 10–30% prevalence of RLS; pregnancy exacerbates existing RLS
- Symptoms usually start in the 3rd trimester and resolve after delivery
- May be secondary to iron or folate deficiency

RISK FACTORS
- Genetic predisposition if RLS starts >45 years and no other causative factors exist.
- Iron deficiency and conditions associated with iron deficiency
- Aging
- See "Associated Conditions."

Genetics
- Primary RLS: Positive family history in ~50% of patients
- RLS susceptibility locus on chromosome 12q; likely dominant inheritance.

ETIOLOGY
- For primary RLS, evidence suggests localized CNS dopamine deficiency.
- RLS may occur secondary to
  - Iron deficiency and associated conditions
  - Any source of chronic extremity tissue irritation.
  - Medications that may precipitate/worsen RLS
    - Most antidepressants (exception: bupropion)
    - Dopamine-blocking antiemetics (e.g., metoclopramide)
    - Some antiepileptic agents (e.g., phenytoin)
    - Phenothiazine antipsychotics
    - Theophylline
    - Antihistamines/OTC cold preparations

ASSOCIATED CONDITIONS
- Periodic limb movements of sleep (common)
- Pregnancy (common)
- Iron deficiency (common)
- End-stage renal disease/dialysis (common)
- CNS dopaminergic dysfunction, including Parkinson disease
- Venous insufficiency
- Peripheral neuropathy secondary to other causes (i.e., diabetes)
- Extremity orthopedic problems/surgery
- Insomnia, sleepwalking, other parasomnias
- ADHD
- Depression
- "Sundowning" in elderly

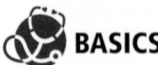 **DIAGNOSIS**

SIGNS AND SYMPTOMS
- Unpleasant sensation, often hard to describe
- Example descriptions: Burning, creepy-crawly feeling, achy, itching, urge to move
- Paresthesias in the muscles or under the skin
- Symptoms painful in ~35% of patients
- May also involve the arms
- Periodic movements persist in sleep in ~80% of patients
- Insomnia, daytime fatigue, sleepiness
- Severe RLS challenges ability to ride in cars, airplanes, and attend activities where people are expected to sit still, especially in evening.
- Severity and frequency of symptoms varies from a minor problem a few days per month to a daily problem with severe impact on quality of life.

History
Diagnosis made by history consistent with above signs and symptoms alone.

TESTS
- Sleep study is not required.
- Suggested immobilization test (SIT)
  - Conducted in evening before nocturnal polysomnography (NPSG)
  - Patient sits still, upright in bed with legs outstretched for 1 hour
  - >40 leg movements per hour suggests RLS.
- Electromyography and nerve conduction studies may be indicated to check for peripheral neuropathy and radiculopathy.

Lab
Hemoglobin/hematocrit, serum iron studies (including ferritin), vitamin B$_{12}$, folate

DIFFERENTIAL DIAGNOSIS
- Limb pain: Movement does not relieve pain, and may worsen it (RLS may be painful)
- Fasciculation and tremor from motor neuron disease: No discomfort or circadian pattern
- Sleep-related leg cramps: Routinely painful; relief requires aggressive stretching and massage
- Periodic limb movement disorder: No wakeful symptoms nor movement
- Sleep starts or hypnic jerks: Isolated involuntary events at sleep onset: No discomfort
- ADHD: No association with leg discomfort, and urge to move not limited to extremities. However, RLS may present as ADHD. (2)[B]
- Growing pains: Not associated with need to move nor are they quickly relieved by movement.

TREATMENT

GENERAL MEASURES
- Appropriate health care: Outpatient
- Daily physical activity
- Regular sleep pattern
- Hot bath, leg massage
- Warming the legs with long socks, leg warmers, or an electric blanket
- Intense mental activity such as complex games, video games, puzzles, or conversation

Diet
- Avoid caffeine, alcohol, tobacco late in day.
- Supplements correct deficiencies in iron, folate, and magnesium.

SPECIAL THERAPY
- Iron supplementation: 200–300 mg FeSO₄ with 200 mg vitamin C between meals. Monitor for side effects. May take months for iron repletion; RLS symptoms usually continue without other treatment. (3,4)[B]
- Vitamin and mineral supplements, including magnesium, B₁₂, and folate. (3,4)[B]
- Quinine (3,4)[B]
- Clonidine: 0.1–0.7 mg/d (3,4)[C]
- Baclofen: 20–80 mg/d (3,4)[C]

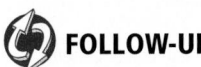 **MEDICATION (DRUGS)**

Four classes of drugs (dopamine agonists, anticonvulsants, benzodiazepines, opioids) are used. (3–5)[A]

First Line
- Dopamine agonists
  - Ropinirole (Requip): FDA-approved for RLS, 0.25–4.0 mg 1 hour before bed; increase by 0.25 mg every 3 days to determine optimal dose; dose may be divided to treat afternoon/evening and bedtime symptoms.
  - Pramipexole (Mirapex): FDA-approved; start at 0.125 mg and increase by 0.125 mg steps every 3 days; usual maximum 1.5 mg.
  - Carbidopa-levodopa (Sinemet): Use only as needed for intermittent symptoms to avoid augmentation of symptoms; dose range 25/100–100/400/d.
- Augmentation of symptoms (increased severity, occurrence earlier in the day, and/or spreading to arms or torso) can occur with prolonged use of dopamine agonists.
  - Daily levodopa or Sinemet carry highest risk for augmentation.
  - Requires reduction of dopaminergic agent and addition of adjunct medication. Watch for rebound while reducing dopaminergics.

Second Line
- Anticonvulsants
  - Gabapentin (Neurontin): 300–1,800 mg/d; particularly useful for painful or neuropathic RLS
  - Carbamazepine: 200–800 mg/d
- Benzodiazepines and agonists: Useful for patients with major complaint of insomnia.
  - Clonazepam (Klonopin): 0.5–3.0 mg/d
  - Other potentially useful benzodiazepines include temazepam, triazolam, alprazolam, zaleplon, zolpidem, and diazepam.
- Opioids: Use with caution
  - Hydrocodone: 5–20 mg/d
  - Tramadol: 50 mg at bedtime
  - Oxycodone: 2.5–20 mg/d
- Severe or refractory cases and augmentation require combination therapy.
- Most of the above medications may cause daytime sleepiness as a side effect, but this is unusual with the doses and timing used for RLS.

ALERT
Pregnancy Considerations
- 1st-line medications are either Class C or D in pregnancy, and should not be used.
- Most RLS in pregnancy should not be treated until the 3rd trimester.
- If needed, opioids at the lowest effective dose may be used along with iron supplementation and nonpharmacologic means.

Pediatric Considerations
- Medications are less studied in children; nonpharmacologic route is 1st-line treatment.
- Klonopin and clonidine at low doses have been used with some effect in children.
- Neurontin (gabapentin) may also be used.

 FOLLOW-UP

Issues for Referral
Daily RLS refractory to treatment with dopamine agonists, augmentation despite change in therapy, or intolerable side effects are indications for referral to an RLS specialist.

PROGNOSIS
- Primary RLS: Lifelong condition with no current cure.
- Secondary RLS: May partially or completely subside with resolution of precipitating factors. Symptoms usually worsen with age.
- Current therapies usually control symptoms and permit normal functioning.

COMPLICATIONS
- Tolerance to medications requiring increased dose or alternatives
- Augmentation of symptoms in response to chronic dopaminergic therapy

PATIENT MONITORING
- At 2-week intervals until stable
- Annual and as needed follow-up thereafter

REFERENCES
1. Sateia MJ. Restless legs syndrome. In: *International Classification of Sleep Disorders Diagnostic & Coding Manual*, 2nd ed. Westchester, IL: American Academy of Sleep Medicine, 2005; 178–181.
2. Cortese S, et al. Restless legs syndrome and attention-deficit/hyperactivity disorder: A review of the literature. *Sleep.* 2005;28(8):1007–1013.
3. Hening W, et al. Impact, diagnosis and treatment of restless legs syndrome (RLS) in a primary care population: The REST (RLS epidemiology, symptoms, and treatment) primary care study. *Sleep Med.* 2004;5(3):237–246.
4. Silber MH, et al. An algorithm for the management of restless legs syndrome. *Mayo Clin Proc.* 2004;79(7):916–922.
5. Hening WA, et al. An update on the dopaminergic treatment of restless legs syndrome and periodic limb movement disorder. *Sleep.* 2004;27(3):560–583.

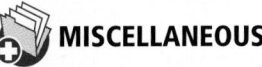 **MISCELLANEOUS**

See also: Periodic limb movement disorder

CODES

ICD9-CM
333.99

PATIENT TEACHING
- Wilson V. Sleep Thief. Orange Park, FL: Galaxy Books Inc.
- Restless Legs Syndrome Foundation http://www.rls.org; Tel: 507-287-6465; Fax: 507-287-6312
- National Sleep Foundation http://www.sleepfoundation.org; Tel: 202-347-3471; Fax: 202-347-3472
- NIH Neurological Institute
- http://www.ninds.nih.gov/disorders/restless_legs/restless_legs/htm; (800) 352-9424

 See Corresponding Diagnostic Algorithm

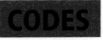 **See Patient Handout on CD**

RESTLESSNESS

Mark R. Dambro, MD

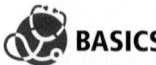

BASICS

DESCRIPTION
Excess physical or psychologic agitation often associated with specific physical abnormalities or existential conflict. When associated with preterminal events, it is sometimes called terminal restlessness.
- System(s) Affected: Nervous

GENERAL PREVENTION
See "General Measures" and "Patient Education."

EPIDEMIOLOGY
Predominant sex: Male = Female

ETIOLOGY
- Delirium
  - Medications (especially polypharmacy; also steroids, narcotics, anticholinergics)
  - Sensory deprivation (e.g., ICU psychosis)
  - Alzheimer disease
  - AIDS (57% have delirium at the time of death)
  - Brain tumor, primary or metastatic
  - Endocrinopathies (thyroid, adrenal dysfunction)
  - Electrolyte imbalance
  - Hepatic encephalopathy
  - Korsakoff syndrome
  - Neurosyphilis and other central nervous system (CNS) infections
  - Nutritional deficiency
- Myoclonus
  - High-dose morphine
  - Prolonged meperidine use
  - Lowered seizure threshold (metoclopramide, phenothiazines, haloperidol, antihistamines, tricyclic antidepressants, anticholinergics, hypoxia, dehydration, electrolyte abnormalities)
- Extrapyramidal symptoms (EPS)
  - Phenothiazines
  - Haloperidol
  - Metoclopramide
- Hypoxia
- Inadequately treated pain, especially in the nonverbal patient
- Anxiety
- Pruritus
- Urinary or fecal retention
- Medication/drug effects
  - Benzodiazepine withdrawal
  - Corticosteroids
  - Cocaine
  - Alcohol
  - Narcotics
- Existential issues
  - Unresolved existential issues
  - Death anxiety: Past-related regret (unfulfilled aspirations, low self-esteem), future-related regret (anticipation of failure to achieve important goals), meaningfulness of death (fear of unknown, concept of death)

ALERT
Geriatric Considerations
EPS more frequent in this group

ASSOCIATED CONDITIONS
- Depression
- Dementia
- Terminal anguish (suspect this as a cause of restlessness in patients without cognitive failure, hallucinations, or delusions)

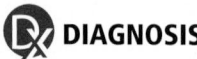

DIAGNOSIS

SIGNS AND SYMPTOMS
- Sleep disturbances
- Inability to concentrate
- Nonpurposeful motor activity
- Inability to relax
- Some clinicians include delirium (a change in level of consciousness)

Physical Exam
- Rectal examination for fecal impaction
- Abdominal examination and/or bladder catheterization for urinary retention

TESTS
- Restlessness scale (to be completed by patient, family, and/or staff)
  - 0—no restlessness
  - 1—mild agitation
  - 2—moderate agitation
  - 3—severe agitation without delirium
  - 4—moderate agitation with delirium
  - 5—severe agitation with delirium
- Mini-Mental Status Examination
- Delirium Rating Scale
- Review unfinished spiritual and/or interpersonal conflicts.
- Pain assessment

Lab
- Electrolytes, calcium, glucose, oxygen (hyponatremia, hypercalcemia, hypoglycemia, oximetry)
- Venereal Disease Research Laboratory, thyroid-stimulating hormone, HIV, and liver function tests; drug screen if cause of restlessness is not obvious

Imaging
MRI/CT of brain

ALERT
Pediatric Considerations
Pain, psychologic, and existential issues may be more difficult to assess in this age group.

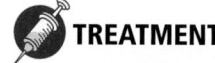

TREATMENT

INITIAL STABILIZATION
Terminal restlessness is best cared for in a quiet, supportive environment, often in the patient's home. Hospice team care is often helpful.

GENERAL MEASURES
- Treatment goals
  - Identify and address physical and/or existential issues to reduce restlessness.
  - Support family members and caregivers in dealing with restlessness, especially terminal restlessness.
- Eliminate unnecessary medications
  - CNS stimulants (e.g., albuterol, theophylline)
  - Anticholinergics (e.g., scopolamine, tricyclic antidepressants)
- Physical modalities
  - Limit extraneous stimuli, including loud noises and bright lights.
  - Teach rhythmic breathing and relaxation techniques.
  - Provide a quiet, well-lit room with familiar objects (e.g., pictures of family or friends, keepsakes).
- Psychosocial modalities
  - Frequent reorientation to person, place, and time
  - Supportive listening
  - Guided imagery
  - Music therapy
  - Massage; gentle touch
  - Recognize caregiver fatigue and provide appropriate respite care.
- Spiritual modalities: Provide for clergy visits for prayer or exploration of spiritual and other existential issues
  - Spiritual assessment
  - Patient and family counsel
  - Offer prayer for existential resolution (e.g., sinner's prayer for Christians, confession).
  - Preparation for death (e.g., last rites for Catholics)

ALERT
Geriatric Considerations
Anticholinergic effects (e.g., dry mouth, urinary retention, delirium, etc.) may be troublesome.

Diet
Avoid caffeine and other CNS stimulants.

Activity
- Rarely, physical restraint or 24-hour bedside assistance is needed.
- Indwelling urinary bladder catheter, for persistent urinary retention

MEDICATION (DRUGS)

First Line

- Antipsychotics
  - Haloperidol (Haldol) 0.5–5 mg q6–12h PO, PR, IM, or SC
  - Risperidone (Risperdal) 1 mg PO b.i.d.
- Narcotics for pain control as needed
  - Hydrocodone
  - Morphine
- Oxygen, when hypoxia is present
- Precautions
  - Use caution when combining CNS–acting drugs
  - Barbiturates increase benzodiazepine levels.
  - Antipsychotics may induce EPS, which may be mistaken for primary restlessness. Treat EPS with benztropine (Cogentin) 1–4 mg b.i.d. if the antipsychotics are relieving disturbing hallucinations or other symptoms causing restlessness.
  - Risperidone may be associated with hyperglycemia and ketoacidosis.

Second Line

- Benzodiazepines: Induce quiet sedation but do not improve cognition or sensorium
  - Lorazepam (Ativan) 1–2 mg q4h PO, PR, or IV
  - Midazolam (Versed) 0.25–3 mg/h via SC infusion
- β-Blockers reduce physical manifestations of autonomic hyperactivity: Atenolol (Tenormin) 25–50 mg/d
- Methotrimeprazine (Levoprome) 12.5–50 mg q4–8h is more sedating than haloperidol (oral form is not available in the US).
- Barbiturates in sedative or hypnotic doses may be helpful, but have a low safety margin, especially when used with narcotics: Pentobarbital (Nembutal) 100 mg IM or PR

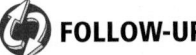 ## FOLLOW-UP

PROGNOSIS

- Terminal restlessness, by definition, is a preterminal event.
- Causes other than the preterminal condition will determine the response to therapy and course.

PATIENT MONITORING

Regular assessment and re-evaluation of the causes of restlessness

REFERENCES

1. Doyle D, Hanks GWC, MacDonald N, eds. *Oxford Textbook of Palliative Medicine*. 2nd ed. New York, NY: Oxford University Press; 1998.
2. Johanson GA. *Physicians Handbook of Symptom Relief in Terminal Care*. 4th ed. Santa Rosa, CA: Sonoma County Academic Foundation of Excellence in Medicine; 1994.
3. Kuebler KK. *The Hospice and Palliative Care Clinical Practice Protocols: Terminal Restless*. Pittsburgh, PA: Hospice and Palliative Nurses Association; 1997.
4. Tomer A, Eliason G. Toward a comprehensive model of death anxiety. *Death Stud*. 1996;20:343–365.
5. Trzepacz PT, Baker RW, Greenhouse J. A symptom rating scale for delirium. *Psychol Res*. 1988;23:89–97.

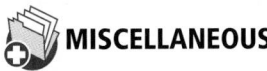 ## MISCELLANEOUS

See also: Anxiety; Delirium

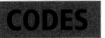 ### CODES

ICD9-CM

799.2 Nervousness

PATIENT TEACHING

Education of family and patient regarding the events surrounding the terminal patient, prior to terminal events, may reduce the severity of restlessness.

RETINAL DETACHMENT

Richard W. Allinson, MD

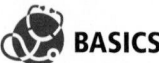 **BASICS**

DESCRIPTION
- Separation of the sensory retina from the underlying retinal pigment epithelium
- Rhegmatogenous retinal detachment (RRD): Most common type; occurs when the fluid vitreous gains access to the subretinal space through a break in the retina (Greek *rhegma*, rent)
- Exudative or serous detachment: Occurs in the absence of a retinal break, usually in association with inflammation or a tumor
- Traction detachment: Vitreoretinal adhesions mechanically pull the retina from the retinal pigment epithelium. The most common cause is proliferative diabetic retinopathy.
- System(s) Affected: Nervous

GENERAL PREVENTION
Patients at risk for retinal detachment should have regular ophthalmologic examinations.

EPIDEMIOLOGY
- Predominant age: Incidence increases with age
- Predominant sex: Male > Female (3:2)

Incidence
Per year: 1/10,000 in patients who have not had cataract surgery

Prevalence
After cataract surgery, 1–3% of patients will develop a retinal detachment.

RISK FACTORS
- Myopia (>5 diopters)
- Aphakia or pseudophakia
- Posterior vitreous detachment (PVD) and associated conditions (aphakia, inflammatory disease, and trauma)
- Trauma
- Retinal detachment in fellow eye
- Lattice degeneration: A vitreoretinal abnormality found in 6–10% of the general population
- Glaucoma: 4–7% of patients with retinal detachment have chronic open-angle glaucoma.
- Vitreoretinal tufts: Peripheral retinal tufts are caused by focal areas of vitreous traction.
- Meridional folds: Redundant retina usually found in the supranasal quadrant

Genetics
Most cases are sporadic.

ETIOLOGY
- Traction from a PVD causes most retinal tears. With aging, vitreous gel liquefies, leading to the separation of the vitreous from the retina. The vitreous gel remains attached at the vitreous base, in the retinal periphery, resulting in vitreous traction producing tears in the retinal periphery. There is an ~15% chance of developing a retinal tear from a PVD.
- PVD associated with vitreous hemorrhage has a high incidence of retinal tears.
- Exudative detachment
  - Tumors
  - Inflammatory diseases (Harada, posterior scleritis)
  - Miscellaneous (central serous retinopathy, uveal effusion, malignant hypertension)

- Traction detachment
  - Proliferative diabetic retinopathy
  - Cicatricial retinopathy of prematurity
  - Proliferative sickle cell retinopathy
  - Penetrating trauma

ALERT
Geriatric Considerations
- Posterior vitreous detachment
- Cataract surgery

Pediatric Considerations
Usually associated with underlying vitreoretinal disorders and/or retinopathy of prematurity

ASSOCIATED CONDITIONS
- Lattice degeneration
- High myopia
- Cataract surgery
- Glaucoma
- History of retinal detachment in the fellow eye
- Trauma

Pregnancy Considerations
Preeclampsia/eclampsia may be associated with exudative retinal detachment. No intervention is indicated, provided hypertension is controlled. Prognosis is usually good.

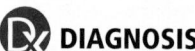 **DIAGNOSIS**

SIGNS AND SYMPTOMS
- Flashes (photopsia)
- Floaters
- Visual field loss
- Pigmented cells within the vitreous "tobacco dust"
- Central vision will be preserved if the macula is not detached.
- Poor visual acuity (20/200 or worse), with loss of central vision when macula is detached
- Elevation of retina associated with one or more retinal tears in RRD or elevation of the retina without tears in exudative detachment
- In 3–10% of patients with presumed RRD, no definite retinal break is found.
- Tenting of the retina without retinal tears in traction detachment

Physical Exam
- Slit lamp examination
- Dilated fundus examination with binocular indirect ophthalmoscopy

TESTS
Visual field testing: Differentiates RRD from retinoschisis. An absolute scotoma is seen in retinoschisis, whereas RRD causes a relative scotoma.

Imaging
- Ultrasonography can demonstrate a detached retina and may be helpful when the retina cannot be visualized directly (e.g., with cataracts).
- Fluorescein dye leakage can be seen in exudative retinal detachment; caused by central serous retinopathy and other inflammatory conditions

Pathological Findings
Elevation of the neurosensory retina from the underlying retinal pigment epithelium

DIFFERENTIAL DIAGNOSIS
Retinoschisis (splitting of the retina)
- Vitreous cell and vitreous hemorrhage are rarely found in the vitreous with retinoschisis, whereas they are commonly seen in RRD.
- Retinoschisis usually has a smooth surface and is dome shaped, whereas RRD often has a corrugated, irregular surface.

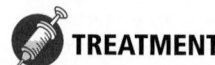 **TREATMENT**

INITIAL STABILIZATION
Referral to an ophthalmologist for examination and treatment, if indicated

GENERAL MEASURES
- Not all retinal tears or breaks need to be treated
  - Flap tears or horseshoe tears in symptomatic patients (e.g., patients with flashes or floaters) frequently are treated. (1)[A]
  - Operculated holes in symptomatic patients are sometimes treated.
  - Atrophic holes in symptomatic patients are rarely treated.
- Lattice degeneration with or without holes within the lattice in an asymptomatic patient with prior retinal detachment in the fellow eye may be treated prophylactically.
- Flap retinal tears in asymptomatic patients are frequently treated prophylactically.
- Exudative detachments are usually managed by treatment of the underlying disorder.
- Traction detachments are usually managed by observation. If the fovea is involved, a vitrectomy is needed.

Diet
NPO if surgery is imminent

Activity
- Bed rest prior to surgery
- Postoperatively, if an intraocular gas has been used, the patient may need specific head positioning and should not travel to high altitudes.

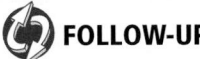 **MEDICATION (DRUGS)**

First Line
- Intraocular gases
  - Air
  - Perfluoropropane (C_3F_8)
  - Sulfur hexafluoride (SF_6)
- Perfluorocarbon liquids
- Silicone oil
- Contraindications: Patients with poorly controlled glaucoma
- Precautions: Expanding intraocular gas bubble increases intraocular pressure; therefore, avoid higher altitudes.
- Significant possible interactions: Nitrous oxide used in general anesthesia can expand an intraocular gas bubble.

Second Line
Steroids may cause worsening of central serous retinopathy.

SURGERY
- Timing of repairs
  - Macula attached: Within 24 hours. If the detachment is peripheral and does not have features suggestive of rapid progression (e.g., large and/or superior tears), repair can be performed within a few days.
  - Macula recently detached: Within 10 days of development of a macula-off retinal detachment (2)[B]
  - Old macular detachment: Elective repair within 2 weeks (3)[B]
- If a retinal break has led to the development of a retinal detachment, surgery is needed. Surgical options (and combinations) include
  - Demarcation laser treatment (4)[C]
  - Pneumatic retinopexy: Head positioning is required postoperatively.
  - Scleral buckle
  - Vitrectomy
  - Perfluorocarbon liquids for giant tears (circumferential tears ≥90)
  - Silicone oil for complex repairs
- Anesthesia: Local or general
- RRD may have more than 1 break. If any retinal break is not closed at the time of surgery, the surgery will fail.
- Additional surgery may be required if the retina redetaches secondary to a new retinal break or because of proliferative vitreoretinopathy (PVR).

 FOLLOW-UP

PROGNOSIS
- RRD
  - 90% of retinal detachments can be reattached successfully after 1 or more surgical procedures. Postoperative visual acuity depends primarily on the status of the macula preoperatively. Also important is the length of time between the detachment and the repair (75% of macular detachments of <1 week will obtain a final visual acuity of 20/70 or better).
  - 87% of eyes with a retinal detachment not involving the macula attain a visual acuity of 20/50 or better postoperatively. 37% of eyes with a detached macula preoperatively attain 20/50 or better vision postoperatively.
  - In 10–15% of successfully repaired retinal detachments not involving the macula preoperatively, visual acuity does not return to the preoperative level. This decrease is secondary to complications such as macular edema and macular pucker.
- Tractional retinal detachment: When it does not involve the fovea, the patient can usually be observed, as it is uncommon for these to extend into the fovea.
- Exudative retinal detachment
  - Management is usually nonsurgical.
  - The presence of shifting fluid is highly suggestive of an exudative retinal detachment. Fixed retinal folds, which are indicative of PVR, are rarely seen in exudative retinal detachment. If the underlying condition is treated, the prognosis is generally good.

COMPLICATIONS
- PVR is the most common cause of failed retinal detachment repair; 10–15% of retinas that reattach initially after retinal surgery will subsequently redetach, usually within 6 weeks, as the result of cellular proliferation and contraction on the retinal surface.
- Partial or total loss of vision due to macular detachment and/or PVR
- Moderate to severe forms of PVR are usually treated with pars plana vitrectomy and fluid-gas exchange. (5)[A] If a segmental scleral buckle was placed at the initial procedure, it must be revised.
- Scleral buckles may erode the overlying conjunctiva and lead to an infection.

PATIENT MONITORING
- Alert ophthalmologist immediately if there are symptoms of PVD and detachment (new onset of floaters or flashes, increase in floaters or flashes, sudden shower of floaters, curtain or shadow in the peripheral visual field, or reduced vision).
- Patients with acute symptomatic PVD associated with mild vitreous hemorrhage should be reexamined by the ophthalmologist in 3–4 weeks. The development of a retinal detachment is unlikely if no retinal tears are present on reexamination in 3–4 weeks.
- A patient with acute symptomatic PVD, even in the absence of vitreous hemorrhage, vitreous pigment, or detectable retinal break, may need to be reexamined by the ophthalmologist in 3–4 weeks, depending on clinical circumstances such as aphakia or myopia, because retinal breaks may develop over time.
- If acute symptomatic PVD is associated with gross vitreous hemorrhage that interferes with complete visualization of the retinal periphery by indirect ophthalmoscopy, the patient should be re-examined at short intervals with indirect ophthalmoscopy until the entire retinal periphery can be observed.
- If the examiner is not certain whether the retina is detached in the presence of opaque media, ultrasonography should be performed.

REFERENCES
1. American Academy of Ophthalmology. *Preferred Practice Pattern: Management of Posterior Vitreous Detachment, Retinal Breaks, and Lattice Degeneration*. San Francisco, CA: American Academy of Ophthalmology.2003;1–17.
2. Hassan TS, et al. The effect of duration of macular detachment on results after the scleral buckle repair of primary, macula-off retinal detachments. *Ophthalmology*. 2002;109:146–152.
3. American Academy of Ophthalmology. Ophthalmic procedure assessment: The repair of rhegmatogenous retinal detachments. *Ophthalmology*. 1996;103:1313–1324.
4. Vrabec TR, Baumal CR. Demarcation laser photocoagulation of selected macula-sparing rhegmatogenous retinal detachments. *Ophthalmology*. 2000;107:1063–1067.
5. Vitrectomy with silicone oil or perfluoropropane gas in eyes with severe proliferative vitreoretinopathy: Results of a randomized clinical trial. Silicone Study Report 2. *Arch Ophthalmol*. 1992;110:780–792.

 MISCELLANEOUS

See also: Retinopathy, Diabetic

CODES

ICD9-CM
- 361.00 Retinal detachment with retinal defect, unspecified
- 379.21 Vitreous degeneration
- 361.2 Serous retinal detachment
- 361.30 Retinal defect, unspecified
- 361.81 Traction detachment of retina
- 362.63 Lattice degeneration of retina

PATIENT TEACHING
American Academy of Ophthalmology, 655 E. Beach Street, San Francisco, CA 94109-1336

See Corresponding Diagnostic Algorithm

RETINITIS PIGMENTOSA (RP)

Richard W. Allinson, MD

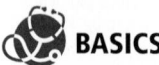 **BASICS**

DESCRIPTION
- Characterized by poor night vision, constricted visual fields, bone spiculelike pigmentation of the fundus, and electroretinographic evidence of photoreceptor cell dysfunction
- System(s) Affected: Nervous
- Synonym(s): Rod-cone dystrophy; Retinal dystrophy

GENERAL PREVENTION
- Genetic counseling
- There is no conclusive evidence demonstrating that the amount of light modifies the course of retinitis pigmentosa. A study in which 1 eye was covered with an opaque lens did not show any difference in disease progression compared with that in the fellow eye.
- UV-absorbing sunglasses and brimmed hats are recommended when patients are at the beach or in the snow.

EPIDEMIOLOGY
- Predominant age
  - X-linked RP has the earliest onset of the major hereditary types; many X-linked patients are legally blind by age 30 years.
  - Autosomal dominant RP has a later onset than autosomal recessive or X-linked recessive RP.
  - Leber congenital amaurosis, which is a variant of RP, presents at birth.
  - Late-onset RP typically is asymptomatic and unrecognized until age 40–50 years.
- Predominant sex: Male > Female

Prevalence
Affects ~1/4,000 people in the US

ALERT
Pediatric Considerations
Leber congenital amaurosis is characterized by severely reduced vision from birth and impaired electroretinogram responses from both cones and rods. Most cases are autosomal recessive.

Geriatric Considerations
Late-onset RP is asymptomatic; generally unrecognized until age >40 years

RISK FACTORS
Family history

Genetics
- Autosomal dominant: 20%
- Autosomal recessive: 37%
- X-linked recessive: 4.5%
- Sporadic: 38.5%

ETIOLOGY
- The genetic mutations responsible for RP have been identified in some families with RP, primarily those with the autosomal dominant form.
- Mutations in the rhodopsin gene account for ~30% of cases of autosomal dominant RP.
- Another 4–6% of autosomal dominant RP are caused by a mutation in the gene for a photoreceptor protein, peripherin/rds.

ASSOCIATED CONDITIONS
With systemic disorders
- Usher syndrome: RP and congenital sensorineural hearing impairment
- Laurence-Moon-Biedl syndrome (also called *Bardet-Biedl syndrome*): Autosomal recessive disorder associated with retinal dystrophy, mental retardation, obesity, hypogonadism, and postaxial polydactyly
- Cockayne syndrome: Autosomal recessive disorder in which children at the age of 1–2 years present with retinal dystrophy, sensorineural deafness, cerebellar dysfunction, dementia, and UV light photosensitivity

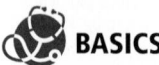 **DIAGNOSIS**

SIGNS AND SYMPTOMS
- Headache and light flashes are the most common initial complaints.
- Night blindness (nyctalopia)
- Bone spicule pigmentation in the retina
- Retinal arteriolar narrowing
- Optic nerve head pallor, "waxy pallor"
- Progressive visual field loss
- Central visual acuity is usually preserved until the end stages.
- Most patients are myopic.
- Posterior subcapsular cataracts are common in all forms.
- Cystoid macular edema
- Optic nerve head drusen
- Electroretinogram changes
- Retinal neovascularization
- RP is associated with an exudative retinal vasculopathy. Fundus findings include serous retinal detachment, lipid deposition in the retina, and telangiectatic vascular anomalies.
- Variants of RP exist with unusual or regional distribution, including
  - Sectorial RP
  - Pigmented paravenous atrophy
  - Unilateral RP

TESTS
- Electroretinography: Photoreceptors generate reduced amplitude A and B waves in RP. Rod and cone responses may be undetectable in advanced RP. (1)[A]

- Visual field testing: A ring scotoma in the midperiphery may be identified. The ring scotoma generally starts as a group of isolated scotomas in the area 20–25 from fixation. Long after the entire peripheral field is gone, there remains a small island of intact central visual field.
- Fluorescein angiography can demonstrate cystoid macular edema.
- Fundus photography to document the status of the retina
- Hearing tests in patients complaining of hearing loss, such as those with Usher syndrome (RP with hearing loss)
- Optical Coherence Tomography can be used to monitor cystoid macular edema.

Lab
- Elevated plasma levels of phytanic acid in Refsum disease
- Acanthocytosis of RBCs in peripheral blood smear in abetalipoproteinemia, an autosomal recessive disorder in which abetalipoprotein B is not synthesized, leading to fat malabsorption and deficiencies of fat-soluble vitamins. Therapy with vitamins A and E may improve retinal function.
- Syphilitic neuroretinitis can be diagnosed by performing a fluorescent treponemal antibody-absorption or microhemagglutination *Treponema pallidum* test.
- Elevated plasma ornithine levels in gyrate atrophy of the choroid and retina; usually a 10–20-fold elevation of plasma ornithine levels

Pathological Findings
- Disappearance of the rods, cones, and outer nuclear layers of the retina
- Bone spicule formation in the retina is secondary to the migration of retinal pigment epithelial cells into the overlying retina.

DIFFERENTIAL DIAGNOSIS
Bone spiculelike retinal pigmentation and retinal atrophy are nonspecific findings and may result from conditions other than RP
- Infections
- Syphilis
- Rubella
- Inflammation (severe uveitis)
- Choroidal vascular occlusion
- Toxicity (chloroquine or thioridazine)
- Choroideremia
- Gyrate atrophy of choroid and retina (10–20-fold elevation of plasma ornithine levels)
- Systemic metabolic disorders such as Refsum disease and abetalipoproteinemia
- Kearns-Sayre syndrome: Usually presents in adolescents; characterized by progressive external ophthalmoplegia—the 1st sign usually being ptosis—pigmentary degeneration of the retina, and a cardiac conduction defect, which may cause complete heart block
- Cone-rod dystrophy: Characterized by bilateral and symmetric loss of cone function in the presence of reduced rod function
- Cone dystrophy: Characterized by marked abnormality in cone function with some or no rod involvement
- Congenital stationary night blindness
- Oguchi disease
- Fundus albipunctatus
- Trauma

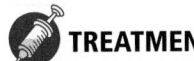 **TREATMENT**

INITIAL STABILIZATION
Outpatient care

GENERAL MEASURES
- Supportive care
- Genetic counseling
- Low-vision aids
- Patient education

Diet
No special diet

Activity
Full; caution should be exercised because of reduced peripheral vision and poor night vision.

 MEDICATION (DRUGS)

- Vitamin A 15,000 IU/d (retinal degeneration slowed as measured by electroretinogram/visual fields). NOTE: β-Carotene is not a suitable substitute; has not been studied in patients <18 years of age. (2)[A]
- Vitamin E 400 IU/d results in faster retinal degeneration and is not recommended (2)[A]
- Acetazolamide may be of benefit in the treatment of cystoid macular edema, which may occur in RP; 500 mg/d in a sustained-release capsule was found to be more effective than 250 mg/d (3)[C]
- Contraindications: Women who are pregnant or considering pregnancy should not take >8,000 IU of vitamin A per day. There is an increased incidence of birth defects in babies born to women who ingest higher dosages of vitamin A during pregnancy. Women should consult their obstetrician (4)[A]
- Precautions: Avoid vitamin A supplement dosages >15,000 IU/d, as higher dosages may cause liver damage.

ALERT
Pregnancy Considerations
Remember the risk of teratogenicity with a high intake of vitamin A during pregnancy.

SURGERY
- The efficacy of the "Cuban" therapy—electric stimulation, autotransfused ozonized blood, and ocular surgery—has not been proven to be of benefit (5)[B]
- Macular grid laser photocoagulation may be of benefit for patients with cystoid macular edema secondary to RP. (6)[C]
- Research is being done on photoreceptor transplantation, gene therapy, and implantation of a visual prosthesis. The inner retinal neurons may be preserved after death of photoreceptors in RP, which could make some of these experimental procedures feasible someday. (7)[C]

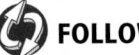 **FOLLOW-UP**

PROGNOSIS
- Reassurance about the slow course of RP
- Most of the deafness in Usher syndrome is congenital. It is unlikely that an RP patient who is not born deaf will become deaf later in life.
- RP severity varies with inheritance pattern.
- Autosomal recessive form has an early age of onset and may have severely constricted visual fields by age 20 years. Tends toward more rapid progression as compared with autosomal dominant RP; also increased incidence of cataracts
- X-linked RP is similar in clinical presentation to autosomal recessive RP.
- Autosomal dominant RP generally has less severe findings initially than does autosomal recessive RP; symptoms may not occur until 30 years of age.
- Good central vision is usually preserved. If the central visual field radius is >30, >90% of patients will have visual acuities of 20/40 or better. If the central visual field radius is <10, 30% of patients will have a visual acuity of 20/40 or better. (8)[C]

COMPLICATIONS
- Cataract
- Cystoid macular edema
- Loss of visual field
- Poor night vision
- Blindness

PATIENT MONITORING
- Ophthalmic examinations every 1–2 years
- Check for complications (e.g., cataracts).

REFERENCES
1. Pagon RA. Retinitis pigmentosa. *Surv Ophthalmol*. 1988;33:137–177.
2. Berson EL, et al. A randomized trial of vitamin A and vitamin E supplements for retinitis pigmentosa. *Arch Ophthalmol*. 1993;111:751–772.
3. Fishman GA, et al. Acetazolamide for treatment of chronic cystoid macular edema in retinitis pigmentosa. *Arch Ophthalmol*. 1989;107:1445–1452.
4. Rothman KJ, et al. Teratogenicity of high vitamin A intake. *N Engl J Med*. 1995;333:1369–1373.
5. Berson EL, et al. Evaluation of patients with retinitis pigmentosa receiving electric stimulation, ozonated blood, and ocular surgery in Cuba. *Arch Ophthalmol*. 1996;114:560–563.
6. Newsome DA, Blacharski P. Grid photocoagulation for macular edema in patients with retinitis pigmentosa. *Amer J Ophthalmol*. 1987;103:161–166.
7. Santos A, et al. Preservation of the inner retina in retinitis pigmentosa: A morphometric analysis. *Arch Ophthalmol*. 1997;115:511–515.
8. Madreperla SA, Palmer RW, Massof RW, Finkelstein D. Visual acuity loss and retinitis pigmentosa: Relationship to visual field loss. *Arch Ophthalmol*. 1990;108:358–364.

 MISCELLANEOUS

See also: Cataract

 CODES

ICD9-CM
362.74 Pigmentary retinal dystrophy

PATIENT TEACHING
- Counsel patients to help them understand RP and its genetics.
- RP is a slowly progressive, chronic disease; patients do not go blind rapidly, and total blindness is not a frequent end point of this disease.
- RP Foundation Fighting Blindness, Executive Plaza One, Suite 800, 11350 McCormick Road, Hunt Valley, MD 21031-1014; (800) 683-5555
- The American Academy of Ophthalmology, 655 E. Beach Street, San Francisco, CA 94109-1336; (415) 561-8540

 See Corresponding Diagnostic Algorithm

RETINOPATHY OF PREMATURITY (ROP)

Richard W. Allinson, MD

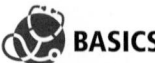 **BASICS**

DESCRIPTION
Proliferative disorder of the retinal blood vessels in premature infants. The normal retinal vascularization occurs nasally at ~36 weeks, gestational age and temporally at ~40 weeks, gestational age.
- System(s) Affected: Nervous
- Synonym(s): ROP; Retrolental fibroplasia

GENERAL PREVENTION
See "Patient Education."

EPIDEMIOLOGY
- Predominant age: Premature infants
- Predominant sex: Male = Female

Incidence
65.8% of infants weighing <1,251 g at birth, and 81.6% of those weighing <1,000 g

RISK FACTORS
- Low birth weight
- Prematurity
- Supplemental oxygen. Once the retina becomes fully vascularized, oxygen does not affect the retina.
- Supplemental oxygen given to premature infants with moderate ROP will not make the retinopathy worse.

Genetics
African American infants appear less susceptible.

ETIOLOGY
Oxidative processes (influenced by high levels of arterial oxygen) in immature retina may be an important causative factor.

ASSOCIATED CONDITIONS
Neonatal respiratory distress syndrome

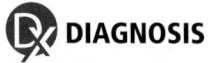 **DIAGNOSIS**

SIGNS AND SYMPTOMS
- Acute ROP is classification
  - Location
    - Zone I: Posterior retina within a 60° circle centered on the optic nerve
    - Zone II: Extends from the edge of zone I to the nasal ora anteriorly
    - Zone III: The residual temporal crescent of retina anterior to zone II
  - Extent
    - Number of clock hours involved
  - Degree of abnormal vascular response observed
    - Stage 1: The development of a demarcation line between the vascularized and nonvascularized retina
    - Stage 2: The presence of a demarcation line that extends out of the plane of the retina (ridge)
    - Stage 3: A ridge with extraretinal fibrovascular proliferation
    - Stage 4: Subtotal retinal detachment
    - Stage 5: Total retinal detachment (1)[A]
  - "Plus" disease is characterized by the tortuosity of the retinal vasculature in the posterior fundus
    - Pre-plus disease denotes retinal vascular abnormalities not of sufficient degree for "plus" disease, but demonstrating more arterial tortuosity and more venous dilatation than normal. (2)[A]

- AP-ROP represents an uncommon aggressive, posterior ROP that is rapidly progressive. (2)[A]

TESTS
Diagnostic Procedures/Surgery
- An ophthalmologist skilled in the detection of this disorder should examine all infants with a birth weight ≤1,500 g or with a gestational age of ≤28 weeks.
- Infants with a birth weight >1,500 g who are clinically unstable and are felt to be at high risk by their pediatrician or neonatologist should have an ophthalmologic examination to detect ROP.
- The American Academy of Pediatrics, the American Association for Pediatric Ophthalmology and Strabismus, and the American Academy of Ophthalmology produced a joint statement recommending the initial eye examination be performed between 4 and 6 weeks of chronologic age or between 31 and 33 weeks postconceptional age (gestational age at birth plus chronologic age). (3)[A]
- The above joint statement had its limitations, and some cases would have been diagnosed with threshold disease at their initial examination if postconceptional age criteria from the joint statement would have been followed. Analysis of the natural history data from the Multicenter Trial of Cryotherapy for Retinopathy of Prematurity (CRYO-ROP) and the Light Reduction in Retinopathy study provided evidenced-based screening criteria and have provided the following updated recommendations
  - Eye examinations for infants at risk for ROP should commence by 31 weeks postmenstrual age or 4 weeks chronologic age, whichever is later. (4)[A]
  - Acute-phase ROP screening may be terminated when 1 of the following 3 end points has been achieved: (i) Infant's attainment of 45 weeks postmenstrual age without the development of prethreshold ROP or worse, (ii) progression of retinal vascularization into zone III without previous zone I or zone II ROP, or (iii) full retinal vascularization.
- Follow-up examinations are performed until the retina is fully vascularized.

Pathological Findings
- Peripheral retinal nonperfusion
- Retinal neovascularization
- Retinal hemorrhages
- Retinal detachment

DIFFERENTIAL DIAGNOSIS
- Retinoblastoma
- Congenital cataracts
- Norrie disease
- Incontinentia pigmenti
- Familial exudative vitreoretinopathy
- Ocular toxocariasis
- Coats disease
- Persistent hyperplastic primary vitreous
- X-linked retinoschisis

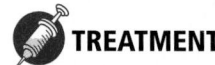 **TREATMENT**

INITIAL STABILIZATION
Treatment usually is performed in the neonatal ICU or as an outpatient or inpatient as the child grows older.

GENERAL MEASURES
- The CRYO-ROP study demonstrated a favorable outcome for eyes treated at threshold (stage 3+ retinopathy of prematurity) vs. control eyes.
- Stage 3 retinopathy is defined as a ridge of extraretinal fibrovascular proliferation.
- A plus sign is added to the ROP stage number when retinal vascular tortuosity is noted in the posterior fundus.
- *Threshold disease* was defined as at least 5 contiguous or 8 cumulative clock hours of stage 3 associated with retinal vascular tortuosity in the posterior segment of the eye ("plus" disease).
- When threshold disease is detected in infants, ablative therapy should be considered in at least 1 eye within 72 hours of diagnosis.
- The The Multicenter Study of Early Treatment for Retinopathy of Prematurity demonstrated that premature infants at high risk of vision loss from ROP retain better vision when therapy is administered early than when treatment is held until the traditional threshold. (5)[A] The eyes assigned to early treatment had a significantly reduced likelihood of poor vision, from 19.5–14.5%, at about 1 year of age
  - In the ETROP study, patients received treatment with laser therapy, but cryotherapy was also allowed.
  - Eyes with high-risk pre-threshold ROP or type 1 ROP were treated. Type 1 ROP was defined as zone I with any stage of ROP with plus disease (dilation and tortuosity of posterior pole retinal vessels in at least 2 quadrants, usually 6 or more clock hours); zone I, stage 3 ROP with or without plus disease; or zone II, stage 2 or 3 ROP with plus disease.
  - Serial examinations should be performed on eyes with type 2 ROP, which is defined as zone I, stage 1 or 2 ROP without plus disease, or zone II, stage 3 ROP without plus disease. Treatment should be considered for an eye with type 2 ROP when progression to type 1 ROP or threshold ROP occurs. Eyes with low-risk prethreshold type 2 ROP received follow-up every 2–4 days for at least 2 weeks until the ROP regressed or progressed to high-risk prethreshold disease.

SURGERY

- Transscleral cryotherapy to the avascular retina when applied to high-risk eyes may reduce the incidence of sight-threatening complications. The CRYO-ROP study has shown that treatment of high-risk eyes reduces the incidence of unfavorable outcomes by 46%.
- The results at 1 year from CRYO-ROP demonstrated an unfavorable outcome in 25.7% of eyes that received cryotherapy compared with 47.4% of control eyes. (6)[A]
- The results at 15 years from CRYO-ROP for retinopathy of prematurity demonstrated the following
  - Vision rated 20/200 or worse occurred in 44.7% of treated eyes vs. 64.3% of control eyes, and an unfavorable outcome for the fundus status was found in 30% of treated eyes vs. 51.9% of control eyes. (7)[A]
- Laser treatment applied to the avascular retina in high-risk eyes may reduce the incidence of sight-threatening complications; cataract formation and serous retinal detachment are possible complications of laser treatment.
- Diode laser treatment is becoming the primary treatment modality, because it may be better tolerated and probably results in better vision, less myopia, and less retinal dragging compared with eyes treated with cryotherapy.
- Threshold ROP had a reduced rate of progression in eyes with zone 2 disease when a dense, near-confluent pattern of diode laser treatment was applied vs. a less-dense pattern of diode laser treatment.
- IV fentanyl is a good analgesic agent to use when performing laser treatment with scleral depression on preterm infants.
- After 10 years of follow-up, eyes treated with laser were 5.2 times more likely to have 20/50 or better vision than eyes treated with cryotherapy.
- Scleral buckling may reduce progression from stage 4 to 5 ROP. The encircling 240 band can be divided at 3 months after surgery if it is felt the retina will remain attached.
- Vitrectomy and/or scleral buckling may be used to treat retinal detachment associated with ROP. Lens-sparing vitrectomy may be used to treat stage 4 ROP. Emphasis should be placed on prevention of retinal detachment in premature infants because of the poor visual outcome after a lensectomy/vitrectomy procedure for retinal detachment due to ROP.

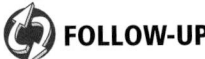 **FOLLOW-UP**

PROGNOSIS

- Spontaneous regression occurs over a period of weeks or months in most cases; occurs in ~85% of eyes.
- The earliest sign of regression is the growth of blood vessels beyond the demarcation line into previously avascular retina.
- Some cases of ROP do not regress spontaneously without sequelae, but progress. A gradual transition then occurs from active ROP to cicatricial ROP, which is associated with varying degrees of fibrosis and vitreoretinal traction that may lead to retinal detachment.

COMPLICATIONS

- Retinal detachment
- Retinal fold involving the macula
- Vitreous hemorrhage
- Angle-closure glaucoma
- Amblyopia
- Strabismus
- Myopia

PATIENT MONITORING

- Close follow-up of patients with ROP is required.
- Eyes with low-risk prethreshold type 2 ROP received follow-up every 2–4 days for at least 2 weeks until the ROP regressed or progressed to high-risk prethreshold disease. (5)[A]
- At least weekly examinations for infants with the following
  - Zone I ROP, less than threshold
  - Zone II ROP including
    - Stage 2 ROP with plus disease
    - Stage 3 ROP without plus disease
    - Stage 3 ROP with plus disease, not extensive enough for ablation therapy (8)[A]
- Follow-up every 1–2 weeks for the following
  - Zone II ROP with less severe findings
  - Incomplete retinal vascularization in zone I and no ROP
- No ROP, but with incomplete retinal vascularization in zone II should be examined at 2–3 week intervals.
- In some cases of regressed ROP, cicatrization may develop and is associated with variable degrees of fibrosis. This may lead to vitreoretinal traction and subsequent retinal detachment from formation of a retinal hole.
- Retinal detachment secondary to cicatricial ROP may occur during the midteens; long-term follow-up of ROP cicatricial cases is indicated.

REFERENCES

1. Committee for the Classification of Retinopathy of Prematurity. An international classification of retinopathy of prematurity. *Arch Ophthalmol*. 1984;102:1130–1134.
2. An International Committee for the Classification of Retinopathy of Prematurity. The international classification of retinopathy of prematurity revisited. *Arch Ophthalmol*. 2005;123:991–999.
3. Screening examination of premature infants for retinopathy of prematurity: A joint statement of the American Academy of Pediatrics, the American Association for Pediatric Ophthalmology and Strabismus, and the American Academy of Ophthalmology. *Ophthalmology*. 1997;104:888–889.
4. Reynolds JD, et al. Evidence-based screening criteria for retinopathy of prematurity: Natural history data from the CRYO-ROP and LIGHT-ROP studies. *Arch Ophthalmol*. 2002;120:1470–1476.
5. Good WV, Hardy RJ. The multicenter study of early treatment for retinopathy of prematurity (ETROP). *Ophthalmology*. 2001;108:1013–1014.
6. Cryotherapy for Retinopathy of Prematurity Cooperative Group. Multicenter trial of cryotherapy for retinopathy of prematurity: One year outcome—structure and function. *Arch Ophthalmol*. 1990;108:1408–1416.
7. Cryotherapy for Retinopathy of Prematurity Cooperative Group. 15-Year Outcome Following Threshold Retinopathy of Prematurity. Final Results From the Multicenter Trial of Cryotherapy for Retinopathy of Prematurity. *Arch Ophthalmol*. 2005;123:311–318.
8. Palmer EA, et al. Incidence and early course of retinopathy of prematurity. The Cryotherapy for Retinopathy of Prematurity Cooperative Group. *Ophthalmology*. 1991;98:1628–1640.

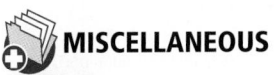 **MISCELLANEOUS**

CODES

ICD9-CM

362.21 Retrolental fibroplasia

PATIENT TEACHING

Expectant mothers should avoid behavioral and environmental risk factors associated with low birth weight, including smoking, alcohol and other substance abuse, and poor nutrition.

RETINOPATHY, DIABETIC

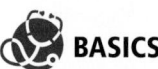

Diane M. Haleem, PhD, RN

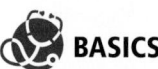 BASICS

DESCRIPTION

- Noninflammatory retinal disorder characterized by retinal capillary closure and microaneurysms. Retinal ischemia leads to release of a vasoproliferative factor stimulating neovascularization on retina, optic nerve, or iris.
- Most patients with diabetes mellitus (DM) will develop diabetic retinopathy. It is the leading cause of new cases of legal blindness among residents in the US between the ages of 20 and 74 years.
- Diabetic retinopathy can be divided into 3 stages
  - Nonproliferative (background) diabetic retinopathy
  - Preproliferative diabetic retinopathy
  - Proliferative diabetic retinopathy
- System(s) Affected: Nervous

ALERT

Geriatric Considerations
Prevalence will increase as population generally ages and patients with diabetes live longer.

Pregnancy Considerations
- Pregnancy can exacerbate condition.
- Pregnant diabetic women should be examined in 1st trimester, then every 3 months until delivery.

GENERAL PREVENTION
Monitoring and control of blood glucose

EPIDEMIOLOGY

Incidence
- Peak incidence of type I, juvenile onset DM, is between the ages of 12 and 15.
- Peak incidence of type II, adult onset, is between the ages of 50 and 70.
- Incidence of diabetic retinopathy is directly related to the duration of diabetes.
- <10 years of age, it is unusual to see diabetic retinopathy, regardless of diabetes duration.

Prevalence
- 6.6% of US population between age 20 and 74 has diabetes.
- ~25% of the diabetic population has some form of diabetic retinopathy.
- Predominant age
  - The risk of developing diabetic retinopathy increases after puberty.
  - Almost all diabetic patients with type I diabetes and >60% of patient's with type II diabetes will develop background retinopathy if they have had diabetes for at least 20 years.
  - 2/3 of juvenile-onset diabetics who have diabetes for at least 35 years will develop proliferative diabetic retinopathy, and 1/3 will develop macular edema. Proportions are reversed for adult-onset diabetes.
- Male = Female (juvenile onset DM); Female > Male (type II)
- 10–50% "preproliferative" retinopathy will develop proliferative retinopathy in 1 year.

RISK FACTORS
- Duration of DM (usually >10 years)
- Poor glycemic control
- Pregnancy
- Renal disease
- Systemic hypertension
- Smoking
- Elevated lipid levels associated with increased risk of retinal lipid deposits (hard exudates)

ETIOLOGY
Related to development of diabetic microaneurysms and microvascular abnormalities

ASSOCIATED CONDITIONS
- Glaucoma
- Cataracts
- Retinal detachment
- Vitreous hemorrhage
- Disk edema (diabetic papillopathy); may occur in type I or type II diabetes.

DIAGNOSIS

SIGNS AND SYMPTOMS
- Nonproliferative (background) diabetic retinopathy
  - Microaneurysms
  - Intraretinal hemorrhage causing sudden visual changes to include spotting
  - Macular edema causing loss of central vision
  - Lipid deposits causing focal capillary closure
- Preproliferative diabetic retinopathy
  - Nerve fiber layer infarctions (cotton wool spots)
  - Venous beading
  - Venous dilation
  - Intraretinal microvascular abnormalities
  - Extensive retinal hemorrhage
- Proliferative diabetic retinopathy
  - New blood vessel proliferation (neovascularization) on the retinal surface, optic nerve, and iris
  - Visual loss is caused by vitreous hemorrhage, which causes the vitreous to become clouded, not allowing light to transmit; also the resorption of the blood in the vitreous leads to the formation of fibrous scar tissue. The scar tissue can cause pulling on the retina, resulting in retinal detachment.

Diagnostic Procedures/Surgery
- Eye examination: Measurement of visual acuity and documentation of the status of the iris, lens, vitreous, and fundus
- Fluorescein angiography visualizes retinal vessels not visualized by the ophthalmoscope, it demonstrates retinal nonperfusion, retinal leakage, and proliferative diabetic retinopathy.
- Optical coherence tomography can be used to help detect diabetic macular edema by measuring retinal thickness.

Pathological Findings
- Increased capillary permeability
- Microaneurysms
- Hemorrhages in retina
- Exudates in retina
- Capillary nonperfusion

DIFFERENTIAL DIAGNOSIS
Other causes of retinopathy (e.g., radiation, retinal venous obstruction, hypertension)

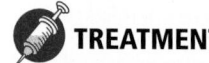 TREATMENT

GENERAL MEASURES
- The Early Treatment Diabetic Retinopathy Study demonstrated that aspirin therapy did not prevent the development of proliferative diabetic retinopathy, nor reduce the risk of visual loss associated with diabetic retinopathy.
- Microvascular complications, including proliferative diabetic retinopathy, are increased when blood sugar levels are ≥200 mg/dL.
- Poor glycemic control is associated with an increased risk both for developing diabetic retinopathy and with its progression, regardless of the type of diabetes.
- Cataracts are more common among those with diabetes. Try to delay cataract surgery in diabetic patients with retinopathy until the symptoms are severe; cataract surgery can cause retinopathy to worsen.
- Hypertension has detrimental effect on diabetic retinopathy and must be controlled. (1)[A]

Diet
Follow prescribed diet for patients with diabetes

Nursing
Patient education to include
- Regular ophthalmic examinations
- Blood glucose control
- If visual loss, identify adaptive devices for ADLs. Consult occupational therapist.
- Psychosocial support to the person with visual loss and family members.
- Cessation of smoking

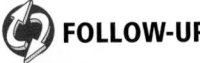

MEDICATION (DRUGS)

First Line

- None is specific for retinopathy. See "Miscellaneous." Lisinopril, an angiotensin-converting enzyme inhibitor, was found to slow the progression of retinopathy in insulin-dependent diabetes. It is used to control hypertension.
- Under evaluation: Protein kinase C-beta is activated by hyperglycemia and is associated with the development of vascular dysfunction. Inhibition of this enzyme could help reduce the retinal vascular complications from diabetes.
- Nutritional antioxidant intake of vitamins C and E and of beta-carotene has no protective effect on diabetic retinopathy.
- Atorvastatin may reduce the severity of lipid deposits with clinically significant diabetic macular edema with type II diabetes and dyslipidemia.

SURGERY

- Laser photocoagulation treatment: Recommended for patients with proliferative diabetic retinopathy and for those with clinically significant macular edema; destroys leaking blood vessels and areas of neovascularization.
- The Diabetic Retinopathy Study demonstrated panretinal photocoagulation overall reduced rate of severe visual loss from 15.9% in untreated eyes to 6.4% in treated eyes. In subgroups; incidence of severe visual loss in untreated eyes was as high as 36.9% within 2 years.
- The Early Treatment Diabetic Retinopathy Study demonstrated eyes with significant diabetic macular edema benefited from focal laser treatment. (2)[A] Clinically significant diabetic macular edema is defined as
  - Thickening of the retina within 500 microns of the center of the macula
  - Hard exudates within 500 microns of the center of the macula associated with thickening of the adjacent retina
  - Zone of retinal thickening 1 disc area or larger within 1 disc diameter of center of macula
- Patients with clinically significant diabetic macular edema and high-risk proliferative disease can have simultaneous focal and panretinal photocoagulation without adversely affecting the visual outcome. (3)[C]
- Vitrectomy may benefit some with diffuse macular edema.
- Intravitreal triamcinolone may be used for DM-related macular edema that fails laser treatment. (4)[B]
- Vascular endothelial growth factor (VEGF) may increase vascular permeability. VEGF is blocked by pegaptanib. Intravitreal injection of pegaptanib is being evaluated in the treatment of diabetic macular edema. (5)[C]
- Cryoretinopexy can be used instead of laser treatment in certain cases to decrease the neovascular stimulus and treat proliferative diabetic retinopathy.
- Vitrectomy: Recommended for patients with severe proliferative diabetic retinopathy, traction retinal detachment involving the macula, and nonclearing vitreous hemorrhage.
- Vitrectomy can be considered after 1 month for a vitreous hemorrhage decreasing the vision to the 5/200 level or worse. (6)[A]

FOLLOW-UP

PROGNOSIS

If the condition is diagnosed and treated early in its development, the outlook is good. If treatment is delayed, blindness may result.

COMPLICATIONS

Blindness

PATIENT MONITORING

Scheduled ophthalmologic eye examinations

- Yearly follow-up if no retinopathy.
- Every 6 months with background diabetic retinopathy
- At least every 3–4 months with preproliferative diabetic retinopathy
- Every 2–3 months with active proliferative diabetic retinopathy

REFERENCES

1. UK Prospective Diabetes Study (UKPDS) Group. Risks of progression of retinopathy and vision loss related to tight blood pressure control in type 2 DM. *Arch Ophthalmol.* 2004;122:1631–1640.
2. Early Treatment Diabetic Retinopathy Study Research Group. Photocoagulation for diabetic macular edema. ETDRS Report No. 1. *Arch Ophthalmol.* 1985;103:1796–1806.
3. Browning DJ, et al. The effect of patient characteristics on response to focal laser treatment for diabetic macular edema. *Ophthalmol.* 1997;104:466–472.
4. Martidis A, et al. Intravitreal triamcinolone for refractory diabetic macular edema. *Ophthalmol.* 2002;109:920–927.
5. Macugen Diabetic Retinopathy Study Group. A Phase II randomized double-masked trial of pegaptanib, an anti-vascular endothelial growth factor aptamer, for diabetic macular edema. *Ophthalmol.* 2005;112:1747–1757.
6. Diabetic Retinopathy Vitrectomy Study Research Group. Early vitrectomy for severe vitreous hemorrhage in diabetic retinopathy: 2 year results of a randomized trial. Diabetic Retinopathy Vitrectomy Study Report 2. *Arch Ophthalmol.* 1985;103:1644–1651.
7. The Diabetes Control and Complications Trial Research Group. The effect of intensive diabetes treatment on the progression of diabetic retinopathy in insulin-dependent DM. *Arch Ophthalmol.* 1995;113:36–51.
8. ADA. Retinopathy in diabetes. *Diabetes Care.* 2004;27(Suppl 1):84–87.
9. Tesfay S, Chaturvedi N, Eaton SEM, et al. Vascular risk factors and diabetic neuropathy. *N Engl J Med.* 2005;352(4):341–350.
10. ADA. Smoking and diabetes (position statement). *Diabetes Care.* 2004;27(1):74–75.
11. Diabetes Control and Complications Trial/Epidemiology of Diabetes Interventions and Complications Research Group Writing Team. Effect of intensive therapy on the microvascular complications of type 1 DM. *JAMA.* 2002;287(19):2563–2569.
12. Fischbach F. *Nurse's Quick Reference to Common Laboratory and Diagnostic Tests*, 3rd ed. Philadelphia: Lippincott, 2002.
13. Smeltzer SC, Bare BG, Hinkle JL, Cheever KH. (2008). *Brunner & Suddarth's Textbook of Medical–Surgical Nursing*, 11 ed. Philadelphia: Lippincott Williams & Wilkins, 2007.

ADDITIONAL READING

- American Association of Diabetes Educators, 444 N. Michigan Ave., Suite 1240, Chicago, IL 60611: 800 332-6874; http://www.aadenet.org/.
- Centers for Disease Control and Prevention, 1600 Clifton Rd., Atlanta GA 30333; 404-639-3311; http://www.cdc.gov/diabetes/pubs/factsheet.htm.

MISCELLANEOUS

- See also: Diabetes mellitus, type I; Diabetes mellitus, type II.
- The Diabetes Control and Complications Trial (DCCT) recommendations
  - For most patients with insulin-dependent DM, blood glucose levels should be as close to the nondiabetic range as safe to reduce the risk and rate of progression of the diabetic retinopathy. (7)[A]
  - Insulin-dependent diabetic patients were randomly assigned into either conventional or intensive insulin treatment. Conventional treatment consisted of 1 or 2 daily insulin injections, with daily self-monitoring of urine or blood glucose. Intensive treatment consisted of insulin administered ≥ 3 daily by injection or an external pump, with self-monitored blood glucose levels measured at least 4 q.i.d.
  - Intensive insulin therapy reduced the risk of macular edema and retinal neovascularization.
  - Intensive insulin therapy was more effective in reducing the risk of progression of diabetic retinopathy in the less advanced stages. However, advanced diabetic retinopathy also benefited from the intensive insulin.
  - Improvement in diabetic retinopathy was more likely to occur with intensive insulin therapy in insulin-dependent diabetes

CODES

ICD9-CM

- 362.01 Background diabetic retinopathy
- 362.02 Proliferative diabetic retinopathy

PATIENT TEACHING

Stress importance of strict blood glucose control through diet, exercise, drugs/insulin, and monitoring of blood glucose.

See Patient Handout on CD

REYE SYNDROME

William A. Primack, MD

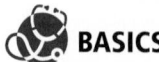 **BASICS**

DESCRIPTION
Acute encephalopathy with cerebral edema and fatty infiltration of the liver

- Occurs in previously healthy children and is often associated with an antecedent viral infection such as varicella or influenza
- Markedly decreased in incidence since the late 1970s, when association with aspirin use was made (1)[B]
- Most cases currently seen are "Reyelike" syndrome caused by inborn error of metabolism or toxin (see "Differential Diagnosis").
- System(s) Affected: Gastrointestinal; Nervous
- Synonym(s): White liver disease

GENERAL PREVENTION
- Avoidance of salicylates in children with viral illness
- Recognition of early symptoms of the disease

EPIDEMIOLOGY
- Predominant age
  - Infants, children, adolescents
  - Peak incidence at 6 years of age
  - Most cases between 4 and 12 years of age
- Predominant sex: Male = Female

Incidence
Currently very rare

RISK FACTORS
- Pediatric age group
- Viral illness, especially varicella, influenza A
- Use of preparations containing aspirin, salicylates, and/or salicylamides
- More common in rural and suburban areas

Genetics
No known genetic pattern

ETIOLOGY
Unknown; mitochondrion is major site of injury.

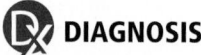 **DIAGNOSIS**

SIGNS AND SYMPTOMS
Symptoms reflected in clinical staging system
- I: Vomiting, sleepiness, lethargy
- II: Confusion, delirium, hyperpnea, irritability, combativeness, hyperreflexia, altered muscle tone
- III: Obtundation, light coma and seizures, decorticate rigidity, loss of oculocephalic reflexes, intact pupillary reflex
- IV: Coma, decerebrate posturing spontaneously or in response to painful stimuli, seizures, fixed pupils
- V: Coma, flaccid paralysis, loss of deep tendon reflexes, seizures, respiratory arrest, isoelectric electroencephalogram (2)[C]

TESTS
EEG

Lab
- Usually severe elevations of aspartate aminotransferase (serum glutamic-oxaloacetic transaminase) and alanine aminotransferase (serum glutamic-pyruvic transaminase)
- Hypoglycemia
- Normal or slightly elevated bilirubin or alkaline phosphatase
- Elevated ammonia
- Prolonged prothrombin time: Often not responsive to vitamin K
- Increased cerebrospinal fluid pressure without pleocytosis (<8 leukocytes per cubic millimeter)
- Mixed respiratory alkalosis and metabolic acidosis
- Hyperaminoacidemia (glutamine, alanine, lysine)

Diagnostic Procedures/Surgery
- Liver biopsy
- Cerebrospinal fluid pressure measurement

Pathological Findings
- Slightly enlarged, firm, yellow liver with fat droplets throughout
- Characteristic liver biopsy with foamy cytoplasm with microvesicular fat—may need special preparation
- Uniformly severe mitochondrial injury

DIFFERENTIAL DIAGNOSIS
- Acute encephalopathy without hepatic abnormalities
  - Encephalitis
  - Meningitis
  - Diabetes mellitus
  - Drug overdose
  - Poisoning
  - Psychiatric illness
- Acute toxic encephalopathy with hepatic abnormalities (Reyelike syndrome)
  - Inherited metabolic disorders: Organic acidurias with defects in hepatic fatty acid oxidation; fatty acid metabolism defects—Acyl-CoA dehydrogenase, carnitine deficiency—urea cycle defects—carbamyl phosphate synthetase, ornithine transcarbamylase—fructosemia
  - Drug ingestions: Valproate, aspirin
  - Toxin ingestion (produces Reyelike syndrome): Margosa oil, hopantenate, aflatoxin, hypoglycin (akee fruit; Jamaican vomiting sickness)

ALERT
Pediatric Considerations
Especially in infants <2 years of age, it is essential to make the correct diagnosis; rule out other causes of Reyelike syndrome. (3,4)[C]

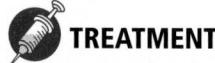 **TREATMENT**

INITIAL STABILIZATION
Medical emergency requiring immediate hospitalization

GENERAL MEASURES
- Supportive care, depending on severity of illness
- Intravenous glucose and close monitoring of blood or serum glucose (to prevent severe hypoglycemia)
- Hyperventilation, mannitol, and barbiturates to reduce intracranial pressure
- Minimization of noise and other CNS stimulation (to prevent increases in intracranial pressure)
- Vitamin K, fresh frozen plasma, and platelets as needed
- Mechanical ventilation
- Dialysis to reduce high ammonia levels and/or residual salicylate

Diet
NPO

Activity
Complete bed rest

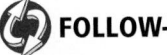 **MEDICATION (DRUGS)**

All treatment is supportive.
- Glucose 10–15% IV
- Vitamin K
- For increased intracranial pressure, e.g.
  - Mannitol 0.5–1.0 g/kg IV, as long as there is urine output
  - Dexamethasone 0.5 mg/kg/d
  - Barbiturates
- Contraindications: Mannitol: Do not use if patient has no renal output.
- Precautions: Mannitol and poor renal output may result in vascular overload and pulmonary edema.
- Significant possible interactions: Refer to the manufacturer's literature.

SURGERY

Decompression craniotomy may be necessary.

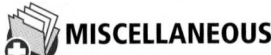 **FOLLOW-UP**

PROGNOSIS
- Most will have mild illness without progression. Prognosis related to degree of cerebral edema and ammonia level on admission
- Possible neurologic sequelae include problems with attention, concentration, speech, language, and fine and gross motor skills—more common with higher stages

COMPLICATIONS
- See also "Signs and Symptoms."
- Aspiration pneumonia
- Respiratory failure
- Cardiac dysrhythmia/arrest
- Inappropriate vasopressin excretion
- Diabetes insipidus
- Cerebral edema
- Seizures

PATIENT MONITORING

Depends on specific residual effects; may require care of physicians, nurses, psychologists, and/or physical, occupational, and/or speech therapists

REFERENCES

1. Monto J. The disappearance of Reye's syndrome—a public health triumph. *N Engl J Med*. 1999;340:1423–1424.
2. Balistreri W. Reye syndrome and "Reye-like" diseases. In: Behrman RE, Kliegman RM, Arvin A, eds. *Nelson Textbook of Pediatrics*. Philadelphia, PA: WB Saunders; 2000;1214–1216.
3. Green A, Hall S. Investigation of metabolic disorders resembling Reye's syndrome. *Arch Dis Child*. 1992;67:1313–1317.
4. Visentin M, Salmona M, Tacconi MT. Reye's and Reye-like syndrome, drug related diseases? *Drug Met Rev*. 1995;27:517–539.
5. Belay E, et al. Reye's syndrome in the United States from 1981 through 1997. *N Engl J Med*. 1999;340:1377–1382.
6. Glasgow JF, Middleton B. Reye syndrome—insights on causation and prognosis. *Arch Dis Child*. 2001;85:351–353.

MISCELLANEOUS

See also: Encephalitis, Viral; Hepatic Encephalopathy

CODES

ICD9-CM
331.81 Reye syndrome

PATIENT TEACHING

Printed material from the National Reye Syndrome Foundation, P.O. Box 829, Byron, OH 43506-0829; (800) 233-7393

RH INCOMPATIBILITY

Donald A. F. Nelson, MD

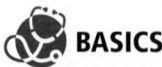 **BASICS**

DESCRIPTION
Antibody-mediated destruction of red blood cells that bear Rh surface antigens by individuals who lack the antigens and have become isoimmunized (sensitized) to them
- System(s) Affected: Hemic/Lymphatic/Immunologic
- Synonym(s): Rh isoimmunization; Rh alloimmunization; Rh sensitization

GENERAL PREVENTION
- Blood typing (ABO and Rh) on all pregnant women
- Antibody screening early in pregnancy
- Rh immune globulin prevents only sensitization to the D antigen.
- Follow prophylaxis routine listed in "Medications" for unsensitized, Rh-negative women.

EPIDEMIOLOGY
- Predominant age: Childbearing
- Predominant sex: Female only

Incidence
- Risk of isoimmunization during or after an Rh-positive pregnancy (without the use of Rh immune globulin had been ≤15%, but seems to be decreasing.
- Risk of isoimmunization antepartum is only 1–2%.
- Risk of isoimmunization is 1–2% after spontaneous abortion, 4–5% after induced abortion. (1)

Prevalence
Fifteen percent of white population and smaller fractions of other races are Rh negative. (2)

RISK FACTORS
- Any Rh-positive pregnancy in an Rh-negative woman. With Rho(D) immune globulin prophylaxis, risk of sensitization is reduced to <1% of susceptible pregnancies.
- Induced abortion
- Spontaneous abortion
- Ectopic pregnancy
- Amniocentesis, chorionic villus sampling
- Fetomaternal hemorrhage (fetal death in utero)
- Fetal manipulation, external version
- Casarean delivery
- Maternal trauma
- Placental abruption
- Placenta previa
- Manual placental removal

Genetics
Complex autosomal inheritance of polypeptide Rh antigens. 2 closely related genes, RHD and RHCE, carry an assortment of alleles: Dd, Cc, Ee. Individuals who express the D antigen (also called *Rho* or *Rho[D]*) are considered Rh positive, as are those expressing the weak D (Du) variant. Individuals lacking the D antigen are Rh negative. Antibodies may be produced to C, c, D, E, or e in individuals lacking the specific antigen; only D is strongly immunogenic. (3) Isoimmunization to Rh antigens is not inherited.

PATHOPHYSIOLOGY
See "Description."

ETIOLOGY
- Transfusion of Rh-positive blood to Rh-negative recipient
- Maternal exposure to fetal Rh antigens, either antepartum or intrapartum
- More commonly seen in the Rh-positive fetus or infant of an Rh-negative mother

ASSOCIATED CONDITIONS
- Hemolytic disease of newborn
- Hydrops fetalis
- Neonatal jaundice
- Kernicterus

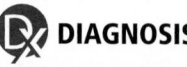 **DIAGNOSIS**

SIGNS AND SYMPTOMS
- Hemolytic transfusion reaction in recipient of Rh-incompatible blood
- Jaundice of newborn
- Kernicterus
- Congenital or fetal anemia
- Fetal hydrops
- Fetal death in utero

TESTS
Lab
- Positive indirect Coombs test (antibody screen) during pregnancy
- Paternal blood typing (new born—in the US, 10% of infants born to married women are not genetically related to the husband)
- Kleihauer–Betke test to quantify an acute fetal-maternal bleed
- Drugs that may alter lab results
  - Prior administration of D immune globulin may lead to weakly (false) positive indirect Coombs test in mother and direct Coombs test in infant.

DIFFERENTIAL DIAGNOSIS
- ABO incompatibility
- Other blood group (non-Rh) isoimmunization
- Nonimmune fetal hydrops
- Hereditary spherocytosis
- Red cell enzyme defects

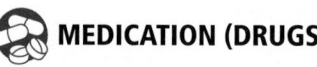 **TREATMENT**

GENERAL MEASURES
- See "Patient Monitoring."
- Depending on severity of involvement, treatment of newborn or fetus may include the following
  - Intrauterine transfusion
  - Early delivery
  - Exchange transfusion
  - Transfusion after delivery
  - Phototherapy
  - Diuretics and digoxin for hydrops
  - Immunoglobulin infusion has reduced the need for exchange transfusion in a few studies. (4)[C]
  - Erythropoetin has been used experimentally to reduce the need for intrauterine transfusion. (5)[C]

MEDICATION (DRUGS)

- For prophylaxis, Rho(D) immune globulin (RhIG, RhoGAM, Gamulin Rh) given to unsensitized, Rh-negative women after the following
  - Spontaneous abortion
  - Induced abortion
  - Ectopic pregnancy
  - Antepartum hemorrhage
  - Amniocentesis
  - Chorionic villus sampling
  - Routinely at 28 weeks' gestation
  - Within 72 hours after delivery of Rh-positive infant
- Dose
  - 50-μg dose for events up to 12 weeks' gestation
  - 300-μg dose for events after 12 weeks' gestation
  - Higher doses may be required in the event of a large fetal-maternal hemorrhage (>30 mL of whole blood).
- Contraindications
  - Patient with known severe reaction to human globulin
  - Refer to the manufacturer's profile.
- Precautions: Refer to the manufacturer's profile.

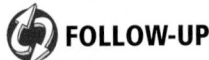 **FOLLOW-UP**

DISPOSITION
Outpatient, ambulatory management in most cases

Issues for Referral
Because of the specialized, somewhat hazardous treatment measures involved, pregnancies in Rh-sensitized women are usually managed at tertiary care level.

PROGNOSIS
- With appropriate monitoring and treatment, infants born of severely affected pregnancies have a survival rate of >80%. (6)
- Fetuses with hydrops have a higher mortality rate.
- Disease is likely to be more severe in affected subsequent pregnancies.
- Even with severe disease, the neurologic outcome of survivors is generally good.

COMPLICATIONS
- Pregnancy loss from umbilical blood sampling
- Pregnancy loss from intrauterine transfusion
- Fetal distress requiring emergent delivery (6)

PATIENT MONITORING
- Antibody titer measured at 20 weeks and every 4 weeks thereafter during pregnancy (6)
  - A titer of $\geq$1:16 indicates need for further testing. [C]
- Amniocentesis for amniotic fluid bilirubin levels [C]
- Umbilical blood sampling (cordocentesis) for fetal blood type, hematocrit, reticulocyte count, and presence of erythroblasts [C]
- Fetal heart rate testing/ultrasonography to assess fetal status
- Amniocentesis for fetal lung maturity if early delivery is a treatment option (6)[C]

REFERENCES

1. Bowman J. Thirty-five years of Rh prophylaxis. *Transfusion.* 2003;43:1661–1666.
2. Bianchi DW, et al. Noninvasive prenatal diagnosis of fetal rhesus D ready for prime(r) time. *Obstetr Gyneco.* 2005;106(4):841–844.
3. Agre P, Cartron J. Molecular biology of the Rh antigens. *Blood.* 1991;78:551–563.
4. Alcock GS, Liley H. Immunoglobulin infusion for isoimmune haemolytic jaundice in neonates. *Cochrane Database of Systematic Reviews.* 2006;1.
5. Ovali F, Samanci N, Dagoglu T. Management of late anemia in Rhesus hemolytic disease: Use of recombinant human erythropoietin (a pilot study). *Pediatri Res.* 1996;39(5):831–834.
6. Management of isoimmunization in pregnancy. ACOG Educational Bulletin *227.* Aug 1996.
7. Prevention of Rh D alloimmunization. ACOG Practice Bulletin 4. May 1999.

 MISCELLANEOUS

See also: Anemia, Autoimmune Hemolytic; Erythroblastosis Fetalis; Jaundice

CODES

ICD9-CM
- 656.10 Rh isoimmunization in pregnancy, unspecified
- 656.11 Rh isoimmunization in pregnancy, delivered
- 656.13 Rh isoimmunization in pregnancy, antepartum
- 656.20 Isoimmunization in pregnancy from other and unspecified blood-group incompatibility, unspecified
- 773.0 Rh hemolytic disease in fetus or newborn
- 773.1 ABO hemolytic disease in fetus or newborn
- 773.2 Other hemolytic disease in fetus or newborn
- 773.3 Isoimmune hydrops fetalis
- 773.4 Kernicterus due to isoimmunization
- 773.5 Isoimmune late anemia
- V28.5 Antenatal screening for isoimmunization

R

RHABDOMYOLYSIS

Scott Kinkade, MD, MSPH

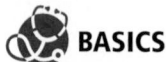 **BASICS**

DESCRIPTION

- Rhabdomyolysis is the breakdown (necrosis) of skeletal muscle cells and release of the intracellular contents into the circulation.
- Rhabdomyolysis typically manifests with muscle aches, pains and weakness, and reddish-brown (tea-colored) urine.
  - Myoglobin from the muscle cells can damage the kidney and cause acute renal failure.
  - System(s) Affected: Musculoskeletal; Renal; Cardiac.

GENERAL PREVENTION

- Avoidance of traumatic or exertional muscle injury (see "Causes")
- Avoidance of precipitating drugs and metabolic states (see "Causes")

EPIDEMIOLOGY

- Male predilection, because higher incidence of trauma
- Depends on the etiology for rhabdomyolysis, i.e., inherited disorders lead to rhabdomyolysis at a younger age but other etiologies may occur at any time, as in trauma or rhabdomyolysis due to infection.

Incidence

Annually: 26,000 hospitalized cases

RISK FACTORS

See "Etiology."

Genetics

Hereditary causes of rhabdomyolysis are infrequent, but should be suspected in the following groups presenting with rhabdomyolysis: Children, recurrent attacks, or attacks after minimal exertion, mild illness, or starvation. Muscular dystrophies have various modes of genetic transmission. Certain inherited disorders of lipid metabolism (e.g., carnitine palmitoyltransferase deficiency and carnitine deficiency) or carbohydrate metabolism (i.e., phosphofructokinase deficiency, phosphoglycerate mutase, myophosphorylase deficiency, for example McArdle disease) can lead to rhabdomyolysis.

ETIOLOGY

- Drugs and toxins
  - Alcohol
  - Cocaine, methamphetamine, phencyclidine
  - Antipsychotics
  - Zidovudine
  - Antimalarials
  - Heroin
  - HMG-CoA reductase inhibitors (statins)
  - Fibrates
  - Colchicine
  - Corticosteroids
  - Carbon monoxide
  - Snake envenomation

- Muscle exertion
  - Intense physical exercise
  - Seizures
  - Delirium tremens
- Direct muscle trauma
  - Crush injuries
  - Contact sports, boxing, physical torture
  - Extended periods of muscle pressure (during surgery, unconscious from alcohol)
  - Burns, electrocution, lightning strike
- Muscle ischemia
  - Thrombosis, embolism, sickle cell disease
  - Compartment syndrome
  - Tourniquets
- Infections
  - Viral: Influenza A and B, coxsackie, HIV, varicella
  - Bacterial: Streptococcus or staphylococcus sepsis, gas gangrene, necrotizing fasciitis, salmonella, Legionella
  - Malaria
- Hypothermia
- Hyperthermia
  - Heat stroke
  - Neuroleptic malignant syndrome
  - Malignant hyperthermia
- Autoimmune and genetic disorders
  - Polymyositis, dermatomyositis
  - Muscular dystrophies
  - Disorders of lipid metabolism (e.g., carnitine palmitoyltransferase deficiency and carnitine deficiency)
  - Disorders of carbohydrate metabolism (i.e., phosphofructokinase deficiency, phosphoglycerate mutase, myophosphorylase deficiency aka McArdle disease/deficiency)
  - Glycogen storage diseases (e.g., phosphorylase b-kinase deficiency) and others (e.g., lactate dehydrogenase A deficiency)
- Metabolic and endocrinologic
  - Hypothyroidism or thyrotoxicosis
  - Electrolyte imbalances (hyponatremia, hypernatremia, hypokalemia, hypocalcemia, hypophosphatemia)
  - Diabetic ketoacidosis
  - Hyperosmolar states
- Inflammatory conditions
  - Polymyositis
  - Dermatomyositis

ASSOCIATED CONDITIONS

See "Etiology."

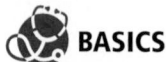 **DIAGNOSIS**

SIGNS AND SYMPTOMS

Patients often note muscle aches, cramps, or fatigue. They may report tea-colored urine indicative of myoglobinuria. Rhabdomyolysis may present with obvious muscle injury and swelling on examination (e.g., crush injury, compartment syndrome; or muscle exam may be completely negative despite severe rhabdomyolysis/myoglobinuria). The signs and symptoms with renal failure are the same as those for acute tubular necrosis from other causes.

TESTS

Lab

- Muscle enzyme elevations (e.g., creatinine kinase [CK] aldolase, and lactic dehydrogenase). A CK more than 5 times the upper limit of normal or >1,000 U/L is usually used for diagnosis of rhabdomyolysis. Commonly CK is elevated into the tens of thousands and sometimes into the hundreds of thousands.
- Marked elevations of potassium from the muscle injury sometimes are compounded by acute renal failure.
- Initial hypocalcemia as calcium deposits in the injured muscle cells; hypercalcemia occasionally during the recovery phase from acute tubular necrosis
- Urinalysis: Dipstick test positive for blood without erythrocytes in sediment is suggestive of injury from either hemoglobin or myoglobin.
- Urine or serum myoglobin levels may be helpful, but normal levels do not rule out rhabdomyolysis as myoglogin is rapidly filtered from the blood stream.
- Extreme hyperuricemia may be present and can cause acute uric acid nephropathy in the setting of rhabdomyolysis.
- Elevations in blood urea nitrogen (BUN) and creatinine indicative of acute renal failure
- Reversible hepatic dysfunction can occur. However, elevations in ALT, AST, and LDH may be due to muscle injury and may not indicate any hepatic injury.
- Disseminated intravascular coagulation can occur with increase in coagulation times, fibrin degradation products, and D-dimer. Decreases in platelets and fibrinogen

Imaging

Any renal imaging is similar to other evaluations of acute renal failure.

Diagnostic Procedures/Surgery

Fasciotomies are occasionally required for acute compartment syndrome causing rhabdomyolysis.

Pathological Findings

- Muscle necrosis
- Myoglobin-related renal injury may resemble acute tubular necrosis from other causes.

DIFFERENTIAL DIAGNOSIS

- For acute renal failure with rhabdomyolysis: Any disease that causes acute tubular necrosis may be confused with rhabdomyolysis.
- Renal pigment injury from hemoglobin resembles pigment injury from myoglobin.

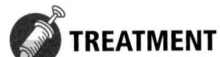 **TREATMENT**

INITIAL STABILIZATION
Inpatient

GENERAL MEASURES
- Aggressive hydration is often necessary. With severe muscle trauma (crush injuries) 10 or more liters of fluid may be sequestered in the muscles leading to intravascular volume depletion which increases the risk for renal failure.
- Dialysis will be necessary for severe renal failure.
- Caution: Diagnose muscle entrapment or compartment syndromes as surgical intervention may be required to stop rhabdomyolysis.
- Severe hypocalcemia with symptoms (Chvostek and Trousseau syndromes) during the oliguric phase may benefit from IV calcium gluconate. Symptomatic hypocalcemia is rare.

Diet
When rhabdomyolysis causes renal failure, restrict protein intake to lower BUN level. Potassium intake must be limited. With anuria, essential to restrict volume intake

Activity
Physical exertion can lead to rhabdomyolysis, and less exertion is tolerated in patients with the metabolic myopathies mentioned in this topic (See "Etiology" and "Genetics").

 MEDICATION (DRUGS)

First Line
- When rhabdomyolysis is identified, appropriate intervention may prevent renal failure.
  - Volume expansion with normal saline to increase urine output to at least 150 mL/h, strong support for aggressive and early fluid replacement
  - Alkalinization of the urine is thought to decrease myoglobin tubular injury (sodium bicarbonate to increase urine pH >6.5). Its use is controversial without strong evidence of efficacy. Side effects include worsening hypocalcemia. Sodium bicarbonate may be of use in cases with very high CK levels, an acidotic state, or with coexisting hyperkalemia.
  - IV mannitol as a bolus: 12.5–25 g (0.25–0.5 g/kg); not to exceed ~50 g/d is used by some to prevent acute renal failure. It is thought to cause renal vasodilation and a diuresis that makes the kidney less susceptible to myoglobin injury. The use of mannitol is controversial in this setting as there is not good evidence that it improves outcomes more than aggressive IV hydration. It should not be used in anuric renal failure.
- Hyperkalemia can result from massive release of intracellular potassium stores or acute renal failure. Severe hyperkalemia may be life threatening. Treatment is warranted when electrocardiographic changes are present (tall, thin T waves; P-R prolongation; QRS widening; P wave flattening).
  - Calcium gluconate: IV 1–2 ampules (0.5 mL of 10% calcium gluconate = 4 mg elemental calcium; give 4 mg/kg/h×4 h).
  - If acidosis is present: 1–2 ampules (2–3 mL/kg) sodium bicarbonate IV. Remember that bicarbonate administration may lead to alkalosis and worsening hypocalcemia.
  - If tolerated: Oral sodium polystyrene sulfonate (Kayexalate) as much as 20 g (1 g/kg). Can also be given via enema if oral intake not tolerated or not indicated.
  - Insulin will transiently drive potassium into the cells. Administration of glucose can prevent the hypoglycemic effects of insulin.
  - Dialysis may become necessary to remove potassium.
- Calcium as already mentioned for severe, symptomatic hypocalcemia
- Contraindications: See the manufacturer's literature.
- Precautions: See "Etiology," especially drug combinations.

Second Line
- Monitoring of CK levels to assure that rhabdomyolysis has ended
- Monitoring of renal function and electrolytes
- If DIC or hepatic dysfunction occurs, they will need treatment and monitoring.

SURGERY
Relief of compartment syndrome by fasciotomy to preserve muscle viability and nerve function

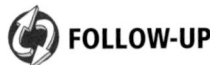 **FOLLOW-UP**

DISPOSITION
Admission Criteria
Patients with significant elevations of CK should be admitted for IV hydration and serial laboratory monitoring.

Discharge Criteria
CK usually peaks 24–36 hours after muscle injury, so monitoring should confirm that the CK is trending down. Renal function should be stable or improving. Electrolytes should be normal.

PROGNOSIS
Contingent on primary cause of rhabdomyolysis and on recovery from acute renal failure without complications

COMPLICATIONS
Death, especially from hyperkalemia or renal failure
With dialysis and supportive care, the prognosis is very good.

PATIENT MONITORING
- Contingent on primary disease. Some cases (e.g., those involving crush injury) are accidental and will not occur again.
- Contingent on disease: Essential for metabolic myopathies
- Myotoxic drugs should be discontinued or monitored closely.

REFERENCES

1. Melli G, Chaudhry V, Cornblath DR. Rhabdomyolysis. An evaluation of 475 hospitalized patients. *Medicine*. 2005;84:377–385.
2. Singh D, Chander V, Chopra K. Rhabdomyolysis. *Methods Find Exp Clin Pharmacol*. 2005;27:39–48.
3. Allison RC, Bedsole DL. The other medical causes of rhabdomyolysis. *Am J Med Sci*. 2003;326:79–88.
4. Huerta-Alardin AL, Varon J, Marik PE. Bench-to-bedside review: Rhabdomyolysis—an overview for clinicians. *Crit Care*. 2005;9:158–169.
5. Brown CVR, et al. Preventing renal failure in patients with rhabdomyolysis: Do bicarbonate and mannitol make a difference? *J Trauma*. 2004;56:1191–1196.
6. Fernandez WG, et al. Factors predictive of acute renal failure and need for hemodialysis among ED patients with rhabdomyolysis. *Am J Emerg Med*. 2005;23:1–7.
7. Malinoski DJ, Slater MS, Mullins RJ. Crush injury and rhabdomyolysis. *Crit Care Clin*. 2004;20:171–192.

 MISCELLANEOUS

See also: Renal Failure, Acute (ARF)

CODES

ICD9-CM
722.88 Rhabdomyolysis

PATIENT TEACHING

 See Corresponding Diagnostic Algorithm

RHEUMATIC FEVER

Frank J. Domino, MD

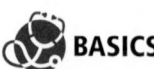 **BASICS**

DESCRIPTION
- An inflammatory disease, possibly autoimmune in nature, that involves many tissues, including the heart, joints, skin, and central nervous system
- Can cause permanent cardiac valvular disease as well as acute cardiac decompensation
- Recurrences are common if not prevented with prophylactic antibiotic treatment. In recent years, there have been multiple reports of recurrences in adults as well as children.
- System(s) Affected: Cardiovascular; Hemic/Lymphatic/Immunologic; Musculoskeletal; Nervous; Skin/Exocrine

ALERT
Pediatric Considerations
More common in children

GENERAL PREVENTION
- Patients must be on prophylactic penicillin throughout childhood and possibly indefinitely during adulthood
  - Monthly IM injections of 1.2 MU of benzathine penicillin are the preferred treatment.
- Adults should be treated for a minimum of 5 years after an attack. Some treat adults indefinitely if there has been valvular disease. Oral penicillin V-K, 125 mg b.i.d., is an alternative to monthly injections. In the event of penicillin allergy, sulfadiazine, 500 mg/d for children weighing <30 kg or 1 g/d for all others may be used.
- If patients have valvular damage from acute rheumatic fever, they require bacterial endocarditis prophylaxis for dental and other high-risk procedures.

EPIDEMIOLOGY
- Predominant age
  - Most common in children ages 5–15 years
  - Recurrences can be seen in adulthood.
- Predominant sex: Male = Female

Incidence
- The incidence of rheumatic fever in the US has been showing an overall decline for decades. In the 1970s, it was a rare disease with an incidence of 0.5–1.88 cases per 100,000. However, since the mid-1980s, a resurgence of cases has occurred, with multiple outbreaks having been reported.
- The incidence calculated on the basis of recent outbreaks has been as high as 18.1 per 100,000 in children aged 5–17 years.

RISK FACTORS
Genetics
A specific genetic marker that correlates with susceptibility to rheumatic fever has not been found, but the disease is known to occur in families.

ETIOLOGY
- Autoimmune mechanisms
- Preceding infection of the upper respiratory tract with group A *Streptococcus* organisms is a prerequisite to the development of acute rheumatic fever.

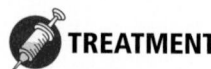 **DIAGNOSIS**

SIGNS AND SYMPTOMS
- Joint symptoms ranging from arthralgias to frank arthritis (75%)
- Joints involved are medium to large (e.g., ankles, knees, wrists).
- Joint involvement is classically migratory.
- Joint symptoms usually disappear in 3–4 weeks without permanent deformities.
- Carditis (65%), mild or severe, with murmurs
- Cardiac involvement may include pericarditis, myocarditis, and/or valvular insufficiency. Appears within 2 weeks and lasts 6 weeks–6 months.
- Valvular damage may be permanent.
- P-R prolongation on ECG
- Erythema marginatum (classic rash; <5%)
- Subcutaneous nodules (painless, hard swellings overlying bony prominences; 5–10%)
- Chorea is often a late finding, but may be a presenting complaint. It occurs in 10–15% of patients, and its duration is not altered by treatment.
- Fever 38.3–40°C (101–104°F)
- Abdominal pain is common and may be severe.
- Epistaxis (historically important, but rarely seen in acute rheumatic fever)
- Facial tics
- Facial grimace

TESTS
Lab
- Increased acute-phase reactants, including ESR and C-reactive protein (CRP)
- Bacteriologic or serologic evidence of group A streptococcal infection, antistreptolysin O (ASO), streptozyme, or antideoxyribonuclease B (DNAse)
- Anemia
- Drugs that may alter lab results: Prior treatment with aspirin or steroids

Imaging
- Chest radiograph
- ECG (reveals pericardial effusion and documents valvular disease)

Diagnostic Procedures/Surgery
- Throat cultures for group A-hemolytic streptococci
- Diagnosis depends on fulfilling the modified Jones criteria of 2 major manifestations or 1 major and 2 minor manifestations. In either case, evidence must exist of preceding group A streptococcal infection. The 5 major criteria are carditis, arthritis, chorea, erythema marginatum, and subcutaneous nodules. The minor criteria include fever, arthralgia (cannot use if arthritis was used as a major criteria), previous rheumatic fever, acute-phase laboratory results, and prolonged P-R interval on ECG.

Pathological Findings
- SQ nodules have a characteristic histologic appearance.
- Pericardial effusion
- Fibrinous pericardium

DIFFERENTIAL DIAGNOSIS
- Lupus
- Juvenile rheumatoid arthritis
- Infectious arthritis
- Viral myocarditis
- Innocent murmurs
- Tourette syndrome
- Kawasaki syndrome

TREATMENT

INITIAL STABILIZATION
- Outpatient care
- Initial hospitalization may be helpful to diagnose and establish stability of the patient.

GENERAL MEASURES
- Mainstay of therapy is anti-inflammatory.
- Patients with arthritis: Therapy for relief of pain
- Patients with carditis: Suppress inflammation.
- Patients with arrhythmias: Treat with appropriate agents.

Diet
- Regular diet
- Low-sodium diet initially, if the patient has carditis

Activity
- Initial bed rest with activity increasing gradually as tolerated
- Advance activity cautiously if evidence of carditis is present.

MEDICATION (DRUGS)

First Line

- If patient has carditis with cardiomegaly, start prednisone, 2 mg/kg/d (maximum 60 mg) for 2 weeks, then taper over 2 weeks. Start aspirin at beginning of steroid taper, and continue aspirin for 6 weeks.
- If no cardiomegaly, start aspirin 60 mg/kg/d (to maintain salicylate level of 20–25 g/mL), 75–100 mg/kg/d for children, for 4–6 weeks.
- Treat initially with penicillin as if active streptococcal infection is present, then begin prophylaxis (see "Follow-up").
- Chorea may require treatment with haloperidol.
- Contraindications: Specific drug allergies
- Precautions
  – Usual steroid side effects
  – Extrapyramidal effects can occur with haloperidol.
- Significant possible interactions: Refer to the manufacturer's profile of each drug.

Second Line

- Sulfadiazine may be used for prophylaxis in penicillin-allergic patients. Patients who take sulfadiazine should take at least 2 L of fluid daily to guard against sulfadiazine crystalluria.
- Naproxen at a dose of 15–20 mg/kg/d, divided b.i.d., for children, has been found to be safe and effective in rheumatic fever and has fewer adverse reactions than aspirin.

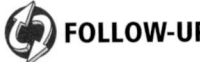 **FOLLOW-UP**

ALERT

Pregnancy Considerations
Residual valvular disease may be exacerbated by pregnancy. Refer pregnant patient to cardiologist for assistance in management.

PROGNOSIS

Sequelae is limited to the heart and depends on severity of carditis during an acute attack.

COMPLICATIONS

- Subsequent attacks of acute rheumatic fever secondary to streptococcal reinfection
- Carditis
- Mitral stenosis
- CHF

PATIENT MONITORING

Each week initially, then every 6 months

REFERENCES

1. Behrman RE, Kliegman RM, Jenson HB, eds. *Nelson Textbook of Pediatrics*, 17th ed. Philadelphia: WB Saunders, 2003.
2. daSilva NA. Acute rheumatic fever: Still a challenge. *Rheumatol Dis Clin North Am*. 1997;23:545–568.
3. Ferrieri P. Acute rheumatic fever: The come-back of a disappearing disease. *Am J Dis Child*. 1987;141: 725–727.
4. Hashkes PJ, et al. Pediatric Rheumatology Study Group of Israel. Naproxen as an alternative to aspirin for the treatment of arthritis of rheumatic fever: A randomized trial. *J Pediatr*. 2003;143: 399–401.
5. Milojevic DS, Ilowite NT. Treatment of rheumatic diseases in children: Special considerations. *Rheum Dis Clin North Am*. 2002;28:461–482.
6. Quinn RW. Comprehensive review of morbidity and mortality trends for rheumatic fever, streptococcal disease, and scarlet fever: The decline of rheumatic fever. *Rev Infect Dis*. 1989;11:928–953.

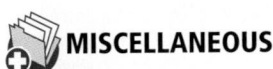 **MISCELLANEOUS**

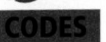

ICD9-CM
390 Rheumatic fever without mention of heart involvement

PATIENT TEACHING

Patient information is available from the American Heart Association (www.americanheart.org)

RHINITIS, ALLERGIC

Stanley Fineman, MD
Frank J. Domino, MD

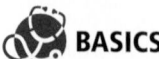 **BASICS**

DESCRIPTION

- Immediate and delayed reactions to airborne allergens, beginning with the presence of specific antigen-responsive IgE antibody receptors on mast cells of the nasal mucosa
- An antigen–antibody reaction initiates a cascade of events in the mast cell culminating in its degranulation and production of a melange of inflammatory mediators including histamine, heparin, leukotrienes, prostaglandins, proteases, and platelet-activating factor.
- An immediate symptomatic response occurs followed by a more prolonged, persistent late-phase reaction. This involves the infiltration into the reactive region of eosinophils, neutrophils, basophils, and mononuclear cells.
- Allergies may be seasonal or perennial, depending on the patient's response to the offending antigens.
- Seasonal responses usually are associated with pollen sensitivity to grasses, trees, and/or weeds.
- Perennial responses occur with house dust mites, mold antigens, and animal products (i.e., dander).
- System(s) Affected: Hemic/Lymphatic/Immunologic; Pulmonary; Dermatologic/Exocrine
- Synonym(s): Hay fever, Rose fever, Pollinosis, and IgE-mediated rhinitis

ALERT

Geriatric Considerations
- Increased medication side effects are possible.
- Number and specific types of allergens causing symptoms may change.
- IgE-mediated symptoms may decrease by 4th–5th decade, but nonallergic triggers may cause similar symptoms, particularly atrophic rhinitis.

Pediatric Considerations
- Consider allergy with persistent rhinitis.
- Family involvement is important.
- Environmental control requires a cooperative effort and may include dust mite–proof mattress encasements, carpet and drape removal, removal of plants in the home, pet control, avoidance of smoke, and other measures.

Pregnancy Considerations
Physiologic changes of pregnancy may aggravate all types of rhinitis including allergic, vasomotor, nonallergic rhinitis with eosinophilia and chronic irritable airways. This frequently presents in the 2nd trimester.

GENERAL PREVENTION

- Avoidance: Most patients with inhalant allergies cannot control symptoms completely by solely avoiding the allergy source.
- Air conditioning and limited outside exposure during allergy season are helpful.
- Instructions as to the best housekeeping tactics and control for dust mites in patients sensitive to this allergen are helpful.
- Exposure to all animal contacts should be minimized. Discourage house pets.
- Avoid environmental irritants (smoke and fumes).
- HEPA air cleaners may be helpful.
- Use of allergy control covers, especially on mattresses and pillows, is of unclear benefit.

EPIDEMIOLOGY

- Onset usually in 1st 4 decades with tendency declining with advancing age
- No gender predilection

Prevalence
~10–25% of the US population is affected.

RISK FACTORS

- Family history
- Repeated exposure to offending antigen
- Exposure to multiple offending allergens
- Presence of other allergies (e.g., atopic dermatitis, asthma, urticaria)

Genetics
Complex, but strong genetic predilection present

ETIOLOGY
Inhalant allergens
- Perennial: House dust mites, molds, animal dander, cockroach detritus.
- Seasonal: Tree, grass, and weed pollens
- Occupational: Latex, plant products (e.g., baking flour), sensitizing chemicals

ASSOCIATED CONDITIONS
Other IgE-mediated conditions (e.g., asthma and atopic dermatitis)

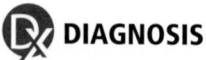 **DIAGNOSIS**

SIGNS AND SYMPTOMS
- Nasal stuffiness and congestion
- Rhinorrhea usually with clear discharge
- Pruritus of nose, eyes, and palate
- Sneezing, often paroxysmal
- Injection, itching, and watering of eyes
- Postnasal drainage
- Mouth breathing
- Fatigue or malaise
- Dark circles under eyes, "allergic shiners"
- Transverse nasal crease from rubbing nose upward typically seen in children

TESTS

Lab
- CBC with differential may show a slight increase in eosinophils.
- Nasal probe smear for eosinophils
- Increased IgE level. Determine specific allergen sensitivity with allergen skin testing or radioallergosorbent testing (poor PPV)
- Drugs that may alter lab results
  - Corticosteroids will palliate eosinophilia.
  - Antihistamines inhibit skin testing response.
- Disorders that may alter lab results
  - Secondary infections may alter differential.
  - Parasitic infection shows greater eosinophilia.

Imaging
Sinus films when indicated. Check for complete opacity, fluid level, and mucosal thickening. Sinus imaging with CT may be preferable.

Diagnostic Procedures/Surgery
- Appropriate diagnostic allergen prick test kits are used to determine agent for immunotherapy, but of limited diagnostic value (PPV = 60%).
- Skin tests using suspected antigens produce a positive reaction by inducing an expanding wheal-and-flare reaction. Special training is recommended, and available treatment for anaphylaxis is mandatory
  - Prick or puncture: Superficial injury to epidermis with application of test antigen
  - Intradermal: Introduction of diluted material between layers of skin raising a 4 mm wheal using a 25- or 27-gauge needle
- Radioallergosorbent test
  - More expensive and used especially in cases where skin testing not practical (e.g., in atopic dermatitis and dermatographia)
- Audiometry
  - For deficits and baseline evaluation
  - Rhinoscopy: Useful to visualize intranasal anatomy, posterior pharyngeal structures including adenoids, polyps, and larynx

Pathological Findings
- Nasal washing/scraping
  - Eosinophils predominate
  - Basophils
  - May see mast cells
- Nasal mucosa
  - Submucosal edema but without destruction
  - Eosinophilic infiltration
  - Granulocytes to lesser extent
  - Increased amount of tissue water with poor staining of ground substance
  - Congested mucous glands and goblet cells

DIFFERENTIAL DIAGNOSIS
- Nonallergic rhinitis with eosinophilia syndrome (NARES)
- Vasomotor rhinitis
- Chronic sinusitis
- IgA deficiency with recurrent sinusitis
- Nasal polyps and tumor
- Reactive rhinitis of recumbency
- Cribriform plate defect with cerebrospinal fluid leakage (test watery discharge for glucose)
- Foreign body
- Hormonal: Pregnancy, thyroid, oral contraceptives
- Medications
  - Rebound effect associated with continued use of topical decongestant drops and sprays
  - Aldosterone-converting enzyme inhibitors
  - Aspirin use in patients with aspirin sensitivity
- Septal/anatomic obstruction

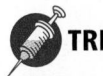

TREATMENT

GENERAL MEASURES
- Limit exposure to offending allergen.
- Try to establish specific cause(s) by history.
- Treatment determined by severity of disease
- Allergen immunotherapy (allergy shots/desensitization)
  - Usually reserved for patients with allergic rhinitis when symptoms are uncontrollable with medical therapy or have a comorbidity such as asthma or chronic sinusitis.
  - Specific allergen extract is injected SC in increasing doses to induce tolerance.
  - Repeat allergen skin testing is not helpful.

Diet
No special diet unless concomitant food reactions are suspected and evaluated. Some patients with severe sensitivity to seasonal pollens may have oral allergy syndrome, which is associated with itching in mouth with ingestion of fresh fruits, which may cross-react with the sensitizing allergen.

Activity
No specific restrictions; emphasize avoiding activity where exposure to the allergen is likely.

MEDICATION (DRUGS)

First Line
- Most patients present because of inability to control symptoms with avoidance or with OTC medications. Antihistamines are 1st-line therapy. Topical nasal corticosteroids are 2nd-line, but should be used in patients with more severe nasal symptoms. Consider immunotherapy when usual pharmaceutical therapy fails or in patients with comorbidities or complications.
- Antihistamines (H_1 antagonists)
- 1st-generation: Side effects include sedation, performance impairment, anticholinergic effects. Includes 5 major classes
  - Ethanolamines: Diphenhydramine (Benadryl), clemastine (Tavist)
  - Alkylamine: Chlorpheniramine, brompheniramine
  - Ethylenediamines: Tripelennamine (PBZ)
  - Piperazines: Hydroxyzine (Atarax)
  - Phenothiazines: Promethazine (Phenergan), methdilazine (Tacaryl)
- 2nd-generation (considered nonsedating)
  - Loratadine 10 mg/d (Claritin)
  - Desloratadine 5 mg/d (Clarinex)
  - Fexofenadine 60 mg b.i.d. (Allegra)
  - Cetirizine 10 mg/d (Zyrtec)
  - Intranasal: Azelastine 2 P/nostril b.i.d. (Astelin)
- Decongestants
  - Oral (e.g., pseudoephedrine)
  - Topical drops or sprays (e.g., phenylephrine)
  - Topical ophthalmic agents for conjunctival itching and watering. These may include mast cell stabilizers or antihistamines or products that have dual action, such as antihistamine and mast cell stabilizer activity.
- Mast cell stabilizers
  - Cromolyn (NasalCrom)
  - Olopatadine (Patanol), azelastine (Optivar) cromolyn (Opticrom)
- Leukotriene antagonist
  - Montelukast (Singulair)
- Steroids
- Intranasal (effective for both nasal and systemic symptoms)
  - Beclomethasone (Beconase, Vancenase AQ)
  - Flunisolide (Nasalide, Nasarel)
  - Triamcinolone (Nasacort)
  - Budesonide (Rhinocort)
  - Mometasone (Nasonex)
  - Fluticasone (Flonase)
- Systemic steroids should only be considered in urgent cases and only for short-term use.
- Contraindications
  - Antihistamines may precipitate urinary retention in men with prostatism or BPH.
  - Topical decongestants, if "rebound" phenomenon
  - Discourage oral decongestants if hypertension or cardiac arrhythmia
- Precautions: 1st-generation antihistamines are associated with somnolence and may impair performance, particularly if operating machinery.
- Significant possible interactions: Refer to the manufacturer's literature.

Second Line
Combinations with decongestants

SURGERY
Nasal surgery may be necessary when septal deviation is significant enough to interfere with medications or if nasal polys are present.

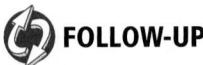

FOLLOW-UP

PROGNOSIS
- Acceptable control of symptoms is the goal.
- Treatment is helpful to reduce the risk of comorbidities such as sinusitis and asthma.
- Immune system changes over time often are associated with lessening of rhinitis symptoms.

COMPLICATIONS
- Secondary infection
- Otitis media
- Sinusitis
- Epistaxis
- Nasopharyngeal lymphoid hyperplasia
- Airway hyper-reactivity with allergen exposure
- Asthma
- Facial changes (see "Signs and Symptoms")

PATIENT MONITORING
Initiation of patient education is critical.

REFERENCES
1. Dykewicz MS. Rhinitis and sinusitis. *J Allergy Clin Immunol*. 2003;111(Suppl. 2):S520–S529.
2. Dykewicz MS, et al. Diagnosis and management of rhinitis: Complete Guidelines of the Joint Task Force on Practice Parameters in Allergy, Asthma, and Immunology. American Academy of Allergy, Asthma, and Immunology. *Ann Allergy Asthma Immunol*. 1998;81:478–518.
3. Bousquet J, et al. *J Allergy Clin Immunol*. 2001;108:147s–334s.
4. Wilson AM, O'Byrne PM, Parameswaran K. Leukotriene receptor antagonists for allergic rhinitis: A systematic review and meta-analysis. *Am J Med*. 2004;116:338–344.
5. Plaut M, Valentine M. Allergic rhinitis. *N Engl J Med*. 2005;353:1934–1944.

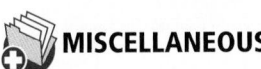

MISCELLANEOUS

See also: Conjunctivitis, acute

CODES

ICD9-CM
477.9 Allergic rhinitis, cause unspecified

PATIENT TEACHING
- Printed material available from many sources, including: Asthma & Allergy Foundation of America, 1717 Massachusetts Ave., Suite 305, Washington, DC 20036; (800) 7-ASTHMA; web site www.aafa.org.
- Other helpful information available: www.acaai.org and www.aaaai.org

 See Corresponding Diagnostic Algorithm

 See Patient Handout on CD

ROCKY MOUNTAIN SPOTTED FEVER

Brock D. Lutz, MD
Ronald A. Greenfield, MD

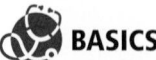 **BASICS**

DESCRIPTION
Rocky Mountain spotted fever (RMSF) is an acute, potentially fatal febrile illness caused by *Rickettsia rickettsii* and transmitted by tick bite.

- System(s) Affected: Cardiovascular; Musculoskeletal; Nervous; Skin/Exocrine

GENERAL PREVENTION
People who go into tick-infested areas can take measures to prevent infection.

- Occlusive clothing should be worn and insect repellants applied.
- After possible exposure, all body areas should be carefully inspected for ticks, especially legs, groin, external genitalia, and belt lines. Likelihood of infection increases with the duration of tick attachment.
- Ticks should be removed from humans or animals with caution; gloves should be worn or instruments used to minimize direct contact. Place a drop of oil, alcohol, gasoline, or kerosene on the tick first. Hands should be washed thoroughly after tick removal.

EPIDEMIOLOGY
- Predominant age: Highest incidences occur among children and young adults, primarily owing to environmental exposure patterns. All ages are susceptible.
- Predominant sex: Male > Female (owing to more frequent outdoor activity by males).
- Peak incidence is in late spring and summer.

Incidence
- In the US, 0.22 per 100,000 persons per year. 56% of cases are reported from 5 states: North Carolina, South Carolina, Tennessee, Oklahoma, and Arkansas.
- Also endemic in several countries in Central and South America

RISK FACTORS
- History of tick bite in preceding 14 days (60%)
- Outdoor activity, particularly although not exclusively during spring and summer months in an endemic area
- Contact with outdoor pets or wild animals
- Similar illness in family members, coworkers, or pets

PATHOPHYSIOLOGY
The primary pathology is a vasculitis owing to direct endothelial cell invasion by rickettsiae. This leads to life-threatening damage to brain, lungs, and other viscera.

ETIOLOGY
- RMSF is caused by *R. rickettsii*, which is transmitted by the bite of ticks (principally, *Dermacentor andersoni* or *Dermacentor variabilis* in the US).
- Rarely, RMSF is caused by direct inoculation of tick blood into open wounds or conjunctivae.

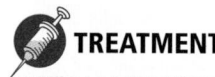 **DIAGNOSIS**

SIGNS AND SYMPTOMS
The cardinal clinical features are headache, fever, and a centripetal rash (involves the palms and soles and spreads centrally to arms, legs, and trunk), which is often petechial.

- Patients do not typically have this characteristic rash at initial presentation, but may have a maculopapular rash.
- Fever (100%)
- Rash (macular, maculopapular, petechial; 90–100%)
- Headache (65%)
- Rash (petechial; 50%)
- Headache, fever, rash (50–60%)
- Other neuropsychiatric symptoms (40–50%)
- Nausea, vomiting (30–50%)
- Headache, fever, petechial rash (33%)
- Abdominal pain (30%)
- Myalgias (30%)
- Hepatosplenomegaly (30%)
- Lymphadenopathy (25%)
- Arthralgias (10%)
- Cough (15%)
- CNS dysfunction (stupor, confusion, coma, focal abnormalities; 10–30%)

TESTS
Lab
- Specific laboratory diagnosis
  - Serum indirect fluorescent antibody (IFA): 4-fold increase or solitary titer >1:64.
  - Polymerase chain reaction testing by CDC
- Nonspecific laboratory changes
  - Thrombocytopenia
  - White blood cell (WBC) count: Normal, increased, or decreased
  - Anemia (mild)
  - Hyponatremia (usually mild)
  - CSF protein and WBC modestly elevated (lymphocytic predominance), glucose usually normal
  - Prolonged prothrombin time (PT) and partial thromboplastin time (PTT); decreased fibrinogen; elevated fibrin degradation products (FDPs; uncommon)
- Drugs that may alter lab results: Early treatment may blunt antibody response.

Imaging
Other than nonspecific pneumonic infiltrates, which may be seen on routine chest radiograph, imaging procedures are rarely helpful.

Diagnostic Procedures/Surgery
- Tissue (primarily skin) biopsy can be helpful if rapid DFA or nucleic acid amplification testing or electron microscopy is available.
- Diagnosis is usually presumptive and based on a compatible syndrome in a patient with exposure history in an endemic area.
  - Confirmation is obtained by subsequent serology.

Pathological Findings
- The principle pathologic abnormality is a systemic vasculitis.
- Rickettsiae may be demonstrated within endothelial cells by DFA, PCR, or electron microscopy.
- Petechiae owing to the vasculitis may be seen on various organ surfaces (e.g., liver, brain, epicardium).
- Secondary thromboses and tissue necrosis may be seen.

DIFFERENTIAL DIAGNOSIS
- Viral exanthems (e.g., measles, rubella)
- Meningoencephalitis (viral meningitis or encephalitis, bacterial meningitis)
- Typhus
- Rickettsialpox
- Ehrlichiosis
- Lyme disease
- Meningococcemia
- Leptospirosis

TREATMENT

GENERAL MEASURES
Treatment should be initiated on the basis of clinical diagnosis or skin biopsy and should not be delayed for serologic confirmation or development of the characteristic rash.

- Monitor patient's arterial oxygen saturation. Oxygen therapy and assisted ventilation for pulmonary complications, if necessary
- Good mouth care
- Blood transfusions for anemia
- Turn bed-confined patient frequently.
- Monitor patient carefully for signs of renal failure.

Diet
- Critically ill patients will require IV fluids and may require parenteral nutrition.
- In others, small frequent meals may be necessary to maintain nutritional levels.

Activity
Bed rest until symptoms subside

MEDICATION (DRUGS)

First Line

- Doxycycline is the treatment of choice in children and adults. (A)[3]
  - For adults, doxycycline 200 mg PO initially, followed by 100 mg PO b.i.d. for 5–7 days including 3 days after fever resolution; same dosage IV; 100 mg q24h in renal failure
  - For children <100 lbs, 2.2 mg/kg/dose given q12h
- Pregnant women
  - Brief course of doxycycline is appropriate for this life-threatening infection if suspicion is high, despite potential risk to fetal bones and teeth.
  - Chloramphenicol may be preferred during the 1st 2 trimesters but should be avoided in the 3rd trimester because of potential grey baby syndrome.
- Precautions
  - Patients taking doxycycline should minimize sun exposure to avoid photosensitization.
  - Chloramphenicol may rarely cause idiosyncratic, nonreversible, aplastic anemia.
  - Doxycycline may cause staining of permanent teeth when given to children <9 years of age. This risk appears to be minimal if no more than 5 courses of therapy are administered prior to age 9.
- Significant possible interactions
  - Absorption of doxycycline may be inhibited if it is ingested with milk products, iron preparations, or antacids containing aluminum or magnesium.

Second Line

- Chloramphenicol 20 mg/kg IV q6h (4 g/d maximum); same dose in renal failure (oral chloramphenicol is not available in the US). Chloramphenicol may be less effective than doxycycline.
- Modern fluoroquinolones have in vitro activity against *R. rickettsii* and have been evaluated in other spotted fever group rickettsioses but have not been clinically evaluated in Rocky Mountain spotted fever.

ALERT

Pregnancy Considerations

- See above for special therapeutic considerations.
- Transplacental transmission of infection has not been demonstrated.

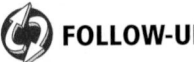 **FOLLOW-UP**

DISPOSITION

- Patients with the full clinical presentation or who are moderately ill should usually be hospitalized.
- Patients with mild disease are treated presumptively as outpatients. Close follow-up is important in identifying complications.

Admission Criteria

- Severe illness
- Obtundation
- Nausea/vomiting precluding oral antibiotic therapy

PROGNOSIS

- When treated promptly, the usual prognosis is excellent with resolution of symptoms over several days and no sequelae.
- Mortality is rare with prompt institution of appropriate therapy.
- If complications develop (see "Complications"), the course may be more severe and long-term sequelae may be present, particularly neurologic sequelae.

ALERT

Geriatric Considerations

Mortality risk is higher in the elderly.

COMPLICATIONS

- Encephalopathy, usually transient (30–40%)
- Seizures, focal neurological signs (10%)
- Renal insufficiency (10%)
- Hepatitis (10%)
- CHF (5%)
- Respiratory failure (5%)

PATIENT MONITORING

- If patients are not hospitalized, they should be seen every 2–3 days until symptoms have fully resolved.
- CBC, creatinine, and electrolytes should be monitored.

REFERENCES

1. Archibald LK, Sexton DJ. Long-term sequelae of Rocky Mountain spotted fever. *Clin Infect Dis.* 1995;20:1122–1125.
2. Buckingham SC. Rocky Mountain spotted fever: A review for the pediatrician. *Pediatr Ann.* 2002;3:163–168.
3. Centers for Disease Control and Prevention. Diagnosis and management of tick-borne rickettsial diseases: Rocky Mountain spotted fever, ehrlichiosis and anaplasmosis—United States. A practical guide for physicians and other health-care and public health professionals. *Morbid Mortal Weekly Rep.* 2006;55(No. RR-4):1–29.
4. Masters EG, et al. Rocky Mountain spotted fever. *Arch Intern Med.* 2003;163:769–774.
5. Sexton DJ, Kaye KS. Rocky Mountain spotted fever. *Med Clin North Am.* 2002;86:351–360.
6. Stallings SP. Rocky Mountain spotted fever and pregnancy: A case report and review of the literature. *Obstet Gynecol Surv.* 2001;56:37–42.

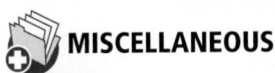 **MISCELLANEOUS**

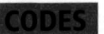 **CODES**

ICD9-CM

082.0 Spotted fevers

PATIENT TEACHING

Prevention

With early appropriate therapy, antibody response may be blunted and recurrent infection has been reported. Patients should therefore be educated about general preventive measures presented above.

 See Corresponding Diagnostic Algorithm

ROSEOLA

Jeffery T. Kirchner, DO

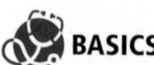 **BASICS**

DESCRIPTION

Acute disease of infants or very young children. Characteristically, it causes 1st a high fever, followed by the appearance of an eruption (appearance of which is similar to that of measles) simultaneously with, or following, defervescence. Transmission now believed to be via contact of salivary secretions from adults shedding HHV-6. Incubation period of ~5–15 days

- System(s) Affected: Endocrine/Metabolic; Skin/Exocrine
- Synonym(s): Exanthem subitum; Pseudorubella; Sixth disease

ALERT

Pediatric Considerations

A disease of infants and very young children

GENERAL PREVENTION

None

EPIDEMIOLOGY

- Predominant age: Infants and very young children (6 months to 3 years); 90% before age 2 years (1,2)
- Predominant sex: Male = Female

Incidence

- Unknown
- More likely to occur in spring and fall

Prevalence

Unknown

RISK FACTORS

- Day care center
- Exposure to infected infant

Genetics

No known genetic pattern

ETIOLOGY

A communicable DNA virus: human herpesvirus-6B (HHV-6B) (1,3)

DIAGNOSIS

SIGNS AND SYMPTOMS (2,4,5)

- Abrupt fever without apparent cause (39.4–40.5°C [103–105°F]) for 3–5 days
- Sudden drop of fever
  - As fever disappears, skin rash begins (lasts hours to days).
- Anorexia
- Irritability
- Inflammation of the tympanic membranes
- Listlessness
- Does not appear seriously ill
- Maculopapular, nonpruritic rash, first appearing on the trunk, that blanches on pressure
- Rash appears as very slightly elevated, rose-pink papules that appear profusely on trunk, arms, and neck; mild on face and legs.
- Rash fades within a few hours to 2 days.
- Febrile convulsions during height of fever (10–15%)
- Lymphadenopathy in cervical and posterior auricular regions
- Spleen enlarged (uncommon)

TESTS

Lab

- CBC
  - Leukopenia with relative lymphocytosis
  - Thrombocytopenia
- Urinalysis
- Immunoglobulin M (IgM), IgG (4-fold increase IgG for diagnosis) for HHV-6
- Polymerase chain reaction (PCR; serum) for HHV-6–qualitative and –quantitative can be performed.
- Blood culture for HHV-6

Imaging

Chest radiograph: Negative findings

Diagnostic Procedures/Surgery

- Careful physical examination
- Roseola should be suspected if it is known to be in the community and the child presents with a high temperature.
- HHV-6-IgM: Diagnostic for acute infection
- HHV-6 by PCR found in CSF and saliva

Pathological Findings

None

DIFFERENTIAL DIAGNOSIS

- Enterovirus infection
- Fifth disease
- Rubella
- Measles
- Sepsis
- Otitis media
- Urinary tract infection
- Meningitis
- Drug eruption

TREATMENT

GENERAL MEASURES

- Symptomatic
- Tap water baths to cool excess temperature elevation
- Lightweight clothing
- Maintain normal room temperature.

Diet

Encourage fluids.

Activity

Rest until rash appears and fever breaks.

 **MEDICATION (DRUGS)**

First Line

- Antipyretics for excessively high fever. Avoid aspirin. Instead, use acetaminophen, 10–15 mg/kg q4h to a maximum of 2.6 g per 24-hour period. (Aspirin may enhance the risk of Reye syndrome). (1)[C]
- Phenobarbital may be considered for seizure. (1)[C]

Second Line

No clinical trials evaluating antiviral agents, but in vitro data do exist.

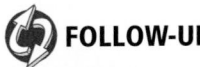 **FOLLOW-UP**

DISPOSITION

Outpatient care

PROGNOSIS

- Course: Acute, benign, complete recovery without sequelae
- 1 attack usually confers permanent immunity.
- Reactivation in immunocompromised patients is possible.

COMPLICATIONS

- Febrile seizures
- Encephalitis (rare)
- Meningitis
- Hepatitis

PATIENT MONITORING

None after typical rash appears

REFERENCES

1. Leach CT. Human herpesvirus-6 and -7 infections in children: Agents of roseola and other syndromes. *Curr Opin Pediatr*. 2000;12:269–274.
2. Zerr DM. A population-based study of primary human herpes virus 6 infection. *N Engl J Med*. 2005;353:768–776.
3. Caserta MT, Mock DJ, Dewhurst S. Human herpesvirus 6. *Clin Infect Dis*. 2001;33:829–833.
4. Asano Y, et al. Clinical features of infants with primary human herpesvirus 6 (roseola infantum). *Pediatrics*. 1994;93:104–108.
5. Dockrell DH, Smith TF, Paya CV. Human herpesvirus 6. *Mayo Clin Proc*. 1999;74:163–170.

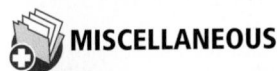 **MISCELLANEOUS**

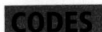 **CODES**

ICD9-CM

057.8 Other specified viral exanthemata

PATIENT TEACHING

- Infection is self-limiting.
- If seizures occur, they will not cause brain damage and will cease after fever subsides.

ROTATOR CUFF (IMPINGEMENT) SYNDROME

Justin Dorfman, DO
Gregory R. Czarnecki, DO
John Herbert Stevenson, MD

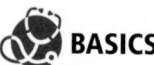 **BASICS**

DESCRIPTION

Impingement syndrome is the result of the rotator cuff (primarily supraspinatus) or biceps tendon being impinged or irritated along the undersurface of the acromion and coracoacromial ligament. This results in shoulder pain and decreased range of motion. There are 3 stages of impingement syndrome

- Stage I: Inflammation and/or tendonosis of the underlying tendons
- Stage II: Partial rotator cuff tear along with underlying thickening or fibrosis of surrounding structures
- Stage III: Full thickness rotator cuff tendon tear

GENERAL PREVENTION

- Proper throwing and lifting techniques
- Well-developed and strong rotator cuff and scapula stabilizer muscles

EPIDEMIOLOGY

- Predominant age: >25
  - Most common in middle-aged people,
- Predominant sex: Males > Females
- Shoulder pain 3rd most common musculoskeletal complaint in the general population
- 50–70% of shoulder pain in adults >25 due to impingement syndrome (5)[B]
- Shoulder pain in people <25 years old usually due to trauma or underlying shoulder instability (5)[B]

Incidence

- The incidence of shoulder pain is 6.6–25 cases per 1,000 patients; peak incidence in the 4th through 6th decades (5)[B]
- Age is greatest predictor of impingement syndrome stage (5)[B]
  - Age 25–40 most frequently Stage I impingement (tendonosis/tendonitis)
  - Age 40–60 most frequently Stage II impingement (partial tear of rotator cuff tendon)
  - Age >60 most frequently Stage II impingement (partial tear of rotator cuff tendon)

Prevalence

In adults 50–70% of shoulder pain >25 due to impingement syndrome (5)[B]

RISK FACTORS

- Repetitive overhead motions, including throwing
- Multidirectional instability of the shoulder
- Hooked acromion
- AC spurring
- Thickened coricoacromial ligament
- Shoulder trauma
- Os acromiale

PATHOPHYSIOLOGY

The rotator cuff tendons run between the coracoacromial arch and the greater tubercle of the humeral head. The rotator cuff tendons (most commonly supraspinatus) and subacromial bursa are compressed and inflamed by the anterior aspect of the acromion, coracoacromial ligament, and humeral head with repetitive overhead arm activity. As the impingement advances, thinning of the rotator cuff may result until a partial or complete tear results.

ETIOLOGY

- Repetitive overhead activities (throwing, swimming, etc.) and shoulder instability can result in recurrent compression and irritation of the tendon and subacromial bursa.
- Direct trauma can compress the humerus and the coracoacromial arch resulting in inflammation of the subacromial bursa and rotator cuff tendons.
- Narrowing of the subacromial space secondary to AC joint/spurring, thickened coracoacromial ligament, or sloped acromion are additional etiologies.
- Acute rotator cuff tears can create impingement syndrome as the humeral head depressors (rotator cuff muscles) fail to keep the humeral head from riding up into the coracoacromial arch.

DIAGNOSIS

SIGNS AND SYMPTOMS

- Patients will usually complain of anterolateral shoulder pain worse with overhead activities.
- Pain may present at night and wake from sleep.
- Pain may radiate down to the elbow.
- May complain of weakness or stiffness
- Associated clicking or popping may be felt with certain movements in the shoulder.

History

Symptoms are usually insidious in onset with gradual worsening over time. Many patients do not present until significant impedance in their activities of daily living.

Physical Exam

- Painful arc with abduction between 60° and 120°
- Tenderness to palpation along biceps tendon and greater tuberosity of the humerus
- Decreased shoulder strength and/or pain with "Empty Can Test"
- Positive Impingement Tests (Neer's and/or Hawkins-Kennedy)
- Weakness with "Empty Can Test", external rotation, and positive impingement test associated with 98% chance rotator cuff tear (Stage II or III impingement syndrome) (5)[B]
- Positive drop arm test associated with 98% chance rotator cuff tear (Stage II or III impingement syndrome) (5)[B]
- Atrophy of the supraspinatus and infraspinatus may be observed late in disease.
- Evaluate C-spine and rule out cervical pathology.

TESTS

- Neer impingement sign is done by stabilizing the patient's scapula and with passive flexion of the arm until the patient reports pain or has full elevation.
- Hawkins-Kennedy impingement sign: The patient's arm is placed in 90° of forward flexion, the examiner stabilizes the scapula, and internally rotates the shoulder. Pain signifies a positive test.
- Drop arm test: Have the patient hold his/her arm at 90° of abduction (an inability to do this can represent rotator cuff tear).

Imaging

- X-ray may reveal osteophytes or hooked acromion. Include AP, axillary lateral, supraspinatus outlet views
- Ultrasound well validated but limited by operator experience and patient factors
- MRI to assess integrity of rotator cuff and possible source of impingement, bony and/or soft-tissue structures
- MR arthrogram increases sensitivity for detecting partial-thickness tears of the rotator cuff and labral pathology.

Diagnostic Procedures/Surgery

Lidocaine or bupivicaine can be injected into the subacromial space, and if a decrease in pain is elicited then impingement is the primary cause.

Pathological Findings

May have tendinosis, tendonitis, or tear of muscle/tendon

DIFFERENTIAL DIAGNOSIS

- Acromioclavicular arthritis
- Adhesive capsulitis
- Anterior shoulder instability
- Multidirectional instability
- Biceps or calcific tendonitis
- Cervical disc disease or herniation
- Glenohumeral arthritis
- Labral Injury
- Spinal or foraminal stenosis
- Suprascapular nerve entrapment
- Thoracic outlet syndrome

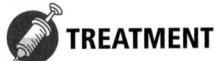 TREATMENT

INITIAL STABILIZATION
- Rest
- Avoidance of aggravating activities

GENERAL MEASURES
- Activity modification initially limiting overhead activities
- Range of motion exercises, rotator cuff and parascapular strengthening
- Ice/heat for symptom relief

Activity
As tolerated

SPECIAL THERAPY
Subacromial injection of corticosteroid for pain relief may allow progression with therapy. (1)[B]

Physical Therapy
- Mainstay of treatment, involves parascapular stabilization and rotator cuff strengthening
- Initial goal to restore range of motion, then gradual addition of strengthening followed by advancement to full activities.
- May take up to 6–12 weeks to note significant improvement

Complementary and Alternative Therapies
- ICE
- Ultrasound via physical therapy
- Iontopheresis via physical therapy
- Phonopheresis via physical therapy

 MEDICATION (DRUGS)

First Line
NSAIDs or other analgesic

Second Line
Corticosteroid (injection)

SURGERY
- Consider for failed conservative treatment or early for complete rotator cuff tear
- Subacromial decompression, open or arthroscopic
- Arthroscopy (or open) to assess integrity of rotator cuff and for definitive treatment

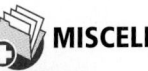 FOLLOW-UP

Follow-up every 1–2 months initially to assess progress, review goals, and encourage continued therapy.

DISPOSITION
Issues for Referral
Failure of conservative treatment, persistent pain, weakness, complete tear of rotator cuff

PROGNOSIS
- Variable
- Majority of patients improve with conservative management.

COMPLICATIONS
- Progression of injury
- Tendon retraction in complete rotator cuff tear

PATIENT MONITORING
Frequent follow-up to monitor progress

REFERENCES
1. Browning DG, Desai MM. Rotator cuff injuries and treatment. *Primary Care: Clinics in Office Practice.* 2004;31:807–829.
2. Gordski JM, Schwartz LH. Shoulder impingement presenting as neck pain. *J Bone Joint Surg.* 2003;85:635–638.
3. Lewis JS, Green A, Wright C. Subacromial impingement syndrome: The role of posture and muscle imbalance. *J Shoulder Elbow Surg.* 2005;14(4):385–392.
4. Park HB, et al. Diagnostic accuracy of clinical tests for the different degrees of subacromial impingement syndrome. *J Bone Joint Surg.* 2005;87:1446–1455.
5. Stevenson JH, Trojian T. Evaluation of shoulder pain. *J Fam Pract.* 2002;51(7):605–611.
6. Woodward TW, Best TM. The painful shoulder: Part II. Acute and chronic disorders. *Am Fam Physician.* 2000;61(11):3291–3300.

ADDITIONAL READING
Henrichs J, Stone D. Shoulder impingement syndrome. *Primary Care: Clinics in Office Practice.* 2004;31:789–805.

 MISCELLANEOUS

CODES

ICD9-CM
726.10 Disorders of bursae and tendons in shoulder region, unspecified

PATIENT TEACHING
- Symptoms often recur.
- Early presentation and treatment usually better prognosis

Activity
- Continue maintenance therapy, home or formal, for shoulder stabilization.
- Activity modification when symptoms flare including relative rest and limit of overhead activities.

Prevention
See "General Prevention."

 See Corresponding Diagnostic Algorithm

See Patient Handout on CD

ROUNDWORMS, INTESTINAL

James F. Broomfield, MD

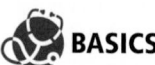 **BASICS**

DESCRIPTION
- Intestinal roundworms (nematodes) have adult stages infecting the intestinal tract of humans. Larval stages may exist elsewhere in the body. Except for *Trichinella spiralis*, which is encysted in muscle, egg and/or larval stages can be isolated from the intestinal canal.
- Nematodes parasitizing the intestinal tract of man
  - *Enterobius vermicularis* (pinworm)
  - *Trichuris trichiura* (whipworm)
  - *Ascaris lumbricoides* (large roundworm of man)
  - *Necator americanus* (hookworm)
  - *Ancylostoma duodenale* (hookworm)
  - *Strongyloides stercoralis*
  - *Trichostrongylus*
  - *T. spiralis* (trichinosis)
- System(s) Affected: Cardiovascular; Gastrointestinal; Musculoskeletal; Nervous; Pulmonary; Renal/Urologic

ALERT
Pediatric Considerations
Children commonly are infected.

GENERAL PREVENTION
Good hygiene and sanitation

EPIDEMIOLOGY
- Predominant age
  - All ages
  - Pinworm infestations more common in children
- Predominant sex: Male = Female

Incidence
- Incidence of intestinal obstruction with ascaris is 2/1,000.
- Incidence of ascariasis reportedly is decreasing in the US, presumably owing to improved sanitation.

Prevalence
- Up to 40% of children may have pinworms in their lifetime.
- Trichinella 4–20%
- Others mostly in southern regions

RISK FACTORS
- Low standard of hygiene
- Poor sanitation
- Human feces fertilizer

ETIOLOGY
- Ingestion of mature eggs in fecally contaminated food or drink
- Larval penetration of skin (hookworm)

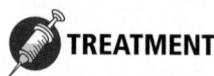 **DIAGNOSIS**

SIGNS AND SYMPTOMS
- Lung invasion
  - Fever
  - Cough
  - Blood-tinged sputum
  - Wheezing
  - Rales
  - Dyspnea
  - Substernal pain
  - Pulmonary consolidations
  - Eosinophilia
  - Urticaria
  - Asthma
  - Angioneurotic edema
  - Brain, kidney, eye, spinal cord, and so forth (rare)
- Intestinal invasion
  - May be asymptomatic (small number)
  - Abdominal pain (usually vague)
  - Abdominal cramps/colic
  - Diarrhea
  - Rarely vomiting
  - Occasionally constipation
- Muscle and other tissue invasion (trichinosis)
  - Myalgias
  - Fever
  - Edema and spasm
  - Periorbital and facial edema
  - Photophobia
  - Sweating
  - Conjunctivitis
  - Weakness or prostration
  - Pain on swallowing
  - Subconjunctival, retinal and nail hemorrhages
  - Rashes and formication
  - Encephalitis, myocarditis, nephritis
  - Pneumonia, meningitis, neuropathy

TESTS
Serologic tests not useful

Lab
- Based on characteristics of eggs or larvae in stool or adult worm, if passed
- Eosinophilia
- Larvae in sputum or adult worms seen on radiologic studies (uncommon)

Imaging
Ultrasound is useful in the diagnosis of ascariasis as cause of biliary tract disease.

Diagnostic Procedures/Surgery
- Stool exams
- Cellophane-tape impression for pinworms

Pathological Findings
Characteristic eggs/worms

DIFFERENTIAL DIAGNOSIS
- Pulmonary ascariasis with eosinophilia
  - Consider asthma, Löffler syndrome, eosinophilic pneumonia, systemic lupus erythematosus, Hodgkin disease, and other parasitic causes (tropical pulmonary eosinophilia, toxocariasis, strongyloidiasis, hookworm, paragonimiasis)
- Worm-induced gastrointestinal diseases
  - Consider other causes of pancreatitis, appendicitis, diverticulitis, duodenitis, esophagitis, and cholecystitis.
- Anemia/hypoproteinemia (hookworm)
  - Consider other etiology.
- Neurohelminthiasis
  - Consider other causes of central nervous system infection or mass lesion.

TREATMENT

GENERAL MEASURES
None other than medications to eradicate the worms

Diet
No special diet

Activity
No restrictions

MEDICATION (DRUGS)

First Line

- *E. vermicularis* (pinworm)
  - Mebendazole (Vermox) 100 mg single dose, albendazole 400 mg once, or pyrantel pamoate 11 mg/kg once (maximum of 1 g); repeat drug chosen after 2 weeks (all dosages for adult and children)
- *T. trichiura* (whipworm)
  - Mebendazole 100 mg b.i.d. for 3 days or 500 mg once (all dosages for adults and children)
- *A. lumbricoides* (large roundworm of man)
  - Mebendazole 100 mg b.i.d. for 3 days or 500 mg once, pyrantel pamoate 11 mg/kg once (maximum of 1 g; all dosages for adult and children), or albendazole 400 mg once
- *N. americanus* (hookworm), *Ancylostoma duodenale* (hookworm)
  - Mebendazole 100 mg b.i.d. for 3 days, pyrantel pamoate 11 mg/kg (maximum of 1 g) for 3 days (all dosages for adult and children), or albendazole 400 mg once
- *Trichostrongylus* species
  - Pyrantel pamoate 11 mg/kg once (maximum of 1 g) or mebendazole 100 mg b.i.d. for 3 days (all dosages for adult and children)
- *T. spiralis*
  - Mebendazole 200–400 mg t.i.d. for 3 days, then 400–500 mg t.i.d. for 10 days (adult dosage) plus steroids if severe symptoms (same dosages for adults and children)
- *S. stercoralis*
  - Thiabendazole 50 mg/kg/d in 2 doses (maximum of 3 g/d) for 2 days (adult and children), or ivermectin (Mectizan) 200 g/kg/d for 1–2 days (also effective against coexisting infection with *Ascaris*, *Trichuris*, and *Enterobius* species). Superior to benzimidazoles for this indication.
- Note: The US FDA may consider certain uses of these drugs investigational. Consult Medical Letter or appropriate drug reference.
- Contraindications: Refer to the manufacturer's profile of each drug.
- Precautions: Refer to the manufacturer's profile of each drug.
- Significant possible interactions: Refer to the manufacturer's profile of each drug.

Second Line

- *T. trichiura* (whipworm)
  - Albendazole 400 mg once (adults and children)
  - Note: albendazole investigational for this purpose
- *S. stercoralis*: Albendazole 400 mg/d for 3 days

ALERT

Pregnancy Considerations

- Benzimidazoles (mebendazole, albendazole, thiabendazole) should not be used.
- Ivermectin has shown little teratogenic potential and has provided an effective therapy, although benefits should clearly outweigh risks.

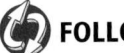 ## FOLLOW-UP

DISPOSITION

Outpatient care

PROGNOSIS

- Good for light to moderate infections
- Ascariasis should always be treated owing to the risk of migrating adult worms.

COMPLICATIONS

- Vomiting worms
- Cholangitis: Migration to common bile duct
- Pancreatitis: Migration to pancreatic duct
- Appendicitis: Migration to appendix
- Diverticulitis: Migration to diverticula
- Liver abscess
- Intestinal obstruction
- Volvulus
- Intussusception
- Bowel penetration
- Anemia (hookworm)
- Hypoproteinemia (hookworm)
- CNS infection (*Strongyloides* species)
- HIV-infected patients have a higher risk of dissemination (e.g., strongyloides) and "standard" treatment failure; therefore, they may require prolonged, repeated, or alternative therapies.

PATIENT MONITORING

Follow-up stool studies at 2 weeks and retreat if necessary.

REFERENCES

1. Drugs for parasitic infections. *Med Lett Drugs Ther*. 1998;40:1–12.
2. Hardman JG, et al., eds. Goodman & Gilman's: The Pharmacological Basis of Therapeutics, 10th ed. New York: McGraw-Hill, 2001.
3. Jensenius M. Hookworm disease: A differential diagnosis in iron deficiency anemia. *Tidsskrift for den Norske Laegeforening*. 1995;115:367–369.
4. Jong EC. Travel and Tropical Medicine Manual, 3rd ed. Philadelphia: WB Saunders, 2003.
5. Steffen R. Manual of Travel Medicine & Health, 2nd ed. Ontario, Canada: BC Decker, 2003.
6. Strickland GT. Hunter's Tropical Medicine, 8th ed. Philadelphia: WB Saunders, 2000.

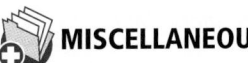 ## MISCELLANEOUS

See also: Intestinal parasites; Roundworms, tissue

CODES

ICD9-CM

127.0 Ascariasis

PATIENT TEACHING

Avoid fecally contaminated food, water, and soil.

ROUNDWORMS, TISSUE

Jeremy Golding, MD
James F. Broomfield, MD

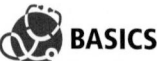 **BASICS**

DESCRIPTION
- Tissue roundworms (nematodes) affect humans when the adults or larval stages infect certain tissues.
- Filarial infections
  - *Wuchereria bancrofti* (bancroftian filariasis)
  - *Brugia malayi* (Malayan filariasis)
  - *Brugia timori* (Timorian filariasis)
  - *Loa loa* (eye worm)
  - *Onchocerca volvulus* (river blindness, onchocerciasis)
  - *Mansonella perstans*
  - *Mansonella ozzardi* (Ozzard filariasis)
  - *Mansonella streptocerca*
- Other tissue nematode infections
  - *Dracunculus medinensis* (guinea worm, dracunculosis)
  - *Ancylostoma braziliense* (cutaneous larva migrans, creeping eruption)
  - *Toxocara canis* or *T. cati* (visceral larva migrans, toxocariasis)
- System(s) Affected: Cardiovascular; Gastrointestinal; Hemic/Lymphatic/Immunologic; Musculoskeletal; Nervous; Renal/Urologic; Skin/Exocrine
- Synonym(s): Nematodes

GENERAL PREVENTION
- Avoid sources of infection (arthropod bites, rivers/streams, or contaminated soils).
- Diethylcarbamazine (DEC) 300 mg once weekly has been used successfully in Peace Corps workers for prophylaxis against *L. loa*.
- Prophylaxis with ivermectin is under investigation.
- Undertake public health activities, such as vector control

EPIDEMIOLOGY
- Predominant age: All ages, but children more commonly infected
  - Presence of onchocerciasis increases with age.
- Predominant sex: Male = Female
- Distribution
  - >300 million people are exposed to lymphatic filariasis in India and Southeast Asia; 30 million exposed to onchocerciasis
  - *W. bancrofti*: Tropics worldwide
  - *B. malayi*: Southeast Asia
  - *B. timori*: Indonesia
  - *L. loa*: Africa
  - *O. volvulus*: Africa and Central and South America
  - *M. perstans*: Africa and South America
  - *M. ozzardi*: Africa
  - *M. streptocerca*: Central and South America
  - *D. medinensis*: Africa and Asia
  - *A. braziliense*: tropics and subtropics worldwide
  - *T. canis/cati*: >50 countries worldwide, especially warmer tropical and subtropical regions

ALERT
Pediatric Considerations
Children commonly are infected.

Prevalence
- Visceral larva migrans
  - 4–30% seroprevalence has been reported.
  - In US, highest prevalence is in the coastal southeast
- Others: Unknown

RISK FACTORS
- Geographic exposure to arthropod vectors
- Fishermen or women washing clothes have increased risk of river blindness.
- Contact with infected soil in cutaneous larva migrans (hence plumber's itch, sandworm, duck hunter's itch)

PATHOPHYSIOLOGY
Infective larval stages are transmitted to humans by arthropod vectors or from the soil. Once in human tissue, worms mature over 6–12 months and survive as long as 15 years. Symptoms depend on tissue infected.

ETIOLOGY
Larvae introduced into human host by arthropod vector or infected soil

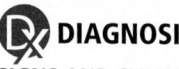 **DIAGNOSIS**

SIGNS AND SYMPTOMS
- Lymphatic filariasis (*W. bancrofti, B. malayi, B. timori*)
  - Inflammatory signs: Pain, tenderness, swelling, erythema
  - Filarial adenolymphangitis
  - Filarial orchitis
  - Funiculitis and epididymitis
  - Filarial and elephantoid fever
  - Filarial abscess
  - Obstructive signs: Lymph varices, lymph scrotum, hydrocele
  - Lymphedema and elephantiasis
  - Chyluria
  - Filarial hypereosinophilia (tropical pulmonary eosinophilia)
- Loiasis (*L. loa*)
  - Calabar swellings: Recurrent subcutaneous inflammation/swelling
  - Eye worm: Adult or larvae migrate under conjunctiva.
  - Eosinophilia (may be >70%)
  - Fever, irritability, urticaria, and pruritus
- Onchocerciasis (*O. volvulus*)
  - Dermatitis
  - Nodules
  - Lymphadenitis
  - Ocular changes: Intraocular microfilariae, punctate keratitis, sclerosing keratitis, anterior uveitis chorioretinitis, optic neuritis, optic atrophy, glaucoma, and blindness (river blindness)
- Other filarial syndromes (*M. ozzardi, M. perstans, M. streptocerca*)
  - Headaches, coldness, pruritus, and articular swelling/arthritis
  - Eosinophilia and vague allergic signs
  - Chronic dermatitis and macules can be confused with leprosy.
  - Lymphadenopathy

- Dracunculiasis (*D. medinensis*, guinea worm disease)
  - Allergic manifestations: Erythema, urticaria, pruritus, nausea, vomiting, giddiness, syncope, and occasional fever
  - Local lesions: Papule, sterile blister, ulceration, abscesses
  - Worm protrusion
- Toxocariasis (*T. canis/cati*, visceral or ocular larva migrans)
  - Eosinophilia
  - Visceral larva migrans
  - Ocular larva migrans
- Cutaneous larva migrans (*A. braziliense*, creeping eruption)
  - Itching and red papules
  - Serpiginous track
  - Edema and acute inflammation
  - Secondary infection
  - Very rare dissemination may occur

TESTS
Lab
- Examination of larvae or adult worms taken from the tissue
  - Characteristic microfilariae on blood smear
  - Eosinophilia
- Distinction of species by larval examination is challenging and may require expert examination.

Imaging
Occasional worms seen on radiographs

Diagnostic Procedures/Surgery
- Onchocerciasis is identified by skin snip/biopsy showing larvae
  - Skin snip, nodulectomy, slit-lamp exam, and Mazzotti test may be helpful in onchocerciasis.
- Microfilariae on blood smear or other body fluids, clinical observations, and serologies (e.g., enzyme-linked immunosorbent assay [ELISA])

Pathological Findings
Characteristic eggs/worms/larvae in tissue

DIFFERENTIAL DIAGNOSIS
- Other causes of tissue inflammation (i.e., lymphangitis, epididymitis, dermatitis, conjunctivitis, blisters, pleuritis, peritonitis, pericarditis, encephalitis, nephropathy, cardiomyopathy, and so forth)
- Nonfilarial causes of lymphangitis
  - Acute bacterial lymphangitis
  - Phlebitis
  - Unusual: Plague, anthrax, tuberculosis, lymphogranuloma inguinale
- Nonfilarial causes of lymphedema, chyluria, and elephantiasis
  - Infiltrative or granulomatous process: Tumor, fungus, tuberculosis, leprosy
  - Chronic venostasis or phlebitis
  - Cardiac insufficiency
  - Nutritional deficiencies
  - Hereditary (Milroy disease)
  - Lateritious soil obstructing lymphatics

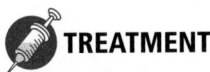

TREATMENT

GENERAL MEASURES
- Identify cause and treat accordingly.
- Best treatment: Direct removal of worm from tissue with caution not to break the worm
- Treat secondary infections.

Diet
No special diet

Activity
- No restrictions
- If edema is a problem, patient should elevate legs while sitting.

MEDICATION (DRUGS)

First Line
- Visceral larva migrans (*Toxocara* species)
  - Diethylcarbamazine (DEC) 6 mg/kg/d in 3 doses for 7–10 days for adults and children
- Cutaneous larva migrans (*A. braziliense*)
  - Ivermectin 200 μg/kg once
  - Albendazole 400 mg b.i.d. for 3 days
  - Topical thiabendazole 10% cream is a good alternative for young children or if oral therapy should be avoided.
- Filariasis (*W. bancrofti, B. malayi*)
  - DEC: Adult: day 1: 50 mg PO after meals; day 2: 50 mg t.i.d.; day 3: 100 mg t.i.d.; days 4–14: 6 mg/kg/d in 3 doses. Children; day 1: 1 mg/kg PO after meals; day 2: 1 mg/kg t.i.d.; day 3: 1–2 mg/kg t.i.d.; days 4–14: 6 mg/kg/d in 3 doses
- *L. loa*
  - DEC: As for filariasis except days 4–21: 9 mg/kg/d in 3 doses (adults and children)
  - Antihistamines and steroids: May be useful to reduce allergic response to disintegration of microfilaria.
- Onchocerciasis: Ivermectin (Mectizan)
  - 150 μg/kg PO once
  - If repeated every 6–12 months for adults and children, it can prevent blindness.
  - Treatment with ivermectin kills only the larval worms responsible for pathology, not the adult worms producing the larvae. Thus, treatment must be continued over a period of years until the adult worms die.
- *M. ozzardi*
  - Ivermectin 6 mg in single dose has been effective.
  - DEC is not effective.
- *M. perstans*
  - Mebendazole 100 mg b.i.d. for 30 days (approved drug, but considered investigational for this condition)

- *D. medinensis* (guinea worm)
  - Metronidazole 250 mg t.i.d. for 10 days for adult; 25 mg/kg/d (maximum, 750 mg/d) in 3 doses for 10 days for children
  - Metronidazole does not cure the infection, but rather, decreases the reaction to worm products.
  - Cure is achieved only through physical removal of the adult worm.
- Note: The US FDA may consider certain uses of these drugs investigational, and some may not be available in the US. Contact Parasitic Disease Drug Service (Parasitic Diseases Branch, Centers for Disease Control and Prevention [CDC], Atlanta, GA 30333; 404-488-4240) for information.
- Contraindications: Refer to the manufacturer's information.
- Precautions: Children, pregnancy, lactation
- Significant possible interactions: Refer to the manufacturer's profile of each drug.

Second Line
- Visceral larva migrans (*Toxocara* species)
  - Albendazole 400 mg b.i.d. for 3–5 days for adults and children or mebendazole 100–200 mg b.i.d. for 5 days for adults and children
- Filariasis (*W. bancrofti, B. malayi*)
  - Ivermectin (available from the CDC Drug Services; Tel. No.: 404-639-3670) 150 g/kg as a single dose is highly effective against microfilaria, but does not kill adult worms. More effective when combined with albendazole 400 mg
- Onchocerciasis
  - DEC has been used, but causes bad reactions, likely owing to rapid killing of the larval worms with sudden release of large amounts of worm antigens; thus, DEC is obsolete for this indication.
  - Suramin, a drug used in the treatment of trypanosomiasis, is effective at killing the adult worms, but severe side effects prevent its use for onchocerciasis.

SURGERY
Long-standing lymphatic filariasis owing to *W. bancrofti* and *B. malayi* may require surgical intervention to increase lymphatic drainage. This is unusual and is likely seen in long-term residents of endemic areas who are subjected to extensive exposure to parasite.

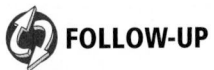

FOLLOW-UP

DISPOSITION
Outpatient care

PROGNOSIS
- Good for light to moderate infections
- Depends on organ infected and extent of infection

COMPLICATIONS
- Depends on type of worm
- Onchocerciasis: Blindness
- Visceral worms: Hepatitis, splenomegaly, pleuritis, peritonitis, eosinophilic granuloma, or other organ damage as larvae migrate for up to 6 months
- Filariasis: Lymphatic destruction leading to severe edema (elephantiasis)
- Neurohelminthiasis: CNS migrations and infection

PATIENT MONITORING
- As needed:
  - Long-term DEC treatment and immunomonitoring of patients with filaria infection are essential in endemic areas to arrest and prevent pathology.

REFERENCES
1. Cook GC. Manson's Tropical Diseases, 21st ed. Philadelphia: WB Saunders, 2002.
2. Drugs for parasitic infections. *Med Lett Drugs Ther.* 1998;40:1–12.
3. Jong EC. Travel and Tropical Medicine Manual, 3rd ed. Philadelphia: WB Saunders, 2003.
4. Padrigel UM, et al. Immunomonitoring of filarial patients during DEC therapy in an endemic area: A seven year followup. *J Trop Med Hyg.* 1995;98:52–56.
5. Steffen R. Manual of Travel Medicine and Health, 2nd ed. Ontario, Canada: BC Decker, 2003.
6. Strickland GT. Hunter's Tropical Medicine, 8th ed. Philadelphia: WB Saunders, 2000.
7. Warren KS, Mahmoud AAF. Tropical and Geographic Medicine. New York: McGraw-Hill, 1990.

MISCELLANEOUS

See also: Roundworms, intestinal

CODES

ICD9-CM
127.0 Ascariasis

PATIENT TEACHING
- Avoid bites by arthropod vectors.
- Use insect repellants and other protective measures (e.g., proper clothing).
- Avoid infected rivers, streams, and soil .

SALICYLATE POISONING

Lars C. Larsen, MD

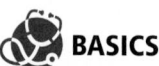 BASICS

DESCRIPTION

Systemic disorder caused by acute and/or chronic intoxication from salicylate-containing medications

- Following accidental or intentional exposure, toxic actions of salicylates include
  - Stimulation of CNS respiratory center
  - Uncoupling of oxidative phosphorylation
  - Inhibition of Krebs cycle dehydrogenases
  - Stimulation of gluconeogenesis
  - Increased lipolysis and lipid metabolism
  - Inhibition of aminotransferases
  - Cyclooxygenase inhibition and decreased production of clotting factors
  - Irritation of the gastric mucosa and stimulation of the CNS chemoreceptor trigger zone
- These actions cause sequential and progressively severe physiologic abnormalities with increasing doses of salicylates, time following exposure, duration of chronic exposure, extremes of age, and presence of concurrent medical conditions; abnormalities include
  - Respiratory alkalosis accompanied by progressive metabolic acidosis
  - Hyperpyrexia
  - Gastrointestinal, renal, pulmonary, and skin losses of body fluids and electrolytes
  - Initial hyperglycemia followed by hypoglycemia, particularly CNS hypoglycemia
  - Abnormal hemostasis and coagulation
- Clinical presentation of patients with salicylate toxicity can range from minor symptoms to a syndrome initially indistinguishable from septic shock with multiple organ failure, including encephalopathy and adult respiratory distress syndrome.
- The very young and elderly are particularly prone to develop severe toxicity, as are those with chronic intoxication.
- Conditions causing concurrent acidosis may increase tissue concentrations of salicylate and result in greater morbidity and mortality.
- System(s) Affected: Cardiovascular; Endocrine/Metabolic; Gastrointestinal; Hemic/Lymphatic/Immunologic; Musculoskeletal; Nervous; Pulmonary; Renal/Urologic; Skin/Exocrine.

ALERT

Geriatric Considerations
- Increased risk for chronic toxicity because of decreased renal function
- Increased risk for bleeding or perforated gastric ulcers in patients >70 years

Pediatric Considerations
Acidosis is often more severe in the very young, particularly in chronic or repeated therapeutic dose poisonings.

Pregnancy Considerations
- Salicylates may cause premature closure of ductus arteriosus in the fetus.
- Increased risk of ante- and intrapartum hemorrhage

GENERAL PREVENTION
- Patient and parent/caregiver education essential. See "Patient Education."
- Emergency telephone numbers (poison control centers)

EPIDEMIOLOGY
Incidence/prevalence in the US

- >20,300 ingestions of salicylate-containing medications reported to poison control centers in 2004
- 60 deaths in 2004, none in children <6
- Predominant age: Occurs in children and adults at any age; >73% of cases are in children >5 and adults
- Predominant sex: Male = Female

RISK FACTORS
- Dehydration
- Conditions causing metabolic or respiratory acidosis
- Extremes of age—very young and elderly
- Psychiatric illness
- History of previous toxic ingestions or suicide attempts
- Concurrent oral poisoning with other substances
- Concurrent use of acetazolamide (Diamox)

ETIOLOGY
- Accidental or intentional ingestion of salicylates or salicylate-containing medications
- Percutaneous absorption of dermatologic medications containing salicylate
- Breast-feeding by mothers ingesting salicylate-containing medications
- Teething gels containing salicylates

ASSOCIATED CONDITIONS
Reye syndrome with salicylate use and varicella or influenza viral infection

DIAGNOSIS

SIGNS AND SYMPTOMS
- Acute intoxication
  - Symptoms vary with amount ingested, usually begin within 3–8 hours of ingestion, and progress more rapidly in children
    - <150 mg/kg, minimal symptoms
    - 150–300 mg/kg, moderate symptoms
    - 300–500 mg/kg, severe symptoms
    - >500 mg/kg, potentially fatal
  - Nausea and vomiting
  - Hyperpnea
  - Tachypnea
  - Hyperpyrexia
  - Tinnitus
  - Disorientation
  - Coma
  - Convulsions
  - Cardiac arrhythmias
  - Hypotension
  - Pulmonary edema
- Chronic intoxication
  - Signs and symptoms similar to acute intoxication may occur.
  - Onset of symptoms is usually gradual.
  - Signs and symptoms may be advanced at diagnosis and include severe hypotension and adult respiratory distress syndrome.
  - Neurologic symptoms often predominate, particularly in the elderly, and include agitation, confusion, stupor, hyperactivity, paranoia, bizarre behavior, dysarthria, and restlessness.

TESTS

Lab
- Serum salicylate levels initially on all patients to confirm diagnosis. Following acute ingestions, check levels ≥6 hours after ingestion and repeat q2h until the levels are declining and patient's condition has stabilized.
- Acid–base abnormalities common
  - Usually respiratory alkalosis or mixed respiratory alkalosis and metabolic acidosis
  - Metabolic acidosis often predominates in chronic or severe acute poisonings and in poisonings in young children.
- Increased anion gap, especially in acute poisonings and salicylate-only poisonings
- Initial hyperglycemia may be followed by hypoglycemia.
- Electrolyte abnormalities such as hypernatremia or hyponatremia and hypokalemia are common.
- Findings consistent with dehydration are common, including an increased BUN/creatinine ratio.
- PTT may be increased.
- Liver function abnormalities may be present.
- Proteinuria, renal function abnormalities may be present.
- Stool guaiac testing may be positive.
- Occasional hypouricemia
- Drugs that may alter lab results
  - Diflunisal (Dolobid) may cross-react with assay of salicylate concentration.
  - Medications affecting similar organ systems including oral anticoagulants and hypoglycemic agents
- Disorders that may alter lab results: Concurrent medical conditions involving similar organ systems

Imaging
- Chest radiograph
  - Noncardiogenic pulmonary edema
  - Variable severity, from mild to adult respiratory distress syndrome
- Abdominal plain film: Nonspecific bowel gas pattern with retained contrast in chronic bismuth subsalicylate ingestion

Diagnostic Procedures/Surgery
- None, other than correlating serum salicylate concentration with clinical presentation
- The usefulness of the Done nomogram in managing patients following acute ingestion is limited because it may underestimate the severity of poisonings in patients with
  - Illnesses accompanied by dehydration and/or acidosis
  - Chronic exposure to salicylates
  - Ingestion of enteric-coated or sustained-release medications
  - Unknown time of ingestion

Pathological Findings

None specific for salicylate intoxication; associated findings include

- Gastrointestinal
  - Antral and prepyloric ulcers
  - Small bowel ulcerations with enteric-coated salicylates
- Renal
  - Interstitial nephritis
  - Acute tubular necrosis
  - Minimal change nephrotic syndrome
- Pulmonary: Noncardiogenic pulmonary edema

DIFFERENTIAL DIAGNOSIS

- All ages
  - Infection
  - Sepsis
  - Diabetic ketoacidosis
  - Other causes of metabolic acidosis
- In the elderly
  - Delirium
  - Cerebral vascular accident
  - Myocardial infarction
  - Ethyl alcohol intoxication
  - CHF

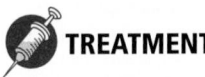

TREATMENT

- Evaluate all patients at a health care facility.
- Outpatient for nontoxic accidental ingestions
- Inpatient for toxic and intentional ingestions

GENERAL MEASURES

- Prevent further absorption if the ingestion is felt to be life-threatening
  - Gastric lavage, within 1 hour of ingestion
  - Activated charcoal after gastric emptying (1,2)[C]
  - Ipecac no longer recommended for routine use at home or in health care facilities (3)[C]
- Fluid/electrolyte balance: IV fluids to restore intravascular volume and prevent hypoglycemia
  - With hypotension give isotonic fluid until orthostatic changes no longer present
  - Fluids should contain ≥5% dextrose unless hyperglycemia is a problem.
  - Normal saline or a mixture of 0.45% NaCl with 1 ampule of sodium bicarbonate (50 mEq NaHCO$_3$) may be administered at 10–15 mL/kg/h for 1–2 hours, depending on the degree of acidosis.
  - When blood pressure stable, fluid management is directed toward alkalinizing the urine to enhance salicylate excretion, preventing CNS hypoglycemia, and treating fluid and electrolyte abnormalities
- Enhance elimination by alkaline diuresis (4)[C]
  - Alkaline diuresis (urine pH >7.5) and prevention of hypoglycemia can usually be maintained by initial bolus of NaHCO$_3$, 1–2 mEq/kg IV, followed by infusion of 1,000 cc D$_5$W plus 3 ampules of NaHCO$_3$ (50 mEq NaHCO$_3$/ampule) at 1.5–2 times maintenance rate.
  - Potassium should be added for potassium levels <4.0 mEq/L.
  - Serum electrolytes and glucose should be monitored frequently and urine pH checked hourly until stable at >7.5.
  - Arterial blood gases should be monitored >2–4 hours to ensure blood pH is ≤7.5
  - Patients with cardiovascular compromise should be monitored closely for fluid overload.
  - Alkalinization can be discontinued when the salicylate level decreases into the therapeutic range.

- Hemodialysis should be considered in poisonings with markedly elevated salicylate levels (>100 mg/dL in acute poisonings, >40–60 mg/dL in chronic poisonings), acidosis unresponsive to alkalinization and diuresis, renal and/or hepatic dysfunction with impaired salicylate clearance, noncardiac pulmonary edema, and persistent, severe CNS symptoms.

Diet

No special diet

 ## MEDICATION (DRUGS)

First Line

Emergency facility/hospital

- Activated charcoal 1–2 g/kg, single dose
- Bicarbonate to alkalinize the urine (pH >7.5) and, when appropriate, to correct severe systemic acidosis (for pH <7.1)
- Dextrose-containing IV solution to prevent hypoglycemia; CNS hypoglycemia may be present despite normal serum glucose.
- Contraindications: Medication allergies
- Precautions
  - Intravascular overload may result from injudicious use of sodium bicarbonate.
  - Dextrose should not be given to patients with severe hyperglycemia.

PROGNOSIS

- Complete recovery with early therapy
- Clinical course and prognosis are worse in very young and elderly, chronic intoxications, and in patients with concurrent conditions that cause dehydration and/or acidosis.

COMPLICATIONS

- Noncardiogenic pulmonary edema, including development of adult respiratory distress syndrome
- Rare following recovery from poisoning

PATIENT MONITORING

- Fluid, acid–base, blood glucose, and electrolyte status until stable; urine pH (to enhance elimination of salicylate)
- Psychiatric follow-up after intentional ingestions

REFERENCES

1. Gaudreault P. Activated charcoal revisited. *Clin Pediatr Emerg Med*. 2005;6:76–80.
2. Heard K. Gastric decontamination. *Med Clin N Am*. 2005;89:1067–1078.
3. American Academy of Pediatrics Committee on Injury, Violence, and Poison Prevention. Poison treatment in the home. *Pediatrics*. 2003;112:1182–1185.
4. Proudfoot AT. Position paper on urine alkalinization. *J Toxicol Clin Toxicol*. 2004;42(1):1–26.
5. Watson WA, et al. 2004 annual report of the American Association of Poison Control Centers Toxic Exposure Surveillance System. *Am J Emerg Med*. 2005;23(5):589–666.

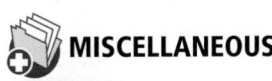 ## MISCELLANEOUS

CODES

ICD9-CM
965.1 Poisoning by salicylates (aspirin)

PATIENT TEACHING

- Education of parents/caregivers during well-child visits
- Education of patients on chronic salicylate therapy
- Anticipatory guidance for caregivers, family, and cohabitants of potentially suicidal patients
- Patient brochure (item 1515): Child safety: Keeping your home safe for your baby. American Academy of Family Physicians, 11400 Tomahawk Creek Parkway, Leawood, KS 66211-2672.

 See Corresponding Diagnostic Algorithm

SALIVARY GLAND CALCULI

Felix B. Chang, MD

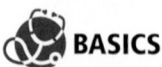 **BASICS**

DESCRIPTION
- Formation of calculi in the ductal system of the salivary glands.
- The submandibular gland is the most common affected.
  - 80–90% Wharton duct
  - 10–20% Stensen parotic duct
  - 1–2% sublingual duct
- System(s) Affected: Gastrointestinal
- Synonym(s): Sialolithiasis

ALERT
Geriatric Considerations
Multiple chronic illnesses, multiple anticholinergics, dehydration

GENERAL PREVENTION
- Treat any associated conditions.
- Avoid anticholinergics.
- Maintain good hydration.
- Maintain good oral hygiene.

EPIDEMIOLOGY
- Predominant age
  - Middle to old age; 5th–8th decade of life
  - Uncommon in children
- Male > Female (slight predominance)

Incidence
Not uncommon; reliable figures not available

Prevalence
One percent in autopsy series, most of these asymptomatic

RISK FACTORS
- Alterations in gland function and duct anatomy
- Previous stone formation
- Local irradiation
- Chronic, debilitating illness
- Poor oral hygiene

Genetics
No known genetic pattern

PATHOPHYSIOLOGY
- Salivary stasis, ductal inflammation, and injury are factors contributing to stones formation.
- Intermittent salivary stasis results in an alteration of the mucoid elements of saliva, forming an organic gel.
- The gel becomes framework for the deposition of salts, which leads to development of calculi.
- Salivary stones are composed predominantly of calcium phosphate and carbonate in combination with an organic matrix of glycoproteins and mucopolysaccharides.
- Magnesium, potassium, and ammonium salts also are involved.

ETIOLOGY
- In past, stones were thought to be secondary to altered calcium metabolism, but this has not been demonstrated.
- Submandibular gland/ducts are involved in >80% of cases, thought to be due to
  - Tortuous course of these ducts
  - Flow of saliva in these ducts is "uphill."
  - Submandibular saliva has higher calcium concentration and is more viscous.
- General causes of salivary gland stones
  - Any hindrance to normal saliva flow
    ○ Acute or chronic inflammation near duct
    ○ Scarring or stenosis of duct (trauma, surgery, past stone damage)
    ○ Altered or tortuous duct path (extrinsic masses, surgery, or previous obstruction)
    ○ Presence of food particles or organic debris in duct as an obstruction and/or nidus of stone formation
  - Alteration of saliva quality
    ○ Dehydration
    ○ Anticholinergic medications (including those with anticholinergic side effects such as tricyclic antidepressants and phenothiazines)
    ○ Chronic parotitis, Sjögren syndrome, cystic fibrosis

ASSOCIATED CONDITIONS
- Sialadenitis
- Chronic anticholinergics
- Poor oral hygiene
- Sjögren syndrome
- Cystic fibrosis
- Oral trauma
- Gout and nephrolithiasis
- Sarcoidosis

DIAGNOSIS

SIGNS AND SYMPTOMS
- Initial symptoms, consistent with partial duct obstruction
  - Episodic or variable unilateral swelling and tenderness of the affected gland, worse just before meals, then tapering off until the next meal
- Symptoms of complete duct obstruction
  - Persistent swelling and pain
- Symptoms of commonly associated sialadenitis
  - Fever, sweats, chills
  - Acute and severe worsening of localized pain and swelling
  - Acute general malaise
- Signs when not associated with sialadenitis
  - Unilateral localized swelling
  - Boggy, tender mass associated with affected gland in acute obstruction
  - Firm to hard mass associated with gland fibrosis in chronic obstruction
  - Palpable and/or visible stone in distal duct (in 1/2–1/3 of cases and more often with submandibular stones than parotid stones)
  - No saliva expressed or scant, cloudy, thick, mucinous saliva expressed on milking duct
- Signs in association with sialadenitis
  - Fever, tachycardia
  - Generalized toxicity
  - Diffuse, tender, hot swelling
  - Otherwise palpable stone now obscured by swelling and acute pain

History
Pain and swelling in the involved gland, aggravated by eating or with anticipation of eating

Physical Exam
- Bimanual palpation will reveal the presence of a palpable stone in most cases involving the submandibular gland.
- Parotid stones might be noted at the orifice of Stensen duct or along the course of the duct.
- If a stone cannot be palpated, high resolution noncontrast CT should be performed

TESTS
Lab
WBC count and serum amylase may be elevated if associated with sialadenitis.

Imaging
- Owing to differences in mineralization, 80% of submandibular gland stones are radiopaque, but 80% of parotid stones are radiolucent.
- Plain head and neck radiographs
- Intraoral or dental occlusal films
- Ultrasound (particularly useful in acute parotid sialadenitis with swelling and pain)
  - Detect 90% of stones >2 mm
- MRI
  - Does not visualize stones, but shows ducts as with sialography
- High resolution CT is currently the imaging modality of choice.
  - CT reconstruction is most sensitive technique, showing presence of stones or differentiating multiple stones.
- Xerography
  - Digital subtraction sialography

Diagnostic Procedures/Surgery

- Fine-needle aspiration if glandular neoplasm is high in the differential diagnosis
- Surgical excision may be needed to differentiate chronic ductal squamous metaplasia from low-grade mucoepidermoid carcinoma.
- Sialoendoscopy is under development.

Pathological Findings

- Submandibular glands/ducts involved in 80% of cases, parotid in 15%, and remainder in sublingual and minor salivary glands
- In acute cases without sialadenitis
  - Acute ductal and glandular inflammation
- In chronic cases
  - Ductal ectasia, stenosis, scarring, thickening
  - Metaplasia of duct lining
  - Periductal chronic inflammation
  - Glandular fibrosis and atrophy
  - Multiple stones in intraglandular and extraglandular ducts
- Stones vary in size from <1 mm to >10 mm and show alternating layers of mineralization (predominantly calcium salts) and organic material (mucinous material, lipids, cellular debris).
- Multiple stones in 20% of cases

DIFFERENTIAL DIAGNOSIS

- Sialadenitis
- Lymphadenitis
- Salivary neoplasms (80% benign in parotid, 50% benign in submandibular gland)
- Foreign body in duct or soft tissue
- Neoplasms of adjacent oral or neck tissues
- Other facial/dental soft tissue infections (e.g., dissecting dental abscess)

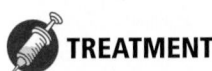

TREATMENT

GENERAL MEASURES

- Small stones close to the ductal orifice are often removed with a conservative approach
  - Sialagogues (e.g., hard sour candy) to stimulate salivary flow
  - Gentle ductal massage, from gland to ductal orifice; "milk the duct"
  - Ductal dilatation (lacrimal probe and/or lacrimal punctum dilator)
  - Incision of ductal papilla if stone is hung up just inside the orifice
  - For more proximal submandibular gland stones still ≤1.25 cm from orifice (Wharton duct), the duct may be incised longitudinally from the orifice and the stone expressed by massage.
  - Penicillinase-resistant staphylococcal antibiotic coverage, particularly if duct instrumented or incised
- In setting of acute sialadenitis
  - Hydration
  - Sialagogues
  - Local heat
  - Release of a obstructing stone, if palpable
  - Attempted proximal-to-distal expression of pus after release of obstruction
  - Full course of penicillinase-resistant staphylococcal coverage (IV therapy in hospital for severely ill or elderly)
  - Extracorporeal shock-wave lithotripsy (ECSWL) has been effective in treating >50% of the parotid stones not cleared with conservative measures.

Diet

- Until specific therapy is initiated
  - Liberal oral water intake for hydration
  - Reduce other oral intake to reduce pain
  - Particularly avoid sialagogues to reduce pain
- No dietary measures required after therapy

 ## MEDICATION (DRUGS)

First Line

- Antibiotics, if infection present
  - Amoxicillin clavulanate (Augmentin) 500 mg PO t.i.d. for 10 days
  - Cefuroxime (Ceftin) 250 mg PO b.i.d. for 10 days
- Analgesic: Codeine, NSAIDs
- Contraindications: Hypersensitivity to drugs chosen
- Precautions
  - Refer to the manufacturer's literature for drugs chosen.
  - Prescribed or OTC anticholinergics may predispose to, or accelerate, stone formation.
- Significant possible interactions: Refer to the manufacturer's literature.

Second Line

Erythromycin 250 mg PO q.i.d. for 10 days

SURGERY

A more extensive procedure by a surgical specialist, such as proximal duct dissection or gland excision, is appropriate for the following

- Any but most distal parotid stones, particularly if ECSWL is not available or ineffective.
- Proximal stone with high-grade obstruction
- Chronic or recurrent sialadenitis with glandular fibrosis or ductal scarring and stenosis
- Multiple stones
- If neoplasm is a consideration

 ## FOLLOW-UP

DISPOSITION

- Outpatient care for conservative treatment or minor surgical procedures
- Inpatient care for salivary gland excision or for treating associated severe sialadenitis

Issues for Referral

- Driven by symptoms
- Symptoms lasting more than a few days
- Frequently recurrent symptoms
- Recurrent episodes of infections
- Infection that worsens or does not respond to antibiotics within 7 days requires urgent referral.

PROGNOSIS

- Most patients with uncomplicated stones who are successfully treated early in the process do not have recurrences.
- A previous stone may damage the duct, setting up conditions for more stones.
- Recurrence, particularly with multiple proximal stones, may warrant gland excision.

COMPLICATIONS

- Ductal scarring after stone passage, instrumentation, or surgery
- Infection associated with stone itself or with surgical procedures
- Salivary gland fibrosis and atrophy from duct obstruction or infection
- Salivary fistula after surgical procedure

PATIENT MONITORING

- Close postprocedure or postoperative surveillance for infection
- Close follow-up during treatment of sialadenitis to ensure resolution of infection
- Educate patient to seek early medical attention for symptoms of recurrence.

REFERENCES

1. Yousem DM, Kraut MA, Chalian AA. Major salivary gland imaging. *Radiology*. 2000;22116:19–20.
2. McGurk M, Escudier MP, Brown JE. Modern management of salivary calculi. *Br J Surg*. 2005;92:107.
3. Alyas F, Lewis K, Williams M, et al. Diseases of the submandibular gland as demonstrated using high resolution ultrasound. *Br J Radiol*. 2005;78:362.
4. Marchal F, Dulguerov P. Sialolithiasis management: The state of the art. *Arch Otolaryngol Head Neck Surg*. 2003;129:951.
5. Williams MF. Sialolithiasis. *Otolaryngol Clin North Am*. 1999;32:819–834.

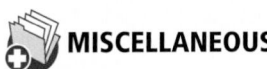 ## MISCELLANEOUS

See also: Sialadenitis

CODES

ICD9-CM
527.5 Sialolithiasis

PATIENT TEACHING

- General management principles and diet as described (see "Diet")
- Avoid OTC anticholinergic medications as discussed in "Medication," "Drugs."
- Bring early signs of recurrence to medical attention.

SALIVARY GLAND TUMORS

Bruce T. Vanderhoff, MD
Frank Moskos, MD

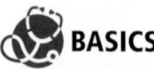 **BASICS**

DESCRIPTION

Benign or malignant neoplasms of major (parotid, submaxillary, sublingual) salivary glands or minor (intraoral, pharyngeal, nasal) salivary glands

- Types
  - Pleomorphic adenoma (most common tumor): 45% overall
  - Monomorphic adenoma: 12% overall
  - Mucoepidermoid carcinoma: 12% overall
  - Adenoid cystic: 6% overall
  - Uncommon are adenocarcinoma, squamous cell carcinoma, acinic cell carcinoma, oxyphilic adenomas, Warthin tumor
- Distribution
  - Generally, the smaller the salivary gland, the higher the probability of malignancy if a tumor is found in it.
  - Parotid (80% benign, 20% malignant): 70% are pleomorphic adenoma, 10% monomorphic adenoma, 12% mucoepidermoid carcinoma, and 5% are adenoid cystic.
  - Submandibular (60% benign, 40% malignant): 40% are pleomorphic adenoma, 10% are mucoepidermoid carcinoma, and 20% are adenoid cystic carcinoma.
  - Minor salivary glands (40% benign, 60% malignant): 40% are pleomorphic adenoma, 25% are mucoepidermoid carcinoma, and 25% are adenoid cystic carcinoma.
- Staging
  - Based on tumor size (T0–T4), nodal status (N0–N3), and metastasis (M0–M1).
  - Ranges from stage I (T0, N0, M0) to stage IVC (any T, any N, M1)
- System(s) Affected: Gastrointestinal; Nervous

ALERT

Pediatric Considerations
- Mucoepidermoid and acinic cell carcinomas account for 60% of these malignancies. (9)
- Total or superficial parotidectomy or gland removal achieves good cure rates. (9)

Pregnancy Considerations
Not affected

GENERAL PREVENTION
- Tobacco cessation
- Alcohol cessation

EPIDEMIOLOGY
- Predominant age
  - Malignant: 55 years
  - Benign: 45 years
- Predominant sex
  - Pleomorphic adenoma: Female > Male
  - Other adenomas: Male = Female

Incidence
- 1–3/100,000 per year
- 3% of new tumors

Prevalence
Three percent to 4% of all head and neck neoplasms (6)

RISK FACTORS
- Tobacco smoke and excess alcohol intake associated with Warthin tumor
- Alcohol increases likelihood ratio by 2 : 11. (7,8)
- Radiation has shown a 4.5-fold increased dose related response in salivary gland cancer. (7,8)
- EBV has been associated with lymphoepithelial carcinoma in Asians. (7,8)
- Silica dust has been associated with a 2.5-fold increase in salivary gland neoplasia. (7,8)
- Kerosene cooking fuel exposure (7,8)
- Nitrosamine exposure (7,8)
- Early menarche and nulliparity in women (7,8)

Genetics
Increased incidence of adenocarcinoma of parotid in Eskimos, otherwise no known genetic pattern

ETIOLOGY
Unknown

ASSOCIATED CONDITIONS
None known

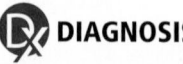 **DIAGNOSIS**

SIGNS AND SYMPTOMS

Most tumors are discrete masses, although some manifest as diffuse enlargement of the gland or submucosal intraoral swelling. Malignant tumors are characterized by local recurrence and perineural spread (adenoid cystic) or local recurrence and lymph node metastases (mucoepidermoid, adenocarcinoma, squamous cell carcinoma).

- Discrete mass in anatomic area: 96%
- Elevation of earlobe
- Pain: 12%–25% (malignant); 2.5% (benign)
- Trigeminal paresthesias
- Facial nerve palsy or dysfunction: 8–26%
- Fixation to masseter and pterygoids: 17%
- Skin ulceration: 9% (malignant)
- Cervical lymph node metastases: 20%
- Pharyngeal mass

TESTS
- Technetium-99 (Warthin tumor)
  - Follow patient closely as Warthin tumor has low chance of metastatizing (6)
- Sialography (for calculi or chronic parotitis)

Lab
- Autoimmune studies
- Fractionated amylase (inflammation)
- Drugs that may alter lab results
  - None known
- Disorders that may alter lab results
  - None known

Imaging
- Chest radiograph
  - Sjögren syndrome
  - Metastases
- Ultrasound: Inflammatory or malignant
- CT: Provides detail of tumor invasion and temporal bone or mandibular destruction

- MRI
  - Provides definition of soft tissue and any evidence of perineural invasion or intracranial extension
  - Discriminates tumor from mucus and bone marrow invasion
- PET
  - Useful for detecting malignancy in early stages, and for detecting recurrences and differentiating soft tissue damage secondary to radiation from inflammatory changes

Diagnostic Procedures/Surgery
- Fine-needle aspiration
  - There is concern as there may be tumor seeding via the needle track. However, tumor spread from tumor seeding is rare.
  - Sensitivity of 92%, sensitivity of 100%, but a false-negative rate of up to 53%. (10)
- Superficial lobectomy

Pathological Findings
Of 100 parotid masses, 70 will be nonneoplastic, 21 will be benign neoplasms, and 9 will be malignant neoplasms.

DIFFERENTIAL DIAGNOSIS
- Metabolic causes (diabetes, vitamin deficiencies, alcohol, gout)
- Drugs (thiourea, iodine)
- Inflammatory masses
- Parotid and submandibular lymph nodes
- Mikulicz syndrome
- Salivary gland stones
- Torus palatinus (minor)
- Necrotizing sialometaplasia (minor)
- Cervical lymph nodes
- Sjögren syndrome
- Sarcoidosis
- Lymphadenopathy with AIDS
- Actinomycosis
- Cat-scratch disease
- Tuberculosis

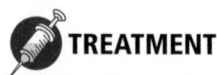 **TREATMENT**

INITIAL STABILIZATION
Inpatient care

GENERAL MEASURES
- Postoperative care (see "Surgery")
  - Elevate head of bed postoperatively.
  - Suction drainage for 1–2 days
  - Suture line care with antibiotic ointment
- Drain parotid bed
- Usually 1–2-day hospitalization

Diet
Nonstimulating liquid diet

Activity
Moderate restriction for 1 day postoperatively.

SPECIAL THERAPY
Radiation and oncological measures

- Postoperative irradiation (via fast neutron beam) for larger and high-grade carcinomas
- Chemotherapy reserved for metastases, or locally advanced and unresectable tumors

MEDICATION (DRUGS)

First Line
Cisplatin based regimens for recurrent or nonoperable disease (6)

SURGERY
- Benign tumors
  - Superficial or total conservative (nerve-sparing) parotidectomy
- Malignant tumors
  - Total parotidectomy or sialadenectomy with adjuvant radiotherapy to parotid base of skull with or without neck
  - Preservation of facial nerve unless involved by tumor
- Cervical lymphadenectomy if palpable nodes or elective neck dissection in squamous cell carcinoma, high-grade mucoepidermoid carcinoma, or high-grade adenocarcinoma

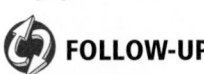 **FOLLOW-UP**

Admission Criteria
Airway impingement

PROGNOSIS
- By tumor type
  - Parotid pleomorphic adenoma: Untreated will demonstrate malignant degeneration in 2–10% over 20 years. Treated adequately, parotid pleomorphic adenoma has 1.5% recurrence rate. Extension of pseudopods of tumor beyond the tumor mass increases the risk of recurrent disease.
  - Adenoid cystic: Parotid 5-year survival, 73%; 15-year survival, 21%; submandibular 5-year survival, 50%; 15-year survival, 0%; palate 5-year survival, 80%; 15-year survival, 38%
  - Adenocarcinoma: Aggressive tumors with a tendency for local recurrence (38%), regional lymph node metastasis (33%), and dissemination to lungs, bone, and liver. 5-year survival, 78%; 20-year survival, 41%
  - Mucoepidermoid: Low-grade 5-year survival, 81%; 15-year survival, 48%; high-grade 5-year survival, 46%, 15-year survival, 25%
  - Squamous cell carcinoma: Rare tumor with 50% incidence of cervical lymph node metastasis and local recurrence. 5-year survival, 18%; 15-year survival, 0%
  - Lymphoma: Rare accounting for 1.7% of salivary neoplasms. 5 year survival: Hodgkin's type: 90%; Non-Hodgkin's 43%. (6)
- 5-year survival rate for stages I–IV and cause-specific survival (CSS):
  - Stage I: 75% (CSS, 86%)
  - Stage II: 59% (CSS, 66%)
  - Stage III: 57% (CSS, 53%)
  - Stage IV: 28% (CSS, 32%)

COMPLICATIONS
- Frey syndrome (gustatory sweating) occurs symptomatically in ~20% of patients undergoing parotidectomy.
- Hematoma with possible posterior displacement of tongue and airway obstruction
- Facial neurapraxia from surgery should resolve within 6 months even with radiotherapy.
- Cosmetic deformity of moderate facial flattening on side of parotidectomy
- Injury to hypoglossal or lingual
- If inadequately excised, pleomorphic adenoma may recur due to pseudopods in the lobe.
- Wound infection of surgical site

PATIENT MONITORING
- For malignancy
  - Once every 6–8 weeks the 1st year, every 8–12 weeks the 2nd year, every 4 months the 3rd year, every 6 months the 4th year, then yearly visits. (6)
- For benign tumors
  - Once per year for 5 years

REFERENCES
1. Batsakis JG. *Tumors of the Head and Neck: Clinical and Pathological Considerations*. 3rd ed. Baltimore, MD: Lippincott Williams & Wilkins; 2000.
2. Coleman JJ. Salivary gland disorders. In: Jurkiewicz MJ, et al., eds. *Plastic Surgery: Principles & Practices*. St. Louis, MO: Mosby; 1991.
3. Lorenz RR, Nutterville JL, Burkey BB. Head and neck. In: Sabiston D Jr, ed. *Textbook of Surgery: The Biological Basis of Modern Surgical Practice*. 17th ed. Philadelphia, PA: WB Saunders; 2004.
4. Rankow RM. *Diseases of the Salivary Glands*. Philadelphia, PA: WB Saunders; 1976.
5. Ward MJ, Levine PA. Salivary gland tumors. In: Close LG, Larson DL, Shah JP, eds. *Essentials of Head & Neck Oncology*. New York, NY: Thieme; 1998.
6. Cummings CW. *Otolaryngology: Head & Neck Surgery*, 4th ed. Philadelphia, PA: Mosby; 2005.
7. Spitz MR. Epidemiology and risk factors for head and neck cancer. *Semin Oncolo*. 1994;21:281.
8. Zheng W, et al. Diet and other risk factors for cancer of the salivary glands: A population-based case-control study. *Intern J Cancer*. 1996;67(2): 194–198.
9. Guzzo M, et al. Salivary gland neoplasms in children: The experience of the Istituto Nazionale Tumori of Milan. *Pediatr Blood & Cancer*. 2006;
10. Cohen EG, et al. Fine-needle aspiration biopsy of salivary gland lesions in a selected patient population. *Archi Otolaryngo: Head Neck Sur*. 2004;130:773–778.

 MISCELLANEOUS

See also: Sjögren syndrome

CODES

ICD9-CM
- 142.0 Malignant neoplasm of parotid gland
- 142.1 Malignant neoplasm of submandibular gland
- 142.2 Malignant neoplasm of sublingual gland
- 142.9 Malignant neoplasm of salivary gland, unspecified
- 145.9 Malignant neoplasm of mouth, unspecified
- 210.2 Benign neoplasm of major salivary glands
- 210.3 Benign neoplasm of floor of mouth

ICD10
- C06.9 Malignant neoplasm of mouth, unspecified
- C07 Malignant neoplasm of parotid gland
- C08.0 Malignant neoplasm of submandibular gland
- C08.1 Malignant neoplasm of sublingual gland
- C08.8 Malignant neoplasm, overlapping lesion of major salivary glands
- C08.9 Malignant neoplasm of major salivary gland, unspecified
- D10.3 Benign neoplasm of mouth, unspecified
- D11.0 Benign neoplasm of parotid gland
- D11.7 Benign neoplasm of major salivary glands
- D11.9 Benign neoplasm of other salivary glands

PATIENT TEACHING
- Trigeminal nerve symptoms
- Frey syndrome (gustatory sweating)
- Facial nerve symptoms (paresis)
- Xerostomia treatment and mouth care
- Tobacco cessation
- Alcohol abstinence

SALMONELLA INFECTION

Richard Viken, MD

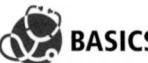

BASICS

DESCRIPTION
- Disease caused by any serotype of the genus *Salmonella*
- Clinical syndromes include enterocolitis (75%), bacteremia (10%), enteric fever (10%) (see "Typhoid Fever"), localized infection outside gastrointestinal tract (5%), and an asymptomatic carrier state (<1%).
- Organisms invade gut mucosa, producing inflammatory, cytotoxic response.
- Organisms can then disseminate into systemic circulation via lymphatics.
- Infective dose and host defenses dictate extent of disease.
- Molecular studies have determined the total genome DNA sequence for a particular multidrug resistant human *Salmonella* serotype.
- System(s) Affected: Gastrointestinal

ALERT
Geriatric Considerations
Patients >60 have high carrier rate presumably due to biliary sequestration of organisms.

Pediatric Considerations
Children, especially neonates, are more likely to become chronic carriers.

Pregnancy Considerations
- Consult obstetrician regarding antibiotics.
- Keep a low threshold for hospital admission.

GENERAL PREVENTION
- Proper hygiene in production, transport, and storage of food
- Control of animal reservoir, especially by avoiding contact with animal feces
- Hand washing emphasized
- No vaccine available to oppose salmonellosis

EPIDEMIOLOGY
- Predominant age
  - High prevalence in persons >70 or <20
  - Highest in infants <1 year
- Predominant sex: Male = Female

Incidence
In the US
- 800 cases/100,000 population/year
- Peak frequency July–November
- *Salmonella* isolations represent only 1–10% of the actual yearly incidence.
- 2nd only to *Campylobacter* as the cause of bacterial diarrheal illness
- Each year, an average of 55 outbreaks of *Salmonella* infections are reported to the Centers for Disease Control and Prevention.

Prevalence
In the US
- Infants: 130/100,000
- Adults: 6/100,000

RISK FACTORS
- Impaired gastric acidity—histamine-2 receptor blockers, antacids, gastrectomy, achlorhydria
- Hemolytic anemias—sickle-cell, malaria, bartonellosis
- Malignancy—lymphoma, leukemia, disseminated carcinoma (1)[C]
- Immunosuppression—AIDS, diabetes mellitus, steroids, other immunosuppressants, chemotherapy, radiation (1)[C]
- Pets with high fecal carriage rates for *Salmonella*, especially reptiles. Antibiotic treatment of the animal is not recommended, due to temporary effect only.

ETIOLOGY
- Ingestion of contaminated food—(poultry, beef, eggs, dairy products)—or water accounts for 95% of cases. (2)[C]
- Person-to-person and/or fecal–oral spread
- Iatrogenic contamination—blood transfusion, endoscopy
- Contact with asymptomatic chronic carrier (e.g., day care center)
- Ulcerative colitis
- Systemic lupus erythematosus
- Schistosomiasis
- Cholelithiasis
- Nephrolithiasis
- Intentional contamination of restaurant food through criminal mischief has been reported.
- Contaminated marijuana is important source of infection, particularly in young adults.

ASSOCIATED CONDITIONS
The frequency of reactive arthritis after various *Salmonella* outbreaks is <10%.

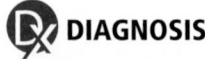

DIAGNOSIS

SIGNS AND SYMPTOMS
- Acute uncomplicated illness
  - Nausea, vomiting, diarrhea
  - Abdominal cramps
  - Headache, myalgias
  - Fever to 102°F (39°C)
- Protracted disease
  - Persistent fever
  - Arthritis, reactive or septic
  - Osteomyelitis
  - Sacroiliitis
  - Wound infection, soft tissue abscesses
  - Meningitis
  - Arteritis
  - Endocarditis, pericarditis
  - Pneumonia, lung abscess, empyema
  - Hypovolemia
  - Splenic (abscess)
  - Hepatic (abscess)
  - Urogenital tract infection

TESTS
A rapid test (TUBEX) used in children to detect anti-*Salmonella* IgM antibodies was found to be 92.6% sensitive and 94.8% specific.

Lab
- Enterocolitis
  - Fecal leukocytes positive
  - Stool culture positive for *Salmonella* species
  - WBC normal or decreased
  - Blood cultures negative
- Bacteremia
  - Blood cultures positive
  - Stool cultures negative
- Local infections
  - Polymorphonuclear leukocytosis
  - Tissue site culture positive
- Asymptomatic carrier state
  - Stool culture positive for >1 year
  - Urine culture may be positive with certain serotypes.
- Drugs that may alter lab results
  - Antibiotics used early may lead to false-negative cultures and blunted immunologic response.

Imaging
Angiography in patients >50 with bacteremia; to rule out presence of infected aneurysm, particularly of aorto-iliac vessels

Pathological Findings
- Mucosal ulceration, hemorrhage, and necrosis
- Reticuloendothelial hyperplasia and hypertrophy
- Focal organ and soft-tissue abscesses

DIFFERENTIAL DIAGNOSIS
- Viral gastroenteritis
- Other bacterial enteritis (e.g., shigellosis, cholera)
- Other bacterial sources or systemic and localized sepsis (e.g., meningococci, staphylococci)
- Pseudomembranous colitis
- Inflammatory or granulomatous bowel disease
- Appendicitis
- Cholecystitis
- Perforated viscus

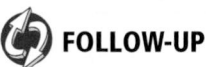

TREATMENT

- Outpatient for uncomplicated enterocolitis and carrier state
- Inpatient for bacteremia and extraintestinal infection (11% hospitalization rate)
- Do not wait for stool culture results before initiating therapy. (1)[C]

GENERAL MEASURES
- Correct fluid and electrolyte deficits.
- Control symptoms (pain, nausea, vomiting).

Diet
Oral rehydration solution during diarrhea phase; advance to normal diet as tolerated

Activity
As tolerated

MEDICATION (DRUGS)

First Line

- Enterocolitis, uncomplicated: None recommended (3)[B]

- Enterocolitis, complicated (by age extremes, immunosuppression, underlying cardiovascular abnormalities, prosthetic orthopedic devices, hemolytic anemia):
  - Adults (3)[B]
    ○ Ciprofloxacin (Cipro): 500 mg PO b.i.d. for 5–7 days; or
    ○ Azithromycin (Zithromax): 1.0 g PO once, then 500 mg PO every day for 6 days
  - Children
- Ampicillin: 50–100 mg/kg/d in 4 divided doses for 10–14 days; or
- Trimethoprim-sulfamethoxazole (Bactrim, Septra): 10–50 mg/kg/d in 2 divided doses for 10–14 days
- Bacteremia
  - Adults (1)[C]
    ○ Ciprofloxacin (Cipro): 400 mg IV b.i.d. or 500 mg PO b.i.d. for 7 days; or
    ○ Ceftriaxone (Rocephin): 2 g IV and IM every day for 7 days
  - Children
    ○ Ampicillin: 200 mg/kg/d in 4 divided doses for 10–14 days; or
    ○ Trimethoprim-sulfamethoxazole (Bactrim, Septra): 10–50 mg/kg/d in 2 divided doses for 10–14 days; or
    ○ Chloramphenicol: 75 mg/kg/d in 4 divided doses for 10–14 days
- Localized infection
  - Same as for bacteremia
  - In sustained bacteremia or prolonged local infection, antibiotics can be given PO for 4–6 weeks (substitute trimethoprim–sulfamethoxazole for cefotaxime, using 2–4 double strength tablets given t.i.d.)

- Chronic carrier state
  - Ampicillin: 2–4 g/d plus probenecid 1–2 g/d, both divided into 4 PO doses, for 6 weeks; or
  - Trimethoprim: 40–160 mg/d and 200–800 mg/d sulfamethoxazole divided into 2 doses for 6 weeks
  - Consider ciprofloxacin 500 mg PO b.i.d. for 4 weeks, or norfloxacin (Noroxin) 400 mg PO b.i.d. for 4 weeks, if gallstones are present.
  - Contraindications: Known drug allergy
  - Precautions
    ○ Use bowel motility inhibitors (Lomotil, Imodium) with caution, if at all.
    ○ Monitor blood levels of chloramphenicol in neonates and infants.
    ○ Ampicillin-resistant strains increasing; now at 15–30% in the US. Some strains are rapidly becoming multidrug resistant. (1)[C]
  - Significant possible interactions
- Ampicillin failure rate is 75% in chronic carriers with gallbladder disease.
- Fluoroquinolone resistance has been observed in some *Salmonella* serotypes common to swine and humans. Use of fluoroquinolones in food animals is implicated. (1)[C]
- Ceftriaxone resistance has been reported in the US with increasing frequency. (2)[C]

Second Line
Fluoroquinolones

- Ciprofloxacin (Cipro) and ofloxacin (Floxin) are gaining favor for use in the management of gastroenteritis, osteomyelitis, and the carrier state.
- Routinely given to children for 5–7 days in areas of the world where multidrug-resistant *Salmonella typhi* is common. (1)[C]

SURGERY
- Surgical excision, drainage and vascular bypass procedures for infected tissue sites, particularly endocarditis (1)[C]
- When biliary tract disease is present, the best results are obtained with the combination of cholecystectomy and a 10-day to 14-day course of parenteral antibiotics (see "First Line—bacteremia") initiated before surgery.

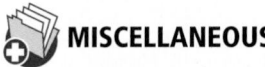

FOLLOW-UP

PROGNOSIS
- Prognosis for enterocolitis is excellent. Exceptions
  - The very young (7.0% fatal)
  - The very old (8.7% fatal)
  - The debilitated and/or institutionalized (2.3% fatal)
- Prognosis for meningitis or endocarditis is poor, unless effective treatment given early
- Mortality increased with multidrug-resistant strain

COMPLICATIONS
- Toxic megacolon
- Hypovolemic shock
- Metastatic abscess formation
- Acute or chronic hydrocephalus

PATIENT MONITORING
- Repeat stool culture at 5 months (40% of children negative, 90% of adults negative) and at 1 year (>99% of all patients negative).
- Check state law regarding health care professional infection and return to work rules.

REFERENCES
1. Hohmann EL. Nontyphoidal salmonellosis. *Clin Infect Dis*. 2001;32:263–269.
2. Pitout JDD, Church DL. Emerging gram-negative enteric infections. *Clin Lab Med*. 2004;24: 605–626.
3. Gilbert DN, Moellering RC, Eliopoulos GM, Sande MA. *The Sanford Guide to Antimicrobial Therapy*. 35th ed. Dallas, TX: Antimicrobial Therapy; 2005.

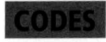

MISCELLANEOUS

Other notes
- If 1 member of a household becomes infected with salmonellosis, the chance of at least 1 other member becoming infected is 60%.
- The Centers for Disease Control and Prevention has identified *Salmonella* as a Category B biological terrorism agent: Moderately easy to disseminate, causing moderate morbidity/low mortality, requiring specific enhancements of the CDC's diagnostic capacity and disease surveillance capabilities.
- See also: Gastroenteritis, viral; Typhoid fever

CODES

ICD9-CM
003.0 Salmonella gastroenteritis

PATIENT TEACHING
Food Safety and Inspection Service, Office of Public Awareness, Department of Agriculture, Room. 1165-S, Washington, DC 20205; (202) 447-9351

 See Corresponding Diagnostic Algorithm

SARCOIDOSIS

Donnah Mathews, MD

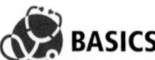 **BASICS**

DESCRIPTION (1)[B]
- Noninfectious multisystem granulomatous disease of unknown cause, commonly affecting young and middle-age adults
- Frequently presents with bilateral hilar adenopathy, pulmonary infiltrates, ocular and skin lesions
- Can also be diagnosed in asymptomatic patients with abnormal chest radiographs
- Almost any other organ may be involved, including liver, spleen, lymph nodes, heart, and CNS.
- System(s) Affected: Primarily Pulmonary but also Cardiovascular; Gastrointestinal; Heme/Lymphatic/Immunologic; Endocrine; Renal; Neurologic; Dermatologic; Ophthalmologic
- Synonym(s): Löfgren syndrome (erythema nodosum; hilar adenopathy plus uveitis); Heerfordt syndrome (uveitis, parotid enlargement, facial palsy, fever); Besnier-Boeck disease; Boeck sarcoid; Schaumann disease

ALERT
Geriatric Considerations
<15% of patients with active disease are ≥60 years old

Pediatric Considerations
Rare

Pregnancy Considerations
No increased incidence

GENERAL PREVENTION
None known

EPIDEMIOLOGY (1,2)[C]
- Incidence/prevalence in the US: Estimated 10–20 per 100,000.
- Predominant age: 20–60 years; sarcoidosis is a disease of youth to middle age
- Predominant sex: Female > Male (slight)

RISK FACTORS
None known

Genetics (1,2)[C]
Although worldwide in distribution, increased prevalence is found in Scandinavians, Japanese, and African American women.

ETIOLOGY
Unknown

ASSOCIATED CONDITIONS
None known

DIAGNOSIS

SIGNS AND SYMPTOMS
- Patients may be asymptomatic.
- Cough
- Shortness of breath
- Skin (new lesions)
- Pain or irritation of eyes
- General fatigue, malaise
- Fever
- Night sweats
- Bell palsy

TESTS (1,2)[B]
- No definitive test for diagnosis, but diagnosis suggested by the following
  - Clinical and radiographic manifestations
  - Exclusion of other diagnoses
  - Histopathologic detection of noncaseating granulomas
- Chest radiograph or CT scan may reveal granulomas
- Serum angiotensin-converting enzyme (ACE) is elevated in >60% of patients but is not diagnostic or exclusionary.
- Gallium scan uptake in chest, lymph nodes, and parotids may be seen in active disease.
- Characteristically in active disease, bronchoalveolar lavage fluid has an increased percentage of lymphocytes, specifically CD4-positive (T-helper/inducer lymphocytes).
- Biopsy of lesions should reveal noncaseating granulomas. (Note: It is not necessary to biopsy if signs indicate classic Löfgren syndrome, because prognosis is good with observation alone and biopsy would not change management.)
- Ophthalmologic examination
- ECG

Labs (1,3)[C]
- Anemia or leucopenia with or without eosinophilia can be seen.
- Abnormal liver function, especially >alkaline phosphatase, is frequently encountered.
- Hypercalciuria occurs in up to 10% of patients, with hypercalcemia less frequent.
- Drugs that may alter lab results: Prednisone will lower serum ACE and normalize gallium scan. ACE inhibitors will lower serum ACE level.
- Disorders that may alter lab results: Hyperthyroidism and diabetes will increase serum ACE level

Imaging (1,3,4)[B]
- Routine chest radiographs are staged using Scadding classification
  - Stage 0 = normal
  - Stage 1 = hilar adenopathy alone
  - Stage 2 = hilar adenopathy plus parenchymal infiltrates
  - Stage 3 = parenchymal infiltrates alone
  - Stage 4 = pulmonary fibrosis
- Gallium scan will be positive in areas of acute disease or inflammation.
- CT may enhance appreciation of lymph nodes, and high-resolution CT scan shows peribronchial disease.
- PET scan can indicate areas of disease activity in lungs, lymph nodes, and other areas of the body. Cardiac PET scan may detect cardiac sarcoidosis.

Diagnostic Procedures/Surgery
- Bronchoscopy with transbronchial biopsy and bronchoalveolar lavage is often performed to diagnose lung disease.
- Mediastinoscopy, skin or lymph-node biopsy (if needed to establish diagnosis)

Pathological Findings
Noncaseating epithelioid granulomas without evidence of fungal or mycobacterial infection

DIFFERENTIAL DIAGNOSIS
- Infectious granulomatous disease such as tuberculosis and fungal infections
- Foreign body reactions
- Lymphoma
- Other malignancies associated with lymphadenopathy
- Berylliosis

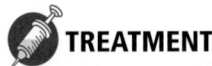 **TREATMENT**

INITIAL STABILIZATION
Outpatient

GENERAL MEASURES
- Disease may require no specific therapy in the asymptomatic individual or may treat for specific indications, such as cardiac, CNS, ocular, or hypercalcemia
- Treatment of pulmonary and skin manifestations usually done on the basis of impairment

Diet
- Avoid high-calcium diets.
- In patients on corticosteroids, avoid high-salt foods

Activity
Generally no limitations

 MEDICATION (DRUGS) (1,2,3)[C]

First Line
- Systemic corticosteroids in the symptomatic individual
  - Usually prednisone initially 40–60 mg/d for 1st 6 weeks
  - If stable, taper by 5 mg/wk to 15–20 mg/d over the next 6 weeks
  - If no relapse, treat with 15–20 mg/d of prednisone for 8–12 months
  - Relapse is common
- In patients with skin or ocular disease, topical steroids may be effective.
- Contraindications: Patients with known problems with corticosteroids
- Precautions: Careful monitoring in patients with diabetes mellitus and/or hypertension
- Significant possible interactions: Refer to the manufacturer's profile of each drug.

Second Line (5)[C]
- Methotrexate: 10 mg/wk
- Hydroxychloroquine (Plaquenil): 100–400 mg/d
- Azathioprine: 50–100 mg/d
- Use of immunosuppressants such as methotrexate or azathioprine will require careful, regular monitoring of CBC.
- Infliximab, a chimeric monoclonal antibody, has been useful in refractory cases. Dose is 3–5 mg/kg IV initially, 2 weeks later, then every 4–6 weeks.
- Thalidomide has been used for chronic skin lesions. The anti-TNF agent infliximab has also been used in some refractory cases.

 FOLLOW-UP

PROGNOSIS
- 50% of patients will have spontaneous resolution within 2 years.
- 25% of patients will have significant fibrosis, but no further worsening of the disease after 2 years.
- 25% of patients (higher in some populations, including African Americans) will have chronic disease.
- Patients on corticosteroids for >6 months have a greater chance of having chronic disease.

COMPLICATIONS
- Patients may develop significant respiratory involvement including cor pulmonale.
- Other organs, especially the heart (CHF, arrhythmias), eyes (rarely blindness), and CNS can be involved with serious consequences. Fortunately, cardiac, ocular, and CNS involvement usually manifests itself early on in patients with these manifestations of the disease.

PATIENT MONITORING
- Patients on prednisone for symptoms should be seen every month or 2 while on therapy.
- Patients not requiring therapy should be seen regularly (every 3 months) for at least the 1st 2 years after diagnosis.
- Chest radiograph and pulmonary function tests are useful for monitoring for pulmonary changes.
- The serum ACE level is used by some to follow the disease activity. In patients with an initially elevated ACE level, it should fall toward normal while on the therapy or when the disease resolves.

REFERENCES

1. Statement on sarcoidosis. Joint Statement of the American Thoracic Society (ATS), the European Respiratory Society (ERS) and the World Association of Sarcoidosis and Other Granulomatous Disorders (WASOG) adopted by the ATS Board of Directors and by the ERS Executive Committee, February 1999. *Am J Respir Crit Care Med*. 1999;160: 736–755.
2. Weinberger SE, et al. A 47-year-old woman with sarcoidosis. *JAMA*. 2006;296(17):2133–2140.
3. Baughman RP, et al. Pulmonary sarcoidosis. *Clin Chest Med*, 2004;25:521.
4. Baughman RP, et al. Sarcoidosis. *Lancet*. 2003;361: 1111.
5. Baughman RP, et al. Steroid-sparing alternatives for sarcoidosis. *Arch Intern Med*. 1997;18:853–864.

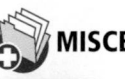 **MISCELLANEOUS**

CODES

ICD9-CM
135 Sarcoidosis

PATIENT TEACHING

Sarcoidosis is generally benign. It is not contagious, and it is not a malignancy.

 See Corresponding Diagnostic Algorithm

 See Patient Handout on CD

SCABIES

Gary J. Silko, MD, MS

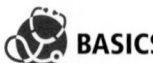 **BASICS**

DESCRIPTION
A contagious disease caused by infestation of the skin by the mite *Sarcoptes scabiei*, var. hominis

- System(s) Affected: Skin/Exocrine

EPIDEMIOLOGY
- Predominant age: Children and young adults
- Predominant sex: Male = Female

Incidence
Worldwide incidence is 300 million cases per year.

Prevalence
Common in the US, although number of cases per year is declining as the epidemic, which began in 1971, passed its peak (1986).

RISK FACTORS
- Personal skin-to-skin contact (e.g., sexual promiscuity, crowding, poverty, nosocomial infection)
- Immunocompromised patients including those with HIV/AIDS
- Atopic eczema

ETIOLOGY
Sarcoptes scabiei, var. hominis

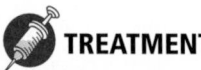 **DIAGNOSIS**

SIGNS AND SYMPTOMS
- Generalized itching (often severe)
- Nocturnal pruritus
- Burrows in finger webs and sides of fingers
- Excoriated and nonexcoriated papules on hands, waistline, penis, scrotum, buttocks, and flexor surfaces of wrist, elbow, and anterior axillary folds
- Vesicles and papules (discrete)
- Secondary erosions or excoriations
- Pustules (if secondarily infected)
- Scaling
- Erythema
- Nodules in covered areas (buttocks, groin, axillae)
- Atypical infestations in immunosuppressed patients

ALERT
Geriatric Considerations
The elderly often itch more severely, despite fewer cutaneous lesions, and are at risk for extensive infestations, perhaps related to a decline in cell-mediated immunity. May see back involvement in those who are bedridden

Pediatric Considerations
Infants often have more widespread involvement. They are occasionally infested on the face and scalp (rare for adults). Vesicular lesions on the palms and soles are also more commonly seen. When treating infants with permethrin, the entire body should be treated.

TESTS
Lab
CBC, although rarely needed, will frequently demonstrate eosinophilia.

Diagnostic Procedures/Surgery
- Examination of skin with magnifying lens
  - Look for typical burrows in finger webs, on flexor aspects of the wrists, and penis.
  - Look for a dark point at the end of the burrow (the mite).
  - The mite can be extracted with a 25-gauge needle and examined microscopically.
- Mineral oil mounts
  - Place a drop of mineral oil over a suspected lesion. Nonexcoriated papules or vesicles may also be sampled.
  - Scrape the lesion with a no. 15 surgical blade.
  - Examine under a microscope for mites, eggs, egg casings, or feces.
  - Scraping from under fingernails may often be positive.
- Potassium hydroxide (KOH) wet mount
  - Transfer skin scrapings directly to a glass slide, add a drop of KOH, and apply a cover slip.
  - Examine the slide for diagnostic material.
  - If none is evident, heat slide gently to separate squamous cells and re-examine.
- Burrow ink test
  - If burrows are not obvious, apply blue-black ink to an area of rash. Wash off the ink with alcohol. A burrow should remain stained and become more evident.
  - Then apply mineral oil, scrape, and observe microscopically as previously noted.

Pathological Findings
Skin biopsy of a nodule (although rarely performed) will reveal portions of the mite in the corneal layer.

DIFFERENTIAL DIAGNOSIS
- Atopic dermatitis
- Dermatitis herpetiformis
- Eczema
- Insect bites
- Papular urticaria
- Pediculosis corporis
- Pityriasis rosea
- Prurigo
- Pyoderma
- Seborrheic dermatitis
- Syphilis

TREATMENT

GENERAL MEASURES
- Treat all intimate contacts and close household and family members.
- Wash all clothing, bed linen, and towels in a normal wash cycle.

Diet
No special diet

Activity
Full activity

MEDICATION (DRUGS)

First Line
- Permethrin ((Elimite, Acticin) 5% cream (Nix) 1% cream rinse)
  - Considered by many to be the drug of choice for scabies
  - Cream is applied into the skin from the neck to the soles of the feet with particular attention given to skin creases. It is left on for 8–14 hours, and then thoroughly washed off. Thirty grams is usually adequate for an adult. A 2nd application 1 week later is sometimes recommended. (1)[C]
- Lindane (Kwell, Scabene) 1%
  - Available in lotion, cream, and shampoo. The cream or lotion should be applied to all skin surfaces from the neck down and washed off 8–12 hours later. 2 applications 1 week apart are recommended by some physicians. (1)[C]
- Crotamiton (Eurax) 10%
  - Cream is applied into the skin from the head to the soles of the feet, left on for 8–14 hours, and then thoroughly washed off. It is believed to be less toxic than Lindane, but perhaps slightly less effective; therefore, application 5 nights in a row is advised. (2)[C]
- Contraindications
  - Lindane should be avoided in children who are premature, malnourished, or emaciated and those with severe underlying skin disease or a history of seizure disorders.
- Precautions
  - Patients should be cautioned not to overuse the medication when applying it to the skin.
  - For medications other than permethrin, patients should use a 2nd application only when specifically advised to do so by their physician.
  - Lindane should be used cautiously in immunocompromised patients.
- Significant possible interactions
  - Avoid lindane for patients on medications that lower the seizure threshold, such as tricyclic antidepressants.

ALERT
Pregnancy Considerations
Permethrin and lindane are category B drugs. Until more information is available, precipitated sulfur appears to be the safest treatment in pregnant or lactating women.

Pediatric Considerations
The US Food and Drug Administration (FDA) recommends caution when using lindane in patients who weigh <50 kg. It is not recommended for infants and is contraindicated in premature infants.

Second Line
- Precipitated sulfur 6% in petroleum
  - Applied to the entire body from the neck down for 3 nights. It is malodorous and messy, but is thought to be safer than lindane, especially in infants <6 months and safer than permethrin in infants <2 months.
- Ivermectin (Mectizan)
  - 100–200 μg/kg in 1 or 2 divided doses.
  - May need higher doses or in combination with topical scabicide for HIV-positive patients. (1)[B]

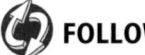 **FOLLOW-UP**

DISPOSITION
Outpatient care

PROGNOSIS
- Lesions begin to regress in 1–2 days along with the worst itching.
- Some itching and dermatitis commonly persists for 10–14 days and can be treated with antihistamines and/or topical or oral corticosteroids.
- Nodular lesions may persist for several weeks, perhaps necessitating intralesional or systemic steroids.
- Some instances of lindane-resistant scabies have now been reported. These do respond to permethrin.

COMPLICATIONS
- Eczema
- Pyoderma
- Postscabetic pruritus
- Nodular scabies

PATIENT MONITORING
Recheck patient at weekly intervals only if rash or itching persists. Scrape new lesions and retreat if mite or products found.

REFERENCES
1. Freedberg IM et al. *Fitzpatrick's Dermatology in General Medicine*. 6th ed. New York, NY: McGraw-Hill; 2003: 2283–2285.
2. James WD, Berger TG, Elston DM. *Andrews' Diseases of the Skin*. 10th ed. Philadelphia, PA: WB Saunders; 2006;452–453.

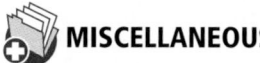 **MISCELLANEOUS**

See also: Insect bites and stings

CODES

ICD9-CM
133.0 Scabies

PATIENT TEACHING
For information on patient teaching, please see the following
- Patient instruction sheet, "Scabies." In: Epstein E. *Common Skin Disorders*. 5th ed. Philadelphia: WB Saunders; 2001:95.
- Schmitt BD, Jacobs JT. *Instructions for Pediatric Patients*. Philadelphia: WB Saunders.

 See Corresponding Diagnostic Algorithm

 See Patient Handout on CD

S

SCARLET FEVER

Felix B. Chang, MD
Smitha Nair, MD

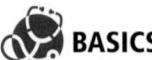 **BASICS**

DESCRIPTION
- "Streptococcal sore throat with a rash." A childhood disease characterized by high fever, pharyngitis, and rash caused by group A β-hemolytic streptococci (GAS) pyogenes that produce erythrogenic toxin.
- Incubation period 1–7 days
- Duration of illness 4–10 days
- Rash usually appears on the 2nd day of illness.
- Rash clears at the end of the 1st week and is followed by several weeks of desquamation.
- 1st appears in the upper chest and spread rapidly all over the body, including hands and feet.
- System(s) Affected: Gastrointestinal; Skin/Exocrine
- Synonym(s): Scarlatina

ALERT
Pediatric Considerations
Rare in infancy

GENERAL PREVENTION
- GAS is spread by contact with respiratory secretions. Avoid if possible.
- Children should not return to school or day care until >24 hours of antibiotic therapy.
- Prophylactic penicillin is not recommended after exposure to scarlet fever.

EPIDEMIOLOGY
- Predominant age: 6–12 years
- Predominant sex: Male = Female

Incidence
Up to 10% of GAS pharyngitis in the US

Prevalence
Fairly common, rare in infancy

RISK FACTORS
- Winter/spring seasons
- Age: School-aged children: By age 10, 80% have antibodies to erythrogenic toxin.
- Contact with infected individual
- Crowded living conditions (e.g., lower socioeconomic status, military, child care)

PATHOPHYSIOLOGY
- Erythrogenic toxin produced by phage is necessary for scarlet fever.
- Others virulent factors: DNAse, fibrinolysin, M protein, hyaloridase, streptolysin-O or -S, hyaluronidase capsule

ETIOLOGY
- Hypersensitivity to erythrogenic toxins produced by GAS
- Site of GAS infection usually tonsils; may occur with skin infection
- *Staphylococcus aureus* may also produce erythrogenic toxin: Staphylococcal scarlet fever
  – May be mild form of toxic shock syndrome or scalded skin syndrome

ASSOCIATED CONDITIONS
- Pharyngitis
- Impetigo
- Puerperal sepsis

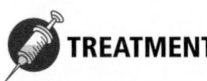 **DIAGNOSIS**

SIGNS AND SYMPTOMS
- Prodrome 1–2 days
  – Sore throat
  – Headache
  – Vomiting
  – Abdominal pain (may mimic acute abdomen)
  – Fever ($\leq 40°$C [103.6°F])
- Oral exam
  – Beefy red tonsils and pharynx with or without exudate
  – Petechiae on palate
  – White coating on tongue: "White strawberry tongue" appears on days 1–2. This sheds by days 4–5 leaving a "red strawberry tongue," which is shiny and red with prominent papillae.
- Exanthem (appears within 1–5 days)
  – Orange-red punctate skin eruption with sandpaper like texture: "Sunburn with goose pimples"
  – Initially, chest and axillae, then spreads to abdomen and extremities; prominent in skin folds (axillae, groin, buttocks)
  – Flushed face with circumoral pallor, red lips
  – Pastia lines: Transverse red streaks in skin folds of abdomen, antecubital space, and axillae
  – Desquamation begins on face after 7–10 days and proceeds over trunk to hands and feet; may persist for 6 weeks
  – In severe cases, small vesicular lesions (miliary sudamina) may appear on abdomen, hands, and feet.
  – Rash: Blanches if pressed

TESTS
Lab
- Throat culture definitive diagnosis
- Rapid strep antigen tests
  – Diagnostic if positive, but sensitivity only 50–90%, so do throat culture if result is negative.
- Serologic tests (includes antistreptolysin O titer and streptozyme tests, antihyaluronidase)
  – Confirm recent GAS infection; not helpful for diagnosis of acute disease
- Drugs that may alter lab results
  – Prior antibiotic therapy may result in negative throat culture.
  – Within 5 days of symptoms, antibiotics can delay/abolish antistreptolysin O response.
  – Gram stain: Positive cocci in chains
  – Culture B-hemolytic colonies, catalase negative, sensitive to bacitracin
  – Dick test: Injection of skin test dose of erythrogenic toxin is positive in persons lacking antitoxin

DIFFERENTIAL DIAGNOSIS
- Measles
- Rubella
- Infectious mononucleosis
- Roseola
- Severe sunburn
- Secondary syphilis
- *Arcanobacterium haemolyticum*
- Toxic shock syndrome
- Staphylococcal scalded skin syndrome
- Kawasaki disease
- Drug hypersensitivity
- Mycoplasma pneumonia
- Viral exanthem

TREATMENT

GENERAL MEASURES
Supportive care

Diet
No special diet

Activity
Fully active

MEDICATION (DRUGS)

First Line
- Acetaminophen for fever and comfort
- Penicillin (oral; penicillin V and others) for 10 days
  - 125 mg PO t.i.d. for <27 kg (60 lb); 250 mg t.i.d. for others; b.i.d. dosing may also be effective.
  - If compliance is questionable, use penicillin, benzathine (Bicillin LA): Single IM dose 600,000 U for <27 kg (60 lb); 1.2 mU for others
- Contraindications: Penicillin allergy
- Precautions: Refer to the manufacturer's profile of each drug.
- Significant possible interactions: Refer to the manufacturer's profile of each drug.

Second Line
- Erythromycin estolate (20–40 mg/kg/d divided t.i.d. or q.i.d. or erythromycin ethyl succinate (40–50 mg/kg/d divided t.i.d. or q.i.d.) for 10 days. Maximum dose: 1 g/d
- Newer macrolides
  - Azithromycin (Zithromax, Z pack): Adults: 500 mg the 1st day, then 250 mg daily for 4 days; children >2 years: 12 mg/kg/d (maximum of 500 mg) for 5 days
  - Clarithromycin (Biaxin): Adults: 250 mg b.i.d. for 10 days; children >6 months: 7.5 mg/kg b.i.d. for 10 days
- Oral cephalosporins: Many are effective, but 1st-generation cephalosporins are less expensive.
  - Cephalexin 40 mg/kg/d divided t.i.d. Maximum: 250 mg t.i.d. for 10 days
  - Cefadroxil 30 mg/kg/d divided b.i.d. Maximum: 500 mg b.i.d. for 10 days
- Clindamycin 20 mg/kg/d divided t.i.d. for 10 days
- Tetracyclines and sulfonamides should not be used.

SURGERY
Tonsillectomy may be recommended with recurrent bouts of pharyngitis.

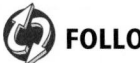 FOLLOW-UP

DISPOSITION
Outpatient care except for severe suppurative complications

PROGNOSIS
- Course may be shortened by 12–24 hours with penicillin.
- Recurrent attacks are possible.
- Mild disease usually responds well to antibiotics.

COMPLICATIONS
- Suppurative
  - Sinusitis
  - Otitis media/mastoiditis
  - Cervical adenitis
  - Peritonsillar abscess/retropharyngeal abscess
  - Pneumonia
  - Septicemia/meningitis/osteomyelitis/septic arthritis
- Nonsuppurative
  - Rheumatic fever: Prevents rheumatic fever when started as long as 10 days after onset of acute GAS infection.
  - Glomerulonephritis: Prevention even after adequate treatment of GAS is less certain.
  - Streptococcal toxic shock syndrome: Fever, hypotension, disseminated intravascular coagulation (DIC), and cardiac, liver, and/or kidney dysfunction
  - Cellulitis

PATIENT MONITORING
- Routine follow-up throat cultures is not needed unless patient is symptomatic.
- Because GAS is uniformly susceptible to penicillin, bacteriologic treatment failures are possibly owing to
  - Poor compliance
  - β-Lactamase oral flora hydrolyzing penicillin
  - GAS carrier state and concurrent viral rash (requires no treatment)

REFERENCES
1. Committee on Infectious Diseases of American Academy of Pediatrics. Red Book. *Elk Grove Village, American Academy of Pediatrics*; 2003;573–589.
2. Hahn R, Knox L, Forman T. Evaluation of poststreptococcal illness. *Am Fam Phys*. 2005; 71(10):1949–1954.
3. Del Mar CB, Glasziou PP, Spinks AB. Antibiotics for sore throat. *Cochrane Database Sys Rev*. 2005;4:CD00023.

ADDITIONAL READING
McKinnon H, Howard T. Evaluating febrile patients with rash. *Am Fam Phys*. 200015;62(4):804.

 MISCELLANEOUS

See also: Pharyngitis

CODES

ICD9-CM
034.1 Scarlet fever

ICD10
A38 Scarlet fever

PATIENT TEACHING
- Must take antibiotics for full course.
- Brief delay in initiating treatment awaiting throat culture results does not increase the risk of rheumatic fever.

Diet
No restriction

Activity
As tolerated

Prevention
- Can spread person to person.
- Avoid contact. Wash hands.

 See Corresponding Diagnostic Algorithm

 See Patient Handout on CD

S

SCHIZOPHRENIA

Jeffrey Stovall, MD

 BASICS

DESCRIPTION
- Major psychiatric disorder with prodrome, active, and residual symptoms involving disturbances (lasting ≥6 months) in appearance (deteriorated), speech (loosened association), behavior (grossly disorganized), perception (hallucinations), or thinking (delusions).
- System(s) Affected: Nervous

ALERT
Geriatric Considerations
Those who survive enter into a chronic phase marked by social and cognitive decline.

Pediatric Considerations
Unusual before puberty

Pregnancy Considerations
Use haloperidol if necessary. Newer, less-studied, atypical antipsychotics may also be used.

EPIDEMIOLOGY
- Predominant age: Onset typically <45 years
- Predominant sex: Male = Female
  - Onset earlier in males (early to mid-20s) than females (late 20s)

Prevalence
- Lifetime (1%): Highest prevalence in lower socioeconomic classes
- 1.1% of the population >18 years: Similar rates in all countries

RISK FACTORS
Biologic relative with schizrenia: If 1st-degree relative, risk is 8%.

Genetics
Genetic predisposition

ETIOLOGY
- Unknown: Not initiated or maintained by an organic factor
- Probably a complex interaction between inherited and environmental factors

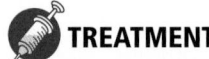 **DIAGNOSIS**

SIGNS AND SYMPTOMS
- Withdrawal from usual activities
- Delusions (false personal beliefs)
- Reference (people or things have unusual significance)
- May believe others can hear their thoughts, put thoughts into their mind, or control them
- May have grandiose or religious delusions
- Hallucinations: Usually auditory
- Illusions: Incorrectly interpreted sensory stimuli
- Affect: Flat or blunted, although may be anxious or irritable
- Thought processes: Loose associations, illogical
- Extremes of overactivity to stupor with mutism
- Onset in 20s

TESTS
Lab
- No test are available to indicate schizophrenia.
- Laboratory tests are needed to rule out other causes; these may include
- CBC, blood chemistries
- TSH
- RPR
- URINALYSIS
- Vitamin levels (B$_{12}$, folate, thiamine)
- Drug/alcohol screen of blood and urine
- Heavy metal exposure: Ceruloplasmin, urine porphobilinogen as indicated

Imaging
CT and MRI to rule out other causes

Diagnostic Procedures/Surgery
- Psychological: Not a routine part of assessment
- EEG to rule out seizure disorder
- Lumbar puncture if indicated by clinical presentation

DIFFERENTIAL DIAGNOSIS
- Mental disorder due to medical illnesses
  - Characterized by impaired judgment, orientation, memory, affect, and concentration, in association with a known medical illness
  - Disorientation, in particular, indicates delirium.
  - Possible medical illnesses include trauma, infection, tumor, metabolic, endocrine, intoxication (psychoactive substance use), epilepsy, withdrawal states.
- Organic delusional syndrome
  - Secondary to substance use/abuse including cocaine, amphetamines, lysergic acid diethylamide [LSD], phencyclidine, and alcohol, which may have identical symptoms
- Mood disorders
  - Especially bipolar disorder (manic-depressive disorder), schizoaffective disorder; mood disorders with psychotic features
- Cultural belief system

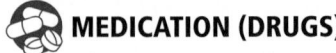 **TREATMENT**

GENERAL MEASURES
- Ensure safety of patient and others
- Patient may act on delusional thinking, or agitation
- Suicide risk is significant (10% of individuals with schizophrenia die by suicide).

Diet
No special diet, although metabolic syndrome and obesity are common in people with schizophrenia treated with atypical antipsychotics.

Activity
Establish safe hospital environment.

MEDICATION (DRUGS)

First Line
- 2 main groups
  - Conventional: Chlorpromazine, fluphenazine, trifluoperazine, perphenazine, thioridazine, haloperidol, thiothixene
  - Atypical: Risperidone, clozapine, olanzapine, quetiapine, ziprasidone, aripiprazole
- Medication choice is based on clinical and subjective response, and side effect profile
  - For sensitivity to extrapyramidal adverse effects: Atypical
  - For tardive dyskinesia: Clozapine
  - For poor compliance/high risk of relapse: Injectable form of long-acting antipsychotic, such as haloperidol, fluphenazine, or risperidone
- Usual oral daily dose (initial dose may be lower):
  - Chlorpromazine 200 mg b.i.d.
  - Fluphenazine 10 mg/d
  - Trifluoperazine 10 mg b.i.d.
  - Perphenazine 25 mg/d divided b.i.d. or t.i.d.
  - Thioridazine 150 mg b.i.d.
  - Haloperidol 5 mg b.i.d.
  - Thiothixene 10 mg b.i.d.
  - Risperidone 4 mg/d
  - Clozapine 100–200 mg t.i.d.
  - Olanzapine 15–25 mg/d
  - Quetiapine 200–300 mg b.i.d.
  - Ziprasidone 40–80 mg b.i.d.
  - Aripiprazole 10–30 mg/d
- Contraindications: Refer to the manufacturer's profile of each drug.
- Precautions
  - For acute side effects of antipsychotics: Dystonic reaction (especially of head and neck): Give diphenhydramine (Benadryl) 25–50 mg IM.
  - For pseudoparkinsonism reaction: Trihexyphenidyl (Artane) 2 mg b.i.d. (may be increased to 15 mg/d if needed) or benztropine (Cogentin) 0.5 b.i.d. (range, 1–4 mg/d)
  - For neuroleptic malignant syndrome: Hyperthermia, severe extrapyramidal effect, and autonomic dysfunction (hypertension, tachycardia, diaphoresis, and incontinence). Acute hyperthermia treated with Dantrolene 1 mg/kg IV push and continued as needed until cumulative total dose is up to 10 mg/kg. Stop antipsychotic. Post crisis management with Dantrolene 4–8 mg/kg/d PO in 4 divided doses for 1–3 days to prevent recurrence. Extrapyramidal effects treated with bromocriptine 2.5 mg t.i.d. to q.i.d. PO/NG

- Risperidone, olanzapine, quetiapine and clozapine are associated with weight gain and development of metabolic syndrome.
- Significant possible interactions: Refer to the manufacturer's profile of each drug.

Second Line
- Clozapine (Clozaril) 25 mg/d
  - Increase slowly to dose of 300–400 mg given t.i.d.; do not exceed 900 mg/d.
  - Serious toxicity of agranulocytosis mandates weekly CBC; reserve for therapy-resistant patients.
  - Effective in treatment of refractory patients
- Benzodiazepines
  - May be effective adjuncts to antipsychotics during acute phase of illness
  - Withdrawal reactions can include psychosis or seizures.
  - Schizophrenic patients are vulnerable to abuse/addiction.
- Anticonvulsants
  - May be effective adjuncts to patients with EEG abnormalities suggestive of seizure activity and those with agitated/violent behavior

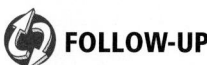 FOLLOW-UP

DISPOSITION
- Outpatient care if patient is not dangerous to self or others, able to cooperate with treatment, and has a supportive family: Community treatment and case management often are integrated into community support teams.
- Family intervention: Psychoeducation

Admission Criteria
Usually hospitalize initially for organic workup and for treatment of psychotic symptoms.

PROGNOSIS
- Chronic course: Remission and exacerbations
- Guarded prognosis
  - Complete remission not common
- The negative symptoms (consisting of decreased ambition, energy, and emotional responsiveness and social withdrawal) are often most difficult to treat.
- Excessive mortality occurs due to suicide, accidents, coronary artery disease, nicotine dependence, substance abuse..

COMPLICATIONS
- Side effects of neuroleptics, especially risk of tardive dyskinesia and metabolic syndrome with chronic use
- Self-inflicted trauma
- Combative behavior toward others
- High risk of suicide
- Comorbid addictions, including nicotine

PATIENT MONITORING
Continue medication as well as psychiatric therapies (individual, group, family), vocational rehabilitation, social skills training, day treatment.

REFERENCES
1. AACAP practice parameters for the assessment and treatment of children and adolescents with schizophrenia. American Academy of Child and Adolescent Psychiatry. *J Am Acad Child Adolesc Psychiatry.* 1997;36(Suppl):1775–1935.
2. American Psychiatric Association. Practice guidelines for the treatment of patients with schizophrenia. *Am J Psychiatry.* 1997;154(Suppl): 1–63.
3. Bustillo JR, Lauriello J, Horan WP, Keith SJ. The psychosocial treatment of schizophrenia: An update. *Am J Psychiatry.* 2001;158:163–175.
4. Diagnostic and Statistical Manual of Mental Disorders, Text Revised, 4th ed. (DSM-IV-TR). Washington, DC: American Psychiatric Association, 2000.
5. Kaplan HI, Sadock BJ, eds. Comprehensive Textbook of Psychiatry, 7th ed. Baltimore: Williams & Wilkins, 2000.
6. Lieberman JA, Stroup TS, McEvoy JP, et al. Effectiveness of antipsychotic drugs in patients with chronic schizophrenia. *N Engl J Med.* 2005;353:1209–1223.
7. Miller BJ, Paschall CB, Svenden DP. Mortality and medical comorbidity among patients with serious mental illness. *Psych Serv.* 2006;57:1482–1487.
8. Mojtabai R, Nicholson RA, Carpenter BN. Role of psychosocial treatments in management of schizophrenia: A meta-analytic review of controlled outcome studies. *Schizophr Bull.* 1998;24:569–587.

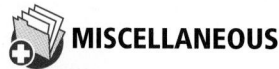 MISCELLANEOUS

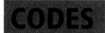 CODES

ICD9-CM
295.90 Unspecified schizophrenia, unspecified

PATIENT TEACHING
Information is available from the following organizations
- Education and support groups for patient and are family available from National Alliance for the Mentally Ill (NAMI; 2101 Wilson Blvd., Suite 302, Arlington, VA 22201; 703-524-7600).
- National Mental Health Association, National Mental Health Information Center (1021 Prince St., Alexandria, VA 22314-2971; 800-969-6642)
- Smoking cessation: American Cancer Society (www.cancer.org) and American Lung Association (www.lungusa.org)

Diet
Diet is not important in terms of prevention or treatment. However, given the high rates of metabolic abnormalities and obesity that develop in people with schizophrenia, early teaching in this area is important

Activity
As with diet, teaching the importance of exercise and smoking prevention can address the secondary complications of schizophrenia and its treatment.

Prevention
No primary prevention interventions are known. Patient teaching should focus on the importance of adherence to treatment, and preventing and managing comorbidities.

 See Corresponding Diagnostic Algorithm

 See Patient Handout on CD

S

SCLERITIS

Benjamin L. Sapers, MD

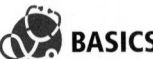 **BASICS**

DESCRIPTION
- Inflammation of the sclera, part of the eye's outer coat
- System(s) Affected: Nervous

GENERAL PREVENTION
None

EPIDEMIOLOGY
Predominant age: Most frequently occurs in 4th and 5th decades; mean age for all types of scleritis is 52 years.
- Predominant sex: Female > Male (1.6:1)

Incidence
Uncommon in the US In 1 study 0.08% of new patients presenting to an ophthalmology department were diagnosed with scleritis. 94% of patients will have anterior scleritis; the remaining 6% have posterior.

Prevalence
Uncommon in US

RISK FACTORS
Individuals with autoimmune disorders or chronic rheumatoid arthritis are most at risk.

Genetics
None

ETIOLOGY
- ~50% of cases of scleritis are associated with autoimmune diseases such as rheumatoid arthritis. In 15% of cases, scleritis is the presenting manifestation of a systemic disorder appearing 1 or more months before other symptoms of the condition.
- Scleritis has been reported in patients taking bisphosphonate therapy.

ASSOCIATED CONDITIONS
- Sjögren syndrome
- Ankylosing spondylitis
- Systemic lupus erythematosus
- Polyarteritis nodosa
- Wegener granulomatosis
- Gout
- Sarcoid
- Varicella zoster virus
- Syphilis

DIAGNOSIS

SIGNS AND SYMPTOMS
- Redness and inflammation of the sclera
- Pain ranging from mild discomfort to extreme localized tenderness. May be described as constant, deep, boring, or pulsating.
- Pain may be referred to the eyebrow, temple, or jaw.
- Photophobia and lacrimation may occur, but discharge is uncommon.

Physical Exam (1)[C]
- Visual acuity
- Examine for pain with consensual constriction, which suggests uveal involvement.
- Inspect for breadth and degree of injection.
- A bluish hue may suggest thinning of the sclera.
- Deeper scleral blood vessels appear darker, follow a radial pattern, and do not move when manipulated with a cotton swab.
- Complete physical examination, particularly of the skin, joints, heart, and lungs, may be done to evaluate for associated conditions

TESTS
Lab (1)[C]
- Consider further testing if history, physical examination, CBC and/or ESR suggest a systemic cause
- Rheumatoid factor
- Antinuclear antibody (ANA) and human leukocyte antigen (HLA) serotyping may help aid in the diagnosis.
- Chest radiograph (CXR) and sacroiliac joint films
- FTA-ABS and Lyme titers
- Uric acid

Imaging
CT scan of the orbit to determine the extent and location of scleritis

Pathological Findings (2)[B]
- Adjacent inflammation may or may not be present.
- The scleritis may be diffuse, nodular, or necrotizing (with or without associated inflammation).
- If the posterior region of the globe is involved, adjacent swelling of orbital tissues may occur.

DIFFERENTIAL DIAGNOSIS
- Conjunctivitis
- Episcleritis
- Pink eye
- Iritis (anterior uveitis)
- Trauma

TREATMENT

GENERAL MEASURES (3)[C]
- Treatment of the inflammation, usually with systemic steroids, is required.
- Immunosuppressants used for autoimmune and collagen vascular disorders may be of help in active scleritis.

Diet
No special diet

Activity
No restrictions

MEDICATION (DRUGS)

First Line (3)[C]
- Prednisone is the mainstay of treatment including topical, periocular, and systemic administration.
- Contraindications: None
- Precautions: Scleritis can progress to ocular perforation, which may be hastened with periocular steroid injection.
- Significant possible interactions: Refer to the manufacturer's literature.

Second Line
NSAIDs

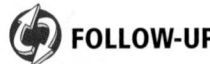 ## FOLLOW-UP

DISPOSITION
Outpatient care

PROGNOSIS
- Scleritis is indolent, chronic, and often progressive.
- Recurrent bouts of inflammation occur.

COMPLICATIONS
- Increased intraocular pressure
- Cataract and glaucoma can result from treatment.
- Ocular perforation can occur in severe stages.

PATIENT MONITORING
The patient should be followed very closely in the active stage of inflammation to assess the effectiveness of therapy.

REFERENCES

1. Merril IGM. Diseases of the Cornea. Boston: Little, Brown and Company, 1990.
2. Fong LP, Sainz de la Maza M, Rice BA, et al. Immunopathology of scleritis. *Ophthalmology*. 1991;98(4):472–479.
3. McCluskey P, Wakefield D. Current concepts in the management of scleritis. *Aust N Z J Ophthalmol*. 1988;16(3):169–176.

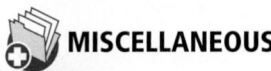 ## MISCELLANEOUS

CODES

ICD9-CM
379.00 Scleritis, unspecified

SCLERODERMA

Jeremy Golding, MD

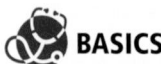 **BASICS**

DESCRIPTION

- Scleroderma (systemic sclerosis [SSc]) is a chronic disease of unknown cause, characterized by diffuse fibrosis, degenerative changes, and vascular abnormalities in the skin, articular structures, and other organs (kidneys, lung, heart, gastrointestinal and skeletal muscles).
- Most manifestations have vascular features (e.g., Raynaud phenomenon), but frank vasculitis is rarely seen. It can range from a mild disease, affecting the skin, to a systemic disease that can cause death in a few months.
- The disease is categorized into 2 major clinical variants
  - Diffuse
    ○ Distal and maximal extremity and truncal skin thickening
  - Limited
    ○ Restricted to the fingers, hands, and face
    ○ CREST syndrome (calcinosis, Raynaud phenomenon, poor esophageal mobility, sclerodactyly, telangiectasia) closely analogous with limited scleroderma
- System(s) Affected: Cardiovascular; Gastrointestinal; Musculoskeletal; Pulmonary; Renal/Urologic; Skin/Exocrine
- Synonym(s): Progressive systemic sclerosis (PSS); Morphea

ALERT

Geriatric Considerations
Uncommon >75 years of age

Pediatric Considerations
Rare in this age group

GENERAL PREVENTION
None

EPIDEMIOLOGY
- Predominant age
  - Young adult (16–40 years); middle-aged (40–75 years)
  - Symptoms usually appear in the 3rd–5th decades.
- Predominant sex: Female > Male (4:1)

Incidence
In the US: 1–2 per 100,00

Prevalence
In the US: 1–25 per 100,000

RISK FACTORS
Unknown

Genetics
Familial clustering is rare, but has been seen.

ETIOLOGY
- Unknown
- Possible alterations in immune response
- Possibly some association with exposure to quartz mining, quarrying, vinyl chloride, hydrocarbons, toxin exposure, and rapeseed oil
- Treatment with bleomycin has caused a sclerodermalike syndrome.

ASSOCIATED CONDITIONS
- Rheumatoid arthritis
- Systemic lupus erythematosus
- Polymyositis
- Overlap (and mixed) connective tissue disease

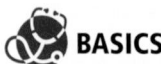 **DIAGNOSIS**

SIGNS AND SYMPTOMS
- Skin
  - Digital ulcerations
  - Tightness, swelling, thickening of digits
  - Hyperpigmentation
  - Hypopigmentation
  - Narrowed oral aperture
  - Pruritus
  - Scaling of skin
  - Subcutaneous calcinosis
- Peripheral vascular system
  - Raynaud phenomenon (differentiate from Raynaud disease, generally affecting younger individuals, and without digital ulcers)
  - Telangiectasia
- Joints, tendons, and bones
  - Flexion contractures
  - Friction rub on tendon movement
  - Hand swelling
  - Joint stiffness
  - Polyarthralgia
  - Sclerodactyly
- Muscle
  - Proximal muscle weakness
  - Weakness
- Gastrointestinal tract
  - Dysphagia
  - Esophageal reflux due to dysmotility (most common systemic sign in diffuse disease)
  - Malabsorptive diarrhea
  - Nausea and vomiting
  - Weight loss
  - Xerostomia
- Kidney
  - Hypertension
  - May develop scleroderma renal crisis: Acute renal failure
- Pulmonary
  - Dry crackles at lung bases
  - Dyspnea
- Nervous system
  - Peripheral neuropathy
  - Trigeminal neuropathy

TESTS
- ECG
  - Low voltage; possibly nonspecific abnormalities
- Lung function tests
  - Decreased diffusion and vital capacity
- Nail fold capillary loop abnormalities

Lab
- Increased ESR
- Normocytic anemia
- Normochromic anemia
- Positive antinuclear antibody (ANA), often with a nucleolar pattern
- Anticentromere antibody (usually associated with limited cutaneous disease)
- Anti–Scl-70 (topoisomerase antibody) is highly specific for systemic disease.
- Albuminuria
- Microscopic hematuria
- Eosinophilia
- Hemolysis
- Hypergammaglobulinemia
- Decreased maximum breathing capacity
- Increased residual volume
- Diffusion defect
- Positive rheumatoid factor test (33%)

Imaging
- Hand radiograph
  - Actor-osteolysis
  - Soft tissue atrophy
  - Subcutaneous calcinosis
- Upper gastrointestinal
  - Distal esophageal dilatation
  - Atonic esophagus
  - Esophageal dysmotility
  - Duodenal diverticula
- Barium enema
  - Colonic diverticula
  - Megacolon
- Chest radiograph
  - Diffuse reticular pattern
  - Bilateral basilar pulmonary fibrosis
- Gallium^{67} lung scan
  - Can be positive in early interstitial disease
- High-resolution CT scan for detecting alveolitis
  - Ground-glass appearance or honeycomb pattern in fibrosis

Diagnostic Procedures/Surgery
- Skin biopsy
  - Compact collagen fibers in the reticular dermis and hyalinization and fibrosis of arterioles
  - Thinning of epidermis with loss of rete pegs and atrophy of dermal appendages
  - Accumulation of mononuclear cells is also seen.
- Right heart catheterization
  - Pulmonary hypertension is an ominous prognostic feature.

Pathological Findings

- Skin
  - Edema, fibrosis, or atrophy (late stage)
  - Lymphocytic infiltrate around sweat glands
  - Loss of capillaries
  - Endothelial proliferation
  - Hair follicle atrophy
- Synovium
  - Pannus formation
  - Fibrin deposits in tendons
- Kidney
  - Small kidneys
  - Intimal proliferation in interlobular arteries
- Heart
  - Endocardial thickening
  - Myocardial interstitial fibrosis
  - Ischemic band necrosis
  - Enlarged heart
  - Cardiac hypertrophy
- Lung
  - Interstitial pneumonitis
  - Cyst formation
  - Interstitial fibrosis
  - Bronchiectasis
- Esophagus
  - Esophageal atrophy
  - Fibrosis

DIFFERENTIAL DIAGNOSIS

- Sclerodermatomyositis
- Mixed connective tissue disease
- Toxic oil syndrome (Madrid, 1981, affecting 20,000 people)
- Eosinophilia–myalgia syndrome
- Diffuse fasciitis with eosinophilia
- Scleredema of Buschke

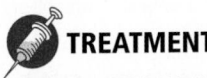 **TREATMENT**

GENERAL MEASURES

- Treatment is symptomatic and supportive.
- Esophageal dilatation may be used for strictures.
- Avoid cold; dress appropriately for the weather; be wary of air conditioning.
- Avoid smoking (crucial)
- For chronic digital ulcerations
  - Débridement after soaking in 1/2-strength hydrogen peroxide solution
  - Digital plaster to immobilize
- Avoid finger sticks (e.g., blood tests).
- Elevate of the head of the bed during sleep to help relieve gastrointestinal symptoms.
- Skin
  - Use softening lotions, ointments, and bath oils to help prevent dryness and cracking.
- Dialysis may be necessary in renal crisis.

Diet

- Soft, bland diet with frequent small meals
- Drink plenty of fluids with meals.

Activity

Stay as active as possible, but avoid fatigue.

Physical Therapy

- Physical therapy to maintain function and promote strength
- Heat therapy to relieve joint stiffness

 MEDICATION (DRUGS)

First Line

- Few drug therapies have proven value, except for angiotensin-converting enzyme (ACE) inhibitors for hypertensive renal crisis.
- Corticosteroids: For disabling myositis, pulmonary alveolitis, or mixed connective tissue disease
- NSAIDs: For joint or tendon symptoms
- Antibiotics: For secondary infections in bowel
- Antacids or cimetidine: For gastric reflux
- Dipyridamole (Persantine) or aspirin: Antiplatelet therapy
- Hydrophilic skin ointments: Skin therapy
- Topical clindamycin or erythromycin or silver sulfadiazine (Silvadene) cream may prevent recurrent infectious cutaneous ulcers.
  - Use systemic antibiotic therapy for active infections.
- Consider immunosuppressives
  - Used alone or with plasmapheresis for treatment of life-threatening or potentially crippling scleroderma or interstitial pneumonitis
- Avoidance of caffeine, nicotine, and sympathomimetics may ease Raynaud symptoms
- Vasoactive agents (nitrates) and antihypertensives (dihydropyridine calcium channel blockers): For Raynaud phenomenon
- Penicillamine (D-penicillamine): To reduce skin thickening and delay the rate of new visceral involvement (anecdotally)
- ACE (captopril): For kidney disease
- PDE-5 antagonists (e.g., sildenafil), prostanoids, and endothelin-1 antagonists are changing management of pulmonary hypertension
- Contraindications: Refer to the manufacturer's literature.
- Precautions: Refer to the manufacturer's literature.
- Significant possible interactions: Refer to the manufacturer's literature.

Second Line

Many other drugs are currently under investigation, but no evidence of real benefits have emerged yet.

SURGERY

- Some success with gastroplasty for correction of gastroesophageal reflux
- Limited role for sympathectomy for Raynaud

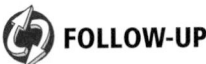 **FOLLOW-UP**

DISPOSITION

Outpatient care

Admission Criteria

Inpatient may be considered possibly for some surgical procedures.

PROGNOSIS

- Variable
- Possible improvement, but incurable
- Prognosis is poor if cardiac, pulmonary, or renal manifestations present early.

COMPLICATIONS

- Renal failure
- Respiratory failure
- Flexion contractures
- Disability
- Esophageal dysmotility
- Reflux esophagitis
- Arrhythmia
- Megacolon
- Pneumatosis intestinalis
- Obstructive bowel
- Cardiomyopathy
- Possible association with lung and other cancers
- Death

PATIENT MONITORING

Frequent monitoring of end-organ involvement and medications, and encouragement

REFERENCES

1. Kelley WN, et al., eds. *Textbook of Rheumatology*, 7th ed. Philadelphia: WB Saunders, 2005.
2. Reveille JD. Evidence-based guidelines for the use of immunologic tests: Anticentromere, SCL-70, and nucleolar antibodies. *Arthritis Rheum.* 2003;49(3):399–412.
3. Kippel JH, Dippe PR, eds. *Rheumatology*. St. Louis, MO: Mosby, 1994.
4. Koopman WJ, ed. *Arthritis and Allied Disorders*, 13th ed. Philadelphia: Lea & Febiger, 1997.

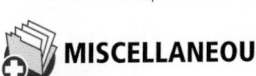 **MISCELLANEOUS**

CODES

ICD9-CM

710.1 Systemic sclerosis

PATIENT TEACHING

- Printed patient information available from the Scleroderma Federation (1725 York Avenue, No. 29F, New York, NY 10128; 212-427-7040).
- Advise patient to report any abnormal bruising or nonhealing abrasions.
- Assist patient in smoking cessation, if needed.

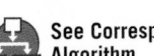 **See Corresponding Diagnostic Algorithm**

S

SEASONAL AFFECTIVE DISORDER

Christopher C. White, MD, JD

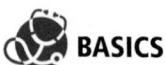 **BASICS**

DESCRIPTION
- Seasonal Affective Disorder (SAD) is a heterogeneous mood disorder with depressive episodes associated with winter months (possibly due to changes in light) with full remissions in the spring and summer.
- Although noted to occur decades ago, it was not formally named until the 1980s.
- Ranges from a milder form causing discomfort often called "winter blues" or sub-syndromal SAD to a seriously disabling illness
- Must separate out patients with other mood disorders (such as major depressive disorder and bipolar affective disorder) whose symptoms persist during spring and summer months

GENERAL PREVENTION
- Individuals with prior episodes should either begin daily light therapy in October or spend increased time outside during winter.
- Patients may consider moving to a more southern location to decrease symptoms.

EPIDEMIOLOGY
- Predominant age: Can occur at any age, but peak is 20s–30s (1)
- Predominant sex: Female > Male (3:1)

Incidence
- Affects up to 500,000 people every winter
- Up to 30% of patients visiting a PCP during winter may report winter depressive symptoms.

Prevalence
- 1–2% of the general population (2)
- 10–20% of patients identified as having mood symptoms will have a seasonal component.

RISK FACTORS
- Most common during winter months of January and February
  - Patients frequently visiting PCP during winter months complaining of recurrent flu, chronic fatigue, and unexplained weight gain should be screened for SAD.
- Women and young people at increased risk
- Decreased risk for those who live within 30° of equator
- Working in a building without windows or other environment without exposure to sunlight

Genetics
- Some twin studies have suggested a genetic component, but further study is needed.
- Increased incidence of depression and alcoholism in close relatives

PATHOPHYSIOLOGY
The major theories currently involve the interplay of phase-shifted circadian rhythms, genetic vulnerability, and serotonin dysregulation. (3)

ETIOLOGY
- Melatonin produced by the pineal gland at increased levels in the dark has been linked to depressive symptoms.
  - Light therapy on the retina acts to inhibit melatonin secretion.
- Serotonin dysregulation, because it is secreted at lower levels during winter months, must be present for light therapy to work, and treatment with SSRIs appears to reverse SAD symptoms.

ASSOCIATED CONDITIONS
Some with SAD have a weakened immune system and may be more vulnerable to infections.

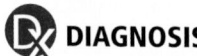 **DIAGNOSIS**

SIGNS AND SYMPTOMS
- Symptoms of depression (SIGECAPS) meeting the criteria for major depressive disorder
  - Sleep disturbance—either too much or too little
  - Interest (lack of)—in life and absence of pleasure from hobbies/activities
  - Guilt—feelings of guilt or worthlessness
  - Energy—fatigue or constantly feeling tired
  - Concentration—difficulty with concentration and memory
  - Appetite—changes in appetite and weight
  - Psychomotor retardation—patients may feel slowed down with decreased activity
  - Suicidal thoughts—patients may report thoughts of suicide
- In SAD hypersomnia, hyperphagia (craving for carbohydrates and sweets), and weight gain usually predominates. Despite sleeping more, patients report daytime sleepiness and fatigue. Cravings may lead to binge eating and weight gains >20 lbs.
- Remission of symptoms during spring and summer
  - Patients may report hypomanic episodes upon re-exposure to sunlight during spring.
- Symptoms have occurred the past 2 years
- Seasonal episodes associated with winter months substantially outnumber any nonseasonal depressive episodes.

History
- Obtain collateral history if patient is unable to provide insight into the seasonal component.
- Carefully document the presence or absence of prior manic episodes.
- Screen for the existence of any suicidal ideation and safety risk factors.

Physical Exam
Use the physical exam to exclude other organic causes for the symptoms. Focal neurological deficits, signs of endocrine dysfunction, or stigmata of substance abuse should prompt further testing and examination.

TESTS
Lab
- TSH to rule out hypothyroidism
- CBC to rule out anemia
- Renal to examine electrolytes and glucose dysregulation
- 25 OH Vitamin D level
- BHCG for women of childbearing potential
- Urine tox screen if substance abuse is a concern

Imaging
Generally not very useful unless focal neurological finding on physical exam or looking to exclude an organic cause

DIFFERENTIAL DIAGNOSIS
- Similar to that of major depressive disorder meaning organic causes of low energy and fatigue such as hypothyroidism, anemia, and mononucleosis (or other viral syndromes) accounting for the low energy and fatigue need to be considered
- Other mood disorders without a seasonal component such as major depression, bipolar disorder, adjustment disorder, or dysthymia
- Symptoms should not be better accounted for by seasonal psychosocial stressors, which often accompany the winter holiday seasons.
- Substance abuse

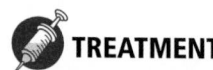 **TREATMENT**

GENERAL MEASURES
Work to reduce stress levels through meditation, progressive relaxation exercises, and/or lifestyle modification.

Activity
- Increase time outdoors during daylight.
- Rearrange home or work environment to get more direct sunlight through windows.

SPECIAL THERAPY
Vitamin D supplementation has been found to be more effective than phototherapy in small studies.

- Phototherapy using special light sources has been shown to be effective in 60–90% of patients often providing relief within a few sessions. (2,4)[B]
  - Variables which can regulate effect are
    - Light intensity—Although the minimum light source intensity is under investigation, 2,500 lux is suggested (domestic lights emit on average 200–500 lux). There is good evidence for 10,000 lux as the recommended source. (4)[A]
    - Treatment duration—exposure time varies on intensity of light source with daily sessions of 30 minutes to a few hours.
    - Time of treatment—most patients respond better by using the light therapy early in the morning.
  - Light box is placed on table several feet away and the light is allowed to shine onto the patient's eyes (sunglasses should be avoided). Ensure light box has a UV filter.
  - Most common side effects are eye strain and headache. Insomnia can result if the light box is used too late in the day.
  - Dawn simulation machines gradually increase illumination while the patient sleeps simulating sunrise while using a significantly less intense light source.

MEDICATION (DRUGS)

There is a lack of evidence to determine whether light therapy or medication should be the 1st-line agent. It depends on the acuity of the patient and the comfort level of the prescribing clinician with each treatment modality, [C].

First Line
Vitamin D supplementation may be beneficial.

- SSRIs such as sertraline (Zoloft), paroxetine (Paxil), fluoxetine (Prozac), citalopram (Celexa) in their traditional antidepressant doses (2)[B]

 FOLLOW-UP

Regular monitoring by PCP or psychiatrist for response to treatment. Patients may become manic when treated with SSRIs or light therapy.

DISPOSITION
Admission Criteria
If the patient develops suicidal ideation as part of their depression or mania after treatment is initiated, hospitalization should be considered.

Issues for Referral
- Patients with a history of ocular disease should be referred for an ophthalmologic exam before phototherapy and for serial monitoring.
- Patients who fail to respond to a medication trial or phototherapy should be considered for psychiatric referral.

PROGNOSIS
Symptoms, if untreated, generally remit within 5 months with exposure to spring light only to return in subsequent winters. If treated, patients usually respond within 2–3 weeks.

COMPLICATIONS
Development of suicidal ideation or mania are 2 outcomes which the clinician needs to monitor.

PATIENT MONITORING
Patients should be seen in the outpatient clinic weekly to bi-weekly when initiating light or pharmacotherapy to monitor treatment results, side effects, and any increased suicidal thoughts if using SSRIs. [B]

REFERENCES

1. Saeed SA, Brucw TJ. Seasonal affective disorders. *American Family Physician*. 1998: 57.
2. Lam RW. Seasonal affective disorder: Diagnosis and management. *Primary Care Psychiatry*. 1998;4:63–74.
3. Lam RW, Levitan RD. Pathophysiology of seasonal affective disorder: A review. *J Psychiatry Neurosci*. 2000;25:469–480.
4. Terman M, Terman JS. Light therapy for seasonal and nonseasonal depression: Efficacy, protocol, safety, and side effects. *CNS Spectr*. 2005;10:647–663.

 MISCELLANEOUS

See also: Bipolar disorder

CODES

ICD9-CM
The seasonal specifier can be applied to either recurrent major depressive disorder or bipolar disorder.

- 296.30 Major depressive episode, recurrent
- 296.80 Bipolar disorder NOS

PATIENT TEACHING

Diet
No specific diet modification needed

Activity
Increase time spent outside during sunlight.

Prevention
Consider use of light therapy at start of winter, increasing time outside during daylight, or moving to a more southern location.

S

SEIZURE DISORDER, ABSENCE

Wyley Hall, MD

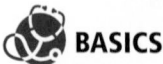 **BASICS**

DESCRIPTION
- Pediatric epilepsy type with brief seizures characterized by lapses of consciousness
- Often mistaken for daydreaming/inattention
- Childhood absence: 80% of cases
  - Onset age 4–8
  - 30% develop tonic–clonic seizures
  - 10–20% experience status epilepticus
- Juvenile absence: 20% of cases
  - Onset averages age 12
  - 80% develop tonic–clonic seizures
  - 40% experience status epilepticus
- Also divided into typical and atypical absence
- Typical absence
  - Abrupt onset unresponsiveness/behavior arrest without aura or postictal state
  - Rarely last >0 seconds
  - May occur hundreds of times daily
  - May include automatisms, tonic or atonic features, eyelid or facial clonus
- Atypical absence
  - More gradual on and offset
  - Often last >0 seconds
  - Often with tonic, atonic, myoclonic features
  - Associated with more severe epilepsy syndromes such as Lennox-Gastaut

EPIDEMIOLOGY
Incidence
1.9–8 per 100,000 Population

Prevalence
Accounts for 3–4% of epilepsies

RISK FACTORS
Genetics
- 64% concordance occurs in monozygotic twins or clinical epilepsy; 82% share EEG features.
- 33% concordance among 1st-degree relatives.
- 16–45% have family history of epilepsy.
- Girls are affected twice as often as boys.
- Likely autosomal dominant inheritance with incomplete penetrance
- For childhood absence, genes/loci implicated include 6q, 8q24, 5q14.
- For juvenile absence, chromosomes 5, 8, 18, 21 may have genes involved.
- Mutations of GABA-A receptor also are implicated.

PATHOPHYSIOLOGY
Corticoreticular theory implicates abnormal activity in thalamocortical circuits
- Reticular nucleus sends γ-aminobutyric acid (GABA)ergic neurons to thalamic relay nuclei.
- These neurons affect low-threshold calcium currents.
- These circuits can fire in oscillatory/rhythmic fashion or tonic bursts
  - Tonic firing present during awake state
  - Alertness suppressed by oscillatory firing
- Absence seizure potentiates rhythmic firing and produces lapse of consciousness.

ASSOCIATED CONDITIONS
- Multiple genetic syndromes exist
  - Lennox-Gastaut most recognizable, severe
- May evolve into juvenile myoclonic epilepsy

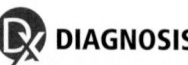 **DIAGNOSIS**

PRE HOSPITAL
Seizures are often so brief that untrained observers are not aware of diagnosis

SIGNS AND SYMPTOMS
History
Frequently diagnosed in children being evaluated for poor school performance
- Teachers report child seems to daydream or "zone out" frequently
- Child will forget portions of conversations
- Child with normal IQ underperforms in school

Physical Exam
- Unless child has other genetic or acquired abnormality, neurologic examination is usually normal
- Seizures may be frequent enough to be observed during physical examination
  - Manifest by behavior arrest: Child will stop speaking in mid-sentence, stare blankly, etc.
  - Automatisms (repetitive stereotyped behaviors) may be present.
  - Child resumes previous activity and may attempt to "cover up" lapse in awareness.
- Seizures may be induced by hyperventilation
  - Have child blow on a piece of paper or similar exercise until seizure occurs.
  - Photic stimulation may also evoke seizure although less frequently than hyperventilation.
- Patient manifests unresponsiveness, but retains postural tone in a typical absence seizure.
- Patients with associated tonic–clonic seizures are at risk of injury due to falls, similar to patients with partial and generalized epilepsy subtypes.

TESTS
- EEG is standard for diagnosis.
- Typical absence features 3.0-Hz spike-and-wave activity on normal EEG background
  - Seizures feature bursts of 3–4 Hz spike-and-wave activity, which may slow to 2.5–3 Hz during seizure
  - Seizure is usually evident clinically if bursts last >3 seconds; subtle changes of "transient cognitive impairment" may be evident with briefer seizures.
- Atypical absence seizures feature 0.5–2.5 Hz slow spike-and-wave activity superimposed on an abnormal background EEG pattern.
- Hyperventilation and occasionally photic stimulation are performed and may induce seizure, thus confirming diagnosis of typical absence epilepsy
  - Atypical absence seizures generally are not inducible.

Lab
- No specific hematological workup
- Follow blood chemistry, hepatic function, blood counts specific to drug regimen.
- Drug levels useful to evaluate symptoms of toxicity or for breakthrough seizures; less useful for routine monitoring

Imaging
- Not routinely indicated in children with typical absence and normal neurologic examination and IQ
- Brain MRI is indicated in atypical absence and in children with mixed seizure types when combined with abnormal neurologic examination or low IQ.

DIFFERENTIAL DIAGNOSIS
- Temporal lobe epilepsy with complex partial seizures
  - Differentiate by longer duration (>30 seconds vs. <10 in absence) and presence of postictal confusion
- Frontal lobe complex partial seizures
  - More difficult to distinguish on EEG due to rapid spread to bilateral cortex
  - Difference in duration and postictal state applies as in temporal lobe seizures

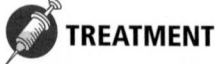 **TREATMENT**

GENERAL MEASURES
Activity
- Patients with associated tonic–clonic seizures should avoid high places, swimming alone.
- Absence rarely persists into adulthood, but affected adults may be restricted from driving, working over open flames, etc., as with other generalized and partial epilepsy subtypes.

MEDICATION (DRUGS)

Certain common anticonvulsants may exacerbate absence: Carbamazepine, tiagabine, vigabatrin, and gabapentin.

First Line
- Ethosuximide blocks T-type calcium channels
  - 1st line, except in absence patients with tonic–clonic seizures (lacks efficacy).
  - Side effects: Headache, hiccups, behavior changes, tremor
  - Adverse effects: Rare blood dyscrasias (monitor CBC)
- Lamotrigine affects sodium channels
  - Side effects: Headache, insomnia, dizziness
  - Adverse effects: Rare Stevens-Johnson rash, more often when coadministered with valproic acid
- Valproic acid has multiple mechanisms
  - 1st choice in absence patients with tonic–clonic, myoclonic, mixed seizure types
  - Side effects: Weight gain, alopecia, sedation
  - Adverse effects: Thrombocytopenia, rare fulminant hepatic failure (especially in children <2 years)

Second Line
- Topiramate affects GABA and excitatory neurotransmission
  - FDA approved for Lennox-Gastaut syndrome
  - Side effects: Psychomotor slowing
  - Adverse effects: Weight loss, renal stones, myopia, glaucoma (rare), anhidrosis
- Zonisamide, Levetiracetam also are used off label

ALERT
Pregnancy Considerations
Anticonvulsants, especially valproic acid, are associated with an increase in fetal malformations. Use of valproic acid in women who are or are likely to become pregnant generally is contraindicated. Obtain specialty consultation.

 FOLLOW-UP

Patients should be monitored periodically by a neurologist for evolution of absence epilepsy into tonic–clonic or other seizure types.

DISPOSITION
Admission Criteria
- Absence epilepsy rarely requires admission.
- Tonic–clonic status epilepticus requires inpatient management.

DISCHARGE CRITERIA
Resolution of status epilepticus

PROGNOSIS
- In typical absence epilepsy without tonic–clonic seizures, 65–70% remit by adulthood.
- 35% of patients with tonic–clonic seizures experience complete remission of absence.
- 15% of patients develop juvenile myoclonic epilepsy (JME).
- Decreased IQ, abnormal EEG background, resistance to medications, positive family history of epilepsy, presence of myoclonic seizures all associated with poorer prognosis for remission.

REFERENCES
1. Bouma PA, Westendorp RG et al. The outcome of absence epilepsy: A meta-analysis. *Neurology*. 1996;47:802–808.
2. Camfield P, Camfield C. Epileptic syndromes in childhood: Clinical features, outcomes, and treatment. *Epilepsia*. 2002;43(3):27–32.
3. Crunelli V, Leresche N. Childhood absence epilepsy: Genes, channels, neurons, and networks. *Nat Rev Neuro*. 2002;3:371–382.
4. Delgado-Escueta AV, Treiman DM, Walsh GO. The treatable epilepsies. *N Engl J Med*. 1983;308: 1508–1514.
5. Nordli DR. Idiopathic generalized epilepsies recognized by the International League Against Epilepsy. *Epilepsia*. 2005;46(9):48–56.

 MISCELLANEOUS

Other uncommon absence subtypes exist
- Micturition absence
  - Detrusor spasm during seizures
  - Problematic due to frequency of seizures Children are always wet, causing social issues.
- Myoclonic absence
  - Arms ratchet upwards at 3 Hz, retain posture
  - Associated with mental retardation
  - Resistant to therapy
- Absence with eyelid myoclonia
  - Prominent upper facial spasm
  - Resistant to therapy, autosomal dominant

S

SEIZURE DISORDER, PARTIAL

Sarah Guzofski, MD
Wylie Hall, MD
Ruben Peralta, MD, FACS

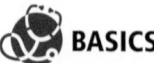 BASICS

DESCRIPTION
- Seizures occur when abnormal synchronous neuronal discharges cause transient cortical dysfunction.
- Generalized seizures involve bilateral cerebral cortex from the seizure's onset.
- Partial seizures originate from a discrete focus in the cerebral cortex.
- Partial seizures are further divided into simple and complex subtypes. If consciousness is impaired during a partial seizure, it is classified as complex; if consciousness is preserved, it is a simple partial seizure.

EPIDEMIOLOGY
Incidence
Partial seizures occur in 20/100,000 in US

RISK FACTORS
Genetics
One form of partial seizure, benign rolandic epilepsy, has an autosomal dominant inheritance pattern with penetrance dependant on multiple factors.

ETIOLOGY
- Partial seizures begin when a localized seizure focus produces an abnormal, synchronized depolarization, which spreads to a discrete portion of the surrounding cortex.
- The area of cortex involved in the seizure determines the symptoms; for example, an epileptogenic focus in motor cortex produces contralateral motor symptoms.
- Some conditions lead to structural abnormalities, which are prone to epileptogenesis. Some common examples include
  - Early childhood: Developmental/congenital malformation, trauma
  - Young adults: Developmental, infection, trauma
  - Adults 40–60: Cerebrovascular, infection, trauma
  - Adults >60: Cerebrovascular, trauma, neoplasm
- Complex partial seizures: A common cause is mesial temporal sclerosis

ASSOCIATED CONDITIONS
Epilepsy patients have a higher incidence of depression than does the general population.

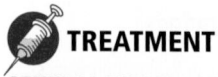 DIAGNOSIS

SIGNS AND SYMPTOMS
- Seizure activity usually stereotyped.
- Duration: Seconds to minutes unless status epilepticus develops. Status epilepticus may present as focal or generalized convulsion or altered mental status without convulsion.
- Simple partial seizure
  - Simple partial seizures are characterized by localized symptoms. The patient is conscious. Symptoms may involve motor, sensory, or psychic systems.
  - Motor: Seizure activity in motor strip causes contraction (tonic) or rhythmic jerking (clonic) movements that may involve 1 entire side of body or may be more localized (i.e., hands, feet, face).
  - "Jacksonian march": As discharge spreads through motor cortex, tonic-clonic activity spreads in predictable fashion (i.e., beginning in hand, progressing up arm, to face).
  - Sensory/psychic
    - Todd's paresis: Residual, temporary weakness in the area affected by a motor seizure
    - Parietal lobe: Sensory loss or paresthesias, dizziness
    - Temporal lobe: Déjà vu, rising sensation in epigastrium, auditory hallucinations or forced memories, unpleasant smell or taste
    - Occipital: Visual hallucinations
- Complex partial seizure
  - May have aura; this is start of seizure.
  - Impaired consciousness by definition
  - Amnesia for the event, postictal confusion
  - Most often, focus in complex partial seizures is temporal or frontal.
  - Motor manifestations may include dystonic posturing or automatisms (simple, repetitive movements of face and hands such as lip smacking, picking or more complex actions such as purposeless walking).
  - Frontal lobe seizure is characterized by brief, bilateral complex movements, vocalizations, often with onset during sleep.

History
- A detailed description of the seizure should be obtained from an observer.
- Review medication list for drugs that lower seizure threshold
  - Tramadol (Ultram), bupropion, theophylline

Physical Exam
Include neurologic exam with attention to lateralizing signs suggestive of structural lesion.

TESTS
EEG: Spikes/sharp waves over seizure focus
- Yield of EEG increased by obtaining in 1st 24 hours following seizure and by sleep deprivation.
- Frontal lobe seizure focus may be difficult to detect by routine EEG.
- If difficulty with diagnosis, continuous video-EEG monitoring may be appropriate.

Lab
- Serum electrolytes including calcium, magnesium, and phosphorus; hepatic function panel, CBC, drugs of abuse
- If measured within 10–20 minutes after suspected seizure, prolactin level may help differentiate generalized or complex partial seizure from psychogenic seizure.
- CSF exam if infection is suspected
- Urinalysis, chest radiogram, levels of antiepileptic drugs for breakthrough seizure

Imaging
- Emergency evaluation of new seizure: CT to screen for hemorrhage, stroke
- After emergency evaluation, MRI with thin cuts through area of interest
- If planning epilepsy surgery; PET scan and/or interictal SPECT may be of value.
- Magnetoencephalography is an evolving technology for localizing seizure focus.

DIFFERENTIAL DIAGNOSIS
- Nonepileptic seizure
- Syncope/post-anoxic myoclonus
- Hypoglycemia
- For hemiparesis following event
  - TIA
  - Hemiplegic migraine

TREATMENT

GENERAL MEASURES
- Ask patient to maintain a seizure diary.
- Note potential triggers such as stress, sleep deprivation, drug use, discontinuation of alcohol or benzodiazepines, menses.

Diet
Ketogenic or low-glycemic-index diet may improve seizure control in some patients.

Activity
- Most states have restrictions on driving for those with seizure disorders.
- Depending on seizure manifestation, may recommend against activities such as swimming, climbing to heights, working over open flames, or operating heavy machinery.

SPECIAL THERAPY
- Vagal nerve stimulator: Implanted in neck; provides periodic stimulation to vagus nerve. May induce hoarseness, cough, and dysphagia.
- New technologies being developed include deep brain stimulation.

MEDICATION (DRUGS)

- Some physicians do not start medication after a single seizure if EEG and MRI are normal, and/or a precipitant is clear and avoidable.
- Antiepileptic drugs (AEDs) act on voltage-gated ion channels, affect neuronal inhibition via enhancement of GABA (an inhibitory neurotransmitter), or decrease neuronal excitation. End result is to decrease the abnormal synchronized firing and to prevent seizure propagation.
- ~50% of those with newly diagnosed partial seizures will respond to and tolerate the 1st AED trial (1).
- Choose AED based on seizure type, side effect profile, and patient characteristics
  – Increase dose until seizure control obtained or side effects become unacceptable.
- Attempt monotherapy, but many patients will require adjunct agents.
- "Refractory to medications" is defined as failure of at least 3 anticonvulsants to achieve adequate control.
- Several AEDs induce or inhibit cytochrome P450 enzymes (watch for drug interactions).

First Line
- Carbamazepine: Affects sodium channels
  – Side effects: GI distress, hyponatremia, diplopia, dizziness; rare pancytopenia/marrow suppression, exfoliative rash
- Oxcarbazepine: Affects sodium channels
  – Side effects: Dizziness, diplopia, hyponatremia, headache
- Lamotrigine: Affects sodium channels
  – Side effects: Insomnia, dizziness, ataxia
  – Risk of Stevens-Johnson reaction (potentially fatal exfoliative rash) especially when given with valproate—requires slow titration
- Levetiracetam: Multiple mechanisms
  – Side effects: Sedation, ataxia, irritability

Second Line
- Phenytoin: Affects sodium channels
  – Side effects: Ataxia, dizziness, diplopia, tremor, GI upset, gingival hyperplasia, fever
- Phenobarbital: Multiple mechanisms
  – Side effects: Sedation, withdrawal seizures
- Valproate: Multiple mechanisms
  – Side effects: GI upset, weight gain, alopecia, tremor; less common thrombocytopenia, hepatitis, pancreatitis
- Topiramate: Multiple mechanisms
  – Side effects: Anorexia, cognitive slowing, sedation, nephrolithiasis, anhidrosis
- Gabapentin: Multiple mechanisms
  – Side effects: Sedation, dizziness, ataxia
- Pregabalin: Affects calcium channels
  – Side effects: Sedation, dizziness, weight gain
- Zonisamide: Affects sodium channels
  – Side effects: Sedation, anorexia, nausea, dizziness, ataxia, anhidrosis, nephrolithiasis
  – Cross reaction with sulfa allergy

ALERT
Pregnancy Considerations
- Several antiepileptic medications induce hepatic metabolism of oral contraceptives, decreasing their efficacy. AED therapy during 1st trimester is associated with doubled risk for major fetal malformations (6% vs. 3%) (2). Phenytoin in pregnancy may result in fetal hydantoin syndrome.
- Fetal insult from seizures following withdrawal of therapy also may be severe. Risk/reward balance should be evaluated with high-risk pregnancy and epileptology consultations. Most patients remain on anticonvulsants.

SURGERY
For refractory partial complex seizures
- Should have identifiable focus
- Preoperative testing, such as Wada test, should be done to decrease likelihood of inducing aphasia and memory loss.
- Workup also may include MRI, video-EEG monitoring, electrocorticography, MEG, ictal SPECT.
- 64% will be seizure free after surgery (with continued medication treatment); 25% will have significant decrease in frequency. 1/3 continue to have disabling seizures (3)[B]
- Goal of surgical intervention is to reduce reliance on medications; most remain on anticonvulsants postoperatively.

 FOLLOW-UP

Outpatient follow-up with neurologist

DISPOSITION
Admission Criteria
Generally, outpatient treatment; admission for unremitting seizure (partial or secondary generalized status epilepticus)

Issues for Referral
For refractory seizures, consider referral to an epilepsy specialist.

PROGNOSIS
- Risk of seizure recurrence is ~30% after 1st seizure; 50% of these recurrences will occur in the 1st 6 months; 90% in the 1st 2 years. (4)[B]
- Depends on seizure type. Rolandic epilepsy has a good prognosis; temporal lobe epilepsy more likely to be persistent. (5)[A]
- Long duration of uncontrolled seizure disorder associated with increased cognitive and functional impairments. Early pharmacologic intervention is encouraged. (5)[A]

COMPLICATIONS
- Risk of accidental injury
- SUDEP (Sudden Death in Epilepsy Patients)

PATIENT MONITORING
AED levels if concern over toxicity, noncompliance, or for breakthrough seizures

REFERENCES
1. Kwan P and Brodie MJ. Effectiveness of first anticonvulsant drug. *Epilepsia* 2001;42:1255–1260.
2. Bromfield EB. Clinical use of anticonvulsants: A neurologist's perspective. *Harv Rev Psychiatry* 2003;11:257–268.
3. Schmidt D, Loscher W. How effective is surgery to cure epilepsy in drug-resistant temporal lobe epilepsy? *Epilepsy Res* 2003;56:85–91.
4. Pohlmann-Eden B, Beghi E, Camfield C et al. The first seizure and its management in adults and children. *BMJ* 2006;322:339–342.
5. Wolf P. Determinants of outcome in childhood epilepsy. *Acta Neurol Scand* 2005;112:5–8.

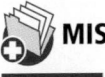 **MISCELLANEOUS**

CODES
ICD9-CM
- 345.4 Partial epilepsy with impairment of consciousness
- 345.5 Partial epilepsy without mention of impairment of consciousness

PATIENT TEACHING
Avoid potential triggers such as alcohol or drug use, sleep deprivation.

 See Corresponding Diagnostic Algorithm

S

SEIZURE DISORDERS

Shawn H. Blanchard, MD
William L. Toffler, MD

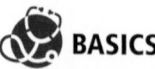 **BASICS**

DESCRIPTION
A seizure is a sudden change in cortical electrical activity, manifested through motor, sensory, or behavioral changes, with or without an alteration in consciousness.

- System(s) Affected: Nervous
- Synonym(s): Convulsions; Epilepsy; Fits; Spells; Attacks

ALERT
Geriatric Considerations
Fractures from falls are more common in the osteopenic age range.

Pediatric Considerations
- Breast-feeding is not contraindicated in mothers taking anticonvulsant medication; however, drug levels can be measured if sedation occurs in the infant.
- Pharmaceutical labeling is 1C or 1D, and consideration toward consultation should be entertained.

Pregnancy Considerations
- Serum levels of anticonvulsants may decline; frequent monitoring recommended
- 2-fold increased risk of congenital malformation in mothers taking anticonvulsant medications
- All anticonvulsants recommend against use both during pregnancy and while nursing

GENERAL PREVENTION
Maintain adequate epileptic drug therapy; continue efforts at insuring compliance and/or access to medication.

EPIDEMIOLOGY
- Predominant age: Pediatric and geriatric populations most commonly present with new-onset seizure disorder. Drug and or drug withdrawal seizures should be strongly considered in the adult population.
- Predominant sex: Male = Female

Incidence
In the US
- 181,000 people with lst seizure per year
- 45,000 new cases <15 years of age per year

Prevalence
In the US
- 4 million people have had 1 or more seizures; 2.5 million have a seizure disorder.
- ~600,000 people >65 years of age have a seizure disorder.
- 33% >75 years of age have had at least 1 lifetime seizure.

RISK FACTORS
- Susceptibility to seizures determined by a complex interplay between genetic factors and acquired brain disorders
- Children delivered breech have a prevalence rate of 3.8% compared with 2.2% in children delivered vertex.

Genetics
- Genetically predisposed with variable penetrance
- Family history increases risk 3-fold.
- Much will be understood concerning genetics and seizure disorder in the near future.

ETIOLOGY
- Brain tumor
- Cerebral hypoxia (breath holding, carbon monoxide poisoning, anesthesia)
- Cerebrovascular accident (infarct or hemorrhage)
- Convulsive or toxic agents (lead, alcohol, picrotoxin, strychnine)
- Drug overdose/withdrawal
- Eclampsia
- Exogenous factors (sound, light, cutaneous stimulation)
- Fever (see topic on Febrile seizures)
- Head injury
- Heat stroke
- Infection
- Metabolic disturbances
- Withdrawal from, or hereditary intolerance of, alcohol

ASSOCIATED CONDITIONS
- Infections
- Tumors
- Drug abuse
- Alcohol and drug withdrawal
- Metabolic disorders
- Trauma

DIAGNOSIS

SIGNS AND SYMPTOMS
- General
  - Fever: Indicative of infectious etiology
  - Focal neurologic finding: May indicate tumor or localized injury to the brain
  - Papilledema: Suggestive of increased intracranial pressure
  - Hemorrhagic eye grounds: Suggests underlying hypertension
  - Meningismus: May be present with meningitis
  - Headache: Sometimes associated with infectious or hemorrhagic causes of seizures
- Generalized seizures
  - Absence: Loss of consciousness or posture
  - Myoclonic: Repetitive muscle contractions
  - Tonic-clonic: Sustained contraction followed by rhythmic contractions of all four extremities
- Partial seizures
  - Simple: Focal seizures without alteration of awareness/consciousness
  - Complex: Focal seizures with alteration of awareness/consciousness
- Febrile seizures (see separate topic)
  - Occurs between 3 months and 5 years of age
  - Fever without evidence of any other defined cause for seizures
  - If febrile seizures occur in the 1st year, the recurrence rate is 51%.
  - If febrile seizures occur in the 2nd year, the recurrence rate is 25%.

- 88% of all recurrences of febrile seizures occur in the 1st 2 years.
  - The earlier the age of onset, the more likely repetitive febrile seizures will occur.
  - Recurrent febrile seizures probably do not increase the risk of epilepsy.
- Status epilepticus (see separate topic)
  - Repetitive generalized seizures without return to consciousness between seizures
  - Considered a neurological emergency

TESTS
- ECG: A negative ECG does not rule out a seizure disorder. Sleep deprivation is helpful prior to ECG to identify positive spike wave formations.
- Video ECG monitoring is helpful in differentiating psychomotor nonepileptiform seizures.

Lab
- Serum tests: Glucose, sodium, potassium, calcium, phosphorus, magnesium, BUN, ammonia
- Anticonvulsant levels: Inadequate level of anticonvulsant medication is the most common cause of recurrent seizures in children and many adults.
- Drug and toxic screens, include alcohol
- CBC helpful in evaluating infection
- Drugs that may alter lab results
  - Anticonvulsant therapy may dramatically affect the ECG results.
  - Levels of anticonvulsants may be altered by a variety of common medications such as erythromycin, sulfonamides, warfarin, and cimetidine, as well as alcohol.
- Disorders that may alter lab results: Pregnancy decreases serum concentration. Frequent monitoring and dosage adjustments are necessary.

Imaging
- MRI of brain: Superior in evaluation of the temporal lobes
- CT scan of brain: Indicated routinely in workup of tonic–clonic seizures

Diagnostic Procedures/Surgery
Stereotactic investigation may prove beneficial for the 10% of seizures recalcitrant to pharmaceutical therapy.

Pathological Findings

MRI may identify a lesion responsible (i.e., a nidus) for seizure activity.

DIFFERENTIAL DIAGNOSIS

- Infancy (0–2)
  - Perinatal hypoxia
  - Birth injury
  - Metabolic—hypoglycemia, hypocalcemia, hypomagnesemia, vitamin B_6 deficiency, phenylketonuria
  - Acute infection
- Childhood (2–10)
  - Febrile seizure
  - Idiopathic
  - Acute infection
  - Trauma
- Adolescent (10–18)
  - Idiopathic
  - Trauma
  - Drug and alcohol withdrawal
  - Arteriovenous malformations
  - Conversion disorder—pseudoseizure
- Early adulthood (18–25)
  - Idiopathic
  - Drug and alcohol withdrawal
  - Trauma
  - Conversion disorder—pseudoseizure
- Middle age (25–60)
  - Drug and alcohol withdrawal
  - Trauma
  - Tumor
  - Vascular disease
  - Conversion disorder—pseudoseizure
- Late adulthood (>60)
  - Vascular disease
  - Tumor
  - Degenerative disease
  - Metabolic: Hypoglycemia, uremia, hepatic failure, electrolyte abnormality

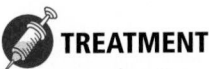 TREATMENT

INITIAL STABILIZATION

Outpatient therapy is usually sufficient except for status epilepticus.

GENERAL MEASURES

- Protect the patient's airway.
- If possible, protect the patient from physical harm.

Diet

Regular

Activity

- Individuals with uncontrolled seizures should avoid heights and swimming.
- State driving laws can be located at www.epilepsyfoundation.org

 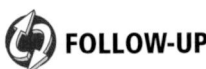 MEDICATION (DRUGS)

First Line

Selection of medications from following seizure groups, with attention toward potential side effects, is preferred, as is monotherapy whenever possible. Systemic reviews found insufficient evidence on which to base a choice among these drugs in terms of seizure control.

- Generalized seizures: Tonic–clonic
  - Phenytoin (Dilantin): 200–400 mg/d in 1–3 doses; therapeutic range 10–20 μg/mL
  - Carbamazepine (Tegretol) 100–200 mg/d in 1–2 doses; therapeutic range: 4–12 μg/mL
  - Valproic acid (Depakene): 750–3,000 mg/d in 1–3 doses; begin at 15 mg/kg/d; therapeutic range 50–150 μg/mL
- Generalized seizures—absence
  - Ethosuximide (Zarontin): 250–1,500 mg/d in 1–2 doses; therapeutic range 40–100 μg/mL
  - Valproic acid (see information provided previously)
- Partial seizures
  - Phenytoin (Dilantin)
  - Carbamazepine (Tegretol)
  - Phenobarbital
    - There is evidence to suggest long-term use of phenobarbitol may impair cognative ability. (1)[C]
- Contraindications: Refer to the manufacturer's profile of each drug.
- Precautions: Doses should be based on individual's response and drug levels where available.
- Significant possible interactions: Refer to the manufacturer's profile of each drug.

Second Line

- Felbamate (Felbatol): 1,200 mg/d in 3–4 divided doses. max 3,600 mg/d
- Gabapentin (Neurontin): 300 mg at bedtime, then 2–3 divided doses, max. 2,400–3,600 mg/d
- Lamotrigine (Lamictal): 25–50 mg/d. Adjust in 100-mg increments every 1–2 weeks to 300–500 mg/d in 2 divided doses.
- Levetiracetam (Kepra) 500 mg b.i.d. with a max. of 3000 mg/d
- Methsuximide (Celontin): 300 mg/d for 1st week, increase 300 mg/3 weeks, max. 1,200 mg/d
- Oxcarbazepine (Trileptal): 300 mg b.i.d., increase 300 mg/3 days; maintenance 1,200 mg/d
- Pregabalin (Lyrica) 150–600 mg/d in divided doses
- Primidone (Mysoline): 100–125 mg at bedtime adjust to max. 2,000 mg/d in 2 doses
- Tiagabine (Gabitril): 4 mg/d, adjust weekly to max. 56 mg/d
- Topiramate (Topamax): 50 mg/d, adjust weekly to effective 400 mg/d in 2 doses, max. 1,600 mg/d
- Zonisamide (Zonegran) 100 mg/d for 2 weeks, increase 100 mg/d each 2 weeks to a max. of 400 mg/d

SURGERY

Many academic centers are finding success with stereotactic surgery for seizures that fail traditional therapy.

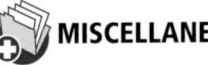 FOLLOW-UP

PROGNOSIS

- Dependent on type of seizure disorder
- Seizure activity may become quiescent.
  - After a seizurefree 2-year period, withdrawal of therapy may be considered.
  - 33% relapse rate should be expected in the following 3 years.

COMPLICATIONS

Drug toxicity

PATIENT MONITORING

- Regular monitoring of anticonvulsant levels and seizure frequency
- CBC as indicated
- Monitor medication side effects and adverse reactions.

REFERENCES

1. Marson A, Ramaratnam S. *Epilepsy Clin Evid Concise*. 2005;13:362–364.
2. Chang BS, Lowenstein DH. Epilepsy. *N Engl J Med*. 2003;349:1257–1266.
3. Annegers JF. The epidemiology of epilepsy. In: Wyllie E, ed. *The Treatment of Epilepsy: Principles and Practice*. 3rd ed. Philadelphia, PA: Lippincott Williams & Wilkins; 2001:131–138.
4. Mengel MB, Schwiebert LB, eds. *Ambulatory Medicine: Primary Care Families*. 4th ed. New York, NY: McGraw-Hill; 2004.
5. Goldstein LH. Assessment of patients with psychogenic non-epileptiform seizures. *J Neurol Neurosurg Psychiatry*. 2004;75:667–668.

MISCELLANEOUS

- See also: Seizures, Febrile; Status epilepticus
- Other notes: The International League Against Epilepsy (ILAE) is currently making progress in a new 5-axis classification system for seizure disorder, which will include genetics, characterization, and disability for seizure disorder syndromes.

CODES

ICD9-CM

- 345.10 Generalized convulsive epilepsy without mention of intractable epilepsy
- 779.0 Convulsions in newborn
- 780.39 Other convulsions

PATIENT TEACHING

Stress the importance of medication compliance and the avoidance of alcohol and recreational drugs, and refer to the web sights referenced below.

- www.epilepsy.org
- www.epilepsyfoundation.org
- www.ninds.nih.gov/health_and_medical/disorders/epilepsy.htm

 See Corresponding Diagnostic Algorithm

 See Patient Handout on CD

SEIZURES, FEBRILE

Malgorzata E. Klonowska, MD
Wyley Hall, MD

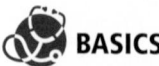 **BASICS**

DESCRIPTION
- A seizure that occurs in children between 6 months and 5 years of age, in association with fever and in the absence of CNS infection or previous diagnosis of epilepsy
- Simple febrile seizure (FS) (~80%)
  - Duration <15 minutes
  - Generalized seizure with no focal features
  - No recurrence in 24 hours
- Complex FS (~20%)
  - Duration >15 minutes
  - Focal features
  - >1 seizure in 24 hours

EPIDEMIOLOGY
- FS are the most common seizures in children.
- ~3% of children affected (1,2)[B]
- Average age of onset is 18–22 months, usually before the age of 3 years.
- Males have a slightly higher incidence.

RISK FACTORS
- For 1st FS
  - Family history of FS
  - Neurodevelopmental abnormality
  - >50% of children will have no identifiable risk factors
- For recurrent FS
  - Onset at age <18 months
  - Family history of FS
  - Temperature <40°C (104°F) with prior FS
- For subsequent epilepsy after FS
  - Family history of epilepsy
  - Complex FS
  - Neurodevelopmental abnormality

Genetics
- Complex polygenic basis
- A history of FS in immediate family members is present in 10–40% of cases.
- Monozygotic twins have a much higher concordance rate than dizygotic twins, supporting a genetic contribution.
- Susceptibility of FS has been linked to several genetic loci in different families.
- The syndrome of generalized epilepsy with FS plus (GEFS+) is characterized by heterogeneous epilepsy phenotypes with complex inheritance. (3)
- The most common phenotype is a continuation of FS >6 years of age associated with afebrile tonic–clonic seizures as well as other seizure types.
- Sodium channel and GABA$_A$ receptor genes have been associated with FS and GEFS+. (3)

PATHOPHYSIOLOGY
The underlying pathophysiology is unknown.

ASSOCIATED CONDITIONS
- Any viral or bacterial infections can provoke FS.
- Human herpesvirus-6 and herpes simplex virus have been associated with increased risk.
- The risk of FS is increased on the day of administration of diphtheria, tetanus toxoid, and whole-cell pertussis vaccine and 8–14 days after measles, mumps, rubella vaccine, but these are not associated with any long-term adverse effects.

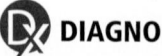 **DIAGNOSIS**

PRE HOSPITAL
FS may be the 1st sign of illness.

SIGNS AND SYMPTOMS
- Temperature >38°C (100.5°F), usually ≥39°C (102.2°F), average 40°C (104°F)
- Pyrexia may follow an FS, although this will rarely exceed 38°C (100.5°F)

History
- Description of seizure, presence of fever, character of illness
- Lethargy, irritability, decreased feeding, vomiting
- Recent treatment with antibiotics (meningitis can be masked if partially treated)
- Recent immunization
- Patient and family history of seizures
- Evaluate for other causes of seizures, such as trauma or toxin exposure

Physical Exam
- Usually normal neurologic exam
- Further workup indicated if evidence of meningitis (nuchal rigidity, drowsiness, bulging fontanelle, papilledema, petechiae)
- Focal neurologic signs
- Postictal (Todd) paralysis may be observed after a focal seizure.
- Stigmata of a neurocutaneous or metabolic disorder

TESTS
- The most urgent diagnostic decision is whether to perform a lumbar puncture (LP)
  - The incidence of meningitis in children with FS is no higher than in febrile children without seizure.
  - The earliest sign of meningitis (in 13–16% of children) can be a seizure and fever.
- LP in <12-month-olds with FS should be strongly considered, in 12–18-month-olds with FS should be considered, and in >18-month-olds is not routinely warranted but recommended in the presence of meningismus or other clinical suspicion of meningitis. (4)
- Cerebrospinal fluid is more likely to be abnormal in children with FS if
  - Complex FS
  - Prolonged postictal state
  - Initial seizure >3 years of age
- A recognized source of fever (e.g., otitis media) does not exclude the presence of meningitis. (4)
- In practice, the decision to perform LP should be tailored to each individual child's presentation.

ALERT

Pediatric Considerations
In infants <2 years, clinical signs and symptoms of meningitis may be minimal or absent.

Lab
- Routine measurement of serum electrolytes, calcium, phosphorous, magnesium, CBC, and serum glucose are low-yield and should not be routinely performed unless clinically indicated. (2,4)
- Serum glucose should be obtained if there is a prolonged postictal state or recurrent seizures.
- Laboratory testing should be directed at identifying source of fever.

Imaging
- Routine neuroimaging is not indicated in the evaluation of simple or complex FS. (4,5)
- Neuroimaging should be performed if the physical examination points to a possible structural lesion (e.g., micro/macrocephaly, focal neurologic signs, symptoms of increased intracranial pressure).

Diagnostic Procedures
- Electroencephalography (EEG) is not recommended as part of evaluation of a neurologically healthy child with a 1st simple FS. (4)
- EEG is recommended in children with complex FS who have developmental delay or abnormal neurologic signs and symptoms.
- EEG does not predict the recurrence of FS or the development of epilepsy. (4)

DIFFERENTIAL DIAGNOSIS
- Rigors
- Syncope
- Febrile delirium (acute and transient confusional state associated with high fever)
- Breath-holding spell

TREATMENT

PRE HOSPITAL

- During seizure, protect child from injury. Place child in lateral position to maintain airway and allow drainage of secretions/vomitus if present.
- Observe seizure closely.

INITIAL STABILIZATION

- Assessment of airway, breathing, and circulatory status
- Seizures >5 minutes duration should be treated, usually with a benzodiazepine as 1st-line therapy (e.g., lorazepam [0.05–0.1 mg/kg]), which may be repeated if seizure persists; then proceed to fosphenytoin 15–20 mg/kg IV if needed.

GENERAL MEASURES

- Identify whether an underlying illness exists.
- Evaluate source of fever (e.g., meningitis, otitis media, upper or lower respiratory tract infection, urinary tract infection, gastroenteritis, post-immunization). (5)
- Supportive care

Activity

No activity restrictions are necessary

 MEDICATION (DRUGS)

- Although anticonvulsants may be effective in reducing FS, the potential side effects outweigh the benefits. (1)
- Therefore, anticonvulsant therapy is not generally recommended for children with FS. (1)
- In situations of parental anxiety or frequent or prolonged FS, diazepam may be effective in preventing recurrence, but appropriate education and emotional support is more beneficial. (1)
- Diazepam may be administered as
  - Oral diazepam intermittently during febrile illness (e.g., 0.3 mg/kg q8h)
  - Diazepam rectal gel (Diastat) 0.5 mg/kg acutely for seizures of >5 minutes in duration
- Note: Diazepam can lead to significant lethargy and possibly mask signs of a serious illness such as meningitis.
- Antipyretics may be given for comfort, but have not been shown to reduce the risk of FS. (1)

FOLLOW-UP

PROGNOSIS

- Excellent prognosis
- Extremely low morbidity and mortality rate
- There is no known risk of neurologic sequelae including neurologic deficits and intellectual impairment. (1)
- Children with FS are at risk for developing recurrent FS.
- The major factor increasing recurrence rate is younger age at time of 1st seizure.
- Risk of developing further FS after 1st FS at
  - <1 year of age is ~50%(1)
  - >1 year of age is ~30%(1)
  - Risk of at least 1 additional recurrence after 2nd FS is 50%
- ~50–75% of recurrence is within 1 year of initial seizure, ~90% within 2 years
- Risk of epilepsy after a simple FS is slightly greater than the 1% risk of FS in the general population (1)
  - Risk of epilepsy after multiple FS with 1st seizure at <1 year of age is 2.4% (1)
  - Risk of epilepsy after a complex FS has been reported to be 4.1–6%. (2)[B]
  - Factors that increase risk of epilepsy include neurodevelopmental abnormality, increased number of characteristics of complex partial seizures, and family history of epilepsy.

COMPLICATIONS

- It remains controversial whether FS cause the later development of mesial temporal sclerosis.
- Retrospective studies show an association between temporal lobe epilepsy and FS, but prospective, controlled, population-based studies failed to confirm this association.
- The association may represent an inherent susceptibility in some children to both FS and epilepsy resulting from complex interactions between several genetic and environmental factors.

PATIENT MONITORING

Depends on clinical status of patient

REFERENCES

1. American Academy of Pediatrics, Provisional Committee on Quality Improvement and Subcommittee on Febrile Seizures. Practice parameter: Long-term treatment of the child with simple febrile seizures. *Pediatrics*. 1999;103(6): 1307–1309.
2. Baumer JH. Evidence based guideline for post-seizure management in children presenting acutely to secondary care. *Arch Dis Child*. 2004;89:278–280.
3. Scheffer IE, et al. Neonatal epilepsy syndromes and generalized epilepsy with febrile seizure plus (GEFS+). *Epilepsia*. 2005;46(10):41–47.
4. American Academy of Pediatrics, Provisional Committee on Quality Improvement and Subcommittee on Febrile Seizure. Practice parameter: the neurodiagnostic evaluation of the child with a first simple febrile seizure. *Pediatrics*. 1996;97(5):769–772.
5. DiMario FJ, Jr. Children presenting with complex febrile seizures do not routinely need computer tomography scanning in the emergency department. *Pediatrics*. 2006;117:528–530.

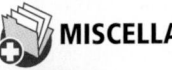 MISCELLANEOUS

CODES

ICD9-CM

780.31 Febrile convulsions

PATIENT TEACHING

- FS are common.
- There is no evidence that FS cause neurologic sequelae or death.
- There is no indication for routine investigations in patients presenting with a FS.
- Treatment of FS is not generally recommended and has not been shown to prevent the development of epilepsy.

SEPSIS

Suzanne Klainer, MD

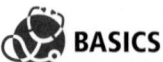 **BASICS**

DESCRIPTION
- Sepsis is the systemic response to infection; it is defined as systemic inflammatory response syndrome (SIRS) with documented infection.
- SIRS is an inflammatory reaction to various clinical insults (e.g., severe trauma or burn) manifested by 2 of the following
  - Temperature >38°C or <36°C
  - Heart rate >90/min
  - Respiratory rate >20/min or $Paco_2$ <32 mm Hg
  - WBC count >12,000/mm³, <4,000/mm³, or >10% immature forms (bands)
- Severe sepsis: When associated with organ dysfunction or hypotension
- Septic shock: Sepsis induced hypotension (systolic BP <90 mm Hg or ≥40 mm Hg drop from baseline) despite adequate fluid resuscitation plus hypoperfusion abnormalities (oliguria, lactic acidosis, acute change in mental status)
- MODS: Multiple organ dysfunction syndrome
- Bacteremia: Bacteria in the blood; may have no accompanying symptoms
- Synonym(s): Septicemia; Sepsis neonatorum

ALERT
Geriatric Considerations
- Often more difficult to diagnose clinically in the elderly
- Change in mental status/behavior may be only early manifestation

Pediatric Considerations
Screen newborns for infection due to prolonged rupture of membranes (>24 hours), maternal fever, and prematurity.

Pregnancy Considerations
β-Lactam antibiotics, aminoglycosides, and erythromycin are considered safe.

GENERAL PREVENTION
- Vaccination: Pneumococcal (geriatric patients, patients with certain chronic diseases), *Haemophilus influenzae* type B (infants, young children)
- γ-Globulin (for hypo- or agammaglobulinemic patients)
- Hand washing by hospital personnel, appropriate catheter care, and so forth, for hospitalized patients

EPIDEMIOLOGY
Predominant age: All ages

Incidence
- 3 cases per 1,000 population
- 2 cases per 100 patients admitted to hospital (1)

RISK FACTORS
- Positive blood cultures
- Age extremes (very old and very young)
- Impaired host (see "Associated Conditions")
- Critically ill patients
- Indwelling catheters: Intravascular, urinary, biliary
- Complicated labor and delivery: Premature and/or prolonged rupture of membranes, other complications
- Certain surgical procedures

Genetics
Single-nucleotide polymorphisms (i.e., cytokine and cytokine receptor genes) influence the risk for the development of sepsis and the risk of mortality from sepsis.

PATHOPHYSIOLOGY
In sepsis, the dysregulation of the inflammatory process is precipitated by an imbalance between pro- and anti-inflammatory mediators, resulting in widespread systemic tissue destruction and organ dysfunction.

ETIOLOGY
- Specific etiologic agents include
  - Gram-positive organisms: Most commonly *Staphylococcus* spp., *Streptococcus* spp., *Enterococcus* spp.
  - Gram-negative organisms: Most commonly *Escherichia coli*, *Klebsiella* spp., *Proteus* spp., *Pseudomonas* spp.
  - Fungi: Most commonly *Candida* spp.
  - Other agents: Anaerobes. See also "Differential Diagnosis."
- Common sources of septicemia include
  - Lungs
  - Urinary tract
  - Intra-abdominal focus: Biliary tree, abscess, peritonitis
  - Intravascular catheters
  - Skin: Cellulitis, decubitus ulcer, gangrene
  - Heart valves

ASSOCIATED CONDITIONS
- Immunologic disorders
  - Neutropenia, HIV, hypo-/agammaglobulinemia, complement deficiency, splenectomy
- Diabetes mellitus
- Alcoholism
- Malignancy
- Cirrhosis
- Burns
- Multiple trauma
- IV drug abuse
- Malnutrition

DIAGNOSIS

SIGNS AND SYMPTOMS
- Fever
- Chills, rigors
- Myalgias
- Changes in mental status: Restlessness, agitation, confusion, delirium, lethargy, stupor, coma
- Tachycardia
- Tachypnea
- Hypotension
- Skin lesions: Erythema, petechiae, ecthyma gangrenosum, embolic lesions, purpura
- Signs and symptoms related to site of primary infection
  - Respiratory tract: Cough, sputum production, dyspnea, chest pain
  - Urinary tract: Dysuria, flank pain, frequency, urgency
  - Intra-abdominal source: Nausea, vomiting, diarrhea, constipation, abdominal pain
  - CNS: Stiff neck, headache, photophobia, focal neurologic signs
- Signs and symptoms related to end-organ failure
  - Pulmonary: Cyanosis
  - Renal: Oliguria, anuria
  - Hepatic: Jaundice
  - Cardiac: CHF

TESTS
- Antigen detection systems Counterimmunoelectrophoresis and latex agglutination tests (pneumococcus, *H. influenzae* type B, group B streptococcus, meningococcus)
- Gram stain of buffy coat smears occasionally useful

Lab
- Positive blood cultures (not required for diagnosis)
- Positive cultures from other sites (sputum, urine, CSF, wound)
- Gram stain of clinical specimens (sputum, urine, CSF, wound)
- Common
  - Leukocytosis
  - Proteinuria
  - Hypoxemia
  - Hyperglycemia
  - Hypocalcemia
  - Mild hyperbilirubinemia
- Less common (more severe cases)
  - Lactic acidosis
  - Leukopenia
  - Azotemia
  - Thrombocytopenia
  - Prolonged prothrombin time
  - Anemia
  - Hypoglycemia
- Drugs that may alter lab results: Prior antibiotic use

Imaging
- Radiographs (e.g., chest)
- Ultrasound, CT scan, or MRI may be useful in delineating sites of infection.

Diagnostic Procedures/Surgery
- Aspiration of potentially infected body fluids (pleural, peritoneal, CSF) when appropriate
- Biopsy, drainage of potentially infected tissues (abscess, biliary tree, others) when appropriate

Pathological Findings
- Inflammation at primary site of infection
- Disseminated intravascular coagulation
- Noncardiogenic pulmonary edema

DIFFERENTIAL DIAGNOSIS
- Shock of other etiology
- Bacteremia without sepsis
- Localized infection
- SIRS
- Viral diseases (influenza, dengue and other hemorrhagic viruses, West Nile)
- Rickettsial diseases (Rocky Mountain spotted fever, endemic typhus)
- Spirochetal diseases (leptospirosis, relapsing fever [*Borrelia* sp.], Jarisch-Herxheimer reaction in syphilis)
- Protozoal diseases (*Toxoplasma gondii*, *Trypanosoma cruzi*, *Pneumocystis carinii*, *Plasmodium falciparum*)
- Collagen vascular diseases, vasculitides, myocardial infarction, pulmonary embolus, thrombotic thrombocytopenic purpura/hemolytic-uremic syndrome, thyrotoxicosis, adrenal insufficiency (Addison disease)

TREATMENT

INITIAL STABILIZATION
- Hospitalization
- Intensive care treatment of patients with shock, respiratory failure

GENERAL MEASURES
- ABCs
  - Oxygen supplementation, monitoring
    - Intubation and invasive monitors if necessary for respiratory failure/hemodynamic instability
- Initial resuscitation targeted at
  - CVP: 8–12 mm Hg
  - MAP $\geq$65 mm Hg
  - Urine output $\geq$ 0.5 mL/kg/h
  - Central venous/mixed venous oxygen saturation $\geq$70% (2)[A]
- Identification of etiology
  - Removal or drainage of septic foci
- Transfusion of RBCs, platelets, and/or fresh frozen plasma for coagulopathy
- Stress ulcer and deep venous thrombosis prophylactic measures
- Tight glucose control (3)[B]

Diet
- NPO initially
- Enteral feeds beneficial when possible however, IV alimentation is appropriate in severely malnourished patients and in patients who will be unable to receive enteral alimentation within the week.

SPECIAL THERAPY
Ventilatory support: See "Acute Respiratory Distress Syndrome (ARDS)"

IV Fluids
No evidence to support 1 type of fluid over another (colloid/crystalloid) (2)[B]

 # MEDICATION (DRUGS)

First Line
- Pressors
  - Norepinephrine/dopamine 1st line (2)[C]
  - Renal dose dopamine not recommended (2)[B]
- Antibiotic coverage immediately after cultures are obtained (1)[C]
  - Should be broad-spectrum initially, with emphasis on most likely pathogen.
  - After culture results are available, treatment should be organism-specific.
  - Knowledge of antibiotic susceptibility patterns of local pathogens is extremely important.
- Neonatal (<7 days old) sepsis: Ampicillin 300 mg/kg/d in 3 divided doses and gentamicin (Garamycin) 5 mg/kg/d in 2 divided doses
- Nonimmunocompromised child: Cefotaxime (Claforan): 200 mg/kg/d in 4 divided doses
- Adult (pseudomonas not suspected): Vancomycin plus gram-negative coverage (cefepime 1–2 g q12h or gentamicin 3–5 mg/kg/d divided over 2–3 doses)

- Adult in whom pseudomonas is suspected (neutropenic/burn, e.g.): Vancomycin plus double pseudomonal coverage (ceftazidime 1–2 g IV/IM q8–12h; gentamicin, piperacillin-tazobactam 3.375 g IV q6h, ciprofloxacin 400 mg IV q8–12h, e.g.)
- Antifungal: When fungal infection is suspected
- Contraindications: History of anaphylaxis or other allergic reaction to the antibiotic

ALERT
Dose adjustments are required for renal function.
- Significant possible interactions
  - Aminoglycosides: Increased nephrotoxicity with enflurane, cisplatin, and possibly vancomycin; increased ototoxicity with loop diuretics; increased paralysis with neuromuscular blocking agents
  - Ampicillin: Increased frequency of rash with allopurinol

Second Line
- IV hydrocortisone (2)[A]
  - May benefit patients who require vasopressor therapy to maintain BP
  - Long-term mortality benefit not proven
- Drotrecogin alfa (Xigris) (2)[B]
  - 24 μg/kg/h for 96 hours in patients with severe sepsis (APACHE score >24)

ALERT
- Increases risk of bleeding
- Not recommended in children
- Polyclonal IVIG as adjuvant therapy in bacterial sepsis or septic shock (4)[B]

SURGERY
- Drainage of infected sites
- Débridement of necrotic tissues

 # FOLLOW-UP

PROGNOSIS
Even with optimal care, mortality is 10–50% overall; this is increased in patients with
- Neutropenia
- Diabetes
- Alcoholism
- Renal failure
- Respiratory failure
- Hypogammaglobulinemia
- Certain etiologic agents (e.g., *Pseudomonas aeruginosa*)
- Delay in appropriate antimicrobial therapy
- Patients at the age extremes

COMPLICATIONS
- Death
- Adult respiratory distress syndrome
- Multiorgan failure (cardiac, pulmonary, renal, hepatic)
- Disseminated intravascular coagulation
- Gastrointestinal hemorrhage

PATIENT MONITORING
- Depends on source of infection, underlying disease(s)
- Drug levels if necessary
- BUN, creatinine, electrolytes and CBCs at least twice weekly; more frequently if unstable
- In unstable patients: Invasive hemodynamic monitoring, arterial blood gas, venous gas, frequent electrolytes.

REFERENCES
1. Angus DC, et al. Epidemiology of severe sepsis in the United States: Analysis of incidence, outcome, and associated cost of care. *Crit Care Med.* 2001;29:1303.
2. Dellinger RP, Carlet JM, Masur H, et al. Surviving Sepsis Campaign Management Guidelines Committee. Surviving sepsis campaign guidelines for management of severe sepsis and septic shock. *Crit Care Med.* 2004;32:858–873.
3. Bone RC, Balk RA, Cerra FB, et al. Definitions for sepsis and organ failure and guidelines for the use of innovative therapies in sepsis. *Chest.* 1992;101:1644–1655.
4. Alejandria et al. Intravenous immunoglobin for treating sepsis and septic shock. *Cochrane Database of Systematic Rev.* 1, 2006.
5. Bochud et al. Antibiotics in sepsis. *Intensive Care Med.* 2001;27:14.

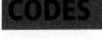 # MISCELLANEOUS

- High-dose steroids are of no benefit.
- See also: Candidiasis; Endocarditis, infective; Listeriosis, Meningitis, bacterial; Pneumonia, bacterial; Pyelonephritis, Rocky Mountain spotted fever; Toxic shock syndrome; Tularemia

CODES

ICD9-CM
038.9 Unspecified septicemia

 See Corresponding Diagnostic Algorithm

SERUM SICKNESS

Brian P. Vickery, MD

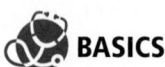 **BASICS**

DESCRIPTION

An acute Type III hypersensitivity reaction, classically described 1–3 weeks following administration of nonhuman serum or with exposure to certain medications. Reactions tend to peak around day 10 postexposure. Serum sicknesslike reactions (SSLR) occur after administration of certain drugs, especially antibiotics.

- System(s) Affected: Heme/Lymphatic/Immunologic; Musculoskeletal; Skin/Exocrine; Cardiovascular; Gastrointestinal; Genitourinary

EPIDEMIOLOGY

No gender or age predominance

RISK FACTORS

Preceding exposure to drugs or serum

PATHOPHYSIOLOGY

- Immunoglobulin G (IgG) antibodies form immune complexes with the antigen in circulation.
- When an excess of antibody or antigen occurs, small complexes are formed which are cleared rapidly and do not generally cause reactions.
- When concentrations of antibody and antigen are approximately equal, intermediate size immune complexes are formed which are deposited in tissues and efficiently activate complement.
- Complement activation causes release of inflammatory mediators, recruitment of leukocytes, and vascular leak.

ETIOLOGY

- Anti-thymocyte globulin (ATG)
- Antimicrobials
  - Cephalosporins, esp. Cefaclor
  - Minocycline
  - TMP/SMX
  - Rifampin
  - Penicillins
  - Streptokinase
- Monoclonal antibodies
- SSRIs
- Propranolol
- Vaccines
- Equine diptheria antiserum
- Rabies antiserum
- Rabbit antiserum
- Crotalidae antivenin

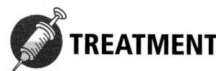 **DIAGNOSIS**

SIGNS AND SYMPTOMS

Characterized by an ill-appearing patient with fever, arthralgias, morbilliform or urticarial skin rash, and lymphadenopathy

- Fever
- Arthralgia/myalgia
- Morbilliform or urticarial rash, especially at injection site
- Malaise
- Pruritus
- Nausea
- Vomiting
- Abdominal pain
- Hepatomegaly or splenomegaly
- Lymphadenopathy, especially in location draining injection site
- Headache (usually due to TMJ arthralgia)
- Arthritis

History

- History of exposure to medication or serum in preceding 1–3 weeks
- Absence of chronic constitutional symptoms

TESTS

Lab

Detection of immune complexes in serum is not widely available and of limited clinical value.

- C3/C4: Helpful if low but can be normal
- ESR/CRP: Usually elevated
- CBC with differential: Leukocytosis
- Liver enzymes: Transaminitis
- Serum electrolytes: Renal insufficiency (rare)
- Urinalysis: Nephritis (rare)

ALERT

Special Considerations

If rash is atypical or does not improve after withdrawing suspected drug, consider

- Antinuclear antibodies (ANA)
- Antineutrophil cytoplasmic antibodies (ANCA)
- Rheumatoid factor (RF)
- Cryoglobulins
- Skin biopsy with immunofluorescence

DIFFERENTIAL DIAGNOSIS

- Systemic vasculitis
  - Periarteritis nodosa
  - Wegener granulomatosis
  - Cryoglobulinemia
  - Juvenile idiopathic arthritis
  - Kawasaki syndrome
  - Henoch-Schonlein purpura
  - Hypersensitivity vasculitis
- Sepsis
- Rheumatic fever
- Viral syndrome
- Anaphylaxis
- Drug hypersensitivity
- Stevens-Johnson/TEN

TREATMENT

GENERAL MEASURES

- Mainstay of treatment is to remove the offending antigen.
- Reticuloendothelial system removes immune complexes, leading to improvement and resolution within 48–72 hours (depending upon half-life of antigen).

Activity

Bed rest during acute illness if arthralgia/myalgia severe

MEDICATION (DRUGS)

First Line
- Diphenhydramine or hydroxyzine 25–50 mg IV/PO q4–6h for urticaria and generalized pruritus
- NSAIDs may offer relief of arthralgia/myalgia.

Second Line
Prednisone
- 40 mg/d PO 5–7 days if inflammation is severe or 1st-line drugs fail

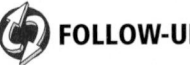 **FOLLOW-UP**

Admission Criteria
Most patients with acute serum sickness or SSLR will require admission for observation and exclusion of other diagnoses.

Discharge Criteria
- When significant improvement in inflammation occurs after stopping suspected drug
- When ambulatory and tolerating PO

PROGNOSIS
Favorable
- Self-limiting with improvement in 48–72 hours once offending antigen removed

COMPLICATIONS
- Vasculitis
- Neuropathy
- Hepatitis
- Glomerulonephritis
- Anaphylaxis
- Shock
- Death

REFERENCES

1. Friedmann PS, et al. Mechanisms in cutaneous drug hypersensitivity reactions. *Clin Exp Allergy*. 2003;33(7):861–872.
2. Jancar S, et al. Immune complex-mediated tissue injury: A multistep paradigm. *Trends Immunol*. 2005: 26(1):48–55.
3. Roujeau JC, et al. Severe adverse cutaneous reactions to drugs. *N Engl J Med*. 1994;331:1272–1285.

ADDITIONAL READING

- Pichler WJ. Immune mechanism of drug hypersensitivity. *Immunol Allergy Clin N Am*. 2004;24:373–397.
- Frank MM, Hester CG. Immune complexes and allergic disease. In: Adkinson NF, et al. *Middleton's Allergy: Principles and Practice*. 6th ed. Philadephia, PA: Elsevier; 2003:997–1014.

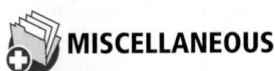 **MISCELLANEOUS**

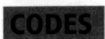 **CODES**

ICD9-CM
999.5 Other serum reaction

SEXUAL DYSFUNCTION IN WOMEN

Lisa M. Schroeder, MD

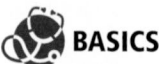 **BASICS**

DESCRIPTION

Difficulty getting or staying sexually aroused, reaching orgasm too quickly, difficulty or inability to reach orgasm, inability to relax, lack of interest in sex, distaste or revulsion with sex, too little foreplay, too little tenderness after intercourse

- Most women who have orgasms do not do so during intercourse, and mistakenly think this is dysfunction.
- 4 major types
  - Disorder of desire: Both hypo- and hyper- (initiation and response), global desire disorder, couple desire discrepancy, situational desire disorder—these must be evaluated in the context of the relationship overall
  - Disorder of arousal
  - Dyspareunia, vaginismus
  - Disorders of orgasm: Primary and secondary, during masturbation or coitus, situational or partner specific
- System(s) Affected: Nervous; Reproductive; Genitourinary; Psychiatric
- Synonym(s): Hypoactive sexual desire disorder; Sexual aversion disorder; Female sexual arousal disorder; Inhibited female orgasm

ALERT

Geriatric Considerations

- Societal expectations about geriatric sexuality (especially the myth older women are not sexually active) can cause distress if the patient has sexual desires or sexual experience.
- Normal physiologic changes in aging are misinterpreted as dysfunction.

Pregnancy Considerations

Often affects sexual function in women, but the effect varies depending on the patient and couple's beliefs about pregnancy and the problem.

EPIDEMIOLOGY

- Predominant age
  - Postpubertal age group
  - Women's ability to experience orgasm increases gradually from puberty.
  - In later, teens, nearly 1/2 have not had orgasm; by mid-30s, about 10% have not.
  - Sex role stereotypes can be a factor.
- Predominant sex: Female (heterosexual, homosexual, and bisexual women)

Prevalence

- 1:5 women are sexually dissatisfied, and 2/3 of women report some degree of sexual dysfunction. Only 1/3 of anorgasmic women in general think it is a problem.
- Overall prevalence for dysfunction is 15–30% of all women. Desire disorders are complaint of 30–55% of individual patients presenting to clinics, and 31% of couples; arousal disorders present in <14–48% in community studies. Orgasmic disorders probably the most common; <10% primary, and up to 65–80% secondary in community studies.
- There are many barriers to seeking help, so data for prevalence incomplete; barriers include stigma of exposing sexual inadequacy, fear of unknown therapy, e.g., of having to perform before a therapist.

RISK FACTORS

- Couple discrepancies in expectations, cultural backgrounds
- Attitudes toward sexuality in family of origin
- Previous sexual trauma
- Chronic medical problems
  - Cardiovascular disease
  - Endocrine disorders
  - HTN
  - Neurologic disorders
- Smoking

ETIOLOGY

- Interrelational difficulties and conflict regarding intimacy
- Anxiety
- Survivor of sexual abuse, including incest
- Alcohol
- Drug use, including prescription medications (e.g., monoamine oxidase inhibitors, tricyclic antidepressants, especially selective serotonin reuptake inhibitor antidepressants, beta blockers)
- Proximity of other people in household
- Anorgasmia can be due to diabetes.
- Spinal cord damage
- Hormonal imbalance
- Thyroid disease
- Sexual frequency myths
- Control issues in the relationships
- Dyspareunia, including vaginal dryness causing interference with lubrication, secondary to infection or endocrine
- There are few endocrine data on women with sexual dysfunction.

ASSOCIATED CONDITIONS

Marital stress

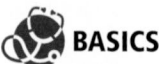 **DIAGNOSIS**

SIGNS AND SYMPTOMS

- Complaint to health care provider (if the clinician inquires, over twice as many are revealed than if clinician waits for patient to mention)
- Infertility
- Marital conflict
- Family dysfunction

Physical Exam

Most commonly a normal exam

- Assess for vaginal atrophy, adequate estrogenization
- Assess for infection
- Recognize signs of anxiety, apprehension, and pain during speculum and pelvic exam.

TESTS

Special tests: May need life experiences or some other psychological inventory to evaluate couple. (Alcohol, marijuana, or other illicit drug use may make these evaluations unreliable.)

Lab

As needed to identify infections and other medical causes

Pathological Findings

Varied if any

DIFFERENTIAL DIAGNOSIS

- Medication side effects
  - Psychotropics
  - Monoamine oxidase inhibitors
  - Tricyclic and other antidepressants
- Marital dysfunction including domestic violence
- Decreased sensation secondary to back or nerve disease
- Multiple sclerosis
- Abdominal surgery (can interfere with pelvic innervation)
- Depression
- Vaginitis
- Decreased vaginal lubrication secondary to hormonal imbalance
- Pregnancy
- Anatomic or congenital abnormalities
- Pseudodyspareunia (use of complaint of pain to distance from partner)

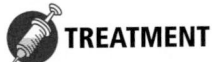

TREATMENT

GENERAL MEASURES
- For childhood trauma: Scripting, psychotherapy, cognitive restructuring
- For anorgasmia: Directed masturbation and "homework" with partners
- For prescription drug causes: Reduced dosages or change to different medication
- Other: Family therapy, sensate conditioning; referral to specialized sex therapy

Diet
Weight reduction if needed for either partner

Activity
Varies with couple

SPECIAL THERAPY
Complementary and Alternative Medicine
- Yohimbe-not recommended, potentially dangerous
- DHEA-androgenic effects, will decrease HDL cholesterol

MEDICATION (DRUGS)

These are usually multifactorial psychosocial conditions. Using medications doesn't address the cause of the problem and can make it worse. Sildenafil: Some evidence on the effectiveness for arousal and orgasm disorders (1,2)[B]

ALERT
Do not use with nitrates

- Bupropion: May be useful in treating sexual dysfunction, or as an adjunct for SSRI induced sexual dysfunction (3–5)[B]

- Postmenopausal women

  – Adding testosterone to hormone replacement therapy may increase sexual desire. (6)[A]
    ○ Several RCT show an improvement in sexual desire.

  – Estrogen replacement may help to improve vaginal atrophy and clitoral sensitivity.
- Premenopausal women
  – Some data suggest that testosterone may be low with decreased libido.
  – No clear studies indicate testosterone replacement as beneficial.

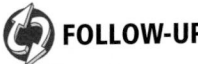

FOLLOW-UP

DISPOSITION
Issues for Referral
- Sexual abuse, partner violence
- Marital counseling

PROGNOSIS
- Lack of desire is the most difficult to treat (<50% successful by patient report), and success is sometimes less optimal than patient's initial wish.
- Best predictors are desire to change and overall healthy relationship.

COMPLICATIONS
Marital or family stress, breakup, and divorce.

PATIENT MONITORING
Varies with patient

REFERENCES

1. Basson R, Brotto L. Sexual psychophysiology and effects of sildenafil citrate in oestrogenised women with acquired genital arousal disorder and impaired orgasm: A randomized controlled trial. *Br J Obstect Gynaecol*. 2003;11:1014–1024.
2. Caruso S, et al. Premenopausal women affected by sexual arousal disorder treated with sildenafil: A double blind, crossover, placebo-controlled study. *Br J Obstect Gynaecol*. 2001;108(6):623–628.
3. Segraves RT, Clayton A, Croft H, et al. Bupropion sustained release for the treatment of hypoactive sexual desire disorder in premenopausal women. *J Clin Psychopharmacol*. 2004;24(3):339–342.
4. Rudkin L, Taylor MJ, Hawton K. Strategies for managing sexual dysfunction induced by antidepressant medication. *Cochrane Database Syst Rev*. 2004;(4):CD003382.
5. Ginzburg R, Wong Y, Fader JS. Effect of bupropion on sexual dysfunction. *Ann Pharmacother*. 2005;39(12):2096–2099.
6. *Mayo Clin Proc*. 2004;79(Suppl):S19–S24.

ADDITIONAL READING

- Bancroft J. *Human Sexuality and Its Problems*. 2nd ed. New York, NY: Churchill Livingstone; 1989.
- Leiblum SR, Rosen RC. *Principles and Practice of Sex Therapy: Update for the 1990s*. New York, NY: The Guilford Press; 1989.
- Wincze JP, Carey MP. *Sexual Dysfunction: A Guide for Assessment and Treatment*. New York, NY: The Guilford Press; 1991.
- Basaria S, Dobs A. Safety and advere effects of androgens: How to counsel patients. *Mayo Clin Proc*. 2004;79(Suppl):S25–S32.

MISCELLANEOUS

- See also: Vaginismus
- Other notes
  – Women must feel safe in order to let go and lose some control to experience orgasm.
  – Performance anxiety makes males ejaculate prematurely, whereas it inhibits orgasm in women.
  – Simple lack of knowledge about anatomy and physiology of sex can lead to problems.

CODES

ICD9-CM
- 302.70 Psychosexual dysfunction, unspecified
- 302.71 Hypoactive sexual desire disorder
- 302.72 Psychosexual dysfunction with inhibited sexual excitement
- 302.73 Psychosexual dysfunction with inhibited female orgasm
- 302.76 Psychosexual dysfunction with functional dyspareunia
- 799.81 Decreased sexual desire NOS

PATIENT TEACHING

Information about normal sexual function and human reproductive anatomy and function and changes expected with aging

 See Patient Handout on CD

S

SHOCK, CIRCULATORY

Felix Chang, MD

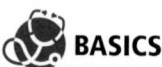 **BASICS**

DESCRIPTION

Inadequate tissue perfusion resulting in organ dysfunction. Classified as

- Hypovolemic shock
  - Cardiac output is severely reduced due to loss of intravascular volume.
  - Blood loss is most common cause.
- Cardiogenic shock
  - Cardiac output is severely compromised by loss of myocardial muscle function, valvular dysfunction, or arrhythmia.
  - Myocardial infarction is most common cause.
- Obstructive shock
  - Cardiac output reduced due to obstruction of venous return to the heart (vena cava syndrome), compression of the heart, (pericardial tamponade, tension pneumothorax), or disrupted cardiac outflow (aortic dissection, pulmonary embolism).
- Distributive shock
  - Reduced systemic vascular resistance and effective circulating volume. Dilated peripheral vessels shunt blood flow away from perfusion of critical organs.
  - Most commonly due to sepsis and inflammation, which cause vasodilation and increased capillary permeability.
- Neurogenic
  - Venous pooling in periphery (most often owing to spinal shock or drug overdose); behaves much like hypovolemic shock.

GENERAL PREVENTION

Prompt treatment of underlying condition.

EPIDEMIOLOGY

- Predominant age: Increased in elderly, somewhat dependent on underlying cause
- Predominant sex: Male = Female

ETIOLOGY

- Hypovolemic shock
  - Hemorrhagic: Blood loss owing to trauma or gastrointestinal bleeding
  - Nonhemorrhagic: 3rd-space loss of plasma volume (pancreatitis, bowel obstruction, infarction, anaphylaxis, diarrhea, burns)
- Cardiogenic shock
  - Acute myocardial infarction (>40% of left ventricular myocardium)
  - Arrhythmia (heart block, ventricular tachycardia, atrial fibrillation with rapid ventricular response, etc.)
  - Acute valvular dysfunction: Mitral valve due to papillary muscle rupture following inferior myocardial infarctions or after rupture of chordae; aortic or mitral valve dysfunction, for example in bacterial endocarditis
  - Ventricular septal rupture following anterior/septal myocardial infarction
- Obstructive shock
  - Pericardial tamponade
  - Inferior/superior vena caval obstruction usually owing to neoplasms
  - Aortic dissection
  - Massive pulmonary embolism
- Distributive shock: High-output shock is a result of sepsis, toxic shock, burns, or anaphylaxis. Severe noninfectious systemic inflammatory response can be due to sepsis, but also can independently cause distributive shock.
- Neurogenic: Venous pooling when loss of sympathetic innervation causes loss of venous tone (e.g., acute spinal injury, general or spinal anesthesia, or overdose of sedative drugs)

ASSOCIATED CONDITIONS

See "Etiology."

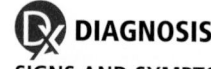 **DIAGNOSIS**

SIGNS AND SYMPTOMS

- Signs/symptoms of underlying disease
  - Upper gastrointestinal (UGI) tract bleeding (hematemesis, melena)
  - Sepsis (fever, chills, symptoms of underlying infection such as dysuria, costovertebral angle tenderness in urosepsis)
  - Myocardial infarction (chest pain, diaphoresis, nausea, vomiting, S_4 or S_3 gallop, new heart murmur, rales)
  - Jugular-venous distention (JVD), pulsus paradoxus in pericardial tamponade
- Signs/symptoms of underperfusion of organ systems
  - Brain: Confusion, anxiety, agitation, coma
  - Kidney: Oliguria
  - Skin: Peripheral cyanosis, sluggish capillary refill, mottling, and/or coolness; may be overly perfused (flushed and warm) in high-output (septic) shock
  - Gastrointestinal tract: Absence of bowel sounds
  - Circulation: Thready pulses, tachycardia, hypotension, secondary cardiac ischemia (ST depression), or heart failure.

TESTS

- Pulmonary artery (Swan-Ganz) catheterization
  - Serial measurement of cardiac output; central venous, pulmonary arterial, and pulmonary arterial occlusion pressures (left atrial pressure); and vascular resistance
  - Mixed venous blood gases can be drawn from the catheter.
  - Was standard of care, but recent studies suggest increased mortality with use, thus this practice is currently controversial. (1)[B]
- ECG
  - Valvular failure
  - Pericardial effusions
  - Echo-guided pericardiocentesis
- Endoscopy if suspect GI bleed

Lab

- Specific to shock
  - Elevated lactate (>2 mmol/L) suggests anaerobic metabolism from underperfusion.
  - Reduced mixed venous Po_2 obtained from the pulmonary artery indicates vigorous extraction of oxygen from tissues owing to underperfusion.
- For underlying diseases responsible for shock
  - ECG, creatine kinase levels (serial), troponin levels (serial)
  - Arterial blood gases
  - Gram stain and culture of infected sites
  - Blood cultures
  - CBC (serial determination of hemoglobin and hematocrit in bleeding patients)
  - Type and cross bleeding patients

Imaging

Depends on suspected underlying etiology

TREATMENT

INITIAL STABILIZATION
- Support airway, breathing, circulation
- Continuous ECG monitoring with frequent assessment of BP, respiratory status, and urine output

GENERAL MEASURES
- Therapy involves aggressive volume resuscitation with control of the underlying etiology and monitoring of end-organ perfusion.
- Maintain Sao_2 >92% with supplemental oxygen. Intubate and mechanically ventilate if patient cannot oxygenate adequately or has markedly increased breathing effort.
- Correct plasma volume deficits rapidly with crystalloids and/or packed RBCs.
- Correction of coagulation derangement by administration of coagulation factors (fresh frozen plasma, cryoprecipitate) and platelets if coagulopathy (prolonged prothrombin time, partial thromboplastin time, or platelet count <50 X 10^9/L) is present in a patient who is bleeding.
- Tachyarrhythmias (other than sinus tachycardia) should be promptly corrected by electrocardioversion. Insert transvenous pacemaker to correct bradyrhythmias.
- Vasopressors to correct hypotension or low cardiac output owing to myocardial failure or hypotension caused by low vascular resistance
- Treat underlying conditions, for example
  - Hemorrhagic
    ○ Trauma
    ○ GI blood loss may require endoscopic or surgical intervention
  - Sepsis
    ○ Empiric antibiotic therapy.
    ○ Hydrocortisone and vasopressin improve BP. Consider when patients do not improve in response to fluids, antibiotics, and low doses of vasopressors.
  - Cardiogenic shock
    ○ Therapy should help reduce cardiac ischemia (oxygen, nitrates) and accomplish rapid reperfusion of injured, but potentially viable, myocardium. A balloon pump may temporize by providing improved coronary blood flow during and after diagnostic testing and revascularization therapy.
    ○ If shock is a result of acute failure of the mitral or aortic valve, surgical valve replacement may be lifesaving.

Diet
NPO

Activity
Bed rest

SPECIAL THERAPY
IV Fluids
Infusion of crystalloids to support BP

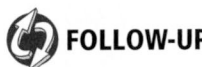 **MEDICATION (DRUGS)**

- In addition to specific treatment of underlying condition, use medications to support perfusion. (2)[B]
- Dopamine IV effects depend on dosing
  - Augments contractility, cardiac output and heart rate at moderate doses via β-1 effects. Increases BP by a combination of increased cardiac output and, at higher doses, vasoconstriction (via α-effects).
- Norepinephrine IV: Augments BP by increasing vascular resistance (α). Cardiac output in septic shock maintained/ increased (β-1).
- Phenylephrine IV: Pure α-agonist that increases BP via vasoconstriction
- Dobutamine IV: Inotropic agent with β-1 effects
  - Augments contractility and cardiac output (β-1); does not raise BP because of vasodilation (β-2).

- Vasopressin: Used in patients refractory to inotropic agents. Increases vascular smooth muscle tone, may increase mean arterial pressure (3)[B]
- Activated protein C: In the PROWESS study, APC was shown to reduce mortality from severe sepsis at 28 days from 31–25%. (4)[B] Treatment of DIC is critical to prevent sepsis-related organ failure. Activated protein C may help by effects on microcirculation. (5,6)[B]
- Corticosteroids: Low doses of hydrocortisone and fludrocortisone may reduce mortality in shock from sepsis. (7,8)[B]

- Precautions
  - Myocardial oxygen consumption is increased by increased heart rate, afterload, and contractility.
  - Pressors can increase myocardial ischemia if present and may precipitate or worsen tachyarrhythmias. Use in lowest possible dose for as limited period as possible.

SURGERY
In hemorrhagic and septic shock, surgery may be indicated to correct the underlying pathology.

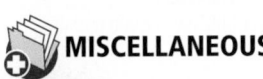 **FOLLOW-UP**

DISPOSITION
ICU care

PROGNOSIS
Mortality is determined by a complex interaction of primary disease causing shock, age, coexisting chronic disease, and shock severity as marked by the number of acute organ system failures that follow shock.

ALERT
Geriatric Considerations
Prognosis guarded

COMPLICATIONS
- Multiple organs may be damaged by underperfusion during shock.
- Acute tubular necrosis
- Ischemic hepatitis
- Ischemic bowel
- Abdominal compartment syndrome
- Adult respiratory distress syndrome
- Encephalopathy and/or cerebrovascular accident

PATIENT MONITORING
Careful monitoring in intensive care

REFERENCES
1. Shah MR, Hasselad V, Binany C. Impact of the pulmonary artery catheter in critically ill patients. *JAMA* 2005;294:1664–1670.
2. Holmes CL. Vasoactive drugs in the intensive care unit. *Curr Opin Crit Care* 2005;11:413–417.
3. Holmes CL, Patel BM, Russell JA, et al. Physiology of vasopressin relevant to management of septic shock. *Chest* 2001;120:989–1002.
4. Bernard GR, Vincent JL, Laterre PF, et al. Efficacy and safety of recombinant human activated protein C for severe sepsis. *N Engl J Med* 2001;344:699–709.
5. Ince C: The microcirculation is the motor of sepsis. *Crit Care* 2005;S13–19.
6. Zeerleder S, Hack CE, Wuillemin WA. Disseminated intravascular coagulation in sepsis. *Chest* 2005;128:2864–2875.
7. Cooper MS, Stewart PM. Corticosteroid insufficiency in acutely ill patients. *N Engl J Med* 2003;348:727–734.
8. Annane D, Sebill V, Charpentier C et al. Effect of treatment with low does of hydrocortisone and fludrocortisones on mortality of patients with septic shock. *JAMA* 2002;862–871.

 MISCELLANEOUS

CODES

ICD9-CM
- 785.50 Shock, unspecified
- 785.51 Cardiogenic shock
- 785.59 Shock without mention of trauma, other

See Corresponding Diagnostic Algorithm

SIALADENITIS

Felix B. Chang, MD
Thomas Jaquith-Houston, MD

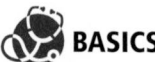 **BASICS**

DESCRIPTION

- Sialadenitis is an inflammation of the salivary glands, most commonly from bacteria or virus infection. Inflammation often arises in the excretory duct.
- The parotid or submandibular glands are most frequently affected.
- Inflammation is likely caused by salivary stasis allowing retrograde passage of organisms.
- Inflammation may also follow trauma, spread of infection from adjoining tissues, and via hematogenous routes during bacteremia.
- Inflammation may lead to stone formation (sialolithiasis), or an obstructed duct may lead to inflammation of the gland. Stones are more commonly associated with the submaxillary glands.
- Recurrent infections or other chronic inflammatory processes may lead to decreased gland function, resulting in xerostomia.
- System(s) Affected: Gastrointestinal; Skin/Exocrine
- Synonym(s): Sialadenosis

EPIDEMIOLOGY

- Most commonly seen in debilitated patients
- 50–60 years of age
- Male = Female
- Immune-compromised patients
- Postoperative patients
- Of the medically ill patient with sialoadenitis
  - 25% have a malignant lesion
  - 50% have a pre-existing infection elsewhere than head and neck

ALERT
Pediatric Considerations
- Rare in children
- Cases have been reported in premature neonates: Neonatal suppurative parotitis
  - *Staphylococcus aureus*
  - *Escherichia coli*
  - *Pseudomonas aeruginosa*
  - B Streptococci
- Recurrent parotitis of childhood
  - Age of onset 8 months–16 years
  - Male > Female
  - *S. aureus*
  - *S. viridans*

Incidence
- ~0.02% of hospital admission
- Occurs between 1/1,000 and 1/2,000 operative procedures

RISK FACTORS
- Dehydration
- Fever
- Hypercalcemia
- Severely debilitated patient
- Diabetes mellitus
- Hypothyroidism
- Lack of salivary stimulation (postoperative patients)
- Treatment with radiation or chemotherapy for underlying malignant disease
- Patients undergoing major abdominal and hip repair surgery have been identified as being at increased risk for acute suppurative sialadenitis.
- Bulimia and anorexia nervosa
- Sjögren syndrome
- Chronic illness
- Immune compromise
- Cachexia

Genetics
A familial form of recurrent parotitis of childhood has been described with autosomal inheritance.

PATHOPHYSIOLOGY
- Acute infection of the salivary glands is caused by retrograde bacterial contamination of the salivary ducts from the oral cavity.
- Mechanical impairment of salivary flow also predisposes to acute infection (trauma, foreign body).
- Ductal obstruction is generally secondary to mucous plug caused by stasis of saliva with increased viscosity with subsequent stasis and infection.

ETIOLOGY
- Bacteria from the oral cavity are the most common infectious cause of sialadenitis
  - *Staphylococcus aureus*
  - *Streptococcus*
  - *Haemophilus Influenzae*
  - *Pseudomonas*
  - *Enterobacter*
  - *Klebsiella*
  - *Enterococcus*
  - *Proteus*
  - *Candida* spp.
  - Anaerobic bacteria
    ○ *Peptostreptococcus*
    ○ *Bacteroides* spp.
    ○ *Fusobacterium*
- The causative agents of the following diseases may also infect a salivary gland, resulting in sialadenitis
  - Mumps
  - Actinomycosis
  - Tuberculosis
  - Syphilis
  - Cytomegalovirus
  - Cat scratch disease
- Drug: Terbinafine

ASSOCIATED CONDITIONS
- Rheumatoid arthritis (Sjögren syndrome)
- Sarcoidosis (Heerfordt syndrome)
- Sicca syndrome
- HIV
- Kuttner tumor
- Malnutrition

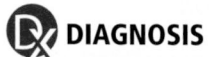 **DIAGNOSIS**

SIGNS AND SYMPTOMS
- Enlarged, painful salivary gland
- Increase pain with meals
- Purulent discharge from duct orifice
- Red, painful duct orifice
- Fever
- Malaise
- Xerostomia
- Decreased salivary secretion (aptyalism)

History
Check for recent dehydration.

Physical Exam
- Erythema, tenderness at the duct opening
- Induration and pitting of the skin with involvement of the masseteric and submandibular spatial planes in severe cases
- Bimanual palpation of the gland results in suppurative discharge from the duct orifice in 3/4 of cases of acute suppurative sialadenitis.
- Bilateral involvement in up to 25% of cases

TESTS
Lab
- Not often warranted. WBC; leukocytosis with predominant of neutrophils if bacterial or lymphocytosis if viral
- Serum amylase normal
- Culture of the purulent discharge from the duct (suppurative sialadenitis)

Imaging
- Consider ultrasound or CT scan in patients not responding to treatment in 48–72 hours.
- Radiographs may reveal a stone in sialolithiasis.
- Ultrasound may show ductal dilatation and a stone.
- CT may show abscess in advanced infection.
- Sialography is contraindicated in acute infection.
- MRI may be used to evaluate the salivary duct architecture noninvasively.

Diagnostic Procedures/Surgery
- Digital manipulation of the duct may express pus from the ductal orifice.
- Percutaneous needle aspiration of the involve duct in cases of suppurative sialadenitis, limit the amount of contamination by means of an intraoral route.

Pathological Findings
With chronic infection of the gland
- Enlarged gland
- Ductal dilatation with retention of saliva
- Acinar atrophy, or acinus dilated and filled with mucus
- Purulent/seropurulent exudate within the duct
- Glandular replacement by fibrotic tissue
- Infiltration with leukocytes

DIFFERENTIAL DIAGNOSIS

- Decreased salivary secretion is associated with
  - Drugs
    - Tricyclic antidepressants (e.g., amitriptyline), phenothiazines (e.g., chlorpromazine, fluphenazine, thioridazine, prochlorperazine)
    - Anticholinergics
    - Antihistaminics: Diphenhydramine
  - Myxedema
  - Plummer-Vinson disease
  - Pernicious anemia
  - Febrile diseases
  - Neuropsychiatric disorders
  - Mikulicz disease (benign lymphoepithelial lesion)
- Enlarged glands may be the result of a variety of neoplasms, including
  - Pleomorphic adenoma
  - Mucoepidermoid carcinoma
  - Other tumor types may occur very rarely (e.g., lipoma, neurofibroma, fibrosarcoma, melanoma, lymphocytoma, Hodgkin)
  - Lymphangitis external otitis
  - Bezold abscess
  - Cervical adenitis
  - Dental abscesses
  - Infected brachial cleft or sebaceous cyst.
- Also, obesity results in what appears to be enlarged parotids, but the bilateral nature and nonprogressive course should help differentiate this from malignant neoplasms.

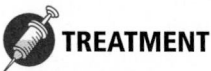 TREATMENT

INITIAL STABILIZATION
Outpatient care

GENERAL MEASURES
- A heating pad and/or cool compresses may be comforting.
- Massaging the gland may express pus and relieve some of the pressure.
- Rehydration
- Oral cavity irrigations

Diet
Avoid pain-producing sialagogues (e.g., lemon) during an acute episode.

Activity
Unrestricted

SPECIAL THERAPY
IV Fluids
Fluid and electrolyte replacement

 MEDICATION (DRUGS)

- Antibiotics
  - Penicillin V (Pen-Vee K) 250–500 mg q.i.d.
  - Erythromycin 250 mg q.i.d.
  - Amoxicillin-clavulanate (Augmentin) 500 mg t.i.d.
  - Cefuroxime (Ceftin) 750–1500 mg/IM/IV q8h Children: 20–30 mg/kg/d suspension PO divided b.i.d.
  - Clindamycin in patients allergic to penicillin
  - IV antibiotics in severe cases
  - Methicillin–resistant *S. aureus* may require vancomycin or linezolid
- Analgesics, e.g., codeine, hydrocodone, NSAIDs

SURGERY
Superficial parotidectomy in patients with chronic nonspecific sialadenitis. Complications include temporary (or permanent) facial nerve weakness and neuromas, but a reduction in symptoms may be expected.

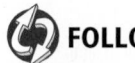 FOLLOW-UP

DISPOSITION
Complete recovery unless the patient has underlying obstruction (ductal stricture, tumor or stone)

Admission Criteria
- Severely ill
- Dehydration
- IV antibiotics
- Intractable pain
- Complications

Discharge Criteria
Response to antimicrobial therapy is seen within 48–72 hours of initiating treatment; treatment should continue for 1 week after resolution of symptoms.

Issues for Referral
Refer cases that do not resolve despite appropriate antibiotic therapy to ENT.

PROGNOSIS
Good; complete recovery

COMPLICATIONS
- Suppurative sialadenitis
  - Abscess
  - Bacteremia
  - Osteomyelitis
  - Thrombophlebitis of the jugular vein
  - Septicemia
  - Respiratory obstruction
  - Facial nerve paralysis
  - Death
- Occasional loss of salivary function

REFERENCES

1. Bhatty MA, et al. Chronic non-specific parotid sialadenitis. *Br J Plast Surg*. 1998;517–521.
2. Chitre VV, Premchandra DJ. Review: Recurrent parotiditis. *Arch Dis Child*. 1997;77:559–363.
3. Salivary gland infections: MedlinePlus, US National Institutes of Health web site. http://www.nim.nih.gov/medlineplus/ency/article/001041.htm.

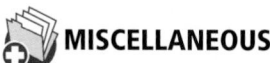 MISCELLANEOUS

See also: Sjögren syndrome

CODES

ICD9-CM
527.2 Sialadenitis

S

PATIENT TEACHING

Diet
Avoid pain-producing sialogogues (lemon) during attacks.

Prevention
- Oral hygiene
- Avoid dehydration
- Stimulation of salivary flow using sialogogues such as lemon drops or orange juice
- Regular external and bimanual massage

SILICOSIS

Robert P. Baughman, MD

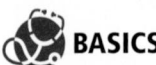 **BASICS**

DESCRIPTION
Pneumoconiosis (fibrogenic) caused by inhaling silica dust (in the form of quartz, cristobalite, or tridymite)

- Chronic (classical) silicosis can be simple or complicated.
- Chronic simple silicosis is asymptomatic, nonprogressive after the exposure ends, and consists solely of small round radiographic pulmonary opacities.
- Chronic complicated silicosis has progressively worsening symptoms and enlarging pulmonary opacities, even after exposure ends.
- Subacute silicosis develops after 3–6 years of high exposure, and resembles chronic complicated silicosis.
- Acute silicosis develops within a couple years of massive exposure and is clinically distinct from the other forms.
- System(s) Affected: Pulmonary

ALERT
Geriatric Considerations
Symptoms and complications more severe

Geriatric Considerations
Unusual

GENERAL PREVENTION
- Avoid dust exposure.
- Substitute other materials for silica.
- Respiratory protective devices for unavoidable short-term exposure

EPIDEMIOLOGY
- Predominant age: 40–75
- Predominant sex: Male > Female

Incidence
Unknown

Prevalence
Unknown

RISK FACTORS
Industrial activities that involve cutting, polishing, or shearing rock, or involve the use of sand, including
- Metal mining (copper, silver, gold, lead, hard coal)
- Foundries
- Pottery making
- Sandstone cutting
- Granite cutting

Genetics
No known genetic pattern

ETIOLOGY
- Chronic simple silicosis: 10–12 years of exposure to silica dust
- Chronic complicated silicosis: >20 years of exposure
- Subacute silicosis: 3–6 years of heavy exposure
- Acute silicosis: <2 years of massive exposure

ASSOCIATED CONDITIONS
- Tuberculosis
- Caplan syndrome (coexistence of rheumatoid arthritis with a pneumoconiosis)

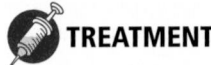 **DIAGNOSIS**

SIGNS AND SYMPTOMS
- Chronic simple silicosis
  - Asymptomatic
  - Cough and mild dyspnea typically accompany, and are due to smoking or occupational bronchitis.
- Chronic complicated silicosis; subacute silicosis
  - Chest tightness
  - Cough
  - Dyspnea
  - Expectoration
  - Signs and symptoms of right heart failure as cor pulmonale develops
- Acute silicosis
  - Dry cough
  - Fever
  - Severe dyspnea

TESTS
Special tests
- Pulmonary function testing is normal in simple silicosis. Other forms show decreased pulmonary compliance, decreased lung volumes, and decreased diffusing capacity.
- International Labor Office (ILO) classification system for quantification of chest radiograph abnormalities
- Yearly purified protein derivative (PPD) test

Lab
- Hypoxemia
- Hypercarbia

Imaging
Chest radiograph
- Chronic simple silicosis
  - Eggshell calcification in hilar and mediastinal lymph nodes
  - Small round opacities, initially in upper lobes
- Chronic complicated silicosis, subacute silicosis
  - Pulmonary opacities >1 cm
  - Opacities form bilateral conglomerate shadows (progressive massive fibrosis)
  - Opacities initially peripheral, later migrate toward hilum
  - Opacities may cavitate. (Rule out tuberculosis!)
  - High-resolution CT scan provides more definition of infiltrates and is helpful in identifying nodules.

Diagnostic Procedures/Surgery
- Bronchoscopy
- Detailed occupational history
- Open lung biopsy

Pathological Findings
Lung
- Pleural adhesions
- Pleural thickening
- Gray-black subpleural nodules
- Blackened lung
- Leathery lung
- Concentric layers of dense connective tissue
- Cellular infiltrate
- Ischemic degeneration of central nodule
- Metachromatic silica particles

DIFFERENTIAL DIAGNOSIS
- Chronic simple silicosis
  - Sarcoidosis
  - Radiographic eggshell calcifications also seen in sarcoidosis and Hodgkin's disease
- Chronic complicated silicosis, subacute silicosis
  - Coal worker pneumoconiosis
  - Consider especially when consolidations are rapidly progressive, unilateral, or cavitating—tuberculosis, neoplasia, fungal pneumonia
- Acute silicosis: Alveolar proteinosis

TREATMENT

GENERAL MEASURES
- No known effective treatment
- Postural drainage
- Mist inhalation
- Chest physical therapy
- Breathing exercises

Diet
- No special diet
- Increase fluid intake

Activity
Maintain regular exercise program.

MEDICATION (DRUGS)

First Line
- None specific for silicosis
- Isoniazid: 300 mg/d for 1 year, if tuberculin skin test is positive
- Silicotuberculosis requires at least 3 antituberculous drugs initially, including rifampin.
- Contraindications: Avoid sedatives and hypnotics.
- Precautions: Refer to the manufacturer's literature.
- Significant possible interactions: Refer to the manufacturer's literature.

Second Line
Antifibrinogenic agents remain investigational.

SURGERY
- Lung transplantation
- Whole lung lavage remains investigational.

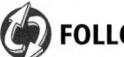 **FOLLOW-UP**

PROGNOSIS
- Chronic simple silicosis: Remains asymptomatic and does not progress if exposure ends.
- Chronic complicated silicosis; subacute silicosis: Progressive pulmonary fibrosis with cor pulmonale and right heart failure, even after exposure ends

COMPLICATIONS
- Progressive massive fibrosis
- Respiratory infection
- Pneumothorax
- Emphysema
- Cor pulmonale
- Right heart failure
- Mycobacterial infections
- Fungal infections

PATIENT MONITORING
- Monitor for heart failure and hypoxemia.
- Treat intercurrent infections aggressively.

REFERENCES

1. Banks DE, et al. Strategies for the treatment of pneumoconiosis. *Occup Med*. 1993;8:205–232.
2. Silicosis and Silicate Disease Committee. Diseases associated with exposure to silica and non-fibrous silicate materials. *Arch Pathol Lab Med*. 1988;112:673.

 MISCELLANEOUS

Other notes
- Silica: Formula for calculating the threshold limit value for respirable dust: Threshold limit value $= (10$ mg per m^2/% SiO$_2) + 2$
- See also: Chronic obstructive pulmonary disease and emphysema; Cor pulmonale; Pneumothorax; Tuberculosis

CODES

ICD9-CM
502 Pneumoconiosis due to other silica or silicates

PATIENT TEACHING

Printed patient information available from American Lung Association, 1740 Broadway, New York, NY 10019; (212) 315-8700

S

SINUSITIS
Rebecca Musher Gross, MD

 BASICS

DESCRIPTION
- Acute rhinosinusitis (generally called sinusitis) is a symptomatic inflammation of the paranasal sinuses of <4 weeks duration resulting from impaired drainage and retained secretions. Disease is subacute when symptomatic for 4–12 weeks; chronic when symptomatic for >12 weeks
- System(s) Affected: HEENT; Pulmonary

GENERAL PREVENTION
No documented preventive measures

EPIDEMIOLOGY
- Of ~1 billion viral respiratory illnesses in the US each year, perhaps 200 million (10%) are associated with inflammation, impaired drainage and retained secretions in sinuses; ~20 million cases are secondarily infected by bacteria.
- Diagnosis of acute bacterial rhinosinusitis is 5th leading reason for prescribing antibiotics, accounting for 9% of all pediatric and 21% of all adult antibiotic prescriptions in 2002.
- Many of these diagnoses are erroneous.
- Incidence highest in early fall through early spring (related to incidence of viral URI)

RISK FACTORS
- Viral upper respiratory infection
- Allergic rhinitis
- Asthma
- Cigarette smoking
- Trauma
- Dental infections and procedures
- Anatomical variations
  - Tonsillar and adenoid hypertrophy
  - Turbinate hypertrophy, nasal polyps
  - Deviated septum
  - Cleft palate
- Immunodeficiency (e.g., HIV)
- Cystic fibrosis

Genetics
No known genetic pattern

PATHOPHYSIOLOGY
- Important features
  - Inflammation and edema of the sinus mucosa
  - Obstruction of the sinus ostia
  - Impaired mucociliary clearance
- Secretions that are not cleared become hospitable to bacterial growth.
- Inflammatory response (neutrophil influx and release of cytokines) damages mucosal surfaces.

ETIOLOGY
- Viral: Vast majority of cases (rhinovirus, influenza A and B, parainfluenza virus, respiratory syncytial, adeno-, corona-, and entero-viruses
- Bacterial (complicates 0.2–2% of viral cases)
  - More likely if symptoms worsen >5–7 days or do not improve >10 days
  - *Streptococcus pneumoniae, Haemophilus influenzae*, and *Moraxella catarrhalis* are the most common bacterial etiologies.
  - Often overdiagnosed, which leads to overuse of, and increasing resistance to, antibiotics
- Fungal infection seen In immunocompromised hosts (uncontrolled diabetes, neutropenia, glucocorticosteroids) or as nosocomial infection

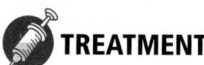 **DIAGNOSIS**

History and physical exam suggest the diagnosis in the majority of cases.

SIGNS AND SYMPTOMS
- Major challenge is to distinguish between viral and bacterial disease; use constellation of symptoms rather than a particular sign or symptom.
- Symptoms predictive of bacterial sinusitis
  - Persistent symptoms for ≥10 days
  - Worsening of symptoms >5–7 days after initial improvement
  - Persistent purulent nasal discharge
  - Unilateral maxillary tooth or facial pain
  - Unilateral maxillary sinus tenderness
  - Appearance of fever (usually low-grade)
- Associated symptoms
  - Headache
  - Nasal congestion
  - Retro-orbital pain
  - Otalgia
  - Hyposomia
  - Halitosis
  - Chronic cough
- Symptoms requiring urgent attention
  - Visual disturbances, especially diplopia
  - Periorbital swelling or erythema
  - Altered mental status

Physical Exam
- Fever
- Edema and erythema of nasal mucosa
- Purulent discharge
- Tenderness to palpation over sinus(es)

TESTS
- None indicated in routine evaluation
- Transillumination of the sinuses
  - May confirm fluid in sinuses
  - Value is limited as it does not distinguish between viral and bacterial etiology.

Lab
None indicated in routine evaluation

Imaging
- Routine use of sinus radiography discouraged because: (i) ≥3 clinical findings may have similar diagnostic accuracy as imaging and (ii) imaging does not distinguish viral from bacterial etiology.
- Limited coronal CT can be useful in recurrent infection or failure to respond to medical therapy.

Diagnostic Procedures/Surgery
- Gold standard = transnasal endoscopic or sublabial maxillary antrum aspiration culture; generally performed only in recurrent and/or complicated cases (1,2)[A]

Pathophysiological Findings
- Inflammation
- Edema
- Thickened mucosa
- Impaired ciliary function
- Metaplasia of ciliated columnar cells
- Relative acidosis and hypoxia within sinuses
- Polyps

DIFFERENTIAL DIAGNOSIS
- Dental disease
- Cystic fibrosis
- Wegener granulomatosis
- HIV infection
- Kartagener syndrome
- Immotile cilia syndrome
- Neoplasm

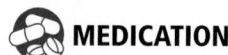 **TREATMENT**

- Majority of cases treated in outpatient setting
- Hospitalization for complications (meningitis, orbital cellulitis or abscess, brain abscess)

GENERAL MEASURES
- Adequate hydration
- Steam inhalation 20–30 minutes t.i.d.
- Saline irrigation or saline nose drops
- Sleep with head of bed elevated.
- Avoid exposure to cigarette smoke, fumes.
- Avoid dehydrants (caffeine and alcohol).
- Antibiotics indicated only when findings suggest bacterial infection
- Analgesics, NSAIDs (see below)
- Acute viral sinusitis is self-limiting, and antibiotics should not be used.

Diet
No special diet

Activity
Adequate rest, otherwise no restrictions

 MEDICATION

First Line
- Decongestants
  - Pseudoephedrine HCl
  - Phenylephrine (limited use)
  - Oxymetazoline (i.e., Afrin) (limited use)
- Analgesics
  - Acetaminophen
  - Aspirin
  - NSAIDs
  - Acetaminophen–codeine
- Antibiotics
  - Antibiotics appear to have a slight advantage over placebo, yet most patients improve without therapy.
  - Major issue: Distinguish bacterial from viral
  - Reserve antibiotic use for patients with moderate to severe disease.
  - Treat 10–14 days unless otherwise specified.
  - Choice should be based on understanding of antibiotic resistance in the community.
  - Multiple meta-analyses have demonstrated NO benefit of newer antibiotics over Amoxicillin, Trimethoprim-sulfamethoxazole, or Doxycyclin.

  - Initial therapy (2)[A]

  - Amoxicillin: 500 mg–1 g t.i.d. (adults); 80–90 mg/kg/d divided q8h (children)
  - Trimethoprim-sulfamethoxazole: 160 mg/800 mg q12h in adults and 8–12 mg/kg/d of trimethoprim component divided q12h for children
  - Doxycyline 100 mg PO b.i.d.

Second Line

- Amoxicillin-clavulanate (Augmentin) 875 mg/ 125 mg q12h (adults); 30 mg/kg/d of amoxicillin component divided b.i.d. in children
- Cefpodoxime (Vantin): 200 mg q12h in adults and 10 mg/kg/d divided b.i.d. in children
- Cefuroxime axetil (Ceftin): 250 mg q12hrs in adults and 30 mg/kg/d divided q12h in children
- Telithromycin: 800 mg/d × 5 days in adults, no pediatric indication
- Azithromycin (Zithromax): 500 mg on day 1 and 250 mg on days 2–5 in adults; 10 mg/kg on day 1 and 5 mg/kg on days 2–5 in children
- Clarithromycin: 500 mg b.i.d. (regular) or 1000 mg/d (extended release) in adults; 15 mg/kd/d divided b.i.d. in children
- Levofloxacin (Levaquin): 500 mg/d in adults; if patients have had antibiotics within past 4–6 weeks or if no response to above therapy within 72 hours, change to
  - High dose amoxicillin/clavulanate
  - Cephalosporins as above
  - Fluoroquinolones as above
- NOTE: Bacteriologic failure rates up to 20–25% are possible with use of azithromycin and clarithromycin (2)[C]
- If lack of response to 3 weeks of antibiotics, consider
  - CT scan of sinuses
  - Ear, nose, and throat referral
- Precautions
  - Decongestants can exacerbate hypertension.
  - Prolonged use of topical decongestants (>4 days) may precipitate rhinitis medicamentosa.
  - Sulfonamides may induce Stevens-Johnson syndrome (risk ~1 in 2,000): Inform patients to report any mucous membrane ulcerations.
- Significant possible interactions
  - Warfarin (Coumadin): Increased effect of warfarin with macrolides or TMP/SMX, resulting in marked increase in INR and PT
  - Statins should be stopped when macrolides or telithromycin are prescribed due to increased risk of myopathy, rhabdomyolysis.

Other Medications

- As allergies may be a predisposing factor, some patients may benefit from use of oral antihistamines or nasal steroids.
- Oral antihistamines
  - Loratadine (Claritin)
  - Fexofenadine (Allegra)
  - Cetirizine (Zyrtec)
  - Chlorpheniramine (Chlor-Trimeton)
  - Diphenhydramine (Benadryl)
- Leukotriene inhibitors (Singulair, Accolate) may be indicated in patients with concomitant asthma.
- Nasal steroids (i.e., fluticasone [Flonase])

ALERT

Pediatric Considerations

- Sinuses are not fully developed until age 20, but the maxillary and ethmoid sinuses, although small, are present from birth.
- As children have an average of 6–8 colds per year, they are at risk for development of sinusitis.
- Diagnosis can be more difficult than in adults, as symptoms are often more subtle.

Pregnancy Considerations

- Rhinitis of pregnancy predisposes to sinusitis.
- Nasal irrigation with saline as well as pseudophedrine are safe during pregnancy and lactation.
- Antibiotics considered to be safe in pregnancy and lactation
  - Amoxicillin and amoxicillin-clavulanate (B)
  - Cephalosporins (B)
  - Azithromycin (B)
- Contraindicated in pregnancy and lactation
  - Clarithromycin
  - Telithromycin
- Safe in lactation but not during pregnancy
  - Levofloxacin

SURGERY

- If medical therapy fails, consider sinus irrigation.
- Functional endoscopic sinus surgery is the preferred treatment for medically recalcitrant cases (2)[C]
- Absolute surgical indications
  - Massive nasal polyposis
  - Acute complications: Subperiosteal or orbital abscess, frontal soft tissue spread of infection
  - Mucocele or mucopyocele
  - Invasive or allergic fungal sinusitis
  - Suspected obstructing tumor
  - CSF rhinorrhea

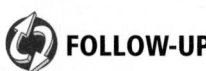 FOLLOW-UP

DISPOSITION
Admission Criteria
Complications as below

Issues for Referral
- Complications as below
- Failure of treatment

PROGNOSIS
Alleviation of symptoms within 72 hours with complete resolution within 10–14 days

COMPLICATIONS
- Meningitis
- Orbital cellulitis
- Brain abscess
- Cavernous sinus thrombosis
- Osteomyelitis
- Subdural empyema

PATIENT MONITORING
- Instruct for proper use of all medications.
- Return if no improvement after 72 hours or no resolution of symptoms after 10 days of antibiotics.
- If symptoms resolve, no routine follow-up, is needed.

REFERENCES

1. Sande MA, Gwaltney JM. Acute community-acquired bacterial sinusitis: Continuing challenges and current management. *Clin Infect Dis*. 2004;39:S151–S158.
2. Varonen H, et al. Comparison of ultrasound, radiography, and clinical examination in the diagnosis of acute maxillary sinusitis: A systematic review. *J Clin Epidemiol*. 2000;53:940–948.
3. Sinus and Allergy Health Partnership. Antimicrobial treatment guidelines for acute bacterial rhinosinusitis. *Otolaryngol Head Neck Surg*. 2004;130:1–45.
4. Williams JW Jr, et al. Antibiotics for acute maxillary sinusitis. *Cochrane Database Syst Rev*. 2003;2:CD000243.

 MISCELLANEOUS

CODES

ICD9-CM
- 117.9 Other and unspecified mycoses
- 461.0 Acute maxillary sinusitis
- 461.1 Acute frontal sinusitus
- 461.2 Acute ethmoidal sinusitis
- 461.3 Acute sphenoidal sinusitus
- 461.8 Other acute sinusitis
- 461.9 Acute sinusitis, unspecified
- 473.0 Chronic maxillary sinusitis
- 473.9 Unspecified sinusitis (chronic)

PATIENT TEACHING

- Call back if no significant improvement within 1 week, if symptoms worsen, or for symptoms such as headache, neck stiffness, visual changes, nausea, or vomiting.
- Educate the patient on the potential major side effects of selected medications.
- For patient education on this topic
  - www.familydoctor.org
  - www.medlineplus.gov

 See Corresponding Diagnostic Algorithm

 See Patient Handout on CD

SLEEP APNEA, OBSTRUCTIVE

Anjali Koka, MD
Frank J. Domino, MD

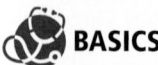 **BASICS**

DESCRIPTION

- Obstructive sleep apnea (OSA) is defined as repetitive episodes of cessation of airflow at nose and mouth during sleep due to obstruction at level of the pharynx.
  - Associated with oxygen desaturation and nocturnal asphyxia
  - 60% of people with OSA snore
  - Apneas often terminate with a snort or gasp.
  - Repetitive apneas produce sleep disruption, leading to excessive daytime sleepiness.
  - Usual course is chronic
- System(s) Affected: Cardiovascular; Nervous; Pulmonary
- Synonym(s): Pickwickian syndrome; Sleep apnea syndrome; Nocturnal upper airway occlusion

GENERAL PREVENTION
See "Patient Education."

EPIDEMIOLOGY
- Predominant age: Middle age
- Predominant sex: Male > Female (2–3:1)

Incidence
Undetermined

Prevalence
- 4% for males and 2% for females (estimated)
- Prevalence increases with age.

RISK FACTORS
- Obesity
- Male sex
- Postmenopausal female
- Age >40 years old
- Nasal obstruction (due to polyps, rhinitis, or deviated septum)
- Anatomic narrowing (tonsillar hypertrophy, macroglossia, micrognathia, retrognathia, craniofacial abnormalities)
- Acromegaly
- Hypothyroidism
- Neurologic syndromes (muscular dystrophy, cerebral palsy)
- Alcohol/Sedative intake before bedtime
- Smoking

Genetics
Hereditary factors unknown; familial patterns seen

PATHOPHYSIOLOGY
OSA occurs when the naso- or oropharynx collapses passively during inspiration. A balance of anatomic and neuromuscular factors contribute to pharyngeal collapse.

- Anatomic abnormalities predispose the airway to collapse by decreasing the area of the upper airway or increasing the pressure surrounding the airway.
- Abnormal pharyngeal muscle control during sleep can decrease tonic input to upper airway muscles and can reduce reflexes to keep the upper airway open.

ETIOLOGY
Upper airway narrowing may be due to

- Obesity
- Enlarged tonsils or uvula
- Low soft palate
- Redundant tissue in soft palate or tonsillar pillars
- Large or posteriorly located tongue
- Craniofacial abnormalities
- Alcohol or sedative use before bedtime

ASSOCIATED CONDITIONS
- Hypertension
- Stroke
- Cardiovascular disease
- Cardiac arrythmias
- CHF
- Nasal obstructive problems
- Insulin resistance

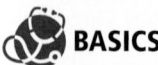 **DIAGNOSIS**

SIGNS AND SYMPTOMS
- Daytime symptoms
  - Excessive daytime sleepiness (cardinal symptom)
  - Tired or unrefreshed upon morning awakening
  - Sore or dry throat
  - Complaints of poor concentration, memory problems, irritability, mood changes
  - Morning headaches
  - Decreased libido
  - Depression
  - Daytime fatigue or tiredness
  - Systemic and pulmonary hypertension
- Nighttime symptoms
  - Loud snoring
  - Snort or gasp that arouses patient from sleep
  - Disrupted sleep, nocturia
  - Witnessed apneic episodes at night

History
Be sure to elicit a complete history of daytime and nighttime symptoms. Symptoms can be insidious and present for years.

- Evaluation of EDS
  - Mild symptoms begin during quiet activities (reading, watching television).
  - Severe symptoms begin during dynamic activities (work, driving).

Physical Exam
Most patients have a normal physical exam or may have hypertension, obesity, or appear sleepy.

- Focus of head and neck exam
  - Oropharynx
    ○ Narrowing of the lateral airway wall
    ○ Tonsillar hypertrophy
    ○ Micrognathia or retrognathia
    ○ Long or thick uvula
    ○ High, arched hard palate
    ○ Soft palate edema
    ○ Macroglossia
  - Nasopharynx
    ○ Deviated nasal septum
    ○ Poor nasal airflow
  - Short neck with large circumference

TESTS
Lab
When clinically indicated

- TSH to rule out hypothyroidism
- Hct to evaluate polycythemia which can indicate nocturnal hypoxemia
- ABG to evaluate daytime hypercapnia

Imaging
Cephalometric measurements from lateral head and neck radiographs can aid in surgery treatments.

Diagnostic Procedures/Surgery
- Gold standard remains polysomnography (PSG), a nighttime sleep study
  - Demonstrates severity of hypoxemia, sleep disruption, and cardiac arrhythmias associated with obstructive sleep apnea and elevated end tidal CO_2
  - Shows repetitive episodes of cessation or marked reduction in airflow despite continued respiratory efforts
  - These apneic episodes must last at least 10 seconds and occur 10–15 times per hour to be considered clinically significant.
  - Complete PSG is expensive, and health insurance may not cover the cost. In the future, portable monitoring will diagnose OSA once standards are established.
- Multiple sleep latency testing provides an objective measurement of daytime sleepiness.
- The apnea/hypoapnea index is defined as the total number of apneas and hypopneas divided by the total sleep time.
  - Mild OSA: AHI = 5–15
  - Moderate OSA: AHI = 15–30
  - Severe OSA: AHI >30
- Drugs that may alter lab results: Benzodiazepines and other sedatives can amplify the severity of apnea seen on sleep study.

DIFFERENTIAL DIAGNOSIS
- Other causes of excessive daytime sleepiness such as
  - Narcolepsy
  - Idiopathic daytime hypersomnolence
  - Inadequate sleep time
  - Depressive episodes with excessive daytime sleepiness
  - Periodic limb movements disorder
- Respiratory disorders with nocturnal awakenings such as asthma, chronic obstructive pulmonary disease, CHF
- Central sleep apnea may mimic obstructive sleep apnea.
- Sudden nocturnal awakenings due to panic attacks
- Sleep-related choking or laryngospasm
- Gastroesophageal reflux may also present with similar symptoms.
- Sleep-associated seizures (temporal lobe epilepsy)

TREATMENT

Outpatient for treatment or sleep study; inpatient for surgery

GENERAL MEASURES

- Continuous positive airway pressure (CPAP) treatment that restores regular nighttime breathing not only reduces snoring and ESD, but also decreases the risk for stroke (1)[B] and CHF and lowers blood pressure over the short-term. (2)[A]
- The most effective treatment for OSA is nasal CPAP. CPAP prevents the soft tissue in pharynx from collapsing, thus eliminating apneas and restoring oxygen saturation.
  – Mild to moderate obstructive sleep apnea: CPAP, surgery, dental appliances
  – Moderate to severe obstructive sleep apnea: CPAPA or BiPAP is the standard therapy.
- If OSA is present only when supine, keep the patient off his back (e.g., tennis ball in pocket sewn on back of nightshirt; fanny-pack with tennis balls worn at back).
- Avoid driving, if excessive daytime sleepiness is significant.
- No alcohol within 6 hours of bedtime
- Avoid sedatives and sleeping pills.

Diet

Overweight patients must lose weight, and all patients must avoid weight gain. Weight loss alone can relieve symptoms of OSA. (3)[A]

Activity

- Significantly sleepy patients should not drive a motor vehicle or operate dangerous equipment.
- Avoid alcohol, smoking, and sedatives.

 MEDICATION (DRUGS)

First Line

Medications are generally not effective in treating OSA except in patients with rapid eye movement (REM) sleep–related apnea in whom protriptyline or fluoxetine may be helpful.

SURGERY

Surgical correction of the upper airway is not first line treatment and should only be considered in OSA that is not controllable with CPAP or weight loss. Surgeries: Uvulopalatopharyngoplasty (effective in 40% patients), tracheostomy, craniofacial surgery

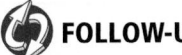 FOLLOW-UP

PROGNOSIS

- With appropriate control of apneas, excessive daytime sleepiness dramatically improves quickly.
- Lifelong compliance with weight loss or nasal CPAP is necessary for therapy of obstructive sleep apnea.
- Untreated, obstructive sleep apnea appears to progress in severity.
- Significant morbidity and mortality due to OSA is usually secondary to arrhythmias, cardiac ischemia or hypertensive complications, or motor vehicle accidents.

COMPLICATIONS

Untreated OSA increases the risk for development of hypertension, stroke, myocardial infarction, diabetes, cardiovascular disease, and work-related and driving accidents

PATIENT MONITORING

- Physician follow-up improves compliance with CPAP therapy.
- Observe for return of snoring, EDS, or sleep disruption, which may indicate inadequate control of apneas.

ALERT

Pediatric Considerations

- The prevalence of pediatric OSA is 1–2% in children 4–5 years of age, and the peak incidence is between 3 and 6 years of age. Gender ratio: M = F
- Etiology: The most common cause is tonsillar hypertrophy. Additional causes are obesity and craniofacial abnormalities. OSA is also seen in children with neuromuscular diseases, such as cerebral palsy, spinal muscular atrophy due to abnormal pharyngeal muscle control.
- Sign and symptoms: Nighttime: Loud snoring, restlessness, and sweating. Daytime: Hyperactivity and decreased school performance. EDS is not a significant symptom.
- Diagnosis: Gold standard is PSG. Abnormal apnea/hypopnea index is different in children; >1–2 per hour is abnormal.
- Treatment: Surgery is the 1st-line treatment in cases due to tonsillar enlargement (improves symptoms in 70%). For cases due to obesity or craniofacial abnormalities, patients can use CPAP.

Pregnancy Considerations

Rare

REFERENCES

1. Yaggi HK, et al. Obstructive sleep apnea as a risk factor for stroke and death. *N Engl J Med.* 2005;353:2034–2041.
2. Giles T, et al. Continuous positive airways pressure for obstructive sleep apnoea in adults. *Cochrane Database Syst Rev.* 2006;(1):CD001106.
3. Ryan CF. Sleep x 9: an approach to treatment of obstructive sleep apnoea/hypopnoea syndrome including upper airway surgery. *Thorax.* 2005;60(7):595–604.

ADDITIONAL READING

- Kryger MH. *Principles and Practice of Sleep Medicine.* 3rd ed. Philadelphia, PA: WB Saunders; 2000.
- Thorpy MJ. *Handbook of Sleep Disorders.* New York, NY: Marcel Dekker; 1990.

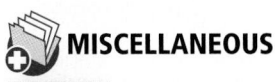 MISCELLANEOUS

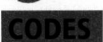 CODES

ICD9-CM
780.57 Other and unspecified sleep apnea

PATIENT TEACHING

Diet

Weight loss and avoidance of alcohol and sedatives can prevent OSA symptoms.

Activity

Avoid driving if excessive daytime sleepiness is significant.

 See Corresponding Diagnostic Algorithm

S

SMELL AND TASTE DISORDERS

Steven M. Bromley, MD

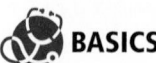 **BASICS**

DESCRIPTION

- The senses of smell and taste allow full appreciation of the flavor and palatability of foods and also serve as an early-warning system against toxins, polluted air, smoke, and spoiled food products. Physiologically, the chemical senses aid in normal digestion by triggering gastrointestinal secretions. Smell or taste dysfunction may have a significant impact on quality of life.
- Loss of smell occurs more frequently than loss of taste, and patients frequently confuse the concepts of flavor loss (as a result of smell impairment) with taste loss (impaired ability to sense sweet, sour, salty, or bitter).
- Smell depends on the functioning of cranial nerve I (olfactory nerve) and cranial nerve V (trigeminal nerve).
- Taste depends on the functioning of cranial nerves VII, IX, and X. Because of these multiple pathways, total loss of taste (ageusia) is rare.
- System(s) Affected: Nervous
- Synonym(s): Burning mouth syndrome

GENERAL PREVENTION

- Avoid exposure to chemicals, smoke, and radiation.
- Maintain good oral and nasal health, with routine visits to the dentist.
- Eat a well-balanced diet for optimal nutrition.

EPIDEMIOLOGY

- Predominant age: Chemosensory loss is age dependent.
- Predominant sex: Male > Female (Men also begin to lose ability to smell earlier in life than do women.)

Incidence

Estimated >2 million; 200,000 visit a physician each year.

Prevalence

- Age >80 years: 80% have major olfactory impairment; nearly 50% are anosmic.
- Ages 65–80 years: 60% have major olfactory impairment; nearly 25% are anosmic.
- Age <65 years: 1–2% have smell impairment.

RISK FACTORS

Genetics

Smell and taste disturbances may be related to genetically associated underlying diseases (e.g., Kallmann syndrome, Alzheimer disease, migraine, and rheumatologic and endocrine disorders).

ETIOLOGY

- Smell and/or taste disturbances
  - Nutritional factors (malnutrition, vitamin deficiencies, liver disease, anemia)
  - Endocrine disorders (thyroid disease, diabetes mellitus, renal disease)
  - Head trauma
  - Migraine headache (gustatory aura, olfactory aura)
  - Sjögren syndrome
  - Toxic chemical exposure
  - Industrial agent exposure
  - Aging
  - Medications (see below)
  - Neurodegenerative diseases (multiple sclerosis, Alzheimer disease, cerebrovascular accident, Parkinson disease)
  - Infections (upper respiratory infection, oral and perioral infections, candidiasis, coxsackievirus, AIDS, viral hepatitis, herpes simplex virus)
- Possible causes of smell disturbance
  - Nasal and sinus disease (allergies, rhinitis, rhinorrhea)
  - Cigarette smoking
  - Cocaine abuse (intranasal)
  - Radiation treatment of head and neck
  - Congenital conditions
  - Neoplasm (brain tumor, nasal polyps, intranasal tumor)
  - Systemic lupus erythematosus
  - Bell palsy
  - Oral or perioral skin lesion
  - Damage to cranial nerve I or V
- Possible causes of taste loss
  - Oral appliances
  - Dental procedures
  - Intraoral abscess
  - Gingivitis
  - Damage to cranial nerve VI, IX, or X
- Selected medications that reportedly alter smell and taste
  - Antibiotics: Ampicillin, azithromycin (Zithromax), ciprofloxacin (Cipro), clarithromycin (Biaxin), griseofulvin (Grisactin), metronidazole (Flagyl), ofloxacin (Floxin), tetracycline, terbinafine (Lamisil)
  - Anticonvulsants: Carbamazepine (Tegretol), phenytoin (Dilantin)
  - Antidepressants: Amitriptyline (Elavil), clomipramine (Anafranil), desipramine (Norpramin), doxepin (Sinequan), imipramine (Tofranil), nortriptyline (Pamelor)
  - Antihistamines and decongestants: Chlorpheniramine, loratadine (Claritin), pseudoephedrine
  - Antihypertensives and cardiac medications: Acetazolamide (Diamox), amiloride (Midamor), betaxolol (Betoptic), captopril (Capoten), diltiazem (Cardizem), enalapril (Vasotec), hydrochlorothiazide (Esidrix) and combinations, nifedipine (Procardia), nitroglycerin, propranolol (Inderal), spironolactone (Aldactone)
  - Anti-inflammatory agents: Auranofin (Ridaura), colchicine, dexamethasone (Decadron), gold (Myochrysine), hydrocortisone, penicillamine (Cuprimine)

- Antimanic drugs: Lithium
- Antineoplastics: Cisplatin (Platinol), doxorubicin (Adriamycin), methotrexate (Rheumatrex), vincristine (Oncovin)
- Antiparkinsonian agents: Levodopa (Larodopa; with carbidopa: Sinemet)
- Antipsychotics: Clozapine (Clozaril), trifluoperazine (Stelazine)
- Antithyroid agents: Methimazole (Tapazole), propylthiouracil
- Lipid-lowering agents: Fluvastatin (Lescol), lovastatin (Mevacor), pravastatin (Pravachol)
- Muscle relaxants: Baclofen (Lioresal), dantrolene (Dantrium)

ALERT

Pregnancy Considerations

Uncommon cause of smell and taste disturbances. Many women report increased sensitivity to odors during pregnancy as well as an increased dislike for bitter and a preference for salty substances.

ASSOCIATED CONDITIONS

Smell and taste disturbances are primarily symptoms; it is essential to look for possible underlying cause.

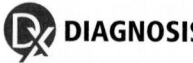 **DIAGNOSIS**

SIGNS AND SYMPTOMS

- Problems with smell and taste
- Weight loss
- Malnutrition
- Impaired immunity
- Worsening of medical illness
- Increased use of sugar and salt to compensate for diminished senses of smell and taste

TESTS

- Olfactory tests
  - Smell identification test: Evaluates the ability to identify 40 microencapsulated "scratch and sniff" odorants
  - 3-item forced-choice microencapsulated Pocket Smell Test
  - Brief smell identification test
  - Squeeze-bottle odor threshold test kit
- Taste tests (more difficult because no convenient standardized tests are presently available)
  - Solutions containing sucrose (sweet), sodium chloride (salty), quinine (bitter), and citric acid (sour) are helpful.
  - Electrogustometry: A portable battery-powered device delivers small currents to different parts of the tongue to obtain threshold and suprathreshold measures.

Lab
- Hematocrit
- Hemoglobin
- WBC count
- BUN
- Blood glucose
- Creatinine
- Bilirubin
- Alkaline phosphatase
- Prothrombin time
- ESR
- Altered thyroid function tests
- Eosinophil count
- IgE

Imaging
- Plain radiographs have substantial limitations (rarely useful).
- CT scanning is the most useful and cost-effective technique for assessing sinonasal disorders and is superior to MRI in evaluating bony structures. Coronal CT scans are particularly valuable in assessing paranasal anatomy.
- MRI is useful in defining soft tissue disease; therefore, it is the technique of choice to image the olfactory bulbs, tracts, and cortical parenchyma.

Diagnostic Procedures/Surgery
- Medical history
- Physical examination

DIFFERENTIAL DIAGNOSIS
- Epilepsy (gustatory aura)
- Epilepsy (olfactory aura)
- Memory impairment
- Psychiatric conditions

ALERT
Geriatric Considerations
Aging is a cause of smell/taste deficits; consider a diagnosis of exclusion.

Pediatric Considerations
Delayed puberty in association with anosmia (with or without midline craniofacial abnormalities, deafness, or renal abnormalities) suggests the possibility of Kallmann syndrome.

TREATMENT

INITIAL STABILIZATION
Outpatient care usually

GENERAL MEASURES
- Appropriate treatment for underlying cause
- Quit smoking.
- Some drug-related dysgeusias can be reversed with cessation of the offending agent.
- Eliminate exposures (e.g., volatile gases, toxins, repeated use of oxygen-liberating mouthwashes).
- Stop repeated oral trauma (e.g., appliances, tongue-biting behaviors).
- Proper nutritional and dietary assessment
- Formal dental evaluation

Diet
- Caution patients not to overindulge as compensation for the bland taste of food. For example, patients with diabetes may need help in avoiding excessive sugar intake as an inappropriate way of improving food taste.
- Patients with chemosensory impairment should use measuring devices when cooking and should not "cook by taste."
- Optimizing food texture, aroma, temperature, and color may improve the overall food experience when taste is limited.

MEDICATION (DRUGS)

- Corticosteroids topically (e.g., aqueous nasal spray) or systemically (e.g., oral prednisone) may be helpful. Prednisone 60 mg/d for 4 days, with the dosage tapered by 10 mg/d thereafter
- Artificial saliva (e.g., Xero-Lube) may be helpful in patients with xerostomia.
- Pilocarpine (Salagen) 5–10 mg PO t.i.d. may help with dry mouth/xerostomia. Response may take 6–12 weeks.
- Chlorhexidine (Peridex) 0.12% oral rinse may help with gingivitis or dysgeusia.
- Zinc and vitamins (A, B complex) when deficiency is suspected

SURGERY
If needed for treatment of underlying cause

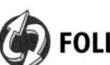

FOLLOW-UP

PROGNOSIS
- In general, the olfactory system regenerates poorly after a head injury. Most patients who recover smell function subsequent to head trauma do so within 12 weeks of injury.
- Patients who quit smoking typically have improved olfactory function and flavor sensation over time.
- Many taste disorders (dysgeusias) resolve spontaneously within a few years of onset.
- Conditions such as radiation-induced xerostomia and Bell palsy generally improve over time.

COMPLICATIONS
Permanent loss of ability to smell or taste

PATIENT MONITORING
Patients with persistent smell and taste complaints may need to be referred to otolaryngologist, neurologist, or subspecialist at a smell and taste center.

REFERENCES
1. Bromley SM. Smell and taste disorders: A primary care approach. *Am Fam Phys*. 2000;61:427–436.
2. Deems DA, et al. Smell and taste disorders, a study of 750 patients from the University of Pennsylvania Smell and Taste Center. *Arch Otolaryngol Head Neck Surg*. 1991;117:519–528.

MISCELLANEOUS

PATIENT TEACHING
- Patients with permanent smell dysfunction must develop adaptive strategies for dealing with hygiene, appetite, safety, and health.
- Check smoke detectors frequently.
- Use electric instead of gas appliances (if anosmic).
- Check food expiration dates frequently; discard old food.

SNAKE ENVENOMATIONS: CROTALIDAE

Alan L. Williams, MD
Pamela M. Williams, MD

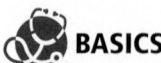 BASICS

DESCRIPTION
- Symptom complex following envenomation by a snake of the family Crotalidae (pit vipers)
- Includes snakes of the genera *Crotalus* (rattlesnakes), *Agkistrodon* (moccasins), and *Sistrurus* (pygmy rattlesnakes)
- Occur most commonly in the southeastern and southwestern US
- North American crotalid characteristics: Triangular-shaped heads, eyes with elliptical pupils, and small heat-sensing facial pits located between the nostril and the eye
  - In contrast, nonpoisonous snakes in the US generally have small round heads and round pupils, except coral snakes, which are brightly colored.
- System(s) Affected: Cardiovascular; Hemic/Lymphatic/Immunologic; Nervous; Skin/Exocrine
- Synonym(s): Snakebite; Venomous snakebite; Pit viper snakebite

GENERAL PREVENTION
- Use preventive measures if handling snakes.
- In snake-infested areas
  - Wear protective shoes and clothing when walking.
  - Do not insert hands or feet into cracks, crevices, or hollow logs.
  - Carry a flashlight if walking at night.

EPIDEMIOLOGY
- Predominant age: 19–30 years
- Predominant sex: Male > Female

Incidence
- ~2,400 reported crotalid snakebites in the US annually accounting for 92% of reported identified snakebites US
  - 2,000 additional reported bites from unknown snakes.
- The actual incidence of envenomation may be higher due to underreporting or lower due to dry bites.

RISK FACTORS
- Risk-taking behaviors
- Acute ethanol intoxication or intoxication with other drugs that impair judgment

PATHOPHYSIOLOGY
Clinical problems related to envenomation include tissue damage, coagulopathy, thrombocytopenia, hypovolemia, and neruotoxicity.

ETIOLOGY
- Pit viper venom is a complex mixture that contains cytotoxins, hemotoxins, neurotoxins, and cardiotoxins.
- Toxin composition varies from bite to bite even with the same snake.
- Envenomation can affect all major organ systems.
- Mojave Rattlesnake venom is more neurotoxic than that of other crotalids, and can cause respiratory depression.

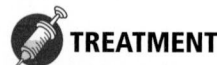 DIAGNOSIS

SIGNS AND SYMPTOMS
- Vary from minor local injury to severe systemic illness
- Fang marks may be 2 or only 1 (>90%)
- Pain out of proportion to puncture wound (usually within minutes of the bite) (>50%)
- Edema of site, progressing proximally up extremity (>50%)
- Weakness, dizziness (>50%)
- Numbness/tingling in extremity, mouth, tongue (>50%)
- Ecchymosis of skin, vesicles around bite (may take hours to develop) (>50%)
- Tachycardia (>50%)
- Nausea/vomiting (<50%)
- Hypo- or hypertension (<50%)
- Muscle fasciculations (<50%)
- Mental status changes, including coma (<25%)
- Change in sensation of taste

History
- Snake identification is helpful, but should not place others at risk for being bitten.
- A digital photo may be a safe means to identify the snake.

TESTS
Lab
- Complete blood count (hemoglobin/hematocrit decreased in <50%) (decrease in platelets <50%)
- Prothrombin time/international normalized ratio, A-PTT (prolonged in >50%)
- Fibrinogen (decreased in <50%), fibrin degradation products (increased in <50%)
- Urinalysis: glycosuria (<50%), proteinuria (<25%), hematuria (<25%)
- Type and cross-match "to hold" in severe envenomations
- Electrolytes, BUN, creatinine
- Liver function tests
- Creatine kinase in severe envenomations
- Serum ethanol level if suspicious
- Disorders that may alter lab results
  - Preexisting anemia or polycythemia
  - Advanced liver disease
  - Kidney disease
  - Platelet disorders
- Drugs that may alter lab results
  - Anticoagulants

DIFFERENTIAL DIAGNOSIS
- Bite of nonvenomous snake
- Bite of venomous species other than those of Crotalidae family

TREATMENT

PRE HOSPITAL
- Patients with true envenomations need emergency department evaluation.
- Rapid transportation should take priority over all but the most basic first aid.
  - Most field snakebite treatments (cutting the bite, attempting to remove poison with suction, and constriction bandages) have been shown to be ineffective and potentially harmful.
- Reassure patient, minimize patient movement during transport
- Splint area of bite allowing room for swelling.
  - Position affected extremity at or below level of heart.

INITIAL STABILIZATION
- Support vital signs, place on monitor, O_2 as needed, obtain IV access
- Reassurance
- Remove rings and constrictive items.

GENERAL MEASURES
- Evaluate all prehospital care. Use of tourniquet and pressure dressings are controversial. If tourniquet has been placed in prehospital setting, sudden removal could bolus patient with venom. The tourniquet or constriction band should be removed only after beginning treatment with antivenom.
- Obtain toxicology consultation by contacting American Association of Poison Control Centers (AAPCC) Regional Poison Information Center.
- Level 1
  - If local signs of edema are confined to area of bite, without any other symptom of envenomation, place IV line of crystalloid at maintenance rates and draw baseline laboratory studies.
  - Place reference marks for measuring circumference of extremity at 10 cm and 20 cm proximal to site of envenomation.
    - Measure every 15 minutes and trace leading edge of swelling.
  - Give tetanus toxoid if needed.
  - Provide pain relief.
  - Repeat laboratory studies in 6 hours. If all remain normal and swelling does not progress, observe 8–12 hours then follow up as outpatient.
  - If swelling progresses or systemic signs and symptoms appear, patient needs admission and further therapy (progresses to Level 2).
- Level 2
  - If edema, vesicles, erythema progress beyond the immediate bite area or there are associated systemic signs/symptoms or laboratory abnormalities, give IV antivenom plus all Level 1 management.
  - Intensive care monitoring may be necessary.
  - Repeat laboratory evaluations q6h initially until stable, then less frequently.
  - Blood products are necessary only for coagulopathies with clinical bleeding, not for treatment of laboratory abnormalities.
    - Antivenom treatment may reverse hematologic abnormalities and should be given 1st.
  - Have equipment and medications readily at hand to treat allergic reactions to antivenom.

Diet
Nothing by mouth initially

Activity
Bed rest, with extremity elevated

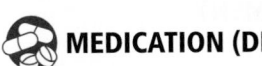 **MEDICATION (DRUGS)**

First Line

- Crotalidae polyvalent immune Fab (Ovine) (1)[B]
  - No skin test necessary
  - Initial dose: 5 reconstituted vials added to normal saline to make total volume of 250 mL
    - 10 mL of sterile water added to each vial. Swirl only (do not shake), so as to not denature proteins.
    - Infuse IV slowly for the 1st 10 minutes, then increase rate to 250 mL/h to run remainder over 60 minutes.
    - After 1st infusion is complete, if all signs/symptoms of envenomation have not ceased, give up to two more doses of 4–6 vials until initial control is achieved.
  - Maintenance: After initial control of symptoms, administer 3 maintenance doses of 2 vials at 6, 12, and 18 hours following time of initial control.

- Precautions: Papain is used in the manufacturing process of Crotalidae polyvalent immune Fab; patients with papaya allergies may be at risk for allergic reaction.
- Adverse reactions: Anaphylaxis, serum sickness

Second Line
Pain relief with opiate (e.g., morphine sulfate 0.1–0.2 mg/kg per dose q2–6h as needed) or acetaminophen (10–15 mg/kg per dose q4–6h as needed; maximum 4 g/d in adults)

ALERT
Avoid aspirin and other anticoagulants.

SURGERY
- Fasciotomy is rarely needed in snake envenomations.
- Envenomation may mimic compartment syndrome, making clinical distinction difficult.
- Decision to perform a fasciotomy should be based on measured compartmental pressures.

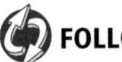 **FOLLOW-UP**

DISPOSITION
Admission Criteria
- Dry bites may be observed for 8–12 hours and the patient discharged if there is no evidence of envenomation.
- Anyone receiving antivenom should be admitted, likely to the ICU.

PROGNOSIS
Mortality: <0.1% in reported bites

ALERT
Geriatric Considerations
- Course may be more severe.
- Consider EKG, CXR, ABG if underlying conditions may be exacerbated by stress of envenomation.

Pediatric Considerations
- Course may be more severe.
- CroFab dosing is the same as for adults. (2)[C]

Pregnancy Considerations
- Limited data, but there have been reports of miscarriage following snakebite
- Treatment that optimizes maternal health is presumed to be the best available treatment for the fetus.
- There are no studies of CroFab in pregnant women.

COMPLICATIONS
- Local wound infection (rare)
- Bleeding after discharge from hospital
  - Patients should be told to report nosebleeds, excessive bleeding after brushing teeth, blood in stools or vomitus, or excessive menstrual bleeding.

PATIENT MONITORING
- Phone follow up in 12–24 hours for discharged dry bites.
- 1st return visit within 48 hours after hospital discharge, then as clinically indicated
- Physical therapy referral should be made early for optimal outpatient intervention.

REFERENCES

1. Dart RC, et al. A randomized multicenter trial of crotalinae polyvalent immune Fab (ovine) antivenom for the treatment for crotaline snakebite in the United States. *Ann Emerg Med*. 2001;161:2030–2036.
2. Schmidt JM. Antivenom therapy for snakebites in children: Is there evidence? *Curr Opin Pediatr*. 2005;17:234–238.
3. Gold BS, Barish RA, Dart RC. North American snake envenomation: Diagnosis, treatment, and management. *Emerg Med Clin North Am*. 2004;22:423–443.

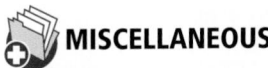 **MISCELLANEOUS**

See also: Snake envenomations: elapidae

CODES

ICD9-CM
989.5 Bites of venomous snakes, lizards, and spiders

PATIENT TEACHING
- Snake bite prevention and first aid
- Avoid elective surgery, dental work, contact sports, and anticoagulant medications (including aspirin) after discharge.

SNAKE ENVENOMATIONS: ELAPIDAE (CORAL SNAKE)

Alan L. Williams, MD
Pamela M. Williams, MD

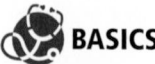 **BASICS**

DESCRIPTION
- Symptom complex following envenomation by a snake of the family Elapidae
  - Local signs and symptoms are mild in envenomation of Elapidae, even those that prove to be severe envenomations.
  - Neurologic symptoms may be delayed; they have been reported to develop up to 12 or more hours after the envenomation.
- In the US, these snakes include the genera *Micrurus* and *Micruroides*, commonly called "coral snakes."
  - The Sonoran or Arizona coral snake is found mainly in Arizona (*Micruroides euryxanthus*)
  - Texas coral snake (*Micrurus fulvius tenere*) in Texas, Arkansas, and Louisiana
  - Eastern coral snake (*Micrurus fulvius fulvius*) throughout the southeast.
- Coral snakes have a characteristic rounded head with round pupils.

ALERT
- Coloration is important: North American coral snakes have broad rings of red and black separated by narrow rings of yellow.
  - In contrast, milk snakes are nonpoisonous snakes with similar coloration. The areas of orange/red and yellow/white are separated by bands of black.
- "Red on yellow, kill a fellow; red on black, friend of Jack."
- System(s) Affected: Nervous; Skin/Exocrine
- Synonym(s): Neurotoxic snakebite; Snakebite

GENERAL PREVENTION
- Use preventive measures if handling snakes.
- In snake-infested areas
  - Wear protective shoes and clothing when walking.
  - Do not insert hands or feet into cracks, crevices, or hollow logs.
  - Carry a flashlight if walking at night.

EPIDEMIOLOGY
- Predominant age: 19–30 years
- Predominant sex: Male > Female

Incidence
- Coral snake bites comprise ~4% of identified snakebites reported to American Association of Poision Control Centers (AAPCC).
- <100 reported each year in the US

RISK FACTORS
Coral snakes are nocturnal and timid; therefore, they rarely bite humans. They must be deliberately provoked to bite.

ETIOLOGY
Venom is primarily a neurotoxin; little or no cytotoxin to cause local tissue reaction

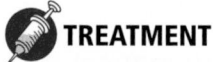 **DIAGNOSIS**

SIGNS AND SYMPTOMS
- Fang marks; may be shallow or appear as scratch (>75%)
- Onset of symptoms following envenomation may be delayed 10–12 hours.
  - Local swelling (<50%)
  - Numbness/change in sensation (<50%)
  - Nausea/vomiting (<50%)
  - Weakness (<25%)
  - Dizziness (<15%)
  - Diplopia (<15%)
  - Muscle fasciculations (<15%)
  - Dysarthia
  - Dysphagia with increased salivation

History
- Snake identification is helpful, but should not place others at risk for being bitten.
- A digital photo may be a safe means to identify the snake.
- Determine previous snakebite history, any allergy to horse serum.

TESTS
- Baseline and serial pulmonary function with special attention to peak flow and vital capacity as well as oxygen saturation may help in early recognition of decreasing ventilatory function.
- Skin test for horse serum sensitivity

Lab
- Creatine phosphokinase often elevated
- Consider blood ethanol level.

DIFFERENTIAL DIAGNOSIS
- Bite of other venomous snake (Crotalidae) without envenomation ("dry bite")
- Bite of a nonvenomous snake

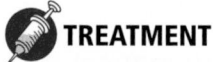 **TREATMENT**

PRE HOSPITAL
- Pressure/immobilization of the affected limb is under study, but currently there are insufficient data to determine its efficacy.
- Transportation of a calm and still patient to a treatment facility is the primary goal.
- Administer O_2.
- Obtain IV access.

INITIAL STABILIZATION
ABCs, O_2, monitored bed

GENERAL MEASURES
- All patients with any of the following should be admitted to hospital for intensive care monitoring
  - Confirmed bite by a snake identified as a coral snake
  - History of the snake having chewed on the person
- Perform a skin test for horse serum sensitivity.
  - If negative, give antivenin to *Micrurus fulvius fulvius* early, even when there are no neurologic signs or symptoms.
  - If skin test is positive, contact the AAPCC to help coordinate care with experienced consultants.
- Give tetanus toxoid if needed.
- Support vital signs; intubation may be necessary if respiratory compromise ensues.
- Good supportive care with cardiac, respiratory, neurologic monitoring
- Reassurance
- Immobilize extremity and keep at level of heart.
- Contact the AAPCC Regional Center for your area.

Diet
NPO initially

Activity
Bed rest initially. May need physical therapy in severe cases of envenomation

MEDICATION (DRUGS)

First Line
- No antivenin is available for *Micruroides euryxanthus*.
- Antivenin to the North American coral snake (*Micrurus fulvius fulvius* antivenin) (1)[C]
  - Horse serum product effective only for the envenomation of the Texas and eastern coral snakes (*Micrurus fulvius tenere* and *Micrurus fulvius fulvius*)
  - Perform skin testing 1st.
  - Initial dose: 4–6 reconstituted vials added to 250 mL of normal saline
    - Begin infusion at 3–5 mL/h; if no systemic reaction occurs, increase until a rate of 1 diluted vial is being given every 30 minutes.
    - Because of the low numbers of patients treated with antivenin, an exact dosing schedule has not been determined.
  - If a patient has been treated with antivenin and starts to develop neurologic symptoms, an additional 10–15 vials may be necessary. (2)[C]
  - If skin test is positive, the literature is not clear regarding specific recommendations; however, pretreatment with diphenhydramine (Benadryl; 1 mg/kg per dose q6h IV; adults 25–50 mg IV), steroids (e.g., methylprednisolone [Solu-Medrol] 1–2 mg/kg per dose q8h IV), and other antihistamines (e.g., cimetidine 10 mg/kg per dose IV; adults 300 mg IV) may allow for infusion of antivenin. In this instance, obtain toxicology consultation from the AAPCC-certified Poison Information Center for your area.
- Contraindication: History of allergy to horse serum
- Precautions: Have equipment and medications readily at hand to treat anaphylaxis.
- Adverse reactions: Anaphylaxis, serum sickness

ALERT
Avoid sedatives and opioids, which may compound any respiratory compromise. (2)[C]

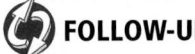 **FOLLOW-UP**

DISPOSITION
Admission Criteria
All suspect coral snake bites warrant admission for observation and treatment.

Discharge Criteria
- Discharge should not occur until the patient has made neurologic recovery to the point at which there is no concern of respiratory failure.
- Asymptomatic patients admitted for observation may be discharged after 24–48 hours.

PROGNOSIS
- Neurologic deterioration may progress despite antivenin administration. Complete paralysis may occur.
- Early, elective intubation during progression of paralysis may help to prevent aspiration pneumonia.
- Neurologic symptoms can last 3–6 days despite treatment with antivenin.
- Muscle strength may not return to normal for 4–6 weeks.
- Long-term morbidity is rare.
- Mortality does occur even with antivenin therapy.

ALERT
Pregnancy Considerations
- Limited data, but there have been reports of miscarriage following snakebite
- Treatment that optimizes maternal health is presumed to be the best available treatment for the fetus.

COMPLICATIONS
- Local wound infection
- Aspiration pneumonia

PATIENT MONITORING
First return visit within 48 hours, then as clinically indicated

REFERENCES
1. Kitchens CS, Van Mierop LHS. Envenomation by the eastern coral snake (*Micrurus fulvius fulvius*). *JAMA*. 1987;258:1615–1618.
2. Gold BS, Barish RA, Dart RC. North American snake envenomation: Diagnosis, treatment, and management. *Emerg Med Clin North Am*. 2004;22:423–443.

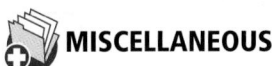 **MISCELLANEOUS**

See also: Snake envenomations: crotalidae

CODES

ICD9-CM
989.5 Bites of venomous snakes, lizards, and spiders

S

SOMATIZATION DISORDER

Laurie A. Carrier, MD

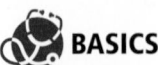 **BASICS**

DESCRIPTION

- A pattern of recurring, multiple, clinically significant somatic complaints beginning <30 years of age that occur over a period of several years and result in treatment being sought or significant impairment in social, occupational, or other important areas of functioning.
- Each of the following criteria must be met, with individual symptoms occurring at any time during the course of the disturbance
  - 4 pain symptoms: Different sites or functions
  - 2 gastrointestinal symptoms: Other than pain
  - 1 sexual symptom
  - 1 pseudoneurological symptom
- The above symptoms are not intentionally produced or feigned.
- Chronic course, fluctuating in severity
- Affected individual rarely goes 1 year without seeking medical attention prompted by unexplained somatic complaints
- System(s) Affected: Multiple
- Synonym(s): Briquet syndrome

EPIDEMIOLOGY

- Predominant age: Usually, the 1st symptoms appear in adolescence and the full criteria are met by 30 years of age
- Predominant sex: Female > Male (10:1)
  - 10× more common in women than in men
- The type and frequency of somatic complaints may differ among cultures, so symptom reviews should be adjusted by culture.

Prevalence

- Ranges from 0.2–2% among women and <0.2% in men
- 1 in 500 adults in the US
- 544,000 people affected in the US

RISK FACTORS

- Child abuse, particularly sexual abuse, has been shown to be a risk factor.
- Symptoms begin or worsen after losses (for example, job, close relative, or friend).
- Greater intensity of symptoms often occurs with stress.

Genetics

- Observed in 10–20% of female 1st-degree biological relatives of women with Somatization Disorder (SD)
- Male relatives of woman with this disorder show an increased risk of Antisocial Personality Disorder and substance-related disorders.

ETIOLOGY

- The exact cause of this disorder is unknown.
- Adoption studies indicate that both genetic and environmental factors contribute to the risk of SD.

ASSOCIATED CONDITIONS

- Comorbid with other psychiatric conditions, including major depression (55% of patients), anxiety disorders (34%), personality disorders (61%), and panic disorders (26%)

DIAGNOSIS

SIGNS AND SYMPTOMS

- Pain symptoms (4 or more) related to different sites, such as head, abdomen, back, joints, extremities, chest, or rectum, or related to body functions such as menstruation, sexual intercourse, or urination
- Gastrointestinal symptoms (2 or more, excluding pain) such as nausea, bloating, vomiting (not during pregnancy), diarrhea, intolerance of several foods
- Sexual symptoms (at least 1, excluding pain) including indifference to sex, difficulties with erection or ejaculation, irregular menses, excessive menstrual bleeding, or vomiting throughout all 9 months of pregnancy
- Pseudoneurological symptoms (at least 1) including impaired balance or coordination, weak or paralyzed muscles, lump in throat or trouble swallowing, loss of voice, retention of urine, hallucinations, numbness (to touch or pain), double vision, blindness, deafness, seizures, amnesia or other dissociative symptoms, loss of consciousness (other than with fainting). None of these are limited to pain.

History

- Multiple somatic complaints including pain symptoms, gastrointestinal symptoms, a sexual symptom, and neurological symptoms
- Patients usually have a grossly positive review of symptoms.

Physical Exam

Remarkable for absence of objective findings to fully explain the many subjective complaints

TESTS

Several screening tools are available which help to identify symptoms as somatic.

- PHQ-15 (screens and monitors symptoms) (1)[C]
- MMPI (identifies somatization) (2)[C]
- Perley-Guze Checklist (helps the physician identify SD)

Lab

Laboratory test results do not support the subjective complaints.

Imaging

Imaging studies do not support the subjective complaints.

Pathological Findings

None are identified.

DIFFERENTIAL DIAGNOSIS

- Other psychiatric illnesses must be ruled out
  - Depressive disorders
  - Anxiety disorders
  - Schizophrenia
  - Other somatoform disorders: Conversion disorder, Factitious disorders, Hypochondriasis, Pain disorder
- General medical conditions, with vague, multiple, confusing symptoms, must be ruled out
  - Systemic Lupus Erythematosus
  - Hyperpartathyroidism
  - Hyper- or Hypothyroidism
  - Lyme disease
  - Porphyria

TREATMENT

GENERAL MEASURES

- The goal of treatment is to help the person learn to control the symptoms.
- A supportive relationship with a sympathetic health care provider is the most important aspect of treatment. (3)[C]
  - Regularly scheduled appointments should be maintained to review symptoms and the person's coping mechanisms (at least 15 minutes once a month). (3)[C]
  - Acknowledgment and explanation of test results should occur.
- The involvement of a single physician is important, as a history of seeking medical attention and "doctor shopping" is common.
- Antidepressant or antianxiety medication and referral to a support group or psychiatrist can help patients who are willing to participate in their treatment.
- Patients usually receive the most benefit from primary care physicians who accept the limitations of treatment, listen to their patient's concerns, and provide reassurance.
- It is not helpful to tell patients that their symptoms are imaginary.

SPECIAL THERAPY

Treatment typically includes long-term therapy which has been shown to decrease the severity of symptoms.

- Cognitive behavioral therapy has been shown to be the most efficacious treatment in SD. (4–6)[C]
- Psychotherapy
- Supportive therapy

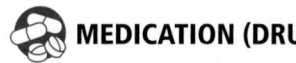 MEDICATION (DRUGS)

Antidepressants (e.g., SSRIs) help in some cases.

 FOLLOW-UP

Patients should have regularly scheduled follow-up with a primary care doctor, psychiatrist, or therapist.

Issues for Referral

- Referrals to specialist for further investigation of somatic complaints should be discouraged.
- Referrals to support groups or to a psychiatrist may be helpful.

PROGNOSIS

- Chronic course, fluctuating in severity
- Full remission is rare.
- Individuals with this disorder do not experience any significant difference in mortality rate or significant illness.

COMPLICATIONS

- May result from invasive testing and from multiple evaluations that are performed while looking for the cause of the symptoms
- A dependency on pain relievers or sedatives may develop.

REFERENCES

1. Kroenke K, Spitzer R, Williams J. The PHQ-15: Validity of a new measure for evaluating the severity of somatic symptoms. *Psychosom Med*. 2002;64:258–266.
2. Wetzel RD, et al. MMPI screening scales for Somatization Disorder. *Psychol Rep*. 1999; 85(1):341–348.
3. Servan-Schreiber NR, Tabas G, Kolb D. Somatizing patients: Part II. Practical management. *Am Fam Physician*. 2000;61(5):1423–1430.
4. Kroenke K, Swindle R. Cognitive-Behavioral therapy for somatization and symptom syndromes: A critical review of controlled clinical trials. *Psychother Psychosom*. 2000;69:205.
5. Mai F. Somatization disorder: A practical review. *Can J Psychiatry*. 2004;49:652–662.
6. Speckens AE, van Hemert AM, Spinhoven P, Hawton KE, Bolk JH, Rooijmans HG. Cognitive behavioural therapy for medically unexplained physical symptoms: A randomised controlled trial. *BMJ*. 1995;311:1328–1332.
7. American Psychiatric Association. *Diagnostic and Statistical Manual of Mental Disorders*. 4th ed. Text revision. Washington, DC: American Psychiatric Association, 2000.

 MISCELLANEOUS

See also: Somatoform disorders

CODES

ICD9-CM
300.81 Somatization Disorder

S

PATIENT TEACHING

Activity

Interventions that decrease stressful elements of the patient's life should be encouraged.

- Psychoeducational advice
- Increase in exercise
- Pleasurable private time

SPINAL STENOSIS

Dhruv B. Pateder, MD
Donald S. Corenman, MD, DC

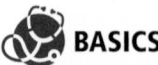 **BASICS**

DESCRIPTION

Spinal stenosis is a condition in which a narrowing of the spinal canal and foramen occurs. Although myriad of etiologies exist, in the most generic sense, it refers to compression of the lumbar spinal elements secondary to arthritic changes (bone spurs, hypertrophied ligamentum flavum, disc space narrowing). This condition generally causes back/buttock pain with possible radiation in the lower extremities if foraminal stenosis also is present.

GENERAL PREVENTION

There is no known way to prevent spinal stenosis but symptoms can be alleviated by any means that "open up" the spinal canal and foramen, such as leaning forward when walking.

EPIDEMIOLOGY

The prevalence of spinal stenosis increases with age, because it is essentially an arthritic condition from "wear and tear" on the normal spine.
- Symptoms develop in 5th and 6th decades
- No sex predominance
- Degenerative spondylolisthesis with spinal stenosis is 4 times more common in women.

Incidence

The incidence of symptomatic spinal stenosis is as high as 8% of the population.

Prevalence

The prevalence increases with age and can be as high as 100% on assessment by radiographic studies on elderly patients; however, it is important to remember that not all patients with radiographic spinal stenosis are symptomatic.

RISK FACTORS

Increasing age and spinal arthritis

Genetics

No definitive genetic links

PATHOPHYSIOLOGY

Disc dehydration leads to loss of height with bulging of annulus and ligamentum flavum into the spinal canal, thus increasing joint loading of facets. This leads to reactive sclerosis and osteophytic bone growth, leading to further compression of neural elements in the spinal canal and the foramen.

ETIOLOGY

- Congenital
- Chondrodystrophy
- Idiopathic
- Acquired
- Degenerative
- Spondylolytic
- Iatrogenic
- Posttraumatic
- Tumorous (primary or metastatic)

ASSOCIATED CONDITIONS

Spinal stenosis can be associated with a congenitally narrowed spinal canal and osteoarthritic changes of the lumbar spine.

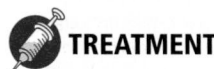 **DIAGNOSIS**

SIGNS AND SYMPTOMS

- Longstanding back pain that progresses to buttock and lower extremity pain
- Neurogenic claudication (pain, tightness, numbness, and subjective weakness of lower extremities)
- Symptoms worsen with standing, walking, back extension
- Symptoms improve with sitting or leaning forward

History

- Insidious onset
- Progresses slowly
- Symptoms worse when walking "uphill" and improve with leaning forward ("while pushing cart in grocery store")

Physical Exam

There maybe few physical findings even in effected patients
- Gait alteration (rule out cervical myelopathy or intracranial pathology)
- Loss of lumbar lordosis
- Decreased ROM of lumbar spine
- Pain with extension of the lumbar spine
- Straight-leg-raise test maybe positive if nerve root entrapment is present.
- Muscle weakness most commonly present in L5 distribution

TESTS

Spinal stenosis is generally diagnosed with a combination of history, physical examination, and imaging studies (MRI is best).

Lab

CBC, ESR, CRP if infection or cancer are in differential

Imaging

- AP and lateral radiographs of spine show degenerative changes or spondylolisthesis and rule out fractures, infection, or tumor; flexion/extension views help evaluate instability
- MRI will demonstrate compression of neural elements
- CT myelography is comparable to MRI in demonstrating neural compression but is an invasive procedure (dye injection associated with post spinal headache)

Diagnostic Procedures/Surgery

Selective injections can be used to localize source of pain in patients with multiple sites of neural compression and unclear findings. Surgical decompression is the only definitive treatment in patients who continue to be symptomatic after nonoperative treatment

Pathological Findings

- Decreased disc height
- Facet hypertrophy
- Spinal canal and/or foraminal narrowing
- Possible intervertebral instability

DIFFERENTIAL DIAGNOSIS

- Vascular claudication can also cause calf pain after ambulation; however, no back/buttock pain is present in vascular claudication. Also, the symptoms of vascular claudication do not improve with leaning forward.
- Disc herniation
- Cervical myelopathy
- Spinal stenosis in thoracic spine

TREATMENT

No good, randomized, controlled studies have examined operative versus nonoperative treatment for spinal stenosis. The general protocol among spinal surgeons is to treat spinal stenosis nonoperatively unless the symptoms impede patient's life. Decompressive surgery is quite successful in alleviating symptoms of spinal stenosis; there is controversy whether a fusion should be performed along with the decompression, because of risk of future spondylolisthesis.

PRE HOSPITAL

Spinal stenosis generally does not lead to neurologic damage. Surgery is essentially for pain relief, allowing patients to become more mobile, thus improving overall health.

INITIAL STABILIZATION

- Brace or corset may help for short time but not recommended long-term, because it leads to paraspinal muscle weakness.
- Patient should be encouraged to continue to be active despite pain to prevent deconditioning.
- Weight loss

Diet

If undergoing surgery, optimize nutritional status.

Activity

As tolerated, as long as no other pathology is present (e.g., fractures, gross instability, etc.)

SPECIAL THERAPY

Aquatic therapy is generally helpful for muscle and general conditioning.

Physical Therapy

- General conditioning (these patients are able to ride an exercise bicycle without many problems, because they can lean forward and relieve symptoms).
- Aquatic therapy
- Back extensor muscle strengthening
- Abdominal muscle strengthening
- Gait training

MEDICATION (DRUGS)

No role for maintenance opiates

First Line
- Anti-inflammatory medications (unless GI side-effects)
- Enteric coated aspirin (less GI side-effects)
- Acetaminophen

Second Line
- COX-2 inhibitors (be aware of changing side-effect profile)
- Lumbar epidural steroids

SURGERY
- Indicated when patient fails nonoperative treatment and cannot attain a tolerable quality of life. Preoperative clearance by an internist, cardiologist and/or anesthesiologist is necessary.
- Decompression of neural elements is mainstay of treatment. This generally entails a laminectomy, but foraminotomies and discectomy should also be performed if they are involved in neural compression.
- X STOP is a new device that is lodged between spinous process and indirectly decompresses the spinal canal with minimal surgery; significantly better outcomes compared to nonoperative treatment.
- Fusion is necessary when instability is present or an extensive decompression (with disruption of the pars interarticularis and/or >50% or articular facets) results in instability.
- Instrumentation with pedicle screws is commonly used to achieve fusion.

 ## FOLLOW-UP

Routine follow-up is at 6 weeks, 3 months, 6 months, 1 year, 2 years, then every 2 years.

DISPOSITION
Admission Criteria
Unremitting pain that prevents the ability to perform activities of daily living or acute or progressive neurologic deficit.

Discharge Criteria
Improved pain or after neurologic deficit has been addressed (usually via surgical decompression)

Issues for Referral
Refer to a spine surgeon when patients are unwilling to live with the pain, have a worsening spinal deformity, or have a neurologic deficit (rare in arthritic spinal stenosis).

PROGNOSIS
- Spinal stenosis generally worsens with time.
- Surgery is successful in improving pain and symptoms in patients who fail nonoperative treatment.

COMPLICATIONS
- Severe spinal stenosis can lead to bowel and/or bladder dysfunction.
- Surgical complications include infection, neurologic injury, pseudarthrosis, chronic pain, and disability.

PATIENT MONITORING
Patients are monitored for improvement of symptoms, fusion (if one was performed), and development of any complications after nonoperative or operative care.

REFERENCES

1. Noponen-Hietala N, Kyllonen E, Mannikko M, et al. Sequence variations in the collagen IX and XI genes are associated with degenerative lumbar spinal stenosis. *Ann Rheum Dis*. 2003;62(12):208–214.
2. Hilibrand AS, Rand N. Degenerative lumbar stenosis: Diagnosis and management. *J Am Acad Orthop Surg*. 1999;7(4):239–249.
3. Amundsen T, Wever H, Lilleas F, et al. Lumbar spinal stenosis: Clinical and radiologic stenosis. *Spine*. 1995;20:1178–1186.
4. Zucherman JF, Hsu KY, Hartjen CA, et al. A multicenter, prospective, randomized trial evaluating the X STOP interspinous process decompression system for the treatment of neurogenic intermittent claudication: Two-year follow-up results. *Spine*. 2005;30(12):1351–1358.
5. Yuan HA, Garfin SR, Dickman CA, et al. A historical cohort study of pedicle screw fixation in thoracic, lumbar and sacral spinal fusions. *Spine*. 1994;19(Suppl 20):2279S–2296S.

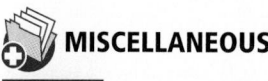 ## MISCELLANEOUS

CODES
ICD9-CM
- 723.00 Cervical spinal stenosis
- 724.00 Spinal stenosis
- 724.02 Lumbar spinal stenosis

PATIENT TEACHING
- Patients should be alerted to possibility of progressive motor weakness and bladder/bowel dysfunction.
- Patients should be educated about the natural history of the condition.

Diet
A generally healthy diet

Activity
No limitations to activity; patients may be as active as tolerated. Exercise should be encouraged.

Prevention
Avoid provocative maneuvers that can cause pain (e.g., back extension, ambulating long distances without resting).

 See Corresponding Diagnostic Algorithm

SPOROTRICHOSIS

Linda J. Machado, MD
Ronald A. Greenfield, MD

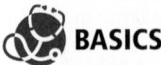 **BASICS**

DESCRIPTION
- Subacute or chronic fungal infection
- Occurs in the following forms
  - Cutaneous or lymphocutaneous
  - Pulmonary
  - Osteoarticular
  - Disseminated
- Most likely to occur in farmers, horticulturists, and gardeners
- System(s) Affected: Hemic/Lymphatic/Immunologic; Musculoskeletal; Skin/Exocrine
- Synonym(s): Schenck disease; Rose gardener disease

GENERAL PREVENTION
- Avoid areas where sporotrichosis is endemic.
- Wear gloves when working in soil.

EPIDEMIOLOGY
- Predominant age: Adults
- Predominant sex: Male > Female (mostly as a result of occupational exposure)

ALERT
Pediatric Considerations
Rare

Incidence
<1:100,000 person/year

RISK FACTORS
- Gardening: Contact with mulch, sphagnum moss, hay, timber, or thorny bushes
- Occupations involving the handling of gardening materials: Nursery workers, landscapers, florists, carpenters
- Animal handlers (transmission from animals, especially cats, to humans has been documented)
- Immunocompromised patient (e.g., because of drugs or HIV infection)
- Alcoholism (factor for pulmonary and disseminated forms)
- HIV/AIDS patients are at increased risk for disseminated disease involving the CNS.

Genetics
No known genetic pattern

PATHOPHYSIOLOGY
- Lymphocutaneous
- Primary lesion forms 1–10+ weeks following direct inoculation and spreads along lymphatic channels.
- Osteoarticular
- Results from direct extension of a cutaneous lesion or dissemination
- Pulmonary
- Pathogenesis unclear, likely inhalation or dissemination
- Disseminated disease results from hematogenous spread

ETIOLOGY
Infection with *Sporothrix schenckii*, a fungus found in soil, sphagnum peat moss, and decaying vegetation

ASSOCIATED CONDITIONS
See "Risk Factors".

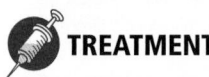 **DIAGNOSIS**

SIGNS AND SYMPTOMS
- Cutaneous or lymphocutaneous
  - Characteristic skin lesions beginning as an inoculation chancre, or erythematous plaque with satellite, small papule, painless, movable, subcutaneous nodules in a linear distribution. Lesions progress to larger nodules, which may ulcerate and drain. Affects primarily upper extremities.
  - Additional lesions spread proximally along lymphatics.
- Pulmonary
  - Cough, occasionally productive
  - Rare hemoptysis
  - Cavitary lung disease
  - Hilar adenopathy
  - Signs and symptoms indistinguishable from other chronic pneumonias
- Osteoarticular
  - Subacute or chronic inflammatory arthritis, often monoarticular; may persist for many years
  - Signs and symptoms of osteomyelitis
  - Generally afebrile
- Disseminated
  - Multifocal skin lesions
  - Polyarticular arthritis
  - Weight loss
  - Chronic lymphocytic meningitis

History
Skin trauma–associated involving contact with plants or plant products. Animal-to-human transmission documented (dogs, cats, horses, squirrels, pigs, and insects) (2)

Physical Exam
See "Signs and Symptoms".

TESTS
Immunohistochemical staining of biopsy specimens

Lab
- Culture of *S. schenckii* in sputum, pus, synovial fluid, or bone drainage
- Organism found with difficulty with periodic acid–Schiff and Gomori stains of skin or other biopsied lesions
- Drugs that may alter lab results: Antifungal drugs

Imaging
Chest and skeletal x-rays

Diagnostic Procedures/Surgery
- Careful history and physical examination
- Culture of draining lesions
- Culture of inflammatory joint effusions or sputum
- Biopsy if diagnosis not confirmed

Pathological Findings
Granulomas with central necrosis

DIFFERENTIAL DIAGNOSIS
- Cutaneous or lymphocutaneous (2)
  - Sporotrichoid nocardiosis
  - Leishmaniasis
  - Chromomycosis
  - Atypical mycobacterial infection (*Mycobacterium marinum*, *M. chelonae*, *M. kansasii*)
  - Tularemia
  - Plague
- Pulmonary
  - Tuberculosis
  - Sarcoidosis
  - Chronic fungal pneumonia
  - Neoplasm
  - Atypical mycobacterial infection (*M. avium complex*, *M. kansasii*)
  - *Rhodococcus equi* infection
  - *Nocardia* spp. infections
- Osteoarticular
  - Rheumatoid arthritis
  - Bacterial arthritis/osteomyelitis

TREATMENT

INITIAL STABILIZATION
- Many patients can be managed on an outpatient basis.
- Hospitalization for adjunctive surgical procedures or initiation of amphotericin B therapy

GENERAL MEASURES
- Local heat application is useful for cutaneous and lymphocutaneous disease.
- Keep cutaneous lesions clean.
- Repeated drainage of infected joints may be indicated.

Diet
No special diet

Activity
No restrictions

MEDICATION (DRUGS)

First Line

- Cutaneous or lymphocutaneous disease

  – Itraconazole 100–200 mg/d for 3–6 months (3)[A]
  – Fluconazole 400 mg/d for 6 months (3)[B]
  – Potassium iodide saturated solution (SSKI) is an alternative treatment. Initially, 5 drops orally t.i.d., increased by 1 drop each dose to 40–50 drops t.i.d. as tolerated for 3–6 months. (3)[B] Dilute in a beverage to disguise taste.

- Pulmonary

  – Amphotericin B for extensive or life-threatening disease (0.5 mg/kg/d up to 1–2 g total dose) (3)[B]
  – Itraconazole 200 mg b.i.d. for non–life-threatening disease (3)[B]
  – Surgical resection combined with antifungals when feasible (3)[B]
- Osteoarticular: Itraconazole 200 mg b.i.d. for 12 months (3)[A]
- Fluconazole 800 mg/d for 12 months (3)[B]
- Meningeal and disseminated: Amphotericin B, total dose, 1–2 g (3)[A]

- AIDS: Amphotericin B until clinical improvement, (3)[B] then itraconazole 200 mg b.i.d (3)[C]

- Pregnancy: Local hyperthermia for lymphocutaneous infection (3)[B]; amphotericin B for serious infection (3)[A]

- SSKI is contraindicated in tuberculosis.
- Precautions
  – Amphotericin B may cause fever, chills, nausea, and vomiting. Refer to manufacturer's literature for precautions, adverse effects, and interactions.
  – SSKI requires extra care if patient also has tuberculosis, kidney disease, renal dysfunction, or hyperthyroidism. May cause folliculitis and tender, swollen salivary glands
  – Itraconazole capsule absorption may be decreased with concomitant administration of antacids or gastric acid secretion suppressors.
- Significant possible interactions
  – SSKI taken concurrently with amiloride, spironolactone, or triamterene may result in hyperkalemia.
  – Itraconazole taken with terfenadine or astemizole may result in life-threatening cardiac dysrhythmias.

Second Line

Terbinafine, though not approved for treatment of sporotrichosis, may be a reasonable alternative to itraconazole for lymphocutaneous disease. (3)[C],(4)

SURGERY

- Synovectomy of infected joints may be indicated.
- Surgical débridement of osteomyelitis is usually indicated.

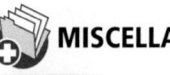 **FOLLOW-UP**

DISPOSITION

Issues for Referral

Infectious diseases consultation suggested for optimal management

PROGNOSIS

- Excellent for complete recovery from cutaneous or lymphocutaneous infections
- Other disease forms demonstrate a chronic indolent course and are variably responsive to therapy.
- AIDS patients often have a poor outcome.

COMPLICATIONS

- Secondary bacterial infection
- Bone and joint deformities from osteoarticular disease
- Rare ocular disease due to direct inoculation

PATIENT MONITORING

- Check for compliance with long-term drug therapy (SSKI should be continued for 1–2 months after lesions heal).
- Hepatic enzyme tests should be monitored periodically in patients receiving itraconazole treatment for >1 month.

REFERENCES

1. Pappas PG. Sporotrichosis. In: Dismukes WE, Pappas PG, Sobel JD, eds. *Clinical Mycology*. New York, NY: Oxford University Press; 2003: 346–354.
2. Rex JH, Okhuysen PC. *Sporothrix schenckii*. In: Mandell GL, Bennett JE, Dolin R, eds. *Mandell, Douglas, and Bennett's Principles and Practice of Infectious Diseases*. 6th ed. New York, NY: Elsevier Churchill Livingstone; 2005: 2984–2988.
3. Kauffman CA, Haijeh R, Chapman SW, for the Mycoses Study Group. Practice guidelines for the management of patients with sporotrichosis. *Clin Infect Dis*. 2000;30:684–687.
4. Greenfield RA. *Sporothrix schenckii*. In: Gorbach SL, Bartlett JG, Blacklow NR, eds. *Infectious Diseases*. 3rd ed. Philadelphia, PA: Lippincott Williams; & Wilkins; 2004: 2246–2249.

MISCELLANEOUS

CODES

ICD9-CM

117.1 Sporotrichosis

PATIENT TEACHING

Advise patients of the nature of the infection, the toxicities associated with therapy, and the need for sustained therapy.

Diet

No restrictions

Activity

No restrictions

Prevention

There is no vaccine. Prevention involves avoidance of exposure.

S

SPRAINS AND STRAINS

John Herbert Stevenson, MD
Christopher Lutryzkowski, MD
Peter L. Hoth, MD

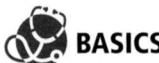 **BASICS**

DESCRIPTION
- Sprains are complete or partial ligamentous injuries either within the body of the ligament or at the site of attachment to bone.
  - May be classified as Grade I, II, or III (AMA Ligament Injury Classification) (4)
  - Grade I: Stretch injury without ligamentous laxity
  - Grade II: Partial tear with increased ligamentous laxity but firm end-point on exam
  - Grade III: Complete tear with increased ligamentous laxity and no firm end-point on exam
  - Physical exam is the key to the diagnosis.
  - Usually secondary to trauma (falls, twisting injuries or motor vehicle accidents)
- Strains are partial or complete disruptions of the muscle, muscle/tendon junction, or tendon; they can be associated with overuse injuries. May be classified as
  - 1st degree: Minimal damage to muscle, tendon or musculotendinous unit.
  - 2nd degree: Partial tear to the muscle, tendon, or musculotendinous unit
  - 3rd degree: Complete disruption of the muscle, etc. (4)
- System(s) Affected: Musculoskeletal

ALERT
Geriatric Considerations
More likely to see associated bony injuries due to decreased joint flexibility and prevalence of osteoporosis and osteopenia

Pediatric Considerations
- Sprains and strains have been found to account for 24% of injuries in pediatric patients.
- 3 million pediatric sports injuries occur annually.
- Must be concerned about physeal/apophyseal injuries in the skeletally immature.

GENERAL PREVENTION
- Maintain a reasonable level of physical conditioning.
- Avoid excessive physical stresses, and wear proper exercise gear (particularly shoes).
- Use proper equipment for the activity.
- Know the risks associated with the intended activity.
- Use appropriate conditioning, warm-up, and cool-down exercises.
- Single leg balancing may help prevent ankle sprains. (1)
- Taping/bracing postinjury may be of short-term benefit for future injury prevention of ankle sprains. (5)[B]

EPIDEMIOLOGY
Incidence
~80% of all US athletes at sometime in their career will experience a sprain or strain that involves the upper or lower extremities, or spine.

Prevalence
- Ankle sprains are one of the most common injuries seen in the primary care setting, making up to 30% of sports medicine clinic visits. (7)
- Predominant age
  - Sprains: Any age when patient is physically active
  - Strains: Usually 15–40 years
- Predominant sex: Male > Female

RISK FACTORS
- Change in or improper shoe gear, protective gear, or environment (e.g., surface)
- Inappropriate sudden increase in training schedule
- Prior history of sprain or strain

ETIOLOGY
- Falls
- Motor vehicle accident
- Trauma
- Excessive exercise
- Inadequate warm-up and stretching prior to activity
- Poor conditioning

ASSOCIATED CONDITIONS
- Hemarthrosis
- Stress, avulsion, or other fractures
- Syndesmotic injuries
- Contusions
- Wounds
- Dislocations
- Subluxations

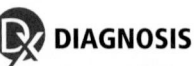 **DIAGNOSIS**

SIGNS AND SYMPTOMS
- Swelling
- Pain
- Ecchymosis (usually late)
- Tenderness
- Gait disturbances if severe
- Decreased ROM of joint and joint instability

History
- May describe feeling or hearing pop or snap
- May remember mechanism (key in diagnosis)

Physical Exam
Sprains
- Grade I: Tenderness without laxity
- Grade II: Tenderness, with increased laxity on exam but firm endpoint
- Grade III: Tenderness, with increased laxity on exam and no firm endpoint

TESTS
Special tests
- Examination under anesthesia and/or arthroscopy may be required in some cases.
- For ankle, use the anterior drawer test, which tests the integrity of the anterior talofibular ligament.
- Apprehension test may indicate glenohumeral ligament sprain of the shoulder.
- Lachman test assesses integrity of ACL.

Imaging
- Radiographs may be needed to rule out bony injury; stress views may be helpful.
- Ankle films (Ottawa ankle rules) [A]
  - Bone tenderness in posterior aspect distal 6 cm of tibia/fibula
  - Inability to bear weight, both immediately or in emergency department/office
  - Age >18 and <55 (8)

- Foot films: Only required if midfoot zone pain is present *and*
  - Bone tenderness at base of 5th metatarsal; *or*
  - Bone tenderness at navicular: *or*
  - Inability to bear weight, immediately or in emergency department
- CT scan of the affected area may be required if occult fracture is suspected, with negative films.
- MRI is gold standard for imaging soft-tissue structures including muscle, ligamentous, and intra-articular structures.
- Exam under anesthesia in difficult cases.

Diagnostic Procedures/Surgery
Surgery may be required for some partial and complete sprains. Need for surgery depends on the ability of ligaments or muscle to heal on their own or ability to attain full ROM and stability of the affected joint.

DIFFERENTIAL DIAGNOSIS
- Tendonitis
- Bursitis
- Contusion
- Hematoma
- Fracture
- Rheumatologic process

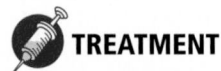 **TREATMENT**

INITIAL STABILIZATION
Outpatient

GENERAL MEASURES
- History and physical exam along with treatment of the worst possible suspected injury
- Acutely: PRICEMM therapy: Protection, relative rest, ice, compression, elevation, medications, modalities. For cryotherapy, see (9)[B].
  - Elastic bandage wrap (Ace) if comfortable
  - Jones dressing for more severe injuries
- Orthosis (splint) for pain relief and stability; air cast–type devices provide effective stability and pain relief for ankle sprains.
- Crutches and crutch gait training
- Stirrup-type ankle brace (3)[A]

Diet
Weight loss if obesity is etiologic.

Activity
If affected joint has full strength and ROM, patient can advance activity as tolerated.

SPECIAL THERAPY
Physical Therapy
- Useful adjunct after injury (6)[B]
- Proprioception retraining (2)[C]
- Core strengthening (2)[C]
- Eccentric exercises (2)[C]

MEDICATION (DRUGS)

First Line
- NSAIDs (9)[C]
  - Ibuprofen: 200–800 mg t.i.d.
  - Naproxen: 375–500 mg b.i.d.
  - Indomethacin: 25–50 mg t.i.d.
  - Acetaminophen (11)[B]
  - Narcotics for severe pain (e.g., acetaminophen–hydrocodone)
- Contraindications: Refer to the manufacturer's profile of each drug.
- Precautions: Refer to the manufacturer's profile of each drug.
- Significant possible interactions: Refer to the manufacturer's profile of each drug.

SURGERY
Casting and surgery are reserved for select grade III injuries.

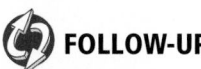

FOLLOW-UP

DISPOSITION
Issues for Referral
- ACL sprain in athletes/physically active
- Salter-Harris physeal fractures
- Lack of improvement with conservative measures
- Joint instability
- Tendon disruption (i.e., Achilles, biceps).

PROGNOSIS
With appropriate treatment and rest, 1–8 weeks or longer for recovery, depending on severity of injury

COMPLICATIONS
- Chronic joint instability
- Arthritis
- Muscle contracture

PATIENT MONITORING
After initial treatment, consider rehabilitation. Direct emphasis toward limiting swelling and providing a painfree full ROM.

REFERENCES

1. McGuine TA, Keene JS. The effect of a balance training program on the risk of ankle sprains in high school athletes. *Am J Sports Med.* 2006;34(7):1103–1111.
2. Brukner PD, Crossley KM, Morris H, et al. Recent advances in sports medicine. *Med J Aust.* 2006;184(4):188–193.
3. Boyce SH, Quigley MA, Campbell S. Management of ankle sprains: A randomized controlled trial of the treatment of inversion ankle sprains using an elastic support bandage or an Aircast ankle brace. *Br J Sports Med.* 2005;39(2):91–96.
4. O'Connor F, et al. Sports medicine: Just the facts. New York: McGraw-Hill, 2005;34.
5. Handoll HHG, Rowe BH, Quinn KM, et al. Interventions for preventing ankle injuries. Cochrane Database of Systematic Rev. 5/26/2005 review.
6. Kerkhoffs, et al. Immobilisation and functional treatment for acute lateral ankle ligament injuries in adults. Cochrane Database of Systematic Rev.12/16/2004 review.
7. Mahaffey D, Hilts M, Fields KB. Ankle and foot injuries in sports. *Clin Fam Pract.* 1999; 1:233–250.
8. Stiell IG, McKnight RD, Greenberg GH, et al. Implementation of the Ottawa ankle rules. *JAMA.* 1994;271:827–832.
9. Nyland J. Therapeutic modality: Rehabilitation of the injured athlete. *Clin Sports Med.* 2004;23(2): 299-313, vii.
10. Mehallo CJ. Practical management: Nonsteroidal anti-inflammatory drug use in athletic injuries. *Clin J Sport Med.* 2006;16(2):170–174.
11. Dalton JD Jr., Schweinle JE. Randomized controlled noninferiority trial to compare extended release acetaminophen and ibuprofen for the treatment of ankle sprains. *Ann Emerg Med.*2006;48(5):615–623.

MISCELLANEOUS

See also: Tendonitis

 CODES

ICD9-CM
- 840.4 Rotator cuff, shoulder
- 844.9 Unspecified site, knee
- 845.00 Ankle sprain, unspecified
- 845.1 Foot sprain, unspecified
- 848.9 Sprain and strain, site unspecified

PATIENT TEACHING
- Instructions on how to wrap with elastic bandage
- Prevention of injury

See Corresponding Diagnostic Algorithm

S

STATUS EPILEPTICUS

Jeff Ray Gibson Jr., MD

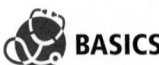 **BASICS**

DESCRIPTION

Epileptic seizure >30 minutes or absence of full recovery of consciousness between seizures. Tonic/clonic (grand mal or generalized convulsive) status epilepticus is the most common and most serious form. For description and treatment of additional types of status (focal, nonconvulsive, and neonatal) see "References".

- System(s) Affected: Nervous
- Synonym(s): Status convulsivus

ALERT

Status epilepticus is a life-threatening emergency; begin treatment if seizure lasts >5 minutes. Rapid control of seizure is critical to success.

GENERAL PREVENTION

Establish maintenance regimen of anticonvulsant.

EPIDEMIOLOGY

- Predominant age: >50% of new cases of status epilepticus occur in young children.
- Predominant sex: Male > Female

Incidence

- 18–50 cases per 100,000 per year; 1/3 as unprovoked 1st seizure, 1/6 in patients with known epilepsy, 1/2 secondary to acute CNS insult.
- Incidence is 2 times higher in elderly.

RISK FACTORS

- Seizure disorder plus any precipitating insult
- Prior history of status epilepticus (recurrence rate is 17% in children; 50% in those with neurologic abnormality)
- Porphyria

Genetics

Unknown

PATHOPHYSIOLOGY

- Direct neuronal injury: Probably an excitotoxic mechanism related to prolonged depolarization-induced apoptosis or necrotic cell death
- Associated autonomic phenomena: Excess catecholamine secretion resulting in glandular hypersecretion, piloerection, hyperthermia, cyclic pupillary dilation, and prolonged apnea/cyanosis
- Metabolic changes: Lactic acidosis, carbon dioxide narcosis, hyperkalemia, hyperglycemia followed by hypoglycemia
- Cardiac changes: Hypertension (followed by hypotension), arrhythmias, high output failure
- Respiratory changes: Increased secretions, lax tongue, possible airway obstruction, pulmonary edema, aspiration
- Renal complications: Acute tubular necrosis from myoglobinuria after rhabdomyolysis. Cerebrovascular changes: Loss of autoregulation, focal ischemia, cerebral edema; Todd paralysis may occur.
- Postictal findings: Fever, tachycardia, mydriasis, conjugate deviation of eyes, decreased corneal reflex, positive Babinski sign; fecal and urinary incontinence; tongue, cheek, or lip injury

ETIOLOGY

Etiology varies by age group

- In adults: Usually related to a known condition, for example, established epilepsy, alcohol withdrawal, anticonvulsant withdrawal/noncompliance, or acquired CNS lesion (especially frontal)
- In children: May present in status epilepticus as their 1st seizure owing to febrile seizure, new-onset epilepsy, CNS infection, metabolic derangement
- Neonatal status: Most often related to meningitis or metabolic disorders (deficiencies of calcium, magnesium, or pyridoxine); needs careful workup for cause
- Acute or chronic CNS injury-trauma, infection, stroke, mass/vascular lesion, metabolic disorder, encephalopathy (hypoxic or degenerative type)
- Intoxication: Cocaine, tricyclic antidepressants, isoniazid, chloroquine, cephalosporins, penicillins, ciprofloxacin, cyclosporin, theophylline, tacrolimus, tiagabine, and nerve agent poisoning
- Idiopathic

 **DIAGNOSIS**

SIGNS AND SYMPTOMS

Depends on the duration and type of seizure

- Recurrent generalized (tonic/clonic) convulsions are most common.
  - May be preceded by aura
  - Tonic phase (stiffening) for 30–45 seconds
  - Clonic phase (rhythmic jerking) for 2–5 minutes
  - No intervening consciousness; seizure recurs

History

- Pursue available drug history.
- Must search for the primary pathology

Physical Exam

Neurologic exam: Confirm true seizure (pseudo status usually atypical); look for localizing signs.

TESTS

Lab

- Glucose (rapid determination)
- Electrolytes, CBC, osmolarity
- Creatine phosphokinase
- Calcium, magnesium, phosphate
- Arterial blood gases, carboxyhemoglobin
- Toxicology screen, anticonvulsant levels
- Liver/renal function
- Coagulation profile

Imaging

- Noncontrast CT scan in new-onset seizure
- MRI or PET if more detail needed
- CXR for endotracheal tube position or suspicion of aspiration pneumonitis

Diagnostic Procedures/Surgery

- Lumbar puncture (if meningitis is suspected) NOTE: Intracranial pressure may be increased.
- EEG: Use to differentiate pseudoseizures, reveal nonconvulsive status, and confirm successful treatment. Check EEG on any patient not awake 30 minutes after seizure.

Pathological Findings

Variable

DIFFERENTIAL DIAGNOSIS

- Pseudostatus may occur with pseudoseizures. Check EEG; avoid dangerous therapy.
- Comatose or paralyzed patients and other forms of status require neurologic exam and EEG.

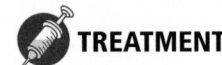 **TREATMENT**

PRE HOSPITAL

- Support ABCs and protect patient from injury.
- Out of hospital treatment by paramedics or caretakers using buccal midazolam or rectal diazepam has been recommended (doses below).

INITIAL STABILIZATION

Begin treatment if seizure lasts >5 minutes. Simultaneous goals are

- Stop seizure.
- Find cause.
- Treat secondary complications.

GENERAL MEASURES

- Manage airway, breathing, and circulation.
- Monitor pulse oximetry, end-tidal CO_2, BP, ECG, and temperature.
- Observe and confirm fit is status epilepticus.
- Give oxygen (intubate and hyperventilate if hypoventilation, hypoxia, and/or hypercarbia occur or if aspiration is a concern. If intubation is needed, use rocuronium bromide 0.6 mg/kg—a short-acting nondepolarizer)
- Establish 2 IV lines.
- Draw blood for initial lab studies.
- Protect patient from injury: Place on side, clear/suction airway, prevent tongue laceration.
- Place nasograstric tube in comatose patient.
- Treat any fever.
- Stop the seizure (see "Medication" below).

Diet

NPO

Activity

Bed rest

SPECIAL THERAPY

IV Fluids

- Give maintenance fluids.
- Hemodynamic instability may require fluid boluses or vasopressors (e.g., dopamine).

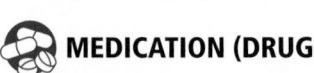 **MEDICATION (DRUGS)**

Drug(s) of choice depend on the type of seizure. Approach tonic/clonic status epilepticus as follows

- Thiamine: 100 mg IV or IM (adults only)
- 50% dextrose: If blood sugar low or cannot be measured, give 50 mL IV (for child use $D_{25}W$; give 2 mL/kg slowly).
- Naloxone (Narcan): If pupils are myotic or drug overdose is suspected, give 2 mg IV (for child—0.1 mg/kg IV, up to 2 mg slowly).
- Pyridoxine: If isoniazid poisoning is suspected
- Antibiotics: If meningitis is strongly suspected
- For nerve agent poisoning, give atropine, benzodiazepines, and pralidoxime (2-PAM).

First Line

- To stop seizures if IV access available

  – Start with lorazepam (Ativan) (1)[A]
  - Give 0.05–0.15 mg/kg IV at 1–2 mg per minute to maximum of 8 mg (for child, 0.05–0.1 mg/kg IV at <2 mg/min to maximum of 4 mg)
  - May repeat every 10 minutes ×2

  – After 5 minutes, if seizure persists, add 2nd agent, fosphenytoin (Cerebyx) (2)[B], prodrug of phenytoin
  - 15–20 mg phenytoin equivalents (PE)/kg IV at <150 mg PE per minute
  - May add 5–10 mg PE/kg IV
  - Maintenance 4–6 mg PE/kg/d IV or IM (child dose same as adult)

  – If these fail, treat as refractory status epilepticus (see below).

- To stop seizures if IV access not available
  – In small children, use intraosseous infusion of IV doses of benzodiazepine and fosphenytoin.
  – *Or use* rectal diazepam (Valium)
  - 0.2–0.5 mg/kg (child —20 mg maximum)
  - Use the gel form (Diastat) or IV solution.
  – *Or,* Lorazepam (sublingual): Use IV dose.
  – *Or,* Midazolam (Versed): 0.2 mg/kg IM or 0.5 mg/kg intranasal or buccal (onset 5–10 minutes)
  – *And* Fosphenytoin IM: Use IV dose (slowly).

- If seizures persist (refractory status)

  – Admit to ICU and induce anesthesia/drug coma (2)[B], give infusion of short-acting agent to stop seizures (see choices below).
  - Requires intubation, ventilation, and monitoring of EEG, ECG, pulse oximetry, and (often) BP support.
  - Monitor temperature and treat/cool if febrile.
  - Adjust to keep EEG at burst suppression.
  - Maintain infusion for 12–24 hours, then withdraw anesthetic infusion gradually while continuing anticonvulsant therapy.

  – *Use* midazolam (Versed): 0.2–0.5 mg/kg slow IV bolus injection, followed by 0.5–10 μg/kg/min IV drip, titrated to burst suppression
  - Tachyphylaxis may develop.
  – *Or* propofol (Diprivan): 3–5 mg/kg IV (in elderly, halve initial dose), follow with 30–150 μg/kg/min IV titrated to burst suppression
  – *Or* thiopental (Pentothal): To 6 mg/kg in divided doses, then add 50 mg IV every 2–5 minutes to produce burst suppression, maintain with IV drip of 0.2% solution; start at 2–5 mg/kg/h and adjust based on EEG
  – Contraindications: See package inserts.
  - Benzodiazepines (diazepam, lorazepam, midazolam) in narrow-angle glaucoma
  - Barbiturates in acute intermittent porphyria
  - Propofol in allergy to soybean oil, egg, lecithin, or glycerol
  - Valproic acid in hepatic disease and pregnancy (risk of neural tube defects)

– Precautions
  - Reduce dosage of depressants in patients with shock, coma, or alcohol intoxication.
  - Most drugs listed may exacerbate porphyria; exceptions: Lorazepam, midazolam, propofol.
  - Benzodiazepines: Apnea may occur with rapid IV injection. Reduce dose in the chronic pulmonary patient, renal failure, the elderly, and hepatic insufficiency.
  - Diazepam: Venous thrombosis/phlebitis
  - Propofol: Strict aseptic technique required. May cause stinging discomfort on injection. Prolonged use may cause lactic acidosis, lipemia, heart failure, systemic collapse, and death in both children and adults. Safety not established for child <3 years old
  - Fosphenytoin (Cerebyx)/Phenytoin: Safety is not established for children. Monitor for arrhythmias, prolonged QT interval, and hypotension. If these occur, decrease rate of administration. Use with caution in liver disease, hyperglycemia, the elderly, and pregnancy (increased risk of malformations, may lead to vitamin K deficiency bleeding problems in both mother and newborn). Abrupt withdrawal may precipitate status. Overdose may cause paradoxical inefficacy.
  - Valproic acid: May decrease platelet function; may cause hyperammonemic encephalopathy.
  – Significant possible interactions
  - Fosphenytoin/phenytoin: Increased serum levels and toxicity of warfarin, disulfiram, phenylbutazone, and isoniazid. Decrease dose with renal insufficiency.
  - Valproic acid: Increased toxicity of phenytoin/fosphenytoin

Second Line

- Diazepam (Valium): (2)[B] Use for lorazepam
  – 0.2–0.5 mg/kg IV at 5 mg/min up to a dose of 30 mg (for child 0.3 mg/kg at <2 mg/min IV up to 10 mg total)

  – Repeat q5min 3, wears off quickly

- Phenytoin: (2)[B]—Use for fosphenytoin. Doses are the same (mg for mg Phenytoin equivalents), but must be given more slowly (<1 mg/kg/min) to lessen toxicity and cardiovascular depression

- Other 2nd-line drugs
  – Pentobarbital: 10–15 mg/kg IV loading dose over 1 hour, followed by continuous infusion of 0.5–1 mg/kg/h; adjust based on EEG
  – Lidocaine (Xylocaine): 1–3 mg/kg IV bolus. If effective, drip at 3–10 mg/kg/h IV.
  – Valproic acid: Clinical pilot studies have used 15–40 mg/kg IV loading dose over 5–10 minutes, followed by 1–5 mg/kg/h.
- Investigational drugs: Isoflurane or desflurane (by inhalation), ketamine, etomidate, nimodipine, chlormethiazole, topiramate (PO), levetiracetam, lamotrigine

SURGERY

Experimental—excision of epileptic focus or propagation pathways

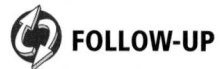 **FOLLOW-UP**

DISPOSITION

Admission Criteria

Admit to stop seizures and stabilize medical condition. Refractory status needs ICU care.

Discharge Criteria

Control of seizures and therapeutic levels of maintenance anticonvulsants

Issues for Referral

Refractory or nonconvulsive status is best referred to a neurologist.

PROGNOSIS

- Prolonged seizures (>30 minutes) may cause neurologic injury or death. For seizure >4 hours, mortality is 50%; >12 hours, mortality is 80%.
- Mortality is 16–25% in adults, 3–19% in children, extremely high in neonates, and up to 76% in the elderly. Morbidity/mortality may be related to acute CNS insult, stress from repeated seizures, cardiopulmonary arrest, renal failure, hyperthermia, aspiration pneumonia, the underlying pathology, or the treatment instituted.

PATIENT MONITORING

Therapeutic blood levels of anticonvulsants

REFERENCES

1. Prasad K, et al. Anticonvulsant therapy for status epilepticus. *Cochrane Database Syst Rev.* 2005, Issue 4: CD003723. DOI:10.1002/14651858.CD003723.pub2.
2. Walker M, Status epilepticus: An evidence based guide. *BMJ.* 2005;331:673–677.
3. Marik P, Varon J. The management of status epilepticus. *Chest.* 2004;126(2):582–591.

 MISCELLANEOUS

See also: Seizure disorders; Seizures, Febrile

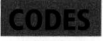 **CODES**

ICD9-CM

- 345.2 Epilepsy, petit mal status
- 345.3 Epilepsy, grand mal status
- 345.71 Epilepsia partialis continua, with intractable epilepsy, so stated

PATIENT TEACHING

- Epilepsy Foundation (800) EFA-1000; www.efa.org
- Epilepsy Therapy Development Project: www.epilepsy.com

 See Corresponding Diagnostic Algorithm

STEVENS-JOHNSON SYNDROME

Matthew Silva, PharmD, RPh, BCPS
Pablo I. Hernandezz, MD

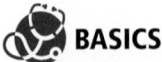

BASICS

DESCRIPTION
- Stevens-Johnson syndrome (SJS) is a generalized hypersensitivity reaction, usually to a drug, in which skin and mucous membrane lesions are an early manifestation.
- Once considered to be the same as erythema multiforme major, a severe form of erythema multiforme in which >1 mucosal surface was involved.
- Erythema multiforme spectrum is now thought to be a single entity
  – Milder form, also known as erythema multiforme-Hebra, either has no mucous membrane involvement, or may involve 1 mucous membrane
  – More severe form, erythema multiforme major, involves >1 mucous membrane
  – In both variants, it is a self-limited hypersensitivity reaction, usually to a preceding viral infection, and has an excellent prognosis.
- May progress to its more severe form, toxic epidermal necrolysis (TEN), which has a high morbidity and up to 70% mortality (2).
- System(s) Affected: Cardiovascular; Hemic/Lymphatic/Immunologic; Nervous; Renal/Urologic; Skin/Exocrine
- Synonym(s): Ectodermosis erosiva pluriorificialis; Febrile mucocutaneous syndrome; Herpes iris; Erythema polymorphe; Toxic epidermal necrolysis (TEN).

ALERT
Geriatric Considerations
Toxic epidermal necrolysis has a greater mortality in older patients.

Pediatric Considerations
- Rare in children <3 years
- More common in children and young adults

Pregnancy Considerations
Pregnancy is possible predisposing condition

GENERAL PREVENTION
- Rarely possible to anticipate a 1st attack
- Avoid re-exposure to presumed cause.
- Although not FDA approved, IV immune globulin may be beneficial for both treatment and prophylaxis.

EPIDEMIOLOGY
Incidence
- Incidence/prevalence in the US is difficult to estimate because there is no universally accepted definition of SJS.
- 1.1–7.1 and 0.4–1.2 cases per million person-years for SJS and TEN, respectively (2)

Prevalence
- Predominant age: SJS is more common in children and young adults.
- Males > Females (2:1)
- Sex (% range of females): 33–62% for SJS and 61.3–64.3% for TEN (2)
- Age (average range): 25–47 years for SJS and 46–63 years for TEN (2)

RISK FACTORS
- Patients with HIV infection may be predisposed to developing SJS in response to their medications.
  – HLA subtypes A, B, and D
  – Disease that cause immune compromise (deficiencies, malignancy, etc)
  – Possibly radiation therapy or UV light
- Previous history of SJS

Genetics
Possibly associated with HLA-B15, HLA-Bw44, part of HLA-B12, and HLA-DQB1*0601

ETIOLOGY
- 50% of cases are idiopathic.
- Associated with metabolism of parent drugs and metabolites
- Sulfonamides are the drug most strongly associated with SJS and TEN, then
  – Cephalosporins
  – Quinolones
  – Aminopenicillins
  – Tetracyclines
  – Macrolides
  – Imidazole antifungals
  – Anticonvulsants
  – NSAIDs, especially oxicam
  – Vaccines—dPT, bCG, oral polio
- Mycoplasma pneumonia infection
- Viruses (HSV, EBV, coxsackie)

ASSOCIATED CONDITIONS
- SJS and toxic epidermal necrolysis are associated conditions.
- Mycoplasma pneumonia may be an infectious precursor.

DIAGNOSIS

History
- Usually a preceding illness for which the medication was given 1–3 weeks before initial cutaneous manifestations
- Sudden onset with rapid progressive pleomorphic rash that includes petechiae, vesicles, bullae.
- Seen in SJS if epidermal detachments affects <10% of the skin
- Seen in TEN if epidermal detachments >30% or if it >10% in the absence of discrete skin lesions
- Cases with discrete skin lesions and 10–30% epidermal detachment are in the overlap between SJS ad TEN

Physical Exam
The condition is classified as follows
- Vesicles and ulcers on the mucous membranes, especially of the mouth and throat
- Burning sensation of the skin and sometimes of the mucous membranes
- Usually no pruritus
- Fever 39–40°C (102–104°F)
- Headache
- Malaise
- Arthralgias
- Epistaxis
- Crusted nares
- Conjunctivitis
- Corneal ulcerations
- Erosive vulvovaginitis or balanitis

- Cough productive of thick purulent sputum
- Tachypnea/respiratory distress
- Arrhythmias
- Pericarditis
- CHF
- Mental status changes
- Seizures
- Coma
- Sepsis
- Seen in SJS if epidermal detachment affects <10% of the skin
- Seen in TEN, if epidermal detachment exceeds 30% or if it exceeds 10% in the absence of discrete skin lesions
- Cases with discrete skin lesions and 10–30% epidermal detachment are in the overlap between SJS and TEN.

TESTS
Lab
- Culture or serological tests for suspected sources of infection
- Electrolyte disturbance
- Albuminuria/hematuria

Diagnostic Procedures/Surgery
Skin biopsy

Pathological Findings
- Compared with the mainly inflammatory changes in erythema multiforme, necrotic changes predominate in SJS and toxic epidermal necrolysis.
- A cell-poor infiltrate is present, in which macrophages and dendrocytes predominate, with a strong immunoreactivity for tumor necrosis factor (TNF)-α.

DIFFERENTIAL DIAGNOSIS
- Exfoliative dermatitis
- Linear IgA bullous dermatosis
- Staphylococcal scalded skin syndrome
- Pemphigus (paraneoplastic)
- Generalized fixed drug eruption
- Erythema multiforme major
- Burns
- Pressure blisters (coma, barbiturates)

TREATMENT

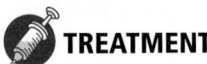

- This disease progresses rapidly, all patients should be admitted.
- Consider admission to a burn unit when sloughed skin >10% of the body surface area.
- ICU for bronchiolitis, ARDS, or multiorgan damage

GENERAL MEASURES
- Withdraw all suspected medication and treat any underlying disease.
- Meticulous care of damaged skin
- Catheter changing and culturing
- Reverse isolation and temperature control with extensive epidermal loss
- Maintenance of fluid, electrolyte, and protein balance
- Plasmapheresis
- Adequate calorie intake; parenteral nutrition, if necessary
- Mouthwashes of warm saline or a solution of diphenhydramine, lidocaine, and kaolin suspension

- Ophthalmologic consultation and monitoring for corneal damage
- Venous thromboembolism prophylaxis with unfractionated heparin or low-molecular-weight heparin

Diet
- Oral fluid intake is recommended.
- Early oral nutrition by nasogastric tube as tolerated
- IV nutritional support with increased protein requirements; may need insulin for glycoregulation in this hypercatabolic state.

Activity
Bed rest until clinically stabilized

Nursing
Avoid administration of topical silver sulfadiazine due to association with sulfonamides and SJS.

SPECIAL THERAPY
IV Fluids
Fluid management with saline and macromolecules are necessary in the 1st 24 hours, with decreasing IV fluid requirements as oral intake proceeds with NG tube.

 ## MEDICATION (DRUGS)

First Line
- Corticosteroids are controversial. Early, high-dose IV steroids may attenuate disease progression, reduce skin detachment, decrease inflammatory cytokine activity, and improve patient comfort. Withdraw if no benefit is seen in the 1st few days.
- Experimental treatments that appear to have been useful include
  - Recombinant granulocyte colony stimulating factor
  - Cyclophosphamide
  - Cyclosporine
  - —IV immune globulin in HIV-positive patients
    ○ IV immune globulin considered beneficial treatment and prophylaxis, although not FDA approved
- Contraindications: Avoid steroids in diabetic or immunosuppressed patients or those with chronic infections.
- Precautions: Refer to the manufacturer's profile for each drug.
- Significant possible interactions: Refer to manufacturer's profile of each drug.

Second Line
- Acyclovir for herpetic infections
- Erythromycin or related antibiotic for *Mycoplasma* infections (empiric use of antibiotics is not recommended)

SURGERY
- Sterile debridement of areas of extensive epidermal loss
- Application of biosynthetic dressings, such as Biobrane to denuded areas
- Damage to the vulva, vagina, or cornea; consider surgical repair

 ## FOLLOW-UP

PROGNOSIS
- Disease may have a rapid onset or may evolve slowly over 1–2 weeks with resolution over 4–6 weeks.
- Often scarring of the skin or mucous membranes occurs, especially of the vulva.
- Blindness or corneal opacities occur in 7–20% of patients.
- The risk of recurrence as high as 37%.
- Death occurs in 5–15% of the patients with SJS, and up to 40% of patients with TEN.

COMPLICATIONS
- Secondary infections
- Sepsis
- Pneumonia
- ARDS
- Bronchiolitis obliterans in children
- Dehydration/electrolyte disturbance
- Acute tubular necrosis
- Corneal ulceration or iritis
- Arrhythmias
- Venous thromboembolism
- Disseminated intravascular coagulation
- Death in 15% of untreated cases of SJS and up to 40% of TEN

PATIENT MONITORING
- Secondary or concurrent infections
- Dehydration
- Electrolyte imbalance
- Malnutrition
- End-organ damage

REFERENCES
1. French LE, Trent JT, et al. Use of intravenous immunoglobulin in toxic epidermal necrolysis and Stevens-Johnson syndrome: Our current understanding. *Int Immunopharmacol.* 2006;6:543–549.
2. Letko E, Papaliodis DN, et al. Stevens-Johnson syndrome and toxic epidermal necrolysis: A review of the literature. *Ann Allergy Asthma Immunol.* 2005;94:419–436.
3. Wolf R, et al. Life-threatening acute adverse cutaneous drug reactions. *Clin Dermatol.* 2005;23:171–181.

 ## MISCELLANEOUS

See also: Burns, Erythema multiforme, Pemphigoid, bullous, Pemphigus vulgaris, Acute respiratory distress syndrome, cutaneous drug reactions, dermatitis herpetiformis

CODES

ICD9-CM
695.1 Erythema multiforme

PATIENT TEACHING
- The patient should be kept informed of the progress of the disease and the treatment options available.
- Recurrences are possible. Etiologic agents should be identified if possible and avoided indefinitely.

STOKES-ADAMS ATTACKS

Jeremy Golding, MD

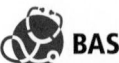 **BASICS**

DESCRIPTION
- Syncope due to transient complete heart block and resulting severe bradycardia or asystole with hypotension
- System(s) Affected: Cardiovascular; Nervous
- Synonym(s): Drop attacks

GENERAL PREVENTION
Avoid negative chronotropic drugs (e.g., β-blockers, calcium channel blockers, digoxin) in at-risk patients.

EPIDEMIOLOGY
- Predominant age: Most common >40 years of age
- Predominant sex: Male = Female

ALERT
Pregnancy Considerations
Rare during pregnancy

Incidence
Undocumented

Prevalence
Undocumented

Geriatric Considerations
Prevalence increases with age

RISK FACTORS
- Use of the medications listed under "Etiology"
- Coronary artery disease
- History of previous atrioventricular nodal dysfunction
- Bundle branch and/or fascicular block
- Acute myocardial infarction (MI) (especially acute right coronary artery occlusion)
- Amyloidosis
- Chagas disease
- Connective tissue diseases involving the heart (e.g., systemic lupus erythematosus, rheumatoid arthritis, sarcoidosis)

Genetics
No known genetic pattern

ETIOLOGY
- Medications
  - Calcium channel blockers
  - β-blockers
  - Sotalol
  - Digoxin
  - Clonidine
  - Propafenone (Rythmol); a class IC antiarrhythmic
- Other causes
  - Myocardial ischemia involving the atrioventricular node
  - Degenerative (fibrosing) and infiltrative diseases involving the heart and its conduction system (e.g., Lenègre)
  - Degeneration of the atrioventricular node secondary to aging
  - Neuromuscular diseases (e.g., myotonic muscular dystrophy or Kearns-Sayre syndrome)

ASSOCIATED CONDITIONS
- Myocardial ischemia
- Acute MI
- Systemic manifestations of connective tissue disease
- Unreliable self-administration of medications
- Neuromuscular disease

 DIAGNOSIS

SIGNS AND SYMPTOMS
- Acute bradycardia
- Hypotension
- Paleness
- Altered sensorium or loss of consciousness, unrelated to position or exertion
- Acute onset of syncopal or near-syncopal symptoms (with or without palpitations)

TESTS
Lab
- Serum digoxin level
- Cardiac enzymes
- Transient or long-standing renal failure may falsely elevate cardiac enzymes (creatine kinase).

Imaging
Transthoracic cardiac 2-D echocardiogram if infiltrative disease is suspected

Diagnostic Procedures/Surgery
- Cardiac coronary catheterization to rule out coronary ischemia
- Electrophysiologic testing to assess status of atrioventricular nodal conduction
- Myocardial biopsy if infiltrative disease is suspected
- ECG, event monitor, or Holter monitor demonstrating (transient) complete heart block with slow or no ventricular escape
- Tilt table testing to rule out a neurogenic etiology for bradycardia and syncope

DIFFERENTIAL DIAGNOSIS
- Seizures
- Transient ischemic attacks
- Orthostatic hypotension
- Vasovagal attacks
- Neurocardiogenic syncope
- Cardiac arrhythmias
  - Ventricular tachycardia
  - Supraventricular tachycardia
  - Reentrant tachycardia
  - Wolff-Parkinson-White syndrome
  - Sinus arrest
  - Sinus exit block
  - Sick sinus syndrome
  - Transition from normal sinus rhythm to atrial fibrillation or from atrial fibrillation to normal sinus rhythm

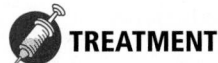 **TREATMENT**

INITIAL STABILIZATION
- Inpatient assessment in a monitored setting
- Continuing treatment ambulatory

GENERAL MEASURES
- Cardiac monitoring
- Transthoracic pacer availability
- Atropine by the bedside

Diet
Regular

Activity
As tolerated after assessment

MEDICATION (DRUGS)

- For symptomatic bradyarrhythmias
  - For acute bradyarrhythmias: Atropine 1 mg IV push, to be given during the complete heart block with hypotension; may be repeated once for a total dosage of 2 mg
  - Epinephrine: 1 mg 1:10,000 IV push, to be given during the complete heart block if associated with asystole; may be repeated every 5 minutes
  - Isoproterenol: Drip 1 mg in 250 cc D_5W or normal saline to be started at 2–20 mcg/min if patient maintains bradycardia and is hypotensive after atropine is given; may titrate drip as necessary
- Contraindications
  - Use of epinephrine in a patient with bradycardia and a normal BP may precipitate hypertensive crisis.
- Precautions: Possible tachycardiac response to the above-mentioned medications

SURGERY

- Consider temporary pacemaker placement.
- Permanent pacemaker placement if etiology of transient complete heart block is not reversible.

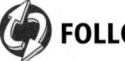 FOLLOW-UP

PROGNOSIS
After diagnosis is made and appropriate treatment is implemented (e.g., pacemaker insertion), prognosis is excellent and further difficulty is not expected.

COMPLICATIONS
- Protracted bradycardia with hypotension, leading to end-organ damage or death
- Loss of consciousness while operating machinery or at unprotected heights

PATIENT MONITORING
- Routine pacemaker checks if permanent pacemaker has been implanted
- Follow-up Holter and/or event monitoring within 2 weeks after causal medications have been discontinued
- Discontinuation of driving, heavy-machinery operation, and being at unprotected heights pending normal follow-up

REFERENCES

1. Brandenburg RO, et al. *Cardiology: Fundamentals and Practice*. Chicago: Year Book Medical Publishers, 1987.
2. Braunwald E, ed. *Heart Disease: A Textbook of Cardiovascular Medicine*, 5th ed. Philadelphia: WB Saunders, 1996.

 MISCELLANEOUS

See also: Amyloidosis; Myocardial infarction; Seizure disorders

CODES

ICD9-CM
426.9 Conduction disorder, unspecified

S

PATIENT TEACHING

After the diagnosis has been made and a pacemaker has been implanted (if indicated), instruct the patient in pacemaker guidelines.

STOMATITIS

Mark R. Dambro, MD

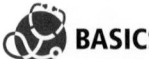 **BASICS**

DESCRIPTION
- Generalized inflammation of the oral mucosa, of many possible etiologies
- System(s) Affected: Skin/Exocrine

GENERAL PREVENTION
Avoid causative factors.

EPIDEMIOLOGY
- Predominant age
  - Primary herpetic infections (children)
  - Hand-foot-and-mouth disease (children)
  - Vincent stomatitis (also known as Vincent disease or acute necrotizing ulcerative gingivitis) (teenagers and young adults)
  - Behçet disease (young adults)
  - Herpangina (children)
  - Other types N/A
- Predominant sex: Male = Female

Prevalence
- Herpetic stomatitis, hand-foot-and-mouth disease, and recurrent aphthous stomatitis are very common.
- Herpangina is fairly common, as are nicotinic and denture-related stomatitis. The remaining causes are uncommon or rare.

ETIOLOGY
- Allergy: Foods, drugs, contact (some erythema multiforme)
- Vitamin deficiency: Riboflavin (angular stomatitis)
- Viral: herpes simplex I and II (herpetic stomatitis), Coxsackie A (herpangina and hand-foot-and-mouth disease)
- Smoking (nicotinic stomatitis)
- Hormonal (possibly recurrent ulcerative stomatitis)
- Uncertain (recurrent aphthous stomatitis, Vincent stomatitis, recurrent scarifying stomatitis, Behçet disease, angular stomatitis, gangrenous stomatitis, erythema multiforme)
- Bacterial (scarlatina)
- Uremic (uremic/nephritic)
- Dentures

ALERT
Pediatric Considerations
Certain etiologies more likely in the pediatric population: Herpetic-primary, hand-foot-and-mouth disease, herpangina

Geriatric Considerations
Certain etiologies more likely in the geriatric population, e.g., dentures

ASSOCIATED CONDITIONS
- AIDS: Associated with severe lesions
- Pregnancy may bring on recurrent ulcerative stomatitis.

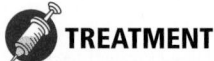 **DIAGNOSIS**

SIGNS AND SYMPTOMS
- General
  - Depends on etiology
  - Varies from minimal to severe pain
  - Many have multiple intraoral ulcers from 1 mm to several centimeters in diameter
  - Some with constitutional symptoms: Fever, malaise, headache
- Allergic stomatitis
  - Intense shiny erythema
  - Slight swelling
  - Itching
  - Dryness
  - Burning
- Vincent infection
  - Necrotic ulceration of interdental papillae and mucous membrane
- Thrush (candidiasis)
  - White patches, slightly raised (resembling milk curds)
  - Distribution: Tongue, buccal mucosa, palate, gums, tonsils, larynx, pharynx, gastrointestinal tract, skin; commonly seen in infants, immunocompromised patients, and patients on long-term antibiotics, corticosteroids, and antineoplastic treatment
- Pseudomembranous stomatitis: Membranelike exudate
- Mucous lesions accompanying systemic disease
  - Mucous patches (syphilis)
  - Strawberry (measles)
  - Koplik spots (measles)
  - Ulcers (erythema multiforme)
  - Smooth, fire-red, painful (pellagra)

TESTS
Lab
- Hematologic profile
- Tzanck test of historic interest only
- Serologic test for syphilis

Diagnostic Procedures/Surgery
Biopsy if persistent/recurrent/suspicious

Pathological Findings
Biopsy suspicious lesions or lesions that fail to heal or chronically recur, to rule out cancer or vasculitis.

DIFFERENTIAL DIAGNOSIS
- Squamous cell cancer
- Herpetic stomatitis
- Hand-foot-and-mouth disease
- Recurrent aphthous stomatitis
- Vincent stomatitis
- Nicotinic stomatitis
- Denture-related stomatitis
- Erythema multiforme/Stevens-Johnson syndrome
- Recurrent ulcerative stomatitis
- Recurrent scarifying stomatitis
- Behçet disease
- Angular stomatitis
- Noma (gangrenous stomatitis)
- Scarlatina (scarlet fever)
- Herpangina
- Uremic stomatitis
- Pemphigus/pemphigoid

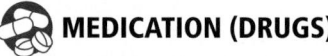 **TREATMENT**

INITIAL STABILIZATION
Outpatient care, unless severe

GENERAL MEASURES
- In most cases, treatment of symptoms only
- Severe cases may require parenteral fluids, particularly in children.
- Topical anesthesia
- Analgesics
- Oral rinses such as half-strength hydrogen peroxide
- Mycostatin, if superinfected with *Candida*
- Smoking cessation

Diet
May need to avoid spicy, sharp, hard, and dry foods

Activity
As tolerated by patient

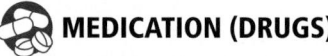 **MEDICATION (DRUGS)**

First Line
- Steroids and cytotoxic drugs for Behçet disease
- 2% viscous lidocaine (Xylocaine) for local discomfort
- Liquid diphenhydramine (Benadryl) by mouth, or swish and spit
- Antibiotics for gangrenous stomatitis
- Antifungal ointment, e.g., nystatin (Mycostatin) for candidiasis complicating angular stomatitis
- For candidiasis: Nystatin oral suspension 400,000 U (4 mL) q.i.d. for 10 days. Use as oral rinse, then swallow.
- Acyclovir 200–800 mg 5 times a day for 7–14 days for herpetic stomatitis
- Sucralfate (Carafate) suspension 1 tsp, swish in mouth or place on ulcers q.i.d. (helpful)
- Contraindications: Allergy to specific medication
- Precautions
  - Toxic dose of topical lidocaine uncertain, but likely only 25–33% of infiltration dose may have significant absorption from open ulcers or mucous membrane
- Significant possible interactions: Refer to manufacturer's literature for each drug.

Second Line
Steroid oral rinses or topical preparations for aphthous ulcers

FOLLOW-UP

PROGNOSIS
- Herpetic: Self-limited, with resolution in 7–14 days
- Hand-foot-and-mouth disease: Same as for herpetic
- Recurrent aphthous ulcers: 7–14-day course per episode
- Vincent: May progress to fascial space infection with airway compromise or sepsis
- Nicotinic: Resolves with cessation of smoking
- Denture: Resolves with careful oral hygiene and daytime-only denture wear
- Erythema multiforme: Resolution in 2–3 weeks
- Stevens-Johnson: Resolution in ~6 weeks with adequate supportive care
- Recurrent ulcerative: As the name implies, recurs over time, but the overall prognosis is good.
- Recurrent scarifying: Occasional patients suffer continuous ulcers, others have recurrence with eventual scarring. The prognosis is otherwise good.
- Behçet disease may recur for several years. Prognosis for vision is poor. Overall prognosis is related to other aspects of the disease.
- Angular: After correction of mechanical problems, allergic disorders, and nutritional deficiencies, the prognosis is good.
- Gangrenous: The most serious stomatitis, requiring aggressive treatment with IV antibiotics and débridement to avoid death
- Scarlatina: The prognosis is related to other manifestations of the disease.
- Herpangina: 7–14-day course, with total resolution
- Uremic: Depends on the underlying renal disease

COMPLICATIONS
- Recurrent scarifying stomatitis may result in intraoral scarring with restriction of oral mobility.
- Behçet disease may result in visual loss, pneumonia, colitis, vasculitis, large artery aneurysms, thrombophlebitis, or encephalitis.
- Gangrenous stomatitis may lead to death.
- Scarlet fever may result in cardiac disease.
- Herpetic stomatitis may be complicated by ocular or CNS involvement.

PATIENT MONITORING
Lesions need to be followed until resolved. If they fail to resolve, continuously recur, or appear suspicious, biopsy may be needed to establish a diagnosis.

REFERENCES
1. Moran WJ. Diseases of the mouth. In: Rakel E, ed. *Conn's Current Therapy*. Philadelphia, PA: WB Saunders; 1990.
2. Teele DW. Inflammatory diseases of the mouth and pharynx. In: Paparella MM, Shumrick DA, eds. *Otolaryngology*. Philadelphia, PA: WB Saunders; 1980: 974–1017.

 MISCELLANEOUS

CODES

ICD9-CM
- 054.2 Herpetic gingivostomatitis
- 101 Vincent angina
- 528.0 Stomatitis
- 528.2 Oral aphthae

S

PATIENT TEACHING

See Corresponding Diagnostic Algorithm

STROKE (BRAIN ATTACK)

William A. Tosches, MD
Michael Previti, MD

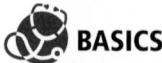 BASICS

DESCRIPTION

- The sudden onset of a focal neurologic deficit resulting from either infarction or hemorrhage within the brain.
- Adults <45 years old are most likely to have a cardiac source of embolism.
- 2 broad categories: Hemorrhagic and ischemic
- System(s) Affected: Cardiovascular; Nervous
- Synonym(s): Cerebrovascular accident; Reversible ischemic neurologic accident

ALERT

Geriatric Considerations
Amyloid (congophilic) angiopathy is most prevalent in the elderly, especially if the patient also has dementia.

Pediatric Considerations
- Cardiac (especially developmental abnormalities)
- Metabolic: Homocystinuria, Fabry disease

Pregnancy Considerations
- Parturition may increase the risk of rupture for aneurysm; amniotic fluid embolism may cause stroke at the time of delivery.
- The postpartum period is associated with an increased risk for cerebral venous thrombosis.

GENERAL PREVENTION

- Stop smoking.
- Control BP, diabetes, hyperlipidemia.
- Use alcohol in moderation, if at all.
- Exercise regularly.
- Maintain positive psychologic outlook.
- Seek professional dietary advice on weight control.
- Antiplatelet drugs
- Angiotensin-converting enzyme (ACE) inhibitors
- Statins
- Treat homocystinemia with vitamin B_6, vitamin B_{12}, and folic acid.
- Nonvalvular atrial fibrillation should be treated with dose-adjusted heparin to achieve an INR of 2–3 to prevent stroke. (1)[A]
- Women >45 years on ASA 100 mg/d have decreased risk of ischemic stroke and TIA but increased risk of GI bleed needing transfusion. (2)[B]

EPIDEMIOLOGY

Incidence
Incidence in the US: 150/100,000

Prevalence
- Prevalence in the US: 550/100,000
- Predominant age: Risk increases >45, and is highest in the 7th and 8th decades.
- Predominant sex: Male > Female (3:1), but equalizes after menopause

RISK FACTORS

- Uncontrollable
  - Age
  - Sex
  - Race
  - Family history
- Controllable
  - Hypertension
  - Diabetes mellitus
  - Hypercholesterolemia
  - Cardiac disease
  - History of stroke or TIA
  - Atrial fibrillation
  - Valvular heart disease
  - Severe carotid stenosis
  - Intracranial arterial stenosis
  - Hypercoagulable states (antiphospholipid antibodies)
  - Homocystinemia
  - Obesity
  - Smoking

Genetics
Inheritance is polygenic, with a tendency to clustering of risk factors within families.

ETIOLOGY

- Ischemic: Carotid atherosclerotic disease with artery-to-artery thromboembolism
- Cardiac
  - Cardioembolism secondary to valvular (mitral valve) pathology
  - Mural hypokinesias or akinesias with thrombosis (acute anterior myocardial infarctions (MIs) or congestive cardiomyopathies)
  - Cardiac arrhythmia (atrial fibrillation)
- Hypercoagulable states
  - Antiphospholipid antibodies, factor V Leiden deficiency, deficiency of protein S, protein C, antithrombin III deficiency
  - Estrogen use (HRT, OCP, etc.)
- Other causes
  - Spontaneous and posttraumatic (i.e., chiropractic manipulation) artery dissection
  - Fibromuscular dysplasia
  - Vasculitis
  - Drugs (cocaine, amphetamines)
- Hemorrhagic
- Hypertension: May cause damage to putamen, internal capsule, cerebellum, brainstem, corona radiata
- Amyloid (congophilic) angiopathy: Lobar (cortical) hemorrhages in the elderly
- Vascular malformations: Arteriovenous malformation, cavernous angioma, venous angioma and capillary angioma

ASSOCIATED CONDITIONS
Cardiac disease is the major cause of death in the 1st 5 years after a stroke.

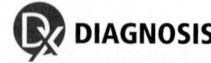 DIAGNOSIS

SIGNS AND SYMPTOMS

- Carotid circulation (hemispheric): Hemiplegia, hemianesthesia, neglect, aphasia, visual field defects; less often headaches, seizures, amnesia, confusion
- Vertebrobasilar (brainstem or cerebellar): Diplopia, vertigo, ataxia, facial paresis, Horner syndrome, dysphagia, dysarthria
- Impaired level of consciousness
- Cerebellar lesion in patients with headache, nausea, vomiting, and ataxia

Physical Exam
- Early mortality increases among those with any combination of impaired consciousness, hemiplegia, and conjugate gaze palsy
- Symptoms associated with the diagnosis of stroke or transient ischemic attack (TIA) are a sudden change in speech, visual loss, diplopia, numbness or tingling, paralysis or weakness, and nonorthostatic dizziness

TESTS

- Duplex carotid ultrasonography
- Cerebral angiography
- ECG
- Transthoracic ECG; if normal and a cardiac source is suspected, follow-up with transesophageal ECG.
- Holter monitoring
- EEG for suspected seizure
- Prothrombin time (PT) and partial thromboplastin time (PTT)
  - Coumadin prolongs PT.
- Antiphospholipid antibodies
- Cardiac enzymes

Imaging
Acute phase
- Multimodal CT of head
- MRI scan of brain with diffusion weighted imaging (DWI) remains the most powerful and accurate method for stroke identification.
- Arterial occlusions are seen with CTA as well as with MRA.
- Both CTA and MRA are highly reliable, noninvasive methods to verify the results of thrombolytic therapy.
- Quantitative CT perfusion and DWI/PWI (perfusion-weighted imaging) can rapidly provide functional information about brain perfusion and thus guide antithrombotic and neuroprotective strategies.
- Quantitative CTP is limited to a single slab of tissue per bolus, whereas MRI can provide whole-brain cerebral blood flow (CBF), cerebral blood volume (CBV), and mean transit time (MTT).
- The goal of perfusion imaging is to reliably identify and distinguish brain tissue that is ischemic and will develop infarction without a specific intervention from brain tissue that is already damaged and cannot escape infarction.

DIFFERENTIAL DIAGNOSIS

- Migraine
- Focal seizure
- Tumor
- Subdural hematoma
- Hypoglycemia; hyperglycemia; hypercalcemia

TREATMENT

- Acute phase: Inpatient care
- Surgical therapy
  - In medically fit patients with nondisabling stroke, carotid endarterectomy is indicated for stenosis of >70% on side ipsilateral to stroke.
  - Medical therapy for <50% stenosis, 50–69% depends on risk factors

GENERAL MEASURES
- Maintain oxygenation.
- Monitor cardiac rhythm for 48 hours.
- Control hyperglycemia (keep glucose <220 mg/dL [12.1 mmol/L]).
- Treat blood pressure >185/110 if patient will be or has been treated with IV tissue plasminogen activator.
- Do not treat elevated BP unless acute end-organ dysfunction (encephalopathy, myocardial ischemia, aortic dissection, acute renal failure) is suspected.
- Prevent hyperthermia.
- Introduce physiotherapy and ambulation early.
- Subcutaneous heparin 5,000 units SC q12h

Diet
- Alert with no dysphagia: Diet as tolerated (no added salt if hypertensive)
- Alert with dysphagia: Pureed dysphagia diet or nasogastric feeding tube if indicated

Activity
Ambulate as soon as possible.

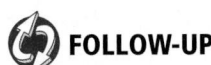 **MEDICATION (DRUGS)**

First Line
- IV tissue plasminogen activator (tPA) 0.9 mg/kg in highly selected cases within 3 hours of ischemic stroke symptom onset
- Enteric-coated aspirin 50–325 mg/d or
- Dipyridamole-aspirin (Aggrenox): Extended release, 200 mg/25 mg capsule PO b.i.d.; more efficacious than aspirin or dipyridamole alone. (3)[A]
- Clopidogrel (Plavix): 75 mg/d; fewer side effects, but shows only slight advantage over aspirin
- Warfarin: INR adjusted dose 2–4 for patients with atrial fibrillation and cardioembolic stroke has shown decreased risk of recurrent stroke compared to ASA 300 mg/d at 2.3 years. (1)[A]
- Contraindications
  - Enteric-coated aspirin: Active peptic ulcer disease, hypersensitivity to aspirin, patients who had bronchospastic reaction to aspirin or other NSAIDs
  - Warfarin: Intolerance or allergy, dementia, liver disease, active bleeding, pregnancy, recent head injury
- Precautions
  - Enteric-coated aspirin: May aggravate pre-existing peptic ulcer disease, may worsen symptoms in some patients with asthma
  - Clopidogrel and ticlopidine: Thrombotic thrombocytopenic purpura can occur.
  - Warfarin: Poor balance, alcohol/drug abuse, age >80

- Significant possible interactions
  - Enteric-coated aspirin: May potentiate effects of anticoagulants and sulfonylurea, hypoglycemic agents
  - Ticlopidine: Digoxin plasma levels decreased 15%, theophylline half-life increased from 8.6–12.2 hours
  - Warfarin: Aspirin, NSAIDs, antibiotics, tranquilizers

Second Line
Ticlopidine (Ticlid): The treatment of 250 mg PO b.i.d. has fallen out of favor, because of an unfavorable side-effect profile, risk of neutropenia, and need for CBC monitoring.
- Caution: 2.4% of patients develop neutropenia (0.8% severe neutropenia) that is reversible with cessation of drug; monitor blood counts every 2 weeks for the 1st 3 months

 FOLLOW-UP

PROGNOSIS
- Variable depending on severity of stroke
- Posterior circulation strokes have a higher acute mortality rate, but generally make a better functional recovery than do hemispheric strokes.

COMPLICATIONS
- Shoulder subluxation
- Hyperextension knee injury
- Depression
- Sympathetic dystrophy

PATIENT MONITORING
Follow the patient every 3 months for the 1st year, then yearly.

REFERENCES
1. Saxena R, Koudstaal PJ. Cochrane Stroke Group. Anticoagulants versus antiplatelet therapy for preventing stroke in patients with nonrheumatic atrial fibrillation and a history of stroke or transient ischemic attack. *Cochrane Database of Systematic Rev.* 1, 2006.
2. ACP Journal Club. Low-dose aspirin lowered stroke risk but not risks for MI or cardiovascular deaths in women. *ACP Journal Club.* 2005;143(2):33.
3. ACP Journal Club Dipyridamole given with or without aspirin reduces recurrent stroke. *ACP Journal Club.* 2005;143(1):10.
4. Aguilar MI, Hart R. Cochrane Stroke Group. Oral anticoagulants for preventing stroke in patients with non-valvular atrial fibrillation and no previous history of stroke or transient ischemic attacks. *Cochrane Database of Systematic Rev.* 1, 2006.

 MISCELLANEOUS

See also: Stroke rehabilitation, Transient ischemic attack (TIA)

CODES

ICD9-CM
- 431 Intracerebral hemorrhage
- 434.11 Cerebral embolism with cerebral infarction
- 436 Acute, but ill-defined, cerebrovascular disease

PATIENT TEACHING
National Stroke Association, 9707 E. Easter Lane, Englewood, CO 80112; (800-STROKES).

See Corresponding Diagnostic Algorithm

See Patient Handout on CD

S

STROKE REHABILITATION

Jeremy Collins, MD
Frank J. Domino, MD

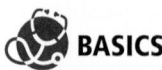 BASICS

DESCRIPTION
- Restoration of function after medical and neurologic stability have been achieved following cerebral compromise.
- Cerebrovascular diseases or disorders that affect CNS compromise delivery of blood or cause hemorrhage, resulting in ischemia, necrosis, and gliosis.
- Anterior lesions in the cerebrovascular system affect the arteries that supply the cerebral hemispheres and cause thrombotic strokes.
- Posterior lesions affect arteries that supply the brainstem and yield the crossed motor and/or sensory signs and symptoms of hemorrhagic strokes.
- Both anterior and posterior lesions can cause sudden death, but the lower in the CNS the lesion, or the more incomplete the lesion, or the more hemorrhagic the lesion, the higher the chance for neurologic return and also for 2nd and subsequent strokes.
- System(s) Affected: Cardiovascular; Nervous

ALERT
Geriatric Considerations
Heart disease, vascular disease, hypertension can lead to stroke.

Pediatric Considerations
Aneurysms, hypertension, tumors, trauma can lead to stroke.

Pregnancy Considerations
Hypertension in pregnancy can lead to stroke.

EPIDEMIOLOGY
- Predominant age: >45
- Predominant sex: Male > Female

Incidence
Annually: 150/100,000

Prevalence
Annually: 550/100,000

RISK FACTORS
- Many are lifestyle-oriented and preventable. Factors include: Coffee ingestion, cigarette smoking, obesity, inactivity, hyperactivity to the point of exhaustion, emotional lability, sexual hyperactivity, starvation, antidepressant or diet reduction medication, alcohol or recreational drug habituation, unusual stress states
- Ethnicity may be a risk factor, but relationships to factors above 1st must be clarified.
- Overly aggressive treatment of diabetes with insulin, hypoglycemia
- Vasculitis; immune, infections, associated with malignancy

Genetics
Similar to the probability of developing hypertension or coronary artery disease

ETIOLOGY
- Coronary artery disease
- Hypertension
- Cerebral arteriosclerosis
- Cardiac thrombus embolus
- Foreign body embolus
- Combination of gout, diabetes, hypertension untreated for 5–10 years before onset of stroke disorder
- Aneurysms and arteriovenous malformations

ASSOCIATED CONDITIONS
- Hypertension
- Coronary artery disease
- Diabetes mellitus
- Gout
- Atherosclerosis
- Smoking
- Alcoholism

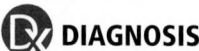 DIAGNOSIS

SIGNS AND SYMPTOMS
- Variable: Depends on the arterial system affected
- Hemiparesis
- Hemianesthesia
- Unilateral central facial palsy
- Homonymous hemianopsia
- Aphasia, apraxia (if the dominant cerebral hemisphere is involved)

TESTS
- Somatosensory, auditory, and visual evoked potential technology can monitor neurologic recovery.
- EEG sometimes useful in evaluating seizure disorders
- Cardiovascular stress testing to evaluate the extent of coronary artery disease
- Serum glucose level

Lab
- CBC
- Blood alcohol level
- Spinal fluid for routine studies (only if indicated)
- Urinalysis
- Rapid plasma reagent test
- Antinuclear antibody for collagen vascular disorders
- Consider quantitative immunoelectrophoresis with the combination of stroke disorders, anemia, hypertension
- Carotid flow studies

Imaging
- CT, MRI, and PET scanning give good data about anatomy, blood flow, and metabolic activity.
- Serial exams can delineate the course of this disease and reveal hydrocephalus or brain tumors.
- Total body bone scans can help diagnose reflex sympathetic dystrophy (hand–shoulder syndrome).

Diagnostic Procedures/Surgery
- Spinal taps, myelography, pneumoencephalography, angiography all have special indications and contraindications at this time. None is routinely used.
- Electrodiagnosis for neuritis, radiculitis in specialized centers if available
- Endovascular procedures have great diagnostic implications.

Pathological Findings
Thrombotic, hemorrhagic, mixed combinations can be present.

DIFFERENTIAL DIAGNOSIS
- Infection, tumor, bleeding disorders, endocrinologic, metabolic, gastrointestinal, toxic
- Different types of stroke disorders can occur in 1 patient.
- Liver failure with or without transplantation can be associated with cognitive deficits that persist even after transplantation.
- Brain tumors often present as stroke syndromes with significant personality and/or aphasic disorders and relatively less obvious weakness or spasticity on examination.

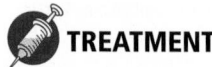 TREATMENT

INITIAL STABILIZATION
- Referral to a full-service rehabilitation center—a rehabilitation medicine team can make the difference between independence and dependency.
- Refer when medically and neurologically stable.

GENERAL MEASURES
- Full-service rehabilitation center characteristics
  - Comparison with national standards for admission, process, discharge, and follow-up care
  - Closed units
  - Regular team meetings to discuss long- and short-term objectives
  - Quality-assurance system in place
  - Accreditation by Commission on Accreditation of Rehabilitation Facilities
- Use deep heat (e.g., ultrasound, prolonged hydrotherapy) with caution in patients with reduced sensation and/or taking anticoagulants.
- Use hydrotherapy and/or isometric exercise cautiously in patients with limited cardiopulmonary reserve.
- In patients able to respond to the protocols after surgery, restorative, tendon transplant, or nerve transplants may be of value.
- Cardiac precautions and a CPR team may be required during exercise programs, because patients who are obese, hypertensive, or have coronary artery disease are at increased risk. Real-time monitoring might be required.
- Open units, especially in investor-owned, private rehabilitation centers, must be closely monitored for outcome and cost/benefit ratio type productivity quality.
- Inpatient rehab in acute rehab units is probably not necessary for stable, uncomplicated strokes (can be done as outpatient).
- Check and adjust serum glucose level if necessary.

Diet
Depends on other medical conditions, but control of hypertension and diabetes is important.

Activity
- Physical therapy, occupational therapy, speech pathology, psychology, and nursing therapy should be delivered to the patient for ≥3 hours/d throughout the inpatient stay.
- Patient must be able to tolerate this vigorous activity level.
  - If patient becomes medically or neurologically unstable during the inpatient stay, 48-hour leeway is usually built into the system. After that period, therapy must resume or the patient must be returned to an acute hospital bed.
  - Most stroke acute rehabilitation units can deliver this type of functional return within 1 month of inpatient stay, although length of stay is individually determined.
- Although most rehabilitative efforts take place within a very short time after ictus, successful rehabilitative efforts have taken place as long as 5 years later. This delayed response is frequent but partial.

MEDICATION (DRUGS)

First Line
- Use only what is absolutely necessary. Sleeping medications, such as flurazepam, can accumulate over time in stroke patients.
- As needed for underlying disorders (e.g., hypertension, heart disease) or for complications (e.g., seizures, deep vein thrombosis, pneumonitis)
- When neurologic and medical stability have been achieved, depression can be treated with a serotonin inhibitor antidepressant, for example, sertraline HCl 50 mg every morning.
- For thrombotic strokes or for patients with a high risk of this type of stroke, anticoagulant medications are important.
- Contraindications: Refer to the manufacturer's profile of each drug.
- Precautions
  - 4 or more medications will often have interactions; polypharmacy is frequent.
  - Antihypertensive medication can generate orthostatic hypotension.
  - Antidepressant medication can lower seizure threshold and interact with antihypertensive medications.
  - Muscle relaxants, tranquilizers, and major neuroleptic medication can confuse, delay return of memory and cognition, sedate, occasionally agitate, and obliterate spontaneous thought.
  - Unnecessary medications, such as antihistamines, should be withdrawn owing to risk of hypertension.
  - Elderly patients regularly require lower dosages of the above medications.
  - Most common cause of resistance to hypertensive medication is patient's failure to take medicine.
- Significant possible interactions
  - NSAIDs can adversely interact with psychotropic medication and can generate hypertension/GI bleeding.
  - Some NSAIDs contain sulfa drugs that will cause allergic reactions.
  - COX-2 NSAIDs should not be used.
  - Overly aggressive treatment of hypertension can yield hypotension and extend the stroke.

Second Line
- Reflex sympathetic dystrophy (shoulder–hand syndrome) can be treated with tizanidine (Zanaflex) 4–8 mg at bedtime and botulinum (Myobloc) injections.
- Flexor spasms in spasticity: To help control, tizanidine 4–8 mg at bedtime, diazepam 5 mg b.i.d. and/or baclofen 10 mg t.i.d.
- For spasticity in those not tolerating systemic medication: Either intrathecal baclofen by pump or botulinum toxin IM administration

SURGERY
- Microcatheter and microsurgical technology have been used to clip, embolize, or reset aneurysms and other lesions.
- Applied cardioangiographic technology has generated new endovascular treatment procedures.

FOLLOW-UP

PROGNOSIS
- Generally good, although pneumonia, respiratory failure, heart failure, and myocardial infarction occur more frequently after stroke
- Outcome studies: Acute rehab center programs generate 33% more functional improvement than comparable skilled nursing facilities, but tend to cost more.
- Premature discharges can often be associated with suboptimal functional recovery.

COMPLICATIONS
- Reflex sympathetic dystrophy syndromes—such as hand–shoulder syndrome—are nonspecific complications and last for 12 weeks before subsiding to adhesive capsulitis.
- Tendonitis–bursitis–capsulitis may coexist with prolonged paralysis
  - Prolonged range-of-motion and neuromuscular re-education exercises help retard functional deterioration of the limb.
  - Electrical stimulation and biofeedback for control and relaxation have also been used, but the treatment of choice is restoration of function.
- Diabetes and alcohol intake will add peripheral neuritis. Diabetes could also be associated (especially in males) with gout and hypertension.
- Many patients develop osteoporosis—especially on side of paresis. The normal side can develop osteoarthritis.
- Repeat strokes from lack of hypertension and/or artery disease control

PATIENT MONITORING
- Within the month following discharge, patient and family should be seen in outpatient group "alumni" day coordinated with an interdisciplinary outpatient clinic appointment.
- If outpatient therapy is rendered, team therapist(s) should meet with the physician regularly to rate progress and discuss long- and short-term objectives.
- For 1st uncomplicated stroke patients: When the acute rehab is completed, the rest of the rehab can be accomplished as an outpatient or in a day care program.

REFERENCES

1. Clinchot DM, Bogner JA, Kaplan PE. Cerebral aneurysms. *Arch Phys Med Rehabil.* 1997;78: 346–349.
2. Clinchot DM, et al. Cerebral aneurysms and arteriovenous malformations. *Arch Phys Med Rehabil.* 1994;75:1342–1351.
3. Kaplan PE, Cailliet R, Kaplan C. Stroke Rehabilitation. Boston: Butterworth, 2002.
4. Kaplan PE, Clinchot DM, Firnett JA. Cognitive deficits after hepatic transplantation. *Brain Inj.* 1996;10:599–607.

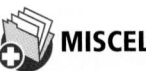 **MISCELLANEOUS**

See also: Brain injury-post acute care issues; Stroke (brain attack)

CODES

ICD9-CM
438.9 Unspecified late effects of cerebrovascular disease

PATIENT TEACHING
- Stroke is usually an unnecessary illness. Major risk factors are nearly all preventable. The difficulty that arises is that the patient's lifestyle must be changed. Aerobic daily exercise, diet, and a balanced conditioning program will significantly lower stroke risk. Patients mount a great deal of active and passive resistance.
- The progressive physical and mental deterioration noted with hypertension and/or coronary artery disease is not inevitable.
- Family pressure and support are helpful in interesting the patient in his health in a consistent and sustained manner.
- Disuse will add subsequent complications and sequelae.
- 2nd complex strokes—patients with 2nd ictus and/or renal failure, heart failure, or cor pulmonale—might require 20–30 days of inpatient rehab in a skilled nursing facility before disposition.

S

SUBARACHNOID HEMORRHAGE

Michael Previti, MD

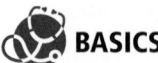 **BASICS**

DESCRIPTION
- Extravasation of blood into subarachnoid space, particularly of basal cisterns, and into CSF pathways including ventricles.
- Accounts for 2–5% of new strokes.
- Traumatic: More common; related to head trauma
- Spontaneous: 80% due to ruptured intracranial saccular aneurysms and have a much worse prognosis than nonaneurysmal subarachnoid hemorrhages (SAHs).
- May also occur from rupture of arteriovenous malformations (AVMs).
- System(s) Affected: Nervous

ALERT
Pregnancy Considerations
Increased BP and blood volume may predispose pregnant women to hemorrhages.

GENERAL PREVENTION
- Incidental aneurysms have risk of hemorrhage according to size; therefore, endovascular coiling or surgical clipping may be indicated.
- The 5-year cumulative rate of aneurysmal rupture in the internal carotid artery, anterior cerebral artery, middle cerebral artery, or anterior communicating artery based on size
  - <7 mm: 0%
  - 7–12 mm: 2.6%
  - 13–24 mm: 14.5%
  - >25 mm: 40%
- The 5-year cumulative rate of aneurysmal rupture in the vertebral, basilar, posterior communicating arteries by size
  - <7 mm: 2.5%
  - 7–12 mm: 14.5%
  - 13–24 mm: 18.4%
  - >25 mm: 50%
- In younger age groups, incidentally found AVMs have a 2% risk of rupture per year.

EPIDEMIOLOGY
- Mean age of presentation is 55 years.
- Majority occur in 4th–7th decades.
- SAHs due to AVMs occur in 2nd–4th decades.
- Female > Male (1.6:1)
- Blacks > Whites (2.1:1)

Incidence
Spontaneous: 10.5/100,000 person years

Prevalence
In the US: 21,000–33,000 new cases each year

RISK FACTORS
- Cigarette smoking
- Cocaine use
- Heavy alcohol use
- Hypertension associated with rupture of aneurysm, but not with saccular aneurysms
- 1st-degree relatives with SAH
- AVMs

ETIOLOGY
- Trauma
- Intracranial saccular aneurysm
- Intracranial AVM
- Hypertension
- Rarely, tumors and blood dyscrasias

ASSOCIATED CONDITIONS
- Morbidity and mortality of SAH are determined by complications that develop after the initial bleed.
- Outcome predicted by the World Federation of Neurological Surgeons clinical grading.
- Blood volume on initial CT is predictive of vasospasm.
- The following complications are common
  - Cerebral vasospasm occurs within 4–12 days of initial bleed, and is seen angiographically in 67%.
  - Cardiac arrhythmias occur in 35% of patients.
  - Seizures occur in up to 33% of patients.
  - Electrolyte disturbances (including SIADH and cerebral salt wasting) occur in 28% of patients.
  - Pulmonary edema occurs in 23% of patients.
  - Hydrocephalus occurs in 20% of patients.
  - Rebleeding occurs in 7% of patients and has a 50% risk of permanent neurologic damage.

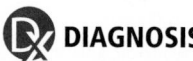 **DIAGNOSIS**

SIGNS AND SYMPTOMS
- Abrupt onset of headache ("worst headache of life") associated with stiff neck, nausea, vomiting, photophobia, and/or LOC.
- Headache may be the only presenting symptom in up to 40% of patients and may disappear within hours (so called *thunderclap headaches*, *sentinel bleeds*, or *warning leaks*).

History
Assess for recent head trauma, perimesencephalic hemorrhage of SAH, hypertension, nicotine/EtOH/cocaine use, AVMs, family history of SAH, and current use of anticoagulants.

Physical Exam
- Retinal hemorrhages
- Meningismus
- Diminished consciousness, calculate Glasgow Coma Scale on all patients
- Focal neurologic signs, such as 3rd-nerve palsy (p. comm. aneurysm), 6th-nerve palsy (increased intracranial pressure [ICP]), bilateral leg weakness and/or abulia (a. comm. aneurysm), hemiparesis and/or aphasia and/or visuospatial neglect (MCA aneurysm).
- Perform lumbar puncture if CT is negative and suspicion is high. Elevated opening pressure, xanthochromia (takes 12 hours to develop), or RBCs unchanged in tubes 1–4 are consistent with SAH.

TESTS
Imaging
- Noncontrast head CT with thin cuts through the base of the brain. Sensitivity drops to 50% at 7 days, but is 100 at 12 hours and 93% at 24 hours.
- CT may show hydrocephalus, cerebral edema, intraparenchymal bleeds, and can predict the site of rupture (particularly in the anterior circulation).
- CT is the most reliable prediction of vasospasm and poor outcome using Fisher Scale.
- CT can rule out mass effect in order to safely perform a necessary lumbar puncture.
- If CT or LP are positive, check cerebral angiography (gold standard) or CT angiography; they have similar sensitivity and specificity.
- If 2nd study is negative, high-definition MRI should be performed. MRA can be used but is not the standard for surgical planning.
- Important: If no source of SAH is found intracranially, obtain MRI spinal or myelography.

DIFFERENTIAL DIAGNOSIS
- Traumatic SAH
- Aneurysmal rupture (including mycotic aneurysms associated with bacterial endocarditis)
- AVM
- Arterial dissection with intracranial extension
- Pituitary apoplexy
- Drug abuse (e.g. cocaine) with or without aneurysm as a result of vasculitis
- Coagulopathies
- Migraine (especially with aura)

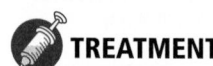 **TREATMENT**

PRE HOSPITAL
- Stabilize ABCs, IV, O₂ monitor
- After stabilized, consider transfer to neurovascular center

GENERAL MANAGEMENT
- Initial therapy in ICU. Treatment is directed to prevent complications, including rebleeding, hydrocephalus, and cerebral vasospasm.
- BP is maintained within normal limits with IV labetalol and nicardipine.
- Maintain euvolemia (CVP 5–8 mm Hg) *unless* cerebral vasospasm is present (see below).
- Evaluate and treat myocardial injury and/or arrhythmias.
- Distinguish cardiogenic vs. neurogenic pulmonary edema and treat appropriately.
- Control pain with morphine sulfate 2–4 mg IV q2–4h.
- Maintain serum glucose at 80–120 mg/dL with insulin sliding scale or continuous infusion.
- Maintain core body temperature ≤37.2°C.
- DVT prophylaxis with thigh-high stockings and compressive devices; *after* aneurysm is secured; subcutaneous heparin 5,000 U SC t.i.d.
- GI prophylaxis with ranitidine 150 mg PO b.i.d. (50 mg IV q8–12h) or lansoprazole 30 mg/d PO
- Stool softeners may also be used.

Diet
If swallow evaluation allows, give PO diet.

Activity
Strict bed rest, reduced noise level, and limited visitors until source of bleeding is secured.

SPECIAL THERAPY
Perform neuropsychological testing before discharge, and schedule cognitive rehabilitation

Physical Therapy
Aggressive physical, occupational and, speech evaluation.

MEDICATION (DRUGS)

- Nimodipine 60 mg PO (via nasogastric tube if necessary) q4h for 21 days for prevention of cerebral vasospasm; start immediately.
- Antifibrinolytic agents may be used *before* aneurysm treatment (aminocaproic acid 5 g IV in the 1st 24–48 hours with a 1.5 g/h infusion thereafter).
- Phenytoin 3–5 mg/kg/d PO or IV, valproic acid 15–45 mg/kg/d PO or IV, or phenobarbital 4 mg/kg IV may be used as seizure prophylaxis.
- Treat seizures with lorazepam 0.1 mg/kg IV at a 2 mg/min rate followed by phenytoin 20 mg/kg IV bolus at <50 mg/min up to 30 mg/kg.
- SIADH vs. cerebral salt wasting *must* be distinguished with serum and urine electrolytes.
- Symptomatic vasospasm is currently treated with hypervolemia (CVP 8–12 mm Hg, PCWP 12–16 mm Hg) and/or induced hypertension

SURGERY
- Endovascular coiling and surgical clipping are options for securing aneurysms. Aneurysmal securing should be performed within 1st 72 hours.
- Rebleeding should be dealt with immediately by treatment of aneurysm.
- 25–30% of aneurysms will be multiple.
- Hydrocephalus should be treated with external ventricular drain (EVD), lumbar drain, or permanent CSF drainage.
- Arteriovenous malformations may be obliterated with embolization and surgery.

PROGNOSIS
- Average case fatality rate is 51% overall: 10% before receiving care, 25% within the 1st 24 hours
- 25–30% of patients die from spontaneous SAH due to aneurysm. Highest morbidity secondary to cerebral vasospasm.
- If aneurysm can be successfully obliterated and vasospasm treated effectively, satisfactory outcome occurs in 50–65% of patients.
- 45–50% of survivors report long-term cognitive impairment of varying degrees.
- 50–75% of survivors return to work after 1 year.

COMPLICATIONS
- Temporary and permanent neurologic deficits and/or disorders (e.g., seizures, headache, SIADH)
- Death

PATIENT MONITORING
As needed

REFERENCES

1. Suarez JI, Tarr RW, Selman WR. Aneurysmal subarachnoid hemorrhage. *N Engl J Med*. 2006;354:387–396.
2. Whitfield PC, Kirkpatrick PJ. Timing of surgery for aneurysmal subarachnoid haemorrhage. *Cochrane Database Sys Rev*. 2006;1.
3. Lapointe M, Haines S. Fibrinolytic therapy for intraventricular hemorrhage in adults. *Cochrane Database Sys Rev*. 2006;1.
4. van der Schaaf I, Algra A, Wermer M, et al. Endovascular coiling versus neurosurgical clipping for patients with aneurysmal subarachnoid haemorrhage. *Cochrane Database Sys Rev*. 2006;1.
5. Rinkel GJE, Feigin VL, Algra A, et al. Calcium antagonists for aneurysmal subarachnoid haemorrhage. *Cochrane Database Sys Rev*. 2006;1.
6. Roos YBWEM, Rinkel GJE, Vermeulen M, et al. Antifibrinolytic therapy for aneurysmal subarachnoid haemorrhage. *Cochrane Database Sys Rev*. 2006;1.
7. Intensive insulin therapy reduced the incidence of neurologic complications in critically ill patients. *ACP Journal Club*. 2006;144(1):20.
8. Review: Computed tomographic angiography and magnetic resonance angiography accurately detect intracranial aneurysms. *ACP Journal Club*. 2001;134(3):113.
9. Mustonen T, Koivisto T, Vanninen E, et al. Cerebral perfusion heterogeneity and complexity in patients with acute subarachnoid haemorrhage. *Nucl Med Commun*. 2006;27(2):157–164.
10. Wijdicks EF. Induced hypothermia in neurocatastrophes: Feeling the chill. *Rev Neurol Dis*. 2004;1(1):10–15. Review.

ADDITIONAL READING

Rinkel GJE, Feigin VL, Algra A, van Gijn J. Circulatory volume expansion therapy for aneurysmal subarachnoid haemorrhage. *Cochrane Database Sys Rev*. 2006;1.

 MISCELLANEOUS

CODES

ICD9-CM
- 430 Subarachnoid hemorrhage
- 852.00 Subarachnoid hemorrhage following injury without mention of open intracranial wound, unspecified state of consciousness

PATIENT TEACHING

See Corresponding Diagnostic Algorithm

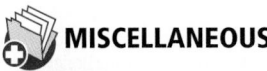

SUBCLAVIAN STEAL SYNDROME

Frederico Milla, MD
Ruben Peralta, MD, FACS

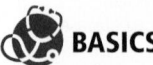 **BASICS**

DESCRIPTION

Origin of the subclavian artery becomes occluded, compromising blood flow to the ipsilateral upper extremity. To supplement this perfusion, blood flow from the vertebral artery reverses, leading to vertebral-basilar insufficiency. Symptoms may be especially prominent when demand increases, for example during upper extremity exercise.

EPIDEMIOLOGY

- Predominant age
  - Age >55 years—atherosclerotic etiology
  - Age <30 years—90% of patients with Takayasu arteritis
- Predominant sex: Male > Female (2:1)

Incidence

Unknown

RISK FACTORS

- Smoking
- Hypertension
- Diabetes
- Hyperlipidemia

ETIOLOGY

- Arteriosclerosis obliterans of the proximal subclavian artery in 95% of cases
- Less common causes of obstruction
  - Dissecting aneurysm of aortic arch
  - Trauma
  - Embolus
  - Takayasu arteritis

ASSOCIATED CONDITIONS

- Carotid artery disease
- Heart disease
- Arteriosclerosis

ALERT

Geriatric Considerations

Older patients are more likely to have arteriosclerosis.

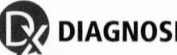 **DIAGNOSIS**

SIGNS AND SYMPTOMS

- Most common: Vertigo or presyncope following upper extremity exercise. The reversal of flow down the ipsilateral vertebral artery results in a relative vertebral-basilar insufficiency.
- Less common: Weakness and clumsiness of an extremity, loss of vision, homonymous hemianopsia, ataxia, and drop attacks
- Arm claudication following minimal exercise
- Reduced blood pressure of >20 mm Hg in involved arm
- Symptoms should be reproducible by exercising the arm

Physical Exam

- Absent or diminished pulses in ipsilateral arm
- Reduced blood pressure (>20 mm Hg) when compared to the contralateral arm

TESTS

- Noninvasive measurement of BP in upper extremities
- Pulse volume recording of upper extremities

Lab

- No labs findings are pathognomonic for subclavian steal syndrome.
- If Takayasu arteritis is suspected
  - Erythrocyte sedimentation rate (elevated)
  - Complete blood count (thrombocytosis)
  - Electrocardiogram (ischemic pattern)
  - Chest radiograph (widening of thoracic aorta)

Imaging

- Duplex scanning of extracranial vessels
- Magnetic Resonance Angiography (1)[B]
- Arteriogram of arch vessels with delayed films of vertebral arteries

Diagnostic Procedures/Surgery

Arteriography

DIFFERENTIAL DIAGNOSIS

- Vascular: Intracranial vascular disease, carotid artery disease, vertebral artery disease
- Neurogenic: Brain tumor, seizures, subdural hematoma
- Cardiac arrhythmias

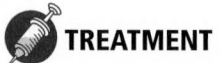 **TREATMENT**

INITIAL STABILIZATION

Outpatient care unless vascular surgery is anticipated

GENERAL MEASURES

Reduce cholesterol levels, if appropriate, using diet or medication.

Diet

Low-cholesterol diet, if appropriate

Activity

Reduced exercise of arms

MEDICATION (DRUGS)

None

SURGERY

Treatment options include

- Balloon angioplasty. Stent insertion may increase long-term patency rates. (2,3)[B]

- Carotid-subclavian bypass

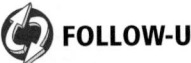 **FOLLOW-UP**

PROGNOSIS

Good

COMPLICATIONS

Completed stroke

PATIENT MONITORING

Annual physical examination including BP reading in both arms

REFERENCES

1. Wu C, Zhang J, Ladner CJ, et al. Subclavian steal syndrome: Diagnosis with perfusion metrics from contrast-enhanced MR angiographic bolus-timing examination-initial experience. *Radiology* 2005;235:927–933.
2. Taylor CL, Selman WR, Ratcheson RA. Steal affecting the central nervous system. *Neurosurgery.* 2002;51:856–857.
3. White CJ. Non-surgical treatment of patients with peripheral vascular disease. *Br Med Bull* 2001;59:173–192.
4. Valadez ER, Martinez PH, Peralta SO, et al. Imaging diagnosis of subclavian steal syndrome secondary to Takayasu arteritis affecting a left-side subclavian artery. *Arch Med Res* 2003;34:433–438.

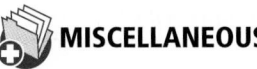 **MISCELLANEOUS**

See also: Arteriosclerosis obliterans, Takayasu syndrome

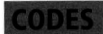 **CODES**

ICD9-CM

435.2 Subclavian steal syndrome

PATIENT TEACHING

- Prevent injury to arm
- Reduce exercise of arm

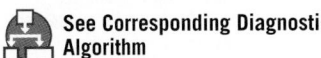 **See Corresponding Diagnostic Algorithm**

S

SUBDURAL HEMATOMA

Oren N. Gottfried, MD
Martin E. Weinand, MD

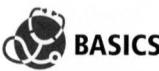 **BASICS**

DESCRIPTION
- Accumulation of blood in subdural space
  - Acute: Most severe form, usually result of trauma involving acceleration or deceleration head injury and commonly associated with parenchymal brain injury. Hematoma age is ≤3 days.
  - Chronic: Often result of trivial head injury in older patients; 25–50% have no history of head trauma. Hematoma is classically >3 weeks and associated with encapsulating membrane.
  - Subacute: Appearing 4–21 days from maturation of acute subdural hematoma
- System(s) Affected: Cardiovascular; Nervous
- Synonym(s): Subdural hemorrhage

GENERAL PREVENTION
- Acute: Trauma-prevention programs
- Chronic
  - Alcoholism prevention
  - Medical and surgical management of epilepsy
  - Conservative use of anticoagulation therapy
  - Medium-pressure or high-pressure ventriculoperitoneal shunt valves in at-risk patients with hydrocephalus

EPIDEMIOLOGY
- Predominant age
  - Acute: <60 years. Relatively infrequent in newborns and children, occurring 25% as often as in adults.
  - Chronic: >50 years. Occurs in children of all ages
- Predominant sex: Male > Female

Incidence
Chronic: Peak incidence at ~6 months and rarely after 1 year of age

Prevalence
- Acute
  - 1–2/100,000
  - Present with 5–22% of episodes of severe head trauma
- Chronic: 1–2/100,000

RISK FACTORS
- Acute
  - Severe head trauma
  - High-velocity acceleration or deceleration head injury (motor vehicle accidents, falls, blunt head trauma)
  - Suspected nonaccidental trauma in infants
- Chronic
  - Chronic alcoholism
  - Epilepsy
  - Coagulopathy/anticoagulation therapy
  - CSF shunt for hydrocephalus
  - Rarely, metastatic carcinoma to subdural space

ALERT
Cerebral atrophy common and predisposes to subdural hematomas

ETIOLOGY
- Acute
  - High-velocity acceleration or deceleration head injury resulting in tearing of bridging veins between cerebral cortex and dural venous sinuses
  - Injury to surface of brain with bleeding from injured cortical vessels
- Chronic
  - Adults: Often from trivial head injury
  - Children: May be caused by unrecognized/unreported trauma, abuse, or, rarely, birth trauma
  - Balance between recurrent bleeding from hematoma membrane and resorption determines ultimate size of hematoma.

ASSOCIATED CONDITIONS
- Acute
  - Multisystem trauma
  - Cervical spinal cord injury
  - Injury to the thoracic, lumbar, or sacral spine
  - Disseminated intravascular coagulation
  - Epilepsy
- Chronic
  - Alcoholism
  - Epilepsy
  - Coagulopathy
  - CSF shunt
  - Birth trauma
  - Child abuse
  - Rarely, metastatic carcinoma

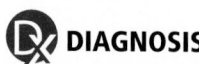 **DIAGNOSIS**

SIGNS AND SYMPTOMS
- Acute
  - Altered level of consciousness: 99%
  - Pupillary irregularity (usually unilateral to hematoma): 47–53%
  - Hemiparesis (usually contralateral to hematoma): 34–47%
  - Decerebrate posturing or flaccid motor exam: 47%
  - Papilledema: 16%
  - Cranial nerve VI palsy: 5%
- Chronic
  - Impaired consciousness: 53%
  - Hemiparesis: 45%
  - Papilledema: 24%
  - Cranial nerve III abnormality: 11%
  - Hemianopsia: 7%
  - Infants often present with accelerated increase in head size with or without irritability, poor feeding, occasional vomiting, or tension of anterior fontanelle (60% of cases).
  - Infants may present with seizures.

TESTS
- EEG for seizures
- ICU: Continuous cardiac monitoring often in conjunction with continuous monitoring of intra-arterial pressure and intracranial pressure (ventriculostomy or intraparenchymal or subdural pressure–monitoring probe)

Lab
- Acute: Consumptive coagulopathy due to underlying parenchymal injury diagnosed with
  - Elevated PT and PTT
  - Elevated fibrin degradation products
  - Decreased fibrinogen
  - Decreased platelet level
  - Extended bleeding time
- Chronic
  - Bleeding time or coagulation parameters: Appropriate abnormalities produced by predisposing factors such as coagulopathy or anticoagulation therapy
  - Subtherapeutic anticonvulsant levels in patients with epilepsy
  - Serum ethanol level in alcoholics
- Drugs that may alter lab results: Anticoagulants (e.g., warfarin)
- Disorders that may alter lab results: DIC and other coagulopathies (e.g., hemophilia)

Imaging
- Acute
  - Imaging study of choice: CT head scan (with intravascular contrast if hemoglobin ≤9 g/d)
  - Axial view demonstrates hyperdense, cresenteric, extra-axial collection usually adjacent to inner table
- Chronic
  - Imaging study of choice: CT head scan
  - Hematomas usually evolve from isodense to hypodense by 3 weeks.
  - MRI head scan: Often necessary for hematomas isodense with brain due to mixture of chronic hematoma with recurrent hemorrhage

Pathological Findings
- Acute: Fresh hemorrhage
- Chronic
  - Liquefied hematoma
  - Outer membrane beneath dura after 1 week
  - Inner membrane between hematoma and arachnoid after 3 weeks
  - On rare occasions, cytology examination may reveal association between metastatic carcinoma cells and hemorrhage

DIFFERENTIAL DIAGNOSIS
- Acute versus chronic
- Other forms of intracranial hematoma (e.g., epidural hematoma, cerebral contusion/hematoma)
- Dementia
- Stroke
- Transient ischemic attack
- Brain tumor
- Subdural empyema
- Meningitis

ALERT
The insidious onset of symptoms may lead to misdiagnosis of dementia, tumor, or depression.

TREATMENT

GENERAL MEASURES

- Inpatient
- Acute: medical management
  - Control of elevated intracranial pressure with osmotic and loop diuretics
  - Hyperventilation to induce hypocapnia ($PaCO_2$ of 22–28 mm Hg [2.9–3.7 kPa])
  - Elevate head of bed to reduce intracranial pressure.
  - Avoid flexion of lower body until thoracic, lumbar, or sacral spine injuries are ruled out.
  - Maintain patient in rigid cervical collar until cervical spine is cleared radiographically.
- Subacute
  - Maintenance of adequate airway and ventilation and support of cardiovascular system to promote normal cerebral perfusion
  - Treatment of multisystem trauma and precautions for cervical and other spine injury
- Chronic
  - Keep head of bed flat.
  - Take appropriate precautions if spinal injury is present.

Diet

- Acute: Most patients require enteral or total parenteral nutrition initially.
- Chronic: Depending on level of consciousness, patients can usually have diet advanced to regular food as tolerated.

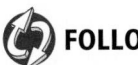 MEDICATION (DRUGS)

First Line

- Acute
  - Prior to surgery, management of cerebral edema and elevated intracranial pressure may require mannitol 20% solution 0.5–1.0 g/kg followed by 0.25–0.75 g/kg q4–6h. If loop diuretic used in conjunction with mannitol, administer furosemide (Lasix) 0.5 mg/kg IV. Check serum osmolality q8h and serum electrolytes at least daily. A 5% or 25% albumin preparation (Plasmanate) may be used either as continuous or intermittent infusion to augment osmotherapy as needed.
  - Seizure prophylaxis includes phenytoin (Dilantin) 1000 mg load (50 mg/min IV) with ECG monitoring, followed by 100 mg IV q8h or as needed to maintain therapeutic blood levels (10–20 μg/mL [40–79 μmol/L]). Convert Dilantin therapy to oral route as soon as possible to avoid cardiovascular complications of IV Dilantin administration.
- Chronic
  - Medical management alone is frequently unsuccessful and entails risks of neurological deterioration.
  - However, when small and asymptomatic, may be appropriate to treat conservatively with observation, as some chronic subdural hematomas have been known to resolve spontaneously.
  - Steroids may be helpful in some patients, if not otherwise contraindicated.
- Contraindications, precautions, and significant possible interactions: Refer to the manufacturer's literature.

SURGERY

- Acute: Emergent craniotomy indicated for evacuation of hematomas causing significant mass effect
- Subacute
  - If patient is neurologically stable, surgery may be delayed until hematoma matures and becomes chronic, at which time a burr hole drainage can be performed.
  - If causing significant mass effect and neurological deficit, may require craniotomy for evacuation
- Chronic: Burr hole drainage; some neurosurgeons leave a catheter in subdural space for 24 hours after operation

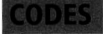 FOLLOW-UP

PROGNOSIS

Outcome highly dependent on presurgical neurological status

- Acute
  - Mortality >50%; lower in patients <40 years old than in those >40 years old
  - Significant neurological disability and impairment of function seen in most surviving patients
  - Seizure prophylaxis usually required for ≥1 year
- Chronic
  - Mortality <10%
  - Most patients resume preoperative functional status.

COMPLICATIONS

- Acute: Immediate postoperative complications include
  - Elevated intracranial pressure and brain edema
  - New or recurrent hematoma
  - Infection
  - Seizures (in ~1/3 of cases)
- Chronic:
  - Recurrent hematoma in up to 50% of cases (can be alleviated by use of subdural drainage catheters)
  - Infection (subdural empyema, wound)
  - Seizures in up to 10% of cases

PATIENT MONITORING

- Anticonvulsant levels should be checked approximately every 3–6 months after initiation.
- Consider discontinuing anticonvulsant if patient has no seizures for ≥1 year.
- EEG may complement decision-making process for discontinuation of anticonvulsants.

REFERENCES

1. Francel et al. Diagnosis and treatment of moderate and severe head injuries in infants and children. In: Youmans JR, ed. *Neurological Surgery*. 4th ed. Philadelphia, PA: WB Saunders; 1996: 1730–1766.
2. Greenberg MS. *Handbook of Neurosurgery*. 4th ed. Lakeland, FL: Greenberg Graphics; 1997.
3. Samudrala S, Cooper PR. Traumatic intracranial hematomas. In: Wilkins RH, Rengachary SS, eds. *Neurosurgery*. 2nd ed. New York, NY: McGraw-Hill; 1996: 2797–2807.

S

 MISCELLANEOUS

CODES

ICD9-CM

852.30 Subdural hemorrhage following injury with open intracranial wound, unspecified state of consciousness

PATIENT TEACHING

The National Institute of Neurological and Communicative Disorders and Stroke (NINDS), the National Institutes of Health, Bethesda, MD 20892

See Corresponding Diagnostic Algorithm

SUBPHRENIC ABSCESS

Ruben Peralta, MD, FACS
Sarah Guzofski, MD

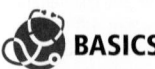 **BASICS**

DESCRIPTION
Any localized collection of pus below the diaphragm.
- Synonym(s): Subdiaphragmatic abscess

RISK FACTORS
- Operative procedure with significant contamination
- Patients with chronic disease: Diabetes, cirrhosis, renal failure, malnutrition
- Patients receiving corticosteroids, chemotherapy, radiotherapy
- Immunosuppression

ETIOLOGY
- Complications of abdominal surgery cause 50% of cases.
- Abdominal trauma
- Gastrointestinal perforations: Appendicitis, diverticulitis, duodenal or gastric ulcer
- Neoplastic disease
- Iatrogenic, for example, after cholecystectomy, retained stone
- Organisms: Ptolymicrobial, mixed aerobic and anaerobic
  - Aerobic
    ○ Escherichia
    ○ Enterococcus
  - Anaerobic
    ○ Bacteroides fragilis
    ○ Peptostreptococcus
    ○ Clostridium

ASSOCIATED CONDITIONS
- Multisystem organ failure
- Sepsis
- Fistula

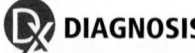 **DIAGNOSIS**

SIGNS AND SYMPTOMS
- High-spiking fever with chills and diaphoresis
- Ileus
- Abdominal pain
- Nausea
- Tachycardia
- Hypotension
- Chest pain
- Dyspnea
- Shoulder pain
- Hiccups

Physical Exam
- Localized abdominal tenderness with or without rebound
- Anterior abdominal wall erythema
- Rales at lung base

TESTS
Lab
- WBC
- Blood cultures
- Serum chemistry

Imaging
- CT scan
- Ultrasound
- Plain films of chest and abdomen display elevation and immobility of right diaphragm and fluid in right costophrenic sulcus; air–fluid level in subphrenic space, pleural effusion

Diagnostic Procedures/Surgery
CT- or ultrasound-guided percutaneous drainage (1)[B]

DIFFERENTIAL DIAGNOSIS
- Other intra-abdominal abscesses
- Empyema

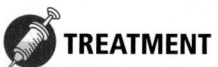 **TREATMENT**

Inpatient care

GENERAL MEASURES
- IV fluid resuscitation
- Drainage of abscess
- Antibiotics
- Supportive care: nutrition, monitoring, oxygenation, hydration
- Swan-Ganz catheter if condition unstable
- Mechanical ventilation if necessary
- Vasopressors if indicated

Diet
NPO until intestinal function returns

Activity
As tolerated

MEDICATION (DRUGS)

First Line

Broad-spectrum antibiotics based on culture and sensitivity (2)[B]

SURGERY

- Adequate drainage of abscess: Percutaneous and/or surgical
- Percutaneous drainage is not advised if
  - Abscess is multiloculated.
  - Drainage route would traverse bowel or uncontaminated peritoneal or pleural space.
  - Source of continued contamination is still present.
  - Fungal infection
  - Pus is too viscous.
- Surgical drainage is mandated if patient fails to respond to percutaneous drainage in 24–48 hours.

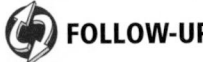 ## FOLLOW-UP

PROGNOSIS

Simple abscess, i.e., perforated appendicitis treated with drainage and antibiotics has a low mortality rate. High mortality rate should be expected in elderly patients with complex abscess who develop multiorgan failure.

COMPLICATIONS

- Mortality with treatment: Range 5–65%
- Multisystem organ failure
- Recurrent abscess
- Hemorrhage
- Bowel obstruction
- Wound dehiscence
- Continuing sepsis
- Pneumonia
- Pleural effusion
- Suppurative pylephlebitis

PATIENT MONITORING

Follow labs and radiographic studies as clinically indicated.

REFERENCES

1. Cinat ME, Wilson SE, Din AM. Determinants for successful percutaneous image-guided drainage of intra-abdominal abscess. *Arch Surg.* 2002; 137:845–849.
2. Solomkin JS, et al. Guidelines for the selection of antiinfective agents for complicated intraabdominal infection. *CID.* 2003;37:997–1005.
3. Men S, et al. Percutaneous drainage of abdominal abscess, 2002. *Euro J Radiol.* 2002;43:204–215.

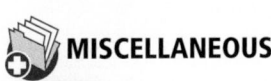 ## MISCELLANEOUS

CODES

ICD9-CM

- 567.22 Peritoneal abscess
- 998.59 Other postoperative infection

S

SUBSTANCE USE DISORDERS

S. Lindsey Clarke, MD

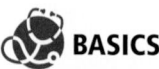 **BASICS**

DESCRIPTION

- Any pattern of substance use causing significant physical, mental, or social dysfunction
- Substances of abuse include
  - Alcohol
  - Amphetamines (black beauties, truck drivers, hearts, uppers, speed)
  - Anabolic steroids (nandrolone [Durabolin], oxandrolone); testosterone (Depo-Testosterone)
  - Barbiturates (barbs, red birds, yellow jackets)
  - Benzodiazepines (downers, candy, tranks)
  - Cannabinoids: Hashish, marijuana (dope, grass, joint, pot, reefer, sinsemilla, weed)
  - Cocaine (coke, crack, blow, rocks, snow)
  - Codeine (Cody, school boy)
  - Fentanyl (Apache, China girl, dance fever)
  - Flunitrazepam (Mexican Valium, roofies)
  - γ-Hydroxybutyrate (GHB, liquid ecstasy, woman's Viagra)
  - Heroin (diacetylmorphine; horse, junk, smack, white horse, brown sugar)
  - Inhalants (gasoline, glue, paint thinners, nitrous oxide)
  - Ketamine (cat Valium, Special K, vitamin K)
  - Lysergic acid diethylamide (LSD; acid, microdot, cubes, yellow sunshine)
  - Mescaline, psilocybin (mushrooms, peyote)
  - Methadone (Methadose)
  - Methamphetamines (crank, crystal, ice, fire, speed; and "designer drugs": Adam, clarity, ecstasy, Eve, MDMA, XTC, lover's speed)
  - Methaqualone (Quaalude, mandrex)
  - Methylphenidate (Ritalin, JIF, Skippy, MPH)
  - Morphine (M, Miss Emma, monkey)
  - Nicotine (tobacco)
  - Opium (Paregoric, big O, block)
  - Oxycodone, hydrocodone, hydromorphone, meperidine, propoxyphene
  - Phencyclidine (PCP; angel dust, hog, love boat, peace pill, supergrass, ozone, wack)
- System(s) Affected: Cardiovascular; Endocrine/Metabolic; Nervous
- Synonym(s): Drug abuse; Drug dependence; Substance abuse

ALERT

Geriatric Considerations
- Alcohol is the most commonly abused substance and often goes unrecognized.
- Higher potential for drug interactions

Pregnancy Considerations
Pregnant women: Substance abuse may cause major problems that can lead to fetal abnormality, morbidity, and death of infant and mother.

GENERAL PREVENTION
Early identification and aggressive early intervention (mild substance use disorders respond better to treatment intervention)

EPIDEMIOLOGY
- Predominant age: Age 16–25
- Predominant sex: Male > Female

Prevalence
- 19.1 million or 7.9% of Americans reported use of an illicit substance in past month in 2004; rates: 10.6% for 12–17; 21.7% for 18–20 years
- 1 in 6 males 18–25 years uses marijuana.
- 36% in the US used a drug at least once.

RISK FACTORS
- Male gender, young adult
- Depression, anxiety
- Other substance use disorders
- Family history
- Peer or family use or approval
- Low socioeconomic status
- Unemployment
- Accessibility of substances of abuse
- Family dysfunction or trauma
- Antisocial personality disorder
- Academic problems, school dropout
- Criminal involvement

Genetics
Substances of abuse affect dopamine, acetylcholine, γ-aminobutyric acid, norepinephrine, opioid, and serotonin receptors. Variant alleles may account for differences in susceptibility to substance use disorders.

ETIOLOGY
Multifactorial, including genetic, environmental

ASSOCIATED CONDITIONS
- Depression
- Personality disorders
- Bipolar affective disorder

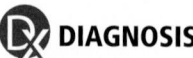 **DIAGNOSIS**

SIGNS AND SYMPTOMS
History
- History of infections, e.g., endocarditis, hepatitis B or C, tuberculosis, sexually transmitted diseases, or recurrent pneumonia
- Social or behavioral problems, including chaotic relationships and/or employment
- Frequent visits to emergency department
- Criminal incarceration
- History of blackouts, insomnia, mood swings, chronic pain, repetitive trauma
- Anxiety, fatigue, depression, psychosis
- Sexual assault with GHB, Rohypnol

Physical Exam
- Dilated or constricted pupils, response to light
- Needle marks on skin
- Nasal septum perforation (with cocaine use)
- Cardiac dysrhythmias, pathologic murmurs

TESTS
- TICS (2-Item Conjoint Screen): At least 1 positive response is 79% sensitive, 78% specific for current substance use disorder (5)[B]
  - In the last year, have you ever drunk or used drugs more than you meant to?
  - Have you felt you wanted or needed to cut down on your drinking or drug use in the past year?

- CAGE-AID (CAGE Adapted to Include Drugs): (5)[B] More than 2 "yes" answers on original CAGE is ~85% sensitive, 90% specific for alcohol use disorder
  - Have you ever tried to Cut down on your alcohol or drug use?
  - Do you get Annoyed when people comment on your drinking or drug use?
  - Do you feel Guilty about things you have done while drinking or using drugs?
  - Do you need an Eye-opener to get started in the morning?

Lab
- Blood alcohol concentration
- Urine drug screen, confirmatory tests
- Approximate detection limits
  - Alcohol: 6–10 hours
  - Amphetamines and variants: 2–3 days
  - Barbiturates: 2–10 days
  - Benzodiazepines: 1–6 weeks
  - Cocaine: 2–3 days
  - Heroin: 1–1.5 days
  - LSD, psilocybin: 8 hours
  - Marijuana: 1 day to 4 weeks
  - Methadone: 1 day to 1 week
  - Opioids: 1–3 days
  - PCP: 7–14 days
  - Anabolic steroids: Oral, 3 weeks; injectable, 3 months; nandrolone, 9 months
- For altered mental status consider: CBC, glucose, chemistry panel, TSH, RPR, urinalysis, head CT scan, chest x-ray, ECG, lumbar puncture, arterial blood gas, blood cultures
- HIV, hepatitis B and C screens

Imaging
ECG for endocarditis

DSM-IV TR Criteria
- Substance abuse: A maladaptive pattern of substance use manifested by one (or more) of the following
  - Failure to fulfill major obligations at work, school, or home
  - Recurrent use in hazardous situations
  - Recurrent substance-related legal problems
  - Continued substance use despite substance-related social or interpersonal problems
- Substance dependence: A maladaptive pattern of substance use manifested by 3 (or more) of the following
  - Tolerance
  - Withdrawal
  - Using the substance more than intended
  - Persistent desire or attempts to cut down/stop
  - Much time spent obtaining, using, or recovering from the substance
  - Social, occupational, or recreational activities sacrificed for substance use
  - Continued use despite substance-related physical or psychological problems

DIFFERENTIAL DIAGNOSIS
- Depression, anxiety, or other mental states
- Metabolic causes of altered mental status (hypoxia, hypoglycemia, infection, thiamine deficiency, hypothyroidism, thyrotoxicosis)
- Delirium, agitation
- Attention deficit hyperactivity disorder
- Medication toxicity

TREATMENT

PRE HOSPITAL
Determine substances abused early (may influence disposition).

INITIAL STABILIZATION
Look for signs of severe infection (e.g., bacterial endocarditis).

GENERAL MEASURES
- Behavioral and cognitive therapy
- Community reinforcement
- Interventional counseling
- Nonjudgmental, medically oriented attitude
- Self-help groups to aid recovery (Alcoholics Anonymous, other 12-step programs)
- Support groups for family (Al-Anon and Alateen)
- Monitoring for infectious diseases and other complications

Diet
Patients often are malnourished.

Activity
Restricted if dangerous, psychotic, or disoriented

Nursing
- Frequent vital signs during withdrawal
- Monitor for signs of drug use in hospital.

IV Fluids
Maintenance until taking fluids well PO

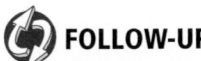

MEDICATION (DRUGS)

First Line
- Alcohol withdrawal: See "Alcohol Use Disorders" chapter.
- Benzodiazepine or barbiturate withdrawal:
  - Substitution of longer-acting benzodiazepine or phenobarbital (3)[C]
  - Tapering doses of the agent of dependence
  - Buspirone 5–15 PO b.i.d.
- Cocaine or stimulant withdrawal: No agent with clear benefit (3)[A]
- Nicotine withdrawal
  - Bupropion 150 mg PO b.i.d. (3)[B]
  - Nicotine replacement systems (patches, gum)
- Opioid withdrawal
  - Methadone 20–35 mg/d PO, use restricted to inpatient settings and specially licensed clinics (2,3)[A]
  - Buprenorphine 2–16 mg SL daily, use restricted to licensed clinics and qualified physicians (see www.buprenorphine.samhsa.gov/howto.html) (1,2,3)[A]
  - Naltrexone 50 mg/d PO or 100 mg PO thrice weekly (2,3)[A]
  - Clonidine 0.1–0.2 mg PO q4h for 5–10 days, often used in combination with other agents (2,3)[A]
- Adjuncts to therapy
  - Antiemetics, nonaddictive analgesics for opioid withdrawal
  - Fluoxetine, desipramine for comorbid depressive states or symptoms that persist 1 week after acute stimulant withdrawal (3)[B]
  - Lithium for comorbid bipolar affective states

- Nonaddictive anxiolytics (buspirone, hydroxyzine) or clonazepam (4)[C]
- Trazodone or nonaddictive hypnotics (eszopiclone, zolpidem) for insomnia (4)[C]
- Use all medications in conjunction with psychosocial, behavioral interventions (2–4)[C]
- Contraindications
  - Buprenorphine in lactation
  - Naltrexone in pregnancy, liver disease
- Precautions
  - Clonidine may cause hypotension.
- Significant possible interactions
  - Buprenorphine and ketoconazole, erythromycin, or HIV protease inhibitors
  - Naltrexone and opioid medications (may precipitate or exacerbate withdrawal)

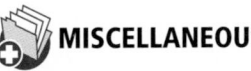

FOLLOW-UP

DISPOSITION
Admission Criteria
- Indications for inpatient detoxification
  - History of withdrawal symptoms, e.g., seizures
  - Disorientation
  - Threat of harm to self or others
  - Obstacles to close monitoring (follow-up)
  - Comorbid medical illness
  - Pregnancy
- For inpatient narcotic or polysubstance detoxification, strongly consider admission to a qualified substance abuse treatment facility.

Discharge Criteria
Detoxification complete

Issues for Referral
- Consider addiction specialist, especially for opioid and polysubstance abuse.
- Maintenance therapy for opioid dependence (e.g., methadone) only in specially licensed clinics
- Psychiatry for comorbid psychiatric disorders
- Social services

PROGNOSIS
- Patients in treatment for longer periods of time (at least a year) have higher success rates.
- Counseling combined with drug therapy is more successful than either 1 alone.

COMPLICATIONS
- Hepatitis, HIV, tuberculosis, syphilis
- Subacute bacterial endocarditis
- Malnutrition
- Social problems, including arrest
- Poor marital adjustment and violence
- Depression, schizophrenia
- Serious harm to self and others
- Sexual assault with GHB, Rohypnol
- Overdoses resulting in seizures, arrhythmias, cardiac and respiratory arrest, coma, death

PATIENT MONITORING
- Verify patient's compliance with the substance abuse treatment program.
- Following treatment, follow-up on medical issues and provide support for continued abstinence.

REFERENCES

1. Abramowicz M, ed. Buprenorphine. *Med Lett.* 2003;45(1150):13–15.
2. Fiellin DA. Office-based treatment of opioid-dependent patients. *N Engl J Med.* 2002;347(11)
3. Kosten TR. Management of drug and alcohol withdrawal. *N Engl J Med.* 2003;348(18):1786.
4. Jones EM. Common problems in patients recovering from chemical dependency. *Am Fam Physician.* 2003;68(10):1971–1978.
5. Brown RL. A two-item conjoint screen for alcohol and other drug problems. *J Am Board Fam Pract.* 2001;14(2):95–106.

MISCELLANEOUS

See also: Alcohol use disorders

CODES

ICD9-CM
- 304.00 Opioid type dependence, unspecified
- 304.10 Barbiturate and similarly acting sedative or hypnotic dependence, unspecified
- 304.20 Cocaine dependence, unspecified
- 305.20 Cannabis abuse, unspecified
- 305.40 Barbiturate and similarly acting sedative or hypnotic abuse, unspecified
- 305.50 Opioid abuse, unspecified
- 305.60 Cocaine abuse, unspecified

PATIENT TEACHING
- American Council on Alcoholism: (800) 527–5344 or www.aca-usa.org (treatment facility locator, educational information)
- National Clearinghouse for Alcohol and Drug Information: (800) 729–6686 or www.health.org
- Center Sub Abuse Treatment: (800) 662-HELP, www.csat.samhsa.gov (facility locator)
- National Families in Action: (404) 248-9676 or www.nationalfamilies.org
- Alcoholics Anonymous: contact local chapter or www.aa.org
- Cocaine Anonymous: www.ca.org
- Narcotics Anonymous: www.na.org
- Rational Recovery: www.rational.org
- Secular Organizations for Sobriety: www.secularsobriety.org

 See Corresponding Diagnostic Algorithm

 See Patient Handout on CD

SUDDEN INFANT DEATH SYNDROME (SIDS)

Fern R. Hauck, MD, MS

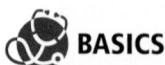 **BASICS**

DESCRIPTION

- The sudden death of an infant <1 year of age that remains unexplained after a thorough case investigation, including performance of a complete autopsy, examination of the death scene, and review of the clinical history. Sudden infant death syndrome (SIDS) was 1st formally defined in 1969, and the definition was revised in 1989.
- System(s) Affected: Cardiovascular; Endocrine/Metabolic; Nervous; Pulmonary
- Synonym(s): Crib death; Cot death

GENERAL PREVENTION

Because a SIDS death is sudden and the cause is unknown, SIDS cannot be "treated." However, there are some measures that may be effective in reducing the risk of SIDS. (1)[B]
- Maternal avoidance of cigarette smoking and illicit drug use during pregnancy
- Avoidance of the prone and side sleep positions, excessive bed clothing, and soft bedding such as pillows and comforters or a soft mattress
- Avoidance of overheating
- A crib, bassinet, or cradle conforming to federal safety standards is the recommended sleeping location.
- Avoidance of bed sharing with the infant, particularly by adults other than the parent(s) or by other children. Bed sharing should be avoided if mother or father has used cigarettes, drugs, or alcohol. Bed sharing on couches is very dangerous and should never be done.
- Infants who sleep in the same room as their parents (without bed sharing) have a lower risk of SIDS. It is recommended that infants sleep in a crib or bassinet in their parents' bedroom, which when placed close to their bed will allow for more convenient breastfeeding and contact.
- Pacifier use is associated with reduced risk of SIDS. Consider offering a pacifier at bedtime and nap time. Delay introduction of the pacifier among breastfed infants until 1 month of age. (2)[B]
- Avoidance of commercial devices marketed to reduce the risk of SIDS
- Avoidance of passive cigarette smoke exposure
- It is critical that all people caring for infants, including day care providers, be instructed in these risk-reduction measures.
- Newborn nurseries should implement these recommendations well before discharge.

EPIDEMIOLOGY

- Predominant age: Uncommon in 1st month of life; peak occurs in infants between 2 and 4 months of age; 80% of deaths occur by 6 months of age
- Predominant sex: Males > Females (52–60% of SIDS cases are boys)

Incidence
For 2002
- All races: 0.57 in 1,000 live births (2,295 cases/year)
- White non-Hispanic: 0.55 in 1,000 live births (1,269 cases/year)
- Black non-Hispanic: 1.11 in 1,000 live births (642 cases/year)
- Hispanic: 0.30 in 1,000 live births (260 cases/year)
- Native American: 1.23 in 1,000 live births (52 cases/year)

ALERT
Pediatric Considerations
Occurs in infants only

RISK FACTORS
- Most SIDS deaths occur in children who are "low risk." However, there are several risk factors associated with SIDS
  - Race: Native Americans and African Americans have highest incidence.
  - Season: Late fall and winter months
  - Time of day: Between midnight and 6 a.m.
  - Activity: During sleep
  - Low birth weight; intrauterine growth retardation (IUGR)
  - Poverty
- Maternal factors
  - Decreased age
  - Decreased education
  - Maternal use of cigarettes or drugs (cocaine, opiates) during pregnancy
  - Higher parity
  - Inadequate prenatal care
- Respiratory or gastrointestinal infection in recent past
- Sleep practices
  - Prone and side sleep position
  - Overheating from heavy clothing and bedding, and/or elevated room temperature
  - Soft bedding
  - Bed sharing
- Passive cigarette smoke exposure after birth
- No pacifier use

Genetics
Emerging evidence for genetic risk factors, especially related to impaired brainstem regulation of breathing or other autonomic control

ETIOLOGY
- There are many theories about the cause of SIDS. There may be subtle developmental abnormalities resulting from pre- and/or perinatal brain injury.
- Possible causes
  - Abnormalities in respiratory control and arousal responsiveness
  - Central and peripheral nervous system abnormalities
  - Cardiac arrhythmias
  - Rebreathing in face-down position on soft surface, leading to hypoxia and hypercarbia
  - SIDS may occur when 1 or more environmental risk factors interact with one or more genetic risk factors.

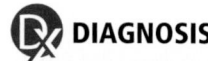 **DIAGNOSIS**

SIGNS AND SYMPTOMS
These babies generally appear healthy or may have had a minor upper respiratory or gastrointestinal infection in the last 2 weeks of life.

History
Infant usually found unresponsive by parent or other caregiver without any warning

TESTS
Lab
- Pneumocardiograms have been abandoned in the workup.
- Postmortem laboratory tests are done to rule out other cause of death (e.g., electrolytes to rule out dehydration and electrolyte imbalance). In SIDS, there are no consistently abnormal laboratory tests.

Imaging
X-rays to rule out possible child abuse

Diagnostic Procedures/Surgery
Because the diagnosis of SIDS is often one of "exclusion," it is crucial to do a thorough death-scene investigation and case review in addition to the autopsy and laboratory tests.

Pathological Findings
Characteristic findings on postmortem examination
- Frothy discharge, sometimes blood tinged, from nostrils and mouth in majority
- Petechiae on surface of lungs, heart, and thymus gland in 50–85% (but not unique to SIDS)
- Pulmonary congestion and edema often present
- Morphologic markers of hypoxia: Increased gliosis in brainstem, retention of periadrenal brown fat, and hematopoiesis in the liver—present to varying degrees; not confirmed by all studies

DIFFERENTIAL DIAGNOSIS
- Suffocation/accidental asphyxia
- Abnormalities of fatty acid metabolism (e.g., deficiency of medium-chain acyl–coenzyme A dehydrogenase or of carnitine)
- Homicide
- Dehydration/electrolyte disturbance

FOLLOW-UP

PROGNOSIS

- SIDS deaths have a powerful impact on families and their functioning. Physicians play an important role in providing immediate information about SIDS and sensitive counseling to limit parents' misinformation and feelings of guilt.
- Counseling needs of families vary from short term to long term; support groups are helpful to many couples. Physicians need to be familiar with resources available in their communities to help families mourning a SIDS death. Parents need to be counseled about subsequent pregnancies. Genetic testing and counseling may be indicated to rule out a metabolic or other genetically acquired disorder. They need to be advised of the most current recommendations regarding sleep position and other infant care practices during subsequent pregnancies.
- Follow-up counseling, including review of the autopsy report with the family after some time has passed, is important to help with understanding this condition and to alleviate the tremendous guilt these families experience.

PATIENT MONITORING

Some authorities recommend cardiopulmonary monitoring in siblings of prior SIDS victims. There is no evidence that use of monitors prevents SIDS, and they should not be prescribed for that purpose. (3)[B]

REFERENCES

1. American Academy of Pediatrics, Task Force on Sudden Infant Death Syndrome. The changing concept of sudden infant death syndrome: Diagnostic coding shifts, controversies regarding the sleeping environment, and new variables to consider in reducing risk. *Pediatrics*. 2005;116:1245–1255.
2. Hauck FR, Omojokun OO, Siadaty MS. Do pacifiers reduce the risk of sudden infant death syndrome? A meta-analysis. *Pediatrics*. 2005;116. Available at: www.pediatrics.org/cgi/content/full/116/5/e716.
3. American Academy of Pediatrics, Committee on Fetus and Newborn. Apnea, sudden infant death syndrome, and home monitoring. *Pediatrics*. 2003;111:914–917.

ADDITIONAL READING

Horchler JN, Morris RR. The SIDS and Infant Death Survival Guide. Information and Comfort for Grieving Family and Friends and Professionals Who Seek to Help Them. Hyattsville, MD: SIDS Educational Services; 2003.

MISCELLANEOUS

CODES

ICD9-CM
798.0 Sudden infant death syndrome

ICD10
R95 Sudden infant death syndrome

PATIENT TEACHING

- Family counseling (see "Prognosis")
- Back to Sleep Information Line, (800) 505-CRIB (2742) (sponsored by the U.S. Public Health Service to provide information to parents and health providers about their recommendations to place infants on back, and general information about SIDS)
- National SIDS/Infant Death Resource Center, McLean, VA; (866) 866-SIDS (7437)
- Association of SIDS and Infant Mortality Programs, Stony Brook, NY; (631) 444–3690
- CJ Foundation for SIDS, Hackensack, NJ; (888) 8CJ-SIDS (825–7437)
- First Candle/SIDS Alliance, Baltimore, MD; (800) 221-SIDS (7437)
- SIDS Network, Ledyard, CT; (800) 560–1454

S

SUICIDE

Sarah Guzofski, MD
Ruben Peralta, MD, FACS

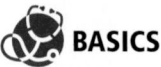 **BASICS**

DESCRIPTION
Suicide, or death due to self-injury and attempted suicide are significant causes of morbidity and mortality. There are ~30,000 completed suicides in the US annually, and 10 suicide attempts for every completed suicide.

GENERAL PREVENTION
- >50% of those who commit suicide saw PCP in month prior to death. Insufficient evidence that routine screening in primary care reduces suicide. (1)[A]

- Look for and treat underlying mental illness.
- Provide risk reduction counseling for alcohol and other drug use.
- For those at risk for suicide, create a safety plan with patient and family, including education about how to access emergency care.
- Screen at-risk patients for gun ownership; encourage these patients to remove guns from their homes and to relinquish gun license.

EPIDEMIOLOGY
- Predominant age: Highest in older people (>65 years old) and adolescent age period (15–24 years old)
- Predominant sex
  - Complete suicide: Male > Female (3:1)
  - Attempted suicide: Female > Male (3:1)
- Rates vary globally; higher rates in Eastern Europe, lower rates in Latin American and Muslim countries.

Incidence
- 10–12 in 100,000.
- In 2000, 11th leading cause of death in adults in the US.

ALERT
Geriatric Considerations
Increasing rate with increasing age (women peak at 55 years of age, men peak at 75 years of age)

Prevalence
In the US, 80 suicide deaths per day and US 10–20 attempts for every death

RISK FACTORS
- Past suicide attempt
- Axis I or II Psychiatric Disorders: 90% who complete suicide meet DSM criteria for Axis I or II disorder
  - Mood disorders: 60% of suicide completers have depression or bipolar disorder. 15–20% with mood disorder die from suicide.
  - Substance use (especially alcohol): 25% of all completed suicides
  - Schizophrenia: 10% die from suicide, especially, young males who recognize a loss of functioning
  - Personality disorders: Especially borderline and antisocial personality disorders
  - Anorexia nervosa
  - Panic disorder
- Family history of suicide
- Physical illness: Multiple sclerosis, brain and spinal cord injury, seizure disorder, stroke, Huntington disease, cancer, HIV/AIDS, COPD, chronic hemodialysis-dependent renal failure, chronic pain

- Hopelessness
- Epidemiologic
  - Sex: Men complete suicide 3× more often than women, women attempt suicide 3× more often than men. Women more likely to choose ingestions which have higher rescue potential than higher lethality methods chosen by males.
  - Age: Adolescent and geriatric population (males peaking at 75 years old, females peaking at 55 years old)
  - Race: 75% of completed suicides are by white males. Native Americans have highest rate in US. Caucasians have twice greater risk than African Americans.
  - Immigration: In 1st generation, mirrors country of origin
  - Marital status: Single > divorced, widowed > married
- Psychologic
  - Recent loss (e.g., loved one, job)
  - Social isolation
  - Anniversaries, holidays
- Access to lethal means
- Mnemonic: SAD PERSONS. If 5 risk factors are present, high suicide risk
  - S—sex (male)
  - A—age
  - D—depression
  - P—previous attempt
  - E—ethanol abuse
  - R—rational thinking loss
  - S—social support loss
  - O—organized plan
  - N—no spouse
  - S—sickness

ETIOLOGY
Combination of psychiatric illness, social circumstances, and other stressors

ASSOCIATED CONDITIONS
- Axis I and II psychiatric illness
- Medical illnesses as above

℞ DIAGNOSIS

SIGNS AND SYMPTOMS
- Hopelessness about the future
- Suicidal thoughts with organized plan and intent to act
- Major depression (screen for symptoms)
  - Change in sleep
  - Loss of interest
  - Loss of energy
  - Loss of concentration
  - Loss of appetite
  - Diminished psychomotor activity
  - Guilt
  - Suicidal ideation

- Psychosis: Ask about command auditory hallucinations to kill oneself, delusional guilt, and persecutory delusions.

History
- Suicide is a statistically rare event, and no reliable method of predicting who will or will not attempt suicide has been devised. Screen for risk factors, and consider overall clinical picture.
- Detailed history of current suicide plans
- Intention to act on plans
- Availability and lethality of means
- Prior attempts: Lethality, intent to die, precipitants, substance use, precautions taken to avoid being rescued
- After an attempt, patient's feelings about surviving
- Detailed history of psychiatric symptoms, especially high risk disorders above
- Substance use history
- Reasons to live, hope for future
- Social supports
- Review risk factors.
- Collateral history is often essential (from friends, family, physicians); it may be appropriate to break confidentiality if patient is at imminent risk of suicide.

TESTS
Lab
- There are no laboratory tests to determine who will commit suicide.
- Patients who have completed violent suicides found to have low levels of 5-hydroxyindoleacetic acid (5-HIAA), a serotonin metabolite, in the CSF and brainstem

DIFFERENTIAL DIAGNOSIS
- Psychiatric
  - Look for high risk disorders: Mood disorders, schizophrenia, panic, axis II, substance abuse and dependence, anorexia nervosa.
  - Consider presence of delirium or dementia.
- Medical illness presenting with depression, mania, psychosis (e.g., hypothyroid, delirium)
- Medication effects causing psychiatric symptoms, (e.g., beta blockers and depression)
- Substance intoxication and substance-induced mood, psychotic and anxiety disorders

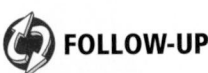

TREATMENT

INITIAL STABILIZATION

- Determine appropriate level of care.
- After a suicide attempt, consider need for medical care before psychiatric care.
- Inpatient if suicidal with a plan to act or otherwise at high risk. If immediate risk for self-harm, may be hospitalized involuntarily
- Intensive outpatient follow-up may be appropriate if not at immediate risk to harm self, adequate social supports, able to seek help when needed

GENERAL MEASURES

- Patients expressing active suicidal thoughts or who made an attempt should be screened for suicide risk factors and have a full mental status examination and psychiatric consultation.
- Ensure patient safety by least restrictive method (i.e., remove potentially dangerous objects, provide one-to-one constant observation, medication, four-point restraints, chemical restraint).
- Search patient for dangerous objects.
- Diagnose and treat underlying psychiatric and medical disorders using standard algorithms.
- Electroconvulsive therapy provides rapid, safe, and effective treatment option for severely depressed, acutely suicidal patients.
- Therapy for suicidal patients
  - Insufficient evidence to recommend, but Dialectical Behavioral Therapy for Borderline Personality Disorder may reduce suicide risk (1,2)[A]
  - Cognitive therapy decreased re-attempt rate in prior suicide attempters by 1/2. (3)[B]

Activity
Assess for less restrictive, yet safe suicide precautions; every-15-minute checks; one-to-one observation; 4-point restraints

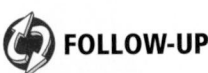

MEDICATION (DRUGS)

- Use standard algorithms to treat underlying psychiatric conditions.
- Anxiety and agitation are risk factors for suicide and should be treated aggressively (e.g., benzodiazepines).
- No evidence that SSRIs decrease suicide risk, although they are proven to decrease depression, a major risk factor for suicide (4)[B]

ALERT

Pediatric Considerations
- FDA has issued a black box warning for SSRIs in pediatric population after increased suicidality noted. If risk of untreated depression is sufficient to warrant treatment with SSRIs, children must be very closely monitored for suicidality.
- Lithium and clozapine have some efficacy in reducing rate of suicide.
  - In patients with mood disorders, a meta-analysis of randomized controlled trials found that lithium reduced risk of death by suicide by 60%. (5)
  - Long-term treatment for psychosis with clozapine shows some benefit for reducing rate of suicide. (6)[A]

- Agitated or combative, patients
  - May require sedation with benzodiazepines (e.g., lorazepam 2 mg IM/IV) and/or antipsychotics (e.g., haloperidol 2–5 mg IM/IV)
  - Clinical response typically seen within 20–30 minutes if given IM/IV
- Precautions
  - Use smaller doses in older patients.
  - Monitor for drug toxicities.
    - Lithium intoxication (includes delirium, ataxia, dysarthria, hyperreflexia)
    - Serotonin syndrome (delirium, diarrhea, myoclonus, autonomic instability)
    - Neuroleptic malignant syndrome (delirium, autonomic instability, rigidity, tremor)
- Significant possible interactions
  - Monoamine oxidase inhibitors (antidepressants) interact with tyramine-containing foods and sympathomimetic medications to cause hypertensive crisis. Washout period required before using other psychoactive medications.
  - Check for cytochrome P450 interactions.
  - Medications such as NSAIDs and diuretics increase lithium levels, and can cause toxicity.

First Line
- Choose medication based on underlying disorder.
- Consider toxicity of medication in overdose (e.g., cardiac toxicity of TCA overdose, compared to safer SSRIs) versus therapeutic benefit.

FOLLOW-UP

DISPOSITION

Discharge Criteria
- No longer considered a danger to self/others
- At discharge, patient must be provided with contact information for emergency mental health services in their community.

PROGNOSIS
The key to a favorable course and prognosis is early recognition of risk factors, early diagnosis and treatment of a psychiatric disorder, and appropriate intervention and follow-up.

PATIENT MONITORING
- Brief period of increased suicide risk as depression resolves and patient's energy and initiative return
- Increased rate of suicide attempts in period following psychiatric hospitalization
- Frequent outpatient follow-up appointments
- Prescribe only a small supply of antidepressants or other psychotropic medications at each appointment.

REFERENCES

1. Gaynes BN, et al. Screening for suicide risk in adults: A summary of the evidence for the U.S. Preventive Services Task Force. *Ann Intern Med*. 2004;140:822–835.
2. Mann JJ, Apter A, Bertolote J. Suicide prevention strategies: A systematic review. *JAMA*. 2005;294:2061–2074.

3. Brown GK, et al. Cognitive therapy for the prevention of suicide attempts: A randomized controlled trial. *JAMA*. 2005;295:563–570.
4. Mann J, et al. The neurobiology of suicide risk: A review for the clinician. *J Clin Psychiatry*. 1999;60(suppl 2):7–11.
5. Cipriani A, et al. Lithium in the prevention of suicidal behavior and all-cause mortality in patients with mood disorders: A systematic review of randomized trials. *Am J Psychiatry*. 2005;162:1805–1819.
6. Hennen J, Baldessarinin RJ. Suicide risk during treatment with clozapine: A meta-analysis. *Schizophrenia Res*. 2004;73:139–145.
7. Patterson WM, et al. Evaluation of suicidal patients: The SAD PERSONS scale. *Psychosomatics*. 1983;24:348–349.

ADDITIONAL READING
American Psychiatric Association Practice Guidelines for the Assessment and Treatment of Patients with Suicidal Behaviors

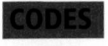

MISCELLANEOUS
Other notes

- Overdose is the most common method for suicide attempts.
- Most common method for completed suicide is self-inflicted gunshot.
- Decrease in suicide rates have been noted where access to lethal means (i.e., firearms, toxic gas) is restricted.

CODES

ICD9-CM
E950.5 Suicide and self-inflicted poisoning by unspecified drug or medicinal substance

PATIENT TEACHING

Prevention
Patients should be educated about the availability of emergency mental health resources to contact if they feel suicidal.

 See Patient Handout on CD

SUPERFICIAL THROMBOPHLEBITIS

Abdulrazak Abyad, MD, PhD, MBA, MPH, AGSF

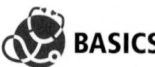 **BASICS**

DESCRIPTION
- Superficial thrombophlebitis is an inflammatory condition of the veins with secondary thrombosis.
- Septic (suppurative) thrombophlebitis types
  - Iatrogenic
  - Infectious, mainly syphilis and psittacosis
- Aseptic thrombophlebitis types
  - Primary hypercoagulable states—disorders with measurable defects in the proteins of the coagulation and/or fibrinolytic systems
  - Secondary hypercoagulable states—clinical conditions with a risk of thrombosis
- System(s) Affected: Cardiovascular
- Synonym(s): Phlebitis; Phlebothrombosis

ALERT
Geriatric Considerations
Septic thrombophlebitis is more common, prognosis is poorer.

Pediatric Considerations
Subperiosteal abscesses of adjacent long bone may complicate.

Pregnancy Considerations
- Associated with increased risk of aseptic superficial thrombophlebitis
- Warfarin and NSAIDs are contraindicated.

GENERAL PREVENTION
- Use of scalp vein cannulae
- Avoidance of lower-extremity cannulations
- Insertion under aseptic conditions
- Secure anchoring of the cannulae.
- Replacement of cannulae, connecting tubing, and IV fluid q48–72h
- Neomycin–polymyxin B-bacitracin ointment in cutdown

EPIDEMIOLOGY
- Predominant age
  - Septic: More common in childhood
  - Aseptic primary hypercoagulable state
    - Antithrombin III and heparin cofactor II deficiency—neonatal period, but 1st episode usually at age 20–30 years
    - Proteins C and S—<30 years of age
  - Aseptic secondary hypercoagulable state
    - Mondor disease: women, ages 21–55 years
    - Thromboangiitis obliterans onset: ages 20–50 years
- Predominant sex
  - Suppurative: Male = Female
  - Aseptic
    - Mondor: Female > Male (2:1)
    - Thromboangiitis obliterans: Female > Male (1–19% of clinical cases)

Incidence
- Septic
  - Up to 10% of all nosocomial infections
  - Incidence of catheter-related thrombophlebitis is 88/100,000
  - Develops in 4–8% if cutdown is performed.
- Aseptic primary hypercoagulable state: Antithrombin III and heparin cofactor II deficiency incidence is 50/100,000.
- Aseptic secondary hypercoagulable state
  - Trousseau incidence in malignancy 5–15%
  - Trousseau in pancreatic carcinoma 50%

- In pregnancy, 49-fold increased incidence of phlebitis
- Superficial migratory thrombophlebitis in 27% of patients with thromboangiitis obliterans

RISK FACTORS
- Nonspecific
  - Immobilization
  - Obesity
  - Advanced age
  - Postoperative states
- Septic
  - IV catheter
  - Duration of IV catheterization (68% of cannulae have been left in place for 2 days)
  - Cutdowns
  - Cancer, debilitating diseases
  - Steroid
  - Incidence is 40 times higher with plastic cannula (8%) than with steel or scalp cannulas (0.2%).
  - Thrombosis
  - Dermal infection
  - Burned patients
  - Lower-extremities IV catheter
  - IV antibiotics
  - AIDS
  - Varicose veins
- Antithrombin II and heparin cofactor II deficiency
  - Pregnancy
  - Oral contraceptives
  - Surgery; trauma; infection
- In pregnancy
  - Increased age
  - Hypertension
  - Eclampsia
  - Increased parity
- Thromboangiitis obliterans: Persistent smoking
- Mondor disease
  - Breast abscess
  - Antecedent breast surgery
  - Breast augmentation
  - Reduction mammoplasty

Genetics
- Septic: No known genetic pattern
- Antithrombin III deficiencies: Autosomal dominant
- Proteins C and S deficiency: Autosomal dominant with variable penetrance
- Disorders of fibrinolytic system: Congenital defects inheritance variable
- Dysfibrinogenemia: Autosomal dominant
- Factor XII deficiency: Autosomal recessive

ETIOLOGY
- Septic
  - *Staphylococcus aureus* in 65–78%
  - Enterobacteriaceae, especially *Klebsiella*
  - Multiple organisms in 14%
  - Anaerobic isolate rare
  - *Candida* spp.
  - Cytomegalovirus in AIDS patients
- Aseptic primary hypercoagulable state
  - Antithrombin III and heparin II deficiency
  - Protein C and protein S deficiency
  - Disorder of tissue plasminogen activator
  - Abnormal plasminogen and co-plasminogen
  - Dysfibrinogenemia
  - Factor XII deficiency
  - Lupus anticoagulant and anticardiolipin antibody syndrome

- Aseptic secondary hypercoagulable states
  - Malignancy (Trousseau syndrome: Recurrent migratory thrombophlebitis): Most commonly seen in metastatic mucin or adenocarcinomas of the gastrointestinal tract (pancreas, stomach, colon, and gall bladder), lung, prostate, ovary
  - Pregnancy
  - Oral contraceptive
  - Infusion of prothrombin complex concentrates
  - Behçet disease
  - Buerger disease
  - Mondor disease

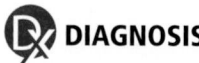 **DIAGNOSIS**

SIGNS AND SYMPTOMS
- Swelling, tenderness, redness along the course of the veins
- May look like cellulitis or erythema nodosa
- Fever in 70% of patients
- Warmth, erythema, tenderness, or lymphangitis in 32%
- Sign of systemic sepsis in 84% in suppurative
- Red, tender cord
- Pain

TESTS
Leukocyte imaging

Lab
- Septic
  - Bacteremia in 80–90%
  - Culture of IV fluid bag
  - Leukocytosis
- Aseptic
  - Acute-phase reactant
  - Factor levels
  - Thrombin activity
  - Platelet function test
- Drugs that may alter lab results
  - In septic, broad-spectrum antibiotics

Imaging
Septic and aseptic

- Ultrasound of veins reveals an increase in the diameter of the lumen.
- Chest x-ray: Multiple peripheral densities or a pleural effusion consistent with pulmonary embolism, abscess, or empyema
- Bone and gallium scan: For associated subperiosteal abscess in septic thrombophlebitis
- Evaluation of complications (deep vein thrombosis and others)

Diagnostic Procedures/Surgery
Skin biopsy

Pathological Findings
- The affected vein is enlarged, tortuous, and thickened.
- Associated perivascular suppuration and/or hemorrhage
- Vein lumen may contain pus and thrombus.
- Endothelial damage, fibrinoid necrosis, and thickening of the vein wall

DIFFERENTIAL DIAGNOSIS
- Cellulitis
- Erythema nodosa
- Cutaneous polyarteritis nodosa
- Sarcoid
- Kaposi sarcoma
- Hyperalgesic pseudothrombophlebitis

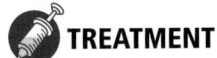 TREATMENT

INITIAL STABILIZATION
- Septic: Inpatient
- Aseptic: Outpatient

GENERAL MEASURES
- Heat application
- Extremity elevation

Diet
No restrictions

Activity
Bed rest

 MEDICATION (DRUGS)

First Line
- Septic
  - Initially: semisynthetic penicillin (e.g., nafcillin 2 g IV q6h) plus an aminoglycoside (e.g., gentamicin, 1.0–1.7 mg/kg IV)
  - Duration of therapy is empiric.
  - If due to *Candida albicans*, consider a short course of amphotericin B, ~200 mg cumulative dose
  - If osteomyelitis documented, antibiotic therapy for at least 6 weeks
- Aseptic general
  - NSAIDs
  - Oral anticoagulant warfarin
  - Systemic anticoagulant heparin
  - Low-molecular-weight heparin
- Antithrombin III and heparin cofactor II deficiency
  - IV heparin
  - Antithrombin III concentrate
  - Prophylaxis: Warfarin, oxymetholone
- Proteins C and S: Long-term warfarin, lower dose, no loading
- Disorder of tissue plasminogen activator
  - Phenformin and ethylestrenol
  - Stanozolol and phenformin
  - Stanozolol alone
  - Ethylestrenol alone
- Dysfibrinogenemia
  - Acute attack: Anticoagulation
  - Prophylaxis: Stanozolol
- Abnormal plasminogen and plasminogenemia
  - Acute attack: Anticoagulation
  - Prophylaxis: Warfarin
- Factor XII deficiency: Standard therapy
- Lupus anticardiolipin: Prophylaxis: Warfarin
- Trousseau syndrome: Heparin
- For pregnancy: Heparin
- Behçet disease
  - Phenformin
  - Ethylestrenol
  - Stanozolol
- Thromboangiitis obliterans
  - Stop smoking.
  - Pentoxifylline
- Contraindications: Refer to the manufacturer's literature.
- Precautions: Refer to the manufacturer's literature.
- Significant possible interactions: Refer to the manufacturer's literature.

Second Line
- Factor XII deficiency—streptokinase or alteplase (tissue plasminogen activator [tPA])
- Behçet—oral anticoagulants plus cyclosporine
- Thromboangiitis obliterans—corticosteroid, antiplatelets, and vasodilating drugs

SURGERY
- Septic
  - Excision of the involved vein segment and all involved tributaries
  - Excision from ankle to groin may be required in some burn patients.
  - If systemic symptoms persist after vein excision, re-exploration is necessary, with removal of all involved veins.
  - Drainage of contiguous abscesses
  - Remove all cannulae.
- Aseptic
  - Mondor disease, consider surgical transection of the phlebitic cord
  - Management of underlying conditions

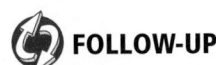 FOLLOW-UP

PROGNOSIS
- Septic: High mortality (50%) if untreated
- Aseptic
  - Usually benign course; recovery in 7–10 days
  - Antithrombin III and heparin cofactor deficiency: recurrence rate 60%
  - Proteins C and S: Recurrence rate 70%
  - Prognosis depends on development of deep vein thrombosis and early detection of complications.
  - Aseptic thrombophlebitis can be isolated, recurrent, or migratory.

COMPLICATIONS
- Septic: Systemic sepsis, bacteremia (84%); septic pulmonary emboli (44%); metastatic abscess formation; pneumonia (44%); subperiosteal abscess of adjacent long bones in children
- Aseptic: Deep vein thrombosis; thromboembolic phenomena

PATIENT MONITORING
- Septic
  - Routine WBC and differential and culture
  - Repeat culture from the phlebitic vein.
- Aseptic
  - Clinical follow-up to rule out secondary complications
  - Repeat of blood studies for fibrinolytic system, platelets, and factors

REFERENCES

1. Mandell GL, ed. *Principles and Practice of Infectious Diseases*. 4th ed. New York, NY: Churchill Livingstone; 1995.
2. Samlaskie CP, James WD. Superficial thrombophlebitis I. Primary hypercoagulable states. *J Am Acad Dermatol*. 1990;22:975–989.
3. Samlaskie CP, James WD. Superficial thrombophlebitis II. Secondary hypercoagulable states. *J Am Acad Dermatol*. 1990;23:1–18.

 MISCELLANEOUS

See also: Thrombosis, deep vein

CODES

ICD9-CM
- 451.0 Phlebitis and thrombophlebitis of superficial vessels of lower extremities
- 451.2 Phlebitis and thrombophlebitis of deep vessels of lower extremities, unspecified

PATIENT TEACHING
- Avoid trauma.
- Be alert to change in skin color.
- Be alert to tenderness over extremities.

 See Patient Handout on CD

SUPERIOR VENA CAVA SYNDROME

Ruben Peralta, MD, FACS
Sarah Guzofski, MD

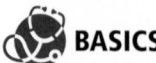 BASICS

DESCRIPTION
- Partial or complete obstruction of the superior vena cava
  - 90% extrinsic
  - 90% from neoplasm (most frequently bronchogenic carcinoma)
- Usual course: Acute; usually 28 days from onset of symptoms to diagnosis
- Synonym(s): Superior mediastinal syndrome; Superior vena cava obstruction

GENERAL PREVENTION
No preventive measures known

EPIDEMIOLOGY
- Predominant age: Young adult (16–40 years old); middle age (40–60 years old)
- Predominant sex: Male > Female

RISK FACTORS
- HIV infection
- History of mediastinal tumor

PATHOPHYSIOLOGY
Increased pressure in the venous system draining into the superior vena cava

ETIOLOGY
- Obstruction of venous drainage of upper part of chest and neck. Sudden occlusion may cause rapid development of cerebral edema, intracranial thrombosis, and death.
- In adults, may be primary tumor or lymph node metastasis; most frequent cause is bronchogenic carcinoma; lymph node metastasis most common from breast and testicular cancer
- In children, most common after cardiac surgical procedures
- Lymphoma
- Thymoma
- Germ cell tumors
- Fungal infections
- Other malignancies
- Iatrogenic (including catheter induced)
- Thyroid goiter
- Primary superior vena caval thrombosis
- Pericardial constriction
- Idiopathic sclerosing mediastinitis

ASSOCIATED CONDITIONS
- Breast cancer
- Lung cancer
- HIV infection
- Hyperthyroidism
- Tuberculosis
- Histoplasmosis
- Lymphoma

DIAGNOSIS

Made on clinical grounds in almost all cases

SIGNS AND SYMPTOMS
- Neck and anterior chest wall venous distension
- Tachypnea, dyspnea
- Cyanosis and edema of upper extremities and face
- Feeling of fullness in the head (ears and eyes)
- Jugular venous distention
- Prominent veins over chest
- Cough
- Dilated retinal vessels, conjunctival edema, proptosis
- Horner syndrome
- Stridor, paralyzed vocal cord
- Nonpitting edema in neck (Stoke's collar)
- Truncal swelling
- Altered consciousness
- Dysphagia, hoarseness
- Easy fatigability
- Chest pain
- Orthopnea

TESTS
Increased central venous pressure; usually 20–50 mm Hg

Lab
Sputum cytology: Malignant cells

Imaging
- Abnormal chest x-ray
- Contrast-enhanced CT or MRI usually adequate to establish diagnosis.
- Venography: Superior vena cava obstruction

Diagnostic Procedures/Surgery
- Percutaneous needle biopsy used to establish histological diagnosis; should be prior to initiation of therapy
- Open biopsy may be necessary; however, these patients are at increased risk for cardiorespiratory compromise under generalized anesthesia.
- Bronchoscopy
- Thoracentesis, thoracotomy, lymph node biopsy, as indicated

Pathological Findings
Sputum cytology, occasionally thoracentesis, bone marrow, lymph node biopsy, bronchoscopy, or thoracotomy confirms malignant cells.

DIFFERENTIAL DIAGNOSIS
- Aortic aneurysm
- Tuberculosis
- Histoplasmosis
- Fungal infections

TREATMENT

INITIAL STABILIZATION
- Inpatient, intensive care
- Institute supportive therapy.

GENERAL MEASURES
- Depending on etiology (1)[B]

- Chemotherapy (treatment of choice for high-grade lymphomas, and small cell lung cancer)
- Percutaneous stenting
- Radiotherapy
- Corticosteroids
- Neoadjuvant chemoradiotherapy and then resection
- Anticoagulation or fibrinolytic therapy
- Benign causes usually respond to medical therapy including diuretics, upright positioning, and fluid restriction until adequate collateral circulation is established and clinical regression is noted.
- In pregnancy: Must treat underlying condition despite pregnancy

Diet
As tolerated; possibly, salt restriction

Activity
Bed rest (head of bed elevated)

MEDICATION (DRUGS)

First Line
Determined by underlying cause

SURGERY
- Superior vena cava reconstruction for benign processes may be considered, but is rarely done.
- Spiral saphenous vein bypass grafting may also be useful in some patients.

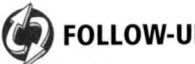 **FOLLOW-UP**

PROGNOSIS
- High probability of response
- Linked to cause
  - Lung cancer: 1-year survival in 20%
  - Lymphoma: 2-year survival in 50%
  - Neoplastic cases: 85% better in 3 weeks with radiation therapy, but symptoms usually recur

COMPLICATIONS
Complications of underlying disease

PATIENT MONITORING
Linked to cause
- If infection, monitor for evaluation of antimicrobial treatment
- If malignant, monitor response to radiotherapy or chemotherapy

REFERENCES
1. Rowell NP, Gleeson FV. Steroids, radiotherapy, chemotherapy and stents for superior vena caval obstruction in carcinoma of the bronchus: A systematic review. *Clin Oncol.* 2002;14:338–351.
2. Hochrein J, et al. Percutaneous stenting of superior vena cava syndrome: A case report and review of the literature. *Am J Med.* 1998;104:78–84.
3. Thirlwell C, Brock CS. Emergencies in oncology. *Clin Med.* 2003;3:306–310.

S

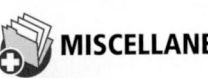 **MISCELLANEOUS**

CODES

ICD9-CM
459.2 Compression of vein

PATIENT TEACHING

 See Corresponding Diagnostic Algorithm

SURGICAL COMPLICATIONS

Michael Ford, MD
Mitchell Cahan, MD

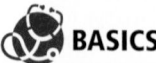 **BASICS**

DESCRIPTION
- When defined broadly, most patients have some form of complication.
- Most common complications are fever and infection.
- Rarely, death or other morbidity occurs.

GENERAL PREVENTION
Operative complications are prevented during the entire perioperative period.
- Imaging to delineate anatomy/recognize aberrancy
- Appropriate resuscitation
- Assessment of underlying risk factors
- Sterile technique
- Preoperative antibiotics

Incidence
- Fever is seen in 27–58% of post-op patients.
- Infection occurs in 3.3–28.3% of operations depending on level of bacterial contamination.
- Dehiscence occurs in 0.5–5% of abdominal operations.
- Renal failure can occur in up to 10% of patients when contrast is used, 4% for all patients.
- Respiratory complications occur in >50% of patients (mostly self-limited atelectasis), and are responsible for 35% of deaths.
- Perioperative myocardial infarction (MI) occurs in between 0.1% and 27%, based on risk factors including age, date of prior MI, and coronary artery disease; 9% risk exists for all patients.
- Fistula/intestinal leaks occur in ~1% of cases.
- Urinary retention occurs in 4–5%.

RISK FACTORS
- Poorly controlled diabetes
- Heart disease (especially recent MI)
- Bleeding disorders
- Malnutrition
- Renal failure
- Liver disease
- Pulmonary disease

Genetics
Malignant hyperthermia; 1 in 100,000, treated with dantrolene

PATHOPHYSIOLOGY
- Fever is caused by pyrogens (bacteria, viruses, antigen–antibody complexes) mediated by interleukin-1.
- Local infection at wound
- Hematoma: Inadequate hemostasis/bleeding disorder
- Seroma: Disruption of lymphatics
- Wound dehiscence: Poor wound healing (malnutrition) or increased abdominal pressure
- Renal failure: Drug toxicity (commonly antibiotics) or inadequate resuscitation leads to poor perfusion (catecholamine release at operation and renin-angiotensin-aldosterone system activation) results in acute tubular necrosis (ATN).
- Respiratory: Decreased vital capacity leads to atelectasis, pneumonitis, and adult respiratory distress syndrome. Aspiration can occur at induction of anesthesia, if stomach acid/particulate matter cause an inflammatory reaction leading to cyanosis, or death. Pulmonary edema is due to fluid transudation to the alveolus, from fluid overload, or heart failure.

- Cardiac: MI generally occurs within 3 days of operation and is caused by anesthetics and blood loss (shock, as little as 500 cc). Arrhythmia is due to destabilization of cardiac membranes or prolongation of conduction.
- Small bowel obstruction: Adhesive bands (scar tissue) form intra-abdominally and can constrict the bowel.
- Urinary retention: Males are affected much more commonly than females; impaired coordination between a-receptors in the bladder neck and parasympathetic stimulation to the bladder.

ETIOLOGY
- Fever in the 1st 24 hours is due to atelectasis.
- *Staphylococcus aureus* is the most common cause of wound infection. Others include *Pseudomonas*, *Proteus*, and *Klebsiella*.
- Hematoma: Inadequate hemostasis
- Dehiscence: Increased abdominal pressure, interrupted fascial closure, malnutrition, contamination, and chemotherapy
- Renal failure: Hypovolemia, drug toxicity (commonly due to antibiotics)
- Respiratory: Many causes including volume overload, aspiration, and decreased vital capacity, leading to decreased diffusion capacity
- Cardiac: Arrhythmia occurs due to electrolyte abnormalities, catecholamine release (due to pain), hypercapnia, and digitalis
- Small bowel obstruction: Occurs remotely after abdominal operation
- Fistula/intestinal leak: Generally occur at site of bowel anastomosis due to suture line breakdown. Can follow local abscess.
- Stomal complications: Increased in obese patients, include fibrosis of bowel at stoma, necrosis, retraction, skin breakdown, and stomal stricture. Most complications are due to technical errors at time of operation.
- Urinary retention: Due to anesthetics

ASSOCIATED CONDITIONS
- Adrenal insufficiency if steroids used
- Liver failure in patients with pre-existing disease
- Delirium tremens in alcoholics
- Thyroid storm in patients with undiagnosed hyperthyroidism
- Parotitis in elderly, under-resuscitated patients
- Depression can occur
- "Sundowning" in the elderly

ALERT
Pediatric Considerations
Operative procedures can lead to severe anxiety in children, with lasting emotional disturbance in 20%, most pronounced between 1 and 2 years old.

Geriatric Considerations
Ninety percent of patients >65 experience depression after surgery, with activities of daily living impaired in 50%. Increased human contact to prevent withdrawal can reduce these symptoms.

Dx **DIAGNOSIS**

SIGNS AND SYMPTOMS
- Low fevers are not significant until 48 hours post-op. Wound infection is the most common cause of fever after 72 hours.
- High fever, mental status changes, hypotension, and rigors are associated with severe wound complications or intestinal leak.
- Dolor, tumor, rubor, and calor indicate a wound infection.
- Hematoma is an expanding, tender mass. Seroma is a slowly expanding, nontender mass.
- Dehiscence is indicated by "salmon" colored drainage post-op day 4–5, evisceration, or later as ventral hernia. Some patients feel sutures "pop." Complain of palpable bulge.
- Renal failure is indicated by persisting oliguria, $FE_{NA} > 1$.
- Pulmonary complications are indicated by dyspnea, cough, fever may be present.
- Cardiac complications present with chest pain (seen in 27% of perioperative MI); ST depression and T-wave flattening; elevated CPK-MB; arrhythmia on telemetry/EKG.
- Small bowel obstruction is heralded by nausea, bilious vomiting, abdominal pain, cessation of flatus.
- Fistula/intestinal leak present with feces protruding from skin opening, acute abdomen, pain, fever, nausea, vomiting.
  - Stomal complications are evident when the ostomy appliance is removed.
  - Urinary retention is indicated by suprapubic pain, inability to void.

History
- Pain is a common complaint
- Wound infection: Operation several days ago, pain, redness at incision
- Expanding mass is consistent with seroma/hematoma. Surgery within 2–3 days is more likely hematoma, further out is likely seroma.
- Dehiscence/hernia: Some patients feel sutures "pop"; caused by lifting within 6 weeks of operation, or increased abdominal operation (i.e., coughing).
- Renal failure: Oliguria, or anuria, fatigue
- Pulmonary: Witnessed aspiration, no incentive spirometry use, narcotic use, fluid retention, advanced age
- Cardiac: Elderly, prior cardiac dysfunction
- Ileus/small bowel obstruction: Progressive nausea/vomiting, inability to tolerate PO, abdominal pain
- Fistula/intestinal leak: Severe abdominal pain (leak), fever, nausea/vomiting
- Stomal complications: Pain at stoma site, change in color of stoma
- Urinary retention: Inability to void, suprapubic pain

Physical Exam
- Wound infection: Dolor, rubor, calor, and tumor at incision, pus or foul-smelling discharge, may be febrile
- Expanding mass is consistent with seroma/hematoma, may have tenderness at site.
- Dehiscence/hernia: Open incision or palpable fascial edge, rarely tender

- Renal failure: Can have pericardial rub, bleeding/hematoma if uremic
- Pulmonary: Basilar crackles, poor inspiratory effort, egophony, dullness to percussion at bases
- Cardiac: Peripheral edema, irregularly irregular heartbeat
- Ileus/small bowel obstruction: "Tinkling" vs. absent bowel sounds, tympanitic abdomen, tenderness to palpation, guarding
- Fistula/intestinal leak: Firm abdomen, guarding, peritoneal signs, possible feculent discharge from site at skin, fever, hypotension
- Stomal complications: Skin irritation, black/discolored intestinal mucosa, retracted ostomy
- Urinary retention: Suprapubic tenderness, palpable bladder

TESTS
Lab
- Elevated WBC count is seen in wound infections, atelectasis, pneumonia, infected hematoma/seroma, bowel leak, and stomal complications.
- BUN and creatinine, along with urine chemistries, are used to diagnose renal failure.
- Pulmonary: Hypoxia, hypercarbia on ABG
- Cardiac: Elevated troponins, CK, CK-MB

Imaging
- SC gas can be seen in necrotizing fasciitis on radiographs or CT.
- CT or ultrasound can be used to diagnose hernia or fascial disruption.
- Small bowel obstruction/ileus: Upright abdominal film shows air fluid levels, dilated small bowel. Transition point may be seen on CT.
- Fistula: Fistulogram aids in diagnosis and is critical for treatment planning.
- Intestinal leak: Chest radiograph reveals free air under the diaphragm.
- Bladder scan can help diagnose urinary retention if the diagnosis is in doubt.

Diagnostic Procedures/Surgery
Exploratory laparotomy/laparoscopy if the patient is extremely ill/septic and diagnosis is unknown, but abdominal cause is suspected

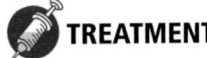

TREATMENT
INITIAL STABILIZATION
- Fluid resuscitate as needed
- Broad spectrum antibiotics, if septic
- IV antibiotics for infections

GENERAL MEASURES
- Surgical site infections are decreased by using clipping to remove hair vs. shaving. Appropriate antibacterial prep should be utilized to decrease bacterial counts. (2)[A]
- Identify the complication.
- Appropriate antibiotics as needed
- Nasogastric tube for bowel obstruction/leak

Diet
- NPO for fistula, intestinal leak, or small bowel obstruction
- Diet as tolerated for other listed complications

Activity
Patients should be out of bed as tolerated.

Nursing
- Monitor vital signs at least every 4 hours
- Strict I & Os
- DVT prophylaxis

IV Fluids
Use D5 1/2 normal saline or lactated Ringer's at a fluid replacement rate.

MEDICATION (DRUGS)
First Line
- Opiates for pain control
- Broad-spectrum antibiotics for sepsis/severe infection (piperacillin/tazobactam and vancomycin)
- Simple wound infections and stomal complications: 1st- or 2nd-generation cephalosporins
- Intestinal leak: Gram-negative and Gram-positive coverage (Levaquin and metronidazole)
- Pneumonia should be treated empirically with antibiotics to cover local flora
- Cardiac complications: Avoided/treated with β-blockade for rate control; angiotensin converting enzyme (ACE) inhibitors and calcium channel blockers also useful.
  – Urinary retention: α-Blockers (tamsulosin)

SURGERY
- Wound infections may need surgical debridement if no response to antibiotics.
- Hematomas may need re-exploration and hemostasis if large and progressing.
- Dehiscence/hernia should be repaired. Evisceration is a surgical emergency.
- Small bowel obstruction that fails to resolve with nasogastric decompression should be explored with lysis of adhesions.
- Intestinal leak is a surgical emergency and needs exploration and repair immediately. Fistulas generally need surgical intervention to resolve.
- Some stomal complications (necrosis, retraction) need surgical revision.

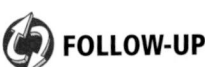

FOLLOW-UP
All complications should be seen by the surgeon responsible for the procedure when they are identified.

Admission Criteria
- Need for IV antibiotics
- Need for surgical procedure
- Need for NG decompression

Discharge Criteria
- Infection resolved/responding to antibiotics
- Able to tolerate PO intake
- Pain controlled
- Patient has bowel function
- Recovered adequately from operation

Issues for Referral
All complications should be seen by the physician performing the operation.

PROGNOSIS
With prompt and appropriate treatment, most patients with complications recover well.

REFERENCES
1. Schwartz S, Shires G, Spencer F, eds. *Principles of Surgery*, 7th ed. New York: McGraw-Hill; 1999:441–483.
2. Tanner J, Woodings D, Moncaster K. Preoperative hair removal to reduce surgical site infection. Cochrane Database Sys Rev. *Cochrane Wound Group*. 2006;3:.

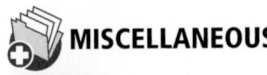

MISCELLANEOUS
CODES
ICD9-CM
- 560.0 Intestinal obstruction without mention of hernia
- 998.1 Hemorrhage or hematoma or seroma complicating a procedure
- 998.3 Disruption of operation wound
- 998.5 Post operative infection

PATIENT TEACHING
Diet
Patient should tolerate clear diet at discharge; advance to regular as tolerated.

Activity
- Cardiac complications: Minimize exertion
- No heavy lifting for dehiscence or hernia
- Unrestricted for all other complications

SYNCOPE

Ricardo A. Samson, MD

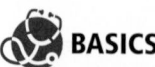 **BASICS**

DESCRIPTION
- Transient loss of consciousness characterized by unresponsiveness, loss of postural tone, and spontaneous recovery
- System(s) Affected: Cardiovascular; Nervous

GENERAL PREVENTION
Avoid risk factors (see "Risk Factors").

EPIDEMIOLOGY
- Predominant age: Elderly
- Rare in infancy, though increasing occurrence during adolescence

Incidence
- Up to 20% of adults will have ≥1 episode by age 75; 15% of children <18 years of age
- Accounts for 1–6% of hospital admissions and about 3% of emergency room visits

Prevalence
In institutionalized elderly (>75 years), 6%

RISK FACTORS
- Heart disease
- Drugs
  - Antihypertensives
  - Vasodilators (including calcium channel blockers, angiotensin-converting enzyme (ACE) inhibitors, and nitrates)
  - Phenothiazines
  - Antidepressants
  - Antiarrhythmics
  - Diuretics

Genetics
Specific cardiomyopathies and arrhythmias may be familiial.

PATHOPHYSIOLOGY
Systemic hypotension secondary to decreased cardiac output and/or systemic vasodilation leads to a drop in cerebral perfusion and resultant loss of consciousness.

ETIOLOGY
- Cardiac: Obstruction to outflow
  - Aortic stenosis
  - Hypertrophic cardiomyopathy
  - Pulmonary embolus
- Cardiac: Arrhythmias
  - Sustained ventricular tachycardia (probable cause)
  - Sick-sinus syndrome
  - Sinus node recovery time ≥3 seconds (probable cause)
  - 2nd-degree and 3rd-degree AV block
  - Pacing-induced infranodal block (probable cause)
  - H-V interval >100 m (probable cause)
- Noncardiac
  - Reflex-mediated vasovagal ("drop atttack") (neurocardiogenic/neurally mediated), situational (micturition, defecation, cough)
  - Orthostatic hypotension
  - Drug induced
  - Neurologic: Seizures, transient ischemic attack
  - Carotid sinus
  - Psychogenic

ASSOCIATED CONDITIONS
See "Etiology."

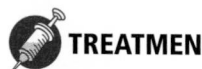 **DIAGNOSIS**

- Careful history, physical examination, and an ECG are more important than other investigations in determining the diagnosis.
- Make sure patient or witness (if present) is not talking about vertigo, coma, or drop attacks.
- After careful evaluation, including diagnostic procedures and special tests, the cause of syncope will be found in only 50–60% of the patients.

PRE HOSPITAL
Support ABCs.

SIGNS AND SYMPTOMS
- Transient loss of consciousness is characterized by unresponsiveness, loss of postural tone, and spontaneous recovery.
- Vasovagal
  - Prodromal manifestations of sudden weakness, nausea, and sweating, especially in circumstances provoking strong emotion
  - Does not occur when patient is horizontal
- Cardiac
  - Suggested by: (a) syncope of sudden onset with no prodrome or brief premonitory symptoms and (b) occurrence with exertion
  - Can occur in any position

History
Onset of syncope is usually rapid, and recovery is spontaneous, rapid, and complete. Duration of episodes are typically brief (<60 s). Presence of underlying cardiac or neurologic conditions provides key to diagnosis.

Physical Exam
- Direct to BP and pulse, both lying and standing.
- Check for cardiac murmur or focal neurologic abnormality.

TESTS
- If history and physical suggest ischemic, valvular, or congenital heart disease
  - ECG
  - Cardiac catheterization
- If CNS disease suspected
  - EEG
  - Head CT
  - Head MRI
  - Do not order these tests unless hints of CNS disease on history or physical examination
- ECG monitoring, either in hospital or ambulatory (Holter)
  - Useful in 4–15% of patients
  - Should be done in patients with heart disease or recurrent syncope
  - Arrhythmias frequently documented, but rarely associated with syncope
- Electrophysiologic studies
  - Have been positive in 18–75% of patients
  - Induction of ventricular tachycardia and dysfunction of His-Purkinje system are the 2 most common abnormalities.
  - Should be done in patients with heart disease or recurrent syncope, although problem exists of knowing whether arrhythmia noted or induced during study is cause of syncope

- Carotid hypersensitivity evaluation
  - Carotid hypersensitivity should be considered in patients with syncope during head turning, especially with head turning while wearing tight collar, and in patients with neck tumors and neck-tissue scars.
  - The technique is not standardized; 1 side should be massaged at a time for 20 seconds with constant monitoring of pulse and BP.
  - Atropine should be readily available.
- Tilt table testing, with and without isoproterenol infusion
  - Provocative test for vasovagal syncope
  - Should be done only if cardiac causes have been excluded; role of test in workup of patients with syncope of unknown origin is not known
  - Not standardized, but has been reported positive (symptomatic hypotension and bradycardia) in 26–87% of patients; however, also reported positive in 0–45% of control subjects
- Psychiatric evaluation
  - Anxiety, depression, alcohol, and drug abuse can be associated with syncope.

Lab
Rarely helpful; <2% have hyponatremia, hypocalcemia, hypoglycemia, or renal failure causing seizures.

Imaging
Lung scan or helical CT of thorax if history and physical examination suggest pulmonary embolism

Diagnostic Procedures/Surgery
Patient-activated implantable loop recorders, which patient activates after regaining consciousness, can record 4–5 minutes of retrograde ECG rhythm. Helpful in patients with recurrent syncope, with diagnostic yield of 24–47%.

Pathological Findings
Depends on etiology and presence of underlying cardiac or neurologic conditions

DIFFERENTIAL DIAGNOSIS
- Drop attacks
- Coma
- Vertigo

TREATMENT

PRE HOSPITAL
Support ABCs.

INITIAL STABILIZATION
Aimed at stabilization of heart rate and blood pressure, typically with IV fluids

GENERAL MEASURES
- Patients with heart disease should be admitted to the hospital for evaluation.
- Elderly patients without previously recognized heart disease should be admitted if the physician thinks that the cause of syncope is likely cardiac.
- Patients without heart disease, especially young patients (<60 years old), can be safely worked up as outpatients.
- Prescribe antiarrhythmic drugs for documented arrhythmias occurring simultaneously with syncope or symptoms of presyncope. Asymptomatic arrhythmias do not require treatment.

- The decision to treat patients on basis of arrhythmias or conduction abnormalities provoked or detected during EPS is even more problematic: Does the arrhythmia or conduction abnormality have anything to do with patient's symptoms?
- Most would treat patient with provoked sustained ventricular tachycardia with antiarrhythmic drug that suppressed arrhythmia during study.
- Many recommend pacemaker implantation in patients with
  – H-V intervals >100 m
  – Pacing-induced infranodal block
  – Sinus node recovery time of ≥3 s
- Rationale for such treatment: Recurrent syncope less frequent in patients with positive EPS who are treated than it is in those who have negative EPS

Diet
- No specific diet unless heart disease
- Increased fluid and salt intake to maintain intravascular volume in cases of recurrent vasovagal syncope

Activity
Full activity unless severe cardiac disease, with avoidance of specific triggers or stimuli

Nursing
Close monitoring of BP, HR during initial presentation

SPECIAL THERAPY
IV Fluids
Use isotonic crystalloids fluids for fluid resuscitation if needed.

 ## MEDICATION (DRUGS)

- Geared towards specific underlying cardiac or neurologic abnormalities
- In cases of recurrent vasovagal/neurocardiogenic/neurally-mediated syncope, the following have been shown to be effective in various placebo-controlled trials
  – Beta-adrenergic blockers
  – Mineralocorticoids (fludrocortisone)
  – Vagolytics (disopyramide)
  – Alpha-adrenergic agonsists (midodrine)
  – Serotonin-reuptake inhibitors (paroxetine, sertraline, fluoxetine)

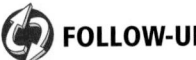 ## FOLLOW-UP

DISPOSITION
Admission Criteria
See "General Measures."

Discharge Criteria
- Attainment of hemodynamic stability
- Satisfactory completion of workup for etiology
- Adequate control of specific arrhythmia or seizure, if present

Issues for Referral
Where cardiac or neurologic etiologies are suspected, appropriate expert consultation is indicated.

PROGNOSIS
Cumulative mortality at 2 years
- Low (25%): Young patients (<60) with noncardiac or unknown cause of syncope
- Intermediate (20%): Older patients (>60) with noncardiac or unknown cause of syncope
- High (32–38%): Patients with cardiac cause of syncope

COMPLICATIONS
- Trauma from falling
- Death (see "Prognosis")

PATIENT MONITORING
- Frequent follow-up visits for patients with cardiac causes of syncope, especially patients on antiarrhythmic drugs
- Patients with an unknown cause of syncope rarely (5%) are diagnosed during the follow-up.

REFERENCES

1. Schnipper JL, Kapoor WN. Diagnostic evaluation and management of patients with syncope. *Med Clin North Am.* 2001;85:423–456.
2. Brignole M, et al. Task Force Report: Guidelines on management (diagnosis and treatment) of syncope. *Eur Heart J.* 2001;22:1256–1306.
3. Goldschlager N, et al. Etiologic considerations in the patient with syncope and an apparently normal heart. *Arch Intern Med.* 2003;163:151–162.

 ## MISCELLANEOUS

See also: Aortic valvular stenosis; Atrial septal defect (ASD); Carotid sinus syndrome; Idiopathic hypertrophic subaortic stenosis (IHSS); Patent ductus arteriosus; Primary pulmonary hypertension; Pulmonary embolism; Seizure disorders; Stokes-Adams attacks

S

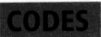 **CODES**

ICD9-CM
780.2 Syncope and collapse

PATIENT TEACHING

Reassure patient that most cardiac causes of syncope can be treated and patients with noncardiac causes do well, even if the cause of syncope is never discovered.

Activity
Physician and patient should carefully consider whether patient should continue to drive while syncope is being evaluated. Physicians should be aware of pertinent laws in their own state.

 See Corresponding Diagnostic Algorithm

 See Patient Handout on CD

SYNDROME OF INAPPROPRIATE ANTIDIURETIC HORMONE (SIADH)

Ruben Peralta, MD, FACS
Jacqueline J. Wu, MD

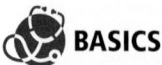 BASICS

DESCRIPTION

- Form of hyponatremia with decreased serum sodium, low serum osmolality, and inappropriately elevated urine osmolality
  - The resulting abnormal urinary water retention and normal sodium excretion lead to dilutional hyponatremia. Total body sodium levels may be normal or near normal. The patient's total body water usually is increased.
  - Associated with an underlying disorder such as neoplasm, pulmonary disorder, or CNS system disease
- Synonym(s): Syndrome of inappropriate secretion of ADH

GENERAL PREVENTION

- Search for cause, if unknown
- Monitor electrolytes in postoperative patients to determine if fluid intake needs restriction
- Reduce or change medications, if caused by drug
- Life-long restriction of fluid intake

EPIDEMIOLOGY

Predominant age: Elderly
Predominate sex: Females > Males

Incidence

Usually found in the hospital setting, where incidence can be as high as 35%

RISK FACTORS

- Use of predisposing drugs
- Advanced age
- Postoperative status
- Institutionalization

Genetics

No known genetic pattern

ETIOLOGY

- Drugs (1)[B]
  - Antidepressants (MAOIs, tricyclics, SSRIs)
  - Oral hypoglycemics (chlorpropamide, metformin)
  - Antineoplastic drugs (vincristine, vinblastine, cisplatin, cyclophosphamide)
  - Antipsychotic agents (phenothiazines, thioridazine, haloperidol)
  - Analgesics (NSAIDs)
  - Antiepileptics (carbamazepine, valproic acid)
  - Diuretics (thiazides and loop)
  - Others (vasopressin, DDAVP, Ecstasy, oxytocin, alpha interferon)
- Neoplasms (ectopic ADH production)
  - Small cell carcinoma of the lung
  - Oat-cell carcinoma of the lung
  - Hodgkin disease
  - Pancreatic carcinoma
  - Thymoma
  - Mesothelioma
  - Bronchogenic carcinoma
- Infectious diseases
  - Meningitis
  - Encephalitis
  - Pneumonia
  - Pulmonary tuberculosis
  - Rocky Mountain spotted fever
  - HIV
- Miscellaneous cardiopulmonary conditions
  - Asthma
  - Atelectasis
  - Myocardial infarction
  - Vascular diseases
- Other
  - CNS injury
  - Mechanical ventilation
  - Multiple sclerosis
  - Guillain-Barré syndrome
  - Lupus erythematosus
  - Porphyria
  - Hypothyroidism, myxedema
  - Idiopathic

ASSOCIATED CONDITIONS

See "Etiology."

DIAGNOSIS

SIGNS AND SYMPTOMS

- Early symptoms
  - Fatigue
  - Anorexia
  - Nausea
  - Vomiting
  - Diarrhea
  - Headaches
  - Myalgias
  - Increased thirst
- Late/severe hyponatremia (serum sodium <100–115 mEq/L)
  - Altered mental status
  - Confusion
  - Lethargy
  - Seizures
  - Psychosis
  - Coma
  - Death

TESTS

Oral water-loading test

- May be helpful in diagnosing some patients.
- Response to water-load will be impaired in SIADH.
- May be unsafe and often not necessary to establish diagnosis.

Lab

- Serum sodium level (low)
- Serum osmolality (low <280)
- BUN
- Creatinine
- Urine osmolality (100+ mOsm/kg)
- Urinary sodium concentration >40 mEq/L (>40 mmol/L)
- Serum glucose
- Thyroid function
- Morning cortisol
- Elevated serum ADH level
- Uric acid

Imaging

Not usually required for diagnosis

DIFFERENTIAL DIAGNOSIS

- Postoperative complication
  - Usually after major abdominal or thoracic surgery
  - Caused by nonosmotic release of ADH, probably mediated by pain afferents
  - ADH increased by pain and narcotics
- Postprostatectomy syndrome
  - Irrigating solution must be nonconducting (i.e., electrolyte free)
  - D5W absorbed
- Psychogenic polydipsia
  - Active therapy rarely is needed.
  - Diuresis occurs when intake is stopped.
  - Intake usually over 10 L/d
  - Interaction with other psychotropic drugs
- Acute (usually in children)
  - Swallowing water during swimming
  - Diluted formula
  - Tap-water enemas
- Endocrine
  - Addison disease
  - Hypothyroidism
- Factitious hyponatremia: Caused by increased serum glucose, cholesterol, or proteins
- "Appropriate" ADH secretion and hyponatremia with decreased effective arterial blood volume (e.g., CHF, nephrotic syndrome, cirrhosis)

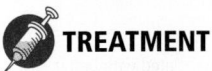

TREATMENT

GENERAL MEASURES

- Fluid restriction: 800–1000 mL/d. This is the main form of treatment.
- Mildly symptomatic (serum sodium >125 mEq/L [>125 mmol/L]): Restrict fluid to 800–1000 mL/d (1)[B]
- Acute (<48 h duration) or symptomatic (altered mental status, seizure, coma)
  - Hypertonic saline (3% normal saline) bolus
  - Diuresis with loop diuretics
  - Decrease oral free water to 2/3 maintenance
  - Increase oral salt
  - Correct serum sodium deficit (mEq sodium deficit = [desired sodium − actual sodium] × 0.5 times body weight [kg])
  - Increase serum sodium slowly with hypertonic saline by 0.5 mEq/L/h until it reaches 120 mEq/L

ALERT

Increase sodium levels slowly, no greater than 0.5–1 mEq/L/h to prevent complications such as central pontine myelinosis (CPM)

Diet

May need increased salt or decreased water intake, depending on cause

Activity

As tolerated

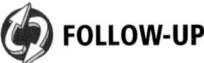 MEDICATION (DRUGS)

First Line

- Diuretics: Furosemide (Lasix) plus hourly sodium chloride and potassium chloride replacement
  - Requires frequent monitoring (see "Patient Monitoring")
  - Treatment of choice for acute management
- Hypertonic (3%) saline; to cautiously increase serum sodium (2)[B]
  - By 10–12 mEq/L (10–12 mmol/L) q24h (in chronic hyponatremia)
  - 5% over 1st few hours
  - To only 120 mEq/L (120 mmol/L), acutely
  - By 0.5 mEq/h (0.5 mmol/h)
- Contraindications: Avoid fluids in CHF, nephrotic syndrome, or cirrhosis
- Precautions: Overly rapid correction (>12m Eq/L/d [>12 mmol/d]) can cause
  - CHF
  - Subdural and intracerebral hemorrhage
  - Permanent CNS damage, especially with serum sodium <120 mEq/L (<120 mmol/L)
  - Demyelination syndrome
- Demeclocycline
  - Blocks ADH at renal tubule, produces nephrogenic diabetes insipidus
  - Dosage for long-term management: 600–1,200 mg/d
  - Onset of action within 1 week, therefore not best for acute management
- Lithium
  - Blocks ADH at renal tubule
  - Use with caution to avoid lithium toxicity.

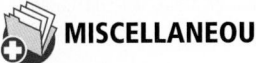 FOLLOW-UP

PROGNOSIS

- Depends on underlying cause
- If symptomatic (seizure, coma): High mortality due to cerebral edema if serum sodium <120 mEq/L (<120 mmol/L)

COMPLICATIONS

- Central pontine myelinosis
- Chronic hyponatremia: Usually <120 mEq/L (<120 mmol/L)
- Complications of overly rapid correction (see "Treatment, Precautions")

PATIENT MONITORING

- Careful, continuous clinical and laboratory monitoring of hyponatremic state during acute phase
  - Hourly urine output
  - Urine sodium
  - Serum sodium and potassium
- Chronic management: Monitor underlying cause as needed.

REFERENCES

1. Yeates KE, Singer M, Morton AR. Salt and water: A simple approach to hyponatremia. *CMAJ* 2004;170(3):365–369.
2. Arvanitis ML, Pasquale JL. External causes of metabolic disorders. *Emerg Med Clin North Amer* 2005:827–841.
3. Adrogue HJ, Madias NE. Hyponatremia. *N Engl J Med* 2000;342:1581–1589.

 MISCELLANEOUS

See also: Hyponatremia

CODES

ICD9-CM

- 253.6 Syndrome of inappropriate secretion of antidiuretic hormone
- 276.9 Electrolyte and fluid disorders NEC

PATIENT TEACHING

Diet

Diet and fluid restrictions

See Corresponding Diagnostic Algorithm

SYNOVITIS PIGMENTED VILLONODULAR

Brian Busconi, MD
Adam Harner, MD

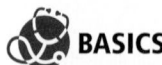 BASICS

DESCRIPTION
- Pigmented villonodular synovitis (PVNS) is a condition of the synovial membrane that is characterized by the presence of inflammation and hemosiderin deposition in the synovium.
- 2 forms of PVNS exist: Diffuse (DPVNS) and localized (LPVNS).

EPIDEMIOLOGY
- Predominant age: 3rd and 4th decades
- Predominant sex: Male = Female

Incidence
1.8 per million

PATHOPHYSIOLOGY
- Histologically, LPVNS and DPVNS are similar
  - Lipid-laden macrophages
  - Multinucleated giant cells
  - Hemosiderin deposition in the synovium
  - Stromal and fibroblast cell proliferation
- DPVNS and LPVNS differ in their disease course
  - DPVNS
    - Characterized by involvement of most or all of the joint synovium
    - More common
    - More rapidly destructive course with poorer prognosis
    - Can encroach on major neurovascular structures
    - Higher occurrence rate
    - Continued inflammation and joint erosions lead to articular cartilage destruction and subsequent osteoarthritis
  - LPVNS
    - Characterized by a pedunculated, lobular lesion localized to one area of the synovium
    - Favorable prognosis secondary to its localized nature
    - Low recurrence rate following surgical intervention

ETIOLOGY
- Still largely unknown
- Possibly the result of trauma and subsequent recurrent local hemorrhage in the affected joint
  - <1/3 of patients report a history of trauma.
- Possibly secondary to abnormal local metabolic activity
- Possibly a neoplastic process with rare reports of malignant transformation and metastasis
  - Demonstrates neither cellular atypia nor abnormal mitotic activity
  - Exhibits some cytogenetic abnormalities
- Possibly a chronic inflammation process

DIAGNOSIS

SIGNS AND SYMPTOMS
- Typically a monoarticular process that often involves the large joints.
- Knee is most commonly involved.
- Hip, ankle, shoulder, and elbow also are possibilities.

History
- Slow and insidious onset of pain, swelling, and stillness
- History of locking, catching, or instability is more common with LPVNS.
- Symptoms are often intermittent

Physical Exam
- Tenderness to palpation of involved joint
- Joint effusion
- Loss of range of motion

Imaging
- Plain radiographs
  - Periarticular erosions with thin rim of reactive bone
  - Reciprocal bony lesions on opposite sides of the joint
  - Joint space narrowing is a late finding.
  - Majority of cases have no findings.
- CT
  - Appears as a soft tissue mass of high density
  - Underlying bone erosions or cysts
- MRI
  - Modality of choice
  - Helpful for determining the extent of disease and differentiation DPVNS from LPVNS
  - DPVNS
    - Poorly localized mass or synovial thickening with varying degrees of periarticular erosions
    - Low signal on T1 and T2 weighted images
    - Joint effusion
  - LPVNS
    - Periarticular or synovial nodular mass with varying degrees of bond erosion
    - High hemosiderin content causes low signal on T1- and T2-weighted images
    - Joint effusion

Diagnostic Procedures/Surgery
Synovial fluid aspiration
- Brownish-stained bloody fluid is indicative of PVNS.
- Lacks sensitivity and specificity

DIFFERENTIAL DIAGNOSIS
- Rheumatoid arthritis
- Osteoarthritis
- Synovial sarcoma
- Hemophilia
- Lipoma arborescens
- Hematoma
- Hemangioma
- Giant cell tumor of the tendon sheath

TREATMENT

GENERAL MEASURES
- The goal is to eradicate all abnormal synovial tissue, thus removing the source of pain and reducing the risk of joint destruction and recurrence.
- The treatment of PVNS is largely surgical.

Activity
As tolerated

Radiotherapy
- An alternative to surgical synovectomy
- Serious potential complications
  - Skin reactions
  - Poor wound healing
  - Joint stiffness
  - Sarcomatous transformation
- Highly useful in managing refractory cases or in those with extensive extra-articular involvement
- May be used as an adjuvant to surgical synovectomy, especially in challenging cases with persistently recurrent disease and involvement of critical anatomic structures.

SURGERY
- The mainstay of treatment
- Arthroscopy has been associated with better functional results and lower rates of postoperative stiffness than have open techniques.
- Arthroscopic partial synovectomy is the standard care for LPVNS.
  - Recurrence is rare after limited local treatment of LPVNS.
- Arthroscopic treatment of DPVNS is associated with a significantly higher recurrence rate.
- Patients with large popliteal masses or extra-articular involvement generally are not candidates for an exclusively arthroscopic approach.
- A thorough, complete synovectomy is the treatment of choice for DPVNS.
  - This is most easily accomplished through an open surgical procedure.
  - A combined arthroscopic and open approach is also a commonly utilized alternative.
- Joint replacement is indicated in cases with significant joint destruction.

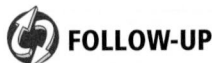 FOLLOW-UP

PROGNOSIS
- Patients presenting with recurrent disease have much more extensive involvement and a poorer likelihood of successful treatment.
- DPVNS is more rapidly destructive and has a poorer prognosis.
- Recurrence rates after adequate synovectomy are in the range of 5–20%.
  - Rates are higher with DPVNS.
  - Rates are also increased with extra-articular involvement.
- Articular cartilage destruction and the development of osteoarthritis requires joint replacement surgery.
- Malignant transformation has been reported but is exceedingly rare.
- Extensive joint involvement and extra-articular spread may result after failed arthroscopic management.
- Postoperative stiffness occurs in ~25% of patients treated with an open procedure.

REFERENCES
1. Tyler WK, Vidal AF, Williams RJ, Healey JM. Pigmented villonodular synovitis. *J Am Acad Orthopaed Surg.* 2006;14:376–385.
2. Al-Nakshabandi NA, Ryan AG, Choudur H, Al-Ismail K. Pigmented villonodular synovitis. *Clin Radiol.* 2004;59:414–420.

ADDITIONAL READING
Flandry F, Hughston JC. Pigmented villonodular synovitis. J Bone Joint Surg Am. 1987;69:942–949.

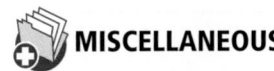 MISCELLANEOUS

PATIENT TEACHING
Resources and education are important when dealing with patients with PVNS

S

SYPHILIS

Milisa K. Rizer, MD, MPH

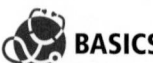 **BASICS**

DESCRIPTION

- Infectious disease caused by the spirochete, *Treponema pallidum*. Transmitted sexually, maternal-fetal, and via blood transfusions
- Primary
  - Painless ulcer at site of infection (chancre)
- Secondary
  - Rash, usually palms and soles, can be whole body.
- Latent
  - Seroreactive without evidence of disease.
  - Early latent: Acquired within the past year
  - Late latent or latent of unknown duration
    - Exposure >12 months prior
- Tertiary (late)
  - Serology may be negative
  - Damage to multiple systems
    - Cardiovascular
    - CNS
    - Musculoskeletal
  - May result in death
  - Mental status may be altered
- Neurosyphilis
  - May occur at any stage of syphilis
- Congenital
  - Syphilis acquired in utero

ALERT

Pediatric Considerations

In noncongenital cases, must consider possibility of child abuse

Pregnancy Considerations

- All expectant mothers should have VDRL or RPR at 1st prenatal visit. If high exposure risk, repeat the tests at 28 weeks and at delivery.
- Jarisch-Herxheimer reaction (acute febrile reaction of headache, myalgia, rash, and hypotension) may induce preterm labor or fetal distress, but is not a reason to delay treatment.

GENERAL PREVENTION

Safe sex; use of condoms

EPIDEMIOLOGY

Predominant age: Sexually active years
Predominant sex: Male > Female (5.9:1)

Incidence

In 2004: 2.7/100,000 population

- White, non-Hispanic: 1.6/100,000
- Black: 9.0/100,000
- Hispanic: 3.2/100,000
- Asian/Pacific Islander: 1.2/100,000
- American Indian/Alaska Native: 3.2/100,000

RISK FACTORS

- Men having sex with men
- Multiple sexual partners
- Exposure to infected body fluids
- IV drug use
- Transplacental transmission

ETIOLOGY

Treponema pallidum

ASSOCIATED CONDITIONS

- HIV infection
- Hepatitis B
- Other sexually transmitted diseases

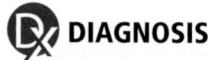 **DIAGNOSIS**

SIGNS AND SYMPTOMS

- Primary
  - Small, round, firm ulcer at the place where the bacteria enter (chancre). Typically on penis, vulva, or vagina but can be lips, tongue, and cervix. Occurs 9–90 days after exposure (mean of 21–28 days).
  - Lymphadenopathy often present locally.
  - Chancre heals spontaneously within 28 days.
  - ~3/4 of the patients have no further symptoms; 1/4 progress.
- Secondary
  - Occurs ~28–70 days after the chancre
  - May have fever, lymphadenopathy, malaise, myalgias, and arthralgias
  - Patchy alopecia: Scalp, eyebrows, and beard
  - Nickel and dime lesions: Hyperpigmented annular lesions with raised depigmented border.
  - Often characterized by generalized body rash: Polymorphic, nonpruritic; usually not bullous or vesicular.
  - Papules may coalesce to form highly infectious lesions called *condylomata lata;* these start as red, vesicular, and painful, and progress to gray. Often in perineal region.
  - Active spirochetes are present in lesions; contact with broken skin or mucous membrane can spread infection.
  - Rash resolves spontaneously in <49 days.

- Latent syphilis
  - Characterized by positive serology but no signs or symptoms
  - Early latent: Acquired within the past year; within the past year patient had to have
    - 4-fold seroconversion in nontreponemal test titer, or
    - Unequivocal symptoms of primary or secondary syphilis, or
    - Sex partner with primary, secondary, or early latent syphilis, or
    - Reactive nontreponemal and treponemal tests with only possible exposure within the last 12 months.
  - Late latent or latent of unknown duration
    - Exposure >12 months prior
- Tertiary syphilis
  - Serologies often are negative.
  - Gummatous lesions that usually affect skin, bone, and mucous membranes, but may involve any organ and cause local destruction of the affected organ system.
  - Cardiovascular symptoms result from endarteritis of the aorta resulting in aortitis and aneurysm formation
    - Asymptomatic murmur, aortic insufficiency, left heart failure, aneurysms of ascending thoracic aorta, aortic-valve regurgitation
  - Orthopedic complications
    - Rare with antibiotics
    - Charcot joints, osteomyelitis
- Neurosyphilis
  - May be symptomatic or asymptomatic
  - Personality change, ataxia, stroke
  - Blurred vision, photophobia
  - Urinary incontinence, meningitis
  - Headache, nausea, and vomiting
  - Cranial nerve involvement, paresthesias
  - Loss of position, vibratory, pain, and temperature sensation

- Congenital syphilis
  - Young infants
    - Rash: Hallmark similar to secondary syphilis in adults, may be bullous or vesicular
    - Snuffles (mucopurulent rhinitis)
    - Failure to thrive
    - Nonimmune hydrops
    - Osteochondritis
    - Lymphadenopathy
    - Jaundice
    - Anemia
    - Hepatosplenomegaly
    - Nephrosis
    - Meningitis
    - Saddle nose
    - Iritis
    - Pseudoparalysis of a limb
  - Children
    - Hutchinson teeth
    - Saber shins
    - Charcot joints
    - Deafness
    - Interstitial keratitis

History
Exposure

TESTS
- Dark-field microscopy demonstrating *T. pallidum* spirochetes is gold standard for definitive diagnosis.
- Direct florescent antibody test
- Skin biopsy to demonstrate *Treponema pallidum* in tissue

Lab
- Nontreponemal tests: VDRL or RPR
  - Primary screening test
  - Relatively inexpensive
  - Positive within 7 days of exposure
  - Positive test should be quantified and titers followed at regular intervals after treatment.
  - Titers usually correlate with disease activity.
  - Titer decreases with time or treatment; following adequate treatment for primary or secondary a 4-fold decline should be noted by 4 months and an 8-fold decline by 8 months. Titer eventually should be negative (see "Serofast Reaction"). Titers of patients treated in latent stages will decline more gradually.
  - Failure of nontreponemal test titers to decline 4-fold within 6 months after therapy for primary or secondary might indicate treatment failure.
  - Nonspecific; must confirm diagnosis with treponemal test (false-positive common)
  - Prozone phenomenon: Negative results due to very high titers of antibody; test diluted serum sample
  - Serofast reaction: Persistently positive results years after successful treatment; new infection is diagnosed by 4-fold rise in titer
  - Drugs that may alter lab results
    - Recent immunization (e.g., smallpox)
    - Many reported to cause false positive, but uncommon with a good history
  - Disorders that may alter lab results
    - Pregnancy
    - Autoimmune disease
    - Systemic lupus erythematosus
    - Mononucleosis
    - Malaria
    - Leprosy
    - Viral pneumonia
    - Presence of cardiolipin antigens
    - Drug addiction
    - Acute febrile illness
    - HIV infection
    - Elderly can be false positive

S

- Treponemal tests: FTA-ABS, TP-PA
  - Confirmatory test, not used for screening
  - More expensive
  - Usually positive for life after treatment
  - Titers of no benefit
  - 15–20% of patients treated during the primary stage revert to being serologically nonreactive after 2–3 years.
  - Drugs that may alter lab results: See "Nontreponemal Tests"
  - Disorders that may alter lab results: See "Nontreponemal Tests"
- Lumbar puncture
  - Indicated for any patient who has clinical evidence of neurologic involvement or has syphilitic ocular or auditory manifestations
  - Some experts advise in all secondary and early latent cases without neuro symptoms
  - In HIV-positive patients with late latent or latent of unknown duration
  - In cases of late latent or latent of unknown duration, or when nonpenicillin therapy is planned
  - In treatment failures
  - If other evidence of active syphilis is present (aortitis, gumma, iritis)
  - In children with syphilis, after the newborn period, to rule out neurosyphilis
  - VDRL, not RPR, used on CSF; may be negative in neurosyphilis; highly specific but insensitive
  - Send fluid for protein, glucose and cell count
  - Monitor resolution by cell count at 6 months along with serologies as recommended (see Patient Monitoring)
  - Negative FTA-ABS or MHA-TP on CSF excludes neurosyphilis, highly sensitive
  - Positive FTA-ABS or MHA-TP on CSF not diagnostic because high false-positive rate
  - Bloody tap, tuberculosis, pyogenic or aseptic meningitis can result in false-positive VDRL

Imaging
Only in late cases as indicated

Pathological Findings
- Aneurysm
- Osteomyelitis
- Gummas in late cases

DIFFERENTIAL DIAGNOSIS
- Primary
  - Chancroid
  - Lymphogranuloma venereum
  - Granuloma inguinale
  - Condyloma Acuminata
  - Herpes Simplex
  - Behçet syndrome
  - Trauma
  - Carcinoma
  - Mycotic infection
  - Lichen planus
  - Psoriasis
  - Fungal infection
- Secondary
  - Pityriasis rosea
  - Drug eruption
  - Psoriasis
  - Lichen planus
  - Viral exanthema
  - Stevens-Johnson syndrome
- Positive serology, asymptomatic
  - Previously treated syphilis
  - Other spirochetal disease (yaws, pinta)
  - Biological false positive: See "Disorders that May Alter Lab Results"

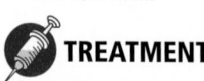 **TREATMENT**

GENERAL MEASURES
- Outpatient, except for initiating IV penicillin or desensitization
- Baseline serologies prior to treatment

Diet
No special diet

Activity
Full activity, but no sexual contacts until 4-fold drop in nontreponemal test titer

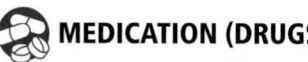 **MEDICATION (DRUGS)**

First Line
Parenteral penicillin G is drug of choice for all stages. (2)[A] Choice of penicillin formulation is determined by the disease stage and clinical manifestations.

ALERT
Bicillin L-A should be used and *not* Bicillin C-R when penicillin G benzathine is indicated. (4)[A]

- Primary, secondary, and early latent <1 year
  - Benzathine penicillin G 2.4 million units IM for 1 dose (2)[A]
  - Penicillin-allergic patients: Doxycycline 100 mg PO b.i.d. for 2 weeks or tetracycline 500 mg PO q.i.d. for 2 weeks; Ceftriaxone 1 g IM or IV daily for 8–10 days is used by some
- Late latent or latent of unknown duration and tertiary without evidence of neurosyphilis
  - Benzathine penicillin G 2.4 million units IM weekly for 3 doses (2)[A]
  - Penicillin-allergic patients: Attempt desensitization and treatment with penicillin; doxycycline 100 mg PO 2 b.i.d. for 28 days or tetracycline 500 mg PO for 28 days; compliance may be an issue
- Neurosyphilis
  - Aqueous crystalline penicillin G 3–4 million units IV q4h, or continuous infusion for 10–14 days, or procaine penicillin G 2.4 million units IM daily and probenecid 500 mg PO q.i.d. for 10–14 days (if compliance can be ensured) (2)[A]
  - Penicillin-allergic patients: Attempt desensitization and treatment with penicillin; Ceftriaxone 2 g daily IM or IV for 10–14 days
  - If late latent, latent of unknown duration, or tertiary in addition to neurosyphilis, consider also treating as recommended for late latent after completion of neurosyphilis treatment
- Congenital
  - Aqueous crystalline penicillin G 50,000 units/kg/dose IV q12h for 1st 7 days of life and q8hs thereafter for a total of 10 days, or procaine penicillin G 50,000 units/kg/dose IM daily for 10 days (2)[A]
  - If negative CSF serologies, normal physical exam, and titer ≤ maternal titer then 50,000 units/kg benzathine penicillin G IM in single dose is also alternative (2)[A]
  - If >1 day of therapy is missed, restart entire course.
- Children (after newborn period)
  - Aqueous crystalline penicillin G 50,000 units/kg/dose IV q4–6h for 10 days; late latent: 50,000 units/kg IM as 3 doses at 1-week intervals (2)[A]

- Pregnancy
  – Treatment same as for nonpregnant patients;
  – Some specialists recommend 2nd dose of 2.4 million units benzathine penicillin G 1 week after initial dose, especially in 3rd trimester or with primary, secondary, or early latent syphilis.
  – Penicillin sensitivity: No proven alternatives to penicillin exist for treatment during pregnancy; consider desensitization and treat with penicillin (2)[A]
- Epidemiologic treatment for contacts without symptoms, treat as primary after baseline serologies obtained
- Contraindications: Allergy to penicillin
- Precautions
  – HIV-infected and pregnant patients may show poor response to recommended IM doses. Use IV therapy for all treatment failures in these patients.
  – *Do not* give benzathine or procaine penicillins IV.
- Significant possible interactions: Refer to manufacturer's literature.

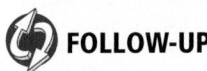 ## FOLLOW-UP

Follow-up is very important

DISPOSITION

Issues for Referral
Sonographic signs of fetal or placental syphilis indicate a greater risk for treatment failure and should be managed in consult with obstetric specialist.

PROGNOSIS

- Excellent in all cases except patients with late-syphilis complications and a few with HIV infection
- Syphilis in HIV-infected patient
  – Test for HIV in any patient with syphilis.
  – Treatment recommendations are same as HIV negative.
  – More often false-negative treponemal and nontreponemal tests or unusually high titers (see "Prozone Phenomenon")
  – Serologic response to therapy sometimes less predictable
  – Early syphilis: Increased risk of neurosyphilis and might have higher rates of treatment failure
  – Neurosyphilis: Harder to treat; can occur up to 20 years after infection

COMPLICATIONS

- Cardiovascular disease
- CNS disease
- Membranous glomerulonephritis
- Paroxysmal cold hemoglobinemia
- Meningitis
- Tabes dorsalis
- Irreversible organ damage
- Jarisch-Herxheimer reaction
  – Marked by fever, chills, headache, myalgias, new rash
  – Common on starting treatment (of primary or secondary disease; less common with tertiary) due to lysis of treponemes
  – Should not be confused with reaction to antibiotics
  – Managed with analgesics and antipyretics

PATIENT MONITORING

- Use VDRL or RPR to monitor therapy: 4-fold rise in titer indicates new infection, whereas failure to decrease 4-fold within 6 months is treatment failure (although definitive criteria for cure not established); always use same test (VDRL or RPR).
- Re-treat for persistent clinical signs or recurrence, 4-fold rise in titers, or failure of initially high titer to decrease 4-fold by 6 months.
- Labs must titer tests to final end point (e.g., not report as ">1:512") to make best use of results in monitoring therapy response.
- Repeat serologies at 3, 6, 9, and 12 months after treatment; if >1 year's duration, check at 24 months also.

REFERENCES

1. CDC. Sexually transmitted disease surveillance, 2004. Atlanta, GA: US Department of Health and Human Services.
2. CDC Sexually Transmitted Diseases Treatment Guidelines, 2006. *MMWR Weekly*. 2006; 55(RR-11):22–34.
3. Drugs for sexually transmitted infections. *Med Lett.* 2004;2(26).
4. Palacioz K. Syphilis treatment errors. *Prescriber's Letter*. 2004;11(5):200513.
5. CDC. Primary and Secondary Syphilis—United States, 2003–2004. *MMWR Weekly*. 2006;55(10): 269–273.
6. McGregor T. Syphilis. www.emedicine.com/emerg/topic563.htm. Accessed 8/26/2006.
7. Knudsen R. Neurosyphilis. www.emedicine.com/neuro/topic684.htm Accessed 8/28/2006.
8. Larson S. *A Manual of Tests for Syphilis*. Washington, DC: American Public Health Association, 1990.

 ## MISCELLANEOUS

- See also: Chlamydial sexually transmitted diseases; Gonococcal infections
- Many experts urge more aggressive treatment than standard regimens in all patients especially HIV-positive and pregnant patients, and strongly advocate use of penicillin rather than any alternative antibiotic.
- Penicillin-allergic patients, particularly with neurosyphilis, HIV infection, and pregnancy, should undergo desensitization.

CODES

ICD9-CM
097.9 Syphilis, unspecified

PATIENT TEACHING

- Advise patient to
  – Trace all sexual contacts so they can be treated.
  – Keep follow-up appointments to monitor the success of therapy.
- Local health department can provide literature and contact tracing.

Activity
Advise patient to avoid intercourse until treatment is complete.

Prevention
Discuss safe sex and use of condoms.

 See Corresponding Diagnostic Algorithm

SYSTEMIC LUPUS ERYTHEMATOSUS (SLE)

Michael Tutt, MD

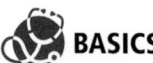 **BASICS**

DESCRIPTION

Multisystem, autoimmune inflammatory condition characterized by fluctuating, chronic course; varies from mild to severe and may be lethal (CNS and renal forms)

- System(s) Affected: Endocrine/Metabolic; Gastrointestinal; Hemic/Lymphatic/Immunologic; Musculoskeletal; Nervous; Renal/Urologic; Skin/Exocrine
- Synonym(s): SLE; Disseminated lupus erythematosus

ALERT

Stroke syndromes frequently seen in children

Pregnancy Considerations

- The onset of lupus and lupus flares more common during pregnancy.
- Fetal loss increased for mothers with lupus
- Newborns of mothers who have lupus are more likely to have cardiac arrhythmias.
- Specialists' collaboration during pregnancy is indicated.

GENERAL PREVENTION

- Avoiding sun exposure is only necessary for ~1/6 of SLE patients (those who report such sensitivity).
- Routine vaccinations are safe and appropriate for SLE patients.
- Drugs known to induce SLE in normal individuals are not necessarily contraindicated in patients who have idiopathic SLE.

EPIDEMIOLOGY

- Predominant age: All ages, but 30–50 most common
- Predominant sex: Female > Male (10:1)
- Higher percentage of males involved among elderly

Prevalence

20/100,000

RISK FACTORS

- Race: African Americans, Hispanics, Asians, and Native Americans have a higher prevalence than whites.
- Genetic markers (see "Genetics")
- Hereditary complement deficiency, especially C1q, C1r, C1s, C4, and C2
- Polymorphisms in the FCGR2A and FCGR3A genes may be important.

Genetics

Markers: HLA-B8, HLA-DR2, HLA-DR3

ETIOLOGY

- Most cases are idiopathic.
- Drugs: Drug-induced lupus is clinically different from idiopathic SLE.

ASSOCIATED CONDITIONS

Other autoimmune diseases

- Rheumatoid arthritis
- Hypothyroidism
- Diabetes

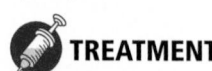 **DIAGNOSIS**

SIGNS AND SYMPTOMS

- Arthritis
- Fever
- Anorexia
- Malaise
- Weight loss
- Skin lesions
- Oral ulcers
- Eye pain and/or redness
- Chest pain and/or shortness of breath
- Pallor
- Nausea, vomiting, diarrhea
- Muscles: Tenderness, aching, and stiffness
- Headaches and visual problems
- Psychosis/delirium

TESTS

Special tests

- Complement levels, immune complex assays (cryoglobulins, Raji cell test, C1q precipitins)
- Coagulation studies (lupus anticoagulant)
- Biopsy of skin, kidney, and peripheral nerves may reveal typical histopathology.

Lab

- Positive antinuclear antibody
  - "False-positive ANA" occurs in 15% of the elderly tested, so caution is required when interpreting the lab results for patients in this age group.
- Anti-double standard DNA (dsDNA), anti-Sm, false-positive VDRL, or positive LE preparation. These tests have either high sensitivity (ANA, false-positive VDRL) or specificity (anti-dsDNA, anti-Sm, and LE preparation) and are included as American Rheumatology Association criteria for diagnosis along with clinical features.
- Sedimentation rate nonspecific, but valuable in assessing SLE activity
- Anemia
- Anticardiolipin antibody
- Leukopenia
- Lymphopenia
- Abnormal urinary sediment
- Proteinuria
- Increased prothrombin time
- Hypoalbuminuria
- Thrombocytopenia
- Increased serum creatinine
- Positive Coombs test

Imaging

- Cerebral angiography in CNS lupus
- Chest x-ray for pulmonary infiltration, pleural effusion
- MRI to detect CNS lupus
- ECG for pericardial effusion

Diagnostic Procedures/Surgery

The American Rheumatology Association criteria (any 4 manifestations of the 11 listed)

- Malar (butterfly) rash
- Discoid rash
- Photosensitivity
- Oral/nasopharyngeal ulcers
- Nonerosive arthritis
- Pleuritis or pericarditis
- Renal disorder: Proteinuria or cylindruria
- Neurologic disorder: Psychosis or seizures
- Hematologic disorder: Hemolytic anemia, leukopenia (<4000), lymphopenia (<1500), thrombocytopenia (<100,000)
- Immunologic disorder
- Positive ANA in absence of drugs known to cause positive ANA

Note: Although the above criteria are required for proper epidemiologic classification of SLE, in practical situations, a combination of a multisystem inflammatory illness, a positive ANA, and the absence of a better diagnosis often represents the most practical way to make a clinical diagnosis.

Pathological Findings

Connective-tissue disorders affecting skin, blood vessels, and serous and synovial membranes

- Collagenous swelling
- Fibrinoid change
- Cellular necrosis
- Periarterial sclerosis
- Granulomatous reaction
- Infiltration of polymorphonuclear leukocytes, plasma cells, lymphocytes in walls of small vessels, arterioles of skin, spleen, glomeruli, endocardium pericardium, brain
- Hematoxylin bodies resembling those in LE cells
- Vegetation on heart valves

DIFFERENTIAL DIAGNOSIS

- SLE mimics numerous systemic conditions, especially those involving inflammation.
- Many other disorders mimic SLE: Rheumatoid arthritis, mixed connective tissue disease, scleroderma, metastatic malignancy, fever of unknown origin, psychogenic rheumatism, and many cutaneous rashes. No one test or biopsy is pathognomonic.

TREATMENT

GENERAL MEASURES

- Outpatient with regular monitoring
- Avoidance of, or protection from, ultraviolet light by using sunscreens, hats, and so on
- Early intervention when infections occur
- Energy conservation
- Stress avoidance/management

Diet

No special diet unless for complications, such as renal failure

Activity

- As active as possible
- Those with arthritis may be limited by pain, but active exercises are to be encouraged.

MEDICATION (DRUGS)

Treatment is symptomatic with certain exceptions. No 1 drug of choice is available. Local steroids for cutaneous manifestations, NSAIDs for minor arthritis symptoms, low-dose steroids for minor discomfort, and high-dose steroids for major inflammatory disease

- Renal disease and severe disease in other organs: Immunosuppressants
- Minor arthritis: NSAIDs
- Cutaneous lupus: Sunscreen and topical steroids
- More significant arthritis or dermal lupus: Hydroxychloroquine 310 mg/d (400 mg/d of the sulfate salt)
- Major symptoms in one or more organ systems: Prednisone 30–60 mg/d
- Glomerulonephritis: Cyclophosphamide 0.5 g/m^2 IV on a monthly basis together with prednisone 60 mg/d PO tapering to 10 mg every other day after 4 months
- Arthritis, rash, serositis, or fever: Methotrexate 5–25 mg PO or SC weekly in a single dose has been effective as a "steroid sparer."
- SLE thrombocytopenia: Immune globulin IV pulse has been effective in temporary treatment.
- Obvious thrombotic disease and/or CNS symptoms, when associated with a positive "lupus anticoagulant" test or anticardiolipin antibody: Heparin or warfarin (Coumadin)
- Contraindications: Refer to the manufacturer's profile of each drug.
- Precautions: Ensure good hydration when administering cyclophosphamide, due to possibility of hemorrhagic cystitis.
- Significant possible interactions: Refer to the manufacturer's profile of each drug.

 ## FOLLOW-UP

PROGNOSIS

- Most patients with lupus follow a course of remissions and exacerbations. Many experience spontaneous permanent remission.
- Treatment of renal lupus (the most serious form) with immunosuppressors, renal dialysis, and renal transplantation has increased the 5-year life expectancy to >90%. For those patients surviving the 1st 2 years of the disease, life expectancy is essentially normal.
- In patients with drug-induced lupus, symptoms should gradually decrease upon the discontinuation of the suspected agent.

COMPLICATIONS

- Fever
- Vasculitis
- Panniculitis
- Myositis
- Avascular necrosis of bone
- Endocarditis
- Pulmonary fibrosis
- Renal failure
- Organic brain syndromes
- Peripheral neuropathy
- Stroke syndromes
- Pancreatitis and elevated liver enzymes
- Infertility
- Ascites
- Venous thrombosis
- Seizures

PATIENT MONITORING

- Follow acute flares frequently (weekly to monthly) in order to adjust the medication based on the clinical impression.
  – Laboratory parameters are of limited value.
  – CBC useful in hematologic lupus
  – Serum creatinine or renal clearance tests of value in renal lupus
  – The sedimentation rate often helps determine adequate suppression of the symptoms or the development of remission.
- Confirming tests for lupus (e.g., ANA titers, anti-DNA titers, complement levels) are usually not helpful in the follow-up assessment.
- The value of continuing the medication depends upon the symptoms. The exception is in the case of renal lupus, for which it has been shown that a defined course of monthly IV cyclophosphamide has been of value.
- Baseline ophthalmological exam and yearly exam while on hydroxychloroquine

REFERENCES

1. Kelley WN, Harris ED, Ruddy S, Sledge CB. *Textbook of Rheumatology.* 4th ed. Philadelphia, PA: WB Saunders Co.1993.
2. Kippel JH, Dippe PA, eds. *Rheumatology.* St. Louis, Mo: Mosby; 1994.
3. Tan FK, Arnett FC. The genetics of lupus. *Curr Opin Rheumatol.* 1998;10:399–408.
4. Godfrey T, et al. Therapeutic advances in SLE. *Curr Opin Rheumatol.* 1998;10:435–441.

 ## MISCELLANEOUS

See also: Anemia, autoimmune hemolytic

 CODES

ICD9-CM
710.0 Systemic lupus erythematosus

PATIENT TEACHING

Printed materials available from
- Arthritis Foundation, 1314 Spring Street NW, Atlanta, GA 30309; (404) 872–7100.
- Lupus Foundation of America, 1717 Massachusetts Avenue, NW, Suite 203, Washington, DC 20036; (800) 558–0121

 See Corresponding Diagnostic Algorithm

 See Patient Handout on CD

S

TAPEWORM INFESTATION

Kenton Voorhees, MD, FAAFP

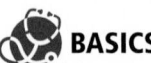 **BASICS**

DESCRIPTION

- Tapeworms (cestodes, flatworms) can be parasitic in humans.
- Adult worms consist of a head (scolex), which attaches to the host's gastrointestinal (GI) tract; a neck; and a segmented body (strobila), with individual segments (proglottid) containing sets of male and female reproductive organs that produce eggs.
- The life cycle of all but *Hymenolepis nana* requires an intermediate host, where they grow as larval forms in tissue that is then ingested by the final host, where it subsequently develops into an adult. *H. nana* can complete all stages of development in humans, helping to make it the most common tapeworm in humans.
- Most tapeworm infections are confined to the GI tract, except in *Taenia solium* (causing cysticercosis), or with *Echinococcus* infections, making infections with these more serious.
- Neurocysticercosis is the most common inpatient disorder due to parasite infection.
- Common tapeworms and their usual intermediate hosts and type of infection in humans include

Tapeworm intermediate hosts

Name	Host
D. latum	Freshwater fish
D. caninum	Dog, cat, fleas
E. granulosis	Human, sheep, cow, dog
E. multilocularis	Fox, coyotes, cats, rodents
H. diminuta	Rodent, insects
H. nana	Human, rodent, insects
T. saginata	Cow
T. solium	Pig

- *Taenia saginata:* Beef causing an intestinal worm; 2–4 months from ingestion to adult; 3–10 m long; usually single tapeworm. Proglottids are motile; may crawl out of anus. May live 30 years
- *Taenia solium:* Pork; Intestinal worm or cysticercosis 2–4 months to become adult worm; 3 m long, occasionally multiple. Proglottids not motile. May live up to 25 years. Ingestion of encysted larvae (cysticerci) causes intestinal tapeworm. Ingestion of *T. solium* eggs causes cysticercosis. Eggs look identical to *T. saginata* eggs.
- *Diphyllobothrium latum* and other species: Freshwater fish; Intestinal worm. Longest adult tapeworm—up to 25 m. Matures to adult in 3–5 weeks
- *H. nana:* Rodent, insects, or humans; intestinal worm. Mature to adult worms in 10–12 days. Seldom exceeds 40 mm long. Proglottids rarely seen in stool. Eggs can autoinfect individual, or occasionally insects (especially meal worms). Fecal–oral transmission possible. Life span 4–10 weeks, but autoinfection can perpetuate infection. Usually self-cleared by adolescence

- *Echinococcus granulosis* and *E. multilocularis:* Humans, sheep, and cattle are intermediate hosts, with dogs the definitive hosts for *E. granulosis.* Foxes, coyotes, or cats are definitive hosts for *E. multilocularis,* with rodents the intermediate hosts. *E. granulosis*—cystic Echinococcus. *E. multilocularis*—alveolar Echinococcus. Hydatid disease of liver, spleen, etc., or alveolar hydatid disease Adult worm lives in dogs (or rodents). Human ingests eggs; larvae hatch and are carried through circulation to various organs such as liver and lungs, where they develop into hydatid cysts that enlarge, causing symptoms perhaps 5–20 years later.
- *H. diminuta:* Rodents and insects; intestinal worm. 90 cm long. Humans rare accidental hosts, by swallowing mealworms or grain beetles from grain.
- *Dipylidium caninum:* Dogs and cats, and fleas; intestinal worm. 10–70 cm long. Motile proglottids, shape of cucumber seeds, can crawl out anus. Rare accidental infection by ingesting infected flea that came from dogs or cats
- System(s) Affected: Gastrointestinal; Nervous

ALERT
Pediatric Considerations
- *H. nana,* highest among children with fecal–oral spread
- *H. diminuta* and *D. caninum* more common in children, as more likely to ingest insects accidentally

GENERAL PREVENTION
- Treatment of infected animals, populations, and screening household contacts, immigrants
- Improved sewage treatment
- See Patient Teaching

EPIDEMIOLOGY
- Predominant age: All ages affected
  – *H. nana* and *H. diminuta* more common in children
- Predominant sex: Male = Female

Incidence
- Occurs infrequently
- More often associated with immigrant populations with cultural eating habits
- Can be endemic when fecal contamination enters water or food supplies

RISK FACTORS
- Taenias: Eating raw beef or pork, particularly in Africa, Central America, Asia
- Cysticercosis: A tapeworm carrier in close environment. Water contaminated with sewage
- *Diphyllobothrium:* Eating raw or undercooked fish, particularly in northern Europe
- *H. nana:* More frequent in children, the institutionalized, malnourished, and immunodeficient
- *E. granulosis:* Keeping dogs around sheep and goats; highest risk for hydatid cyst disease
- *E. multilocularis:* Contact with foxes, coyotes; mostly found in northern latitudes

ETIOLOGY
Eating the infective form of the parasite, either by eating contaminated food (meat, fish) or infected insects in cereals or grains, or through fecal–oral contamination

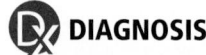 **DIAGNOSIS**

SIGNS AND SYMPTOMS
- *T.* saginata (beef tapeworm): Often noted by passing eggs or proglottids, which can be felt crawling out of anus. Mild gastrointestinal symptoms may occur: Nausea, abdominal pain, change in appetite, weakness, weight loss, allergic symptoms, urticaria, pruritus
- *T. solium* (pork tapeworm): Intestinal worm—noted passing eggs or proglottids. Occasional minor abdominal complaints similar to *T. saginata*. Larval migration—cysticercosis—most common to brain and skeletal muscle. Neurologic manifestations such as new onset of seizures, focal neurologic deficits, hydrocephalus, headache, vomiting, visual changes, dizziness
- *D. latum* (fish tapeworm): Noted passing eggs, or proglottid segments or vomiting segment of worm. Occasionally mild abdominal discomfort, weight loss. Worm has marked affinity for vitamin B$_{12}$; 40% decreased B$_{12}$ levels, 2% megaloblastic anemia with glossitis
- *H. nana* (dwarf tapeworm): Anorexia, abdominal pain, and diarrhea
- Echinococcosis (hydatid disease): *E. granulosis* often asymptomatic for years. Liver cysts—abdominal pain, right upper quadrant mass, obstructive jaundice. Cyst rupture—fever, urticaria, pruritus, anaphylaxis. Pulmonary cyst—cough, chest pain, hemoptysis. Other organs possible—bone with pathologic fractures, CNS, cardiac conduction defects, pericarditis
- *H. diminuta* (rodent tapeworm): Pass eggs in stool, proglottids disintegrate. Headache, mild GI symptoms—anorexia, nausea, cramps, diarrhea
- *D. caninum* (dog tapeworm): Occasionally abdominal pain, diarrhea, anal pruritus, urticaria. May observe proglottid in diaper or stool

TESTS
- Stool evaluation of ova and parasites
- Microscopic evaluation of proglottid collected in water or saline
- Antibody testing by ELISA to differentiate *T. saginata* eggs from *T. solium*
- Enzyme-linked immunoelectrotransfer blot: Test of choice for cysticercosis, *Echinococcus* (1)[C]
- DNA probes for *T. saginata* or *T. solium*

Lab
- Mild to moderate eosinophilia, increased IgE
- Microscopic analysis of eggs or proglottids
- Macrocytic, megaloblastic anemia rarely with diphyllobothriasis

Imaging
- Intestinal tapeworms occasionally seen by small bowel enteroclysis
- Cysticercosis: MRI preferred, CT OK (1)[C]
- Echinococcus cysts: Start with ultrasound

Diagnostic Procedures/Surgery
- Excisional biopsy of cysticercosis cyst
- Perianal inspection for eggs or proglottids

Pathological Findings
- Intestinal tapeworms: No pathologic findings
- Cysticerosis: Cysts, 5–10 mm in soft tissue. Calcified cysts in CNS, muscle
- Echinococcus: Hydatid cyst in liver, lung, other

DIFFERENTIAL DIAGNOSIS
- Nontapeworm gastroenteritis
- Irritable bowel syndrome
- Intestinal obstruction
- Cholecystitis or biliary obstruction
- B_{12} deficiency from nontapeworm etiologies
- Tumors (abscesses, malignant, benign)
- Idiopathic epilepsy

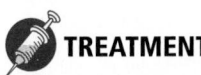 TREATMENT

Outpatient unless complications from cysts

GENERAL MEASURES
- Treatment of population in endemic area
- Treatment of all immigrants from endemic countries with albendazole is being evaluated.
- General supportive care during treatment
- Good hygienic measures should be employed.
- Asymptomatic cysticercosis may resolve spontaneously without treatment; however, antiparasitic therapy of parenchymal cysts may reduce the number of seizures with generalization. Treatment may induce an inflammatory response and symptoms. (2)[C]

Diet
As tolerated

Activity
As tolerated

 MEDICATION (DRUGS)

First Line
- Praziquantel (Droncit): (1,3,4)[C]
  - Single dose of 5–10 mg/kg (generally 10 mg/kg) for taeniasis, diphyllobothriasis, dipylidium infection, and most other intestinal cestodes (cure rate >95%)
  - Single dose of 25 mg/kg for *H. nana* adults or children (cure rate >95%)
  - 50–100 mg/kg/d t.i.d. × 14–30 days for children and adults for cysticercosis
- Albendazole (Zentel): (1,3,4)[C]
  - Dose: Weight >60 kg, 400 mg b.i.d. with meals; weight <60 kg, 15 mg/kg/d b.i.d. (maximum 800 mg/d)
  - For *Echinococcus* hydatid cysts, give for 28 days, 14 days off, repeat for 3 cycles; can be 1–6 months
  - For neurocysticercosis, drug of choice, give for 8–30 days, but examine for retinal lesions first; may repeat
- Neurocysticercosis: Steroids, anticonvulsants. Dexamethasone 4.5–12 mg/d (4)[C]
- PAIR therapy (puncture, aspiration, injection of a scolicidal, reaspiration) compares favorably with surgery for cystic echinococcosis.
- Contraindications
  - Prior sensitivity

- Precautions
  - Niclosamide: Occasional nausea and abdominal pain, diarrhea, dizziness
  - Praziquantel: Mild but frequent dizziness, myalgias, nausea, diarrhea, abdominal pain
  - Albendazole: Diarrhea and abdominal pain; leukopenia, increased transaminase levels
- Significant possible interactions
  - Phenytoin and carbamazepine can induce metabolism of praziquantel by cytochrome P-450, causing treatment failure.
  - Cimetidine, dexamethasone, and praziquantel can increase concentration of albendazole.
  - Corticosteroids may decrease concentration of praziquantel.

Second Line
Niclosamide (Nicloside) (not available in the United States)
- Single dose of 2 g for adult or 50 mg/kg for children for diphyllobothriasis, taeniasis, and dipylidium infection (cure rate 90% for taeniasis and slightly less for diphyllobothriasis)
- 2 g, then 1 g/d for 5 more days for *H. nana*

SURGERY
- Cysticercosis and hydatid cysts have been removed surgically, with care not to leak fluid.
  - Shunts for hydrocephalus (4)[C]
- Echinococcus hydatid cysts: (5)[C]
  - Surgery based upon location of cyst
  - Surgical risks may make medical therapy preferred.
  - Surgery generally involves total pericystectomy or partial resection of the affected organ, with albendazole pretreatment for 1 month.
  - Follow surgery with albendazole.

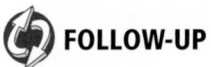 FOLLOW-UP

PROGNOSIS
- Cure of >95% of intestinal tapeworms with medications
- *H. nana* often self-cured by adolescence
- *E. multilocularis* often severe or fatal
- Prognosis of systemic cysts by location
- Neurocysticercosis—Intraparenchymal cysts often benign. Extraparenchymal (subarachnoid, ventricular, cisternal) more serious (1)[C]

COMPLICATIONS
- Larval form of *T. solium* can cause system-wide cysticercosis, including neurocysticercosis (etiologic in up to 25% of cases of new-onset seizures in indigenous areas).
- Echinococcus hydatid cysts may cause abnormalities in the organ involved. Cyst rupture can cause spread of disease and anaphylaxis.
- B_{12} deficiency with *D. latum*
- Proglottid of *T. saginata* can rarely obstruct appendix and pancreatic and bile ducts.
- *D. latum* can occasionally cause intestinal obstruction, cholangitis, and cholecystitis.

PATIENT MONITORING
- Examine several stool specimens for ova and parasites at 3 months for *Taenia* species and 1 month for others.
- Follow neurocysticercosis with CT.

REFERENCES
1. Garcia HH, et al. Diagnosis, treatment and control of Taenia solium cysticercosis. *Curr Opin Infect Dis.* 2003;16:411–419.
2. Garcia HH, et al. A trial of antiparasitic treatment to reduce the rate of seizures due to cerebral cysticercosis. *N Engl J Med.* 2004;350:249–258.
3. Abramowicz M, ed. *The Medical Letter on Drugs and Therapeutics. Drugs for Parasitic Infections.* New Rochelle, NY: The Medical Letter; August, 2004.
4. Garcia HH, et al. Current consensus guidelines for treatment of neurocysticercosis. *Clin Microbiol Rev.* 2002;15(4):747–756.
5. Guidelines for treatment of cystic and alveolar echinococcosis in humans. WHO Informal Working Group on Echinococcosis. *Bull World Health Organ.* 1996;74:231–242.

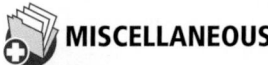 MISCELLANEOUS

CODES

ICD9-CM
- 122.9 Echinococcosis, other and unspecified
- 123.8 Other specified cestode infection
- 123.9 Cestode infection, unspecified

PATIENT TEACHING
- Proper cooking of beef, pork, fish
- Proper freezing of meat or fish
- Good hand washing
- Treatment of infected animals and flea prevention

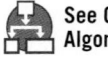 **See Corresponding Diagnostic Algorithm**

T

TARDIVE DYSKINESIA

Lawrence E. Udom, MD, MPH

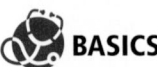 **BASICS**

DESCRIPTION

- Tardive dyskinesia (TD) is a neurologic syndrome that possesses the essential features of abnormal, involuntary movements of the tongue, lips, face, trunk, and extremities. It is most commonly associated with long-term treatment with neuroleptic medications. The movements can include grimacing, sticking out the tongue, and smacking and sucking the lips. They have choreiform characteristics (rapid, jerky, or nonrepetitive); athetoid characteristics (slow, sinuous, continual); or rhythmic characteristics. TD symptoms can begin during treatment with neuroleptics or within 4 weeks of discontinuing neuroleptics. TD can be mild, moderate, or severe.
- System(s) Affected: Nervous; Musculoskeletal
- Synonym(s): Orofacial dyskinesia

GENERAL PREVENTION

Choosing an "atypical" [newer] neuroleptic statistically makes the chance of TD less likely.

EPIDEMIOLOGY

- TD rates for patients beginning treatment with conventional antipsychotics in their 5th decade or later are 3 to 5 times those found for younger patients, despite treatment with lower doses. (1)
- Predominant age: Occurs in all ages; however, advanced age is a major risk factor for TD.
- Predominant sex: No difference in susceptibility between the genders until advanced years when females become more susceptible.

Incidence

In studies that used Haloperidol as their predominant classical antipsychotic

- Younger patients (<55 years old) on the classical antipsychotics have a 5% incidence of developing TD per year of use with a 50–60% development over their lifetime.
- Older patients (>60 years old) had an approx. 20% incidence rate after 1 year of exposure, to 30%, and near 50% at 2- and 3-year exposures, respectively. (1)

Prevalence

There is overall estimated prevalence of 15–25% of TD within 5 years of continuous classical antipsychotic use.

RISK FACTORS

- Use of classical antipsychotics
  - Haloperidol (Haldol)
  - Chlorpromazine (Thorazine)
  - Fluphenazine (Permitil, Prolixin)
  - Thioridazine (Mellaril)
  - Perphenazine (Trilafon)
  - Trifluoperazine (Stelazine)
  - Pimozide (Orap)
  - Thiothixene (Navane)
  - Molindone (Moban)
  - A few of the new class of atypical antipsychotics have been linked to TD although in much lower incidences than noted with the older medications
    ○ Quetiapine (Seroquel)
    ○ Olanzapine (Zyprexa)
    ○ Risperidone (Risperdal)
- Length of neuroleptic use
- Older age
- Postmenopausal females
- Mental retardation
- Alcoholism and substance abuse
- Extrapyramidal symptoms early in the course of neuroleptic treatment
- Presence of other movement disorders
- Diabetes mellitus
- Mood disorders (particularly MDD)

ALERT

Geriatric Considerations

Occurs in all ages; however, advance age is a major risk factor for TD.

Genetics

No definitive data indicate a genetic basis for TD; however, recent research suggests a possible association with a polymorphic variant of the Ser9Gly DRD3 gene and severe TD. Also, the absence of a glutathione S-transferase gene (GSTM1) was associated with TD, particularly in white women. (2)

PATHOPHYSIOLOGY

The mechanism by which TD occurs is still under debate. Antipsychotics (both traditional and atypical) have a high affinity for the dopamine-2 (D2) receptors. It is postulated that the long-term blockade of these D2 receptors leads to an up-regulation in the number and sensitivity of D2 receptors in the striated region of the brain (which controls muscle coordination). This up-regulation is associated with involuntary movements and hence TD. It has also been postulated that the depletion of GABA in the substantia nigra may lead to orofacial dyskinesia, as may excess free radicals.

ETIOLOGY

Prolonged use of dopamine antagonist drugs, e.g.

- Traditional antipsychotics
- Atypical antipsychotics
- Metoclopramide (Reglan), an antiemetic with potent D2 antagonism

ASSOCIATED CONDITIONS

- Presence of movement disorder
- Psychiatric disorders commonly treated with neuroleptics

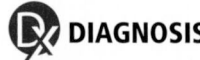 **DIAGNOSIS**

SIGNS AND SYMPTOMS

- Abnormal, involuntary movements of the tongue, lips, face, trunk, and extremities. In one major report
  - 75% of individuals with TD have orofacial dyskinesia
  - 50% have limb dyskinesia
  - 25% have axial dyskinesia
  - 10% have total body involvement
- Orofacial dyskinesia is common in the 60 years and older population
- Limb + axial dyskinesia is more common in the younger population. (3)
- These signs and symptoms must occur while taking neuroleptics or within 4 weeks or 8 weeks of withdrawal from an oral or depot neuroleptic medication, respectively.
- The signs typically begin minimal to mild in nature, and progress in severity with prolonged use.

History

- There must be a history of neuroleptic use for at least 3 months (or 1 month if individual's age is 60 years or older). TD must be distinguished from other movement disorders. The abnormal movements must not be due to a neurological condition or other general medical conditions (e.g., Huntington disease, Sydenham chorea, spontaneous dyskinesia, hyperthyroisim, heavy metal poisoning, Wilson disease), to ill-fitting dentures, or exposure to other medications that can cause acute reversible dyskinesia (l-dopa, bromocriptine, amantadine, Sinemet, Adderall, Ritalin, and Compazine). Other neuroleptic-induced movement disorders must be ruled out (e.g., tardive tourettism, blepharospasm, tardive akathisia, tardive myoclonus, tardive tremor, and tardive dystonia), as well as spontaneous dyskinesias and mental disorders.
- Question patient about a history of neurologic disorders that may involve the basal ganglia (e.g., cerebral vascular accident, encephalitis, head trauma, neoplasms).
- Attempt to illicit a family history for hereditary dyskinesias (e.g., Huntington disease).
- Ask about medication usage, particularly aforementioned medications.
  - Note: Neuroleptics can also mask TD. Thus, the reason one may see onset after medication discontinuaton

Physical Exam
- Previously mentioned abnormal movements: Random movements in the tongue, lips, or jaw as well as facial grimacing; movements of arms, legs, fingers, and toes; or swaying movements of the trunk or hips
- See "Diagnosis" for possible rule out criteria

TESTS
There are several questionnaires created to illicit this information and rate TD on a severity scale; Most commonly used is the Abnormal Involuntary Movement Scale (AIMS) [A].

Lab
Only used to rule out other causes

Imaging
May be done to rule out other causes.

DIFFERENTIAL DIAGNOSIS
- Huntington disease
- Sydenham chorea
- Spontaneous dyskinesia
- Wilson disease
- Thyrotoxicosis
- Blepharospasm
- Tardive akathisia
- Tardive dystonia
- Physical signs may point the way to another diagnosis.
  - Tachycardia, sweating, and a goiter suggests thyrotoxicosis.
  - Jaundice, hepatomegaly, or Kayser-Fleischer rings suggest a work-up for Wilson disease.
- Dementia in addition to the movement disorder (chorea) and postural instability requires a workup for Huntington disease.

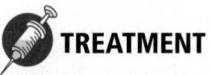

TREATMENT

INITIAL STABILIZATION
Cessation of neuroleptic use

MEDICATION (DRUGS)

No definitive treatment for TD
- Replacement of traditional antipsychotic with an atypical (Risperidal, Olanzapine, Quetiapine, Ziprasidone, and Clozapine) (4)

- There has been some evidence that the use of Clozapine has been effective in diminishing involuntary movements in patients with TD. Some studies have shown remission of TD in up to 34% of cases after treatment with Clozapine. (5)[A] However, the side-effect of Clozapine (agranulocytosis) prevents it from being a first-line medication.
- Vitamin E, a free-radical scavenger, has been found in a number of studies to reduce the severity of TD. (6)[A] Supplementation seems to be most effective when started within the first 5 years of neuroleptic treatment. The most effective dosage is in question; one study reported that 1,600 IU of vitamin E per day may be the optimal amount (7,8)[B] but many studies have found this dose to be toxic. Therefore, vitamin E levels in patients must be monitored closely.

FOLLOW-UP

PROGNOSIS
TD can be mild to moderate with resolution of symptoms after a period of discontinuation from offending drug. There are rare incidences where TD may be severe and irreversible.

REFERENCES

1. Woerner MG, et al. Prospective study of tardive dyskinesia in the elderly: Rates and risk factors. *Am J Psychiatry*. 1998;155:1521–1528.
2. de Leon J, et al. Polymorphic variations in GSTM1, GSTT1, PgP, CYP2D6, CYP3A5, and dopamine D2 and D3 receptors and their association with tardive dyskinesia in severe mental illness. *J Clin Psychopharmacol*. 2005;25(5):448–456.
3. American Psychiatric Association. *DSM-IV-TR 2000: Diagnostic & Statistical Manual of Mental Disorders*. 4th ed. American Psychiatric Publishing Inc; 2000.
4. Caroff SN, et al. Movement disorders associated with antipsychotic drugs. *J Clin Psychiatry*. 2002;63(suppl 4):12–19.
5. Lieberman JA, et al. The effects of clozapine on tardive dyskinesia. *Br J Psychiatry*. 1191;158: 503–510.
6. Adler LA, et al. Vitamin E treatment of tardive dyskinesia. *Am J Psychiatry*. 1993;150:1405–1407.
7. Hashim S, Sajjad A. Vitamin E in the treatment of tardive dyskinesia: A preliminary study over 7 months at different amounts. *Int Clin Psychopharmacol* 1988;13:147–155.
8. Egan MF, et al. Treatment of tardive dyskinesia with vitamin E. *Am J Psychiatry*. 1992;149:773–777.

ADDITIONAL READING
DSM-IV-TR

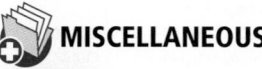

MISCELLANEOUS

CODES

ICD9-CM
333.82 Orofacial dyskinesia

PATIENT TEACHING
- Instruct patients and family members to watch for the subtle early signs.
- Warn that TD may be exacerbated by stimulant use (Ritalin, Adderall), neuroleptic withdrawal, and anticholinergics.
- Symptoms are affected by emotional states and stress.

Prevention
- Use of an atypical antipsychotic as a first-line antipsychotic. (3)[A]
- If traditional neuroleptics must be used, limit long-term use and use lowest effective doses with frequent patient assessments.

TEETHING

Alan M. Ehrlich, MD

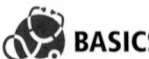 ## BASICS

DESCRIPTION
- Teething is the eruption of the deciduous teeth, which most children experience without difficulty. It is a natural, gradual, and predictable process, but the timetable varies from baby to baby.
- Deciduous teeth
  - Most deciduous teeth begin to erupt at 5–7 months of age, and teething is completed by 2–3 years of age.
  - The mandibular central incisors erupt 1st, then the 2 or 4 maxillary incisors, followed by the lower lateral incisors.
  - After a few months, the 4 molars appear (the lower ones at 12 months of age, the upper ones at 14 months of age).
  - After the cuspid teeth appear at 16–18 months of age, the 2nd molars erupt at 25–33 months of age.
  - <25% normal babies may have delayed eruption of teeth until 4 or 6 teeth appear simultaneously after their 1st birthday.
  - Premature babies erupt teeth according to their gestational age rather than their chronological age. If teething seems particularly delayed, refer patient to a pediatric dentist.
- Teeth in neonates
  - 1 in 2,000 neonates are born with a tooth (appears to be familial).
  - These neonatal teeth may be loose, but most are the normal deciduous lower central incisors and can persist.
  - Mild ulceration in the sublingual area has been reported in 18% of these babies.
  - Because of the potential for aspiration, there is some controversy about elective removal of the loose teeth (most pediatric dentists will remove these teeth if they are loose).
- System(s) Affected: Gastrointestinal

EPIDEMIOLOGY
Predominant age: Birth to 2 1/2 years of age

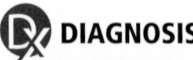 ## DIAGNOSIS

SIGNS AND SYMPTOMS
- A large percentage of babies have no signs or symptoms of teething.
- Excessive drooling and chewing on fingers begins at 3–4 months of age. This is also the time that normal hand–mouth stimulation increases salivation.
- Discomfort may be noted more with the eruption of the 1st tooth, the molars, and/or with the simultaneous eruption of multiple teeth.
- Restlessness, irritability, disturbed sleep, changes in feeding patterns, nasal discharge, mild cough, chin rash, fever, diarrhea, pulling of ear, and rubbing of the cheeks have been reported by parents. In any given infant, it is impossible to document that these are caused by teething, so parents and health providers should always consider other possible etiologies so as not to miss or delay diagnosing an illness.

History
- Biting
- Drooling
- Gum rubbing
- Sucking
- Irritability
- Wakefulness
- Ear rubbing
- Facial rash
- Decreased appetite for solid foods

Physical Exam
- A small red or white spot may appear over the swollen gum just prior to tooth eruption
- Local inflammation, swelling, and occasional hemorrhage can be found on the involved gums

DIFFERENTIAL DIAGNOSIS
Herpetic gingivostomatitis: Infants with fever, irritability, sleeplessness, and difficulty feeding may have underlying infection caused by herpes simplex virus. Some of these infants with positive culture may not have evidence of inflammation or ulceration expected in gingivitis.

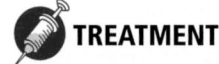 ## TREATMENT

INITIAL STABILIZATION
Outpatient

GENERAL MEASURES
- Treatment for teething includes reassurance for the parents and symptomatic relief, if needed.
- Provide the infant with a safe, 1-piece teething ring, clean cloth, or pacifier for gumming.
- Rub the involved swollen gums if the baby appears to be comforted by this.
- Cool fluids may be offered, but avoid frozen foods or objects. These could cause thermal damage to the tissues.
- Toast, cookies, bagels, and crackers are offered by some parents for teething, but parents must observe carefully to prevent choking.
- Avoid OTC preparations for teething such as lidocaine (Xylocaine 2%, Baby Ora-Gel, Num-zit Gel, Num-zit Liquid, Anbesol). Misuse, overuse, and sensitivity have been reported.
- Avoid the use of alcohol.
- For an infant with low-grade fever, irritability, and/or inflamed gums (where other comforting measures have not been of help), acetaminophen, in proper doses (10–15 mg/kg/dose q4h p.r.n.), can be used intermittently.
- Gum hematomas that erupt appear as blue cysts. Most do not require medical intervention. Be sure there are no other signs of a bleeding disorder.
- Breast-feeding babies may attempt to chew on the nipple at the end of sucking while teething but can be taught not to bite. Breast-feeding can continue after teeth are present.
- Advise parents to avoid sugared pacifiers, tying teething ring with cord around the infant's neck, and imported fluid-filled teething rings. They should remove painted furniture that may contain lead.

Diet
No special diet

Activity
No restrictions

MEDICATION (DRUGS)

First Line
Acetaminophen 10–15 mg/kg q4h as needed

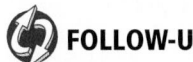 **FOLLOW-UP**

PROGNOSIS
Normal progression through the teething process without illness

REFERENCES

1. Macknin ML, et al. Symptoms associated with infant teething. *Pediatrics*. 2000;105:747–752. [B]
2. Wake M et al. Teething and tooth eruption in infants. *Pediatrics*. 2000;106(6):1374–1379. [B]
3. Falkner F. Deciduous tooth eruption. *Arch Dis Childhood*. 1957;32:386–391.
4. Gardiner J. Erupted teeth in the newborn. *Proc R Soc Med*. 1961;4:504.
5. Golden N, Takieddine F, Hirsch V. Teething age—prematurely born infants. *Am J Dis Child*. 1981;135:903–904.
6. King DL, et al. Herpetic gingivostomatitis and teething difficulty in infants. *Pediatr Dent*. 1992;14:82–85.
7. King NM, Lee A. Prematurely erupted teeth in the newborn infant. *J Pediatr*. 1989;114:807.
8. McDonald RE. Eruption of the teeth, local, systematic and congenital factors that influence the process. In: *Dentistry for the Child and Adolescent*, 5th ed. St. Louis: Mosby; 1987:189–196.
9. Seward M. General disturbances attributed to the eruption of human primary dentition. *J Dent Child*. 1972;39:178–183.

ADDITIONAL READING

http://www.ada.org/public/topics/teething.asp

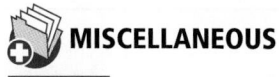 **MISCELLANEOUS**

CODES

ICD9-CM
520.7 Teething syndrome

PATIENT TEACHING

- Parents should be cautioned not to misinterpret teething as the cause of any systemic manifestation. The health provider should be consulted for any systemic complaints.
- American Academy of Pediatric Dentistry, *The ABC's of Teething*, Public Relations Manual.

T

TEMPOROMANDIBULAR JOINT (TMJ) SYNDROME

Scott A. Fields, MD

 BASICS

DESCRIPTION
- Syndrome characterized by
  - Pain and tenderness in jaw muscles
  - Sound and/or pain over temporomandibular joint
  - Limitation of mandibular movement
- System(s) Affected: Musculoskeletal
- Synonym(s): Myofascial pain-dysfunction syndrome

ALERT
Pregnancy Considerations
No association

GENERAL PREVENTION
- Elimination of tension-relieving oral habits
- Reduction in overall muscle tension

EPIDEMIOLOGY
- Predominant age: Symptoms more common age 30–50
- Predominant sex: Female > Male (3:1)

Prevalence
Symptoms or signs of TMJ dysfunction are present in up to 1/2 of the population, but only 5–25% seek treatment.

RISK FACTORS
- Chronic oral habit, such as clenching or grinding of the teeth
- Osteoarthritis, rheumatoid arthritis
- Dental malocclusion
- Fibrositis
- Psychosocial stress

ETIOLOGY
- TMJ synovitis
- TMJ disc derangement
- Hypermobile or hypomobile TMJ
- Occluso-muscular dysfunction (bruxism)
- Masticatory muscle spasm
- Trauma
- Poorly fitting dentures

ASSOCIATED CONDITIONS
Cranio-mandibular disorders

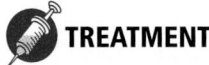 **DIAGNOSIS**

SIGNS AND SYMPTOMS
- Facial and/or TMJ pain
- Locking or catching of jaw
- TMJ noises: Clicking, grinding, popping
- Headache
- Earache
- Neck pain

Physical Exam
Jaw range of motion (opening, closing, lateral, protrusive) and masticatory muscle strength

TESTS
Imaging
- Single-contrast videoarthrography: Demonstrates joint dynamics and disc movement
- Panoramic dental radiographs
- MRI: Noninvasive study for disc position; information gained helps in deciding conservative versus surgical management

Pathological Findings
- Condylar head displacement
- Anterior disc displacement
- Posterior capsulitis
- Loosening of disc and capsular attachments
- Chondroid metaplasia of disc leading to disc perforation and degeneration

DIFFERENTIAL DIAGNOSIS
- Condylar fracture/dislocation
- Trigeminal neuralgia
- Dental or periodontal conditions
- TMJ neoplasm

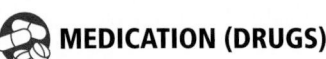 **TREATMENT**

GENERAL MEASURES (1)[C]
- Jaw rest
- Local heat therapy
- Anti-inflammatory medications
- Muscle relaxants
- Analgesics
- Correction of malocclusion with orthodontic appliance
- Stress reduction
- Behavior modification to eliminate tension-relieving oral habits
- Buccal separator orthodontic appliance
- Linearly polarized, near-infrared irradiation

Diet
Soft diet to reduce chewing

MEDICATION (DRUGS)

First Line
- NSAIDs: No single drug more efficacious than another (1)[C]
- Botulinum toxin (2)[C]
- Contraindications
  - History of anaphylaxis to aspirin
  - Peptic ulcer disease
  - Renal insufficiency
- Precautions
  - Peptic ulcers, gastritis, or GI bleeding may occur with chronic use.
  - May cause acute interstitial nephritis
  - Drug accumulation with renal insufficiency
  - Liver function abnormalities in up to 15% of patients
- Significant possible interactions
  - Albumin-bound drugs: Displacement of either drug
  - Warfarin: Increased prothrombin time
  - Lithium: Increased lithium plasma level
  - Furosemide: Decreased natriuretic effect
  - Propranolol: Decreased antihypertensive effect

Second Line
- Analgesic agents (1)[C]
- Muscle relaxants (1)[C]

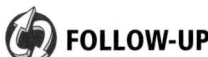 **FOLLOW-UP**

PROGNOSIS
- With conservative therapy, symptoms resolve in 3/4 of cases within 3 months.
- Patients benefit the most from a comprehensive treatment approach, including
  - Correction of occlusal discrepancies
  - Restoration of normal muscle function
  - Pain control
  - Stress management
  - Behavior modification

COMPLICATIONS
- Secondary degenerative joint disease
- Chronic TMJ dislocation
- Loss of joint range of motion
- Depression and chronic pain syndromes

PATIENT MONITORING
- Ongoing assessment of clinical response to conservative therapies (NSAIDs, behavior modification, occlusal splints) is necessary.
- Surgical procedure to correct disc displacement or replace a damaged disc may be indicated only if the patient has not responded to conservative treatment.

REFERENCES
1. Laskin DM. Putting order into temporomandibular disorders. *J Oral Maxillofac Surg*. 1998;56:121.
2. Schwartz MB, Freund BB. Treatment of temporomandibular disorders with botulinum toxin. *Clin J Pain*. 2002;18(suppl 6):S198–S203.
3. Mock D. The differential diagnosis of temporomandibular joint disorders. *J Orofac Pain*. 1999;13:246–250.
4. Kuttila S, et al. Aural symptoms and signs of temporomandibular disorder in association with treatment need and visits to a physician. *Laryngoscope*. 1999;109:1669–1673.
5. Pankhurst CL. Controversies in the aetiology of temporomandibular disorders. Part 1. Temporomandibular disorders: All in the mind? *Prim Dent Care*. 1997;4:25–30.
6. Bush FM, Harkins SW, Harrington WG. Otalgia and aversive symptoms in temporomandibular disorders. *Ann Otol Rhinol Laryngol*. 1999;108:884–892.
7. Yokoyama K, Sugiyama K. Temporomandibular joint pain analgesia by linearly polarized near-infrared irradiation. *Clin J Pain*. 2001;17:47–51.
8. Dimitroulis G. The role of surgery in the management of disorders of the temporomandibular joint: A critical review of the literature. Part 1. *Int J Oral Maxillofac Surg*. 2004;33.
9. Dimitroulis G. The role of surgery in the management of disorders of the temporomandibular joint: A critical review of the literature. Part 2. *Int J Oral Maxillofac Surg*. 2005;34(3):231–237.
10. Al-Ani MZ, et al. Stabilisation splint therapy for temporomandibular pain dysfunction syndrome. *Cochrane Oral Health Group Cochrane Database of Systematic Reviews*. 1,2006.
11. Koh H, Robinson PG. Occlusal adjustment for treating and preventing temporomandibular joint disorders. *Cochrane Oral Health Group Cochrane Database of Systematic Reviews*. 1,2006.

 MISCELLANEOUS

See also: Bruxism

 CODES

ICD9-CM
524.60 Temporomandibular joint disorders, unspecified

PATIENT TEACHING

Diet
Softer diet content is helpful.

Activity
- Be aware of any teeth-clenching or grinding habits.
- Relax jaw by disengaging teeth.
- Avoid wide, uncontrolled opening, such as yawning.

Prevention
Stress management and behavior-modification counseling may be helpful.

 See Corresponding Diagnostic Algorithm

 See Patient Handout on CD

T

TENDINITIS

Mathew J. Devine, DO
Matthew J. Fleig, MD
E. James Swenson, MD

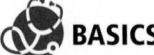 **BASICS**

DESCRIPTION
- Inflammation of a tendon and/or tendinous sheath
- System(s) Affected: Musculoskeletal

ALERT
- The term tendinopathy has replaced the term tendinitis as a generic descriptor of clinical conditions associated with pain, swelling, and impaired performance in and around tendons arising from overuse.
  - The labels "tendinitis" and "tendinosis" are reserved for the condition after histological examination is performed. (1)
- Tendinopathies can be subdivided into the following categories
  - Tendinitis: Acute inflammation of the tendon
  - Tendinosis: Chronic degeneration of the tendon. Can also be related to partial tendon rupture.
  - Tenosynovitis: Inflammation of the tendon sheath
- Common sites of overuse tendon injuries
  - Knee: Patella or "jumper's knee," medial plica, and pes anserine
  - Shoulder: Rotator cuff muscles
  - Ankle: Achilles and posterior tibialis
  - Hip: Hamstring muscles and iliotibial tract
  - Elbow: Lateral epicondylitis or "tennis elbow," medial epicondylitis or "golfer's or thrower's elbow," and triceps (2)

GENERAL PREVENTION
For prevention of future injuries, the following have been shown to be useful
- Pre-participation screening, warm-up sessions, core and supporting muscle strengthening, safe environment, protective equipment using braces or taping, and health education

EPIDEMIOLOGY
- Predominant age: Rotator cuff, Achilles tendon, and patellar injuries are more common in adolescent and in middle-aged groups.
- Predominant sex: Male = Female
- Overuse injuries are more common in high risk populations; athletes and geriatric populations

Pediatric Considerations
Tendons in children tend to be stronger than the epiphyseal plate. Therefore, consider growth plate, avulsion fractures versus overuse apophysitis following trauma in children. (2)

Prevalence
Tendinopathy is commonly seen.

RISK FACTORS
- Extrinsic factors
  - Training errors (most common)
  - Footwear and equipment (2nd most common)
  - Training surfaces
  - Environmental conditions
- Intrinsic factors
  - Malalignment
  - Limb length discrepancy
  - Muscular imbalance
  - Muscular insufficiency

PATHOPHYSIOLOGY
- Overuse injuries involve incomplete and disorganized repair mechanisms. These result in a defective "repaired" tendon which lacks extra cellular tissue organization and has decreased strength making the tendon more susceptible to further injury. (1)
- Healing response of an acute tendon injury has a triphasic response of inflammation, proliferation, and maturation.

ETIOLOGY
- Increased repetitive stress and force on the tendon cause an increased risk of injury. Over time with intrinsic and extrinsic factors listed above tendinopathies can develop.
- Etiologic causes are still unknown and have only been theorized. (3)

ASSOCIATED CONDITIONS
- Bursitis (common)
- Arthritis

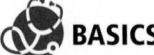 **DIAGNOSIS**

SIGNS AND SYMPTOMS
- Pain at the specific point of the affected tendon is the most common symptom.
- Reproducible pain on muscle group activity
- Thickening of tendon(s) involved
- Decreased active range of motion of the muscle group involved

ALERT
- Excessive post-traumatic tension or pain in lower extremity, should consider urgent care for acute compartment syndrome
- With excessive swelling in traumatic injury, must also consider tendon rupture

History
- In general population, history of repetitive use with onset of pain in area of muscle origin or insertions
- History of overuse or overtraining in the case of an athlete

Physical Exam
- Precise physical exam is key to the diagnosis.
- Palpable pain over muscle tendon unit
- Warmth and redness in acute tendinopathies
- Note asymmetry and tendon thickness in chronic tendinopathies.
- Pain may limit range of motion.

TESTS
- Full musculoskeletal exam
- Neurological exam as needed

Lab
If arthritis suspected—ANA, sed rate

Imaging
- Imaging only to be used as adjunct as needed
- Ultrasound: Can measure tendon width, water content within the tendon and peritendon, and collagen integrity.
  - Abnormal tendons on sonogram have the following findings: Increased tendon diameter, focal hypoechoic intratendinous areas, localized tendon swelling and thickening, collagen discontinuity, and tendon sheath swelling of calcifications. (4)
- MRI
  - Indicated only in specific causes
  - Reveals tendon thickening and increased signal of tendons
  - Areas of mucoid degeneration seen as high intensity on T1- and T2- weighted images

ALERT
- Areas of increased signal on MRI need to be correlated with clinical pathology because these could represent asymptomatic areas of degeneration.
- MRI is unreliable in changes of paratendinitis.

Pathological Findings
- Tendinitis: Symptomatic degeneration of the tendon with an inflammatory response
- Tendinosis: Intratendinous degeneration. Common findings are collagen disorientation, fiber separation with increased mucoid ground substance
- Paratendinitis: Inflammation of the outer layer of the tendon alone
- Paratendinitis with tendinosis: Paratendinitis with intratendinous degeneration

DIFFERENTIAL DIAGNOSIS
- Knee
  - Patellofemoral pain syndrome: Lateral tracking of patella causing irritation and abrasion of the cartilage of the patella resulting in pain
  - Exertional compartment syndrome: A reversible ischemia secondary to a noncompliant osseofascial compartment that is unresponsive to the expansion of muscle volume that occurs with exercise. (1) Most common in anterior compartment of lower extremities
  - Stress fractures: Partial or complete bone fracture from repeated force lower than the force required to fracture the bone in a single loading. Most common areas are the tibia, metatarsals, and the fibula. (1)[A]

- Shoulder
  - Bursitis: Often is present with a tendinopathy
  - Frozen shoulder
  - Arthritis: An inflammation within a specific joint of the body. Should be differentiated from tendinopathy, which is isolated to the muscle insertion site and not within the joint spaces
  - Cervical radiculopathy
- Ankle
  - Rupture: Achilles rupture is uncommon and is not a cause of tendinitis.
  - Sprains: In acute sprains, tendinitis can develop if too much stress is placed on noninjured musculature.
- Hip
  - Stress fracture: With excessive pain on internal rotation of hip, place the patient on crutches until femoral fracture is ruled out.

Pediatric Considerations
- Osgood-Schlatter lesion (common)
- Sever's disease: Calcaneal apophysitis
- Pelvic apophysitis
- Little league elbow/Little league shoulder

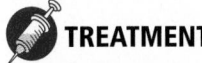 ## TREATMENT

INITIAL STABILIZATION
Avoid extrinsic factors.

GENERAL MEASURES
Treat as outpatient

Diet
No special diets recommended

Activity
During acute phase: Rest of tendon involved

SPECIAL THERAPY
Cryotherapy
Icing very beneficial in treatment (A)

Physical Therapy
Muscle strengthening and intrinsic factor recognition is critical to continue healing process. Patient progress should be monitored with pain threshold. If pain continues, then the activity needs to be decreased.

Radiotherapy
Current research shows no benefit using laser therapy or other radiotherapies. (3)[C]

Complementary and Alternative Therapies
Orthotics: OTC or prescription as needed

 ## MEDICATION (DRUGS)

First Line
NSAIDs provide good analgesic effects.
- Piroxicam (Feldene): 10–20 mg/d
- Naprosyn: OTC; 500 mg b.i.d. with food
- Ibuprophen: OTC: Up to 800 mg t.i.d. with food

Second Line
Corticosteroids
- Medrol dose pack (PO)
- Injectable
  - Methylprednisolone (Depo-medrol): 40 mg used with 1 or 2% lidocaine (Xylocaine) 4–6 cc
  - Contraindication: Tendons should never be injected with local anesthetic and/or cortisone to allow participation in an athletic event. This can lead to complete rupture of the tendon.
- Topical: Research in progress

ALERT
- Recently, some of the COX-2 inhibitors have been removed from the market. Current literature supports the use of Celecoxib for tendinopathy in individuals without cardiovascular risk.
- Contraindication: Do not use NSAIDs in patient with recent history of GI bleed or ulcer.
- Precautions: Compare medications for any drug interactions. See manufacturer's profile of each drug.
- Use caution with renal disease.
- A rare side effect of fluoroquinolones has been tendon rupture and tendinopathy. (3)[A]

SURGERY
- For chronic tendinopathy, surgical treatment is an option if conservative treatment fails after 4–6 months. Patellar tendinitis most commonly operated on. (3)
- Long-standing tendinopathies are associated with poorer surgical outcomes.

 ## FOLLOW-UP

- Advise patient of susceptibility of exacerbation of injury up to 3 weeks after resolution of symptoms with increased activity.
- Treatment plans vary on site of injury.
- Most plans include rest, medications, cryotherapy, and physical therapy.

DISPOSITION
Most individuals recover to full strength and normal activity.

Issues for Referral
Orthopedics/Sports medicine referral in cases of highly competitive athlete, continued pain greater than 4 weeks, radiological finding of avulsion/stress fractures, or uncertainty of diagnosis.

PROGNOSIS
Symptoms usually subside with rest and proper therapy. Most tendinopathies improve without any major complications.

COMPLICATIONS
Exacerbation of pain in affected area

REFERENCES
1. Wilder RP, Sethi S. Overuse injuries: Tendinopathies, stress fractures, compartment syndrome, and shin splints. *Clin Sports Med*. 2004;23:55–81.
2. Maffulli N, et al. Types and epidemiology of tendinopathy. *Clin Sports Med*. 2003;22:675–693.
3. Sharma P, Maffulli N. Tendon injury and tendinopathy: Healing and repair. *J Bone Joint Surg*. 2005;87:187–202.
4. Warden S, Brukner P. Patellar tendinopathy. *Clin Sports Med*. 2003;22:743–760.
5. Cook JL, Purdam CR. Rehabilitation of lower limb tendinopathies. *Clin Sports Med*. 2003;22: 777–789.

 ## MISCELLANEOUS

CODES
ICD9-CM
Knee
- 726.64 Patellar tendinitis
- 717.9 IT band syndrome
- 727.09 Tenosynovitis/synovitis

Shoulder
- 726.10 Bursitis/tendinitis

Ankle
- 726.71 Achilles tendinitis/bursitis
- 726.79 Peroneal tendinitis
- 727.06 Tenosynovitis elbow

Elbow
- 726.32 Lateral epicondylitis
- 726.31 Medial epicondylitis

PATIENT TEACHING
Explanation of problem with precise treatment plans outlined to them

Activity
- Increase activity in stepwise fashion as long as pain-free
- Scales such as the Victorian Institute of Sports Assessment (VISA) for patellar and Achilles tendons may provide some quantification of progress. (5)

Prevention
Strengthening and stretching of muscle group involved

 See Corresponding Diagnostic Algorithm

See Patient Handout on CD

TESTICULAR MALIGNANCIES

Eric Nelson, MD
Leonard G. Gomella, MD

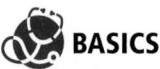 **BASICS**

DESCRIPTION
Testicular cancer is relatively rare, but is the most common malignancy among 20- 34-year-old men. Fortunately, it is one of the most curable solid organ cancers (93% 5-year survival). Testicular neoplasms may arise from any testicular or adnexal cell component and are divided into germinal (90–95%) and nongerminal tumors (5–10%). The germinal tumors, discussed here, are further divided into seminomatous and nonseminomatous types (embryonal, teratoma, choriocarcinomas, yolk sac).

- Clinical staging (based on 1997 AJCC TNMS)
  - Stage 0: Carcinoma in situ
  - Stage Ia: Tumor limited to testis and epididymis without vascular/lymphatic invasion
  - Stage Ib: Tumor limited to testis and epididymis with vascular/lymphatic invasion or tumor extending through the tunica albuginea with involvement of tunica vaginalis
  - Stage Ic: Any tumor with elevated markers
  - Stage IIa: Any tumor with lymph node mass/masses no more than 2 cm
  - Stage IIb: Any tumor with lymph node mass/masses 2–5 cm
  - Stage IIc: Any tumor with lymph node mass greater than 5 cm
  - Stage IIIa: Any tumor/lymph node presence with evidence of nonregional nodal or pulmonary metastases
  - Stage IIIb: Any tumor/lymph node presence with moderately elevated serum tumor markers
  - Stage IIIc: Any tumor/lymph node presence with greatly elevated serum tumor markers
- System(s) Affected: Reproductive

ALERT
Pediatric Considerations
Rare (2% of all solid tumors in childhood)

EPIDEMIOLOGY
- Predominant age: Peak incidence: Age 20–40 years; smaller peaks between age 0–10 years and >60 years
- Predominant sex: Male only

Incidence
- 1–2% of all neoplasms in men
- Increased incidence in last 40 years with substantial differences among countries; etiology unclear
- In adults, 95% are Germ Cell Tumors (GCT); In children, 65% are GCTs. Half of GCTs are seminomas; half are nonseminomatous.

Prevalence
- 2.3–6.3 cases/year per 100,000 men (less common in African Americans—0.9 cases/year per 100,000)
- Trimodal distribution: Predominant peak at 20–40 years; slight peak in children younger than 5 years; slight peak in men older than 60 years
- Seminoma rare before 10 years or after age 60 years, but most common histologic type overall

RISK FACTORS
- Crytporchidism: The only proven risk factor with 2.5- to 11-fold incidence increase
- Caucasian race: Especially Scandinavian and Swiss
- Family history
- Higher socioeconomic status
- Increased maternal hormones during pregnancy
- Infertility or abnormal semen parameters
- Preterm birth
- Testicular atrophy
- Trauma

Genetics
- Familial clustering observed
- All cases show chromosome 12 alteration (12p)

ETIOLOGY
Cryptorchidism increased risk

ASSOCIATED CONDITIONS
Weak association with testicular microlithiasis

DIAGNOSIS

SIGNS AND SYMPTOMS
History
In adults
- Testicular nodule/painless swelling (most common presentation)
- Dull ache/heavy sensation (30–40%)
- Hydrocele (10–20%)
- Acute pain (10%), especially with epididymitis/acute hemorrhage
- Gynecomastia (may or may not be due to elevated hormones) (5%)
- Enlargement of a small or atrophic testicle
- Infertility
- Symptoms due to metastases: Supraclavicular mass, respiratory symptoms (lung metastasis), low back pain (nerve root or psoas irritation), lower extremity swelling (iliac or caval thrombosis or obstruction), GI disturbances (retroduodenal metastasis), bone pain (skeletal metastasis)
- In children: Painless testicular mass most common; can be seen in association with torsion

TESTS
Lab
- Markers are useful in the following settings
  - To diagnose and stage disease
  - To monitor the therapeutic response
  - To detect tumor recurrence
- Levels should be drawn pre- and postoperatively
- Elevated markers postorchiectomy generally indicates systemic metastases rather than tumor confined to retroperitoneal nodes.
- Half-life important to evaluate therapeutic responses
- Alpha-fetoprotein (AFP)
  - Half-life 5–7 days
  - Increased in yolk sac tumors, teratoma, embryonal carcinoma, or combined tumors
  - Not increased in pure choriocarcinoma or pure seminoma
  - Levels also increased with liver disease

- Human chorionic gonadotropin (hCG)
  - Half-life 24–36 hours
  - Increased in pure choriocarcinoma, but found in 5–10% pure seminomas
  - Beta subunit measured; alpha subunit shared with FSH, LH, TSH
- Lactate dehydrogenase (LDH)
  - Reflects "tumor burden"
  - Too ubiquitous to be specific, but proven prognostic factor
- Placental alkaline phosphatase (PLAP) and Gamma-glutamyl-transpeptidase (GGTP): Individual sensitivities low, but simultaneous determinations revealed elevation of one or both in 80% of patients with active disease
- Drugs that may alter lab results
  - AFP may be elevated with chemotherapy, anesthetics, antiepileptics, alcohol abuse
  - hCG may be elevated by marijuana use.
- Disorders that may alter lab results
  - AFP may be altered by liver damage by drugs (above), viral hepatitis, alcohol abuse, benign or malignant liver conditions
  - hCG may be altered by hypogonadism and malignancies of pancreas, stomach, kidney, breast, and bladder.

Imaging
- Scrotal ultrasound is the gold standard for testicular imaging; any hypoechoic area within the tunica albuginea is markedly suspicious for testicular cancer; also used for patients with palpably normal testes and evidence of extragonadal metastases.
- For staging
  - Chest x-ray: PA/Lat to assess lung parenchyma and mediastinal structures
  - Chest CT: More sensitive than x-ray, but must have high index of suspicion because high incidence of false positives
  - Abdomen/Pelvis CT: Most effective to identify retroperitoneal lymph node involvement; replaced IV urography and pedal lymphangiography; is excellent at identifying retrocrural nodes
  - MRI: No real advantage over CT
  - PET: No real advantage over CT

Diagnostic Procedures/Surgery
- Radical inguinal orchiectomy: Definitive procedure for pathologic diagnosis
- Transscrotal biopsy/orchiectomy contraindicated as lymphatic drainage violated and inguinal portion of spermatic cord left
- Open biopsy rarely done except in highly selected cases of pediatric tumors that may be benign

Pathological Findings
Basically, two different groups based on germinal versus nongerminal and seminomatous versus nonseminomatous types

DIFFERENTIAL DIAGNOSIS
- Epididymitis
- Hernia
- Hydrocele
- Hematoma
- Spermatocele
- Syphilitic gumma
- Varicocele
- In children: Epidermoid/dermoid cyst, paratesticular rhabdomysocarcoma, macroorchidism, torsion

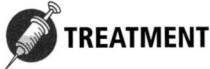 **TREATMENT**

Inpatient and outpatient

GENERAL MEASURES

- Germ cell cancers are divided into seminoma and nonseminoma types for treatment planning.
- Tumors with a mixture of seminomatous and nonseminomatous components should be managed as nonseminoma.
- All patients should be treated on an intent-to-cure basis, even if metastatic.
- Surgery
  - Radical inguinal orchiectomy for all patients
  - Prosthesis can be inserted at this time.
- Pure seminoma
  - General principles
    ○ Highly radiosensitive
    ○ Relatively slow growth of micrometastases
  - Stage IS (carcinoma in situ): Chemotherapy
    ○ Spermatocytic: Age usually over 65 years; no adjuvant therapy
    ○ Typical and anaplasatic: If patient has risk factors (tumor >6 cm; vascular/lymphatic invasion), low-dose abdominal/pelvic radiation with single-agent chemotherapy with carboplatin. If no risk factors, follow with surveillance in a motivated patient.
  - Stage IIa and IIb: Radiation; chemotherapy if involved nodes close to kidney
  - Stage IIc and III: Cisplatin-based chemotherapy; if residual mass: Observe if desmoplastic; if mass >3 cm and well-delineated: Do surgical resection; if histology positive: Do salvage chemotherapy
- Nonseminomatous germ cell tumors
  - Stage IS: Chemotherapy with bleomycin, etoposide, cisplatin (BEP) (3 cycles)
  - Stage I: If risk factors (T2, embryonal >40%, vascular/lymphatic invasion) absent, can do surveillance in motivated patient; if risk factors present or unreliable patient, do modified (template) RPLND and primary chemo with 3 cycles BEP. Then observe for N0-N1; for N2, give adjuvant chemotherapy, BEP
  - Stage IIa, IIb: Bilateral RPLND and chemotherapy with BEP ×3 cycles. If minimal nodal involvement (<2 cm), no adjuvant chemo; if nodal involvement (>2 cm), give adjuvant chemo and BEP (2 cycles).
  - Stage IIc, III: For good-risk disease, chemotherapy with BEP ×3 cycles. RPLND if residual retroperitoneal mass. Salvage chemotherapy for recurrent disease after chemo, RPLND, or persistently elevated tumor markers. For poor-risk disease, primary chemotherapy with ifosfamide and possible bone marrow transplant; salvage chemo if poor response. "Desperation surgery" for tumor unresponsive to salvage chemo.

Diet
No special diet

Activity
As tolerated

SPECIAL THERAPY
Radiotherapy
Selective cases of seminoma

 MEDICATION (DRUGS)

First Line
- Commonly used chemotherapeutic agents include BEP. Other regimens include vinblastine which has greater toxicity.
- Salvage chemotherapy includes vinblastine, ifosfamide, and cisplatin.
- Precautions
  - Cisplatin: Nephrotoxicity, ototoxicity, neurotoxicity
  - Etoposide: Marrow suppression, leukemia
  - Cyclophosphamide/ifosfamide: Hemorrhagic cystitis (prevent with Mesna)
  - Bleomycin: Pulmonary fibrosis
  - Vincristine: Marrow suppression, neuromuscular toxicity
  - Carboplatin: Ototoxicity
  - Taxol: Neuropathy
- Refer to the manufacturer's literature for each drug.

Second Line
Ondansetron (Zofran), dronabinol (Marinol), metoclopramide (Reglan), and others for nausea control

SURGERY
- All patients receive radical orchiectomy for diagnosis and excellent local control.
- Retroperperitoneal lymph node dissection (open or laparoscopic) based on treatment algorithm

 FOLLOW-UP

PROGNOSIS
- More than 90% of patients with newly diagnosed GCT are cured.
- Seminoma has a cure rate greater than 90% (near 100% for low-stage disease).
- For nonseminomatous tumors, cure rate is >95% in stages I and II; it is approximately 70% with chemotherapy and resection of residual disease in stages III and IV.

COMPLICATIONS
- Orchiectomy: Intrascrotal hematoma, retroperitoneal hematoma
- RPLND: Intraoperative hemorrhage, lymphocele, loss of seminal emission/infertility
- Radiation: Radiation enteritis, nephritis

PATIENT MONITORING
- Intensity and details of follow-up are evolving.
- General guidelines below
  - For seminomatous tumors
    ○ Clinical examination/tumor markers and CXR: At one month; every 3 months for 2 years; then every 6 months until 5 years
    ○ Pelvic CT at years 1, 2, and 5 (every 6 months if abnormal post-treatment CT)
  - For nonseminomatous tumors
    ○ Clinical examination/tumor markers and CXR: Every 2 months for first year; every 3 months for second year; then every 6 months until 5 years
    ○ Pelvic CT at 3, 6, 9, 12, 24 months for surveillance and only when clinically indicated for postchemotherapy patients

REFERENCES

1. Gori S, et al. Germ cell tumours of the testis. *Crit Rev Oncol Hematol*. 2005;53:141–164.
2. Gosse ON, et al. Testicular tumours (nonseminomatous). *BJU Int*. 2004;94:1196–1201.
3. Huyghe E, et al. Increasing incidence of testicular cancer worldwide: A review. *J Urol*. 2003;170: 5–11.
4. Richie JP. In: Walsh PC, et al. eds. *Campbell's Urology*. Philadelphia, PA: W.B. Saunders Co.; 2002.

 MISCELLANEOUS

CODES

ICD9-CM
- 186.0 Malignant neoplasm of undescended testis
- 186.9 Malignant neoplasm of testis, other and unspecified

PATIENT TEACHING
- Testicular self-exams and awareness of signs/symptoms should be encouraged at primary care level. There is often a delay in diagnosis from lack of knowledge or embarrassment
- Infertility possible after chemotherapy and RPLND; sperm banking must be discussed with patient prior to treatment initiation
- Well-reputed websites with educational materials
  - www.urologyhealth.org (American Urological Association)
  - www.cancer.org (American Cancer Society)

Prevention
Testicular self-exam

 See Corresponding Diagnostic Algorithm

See Patient Handout on CD

T

TESTICULAR TORSION

Timothy L. Black, MD

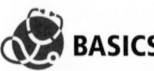 **BASICS**

DESCRIPTION
- Twisting of testis and spermatic cord, resulting in acute ischemia
  - Intravaginal torsion: Occurs within tunica vaginalis
  - Extravaginal torsion: Involves twisting of testis, cord, and processus vaginalis (especially in newborns) and in undescended testes
- System(s) Affected: Reproductive

ALERT
Geriatric Considerations
Rare in this age group

Pediatric Considerations
Most common at age 14 years

EPIDEMIOLOGY
- Predominant age
  - Occurs from newborn period to seventh decade
  - Two thirds of cases occur in second decade, with peak at age 14 years. (1)[C]
  - Second peak in neonates
- Predominant sex: Males only

Incidence
1:160 males

RISK FACTORS
- May be more common in winter
- Paraplegia
- Previous contralateral testicular torsion

Genetics
Unknown

ETIOLOGY
- Torsion is usually spontaneous and idiopathic.
- History of trauma in 20% of patients
- One third have had prior episodic testicular pain.
- Contraction of cremasteric muscle or dartos may play a role and is stimulated by trauma, exercise, cold, and sexual stimulation.
- Possible alterations in testosterone levels during nocturnal sex response cycle; possible elevated testosterone levels in neonates
- Testis must have inadequate, incomplete, or absent fixation within scrotum.
- Torsion may occur in either clockwise or counter-clockwise direction. (2)[C]

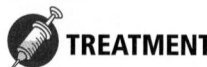 **DIAGNOSIS**

SIGNS AND SYMPTOMS
- Scrotum is enlarged, red, edematous, and painful.
- The first symptom is pain (usually sudden, but may have a gradual onset, with subsequent increase in severity).
- Nausea and vomiting are common.
- Fever may occur, but is not typical.
- Testicle exquisitely tender
- Testis may be high in scrotum with a transverse lie.
- Absence of cremasteric reflex

History
- Acute onset of pain, often during period of inactivity
- Prior history of multiple episodes of testicular pain with spontaneous resolution may indicate intermittent testicular torsion. (1)

Physical Exam
Tender, swollen, erythematous testicle

TESTS
Lab
Urinalysis usually not helpful

Imaging
Doppler ultrasound may confirm testicular swelling, but is diagnostic by demonstrating lack of blood flow to the testicle.

Diagnostic Procedures/Surgery
- Doppler ultrasonic flow detection demonstrates absent or reduced blood flow with torsion, increased flow with inflammatory process (reliable only in first 12 hours). (2)[C]
- Radionuclide testicular scintigraphy with technetium-99m pertechnetate demonstrates absent/decreased vascularity in torsion, increased vascularity with inflammatory processes (including torsion of appendix testes).
- In boys with intermittent, recurrent testicular torsion, both Doppler ultrasound and radionuclide scintigraphy will be normal. (3)[C]

Pathological Findings
- Venous thrombosis
- Tissue edema and necrosis
- Arterial thrombosis

DIFFERENTIAL DIAGNOSIS
- Epididymo-orchitis
- Incarcerated/strangulated inguinal hernia
- Acute hydrocele
- Traumatic hematoma
- Idiopathic scrotal edema
- Torsion appendix testis
- Acute varicocele
- Testicular tumor
- Henoch-Schönlein purpura
- Scrotal abscess
- Leukemic infiltrate

TREATMENT

- Manual reduction: May be successful, facilitated by lidocaine 1% (plain) injection at level of external ring. Must always be followed by orchidopexy
- Surgical exploration via scrotal approach with detorsion, evaluation of testicular viability, orchidopexy of viable testicle, orchiectomy of nonviable testicle
- In boys with history of intermittent episodes of testicular pain, scrotal exploration warranted with testicular fixation if abnormal testicular attactments confirmed. (3)[C]

GENERAL MEASURES
Early examination crucial as necrosis of the testicle usually occurs after 6–8 hours

Diet
Regular

SURGERY

- Bilateral testicular fixation is recommended by many surgeons.
- At least 3- to 4-point fixation with nonabsorbable sutures between the tunica albuginea and the tunica vaginalis.
- Excision of window of tunica albuginea with suture to dartos fascia
- Any testis that is not clearly viable (and obvious) should be removed.
- Testes of questionable viability which are preserved and pexed invariably atrophy.
- Requires general anesthesia
- Usually can be done as an outpatient

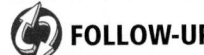 FOLLOW-UP

PROGNOSIS

- Testicular salvage is related directly to duration of torsion (85–97% if <6 hours, less than 10% if >24 hours).
- 80–94% may have depressed spermatogenesis related to duration of ischemic injury (possibly related to autoimmune-mediated injury).
- As many as 2/3 of salvaged testicles may atrophy in first 2–3 years after torsion.

COMPLICATIONS

- Possible testicular atrophy
- Abnormal spermatogenesis
- Infertility

PATIENT MONITORING

- Postoperative visit at 1–2 weeks
- Yearly visits until puberty, to evaluate for atrophy

REFERENCES

1. Van Glubeke E, et al. Acute scrotal pain in children: Results of 543 surgical explorations. *Pediatr Surg Int*. 1999;15:353–357.
2. Sessions AE, et al. Testicular torsion: Direction, degree, duration and disinformation. *J Urol*. 2003;169:663–665.
3. Eaton SH, et al. Intermittent testicular torsion: Diagnostic features and management outcomes. *J Urol*. 2005;174:1532–1535.

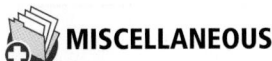 MISCELLANEOUS

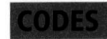

ICD9-CM
608.2 Torsion of testis.

PATIENT TEACHING

Possibility of testicular atrophy in salvaged testis with depressed sperm counts

T

TETANUS

Abdulrazak Abyad, MD, PhD, MBA, MPH, AGSF

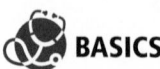 **BASICS**

DESCRIPTION
- Severe illness characterized by intermittent tonic spasms of voluntary muscles
- Toxin enters the central nervous system along the peripheral nerves or is blood borne.
- Tetanospasmin binds at synapses and blocks inhibitors.
- Usual course is acute
- System(s) Affected: Nervous
- Synonym(s): Lockjaw

ALERT
Geriatric Considerations
Mortality high in elderly, and this group may not have adequate immunizations.

Pediatric Considerations
- Mortality high in young
- Infection may enter through umbilical cord.

Pregnancy Considerations
- Must treat vigorously despite pregnancy
- Infection may enter uterus postpartum.
- Tetanus toxoid probably safe, but few data available

GENERAL PREVENTION
- Active immunization with tetanus toxoid
- Wound débridement
- Passive immunization with tetanus immune globulin (TIG)
- Acellular vaccine
- Benzathine penicillin
- Penicillin G
- Erythromycin

EPIDEMIOLOGY
- Predominant age: >70% of cases in persons >50 years of age
- Predominant sex: Male = Female

Incidence
Rare

Prevalence
Rare

RISK FACTORS
- Burns
- Drug addiction (parenteral)
- Ear infection (with tympanic membrane perforation)
- Early postpartum with an infected uterus
- Exposure of open wounds to soil and animal feces
- Frostbite
- Newborn (umbilicus stump entry)
- Skin ulcers
- Surgical wounds
- Age >50 years
- Traumatic wound

ETIOLOGY
- Infection with *Clostridium tetani*
- Neurotoxin produced by *C. tetani*
- Tetanospasmin (an exotoxin)

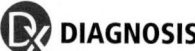 **DIAGNOSIS**

SIGNS AND SYMPTOMS
- Arrhythmias
- Asphyxia
- Convulsions
- Cyanosis
- Drooling
- Dysphagia
- Fluctuating hypertension
- Hydrophobia
- Hyperhidrosis
- Hyperpyrexia
- Hyperreflexia
- Hypotension
- Irritability
- Low-grade fever
- Muscular rigidity
- Muscular spasticity
- Nuchal rigidity
- Opisthotonos
- Pain at wound site
- Painful tonic convulsions
- Risus sardonicus (fixed smile)
- Stiffness of the jaw
- Sudden bradycardia
- Sudden cardiac arrest
- Tachycardia
- Tingling at wound site
- Trismus
- Wound history (may be absent)

TESTS
- ECG: Supraventricular tachycardia
- Multifocal ventricular ectopia
- Bradycardia
- EEG sleeping pattern
- Culture of wound infrequently recovers *C. tetani*

Lab
- Polymorphonuclear leukocytosis
- Culture of *C. tetani* from wound (may not be positive even if tetanus is the problem)

DIFFERENTIAL DIAGNOSIS
- Dental abscess
- Subarachnoid hemorrhage
- Seizure disorder
- Meningoencephalitis
- Peritonsillar abscess
- Dystonic reaction to phenothiazines
- Hypocalcemic tetany
- Strychnine poisoning
- Alcohol withdrawal

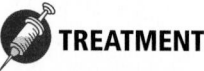 **TREATMENT**

INITIAL STABILIZATION
Intensive care

GENERAL MEASURES
- Wound excision
- Quiet observation
- Intubation
- IV hydration
- Catheterize the bladder.
- Prevent jarring of bed or drafts.

Diet
Nothing by mouth until well

Activity
Absolute bed rest with sedation

MEDICATION (DRUGS)

First Line

- Anticonvulsants
- Diazepam for muscle rigidity
- Pancuronium bromide (administered by anesthesiologist) plus ventilation
- Tetanus toxoid in a previously immunized patient
- TIG: 3,000–6,000 U IM. May infiltrate the area around the wound with a portion of the dose
- Penicillin G: 2 million U IV q6h. In a penicillin-allergic patient, use doxycycline 100 mg q12h, or clindamycin 150–300 mg IV q6h.
- Contraindications: Refer to the manufacturer's literature for each drug.
- Precautions
  - Refer to the manufacturer's literature for each drug.
  - Do not use TIG IV.
- Significant possible interactions: Refer to the manufacturer's literature for each drug.

Second Line

Equine tetanus antitoxin: 50,000 U IM, but only if TIG (human) is not available.

SURGERY

Tracheostomy if needed

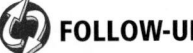 **FOLLOW-UP**

PROGNOSIS

- 25–50% mortality
- Poor prognostic factors
  - Form of tetanus
  - Incubation period
  - Onset period
  - Patient's age
  - Severity of symptoms
  - Heart wound
- Recovery is complete if patient survives.

COMPLICATIONS

- Respiratory arrest
- Cardiac failure
- Pulmonary emboli
- Bacterial infection
- Dehydration
- Vertebral fractures
- Airway obstruction
- Anoxia
- Urinary retention
- Constipation
- Pneumonia
- Rhabdomyolysis

PATIENT MONITORING

Careful observation in intensive care

REFERENCES

1. Centers for Disease Control. Tetanus: United States 1981–1984. *Morbid Mortal Weekly Rep*. 1985;34:602.
2. Lugauer S, et al. Long-term clinical effectiveness of an acellular pertussis component vaccine and a whole cell pertussis component vaccine. *Eur J Pediatr*. 2002;161:142–146.
3. Mandell GL, ed. *Principles and Practice of Infectious Diseases*. 4th ed. New York: Churchill Livingstone; 1995.
4. von Behring E, Kitasato S. Über das Zustandelkommen der Diphtherie-Immunität und der Tetanus-Immunität bei Thieren. *Deutsch Med Wochenschr*. 1890;16:1113.

 MISCELLANEOUS

See also: Anaerobic and necrotizing infections; Immunizations; Meningitis, Bacterial

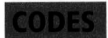 **CODES**

ICD9-CM
037 Tetanus

T

TETRALOGY OF FALLOT

Maya Roberts, BA
Mark R. Dambro, MD

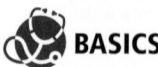 **BASICS**

DESCRIPTION

- Large ventricular septal defect associated with right ventricular outflow obstruction (infundibular and/or valvular pulmonic stenosis), concentric right ventricular hypertrophy, and overriding aorta
- Pathophysiology depends primarily on severity of right ventricular outflow tract obstruction.
- Right and left ventricular pressures are generally equal.
- Right ventricular pressures are elevated with ventricular septal defect proximal to level of right ventricular obstruction.
- Right-to-left shunting predominates, resulting in varying degrees of arterial hemoglobin desaturation.
- System(s) Affected: Cardiovascular; Pulmonary

ALERT

Pediatric Considerations
Congenital disorder

Pregnancy Considerations
Pregnancy is usually well tolerated after successful surgical repair.

EPIDEMIOLOGY
- Predominant age: Newborn
- Predominant sex: Male > Female (slightly)

Incidence
- 5–10% of all congenital heart disease.
- Most common cardiac anomaly within 1st year of life requiring intervention.

Prevalence
In the US: 3.9/10,000 live births.

RISK FACTORS
- Predominately sporadic
- Increased incidence with increasing maternal age

Genetics
- Occasional familial occurrence, dominant mode of inheritance
- Reports of "incomplete penetrance" as asymptomatic mitral valve malpositioning in family members

ETIOLOGY
Unknown

ASSOCIATED CONDITIONS
- Stenotic pulmonary artery
- Patent ductus arteriosus
- Atrial septal defect
- Iron deficiency anemia
- 15% have extracardiac anomalies including Down syndrome, Alagille, DiGeorge, and velocardiofacial syndromes

DIAGNOSIS

SIGNS AND SYMPTOMS
- Presentation depends on the severity of pulmonic stenosis.
- "Pink" tetralogy of Fallot: Occurs in patients in whom mild right ventricular outflow tract obstruction results in left-to-right shunt (thus acyanotic)
- Cyanosis, particularly in the nail beds and lips, with severe right ventricular outflow tract obstruction (generally recognized early)
- Delayed development
- Retarded growth
- Clubbing and polycythemia in children secondary to hypoxia
- Exertional dyspnea, poor exercise tolerance
- Acute hypercyanotic episodes or "Tet spells" (caused by increased right-to-left shunt)
- Squatting position, typically following exertion and during "Tet spells" (reduces right-to-left shunting by increasing systemic vascular resistance)
- Normal arterial and jugular venous pulses
- Systolic thrill along the left sternal border
- Early systolic ejection sound (aortic)
- Single S2 (decreased P2)
- Crescendo–decrescendo systolic ejection murmur results from flow across narrowed right ventricular outflow tract.
- Continuous soft murmur of bronchial collateral vessels
- Retinal ischemia
- Right sided aortic arch: 25%
- Atrial septal defect: 15%
- Anomalous coronary arteries: 9%

TESTS
ECG
- Sinus rhythm in general; however, some may develop atrial fibrillation or flutter
- Right atrial enlargement and right ventricular hypertrophy
- Right axis deviation and right ventricular conduction abnormality may also be seen.

Imaging
- Chest radiograph
  - Classic boot-shaped heart (coeur en sabot) with diminished pulmonary blood flow
  - Prominent right ventricle
  - Right-sided aortic arch and knob in 25% of patients
  - Normal (or decreased) pulmonary vascularity in <50% of adults

- Transthoracic echocardiogram (occasionally transesophageal)
  - 2-D images outline
    - Ventricular septal defect, atrial septum, right ventricular hypertrophy and extent and location of the infundibular obstruction.
    - Overriding aorta and assessment of pulmonic valve.
    - Coronary anatomy and peripheral branch pulmonic arteries.
  - Doppler echocardiogram allows quantification of the outflow gradient.
  - Color-flow Doppler mapping provides detailed assessment of the ventricular septal defect.

Diagnostic Procedures/Surgery
Cardiac catheterization
- Details anatomic structure
- Assesses pulmonary annulus size and pulmonary artery hypoplasia
- Assesses severity of right ventricular outflow obstruction
- Locates position of primary ventricular septal defect and its size, identifies possible additional ventricular septal defects
- Rules out coronary artery anomalies
- Balloon valvuloplasty to reduce pulmonary stenosis

Pathological Findings
- Anterior and cephalad deviation of the infundibular septum, resulting in malalignment with the muscular septum, creating a ventricular septal defect
- Malposition of the infundibular septum encroaching on the right ventricular outflow tract, resulting in an increased aortic root size
- Aortic root rotated into overriding position

DIFFERENTIAL DIAGNOSIS
- Fallot tetralogy with absent pulmonic valve
- Fallot tetralogy with absent pulmonary artery
- Pseudotruncus arteriosus

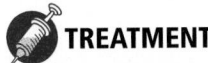 **TREATMENT**

INITIAL STABILIZATION
Inpatient for diagnosis and surgery

GENERAL MEASURES
• Good dental hygiene
• Endocarditis prophylaxis

Diet
Salt restriction

Activity
As tolerated

 MEDICATION (DRUGS)

No specific drug therapy in the absence of heart failure

SURGERY
• Total corrective surgical therapy includes patch closure of ventricular septal defect and pulmonary valvulotomy to relieve right ventricular outflow obstruction.
• Palliative surgical therapy (complete repair with a systemic-to-pulmonary shunt is the preferred modality of treatment).
   – Blalock-Taussig shunt or modified shunt with Gore-Tex tubing: Subclavian to pulmonary artery
   – Pott procedure (descending aorta to pulmonary artery and Waterston shunt (ascending aorta to pulmonary artery) no longer used because of high pulmonary blood flow and development of pulmonary hypertension

 FOLLOW-UP

PROGNOSIS
Without surgery, survival was 40% at 3 years and 3% at 40 years. Surgical correction yields a survival of 92% at 10 years, 76% at 40 years.

COMPLICATIONS
• Postoperatively
   – Residual right ventricular outflow obstruction
   – Residual ventricular septal defect
   – Chronic pulmonary regurgitation (with subsequent valve replacement occasionally required)
   – Ventricular and atrial tachyarrhythmias
   – Right bundle branch block (common)
   – Left anterior hemiblock
   – Infective bacterial endocarditis
   – Hemoptysis
• Erythrocytosis secondary to chronic hypoxemia (increased risk for thrombosis, thrombotic cerebrovascular accident, and paradoxical emboli).
• Increased risk for brain abscess
• Acute gouty arthritis
• Infective endocarditis
• Delayed puberty

PATIENT MONITORING
• Postprocedure echocardiography suggested after 1 year
• Good dental hygiene and subacute bacterial endocarditis prophylaxis
• Regular follow-up assessment for patients not undergoing surgical correction

REFERENCES
1. Shinebourne E, Babu-Narayan S, Carvalho J. Tetralogy of Fallot: From fetus to adult. *Heart.* 2006;92:1353–1359.
2. Doyle T, Kavanaught-McHugh A, Graham T. Pathophysiology; clinical features; and diagnosis of tetralogy of Fallot & overview of the management of tetralogy of Fallot. UpToDate. 2006.
3. Pham P, Silberbach M. What's new in pediatric cardiology. *Pediatr Rev.* 2004;25(11):381–387.
4. Ramaswamy P. Systemic to pulmonary artery shunting for palliation. eMedicine. 12 Dec, 2006
5. Braunwald E, ed. *Heart Disease:* A Textbook of Cardiovascular Medicine, 5th ed. Philadelphia: WB Saunders, 1996
6. Bertranou EG, Blackston EH, Hazelrig JB, et al. Life expectancy without surgery in tetralogy of Fallot. *Am J Cardiol.* 1978;42(3):458–466.
7. Liberthson R. Congenital Heart Disease: Diagnosis & Management in Children and Adults. Boston: Little, Brown, and Company, 1989.
8. Perloff J. Clinical Recognition of Congenital Heart Disease, 4th ed. Philadelphia: WB Saunders, 1994.

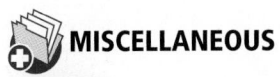 **MISCELLANEOUS**

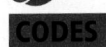 **CODES**

ICD9-CM
745.2 Tetralogy of Fallot

PATIENT TEACHING
American Heart Association, 7320 Greenville Avenue, Dallas, TX 75231; (214) 373-6300

THALASSEMIA

Herbert L. Muncie, Jr., MD

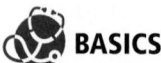 **BASICS**

DESCRIPTION
- A group of inherited disorders that affect the synthesis of adult hemoglobin tetramer (Hb A)
- α-Thalassemia is due to a deficient synthesis of α-globin, while β-thalassemia is due to a deficient synthesis of β-globin.
  - The synthesis of the unaffected globin chain proceeds normally.
  - This leads to inadequate hemoglobin and unbalanced accumulaton of goblin sythesis, which then results in hypochromic, microcytic red cells and hemolytic anemia.
- Thalassemia is prevalent in the Mediterranean region, the Middle East, Southeast Asia, and among ethnic groups originating from these areas.
- β-Thalassemia is more common in persons of Mediterranean, African, or Southeast Asian descent, whereas α-thalassemia is increased in patients of African and Southeast Asian descent.
- Types
  - Thalassemia trait (α- or β-): Mild anemia with microcytosis and hypochromia. No transfusion therapy is needed.
  - β-Thalassemia intermedia: Milder form. Transfusion therapy may not be needed.
  - β-Thalassemia major: Severe anemia, growth retardation, hepatosplenomegaly, bone marrow expansion, and bone deformities. Transfusion therapy is necessary to sustain life.
- Varieties unique to Southeast Asians include hemoglobin H disease (a more severe form of α-thalassemia) and hemoglobin E/β-thalassemia, which often mimics β-thalassemia major in its severity.
- System(s) Affected: Hematologic/Lymphatic/Immunologic; Cardiac; Hepatic
- Synonym(s): Mediterranean anemia; Hereditary leptocytosis; Thalassemia major and minor; Cooley anemia

ALERT
Pediatric Considerations
- Severe forms cause symptoms during early childhood and require treatment to sustain life.
- Newborns' cord blood or heel stick should be screened for hemoglobinopathies with hemoglobin electrophoresis or comparably accurate test. (1)[A]

Pregnancy Considerations
- Genetic counseling is advised for parents or other relatives of a child with thalassemia and for any individual with β-thalassemia minor.
- During the first trimester, test chorionic-villus samples with polymerase chain reaction (PCR) technology to detect point mutations or deletions.

GENERAL PREVENTION
- Prenatal information
  - Genetic counseling regarding partner selection and information on the availability of diagnostic tests in the event of pregnancy
- Complication prevention
  - For offspring of adult thalassemia patients, evaluation for thalassemia by 1 year of age
  - Severe forms
    - Avoid exposure to sick contacts.
    - Keep immunizations up-to-date, including pneumococcal vaccine and annual influenza vaccine.
  - Prompt treatment of bacterial infections (after splenectomy, patients should maintain a supply of an appropriate antibiotic to take at the onset of symptoms of a bacterial infection.)
  - Dental checkups every 6 months.
  - Avoid activities that could increase the risk of bone fractures.

EPIDEMIOLOGY
- Predominant age: Symptoms start to appear 3–6 months after birth with severe form
- Predominant sex: Male = Female

Incidence
Occurs in 4.4/10,000 live births

Prevalence
- <1,000 patients in the United States are affected with β-thalassemia major.
- The prevalence of thalassemia trait within the involved ethnic groups ranges from 5–30%.

RISK FACTORS
Family history

Genetics
- Inherited in an autosomal recessive pattern
- α-Thalassemia results from deletion of one or more of the four genes responsible for α-globin synthesis. Four-gene deletions results in fatal hydrops fetalis. Three-gene deletions results in hemoglobin H. Two-gene deletions is trait and one-gene deletion is a "silent" carrier state.
- β-Thalassemia is caused by any of more than 200 point mutations and very rarely deletions.
- Significantly disparate phenotype with the same genotype is unexplained by variability of known loci

ETIOLOGY
Genetic

ASSOCIATED CONDITIONS
See Complications

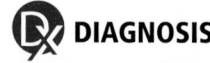 **DIAGNOSIS**

SIGNS AND SYMPTOMS
Thalassemia trait has no signs or symptoms.

History
- Poor growth
- Inadequate food intake
- Fatigue
- Cholelithiasis
- Pathologic fractures
- Shortness of breath

Physical Exam
- Pallor
- Splenomegaly
- Jaundice
- Maxillary hyperplasia
- Dental malocclusion

TESTS
Special tests
- Bone marrow aspiration
- For children, calculate Mentzer index (MCV/RBC count)
  - <13, thalassemia more likely
  - >13, iron deficiency more likely. (2)

Lab
- Hemoglobin: Usual range 10.0–12.0 g/dL with thalassemia trait
- Hematocrit
  - 28–40% in thalassemia trait
  - May fall to <10% in β-thalassemia major
- Peripheral blood
  - Microcytosis
  - Hypochromia
  - High percentage of target cells
  - Reticulocyte count elevated
- Hemoglobin electrophoresis
  - In β-thalassemia trait elevated Hb A2 levels
  - In β-thalassemia major or intermedia elevated Hb A2, elevated Hb F, reduced or absent Hb A1
  - In α-thalassemia, no recognizable electrophoretic pattern occurs.

Pathological Findings
- Bone marrow erythroid hyperplasia
- Iron deposits in heart muscle
- Hepatic siderosis

DIFFERENTIAL DIAGNOSIS
- Iron deficiency
- Other hemoglobinopathies
- Other hemolytic anemias

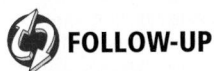

TREATMENT

- Outpatient for mild cases
- Inpatient for transfusion therapy

GENERAL MEASURES

- Mild cases require no therapy.
- Thalassemia intermedia: Normally no therapy necessary unless hemoglobin levels fall to a level that causes symptoms, then transfusion therapy may be needed
- Thalassemia major
  - Maintain a mean hemoglobin level of at least 9.3 g/dL (1.4 mmol/L) with a regular transfusion schedule.
  - Folate supplementation daily
  - Treat bacterial infections promptly.
- Iron overload
  - Patients receiving transfusion therapy increase total body iron 4 times over the normal amount.
  - Therapy is iron chelation.

Diet

- Thalassemia minor requires no restrictions.
- β-Thalassemia major
  - Avoid iron-rich foods (red meats such as liver, and some cereals).
  - Drinking tea may possibly help reduce iron absorption.

Activity

- Thalassemia minor requires no restrictions
- β-Thalassemia major
  - Avoid strenuous activities (e.g., football, soccer).
  - Acceptable activity levels will be determined on an individual basis depending on severity of disorder.

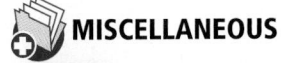

MEDICATION (DRUGS)

- Antibiotics for bacterial infections
- Thalassemia intermedia
  - Folic acid supplements

First Line

Thalassemia major

- Iron chelation with deferoxamine (Desferal)
  - SC or continuous IV infusion (3)[C]
  - Usually started before 5–8 years of age

Second Line

- Deferiprone, PO, acceptable alternative for patients unable to receive deferoxamine (3)[C]
- Contraindications to chelation therapy Refer to manufacturer's literature.
- Precautions with chelation therapy Refer to manufacturer's literature.
- Possible significant interactions with chelation therapy Refer to manufacturer's literature.

SURGERY

- Splenectomy
  - May be needed if hypersplenism causes a marked increase in the transfusion requirement
  - Defer surgery until patient is 4–6 years of age (due to increased infection risk).
  - Administer polyvalent pneumococcal vaccine 1 month prior to splenectomy.
  - Daily penicillin prophylaxis post splenectormy
- Bone marrow transplantation in childhood
  - Only curative therapy and generally excellent outcome for low-risk patients

FOLLOW-UP

DISPOSITION

Issues for Referral

Thalassemia major usually requires hematology consult.

PROGNOSIS

- Outlook varies depending on type.
- Thalassemia minor patients live a normal life span.
- Thalassemia major patients live an average of 17 years and usually die by age 30.
- Iron overload causes most of the morbidity and mortality.
  - Cardiac events are the primary cause of death.
  - Effective iron chelation is improving longevity.

COMPLICATIONS

- Chronic hemolysis
- Susceptibility to infections after splenectomy
- Infections from blood transfusion
- Jaundice
- Leg ulcers
- Cholelithiasis
- Osteoporosis and low-trauma fractures
- Impaired growth rate
- Delayed or absent puberty
- Hypogonadism
- Hepatic siderosis
- Splenomegaly
- Cardiac disease from iron overload
- Thromboembolic phenomenon
- Aplastic and megaloblastic crises

PATIENT MONITORING

- For β-thalassemia major, life-long monitoring is necessary because the therapy and disease progression have numerous potential complications.
- Thalassemia minor patients require no special follow-up.

REFERENCES

1. Andrews J, Wilson M. Screening for hemoglobinopathies. United States Preventive Services Task Force,1996;485–492.
2. Irwn JJ, Kirchner JT. Anemia in children. *Am Fam Physician*. 2001;64:1379–1386.
3. Rund D, Rachmilewitz E. β-Thalassemia. *N Engl J Med*. 2005;353:1135–1146.
4. Dhaliwal G, Cornett PA, Tierney LM. Hemolytic anemia. *Am Fam Physician*. 2004;69:2599–2606.

MISCELLANEOUS

CODES

ICD9-CM

- 282.49 Thalassemia (alpha, beta, intermedia, major, minor, trait)

PATIENT TEACHING

Prevention

- Genetic counseling
- Teach parents signs of hepatitis, iron overload
- Printed patient information available from: Cooley Anemia Foundation, 330 Seventh Ave. Suite 900, New York, NY 10001 (www.cooleyanemia.org)

See Corresponding Diagnostic Algorithm

THORACIC OUTLET SYNDROME

Frederico Milla, MD
Ruben Peralta, MD, FACS

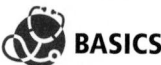 **BASICS**

DESCRIPTION
- A constellation of symptoms that affect the head, neck, shoulders, and upper extremities, caused by compression of the neurovascular structures (i.e., brachial plexus and subclavian vessels) at the thoracic outlet
- Resulting from congenital bony, muscular, or tendon anomalies; posttraumatic, following clavicular or cervical spine injures; or idiopathic.
- Synonym(s): Scalenus anticus syndrome; Cervical rib syndrome; Costoclavicular syndrome; Thoracic outlet syndrome

ALERT
Pregnancy Considerations
Generalized tissue fluid accumulations and postural changes could aggravate symptoms.

EPIDEMIOLOGY
- Predominant age
  - Neurologic type (95%): 20–60 years
  - Venous type (4%):20–35 years
  - Arterial type (1%; atherosclerosis): Young adult or >50
- Predominant sex
  - Neurologic type: Female > Male (3.5:1)
  - Venous type: Male > Female
  - Arterial type: Male = Female

Incidence
3–80/1,000 population

RISK FACTORS
- Posttraumatic
- Exostosis of clavicle or first rib
- Postural abnormalities (e.g., drooping of shoulders, scoliosis)
- Body building, with increased muscular bulk in thoracic outlet area
- Rapid weight loss combined with vigorous physical exertion and/or exercise
- Occupational exposure
  - Computer users
  - Musicians
  - Repetitive work involving shoulders, arms, hands
  - Young thin females with long necks and drooping shoulders

ETIOLOGY
Compression of upper thoracic neurovasculature by
- Cervical rib
- Taut anomalous scalene muscles
- Elongated C7 transverse process
- Poor posture
- Pancoast tumor
- Atherosclerotic plaques within vessels
- Subclavian muscle
- Fibrous and ligamentous bands
- Costocoracoid tendon
- Callous bone formation from fractured clavicle or 1st rib
- Aberrant tissue
- Neck trauma

ASSOCIATED CONDITIONS
- Paget-von Schrötter syndrome: Thrombosis of subclavian vein
- Gilliatt-Sumner hand: Neurogenic atrophy of abductor pollicis brevis

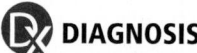 **DIAGNOSIS**

SIGNS AND SYMPTOMS
- Neurologic type, upper plexus (C4–C7)
  - Pain and paresthesias in head, neck, mandible, face, temporal area, upper back/chest, outer arm, and hand in a radial nerve distribution
  - Occipital and orbital headache
- Neurologic type, lower plexus (C8–T1)
  - Pain and paresthesias in axilla, inner arm, and hand in an ulnar nerve distribution, often nocturnal
  - Hypothenar and interosseous muscle atrophy
- Venous type
  - Arm claudication
  - Cyanosis
  - Swelling
  - Distended arm veins
- Arterial type
  - Digital vasospasm
  - Thrombosis/embolism
  - Aneurysm
  - Gangrene
- Positive Adson maneuver (head rotation to the affected side with cervical extension then deep inhalation. Test is positive if paresthesias or if radial pulse not palpable during maneuver)
- Tenderness to percussion or palpation of supraclavicular area
- Worsening of symptoms with elevation of arm, overhead extension of arms, or with arms extended forward (e.g., driving a car, typing, carrying objects). Prompt disappearance of symptoms with arm returning to neutral position
- Morley test
  - Brachial plexus compression test in the supraclavicular area from the scalene triangle
  - A positive response is the reproduction of an aching sensation and typical localized paresthesia
- 1-minute Roos test
  - A thoracic outlet shoulder girdle stress test
  - Shoulders and arms are braced in a 90° abducted and externally rotated position; patient is required to clench and relax fists repetitively for 1 minute.
  - A positive test reproduces the symptom.

TESTS
- Plethysmography with previously mentioned maneuvers.
- Doppler and duplex ultrasound if venous obstruction suspected
- Ulnar and median nerve conduction velocity studies (<70 m/sec is abnormal)
- Venogram and arteriogram if presents with edematous changes in upper extremity

Imaging
- Radiograph (chest, C-spine, shoulders) may reveal elongated C7 transverse process or a cervical rib, Pancoast tumor, or healed clavicle fracture.
- Arteriogram or venogram, if arterial or venous obstruction, aneurysm, or emboli are suspected
- CT scan, if cord compression lesions (disc and/or tumor) are suspected
- Helical CT
- 3D MR angiography

Diagnostic Procedures/Surgery
- Thoracic outlet syndrome is a clinical diagnosis.
- Anterior scalene muscle injections are useful in confirming the diagnosis and in determining which patients may respond favorably to surgery.

DIFFERENTIAL DIAGNOSIS
- Cervical disk syndrome
- Carpal tunnel syndrome
- Orthopedic shoulder problems (shoulder strain, rotator cuff injury, tendinitis)
- Cervical spondylitis
- Ulnar nerve compression at elbow and hand
- Multiple sclerosis
- Spinal cord tumor or disease
- Angina pectoris
- Migraine
- Reflex sympathetic dystrophy
- C8 radiculopathies

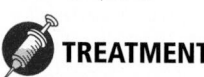 **TREATMENT**

INITIAL STABILIZATION
- Outpatient for conservative treatment
- Inpatient if surgery required

GENERAL MEASURES
- Conservative therapy
  - If no vascular involvement is present and/or if no loss of function or lifestyle is present owing to severity of symptoms, conservative therapy may be undertaken for 2–3 months.
  - Improvement can be expected in 60% of patients.
  - Exercise program to promote shoulder muscle function
  - Physical therapy for postural faults
  - Cervical collar, traction
  - Weight loss if axillary folds are causing compression
- Consultation with vascular surgeon or neurosurgeon if vascular or neurologic involvement is suspected.

Activity
- Light activity with arm and hand is encouraged.
- No straining or heavy activity for 3 months.

SPECIAL THERAPY
Physical Therapy
- Exercise program
- Postural correction

MEDICATION (DRUGS)

- Analgesics
- Muscle relaxants
- Antispasmodics

SURGERY

- Operative if vascular involvement is present and/or loss of function or lifestyle occurs secondary to severity of symptoms, and if conservative therapy fails after 2–3 months (1)[B].
- Resection of 1st rib or cervical ribs (transaxillary, supraclavicular, posterior approaches) (2)[B]
- Excision of adhesive bands via transaxillary approach
- Anterior scalenectomy

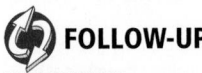 **FOLLOW-UP**

PROGNOSIS

- 60% improve with appropriate physiotherapy program.
- 90% have excellent or good early results with surgery (3)[B].
- 70–80% have no recurrence at 5 and 10 years.

COMPLICATIONS

- Postoperative shoulder, arm, hand pain, and paresthesias in 10%; usually responds to physiotherapy
- 1.5–2% of patients will have symptomatic recurrences 1 month–7 years postoperatively (usually within 3 months).
- 0.5–1% of patients have brachial plexus injury, probably owing to intraoperative traction
- Reoperation indicated for symptomatic recurrence with long posterior remnant of 1st rib (posterior approach) or with disrupted fibrous adhesions (transaxillary approach)
- Venous obstruction or arterial emboli; usually responds to thrombolytics

PATIENT MONITORING

Office follow-up visits, e.g., every 3 weeks

REFERENCES

1. Huang JH, Zager EL. Thoracic outlet syndrome. *Neurosurgery.* 2004;55:897–903.
2. Sanders RJ, Hammond SL. Management of cervical ribs and anomalous first ribs causing neurogenic thoracic outlet syndrome. *J Vasc Surg.* 2002;36:51–56.
3. Axelrod DA, Proctor MC, Geisser ME, et al. Outcomes after surgery for thoracic outlet syndrome. *J Vasc Surg.* 2001;33:1220–1225.
4. Mackinnon SE, Patterson GA, Novak CB. Thoracic outlet syndrome: A current overview. *Semin Thoracic Cardiovasc Surg.* 1996a;8:176–182.
5. Cooke RA. Thoracic outlet syndrome-aspects of diagnosis in the differential diagnosis of hand-arm vibration syndrome. *Occupation Med.* 2003;53:331–336

 MISCELLANEOUS

2–3 months trial of physiotherapy is always indicated, except in presence of obvious bony abnormality.

 CODES

ICD9-CM
353.0 Brachial plexus lesions

PATIENT TEACHING

- Physical therapy following surgery
- Postural exercises
- NSAIDs may improve pain.
- Ergonomic workstation

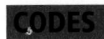 **See Corresponding Diagnostic Algorithm**

T

THROMBOANGIITIS OBLITERANS (BUERGER DISEASE)

Rick Kellerman, MD

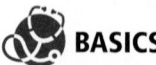 BASICS

DESCRIPTION
- Nonatherosclerotic segmental occlusion of small- and medium-sized arteries and veins caused by inflammatory changes in these vessels
- Primarily occurs in men who smoke
- System(s) Affected: Cardiovascular
- Synonym(s): Buerger disease

GENERAL PREVENTION
Never smoke.

EPIDEMIOLOGY
- Predominant age: 20–40 years
- Predominant sex: Male > Female (3:1). Increasing numbers of women are being diagnosed, possibly due to increased smoking.

Incidence
13 per 100,000 in U.S.

Prevalence
Among those with peripheral artery disease, prevalence ranges from 0.5–5.5% in Western Europe, to 45–63% in India, to 80% in Jews of Ashkenazi ancestry.

ALERT
Geriatric Considerations
Not common in this age group, but diagnosis in the elderly is increasing.

Pediatric Considerations
Not a problem in this age group

RISK FACTORS
- Smoking tobacco
- Occasional cases in users of smokeless tobacco and snuff
- Incidence higher in Israel, Middle East, Eastern Europe, Japan, India, Far East than in North America and Western Europe
- More common in countries with heavy tobacco use

Genetics
- Greater prevalence of HLA-A54, HLA-A9, and HLA-B5
- Familial cases reported rarely

ETIOLOGY
Postulated
- Smoking
- Genetic factors
- Autoimmune disorder with cell-mediated sensitivity to types I and III human collagens (both are normal constituents of blood vessels)
- Impaired peripheral endothelium-dependent vasodilation. Nonendothelium mechanisms of vasodilation are intact.
- Arsenic content of tobacco
- Chronic anaerobic periodontal infection

DIAGNOSIS

PRE HOSPITAL
- Point scoring systems may help clarify clinical diagnosis
- 1 set of criteria includes age <45; current or recent use of tobacco; distal extremity ischemia; exclusion of autoimmune and hypercoagulable disease

SIGNS AND SYMPTOMS
Symptoms tend to wax and wane in early disease and are often asymmetric. Symptoms may be gradual or have a sudden onset related to impaired vasculature. Usually more than 1 limb is involved.

History
- Coldness in feet and/or fingers
- Cold sensitivity
- Paresthesias (numbness, tingling, burning, hypoesthesia) of feet and/or fingers
- Intermittent claudication in arch of foot or leg (rarely hand, forearm)
- Persistent extremity pain (may be worse at rest); pain may be disabling
- Paroxysmal "electric shock" pain of ischemic neuropathy
- Migratory superficial phlebitis

Physical Exam
- Ulceration of digits
- Raynaud phenomenon
- Postural color changes: Pallor on elevation; rubor on dependency
- "Buerger color": Cyanosis of hands and feet
- Tender skin nodules on extremities
- Impaired distal pulses
- Proximal pulses normal; Allen test may be abnormal
- Foot edema
- Gangrene

TESTS
Lab
- Routine laboratory studies show no changes characteristic of this disorder.
- Autoantibodies to collagen and circulating immune complexes may be present, but are strictly for research purposes.
- Homocysteine may be elevated, but lacks specificity.

Imaging
- Doppler ultrasound (not specific)
- Arteriogram or digital-subtraction angiography
  - Multiple areas of segmental occlusion of small to medium arteries of arms and legs
  - "Skip" areas may be demonstrated.
  - Numerous collateral vessels around occluded segments may give a characteristic corkscrew appearance
  - Larger arteries are spared. More serious disease occurs distally.
  - No apparent source of emboli

Diagnostic Procedures/Surgery
- History and physical examination
- Studies of nerve conduction velocity (to exclude neuropathy)
- Echocardiography (to exclude emboli)

Pathological Findings
- Segmental inflammatory thrombosis of both arteries and veins
- Histologic findings may vary between acute, intermediate, and chronic stages of the disease.
- Histologic sine qua non: Granulomas with collections of neutrophils in the organizing thrombus
  - The vessel wall is relatively spared.
  - Wall-sparing distinguishes thromboangiitis obliterans from arteriosclerosis and other systemic vasculitis, which show striking wall disruption.
- Acute lesions show occlusive, highly cellular inflammatory thrombi with less inflammation in vessel wall. Polymorphonuclear leukocytes, microabscesses, and multinucleated giant cells may be present.
- Intermediate lesions show organizing thrombus.
- Chronic lesions show recanalized thrombus and perivascular fibrosis.

DIFFERENTIAL DIAGNOSIS
- Peripheral neuropathy
- Peripheral atherosclerotic disease
- Arterial embolus and thrombosis
- Idiopathic peripheral thrombosis
- Hypercoagulable states
- Other causes of vasculitis
- Systemic lupus erythematosus
- Scleroderma
- Occupational trauma
- Repetitive trauma
- Cervical rib
- Livedo reticularis
- Raynaud disease
- Acrocyanosis
- Ergotism
- Frostbite
- Neurotrophic ulcers
- Reflex sympathetic dystrophy
- Metatarsalgia
- Gout
- Periarteritis nodosa
- Juvenile temporal arteritis with eosinophilia
- Polyarteritis
- Carpal tunnel syndrome
- Takayasu arteritis (young Japanese women)
- CREST syndrome (calcinosis, Raynaud phenomenon, poor esophageal mobility, sclerodactyly, telangiectasia)

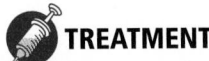 ## TREATMENT

INITIAL STABILIZATION
- Outpatient
- Inpatient if surgery needed for gangrene
- Inpatient for dorsal or lumbar sympathectomy if indicated

GENERAL MEASURES
- Stop smoking (mandatory).
- Protect against trauma (poor fitting shoes).
- Protect against infections.
- Protect against vasoconstriction from cold or drugs.
- Eliminate exposure to thermal damage.
- Eliminate exposure to chemical damage (iodine, carbolic acid, salicylic acid).
- Thrombolytic therapy of occlusive thrombus and angioplasty are experimental.

Diet
No restrictions

Activity
- Restricted by symptoms
- Use a bed cradle (nonheated) to prevent pressure from bed linens.

 ## MEDICATION (DRUGS)

First Line
- Medications are not a substitute for discontinuing smoking.
- Antibiotics for infected digital ulcers and osteomyelitis
- Iloprost, a prostacyclin analog, promotes ulcer healing (available in Europe).
- Urokinase or streptokinase selectively infused into occluded artery
- Intramuscular endothelial growth factor gene therapy
- No form of medical treatment has been shown to be effective (including steroids, calcium channel blockers, reserpine, pentoxifylline, vasodilators, antiplatelet drugs, anticoagulants).
- Contraindications: Refer to manufacturer's literature.
- Precautions: Refer to manufacturer's literature.
- Significant possible interactions: Refer to manufacturer's literature.

Second Line
Calcium channel blocking agents, such as nifedipine, may allow vasodilatation, but have not been proven effective.

SURGERY
- Amputation
  - For nonhealing ulcers, gangrene, or intractable pain
  - Should preserve as much limb as possible
  - Rarely required
- Omental autotransplantation has been successful in treating ulcers.
- Infrainguinal bypass
- In severe disease, a lumbar sympathectomy to increase blood supply to the skin
- Spinal cord stimulator
- Direct revascularization of distal arteries is not practical. Distal target vessel is usually not available.

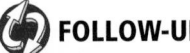 ## FOLLOW-UP

PROGNOSIS
- Occasional remissions
- Unremitting progression if patient continues to smoke
- Death rare; normal survival curve

COMPLICATIONS
- Ulcerations
- Gangrene
- Need for amputation
- Rare occlusion of cerebral, coronary, renal, splenic, mesenteric, pulmonary, iliac arteries, and aorta

PATIENT MONITORING
Frequent history and physical examinations

REFERENCES

1. Case records of the Massachusetts General Hospital. Weekly clinicopathological exercises. Case 16-1989. A 36-year-old man with peripheral vascular disease. *N Engl J Med*. 1989;320:1068–1076. (C)
2. Olin JW. Thromboangiitis obliterans (Buerger's disease). *N Engl J Med*. 2000;343:864–869. (C)
3. Olin JW, et al. The changing clinical spectrum of thromboangiitis obliterans (Buerger's disease). *Circulation*. 1990;82(Suppl):IV3–8.
4. Iwai T, Inoue Y, Umeda M, et al. Oral bacteria in the occluded arteries of patients with Buerger disease. *J Vasc Surg*. 2005;42:107. (C)

 ## MISCELLANEOUS

May be difficult to differentiate from some types of atherosclerosis, systemic emboli, or idiopathic peripheral thromboses

CODES

ICD9-CM
443.1 Thromboangiitis obliterans (Buerger disease)

PATIENT TEACHING
- Must stop smoking
- Remove possibilities of exposure to others in the environment who smoke.
- Nicotine replacement may keep the disease active.
- Use heel pads or foam rubber boots.

 See Corresponding Diagnostic Algorithm

T

THROMBOTIC THROMBOCYTOPENIC PURPURA

Rimini Varghese, MD
James N. Butera, MD

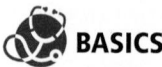 **BASICS**

DESCRIPTION
- An acute syndrome hallmarked by consumptive thrombocytopenia and microangiopathic hemolytic anemia with deposition of hyaline thrombi in arterioles, leading to ischemic multiorgan damage.
- Thrombotic thrombocytopenic purpura (TTP) syndrome is characterized by a pentad
  - Thrombocytopenia
  - Microangiopathic hemolytic anemia
  - Renal insufficiency
  - CNS symptoms
  - Fever

EPIDEMIOLOGY
- Predominant age: Most common in patients 30–60 years old
- Predominant sex: Females > Males (2:1)
- Incidence ratio in blacks to non-blacks is 9:3

Incidence
11 cases/million/year

RISK FACTORS
- Pregnancy and oral contraceptives
- AIDS and early symptomatic HIV infection
- Autoimmune disease
  - Antiphospholipid antibody syndrome
  - Systemic lupus erythematosus
  - Scleroderma
- Drug toxicity
  - Cancer chemotherapy
    ○ Mitomycin C, gemcitabine
    ○ Bleomycin and cisplatin
    ○ Tacrolimus and cyclosporine
  - Immune mediated
    ○ Quinine
    ○ Ticlopidine and clopidogrel
- Hematopoietic cell transplantation

Genetics
Mutation at the ADAMTS13 metalloproteinase gene locus on chromosome 9q34 has been described as the cause of familial TTP.

PATHOPHYSIOLOGY
- In TTP, the aggregating agent responsible for platelet thrombi is unusually large von Willebrand factor (ULvWF) multimers, which are far larger than those found in normal plasma.
- A metalloproteinase, ADAMTS13, which normally enzymatically cleaves the ULvWF multimers to prevent clumping within vessels is deficient, defective, or absent, allowing UlvWF to react with platelets. This leads to endothelial cell damage and disseminated thrombi characteristic of TTP.
- Arterioles most often affected are in the brain, kidney, pancreas, heart, and adrenal glands.
  - Lungs and liver are relatively spared.

ETIOLOGY
- In familial TTP, patients have very low or absent levels of ADAMTS13.
- In acquired idiopathic TTP, some studies have demonstrated IgG autoantibodies are made to the metalloproteinase ADAMTS13, to receptors on the surface of platelets, or to the surface of the endothelial cell (1)[A]. Trigger is unknown.
- Especially in those without ADAMTS13 deficiency, endothelial injury, either directly from a drug/toxin or indirectly via platelet/neurophil activation, has been proposed as a cause of TTP.
  - Drug-induced (see Risk Factors)

ASSOCIATED CONDITIONS
TTP and hemolytic-uremic syndrome (HUS) have very similar presentations and are often described as a continuum of the same pathophysiologic process, with some notable distinctions
- TTP generally presents with prominent neurologic symptoms and minimal renal involvement, whereas the opposite tends to be more characteristic of HUS.
- However, patients with HUS and TTP may have both prominent renal and neurologic manifestations, often making the distinction unclear.
- ADAMTS13 levels are diminished in adults with TTP but are normal in children diagnosed with HUS following infection with *E. coli* (particularly type O157:H7).

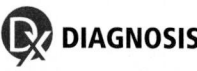 **DIAGNOSIS**

SIGNS AND SYMPTOMS
- Most commonly nonspecific
  - Nausea, vomiting, weakness, abdominal pain, fatigue
- Related to thrombocytopenia
  - Easy bruising, purpura or petechiae
  - Epistaxis, menorrhagia
  - Gastrointestinal bleeding
  - Intracranial Hemorrhage
  - Visual symptoms due to retinal hemorrhage
- Related to hemolytic anemia (microangiopathic hemolytic anemia [MAHA])
  - Jaundice
- Related to end-organ ischemia
  - Neurologic: CNS symptoms occur in 90%; presenting complaint in 60%
    ○ Often fluctuating symptoms
    ○ Headache
    ○ Altered mental status; spectrum runs from behavioral/personality changes to obtundation/stupor or coma
    ○ Seizures

History
- Generally acute onset of symptoms
- It is important to assess for cause or risk factors (see above).
- 58% of patients die within the 1st 48 hours without treatment.
- 90% mortality without treatment
- Patients often do not present with the classic presentation because the treatment is initiated before the pentad can develop.

Physical Exam
- Mental status/neurologic: Confusion, coma, stupor, weakness
- HEENT: Retinal hemorrhage, scleral icterus, epistaxis
- Abdomen/GI
  - Nonspecific tenderness
- Skin: Jaundice, petechiae, purpura, ecchymoses

TESTS
Lab
- CBC/Reticulocyte count/peripheral smear
  - Hemoglobin < 10 g/dL
    ○ Average is 8–9 g/dL; <6 g/dL in 40%
  - Platelets <25,000/mm³
    ○ Range 5,000–120,000/mm3
  - Reticulocyte count increased
  - Peripheral smear
    ○ Schistocytes (prominent)
    ○ Helmet cells, RBC fragments
    ○ Nucleated RBCs
    ○ Polychromasia
- Coagulation studies
  - Normal in most; mild elevation in 15%
  - Fibrinogen normal
- Coombs test: Negative direct Coombs test
- Electrolytes, BUN/creatinine: Mild elevation of BUN and creatinine (Creatinine <3)
- Liver function studies: Increased indirect bilirubin (hemolysis)
- LDH: 5–10 times normal
- Urinalysis
  - Proteinuria, microscopic hematuria
  - Positive dipstick for large blood but minimal RBCs on microscopic examination
- Haptoglobin decreased (hemolysis)
- EKG: Sinus tachycardia, heart block
- No utility of ADAMTS13 assay in diagnosis

Imaging
CT scan of the head: Often performed due to mental status changes to rule out possible intracranial hemorrhage or ischemic changes

Pathological Findings
Biopsy confirms the diagnosis, because diagnosis is made on clinical grounds and laboratory findings (2, 3)[A].

DIFFERENTIAL DIAGNOSIS

- HUS: (see "Associated Conditions")
- Antiphospholipid antibody syndrome: Prolonged PTT and presence of lupus anticoagulant
- Malignant hypertension: Diastolic >130, papilledema, retinal hemorrhages
- Pregnancy associated Preeclampsia/eclampsia or HELLP
  - Low ATIII levels
- Disseminated intravascular coagulation
  - Prolonged PT/PTT, low fibrinogen
  - Low factor V and VIII
  - Secondary to sepsis/shock or widely disseminated malignancy
- Idiopathic thrombocytopenic purpura
  - No hemolysis, normal LDH and bilirubin
  - Presence of anti-platelet antibodies
- Malignancy-associated microangiopathy
- Autoimmune hemolytic anemia: Positive direct Coombs test
- Sclerodermal kidney

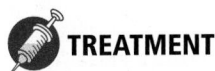

TREATMENT

INITIAL STABILIZATION

- ABCs, oxygen, IV access, telemetry
- Volume resuscitation if hypotensive/active bleeding
- Platelet transfusions may exacerbate end organ ischemia and should only be used in the setting of life-threatening hemorrhage (1, 4, 5)[B].

SPECIAL THERAPY

- In the absence of another apparent cause, the following dyad is sufficient to begin treatment for TTP while the workup proceeds (1)[B]
- Thrombocytopenia
  - MAHA emergent plasma exchange transfusion (PET) (1, 4, 5)[A]
    ○ Cornerstone of treatment of classic TTP
    ○ Thought to replace a deficient or defective metalloproteinase and remove ULvWF and anti metalloproteinase antibodies.
    ○ 1–1.5 plasma volumes/day should begin immediately and continue daily.
    ○ Continue daily until LDH, platelets, neurologic symptoms and renal function normalize (1,5)[A]
  - Fresh frozen plasma: (1, 5)[A]
    ○ Temporary measure until plasma exchange transfusion can begin

 MEDICATION (DRUGS)

First Line

- Utility of glucocorticoid therapy is still debated, with the majority of data derived from case series and clinical experience; British Guidelines recommend its use for all patients (6)[C]. In general, its use seems most beneficial in setting of exacerbation when PET is stopped, or in relapse after remission.
- Doses: Prednisone 1 mg/kg/d and taper once in remission (1, 6)[C] or methylprednisolone 1g IV per day for 3 days (6)[C]

Second Line

The following are used in refractory cases

- Rituxan (7)[C]
- Vincristine, cyclophosphamide, azathioprine
- IV immunoglobulin (IVIG)

SURGERY

Splenectomy is reserved severe, refractory cases; ambiguous results (5)[C].

 FOLLOW-UP

- No maintenance therapy. After plasma exchange is discontinued, CBC and LDH should be frequently monitored. If testing remains normal, interval testing can be lengthened (2, 4)[C].
- Estimated 10-year relapse rate is 36%, and most often occur in patients with severe deficiency of ADAMTS13 activity.
- Promptly evaluate at manifestation of any symptoms of relapse (see "Signs and Symptoms") (8).

Issues for Referral

Nephrology or hematology for plasma exchange, cardiology for presence of significant heart block, neurosurgery for intracranial hemorrhage

PROGNOSIS

- Initial LDH and platelet counts are not predictive of the patient's response to treatment.
- Final platelet count and LDH or the length or intensity of treatment does not predict relapse.
  - 30-day mortality is 10% in those who receive PET.
  - 70% respond within 14 days; 90% within 28 days

COMPLICATIONS

- Central line infections and hemorrhage
- Citrate toxicity
- Hypersensitivity reactions to frequent plasma

REFERENCES

1. George JN. Clinical practice. Thrombotic thrombocytopenic purpura. N Engl J Med. 2006;354:1927.
2. Sadler JE, et al. Recent advances in thrombotic thrombocytopenic purpura. Hematology. 2004;407–421.
3. Rose BD, George JN. Causes of thrombotic thrombocytopenic purpura-hemolytic uremic syndrome in adults. Uptodate.com.
4. Yarranton H, Machin S. An update on the pathogenesis and management of acquired thrombotic thrombocytopenic purpura. Curr Opin Neurol. 2003;16:367–373.
5. Rose BD, George JN. Diagnosis of thrombotic thrombocytopenic purpura-hemolytic uremic syndrome in adults. Uptodate.com.
6. Allford SL, Hunt BJ, Rose P, Machin SJ. Guidelines on the diagnosis and management of the thrombotic microangiopathic haemolytic anaemias. Br J Haematol. 2003;120:556.
7. Darabi K, Berg AH. Rituximab can be combined with daily plasma exchange to achieve effective B-cell depletion and clinical improvement in acute autoimmune TTP. Am J Clin Pathol. 2006;125: 592–597.
8. Ruggenenti P, Galbusera M, Cornejo RP, et al. Thrombotic thrombocytopenic purpura: Evidence that infusion rather than removal of plasma induces remission of the disease. Am J Kidney Dis. 1993;21:314.

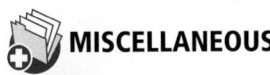 MISCELLANEOUS

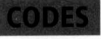 CODES

ICD9-CM

446.6 Thrombotic microangiopathy

 See Corresponding Diagnostic Algorithm

T

THYROGLOSSAL DUCT CYST

Maryellen Antonetti, MPH, PA-C, RN

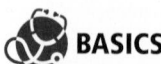 **BASICS**

DESCRIPTION
- Persistence of thyroglossal duct or remnant with fluid accumulation (cyst) following embryologic thyroid descent in the neck
- Usually midline, single, smooth, and mobile
- Reported to be the most common congenital thyroid malformation seen on ultrasound.
- System(s) Affected: Endocrine/Metabolic; Skin/Exocrine

EPIDEMIOLOGY
- Predominant age: 50% <10 years, 65% <20 years
- Predominant sex: Male = Female

RISK FACTORS
None

Genetics
Familial inheritance is rare, with dominance being the most common.

ETIOLOGY
Failure of the thyroglossal duct to obliterate after descent of the thyroid in the 6th gestational week

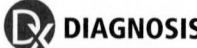 **DIAGNOSIS**

SIGNS AND SYMPTOMS
History
- Swelling
- Pain
- Redness
- Palpable neck mass

Physical Exam
- Midline neck mass
- Nontender, unless infected
- Rises in the neck with tongue protrusion and swallowing
- 80% juxtaposed to the hyoid bone
- Palpate cervical and supraclavicular nodes
- Doppler to evaluate vascularity

TESTS
Lab
Thyroid stimulating hormone

Imaging
- Ultrasound
- Thyroid scan if midline ectopic thyroid or thyroid nodule is suspected
- Small roll under shoulders allows exposure of neck in infants.

Diagnostic Procedures/Surgery
If infected, may need initial drainage before definitive resection

Pathological Findings
- Cyst lined with stratified squamous or pseudostratified ciliated columnar epithelium
- Thyroid tissue seen in 10–45% of cysts
- Reports show traces of the thyroglossal duct located near the hyoid bone, superior to thyroid isthmus or lingually.

DIFFERENTIAL DIAGNOSIS
- Ectopic midline thyroid
- Dermoid cyst
- Thyroid adenoma of isthmus or pyramidal lobe
- Lymphadenitis
- Cervical thymic cyst

 TREATMENT

Outpatient surgery under general anesthesia

GENERAL MEASURES
Diet
Unrestricted

Activity
Unrestricted

MEDICATION (DRUGS)

None. All thyroglossal duct cysts should be surgically removed.

SURGERY
- Once diagnosed, the excision can be done using the Sistrunk procedure. This requires removal of the center portion of the hyoid bone to minimize recurrence.
- If the cyst is infected, it should be initially treated (antibiotics and local heat) and/or drained. After resolution of the inflammation, excision should be performed (1,2)[C].

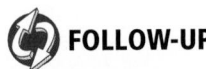 **FOLLOW-UP**

DISPOSITION
Admission Criteria
Drainage of abscess

PROGNOSIS
Resolution with resection (<5% recurrence using the Sistrunk procedure)

COMPLICATIONS
- Infection and malignant degeneration may occur if cyst is not excised.
- Reports demonstrate that the location of such masses (lingual) can cause not only various respiratory problems but also infant death.
- Wide local excision is a valuable extension of the Sistrunk operation for the management of recurrent disease (4)[A].

PATIENT MONITORING
One to 2 weeks after drainage or resection

REFERENCES

1. Ostlie DJ, et al. Thyroglossal duct infections and surgical outcomes. *J Pediatr Surg.* 2004;39:396–399.
2. Kaselas CH, et al. Thyroglossal duct cyst's inflammation. When do we operate? *Pediatr Surg Int.* 2005;21:991–993.
3. Schader I, et al. Hereditary duct cyst. *Pediatric Surg Int.* 2005;21(7):593–594.
4. Patel NN, Hartley BEJ, Howard DJ. Management of thyroglossal tract disease after failed Sistrunk's procedure. *J Laryngol Otol.* 2003;117(9):710–712.[A]

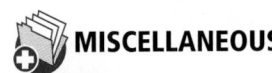 **MISCELLANEOUS**

 CODES

ICD9-CM
759.2 Congenital anomalies of other endocrine glands

PATIENT TEACHING
- Reassurance to family about absence of malignancy
- Patient may require thyroid medication for life, if ectopic, midline thyroid is mistakenly removed.

 See Corresponding Diagnostic Algorithm

T

THYROID MALIGNANT NEOPLASIA

James P. Miller, MD
Timothy L. Black, MD

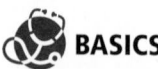 **BASICS**

DESCRIPTION

Autologous growth of thyroid nodules with potential for metastases

- Papillary carcinoma
  - Most common variety, 60–70% of thyroid tumors
  - May be associated with radiation exposure
  - Tumor contains psammoma bodies
  - Metastasizes by lymphatic route (30% at time of diagnosis)
  - Multicentric
- Follicular carcinoma
  - 10–20% of thyroid tumors
  - Incidence has been decreasing since the addition of dietary iodine.
  - Occurs usually in females >40 years of age
  - Metastasizes by the hematogenous route
- Hürthle cell carcinoma
  - Usually in patients >60 years of age
  - Radioresistant
  - Composed of distinct large eosinophilic cells with abundant cytoplasmic mitochondria
- Medullary carcinoma (MTC)
  - Arises from parafollicular cells, C-cells
  - 2–5% of all thyroid tumors
  - 25–35% are associated with multiple endocrine neoplasia syndromes, which can be familial or sporadic.
  - Calcitonin is a chemical marker.
- Anaplastic carcinoma
  - 3% of thyroid tumors
  - Usually in patients >60 years of age
- Other: Lymphoma, sarcoma, or metastatic (renal, breast, or lung)
- System(s) Affected: Endocrine/Metabolic
- Synonym(s): Follicular carcinoma of the thyroid; Papillary carcinoma of the thyroid; Hürthle cell carcinoma of the thyroid; Anaplastic cell carcinoma of the thyroid

ALERT

Geriatric Considerations
Risk of malignancy increases over age 60.

Pediatric Considerations
>60% of thyroid nodules are malignant.

GENERAL PREVENTION

- Physical exam in high-risk group
- Calcium infusion or pentagastrin stimulation test in high-risk multiple endocrine neoplasia patients

EPIDEMIOLOGY

- Predominant age: Usually > 40 years of age
- Predominant sex: Female > Male (2.6:1)

Incidence

- 10/100,000/yr in United States
- 6 deaths/1,000,000/yr in United States

RISK FACTORS

- Family history
- Neck irradiation (6–2,000 rads): Papillary carcinoma
- Iodine deficiency: Follicular carcinoma
- Multiple endocrine neoplasia syndrome: Medullary carcinoma
- Previous history of less than a total thyroidectomy for malignancy: Anaplastic carcinoma

Genetics

- Medullary: Autosomal dominant with multiple endocrine neoplasia syndrome
- BRAF mutation
- RET oncogene

ETIOLOGY

Unknown

ASSOCIATED CONDITIONS

Medullary carcinoma: Pheochromocytoma, hyperparathyroidism, ganglioneuroma of the gastrointestinal tract, neuromata of mucosal membranes

 DIAGNOSIS

SIGNS AND SYMPTOMS

History
- Change in voice
- Positive family history
- Neck mass
- Dysphagia
- Dyspnea

Physical Exam
- Neck mass, if fixed suggest advanced disease
- Cervical adenopathy

TESTS

- Medullary carcinoma: Calcitonin level (normal is <30 pg/mL [300 ng/L]), Pentagastrin stimulation test
- Thyroglobulin level (TG): Postoperative tumor marker
- DNA content of tumors from biopsy specimen; diploid content has a better prognosis

Lab
Thyroid function tests usually normal

Imaging

- Thyroid scan: Cold nodules are more suspicious of malignancy.
- Ultrasound: Solid mass is more suspicious of malignancy
- CT and MRI can be useful to evaluate large substernal masses and recurrent soft tissue masses.
- ^{18}F-FDG positron emission tomography scan can help if the cytology is inconclusive. Helpful with recurrent disease when patient has negative I^{131} scan and an elevated TG level (1)[C]

Diagnostic Procedures/Surgery

- Fine-needle aspiration
- Surgical biopsy/excision
- Laryngoscopy, if vocal cord paralysis is suspected

Pathological Findings

- Papillary: Psammoma bodies, anaplastic epithelial papillae
- Follicular: Anaplastic epithelial cords with follicles
- Hürthle cell: Large eosinophilic cells with granular cytoplasm
- Medullary: Large amounts of amyloid stroma
- Anaplastic: Small cell and giant cell undifferentiated tumors

DIFFERENTIAL DIAGNOSIS

- Multinodular goiter
- Thyroid adenoma
- Thyroglossal duct cyst
- Thyroiditis
- Thyroid cyst
- Ectopic thyroid
- Dermoid cyst

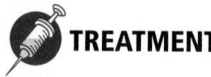 **TREATMENT**

Inpatient

GENERAL MEASURES

Diet
Avoid iodine deficiency.

Activity
As tolerated

SPECIAL THERAPY

Radiotherapy
- I^{131} thyroid remnant ablation
- External beam radiation for advanced disease

MEDICATION (DRUGS)

- Postoperatively will require thyroid replacement to suppress serum thyroid-stimulating hormone (TSH) level
  - Levothyroxine (T4, Synthroid) 100–200 μg/d *or*
  - Liothyronine (T3, Cytomel) 50–100 μg/d
- Significant possible interactions
  - Amphetamines
  - Anticoagulants
  - Tricyclic antidepressants
  - Antidiabetic medications
  - Aspirin
  - Barbiturates
  - β-Adrenergic blockers
  - Cholestyramine
  - Colestipol
  - Oral contraceptives
  - Digitalis preparation
  - Ephedrine
  - Estrogens
  - Methylphenidate
  - Phenytoin

SURGERY
- Papillary carcinoma: Lobectomy with isthmectomy (if lesion <1.5 cm) or total thyroidectomy and removal of suspicious lymph nodes
- Follicular carcinoma and Hürthle cell: Total thyroidectomy and removal of suspicious lymph nodes
- Medullary carcinoma: Total thyroidectomy with central node dissection. Unilateral or bilateral modified radical neck dissection if lateral nodes are histologically positive
- Anaplastic carcinoma: Aggressive en bloc thyroidectomy; tracheostomy often required

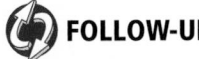 ## FOLLOW-UP

PROGNOSIS
- Papillary carcinoma: Overall mortality 3–8%
- Follicular carcinoma: Overall 80% 5-year survival rate, 77% 10-year survival rate. Histologically microinvasive tumors parallel papillary tumor results, whereas grossly invasive tumors do far worse.
- Hürthle cell carcinoma: 93% 5-year survival rate and 83% survival rate overall. Grossly invasive tumors—survival is <25%.
- Medullary carcinoma: Negative nodes 90% 5-year survival rate and 85% 10-year survival rate; with positive nodes 65% 5-year survival rate and 40% 10-year survival rate
- Anaplastic carcinoma: Survival unexpected

COMPLICATIONS
Recurrence of tumor

PATIENT MONITORING
- Thyroid scan at 6 weeks and administration of iodine-131 for any visible uptake evidence of residual thyroid tissue (after total thyroidectomy) or lymph node disease is treated with radioactive iodine
- At 6 months and then yearly, the patient should have a thyroid scan and chest radiograph.
- Papillary and follicular: A thyroglobulin level should be done yearly. rhTSH stimulated thyroglobulin level may be more sensitive. (2,3)[B]
- Medullary: Calcitonin level should be done yearly with pentagastrin stimulation.
- The thyroid scan and thyroglobulin level should be done with the patient in the hypothyroid state induced by 6-week withdrawal of levothyroxine or 2- to 3-week withdrawal of liothyronine.

REFERENCES
1. Wang W, et al. Prognostic value of [18F]-Fluorodeoxyglucose positron emission tomographic scanning in patients with thyroid cancer. *J Clin Endocrinol Metab*. 2000;85:1107–1113.
2. Blamey S, et al. Using recombinant Human TSH for the diagnosis of recurrent thyroid cancer. *ANZ Journal of Surg*. 2005;75:10–20.
3. Haugen BR, et al. A comparison of recombinant human thyrotropin and thyroid hormone withdrawal for the detection of thyroid remnant or cancer. *J Clin Endocrinol Metab*. 1999;84:3877–3885.
4. www.thyroidmanager.org/chapter18/18-nodu-cancer.htm
5. Gagel RF, Goepfert H, Callender RL. Changing concepts in the pathogenesis and management of thyroid carcinoma. *CA Cancer J Clin*. 1996;46:261–283.

 ## MISCELLANEOUS

See also: Multiple endocrine neoplasia (MEN).

CODES

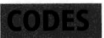 *ICD9-CM*
- 193 Malignant neoplasm of thyroid gland
- 198.89 Secondary malignant neoplasm of other specified sites, other

PATIENT TEACHING
National Cancer Institute Building 31, Room 101-18 9000 Rockville Pike, Bethesda, MD 20892; (301) 496-5583.

 See Corresponding Diagnostic Algorithm

T

THYROIDITIS

Richard P. Levy, MD

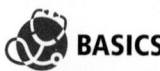 **BASICS**

DESCRIPTION

Variety of inflammatory thyroid disorders that can cause thyroid enlargement and thyroid atrophy; may lead to hypothyroidism or hyperthyroidism; complete resolution can occur (1)[B]

- Hashimoto disease
  - Most common form
  - Autoimmune disease, often presenting as asymptomatic diffuse goiter
  - Often first detected after thyroid atrophy and hypothyroidism have occurred
  - Can present as hyperthyroidism (Hashitoxicosis)
- Granulomatous thyroiditis (subacute)
  - Probably related to viral infection
  - Usually presents with thyroid pain, which may be severe
  - Involves 1 or both thyroid lobes
  - Accompanied by hyperthyroidism, followed by phase of mild hypothyroidism, then by permanent resolution to normal
- "Silent" thyroiditis
  - Characterized by lack of pain
  - One form is characterized by spontaneously resolving hypothyroidism and/or hyperthyroidism often associated with pregnancy. (2)[B]
  - Another form has characteristics of granulomatous thyroiditis without the pain.
- Rare forms
  - Suppurative: Due to bacterial infection of thyroid
  - Radiation-induced: Due to ingested radionuclides or external irradiation
  - Riedel: Dense infiltration of fibrous tissue into thyroid gland and surrounding structures; cause unknown
- Other forms
  - Lymphocytic thyroiditis
  - Postpartum onset of goiter and/or hypothyroidism that may resolve spontaneously
- System(s) Affected: Endocrine/Metabolic

ALERT

Pregnancy Considerations
- Avoid radioisotope scanning.
- Avoid hypothyroidism.
- Minimize use of antithyroid drugs. (3)[B]

EPIDEMIOLOGY
- Incidence/prevalence not known definitively
- Lymphocytic thyroiditis incidence increases with age, probably up to 10% > age 65
- Granulomatous thyroiditis is much less common and has an epidemic pattern.
- Predominant age: All ages, but predominantly postpuberty
- Predominant sex: Female > Male

RISK FACTORS
- Hashimoto disease
  - Positive family history of thyroid disease or other autoimmune disease
  - Preceding autoimmune diseases, including type I diabetes, primary adrenal insufficiency, rheumatoid arthritis, pregnancy/delivery
- Granulomatous thyroiditis
  - Recent viral respiratory infection
  - Other known cases in community

ETIOLOGY
- Hashimoto disease
  - Autoimmune response of thyroid tissue
  - Genetic susceptibility
- Granulomatous thyroiditis
  - Chronic inflammatory response of thyroid tissue
  - Preceding infection with any of a variety of viruses

ASSOCIATED CONDITIONS
Hashimoto disease: Other autoimmune diseases including
- Type I diabetes
- Primary adrenal insufficiency
- Premature ovarian failure

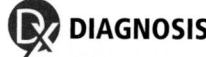 **DIAGNOSIS**

SIGNS AND SYMPTOMS
- Lymphocytic thyroiditis
  - Insidious onset of goiter, often detected incidentally
  - Slow onset of hypothyroidism
  - Association with other autoimmune diseases
- Granulomatous thyroiditis
  - Pain, tenderness, and enlargement of one or both thyroid lobes
  - Malaise, fever
  - Mild to moderate symptoms of hyperthyroidism
  - History of recent respiratory infection

TESTS
Lab
- Hashimoto disease
  - Elevated antithyroid antibodies (especially high titers of anti-thyroid peroxidase antibodies)
  - Free thyroxine index <5 (normal 4.5–12) with thyroid-stimulating (TSH) >5 μg/dL (normal 0.5 to 5 μg/dL)
  - Thyroid radioactive iodine uptake variable with scintiscan showing patchy distribution of radioiodine
  - Positive cytopathology of fine needle aspirate or positive formal biopsy
- Granulomatous thyroiditis
  - Elevated erythrocyte sedimentation rate
  - Normal or moderately elevated WBC without a granulocyte shift to band forms
  - Free thyroxine index >12, TSH undetectable, radioactive iodine uptake <5% in 24 hours (often nil) early in course
  - Free thyroxine index <4.5 with radioactive iodine uptake above normal (>35% in 24 hours in the United States) late in course
- Immunometric assays
- CBC with differential count
- Drugs that may alter lab results
  - Thyroid
  - Corticosteroids
  - Iodine-containing drugs and contrast media
  - Lithium
  - Amiodarone
- Disorders that may alter lab results
  - Iodine deficiency
  - Nonthyroidal illness

Imaging
- Thyroid radioiodine uptake and scan in granulomatous thyroiditis
- Ultrasonography if hemorrhage into thyroid cyst suspected

Diagnostic Procedures/Surgery
Needle biopsy in confusing cases

Pathological Findings
- Hashimoto disease
  - Lymphocytic infiltration
  - Oxyphilic changes in follicular cells
  - Fibrosis
  - Thyroid atrophy
- Granulomatous thyroiditis
  - Giant cells
  - Mononuclear cell infiltrate

DIFFERENTIAL DIAGNOSIS
- Hashimoto disease
  - Simple goiter
  - Iodine-deficient goiter (especially in endemic areas)
  - Early Graves disease
  - Lithium-induced goiter
- Granulomatous thyroiditis
  - Infections of oropharynx and trachea
  - Hemorrhage into a thyroid cyst
  - Subacute systemic illness
  - Suppurative thyroiditis

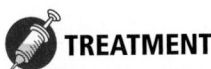 TREATMENT

GENERAL MEASURES
- Outpatient
- Analgesics for pain
- Corticosteroids for severe granulomatous thyroiditis

Diet
No special diet

Activity
Fully active

 MEDICATION (DRUGS)

First Line
- Hashimoto disease
  - If hypothyroid or goitrous: Levothyroxine (Synthroid, Levoxyl); generic may not be bioavailable; begin with 25 or 50 μg/d and titrate to TSH suppression to lower limit of assay normal range
  - If thyrotoxic and symptomatic: Propylthiouracil and propranolol
- Granulomatous thyroiditis
  - Pain: Analgesics, (e.g., codeine)
  - Symptomatic hyperthyroidism: Propranolol 40 mg q6h
  - Symptomatic hypothyroid phase: Levothyroxine 80 μg/100 lbs (45.5 kg) body weight per day
  - Severe symptoms: Prednisone once daily in lowest effective dose
- Maintenance: Optimal levothyroxine dose can be established by measuring TSH at 6- to 8-week intervals until the TSH is at a lower level of normal for the assay used
- Contraindications
  - Propylthiouracil: Allergy or hypersensitivity to analgesics/narcotics
  - Propranolol: Insulin therapy, asthma
  - Prednisone: Adverse reactions
  - Levothyroxine: None
- Precautions: Reduce doses of corticosteroids, propranolol, and narcotics as soon as feasible
- Significant possible interactions: Sucralfate (Carafate) and iron preparations may decrease levothyroxine availability

Second Line
Methimazole for propylthiouracil

 FOLLOW-UP

PROGNOSIS
- Hashimoto disease: Persistent goiter, eventual thyroid failure
- Granulomatous thyroiditis: Eventual return to normal over weeks or months; remission may be slower in elderly

COMPLICATIONS
Treatment-induced hypothyroidism or hyperthyroidism

PATIENT MONITORING
- Hashimoto disease: Repeat thyroid function tests every 3–12 months
- Granulomatous thyroiditis: Repeat thyroid function tests every 3–6 weeks until permanently euthyroid and check every 6–12 months

REFERENCES
1. Burman KD. *Thyroiditis*. Wellesley, MA: UpToDate; 2004.
2. Muller AF, Drexhage HA, Berghout A. Postpartum thyroiditis and autoimmune thyroiditis in women of childbearing age: Recent insights and consequences for antenatal and postnatal care. *Endocr Rev.* 2001;22:605–630.
3. StagnaroGreen A. Recognizing, understanding, and treating postpartum thyroiditis. *Endocrinol Metab Clin North Am.* 2000;29:417–430.

 MISCELLANEOUS

See also: Hyperthyroidism; Hypothyroidism, adult

 CODES

ICD9-CM
245.0 Acute thyroiditis

 See Corresponding Diagnostic Algorithm

T

TINEA CAPITIS

George R. Bergus, MD

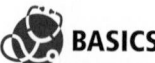 **BASICS**

DESCRIPTION

- A fungal infection of the scalp and hair; often called "ringworm"
- Infection results from contact with infected persons or animals.
- Contagious and may become epidemic
- Affected areas of the scalp can show characteristic black dots resulting from broken hairs.
- System(s) Affected: Skin/Exocrine
- Synonym(s): Scalp ringworm

GENERAL PREVENTION

- Good personal hygiene
- Don't share headwear.
- Identification and treatment of infected individuals and household pets

EPIDEMIOLOGY

- Predominant age: Children, particularly ages 3–9 years. Adult infection is rare.
- Predominant sex: Male = Female

Incidence

Although still common, incidence and prevalence have dropped markedly over the past 30 years.

ALERT

Pediatric Considerations

Highest incidence in this age group

RISK FACTORS

- Day care centers or schools
- Living in confined quarters
- Poor hygiene
- Immunosuppression

ETIOLOGY

- 90% *Trichophyton tonsurans*
- 10% *Microsporum* species (*canis, audouinii, gypseum*)

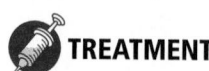 **DIAGNOSIS**

SIGNS AND SYMPTOMS

- Infection commonly begins with round patches of scale (alopecia less common).
- Frequently, infection will take on the patterns of chronic scaling with little inflammation or marked inflammation and alopecia.
- Less frequently, patients will present with multiple patches of alopecia and characteristic black-dot pattern of broken hairs.
- Extreme inflammation results in kerion (exudative pustular nodulation).

TESTS

Viewed under a Wood lamp, the 10% of infections caused by *Microsporum* species will fluoresce a light green. 90% of tinea capitis infections, those caused by *Trichophyton*, will *not* fluoresce.

Lab

- Microscopy of a Potassium hydroxide preparation of hairs from affected area can show arthrospores that appear within hair shafts.
- Fungal culture of hairs from affected areas allows the infection to be confirmed and the causative organism to be identified.

Pathological Findings

- Chronic inflammation
- Superficial infection producing lesions with follicular pustules, abscess
- Hyphae in follicles, keratin of skin

DIFFERENTIAL DIAGNOSIS

- Psoriasis and seborrhea dermatitis are most often confused with tinea capitis.
- Pyoderma
- Alopecia areata and trichotillomania
- Aphasia cutis congenita

TREATMENT

Outpatient

GENERAL MEASURES

- Careful hand washing
- Launder towels, clothing, headwear of infected individual
- Check other family members

Diet

No special diet, except persons treated with griseofulvin should not be on a restricted-fat diet.

Activity

No restrictions

MEDICATION (DRUGS)

First Line

- Griseofulvin (Fulvicin P/G, Fulvicin U/F, Gris-PEG)—(1,2A for Trichophyton and Microsporum)
  - Microsized preparation
  - Available in 125-mg, 250-mg, and 500-mg tablets and 125-mg/5-mL suspension
  - Standard dose for griseofulvin used in trials is 125 mg/d in patients weighing 10–20 kg; 250 mg/d for 20–40 kg, and 500 mg/d > 40 kg taken b.i.d. or as a single daily for 6–12 weeks
- Oral terbinafine (Lamisil)—(1A for Trichophyton) standard dosing for terbinafine is 62.5 mg/d in patients weighing 10–20 kg; 125 mg/d for 20–40 kg, and 250 mg/d > 40 kg for 2–4 weeks
- Itraconazole (Sporanox) (2A for Microsporum)
  - Matches griseofulvin in treatment and is better tolerated
  - 3–5 mg/kg/d, but most studies have used 100 mg/d for 6 weeks in children >2 years of age
- Contraindications
  - Griseofulvin is contraindicated in patients with porphyria because of increased risk of hepatotoxicity.
- Precautions
  - Griseofulvin: Headache in up to 10% of patients initially, but generally resolves after 1st week of treatment. Abdominal bloating, dyspepsia, and diarrhea also common. Hypersensitivity and liver toxicity rare. The manufacturer recommends monitoring liver functions while on griseofulvin.
  - Terbinafin: Gastrointestinal symptoms (including diarrhea, dyspepsia, and abdominal pain), liver test abnormalities, and taste disturbances. In general, the adverse events were mild and transient
  - Itraconazole: Nausea, vomiting, diarrhea, headache, dizziness, abnormal hepatic function tests, rare significant liver toxicity
- Significant possible interactions
  - Griseofulvin accentuates the effect of alcohol and increases the metabolism of warfarin and oral contraceptives.
  - Terbinafine clearance is increasedby rifampin, decreased by cimetidine.

Second Line

If kerion is present, prednisone 1 mg/kg/d can be added to antifungal therapy for 5–10 days. (3)[C]

ALERT

Pregnancy Considerations

Oral antifungals are contraindicated in pregnancy.

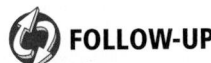 **FOLLOW-UP**

PROGNOSIS

- Without treatment, lesions will usually heal spontaneously in 6 months.
- Lesions with marked inflammation will resolve spontaneously much more rapidly but are more likely to leave scarring

COMPLICATIONS

Permanent scarring and hair loss from kerion

PATIENT MONITORING

- Recheck after 2 weeks of therapy to document improvement and after the 6-week course of therapy
- Patients might need liver function monitoring—see medication precautions

REFERENCES

1. Fuller LC, et al. A randomized comparison of 4 weeks of terbinafine vs. 8 weeks of griseofulvin for the treatment of tinea capitis. *Br J Dermatol*. 2001;144(2):321–327.
2. Gupta AK, et al. Therapeutic options for the treatment of tinea capitis caused by *Trichophyton* species: Griseofulvin versus the new oral antifungal agents, terbinafine, itraconazole, and fluconazole. *Pediatr Dermatol*. 2001;18:433–438.
3. Hussain I, et al. A randomized, comparative trial of treatment of kerion celsi with griseofulvin plus oral prednisolone vs. griseofulvin alone. *Med Mycol*. 1999;37(2):97–99.
4. Fuller LC, et al. Diagnosis and management of scalp ringworm. *BMJ*. 2003;326(7388):539–541.
5. Friedlander SF. The evolving role of itraconazole, fluconazole and terbinafine in the treatment of tinea capitis. *Pediatr Infect Dis J*. 1999;18:205–210.
6. Friedlander SF, et al. Terbinafine in the treatment of *Trichophyton tinea capitis*. *Pediatrics*. 2002;109:602–607.
7. Temple ME. Pharmacotherapy of tinea capitis. *J Amer Board Fam Pract*. 1999;12:236–242.

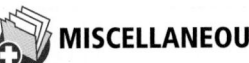 **MISCELLANEOUS**

See also: Alopecia; Tinea corporis

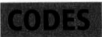 **CODES**

ICD9-CM

110.0 Dermatophytosis of scalp and beard

PATIENT TEACHING

- KidsHealth at the American Medical Association: www.ama-assn.org/insight/h´focus/nemours/infectio/childhd/fungi.htm
- Information from your family doctor: http://familydoctor.org/handouts/316.html

 See Corresponding Diagnostic Algorithm

 See Patient Handout on CD

T

TINEA CORPORIS

Elizabeth L. Backer, MD

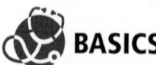 BASICS

DESCRIPTION
- Scaling, pruritic plaques characterized by a sharply defined annular pattern with peripheral activity and central clearing
- Ringlike shaped lesions (hence called *ringworm*)
- Papules and occasionally pustules/vesicles present at border, and less commonly in center
- Affects face, trunk, and extremities
- Zoophilic infections are acquired from animals.
- Anthropophilic infections are acquired from personal contact (e.g., wrestling) (1)[C] or fomites.
- System(s) Affected: Skin/Exocrine
- Synonym(s): Ringworm; Tinea circinata

GENERAL PREVENTION
- Avoid contact with suspicious lesions
- Some evidence for using fluconazole or itraconazole in suppressive doses in wrestlers to prevent outbreaks during competitive season (2)[C].]

EPIDEMIOLOGY
- Predominant age: All ages
- Predominant sex: Male = Female

Incidence
Fairly common

RISK FACTORS
- Warm climates
- Direct contact with an active lesion on a human, an animal, or rarely from soil
- Working with animals
- Immunosuppression (such as in diabetes and HIV, or with prolonged use of topical steroids)

Genetics
Evidence suggests a genetic susceptibility in some people.

ETIOLOGY
- Fungal infection due to dermatophyte (e.g., *Trichophyton rubrum* [most common])
- *Microsporum canis* often results in multiple lesions.

ASSOCIATED CONDITIONS
Other tinea infections such as tinea pedis, cruris, capitis, barbae, and manus

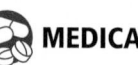 DIAGNOSIS

SIGNS AND SYMPTOMS
- Characteristic rash and pruritus
- Scaling plaques that are circular/ovale, bright red, sharply marginated, occurring singly or in groups of 3–4 (lesions may run together)
- Each plaque is <5 cm in diameter.
- Plaques are solid, but annular forms occur.
- Occasional hyperpigmentation

TESTS
- Tinea corporis does not fluoresce under Wood's lamp.
- Culture on Sabouraud's medium: Sample by scraping or vigorous rubbing of a cotton swab on the lesion, then rolling/rubbing it on the medium.

Lab
- Potassium hydroxide preparation of skin scrapings
- Fungal culture may be obtained, but not generally necessary

Diagnostic Procedures/Surgery
Skin scraping
- Use No. 15 blade and place several small scrapings of the active border on glass slide with coverslip.
- Apply 10–20% potassium hydroxide and heat gently without boiling.
- Let stand for 5 minutes and examine for septate, branching hyphae
  - Use lowered condenser and dim light to enhance contrast.
  - Hyphae may be accentuated with a commercial fungal stain or a drop of blue ink.

Pathological Findings
Branching hyphae with septa on potassium hydroxide preparation

DIFFERENTIAL DIAGNOSIS
- Pityriasis rosea
- Eczema (nummular)
- Contact dermatitis
- Syphilis
- Psoriasis
- Subacute lupus erythematosus
- Erythema annulare
- Erythema multiforme
- Erythema migrans

TREATMENT

INITIAL STABILIZATION
Outpatient

GENERAL MEASURES
Proper hygiene

Diet
Unrestricted diet

Activity
Avoid contact sports (e.g., wrestling) temporarily while starting treatment.

MEDICATION (DRUGS)

- Topical antifungal creams: (3, 4)[C]
  - Miconazole (Monistat-Derm) or clotrimazole (Lotrimin, Mycelex) applied b.i.d. for 2 weeks. Also ketoconazole (Nizoral) applied daily for 2 weeks.
  - To prevent relapse, use for 1 week after resolution.
  - Also econazole (Spectazole) and allylamines, such as naftifine (Naftin, Lamisil)
  - For added benefit, wash with antifungal shampoo ketoconazole (Nizoral shampoo) prior to use of cream.
- For resistant, extensive, and/or invasive infections, or in immunocompromised patients, oral agents are recommended
  - Oral ultramicrosize griseofulvin (e.g., Gris-PEG) 7 mg/kg/d in children >2 years of age; 375 mg/d in adults for 4 weeks
  - Oral itraconazole, in lieu of ketoconazole: Less toxic and fewer drug side effects. Although not indicated, itraconazole (Sporanox) is effective at 200 mg/d for 7–14 days.
- Terbinafine(Lamisil) 250 mg/d for 1–2 weeks
- Fluconazole (Diflucan) 150–300 mg (1 dose weekly for 2–4 weeks)
- Contraindications: Known hypersensitivity to agent
- Precautions: Terbinafine—gastrointestinal side effects; rare hepatotoxicity and hematologic changes
- Griseofulvin induces hepatic enzymes that metabolize warfarin and other drugs.

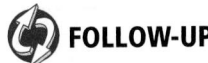 **FOLLOW-UP**

PROGNOSIS
Resolution without sequelae in 1–2 weeks of therapy

COMPLICATIONS
- Bacterial superinfection
- Generalized, invasive dermatophyte infection

PATIENT MONITORING
Necessary for invasive disease or prolonged treatment with oral ketoconazole

REFERENCES

1. Adams BB, et al. Tinea corporis gladiatorum. *J Am Acad Dermatol* 2002;47:286.
2. Kohl TD, Martin DC, Nemeth R, et al. Fluconazole for the prevention and treatment of tinea gladiatorum. *Pediatr Infect Dis J* 2000;19(8):717–722.
3. Bonifaz A, et al. Comparative study between terbinafine 1% emulsion-gel versus ketoconazole 2% cream in tinea cruris and tinea corporis. *Eur J Dermatol* 2000;10:107.
4. Kohl TD, et al. Comparison of topical and oral treatments for tinea gladiatorum. *Clin J Sport Med* 1999;9:161.
5. www.uptodate.com

 MISCELLANEOUS

See also: Tinea capitis, Tinea cruris, Tinea pedis

CODES

ICD9-CM
110.5 Dermatophytosis of the body

PATIENT TEACHING
- Avoid contact with suspected lesions.
- Be careful with animal contacts.
- Wrestlers may need to temporarily withdraw from competition (10–15 day restriction from participation may be reasonable).

 See Patient Handout on CD

TINEA CRURIS

Elizabeth L. Backer, MD

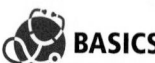 **BASICS**

DESCRIPTION

- Superficial fungal infection of groin area
- Most common cause in North America: *Trichophyton rubrum* (rare cases caused by *Epidermophyton floccosum* and *Trichophyton mentagrophytes*)
- Characterized by development of well-marginated, erythematous, half-moon–shaped plaques in crural folds that spread to upper thighs
- Advancing border is well defined, often with fine scaling and sometimes vesicular eruptions.
- Lesions are usually bilateral and do not include scrotum or penis (unlike *Candida* infections), but may migrate to perineum, perianal area, gluteal cleft, and onto buttocks in chronic/progressive cases
- System(s) Affected: Skin/Exocrine
- Synonym(s): Jock itch; Ringworm

GENERAL PREVENTION
Avoidance of risk factors

EPIDEMIOLOGY
- Predominant age: Any age, but rare in children
- Predominant sex: Male > Female

Incidence
Common

ALERT
Pediatric Considerations
Rare prior to puberty

Geriatric Considerations
More common in geriatric population, due to increase in risk factors

Pregnancy Considerations
Rare in pregnancy

RISK FACTORS
- Summer months and/or increased sweating
- Wearing wet clothing
- Wearing multiple layers of clothing
- Depression of cell-mediated immune response (e.g., individuals with atopy or AIDS)
- Obesity

ETIOLOGY
- Source of infection usually the patient's own tinea pedis.
- Most common causative dermatophyte is *Trichophyton rubrum*
- Rare cases caused by *Epidermophyton floccosum* and *Trichophyton mentagrophytes*

ASSOCIATED CONDITIONS
Tinea pedis

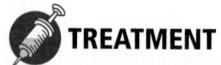 **DIAGNOSIS**

SIGNS AND SYMPTOMS
- Lesions may be asymptomatic, but more frequently are quite pruritic.
- Acute inflammation may result from wearing occlusive clothing.
- Chronic scratching may result in an eczematous appearance.
- Previous application of topical steroids may alter appearance, causing a more extensive eruption with irregular borders and erythematous papules. This modified form is called *tinea incognito* (1)[C].

TESTS
Wood's lamp exam reveals no fluorescence.

Lab
- Fungal culture using Sabouraud's dextrose agar or dermatophyte test medium
- Potassium hydroxide preparation of skin scrapings from dermatophyte leading border shows translucent, branching, rod-shaped hyphae

Pathological Findings
Skin biopsy showing fungal hyphae in epidermis

DIFFERENTIAL DIAGNOSIS
- Intertrigo: Inflammatory process of moist opposed skin folds, often including infection with bacteria, yeast, and fungi. Painful longitudinal fissures occur in creases of skin folds.
- Erythrasma: Diffuse brown, scaly, noninflammatory plaque with irregular borders, often involving groin. Caused by bacterial infection with *Corynebacterium minutissimum*. Fluoresces coral-red with Wood's lamp.
- Seborrheic dermatitis of groin
- Psoriasis of groin
- Candidiasis of groin
- Acanthosis nigricans

TREATMENT

INITIAL STABILIZATION
Outpatient

GENERAL MEASURES
- Avoid predisposing conditions such as hot baths and tight-fitting clothing (boxer shorts better than briefs) (2)[C].
- Keep area as dry as possible (talcum/powders may be beneficial) (2)[C].
- Topical steroid preparations should not be used (see "Tinea incognito") (1)[C].

Diet
No restrictions

Activity
Full activity

MEDICATION (DRUGS)

First Line
Topical azole antifungal compounds (3)[C]:

- Econazole (Spectazole), ketoconazole (Nizoral), usually applied b.i.d. for 2–3 weeks
- Terbinafine (Lamisil) is an OTC compound; can be applied once daily or b.i.d. for 1–2 weeks
- Butenafine (Mentax): Applied once daily for 2 weeks; also very effective

Second Line
- Oral antifungal agents are effective, but not indicated in uncomplicated tinea cruris. If topical therapy fails, consult a dermatologist for possible oral therapy. Griseofulvin can be given 500 mg/d PO for 1–2 weeks.
- The following oral regimens have been reported in medical literature as being effective, but currently are not specifically approved by the FDA for tinea cruris
  - Oral terbinafine (Lamisil) 250 mg/d for 1 week
  - Oral itraconazole (Sporanox) 100 mg b.i.d. once and repeated 1 week later
  - Oral fluconazole (Diflucan) 150 mg once per week for 4 weeks
- Topical terbinafine 1% solution has recently been studied and appears effective as a once-daily application for 1 week.
- Contraindications: Oral itraconazole (Sporanox) is contraindicated with astemizole (Hismanal), triazolam (Halcion), lovastatin (Mevacor), simvastatin (Zocor). But pravastatin (Pravachol) can be given with itraconazole. These compounds should not be given during pregnancy.

 FOLLOW-UP

PROGNOSIS
Excellent prognosis for cure with therapy

COMPLICATIONS
Secondary bacterial infection

PATIENT MONITORING
Liver function testing prior to therapy and at regular intervals during course of therapy for patients requiring oral terbinafine, fluconazole, itraconazole, and griseofulvin

REFERENCES

1. Smith ES, et al. Nondermatologists are more likely to prescribe antifungal/corticosteroid products. *J Am Acad Dermatol*. 1998;39:43.
2. Akinwale SO. Personal hygiene as an alternative to griseofulvin in the treatment of tinea cruris. *Afr J Med Sci*. 2000;29:41.
3. Bonifaz A, et al. Comparative study between terbinafine 1% emulsion-gel versus ketoconazole 2% cream in tinea cruris and corporis. *Eur J Derm*. 2000;10:107.
4. www.uptodate.com

 MISCELLANEOUS

See also: Acanthosis nigricans

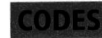 **CODES**

ICD9-CM
110.3 Dermatophytosis of groin and perianal area

PATIENT TEACHING
Explain the causative agents, predisposing factors, and prevention measures.

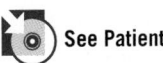 **See Patient Handout on CD**

T

TINEA PEDIS

Elizabeth L. Backer, MD

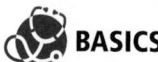 **BASICS**

DESCRIPTION
- Superficial infection of feet caused by dermatophytes. Most common dermatophyte infection encountered in clinical practice.
- 2 clinical forms: Acute and chronic
- System(s) Affected: Skin/Exocrine
- Synonym(s): Athlete's foot

GENERAL PREVENTION
- Good personal hygiene
- Wearing rubber or wooden sandals in community showers or bathing places
- Careful drying between toes after showering or bathing. (Blow drying feet with hair dryer may be more effective than drying with towel.)
- Changing socks and shoes frequently
- Applying drying or dusting powder
- Applying topical antiperspirants
- Putting on socks before underwear, to prevent infection from spreading to groin

EPIDEMIOLOGY
- Predominant age: 20–50 years, although can occur at any age
- Predominant sex: Male > Female

Prevalence
~4% of population

ALERT
Pediatric Considerations
Rare in younger children; common in teens

Geriatric Considerations
Elderly are more susceptible to outbreaks because of immunocompromise and impaired perfusion of distal extremities.

RISK FACTORS
- Hot, humid weather
- Occlusive/tight-fitting footwear
- Immunosuppressed patients
- Prolonged application of topical steroids

Genetics
No known genetic pattern

ETIOLOGY
- *Trichophyton mentagrophytes* (acute)
- *Trichophyton rubrum* (chronic)
- *Trichophyton tonsurans*
- *Epidermophyton floccosum*

ASSOCIATED CONDITIONS
- Hyperhidrosis
- Onychomycosis
- Tinea manum/cruris/corporis

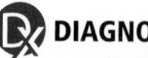 **DIAGNOSIS**

SIGNS AND SYMPTOMS
- Acute form: Self-limited, intermittent, recurrent vesicular/bullous lesions between toes or on soles
- Chronic form: Most common; slowly progressive pruritic erythematous lesions between toes; interdigital fissures opaque white scales with extension onto soles, sides/dorsum of feet (moccasin distribution)
- Other features: Strong odor, hyperkeratosis, maceration, ulceration
- May be associated with onychomycosis and other tinea infections.

TESTS
Wood's lamp exam will not fluoresce unless complicated by another fungus, which is very uncommon; M. furfur (yellow to white), coryne bacterium (red), or Microsporum (blue green).

Lab
- Direct microscopic examination (potassium hydroxide)
- Culture (Sabouraud's medium)

Pathological Findings
- Potassium hydroxide preparation: Septate and branched mycelia
- Culture: Dermatophyte

DIFFERENTIAL DIAGNOSIS
- Interdigital type: Erythrasma, impetigo, pitted keratolysis, candida intertrigo
- Moccasin type: Psoriasis vulgaris, eczematous dermatitis, pitted keratolysis
- Inflammatory/bullous type: Impetigo, allergic contact dermatitis, dyshidrotic eczema, bullous disease

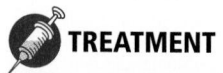 **TREATMENT**

INITIAL STABILIZATION
Outpatient

GENERAL MEASURES
- Treatment is generally with topical antifungal medications for up to 4 weeks (1)[A].
- Soak with aluminum chloride 30% or aluminum subacetate for 20 minutes b.i.d.
- Careful removal of dead/thickened skin after soaking or bathing
- Chronic or extensive disease or nail involvement requires oral antifungal medication, systemic therapy.

Diet
No restrictions

Activity
Avoid sweating feet

MEDICATION (DRUGS)

First Line
- Acute treatment
  - Aluminum acetate soak (Burow's solution; Domeboro, 1 pack to 1 quart warm water)
  - Antifungal cream of choice b.i.d. after soaks.
- Chronic treatment
  - Antifungal cream b.i.d. (1)[A]
  - May try systemic antifungal therapy (consider if concomitant onychomycosis or after failed topical treatment)
- Systemic antifungals (2)[A]
  - Itraconazole (Sporanox) 200 mg PO b.i.d. for 14 days (cure rate >90%)
  - Terbinafine (Lamisil) 250 mg PO daily for 14 days
- If concomitant onychomycosis
  - Itraconazole 200 mg PO b.i.d. for 1st week of month for 3 months. Monitoring liver function testing is recommended.
  - Terbinafine 250 mg PO daily for 12 weeks, or pulse dosing: 500 mg PO daily for 1st week of month for 3 months. Not recommended if creatinine clearance <50 mL/min.
- Contraindications: Itraconazole, pregnancy category C
- Precautions: All systemic antifungal drugs may have potential hepatotoxicity.
- Significant possible interactions: Itraconazole requires gastric acid for absorption; effectiveness is reduced with antacids, H_2 blockers, proton pump inhibitors, etc. Take with acidic beverage such as soda if on antacids.

Second Line
- Systemic antifungals
  - Fluconazole 150 mg, 1 tablet every week for 1–4 weeks. (Noted in 1997 Sanford Guide: 70% cure; however, not an FDA-approved indication)
  - Griseofulvin 660–750 mg/d for 21 days
- Contraindications: Griseofulvin
  - Patients with porphyria, hepatocellular failure
  - Patients with history of hypersensitivity to griseofulvin
- Precautions: Griseofulvin
  - Should be used only in severe cases
  - Periodic monitoring of organ-system functioning, including renal, hepatic, and hematopoietic
  - Possible photosensitivity reactions
  - Lupus erythematosus, lupuslike syndromes, or exacerbation of existing lupus erythematosus have been reported.
- Significant possible interactions: Griseofulvin
  - Decreases activity of warfarin-type anticoagulants
  - Barbiturates usually depress griseofulvin activity.
  - May potentiate effect of alcohol, producing such effects as tachycardia and flush.

 ## FOLLOW-UP

PROGNOSIS
- Control, but not complete cure.
- Infections tend to be chronic with exacerbations (e.g., in hot weather).

COMPLICATIONS
- Secondary bacterial infections (portal of entry for streptococcal infections, producing lymphangitis/cellulitis)
- Eczematoid changes

PATIENT MONITORING
As needed

REFERENCES

1. Crawford F, et al. Athlete's foot and fungally infected toe nails. *Clin Evid.* 2000;4:939.
2. Bell-Syer SE, et al. Oral treatments for fungal infections of the skin of the foot. *Cochrane Database Syst Rev.* 2002;CD003584.
3. www. uptodate.com.

 ## MISCELLANEOUS

See also: Dermatitis, Contact, Dyshidrosis

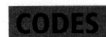 ## CODES

ICD9-CM
110.4 Dermatophytosis of foot

PATIENT TEACHING

See "General Prevention"

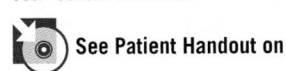 See Patient Handout on CD

TINEA VERSICOLOR

Elisabeth L. Backer, MD

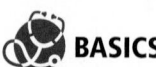 ## BASICS

DESCRIPTION
- Common superficial mycosis with variety/changing shades of colors. Macules usually hypopigmented, light brown or salmon colored. Fine scale often apparent.
- System(s) Affected: Skin/Exocrine
- Synonym(s): Pityriasis versicolor

EPIDEMIOLOGY
- Predominant age: Teenagers and young adults
- Predominant sex: Male = Female

Prevalence
Common

ALERT

Pregnancy Considerations
Usually occurs after puberty (except in tropical areas). Facial lesions are more common in children.

Geriatric Considerations
Not common in geriatric population

RISK FACTORS
- Hot, humid weather
- Use of oils
- Hyperhydrosis
- HIV infection/immunosuppression (1)[C]
- High cortisol levels (Cushings, prolonged steroid administration)
- Pregnancy
- Malnutrition
- Oral contarceptives

Genetics
No known genetic pattern

ETIOLOGY
- Saprophytic yeast: Pityrosporum orbiculare (also known as Pityropsporum ovale, Malassezia furfur or Malassezia ovalis)
- Variations in skin lipid formation

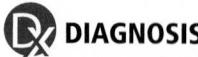 ## DIAGNOSIS

SIGNS AND SYMPTOMS
- Color
  - Sun-exposed areas: Lesions usually white
  - Covered areas: Lesions often brown or red-brown
- Distribution (sebum-rich areas): Chest, shoulders, back (also face and intertriginous areas)
- Appearance: Small individual lesions that frequently coalesce
- Scale: Fine, more visible with scraping
- Pruritus (mild)
- More prominent in summer
- Periodic recurrence

TESTS
Wood's lamp: Golden fluorescence or pigment changes

Lab
- Direct microscopy of scales with 10% potassium hydroxide preparation to visualize hyphae and spores
- Routine lab not usually necessary

Pathological Findings
- Short, stubby, or Y-shaped hyphae
- Small, round spores in clusters on hyphae

DIFFERENTIAL DIAGNOSIS
Other skin diseases with discolored macules and plaques, including
- Pityriasis alba/rosea
- Vitiligo
- Seborrheic dermatitis
- Nummular eczema
- Secondary syphilis

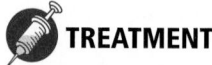 ## TREATMENT

GENERAL MEASURES
- Outpatient
- Apply prescribed topical medications to affected parts with cotton balls.
- Repeat treatment each spring prior to sun exposure.

Diet
No special diet

Activity
No restrictions

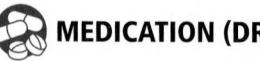 ## MEDICATION (DRUGS)

First Line
- Ketoconazole 2% shampoo applied to damp skin and left on for 5 minutes for 1–3 days *or*
- Selenium sulfide shampoo 2.5% (Selsun)
  - Allowed to dry for 10 minutes prior to showering: Daily for 1 week *or*
  - Allowed to remain on body for 12–24 hours prior to showering: Once a week for 4 weeks *or*
- Clotrimazole topical (Lotrimin) b.i.d. for 2–4 weeks, *or*
- Miconazole (Micatin, Monistat) b.i.d. for 2–4 weeks, *or*
- Ketoconazole 2% (Nizoral) cream b.i.d. for 2–4 weeks, *or*
- Terbinafine (Lamisil) 1% solution b.i.d. for 1 week *or*
- Terbinafine (Lamisil DermGel) once daily for 1 week
- Cure rates of topical anti-yeast preparations typically 70–80%. (2,3)[C] Healing continues post active treatment. Resumption of even pigmentation may take months.
- Contraindications: Ketoconazole contraindicated in pregnancy

Second Line
- Use for extensive disease or non-responders
- Ketoconazole (rarely needed and has significant adverse reactions) 400 mg in single dose or 200 mg/d for 1 week. Cure rate >90% (4)[C]
- Itraconazole 200 mg/d for 1 week. Cure rate >90% (5)[C]
- Ketoconazole shampoo can be used weekly for maintenance.
- Sulfur-salicylic acid (Sebulex) soap or shampoo can be used chronically for prophylaxis.

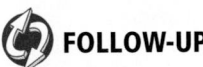 **FOLLOW-UP**

PROGNOSIS
- Duration of lesions months/years
- Recurs almost routinely

COMPLICATIONS
None expected

PATIENT MONITORING
- Recheck and treat again each spring prior to tanning season.
- Avoid skin oils.
- Suntanning accentuates lesions.

REFERENCES

1. Gulec AT, et al. Superficial fungal infections in 102 renal transplant recipients. *J Am Acad Dermatol*. 2003;49:187.
2. Lange DS, et al. Ketoconazole 2% shampoo in the treatment of tinea versicolor. *J Am Acad Dermatol*. 1998;39:944.
3. del Pacio et al. Randomized comparative trial of itraconazole and selenium shampoo for the treatment of P. versicolor. *Rev Infect Dis*. 1987;9(Suppl 1):S121.
4. Goodless, DR, et al. Ketoconazole in the treatment of Pityriasis Versicolor: International review of clinical trials. *DICP*. 1991;25:395.
5. Kose, O, et al. Comparison of single 400 mg dose versus a 7 day 200 mg daily dose of itraconazole in the treatment of tinea versicolor. *J Derm Treat*. 2002;13:77.
6. Habif TP. Clinical Dermatology, *Third edition*. 1996.
7. Faergemann J. Pityriasis versicolor. *Semin Dermatol*. 1993;12:276.
8. Drake LA, et al., and the Guidelines/Outcomes Committee of the American Academy of Dermatology. Guidelines of care for superficial mycotic infections of the skin: Pityriasis (tinea) versicolor. *J Amer Acad Dermatol*. 1996; 34(2 pt 1):287–289.
9. Lynch PJ. *Dermatology for the House Officer*. 3rd ed. Baltimore, MD: Williams & Wilkins; 1994.
10. Savin R. Diagnosis and treatment of tinea versicolor. *J Fam Pract*. 1996;43:127.

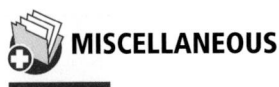 **MISCELLANEOUS**

ICD9-CM
111.0 Pityriasis versicolor

PATIENT TEACHING
- Warn patients that whiteness will remain for several months after treatment.
- For patient education materials favorably reviewed on this topic, contact: American Academy of Dermatology, 930 N. Meacham Rd., P.O. Box 4014, Schaumberg, IL 60168-4014; (708) 330-0230

See Patient Handout on CD

T

TINNITUS

David M. Holmes, MD

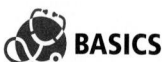 **BASICS**

DESCRIPTION

Tinnitus is derived from the Latin word tinnire meaning "to ring." Tinnitus is the perception of sound in the absence of an acoustic stimulus. The sound may be of a buzzing, ringing, roaring, chirping, whistling or hissing quality.

- Subjective tinnitus can be heard only by the patient.
- Objective tinnitus can be heard through a stethoscope placed on the head and neck near the patient's ear.
- Tinnitus >6 months is chronic.

GENERAL PREVENTION

- Avoid prolonged exposure to loud noises.
- Wear hearing protection when loud noises can't be avoided, such as when using a lawn mower, power tools, guns, and machinery.
- Avoid overuse of ototoxic medications.

EPIDEMIOLOGY

- Predominant age: 40–70 years old (prevalence increases with age)
- Predominant sex: Males > Females (due to males traditionally having greater noise exposure in military, occupational, and recreational activities). 27% of males and 15% of females ≥45 yrs experience tinnitus.

Incidence

About 50 million people in United States have tinnitus. About 12 million people seek medical attention.

Prevalence

- Affects up to 17% of general population in the United States
- 25% of people with chronic tinnitus consider it to be a significant problem.
- 4% of people with tinnitus experience impairment in their day-to-day functional abilities.

RISK FACTORS

- Advanced age
- Renal impairment
- Hepatic impairment
- Pregnancy
- Hearing loss
- Excessive noise exposure
- Use of ototoxic medications

Genetics

There appears to be a genetic predisposition, but a tinnitus gene has not yet been discovered. Genes have been identified for temporal mandibular joint (TMJ) dysfunction, Ménière's Disease, acoustic neuroma and a few rare causes of hearing loss.

PATHOPHYSIOLOGY

- Moderate sounds cause tiny movements of the stereocilia, which are attached to hair cells in the cochlea. This triggers neuronal transmission in the 8th cranial nerve. Loud sounds (≥85 decibels) cause stereocilia to bend more than they should. Hair cells that respond to higher-frequency sounds are located at the base of the cochlea and are the first to be damaged. This causes high-pitched ringing. If loud noise exposure is excessive, then stereocilia cannot recover and permanent damage occurs. This results in hearing loss and possibly tinnitus.
- Other causes of hearing loss or damage to the auditory system can also cause tinnitus.

ETIOLOGY

- Subjective Tinnitus
  - "My AAAA NOISE PAIN"
    - **M**edications and heavy **M**etals that cause or exacerbate tinnitus: Aspirin, aminoglycosides, benzodiazepines, calcium channel blockers, chloroquine, cisplatin, erythromycin, fluoroquinolones, lead, lidocaine, loop diuretics, mercury, methotrexate, NSAIDs, proton pump inhibitors, quinine, sertraline, tetracycline, tricyclic antidepressants (TCAs), valproate, vancomycin
    - **M**eniere disease (estimated 1% prevalence in the United States) or other forms of endolymphatic hydrops (abnormally high inner ear pressure)
    - **A**coustic trauma (one-time exposure to very loud noise)
    - **A**ging-related hearing loss (presbycusis)
    - **A**nemia
    - **A**rterial problems (high blood pressure [HTN], arteriosclerosis, cerebral aneurysm, cerebrovascular accident [CVA])
    - **N**oise-induced hearing loss
    - **O**tosclerosis and **O**steogenesis Imperfecta
    - **I**nfections (otitis media/externa, meningitis, lyme disease, neurosyphillis, rubella) and **I**mpaction (cerumen)
    - **S**clerosis (multiple sclerosis)
    - **E**ndocrine (diabetes mellitus, hypothyroid, hyperthyroid)
    - **P**sychogenic (depression, anxiety, fibromyalgia, psychosis)
    - **A**utoimmune disease of inner ear
    - **I**njury (head and neck) and **I**diopathic
    - **N**eoplasms (acoustic neuroma or cholesteatoma)
- Objective Tinnitus (< 1% of all cases of tinnitus) "CAGED PETS"
  - Vascular abnormalities
    - **C**arotid stenosis
    - **A**-V shunt/fistula (congenital and acquired)
    - **G**lomus jugulare
    - **E**xisting stapedial artery
    - **D**ehiscent jugular bulb or a vascular loop
  - Mechanical abnormalities
    - **P**alatal myoclonus
    - **E**ustachian tube is abnormally patent
    - **T**emporo-mandibular joint disorder
    - **S**tapedial muscle spasticity

ASSOCIATED CONDITIONS

- Hearing loss (approx. 90% of chronic tinnitus is associated with sensorineural hearing loss) (5)
  - Causes of sensorineural hearing loss: Loud noise, presbycusis, ototoxic medications, Meniere disease, acoustic neuroma
  - Causes of conductive hearing loss: Cerumen, ear infection/effusion, trauma, tumor
- TMJ dysfunction
- Depression, anxiety, insomnia, fibromyalgia

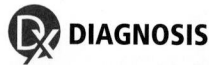 **DIAGNOSIS**

SIGNS AND SYMPTOMS

- Onset and duration: Gradual (presbycusis), sudden (recent loud noise exposure)
- Location: Unilateral (cerumen impaction, otitis media), unilateral plus hearing loss (acoustic neuroma, CVA)
- Pattern: Continuous (hearing loss), episodic (Meniere disease), pulsatile (vascular)
- Pitch: Low-pitch, rumbling (Meniere disease), high-pitched (sensorineural hearing loss)
- Severity: Use 1–10 scale (10 = most severe), Visual Analog Scale, Tinnitus Severity Index, or Tinnitus Handicap Inventory
- Excerbated by fatigue, stress, noise exposure, medications
- Alleviated by lying down with head in dependent position (patent eustachian tube), medications, masking sounds (e.g., water running)

Other Associated Signs and Symptoms

- Hearing loss
- Sudden hearing loss in one ear that progresses to the other ear (autoimmune)
- Ear pain
- Sinus congestion, allergies
- Vertigo (Meniere disease)
- Vestibular disturbances
- Facial muscle paralysis (cholesteatoma)
- High blood pressure
- Symptoms of hyper or hypo-thryoidism
- Symptoms of hyperglycemia
- Symptoms of depression or anxiety
- Insomnia
- Difficulty concentrating
- Suicidal thoughts

History

- Noise exposure >85 dB (normal traffic = 85 dB)
- Upper respiratory infection, ear infection
- Otalgia
- Otorrhea
- Head trauma
- Surgery
- Family history of hearing loss or tinnitus
- Hearing history: Type of hearing loss (congenital, sensorineural, conductive, or mixed)
- Medical history: Hypo/hyperthyroidism, HTN, diabetes mellitus, arteriosclerosis, autoimmune disorders
- Medications
- Exposure to heavy metals (lead or mercury)
- Psychosocial history: Employment, recreational activities, insomnia, anxiety, depression, obsessive compulsive disorder, psychosis, fibromyalgia

Physical Exam

- Otoscopy: Otitis media/externa, cerumen
- Auscultation close to ear for objective tinnitus
- Auscultation of blood vessels in the neck (bruits, venous hum)
- Tinnitus of venous origin is suppressed by compression of ipsilateral jugular vein
- Examine temporal mandibular joint
- Air and bone conduction testing with 512 or 1024 Hz tuning fork (Weber and Rinne tests)

- Neurological exam: Romberg test, Dix-Hallpike maneuver (if patient has vertigo), gait testing, cranial nerves
- Test hearing
- Refer to audiologist for complete evaluation.

TESTS
- Audiometry
- Tympanometry
- Auditory Brainstem Response (to diagnose retrocochlear pathology such as acoustic neuroma)
- Electrocochleography (to diagnose endolymptic hydrops)
- Electronystagmography (to diagnose vestibular disorders)

Lab
- Western blot immunoassay for HIV, renal failure, anaphylaxis, double strand DNA
- Thyroid-stimulating hormone, free T4
- Glucose
- Lipid profile
- CBC

Imaging
- Gadolinium-enhanced MRI (if tinnitus is continuous)
- Contrast-enhanced CT or MRI (if tinnitus is pulsatile)
- Sonography, angiography, or MRA (to asses vascular abnormalities in the neck)
- SPECT may be more sensitive than CT, MRI or magnetic resonance angiography and it identifies dynamic changes within the brain at the neurotransmitter level

DIFFERENTIAL DIAGNOSIS
Auditory hallucinations

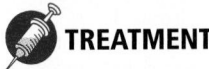 TREATMENT

GENERAL MEASURES
- Teat the underlying cause
- Discharge and continue ototoxic medications, if possible
- Use a combination of measures. (5)[B]
- Management depends on tinnitus severity and how it affects the patient's quality of life.
- Anxiety, insomnia, and depression may exacerbate tinnitus, which may in turn exacerbate the anxiety, insomnia, and/or depression. Treat these conditions to stop this vicious cycle. (5)[B]
- Hearing aids/cochlear implants (7)[C]
- Hearing protection for loud noise exposure (5)[A]
- Refer patients to a comprehensive tinnitus management program (audiologist) (5)[B]

Diet
Normal

SPECIAL THERAPY
- Tinnitus retraining therapy and masking: Counseling and wearable low-level, broad-band noise generators. It may require 1–2 yrs of therapy. Significant improvement has been reported in up to 80% of patients with high-pitched tinnitus. (7) However, clinical evidence concluded masking devices have unknown effectiveness. (6)
- Acoustic therapy: Listening to relaxing music or other sounds through head phones when the environment is too quiet. (5)[B]
- Biofeedback and stress reduction: Relaxation technique that helps people manage stress by changing the body's reaction to it. This in turn helps reduce the severity of the tinnitus. (7)[B]
- Psychotherapy: May reduce severity (5)[B]

Complementary and Alternative Therapies
- Acupuncture (unknown effectiveness) (6)
- Hypnosis (unknown effectiveness) (6)
- Low-power laser to mastoid bone (unknown effectiveness) (6)
- Ginko biloba, melatonin, lecithin, (all are ineffective) (6)

 MEDICATION (DRUGS)

First Line (Likely to be effective)
- TCAs such as Amitriptyline (50 mg qhs X 1 wk followed by 100 mg at bedtime) (3,6)[A]
- Antiepileptics
- Baclofen
- Benzodiazepines
- Cinnarizine
- Hyperbaric oxygen
- Nicotinamide
- Zinc

SURGERY
- Otosclerosis: Stapedectomy surgery with implantation of ossicular prostheses (5)[C]
- Severe Meniere disease or other forms of endolymphatic hydrops that are not alleviated with medications: Installation of endolyphatic shunt, labyrinthectomy, or vetibular neurectomy (5)[C]
- Auditory neoplasms: Surgical resection or radiation (5)[C]

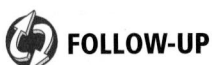 FOLLOW-UP

DISPOSITION
Admission Criteria
Hospitalization is rarely indicated

Issues for Referral
- Audiologist for complete evaluation/therapy
- Otolaryngologist, neurologist, or neurosurgeon, depending on etiology

PROGNOSIS
Most cases of chronic tinnitus cannot be cured (due to association with irreversible sensorinerual hearing loss). Therefore, focus is on managing the tinnitus and reducing its severity, not curing it. (5)

REFERENCES
1. Adams PF, Hendershot GE, Marano MA. *Current estimates from the National Health Interview Survey, 1996.* Hyattsville, MD: National Center for Health Statistics, 1999.
2. Bayar N, et al. Efficacy of amitriptyline in the treatment of subjective tinnitus. *J Otolaryngol.* 2001;30:300–303.
3. Crummer RW, Hassan GA. Diagnostic approach to tinnitus. *Am Fam Physician.* 2004;69:1:121–126.
4. Folmer RL, Martin WH, Shi Y. Tinnitus: Questions to reveal the cause, answers to provide relief. *J Fam Prac.* 2004;53:7.
5. Waddell A, Canter R. Tinnitus. *Clinical Evidence.* 2003;10:634–643.

ADDITIONAL READING
Review references above and Web sites below.

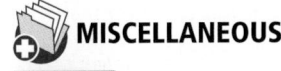 MISCELLANEOUS

CODES

ICD9-CM
388.30 Tinnitus, unspecified

PATIENT TEACHING
- Once underlying conditions have been treated or ruled out, help patients understand that tinnitus is nothing more than a perception of sound and is not a threat to their physical health.
- Sources of information for patients
  - American Tinnitus Association: (800) 634-8978, Web site: www.ata.org
  - National Institute on Deafness and Other Communication Disorders: (800) 241-1044, Web site: www.nidcd.nih.gov
  - American Academy of Otolaryngology: (703) 836-4444, Web site: www.entnet.org
- American Tinnitus Association Web site: Available at: www.ata.org (accessed February 11, 2006.)
- Up To Date Web site: www.uptodate.com (accessed 2/7/06)

Prevention
Avoid causes such as exposure to loud sounds, ototoxic medications, and heavy metals

 See Patient Handout on CD

TORTICOLLIS

Mark L. Shatsky, DO

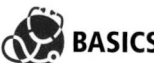 **BASICS**

DESCRIPTION
- Torticollis (L. *tortus*, twisted + *collum*, neck) used generically to describe a broad spectrum of disorders characterized by head tilt and rotation or involuntary movement.
- Adult spectrum includes
  - Spasmodic torticollis (cervical dystonia; dystonia is a muscle contraction causing twisting and repetitive movements)
  - Acute wryneck
- Childhood spectrum includes
  - Congenital muscular torticollis; the most common cause of torticollis in 1st year of life. 3 types are described (1)
    - Most common: Sternocleidomastoid (SCM) tumor (fibromatosis colli)
    - Muscular torticollis: Tightness and no mass
    - Postural torticollis: No mass or tightness
  - Acquired torticollis of childhood
- Other forms (oculogyric, gastroesophageal reflux, arthritis-related, scoliosis-related and hysterical torticollis) are not discussed here.
- Types
  - Rotational (twisting)
  - Anterocollis (flexion)
  - Laterocollis (side bending)
  - Retrocollis (extension)
- System(s) Affected: Musculoskeletal; Nervous
- Synonym(s): Adult acute: Wryneck; Congenital: Idiopathic generalized torticollis, sternocleidomastoid torticollis, neonatal torticollis; Spasmodic: Idiopathic cervical dystonia, focal dystonia, nuchal dystonia

GENERAL PREVENTION
No preventive measures known

EPIDEMIOLOGY
- By age
  - Congenital muscular torticollis: Newborn and infants
  - Acquired torticollis of childhood: <10 years
  - Acute wryneck: 30–60 years
  - Spasmodic torticollis: 30–50 years, mean age 40–43 years (2, 3)
- By gender
  - Spasmodic torticollis: Female > Male (1.6:1) (2)
  - Congenital muscular: Male > Female (3:2) (1)

Incidence
- Congenital: Up to 1:250 live births (1)
- Spasmodic: ~1:100,000
- Annual incidence for all focal dystonias combined 24:1,000,000 persons

Prevalence
- Prevalence for all focal dystonias combined: 295:1,000,000 persons
- No reliable evidence for acute wryneck and childhood acquired torticollis

RISK FACTORS
- Congenital muscular torticollis
  - Intrauterine crowding
  - Breech position in utero
  - Ischemia or injury of muscle fibers during traumatic birth

- Acute wryneck
  - Stress
  - Unusual positioning of neck
  - Localized exposure to cold
  - Medication reaction
- Acquired torticollis of childhood
  - Inflammation
  - Neurologic disorder
  - Optical disorder
  - Rotatory force
- Spasmodic
  - Family history of dystonia ~10% (2)
  - Inflammation
  - Neurologic disorder
  - Optical disorder
  - Rotatory force
  - Link between spasmodic torticollis and psychological factors is unclear

Genetics
Some forms may have genetic basis (3)

ETIOLOGY
- Congenital muscular torticollis
  - Prenatal or birth trauma
  - Sternocleidomastoid may appear normal at birth, then swelling and tightness develop
- Acquired torticollis of childhood
  - Onset of unilateral muscle pain, spasm and/or decreased range of motion without known trauma
  - Look for underlying causes
- Acute wryneck
  - Onset of unilateral muscle pain, spasm and/or decreased range of motion
  - Precipitating factors include tension, stress, postural factors (work, sleep, lying while reading or watching TV, prolonged unusual positioning of neck), or localized exposure to cold (sleeping in draft, open car window)
  - Medication reaction (amphetamines, cocaine, haloperidol, chlorpromazine, prochlorperazine, ketamine, etc.)
- Spasmodic torticollis
  - Muscular damage from inflammatory disease (myositis, lymphadenitis)
  - Cervical spine injuries
  - Ocular disorder
  - Organic CNS disorder
  - Psychogenic
  - Tumor
  - Cervical spondylosis
  - Vestibular dysfunction

ALERT

Pediatric Considerations
Congenital
- Associated with birth injury that, without treatment, becomes fibrous cord
- If untreated, is associated with craniofacial deformities

Pregnancy Considerations
- Difficult delivery in congenital cases
- Associated with breech birth

ASSOCIATED CONDITIONS
- Congenital: Consider Klippel-Feil syndrome
- Acquired torticollis in childhood: Consider Klippel-Feil syndrome
- Spinal abnormalities
- Spasmodic: Consider psychiatric disorder

DIAGNOSIS

SIGNS AND SYMPTOMS
- Head tilt to affected side (80% right side); chin rotates to opposite side
- Intermittent painful spasms of sternocleidomastoid, trapezius, and other neck muscles
- Congenital: 1st sign at birth may be firm, nontender, palpable enlargement of sternocleidomastoid muscle (1, 4).
- Acquired in childhood: Unilateral neck stiffness, pain, or decreased range of motion
- Acute wryneck: Unilateral neck stiffness, pain, or decreased range of motion
- Spasmodic: Features include initial neck stiffness progressing to pain, head jerking, and neck spasms (2,3).

History
- Abnormal head posture
- Neck pain
- Neck mass or swelling
- Birth history
- Family history
- Medication history
- Trauma

Physical Exam
- Tenderness over cervical spine
- Neck mass, lymphadenopathy
- Craniofacial asymmetry (plagiocephaly)
- Range of motion for restrictions or pain; flexion (normal 45°), extension (normal 55°), rotation (normal 70°), sidebending (normal 40°)
- Phasic jerking or tremor of antagonist muscles
- Sensory tricks (*geste antagoniste*) such as touching face or chin reduces severity in most patients (pathognomonic for spasmodic torticollis) (3, 5).
- Ocular irregularities
- Spinal abnormality (short neck with low posterior hair line may indicate occipitocervical synostosis)
- Extremities: Check sensation, strength, reflexes, pulses
- Clicks/clunks/dislocation of hips
- Structural abnormalities of feet

TESTS
Imaging
- Radiographs to rule out spinal pathology
- Consider CT or MRI of cervical spine to aid in differential diagnosis, especially for acquired cases.
- Consider ultrasound and biopsy for congenital cases to rule out tumor.

DIFFERENTIAL DIAGNOSIS
- Osseous
  - Atlantoaxial rotatory subluxation
  - Atlanto-occipital subluxation
  - Post-traumatic fracture or dislocation
  - Cervical disk disorder
  - Congenital scoliosis
  - Klippel-Feil syndrome (congenital fusion of cervical vertebrae)
  - Occipitocervical synostosis
  - Grisel syndrome (unilateral or bilateral subluxation of C1 on C2, associated with infectious condition in the head or neck)
  - Syringomyelia
  - Arnold-Chiari malformation

- Nonosseous
  - Myositis involving cervical muscles
  - Soft-tissue trauma
  - Neoplastic: Spinal cord tumor, acoustic neuroma, osteoblastoma, orbital tumor, fibromatosis, metastasis
  - Infection: Upper respiratory tract infection, cervical lymph node abscess, epidural abscess, retropharyngeal abscess, vertebral osteomyelitis
  - Vestibular disorders
  - Essential head tremor
  - Basal ganglia disease
  - Cranial nerve palsy
  - Psychiatric disorders
  - Drug or toxin induced
  - Down syndrome
  - Sandifer syndrome (association of gastroesophageal reflux disease with spastic torticollis and dystonic body movements)
  - Myasthenia gravis

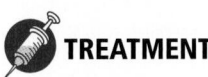 **TREATMENT**

Issues for Referral
Specialty consultation as appropriate (neurologist, neurosurgeon, ophthalmologist, orthopedist, otolaryngologist)

GENERAL MEASURES
- Congenital
  - Physical therapy and aggressive stretching program if started before age 3–6 months (1, 6)[B]
  - Place TV/toys on opposite side of bed from rotational deformity (4)[B]
- Acquired in children
  - Place TV on opposite side of bed from rotational deformity
- Acute wryneck
  - Conservative management includes soft cervical collar, intermittent heat or ice, and/or bed rest
  - Analgesics for temporary relief and to break pain/spasm cycle
  - Benztropine reported to relieve acute muscle spasm
- Spasmodic
  - Conservative management includes soft cervical collar, intermittent heat or ice, and/or bed rest
  - Botulinum toxin type A or B is effective and safe for treating adults with cervical dystonia.

Diet
No special diet

Activity
No restrictions

Physical Therapy
If detected early, 90% of congenital muscular torticollis can be managed by stretching exercises performed by parents after receiving physical therapy instructions.

Complementary and Alternative Therapies
Evidence lacking for
- Acupuncture
- Behavior modification
- Spinal manipulation

 MEDICATION (DRUGS)

- Congenital muscular: Botulinum toxin type A effective in case series (1, 7)[C]
- Analgesics for temporary relief of pain
- Anticholinergics (benztropine, trihexyphenidyl) may relieve acute muscle spasm (3)[C].
- Diphenhydramine or diazepam for torticollis caused by medication (3)[C]
- Single injection cycle of botulinum toxin type A is effective and safe for treating adults with cervical dystonia (3)[B].
- Botulinum toxin type A and B injections may be more effective than anticholinergic drugs for cervical dystonia (3)[B].
- Patients with focal dystonia of unknown cause: Trial of carbidopa-levodopa (3)[C]

SURGERY
Congenital: Surgical release of involved muscle if physical therapy unsuccessful by 1 year of age (4)[C]

 FOLLOW-UP

PROGNOSIS
- Congenital: Good for correctable pathology
  - 50–70% resolve spontaneously by 1st year of life
- Child acquired: Good if underlying pathology is discovered
- Acute wryneck: Typically resolves in a few days to weeks
- Spasmodic: May wax and wane for years

COMPLICATIONS
- Facial asymmetry in congenital cases
- May have developmental dysplasia of hip in congenital cases
- Movement disorders
- Postural disorders
- Dental malocclusion
- Psychosocial: May have negative impact on quality of life

PATIENT MONITORING
- Periodic follow-up to assess progress
- Frequent assessment in acquired form

REFERENCES

1. Do TT. Congenital muscular torticollis: Current concepts and review. *Curr Opin Pediatr.* 2006;18(1):26–29.
2. Chan J, Brin MF, Fahn S. Idiopathic cervical dystonia: Clinical characteristics. *Mov Disorder.* 1991;6:119–126.
3. Tarsay D, Simon DK. Current concepts dystonia. *N Engl J Med.* 2006;355(8):818–829.
4. Epps HR, Salter RB. Orthopedic conditions of the cervical spine and shoulder. *Pediatr Clin N Am.* 1996;43(4):919–931.
5. Consky EA, Lang AE. Clinical assessments of patients with cervical dystonia. In: Jancovic J, Hallet M, eds. *Therapy with Botulinum Toxin.* New York: Marcel Dekker; 1994:211–237.
6. Demirbilek S, Atayurt HF. Congenital muscular torticollis and sternomastoid tumor: Results of nonoperative treatment. *J Pediatr Surg.* 1999;34(4):549–551.
7. Olexzek JL, Chang N, Apkon SD, Wilson PE. Botulinum toxin Type A in the treatment of children with congenital muscular torticollis. *Am J Phys Med Rehabil.* 2005;84(10):813–816.
8. Alper BS. Torticollis. DynaMed. Available from: http://www.DynamicMedical.com. Accessed Sept 4, 2006.

 MISCELLANEOUS

CODES

ICD9-CM
- 333.83 Spasmodic torticollis
- 306.00 Psychogenic torticollis
- 300.1 Hysterical torticollis
- 300.11 Conversion disorder
- 723.5 Torticollis not otherwise specified
- 754.1 Certain congenital musculoskeletal deformities of sternocleidomastoid muscle

PATIENT TEACHING
Congenital: Train parents to perform massage and range-of-motion exercises.

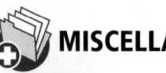 **See Patient Handout on CD**

T

TOURETTE SYNDROME

Cheryl A. Wehler, MD

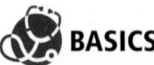 BASICS

DESCRIPTION
- Tourette syndrome (TS) is a childhood onset neurobehavioral disorder characterized by the presence of multiple motor and at least 1 phonic tics (see "Physical Exam") (1).
  - Tics are sudden, brief, repetitive, stereotyped motor movements (motor tics) or sounds produced by moving air through the nose, mouth, or throat (phonic tics).
  - Tics tend to occur in bouts.
  - Tics can be simple or complex; motor tics precede vocal tics, and simple tics precede complex tics.
  - Tics often are preceded by sensory symptoms, especially a compulsion to move; patients are able to suppress their tics but voluntary suppression is associated with an inner tension that results in more forceful tics when suppression ceases.
- System(s) Affected: Nervous

EPIDEMIOLOGY
- Predominant age
  - By definition, TS onset is in 1st 2 decades
  - In TS, simple motor tics typically begin at age 5–6 years (phonic tics usually appear a few years later), and reach peak severity between 10 and 12 years.
  - 1/2 to 3/4 of children with TS experience a substantial decrease in tics by late adolescence or early adulthood.
- Predominant sex: Male > Female (3–4:1)
- Predominant race/ethnicity: Clinically heterogeneous disorder, but main characteristics independent of culture

Prevalence
Prevalence of TS estimated at 1–10:1000 children and adolescents

RISK FACTORS
- Inherited developmental disorder; frequency and severity of tics exacerbated by environmental factors
- Morbid risk for TS among relatives range between 9.8% and 15%; 1st-degree relatives of individuals with TS have a 10- to 100-fold increased risk of developing TS compared with general population.

Genetics
- Genetic predisposition, frequent familial history of tic disorders and OCD
- Precise pattern of transmission and identification of genes are unknown; recent studies suggest polygenic inheritance with evidence for a locus on chromosome 17q; sequence variants in SLITRK1 gene on chromosome 13q also are associated with TS.
- Higher concordance in monozygotic compared to dizygotic twins; wide range of phenotypes

ETIOLOGY
- Abnormality of basal ganglia development
- Mechanism uncertain; probably involves dysfunction of basal ganglia-thalamo-cortical circuits likely involving decreased inhibitory output from the basal ganglia, which results in an imbalance of inhibition and excitation in the motor cortex.
- Research suggests that abnormalities of dopamine neurotransmission, most likely in the ventral striatum, play a primary role in the pathophysiology.

ASSOCIATED CONDITIONS
- Most common comorbid conditions are ADHD, OCD (symptoms peak later than tics), and depression
- Impairments of visual perception, sleep disorders, restless leg syndrome, and migraine headaches higher than in general population
- Disruptive behavior problems, aggression, anxiety disorders, social difficulties, and/or learning problems

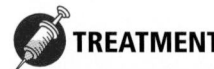 DIAGNOSIS

Often retrospective; no sensitive and specific diagnostic tests for TS

SIGNS AND SYMPTOMS
- Motor and vocal tics are the clinical hallmark
- Tics fluctuate in type, frequency, and anatomic distribution over time
- Multiple motor tics such as facial grimacing, blinking, head or neck jerking, tongue protruding, sniffing, touching
- Vocal tics such as grunts, snorts, throat clearing, barking, yelling, hiccupping
- Tics are exacerbated by anticipation, emotional upset, anxiety, or fatigue.
- Tics subside when patient is concentrating or absorbed in activities.
- Motor and vocal tics may persist during all stages of sleep, especially light sleep.

History
Diagnosis of TS is based on history and clinical presentation (i.e., observation of tics with or without presence of coexisting disorders).

Physical Exam
- Typically normal; blink reflex abnormalities may be observed.
- Motor and vocal tics are diagnostic sine qua non of TS.
- No clinical measures known to reliably predict children who will continue to express tics in adulthood; severity of tics in late childhood is associated with future tic severity.
- DSM criteria
  - A. Both multiple motor and ≥1 vocal tics have been present at some time during the illness, although not necessarily concurrently.
  - B. These may appear simultaneously or at different periods during the illness. The tics occur many times a day (usually in bouts) nearly every day or intermittently throughout a period of >1 year, with no tic-free period of >3 consecutive months.
  - C. The anatomic location, number, frequency, complexity, type, and severity of tics change over time.
  - D. Onset before age 18 years.
  - E. The tics are not due to the direct physiologic effects of a substance (e.g., stimulants) or a general medical condition (e.g., Huntington disease or post-viral encephalitis).

TESTS
Lab
- No definitive laboratory tests for diagnosis of TS.
- TSH should be measured because of association of tics with hyperthyroidism

Imaging
- No useful imaging studies available for diagnosis of TS.
- EEG shows nonspecific abnormalities; useful only to differentiate tics from epilepsy.

Pathological Findings
- Smaller caudate volumes in TS patients
- Striatal dopaminergic terminals are increased, as is striatal dopamine transporter (DAT) density.

DIFFERENTIAL DIAGNOSIS
- Chronic motor or vocal tic disorder
- Transient tic disorder
- Tic disorder not otherwise specified
- Huntington disease
- Stroke
- Lesch-Nyhan syndrome
- Wilson disease
- Sydenham's chorea
- Multiple sclerosis
- Post-viral encephalitis
- Head injury
- Drug effects (e.g., dopamine agonists)

TREATMENT

GENERAL MEASURES
- Neurologic and psychiatric evaluation for diagnosis of primary disorder and comorbid psychiatric conditions (especially ADHD, OCD, and depression)
- Educate patient, family, teachers, and friends to identify and address psychosocial stressors and environmental triggers.
- Many patients require no treatment for tics; patient should play active role in treatment decisions.
- No cure for tics: Treatment is purely symptomatic, and multimodal treatment usually is indicated.
- TS clusters with several comorbidities; each disorder must be evaluated for associated functional impairment, because patients often are more disabled by their psychiatric conditions than tics; choice of initial treatment largely depends on worst symptoms (tics, obsessions, impulsivity).
- Monotherapy at low doses is preferred to polytherapy.
- Taper medications known to exacerbate tics (e.g., dopamine agonists).

Diet
No restrictions

Activity
No restrictions, encourage exercise and activities

SPECIAL THERAPY
Behavioral treatment of tics

- Habit reversal training (HRT) provides a viable tic-suppression treatment (2)[A].
  - HRT is equally effective for motor and vocal tics.

MEDICATION (DRUGS)

First Line
α-Adrenergic medications

- Clonidine is a first-line agent for tic suppression; an α₂-adrenergic receptor agonist, it is drug of choice (3)[A].
  - Ameliorate both tics and ADHD (4)[A]
  - Efficacious and safe in children with average dose of 0.3 mg/d
  - Clonidine causes sedation and hypotension, but not EKG abnormalities.
- Guanfacine, also an α₂-adrenergic receptor agonist, is useful in controlling tics and ADHD at 0.5–1.5 mg b.i.d. (5)[A].
  - Guanfacine is less sedating and has a longer duration of action.

Second Line
- Dopamine receptor antagonists

  - Typical antipsychotics (e.g., haloperidol 0.5–5 mg at bedtime; pimozide 1–8 mg at bedtime; and chlorpromazine) (3)[A]
  - Atypical antipsychotics (e.g., risperidone 0.5–3 mg b.i.d.; olanzapine and quetiapine) (6)[A]

  - Only haloperidol, pimozide, and risperidone proven effective in controlled studies
  - Olanzapine (5–20 mg/d) also has been shown to reduce tics and aggression.
  - No controlled trials evaluating clozapine for TS treatment; does not cause tardive dyskinesia, but risk of agranulocytosis necessitates weekly CBCs for 6 months, and monthly CBCs thereafter.
  - Shared side effects include sedation, weight gain, anxiety, orthostatic hypotension, restlessness, extrapyramidal movements, Parkinsonism, tardive dyskinesia, lowered seizure threshold (especially clozapine), and QTc prolongation (especially pimozide).
    ○ Haloperidol used in range of 0.5–4 mg at bedtime
    ○ Pimozide is dosed at 1–8 mg at bedtime; must be given under EKG monitoring because of risk of cardiac arrhythmias.
    ○ Risperidone 1–2 mg b.i.d. or t.i.d.; causes tardive dyskinesia at doses exceeding 6 mg/d.
    ○ EKG abnormalities are common and dose-dependent with olanzapine, clozapine, haloperidol.
    ○ Typical neuroleptics (e.g., haloperidol and pimozide) are more prone to cause extrapyramidal side effects.
    ○ Atypical antipsychotics (e.g., olanzapine and risperidone) are less likely to result in extrapyramidal side effects (e.g., akathisia) but may be associated with metabolic abnormalities such as weight gain, diabetes, hypertriglyceridemia, and dyslipidemia.

    ○ Use of risperidone in TS is associated with dysphoria and depression (6)[A].

- Benzodiazepines
  - Better tolerated than neuroleptics, but less efficacious
  - Side effects include sedation, weight gain, irritability, oppositional behavior, mood changes, and cognitive impairment

- Presynaptic dopamine-depleting agents
  - Tetrabenazine (not yet available in U.S.) is very effective for tic control but has some side effects associated with postsynaptic dopamine blockade.
- Miscellaneous medications
  - Botulinum toxin injections may be used for severe dystonic tics.
- Treatment of ADHD in patients with tics
  - Stimulants such as methylphenidate and dextroamphetamine are most effective and safe treatments of ADHD (7)[A].
    ○ Comorbid tic disorder is not a serious contraindication as previously held; exacerbation of tics is neither clinically significant nor common (7)[A].
    ○ Guanfacine or clonidine is safe and effective for ADHD treatment (5)[A].
- Treatment of OCD in patients with tics
  - Selective serotonin reuptake inhibitors (SSRIs) are most effective and safe; the 1st-line treatment of OCD (8)[A].
    ○ Comorbid tic disorder not a contraindication; exacerbation of tics neither clinically significant nor common.
    ○ Side effects of SSRIs include gastrointestinal distress, agitation, sexual dysfunction, akathisia, and headache.
    ○ Some risk of suicidality noted with SSRIs and other antidepressants.
    ○ Clomipramine, a tricyclic antidepressant, is also effective in reducing OC behaviors.
    ○ It can be used in place of SSRIs in patients refractory to that treatment or to augment SSRI treatment in partial responders.
    ○ Clomipramine side effects include weight gain, dry mouth, constipation, and lowering of seizure threshold.
    ○ EKG changes including QTc interval prolongation and tachycardia are the more serious side effects of clomipramine and require monitoring.
    ○ Other effective augmentation agents include atypical neuroleptics, such as clonazepam or buspirone.

SURGERY
Thalamic ablation and deep brain stimulation (DBS) have been used experimentally for tic reduction.

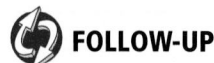 **FOLLOW-UP**

PROGNOSIS
In 1/2–2/3 of children with TS, severity of tics attenuate during adolescence, often remitting completely by early adulthood. However, OCD symptoms tend to increase during this same period in many individuals.

PATIENT MONITORING
Observe for associated psychiatric disorders.

REFERENCES
1. American Psychiatric Association. Diagnostic and Statistical Manual of Mental Disorders (DSM-IV-TR), 4th ed. Washington, DC: American Psychiatric Association; 2000.
2. Wilhelm S, Deckersbach T, Coffey BJ, et al. Habit reversal versus supportive psychotherapy for Tourette's disorder: a randomized controlled trial. *Am J Psychiatry.* 2003;160(6):1175–1177.
3. Scahill L, Erenberg G, Berlin CM, et al. Contemporary assessment and pharmacotherapy of Tourette syndrome. *NeuroRx.* 2006;3(2):192–206.
4. Tourette Syndrome Study Group. Treatment of ADHD in children with tics: a randomized controlled trial. *Neurology.* 2002;58(4):527–536.
5. Scahill L, Chappell OB, Kim YS, et al. A placebo-controlled study of guanfacine in the treatment of children with tic disorders and attention deficit hyperactivity disorder. *Am J Psychiatry.* 2001;158(7):1067–1074.
6. Dion Y, Annable L, Stat D, et al. Risperidone in the treatment of Tourette syndrome: a double-blind, placebo-controlled trial. *J Clin Psychopharmacol.* 2002;22(1):31–39.
7. Spencer T, Biederman, J, Wilens, T, et al. A large, double-blind, randomized clinical trial of methylphenidate in the treatment of adults with attention-deficit/hyperactivity disorder. *Biolog Psychiatry.* 2005;57(5):456–463.
8. Eapen V, MM Robertson. Co-morbid obsessive-compulsive disorder and Tourette syndrome. *CNS Drugs.* 2000;13(3):173–183.

 MISCELLANEOUS

CODES

ICD9-CM
307.23 Gilles de la Tourette disorder

PATIENT TEACHING
Printed patient information available from: Tourette Syndrome Association (TSA), 42-40 Bell Blvd., Bayside, NY 11361-2861; 718-224-2999 National Hotline (800) 237-0717; http://www.tsa-usa.org

T

TOXIC SHOCK SYNDROME (TSS)

Anthony W. Chow, MD

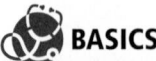 **BASICS**

DESCRIPTION

Acute multisystem illness associated with *Staphylococcus aureus* infections and characterized by sudden onset of high fever, peculiar skin rash with desquamation, and shock

- Menstrual: Associated with menstruation and tampon use
- Nonmenstrual: Associated with postoperative wounds and barrier contraception; more common than menstrual form
- Can occur in children, men, and women
- System(s) Affected: All organ systems can be affected, particularly: Cardiovascular/Pulmonary; Renal/Hepatic; Neurologic/Muscular; Endocrine/Metabolic; Skin/Exocrine
- Synonym(s): Staphylococcal scarlet fever

GENERAL PREVENTION

- Avoidance of continuous tampon use during menstruation
- Avoidance of super-absorbency tampons
- Frequent tampon changes during day
- Use of sanitary napkins at night
- Early medical attention to infected wounds

EPIDEMIOLOGY

- Predominant age: 30–60 years, but can occur in all ages
- Predominant sex: Female > Male (3:2)

Prevalence

Approximately 0.22–1.23 cases per 100,000 in the United States (1)

RISK FACTORS

- High
  - Absence of antibody to TSS toxin-1 (TSST-1)
  - Infection with *S. aureus,* which produces TSST-1
  - Continuous use of super-absorbency tampons during menstruation
  - Nasal surgery with packing
- Moderate
  - Use of regular-absorbency tampons during menstruation
  - Use of contraceptive sponge
- Low
  - Alternating use of tampons and pads during menstruation
  - Intrauterine contraceptive device
  - Surgical-wound infections
  - Early postpartum state

Genetics

No specific mode of inheritance is recognized.

ETIOLOGY

- *S. aureus* exotoxins, especially
  - TSST-1
  - Staphylococcal enterotoxins A, B, and C
  - Other staphylococcal superantigens including enterotoxins D, E, and H
- Pediatric population: May occur as complication of chickenpox
- Geriatric population: Cellulitis or surgical-wound infections
- Pregnancy: Postpartum infections, especially post-cesarean section wound infection, or episiotomy infections

ASSOCIATED CONDITIONS

Staphylococcal infections

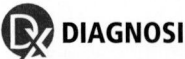 **DIAGNOSIS**

SIGNS AND SYMPTOMS

- Almost always present (>80%)
  - Temperature >38.9°C (>102°F)
  - Erythroderma
  - Diffuse macular rash
  - Skin desquamation a few days after rash appears
  - Shock, orthostatic hypotension, or syncope
  - Nausea or vomiting
- Commonly present (20–80%)
  - Headache
  - Confusion or agitation
  - Acute respiratory distress syndrome
  - Meningismus
  - Pharyngeal erythema
  - Vaginitis or vaginal discharge
  - Conjunctivitis
  - Periorbital edema
  - Strawberry tongue
  - Non-pitting edema
  - Myalgia
  - Oliguria
  - Arthralgia
  - Diarrhea
- Rarely present (<20%)
  - Arthritis
  - Lymphadenopathy
  - Hepatosplenomegaly
  - Cardiomyopathy
  - Pericarditis
  - Photophobia
  - Seizure

TESTS

Lab

- Microbiologic
  - Isolation of *S. aureus* strains that produce TSST-1 or other toxins in a patient who does not have acute phase serum antibodies to these superantigens. (2)[B]
  - Positive culture for *S. aureus* from vagina or surgical wound (>90%)
  - Nasal or perineal carriage of *S. aureus*
  - Positive blood culture for *S. aureus* (uncommon)
- Hematologic (50–90%)
  - Granulocytosis with increased band forms
  - Lymphopenia
  - Normocytic, normochromic anemia
  - Thrombocytopenia
  - Coagulopathy
- Biochemical (50–90%)
  - Hypoalbuminemia
  - Abnormal electrolytes
  - Hypocalcemia
  - Hypomagnesemia
  - Hypophosphatemia
  - Increased serumglutamic-oxalcacetic transaminase
  - Increased serumglutamic pyruric transaminase
  - Increased creatine phosphokinase
  - Increased blood urea nitrogen
  - Increased serum creatinine
  - Increased calcitonin
  - Increased serum bilirubin
  - Abnormal urine sediment

Imaging

No unusual or characteristic findings

Diagnostic Procedures/Surgery

No specific diagnostic test is currently available.

Pathological Findings

- Subepidermic cleavage plane in skin
- Minimal inflammatory reaction in tissues
- Lymphocyte depletion in lymph nodes
- Cervico-vaginal ulcerations

DIFFERENTIAL DIAGNOSIS

- Streptococcal scarlet fever
- Streptococcal TSS
  - More often associated with severe pain and tenderness at a site of local trauma and infection, and more frequently accompanied by bacteremia
- Drug reactions
- Rocky Mountain spotted fever
- Leptospirosis
- Kawasaki disease
- Staphylococcal scalded-skin syndrome
- Meningococcal or possibly Gram-negative sepsis
- Measles, rubeola

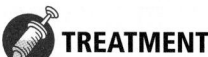 **TREATMENT**

INITIAL STABILIZATION
Inpatient, admission to intensive care for monitoring

GENERAL MEASURES
- Removal of tampon or other vaginal foreign bodies
- Removal of nasal packings
- Local wound care
- Fluid resuscitation
- Management of renal or cardiac insufficiency
- Mechanical ventilation if necessary

Diet
As tolerated

Activity
Bed rest throughout acute illness

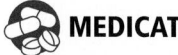 **MEDICATION (DRUGS)**

First Line
- Treatment of shock or hypotension
  - Fluid replacement
  - Dopamine
  - Steroids or naloxone have not been proven to be of value
- Eradication of *S. aureus* and inhibition of toxin production
- Oxacillin or nafcillin 100 mg/kg/d q4h (bactericidal against susceptible *S. aureus*, but may release more toxins by bacterial lysis) (3)[B]
- Clindamycin 25 mg/kg/d q8h (more efficacious than betalactams in suppressing *in vitro* production of TSST-1) (3)[B]
- Combination of clindamycin 25 mg/kg/d q8h plus oxacillin or nafcillin 100 mg/kg/d q4h (recommended for patients with deep-seated infections or bacteremia) (3)[B]
- Contraindications: Penicillin allergy
- Precautions
  - Rash, diarrhea, seizures
  - Reduce oxacillin dosage in patients with severe renal failure. It is not necessary to reduce the nafcillin dose for renal dysfunction.
- Significant possible interactions: See the manufacturer's profile of each drug.

Second Line
- Vancomycin: 30 mg/kg/d q6h for patients infected with methicillin-resistant *S. aureus* (MRSA)
- Linezolid: 10 mg/kg or 600 mg q12h for patients infected with MRSA
- Toxin neutralization
  - Benefit in humans unproven, but animal and *in vitro* studies support this approach (4)[B]
  - Immune globulin IV: 0.4 g/kg over 6 hours (5)[B]

SURGERY
- Surgical drainage of loculated infections
- Exploration and debridement of surgical wounds, which may not appear purulent or infected due to a decreased local inflammatory response in a patient with nonmenstrual TSS

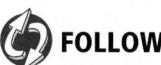 **FOLLOW-UP**

PROGNOSIS
- Mortality: 3–9%
- Recurrence: 10–15%

COMPLICATIONS
- Common (>20%)
  - Acute renal failure
  - Adult respiratory distress syndrome
  - Menorrhagia
  - Alopecia
  - Nail loss
- Rare (<20%)
  - Disseminated intravascular coagulation
  - Ataxia, toxic encephalopathy
  - Memory impairment
  - Cardiomyopathy
  - Protracted malaise

PATIENT MONITORING
- Admit to intensive care if in shock
- Daily vital signs until patient is afebrile and normotensive

REFERENCES
1. Hajjeh RA, et al. Toxic shock syndrome in the United States: Surveillance update, 1979-1996. *Emerg Infect Dis*. 1999;5:807–810.
2. Whiting JL, Rosten PM, Chow AW. Determination by Western blot (immunoblot) of seroconversions to toxic shock syndrome toxin 1 and enterotoxin A, B, or C during infection with TSS- and non-TSS-associated Staphylococcus aureus. *Infect Immun*. 1989;57:231–234.
3. Parsonnet J, Modern PA, Giacobbe KD. *Effect of subinhibitory concentrations of antibiotics on production of TSST-1 [abstract 29], Program and Abstracts of the 32nd Meeting of the IDSA, Orlando*. 1994:6A.
4. Barry W, et al. Intravenous immunoglobulin therapy for Toxic Shock Syndrome. *JAMA*. 1992;267:3315–3316.
5. Keller MA, Stiehm ER, Passive immunity in prevention and treatment of infectious diseases. *Clin Microbiol Rev*. 2000;13:602–614.
6. Darenberg J, et al. Intravenous immunoglobulin G therapy in streptococcal toxic shock syndrome: A European randomized double-blind, placebo-controlled trial. *Clin Infect Dis*. 2003;37:333–340.

 MISCELLANEOUS

See also: Measles, rubeola; Pancreatitis; Rocky Mountain spotted fever; Scarlet fever

CODES

ICD9-CM
40.82 Toxic shock syndrome

PATIENT TEACHING
Advise patient regarding possible sequelae or recurrence.

TOXOPLASMOSIS

William G. Gardner, MD, MACP

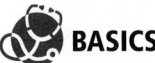 **BASICS**

DESCRIPTION

Infection with the protozoan parasite *Toxoplasma gondii* resulting in one of the following conditions

- Acute self-limited infection in immunocompetent persons
- Acute often symptomatic infection in immunocompromised persons
- Reactivation of latent infection in immunocompromised persons
- Congenital infection due to acute infection or reactivation of latent infection in the mother during pregnancy

ALERT

Pediatric Considerations

- Transmission to fetus in early pregnancy is less common but results in more severe disease
  - Risk of perinatal death 5% if infected during 1st trimester
- The majority of infected children who are asymptomatic at birth eventually develop manifestations unless treated
- Early recognition and treatment of disease in the infant improves prognosis

Pregnancy Considerations

- Immunocompromised and HIV-infected women should undergo serologic testing in pregnancy
- Seronegative pregnant women should take precautions to avoid contact with cats, not eat raw or undercooked meat, and wash all fruits and vegetables carefully

GENERAL PREVENTION

Prevention important in seronegative pregnant women and immunodeficient patients

- Avoid eating raw or undercooked meat
- Wear gloves while handling, and wash hands after handling, raw meat
- Avoid contact with cat feces; wear gloves and wash hands immediately after changing cat litter

EPIDEMIOLOGY

- Predominant age: All ages
- Predominant sex: Male = Female

Incidence

- Incidence of congenital toxoplasmosis in the United States is 1/1,000–8,000 live births
- Affects ~4,000 newborns in the United States each year

Prevalence

- Overall 22.5% in the United States
- 15% among women of childbearing age

RISK FACTORS

- Immunocompromised patients, especially AIDS, lymphoma, high-dose corticosteroids
- Risk of transplacental transmission greatest during 3rd trimester, but disease more severe if acquired during 1st trimester

Genetics

Human leukocyte antigen DQ3 is a genetic marker of susceptibility to development of toxoplasma encephalitis in AIDS patients

ETIOLOGY

- Etiologic agent for each of the clinical syndromes is *T. gondii.*
- Transmission to humans
  - Ingestion of raw or undercooked meat, food, or water containing tissue cysts or oocytes
  - Transplacental to fetus from infected mother
  - Blood product transfusion
  - Solid organ transplantation
- Clinical syndromes
  - Acute infection in immunocompetent host
  - Acute or reactivation infection in immunocompromised host
  - Congenital toxoplasmosis
  - Ocular toxoplasmosis
- Not transmitted by breast feeding

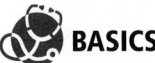 **DIAGNOSIS**

SIGNS AND SYMPTOMS

- Congenital toxoplasmosis
  - Clinical presentation varies widely
  - No signs or symptoms of infection (67%)
  - Classic triad uncommon: Chorioretinitis, hydrocephalus, cerebral calcifications
  - Cerebrospinal fluid (CSF) pleocytosis and elevated protein (20%)
  - Anemia, thrombocytopenia, jaundice at birth
  - Microcephaly
  - Mental retardation, seizures, visual defects, spasticity, other severe neurologic sequelae
- Ocular toxoplasmosis
  - Chorioretinitis: Focal necrotizing retinitis
  - Yellowish-white elevated cotton patch
  - Congenital disease usually bilateral
  - Acquired disease usually unilateral
  - Symptoms include blurred vision, scotoma, pain, photophobia
- Acute toxoplasmosis: Immunocompetent host
  - Approximately 80–90% are asymptomatic
  - Cervical lymphadenopathy with discrete, usually nontender nodes <3 cm in diameter
  - Fever, malaise, night sweats, myalgias
  - Sore throat, maculopapular rash
  - Visual disturbance due to chorioretinitis
  - Hepatosplenomegaly, mesenteric, and retroperitoneal adenopathy
  - Atypical lymphocytosis
  - Most infected pregnant women are asymptomatic
- Acute toxoplasmosis: Immunocompromised host
  - CNS disease (50%)
    - Encephalitis, meningoencephalitis, or mass lesions, hemiparesis, seizures, mental status changes, CSF with elevated protein, normal glucose, and mononuclear pleocytosis
  - Chorioretinitis
  - Myocarditis
  - Pneumonia with high mortality rate

TESTS
Lab
- Lab diagnosis is made by polymerase chain reaction (PCR), histology, isolation, and indirect (serologic) methods
- PCR on blood, body fluids, and tissue
  - Sensitive and specific
  - Indicates current infection
- Direct demonstration of parasite in tissue or body fluid by histology or culture
- Serologic methods
  - Does not distinguish time of infection
  - IgG antibody is useful to indicate prior infection in immunocompromised persons and pregnant women; indicates risk for reactivation disease. If negative, indicates risk for acquiring; maternal antibodies persist in infants up to 1 year
  - IgG avidity test: High avidity antibodies exclude recent infection
  - IgM antibody may persist >1 year, so does not always indicate recent infection
  - Absence of IgM antibody excludes infection
- Amniocentesis at 20–24 weeks in suspected congenital disease with PCR on amniotic fluid
- Amniotic fluid PCR before week 18 unreliable; isolation of toxoplasma from the placenta is diagnostic of a congenital infection.
- Newborn suspected of having congenital disease should have PCR testing on blood, CSF, and urine
- Several serologic tests used in diagnosis, some measuring IgM and other IgG antibodies
  - The Sabin-Feldman dye test is a sensitive and specific neutralization test that measures the IgG antibodies and is a standard reference test for toxoplasmosis.
  - Indirect fluorescent antibody test measures same antibodies as dye test. Titers parallel dye-test titers.
  - IgM fluorescent antibody test detects IgM antibodies within 1st week of infection
- Double-sandwich IgM enzyme linked immunosorbent assay is more sensitive and specific than other IgM tests
  - Negative results for IgM antibodies during the first 2 trimesters excludes a recently acquired infection.

Imaging
- Cerebral toxoplasmosis
  - CT scan of head
  - MRI scan of head
- Ultrasound of fetus at 20–24 weeks

Diagnostic Procedures/Surgery
- Lymph-node biopsy showing characteristic pathologic triad, as described subsequently
- Brain biopsy in CNS disease and demonstration of organisms by peroxidase-antiperoxidase technique
- Empiric therapy for CNS mass lesions in toxoplasma antibody–positive HIV patients with response on 2-week follow-up imaging study is presumptive evidence for a diagnosis.

Pathological Findings
Lymph-node histology shows triad of
- Reactive follicular hyperplasia
- Irregular clusters of epithelioid histiocytes on and blurring margins of germinal centers
- Distention of sinuses with monocytoid cells

DIFFERENTIAL DIAGNOSIS
- Congenital toxoplasmosis
  - Other members of TORCH syndrome (rubella, cytomegalovirus, herpes simplex)
  - Syphilis
  - Listeria
  - Other infectious encephalopathies
  - Erythroblastosis fetalis
  - Sepsis
- Ocular toxoplasmosis
  - Tuberculosis
  - Syphilis
  - Leprosy
  - Ocular histoplasmosis
- Acute toxoplasmosis (normal and immunocompromised)
  - Lymphoma
  - Infectious mononucleosis
  - Cytomegalovirus
  - Cat scratch disease
  - Sarcoidosis
  - Tuberculosis (TB)
  - Tularemia
  - Metastatic carcinoma
  - Leukemia

- Toxoplasma encephalitis
  - TB
  - Fungal diseases
  - Vasculitis
  - Progressive multifocal leukoencephalopathy
  - Brain abscess
  - Tumor
  - Herpes encephalitis
  - CNS lymphoma
  - *Nocardia* species

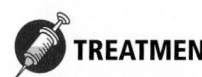

TREATMENT

INITIAL STABILIZATION
- Outpatient for acquired disease in immunocompetent host and ocular toxoplasmosis
- Inpatient initially for CNS toxoplasmosis and acute disease in immunocompromised host

GENERAL MEASURES
Immunocompetent children and adults with toxoplasma lymphadenopathy usually require no treatment unless symptoms severe or prolonged
- If fetal infection add pyrimethamine, sulfadiazine, and leucovorin
- Infants with congenital toxoplasmosis should be treated for one year

Diet
No special diet

Activity
Level of activity dependent on organ systems involved and severity of disease

MEDICATION (DRUGS)

First Line

- Acute asymptomatic acquired infection in immunocompetent host requires no treatment
- Acute toxoplasmosis in pregnant woman
  - Spiromycin 1 g t.i.d.
    - Without food
    - Continue until term
    - If documented fetal infection, after 18 weeks add pyrimethamine, sulfadiazine, and leucovorin
- Congenital toxoplasmosis
  - Sulfadiazine 100 mg/kg/d plus
  - Pyrimethamine 2 mg/kg/d for 2 days, then 1 mg/kg/d for 2–6 months, then same dose every Mon, Wed, and Friday *plus*
  - Leucovorin (folinic acid) 10 mg 3 times a week while on pyrimethamine
  - Treat for 1 year
- Ocular toxoplasmosis in adults
  - Sulfadiazine 1–1.5 g/d *plus*
  - Pyrimethamine loading dose 200 mg 1st day, then 50–75 mg/d *plus*
  - Leucovorin 5–20 mg 3 times a week
  - Treat 1–2 weeks after resolution of symptoms

- Toxoplasma encephalitis in AIDS patients
  - Sulfadiazine 1–1.5 g q6h *plus*
  - Pyrimethamine 200 mg 1st day then 50–75 mg/d *plus*
  - Leucovorin 10–20 mg/d
  - Cilndamycin 600–1200 mg IV q6h plus pyrimethamine and leucovorin for those who cannot tolerate sulfonamide
  - Treat for at least 6 weeks
  - After acute treatment continue suppression therapy indefinitely
    - Sulfadiazine 500 mg q6h *plus*
    - Pyrimethamine 25–50 mg/d *plus*
    - Leucovorin 10 mg/d
- Contraindications: Known hypersensitivity to pyrimethamine or sulfadiazine (NOTE: Many HIV-positive patients have a sulfa sensitivity)
- Precautions
  - Monitor for bone marrow toxicity
  - Use with caution in patients with renal or hepatic dysfunction
  - Adequate hydration is essential, because sulfadiazine is poorly soluble and may crystallize in the urine.
  - Watch for diarrhea especially if on clindamycin
- Significant possible interactions: Sulfonamides may increase
  - Phenytoin (dilantin) levels
  - Anticoagulant effect of warfarin (coumadin)
  - Hypoglycemic effect of oral hypoglycemic agents

Second Line

- Clindamycin: 900–1,200 mg t.i.d. IV used for ocular and CNS toxoplasmosis alone and in combination with pyrimethamine. As effective as the sulfa + pyrimethamine, but fewer adverse effects.
- Corticosteroids (prednisone 1–2 mg/kg/d) added for macular chorioretinitis or CNS infection.
- Alternative atovaquone (mepron), azithromycin (zithromax), clarithromycin (biaxin), or dapsone plus pyrimethamine and leucovorin
- Trimethoprim/sulfamethoxazole appears to be equivalent to pyrimethamine/sulfadiazine in AIDS patients wih CNS disease

SURGERY

- Lymphnode biosy for presistantly enlarged lymphnodes to secure diagnosis
- Biopsy of brain lesion for diagnosis

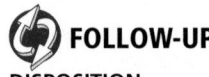

FOLLOW-UP

DISPOSITION

Admission Criteria

- Acutely ill patients
- Neurologic abnormalities

Discharge Criteria

- Symptoms improving
- Taking oral medications

Issues for Referral

- Ophthalmologist if ocular disease
- Neurology consult for CNS disease
- Infectious diseases consult for systemic disease or HIV

PROGNOSIS

- Immunodeficient patients often relapse if treatment is stopped.
- Treatment may prevent the development of untoward sequelae in both symptomatic and asymptomatic infants with congenital toxoplasmosis.

COMPLICATIONS

- CNS toxoplasmosis: Seizure disorder or focal neurologic deficits
- Ocular toxoplasmosis: Partial or complete blindness
- Congenital toxoplasmosis: Multiple complications may occur, including
  – Mental retardation
  – Seizures
  – Deafness and blindness

PATIENT MONITORING

- Follow-up visits every 2 weeks until stable, then every 1–3 months during therapy
- CBC weekly for 1st month, then every 2–4 weeks
- Renal and liver function tests monthly

REFERENCES

1. Benson CA, et al. Treating opportunistic infections among HIV infected adults and adolescents. *Clin Infect Dis.* 2005;40:S138–S140.
2. Mofenson LM, et al. Treating opportunistic infections among HIV-exposed and infected children. *Clin Infect Dis.* 2005;40:S6–S8.
3. Katkama C, et al. Pyrimethamine-clindamycin vs pyrimethamine-sulfadiazine in acute and long term therapy for toxoplasmic encephalitis in patients with AIDS. *Clin Infect Dis.* 1996;22:268.
4. Montoya JG, Liesenfeld O. Toxoplasmosis. *Lancet.* 2004;363:1965–1976.

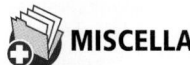 **MISCELLANEOUS**

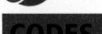

ICD9-CM

- 130.9 Toxoplasmosis, unspecified
- 771.2 Other congenital infections

PATIENT TEACHING

- Avoid raw or undercooked meats
- Pregnant women
  – Avoid raw meat products
  – Wash hands thoroughly after handling raw meats or cleaning cat litter boxes
  – Keep pet cats indoors and feed commercial cat food
  – Consider serologic testing in pregnancy
  – Counsel women who seroconvert in pregnancy of need for amniocentesis to assess fetal infection
- Immunocompromised patients
  – Prophylaxis is important because most cases represent reactivation of latent infection
  – Prophylaxis is important after treatment of acute infection to prevent recurrence
  – AIDS patients
    ○ Avoid raw meats
    ○ Glove and hand washing when cleaning litter box
    ○ Keep pet cats indoors and feed commercial cat food

 See Corresponding Diagnostic Algorithm

T

TRACHEITIS, BACTERIAL

Bruce T. Vanderhoff, MD
Ramon F. Fakhoury, MD

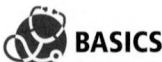 BASICS

DESCRIPTION

Acute, potentially life-threatening infraglottic bacterial infection following a primary viral infection, usually parainfluenzae or influenza viruses

- Direct laryngoscopy reveals subglottic edema compounded by thick, purulent exudate in larynx, trachea, and bronchi, sometimes causing pseudomembranes.
- System(s) Affected: Pulmonary
- Synonym(s): Pseudomembranous croup; Membranous tracheitis

EPIDEMIOLOGY

- Predominant age: Mean age 54 months; range 3 weeks to 168 months. Infections in adolescents and adults have been reported.
- Predominant sex: Male > Female some studies have shown a ratio as high as 5:1; others, 1:1)

ALERT

Pediatric Considerations

Typically affects children ages 3–5 years.

Incidence

- True incidence unknown
- First cases described prior to 1950; resurgence of cases has been noted since 1979
- Fall/winter predominance

RISK FACTORS

- Periods of increased seasonal activity of respiratory viruses
- Case reports following adenoidectomy

Genetics

No known genetic predisposition

ETIOLOGY

- *Staphylococcus aureus* (most common pediatric cause): Consider methicillin resistance (MRSA)
- *Haemophilus influenzae* type b
- *Streptococcus pyogenes*/group A streptococcus
- *Moraxella catarrhalis*
- Peptostreptococcus
- *Streptococcus pneumoniae*
- *Klebsiella pneumoniae*
- *Neisseria gonorrhea*

ASSOCIATED CONDITIONS

Consider anatomic abnormalities or foreign body as well as recent pharyngeal or laryngeal surgery.

DIAGNOSIS

SIGNS AND SYMPTOMS

- Barking, "brassy" cough
- Inspiratory stridor
- Variable degree of respiratory distress
- Child is usually lying flat
- Fever >38°C (100.4°F)
- Toxic appearing
- Gradual progression of mild upper airway symptoms over 1 hour to 6 days to an acute, febrile phase of rapid respiratory decompensation
- Voice and cry usually normal
- Absence of drooling and dysphagia help distinguish it from epiglottitis.
- Does not respond to aerosolized epinephrine (unlike patients with croup)
- Subglottic edema
- If intubated for viral croup, premembranous tracheitis "web" can obstruct distal airway beyond endotracheal tube

TESTS

Rapid antigen tests are available for bacteria and viruses in some centers.

Lab

- Elevated WBC count with predominance of polymorphonuclear leukocytes
- Band cells often present
- Blood cultures usually negative

Imaging

- Anterior-posterior and lateral neck x-rays show subglottic and tracheal narrowing with haziness and radio-opaque linear or particulate densities (crusts)
- In patients with risk of acute respiratory obstruction, either do not obtain x-rays or monitor carefully.
- Often see pneumonic infiltrates

Diagnostic Procedures/Surgery

- Endoscopy is diagnostic and demonstrates severe inflammation of subglottic region and trachea with copious mucopurulent secretions and sloughed epithelium that separates from tracheal wall in sheets
- Obtain Gram stain, aerobic and anaerobic cultures of tracheal secretions

Pathological Findings

- Mucosal destruction and/or local immunodeficiency caused by viral infection may predispose to bacterial infection.
- Intense inflammation, sloughing of subglottic epithelium, and profuse mucopurulent secretions, which compromise airway and make airway management difficult

DIFFERENTIAL DIAGNOSIS

- Laryngotracheobronchitis (viral)
- Epiglottitis
- Foreign-body aspiration
- Retropharyngeal abscess
- Pneumonia
- Asthma
- Spasmodic croup
- Diphtheritic laryngitis

TREATMENT

GENERAL MEASURES

- Admission to ICU
- Constitutes true pediatric emergency
- Maintain airway: Often difficult due to copious secretions
- Hydration, humidification, antibiotics
- Endotracheal or nasotracheal intubation usually needed, especially in infants and children <4 years. Much less likely to need intubation if child >8 years. Advantage of intubation is ability to clear trachea and bronchi of secretions and pseudomembranes.
- Vigorous pulmonary toilet to clear airway of secretion
- Does not respond to epinephrine

ALERT

Pregnancy Considerations

Scrupulous hand washing is recommended for prevention.

Diet

Parenteral nutrition or nasogastric tube feeding if intubated; oral nutrition otherwise

Activity

Complete bed rest

MEDICATION (DRUGS)

First Line
- Nafcillin 150 mg/kg/d q.i.d. *plus* cefotaxime 150 mg/kg/d in 4–6 divided doses; maximum of 2 g q6h
- Vancomycin for MRSA
- Ceftriaxone 75 mg/kg/d b.i.d. *plus* ampicillin-sulbactam 300 mg/kg/d q.i.d.
- Best single drug choice: Ticarcillin-clavulanate 3.1 g IV q4–6h for adults, 150 mg/kg/d IV q12h for children (maximum 18–24 g/d)
- Does not respond to epinephrine
- Narrow regimen when pathogens and sensitivities available
- Contraindications: Refer to the manufacturer's literature for each drug.
- Precautions: Refer to the manufacturer's literature for each drug.
- Significant possible interactions: Refer to the manufacturer's literature for each drug.

Second Line
For patients with penicillin allergy: Clindamycin 40 mg/kg/d q.i.d. *plus* chloramphenicol 75 mg/kg/d q.i.d.

SURGERY
- Tracheotomy may be necessary
- Membrane may require surgical removal

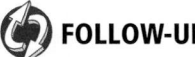 **FOLLOW-UP**

PROGNOSIS
- With vigorous airway management with or without intubation for up to 7 days, complete recovery is expected.
- Cardiopulmonary arrest and death have occurred.

COMPLICATIONS
- Postintubation subglottic stenosis
- Cardiopulmonary arrest
- Pneumonia
- Toxic shock syndrome secondary to enterotoxin-producing staphylococci

PATIENT MONITORING
ICU care with cardiopulmonary monitoring

REFERENCES

1. Ang JY, Ezike E, Asmer BI, Antibacterial resistance. *Indian J Pediatr*. 2004;71:229–239.
2. Berhman RE, Kliegman RM, Jenson HB, eds. *Nelson Textbook of Pediatrics*. 16th ed. Philadelphia, PA: WB Saunders; 2000.
3. Bernstein T, Brilli R, Jacobs B. Is bacterial tracheitis changing? A 14-month experience in a pediatric intensive care unit. *Clin Infect Dis*. 1998;27:458–462.
4. Brook I. Aerobic and anaerobic microbiology of bacterial tracheitis in children. *Clin Infect Dis*. 1995;20(suppl 2):S222–S223.
5. Burns JA, Brown J, Ogle JW. Group A streptococcal tracheitis associated with toxic shock syndrome. *Pediatr Infect Dis J*. 1998;17:933–935.
6. Cunningham MJ. The old and new of acute laryngotracheal infections. *Clinical Pediatr*. 1992;31:56–64.
7. Eid NS, Jones VF. Bacterial tracheitis as a complication of tonsillectomy and adenoidectomy. *J Pediatr*. 1994;125:401–402.

 MISCELLANEOUS

See also: Bronchiolitis; Common cold; Epiglottitis

CODES

ICD9-CM
- 464.10 Acute tracheitis without mention of obstruction
- 464.20 Acute laryngotracheitis without mention of obstruction
- 464.11 Acute tracheitis with obstruction
- 464.21 Acute laryngotracheitis with obstruction

PATIENT TEACHING

Usually requires 3–7 days of hospitalization, with complete recovery expected

T

TRANSFUSION REACTION

Ruben Peralta, MD, FACS
Sarah Guzofski, MD

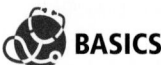 **BASICS**

DESCRIPTION
The transfusion of blood products can cause numerous serious complications, even death. Adverse reactions to blood products may occur by immune or non-immune mechanisms.

- Immune: Acute, febrile, allergic, transfusion-related acute lung injury (TRALI)
- Non-immune
  - Acute: Circulatory overload, bacterial contamination, and other effects, including hyperkalemia, hypocalcemia, acidosis, coagulopathy, hypothermia
  - Chronic: Viral infection (cytomegalovirus human T-cell leukemia virus, HTLV, HIV, hepatitis), hemosiderosis

ALERT
Pediatric Considerations
Reaction greater and outlook poorer in the very young

Geriatric Considerations
Higher risk of complications in the elderly

GENERAL PREVENTION
- Follow procedures for sample and blood labeling and patient identification. Two practitioners, and if possible, patient should verify that blood product and patient identity match. (1)[C]
- Obtain detailed history of patient's responses to previous transfusions
- Risk/benefit of any transfusion needs to favor benefit
- Autologous transfusion
- Use matched blood whenever possible; if not possible, thoroughly check universal blood for agglutination titer
- Observe patient closely during transfusion with serial vital signs
- Consider leukocyte-depleted blood in people with history of recurrent febrile reactions
- Avoid prophylactic antipyretics
- Use genotype-specific RBCs in sickle cell anemia
- Blood bank screening for bacteria and viruses

EPIDEMIOLOGY
- Frequency of immunologic reaction per unit of blood
  - Allergic 1:100
  - Febrile 1:100
  - Delayed hemolytic 1:1600
  - Acute hemolytic 1:50,000
  - Fatal hemolytic reaction 1:500,000
- Infectious complications per unit of blood
  - Hepatitis B 1:81,000
  - HTLV-1 1:642,000
  - Hepatitis C: 1:1,600,000
  - HIV-1 1:2,000,000

RISK FACTORS
- Multiple blood transfusions
- Rh-negative mother
- Multiple pregnancies

Genetics
No known genetic pattern

ETIOLOGY
- Acute hemolytic transfusion reaction
  - When ABO-incompatible blood is transfused, donor erythrocytes are destroyed by recipient's pre-formed antibodies causing intravascular hemolysis.
  - Most commonly, when group O recipients receive non-group O blood; IgM antibodies to group A and B antigens fix complement and cause rapid hemolysis
  - Often due to clerical error, misidentification of blood product or patient
- Febrile nonhemolytic transfusion reaction: Caused by recipient antibodies to leukocytes in unit of red cells, prevented by leukoreduction
- Anaphylactic: Reaction to a transfusion that contains plasma, theory that this is a reaction to IgA in donor blood in IgA-deficient patient has been called into question (2)[C]
- Urticarial: IgE antibodies in recipient react with allergen in donor's plasma
- Delayed reactions can occur in patients sensitized to an antigen by prior transfusions or pregnancy. It may be difficult to detect because antibody titer falls after initial sensitization, reaction 2–10 days after transfusion.
- TRALI: Begins with neutrophil adhesion to pulmonary endothelium, leading to endothelial damage and increased capillary permeability

ASSOCIATED CONDITIONS
- Disseminated intravascular coagulation
- Shock
- Acute renal failure

DIAGNOSIS

SIGNS AND SYMPTOMS
- Acute hemolytic transfusion reaction
  - Anxiety
  - Flushing
  - Tachycardia
  - Hypotension
  - Chest, back, or flank pain
  - Tachypnea
  - Dyspnea
  - Fever
  - Chills
  - NOTE: Symptoms masked in anesthetized patient, may see red-tinged urine
- Delayed (extravascular) hemolytic transfusion reaction
  - Fever
  - Anemia (2–14 days after transfusion)
  - Jaundice
- TRALI: Range of symptoms from cough to life-threatening respiratory distress, can appear similar to acute respiratory distress syndrome

TESTS
Lab
Acute hemolytic transfusion reaction

- Positive direct antiglobulin test (Coombs)
- Plasma obtained 2–4 hours after lysis is red or pink, indicating free hemoglobin
- Elevated serum bilirubin (mild)
- Elevated lactate dehydrogenase
- Reduced serum haptoglobin
- Wine-colored urine indicating hemoglobinuria
- Additional lab tests for immune reactions, including blood bank incompatibility evaluation
- Tissue factor released from lysed RBCs can initiate disseminated intravascular coagulation; platelet count and coagulation studies should be monitored
- Monitor blood urea nitrogen, creatinine given risk of renal failure

DIFFERENTIAL DIAGNOSIS
Other causes of acute hemolysis

- Autoimmune diseases
- Hemoglobinopathies
- RBC enzyme defects
- Bacterial contamination of stored blood

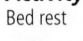

TREATMENT

GENERAL MEASURES

- Follow hospital protocol for evaluation of transfusion reactions
- Stop transfusion immediately upon first sign of reaction
- IV normal saline to support blood pressure and adequate urine output, especially in DIC
- Avoid lactated Ringer's solution
- Repeat thorough evaluation of transfusion paperwork to rule out any clerical error (a common cause of an ABO-incompatible transfusion)
- Monitor vital signs.
- Recognize and treat disseminated intravascular coagulation if it occurs.
- Supportive therapy, maintain blood pressure using vasopressors in indicated airway
- For TRALI, patients may require ventilatory support. Use of corticosteroids and diuretics is controversial. (3)[C]

Diet
As tolerated

Activity
Bed rest

MEDICATION (DRUGS)

First Line
- Oxygen and ventilation support, as needed
- Epinephrine for anaphylaxis
- Corticosteroids may be helpful to reduce inflammation
- Normal saline and/or vasopressors to maintain systolic blood pressure
- Treat DIC if present, including supportive therapy and possibly heparin
- Diphenhydramine for urticarial reaction

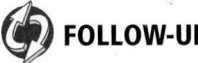

FOLLOW-UP

PROGNOSIS
- Usual course: Acute
- Usually no harm if transfusion stopped at onset of manifestations
- TRALI: Can appear similar to acute respiratory distress syndrome but has a better prognosis; 10% mortality, generally self-limited with supportive care

COMPLICATIONS
- Uremia, oliguria, anuria
- Right heart failure
- Respiratory failure
- Multiorgan dysfunction syndrome

PATIENT MONITORING
Until hemolytic signs are gone

REFERENCES

1. Bryan S. Hemolytic transfusion reaction: Safeguards for practice. *J Perianesth Nurs*. 2002;17:399–403.
2. Gilstad CW. Anaphylactic transfusion reactions. *Curr Opin Hematol*. 2003;10:419–423.
3. Bux J. Transfusion-related acute lung injury (TRALI): A serious adverse event of blood transfusion. *Vox Sanguinis*. 2005;89(1);1–10.
4. Herbert PC, et al. Is a low transfusion threshold safe in critically ill patients with cardiovascular disease? *Crit Care Med*. 2001;29:227–234.

MISCELLANEOUS

Post-transfusion Purpura: Delayed thrombocytopenia (7–10 days after platelet transfusion), due to production of antibodies to donor or recipient platelets, more common in women. Treat with IV immunoglobulin or plasmapheresis. Avoid additional platelet transfusions, which may worsen thrombocytopenia

CODES

ICD9-CM
- 999.6 ABO Incompatibility reaction
- 999.8 Other transfusion reaction

PATIENT TEACHING

Before starting a transfusion, give the patient instructions to report any unusual symptoms (e.g., rash, itching, or fever) to the nursing staff immediately.

T

TRANSIENT ISCHEMIC ATTACK (TIA)

Vladimir Hachinski, MD, DSc
Vivek Jain, MD

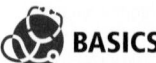

BASICS

DESCRIPTION
Sudden onset of focal and transient (<24 hours) neurological deficit due to brain ischemia
- System(s) Affected: Nervous
- Synonym(s): Mini-stroke

GENERAL PREVENTION
- Counseling toward cessation of smoking
- Strict control of medical risk factors (e.g., diabetes, hypertension, hyperlipidemia, cardiac disease)
- Antiplatelet therapy
- Angiotensin-converting enzyme inhibitors
- Statins
- Treat homocystinemia with vitamin B_6, vitamin B_{12}, and folic acid
- Anticoagulation when high risk of cardioembolism (e.g., atrial fibrillation)

EPIDEMIOLOGY
- Predominant age: Risk increases >45 years; highest in 7th and 8th decades
- Predominant sex: Male > Female (3:1)

Incidence
30/100,000

RISK FACTORS
- Hypertension
- Cardiac disease
- Smoking
- Diabetes
- Antiphospholipid antibodies
- Family history
- Hypercholesterolemia
- Atrial fibrillation
- Homocystinemia

Genetics
Inheritance is polygenic with tendency to clustering of risk factors within families

ETIOLOGY
- Carotid atherosclerotic disease with artery-to-artery thromboembolism
- Small, deep vessel disease associated with hypertension
- Cardiac
  - Cardioembolism secondary to valvular (mitral valve) pathology
  - Mural hypokinesias or akinesias with thrombosis (acute anterior myocardial infarctions or congestive cardiomyopathies)
  - Cardiac arrhythmia (atrial fibrillation)
- Hypercoagulable states
  - Antiphospholipid antibodies
  - Deficiency of protein S, protein C
  - Presence of antithrombin 3
  - Oral contraceptives
  - Associated with pregnancy and parturition
- Other causes
  - Spontaneous and posttraumatic (e.g., chiropractic manipulation) arterial dissection
  - Fibromuscular dysplasia

ALERT
Pediatric Considerations
- Cardiac (especially developmental abnormalities)
- Metabolic: Homocystinuria, Fabry disease
- Atrial fibrillation is frequent cause among the elderly

ASSOCIATED CONDITIONS
- Atrial fibrillation
- Other cardiac disease

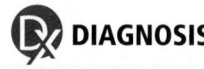

DIAGNOSIS

SIGNS AND SYMPTOMS
- Carotid circulation (hemispheric): Monocular visual loss, hemiplegia, hemianesthesia, neglect, aphasia, visual field defects (less often: Headaches, seizures, amnesia, confusion)
- Vertebrobasilar (brainstem or cerebellar): Bilateral visual obscuration, diplopia, vertigo, ataxia, facial paresis, Horner syndrome, dysphagia, dysarthria; also headache, nausea, vomiting, and ataxia

TESTS
Lab
- International normalized ratio (INR) and partial thromboplastin time (PTT) (coumadin prolongs INR)
- Antiphospholipid antibodies

Imaging
- Duplex carotid ultrasonography
- ECG
- Angiography
  - Cerebral
  - Carotid arterial stenosis
- Transthoracic echocardiogram; if normal and cardiac source is suspected, follow with transesophageal echocardiogram
- Holter monitoring
- CT of head: Acute phase
- Brain MRI, include diffusion-weighted imaging
- MR angiography: Brain and blood vessels
- EEG, if suspecting seizure

DIFFERENTIAL DIAGNOSIS
- Migraine (hemiplegic)
- Focal seizure (Todd paralysis)
- Hypoglycemia

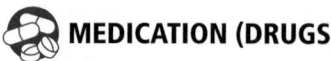

TREATMENT

GENERAL MEASURES
- Acute phase
  - Outpatient for investigations
  - Inpatient for surgery and high-risk groups
- Antithrombotic therapy

Diet
As appropriate to underlying medical problems (e.g., diabetic, low-fat, or low-salt diet)

Activity
No restrictions

MEDICATION (DRUGS)

First Line
- Enteric coated aspirin: 50–325 mg/d *or*
- Clopidogrel (Plavix): 75 mg/d
  - Ticlopidine's descendent
  - Has fewer side effects than Ticlopidine
  - Shows slight advantage over aspirin
- Dipyridamole-aspirin (Aggrenox): 1 capsule PO b.i.d.
  - Each capsule contains 200 mg extended-release dipyridamole and 25 mg immediate-release aspirin
  - More efficacious than aspirin alone, but more costly
- Warfarin (INR-adjusted dose): For patients with atrial fibrillation and cardioembolic stroke

Second Line
- Ticlopidine (Ticlid): 250 mg PO b.i.d.; fallen out of favor due to unfavorable side-effect profile
- Contraindications
  - Enteric coated aspirin: Active peptic ulcer disease, hypersensitivity to aspirin, previous bronchospastic reaction to aspirin or other NSAIDs
  - Warfarin: Intolerance or allergy, dementia, liver disease, active bleeding, pregnancy, recent head injury
  - Ticlopidine: Known hypersensitivity to the drug, presence of hematopoietic disorders, presence of hemostatic disorder, conditions associated with active bleeding, severe liver dysfunction

- Precautions
  - Enteric coated aspirin: May aggravate pre-existing peptic ulcer disease; may worsen symptoms in some patients with asthma
  - Warfarin: May cause poor balance, which can be dangerous for people with alcohol/drug problems or >80 years
  - Clopidogrel and ticlopidine: TTP can occur
  - Ticlopidine: 2.4% of patients develop neutropenia (0.8% severe), which is reversible with cessation of drug. Monitor blood counts every 2 weeks for first 3 months.
- Significant possible interactions
  - Enteric coated aspirin: May potentiate effects of anticoagulants and sulfonylurea, hypoglycemic agents
  - Warfarin: Aspirin, NSAIDs, antibiotics, tranquilizers
  - Ticlopidine: Digoxin plasma levels decreased 15%, theophylline half-life increased from 8.6–12.2 hours

SURGERY
In medically fit patients with nondisabling stroke: Carotid endarterectomy

- Carotid artery stenosis 70–99%: Indicated on side ipsilateral to stroke
- Carotid artery stenosis 50–69%: Of modest benefit; depends on risk factors
- Carotid artery stenosis <50%: North American Symptomatic Carotid Endarterectomy Trial showed no benefit above medical therapy alone

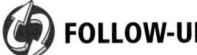 **FOLLOW-UP**

PROGNOSIS
- The risk of stroke on the ipsilateral side within 1 year and cumulative thereafter is 5–20%.
- Frequency increases with addition of multiple risk factors and severity of carotid stenosis
- The major cause of death in the first 5 years is cardiac disease.

COMPLICATIONS
- Stroke
- Seizure
- Trauma if patient experiences sudden fall due to weakness

PATIENT MONITORING
Follow-up every 3 months for 1st year, then yearly

REFERENCES
1. Hachinski V. Stroke. *Lancet*. 1998;352(Suppl 3):S1S30.
2. Hachinski V. *Brain Attack: The Clinical Handbook*. Guelph, Canada: Meducom International; 1999.

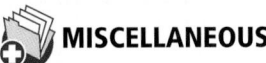 **MISCELLANEOUS**

See also: Stroke (Brain Attack)

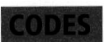 **CODES**

ICD9-CM
435.9 Unspecified transient cerebral ischemia

PATIENT TEACHING
National Stroke Association, 9707 East Easter Lane, Englewood, CO 80112; (800) STROKES.

 See Corresponding Diagnostic Algorithm

 See Patient Handout on CD

T

TRICHINELLOSIS

Kenton I. Voorhees, MD, FAAFP

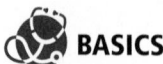 **BASICS**

DESCRIPTION

Trichinellosis is a parasitic disease that develops after ingesting infected pork or other meat containing viable cysts of *Trichinella spiralis*, a nematode, with rarer cases attributable to several different species of *Trichinella*. Cysts remain viable and can cause disease when infected meat is undercooked. Most common outbreaks are attributable to undercooked pork, homemade and commercial sausage, wild boar, bear, walrus, and other wild-animal meats. Horsemeat has become another important source in the European Union.

- Enteric phase: Phase I
  - Cysts broken down by digestive acid and pepsin in stomach, freeing larvae, which develop into mature adult worms in upper to middle small intestine
  - Takes about 1 week after ingestion; may last 3–5 weeks
- Systemic phase: Phase II
  - Female worms then release newborn larvae that migrate through blood vessels and lymphatics to multiple organ systems
  - Occurs 2–3 weeks after ingestion; may last for 2 months
- Muscular encystment phase: Phase III
  - Larvae become encysted in striated skeletal and sometimes cardiac muscle, where they form a nurse cell that functions to nourish them and protect them from host immunity
  - Complex can survive in humans up to 30 years
  - Intramuscular cysts usually eventually calcify
- System(s) Affected: Gastrointestinal; Musculoskeletal
- Synonym(s): Trichinelliasis

ALERT

Pregnancy Considerations

Although not much information is available, 1 case has been reported of an infected woman 16 weeks pregnant who delivered a normal child without complications or evidence of problems.

GENERAL PREVENTION

- Avoid eating undercooked pork and game meat
- Prolonged freezing may be effective, but less so for wild-game meat

EPIDEMIOLOGY

- Predominant age: 20–49, although cases reported from all age groups
- Predominant sex: Male = Female

Incidence

- From 1997–2001, on average, 12 cases were reported annually in the United States. (1)
- Higher incidence in Alaska and northeastern United States
- Most mild cases probably undiagnosed, based on autopsy studies.

RISK FACTORS

- Access to wild game, homemade pork products, noncommercial sources of meat
- Eating pigs that were fed uncooked garbage
- Undercooking pork
- Eating inadequately cooked or frozen wild game
- Ethnic groups from Southeast Asia raising their own pork or favoring partially cooked pork products
- Residence in Alaska and northeastern United States

ETIOLOGY

Eating undercooked meat that is infected with viable *Trichenella* cysts

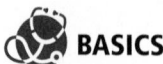 **DIAGNOSIS**

SIGNS AND SYMPTOMS

Signs and symptoms begin within 1 week of ingesting infected meat

- Common symptoms (can occur concurrently)
  - Diarrhea: Mostly phase I
  - Abdominal cramping: Mostly phase I
  - Fever: Mostly phase II and III
  - Myalgias: Mostly phase II and III
  - Eosinophilia: Mostly phase II and III
  - Periorbital edema: Mostly phase II and III
  - Weakness: Mostly phase II and III
- Less common symptoms: Mostly phase II and III
  - Conjunctivitis
  - Subconjunctival hemorrhage
  - Retinal hemorrhages
  - Maculopapular rash
  - Splinter hemorrhages
  - Headache
  - Photophobia
  - Pneumonitis
  - Tachycardia
  - Heart failure
  - Pericardial effusion
  - CNS involvement
- Symptoms depend on number of ingested infective larvae and phase of parasitic invasion
  - Light infections: <10 larvae per gram of muscle; usually asymptomatic
  - Heavy infections: >50 larvae per gram of muscle; can be life threatening
  - Skeletal muscle (gastrocnemius, masseter, diaphragm, biceps, lower back, extraocular muscles, jaw and neck) is most frequent site of symptoms due to larval migration; however, in severe cases myocardial damage, pulmonary infiltration, and focal neurologic damage can occur

History

A history of having eaten undercooked pork or wild game meat.

TESTS

Lab

- Serologic tests for *T. spiralis*, IgM, and IgG
- Enzyme linked immunosorbent assay IgM and IgG
- Bentonite flocculation after 3rd week for parasite-specific antibody
- Indirect immunofluorescence
- Complement fixation
- DNA testing: Random amplified polymorphic DNA, polymerase chain reaction
- Antibody levels
  - Often not detectable until 3–5 weeks post infection, high false negative rate in phase I
  - Peak 3rd month
  - Remain detectable 2–3 years
- Antibody testing
  - Testing 15–22% false negative in phase I
  - Paired specimens helpful, 1–2 months apart; look for 4-fold increase in titer
- Eosinophilia (>600/mm^3), with leukocytosis
- Increased creatine phosphate kinase
- Increased lactate dehydrogenase
- Hypergammaglobulinemia
- Elevated erythrocyte sedimentation rate (several weeks)
- Urinalysis may show myoglobinuria
- Drugs that may alter lab results: Rare increases in serum glutamic-oxaloacetic transaminase with thiabendazole

Imaging

- CT may help see calcified muscle cysts
- MRI may help in evaluation of neurologic complications
- Chest x-ray may detect patchy infiltrates
- Extremity x-ray may show calcified densities

Diagnostic Procedures/Surgery

Muscle biopsy of gastrocnemius or deltoid with ≥1 gram of muscle, including examination between compressed slides (higher detection rate)

Pathological Findings

Larvae on muscle biopsy (often gastrocnemius); absence of larvae does not exclude diagnosis; rarely find worm in stool

DIFFERENTIAL DIAGNOSIS

- Acute rheumatic fever
- Arthritis
- Angioedema
- Botulism
- Collagen vascular disease
- Dermatomyositis
- Encephalitis
- Eosinophilia-myalgia syndrome
- Gastroenteritis
- Idiopathic hypereosinophilic syndrome
- Idiopathic polymyositis
- Influenza
- Meningitis
- Pneumonitis
- Polyarteritis nodosa
- Polymyositis
- Typhoid fever
- Tuberculosis

TREATMENT

GENERAL MEASURES
- Outpatient unless complications such as cardiac, pulmonary, or neurological
- May call the centers for disease control and prevention (CDC) for appropriate diagnostic tests: (404) 639-3311
- Bedrest
- Antipyretics
- Analgesics

Diet
As tolerated

Activity
- As tolerated
- Bed rest may help muscular pain.

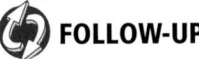 **MEDICATION (DRUGS)**

First Line
- For early intestinal phase (presenting in the 1st 1–2 weeks), to treat adult worms
  – Mebendazole may be used 200–400 mg t.i.d. for 3 days, then 400–500 mg t.i.d. × 10 days, adults and children > 2 years (2)[C]
  – Albendazole: 400 mg b.i.d. for 8–14 days, adults and children > 2 years (2)[C]
  – Pyrantel may be used 10–20 mg/kg body weight, repeated 2–3 days for pregnant women and children (3)[C]
  – No drugs are very effective against larvae once they are encysted in muscle; however, they may halt further dissemination.
- Call the CDC for current dosage and recommendations (404) 639-3311.
- Severe cases: Corticosteroids, such as prednisone 40–60 mg/d for 3–5 days; taper as symptoms subside, particularly to help decrease inflammation when there are signs of myocarditis, neurologic disease, pulmonary insufficiency, or severe myositis
- Analgesics, NSAIDS, anti-pyretics may be helpful as needed
- Contraindications: Corticosteroids have been reported to be contraindicated in the intestinal phase, as they could prolong the phase.
- Precautions: Minimal experience exists with the use of medications in small children and in pregnancy. Mebendazole should not be given during the 1st trimester, and any medications should only be used if absolutely necessary.
- Significant possible interactions
  – Carbamazepine or alcohol may decrease the effect of mebendazole.
  – Cimetidine may increase the level of mebendazole.

Second Line
Thiabendazole: Used to be drug of choice at 25 mg/kg b.i.d. for 1 week, maximum dose 1.5 gm; replaced by the drugs previously mentioned because they have fewer side effects and are equally effective.

SURGERY
Pacemaker has been required on occasion for severe myocarditis

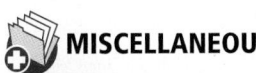 **FOLLOW-UP**

Admission Criteria
- Admit if cardiac, pulmonary or neurologic manifestations
- Pregnancy

PROGNOSIS
- Most infections are asymptomatic, short-lived, and generally have an uneventful recovery without medication.
- Prognosis good in most cases, although 5–10% of the cases can be severe.
- No clear evidence that chronic trichinosis exists.
- <1% of cases can be fatal, generally around 4th–8th week, as a result of cardiac failure or pneumonia

COMPLICATIONS
- Meningitis
- Subcortical infarcts
- Encephalitis
- Myocarditis with congestive heart failure
- Nephritis
- Glomerulonephritis
- Sinusitis
- Pneumonitis
- Ocular
- Prenancy: Abortion, premature delivery
- Death: Typically cardiac or thromboembolic events

PATIENT MONITORING
Monitor the patient for signs and symptoms of complications, such as cardiac, neurological, and pulmonary.

REFERENCES
1. Roy SL, et al. Trichinellosis surveillance—United States, 1997–2001. *MMWR Surveill Summ.* 2003;52(6):1–8.
2. Abramowicz M, ed. *The Medical Letter on Drugs and Therapeutics. Drugs for Parasitic Infections.* New Rochelle, NY: The Medical Letter, 2004
3. Kociecka W. Trichinellosis: Human disease, diagnosis and treatment. *Vet Parisitol.* 2000,93(3–4):365–383.
4. Dupouy-Camet J, et al. Opinion on the diagnosis and treatment of human trichinellosis. *Expert Opin Pharmacother.* 2002;3(8):1117–1130.
5. Bruschi F. New aspects of human trichinellosis: The impact of new Trichinella species. *Postgrad Med J.* 2002;78(915):15–22.

MISCELLANEOUS

CODES

ICD9-CM
124 Trichinosis

PATIENT TEACHING
- Manage complications as appropriate.
- Cook potentially contaminated meat, such as pork, to 170°F (77°C) until no longer pink.
- Freeze at -15°C for 21 days (longer if meat is >15 cm thick); however, *Trichinella* larvae in wild game may be resistant to freezing.
- Do not feed hogs uncooked garbage.

TRICHOMONIASIS

George R. Bergus, MD

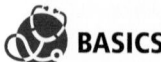 **BASICS**

DESCRIPTION
Infection with *Trichomonas vaginalis*, a pear-shaped protozoan parasite that is a facultative anaerobe
- Found in men and women at genitourinary sites
- Incubation period: 3–28 days
- Transmission rarely seen in female children of infected women
- System(s) Affected: Renal/Urologic; Reproductive
- Synonym(s): Trick; Trichomonal urethritis

GENERAL PREVENTION
Practice safe sex by using condoms.

EPIDEMIOLOGY
- Makes up 10–25% of vaginal infections
- Predominant age: Young and middle-aged adults:
  - Rare until onset of sexual activity
  - Uncommon in prepubertal children; confirmed diagnosis should raise concern of sexual abuse
  - Not uncommon in postmenopausal women; older people remain at risk
- Predominant sex: Both affected, but women more commonly symptomatic

Incidence
- First-time diagnosis: 300/100,000 women/year
- Any diagnosis: 600/100,000 women/year
- Among special populations
  - Sexually active adult women in a family-planning clinic: 2,000/100,000
  - Sexually active adult women in a sexually transmitted disease (STD) clinic: 35,000/100,000

RISK FACTORS
- Multiple sexual partners
- Trichomonas can be identified in 30–40% of the male sexual partners of infected women.

ETIOLOGY
Trichomonas vaginalis: Usually sexually transmitted, although a nonvenereal route is possible, as the organism survives for several hours in a moist environment.

ASSOCIATED CONDITIONS
Other STDs

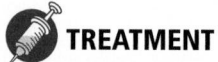 **DIAGNOSIS**

SIGNS AND SYMPTOMS
- Female
  - 40% of patients can be asymptomatic at the time of the diagnosis.
  - Symptoms typically begin or worsen at the time of the menstrual period.
  - Vaginal discharge: 75%; usually copious, and can be frothy; sometimes watery and pooling
  - Vulvovaginal irritation: 50%
  - Dysuria: 50%
  - Vaginal odor: 10%
  - "Strawberry cervix" from punctate hemorrhages: 5%
  - Vaginal hyperemia
  - Dyspareunia
  - Suprapubic discomfort
  - Cervical erosion
- Male
  - Asymptomatic: 80%
  - Symptomatic: 20%; urethral discharge, dysuria, epididymitis (rare)

TESTS
Lab
- Culture: Sensitivity >95% but takes 4–7 days
- Enzyme linked immunosorbent assay and direct fluorescent antibody tests: Sensitivity 80–90%
- Rapid diagnostic kits using polymerase chain reaction DNA probes: Sensitivity 97%, specificity 98%
- Female
  - Wet prep: Sensitivity 60–70%, specificity 100%. Sensitivity reduced with loss of motility due to cooling, low inoculum size, and rapid scanning of the slide. Usually shows many more polymorphonuclear leukocytes (PMNs) than epithelial cells.
  - Pap smear: Sensitivity 60%, specificity 99%
  - The vaginal pH is >4.5 in 90% of women.
- Male: Wet prep and culture of urethral discharge after prostatic exam; sensitivity 50–80%

DIFFERENTIAL DIAGNOSIS
- Female: Vaginal candidiasis, bacterial vaginosis; cervical inflammation can lead to mistaken diagnosis of cervicitis
- Male: *Chlamydia urethritis*

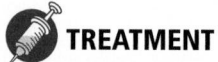 **TREATMENT**

INITIAL STABILIZATION
Outpatient

GENERAL MEASURES
Medication for both patient and partner(s)

Diet
Abstention from alcohol if metronidazole used for therapy

Activity
Sexual activity should not be resumed until patient and partner are both treated.

MEDICATION (DRUGS)

First Line
- Metronidazole
  - Adult dose: 2 g at one time or 500 mg b.i.d. for 7 days
  - Both routines effective in women, but one-time dose has higher failure rate in men
  - All sexual partners need treatment.
- Contraindications: 1st trimester pregnancy or allergy to the antibiotic
- Precautions: Avoid metronidazole or reduce dosage in patients with liver failure
- Significant possible interactions: Ethanol, warfarin, disulfiram, phenobarbital

Second Line
- For treatment failure after first line metronidazole dose, the Centers for Disease Control and Prevention (CDC) recommends 2 g metronidazole daily for 3–5 days. If repeated failure, consider non-compliance, re-infection, or susceptibility testing through the CDC.
- Tinidazole: 2 g at one time (has enhanced activity and fewer side effects)
- Clotrimazole
  - 100 mg vaginal tablets at bedtime for 14 days
  - Cure rate: 20–25%, but will reduce symptoms in most women
- Alternatively, saline or vinegar douching can be tried.

ALERT
Pregnancy Considerations
- Do not use metronidazole in 1st trimester.
- Treatment of the infection during pregnancy does not prevent preterm labor.

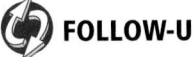 **FOLLOW-UP**

PROGNOSIS
Good, but recurrent infection raises possibility of noncompliance with therapy, reinfection, or infection with resistant organism. If resistance suspected, try metronidazole 2 g daily for 3–5 days.

COMPLICATIONS
Recurrent infections.

PATIENT MONITORING
- Monitor target symptoms.
- No follow-up needed if symptoms resolve with treatment

REFERENCES

1. The Centers for Disease Control and Prevention (CDC). 2002 Sexually transmitted disease treatment guidelines. *MMWR*. 2002;51(RR-6):1–84.
2. Forna F, Gulmezogly AM. Interventions for treating trichomoniasis in women. *Cochrane Database Syst Rev*. 2003:CD000218.
3. Okun N, et al. Antibiotics for bacterial vaginosis or Trichomonas vaginalis in pregnancy: A systematic review. *Obstet Gynecol*. 2005;105(4):857–868.
4. Sobel JK. Vaginitis. *N Engl J Med*. 1997;337: 1896–1903.
5. Klebanoff MA, et al. Failure of metronidazole to prevent preterm labor. *N Engl J Med*. 2001;345:487–493.

 MISCELLANEOUS

See also: Abnormal pap smear; Vulvovaginitis, bacterial

CODES

ICD9-CM
- 131.9 Trichomoniasis, unspecified
- 131.01 Trichomonal vulvovaginitis
- 131.00 Urogenital trichomoniasis, unspecified

PATIENT TEACHING
- Education about the venereal aspect of the infection
- Discussion about safe sex during health maintenance visits
- Internet education resources
  - National Institutes of Health: www.niaid.nih.gov//factsheets/stdvag.htm
  - Planned Parenthood: www.plannedparenthood.org/womenshealth/vaginitis.htm
  - Family Doctor Web site: http://familydoctor.org/handouts/275.html
  - American Social Health Association: www.ashastd.org/std/vaginit.html

 See Corresponding Diagnostic Algorithm

 See Patient Handout on CD

T

TRIGEMINAL NEURALGIA

Michael D. Perloff, MD, PhD

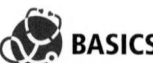 BASICS

DESCRIPTION
Disorder of sensory nucleus of 5th cranial nerve (trigeminal nerve), producing episodic, paroxysmal, severe, lancinating facial pain lasting seconds to minutes, followed by pain-free period in distribution of one or more of nerve divisions.

- Often precipitated by stimulation of well-defined, ipsilateral trigger zones, usually perioral, perinasal, and occasionally intraoral (e.g., washing, shaving)
- System(s) Affected: Nervous
- Synonym(s): Tic douloureux; Fothergill neuralgia; Trifacial neuralgia

EPIDEMIOLOGY
- Predominant age: Over age 50 years, incidence increases with age. (1,2)[A] Rare <35 years (consider another primary disease; *see Etiology*)
- Predominant sex: Female > Male (2:1)[1A]

Incidence
- 4.3/100 000/year (1)[A]
  - 5.9/100 000/year for women (1)[A]
  - 3.4/100 000/year for men (1)[A]
- >70, ~25.6/100 000/year (1)[A]

Prevalence
16/100,000 (1)[B]

ALERT
Pediatric Considerations
Unusual in childhood

RISK FACTORS
Unknown

ETIOLOGY
- Compression of trigeminal nerve by anomalous arteries or veins of posterior fossa, usually superior cerebral artery compressing trigeminal root, with cascade changes of sensory neurons occurring over days to weeks (2,3)
- Etiology classification
  - Idiopathic
  - Secondary: Cerebellopontine angle tumors (e.g., meningioma); tumors of 5th nerve (e.g., neuroma, vascular malformations), trauma, demyelinating disease (e.g., multiple sclerosis [MS])

ASSOCIATED CONDITIONS
- Sjögren syndrome
- Rheumatoid arthritis
- Chronic meningitis
- Facial migraine
- Acute polyneuropathy
- MS
- Hemifacial spasm
- Pretrigeminal neuralgia
- Charcot-Marie-tooth neuropathy
- Glossopharyngeal neuralgia

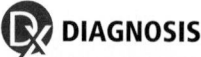 DIAGNOSIS

SIGNS AND SYMPTOMS
- Unilateral (rarely bilateral, unless secondary to MS)
- Symptoms rarely present at night
- Excruciating lip and/or gum and/or facial pain
- Paroxysmal facial pain
- Wincing, facial tic
- Pain elicited by tickle or touch
- Flushing
- Lacrimation
- Salivation
- Pain bursts several seconds to minutes, with refractory period after
- Slight right > left side preference (1)[C]
- 2nd-, 3rd-, 1st (rare) division trigeminal nerve most commonly affected (2,3)[A]

History
- Paroxysmal facial pain
- Pain elicited by tickle or touch

Physical Exam
All exam findings are typically negative due to paroxysmal nature of disorder

TESTS
Imaging
- MRI or CT scan: Neoplasm in cerebellopontine angle must be ruled out. Special MRA technique of collapsed MRA superimposed on routine spin echo T-1-weighted images
- No positive findings are significantly correlated with diagnosis (2,3)

Pathological Findings
- Trigeminal nerve: Inflammatory changes, demyelination, and degenerative changes (2)
- Trigeminal ganglion: Hypermyelination and microneuromata (3)

DIFFERENTIAL DIAGNOSIS
- Other forms of neuralgia usually have sensory loss. Presence of sensory loss nearly excludes diagnosis of trigeminal neuralgia (if younger patient, frequently MS).
- Neoplasia in cerebellopontine angle
- Vascular malformation of brain stem
- Demyelinating lesion (MS is diagnosed in 2–4% of patients with trigeminal neuralgia) (2)
- Vascular insult
- Migraine, cluster headache
- Giant cell arteritis
- Post-herpetic neuralgia
- Chronic meningitis
- Acute polyneuropathy
- Atypical odontalgia
- SUNCT syndrome (short-lasting, unilateral, neuralgiform pain with conjunctival injection)

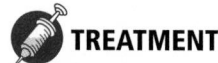 TREATMENT

GENERAL MEASURES
- Outpatient
- Drug treatment is 1st approach. Invasive procedures for patients who cannot tolerate, or fail to respond to, or relapse after chronic, drug treatment
- Avoidance of stimulation (air, heat, cold) of trigger zones (lips, cheeks, gums)

Diet
No special diet

Activity
Full activity

SPECIAL THERAPY
Radiotherapy
Stereotactic radiosurgery has been shown to be effective after drug failure

- Minimal clinically effective dose: 70 Gy
- 75% of patients achieve complete relief within 3 months; by 3 years, 50% maintain complete relief (NNT = 2) (4)[B]
- Most common side effect: Sensory disturbance (corneal numbness)

Complementary and Alternative Medicine
Acupuncture, moxibustion (herb): Poor evidence

MEDICATION (DRUGS)

First Line
- Carbamazepine (Tegretol)
  - Starting dose 100–200 mg b.i.d.; effective dose usually 200 mg q.i.d.; 1,200 mg/d maximum
  - 70–90% of patients initially respond; by 3 years, 30% no longer helped (number needed to treat [NNT] = 1.8) (5)[A]
  - Most common side effect: Sedation
- Contraindications: Monoamine oxidase (MAO) inhibitors, taken concurrently
- Precautions: Use with caution in the presence of liver disease.
- Significant possible interactions: Macrolide antibiotics, oral anticoagulants, anticonvulsants, tricyclics, oral contraceptives, steroids, digitalis, isonazid, monoamine oxidase (MAO) inhibitors, methyprylon nabilone, nizatidine, other H_2 blockers, phenytoin, propoxyphene, benzodiazepines, calcium channel blockers
- Oxacarbazepine (Trileptal)
  - Starting dose 150–300 mg b.i.d.; effective dose usually 375 mg b.i.d.; 1,200 mg/d maximum
  - Efficacy similar to carbamazepine (5)[B]
  - Faster, with less drowsiness and drug interactions than carbamazepine
  - Decreases serum sodium
  - Most common side effect: Sedation

Second Line
- Phenytoin (Dilantin)
  - 300–400 mg/d (synergistic with carbamazepine)
  - Potent P450 inducer (enhanced metabolism of many drugs)
  - Various CNS side effects (sedation, ataxia)
- Baclofen (Lioresal)
  - 10–80 mg/d; start at 5–10 mg t.i.d. with food (as adjunct with phenytoin or carbamazepine)
  - Side effects: Drowsiness, weakness, nausea, vomiting
- Gabapentin (Neurontin)
  - 100 mg t.i.d. or 300 mg at bedtime, increased up to 300–600 mg t.i.d.–q.i.d.
- Lamotrigine
  - Titrate up to 200 mg b.i.d. (over weeks)
  - 10% experience rash.
- Chlorphenesin carbamate (Maolate)
  - 800–2,400 mg/d (as adjunct with phenytoin and/or carbamazepine)
  - Side effect: Drowsiness
- Antidepressants: Amitriptyline, fluoxetine, trazodone
  - Used especially with anticonvulsants
  - Particularly effective for atypical forms of trigeminal neuralgia
- Clonazepam (Klonopin): Frequently causes drowsiness and ataxia
- Capsaicin cream, locally
- Botulinum toxin injection into zygomatic arch
- Valproic acid (Depakene, Depakote)

SURGERY
- Microvascular decompression of 5th cranial nerve at its entrance to (or exit from) brainstem
  - 98% of patients achieve intial pain relief; by 33 months, 73% maintain complete relief (NNT 1.3) (6)[B]
  - Surgical mortality across studies was ~1% (6)
  - Most common side effect: Transient facial numbness and diplopia, headache, nausea, vomiting
  - Mean hospital stay was ~5.4 days (6)[B]
- Peripheral-nerve ablation
  - Radiofrequency thermocoagulation (possibly 90–97% partial or complete relief; recurrence rate unknown) (7)[C]
  - Neurectomy
  - Cryotherapy: High relapse rate
- 4% tetracaine dissolved in 0.5% bupivacaine nerve block (only a few case reports to date)
- Alcohol block or glycerol injection into trigeminal cistern: Unpredictable side effects (dysesthesia and anesthesia dolorosa); temporary relief
- Partial sensory rhizotomy
- Peripheral block or section of 5th nerve proximal to Gasserian ganglion
- Balloon compression of Gasserian ganglion (especially effective for 1st-division trigeminal neuralgia pain) (7)

 FOLLOW-UP

PROGNOSIS
- 50–60% eventually fail pharmacological treatment (5B)
- Of those, relapse is seen in ~50% of stereotactic radiosurgeries and ~27% surgical microvascular decompressions (4,5)[B]

COMPLICATIONS
- Mental and physical sluggishness; dizziness with carbamazepine (5)
- Paresthesiae and corneal reflex loss with stereotactic radiosurgery (4)
- Surigical mortality and morbidity associated with microvascular decompression (6)

PATIENT MONITORING
- Carbamazepine and/or phenytoin serum levels
- If carbamazepine prescribed: CBC and platelets at baseline, then weekly for a month, then monthly for 4 months, then every 6–12 months if dose stable (regimens for monitoring vary)
- Reduce drugs after 4–6 weeks to determine whether condition is in remission; resume at previous dose if pain recurs. Withdraw drugs slowly after several months, again to check for remission or if lower dose of drugs can be tolerated.

REFERENCES
1. Manzoni GC, Torelli P. Epidemiology of typical and atypical craniofacial neuralgias. *Neurol Sci.* 2005; 26(Suppl 2):s65–s67.
2. Scrivani SJ, Mathews ES, Maciewicz RJ. Trigeminal neuralgia. *Oral Surg Oral Med Oral Pathol Oral Radiol Endod.* 2005;100(5):527–538.
3. Nurmikko TJ, Eldridge PR. Trigeminal neuralgia–pathophysiology, diagnosis and current treatment. *Br J Anaesth.* 2001;87(1):117–132.
4. Lopez BC, Hamlyn PJ, Zakrzewska JM. Stereotactic radiosurgery for primary trigeminal neuralgia: State of the evidence and recommendations for future reports. *J Neurol Neurosurg Psychiatry.* 2004;75(7):1019–1024.
5. Beniczky S, Tajti J, Timea Varga E, Vecsei L. Evidence-based pharmacological treatment of neuropathic pain syndromes. *J Neural Transm.* 2005;112(6):735–749.
6. Ashkan K, Marsh H. Microvascular decompression for trigeminal neuralgia in the elderly: A review of the safety and efficacy. *Neurosurgery.* 2004;55(4):840–8; discussion 848–850.
7. Lopez BC, Hamlyn PJ, Zakrzewska JM. Systematic review of ablative neurosurgical techniques for the treatment of trigeminal neuralgia. *Neurosurgery.* 2004;54(4):973–82; discussion 982–983.

 MISCELLANEOUS

See also: Headache, cluster; Migraine

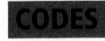 **CODES**

ICD9-CM
350.1 Trigeminal neuralgia

PATIENT TEACHING
Instruct regarding medication dosage and side effects, risk benefit of surgery or radiation therapy

 See Patient Handout on CD

T

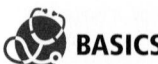

TRIGGER FINGER

Alan M. Ehrlich, MD

BASICS

DESCRIPTION
A clicking, snapping, or locking of a finger or thumb after full flexion, with or without associated pain

GENERAL PREVENTION
Most cases are idiopathic, and no known prevention exists. No clear association with repetitive movements.

EPIDEMIOLOGY
- Predominant age: A childhood form that presents typically with thumb involvement in the 1st decade of life and an adult form that typically presents in the 5th and 6th decades of life
- Predominant sex: Female > Male (adult) (6:1); Female = Male (children)

Incidence
- 28/100,000/year in the general population
- Diabetics have 4 times the risk of the general population.

Prevalence
Lifetime prevalence in the general population is 2.8%

ALERT
Pediatric Considerations
- The thumb is more commonly involved with children.
- When children have a trigger finger instead of trigger thumb, surgery is often more complicated. Release of the A1 pulley alone is often insufficient, and other procedures may need to be done at the time of surgery.

RISK FACTORS
- Diabetes mellitus
- Rheumatoid arthritis
- Hypothyroidism
- Mucopolysaccharide disorders
- Amyloidosis

PATHOPHYSIOLOGY
- Narrowing of the flexor tendon sheath of the A1 pulley due to either thickening from inflammation or protein deposits. With prolonged inflammation, fibrocartilagenous metaplasia of the tendon sheath occurs.
- The flexor tendon may become distorted with a nodule formation, which can give rise to the triggering as the nodule has difficulty passing through the area of narrowing. Because flexors are stronger than extensors, the finger can get stuck in the flexed position.

ETIOLOGY
- Narrowing of the flexor tendon sheath due to either thickening from inflammation or protein deposits
- Most cases are idiopathic, and no known prevention exists.
- No clear association with repetitive movements.

ASSOCIATED CONDITIONS
DeQuervain tenosynovitis, Carpal tunnel syndrome
Dupytren contracture, Diabetes mellitus
Rheumatoid arthritis, Hypothyroidism, Amyloidosis

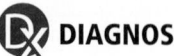 DIAGNOSIS

PRE HOSPITAL
Diagnosis is based on clinical presentation

SIGNS AND SYMPTOMS
- History of clicking, snapping, or locking of a finger or thumb after full flexion, with or without associated pain.
- A palpable nodule may be present. Snapping or locking may be present, but are not necessary for the diagnosis

History
History of clicking, snapping, or locking of a finger or thumb after full flexion, with or without associated pain

Physical Exam
- A palpable nodule may be present.
- Snapping or locking may be present but are not necessary for the diagnosis

TESTS
None

Lab
None

Imaging
None

Diagnostic Procedures/Surgery
None

Pathological Findings
- Thickening of the A1 tendon sheath with fibrocartilagenous metaplasia
- Swelling or nodule formation of flexor tendon

TREATMENT

PRE HOSPITAL
- Splinting the metacarpophalangeal (MCP) joint at 10–15° flexion for 6 weeks with the distal joints free to move has been effective. Splinting is more effective for treating fingers than thumbs (70% vs 50%). Less effective with severe symptoms, symptoms > 6 months, and multiple digits involved
- Long-acting corticosteroids may be injected up to 3 times to achieve relief of symptoms.

GENERAL MEASURES
- Splinting or steroid injection should be tried before surgery.
- Percutaneous release is usually preferred to open release.

Activity
Splinting of the affected digit to minimize flexion/extension of the MCP joint can lead to resolution of symptoms.

SPECIAL THERAPY
Physical Therapy
Physiotherapy has been used in the treatment of trigger digits in children.

MEDICATION (DRUGS)

First Line
Steroid injection of the tendon sheath or surrounding subcutaneous tissue

Second Line
NSAIDs may reduce pain and discomfort but have not been shown to improve the underlying cause. They do not reduce symptoms of snapping or locking.

SURGERY
- Percutaneous release of trigger finger has 90% success rate.
- Open surgery is an alternative to percutaneous release. Success rates are comparable to percutaneous release although complication rates may be higher

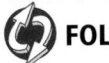 ## FOLLOW-UP

Follow up only needed if symptoms persist or if complications of surgery develop

DISPOSITION
Admission Criteria
Day surgery for trigger finger release

Discharge Criteria
Absence of complications

Issues for Referral
Refer to hand surgeon if not responding to splinting and/or steroid injections

PROGNOSIS
Prognosis for resolution of symptoms is excellent with either conservative or surgical intervention

COMPLICATIONS
- Complications from surgery include infection, bleeding, digital nerve injury, and persistent pain.
- Injury to the A2 pulley may result in bowstringing which is a bulging of the flexor tendon in the palm with flexion. This can be associated with pain.

REFERENCES

1. Akhtar S, Bradley MJ, Quinton DN, Burke FD. Management and referral for trigger finger/thumb. *BMJ*. 2005;331:30–33.
2. Ryzewicz M, Wolf JN. Trigger digits: Principles, management, and complications. *J Hand Surg*. 2006;31A:135–146.
3. Moore JS. Flexor tendon entrapment of the digits (trigger finger and trigger thumb). *J Occup Environ Med*. 2000;42:5
4. Nimigan AS, Ross DC, Gan BS. Steroid injections in the management of trigger fingers. *Am J Phys Med Rehabil*. 2006;85:36–43.
5. Gilberts ECAM, Beekman WH, Stevens HJPD, Wereldsma JCJ. Prospective randomized trial of open versus percutaneous surgery for trigger digits. *J Hand Surgery*. 2001;26A:497–500
6. Cardon LJ, Ezaki M, Carter PR. Trigger finger in children. *J Hand Surgery*. 1999;24A:1156–1161.
7. Tordai P, Engkvist O. Trigger fingers in children. *J Hand Surgery*. 1999;24A:1162–1165.

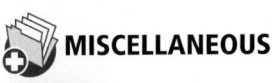 ## MISCELLANEOUS

CODES

ICD9-CM
727.03 Trigger finger (acquired)

 See Patient Handout on CD

TROCHANTERIC BURSITIS

Matthew Pecci, MD

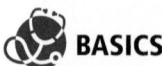 BASICS

DESCRIPTION
The trochanteric bursa is a fluid filled sac overlying the greater trochanter of the femur, and beneath the iliotibial band (IT band).
- Bursitis refers to inflammation of this bursa

GENERAL PREVENTION
- Maintain IT band, hip and low back flexibility
- Avoid direct trauma

EPIDEMIOLOGY
- More common in adults
- Common in runners
- Predominant age: All ages
- Predominant sex: Male = Female

RISK FACTORS
- Tight hip musculature
- Direct contusion
- Abnormal gait
  - Leg length discrepancy
  - Sacroiliac joint dysfunction
  - Knee or hip osteoarthritis
  - Abnormal foot mechanics (e.g., pes planus, overpronation)

PATHOPHYSIOLOGY
- Abnormal gait or poor muscle flexibility leads to friction on bursa causing inflammatory response
- Long-term
  - Fibrosis and thickening of bursal sac due to chronic inflammatory process

ETIOLOGY
See "Risk Factors."

ASSOCIATED CONDITIONS
- Tight IT bands
- Leg length discrepancy
- Sacroillic (SI) joint dysfunction
- Osteoarthritis
- Pes planis

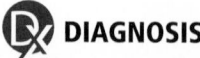 DIAGNOSIS

SIGNS AND SYMPTOMS
History
- Pain localized to the lateral aspect of the hip
  - May radiate to groin or lateral thigh
  - Worse when rising after prolonged sitting
  - Exacerbated by prolonged walking or standing
  - Worse with direct pressure over the greater trochanter. May not be able to lie on the affected side due to pain.
- Possible
  - A fall landing directly on the affected hip
  - Chronic low back pain
  - Chronic leg/knee/ankle/hip pain
- Recent increase in running distance or intensity, or a change in running surfaces

Physical Exam
- Tenderness with direct palpation over the greater trochanter
- May have pain with extremes of internal and external rotation of hip
- May have pain with abduction of the hip against resistance
- May have a positive Ober test, which assesses IT band flexibility
- May have abnormal gait
- May have measurable leg length discrepancy
- May have positive Fabers test for SI joint dysfunction
- May have pes planus or overpronation
- Rarely has palpable fullness over the bursal sac

TESTS
Imaging
- Anteroposterior frog leg lateral of affected hip
- Consider lumbar spine x-rays if back pain thought to be a contributing factor

DIFFERENTIAL DIAGNOSIS
- IT band tendonitis
- Gluteus medius tendonitis/bursititis
- Osteoarthritis of hip
- Lumbo-sacral osteoarthritis/disc disease causing nerve root compression
- If associated trauma: Fracture of hip
- Stress reaction/fracture of femoral neck especially in female runners
- Septic bursitis/arthritis

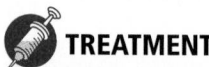 TREATMENT

GENERAL MEASURES
Activity
- Minimize aggravating activities such as prolonged walking, or standing.
- Avoid lying on affected side.
- Runners
  - May need to decrease distance and/or intensity of runs
  - May need a period of cessation from running
  - Avoid banked tracks or roads with excessive tilt.

Physical Therapy
- Ice
- Focus on achieving flexibility of hip musculature, particularly the IT band
- Address contributing factors
  - Low back flexibility and strengthening
  - If leg length discrepancy, may need heel lift
  - If pes planis or overpronation, may need arch support, or custom orthotics

MEDICATION (DRUGS)

First Line
NSAIDs (1)[B]
- Naprosyn 500 mg PO b.i.d.
- Ibuprofen 800 mg PO t.i.d.

Second Line
Intra-bursal steroid injection (2,3)[B]
- 1 cc Dexamethasone 4 mg/cc *or*
- 1 cc Kenalog 40 mg/cc

SURGERY
- Rarely requires surgery
- Bursectomy
- Longitudinal release of the IT band (4)[B]

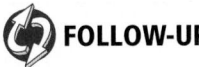 **FOLLOW-UP**

Four weeks post-treatment

PROGNOSIS
Depends on chronicity, with more acute cases having an excellent prognosis

COMPLICATIONS
Bursal thickening and fibrosis

REFERENCES

1. Browning KH. Hip and pelvis injuries in runners. *The Physician and Sports Medicine*. 2001;29.
2. Cardone DA, Tallia AF. Diagnostic and therapeutic injection of the hip and knee. *Am Fam Physician*. 2003;63;2147–2157.
3. Sheeb MI, et al. Evaluation of glucocorticosteroid injection for the treatment of trochanteric bursitis. *J Rheumatol*. 1996;23;2104–2106.
4. Anderson B. Trochanteric bursitis. *UptoDate Online*. 2006.

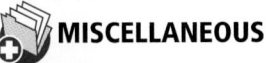 **MISCELLANEOUS**

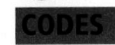 **CODES**

ICD9-CM
726.5 Trochanteric Bursitis

PATIENT TEACHING

Activity
- Avoid lying on affected side
- Minimize prolonged standing or walking.

Prevention
- Maintain hip musculature flexibility.
- Correct issues that may cause abnormal gait
  – Low back pain
  – Leg length discrepancy
  – Foot mechanics

T

TROPICAL SPRUE

Abdulrazak Abyad, MD, PhD, MBA, MPH, AGSF

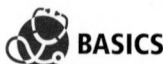 **BASICS**

DESCRIPTION

Malabsorption syndrome of unknown or mutable etiology that occurs primarily in patients in the tropics and subtropics. Characteristics include protein malnutrition and folic acid anemia. Usual course is relapsing without treatment. Symptoms may appear years after leaving an endemic area.

- Endemic areas: Tropic regions only, Far East, India, Caribbean, and the Middle East. Distribution is sporadic.
- System(s) Affected: Gastrointestinal; Hemic; Lymphatic; Immunologic

EPIDEMIOLOGY

Predominant sex: Male = Female

Incidence
Unknown

RISK FACTORS

Parasitic infestation

ETIOLOGY

- Unknown
- Possible dietary deficiency
- Possible infectious agent
- Vitamin deficiency (folate), B_{12}
- Food toxins (rancid fats)
- Toxigenic strains of coliform bacteria

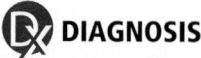 **DIAGNOSIS**

SIGNS AND SYMPTOMS

- Fatigue
- Asthenia
- Weight loss
- Pallor
- Diarrhea
- Abdominal cramps
- Borborygmus
- Night blindness
- Stomatitis
- Glossitis
- Cheilosis
- Anorexia
- Steatorrhea
- Hyperkeratosis
- Edema
- Abdominal distension
- Hyperpigmentation
- Koilonychia

TESTS
Lab
- Megaloblastic anemia in 60% of cases
- Steatorrhea
- Decreased D-xylose
- Decreased serum iron
- Decreased calcium
- Decreased folic acid
- Decreased serum vitamin B_{12}
- Decreased serum carotene
- Decreased cholesterol, albumin
- Deficiency of magnesium
- Deficiency of α-tocopherol

Imaging
- Mild jejunal dilatation
- Jejunal fold coarsening
- Flocculation and segmentation of barium meal

Diagnostic Procedures/Surgery
- The presence of normal result on jejunal biopsy nearly excludes this diagnosis.
- Abnormal results on duodenal/jejunal biopsy: Not specific
- Malabsorption of at least 2 nutrients is considered essential for diagnosis.
- D-Xylose, fat, and radiolabeled vitamin B_{12} are used to test for absorptive capacity.
- Stool microscopy
- Imaging: Not specific

Pathological Findings
- Jejunal biopsy: Mild villous atrophy, increased villous crypts, mononuclear cell infiltration
- Patients may have chronic atrophic gastritis and nonspecific abnormalities of the colonic mucosa.
- Serum motilin and enteroglucagon levels are increased both while fasting and postprandially.

DIFFERENTIAL DIAGNOSIS
- Other causes of megaloblastic anemia
- Other malabsorption syndromes
- Celiac disease
- Inflammatory bowel disease
- Giardiasis
- Strongylosis
- Other infectious causes
  - Coccidial isospora
  - *Capillaria philippinensis*
  - *Cryptosporidium*

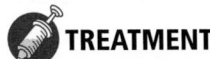 **TREATMENT**

INITIAL STABILIZATION
Outpatient

GENERAL MEASURES
- Replace deficiencies of elements (e.g., vitamin B_{12}, folic acid)
- Control diarrhea
- Replace fluids and blood

Diet
No special diet (glutenfree diets do not improve this disease)

Activity
No restrictions, as tolerated

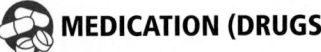 **MEDICATION (DRUGS)**

First Line
- Vitamin B_{12} 1,000 μg SC for several days, then monthly thereafter for 6 months
- Folic acid 5 mg PO daily
- Tetracycline 250 mg q.i.d. for 1–2 months, then 1/2 doses for up to 6 months. Occasionally, longer course required
- Combination folic acid and B_{12} plus tetracycline or sulfonamide
- Contraindications: Allergy to tetracycline or oxytetracycline
- Precautions
  – Use with caution in patients with intercurrent lupus, myasthenia gravis, or kidney or liver disease.
  – Do not take medication with milk, antacids, or with iron preparations.
  – Do not use tetracycline during pregnancy
  – Do not use tetracycline in children <8 years.
- Significant possible interactions
  – Antacids, anticoagulants, bismuth subsalicylate
  – Oral contraceptives
  – Lithium

Second Line
- Oxytetracycline
- Nonabsorbable sulfonamides

ALERT
Pediatric Considerations
Do not treat pediatric patients with tetracycline.

Pregnancy Considerations
Do not treat with tetracycline during pregnancy.

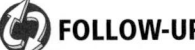 **FOLLOW-UP**

PROGNOSIS
- Good with appropriate treatment
- Recurrences do happen in native residents treated in the tropics.

COMPLICATIONS
- Malabsorption
- Relapse is possible if medication regimen is stopped too soon.

PATIENT MONITORING
As needed for symptoms

REFERENCES
1. Mandell GL, ed. *Principles and Practice of Infectious Diseases*. 5th ed. New York, NY: Churchill Livingstone; 2000.
2. Sleisenger MH, Fordtran JS, eds. *Gastrointestinal and Liver Disease: Pathophysiology, Diagnosis, Management*. 7th ed. Philadelphia, PA: WB Saunders; 2002.

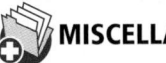 **MISCELLANEOUS**

See also: Celiac disease; Diarrhea, chronic

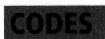 **CODES**

ICD9-CM
579.1 Tropical sprue

PATIENT TEACHING
Written patient information available from: National Digestive Diseases Information Clearinghouse, Box NDDIC, Bethesda, MD 20892; (301) 654-3810

T

TUBERCULOSIS

Katherine Berg, MD

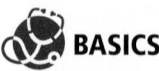 **BASICS**

DESCRIPTION

Common disease transmitted by inhaling airborne bacilli from a person with active tuberculosis. Bacilli multiply in alveoli, are carried by macrophages, lymphatics, and blood to distant sites. Tissue hypersensitivity usually halts infection within 10 weeks.

- Latent infection
  - Asymptomatic, with positive PPD
  - Negative chest radiograph
  - Noninfectious
- Active disease
  - Occurs in 10% of infected individuals without preventive therapy
  - Risk increases with immunosuppression and is highest within 2 years of infection
  - 85% of cases are pulmonary, which is contagious.
- Primary: Disease resulting from initial infection.
- Recrudescent: Active disease occurring after period of latent, asymptomatic infection
- Miliary: Disseminated disease
- Systems Affected: Potentially any via hematogenous spread

ALERT
Pediatric Considerations
- Emphasize DOT (directly observed therapy)
- Caution with ethambutol
- Children on medication may attend school.
- Disseminated TB more common in infants; prompt treatment with 4 drugs if TB suspected
- Congenital infection may occur with miliary TB or endometrial TB in mother. If suspected, get PPD, chest radiograph, lumbar puncture, culture placenta in infant, then start treatment promptly.
- Consider BCG if unavoidable contact with TB

GENERAL PREVENTION
- Treat those with latent TB infection.
- Identify and test all close contacts of infected person.
- BCG vaccine: Live attenuated *Mycobacterium bovis*
  - 50% efficacy preventing pulmonary disease, prevents 80% of TB meningitis and miliary disease in children
  - In the US, consider BCG for children with negative PPD and HIV tests with unavoidable high risk, and for health care workers at high risk for drug-resistant infection (1).
  - Used more commonly in countries where TB is endemic.

EPIDEMIOLOGY
- 1/3 of world's population infected with TB bacillus
- Higher incidence in ethnic minorities and medically underserved populations.

Incidence
- The Americas: 41 per 100,000
- Worldwide: 140 per 100,000
- In US, rate of decline of incidence slowing since 2000 (3.8% decrease per year as opposed to 7.1% per year in years 1993–2000)

Prevalence
- The Americas: 53 per 100,000
- Worldwide: 229 per 100,000

RISK FACTORS
- For infection
  - Demographics: Homeless, minority
  - Institutionalization (e.g., prison, nursing home)
  - Close contact with infected individual
  - Immigrant within 5 years (from Asia, Africa, Latin America, former Soviet Union states)
  - Health care workers
- For development of disease once infected
  - HIV; lymphoma; diabetes mellitus; chronic renal failure; cancer of head, neck, or lung
  - Gastrectomy
  - Steroids, immunosuppressive drugs
  - IV drug abuse, malnutrition

ETIOLOGY
- *Mycobacterium tuberculosis*
- *Mycobacterium bovis*
- *Mycobacterium africanum*

ASSOCIATED CONDITIONS
HIV infection (emphasize DOT; most recommendations remain the same)

DIAGNOSIS

SIGNS AND SYMPTOMS
- Cough
- Hemoptysis
- Fever and night sweats
- Weight loss
- Malaise
- Painless adenopathy
- Pleuritic chest pain
- Hepatosplenomegaly
- Late findings: Renal, bone, or CNS disease

History
- Recent travel to or immigration from high-prevalence country
- Exposure to high-risk populations (see "Risk Factors"), or to known infected person
- HIV status/risk factors

Physical Exam
- Often normal
- May note rales on lung exam.
- Specific findings vary based on organ involvement.

TESTS
Lab
- Persons with TB should be tested for HIV; if positive, get CD4 count.
- Baseline liver enzymes, bilirubin, creatinine, CBC with platelet count
- If using ethambutol: Baseline visual acuity and color discrimination
- If high risk: Test for hepatitis B and C
- If extrapulmonary suspected: Urine, CSF, bone marrow, and liver biopsy for culture
- Nonspecific laboratory findings include
  - Anemia
  - Monocytosis
  - Thrombocytosis
  - Hypergammaglobulinemia
  - SIADH
  - Sterile pyuria
  - Steroids: False-negative skin test

- Factors that may yield false-negative skin test
  - Recent viral infections
  - New (<10 weeks) infection
  - Severe malnutrition
  - HIV
  - Anergy
  - Age <6 months
  - Overwhelming TB

Imaging
- Chest radiograph
  - With primary TB: May show infiltrate with or without effusion, atelectasis, or adenopathy
  - With recrudescent TB: Cavitary lesions and upper-lobe disease with hilar adenopathy common
  - HIV: Atypical findings with primary infection, right upper-lobe atelectasis
- CT chest: Good sensitivity

Diagnostic Procedures/Surgery
- PPD: 5 units (0.1 cc) intermediate-strength intradermal injection into volar forearm. Measure induration at 48–72 h
- PPD positive if induration
  - >5 mm and HIV infection (or suspected), immunosuppressed, recent TB contact, clinical evidence of disease on chest film
  - >10 mm and age <4 years or other risk factors
  - >15 mm and age >4 years and no risk factors
  - 2-step test if patient has no recent PPD, age >55, nursing home resident, prison inmate, or health care worker. Administer second test 1–3 weeks after initial one; interpret as usual.
- Drugs that may alter PPD results
  - BCG: False-positive skin test, but unreliable and should not influence decision to treat latent tuberculosis infection

    ○ QuantiFERON whole blood assay not affected by BCG vaccine (2)[A]

- 3 different morning sputum samples for acid-fast bacilli (AFB) stain and culture; use aerosol induction, gastric aspirate (children), or bronchoalveolar lavage if needed
- If positive AFB, begin treatment immediately
- Culture and sensitivity guide treatment

Pathological Findings
- AFB stains positive
- Biopsy may show granulomas with central caseating necrosis.

DIFFERENTIAL DIAGNOSIS
- Other pneumonias
- Lymphomas
- Fungal infections, especially other atypical *Mycobacteria* or *Nocardia*

TREATMENT

GENERAL MEASURES
- If clinical suspicion, treat immediately
- Prescribing physician responsible for treatment completion.
- Inpatient: Use personal sealed respirators, negative pressure ventilation, ultraviolet
- Ambulatory patients use mask and tissues
- Not infectious if: Favorable clinical response after 2–3 weeks of therapy and 3 negative AFB smears
- Age no longer a factor in the treatment of latent tuberculosis

Activity
Respiratory isolation for infectious pulmonary TB until clinical response and 3 negative AFB smears

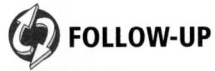 **MEDICATION (DRUGS)**

First Line
- Regimen 1 (preferred)
  - Initial phase: Isoniazid (INH), rifampin (RIF), pyrazinamide (PZA), and ethambutol (EMB) once daily for 8 weeks
  - Continuation phase: INH/RIF daily for 18 weeks. Or INH/RIF twice weekly for 18 weeks (only use for HIV+ if CD4>100) Or INH/ Rifapentine once weekly for 18 weeks (acceptable alternative for HIV− patients only) (1)[A]

- Regimen 2
  - Initial phase: INH/RIF/PZA/EMB daily for 2 weeks, then twice weekly for 6 weeks
  - Continuation phase: INH/RIF twice weekly for 18 wks (HIV+ patients only if CD4>100) or INH/Rifapentine once weekly for 18 weeks (acceptable alternative for HIV− patients only) (1)[A]

- Regimen 3 (acceptable alternative)
  - Initial phase: INH/RIF/PZA/EMB daily for 8 weeks
  - Continuation phase: INH/RIF 3 times weekly for 18 weeks (1)[A]

- Regimen 4 (only when unable to give preferred regimen)
  - Initial phase: INH/RIF/EMB daily for 8 weeks
  - Continuation phase: INH/RIF daily or twice weekly for 31 weeks (1)[B]

  - No studies proving efficacy of 5 times weekly regimen, but clinical evidence suggests it. [C] Directly observed therapy required for nondaily regimens. (1)
- Latent tuberculosis should be treated with Isoniazid 300 mg/d for adults, and 10–15 mg/kg (not to exceed 300 mg/d) in children for 6–12 months with DOT.
  Dosing
- INH: Scored tabs 50/100/300 mg, syrup 10 mg/mL, or aqueous solution 100 mg/mL
  - Daily dose: Adult 5 mg/kg (max 300 mg); pediatric 10–15 mg/kg (max 300 mg)
  - 3 times weekly: Adult 15 mg/kg (max 900 mg)
  - Twice weekly: Adult 15 mg/kg, (max 900 mg); pediatric 20–30 mg/kg (max 900 mg)
  - Weekly: Adult only, 15 mg/kg (max 900 mg);
  - Consider pyridoxine 10–50 mg/d

- RIF: Capsules 150/300 mg, powder for oral suspension, or IV aqueous
  - Daily or twice weekly dose: Adult and pediatric 10–20 mg/kg (maximum 600 mg)
- PZA: Scored tabs 500 mg. Dosed by weight
  - Adults 40–55 kg
    - Daily: 18–25 mg/kg, max 1 g
    - 3 times weekly: 27–37 mg/kg, max 1.5 g
    - Twice weekly: 36–50 mg/kg, max 2 g
  - Adults 56–75 kg
    - Daily: 20–27 mg/kg, max 1.5 g
    - 3 times weekly: 33–45 mg/kg, max 2.5 g
    - Twice weekly: 40–54 mg/kg, max 3 g
  - Adults >75 kg
    - Daily: 22–26 mg/kg, max 2 g
    - 3 times weekly: 33–40 mg/kg, max 3 g
    - Twice weekly: 44–53 mg/kg, max 4 g
  - Pediatric daily: 15–30 mg/kg (maximum 2 g)
  - Pediatric twice weekly: 50 mg/kg (maximum 4 g)
- Rifabutin (Mycobutin): Capsules 150 mg
  - Daily or twice weekly: Adult 5 mg/kg, max 300 mg
- Rifapentine (Priftine): Tablet 150 mg; for continuation phase only
  - HIV− adults: 600 mg once weekly, given with INH. Not effective if HIV+. (1)[A]
- EMB: Tablets 100/400 mg bacteriostatic. Dose based on weight.
  - Adults 40–55 kg
    - Daily: 15–20 mg/kg, max 800 mg
    - 3 times weekly: 22–30 mg/kg, max 1.2 g
    - Twice weekly: 36–50 mg/kg, max 2 g
  - Adults 56–75 kg
    - Daily: 16–22 mg/kg, max 1.2 g
    - 3 times weekly: 27–36 mg/kg, max 2 g
    - Twice weekly: 37–50 mg/kg, max 2.8 g
  - Adults >75 kg
    - Daily: 22–26 mg/kg, max 2.6 g
    - 3 times weekly: 33–40 mg/kg, max 2.4 g
    - Twice weekly: 44–53 mg/kg, max 4 g
  - Pediatrics
    - Daily: 15–20 mg/kg, max 1 g
    - Twice weekly: 50 mg/kg, max 4 g
- Contraindications
  - RIF: Avoid if patient taking antiretrovirals
  - EMB: May cause optic neuritis. Avoid unless patient old enough to cooperate for visual acuity and color testing
- Precautions
  - INH, RIF, PZA: May cause hepatitis. Caution if liver disease.
  - RIF: Colors urine, tears, and secretions orange. Can stain contact lenses.
  - INH: Peripheral neuritis and hypersensitivity possible. Treat with pyridoxine.
  - PZA: May increase uric acid. Unclear safety during pregnancy [C]
- Significant possible interactions: Rifamycins alter level of phenytoin, antivirals, and other drugs metabolized by liver and may inactivate birth control pills (recommend a barrier method).

Second Line
- Steroids: Use only with concurrent anti-TB therapy. Recommended for TB meningitis or pericarditis. (3)[B]

- Streptomycin: Caution—ototoxic and nephrotoxic; do not use in pregnancy.

ALERT
Pregnancy Considerations
- Treat pregnant women with INH, RIF, and EMB; add pyridoxine.
- Avoid streptomycin due to ototoxicity.
- Use pyrazinamide with caution.
- Breast-feeding OK while taking TB drugs.

SURGERY
For extrapulmonary complications (e.g., spinal cord compression, constrictive pericarditis)

 FOLLOW-UP

PROGNOSIS
Generally, few complications and full resolution if drugs taken for full course as prescribed

COMPLICATIONS
- Cavitary lesions can be secondarily infected.
- Drug resistance: Drug resistance declining in US. At risk if HIV+, or treatment taken improperly, or if from area with high incidence of resistance

PATIENT MONITORING
- Assess monthly for treatment adherence and adverse effects.
- Check liver enzymes if symptomatic, HIV+, chronic liver disease, alcohol use, pregnant or postpartum. Temporarily discontinue medications if enzymes are 5 times normal.
- If culture is positive after 2 months of therapy, reassess drug sensitivity and initiate DOT.
- Chest radiograph at 3 months

REFERENCES
1. Potter B. Management of active TB. *Am Fam Physician* 2005;72(11).
2. Centers for Disease Control. Guideline for using the QuantiFERON-TB gold test for detecting mycobacterium tubercular infection. United States. *MMWR* 2005;54(RR15): 49–55.
3. Golden M. Extrapulmonary TB; an overview. *Am Fam Physician* 2005;72(9).

 MISCELLANEOUS

See also: Tuberculosis, CNS; Tuberculosis, latent; Tuberculosis, miliary

CODES

ICD9-CM
011.90 Pulmonary tuberculosis, unspecified

PATIENT TEACHING
- Emphasize importance of drug therapy.
- Identify patient contacts to notify.
- Let patient know that you are obligated to inform the local health department.

See Corresponding Diagnostic Algorithm

TUBERCULOSIS, CNS

Linda M. Spooner, PharmD, BCPS
Edward Liu, MD

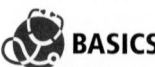 **BASICS**

DESCRIPTION

- Tuberculosis (TB) of the CNS is a granulomatous infection of the brain, meninges, or spinal cord caused by *Mycobacterium tuberculosis*. Clinical forms include tuberculous meningitis, intracranial tuberculoma, spinal tuberculoma, and spinal tuberculous arachnoiditis.
- Uncommon manifestations of CNS TB: En-plaque granulomas, tuberculous abscesses, pituitary TB, and tuberculous ventriculitis. Spinal cord infection is less common but results in arachnoiditis, focal intramedullary tuberculomas, or abscesses.
- System(s) Affected: Endocrine/Metabolic, Nervous

GENERAL PREVENTION

- Treatment of other sites of infection
- Aggressive and complete antitubercular therapy to prevent recurrence or major sequelae

EPIDEMIOLOGY

- Predominant age
  - Tuberculous meningitis: Highest incidence in 1st 3 years of life in TB-endemic areas; highest incidence in adults in countries with low incidence of TB (e.g., U.S.)
  - Intracranial tuberculomas: Majority of patients are <30 years of age
- Predominant sex: Male = Female

Incidence

- In the US: The incidence of TB is 4.8/100,000. CNS involvement: 15% of extrapulmonary TB cases
- Worldwide, the incidence of TB continues to increase, with an overall incidence of 140/100,000. CNS tuberculomas account for ~20% of all intracranial mass lesions.
- In developing countries, intracranial tuberculomas occur in ~ 20% of TB meningitis.

Prevalence

- 1.7 billion worldwide are infected with TB.
- Prevalence of CNS TB varies depending on region of the world, public health infrastructure, and socioeconomic status.

RISK FACTORS

- CNS TB more common in immunosuppressed patients (e.g., old or young, HIV⁺ patients, diabetics, users of steroids or cytotoxic drugs)
- Immigrants from TB-endemic areas
- History of pulmonary TB
- Exposure to population with high rates of TB (e.g., health care professionals, prison workers)

Genetics

Host immune response is related to incompletely understood genetic factors.

PATHOPHYSIOLOGY

- Tuberculous infection spreads hematogenously to the CNS, generally from a pulmonary focus. Infection starts as a subpial or subependymal cortical focus (Rich focus).
- Meningitis results from rupture of a Rich focus into the subarachnoid space. Meningitis causes communicating or obstructive hydrocephalus and cranial neuropathies.
- Tuberculomas result from coalescence of granulomas or as a paradoxical reaction despite adequate drug therapy.

ETIOLOGY

Mycobacterium tuberculosis

ASSOCIATED CONDITIONS

- HIV
- Deep cerebral infarcts
- TB osteomyelitis of spine

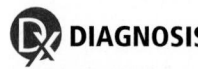 **DIAGNOSIS**

SIGNS AND SYMPTOMS

- Malaise
- Fever
- Headache
- Meningismus
- Vomiting
- Confusion/decreased consciousness
- Cranial nerve palsy
- Coma
- Hemiparesis
- Hyponatremia secondary to syndrome of inappropriate antidiuretic hormone (SIADH)
- Seizures
- Signs of extracranial TB

TESTS

- PCR of CSF has sensitivity of 56% and specificity of 98%. (1)[A]
- Culture (*M. tuberculosis* direct test [MTD]) with Ziehl-Neelsen (ZN) staining of CSF have similar accuracy prior to treatment initiation. (1)[B]

Lab

- General labs
  - Purified protein derivative (PPD) tuberculin skin test may be of limited value in many patients, since active TB infection may suppress reactivity (anergy). (2)[C]
- CSF study in tuberculous meningitis
  - Moderate elevation in protein
  - Lymphocytic predominance
  - Normal or slightly low glucose
  - Tubercle bacilli found on direct smear in 10–20%, depending on quality
  - Cultures grow in 4–8 wks but DNA probes may provide preliminary identification
- CSF study in tuberculomas
  - Isolated from subarachnoid space due to thick capsule, so rare CSF changes seen
- Drugs that may alter lab results
  - Steroids may alter CSF and give false negative skin test results.
  - Antituberculous therapy
- Disorders that may alter lab results
- Immunodeficient states (e.g., HIV) may give false negative skin test results.

ALERT

Geriatric Considerations

May have atypical clinical presentation and CSF findings

Imaging

- CT scan of head with contrast
  - Useful for revealing
    - Hydrocephalus
    - Tuberculomas
    - Cerebral edema
    - Basilar meningeal involvement
    - Response to treatment
  - Can be normal
- MRI scan
  - In tuberculous meningitis, MRI more sensitive in demonstrating early infarcts or brainstem, midbrain, basal ganglion lesions than CT
  - Solid tuberculomas iso- or hypointense on T1-weighted images and hyperintense on T2 with ring enhancement.

Diagnostic Procedures/Surgery

- Need lumbar puncture for diagnosis and monitoring response to therapy. (3)[C]
- CT-guided stereotactic brain biopsy is helpful in differentiating tuberculomas from other space-occupying lesions. (4)[A]

Pathological Findings

- In tuberculous meningitis
  - Thick tubercular exudates seen in the basal cisterns and sylvian fissures
  - Hydrocephalus common
  - Exudates in basal cisterns compress vessels, with subsequent ischemia
- In tuberculoma
  - Well-defined avascular lesions composed of a necrotic caseous center surrounded by a tuberculous granulation tissue; TB bacilli can be present in this granulation tissue.
  - Surrounding brain shows edema.
  - Occurs at any site; may adhere to dura
- Tuberculous bacilli are difficult to culture from tuberculomas.
- Immunohistochemical demonstration of mycobacterial antigen is possible from tuberculoma tissue.

DIFFERENTIAL DIAGNOSIS

- Tuberculous meningitis
  - Meningitis (e.g., chronic, viral, fungal, bacterial, carcinomatous)
  - Sarcoidosis
  - Lymphoma
- Intracranial tuberculoma
  - Granulomas (e.g., sarcoid, fungal)
  - Pyogenic abscess
  - Metastasis
  - Glioma
- Spinal tuberculoma
  - Intramedullary tumors
  - Syringomyelia
  - Spinal abscess
  - Myelitis

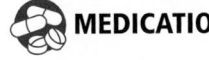

TREATMENT

- Best evidence suggests that Initial treatment should include 4-drug therapy with isoniazid, rifampin, pyrazinamide, and ethambutol for 2 months, followed by isoniazid and rifampin for 7–10 months. Optimal treatment duration is unknown. (3)[B]
- Adjunctive dexamethasone is recommended for tuberculous meningitis and tuberculoma. (5)[A]

INITIAL STABILIZATION
Often inpatient care needed

GENERAL MEASURES
- Look for other foci of infection.
- Seizure precautions.
- Neuropsychological surveillance is essential.
- Concurrent treatment of HIV, if present.

Diet
Pyridoxine supplementation (25 mg/d) in patients may prevent neuropathy (poor nutritional status, diabetes, HIV infection, pregnancy, alcohol use), especially if taking isoniazid. (3)[C]

Activity
- Appropriate restriction if seizures are present
- Isolation required only if pulmonary disease

ALERT
Pregnancy Considerations
Breast-feeding is not contraindicated. (3)[C]

MEDICATION (DRUGS)

First Line
- Antituberculous medications
  - Ist-line agents used in CNS TB are
    o Isoniazid (INH): Adults: 5 mg/kg PO or IM daily (max 300 mg/d) ; children: 10–15 mg/kg/d PO or IM (max 300 mg/d)
    o Rifampin (RIF): Adults: 10 mg/kg/d PO or IV (max 600 mg/d); children: 10–20 mg/kg/d PO or IV (max 600 mg/d)
    o Ethambutol (EMB): Adults: body weight (BW) 40–55 kg, 800 mg/d PO; BW 56–75 kg, 1200 mg/d PO; BW 76–90 kg, 1600 mg; children: 15–20 mg/kg/d (max 1000 mg/d)
    o Pyrazinamide (PZA): Adults: BW 40–55 kg, 1000 mg/d PO; BW 56–75 kg, 1500 mg/d PO; BW 76–90 kg, 2000 mg/d PO; children: 15–30 mg/kg/d (max 2000 mg/d)
  - Usual regimen: INH + RIF + EMB + PZA for 2 months, followed by INH + RIF for 7–10 months (3)[B]
  - Other drugs are added when drug resistance is suspected.
- Corticosteroids
  - Steroids are recommended for patients with meningitis (5)[A] or tuberculoma. (3)[C]
  - Dosing (IV or PO)
    o Adults and children >25 kg: 12 mg/d dexamethasone
    o Children <25 kg: 8 mg/d
  - Continue full-dose steroids for 3 weeks, followed by taper over 3 more weeks.

- Anticonvulsants
  - High incidence of seizures in tuberculomas requires the routine use of anticonvulsants.
  - Phenytoin or carbamazepine
- Diuretics
  - Furosemide or acetazolamide used for communicating hydrocephalus. (6)[C]
- Contraindications
  - INH: Acute liver disease, previous INH-associated hepatitis
  - RIF: Concomitant use of some HIV antiretrovirals, hypersensitivity to RIF
  - EMB: Optic neuritis, patients unable to report visual adverse effects (e.g., young children)
  - PZA: Severe hepatic dysfunction
- Precautions
  - INH: Peripheral neuropathy, rash, elevated liver function tests, psychosis, lupuslike syndrome, hepatitis, seizures, optic neuritis
  - RIF: Hepatotoxicity, red-orange colored body fluids, gastrointestinal distress
  - EMB: Optic neuritis (color blindness, decreased visual acuity), rash, dizziness, hyperuricemia
  - PZA: Transient rash, hyperuricemia, hepatotoxicity, arthralgias
- Significant possible interactions
  - INH inhibits the metabolism of phenytoin, carbamazepine, warfarin, and theophylline, resulting in elevated serum concentrations of these drugs. Monitor closely.
  - RIF has numerous significant drug interactions due to its potent hepatic enzyme-inducing effects. Consult prescribing information for details.
  - Antacids decrease the absorption of EMB.

Second Line
- 2nd-line drugs include streptomycin, ethionamide, kanamycin, capreomycin, cycloserine, and fluoroquinolones.
- Reserved for patients with resistant TB or intolerance to 1st-line agents (3)[C]

ALERT
Pregnancy Considerations
- Streptomycin and fluoroquinolones are not recommended.
- Anticonvulsants must be properly chosen.

SURGERY
- Tuberculous meningitis
  - Surgical diversion of CSF when tuberculous meningitis associated with symptomatic elevated intracranial pressure and noncommunicating hydrocephalus (ventriculoperitoneal shunt preferred) (7)[B]
- Tuberculoma
  - Surgical intervention for decompression or debulking of large, symptomatic tuberculomas is required. (8)[C]
  - Surgery considered for treatment failures or to relieve elevated intracranial pressure. Antituberculous therapy is continued to prevent seeding of meninges. (2)[C]

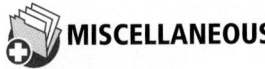

FOLLOW-UP

PROGNOSIS
- In tuberculous meningitis and tuberculomas, prognosis depends on age, duration of symptoms, and neurologic status.
- 10–30% of patients have permanent neurologic deficits.

COMPLICATIONS
- Visual deterioration
- Focal deficits
- Cognitive deterioration
- Paraplegia
- Hormonal deficiencies
- Shunt block
- Shunt infection
- Side effects of antituberculous therapy

PATIENT MONITORING
- Liver function tests
- Uric acid
- Assessment of peripheral neuropathy
- Monthly visual acuity and red-green color discrimination testing if receiving EMB therapy
- Anticonvulsant medication serum levels
- Attention to possible drug–drug interactions.
- Contrast-enhanced CT scan in patients with tuberculoma on medical treatment every 3–6 months until complete resolution of symptoms
- Hormonal evaluation (e.g., thyroid-stimulating hormone, cortisol, prolactin) in pituitary TB

REFERENCES
1. Thwaites GE, Hien TT. Tuberculous meningitis: Many questions, too few answers. *Lancet Neurol* 2005;4:160–170.
2. Afghani B, Lieberman JM. Paradoxical enlargement or development of intracranial tuberculomas during therapy: Case report and review. *Clin Infect Dis* 1994;19:1092–1099.
3. American Thoracic Society, CDC, Infectious Diseases Society of America. Treatment of tuberculosis. *MMWR Recomm Rep* 2003;52(RR–11):1–77.
4. Gropper MR, Schulder M, Sharan AD, Cho E-S. Central nervous system tuberculosis: Medical management and surgical indications. *Surg Neurol* 1995;44:378–385.
5. Prasad K, Volmink J, Menon GR. Steroids for treating tuberculous meningitis. *Cochrane Database Syst Rev* 2000;(3):CD02244.
6. Donald PR, Schoeman JF. Tuberculous meningitis. *N Engl J Med* 2004;351:1719–1720.
7. Thwaites G, Chau TTH, Mai NTH, Drobinewski F, McAdam K, Farrar J. Tuberculous meningitis. *J Neurol Neurosurg Psychiatry* 2000;68:289–299.
8. Jain SK, Kwon P, Moss WJ. Management and outcomes of intracranial tuberculomas developing during antituberculous therapy: Case report and review. *Clin Pediatr* 2005;44:443–450.

MISCELLANEOUS

See also: Tuberculosis

CODES

ICD9-CM
- 013.0 Tuberculous meningitis
- 013.1 Tuberculoma of meninges
- 013.2 Tuberculoma of brain
- 013.4 Tuberculoma of spinal cord

PATIENT TEACHING
Explain the nature of the disease state, importance of adherence to drug therapy, adverse effects, and drug interactions with therapy.

T

TUBERCULOSIS, LATENT

Kay A. Bauman, MD, MPH

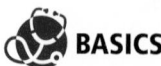 **BASICS**

DESCRIPTION

Tuberculosis (TB) is a common infection transmitted by inhaling airborne bacilli from a person with active tuberculosis. The bacilli multiply in the alveolus and are carried by macrophages, lymphatics, and blood to distant sites (e.g., lung pleura, brain, kidney, bone). Tissue hypersensitivity halts infection within 10 weeks.

- Latent tuberculosis infection (LTBI) is asymptomatic, noninfectious, and usually detected by a positive skin test (evidence of prior TB infection by purified protein derivative [PPD] or chest radiograph, but acid-fast bacilli smear and culture are negative and chest radiograph does not suggest active TB).
- TB: Active disease occurs in 5–10% of infected individuals without preventive therapy. (1) Chance of disease increases with immunosuppression and is highest for all individuals within 2 years after infection; 85% of the cases are pulmonary, which is infectious.
- Recrudescent TB: The active disease occurs after a period of latent asymptomatic infection.
- System(s) Affected: Asymptomatic

GENERAL PREVENTION

Treatment of LTBI is also preventive: To decrease the incidence of TB in both the individuals treated and to decrease the risk to close contacts should active TB occur.

EPIDEMIOLOGY

- TB screening of high risk groups (e.g., recent immigrants from Asia, Latin America, and Africa; pockets of homelessness; history of drug use; history of incarceration). (1)
- Recrudescent disease: Adults and elderly, HIV infected, those newly exposed, including pediatric population
- Predominant sex: Male > Female

Prevalence

In the US, 10–15 million people have the latent infection. (1)

RISK FACTORS

- Immigrant within 5 years (from Asia, Africa, Latin America); including migrant workers
- HIV infection, immunosuppression
- Close contact with infected individual
- Institutional environment (e.g., prison, nursing home)
- Use of illicit drugs
- Lower socioeconomic or homeless
- Health care workers
- Chronic disease such as diabetes mellitus, end-stage renal disease, cancer or silicosis.

ETIOLOGY

Mycobacterium tuberculosis, Mycobacterium bovis, and *Mycobacterium africanum*

ASSOCIATED CONDITIONS

- HIV infection (see "Tests")
- Immune suppression

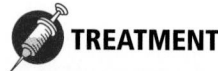 **DIAGNOSIS**

SIGNS AND SYMPTOMS

None

History

History of recent immigration from a high-risk area, history of IV drug use and/or drug treatment, HIV, homelessness, recent incarceration (1)

TESTS

- HIV test recommended to assess risk for active TB in men who have sex with men or persons with a history of IV drug use
- PPD: 5 units (0.1 mL) intermediate strength intradermal volar forearm. Measure induration at 48–72 hours.
  - Positive if induration is >5 mm and patient has HIV infection (or suspected) (2), is immunosuppressed, had recent close TB contact, or has clinical evidence of active or old disease on chest radiograph; induration is >10 mm and patient is <4 years old or has other risk factors noted above; or induration is >15 mm and patient is >4 years old and has no risk factors (3)
  - Negative if induration is <5 mm on initial test and, if indicated, on 2nd test. Utilize the 2-step test if patient has had no recent PPD and is >55 years old, or is a nursing home resident, prison inmate, or health care worker (administer a 2nd intradermal test 1–3 weeks after initial test; measure and interpret as usual). (3)
  - The interferon-gamma blood test or QuantiFERON-TB and QuantiFERON-TB GOLD, measure the release of interferon-gamma by sensitized lymphocytes when exposed to antigens of *M. tuberculosis*. It is unaffected by prior Bacillus Calmette-Guérin (BCG) vaccination, requires only 1 patient visit, has improved sensitivity and specificity, but is costly. (4)
  - Do not use BCG vaccination as a reason to ignore a positive PPD in adults and forego recommendation for treatment.
- The multiple puncture (Tine) test is not recommended.

Lab

- None routinely recommended
  - BCG vaccine: False-positive skin test but unreliable and *should not influence decision* to treat LTBI
  - Steroids: False-negative skin test
  - Measles vaccine: May suppress tuberculin activity; simultaneous PPD and measles vaccine recommended; if not simultaneous, defer PPD 4–6 weeks after measles vaccine
- Disorders that may alter results: False-negative skin test
  - Recent viral infection
  - New (<10 weeks) infection
  - Severe malnutrition
  - HIV
  - Anergy
  - Age <6 months
  - Overwhelming TB

Imaging

- Chest radiography required to rule out TB in asymptomatic infected persons
- CT of the chest—good sensitivity

DIFFERENTIAL DIAGNOSIS

Fungal infections, especially other atypical mycobacteria or nocardia

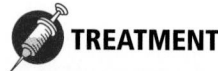 **TREATMENT**

GENERAL MEASURES

- Treat LTBI at any age if patient has HIV, has had close TB contact, is a recent converter (<2 years), is an IV drug user, has an abnormal chest radiograph, has a high-risk medical condition, or is in another high-risk group. (1) Use isoniazid (INH) daily for 9 months [A] or an accepted alternative
  - INH twice weekly for 9 months with directly observed treatment (DOT) [B]
  - INH daily or twice weekly for 6 months with DOT (B)
  - Rifampin (RIF) daily for 4 months [B] RIF plus pyrazinamide (PZA) daily for 2 months or twice weekly for 2–3 months [D]; special monitoring for hepatic toxicity required (preferred if patient is INH resistant). For inactive pulmonary TB on chest radiograph, use INH for 9 months

  - Consider INH resistance
  - DOT is recommended if patient adherence is not assured
- Careful reevaluation required; change to twice weekly dosing only if using DOT
- Treat LTBI during pregnancy if patient has recent infection or is HIV positive (use INH with pyridoxine and monitor liver enzymes); otherwise, treatment may be postponed until postpartum (2)

Diet

Regular, consider pyridoxine supplement: 10–50 mg/d

Activity

- As tolerated
- No isolation required

ALERT

Geriatric Considerations

- Before entering a chronic care facility, patients should have a PPD using 2-step protocols.
- INH side effects are more pronounced.

Pediatric Considerations

- Protocol for newborn with mother/household contact with infection or disease
  - If mother or household contact has LTBI, skin test all household contacts and treat any with positive PPD
  - If contact has abnormal chest radiograph, separate infant until infectious status known; if not contagious, monitor infant PPD (5)
  - If mother has disease and is possibly contagious, evaluate infant for congenital TB and test for HIV; separate newborn until mother is noninfectious (5)
  - If congenital TB is suspected, treat.
  - If there is no congenital disease, start INH and repeat PPD after 3–4 months. If positive, reassess infant and finish 9 months INH. If PPD is negative and source is noninfectious, stop INH and monitor infant. (5)
- Consider BCG

MEDICATION (DRUGS)

- INH scored tablets: 100 mg, 300 mg, or syrup 10 mg/mL
  - Daily: Adult 300 mg; pediatric 10–15 mg/kg (maximum 300 mg) (3,5)
  - Twice weekly: Adult 15 mg/kg; pediatric 20–30 mg/kg (maximum 900 mg) (3,5)
- RIF capsules: 150/300 or syrup 10 mg/mL
  - Daily: Adult 600 mg; pediatric 10–20 mg/kg (maximum 600 mg) (3,5)
  - Twice weekly: Adult 600 mg; pediatric 10–20 mg/kg (maximum 600 mg) (3,5)
- PZA scored tablets: 500 mg
  - Daily: Adult 15–25 mg/kg (maximum 2 g); pediatric 20–40 mg/kg (maximum 2 g) (3,5)
  - Twice weekly: Adult 50 mg/kg; pediatric 50 mg/kg (maximum 4 g)
- Precautions
  - RIF and PZA may cause hepatitis. (3)
  - Follow liver function if the patient has history of liver dysfunction or new signs develop.
  - RIF colors urine, tears, and secretions orange. May permanently stain contact lenses. (3)
  - INH: Peripheral neuritis and hypersensitivity are possible. Consider pyridoxine. (3)
  - PZA may increase uric acid. (3)
  - Avoid PZA during pregnancy.
- Significant possible interactions: RIF alters the level of phenytoin (Dilantin), antivirals (3), and other drugs metabolized by the liver; may inactivate birth control pills (recommend barrier method).
- Women may breast-feed while taking TB drugs.

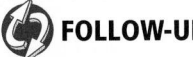 **FOLLOW-UP**

PROGNOSIS
Generally few complications and effective if drugs are taken for full course as prescribed

COMPLICATIONS
Recrudescent TB

PATIENT MONITORING
- During preventive therapy for LTBI: Initial monthly visits to assess adherence to regimen and to monitor for hepatitis and neuropathy; if stable, can monitor less frequently.
- If patient remains asymptomatic, repeat chest radiograph is not needed.
- Check liver enzymes if patient is symptomatic, is HIV positive, has chronic liver disease, uses alcohol, or is pregnant or postpartum, and modify drugs if needed.
- RIF plus PZA treatment of LTBI requires special monitoring. Dispense only 2-week supply of RIF-PZA. Reevaluate in person at 2, 4, 6, and 8 weeks; test liver enzymes and bilirubin at baseline 2, 4, and 6 weeks. Stop treatment if bilirubin is above normal or symptoms of hepatitis with enzymes are above normal or enzymes are 5 times normal. (5)

REFERENCES

1. Centers for Disease Control and Prevention. Controlling Tuberculosis in the United States: Recommendations from the American Thoracic Society, CDC, and the Infectious Diseases Society of America. *MMWR Recomm Rep*. 2005;54(RR-12): 1–80.
2. Centers for Disease Control and Prevention. Prevention and treatment of tuberculosis among patients infected with human immunodeficiency virus: Principles and revised recommendations. *MMWR Recomm Rep*. 1998;47(RR-20):1–58.
3. Blumberg HM, Leonard MK, Jasmer RM. Update on the treatment of tuberculosis. Part II. *Dis Mon*. 1997;43:181–274.
4. Campos-Outcalt D. When, and when not, to use the interferon-gamma TB blood test. *J Fam Pract*. 2005;54:873–875.
5. *American Academy of Pediatrics. Report of the Committee on Infectious Diseases (Red Book)*. Elk Grove Village, IL: American Academy of Pediatrics; 2003.
6. Centers for Disease Control and Prevention. Update: Adverse event data and revised American Thoracic Society/CDC recommendations against the use of rifampin and pyrazinamide for treatment of latent tuberculosis infection United States, 2003. *MMWR*. 2003;52:735–738.

 MISCELLANEOUS

- BCG vaccine, live attenuated *M. bovis*: Used more commonly in developing countries to prevent complications of TB
- See also: Tuberculosis

CODES

ICD9-CM
795.5 Nonspecific reaction to tuberculin skin test without active tuberculosis (PPD positive)

PATIENT TEACHING
- Teach pathogenesis, emphasize importance of drug therapy, warn of effects and/or interactions, and find contacts
- Inform local health department

T

TUBERCULOSIS, MILIARY

Katherine Berg, MD

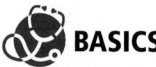 **BASICS**

DESCRIPTION

- Any progressive, disseminated form of TB, resulting from uncontrolled hematogenous spread of *Mycobacterium tuberculosis*. Originally named for "millet seed" appearance of nodules often found in lungs. 3 types
  - Acute: Usually with primary infection. Rapidly progressive, more severe type
  - Late generalized: Occurs after years of latent infection. Chronic, more indolent course
  - Anergic: Rare. Microabscesses form in place of granulomas. Generally a reactivation of old disease, older patients
- System(s) Affected: Most commonly Pulmonary; Lymphatic; CNS (TB meningitis); Hepatic; Splenic; and Bone Marrow.
- Multiorgan failure and ARDS also known to occur
- Synonym(s): Disseminated TB

GENERAL PREVENTION

- BCG vaccine
  - 78% effective preventing severe meningeal and miliary TB in children (1)[B]
- Treatment of latent TB infection with INH (see "Tuberculosis, latent")

EPIDEMIOLOGY

- 1–3% of all TB cases (See "Tuberculosis" chapter)
- 10% of pulmonary TB cases and 38% of extrapulmonary cases in AIDS population (2)
- Gender: Male > Female (as in all types of TB)

RISK FACTORS

Within TB-infected population, risk factors for miliary disease include
- HIV infection/AIDS
- Young age (especially <1 year) or old age
- Iatrogenic immunosuppression (i.e., organ transplant patients, chronic corticosteroid use)
- Diabetes mellitus
- Pregnancy
- Chronic renal failure
- Protein malnutrition

PATHOPHYSIOLOGY

- Lymphatic or hematogenous spread from a local focus, with failure of the body to halt infection by granulomatous encapsulation.
- Commonly affects the more vascular organs (i.e., spleen, liver, brain, bone marrow)
- Iatrogenic disease also reported after solid organ transplants, urethral catheterization, and cardiac valve transplants.

ETIOLOGY

TB infection in the context of impaired cell-mediated immunity
- Primary infection in immunocompromised host, or recrudescent infection in once-healthy host with new health impairment.
- Iatrogenic infection as above.

ASSOCIATED CONDITIONS

HIV/AIDS: See "Special Considerations"

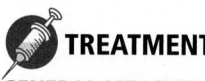 **DIAGNOSIS**

PRE HOSPITAL

- Diagnosis often is impeded by low suspicion and delay in collecting fluid/tissue samples for AFB smear and culture.
- Identify and test any close contacts.

SIGNS AND SYMPTOMS

Presentation extremely variable, but may include
- Night sweats (near 100%)
- Fever (96%)
- Weight loss, anorexia (92%)
- Tachypnea, tachycardia (77%)
- Cough, dyspnea (72%)
- Hepatomegaly (52%)
- Neurological/HA/mental status changes (25%)
- Chills
- Single or multiorgan failure
- Severe disease resulting in septic shock and ARDS has been reported.
- Chest pain

History
Ask about risk factors

Physical Exam
- Vital signs: Fever, tachycardia, tachypnea common
- Pulmonary: Rales (50%)
- Hepatosplenomegaly common
- Should have ophthalmologist do dilated funduscopic exam to look for choroidal tubercles (found in 50% postmortem) (3)[B]
- Evaluate for meningeal signs

TESTS

- PPD positive in <50% of cases
- Sputum for AFB smear and culture
- Gastric washings (especially in children), CSF, blood cxs, or bone and liver biopsy also for smear and culture
- Test for HIV (4)[C]

ALERT

Pediatric Considerations
May need to culture samples from infected adult contact, because samples can be difficult to obtain in pediatric cases.

Lab
Abnormal lab findings may include
- Normochromic anemia
- Leucopenia or leukocytosis
- Elevated ESR
- Hyponatremia

Imaging
- Chest radiograph: Faint, reticulonodular infiltrate, uniform distribution. Often mediastinal/hilar adenopathy
- Chest CT: Numerous 2–3 mm nodules scattered throughout lungs in >85% of patients
- Abdominal/pelvic CT: If suspicious of other organ involvement.
- Brain MRI: Cerebral nodules or tuberculoma
  - Only if neurological symptoms present

Diagnostic Procedures/Surgery
- See "Tuberculosis" chapter.
- Collect samples for AFB/culture. (4)[A] Sampling fluids from multiple sites greatly improves yield for AFB smear and culture.
  - Sputum culture positive in 62% (smear in 33%)
  - BAL culture positive in 55% (smear in 27%)
  - Gastric aspirate culture positive in 100% (smear in 43%)
  - CSF culture positive in 60% (smear in 8%) (5)
- Biopsy organs based on symptoms

Pathological Findings
- Caseating granulomas on tissue biopsy (liver most common site)
- Microabscesses with neutrophilic response in acute type
- Can see mycotic aneurysms if disease affects aorta
- TB pericarditis diagnosed by pericardial biopsy

DIFFERENTIAL DIAGNOSIS

- Other pneumonias
- Lymphoma
- Metastatic carcinoma
- Sarcoidosis

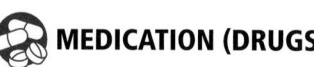 **TREATMENT**

GENERAL MEASURES

- See "Tuberculosis" chapter
- Respiratory isolation until clinically responding and 3 negative AFB smears (4)[B]
- ARDS/organ failure may complicate treatment.
- If CNS involvement, extended treatment is advised (9–12 months). (6)[C]

Diet
Some evidence suggests that high-cholesterol diet accelerates sterilization of sputum in pulmonary TB patients.

Activity
Respiratory isolation if pulmonary disease
- Negative pressure room
- TB mask when out of room

MEDICATION (DRUGS)

- All drug regimens same as those for general tuberculosis.
- Adherence extremely important to prevent drug resistance. Responsibility is the provider's.

First Line
- Regimen 1 (preferred)
  - Initial phase: Isoniazid (INH), rifampin (RIF), pyrazinamide (PZA), and ethambutol (EMB) once daily for 8 weeks
  - Continuation phase: INH/RIF daily for 18 weeks. Or INH/RIF twice weekly for 18 weeks (only use for HIV+ if CD4>100); or INH/ rifapentine once weekly for 18 weeks (acceptable alternative for HIV− patients only) (7)[A]

- Regimen 2
  - Initial phase: INH/RIF/PZA/EMB daily for 2 weeks, then twice weekly for 6 weeks
  - Continuation phase: INH/RIF twice weekly for 18 weeks (HIV⁺ patients only if CD4>100) or INH/rifapentine once weekly for 18 weeks (acceptable alternative for HIV⁻ patients only) (7)[A]
- Regimen 3 (acceptable alternative)
  - Initial phase: INH/RIF/PZA/EMB daily for 8 weeks
  - Continuation phase: INH/RIF 3 times weekly for 18 weeks (7)[A]
- Regimen 4 (only when unable to give preferred regimen)
  - Initial phase: INH/RIF/EMB daily for 8 weeks
  - Continuation phase: INH/RIF daily or twice weekly for 31 weeks (7)[B]
- No studies proving efficacy of 5 times a week regimen, but clinical evidence suggests it. [C]
- Directly observed therapy required for non-daily regimens (7).
- Dosing
- INH: Scored tabs 50/100/300 mg, syrup 10 mg/mL, or aqueous solution 100 mg/mL
  - Daily dose: Adult 5 mg/kg (max 300 mg); pediatric 10 to 15 mg/kg (max 300 mg)
  - 3 times weekly: Adult 15 mg/kg (max 900 mg)
  - Twice weekly: Adult 15 mg/kg (max 900 mg); pediatric 20–30 mg/kg (max 900 mg)
  - Weekly: Adult only, 15 mg/kg (max 900 mg)
  - Consider pyridoxine 10–50 mg/d
- RIF: Capsules 150/300 mg, powder for oral suspension, or IV aqueous
  - Daily or twice weekly dose: Adult and pediatric 10–20 mg/kg (maximum 600 mg)
- PZA: Scored tabs 500 mg. Dosed by weight
  - Adults 40–55 kg
    - Daily: 18–25 mg/kg, max 1 g
    - 3 times weekly: 27–37 mg/kg, max 1.5 g
    - Twice weekly: 36–50 mg/kg, max 2 g
  - Adults 56–75 kg
    - Daily: 20–27 mg/kg, max 1.5 g
    - 3 times weekly: 33–45 mg/kg, max 2.5 g
    - Twice weekly: 40–54 mg/kg, max 3 g
  - Adults > 75 kg
    - Daily: 22–26 mg/kg, max 2 g
    - 3 times weekly: 33–40 mg/kg, max 3 g
    - Twice weekly: 44–53 mg/kg, max 4 g
  - Pediatric daily: 15 to 30 mg/kg (maximum 2 g)
  - Pediatric twice weekly: 50 mg/kg (maximum 4 g)
- Rifabutin (Mycobutin): Capsules 150 mg
  - Daily or twice weekly: Adult 5 mg/kg, max 300 mg
- Rifapentine (Priftine): Tablet 150 mg; for continuation phase only
  - HIV⁻ adults: 600 mg once weekly, given with INH. Not effective if HIV⁺. (7)[A]
- EMB: Tablets 100/400 mg bacteriostatic. Dose based on weight
  - Adults 40–55 kg
    - Daily: 15–20 mg/kg, max 800 mg
    - 3 times weekly: 22–30 mg/kg, max 1.2 g
    - Twice weekly: 36–50 mg/kg, max 2 g
  - Adults 56–75 kg
    - Daily: 16–22 mg/kg, max 1.2 g
    - 3 times weekly: 27–36 mg/kg, max 2 g
    - Twice weekly: 37–50 mg/kg, max 2.8 g

- Adults >75 kg
    - Daily: 22–26 mg/kg, max 2.6 g
    - 3 times weekly: 33–40 mg/kg, max 2.4 g
    - Twice weekly: 44–53 mg/kg, max 4 g
  - Pediatrics
    - Daily: 15–20 mg/kg, max 1 g
    - Twice weekly: 50 mg/kg, max 4 g
- Contraindications
  - RIF: Avoid if patient taking antiretrovirals
  - EMB: May cause optic neuritis. Avoid unless patient old enough to cooperate for visual acuity and color testing
- Precautions
  - INH, RIF, PZA: May cause hepatitis. Caution if liver disease.
  - RIF: Colors urine, tears, and secretions orange. Can stain contact lenses.
  - INH: Peripheral neuritis and hypersensitivity possible. Treat with pyridoxine.
  - PZA: May increase uric acid. Unclear safety during pregnancy [C]
- Significant possible interactions: Rifamycins alter level of phenytoin, antivirals, and other drugs metabolized by liver and may inactivate birth control pills (recommend a barrier method).

Second Line

- Corticosteroids: Use only with concurrent anti-TB therapy. Recommended for TB meningitis, pericarditis, or severe miliary disease (3)[B]
  - Reduce fluid reaccumulation in pericarditis, but no proven mortality benefit. (2)[B]
  - Also for HIV⁺ population (see "Considerations" below)
- Streptomycin: Caution—ototoxic and nephrotoxic; do not use in pregnancy.

ALERT

Geriatric Considerations
See "Tuberculosis" chapter.

Pediatric Considerations
See "Tuberculosis" chapter.

Pregnancy Considerations
See "Tuberculosis" chapter.

SPECIAL CONSIDERATIONS FOR HIV⁺ GROUP

- If CD4, 100, risk of developing resistance to RIF if given <3 times weekly.
- INH/Rifapentine once weekly continuation phase contraindicated.
- Paradoxical worsening of disease may occur during treatment; this is thought due to immune reconstitution while on antiretrovirals.
  - If mild, treat with NSAIDs
  - If severe, prednisone (1–2 mg/kg for 2 weeks, then taper) has been shown helpful) (6)[C]

Second Line

- Corticosteroids shown effective for TB pericarditis and meningitis, and miliary TB (2)[B]
- Streptomycin-resistance has increased in recent years. Contraindicated in pregnancy; it causes ototoxicity in fetus.

SURGERY
Case-specific, depending on location of disease.

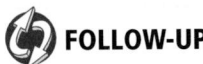

FOLLOW-UP

As for general TB.

Issues for Referral
ID specialist helpful for patients also on antiretrovirals, because doses may need adjusting

PROGNOSIS
- Mortality: 16–38%
- If ARDS develops, mortality is 80–100%

COMPLICATIONS
- ARDS with refractory hypoxemia can occur
- Multidrug resistant TB rare in the US, but increasing elsewhere.

PATIENT MONITORING
See "Tuberculosis" chapter.

REFERENCES

1. Coditz. Efficacy of BCG vaccine in the prevention of TB. *JAMA* 1994;271(9):698–702.
2. Golden M. Extrapulmonary TB; an overview. *Am Fam Physician* 2005;72(9).
3. Slavin. Late generalized TB; a clinical pathologic analysis and comparison of 100 cases in the preantibiotic and antibiotic eras. *Medicine* 1980;59(5):352–366.
4. Horsburgh et al. Treatment guidelines for treatment of TB. *Clin Infect Dis* 2000;31:633–6392000.
5. Maartens. Miliary TB; rapid diagnosis, hematologic abnormalities and outcome in 109 treated adults. *Am J Med* 1990;89(3):291–296.
6. American Thoracic Society, CDC, and Infectious Diseases Society of America. Treatment of tuberculosis. *MMWR* 2003;52(RR11):1–77.
7. Potter B. Management of active TB. *Am Fam Physician* 2005;72(11).

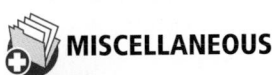

MISCELLANEOUS

CODES

ICD9-CM
018.9- Miliary tuberculosis, unspecified

PATIENT TEACHING
- Emphasize importance of adherence to treatment.
- Educate about adverse effects of medications.

TUBEROUS SCLEROSIS COMPLEX

Nuhad D. Dinno, MD

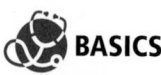

BASICS

DESCRIPTION
- 1 of the neurocutaneous syndromes (phakomatoses).
- A genetic developmental disorder with variable presentations, a broad clinical spectrum, and multiorgan involvement.
- Organ system changes may be few and subtle but can encompass multiple types of cutaneous lesions and tumor formation in the CNS, skin, retina, heart, lung, viscera, liver, kidney, bone, teeth, and nails. Other phakomatoses include neurofibromatosis, Sturge-Weber disease, von Hippel-Lindau syndrome, and ataxia-telangiectasia.
- System(s) Affected: Cardiovascular; Musculoskeletal; Nervous; Pulmonary; Renal/Urologic; Skin/Exocrine
- Synonym(s): Bourneville disease

ALERT
Pregnancy Considerations
- Genetic counseling
- Prenatal testing by ultrasonography for tumors is available, but sensitivity is unknown. Prenatal DNA analysis is available to families previously enrolled in a research protocol.

GENERAL PREVENTION
Genetic counseling

EPIDEMIOLOGY
- Predominant age: Clinical expression is variable, so diagnosis may be delayed. Usually diagnosed during the 1st decade of life.
- Predominant sex: Male = Female (but autism more common in male patients)

Prevalence
Reported to affect 1/5,800–1/30,000 in the general population

RISK FACTORS
Family history

Genetics
- Autosomal dominant with variable penetrance
- 2/3 of cases result from new genetic mutations.
- 2 chromosomal loci have been mapped: Tuberous sclerosis complex 1 (locus 9q34) and tuberous sclerosis complex 2 (locus 16p13.3).

ETIOLOGY
Congenital

DIAGNOSIS

SIGNS AND SYMPTOMS
- Most cases have more than one of the following findings
  - Angiofibromata (termed adenoma sebaceum and ranging from 0.1–1.0 cm) and often present as facial lesions in a "butterfly" distribution (80%)
  - Hypopigmented areas, mainly on trunk and extremities, are often the 1st sign (e.g., ash-leaf spots); present at birth or shortly after (50%)
  - Seizure disorders including myoclonic (90%)
  - Renal cysts (50–80%)
  - Pulmonary lymphangiomatosis (<10%)
  - CNS periventricular calcifications (50–80%)
  - Retinal astrocytomas and hamartomas (50–80%)
  - Cardiac rhabdomyomas (50%)
  - Mental retardation (60–70%)
  - Autism (10–20%)
  - Ungual fibromas, multiple (20%)
  - Dental pits
  - Liver hamartomas (10%)
- Any combination of the above stigmata may be present at, or shortly after, birth or may only become apparent in later childhood or adulthood.

TESTS
Must rely mainly on clinical diagnostic criteria until a reliable molecular marker is found.

Lab
- Abnormal electroencephalographic results
- Research to isolate and determine reliable molecular marker and gene seems promising.

Imaging
- MRI and CT have become primary diagnostic techniques in this disorder.
- With gadolinium enhancement, MRI provides more detailed imaging of characteristic subependymal nodules and cortical white matter tubers.
- Fetal cardiac rhabdomyomas can be seen sonographically during late gestation.
- EEG
- MRI with gadolinium contrast
- Renal CT, ultrasound
- ECG

Diagnostic Procedures/Surgery
- Woods lamp evaluation for ash-leaf spots
- Biopsy of indeterminate lesions
- Molecular testing generally available on research basis only, although now more routinely offered to families with diagnosed tuberous sclerosis complex 1 or tuberous sclerosis complex 2 mutation
- Neurodevelopmental testing as age-appropriate.
- Screening for neurodevelopmental and behavioral difficulties at time of diagnosis

Pathological Findings
- Nodular lesions made up largely of irregular groups of glial fibrils, ganglion cells, and atypical cells thought to result from faults in developing tissue combinations (e.g., hamartomas)
- Lesions may be sparse at birth.
- Calcification of subependymal lesions may not occur until several months after birth.
- Facial angiofibromas, ungual fibromas, and renal angiomyolipomas are specific lesions that may develop months after birth.
- ~1% of affected patients present with tuberous sclerosis lymphangioleiomyomatosis, usually women of reproductive age
- Not practical to have age-specific criteria

DIFFERENTIAL DIAGNOSIS
- Polycystic kidney disease, renal hamartomas
- Other causes of seizure disorders, mental retardation, autistic behavior, or traumatic ungual fibromata
- Other neurocutaneous syndromes (e.g., the phacomatoses)

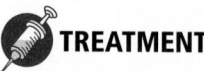

TREATMENT

INITIAL STABILIZATION
Outpatient, except for complications for severely involved manifestations or uncontrolled seizures

GENERAL MEASURES
- Team approach with involvement of primary care providers, neurologic, orthopedic, surgical, and radiologic specialists
- Physical, occupational, and speech therapy
- Social workers for home care

- Vocational training support
- Periodic reassessment in at-risk families
- Genetic counseling for patient and family
- Neurosurgical consideration for uncontrollable seizures

Diet
No restrictions. Special diets, such as a ketogenic diet, have been used for seizure control.

Activity
Determined by degree and complexity of involvement

 ## MEDICATION (DRUGS)

First Line
- Anticonvulsants for seizure control
- Antibiotic prophylaxis for surgery if indicated
- Precautions: Refer to the manufacturer's profile for each drug.
- Significant possible interactions: Knowledge of anticonvulsant used is necessary to avoid drug interactions, especially with antibiotics.
- Refer to the manufacturer's profile for each drug.

Second Line
Refer to http://clinicaltrials.gov

SURGERY
Surgical excision of tumors where and when appropriate

 ## FOLLOW-UP

PROGNOSIS
Variable; shortened longevity compared with expectations in general population

COMPLICATIONS
See "Signs and Symptoms."

PATIENT MONITORING
- Clinical features and symptoms should be reviewed and updated periodically.
- Periodic reassessment of at-risk patients

REFERENCES

1. Aicardi J. Tuberous sclerosis. *Int Pediatr*. 1993;8:2: 171–175.
2. *Perspective* Newsletter, National Tuberous Sclerosis Association, Spring/Summer/Fall/Winter Publications.
3. Roach ES, et al. Tuberous sclerosis consensus conference: Recommendations for diagnostic evaluation. *J Child Neurol*. 1999;14:401–407.
4. Caldemeyer KS, Mirowski GW. Tuberous sclerosis. Part 1: Clinical and central nervous system findings. *J Amer Acad Dermatol*. 2001;45:448–449.
5. Baker P, Piven J, Sato Y. Autism and tuberous sclerosis complex: Prevalence and clinical features. *J Autism Dev Disord*. 1998;28:279–285.
6. Roach ES, Sparagana P. Diagnosis of Tuberous Sclerosis complex. *J Child Neurol*. 2004(9): 643–649.

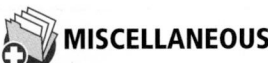 ## MISCELLANEOUS

See also: Neurofibromatosis (Types 1 and 2)

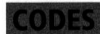 CODES

ICD9-CM
759.5 Tuberous sclerosis

PATIENT TEACHING
- Precautions related to seizures
- Updated information available from National Tuberous Sclerosis Association, Inc., 8181 Professional Place, Suite 110, Landover, MD 20785; (800) 225-6872; e-mail ntsa@ntsa.org; Web site www.ntsa.org

 See Corresponding Diagnostic Algorithm

T

TULAREMIA
Omar A. Khan, MD, MHS

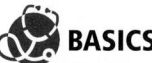 **BASICS**

DESCRIPTION
- Zoonotic infection caused by 2 subspecies of *Francisella tularensis* (subsp. *tularensis* and *holarctica*).
- Incubation averages 3–4 days; range, 1–21 days. May be ulceroglandular, glandular, typhoidal, oculoglandular, or oropharyngeal in manifestation
- System(s) Affected: Cardiovascular; Hemic/Lymphatic/Immunologic; Pulmonary; Skin/Exocrine
- Synonym(s): Rabbit fever; Deer-fly fever; *Pasteurella tularensis*; *Bacterium tularense*; Tick fever; Ohara disease; Francis disease

GENERAL PREVENTION
- Wear tick repellents.
- Avoid contact with material (e.g., water) that may have been in contact with infected animals.
- Remove tick by grasping near its mouth parts.
- Avoid squeezing body of engorged tick.
- Wear gloves while handling game and other animals, especially rabbits and rodents.
- Cook wild game thoroughly.
- Lab workers. Wear protective hoods and use negative-pressure cabinets when working with *F. tularensis*. Follow Biosafety Level 3 precautions
- A live attenuated vaccine applied intradermally to high-risk individuals (e.g., military personnel) is not available for general use.

EPIDEMIOLOGY
- Predominant age: All ages; more likely to occur in young adults with outdoor interests
- Predominant sex: Male > Female

Incidence
0.1/100,000; high rate of asymptomatic infection in endemic areas

Prevalence
~200 cases reported annually in US; likely an under-reported disease.

RISK FACTORS
- Location in endemic area; >50% of US cases in Arkansas, Missouri, Oklahoma, Tennessee, and Texas; also in South Dakota, Montana, Kansas, Colorado, and Illinois
- Non-US cases occur in Eastern Europe, China, Japan, and northern Europe, with predilection for rural areas.
- Outdoor work
- Rural residence
- Handling wild game or infected hay
- Laboratory work with the causative organism

PATHOPHYSIOLOGY
- Acquired through arthropod, fly, or mosquito vector (see "Etiology").
- Depending on route of infection, may cause a respiratory illness ± septicemia, or local ulceration and lymphadenopathy.
- Of the 2 subspecies, *tularensis* is more virulent than *holarctica*.

ETIOLOGY
Inoculation of *F. tularensis* via
- Tick bite (most common)
- Deer fly (*Chrysops*) bite (less common than via tick bites)
- Mosquitoes, especially in Eastern Europe
- Aerosol inhalation, from contaminated dust, hay, or pelts
- Contact of skin or mucous membranes with blood or tissue of infected carcass (e.g., pathogen can penetrate unbroken skin)
- Ingestion of undercooked meat of infected animals
- Ingestion of contaminated water
- Laboratory-acquired infections (usually respiratory)

ASSOCIATED CONDITIONS
- Other arthropod-borne diseases
- Tularemic conjunctivitis
- Bacteremia/septicemia
- Lymphadenopathy
- Pneumonia

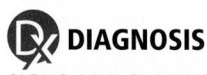 **DIAGNOSIS**

SIGNS AND SYMPTOMS
- Nearly all patients suffer fever, chills, fatigue, and malaise; rash/ulcer may be present.
- Ulceroglandular at bite site (75% of cases)
  - Nonhealing ulcer
  - Regional adenopathy
- Glandular
  - Localized adenopathy, sometimes suppurative
  - Usually no ulcer
- Typhoidal
  - Systemic febrile illness
  - Fulminating sepsis
  - Pleuropulmonary disease
  - Usually no ulcer
- Oropharyngeal
  - Exudative pharyngitis
  - Gastrointestinal symptoms
  - Cervical adenopathy
- Oculoglandular
  - Purulent conjunctivitis
  - Regional adenopathy

History
- Thorough history of patient's contact with known vectors, reservoirs (e.g., game animals, wild rodents), lab exposure, or exposure to infected materials such as water or hay
  Social history including place of residence and leisure activities
- Travel history focusing on known risk factors and countries/states of high prevalence

Physical Exam
Focused exam based on symptoms
- Presence of fever
- Skin: Look for nonhealing ulcer
- Eyes: Conjunctivitis
- Throat: Pharyngitis
- Gastrointestinal: If nausea, vomiting, diarrhea
- Lymphatic system: Lymphadenopathy
- Pulmonary: Findings suggestive of pneumonia

TESTS
- Referral to specialized lab for ELISA-based serological testing or polymerase chain reaction (PCR)
- Pleomorphic Gram-negative coccobacilli
- Culture of ulcer exudate (2 distinct varieties of the organism exist)
  - Jellison Type A biovar tularensis is more virulent and is prevalent in North America.
  - Jellison Type B biovar holarctica is less virulent and is prevalent in Europe and Asia.

Lab
- 4-fold rise in antibody titer (peak, 4–8 weeks)
- Convalescent titer of ≥160
- Elevated ESR
- Normal leukocyte count, left shift
- PCR, if available
- Disorders that may alter lab results: *Brucella* antibodies may cross-react
- ELISA-based serologic testing is more specific.

Imaging
Chest radiograph may show ill-defined infiltrates, lobar consolidation, or pleural effusion.

Diagnostic Procedures/Surgery
- Lymph node aspiration done once antibiotic therapy has been started to avoid bacteremia
- Thoracentesis
- Extreme care should be taken when handling infected material due to concern for aerosolization.

Pathological Findings
- Necrotic areas in liver, spleen, and other organs
- Caseating granulomata
- Microscopic foci with polymorphonuclear leukocytes, macrophages, giant cells

DIFFERENTIAL DIAGNOSIS
- Ulceroglandular/glandular
  - Staphylococcal infections
  - Streptococcal infections
  - Cat-scratch disease
  - Lymphoma
  - *Pasteurella* infections
  - Lymphogranuloma venereum
  - Sporotrichosis
  - Anthrax
  - Plague
  - Toxoplasmosis
- Typhoidal
  - Legionellosis
  - Rocky Mountain spotted fever
  - Ehrlichiosis
  - Borreliosis (including Lyme disease)
  - Infectious mononucleosis
  - Nontyphoid salmonellosis
  - Typhoid fever
  - Brucellosis
  - Q fever
  - Psittacosis
  - Tick-borne typhus
  - Viral pneumonia
  - Tuberculosis
- Oropharyngeal
  - Streptococcal pharyngitis
  - Viral pharyngitis
  - Diphtheric pharyngitis
  - Infectious mononucleosis
- Oculoglandular
  - Bacterial (e.g., gonorrheal) or viral (e.g., HSV) conjunctivitis

TREATMENT

INITIAL STABILIZATION
Inpatient or outpatient, depending on severity

GENERAL MEASURES
- Isolation not needed for patient, but handle secretions carefully
- Hydration, fever control, antibiotics
- Wet saline dressings for skin lesions
- Recovery requires intact cell-mediated immunity
- Bacterium is readily killed off by heat (56°C for 10 minutes). May remain viable frozen 3 years

Diet
As tolerated, high calorie, easily digestible

Nursing
Monitor for fever or shortness of breath (pneumonia risk) or septicemia

 MEDICATION (DRUGS)

First Line
- Aminoglycosides (streptomycin or gentamicin) are the antimicrobials of choice
  - Streptomycin: 15–20 mg/kg/d IM, divided b.i.d., for 7–14 days, not to exceed 2 g/d
  - Gentamicin: 3–5 mg/kg/d; divided b.i.d. dosing may be possible.
  - Fluoroquinolones are gaining acceptance, and may be used as alternative therapy.
- Contraindications
  - Known hypersensitivity, pregnancy
  - Doxycycline or ciprofloxacin are considered drugs of choice in mass-casualty situation (e.g., biowarfare). Prophylactic use in postexposure period is suggested
- Precautions
  - Long-term therapy may damage the 8th cranial nerve.
  - Reduce dosage in patients with known renal dysfunction.
  - Long-term therapy may induce renal dysfunction.
  - Use cautiously, with care postanesthesia (respiratory paralysis), and in patients with myasthenia gravis.
- Significant possible interactions
  - Other aminoglycosides, cephaloridine, polymyxin B, amphotericin B, colistin, muscle relaxants, paralyzing anesthetic agents

- β-Lactams (e.g., penicillin derivatives), most cephalosporins, and many macrolides are ineffective or have resistance.

Second Line
- Chloramphenicol: May be difficult to obtain
- Tetracyclines: Higher relapse rate
- Postexposure prophylaxis (effective if administered within 24 hours of an aerosol exposure in a mass-casualty situation)
  - Ciprofloxacin: 500 mg PO b.i.d. for 10 days
  - Doxycycline (Doryx, Vibra-Tabs, Vibramycin): 100 mg PO b.i.d. for 14–21 days

ALERT
Pregnancy Considerations
Aminoglycosides and quinolones all carry cautions for use in pregnant or pediatric patients

SURGERY
Incision and drainage of abscesses if needed

 FOLLOW-UP

Admission Criteria
- Fever with shortness of breath
- Concern for septicemia
- Need for surgery
- Risk of biowarfare

Discharge Criteria
- Improvement in symptoms
- Ability to tolerate oral antibiotics
- Compliance

Issues for Referral
- Considered infectious disease referral
- Appropriate public health authority (e.g., state, CDC, WHO) notified of suspected cases

PROGNOSIS
- Cure, if disorder is treated early and vigorously
- Immunity is life-long
- Mortality: 1–3%, higher in typhoidal disease

COMPLICATIONS
- Lung abscess
- Adult respiratory distress syndrome
- Hepatic dysfunction
- Rhabdomyolysis
- Renal failure
- Osteomyelitis, meningitis, endocarditis, pericarditis, peritonitis, conjunctivitis
- Mediastinitis
- Drug-induced side effects (e.g., diarrhea, renal failure)

PATIENT MONITORING
- Monitor function of 8th cranial nerve during long-term therapy with aminoglycosides.
- Monitor renal function during long-term therapy with aminoglycosides or quinolones.

REFERENCES
1. Eliasson H, Broman T, Forsman M, Back E. Tularemia: Current epidemiology and disease management. *Infect Dis Clin North Am*. 2006;20(2).
2. Tularemia. In: Darling RG, Woods JB, eds. USAMRIID Medical Management of Biological Casualties Handbook, 5th ed. Fort Detrick, Maryland:, 2004.
3. Sjostedt A. Tularemia. In: Heymann DL, ed. Control of Communicable Diseases Manual. Washington, DC: APHA Press, 2004.
4. Cronquist SD. Tularemia: The disease and the weapon. *Dermatol Clin*. 2004;22(3):313–320.
5. Farlow J, Wagner DM, Dukerich M, et al. *Francisella tularensis* in the United States. *Emerg Infect Dis*. 2005;11(12):1835–1841.

ADDITIONAL READING
Public health response to biological and chemical weapons: WHO guidance. World Health Organization, Geneva, Switzerland, 2004.

MISCELLANEOUS
- See also: *Bartonella* infections; Diphtheria; Ehrlichiosis; Lymphogranuloma venereum; Plague; Psittacosis; Rocky Mountain spotted fever; Toxoplasmosis; Typhus fevers
- Other notes: Incidence is higher in summer and fall; discussed as a possible bioweapon.

CODES

ICD9-CM
021.9 Unspecified tularemia

ICD10
A21 Tularemia

TURNER SYNDROME

Katrina Carter, MD

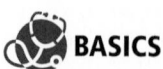**BASICS**

DESCRIPTION
- Most common sex chromosome abnormality in females
- Usually absence of one X chromosome, resulting in an XO genotype
- Edema of hands, feet, and excess skin of the neck (e.g., webbing) are presenting features during infancy.
- As children, girls are short and may have left-sided heart or aortic abnormalities.
- Primary amenorrhea and delayed onset of puberty with short stature are important clues during adolescence.
- System(s) Affected: Cardiovascular; Endocrine/Metabolic; Musculoskeletal; Nervous; Renal/Urologic; Reproductive
- Synonym(s): Ullrich-Turner syndrome; Bonnevie-Ullrich syndrome, XO syndrome, Monosomy X ; Short stature; Sexual infantilism; Gonadal dysgenesis

GENERAL PREVENTION
Prenatal detection is available for high-risk couples (who carry chromosomal translocations or who have had an affected child). No in utero treatment exists, but pregnancy termination is an option if a fetus with Turner syndrome is identified.

EPIDEMIOLOGY
- Predominant age: All ages
- Predominant sex: Female only

Incidence
- 1/1,900 live female births
- 3% of all females conceived
- Accounts for 15% of all spontaneously aborted fetuses (1)

RISK FACTORS
Familial chromosome translocations involving the X chromosome increase the risk of conceiving a child with Turner syndrome.

Genetics
- Usually sporadic deletion
- Usually a deletion of one X chromosome in a female, but may be a deletion of the SRY portion of a Y chromosome in a male. With the SRY portion of the Y gene missing, these individuals develop as females. (1)

ETIOLOGY
Monosomy for all or part of the X chromosome can result in symptoms consistent with Turner syndrome.

ASSOCIATED CONDITIONS
- Hashimoto thyroiditis
- Hypothyroidism
- Alopecia
- Vitiligo
- Gastrointestinal vascular malformations
- Gastrointestinal disorders
- Carbohydrate intolerance
- Aortic dissection in adults
- Deafness

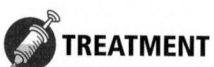**DIAGNOSIS**

SIGNS AND SYMPTOMS
Frequencies are for classic 45, X and vary with other chromosomal abnormalities associated with Turner syndrome:
- Short stature (98%)
- Gonadal dysgenesis (95%)
- Lymphedema of hands and feet present at birth (70%)
- Broad chest (75%)
- Hypoplastic, widely spaced nipples (78%)
- Prominent, anomalous ears with hearing impairment (70%)
- High palate (82%)
- Short neck (80%)
- Webbing of neck (65%)
- Low hairline (80%)
- Cubitus valgus (75%)
- Short 4th metacarpal (65%)
- Nail hypoplasia (75%)
- Excess nevi (70%)
- Renal anomalies (60%)
- Cardiovascular abnormalities (30%)
- Ocular abnormalities
- CNS abnormalities

TESTS
Upper-/lower-extremity BP

Lab
- Chromosome analysis: A buccal smear is not adequate to rule out diagnosis of Turner syndrome, An analysis of at least 20 cells is required, if history and physical exam is highly suspicious, an analysys from 2 cell types should be done, such as from blood and skin.
- At puberty, follicle-stimulating hormone (FSH) and luteinizing hormone levels may approach levels consistent with absence of ovaries. FSH may be transiently high in infancy.
- High incidence of thyroid problems should prompt evaluation of thyroid function annually

Imaging
- Renal ultrasound
- Cardiac ultrasound
- ECG

Pathological Findings
- Ovarian dysgenesis (>90%): Streak gonads, atretic follicles, or no follicles present
- Renal: Horseshoe kidney, double collecting system (60%)
- Cardiac: Bicuspid aortic valve, coarctation of aorta, valvular aortic stenosis (70% of patients with heart defects also have coarctation), hypertension
- Bone dysplasia (>50%), osteoporosis
- Gonadoblastomas in patients with X/XY mosaicism
- Ocular abnormalities: Amblyopia, ptosis, strabismus, red/green color blindness
- Gastrointestinal: Increased incidence of Celiac Disease
- CNS abnormalities: Attention deficit hyperactivity disorder (ADHD), decreased visuospatial organization

DIFFERENTIAL DIAGNOSIS
- Short stature
  - Noonan syndrome
  - Hypothyroidism
  - Familial short stature
  - Dyschondrosteosis (Léri-Weill syndrome)
  - Brachydactyly E
  - Growth hormone deficiency
  - Glucocorticoid excess
  - Klippel-Feil anomaly
  - Short stature due to chronic disease
- Amenorrhea or delayed puberty
  - Pure gonadal dysgenesis
  - Polycystic ovary syndrome (Stein-Leventhal syndrome)
  - Primary/secondary amenorrhea
- Lymphedema
  - Hereditary congenital lymphedema
  - Milroy disease
  - Lymphedema with recurrent cholestasis
  - Lymphedema with intestinal lymphangiectasia
- Other
  - Multiple pterygium syndrome
  - Pseudohypoparathyroid

TREATMENT

INITIAL STABILIZATION
Outpatient

GENERAL MEASURES
After diagnosis has been confirmed by karyotype, the following measures are appropriate
- Cardiology evaluation to include upper- and lower-extremity BPs, and ECG. If an abnormality exists, prophylactic antibiotics may be indicated (e.g., in cases of dental procedures).
- Renal ultrasound or IV pyelography
- Thyroid function test and antithyroid antibodies
- Routine hearing examination
- Treat gonadal failure in girls who do not enter puberty spontaneously
  - Replacement therapy: Begin with 1–2 years of low-dose estrogen, followed by larger-dose estrogens cycled with progesterone.
  - Maintenance therapy: Birth control pills, after menses onset and secondary sexual characteristics are established. Continue into patient's 5th decade.
  - Routine gynecologic evaluation is indicated.
  - Infertility is the general rule, <2% are able to conceive spontaneously (1), but alternatives such as in vitro fertilization and embryo transfer may be options.
  - High risk of maternal mortality secondary to cardiac complications during pregnancy. Aortic root dimensions must be monitored throughout pregnancy by ECG.

- Growth retardation has been managed with sex hormone replacement, anabolic agents, and human recombinant growth hormone (hrGH). Some patients increase final height attainment with hrGH treatment. Start hrGH therapy (0.05 mg/kg SC once daily) before significant growth deceleration occurs (between 3 and 10 years of age).
- Intelligence is usually normal. Problems may exist in nonverbal areas such as evaluating objects in relationship to one another. If concerns about school performance arise, patients should be evaluated and treated. May be at increased incidence for ADHD. (1)
- Regular visits to primary care physician are recommended. Be aware of the social and emotional problems associated with issues such as short stature and infertility.

Diet
Normal, but tendency toward obesity ought to be considered

Activity
Usually normal with no restrictions except specific limitations that may be placed if associated with certain cardiac or renal abnormalities

SURGERY
- Removal of gonads is needed in patients with X/XY syndrome/mosaicism.
- Physical appearance may be enhanced by reconstructive surgery for inner canthal folds, protruding auricles, and webbed neck

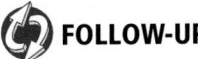 FOLLOW-UP

PROGNOSIS
Most girls with Turner syndrome can be expected to lead reasonably normal lives with appropriate medical management.

COMPLICATIONS
Complications are related to associated abnormalities.

PATIENT MONITORING
- Regularly measure growth parameters.
- Check BP regularly.
- Get annual urinalysis if renal abnormality is present.
- Monitor for signs of hypothyroidism, annual thyroid-stimulating hormone
- Regular hearing testing
- Regular eye exams
- Consider screening for occult blood loss.
- Regular cardiac exams with sonography of the aortic root in adult women

REFERENCES

1. Tyler C. Down syndrome, Turner's syndrome, and Klinefelter's syndrome: Primary care throughout the life span. *Primary Care Clinics in Office Practice*. 2004;31:627–648.
2. Frias JL, Davenport ML. The Committee on Genetics and the Section on Endocrinology. Health supervision for children with Turner syndrome. *Pediatrics*. 2003;111:692–702.
3. Hall JG, Gilchrist DM. Turner's syndrome and its variants. *Pediatr Clin North Amer.* 1990;37:1421–1440.
4. Jones KL. *Smith's Recognizable Patterns of Human Malformation*. Philadelphia, PA: WB Saunders; 1997.
5. Ranke MB, Saenger P. Turner's syndrome. *Lancet*. 2001;358:309–314.
6. Sanger P. Turner syndrome. *N Engl J Med*. 1996;335:1749–1754.

 MISCELLANEOUS

See also: Amenorrhea; Coarctation of the aorta; Hypothyroidism, adult; Thyroiditis

CODES

ICD9-CM
758.6 Gonadal dysgenesis

PATIENT TEACHING

- Families and patients need a thorough explanation of the condition and its management, especially about sexual development and growth. Suggest advising the patient between age 8 years and adolescence that she will probably not be able to bear children without assistance.
- Excellent patient educational materials include
  – Plumridge D. *Good Things Come in Small Packages: The Whys and Hows of Turner Syndrome*. Portland, OR: Crippled Children's Division, University of Oregon Health Sciences Center; year?
  – Rieser PA, Underwood LE: *Turner Syndrome: A Guide for Families*. Turner Syndrome Society, York University, ASB 006, 4700 Keele St., Downsview, ON, M3J1P3, Canada; (416) 667-3773, or Turner Syndrome Society, 3539 Tonkawood Rd., Minnetonka, MN 55345; (612) 938-3118

 See Corresponding Diagnostic Algorithm

T

TYPHOID FEVER

D. W. MacPherson, MD, MSc (CTM), FRCPC

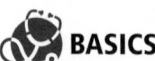 **BASICS**

DESCRIPTION
- Typhoid fever is an acute systemic illness in humans caused by *Salmonella typhi*. It is a classic example of enteric fever caused by the *Salmonella* bacterium.
- It is endemic in some developing nations where sanitation is poor. Most cases in North America and other developed nations are acquired after travel to disease-endemic areas.
- Mode of transmission is fecal–oral through ingestion of contaminated food (commonly poultry), water, and milk. Incubation period varies from 7–21 days.
- System(s) Affected: Gastrointestinal; Pulmonary; Skin/Exocrine
- Synonym(s): Typhoid; Typhus abdominalis; Enteric fever

ALERT

Geriatric Considerations
Disease more serious in elderly

Pediatric Considerations
Disease more serious in infants but may be milder in children

GENERAL PREVENTION
- For high-risk travel to an endemic area, consider vaccination for typhoid
  - Parenteral ViCPS or capsular polysaccharide typhoid vaccine (Typhim Vi) *or*
  - Ty21a or live oral typhoid vaccine (Vivotif Berna), particularly if traveler will be at prolonged risk (>4 weeks)
- Avoid tap water, salad/raw vegetables, unpeeled fruits, and dairy products during tropical travel.
- Avoid poultry or poultry products left unrefrigerated for prolonged periods.
- Consider vaccination for workers exposed to *S. typhi*, or those with household or intimate exposure to a carrier of *S. typhi*
- The parenteral heat-phenol-inactivated vaccine (manufactured by Wyeth-Ayerst) has been discontinued.

EPIDEMIOLOGY
- Predominant age: All ages
- Predominant sex: Male = Female

Incidence
Per year 300–500 new cases

RISK FACTORS
Must be considered in any patient presenting with fever after tropical travel or exposure to chronic carrier

ETIOLOGY
S. typhi

 DIAGNOSIS

SIGNS AND SYMPTOMS
- Fever
- Headache
- Malaise
- Abdominal discomfort/bloating/constipation
- Diarrhea (less common)
- Dry cough
- Confusion/lethargy
- Rose spot (transient erythematous maculopapular rash in anterior thorax or upper abdomen)
- Splenomegaly
- Hepatomegaly
- Cervical adenopathy
- Relative bradycardia
- Conjunctivitis

History
Travel and exposure

Physical Exam
Constitutionally unwell, fever, relative bradycardia, Rose spots, abdominal pain, hepato-splenmegaly

TESTS

Lab
- Definitive diagnosis by isolation of *S. typhi* from blood. Isolation of *S. typhi* in sputum, urine, or stool is presumptive diagnosis in typical clinical presentation.
- Serology is nonspecific and usually not useful.
- If multiple blood cultures have negative result or in patients with prior antibiotic therapy, diagnostic yield is better with bone marrow culture.
- Anemia, leukopenia (neutropenia), thrombocytopenia, or evidence of disseminated intravascular coagulopathy are supportive evidence. Elevated liver enzyme levels are commonly found.
- Drugs that may alter lab results
  - Prior antibiotic therapy
  - Vaccination

Imaging
Consider serial plain abdominal films for evidence of intestinal perforation.

Diagnostic Procedures/Surgery
Bone marrow for culture is rarely indicated

Pathological Findings
Classically, mononuclear proliferation involving lymphoid tissue of intestinal tract, especially Peyer patch in terminal ileum

DIFFERENTIAL DIAGNOSIS
- Malaria
- "Enteric fever-like" syndrome caused by *Yersinia enterocolitica*, pseudotuberculosis, and *Campylobacter* spp.
- Enteric fever caused by nontyphoid *Salmonella* spp.
- Infectious hepatitis
- Atypical pneumonia
- Infectious mononucleosis
- Subacute bacterial endocarditis
- Tuberculosis
- Brucellosis
- Q fever
- toxoplasmosis
- Viral infections: Epstein-Barr virus, cytomegalovirus, viral hemorrhagic agents

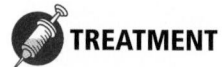 **TREATMENT**

INITIAL STABILIZATION
- Inpatient if acutely ill
- Outpatient for less-ill patient or for carrier

GENERAL MEASURES
- Fluid and electrolyte support
- Strict isolation of patient's linen, stool, and urine
- Monitor clinically and consider serial plain abdominal films for evidence of perforation, usually in the 3rd–4th week of illness.
- Indication for treatment must be determined on an individual basis. Factors to be considered are age, public health risk (e.g., food handler, chronic care facilities, medical personnel), intolerance to antibiotics, and evidence of biliary tract disease.
- For hemorrhage: Blood transfusion and management of shock

Diet
If abdominal symptoms severe, nothing by mouth. With improvement, normal low-residue diet, possibly high calorie

Activity
Bed rest initially, then as tolerated

Nursing
Observe enteric precautions.

Typhoid Fever Vaccinations

Vaccine name	How given	Number of doses necessary	Time between doses	Total time needed to set aside for vaccination	Minimum age for vaccination	Booster needed every...
Ty21a (Vivotif Berna, Swiss Serum and Vaccine Institute)	1 capsule by mouth	4	2 days	2 weeks	6 years	5 years
ViCPS (Typhim Vi, Pasteur Merieux)	Injection	1	N/A	2 weeks	2 years	2 years

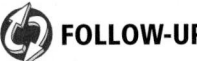 MEDICATION (DRUGS)

First Line
- Chloramphenicol: Pediatric 50 mg/kg/d PO q.i.d. × 2 weeks; adult dose 50 mg/kg/d, divided q6h × 2 weeks; *or*
- Ampicillin: Pediatric 100 mg/kg/d q.i.d. PO × 2 weeks; adults 500 mg q6h × 2 weeks; *or*
- Ciprofloxacin: 500 mg PO b.i.d. × 2 weeks, indicated in multiple drug–resistant typhoid, has been successfully and safely used in children; *or*
- Ceftriaxone: 1–2 g IV once daily × 2 weeks; *or*
- Furazolidone: 7.5 mg/kg/d PO × 10 days; in uncomplicated multiple drug–resistant typhoid; safe in children; efficacy >85% cure
- Chronic carrier state:
  – Ampicillin: 4–5 g/d + probenecid 2 g/d q.i.d. × 6 weeks (for patients with normally functioning gallbladder without evidence of cholelithiasis)
  – Ciprofloxacin: 500 mg PO b.i.d. × 4–6 weeks is also efficacious. NOTE: Chloramphenicol resistance has been reported in Mexico, South America, Central America, Southeast Asia, India, Pakistan, Middle East, and Africa.
- Contraindications: Refer to the manufacturer's profile for each drug.
- Precautions: Rarely, Jarisch-Herxheimer reaction appears after antimicrobial therapy.
- Significant possible interactions: Refer to the manufacturer's profile for each drug.

Second Line
Trimethoprim-sulfamethoxazole

ALERT
Pregnancy Considerations
Ciprofloxacin therapy is relatively contraindicated in pregnant patients.

SURGERY
- Complications: Bowel perforation
- Cholecystectomy may be warranted in carriers with cholelithiasis, relapse after therapy, or intolerance to antimicrobial therapy.

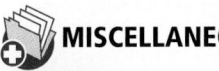 FOLLOW-UP

DISPOSITION
Admission Criteria
Clinical severity

Issues for Referral
Complications of sepsis, bowel perforation

PROGNOSIS
Overall prognosis good with therapy; <2% mortality rate; 15% relapse rate with some antibiotic treatments; 3% bowel perforation

COMPLICATIONS
- Intestinal hemorrhage and perforation in distal ileum
- Patients may become chronic carriers (up to 3%), defined as persistent stool excretor for longer than 1 year
- Predilection for seeding in the biliary tract exists and may become a focus for relapse of typhoid fever. Most common in females and the elderly (>50 years old).
- Osteomyelitis found especially in patients with sickle cell anemia, systemic lupus erythematosus, hematologic neoplasms, and in immunosuppressed hosts
- Endovascular infection in the elderly and in patients with history of bypass operation or aneurysm
- Rarely, endocarditis or meningitis

PATIENT MONITORING
See "General Measures."

REFERENCES

1. Crump JA, et al. Estimating the incidence of typhoid fever and other febrile illnesses in developing countries. *Emerg Infect Dis*. 2003; Available at: http://www.cdc.gov/ncidod/EID/vol9no5/02-0428.htm. Accessed June 18, 2006.
2. Dick L. Travel medicine: helping patients prepare for trips abroad. *Am Fam Physician*. 1998;58:383–398, 401–402.
3. Mandell GL. *Principles and Practice of Infectious Diseases*. 6th ed. New York, NY: Churchill Livingstone; 2004.
4. Peter G, et al. Lessons learned from a review of the development of selected vaccines. *Pediatrics*. 1999;104:942–950.
5. Rowe B, Ward LR, Threlfall EJ. Multidrug-resistant *Salmonella typhi*: A worldwide epidemic. *Clin Infect Dis*. 1997;24(suppl 1):S106–S109.
6. Thompson RF, Bass DM, Hoffman SL. Travel vaccines. *Infect Dis Clin North Amer*. 1999;13:49–67.
7. Yoon J, Segal-Maurer S, Rahal JJ. An outbreak of domestically acquired typhoid fever in Queens, NY. *Arch Intern Med*. 2004;164:565–567.
8. Centers for Disease Control and Prevention. Typhoid Fever. (dated January 10, 2005). Available at: http://www.cdc.gov/ncidod/dbmd/diseaseinfo/files/typhoid_fever_FAQ.pdf

MISCELLANEOUS

CODES
ICD9-CM
- 002.0 Typhoid fever
- 002.9 Paratyphoid fever, unspecified

PATIENT TEACHING
- Discussion of chronic carrier state and its complications
- For family members, travelers, or workers at risk, provide hygiene education, and possibly vaccination

TYPHUS FEVERS

Jeremy Golding, MD

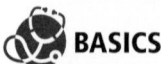 **BASICS**

DESCRIPTION

- Acute infectious diseases caused by 3 species of rickettsiae
  - Epidemic typhus: Human-to-human transmission by body louse vector. Primarily in circumstances such as refugee camps, war, famine, and disaster. Recrudescent disease (Brill-Zinsser Disease), occurring years after initial infection, can be source of human outbreak. Flying squirrels are also a reservoir.
  - Endemic (murine) typhus: Infection by rodents. To humans by rat flea bite.
  - Scrub typhus: Infection and infestation of chiggers and of rodents. To humans by the chigger. Primarily in Asia and Western Pacific areas.
- System(s) Affected: Endocrine/Metabolic; Hemic/Lymphatic/Immunologic; Pulmonary; Skin/Exocrine
- Synonym(s): Louse-borne typhus; Brill-Zinsser disease; Murine typhus

GENERAL PREVENTION

Avoid vectors for each disease

- Scrub typhus: Wear protective clothing and use insect repellents.
- Endemic typhus: Practice ectoparasite and rodent control.
- Epidemic typhus: Delousing and cleaning of clothing; vaccine may be considered for those at high risk of exposure (typhus vaccine production has been discontinued in the US).

EPIDEMIOLOGY

- Epidemic and endemic typhus: Rare in US
- Scrub typhus: Travelers returning from endemic areas only (rare)

Incidence

Endemic typhus: <100 cases annually, primarily in states around Gulf of Mexico, especially south Texas, under-reporting suspected

RISK FACTORS

- Exposure to vectors (e.g., during travel to countries where endemic)
- Elderly may have more severe disease

ETIOLOGY

- Epidemic typhus by *Rickettsia prowazekii*
- Endemic typhus by *R. typhi*
- Scrub typhus by *R. tsutsugamushi*

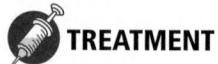 **DIAGNOSIS**

SIGNS AND SYMPTOMS

- General
  - Acute onset
  - Fever
  - Chills
  - Headache
  - Myalgia
  - Malaise
  - Diffuse organ involvement (e.g., intestine, liver, heart, kidneys, brain)
- Epidemic typhus
  - Incubation period ~1 week
  - Macular or maculopapular rash, begins on trunk spreads to extremities about 5th day of illness
  - Nonproductive cough
  - Pulmonary infiltrates
  - Conjunctivitis
  - Neurologic involvement
- Endemic typhus
  - Incubation period 1–2 weeks
  - Macular or maculopapular rash beginning on trunk 3rd–5th day of illness, spreads to trunk ~5th day
  - Duration 12 days untreated
  - Usually milder illness
- Scrub typhus
  - Incubation period 1–3 weeks
  - Eschar at bite site
  - Regional lymphadenopathy
  - Generalized lymphadenopathy
  - Splenomegaly
  - Macular or maculopapular rash beginning on trunk about the 5th day of illness
  - Relative bradycardia early in disease
  - Ocular pain
  - Conjunctival injection

History

Travel or other risk exposure

Physical Exam

As above

TESTS

Specific serologic test showing a rising antibody titer. Isolation of *Rickettsia* should be undertaken only in special laboratories, to minimize risk of laboratory-acquired infection.

Lab

- Leukocyte findings usually normal
- Abnormalities reflecting the particular organs affected
- Weil-Felix serologic reaction may be positive; test value limited to mid-illness or after, and by low sensitivity and specificity. Epidemic and endemic typhus, 4-fold titer rise or titer >1/320 to OX-19. Scrub typhus, 4-fold rise in titer to OX-K.
- Hyponatremia in severe cases
- Hypoalbuminemia in severe cases
- Drugs that may alter lab results: Prior antibiotic use

Pathological Findings

Diffuse vasculitis

DIFFERENTIAL DIAGNOSIS

- Any acute febrile disease
- Rocky Mountain spotted fever
- Meningococcemia
- Bacterial meningitis
- Mediterranean spotted fever (boutonneuse fever) (*R. conorii*)
- Measles
- Rubella
- Toxoplasmosis
- Leptospirosis
- Typhoid fever
- Dengue
- Relapsing fever
- Secondary syphilis
- Viral syndromes: Mononucleosis, acute retroviral syndrome

TREATMENT

INITIAL STABILIZATION

Outpatient care unless severely ill

GENERAL MEASURES

- Protect agitated patient from injury
- Skin and mouth care
- Supportive care for the severely ill, directed at the complications

Diet

As tolerated

Activity

Bed rest during acute stages, otherwise as tolerated

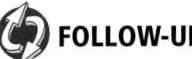 **MEDICATION (DRUGS)**

First Line

- Treatment should begin when diagnosis is reasonably likely and continue until the patient's state is improved and the patient is afebrile for a minimum of 48 hours. Usual treatment course: 5–7 days.
- Children ≥8 years of age and adults
  - Tetracycline, or a congener: 25 mg/kg PO initially, and then 25 mg/kg/d in equally divided doses q6h
  - If severely ill, may use doxycycline IV: Adults 100 mg q12h, children ≥8 years of age 5 mg/kg/d (maximum of 200 mg/d)
- Children ≤8 years of age, pregnant women, or if typhoid fever is possible cause of illness
  - Chloramphenicol: 50 mg/kg PO initially, and then 50 mg/kg daily in equally divided doses q6h
  - If severely ill, chloramphenicol sodium succinate: 20 mg/kg IV initially, infused over 30–45 minutes, and then 50 mg/kg/d infused in equally divided doses q6h until orally tolerable
- Precautions: Refer to the manufacturer's profile for each drug.
- Significant possible interactions: Refer to the manufacturer's profile for each drug.

Second Line

- Doxycycline: Single oral dose of 100 or 200 mg for those in refugee camps, victims of disasters, or in presence of limited medical services
- Isolated reports indicate that erythromycin and ciprofloxacin are effective.

 FOLLOW-UP

DISPOSITION
Admission Criteria
Severely ill or constitutionally unstable (e.g., shock)

PROGNOSIS
- Recovery is expected if treatment is instituted before onset of complications.
- Relapses may follow treatment, especially if initiated within 48 hours of onset (this is *not* an indication to delay treatment). Relapses are treated same as primary disease.
- Without treatment, mortality rate of typhus is 40–60% for epidemic, 1–2% for endemic, and up to 30% for scrub. Mortality is higher among the elderly.

COMPLICATIONS
- Consequences of specific organ system involvement in the 2nd week (e.g., azotemia, meningoencephalitis, seizures, delirium, coma, myocardial failure, hyponatremia, hypoalbuminemia, hypovolemia, and shock)
- Death

PATIENT MONITORING
Severely ill patients should be observed regularly in the hospital. Outpatients should be checked periodically as improvement is evident.

REFERENCES
1. Azad AF, Beard CB. Rickettsial pathogens and their arthropod vectors. *Emerg Infect Dis*. 1998;4: 179–186.
2. Azad AF, et al. Flea-borne rickettsioses: Ecologic considerations. *Emerg Infect Dis*. 1997;3:319–327.
3. Dumlev JS, Taylor JP, Walker DH. Clinical and laboratory features of murine typhus in south Texas, 1980 through 1987. *JAMA*. 1991;266:1365–1370.
4. Jensenius M, Forunier PE, Raoult D. Rickettsioses and the international traveler. *Clin Infect Dis*. 2004;39:1493–1499.
5. Mandell GL, Bennett JF, Dolin R, eds. Principles and Practice of Infectious Diseases, 6th ed. New York: Churchill Livingstone, 2004.
6. Raoult D, Roux V. The body louse as a vector of reemerging human diseases. *Clin Infect Dis*. 1999;29:888–911.
7. Watt G, Parola P. Scrub typhus and tropical rickettsioses. *Curr Opin Infect Dis*. 2003;16: 429–436.

MISCELLANEOUS

- Severe headache is often intractable and not eased by the standard drugs.
- Report case to appropriate health department or other agency.

CODES

ICD9-CM
- 080 Louse-borne [epidemic] typhus
- 081.0 Murine [endemic] typhus
- 081.1 Brill disease

PATIENT TEACHING
Provide prevention information for travelers.

T

ULCERATIVE COLITIS

Venu G. Pillarisetty, MD
Ruben Peralta, MD, FACS

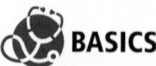 **BASICS**

DESCRIPTION
An idiopathic inflammatory disease of the colon mucosa, affecting the rectum and usually extending proximally to involve the entire colon in a continuous manner.

- At least 95% have rectal involvement
- 50% limited to rectum and sigmoid.
- 30–40% of patients have disease beyond the sigmoid, but not of the entire colon.
- 20% have pancolitis.

EPIDEMIOLOGY
- Predominant age: 15–35. 2nd and smaller peak in the 7th decade.
- Predominant sex: Female slightly > Male

Incidence
US population: 5–12 new cases per 100,000

Prevalence
70–150/100,000

ALERT
Pediatric Considerations
Twenty percent of patients are ≤21 years

Pregnancy Considerations
- Outcome of pregnancy similar to general population. 1 study showed 30% of those with inactive disease at onset of pregnancy relapsed and 14% did so in 1st trimester.
- Treatment with sulfasalazine does not seem to affect outcome of pregnancy.
- Recommend that patient delays pregnancy until time when disease is inactive.

RISK FACTORS
- Better sanitation, artificial work environments (e.g., indoors), and fatty food increase risk
- NSAIDs can activate disease
- Appendectomy is protective against later development of disease
- Negative association with smoking (relative risk of smokers is 40% of nonsmokers)

Genetics
Family history in 5–10% in population surveys and 20–30% in referral-based studies. More common in the Jewish population.

ETIOLOGY
Unknown; major hypotheses include allergy to dietary components and abnormal immune responses to bacterial or self-antigens; final outcome is mucosal inflammation secondary to immune cell infiltration (1)[B].

ASSOCIATED CONDITIONS
- Extracolonic manifestations in 10–15%
- Arthritic conditions including large joint arthritis, sacroiliitis, and ankylosing spondylitis. Infliximab has had a favorable response in treating these conditions.
- Pyoderma gangrenosum and other skin conditions; infliximab has helped.
- Episcleritis and uveal tract disease
- Sclerosing cholangitis; ursodeoxycholic acid is helpful

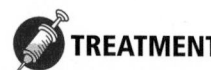 **DIAGNOSIS**

SIGNS AND SYMPTOMS
- Bloody diarrhea (watery stool accompanied by blood, pus, and mucus)
- Tenesmus
- Abdominal pain; tenderness in severe disease
- Rectal urgency, occasional fecal incontinence
- Fever
- Weight loss
- Arthralgias and arthritis: 15–20%
- Spondylitis: 3–6%
- Ocular: 4–10% include episcleritis, uveitis, cataracts, keratopathy, marginal corneal ulceration, and central serous retinopathy
- Erythema nodosum
- Pyoderma gangrenosum
- Aphthous ulcers of mouth: 5–10%
- Asymptomatic fatty liver (common); occasional hepatomegaly
- Pericholangitis (uncommon)
- Primary sclerosing cholangitis: 1–4%
- Cirrhosis of liver: 1–5%
- Bile duct carcinoma
- Thromboembolic disease: 1–6%
- Pericarditis (rare)
- Amyloidosis (rare)

TESTS
Lab
- Anemia may reflect chronic disease as well as iron deficiency from blood loss.
- Leukocytosis during exacerbation
- Elevated ESR and C-reactive protein
- Electrolyte abnormalities, especially hypokalemia
- Hypoalbuminemia
- Elevated liver function tests
- Perinuclear antineutrophil cytoplasmic antibody is elevated in 85% of cases of ulcerative colitis and 15% of Crohn disease.
- Antiglycan antibody is elevated in 75% of Crohn disease and 5% of ulcerative colitis cases.

Imaging
- Plain abdominal films
  - Invaluable in management of acute complications of ulcerative colitis and should be immediately available in all patients who show tenderness of the colon, fever, and leukocytosis
  - Permit the early diagnosis of toxic megacolon and perforation and treatment planning; toxic megacolon is most severe near the cecum and is present when diameter >12 cm.
- Barium enema
  - Mucosal irregularities, effacement of haustra, pseudopolyposis
- Upper gastrointestinal series with small bowel follow-through to rule out Crohn disease

Diagnostic Procedures/Surgery
- Sigmoidoscopy; may include biopsy
  - Should be sufficient to make initial diagnosis
- Colonoscopy; may include biopsy for evaluation for premalignant features
  - To differentiate from Crohn disease
  - To investigate suspected stricture or mass
  - To define the extent and location of involvement and specific segments
  - Full colonoscopy contraindicated in active disease or colonic dilatation because of risk of perforation

Pathological Findings
Inflammation of the colonic mucosa with ulcerations

- Ulcerations are hyperemic and hemorrhagic.
- Rectum is involved 95% of the time.
- The inflammation extends proximally in a continuous fashion but for a variable distance.
- May affect terminal ileum, so-called *backwash ileitis*.

DIFFERENTIAL DIAGNOSIS
- Other sources of rectal bleeding, including hemorrhoids, neoplasms, colonic diverticula, arteriovenous malformation, Crohn disease
- Infectious diarrhea including bacterial (enterotoxigenic *Escherichia coli*, *E. coli* 0157:H7, *Salmonella*, *Shigella*, *Aeromonas*, *Plesiomonas*) and parasitic (*Entamoeba histolytica*)
- *Herpes simplex*, *Chlamydia trachomatis*, *Cryptosporidium*, *Isospora belli*, cytomegalovirus
- Antibiotic-associated diarrhea
- Radiation proctitis
- Ischemic proctitis and colitis

TREATMENT

INITIAL STABILIZATION
Hospitalization for severe exacerbations

GENERAL MEASURES
Control inflammation, prevent complications, and replace nutritional losses and blood volume.

Diet
No specific diet; milk products not withheld unless an associated lactase deficiency exists

Activity
Full activity as tolerated

MEDICATION (DRUGS)

First Line
- Sulfasalazine is treatment of choice both for mild exacerbations and for chronic treatment. Used to decrease the frequency of relapses (dosage range 2–6 g/d).
- Proctitis or proctosigmoiditis may be treated topically with steroid enemas or mesalamine (5-aminosalicylic acid [5-ASA]) enemas and suppositories.
- Oral or parenteral corticosteroids are used for more severe exacerbations (e.g., prednisone 40–60 mg/d, gradual taper over 2 months).
- 10% of patients have chronic disease and require continuous low to moderate steroid doses.
- Newer agents include oral 5-ASA derivatives.
- Immunomodulators, such as azathioprine, mercaptopurine (6-mercaptopurine), methotrexate, and cyclosporine, used in patients unresponsive to steroids and 5-ASA drugs or who cannot be weaned from high-dose steroids.
  - Most experience is with azathioprine and mercaptopurine.
  - Daily plain films of the abdomen are obtained until improvement occurs.
  - If dilatation of colon increases or treatment has failed to attain reversal in 72 hours, emergency colectomy is indicated.
- Antimicrobial agents (antimycobacterials and metronidazole) are sometimes useful in Crohn disease, but not in ulcerative colitis.
- Antidiarrheal agents such as diphenoxylate-atropine and loperamide may be used to help control diarrhea, but require careful monitoring because they may precipitate toxic megacolon.
- Precautions: Use of antidiarrheal agents in severe disease could precipitate toxic megacolon.

Second Line
- Budesonide is a less toxic steroid almost totally cleared by the liver; it may help avoid steroid risks.
- Several preparations of 5-ASA exist, but results seem best with sulfasalazine in full dose.
- Infliximab recently was found to improve long-term outcomes in patients with moderate to severe disease despite treatment with other medications. (2)[B]

SURGERY
- Emergency surgery for massive hemorrhage, perforation, and toxic dilatation of the colon
- Surgery indicated for cancer, persistent multisite mucosal dysplasia, and patients refractory to all other forms of therapy.
- Total colectomy with ileostomy pouch is curative.
- Many patients prefer a continent ileostomy (J-pouch) emptying through the rectum.
- With the continent ileostomy operations, "pouchitis" occurs in ~10% with erratic partial response to antibiotics.
- Subtotal colectomy with the ileum connected to the rectal stump also may be performed.
- Regular proctoscopic surveillance is required because colonic mucosa is retained, thereby leaving a risk of future cancer development.

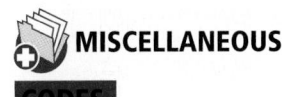 **FOLLOW-UP**

PROGNOSIS
- Variable course; mortality for initial attack is ~5%. 75–85% experience relapse, and up to 20% eventually require colectomy.
- Colon cancer risk is the single most important risk factor affecting long-term prognosis.
- Left-sided colitis and ulcerative proctitis have favorable prognosis with probable normal lifespan.

ALERT
Geriatric Considerations
Increased mortality if 1st presentation after 60 years of age

COMPLICATIONS
- Perforation
- Toxic megacolon
- Liver disease
- Stricture formation (less than Crohn disease)
- Colon cancer (may occur in as many as 30% of those with pancolitis for 25 years). Incidence of cancer is cumulative over time and begins after 7–8 years of the disease; risk may be considerably less in left-sided disease.

PATIENT MONITORING
- Colonoscopy for cancer surveillance with biopsy of the mucosa for evidence of dysplasia every 1–2 years after the disease has been present for 7–8 years. This is particularly important in pancolitis. Low-grade dysplasia warrants more frequent evaluation (e.g., every 3–6 months), and high-grade dysplasia (or low-grade dysplasia within a mass) warrants consideration of colectomy.
- Magnification chromoendoscopy has been shown to be capable of detecting significantly more intraepithelial neoplasias than conventional colonoscopy. (3)[B]
- Annual liver tests
- Cholangiography for cholestasis

Pediatric Considerations
Cancer surveillance is important because occurrence of cancer relates to the duration and extent of disease, whether frequently symptomatic or not.

REFERENCES
1. Hanauer SB. Inflammatory bowel disease: Epidemiology, pathogenesis, and therapeutic opportunities. *Inflamm Bowel Dis* 2006;12:S3–S9.
2. Rutgeerts R, Sandborn WJ, Feagan BG. Infliximab for induction and maintenance therapy for ulcerative colitis. *N Engl J Med* 2005;353:2462–2476.
3. Kiesslich R, Hoffman A, Neurath MF. Colonoscopy, tumors, and inflammatory bowel disease—new diagnostic methods. *Endoscopy* 2006;38(1):5–10.

 MISCELLANEOUS

CODES

ICD9-CM
556.9 Ulcerative colitis, unspecified

PATIENT TEACHING
Self-help organizations such as the National Foundation for Ileitis and Colitis, 444 Park Avenue S., 11th Floor, New York, NY 10016-7374; (800) 343-3637

Prevention
Patients retaining colon are at risk for colon cancer. Daily 300 mg aspirin and, in those with sclerosing cholangitis, daily ursodeoxycholic acid 10 mg/kg have been shown to be preventive.

See Corresponding Diagnostic Algorithm

 See Patient Handout on CD

U

URETHRITIS
Chad M. Braun, MD

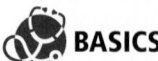

BASICS

DESCRIPTION
Syndrome of urethral inflammation marked by painful urination, urethral pruritis, and discharge
- Usually a sexually transmitted infection (STI); other causes not uncommon
- Untreated cases may gradually resolve, but complications, such as urethral stricture in males or pelvic inflammatory disease (PID) in women, may ensue.
- System(s) Affected: Renal/Urologic

GENERAL PREVENTION
- Safer sex protection techniques
- Sexual abstinence only sure way for complete prevention of STI-related causes
- Treatment of all sexual partners

EPIDEMIOLOGY
- Predominant age: 15–24 years, sexually active
- Predominant sex: Classic symptoms more commonly reported by males; incidence in females probably equal

Incidence
Very common: >830,000 cases of chlamydia and 350,000 cases of gonorrhea reported in 2002 in the US

RISK FACTORS
- Multiple sexual partners
- History of other STI
- Unprotected sexual activity

ETIOLOGY
- Predominantly *Neisseria gonorrhoeae* and *Chlamydia trachomatis* infection, often together
- Less common infectious agents, including
  - *Ureaplasma urealyticum*
  - *Trichomonas vaginalis*
  - Herpesvirus
  - *Mycoplasma genitalium*
- Noninfectious causes (generally rare)
  - Foreign bodies, soaps, shampoos, douches, spermicides, urethral instrumentation

ASSOCIATED CONDITIONS
Other STIs: Patients should be strongly urged to undergo testing for syphilis, hepatitis B, and HIV.

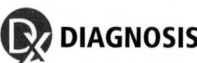

DIAGNOSIS

SIGNS AND SYMPTOMS
- Both sexes may be asymptomatic carriers of the causative organisms.
- In males: Abrupt onset of symptoms 3–5 days after exposure to an infected sexual partner
- In females: Classic urethral syndrome often is not present. Infections that cause simple urethritis in males will often have symptoms other than dysuria, including vaginal discharge and cervicitis.
- Dysuria: Pain throughout urination
- Urethral discharge; may be profuse and purulent in acute gonorrhea, or scanty, evident only with milking of the urethra, with other causes
- Urethral itching or tenderness
- Tenderness, edema, and inflammation of the urethral meatus, especially in women
- Dyspareunia
- Vaginitis, cystitis, cervicitis in women
- Proctitis, pharyngitis, conjunctivitis may also be present (sexual history is important)
- Fever is not part of the syndrome and suggests another diagnosis.
- Bloody discharge: Rarely seen and suggests another diagnosis
- Suprapubic or abdominal pain suggests another diagnosis or presence of complications, e.g., PID, prostatitis, or cystitis.

ALERT
Pediatric Considerations
Proven cases of gonorrhea, chlamydia, and trichomoniasis should raise the question of sexual abuse.

TESTS
For patients who present without symptoms stating that a sexual partner was treated for this problem: Obtain specimens for lab tests, but immediate treatment is recommended.

SCREENING
- The US Preventative Services Task Force (USPSTF) recommends routine screening in all sexually active women 25 years old and younger and all other women at increased risk of infection. (4)[A]
- The optimal screening interval is uncertain.
- They make no recommendation for or against the screening of low-risk women. (4)[A]
- The USPSTF states that the evidence is insufficient to recommend for or against screening in asymptomatic men at increased risk. (4)[I]

Lab (1)[C]
- Gram stain of discharge: Intracellular gram-negative diplococci strongly indicate gonorrhea; 5 or more white blood cells (WBC) per high-power field (HPF) indicate urethritis.
- Cultures or reagin detection: DNA probe is probably the best screening test.
  - Cultures may be difficult to obtain correctly but allow for antimicrobial sensitivity testing.
  - Polymerase chain reaction (PCR) assay on urine is more sensitive and specific, but costly. Can get PCR on sample from ThinPrep test. Negatives may be false results or may indicate another infecting organism.
- Urinalysis: If indicated, sample discharge before patient voids; usually normal in cases of simple urethritis.
  - 1st-void urine is often positive for leukocyte esterase and should have 10 or more WBC per HPF in urethritis.
  - Ideally, men should not have urinated for at least 4 hours prior.
  - Symptomatic patients in whom no urethritis is detected initially should be retested having held their urine overnight.
- Urine culture: Performed only if gram stain of discharge is unremarkable or unobtainable

- Wet prep of discharge: May reveal *Trichomonas*; usually reserved in males who fail adequate treatment for gonorrhea and chlamydia
- Syphilis, HIV, and hepatitis B serology as indicated to rule out concomitant STIs
- Recent treatment with antibiotics may lead to false-negative results.

Diagnostic Procedures/Surgery
Urethrocystoscopy for cases with suspected foreign body, intraurethral warts, urethral stricture

Pathological Findings
Urethral strictures (untreated gonorrhea), intraurethral lesions (venereal warts, congenital anomalies)

DIFFERENTIAL DIAGNOSIS
- Other urinary tract infections
  - Cystitis
  - Epididymitis
  - Prostatitis
  - PID
  - Pyelonephritis
- Atrophy, especially in postmenopausal women
- Stevens-Johnson syndrome
- Reiter syndrome: Arthritis, uveitis, and urethritis
- Wegener granulomatosis may have urethritis as one of its manifestations.

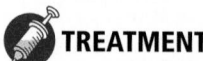

TREATMENT

INITIAL STABILIZATION
- Most cases can be treated in the outpatient setting.
- Single-dose regimens can be directly observed in the office for noncompliant or high-risk patients.
- Antibiotics should not be withheld from symptomatic patients until culture (test) results are known, rather they should be initiated as soon as cultures (samples) have been collected.
- Treatment should cover both gonorrhea and chlamydia because they cause the majority of cases and often coexist.
- Patients with persistent symptoms and signs after adequate treatment should be
  - Evaluated and/or treated for trichomoniasis
  - Retreated with the original regimen if not compliant or re-exposed
  - Retreated with an alternative regimen for 14 days if *U. urealyticum* is suspected (tetracycline resistance in <10% of isolates)
  - Evaluated for HSV

GENERAL MEASURES
Identification and treatment of sexual partners
All sexual partners within the previous 60 days should be investigated and treated.

Diet
Avoid alcohol with metronidazole.

Activity
- Full activity
- No sexual intercourse until 7 days after single dose therapy or completion of 7-day therapy

MEDICATION (DRUGS)

First Line

- Gonorrhea: (1)[C]
  - Cefixime: 400 mg PO single dose
  - Ceftriaxone: 125 mg IM single dose (superior for gonococcal pharynigitis)
- Chlamydia: (5)[A]
  - Azithromycin: 1 g PO single dose
  - Doxycycline: 100 mg PO b.i.d. for 7 days
- Trichomoniasis: Metronidazole 2 g PO single dose or 250 mg t.i.d. for 7 days
- Recurrent and resistant urethritis: (5)[C] Metronidazole 2 mg PO single dose PLUS erythromycin base 500 mg PO q.i.d. for 7 days or erythromycin ethylsuccinate 800 mg PO q.i.d. for 7 days
- Contraindications: Sensitivity to any of the indicated medications. Pregnant patients should not receive tetracyclines, and metronidazole should be avoided in the 1st trimester.
- Precautions: Patients taking tetracyclines need to be told of the possibility of increased sensitivity to sunlight.
- Significant possible interactions
  - Tetracyclines should not be taken with milk products or antacids.
  - Oral contraceptives may be rendered ineffective by oral antibiotics. Patients and partners should use a backup method of birth control for remainder of the cycle.

ALERT

Pregnancy Considerations

- Tetracyclines and quinolones are contraindicated.
- Avoid erythromycin estolate because of an increased risk of cholestatic jaundice; otherwise use the standard treatment recommendations.
- 7-day therapy for chlamydia is favored in pregnancy, but single dose is still recommended.

Second Line

- Gonorrhea
  - Because of the spread of quinolone-resistant *N. gonorrhoeae* from the Pacific and Asia, quinolones are no longer recommended treatment in individuals who have acquired gonorrhea from that area. (2)[C]
  - Fluoroquinolones are also not recommended as 1st-line therapy for people in Hawaii and California and men who have sex with men, because of endemic spread of quinolone-resistant gonorrhea. (2)[C]
  - Resistance to penicillin and tetracycline has been reported in up to 1/3 of isolates of *N. gonorrhoeae*.
  - Ciprofloxacin: 500 mg PO single dose (1)[C]
  - Ofloxacin: 400 mg PO single dose (1)[C]
  - Levofloxacin: 250 mg PO single dose (1)[C]
  - Others drugs are available, but offer no particular advantage over the drugs of choice.

- Chlamydia
  - Erythromycin base: 500 mg PO q.i.d. for 7 days (5)[A]
  - Erythromycin ethylsuccinate: 800 mg PO q.i.d. for 7 days. If intolerant of high-dose erythromycin: Erythromycin base 250 mg PO q.i.d. for 14 days or erythromycin ethylsuccinate 400 mg PO q.i.d. for 14 days
  - Ofloxacin: 300 mg PO b.i.d. for 7 days (5)[A]
  - Levofloxacin: 500 mg PO daily for 7 days

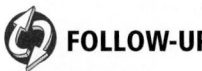

FOLLOW-UP

DISPOSITION
Outpatient management

PROGNOSIS
If the diagnosis is firmly established, appropriate medications are prescribed, and the patient is compliant with treatment, there will be relief of symptoms within days and the problem will resolve without sequelae.

COMPLICATIONS

- Stricture formation
- Epididymitis
- PID in women
- Disseminated gonococcal infection
- Gonococcal meningitis
- Gonococcal endocarditis
- Perinatal transmission (chlamydial conjunctivitis, chlamydial pneumonia, ophthalmia neonatorum)
- Reiter syndrome

PATIENT MONITORING
Instruct patients to return if symptoms persist or recur after completing treatment. Test of cure cultures is not usually required unless patient is pregnant.

REFERENCES

1. Centers for Disease Control and Prevention. Sexually transmitted diseases treatment guidelines for 2002. *MMWR Recomm Rep.* 2002;51(RR-06):1–80.
2. Centers for Disease Control and Prevention. Increases in fluoroquinolone-resistant Neisseria gonorrhoeae among men who have sex with men—United States, 2003, and revised recommendations for gonorrhea treatment, 2004. *MMWR Morb Mortal Wkly Rep.* 2004;53:335–338.
3. Groseclose SL et al. Centers for Disease Control and Prevention. Summary of notifiable diseases—United States, 2002. *MMWR Morb Mortal Wkly Rep.* 2004;51:1–84.
4. Berg AO. Screening for chlamydia infections: Recommendations and rationale. *Am J Prev Med.* 2001;20:90–4.
5. 2002 National Guideline on the Management of Non-gonoccal urethritis, Association for Genitourinary Medicine.

MISCELLANEOUS

See also: Chlamydial sexually transmitted diseases; Epididymitis; Gonococcal infections; Pelvic inflammatory disease (PID); Prostatitis; Urinary tract infection in females; Urinary tract infection in males; Vulvovaginitis, bacterial; Vulvovaginitis, candidal

CODES

ICD9-CM

- 098.0 Acute gonococcal infection of lower genitourinary tract
- 098.2 Chronic gonococcal infection of lower genitourinary tract
- 099.3 Reiter disease
- 099.40 Other nongonococcal urethritis (NGU), unspecified
- 099.41 Chlamydia trachomatis
- 099.49 Other nongonococcal urethritis (NGU), other specified organism
- 131.02 Trichomonal urethritis
- 597.80 Urethritis, unspecified
- 597.81 Urethral syndrome NOS

PATIENT TEACHING

- Handouts available online at www.familydoctor.org.
- Most important to emphasize the need for compliance with therapy, treatment of sexual partners, and use of safer sex practices. Patients should be urged to undergo screening for other STIs.

 See Corresponding Diagnostic Algorithm

 See Patient Handout on CD

U

URINARY INCONTINENCE
Pamela I. Ellsworth, MD

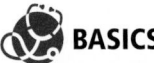 **BASICS**

DESCRIPTION
Involuntary loss of urine from the bladder
- May occur while asleep or awake
- Amount of urine lost may vary greatly.
- Condition comes to medical attention when it is perceived to be a social and/or hygiene problem by the patient or caregiver
- System(s) Affected: Renal/Urologic; Skin/Exocrine
- Synonym(s): Transient incontinence; Urge incontinence; Overflow incontinence; Stress incontinence; Overactive bladder

GENERAL PREVENTION
- Routine Kegel exercises after childbirth
- Regular pelvic examination of female patients to detect pelvic pathology

EPIDEMIOLOGY
- Predominant age: Elderly
- Predominant sex: Female > Male

Prevalence
- 1 in 20 people in the US
- Women (community dwelling)
  - Aged <65 years: 10%
  - Aged >65 years: 35%
- Men (community-dwelling)
  - Aged <65 years: 1.5%
  - Aged <65: 1.5%
- Institutionalized men and women aged >65 years: 30–50%

ALERT

Geriatric Considerations
This problem is most commonly seen in older patients.

Pediatric Considerations
Neurogenic, congenital, and idiopathic overactive bladder also occurs in children.

RISK FACTORS
- Increasing age
- Female sex/estrogen deficiency
- Prostatic hypertrophy (males)
- Multiparity (females)
- Dementia
- Stroke
- Diabetes
- Spinal cord injury
- Multiple sclerosis
- Obesity
- Hysterectomy
- Vaginal childbirth
- Functional impairment

Genetics
Unknown

ETIOLOGY
- Urgency urinary incontinence (UUI)
  - Idiopathic
  - Neurogenic (stroke, dementia, Parkinson disease, multiple sclerosis)
  - Inflammatory (infection, tumors, stones, diverticula)
- Stress urinary incontinence (SUI)
  - Genuine (types 0, 1, 2): pelvic floor muscle weakness, urethral hypermobility
  - Intrinsic sphincteric deficiency (type 3): Post transurethral resection of the prostate (TURP), post radical prostatectomy, prior urethral/pelvic surgery
  - May occur during pregnancy
- Mixed (MUI): Stress plus urge incontinence
- Overflow incontinence
  - Bladder outlet obstruction (benign prostatic hyperplasia, urethral stricture, pelvic prolapse)
  - Neurogenic bladder (diabetes, spinal cord injury, multiple sclerosis)
- Transient/reversible: Delirium, infection, atrophic urethritis/vaginitis, excessive urine output, restricted mobility, stool impaction (DIAPPERS)

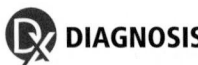 **DIAGNOSIS**

SIGNS AND SYMPTOMS
- Involuntary loss of urine
- May be associated with urinary urgency, or exertion

History
The diagnosis is often made by history.

Physical Exam
- Men: Palpate abdomen (for distended bladder), digital rectal exam (for prostatic hypertrophy/cancer/fecal impaction), and neurologic exam
- Women: Palpate abdomen (for distended bladder), pelvic exam (for gynecologic pathology), rectal exam (for fecal impaction), and neurologic exam
- Assess lower extremities for edema.
- Helpful to ask the patient to reproduce the activities (e.g., coughing, sneezing, laughing) that result in loss of urine
- Urinary diaries over 2–3 days

TESTS
Urodynamic evaluation may be indicated in select patients.
- Uroflowmetry: Poor flow rate may be indicative of obstruction or poor detrusor contractility.
- Cystometrogram: May show abnormal sphincter pressure or bladder function
- Pressure flow: High pressure with low flow may indicate obstruction.
- Video: Visualization to rule out diverticulum, reflux
- Electromyogram: Assesses sphincteric activity

Lab
- Urinalysis: R/0 glycosuria (diabetes), proteinuria (glomerular disease), white blood cells (infection), red blood cells (tumor), or bacteria (infection)
- Urine culture: Positive if urinary tract infection
- Drugs that may alter lab results
  - Diuretics (low urine specific gravity)
  - Antibiotics (negative urine culture)
- Disorders producing abnormal lab results generally contribute to the problem of incontinence.

Imaging
May be indicated in some patients
- Renal ultrasound to rule out hydronephrosis
- Bladder scan or ultrasound postvoid residual: May show increased residual urine (normally <50 mL); ultrasound can assess bladder wall thickness and rule out bladder stones
- Voiding cystourethrogram: May show bladder and/or urethral pathology

Pathological Findings
- Relate to the primary cause of incontinence
- Intrinsic urinary sphincter disorder
- Prostatic hypertrophy
- Neurogenic bladder
- Bladder tumors

DIFFERENTIAL DIAGNOSIS
- Urinary tract infection
- Vaginal discharge (women)
- Urethral discharge (men)
- Medication effect (diuretics, alcohol, caffeine, anticholinergics, β-agonists, calcium channel blockers, α-adrenergic blockers, antiparkinson drugs, angiotensin-converting enzyme inhibitors)
- Polyuria (diabetes, excessive water intake)
- Bladder tumor

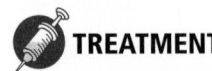 **TREATMENT**

INITIAL STABILIZATION
Outpatient evaluation and management

GENERAL MEASURES
Identification and specific treatment of all primary conditions relating to urinary incontinence (e.g., urinary tract infection, bladder tumors, prostatic hypertrophy, diabetes)
- Pelvic floor muscle therapy (PFMT) should be offered as 1st line therapy to all women with SUI, UUI, or MUI.
- Females with SUI or MUI combination of PFMT/bladder training may be more effective than PFMT alone in the short term.
- PFMT in men with post RRPX incontinence
- Biofeedback/behavioral training
- Behavioral therapy in men with incontinence
- Intermittent catherization if overflow incontinence
- Incontinence pads
- Indwelling catheterization (selected patients); rarely
- Condom catheters (male patients)
- Treatment for fecal impaction
- Weighted vaginal cones and electrical stimulation appear to be equally effective for women with SUI, but these may have side effects.

Diet
- In situations in which access to bathroom facilities is limited, patients should avoid high-volume fluid intake.
- Caffeine may aggravate overactive bladder symptoms by increasing urine volume and by having an irritant effect on the bladder.
- Weight loss: Obesity is an independent risk factor for urinary incontinence.

Activity
Encourage full activity.

MEDICATION (DRUGS)

First Line

- UUI (A, level of evidence 1)
  - Oxybutynin (Ditropan XL): 5–30 mg/d
  - Oxybutynin (Ditropan): 2.5–5 mg q.i.d.
  - Tolterodine (Detrol IR): 1–2 mg b.i.d.
  - Tolterodine (Detrol LA): 2–4 mg/d
  - Trospium chloride (Sanctura): 20 mg b.i.d
  - Topical estrogen
  - Flavoxate (Urispas): 100–200 mg t.i.d.
  - Imipramine (Tofranil): 25–50 mg t.i.d.
- SUI
  - Pseudoephedrine (Sudafed): 30–60 mg t.i.d.): Weak evidence to suggest alpha-adrenergic agent is better than PBO
  - Imipramine (Tofranil): 25–50 mg t.i.d.
  - Topical estrogen
- Overflow incontinence secondary to BPH
  - Doxazosin (Cardura): 1–8 mg/d
  - Terazosin (Hytrin): 1–10 mg/d
  - Tamsulosin (Flomax): 0.4–0.8 mg/d
  - 5-alpha reductase inhibitors
  - Finasteride (Proscar): 5 mg/d
  - Dutasteride (Avodart): 0.5 mg/d
- Contraindications
  - Review each medication before initiation.
  - Anticholinergic agents are contraindicated in patients with glaucoma, decreased gastrointestinal motility, or bladder outlet obstruction (e.g., prostatic hypertrophy).
- Precautions
  - Use the smallest dose possible in elderly
  - Common side effects include dry mouth, blurred vision, constipation, postural hypotension (alpha-blockers), and cognitive dysfunction.
- Significant possible interactions: These vary for each of the drugs listed.

Second Line

Desmopressin (DDAVP) nasal spray (nocturnal enuresis)

SURGERY

- Male patients with overflow incontinence secondary to prostatic hypertrophy benefit from prostatic reduction (e.g., TURP). Men with post-radical prostatectomy incontinence and post-TURP incontinence may benefit from bulking agents (4–20% report being dry), artificial sphincter (success rates range from 59–85%), or male sling (cure rate ranging from 76–86%).
- Female patients with stress incontinence may benefit from open colposuspension (cure rate 85%, A), autologous sling, transvaginal tape procedure (cure rate 81%, level of evidence 2)
- Female patients with poor urethral tone may benefit from periurethral bulking agents (low morbidity but low long-term success rate), or sling procedures.
- Neuromodulation for women with refractory UUI.
- Rarely with refractory UUI augmentation cystoplasty

 ## FOLLOW-UP

DISPOSITION

Discharge Criteria

Most surgical procedures are outpatient procedures or overnite stay. Most patients are taught clean intermittent catheterization prior to surgical intervention.

Issues for Referral

- Recurrent UTIs
- Microscopic hematuria

PROGNOSIS

- Generally good; most patients can achieve an increase in bladder control with appropriate medical/behavioral management
- Some experts feel sphincter incompetence is best treated surgically.

COMPLICATIONS

- Urinary tract infections
- Hydronephrosis (with atonic bladder or outlet obstruction)
- Renal failure (with obstructive hydronephrosis)
- Bladder calculi
- Skin irritation or infection
- Increased incidence of falls and fractures in elderly with overactive bladder
- Adverse drug events

PATIENT MONITORING

- With medical, behavioral, and PFMT regular follow-up is indicated to ensure proper technique and compliance and to assess response.
- Ask about side effects of medication.
- Check for orthostatic hypotension (in patients using alpha-blockers).

REFERENCES

1. Abrams P, Cardozo L, Khoury S, Wein A, eds. *Incontinence*. 3rd ed. Plymouth, UK: Health Publication Ltd; 2005.
2. Alhasso A, Glazener CMA, Pickard R. N'Dow Adrenergic drugs for urinary incontinence in adults. *Cochrane Database of Systematic Reviews*. 2005;(4).
3. Hay-Smith J, Herbison P, Ellis G, Moore K. Anticholinergic drugs versus placebo for OAB syndrome in adults. *Cochrane Database of Systematic Reviews*. 2002;(3):CD003781.
4. Herbison P, Plevnik S, Mantle J. Weighted vaginal cones for urinary incontinence. *Cochrane Database of Systematic Reviews*. 2002;(1):CD002114.
5. Borello-France D, Burgio KL. Nonsurgical treatment of urinary incontinence. *Clin Obstet Gynecol*. 2004;47:70–82.
6. Fine P, Antonini TG, Appell R. Clinical evaluation of women with lower urinary tract dysfunction. *Clin Obstet Gynecol*. 2004;47:44–52.

 ## MISCELLANEOUS

See also: Prostatic hyperplasia, benign (BPH); Urethritis; Urinary tract infection in females; Urinary tract infection in males;

CODES

ICD9-CM
788.30 Urinary incontinence, unspecified

PATIENT TEACHING

- Direct toward the general problem as well as underlying diseases
- Include instructions regarding good general nutrition and exercise practices.
- Encourage a rational toileting schedule, based on the pattern of incontinence.
- Stress the need for easy access to toilet facilities.
- Recommend pelvic floor (Kegel) exercises.
- Recommend bladder training—timed voiding and double voiding to ensure regular and complete bladder emptying.

 See Patient Handout on CD

U

URINARY TRACT INFECTION IN FEMALES

Barry D. Weiss, MD

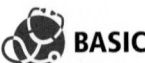 BASICS

DESCRIPTION
- Inflammation of the bladder mucosa
- This topic refers primarily to infectious cystitis; other urinary tract infections (UTIs) are discussed elsewhere.
- System(s) Affected: Renal/Urologic
- Synonym(s): Cystitis

GENERAL PREVENTION
- Maintain good hydration.
- Women with frequent or intercourse-related UTI should empty bladder immediately before and following intercourse and consider postcoital antibiotic treatment.
- Avoid feminine hygiene sprays and scented douches.
- Wipe urethra from front to back.

EPIDEMIOLOGY
- Predominant age: Young adults and older
- Predominant sex: Female only (for this discussion)

Incidence
Accounts for 7 million doctor visits a year

Prevalence
- ~3–8% of women have bacteriuria at any given time.
- ~30% of females have at least one UTI.

RISK FACTORS
- Previous UTI
- Diabetes mellitus
- Pregnancy
- More frequent or vigorous sexual activity than usual
- Use of spermicides or diaphragm
- Underlying abnormalities of the urinary tract, such as tumors, calculi, strictures, incomplete bladder emptying

ETIOLOGY
Acute infection, usually with Gram-negative bacteria (*Escherichia coli* in >90% of uncomplicated cystitis)

ASSOCIATED CONDITIONS
Described under "Risk Factors"

ALERT
Geriatric Considerations
- Elderly are more apt to have underlying urinary tract abnormality.
- Acute UTI is sometimes associated with incontinence or mental status changes in the elderly.

Pediatric Considerations
UTI in children, especially in those <1 year of age should prompt workup for urinary tract anomalies.

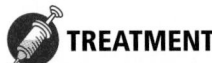 DIAGNOSIS

SIGNS AND SYMPTOMS
Note: Any or all may be present.
- Burning during urination
- Pain during urination
- Urgency (sensation of need to urinate frequently)
- Frequency
- Sensation of incomplete bladder emptying
- Blood in urine
- Lower abdominal pain or cramping
- Offensive odor of urine
- Nocturia

TESTS
Some recent research suggests the most cost-effective approach is empiric treatment without lab tests in nonpregnant premenopausal women with symptoms of UTI and no risks for complicated infection.

Lab
- Urinalysis demonstrating pyuria (>10 neutrophils/high power field [HPF] on microscopic exam). Leukocyte esterase dipsticks are also useful for detecting pyuria, but fail to detect pyuria in up to 20% of patients, and false positives occur from vaginal leukocytes.
- Urinalysis demonstrating bacteriuria (any amount on unspun urine, or 10 rod-shaped bacteria/HPF on centrifuged urine). Nitrite dipsticks are also useful (and 94% specific), but fail to detect bacteriuria in 30–50% of patients. Nitrite dipsticks may be negative in patients who do not eat meat.
- Urine culture demonstrating growth of single species of bacteria. Suspect contaminated specimen when culture shows multiple types of bacteria.
- Classic symptoms in nonpregnant young adult female with first episode of UTI require no urine culture for diagnosis. Obtain urinalysis and culture in other age groups, if it is a repeat episode, if the patient is pregnant, or if the symptoms are not classic.

Imaging
For all infants; may be indicated for older patients with recurrent infections
- Ultrasound imaging is the 1st-choice test.
- For infants and children, obtain ultrasound; if ureteral dilation is detected, obtain either voiding cystourethrogram or isotope cystogram to detect reflux.

Diagnostic Procedures/Surgery
- Suprapubic bladder aspiration or urethral catheterization to obtain urine specimen from infants
- Urethral catheterization to obtain urine specimen from children and adults if voided urine is suspected of being contaminated

DIFFERENTIAL DIAGNOSIS
- Vaginitis
- Sexually transmitted diseases causing urethritis or pyuria
- Hematuria from causes other than infection (e.g., neoplasia, calculi)
- Interstitial cystitis
- Psychologic dysfunction

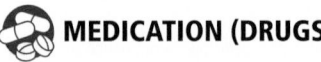 TREATMENT

INITIAL STABILIZATION
Outpatient treatment, except for complicated or upper tract infections

GENERAL MEASURES
- Maintain good hydration.
- 1/4 of women with simple UTI experience a second UTI within 6 months, and 1/2 at some time during their lifetime. Patients with multiple recurrent UTI and no underlying urinary tract abnormality may receive long-term prophylactic antibiotic treatment. Trimethoprim-sulfamethoxazole (TMP-SMX) and nitrofurantoin are commonly used.
- Patients with chronic indwelling urinary catheters always have colonization of urine, usually with multiple bacterial species. This should not be treated unless symptomatic with fever, sepsis, or other systemic symptoms.
- Preliminary studies indicate that *Vaccinium macrocarpon* (cranberry juice) may help prevent and treat UTIs by inhibiting bacterial adherence to the bladder epithelium.
- UTI during pregnancy always requires culture/sensitivity and usually requires a 10–14-day treatment. Following the treatment of acute infection, pregnant women often receive prophylactic antibiotics for the remainder of pregnancy.

Diet
No special diet

Activity
Avoid sexual intercourse when symptoms are present.

ALERT
Elderly may have bacteriuria without symptoms; generally this does not require treatment, if the urinary tract is otherwise normal.

MEDICATION (DRUGS)

- 1st, rare, or infrequent UTIs in older children, adolescents, and adults who are nonpregnant, nondiabetic, afebrile, nonimmunocompromised, and have no abnormality of the urinary tract (i.e., uncomplicated)
  - 3-day treatment with fluoroquinolone or TMP-SMX. Increasing resistance being reported to TMP-SMX. It is the preferred treatment if local sensitivity patterns indicate low resistance rates.
  - New studies show 3-day therapy may be used in children.
- Postcoital: Single-dose TMP-SMX or cephalexin may reduce frequency of UTI in sexually active women.
- Pregnant patients: 10–14-day or longer treatment with pregnancy-safe antibiotic chosen based on culture/sensitivity results. May begin with cephalosporin, amoxicillin, or other antibiotic while awaiting culture/sensitivity results.
- All other patients: 10–14-day treatment with antibiotic chosen based on culture/sensitivity results. May begin with fluoroquinolone, TMP-SMX, cephalosporin, or other antibiotic while awaiting culture/sensitivity results.

- Contraindications
  - Refer to the manufacturer's literature.
  - Fluoroquinolones are not safe during pregnancy or for treatment of children.
  - TMP-SMX use in pregnancy is not desirable (especially in the 3rd trimester), but is appropriate in some circumstances.
- Precautions: Refer to the manufacturer's literature.
- Significant possible interactions: Refer to the manufacturer's literature.
- Change the antibiotic if it is indicated by the culture/sensitivity results.

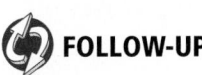

FOLLOW-UP

PROGNOSIS
Symptoms resolve within 2–3 days after starting a treatment in almost all patients.

COMPLICATIONS
- Pyelonephritis or sepsis
- Renal abscess
- Acute urinary outlet obstruction

ALERT
Infants and young children with cystitis are at higher risk of pyelonephritis.

PATIENT MONITORING
- 1st or rare UTI: In young or middle age, nonpregnant adult females require no follow-up if cured after 3-day therapy. If not resolved within 2–3 days, obtain culture/sensitivity and change antibiotic accordingly.
- All other patients should have post-treatment urine culture to document eradication of infection.

REFERENCES

1. Barry HG, Ebell MH, Hickner J. Evaluation of suspected urinary tract infection in ambulatory women: A cost-utility analysis of office-based strategies. *J Fam Pract*. 1997;44:49–60.
2. Bent S, et al. Does this woman have an acute uncomplicated urinary tract infection. *JAMA*. 2002;287:2701–2710.
3. Ebell MH, Barry NC. Urinary tract infection. In: Weiss BD, ed. *20 Common Problems in Primary Care*. New York, NY: McGraw-Hill; 1999.
4. Gupta K, Scholes D, Stamm WE. Increasing prevalence of antimicrobial resistance among uropathogens causing acute uncomplicated cystitis in women. *JAMA*. 1999;281:736–738.
5. Huang ES, Stafford RS. National patterns in the treatment of urinary tract infections in women by ambulatory care physicians. *Arch Intern Med*. 2002;162:41–47.
6. Stamm WE, Hooton T. Management of urinary tract infections in adults. *N Engl J Med*. 1993;329:1328–1334.

 MISCELLANEOUS

See also: Pyelonephritis

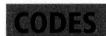 **CODES**

ICD9-CM
595.0 Acute cystitis

PATIENT TEACHING
- Take antibiotic as directed.
- Return if symptoms are not resolved or markedly improved within 48 hours.
- Return if fever, chills, or flank pain develop.
- If taking prophylactic antibiotics, take at bedtime.

 See Corresponding Diagnostic Algorithm

 See Patient Handout on CD

U

URINARY TRACT INFECTION IN MALES

Scott A. Fields, MD

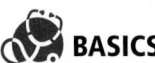 **BASICS**

DESCRIPTION
Cystitis is an infection of the lower urinary tract, usually resulting from a single gram-negative enteric bacteria. (See separate chapters for information on prostatitis, pyelonephritis, and nongonococcal urethritis.)
- System(s) Affected: Renal/Urologic
- Synonym(s): UTI; Cystitis

GENERAL PREVENTION
- Prompt treatment of predisposing factors
- Catheter use only when necessary; if needed, use aseptic technique and closed system, with removal as soon as possible

EPIDEMIOLOGY
- Predominant age: Increases with age. Uncommon in men <50 years old; 8 infections/10,000 men, ages 21–50 years
- Predominant sex: Male only (for this discussion)

Prevalence
Not common

RISK FACTORS
- Benign prostatic hypertrophy
- Cognitive impairment
- Fecal incontinence
- Urinary incontinence
- Anal intercourse
- Recent urologic surgery, catheterization
- Infection of the prostate or kidney
- Urinary tract instrumentation
- Immunocompromised host
- Outlet obstruction

Genetics
No specific genetic pattern

ETIOLOGY
- *Escherichia coli* (80% of infections)
- *Klebsiella*
- *Enterobacter*
- *Proteus*
- *Pseudomonas*
- *Serratia*
- *Streptococcus faecalis* and *Staphylococcus*

ASSOCIATED CONDITIONS
- Acute bacterial pyelonephritis
- Chronic bacterial pyelonephritis
- Urethritis
- Prostatitis
- Prostatic hypertrophy
- Prostate cancer

ALERT
Geriatric Considerations
Bacteriuria is common in the elderly, appears related to functional status, and is usually transient. If asymptomatic bacteriuria is noted, no treatment is needed.

Pediatric Considerations
Usually associated with obstruction to normal flow of urine, such as vesicoureteral reflux

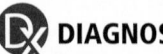 **DIAGNOSIS**

SIGNS AND SYMPTOMS
- Urinary frequency
- Urinary urgency
- Dysuria
- Hesitancy
- Slow urinary stream
- Dribbling of urine
- Nocturia
- Suprapubic discomfort
- Low back pain
- Hematuria
- Systemic symptoms (chills, fever) present with concomitant pyelonephritis or prostatitis

History
Careful history and physical exam

TESTS
Urologic investigations are necessary to rule out other disorders.

Lab
- Pyuria
- Bacteriuria
- Urine dipstick leukocyte esterase (75–90% sensitivity, 95% specificity) and nitrate (35–85% sensitivity, 70% specificity)
- Urine culture: 10 high-power colonies of pathogens (or counts >100,000 bacteria/mL of urine) confirm diagnosis (*E. coli*, *Klebsiella*, *Pseudomonas*, other agents). Lower counts may also be indicative of infection, especially in presence of pyuria.
- Segmented bacteriologic localization cultures
  - Variable block 1 (VB1): Collect 5–10 mL of urine from patient's initial voiding.
  - VB2: Then a sample of sterile midstream urine is obtained.
  - Expressed prostatic secretion (EPS): Prostatic massage is performed and EPS is collected from the meatus.
  - VB3: Patient completes voiding, and fourth sample is collected.
  - Cultures and sensitivity are collected from each specimen.
- Drugs that may alter lab results: Antibiotics prior to culture

Imaging
- IV pyelography
- Cystoscopy
- Ultrasound

Pathological Findings
Depends on site of infection

DIFFERENTIAL DIAGNOSIS
- Anatomic or functional pathology
- Urethritis
- Infections in other sites of the genitourinary tract (e.g., epididymis)

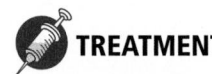 **TREATMENT**

INITIAL STABILIZATION
Outpatient treatment, except for acute illness with toxicity or kidney failure

GENERAL MEASURES
- Hydration; analgesia if required
- Discontinue sexual activity until cured.
- Patient with indwelling catheters
  - If asymptomatic bacterial colonization, no need to treat (sterilization of urine is not possible and resistant organisms may take up residence)
  - If symptomatic of acute infection, institute treatment

Diet
No special diet

Activity
As tolerated

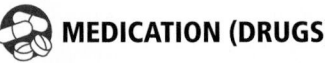 **MEDICATION (DRUGS)**

First Line
- Acute infection, 1st infection, no risk factors for treatment: Prescribe 7–10 days of oral antibiotics, either empirically or based on culture and sensitivity results. For empiric therapy, trimethoprim-sulfamethoxazole (SMX-TMP) b.i.d. will usually treat the most likely pathogens. (1–4,6–8)[C]
- Complicated or recurrent infection: Prescribe 14–21 days of antibiotics based on antimicrobial sensitivities with repeat urine check after the treatment. (1–4,6–8)[C]
- For contraindications, precautions, and possible significant interactions, refer to the manufacturer's information.

Second Line
According to culture and sensitivity results and patient's history

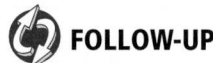

FOLLOW-UP

PROGNOSIS
Clearing of infections with appropriate antibiotic treatment

COMPLICATIONS
- Pyelonephritis
- Ascending infection
- Recurrent infection

PATIENT MONITORING
- Close follow-up until clinically well
- Repeat urinalysis after treatment.

REFERENCES

1. Finn SD. Urinary tract infections—diagnosis and treatment in women and men. *Consultant*. 1992;10:43–58.
2. Hooton TM, Stamm WE. Management of acute uncomplicated urinary tract infection in adults. *Med Clin North Am*. 1991;75:339–357.
3. Harrington RD, Hooton TM. Urinary tract infection risk factors and gender. *J Gend Specif Med*. 2000;3:27–34.
4. Hatton J, Hughes M, Raymond CH. Management of bacterial urinary tract infections in adults. *Ann Pharmacother*. 1994;28:1264–1272.
5. Khan AJ, Schaeffer HA, Evans H. Urinary tract infections in adolescent boys. *J Natl Med Assoc*. 1996;88:25–26.
6. Lipsky BA. Urinary tract infections in men. Epidemiology, pathophysiology, diagnosis, and treatment. *Ann Intern Med*. 1989;110:138–150.
7. Lipsky BA. Managing urinary tract infections in men. *Hosp Pract (Off Ed)*. 2000;35:53–59, discussion 59–60.
8. Naber KG, et al. Urinary Tract Infection (UTI) Working Group of the Health Care Office (HCO) of the European Association of Urology (EAU). EAU guidelines for the management of urinary and male genital tract infections. Urinary Tract Infection (UTI) Working Group of the Health Care Office (HCO) of the European Association of Urology (EAU). *Eur Urol*. 2001;40:576–588.

MISCELLANEOUS

See also: Prostatic cancer; Prostatic hyperplasia, benign (BPH); Prostatitis; Pyelonephritis

CODES

ICD9-CM
- 595.0 Acute cystitis
- 595.1 Chronic interstitial cystitis
- 595.2 Other chronic cystitis

PATIENT TEACHING

For patient education materials favorably reviewed on this topic, contact the National Kidney Foundation, 30 E. 33rd Street, Suite 1100, New York, NY 10016; (212) 889–2210.

Diet
Pushing fluids, especially those that acidify the urine

Prevention
Pushing fluids

 See Corresponding Diagnostic Algorithm

U

UROLITHIASIS

Alison H. Blatt, MD

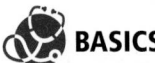 **BASICS**

DESCRIPTION
- Stone formation within the urinary tract: Urinary crystals bind to form a nidus, which grows to form a calculus (stone).
- Calculus may be asymptomatic or obstructive, or may be a source of chronic infection.

GENERAL PREVENTION
Increased water intake reduces the risk of recurrence and time to recurrence of urinary calculi.

ALERT
Pediatric Considerations
Rare; more common in males; low socioeconomic status

Pregnancy Considerations
- Pregnant women have the same incidence of renal colic as do nonpregnant women.
- Diagnosis is challenging: Most common differential is physiological hydronephrosis of pregnancy.
- Ultrasound; avoid irradiation
- Aim of treatment is pain control, renal function preservation and aseptic urine until birth or stone passage. Only 30% require some form of intervention.
- NSAIDs must be avoided; therefore, acetaminophen ± codeine is the mainstay.

EPIDEMIOLOGY
- Predominant age: Mean age is 40–50 years
- Predominant sex: Male > Female (~2:1)
- High frequency of urolithiasis worldwide although rare in a few parts of the world (e.g., in Greenland in the coastal areas of Japan)
- The worldwide epidemiology differs according to both geographical area and socioeconomic conditions (dietary intake and lifestyle).
  - Radiolucent and infection stones are less influenced by environmental conditions.
- Vesical calculus (bladder stones), due to malnutrition in early life, is frequent in Middle Eastern and Asian countries. The incidence is improving as social conditions gradually improve.
- Incidences in industrialized countries appear to be increasing, probably due to improved diagnostics, as well as increasingly rich diets and altered environmental conditions.

Incidence
In industrialized countries: 100–200 per 100,000

Prevalence
In industrialized countries: 5–10%

RISK FACTORS
- White > African American in regions with both populations
- Family history
- Diet rich in protein, refined carbohydrates, and sodium
- Occupations associated with a sedentary lifestyle or with a hot, dry workplace
- Incidence rates peak in summer.

Genetics
- Up to 20% of patients have a family history. However, spouse of stone formers have higher calcium excretion rates than controls, suggesting strong dietary-environmental factors.
- Autosomal dominant: Idiopathic hypercalciuria
- Autosomal recessive: Cystinuria, Lesch-Nyan syndrome, hyperoxaluria types I and II
- Ehler-Danlos syndrome, Marfan syndrome, Wilson disease, familial renal tubular acidosis

PATHOPHYSIOLOGY
- Supersaturation and dehydration
- Stasis of urine
  - Renal malformation (e.g., horseshoe kidney)
  - Incomplete bladder emptying (e.g., neuropathic bladder, prostate enlargement)
- Nucleation and epitaxy: Crystals may form in pure solutions or on existing surfaces (other crystals, cellular debris, etc.).
- Balance of promoters and inhibitors: Organic (Tamm-Horsfall protein, GAG, uropontin, nephrocalcin) and Inorganic (citrate, pyrophosphate)

ETIOLOGY
- Calcium oxalate and/or phosphate stones (80%)
  - Idiopathic hypercalciuria
    - Autosomal dominant trait; present in 50% of calcium stone formers and 10% of the normal population
    - Absorptive hypercalciuria: Increased jejunal calcium absorption
    - Renal leak: Increased calcium excretion from renal proximal tubule
    - Resorptive hypercalciuria: Subtle hyperparathyroidism
  - Hypercalcemia
    - Hyperparathyroidism
    - Sarcoidosis
    - Malignancy
    - Pagets disease
    - Multiple myeloma
  - Hyperoxaluria
    - Enteric hyperoxaluria: Bowel disease, acidosis, or hypokalaemia; bile salt malbsorption leads to formation of calcium soaps, thus leaving increased oxalate available for colon absorption and subsequent increased renal excretion
    - Primary hyperoxaluria: Autosomal recessive, types I and II
    - Dietary hyperoxaluria
  - Hyperuricemia
    - Seen in 10% of calcium stone formers
    - Acidosis, malbsorption, myeoloproliferative diseases, gout, chemotherapy, Lesch-Nyan syndrome (rare autosomal recessive disorder)
    - Thiazides, probenicid
  - Hypocitraturia
    - Caused by acidosis: Infection, malabsorption, thiazides, hypokalaemia, dietary salt and protein
- Uric acid stones (10–15%): Hyperuricemia causes as above
- Struvite stones (5–10%): Infected urine with urease-producing organisms (most commonly proteus)
- Cystine stones (<1%): Autosomal recessive disorder of renal tubular reabsorption of cystine
- Bladder stones
  - Inadequate bladder emptying in adults
  - In children, it is usually due to malnutrition.

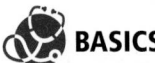 **DIAGNOSIS**

SIGNS AND SYMPTOMS
- Pain
  - Renal colic: Acute onset of severe loin to groin pain; typically patient cannot lie still.
  - Distal stones may present with referred pain in labia, penile meatus, or testis.
  - Tender renal angle and/or iliac fossa
- Microscopic or gross hematuria occurs in 95% of patients.
- Nonspecific symptoms of nausea, vomiting, tachycardia, diaphoresis
- Low grade fever without infection
- High grade fever, cloudy urine. Infection requires urgent treatment (see below).
- Irritative lower urinary tract symptoms such as frequency and dysuria especially occur with stones at the vesico-ureteric junction.
- Asymptomatic. Particularly nonobstructing stones within the renal calyces

TESTS
Lab
- Urinalysis for red cells, leukocytes, nitrates, pH (acidic urine <5.5 is associated with uric acid stones, alkaline >7.0 with struvite stones)
- Midstream urine for microscopy, culture, and sensitivity.
- Bloods: FBC, urea, creatinine, electrolytes, calcium, and urate
- Blood culture if suspect sepsis
- Parathyroid hormone only if calcium elevated
- Stone analysis if/when stone passed

Imaging
- Noncontrast helical CT of the abdomen and pelvis is the investigation of choice where available.
  - Stone is most commonly found at levels of ureteric luminal narrowing: The pelvi-ureteric junction, the pelvic brim, and the vesico-ureteric junction.
  - If the obstruction is acute, proximal ureter and renal pelvis is dilated to the level of obstruction and perinephric "stranding" is seen.
  - If chronic, renal atrophy may be noted.
- KUB is necessary when a stone is diagnosed to determine whether the stone is radio-opaque or lucent (determines treatment as well as type of follow-up imaging).
  - Calcium oxalate/phosphate stones are radio-opaque.
  - Uric acid stones are radiolucent.
  - Staghorn calculi (that fill the shape of the renal calyces) are usually struvite and opaque.
  - Cystine stones are faintly opaque ("ground-glass" appearance).
- IVP has been largely replaced by CT in the initial diagnostic workup.
- Ultrasound has no role in diagnosis due to its low sensitivity and specificity; exceptions are pregnancy and pediatrics.

DIFFERENTIAL DIAGNOSIS
- Appendicitis
- Ruptured aortic aneurysm
- Musculoskeletal strain
- Pyelonephritis (upper urinary tract infection)
- Pyonephrosis (obstructed upper urinary tract infection–emergency)
- Perinephric abscess
- Ectopic pregnancy
- Salpingitis

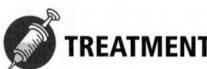 **TREATMENT**

PRE HOSPITAL
- Analgesia
  - Combination of NSAIDs (indomethacin suppository 100 mg) and acetaminophen-codeine orally
  - Parenteral narcotic if above fails to control pain (morphine 5–10 mg IV or IM q4h)
  - Antiemetic if required or prophylactically with parenteral narcotics
- Antibiotics only if patient septic and after urine and blood cultures taken
- Pushing fluids during an acute episode is not advised. It increases pain and probably does not improve stone passage rates.

INITIAL STABILIZATION
Septic patients with pyonephrosis may require intravenous fluids, and in severe cases, cardiorespiratory support in intensive care even after relief of obstruction.

GENERAL MEASURES
- 75% of patients are successfully treated conservatively and pass the stone spontaneously
- Advise patient to strain urine and take regular analgesia. Present to hospital if pain is uncontrolled or fevers develop.

Diet
- Increased fluid intake for life cannot be overemphasized for decreasing recurrence.
  - Encourage 2–3 L/d intake; advise patient to have "clear" urine rather than yellow.
- Diet modification has less effect than fluid intake on urine concentrations of stone substrates, and has low compliance rates.
- Calcium stone formers should minimize high oxalate foods such as spinach, rhubarb, peanuts, chocolates, and parsley.
- Decrease protein and salt intake.
- Lowering calcium intake is inadvisable and may even increase urine calcium excretion.

SPECIAL THERAPY
- Uric acid stone dissolution therapy
  - Ural sachet 3x/d OR potassium citrate OR sodium bicarbonate to alkalinize the urine; keep pH >6.5
  - Allopurinol 100–300 mg/d PO
- Cystine stone dissolution/prevention
  - Captopril, D-penicillamine, alkalinizers
- Consider altering medications that increase risk of stone formation: Probenicid, loop diuretics, salicylic acid, salbutamol, indinavir, triamterine, acetazolamide
- Recurrent calcium stone formers may improve with thiazides; however, long-term use is limited by side effects such as hypotension, hypokalemia, weakness, and impotence.
- Orthophosphate is required in large daily doses to significantly reduce urine calcium excretion causing side effects of diarrhea, flatus, and bloating.

SURGERY
- Immediate relief of obstruction is imperative in 2 groups of patients
  - Patients with signs of sepsis
  - Renal failure (obstructed solitary kidney, bilateral obstruction)
- Uncontrolled pain despite adequate analgesia is the most common indication for semi-urgent endoscopic stenting.
- Emergency surgery to unobstruct kidney
  - Placement of a retrograde stent (i.e., endoscopic surgery, usually requiring an anesthetic)
  - Radiological placement of a percutaneous nephrostomy tube, usually performed in emergencies under local anesthetic
- Elective surgery for stone treatment
  - Extracorporeal shock-wave lithotripsy (ESWL)
  - Ureteroscopy with basket extraction orlithotripsy (laser or pneumatic)
  - Percutaneous nephrolithotomy (PCNL)
  - Open surgery uncommon

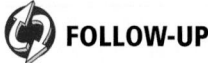 **FOLLOW-UP**

- Patients being treated conservatively with ureteric stones should be followed until imaging is clear (KUB 2nd weekly if stone is visible) or stone is visibly passed.
  - These patients should be advised to strain their urine.
  - If pain management is suboptimal or stone does not progress or pass within 2–4 weeks, patient should be referred to a urologist.
- Recurrent stone formers should have follow-up with a urologist for a full biochemical screen to identify reversible risk factors.
  - 24 hour urine for volume, pH, creatinine, calcium, cystine, phosphate, oxalate, uric acid, magnesium

DISPOSITION
Issues for Referral
- Urgent referral of patients with urine infection/sepsis, or acute renal failure/solitary kidney
- Early referral of pregnant patients, large stones (>8 mm), chronic renal failure, children
- Referral if stone not passing at 2–4 weeks or pain is poorly controlled
- All patients with >1 stone or stone episode require referral for metabolic screening.

PROGNOSIS
- Spontaneous stone passage depends on stone location (proximal vs. distal) and stone size (<5 mm 90% pass, >8 mm 10% pass)
- Stone recurrence: 50% of patients at 10 years

REFERENCES
1. Qiang W, Ke Z. Water for preventing urinary calculi. *Cochrane Database of Systematic Reviews*. 2004;3: CD004292.
2. Tiselius HG. Epidemiology and medical management of stone disease. *BJU Int*. 2003;91: 758–767.
3. Worster A, Preyra I, Weaver B, Haines T. The accuracy of noncontrast helical computed tomography versus intravenous pyelography in the diagnosis of suspected acute urolithiasis: A meta-analysis. *Ann Emerg Med*. 2002;40(3): 280–286.

 MISCELLANEOUS

CODES

ICD9-CM
592.9 Urinary calculus, unspecified

 See Corresponding Diagnostic Algorithm

 See Patient Handout on CD

U

URTICARIA
Weily Soong, MD

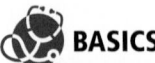 **BASICS**

DESCRIPTION

A rapid eruption of polymorphic-shaped cutaneous wheals with central swelling, erythema, and blanching; size ranges from a few millimeters to several centimeters; single or multiple superficial papules and plaques; associated with itching or burning; subsides within 24 hours with no scars or change in pigmentation; may be recurrent; often associated with angioedema (swelling of the lower dermis and subcutis); also known as hives.

- Spontaneous urticaria
  - Acute: Persists <6 weeks
    - Vast number of possible triggers, e.g., foods, medications, insect stings/bites, infections, physical stimuli, and occupational exposures
    - Etiology is usually obvious to the patient and physician.
  - Chronic: Persists >6 weeks
    - Can be either continuous (daily symptoms) or recurrent (periods with flares and periods with no symptoms)
    - The longer the urticaria persists, the more difficult to find the etiology
    - Usually not IgE mediated
    - Most likely idiopathic (~80% of cases), but reported associations with psychological stress, pseudoallergenic foods/additives, autoimmunity, chronic indolent infections, or malignancy
- Physical urticaria
  - Dermatographism: Linear, itchy, red wheal and flare from scratching or rubbing the skin
  - Cold urticaria: From exposure to cold; usually idiopathic but can be due to infections, neoplasia, or autoimmune diseases. The familial form, called Familial Cold Autoinflammatory Syndrome, is characterized by recurrent bouts of fever, urticaria, and joint pain triggered by cold, and is caused by mutations in the Cryopyrin gene resulting in the release of interleukin 1.
  - Delayed pressure urticaria: Deeper and more painful urticaria; occurs 2–6 hours after pressure to skin (e.g., from elastic or shoes)
  - Solar urticaria: From exposure to sunlight of different wavelengths, usually ultraviolet light; onset in minutes; subsides within 2 hours
  - Heat urticaria: From direct contact with warm objects or air; rare
  - Vibratory urticaria/angioedema: From strong vibrating mechanical forces; rare
- Special forms of urticaria
  - Cholinergic urticaria: Due to brief increase of core body temperature; small pin-sized (5–10 mm) wheals surrounded by an erythema but can also have larger wheals; from physical exercise, stress, and hot showers
  - Adrenergic urticaria: Caused by stress; extremely rare; has pinpoint-sized red wheals with a white halo
  - Contact urticaria: Wheals at sites where chemical substances contact with the skin
  - Aquagenic urticaria: Small wheals after contact with water at any temperature; rare
  - Urticarial vasculitis: A leukocytoclastic vasculitis looking like urticaria and tending to last >24 hours; more painful than puritic; maybe palpable and purpuric

GENERAL PREVENTION

- Acute, physical, and special forms of urticaria: Avoidance of the potential trigger
- Chronic urticaria: Usually unable to prevent

EPIDEMIOLOGY

- Predominant in all ages: Acute form mainly in children; chronic form mainly in adults
- Predominant sex: Male = Female
- 50% of patients have urticaria with angioedema, 40% with urticaria only, 10% with angioedema only
- <20% of chronic urticaria have known causes.

Prevalence

- Affects 15–25% of population during lifetime
- In the US population: 1 in 1000

ALERT

Pediatric Considerations

- Acute isolated incidents are more frequent; affects 6–7% of preschool children; 17% of children have a history of atopic dermatitis
- In childhood acute urticaria, infection (especially respiratory and urinary tract) is the most frequently documented cause (49%), followed by drug (5%) and food allergies (3%)

RISK FACTORS

History of atopic diseases: Allergic rhinitis, asthma, atopic dermatitis, food and drug allergies

Genetics

No consistent pattern known

PATHOPHYSIOLOGY

- Caused by a degranulation of mast cells which triggers a release of inflammatory mediators (e.g., histamine and leukotrienes) to cause local vasodilatation, cellular infiltration (lymphocytes, eosinophils, mast cells, basophils, neutrophils), vascular permeability, and edema of the dermis of the skin (urticaria) or of subcutaneous skin tissue (angioedema)
- May be immune-mediated (IgE-mediated), complement-mediated, nonimmune-mediated (e.g., degranulation of mast cells by physical stimuli), autoimmune-mediated, or idiopathic

ETIOLOGY

- Spontaneous urticaria
  - Acute
    - Viral infections: Upper respiratory tract (most common cause, especially in children), mononucleosis, viral hepatitis
    - Bacterial infections: Strep throat, sinusitis, dental caries, otitis, urinary tract
    - Foods, especially in children: Most common are peanut, tree nuts, seafood, milk, soy, fish, wheat, and eggs. Tend to be IgE mediated. Allergies to food preservatives and additives are possible but not common.
    - Drugs: Can be IgE-mediated (e.g., penicillin), nonIgE-mediated (e.g., aspirin and NSAIDs), or idiosyncratic
    - Inhalant, contact, ingestion, or occupational exposure
    - Insect bite or sting
    - Transfusion reaction
  - Chronic: >80% of cases idiopathic; usually nonIgE-mediated
    - Chronic indolent infections: *Helicobacter pylori*, vaginitis, fungal or tinea, parasitic, chronic sinusitis, dental cavities, and chronic viral infections (hepatitis)
    - Collagen vascular disease (cutaneous vasculitis, serum sickness, lupus)
    - Thyroid autoimmunity
    - Autoimmune antibodies to the IgE receptor on mast cells and to the IgE antibody causing mast cell degranulation
    - Malignancy; rare
    - Emotional stress (little supporting evidence)
- Physical and special forms of urticaria: Nonimmune-mediated mast cell degranulation caused by a specific physical stimuli, body temperature changes, stress, chemical substances, and water

ASSOCIATED CONDITIONS

- Angioedema
- Anaphylaxis

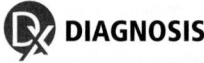 **DIAGNOSIS**

SIGNS AND SYMPTOMS

- Seen alone or with angioedema
- Urticaria may be an initial symptom of a generalized anaphylactic reaction, potentially fatal.
- Single or multiple raised, blanched, central wheals surrounded by red flare anywhere on body
- Intensely pruritic
- Variably sized, 1–2 mm to 15–20 cm or larger; sometimes confluent
- Fast onset, resolves spontaneously in <48 hours

History

The most important: A detailed history and review of symptoms, including the timing/duration of the symptoms, potential triggers, and history of atopic diseases and autoimmune diseases

Physical Exam

A complete physical exam to detect any associated conditions (autoimmune; malignancy; and viral, bacterial, and fungal/tinea infections)

TESTS

Lab

- Acute urticaria: Testing depends on the history and the potential triggers.
  - Allergy skin tests and radioallergosorbent test (RAST) for inhaled allergens, insects, drugs, or foods and for assessing other atopic conditions
  - Infection: Pharyngeal culture, liver function tests, mononucleosis test, urine analysis
  - Food and drug reactions: Elimination of or challenges with suspected agents
- Chronic urticaria: Depending on diagnostic suspicions
  - CBC with differential
  - Tests for *H. pylori* (e.g., antibodies)
  - Thyroid function tests and anti-thyroid antibodies (anti-thyroperoxidase and anti-thyroglobulin)
  - Autoimmune: ESR, antinuclear antibody (ANA), rheumatoid factor, complement (such as CH50), cryoglobulins
  - Stool for ova and parasites
  - Urine analysis

– Autologous serum skin testing
– Food and drug reactions: Elimination of or challenges with suspected agents
– Malignancy work-up, including serum protein electrophoresis and immunofixation assay
• Physical and special forms of urticaria
– Dermatographism: Scratch skin with a tongue blade, observe for surrounding uricaria.
– Cold urticaria: Ice cube test—place ice cube on skin 5 minutes, observe 10–15 minutes
– Cholinergic: Exercise challenge
– Solar: Expose skin to wavelengths of light.
– Delayed pressure: Apply 5–10-lb sandbag for 3 hours, observe
– Aquagenic: Apply water at various temperatures.
– Vibratory: Apply vibration 4–5 minutes with a lab mixing device, observe.

Imaging
Any imaging necessary to rule out chronic indolent infections (e.g., sinus CT) or malignancy

Diagnostic Procedures/Surgery
• Skin biopsy to rule out urticarial vasculitis
• Routine dental care to rule out dental caries

DIFFERENTIAL DIAGNOSIS
• Anaphylaxis (a potentially fatal generalized systemic allergic disorder with urticaria, angioedema, respiratory distress, abdominal pain, hypotension; may present initially with urticaria)
• Insect bites
• Morbilliform drug eruptions
• Erythema multiforme
• Systemic lupus erythematosus
• Vasculitis and polyarteritis
• Angioedema without urticaria (related to complement and bradykinin disorders, such as familial hereditary angioedema, angiotensin converting enzyme (ACE) inhbitor angioedema, complement deficiencies)
• Urticaria pigmentosa (mastocytosis). Pink lesions urticate when scratched (Darier sign).
• Bullous pemphigoid (urticarial stage)

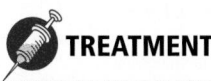

TREATMENT

GENERAL MEASURES
Avoidance or elimination of the eliciting stimulus

Diet
If a particular food is implicated, avoidance of the food or a trial of avoiding the food for 2–3 weeks

Activity
Depends on the urticarial trigger
• Cold and heat urticaria: Avoid sudden changes in temperature (e.g., slowly getting into a cold swimming pool).
• Dermatographic and delayed-pressure urticaria: Spread out the amount of force per area applied to the skin.
• Solar urticaria: Avoid the sun; use sunscreen.
• Cholinergic urticaria: Avoid sudden changes in body temperature (e.g., slow warm-ups and cooldowns during exercise).

Complementary and Alternative Medicine
• Avoid use of alternative medicine drugs. Herbal and vitamin supplements may make the urticaria worse, because trace contaminants in the supplements might be allergenic.
• Beware of certain "experts" in alternative medicine who might place chronic urticarial patients on severe food and activity restrictions based on lab tests that have little scientific basis.

 ## MEDICATION (DRUGS)

First Line
• 1st-generation antihistamines—mainly for short, intermittent attacks of urticaria; use is limited by its sedation and short half-life) (1,2)[A]
– Older children and adults: Hydroxyzine or diphenhydramine 25–50 mg q6h
– Children <6 years old: Diphenhydramine 12.5 mg (elixir) q6–8h (5 mg/kg/d) or hydroxyzine elixir (10 mg/5 mL) 2 mg/kg/d divided q6–8h
• 2nd-generation H_1-blockers—more expensive; effectiveness like older antihistamines but less sedating; a longer half-life. (1,2)[A]
– Fexofenadine (Allegra): 180 mg/d
– Loratadine (Claritin): 10 mg/d
– Desloratadine (Clarinex): 5 mg/d
– Cetirizine (Zyrtec): 10 mg/d

• May need higher doses of antihistamines or a combination of multiple antihistamines for control
• Precautions
– Drowsiness and dry mouth and eyes
– Should be used with caution in the elderly and during pregnancy

Second Line
• Doxepin (Sinequan): Tricyclic antidepressant with strong H_1- and H_2-blocking properties; 10–25 mg at bedtime; sedation limits usefulness (2)[C]
• H_2-blockers: mildly helpful (1,2)[C]
• Corticosteroids: For unresponsive cases, e.g., prednisone 40 mg/d for 5–7 days, taper as antihistamines are introduced; avoid chronic use due to the severe side effects which might be worse than the effects of the urticaria (2)[C]
• Cyproheptadine: Antihistamine and antiserotonergic agent (2)[C]
• Cyclosporine: Best-studied immunosuppressive therapy; effective (2.5–5 mg/kg/d) and steroid sparing (3)[C]
• Leukotriene antagonists: Safe and worth trying in chronic, unresponsive cases (2)[C]
• Intravenous immune globulin, plasmapheresis, sulfasalazine, dapsone, danazol, and hydroxychloroquine require further study. (3)
• Administering thyroid hormone may alleviate chronic urticaria in hypothyroid patients with autoantibodies. (3)[C]

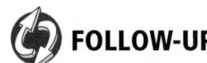 ## FOLLOW-UP

DISPOSITION
Admission Criteria
If urticaria and angioedema progress into anaphylaxis or threaten the airway. Will need to be discharged with an EpiPen

Issues for Referral
• Referral to an allergist and immunologist for elucidating and testing of potential triggers, life-threatening reactions, and complex management
• Referral to a dermatologist for skin biopsy
• Referral to a rheumatologist for treatment of autoimmune causes of urticaria

PROGNOSIS
• 70% of acute symptoms are better in <72 hours.
• 30% of the patients are chronic.
• >50% of chronic idiopathic urticaria resolve in 3–5 years but are at risk for a reoccurrence many years later.

PATIENT MONITORING
If symptoms persist or recur, patient may need to keep a daily diary of potential triggers (foods, activities, etc.). Pictures of the urticarial lesions are helpful.

REFERENCES

1. Baxi S, Dinakar C. Urticaria and angioedema. *Immunol Allergy Clin N Am*. 2005;25:353–367.
2. Zuberbier T. Urticaria. *Allergy*. 2003;58: 1224–1234.
3. Kaplan AP. Chronic urticaria: Pathogenesis and treatment. *J Allergy Clin Immunol*. 2004;114: 465–474.
4. Joint Task Force on Practice Parameters. The diagnosis and management of urticaria: A practice parameter. *Ann Allergy Asthma Immunol*. 2000; 85:521–544.
5. Wedi B, Raap U, Kapp A. Chronic urticaria and infections. *Curr Opin Allergy Clin Immunol*. 2004;4:387–396.

 ## MISCELLANEOUS

See also: Anaphylaxis; Angioedema

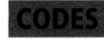 CODES

ICD9-CM
• 708 Urticaria

U

UTERINE MYOMAS

Eric L. Jenison, MD
Michael P. Hopkins, MD, MEd
Summer L. James, MD

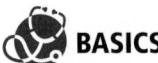 **BASICS**

DESCRIPTION
- Uterine leiomyomas are well-circumscribed, pseudo-encapsulated benign tumors composed mainly of smooth muscle but with varying amounts of fibrous connective tissue.
- 3 major types
  - Submucous: ~5% of all cases, evincing abnormal uterine bleeding and infection, and do occasionally protrude from cervix
  - Subserous: Common; may become pedunculated and rarely parasitic
  - Intramural: Common; may cause marked uterine enlargement
- System(s) Affected: Reproductive
- Synonym(s): Fibroids; Myoma; Fibromyoma; Myofibroma; Fibroleiomyoma

ALERT
Geriatric Considerations
In postmenopausal patients with newly diagnosed uterine myoma or enlarging uterine myomas, high suspicion of uterine sarcoma or other gynecologic malignancy

Pregnancy Considerations
- Pregnant women may need additional fetal testing if placenta is located over or near a fibroid.
- Complications during pregnancy include abortion, premature labor, 2nd-trimester rapid myoma growth leading to degeneration and pain, and 3rd-trimester fetal malpresentation and dystocia during labor and delivery.
- Previous myomectomy patients may develop uterine rupture during labor. Caesarean section is recommended if endometrial cavity has been entered during myomectomy.

GENERAL PREVENTION
Excessive growth may occur with estrogen stimulation (i.e., estrogen-containing birth control, HRT, and pregnancy).

EPIDEMIOLOGY
- Predominant age: 4th and 5th decades
- Predominant sex: Female only

Incidence
- Incidence increases with each decade during reproductive years and is highest in perimenopausal age group.
- Not seen in premenarchal females.

Prevalence
- 4–11% of all women
- 20% of all women ≥35 years of age
- 40% of women ≥50 years of age

RISK FACTORS
- Later reproductive and perimenopausal age groups
- 3–9 times higher among African Americans

ETIOLOGY
- May arise from totipotential cells that normally give rise to muscle and connective tissue cells
- May arise from small immature smooth muscle cell nests
- Positive correlation with estrogen stimulation (i.e., not seen before menarche), may grow rapidly during pregnancy, with use of oral estrogen, and with estrogen-producing tumors
- Myomas usually regress after pregnancy and menopause.

ASSOCIATED CONDITIONS
Endometrial carcinoma is also associated with high unopposed estrogen stimulation.

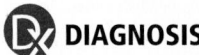 **DIAGNOSIS**

SIGNS AND SYMPTOMS
- Most affected patients: Asymptomatic disease only becomes suspected based on results of pelvic examination.
- Most common symptom is abnormal uterine bleeding. Hypermenorrhea is most common. Symptoms of secondary anemia may result.
- Pressure on bladder may result in suprapubic discomfort, urinary frequency.
- Pressure on rectosigmoid may result in low back pain.
- Edema and varicosities of the lower extremities may result from large tumors.
- Pain may result from twisted, pedunculated myomas or degenerating, hemorrhagic, or infected myomas.
- Infertility may result from submucous myomas or with distortion of uterine cavity.
- Rapid growth, particularly in perimenopausal or postmenopausal patients, may indicate sarcoma.

Physical Exam
Presumptive diagnosis by abdominal and pelvic examination: Firm, smooth nodules or masses arising from uterus. Masses are mobile without pain.

TESTS
Lab
- Pregnancy test
- CBC with differential

Imaging
- Ultrasonography shows characteristic hypoechoic appearance.
- Saline-infusion hysterosonography may help to distinguish submucosal myomas.
- Hysterosalpingogram to evaluate contour of endometrial cavity
- CT scan, MRI may help to differentiate complex cases or used when uterine artery embolization is planned.
- IV pyelogram
- Barium enema

Diagnostic Procedures/Surgery
- Fractional dilation and curettage aids in ruling out cervical or uterine carcinomas.
- Hysteroscopy may help diagnose submucous myomas.
- Laparoscopy may be useful in complex cases and to rule out other pelvic disease or disorder.

Pathological Findings
- Myomas are usually multiple and vary in size and location; have been reported up to 100 lb.
- Gross pathology reveals firm tumors with characteristic whorl-like trabeculated appearance. A thin pseudo-capsular layer is present.
- Microscopic appearance reveals bundles of smooth muscle mixed with varying amounts of connective tissue elements running in different directions.
- Cellular variant has a preponderance of muscle cells. Mitoses are rare.
- May undergo various types of degeneration
  - I. Hyaline degeneration: Very common
  - II. Calcification: Late result of circulatory impairment to myomas
  - III. Infection and suppuration: Most common with submucosal myomas
  - IV. Necrosis: Most common with pedunculated myomas secondary to torsion
  - V. Sarcomatous change: Incidence 1.0–0.1% of clinically apparent myomas

DIFFERENTIAL DIAGNOSIS
- Intrauterine pregnancy
- Ovarian tumor
- Cecal or sigmoid tumor
- Appendiceal abscess
- Diverticulitis
- Pelvic kidney
- Urachal cyst

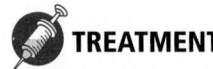 **TREATMENT**

INITIAL STABILIZATION
Outpatient usually; inpatient for some surgical procedures

GENERAL MEASURES
- Treatment must be individualized.
- Patients with minimal symptoms may be managed with iron preparations and analgesics.
- Conservative management: Asymptomatic myomas should be closely observed with pelvic examinations and ultrasonography at 3–6-month intervals, as long as size remains stable. Usually regression occurs after menopause.
- Patients that do not want surgery or pharmacologic therapy may consider uterine artery embolization (UAE).
- UAE averages 30–46% shrinkage of myomas (1); painful, may cause ovarian failure or amenorrhea

Diet
No restrictions

Activity
- After hysteroscopic or laparoscopic myomectomy, bed rest for 24 hours, no sexual intercourse for 2 weeks
- After laparotomy for myomectomy or hysterectomy, 3–5 days inpatient, followed by limited activity and no sexual intercourse for 1 month

MEDICATION (DRUGS)

Patients with minimal symptoms may be managed conservatively with iron preparations for anemia and analgesics.

First Line

- Progestins such as norethindrone, 10 mg/d, or medroxyprogesterone (Depo-Provera) 200 mg IM, once monthly, may reduce overall uterine size. (2)
  - Contraindications: History of thromboembolic events; see the manufacturer's profile
  - Adverse reactions: See the manufacturer's profile.
  - Significant interactions: See the manufacturer's profile.
- Luteinizing hormone-releasing hormone (LHRH) agonists such as nafarelin (Synarel Nasal Spray), goserelin (Zoladex Depot), and leuprolide (Lupron Depot)
  - Induce abrupt, artificial menopause and render patients asymptomatic.
  - Induce atrophy of myomas by up to 40% within 2–3 months (2)
  - May be valuable as a preoperative adjunct to myomectomy or hysterectomy by allowing recovery of anemia, donation of autologous blood, and possibly converting abdominal to vaginal hysterectomy, thereby decreasing postoperative pain, hospitalization, and morbidity (2)
  - Not recommended for use >6 months because of osteoporosis risk
  - Following discontinuation, myomas return within 60 days to pretherapy size
- Contraindications: Osteoporosis; refer to the manufacturer's profile
- Adverse reactions: Acute menopausal symptoms, decreased bone density; refer to manufacturer's profile
- Significant interactions: Refer to the manufacturer's profile.

SURGERY

- Surgical management is indicated in the following situations (2)[B]
  - Excessive uterine size or excessive rate of growth (except during pregnancy)
  - Submucosal location if associated with hypermenorrhea
  - Pedunculated myomas may undergo torsion, pain, necrosis, and hemorrhage.
  - Symptomatic from pressure on bladder or rectum
  - If differentiation from ovarian mass is not possible
  - If associated pelvic disease present (i.e., endometriosis, pelvic inflammatory disease)
  - If infertility or habitual abortion is likely due to the anatomic location of the myoma
- Surgical procedures
  - Hysteroscopic or laparoscopic cautery or laser myoma resection can be performed in selected cases.
  - Endometrial ablation for small submucosal myomas
  - Endometrial sampling should be performed prior to or in conjunction with procedure.
  - Abdominal or laparoscopic myomectomies may be performed in younger women who want to maintain fertility. (2)[B]
  - Hysterectomy, either vaginal or abdominal, is procedure of choice for symptomatic women who do not want to maintain fertility. (2)[B]
  - Preliminary pap smear and endometrial biopsy should be performed to rule out malignant or premalignant conditions. (3)[B]

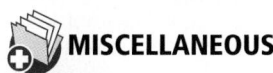 **FOLLOW-UP**

PROGNOSIS

- After abdominal myomectomy, 57% pregnancy rate in previously infertile patients (3)
- At least 10% of myomas recur after myomectomy.

COMPLICATIONS

- May mask other gynecologic malignancies (e.g., uterine sarcoma, ovarian cancer)
- Degenerating fibroid may cause pain.
  - May rarely prolapse through the cervix

PATIENT MONITORING

- Newly diagnosed uterine myoma, if symptomatic or of excessive size: Every 2–3 months with pelvic exam and ultrasonography
- Monitor hemoglobin and hematocrit levels, if uterine bleeding is excessive.
- If uterine size and symptoms are stable, monitor only every 6–12 months.

REFERENCES

1. Gupta JK, Sinha AS, Lumsden MA, Hickey M. Uterine artery embolization for symptomatic uterine fibroids. *Cochrane Database Syst Rev.* 2006;1.
2. Wallach EE, Vlahos NF. Uterine myomas: An overview of development, clinical features and management. *Obstet Gynecol.* 2004;104(2): 393–406.
3. Lefebvre G, et al. The management of uterine leiomyomas. *J Obstet Gynaecol Can.* 2003;25(5): 396–418.

 MISCELLANEOUS

CODES

ICD9-CM

218.0 Submucous leiomyoma of uterus

PATIENT TEACHING

ACOG (American College of Obstetricians and Gynecologists) pamphlet entitled "Uterine Fibroids," ACOG p–074.

See Corresponding Diagnostic Algorithm

U

UTERINE PROLAPSE

Eric L. Jenison, MD
Michael P. Hopkins, MD, MEd
Jennifer L. Savitski, MD

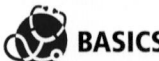 BASICS

DESCRIPTION
- Uterine prolapse occurs when the integrity of supporting structures is lost. This allows the uterus to descend into the vagina. In advanced cases, complete protrusion with inversion of the vagina occurs.
- Before menopause, the degree and severity of prolapse are usually related to the number of children and the difficulty of childbirth. After menopause, atrophy and loss of tissue integrity lead to further prolapse.
- System(s) Affected: Gastrointestinal; Renal/Urologic; Reproductive
- Synonym(s): Uterine prolapse; Genital prolapse; Genital relaxation; Uterine descensus; Total or partial procidentia; Dropped uterus

ALERT
Geriatric Considerations
This is largely a disease of aging, and incidence will be much higher as the median age of the population increases.

Pediatric Considerations
Prolapse in newborns has been reported, but it is rare and usually associated with congenital disorders and neuropathies.

GENERAL PREVENTION
- Kegel exercises will increase the strength of the pelvic diaphragm muscles and may provide some pelvic support.
- Weight loss and proper management of conditions that would increase abdominal pressure help to prevent prolapse.

EPIDEMIOLOGY
- Predominant age: Perimenopausal and postmenopausal women
- Predominant sex: Female only

Prevalence
~30–50% of women experience some degree of prolapse.

RISK FACTORS
- Childbirth, particularly multiple parity
- Advancing age
- White race
- Various connective tissue and neurogenic disorders
- Conditions resulting in increased intra-abdominal pressure (e.g., obesity, abdominal or pelvic tumors, pulmonary disease with chronic coughing, chronic constipation)
- Occupations requiring heavy lifting

Genetics
- Common among white people
- Less common among Asians and African Americans and particularly uncommon in South African Bantus and in West Africans

ETIOLOGY
- Advancing age and vaginal childbirth are the most important factors.
- Incidence of prolapse increases with frequency and difficulty of vaginal deliveries; <2% of prolapse occurs in nulliparous women.
- Although this disorder in large part results from the distention and distortion of supporting tissues with vaginal childbirth, pregnancy regardless of mode of delivery may contribute to prolapse.
- Other causes of prolapse include connective tissue disorders with lax tissue (e.g., Marfan syndrome), neurogenic disorders (e.g., multiple sclerosis), cloacal agenesis, chronic constipation, pelvic tumors or ascites, and chronic coughing resulting from chronic lung disease.
- Patients who have undergone radical vulvectomy with loss of the external supporting structures have a higher rate of prolapse.

ASSOCIATED CONDITIONS
Cystocele, rectocele, enterocele, and vaginal vault prolapse are often associated with uterine prolapse.

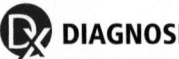 DIAGNOSIS

SIGNS AND SYMPTOMS
- Often asymptomatic
- Pelvic pressure and low back pain
- Bulging sensation in vagina or at introitus.
- Dyspareunia
- Difficulty with urination or defecation

History
- Number of pregnancies, mode of deliveries, episiotomies, extent and repair of vaginal/perineal lacerations.
- Previous pelvic surgery
- Congenital abnormalities
- Medical conditions that chronically increase intra-abdominal pressure (e.g., COPD)

Physical Exam
Diagnosis is confirmed by pelvic examination. With coughing and straining, the cervix will prolapse toward introitus or beyond. The patient may need to be examined standing as well as lying down to confirm diagnosis.

TESTS
Lab
- Evaluation of renal function to rule out ureteral obstruction
- Urinalysis to rule out urinary tract infection

Imaging
- Intravenous pyelogram to rule out ureteral obstruction in complete uterine prolapse (optional)
- Pelvic ultrasound or CT scan to rule out other pelvic pathology, if suspected (optional)

Diagnostic Procedures/Surgery
- If surgical correction is planned, urodynamic studies should be performed to evaluate for potential urinary incontinence masked by the prolapse. (1)[B]
- If ulceration or bleeding is present, Pap smears and appropriate cervical and endometrial biopsies should be done to rule out concomitant malignancies.

Pathological Findings
- Hyperkeratosis of the cervical and vaginal tissues occurs with prolapse beyond the introitus due to chronic irritation and drying. As the irritation becomes more pronounced, bleeding and ulceration occur.
- Degrees of prolapse
  - 1st-degree prolapse: To the ischial spine
  - 2nd-degree prolapse: To the introitus
  - 3rd-degree prolapse: Just beyond the introitus
  - 4th-degree prolapse: Complete uterine and vaginal inversion involving bladder and bowel

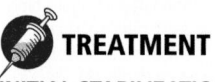 TREATMENT

INITIAL STABILIZATION
- Outpatient
- Inpatient when surgery is necessary

GENERAL MEASURES
- Treatment depends on multiple variables including the severity of prolapse, age, sexual activity, associated pelvic pathology, and desire for future fertility.
- Treatment of 1st- and 2nd-degree prolapse is expectant unless patient is symptomatic.
- Conservative therapies include estrogen replacement (see below), pessary use, and physical therapy (see below).
- Pessaries are indicated for women who are unfit for or decline surgery. Proper fitting and maintenance are required. (2)[C]
- Pessaries may also be used in the preoperative evaluation of prolapse. (2)[C]
- Surgery is indicated for women who fail conservative therapies and/or desire definitive treatment. (1)[B]

Diet
Avoid constipation.

Activity
- Heavy lifting, sexual intercourse, and other activities that increase intra-abdominal pressure should be avoided for 6–12 weeks after surgical correction.
- Maintain ideal body weight.

SPECIAL THERAPY
Physical Therapy
Biofeedback and pelvic muscle training (Kegels) may be an option for women with mild prolapse and/or those wishing conservative therapy. (2)[C]

MEDICATION (DRUGS)

- Estrogen replacement therapy (oral or vaginal cream) can increase blood supply to vaginal tissues and supporting tissue strength. This is especially important in postmenopausal women using pessaries or undergoing reconstructive pelvic surgery. (1,3)[B]
- Contraindications: Those associated with the use of estrogen. Refer to the manufacturer's literature.
- Precautions: If estrogen therapy is used and the uterus is present, progesterone should be prescribed to offset the potential for endometrial carcinoma.
- Significant possible interactions: Refer to the manufacturer's literature.

SURGERY

- Surgically able patients without additional pelvic pathology: Vaginal hysterectomy with or without enterocele, cystocele, rectocele, paravaginal repair, culdoplasty, and vaginal vault suspension depending on coexisting pelvic organ prolapse. (1)[B]
- If vault suspension is necessary in conjunction with hysterectomy, abdominal approach has decreased risk of recurrent prolapse compared to vaginal approach. (4)[A]
- Uterine suspension is an option for patients who desire to maintain reproductive function. (1)[B]
- Older women who are not sexually active can be treated with a colpocleisis or vaginal obliteration procedure.

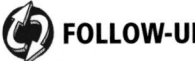 **FOLLOW-UP**

PROGNOSIS

- It is expected that the incidence and severity of prolapse will increase as patients age.
- Although surgical correction is usually successful initially, reoperation rate is ~29%. (1)

COMPLICATIONS

- Ureteral obstruction and renal failure
- Incarceration of bowel herniations
- Pessary use may not always be effective, and may cause discomfort, ulcers, and infection.

PATIENT MONITORING

- Expectant management is appropriate, with periodic follow-up examinations.
- If a pessary is placed, it should be removed, cleaned, and replaced every 3–6 months. (2)[C]

REFERENCES

1. Thakar R, Stanton S. Regular review: Management of genital prolapse. *BMJ*. 2002;324:1258–1262.
2. Trowbridge ER, Fenner DE. Conservative management of pelvic organ prolapse. *Clin Obstet Gynecol*. 2005;48(3):668–681.
3. Drutz HP, Alnaif B. Surgical management of pelvic organ prolapse and stress urinary incontinence. *Clin Obstet Gynecol*. 1998;41(3):786–793.
4. Maher C, et al. Surgical management of pelvic organ prolapse in women. *Cochrane Database Syst Rev*. 2006;1.

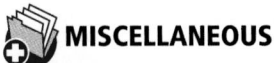 **MISCELLANEOUS**

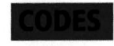 **CODES**

ICD9-CM

- 618.1 Uterine prolapse without mention of vaginal wall prolapse
- 618.4 Uterovaginal prolapse, unspecified
- 618.9 Unspecified genital prolapse

PATIENT TEACHING

- Kegel exercises when applicable
- American College of Obstetricians & Gynecologists (ACOG), 409 12th St., SW, Washington, DC 20024-2188; (800) 762-ACOG.

U

UVEITIS

Teresa A. Everson, MD
William L. Toffler, MD

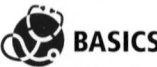 BASICS

DESCRIPTION

- Uveitis is a nonspecific term used to describe any intraocular inflammatory disorder. Symptoms vary depending on depth of involvement and associated conditions.
  - Anterior uveitis: Refers to ocular inflammation limited to the iris (iritis) alone or iris and ciliary body (iridocyclitis)
  - Intermediate uveitis: Refers to inflammation of the structures just posterior to the lens (pars planitis or peripheral uveitis)
  - Posterior uveitis: Refers to inflammation of the choroid (choroiditis), retina (retinitis), or vitreous near the optic nerve and macula
- System(s) Affected: Nervous
- Synonym(s): Iritis; Iridocyclitis; Choroiditis; Retinochoroiditis; Chorioretinitis; Anterior uveitis; Posterior uveitis; Pars planitis; Panuveitis

ALERT

Geriatric Considerations

The inflammatory response to systemic disease may be suppressed.

Pediatric Considerations

Infection should be the primary consideration. Allergies and psychologic factors (depression, stress) may serve as a triggers. Trauma is also a common cause in this population.

Pregnancy Considerations

May be of importance in the selection of medications

EPIDEMIOLOGY

- Predominant age: All ages
- Predominant sex: Male = Female (except for HLA-B27 anterior uveitis: Male > Female [2.5:1])

Incidence

Anterior uveitis most common (8.2 cases/100,000 annual incidence)

Prevalence

Iritis is 4 × more prevalent than posterior uveitis.

RISK FACTORS

No specific risk factors. Higher incidence seen with specific associated conditions

Genetics

- No specific pattern for uveitis in general
- Iritis: Of patients, 50–70% are HLA-B27 positive.

ETIOLOGY

- Infectious: May result from viral, bacterial, parasitic, or fungal etiologies
- Suspected immune-mediated: Possible autoimmune or immune-complex–mediated mechanism postulated in association with systemic (especially rheumatologic) disorders
- Isolated eye disease
- Idiopathic (~25%)
- Masquerade syndromes: Diseases such as malignancies that may be mistaken for primary inflammation of the eye

ASSOCIATED CONDITIONS

- Viral infections: HIV, herpes simplex, herpes zoster, cytomegalovirus
- Bacterial infections: Tuberculosis, leprosy, propionibacterium infection, syphilis, leptospirosis, brucellosis, Lyme disease, Whipple disease
- Parasitic infections: Toxoplasmosis, acanthamebiasis, toxocariasis, cysticercosis, onchocerciasis
- Fungal infections: Histoplasmosis, coccidioidomycosis, candidiasis, aspergillosis, sporotrichosis, blastomycosis, cryptococcosis
- Suspected immune-mediated: Ankylosing spondylitis, Behçet disease, Crohn disease, drug or hypersensitivity reaction, interstitial nephritis, juvenile rheumatoid arthritis, Kawasaki disease, multiple sclerosis, psoriatic arthritis, Reiter syndrome, relapsing polychondritis, sarcoidosis, Sjögren syndrome, systemic lupus erythematosus, ulcerative colitis, vasculitis, vitiligo, Vogt-Koyanagi (Harada) syndrome
- Isolated eye disease: Acute multifocal placoid pigmentary epitheliopathy, acute retinal necrosis, bird-shot choroidopathy, Fuch heterochromatic cyclitis, glaucomatocyclitic crisis, lens-induced uveitis, multifocal choroiditis, pars planitis, serpiginous choroiditis, sympathetic ophthalmia, trauma
- Masquerade syndromes: Leukemia, lymphoma, retinitis pigmentosa, retinoblastoma

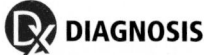 DIAGNOSIS

SIGNS AND SYMPTOMS

- Anterior uveitis (~80% of patients with uveitis)
  - Decreased visual acuity
  - Generally acute in onset
  - Deep eye pain
  - Photophobia (consensual)
  - Conjunctival vessel dilation
  - Perilimbal (circumcorneal) dilation of episcleral and scleral vessels (ciliary flush)
  - Small pupillary size of affected eye
  - Hypopyon or hyphema (white or red blood cells pooled in the anterior chamber)
  - Frequently unilateral (95% of HLA-B27-associated cases)
  - Bilateral involvement and systemic symptoms (fever, fatigue, abdominal pain) may be associated with interstitial nephritis.
  - Systemic disease is most likely to be associated with anterior uveitis (in 1 study, 53% of patients found to have systemic disease).
- Intermediate and posterior uveitis
  - Decreased visual acuity
  - Unresolving floaters
  - Generally insidious in onset
  - More commonly bilateral
  - Posterior inflammation will generally cause minimal pain or redness unless associated with an iritis.

Physical Exam

Slit-lamp examination and indirect ophthalmoscopy are necessary for precise diagnosis.

TESTS

Lab

- No specific test for the diagnosis of uveitis. Tests for etiologic factors or associated conditions should be based on history and physical examination.
- CBC, BUN, creatinine (interstitial nephritis)
- HLA-B27 typing (ankylosing spondylitis, Reiter syndrome)
- Antinuclear antibody, ESR (systemic lupus erythematosus, Sjögren syndrome)
- Venereal Disease Research Lab test, fluorescent titer antibody (syphilis)
- Purified protein derivative (PPD) tuberculin skin test (tuberculosis)
- Lyme serology (Lyme disease)
- Special tests
- Disorders that may alter lab results: Immune deficiency

Imaging

- Chest x-ray (sarcoidosis, histoplasmosis, tuberculosis, lymphoma)
- Sacroiliac x-ray (ankylosing spondylitis)

Diagnostic Procedures/Surgery

Slit-lamp examination

Pathological Findings

Keratic precipitates, inflammatory cells in anterior chamber or vitreous, synechiae (fibrous tissue scarring between iris and lens), macular edema, perivasculitis of retinal vessels

DIFFERENTIAL DIAGNOSIS

- Conjunctivitis
- Episcleritis
- Scleritis
- Keratitis
- Acute angle-closure glaucoma

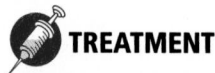 TREATMENT

GENERAL MEASURES

- Appropriate health care: Outpatient with urgent ophthalmologic consultation
- Medical therapy best initiated following full ophthalmologic evaluation
- Treatment of underlying cause, if identified
- Cycloplegia
- Anti-inflammatory therapy

Diet

No special diet

Activity

Full activity

MEDICATION (DRUGS)

First Line

- Caution should be used when using empiric treatment; referral to an ophthalmologist is recommended in most cases.
- Homatropine hydrobromide (Isopto) 2% ophthalmic solution: 2 drops to the affected eye b.i.d., or as often as q3h if necessary; *plus*
- Prednisolone acetate 1% ophthalmic suspension: 2 drops to the affected eye q1h initially, tapering to once a day with improvement
- Contraindications
  - Hypersensitivity to the medication or component of the preparation
  - Cycloplegia is contraindicated in patients known to have, or be predisposed to, glaucoma.
  - Topical corticosteroid therapy is contraindicated in uveitis secondary to infectious etiologies.
- Precautions
  - Homatropine hydrobromide may produce adverse systemic antimuscarinic effects. Use extreme caution in infants and young children because of increased susceptibility to systemic effects.
  - Topical corticosteroids may increase intraocular pressure. Prolonged use may cause cataract formation and exacerbate existing herpetic keratitis which may masquerade as iritis.
- Significant possible interactions
  - Refer to manufacturer's profile for each drug.

Second Line

- Cycloplegia: Scopolamine hydrobromide 0.25% (Isopto Hyoscine) up to t.i.d. or cyclopentolate hydrochloride 1% (Cyclogyl)
- Anti-inflammatory: Prednisolone sodium phosphate 1% (Ocu-Pred Forte), dexamethasone sodium phosphate 0.1% (Ocu-Dex), and dexamethasone suspension
- Systemic NSAIDs may provide some benefit.

 ## FOLLOW-UP

PROGNOSIS

- Dependent on the presence of causal diseases, or associated conditions
- Uveitis resulting from infections (systemic or local) tend to resolve with eradication of the underlying infection.
- Uveitis associated with seronegative arthropathies tend to be acute (lasting <3 months) and frequently recurrent.

COMPLICATIONS

Loss of vision as a result of the following

- Keratic precipitate deposition on the corneal or lens surfaces
- Increased intraocular pressure, acute angle-closure glaucoma
- Formation of synechiae
- Cataract formation
- Vasculitis with vascular occlusion, retinal infarction
- Macular edema
- Optic nerve damage

PATIENT MONITORING

- Ophthalmologic follow-up as recommended by consultant
- Schedule for complete history and physical to evaluate for associated systemic disease.

REFERENCES

1. McCluskey PJ, Towler HM, Lightman S. Management of chronic uveitis. *BMJ.* 2000;320(7234):555–558.
2. Schiffman RM, Jacobsen G, Whitcup SM. Visual functioning and general health status in patients with uveitis. *Arch Ophthalmol.* 2001;119(6):841–849.
3. Smith JR, Rosenbaum JT. Management of uveitis: A rheumatologic perspective. *Arthritis Rheum.* 2002;46(2):309–318.
4. Patel H, Goldstein D. Pediatric uveitis. *Pediatr Clin North Am.* 2003;50(1):125–136.
5. Lee AG, Beaver HA. Painful ophthalmologic disorders and eye pain for the neurologist. *Neurol Clin.* 2004;22(1):75–97.

 ## MISCELLANEOUS

- See also: Conjunctivitis, acute; Glaucoma, primary angle-closure; Scleritis
- Other notes
  - Synonyms are anatomic descriptions of the focus of the uveal inflammation.
  - Severe or unresponsive uveitis may require therapy including periocular injection of corticosteroids, systemic corticosteroids, cytotoxic agents (azathioprine, cyclophosphamide, chlorambucil, and methotrexate), immunosuppressive agents (cyclosporine), immunomodulatory agents (sulfasalazine), or tumor necrosis factor inhibitors (infliximab, etanercept).

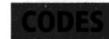 **CODES**

ICD9-CM

364.3 Unspecified iridocyclitis

PATIENT TEACHING

- Instructions on proper method for instilling eye drops
- Wear dark glasses if photophobia a problem
- Medication side effects to watch for and report

 See Corresponding Diagnostic Algorithm

U

VAGINAL ADENOSIS

Michael P. Hopkins, MD, MEd
Jennifer Savitski, MD
Eric L. Jenison, MD

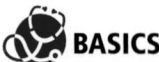 **BASICS**

DESCRIPTION

- Adenosis is a term used to describe nonepithelialized columnar glandular epithelium in the vagina. At ~15th week of embryological development, the Müllerian system, which forms the upper 2/3 of the vagina, fuses with the invaginating cloaca, which forms the lower vagina. Squamous metaplasia from the cloacal region then produces a squamous epithelium through the vagina. Adenosis occurs when this squamous epithelium fails to completely epithelialize the vagina.
- System(s) Affected: Reproductive

ALERT
Geriatric Considerations
- Adenosis is a disorder of the young female. By the time of menopause the vagina and cervix should be completely epithelialized.
- The presence of glandular epithelium in the postmenopausal patient is an indication for excision and close evaluation for the possibility of a well-differentiated adenocarcinoma.

Pregnancy Considerations
Pregnancy produces a wide eversion of the transformation zone of the cervix. This will occasionally become so widely everted that it will extend onto the vaginal fornices, leading to the impression of adenosis. This will resolve after the pregnancy is completed.

EPIDEMIOLOGY
- Predominant age
  - Teenage years: Epithelialization occurs from puberty to 20 years of age.
  - By age 30 years, it is extremely rare for adenosis to be present.
- Predominant sex: Female only

Prevalence
In the US: Adenosis is relatively common, affecting 10–20% of young females studied. As maturation progresses with puberty, epithelialization occurs. (3)

RISK FACTORS
Diethylstilbestrol (DES)-exposed females

Genetics
Unknown

ETIOLOGY
- In the vast majority of young females, the etiology is incomplete squamous metaplasia. This occurs as a natural phenomenon and resolves with age.
- In DES-exposed females, the incidence of adenosis is higher and the etiology presumably is from the effect of the DES on the developing embryologic system.

ASSOCIATED CONDITIONS
DES exposure

- Adenosis from DES exposure should lead to an evaluation of other DES-related abnormalities.
- The greatest risk to the patient is from Müllerian tract anomalies. These include cervical abnormalities with cervical hood, ridges, shortened cervix, and incompetent cervix, T-shaped uterine cavity.
- Patients with known DES exposure should have the reproductive tract evaluated prior to conception.
- The vast majority of patients with adenosis have not been DES exposed and do not require evaluation of the reproductive system.
- DES was last used to prevent spontaneous abortion in ~1970. This is a problem of decreasing importance.

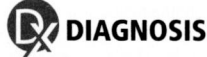 **DIAGNOSIS**

SIGNS AND SYMPTOMS
A clear, watery vaginal discharge, which is the glandular epithelium producing a small amount of mucus

TESTS
Diagnostic Procedures/Surgery
- 4-quadrant Pap smear should be utilized liberally, to isolate quadrants of the vagina which may contain abnormalities. This can be followed by colposcopy and biopsy.
- Colposcopy should be used to outline areas of adenosis and ensure that no malignancy is present.

Pathological Findings
Biopsy will show benign glandular epithelium, which has not yet undergone squamous metaplasia. Biopsies in the areas of ongoing squamous metaplasia will be typical for this process.

DIFFERENTIAL DIAGNOSIS
A thorough evaluation for adenocarcinoma of the vagina arising in adenosis should be done. A biopsy may be necessary to ensure that the process represents only benign adenosis. Colposcopy of the upper vagina aids in choosing the areas for biopsy. On visual inspection, adenosis appears as a fine, raised, reddened, granular-type tissue.

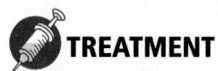 **TREATMENT**

INITIAL STABILIZATION
Outpatient

GENERAL MEASURES
- Unless malignancy is present, conservative treatment is indicated.
- In the vast majority of young females with this condition, it will resolve with expectant management.

Diet
No special diet

Activity
- No limitations
- It is not necessary to avoid intercourse or placing objects in the vagina.

SURGERY
Aggressive therapy such as laser or surgical excision is necessary only if premalignant or malignant changes arise. (1)[C]

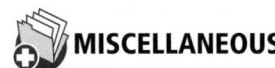
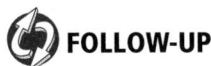 **FOLLOW-UP**

Yearly after a negative initial evaluation

PROGNOSIS

- It is expected that the vast majority of patients will have squamous metaplasia with complete resolution of the adenosis.
- The rare patient, 1:1,000–1:10,000, may develop adenocarcinoma in the adenosis and will require definitive therapy as for vaginal cancer.

COMPLICATIONS

Infertility, miscarriage, dysplasia, cancer

PATIENT MONITORING

- Initial evaluation consists of four-quadrant vaginal Pap smear, cervical Pap smear, and colposcopy of the upper vagina and cervix.
- If the initial colposcopy is normal, a yearly 4-quadrant Pap smear of the vagina and Pap smear of the cervix are all that is necessary.

REFERENCES

1. Chattopadhyay I, Cruickshank DJ, Packer M. Non diethylstilbesterol induced vaginal adenosis—A case series and review of literature. *Eur J Gynaecol Oncol*. 2001;22(4):260–262.
2. Herbst A. Behavior of estrogen-associated female genital tract cancer and its relation to neoplasia following intrauterine exposure to diethylstilbesterol (DES). *Gynecol Oncol*. 2000;76: 147–156.
3. Sandberg EC. The incidence and distribution of occult vaginal adenosis. *Am J Obstet Gynecol*. 1968;101:322–334.

 MISCELLANEOUS

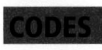

ICD9-CM
752.49 Other congenital anomalies of cervix, vagina, and external female genitalia

PATIENT TEACHING

- The patient should be educated to keep annual pelvic and Pap smear appointments. In the vast majority of situations this is benign, and expectant management is all that is necessary.
- American College of Obstetricians & Gynecologists (ACOG), 409 12th St., SW, Washington, DC 20024-2188; (800) 762-ACOG

 See Corresponding Diagnostic Algorithm

See Patient Handout on CD

V

VAGINAL BLEEDING DURING PREGNANCY

Kimberle Vore, MD

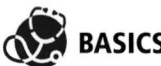 BASICS

DESCRIPTION
- Vaginal bleeding during pregnancy has many causes and ranges in severity from mild (with normal pregnancy outcome) to life threatening for both infant and mother.
- Bleeding can vary from scant to excessive, from brown to bright red, and can be painless or painful.
- Causes can be divided into vaginal, cervical, and uterine factors. The differential diagnosis is guided by the gestational age of the pregnancy.
- System(s) Affected: Cardiovascular; Reproductive

ALERT
Pregnancy Considerations
A complication of pregnancy

EPIDEMIOLOGY
- Predominant age: Childbearing
- Predominant sex: Female only

Prevalence
In the US: Common

RISK FACTORS
- Cervical or vaginal infections
  - Multiple sexual partners
  - Previous history of sexually transmitted disease or pelvic inflammatory disease
- Cervical dysplasia: Previous history of abnormal pap
- Placenta previa
  - Previous history of previa
  - Previous caesarean section
  - History of uterine surgery including dilation and curettage (D&C)
- Placental abruption
  - Previous history of abruption (increases risk by 10%)
  - Hypertension
  - Preeclampsia
  - Multiple gestation
  - Smoking
  - Cocaine use

Genetics
No known genetic pattern

ETIOLOGY
- Vaginal or cervical causes can occur throughout the pregnancy, and usually are no threat to the pregnancy. They include
  - Vaginal infection or trauma
  - Cervicitis (infections or noninfections)
  - Cervical polyp
  - Cervical neoplasia
  - Hyperemia of cervix (increased blood flow from pregnancy)
  - Postcoital bleeding: Usually cervical source
- Bleeding from above the cervix is a concern because it can be life threatening to mother and/or fetus. In determining the cause it is helpful to separate first-trimester bleeding from later-pregnancy bleeding.
  - 1st-trimester bleeding causes include Implantation bleeding—benign; ectopic pregnancy; threatened or spontaneous abortion; molar pregnancy; subchorionic bleed

  - 2nd- or 3rd-trimester bleeding causes include: Placenta previa (nonpainful); placenta abruption (painful, contraction usually present); subchorionic bleed
- Many times the cause is unknown. For up to 50% of 1st-trimester bleeding, no cause is ever found.

ASSOCIATED CONDITIONS
Depends on cause of vaginal bleeding

 DIAGNOSIS

SIGNS AND SYMPTOMS
- Bleeding can vary from scant to excessive.
- Color of blood varies from brown to bright red.
- May be painless or painful
- Patient reports bleeding from vagina.

TESTS
Lab
- Blood work based on dating of pregnancy, previous tests, and need for further diagnosis
- Blood type and screen. If not known already, needs to be done on all women
- Rh-negative patients who bleed during pregnancy will need Rho(d) immune globulin (RhoGAM), to prevent mother from becoming sensitized if exposed to infant's Rh-positive blood. In 3rd-trimester bleeding, the mother may lose significant amounts of blood and require transfusion.
- Quantitative-β-human chorionic gonadotropin (Q hCG) can be used in early pregnancy when ultrasound is not able to diagnose cause. Ultrasound should be able to see an intrauterine pregnancy (IUP) when Q hCG >2,000.
- Levels can be followed serially every 2 days. Levels fall in spontaneous abortion, are extremely high in molar pregnancy, and rise gradually in ectopic or intrauterine pregnancy. This level usually doubles in 48 hours in normal pregnancy, and failure to increase by 50% is concerning for ectopic
- Once Q hCG level is >2,000, an ultrasound should be performed to confirm diagnosis. When spontaneous abortion is suspected but there is no definitive diagnosis by either ultrasound or pathology confirmation of products of conception, then following Q hCG weekly until level is <25 is advised to exclude possible undiagnosed ectopic pregnancy. If dropping levels start to rise, reconsider ectopic pregnancy. In molar pregnancy, after surgical evacuation of productions of conception, monthly Q hCG are followed for 1 year to rule out the possibility of choriocarcinoma. During this time the patient should be instructed not to get pregnant.
- Other labs are based on severity of bleeding:
  - CBC: May be done to assess severity, when bleeding profuse
  - Bleeding time, fibrinogen, fibrin split products: Rarely necessary. Disseminated intravascular coagulation (DIC) reported rarely in missed abortion.

Imaging
- Ultrasound (USN) is the diagnostic test of choice. A gestational sac can be seen at 5–6 weeks, fetal heart tone can be observed by 8–9 weeks. USN is diagnostic of molar pregnancy with 98% accuracy. In later pregnancy USN locates the placenta and may show degree of placental separation in abruption.
- Serial ultrasound may be required in early pregnancy.

Diagnostic Procedures/Surgery
- It is important to evaluate whether bleeding is coming from genital tract or from other nearby structures.
- Association of bleeding with other activities or symptoms may aid in the diagnosis (e.g., following bowel movement, after intercourse, associated with abdominal cramping).
- In 1st-trimester bleeding: Pelvic exam is performed to confirm bleeding from cervical os, and if any adnexal masses. If pregnancy is >8 weeks, USN should be done to confirm IUP. If no IUP and USN not confirmatory for ectopic, then serial Q hCG are followed. If pelvic pain and concern for ectopic pregnancy is high but not confirmed by USN, a laparoscopy or laparotomy may be performed to make a diagnosis.
- In 2nd- or 3rd-trimester bleeding: Locate placenta by ultrasound prior to pelvic exam. If placenta previa, do not perform bimanual or speculum exam unless set up for immediate caesarean delivery.

Pathological Findings
Dependent on cause

DIFFERENTIAL DIAGNOSIS
- Hematuria from urinary tract infection (UTI), kidney stones
- Bleeding hemorrhoids
- Rectal bleeding from lower gastrointestinal bleed: Extremely rare in pregnancy

 TREATMENT

GENERAL MEASURES
- Appropriate health care
  - In 1st-trimester bleeding, most, patients can be managed as outpatients.
  - In late-pregnancy bleeding, most patients need inpatient monitoring.
- In late-pregnancy bleeding, the amount of bleeding and presence of maternal or fetal compromise indicates whether emergent caesarean section is performed or whether conservative measures are appropriate until greater fetal lung maturity can be obtained.
- Threatened abortion: Bed rest and nothing in the vagina. If bleeding is severe, hospitalization and close observation. Type and screen for possible transfusion.

Diet
No restrictions

Activity
Bed rest: no coitus, no douching

MEDICATION (DRUGS)

First Line
Rho(d) immune globulin (Rhogam) if mother Rh-negative and significant bleeding from uterus

Second Line
Tocolytics in suspected premature labor

SURGERY
- If ectopic or molar pregnancy is diagnosed, immediate surgical treatment may be needed in some cases.
- Some early ectopic pregnancies can be treated medically if certain criteria are met.
- Inevitable or incomplete abortion: D&C (usually suction).
- If completeness of abortion is in doubt, then D&C and removal of retained products
- Caesarean section for placenta previa or placental abruption

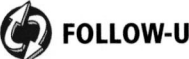 **FOLLOW-UP**

PROGNOSIS
- Depends on the cause of vaginal bleeding, the severity of bleeding, and the rapidity of diagnosis. Maternal mortality is 31.9 per 100,000 of ectopic pregnancies. (4)
- If fetal heart tones present in first trimester bleed, <10% chance of pregnancy loss

COMPLICATIONS
- Anemia
- Shock
- Fetal or maternal death
- Infection
- Choriocarcinoma or invasive mole in the case of hydatidiform mole
- Premature delivery of infant with associated complications
- Coagulopathy (extremely rare)

PATIENT MONITORING
Daily to weekly, depending on diagnosis and severity of bleeding

REFERENCES
1. American College of Emergency Physicians. Clinical policy for the initial approach to patients presenting with a chief complaint of vaginal bleeding. *Ann Emerg Med*. 1997;29(3):435–458.
2. Suspected ectopic pregnancy. *Obstet Gynecol*. 2006;107:399–413.
3. Signore CC. Second trimester vaginal bleeding: Correllation of ultrasonographic findings with perinatal outcome. *Am J Obstet Gynecol*. 1998;179(2):336–340.
4. Estimation of pregnancy-related mortality risk by pregnancy outcome, United States, 1991 to 1999. *Am J Obstet Gynecol*. 2006;194:92–94.

 MISCELLANEOUS

See also: Abnormal Pap Smear; Abortion, Spontaneous; Abruptio Placentae; Cervical Dysplasia; Cervical Malignancy; Cervical Polyps; Cervicitis; Cervicitis, Ectropion and True Erosion; Chlamydial Sexually Transmitted Diseases; Ectopic Pregnancy; Placenta Previa; Preterm Labor; Trichomoniasis; Vaginal Malignancy; Vulvovaginitis, Bacterial; Vulvovaginitis, Candidal

CODES

ICD9-CM
- 630 Hydatidiform mole
- 633.90 Unspecified ectopic pregnancy without intrauterine pregnancy
- 634.90 Spontaneous abortion without mention of complication, unspecified
- 641.10 Hemorrhage from placenta previa, unspecified
- 641.20 Premature separation of placenta, unspecified

PATIENT TEACHING
- Patient should be instructed to report any increase in the amount and frequency of bleeding and should seek immediate care if experiencing abdominal pain or sudden increased bleeding. She should bring for examination any tissue passed vaginally.
- Grief counseling is appropriate if pregnancy loss is inevitable.
- American College of Obstetricians & Gynecologists (ACOG), 409 12th St., SW, Washington, DC 20024-2188; (800) 762-ACOG

 See Corresponding Diagnostic Algorithm

 See Patient Handout on CD

V

VAGINAL MALIGNANCY

Michael P. Hopkins, MD, MEd
Ahntuan T. Huynh, DO
Eric L. Jenison, MD

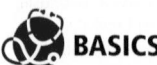 **BASICS**

DESCRIPTION
- Vaginal intraepithelial neoplasia (carcinoma in situ): A premalignant phase with full-thickness neoplastic changes in the superficial epithelium. However, there is no invasion through the basement membrane.
- Invasive malignancies: Vaginal malignancies are squamous cell in 90% of patients; the remaining 10% are adenocarcinomas, sarcomas, and melanomas. The clear-cell carcinoma is a subtype of adenocarcinoma.
- To be classified as a vaginal malignancy, only the vagina can be involved. If the cervix or the vulva is involved, then the tumor is classified as a primary cancer arising from the cervix or the vulva.
- System(s) Affected: Reproductive
- Synonym(s): Bowen disease; Vaginal intraepithelial neoplasia (VAIN)

ALERT
Geriatric Considerations
Older patients, many with a long history of smoking, are at a higher risk for malignancies requiring surgical treatments.

Pediatric Considerations
Childhood sarcomas can be treated in a conservative fashion with multimodality therapy. This avoids the loss of the young child's bladder and/or rectum.

Pregnancy Considerations
This malignancy is not associated with pregnancy.

EPIDEMIOLOGY
Incidence
- Predominant age
  - Carcinoma in situ: Mid-40s–60s
  - Invasive squamous cell malignancy: Mid-60s–70s
  - Adenocarcinoma: Any age range, 50s is mean age
  - Mixed Müllerian sarcomas and leiomyosarcomas in the adult population: Mean age 60 years
  - Sarcoma botryoides and embryonal sarcomas: Occur in the pediatric population
- Predominant sex: Female only

Prevalence
In the US: This is 1 of the rarest of all gynecologic malignancies.

RISK FACTORS
- History of squamous cell cancer of the cervix or vulva
- Smoking
- Multiple sex partners
- Age
- Vaginal adenosis
- HPV infection
- Daughters of mothers who took diethylstilbestrol (DES)

Genetics
No known genetic pattern

ETIOLOGY
- Women with a history of cervical malignancy have a higher probability of developing squamous cell malignancy in the vagina after hysterectomy.
- The human papilloma virus (HPV) has been associated with vulvovaginal, cervical, adenocarcinoma, and squamous cell carcinoma.
- Smokers have a higher incidence.
- Clear-cell adenocarcinoma of the vagina in young women has been associated with DES exposure. The incidence, however, is exceedingly rare, estimated at 1:1,000–1:10,000 DES-exposed females.
- Metastatic lesions can involve the vagina from the other gynecologic organs.
- Renal cell carcinoma and breast cancer can metastasize to the vagina (rarely).

ASSOCIATED CONDITIONS
Due to the field effect, patients with vaginal cancer are more likely to develop malignancy in the cervix or vulva and should be followed closely.

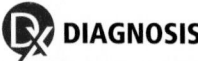 **DIAGNOSIS**

SIGNS AND SYMPTOMS
- Abnormal bleeding is the most common symptom. This results from a fungating tumor present in the vagina.
- Dyspareunia
- Postcoital bleeding can result from direct trauma to the tumor.
- Pain along with symptoms and signs of hydroureter are late findings when the tumor has spread into the paravaginal tissues and extends to the pelvic side wall.
- In the pediatric population, sarcomas can present either as a mass protruding from the vagina or as abnormal genital bleeding.

TESTS
Lab
Cytology will usually be positive when an obvious lesion is present.

Imaging
- Chest x-ray: Lung metastases are a late finding.
- Intravenous pyelogram (IVP): To evaluate for ureteral obstruction
- CAT scan to evaluate the retroperitoneum and especially the lymph nodes in the pelvic and periaortic area
- Lymphangiography is also useful for evaluation of the lymph node status.
- Barium enema to rule out rectal invasion

Diagnostic Procedures/Surgery
- Colposcopy with directed biopsies for small lesions
- Wide excision under anesthesia of superficial disease may be necessary to ensure that invasive cancer is not present.
- Cystoscopy to rule out bladder invasion
- Sigmoidoscopy to rule out rectal invasion

Pathological Findings
- Stage 0: Carcinoma in situ
- Stage I: Infiltrative tumor not involving the paravaginal tissues
- Stage II: Paravaginal extension but not to the side wall
- Stage III: Paravaginal extension to the side wall
- Stage IVA: Tumor involving the bladder or the rectum
- Stage IVB: Distant metastatic disease

DIFFERENTIAL DIAGNOSIS
- VAIN involves premalignant changes that do not infiltrate beyond the basement membrane.
- Adequate biopsies ensure that invasive lesions are not overlooked. Invasive lesions penetrate the basement membrane and cannot be treated conservatively. Other malignancies such as endometrial, cervix, bladder, or colon cancer can invade directly into the vagina or metastasize to the vagina.
- In the childbearing ages, trophoblastic disease should be considered. The vagina is a common site of metastases. Biopsy will usually provide a clue to the primary site.

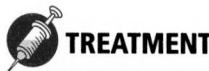 **TREATMENT**

GENERAL MEASURES
- Appropriate health care: Outpatient or inpatient, depending on treatment
- Carcinoma in situ can be treated by a variety of methods: Laser vaporization under microscopic guidance; fluorouracil (Efudex) intravaginal cream; partial vaginectomy
- In all tumor types, metastatic disease from the vagina to other sites is only minimally responsive to chemotherapy.

Diet
Unrestricted unless undergoing radiation

Activity
- Patients are usually ambulatory and able to resume full activity by 6 weeks after surgery.
- Most patients are fully active while receiving radiation therapy.

SPECIAL THERAPY
Radiotherapy
- Treatment with radiotherapy is dependent on the stage of disease. This treatment option should be discussed with physicians experienced with this malignancy. (1,2)[C]

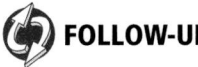

MEDICATION (DRUGS)

First Line

- With 1 exception, there are no chemotherapeutic agents to which this tumor is responsive. The exception is the childhood sarcomas, which have been treated with combinations of
  – Vincristine
  – Dactinomycin (actinomycin-D)
  – Cyclophosphamide (Cytoxan)
  – Cisplatin
  – Etoposide (VP-16)
- Patients with advanced cervical cancer receive concurrent irradiation and cisplatin-based chemotherapy. This may become a treatment option for advanced carcinoma of the vagina. (2)[C]
- Adjuvant chemotherapy has no proven benefit in squamous cell or adenocarcinoma of the vagina.
- Intraepithelial neoplasia of the vagina can be treated with topical chemotherapy (5-fluorouracil cream). (1,3)[C]
- Contraindications
  – The diagnosis must be established with certainty prior to treatment.
  – If there is any doubt that a process beyond in situ disease exists, vaginectomy must be performed. Because these patients are often elderly, aggressive therapy is limited by the patient's performance status and ability to tolerate radical surgery, chemotherapy, or radiation.
- Precautions: Refer to the manufacturer's literature.
- Significant possible interactions: Refer to the manufacturer's literature.

Second Line

Ondansetron (Zofran), dronabinol (Marinol), metoclopramide (Reglan), and others for nausea control

SURGERY

- Whenever there is a doubt as to the presence or absence of invasive disease, vaginectomy must be performed.
- Invasive lesions are usually treated by radiation therapy, but stage I lesions can be treated with radical hysterectomy, radical vaginectomy with pelvic lymph node dissection. (1)[C]
- If the lesion involves the lower vagina, inguinal node dissection must also be done, as cancer involving the lower vagina can metastasize to the groin region.
- Premenopausal women, who desire to retain ovarian function, are better candidates for radical surgery for early-stage disease.
- Younger patients, who have not completed their family, can occasionally be treated with limited resection and localized radiation to the area.
- Sarcomas are treated by radiation therapy followed by pelvic exenteration if persistent disease is present.
- Childhood sarcomas are treated with chemotherapy followed by local resection. Childhood sarcomas are responsive to multiagent combination chemotherapies.

FOLLOW-UP

PROGNOSIS

Stage and 5-year survival
- I: 60%
- II: 40%
- III: 20%
- IVA: 5%
- IVB: 0%

COMPLICATIONS

Those associated with major abdominal surgery or radiation therapy

PATIENT MONITORING

- Pelvic examination and Pap smear every 3 months for 2 years and then every 6 months for subsequent 3 years
- Chest x-ray once a year

REFERENCES

1. Creasman WT. Vaginal cancers. *Curr Opin Obstet Gynecol*. 2005;17:71–76.
2. Grigsby PW. Vaginal cancer. *Curr Treat Options Oncol*. 2002;3:125–130.
3. Cardosi RJ, Bomalaski JJ, Hoffman MS. Diagnosis and management of vulvar and vaginal intraepithelial neoplasia. *Obstet Gynecol Clin North Am*. 2001;28:685–702.
4. Yalcin OT, et al. Vaginal intraepithelial neoplasia: Treatment by carbon dioxide laser and risk factors for failure. *Eur J Obstet Gynecol Reprod Biol*. 2003;106:64–68.

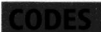

MISCELLANEOUS

This is an uncommon malignancy, and patients should be treated by a physician familiar and experienced with this malignancy.

CODES

ICD9-CM

184.0 Malignant neoplasm of vagina

PATIENT TEACHING

- Printed patient information available from: American College of Obstetricians & Gynecologists, 409 12th St., SW, Washington, DC 20024-2188; (800) 762-ACOG
- American Cancer Society, www.cancer.org

 See Corresponding Diagnostic Algorithm

 See Patient Handout on CD

V

VAGINISMUS

Leena Nathan, MD
Wendy Satmary, MD, FACOG

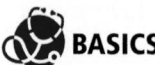 **BASICS**

DESCRIPTION

- Involuntary painful contraction of perineal muscles and levator ani prior to or during vaginal intercourse. The experience of or even the anticipation of pain on vaginal entry causes these muscles to contract, occluding the vaginal opening and causing further pain when penetration is attempted. Repeated dyspareunia (pain with intercourse) can cause vaginismus and vaginismus can cause dyspareunia.
- System(s) Affected: Reproductive

ALERT
Pregnancy Considerations
Pregnancy can occur in patients with vaginismus, via perineal ejaculation.

EPIDEMIOLOGY
Predominant age
- Postpubertal

Prevalence
In the US: 5.1–17% in females presenting to sexual dysfunction clinics. No incidence or prevalence data available for occurrence in general population.

RISK FACTORS
- Previous sexual trauma, but rates appear to be similar in abused and nonabused women
- Often associated with other sexual dysfunctions

ETIOLOGY
- Primary: Often multifactorial
  - Negative messages about sex and sexual relations in upbringing may cause phobic reaction
  - Poor body image of genital area
  - History of sexual trauma, although rates of vaginismus appear to be similar in sexually abused and nonabused populations of women (studies show incidence of sexual abuse of women to be 12–40%)
- Secondary
  - New onset of infection
  - Surgical or postdelivery scarring
  - Endometriosis
  - Inadequate vaginal lubrication
- Can be complete (perineal spasm with attempts to insert anything into vagina) or situational (tampons or pelvic exams permitted)

ASSOCIATED CONDITIONS
- Marital stress, family dysfunction
- Dyspareunia

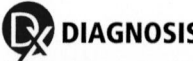 **DIAGNOSIS**

SIGNS AND SYMPTOMS
- Inability to allow entry for vaginal sexual intercourse secondary to involuntary muscle spasms
- Reluctance or avoidance of pelvic examination
- Relationship discord or difficulty
- Infertility
- Sexual satisfaction may be independent of sexual function.

History
General and sexual history

Physical Exam
- At some point, a careful pelvic examination to rule out medical cause
- Lamont classification of degree
  - 1st degree: Perineal and levator spasm relieved with reassurance
  - 2nd degree: Perineal spasm maintained throughout the pelvic exam
  - 3rd degree: Levator spasm and elevation of buttocks
  - 4th degree: Levator and perineal spasm and elevation with adduction and retreat

TESTS
Psychiatric consultation if not responsive to primary physician's therapy or if primary provider not comfortable with caring for sexual problems

Pathological Findings
Rarely found in primary vaginismus, but may be varied, such as endometriosis or scarring, in secondary vaginismus

DIFFERENTIAL DIAGNOSIS
Dyspareunia

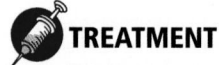 **TREATMENT**

GENERAL MEASURES
- Outpatient care
- Can often treat vaginismus successfully without defining/treating its etiologies
- No published controlled studies on success of psychotherapy for vaginismus
- Patient education as noted on pelvic anatomy and sexual function
- Sexual cognitive behavioral therapy has been found to be very effective
- Kegel exercises to control perineal muscles
- Stepwise vaginal desensitization exercises
  - With vaginal dilators (patient inserts/controls)
  - With woman's own finger(s) (promotes sexual self-awareness)
- Valsalva can help with vaginal entry
- Advance to husband's fingers with patient's control
- Coitus after achieving largest vaginal dilator or 3 fingers; important to begin with sensate-focused exercises/sensual caressing without necessarily a demand for coitus
  - Female superior at 1st; passive (nonthrusting); female directed
  - Later, thrusting may be allowed

Diet
No special diet

Activity
Simple techniques of gentle, progressive, patient-controlled vaginal dilation

SPECIAL THERAPY
Complementary and Alternative Medicine
- Biofeedback
- Functional electrical stimulation

MEDICATION (DRUGS)

- Botulism toxin: 150–400 U of botulism toxin type A injected in the levator ani at 3 points on each side with 23-gauge needle is effective for 3rd- and 4th-degree disease but still experimental.
- Contraindications: Anxiolytics, especially benzodiazepines

SURGERY
Contraindicated

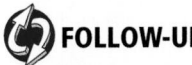 **FOLLOW-UP**

PROGNOSIS
- Some studies show high degrees of success (58–70%) with behavioral interventions.
- History of sexual abuse does not predict outcome negatively or positively.

PATIENT MONITORING
General preventive health care

REFERENCES

1. Lamont J. Vaginismus. *Am J Obstet Gynecol* 1978;131:632–636.
2. Spector IP, Carey MP. Incidence and prevalence of the sexual dysfunctions: A critical review of the empirical literature. *Arch Sexual Behavior* 1990;19:389–405.
3. Biswas A. Vaginismus and outcome of treatment. *Ann Acad Med Singapore* 1995;24:755–758.
4. Heiman JR. Evaluating sexual dysfunctions: Primary care of women. Norwalk, CT: Appleton & Lange, 1995.
5. Read S, King M, Watson J. Sexual dysfunction in primary medical care. *J Public Health Med* 1997;19(4):387–391.
6. Sarwer D, Durlak J. A field trial of the effectiveness of behavioral treatment for sexual dysfunctions. *J Sex Marital Ther* 1997;23(2):87–97.
7. Ghazizadeh S, Nikzad M. Botulism toxin in the treatment of refractory vaginismus. *Obstet Gynecol* 2004;104:922–925.

 MISCELLANEOUS

See also: Dyspareunia; Sexual Dysfunction in Women

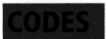 **CODES**

ICD9-CM
306.51 Psychogenic vaginismus

PATIENT TEACHING
- Education about pelvic anatomy, nature of the vaginal spasms, normal adult sexual function
- Hand-held mirror can help the woman learn visually to tighten and loosen perineal muscles
- Important to teach the partner that spasms are not under conscious control and are not a reflection on the relationship or a woman's feelings about her partner
- Instruction in techniques for vaginal dilation
- Resources
  - American College of Obstetricians & Gynecologists (ACOG), 409 12th St., SW, Washington, DC 20024-2188; (800) 762-ACOG
  - Valins L. When a woman's body says no to sex: understanding and overcoming vaginismus. New York: Penguin, 1992.

 See Corresponding Diagnostic Algorithm

 See Patient Handout on CD

V

VARICOSE VEINS

Joseph A. Florence, MD

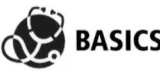 BASICS

DESCRIPTION

- Permanent dilation and tortuosity of superficial veins usually occurring in the legs and feet. May result from congenitally incomplete valves, or valves that have become incompetent. Affects legs where reverse flow occurs when dependent.
- System(s) Affected: Cardiovascular; Skin/Exocrine

ALERT

Ulceration of varicose veins has a high rate of infection which can lead to sepsis.

Geriatric Considerations

- More common, usually valvular degeneration, but may be secondary to chronic venous deficiency
- Recommended therapy: Elastic support hose and frequent rests with legs elevated rather than ligation and stripping

Pregnancy Considerations

- Frequent problem
- Use of elastic stockings recommended for individuals who have a history of varicosities or when activities involve a great deal of standing

EPIDEMIOLOGY

- Predominant age: Middle age
- Predominant sex: Female > Male (5:1)

Incidence

- 45 per 1,000 (National Health Interview Survey NHIS95)
- The National Women's Health Information Center (NWHIC) estimates that 50% of all women are affected by varicose veins.

RISK FACTORS

- Increasing age
- Pregnancy, especially multiple pregnancies
- Occupations requiring prolonged standing, restrictive clothing (e.g., very tight girdles)
- Obesity
- History of phlebitis
- Family history

Genetics

Familial, dominant, X-linked

PATHOPHYSIOLOGY

- Varicose veins are caused by venous insufficiency from faulty valves in 1 or more perforator veins in the lower leg, causing secondary incompetence at the saphenofemoral junction (valvular reflux).
- Valvular dysfunction causing venous reflux and subsequently venous hypertension
- Failed valves allow blood to flow in the reverse direction (away from the heart) from deep to superficial and from proximal to distal veins.
- Deep thrombophlebitis
- Increased venous pressure from any cause
- Congenital valvular incompetence
- Trauma (should consider AV fistula: Listen for bruit)
- In many individuals, no cause or precipitating factor found
- Presumed to be due to a loss in vein wall elasticity with failure of the valve leaflets to coapt (1)[C]

ASSOCIATED CONDITIONS

- Stasis dermatitis
- Stasis ulcer, venous ulcer (large varicose veins may lead to skin changes and eventual ulceration (2)

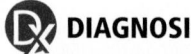 DIAGNOSIS

SIGNS AND SYMPTOMS

History

Symptoms range from minor annoyance or cosmetic problem to a lifestyle-limiting problem.

- Localized symptoms
  - Sometimes asymptomatic or minimal symptoms
  - Pain
  - Burning
  - Itching
- Generalized symptoms
  - Leg muscular cramp, aching
  - Leg fatigue or swelling
- Pain if varicose ulcer develops
- Symptoms often worse at the end of the day, especially with prolonged standing
- Women are more prone to symptoms due to hormonal influences: Symptoms worse during menses (3)[B]
- There is no direct correlation with the severity of the varicose veins and the severity of symptoms.

Physical Exam

- Inspect lower extremities with patient standing. Varicose veins in the proximal femoral ring and distal portion of the legs may not be visible when the patient is supine.
- Varicose veins are
  - Dilatated, tortuose superficial veins, chiefly in the lower extremities
  - Dark purple or blue in color and are raised above the surface of the skin.
  - Often twisted and bulging and can look like cords.
  - Most commonly found on the posterior or medial lower extremity
- Edema of affected limb may be present.
- Skin changes may include
  - Eczema
  - Hyperpigmentation
  - Lipodermatosclerosis
- Spider veins (idiopathic telangiectases)
  - Fine intracutaneous angiectasis
  - May be extensive/unsightly
- Documentation to help with differential diagnosis should include
  - The extent and location of varicose veins
  - Description of the skin including hair distribution
  - Neurological—especially sensory and motor
  - Periferial arterial vasculature—pulses
  - Musculoskeletal system to document associated rheumatologic or orthopedic issues

TESTS

Special tests

- Trendelenburg test (4): Test for varicose veins. Patient lies on his back and raises his leg to empty the veins. A tourniquet is applied just below the saphenous opening. The patient is then stood up and the tourniquet removed in 60 seconds. Normally the vein should fill from below within 35 seconds with the tourniquet in situ. Earlier filling indicates incompetence of a communicating vein. If on release the veins fill rapidly from above it is due to incompetent sapheno-femoral valves.
- Perthes test (5): A clinical test for assessing the patency of the deep femoral veins, used in preparations for operation for varicose veins. With the patient standing and veins filled, a tourniquet is placed around the mid-thigh, and the patient walks for 5 minutes. If the saphenous veins collapse below the tourniquet, the deep veins are patent and the communicating veins are competent; if unchanged, both saphenous and communicating veins are incompetent, and if the veins increase in prominence and pain occurs the deep veins are occluded.

Imaging

- Duplex ultrasound—formal noninvasive imaging of the venous system with duplex ultrasound will confirm the etiology, anatomy, and pathophysiology of segmental venous reflux.
- Duplex scanning, venous Doppler study, photoplethysmography, light-reflection rheography, air plethysmography, and other vascular testing should be reserved for those patients who have venous symptoms and/or large (>4 mm in diameter) vessels or large numbers of spider telangiectasia indicating venous hypertension.

Pathological Findings

- Elongation and tortuosity of veins
- Medial fibrosis of veins
- Disappearance or atrophy of valves

DIFFERENTIAL DIAGNOSIS

- Nerve root compression
- Arthritis
- Peripheral neuritis
- Telangiectasia: Smaller, visible blood vessels that are permanently dilated
- Deep vein thrombosis

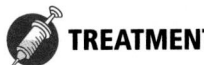 **TREATMENT**

Patients with unsightly varicose veins seek treatment for cosmetic reasons.

GENERAL MEASURES
- Appropriate health care: Outpatient
- Conservative methods
  - Frequent rest periods with legs elevated
  - Lightweight, elastic compression hosiery. Best put on before getting out of bed
  - Graduated compressing stockings are considered 1st-line therapy.
  - Avoid girdles and other restrictive clothing.
  - If stasis ulcers present, use warm, wet dressings

SURGERY
- Challenge to balance a cosmetically acceptable result with a low incidence of recurrence and complications
- Surgery is indicated if there is pain, recurrent phlebitis, skin changes/ulceration, or for cosmetic improvement for severe cases.
- Minimally invasive techniques include (6)[C]
  - Radiofrequency ablation (RFA)
  - Endovenous laser therapy (EVLT)
  - Transilluminated power phlebectomy (TIPP)
  - Foam sclerotherapy is more powerful than a liquid sclerosant. (7)[A]
  - Ambulatory phlebectomy–has a lower risk of recurrence than with sclerotherapy. (7)[A]
- Traditional surgical methods include
  - Ligation and stripping of the varicose vein (Sclerotherapy: Sclerosing solution is injected into varicosities causing vein walls to swell, adhere, and scar. 50–90% improvement expected [American Academy of Dermatology])
  - Stab avulsion phlebectomy
- For extensive fibrosis: Excision of the entire area, followed by skin graft, may be necessary.
- Surgical treatment of clinically symptomatic varicose veins involves treatment of the saphenous vein reflux as well as the varicosities.

PROGNOSIS
- Usual course: Chronic
- Favorable with appropriate treatment
- Quality of surgical treatment is less satisfactory if significant deep venous reflux, history of ulceration, or congenital arteriovenous malformation exists. (6)

COMPLICATIONS
- Petechial hemorrhages
- Chronic edema
- Superimposed infection
- Varicose ulcers
- Pigmentation
- Eczema
- Recurrence after surgical treatment
- Scarring or nerve damage from stripping technique

PATIENT MONITORING
Until surgery or conservative therapy brings maximal benefit

REFERENCES
1. Clarke GH, Vasdekis SN, Hobbs JT, Nicolaides AN. Venous wall function in the pathogenesis of varicose veins. *Surgery.* 1992;111(4):402–408.
2. Hanrahan LM, et al. Distribution of valvular incompetence in patients with venous stasis ulceration. *J Vasc Surg.* 1991;13(6):805–811.
3. Fegan WG, Lambe R, Henry M. Steroid hormones and varicose veins. *Lancet.* 1967;2:1070–1071.
4. Trendelenburg F. *Über die Unterbindung der Vena saphena magna bei Unterschenkelvaricen.* [Brun's] Beiträge zur klinischen Chirurgie,1891;7:195–210.
5. Perthes GC. *Über die Operation der Unterschenkelvarizen nach Trendelenburg.* Deutsche medizinische Wochenschrift. Berlin,1895;16:253–257.
6. Teruya TH, Ballard JL. New approaches for the treatment of varicose veins. *Surg Clin North Am.* 2004;84(5):1397–1417.
7. Sadick NS. Advances in the treatment of varicose veins: Ambulatory phlebectomy, foam sclerotherapy, endovascular laser, and radiofrequency closure. *Dermatol Clin.* 2005;23(3):443–455.

ADDITIONAL READING
- Callam MJ. Epidemiology of varicose veins. *Br J Surg.* 1994;81:167–173.
- Ellis H, Taylor P. *Varicose Veins.* 3rd ed. London: Greenwich Medical Media; 1999.

 MISCELLANEOUS

See also: Hemorrhoids; Dermatitis, Stasis

 CODES

ICD9-CM
454.1 Varicose veins of lower extremities with inflammation

PATIENT TEACHING

For patient education materials favorably reviewed on this topic, contact: National Heart, Lung & Blood Institute, Communications & Public Information Branch, National Institutes of Health, Building 31, Room 41–21, 9000 Rockville Pike, Bethesda, MD 20892, (301) 496-4236.

Diet
- No special diet
- Weight-loss diet recommended, if obesity a problem

Activity
- Avoid long periods of standing.
- If standing is necessary, frequently shift weight from side to side.
- Appropriate exercise routine as part of conservative treatment.
- Walking regimen after sclerotherapy is important to help promote healing.
- Apply elastic stockings before lowering legs from the bed.
- Never sit with legs hanging down.

Prevention
- Exercise regularly to improve leg strength, circulation: Walking and running
- Maintain an appropriate weight.
- Avoid crossing legs when sitting.
- Wear elastic support stockings.
- Avoid clothing that constricts your legs.
- Inform patients that the surgery or sclerotherapy may not prevent development of varicosities and that the procedure may need to be repeated in later years.

 See Corresponding Diagnostic Algorithm

 See Patient Handout on CD

V

VENTRICULAR SEPTAL DEFECT (VSD)

Brent Barber, MD
Brad Friedman, MD

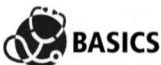

BASICS

DESCRIPTION
- Congenital or acquired defect of the interventricular septum that allows communication of blood between the left and right ventricles
- Other than bicuspid aortic valve, this is the most common congenital heart malformation reported in infants and children. It also occurs as a complication of acute myocardial infarctions (MI).
- Blood flow across the defect is typically left to right and depends on the size of the defect and the pulmonary vascular resistance (PVR).
- Prolonged shunting of blood can lead to pulmonary hypertension and eventually reversal of flow across the defect, and to cyanosis (Eisenmenger complex).
- System(s) Affected: Cardiovascular

ALERT

Geriatric Considerations
In this population, almost entirely associated with myocardial infarction

Pediatric Considerations
Congenital

Pregnancy Considerations
- Pregnancy may exacerbate symptoms and signs of a VSD.
- Tolerated during pregnancy if the septal defect is small

GENERAL PREVENTION
For adults, avoid risk factors for MI and obtain evaluation before pregnancy.

EPIDEMIOLOGY
- Predominant age: Infants and children
- Predominant sex: Male = Female (Male > Female if secondary to myocardial infarction)

Prevalence
In the US
- Congenital: 100–500 of 100,000 live births
- Acute myocardial infarctions: Estimated to complicate 1–3%

RISK FACTORS
- Congenital
  - 4.2% risk of sibling being affected
  - 4.0% of offspring being affected
- Post–acute MI
  - 1st MI
  - Limited coronary artery disease
  - Hypertension
  - Most frequent within 1st week after MI
  - Occur in 1–2% of MI, most commonly after anterior MI

Genetics
Multifactorial etiology; autosomal dominant and recessive transmission have been reported.

ETIOLOGY
- Congenital
- In adults, secondary to MI

ASSOCIATED CONDITIONS
- Congenital
  - Tetralogy of Fallot
  - Aortic valvular deformities, especially aortic insufficiency
  - Down syndrome (Trisomy 21), endocardial cushion defect
  - Transposition of the great arteries
  - Coarctation of the aorta
  - Tricuspid atresia
  - Truncus arteriosus
  - Patent ductus arteriosus
  - Atrial septal defect
  - Pulmonic stenosis
  - Subaortic stenosis
- Adult: Coronary artery disease

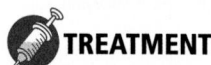

DIAGNOSIS

SIGNS AND SYMPTOMS
- Depend on the degree of shunting across the defect
- Respiratory distress, tachypnea, tachycardia
- Diaphoresis with feeds, poor weight gain in infants
- Forceful apical impulse
- Thrill along the left lower or midsternal borders
- High-frequency holosystolic murmur
- S3
- Increased intensity of P2
- Elevated jugular venous pressure
- Diastolic rumble due to increased flow across the mitral valve
- If pulmonary hypertension exists: Cyanosis with exertion
- If Eisenmenger complex is present: Cyanosis and clubbing

TESTS
Lab
Special tests
- ECG may suggest severity of VSD. Initially, left ventricular hypertrophy and left atrial enlargement may be evident. With pulmonary hypertension, right ventricular hypertrophy and right atrial enlargement may be seen.
- After surgical repair, right bundle branch block and left anterior hemi-block are common.

Imaging
- Chest x-ray may demonstrate increased pulmonary vascularity and/or cardiomegaly.
- 2-dimensional ECG for visualization and size of defect.
- Color-flow Doppler, for direction and velocity of ventricular septal defect jet. May be used to estimate right ventricular pressure

Diagnostic Procedures/Surgery
- Cardiac catheterization (left and right heart) can establish the diagnosis, and quantitate degree of shunting.
- Demonstration of an oxygen saturation step-up from the right atrium to the distal pulmonary artery

Pathological Findings
- Congenital VSDs (4 major anatomical types)
  - Membranous (70%)
  - Muscular (20%)
  - Atrioventricular canal type (5%)
  - Supracristal (5%; higher percentage in Asian populations)
- Post-MI VSDs: Involve predominantly the muscular septum

DIFFERENTIAL DIAGNOSIS
- Any defect with left to right shunt, such as patent ductus arteriosus, atrial septal defect
- Children: Tetralogy of Fallot
- Adults: Mitral regurgitation

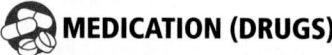

TREATMENT

GENERAL MEASURES
Appropriate health care
- Outpatient, until surgical repair is indicated
- Inpatient in setting of acute MI
- Inpatient for treatment of severe congestive heart failure

Diet
Low sodium

Activity
As tolerated

MEDICATION (DRUGS)

First Line
- Endocarditis antibiotic prophylaxis (1)[A]
- Pediatric
  - Furosemide 1–2 mg/kg PO/IV once to twice a day (2)[A]
  - Digoxin: Infants <2 years old, 10 μg/kg/d PO divided b.i.d.; children 2–10 years old, 5–10 μg/kg/d PO divided b.i.d.; children >10 years old, 2–5 μg/kg/d PO divided b.i.d.
  - Spironolactone: 1–2 mg/kg/d divided b.i.d.
  - Captopril: 0.1–0.4 mg/kg PO given q6–24h (max 6 mg/kg per 24 hours)
- Adult: Digoxin and diuretics may be beneficial in some circumstances.
- Precautions
  - Drugs that increase peripheral vascular resistance may increase left-to-right shunting and cause signs and symptoms of pulmonary overcirculation.
  - Hypotension
- Significant possible interactions: Refer to manufacturer's profile for each drug.

SURGERY
- Surgical closure is generally indicated if the pulmonic-to-systemic flow is >1.5:1.
- Congenital VSD surgery is usually performed before the child enters school or earlier, if hemodynamically indicated. (3)[A]
- Percutaneous transcatheter device closure of muscular and perimembranous is an alternative to surgery which has shown promising results. (4)[B]
- In the post-MI setting, afterload reduction, inotropic support, and intra-aortic balloon pump may be used to stabilize the patient prior to surgery.

FOLLOW-UP

PROGNOSIS

- Congenital:
  - Course is variable, depending on the size of the VSD.
  - Small VSD: 25–45% will close spontaneously by age 3 years. Muscular defects are more likely to close spontaneously.
  - Large VSD: CHF, failure to thrive in infancy, necessitating surgical repair
  - 4% of patients with VSD develop infective endocarditis by the 3rd or 4th decade of life.
  - Progressive pulmonary vascular disease and pulmonary hypertension are the most feared complications of VSD caused by left-to-right shunting, and may eventually lead to reversal of the shunt (Eisenmenger complex). Death usually occurs in the 4th decade of life if untreated.
- Post–MI:
  - With medical management alone, 80–90% mortality in the 1st 2 weeks
  - Prognosis worse with inferior MI compared to anterior MI

COMPLICATIONS

- CHF
- Infective endocarditis
- Aortic insufficiency
- Sudden death
- Hemoptysis
- Chest pain
- Cerebral abscess
- Paradoxical emboli
- Cardiogenic shock
- Heart block may rarely accompany surgical closure.
- Pulmonary hypertension

PATIENT MONITORING

Close follow-up of a congenital VSD is necessary until primary intracardiac repair is performed, to ensure that significant pulmonary hypertension does not develop.

REFERENCES

1. Glen S, Burns J, Bloomfield P. Prevalence and development of additional cardiac abnormalities in 1448 patients with congenital VSD. *Heart.* 2004;90(11):1321–1325.
2. Faris R, et al. *Diuretics for heart failure.* The Cochrane Database of Systemic Reviews: John Wiley and Sons; 2006.
3. Chang RK, Chen A, Klitzner TS. Factors associated with age at operation for children with congenital heart disease. *Pediatrics.* 2000;(105):1073–1081.
4. Hein R, et al. Atrial and septal defects can safely be closed by percutaneous intervention. *J Interventional Cardiol.* 2005;(18):515–522.

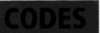 **MISCELLANEOUS**

See also: Down Syndrome; Myocardial Infarction; Tetralogy of Fallot

 CODES

ICD9-CM
745.4 Ventricular septal defect

PATIENT TEACHING

- Endocarditis prophylaxis
- Parents need support and instructions for prevention of complications until the child is ready for surgery.

 See Corresponding Diagnostic Algorithm

See Patient Handout on CD

V

VERTIGO

Michele Matthews, PharmD
Kristy Kedian, DO

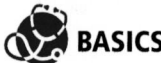 **BASICS**

DESCRIPTION
- Sensation of movement when no movement is actually occurring. Results from peripheral or central causes or, in some instances, may be induced by medications or anxiety disorders.
- System(s) Affected: Nervous
- Synonym(s): Dizziness; Acute vestibular neuronitis; Labyrinthitis; Benign paroxysmal positional vertigo (BPPV)

GENERAL PREVENTION
- Precautions to avoid injuries from falls that may occur secondary to imbalance
- If due to motion sickness, pretreatment with anticholinergics such as scopolamine

EPIDEMIOLOGY
- Women are more likely to experience central causes, particularly vertiginous migraine.
- Patients who are elderly and have risk factors for cerebrovascular disease (CVD) are more likely to experience central causes.

Incidence
Accounts for 54% of cases of dizziness reported in primary care:
- >90% of these patients are diagnosed with peripheral causes, such as BPPV.

Prevalence
Ranges from 5–10% within the general population

RISK FACTORS
- History of migraines
- History of CVD or risk factors for CVD
- Use of ototoxic medications
- Trauma or barotrauma
- Perilymphatic fistula
- Heavy weightbearing
- Psychosocial stress
- Exposure to toxins

Genetics
Family history of CVD or migraines may indicate higher risk of central causes.

PATHOPHYSIOLOGY
Caused by dysfunction of the rotational velocity sensors of the inner ear. Results in asymmetrical central processing. Related to the combination of sensory disturbance of motion and the malfunction of the central vestibular apparatus.

ETIOLOGY
- Peripheral causes
  - Acute labyrinthitis, acute vestibular neuronitis, BPPV, cholesteatoma, herpes zoster oticus, Ménière disease, otosclerosis
- Central causes
  - Cerebellar tumor, CVD, migraine, multiple sclerosis
- Other causes
  - Cervical, drug-induced, psychological

ASSOCIATED CONDITIONS
See "Etiology."

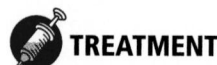 **DIAGNOSIS**

SIGNS AND SYMPTOMS
- Dizziness
- Rotary illusions
- Nystagmus
- Nausea and vomiting
- Hearing loss
- Pallor
- Diaphoresis
- Pain
- Neurologic symptoms (i.e., ataxia)

History
- Determine if true vertigo exists versus other causes of dizziness by asking the patient if they feel lightheaded or if they see the world spinning around them during a dizzy spell. (1)
  - Affirmative answer to spinning is indicative of true vertigo
- Distinguish between peripheral and central causes.
  - Timing and duration
    ○ Seconds to minutes: Peripheral
    ○ Minutes to hours: Peripheral or central
    ○ Days: Peripheral or central
    ○ Weeks: Central or psychological
  - Provoking factors
    ○ Changes in head position: Peripheral or central
    ○ Spontaneous episodes: Peripheral or central
    ○ Recent upper viral respiratory infection: Peripheral
    ○ Stress: Central or psychological
    ○ Immunosuppression: Peripheral
    ○ Changes in ear pressure: Peripheral
  - Associated symptoms
    ○ Rotary illusions with nausea and vomiting: Peripheral
    ○ Horizontal and rotational nystagmus: Peripheral
    ○ Horizontal, vertical, or rotational nystagmus: Central
    ○ Hearing loss: Peripheral
    ○ Neurologic symptoms: Central
- Obtain medical and medication history
  - Recent use of ototoxic medications
  - History of CVD or risk factors for CVD

Physical Exam
- Neurologic (1)
  - Cranial nerves for signs of palsies, nystagmus
  - Balance
    ○ Peripheral: Mild to moderate, able to walk
    ○ Central: Severe, unable to walk
  - Dix-Hallpike maneuver (PPV = 83%, NPV = 52%)
    ○ If induced symptoms subside after repeated maneuvers, consider peripheral causes.
    ○ If induced symptoms do not subside, consider central causes.
- Head and neck (1)
  - Tympanic membranes
    ○ Vesicles: Herpes zoster oticus
    ○ Cholesteatoma
- Cardiovascular (1)
  - Orthostatic changes in BP: Dehydration or autonomic dysfunction

TESTS
Lab
Audiometry if acoustic neuroma or Ménière disease is suspected

Imaging
Consider MRI in the presence of neurologic symptoms, risk factors for CVD, or progressive unilateral hearing loss.

DIFFERENTIAL DIAGNOSIS
- Acoustic neuroma
- Anxiety disorder
- BPPV
- Cerebellar degeneration
- Cerebellar tumor
- Labyrinthine concussion
- Labyrinthitis
- Ménière disease
- Multiple sclerosis
- Perilymphatic fistula
- Syphilis
- Vascular ischemia
- Vertiginous migraine
- Vestibular neuronitis
- Vestibular ototoxicity

TREATMENT

- Epley maneuver for BPPV (2)[A]
- Modified Epley maneuver for BPPV (3)[B]
- Vestibular exercises for acute vestibular neuronitis (3)[B]
- Low-salt diet and diuretics for Ménière disease (3)[B]
- Migraine prophylaxis, migraine abortive medications, and vestibular exercises for vertiginous migraines (3)[B]
- Selective serotonin reuptake inhibitors (SSRIs) when associated with anxiety disorders (3)[B]

- Vestibular suppressant medications for symptom relief in acute vestibular neuronitis (3,4)[C]

GENERAL MEASURES
- Provide an explanation and offer assurance to avoid anxiety that may exacerbate vertigo.
- Treatments depend on cause

  - BPPV: Epley maneuver or modified Epley maneuver (2)[A] (see "Special Therapy")

  - Vestibular neuronitis and labyrinthitis
    ○ Vestibular suppressant medications (3,4)[C] (see "Medications")

    ○ Vestibular rehabilitation exercises (3)[B] (see "Physical Therapy")

  - Ménière disease:

    ○ Low-salt diet (<1–2 g/d) (3)[B]
    ○ Diuretics such as hydrochlorothiazide (3)[B]

  - Vascular ischemia
    ○ Prevention of future events through blood pressure reduction, lipid lowering, smoking cessation, antiplatelet therapy, and anticoagulation if necessary

- Vertiginous migraines
  - Dietary and lifestyle modifications, vestibular rehabilitation exercises, prophylactic and migraine abortive medications (3)[B]
- Drug-induced vertigo
  - Discontinue causative agent
- Psychological
  - SSRIs (3)[B]

Diet
- Restricted salt intake for Ménière disease
- Dietary modifications for vertiginous migraine

SPECIAL THERAPY
Epley maneuver or modified Epley maneuver for BPPV to displace calcium deposits in the semicircular canals (2)[A]

- Improves symptoms and converts patient from positive to negative Dix-Hallpike maneuver
- Contraindications: Carotid stenosis, unstable cardiac disease, severe neck disease

Physical Therapy
Vestibular rehabilitation exercises (3)[B]

- Ball toss
- Lying-to-standing
- Target-change
- Thumb-tracking
- Tightrope
- Walking turns

 MEDICATION (DRUGS)

First Line
- Meclizine (Antivert): 12.5–50 mg PO q4–8h (3,4)[C]
- Dimenhydrinate (Dramamine): 25–100 mg PO, IM, or IV q4–8h (3,4)[C]
  - Precautions: Concomitant use of CNS depressants, prostatic hyperplasia, glaucoma
  - Adverse effects: Sedation, xerostomia
  - Interactions: CNS depressants
- Prochlorperazine (Compazine): 5–10 mg PO or IM q6–8h; 25 mg rectally q12h; 5–10 mg by slow IV over 2 minutes (3,4)[C]
  - Contraindications: Blood dyscrasias, age <2 years, severe hypotension
  - Precautions: Children with acute illness; glaucoma, history of breast cancer, impaired cardiovascular function, pregnancy, prostatic hyperplasia
  - Adverse effects: Sedation, xerostomia, hypotension, extrapyramidal effects
  - Interactions: Phenothiazines, tricyclic antidepressants
- Metoclopramide (Reglan): 5–10 mg PO q6h, 5–10 mg slow IV q6h
  - Contraindications: Concomitant use of drugs with extrapyramidal effects, seizure disorders
  - Precautions: History of depression, Parkinson disease, hypertension
  - Adverse effects: Sedation, fluid retention, constipation
  - Interactions: Linezolid, cyclosporine, digoxin, levodopa

- Benzodiazepines (3,4)[C]
  - Diazepam (Valium): 2–10 mg PO or IV q4–8h
  - Lorazepam (Ativan): 0.5–2 mg PO, IM, or IV q4–8h
    - Contraindications: Glaucoma, age <6 months
    - Precautions: Concomitant use of CNS depressants, hepatic insufficiency, pregnancy
    - Adverse effects: Sedation, respiratory depression, hypotension
    - Interactions: CNS depressants

ALERT
Geriatric Considerations
Use vestibular suppressant medications with caution
- Increased risk of falls
- Urinary retention

Pregnancy Considerations
Meclizine and dimenhydrinate are Pregnancy Category B

 FOLLOW-UP

DISPOSITION
Issues for Referral
Consider referral to otolaryngologist, ENT specialist, or neurologist if patient requires further care.

PROGNOSIS
Depends on diagnosis and response to treatment

COMPLICATIONS
- Anxiety
- Depression
- Disability
- Injuries from falls

PATIENT MONITORING
After 1–2 weeks, assess for
- Recurrence of symptoms
- New-onset symptoms
- Medication-related adverse effects
- Relief from vestibular rehabilitation exercises

REFERENCES
1. Labuguen RH. Initial evaluation of vertigo. *Am Fam Physician*. 2006;73:244–251.
2. Hilton M, Pinder D. The Epley (canalith repositioning) maneuver for benign paroxysmal positional vertigo. *Cochrane Database Syst Rev*. 2004;(3):CD003162.
3. Swartz R, Longwell P. Treatment of vertigo. *Am Fam Physician*. 2005;71:1115–1122.
4. Hain TC, Uddin M. Pharmacological treatment of vertigo. *CNS Drugs*. 2003;(2):85–100.

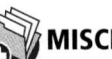 **MISCELLANEOUS**

See also BPPV, Ménière disease, Motion sickness

CODES
ICD9-CM
- 386.2 central origin vertigo
- 386.10 peripheral origin vertigo
- 386.11 BPPV
- 780.4 Vertigo

PATIENT TEACHING
Diet
- Reduce sodium intake (Ménière disease).
- Avoid triggers such as caffeine or alcohol (vertiginous migraine).

Activity
Balance exercises should be adhered to for symptom improvement and return to normal activities of daily living.

 See Corresponding Diagnostic Algorithm

 See Patient Handout on CD

V

VITAMIN D DEFICIENCY

Frank J. Domino, MD
Samir Malkani, MD

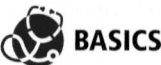 **BASICS**

This topic covers the commonly acquired vitamin D Deficiency and not type II vitamin D–resistant rickets or type I pseudo-vitamin D resistant rickets (both rare autosomal recessive disorders).

DESCRIPTION
- Vitamin D is both a hormone and a vitamin. Cholecalciferol (D3) is synthesized in the skin by exposure to ultraviolet B (UVB) radiation. Ergocalciferol (D2) and D3 are present in foods.
- D2 and D3 are hydroxylated in the liver to 25 vitamin D (calcidiol), which is the major circulating form.
- This is further hydroxylated in the kidney to the active metabolite 1,25 vitamin D (calcitriol). Any insult to this production can result in deficiency.

GENERAL PREVENTION
- Adequate exposure to sunlight and dietary sources of vitamin D (plants, fish). Many foods are fortified with D2 and D3.
- Higher intake of vitamin D recommended for ages >50.
- For age 51–70, recommended intake is 400 IU/day; for ≥71, 600 IU/day.

ALERT
Pediatric Considerations
The American Academy of Pediatrics recommends all breast-fed babies receive 200 I.U. of vitamin D per day.

EPIDEMIOLOGY
- Unclear in general population.
- In the community, a cohort study of asymptomatic adolescents in Boston found 24.1% were deficient, with 4.6% severely deficient. (1)
- A study of hospitalized patients in Massachusetts found 57% vitamin D deficient. (2)
- Women with history of osteoporosis or osteoporotic fracture have high prevalence of vitamin D deficiency. (3)[A]
- A cross-sectional study of patients with persistent, nonspecific pain in an urban Minneapolis primary care clinic found 93% deficient and 28% severely deficient. (4)

RISK FACTORS
- Inadequate sun exposure
- Female
- Dark skin
- Immigrant populations
- Low socioeconomic status
- Latitudes higher than 38°
- Elderly
- Institutionalized
- Medications (phenobarbital, phenytoin)

Genetics
Numerous rare genetic disorders can induce hypoparathyroidism (DiGeorge syndrome)

PATHOPHYSIOLOGY
- Insufficient dietary intake of vitamin D and/or lack of UVB exposure results in low levels of vitamin D; this limits calcium absorption, causing excess parathyroid hormone (PTH) to be released.
- PTH stimulates osteoclast activity, which raises calcium and phosphorous, but results in osteomalacia.

ETIOLOGY
- Dietary deficiency
  - Inadequate vitamin D intake
  - Macrobiotic diet
- Inadequate sunlight exposure
  - Institutionalized patients
  - Hospitalized patients
  - Chronic illness
  - Liver or kidney disease
  - Malabsorptive states

ASSOCIATED CONDITIONS
- Osteomalacia, osteoporosis
- Rickets
- Celiac disease
- Gastric bypass
- Chronic renal disease

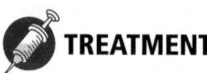 **DIAGNOSIS**

SIGNS AND SYMPTOMS
- Nonspecific musculoskeletal complaints
- Weak antigravity muscles

History
- Renal disease
- Gastrointestinal (malabsorption) disorders
- Liver dysfunction
- Immigration from tropical to colder climates

Physical Exam
- Numerous neurologic signs: Numbness, proximal myopathy, paresthesias, muscle cramps, laryngospasm
- Chvostek sign: Contraction of the muscles of the eye, mouth or nose, by tapping along the facial nerve
- Trousseau phenomenon: Carpal spasms and paraesthesia produced by pressure upon nerves and vessels of the upper arm
- Tetany
- Seizures

TESTS
Lab
- 25 vitamin D (most sensitive vitamin D status)
- Vitamin D Insufficiency
  - 25 D is 15–40 ng/mL
- Vitamin D deficiency
  - <15 ng/mL
- PTH elevation (normal in early vitamin D deficiency)
- Low calcium and phosphorous
- Elevated alkaline phosphatase (in later disease)

Imaging
- Plain radiographs: If atypical fracture, radiographs may show osteomalacia (pseudofractures or Looser zones) in pelvis, femur, and fibula.
- Osteoporosis Screen (5)[C]
  - Women ≥65 years with no risk factors
  - Women ≥60 years at risk: Body weight <70 kg (best predictor); less evidence smoking, low body mass index (BMI), family history, decreased activity, alcohol, or caffeine use.
  - African American women have higher bone density than Caucasians; thus, rarely screen <65

TREATMENT

Diet
- Fatty fish (tuna, salmon)
- Fortified milk, cereal, and foods

Activity
Weightbearing exercise

SPECIAL THERAPY
Aggressive calcium in ICU patients with ionized calcium <3.2 mg/dL or if symptomatic (tetany, seizures, QT prolongation, bradycardia, or hypotension, or ventilated patient with decreased diaphragmatic function)

MEDICATION (DRUGS)

First Line
- Vitamin D Insufficiency
  - Vitamin D 800 IU/d *plus*
  - Elemental calcium 1,200 mg/d
  - *Or*
- Ergocalciferol 50,000 IU/wk for 8 weeks *plus*
- Elemental calcium 1,200 mg/d

Second Line
Vitamin D deficiency
- Ergocalciferol 50,000 IU daily for 3 weeks, followed by 50,000 IU/week *plus*
- Elemental calcium 1,200 mg/d
- Patients with no sun exposure, malabsorption syndromes, and antiepileptic drugs may require more replacement

 ## FOLLOW-UP

Repeat abnormal 25 vitamin D and other abnormal labs at 8 weeks.

DISPOSITION
Admission Criteria
- Symptoms of severe hypocalcemia or
- Malabsorption syndromes

Issues for Referral
Endocrinology if no response to treatment

REFERENCES

1. Prevalence of vitamin D deficiency among healthy adolescents. *Arch Pediatr Adolesc Med*.
2. Hypovitaminosis D in medical inpatients. *N Engl J Med*. 1998;338:777–783.
3. *QJM*. 2005;98(9):667–676. Epub 2005 Jul 8.
4. *Mayo Clin Proc*. 2003;78(12):1463–1470. 2004;158:531–537.
5. www.ahrq.gov

ADDITIONAL READING
Undiagnosed vitamin D deficiency in the hospitalized patient: http://www.aafp.org/afp/20050115/299.html

 ## MISCELLANEOUS

 CODES

ICD9-CM
268.9

See Corresponding Diagnostic Algorithm

See Patient Handout on CD

VITAMIN DEFICIENCY

Samuel N. Grief, MD, FCFP

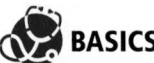 **BASICS**

DESCRIPTION
Vitamin deficiencies

- Vitamins are essential micronutrients required for normal metabolism, growth, and development.
- Deficiencies usually related to disease can occur under healthy conditions.
  NOTE: Deficiencies are rarely diagnosed or documented in the western world. Regulations mandating vitamin supplementation in food products, adequate food supply, availability of vitamin supplements, and lack of physician awareness all play a role.

GENERAL PREVENTION
- Adequate intake of an appropriately balanced diet containing carbohydrates, proteins, and fats
- Avoidance of fad diets
- Vitamin or nutrition supplementation when appropriate

EPIDEMIOLOGY
- Affects mainly geriatric population
- Occurs in select adult demographics: Pregnant women, chronic disease states (see "Etiology")
- Travelers spending extended time in developing nations

Incidence
- Very low for isolated vitamin deficiencies in western world; true incidence unknown
- Vitamin levels rarely measured (exceptions include vitamin B12–incidence increases over age 50; and folate–incidence increases with specific states: Pregnancy, antiepileptic drugs, neoplastic processes, alcoholism)

Prevalence
Varies by
- Age groups (1)[C]
- Comorbid conditions
- Geography
- Setting (i.e., urban, rural)

RISK FACTORS
Poverty, malnutrition, chronic disease states, advanced age

Genetics
- Cystic fibrosis
- Rare genetic predisposition
  - Autoimmune disease (e.g., pernicious anemia)
  - Congenital enzyme deficiencies (e.g., biotinidase deficiency)
  - Transcobalamin II deficiency
  - Ataxia and vitamin E deficiency (AVED)
  - A-β-lipoproteinemia

PATHOPHYSIOLOGY
Various mechanisms, including
- Bleeding diathesis
- Bone disruption
- Cognitive impairment
- Visual distortion
- Skin breakdown
- Anemia
- Alopecia
- Cardiovascular compromise

ETIOLOGY
- Chronic disease states: (e.g., HIV, malabsorption, chronic liver and kidney disease, alcoholism, pernicious anemia)
- Gastric surgeries: (e.g., gastric bypass, gastrectomy, small or large bowel resection)
- Predisposition related to certain medicines: (e.g., prednisone, phenytoin, isoniazid, protease inhibitors, proton pump inhibitors, chronic antibiotic use, penicillamine, hydralazine)
- Malnutrition, imbalanced nutrition, eating disorders: Obesity, bulimia/anorexia, fad diets, extreme vegetarianism
- Dialysis
- Parasitic infestation

ASSOCIATED CONDITIONS
- Osteoporosis, anemia, neuropathies
- Hartnup disease

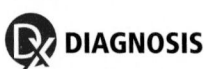 **DIAGNOSIS**

SIGNS AND SYMPTOMS
- Night blindness
- Macular degeneration
- Decreased visual acuity
- Poor wound
- Healing
- Hyperkeratosis of skin
- Neuropathy
- Abnormal food cravings (pica)
- Osteomalacia
- Spina bifida

History
- Previous gastrointestinal or gastric bypass surgery
- Prior or current medical conditions
  - TB
  - HIV
  - Hepatitis
  - Neoplastic condition
  - Hypermetabolic state
    ○ Thyrotoxicosis
    ○ Second or third degree burns
    ○ Wound healing
    ○ Any other systemic infection
  - Any chronic disease requiring steroids or immunosuppressants
  - Any malabsorption or chronic gastrointestinal disorder
    ○ Celiac disease, sprue, Crohn, ulcerative colitis
- Parenteral or enteral nutrition via tube feeding (2)[C]
- Pregnancy
- Medications
- Supplements
- Food allergies or intolerances

Physical Exam
- Breakdown of skin integrity
- Coarse or thinning hair
- Reduced visual acuity
- Beefy red tongue
- Angular cheilitis (perleche)
- Poor dentition and gingivitis
- Cognitive impairment
- Bruising and/or petechiae
- Sensory and motor neuropathies
- Ataxic gait

TESTS
- CBC
- If clinical characteristics are present, consider
  - Prothrombin and partial thromboplastin times
  - Vitamin B12 and folate levels
  - Consider serum homocysteine level if suspect vitamin B12, folate deficiency, and normal serum levels (3)[C]
- Specific vitamin level of choice

Lab
Ancillary tests include
- Blood urea nitrogen
- Albumin
- Pre-albumin
- Calcium
- Phosphorous
- Magnesium
- Liver function tests

Imaging
- X-ray of long bones and spine
- Bone densitometry: Indicated in
  - Women over age 65 years
  - Patients with chronic disease requiring long-standing steroids or immunosuppressants
  - Patients on thyroid medicine
  - Patients on antiepileptic drugs

Pathological Findings
- Rickets/Osteomalacia
  - Osteoid demineralization
  - Osteoporosis
- Scurvy
  - Ecchymoses
  - Bleeding gums
- Beriberi
  - Muscle wasting
  - Neuropathy
  - CHF
- Korsakoff syndrome
  - Confabulation
  - Memory disturbance
- Wernicke encephalopathy: Cognitive impairment
- Macular degeneration: Decreased visual acuity
- Pellagra
  - Dermatitis
  - Diarrhea
  - Dementia
  - Death
- Pernicious anemia
  - Subacute combined degeneration
  - Gait disturbance
  - Cognitive impairment
  - Alopecia

ALERT
Pediatric Considerations
- Hemorrhagic disease of the newborn
  - Deficiency of vitamin K is seen in neonates as they require 1 week of life to establish their intestinal flora (intestinal bacteria manufacture vitamin K) and as breast milk is a poor source of vitamin K.
  - Peaks 2–10 days after birth. Presents with bleeding from the umbilical stump and/or circumcision site along with generalized bruising and gastrointestinal hemorrhage. Routine injection of newborns with vitamin K (1 mg) prevents hemorrhagic disease.
- Vitamin D deficiency: Vitamin D supplementation (200 IU/day) is recommended in all exclusively breast-fed infants for the 1st 2 months of life (AAP recommendations) to prevent rickets.
- Many vitamin deficiencies lead to developmental delay in children.
- Supplemental vitamins in otherwise healthy children, although encouraged, are not mandated by medical authorities.

Pregnancy Considerations
Folate deficiency
- All pregnant women, and women of childbearing age considering pregnancy, should be strongly encouraged to take a multivitamin containing 0.8 mg of folic acid daily.

Geriatric Considerations
- Vitamin B12 deficiency: 25% of the general population age 65 and older has borderline or low levels of vitamin B12 necessitating supplementation. Method of administration for maximum B12 absorption is via sublingual route.
- Concurrent deficiency of other B vitamins often co-exists.

DIFFERENTIAL DIAGNOSIS
Many medical conditions may lead to symptoms and signs that mimic vitamin deficiencies, including
- Diabetes mellitus types 1 and 2
- Hyperparathyroidism
- Thyroid disorders
- Alzheimer disease
- Multiple sclerosis
- Substance abuse
- Toxic ingestion/overdose
- Hematologic malignancies/disorders

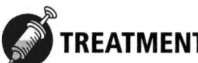

TREATMENT
PRE HOSPITAL
- Obtain prior medical records
- Nutrition history focusing on any food allergies, aversions, or intolerances

INITIAL STABILIZATION
Provide daily B-vitamin complex (folate, B6, B12), including thiamine supplementation (dose = 100 mg) via oral or parenteral route, to all patients with chronic medical conditions admitted to hospital or in postoperative state. (4)[B], (5)[C], (6)[A]

GENERAL MEASURES
Diet
- Obtain dietetics/nutrition consult.
- Monitor nutrient intake.
- Tailor diet to underlying chronic medical condition, such as
  - Diabetes: Carbohydrate counting required
  - Hypertension: DASH diet
  - Obesity: Calorie-controlled diet
  - Chronic kidney disease: Appropriate protein intake and balanced diet
  - Congestive heart failure: Low-salt, free-water restricted diet
  - Inflammatory bowel disease: Low-residue diet
  - Osteoporosis: Calcium-laden diet
- Supplemental enteral nutrition (i.e., Ensure, Boost, Sustacal, etc.) if anorexic or if difficulty eating solids

MEDICATION (DRUGS)
- The abundance of multivitamin formulations makes it very difficult for the medical provider to advise use or avoidance of each product.
- Encourage patients to bring in multivitamin bottle for personal review by a physician or knowledgeable health care practitioner or pharmacist.

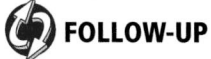

FOLLOW-UP
PROGNOSIS
- Most vitamin deficiencies are fully reversible if treated without undue delay.
- Vitamin repletion or supplementation may be required short term (<3 months) or long term (>3 months) dependent upon cause of deficiency

COMPLICATIONS
Vitamin toxicities
- Liver failure (vitamins A, D, E, K)
- Desquamation of skin (vitamin A)
- Kidney stones (vitamin C)
- Hypercoagulability (vitamin K)
- Facial flushing (vitamin B3)
- Pseudohyperparathyroidism (vitamin D)
- Masking of pernicious anemia (folic acid)
  NOTE: Any vitamin can be taken to excess; refer to the Recommended Dietary Allowance (RDA) for specific intake guidelines.

PATIENT MONITORING
- Symptomatic observation needed in majority of cases
- Semi-annual to annual monitoring of pertinent lab tests, as needed

REFERENCES
1. Van Wayenburg CAM, et al. Nutritional deficiency in Dutch primary care: Data from general practice research and registration networks. *Clin Nutr.* 2005;59(suppl):187–194.
2. Skelton JA, Havens PL, Werlin SL. Nutrient deficiencies in tube-fed children. *Clin Pediatrics.* 2006;45:37–41.
3. Hankey GJ. Is plasma homocysteine a modifiable risk factor for stroke? *Nat Clin Pract Neurol.* 2006;2:26–33.
4. Thomson AD, Marshall EJ. The treatment of patients at risk of developing Wernicke's encephalopathy in the community. *Alcohol Alcoholism.* 2006;41:159–167.
5. Parsons JP, Marsh CB, Mastronade JG. Wernicke's encephalopathy in a patient after gastric bypass surgery. *Chest.* 2005;128(suppl):453–454.
6. Jacques JND. Nutritional implications of weight loss surgery. *Nutrition & the MD.* 2005;31:1–6.

CODES

ICD9-CM
- 264 Vit A deficiency
- 266.1 Vit B6 deficiency
- 266.2 Other B-complex deficiencies
- 266.9 Unspecified vitamin B deficiency
- 267 Ascorbic acid deficiency
- 268 Vitamin D deficiency
- 269.0 Deficiency of vitamin K
- 269.1 Deficiency of other vitamins
- 269.2 Unspecified vitamin deficiency
- 275.3 Rickets/Osteomalacia
- 776.0 Vit K deficiency of newborn

 See Corresponding Diagnostic Algorithm

 See Patient Handout on CD

VITILIGO

Gary J. Silko, MD, MS

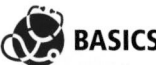 **BASICS**

DESCRIPTION
- An acquired, slowly progressive depigmenting condition in small or large areas of the skin due to the disappearance of previously active melanocytes
  - Focal (including segmental) vitiligo: 1 to a few scattered macules, occasionally in a dermatomal distribution
  - Generalized vitiligo: Many widespread macules (most common form)
  - Universal vitiligo: Little remaining normal pigment
  - Acrofacial: Affects distal fingers and facial orifices
- System(s) Affected: Skin/Exocrine
- Synonym(s): Hypomelanosis; Depigmentation

ALERT
Pediatric Considerations
Childhood vitiligo is a distinct subset of vitiligo. Higher incidence of focal vitiligo. Also higher incidence of autoimmune and endocrine disease. Response is poor to topical psoralen plus ultraviolet exposure (PUVA) therapy, but can be tried. Topical steroids may be prescribed (e.g., desonide 0.05% cream every day for 4 months).

Pregnancy Considerations
Treatment with topical or oral psoralens is contraindicated.

GENERAL PREVENTION
While undergoing all therapies, avoid excessive sun exposure.

EPIDEMIOLOGY
- Predominant age: All ages: 50% begin before age 20 years.
- Predominant sex: Male = Female

Incidence
In the US: 500–1,000/100,000

RISK FACTORS
- Positive family history
- Autoimmune disorders including hemolytic anemia and adrenal insufficiency
- Major life crisis or illness

Genetics
Autosomal dominant with variable expression and incomplete penetrance. Positive family history in 30% of cases

ETIOLOGY
Etiology unclear, but thought to be an autoimmune reaction to preexisting melanocytes

ASSOCIATED CONDITIONS
- Addison disease
- Alopecia areata
- Chronic mucocutaneous candidiasis
- Diabetes mellitus (insulin dependent)
- Hypoparathyroidism
- Melanoma
- Pernicious anemia
- Polyglandular autoimmune syndrome
- Thyroid disorders (hyperthyroidism and hypothyroidism), 30% of patients with vitiligo
- Uveitis
- Halo nevi

DIAGNOSIS

SIGNS AND SYMPTOMS
- Loss of pigment
- Locally increased sunburning
- Predilection for acral areas and around orifices such as eyes, mouth, anus
- Pruritus (10%)
- Premature graying (35%)
- Koebner phenomenon (aggravation by trauma)

TESTS
Lab
- Routine blood and urine studies are usually normal in the absence of associated diseases in adults.
- In children, screen for autoimmune diseases with thyroid-stimulating hormone, CBC, and fasting glucose.

Diagnostic Procedures/Surgery
- Examination under Wood light accentuates the hypopigmented areas, especially in light-skinned individuals.
- Skin scraping and a potassium hydroxide (KOH) preparation can be examined microscopically to rule out tinea versicolor.

Pathological Findings
Complete absence of melanocytes in skin biopsy. At the margins one may see a few lymphocytes and large melanocytes with abnormal melanosomes.

DIFFERENTIAL DIAGNOSIS
Any condition that causes acquired hypomelanosis
- Tinea versicolor
- Leprosy
- Lupus erythematosus
- Pityriasis alba
- Atopic dermatitis
- Albinism
- Alopecia areata
- Chemical exposure (phenols, arsenic, chloroquine, hydroquinone)
- Steroid exposure
- Retinoic acid use
- Tuberous sclerosis
- Neurofibromatosis
- Melanocytic nevi (halo nevi)
- Tumor regression of malignant melanoma
- Piebaldism
- Hypopituitarism
- Hyperthyroidism
- Morphea
- Lichen sclerosis

TREATMENT

GENERAL MEASURES
- Appropriate health care: Outpatient except in rare cases of surgical skin grafting or transplantation
- Sun exposure can accentuate the difference between normal and abnormal skin, so for cosmetic reasons patients may wish to avoid this.
- Skin dyes and cosmetics may be used as cover-ups.

Diet
No special diet

Activity
Full activity

MEDICATION (DRUGS)

First Line
- Focal or segmental vitiligo
  - A midpotency steroid cream can be applied daily for 3–4 months. If no response, advance to high-potency steroids. Clobetasol (Temovate) cream applied daily for 2 months (every other day on the face). Treatment may be resumed following a 1–4-month respite.
  - Phototherapy with narrow band UVB 2 times per week. (1)[C]
- Generalized vitiligo:
  - Oral systemic steroids, e.g., betamethasone 5 mg given 2 days in a row, then held the remainder of the week. This pattern continued for 2–4 months minimizes side effects and is effective in arresting the disease in many patients.
  - Narrow-band UVB therapy is the preferred initial phototherapy, given 2 times per week.
  - Oral trimethylpsoralen or methoxsalen (Oxsoralen-Ultra, 8-MOP) and UVA over a 12–24-month period
  - Alternatively, depigmenting the remaining normal skin with monobenzone, a hydroquinone derivative, 20% cream may be elected. It should be applied b.i.d. for 3–6 months. (1)[C]
- Contraindications
  - Absolute contraindications to use of psoralen compounds: Idiosyncratic reaction to psoralens, photosensitive disease (e.g., systemic lupus erythematosus, albinism, porphyria), invasive squamous cell carcinoma, melanoma, aphakia
  - Relative contraindications to use of psoralen compounds: Cardiac disease, hepatic dysfunction, multiple basal cell carcinomas, prior radiation therapy, prior arsenic therapy
- Precautions
  - Watch for skin atrophy and telangiectasias when using topical steroids, especially on the face.
  - Watch for photosensitizers with UVA treatment.
  - Severe burns possible with topical psoralens. Partially avoided with: 1:10 or 1:50 dilution of psoralens
  - PUVA cannot be used for children <12 years of age due to immaturity of the ocular lens.
  - Patients undergoing PUVA therapy should have a screening ophthalmologic examination to rule out subclinical retinal pigmentary disease, which is frequently associated with vitiligo.
- Significant possible interactions: Other photosensitizers, e.g., tetracyclines and retinoic acid

Second Line
- Patients with unresponsive focal vitiligo may be candidates for minigrafting with or without PUVA therapy.
- Levamisole 150 mg 2 days a week for several months has been effective in patients with limited or slowly spreading disease.

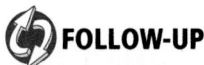

FOLLOW-UP

DISPOSITION
Issues for Referral
Dermatology consultation should be considered for facial or widespread vitiligo or when PUVA therapy may be necessary.

PROGNOSIS
- Only 5% repigment spontaneously.
- Best results are with PUVA therapy, with which 70% have repigmentation of head and neck area, less in other body areas. Lower percentages respond to topical therapy.
- There is no response in at least 20% of cases, especially long-standing cases.
- Once repigmentation occurs, it usually persists.

COMPLICATIONS
- Phototoxic reactions ranging from mild to severe with PUVA
- Skin atrophy and telangiectasias with topical steroids
- Contact dermatitis can occur with use of depigmenting agents and cosmetic covers.

PATIENT MONITORING
- With PUVA therapy, complete blood count, liver, renal function tests, and an antinuclear antibody should be done every 6 months.
- With topical steroids, follow at monthly intervals to avoid steroid-atrophy of the skin.

REFERENCES
1. James WD, Berger TG, Elston DM. *Andrews' Diseases of the Skin*. 10th ed. Philadephia, PA: WB Saunders; 2006: 860–863.
2. Freedberg IM, et al. *Fitzpatrick's Dermatology in General Medicine*, 6th ed. New York, NY: McGraw-Hill; 2003: 839–847.
3. Habif TP. *Clinical Dermatology*. 4th ed. New York, NY: Mosby; 2004.

MISCELLANEOUS

See also: Hyperthyroidism; Hypothyroidism, Adult; Pityriasis Alba; Tinea Versicolor

CODES

ICD9-CM
709.00 Dyschromia, unspecified

PATIENT TEACHING
- Reassure patient that in absence of associated autoimmune illness the problem is purely cosmetic. Successful cosmetic cover-up is usually quite simple. Some areas offer vitiligo support groups.
- Information available through National Vitiligo Foundation, P.O. Box 6337, Tyler, TX 75711; (903) 531-0074

 See Corresponding Diagnostic Algorithm

 See Patient Handout on CD

V

VULVAR MALIGNANCY

Michael P. Hopkins, MD, MEd
Noridelle Gilo, MD
Eric L. Jenison, MD

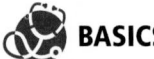 **BASICS**

DESCRIPTION
- Carcinoma in situ (Bowen disease): Premalignant changes involving the squamous epithelium of the vulva
- Squamous cell carcinoma: Invasive squamous cell carcinoma is the most common malignancy involving the vulva (85% of the patients). The malignancy can be well, moderately, or poorly differentiated.
- Other invasive cell types include melanoma, Paget disease, adenocarcinoma, adenocystic carcinoma, small cell carcinoma, and sarcomas. Sarcomas are usually leiomyosarcoma and probably arise at the insertion of the round ligament in the labium majus.
- System(s) Affected: Reproductive
- Synonym(s): Bowen disease; Vulvar cancer

ALERT
Geriatric Considerations
- Older patients with associated medical problems are at high risk for radical surgery. The surgery, however, is external, usually well tolerated, and is the treatment of choice.
- In the very elderly, palliative vulvectomy provides relief of symptoms for ulcerating symptomatic advanced disease.

Pregnancy Considerations
This malignancy is not associated with pregnancy.

GENERAL PREVENTION
- Any woman complaining of symptoms related to the vulva should have a close examination and biopsies made of appropriate areas.
- The vulva can be washed with 3% acetic acid to highlight areas. Areas of white raised epithelium should be biopsied.
- Patients with new onset of pruritus should be biopsied in the area of pruritus.
- Liberal biopsy must be used to diagnose in situ disease prior to invasion and to diagnose early invasive disease.
- The patient should not be treated for presumed benign conditions of the vulva without full examination and biopsy.
- When symptoms persist, re-examination and rebiopsy should be undertaken.
- The treatment of benign condyloma of the vulva has not been shown to decrease the eventual incidence of in situ or invasive disease of the vulva.

EPIDEMIOLOGY
- Predominant age
  - In situ disease: Mean age, 40s
  - Invasive malignancy: Mean age, 60s, with a range of 20s–90s
- Predominant sex: Female only

Incidence
In the US: Invasive vulvar malignancy is a rare gynecologic malignancy, accounting for ~2,000 new cases per year.

RISK FACTORS
- Old age: Invasive disease is rarely seen before age 40 years, and the majority of patients are elderly.
- In situ disease can occur at any age but is rarely seen before the age of 25 years.
- Human papilloma virus (HPV)
- Immunosuppression

Genetics
No known genetic pattern

ETIOLOGY
- Patients with cervical cancer are more likely to develop vulvar cancer at a later date. This is due to the so-called field effect with a carcinogen involving the lower genital tract.
- HPV has been associated with squamous cell abnormalities of the cervix, vagina, and vulva but has not been proven to be the causative agent.
- Smoking is associated with squamous cell disease of the vulva, possibly from direct irritation of the vulva by the transfer of tars and nicotine on the patient's hands or from systemic absorption of carcinogen.

ASSOCIATED CONDITIONS
- Patients with invasive vulvar cancer are often elderly and have associated medical conditions.
- High rate of other gynecologic malignancies. Patients should be evaluated for these.

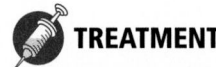 **DIAGNOSIS**

SIGNS AND SYMPTOMS
- In situ disease: A small raised area associated with pruritus
- Invasive malignancy: An ulcerated, nonhealing area; as lesions become large, bleeding occurs with associated pain and foul-smelling discharge
- In far advanced disease: The patients can develop rectal bleeding or urethral obstruction.
- Large involved inguinal lymph nodes are also associated with advanced disease.

TESTS
Lab
- Squamous cell antigen can be elevated with invasive disease.
- Hypercalcemia can occur when metastatic disease is present.

Imaging
- Chest x-ray to evaluate for metastatic disease to lungs
- CAT scan to evaluate pelvic lymph node status and periaortic lymph node status

Diagnostic Procedures/Surgery
- Office vulvar biopsy. Vulvar punch biopsy should be done to establish the diagnosis.
- Wide excision can be performed for carcinoma in situ, and any lesion about which there is doubt should be further excised for definitive diagnosis to ensure that invasive disease is not coexistent with the carcinoma in situ.
- Cystoscopy and sigmoidoscopy should be performed if there is a question of invasion into the urethra, bladder, or rectum.

Pathological Findings
- A surgical staging system is used for vulvar cancer: TNM classification = tumor, node, and metastases
  - T1: Tumor ≤2.0 cm
  - T2: Tumor >2.0 cm
  - T3: Lower urethra or vagina involved
  - T4: Upper urethra, bladder, or rectum involved
  - N0: Nodes negative
  - N1: Unilateral positive lymph nodes
  - N2: Bilateral positive lymph nodes
  - M0: No metastatic disease
  - M1: Distant metastatic disease, positive pelvic lymph node
- International Federation of Obstetrics and Gynecology Classification using TNM
  - Stage I: T1, N0, M0
    - Stage IA: T1a: < 1 mm stromal invasion
    - Stage IB: T1b: > 1 mm stromal invasion
  - Stage II: T2, N0, M0
  - Stage III: T1–3, N1, M0; T3, N0–I, M0
  - Stage IVA: T1–3, N2, M0
  - Stage IVB: Any T, any N, any M

DIFFERENTIAL DIAGNOSIS
- The definitive diagnosis for vulvar lesions is made by biopsy. Infectious processes can present as ulcerative lesions and include syphilis, lymphogranuloma venereum, and granuloma inguinale.
- Crohn disease can present as an ulcerative area on the vulva.
- Rarely, lesions can metastasize to the vulva.

TREATMENT

GENERAL MEASURES
- Appropriate health care: Inpatient for treatment
- In advanced malignancy involving the urethra and rectum, concomitant cisplatin/5-fluorouracil (5-FU) chemotherapy with radiation produces significant decrease in size of the primary tumor, usually obviating the need for pelvic exenteration.

Diet
Unrestricted, unless undergoing radiation

Activity
Patients are usually ambulatory and able to resume full activities by 6 weeks after surgery unless wound breakdown occurs.

SPECIAL THERAPY
Radiotherapy
- Radiation therapy is used as adjuvant therapy for patients with positive inguinal lymph nodes.
- Pre-operative radiation may allow for a less radical surgical procedure in patients with advanced disease. [B]
- Postoperative radiation as an adjuvant treatment in early/intermediate stage disease decreases recurrence frequency and may improve survival. [B]

MEDICATION (DRUGS)

- There are no curative drugs.
- As an adjuvant therapy, fluorouracil (Efudex) cream for in situ disease can produce occasional results, but the regimen is not well tolerated because of the excoriation and irritation of the vulva. Adjuvant chemotherapy has not proven to be effective in this disease.
- Chemoradiotherapy has been successful in limiting spread of locally advanced or recurrent disease, though local morbidity is increased.
- Metastatic disease, especially in the subcutaneous tissues of the leg or abdomen, will produce hypercalcemia, which is treated in the usual medical fashion for hypercalcemia.
- Contraindications
  - Elderly patients: If chemotherapeutic agents are used, pay close attention to the patient's performance status and ability to tolerate aggressive chemotherapy.
- Precautions: The usual precautions for chemotherapy agents. Refer to the manufacturer's literature for each drug.
- Significant possible interactions: Refer to the manufacturer's literature for each drug.

Second Line

- Surgery: In situ disease can be treated with wide excision or laser vaporization of the affected area. Laser vaporization is preferable in the younger patient, where as wide excision is preferable in the elderly patient, in whom the risk of invasive disease is also higher.
- 0.5 mm of negative margin is adequate for in situ disease.
- Invasive disease is treated primarily by radical vulvectomy and bilateral groin node dissection.
- Pelvic exenteration after radiation provides effective therapy for advanced or recurrent malignancies involving the bladder or rectum.
- More limited surgery
  - Has been undertaken for invasive lesions, especially in young patients, to preserve the clitoris and sexual function
  - Radical vulvectomy with bilateral groin node dissection through separate incisions provides better cosmetic results than the en bloc technique.
  - Radical hemivulvectomy and unilateral groin node dissection can also be utilized for smaller lesions.

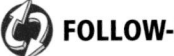 **FOLLOW-UP**

PROGNOSIS
The 5-year survival is based on stages
- Stage I: 90%
- Stage II: 85%
- Stage III: 70%
- Stage IVA: 25%
- Stage IVB: 5%

COMPLICATIONS
The major complications from radical vulvectomy and groin node dissection are wound breakdown, lymphedema, and urinary stress incontinence.

PATIENT MONITORING
- Clinical examination of the groin nodes and vulvar area every 3 months for 2 years, then every 6 months for 3 years.
- Chest x-ray should be obtained once a year.

REFERENCES
1. Cardosi RJ, Bomalaski JJ, Hoffman MS. Diagnosis and management of vulvar and vaginal intraepithelial neoplasia. *Obstet Gynecol Clin North Am*. 2001;28:685–702.
2. Montana GS. Carcinoma of the vulva: Combined modality treatment. *Curr Treat Options Oncol*. 2004;5:85–95.
3. Tyring SK. Vulvar squamous cell carcinoma: Guidelines for early diagnosis and treatment. *Am J Obstet Gynecol*. 2003;189(3 Suppl):S17–S23.
4. Hoffman MS. Squamous-cell carcinoma of the vulva: Locally advanced disease. *Best Pract Res Clin Obstet Gynaecol*. 2003;17:635–647.
5. Hopkins MP, Reid GC, Vettrano I, Morley GW. Squamous cell carcinoma of the vulva: Prognostic factors influencing survival. *Gynecol Oncol*. 1991;43:113–117.

CODES

ICD9-CM
184.4 Malignant neoplasm of vulva, unspecified

PATIENT TEACHING

- 2 complications are common with radical vulvectomy and bilateral groin node dissection.
  - In the immediate postoperative period, ~50% of patients experience breakdown of the wound. This requires aggressive wound care by visiting nurses approximately twice a day. The wounds usually granulate and heal over a period of 6–10 weeks.
  - ~15–20% of patients experience some form of mild to moderate lymphedema after the groin node dissection. These patients should be instructed in the use of leg elevation and support hose. <1% of patients experience severe, debilitating lymphedema.
- American College of Obstetricians & Gynecologists (ACOG), 409 12th St., SW, Washington, DC 20024-2188; (800) 762-ACOG
- American Cancer Society, www.cancer.org

 See Corresponding Diagnostic Algorithm

 See Patient Handout on CD

V

VULVOVAGINITIS, BACTERIAL

J. C. Chava-Zimmerman, MD

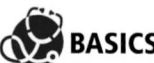

BASICS

DESCRIPTION
A syndrome in which H_2O_2–producing lactobacilli are replaced by anaerobic bacteria
- System(s) Affected: Reproductive
- Synonym(s): Gardnerella vaginosis; Bacterial vaginosis; Nonspecific vaginitis; Haemophilus vaginitis; Corynebacterium vaginitis

GENERAL PREVENTION
- Good hygiene
- Use of condoms for sexual intercourse

EPIDEMIOLOGY
Predominant sex: Female

Prevalence
- As low as 4% in unselected populations
- Up to 33% in sexually transmitted disease clinics
- Up to 44% in patients with vaginitis

RISK FACTORS
- Controversial regarding multiple sexual partners
- Intrauterine device use

ETIOLOGY
- Polymicrobial: *Gardnerella vaginalis*, *Mobiluncus* species, *Mycoplasma hominis*, *Peptostreptococcus*, other various anaerobes, including *Prevotella*, *Bacteroides*, and *Fusobacterium*
- Shift from a healthy lactobacilli-based endogenous flora to an anaerobically based endogenous flora
- Rectal reservoir of organisms leading to autoinfection

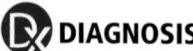

DIAGNOSIS

SIGNS AND SYMPTOMS
- Unpleasant musty or fishy vaginal odor, exacerbated immediately after intercourse
- Thin gray-white vaginal discharge, mildly adherent to vaginal walls
- 10–30% with vaginal/vulvar irritation
- 10% with frothy discharge

TESTS
Lab
- Affirm VP Microbial Identification Test
- pH paper test (pH >4.5)
- Wet prep: Clue cells in >10–20% of epithelial cells; fewer white blood cells than epithelial cells
- 10% potassium hydroxide (KOH); "whiff test"—transient but potent amine or fishy odor
- Gram stain indicating absence of lactobacilli
- May be seen on cytology
- Culture difficult for mycoplasma; not useful
- Lab results may be altered by recent douching

DIFFERENTIAL DIAGNOSIS
- Gonorrhea
- Chlamydial infection
- Trichomoniasis
- *Escherichia coli* vaginitis
- Staphylococcal vaginitis
- Fungal vaginitis
- Atrophic vaginitis

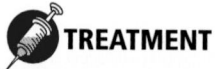

TREATMENT

INITIAL STABILIZATION
Outpatient treatment

GENERAL MEASURES
Consider repletion of lactobacilli.

Diet
No restrictions

Activity
No restrictions

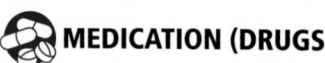

MEDICATION (DRUGS)

First Line
- Metronidazole (Flagyl): 500 mg PO 2 b.i.d. for 7 days, or
- Metronidazole vaginal gel: 0.75% 5 g intravaginally daily for 7 days, or
- Clindamycin: 2% vaginal cream 5 g intravaginally daily for 7 days
- Contraindications: Refer to the manufacturer's literature.
- Precautions: Refer to the manufacturer's literature.
- Significant possible interactions: Metronidazole and alcohol

ALERT

Pregnancy Considerations
All symptomatic women and those who have had preterm delivery should be treated. Avoid creams; Metronidazole 250 mg PO t.i.d. for 7 days or clindamycin 300 mg PO 2 b.i.d. for 7 days

Second Line
- Metronidazole: 2 g PO single dose
- Clindamycin: 300 mg PO daily for 7 days
- Clindamycin ovules: 100 g intravaginally at bedtime for 3 days (clindamycin creams are less effective than metronidazole)

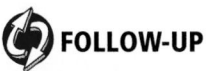 **FOLLOW-UP**

PROGNOSIS

Relapses are fairly common; may be decreased by increased colonization of lactobacilli

COMPLICATIONS

- Uncommon but include:
  - Adnexal tenderness
  - Pelvic inflammatory disease (PID)
  - Intrauterine infections
  - Chorioamnionitis
  - Postabortion PID
  - Postpartum endometritis
  - Pelvic abscesses
  - Vaginitis emphysematosa
  - Rare extravaginal disease
  - Preterm labor
  - Premature rupture of membranes
  - Chorioamnionitis
  - Newborn infections, including scalp electrode sites, abscesses, and one reported case of meningitis
  - Fetal loss
- Posthysterectomy infection, septicemia, gaseous crepitation in wound

PATIENT MONITORING

None indicated

REFERENCES

1. Briselden AM, Hillier SL. Evaluation of affirm VP microbial identification test for *Gardnerella vaginalis* and *Trichomonas vaginalis*. *J Clin Microbiol*. 1994;32:148–152.
2. Caitlin BW. *Gardnerella vaginalis*: Characteristics, clinical considerations and controversies. *Clin Microbiol Rev*. 1992;5:213–217.
3. Centers for Disease Control and Prevention. Sexually transmitted diseases treatment guidelines, 2002. *MMWR Recomm Rep*. 2002;51(RR-06):1–80.
4. Curry SL, Barclay DL. Benign disorders of the vulva-vagina. In: DeCherney AH, Perroll ML, eds. *Current Obstetric and Gynecologic Diagnosis and Treatment*. 8th ed. Norwalk, CT: Appleton & Lang; 1994.
5. Herbst A, Mishell D Jr, Stenchever A, Droegemueller W. *Comprehensive Gynecology*. 2nd ed. St. Louis, MO: Mosby-Year Book; 1992.
6. Kharsany AB, Hosen AA, Vanden Ende J. Antimicrobial susceptibility of Gardnerella vaginalis. *Antimicrob Agents Chemother*. 1993;37:2733–2735.
7. Majeroni BA. Bacterial vaginosis: An update. *Am Fam Physician*. 1998;57:1285–1289.
8. Ray A, Gulati AK, Pandey LK, Pandey S. Non-specific vaginitis vis-a-vis Gardnerella vaginalis. *J Commun Dis*. 1990;22:274–276.
9. Reed B, Eyler A. Vaginal infections: Diagnosis and management. *Am Fam Physician*. 1993;47:1805–1818.

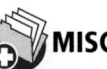 **MISCELLANEOUS**

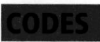 **CODES**

ICD9-CM
616.10 Vaginitis and vulvovaginitis, unspecified

 See Corresponding Diagnostic Algorithm

 See Patient Handout on CD

V

VULVOVAGINITIS, CANDIDAL

Martha H. McLoughlin, MD

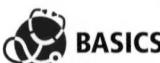 **BASICS**

DESCRIPTION
Vulvar pruritus and/or burning, often with abnormal vaginal discharge
- System(s) Affected: Reproductive; Skin/Exocrine
- Synonym(s): Monilial vulvovaginitis

GENERAL PREVENTION
- Follow instructions under "Patient Teaching".
- For recurrences, consider reinfection from sexual partner(s). Examine and treat the sex partner for *Candida balanitis* and oral *Candida* if vaginitis recurs.
- Review "Risk Factors."

EPIDEMIOLOGY
- Predominant age: Menarche to menopause
- Predominant sex: Female only

Prevalence
- 10–20% of nonpregnant premenopausal women are asymptomatic carriers
- Common in pregnancy

ALERT
Pediatric Considerations
Less common before puberty

RISK FACTORS
- Pregnancy
- Diabetes mellitus
- Antibiotic therapy
- Corticosteroid therapy
- Immunosuppressed states
- HIV infection
- Occlusive synthetic underpants and undergarments
- Hypothyroidism
- Oral contraceptive medications (low dose formulations usually not a cause of increased infection risk)
- Anemia
- Zinc deficiency
- Other contraceptives: Sponge, diaphragms, intrauterine devices

ETIOLOGY
- 40% of vulvovaginitis is caused by *Candida*.
- Overgrowth of *Candida* species (*C. albicans, C. glabrata, C. tropicalis*) in vagina

ASSOCIATED CONDITIONS
Sexually transmitted diseases

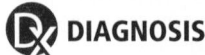 **DIAGNOSIS**

SIGNS AND SYMPTOMS
- Intense vulvar pruritis
- Thick curdlike vaginal discharge
- Dyspareunia at times
- Erythema and/or edema of vulva
- Erythema, pain, and pruritus of crural and perineal area
- Thick white patches appear attached to vaginal mucosa.
- Inflamed vulvar skin

TESTS
Lab
- Yeast, spores, and/or pseudohyphae on smear with 10% potassium hydroxide (KOH) solution
- Vaginal pH <4.5
- Culture findings on Nickerson or Sabouraud medium; usually only indicated for recurrent infections
- Pap smear

DIFFERENTIAL DIAGNOSIS
- *Trichomonas* vaginitis
- Gonorrheal vaginitis—in prepubertal girls
- Pinworm vaginitis
- Contact dermatitis/vaginitis
- Allergic vulvitis/hypersensitivity
- Mechanical/chemical irritation

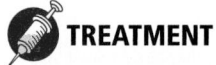 **TREATMENT**

INITIAL STABILIZATION
Outpatient treatment

GENERAL MEASURES
- Remove foreign body if one present
- Consider recommending that the patient use a povidone-iodine (Betadine, Operand) douche (15–30 mL/L [2 tbsp/qt] of water) for symptomatic relief until the specific therapy is effective.
- If urination causes burning, have the patient
  - Urinate through a tubular device such as a toilet-paper roll or plastic cup with the end cut out
  - Pour warm water over vaginal area while urinating
- Insist on strict diabetic control if patient is diabetic.

Diet
Limit sweets (sucrose) and dairy products (lactose for a patient with recurrent infections.

Activity
- Avoid overexertion, heat, and excessive sweating.
- Delay sexual relations until the symptoms clear/discomfort resolves.

MEDICATION (DRUGS)

First Line
- Fluconazole (Diflucan): 150 mg PO once; use with caution in patients with liver disease.
- Miconazole nitrate (Monistat): 1 200 mg suppository at bedtime for 3 days or miconazole vaginal cream at bedtime for 7 days, or
- Butoconazole nitrate (Femstat): 2% vaginal cream at bedtime for 3 days, or
- Terconazole (Terazol): 1 suppository or 0.8% vaginal cream at bedtime for 3 days, or
- Clotrimazole (Gyne-Lotrimin): 2 100 mg tablets intravaginally for 3 days or cream at bedtime for 7–14 days
- Significant possible interactions: Refer to the manufacturer's profile of each drug.

Second Line
- Retreat with different agent, if recurrence
- Course of oral nystatin; 100,000 units t.i.d. for 2 weeks
- Topical gentian violet 1% aqueous solution painted onto vagina weekly until infection resolves (usually 2–3 weeks)
- Boric acid 600 mg in gelatin capsule inserted vaginally daily for 2 weeks

ALERT
Pregnancy Considerations
Oral azoles are contraindicated in pregnancy. A topical azole may be used with no adverse outcomes.

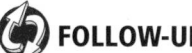 **FOLLOW-UP**

PROGNOSIS
- Complete cure with vigorous treatment
- Recurrences are common.

COMPLICATIONS
Secondary bacterial infections of the vagina or vulva

PATIENT MONITORING
Generally no specific follow-up is needed. If symptoms persist, repeat pelvic exam and culture.

REFERENCES

1. Fong IW. The value of treating the sexual partners of women with recurrent vaginal candidiasis with ketoconazole. *Genitourin Med*. 1992;68:174.
2. Jones HW, Wentz-Colston A, eds. *Novak's Textbook of Gynecology*.11th ed. Baltimore, MD: Williams & Wilkins Co.; 1988.
3. Kaufman RH, Faro S, eds. *Benign Diseases of the Vulva and Vagina*.4th ed. St. Louis, MO: Mosby-Year Book; 1994.
4. National guideline for the management of vulvovaginal candidiasis. *Sex Transm Infect*. 1999;75(Suppl 1):S19.
5. Sobel J. Vulvovaginitis, when candida becomes a problem. *Clin Dermatol*. 1998;16:763–769.
6. Spinillo A, Carratta L, Pizzoli G. Recurrent vaginal candidiasis. *J Reprod Med*. 1992;37:343.

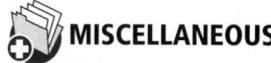 **MISCELLANEOUS**

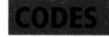 **CODES**

ICD9-CM
112.1 Candidiasis of vulva and vagina

PATIENT TEACHING
American College of Obstetricians & Gynecologists (ACOG), 409 12th St., SW, Washington, DC 20024-2188; (800) 762-ACOG

Prevention
- Keep the genital area clean; use plain, unscented soap.
- Take showers rather than tub baths.
- Wear cotton underpants with a cotton crotch. Avoid clothing made from nonventilating materials, including most synthetic underclothing. Avoid tight-fitting jeans or pants.
- Sleep in loose gown without underpants.
- Avoid prolonged wear of wet clothing, especially a wet bathing suit.
- Avoid frequent douches.
- Avoid broad-spectrum antibiotics, when possible.
- After urinating or bowel movements, cleanse by wiping or washing from front to back (vagina toward anus).
- Lose weight, if obese, and maintain euglycemia in diabetic patients.

 See Corresponding Diagnostic Algorithm

 See Patient Handout on CD

V

VULVOVAGINITIS, ESTROGEN DEFICIENT

Michael P. Hopkins, MD, Med
Jamie Byler, MD
Eric L. Jenison, MD

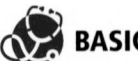 BASICS

DESCRIPTION
- Decreased blood flow with thinning and atrophy of the female genital tissue
- Changes from estrogen deficiency occur throughout the body; the genital tissues are especially hormone responsive.
- Estrogen-deficient vulvovaginitis is frequently associated with urinary incontinence.
- System(s) Affected: Reproductive

EPIDEMIOLOGY
- Predominant age: Predominantly a problem of the postmenopausal female. The average age of menopause in the US is 52.5 years.
- Predominant sex: Female only

Prevalence
This disorder will affect all women to some degree unless estrogen replacement therapy (ERT) is provided.

RISK FACTORS
- Estrogen-deficient states accompanying metabolic disorders
- Vaginal infections with bacteria and fungi

Genetics
No known pattern

ETIOLOGY
Estrogen deficiency due to
- Menopause (surgical or natural)
- Ovariectomy
- Radiation of the pelvis

ASSOCIATED CONDITIONS
- Incontinence
- Pelvic organ prolapse
- Frequent urinary tract infections

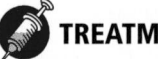 DIAGNOSIS

SIGNS AND SYMPTOMS
- Vaginal dryness
- Decreased vaginal secretions
- Dyspareunia
- Vulva undergoes a thinning of the epidermis along with decreased integrity of the supporting structures; the thinning and atrophy often produce pruritus.
- Obese patients, especially those weighing > 100 lb (45 kg) over an ideal body weight, have higher levels of circulating estrogen and thus may have fewer symptoms. (Androstenedione is converted to estrone in peripheral adipose tissue, and when there is an abundance of adipose, higher estrone levels are present.)

Physical Exam
Examination of the vagina and the vulva for maturation index

TESTS
Lab
- Cytology for maturation index will show a low maturation index, signifying a decreased turnover of the cells from the decreased estrogen effect.
- Check the follicle-stimulating hormone (FSH) level to confirm menopause. In the perimenopausal or menopausal female, FSH will be elevated and estradiol will be decreased.
- Estradiol level to evaluate circulating estrogen level
- Drugs that may alter lab results
  - Estrogen therapy will alter the maturation index.
  - Digoxin has estrogenlike properties.
  - Tamoxifen (Nolvadex) may produce menopausal-type symptoms, but may also act on genital tissues as a weak estrogen agonist. Symptoms may vary.
  - Drugs used to treat endometriosis or uterine bleeding, such as progestins, danazol, or gonadotropin-releasing hormone agonists, may produce a pseudomenopause, which is reversible.

Pathological Findings
Thinning of the cornified squamous layer of both the vulva and the vagina

DIFFERENTIAL DIAGNOSIS
- Malignancy
- Vulvar dystrophies

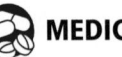 TREATMENT

INITIAL STABILIZATION
Outpatient treatment

GENERAL MEASURES
- ERT will alleviate and reverse the symptoms and the thinning of the squamous epithelial layer. Replacement therapy leads to an increased blood supply to the genital tissues.
- OTC vaginal lubricants
- Symptomatic relief if needed, e.g., cool baths or compresses

Diet
No special diet

Activity
No restriction

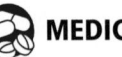 MEDICATION (DRUGS)

First Line (1,2)[A]
- A wide variety of preparations are available.
- Progesterone should be used in women with an intact uterus when given estrogen to decrease risk of endometrial carcinoma.
  - Estrogen, conjugated: 0.625 mg/d
  - Estradiol: 1 mg/d
  - Estradiol patch: 0.05 mg, changed twice weekly
  - Estrogen vaginal preparations
    ○ Cream
    ○ Tablet
    ○ Ring
- Contraindications
  - Estrogen therapy is contraindicated in patients with a history of breast cancer with estrogen-positive tumor receptors.
  - Undiagnosed uterine bleeding
  - A history of uterine malignancy is a relative contraindication.
- Precautions: Refer to the manufacturer's literature.
- Significant possible interactions: Refer to the manufacturer's literature.

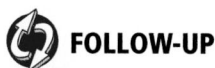 **FOLLOW-UP**

PROGNOSIS

The prognosis is excellent. The vast majority of symptoms will be relieved with ERT.

COMPLICATIONS (2)[A]

Those associated with estrogen replacement
- Postmenopausal bleeding
- Nausea
- Headache
- Libido changes
- Thrombophlebitis
- Thromboembolic events (coronary, stroke)
- Breast cancer
- Gallbladder disease
- Uterine cancer

PATIENT MONITORING

The patient should be instructed that symptoms should resolve within 30–60 days. If they do not, reevaluation and reexamination for other causes should be undertaken.

REFERENCES

1. Suckling J, Lethaby A, Kennedy R. Local oestrogen for vaginal atrophy in postmenopausal women. *Cochrane Database Syst Rev.* 2003;4:CD001500.
2. Farquhar CM, et al. Cochrane HT Study Group. Long term hormone therapy for perimenopausal and postmenopausal women. *Cochrane Database Syst Rev.* 2005;3:CD004143.

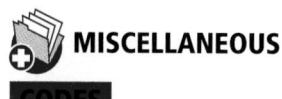 **MISCELLANEOUS**

CODES

ICD9-CM

616.10 Vaginitis and vulvovaginitis, unspecified

PATIENT TEACHING

- American College of Obstetricians and Gynecologists (ACOG), 409 12th St., SW, Washington, DC 20024-2188; (800) 762-ACOG
- Lactating postpartum women with high levels of prolactin are in a hypoestrogenic state. These women should be instructed to use lubrication for symptoms of dyspareunia. The symptoms will resolve when breast-feeding is stopped.

 See Corresponding Diagnostic Algorithm

 See Patient Handout on CD

V

VULVOVAGINITIS, PREPUBESCENT

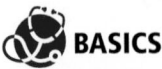

Theresa N. Grabo, PhD, APRN, BC, FNP

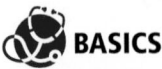

BASICS

DESCRIPTION
- Irritation and/or inflammation of the vulva and/or vagina, associated with vaginal discharge
- In children, the vulva usually becomes inflamed first, with the vagina either not involved, or affected secondarily.
- System(s) Affected: Reproductive; Skin/exocrine
- Synonym(s): Vaginitis; Vulvitis

ALERT
Pediatric Considerations
- Usual adult vulvitis/vaginitis organisms are rare in the prepubertal child.
- Lack of estrogen causes thin vaginal mucosa, which is more susceptible to trauma and infection.

GENERAL PREVENTION
- Perineal hygiene
- Avoidance of irritants and tight or occlusive, nonbreathable clothing
- White, unscented toilet paper

EPIDEMIOLOGY
- Predominant age: Toddlers to menarche
- Predominant sex: Female only

Incidence
Unknown

Prevalence
Common in the US

RISK FACTORS
- Coexisting pharyngitis or other systemic conditions
- Faulty hygiene
- Trauma

Genetics
Not well studied

ETIOLOGY
- Most often due to
  - Poor hygiene, may lead to labial agglutination
  - Primary infection elsewhere (e.g., otitis media, pharyngitis)
- Most common specific organisms
  - Group A α-hemolytic streptococci; *Streptococcus pyogenes*, *S. pneumoniae*
  - *Escherichia coli*
  - *Staphylococcus aureus*
  - *Haemophilus influenzae*
- Less common specific organisms
  - Pinworms
  - *Sarcoptes scabiei* (scabies)
  - *Candida* spp: most common with immunocompromised, antibiotic therapy, or diapers
  - *Shigella flexneri*
- Systemic illnesses
  - Measles
  - Chickenpox
  - Stevens-Johnson syndrome
  - Inflammatory conditions (e.g., Reiter syndrome)

- Localized vulvar disease
  - Seborrheic dermatitis
  - Psoriasis
  - Atopic dermatitis
  - Contact dermatitis
  - Lichen sclerosus et atrophicus
- Other
  - Urethral prolapse
  - Ectopic ureter
  - Sexual abuse (gonorrhea, chlamydia, trichomoniasis, herpes). In 1 study, 4% of girls not suspected to have sexual abuse had positive cultures for gonorrhea.
  - Other trauma
  - Foreign body
  - Tumors or polyps
  - Masturbation
  - Genital tract malformations
  - Polyps or tumors

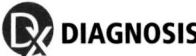

DIAGNOSIS

SIGNS AND SYMPTOMS
- Irritation and erythema of vulva
- Vaginal discharge
- Unpleasant odor
- Itching
- Excoriation of the genital area
- Bleeding
- Dysuria
- Inflammation of the introitus
- Soreness

Physical Exam
- See "Diagnostic Procedures."
- Look for evidence of chronic illness or dermatologic disease
- Inspection of the genital area in the supine position
- Inspection of the vagina and cervix in the knee-chest position
- Rectal examination if vaginal bleeding or abdominal pain

TESTS
Lab
- Culture for bacteria, fungi, or viruses
- Gram stain
- Tape examination for pinworms
- Potassium hydroxide and saline smears
- Special tests: Exploration of vagina for foreign body may be necessary in long-standing foul vaginal discharge.

Diagnostic Procedures/Surgery
Visualization of the vagina may be necessary using a nasal speculum or infant laryngoscope. If blood or foul-smelling discharge is present, visualization is mandatory. Place child in knee-chest position for best result. Hold buttocks apart and slightly upward.

DIFFERENTIAL DIAGNOSIS
- Contact dermatitis
- Eczema
- Psoriasis
- *Shigella* vulvovaginitis

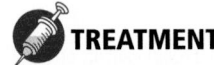

TREATMENT

GENERAL MEASURES
- Appropriate health care: Outpatient (except where systemic illness requires hospital care)
- Hygiene
  - Wipe front-to-back after elimination.
  - Avoid bubble baths and other irritating products.
  - Clean daily with mild soap and water and dry gently with soft towel or cool hair dryer.
  - Apply bland ointments for protection of the skin, if necessary.

Diet
Healthy balanced diet, high in fiber to prevent constipation; adequate fluid intake.

Activity
Normal with regular exercise

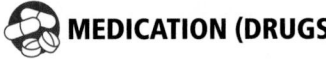

MEDICATION (DRUGS)

First Line
- For empiric treatment, amoxicillin 20 mg/kg/d for 7 days; in areas of high prevalence of resistant *H. influenzae*, amoxicillin–clavulanate (Augmentin) 20 mg/kg/d
- Estrogen deficiency with labial adhesion/agglutination: Estrogen, conjugated cream to fused area nightly for 2 weeks
- Specific organisms on culture
  - Group A -streptococcus, *Streptococcus pneumoniae*: Penicillin V (Pen Vee K) 25–50 mg/kg/d, maximum of 3 g/d, divided q.i.d., for 10 days
  - *H. influenzae*: Amoxicillin 20–40 mg/kg/d for 7 days; amoxicillin–clavulanate 20 mg/kg/d
  - *Staphylococcus aureus*: Cephalexin 25–50 mg/kg/d, divided q.i.d., for 7–10 days; *or* dicloxacillin 12.5–25 mg/kg/d for 7–10 days
  - *Candida* spp: Topical nystatin (Mycostatin), miconazole, clotrimazole, or terconazole
- Contraindications: Allergy to proposed treatment
- Precautions: Avoid potential allergens and topical sensitizers if possible.
- Significant possible interactions: See the manufacturer's profile for each drug.

Second Line
Topical corticosteroids for pruritus; avoid long-term use

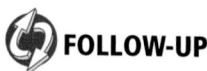 **FOLLOW-UP**

Recurring vulvovaginitis that does not respond to treatment should be referred to a specialist for further evaluation

PROGNOSIS
Usually clears with appropriate treatment with no permanent sequelae (if not due to underlying disease such as psoriasis, etc.)

COMPLICATIONS
Labial agglutination or adhesions

PATIENT MONITORING
Only if symptoms do not respond to treatment

REFERENCES
1. Jones R. Childhood vulvovaginitis and vaginal discharge in general practice. *Fam Pract*. 1996;13(4):369–372.
2. Paek SC, Merritt D, Mallory SB. Pruritus vulvae in prepubertal children. *J Am Acad Dermatol*. 2001;44:795–802.
3. Pierce AM, Hart CA. Vulvovaginitis: Causes and management. *Arch Dis Child*. 1992;67:509–512.
4. Shapiro RA, Schubert CJ, Siegel RM. Neisseria gonorrhea infections in girls younger than 12 years of age evaluated for vaginitis. *Pediatrics*. 1999;104(6):e72.
5. Vandeven AM, Emans SJ. Vulvovaginitis in the child and adolescent. *Pediatr Rev*. 1993;14:141–147.
6. Jasper JM, Ward MA. Shigella vulvovaginitis in a prepubertal child. *Pediatr Emerg Care*. 2006;22(8):585–6. (3) [C].
7. Emans SJ, Goldstein DP. Pediatrics. The gynecologic examination of the prepubertal child with vulvovaginitis: Use of the knee-chest position. *Pediatrics*. 1980;65(4):758–760.
8. Joishy M, Ashtekar CS, Jain A, Gonsalves R. Do we need to treat vulvovaginitis in prepubertal girls? *Br Med J*. 2005;22:330(7484):186–188.
9. Stricker T, Navratil F, Sennhauser FH. *BMJ*. 2002. *Archives of Disease in Childhood*. 2003;88:324–326. (2) [B].

ADDITIONAL READING
• Sultan C, ed. Pediatric and adolescent gynecology. evidence-based clinical practice. *Endocr Dev*. 2004;7:1–8.
• Farrington PF. Pediatric Vulvo-Vaginitis. Clinical Obstetrics & Gynecology. Thyroid Diseases in Pregnancy.1997;40(1):135–140.
• Merkley K. Vulvovaginitis and vaginal discharge in the pediatric patient. *J Emerg Nurs*. 2005;31(4):400–402.

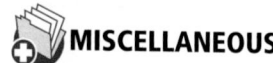 **MISCELLANEOUS**

 CODES

ICD9-CM
616.10 Vaginitis and vulvovaginitis, unspecified

PATIENT TEACHING
See "General Measures."

 See Corresponding Diagnostic Algorithm

 See Patient Handout on CD

V

WARTS

Herbert P. Goodheart, MD

BASICS

DESCRIPTION

Warts (verrucae) are benign growths that are confined to the epidermis. All warts are caused by the human papillomavirus (HPV).

- Warts often vary widely in shape, size, and appearance, and the different names for them generally reflect their clinical appearance, location, or both.
- For example, filiform warts are threadlike, planar warts are flat, and plantar warts are located on the soles of the feet.
- Genital warts, or *condyloma acuminatum*, may be large and cauliflowerlike, or they may consist of small papules.
- 5 types of warts are caused by specific genotypes of HPV
  - Common wart (*verruca vulgaris*)
  - Plantar wart (*verruca plantaris*)
  - Flat wart (*verruca plana*)
  - Venereal wart (*condyloma acuminatum*); see separate topic in this volume
- Epidermodysplasia verruciformis is a very rare, lifelong, hereditary disorder characterized by chronic infection with HPV.
- System(s) Affected: Skin/Exocrine

EPIDEMIOLOGY

- Predominant age: Young adults and children
- Predominant sex: Female = Male

Incidence

An estimated 20% of school-age children will at some time have at least one wart.

Prevalence

- ~7–10% of the US population
- Common warts appear ~2 times as frequently in whites as in African Americans or Asians.

RISK FACTORS

- AIDS and other immunosuppressive diseases (e.g., lymphomas)
- Immunosuppressive drugs that decrease cell-mediated immunity (e.g., prednisone, cyclosporine, and chemotherapeutic agents)
- Pregnancy
- Handling raw meat, fish, or other types of animal matter in one's occupation, e.g., butchers

ETIOLOGY

- Various strains of a DNA HPV virus: To date, >150 different subtypes have been identified.
- Common warts: HPV types 2 and 4 (most common), followed by types 1, 3, 27, 29, and 57
- Palmoplantar warts: HPV type 1 (most common), followed by types 2, 3, 4, 27, 29, and 57
- Flat warts: HPV types 3, 10, and 28
- Butcher warts: HPV type 7
- The virus is passed primarily through skin-to-skin contact or from the recently shed virus kept intact in a moist, warm environment.
- HPV infects epidermal keratinocytes, which stimulates cell proliferation.

DIAGNOSIS

- Most often made on clinical appearance
- Skin biopsy, if necessary

SIGNS AND SYMPTOMS

Common wart: Rough-surfaced, hyperkeratotic, papillomatous, raised, skin-colored to tan papules 5–10 mm in diameter; may coalesce into a mosaic 1–3 cm in diameter

- Most frequently seen on hands, knees, and elbows
- Usually asymptomatic, but may cause cosmetic disfigurement or tenderness

Variant

- Filiform warts: These are long, slender, delicate, fingerlike growths, usually seen on the face around the lips, eyelids, or nares.
- Plantar warts appear on the plantar surface of the feet in children and young adults.
  - Can be tender and painful, and extensive involvement on the sole of the foot may impair ambulation, particularly when present on a weight-bearing surface
  - Most often seen on the metatarsal area, heels, and toes in an asymmetric distribution
  - Frequently attain 2–3 cm in diameter
  - Pathognomonic "black dots" (thrombosed dermal capillaries). Punctate bleeding becomes more evident after paring with a #15 blade.
  - Both common and plantar warts generally demonstrate the following clinical findings:
  - A loss of normal skin markings (dermatoglyphics) such as finger, foot, and hand prints
  - Lesions may be solitary or multiple, or they may appear in clusters (mosaic warts)
- Flat wart: Slightly elevated, flat-topped, skin-colored or tan papules, small (1–3 mm) in diameter
  - Commonly found on the face, arms, dorsa of hands, shins (women)
  - Sometimes exhibit a linear configuration caused by autoinoculation
  - In men, shaving spreads flat warts
  - In women, they often occur on the shins, where leg shaving spreads lesions.
- Epidermodysplasia verruciformis: Widespread flat, reddish-brown pigmented papules and plaques that present in childhood with lifelong persistence on the trunk, the hands, the upper and lower extremities, and the face, are characteristic.
  - Lesions may transform into carcinomas, usually after age 30 years. Skin cancers initially appear on sun-exposed areas.

Physical Exam

Warts may develop anywhere on the body, but they are most often found at sites subject to frequent trauma, such as the hands and feet.

- Distribution is generally asymmetric, and lesions are often clustered.

TESTS

Lab

- HPV cannot be cultured.
- Definitive diagnosis can be achieved by
  - Electron microscopy
  - Viral DNA identification using Southern blot hybridization used to identify the specific HPV type present in tissue
  - Polymerase chain reaction may be used to amplify viral DNA for testing.

Pathological Findings

- Histopathologic features of common warts include digitated epidermal hyperplasia, acanthosis, papillomatosis, compact orthokeratosis, hypergranulosis, dilated tortuous capillaries within the dermal papillae, and vertical tiers of parakeratotic cells with entrapped red blood cells above the tips of the digitations.
- In the granular layer, HPV-infected cells may have coarse keratohyaline granules and vacuoles surrounding wrinkled-appearing nuclei. These koilocytic (vacuolated) cells are pathognomonic for warts.

DIFFERENTIAL DIAGNOSIS

Pediatric

Molluscum contagiosum

Adults/Elderly

- Seborrheic keratosis
- Acrochordon (skin tag)
- Solar keratosis and cutaneous horn
- Squamous cell carcinoma
- Keratoacanthoma
- Subungual squamous cell carcinoma can easily be misdiagnosed as a subungual wart or onychomycosis.
- Plantar warts
- Corns (*clavi*) are sometimes difficult to distinguish from warts. Like calluses, corns are thickened areas of the skin and most commonly develop at sites subjected to repeated friction and pressure, such as the tops and the tips of toes and along the sides of the feet.
  - They are usually hard and circular-shaped, with a polished or central translucent core, like the kernel of corn from which they take their name.
  - Corns do not have "black dots," and skin markings are retained except for the area of the central core.

ALERT

- Melanoma can mimic a plantar wart.
- Verrucous carcinoma, a slow growing, locally invasive, well-differentiated squamous cell carcinoma, may also be easily mistaken for a common or plantar wart.

TREATMENT

GENERAL MEASURES

- The clinical management of verrucae vulgaris is often challenging, and there is no ideal treatment.
- In children, most warts tend to regress spontaneously, which is probably related to a host immune response.
- In many adults and immunocompromised patients, however, warts often prove difficult to eradicate.
- Painful, aggressive therapy should be avoided unless there is a pressing need to eliminate the wart(s).
- For surgical procedures, especially in anxious children, pretreatment with anesthetic cream such as EMLA (emulsion of lidocaine and prilocaine):
  - Benign neglect: Providing no treatment at all is certainly safe and cost effective as most may regress spontaneously within 2 years.
  - If warts are extensive, spreading, or symptomatic, the method of treatment will depend upon the age of the patient, the patient's pain threshold, the type of wart, and its location.
  - A cure is achieved when the skin lines are restored to a normal pattern and there is no recurrence.

Complementary and Alternative Medicine

- Occlusion: Easiest and least expensive. Cover wart with waterproof tape (e.g., duct tape) and leave on for 6 days, then soak, pare with emery board, leave uncovered overnight, then reapply tape cyclically for 8 cycles
- Hyperthermia: Safe and inexpensive approach; immerse affected area into 45°C water bath for 30 minutes 3 times per week

ALERT

Pregnancy Considerations

- The use of many of the following topical chemical approaches may be contraindicated during pregnancy or in women who are likely to become pregnant during the treatment period.
- Refer to the manufacturer's profile of each drug.

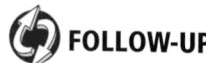 **MEDICATION (DRUGS)**

First Line

The abundance of treatment modalities described below is a reflection of the fact that none of them is uniformly effective.

- Keratolytic (peeling) agents, primarily containing salicylic or salicylic acid plus lactic acid, are available in numerous OTC preparations that are self-administered. Best treatment for small children in whom warts are usually self-limiting. For best results and increased penetration with any of following keratolytic agents, the affected area should be hydrated 1st by soaking it in warm water for 5 minutes before application.
- Duofilm
- Occlusal-HP
- Trans-Ver-Sal
  - Office-based and prescription treatment
- Combination cantharidin; 30% salicylic acid, 2% podophyllin, and 19% cantharidin in flexible collodion: Applied in a thin coat, occluded 4–6 hours, then washed off

- Aldara (imiquimod) 5% cream, a local inducer of interferon, is applied at home by the patient. It is approved for external genital and perianal warts and is used "off-label" and applied under duct tape occlusion applied at bedtime and washed off after 6–10 hours.
- Aldara is applied to flat warts without occlusion.

Second Line

Immunotherapy: Induction of delayed-type hypersensitivity with

- Diphencyprone
- Dinitrochlorobenzene (DNCB)
- Squaric acid dibutylester (SADBE)
- Possible mutagenicity and side effects with these agents
- Bleomycin: Intradermal injection is expensive and causes severe pain.
  - Alpha-2 interferon
  - Intralesional mumps or candida antigen
  - Oral high dose cimetidine: Possibly works better in children
  - Topical retinoids for facial flat warts
  - Acitretin (an oral retinoid)
  - Others: Dichloroacetic acid, trichloroacetic acid, podophyllin, formic acid, 5-fluorouracil, silver nitrate, formaldehyde, levamisole, topical or IV cidofovir for recalcitrant warts in the setting of HIV, glutaraldehyde, have all been used with varying results

SURGERY

- Duct tape: Cover wart with waterproof tape (e.g., duct tape) and leave on for 6 days, then soak, pare with emery board, leave uncovered overnight, then reapply tape cyclically for 8 cycles; 85% resolved compared to 60% efficacy with cryotherapy
- Cryotherapy with liquid nitrogen (LN2) may be applied with a cotton swab or with a cryotherapy gun (Cryogun).
  - Best for warts on hands.
  - Fast; can treat many lesions per visit.
  - Painful; not tolerated well by young children
  - Freezing periungual warts may result in nail deformation.
  - In darkly pigmented skin, treatment can result in hypo- or hyperpigmentation.
- Light electrocautery with or without curettage:
  - Best for warts on the knees, elbows, and dorsa of hands
  - Also good for filiform warts
  - Tolerable in most adults
  - Requires local anesthesia
  - May cause scarring
- Photodynamic therapy
- CO$_2$ or pulse-dye laser ablation: Expensive and requires local anesthesia
- Filifarm warts
  - An almost painless method is to dip a hemostat into LN2 for 10 seconds and then gently grasp the wart for ~5–10 seconds. The frozen wart is generally shed in 7–10 days.

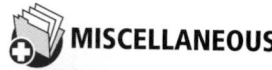 **FOLLOW-UP**

COMPLICATIONS

- Autoinoculation ("pseudo Koebner") reaction
- Scar formation
- Chronic pain after plantar wart removal or scar formation
- Nail deformity after injury to nail matrix

PATIENT MONITORING

One third of the warts of epidermodysplasia may become malignant.

REFERENCES

1. Micali G et al. Use of squaric acid dibutylester (SADBE) for cutaneous warts in children. *Pediatr Dermatol.* 2000;17:315–318.
2. Rogers J, et al. Cimetidine therapy for recalcitrant warts in adults: Is it any better than placebo? *J Am Acad Dermatol.* 1999;41:123–127.
3. Robson KJ, et al. Pulsed-dye laser versus conventional therapy in the treatment of warts: A prospective randomized trial. *J Am Acad Dermatol.* 2000;43(2 pt 1):275–280.
4. Silverberg NB, Lim JK, Paller AS, Mancini AJ. Squaric acid immunotherapy for warts in children. *J Am Acad Dermatol.* 2000;42(5 pt 1):803–808.
5. Stender IM et. al. Photodynamic therapy with 5-aminolevulinic acid or placebo for recalcitrant foot and hand warts: Randomized double-blind trial. *Lancet.* 2000;355:963–966.

 MISCELLANEOUS

CODES

ICD9-CM

078.10 Viral warts, unspecified

PATIENT TEACHING

More often than not (especially in children), warts tend to "cure" themselves over time.

See Corresponding Diagnostic Algorithm

 See Patient Handout on CD

W

WARTS, PLANTAR

Gary J. Silko, MD, MS

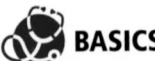 BASICS

DESCRIPTION
- Discrete or grouped firm keratotic masses on the sole of the foot initiated by a viral infection of keratinocytes
- System(s) Affected: Skin/Exocrine
- Synonym(s): Verruca plantaris

ALERT
Pediatric Considerations
Duration of warts is generally shorter in children than in adults.

Pregnancy Considerations
Avoid bleomycin treatments.

GENERAL PREVENTION
Use rubber footwear in communal shower areas.

EPIDEMIOLOGY
- Predominant age: Any age, although more common in children and young adults
- Predominant sex: Female > Male (slightly)

Incidence
In the US: Widespread; 2,000/100,000

RISK FACTORS
- AIDS
- Atopic dermatitis
- Lymphomas
- Patient taking immunosuppressive drugs

Genetics
Unknown

ETIOLOGY
Human papillomavirus type 1; less commonly types 2, 4, 27, and 57

DIAGNOSIS

TESTS
- Foot pain
- Discrete or grouped masses on sole of foot with disruption of normal skin markings
- Generally occur at pressure points
- Rough, hyperkeratotic surface with brown-black dots (thrombosed capillaries)
- Callus formation
- Leg or back pain (distortion of posture)

Diagnostic Procedures/Surgery
- Inspection usually confirms the diagnosis.
- If cannot distinguish between callus and wart, can examine with a magnifying lens. The wart should demonstrate a highly organized mosaic pattern.
- When pared down, have a soft central core and bleeding points (unlike calluses)

Pathological Findings
Acanthotic epidermis with hyperkeratosis, papillomatosis, and parakeratosis

DIFFERENTIAL DIAGNOSIS
- Corns (clavi)
- Calluses
- Black heel (ruptured capillaries)

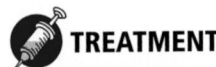 TREATMENT

INITIAL STABILIZATION
- Outpatient cryotherapy at weekly intervals
- Repeated parings at weekly intervals with or without use of a keratolytic is also an option. Most successful appears to be curettage and chemical cautery (with phenol or trichloroacetic acid) or light electrocautery. (Note: Extreme care must be exercised with this procedure, because excessive cautery or curettage can cause a painful scar.)

GENERAL MEASURES
- If warts are asymptomatic, no treatment is necessary. However, patient may be at risk for spread of warts.
- Warm soaks followed by patient's paring of the top layer of skin on repeated occasions may speed disappearance.
- Patient may use pumice stone, emery board. or a blade.
- OTC keratolytics containing salicylic acid in liquid or film may help. The advised procedure is paring of skin followed by warm soaks, and finally application of a few drops of keratolytic daily.
- Hyperthermia: Hot water immersion (113°F) 1/2–3/4 hour 2–3 times per week for 16 treatments is effective for some patients.
- Duct tape: Cut a piece to the size of the wart and apply continuously for 6 days, remove and repeat for up to 2 months. (5)[B]
- Other measures include use of a heel bar or appropriate padding to relieve pressure points where warts tend to aggregate. (1)[C]

Diet
No special diet

Activity
Ambulatory unless warts or treatment are painful

MEDICATION (DRUGS)

First Line
- No effective antiviral wart medications currently exist. Keratolytics (OTC or prescription) and a variety of chemotherapeutic acids may be used.
- Salicylic acid: See "General Measures" for instructions.
- 40% salicylic acid plasters: available as Mediplast. It is supplied in 3 × 4 in sheets which are cut to the size of the wart, and the sticky surface is applied to the wart. They are removed every 1–2 days, the white keratin peeled, and a fresh plaster applied.
- Chemotherapy dichloroacetic acid and trichloroacetic acid kits are available. Callus is pared and the surrounding skin is protected by a ring of petrolatum. The wart(s) are coated with acid, which is then worked into the wart with a sharp toothpick. Procedure should be repeated at weekly intervals.
- Transdermal salicylates (Trans-Plantar)
- Vesicants containing cantharidin (Cantharone, Verrusol), applied in the office, allowed to dry, and are then covered with occlusive tape for 24 hours.
- Contraindications: Infection, vascular insufficiency
- Precautions
  - If the dermis is damaged with any of the above procedures, a scar may result which can be permanently painful.
  - Care should be taken to avoid excessive contact with normal skin when using keratolytics or chemotherapy.
  - Avoid bleomycin treatment during pregnancy.
  - Imiquimod has not been studied in patients <18 years. (1)[C]

Second Line
- Bleomycin injected intralesionally every 2 weeks
- Imiquimod (Aldara) 5% cream applied daily after soaking. It appears to be more effective when occluded and when in combination with other treatments such as cryotherapy or keratolytics.
- Alternative procedures include laser therapies (various).

SURGERY
- Cryotherapy: Application of liquid nitrogen is often effective. It usually requires at least four applications at weekly or biweekly intervals. Aggressive cryotherapy may cause blistering or even scarring, so light applications with 2 freeze–thaw cycles is preferred.
- Blunt dissection: A simple surgical procedure is effective and usually nonscarring. It requires inserting a blunt dissector between the wart and normal skin and separating the wart using short, firm stroke.
- Carbon dioxide laser surgery: used for recalcitrant warts (1)[C]

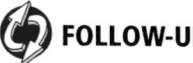 ## FOLLOW-UP

PROGNOSIS
The course of plantar warts is like that of other varieties of warts (i.e., highly variable). Most resolve spontaneously in weeks to months.

COMPLICATIONS
- Scarring with overly aggressive treatment
- A rare type of verrucous carcinoma, epithelioma cuniculatum, is thought to arise from these warts.

PATIENT MONITORING
With any treatment modality, follow-up weekly.

REFERENCES

1. Habif TP. *Clinical Dermatology*. 4th ed. New York, NY: Mosby; 2004: 374–377.
2. Epstein E. *Common Skin Disorders*. 5th ed. Philadelphia, PA: WB Saunders; 2001.
3. Freedberg IM et al. *Fitzpatrick's Dermatology in General Medicine*, 6th ed. New York, NY: McGraw-Hill; 2003;2120–2123, 2129.
4. James WD, Berger TG, Elston DM. *Andrews' Diseases of the Skin*, 10th ed. Philadephia, PA: WB Saunders; 2006;405–407.
5. Focht DR, Spicer C, Fairchok MP. The efficacy of duct tape vs cryotherapy in the treatment of verruca vulgaris. *Arch Pedatr Adolesc Med*. 2002;156: 971–974.

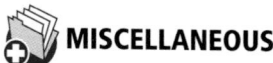 ## MISCELLANEOUS

See also: Condyloma Acuminata; Warts

CODES

ICD9-CM
078.19 Other specified viral warts

PATIENT TEACHING
- In Epstein: *Common Skin Disorders*, patient instructions, P-129 (see: References)
- American Academy of Dermatology, (708) 330–0230

 See Corresponding Diagnostic Algorithm

 See Patient Handout on CD

W

WEGENER GRANULOMATOSIS

Christopher M. Wise, MD

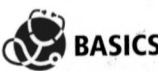 **BASICS**

DESCRIPTION

A disease characterized by granulomatous vasculitis involving multiple organs. The characteristic "triad" of involvement includes the upper airway (otitis, sinusitis, nasal mucosa), lungs, and kidneys. Other organ systems involved include the skin, joints, and nervous system (peripheral or central).

- As the condition progresses untreated, upper airway erosions, necrotic pulmonary nodules, and renal failure are common; without treatment, mortality rate is high.
- System(s) Affected: Upper Airways (sinusitis, otitis); Cardiovascular; Gastrointestinal; Nervous; Pulmonary; Renal/Urologic; Skin/Exocrine

ALERT
Pregnancy Considerations
- Rarely reported
- Should be considered only when patient is disease-free and off therapy
- Cyclophosphamide often causes sterility and is potentially teratogenic.

EPIDEMIOLOGY
- Predominant age: mean age of onset in mid-40s, but has been described in all age groups
- Predominant sex: Male > Female (3:2)

Incidence
Estimated at ~0.4/100,000

Prevalence
Three per 100,000

RISK FACTORS
None identified

Genetics
Increased presence in HLA-B8 and HLA-DR2

ETIOLOGY
The etiology is unknown; the autoimmune phenomena and immune complex deposition in arterial walls are implicated. Triggering infectious agents, yet unidentified, may be involved.

ASSOCIATED CONDITIONS
None

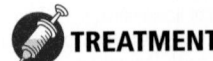 **DIAGNOSIS**

SIGNS AND SYMPTOMS
- Pulmonary infiltrates: 71%
- Sinusitis: 67%
- Arthralgia/arthritis: 44%
- Fever: 34%
- Cough: 34%
- Otitis: 25%
- Rhinitis: 22%
- Hemoptysis: 18%
- Ocular inflammation: 16%
- Weight loss: 16%
- Skin rash: 13%
- Epistaxis: 11%
- Renal failure: 11%
- Chest pain, anorexia, proptosis, dyspnea, oral ulcers, hearing loss, headache (all <10%)

TESTS
Lab
- Anemia, leukocytosis, and thrombocytosis common during active phases of disease
- Erythrocyte sedimentation rate usually markedly elevated (75%)
- Rheumatoid factor present in low to moderate titer in up to 50%
- Hematuria and/or cellular casts with moderate range proteinuria
- Renal insufficiency, mild to moderate at 1st, frequently progresses to end-stage renal disease.
- Antibodies to neutrophilic cytoplasmic antigens with a cytoplasmic pattern of staining (c-ANCA) are detected in 60–90% of patients. c-ANCA is highly specific (90+%); immunoblotting techniques or enzyme-linked immunoassay may detect antibodies to PR3 or MPO (anti-PR3 antibodies are more specific)
- Perinuclear staining (p-ANCA), is nonspecific and seen with other vasculitic syndromes or isolated necrotizing glomerulonephritis.
- Drugs that may alter lab results: Corticosteroids and cytotoxic drugs, used to treat the disease, may cause normalization of most abnormal laboratory findings.
- Disorders that may alter lab results: See disorders listed under "Differential Diagnosis."

Imaging
- Upper airways: Chronic otitis and sinusitis, often with evidence of erosion into bony structures—seen on plain radiographs
- CT scans of sinuses may show mucosal and bony involvement.
- Lungs: Radiographs show nodular pulmonary densities, often with central necrosis and cavitation. Local infiltrates or more diffuse interstitial involvement are also described, as are radiographic findings of pulmonary hemorrhage.

Diagnostic Procedures/Surgery
- Open lung biopsy is most likely to confirm granulomatous arteritis.
- Renal biopsy may give findings consistent with diagnosis, although findings are not always definitive.
- Sinus or upper airway mucosal biopsy is often helpful, although findings are often nonspecific.
- Diagnosis is best made by demonstration of granulomatous arteritis of involved organ, although compatible renal lesion in setting of chronic destructive sinusitis and/or pulmonary nodules may make a presumptive diagnosis.
- A positive serologic test for c-ANCA in the proper clinical setting is often diagnostic.

Pathological Findings
- Upper airways: Granulomatous inflammation frequently seen, although not specific unless showing actual vasculitis
- Lung: Granulomatous arteritis involving vessels; classically medium-sized arteries
- Kidney: Necrotizing and crescentic glomerulonephritis without immunofluorescent staining (pauci-immune) is common; granulomatous vasculitis rarely seen
- Skin: Vasculitic lesions, from leukocytoclastic vasculitis of small vessels; granulomatous arteritis seen occasionally

DIFFERENTIAL DIAGNOSIS
- Infectious otitis and sinusitis (bacterial or fungal)
- Midline granuloma or other upper airway malignancy
- Relapsing polychondritis
- Fungal or tuberculous pulmonary infections (Goodpasture syndrome)
- Other vasculitic syndromes (including polyarteritis nodosa, lymphomatoid granulomatosis, Churg-Strauss vasculitis, and overlap vasculitis syndromes)
- Any disease associated with necrotizing and crescentic glomerulonephritis, sarcoidosis

TREATMENT

INITIAL STABILIZATION
- Patients are usually ill enough with fever, sinus or pulmonary involvement, or renal disease to require hospitalization for diagnostic tests (to rule out infectious causes) and appropriate biopsies.
- An occasional patient can be managed as an outpatient.

GENERAL MEASURES
- Careful attention to upper airway drainage
- Supportive measures for pulmonary, renal, or neurologic involvement

Diet
- Vigorous nutritional support may be needed early in the illness.
- Reduce calories salt in patients on prednisone.
- High fluid intake prevents hemorrhagic cystitis from cyclophosphamide.

Activity
There are no specific restrictions; fatigue, fever, and weight loss usually limit activity.

MEDICATION (DRUGS)

First Line
- Prednisone (1)[C]
  - Given initially in high doses (60–100 mg/d)
  - After the initial 2–4 weeks, may be tapered to alternate-day regimen then gradually discontinued over 2–6 months in most patients, depending on clinical course
- Cyclophosphamide (2,3)[A]
  - In critically ill patient, may be given initially at a dose of 4 mg/kg/d IV for 2–3 days then at 2 mg/kg/d PO
  - In stable patient, start at 2 mg/kg/d PO
  - Dosage may need to be adjusted based on patient response and toxicity (usually bone marrow suppression)
  - Usually continued for 1–2 years after patient is felt to be in remission, then tapered slowly, with careful monitoring for reactivation of disease
  - Give dose in morning to decrease amount of drug present overnight in bladder
- Methotrexate 15–25 g/wk PO has been shown in a recent trial to be successful in maintaining remission in patients treated with cyclophosphamide. Methotrexate may be used in place of cyclophosphamide in some patients without pulmonary or renal involvement. (1,3)[B]
- There are no absolute contraindications, although diabetes, hypertension, and metabolic bone disease are relative contraindications to prednisone.
- Precautions
  - Carefully monitor a patient taking corticosteroids.
  - Consider reducing dose of cyclophosphamide with baseline leukopenia or renal insufficiency.
- Significant possible interactions
  - Prednisone may interfere with hypoglycemics and antihypertensives.
  - Cyclophosphamide may increase risk of other drugs with potential for bone marrow toxicity.

Second Line
- Azathioprine: For patients with history of severe bone marrow toxicity or hemorrhagic cystitis from cyclophosphamide
- Trimethoprim-sulfamethoxazole (TMP-SMX) has been used alone with success in some patients with limited (usually upper airway) disease, and has some potential as an adjunctive therapy with prednisone and cyclophosphamide.
- Methotrexate: For some patients without renal involvement; may be useful in maintaining remission in patients with stable disease, as an alternative to chronic cyclophosphamide therapy
- Rituximab has been reported to be useful in isolated cases or small series of patients.
- Etanercept does not appear to be of benefit, based on information from a recent clinical trial.

 ## FOLLOW-UP

PROGNOSIS
- Without treatment, almost uniformly fatal, with a 10% 2-year survival; mean survival of 5 months
- With aggressive treatment, survival improved to 75–90% at 5 years.
- Treatment-related toxicity is significant, especially from long-term cyclophosphamide. After 1 year of diseasefree interval, cyclophosphamide is usually changed to methotrexate or tapered, although some patients may demonstrate disease reactivation. (4)[A]

COMPLICATIONS
- Disease related
  - Destructive nasal lesions with "saddle nose" deformity
  - Deafness from refractory otitis
  - Necrotic pulmonary nodules with hemoptysis
  - Interstitial lung disease
  - Renal failure
  - Foot drop from peripheral nerve disease
  - Skin ulcers, digital and limb gangrene from peripheral vascular involvement
- Drug related
  - Prednisone: Weight gain, hyperglycemia, hypertension, hypokalemia, skin thinning and bruising, infection, osteoporosis
  - Cyclophosphamide: Bone marrow suppression (especially leukopenia, neutropenia), alopecia, hemorrhagic cystitis, mucosal membrane irritation, sterility and premature gonadal failure, secondary malignancies (especially leukemias) with long-term therapy. Risk of bladder cancer is 5% (10 years) and 16% (15 years) after first treatment, and is related to previous cystitis.

PATIENT MONITORING
- Early, careful monitoring of upper airway, pulmonary, and renal manifestations
- Blood pressure, glucose, potassium for steroid effects
- Frequent (every 2–4 weeks) complete blood count with differential to monitor for bone marrow toxicity from cyclophosphamide. Leukopenia is most common. Dose needs to be reduced if peripheral white blood cell count <3000/mm³.
- Urinalysis for potential of hemorrhagic cystitis from cyclophosphamide. Consider cystoscopy for persistent or recurrent hematuria.
- Acute phase reactants (ESR, CRP) and serum c-ANCA levels may be useful in monitoring disease activity during follow-up. (5)[A]

REFERENCES
1. Specks U. Methotrexate for Wegener's granulomatosis: What is the evidence? *Arthritis Rheum.* 2005;52:2237–2242.
2. Goek ON, Stone ON. Randomized controlled trials in vasculitis associated with anti-neutrophil cytoplasmic antibodies. *Curr Opin Rheumatol.* 2005;17:257–264.
3. DeGroot K, et al. Randomized trial of cyclophosphamide versus methotrexate for induction of remission in early systemic antineutrophil cytoplasmic antibody-associated vasculitis. *Arthritis Rheum.* 2005;52:2461–2469.
4. Seo P, et al. Damage caused by Wegeneris granulomatosis and its treatment: Prospective data from the Wegener's Granulomatosis Etanercept Trial (WGET). *Arthritis Rheum.* 2005;52:2168–2178.
5. Hogan SL, et al. Predictors of relapse and treatment resistance in antineutrophil cytoplasmic antibody-associated small-vessel vasculitis. *Ann Intern Med.* 2005;143:621–631.

 ## MISCELLANEOUS

See also: Polyarteritis Nodosa

CODES

ICD9-CM
446.4 Wegener granulomatosis

PATIENT TEACHING
- Nutritional and drug counseling when patient is able to return home
- Wegener Granulomatosis Support Group, PO Box 28660, Kansas City, MO 64188

Diet
- Vigorous nutritional support may be needed early in the illness.
- Calorie and salt reduction in patients on prednisone
- High fluid intake to prevent hemorrhagic cystitis from cyclophosphamide

Activity
There are no specific restrictions; fatigue, fever, and weight loss usually limit activity.

 See Corresponding Diagnostic Algorithm

 See Patient Handout on CD

W

WILLIAMS SYNDROME

Gene S. Fisch, PhD

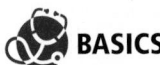

BASICS

DESCRIPTION
- Williams syndrome is an unusual multisystem neurodevelopmental disorder typified by characteristic craniofacial features, mild microcephaly, mild to moderate mental retardation with a distinctive cognitive-behavioral profile, connective tissue abnormalities, growth retardation, supravalvular aortic stenosis, peripheral pulmonary stenosis, renal artery stenosis, limited joint movement, and transient hypercalcemia.
- Occurrence is sporadic, although familial autosomal dominant cases have been infrequently reported.
- System(s) Affected: Cardiovascular; Endocrine/Metabolic; Musculoskeletal; Nervous; Renal/Urologic
- Synonym(s): Williams-Beuren syndrome; Fanconi-type idiopathic infantile hypercalcemia; Elfin facies syndrome

ALERT
Pediatric Considerations
Infantile hypercalcemia

Pregnancy Considerations
Patient and family should receive genetic evaluation and counseling, as prenatal diagnosis is available.

GENERAL PREVENTION
Genetic counseling and evaluation, especially among high-functioning patients, about pregnancies. Prenatal diagnosis is available.

EPIDEMIOLOGY
- Predominant age: Life-long condition
- Predominant sex: Male = Female

Incidence
In the US: Affected individuals have been estimated at 1:20,000 live births.

RISK FACTORS
Possible familial transmission as an autosomal dominant mutation

Genetics
The pattern of occurrence is nearly always sporadic and is observed in both sexes, although there are several reported cases of familial transmission as an autosomal dominant mutation. The phenotypic expression is somewhat varied and associated with a hemizygous microdeletion of ~1.6 Mb in the 7q11.23 region which includes the elastin (ELN) and LIM-kinase (LIMK) gene.

ETIOLOGY
Microdeletion in the 7q11.23 region produced by unequal crossing over

ASSOCIATED CONDITIONS
- Developmental delay
- Growth retardation
- Cardiovascular dysfunction
- Renal dysfunction
- Attention deficit disorder (ADD)
  - Frequently associated with neuropsychologic dysfunction
  - Treatment for ADD is similar to methods used in the general population.

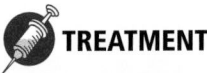

DIAGNOSIS

SIGNS AND SYMPTOMS
- The signs and symptoms observed in the classic case of Williams syndrome may be diagnostic, but the clinical presentation is somewhat varied.
- Early childhood: global developmental delay, albeit with seemingly normal speech and expressive language
  - Hyperacusis
  - Characteristic craniofacial features: Elfin-like facial appearance; medial eyebrow flare and stellate irises; wide mouth; long flat philtrum; upturned nose with a flat nasal bridge; dental anomalies; mild microcephaly
  - Characteristic clinical features: Supravalvula aortic stenosis; peripheral pulmonary stenosis; renal artery stenosis; infantile hypercalcemia; growth retardation and short stature; slender limbs and trunk
  - Characteristic cognitive/behavioral features: Weakness in abstract/visual reasoning; highly developed expressive language skills; low levels of daily living skills; age-related decreases in IQ scores
- Postpubertal males and females
  - Characteristic clinical features: Hypertension; lordosis, and/or limited joint movement
  - Characteristic behavioral features: Anxiety, depression, and suicidal ideation

TESTS
Lab
- Molecular-genetic (DNA) evaluation is the diagnostic test of choice and can determine the size of the deletion.
- Special tests: Affected individuals require cognitive, behavioral, psychologic, and educational evaluations to develop individual education programs.

DIFFERENTIAL DIAGNOSIS
Rule out uncomplicated hypercalcemia or supravalvular aortic stenosis.

TREATMENT

GENERAL MEASURES
- Appropriate health care: Affected individuals will generally need life-long adult supervision. Early intensive educational intervention and behavior modification should be implemented.
- Early detection will permit early intervention and intensive behavioral training.
- Treatment for hypercalcemia by controlling dietary intake of calcium and vitamin D
- Ophthalmologic evaluations are recommended for problems associated with visual acuity.
- Preventive dentistry to reduce risk of malocclusion
- Continual monitoring of cardiovascular anomalies and for hypertension
- Filtered ear protection for hyperacusis

Diet
For hypercalcemia, control intake of calcium and vitamin D.

Activity
Full activity unless cardiovascular stenoses are problematic

MEDICATION (DRUGS)

Medication for hypertension and for hyperparathyroidism

SURGERY
Treatment for aortic, pulmonary, or renal artery stenoses if needed

 FOLLOW-UP

PROGNOSIS
- Individuals may need life-long supervision.
- Life span may be affected by renal dysfunction or hypertension resulting from supravalvuar stenosis and/or peripheral pulmonary stenosis

COMPLICATIONS
- Learning problems, especially in abstract/visual reasoning
- Behavioral problems concerning indifference to personal safety
- Postpubescent anxiety and depression
- Risk of cardiovascular disease and/or renal dysfunction

PATIENT MONITORING
Regular pediatric care and general health maintenance with particular attention to endocrine, renal, and cardiovascular function

REFERENCES
1. Anderson PE, Rourke BP. Williams syndrome. In: White BP, ed. *Syndrome of Nonverbal Learning Disabilities*. New York: Guilford Press; 1995.
2. Bayes M, Perez-Juardo LA. Williams-Beuren syndrome. In: Fisch GS, ed. *Genetics and Genomics of Neurobehavioral Disorders*. Totowa, NJ: Humana Press; 2003.

 MISCELLANEOUS

See also: Attention Deficit/Hyperactivity Disorder; Down Syndrome; Fragile X Syndrome; Hyperparathyroidism; Hypertension, Essential; Mental Retardation

CODES

ICD9-CM
758.9 Conditions due to anomaly of unspecified chromosome

PATIENT TEACHING
- The patient and family should receive genetic evaluation and counseling.
- Patient and family should contact the Williams Syndrome Association, Box 297, Clawson, MI 48017; (800) 806-1871; website http://www.williams-syndrome.org

See Corresponding Diagnostic Algorithm

See Patient Handout on CD

 W

WILMS TUMOR

Timothy L. Black, MD

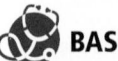 **BASICS**

DESCRIPTION
- An embryonal renal neoplasm containing blastema, stromal, or epithelial cell types, usually affecting children before age 5 years.
- For staging, see "Prognosis" section.
- System(s) Affected: Renal/Urologic
- Synonym(s): Nephroblastoma

ALERT
Pediatric Considerations
- Occurs only in children
- Most common renal malignancy in childhood

EPIDEMIOLOGY
- Predominant age: Median age of 36.5 months
- Predominant sex: Female > Male (1.1:1)

Incidence
- Frequency rarer in East Asian populations than whites (1)[C]
- Frequency higher in black children than whites (1)[C]

Prevalence
US: 0.69/100,000. 7.6 cases/1 million children under 15 years of age

RISK FACTORS
- Aniridia (partial or complete absence of iris) 600 times greater than normal risk
- Hemihypertrophy (100 times greater than normal risk)
- Cryptorchidism
- Hypospadias
- Duplicated renal collecting systems
- Wiedemann-Beckwith syndrome
- Denys-Drash syndrome (nephropathy, renal failure, male pseudohermaphroditism, Wilms tumor)
- Klippel-Trenaunay syndrome
- WAGR complex (Wilms tumor, aniridia, genitourinary malformations, and mental retardation)
- Beckwith-Wiedemann syndrome (visceromegaly, macroglossia, omphalocele, hyperinsulinemic hypoclycemia)
- Familial occurrence (1–2%)
- Paternal occupation (see "Etiology")

Genetics
- Several congenital anomalies are known to be associated with Wilms tumor. A 2-stage mutational model has been proposed: Occurrence in either hereditary form or sporadic form. Patients with aniridia have a deletion of the short arm of chromosome 11 (11p13).
- Abnormalities of chromosome 11 at the 11p15 locus are associated with Beckwith-Wiedemann syndrome
- Wilms tumor suppressor gene (WT1) has been identified as well as additional candidates for another suppressor gene (WT2) (1)[C]
- Chromosome band 17q12-21 has been linked to two kindreds with Wilms tumor and other kindreds are associated with a Wilms tumor predisposition gene at 19q13.3-q13.4 (1)[C]

ETIOLOGY
- Hereditary or sporadic forms of genetic mutation
- Familial form: autosomal dominant trait with incomplete penetrance (1%)
- Potential of paternal occupational exposure (machinists, welders, motor vehicle mechanics, auto body repairmen)

ASSOCIATED CONDITIONS
See "Risk Factors."

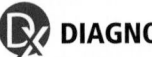 **DIAGNOSIS**

SIGNS AND SYMPTOMS
- Usually asymptomatic
- Palpable upper abdominal mass
- Abdominal pain
- Fever
- Anemia
- Rarely, signs of acute abdomen with free intraperitoneal rupture
- Cardiac murmur
- Hepatosplenomegaly
- Ascites
- Prominent abdominal wall veins
- Varicocele
- Gonadal metastases
- Aniridia

History
History of increasing abdominal size

Physical Exam
Palpable abdominal mass

TESTS
Lab
- Urinalysis (occasional hematuria)
- CBC (anemia)
- Lactate dehydrogenase
- Plasma renin (rarely helpful)
- Urine catecholamines

Imaging
- Chest x-ray
- Kidney, ureter, bladder (presence of linear calcifications)
- Abdominal ultrasound: Gives best information about tumor extension into inferior vena cava
- CT (with IV and oral contrast) of chest and abdomen
- IV pyelogram rarely helpful

Diagnostic Procedures/Surgery
Occasionally, bone marrow aspiration necessary to distinguish from neuroblastoma

Pathological Findings
- Favorable findings (mortality of 7%)
  - Bulky lesion, well encapsulated
  - Focal areas of hemorrhage and necrosis
  - Absence of anaplasia and sarcomatous cell types
  - Presence of blastema, stomal, and epithelial elements
- Unfavorable histology (mortality rate of 57%)
  - Anaplasia: Markedly enlarged and multipolar mitotic figures, 3-fold enlargement of nuclei in comparison with adjacent similar nuclei, hyperchromasia of enlarge nuclei. Anaplasia may be diffuse or focal.
  - Sarcomatous changes: Now considered to be separate from Wilms, not subtypes (mortality 64%)
- Nephroblastomatosis: Considered premalignant

DIFFERENTIAL DIAGNOSIS
- Neuroblastoma
- Hepatic tumor
- Sarcoma
- Rhabdoid tumor
- Cystic nephroma
- Mesoblastic nephroma
- Renal cell carcinoma (generally occurs in older children)

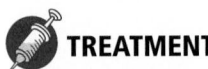 **TREATMENT**

GENERAL MEASURES
- Appropriate health care: Inpatient workup and treatment until stable postoperative and induction chemotherapy completed
- Chemotherapy
- Radiation therapy in Stage II, unfavorable histology, Stage II and Stage IV

Diet
No special diet

Activity
As tolerated

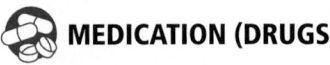 **MEDICATION (DRUGS)**

First Line
- Dactinomycin (actinomycin-D)
- Vincristine
- Doxorubicin
- Cyclophosphamide (Cytoxan)
- Ifosphamide
- Etoposide
- Contraindications: Refer to the manufacturer's literature for each drug.
- Precautions: Refer to the manufacturer's literature for each drug.
- Significant possible interactions: Refer to the manufacturer's literature for each drug.

Second Line
- Doxorubicin (Adriamycin)
- Cyclophosphamide

SURGERY
- Examination (visual and manual) of contralateral kidney
- Radical nephroureterectomy and biopsies as needed to provide precise staging information
- Sampling of any enlarged lymph nodes
- Identification of any retained tumor with titanium clips
- Tumor should be given to pathologist fresh, not in formalin.
- Vertical midline incision if tumor extension to right atrium present (possible use of cardiopulmonary bypass)
- With bilateral Wilms tumors, biopsy, then chemotherapy and 2nd-look operation 6 weeks to 6 months later for partial bilateral nephrectomy if possible
  - Preopoerative treatment also generally accepted in a solitary kidney, horseshoe kidneys, intravascular extension of tumor above the intrahepatic vena cava, and in the case of respiratory distress from extensive metastatic tumor

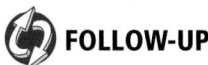 **FOLLOW-UP**

Issues for Referral

Surgical complications have been found to be significantly higher if the radical nephrectomy is done by a general surgeon rather than an pediatric surgeon or a pediatric urologist. (2)[B]

PROGNOSIS

- With favorable histology, 91% survival
- With diffuse anaplasia, 20% survival
- With focal anaplasia, 64% survival
- With rhabdoid features, 19% 3-year survival
- Staging
  - I: Tumor limited to kidney, completely excised
  - II: Tumor extends beyond kidney, completely excised
  - III: Residual nonhematogenous tumor confined to abdomen (lymph nodes positive, spillage of tumor, peritoneal implants, extension beyond resection region)
  - IV: Hematogenous metastases
  - V: Bilateral renal involvement

COMPLICATIONS

- 1–2% will develop second malignant neoplasms (leukemia, lymphoma, hepatocellular carcinoma, soft tissue sarcoma)
- High risk of low-birth-weight infants, perinatal mortality in offspring of female survivors of Wilms tumor
- Chest is usual site of recurrence.
- Occurrence of second malignant neoplasms in 2% of patients 7–34 years after treatment
- Surgical complications: (2)[B]
  - Postoperative hemorrhage
  - Postoperative small bowel obstruction (5–7%)
  - Tumor rupture with spillage in 19%. This may be spontaneous or surgical and results in upstaging the tumor. Only 2.7% of spills are considered avoidable. (3)[B]
- Local tumor recurrence

PATIENT MONITORING

- Multidrug chemotherapy every 3–4 weeks for 16 weeks: 15 months depending on stage
- Every 4 months for 1 year, every 6 months for 2nd to 3rd year, yearly after that
- Complete blood count, CT of chest and abdomen with each visit

REFERENCES

1. Ashcraft KW, Holcomb GW, Murphy JP, eds. *Pediatric Surgery*, 4th ed. Philadelphia, PA: Elsevier Saunders; 2005.
2. Ritchey ML, et al. Surgical complications after primary nephrectomy for Wilms tumor: Report from the national Wilms tumor study group. *J Am Coll Surg*. 2001;192:63–68.
3. Ehrlich PF, et al. Quality assessment for Wilms tumor: A report from the national Wilms study-5. *J Ped Surg*. 2005;40:208–210.

 MISCELLANEOUS

Other notes

- Mesoblastic nephroma: Distinguished only by histology. Age usually <6 months. Essentially benign, although metastases have been reported; tends to be locally invasive. Operative spillage may lead to recurrence. No chemotherapy or radiotherapy needed with complete excision.
- Nephroblastomatosis: Considered premalignant; may present as nodularity of one or both kidneys; treated with biopsy and local excision (renal tissue sparing)

ICD9-CM

189.0 Malignant neoplasm of kidney, except pelvis

PATIENT TEACHING

- Patient and family teaching regarding long-term outlook
- Possibility of second malignancy
- Side effects of chemotherapy, radiation therapy

 See Corresponding Diagnostic Algorithm

 See Patient Handout on CD

W

WISKOTT-ALDRICH SYNDROME

Patricia Borman, MD

BASICS

DESCRIPTION
- Males affected by this rare X-linked genetic disorder display combined immunodeficiency, microcytic thrombocytosis, and eczema leading to life-threatening infections and bleeding complications. Average life span is 11 years. The syndrome has variable expression. X-linked thrombocytopenia (XLT) is a related but milder form with mostly platelet defects.
- System(s) Affected: Hemic/Lymphatic/Immunologic; Skin/Exocrine
- Synonym(s): Aldrich syndrome; Immunodeficiency-2

ALERT
Geriatric Considerations
None have survived this long.

Pediatric Considerations
- Onset at birth
- 1st-year infections with encapsulated bacteria: respiratory, meningitis, sepsis
- Later infections occur with opportunistic organisms and virus.

GENERAL PREVENTION
Genetics counseling
- Identify carriers
- Prenatal diagnosis

EPIDEMIOLOGY
- Predominant age: Onset at birth, most diagnosed by 24 months of age
- Predominant sex: Male > Female
  - Females rarely develop Wiskott-Aldrich syndrome (WAS). Some carriers express disease; others have different but related gene defect.

Incidence
In the US: 1 in 4 million live male births

RISK FACTORS
- Family history of WAS
- History of congenital defects

Genetics
- Family history in >60%
- X-linked recessive trait
- Wiskott-Aldrich syndrome protein (WASP) and XLT genes located at X/11.22
  - Codes for cytoplasmic protein that signals cell membrane structure changes required for activation of blood cells

ETIOLOGY
- Hematopoietic cells express WASP.
  - Defective WASP fails to organize membrane activation.
  - Membranes do not form normal actin cytoskeletons.
  - Altered motility and inability to change cell shapes inhibit normal functions.
- Platelets are intrinsically abnormal.
  - Accelerated destruction, sequestered in spleen
- T cells show decreased responsiveness to antigens.
- B cells show abnormal antibody production.

ASSOCIATED CONDITIONS
Lymphomas, brain is primary site in 50%; nephropathy, other lymphoreticular tumors

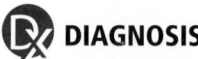

DIAGNOSIS

SIGNS AND SYMPTOMS
Physical Exam
- Neonatal
  - Excessive bleeding from circumcision
  - Bloody diarrhea
  - Petechiae and purpura
- Childhood
  - Eczema with secondary skin infections
  - Recurrent bacterial infections
  - Viral infections
  - Hepatosplenomegaly
  - Autoimmune vasculitis and hemolytic anemia

TESTS
Lab
- Platelets abnormal at birth
  - <30,000 mean platelet volume, 2/3 normal
- B-cell and T-cell changes over time
  - White blood cell count fall by age 6 years
  - Low IgM, normal IgG, high IgA and IgE
  - Decreased response to capsular antigens
  - Low CD 8 counts in 61%
  - Decreased delayed hypersensitivity responses
  - Decreased mitogenic responses
- Special tests
  - Genetic testing for WASP
  - Carrier identification
- Drugs that may alter lab results: Antibiotics
- Disorders that may alter lab results: Infections

Imaging
Not helpful

Diagnostic Procedures/Surgery
- Bone marrow aspiration to exclude leukemia and aplastic conditions and to HLA type for bone marrow transplantation
- Gene mapping of mutation in affected or female carriers
- Chorionic villus sampling for in utero diagnosis

Pathological Findings
- Hyperplasia of lymphoreticular system
- Vasculitic changes with multiple thromboses of small arterioles of kidney, lung, pancreas, brain

DIFFERENTIAL DIAGNOSIS
- May be difficult in infancy, before immune changes present
- Idiopathic thrombocytopenic purpura; other causes of thrombocytopenia
- Severe atopic disease
- Acute lymphoblastic anemia
- Other causes of immunodeficiency: Severe combined immunodeficiency, HIV
- Leukemias or marrow aplasias

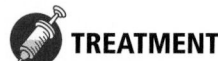

TREATMENT

INITIAL STABILIZATION
- Inpatient for acute infections
- No live virus vaccination

GENERAL MEASURES
- Cross-matched platelets
- Irradiated, cytomegalovirus-negative blood products
- Aggressive antibiotic therapy for infections
- Prophylactic antibiotics

Diet
No special diet

Activity
- Plan activities to help normal development.
- Avoid contact sports and prevent head injuries.
- Avoid crowds.

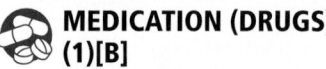

MEDICATION (DRUGS) (1)[B]
- Immunoglobulin infusions
- Prophylactic penicillin after splenectomy
- Antibiotics as indicated by culture
- Topical steroids for eczema
- Parenteral steroids, vincristine, or plasmapheresis for autoimmune complications
- Interleukin-2 can increase platelet counts while awaiting stem cell transplantation.
- Contraindications: Refer to the manufacturer's literature for each drug.
- Precautions: Corticosteroids in immunosuppressed patients. Refer to the manufacturer's literature for each drug.
- Significant possible interactions: Refer to the manufacturer's literature for each drug.

First Line
HLA-typed bone marrow or umbilical cord blood stem cell transplant restores all abnormalities with an 85% cure rate. (2)[B]

SURGERY
Splenectomy can transiently improve thrombocytopenia but increases the risk of infection.

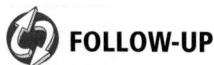 **FOLLOW-UP**

PROGNOSIS
- Usual course is acute and chronic infections with progressive decrease in immune status.
- Average life expectancy is 11 years, with more living past 20 with stem cell transplant. Transplant therapy can restore all abnormalities. Causes of death have been infection (50%), bleeding (27%), and malignancies (12%).

COMPLICATIONS
- Severe infections, especially after splenectomy
- Hemorrhage, cerebral common
- Malignancies (lymphoreticular, leukemia, Kaposi)
- Nephropathy
- Autoimmune disease in 40%, can be aggressive
- Malabsorption syndrome

PATIENT MONITORING
As needed for therapy; monitor for infections, for progression of disease, complications

REFERENCES
1. Ochs HD. The Wiskott-Aldrich syndrome. *Isr Med Assoc J*. 2002;4(5):379–384.
2. Tsuji Y, et al. Hematopoietic stem cell transplantation for 30 patients with primary immunodeficiency diseases: 20 years experience of a single team. *Bone Marrow Transplant*. 2006;1–9.
3. Klein C, et al. Gene therapy for Wiskott-Aldrich syndrome: Rescue of T-cell signaling and amelioration of colitis upon transplantation of retrovirally transduced hematopoietic stem cells in mice. *Blood*. 2003;101(6):2159–2166.
4. Braithwaite K, Abu-Ghosh A, Anderson L, Cairo MS. Treatment of severe thrombocytopenia with IL-11 in children with Wiskott-Aldrich syndrome. *J Pediatr Hematol Oncol*. 2002;24(4):323–326.
5. Ming JE. Syndromic immunodeficiencies with humoral defects. *Immunol Allergy Clin North Am*. 2001;21(1):91–111.

 MISCELLANEOUS

See also: Idiopathic Thrombocytopenic Purpura (ITP); Immunodeficiency Diseases; Leukemia

 CODES

ICD9-CM
279.12 Wiskott-Aldrich syndrome

PATIENT TEACHING
- Patient/parent counseling to cope with disease and outcome
- Genetic testing and counseling for family

 See Corresponding Diagnostic Algorithm

 See Patient Handout on CD

W

ZINC DEFICIENCY

Jeremy Golding, MD

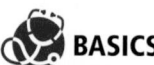 **BASICS**

DESCRIPTION
- Condition whose manifestations may involve growth retardation, hypogonadism, cell-mediated immune dysfunction, and skin changes related to decreased zinc levels
- System(s) Affected: Endocrine/metabolic; Nervous; Skin/exocrine

ALERT
Geriatric Considerations
- Zinc deficiency may cause poor night vision, leading to falls; poor wound healing or chronic ulcer; or loss of smell and taste, which may cause worsening nutrition.
- Elderly persons living in institutions may have low zinc intake.

Pediatric Considerations
Zinc deficiency may cause failure to thrive, and impair growth and development of secondary sexual characteristics.

Pregnancy Considerations
Requirements increase; deficiency may cause spontaneous abortion, inadequate weight gain.

GENERAL PREVENTION
- Adequate diet
- Supplementation when indicated (see "Medication")

EPIDEMIOLOGY
- Predominate age: All ages
- Predominant sex: Male = Female

Prevalence
In the US: Unknown

RISK FACTORS
- High milk consumption
- Low socioeconomic status
- Malabsorption syndromes
- Living in developing nations
- Strict vegetarian diet

Genetics
Usually acquired, but rarely caused by acrodermatitis enteropathica (autosomal recessive) and associated with sickle cell anemia (autosomal recessive).

ETIOLOGY
- Increased requirements
  - Pregnancy
  - Lactation
  - Rapid growth phase in childhood
  - Burns
  - Major trauma
- Increased losses
  - Diabetes
  - Cirrhosis
  - Renal disease
  - Malabsorption states (e.g., inflammatory bowel diseases)
  - Sickle cell anemia
- Decreased absorption
  - Acrodermatitis enteropathica, an autosomal recessive deficiency in the enzyme required for intestinal absorption
  - Geophagia
  - Chelating agents
  - Parasitism
  - Diet high in phytates (plant fiber)
- Insufficient dietary intake
  - Vegetarianism
  - Parenteral hyperalimentation without supplementation
  - Breast-feeding
  - Suboptimal zinc conditions in diet (rare)
  - Alcoholism

ASSOCIATED CONDITIONS
- Sickle cell anemia
- Malabsorption
- Parenteral hyperalimentation
- In the older patient, diabetes, cirrhosis, those taking diuretics

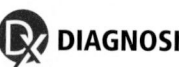 **DIAGNOSIS**

SIGNS AND SYMPTOMS
- Mild deficiency
  - Hypogeusia
  - Decreased dark adaptation
  - Decreased lean body mass
- Moderate deficiency
  - All the above
  - Diarrhea
  - Growth retardation
  - Hypogonadism (especially male)
  - Mental lethargy
  - Anergy
  - Rough skin
  - Delayed wound healing
  - Glucose intolerance
  - Impaired cell-mediated immunity
- Severe deficiency
  - All the above
  - Bullous pustular dermatitis
  - Weight loss
  - Dwarfism
  - Emotional instability
  - Tremors
  - Ataxia
  - Alopecia
  - Death

TESTS
Lab
- Plasma zinc levels decreased (in moderate to severe zinc deficiency). Levels <60 μg/L are strongly suggestive, but correction may be needed for low albumin, because most serum zinc is bound to albumin.
- Erythrocyte or leukocyte zinc levels more adequately assess tissue stores, but these are more costly and not widely available.
- Hair and fingernail levels are not useful.

DIFFERENTIAL DIAGNOSIS
- Congenital dwarfism
- Failure to thrive in infants
- Multiple micronutrient deficiencies
- Primary hypogonadism
- Mental retardation

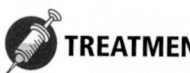 **TREATMENT**

GENERAL MEASURES
Diet
- Balanced omnivorous diet, or vegetarian diet with supplementation
- Avoid excessive intake of foods with high phytate content (e.g., raw cereals, but ready-to-eat cereal may be the richest source of zinc from a plant product).
- Meat, seafood, milk, eggs, grains, legumes, nuts, and seeds are rich in zinc.

Activity
Full activity

MEDICATION (DRUGS)

- Zinc gluconate or zinc sulfate 25–50 mg PO q.i.d. for 6–9 months
- In adult patient, 4–6 mg of elemental zinc daily added to hyperalimentation, may increase to 12 mg q.i.d. if suspect ongoing heavy zinc losses (e.g., burns or major trauma)
- In pediatric patients, 0.02–0.04 mg zinc/kg/d in hyperalimentation
- Prenatal vitamins with minerals during pregnancy and lactation to prevent deficiency
- Precautions: Avoid large (>20 mg elemental zinc) parenteral doses
- Recommended daily intake is 15 mg, assuming no excessive losses

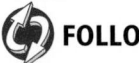 FOLLOW-UP

PROGNOSIS
Immediate improvement in clinical status with treatment. Full resolution in signs and symptoms

PATIENT MONITORING
Clinical status such as improved energy, weight gain, resolution of symptoms

REFERENCES

1. Abrams S. zinc deficiency and supplementation in children and adolescents. UpToDate; 2006.
2. Ronaghy H. The role of zinc in human nutrition. *World Rev Nutr Diet*. 1987;54:237–254.
3. Tasman-Jones C. Disturbances of trace mineral metabolism. In: Wyngaarden JB, Smith LH Jr, Bennet JC, eds. *Cecil Textbook of Medicine*, 19th ed. Philadelphia: WB Saunders, 1992.

 MISCELLANEOUS

See also: Alcohol use disorders; Anemia, sickle cell; Failure to thrive (FTT)

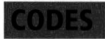 CODES

ICD9-CM
- 269.3 Mineral deficiency, NEC
- 686.8 Other specific local infections of skin and subcutaneous tissue

 See Corresponding Diagnostic Algorithm

 See Patient Handout on CD

Z

ZOLLINGER-ELLISON SYNDROME

Douglas S. Parks, MD

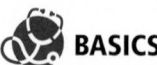

BASICS

DESCRIPTION
- A triad of
  - Markedly elevated gastric acid secretion
  - Peptic ulcer disease
  - A gastrinoma or non-beta islet cell tumor of the pancreas or duodenal wall that produces gastrin
- Gastrinomas (at time of diagnosis) may be single or multiple (1/2–2/3), large or small, benign or malignant (two thirds), sporadic (70–75%) or associated with multiple endocrine neoplasia type 1 (MEN1; 25–30%)
- System(s) Affected: Endocrine/Metabolic; Gastrointestinal
- Synonym(s): Z-E syndrome; Pancreatic ulcerogenic tumor syndrome; Multiple endocrine neoplasia, partial; Ulcerogenic islet cell tumor

GENERAL PREVENTION
Screen 1st-degree relatives of patients with MEN1.

EPIDEMIOLOGY
- Predominant age: Middle age (30–65 years)
- Predominant sex: Male > Female (3:2)

Incidence
Per year: 1–3 per million

ALERT
Pediatric Considerations
Very aggressive cases have been reported in teenagers.

Pregnancy Considerations
Cases reported; influences medication choices and surgical timing

RISK FACTORS
- MEN1
- Family history of ulcer disease

Genetics
~25–30% occur in association with the MEN1 syndrome.

ETIOLOGY
Gastrinoma equally distributed between the head of the pancreas and the 1st or 2nd portion of the duodenum. If in the pancreas is more likely to metastasize to liver. May also be found rarely in the mesentery, peritoneum, spleen, skin, or mediastinum (possibly metastasis with primary not identified).

ASSOCIATED CONDITIONS
- MEN1: hyperparathyroidism, prolactinomas, other pituitary tumors
- Insulinoma
- Carcinoid tumors

DIAGNOSIS

SIGNS AND SYMPTOMS
- Abdominal pain 80%
- Diarrhea, including while fasting 70%
- Heartburn 60%
- Nausea 30%
- Reflux esophagitis
- Vomiting unresponsive to standard therapy
- Peptic ulcer disease
- Weight loss
- Hepatomegaly with metastasis
- Steatorrhea
- Endoscopic findings including esophagitis, duodenal ulceration with multiple ulcers, and prominent gastric and duodenal folds
- Complications of severe peptic ulcer disease including hemorrhage, perforation, and obstruction
- Signs of MEN1, including those of hypercalcemia hyperparathyroidism and Cushing syndrome

Geriatric Considerations
Consider diagnosis in patient with persistent or recurring peptic ulcer disease; less aggressive disease if it appears after 65 years

History
Average of 5 years of symptoms including recurrent ulcers before diagnosis of Zollinger-Ellison syndrome (ZE) made

TESTS
- Preferred test is secretion stimulation test: Gastrin level increases >200 pg/mL (>200 ng/L)
- Gastric secretory studies: Basal acid output
- Alternative test is calcium infusion test: Gastrin level increases >400 pg/mL (test is less specific and is more dangerous because of IV calcium infusion)

Lab
- Elevated serum gastrin fasting level: >1000 pg/mL with ulcers diagnostic; >200 pg/mL with ulcers suggestive
- Elevated basal gastric acid output: >15 mEq/h (>15 mmol/h)
- Gastric pH <2.0 with elevated gastrin
- Check serum calcium, phosphorus, cortisol, and prolactin to rule out MEN1
- Drugs that may alter lab results: Histamine$_2$ (H$_2$)-blockers and proton pump inhibitors (PPIs) may increase gastric pH and serum gastrin. Need to hold PPIs 7 days and H$_2$-blockers 2 days prior to drawing gastrin level.

Imaging
- Used to localize tumor for possible resection
- Much more likely to find tumors >3 cm (95%) than <1 cm (<15%) (1)[B]
- Abdominal computed tomography (CT) scan: Most useful for pancreatic tumors and metastasis >3 cm
- Abdominal ultrasound: Not very useful except in large tumors
- Abdominal angiography not very useful except in large tumors
- Endoscopic ultrasound: Finds 24–38% of primary tumors
- Abdominal magnetic resonance imaging (MRI: Not very useful except in large tumors
- Somatostatin receptor scintigraphy (SRS), more sensitive than radiological studies but still only finds 30% of small tumors
- Portal venous sampling and selective venous sampling for gastrin can localize area of tumor and metastasis (80–90% sensitivity).
- Sella turcica imaging may help if MEN1 is suspected, to look for pituitary tumors.
- Because pancreatic tumors are most likely to be large and to metastasize to the liver which worsens prognosis, it is suggested to get SRS and CT abdomen to look for resectable tumors. Both studies are much more sensitive for pancreatic tumors, and surgical resection may improve prognosis considerably. (2,3)[B]

Diagnostic Procedures/Surgery
Endoscopy may reveal tumors in duodenal wall; multiple ulcers, including jejunal ulcers; and prominent gastric and duodenal folds.

Pathological Findings
- 90% of gastrinomas are found in the gastric triangle (borders are bile duct, junction of second and third portion of duodenum, and junction of head and body of pancreas).
- ~50% in head of pancreas (more likely to be >3 cm, metastasis to liver)
- ~50% in wall of 1st or 2nd portion of duodenum (more likely to be small, solitary)
- Two thirds malignant in both sites (defined by behavior not histology)
- Fifty percent of gastrinomas stain positive for adrenocorticotropic hormone (ACTH), vasoactive intestinal polypeptide, insulin, or neurotensin (in decreasing order of incidence)
- One third of patients have metastasis on presentation with regional nodes > liver > bone. Rarely to peritoneum, spleen, skin, and mediastinum.
- Duodenal, jejunal, and gastric ulcers, often multiple
- Gastric and duodenal mucosal fold thickening
- Hyperplasia of antral gastrin-producing cells
- Histology similar in appearance to carcinoid

DIFFERENTIAL DIAGNOSIS

- Elevated serum gastrin with hypochlorhydria/achlorhydria
  - Atrophic gastritis
  - Drug induced (associated with proton pump inhibitors)
  - Gastric cancer
  - Pernicious anemia
  - Post-vagotomy
- Elevated serum gastrin with normal or increased gastric acid
  - Antral G cell hyperfunction
  - Chronic renal failure
  - *Helicobacter pylori* infection
  - Gastric outlet obstruction
  - Retained gastric antrum
- Consider gastrinoma in all patients with
  - Recurrent or refractory ulcer disease
  - Gastric hypertrophy and ulcers
  - Duodenal and jejunal ulcers
  - Ulcers and diarrhea
  - Ulcers and kidney stones
  - Hypercalcemia and ulcers
  - Pituitary disease
  - Family history of ulcer disease or endocrine tumors suggestive of MEN1

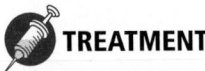 TREATMENT

INITIAL STABILIZATION

- Advise daily care based on symptoms
- Appropriate surveillance of basal gastric acid output to monitor anti–acid secretory therapy
- Appropriate surveillance postoperatively to look for metastasis

GENERAL MEASURES

- Advanced imaging initially to assess for possible resection
- Surgical removal when primary tumor can be identified and as an adjunct to symptom control
- Medical treatment for symptom control when primary tumor is not found or metastasis is present on diagnosis

Diet
Restrict foods that aggravate symptoms.

Activity
As tolerated

 MEDICATION (DRUGS)

General guidelines
- Drugs heal 80–85% of ulcers.
- Although medications heal ulcers, they nearly always recur. Although doses may be adjusted, plan on lifelong medication use.
- Dosages frequently exceed usual doses for treatment of ulcers by 4-fold to 8-fold. Start at lower recommended dose given below, and titrate up to resolution of symptoms or maximum listed subsequently.
- If hyperparathyroidism is present because of MEN1, hypercalcemia must be corrected.
- PPIs are the 1st-line treatment; H₂-blockers may need to be added.

First Line
- PPIs
  - Omeprazole: 60–120 mg/d
  - Lansoprazole: 60–180 mg/d (doses >120 mg need to be divided b.i.d.)
  - Rabeprazole: 60–100 mg/d up to 60 mg b.i.d.
  - Pantoprazole: 40–240 mg/d PO; 80–120 mg q12h IV
- H₂-blockers
  - Cimetidine: 300 mg q6h up to 1.25–5 g/d
  - Ranitidine: 150 mg q12h up to 6 g/d
  - Famotidine: 20 mg at bedtime up to 800 mg/d
- Contraindications
  - Known hypersensitivity to the drug
  - H₂-blockers: Androgen effects, drug interactions due to cytochrome P-450 stimulation
  - PPIs: None
- Precautions
  - Adjust the doses for renal and geriatric patients depending on the drug.
  - Gynecomastia reported with high-dose cimetidine (>2.4 g/d)
  - PPIs may induce a profound and long-lasting effect on gastric acid secretion, thereby affecting the bioavailability of drugs dependent on low gastric pH (e.g., ketoconazole, ampicillin, iron).
- Significant possible interactions: Refer to the drug manufacturer's literature.

Second Line
- Octreotide appears helpful in slowing the growth of a liver metastasis. May produce regression in some cases. Octreotide-LAR (long-acting release) can be given every 28 days. (1)[B]
- Chemotherapy regimens of streptozocin, 5-fluorouracil, and doxorubicin show only limited response.
- Interferon shows a limited response, but may be useful in combination with octreotide.

SURGERY
- Laparotomy to search for resectable tumors (especially in the pancreas and duodenal wall), unless patient has liver metastasis on presentation or MEN1
- Definitive therapy: Removal of gastrinomas when found (surgery finds 95% of tumors; 5-year cure 40% when all can be removed)
- Total gastrectomy was formerly used to stop acid production before pharmacologic therapy became available; now is seldom done
- In MEN1, parathyroidectomy, by lowering calcium, may decrease acid production and decrease antisecretory drug use. Gastrinomas are generally small, benign, and multiple and not usually cured by surgery.

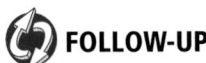 FOLLOW-UP

PROGNOSIS
- Overall survival rate: 5-year to 10-year 69–94%
- Prognosis improves if complete surgical removal of tumor is possible.
- If liver metastasis is present on initial surgery, 5-year survival is 30–40%, 10-year 25%
- Mortality directly related to liver metastasis, associated with larger tumors and pancreatic tumors (1–3)[B]

COMPLICATIONS
- Complications of peptic ulcer disease (bleeding, perforation, obstruction)
- 2/3 of gastrinomas are malignant with metastasis.
- Tumor may produce other substances, such as ACTH (5–8% of patients), with resulting Cushing syndrome
- Decrease in vitamin B12 levels possible with long-term PPI use (4)[B]

PATIENT MONITORING
- Patient must be monitored over time for evidence of metastasis.
- Careful dose titration of medical therapy is necessary to control symptoms.
- Gastric acid analysis to maintain basal gastric acid output to <10 mEq/h (<2 mEq/h if patient has complications such as perforation or esophagitis)

REFERENCES

1. Hoffman K, Furukawa M, Jensen R. Duodenal neuroendocrine tumors: Classification, functional syndromes, diagnosis and medical treatment. *Best Practice & Research Clinical Gastroenterology.* 2005;19(5):675–697.
2. Jensen R. Gastrinomas: Advances in diagnosis and management. *Neuroendocrinology.* 2004;80(suppl 1):23–27.
3. Ellison E, Sparks J. Zollinger-Ellison syndrome in the era of effective acid suppression: Are we unknowingly growing tumors? *Am J Surg.* 2003;186:245–248.
4. Hirshowitz B, Simmons J, Mohnen J. Clinical outcome using lansoprazole in acid hypersecretors with and without Zollinger-Ellison syndrome: A 13-year prospective study. *Clin Gastroenterol Hepatol.* 2005;3:39–48.

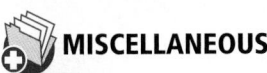 MISCELLANEOUS

CODES

ICD9-CM
251.5 Abnormality of secretion of gastrin

PATIENT TEACHING
Inform as to nature of disease and prognosis.

 See Corresponding Diagnostic Algorithm

 See Patient Handout on CD

APPENDIX

U.S. Preventive Services Task Force Recommendations

These pages are designed to be a quick reference to the recommendations of the leading organizations on screening and prevention. Included are the United States Preventive Services Task Force (USPSTF), the United States Centers for Disease Control (CDC), the American Academy of Pediatrics, and the American Academy of Family Physicians.

Each intervention receives an evidence-based grading of the recommendations based on the standard set by the USPSTF. These are:

2005 TASK FORCE RATINGS
Strength of Recommendations

The U.S. Preventive Services Task Force (USPSTF) grades its recommendations according to one of five classifications (A, B, C, D, I) reflecting the strength of evidence and magnitude of net benefit (benefits minus harms).

A. The USPSTF strongly recommends that clinicians provide [the service] to eligible patients. *The USPSTF found good evidence that [the service] improves important health outcomes and concludes that benefits substantially outweigh harms.*

B. The USPSTF recommends that clinicians provide [this service] to eligible patients. *The USPSTF found at least fair evidence that [the service] improves important health outcomes and concludes that benefits outweigh harms.*

C. The USPSTF makes no recommendation for or against routine provision of [the service]. *The USPSTF found at least fair evidence that [the service] can improve health outcomes but concludes that the balance of benefits and harms is too close to justify a general recommendation.*

D. The USPSTF recommends against routinely providing [the service] to asymptomatic patients. *The USPSTF found at least fair evidence that [the service] is ineffective or that harms outweigh benefits.*

I. The USPSTF concludes that the evidence is insufficient to recommend for or against routinely providing [the service]. *Evidence that the [service] is effective is lacking, of poor quality, or conflicting and the balance of benefits and harms cannot be determined.*

These recommendations should be tailored to patients' preferences. For example, screening for carcinoma of the prostate receives an "I" recommendation, yet many providers (and their patients) are concerned. Use of a detailed Informed Consent discussion of prostate cancer screening empowers the patient and the clinician to use these recommendations in a patient-centered manner.

Another area of note is the absence of "vested interests" in these recommendations. Many groups have suggested screening all women for osteoporosis at age 50 years or the onset of menopause; yet there are no data to support the benefit of this action, and emerging data showing harm.

Feel free to copy these recommendations for posting in the office, incorporation into patients' charts, and/or distribution as a patient education tool.

Frank J. Domino, MD

HEALTH MAINTENANCE: BIRTH TO 10 YEARS

(www.ahrq.gov/clinic/prevenix.htm)

Common Causes of Death

Perinatal Infections

Congenital Anomalies

Sudden Infant Death Syndrome (SIDS)

Accidents (Drowning, Abuse)

Motor Vehicle related Accidents

A. USPSTF Strongly Recommend this service; Good Evidence Found

B. USPSTF Recommends this service; Fair Evidence Found

C. USPSTF makes no recommendation about this service; balance of risks and benefits too close recommend

D. USPSTF recommends AGAINST this service; Good Evidence Found

I. USPSTF found insufficient evidence to support this service.

HR   High Risk

HTN   Hypertension

IUD   Injection Drug Users

MSM   Men who have sex with Men

MSP   Multiple Sexual Partners

SA   Sexually Active

Recommended Counseling, Testing or Intervention

Height, Weight, Growth Chart

Immunizations	DPaT, IPV, Hib, Hepatitis B, MMR, Pneumococcal, Varicella, Influenza (*www.immunizationed.org*)

Influenza Vaccine indicated for:
1) All children aged 6–24 months
2) High risk children with:
    (a) Asthma or chonic pulmonary disease (cystic fibrosis)
    (b) Significant cardiac disease
    (c) Immunosuppressive disorder or therapy
    (d) HIV infection
    (e) Sickle cell anemia or other hemoglobinopathies
    (f) Diseases requiring long term aspirin treatment (e.g. rheumatoid arthritis or Kawasaki disease)
    (g) Chronic renal dysfunction
    (h) Chronic metabolic disease (e.g. diabetes mellitus)

Counseling	Injury Prevention (Car Seats, Seat Belts, Bicycle Helmets, Smoke Detector, Carbon Monoxide Detector, Window/Stair guards, Firearm Storage) Breast Feeding Low Saturated Fat diet Physical Exercise Substance Abuse Tobacco, Alcohol
Dental Counseling (Regular Visits, Brushing)	B
Tuberculosis Screening	HR
Vision Screening	B

Not Recommended

Scoliosis Screening	D

HEALTH MAINTENANCE: 11–24 YEARS

(www.ahrq.gov/clinic/prevenix.htm)

Leading Causes of Death

Motor Vehicle Accidents

Unintentional Injuries

Homicide

Suicide

Malignant Neoplasms

A. USPSTF Strongly Recommend this service; Good Evidence Found

B. USPSTF Recommends this service; Fair Evidence Found

C. USPSTF makes no recommendation about this service; balance of risks and benefits too close recommend

D. USPSTF recommends AGAINST this service; Good Evidence Found

I. USPSTF found insufficient evidence to support this service.

HR High Risk

HTN Hypertension

IUD Injection Drug Users

MSM Men who have sex with Men

MSP Multiple Sexual Partners

SA Sexually Active

Tdap Tetanus, Diptheria, Pertussis

Recommended Counseling, Testing or Intervention

Height, Weight, Growth Chart	
Immunizations	Tdap, Meningococcal Vaccine (*www.immunizationed.org*)
Alcohol	B
Cervical Cancer Screening	
via Papanicolaou Smear	A: SA or Age >/= 21 years
Chlamydial Infection Screening	A-HR: IDU, SA, Pregnancy
Gonorrhea Screening	A-HR: IDU, SA, Pregnancy
Vision Screening	B
HIV Screening	A-HR: IDU, SA, Pregnancy
Hepatitis B	HR: IDU, SA, Pregnancy
Syphilis Screening	A-HR: IDU, SA, Pregnancy
Tuberculosis Screening	A-HR: IDU, Foreign Travel, Recent Immigrant
Dental Counseling (Regular Visits, Brushing)	B
Domestic Violence	I: SA
Obesity	B
Tobacco Abuse	A
Suicide Screening	I
General Counseling	Injury Prevention (Seat Belts, Bicycle Helmets, Firearm Storage)
	Low Saturated Fat diet
	Physical Exercise

Domestic Violence — Screen all at risk patients (all women, especially when pregnant) "Do you feel safe in your present relationship?" "Have you been hit, kicked, punched or otherwise hurt by someone in the last year?")

Suicide — Strongest risk factors of attempted suicide include history of mood disorder or other mental disorders, comorbid substance abuse, history of "Deliberate Self-Harm" (DSL intentionally initiated acts with non-fatal outcomes)

Alcohol Abuse: — "Risky" or "hazardous" alcohol use has been defined as more than 7 drinks per week or more than 3 drinks on any on occasion for women, and more than 14 drinks per week or more than 4 drinks on any one occasion for men.

- Screening question: "on any occasion during the last 3 months, have had more than 5 alcohol drinks" or
- CAGE: tried to CUT down, been ANGERED by questions about your drinking, felt GUILTY about your drinking, had an EYE OPENER (drink in the morning)

Substance Abuse — Although there is insufficient evidence currently exisits to recommend routine screening for drug abuse with standardized tools, questioning about drug use and drug-related problems when taking a history from all adolescent and adult patients is felt to be recommended on empiric grounds.

Not Recommended

Scoliosis Screening	D
Testicular Cancer	D

HEALTH MAINTENANCE: 25–44 YEARS

(www.ahrq.gov/clinic/prevenix.htm)

Leading Causes of Death

Motor Vehicle Accidents

Cardiovascular Disease

Malignant Neoplasm

HIV

A. USPSTF Strongly Recommend this service; Good Evidence Found

B. USPSTF Recommends this service; Fair Evidence Found

C. USPSTF makes no recommendation about this service; balance of risks and benefits too close recommend

D. USPSTF recommends AGAINST this service; Good Evidence Found

I. USPSTF found insufficient evidence to support this service.

HR High Risk

HTN Hypertension

IUD Injection Drug Users

MSM Men who have sex with Men

MSP Multiple Sexual Partners

SA Sexually Active

Recommended Counseling, Testing or Intervention

Height, Weight, Blood Pressure	A
Alcohol	B
Aspirin	HR: Male > 40, post menopausal female, younger if CHD risk factors (DM, HTN, Tobacco Abuse, Hyperlipidemia, family history of premature CHD)
Breast/Ovarian BRCA Mutation Testing	HR: Maternal &/or Paternal History of Breast and/or Ovarian Cancer
Breast Cancer Screening (mammography)	B-HR: Age >/= 40 every 1–2 years
Breast Cancer Prophylaxis	HR: Family History of Breast Cancer or atypia on Breast Biopsy
Cervical Cancer Screening	A
Chlamydia Infection Screening	HR: IDU, MSP, MSM, Preg.
Dental Counseling (Regular Visits, Brushing)	B
Depression	B
Diabetes mellitus	B-HR: HTN, Hyperlipidemia
Domestic Violence	I: SA
Diet/Obesity	B
Gonorrhea Screening	HR: IDU, MSP, MSM, Preg.
HIV Screening	HR: IDU, MSP, MSM, Preg.
Hepatitis B	HR: IDU, MSP, MSM, Preg.
Hepatitis C	HR: IDU, MSP, MSM, Preg.
Lipid Disorders	HR: Age >/= 20 with any CHD risk factors (HTN, Tobacco abuse, Diabetes Mellitus, Family History of Premature CHD)
Suicide Screening	I
Syphilis Screening	HR: IDU, MSP, MSM, Preg.
Tobacco Abuse	A
Tuberculosis Screening	A-HR: IDU, Foreign Travel, Low Income, Immigrant, Alcohol Abuse
Vision Screening	B
General Counseling:	Injury Prevention (Seat Belts, Bicycle Helmets, Firearm Storage) Low Saturated Fat diet, Physical Exercise
Immunizations	Tetanus: every 10 years or just at age 50 (if completed primary series) Influenza: all age >/= 50 years, all pregnant women, any adult with chronic disease or recurrent exposure to those with chronic disease) (www.immunizationed.org/)

Not Recommended

Bladder Cancer	D
Testicular Cancer	D
Vitamin Supplementation	D

Leading Causes of Death

Malignant Neoplasm

Cardiovascular Disease

Accidents

Cirrhosis

A. USPSTF Strongly Recommend this service; Good Evidence Found

B. USPSTF Recommends this service; Fair Evidence Found

C. USPSTF makes no recommendation about this service; balance of risks and benefits too close recommend

D. USPSTF recommends AGAINST this service; Good Evidence Found

I. USPSTF found insufficient evidence to support this service.

HR: High Risk

HTN: Hypertension

IUD: Injection Drug Users

MSM: Men who have sex with Men

MSP: Multiple Sexual Partners

SA: Sexually Active

Recommended Counseling, Testing or Intervention

Height, Weight, Blood Pressure	A
Alcohol	B
Aspirin	HR: Male > 40, post menopausal female, younger if CHD risk factors (DM, HTN, Tobacco Abuse, Hyperlipidemia, family history of premature CHD)
Breast/Ovarian BRCA Mutation Testing	HR: Maternal &/or Paternal History of Breast and/or Ovarian Cancer
Breast Cancer Screening (mammography)	B-HR: Age >/= 40 every 1-2 years
Breast Cancer Prophylaxis	HR: Family History of Breast Cancer or atypia on Breast Biopsy
Cervical Cancer Screening	A
Chlamydia Infection Screening	HR: IDU, MSP, MSM, Preg.
Colorectal Cancer	A: (FOBT-yearly of colonoscopy every 10 years)—start age >/= 50
Dental Counseling (Regular Visits, Brushing)	B
Depression	B
Diabetes mellitus	HR: HTN, Hyperlipidemia
Domestic Violence	I: SA
Gonorrhea Screening	HR: IDU, MSP, MSM, Preg.
HIV Screening	HR: IDU, MSP, MSM, Preg.
Hepatitis B	HR: IDU, MSP, MSM, Preg.
Hepatitis C	HR: IDU, MSP, MSM, Preg.
Lipid Disorders	A
Obesity	B
Prostate Cancer	I: Inconclusive evidence, early detection, improved outcome
Suicide Screening	I
Syphilis Screening	HR: IDU, MSP, MSM, Preg.
Tobacco Abuse	A
Tuberculosis Screening	HR: IDU, Foreign Travel, Low Income, Immigrant, Alcohol Abuse
Vision Screening	B
General Counseling:	Injury Prevention (Seat Belts, Bicycle Helmets, Firearm Storage) Low Saturated Fat diet, Physical Exercise
Immunizations	Tetanus: every 10 years or just at age 50 (if completed primary series) Influenza: all age >/= 50 years, all pregnant women, any adult with chronic disease or recurrent exposure to those with chronic disease) (www.immunizationed.org/)

Not Recommended

Bladder Cancer	D
Ovarian Cancer	D
Pancreatic Cancer	D
Peripheral Artery Disease	D
Testicular Cancer	D
Vitamin Supplementation	D

HEALTH MAINTENANCE: 65–75 YEARS

(www.ahrq.gov/clinic/prevenix.htm)

Leading Causes of Death

Cardiovascular Disease

Malignant Neoplasm

Cerebrovascular Accident

Chronic Obstructive Pulmonary Disease

Pneumonia

A. USPSTF Strongly Recommend this service; Good Evidence Found

B. USPSTF Recommends this service; Fair Evidence Found

C. USPSTF makes no recommendation about this service; balance of risks and benefits too close recommend

D. USPSTF recommends AGAINST this service; Good Evidence Found

I. USPSTF found insufficient evidence to support this service.

HR High Risk

HTN Hypertension

IUD Injection Drug Users

MSM Men who have sex with Men

MSP Multiple Sexual Partners

SA Sexually Active

Recommended Counseling, Testing or Intervention

Height, Weight, Blood Pressure	A
Abdominal Aortic Aneurysm	HR: Ultrasound only in men aged 65 to 75 who have ever smoked
Alcohol	B
Aspirin	A
Breast/Ovarian BRCA Mutation Testing	HR: Maternal &/or Paternal History of Breast and/or Ovarian Cancer
Breast Cancer Screening (mammography)	B
Breast Cancer Prophylaxis	HR: Family History of Breast Cancer or atypia on Breast Biopsy
Cervical Cancer Screening	D
Chlamydia Infection Screening	HR: IDU, MSP, MSM
Colorectal Cancer	A: (FOBT-yearly or colonoscopy every 10 years)—start age >/= 50
Dental Counseling (Regular Visits, Brushing)	B
Depression	B
Diabetes mellitus	HR: HTN, Hyperlipidemia
Domestic Violence	I: SA
Gonorrhea Screening	HR: IDU, MSP, MSM
HIV Screening	HR: IDU, MSP, MSM
Hepatitis B	HR: IDU, MSP, MSM
Hepatitis C	HR: IDU, MSP, MSM
Lipid Disorders	A
Obesity	B
Osteoporosis	B: Women aged >/=65 years or at 60 years if high risk < Low BMI or chronic corticosteroid use
Prostate Cancer	I: Inconclusive evidence, early detection, improved outcomes
Suicide Screening	HR: Isolation
Syphilis Screening	HR: IDU, MSP, MSM
Tobacco Abuse	A
Tuberculosis Screening	HR: IDU, Foreign Travel, Low Income, Immigrant, Alcohol Abuse
Vision Screening	B
General Counseling:	Injury Prevention (Seat Belts, Bicycle Helmets, Firearm Storage) Low Saturated Fat diet, Physical Exercise
Immunizations	Tetanus: every 10 years or just at age 50 (if completed primary series) Influenza: all age >/= 50 years, all pregnant women, any adult with chronic disease or recurrent exposure to those with chronic disease) (www.immunizationed.org/)

Not Recommended

Bladder Cancer	D
Ovarian Cancer	D
Pancreatic Cancer	D
Peripheral Artery Disease	D
Testicular Cancer	D
Vitamin Supplementation	D

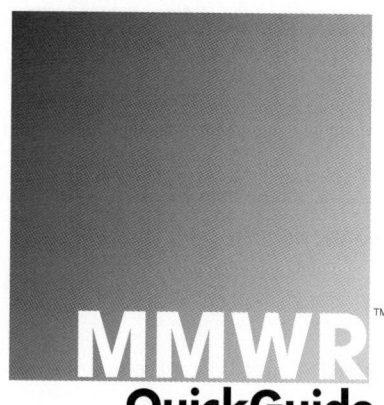

MMWR™

QuickGuide

Weekly   **January 5, 2007 / Vol. 55 / Nos. 51 & 52**

Recommended Immunization Schedules for Persons Aged 0–18 Years — United States, 2007

The Advisory Committee on Immunization Practices (ACIP) periodically reviews the recommended immunization schedule for persons aged 0–18 years to ensure that the schedule is current with changes in vaccine formulations and reflects revised recommendations for the use of licensed vaccines, including those newly licensed.

The changes to the previous childhood and adolescent immunization schedule, published January 2006 (*1*), are as follows:

- The new rotavirus vaccine (Rota) is recommended in a 3-dose schedule at ages 2, 4, and 6 months. The first dose should be administered at ages 6 weeks through 12 weeks with subsequent doses administered at 4–10 week intervals. Rotavirus vaccination should not be initiated for infants aged >12 weeks and should not be administered after age 32 weeks (*2*).

- The influenza vaccine is now recommended for all children aged 6–59 months (*3*).

- Varicella vaccine recommendations are updated. The first dose should be administered at age 12–15 months, and a newly recommended second dose should be administered at age 4–6 years (*4*).

- The new human papillomavirus vaccine (HPV) is recommended in a 3-dose schedule with the second and third doses administered 2 and 6 months after the first dose. Routine vaccination with HPV is recommended for females aged 11–12 years; the vaccination series can be started in females as young as age 9 years; and a catch-up vaccination is recommended for females aged 13–26 years who have not been vaccinated previously or who have not completed the full vaccine series (*5*).

The recommended immunization schedules for persons aged 0–18 years and the catch-up immunization schedule for 2007 have been approved by the Advisory Committee on Immunization Practices, the American Academy of Pediatrics, and the American Academy of Family Physicians. The standard *MMWR* footnote format has been modified for publication of this schedule.

Suggested citation: Centers for Disease Control and Prevention. Recommended immunization schedules for persons aged 0–18 years—United States, 2007. MMWR 2006;55(51&52):Q1–Q4.

- The main change to the format of the schedule is the division of the recommendation into two schedules: one schedule for persons aged 0–6 years (Figure 1) and another for persons aged 7–18 years (Figure 2). Special populations are represented with purple bars; the 11–12 years assessment is emphasized with the bold, capitalized fonts in the title of that column. Rota, HPV, and varicella vaccines are incorporated in the catch-up immunization schedule (Table).

Vaccine Information Statements

The National Childhood Vaccine Injury Act requires that health-care providers provide parents or patients with copies of Vaccine Information Statements before administering each dose of the vaccines listed in the schedule. Additional information is available from state health departments and from CDC at http://www.cdc.gov/nip/publications/vis.

Detailed recommendations for using vaccines are available from package inserts, ACIP statements on specific vaccines, and the *2003 Red Book* (*6*). ACIP statements for each recommended childhood vaccine are available from CDC at http://www.cdc.gov/nip/publications/acip-list.htm. In addition, guidance for obtaining and completing a Vaccine Adverse Event Reporting System form is available at http://www.vaers.hhs.gov or by telephone, 800-822-7967.

References
1. CDC. Recommended childhood and adolescent immunization schedule—United States. MMWR 2006;54(52):Q1–Q4.
2. CDC. Prevention of rotavirus gastroenteritis among infants and children. Recommendations of the Advisory Committee on Immunization Practices (ACIP). MMWR 2006;55(No. RR-12):1–13.
3. CDC. Prevention and control of influenza. Recommendations of the Advisory Committee on Immunization Practices (ACIP). MMWR 2006;55(No. RR-10):1–42.
4. CDC. ACIP provisional recommendations for the prevention of varicella. Available at http://www.cdc.gov/nip/vaccine/varicella/varicella_acip_recs_prov_june_2006.pdf.
5. CDC. ACIP provisional recommendations for the use of quadrivalent HPV vaccine. Available at http://www.cdc.gov/nip/recs/provisional_recs/hpv.pdf.
6. American Academy of Pediatrics. Active and passive immunization. In: Pickering LK, ed. 2003 red book: report of the Committee on Infectious Diseases. 26th ed. Elk Grove Village, IL: American Academy of Pediatrics; 2003.

FIGURE 1. Recommended immunization schedule for persons aged 0–6 years — United States, 2007

Vaccine ▼ / Age ▶	Birth	1 month	2 months	4 months	6 months	12 months	15 months	18 months	19–23 months	2–3 years	4–6 years
Hepatitis B[1]	HepB	HepB		See footnote 1	HepB					HepB Series	
Rotavirus[2]			Rota	Rota	Rota						
Diphtheria, Tetanus, Pertussis[3]			DTaP	DTaP	DTaP		DTaP				DTaP
Haemophilus influenzae type b[4]			Hib	Hib	*Hib*[4]	Hib		Hib			
Pneumococcal[5]			PCV	PCV	PCV	PCV				PCV / PPV	
Inactivated Poliovirus			IPV	IPV		IPV					IPV
Influenza[6]						Influenza (Yearly)					
Measles, Mumps, Rubella[7]						MMR					MMR
Varicella[8]						Varicella					Varicella
Hepatitis A[9]						HepA (2 doses)				HepA Series	
Meningococcal[10]										MPSV4	

■ Range of recommended ages

▨ Catch-up immunization

▨ Certain high-risk groups

This schedule indicates the recommended ages for routine administration of currently licensed childhood vaccines, as of December 1, 2006, for children aged 0–6 years. Additional information is available at http://www.cdc.gov/nip/recs/child-schedule.htm. Any dose not administered at the recommended age should be administered at any subsequent visit, when indicated and feasible. Additional vaccines may be licensed and recommended during the year. Licensed combination vaccines may be used whenever any components of the combination are indicated and other components of the vaccine are not contraindicated and if approved by the Food and Drug Administration for that dose of the series. Providers should consult the respective Advisory Committee on Immunization Practices statement for detailed recommendations. Clinically significant adverse events that follow immunization should be reported to the Vaccine Adverse Event Reporting System (VAERS). Guidance about how to obtain and complete a VAERS form is available at http://www.vaers.hhs.gov or by telephone, 800-822-7967.

1. **Hepatitis B vaccine (HepB).** *(Minimum age: birth)*
   At birth:
   - Administer monovalent HepB to all newborns before hospital discharge.
   - If mother is hepatitis surface antigen (HBsAg)-positive, administer HepB and 0.5 mL of hepatitis B immune globulin (HBIG) within 12 hours of birth.
   - If mother's HBsAg status is unknown, administer HepB within 12 hours of birth. Determine the HBsAg status as soon as possible and if HBsAg-positive, administer HBIG (no later than age 1 week).
   - If mother is HBsAg-negative, the birth dose can only be delayed with physician's order and mothers' negative HBsAg laboratory report documented in the infant's medical record.
   After the birth dose:
   - The HepB series should be completed with either monovalent HepB or a combination vaccine containing HepB. The second dose should be administered at age 1–2 months. The final dose should be administered at age ≥24 weeks. Infants born to HBsAg-positive mothers should be tested for HBsAg and antibody to HBsAg after completion of ≥3 doses of a licensed HepB series, at age 9–18 months (generally at the next well-child visit).
   4-month dose:
   - It is permissible to administer 4 doses of HepB when combination vaccines are administered after the birth dose. If monovalent HepB is used for doses after the birth dose, a dose at age 4 months is not needed.

2. **Rotavirus vaccine (Rota).** *(Minimum age: 6 weeks)*
   - Administer the first dose at age 6–12 weeks. Do not start the series later than age 12 weeks.
   - Administer the final dose in the series by age 32 weeks. Do not administer a dose later than age 32 weeks.
   - Data on safety and efficacy outside of these age ranges are insufficient.

3. **Diphtheria and tetanus toxoids and acellular pertussis vaccine (DTaP).** *(Minimum age: 6 weeks)*
   - The fourth dose of DTaP may be administered as early as age 12 months, provided 6 months have elapsed since the third dose.
   - Administer the final dose in the series at age 4–6 years.

4. *Haemophilus influenzae* **type b conjugate vaccine (Hib).** *(Minimum age: 6 weeks)*
   - If PRP-OMP (PedvaxHIB® or ComVax® [Merck]) is administered at ages 2 and 4 months, a dose at age 6 months is not required.
   - TriHiBit® (DTaP/Hib) combination products should not be used for primary immunization but can be used as boosters following any Hib vaccine in children aged ≥12 months.

5. **Pneumococcal vaccine.** *(Minimum age: 6 weeks for pneumococcal conjugate vaccine [PCV]; 2 years for pneumococcal polysaccharide vaccine [PPV])*
   - Administer PCV at ages 24–59 months in certain high-risk groups. Administer PPV to children aged ≥2 years in certain high-risk groups. See *MMWR* 2000;49(No. RR-9):1–35.

6. **Influenza vaccine.** *(Minimum age: 6 months for trivalent inactivated influenza vaccine [TIV]; 5 years for live, attenuated influenza vaccine [LAIV])*
   - All children aged 6–59 months and close contacts of all children aged 0–59 months are recommended to receive influenza vaccine.
   - Influenza vaccine is recommended annually for children aged ≥59 months with certain risk factors, health-care workers, and other persons (including household members) in close contact with persons in groups at high risk. See *MMWR* 2006;55(No. RR-10):1–41.
   - For healthy persons aged 5–49 years, LAIV may be used as an alternative to TIV.
   - Children receiving TIV should receive 0.25 mL if aged 6–35 months or 0.5 mL if aged ≥3 years.
   - Children aged <9 years who are receiving influenza vaccine for the first time should receive 2 doses (separated by ≥4 weeks for TIV and ≥6 weeks for LAIV).

7. **Measles, mumps, and rubella vaccine (MMR).** *(Minimum age: 12 months)*
   - Administer the second dose of MMR at age 4–6 years. MMR may be administered before age 4–6 years, provided ≥4 weeks have elapsed since the first dose and both doses are administered at age ≥12 months.

8. **Varicella vaccine.** *(Minimum age: 12 months)*
   - Administer the second dose of varicella vaccine at age 4–6 years. Varicella vaccine may be administered before age 4–6 years, provided that ≥3 months have elapsed since the first dose and both doses are administered at age ≥12 months. If second dose was administered ≥28 days following the first dose, the second dose does not need to be repeated.

9. **Hepatitis A vaccine (HepA).** *(Minimum age: 12 months)*
   - HepA is recommended for all children aged 1 year (i.e., aged 12–23 months). The 2 doses in the series should be administered at least 6 months apart.
   - Children not fully vaccinated by age 2 years can be vaccinated at subsequent visits.
   - HepA is recommended for certain other groups of children, including in areas where vaccination programs target older children. See *MMWR* 2006;55(No. RR-7):1–23.

10. **Meningococcal polysaccharide vaccine (MPSV4).** *(Minimum age: 2 years)*
    - Administer MPSV4 to children aged 2–10 years with terminal complement deficiencies or anatomic or functional asplenia and certain other high-risk groups. See *MMWR* 2005;54(No. RR-7):1–21.

The Recommended Immunization Schedules for Persons Aged 0–18 Years are approved by the Advisory Committee on Immunization Practices (http://www.cdc.gov/nip/acip), the American Academy of Pediatrics (http://www.aap.org), and the American Academy of Family Physicians (http://www.aafp.org).

FIGURE 2. Recommended immunization schedule for persons aged 7–18 years — United States, 2007

Vaccine ▼　　　　　Age ▶	7–10 years	11–12 YEARS	13–14 years	15 years	16–18 years	
Tetanus, Diphtheria, Pertussis[1]	See footnote 1	Tdap	Tdap	Tdap	Tdap	**Range of recommended ages**
Human Papillomavirus[2]	See footnote 2	HPV (3 doses)	HPV Series	HPV Series	HPV Series	
Meningococcal[3]	MPSV4	MCV4	MCV4	MCV4[3] / MCV4	MCV4	
Pneumococcal[4]		PPV				
Influenza[5]		Influenza (Yearly)				**Catch-up immunization**
Hepatitis A[6]		HepA Series				
Hepatitis B[7]		HepB Series				
Inactivated Poliovirus[8]		IPV Series				
Measles, Mumps, Rubella[9]		MMR Series				**Certain high-risk groups**
Varicella[10]		Varicella Series				

This schedule indicates the recommended ages for routine administration of currently licensed childhood vaccines, as of December 1, 2006, for children aged 7–18 years. Additional information is available at http://www.cdc.gov/nip/recs/child-schedule.htm. Any dose not administered at the recommended age should be administered at any subsequent visit, when indicated and feasible. Additional vaccines may be licensed and recommended during the year. Licensed combination vaccines may be used whenever any components of the combination are indicated and other components of the vaccine are not contraindicated and if approved by the Food and Drug Administration for that dose of the series. Providers should consult the respective Advisory Committee on Immunization Practices statement for detailed recommendations. Clinically significant adverse events that follow immunization should be reported to the Vaccine Adverse Event Reporting System (VAERS). Guidance about how to obtain and complete a VAERS form is available at http://www.vaers.hhs.gov or by telephone, 800-822-7967.

1. **Tetanus and diphtheria toxoids and acellular pertussis vaccine (Tdap).** *(Minimum age: 10 years for BOOSTRIX® and 11 years for ADACEL™)*
   - Administer at age 11–12 years for those who have completed the recommended childhood DTP/DTaP vaccination series and have not received a tetanus and diphtheria toxoids (Td) booster dose.
   - Adolescents aged 13–18 years who missed the 11–12 year Td/Tdap booster dose should also receive a single dose of Tdap if they have completed the recommended childhood DTP/DTaP vaccination series.
2. **Human papillomavirus vaccine (HPV).** *(Minimum age: 9 years)*
   - Administer the first dose of the HPV vaccine series to females at age 11–12 years.
   - Administer the second dose 2 months after the first dose and the third dose 6 months after the first dose.
   - Administer the HPV vaccine series to females at age 13–18 years if not previously vaccinated.
3. **Meningococcal vaccine.** *(Minimum age: 11 years for meningococcal conjugate vaccine [MCV4]; 2 years for meningococcal polysaccharide vaccine [MPSV4])*
   - Administer MCV4 at age 11–12 years and to previously unvaccinated adolescents at high school entry (at approximately age 15 years).
   - Administer MCV4 to previously unvaccinated college freshmen living in dormitories; MPSV4 is an acceptable alternative.
   - Vaccination against invasive meningococcal disease is recommended for children and adolescents aged ≥2 years with terminal complement deficiencies or anatomic or functional asplenia and certain other high-risk groups. See *MMWR* 2005;54(No. RR-7):1–21. Use MPSV4 for children aged 2–10 years and MCV4 or MPSV4 for older children.
4. **Pneumococcal polysaccharide vaccine (PPV).** *(Minimum age: 2 years)*
   - Administer for certain high-risk groups. See *MMWR* 1997;46(No. RR-8):1–24, and *MMWR* 2000;49(No. RR-9):1–35.
5. **Influenza vaccine.** *(Minimum age: 6 months for trivalent inactivated influenza vaccine [TIV]; 5 years for live, attenuated influenza vaccine [LAIV])*
   - Influenza vaccine is recommended annually for persons with certain risk factors, health-care workers, and other persons (including household members) in close contact with persons in groups at high risk. See *MMWR* 2006;55 (No. RR-10):1–41.
   - For healthy persons aged 5–49 years, LAIV may be used as an alternative to TIV.
   - Children aged <9 years who are receiving influenza vaccine for the first time should receive 2 doses (separated by ≥4 weeks for TIV and ≥6 weeks for LAIV).

6. **Hepatitis A vaccine (HepA).** *(Minimum age: 12 months)*
   - The 2 doses in the series should be administered at least 6 months apart.
   - HepA is recommended for certain other groups of children, including in areas where vaccination programs target older children. See *MMWR* 2006;55 (No. RR-7):1–23.
7. **Hepatitis B vaccine (HepB).** *(Minimum age: birth)*
   - Administer the 3-dose series to those who were not previously vaccinated.
   - A 2-dose series of Recombivax HB® is licensed for children aged 11–15 years.
8. **Inactivated poliovirus vaccine (IPV).** *(Minimum age: 6 weeks)*
   - For children who received an all-IPV or all-oral poliovirus (OPV) series, a fourth dose is not necessary if the third dose was administered at age ≥4 years.
   - If both OPV and IPV were administered as part of a series, a total of 4 doses should be administered, regardless of the child's current age.
9. **Measles, mumps, and rubella vaccine (MMR).** *(Minimum age: 12 months)*
   - If not previously vaccinated, administer 2 doses of MMR during any visit, with ≥4 weeks between the doses.
10. **Varicella vaccine.** *(Minimum age: 12 months)*
   - Administer 2 doses of varicella vaccine to persons without evidence of immunity.
   - Administer 2 doses of varicella vaccine to persons aged ≤13 years at least 3 months apart. Do not repeat the second dose, if administered ≥28 days after the first dose.
   - Administer 2 doses of varicella vaccine to persons aged ≥13 years at least 4 weeks apart.

The Recommended Immunization Schedules for Persons Aged 0–18 Years are approved by the Advisory Committee on Immunization Practices (http://www.cdc.gov/nip/acip), the American Academy of Pediatrics (http://www.aap.org), and the American Academy of Family Physicians (http://www.aafp.org).

TABLE. Catch-up immunization schedule for persons aged 4 months–18 years who start late or who are ≥1 month behind — United States, 2007

The table below provides catch-up schedules and minimum intervals between doses for children whose vaccinations have been delayed. A vaccine series does not need to be restarted, regardless of the time that has elapsed between doses. Use the section appropriate for the child's age.

CATCH-UP SCHEDULE FOR PERSONS AGED 4 MONTHS–6 YEARS

Vaccine	Minimum age for Dose 1	Minimum interval between doses			
		Dose 1 to Dose 2	Dose 2 to Dose 3	Dose 3 to Dose 4	Dose 4 to Dose 5
Hepatitis B[1]	Birth	4 weeks	8 weeks (and 16 weeks after first dose)		
Rotavirus[2]	6 weeks	4 weeks	4 weeks		
Diphtheria, Tetanus, Pertussis[3]	6 weeks	4 weeks	4 weeks	6 months	6 months[3]
Haemophilus influenzae type b[4]	6 weeks	4 weeks if first dose administered at age <12 months / 8 weeks (as final dose) if first dose administered at age 12–14 months / No further doses needed if first dose administered at age ≥15 months	4 weeks[4] if current age <12 months / 8 weeks (as final dose)[4] if current age ≥12 months and second dose administered at age <15 months / No further doses needed if previous dose administered at age ≥15 months	8 weeks (as final dose) This dose only necessary for children aged 12 months–5 years who received 3 doses before age 12 months	
Pneumococcal[5]	6 weeks	4 weeks if first dose administered at age <12 months and current age <24 months / 8 weeks (as final dose) if first dose administered at age ≥12 months or current age 24–59 months / No further doses needed for healthy children if first dose administered at age ≥24 months	4 weeks if current age <12 months / 8 weeks (as final dose) if current age ≥12 months / No further doses needed for healthy children if previous dose administered at age ≥24 months	8 weeks (as final dose) This dose only necessary for children aged 12 months–5 years who received 3 doses before age 12 months	
Inactivated Poliovirus[6]	6 weeks	4 weeks	4 weeks	4 weeks[6]	
Measles, Mumps, Rubella[7]	12 months	4 weeks			
Varicella[8]	12 months	3 months			
Hepatitis A[9]	12 months	6 months			

CATCH-UP SCHEDULE FOR PERSONS AGED 7–18 YEARS

Vaccine	Minimum age for Dose 1	Dose 1 to Dose 2	Dose 2 to Dose 3	Dose 3 to Dose 4	
Tetanus, Diphtheria/ Tetanus, Diphtheria, Pertussis[10]	7 years[10]	4 weeks	8 weeks if first dose administered at age <12 months / 6 months if first dose administered at age ≥12 months	6 months if first dose administered at age <12 months	
Human Papillomavirus[11]	9 years	4 weeks	12 weeks		
Hepatitis A[9]	12 months	6 months			
Hepatitis B[1]	Birth	4 weeks	8 weeks (and 16 weeks after first dose)		
Inactivated Poliovirus[6]	6 weeks	4 weeks	4 weeks	4 weeks[6]	
Measles, Mumps, Rubella[7]	12 months	4 weeks			
Varicella[8]	12 months	4 weeks if first dose administered at age ≥13 years / 3 months if first dose administered at age <13 years			

1. **Hepatitis B vaccine (HepB).** *(Minimum age: birth)*
   - Administer the 3-dose series to those who were not previously vaccinated.
   - A 2-dose series of Recombivax HB® is licensed for children aged 11–15 years.
2. **Rotavirus vaccine (Rota).** *(Minimum age: 6 weeks)*
   - Do not start the series later than age 12 weeks.
   - Administer the final dose in the series by age 32 weeks. Do not administer a dose later than age 32 weeks.
   - Data on safety and efficacy outside of these age ranges are insufficient.
3. **Diphtheria and tetanus toxoids and acellular pertussis vaccine (DTaP).** *(Minimum age: 6 weeks)*
   - The fifth dose is not necessary if the fourth dose was administered at age ≥4 years.
   - DTaP is not indicated for persons aged ≥7 years.
4. ***Haemophilus influenzae* type b conjugate vaccine (Hib).** *(Minimum age: 6 weeks)*
   - Vaccine is not generally recommended for children aged ≥5 years.
   - If current age <12 months and the first 2 doses were PRP-OMP (PedvaxHIB® or ComVax® [Merck]), the third (and final) dose should be administered at age 12–15 months and at least 8 weeks after the second dose.
   - If first dose was administered at age 7–11 months, administer 2 doses separated by 4 weeks plus a booster at age 12–15 months.
5. **Pneumococcal conjugate vaccine (PCV).** *(Minimum age: 6 weeks)*
   - Vaccine is not generally recommended for children aged ≥5 years.
6. **Inactivated poliovirus vaccine (IPV).** *(Minimum age: 6 weeks)*
   - For children who received an all-IPV or all-oral poliovirus (OPV) series, a fourth dose is not necessary if third dose was administered at age ≥4 years.
   - If both OPV and IPV were administered as part of a series, a total of 4 doses should be administered, regardless of the child's current age.

7. **Measles, mumps, and rubella vaccine (MMR).** *(Minimum age: 12 months)*
   - The second dose of MMR is recommended routinely at age 4–6 years but may be administered earlier if desired.
   - If not previously vaccinated, administer 2 doses of MMR during any visit with ≥4 weeks between the doses.
8. **Varicella vaccine.** *(Minimum age: 12 months)*
   - The second dose of varicella vaccine is recommended routinely at age 4–6 years but may be administered earlier if desired.
   - Do not repeat the second dose in persons aged <13 years if administered ≥28 days after the first dose.
9. **Hepatitis A vaccine (HepA).** *(Minimum age: 12 months)*
   - HepA is recommended for certain groups of children, including in areas where vaccination programs target older children. See *MMWR* 2006;55(No. RR-7):1–23.
10. **Tetanus and diphtheria toxoids vaccine (Td) and tetanus and diphtheria toxoids and acellular pertussis vaccine (Tdap).** *(Minimum ages: 7 years for Td, 10 years for BOOSTRIX®, and 11 years for ADACEL™)*
    - Tdap should be substituted for a single dose of Td in the primary catch-up series or as a booster if age appropriate; use Td for other doses.
    - A 5-year interval from the last Td dose is encouraged when Tdap is used as a booster dose. A booster (fourth) dose is needed if any of the previous doses were administered at age <12 months. Refer to ACIP recommendations for further information. See *MMWR* 2006;55(No. RR-3).
11. **Human papillomavirus vaccine (HPV).** *(Minimum age: 9 years)*
    - Administer the HPV vaccine series to females at age 13–18 years if not previously vaccinated.

Information about reporting reactions after immunization is available online at http://www.vaers.hhs.gov or by telephone via the 24-hour national toll-free information line 800-822-7967. Suspected cases of vaccine-preventable diseases should be reported to the state or local health department. Additional information, including precautions and contraindications for immunization, is available from the National Center for Immunization and Respiratory Diseases at http://www.cdc.gov/nip/default.htm or telephone, 800-CDC-INFO (800-232-4636).

Recommended Adult Immunization Schedule, by Vaccine and Age Group
UNITED STATES • OCTOBER 2006–SEPTEMBER 2007

Vaccine / Age group	19–49 years	50–64 years	≥65 years
Tetanus, diphtheria, pertussis (Td/Tdap)[1],*	1-dose Td booster every 10 yrs — Substitute 1 dose of Tdap for Td		
Human papillomavirus (HPV)[2]	3 doses (females)		
Measles, mumps, rubella (MMR)[3],*	1 or 2 doses	1 dose	
Varicella[4],*	2 doses (0, 4–8 wks)	2 doses (0, 4–8 wks)	
Influenza[5],*	1 dose annually	1 dose annually	
Pneumococcal (polysaccharide)[6,7]	1–2 doses		1 dose
Hepatitis A[8],*	2 doses (0, 6–12 mos, or 0, 6–18 mos)		
Hepatitis B[9],*	3 doses (0, 1–2, 4–6 mos)		
Meningococcal[10]	1 or more doses		

*Covered by the Vaccine Injury Compensation Program. NOTE: These recommendations must be read with the footnotes (see reverse).

For all persons in this category who meet the age requirements and who lack evidence of immunity (e.g., lack documentation of vaccination or have no evidence of prior infection)

Recommended if some other risk factor is present (e.g., on the basis of medical, occupational, lifestyle, or other indications)

This schedule indicates the recommended age groups and medical indications for routine administration of currently licensed vaccines for persons aged ≥19 years, as of October 1, 2006. Licensed combination vaccines may be used whenever any components of the combination are indicated and when the vaccine's other components are not contraindicated. For detailed recommendations on all vaccines, including those used primarily for travelers or that are issued during the year, consult the manufacturers' package inserts and the complete statements from the Advisory Committee on Immunization Practices (www.cdc.gov/nip/publications/acip-list.htm).

Report all clinically significant postvaccination reactions to the Vaccine Adverse Event Reporting System (VAERS). Reporting forms and instructions on filing a VAERS report are available at www.vaers.hhs.gov or by telephone, 800-822-7967.

Information on how to file a Vaccine Injury Compensation Program claim is available at www.hrsa.gov/vaccinecompensation or by telephone, 800-338-2382. To file a claim for vaccine injury, contact the U.S. Court of Federal Claims, 717 Madison Place, N.W., Washington, D.C. 20005; telephone, 202-357-6400.

Additional information about the vaccines in this schedule and contraindications for vaccination is also available at www.cdc.gov/nip or from the CDC-INFO Contact Center at 800-CDC-INFO (800-232-4636) in English and Spanish, 24 hours a day, 7 days a week.

Recommended Adult Immunization Schedule, by Vaccine and Medical and Other Indications
UNITED STATES • OCTOBER 2006–SEPTEMBER 2007

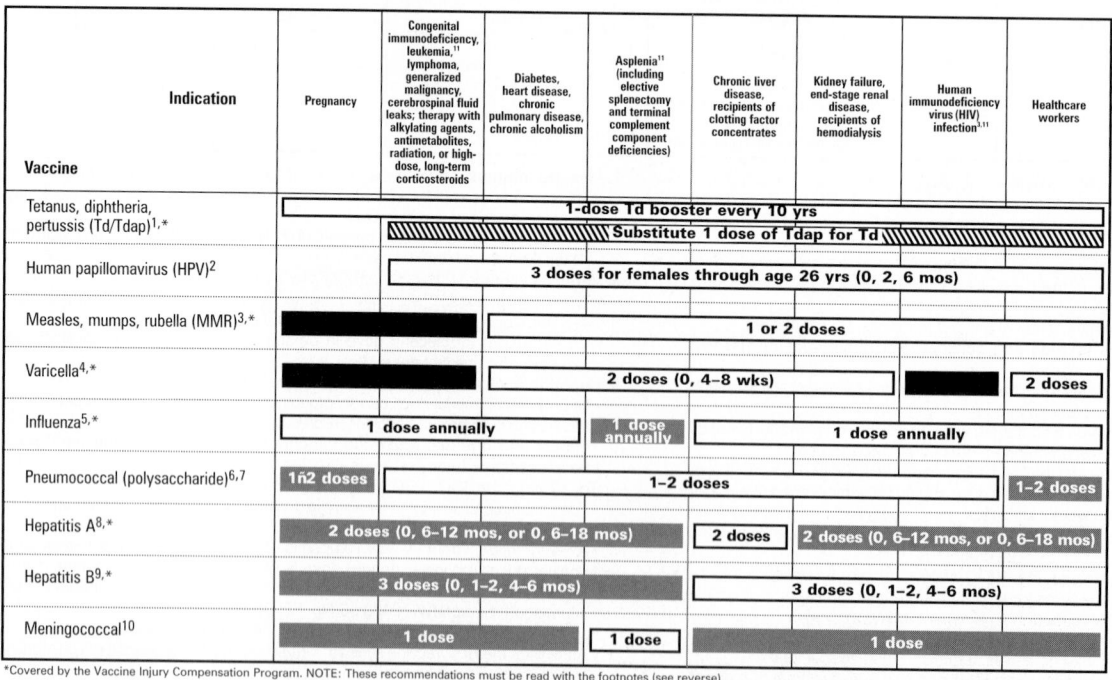

Vaccine / Indication	Pregnancy	Congenital immunodeficiency, leukemia,[11] lymphoma, generalized malignancy, cerebrospinal fluid leaks; therapy with alkylating agents, antimetabolites, radiation, or high-dose, long-term corticosteroids	Diabetes, heart disease, chronic pulmonary disease, chronic alcoholism	Asplenia[11] (including elective splenectomy and terminal complement component deficiencies)	Chronic liver disease, recipients of clotting factor concentrates	Kidney failure, end-stage renal disease, recipients of hemodialysis	Human immunodeficiency virus (HIV) infection[3,11]	Healthcare workers
Tetanus, diphtheria, pertussis (Td/Tdap)[1],*	1-dose Td booster every 10 yrs — Substitute 1 dose of Tdap for Td							
Human papillomavirus (HPV)[2]	3 doses for females through age 26 yrs (0, 2, 6 mos)							
Measles, mumps, rubella (MMR)[3],*	(Contraindicated)		1 or 2 doses					
Varicella[4],*	(Contraindicated)		2 doses (0, 4–8 wks)				(Contraindicated)	2 doses
Influenza[5],*	1 dose annually			1 dose annually	1 dose annually			
Pneumococcal (polysaccharide)[6,7]	1–2 doses		1–2 doses					1–2 doses
Hepatitis A[8],*	2 doses (0, 6–12 mos, or 0, 6–18 mos)			2 doses	2 doses (0, 6–12 mos, or 0, 6–18 mos)			
Hepatitis B[9],*	3 doses (0, 1–2, 4–6 mos)			3 doses (0, 1–2, 4–6 mos)				
Meningococcal[10]	1 dose		1 dose	1 dose				

*Covered by the Vaccine Injury Compensation Program. NOTE: These recommendations must be read with the footnotes (see reverse).

For all persons in this category who meet the age requirements and who lack evidence of immunity (e.g., lack documentation of vaccination or have no evidence of prior infection)

Recommended if some other risk factor is present (e.g., on the basis of medical, occupational, lifestyle, or other indications)

Contraindicated

Approved by
the Advisory Committee on Immunization Practices,
the American College of Obstetricians and Gynecologists,
the American Academy of Family Physicians,
and the American College of Physicians

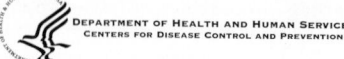
DEPARTMENT OF HEALTH AND HUMAN SERVICES
CENTERS FOR DISEASE CONTROL AND PREVENTION

Footnotes
Recommended Adult Immunization Schedule • UNITED STATES, OCTOBER 2006–SEPTEMBER 2007

1. **Tetanus, diphtheria, and acellular pertussis (Td/Tdap) vaccination.** Adults with uncertain histories of a complete primary vaccination series with diphtheria and tetanus toxoid–containing vaccines should begin or complete a primary vaccination series. A primary series for adults is 3 doses; administer the first 2 doses at least 4 weeks apart and the third dose 6–12 months after the second. Administer a booster dose to adults who have completed a primary series and if the last vaccination was received ≥10 years previously. Tdap or tetanus and diphtheria (Td) vaccine may be used; Tdap should replace a single dose of Td for adults aged <65 years who have not previously received a dose of Tdap (either in the primary series, as a booster, or for wound management). Only one of two Tdap products (Adacel® [sanofi pasteur]) is licensed for use in adults. If the person is pregnant and received the last Td vaccination ≥10 years previously, administer Td during the second or third trimester; if the person received the last Td vaccination in <10 years, administer Tdap during the immediate postpartum period. A one-time administration of 1 dose of Tdap with an interval as short as 2 years from a previous Td vaccination is recommended for postpartum women, close contacts of infants aged <12 months, and all healthcare workers with direct patient contact. In certain situations, Td can be deferred during pregnancy and Tdap substituted in the immediate postpartum period, or Tdap can be given instead of Td to a pregnant woman after an informed discussion with the woman (see www.cdc.gov/nip/publications/acip-list.htm). Consult the ACIP statement for recommendations for administering Td as prophylaxis in wound management (www.cdc.gov/mmwr/preview/mmwrhtml/00041645.htm).

2. **Human papillomavirus (HPV) vaccination.** HPV vaccination is recommended for all women aged ≤26 years who have not completed the vaccine series. Ideally, vaccine should be administered before potential exposure to HPV through sexual activity; however, women who are sexually active should still be vaccinated. Sexually active women who have not been infected with any of the HPV vaccine types receive the full benefit of the vaccination. Vaccination is less beneficial for women who have already been infected with one or more of the four HPV vaccine types. A complete series consists of 3 doses. The second dose should be administered 2 months after the first dose; the third dose should be administered 6 months after the first dose. Vaccination is not recommended during pregnancy. If a woman is found to be pregnant after initiating the vaccination series, the remainder of the 3-dose regimen should be delayed until after completion of the pregnancy.

3. **Measles, mumps, rubella (MMR) vaccination.** *Measles component:* adults born before 1957 can be considered immune to measles. Adults born during or after 1957 should receive ≥1 dose of MMR unless they have a medical contraindication, documentation of ≥1 dose, history of measles based on healthcare provider diagnosis, or laboratory evidence of immunity. A second dose of MMR is recommended for adults who 1) have been recently exposed to measles or in an outbreak setting; 2) have been previously vaccinated with killed measles vaccine; 3) have been vaccinated with an unknown type of measles vaccine during 1963–1967; 4) are students in postsecondary educational institutions; 5) work in ahealthcare facility; or 6) plan to travel internationally. Withhold MMR or other measles-containing vaccines from HIV-infected persons with severe immunosuppression.

   Mumps component: adults born before 1957 can generally be considered immune to mumps. Adults born during or after 1957 should receive 1 dose of MMR unless they have a medical contraindication, history of mumps based on healthcare provider diagnosis, or laboratory evidence of immunity. A second dose of MMR is recommended for adults who 1) are in an age group that is affected during a mumps outbreak; 2) are students in postsecondary educational institutions; 3) work in a healthcare facility; or 4) plan to travel internationally. For unvaccinated healthcare workers born before 1957 who do not have other evidence of mumps immunity, consider giving 1 dose on a routine basis and strongly consider giving a second dose during an outbreak. *Rubella component:* administer 1 dose of MMR vaccine to women whose rubella vaccination history is unreliable or who lack laboratory evidence of immunity. For women of childbearing age, regardless of birth year, routinely determine rubella immunity and counsel women regarding congenital rubella syndrome. Do not vaccinate women who are pregnant or who might become pregnant within 4 weeks of receiving vaccine. Women who do not have evidence of immunity should receive MMR vaccine upon completion or termination of pregnancy and before discharge from the healthcare facility.

4. **Varicella vaccination.** All adults without evidence of immunity to varicella should receive 2 doses of varicella vaccine. Special consideration should be given to those who 1) have close contact with persons at high risk for severe disease (e.g., healthcare workers and family contacts of immunocompromised persons) or 2) are at high risk for exposure or transmission (e.g., teachers of young children; child care employees; residents and staff members of institutional settings, including correctional institutions; college students; military personnel; adolescents and adults living in households with children; nonpregnant women of childbearing age; and international travelers). Evidence of immunity to varicella in adults includes any of the following: 1) documentation of 2 doses of varicella vaccine at least 4 weeks apart; 2) U.S.-born before 1980 (although for healthcare workers and pregnant women, birth before 1980 should not be considered evidence of immunity); 3) history of varicella based on diagnosis or verification of varicella by a healthcare provider (for a patient reporting a history of or presenting with an atypical case, a mild case, or both, healthcare providers should seek either an epidemiologic link with a typical varicella case or evidence of laboratory confirmation, if it was performed at the time of acute disease); 4) history of herpes zoster based on healthcare provider diagnosis; or 5) laboratory evidence of immunity or laboratory confirmation of disease. Do not vaccinate women who are pregnant or might become pregnant within 4 weeks of receiving the vaccine. Assess pregnant women for evidence of varicella immunity. Women who do not have evidence of immunity should receive dose 1 of varicella vaccine upon completion or termination of pregnancy and before discharge from the healthcare facility. Dose 2 should be administered 4–8 weeks after dose 1.

5. **Influenza vaccination.** *Medical indications:* chronic disorders of the cardiovascular or pulmonary systems, including asthma; chronic metabolic diseases, including diabetes mellitus, renal dysfunction, hemoglobinopathies, or immunosuppression (including immunosuppression caused by medications or HIV); any condition that compromises respiratory function or the handling of respiratory secretions or that can increase the risk of aspiration (e.g., cognitive dysfunction, spinal cord injury, or seizure disorder or other neuromuscular disorder); and pregnancy during the influenza season. No data exist on the risk for severe or complicated influenza disease among persons with asplenia; however, influenza is a risk factor for secondary bacterial infections that can cause severe disease among persons with asplenia. *Occupational indications:* healthcare workers and employees of long-term–care and assisted living facilities. *Other indications:* residents of nursing homes and other long-term–care and assisted living facilities; persons likely to transmit influenza to persons at high risk (e.g., in-home household contacts and caregivers of children aged 0–59 months, or persons of all ages with high-risk conditions); and anyone who would like to be vaccinated. Healthy, nonpregnant persons aged 5–49 years without high-risk medical conditions who are not contacts of severely immunocompromised persons in special care units can receive either intranasally administered influenza vaccine (FluMist®) or inactivated vaccine. Other persons should receive the inactivated vaccine.

6. **Pneumococcal polysaccharide vaccination.** *Medical indications:* chronic disorders of the pulmonary system (excluding asthma); cardiovascular diseases; diabetes mellitus; chronic liver diseases, including liver disease as a result of alcohol abuse (e.g., cirrhosis); chronic renal failure or nephrotic syndrome; functional or anatomic asplenia (e.g., sickle cell disease or splenectomy [if elective splenectomy is planned, vaccinate at least 2 weeks before surgery]); immunosuppressive conditions (e.g., congenital immunodeficiency, HIV infection [vaccinate as close to diagnosis as possible when CD4 cell counts are highest], leukemia, lymphoma, multiple myeloma, Hodgkin disease, generalized malignancy, or organ or bone marrow transplantation); chemotherapy with alkylating agents, antimetabolites, or high-dose, long-term corticosteroids; and cochlear implants. *Other indications:* Alaska Natives and certain American Indian populations and residents of nursing homes or other long-term–care facilities.

7. **Revaccination with pneumococcal polysaccharide vaccine.** One-time revaccination after 5 years for persons with chronic renal failure or nephrotic syndrome; functional or anatomic asplenia (e.g., sickle cell disease or splenectomy); immunosuppressive conditions (e.g., congenital immunodeficiency, HIV infection, leukemia, lymphoma, multiple myeloma, Hodgkin disease, generalized malignancy, or organ or bone marrow transplantation); or chemotherapy with alkylating agents, antimetabolites, or high-dose, long-term corticosteroids. For persons aged ≥65 years, one-time revaccination if they were vaccinated ≥5 years previously and were aged <65 years at the time of primary vaccination.

8. **Hepatitis A vaccination.** *Medical indications:* persons with chronic liver disease and persons who receive clotting factor concentrates. *Behavioral indications:* men who have sex with men and persons who use illegal drugs. *Occupational indications:* persons working with hepatitis A virus (HAV)–infected primates or with HAV in a research laboratory setting. *Other indications:* persons traveling to or working in countries that have high or intermediate endemicity of hepatitis A (a list of countries is available at www.cdc.gov/travel/diseases.htm) and any person who would like to obtain immunity. Current vaccines should be administered

   in a 2-dose schedule at either 0 and 6–12 months, or 0 and 6–18 months. If the combined hepatitis A and hepatitis B vaccine is used, administer 3 doses at 0, 1, and 6 months.

9. **Hepatitis B vaccination.** *Medical indications:* persons with end-stage renal disease, including patients receiving hemodialysis; persons seeking evaluation or treatment for a sexually transmitted disease (STD); persons with HIV infection; persons with chronic liver disease; and persons who receive clotting factor concentrates. *Occupational indications:* healthcare workers and public-safety workers who are exposed to blood or other potentially infectious body fluids. *Behavioral indications:* sexually active persons who are not in a long-term, mutually monogamous relationship (i.e., persons with >1 sex partner during the previous 6 months); current or recent injection-drug users; and men who have sex with men. *Other indications:* household contacts and sex partners of persons with chronic hepatitis B virus (HBV) infection; clients and staff members of institutions for persons with developmental disabilities; all clients of STD clinics; international travelers to countries with high or intermediate prevalence of chronic HBV infection (a list of countries is available at www.cdc.gov/travel/diseases.htm); and any adult seeking protection from HBV infection. Settings where hepatitis B vaccination is recommended for all adults: STD treatment facilities; HIV testing and treatment facilities; facilities providing drug-abuse treatment and prevention services; healthcare settings providing services for injection-drug users or men who have sex with men; correctional facilities; end-stage renal disease programs and facilities for chronic hemodialysis patients; and institutions and nonresidential daycare facilities for persons with developmental disabilities. *Special formulation indications:* for adult patients receiving hemodialysis and other immunocompromised adults, 1 dose of 40 μg/mL (Recombivax HB®) or 2 doses of 20 μg/mL (Engerix-B®).

10. **Meningococcal vaccination.** *Medical indications:* adults with anatomic or functional asplenia, or terminal complement component deficiencies. *Other indications:* first-year college students living in dormitories; microbiologists who are routinely exposed to isolates of *Neisseria meningitidis*; military recruits; and persons who travel to or live in countries in which meningococcal disease is hyperendemic or epidemic (e.g., the "meningitis belt" of sub-Saharan Africa during the dry season [December–June]), particularly if their contact with local populations will be prolonged. Vaccination is required by the government of Saudi Arabia for all travelers to Mecca during the annual Hajj. Meningococcal conjugate vaccine is preferred for adults with any of the preceding indications who are aged ≤55 years, although meningococcal polysaccharide vaccine (MPSV4) is an acceptable alternative. Revaccination after 5 years might be indicated for adults previously vaccinated with MPSV4 who remain at high risk for infection (e.g., persons residing in areas in which disease is epidemic).

11. **Selected conditions for which *Haemophilus influenzae* type b (Hib) vaccine may be used.** Hib conjugate vaccines are licensed for children aged 6 weeks–71 months. No efficacy data are available on which to base a recommendation concerning use of Hib vaccine for older children and adults with the chronic conditions associated with an increased risk for Hib disease. However, studies suggest good immunogenicity in patients who have sickle cell disease, leukemia, or HIV infection or who have had splenectomies; administering vaccine to these patients is not contraindicated.

INDEX

A

Abacterial meningitis, 784–785
Abdominal aortic aneurysm (AAA), 60–61
Abdominal cryptorchidism, 320–321
Abdominal pregnancy, 418–419
Abdominal rigidity, signs and symptoms
    algorithm for, A-2
Abnormal uterine bleeding (AUB), 404–405
Abortion
    recurrent, 4–5
      signs and symptoms algorithm for, A-4
    spontaneous, 4–5
Abruptio placentae, 6–7
Abscess
    anorectal, 72–73
    brain, 172–173
    breast, 180–181, 474–475
    lung, 746–747
    mammary, 180–181
    puerperal, 180–181
    pulmonary, 746–747
    subareolar, 180–181
    subdiaphragmatic, 1206–1207
    subphrenic, 1206–1207
    tubo-ovarian, 926–927
Absence seizure disorder, 1150–1151
Abuse
    child, 252–253
    drug, 1208–1209
    laxative, 714–715
Accelerated hypertension, 632–633
Accidental hypothermia, 654–655
Acetaminophen
    dosing of, 8
    poisoning with, 8–9
Acid burn, of eye, 868–869
Acidosis, signs and symptoms algorithm for,
    A-6
Acid phosphatase elevation, signs and
    symptoms algorithm for, A-21
Acne, signs and symptoms algorithm for, A-7
Acne inversa, 582–583
Acne rosacea, 10–11
Acne vulgaris, 12–13
Acoustic neuroma, 14–15
Acquired angioedema (AAE), 64–65
Acquired hypoparathyroidism, 650–651
Acquired immunodeficiency syndrome (AIDS),
    592–593
Actinic keratosis, 700–701
Acute-angle closure glaucoma, 508–509
Acute anterior poliomyelitis, 988–989
Acute bacterial endocarditis, 426–427
Acute confusional state, 346–347
Acute febrile respiratory illness (AFRI), from
    adenovirus, 18
Acute idiopathic polyneuritis, 528–529
Acute immune-mediated polyneuritis,
    528–529

Acute inflammatory demyelinating
    polyradiculoneuropathy,
    528–529
Acute inflammatory neuropathy,
    528–529
Acute intermittent porphyria (AIP),
    1002–1003
Acute interstitial allergic nephritis,
    682–683
Acute interstitial pneumonia (AIP),
    382–383
Acute lateral poliomyelitis, 988–989
Acute lymphoblastic/lymphocytic leukemia
    (ALL)
    in adults, 728–729
    L3 type, 758–759
Acute mental status change, 346–347
Acute mountain sickness (AMS), 28–29
Acute nephritic syndrome, 512–513
Acute non-lymphoblastic leukemia (ANLL),
    726–727
Acute otitis media (AOM), 896–897
Acute pancreatitis, 910–911
Acute pericarditis, 934–935
Acute peripheral vestibulopathy, 702–703
Acute pharyngoconjunctival fever (APC), from
    adenovirus, 18
Acute post-streptococcal glomerulonephritis,
    512–513
Acute renal failure (ARF), 1084–1085
Acute respiratory disease (ARD), from
    adenovirus, 18
Acute respiratory distress syndrome (ARDS),
    846–847, 1090–1091
Acute situational anxiety, 84–85
Acute suppurative pericarditis, 934–935
Acute vestibular neuronitis, 1358–1359
Addison anemia, 54–55
Addison disease, 16–17
Addisonian crisis, 16–17
Adenocarcinoma, of bladder, 156–157
Adenosis, 474–475, 1342
Adenovirus infections, 18–19
Adherent bursitis, 488–489
Adhesive capsulitis, 488–489
Adiposis (adiposity), 864–865
Adnexitis, 926–927
Adrenal crisis, 16–17
Adrenergic urticaria, 1334–1335
Adrenocortical insufficiency
    primary, 16–17
    secondary, 17
    signs and symptoms algorithm for, A-8
    tertiary, 17
Aeromonas hydrophila infection, lymphangitis
    from, 754–755
Aerotitis, 142–143
African kala azar, 722–723
African Kaposi sarcoma, 694–695

African lymphoma, 758–759
Agammaglobulinemia, 666–667
Aganglionic megacolon, 298–299
Age-related macular degeneration (ARMD),
    760–761
Agnogenic myeloid metaplasia, 838–839
Agoraphobia, 954–955
AIDS, 592–593
AIDS-related Kaposi sarcoma, 694–695
Air sickness, 820–821
Albumin, low, signs and symptoms algorithm
    for, A-93
Alcohol abuse, 20–23
Alcohol dependence, 20–23
Alcoholism, 20–23
Alcohol use disorders, 20–23
Aldosterone-producing adenoma (APA),
    24–25
Aldosteronism
    primary, 24–25
    signs and symptoms algorithm for, A-9
Aldosteronoma, 24–25
Aldrich syndrome, 1382–1383
Aleukia hemorrhagica, 48–49
Algorithms, signs and symptoms. *See* Signs
    and symptoms algorithms
Alkaline burn, of eye, 868–869
Alkaline phosphatase elevation, signs and
    symptoms algorithm for, A-10
Alkalosis, signs and symptoms algorithm for,
    A-11
Allergic alveolitis, extrinsic, 628–629
Allergic angiitis, 434–435
Allergic aspergillosis, 116–117
Allergic bowel disease, 480–481
Allergic bronchopulmonary aspergillosis
    (ABPA), 434–435
Allergic contact dermatitis (ACD), 356–357
Allergic interstitial pneumonitis, 628–629
Allergic rhinitis, 1116–1117
Allergy, food, 480–481
Alopecia, 26–27
    signs and symptoms algorithm for, A-12
Alopecia areata, 26–27
α-thalassemia, 1250–1251
ALS, 40–41
ALS-like syndrome, 40
ALS-Parkinson-dementia complex of Guam,
    40–41
Altered mental status, 346–347
Altitude illness, 28–29
Alveolitis, extrinsic allergic, 628–629
Alzheimer dementia (Alzheimer disease, AD),
    30–31, 348–349
Amblyopia, 32–33
Amblyopia ex anopsia, 32
Amebiasis, 34–35
Amebic colitis, 34–35
Amebic dysentery, 34–35